BRAUNWALD'S

Heart Disease

A Textbook of Cardiovascular Medicine

Cover and Spine Illustration:

Fused myocardial perfusion and CT coronary angiography images in a patient with hypertrophic cardiomyopathy presenting with chest pain. The images demonstrate a large area of ischemia in the distribution of the left anterior descending coronary artery and an occluded diagonal branch.

Courtesy of Drs. Marcelo F. DiCarli and Mouaz H. Al-Mallah, Brigham and Women's Hospital, Boston, Massachusetts.

BRAUNWALD'S

Heart Disease

A Textbook of Cardiovascular Medicine

EIGHTH EDITION VOLUME 1

EDITED BY

Peter Libby, MD
Mallinckrodt Professor of Medicine
Harvard Medical School
Chief, Cardiovascular Division
Brigham and Women's Hospital
Boston, Massachusetts

Robert O. Bonow, MD
Max and Lilly Goldberg Distinguished Professor of Cardiology
Northwestern University Feinberg School of Medicine
Chief, Division of Cardiology
Co-Director, Bluhm Cardiovascular Institute
Northwestern Memorial Hospital
Chicago, Illinois

Douglas L. Mann, MD
Don W. Chapman Chair
Professor of Medicine and Molecular Physiology and Biophysics
Chief, Section of Cardiology
Baylor College of Medicine
St. Luke's Episcopal Hospital
Texas Heart Institute
Houston, Texas

Douglas P. Zipes, MD
Distinguished Professor
Professor Emeritus of Medicine, Pharmacology, and Toxicology
Director Emeritus, Division of Cardiology and the Krannert Institute of Cardiology
Indiana University School of Medicine
Indianapolis, Indiana

FOUNDING EDITOR AND E-DITION EDITOR

Eugene Braunwald, MD, MD(HON), SCD(HON), FRCP
Distinguished Hersey Professor of Medicine
Harvard Medical School
Chairman, TIMI Study Group
Brigham and Women's Hospital
Boston, Massachusetts

SAUNDERS
ELSEVIER

SAUNDERS
ELSEVIER

1600 John F. Kennedy Boulevard
Suite 1800
Philadelphia, PA 19103-2899

BRAUNWALD'S HEART DISEASE: A Textbook of Cardiovascular Medicine, Eighth Edition

Two-volume set	978-1-4160-4107-8
Single volume	978-1-4160-4106-1
Two-volume e-dition	978-1-4160-4105-4
Single volume e-dition	978-1-4160-4104-7
International edition	978-0-8089-2385-5
Online edition	978-1-4160-4103-0

Notice

Knowledge and best practice in this field are constantly changing. As new research and experience broaden our knowledge, changes in practice, treatment, and drug therapy may become necessary or appropriate. Readers are advised to check the most current information provided (i) on procedures featured or (ii) by the manufacturer of each product to be administered, to verify the recommended dose or formula, the method and duration of administration, and contraindications. It is the responsibility of the practitioners, relying on their own experience and knowledge of the patient, to make diagnoses, to determine dosages and the best treatment for each individual patient, and to take all appropriate safety precautions. To the fullest extent of the law, neither the Publisher nor the Editors assume any liability for any injury and/or damage to persons or property arising out of or related to any use of the material contained in this book.

The Publisher

Library of Congress Cataloging-in-Publication Data
Braunwald's heart disease : a textbook of cardiovascular medicine / Peter Libby . . . [et al.].—8th ed.
p. ; cm.
Includes bibliographical references and index.
ISBN 978-1-4160-4106-1
1. Heart—Diseases. 2. Cardiology. I. Libby, Peter. II. Title: Heart disease.
[DNLM: 1. Heart Diseases. 2. Cardiovascular Diseases. WG 210 B825 2008]
RC681.H36 2008
616.1′2—dc22 2007009890

Executive Publisher: Natasha Andjelkovic
Developmental Editor: Anne Snyder
Publishing Services Manager: Frank Polizzano
Senior Project Manager: Robin E. Hayward
Multimedia Producer: David Wisner
Design Direction: Steve Stave

Printed in the United States of America.

Last digit is the print number: 9 8 7 6 5 4 3 2

To:

Beryl, Oliver, and Brigitte

Pat, Rob, and Sam

Laura, Stephanie, Jonathan, and Erica

Joan, Debra, Jeffrey, and David

Contributors

Stephan Achenbach, MD
Professor of Medicine, Department of Cardiology, University of Erlangen, Erlangen, Germany
Computed Tomography of the Heart

Philip A. Ades, MD
Professor of Medicine, University of Vermont College of Medicine; Director, Cardiac Rehabilitation and Prevention, Fletcher-Allen Health Care, Burlington, Vermont
Exercise and Sports Cardiology

Elliott M. Antman, MD
Professor of Medicine, Harvard Medical School; Senior Investigator, TIMI Study Group, and Director, Samuel A. Levine Cardiac Unit, Brigham and Women's Hospital, Boston, Massachusetts
ST-Elevation Myocardial Infarction: Pathology, Pathophysiology, and Clinical Features; ST-Elevation Myocardial Infarction: Management

Donald S. Baim, MD
Chief Medical and Scientific Officer, Boston Scientific Corporation, Natick, Massachusetts
Percutaneous Coronary and Valvular Intervention

Gary J. Balady, MD
Professor of Medicine, Boston University School of Medicine; Director, Preventive Cardiology, Boston Medical Center, Boston, Massachusetts
Exercise and Sports Cardiology

Arthur J. Barsky, MD
Professor of Psychiatry, Harvard Medical School; Director of Psychiatric Research, Brigham and Women's Hospital, Boston, Massachusetts
Psychiatric and Behavioral Aspects of Cardiovascular Disease

Joshua A. Beckman, MD, MSc
Assistant Professor of Medicine, Harvard Medical School; Director, Cardiovascular Fellowship Program, Brigham and Women's Hospital, Boston, Massachusetts
Diabetes Mellitus, the Metabolic Syndrome, and Atherosclerotic Vascular Disease

Michael A. Bettmann, MD
Professor of Radiology, Wake Forest University School of Medicine; Vice Chair, Department of Radiology, Wake Forest University Baptist Medical Center, Winston-Salem, North Carolina
The Chest Radiograph in Cardiovascular Disease

Robert O. Bonow, MD
Max and Lilly Goldberg Distinguished Professor of Cardiology, Northwestern University Feinberg School of Medicine; Chief, Division of Cardiology, and Co-Director, Bluhm Cardiovascular Institute, Northwestern Memorial Hospital, Chicago, Illinois
Nuclear Cardiology; Cardiac Catheterization; Care of Patients with End-Stage Heart Disease; Valvular Heart Disease; Guidelines: Management of Valvular Heart Disease

Eugene Braunwald, MD, MD(Hon), ScD(Hon), FRCP
Distinguished Hersey Professor of Medicine, Harvard Medical School; Chairman, TIMI Study Group, Brigham and Women's Hospital, Boston, Massachusetts
ST-Elevation Myocardial Infarction: Pathology, Pathophysiology, and Clinical Features; Unstable Angina and Non-ST Elevation Myocardial Infarction

Hugh Calkins, MD
Professor of Medicine, Johns Hopkins University School of Medicine; Director, Electrophysiology, Johns Hopkins Hospital, Baltimore, Maryland
Hypotension and Syncope

Christopher P. Cannon, MD
Associate Professor of Medicine, Harvard Medical School; TIMI Study Group, Cardiovascular Division, Brigham and Women's Hospital, Boston, Massachusetts
Approach to the Patient with Chest Pain; Unstable Angina and Non-ST Elevation Myocardial Infarction

John M. Canty, Jr., MD
Albert and Elizabeth Rekate Professor of Medicine and Chief of Cardiovascular Medicine, University at Buffalo School of Medicine and Biomedical Sciences, The State University of New York, Buffalo, New York
Coronary Blood Flow and Myocardial Ischemia

John D. Carroll, MD
Professor of Medicine, Division of Cardiology, University of Colorado Health Sciences Center; Director, Cardiac and Vascular Center, and Director, Interventional Cardiology, University of Cardiology Hospital, Denver, Colorado
Clinical Assessment of Heart Failure

Agustin Castellanos, MD
Professor of Medicine, University of Miami Leonard M. Miller School of Medicine; Director, Clinical Electrophysiology, Jackson Memorial Hospital, Miami, Florida
Cardiac Arrest and Sudden Cardiac Death

Bernard R. Chaitman, MD
Professor of Medicine and Director of Cardiovascular Research, St. Louis University School of Medicine; Attending Physician, Division of Cardiology, St. Louis University Hospital, St. Louis, Missouri
Exercise Stress Testing

Danny Chu, MD
Assistant Professor, Baylor College of Medicine; Staff Physician, Michael E. DeBakey VA Medical Center, Houston, Texas
Traumatic Heart Disease

Heidi M. Connolly, MD
Professor of Medicine, Mayo Clinic College of Medicine; Consultant, Cardiovascular Diseases and Internal Medicine, Saint Marys Hospital, Rochester Methodist Hospital, Rochester, Minnesota
Echocardiography

Rebecca B. Costello, PhD
Nutrition Scientist, Office of Dietary Supplements, National Institutes of Health, Bethesda, Maryland
Complementary and Alternative Approaches to Management of Patients with Heart Disease

Mark A. Creager, MD
Professor of Medicine, Harvard Medical School; Simon C. Fireman Scholar in Cardiovascular Medicine and Director, Vascular Center, Brigham and Women's Hospital, Boston, Massachusetts
Diabetes Mellitus, the Metabolic Syndrome, and Atherosclerotic Vascular Disease; Peripheral Arterial Diseases

Werner G. Daniel, MD
Professor of Medicine and Chair, Department of Cardiology, University of Erlangen, Erlangen, Germany
Computed Tomography of the Heart

Charles J. Davidson, MD
Professor of Medicine, Northwestern University Feinberg School of Medicine; Chief, Cardiac Catheterization Laboratories, Northwestern Memorial Hospital, Chicago, Illinois
Cardiac Catheterization

Vasken Dilsizian, MD
Professor of Medicine and Radiology, University of Maryland School of Medicine; Director of Cardiovascular Nuclear Medicine and Cardiac Positron Emission Tomography, University of Maryland Medical Center, Baltimore, Maryland
Nuclear Cardiology

Stefanie Dimmeler, PhD
Professor of Molecular Cardiology, University of Frankfurt Medical School, Frankfurt, Germany
Emerging Therapies and Strategies in the Treatment of Heart Failure

Pamela S. Douglas, MD
Ursula Geller Professor of Research in Cardiovascular Diseases and Chief, Division of Cardiovascular Medicine, Duke University Medical Center, Durham, North Carolina
Cardiovascular Disease in Women

Kim A. Eagle, MD
Albion Walter Hewlett Professor of Internal Medicine, University of Michigan Medical School; Chief, Clinical Cardiovascular Medicine, University of Michigan Health System, Ann Arbor, Michigan
Anesthesia and Noncardiac Surgery in Patients with Heart Disease

Andrew C. Eisenhauer, MD
Assistant Professor of Medicine, Harvard Medical School; Director, Interventional Cardiovascular Medicine Service, Brigham and Women's Hospital, Boston, Massachusetts
Endovascular Treatment of Noncoronary Obstructive Vascular Disease

Linda L. Emanuel, MD, PhD
Professor of Medicine and Director of the Buehler Center on Aging, Health & Society, Northwestern University Feinberg School of Medicine, Chicago, Illinois
Care of Patients with End-Stage Heart Disease

James C. Fang, MD
Associate Professor of Medicine, Case Western Reserve University School of Medicine; Associate Chief of Clinical Affairs and Medical Director of Heart Failure, Transplant, and Circulatory Assistance, University Hospital/Case Medical Center, Cleveland, Ohio
The History and Physical Examination: An Evidence-Based Approach

Stacy D. Fisher, MD
Director, Cardiac Education for Internal Medicine Residency, Johns Hopkins/Sinai Hospital of Baltimore, Baltimore, Maryland
Cardiovascular Abnormalities in HIV-Infected Individuals

Thomas Force, MD
Professor of Medicine, Jefferson Medical College, Thomas Jefferson University; Clinical Director, Center for Translational Medicine, Thomas Jefferson University Hospital, Philadelphia, Pennsylvania
The Cancer Patient and Cardiovascular Disease

Lee A. Fleisher, MD
Robert D. Dripps Professor of Anesthesiology and Critical Care and Professor of Medicine, University of Pennsylvania School of Medicine; Chair, Department of Anesthesiology and Critical Care, University of Pennsylvania Health System, Philadelphia, Pennsylvania
Anesthesia and Noncardiac Surgery in Patients with Heart Disease

Apoor S. Gami, MD
Assistant Professor of Medicine, Division of Cardiovascular Diseases, Mayo Clinic, Rochester, Minnesota
Sleep Apnea and Cardiovascular Disease

J. Michael Gaziano, MD, MPH
Associate Professor of Medicine, Harvard Medical School; Chief, Division of Aging, Brigham and Women's Hospital; Director, Massachusetts Veterans Epidemiology and Research Information Center (MAVERIC), Boston Veterans Affairs Healthcare System, Boston, Massachusetts
Global Burden of Cardiovascular Disease; Primary and Secondary Prevention of Coronary Heart Disease

Jacques Genest, MD
Professor of Medicine, McGill University Faculty of Medicine; Chief, Department of Cardiology, McGill University Health Center, Montreal, Quebec, Canada
Lipoprotein Disorders and Cardiovascular Disease

Bernard J. Gersh, MD, DPhil
Professor of Medicine, Mayo Clinic College of Medicine; Consultant in Cardiovascular Diseases and Internal Medicine and Associate Chair of Academic Affairs and Faculty Development, Division of Cardiovascular Diseases, Mayo Clinic, Rochester, Minnesota
Chronic Coronary Artery Disease

Ary L. Goldberger, MD
Professor of Medicine, Harvard Medical School; Associate Director of Interdisciplinary Medicine and Biotechnology and Director of the Margaret and H. A. Rey Institute for Nonlinear Dynamics in Physiology and Medicine, Boston, Massachusetts
Electrocardiography

Samuel Z. Goldhaber, MD
Professor of Medicine, Harvard Medical School; Senior Staff Cardiologist, Director of the Venous Thromboembolism Research Group, and Director of the Anticoagulation Service, Brigham and Women's Hospital, Boston, Massachusetts
Pulmonary Embolism

Larry B. Goldstein, MD
Professor of Medicine, Division of Neurology, Duke University School of Medicine; Director, Center for Cerebrovascular Disease, Duke University Medical Center; Durham VA Medical Center, Durham, North Carolina
Prevention and Management of Stroke

Richard J. Gray, MD
Medical Director, Sutter Pacific Heart Centers, California Pacific Medical Center, San Francisco, California
Medical Management of the Patient Undergoing Cardiac Surgery

William J. Groh, MD, MPH
Associate Professor of Medicine, Krannert Institute of Cardiology, Indiana University School of Medicine, Indianapolis, Indiana
Neurological Disorders and Cardiovascular Disease

Joshua M. Hare, MD
Louis Lemberg Professor of Medicine, Professor of Cellular and Molecular Pharmacology, Chief of Cardiology, and Director of the Interdisciplinary Stem Cell Institute, University of Miami Leonard M. Miller School of Medicine, Miami, Florida
The Dilated, Restrictive, and Infiltrative Cardiomyopathies

David L. Hayes, MD
Professor of Medicine, Mayo Clinic College of Medicine; Chair, Division of Cardiovascular Diseases, Mayo Clinic, Rochester, Minnesota
Cardiac Pacemakers and Cardioverter-Defibrillators

Otto M. Hess, MD
Professor of Cardiology, Swiss Cardiovascular Center, University Hospital, Bern, Switzerland
Clinical Assessment of Heart Failure

L. David Hillis, MD
Daniel W. Foster Distinguished Chair in Internal Medicine and Vice-Chair of Medicine, University of Texas Southwestern Medical Center, Dallas, Texas
Toxins and the Heart

Mark A. Hlatky, MD
Professor of Health Research and Policy and Professor of Cardiovascular Medicine, Stanford University School of Medicine, Stanford, California
Economics and Cardiovascular Disease

Gary S. Hoffman, MD
Professor of Medicine, Cleveland Clinic Lerner College of Medicine of Case Western Reserve University; Harold C. Schott Chair of Rheumatic and Immunologic Diseases, Cleveland Clinic, Cleveland, Ohio
Rheumatic Diseases and the Cardiovascular System

David R. Holmes, Jr., MD
Professor of Medicine, Mayo Clinic College of Medicine; Consultant, St. Marys Hospital, Mayo Clinic, Rochester, Minnesota
Primary Percutaneous Coronary Intervention in the Management of Acute Myocardial Infarction

Eric M. Isselbacher, MD
Associate Professor of Medicine, Harvard Medical School; Associate Director of the Heart Center and Co-Director of the Thoracic Aortic Center, Massachusetts General Hospital, Boston, Massachusetts
Diseases of the Aorta

Suraj Kapa, MD
Physician, Mayo Clinic College of Medicine, Rochester, Minnesota
Cardiovascular Manifestations of Autonomic Disorders

Norman M. Kaplan, MD
Clinical Professor of Internal Medicine, University of Texas Southwestern Medical Center at Dallas; Attending Physician, Parkland Memorial Hospital, Dallas, Texas
Systemic Hypertension: Mechanisms and Diagnosis; Systemic Hypertension: Therapy

Adolf W. Karchmer, MD
Professor of Medicine, Harvard Medical School; Chief, Division of Infectious Diseases, Beth Israel Deaconess Medical Center, Boston, Massachusetts
Infective Endocarditis

Irwin Klein, MD
Professor of Medicine and Cell Biology, New York University School of Medicine; Associate Chair, Department of Medicine, North Shore University Hospital, Manhasset, New York
Endocrine Disorders and Cardiovascular Disease

Barbara A. Konkle, MD
Professor of Medicine and of Pathology and Laboratory Medicine and Director of the Penn Comprehensive Hemophilia and Thrombosis Program, University of Pennsylvania School of Medicine, Philadelphia, Pennsylvania
Hemostasis, Thrombosis, Fibrinolysis, and Cardiovascular Disease

Ronald M. Krauss, MD
Adjunct Professor, Department of Nutritional Sciences, University of California, Berkeley, Berkeley; Senior Scientist and Director, Atherosclerosis Research, Children's Hospital Oakland Research Institute, Oakland, California
Nutrition and Cardiovascular Disease

Mitchell W. Krucoff, MD
Professor of Medicine, Division of Cardiology, Duke University School of Medicine; Director, CU Devices Unit; Director, ECG Core Lab, Duke Clinical Research Institute, Duke University Medical Center, Durham, North Carolina
Complementary and Alternative Approaches to Management of Patients with Heart Disease

Harlan M. Krumholz, MD
Harold J. Hines, Jr. Professor of Medicine and Epidemiology and Public Health, Yale University School of Medicine; Director, Center for Outcomes Research and Evaluation, Yale-New Haven Hospital, New Haven, Connecticut
Clinical Decision-Making in Cardiology

Gary E. Lane, MD
Assistant Professor of Medicine, Mayo Clinic College of Medicine; Director, Cardiac Catheterization Laboratory, St. Luke's Hospital, Mayo Clinic, Jacksonville, Florida
Primary Percutaneous Coronary Intervention in the Management of Acute Myocardial Infarction

Richard A. Lange, MD
E. Cowles Andrus Professor of Cardiology and Chief of Clinical Cardiology, Johns Hopkins Hospital, Baltimore, Maryland
Toxins and the Heart

Cheng-Han Lee, MD, PhD
Department of Pathology and Laboratory Medicine, University of British Columbia Faculty of Medicine; Vancouver General Hospital, Vancouver, British Columbia, Canada
Primary Tumors of the Heart

Thomas H. Lee, MD
Professor of Medicine, Harvard Medical School; Network President, Partners Healthcare System, Boston, Massachusetts
Measurement and Improvement of Quality of Cardiovascular Care; Guidelines: Electrocardiography; Guidelines: Exercise Stress Testing; Guidelines: Use of Echocardiography; Guidelines: Nuclear Cardiology; Guidelines: Appropriateness Guidelines: Cardiovascular Magnetic Resonance; Guidelines: Appropriateness Guidelines: Cardiac Computed Tomography; Guidelines: Coronary Arteriography; Guidelines: Management of Heart Failure; Guidelines: Ambulatory Electrocardiographic and Electrophysiologic Testing; Guidelines: Cardiac Pacemakers and Cardioverter-Defibrillators; Guidelines: Atrial Fibrillation; Guidelines: Treatment of Hypertension; Approach to the Patient with Chest Pain; Guidelines: Primary Percutaneous Coronary Intervention in Acute Myocardial Infarction; Guidelines: Unstable Angina and Non–ST Elevation Myocardial Infarction; Guidelines: Chronic Stable Angina; Guidelines: Percutaneous Coronary and Valvular Intervention; Guidelines: Management of Valvular Heart Disease; Guidelines: Infective Endocarditis; Guidelines: Pregnancy and Heart Disease; Guidelines: Reducing Cardiac Risk with Noncardiac Surgery

Martin M. LeWinter, MD
Professor of Medicine and Molecular Physiology and Biophysics, University of Vermont College of Medicine; Attending Cardiologist, Fletcher Allen Health Care, Burlington, Vermont
Pericardial Diseases

Peter Libby, MD
Mallinckrodt Professor of Medicine, Harvard Medical School; Chief, Cardiovascular Division, Brigham and Women's Hospital, Boston, Massachusetts
The Vascular Biology of Atherosclerosis; Risk Factors for Atherothrombotic Disease; Lipoprotein Disorders and Cardiovascular Disease; Diabetes Mellitus, the Metabolic Syndrome, and Atherosclerotic Vascular Disease; Peripheral Arterial Diseases

Steven E. Lipshultz, MD
Professor and Chair, Department of Pediatrics, University of Miami, Leonard M. Miller School of Medicine, Miami, Florida
Cardiovascular Abnormalities in HIV-Infected Individuals

Peter P. Liu, MSc, MD
Heart & Stroke/Polo Chair and Professor of Medicine, Toronto General Research Institute, University Health Network; Heart & Stroke/Richard Lewar Centre of Excellence in Cardiovascular Research, Toronto, Ontario, Canada
Myocarditis

Brian F. Mandell, MD, PhD
Professor of Medicine, Cleveland Clinic Lerner College of Medicine of Case Western Reserve University; Vice Chairman of Medicine for Education and Staff, Rheumatic and Immunologic Disease, Center for Vasculitis Care and Research, Cleveland Clinic, Cleveland, Ohio
Rheumatic Diseases and the Cardiovascular System

Douglas L. Mann, MD
Don W. Chapman Chair and Professor of Medicine and Molecular Physiology and Biophysics; Chief, Section of Cardiology, Baylor College of Medicine; St. Luke's Episcopal Hospital, Texas Heart Institute, Houston, Texas
Pathophysiology of Heart Failure; Management of Heart Failure Patients with Reduced Ejection Fraction; Emerging Therapies and Strategies in the Treatment of Heart Failure

JoAnn E. Manson, MD, DrPH
Professor of Medicine and Elizabeth F. Brigham Professor of Women's Health, Harvard Medical School; Chief, Division of Preventive Medicine, Brigham and Women's Hospital, Boston, Massachusetts
Primary and Secondary Prevention of Coronary Heart Disease

Daniel B. Mark, MD, MPH
Professor of Medicine, Division of Cardiology, Duke University School of Medicine; Director, Outcomes Research Group, Duke Clinical Research Institute, Durham, North Carolina
Economics and Cardiovascular Disease

Barry J. Maron, MD
Director, The Hypertrophic Cardiomyopathy Center, Minneapolis Heart Institute Foundation, Minneapolis, Minnesota; Adjunct Professor of Medicine, Tufts University School of Medicine, Tufts–New England Medical Center, Boston, Massachusetts
Hypertrophic Cardiomyopathy

Kenneth L. Mattox, MD
Professor of Surgery, Baylor College of Medicine; Chief of Surgery and Chief of Staff, Ben Taub General Hospital, Houston, Texas
Traumatic Heart Disease

Patrick M. McCarthy, MD
Heller-Sacks Professor of Surgery, Northwestern University Feinberg School of Medicine; Chief, Division of Cardiothoracic Surgery, Co-Director, Bluhm Cardiovascular Institute, Northwestern Memorial Hospital, Chicago, Illinois
Surgical Management of Heart Failure

Peter A. McCullough, MD, MPH
Consultant Cardiologist and Chief, Division of Preventive Medicine, William Beaumont Hospital, Royal Oak, Michigan
Interface Between Renal Disease and Cardiovascular Illness

Vallerie V. McLaughlin, MD
Associate Professor of Medicine, University of Michigan Medical School; Director, Pulmonary Hypertension Program, University of Michigan Health System, Ann Arbor, Michigan
Pulmonary Hypertension

Bruce McManus, MD, PhD
Professor of Pathology and Laboratory Medicine, University of British Columbia Faculty of Medicine; Director of the James Hogg iCapture Centre and Scientific Director of the Heart Centre, St. Paul's Hospital, Providence Health, Vancouver, British Columbia, Canada
Primary Tumors of the Heart

John M. Miller, MD
Professor of Medicine, Krannert Institute of Cardiology, Indiana University School of Medicine, Indianapolis, Indiana
Diagnosis of Cardiac Arrhythmias; Therapy for Cardiac Arrhythmias

David M. Mirvis, MD
Professor of Preventive Medicine, University of Tennessee Health Science Center, Memphis, Tennessee
Electrocardiography

David A. Morrow, MD
Assistant Professor of Medicine, Harvard Medical School; Brigham and Women's Hospital, Boston, Massachusetts
Chronic Coronary Artery Disease; Guidelines: Chronic Stable Angina

Robert J. Myerburg, MD
Professor of Medicine, Division of Cardiology, University of Miami School of Medicine; Jackson Memorial Hospital, Miami, Florida
Cardiac Arrest and Sudden Cardiac Death

Elizabeth G. Nabel, MD
Director, National Heart, Lung, and Blood Institute, National Institutes of Health, Bethesda, Maryland
Principles of Cardiovascular Molecular Biology and Genetics

Yoshifumi Naka, MD, PhD
Associate Professor of Surgery, Columbia University College of Physicians and Surgeons; Director, Cardiac Transplantation and Mechanical Circulatory Support Program, New York–Presbyterian Hospital, Columbia University Medical Center, New York, New York
Assisted Circulation in the Treatment of Heart Failure

Carlo Napolitano, MD, PhD
Senior Scientist, Molecular Cardiology Laboratories, IRCCS Fondazione Salvatore Maugeri, Pavia, Italy
Genetics of Cardiac Arrhythmias

Richard W. Nesto, MD
Associate Professor of Medicine, Harvard Medical School, Boston; Chair, Department of Cardiovascular Medicine, Lahey Clinic Medical Center, Burlington, Massachusetts
Diabetes and Heart Disease

L. Kristin Newby, MD, MHS
Associate Professor of Medicine, Division of Cardiovascular Medicine, Duke University School of Medicine; Duke University Medical Center, Durham, North Carolina
Cardiovascular Disease in Women

Patrick T. O'Gara, MD
Associate Professor of Medicine, Harvard Medical School; Director of Clinical Cardiology and Vice Chair of Medicine, Brigham and Women's Hospital, Boston, Massachusetts
The History and Physical Examination: An Evidence-Based Approach

Jae K. Oh, MD
Professor of Medicine, Mayo Clinic College of Medicine; Consultant of Cardiovascular Diseases, Co-Director of Echocardiography Laboratory, Director of Echocardiography Core Laboratory, Mayo Clinic, Rochester, Minnesota
Echocardiography

Jeffrey E. Olgin, MD
Associate Professor in Residence, Chief of Cardiac Electrophysiology, and Melvin M. Schienman Chair in Electrophysiology, University of California, San Francisco, School of Medicine, San Francisco, California
Specific Arrhythmias: Diagnosis and Treatment

Lionel H. Opie, MD, DPhil
Professor of Medicine, Faculty of Health Sciences, The Hatter Institute for Cardiology Research, University of Cape Town, Cape Town, South Africa
Mechanisms of Cardiac Contraction and Relaxation

Catherine M. Otto, MD
J. Ward Kennedy-Hamilton Endowed Professor of Cardiology, Director of Cardiology Fellowship Programs, and Associate Director of Echocardiography, University of Washington School of Medicine, Seattle, Washington
Valvular Heart Disease

Dudley Pennell, MD
Professor of Cardiology, Imperial College London; Director, Cardiovascular Magnetic Resonance Unit, Royal Brompton Hospital, London, United Kingdom
Cardiovascular Magnetic Resonance

Jeffrey J. Popma, MD
Associate Professor of Medicine, Harvard Medical School; Director, Interventional Cardiology, Brigham and Women's Hospital, Boston, Massachusetts
Coronary Arteriography and Intravascular Imaging; Percutaneous Coronary and Valvular Intervention

Silvia G. Priori, MD, PhD
Associate Professor of Cardiology, University of Pavia; Director, Molecular Cardiology, IRCCS Fondazione Salvatore Maugeri, Pavia, Italy
Genetics of Cardiac Arrhythmias

Reed E. Pyeritz, MD, PhD
Professor of Medicine and Genetics, University of Pennsylvania School of Medicine, Philadelphia, Pennsylvania
General Principles of Genetic Factors in Cardiovascular Disease; Genetic Factors in Myocardial Disease

B. Soma Raju, MD
Professor of Cardiology, Care Institute of Medical Sciences; Chair, Division of Cardiology, Care Hospital, Hyderabad, India
Rheumatic Fever

Margaret M. Redfield, MD
Professor of Medicine, Mayo Clinic College of Medicine; Director, Mayo Heart Failure Clinic, Rochester, Minnesota
Heart Failure with Normal Ejection Fraction

Andrew N. Redington, MD
Professor of Pediatrics, University of Toronto Faculty of Medicine; Head of Cardiology, Hospital for Sick Children, Toronto, Ontario, Canada
Congenital Heart Disease

Frederic S. Resnic, MD
Assistant Professor of Medicine, Harvard Medical School; Director, Cardiac Catheterization Laboratory, Brigham and Women's Hospital, Boston, Massachusetts
Percutaneous Coronary and Valvular Intervention

Stuart Rich, MD
Professor of Medicine, University of Chicago Pritzker School of Medicine; Center for Pulmonary Hypertension, University of Chicago Medical Center, Chicago, Illinois
Pulmonary Hypertension

Paul M. Ridker, MD, MPH
Eugene Braunwald Professor of Medicine, Harvard Medical School; Director, Center for Cardiovascular Disease Prevention, Brigham and Women's Hospital, Boston, Massachusetts
Risk Factors for Atherothrombotic Disease; Primary and Secondary Prevention of Coronary Heart Disease

Dan M. Roden, MD
Professor of Medicine and Pharmacology; Director, Oates Institute for Experimental Therapeutics; Assistant Vice-Chancellor for Personalized Medicine, Vanderbilt University School of Medicine, Nashville, Tennessee
The Principles of Drug Therapy

Eric A. Rose, MD
Professor of Surgery, Columbia University College of Physicians and Surgeons; Director of Surgical Service and Surgeon-in-Chief, New York–Presbyterian Hospital, Columbia University Medical Center, New York, New York
Assisted Circulation in the Treatment of Heart Failure

Michael Rubart, MD
Assistant Professor of Pediatrics, Herman B. Wells Center for Pediatric Research, Indiana University School of Medicine, Indianapolis, Indiana
Genesis of Cardiac Arrhythmias: Electrophysiological Considerations

Andrew I. Schafer, MD
E. Hugh Luckey Distinguished Professor of Medicine and Chair, Department of Medicine, Weill Medical College of Cornell University; Physician-in-Chief, New York-Presbyterian Hospital, Weill Cornell Medical Center, New York, New York
Hemostasis, Thrombosis, Fibrinolysis, and Cardiovascular Disease

Heinz-Peter Schultheiss, MD
Department of Cardiology and Pneumology, Charité–University Medicine Berlin, Campus Benjamin Franklin, Berlin, Germany
Myocarditis

Janice B. Schwartz, MD
Clinical Professor of Medicine, University of California, San Francisco, School of Medicine; Director of Research, Jewish Home, San Francisco, California
Cardiovascular Disease in the Elderly

Peter J. Schwartz, MD
Professor and Chair, Department of Cardiology, University of Pavia; Chief, Coronary Care Unit, IRCCS Fondazione Policlinico S. Matteo, Pavia, Italy
Genetics of Cardiac Arrhythmias

Christine E. Seidman, MD
Thomas W. Smith Professor of Medicine and Genetics, Harvard Medical School; Director, Cardiovascular Genetics Center, Brigham and Women's Hospital, Boston, Massachusetts
General Principles of Genetic Factors in Cardiovascular Disease; Genetic Factors in Myocardial Disease

Jonathan G. Seidman, PhD
Henrietta B. and Frederick H. Bugher Professor of Cardiovascular Genetics, Department of Genetics, Harvard Medical School, Boston, Massachusetts
Genetic Factors in Myocardial Disease

Dhun H. Sethna, MD
Associate Director of Cardiology, Almeda County Medical Center, Oakland, California
Medical Management of the Patient Undergoing Cardiac Surgery

Daniel Simon, MD
Herman K. Hellerstein Professor of Medicine, Case Western Reserve University School of Medicine; Chief of Cardiovascular Medicine, Director of the Heart and Vascular Institute, University Hospitals of Cleveland/Case Medical Center, Cleveland, Ohio
Hemostasis, Thrombosis, Fibrinolysis, and Cardiovascular Disease

Jeffrey F. Smallhorn, MBBS
Professor of Pediatrics, University of Alberta Faculty of Medicine and Dentistry; Head, Section of Echocardiography Laboratory, Stollery Children's Hospital, Edmonton, Alberta, Canada
Congenital Heart Disease

Virend K. Somers, MD, DPhil
Professor of Medicine, Division of Cardiovascular Diseases, Mayo Clinic College of Medicine; Consultant, Cardiovascular Diseases, Mayo Clinic, Rochester, Minnesota
Sleep Apnea and Cardiovascular Disease; Cardiovascular Manifestations of Autonomic Disorders

John R. Teerlink, MD
Associate Professor of Medicine, University of California, San Francisco, School of Medicine; Director of Heart Failure, Director of Clinical Echocardiography, San Francisco Veterans Affairs Medical Center, San Francisco, California
Diagnosis and Management of Acute Heart Failure

Judith Therrien, MD
Assistant Professor of Medicine, McGill University Faculty of Medicine; Cardiologist, Sir Mortimer B. Davis Jewish General Hospital, Montreal, Quebec, Canada
Congenital Heart Disease

Paul D. Thompson, MD
Professor of Medicine, University of Connecticut School of Medicine; Director of Cardiology, Henry Low Heart Center, Hartford Hospital, Hartford, Connecticut
Exercise-Based, Comprehensive Cardiac Rehabilitation

Zoltan G. Turi, MD
Professor of Medicine, Robert Wood Johnson Medical School, University of Medicine and Dentistry of New Jersey; Director of the Structural Heart Disease Program, Director of the Cooper Vascular Center, Cooper University Hospital, Camden, New Jersey
Rheumatic Fever

James E. Udelson, MD
Associate Professor of Medicine and Radiology, Tufts University School of Medicine; Associate Chief of Cardiology, Director of Nuclear Cardiology, and Co-Director of the Heart Failure Service, Tufts-New England Medical Center, Boston, Massachusetts
Nuclear Cardiology; Guidelines: Nuclear Cardiology

Ronald G. Victor, MD
Clinical Professor of Medicine, University of Texas Southwestern Medical School; Chief of Hypertension, Norman and Audrey Kaplan Chair in Hypertension, University of Texas Southwestern Medical Center, Dallas, Texas
Systemic Hypertension: Mechanisms and Diagnosis

John H. K. Vogel, MD
Former Chair, Cardiology, Santa Barbara Cottage Hospital; Former President, American Heart Association, Santa Barbara County, Santa Barbara, California
Complementary and Alternative Approaches to Management of Patients with Heart Disease

Matthew J. Wall, Jr., MD
Professor, Michael E. DeBakey Department of Surgery, Baylor College of Medicine; Deputy Chief of Surgery and Chief of Cardiothoracic Surgery, Ben Taub General Hospital, Houston, Texas
Traumatic Heart Disease

Carole A. Warnes, MD
Professor of Medicine, Mayo Clinic College of Medicine; Consultant in Cardiovascular Diseases and Internal Medicine, Pediatric Cardiology; Director, Adult Congenital Heart Disease Clinic; Dean, Mayo School of Continuing Medical Education, Mayo Clinic, Rochester, Minnesota
Pregnancy and Heart Disease

Gary D. Webb, MD
Professor of Medicine, University of Pennsylvania School of Medicine; Director, Philadelphia Adult Congenital Heart Center, University of Pennsylvania Health System, Children's Hospital of Philadelphia, Philadelphia, Pennsylvania
Congenital Heart Disease

Christopher J. White, MD
Chairman, Department of Cardiology, Ochsner Clinic Foundation, New Orleans, Louisiana
Endovascular Treatment of Noncoronary Obstructive Vascular Disease

Lawson R. Wulsin, MD
Professor of Psychiatry and Family Medicine, University of Cincinnati College of Medicine; Director, Family Medicine Psychiatry Training Program, University Hospital, Cincinnati, Ohio
Psychiatric and Behavioral Aspects of Cardiovascular Disease

Clyde W. Yancy, MD
Medical Director, Baylor Heart and Vascular Institute; Chief, Cardiothoracic Transplantation, Baylor University Medical Center at Dallas, Dallas, Texas
Heart Disease in Varied Populations

Andreas M. Zeiher, MD
Professor of Cardiology and Chair, Department of Medicine, University of Frankfurt, Frankfurt, Germany
Emerging Therapies and Strategies in the Treatment of Heart Failure

Douglas P. Zipes, MD
Distinguished Professor; Professor Emeritus of Medicine, Pharmacology, and Toxicology; and Director Emeritus, Division of Cardiology and the Krannert Institute of Cardiology, Indiana University School of Medicine, Indianapolis, Indiana
Genesis of Cardiac Arrhythmias: Electrophysiological Considerations; Diagnosis of Cardiac Arrhythmias; Therapy for Cardiac Arrhythmias; Cardiac Pacemakers and Cardioverter-Defibrillators; Specific Arrhythmias: Diagnosis and Treatment; Hypotension and Syncope; Cardiovascular Disease in the Elderly; Neurological Disorders and Cardiovascular Disease

Preface

The currents of contemporary cardiovascular disease run swiftly, broadly, and deeply. The Eighth Edition of *Braunwald's Heart Disease: A Textbook of Cardiovascular Medicine,* presented here, serves as the hub of a learning system designed to help physicians and students at all levels, from trainees to highly specialized practitioners, confront the challenge of staying abreast of this rapidly evolving field.

We intend *Heart Disease* to constitute the "core curriculum," an up-to-date, comprehensive, and authoritative ready reference for all practitioners. We strove to make this Eighth Edition an information source of practical clinical utility, grounded in the rapidly expanding evidence base that informs our practice. As in the previous editions of *Heart Disease,* we present the scientific underpinnings that govern cardiovascular pathophysiology and provide a rational basis for understanding therapeutics and management of cardiovascular diseases encountered in clinical practice.

Since the preparation of the last edition of *Heart Disease* much has changed, a reflection of the rapid pace of progress in our specialty. The results of manifold new clinical trials have become available in ways that in many cases profoundly affect our management strategies and practice. Novel therapeutics, both pharmacological and device-based, provide new management options. In the last few years we have not only witnessed striking advances in therapeutics but encountered challenges in the application of drug therapies and cardiovascular devices ranging from drug-eluting stents to implantable devices. The constant change and complexities in therapeutics and management strategies render obsolete textbooks published only a few years ago.

Other rapid shifts are under way in the prevalence of cardiovascular disease. In recent years cardiovascular specialists could congratulate themselves that the epidemic of cardiovascular disease had declined, based on the progress in our specialty. Current demographic trends suggest, however, that the scourge of cardiovascular disease, rather than waning, may indeed be increasing in the years to come. The aging of the population will increase the overall burden of cardiovascular disease in society, even as age-adjusted rates of cardiovascular mortality plateau or decline. We also need to confront a renewed upswing of cardiovascular risk linked to the worldwide epidemic of obesity, insulin resistance, and diabetes rooted in over-nutrition and declining physical activity. This gathering of cardiovascular risk increasingly threatens to extend the burden of cardiovascular disease to developing as well as Western societies. Thus, we cannot presume that the toll of cardiovascular disease will continue to ebb, highlighting the urgency of tools such as the *Heart Disease* Learning System that aim to help the clinician remain abreast of the constantly changing landscape of cardiovascular disease.

We have thoroughly revised this new edition to reflect these multiple changes. Thirty of eighty-nine chapters are entirely new. Thus, more than one third of the Eighth Edition represents completely new material. There are 43 new authors, comparing the Eighth to the Seventh Edition of *Heart Disease.* All of the chapters carried over from the Seventh Edition have undergone extensive revision to update them and heighten their utility. A full description of the changes introduced in this Eighth Edition exceeds the scope of this Preface. Among the major changes, Douglas L. Mann, MD, has joined the editorial team and overseen a recasting of the entire section devoted to heart failure and chapters relating to myocardial disease. As heart failure represents the leading cause of admissions of patients covered by Medicare to hospitals, and comprises an ever-increasing fraction of our patient population given the success of acute interventions, the fresh approach to this important topic should be welcome to readers. In particular, new chapters focus on acute heart failure and heart failure with preserved systolic function, two timely and challenging issues in clinical practice.

Given the growing potential of genetics and expanding knowledge of cardiovascular genetics, Christine E. Seidman, MD, and Jonathan G. Seidman, PhD, have joined the author list of *Heart Disease* and provide a thorough revision with Reed E. Pyeritz, MD, PhD, of the chapter on cardiovascular genetics and an entirely new chapter on the genetics of myocardial disease, complemented by online supplements. A new chapter on evidence-based physical examination has replaced the traditional recitation and cataloguing of signs and symptoms of cardiovascular disease. We are grateful to James C. Fang, MD, and Patrick T. O'Gara, MD, for taking on the assignment of preparing this entirely new approach to the foundation of clinical evaluation, the physical examination. Heidi M. Connolly, MD, and Jae K. Oh, MD, have prepared a new chapter on echocardiography that provides in-depth discussion of the current state-of-the-art applications of this versatile imaging modality for virtually all forms of cardiac disease. A new chapter on stroke by Larry B. Goldstein, MD, highlights what a cardiovascular practitioner needs to know about prevention and treatment of stroke and illustrates the extra-cardiac extensions of contemporary cardiology practice. A new chapter on sleep disorders likewise acknowledges the importance of an integrated multi-system approach to the management of our patients with cardiovascular disease. A new chapter on complementary and alternative approaches to cardiovascular disease reflects the growing interest in this area in patients and doctors alike. For similar reasons, we have added a new chapter on sports cardiology.

The Eighth Edition of *Heart Disease* contains 2275 illustrations, in full color where appropriate, as well as 600 tables. The CD-ROM packaged with the book contains all the figures and tables from the book, available to download to PowerPoint® to facilitate the use of these abundant materials for teaching. We hope thus to multiply the communication value of the content offered by the experts who contributed to *Heart Disease.*

As noted above, we conceive of *Heart Disease* as a family of learning tools intended to help the reader surmount the swift change in cardiovascular knowledge. To keep pace with the rapid evolution of our specialty between editions, we have approached *Heart Disease* as a living book. The *Heart Disease* website personally edited and updated by Eugene Braunwald, MD, on a weekly basis provides the readers of *Heart Disease* with a pulse of progress in cardiovascular medicine on an ongoing and contemporaneous basis. The many special features of the website, such as weekly updates, late-breaking clinical trials, hot-off-the-press topics, abstracts, and focused reviews, in addition to the searchability and functionality of the online medium, offer the interested reader the wealth and breadth of current information that no other online resource in cardiology can provide.

We intend the growing family of *Heart Disease* companion volumes to address the breadth and depth of cardiovascular medicine. Several companions are currently in print, many published or revised in the last few years. Other companions in production or the planning stages include topics such as arrhythmology and lipidology, and mechanical circulatory support will emerge in the coming years. Noteworthy additions to the family of *Heart Disease* companions include a new volume on hypertension edited by Henry R. Black, MD, and William J. Elliott, MD, PhD; an entirely revised and updated version of *Cardiovascular Therapeutics* edited by Elliott M. Antman, MD; a comprehensive volume on vascular medicine edited by Mark A. Creager, MD, Victor J. Dzau, MD, and Joseph Loscalzo, MD, PhD; and a volume on cardiac nursing edited by Debra K. Moser, DNSc, RN, and Barbara Riegel, DNSc, RN. Readers of *Heart Disease* who wish to deepen their knowledge of specific areas can turn to the companion volumes as a convenient source, bearing the hallmark of clinical utility with a clinical evidence foundation and scientific basis common to the *Heart Disease* mission. The companions are intended to complement the core curriculum of this *Heart Disease* volume. In response to the growing importance of imaging in cardiovascular practice, atlases of the emerging and established imaging technologies are currently in preparation under editorial direction of Robert O. Bonow, MD. Finally, a new edition of the *Heart Disease Review and Assessment* book is under way, to help trainees prepare for the certification examinations in the specialty of cardiovascular diseases.

These various key components of the *Heart Disease* Learning System, assembled in a personalized way to meet the needs of each practitioner, should help one navigate the rapidly flowing stream of cardiovascular knowledge. We hope that the readers will find *Heart Disease* and its associated learning tools useful in their quest to stay abreast of this ever-evolving field.

PETER LIBBY
ROBERT O. BONOW
DOUGLAS L. MANN
DOUGLAS P. ZIPES
2007

Preface

Adapted from the First Edition

Cardiovascular disease is the greatest scourge affecting the industrialized nations. As with previous scourges—bubonic plague, yellow fever, and smallpox—cardiovascular disease not only strikes down a significant fraction of the population without warning but also causes prolonged suffering and disability in an even larger number. In the United States alone, despite recent encouraging declines, cardiovascular disease is still responsible for almost 1 million fatalities each year and more than half of all deaths; almost 5 million persons afflicted with cardiovascular disease are hospitalized each year. The cost of these diseases in terms of human suffering and of material resources is almost incalculable. Fortunately, research focusing on the causes, diagnosis, treatment, and prevention of heart disease is moving ahead rapidly.

In order to provide a comprehensive, authoritative text in a field that has become as broad and deep as cardiovascular medicine, I chose to enlist the aid of a number of able colleagues. However, I hoped that my personal involvement in the writing of about half of the book would make it possible to minimize the fragmentation, gaps, inconsistencies, organizational difficulties, and impersonal tone that sometimes plague multiauthored texts.

Since the early part of the 20th century, clinical cardiology has had a particularly strong foundation in the basic sciences of physiology and pharmacology. More recently, the disciplines of molecular biology, genetics, developmental biology, biophysics, biochemistry, experimental pathology, and bioengineering have also begun to provide critically important information about cardiac function and malfunction. Although *Heart Disease: A Textbook of Cardiovascular Medicine* is primarily a clinical treatise and not a textbook of fundamental cardiovascular science, an effort has been made to explain, in some detail, the scientific bases of cardiovascular diseases.

EUGENE BRAUNWALD
1980

Contents

Part X ■ Cardiovascular Disease and Disorders of Other Organs 2033

Look for these other titles in the Braunwald's Heart Disease family!

ANTMAN
Cardiovascular Therapeutics
Third Edition

BLACK *and* ELLIOTT
Hypertension

CHIEN
Molecular Basis of Cardiovascular Disease
Second Edition

CREAGER, LOSCALZO, *and* DZAU
Vascular Medicine

LILLY
Heart Disease Review and Assessment

MANN
Heart Failure

MANSON, BURING, RIDKER, *and* GAZIANO
Clinical Trials in Heart Disease
Second Edition

MOSER *and* RIEGEL
Cardiac Nursing

ST. JOHN SUTTON *and* RUTHERFORD
Clinical Cardiovascular Imaging

PART I

Fundamentals of Cardiovascular Disease

CHAPTER 1

Global Burden of Cardiovascular Disease

J. Michael Gaziano

The 20th century saw unparalleled increases in life expectancy and a major shift in the causes of illness and death throughout the world. During this transition, cardiovascular disease (CVD) became the most common cause of death worldwide. A century ago, CVD accounted for less than 10 percent of all deaths. Today, it accounts for approximately 30 percent of deaths worldwide including nearly 40 percent in high-income countries and about 28 percent in low- and middle-income countries.[1] Driven by industrialization, urbanization, and associated lifestyle changes, this ongoing transition is occurring around the world among all races, ethnic groups, and cultures at an even faster rate than last century. This chapter describes how CVD became the dominant disease in the world, beginning with an explanation of the concept of the epidemiological transition and a synopsis of this transition in the United States. This is followed by a survey of the current burden of cardiovascular disease, as well as related trends both globally and in various regions of the world and changing rates of risk factors and behaviors. The chapter ends with a discussion of the diverse challenges that the increasing burden of CVD poses for the various regions of the world and potential solutions to this global problem.

EPIDEMIOLOGICAL TRANSITIONS

With rates that easily surpass projections made a decade ago, we begin the 21st century with CVD as the leading cause of death worldwide. This global rise in CVD results from a dramatic shift in the health status of individuals around the world during the course of the 20th century and an unprecedented transformation in the distribution of diseases responsible for the majority of death and debility. Before 1900, infectious diseases and malnutrition were the most common causes of death in the world. Thanks largely to improved nutrition and public health measures, both have declined, with a resultant increase in life expectancy. Increased longevity and the impact of smoking, high-fat diets, and other risk factors for chronic diseases have combined to make CVD and cancer the leading causes of death in most countries. These changes began in higher income countries, but as they have gradually spread to low- and middle-income countries, CVD mortality rates have increased globally. In absolute numbers, four to five times as many deaths caused by CVD now occur in developing countries as in developed countries. By 2001, CVD had become the leading cause of death in the developing world, just as it has been in the developed world since about 1950. This rate of increase surpassed predictions made in the 1990s.[2] Between 1990 and 2001, deaths from CVD increased from 26 to 28 percent of all deaths in the low- and middle-income countries, a reflection of the continuing global shift in disease burden from communicable to noncommunicable disease (Fig. 1-1).

National health and disease profiles vary widely by country and by region. For example, life expectancy in Japan (78.4 years for men; 85.3 years for women) is more than twice that in Sierra Leone (31.2 years for men; 35.8 years for women).[3] In their original comprehensive analysis of the global burden of disease, Murray and Lopez[2] defined three categories, or groups, of disease. Group I consists of communicable diseases, maternal and perinatal conditions, and nutritional deficiencies; group II comprises noncommunicable diseases including CVD and cancer; and group III consists of injuries. The World Bank divides the world into two major economic categories: high-income countries and low- and middle-income countries. Today, group I diseases account for just 7 percent of deaths in high-income countries, compared with 36 percent in low- and middle-income countries.[1] This percentage is falling rapidly in all regions except sub-Saharan Africa, where the human immunodeficiency virus/acquired immune deficiency syndrome (HIV/AIDS) epidemic has kept this figure high. It is the group II diseases (the category that includes heart disease and stroke) that are presenting an ever larger disease burden in low- and middle-income countries. Group II diseases now account for more than half of the burden in these countries, an increase of 10 percent between 1990 and 2001.[1] In high-income countries, group II diseases are responsible for 87 percent of all deaths, whereas injuries—group III—cause only 6 percent of deaths compared with 10 percent in the low- and middle-income countries.

The World Bank divides the low- and middle-income countries into six subregions: East Asia and Pacific, (Eastern) Europe and Central Asia, Latin America and the Caribbean, Middle East and North Africa, South Asia, and sub-Saharan Africa. The vast differences in burden of cardiovascular disease are readily apparent across these broad economic and geographic sectors of the world (Fig. 1-2). CVD is the primary source of mortality from noncommunicable, or group II, diseases in both high-income and low- and middle-income countries, but in the high-income category, age-adjusted rates of CVD are falling, whereas CVD is on the rise in the low- and middle-income countries. In Eastern Europe and Central Asia, CVD now accounts for nearly 60 percent of all deaths, whereas that figure is only 10 percent in AIDS-ravaged sub-Saharan Africa, reflecting the great heterogeneity among populations across the world.

This shift in the diseases that account for the lion's share of mortality and morbidity is known as the *epidemiological transition.*[4,5] Omran divides the transition into three basic ages: pestilence and famine, receding pandemics, and degenerative and man-made diseases[4] (Table 1-1). Olshansky and Ault[5] added a fourth stage, *delayed degenerative diseases.* A fifth stage, characterized by an epidemic of inactivity and obesity, discussed later in the chapter, may be emerging in some countries. Although any specific country or region enters these stages at different times, the progression from one to another tends to proceed in a predictable manner. Never occurring in isolation, the epidemiological transition is tightly intertwined with changes in personal and collective wealth (economic transition), social structure (social transition), and demographics (demographic transition).

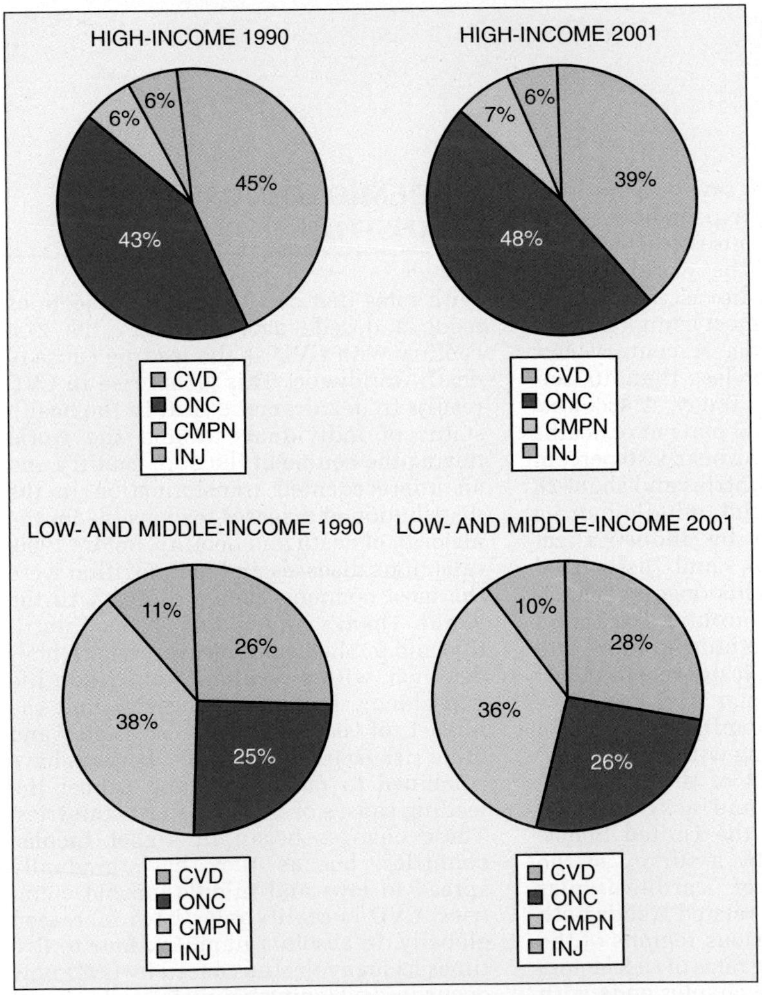

FIGURE 1–1 Changing pattern of mortality, 1990 to 2001. CMPN = communicable, maternal, perinatal, and nutritional diseases; CVD = cardiovascular disease; INJ = injury; ONC = other noncommunicable diseases. *(From Mathers CD, Lopez A, Stein D, et al: Deaths and disease burden by cause: Global burden of disease estimates for 2001 by World Bank Country Groups. Disease Control Priorities Working Paper 18. April 2004, revised January 2005.)*

The Age of Pestilence and Famine

From the epidemiological standpoint, humans evolved under conditions of pestilence and famine and have lived with them for most of recorded history. This age is characterized by the predominance of malnutrition and infectious disease and by the infrequency of CVD as a cause of death. High fertility rates necessitated by high infant and child mortality result in a mean life expectancy on the order of approximately 30 years. In regions that eventually became today's high-income countries, the transition through the age of pestilence and famine was relatively slow, beginning in the late 1700s and progressing throughout the 1800s. Competing influences prolonged the transition—improvements in the food supply early in the Industrial Revolution that by themselves would have reduced mortality were offset by the concentration of the population in urban centers, which led to increases in mortality caused by communicable diseases such as tuberculosis, cholera, dysentery, and influenza.

Although the transition through the age of pestilence and famine has occurred much later in the low- and middle-income countries, it has also occurred more rapidly, driven largely by the transfer of low-cost agricultural products and technologies

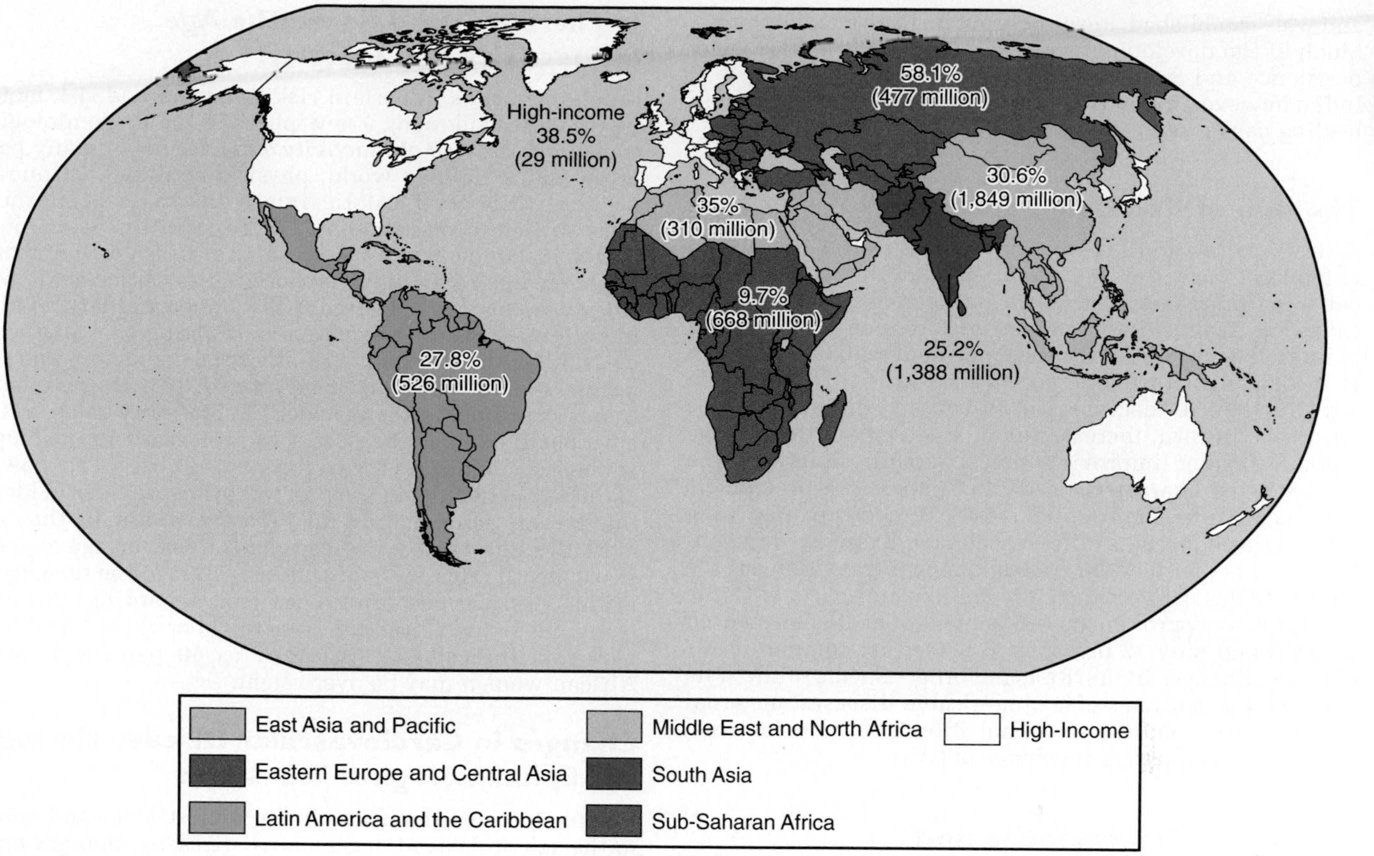

FIGURE 1–2 Cardiovascular disease deaths as a percentage of all deaths in each region and total regional population—2001. *(Based on data from Mathers CD, Lopez A, Stein D, et al: Deaths and disease burden by cause: Global burden of disease estimates for 2001 by World Bank Country Groups. Disease Control Priorities Working Paper 18. April 2004, revised January 2005.)*

TABLE 1–1 Four Typical Stages of the Epidemiological Transition

Stage	Description	Typical Proportion of Deaths Caused by Cardiovascular Disease (%)	Predominant Types of Cardiovascular Disease
Pestilence and famine	Predominance of malnutrition and infectious diseases as causes of death; high rates of infant and child mortality; low mean life expectancy	<10	Rheumatic heart disease, cardiomyopathies caused by infection and malnutrition
Receding pandemics	Improvements in nutrition and public health lead to decrease in rates of deaths caused by malnutrition and infection; precipitous decline in infant and child mortality rates	10-35	Rheumatic valvular disease, hypertension, CHD, stroke
Degenerative and man-made diseases	Increased fat and caloric intake and decreased physical activity lead to emergence of hypertension and atherosclerosis; with increased life expectancy, mortality from chronic, noncommunicable diseases exceeds mortality from malnutrition and infectious diseases	35-65	CHD, stroke
Delayed degenerative diseases	Cardiovascular diseases and cancer are the major causes of morbidity and mortality; better treatment and prevention efforts help avoid deaths among those with disease and delay primary events. Age-adjusted CVD mortality declines; CVD affecting older and older individuals	40-50	CHD, stroke, congestive heart failure

CHD = coronary heart disease; CVD = cardiovascular disease.

Modified from Omran AR: The epidemiologic transition: A theory of the epidemiology of population change. Milbank Mem Fund Q 49:509, 1971; and Olshansky SJ, Ault AB: The fourth stage of the epidemiologic transition: The age of delayed degenerative diseases. Milbank Q 64:355, 1986.

and well-established, lower-cost public health technologies. Much of the developing world has emerged from the age of pestilence and famine. In sub-Saharan Africa and parts of India, however, malnutrition and infectious disease remain leading causes of death.

The Age of Receding Pandemics

Rising wealth and the resultant increase in the availability of food help usher in the second phase of the epidemiological transition. Improved nutrition decreases early deaths caused by malnutrition and may also reduce susceptibility to infectious diseases. Increased personal and public wealth is associated with public health measures that contribute still further to declines in infectious diseases. These advances, in turn, increase the productivity of the average worker, further improving the economic situation. The change most characteristic of this phase is a precipitous decline in infant and child mortality accompanied by a substantial increase in life expectancy. Examples of countries in this phase of the epidemiological transition are the United States early in the 20th century and parts of China today, where approximately 25 percent of deaths are caused by CVD and only 12 percent are caused by communicable disease.[1] Changes in nutrition and other aspects of life style that cause lower rates of communicable diseases, maternal and perinatal conditions, and nutritional deficiencies eventually lead to a greater incidence of CVD.

The Age of Degenerative and Man-Made Diseases

Continued improvements in economic circumstances, combined with urbanization and radical changes in the nature of work-related activities, lead to dramatic life-style changes in diet, activity levels, and behaviors such as smoking. Unlike the age of pestilence and famine when most of the population is deficient in total caloric intake relative to daily caloric expenditure, easier access to less expensive foods and increased fat content increase total caloric intake, as mechanization results in lower daily caloric expenditure. This disparity leads to a higher mean body mass index, blood pressure, and levels of plasma lipids and blood sugar. These changes set the stage for the emergence of hypertensive diseases and atherosclerosis. Cancer rates also rise rapidly during the age of degenerative and man-made diseases. As the average life expectancy increases beyond 50 years, mortality from largely chronic noncommunicable diseases—dominated by CVD—exceeds mortality from malnutrition and infectious diseases.

The Age of Delayed Degenerative Diseases

In the fourth phase of the epidemiological transition, CVD and cancer remain the major causes of morbidity and mortality. In the industrialized nations, however, major technological advances such as coronary care units, bypass surgery, percutaneous coronary interventions, and thrombolytic therapy are available to manage the acute manifestations of CVD, and preventive strategies such as smoking cessation, blood pressure management, and cholesterol management are widely implemented. As a result of better treatment and widespread primary and secondary prevention efforts, deaths are prevented among people with disease and primary events are delayed. Life expectancy continues to creep upward as age-adjusted CVD mortality tends to decline, with the average age of people affected by CVD getting increasingly older.

Is There a Fifth Phase: The Age of Inactivity and Obesity?

Troubling trends in certain risk behaviors and risk factors may be foreshadowing a new phase of the epidemiological transition, the *Age of Inactivity and Obesity*. In many parts of the industrialized world, physical activity continues to decline while total caloric intake increases at alarming rates, with the combination resulting in an epidemic of overweight and obesity. As a result, rates of type II diabetes, hypertension, and lipid abnormalities associated with obesity are on the rise—trends that are particularly evident in children.[6,7] These changes are occurring at a time when measurable improvements in other risk behaviors and risk factors such as smoking have slowed. If these risk factor trends continue, age-adjusted CVD mortality rates, which have declined over the past several decades in developed countries, could increase in the coming years. The slowing of the rate of decline in the past few years provides evidence that we are approaching an inflection point in the CVD mortality curves. This is especially true for age-adjusted stroke death rates. Also of concern, even in the developing world, obesity is becoming a problem. According to a recent study, one in five Chinese is overweight or obese.[8] And other new data indicate that as many as 40 percent of South African women may be overweight.

Changes in Cardiovascular Disease through the Epidemiological Transition

During the transition from the age of pestilence and famine to the age of delayed degenerative diseases, changes occur in both the character of CVD and total rates of CVD.[9] During the age of pestilence and famine, CVD accounts for only 5 to 10 percent of mortality, with the major forms of CVD related to infection and malnutrition, largely rheumatic heart disease and infectious and nutritional cardiomyopathies. Given the potentially long latent period of these diseases, they are apparent well into the age of receding pandemics, when they persist as major causes of death along with emerging hypertensive heart disease and stroke. During the age of receding pandemics, CVD accounts for 10 to 35 percent of deaths. CHD rates tend to be low relative to stroke rates. In addition, risk behaviors and risk factors that foreshadow the next phase become more widespread. During the age of degenerative and man-made diseases, increased caloric intake (particularly from saturated animal fats and processed vegetable fats), reduced daily activity, increased smoking rates, and related changes in the prevalence of hypertension, diabetes, and hyperlipidemia result in further increases in hypertensive diseases and rapid increases in CHD and peripheral vascular disease. During this phase, 35 to 65 percent of all deaths are due to CVD. Typically, the rate of CHD deaths greatly exceeds that of stroke by a ratio of 2 : 1 to 3 : 1.

In the fourth phase of the epidemiological transition, the age of delayed degenerative diseases, age-adjusted death rates from CVD begin to fall, leveling off somewhere below 50 percent of total mortality. The decline in stroke rates tends to precede the decline for CHD; thus the ratio of CHD to stroke deaths increases, typically to between 2 : 1 and 5 : 1 (Fig. 1-3).

The decline in CVD rates results from two factors: better access to health technology and adoption of healthier life styles. Improvements in health technology and better access to it decrease the likelihood of death among patients presenting with acute manifestations of atherosclerotic disease, although better survival means more and more individuals living longer with conditions such as angina pectoris, congestive heart failure, and cardiac arrhythmias.

Reductions in risk behaviors and factors may make even greater contributions to the decline in age-adjusted rates of death. In many cases, these result from concerted efforts by public health and health care communities. In other cases, secular trends also play a role. For example, the widespread availability of fresh fruits and vegetables all year long in developed countries, and thus increased consumption, may have contributed to declining mean cholesterol levels before effective drug therapy was widely available. In general, however, even though *age-adjusted* rates of CVD continue to decline during the final phase of the epidemiological transition, the prevalence of CVD increases as the population ages.

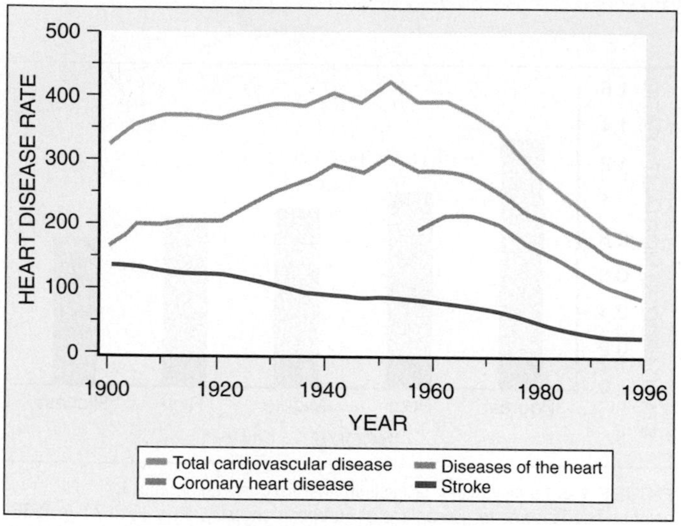

FIGURE 1–3 Increase and decline in age-adjusted heart disease rates through the epidemiological transition in the United States, 1900 to 1996. Rate is per 100,000 population, standardized to the 1940 U.S. population. Diseases are classified according to International Classification of Diseases (ICD) codes in use when the deaths were reported. ICD classification revisions occurred in 1910, 1921, 1930, 1939, 1949, 1958, 1968, and 1979. Death rates before 1933 do not include all states. Comparability ratios were applied to rates for 1970 and 1975. *(From Achievements in public health, 1900-1999: Decline in deaths from heart disease and stroke—United States, 1900-1999. MMWR Morbid Mortal Wkly Rep 48:649, 1999.)*

ECONOMIC, SOCIAL, AND DEMOGRAPHIC TRANSITIONS

As mentioned earlier, several parallel transformations accompany the epidemiological transition. These include economic, demographic, and social transitions that pave the way for major shifts in a population's health and the nature of the diseases that account for most of the mortality and morbidity. The economic transition is characterized by rising levels of personal wealth. This is usually reflected in increasing per capita income, per capita gross domestic product (GDP), or gross national product (GNP). Industrialization tends to spark a large number of social changes that have a significant impact on the epidemiological transition, including urbanization, the development of a public health infrastructure, wider access to health care, and increasing application of health technologies.

Urbanization affects living standards and life style and affords the opportunity to develop organized health care systems. Virtually all regions of the world have shifted from rural to urban life. For example, in the United States, 60 percent of the population lived in rural settings at the beginning of the 20th century compared with only 20 percent at the beginning of the 21st century. In Asia, Africa, and Latin America and the Caribbean, a similar shift has occurred over the second half of the 20th century (Fig. 1-4).

Demographic transition refers to shifts in the age structure of a population because of declining fertility and increased survival. During the age of pestilence and famine, individuals 20 years of age and younger may account for 40 to 50 percent of the population. As child and infant mortality rates decline in the age of receding pandemics, rapid gains accrue in life expectancy, and the proportion of individuals 20 years of age and younger decreases. Reduced mortality rates are generally followed by falling fertility rates, further flattening the shape of the population distribution curve. As population growth rates fall, the mean age of the population continues to rise slowly as individuals live longer.

A demographic profile of the world over the next 25 years shows that the segment of the population aged 65 and older is projected to grow faster than any other segment in all world regions.[10] In 2002, approximately 7 percent of the world's population had reached age 65, a number that is predicted to double by 2020 and more than triple by 2050. By 2040, more than 20 percent of U.S. citizens will be 65 or older. In China and Russia, that number will be approximately 20 percent, whereas in Brazil and India—so-called "young countries"—approximately 8 to 14 percent of residents will have reached 65 years of age. Because cardiovascular disease mortality increases as population longevity increases, there will be economic implications as the disease becomes clinically manifest and more people require treatment.

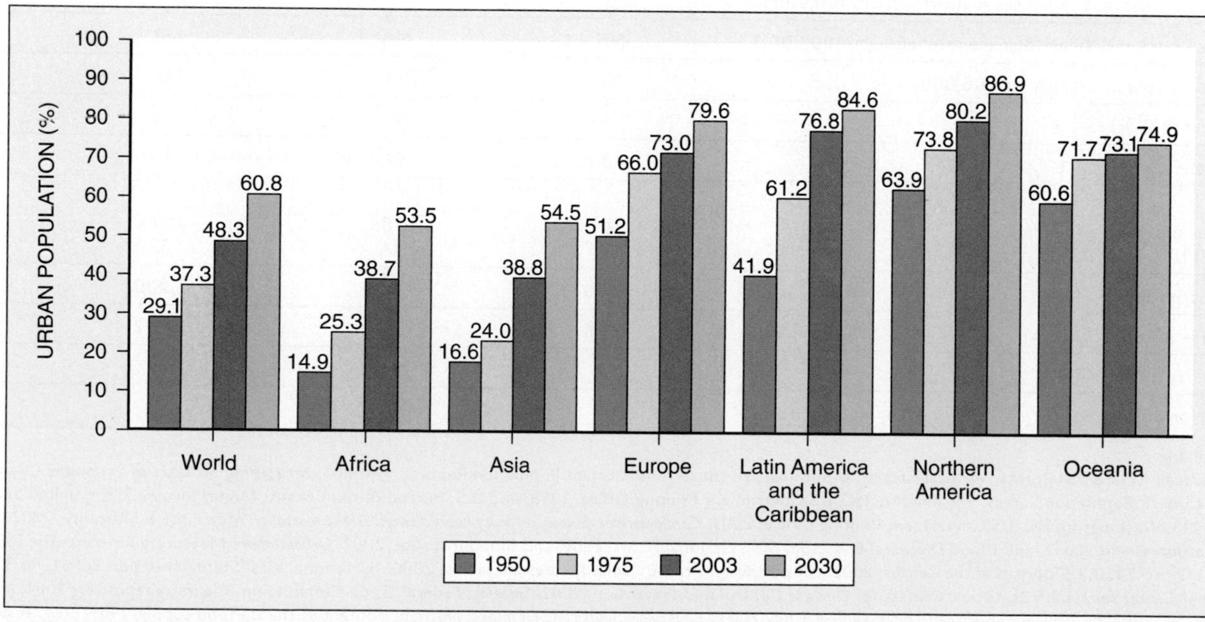

FIGURE 1–4 Number of people living in urban areas, 1950, 1975, 2003, and 2030. *(From United Nations Department of Economic and Social Affairs/Population Division: World Urbanization Prospects: The 2003 Revision. New York, United Nations Population Division, 2004.)*

The life-style changes associated with the economic and social transitions cause shifts in the profile of risk behaviors and risk factors for disease. These include decreased physical activity, increased smoking, and dramatic changes in diet.

RATE OF THE EPIDEMIOLOGICAL TRANSITION

Several factors influence how early or how quickly the epidemiological transition occurs in a given country or region: (1) The rate of economic growth relative to population growth affects the rate of adoption of life styles characteristic of established market economies; (2) Regional economic influences can cause great disparities in the rates of transition within a region; (3) The development of low-cost public health technologies, as well as falling costs of unhealthy aspects of the Western life style such as cigarette smoking and consumption of highly processed food, permits currently developing countries to make transitions more rapidly.

Even within a given country, segments of the population may undergo the transition at varying rates. These factors relate to economic, social, or cultural factors. In fact, epidemiological transitions occur at different rates across economic groups, generally beginning among those with higher socioeconomic status and eventually spreading to those with lower socioeconomic status. The decline in rates of malnutrition and communicable diseases, as well as the rise in coronary risk factors and behaviors, occur first in the privileged classes; increases in rates of stroke and CHD soon follow. Later, as the middle class grows, the epidemiological transition spreads to a broad enough sector of the population to have a measurable impact on population rates. As more and more of the burgeoning middle class passes through the second and third phases of the transition, CVD and cancer rates become the population's dominant causes of death and disability. People in the lower socioeconomic strata tend to acquire the risk factors and behaviors last, in part because of their economic situation and in part because they tend to engage in more physical activity at work. Compared with people in the upper and middle socioeconomic strata, those in the lowest stratum are less likely to have access to advanced treatments and to acquire and apply information on modification of risk factors and behaviors. Thus CVD mortality rates decline later among those with lower socioeconomic status. In a high-income country such as Canada, for example, CVD mortality rates are highest among the poorest individuals (Fig. 1-5).[11]

THE EPIDEMIOLOGICAL TRANSITION IN THE UNITED STATES

Like other high-income countries, the United States has proceeded through four stages of the epidemiological transition. Recent trends, however, suggest that the rates of decline of some chronic and degenerative diseases have slowed, suggesting the possibility that the United States is entering a fifth phase characterized by an epidemic of obesity. Given the large amount of economic, social, demographic, and health data available (Table 1-2), the United States serves as a useful reference point for later comparisons.

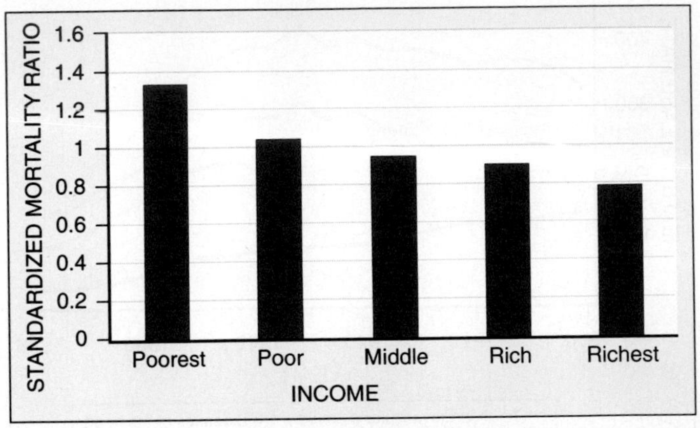

FIGURE 1–5 Cardiovascular disease standardized mortality ratios by neighborhood income for Canadians of European ancestry, ages 35 to 74, in 1986 and 1991. *(From Sheth T, Nair C, Nargundjar M, et al: Cardiovascular and cancer mortality among Canadians of European, South Asian, and Chinese origin from 1979 to 1993: An analysis of 1.2 million deaths. Can Med Assoc J 161:132, 1999.)*

TABLE 1–2 Trends in the United States during the 20th Century

	1900	1930	1970	2000
Population (millions)	76	123	203	281
Median income (real dollars)	NA	$15,050 (1947)	$26,333	$29,058
Age-adjusted cardiovascular disease mortality (n/100,000)	325	390	699	341
Age-adjusted coronary heart disease mortality (n/100,000)	NA	NA	448	186
Age-adjusted stroke mortality (n/100,000)	140	100	148	57
Urbanization (%)	39	56	74	76
Life expectancy (yr)	49.2	59.3	70.8	76.9
Smoking				
Cigarettes per capita (n)	54	1,185	3,969	1,977
Smokers (%)	NA	NA	37.4	23.3
Total caloric intake (kcal)	3,500	3,300	3,200	3,800
Fat intake (% of total calories)	31.6	37.3	41.2	33
Cholesterol level (mg/dl)	NA	NA	216	204
Overweight or obese (%)	NA	NA	47.7	64.5

NA = not available.

Sources: *Population*: US Census Bureau. *Per capita income*: U.S. Bureau of the Census: Current Population Reports, P60-203, Measuring 50 Years of Economic Change Using the March Current Population Survey. Washington, DC, US Government Printing Office, 1998; and U.S. Bureau of the Census: Money Income in the United States, 2000, P60-213. Washington, DC, US Government Printing Office, 2001. *Cardiovascular disease, coronary heart disease, stroke mortality*: Morbidity & Mortality: 2002 Chart Book on Cardiovascular, Lung, and Blood Diseases. Bethesda, Md., National Heart, Lung, and Blood Institute, 2002, *Urbanization*: Measuring America: The Decennial Censuses, 1790 to 2000: US Bureau of the Census, 2002. *Life expectancy*: Arias E: United States life tables, 2000. *In* National Vital Statistics Report vol 51, no 3. Atlanta, GA, National Center for Health Statistics, Centers for Disease Control and Prevention, 2002. *Smoking*: Federal Trade Commission: Cigarette report for 2001. (http://www.ftc.gov/os/2003/06/2001cigreport.pdf) Accessed on 1 July 2003: *Total caloric intake and fat intake*: Nutrient content of the US food supply, 1909-1994: A summary. Washington, DC, US Department of Agriculture, 1998; and Kennedy ET, Bowman SA, Powell R: Dietary-fat intake in the US population. J Am Coll Nutr 18:207, 1999. *Cholesterol level and obesity*: National Center for Health Statistics: Health, United States, 2002. (http://www.cdc.gov/nchs/data/hus/hus02.pdf) Accessed on 15 July 2003.

THE AGE OF PESTILENCE AND FAMINE (BEFORE 1900)

The United States, like virtually all other countries and regions, was born into pestilence and famine. Infectious diseases killed many of the earliest immigrants to the New World. About half of the Pilgrims arriving in the New World in November of 1620 died of infection and malnutrition by the following spring. In addition, the infectious diseases the immigrants brought with them from Europe had a devastating impact on Native American populations.

At the end of the 1800s, the U.S. economy was still largely agrarian, with more than 60 percent of the population living in rural settings. However, industrialization and urbanization were well under way. Per capita income was increasing, and the food supply was improving. Modest gains in life expectancy were apparent throughout the 19th century. By 1900, life expectancy had increased to 47.8 years for men and 50.7 years for women. Infectious diseases—largely tuberculosis, pneumonia, and diarrheal diseases—accounted for more deaths than any other cause. CVD accounted for less than 10 percent of all deaths. Tobacco products were out of the economic reach of a large segment of the population.

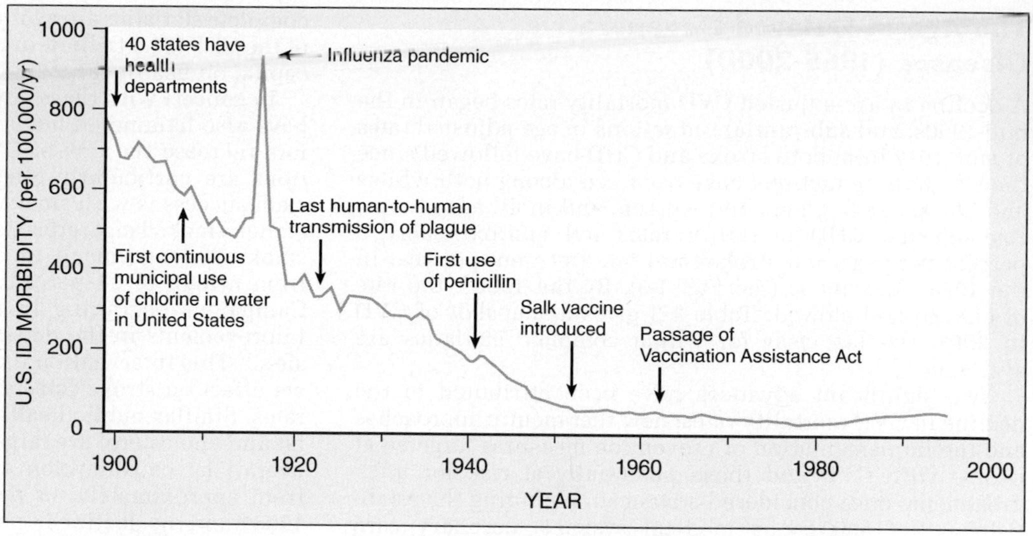

FIGURE 1–6 Decline in mortality due to infectious diseases (ID) in the United States, 1900 to 1996. Rate is per 100,000 population per year. *(From American Water Works Association: Water Chlorination Principles and Practices: AWWA Manual M20. Denver, American Water Works Association, 1973; Achievements in public health 1900-1999: Control of infectious diseases. MMWR Morbid Mortal Wkly Rep 48:621, 1999; and modified from Armstrong GL, Conn LA, Pinner RW: Trends in infectious disease mortality in the United States during the 20th century. JAMA 281:61, 1999.)*

THE AGE OF RECEDING PANDEMICS (1900-1930)

Early in the 20th century, the pace of industrialization accelerated. The shift from a rural, agriculture-based economy to an urban, industry-based economy had a number of consequences on cardiovascular risk behaviors and factors. Food supplies had become abundant, but urbanization required a dramatic shift in dietary staples. The railway network in place at the turn of the century was capable of moving foodstuffs from the farm to the city. But because the trains were not refrigerated, perishable foodstuffs such as fresh fruits and vegetables could not readily be transported, whereas cereal grains and livestock could. Large slaughter houses and meat-packing plants were established in or near urban areas. As a result, consumption of fresh fruits and vegetables declined and consumption of meat and grains increased, resulting in diets that were higher in fat and processed carbohydrates. In addition, the manufacture of factory-rolled cigarettes made them more portable and more affordable for the mass population.[12]

By 1900, a public health infrastructure had emerged: 40 states had health departments and many larger towns had major public works efforts to improve water supply and sewage systems. Municipal use of chlorine to disinfect water was becoming widespread, and improvements in food handling such as pasteurization were introduced. The health care system was growing but still largely comprised general practitioners providing care in the office or home; hospitals were largely for the indigent. The Flexner Report of 1910, which took a careful look at the quality of medical education in the United States and Canada,[13] was the first step toward organized quality improvement in health care personnel that, along with other public health changes, contributed to dramatic declines in infectious disease mortality rates throughout the century (Fig. 1-6).

The population of urban areas outnumbered that of rural areas for the first time by 1920. By 1930, 56 percent of the population was living in or near urban centers. Infectious disease mortality rates had fallen dramatically, from a crude death rate of approximately 800 per 100,000 population in 1900 to approximately 340 per 100,000 people.[14] Largely as a result of rapidly declining infant, childhood, and adolescent mortality from malnutrition and infectious diseases, life expectancy increased by 10 years between 1900 and 1930, to 57.8 years for men and 61.1 years for women. At the same time, cigarette smoking was on the rise. Age-adjusted CVD mortality rates, at approximately 390 per 100,000 people, were in the midst of their steady climb up from slightly more than 300 per 100,000 people in 1900. This increase was largely driven by rapidly rising CHD rates.

THE AGE OF DEGENERATIVE AND MAN-MADE DISEASES (1930-1965)

By the middle of the 20th century, the United States was predominantly an urban, industrial economy, with 64 percent of the population living in urban and suburban settings. With continued mechanization and urbanization, activity levels declined considerably. The rise of suburbs meant that more and more people were driving to work or to shopping rather than walking or bicycling. Prevalence of smoking, one of the major contributors to premature mortality and chronic disease, hit its zenith among adult men at 57 percent in 1955 and among women 10 years later at 34 percent.[15] Annual per capita consumption of cigarettes peaked in 1963 at 4345, or more than half a pack per day for each American.[12]

By 1965, per capita income had risen to approximately $10,000 (in 1997 adjusted dollars).[16] Deaths from infectious diseases had fallen to fewer than 50 per 100,000 population per year, and life expectancy was up to almost 70 years. However, almost 52 percent of men and 34 percent of women were smokers, and fat consumption (much of it saturated) represented 41 percent of total calories. Age-adjusted CHD mortality rates were at their peak, at approximately 225 per 100,000 people. Stroke rates were also high, at 75 per 100,000.

One of the most remarkable changes in the years after World War II was the growth of the health care industry. Only some of this growth was stimulated by rises in per capita GDP. In the private sector, the growth of labor unions propelled a major expansion in private health care insurance. In fact, by the late 1950s, more than two thirds of the working U.S. population had some form of private insurance. The federal government also played an important role. Increases in federal funding (the Hill Burton Act of 1948) led to the construction of more hospitals to deal with the acute manifestations of chronic illnesses. These new hospitals drew on the great successes of the military hospitals. In 1966, two key federal insurance programs, Medicare and Medicaid, provided access to medical care for the medically indigent and the elderly. The Health Professions Education Assistance Act of 1966, which provided capitation grants to medical schools, doubled medical school enrollment over the next two decades through expanded class size and establishment of new medical schools. The establishment of the National Institutes of Health, spurred largely by scientific achievements in medicine made during World War II, not only promoted health-related research but also transformed medical education by providing financial support for the establishment of full-time medical school faculty.

The Age of Delayed Degenerative Diseases (1965-2000)

A decline in age-adjusted CVD mortality rates began in the mid-1960s, and substantial reductions in age-adjusted rates of mortality from both stroke and CHD have followed since then.[17] These reductions have occurred among both whites and blacks, among men and women, and in all age groups. Age-adjusted CHD mortality rates fell approximately 2 percent per year, and stroke rates fell 3 percent per year in the 1970s and 1980s (see Fig. 1-3). By the 1990s, the rate of change had slowed. Table 1-3 gives a snapshot of CVD in 2003, the last year for which complete statistics are available.

Two significant advances have been attributed to the decline in CVD mortality rates: new therapeutic approaches and the implementation of prevention measures targeted at people with CVD and those potentially at risk for it.[18,19] Treatments once considered advanced, including the establishment of emergency medical systems, coronary care units, and the widespread use of new diagnostic and therapeutic technologies such as echocardiography, cardiac catheterization, angioplasty, bypass surgery, and implantation of pacemakers and defibrillators, are now considered the standard of care. Advances in drug development have also had a major beneficial impact on both acute and chronic outcomes. Efforts to improve the acute management of myocardial infarction led to the application of life-saving drugs such as beta blockers, percutaneous coronary intervention, thrombolytics, angiotensin-converting enzyme inhibitors, and others (see Chaps. 51, 52, and 53). The widespread use of an "old" drug, aspirin, has also reduced the risk of dying of acute or secondary coronary events. Low-cost pharmacological treatment for hypertension (see Chap. 41) and the development of highly effective cholesterol-lowering drugs such as statins have also made major contributions to both primary and secondary prevention by reducing deaths from CVD (see Chap. 45). Such shifts are reflected in the burgeoning cost of medical care. In 1965, Americans spent approximately 5.9 percent of the GDP ($42 billion in unadjusted dollars) on health care.[20] In 2004, the last year for which complete statistics are available, Americans spent 16 percent of the GDP ($1.9 trillion in unadjusted dollars), or $6280 per capita, on health care.[21]

In concert with these advances, public health campaigns have also hammered home the message that certain behaviors increase the risk of CVD and that life-style modifications are particularly effective ways to reduce risk. One such success is with smoking cessation. In 1955, 57 percent of men smoked cigarettes,[15] whereas today 23 percent of men smoke. Among women, the prevalence of smoking has fallen from a high of 34 percent in 1965 to 18.5 percent today. Campaigns beginning in the 1970s resulted in dramatic improvements in the detection and treatment of hypertension.[17] This intervention likely had a profound and immediate effect on stroke rates and a more subtle effect on CHD rates. Similar public health messages concerning saturated fat and cholesterol are largely responsible for the decline in overall fat consumption as a percentage of total calories from approximately 45 percent in 1965 to 34 percent in 1995[22] and the decline in population mean cholesterol levels from 220 mg/dl in the early 1960s to 203 mg/dl in the early 1990s.[17]

A main characteristic of the age of delayed degenerative diseases is the steadily rising age at which a first CVD event occurs or at which people die of CVD (Fig. 1-7). Despite declines in age-adjusted mortality, the aging of the population will maintain CVD as the predominant cause of morbidity and mortality. This, in turn, leads to ever-increasing numbers of individuals with CVD, as well as ever-increasing health expenditures related to its treatment. From 1979 to 2003, the number of short-stay hospital patients discharged with CVD as the first-listed diagnosis increased 31 percent.[23] In 2003, hospital discharges included 767,000 for acute myocardial infarction; 799,000 for cardiac dysrhythmias; 1,088,000 for congestive heart failure; 1,257,000 for cardiac catheterizations; 470,000 for bypass surgery; 664,000 for balloon angioplasty and coronary atherectomy, 574,000 for insertion of a stent, and 413,000 for insertions or revision of a pacemaker.[24]

At the beginning of the 21st century, the nation is fully industrialized, with only 2 percent of the population

TABLE 1–3 Cardiovascular Disease in the United States, 2003

Type	Prevalence* (Millions)	Crude Mortality (Thousands)†	Percentage of Total Deaths†	Rate/100,000†
Cardiovascular disease	71.3	902.4	36.9	310.3
Hypertension	65.0	53.4	2	18.3
Ischemic heart disease	13.2	480	19.6	165.1
Stroke	5.5	157.7	6	54.2
Congestive heart failure	5.0	57.4	2	19.8
Rheumatic heart disease	NA	3.6	.15	1.2

Type	Annual Events* (Thousands)	Type	Annual Events* (Thousands)
Myocardial infarction	1200	CABG	467
New	700	PTCA	664
Recurrent	500	Valve surgery	95
Stroke	700	Total costs	$403.1 billion
New	500	Direct	$257.6 billion
Recurrent	200	Indirect	$145.5 billion

*From American Heart Association: 2006 Heart and Stroke Statistical Update. Dallas, AHA, 2006.

†From Hoyert DL, Heron MP, Murphy SL, Kung H: Deaths: Final Data for 2003. National Vital Statistics Reports; vol. 54 no. 13. Hyattsville, Md., National Center for Health Statistics, 2006.

CABG = coronary artery bypass grafting; CDC = Centers for Disease Control and Prevention; NA = not available; PTCA = percutaneous transluminal coronary angioplasty.

involved in farming and a per capita GDP of approximately $37,800. Life expectancy at birth is 74.8 years for men and 80.1 years for women, and at age 65 is 16.8 years for men and 19.8 for women.[25] CVD continues to be the predominant cause of morbidity and mortality, but it afflicts an older population than it did in the middle of the century.

The Age of Inactivity and Obesity

Age-adjusted rates of CHD and stroke death fell 2 to 3 percent per year through the 1970s and 1980s and, although they have continued to decline, the rate has slowed.[19] In contrast to these decreases, starting in the 1990s, the age-standardized death rate has decreased an average of less than 2 percent per year for CHD and stroke. In 2003, the age-adjusted death rate for CHD was 163 per 100,000, whereas the rate for stroke was 54 per 100,000, and the age-standardized death rate for total CVD was 306 per 100,000.[26]

The slowing of the decline may be caused in part by a slowing in the rate of decline in risk factors such as smoking and increases in other risk factors such as obesity and physical inactivity. Rates of detection and treatment of hypertension are stagnant.[27] The decline in smoking rates has leveled off, with approximately 21 percent of adults classified as current smokers.[28] Overweight and obesity are increasing at an alarming pace, and only a minority of the population meets minimal physical activity recommendations, resulting in increases in diabetes and hypertension. Even more troubling are increases in childhood obesity and physical inactivity, leading to large increases in diabetes and hypertension among younger individuals.[6,7] These worrisome changes in CVD risk behaviors and factors may slow the rate of decline and could even contribute to increases in age-adjusted rates of CVD in the coming years. However, continued progress in the development and application of therapeutic advances may offset the effects from an uptick in risk factors.

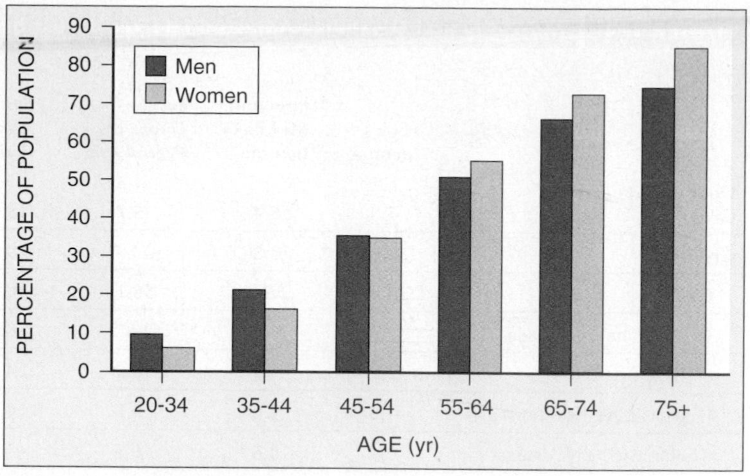

FIGURE 1–7 Estimated prevalence of cardiovascular disease in Americans 20 years of age and older. *(From American Heart Association: Heart Disease and Stroke Statistics—2006 Update. Dallas, AHA, 2006.)*

CURRENT WORLDWIDE VARIATIONS IN THE GLOBAL BURDEN OF CARDIOVASCULAR DISEASE

An epidemiological transition much like the one that occurred in the United States is occurring throughout the world. However, the rate of transition varies widely, leading to large discrepancies in disease burden around the world.

These wide variations began to appear early in the 20th century. Although most of the world remained in the phase of pestilence and famine, economic circumstances in several relatively confined regions changed rapidly, accelerating the pace of their epidemiological transition. Thus the global burden of CVD is best understood by examining the differential rates of change in each economic region. In addition to variability in the rate of the transition, there are unique regional features that have modified aspects of the U.S.-style transition in various parts of the world.

In terms of economic development, as described earlier, the world can be divided into two broad categories, (1) high-income countries and (2) low- and middle-income countries, which can be further subdivided into six distinct economic/geographic regions. Currently, 85 percent of the world's population lives in low- and middle-income countries, and it is these countries that are driving the rates of change in the global burden of CVD. About 30 percent of the world's population lives in East Asia and the Pacific islands, and another 22 percent live in South Asia.

Like the United States, the rest of the high-income countries are largely in the fourth or perhaps the fifth phase of the epidemiological transition, with CVD accounting for 39 percent of all deaths in 2001 and communicable diseases accounting for 7 percent. Across the six regions that constitute the low- and middle-income countries, however, there remains a high degree of heterogeneity with respect to the phase of the epidemiological transition, as illustrated by the dominant disease rates in each region (Table 1-4).

In sub-Saharan Africa, communicable disease rates still far exceed those of chronic diseases, placing it in the first phase (pestilence and famine). Plagued by HIV/AIDS and other communicable diseases, as well as an emerging epidemic of CVD, this region and many low-income countries are facing a "double burden" of disease that is stretching already limited resources. In these developing countries with a high proportion of citizens younger than 65, the onset of CVD will occur among ever-younger people, posing a threat to economic and social development.[29] The level of death and disability attributable to cardiovascular disease in the labor force will be much greater than in Western nations, now or even in the past.

Within regions, there is a great deal of variability. Some regions of India, for example, appear to be in the first phase, characterized by high rates of infectious and communicable disease, whereas others are in the second or even the third phase. The Middle East and North Africa also appear to be entering the third phase of the epidemiological transition. This section briefly discusses the regional rates and describes the difficulties in assessing and comparing disease rates around the world, as well as highlighting within-region variations.

High-Income Countries

Approximately 940 million people (15 percent of the world's population) live in the high-income countries of the United States, Canada, Australia, New Zealand, the European Union, and Japan. In these countries, CHD is the dominant form of CVD with rates that tend to be twofold to fivefold higher than stroke rates. (Table 1-5 demonstrates this tendency in selected European countries.) Two notable exceptions are Portugal and Japan. In Portugal, stroke rates for both men and women are higher than CHD rates. The same is true for Japan, where stroke is responsible for far more fatalities than CHD. In both Portugal and Japan, the pattern seems to be moving toward that in other

TABLE 1–4 Mortality and Disability-Adjusted Life Years Lost by Disease Category

			Low- and Middle-Income Regions					
	High Income	Low and Middle Income	*Eastern Europe & Central Asia*	*East Asia & Pacific*	*South Asia*	*Sub-Saharan Africa*	*Middle East & North Africa*	*Latin America & Caribbean*
Deaths (%)								
Group I	7.0	36.4	5.7	18.9	43.4	71.5	24.2	21.8
Group II	87.0	53.8	83.5	70.5	46.8	21.1	64.5	66.7
CVD	38.5	27.6	58.1	30.6	25.2	9.7	35.0	27.8
Ischemic heart disease	17.3	11.8	29.7	8.9	13.5	3.2	16.9	10.9
Stroke	9.9	9.5	18.2	14.6	6.8	3.3	6.8	8.1
Hypertensive heart disease	1.6	1.6	1.9	0.92	0.7	0.6	3.9	2.6
Rheumatic heart disease	0.2	0.6	0.3	1	0.9	0.2	0.5	0.2
Other CVD	9.5	4.1	7.9	4	3.3	2.4	7.0	5.8
Other non-CMPN	4.8	26.2	25.4	39.9	21.6	11.4	29.5	39.0
Group III	6.0	9.8	10.7	10.5	9.8	7.4	11.3	11.4
DALYs (%)								
Group I	5.7	39.8	9.4	22.2	44.3	70.4	27.0	21.8
Group II	86.7	48.9	76.4	65.9	44.4	21.2	59.3	65.0
CVD	20.0	12.9	32.8	15.3	12.5	4.4	14.5	11.3
Ischemic heart disease	8.3	5.2	15.6	4.1	6.3	1.3	6.6	4.2
Stroke	6.3	4.5	10.8	7.5	3.2	1.5	3.0	3.8
Hypertensive heart disease	0.8	7.2	1.0	1.2	0.4	2.7	1.4	1.0
Rheumatic heart disease	0.1	4.4	0.4	0.6	0.6	0.1	0.4	0.1
Other CVD	4.5	2.0	4.6	1.8	2.0	1.1	3.2	2.3
Other non-CMPN	66.7	36.0	43.5	50.6	31.8	16.8	44.7	53.7
Group III	7.5	11.2	14.3	12.0	11.3	8.4	13.7	13.2

CMPN = communicable diseases, maternal and perinatal conditions, and nutritional deficiency; CVD = cardiovascular disease; DALYs = disability-adjusted life years; Group I = communicable diseases, maternal and perinatal conditions, and nutritional deficiencies; Group II = noncommunicable diseases; Group III = injuries.

high-income countries with more rapid declines in stroke than CHD rates.

The rates of CVD in Western Europe tend to be similar to those in the United States. However, the absolute rates vary threefold among the countries of Western Europe, with a clear north/south gradient of higher CHD and stroke rates in the north. The highest CVD rates in the European high-income countries (two to three times higher than the median rates) are in Finland, Ireland, and Scotland. Although still high, deaths from CHD among Finnish men of working age have decreased by nearly 80 percent over the past 30 years, from 508 deaths per 100,000 in 1967 to 126 per 100,000 in 2003. A program called "Success in Finland" has contributed to this decline, including a more than 40 percent decrease in CHD death rates in both men and women between 1989 and 1999. The Scottish government is also taking measures to drive down rates, including banning smoking in all enclosed places as of spring 2006. The lowest CVD rates in Europe are in the Mediterranean countries of France, Spain, and Italy, where age-adjusted CHD rates are less than 125 and 40 per 100,000 for men and women, respectively.[30] Although both stroke and CHD rates are higher in northern Europe, the disparity in CHD rates is much greater. For example, male CHD rates are 222 percent higher in Finland than in Spain, whereas stroke rates are only 21 percent higher.

CVD rates in Canada, New Zealand, and Australia are similar to rates in the United States. Rapid declines in CHD and stroke rates since the early 1970s signaled that the high-income countries were in the fourth phase of the epidemiological transition, the age of delayed degenerative diseases. But throughout the high-income countries, the rapidly increasing rate of obesity seems to indicate that many may be entering a fifth phase. CVD death rates continue to fall at least in part because of the technical advances in treating CVD.

JAPAN. This country is unique among the high-income countries. As its rates of communicable diseases fell in the early part of the 20th century, stroke rates increased dramatically; and by the middle of the century they were the highest in the world. CHD rates, however, did not rise as sharply as they did in other industrialized nations and have remained lower than in any other industrialized country. Overall CVD rates have fallen 60 percent since the 1960s, largely because of a decrease in age-adjusted stroke rates. Japanese men and women currently have the highest life expectancies in the world: 85.3 years for women and 78.4 years for men. The difference between Japan and other industrialized countries may stem in part from genetic factors, but it is more likely that the fish- and plant-based, low-fat diet and resultant low cholesterol levels have played a more important role. As is true for so many countries,

TABLE 1–5	Age-Adjusted Cardiovascular Mortality (Deaths/100,000) in Europeans 35–74 Years of Age	
Country	**CHD**	**Stroke**
Spain		
Men	120	51
Women	31	27
France		
Men	83	40
Women	20	21
Portugal		
Men	103	123
Women	38	68
Finland		
Men	267	62
Women	68	40
United Kingdom		
Men	229	54
Women	80	43
Economies in Transition		
Russian Federation		
Men	771	429
Women	267	253
Ukraine		
Men	839	292
Women	373	181
Kazakhstan		
Men	703	343
Women	289	234

CHD = coronary heart disease.

Modified from European Cardiovascular Disease Statistics, 2005 edition (http://www.heartstats.org/uploads/documents%5CPDF.pdf).

Japanese dietary habits are undergoing substantial changes. In the last half of the 20th century, there was an estimated 9.3-fold increase in annual per capita consumption of meat, a 5.2-fold increase in egg consumption, a 7.4-fold increase in milk and dairy consumption, and a 5.3-fold increase in consumption of fats and oils.[31] These changes may explain possible recent increases in CHD. Since the late 1950s, cholesterol levels have progressively increased. A study that analyzed diet and cholesterol levels in a cohort of rural Japanese men found that from 1958 to 1999, their carbohydrate intake decreased significantly, from 84 percent to 62 percent, whereas protein and fat intake increased dramatically, from 11 percent to 18 percent for protein and 5 percent to 20 percent for fat.[32] Although cholesterol levels rose from 152.5 mg/dl to 194.2 mg/dl, the incidence of coronary artery disease in this population remains low. This could change, however, as there seems to be a long lag phase before dietary changes are reflected as CHD events.

Low- and Middle-Income Countries

Approximately 85 percent of the world's inhabitants live in low- and middle-income countries, and this percentage is increasing. Consequently, most people with CVD reside in low- and middle-income parts of the world. Three million CVD deaths occurred in high-income countries in 2001, compared with 13 million in the rest of the world. Although communicable diseases continue to be a major cause of death, CVD has emerged as a major health concern in the low- and middle-income countries. Overall, in 2001, CVD mortality rates were approximately 28 percent; however, this represents only 13 percent of total lost disability-adjusted life years (DALYs) because cardiovascular diseases tend to affect an older segment of the population than communicable diseases. An infant death due to malnutrition, for example, results in more lost DALYs than a CHD death in the fifth decade of life. Although CVD rates are rapidly rising, there are vast differences within and between the regions, and even within and between the countries themselves that make up the low- and middle-income countries, both in the rates of CVD and in the resources available to deal with this epidemic. The character of CVD varies greatly by region. In China, for example, stroke rates exceed CHD rates, whereas in India the reverse is true. Rheumatic heart disease remains a major problem in India, China, and sub-Saharan Africa but is less of a problem in other Asian countries and Latin America. Reporting of CVD event rates is often based on sampling rather than on true national data collection efforts.

Many factors contribute to the heterogeneity between and within regions of the low- and middle-income countries. First, the distinct regions are at various stages of the economic and social transitions—some are still in the age of pestilence and famine, whereas others are in the second or even third phase of the epidemiological transition or, as is the case in parts of Latin America and the Caribbean, even the fourth stage of the epidemiological transition. Second, vast differences in life style and behavioral risk factors exist. For example, per capita consumption of dairy products (and thus consumption of saturated fat) is much higher in India than it is in China. Third, racial and ethnic differences may lead to altered susceptibilities to various forms of CVD. Finally, social, cultural, political, and economic differences result in vast disparities in the health care structure in each region.

EASTERN EUROPE AND CENTRAL ASIA. Sometimes referred to as the "emerging market economies," this group of countries has the highest rates of CVD mortality in the world—58 percent of deaths are the result of CVD, with 48 percent due to ischemic heart disease and cerebrovascular disease.[1] However, there is substantial variability, with some countries experiencing increasing CVD mortality and others experiencing a decline. Overall rates are similar to those seen in the United States in the 1960s, when CVD was at its peak. CHD is generally more common than stroke. This suggests that the countries that constitute Eastern Europe and Central Asia are largely in the third phase of the epidemiological transition. As expected in this phase of the transition, the average age of people who develop and die of CVD is lower than that in the high-income economies.

Within this group of countries, nearly all of which are former socialist states, CVD mortality rates vary widely. Since the dissolution of the Soviet Union, there has been a surprising increase in CVD rates in some of these countries with the highest rates in Ukraine, Bulgaria, Belarus, and Russia.[33] In Russia, increased CVD rates have contributed to falling life expectancy, particularly for men, whose life expectancy has dropped from 71.6 in 1986 to 59 years today. For Russian women, life expectancy has declined only slightly over the same period, now standing at 72 years. The causes of this decline in life expectancy are not entirely clear, but Russia's overall death rate jumped by nearly a third during the 1990s, in large part because of heart disease. Nearly two thirds of Russian men smoke. Rapid increases in per capita alcohol consumption have been reported in the wake of economic, political, and social instability in the aftermath of the dissolution of the Soviet Union and may represent one possible cause for the increasing CVD rates that underlie this decline. Inadequate health care infrastructure and lack of preventive public health measures also may contribute to worsening CVD mortality rates.

During the 1990s, age-adjusted CVD rates declined in the Czech Republic, Hungary, and Poland. Even so, CVD rates in these countries remain generally higher than in Western European countries (Fig. 1-8). In Poland, the age-adjusted mortality rate decreased about 30 percent for men during the 1990s, and slightly more among women. Lower smoking rates among Polish men and dietary changes including a 19 percent decrease in saturated fat consumption and a 32 percent increase in polyunsaturated fat, as well as a significant increase in fruit consumption, may be responsible for some of the improvement.[34]

EAST ASIA AND PACIFIC. In their new book, Lopez and colleagues[1] deemed East Asia and the Pacific the "healthiest of all low- and middle-income regions." The diversity of economic circumstances in the countries of the East Asia and Pacific region is reflected in the status and character of the epidemiological transition across the region. In South Korea, for example, about 60 percent of the population resides in urban centers and the mean annual per capita GDP is now $20,400, making it a high-income country, according to the World Bank. By contrast, in Cambodia, approximately three quarters of the population is still engaged in subsistence farming, and the per capita GDP is $2200. Average life expectancy in South Korea is 77 years, compared with 59 years in Cambodia.

The rapid economic expansion and urbanization occurring in several Southeast Asian countries has been accompanied by the expected life-style changes. CVD is a major cause of death in this region, but unlike most other regions, stroke causes more deaths than CHD.[1] However, in the most industrialized countries, such as Singapore, CVD rates mirror those in the high-income countries, with CHD mortality rates twice as high as stroke mortality rates. This is likely because of the greater time since industrialization and a lag in the emergence of CHD as the dominant form of CVD. In other less developed parts of Asia, such as Indonesia and Sri Lanka, they are moving through the epidemiological transition with parts in the first, second, and third phases. Other countries, such as Vietnam and Cambodia, are just emerging from pestilence and famine.

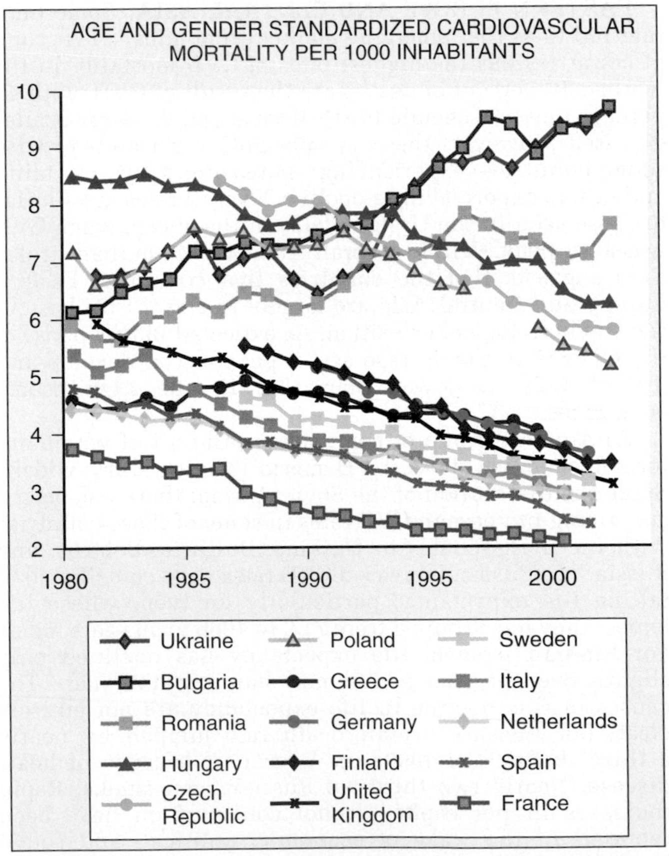

FIGURE 1–8 Trends in age- and gender-standardized cardiovascular mortality in selected European countries. *(From European Society of Cardiology: Cardiovascular Diseases in Europe: Euro Heart Survey and National Registries of Cardiovascular Diseases and Patient Management 2004.)*

CHINA. The People's Republic of China accounts for one fifth of the world's population, and half of the population makes its living from some form of agriculture. Since the 1950s, life expectancy in China has more than doubled from 35 years to 72 years. During the four decades between 1950 and 1990, the rate of mortality from CVD increased threefold as a percentage of total deaths, from 12 to 36 percent.[35]

In the country as a whole, China appears to be straddling the second and third stages of a Japanese-style epidemiological transition. As in Japan, CVD deaths account for more than 35 percent of all deaths, and, in contrast to nearly all high-income countries, stroke is the dominant form. In 2001, stroke resulted in 18 percent of all Chinese deaths, as compared with CHD, which caused 8 percent of all deaths. Hemorrhagic stroke predominates over ischemic stroke, and stroke rates are higher among women than men. These lower rates of CHD and high rates of stroke may be caused by genetic factors; however, some have hypothesized that overall low serum cholesterol levels may contribute to high rates of hemorrhagic stroke.[36] However, in urban centers the transition appears to be much like that in the United States with CHD rates rising rapidly as hemorrhagic stroke rates are falling.

Regional differences exist in CVD rates, although they are not as great as those seen in India and sub-Saharan Africa. This is likely because of the system of resource distribution that results in greater improvements in rural areas in the standard of living and health care infrastructure compared with Africa or India. In China, as in Europe, there appears to be a north/south gradient, with higher CVD rates in northern China than in southern China. As is the case in most low- and middle-income countries, there is also an urban/rural gradient for CHD, stroke, and hypertension, with higher rates in urban centers. In urban China, the death rate from coronary disease rose by 53 percent from 1988 to 1996.

Major features of the transition in China are the rapidly rising rates of cigarette smoking—approximately 60 percent of men smoke—and hypertension, much of which remains untreated. Dietary changes may also be having an impact. In Beijing, between 1982 and 1992, the intake of food from animal sources increased by 6 percent, animal sources of protein increased 18 percent, and fat intake increased from 21.6 percent of total energy to 30.6 percent.[37] Obesity is beginning to emerge in China earlier than it did in Japan's transition.

SOUTH ASIA/INDIA. Most people in South Asia live in India, where one sixth of the world's population lives, with the majority of its more than 1 billion inhabitants residing in rural settings. Accurate country-wide data on cause-specific mortality are not available because death certificate completion is not uniform, and the country does not have a centralized registry for CVD deaths. India is experiencing an alarming increase in heart disease. CVD accounted for 32 percent of all deaths in 2000,[38] and the World Health Organization (WHO) estimates that 60 percent of the world's cardiac patients will be Indian by 2010. As expected, CVD mortality rates tend to be higher in urban than in rural areas, and CVD is much more prevalent among the upper and middle classes.[39,40]

In contrast to China and much of the rest of Asia, the transition appears to be more Western style, with CHD being the dominant form of CVD in India. In 1960, CHD represented 4 percent of all CVD deaths, whereas in 1990 the proportion was greater than 50 percent.[41] In 1990, CHD was responsible for 1.17 million deaths; by 2000, that figure had risen to 1.59 million. Currently, CHD death rates are twice as high as stroke rates.[33] This statistic is somewhat unexpected because stroke tends to be a more dominant form of CVD early in the epidemiological transition. This finding may reflect inaccuracies in cause-specific mortality estimates. However, it may suggest metabolic differences in response to the Western life style of higher-fat diets and lower levels of activity. Diabetes is a major health issue; India has 31.6 million diabetics, more than any other country. On the basis of migration studies, it has been suggested that Indians have an exaggerated insulin insensitivity in response to the Western life-style pattern that may differentially increase rates of CHD and stroke. Furthermore, the proportion of calories derived from fat, much of which comes from dairy products, is significantly higher in India than in other parts of the developing world.

Concerns have been raised that the rising rates of death and disability because of CVD among relatively young Indians will seriously affect productivity and impose economic burdens on the country. Today, approximately 50 percent of CVD-related deaths occur in those younger than the age of 70, compared with approximately 22 percent in the West. Rates of communicable disease remain high, but major noncommunicable diseases account for about 60 percent of all deaths.[38] Thus much of India appears to be early in the second phase of the transition, with the urban upper classes in the third phase. As in China, rheumatic heart disease continues to be a major cause of morbidity and mortality. Certain remote areas, however, are still emerging from the age of pestilence and famine, with CVD accounting for less than 10 percent of total deaths.[42]

SUB-SAHARAN AFRICA. Despite large regional variations, much of sub-Saharan Africa remains largely in the first phase of the epidemiological transition, with approximately 70 percent of all deaths due to infectious and parasitic diseases (see Table 1-4). As is the case in India, accurate country-wide data are not generally available, and most data come from urban centers and sampling in rural areas. Nearly three quarters of the 40 million adults and children living with HIV/AIDS reside in sub-Saharan Africa, an epidemic that will definitely influence the natural history of the epidemiological transition. This devastating disease is having significant effects on virtually all aspects of health and health care in the region. Life expectancy has decreased by an average of 5 years since the early 1990s because of the double burden of HIV/AIDS and other chronic diseases, according to the World Bank. As a result, life expectancies are the lowest in the world.[43]

Overall, CVD was responsible for approximately 10 percent of all deaths in sub-Saharan Africa in 2001, evenly split between CHD and stroke.[44] Even in urban centers, CHD was rare in the middle part of the 20th century. However, with increasing urbanization, average daily physical activity among urban dwellers is falling and smoking rates are increasing. Hypertension has emerged as a major public health concern and accounts for the dominance of stroke and hypertensive heart disease among types of CVD.[42] Rheumatic heart disease and cardiomyopathies, the latter due mostly to malnutrition, various viral illnesses, and parasitic organisms, are also important causes of CVD mortality and morbidity.

Cardiac involvement is a common sequela of infection with HIV (see Chaps. 66 and 67). In an autopsy study of adults who died of AIDS, 19 percent had cardiac abnormalities related to HIV infection.[45] Cardiac manifestations can become apparent even earlier in the course of HIV infection. In a prospective study of 952 asymptomatic HIV-infected adults, 8 percent had significant left ventricular dysfunction over 60 months of follow-up.[46] Other cardiovascular-related manifestations of HIV/AIDS include pericardial effusion, infective endocarditis, malignancies such as myocardial Kaposi sarcoma and myocardial B-cell immunoblastic lymphoma, arrhythmias, and right ventricular and pulmonary disease.

Children with HIV/AIDS are also prone to fetal and congenital cardiovascular malformations, left ventricular dysfunction, myocarditis, vascular disease, dysrhythmias, pericardial disease, cardiovascular tumors, and pulmonary hypertension, as well as infection-related cardiovascular disease.[47] In a retrospective study of 68 children with AIDS, predictors of serious cardiac events included recurrent bacterial infections, AIDS-related wasting, encephalopathy, and male gender.[48]

Although much of this research has been conducted in developed countries, reports from Africa describe similar cardiac manifestations of HIV infection.[49,50] At present, few countries in sub-Saharan Africa have the resources to cope adequately with the AIDS epidemic, and few patients receive medications proven to slow the progression of the disease. Thus opportunistic infections will continue to overshadow cardiac manifestations of AIDS. With the development of public health infrastructures capable of dealing with this disease, cardiac abnormalities should be expected with greater frequency in clinical practice. Use of highly active antiretroviral therapy may further increase the cardiovascular complications of HIV infection.[51]

LATIN AMERICA AND THE CARIBBEAN. In general, Latin America appears to be in the third phase of the epidemiological transition, although as in other low- and middle-income regions, there is vast regional heterogeneity, with some areas in the second phase of the transition and others in the fourth phase. In recent decades average life expectancy has risen by 20 years to 71 years of age, and the quality of nutrition has steadily improved. Over a similar time period, the region has seen a switch to animal from vegetable as a source of protein and an increase in fat intake as a percentage of energy. CVD rates declined overall in this region in the 1990s. Today, approximately 28 percent of all deaths are attributable to CVD,[1] with CHD rates higher than stroke rates (although not to the degree seen in high-income countries). CHD and stroke account for nearly 70 percent of CVD in this region. CVD rates are beginning to decline in some countries in Latin America and the Caribbean. However, those countries with the lowest CVD rates are facing the steepest increases in CVD mortality rates.

Approximately one quarter of the citizens live in poverty, and many are still at risk of contacting malaria or dengue. Although rheumatic heart disease appears to be declining in most countries in this region, Chagas disease remains a major problem in certain regions, with as much as 30 percent of the population infected with the parasite that causes it. In addition, parts of Latin America and the Caribbean have the world's highest HIV prevalence rate outside of sub-Saharan Africa.

MIDDLE EAST AND NORTH AFRICA. In this region, increasing economic wealth has been characteristically accompanied by urbanization but uncharacteristically accompanied by increasing fertility rates as infant and childhood mortality rates declined. This has resulted in rapid population growth and a young mean age of the population (i.e., 44 percent younger than 15 years of age). The rate of mortality from CVD is increasing rapidly, and CVD is now the leading cause of death, accounting for 25 to 45 percent of total deaths. The traditional high-fiber diet, low in fat and cholesterol, has rapidly changed to a Western diet. Over the past few decades, daily fat consumption has increased in most of these countries, ranging from 13.6 percent in Sudan to a 143.3 percent increase in Saudi Arabia.[52] According to national surveys in Iran, the prevalence of overweight and obesity was as high as 50 percent among middle-aged men and 66 percent among women of the same age.[53] In the region overall, as in the higher income countries, CHD is the predominant cause of CVD, with about 2.5 CHD deaths for each stroke death. Rheumatic heart disease remains a major cause of morbidity and mortality, but the number of related hospitalizations is rapidly declining. This region is entering the third phase of the transition.

GLOBAL TRENDS IN CARDIOVASCULAR DISEASE

Estimating global trends in the burden of disease, particularly CVD, is aided by examining regional trends. Because 85 percent of the world's population lives in the low- and middle-income countries, global rates of CVD are largely driven by rates in these countries. Even as rates fall in high-income countries, worldwide CVD rates are accelerating because most low- and middle-income countries are entering the second and third phases of the epidemic transition, marked by rising CVD rates. The economic impact of chronic diseases could be substantial as this transition proceeds. Over the next decade or so, countries such as China, India, and Russia could forego between $200 billion and $550 billion in national income as a result of heart disease, stroke, and diabetes.[54]

In 1990 CVD accounted for 28 percent of the world's 50.4 million deaths and 9.7 percent of the 1.4 billion lost DALYs.[2] By 2001, CVD was responsible for 29 percent of all deaths and 14 percent of the 1.5 billion lost DALYs.[44] By 2020, the population will grow to 7.8 billion and 32 percent of all deaths will be due to CVD, and by 2030, when the population is expected to reach 8.2 billion, 33 percent of all deaths will be caused by CVD (Table 1-6).[33] By 2030, the WHO predicts that worldwide CVD will cause 24.2 million deaths.[33] Of these, 14.9 percent of deaths in men and 13.1 percent of deaths in women will be due to CHD. Stroke will be responsible for 10.4 percent of all male deaths and 11.8 percent of all female deaths.

HIGH-INCOME COUNTRIES. In the high-income countries, population growth will be fueled by emigration from the low- and middle-income countries, but as a proportion of the world's population, the high-income segment is gradually shrinking. In the high-income countries, the modest decline in CVD death rates begun in the latter third of the 20th century will continue, but the rate of decline appears to be slowing. However, these countries are expected to see an increase in the prevalence of CVD, as well as the absolute number of deaths, predicted to increase between 30 percent and 60 percent, as populations age.[37]

LOW- AND MIDDLE-INCOME COUNTRIES. Of the 7.1 million individuals who died from ischemic heart disease in 2001, 5.7 million lived in low- and middle-income countries. And of the 5.4 million people who died from a stroke in 2001, less than 1 million lived in high-income countries. From 1990 to 2001, the percentage of deaths from communicable diseases decreased from 38.7 percent to 36.4 percent and continued substantial declines are expected. Although some countries are still in the first and second phases of the epidemiological transition, large portions of the population living in low- and middle-income countries have entered the third phase and some are entering the fourth. Today, in most of the regions, the pattern is typical, with CHD rates exceeding stroke rates. Exceptions include sub-Saharan Africa and China, home to the vast majority of East Asia and Pacific residents. In sub-Saharan Africa, which is in an earlier stage of the transition, this ratio is currently about 1 : 1, but the balance is likely to shift in favor of CHD over time. In China, however, the ratio is reversed, with stroke rates exceeding CHD rates, but this is also likely to change. In urban China, CHD rates are rapidly increasing as stroke rates fall. Changing demographics play a significant role in future predictions for CVD throughout the world. For example, between 1990 and 2001, the population of Europe and Central Asia grew by 1 million people per year, whereas South Asia added 25 million people each year.[1]

In their report *A Race Against Time: The Challenge of Cardiovascular Disease in Developing Economies,* Leeder and colleagues[55] compare the role of CVD in the death patterns of one low-income country (India) and four middle-income countries (Russia, Brazil, China, and South Africa) in 2000 and in the future.[55] Portugal and the United States were used as high-income comparator countries. Even assuming no increase in CVD risk factors, the authors predict that all five study countries, but especially India and South Africa, will see a dramatic number of working-age people (35 to 64 years old) die of CVD over the next 30 years, as well as an increasing level of morbidity among middle-aged people related to heart disease and stroke. In China, they estimate that there will be 9 million deaths from CVD in 2030—up from 2.4 million in 2002—with half occurring in individuals between 35 and 64 years old. Because of a growing population of younger people at risk for CVD in the five study countries, they predict that the proportion of CVD deaths occurring in the prime labor years will greatly exceed the experience of the United States and Portugal. Predictions of the increase in the number of productive years lost due to CVD between 2000 and 2030 are: South Africa, 28 percent; China, 57 percent; Brazil, 64 percent; and India, 95 percent. (In South Africa and Brazil, the predicted rates per 100,000 population actually decrease slightly as a result of anticipated demographic changes.) In Russia, the

TABLE 1–6 Contribution of Various Disease Categories to Global Mortality

			Total Deaths (%)					
	Population (Millions)	Total Deaths (Millions)	*CMPN*	*Injury*	*Non-CMPN Non-CVD*	*All CVD*	*CHD*	*Stroke*
1990								
World	5267	50.4	34.2	10.1	27.4	28.4	12.4	8.7
High income	798	7.12	6.4	6.2	42.8	44.6	23.4	11.1
Low and middle income	4470	43.3	38.7	10.7	24.8	25.7	10.6	8.3
2001								
World	6148	56.2	32.3	9.2	29.3	29.1	12.5	9.6
High income	929	7.9	7.0	6.0	48.5	38.5	17.3	9.9
Low and middle income	5219	48.3	36.4	9.7	26.2	27.6	11.8	9.5
2020*								
World	7800	65.1				31.5	13.6	10.6
2030*								
World	8200	74.5				32.5	14.0	11.1

CHD = coronary heart disease; CMPN = communicable diseases, maternal and perinatal conditions, and nutritional deficiency; CVD = cardiovascular disease.

*Modified from Mackay J, Mensah G: Atlas of Heart Disease and Stroke. Geneva, World Health Organization, 2004.

number is predicted to decrease because the size of the population at risk is falling. For comparison, the number of years of productive life lost is expected to increase by 20 percent in the United States and by 30 percent in Portugal by 2030.

REGIONAL TRENDS IN RISK FACTORS

As indicated earlier, the global variation in CVD rates is related to temporal and regional variations in known risk behaviors and factors. Discussions of the strength of the associations of the various factors with CVD are found elsewhere in this text (see Chap. 39). Ecological analyses of major CVD risk factors and mortality demonstrate high correlations between expected and observed mortality rates for the three main risk factors—smoking, serum cholesterol, and hypertension[56]—and suggest that many of the regional variations are based on differences in conventional risk factors. The Interheart study, which looked at risk factors in 52 countries, has demonstrated that the same risk factors are causing heart attacks worldwide at all ages.[57] This section focuses on regional differences in these risk factors that help explain regional variations in the rate and character of the epidemiological transition. The adoption of risky behaviors such as smoking, eating a Western-type diet, and decreased physical activity has preceded the development of advanced health care delivery systems because of economic realities in the low- and middle-income countries.

Behavioral Factors: Tobacco, Diet, and Physical Inactivity

TOBACCO. Smoking represents an important and rapidly growing avoidable global cause of CVD and total death. Worldwide, 1.2 billion people smoked in 2000, a number that is projected to increase to 1.6 billion by 2030.[58] Slightly more than 80 percent of current smokers live in low- and middle-income countries. Tobacco currently causes an estimated 5 million deaths annually (9 percent of all deaths). This represents 1 million more tobacco-related deaths than in 1990, with the increase being most marked in developing countries.[43] If current smoking patterns continue, by 2030 the global burden of disease attributable to tobacco will reach 10 million deaths annually, with the majority in low-income countries.[59]

Every year, more than 5.5 trillion cigarettes are produced—enough to provide every person on the planet with 1000 cigarettes.[60] In the world as a whole, the highest per capita cigarette consumption rates are in Europe, at 2060 per year, followed closely by the countries of the Western Pacific with 1897 per year and the Americas with 1408; they are the lowest in Southeast Asia, where annual per capita consumption is 355 cigarettes.[61] However, this number may not accurately capture tobacco consumption in this region because many Indians roll their own cigarettes rather than buying them.

In the high-income economies, smoking rates are declining. In the United States, for example, 42 percent of adults smoked in 1965, whereas only 21 percent currently smoke, with little difference between genders.[15] Among young men and women, smoking rates increased through the 1990s but now appear to be declining.[62] In Western Europe, rates are falling but not as fast as in the United States.

In the low- and middle-income countries, smoking rates are extremely high—and in some countries are still increasing (Fig. 1-9). On the Pacific islands of Samoa, more than 67 percent of men and 29 percent of women smoke. The Eastern Europe and Central Asia region has the highest prevalence, with 35 percent of all adults smoking.[59] Smoking rates among men in some countries in Eastern Europe and the former Soviet economies top 50 percent: Kyrgyzstan, 64 percent; Georgia, 61 percent; Kazakhstan, 57 percent; and Bosnia and Herzegovina, 55 percent.[33] In addition, according to the Global Youth Tobacco Survey, this region also has one of the highest numbers of young smokers.[63] Youth smoking is also prevalent in parts of India and some of the Western Pacific islands, according to the survey, which includes data from 43 countries. In more than 30 percent of these countries, girls reported smoking as much as boys.

In other low- and middle-income countries, tobacco represents an important cash crop and source of employment, two things that are often in short supply. In some of these countries, smoking rates among men are staggeringly high, reaching 69 percent in Laos and 60 percent in Indonesia and the Philippines.[33] Throughout the developing world, women have traditionally represented only a small proportion of the number of smokers—currently about 9 percent.[64] That is certain to change. As women's spending power increases, tobacco companies are targeting them as customers, and woman-specific health education and quitting programs are rare.

A unique feature of the low- and middle-income countries is easy access to smoking during the early stages of the epidemiological transition because of the availability of relatively inexpensive tobacco products. In the high-income countries, cigarette smoking peaked in the third phase of the transition. In many developing countries that are in the first or second stages, however, male smoking rates already exceed the peak rates of the high-income countries, and are expected to continue rising among both men and women. The impact of more widespread smoking earlier in the epidemiological transition means a more rapid increase in CVD rates as the developing countries enter the third phase of the transition. In China, which is in the early stages of the epidemiological transition, 59 percent of men (but only 3.6 percent of women) are current smokers.[33] A massive retrospective study of 1 million deaths estimated that tobacco

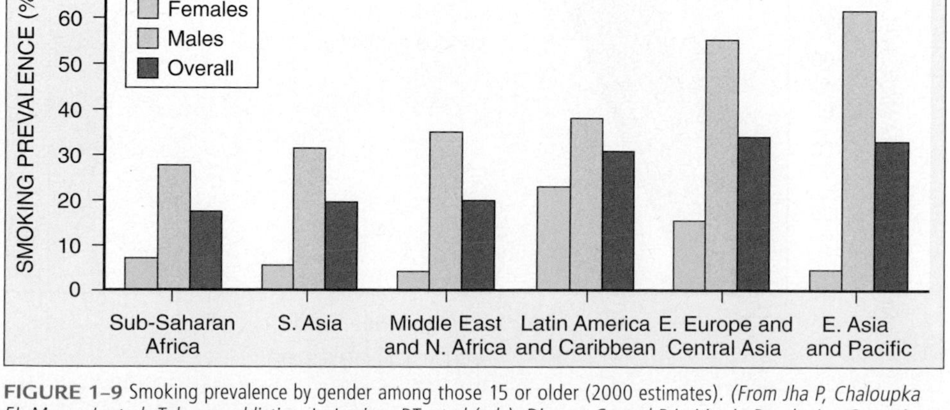

FIGURE 1–9 Smoking prevalence by gender among those 15 or older (2000 estimates). *(From Jha P, Chaloupka FJ, Moore J, et al: Tobacco addiction. In Jamison DT, et al (eds): Disease Control Priorities in Developing Countries. 2nd ed. New York, Oxford University Press, 2006.)*

was responsible for 13 percent (600,000 deaths) of total mortality in China in 1990 and will account for 3 million deaths a year by 2025.[65]

DIET (see Chap. 44). As countries develop, total caloric intake per capita increases. From 1971 to 2000, the daily caloric intake of the typical American woman rose 22 percent, from 1542 kcal to 1877 kcal, and the typical man increased his intake by 7 percent, from 2450 kcal to 2618 kcal.[66] With regard to cardiovascular disease, a key element of dietary change is an increase in intake of saturated animal fats and hydrogenated vegetable fats, which contain atherogenic trans fatty acids, along with a decrease in intake of plant-based foods and an increase in simple carbohydrates. Although dietary habits clearly vary from country to country, intake of dietary fat tends to be low in many less-developed countries and high in many high-income countries and generally increases with annual per capita income (Fig. 1-10). Fat contributes less than 20 percent of calories in rural China and India,[67] less than 30 percent in Japan,[68] and well above 30 percent in the United States. Caloric contributions from fat appear to be falling in the high-income countries. In the United States, for example, the percent of calories from fat has steadily declined over the past 30 years, from 45 percent of calories in 1965 to 33 percent in 2000, although the total amount of fat in the diet has increased slightly since 1989.[66,69] In addition, from 1971 to 2000, the percentage of calories derived from saturated fat decreased from 13 to 11 percent. This decline in fat intake was accompanied by an increase in consumption of simple carbohydrates.

Even in the low-income countries, which are broadly characterized by low fat intake, fat intake varies greatly and tends to increase with industrialization and urbanization. For example, although dietary fat accounts for less than 20 percent of total calories in rural China, in urban areas it contributes more than 30 percent of calories.[70]

PHYSICAL INACTIVITY. One byproduct of the increased mechanization that accompanies the economic transition is decreased physical activity. In the high-income economies, the widespread prevalence of physical inactivity produces a high population-attributable risk of cardiovascular consequences. In the United States, approximately 25 percent of the population does not participate in any leisure-time physical activity and only 22 percent report engaging in sustained physical activity for at least 30 minutes on 5 or more days a week (the current recommendation).[71] The shift from physically demanding, agriculture-based work to largely sedentary service industry- and office-based work is occurring throughout the developing world. This is also accompanied by a switch from physically demanding transportation to mechanized transportation.

In China, physical activity is still integral to everyday life. Approximately 90 percent of the urban population walks or rides a bike to work, shopping, or school daily. And, unlike the United States, where "gym" class has become the exception rather than the rule, school-based physical education is prevalent; 72 percent of Chinese children age 6 to 18 engage in moderate to vigorous physical activity for a median of 90 to 100 minutes a week.[72] Nonetheless, more than 20 percent of children between the ages of 7 and 17 living in big cities are now overweight or obese.[73]

Among five major risk factors for CHD in the United States—diabetes, high blood pressure, high cholesterol, smoking, and physical inactivity—lack of exercise dwarfs the other four in prevalence by a wide margin.[74] Because the contribution of these five factors is approximately equal in the CHD risk equation, there may be a much greater opportunity to lower CHD rates by changing the activity patterns in the population than by lowering blood pressure, improving cholesterol levels, treating diabetes, or helping people to stop smoking.

Metabolic Factors: Lipid Levels, Obesity, Hypertension, and Diabetes Mellitus

LIPID LEVELS. The causal association between plasma cholesterol levels and risk of CVD is indisputable. Low levels of high-density lipoproteins and elevated triglycerides are also clearly associated with excess risk of CVD, and this association holds across racial and ethnic divisions. Interheart, the large, international case-control study, found that worldwide, abnormal lipid levels and smoking are the two most important risk factors for having a heart attack.[57] The lipid profile appears to have a greater impact on CHD than on stroke. Worldwide, high cholesterol levels are estimated to cause 56 percent of global ischemic heart disease and 18 percent of strokes, amounting to 4.4 million deaths annually.[43]

As countries move through the epidemiological transition, mean population plasma cholesterol levels tend to rise. Social and individual changes that accompany urbanization clearly play a role because plasma cholesterol levels tend to be higher among urban residents than among rural residents. This shift is largely driven by greater consump-

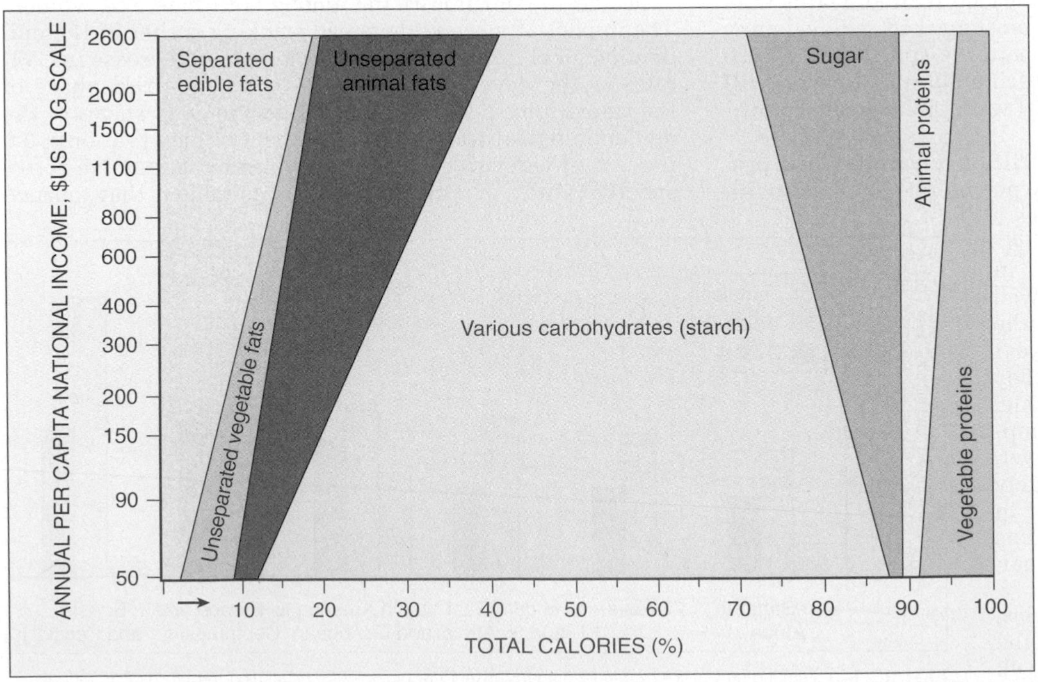

FIGURE 1–10 Association between income and dietary intake, based on country-level sources of energy. *(From Drwenowski A, Popkin BM: The nutrition transition: New trends in the global diet. Nutr Rev 55:31, 1997.)*

tion of dietary fats—primarily from animal products and processed vegetable oils—and decreased physical activity. Cross-cultural differences in mean cholesterol levels reflect this pattern. In rural Nigeria, which is early in the epidemiological transition, mean cholesterol levels are 120 mg/dl (3.1 mmol/liter),[75] whereas in the heavily industrialized United States, which is in the fifth phase, mean cholesterol levels are now 203 mg/dl (5.26 mmol/liter). Currently, 50 percent of Americans have a total cholesterol level of 200 mg/dl or higher, and 17 percent have a level that is 240 mg/dl or higher, down from 20 percent during the 1988 to 1994 period.[76] For comparison, in England, the mean cholesterol level for men is 213 mg/dl (5.5 mmol/liter) and is slightly higher for women, 217 mg/dl (5.6 mmol/liter). Data from the WHO MONICA Project demonstrated considerable variation in the prevalence of high cholesterol among the 19 participating countries, as well as within countries. On average, the prevalence of hypercholesterolemia (>251 mg/dl [>6.5 mmol/liter]) was 27 percent among men and 25 percent among women.

In the high-income countries, mean population cholesterol levels are generally falling. Japan is something of an exception to this pattern, with only relatively recent increases in average serum cholesterol levels.[77] This may help explain why CHD rates did not increase in the third phase of Japan's epidemiological transition. If plasma cholesterol levels continue to rise, however, CHD rates may increase in the coming years. In the emerging market economies, mean population cholesterol levels also tend to be high, but levels are stable or rising.

The low- and middle-income countries exhibit wide variation in mean population cholesterol levels. In Asia, cholesterol levels rose steadily in the last decades of the 20th century, generally faster in urban areas than in rural areas.[78] Once as low as 115 mg/dl (3 mmol/liter), mean total cholesterol levels now tend to be at or above 190 mg/dl (5 mmol/liter). In Singapore, mean population levels reached 250 mg/dl (6.5 mmol/liter) in the mid-1980s but have since fallen. In many countries in Latin America and the Caribbean, cholesterol levels approach those of northern Europe. A population survey in Bogotá, Colombia, for example, found that 46 percent of men had serum cholesterol levels greater than 250 mg/dl (6.5 mmol/liter).[79] In sub-Saharan Africa, mean cholesterol levels in rural areas are similar to the low levels seen in China, whereas levels are considerably higher in urban centers.[80] Given the high level of global capacity to produce Western-style food products at low cost, developing countries can now afford to adopt a Western dietary life style earlier in the economic transition than was possible in the past.

As is true for hypertension, rates of hypercholesterolemia are increasing far faster than the resources necessary for widespread detection and treatment. Thus the impact of both of these on atherosclerosis may be far greater than it has been in developed economies.

OBESITY (see Chaps. 43 and 44). Obesity is clearly associated with increased risk of CHD. However, much of this risk may be mediated by other CVD risk factors including hypertension, diabetes mellitus, and lipid profile imbalances. Whereas rates of smoking and hypertension tend to increase early in the epidemiological transition, obesity tends to increase later, as seen in high-income countries. Worldwide, obesity accounts for approximately 58 percent of diabetes cases, 21 percent of ischemic heart disease cases, 8 to 42 percent of certain cancers, and more than 10 percent of deaths.[43]

In the mid-1980s, the WHO's MONICA Project sampled 48 populations for cardiovascular risk factors. In all but one male population (China), and in most of the female populations, between 50 and 75 percent of adults aged 35 to 64 years were overweight or obese.[81] A later follow-up study showed that the prevalence of obesity has continued to increase.[82]

In many high-income countries, mean body mass index is rising at an alarming rate even as mean plasma cholesterol levels are falling and age-adjusted hypertension levels remain fairly stable during the fourth phase (the age of delayed degenerative diseases). In the United States, weight gain is occurring among all sectors of the population; however, rates are increasing faster among minorities and women. The percentage of adults classified as overweight in the United States has been stable since the 1960s, but the prevalence of obesity doubled between 1980 and 2002, rising from 15 to 30 percent (Fig. 1-11).[83,84] In addition, the prevalence of extreme obesity (BMI > 40 kg/m^2) more than tripled, increasing from 1.3 to 4.9 percent.

Overweight and obesity are not limited to high-income economies. Since 1980, obesity rates have tripled in some parts of Eastern Europe, the Middle East, the Pacific Islands, and China.[43] In many of the low- and middle-income countries, obesity appears to coexist with undernutrition and malnutrition. Although the prevalence of obesity in the low- and middle-income countries is certainly less than among the high-income countries, it is on the rise there as well. A study in Mauritius, for example, documented rapid increases in obesity between 1987 and 1992,[85] whereas a survey undertaken in 1998 found that as many as 58 percent of African women living in South Africa may be overweight or obese.[86]

Excess weight early in life not only increases the likelihood of adult obesity but also increases the prevalence of weight-related disorders, including CVD, diabetes, and hypertension. Further increases in the prevalence of overweight and obesity are to be expected if data on childhood and adolescent obesity are any indication. In Great Britain, for example, waist size and body mass index among youths aged 11 to 16 years increased significantly between 1977 and 1997.[87] But increasing BMI among children is also a problem in low- and middle-income countries. Studies show that obesity levels in children are increasing markedly in countries as diverse as Brazil, China, India, and almost all island states.[55] Because of the lag time associated with CVD risk factors, especially in children, the full effect of this will only be seen in the future.

HYPERTENSION. Hypertension is clearly a risk factor for CHD and stroke (see Chaps. 39, 40, and 41). Elevated

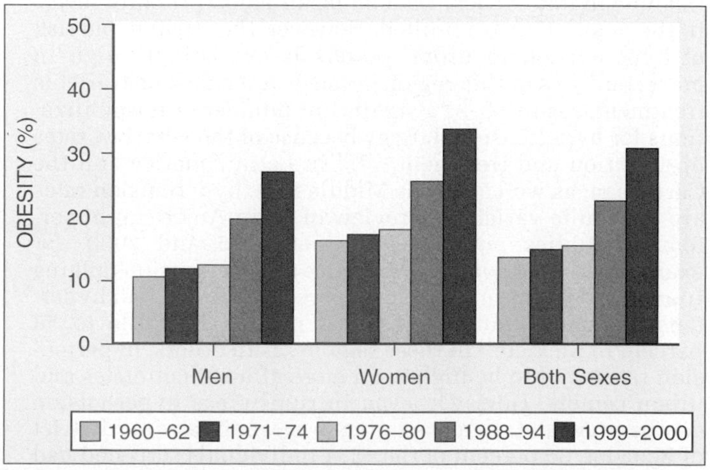

FIGURE 1–11 Trends in obesity (body mass index >30) among Americans aged 20 to 74. *(From the National Health Examination Survey and the National Health and Nutrition Examination Surveys [http://www.cdc.gov/nchs/data/nhanes/databriefs/adultweight.pdf].)*

blood pressure is an early hallmark of the epidemiological transition. Rising mean population blood pressure is apparent as countries industrialize; emigration from less developed to more developed countries, as well as emigration from rural to urban settings, results in increasing blood pressure levels among emigrants. Among urban-dwelling men and women in India, for example, the prevalence of hypertension is 25.5 and 29.0 percent, respectively, whereas it is just 14 and 10.8 percent, respectively, among those living in rural communities.[40] Although the relative increase in mortality associated with a given increase in blood pressure is similar in various regions of the world, the absolute risk at the same blood pressure level varies greatly.[88] In addition, the overall impact of hypertension may vary depending on the proportion of individuals in a country who have untreated hypertension. Worldwide, approximately 62 percent of strokes and 49 percent of cases of ischemic heart disease are attributable to suboptimal (>115 mm Hg systolic) blood pressure, and it is thought to account for more than 7 million deaths annually.[43]

In the high-income countries, hypertension remains a major cause of CVD morbidity and mortality despite high rates of detection and treatment. Given the relationship of increasing blood pressure with advancing age, the prevalence of hypertension is increasing in most of these (aging) established market economies. In most of the high-income countries, the proportion of the population with untreated hypertension is declining, although the United States has witnessed a slight reversal of this trend.[27] In Europe and Central Asia, the prevalence of hypertension is at least as high as it is in the high-income countries, whereas rates of treatment are much lower.

Across the developing countries, hypertension rates are quite variable. One major concern in these countries is the high rate of undetected, and therefore untreated, hypertension. This may explain, at least in part, the higher stroke rates, particularly hemorrhagic, in these countries in relation to CHD rates. In northern Asian countries such as China and South Korea, hypertension is rapidly increasing,[89] with higher rates in urban areas than rural areas. An analysis of several large cohort studies from mainland China, Hong Kong, Japan, Singapore, South Korea, Taiwan, Australia, and New Zealand with more than 3 million person-years of follow-up demonstrated continuous log-linear associations between systolic blood pressure and risks of stroke, ischemic heart disease, and total cardiovascular death.[90]

In contrast, rates of hypertension remain relatively low in sub-Saharan Africa. Data on mean blood pressure levels in the population are limited. However, the attributable risk of hypertension in urban centers is exceedingly high in most countries of this region because of the lack of available treatment, resulting in a significant number of hospitalizations for hypertension, largely because of the very low rates of detection and treatment.[42,90,91] In Latin America and the Caribbean, as well as in the Middle East, hypertension rates are also quite variable. A review of Latin American hypertension studies published between 1995 and 2000, for example, showed overall prevalence of hypertension ranging from 11.1 percent in Chile to 43 percent in Cuba, and hypertension control ranging from 22 percent in Chile to 58 percent in Mexico.[92] In these regions, as in others, hypertension rates tend to be highest in more affluent countries and urban centers. However, even in rural areas hypertension can be prevalent. In a screening program in a rural district of Ecuador, 36 percent of the 4284 individuals screened had hypertension; only 4 of these cases were well controlled by treatment.[93] During 2.5 years of follow-up, hypertension-related cardiovascular disease was the main cause of death.

DIABETES MELLITUS (see Chaps. 39, 43, and 60). Diabetes and impaired glucose tolerance represent strong risk factors for vascular disease, including CHD, cerebrovascular disorders, and peripheral vascular disease. As a consequence of, or in addition to, increasing body mass index and decreasing levels of physical activity, worldwide rates of diabetes—predominantly type II diabetes, or non–insulin-dependent diabetes mellitus—are on the rise.

In 2003, 194 million adults, or 5 percent of the world's population, had diabetes, with nearly three quarters living in high-income countries. By 2025, this number is predicted to increase to 333 million, a 72 percent increase.[94] In 2001, according to WHO estimates, diabetes resulted in 20 million lost DALYs worldwide. More than 80 percent of the lost DALYs were in developing countries, with East Asia and the Pacific bearing the largest burden and the Middle East and the Pacific bearing the smallest burden. By 2025, the number of people with diabetes is projected to double in three of the six low-and middle-income regions: Middle East and North Africa, South Asia, and sub-Saharan Africa, although the prevalence will still be low in sub-Saharan Africa.[94] Not so in South Asia: India already has more diabetics than any other country—31.6 million. This number is expected to reach 57.2 million by 2025 and contribute significantly to that country's alarming increase in heart disease.[38]

The prevalence of diabetes varies greatly by geographic region, race, and ethnic composition. Clear genetic susceptibilities of various racial and ethnic groups are apparent. For example, Pima Indians living in the southwestern United States are many times more likely to develop diabetes than the general U.S. population. Hispanic Americans also tend to have higher rates than white Americans. Migration studies suggest that South Asians and Indians also tend to be at higher-risk than those of European extraction.

Diabetes mellitus is associated with a number of other CVD risk factors including high triglyceride levels, low high-density lipoprotein levels, central obesity, and hypertension. In relative terms, the attributable risk of diabetes is higher in women than in men.

FUTURE CHALLENGES

Although the concept of the epidemiological transition offers tremendous insight into how and why CVD is emerging as the predominant global cause of morbidity and mortality, it also provides great insight about how to alter this course. As has been seen from the experience of high-income countries, CVD rates rise in a predictable fashion with increasing rates of risk factors and risky behaviors. It is equally true that population-based and individual interventions can have an impact on both the rates and the consequences of CVD. This raises the possibility of altering the epidemiological transition to blunt the increase in regional CVD rates or to hasten their decline. The transfer of lower-cost health and food technologies to the low- and middle-income countries has produced great gains in the fight against communicable diseases and clearly helped hasten the transition out of the age of pestilence and famine. It is possible that similar interventions could alter the course of later stages.

Given the multifactorial nature of CVD, and social, economic, and cultural heterogeneity, no single solution will be generally applicable to all geographic and economic regions of the world. In this section are outlined the major challenges facing the high- and low- and middle-income countries, and various strategies to address these problems are discussed. Appropriate regional strategies depend on a number of factors, including a country's or region's stage in the epidemiological transition, the rate of change of the

TABLE 1–7	Complementary Strategies to Reduce Morbidity and Mortality Caused by Cardiovascular Disease
Lower overall burden of risk factors in the entire population through population-wide public health measures such as detection and surveillance strategies; public education campaigns; and the institution of low-cost, population-wide preventive interventions.	
Identify and target higher-risk subgroups of the population who stand to benefit the most from moderate, cost-effective prevention interventions through screening and targeting preventive interventions such as treatment of hypertension and cholesterol.	
Allocate resources to acute and chronic higher-cost treatments and secondary prevention interventions for those with clinically manifest disease.	

epidemiological transition, individual and collective resources, and cultural and political factors.

Three complementary strategies can reduce morbidity and mortality from CVD (Table 1-7). First, population-wide public health measures can lower the overall burden of CVD risk factors in the entire population. These include surveillance strategies, public education campaigns, and the institution of low-cost, population-wide preventive interventions. National campaigns against cigarette smoking are an example of the public health approach. The second approach involves identifying and targeting higher-risk subgroups of the population who stand to benefit the most from specific, low-cost prevention interventions. This involves screening and targeting preventive interventions, such as treatment of hypertension and high cholesterol. Third, resources can be allocated to acute and chronic higher-cost treatments, as well as secondary prevention interventions, such as for those with clinically manifest disease. Typically, some resources simultaneously support all three strategies; however, this three-pronged approach has been implemented mostly in high-income countries with abundant financial resources for health care. Whether or not this makes sense in a given country depends on resources, social norms, and competing priorities. In the following sections are outlined the major challenges and possible solutions for each region.

High-Income Countries

Although CVD mortality rates have fallen in most high-income countries, several important challenges remain. First, socioeconomic and racial disparities in CVD rates continue to linger. In the United States, for example, although rates of CVD mortality have fallen across the population, there are still wide disparities among racial and ethnic groups. Thus a major goal will be to accelerate the widespread application of preventive and therapeutic technologies to all racial, ethnic, and socioeconomic groups.

Second, the rate of declining CVD mortality appears to be stagnating. We are entering the Age of Inactivity and Obesity. This may be the result of troubling trends in a number of coronary risk factors: although older men and women continue to stop smoking, young adults and teenagers continue to take up smoking; the rate of those appropriately treated for hypertension has decreased slightly in the past decade; and the biggest concern is the increase in obesity and diabetes rates. Perhaps most troubling are observations of increasing rates of obesity and decreasing rates of physical activity in children. Taken together, these trends may explain the flattening of mortality curves and may also explain why mortality rates have fallen faster than CVD incidence rates.

In the absence of efforts to reverse these trends in risk factors, we may see increasing rates of CVD once again. More public health dollars need to be directed at antismoking efforts that target high-risk groups such as teenagers and at broader application of guidelines for detecting and managing hypertension and hyperlipidemia. Effective strategies to increase activity and reverse trends in obesity and diabetes must be developed and implemented.

Third, because of the aging of the population, the prevalence of CVD will continue to rise with the increasing mean age of a population even if that population's age-adjusted mortality rates continue to decline. In addition, incremental advances in therapeutic health technology and secondary prevention have led to increasing numbers of people surviving with CVD, which consumes increasing amounts of resources. With the institution of many life-saving strategies among those who present with acute manifestations of atherosclerotic disease, more and more individuals are surviving acute events such as myocardial infarction. For example, approximately one third of those who presented to hospitals with acute myocardial infarction in the 1950s died. Today, in-hospital mortality is less than half that, although sicker and older patients now present to the hospital. Furthermore, CHD is being diagnosed in increasing numbers of individuals before cardiovascular events. Thousands of pacemakers and defibrillators are implanted each year. Because more and more individuals survive longer with CVD, the prevalence of congestive heart failure increases, even as mortality from congestive heart failure is declining.[95] Thus the management of congestive heart failure will consume more and more health care resources. A major challenge for most established market economies will be the increasing financial burden of the management of CVD. More efficient and cost-effective strategies for treating CVD will have to be developed.

Low- and Middle-Income Countries

EASTERN EUROPE AND CENTRAL ASIA. This region is largely in the third phase of the epidemiological transition, although some countries are entering the fourth phase. However, the resources available are considerably less than those available in the high-income countries. This mandates making careful choices in terms of allocating health care dollars to each of the three strategies outlined earlier (see Table 1-7).

In Europe and Central Asia, the two overarching goals are to manage the increasing number of people with CVD and to hasten the transition from the third to the fourth phase of the epidemiological transition. This will likely enhance overall productivity in the region because during the third phase of the transition, CVD, and particularly CHD, often afflict individuals at the age of highest productivity. In terms of challenges facing the former socialist countries, the region can be divided into two categories: those countries with stable or declining rates and those countries with increasing CVD rates. For countries with stable or declining rates, the three-pronged approach used in the high-income countries should serve as a model. For those countries experiencing rapid rises in CVD rates, an important first step will be implementing more centralized efforts at compiling data on rates of disease and risk factors and then determining the major country-specific contributors to the rise. All countries in this economic sector need more careful tracking and assessment of risk factors in terms of population-attributable risk. Better tracking of CVD rates and risk factors will allow for more careful allocation of scarce preventive resources.

National guidelines that have been developed in the high-income countries need to be adapted for this region.

However, Western guidelines should be modified, taking into account public health and health care infrastructure and economic realities. Governments should initiate major public health initiatives aimed at life-style factors including lowering rates of smoking and drinking, modifying diet, and increasing physical activity. Major public health priorities should also include the detection and control of hypertension and high cholesterol, both of which are highly cost effective. The targeting of higher-risk individuals for higher-cost preventive strategies such as pharmacological lowering of cholesterol and blood pressure will initially need to be confined to areas such as urban centers, where the burden is high and the necessary laboratory-based health care infrastructure is available.

Throughout this economic sector, improvements in health care delivery systems will be needed to manage the already high rates of CVD prevalent in these countries. Careful attention must be paid to the transfer of lower-cost health technology, keeping in mind the considerably lower annual health care expenditures in Eastern Europe and Central Asia compared with those in the high-income countries. An intervention such as the more widespread and appropriate use of aspirin and beta blockers during acute myocardial infarction is an example of an extremely cost-effective life-saving therapy that should be implemented universally before extensive resources are directed at higher-cost interventions such as angioplasty. Personnel issues must also be addressed, given the general shortage of health care professionals in this region.

OTHER LOW- AND MIDDLE-INCOME REGIONS. Many low- and middle-income countries may face the most challenging problems. These countries have rapidly increasing burdens of CVD early in their economic transitions. They often do not have the per capita resources needed to create the three-pronged type of public health and health care infrastructure currently available in the high-income countries. In many low- and middle-income countries, per capita health care expenditures are less than $50 per year. In addition, there are a number of competing national priorities, including the stimulation of economic growth, social and political change, and the devastation wrought by communicable diseases, such as HIV/AIDS in sub-Saharan Africa.

Rising CVD rates will eventually exert a drag on economic growth. Early in the epidemiological transition, CVD deaths occur among younger individuals as opposed to later in the transition. Thus the economic impact on both the family and national productivity is greater in developing economies than in established market economies. The loss of the head of a household from CVD (or any other disease) has a devastating impact on the health and well-being of the entire family. In Bangladesh, for example, when there is an adult death, a child who depends on that adult has a 12-fold higher probability of death.[96] At present, the data on the economic consequences of CVD in the low- and middle-income countries are limited. Much more work is necessary to refine estimates that would permit more thoughtful allocation of health care resources.

As mentioned earlier, the epidemiological transition has been accelerated at least in part by an efficient translation of risk behaviors and the rise in risk factors from the high-income countries to the low- and middle-income countries early in the economic transition. The rapid spread of cigarette smoking is a prime example of this. A major challenge for developing countries is to attempt to change the natural history of the epidemiological transition. That such alterations are possible is evident from the experience of Japan, in which CHD rates were kept relatively low during a fairly rapid economic transition to an industrial-based economy. Although embedded cultural practice such as diet likely played a large role, the Japanese experience illustrates that the nature of the transition is variable.

As is true for Eastern Europe and Central Asia, a critical first step in developing a comprehensive plan for many of the low- and middle-income countries is better assessment of cause-specific mortality and morbidity, as well as the prevalence of the major preventable risk factors for CVD. In many areas of the low- and middle-income countries, reliable estimates of the prevalence and incidence of CVD, as well as risk behaviors and factors, are not available. Improved estimates would enable better allocation of resources on the basis of country-wide burdens of disease. Beginning first in the urban centers and then moving out to rural areas, government agencies will need to make careful assessments of, and create longitudinal surveillance of, rates of disease and risk factors for which low-cost strategies are available. High priorities include smoking and hypertension, for which the population-attributable risks are likely to be high and the cost efficacy for intervention is favorable. The strategy for the detection and management of high cholesterol must be carefully tailored for each region because of higher costs of screening. Drug therapy for cholesterol lowering is likely less cost effective than short-term smoking cessation programs or managing hypertension with low-cost medications, though this is changing as statins become available in generic form. Public health approaches aimed at educating the general population about diet and exercise may be useful, but precise estimates of cost efficacy are not available on these even for high-income countries. Simple, low-cost interventions, such as the "polypill," need to be explored as alternatives to more costly approaches developed in high-income countries.

Generic drugs were used in a recent study that examined the prevalence of risk factors for CVD and the cost of treatment in a middle-income country that has experienced rapid social and economic changes.[97] The Seychelles are a group of islands in the Indian Ocean, where per capita GDP has increased from $600 in 1976 to $8432 in 2003 and CVD currently accounts for approximately 38 percent of mortality. A high prevalence of major risk factors (high blood pressure—the most common risk factor—high cholesterol, overweight, and obesity) was observed among men and women, as well as a prevalence of 9 percent for diabetes and a high prevalence of smoking (31 percent) among men. A minimum of $68 per capita was necessary for medications and basic medical follow-up for all high-risk individuals, which represented a major burden on the country's health budget. The authors concluded that treating these risk factors—even earlier in the epidemiological transition when the prevalence is low—would not be possible for many developing countries.

Once these initial assessments have been made, resources should be carefully allocated to each prong of the overall strategy (see Table 1-7), with most resources dedicated to the first two—national programs for population-wide prevention and guidelines for screening and targeted interventions. Guidelines for high-income countries should not be adopted wholesale because they reflect economic realities of cost efficacy that are specific to the country where they are developed. Instead, these programs must be based on the population-attributable risk and the available resources, and guidelines must be developed and implemented with low-cost campaigns. Such prevention-directed efforts could blunt the rise in disease rates already apparent in many developed countries. Given the extreme limitations in per capita health care resources in many low- and middle-income countries, the allocation of resources to higher-cost strategies for treating CVD may divert resources from the potentially more effective population-wide efforts. Thus efforts targeted at interventions and high-technology therapeutics may require parsimonious implementation only in those urban areas where risk is highest. Assistance in the transfer of health care and preventive technologies from high-income countries will greatly enhance regional efforts in countries with developing economies.

SUMMARY AND CONCLUSIONS

We are now halfway through a two-century transition in which CVD will dominate as the major cause of death and disease worldwide. Although CVD rates are declining in the high-income countries, they are increasing in virtually every other region of the world. From a worldwide perspective, the rate of change in the global burden of CVD is accelerating, reflecting the changes in the low- and middle-income economies, which represent 85 percent of the world's population, as they move rapidly through the second and third phases of the epidemiological transition, and in rare cases, the fourth phase. The consequences of this preventable epidemic will be substantial on many levels—individual mortality and morbidity, family suffering, and staggering economic costs, both the direct costs of diagnosis and treatment and the indirect costs of lost productivity.

Each region of the world faces major challenges presented by the epidemic of CVD. There is no single global solution to the rising burden of CVD, given the vast differences in social, cultural, and economic circumstances. The high-income countries must minimize disparities, reverse unfavorable trends in CVD risk factors and behaviors, and deal with the increasing prevalence of CVD in an aging population. The most complex challenges are those facing the low- and middle-income countries. They must dedicate often minuscule resources to better assess rates of death, disease, and CVD risk factors. To hasten the transition from the third to the fourth phase of the epidemiological transition, Eastern Europe and Central Asia must find ways to care efficiently for increasing numbers of individuals with CVD, as well as to deploy lower-cost prevention strategies. The allocation of resources to lower-cost strategies will likely be more cost effective than dedicating resources to high-cost management of CVD in the long run.

The high-income countries must continue to bear the burden of research and development into every aspect of prevention and treatment. Through further expansion of the knowledge base, particularly regarding the economic consequences of various treatment and prevention strategies, it is possible that the efficient transfer of low-cost preventive and therapeutic strategies may alter the natural course of the epidemiological transition in every part of the world and thus reduce the excess global burden of preventable CVD.

REFERENCES

Epidemiologic Transitions

1. Lopez AD, Mathers CD, Ezzati M, et al (eds): Global Burden of Disease and Risk Factors, Oxford, England, Oxford University Press and Washington, DC, The World Bank, 2006.
2. Murray CJL, Lopez AD: The Global Burden of Disease. Cambridge, Mass, Harvard School of Public Health, 1996.
3. World Health Report 2003: Shaping the Future. Geneva, World Health Organization, 2003.
4. Omran AR: The epidemiologic transition. A theory of the epidemiology of population change. Milbank Mem Fund Q 49:509, 1971.
5. Olshansky SJ, Ault AB: The fourth stage of the epidemiologic transition: The age of delayed degenerative diseases. Milbank Q 64:355, 1986.
6. Hannon TS, Rao G, Arslanian SA: Childhood obesity and type 2 diabetes mellitus. Pediatrics 116:473, 2005.
7. Muntner P, He J, Cutler JA, et al: Trends in blood pressure among children and adolescents. JAMA 291:2107, 2004.
8. Wu Y: Overweight and obesity in China. BMJ 333:362, 2006.
9. Pearson TA: Global perspectives on cardiovascular disease. Evid Based Cardiovasc Med 1:4, 1997.
10. US Census Bureau Global Population Profile: 2002. Washington, DC, US Government Printing Office, 2004.
11. Sheth T, Nair C, Nargundkar M, et al: Cardiovascular and cancer mortality among Canadians of European, South Asian and Chinese origin from 1979 to 1993: An analysis of 1.2 million deaths. CMAJ 161:132, 1999.

The Epidemiologic Transition in the United States

12. Reducing the health consequences of smoking: 25 years of progress. A report of the Surgeon General. Rockville, Md, US Department of Health and Human Services, Public Health Service, Centers for Disease Control, Office on Smoking and Health, 1989.
13. Flexner A: Medical education in the United States and Canada: A report to the Carnegie Foundation for the Advancement of Teaching. Boston, Merrymount Press, 1910.
14. Centers for Disease Control and Prevention: Control of infectious diseases. MMWR Morb Mortal Wkly Rep 48:621, 1999.
15. Centers for Disease Control and Prevention: Smoking prevalence among U.S. adults. Washington, DC, Office on Smoking and Health, Centers for Disease Control and Prevention, 2005.
16. U.S. Bureau of the Census: Measuring 50 years of economic change using the March Current Population Survey. Washington, DC: US Government Printing Office, 1998.
17. Decline in deaths from heart disease and stroke—United States, 1900-1999. MMWR Morb Mortal Wkly Rep 48:649, 1999.
18. Hunink MG, Goldman L, Tosteson AN, et al: The recent decline in mortality from coronary heart disease, 1980-1990. The effect of secular trends in risk factors and treatment. JAMA 277:535, 1997.
19. Cooper R, Cutler J, Desvigne-Nickens P, et al: Trends and disparities in coronary heart disease, stroke, and other cardiovascular diseases in the United States: Findings of the national conference on cardiovascular disease prevention. Circulation 102:3137, 2000.
20. Levit KR, Cowan CA, Lazenby HC, et al: National health spending trends, 1960-1993. Health Aff (Millwood) 13:14, 1994.
21. Smith C, Cowan C, Heffler S, Catlin A: National health spending in 2004: Recent slowdown led by prescription drug spending. Health Aff (Millwood) 25:186, 2006.
22. Anand RS, Basiotis PP: Is total fat consumption really decreasing? Washington, DC, US Department of Agriculture, Center for Nutrition Policy and Promotion, 1998.
23. Thom T, Haase N, Rosamond W, et al: Heart disease and stroke statistics—2006 update: A report from the American Heart Association Statistics Committee and Stroke Statistics Subcommittee. Circulation 113:e85, 2006.
24. Kozak LJ, DeFrances CJ: National Hospital Discharge Survey: 2003 annual summary with detailed diagnosis and procedure data. National Center for Health Statistics. Vital Health Stat Series 13(160), 2006.
25. Arias E: United States life tables, 2003. Hyattsville, Md, National Center for Health Statistics, Centers for Disease Control and Prevention, 2003.
26. Hoyert DL, Heron MP, Murphy SL, Kung HC: Deaths: Final data for 2003. Natl Vital Stat Rep 54:1, 2006.
27. Chobanian AV, Bakris GL, Black HR, et al: The Seventh Report of the Joint National Committee on Prevention, Detection, Evaluation, and Treatment of High Blood Pressure: The JNC 7 Report. JAMA 289:2560, 2003.
28. (CDC) CfDCaP: Cigarette smoking among adults—United States, 2003. MMWR 54:1121, 2004.

Current Worldwide Variations

29. Gaziano TA, Gaziano JM: Historical perspective on heart disease and worldwide trends. *In* Gaziano JM (ed): Atlas of Cardiovascular Risk Factors. Philadelphia, Current Medicine, 2006.
30. European Cardiovascular Disease Statistics, 2005 edition. (http://www.heartstats.org/uploads/documents%5CPDF.pdf).
31. Drewnowski A, Popkin BM: The nutrition transition: New trends in the global diet. Nutr Rev 55:31, 1997.
32. Adachi H, Hino A: Trends in nutritional intake and serum cholesterol levels over 40 years in Tanushimaru, Japanese men. J Epidemiol 15:85, 2005.
33. Mackay J, Mensah G: Atlas of Heart Disease and Stroke. Geneva, World Health Organization, 2004.
34. Szostak WB, Sekula W, Figurska K: Reduction of cardiovascular mortality in Poland and changes in dietary patterns. Kardiol Pol 58:173, 2003; discussion 180.
35. Yao C, Wu Z, Wu Y: The changing pattern of cardiovascular diseases in China. World Health Stat Q 46:113, 1993.
36. Okumura K, Iseki K, Wakugami K, et al: Low serum cholesterol as a risk factor for hemorrhagic stroke in men: A community-based mass screening in Okinawa, Japan. Jpn Circ J 63:53, 1999.
37. Yusuf S, Reddy S, Ounpuu S, Anand S: Global burden of cardiovascular diseases: Part I: General considerations, the epidemiologic transition, risk factors, and impact of urbanization. Circulation 104:2746, 2001.
38. Ghaffar A, Reddy KS, Singhi M: Burden of non-communicable diseases in South Asia. BMJ 328:807, 2004.
39. Singh RB, Niaz MA, Thakur AS, et al: Social class and coronary artery disease in an urban population of North India in the Indian Lifestyle and Heart Study. Int J Cardiol 64:195, 1998.
40. Singh RB, Sharma JP, Rastogi V, et al: Social class and coronary disease in rural population of north India. The Indian Social Class and Heart Survey. Eur Heart J 18:588, 1997.
41. Reddy KS: Cardiovascular diseases in India. World Health Stat Q 46:101, 1993.
42. Bertrand E: Cardiovascular disease in developing countries. *In* Dalla Volta S (ed): Cardiology. New York, McGraw-Hill, 1999.

43. World Health Report 2002: Reducing risks, promoting healthy life. Geneva, World Health Organization, 2002.
44. Mathers CD, Lopez A, Stein D, et al: Deaths and disease burden by cause: Global burden of disease estimates for 2001 by World Bank country groups. Disease Control Priorities Project Working Paper 18. April 2004, Revised January 2005 (http://www.dcp2.org/file/33/wp18.pdf).
45. Barbaro G, Di Lorenzo G, Grisorio B, Barbarini G: Cardiac involvement in the acquired immunodeficiency syndrome: A multicenter clinical-pathological study. Gruppo Italiano per lo Studio Cardiologico dei pazienti affetti da AIDS Investigators. AIDS Res Hum Retroviruses 14:1071, 1998.
46. Barbaro G, Di Lorenzo G, Grisorio B, Barbarini G: Incidence of dilated cardiomyopathy and detection of HIV in myocardial cells of HIV-positive patients. Gruppo Italiano per lo Studio Cardiologico dei Pazienti Affetti da AIDS. N Engl J Med 339:1093, 1998.
47. Starc TJ, Lipshultz SE, Easley KA, et al: Incidence of cardiac abnormalities in children with human immunodeficiency virus infection: The prospective P2C2 HIV study. J Pediatr 141:327, 2002.
48. Al-Attar I, Orav EJ, Exil V, et al: Predictors of cardiac morbidity and related mortality in children with acquired immunodeficiency syndrome. J Am Coll Cardiol 41:1598, 2003.
49. Danbauchi SS, Okpapi JU: Cardiovascular involvement in HIV/AIDS: Report of three cases. West Afr J Med 20:261, 2001.
50. Nzuobontane D, Blackett KN, Kuaban C: Cardiac involvement in HIV infected people in Yaoundo, Cameroon. Postgrad Med J 78:678, 2002.
51. Barbaro G: Cardiovascular manifestations of HIV infection. Circulation 106:1420, 2002.
52. Musaiger AO: Diet and prevention of coronary heart disease in the Arab Middle East countries. Med Princ Pract 11(Suppl): 9, 2002.
53. Sheikholeslam R, Mohamad A, Mohammad K, Vaseghi S: Non communicable disease risk factors in Iran. Asia Pac J Clin Nutr 13:S100, 2004.

Global Trends in Cardiovascular Disease

54. Preventing chronic diseases: A vital investment. Geneva, World Health Organization, 2005.
55. Leeder S, Raymond S, Greenberg H, et al: A Race Against Time: The Challenge of Cardiovascular Disease in Developing Economies. New York, Columbia University, 2004.

Regional Trends in Risk Factors

56. Kuulasmaa K, Tunstall-Pedoe H, Dobson A, et al: Estimation of contribution of changes in classic risk factors to trends in coronary-event rates across the WHO MONICA Project populations. Lancet 355:675, 2000.
57. Yusuf S, Hawken S, Ounpuu S, et al: Effect of potentially modifiable risk factors associated with myocardial infarction in 52 countries (the INTERHEART study): Case-control study. Lancet 364:937, 2004.
58. World Health Organization Tobacco Free Initiative: Building Blocks for Tobacco Control: A Handbook. Geneva, World Health Organization, 2004.
59. Jha P, Chaloupka JM, Gajalakshmi V, et al: Tobacco Addiction. Disease Control Priorities in Developing Countries. 2nd ed. New York, Oxford University Press, 2006.
60. World Health Organization: Building Blocks for Tobacco Control: A Handbook. Geneva, WHO, 2004.
61. Guindon GE, Bosclair D: Past, current and future trends in tobacco use. Washington, DC, The World Bank (Health, Nutrition, and Population Discussion Paper, Economics of Tobacco Control, paper no. 6), 2003.
62. Trends in cigarette smoking among high school students—United States, 1991-2001. MMWR Morb Mortal Wkly Rep 51:409, 2002.
63. The Global Youth Tobacco Survey Collaborative Group. Tobacco Use Among Youth: A Cross Country Comparison. Tobacco Control 11:252, 2002.
64. World Health Organization: Building Blocks for Tobacco Control. Geneva, WHO, 2004.
65. Liu BQ, Peto R, Chen ZM, et al: Emerging tobacco hazards in China: 1. Retrospective proportional mortality study of one million deaths. BMJ 317:1411, 1998.
66. Trends in intake of energy and macronutrients—United States, 1971-2000. MMWR Morb Mortal Wkly Rep 53:80, 2004.
67. Janus ED, Postiglione A, Singh RB, Lewis B: The modernization of Asia. Implications for coronary heart disease. Council on Arteriosclerosis of the International Society and Federation of Cardiology. Circulation 94:2671, 1996.
68. Egusa G, Yamane K: Lifestyle, serum lipids and coronary artery disease: Comparison of Japan with the United States. J Atheroscler Thromb 11:304, 2004.
69. Kennedy ET, Bowman SA, Powell R: Dietary fat intake in the US population. J Am Coll Nutr 18:207, 1999.
70. Du S, Lu B, Zhai F, Popkin BM: A new stage of the nutrition transition in China. Public Health Nutr 5:169, 2002.
71. Physical activity trends—United States, 1990-1998. MMWR Morb Mortal Wkly Rep 50:166, 2001.
72. Tudor-Locke C, Ainsworth BE, Adair LS, et al: Physical activity and inactivity in Chinese school-aged youth: The China Health and Nutrition Survey. Int J Obes Relat Metab Disord 27:1093, 2003.
73. Wang L, Kong L, Wu F, Bai Y, Burton R. Preventing chronic diseases in China. Lancet 366:1821, 2005.
74. American Heart Association: Heart Disease and Stroke Statistics: 2004 Update. Dallas, AHA, 2003.
75. Erasmus RT, Uyot C, Pakeye T: Plasma cholesterol distribution in a rural Nigerian population—relationship to age, sex and body mass. Cent Afr J Med 40:299, 1994.
76. Carroll MD, Lacher DA, Sorlie PD, et al: Trends in serum lipids and lipoproteins of adults, 1960-2002. JAMA 294:1773, 2005.
77. Kuzuya M, Ando F, Iguchi A, Shimokata H: Changes in serum lipid levels during a 10 year period in a large Japanese population. A cross-sectional and longitudinal study. Atherosclerosis 163:313, 2002.
78. Khoo KL, Tan H, Liew YM, et al: Lipids and coronary heart disease in Asia. Atherosclerosis 169:1, 2003.
79. INCLEN Multicentre Collaborative Group: Risk factors for cardiovascular disease in the developing world. A multicentre collaborative study in the International Clinical Epidemiology Network (INCLEN). J Clin Epidemiol 45:841, 1992.
80. Walker AR, Sareli P: Coronary heart disease: Outlook for Africa. J R Soc Med 90:23, 1997.
81. Keil U, Kuulasmaa K: WHO MONICA Project: Risk factors. Int J Epidemiol 18:S46, 1989.
82. Dobson AJ, Evans A, Ferrario M, et al: Changes in estimated coronary risk in the 1980s: Data from 38 populations in the WHO MONICA Project. World Health Organization. Monitoring trends and determinants in cardiovascular diseases. Ann Med 30:199, 1998.
83. Hedley AA, Ogden CL, Johnson CL, et al: Prevalence of overweight and obesity among US children, adolescents, and adults, 1999-2002. JAMA 291:2847, 2004.
84. Flegal KM, Carroll MD, Ogden CL, Johnson CL: Prevalence and trends in obesity among US adults, 1999-2000. JAMA 288:1723, 2002.
85. Hodge AM, Dowse GK, Gareeboo H, et al: Incidence, increasing prevalence, and predictors of change in obesity and fat distribution over 5 years in the rapidly developing population of Mauritius. Int J Obes Relat Metab Disord 20:137, 1996.
86. Puoane T, Steyn K, Bradshaw D, et al: Obesity in South Africa: The South African demographic and health survey. Obes Res 10:1038, 2002.
87. McCarthy HD, Ellis SM, Cole TJ: Central overweight and obesity in British youth aged 11-16 years: Cross sectional surveys of waist circumference. BMJ 326:624, 2003.
88. van den Hoogen PC, Feskens EJ, Nagelkerke NJ, et al: The relation between blood pressure and mortality due to coronary heart disease among men in different parts of the world. Seven Countries Study Research Group. N Engl J Med 342:1, 2000.
89. Gu D, Reynolds K, Wu X, et al: Prevalence, awareness, treatment, and control of hypertension in China. Hypertension 40:920, 2002.
90. Lawes CM, Rodgers A, Bennett DA, et al: Blood pressure and cardiovascular disease in the Asia Pacific region. J Hypertens 21:707, 2003.
91. Seedat YK: Hypertension in developing nations in sub-Saharan Africa. J Hum Hypertens 14:739, 2000.
92. Ordunez P, Silva LC, Rodriguez MP, Robles S: Prevalence estimates for hypertension in Latin America and the Caribbean: Are they useful for surveillance? Rev Panam Salud Publica 10:226, 2001.
93. Anselmi M, Avanzini F, Moreira JM, et al: Treatment and control of arterial hypertension in a rural community in Ecuador. Lancet 361:1186, 2003.
94. Narayan KM, Zhang P, Kanaya AM, et al: Diabetes: The Pandemic and Potential Solutions. Disease Control Priorities in Developing Countries. 2nd ed. Washington, DC, The International Bank for Reconstruction and Development/The World Bank, 2006.

Future Challenges

95. Changes in mortality from heart failure—United States, 1980-1995. MMWR Morb Mortal Wkly Rep 47:633, 1998.
96. Howson CP, Reddy KS, Ryan TJ, Bale JR (eds): Control of Cardiovascular Disease in Developing Countries. Washington, DC, National Academy Press, 1998.
97. Bovet P, Shamlaye C, Gabriel A, et al: Prevalence of cardiovascular risk factors in a middle-income country and estimated cost of a treatment strategy. BMC Public Health 6:9, 2006.

CHAPTER 2

Heart Disease in Varied Populations

Clyde W. Yancy

THE CHANGING DEMOGRAPHICS OF THE U.S. POPULATION

Cardiovascular disease (CVD) remains the leading cause of death and disability in the United States, and its burden permeates the entirety of the U.S. population. In the past, data extracted from large epidemiological surveys (e.g., The Framingham Study) and major clinical trials have been applied to assess risk and describe the natural history of CVD in all persons at risk for heart disease. Unfortunately, these databases do not represent the overall patient population and have typically included predominantly white males. Clinically naïve extrapolations have extended the findings to all, irrespective of gender, race, or ethnicity. However, current literature would suggest that CVD may indeed vary significantly among populations. Reduction of the burden of heart disease in all persons requires better understanding of CVD in varied populations.

The necessity to focus on these variances has less to do with inclusiveness and more to do with the changing U.S. demographics. The United States is in the midst of a remarkable shift in demographics. Currently, African Americans account for 14 percent of the U.S. population, whereas Hispanic Americans account for 13 percent. Asian Americans and Native Americans make up a smaller cohort of the U.S. population, but together these racial/ethnic or "varied" groups account for approximately 30 percent of the U.S. population. The diversity of the American population is expected to further increase over the next two to three decades. By 2050, the white non-Hispanic population may reach a nadir of 52.5 percent, compared with 75.7 percent in 1990, whereas Hispanic Americans may account for 22.5 percent and African Americans, 15.7 percent. Asian and Pacific Islanders will account for 10.3 percent, and American Indians and Alaska Natives will add 1.1 percent.[1] Thus the epidemiology, pathophysiology, and treatment of heart disease in varied populations will have a major impact on the cardiovascular health of the United States (Fig. 2-1).

DISTRIBUTION OF KNOWN RISK FACTORS FOR HEART DISEASE IN VARIED POPULATIONS

Within the varied populations, the incidence of known risk factors for CVD is alarmingly high. The Third National Health and Nutrition Examination Survey (NHANES III) contains data on the distribution of hypertension among non-Hispanic white, non-Hispanic black, and Hispanic American groups. At least 33 million whites are hypertensive; nearly 6 million African Americans and 1.3 million Hispanic Americans are also affected with hypertension. Crude prevalence rates of hypertension for African Americans are 29.9 percent for men and 27.3 percent for women. For non-Hispanic whites, hypertension affects 25.6 and 23.8 percent, respectively, for men and women, and for Hispanic Americans, 14.6 and 14 percent, respectively, for men and women. The higher prevalence of hypertension in African Americans is also accompanied by a worse disease severity. The prevalence of severe hypertension (>180/110 mm Hg) is 8.5 percent for African Americans and 1 percent for whites. The mean systolic blood pressure (BP) and diastolic BP for all African Americans is 125/75, which compares to 122/74 for all whites. For hypertensive African Americans, the difference in BP versus normotensive African Americans is 30/20 mm Hg, whereas for hypertensive whites the difference in BP is 23/15 mm Hg.[2]

Diabetes is a deadly risk factor for CVD and currently affects 17 million Americans. The incidence of the disease has increased 49 percent in the past decade—this is likely attributable to the alarming incidence of obesity. Among patients 40 to 74 years of age, the prevalence of diabetes is 11.2 percent for whites, 18.2 percent for African Americans, and 20.3 percent for Hispanic Americans. Despite the higher incidence of diabetes in Hispanic Americans, mortality rates due to diabetes are highest in African Americans, 28.4 per 100,000 for men and 39.1 per 100,000 for women. This compares with 23.4 and 25.7 for white men and women, respectively.[3] Hypertension is concomitantly present in 75.4 percent of African Americans with diabetes, 70.7 percent of Hispanic Americans with diabetes, and 64.5 percent of whites affected with diabetes.[4]

Insulin resistance along with obesity, hypertension, and dyslipidemia constitutes key elements of the metabolic syndrome, which is associated with excessive cardiovascular disease. (See also Chap. 43.) Using the National Cholesterol Education Program Adult Treatment Panel III criteria applied to the NHANES III database, the incidence of the metabolic syndrome is 22 percent overall for the U.S. population older than the age of 20 but increases to more than 40 percent in elderly populations[5] and is highest in the varied populations. Hispanic Americans have the highest incidence of the metabolic syndrome, 31.9 percent overall, and 35 percent in Hispanic American women. Of note, despite the high incidence of insulin resistance and the metabolic syndrome, Hispanic Americans have a lower prevalence of hypertension than African Americans. When the influence of obesity, body fat distribution, and insulin concentrations is followed prospectively in whites and Hispanic Americans, each factor associates independently with the development of hypertension, with the greatest risk in subjects with the highest body mass index (BMI) (>30 kg/m^2) and the highest insulin concentration (>95 pmol/liter). However, there does not appear to be an additional CVD risk for Hispanic ethnicity versus whites.[6]

The incidence of obesity, defined by a BMI greater than 25 kg/m^2 as overweight and greater than 30 kg/m^2 as frank obesity, in the U.S. population is alarming and the varied populations are disproportionately affected by this crisis. The prevalence of obesity is anticipated to be 40 percent by 2015.[7] The prevalence of both over-

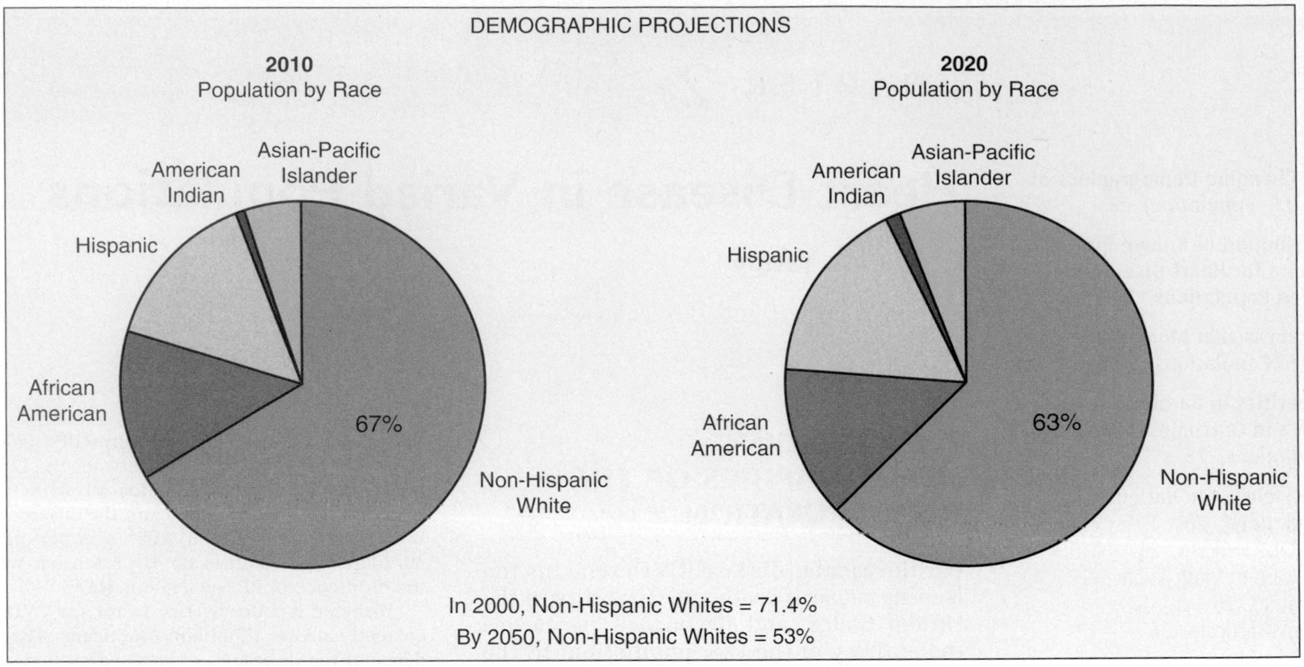

FIGURE 2–1 Changing demographics of the U.S. population. Profile of general demographic characteristics: 2000.

weight and obesity is higher in African Americans than in whites and higher in Hispanic Americans than in whites. The mean BMI for African Americans, Hispanic Americans, and whites is 29.2, 28.6, and 26.3 kg/m^2, respectively. African American women are on average 17 pounds heavier than white women of comparable age and socioeconomic status. Six of the 15 states with the highest prevalence of hypertension are in the southeastern region of the United States (corresponding with the "stroke belt"). The highest prevalence of obesity is in African American women, 44 percent, and in the Southeast, 71 percent of African American women are obese.[7,8]

The International Collaborative Study on Hypertension in Blacks demonstrated an important interaction of BMI and hypertension across the course of the African Diaspora. Seven populations of West African origin were identified. A striking linear relationship was noted between BMI and the percent of the respective population with hypertension varying from less than 15 percent incidence of hypertension in Africans in Nigeria with a mean BMI of less than 24 kg/m^2, to a hypertension incidence of nearly 35 percent in the Chicago area, where the mean BMI was 29 kg/m^2.[9] Overall, 22 percent of the U.S. population is physically inactive but 40 percent of African American women are physically inactive. Data taken from the Coronary Artery Risk Development in Young Adults (CARDIA) study demonstrate that African American women have a higher BMI ($\geq$2.7 kg/m^2), higher energy intake, lower levels of physical activity, and lower overall physical fitness than white women.[10] Thus the influence of obesity and physical inactivity on the development of hypertension and subsequent heart disease in African Americans is great.

Dyslipidemia is an important modifiable risk factor for heart disease in the United States, and correction of lipid disorders results in a decrease in heart disease. Several reports have suggested that African Americans have lower low-density lipoprotein cholesterol concentrations and less hypercholesterolemia. The CARDIA study identified the prevalence of LDL levels in young adults. An LDL cholesterol level greater than 160 mg/dl was seen in 10 percent and 5 percent of young African American men and women, respectively, which compared with 9 percent and 4 percent for young white men and women. High-density lipoprotein levels were higher in African American men than in white men.[10]

In addition to increased energy intake, individuals in varied populations have several important dietary variations that are potentially associated with an increased incidence of cardiovascular disease. These dietary alterations include an increase in sodium consumption, reduced potassium consumption, and decreased calcium intake. The Treatment of Mild Hypertension Study demonstrated dissimilar urinary Na^+ and Na^+/K^+ ratios for African Americans versus whites, especially in lower socioeconomic levels. This difference is related to dietary electrolyte intake, and the higher intake of dietary sodium is linked to the incidence of hypertension.[11] (See also Chaps. 40 and 41.) The required intake of daily sodium is quite low at 20 to 40 mmol sodium per day. Sodium consumption in the United States averages 140 to 150 mmol/day (8 to 10 gm/day) and is highest in African Americans and Hispanic Americans. A direct relationship exists between sodium intake and hypertension, whereas an inverse relationship exists between potassium intake and hypertension.[12] African Americans consume a diet low in potassium. Diets low in potassium are typically associated with concurrent increases in sodium intake, caloric intake, and alcohol consumption and are common in industrialized countries. African Americans also consume a diet low in calcium and perhaps lower in magnesium as well. The intake of calcium and magnesium is associated with lower BPs. The Dietary Approaches to Stop Hypertension (DASH) trial tested the potential benefit of a diet rich in fruits, vegetables, and low-fat dairy products and reduced in saturated and total fats in controls and patients with known hypertension. (See also Chap. 44.) The diet led to an increase in potassium intake from 1700 mg/day to 4100 mg/day and a corresponding drop in sodium intake. The impact of the DASH diet was greatest in those with the highest sodium intake, achieving a 12 mm Hg reduction in BP in African Americans—equivalent to the results expected from pharmacological intervention with a single drug to control BP.[13]

In the setting of hypertension, the rates of left ventricular (LV) hypertrophy as determined by electrocardiography are highest in African Americans, 31 versus 10 percent in whites, and the pattern of hypertrophy as determined by echocardiography is more of the concentric type—a type known to be associated with increased cardiovascular events.[14] These findings have been confirmed using cardiac magnetic resonance imaging. African American men and women have a twofold to threefold higher incidence of LV hypertrophy compared with whites even after controlling for body surface area, fat-free mass, height, systolic BP, and socioeconomic status.[15]

LV mass correlates with systolic BP and with risk of cardiovascular events. The CARDIA study demonstrated a higher incidence of increased LV mass in young adult African Americans and a close relationship among obesity, systolic BP elevation, and LV mass. Smoking rates are generally higher in African Americans and Hispanic Americans and may be increasing in teens and young adults.

Other risk factors for heart disease such as hypertriglyceridemia, hyperuricemia, microalbuminuria, and elevated tissue plasminogen activator inhibitor-1 levels may demonstrate subtle differences in these varied populations, but adequate data are not available to make definitive comment.

CARDIOVASCULAR MORTALITY IN VARIED POPULATIONS

Heart disease is the leading cause of death for all segments of the U.S. population including the varied population. Of these groups, African Americans experience the highest rates of mortality from heart disease. The mortality rate for African Americans is 1.6 times that of whites—a ratio that is identical to the black/white mortality ratio in 1950.[16] Hispanic Americans are twice as likely as all others to die from diabetes, and Native Americans die disproportionately from diabetes as well. The average annual death rate due to heart disease expressed as deaths per 100,000 in the 45 to 64 age range is 404 for African Americans, 219 for whites, 188 for Native Americans, 143 for Hispanic Americans, and 90 for Asian/Pacific Islanders. For the 65 to 74 age range, the corresponding numbers are 1278 for African Americans, 871 for whites, 650 for Native Americans, 614 for Hispanic Americans, and 443 for Asian/Pacific Islanders. In women, cardiovascular disease is the leading cause of death, affecting 41 percent of white women, 41 percent of African American women, 33 percent of Hispanic American women, and 37 percent of Asian American women.[17,18]

The prevalence of coronary heart disease is higher in African Americans, with a prevalence of 7.1 and 9 percent, respectively, for men and women, compared with 6.9 and 5.4 percent for white men and women. Death rates due to CHD are 272 and 193 for African American men and women compared with 249 and 153 for white men and women.[17,18] In fact, death rates due to CHD in African Americans are the highest in the world.[19] Death rates from stroke are also higher in African Americans. Compared with whites, young African Americans have a threefold increased risk of ischemic stroke and a fourfold higher increase in the risk of stroke death. The death rate due to stroke is highest in the Southeastern United States.[17] In addition, the five states with the highest death rates due to congestive heart failure are also in the Southeastern United States and of the 15 states with the highest rates of end-stage renal disease (ESRD), 10 are in the Southeast.[8]

The prevalence of coronary heart disease in Mexican Americans is 7.2 and 6.8 percent for men and women, respectively. The prevalence of myocardial infarction (MI) is 4.1 and 1.9 percent, respectively, for Mexican American men and women, which compares with 5.2 and 2 percent for white men and women, respectively, and 4.3 and 3.3 percent for African American men and women, respectively, experiencing a MI. Death rates are similar for Hispanic Americans and whites.[17]

DISPARITIES IN CARDIOVASCULAR CARE AND OUTCOMES IN VARIED POPULATIONS

The foregoing information clearly establishes important population differences regarding risk and outcomes for cardiovascular disease. The complete explanation for these differential outcomes is lacking but likely reflects a complex interplay of social, political, physiological, and genetic variances in these populations. These differences are best captured by an evaluation of the *disparities* in racial and ethnic health care. Disparities in health care refer to differences in the quality of health care that are not due to access-related factors or clinical needs, preferences (i.e., patient choices), or appropriateness of the intervention (Fig. 2-2).[20] Disparities may emanate from decisions made by the patient, provider, or health care system and may reflect language barriers, cultural insensitivities, or bias.

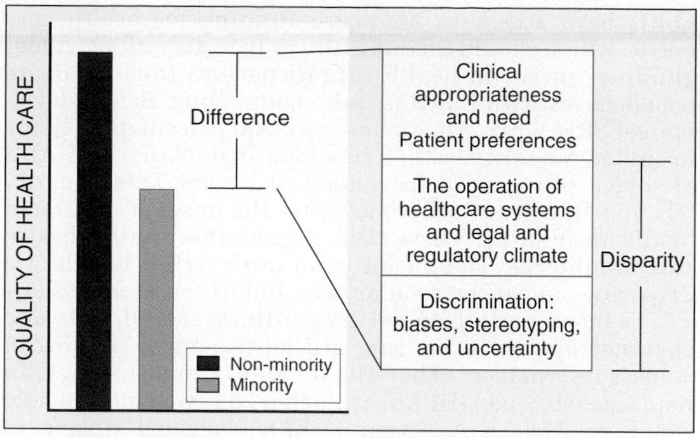

FIGURE 2–2 Differences, disparities, and discrimination: Populations with equal access to health care. Disparities are racial or ethnic differences in health care that are not due to access-related factors, clinical needs, patient preferences, or the appropriateness of the intervention. *(From Gomes C, McGuire TG.* In *Smedley BD, Stith AY, Nelson AR (eds): Unequal Treatment. Washington, DC, Institute of Medicine, 2003.)*

Minorities refuse coronary artery bypass surgery at a higher rate than others but not sufficiently so to account for major differences in outcomes.[21] Greater issues are pertinent at the level of the health care delivery system. Language barriers are important obstacles for many patients. Nearly 14 million Americans are not proficient in English, and 1 in 5 Spanish-speaking persons report that they do not seek health care due to language issues. Nearly 8 million Hispanic Americans do not speak English well. One in 20 Native Americans do not speak English well, and among Asian Americans the language barrier varies from 1 percent in persons of Hawaiian origin to 15 percent for Japanese origin to 55 percent for Cambodian origin.[22] In addition to language barriers, lack of health insurance and geographical isolation both contribute further to disparities.

Providers may contribute to disparities in health care, as well as through subconscious stereotyping, clinical uncertainty due to cultural ignorance, and delay in referral for indicated procedures. Physicians exhibit lesser rates of referrals for cardiac catheterization in African American women compared with white men or women and African American men despite similar articulation of symptoms and reasonable indications for further evaluation.[23]

Because of the interdigitation of these patient, system, and provider issues, ethnic Americans undergo cardiovascular procedures at a lower rate. A survey of 4 million patients with acute MI as indexed in the National Hospital Discharge Survey revealed that African American men and women undergo coronary angiography and coronary artery bypass surgery at much lower rates.[24] A separate Medicare survey suggested that the rate of coronary artery bypass grafting (CABG) was fourfold different between whites and African Americans even after adjusting for age and gender. These differences were most striking in the Southeastern United States.[24] An analysis of Hispanic Americans and whites with a diagnosis of MI revealed that Hispanic Americans were discharged on 38 percent *fewer* medications. Similarly, they were less likely to receive percutaneous coronary interventions.[25] Studies done at Veterans Affair hospitals are quite intriguing because these facilities theoretically have removed any access to care issues. Yet referral for cardiac procedures was higher for whites. Of note, African Americans refused invasive procedures twice as often. Differences in rates of thrombolytic therapy use and CABG were also observed, with African Americans much less likely to receive either strategy.[26] Patients with

ESRD have access to Medicare funding for health care needs, which should theoretically reduce disparities. A longitudinal survey of health care disparities from Medicare beneficiaries with ESRD is quite compelling. Before developing ESRD, white Americans were 300 percent more likely to undergo cardiac catheterization, angioplasty, or CABG after controlling for socioeconomic variables. This disparity fell to a 40 percent difference after the onset of ESRD and Medicare funding. These data suggest that similar health care funding may significantly diminish certain health care disparities in cardiovascular care, but differences persist.

The disproportionate risk for cardiovascular disease and apparent disparities in care are most evident in African American women. The Heart and Estrogen/progestin Replacement Study (HERS) evaluated 2699 women, of whom 218 were African American. HERS evaluated women in a longitudinal study over 4 years to determine the health risks/benefits of hormone replacement therapy. Despite twofold higher cardiovascular event rates, African American women had worse control of hypertension and LDL cholesterol and lesser use of aspirin and statins.[27]

HYPERTENSION IN VARIED POPULATIONS

The excessive cardiovascular risk due to the consequences of hypertension applies especially to the varied populations (Fig. 2-3).

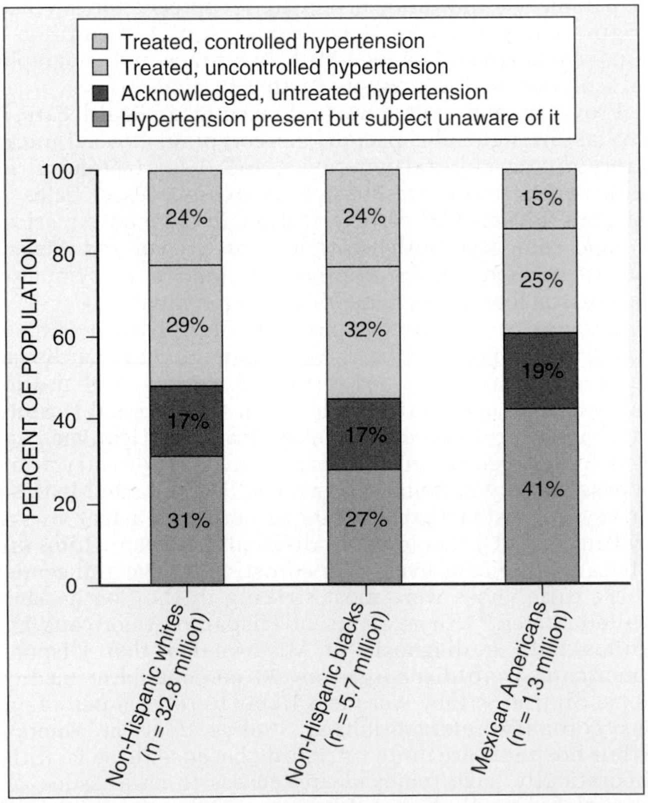

FIGURE 2–3 Extent of awareness, treatment, and control of hypertension among non-Hispanic whites, non-Hispanic blacks, and Mexican Americans with hypertension in the Third National Health and Nutrition Examination Survey. Sample sizes for other racial and ethnic groups were too small to analyze separately. Percentages may not sum to 100 because of rounding.

Hispanic Americans

A paradox exists in Hispanic Americans. Despite a higher incidence of diabetes and obesity, the prevalence of hypertension in Hispanic Americans is *lower* than that in the general population. Hypertension among Hispanic Americans varies by gender and by the country of origin. Puerto Rican origin is associated with the highest incidence of hypertension, followed by Cuban origin and Mexican origin. When Hispanic Americans of Mexican origin do have hypertension, control of BP can be more difficult.[28] The lower incidence of hypertension in Hispanic Americans of Mexican origin versus other Hispanic Americans is postulated to be due to a modernization phenomenon implicating acclimatization to a Western lifestyle as a factor in the development of hypertension. In Puerto Rico, urban men with a high school education have a BP 8 mm Hg higher than less educated men. This is not the same experience seen in other North American ethnic groups, in whom education associates with lower BP. For persons younger than 45, the prevalence of hypertension is twice the rate seen in the mainland United States. Death rates due to heart disease have increased by 72 percent over the past three decades while otherwise falling in the remainder of the United States. The incidence of ESRD is higher in Puerto Rico than in any other region of Latin America.[29]

Americans of South Asian Descent

Americans with ancestry from the Indian subcontinent have a major health problem with hypertension. Hypertension is a significant concern in the Indian subcontinent and is an important cardiovascular risk for South Asians worldwide. The World Health Organization has reported that Indian men in the age range of 40 to 55 have the highest BP among 20 other developing countries. The prevalence of hypertension in Indian countries has increased from less than 2 percent in 1950 to nearly 20 percent currently. This increased risk is further exacerbated with emigration to North America and varies directly with the degree of urbanization. The Study of Health Assessment and Risk in Ethnic Groups done in Canada reported that South Asians had the highest self-reported incidence of hypertension.[30] Coincident with the hypertension risk is a growing risk of diabetes, dyslipidemia (perhaps related to a genetic predisposition to a low HDL level), and obesity. Tobacco consumption is likewise increasing in South Asians, and per capita fat consumption has increased. The confluence of these risk factors not only contributes to the alarming rate of hypertension but also to the increasing rate of symptomatic coronary artery disease (CAD).[31]

African Americans

Hypertension in African Americans represents the most prolific variance in heart disease and CVD risk factors in the varied populations. African Americans experience the highest prevalence of hypertension, perhaps in the world, with nearly 35 percent of them affected by hypertension.[32] Some 5.6 million African Americans have hypertension—a number that eclipses the *total number* of persons affected with congestive heart failure. The Hypertension and Detection Follow-up Program found that severe hypertension (diastolic BP > 115 mm Hg) was 5 to 7 times more likely to be present in African Americans than white Americans.[32] The differential experience of hypertension is evident in childhood with higher recorded BPs noted before the age of *10* in black versus white children.[33] Hypertension in African Americans has serious consequences with a 50 percent higher frequency of heart failure,[34] sixfold higher incidence of developing ESRD due to hypertension,[32] a 38 percent higher risk of stroke, and a higher risk of death due to stroke.[18] Overall, mortality due to hypertension and its consequences is four to five times more likely in African Americans compared with whites.[32]

Hypertensive heart disease promotes LV hypertrophy, a risk factor for sudden death and coronary events. The Coronary Artery Risk Development in Young Adults (CARDIA) study demonstrated that LV mass is higher and independently correlated with systolic BP in young African American males.[32,35] The Veterans Affairs Cooperative Monotherapy Hypertension Trial found LV hypertrophy diagnosed by ECG criteria in 31 percent of African American hypertensives compared with 10 percent of white hypertensives.[36] Increased LV mass associates with an increased rate of death and thus contributes to the excess rate of morbidity and mortality due to CVD seen in African Americans. CAD is the leading cause of heart failure in whites, but pooled data from published clinical trials suggest that hypertension may be the leading imputed cause of heart failure in blacks.[34]

Variances in the pathophysiology of stroke may also pertain. African Americans typically have more occlusive disease in the large- and medium-sized intracranial arteries, whereas whites typically have more occlusive disease in the extracranial arteries. African Americans also have a higher incidence of hemorrhagic stroke. Similar observations have been made in the setting of ESRD. Hypertensive nephrosclerosis is the leading cause of ESRD for African Americans, and they disproportionately populate the hemodialysis cohort. For African Americans aged 20 to 44, hypertension-related ESRD is *20-fold* higher than in whites. African Americans have been noted to lack the nocturnal dip in BP and to have an earlier onset of proteinuria. Both of these observations associate with a higher incidence of hypertension-induced nephrosclerosis.[37]

Several mechanisms may contribute to the excess burden of hypertension in African Americans. Peripheral vascular resistance may be higher in some African Americans with hypertension. Small studies have also demonstrated that vasodilatory responses are blunted in African Americans in a manner suggesting subtle differences in nitric oxide homeostasis.[38] Plasma renin activity is lower in age-matched African American versus white hypertensives,[39] urinary kallikrein excretion is lower, and insulin levels are higher in African Americans.[34]

Much has been written about salt sensitivity in African Americans including a theoretical assertion that genetic pressure, during the African Diaspora (active slave trading from West Africa to North America), led to selective expression favoring genes that promote salt retention that now predispose to hypertension. This is an unproven but nevertheless prevalent theory.[40,41] Rates of hypertension in rural West Africa are the lowest in the world, but populations of West African origin in the Caribbean and in North America demonstrate dramatic rises in BP that are linearly related to increases in BMI (Fig. 2-4).[41] Some African Americans do appear to be more salt sensitive than others, and salt restriction leads to a greater reduction in systolic BP in African Americans (≈12 mm Hg) than in whites.[42] A genetic basis for sodium sensitivity may exist. The epithelial sodium channel is responsible for the final reabsorption of filtered sodium from the distal nephron and has now been found to have at least eight single nucleotide polymorphisms. (See also Chap. 40.) One of these polymorphisms (T594M) is found only in people of West African descent and is four times more likely in African American hypertensives than in normotensive African Americans.[43] Unfortunately, variations in a single gene likely account for only 2 to 4 percent of the difference in hypertension seen between races.[41] Yet another attractive candidate polymorphism related to the excess risk of hypertension-related cardiovascular disease in African Americans is noted within the inflammatory cytokines. Transforming growth factor beta-1 (TGFβ-1) stimulates fibrosis, extracellular matrix turnover, glomerular hyperplasia, and LV hypertrophy. TGFβ-1 is overexpressed in African Americans with higher circulating levels noted. A described polymorphism at codon 25 of the TGFβ-1 gene that involves the substitution of arginine for proline is associated with higher TGFβ-1 levels and is seen more frequently in African Americans.[44] ACE inhibitors and angiotensin-receptor blockers (ARBs) both reduce angiotensin II–mediated stimulation of TGFβ-1, and this may be of clinical importance in the treatment of hypertension in African Americans. Beta blockers are reportedly less effective as monotherapy for hypertension in African Americans,[45] but data exist that suggest a strong correlation between visceral obesity in African American women and exaggerated sympathetic nervous system activity.[46]

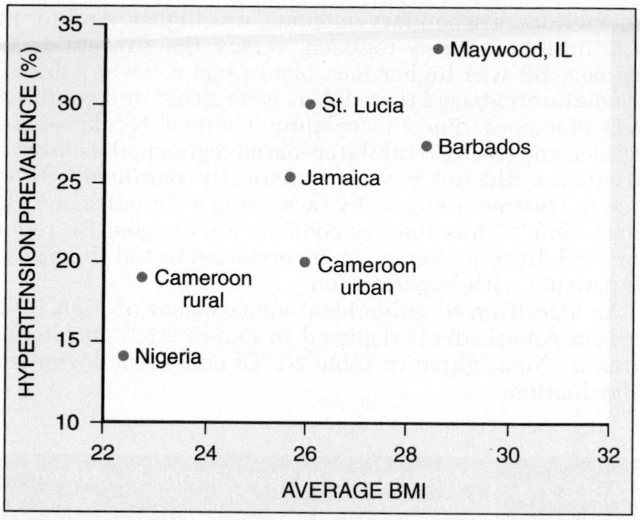

FIGURE 2–4 Hypertension prevalence among the African Diaspora. Body mass index (BMI) measures a person's weight-to-height ratio; a BMI higher than 25 is generally considered a sign of being overweight. In the authors' study of people of African descent, a low average BMI in a population corresponded to a low rate of hypertension in that community. As average BMI increased, so did the prevalence of hypertension. The findings support the view that obesity contributes to high blood pressure. *(From Cooper R, Rotimi C, Ataman S: The prevalence of hypertension in seven populations of West African origin. Am J Public Health 87:160, 1997.)*

Therapy of Hypertension in African Americans (see also Chap. 41)

The therapy of hypertension for all persons should focus clearly on goal BP reduction and the prevention of CVD related to hypertension. The treatment of hypertension is similar for all demographic groups and should follow published guideline-based recommendations for optimal care.[45] Within the African American group the responsiveness to monotherapy with ACE inhibitors, ARBs, and beta blockers may be less compared with diuretics and calcium channel blockers, but these differences are corrected when diuretics are added to the neurohormonal antagonists. The African American Study of Kidney Disease and Hypertension prospectively addressed the impact of three antihypertensive drug classes on glomerular filtration rate decline in hypertension. Diabetic patients were excluded. In patients with established hypertension-induced nephrosclerosis and reduced GFR (20 to 60 ml/min per 1.73 m^2), a clinical composite that included a 50 percent reduction in GFR, ESRD, or death was most favorably decreased by an ACE inhibitor compared with either a beta blocker or calcium channel blocker. This study noted that African American patients with hypertension uniformly required a multidrug regimen to achieve adequate BP control.[47]

The Antihypertensive and Lipid Lowering Trial to Prevent Heart Attack (ALLHAT) was a large 33,357-patient trial that tested the ability of a calcium channel blocker–based and ACE inhibitor–based antihypertensive regimen to lower cardiovascular morbidity and mortality compared with a diuretic-based regimen. Thirty-five percent or 11,674 were African American. All patients had at least one other cardiovascular risk factor in addition to hypertension. The primary outcome was an aggregate of fatal coronary heart disease or nonfatal MI. Secondary outcomes included all-cause mortality; stroke; combined cardiovascular disease (including CHD death, nonfatal MI, stroke, angina, coronary revascularization, heart failure, and peripheral vascular disease); and ESRD. No difference as a function of race existed between the treatment groups on the primary outcome. For the calcium channel blocker–based regimen compared with the diuretic-based regimen, the incidence of heart failure, a secondary outcome, was higher. And for the ACE inhibitor–based regimen versus the diuretic-based regimen, BP was higher (i.e., blacks had a lower achieved BP on diuretic-based therapy), as were stroke and combined CVD outcomes. For the calcium channel blocker–based regimen and the ACE inhibitor–based regimen, the observed differences did not yield a statistically significant difference in treatment effects by race using a statistical test for interaction.[48] Thus the key consideration is goal BP reduction, and diuretic therapy is the preferred initial therapy for *all* patients with hypertension.

An algorithm to guide ideal management of high BP in African Americans is depicted in Figure 2-5,[49] and its features are highlighted in Table 2-1. Of note is the lower goal BP reduction.

TABLE 2–1 Management of Hypertension in African Americans
Increase dietary potassium intake
Limit dietary sodium intake to <2.4 gm/day
Increase physical activity
Weight loss
All antihypertensive medications and combinations are effective
Multiple drug combinations may be required to achieve control
Angiotensin-converting enzyme (ACE) inhibitors and beta blockers as monotherapy may be less effective but should be used when indicated (e.g., renal disease, heart failure, post-myocardial infarction)
Thiazide diuretics and calcium channel blockers may have greater blood pressure–lowering efficacy
A higher incidence of angioedema occurs when using ACE inhibitors

From Douglas JG, Bakris GL, Epstien M, et al: Management of high blood pressure in African Americans; Consensus statement of the Hypertension in African Americans Working Group of the International Society of Hypertension in Blacks. Arch Intern Med 163:525, 2003.

ISCHEMIC HEART DISEASE IN VARIED POPULATIONS (see also Chaps. 51, 53, and 54)

All of the varied populations are experiencing increasing rates of ischemic heart disease related to the concurrent and oftentimes disproportionate presence of risk factors for CAD. Rates for CAD are increasing in Asian Americans, Hispanic Americans, Native Americans, and Americans of South Asian origin. Importantly, the rates of CAD in these groups are approaching but do not exceed those seen in whites. This is, however, not the case for African Americans (Fig. 2-6).

African Americans have the highest overall mortality rate due to coronary artery disease of any ethnic group in the United States. The risk for sudden cardiac death is higher, and the onset of disease occurs approximately 5 years earlier. The usual presentation is more likely to be unstable angina or a non-ST elevation infarct rather than a typical ST-elevation event.[50] Despite this increased incidence of disease, the presence of obstructive epicardial CAD on angiography is less. Not infrequently, angiographic studies show normal epicardial vessels. Yet autopsy studies have demonstrated a greater extent of atherosclerosis in African Americans despite a lesser degree of obstructive CAD.[51] As described earlier, interventions with thrombolytic therapy, percutaneous coronary interventions, and coronary artery bypass surgery are all less frequently administered.

The rationale for the excess prevalence of CAD in African Americans is less likely related to pathophysiological variances, as suggested in the discussion on hypertension, and more likely due to the overabundance of cardiovascular risk factors. Obesity, LV hypertrophy, type II diabetes, and physical activity are all more common in African Americans. Total cholesterol levels may be less in African Americans, and HDL levels higher. Lipoprotein(a) levels are twofold to threefold higher in African Americans, but the relationship of Lp(a) to coronary events remains unclear and may vary according to ethnicity. The relationship between total cholesterol, plaque formation, and coronary events may be weaker in African Americans compared with whites.[52]

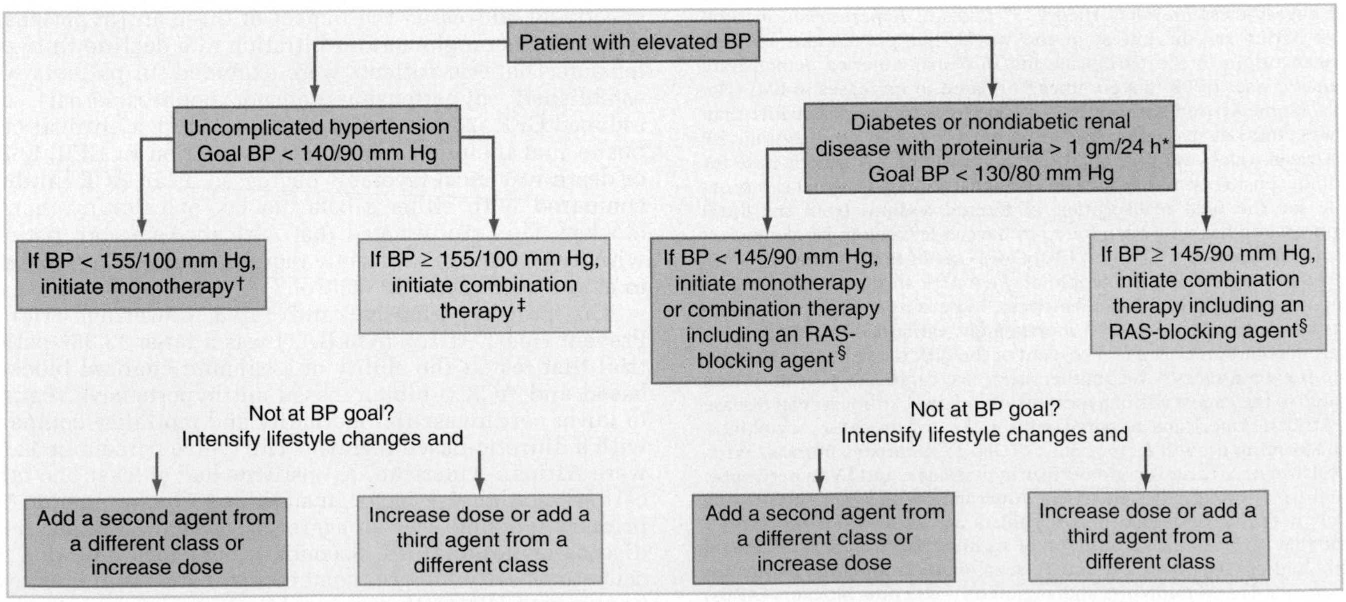

FIGURE 2–5 Algorithm for managing high blood pressure in African Americans. *Preferable blood pressure (BP) goal for patients with renal disease with proteinuria greater than 1 gm/24 hr is less than 125/75 mm Hg. †Initiate monotherapy at the recommended starting dose with an agent from any of the following classes: diuretics, beta blockers, calcium channel blockers (CCBs), angiotensin-converting enzyme (ACE) inhibitors, or angiotensin-receptor blockers (ARBs). ‡To achieve BP goals more expeditiously, initiate low-dose combination therapy with any of the following combinations: beta blocker/diuretic, ACE inhibitor/diuretic, ACE inhibitor/CCB, or ARB/diuretic. §Consider specific clinical indications when selecting agents. *(From Douglas JG, Bakris GL, Epstein M, et al: Management of high blood pressure in African Americans. Arch Intern Med 163:525, 2003.)*

Population Group	Prevalence CHD	Prevalence MI	Incidence CHD	Incidence MI	Mortality CHD	Mortality MI
Total population	12,900,000	7,600,000	1,100,000	540,000	515,204	192,898
Total males	6,300,000	4,700,000	660,000	330,000	260,574	100,306
Total females	6,600,000	2,900,000	440,000	210,000	254,630	92,585
White males	6.9%	5.2%	—	—	230,951	89,383
White females	5.4%	2.0%	—	—	224,449	81,201
Black males	7.1%	4.3%	68,200	—	24,625	9,045
Black females	9.0%	3.3%	47,700	—	26,640	10,067
Mexican-American males	7.2%	4.1%	—	—	—	—
Mexican-American females	6.8%	1.9%	—	—	—	—

FIGURE 2–6 Coronary heart disease and angina pectoris. CHD = coronary heart disease; includes heart attack, angina pectoris (chest pain), or both; MI = myocardial infarction (heart attack). Prevalence: NHANES III (1988-1994), CDC/NCHS; data for white and black males and females are for non-Hispanics. Total population data are for Americans age 20 and older; percentages for racial/ethnic groups are age adjusted for age 20 and older. Incidence: ARIC (1987-1994), NHLBI. Mortality: CDC/NCHS; data for white and black males and females include Hispanics.

The excess prevalence of LV hypertrophy likely confounds the ischemic burden in the setting of CAD and may relate to excess mortality and sudden death. Mechanisms to support this theory are not yet clear. The increase in LV mass with a disproportionately less robust vascular supply may lead to a lower threshold for arrhythmias and more damage due to ischemic events.[50] Higher levels of the potent vasoconstrictor endothelin-1 have been demonstrated in African Americans.[53] Endothelin is stimulated by TGFβ-1, which is higher in hypertensive African Americans. The confluence of LV hypertrophy and endothelial dysfunction may contribute to a greater risk of ischemia-related injury.

Importantly, there are no described differences in the presentation of acute coronary syndromes for any ethnic group, nor any described variations in responses to standard medical and revascularization strategies. As such, no differences should be contemplated in the management of varied populations presenting with symptomatic CAD. The greater concern, however, regards disparate health care for African Americans who present with acute coronary syndromes. The preponderance of data confirms a lower utilization of evidence-based therapies, less frequent use of immediate percutaneous coronary interventions, and lower application of surgical revascularization despite similar disease presentations.[24-26] Overcoming these disparities is now a target for major quality initiatives.

HEART FAILURE IN VARIED POPULATIONS (see also Chaps. 25 and 26)

Heart failure has become one of the most pervasive cardiovascular illnesses in the United States. The prevalence of heart failure is increasing, as is the burden of excess mortality and morbidity—a burden that is once again borne disproportionately by varied populations. Although data for most ethnic groups are lacking in the realm of heart failure, data regarding African Americans are quite compelling and controversial.

Heart failure occurs in African Americans at an increased frequency, perhaps 50 percent higher overall and greater than 100 percent higher in African American women compared with whites. Several differences in the natural history are striking. The disease occurs at an earlier age; there is usually more profound LV systolic dysfunction at the time of onset; and the clinical class is usually more advanced.[34] The overall incidence of heart failure within the U.S. population is 2 percent, but it occurs in 3 percent of the African American population. The issues regarding excess mortality and morbidity in African Americans with heart failure remain unresolved. The original data from the Studies of Left Ventricular Dysfunction (SOLVD) suggested a higher mortality rate,[54] but a reanalysis of African American and white cohorts matched for disease severity and LV dysfunction demonstrated only an excess rate of hospitalization.[55] Data from the SOLVD prevention trial clearly demonstrated a higher incident rate of heart failure, which is consistent with epidemiological surveys, but a similar responsiveness to ACE inhibitors.[56]

On the basis of the foregoing discussion, it is not surprising that the leading putative cause of LV dysfunction in African Americans with heart failure is hypertension. A survey of published clinical trials and registries suggests that the incidence of hypertension as the likely cause of heart failure in this population varies from approximately 30 percent to nearly 60 percent (Fig. 2-7).[34] True cause and effect is lacking because little, if any, mechanistic data support the conversion from hypertensive heart disease to systolic dysfunction. Data from spontaneously hypertensive salt-sensitive animals suggest that the conversion from LV hypertrophy to overt heart failure (with systolic dysfunction) is associated with an increase in the precursors of endothelin.[57] Although data do exist from the Systolic Hypertension in the Elderly Trial (SHEP) to justify therapy of hypertension as an effective means of preventing heart failure, these data are most pertinent for systolic hypertension of the elderly (SHEP included 14 percent African Americans).[58] The ALLHAT experience described earlier also suggests that certain antihypertensive regimens are associated with a lower incidence of heart failure in higher-risk hypertensives.[48] Whether such a regimen retards the development of systolic dysfunction is uncertain. Thus neither SHEP nor ALLHAT provides insight into whether or not treatment of hypertension sufficient to retard the development of heart failure does so by preserving systolic function, diastolic function, or both.

A genomic basis to explain the differential epidemiology and natural history of heart failure in African Americans remains under active investigation. Several candidate polymorphisms have emerged as plausible culprit genetic variations, but the relationship of these genes to the environment and the complex interplay of multiple

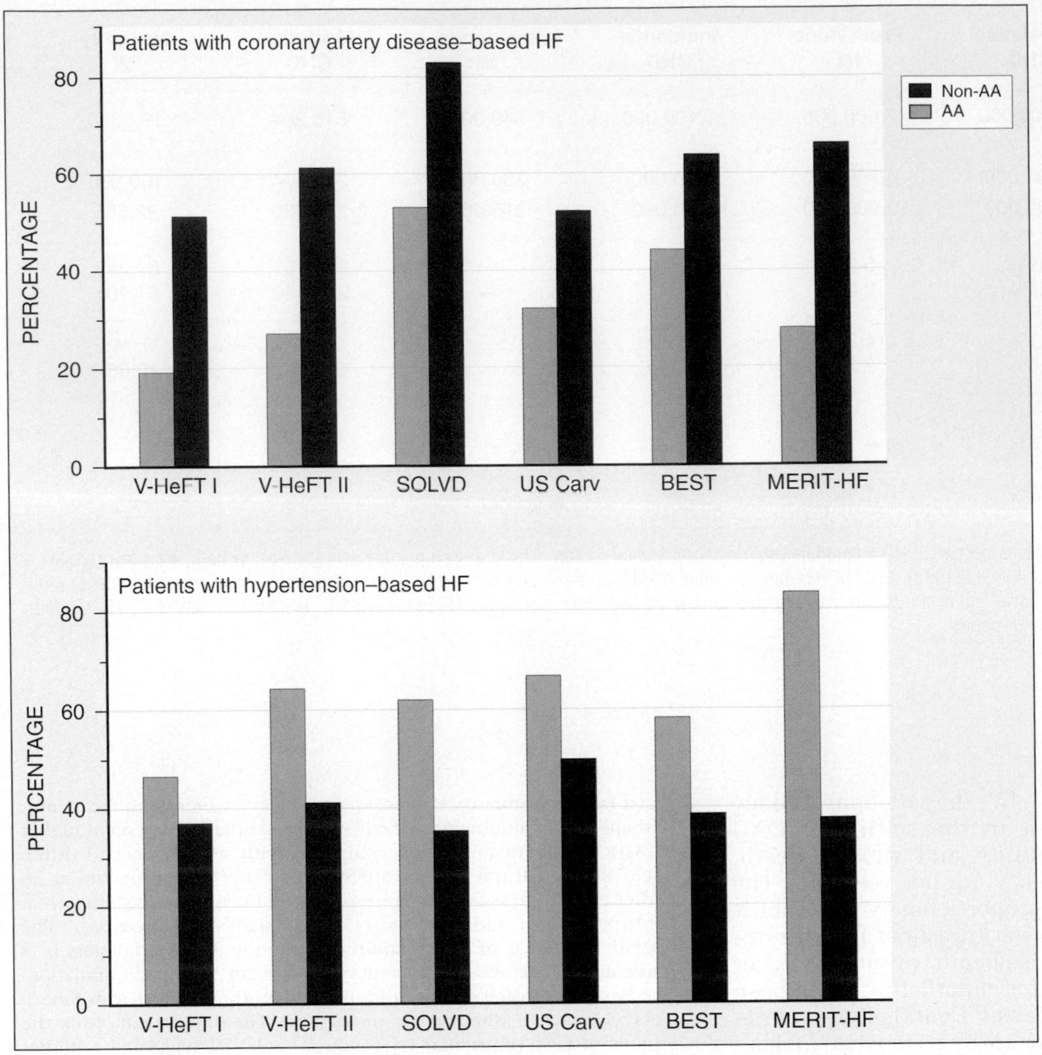

FIGURE 2–7 Etiology of heart failure (HF) in African Americans (AA). (See text and Table 2-3 for abbreviations.) *(Adapted from the BEST Investigators: N Engl J Med 344:1659, 2001; Packer M et al: N Engl J Med 334:1349, 1996; MERIT-HF Study Group: Lancet 353:2001, 1999; Cohn JN et al: N Engl J Med 314:1547, 1986; Cohn JN et al: N Engl J Med 325:303, 1991; The SOLVD Investigators: N Engl J Med 325:293, 1991.)*

physiological systems makes these discussions largely theoretical until additional data from large cohorts of the population are evaluated (Table 2-2).

The majority of the data regarding the response to medical therapy for heart failure affecting African Americans emanate from post hoc analyses of the African American subgroups in major clinical trials in heart failure. These analyses are all compromised by the retrospective nature of the analysis, inconsistent sample sizes of African Americans, and differences in disease expression between the African American and white cohorts. As such, the analyses yield provocative inferences and generate new hypotheses but do not alter current evidence-based guideline recommendations (Table 2-3).[59] In the 2005 ACC/AHA Diagnosis and Management of Chronic Heart Failure in the Adult guidelines, a class I recommendation is given to the following statement: "Groups of patients including (a) high-risk ethnic minority groups (e.g., blacks), (b) groups under-represented in clinical trials, and (c) any groups believed to be underserved should, in the absence of specific evidence to direct otherwise, have clinical screening and therapy in a manner identical to that applied to the broader population. (Level of evidence: B)."[59]

Taken in aggregate, the data from Table 2-3 demonstrate that all approved therapeutic strategies for heart failure are effective and yield improved outcomes. As stated in the guidelines, there should be no reluctance to treat African Americans with heart failure using any of the current treatment modalities. Of note, however, is that data regarding beta-blocker efficacy are inconsistent and potentially confusing. The analysis from the Beta Blocker Evaluation of Survival Trial (BEST) was interpreted to mean that African American patients responded less well to beta-blocker therapy and may have failed to benefit.[67] Given the presence of intrinsic sympathomimetic activity in bucindolol, the agent in BEST, it is more likely that these results are drug specific and not class specific. The number of African Americans exposed to extended-release metoprolol in clinical trials has been insignificant, and subgroup analysis has been unrewarding.[68] However, the experience with carvedilol given in combination with ACE inhibitors to African Americans (U.S. Carvedilol Heart Failure Trials) with all classes of heart failure are quite encouraging and are consistent with salutary outcomes. These data represent the strongest basis for recommended use of ACE inhibitors and beta blockers as primary therapy for heart failure in African Americans, as in all others.[69]

The African American Heart Failure Trial, A-HeFT, recently extended the treatment options for African Americans with heart failure to include the use of combined vasodilator therapy with isosorbide dinitrate and hydralazine. On the basis of a retrospective post hoc analysis of the original Vasodilator in Heart Failure Trials (V-HeFT I & II),[66] a signal of unique responsiveness to combined vasodilator therapy was observed. This signal of efficacy was subsequently studied prospectively in 1040 African Americans with class III heart failure due to systolic dysfunction who were already on evidence-based therapies including ACE/ARB and beta blockers. The study was stopped early due to evidence of significant survival benefit attributed to combined vasodilator therapy. The reduction in mortality was 43 percent, time to first hospitalization was reduced by 39 percent, and quality of life measures were similarly improved (Fig. 2-8).[70,71] Both the American College of Cardiology/American Heart Association and the Heart Failure Society of America guideline statements now strongly recommend the adjunctive use of combined vasodilator therapy in addition to ACE/ARB and beta blockers for African Americans with symptomatic heart failure.[59,72] The imputed but unproven mechanism of benefit targets nitric oxide deficiency and oxidative stress, which have been shown to be abnormal in African Americans[73] but, importantly, not unique to African Americans (Fig. 2-9). A prospective substudy within A-HeFT addressed the corresponding genetic profiles of the patients within A-HeFT and the responsiveness to combined vaso-

TABLE 2–2 Putative Genetic Markers of Cardiovascular Risk in African Americans

Genetic Polymorphism	Clinical Implications
Beta$_1$ adrenergic receptor; Gly-389	Subsensitive beta$_1$ receptor; decreased affinity for agonist and less cAMP generation
Beta$_1$ adrenergic receptor; ARG-389/alpha 2C Del322-325 receptor	Presence of both polymorphisms is associated with increased risk for heart failure in blacks; RR 10.11 when both are present
NOS-3-Glu298Glu	Subsensitive nitric oxide system; ? associated with better responsiveness to ISDN/HYD
Aldosterone synthase [CYP11B2-344-TT allele]	? Excessive fibrosis; associated with better responsiveness to ISDN/HYD
Transforming growth factor beta$_1$, codon 25	40% higher transforming growth factor beta$_1$ levels; higher endothelin levels?; more fibrosis
G Protein 825-T Allele	Marker of low renin hypertension, left ventricular hypertrophy, and stroke

See references 60-65.
ISDN/HYD = isosorbide dinitrate/hydralazine.

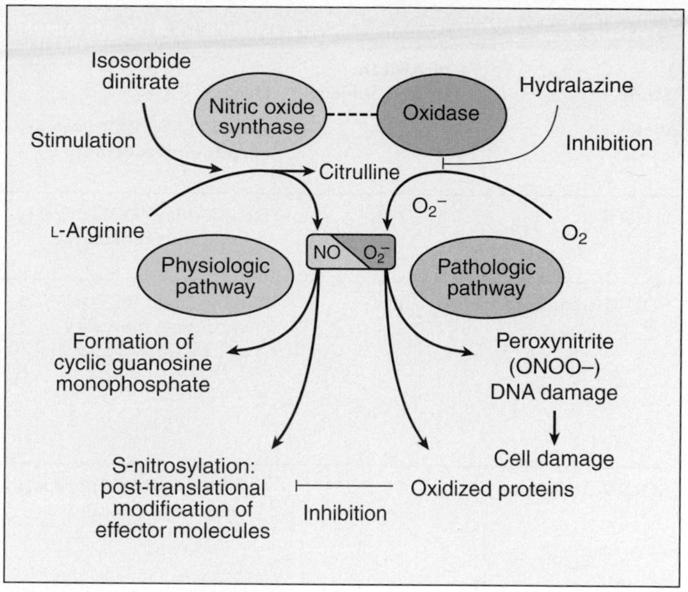

FIGURE 2–9 Consequences of nitric oxide and superoxide balance disruption in heart failure patients.

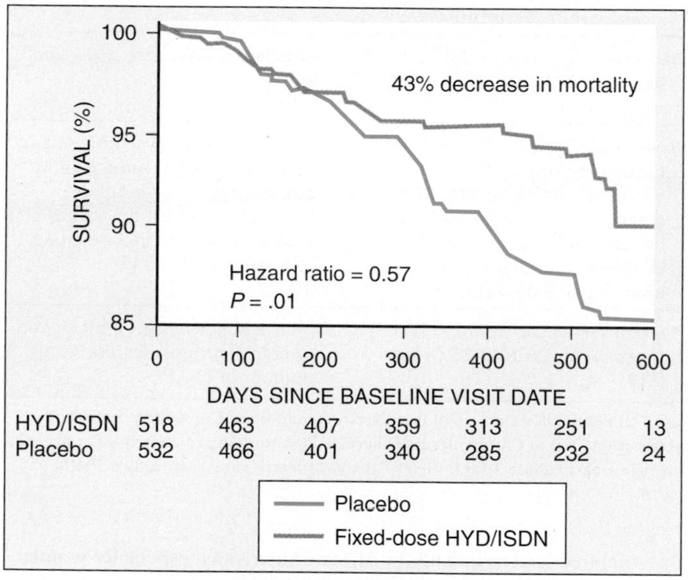

FIGURE 2–8 Overall survival results from the African American Heart Failure Trial.

dilator therapy. Preliminary data outputs implicate potentially important variances in nitric oxide synthase and aldosterone synthase.[65] Confirmation of these results may allow for application of the benefits of combined vasodilator therapy to all appropriate patients irrespective of race and lead to one of the early clinical applications of pharmacogenomics or "personalized medicine."[74]

THE CONSTRUCT OF RACE IN MEDICINE

The inclusion of race or ethnicity in any discussion of medicine is problematic. Race is neither scientific nor physiological. The heterogeneity within race is similar to the heterogeneity among races,[67] and the very requirements for the perpetuation of race (i.e., intermarriage and similar environmental surroundings) are rapidly disappearing in the United States. Even the genomic debates are overshadowed by the observation that all persons share greater than 99 percent of the same genetic code and the variance among races is in approximately 0.1 percent of the code. Whether this one tenth of a percent matters is the crux of many genomic investigations.

The inclusion of race in medicine need always respect the limitations and variability of race-specific data. Race is usually a self-designation, and not all individuals can be easily classified. Some may actually acknowledge more than one racial designation. Race is less likely to be a "risk factor" and much more likely to be a "risk marker" (i.e., a *placeholder* for more pertinent risks). Race provides a clustering of events that occur because of similar environmental factors and physiological variables (e.g., obesity and hypertension) that may affect a given population differentially and not because of race per se. The continued elucidation of nuances in cardiovascular disease as a function of varied populations and the discovery of new pathophysiological considerations is appropriate, but any discussions of race in medicine must rigorously avoid polarization and further perpetuation of disparate health care.[68]

SUMMARY AND CLINICAL MESSAGES

1. The demographic of the U.S. population is changing. Varied populations (e.g., African Americans, Asian Americans, Hispanic Americans, and Native Americans) now make up 30 percent of the population but will soon constitute 50 percent of the U.S. population.
2. Cardiovascular disease affects the varied populations in a striking way. African Americans have the highest mortality rate due to CVD.
3. Risk factors are especially prevalent in the varied populations: African Americans are at risk due to hypertension, obesity, and physical inactivity; Hispanic Americans are at risk due to obesity and diabetes; and emigrant Asian Americans, especially of South Asian origin, are at risk due to hypertension and urbanization. Native Americans are at risk due to diabetes.
4. Disparate outcomes in CVD occur in varied populations due to access to care issues, insurance deficits, and persistent bias in health= care decision-making.

TABLE 2–3 Treatment of Heart Failure in African Americans

Study	% of African American Subjects	Design	Intervention	Results
V-HeFT I	29%	Double-blind RCT; primary endpoint: mortality	Placebo versus hydralazine/isosorbide nitrate Background: diuretics & digoxin	Annual mortality rate decreased from 17.9% to 9.7%; $p = 0.04$
V-HeFT II	27%	Double-blind RCT; primary endpoint: mortality	Hydralazine/isosorbide dinitrate versus enalapril Background: diuretics & digoxin	Annual mortality rate: 12.9% to 12.8%; $p =$ NS
SOLVD-treatment	12%	Double-blind RCT; primary endpoint: mortality	Placebo versus enalapril in NYHA Class II/III HF	No mortality difference blacks versus nonblacks in a matched population, RE: LVEF and clinical trial participation; RR 0.92 versus 0.95; higher hospitalization rate for blacks; RR 0.95 versus 0.54; $p = 0.005$
SOLVD-prevention	9.8%	Double-blind RCT; primary endpoint: mortality	Placebo versus enalapril in NYHA Class I/II HF	No difference in the prevention of heart failure using enalapril; statistically significant difference in the incidence of heart failure; RR 1.81; $p < 0.001$
BEST	23%	Double-blind RCT; primary endpoint: all-cause mortality	Placebo versus bucindolol in NYHA Class III & IV; randomization stratified for women and blacks Background: diuretics, ACE inhibitors; digoxin at investigator's discretion	Nonsignificant 17% increase in risk of death on bucindolol; $p = 0.27$
MERIT-HF	<5%	Double-blind RCT; primary endpoint: mortality	Placebo versus metoprolol succinate in NYHA Class II/IV; mostly II/III	Insufficient numbers to ascertain efficacy
U.S. Carvedilol Trials Program	20%	4 concurrent trials; double-blind RCT design; mortality was not a predetermined endpoint	Placebo versus carvedilol in NYHA Class II/IV; mostly II/III with protocol participation determined by 6-min walk time; background: diuretics, ACE inhibitors and digoxin at investigator's discretion	Similar efficacy between black and nonblack groups; reduction in death for any cause or hospitalization for any cause −48%; reduction in worsening of heart failure −54%
COPERNICUS	5%	Double-blind RCT design; primary endpoint: all-cause mortality	Placebo versus carvedilol in NYHA Class III/IV; LVEF<0.25 (mean 0.19)	Similar efficacy between black and nonblack groups despite small number of blacks

ACE = angiotensin-converting enzyme; BEST = The Beta Blocker Evaluation of Survival Trial; COPERNICUS = Carvedilol Prospective Randomized Cumulative Survival Study; LVEF = left ventricular ejection fraction; MERIT-HF = Metoprolol Randomized Intervention Trial in Chronic Heart Failure; RCT = randomized controlled trial; RR = relative risk; SOLVD = Studies of Left Ventricular Dysfunction; V-HeFT I = Vasodilators in Heart Failure Trial I; V-HeFT II = Vasodilators in Heart Failure Trial II.

Modified from Yancy CW: Does race matter in heart failure? Am Heart J 146:203, 2003.

5. The treatment of hypertension is effective in all individuals; decisions regarding therapy should be based on the absence or presence of compelling indications for aggressive therapy (e.g., renal insufficiency, post-MI and heart failure) and less so on the basis of race.
6. African Americans with hypertension are at high risk for complications due to hypertension, especially renal disease and heart failure, and should be treated aggressively including lower goal BP reductions and earlier use of either combination agents or multiple drug classes. Although the response to ACE inhibitors, ARBs, and beta blockers may be less, these differences are overcome with the concomitant use of diuretics, and these agents should be used preferentially in African Americans to reduce CVD, stroke, and renal disease.
7. Ischemic heart disease occurs at a *lower* frequency in Hispanic Americans and in a similar frequency for Asian Americans as for whites. Ischemic heart disease occurs at a *higher* frequency in African Americans even though epicardial obstructive CAD occurs less frequently. Hypertension and LV hypertrophy are the leading risk factors. Acute coronary syndromes in African Americans more likely present as unstable angina or non-STEMI. Multi-vessel CAD is common when epicardial disease is present. Thrombolytic therapy, percutaneous coronary interventions, and CABG are applied less frequently in African Americans, especially women, thus contributing to disparate outcomes.
8. Heart failure is notably different in African Americans. The disease occurs at an earlier age, with more advanced LV dysfunction and worse clinical class severity. The incidence of heart failure is higher in African Americans, and morbidity is much worse. Yet the mortality risk may be similar. The response to neurohormonal antagonists for heart failure is likely to be similar for all patients, and data regarding the use of beta blockers and ACE inhibitors are consistent with good outcomes in African Americans. The A-HeFT trial now expands the treatment regimen for African Americans with heart failure to include combined vasodilator therapy.
9. A genomic basis for the differential expression of CVD in varied populations may exist, and candidate single nucleotide polymorphisms have been discovered. The exact contribution of these genomic variations to the clinical expression of CVD is not yet clear, and much more investigation is required. But the potential for clinical applications of pharmacogenomics is now apparent.
10. Any use of race/ethnicity in medicine requires caution. The degree of heterogeneity within races resembles that among races. Clinical decision-making should continue to be made on an individual basis.

REFERENCES

General

1. Barnett E, Casper ML, Halverson JA, et al: Men and Heart Disease: An Atlas of Racial and Ethnic Disparities in Mortality. 1st ed. Office for Social Environment and Health Research, Morgantown, WVa, West Virginia University, 2001.
2. Winkleby MA, Kraemer HC, Ahn DK, Varady AN: Ethnic and socioeconomic differences in cardiovascular disease risk factors. JAMA 280:356, 1998.
3. National Center for Health Statistics (NCHS). Fast stats (http://www.cdc.gov/nchc/fastats/). 2002.

Hypertension

4. Geiss LS, Rolka DB, Engelgau MN: Elevated blood pressure among U.S. adults with diabetes, 1988-94. Am J Prev Med 22:42, 2002.
5. Ford ES, Giles WH, Dietz WH: Prevalence of the metabolic syndrome among U.S. adults. JAMA 287:356, 2002.
6. Ferrannini E, Natali A, Capaldo B, et al: Insulin resistance, hyperinsulinemia and blood pressure. Hypertension 30:1144, 1997.
7. Must A, Spadano J, Coakley EH: The disease burden associated with overweight and obesity. JAMA 282:1523, 1999.
8. Hall WD, Ferrario CM, Moore MA: Hypertension related morbidity and mortality in the southeastern United States. Am J Med Sci 313:195, 1997.
9. Cooper R, Rotimi C, Ataman S: The prevalence of hypertension in seven populations of West African origin. Am J Public Health 87:160, 1997.
10. Flack JM, Ferdinand KC, Nasser SA: Epidemiology of hypertension and cardiovascular disease in African Americans. J Clin Hyperten 5(Suppl):5, 2003.
11. Ganguli MC, Grimm RH, Svendsen KH: Higher education and income are related to a better Na:K ratio in blacks. Baseline results of the Treatment of Mild Hypertension Study (TOMHS) data. Am J Hypertens 10:979, 1997.
12. Stamler J, Sacks FM, Svetkey LP: Vollmer WM for the DASH-Sodium Collaborative Research Group. Effects on blood pressure of reduced dietary sodium and the Dietary Approaches to Stop Hypertension (DASH) diet. N Engl J Med 344:3, 2001.
13. INTERSALT Study: Background, methods, findings and implications. Am J Clin Nutr 65:626S, 1997.
14. Kameth S, Markham D, Drazmer MH: Increased prevalence of concentric left ventricular hypertrophy in African Americans: Will an epidenic of heart failure follow? Heart Failure Reviews 11:271, 2006.
15. Drazner MH, Dries DL, Peshock RM, et al: Left ventricular hypertrophy is more prevalent in blacks than whites in the general population: The Dallas Heart Study. Hypertension 46:124, 2005.
16. Williams DR, Rucker TD: Understanding and addressing racial disparities in health care. Health Care Financ Rev 21:75, 2000.
17. American Heart Association: 2002 Heart and Stroke Statistics—Update. Dallas, American Heart Association, 2001.
18. American Heart Association: 2003 Heart Disease and Stroke Statistics—Update. Dallas, American Heart Association, 2002.
19. Gillum RF: The epidemiology of cardiovascular disease in black Americans. N Engl J Med 335:1597, 1996.
20. Gomes C, McGuire TG: Identifying the sources of racial and ethnic disparities in health care use. Washington, DC, Institute of Medicine Report, 2001.
21. Hannan EL, Burke J, et al: Access to coronary artery bypass surgery by race/ethnicity and gender among patients who are appropriate for surgery. Med Care 37:68, 1999.
22. Robert Wood Johnson Foundation: New survey shows language barriers causing many Spanish-speaking Latinos to skip care. *In* Smedley BD, Stith AY, Nelson AR (eds): Unequal Treatment: Confronting Racial and Ethnic Disparities in Healthcare. Washington, DC, U.S. Institute of Medicine, National Academy of Sciences, 2003, pp 88-90.
23. Schulman KA, Berlin JA, Harless W: The effect of race and sex on physicians' recommendations for cardiac catheterization. N Engl J Med 340:618, 1999.
24. Ford E, Cooper R, Costener A, et al: Coronary arteriography and coronary bypass surgery among whites and other racial groups relative to hospital-based incidence rates for coronary artery disease. *In* Smedley BD, Stith AY, Nelson AR (eds): Unequal Treatment: Confronting Racial and Ethnic Disparities in Healthcare. Washington, DC, U.S. Institute of Medicine, National Academy of Sciences, 2003, pp 43-44.
25. Ramsey DJ, Goff DC, Wear ML, et al: Sex and ethnic differences in use of myocardial revascularization procedures in Mexican Americans and Non-Hispanic Whites; The Corpus Christi Heart Project. J Clin Epidemiol 50:603, 1997.
26. Petersen LA, Wright SM, Petersen ED, Daley JL: Impact of race and cardiac care and outcomes in veterans with acute myocardial infarction. Med Care 40(Suppl):I-86, 2002.
27. Jha AK, Varosy PD, Kanaya AM, et al: Differences in medical care and disease outcomes among black and white women with heart disease. Circulation 108:1098, 2003.
28. Haffner SM: Hypertension in the San Antonio Heart Study and the Mexico City Diabetes Study; clinical and metabolic correlates. Public Health Reports 111:11, 1996.
29. Crespo CJ, Smit E, Garcia Palmieri MR: Hypertension in Hispanic Americans. *In* Izzo JL, Black HR (eds): Hypertension Primer. 3rd ed. Philadelphia, Lippincott Williams & Wilkins, 2003.
30. Anand SS, Yusuf S, Vuksan V: Differences in risk factors, atherosclerosis and cardiovascular disease between ethnic groups in Canada; the Study of Health Assessment and Risk in Ethnic Groups (SHARE). Lancet 356:279, 2000.
31. Deewania PC, Gupta R: Hypertension in South Asians. *In* Izzo JL, Black HR (eds): Hypertension Primer, 3rd ed. Philadelphia, Lippincott Williams & Wilkins, 2003.
32. Rahman M, Douglas JG, Wright JT: Pathophysiology and treatment implications of hypertension in the African American population. Endocrinol Metab Clin North Am 26:125, 1997.
33. Berenson GS, Voors AW, Webber LS, et al: Racial differences of parameters associated with blood pressure levels in children: The Bogalusa Heart Study. Metabolism 28:1218, 1979.
34. Yancy CW: Heart failure in African Americans: a cardiovascular enigma. J Card Fail 6:183, 2000.
35. Gardin JM, Wagenknecht LE, Anton-Culver H, et al: Relationship of cardiovascular risk factors to echocardiographic left ventricular mass in healthy young black and white adult men and women: The CARDIA study. Circulation 92:380, 1995.
36. Gottdiener JS, Reda DJ, Materson BJ, et al: Importance of obesity, race and age to the cardiac structural and functional effects of hypertension; The Department of Veterans Affairs Cooperative Study Group on Antihypertensive Agents. J Am Coll Cardiol 24:1492, 1994.
37. Kotchen TA, Piering AW, Cowley AW, et al: Glomerular hyperfiltration in hypertensive African-Americans. Hypertension 35:822, 2000.
38. Stein CM, Lang CC, Nelson R, et al: Vasodilation in black Americans: Attenuated nitric oxide-mediated responses. Clin Pharmacol Ther 62:436, 1997.
39. Kaplan NM: Kaplan's Clinical Hypertension. 8th ed. Philadelphia, Lippincott Williams & Wilkins, 2002.
40. Grim CE, Robinson M: Salt, slavery and survival—hypertension in the African Diaspora. Epidemiology 14:120, 2003.
41. Cooper RS, Rotimi CN, Ward R: The puzzle of hypertension in African Americans. Sci Am 280:56, 1999.
42. Sacks FM, Svetkey LP, Vollmer WM, et al: Effects on blood pressure of reduced dietary sodium and the Dietary Approaches to Stop Hypertension (DASH) diet. DASH-Sodium Collaborative Research Group. N Engl J Med 344:3, 2001.
43. Baker EH: Association of hypertension with T594M mutation in beta subunit of epithelial sodium channels in black people resident in London. Lancet 351:1388, 1998.
44. August P, Leventhal B, Suthanthiran M: Hypertension-induced organ damage in African Americans; transforming growth factor-beta 1 excess as a mechanism for increased prevalence. Curr Hypertens Rep 2:184, 2000.
45. Chobanian AV, Bakris GL, Black HR, et al: The Seventh Report of the Joint National Committee on Prevention, Detection, Evaluation and Treatment of High Blood Pressure. The JNC VII Report. JAMA 289:2560, 2003.
46. Nesbitt S, Victor RG: Pathogenesis of hypertension in African Americans. Congest Heart Fail 10:24, 2004.
47. Wright JT, Bakris G, Green T, et al: Effect of blood pressure lowering and antihypertensive drug class on progression of hypertensive kidney disease. Results from the AASK Trial. JAMA 288:2421, 2002.
48. Wright JT, Dunn JK, Cutler JA, et al; ALLHAT Collaborative Research Group: Outcomes in hypertensive black and nonblack patients treated with chlorthalidone, amlodipine and lisonopril. JAMA 293:1595, 2005.
49. Douglas JG, Bakris GL, Epstein M, et al: Management of high blood pressure in African Americans. Arch Intern Med 163:525, 2003.
50. Clark LT, Ferdinand KC, Flack JM, et al: Coronary heart disease in African Americans. Heart Disease 3:97, 2001.
51. Strong JP, Malcom GT, Oalmann MC, et al: The PDAY study: Natural history, risk factors, and pathobiology. Pathobiological Determinants of Atherosclerosis in Youth. Ann NY Acad Sci 811:226, 1997.
52. Sorlie, PD, Sharrett AR, Patsch W, et al: The relationship between lipids/lipoproteins and atherosclerosis in African Americans and whites: The Atherosclerosis Risk in Communities study. Ann Epidemiol 9:149, 1999.
53. Ergul S, Parish DC, Puett D, et al: Racial differences in plasma endothelin-1 concentrations in individuals with essential hypertension. Hypertension 28:652, 1996.

Heart Failure

54. Dries DL, Exner DV, Gersh BJ, et al: Racial differences in the outcome of left ventricular dysfunction. N Engl J Med 341:298, 1999.
55. Exner DV, Dries DL, Domanski MJ, et al: Lesser response to angiotensin-converting-enzyme inhibitor therapy in black as compared with white patients with left ventricular dysfunction. N Engl J Med 344:1351, 2001.
56. Dries DL, Strong MH, Cooper RS, Drazner M: Efficacy of angiotensin-converting enzyme inhibition in reducing progression from asymptomatic left ventricular dysfunction to symptomatic heart failure in black and white patients. J Am Coll Cardiol 40:311, 2002.
57. Iwanaga Y, Kihara Y, Hasegawa K, et al: Cardiac endothelin-1 plays a critical role in the functional deterioration of left ventricles during the transition from compensatory hypertrophy to congestive heart failure in salt-sensitive hypertensive rats. Circulation 98:2065, 1998.
58. Kostis JB, Davis BR, Cutler J, et al for the SHEP Cooperative Research Group: Prevention of heart failure by antihypertensive drug treatment in older persons with isolated systolic hypertension. JAMA 278:212, 1997.
59. Hunt SA, Abraham WT, Chin MH, et al: ACC/AHA 2005 Guideline Update for the Diagnosis and Management of Chronic Heart Failure in the Adult: A report of the American College of Cardiology/American Heart Association Task Force on Practice Guidelines (Writing Committee to Update the 2001 Guidelines for the Evaluation and Management of Heart Failure): Developed in collaboration with the American College of Chest Physicians and the International Society for Heart and Lung Transplantation: Endorsed by the Heart Rhythm Society. Circulation 112:e154, 2005.
60. August P: TGF Beta-1 overexpressed in African American hypertensives. Proc Natl Acad Sci U S A 97:3479, 2000.
61. McNamara DM, Feldman A, et al: Genetic Risk Assessment of Cardiac Events, GRACE. Circulation 103:1644, 2001.

62. Mason DA, Moore JD, Green SA, Liggett SB: A gain of function polymorphism in a G-protein coupling domain of the human beta-1 adrenergic receptor. J Biol Chem 274:12670, 1999.
63. Small KM, Wagoner LE, Levin AM, et al: Synergistic polymorphisms of beta 1 and alpha 2C adrenergic receptors and the risk of congestive heart failure. N Engl J Med 347:1135, 2002.
64. Turner ST, Schwartz GL, Chapman AB, Boperwinkle E: C825T polymorphism of the G protein beta-3 subunit and antihypertensive response to a thiazide diuretic. Hypertension 37:739, 2001.
65. McNamara DM, Tamm WS, Sabolinski ML, et al: Aldosterone synthase promoter polymorphism predicts outcome in African Americans with heart failure; results from the A-HeFT Trial. J Am Coll Cardiol 48:1277, 2006.
66. Carson P, Ziesche S, Johnson G, et al: Racial differences in response to therapy for heart failure: Analysis of the vasodilator-heart failure trials. Vasodilator-Heart Failure Trial Study Group. J Card Fail 5:178, 1999.
67. The Beta-Blocker Evaluation of Survival Trial Investigators: A trial of the beta-blocker bucindolol in patients with advanced chronic heart failure. N Engl J Med 344:1659, 2001.
68. MERIT-HF Study Group: Effect of metoprolol CR/XL in chronic heart failure: Metoprolol CR/XL Randomised Intervention Trial in Congestive Heart Failure (MERIT-HF). Lancet 353:2001, 1999.
69. Yancy CW, Fowler MB, Colucci WS, et al: Race and the response to adrenergic blockade with carvedilol in patients with heart failure. N Engl J Med 344:1358, 2001.
70. Franciosa JA, Taylor AL, Cohn JN, et al for the A-HeFT Investigators: African American Heart Failure Trial (A-HeFT): Rationale, design, and methodology. J Card Fail 8:128, 2002.
71. Taylor Al, Ziesche S, Yancy CW, et al: Combination of isosorbide dinitrate and hydralazine in blacks with heart failure. N Engl J Med 351:2049, 2004.
72. Adams KF, Lindenfeld, J, Arnold JMO, et al: Heart Failure Society of America 2006 comprehensive heart failure practice guidelines. J Card Fail 12:e1-e22, 2006.
73. Hare JM: Nitroso-redox balance in the cardiovascular system. N Engl J Med 351:2112, 2004.
74. American Anthropological Association: American Anthropological Association statement on race (http://www.aaanet.org/stmts/racepp.htm). 1998.
75. Kaplan JB, Bennett T: Use of race and ethnicity in biomedical publication. JAMA 289:2709, 2003.

CHAPTER 3

Economics and Cardiovascular Disease

Mark A. Hlatky and Daniel B. Mark

Although the United States remains the world leader in spending on health care, medical spending is rising in all major industrialized countries, irrespective of the type of health care system. The decisions made by physicians control the bulk of medical expenditures, and society has increasingly called for greater stewardship of the vast resources that doctors command. This chapter discusses some of the key economic principles that underlie clinical and health policy decision-making and reviews important cardiovascular economic studies that best illustrate those principles.

KEY ECONOMIC PRINCIPLES

Alternative Uses

A key principle of economics is that all resources have alternative uses, so devoting resources to any particular activity makes them unavailable for different and, perhaps better, uses. Society's application of resources to medical care diminishes the resources available for alternative programs such as public safety, assistance to the elderly or the poor, education, or environmental protection. This same principle applies to the resources earmarked to health care: The resources devoted to implantable cardioverter defibrillators (ICDs) (see Chap. 34) might be used to meet alternative health needs such as treatment of heart failure (see Chap. 23), prenatal care programs, or provision of vaccinations. One major goal of health economics is to define the most efficient use of the resources available to provide health care to a population of patients.

Societal Perspective

Economic analyses most often employ the societal perspective: How will society as a whole benefit from the new clinical program and what will society have to pay for it? In contrast, clinicians are focused on individual patients. Their traditional role is to be the patient's advocate and do what is best for that individual, regardless of the value provided to society. Thus economic analysis is a policy tool for informing spending about groups or populations, not a tool for assisting with bedside decision-making.

LAW OF DIMINISHING RETURNS. An economic principle of special relevance to medicine is the so-called "law of diminishing returns," indicated schematically in Figure 3-1. Because resources are initially applied to a particular end, the returns are large, but as additional resources are applied, the returns become progressively smaller to the point that there is no further gain, and perhaps even a loss, with application of yet further resources. This pattern is familiar to clinicians caring for patients; in the case of acute myocardial infarction (MI, see Chap. 50), for example, access to basic defibrillation and hospital care provides great benefits, and the addition of reperfusion therapy further improves patient outcomes (see Chap. 52). The provision of yet more care may improve outcomes further, but eventually maximum benefit is obtained—this point has been termed the "flat of the curve." A key economic insight is that it is not optimal for society to have medical care operate on the flat of the curve, but rather on the upsloping portion of the curve (see Fig. 3-1) because the resources that would be spent in moving along the flat of the curve have better alternative uses. A major goal of economic analysis of cardiovascular care is to find the optimal level of resources for a given clinical problem.

As exemplified in Figure 3-1, a key economic measure of value is the cost of adding another unit of medical benefit, or the slope of the curve.[1,2] In economic analysis, the costs and effects of an intervention are always compared with an explicitly defined alternative. Thus cost-effectiveness analysis assesses the marginal (or incremental) costs required to improve outcomes by one unit. The cost-effectiveness ratio is defined as follows:

$$\frac{\text{Cost}_{\text{new}} - \text{Cost}_{\text{std}}}{\text{Effect}_{\text{new}} - \text{Effect}_{\text{std}}}$$

where cost_{new} is the total cost of the new program, cost_{std} is the total cost of the standard management, and $\text{effect}_{\text{new}}$ and $\text{effect}_{\text{std}}$ indicate the medical effectiveness of the new and standard programs, respectively. The cost of a program should include all relevant costs: the intervention itself; the cost of adverse events induced and averted, and the costs of concomitant treatments. The effectiveness of a medical intervention should be assessed using outcomes directly relevant to patients, such as survival and quality of life. Economic analysis commonly measures effectiveness in "quality-adjusted life years" (QALYs) to assess on a common scale both of these dimensions of improved clinical outcome. Laboratory-based outcome measures (e.g., ejection fraction, serum cholesterol) are intermediate, surrogate markers of ultimate patient benefit, and therefore not useful in economic analysis.

MEDICAL COSTS

Provision of medical care requires resources: the time and energy of physicians, nurses, and other health care professionals; specialized facilities such as intensive care units, angiography suites, and operating rooms; and costly drugs and supplies. Use of these resources has a cost, even if medical care is provided "for free." In principle, the best measure of this cost is what economists term the opportunity cost, or what has been lost by not applying resources to their next best use. As a practical matter, cost is measured by the prices paid in a competitive market. The overall cost of a medical program can then be measured as $\Sigma_i P_i Q_i$, where P_i is the price for resource "i," Q_i is the quantity of resource "i" that is used, and the summation (Σ_i) is overall "i" resources used in care of the patient. Modern hospital cost accounting

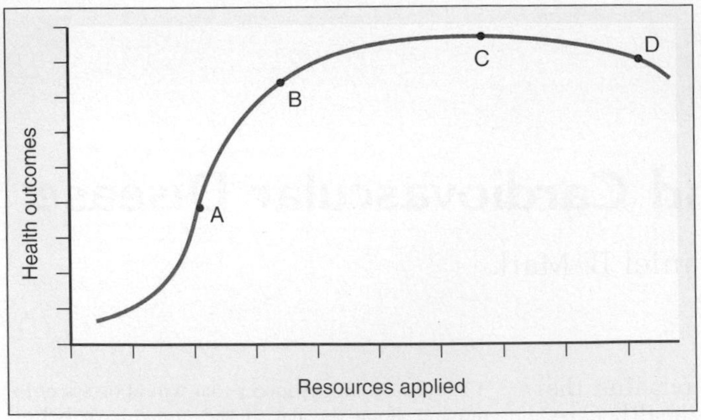

FIGURE 3–1 General relationship between application of health care resources (horizontal axis) and health outcomes (vertical axis). At Point A, outcomes are improving rapidly with increased resources and treatment is cost-effective. At Point B, outcomes are still improving with increased resources, but at a rate that is less cost-effective. At Point C, increased resources are no longer improving outcome (i.e., "flat at the curve"), and at Point D increased resources actually lead to worse outcomes through iatrogenic complications and overtreatment.

systems assist such "microcosting" of medical care services. When microcosting is infeasible, an alternative measure of cost in U.S. fee-for-service hospitals can be calculated by multiplying the charge for the service by a correction factor (the ratio of costs to charges) from the hospital's annual financial report to the Centers for Medicare and Medicaid Services.

In medical economic studies, the cost of an intervention includes all relevant costs, regardless of who pays for them. The cost of percutaneous coronary intervention might be borne in part by the insurance company, in part by the patient (e.g., prescription drugs after discharge), and in part by the hospital (e.g., costs over the contracted insurance payment amount). An expensive new therapy in the interventional laboratory may reduce total costs in the year following the procedure, and therefore be quite economically attractive. Nevertheless, a hospital may resist using the new therapy because its costs are increased. Even programs that save total medical costs can create economic winners and losers whose incentives and disincentives can distort optimal resource allocation from a societal perspective.

Medical costs and benefits occur with varying magnitude over long time intervals, which raises two related issues regarding measurement. Inflation changes the units of measurement, so it is necessary to standardize all costs to a single metric, such as 2007 dollars. A separate issue is that even if there were no cost inflation, it is still preferable to be paid a given amount today rather than that same amount in 5 years, and, conversely, it is preferable to repay a debt sometime in the future than to repay it immediately. To adjust for these time preferences, medical economic studies typically discount future costs and medical benefits by 3% per year.

ANALYSIS OF SPECIFIC INTERVENTIONS

Economic analysis has been applied to treatment of acute illness (e.g., acute MI), specific therapeutic procedures (e.g., coronary bypass surgery; see Chap. 54), treatment of chronic illness (e.g., heart failure), prevention of disease (e.g., reduction of high cholesterol levels; see Chap. 39), or the use of diagnostic tests (e.g., coronary angiography). In the remainder of this chapter, we illustrate the principles of economic analysis by discussing cardiovascular management strategies drawn from each of these areas. Detailed review of the economics of all cardiovascular therapies is beyond the scope of this chapter.

Application of economic analysis to medical care can be illustrated by the use of thrombolytic therapy for acute MI (see Chap. 51). Timely reperfusion of the occluded coronary artery improves survival of the patient with an acute MI, and this survival benefit is maintained over long-term follow-up.[3] The added cost of treating an acute MI patient with reperfusion therapy needs to be weighed against the long-term incremental health benefits in order to assess the value provided by this treatment strategy.

The value of streptokinase administration for acute MI compared with no reperfusion therapy can be analyzed using cost-effectiveness analysis. For the purpose of this example, we assume that streptokinase costs $270 per treatment and that costs of medical care are otherwise equal in treated and untreated MI patients. We further assume that hospital survival is improved from 88% to 92% by streptokinase treatment and that the life expectancy of MI survivors is 15 years, regardless of whether they were treated with streptokinase or not. On the basis of these assumptions, the incremental cost-effectiveness of streptokinase for the treatment of acute MI can be calculated as follows:

$$\frac{\Delta\text{Cost}}{\Delta\text{Life expectancy}} = \frac{\$270-0}{(0.92)(15\,\text{yr})-(0.88)(15\,\text{yr})} = \frac{\$270}{0.6\,\text{yr}} = \$450\,/\,\text{life-year added}$$

Thus the expenditure of $450 adds a year to the life of an average patient with an acute MI. To judge whether streptokinase therapy for acute MI represents a good value for the money spent (i.e., is "economically attractive") requires a standard of comparison. Renal dialysis costs about $50,000 per patient per year in the United States. The cost of dialysis is covered by the publicly funded Medicare program and provides a good benchmark of how much society is willing to spend to add a life-year. Programs that cost up to $50,000 per year of life added are generally considered economically attractive, whereas programs with cost-effectiveness ratios greater than $100,000 per year of life added are generally considered to be economically unattractive. On the basis of these benchmarks, streptokinase therapy for acute MI is a very economically attractive intervention.

ACUTE CORONARY SYNDROMES

(see Chaps. 50-52)

Treatment of acute coronary syndromes (MI, unstable angina) with reperfusion, antithrombotic, and anticoagulant regimens has been extensively investigated. Although clinically diverse, these therapies share common features with respect to economic evaluation. The therapies for acute coronary syndromes are typically short term in duration and expensive, and they provide benefit to patients mainly by reducing the short-term risk of hospital death and/or MI. In addition, the cost-effectiveness of any one of these therapies needs to be judged in the context of available alternatives.

THROMBOLYTIC AGENTS. Tissue plasminogen activator (t-PA) has been extensively studied for the treatment of acute MI. t-PA is much more expensive than streptokinase, the first thrombolytic agent shown to be effective for MI. The cost-effectiveness of t-PA was assessed in the randomized GUSTO-1 trial.[4] In GUSTO-1 the cost of therapy was assessed by assigning standardized costs to each resource consumed (e.g., hospital days, cardiac angiography) and summing the costs over all resources used. Apart from the cost of the thrombolytic agents themselves, hospital and follow-up costs were quite similar in t-PA- and streptokinase-treated patients, and the added cost of t-PA ($2200 vs. $270) was not offset by cost savings in other aspects of the patient's care. The 30-day survival rate of t-PA–treated patients was improved by 1%, and the life expectancy of survivors was projected to be 15.4 years. Using these data, the cost-effectiveness of t-PA relative to streptokinase was $27,100 per year of life saved, which was economically attractive by the previously described benchmarks.[4]

The use of streptokinase and t-PA for acute MI exemplifies the principle of diminishing returns. The greatest gain in clinical outcome comes from using the cheapest effective thrombolytic agent (streptokinase) for acute MI, which improves survival by 4% in absolute terms at a net cost of about $270 per patient. t-PA improves survival by a further 1% in absolute terms but at an added cost of more than $1900 per patient. Thus the cost-effectiveness of streptokinase relative to placebo ($450 per life-year added) is more favorable than the cost-effectiveness of t-PA relative to streptokinase ($27,100 per life-year added). Simple and inexpensive therapies often provide much of the potential improvement in outcomes for a given clinical condition, with smaller and smaller marginal improvements coming at greater and greater cost. This example also illustrates the comparative nature of economic evaluations—the value of a treatment can only be assessed in light of the therapeutic alternatives.

Percutaneous Coronary Intervention

(see Chap. 52)

Primary percutaneous coronary intervention (PCI) for acute MI has been compared with thrombolytic therapy in several clinical trials, some of which also included an economic evaluation. Quantitative overviews of randomized trials show the survival of patients with acute MI treated with angioplasty is better than patients treated with thrombolysis.[5,6] The results of economic analysis have been less consistent, with primary PCI being less expensive than thrombolytic therapy in some studies but more expensive in others.[7,8] The net economic effect of primary PCI depends on the practice patterns of coronary angiography and revascularization among patients who would otherwise be treated with thrombolysis. A strategy of primary PCI lowers overall costs in practice settings where coronary angiography is routinely performed after acute MI: When most patients undergo catheterization anyway, there is relatively little added cost in doing the procedure immediately, and such a practice may allow for shortened hospital stays. By contrast, the strategy of primary PCI increases costs in practice settings in which angiography is used infrequently after acute MI: When catheterization and PCI would not otherwise have been performed, primary PCI is an additional procedure that significantly increases costs. This example highlights the importance of clinical context in evaluating the economic impact of medical therapies—the cost of a new clinical strategy must be judged relative to the cost of the relevant current clinical strategy.

Anticoagulation and Antiplatelet Regimens

Anticoagulant and antiplatelet regimens are now the cornerstone of treatment in acute coronary syndrome (see Chap. 82). Newer agents such as the glycoprotein IIb/IIIa inhibitors and the low-molecular-weight heparins are more expensive than the standard alternatives (aspirin, heparin), so economic evaluation is important to judge their net costs and benefits.

Eptifibatide, a small-molecule glycoprotein IIb/IIIa inhibitor, improves clinical outcomes in patients with acute coronary syndrome. The major benefit of eptifibatide is to reduce the incidence of nonfatal MI rather than reduce 30-day mortality. One randomized trial showed the added cost of eptifibatide (500 Euros) was partially recouped by reducing complications, but total costs were nonetheless increased by 211 to 399 Euros per patient. Because the main effect of eptifibatide is to reduce morbidity rather than mortality, its cost-effectiveness depends on the extent to which preventing a nonfatal MI improves long-term prognosis. The cost-effectiveness ratio for eptifibatide appears to be economically attractive (9600 to 18,000 Euros per life-year added) on the basis of the projection that prevention of a nonfatal MI increases life expectancy by approximately 2 years.[9] This example shows that an expensive therapy may be cost-effective even without a significant effect on short-term mortality.

Cardiac Procedures and Devices

CORONARY BYPASS GRAFTING (see Chap. 54). In 2004, 249,000 patients had coronary bypass surgeries in the United States, and 1,279,000 percutaneous coronary intervention procedures were also performed.[10] With a total cost of roughly 20 billion dollars a year, the use of coronary revascularization has been the subject of extensive economic evaluation.

Coronary artery bypass graft (CABG) surgery is an effective treatment for angina in symptomatic patients and increases life expectancy in patients who have extensive coronary disease. An overview of randomized clinical trials of surgery versus medical therapy estimated that over the first 10 years of follow-up, patients with left main disease live on average 19 months longer after CABG than medical therapy, patients with three-vessel disease live about 6 months longer, and patients with one- or two-vessel disease live about 2 months longer. These data suggest that CABG is more economically attractive in patients with more extensive coronary disease at higher risk of death because the absolute improvement in survival is greatest in these patients while the cost of the surgery is roughly the same.[11] Bypass surgery is also effective in reducing angina and improving quality of life. Bypass surgery is a cost-effective alternative to medical therapy in patients with severe angina because the substantial improvement in quality of life increases the number of quality-adjusted life-years.

PERCUTANEOUS CORONARY INTERVENTION. Despite the extensive use of PCI, there have been few randomized trials that compare it with medical therapy.[12] The RITA-2 trial found that patients with stable angina treated with balloon angioplasty had better angina relief but more cardiac events than patients randomized to medical therapy. RITA-2 documented that the higher initial cost of angioplasty (2793 British pounds) was undiminished after 3 years of follow-up.[13] In contrast, the TIME trial reported that the higher initial costs of elderly patients randomized to PCI were largely balanced by the higher follow-up costs in patients randomized to medical therapy.[14] These findings suggest that the cost-effectiveness of PCI depends in large part on the severity of the patient's angina—in patients with severe symptoms, PCI can improve quality of life and avert some costs, whereas in patients with mild to no symptoms there is less to gain from intervention.

PCI and bypass surgery have been directly compared in several randomized trials conducted in patients with multivessel disease. The clinical results of these studies have been quite consistent in showing significantly less angina and slightly lower mortality in surgery patients.[15] The economic outcomes in the BARI trial[16] were typical of the other trials (EAST, ERACI, RITA) that also collected economic data. The initial cost of coronary angioplasty was significantly lower than that of bypass surgery, roughly one-half to two-thirds the cost. This initial cost advantage was almost completely lost over the subsequent follow-up, however, because of the need for repeat coronary revascularization procedures among patients assigned to angioplasty. At 12 years of follow-up in BARI, the total medical costs were only 2% lower in balloon angioplasty patients than in bypass surgery patients.[16]

In the United States, current practice is for PCI to include coronary stents in almost all cases. The ARTS trial found that patients randomized to receive bare metal stents had 40% lower initial procedure costs than patients randomized to surgery, but this gap narrowed to 20% after 1 year and to only 11% after 3 years.[17] The SOS trial found a similar pattern of costs, with the initial 47% lower costs among stent-assigned patients narrowing significantly to 29% over 1 year.[18] The studies of coronary angioplasty underscore the need for economic evaluations to last long enough to document all relevant costs of an intervention. An initially less expensive therapy may not be a bargain if there are late costs from repeated procedures or complications.

Drug-coated stents (DES) have further reduced the rate of re-peat revascularization procedures in comparison with bare metal stents but are significantly more expensive. The SIRIUS trial suggests that the $2880 higher initial cost of patients assigned to a sirolimus-coated stent was partially offset during follow-up by lowering the need for costly repeat revascularization procedures.[19] The RAVEL trial also reported an equalization of costs 1 year after randomization to either a sirolimus-coated stent or a bare metal stent.[20] Neither of these trials is ideal for economic analysis, however, because they both required follow-up angiography to document restenosis. Prior work in stent trials showed that the repeat revascularization rate was doubled by the requirement for follow-up angiography, due to retreatment of lesions that were otherwise clinically inapparent. By contrast, the BASKET trial evaluated a consecutive group of patients and did not require follow-up angiography. This trial found significantly higher costs after 1 year of follow-up among the patients randomized to a drug-coated stent.[21] The economic impact of drug-coated stents may depend critically on the rate of repeat procedures than can be achieved using alternative therapies—when repeat procedure rates are already quite low, it is difficult to lower them further and thereby recoup the added cost of a drug-coated stent. The cost of the DES is also quite influential in this balance. In the United States the cost of DES—initially $3000 per stent—has dropped significantly since its initial introduction, but the cost of bare metal stents has also dropped dramatically so that there is still a large incremental cost difference between the two stent types.

IMPLANTABLE CARDIOVERTER DEFIBRILLATOR (see Chap. 34). The ICD reduces total mortality by 26% among patients at high risk for sudden cardiac death.[22] Because implantation of an ICD costs $25,000 or more, many have questioned whether it is worth the high cost.

Several randomized trials have reported data on economic and clinical outcomes of ICD implantation including MADIT-I, AVID, CIDS, MADIT-II, and SCD-HeFT. In each study the early costs among ICD patients were considerably higher than those of conventionally treated patients (Table 3-1), and the wide gap in costs was maintained over the next 3 to 5 years of follow-up. Lifetime costs and survival were projected for patients with life-threatening ventricular arrhythmias by Sanders and coworkers[23] using data from seven randomized trials of prophylactic

TABLE 3–1 Costs in Implantable Cardiac Defibrillator (ICD) and Conventionally Treated Patients in Secondary Prevention Trials

	Costs ($)		
Study	***ICD***	***Conventional***	***Difference***
MADIT-I[35]			
Initial therapy	44,565	18,880	25,685
4 year follow-up	52,995	57,100	−4,105
Total	97,560	75,980	21,580
AVID[36]			
Initial therapy	66,629	34,059	32,570
Follow-up	9,604	14,594	−4,990
Total	76,233	48,653	27,580
CIDS[37]			
Initial therapy	48,874	7,927	40,948
Follow-up	38,840	30,673	8,167
Total	87,715	38,600	49,115

ICD placement. Studies in which the ICD significantly reduced mortality led to an acceptable cost-effectiveness ratio of less than $50,000 per life-year added, whereas studies in which the ICD did not reduce mortality led to higher costs and worse outcomes among ICD patients. A major health policy dilemma is whether widespread prophylactic ICD placement is worth the expenditure of more than a billion dollars per year.[24]

These studies illustrate several general points about the economic evaluation of procedures and devices. The initial cost of procedures and devices is often quite high, but long-term follow-up is necessary to assess the total net cost of the procedure relative to alternative therapies. An expensive procedure may have all, some, or none of its incremental costs recouped through prevention of costly adverse events. The higher cost may be only partially offset by later savings (e.g., coronary stents) or barely recovered at all (e.g., ICDs). Nevertheless, high initial costs of procedures and devices may be justified if survival is sufficiently improved or if quality of life is clearly and persistently enhanced. These considerations emphasize the importance of a long-term perspective in the economic evaluation of devices and procedures so that their full costs and benefits can be assessed.

Chronic Disease: Heart Failure

(see Chap. 23)

Economically efficient management of a chronic disease such as heart failure is different from that of an acute illness or a surgical procedure. In chronic diseases, the cost of care is spread over many years instead of being concentrated at the outset of treatment. Similarly, the benefits of treatment accrue only over a period of prolonged follow-up. Most medical care for chronic disease is delivered in an ambulatory, outpatient setting, and patient adherence to prescribed regimens has a substantial impact on the efficacy of therapy. Improvements in clinical and economic outcomes may come from either better therapies or better ways to deliver established therapies, or both.

Angiotensin converting enzyme (ACE) inhibitors have significantly improved survival of patients with heart failure (see Chaps. 26-29).[25] An economic appraisal of enalapril therapy based on the SOLVD trial results suggested that the added cost of enalapril was completely offset by the cost savings from fewer hospitalizations for heart failure. Projections of lifetime costs and life expectancy performed using a model suggested that the net lifetime cost per patient was only $25 and that life expectancy was increased by 0.30 life-years, yielding an extremely favorable cost-effectiveness ratio of $83 per life-year added. An overview of economic analyses of heart failure treatment[26] suggests use of ACE inhibitors is generally economically attractive.

An overview of randomized trials shows that beta-blockade reduces mortality among patients with congestive heart failure by 35% and reduces hospital admissions for heart failure to a similar degree. A cost-effectiveness model based on published data from clinical trials found beta blockers for heart failure improved survival and reduced societal costs.[27]

Aldosterone blockade with eplerenone reduced mortality in the EPHESUS trial. A cost-effectiveness analysis based on the trial data found higher net costs in eplerenone-treated patients but an acceptable cost-effectiveness ratio of $13,700 per life-year added.[28]

Most hospital admissions for heart failure result from lack of patient adherence to drug or dietary regimens, which suggests that disease management programs might improve both clinical outcomes and economic outcomes. An overview of randomized trials found hospitalizations were reduced and overall costs were generally lowered by various disease management programs.[29] Disease management programs have not been widely adopted, however, because economic incentives are misaligned in the fragmented U.S. healthcare reimbursement system. Hospitals lose revenue by preventing heart failure admissions, so only

TABLE 3–2 Clinical and Economic Outcomes of Randomized Trials of Lipid-Lowering Therapy

	Reductions per 1000 Patients			Cost per Patient ($)		
Study	*Deaths*	*Myocardial Infarction*	*Revascularization*	*Drug Treatment*	*Complications Prevented*	*Net*
Primary Prevention						
WOSCOPS	5	19	8	3700	100	3600
AFCAPS	4	26	31	4654	524	4130
Secondary Prevention						
4S	32	47	59	4650	3900	780
CARE	11	18	47	5550	1660	3890

integrated care systems have an incentive to pay the up-front cost of heart failure programs and recoup the later savings from reduced admissions.

Disease Prevention

Some disease prevention programs are both effective and inexpensive, as exemplified by vaccination for common infectious diseases that cut risk by more than 90% at the cost of only a few dollars. Unfortunately, most preventive measures are less effective in reducing the risk of disease and cost far more to implement. Vaccines are relatively inexpensive because they are given only two or three times in a patient's lifetime, whereas drugs to lower serum cholesterol or high blood pressure need to be taken daily for decades. Thus the cost-effectiveness of preventive programs varies considerably according to the risk level of the patients to be treated, the effectiveness of the intervention, and its cost.[30]

Hypercholesterolemia is a well-established, strong factor for coronary atherosclerosis, and HMG-CoA-reductase inhibitors ("statins"), which reduce low-density lipoprotein–cholesterol levels in a dose-responsive fashion, clearly reduce the risk of death and ischemic nonfatal cardiovascular events (see Chap. 45). Secondary prevention trials have consistently shown substantial reductions in the absolute rate of cardiac events in patients treated with statins. The efficacy of cholesterol lowering in primary prevention (i.e., in subjects without overt evidence of clinical disease) is significantly smaller than in secondary prevention.

The cost-effectiveness of HMG-CoA reductase therapy to prevent CHD varies from extremely favorable values in secondary prevention settings to quite unfavorable in lower-risk primary prevention settings (Table 3-2). The reason for this wide variation is that higher-risk patients have a greater absolute benefit from treatment than lower-risk patients. The Heart Protection Study examined the economic effects of simvastatin in 20,536 patients with vascular disease or diabetes. They examined five risk groups within the trial and found the cost per event averted varied inversely with a patient's 5-year risk. In the highest-risk group (42% 5-year risk), the cost was 4500 British pounds per event averted, whereas in the lowest risk group (12% 5-year risk), the cost was 31,000 British pounds per event averted.[31] Savings from averted revascularization procedures and cardiac hospitalizations offset much of the drug cost of statin treatment in the high-risk group, considerably enhancing the drug's cost-effectiveness. Clinical guidelines stress the importance of tailoring therapy to the patient's risk profile[32] to achieve optimal results.

Aspirin is a low-cost drug that is effective in primary prevention. In a model of 45-year-old men, aspirin therapy lowered overall costs and improved clinical outcomes.[33] Whether the addition of clopidogrel to aspirin is effective in preventing coronary disease at an acceptable risk for bleeding remains controversial. The CHARISMA trial found no evidence of clinical benefit for aspirin plus clopidogrel in 3284 high-risk primary prevention patients.[34] In the secondary prevention subgroup of this study, with 12,153 patients, clopidogrel produced a 12% relative reduction in cardiovascular death, MI, or stroke ($p = 0.046$).

Diagnostic Testing

Economic evaluation of diagnostic tests starts from the premise that the information provided by a test only has value if physicians use the information to change therapy and that the change in therapy then improves clinical outcomes. Thus the effectiveness of a test is gauged not solely by its information content, but by its ultimate, indirect effects on patient outcomes.

Tests that provide clinical value do so by adding to what is already known about the patient. In practical terms, the test needs to add independent information to what is available from the clinical history; physical examination; and simpler, cheaper tests. The information value of myocardial perfusion scans in the diagnosis of coronary artery disease, for example, must be judged by how much unique diagnostic and prognostic information they add to the clinical examination and the simpler stress electrocardiogram (see Chap. 13). The evaluation of diagnostic tests by measuring the incremental value of information they provide is analogous to the way that therapies are evaluated by documenting what they add compared with the best available alternative (e.g., how much better is t-PA than streptokinase for treatment of acute MI?). But the additional requirement placed on diagnostic tests is that they add enough information to modify decision-making. A test that is statistically more accurate does not provide value from an economic perspective unless greater accuracy leads to better clinical decisions. Demonstrations of a statistical improvement in diagnostic accuracy with new tests are common, but evaluations of the effects of this extra accuracy on clinical management are rare.

The use of routine coronary angiography in survivors of acute MI has been controversial, in large part due to conflicting evidence on the efficacy of routine versus selective angiography practices (see Chap. 20).[35] The VANQWISH trial found that routine angiography initially cost $4500 more than a conservative, ischemia-guided strategy and that the cost difference narrowed to $2200 after 2 years.[36] TIMI-18 found a similar pattern of costs with the invasive strategy costing $1667 more initially, narrowing to $670 at 6 months' follow-up.[37] FRISC-II also found the invasive approach to be more costly over 1 year.[38] Thus these randomized clinical trials consistently found the invasive strategy to be more costly than a conservative ischemia-guided approach. The cost-effectiveness of the invasive strategy depended on the clinical outcomes of the trial more than the economic outcomes. Studies that found better clinical results from the invasive strategy (TIMI-18 and FRISC-II) judged it to be cost-effective, whereas the trial that found poorer clinical outcomes from the invasive strategy (VANQWISH) judged it to be not economically attractive. A synthesis of the clinical and economic evaluations has not yet been performed, but these disparate findings underscore that economic assessment must be closely tied to clinical evaluation. Although costs can be readily measured, determination of value requires weighing the added costs against the improvement in outcomes.

Developments in Economic Analysis

Cost-effectiveness analysis has been applied to clinical medicine slightly more than 30 years. The initial studies were based largely on decision models and related analytic methods and were of more interest to researchers than clinicians. After considerable experience, consensus on some aspects of the methodology of economic analysis has been reached, although several areas of controversy remain. The most important recent development in cost-effectiveness analysis has been the inclusion of economic endpoints as part of randomized trials, providing rigorous prospective evaluation of the efficacy and efficiency of therapies. As in all arenas of clinical research, the methods of economic evaluation in clinical trials have become more sophisticated, with application of economic models to extend clinical trial findings. Future developments in cost-effectiveness analysis will include wider application of economic evaluations in international settings, improved cost-identification methods, and continued development of statistical methods appropriate to cost and outcome data from clinical trials.

REFERENCES

Key Economic Principles

1. Mark DB, Hlatky MA: Medical economics and the assessment of value in cardiovascular medicine: Part I. Circulation 106:516, 2002.
2. Mark DB, Hlatky MA: Medical economics and the assessment of value in cardiovascular medicine. Part II. Circulation 106:626, 2002.

Analysis of Specific Interventions

3. van Domburg RT, Sonnenschein K, Nieuwlaat R, et al: Sustained benefit 20 years after reperfusion therapy in acute myocardial infarction. J Am Coll Cardiol 46:15, 2005.
4. Mark DB, Hlatky MA, Califf RM, et al: Cost effectiveness of thrombolytic therapy with tissue plasminogen activator as compared with streptokinase for acute myocardial infarction. N Engl J Med 332:1418, 1995.
5. Keeley EC, Boura JA, Grines CL: Primary angioplasty versus intravenous thrombolytic therapy for acute myocardial infarction: A quantitative review of 24 randomised trials. Lancet 361:13, 2003.
6. Boersma E: Does time matter? A pooled analysis of randomized clinical trials comparing primary percutaneous coronary intervention and in-hospital fibrinolysis in acute myocardial infarction patients. Eur Heart J 27:779, 2005.
7. Hartwell D, Colquitt J, Loveman E, et al: Clinical effectiveness and cost-effectiveness of immediate angioplasty for acute myocardial infarction: Systematic review and economic evaluation. Health Technol Assess 17:1, 2005.
8. Machecourt J, Bonnefoy E, Vanzetto G, et al: Primary angioplasty is cost-minimizing compared with pre-hospital thrombolysis for patients within 60 min of a percutaneous coronary intervention center: The Comparison of Angioplasty and Pre-hospital Thrombolysis in Acute Myocardial Infarction (CAPTIM) cost-efficacy sub-study. J Am Coll Cardiol 45:515, 2005.
9. Brown RE, Henderson RA, Koster D, et al: Cost effectiveness of eptifibatide in acute coronary syndromes; an economic analysis of Western European patients enrolled in the PURSUIT trial. The Platelet IIa/IIb in Unstable Angina: Receptor Suppression Using Integrilin Therapy. Eur Heart J 23:50, 2002.
10. DeFrances CJ, Podgornik MN: 2004 National Hospital Discharge Survey. Advance data from vital and health statistics; no 371. Hyattsville, Md, National Center for Health Statistics, 2006.
11. Wong JB, Sonnenberg FA, Salem DN, Pauker SG: Myocardial revascularization for chronic stable angina. Analysis of the role of percutaneous transluminal coronary angioplasty based on data available in 1989. Ann Intern Med 113:852, 1990.
12. Katritsis DG, Ioannidis JPA: Percutaneous coronary intervention versus conservative therapy in nonacute coronary artery disease. A meta-analysis. Circulation 111:2906, 2005.
13. Sculpher M, Smith D, Clayton T, et al: Coronary angioplasty versus medical therapy for angina. Health service costs based on the second Randomized Intervention Treatment of Angina (RITA-2) trial. Eur Heart J 23:1291, 2002.
14. Claude J, Schindler C, Kuster GM, et al: Cost-effectiveness of invasive versus medical management of elderly patients with chronic symptomatic coronary artery disease. Findings of the randomized trial of invasive versus medical therapy in elderly patients with chronic angina (TIME). Eur Heart J 25:2195, 2004.
15. Hoffman SN, TenBrook JA, Wolf MP, et al: A meta-analysis of randomized controlled trials comparing coronary artery bypass graft with percutaneous transluminal coronary angioplasty: One- to eight-year outcomes. J Am Coll Cardiol 41:1293, 2003.
16. Hlatky MA, Boothroyd DB, Melsop KA, et al: Medical costs and quality of life 10 to 12 years after randomization to angioplasty or bypass surgery for multivessel coronary artery disease. Circulation 110:1960, 2004.
17. Legrand VMG, Serruys PW, Unger F, et al: Three-year outcome after coronary stenting versus bypass surgery for the treatment of multivessel disease. Circulation 109:1114, 2004.
18. Weintraub WS, Mahoney EM, Zhang Z, et al: One year comparison of costs of coronary surgery versus percutaneous coronary intervention in the stent or surgery trial. Heart 90:782, 2004.
19. Cohen DJ, Bakhai A, Shi C, et al: Cost-effectiveness of sirolimus-eluting stents for treatment of complex coronary stenoses: Results from the sirolimus-eluting balloon expandable stent in the treatment of patients with de novo native coronary artery lesions (SIRIUS) trial. Circulation 110:508, 2004.
20. van Hout BA, Serruys PW, Lemos PA, et al: One year cost effectiveness of sirolimus eluting stents compared with bare metal stents in the treatment of single native de novo coronary lesions: An analysis from the RAVEL trial. Heart 91:507, 2005.
21. Kaiser C, Brunner-La Rocca HP, Buser PT, et al: Incremental cost-effectiveness of drug-eluting stents compared with a third-generation bare-metal stent in a real-world setting: Randomised Basel Stent Kosten Effektivitats Trial (BASKET). Lancet 366:921, 2005.
22. Ezekowitz JA, Armstrong PW, McAlister FA: Implantable cardioverter defibrillators in primary and secondary prevention: A systematic review of randomized, controlled trials. Ann Intern Med 138:445, 2003.
23. Sanders GD, Hlatky MA, Owens DK: Cost effectiveness of implantable cardioverter-defibrillators. N Engl J Med 353:1471, 2005.
24. Hlatky MA, Sanders GD, Owens DK: Evidence-based medicine and policy: The case of the implantable cardioverter defibrillator. Health Aff (Millwood) 24:42, 2005.
25. Flather MD, Yusuf S, Køber L, et al: Long-term ACE-inhibitor therapy in patients with heart failure or left-ventricular dysfunction: a systematic overview of data from individual patients. Lancet 355:1575, 2000.
26. Weintraub WS, Cole J, Tooley JF: Cost and cost-effectiveness studies in heart failure research. Am Heart J 143:565, 2002.
27. Cowper PA, DeLong ER, Whellan DJ, et al: Economic effects of beta-blocker therapy in patients with heart failure. Am J Med 116:104, 2004.
28. Weintraub WS, Zhang Z, Mahoney EM, et al: Cost-effectiveness of eplerenone compared with placebo in patients with myocardial infarction complicated by left ventricular dysfunction and heart failure. Circulation 111:1106, 2005.
29. McAlister FA, Stewart S, Ferrua S, McMurray JJJV: Multidisciplinary strategies for the management of heart failure patients at high risk for admission. A systematic review of randomized trials. J Am Coll Cardiol 44:810, 2004.
30. Krumholz HM, Weintraub WS, Bradford WD, et al: Task Force #2—the cost of prevention: Can we afford it? Can we afford not to do it? J Am Coll Cardiol 40:603, 2002.
31. Heart Protection Study Collaborative Group: Cost-effectiveness of simvastatin in people at different levels of vascular disease risk: Economic analysis of a randomised trial in 20,536 individuals. Lancet 365:1779, 2005.
32. Third Report of the National Cholesterol Education Program (NCEP) Expert Panel on Detection, Evaluation, and Treatment of High Blood Cholesterol in Adults (Adult Treatment Panel III) final report. Circulation 106:3143, 2002.
33. Pignone M, Earnshaw S, Tice JA, Pletcher MJ: Aspirin, statins, or both drugs for the primary prevention of coronary heart disease events in men: A cost-utility analysis. Ann Intern Med 144:326, 2006.
34. Bhatt DL, Fox KAA, Hacke W, et al: Clopidogrel and aspirin versus aspirin alone for the prevention of atherothrombotic events. N Engl J Med 354:1706, 2006.

Diagnostic Testing

35. Mehta SR, Cannon CP, Fox KA, et al: Routine vs selective invasive strategies in patients with acute coronary syndromes: A collaborative meta-analysis of randomized trials. JAMA 293:2908, 2005.
36. Barnett PG, Chen S, Boden WE, et al: Cost-effectiveness of a conservative, ischemia-guided management strategy after non-Q-wave myocardial infarction. Results of a randomized trial. Circulation 105:680, 2002.
37. Mahoney EM, Jurkovitz CT, Chu H, et al: Cost and cost-effectiveness of an early invasive vs conservative strategy for the treatment of unstable angina and non-ST-segment elevation myocardial infarction. JAMA 288:1851, 2002.
38. Janzon M, Levin LA, Swahn E, The Fast Revascularization during InStability in Coronary artery disease (FRISC II) Investigators: Cost-effectiveness of an invasive strategy in unstable coronary artery disease. Results from the FRISC II invasive trial. Eur Heart J 23:31, 2002.

CHAPTER 4

Clinical Decision-Making in Cardiology

Harlan M. Krumholz

Clinical decision-making is central to all patient care activities and involves selecting an action from among alternatives. Along with performing procedures and providing comfort, deciding among options for the prevention, diagnosis, and treatment of disease constitutes one of the key competencies in our profession. Clinicians are continuously faced with decisions, some that are made deliberately and others urgently. Some decisions can be made in full partnership with patients; others must be made on behalf of patients. All of these decisions have consequences, and some will ultimately determine whether a patient will survive illness and recover without disability. Knowledge of medical evidence is necessary for physicians, but this knowledge needs to be properly integrated into an effective decision-making strategy that promotes the best interests of the patient.

Clinical decision-making is growing increasingly complex. The array of diagnostic and therapeutic options is expanding rapidly. The number of medical journals and published articles is burgeoning, challenging physicians to keep pace with advances in medical knowledge. The cost of care is escalating, which creates the potentially competing pressure to consider value in selecting among clinical strategies. The time available to make decisions is often brief, particularly with the shortening of the average patient visit.

Perhaps the biggest challenge of clinical decision-making is that decisions are almost always made under circumstances of uncertainty. The effect of a decision on the outcome of an individual patient can rarely be known. Clinical and basic research studies can provide guidance, but the relevance of that literature to an individual patient is often inexact.

Another complicating aspect of clinical decision-making is that the physician is not making choices in isolation. The clinician is more often in partnership with the patient, sharing the decision-making and recommending choices that respect the patient's preferences, values, and goals. Thus in the exact same clinical setting, the optimal decision varies on the basis of the patient. Moreover, especially in nonurgent situations, decision-making often occurs in close partnership with patients' families. This dynamic requires an approach that involves negotiation and advocacy rather than imposition.

The goal of this chapter is to provide an overview in which we highlight key issues in clinical decision-making in cardiology. The true breadth of the science of clinical decision-making is enormous, spanning the disciplines of statistics, sociology, psychology, economics, and political science, among others. Moreover, there are many issues to consider including hypothesis generation and refinement, use and interpretation of diagnostic tests, causal reasoning, diagnostic verification, therapeutic decision-making, and cognitive tools and pitfalls.[1] Nevertheless, clinicians should be familiar with certain key concepts that can assist them in enhancing their decision-making skills.

DIAGNOSTIC DECISION-MAKING

General Considerations

Diagnostic hypotheses are often generated from relatively little information, beginning with the presenting complaint.[2] Testing usually consists of strategies for corroborating or rejecting a given clinical hypothesis.

Many conceptual models of diagnostic reasoning underlie the approach of clinicians in various circumstances. Deductive inference describes the situation in which a clinician has a hypothesis that predicts future events. Then observations are assessed for their consistency with the hypothesis. Knowledge progresses according to the refinement of hypotheses. Inductive inference starts with observations and then develops an applicable hypothesis. Most of medical diagnosis is inductive inference, asking the question: Given the observation of the patient's condition, what is the likelihood of different diseases?

Many types of diagnostic reasoning exist. Kassirer[3] considered three major types: probabilistic, causal, and deterministic. The probabilistic approach relies on estimates of the likelihood of various conditions and outcomes and is usually based on clinical evidence. Causal (physiologic) reasoning is rooted in an extrapolation of an understanding of mechanism from basic science (anatomical, physiological, biochemical). Deterministic (rule-based) reasoning is usually in the form of unambiguous rules that are followed to expedite decision-making. These strategies can be complementary. Rationales for decisions should have strong foundations in mechanism and probability. Rules can assist decisions but must make clinical sense for a given individual.

Occasionally tensions develop among these types of reasoning. Individuals who employ probabilistic reasoning may be at odds with those who employ causal reasoning and are making decisions on the basis of their understanding of physiology or other fields rather than on clinical probabilities and evidence. Evidence indicates that decisions based solely on causal reasoning may not always generate the intended result, although it is commonly the only approach available to clinicians.

EXAMPLE. The decision to use a pulmonary artery catheter in critically ill patients or those with heart failure may evolve from causal reasoning. Knowledge of the pulmonary pressures should have value in managing the hemodynamic status of these patients on the basis of extrapolations of knowledge from pathophysiology. Responding to the catheter measurements should improve the likelihood of survival. However, clinical trials have failed to show benefit from this strategy.[4,5]

Deterministic reasoning can be used to develop rules that assist the implementation of best practice rapidly and reliably. The contrast between deterministic and other forms of reasoning may best be illustrated by the decisions prompted by the care of a patient with a sudden cardiac arrest. The initial resuscitation efforts, which include an assessment of the arrest, may best be reflexive, founded on rules based on the best science and codified by the American Heart Association,[6] because there is little time for deliberate decision-making about the diagnosis. The decisions are largely outlined in advance in explicit algorithms, reducing the cognitive burden. The algorithms, however, cannot be all-encompassing, and the clinical situation may require departure from the rules. The decision to depart from the rules or to end the resuscitation effort requires more complex decision-making and involves other models of reasoning.

Rules and algorithms are enabling structures rather than rigid, inviolable policies. Enabling structures are guides that obviate the need to expend our rather limited cognitive resources for problems that can be addressed quickly and effectively by the use of algorithms. They are intended to ensure that information is not omitted by mistake, rather than restricting the range of decisions that can be made. These rules, when anchored in science and filtered through clinical experts and endorsed by professional organizations, tend to provide a mechanism to elevate care and reduce unnecessary and sometimes harmful and/or wasteful variations in practice.

Employing deterministic reasoning should never supersede the interests of the patient. The rules exist to expedite clinical decisions that will result in proper, high-quality care, not to circumvent the importance of judgment. Thus practitioners delivering care dictated by deterministic reasoning must remain alert for circumstances that do not fit the usual pattern and are not appropriate for the rule.

DIAGNOSTIC TEST DECISION-MAKING

Practitioners use diagnostic tests to reduce uncertainty about the presence of disease. These tests are usually expressed in terms of sensitivity, specificity, likelihood ratio, and positive and negative predictive value. The effect of the diagnostic test results on the probability of disease can be calculated using Bayes' Theorem, which incorporates information about the prior probability and the test results.

In actual practice, however, few physicians employ information about test characteristics and make explicit use of the Bayesian approach. A survey of physicians found that only 3 percent implemented the recommended Bayesian methods[7] in decision-making. Almost 60 percent reported using sensitivity and specificity, but 95 percent did not do so formally. Other studies suggest that it is common for physicians to misuse this approach when asked to calculate probabilities for patients on the basis of the test results.[8,9]

For clinicians to be able to incorporate diagnostic test results into clinical decision-making, they should be familiar with the following definitions.

Sensitivity and Specificity[10]

Sensitivity: among those with disease, the proportion with a positive test (true positive)

Specificity: among those without disease, the proportion with a negative test (true negative)

These test characteristics can assist in the diagnosis. High sensitivity tests have low false-negative rates. A test with a high sensitivity will be positive in almost all individuals with the condition being tested. Thus a negative test with high sensitivity makes the diagnosis highly unlikely, essentially ruling out the condition. Conversely, a test with high specificity will have a low false-positive rate. A test with a high specificity will be negative in virtually all individuals without the condition being tested. Thus a positive test with high specificity makes the diagnosis highly likely. A mnemonic is often used for this relationship: SpPIn (high specificity, positive, rules in) and SnNOut (high sensitivity, negative, rules out).

PREDICTIVE VALUES[11]

Positive Predictive Value: among those with a positive test, the proportion that has the disease

$$PPV = sens*prev/[sens*prev + (1 - spec)*(1 - prev)]$$

Negative Predictive Value: among those with a negative test, the proportion that does not have the disease

$$NPV = spec*(1 - prev)/[(1 - spec)*prev + spec*(1 - prev)]$$

Predictive values are more clinically informative than sensitivity and specificity. This value conveys information about how the test result translates into the likelihood that the patient has or does not have the disease. The key insight about predictive values is that, unlike sensitivity and specificity, they are highly dependent on disease prevalence. If the prevalence is low, a positive highly sensitive and specific test will still not yield a high likelihood of disease (i.e., the test has a low positive predictive value). The implication is that even with a test with high sensitivity and specificity, the screening of a low-risk population will still yield many false-positives.

EXAMPLE. A young woman comes to your office with a test result of a positive exercise stress test because of electrocardiographic changes despite good exercise tolerance. She has no traditional risk factors for coronary artery disease including family history and wonders whether this is likely an indication that she has heart disease. If her risk of disease were to be 1 in 1 million and the stress test were to have a sensitivity and specificity of 75 percent, you could calculate that for every 4 million women in her risk group, 4 would have disease and 3 would have a positive test. Of the almost 4 million without disease, 1 million would have a positive test. Therefore for every 1 million positive tests, only about 3 would represent a true positive. Even if the screening test had a sensitivity and specificity of 99 percent, then for every 10 million women screened, 10 would have disease and 9 would have a positive test. Of the approximately 10 million without disease, 100,000 would have a positive test. Thus for every approximately 100,000 positive tests, only 9 would represent a true positive.

BAYES THEOREM[12]

Bayes Theorem relates the change in probability given new information. The posterior, or post-test, probability is a function of the prior, or pre-test, probability (or disease prevalence) and the likelihood ratio. This theorem provides a way to revise probabilities based on new information. In essence, it relates a conditional probability: the probability of A given B.

LIKELIHOOD RATIO[13-15]

Likelihood Ratio: the ratio of the probability of a certain test result in people with the disease to the probability in people without the disease

$$LR+ = sens/(1 - spec)$$

$$LR- = (1 - sens)/spec$$

The LR, which is an expression of diagnostic accuracy, can range from 0 to infinity. The posttest odds that a patient has the disease can be calculated with the LR: pretest odds * LR. An LR value of 1.0 does not modify the posttest probability, thus indicating a test that provides no useful information. If the LR is much greater than 1, it is providing substantial information. The effect of the LR on pretest probabilities is not linear. Nomograms assist the conversion of pretest to posttest probabilities. Although it would seem that the LR would simplify the calculation of posttest probabilities, at least one study suggests that it is not better than sensitivity and specificity.[16]

Importantly, the likelihood ratio may indicate if the test is useful, but if the prevalence is low, the test may still not be a good indicator of disease, as the pretest probability of disease is low. An important implication of testing patients with very low or high pretest probabilities of disease is that test results may be more likely to mislead than enlighten. False-positives and false-negatives should be expected in these situations.

A memory aid by McGee suggests that for pretest probabilities between 10 and 90 percent, the change in probability can be approximated by a constant.[17] In approximate terms, an LR of 2 increases the probability by about 15 percent; an LR of 5 by 30 percent; and an LR of 10 by 45 percent.

Clinicians commonly misunderstand basic information about risk and benefit, particularly as it relates to testing. Some experts have suggested that the use of probabilities hinders clinicians in making decisions and propose that information be expressed as natural frequencies.[8] When asking physicians to calculate the positive predictive value of a test on the basis of prevalence, sensitivity, and specificity they commonly err. Their success is improved if the problem is restated in natural frequencies, indicating that for every 10,000 people, the number with the disease, the number with a positive test, and for those without the disease, the number with a positive test.

The perceived value of a diagnostic test will depend importantly on the accurate characterization of the test characteristics and the pretest probability. The validity of sensitivity and specificity for a test depends importantly on the quality of the studies that generated these values.[18] In high-quality studies the diagnostic test should be compared with a gold standard that is measured independently. Stable estimates of test characteristics require large study populations. The study of test characteristics may be too small to define with precision the performance of the tests. A recent analysis of published studies of diagnostic accuracy found that only 5 percent reported a priori sample size calculations.[19]

Several types of bias may also threaten the validity of studies of diagnostic tests. Studies of tests in populations that do not resemble those seen in clinical practice (spectrum bias) may artificially inflate estimates of test characteristics. Partial verification bias may occur if the gold standard is applied differentially to individuals on the basis of the results of the test. Some studies have even used the test being evaluated as part of the definition of the reference standard (incorporation bias). In addition, the test in practice may not be performed or interpreted with the skill that was present in published studies, again degrading its performance compared with claims. These biases must be considered in assessing the applicability of published estimates of sensitivity and specificity in practice.

Another important issue in the use of diagnostic tests is the definition of normal. By convention, test results are often characterized in a binary fashion (normal/abnormal), which is a translation from a continuous result. Expert decision-makers appreciate that thresholds are often arbitrary and have no special meaning. In some cases thresholds are based on a Gaussian distribution of results in a nondiseased population and define abnormal as more than two standard deviations from the mean. Alternatively, the threshold may be designated on the basis of a range beyond which disease becomes more probable. In other cases it could be that the cutpoint is based on information about the range in which treatment is effective. In any case, clinicians should appreciate that not all abnormal designations are equivalent and a value that barely crosses the threshold may carry different information than one that is far across the threshold. Clinicians lose information and potentially undermine decisions when they focus on tests as binary instead of continuous outcomes.

The value of a test in discriminating disease in a population is often characterized by its performance across a range of cutpoints, producing what is described as a receiver operator characteristic (ROC) curve. These curves were developed in the 1950s in work to differentiate signal to noise. The area under the ROC curve is a measure of the discrimination of a test, where an area under the ROC curve 0.5 identifies a test with no diagnostic value and 1.0 provides perfect discrimination. These curves are not only often used to determine the overall discrimination of a test across a spectrum of test values but also to determine the optimal cutoff that balances the best combination of sensitivity and specificity.

Test Ordering

Sackett and Haynes[20] have described a sequence of questions that should be answered to assess the value of diagnostic tests. The preliminary questions establish whether test results in affected patients differ from those in normal individuals and whether patients with certain test results are more likely to have a particular disorder. These initial evaluations can establish only the promise of the test, but not whether it is useful. They serve as initial screens, providing information about whether further evaluation is necessary. It is also important to know whether the test results distinguish between people with and without a certain condition from among those in whom the test might reasonably be applied (those in whom the disease might be suspected). Sometimes a test is initially evaluated in a population of patients who have a severe manifestation of a condition and in whom there is little diagnostic uncertainty. It is preferable to evaluate the test in a population with diagnostic uncertainty because that is the group to which the test will likely be applied. Ultimately, though, the key question is whether patients undergoing the test have better outcomes than those who are not tested. Unfortunately, too few tests have been subjected to this full spectrum of scrutiny.

The construct of number needed to treat can also apply to screening tests.[21] The number needed to screen, which is defined as the number of people who need to be screened over a defined period to prevent an adverse event, takes into account the number of people tested to identify those eligible for a treatment and the benefit of that treatment among those identified. The measure highlights the importance of linking screening to actual patient benefit.

In deciding about whether to recommend diagnostic tests, clinicians should envision the actions that would occur on the basis of the results. If findings would not change clinical strategies in ways that are likely to improve outcomes, the test should probably not be ordered.[22] For example, screening asymptomatic patients for coronary calcium may have prognostic value, but there is little information that such an approach will improve survival or avert events, even through behavioral change. Decisions about testing need to consider the risks of the test itself (e.g., radiation exposure or invasive instrumentation), as well as the downstream risks and benefits of the procedures and tests that may occur as a result of a positive test (e.g., cardiac catheterization and revascularization). Prior work has also described a testing cascade whereby initial tests, which may be considered inexpensive and benign, inevitably lead to more interventions.[23]

THERAPEUTIC DECISION-MAKING

Decisions about therapy involve weighing risks and benefits to determine the best course of action. The key question for clinical decision-makers is whether an intervention can improve the quantity and/or quality of the patient's life.

Clinicians are challenged to take into account complex trade-offs among treatment strategies. In some situations a strategy is clearly favored because of its high safety and effectiveness. In these cases, deterministic reasoning strategies, guided by rules, often dominate. In other situations, decisions are less clear and require probabilistic or causal reasoning. Not uncommonly in these situations, no therapeutic strategy is clearly dominant. Ultimately, it is important that decisions are grounded in the best data available and not merely intuition.

Clinicians should be aware of the strength of evidence in support of therapeutic decisions. The strongest evidence derives from well-conducted randomized trials. Observational studies and case series can provide useful information but are usually less definitive. Regardless of design, clinicians should not assume that all published studies including randomized trials are of high quality. Criteria for assessing studies are available, though a description is beyond the scope of this chapter.[24]

Clinical practice guidelines from the American College of Cardiology and the American Heart Association (AHA) grade their recommendations with information about the strength of evidence. Level of evidence A is associated with evidence derived from multiple randomized trials or meta-analyses. Level of evidence B is based on a single trial or nonrandomized trials. Level of evidence C is based solely on the consensus opinion of experts, case studies, or standard-of-care, which may be derived primarily from causal reasoning.

Unfortunately, even if high-quality studies are available, precise estimates of risks and benefits are not often available for individual patients. Although the internal validity of a study may be strong, the external validity, or generalizability, may be less clear, because patients in routine practice often do not resemble those enrolled in trials. The extrapolation of the trial results may be difficult. Moreover, clinicians must reconcile average results from large numbers of patients to the decision about an individual patient who will experience the consequence of the decision only once.

DECISION ANALYSIS

Decision analysis was developed to assist in the quantification of therapeutic decisions. This approach seeks to make explicit the assumptions that underlie recommendations. The method takes into account the probabilities of different outcomes and the value (or utility) of various outcomes from the patient's perspective. With the repeating of the analysis with varying assumptions about probabilities and utilities, this approach can reveal how sensitive the decision is to particular factors and under what conditions a specific strategy is favored. A decision analysis cannot mandate a choice. It is a tool intended to assist in illuminating the trade-offs inherent in a decision occurring under conditions of uncertainty.

EXAMPLE. The decision about whether to administer fibrinolytic therapy to patients who are 80 years and older was controversial when the therapy was first introduced. Some clinicians had concerns that the bleeding risk might offset the benefit of restoring blood flow in the coronary artery. A decision analysis modeled the decision, incorporating estimates of the risks and benefits of therapy.[25] In addition, the analysis evaluated the decision across a range of estimates for risk and benefit. The study demonstrated that across a broad range of estimates of risks and benefits, the decision to treat was, on average, favored. The insight from the analysis was that even a small relative reduction in risk produced a substantial absolute reduction in the number of deaths that overshadowed the risk of bleeding. Using the best estimates for benefit, the decision favored treatment until the risk of hemorrhagic stroke rose to above 4 percent.

Evidence

The interpretation of evidence has many subtleties. Several topics bear particular emphasis because they are commonly the source of misunderstanding and can compromise the quality of decisions.

p VALUES

Statistical issues play a key role in therapeutic decision-making. The *p* value, in particular, has taken on great weight in clinical studies. This value represents the probability that the result observed, or a more extreme one, could have occurred under the null hypothesis. Because the null hypothesis generally proposes that there is no effect, the *p* value represents the probability that the observation occurred by chance in the absence of an effect of the factor studied. If the null hypothesis is rejected, then the alternative hypothesis is usually favored, suggesting the presence of an effect. The *p* value conveys the probability of the data given the null hypothesis is true, but not the probability that the null hypothesis is true given the data. The *p* value is not a measure of the probability that the null hypothesis is false. In fact, under the right conditions, the probability that the null hypothesis is false may be low even with a *p* value less than 0.05.[26,27] Other views about how to approach statistical inference exist. Bayesian statisticians reject *p* values in favor of the approach of using data to update their estimates of a certain parameter. Despite growing support for the Bayesian approach, hypothesis testing continues to dominate.

Because the *p* value is so commonly used in clinical research, clinicians must be aware of several key issues. First, the threshold of 0.05 for statistical significance is arbitrary. A *p* value of 0.04 implies that the data could occur 4 percent of the time if the null hypothesis is true, and a *p* value of 0.06 would suggest that the data would occur 6 percent of the time. Is the difference between 6 and 4 percent enough to reject the null hypothesis in one case and accept it in another? Clinicians should understand that *p* values have continuous values and are one piece of information among many. For example, confidence intervals convey the range of plausible values for a given parameter. Second, *p* values do not inform about clinical importance. A large study sample can produce a small *p* value despite a clinically inconsequential difference between groups. Clinicians need to examine the size of the effects in addition to the statistical tests of whether the results could have occurred by chance. Statistics cannot supplant clinical judgment.

EXPRESSIONS OF RISK AND BENEFIT. Clinical decisions involve the balancing of benefit and risk. The expression of benefit and risk can influence decisions. Clinicians need to have an understanding of these expressions because they are the foundation for making decisions from clinical evidence.

The relative benefit (or risk) of an intervention is often expressed as a relative risk or odds ratio. Risk is the probability of an event and odds is the probability an event will occur against the probability that it will not occur. A probability of 25 percent (1 in 4) represents odds of 1:3 or 1/3. The relative risk ratio of an event conveys the relative probability that an event will occur when two groups are compared. The odds ratio expresses the odds of the event in one group compared with another.

Despite its widespread use, the odds ratio is less helpful than relative risk in clinical decision-making. The expressions are similar when baseline event rates are low (<5 percent) but deviate with higher risk and larger treatment effects. The odds ratio can express associations but, unlike the risk ratio, it cannot express the relative size of the treatment effect; if clinicians assume it to be equivalent to risk, it may lead to overestimates of the treatment effect. The odds ratio is common in clinical research because of its mathematical properties and is good for identifying associations in certain situations, but clinicians need to know its limitations for decision-making.

The relative benefit may vary depending on patient characteristics, which is often explored in subgroup analyses. For example, fibrinolytic therapy was effective in the treatment of suspected acute myocardial infarction (AMI) and subgroup analyses revealed the benefit to be substantial in patients with ST-elevation but not in those without it.[28] The challenge is that subgroup analyses introduce the possibility that associations have occurred only by chance. In ISIS-2 the authors provided perspective on subgroup analyses by demonstrating that patients born under the astrological signs of Gemini or Libra were significantly less likely to benefit from fibrinolytic therapy. Thus subgroup analysis is capable of producing important insights but must be interpreted with caution.[29]

A weakness of relative benefit estimates is that they do not convey information about what is achieved for patients at varying levels of risk. A small relative reduction in risk may be meaningful for a high-risk patient, whereas a large relative reduction may be inconsequential for a low-risk patient. Absolute risk reduction, the difference between two rates, varies with the risk of an individual patient. For example, a risk ratio of 2.0 does not distinguish between baseline risks of 80 and 30 percent and between 0.08 and 0.03 percent. In one case the absolute difference is 50 percent (5000 per 10,000), and in the other it is 0.05 percent (5 per 10,000). In one case 1 of 2 persons is benefited, and in the other 1 of 2000 is benefited.

Number needed to treat (NNT), which can be calculated as the inverse of the absolute risk reduction, represents the number of people who need to be treated to prevent an adverse event. NNTs are a useful approach to express risk and benefit that incorporates the patient's baseline risk[30] and a convenient way to express a trial result. For decision-making with an individual patient, the baseline risk, which cannot be assumed to be the same as that of people in a trial, will strongly influence the estimate. Therefore the NNT from the trial may need to be modified for an individual patient.

EXAMPLE. Physicians and their patients are often in a position to decide whether aspirin should be used for primary prevention of cardiovascular disease. To make the example easier, let us assume the patient is male and a physician, the group for which the most data exists. Some of the best information about this topic is from the Physicians' Health Study (PHS) Research Group, which enrolled 22,071 doctors in a randomized, double-blind, placebo-controlled trial of the effect of 325 mg of aspirin every other day (versus placebo) on cardiovascular risk.[31] The study was terminated early because the findings strongly favored aspirin. The investigators reported a 44 percent reduction in the risk of an AMI. The relative reduction sounds impressive, but the absolute reduction in risk is less compelling. The overall risk of an AMI in this population was low, 440 per 100,000 per year in the placebo group. Thus a 44 percent reduction in a low-risk population only averted about 186 events per 100,000 treated (in the trial 100 AMIs [93 percent nonfatal] were averted with 54,560 person years of treatment]. In other words, about 540 physicians needed to take aspirin every other day for a year for 1 person to avoid an AMI. The other 539 did not experience a benefit. On the other hand, there was a strong trend toward doubling the admittedly small risk of incurring a hemorrhagic stroke (relative risk 2.14; 95 percent confidence interval, 0.96 to 4.77; $p = 0.06$). Overall, there were 11 extra hemorrhagic strokes. For every nine AMIs that were avoided, there was one additional hemorrhagic stroke. The overall risk of stroke was slightly, but insignificantly, elevated in the aspirin group (relative risk 1.22; 95 percent confidence interval, 0.93 to 1.60; $p = 0.15$), which also represented 11 extra strokes in the aspirin group. The risk of death was not significantly different in the two groups (relative risk 0.96; 95 percent confidence interval, 0.80 to 1.14; $p = 0.64$). The expression of the result as an absolute risk reduction provides a perspective for the individual patient that is easier to understand than the relative reduction in risk. The main point is that the reporting of a large relative reduction in risk provides only part of the relevant information to make this decision and that presentation can affect the decision.

The evidence that 540 physicians need to take aspirin every other day for a year for 1 person to benefit, with a cost of an additional stroke for every 9 AMIs averted, is difficult to translate into action without incorporating preferences. Some patients may find that result favorable, and others not. Also, people can be overwhelmed by too much information and information on risk may be difficult to understand.

For perspective on this issue, we can look to guidelines from the American Heart Association and the recommendation from the U.S. Preventive Services Task Force (USPSTF). In 2002 the AHA Guidelines for Primary Prevention of Cardiovascular Disease and Stroke recommended that aspirin be considered in people with a high coronary heart disease risk (10-year risk of 10 percent or higher), much higher than what was observed in the PHS.[32] Also in 2002, the USPSTF endorsed the use of aspirin for primary prevention of cardiovascular events only in patients with a high risk of coronary heart disease (5-year risk ≥3 percent).[33] This rate compares with the 5-year risk of AMI in the PHS of 0.9 percent (see Chap. 54).

Another key concept in considering the effect of interventions is the timing of the risk or benefit. Summary expressions can obscure important differences. Small benefit by a large number of patients may appear the same as large benefits in a few patients. This information may be important to patients. Clinicians should know how benefit (or risk) is accrued to be in the best position to inform patients and make recommendations for interventions.

RISK STRATIFICATION. Risk stratification is often used to estimate patient risk and assist in decision-making. This approach generally employs the results of statistical models that have identified prognostic factors and incorporated them into a tool that may assist clinicians. In recent years many tools have been developed to assist in the rapid assessment of patients. For example, the TIMI risk score for unstable angina/non-ST elevation MI uses seven readily available variables to predict the risk of death and ischemic events.[34] The number of risk factors produced a range of risk from 5 percent (0/1 risk factors) to 41 percent (6/7 risk factors).

In evaluating risk stratification studies, it is important to consider whether the score or approach has been validated in populations similar to the patients to whom it is applied in practice. The predictors should have been collected independently of knowledge of the outcome. The outcome and time frame should be appropriate for clinical decisions. The value of the stratification should also be clear. Improving precision in risk estimates without consequence is like ordering tests that have no implications for treatment.

RISK-TREATMENT PARADOX. Several studies have shown a risk-treatment paradox in which the higher-risk patients are least likely to receive interventions that are expected to provide a benefit.[35,36] This pattern is paradoxical because the high-risk patients would be expected to have the most to gain from an intervention that reduces risk, assuming that the relative reduction in risk is constant across groups defined by their baseline risk.

OUTCOMES AND TIMING. Additional considerations in assessing the potential effect of interventions are the outcome that is evaluated and the time period assessed. Articles about patients with cardiovascular disease often focus on cardiovascular events including cardiovascular death, but patients would be expected to have more interest in all-cause mortality. If averting cardiovascular death merely leads to death from other causes, there is little value to the patient. This issue is particularly important for older patients with other conditions, often called *competing risks*.[37] Moreover, even a short-term advantage in mortality, conferred, for example, by bypass surgery, may not be valued by the patient if other conditions and complications diminish the quality of that time. Quality of life and health status are commonly neglected in clinical studies but are important to patients. Thus narrowly focusing on specific outcomes may obscure important insights about an intervention. The challenge is that evaluating many outcomes in a trial can increase the likelihood of false-positive findings.[38] Another important issue with outcomes is that intermediate or surrogate outcomes, such as change in ejection fraction, do not always correspond to outcomes such as survival.

EFFICACY/EFFECTIVENESS. Efficacy is what can be achieved by interventions under ideal circumstances, such as in the setting of a clinical trial. In contrast, effectiveness describes the effect in actual practice. Therapeutic decisions are often based on the assumption that the efficacy and effectiveness of interventions are identical, which is not always the case.

SHARED DECISION-MAKING. Clinical decisions are not the sole domain of physicians. The principle of autonomy maintains that patients retain control over their bodies and must consent to undergo interventions, except in rare circumstances. Informed consent is the cornerstone of this concept. Unfortunately, there is little consensus about how best to involve patients and about the problem of heterogeneity among patients in their preference to participate actively[39] in decision-making. Nevertheless, given the need to align goals of therapy with the patient's preferences and values, it is important to engage them, if possible. This approach is most appropriate for major decisions, especially those with intermediate or low certainty, and those that are not emergent.

Many aspects of communicating risks and benefits exist. First, this information takes many forms. The dimensions of risk and benefit include their identity, permanence, timing, probability, and value to an individual patient.[40] All should be considered in decision-making.

It is known that patients do not always understand benefit and risk well. For example, in a study of patients who had given consent for elective percutaneous coronary intervention (see Chap. 52), an intervention that does not improve survival or prevent AMI in this context, 75 percent thought it would prevent an AMI and 71 percent thought it would improve survival.[41] Moreover, only 46 percent could identify at least one possible complication. Among this group, 67 percent stated that they should be involved at least equally with the physician in making decisions. These deficiencies in patient understanding need to be addressed for shared decision-making to occur.

The manner in which information is presented may influence patients. Like physicians, patients are also susceptible to framing effects.[42] Patients tend to be more likely to choose a therapy that is presented as having an advantage over an alternative in relative rather than absolute terms. The relative effect is almost always much greater than the absolute change. Patients may also be influenced by the order in which information is provided. For example, patients were more favorable to aspirin therapy if the discussion of risks occurred after the benefits.[43]

Some techniques have been proposed to help clinicians convey risk.[44] First, clinicians should avoid descriptive terms only because they may not have a consistent meaning to patients. Terms such as "low risk" may be difficult for people to interpret. If clinicians express risk as ratios, they should use a consistent denominator (e.g., 40 of 1000 and 5 of 1000 instead of 1 in 25 and 1 in 200). Clinicians should offer multiple perspectives, revealing multiple ways of thinking about risk. They should use absolute numbers, not relative risks. Visual aids are useful because poor numeracy or literacy skills may be a barrier for many patients. Many patients do not understand risk communication formats.[45] In addition, clinicians should recognize that information and data are not the same and it is incumbent on the clinician to communicate health information that is meaningful to the patient.

Shared decision-making can be understood as having five phases: assess, advise, agree, assist, and arrange (the "five As"). First, the clinician must assess the patient. Then, the clinician should advise the patient of the options, with their benefits and risks. Next, the clinician and patient should agree on a plan that is aligned with the patient's preferences and values. The clinician should then assist the patient in implementing the plan. Finally, the patient and clinician arrange follow-up. An example of this approach was described for the care of patients with systolic hypertension, for which there are many issues that remain controversial, such as whether patients with minor elevations in blood pressure should be treated.[46]

Cognitive Errors

Cognitive errors can undermine clinical decisions.[47] Some examples of these errors are described as follows.

HEURISTICS OR RULES OF THUMB. Clinicians tend to rely on heuristics, or rules of thumb, to assess probabilities and support complex cognitive tasks required for decision-making.[48] These heuristics can be useful because they allow shortcuts in reasoning but are also vulnerable to important errors and can undermine decisions.

Many medical heuristics are familiar.[49] Occam's razor suggests that a clinician should choose the simplest explanation for a set of observations. Sutton's law, named for a bank robber who explained his action by stating "that's where the money is" encourages clinicians to focus their attention where they will get the most yield.

Heuristics can be useful but may contribute to errors. The following limited set provides some examples of the heuristics that may be helpful in some settings but can cause cognitive errors in others.

The availability heuristic leads clinicians to estimate probability by how readily they can remember examples. Clinicians may estimate the probability of a disease because of its ease of recall. Thus a more recent experience with a certain illness may make someone believe it is more common than it is.

The anchoring heuristic leads people to stay with their initial impressions. This heuristic can mislead if clinicians do not refine initial impressions. A form of this heuristic, called *premature closure,* can lead clinicians to prematurely stop pursuing alternative explanations.

FRAMING EFFECTS. Like their patients, clinicians are sensitive to the framing of information. That is, the same truth is acted on differently depending on the way the information is presented. Clinicians (and patients) need to recognize their sensitivity to the framing of the data. Clinicians are more likely to use a new therapy when presented with the relative reduction in risk rather than the absolute reduction.[50] When presented trial results, physicians rated treatment effectiveness higher when presented with relative risk reductions compared with absolute risk reductions.[51] Physicians can address this error by reframing decisions and being aware of the effect of the presentation of the data on perceptions of benefit.

BLIND OBEDIENCE. The unwavering acceptance of the diagnosis of an authority (test or person) can lead to ignoring information that is clearly discordant. Wise clinicians have the courage to question authority when the information does not provide a clear answer. The persistence of good decision-makers and their refusal to blindly follow the crowd often leads to important insights. The best interests of the patient should guide clinicians and give them the strength to respectfully question authority, when appropriate.

Accuracy of Evidence

An important aspect of clinical decision-making is the accuracy of the primary information on which the decisions are based. Clinicians need to ensure that the evidence is coherent and consistent. Does the evidence, in its totality, make sense? Clinicians must be prepared to review the primary data, particularly when some information is inconsistent with other information. The clinician should be equipped with the knowledge that errors in reporting and interpretation occur too commonly. Moreover, aside from errors, disagreement in interpretations happens frequently. In 1976 Zir[52] reported a classic article of interobserver variability on the basis of the readings of 20 angiograms by four experienced coronary angiographers at Massachusetts General Hospital. The readers agreed about the significance of a stenosis (defined as greater than 50 percent luminal narrowing) in only 65 percent of the cases. They disagreed about the significance of lesions in the left main coronary artery in 15 percent of the cases. Others have reported similar issues with this test and others. Clinicians need to be willing to re-evaluate primary data in order to ensure that decisions are based on the best information. They should be equipped with the knowledge that information is often imperfect even as it may be reported dogmatically.

ADOPTION OF INNOVATION

In the course of clinical decision-making, physicians are continuously exposed to new information and innovation. Decisions must be made about whether to adopt new practices. The Diffusion of Innovations model, promoted by Everett Rogers, describes an S-shaped curve whereby some people adopt early and others later, with most adopting after an initial delay.[53] In medicine, this type of diffusion is commonly observed.

New information does affect practice.[54] Lamas and colleagues[55] analyzed practice from 1987 through 1990 with patients enrolled in the Survival and Ventricular Enlargement trial and found that the use of medications over this period changed with the publication of other trials. For example, the publication of the Second International Study of Infarct Survival (ISIS-2) was associated with an odds increase of 228 percent compared with the prior period. Nevertheless, rates were still low almost 5 years after ISIS-2, with only 61 percent of Medicare beneficiaries being treated.[56] This pattern is seen for many different interventions. Ten years after pivotal trials showing the efficacy of beta blockers for survivors of an AMI, only 50 percent of Medicare beneficiaries without contraindications were being treated with these medications.[57] A cumulative meta-analysis showed that evidence often becomes conclusive before it is incorporated into authoritative texts and review articles.[58] On the other hand, the experience with spironolactone has shown that even when new therapies are adopted, they may be applied to populations that were excluded from the trials because of concerns about risks.[59] The appreciation of the need to improve the appropriate incorporation of new knowledge into clinical practice has spurred efforts to improve quality of care.

A particular challenge to clinicians is the ever-changing nature of the medical literature. Clinicians must be ready to adopt new information into practice but be skeptical of early findings and claims. Ioannidis[60] examined all original research studies published between 1990 and 2003 in the three general medical journals with the current highest impact factor (*New England Journal of Medicine*, *Journal of the American Medical Association*, and *Lancet*) or in medical specialty journals with an impact factor exceeding 7.0 (according to the *Journal Citation Reports 2003*) that are likely to publish clinical research, and he screened all articles with more than 1000 citations. He then compared the result with subsequent studies with comparable or larger samples and similar or better designs. He identified 49 articles, of which 45 reported that an intervention was effective and 16 percent were contradicted in subsequent studies. His conclusion was that highly cited research of clinical interventions is often contradicted or weakened in subsequent publications.

Another aspect of decision-making is the recognition of our knowledge limitations. Expert medical decision-makers continuously pursue new knowledge and make use of opportunities with patients to learn about new information. The Internet makes it possible to gain rapid access to extensive information. Systematic reviews provide an overview of the literature on particular topics.

The best way to determine if evidence is sufficiently strong to support practice change is by referring to Clinical Practice Guidelines and Performance Measures that are published by the American College of Cardiology and the AHA. Guidelines grade and synthesize the current evidence and provide recommendations about practice. Other trustworthy recommendations on specific topics are available from the USPSTF and the Cochrane Collaboration. Performance measures are distinct from guidelines in that they identify key processes of care that are considered essential for high quality care.[61,62]

Information Technology and Systems

The health care system has increasingly recognized the role of tools and systems to enhance decision-making. With increasing emphasis on systems of care and an ever-expanding evidence base, the role of information technology in assisting decision-making is growing. The challenge is to demonstrate that these systems provide a net benefit for patients at a reasonable cost or cost savings without worsening their outcomes. These new technologies should optimally be exposed to the same scrutiny as new drugs or devices. Studies have already indicated that systems with good face validity may not demonstrate benefit when studied under the rigorous conditions of a randomized trial.[63] Nevertheless, these systems hold the potential of incorporating algorithms that can improve decision-making and decrease errors.

CONCLUSION

Clinical decision-making is the cornerstone of good clinical care. Physicians must not only have knowledge of the field but be prepared to use it in ways that optimize the care and outcomes of patients. Good judgment requires an ability to interpret evidence, weigh risks and benefits, and understand and promote the preferences and values of patients.

CLASSIC READING

Eddy D: Clinical Decision Making: From Theory to Practice: A Collection of Essays from the Journal of the American Medical Association. 1st ed. Boston, Jones & Bartlett Publishers, 1996.

Guyatt GH, Rennie D (eds): Users' Guides to the Medical Literature: A Manual for Evidence-Based Clinical Practice (book and CD-ROM). Chicago, American Medical Association, 2001.

Kassirer J, Kopelman R: Learning Clinical Reasoning. Philadelphia, Lippincott Williams & Wilkins, 1991.

Sox HC, Blatt MA, Higgins M, Marton KI: Medical Decision Making. Philadelphia, Butterworth-Heinemann, 1988.

Strauss SE, Richardson WS, Glasziou P, Haynes RB: Evidence-Based Medicine. 3rd ed. Philadelphia, Churchill Livingstone, 2005.

REFERENCES

Diagnostic Decision-Making

1. Kassirer JP, Kopelman RI: Learning Clinical Reasoning. Baltimore, Williams & Wilkins, 1991.
2. Kassirer JP, Gorry GA: Clinical problem solving: A behavioral analysis. Ann Intern Med 89:245, 1978.
3. Kassirer JP. Diagnostic reasoning. Ann Intern Med 110:893, 1989.
4. Binanay C, Califf RM, Hasselblad V, et al: Evaluation study of congestive heart failure and pulmonary artery catheterization effectiveness: The ESCAPE trial. JAMA 294:1625, 2005.
5. Shah MR, Hasselblad V, Stevenson LW, et al: Impact of the pulmonary artery catheter in critically ill patients: Meta-analysis of randomized clinical trials. JAMA 294:1664, 2005.
6. 2005 American Heart Association Guidelines for Cardiopulmonary Resuscitation and Emergency Cardiovascular Care. Circulation 112:IV1, 2005.

Diagnostic Test Decision-Making

7. Reid MC, Lane DA, Feinstein AR: Academic calculations versus clinical judgments: Practicing physicians' use of quantitative measures of test accuracy. Am J Med 104:374, 1998.
8. Hoffrage U, Lindsey S, Hertwig R, Gigerenzer G: Medicine. Communicating statistical information. Science 290:2261, 2000.
9. Steurer J, Fischer JE, Bachmann LM, et al: Communicating accuracy of tests to general practitioners: A controlled study. BMJ 324:824, 2002.
10. Altman DG, Bland JM: Diagnostic tests. 1: Sensitivity and specificity. BMJ 308:1552, 1994.
11. Altman DG, Bland JM: Diagnostic tests 2: Predictive values. BMJ 309:102, 1994.
12. Gill CJ, Sabin L, Schmid CH: Why clinicians are natural Bayesians. BMJ 330:1080, 2005.
13. Deeks JJ, Altman DG: Diagnostic tests 4: Likelihood ratios. BMJ 329:168, 2004.
14. Goodman SN: Toward evidence-based medical statistics. 2: The Bayes factor. Ann Intern Med 130:1005, 1999.
15. Grimes DA, Schulz KF: Refining clinical diagnosis with likelihood ratios. Lancet 365:1500, 2005.
16. Puhan MA, Steurer J, Bachmann LM, ter Riet G: A randomized trial of ways to describe test accuracy: The effect on physicians' post-test probability estimates. Ann Intern Med 143:184, 2005.

17. McGee S: Simplifying likelihood ratios. J Gen Intern Med 17:646, 2002.
18. Pewsner D, Battaglia M, Minder C, et al: Ruling a diagnosis in or out with "SpPIn" and "SnNOut": A note of caution. BMJ 329:209, 2004.
19. Bachmann LM, Puhan MA, ter Riet G, Bossuyt PM: Sample sizes of studies on diagnostic accuracy: Literature survey. BMJ 332:1127, 2006.
20. Sackett DL, Haynes RB: The architecture of diagnostic research. BMJ 324:539, 2002.
21. Rembold CM: Number needed to screen: Development of a statistic for disease screening. BMJ 317:307, 1998.
22. Chen J, Krumholz HM: How useful is computed tomography for screening for coronary artery disease? Screening for coronary artery disease with electron-beam computed tomography is not useful. Circulation 113:125, 2006; discussion 125-146.
23. Wennberg DE, Kellett MA, Dickens JD, et al: The association between local diagnostic testing intensity and invasive cardiac procedures. JAMA 275:1161, 1996.

Therapeutic Decision-Making

24. Guyatt GH, Rennie D: Users' Guides to the Medical Literature: A Manual for Evidence-Based Clinical Practice (book and CD-ROM). Chicago, American Medical Association, 2001.
25. Krumholz HM, Pasternak RC, Weinstein MC, et al: Cost effectiveness of thrombolytic therapy with streptokinase in elderly patients with suspected acute myocardial infarction. N Engl J Med 327:7, 1992.
26. Browner WS, Newman TB: Are all significant P values created equal? The analogy between diagnostic tests and clinical research. JAMA 257:2459, 1987.
27. Sterne JA, Davey Smith G: Sifting the evidence—what's wrong with significance tests? BMJ 322:226, 2001.
28. Fibrinolytic Therapy Trialists' (FTT) Collaborative Group: Indications for fibrinolytic therapy in suspected acute myocardial infarction: Collaborative overview of early mortality and major morbidity results from all randomised trials of more than 1000 patients. Lancet 343:311, 1994.
29. Schulz KF, Grimes DA: Multiplicity in randomised trials II: Subgroup and interim analyses. Lancet 365:1657, 2005.
30. Laupacis A, Sackett DL, Roberts RS: An assessment of clinically useful measures of the consequences of treatment. N Engl J Med 318:1728, 1988.
31. Steering Committee of the Physicians' Health Study Research Group: Final report on the aspirin component of the ongoing Physicians' Health Study. N Engl J Med 321:129, 1989.
32. Pearson TA, Blair SN, Daniels SR, et al: AHA guidelines for primary prevention of cardiovascular disease and stroke: 2002 update: Consensus panel guide to comprehensive risk reduction for adult patients without coronary or other atherosclerotic vascular diseases. American Heart Association Science Advisory and Coordinating Committee. Circulation 106:388, 2002.
33. U.S. Preventive Services Task Force (http://www.ahrq.gov/clinic/uspstf/uspsasmi.htm). Accessed Sept. 11, 2006.
34. Antman EM, Cohen M, Bernink PJ, et al: The TIMI risk score for unstable angina/non-ST elevation MI: A method for prognostication and therapeutic decision making. JAMA 284:835, 2000.
35. Ko DT, Mamdani M, Alter DA: Lipid-lowering therapy with statins in high-risk elderly patients: The treatment-risk paradox. JAMA 291:1864, 2004.
36. Lee DS, Tu JV, Juurlink DN, et al: Risk-treatment mismatch in the pharmacotherapy of heart failure. JAMA 294:1240, 2005.
37. Welch HG, Albertsen PC, Nease RF, et al: Estimating treatment benefits for the elderly: The effect of competing risks. Ann Intern Med 124:577, 1996.
38. Moye LA: Random research. Circulation 103:3150, 2001.
39. Deber RB, Kraetschmer N, Irvine J: What role do patients wish to play in treatment decision making? Arch Intern Med 156:1414, 1996.
40. Bogardus ST Jr, Holmboe E, Jekel JF: Perils, pitfalls, and possibilities in talking about medical risk. JAMA 281:1037, 1999.
41. Holmboe ES, Fiellin DA, Cusanelli E, et al: Perceptions of benefit and risk of patients undergoing first-time elective percutaneous coronary revascularization. J Gen Intern Med 15:632, 2000.
42. Malenka DJ, Baron JA, Johansen S, et al: The framing effect of relative and absolute risk. J Gen Intern Med 8:543, 1993.
43. Bergus GR, Levin IP, Elstein AS: Presenting risks and benefits to patients. J Gen Intern Med 17:612, 2002.
44. Paling J: Strategies to help patients understand risks. BMJ 327:745, 2003.
45. Sheridan SL, Pignone MP, Lewis CL: A randomized comparison of patients' understanding of number needed to treat and other common risk reduction formats. J Gen Intern Med 18:884, 2003.
46. Chaudhry SI, Krumholz HM, Foody JM: Systolic hypertension in older persons. JAMA 292:1074, 2004.

Cognitive Errors

47. Redelmeier DA. Improving patient care. The cognitive psychology of missed diagnoses. Ann Intern Med 142:115, 2005.
48. Tversky A, Kahneman D: Judgment under uncertainty: Heuristics and biases. Science 185:1124, 1974.
49. McDonald CJ: Medical heuristics: The silent adjudicators of clinical practice. Ann Intern Med 124:56, 1996.
50. Forrow L, Taylor WC, Arnold RM: Absolutely relative: How research results are summarized can affect treatment decisions. Am J Med 92:121, 1992.
51. Naylor CD, Chen E, Strauss B: Measured enthusiasm: Does the method of reporting trial results alter perceptions of therapeutic effectiveness? Ann Intern Med 117:916, 1992.

Accuracy of Evidence

52. Zir LM, Miller SW, Dinsmore RE, et al: Interobserver variability in coronary angiography. Circulation 53:627, 1976.
53. Rogers EM: A prospective and retrospective look at the diffusion model. J Health Commun 9:13, 2004.

Adoption of Innovation

54. Fineberg HV: Clinical evaluation: How does it influence medical practice? Bull Cancer 74:333, 1987.
55. Lamas GA, Pfeffer MA, Hamm P, et al: Do the results of randomized clinical trials of cardiovascular drugs influence medical practice? The SAVE Investigators. N Engl J Med 327:241, 1992.
56. Krumholz HM, Radford MJ, Ellerbeck EF, et al: Aspirin in the treatment of acute myocardial infarction in elderly Medicare beneficiaries. Patterns of use and outcomes. Circulation 92:2841, 1995.
57. Krumholz HM, Radford MJ, Wang Y, et al: National use and effectiveness of beta-blockers for the treatment of elderly patients after acute myocardial infarction: National Cooperative Cardiovascular Project. JAMA 280:623, 1998.
58. Antman EM, Lau J, Kupelnick B, et al: A comparison of results of meta-analyses of randomized control trials and recommendations of clinical experts. Treatments for myocardial infarction. JAMA 268:240, 1992.
59. Masoudi FA, Gross CP, Wang Y, et al: Adoption of spironolactone therapy for older patients with heart failure and left ventricular systolic dysfunction in the United States, 1998-2001. Circulation 112:39, 2005.
60. Ioannidis JP: Contradicted and initially stronger effects in highly cited clinical research. JAMA 294:218, 2005.
61. Krumholz HM, Anderson JL, Brooks NH, et al: ACC/AHA clinical performance measures for adults with ST-elevation and non-ST-elevation myocardial infarction: A report of the American College of Cardiology/American Heart Association Task Force on Performance Measures (Writing Committee to Develop Performance Measures on ST-Elevation and Non-ST-Elevation Myocardial Infarction). Circulation 113:732, 2006.
62. Spertus JA, Eagle KA, Krumholz HM, et al: American College of Cardiology and American Heart Association methodology for the selection and creation of performance measures for quantifying the quality of cardiovascular care. Circulation 111:1703, 2005.

Information Technology and Systems

63. Apkon M, Mattera JA, Lin Z, et al: A randomized outpatient trial of a decision-support information technology tool. Arch Intern Med 165:2388, 2005.

CHAPTER 5

Measurement and Improvement of Quality of Cardiovascular Care

Thomas H. Lee

In recent years, measurement and improvement of quality has become an important focus for cardiovascular leaders and researchers due to a combination of factors including advances in measurement of quality and changes in the health care environment. This trend has been made possible by clinical research that has helped define "evidence-based medicine" for common cardiovascular syndromes (i.e., knowledge of which interventions improve patient outcomes). This growing body of knowledge has made possible the development of guidelines more comprehensive and explicit than those for any other specialty of medicine. The availability of these guidelines has in turn enabled the development of measures to assess the reliability with which the guidelines' recommendations are implemented.

Interest in "report cards" on quality has been intensified by concerns about quality and safety of care. Research has shown that patients fail to receive up to 45% of recommended tests and treatments,[1] and some data on gaps in quality are now publicly reported for hospitals and physicians.[2] The prominence of these data has grown with the advent of new insurance products, in which providers receive bonuses for higher measured quality (pay for performance)[3,4] or larger percentages of health care costs are borne by patients. Data on hospital and physician quality are frequently provided to patients in these "consumer-directed health plans" so that, in theory, they might choose providers of superior efficiency and quality.[5,6]

Measurement of quality of cardiovascular care had been building momentum even before these recent trends in the health care marketplace, and numerous U.S. agencies have been actively involved in the development of measures and dissemination of data for several years (Table 5-1). Statewide report cards on cardiac surgery and percutaneous coronary interventions for hospitals and individual physicians have been introduced in some states.[7,8] The National Committee for Quality Assurance (NCQA) developed measures of quality for the managed care organization known as the *health plan employer and data set* (HEDIS).[9] Measures for cardiovascular quality of care delivered by hospitals have been introduced by the Joint Commission on Accreditation of Healthcare Organizations (JCAHO),[10] and data on the volume of cardiovascular procedures have been disseminated via organizations such as Leapfrog.[11] This phenomenon has not been limited to the United States; detailed data on cardiovascular and other outcomes are available via the Internet for hospitals in the United Kingdom[12] and other countries.

GUIDELINES AND PERFORMANCE MEASURES

Amid calls for caution and expression of concern, health care professionals have responded with a variety of initiatives aimed at improving care. The most prominent of these responses in cardiovascular medicine has been the development of guidelines, particularly those from the American College of Cardiology (ACC) and the American Heart Association (AHA).[13,14] These guidelines often provide the basis for measures of quality (also known as *performance measures*) but serve a different purpose. Guidelines are written to describe a consensus on the diagnostic or therapeutic interventions appropriate for most patients in most circumstances. Guidelines are written with the expectation that individual physicians will use discretion in the treatment of individual patients and *not* follow the guidelines in certain cases. Key guidelines are summarized in this text.

In contrast, performance measures build on the consensus expressed in guidelines to define "rules" or standards of care that should be followed for virtually all patients. When the clinician believes that the "rule" is not appropriate for a patient, the reasons should be documented. When such standards are not met, the implication is that an error has occurred (e.g., failure to recommend aspirin for patients with acute myocardial infarction).

Therefore performance measures tend to be written to define the minimum standards of adequate care, as opposed to the targets that might define excellent care. For example, a 2004 report from the National Cholesterol Education Program supported a low-density lipoprotein (LDL) cholesterol goal of less than 70 mg/dl for high-risk patients,[15] which represented a modification of 2002 guidelines that recommended a target cholesterol level below 100 mg/dl for this population.[16] In contrast, a higher LDL cholesterol target has been used by NCQA for its HEDIS measure for cholesterol management in high-risk patients. Until 2006 the HEDIS measure required managed care organizations to report the percentage of such patients who achieved an LDL level below 130 mg/dl. The NCQA rationale was that although experts agreed that a level below 100 mg/dl reflects excellent care, the strength of evidence was such that physicians should be faulted only if they allowed patients with coronary disease to have a level above 130 mg/dl. In 2006 the HEDIS LDL target was changed to 100 mg/dL, which remains higher than the goal supported in current guidelines.

The practical implication of this relationship between performance measures and guidelines in cardiovascular medicine is that quality measures are usually closely linked to class I indications from the ACC/AHA guidelines (i.e., conditions for which there is evidence or general agreement that a given procedure or treatment is useful and effective). Failure

TABLE 5–1 Key Organizations Involved in Measurement of Quality of Cardiovascular Care

Organization	Major Activity	Focus	Web Site
American College of Cardiology (ACC)	Guidelines Applied in Practice (GAP); ACC/AHA Task Force on Performance Measures	Health care providers	www.acc.org
American Heart Association (AHA)	Get with the Guidelines; ACC/AHA Task Force on Performance Measures	Health care providers	www.americanheart.org
American Medical Association (AMA)	Physician Consortium for Quality Improvement	Physicians	www.ama-assn.org
Centers for Medicare & Medicaid Services (CMS)	Hospital Quality Initiative	Physicians and hospitals	www.cms.org
Joint Commission on the Accreditation of Healthcare Organizations (JCAHO)	ORYX Initiatives	Accreditation of hospitals	www.jointcommission.org
Leapfrog	Publication of volume data for cardiac procedures at hospitals	Hospitals	www.leapfroggroup.org
National Committee for Quality Assurance (NCQA)	Health Plan Employer and Data Set (HEDIS); Heart Stroke Provider Recognition Program	Accreditation of health plans; physician provider recognition programs	www.ncqa.org
National Quality Forum (NQF)	Hospital Performance Measures Project	Hospitals	www.qualityforum.org

TABLE 5–2 Summary of Performance Measurement Development Strategy Recommended by American College of Cardiology/American Heart Association

Phase	Tasks
I. Constructing measurement sets	Defining the target population Identifying dimensions of care that should be quantified (e.g., problem diagnosis, patient education, treatment, patient self-management) Synthesizing and reviewing the literature Defining and operationalizing potential measures Selecting measures for inclusion in the performance measures set
II. Determining measure feasibility	Definition of sample (e.g., document sources of case identification and attrition; develop an algorithm to assign patients to providers) Feasibility of measures—report validity, reliability, and completeness of collected data
III. Measuring performance	Determine reporting unit (i.e., level at which information will be reported) Determine number and range of measures Evaluate performance

Modified from Spertus JA, Eagle KA, Krumholz HM, et al: American College of Cardiology and American Heart Association Methodology for the Selection and Creation of Performance Measures for Quantifying the Quality of Cardiovascular Care. Circulation 111:1703, 2005.

to perform interventions that are less strongly supported by evidence is too often a matter of judgment to use as a quality measure.

The ACC and AHA have articulated basic principles for selecting and creating performance measures.[17] These principles define a first phase in which measurement sets are constructed, followed by a second phase in which measure feasibility is assessed, and a third in which performance is measured (Table 5-2). This statement explores in detail the types of pitfalls that might compromise the usefulness or validity of measures as they are developed or applied. Using these principles, AHA/ACC workgroups have reviewed specific domains for measurement of quality for patients with acute myocardial infarction and heart failure and recommended specific performance measures (Tables 5-3, 5-4, and 5-5).[18,19] The appendices of references 18 and 19 include detailed specifications for the collection of data for these measures.

METHODOLOGICAL ISSUES

Many of the methodological issues that affect clinical research influence the measurement of cardiovascular quality, with two major additional themes. First, the performance data for individual physicians and hospitals may be made public in some cases; as a general rule, the more widely data are disseminated, the greater the demand for methodological rigor. Second, the collection and analysis of data for quality measurement is rarely funded as well as in clinical trials. Thus the desire for methodological rigor must be weighed against the cost of collecting and analyzing the data.

Claims Data

The least expensive type of information used for quality measurement is claims data, which are collected for the purposes of mediating payment, not promoting quality of care; thus there is little or no quality control for claims data regarding issues such as the accuracy of diagnoses. These data have the advantage of being readily available for large populations, but error rates in diagnoses are high, and information that is not required for payment is unavailable (e.g., whether heart failure is due to systolic or diastolic dysfunction, or whether blood pressure levels were controlled).

Retrospective Chart Review

This method can be used to collect more accurate clinical data, but such reviews are expensive and are complicated by the existence of multiple medical records for most patients. Patients generally have separate records at each hospital to which they have been admitted, as well as at the office of their primary care physicians and the specialists from whom they have received care; none of these records is complete unless all of these health care providers are part of an integrated delivery system with a single electronic medical record. Even when all records are available for review, data collection from paper records is limited by the completeness, accuracy, and legibility of record-keeping.

The increasing use of electronic medical records potentially will assist use of measures based on clinical data instead of administrative

TABLE 5–3 American College of Cardiology/American Heart Association Inpatient Heart Failure Performance Measures

Performance Measure	Description
Evaluation of left ventricular systolic (LVS) function	Heart failure (HF) patients with documentation in hospital record that LVS function was assessed before arrival, during hospitalization, or is planned after discharge
ACE inhibitor (ACEI) or angiotensin receptor blocker (ARB) for LVS dysfunction (LVSD)	HF patients with LVSD and without both ACEI and ARB contraindications who are prescribed an ACEI or ARB at hospital discharge
Anticoagulant at discharge for HF patients with atrial fibrillation (AF)	HF patients with chronic/recurrent AF and without warfarin contraindications who are prescribed warfarin at discharge
Discharge instructions	HF patients discharged home with written instructions and educational material addressing *all* of the following: activity level, diet, discharge medications, follow-up appointment, weight monitoring, and what to do if symptoms worsen
Adult smoking cessation advice/counseling	HF patients with a history of smoking cigarettes who are given smoking cessation advice or counseling during hospital stay

Modified from Bonow RO, Bennett S, Casey DE, et al: ACC/AHA clinical performance measures for adults with chronic heart failure: A report of the American College of Cardiology/American Heart Association Task Force on Performance Measures (Writing Committee to Develop Heart Failure Clinical Performance Measures): Endorsed by the Heart Failure Society of America. Circulation 112:1853, 2005.

data. However, significant barriers include the difficulty of integration of data from medical records used by different providers in the absence of a single national patient identification number and the failure of many physicians to use key-coded fields of the electronic record such as problem lists and medication lists reliably.

Prospective Data Collection

Collection of key data for quality measurement is becoming an increasingly common and important tactic for quality improvement. Standard dataforms for patients undergoing cardiac surgery or percutaneous coronary intervention (PCI) are now used at many medical centers. At some institutions the data collected via these protocols are used for institutional databases or for regional collaborations.[20] Many hospitals now report data on specific cardiovascular patient populations to national databases such as the Society of Thoracic Surgery or the American College of Cardiology's National Catheterization Data Registry. Participation in such databases allows comparison of institutional performance to regional and national benchmarks.

Collection of Patient Outcome Data

Collection of patient outcome data (e.g., 1-year mortality or functional status) is expensive and difficult. Administrative sources such as the National Death Index can provide information on whether individual patients have died within the United States; analogous resources are available in many other countries. However, obtaining information on the cause of death or on the status of patients who have not died requires interviews or surveys. Even when such data are available, the results should be adjusted for clinical and socioeconomic factors that are likely to influence the results. Therefore many quality measures focus on processes such as the use of medications (e.g., beta blockers after acute myocardial infarction) or tests (e.g., measurement of LDL cholesterol) that are expected to lead to better outcomes.

TABLE 5–4 American College of Cardiology/American Heart Association Outpatient Performance Measures for Heart Failure

Performance Measure	Description
Initial laboratory tests	Initial laboratory evaluation of patients with newly diagnosed heart failure (HF) (complete blood cell count, blood urea nitrogen, blood glucose, serum electrolytes, serum creatinine, thyroid stimulating hormone)
Left ventricular systolic (LVS) assessment	HF patients with documentation that LVS has been assessed
Weight measurement	Measurement of patient's weight at each outpatient visit to assess change in volume status
Blood pressure measurement	Measurement of patient's blood pressure at each outpatient visit
Assessment of clinical symptoms of volume overload	Assessment of clinical *symptoms* of volume overload at each outpatient visit (e.g., dyspnea, fatigue, orthopnea)
Assessment of clinical signs of volume overload	Completion of a physical examination pertaining to volume status assessment in patients diagnosed with HF at each HF visit (e.g., peripheral edema, rales, hepatomegaly, ascites, jugular venous pressure, S3 or S4 gallop)
Assessment of activity level	Evaluation of the impact of HF on activity level at each outpatient visit using standardized scale or assessment tool
Patient education	Percentage of patients who were provided with patient education on disease management and health behavior changes during one or more visits within the period of assessment
Beta blocker therapy	Prescription of beta blockers in patients with HF and LVS dysfunction (LVSD)
ACE inhibitor (ACEI) or angiotensin receptor blocker (ARB) therapy for patients with HF who have LVSD	Prescription of ACEI or ARB for management of outpatient HF patients with LVSD
Warfarin therapy for patients with atrial fibrillation (AF)	Use of warfarin in patients with both HF and AF

Modified from Bonow RO, Bennett S, Casey DE, et al: ACC/AHA clinical performance measures for adults with chronic heart failure: A report of the American College of Cardiology/American Heart Association Task Force on Performance Measures (Writing Committee to Develop Heart Failure Clinical Performance Measures): Endorsed by the Heart Failure Society of America. Circulation 112:1853, 2005.

DEFINITION OF QUALITY

A variety of definitions of quality have been proposed, reflecting the complexity of the health care system and its heterogeneous stakeholders.

An increasingly popular operational definition of quality is based on error reduction and the recognition that there are three major types of errors in health care: errors of underuse, overuse, and misuse.[21] *Underuse* is the failure to provide a medical intervention when it is likely to produce a favorable outcome for a patient, such as the failure to prescribe an angiotensin-converting enzyme inhibitor for a

TABLE 5–5 American College of Cardiology/American Heart Association ST-Elevation and Non-ST-Elevation Myocardial Infarction Performance Measures

Performance Measures	Description
Aspirin at arrival	Acute myocardial infarction (AMI) patients without aspirin contraindications who received aspirin within 24 hours before or after hospital arrival
Aspirin prescribed at discharge	AMI patients without aspirin contraindications who are prescribed aspirin at hospital discharge
Beta blocker at arrival	AMI patients without beta blocker contraindications who received a beta blocker within 24 hours after hospital arrival
Beta blocker prescribed at discharge	AMI patients without beta blocker contraindications who are prescribed a beta blocker at hospital discharge
Low-density lipoprotein (LDL) cholesterol assessment	AMI patients with documentation of LDL cholesterol level in the hospital record or documentation that testing was done during the hospital stay or is planned for after discharge
Lipid-lowering therapy at discharge	AMI patients with elevated LD cholesterol(≥100 mg/dl) who are prescribed a lipid-lowering medication at hospital discharge
ACEI or ARB for left ventricular systolic dysfunction (LVSD) at discharge	AMI patients with LVSD and without both angiotensin converting enzyme inhibitor (ACEI) and angiotensin receptor blocker (ARB) contraindications who areprescribed an ACEI or ARB at hospital discharge
Time to fibrinolytic therapy	Median time for arrival to administration of fibrinolytic therapy in patients with ST-segment elevation or left bundle branch block (LBBB) on the electrocardiogram (ECG) performed closest to hospital arrival time AMI patients receiving fibrinolytic therapy during the hospital stay and having a time from hospital arrival to fibrinolysis of 30 minutes or less
Time to percutaneous coronary intervention (PCI)	Median time for arrival to PCI in patients with ST-segment elevation or left bundle branch block (LBBB) on the ECG performed closest to hospital arrival time AMI patients receiving PCI during the hospital stay and having a time from hospital arrival to PCI of 90 min or less
Reperfusion therapy	AMI patients with ST-segment elevation on the ECG performed closest to arrival who receive fibrinolytic therapy or primary PCI
Adult smoking cessation advice/ counseling	AMI patients with a history of smoking cigarettes who are given smoking cessation advice or counseling during hospital stay

Modified from Krumholz HM, Anderson JL, Brooks NH, et al: ACC/AHA clinical performance measures for adults with ST-elevation and non-ST-elevation myocardial infarction: A report of the ACC/AHA Task Force on Performance Measures (ST-Elevation and Non-ST-Elevation Myocardial Infarction Performance Measures Writing Committee). Circulation 113:732, 2006.

patient with left ventricular dysfunction. *Overuse* occurs when an intervention becomes common practice even though its benefits do not justify the potential harm or costs, such as performance of exercise testing in asymptomatic patients with a low risk for cardiovascular disease. *Misuse* occurs when a preventable complication eliminates the benefit of an intervention. An example is continued administration of a statin to a patient with muscle tenderness and weakness, suggesting possible myopathy.

The relationship between guidelines and these three types of errors is close and complex. In ACC/AHA guidelines, class I indications sometimes define "rules" that, if not applied for an appropriate patient, would suggest an error of underuse. Class III indications define potential errors of overuse. The ACC/AHA guidelines tend to focus on two aspects of quality:

- Complying with evidence-based medicine (i.e., doing the right thing for the patient)
- Procedural quality (i.e., performing interventions correctly)

Failure to comply with evidence-based medicine may constitute an error of underuse (e.g., failure to use a beta blocker after acute myocardial infarction) or an error of overuse (e.g., performance of coronary angiography in a patient without clinical evidence of coronary artery disease). Failure to perform an intervention correctly can constitute an error of misuse (e.g., continued administration of a statin in a patient with symptoms of myopathy).

Outcomes (e.g., mortality, complication rates) are, of course, the measure of performance of greatest interest to patients and clinicians, but adjusting for the effects of comorbid medical conditions, severity of the underlying disease, and socioeconomic status is a formidable challenge. This challenge is particularly great when analyses are restricted to administrative claims data. Investigators recently published severity adjustment models using Medicare claims data for hospital 30-day mortality for patients with heart failure and acute myocardial infarction and reported performance approaching that of clinical data extracted from medical record review.[22,23] These models have been endorsed by the National Quality Forum and are believed to have performance sufficient for use for public reporting, but it should be noted that similar models are necessary for other outcomes for patients and for other diagnoses.

A surrogate marker for quality that is used by the public and by professional organizations is procedure volume. The relationship between volume and patient outcomes has been demonstrated in numerous studies focusing on hospitals and physicians.[24-27] These relationships are complex; for some procedures, outcomes are associated with the volume for the hospital, whereas for other procedures, outcomes are associated with the volume for the individual physician.[25,27] The relationship between hospital volume and mortality for major cardiac surgical procedures from one major study is shown in Table 5-6 and Figure 5-1.[26] These findings were

TABLE 5–6 Annual Volume Categories for Hospitals Performing Cardiac Surgery		
	Coronary Artery Bypass Graft Surgery (n)	Aortic and Mitral Valve Replacement (n)
Very low	<230	<43
Low	230-348	43-74
Medium	349-549	75-119
High	550-849	120-199
Very high	>849	>199

From Birkmeyer JD, Siewers AE, Finlayon EVA, et al: Hospital volume and surgical mortality in the United States. N Engl J Med 346:1128, 2002.

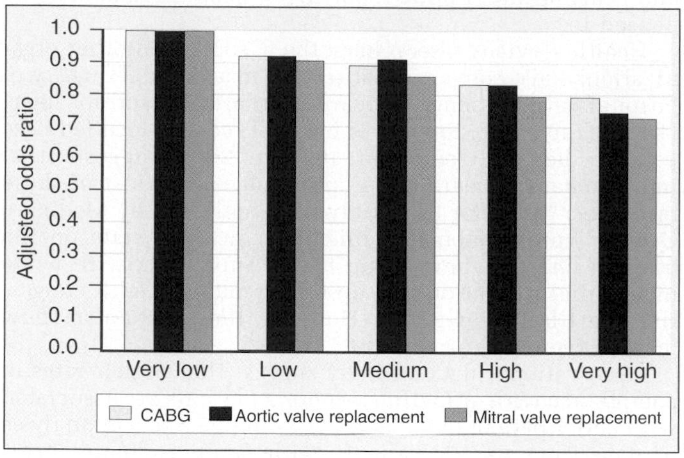

FIGURE 5–1 Relationship of hospital volume and adjusted odds ratio for mortality. See Table 5-6 for definition of volume categories. *(From Birkmeyer JD, Siewers AE, Finlayson EVA, et al: Hospital volume and surgical mortality in the United States. N Engl J Med 346:1128, 2002.)*

based on Medicare claims data from 1994 to 1999, and the study was the largest of its kind to date. A subsequent study by the same investigators found a correlation between higher physician volume (e.g., >42 aortic valve replacements or >162 coronary artery bypass graft operations annually) and lower mortality rates[27] and concluded that surgeon volume was more important for these procedures than hospital volume. On the basis of such research, organizations in the United States and abroad are publishing volume data for major procedures on their Internet sites to help patients choose their hospital for surgery.[11,12]

The ACC/AHA guidelines acknowledge research on the relationship between volume and outcome in guidelines, such as those for the use of PCI for patients with acute myocardial infarction.[28] These guidelines recommend that elective PCI should be performed by experienced operators (at least 75 procedures per year) at high-volume facilities (at least 400 procedures per year).

Current Quality of Cardiovascular Care

Some of the most comprehensive data on the quality of cardiovascular care have come from the Community Quality Index (CQI) study,[1] which draws on medical records and self-reported information from random samples of patients from 12 U.S. metropolitan areas (Boston; Cleveland, Ohio; Greenville, S.C.; Indianapolis, Ind.; Lansing, Mich.; Little Rock, Ark.; Miami; Newark, N.J.; Orange County, Calif.; Phoenix, Ariz.; Seattle; and Syracuse, N.Y.). For this study, investigators selected acute and chronic conditions that represented the leading causes of death and disability and developed indicators to assess potential problems with overuse and underuse of key processes. A sampling of the indicators for cardiovascular conditions and the total number of indicators used are summarized in Table 5-7, along with the percentage of recommendations that had been followed for the 6712 study participants. The full list

TABLE 5–7 Selected Cardiovascular Quality of Care Indicators and Classifications Used in the Community Quality Index Study

Condition	Examples of Selected Indicators	Percentage of Recommended Care Received (95% Confidence Interval)
Atrial fibrillation (10 indicators)	Patients with atrial fibrillation >48 hours' duration or of unknown duration who are undergoing elective electrical or chemical cardioversion should receive anticoagulation for at least 3 weeks before cardioversion unless they have had a transesophageal echocardiogram within 24 hours of cardioversion that indicates no clot. Patients with atrial fibrillation started on warfarin should have an international normalized ratio checked within 1 week of the first dose. Patients with atrial fibrillation >48 hours' duration or of unknown duration who do not have contraindications to warfarin should receive warfarin if they are younger than 65 years, with one or more other risk factors for stroke.	25 (18-31)
Congestive heart failure (36 indicators)	Ejection fraction assessed before medical therapy Angiotensin-converting enzyme inhibitors for patients with congestive heart failure and an ejection fraction <40%	64 (55-72)
Coronary artery disease (37 indicators)	Counseling on smoking cessation Avoidance of nifedipine for patients with an acute myocardial infarction	68 (64-72)
Diabetes (13 indicators)	Diet and exercise counseling Angiotensin-converting enzyme inhibitors for patients with proteinuria	45 (43-48)
Hyperlipidemia (7 indicators)	Treatment of high low-density cholesterol levels in patients with coronary artery disease	49 (44-53)
Hypertension (27 indicators)	Life-style modification for patients with mild hypertension Pharmacotherapy for uncontrolled mild hypertension Change in treatment when blood pressure is persistently uncontrolled	65 (53-67)

For full list, see http://www.rand.org/health/mcglynn_appa.pdf.

From McGlynn EA, Asch SM, Adams J, et al: The quality of health care delivered to adults in the United States. N Engl J Med 348:2635, 2003.

 of measures is available at http://www.rand.org/health/mcglynn_appa.pdf.

Rates of compliance with recommendations ranged from 68 percent for care of coronary disease to 25 percent for atrial fibrillation. For example, only 45 percent of patients presenting with a myocardial infarction received beta blockers, and only 61 percent of participants with a myocardial infarction who were appropriate candidates for aspirin therapy received this drug. It was concluded that patients received about half of the interventions supported by evidence from clinical trials.

TABLE 5–8 Quality Indicators for Inpatient Care for Medicare Patients

Topic	Indicator	Median State Rates* 1998-1999	2000-2001
Acute myocardial infarction	Administration of aspirin within 24 hours of admission	84	85
	Aspirin prescribed at discharge	85	86
	Administration of beta blocker within 24 hours of admission	64	69
	Beta blocker prescribed at discharge	72	79
	Angiotensin-converting enzyme inhibitor prescribed at discharge for patients with left ventricular ejection fraction <0.40	71	74
	Smoking cessation counseling given during hospitalization	40	43
	Time to angioplasty (minutes)	120	107
	Time to thrombolytic therapy (minutes)	41	45
Heart failure	Evaluation of ejection fraction	65	70
	Angiotensin-converting enzyme inhibitor prescribed at discharge for patients with left ventricular ejection fraction <0.40	69	68

*In this study, rates of performance of each measure were calculated from chart reviews in each state. The figures in these columns represent the median performance among the 50 U.S. states.

From Jencks SF, Haft ED, Cuerdon T: Change in the quality of care delivered to Medicare beneficiaries, 1998-1999 to 2000-2001. JAMA 289:305, 2003.

HOSPITALS

For hospitals in the United States, measures of cardiovascular care mandated by the JCAHO have recently become important foci for quality improvement. These measures are part of a program called the *ORYX Initiative,* which integrates outcomes and other performance measurement data into the accreditation process for hospitals. Two of the core foci of the ORYX initiative are acute myocardial infarction and heart failure. Public reporting of hospital data is being phased in.

Health services researchers, the JCAHO, and other organizations have converged on several measures of quality of hospital care for acute myocardial infarction and for heart failure (Table 5-8). Review of medical records for Medicare patients hospitalized from 1998 to 2001 suggests that improvement appears to be taking place for most of these measures.[29] Data for this study were collected by Medicare Quality Improvement Organizations in each state on the basis of chart reviews of up to 750 inpatients with acute myocardial infarction and up to 800 patients with congestive heart failure per state. However, these data also show marked regional variability.

Observational data strongly suggest that higher rates of compliance with guideline recommendations are associated with better patient outcomes. For example, a recent analysis of data from 64,775 patients with acute ischemic heart disease found that adherence to nine ACC/AHA guideline-recommended treatments varied widely (Fig. 5-2).[30] Composite guideline adherence was significantly associated with in-hospital mortality; each 10% increase in composite adherence was associated with a 10% decrease in likelihood of in-hospital mortality (Fig. 5-3).

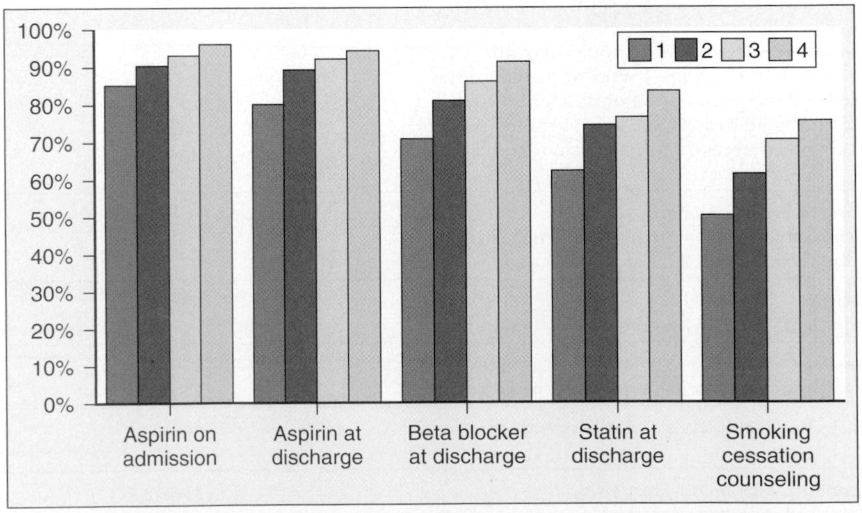

FIGURE 5–2 Compliance by quartile with guidelines for acute myocardial infarction. Bars show percentage compliance for quartiles of hospitals grouped by performance. *(From Peterson ED, Roe MT, Mulgund J, et al: Association between hospital process performance and outcomes among patients with acute coronary syndromes. JAMA 295:1912, 2006.)*

PHYSICIANS

Cardiovascular surgeons and cardiologists who perform PCI are evaluated on their actual outcomes data via public report cards in some states. In these reports, analyses attempt to adjust for the risk of complications and for emergency procedures, allowing calculation of a risk-adjusted mortality rate for individual physicians and hospitals. Thus far, limited data suggest that the public does not use such data extensively,[31] although the public disclosure of performance data is believed to be a powerful driver for individual institutions to improve their care.[7,8]

Nonprocedural care by physicians is often assessed by HEDIS measures developed by NCQA (Table 5-9).[9] These measures were developed for evaluation of health maintenance organizations, and therefore most rely on analyses of medical and pharmacy claims data. In recent years, however, there has been a shift toward measures that are less focused on measuring processes and are more closely tied to patient outcome. Therefore measures that require review of medical records for some data have been introduced (e.g., blood pressure and LDL cholesterol levels).

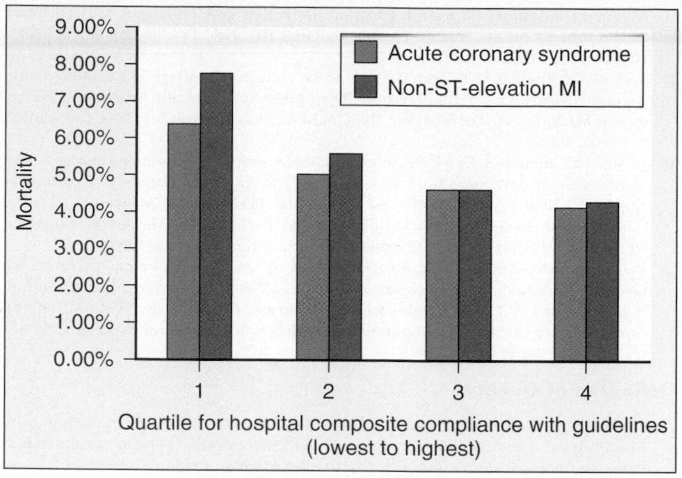

FIGURE 5–3 In-hospital mortality for patients with acute coronary syndrome and non-ST-elevation myocardial infarction correlated with hospital compliance with guidelines. Bars show percentage compliance for quartiles of hospitals grouped by performance. *(From Peterson ED, Roe MT, Mulgund J, et al: Association between hospital process performance and outcomes among patients with acute coronary syndromes. JAMA 295:1912, 2006.)*

TABLE 5–9 Cardiovascular HEDIS Measures

Measure	Description	Mean Performance* (%)
Beta blocker treatment after a heart attack	The percentage of patients ≥35 years old who were hospitalized and discharged alive during the measurement year with a diagnosis of acute myocardial infarction and who received one or more prescriptions for beta blockers covering a period of at least 6 months after discharge.	96.2
Controlling high blood pressure	The percentage of patients 45-85 years old who had a diagnosis of hypertension and whose blood pressure was adequately controlled (≤140/90) during the measurement year.	66.8
Cholesterol screening and management	The percentage of patients 18-75 years old who had evidence of an acute cardiovascular event (hospitalization for acute myocardial infarction, coronary artery bypass graft, or percutaneous transluminal coronary angioplasty) and whose low-density lipoprotein cholesterol was screened and controlled to less than 100 mg/dl in the year following the event.	50.9

*Data are for commercial population for 2004.
From http://www.ncqa.org/Docs/SOHCQ_2005.pdf.

A program called the Heart/Stroke Recognition Program was introduced in 2003 by NCQA in collaboration with the AHA and the American Stroke Association. This program is designed to identify physicians who are providing excellent care to patients who have cardiovascular disease or a history of stroke. In this voluntary program physicians seeking "recognition" must audit a sample of their office records and report on their rates of success in meeting specific performance measures (Table 5-10). A similar physician recognition program for diabetes care has been administered by NCQA for several years, and some employers now pay a bonus to physicians who meet the standards of these two programs.

TABLE 5–10 Measures of the Heart/Stroke Provider Recognition Program of the National Committee for Quality Assurance

Blood pressure testing
Proportion of patients with blood pressure <130/85 mmHg
Lipid testing
Proportion of patients with low-density lipoprotein cholesterol <100 mg/dl
Use of aspirin or other antithrombotics
Smoking status and cessation advice

Improvement Strategies

The American College of Cardiology and a wide range of other organizations are attempting to develop and disseminate tools for improvement in the reliability of delivery of evidence-based cardiovascular care. The ACC's Guidelines Applied in Practice Initiative used tactics known as *continuous quality improvement* (CQI) to help physicians and hospitals improve compliance with guidelines.[32] These CQI tools are based on principles adapted from industrial manufacturers and seek to improve quality and efficiency through repetitive cycles of process and outcomes measurement, design and implementation of interventions to improve the processes of care, and remeasurement to assess the impact of interventions.

Research that has evaluated the impact of CQI programs on quality of cardiovascular care has yielded mixed but encouraging results.[20,33,34] In a large study of CQI for improvement of cardiac surgery,[34] the investigators randomly assigned 359 hospitals that performed coronary artery bypass grafting on 267,917 patients between January 2000 and July 2002 and that participated in the Society of Thoracic Surgeons National Cardiac Database. The hospitals were randomly assigned to a control arm or to one of two groups that used CQI interventions aimed at improving preoperative use of beta blockade in all patients and internal mammary artery graft utilization in elderly patients. The intervention groups received measure-specific information including a call to action to a physician leader, educational products, and periodic longitudinal data with benchmark information. This intervention led to a significant increase in the use of beta blockade at intervention sites (by 7.3 versus 3.6 percent) and a trend toward an increase in use of internal mammary grafts. Both interventions were associated with statistically significant increases in these practices at lower-volume coronary artery bypass grafting sites.

Computerized physician order entry systems are being implemented at many academic medical centers in the United States, as well as a smaller number of community hospitals. These systems have been shown to improve compliance with guidelines to as high as 100 percent for selected quality measures for acute myocardial infarction and congestive heart failure.[35] Other research has shown that administrative and leadership cultures oriented toward quality improvement appear to be important predictors of success in reducing door-to-balloon times for patients with acute myocardial infarction who undergo PCI.[36]

FUTURE PERSPECTIVES

Public reporting on quality and efficiency of cardiac care is likely to become increasingly common in the years ahead due to changes in the U.S. and other health care systems, as well as the availability of new and larger databases of administrative and clinical information. Reporting has thus far been focused on health plans and hospitals but can be expected to focus on groups and even individual physicians. Cardiovascular disease will be among the most prominent areas for such reporting because of the relative wealth of scientific knowledge and guidelines on cardiovascular conditions, as well as the high prevalence and costs of these conditions.

REFERENCES

1. McGlynn EA, Asch SM, Adams J, et al: The quality of health care delivered to adults in the United States. N Engl J Med 348:2635, 2003.
2. Lee TH, Meyer GS, Brennan TA: A middle ground on public accountability. N Engl J Med 350:2409, 2004.
3. Epstein AM, Lee TH, Hamel MB: Paying physicians for high-quality care. N Engl J Med 350:406, 2004.
4. Bufalino V, Peterson ED, Burke GL, et al: Payment for quality: Guiding principles and recommendations. Principles and recommendations from the American Heart Association's Reimbursement, Coverage, and Access Policy Development Workgroup. Circulation 113:1151, 2006.
5. Galvin R, Milstein A: Large employers' new strategies in health care. N Engl J Med 347:939, 2002.
6. Lee TH, Zapert K: Do high-deductible health plans threaten quality of care? N Engl J Med 353:1202, 2005.
7. Jha AK, Epstein AM: The predictive accuracy of the New York State Coronary Artery Bypass Surgery Report-Card system. Health Affairs 25:844, 2006.
8. Chassin MR: Achieving and sustaining improved quality: Lessons from New York State and cardiac surgery. Health Aff (Millwood) 21:40, 2002.
9. National Committee for Quality Assurance (NCQA): Measuring the Quality of America's Health Care: The Health Plan Employer Data and Information Set (HEDIS). vol. 2003. Washington, DC, NCQA, 2003.
10. Joint Commission on Accreditation of Healthcare Organizations (Available at http://www.jcaho.org/).
11. Leapfrog Group (Available at http://www.leapfroggroup.org/).
12. Dr Foster (Available at http://www.drfoster.co.uk/).

Guidelines and Performance Measures

13. Gibbons RJ, Smith S, Antman E: American College of Cardiology/American Heart Association clinical practice guidelines: Part I: Where do they come from? Circulation 107:2979, 2003.
14. Gibbons RJ, Smith S, Antman E: American College of Cardiology/American Heart Association clinical practice guidelines: Part II: Evolutionary changes in a continuous quality improvement project. Circulation 107:3101, 2003.
15. Grundy SM, Cleeman JI, Merz NB, et al: Implications of recent clinical trials for the National Cholesterol Education Program Adult Treatment Panel III Guidelines. Circulation 110:227, 2004.
16. National Cholesterol Education Program: Detection and Treatment of High Blood Cholesterol in Adults (Adult Treatment Panel III). NIH Publication No. 02-5215. Washington, DC, NIH, 2002.
17. Spertus JA, Eagle KA, Krumholz HM, et al: American College of Cardiology and American Heart Association Methodology for the Selection and Creation of Performance Measures for Quantifying the Quality of Cardiovascular Care. Circulation 111:1703, 2005.
18. Bonow RO, Bennett S, Casey DE, et al: ACC/AHA clinical performance measures for adults with chronic heart failure: A report of the American College of Cardiology/American Heart Association Task Force on Performance Measures (Writing Committee to Develop Heart Failure Clinical Performance Measures): Endorsed by the Heart Failure Society of American. Circulation 112:1853, 2005.
19. Krumholz HM, Anderson JL, Brooks NH, et al: ACC/AHA clinical performance measures for adults with ST-elevation and non-ST-elevation myocardial infarction: A report of the ACC/AHA Task Force on Performance Measures (ST-Elevation and Non-ST-Elevation Myocardial Infarction Performance Measures Writing Committee). Circulation 113:732, 2006.

Definition of Quality

20. Moscucci M, Rogers EK, Montoye C, et al: Association of a continuous quality improvement initiative with practice and outcome variations of contemporary percutaneous coronary interventions. Circulation 113:814, 2006.
21. Lee TH: A broader concept of medical errors. N Engl J Med 347:1965, 2002.
22. Krumholz HA, Wang Y, Mattera JA, et al: An administrative claims model suitable for profiling hospital performance based on 30-day mortality rates among patients with acute myocardial infarction. Circulation 113:1683, 2006.
23. Krumholz HA, Wang Y, Mattera JA, et al: An administrative claims model suitable for profiling hospital performance based on 30-day mortality rates among patients with heart failure. Circulation 113:1693, 2006.
24. Epstein AE: Volume and outcome—it is time to move ahead. N Engl J Med 346:1161, 2002.
25. Halm EA, Lee C, Chassin MR: Is volume related to quality in health care? A systematic review and methodologic critique of the medical literature. Ann Intern Med 137:511, 2002.
26. Birkmeyer JD, Siewers AE, Finlayson EVA, et al: Hospital volume and surgical mortality in the United States. N Engl J Med 346:1128, 2002.
27. Birkmeyer JD, Stukel TA, Siewers AE, et al: Surgeon volume and operative mortality in the United States. N Engl J Med 349:2117, 2003.
28. Smith SC Jr, Feldman TE, Hirshfeld JW Jr, et al: ACC/AHA/SCAI 2005 guideline update for percutaneous coronary intervention: A report of the American College of Cardiology/American Heart Association Task Force on Practice Guidelines. ACC/AHA/SCAI Writing Committee to Update the 2001 Guidelines (http://www.americanheart.org).

Current Quality of Care and Improvement Strategies

29. Jencks SF, Huff ED, Cuerdon T: Change in the quality of care delivered to Medicare beneficiaries, 1998-1999 to 2000-2001. JAMA 289:305, 2003.
30. Peterson ED, Roe MT, Mulgund J, et al: Association between hospital process performance and outcomes among patients with acute coronary syndromes. JAMA 295:1912-1920. 2006.
31. Lee TH, Zapert K: Do high deductible health plans threaten quality of care? N Engl J Med 353:1202, 2005.
32. Mehta RH, Montoye CK, Gallogly M, et al: Improving quality of care for acute myocardial infarction: The Guidelines Applied in Practice (GAP) Initiative. JAMA 287:1269, 2002.
33. Krumholz H, Amatruda J, Smith GL, et al: Randomized trial of an education and support intervention to prevent readmission of patients with heart failure. J Am Coll Cardiol 39:83, 2002.
34. Ferguson TB, Peterson ED, Coombs LP, et al: Use of continuous quality improvement to increase use of process measures in patients undergoing coronary artery bypass graft surgery. A randomized controlled trial. JAMA 290:49, 2003.
35. Butler J, Speroff T, Arbogast PG, et al: Improved compliance with quality measures at hospital discharge with a computerized physician order entry system. Am Heart J 151:643, 2006.
36. Bradley EH, Curry LA, Webster TR, et al: Achieving rapid door-to-balloon times: How top hospitals improve complex clinical systems. Circulation 113:1079, 2006.

CHAPTER 6

The Principles of Drug Therapy

Dan M. Roden

IMPORTANCE OF CORRECT DRUG USE

In 2004 Americans spent $244 billion on pharmaceuticals.[1] Adverse drug reactions are estimated to be the fourth to sixth most common cause of death in the United States, to cost $19 to 27 billion annually, and to account directly for 2 to 3 percent of all hospital admissions.[2] The prevalence of heart disease and the increasing utilization of not only acute interventional therapies but also long-term preventive therapies translate into a dominant role of cardiovascular drugs in these costs: 20 percent of all drug costs, a projected $50.1 billion in 2006.[3] Moreover, with increasing success not only in heart disease but also in other therapeutic arenas, cardiovascular physicians are increasingly encountering patients receiving multiple medications with which they may not have complete comfort and familiarity. The goal of this chapter is to outline principles of drug action and interaction that allow the safest and most effective therapy in an individual patient.

The Key Decision in Drug Therapy: Risk versus Benefit

The fundamental assumption underlying administration of any drug is that the real or expected benefit exceeds the anticipated risk. The benefits of drug therapy are initially defined in small clinical trials, perhaps involving several thousand patients, before a drug's marketing and approval. Ultimately, the efficacy and safety profile of any drug is determined after the compound has been marketed and used widely in hundreds of thousands of patients.

When a drug is administered for the acute correction of a life-threatening condition, the benefits are often self-evident; insulin for diabetic ketoacidosis, nitroprusside for hypertensive encephalopathy, or lidocaine for ventricular tachycardia are examples. Extrapolation of such immediately obvious benefits to other clinical situations may not be warranted, however.

The efficacy of lidocaine to terminate ventricular tachycardia led to its widespread use as a prophylactic agent in cases of acute myocardial infarction until it was recognized that, in this setting, the drug does not alter mortality. The outcome of the Cardiac Arrhythmia Suppression Trial (CAST) highlights the difficulties in extrapolating from an incomplete understanding of physiology to chronic drug therapy. CAST tested the hypothesis that suppression of ventricular ectopic activity (a recognized risk factor for sudden death for myocardial infarction) would reduce mortality; this notion was highly ingrained in cardiovascular practice in the 1970s and 1980s. In CAST, sodium channel-blocking antiarrhythmics did suppress ventricular ectopic beats but also unexpectedly increased mortality threefold. In this instance the use of arrhythmia suppression as a "surrogate" marker for a desired drug action, reduction in mortality, was inappropriate because the underlying pathophysiology was incompletely understood. Similarly, reduced contractility in cases of heart failure has led to development of a series of drugs with positive inotropic activity, but these also show an increase in mortality, likely due to drug-induced arrhythmias. Nevertheless, clinical trials with these agents do suggest symptom relief. Thus the prescriber and the patient may elect therapy with positive inotropic drugs, because of this benefit, while recognizing the risk. These examples illustrate the continuing personal relationship between the prescriber and the patient and emphasize the need for a clear understanding of the expected benefit of therapy, as well as a clear understanding of disease pathophysiology and its response to drug therapy, in the drug development and prescribing processes.

The risks of drug therapy may be a direct extension of the pharmacological actions for which the drug is actually being prescribed. Excessive hypotension in a patient taking an antihypertensive agent or bleeding in a patient taking a platelet IIb/IIIa receptor antagonist are examples. In other cases, adverse effects develop as a consequence of pharmacological actions that were not appreciated during a drug's initial development and use in patients. Rhabdomyolysis with HMG-CoA reductase inhibitors, angioedema during angiotensin-converting enzyme (ACE) inhibitor therapy, torsades de pointes during treatment with "noncardiovascular" drugs such as thioridazine or pentamidine, or hyperglycemia and hypoglycemia with gatifloxacin[4] are examples. However, these rarer but serious events may become evident only after a drug has been marketed and extensively used. Even rare adverse effects can alter the overall perception of risk versus benefit and can prompt removal of the drug from the market, particularly if alternate, safer therapies are available. For example, withdrawal of the first insulin-sensitizer, troglitazone, after recognition of hepatotoxicity was further spurred by availability of other new drugs in this class. Further, investigation of the pathophysiology underlying these unusual events can define new mechanisms underlying variable responses to drug therapy.

Variability in Drug Action

Drugs interact with specific molecular targets to effect changes in whole organ and whole body function. The targets with which drugs interact to produce beneficial effects may or may not be the same as those with which drugs interact to produce adverse effects. Drug targets may be in the circulation, at the cell surface, or within cells. Many newer drugs have been developed to specifically interact with a desired drug target; examples of such targets are HMG-CoA reductase, angiotensin-converting enzyme, G-protein coupled receptors (α, β, AT1, histamine, and many others), and platelet IIb/IIIa receptors. On the other hand, many drugs widely used in cardiovascular therapeutics were developed when the technology to identify specific molecular targets simply was not available; digoxin, amiodarone, and aspirin are examples. In some cases, such agents turn out to have rather specific molecular targets: digoxin's actions are mediated primarily by inhibition of Na-K-ATPase.

Aspirin permanently acetylates a specific serine residue on the cyclooxygenase (COX) enzyme, an effect that is thought to mediate both its analgesic effects, as well as its gastrointestinal (GI) toxicity. The recognition of multiple COX isoforms led to the development of specific COX-2 inhibitors to retain the analgesic effects but to reduce GI side effects.[5] However, one of these, rofecoxib, has been withdrawn because of an apparent increase in cardiovascular mortality.[6,7] The COX-2 story has several important implications. First, specificity achieved by targeting a single molecular entity may not necessarily reduce adverse effects. Second, drug side effects may include not only readily identifiable events like rhabdomyolysis or torsades de pointes, but also an increase—that may be difficult to detect—in signs and symptoms that are common in the general population.[8]

MECHANISMS UNDERLYING VARIABILITY IN DRUG ACTION. Two major processes determine how the interaction between a drug and its target molecule can generate variable drug actions in the patient (Fig. 6-1). The first, pharmacokinetics, describes drug delivery to and removal from the target molecule and includes the processes of absorption, distribution, metabolism, and excretion. These are collectively termed "drug disposition." Robust techniques—applicable across drugs and drug classes—to analyze drug disposition have been developed and result in a series of principles that can be used to adjust drug dosages to enhance the likelihood of a beneficial effect and to minimize toxicity.

The second process, pharmacodynamics, describes how the interaction between a drug and its target generates downstream molecular, cellular, whole organ, and whole body effects. Pharmacodynamic sources of variability in drug action arise from the specifics of the target molecule and the biological context in which the drug-target interaction occurs; thus methods for analysis of pharmacodynamics tend to be drug or drug-class specific. In practice, pharmacodynamic variability often arises as a consequence of disease, especially the disease for which the drug is being prescribed.

One source of pharmacodynamic variability is variability in the target molecule itself; this can arise because of genetic factors, discussed subsequently, or because disease alters the number of target molecules or their state (e.g., changes in extent of phosphorylation). A second source of pharmacodynamic variability arises from our increasing understanding of the molecular pathophysiology of disease: The interaction between drugs and their target molecules occurs in a complex biological context, so variability in this biology (often a consequence of disease) can affect the extent to which a drug produces desired or undesired effects. Examples include high dietary salt, which can inhibit the antihypertensive action of beta blockers, or hypokalemia, which increases the risk for drug-induced QT prolongation.

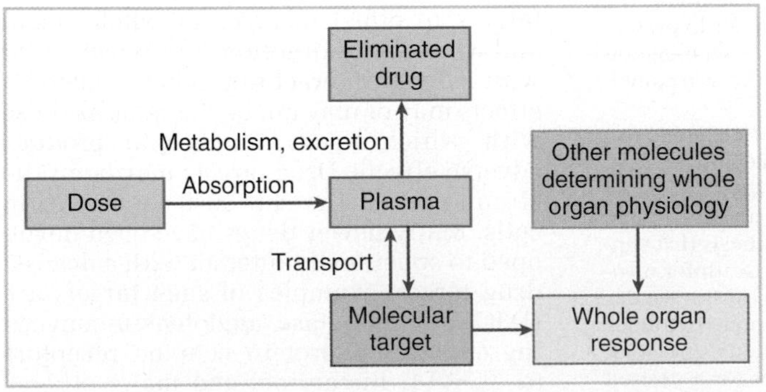

FIGURE 6–1 A model for understanding variability in drug action. When a dose of a drug is administered, the processes of absorption, metabolism, excretion, and transport determine its access to specific molecular targets that mediate beneficial and toxic effects. The interaction between a drug and its molecular target then produces changes in molecular, cellular, whole organ, and ultimately whole patient physiology. This molecular interaction does not occur in a vacuum, but rather in a complex biological milieu modulated by multiple factors (some of which are disturbed to cause disease). DNA variants in the genes responsible for the processes of drug disposition (green), the molecular target (blue), or the molecules determining the biological context in which the drug-target interaction occurs (gold) all can contribute to variability in drug action.

PHARMACOGENETICS AND PHARMACOGENOMICS. This contemporary view of drug actions identifies a series of molecules that mediate drug actions in patients: drug metabolizing enzymes, drug transport molecules, drug targets, and molecules modulating the biology in which the drug-target interaction occurs. The vast majority of these molecules are proteins, so variations in the genes that encode them may therefore contribute to variability in drug actions. Isolated examples of familial aggregation of unusual responses to drug therapy have been recognized for decades and defined the field of pharmacogenetics.[9] Such rare aberrant responses recognized in families generally arise a s a result of mutations, usually defined as rare DNA variants that are associated with a disease phenotype. With the sequencing of the human genome has come the recognition that DNA variants are extremely common, occurring on average in 1 of 300 base pairs; such variants—termed polymorphisms—may or may not alter gene expression or function. The nascent field of pharmacogenomics is attempting to define common polymorphisms, or sets of polymorphisms, that underlie variability in drug action.[10,11] Ultimately, it may be possible to genotype individuals before prescribing medications to ensure that benefit is maximized and risk minimized: the concept of "preprescription genotyping." Indeed, a clinical trial of a new drug targeting cardiovascular risk in a population specifically selected because of a genetic risk marker has now been reported.[12]

PHARMACOKINETICS

Administration of an intravenous drug bolus results in maximal drug concentrations at the end of the bolus and then a decline in plasma drug concentrations over time (Fig. 6-2A). The simplest case is one in which this decline occurs monoexponentially over time. A useful parameter to describe this decline is the half-life ($t_{1/2}$), the time in which 50 percent of the drug elimination occurs; after two half-lives, 75 percent of the drug has been eliminated, after three half-lives 87.5 percent, and so on.

In some cases, the decline of drug concentrations following administration of an intravenous bolus dose is multiexponential. The most common explanation is that drug is not only eliminated (represented by the terminal portion of the time-concentration plot) but also undergoes more rapid distribution to peripheral tissues. Just as elimination may be usefully described by a half-life, distribution half-lives can also be derived from curves such as those shown in Figure 6-2B.

The plasma concentration measured immediately after a bolus dose can be used to derive a volume into which the drug is distributed. When the decline of plasma concentrations is multiexponential, multiple distribution compartments can be defined; these volumes of distribution can be useful in considering dose adjustments in cases of disease but rarely correspond exactly to any physical volume such as plasma or total body water. Indeed, with drugs that are highly tissue bound (such as some antidepressants), volume of distribution can exceed total body volume by orders of magnitude.

Drugs are often administered by nonintravenous routes such as oral, sublingual, transcutaneous, or intramuscular. With such routes of administration, there are two differences from the intravenous route (see Fig. 6-2A). First, concentrations in plasma demonstrate a distinct rising phase as drug slowly enters plasma. Second, the total amount of drug that actually enters the systemic circulation may be less than that achieved by the intravenous route. The relative amount of drug entering by any route, compared with the same dose administered intravenously, is termed *bioavailability.* Bioavailability may be reduced because drug undergoes metabolism before entering the circulation or because drug is simply not absorbed from its site of administration.

Clearance is the most useful way of quantifying drug elimination. Clearance can be viewed as a volume that is "cleared" of drug in any given period. Clearance may be organ specific (e.g., renal clearance, hepatic clearance) or whole body clearance.

With repeated doses, drug levels accumulate to a steady state, the condition under which the rate of drug administration is equal to the rate of drug elimination in any given period. As illustrated in Figure 6-3, the elimination half-life describes not only the disappearance of a drug but also the time course by which a drug accumulates to steady state. It is important to distinguish between steady-state plasma concentrations, achieved in four to five elimination half-lives, and steady-state drug effects, which may take longer to achieve. For some drugs, clinical effects develop immediately on access to the molecular target: nitrates for angina, nitroprusside to lower blood pressure, and sympathomimetics to treat shock are examples. In other situations, drug effects follow plasma concentrations, but with a lag, and several explanations are possible. First, an active metabolite may need to be generated to achieve drug effects. Second, time may be required for translation of the drug effect at the molecular site to a physiological end point: inhibition of synthesis of vitamin K-dependent clotting factors by warfarin ultimately leads to a desired elevation of international normalized ratio, but the development of this desired effect occurs only as levels of clotting factors fall. Third, penetration of a drug into intracellular or other tissue sites of action may be required before development of drug effect. One barrier to such penetration is variable function of specific drug uptake and efflux transport proteins that control intracellular drug concentrations.[13,14] Variable tissue penetration is also widely invoked to explain the lag time between administration of amiodarone and development of its effects, although the precise details underlying this phenomenon remain elusive, and drug transport may not be involved.

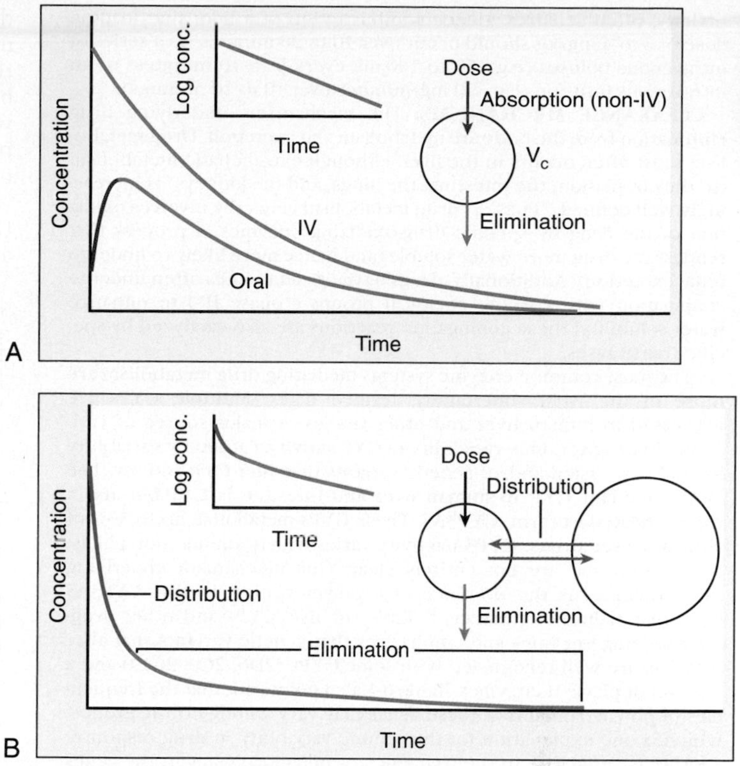

FIGURE 6–2 Models of plasma concentrations as a function of time after a single dose of a drug. **A,** The simplest situation is one in which a drug is administered as a rapid intravenous bolus into a volume (V_c) into which it is instantaneously and uniformly distributed. Elimination then takes place from this volume. In this case, drug elimination is monoexponential; that is, a plot of the logarithm of concentration versus time is linear, as shown in the inset. When the same dose of drug is administered orally, a distinct absorption phase is required before drug entry into V_c. Most absorption (shown here in red) is completed before elimination (shown in green), although the processes overlap. In this example the amount of drug delivered by the oral route is less than that delivered by the intravenous route, assessed by the total areas under the two curves, indicating reduced bioavailability. **B,** In this example, drug is delivered to the central volume, from which it is not only eliminated but also undergoes distribution to the peripheral sites. This distribution process (blue) is more rapid than elimination, resulting in a distinct biexponential disappearance curve, seen best in the inset.

Pharmacokinetic Principles in Managing Drug Therapy

BIOAVAILABILITY AND DOSE ADJUSTMENT. Some drugs undergo such extensive presystemic metabolism that the amount of drug required to achieve a therapeutic effect is much greater (and often much more variable) than that required for the same drug administered intravenously. Thus small doses of intravenous propranolol (5 mg) may achieve heart rate slowing equivalent to that observed with much larger oral doses (80 to 120 mg). Propranolol is actually well absorbed but undergoes extensive metabolism in the intestine and the liver before entering the systemic circulation. Another example is amiodarone, the physicochemical characteristics of which make it only 30 to 50 percent bioavailable when it is administered orally (the drug is highly lipophilic and thus has limited water solubility). Thus an intravenous infusion 0.5 mg/min (720 mg/day) is equivalent to 1.5 to 2 gm/day orally.

DISTRIBUTION. Rapid distribution can alter the way in which drug therapy should be initiated. When lidocaine is administered intravenously, it displays a prominent and rapid distribution phase ($t_{1/2} = 8$ minutes) before slower elimination ($t_{1/2} = 120$ minutes). As a consequence, an antiarrhythmic effect of lidocaine may be transiently achieved but rapidly lost following a single bolus, due not to elimination but to rapid distribution. Administration of larger bolus doses to circumvent this problem results in dose-related

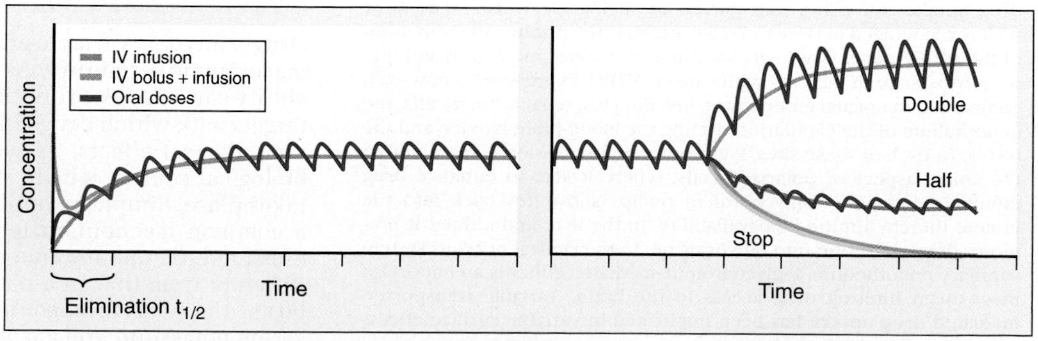

FIGURE 6–3 Time course of drug concentrations when treatment is started or dose changed. **Left,** The hash lines on the abscissa indicate one elimination half-life ($t_{1/2}$). With a constant rate intravenous infusion (gold), plasma concentrations accumulate to steady state in 4 to 5 elimination half-lives. When a loading bolus is administered with the maintenance infusion (blue), plasma concentrations are transiently higher but may dip, as shown here, before achieving the same steady state. When the same drug is administered by the oral route, the time course of drug accumulation is identical (red); in this case the drug was administered at intervals of 50 percent of a $t_{1/2}$. Steady-state plasma concentrations during oral therapy fluctuate around the mean determined by intravenous therapy. **Right,** This plot shows that when dosages are doubled, halved, or drug stopped during steady-state administration, the time required to achieve the new steady-state is 4 to 5 × $t_{1/2}$, and is independent of the route of administration.

toxicity, often seizures. Hence administration of a lidocaine loading dose of 3 to 4 mg/kg should occur over 10 to 20 minutes, as a series of intravenous boluses (e.g., 50 to 100 mg every 5 to 10 minutes) or an intravenous infusion (e.g., 20 mg/minutes over 10 to 20 minutes).

CLEARANCE MECHANISMS. The mechanisms underlying drug elimination from the body are metabolism and excretion. Drug metabolism most often occurs in the liver, although extrahepatic metabolism (in the circulation, the intestine, the lungs, and the kidneys) is increasingly well defined. "Phase I" drug metabolism generally involves oxidation of the drug by specific drug-oxidizing enzymes, a process that renders the drug more water soluble (and hence more likely to undergo renal excretion). Additionally, drugs or their metabolites often undergo conjugation with specific chemical groups ("phase II") to enhance water solubility; these conjugation reactions are also catalyzed by specific transferases.

The most common enzyme systems mediating drug metabolism are those of the P450 superfamily, termed *CYPs.* Multiple CYPs are expressed in human liver and other tissues. A major source of variability in drug action is variability in CYP activity, caused by variability in CYP expression and/or genetic variants that alter CYP activity. The most abundant CYP in human liver and intestine is CYP3A4 and a closely related isoform, CYP3A5. These CYPs metabolize up to 50% of clinically used drugs. CYP3A activity varies widely among individuals, for reasons that are not entirely clear. One mechanism underlying this variability is the presence of a polymorphism in this CYP3A5 gene that reduces its activity.[15] Table 6-1 lists CYPs and other drug-metabolizing enzymes and emphasizes that genetic variants that alter function are well recognized with some CYPs (2D6, 2C9, 2C19) and a number of phase II enzymes. Table 6-1 also points out that the frequencies of polymorphisms in these genes may vary among ethnic groups, which is one explanation for interethnic variability in drug response; another is variability in the frequency of polymorphisms in the genes whose function determines pharmacodynamics, discussed further later.

Reduction in clearance, by disease, drug interactions, or genetic factors, will increase drug concentrations and hence drug effects. An exception is drugs whose effects are mediated by generation of active metabolites. In this case, inhibition of drug metabolism may lead to accumulation of the parent drug but loss of therapeutic efficacy. The anticonvulsant phenytoin is an inhibitor of CYP2C9; when phenytoin is started in a patient receiving the angiotensin receptor blocker losartan, blood pressure control may be lost because of failure of biotransformation of losartan to its active metabolite. This is in contrast to phenytoin effects on CYP3A substrates. In this case, phenytoin acts as a potent inducing agent, increasing gene transcription. Thus administration of phenytoin actually increases CYP3A activity and hence leads to altered effects of CYP3A substrates through this mechanism.

Excretion of drugs, generally into the urine or bile, is accomplished by specific drug-transport molecules, whose level of expression and genetic variation are only now being explored. In fact, drug transporters play a role not only in drug elimination but also in drug uptake into many cells, including hepatocytes and enterocytes. As with CYPs and other drug-metabolizing enzymes, multiple genes encoding multiple drug uptake and efflux transporters are being identified.[14] The most widely recognized of these is P-glycoprotein, the product of expression of the *MDR1* gene. Originally identified as a factor mediating multiple drug resistance in patients with cancer, MDR1 expression is now well recognized in normal enterocytes, hepatocytes, renal tubular cells, the endothelium of the capillaries forming the blood-brain barrier, and the testes. In each of these sites, P-glycoprotein expression is restricted to the apical aspect of polarized cells, where it acts to enhance drug efflux. In intestine, P-glycoprotein pumps substrates back into the lumen, thereby limiting bioavailability. In the liver and kidney, it promotes drug excretion into bile or urine. In the central nervous system capillary endothelium, P-glycoprotein–mediated efflux is an important mechanism limiting drug access to the brain. Variable transporter-mediated drug uptake has been implicated in variable cardiac effects of verapamil and spironolactone.[16]

Clinical Relevance of Polymorphic Drug Metabolism: The Concept of High-Risk Pharmacokinetics

The absence of a specific pathway for drug metabolism, because of genetic factors or the administration of other drugs, has variable clinical consequences. When a drug uses multiple pathways for its elimination, absence of one of these is unlikely to have major clinical consequences because elimination can be accomplished by alternate pathways. On the other hand, a drug eliminated by only a single pathway carries with it the liability that absence of activity of that pathway will lead to marked accumulation of drug in plasma, failure to form downstream metabolites, and thus a risk of unusual drug responses, especially if there is a narrow therapeutic margin (see later).

A classic example was the antihistamine terfenadine, which is eliminated almost exclusively by CYP3A metabolism in the intestine and the liver. Terfenadine itself is a highly potent QT-prolonging agent and is biotransformed to a noncardioactive metabolite (fexofenadine) that mediates the compound's antihistamine actions. Coadministration of terfenadine with CYP3A inhibitors such as ketoconazole or erythromycin led to inhibition of presystemic metabolism, striking elevations of plasma terfenadine concentrations, marked QT prolongation, and torsades de pointes. As a consequence, the drug was withdrawn from the market, and fexofenadine is now marketed as a widely used antihistamine (Allegra).[17]

Similarly, CYP3A inhibition appears to increase the risk of rhabdomyolysis with some but not all HMG-CoA reductase inhibitors, through mechanisms that are not completely understood; fibrates also increase this risk, though the mechanisms are uncertain.

Administration of CYP2D6-metabolized beta blockers to patients with defective enzyme activity (on a genetic basis or because of coadministration of inhibitors) produces exaggerated heart rate slowing. Similarly, the weak beta-blocking actions of the antiarrhythmic propafenone are increased in this setting. The widely used analgesic codeine undergoes CYP2D6-mediated bioactivation to an active metabolite, morphine, and patients with defective CYP2D6 activity display reduced analgesia. A small group of individuals with multiple functional copies of CYP2D6, and hence increased enzymatic activity, has been identified; in this group codeine may produce nausea and euphoria, presumably due to rapid morphine generation. Similarly, some antidepressants are CYP2D6 substrates; for these drugs, cardiovascular adverse effects are more common in CYP2D6 poor metabolizers, whereas therapeutic efficacy is more difficult to achieve in ultra-rapid metabolizers.[11]

The concept of high-risk pharmacokinetics extends from drug metabolism to transporter-mediated drug elimination. The most widely recognized example is digoxin, which is eliminated primarily by P-glycoprotein-mediated efflux into bile and urine. Administration of a wide range of structurally and mechanistically unrelated drugs has been empirically recognized to increase digoxin concentrations, and the common mechanism appears to be inhibition of P-glycoprotein-mediated elimination (see Table 6-1).[11]

PHARMACODYNAMICS AND THE GENETICS OF DRUG RESPONSES

Drugs can exert variable effects, even in the absence of pharmacokinetic variability. As indicated in Figure 6-1, this variability can arise as a function of variability in the molecular targets with which drugs interact to achieve their (beneficial and adverse) effects, as well as variability in the broader biological context within which the drug-target interaction takes place. Simple examples illustrate the point that this is a common mechanism for variability in drug action: the effect of lytic therapy in a patient with no clot is manifestly different from that in a patient with acute coronary thrombosis; the arrhythmogenic effects of digitalis depend on serum potassium; the vasodilating effects of nitrates, beneficial in patients with coronary disease with angina, can be catastrophic in patients with aortic stenosis.

DNA variants in key genes controlling this biological context (as well as genes encoding drug targets themselves) are increasingly recognized as contributors to variability in drug action. Many examples of associations between DNA polymorphisms and disease severity are now reported; there are fewer reports of polymorphisms modulating

TABLE 6-1 Proteins Important in Drug Metabolism and Elimination

Protein	Substrates	Interacting Drugs	Genetics
CYP3A4, CYP3A5	Erythromycin, clarithromycin Quinidine, mexiletine Many benzodiazepines Cyclosporine, tacrolimus Many antivirals HMG CoA reductase inhibitors (atorvastatin, simvastatin, lovastatin; not pravastatin) Many calcium channel blockers	*Inhibitors:* Antivirals: ritonavir and others Amiodarone Erythromycin, clarithromycin (not azithromycin) Ketoconazole, itraconazole Many calcium channel blockers *Inducers:* Rifampin Efavirenz, nevirapine St. John's wort Phenytoin Pioglitazone	Highly variable activity in vivo Common coding region polymorphism in CYP3A5 may contribute; commoner in African-Americans versus Caucasians No common coding region polymorphisms in CYP3A4
CYP2D6	Some beta blockers: Propranolol, timolol, metoprolol, carvedilol Propafenone Desipramine and other tricyclics Codeine Debrisoquine Dextromethorphan	*Inhibitors:* Amiodarone Fluoxetine Quinidine Paroxetine *Inducers:* Rifampin	Multiple loss of function alleles described. Common (25%) in Caucasian and African populations; homozygotes (7%) display the PM phenotype. Reduction of function alleles described in Asian populations, but PMs rare. Ultra-rapid metabolizers due multiple functional copies of CYP2D6 described, especially in Northern Africa.
CYP2C9	Warfarin Phenytoin Tolbutamide Glyburide Losartan, irbesartan	*Inhibitors:* Amiodarone Zafirlukast *Inducers:* Rifampin Barbiturates	Heterozygotes for common (>50% in some populations) loss of function alleles display reduced enzymatic activity and may have lower warfarin dose requirements. Very low warfarin dose requirements in homozygotes.
CYP2C19	Omeprazole Mephenytoin Nelfinavir		PMs common (≈20%) in Asian populations
P-glycoprotein	Digoxin Fexofenadine Cyclosporine, tacrolimus Many anticancer agents Many antivirals	*Inhibitors:* Amiodarone Quinidine Ketoconazole Erythromycin Itraconazole Verapamil Cyclosporine	DNA polymorphisms common; clinical significance uncertain
N-acetyl transferase	Procainamide Hydralazine Isoniazid		Caucasians and Africans: 50% fast acetylators, 50% slow acetylators, no nonacetylators Asians: mostly fast acetylators Slow acetylators: increased risk of the lupus syndrome (procainamide) Slow acetylators: Increased risk of isoniazid hepatotoxicity
Thiopurine methyltransferase	6-mercaptopurine Azathioprine		Homozygous for loss of function mutations (1/300): increased risk for one marrow aplasia at usual doses Rapid metabolizers: suboptimal therapeutic response
Pseudocholinesterase	Succinylcholine		Rare homozygote null individuals: prolonged apnea
UDP-glucuronosyl-transferase	Irinotecan		Polymorphisms cause Gilbert's syndrome Enhanced toxicity of some anticancer drugs[28]

More detailed CYP listing available at http://medicine.iupui.edu/flockhart/
PM = poor metabolizer.

responses to cardiovascular drugs, and examples are listed in Table 6-2.

Polymorphisms in the β_1 and β_2 receptor genes have been associated with variability in heart rate slowing and blood pressure effects with beta blockers and beta agonists.[18] An example of a tumor genotype determining response to therapy is the anticancer drug Herceptin, which is effective only in cancers that do not express the Herceptin receptor; because the drug also potentiates anthracycline-related cardiotoxicity,[19] toxic therapy can be avoided in patients who are receptor negative. The effect of hormone replacement therapy on high-density lipoprotein cholesterol has been linked to a polymorphism in the estrogen receptor, and susceptibility to stroke in patients receiving diuretics to a polymorphism in the alpha-adducin gene whose product plays a role in renal tubular sodium transport. Torsades de pointes during QT-prolonging antiarrhythmic therapy has been linked to polymorphisms in ion channel genes; in addition, this adverse effect

TABLE 6–2 DNA Polymorphisms Implicated in Variable Pharmacodynamics in Cardiovascular Medicine*

Drug	Gene	Reported Association
QT-prolonging drugs	KCNH2/KCNE2 (HERG/MiRP1)†	Increased torsades de pointes risk in patients with KCNE2 T8A
QT-prolonging drugs	KCNQ1 (KvLKQT1)† MinK (KCNE1)† SCN5A†	Increased torsades de pointes risk in patients with KCNE1 D85N, SCN5A S1102Y
Beta blockers	β_1- and β_2-adrenergic receptor	Altered extent of heart rate slowing or blood pressure lowering
ACE inhibitors	ACE	Decreased response in DD subjects
Beta blockers	ACE	Increased response in DD subjects
Fluvastatin	ABCA1 transporter LDL receptor Paraoxonase	Variable LDL lowering
Pravastatin	Cholesteryl ester transfer protein; HMG CoA reductase[25]	Variable regression of atherosclerosis or of LDL lowering
Estrogen	Estrogen receptor	Variable HDL elevation
Lipid-lowering therapy	Hepatic lipase	Variable lipid lowering
Antiplatelet drugs	Platelet glycoprotein IIIa	Variable antiplatelet effects ex vivo
Amiloride	Epithelial sodium channel	Variable antihypertensive effect in African American subjects
Antihypertensive drugs	β_3 G-Protein subunit	Variable BP lowering
Diuretics	α-adducin	Variable MI or stroke incidence during antihypertensive therapy Variable BP response (especially with ACE I/D)
ACE inhibitor	Bradykinin B2 receptor	ACE-inhibitor cough

*DNA variants that modulate pharmacokinetics are listed in Table 6-1.
†Mutations in these genes, causing the long QT syndrome, may be clinically silent until challenged with QT prolonging drugs.
ACE = angiotension-converting enzyme; BP = blood pressure; DD = deletion/deletion genotype; HDL, high-density lipoprotein; LDL, low-density lipoprotein; MI = myocardial infarction.

sometimes arises in patients with clinically latent congenital long QT syndrome, emphasizing the interrelationship among disease, genetic background, and drug therapy.

One of the best-studied human polymorphisms is the insertion/deletion (I/D) variant in the ACE gene that determines ACE activity. DD individuals, homozygous for the D allele, have higher plasma ACE activity and thus are assumed to have higher concentrations of the pressor peptide angiotensin II than do individuals with the II genotype. Many associations have been reported between the DD genotype and worse outcomes in cardiovascular disease. However, a large meta-analysis (almost 38,000 patients) found absolutely no effect of this polymorphism on a range of outcomes like myocardial infarction or death.[20] Thus it is important to recognize that genomic science is in its infancy, and so reported associations—especially in small populations—require independent confirmation and assessment of clinical importance and cost-effectiveness before they can or should enter clinical practice.

Challenges in this area include not only replication but also methods to identify combined effects of multiple genetic variants on disease susceptibility or the outcome of drug therapy. Studies have now identified two genes that contribute to variability in warfarin dose requirements: one is *CYP2C9,* which mediates elimination of the active enantiomer of the drug, and the other is *VKORC1,* part of the vitamin K complex that is the drug target.[21] Technologies to screen hundreds to hundreds of thousands of polymorphisms in large populations are now being developed and are beginning to be applied to identify genes contributing to variability in baseline QT interval,[22] in risk of obesity[23] or diabetes,[24] and in response to HMG-CoA reductase inhibitors[25] and to inhaled β_2 agonists in asthma.[26]

PRINCIPLES OF DOSAGE OPTIMIZATION

The goals of drug therapy should be defined before initiation of drug treatment. These may include acute correction of serious pathophysiology, acute or chronic symptom relief, or changes in "surrogate" endpoints (such as blood pressure or serum cholesterol or international normalized ratio) that have been linked to beneficial outcomes in target patient populations. The lessons of CAST and of positive inotropic drugs should make prescribers skeptical about such surrogate-guided therapy in the absence of controlled clinical trials.

When the goal of drug therapy is to acutely correct a disturbance in physiology, the drug should be administered intravenously, in doses designed to rapidly achieve a therapeutic effect. This approach is best justified when benefits clearly outweigh risks. As discussed earlier with lidocaine, large intravenous drug boluses carry with them a risk of enhancing drug-related toxicity, so even with the most urgent of medical indications, this approach is rarely appropriate. An exception is adenosine, which must be administered as a rapid bolus because it undergoes extensive and rapid elimination from plasma by uptake into virtually all cells; as a consequence, a slow bolus or infusion rarely achieves sufficiently high concentrations at the desired site of action (the coronary artery perfusing the atrioventricular node) to terminate arrhythmias.

The time required to achieve steady-state plasma concentrations is determined by elimination half-life, as discussed earlier. The administration of a loading dose may abbreviate this time, but only if the kinetics of distribution and elimination are known a priori in an individual subject and the correct loading regimen is chosen; otherwise, overshoot or undershoot during the loading phase may occur. Thus the initiation of drug therapy by a loading strategy should be used only when the indication is acute.

Two dose-response curves describe the relationship between drug dose and the expected cumulative incidence of a beneficial effect or an adverse effect (Fig. 6-4). The distance along the X axis describing the difference between these curves, often termed the *therapeutic ratio (or index or window),* provides an index of the likelihood that a chronic dosing regimen that provides benefits without adverse effects can be identified. Drugs with especially wide therapeutic indices can often be administered at infrequent intervals, even if they are rapidly eliminated (Fig. 6-4, left panels).

When expected adverse effects are serious, the most appropriate treatment strategy is to start at low doses and re-evaluate the necessity for increasing drug dosages once steady-state drug effects have been achieved. This approach has the advantage of minimizing the risk of dose-related adverse effects but carries with it a need to titrate doses to efficacy. Only when stable drug effects are achieved should increasing drug dosage to achieve the desired therapeutic effect be considered. An example is sotalol; because the risk of torsades de pointes increases with drug dosage, the starting dose should be low.

In other cases, anticipated toxicity is relatively mild and manageable. It may then be acceptable to start at dosages greater than the minimum required to achieve a therapeutic effect, accepting a greater than minimal risk of adverse effects; some antihypertensives can be administered in this fashion. However, the principle of using the lowest dose possible to minimize toxicity, particularly toxicity that is unpredictable and unrelated to recognized pharmacologic actions, should be the rule.

Occasionally, dose escalation into the high therapeutic range results in no beneficial drug effect and no side effects. In this circumstance the prescriber should be alert to the possibility of drug interactions at the pharmacokinetic or pharmacodynamic level. Depending on the nature of the anticipated toxicity, dose escalation beyond the usual therapeutic range may occasionally be acceptable, but only if anticipated toxicity is not serious and is readily manageable.

PLASMA CONCENTRATION MONITORING. For some drugs, curves such as those shown in Figures 6-4A and B relating drug concentration to cumulative incidence of beneficial and adverse effects can be generated. With such drugs, monitoring plasma drug concentrations to ensure that they remain within a desired therapeutic range (i.e., above a minimum required for efficacy and below a maximum likely to produce adverse effects) may be a useful adjunct to therapy. Monitoring drug concentrations may also be useful to ensure compliance and to detect pharmacokinetically based drug interactions that underlie unanticipated efficacy and/or toxicity at usual dosages. Samples for measurement of plasma concentrations should generally be obtained just before the next dose, at steady state. These "trough" concentrations provide an index of the minimum plasma concentration expected during a dosing interval.

On the other hand, patient monitoring, whether by plasma concentration or other physiological indices, to detect incipient toxicity is best accomplished at the time of anticipated peak drug concentrations. Thus patient surveillance for QT prolongation during therapy with sotalol or dofetilide is best accomplished 1 to 2 hours after administration of a dose of drug at steady state.

A lag between the time courses of drug in plasma and of drug effects may exist, as described earlier. In addition, monitoring plasma drug concentrations relies on the assumption that the concentration measured is in equilibrium with that at the target molecular site. Importantly, it is only the fraction of drug not bound to plasma proteins that is available to achieve such equilibration. Variability in the extent of protein binding can therefore affect the free fraction and the anticipated drug effect, even in the face of apparently therapeutic total plasma drug concentrations. Basic drugs such as lidocaine and quinidine are not only bound to albumin but also bind extensively to α_1-acid glycoprotein, an acute phase reactant whose concentrations are increased in a variety of "stress" situations including acute myocardial infarction. Because of this increased protein binding, drug effects may be blunted despite "therapeutic" total drug concentrations in these situations.

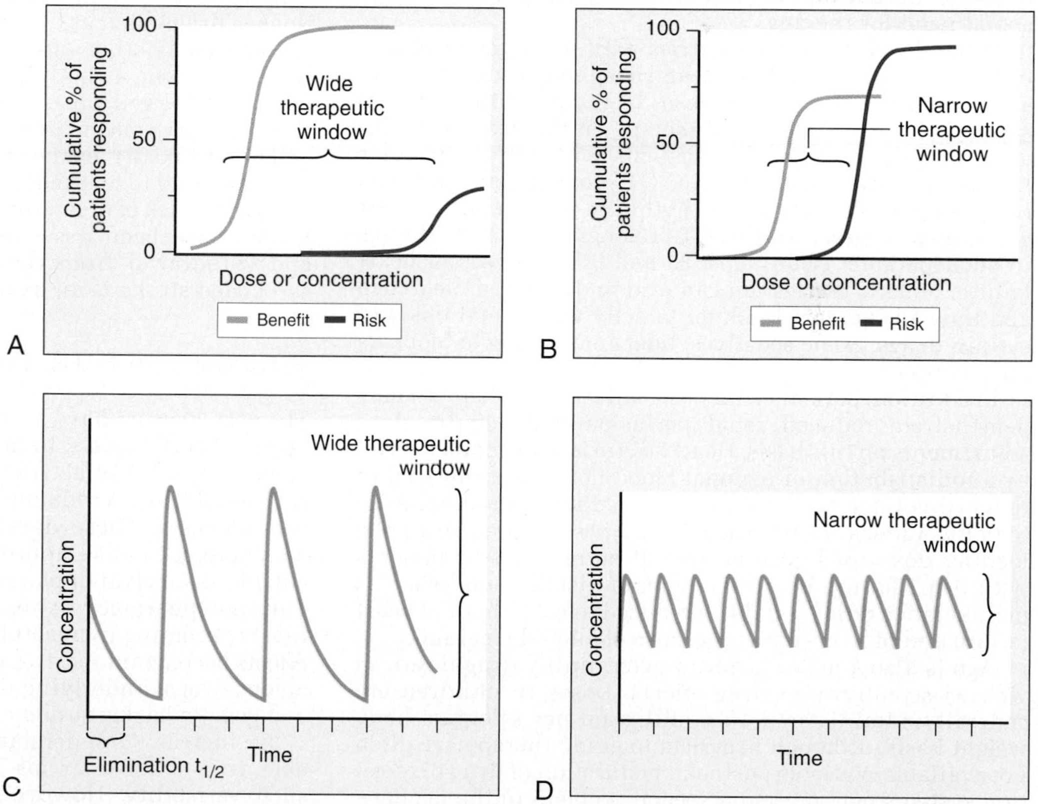

FIGURE 6–4 The concept of a therapeutic ratio. **Panels A** and **B** illustrate two dose- (or concentration-) response curves. The blue line in each panel describes the relationship between dose and cumulative incidence of beneficial effects, and the magenta line the relationship between dose and dose-related adverse effects (risk). A drug with a wide therapeutic ratio displays separation between the two curves, a high degree of efficacy, and low degree of dose-related toxicity **(A).** Under these conditions, a wide therapeutic ratio can be defined. In **(B),** on the other hand, the curves describing cumulative efficacy and cumulative incidence of adverse effects are positioned near each other, the incidence of adverse effects is higher, and the expected beneficial response is lower; these characteristics define a narrow therapeutic ratio. **Panels C** and **D** show steady-state plasma concentrations with oral drug administration as a function of time with wide **(left)** and narrow **(right)** therapeutic ratios. The hash marks on the abscissae indicate one elimination half-life. When the therapeutic window is wide, drug administration every 3 elimination half-lives can produce plasma concentrations that are maintained above the minimum for efficacy and below the maximum beyond which toxicity is anticipated. **Panel D** shows the opposite situation. In order to maintain plasma concentrations within the narrow therapeutic range, the drug must be administered more frequently.

Dose Adjustments

Polypharmacy is common in patients with varying degrees of specific organ dysfunction. Although treatment with an individual agent may be justified, the practitioner should also recognize the risk of unanticipated drug effects, particularly drug toxicity, during therapy with multiple drugs.

The presence of renal disease mandates dose reductions for digoxin, dofetilide, procainamide, and sotalol, drugs eliminated primarily by renal excretion (an example of "high-risk pharmacokinetics, discussed previously). A requirement for dose adjustment in cases of mild renal dysfunction is dictated by available clinical data and the likelihood of serious toxicity if drug accumulates in plasma due to impaired elimination. Renal failure reduces the protein binding of some drugs (e.g., phenytoin); in this instance, a total drug concentration value in the therapeutic range may actually represent a toxic value of unbound drug.

Advanced liver disease is characterized by decreased hepatic drug metabolism and portocaval shunts that decrease clearance (and particularly first-pass clearance). Moreover, such patients frequently have other profound disturbances of homeostasis such as coagulopathy, severe ascites, and altered mental status. These pathophysiological features of advanced liver disease can profoundly affect not only the dose of a drug required to achieve a potentially therapeutic effect but also the perception of risks and benefits, thereby altering the prescriber's assessment of the actual need for therapy.

Heart disease similarly carries with it a number of disturbances of drug elimination and drug sensitivity that may alter either the therapeutic doses or the practitioner's perception of the desirability of therapy on the basis of evaluation of risks and benefits. Patients with left ventricular hypertrophy often have baseline QT prolongation, and thus risks of QT-prolonging antiarrhythmics may increase; most guidelines suggest avoiding QT-prolonging antiarrhythmics in such patients (see Chaps. 33 and 35). In cases of heart failure, hepatic congestion can lead to decreased clearance and thus an increased risk for toxicity with usual doses of certain drugs. Some sedatives, lidocaine, and beta blockers are examples.

In addition, patients with heart failure (see Chap. 23) may demonstrate reduced renal perfusion and require dose adjustments on this basis. Heart failure is also characterized by a redistribution of regional blood flow. This can lead to reduced volume of distribution and enhanced risk for drug toxicity. Lidocaine is probably the best-studied example: loading doses of lidocaine should be reduced in patients with heart failure because of altered distribution, whereas maintenance doses should be reduced in cases both of heart failure and of liver disease because of altered clearance.

Age is also a major factor in determining drug doses, as well as sensitivity to drug effects. Doses in children are generally administered on a milligram per kilogram body weight basis, although firm data to guide therapy are often not available. Variable postnatal maturation of drug disposition systems may present a special problem in the neonate. Elderly persons often have reduced creatinine clearance, even in the face of a normal serum creatinine level, and dosages of renally excreted drugs should be adjusted accordingly (see Chap. 75). Systolic dysfunction with hepatic congestion is more common in the elderly. Vascular disease and dementia are common in the elderly and can lead to increased postural hypotension and risk of falling. Thus therapies such as sedatives, tricyclic antidepressants, or anticoagulants should be initiated only when the practitioner is convinced that the benefits of such therapies outweigh this increased risk.

DRUG INTERACTIONS

Multiple mechanisms, and examples, of interactions on a pharmacokinetic or pharmacodynamic basis have been presented in this chapter. Table 6-3 summarizes these and other mechanisms that may underlie important drug interactions. Drug interactions may be based on altered pharmacokinetics (absorption, distribution, metabolism, and excretion). In addition, drugs can interact at the pharmacodynamic level. A trivial example is coadministration of two antihypertensive drugs leading to excessive hypotension. Similarly, coadministration of aspirin and warfarin leads to an increased risk for bleeding, although benefits of the combination can also be demonstrated.

The most important principle in approaching a patient receiving polypharmacy is to recognize the high potential for drug interactions. *A complete medication history should be obtained from each patient at regular intervals;* patients will often omit topical medications such as eye drops, "health food" supplements, and medications prescribed by other practitioners unless specifically prompted. Each of these, however, carries a risk of important systemic drug actions and interactions. Even high dosages of grapefruit juice, which contains CYP3A and P-glycoprotein inhibitors, can affect drug responses.[27] Beta blocker eye drops can produce systemic beta blockade, particularly with CYP2D6 substrates (e.g., timolol) in patients with defective CYP2D6 activity. St. John's wort induces CYP3A and P-glycoprotein activity and thus can markedly lower plasma concentrations of drugs such as cyclosporine and oral contraceptives. As with many other interactions, this may not be a special problem as long as both drugs are continued. However, if a patient stabilized on cyclosporine stops taking St. John's wort, plasma concentrations of the drug can rise dramatically and toxicity ensue. Similarly, initiation of St. John's wort may lead to markedly lowered cyclosporine concentrations and a risk of organ rejection. A number of other "health foods" have been associated with serious drug toxicity and withdrawal from the market; phenylpropanolamine-associated stroke is an example.

PROSPECTS FOR THE FUTURE

The past 20 years have seen dramatic advances in the treatment of heart disease, in no small part caused by the development of highly effective and well-tolerated drug therapies such as HMG-CoA reductase inhibitors, ACE inhibitors, and beta blockers. These developments, along with improved nonpharmacological approaches, have led to dramatically enhanced survival of patients with advanced heart disease. Thus polypharmacy in an aging and chronically ill population is becoming increasingly common. In this milieu, drug effects become increasingly variable, reflecting interactions among drugs, underlying disease and disease mechanisms, and genetic backgrounds.

An increasing understanding of the genetic basis of variable drug actions carries with it the promise of reducing such variability. However, the logistics of implementing such a strategy and the costs of individualizing therapy on the basis of genetics are major outstanding issues. An alternate view is that effective therapies are available and have not been adequately delivered to populations that would benefit. The two views are not mutually exclusive. In the face of such increasing complexity, the relationship between the individual prescriber and the individual patient remains the centerpiece of modern therapeutics. Each initiation of drug therapy represents a new clinical experiment, and prescribers must be continuously vigilant regarding the possibility of unusual drug effects that may provide initial

TABLE 6–3 Drug Interactions: Mechanisms and Examples

Mechanism	Drug	Interacting Drug	Effect
Decreased bioavailability	Digoxin	Antacids	Decreased digoxin effect due to decreased absorption
Increased bioavailability	Digoxin	Antibiotics	By eliminating gut flora that metabolize digoxin, some antibiotics may increase digoxin bioavailability. NOTE: Some antibiotics also interfere with P-glycoprotein (expressed in the intestine and elsewhere), another effect that can elevate digoxin concentration.
Induction of hepatic metabolism	*CYP3A substrates:* Quinidine Mexiletine Verapamil Cyclosporine	Phenytoin Rifampin Barbiturates St. John's wort	Loss of drug effect due to increased metabolism Similar effects with the CYP2C9 substrate warfarin, except phenytoin
Inhibition of hepatic metabolism	*CYP2C9:* Warfarin Losartan	Amiodarone Phenytoin	Decreased warfarin requirement Diminished conversion of losartan to its active metabolite, with decreased antihypertensive control
	CYP3A substrates: Quinidine Cyclosporine HMG-CoA reductase inhibitors: lovastatin, simvastatin, atorvastatin; not pravastatin Cisapride, terfenadine, astemizole*	Ketoconazole Itraconazole Erythromycin Clarithromycin Some calcium blockers Some HIV protease inhibitors (especially ritonavir) Large quantities of grapefruit juice	Increased risk for drug toxicity
	CYP2D6 substrates: Beta blockers (see Table 6-1), Propafenone Desipramine Codeine	Quinidine (even ultra-low dose) Fluoxetine	Increased beta-blockade Increased adverse effects Decreased analgesia (due to failure of biotransformation to the active metabolite morphine)
Inhibition of drug transport	*P-glycoprotein substrates:* Digoxin	Amiodarone Quinidine Verapamil Cyclosporine Itraconazole Erythromycin	Digoxin toxicity
	Renal tubular transport: Dofetilide	Verapamil Cimetidine	Slightly increased plasma concentration and QT effect
	Monoamine transporter substrates: Guanadrel	Tricyclic antidepressants	Blunted antihypertensive effects
Pharmacodynamic interactions	Aspirin + warfarin		Increased therapeutic antithrombotic effect; increased risk of bleeding
	Nonsteroidal anti-inflammatory drugs	Warfarin	Increased risk of GI bleeding
	Antihypertensive drugs	Nonsteroidal anti-inflammatory drugs	Loss of blood pressure lowering
	QT-prolonging antiarrhythmics	Diuretics	Increased torsades de pointes risk due to diuretic-induced hypokalemia
	Supplemental potassium	ACE inhibitors	Hyperkalemia
	Sildenafil	Nitrates	Increased and persistent vasodilation; risk of myocardial ischemia

*These drugs have been withdrawn or their availability highly restricted because they can produce torsades de pointes, particularly when their metabolism is inhibited.

 clues to unanticipated and important mechanisms of beneficial and adverse drug effects.

REFERENCES

Importance of Correct Drug Use

1. http://www.cms.hhs.gov/NationalHealthExpendData/downloads/proj2005.pdf
2. Pirmohamed M, James S, Meakin S, et al: Adverse drug reactions as cause of admission to hospital: Prospective analysis of 18,820 patients. Br Med J 329:15, 2004.
3. http://www.americanheart.org/downloadable/heart/1140534985281Statsupdate06book.pdf
4. Park-Wyllie LY, Juurlink DN, Kopp A, et al: Outpatient Gatifloxacin Therapy and Dysglycemia in Older Adults. N Engl J Med 354:1352, 2006.
5. FitzGerald GA, Patrono C: The coxibs, selective inhibitors of cyclooxygenase-2. N Engl J Med 345:433, 2001.
6. Bresalier RS, Sandler RS, Quan H, et al: Cardiovascular events associated with rofecoxib in a colorectal adenoma chemoprevention trial. N Engl J Med 352:1092, 2005.
7. Oberholzer-Gee F, Inamdar SN: Merck's recall of rofecoxib—a strategic perspective. N Engl J Med 351:2147, 2004.
8. Roden DM: An underrecognized challenge in evaluating postmarketing drug safety. Circulation 111:246, 2005.

Pharmacogenetics and Pharmacogenomics

9. Weinshilboum R: Inheritance and drug response. N Engl J Med 348:529, 2003.
10. Evans WE, Relling MV: Moving towards individualized medicine with pharmacogenomics. Nature 429:464, 2004.
11. Eichelbaum M, Ingelman-Sundberg M, Evans WE: Pharmacogenomics and individualized drug therapy. Annu Rev Med 57:119, 2006.
12. Hakonarson H, Thorvaldsson S, Helgadottir A, et al: Effects of a 5-lipoxygenase-activating protein inhibitor on biomarkers associated with risk of myocardial infarction: A randomized trial. JAMA 293:2245, 2005.

Pharmacokinetics

13. Kim RB: Transporters and drug discovery: Why, when, and how. Mol Pharm 3:26, 2006.
14. Ho RH, Kim RB: Transporters and drug therapy: Implications for drug disposition and disease. Clin Pharmacol Ther 78:260, 2005.
15. Lamba JK, Lin YS, Schuetz EG, Thummel KE: Genetic contribution to variable human CYP3A-mediated metabolism. Adv Drug Deliv Rev 54:1271, 2002.
16. Grube M, Meyer Zu Schwabedissen HE, et al: Uptake of cardiovascular drugs into the human heart: Expression, regulation, and function of the carnitine transporter OCTN2 (SLC22A5). Circulation 113:1114, 2006.
17. Roden DM: Drug-induced prolongation of the QT Interval. N Engl J Med 350:1013, 2004.

Pharmacodynamics and the Genetics of Drug Responses

18. Johnson JA, Turner ST: Hypertension pharmacogenomics: Current status and future directions. Curr Opin Mol Ther 7:218, 2005.
19. Keefe DL: Trastuzumab-associated cardiotoxicity. Cancer 95:1592, 2002.
20. Arnett DK, Davis BR, Ford CE, et al: Pharmacogenetic association of the angiotensin-converting enzyme insertion/deletion polymorphism on blood pressure and cardiovascular risk in relation to antihypertensive treatment: The Genetics of Hypertension-Associated Treatment (GenHAT) study. Circulation 111:3374, 2005.
21. Rieder MJ, Reiner AP, Gage BF, et al: Effect of VKORC1 Haplotypes on Transcriptional Regulation and Warfarin Dose. N Engl J Med 352:2285, 2005.
22. Arking DE, Pfeufer A, Post W, et al: A common genetic variant in the NOS1 regulator NOS1AP modulates cardiac repolarization. Nat Genet 38:644, 2006.
23. Herbert A, Gerry NP, McQueen MB, et al: A common genetic variant is associated with Adult and Childhood Obesity. Science 312:279, 2006.
24. Grant SFA, Thorleifsson G, Reynisdottir I, et al: Variant of transcription factor 7-like 2 (TCF7L2) gene confers risk of type 2 diabetes. Nat Genet 38:320, 2006.
25. Chasman DI, Posada D, Subrahmanyan L, et al: Pharmacogenetic study of statin therapy and cholesterol reduction. JAMA 291:2821, 2004.
26. Weiss ST, Lake SL, Silverman ES, et al: Asthma steroid pharmacogenetics: A study strategy to identify replicated treatment responses. Proc Am Thorac Soc 1:364, 2004.

Drug Interactions

27. Bailey DG, Dresser GK: Interactions between grapefruit juice and cardiovascular drugs. Am J Cardiovasc Drugs 4:281, 2004.
28. Ratain MJ: From bedside to bench to bedside to clinical practice: An odyssey with irinotecan. Clin Cancer Res 12:1658, 2006.

PART II

Molecular Biology and Genetics

CHAPTER 7

Principles of Cardiovascular Molecular Biology and Genetics

Elizabeth G. Nabel

Molecular biology and genetics now form the solid foundation of cardiovascular science and medicine. In the past two decades, the concepts of molecular biology and genetics have permeated all aspects of medicine. The principles of these disciplines are a cornerstone of medical school curricula. Physician-scientists' laboratories routinely use molecular genetic approaches to test hypotheses about cardiovascular disease. Physicians have access to an array of molecular and genetic tools to guide the diagnosis and treatment of patients. The production of many therapeutic agents now uses recombinant deoxyribonucleic acid (DNA) technology.

The breakthroughs in our understanding of the genetic basis of cardiovascular disease have been equally impressive. Our appreciation of the mechanism by which single genes cause disease, even when the diseases are uncommon, has led to an understanding of the pathogenesis of more common cardiovascular diseases. With completion of sequencing of the Human Genome, genomic discoveries in cardiovascular diseases now occur at a rapid pace. How these discoveries will translate to the care of patients with cardiovascular disease is currently difficult to predict.

This chapter highlights the basic principles of molecular biology and genetics. It is designed as a brief review and reference source, intended to prepare the reader for discussions of specific cardiovascular applications in other chapters in this text and in the contemporary literature. References are provided for a general coverage on a topic, as well as an in-depth coverage of each subject.

PRINCIPLES OF CELL BIOLOGY AND THE CELL CYCLE

All living organisms are composed of cells, and all cells arise from preexisting cells.[1,2] Cells are organized into compartments. Prokaryotes, such as bacteria, contain a single cell compartment bounded by a membrane or membranes. Eukaryotes, such as mammals, are defined by the division of each cell into a nucleus that contains the genetic material, surrounded by a cytoplasm, bounded in turn by the plasma membrane that marks the periphery of the cell. The cytoplasm also contains other discrete compartments, also bounded by membranes. To define the execution of genetic instructions in a cell, we must consider the nature of the various compartments and how they function to create regions with different properties.

The mammalian cell is a highly compartmentalized structure (Fig. 7-1). The outer membrane, called the *plasma membrane,* is a lipid bilayer intended to exclude an aqueous environment, such as extracellular fluid.[3] The plasma membrane is studded with a class of transmembrane proteins called *receptors.* A receptor has a binding site that recognizes some ligand on the exterior side of the membrane. Binding of the ligand usually triggers a change in the protein, which is transmitted to the cytoplasmic face by a conformational change in the receptor protein, or as movement of the whole protein into the interior. This change, in turn, triggers other changes within the cell and thus provides a means for responding to the environment. This type of relationship is called *signal transduction.*[4]

The cytoplasm contains networks of membranes. Membrane sheets make up the endoplasmic reticulum (ER) and the Golgi apparatus.[5] ER consists of a continuous sheet of highly folded membranes extending from the outer nuclear membrane. ER can be divided into two types, which are part of the same membrane sheet. Rough ER has ribosomes, the small particles concerned with the synthesis of proteins, on

All material in this chapter is in the public domain, with the exception of any borrowed figures or tables.

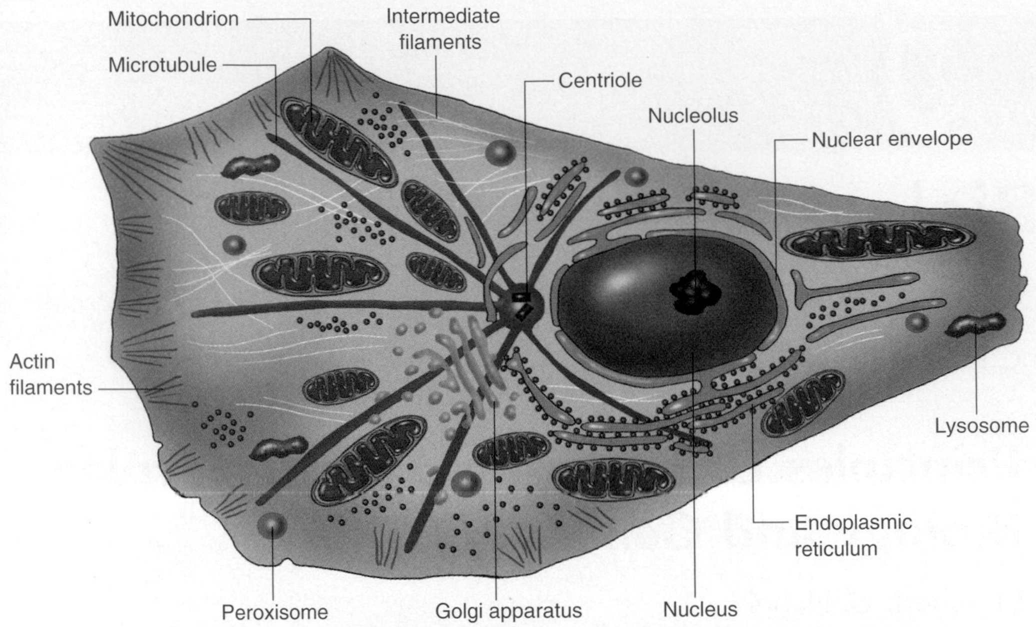

FIGURE 7–1 Structure of a mammalian cell. Schematic illustration of a cell, demonstrating structures common to most cells.

its surface, whereas smooth ER does not. The Golgi apparatus consists of stacks of separate cisternae. Proteins that have been modified in ER enter the Golgi apparatus, undergo further modifications, and then exit. A major function of the ER and Golgi apparatus is to sort proteins according to destination, using signals inherent in the protein sequence. This process of directing proteins to their final destination is called *protein sorting* or *trafficking.*[6] Mitochondria are specialized organelles in the cytoplasm that generate energy stored in the form of adenosine triphosphate from the oxidation of carbon-containing compounds such as sugars or fats. Lysosomes are membrane-enclosed bodies that contain hydrolytic enzymes, which further process proteins and other macromolecules within the cell. Cell shape is determined by the cytoskeleton, which contains networks of protein fibers extending across and around the cell. The three classes of fibers are actin filaments, microtubules, and intermediate filaments.

The most important feature of the nucleus is genetic material. The nucleus has a granular appearance, due to chromatin, which is easily recognized with certain stains. Between cell divisions, chromatin forms a single, dense mass. When a cell divides, its chromatin can be seen to consist of a discrete number of string-like structures, called *chromosomes.*[7] A common feature of cells, except those that have reached a final, specialized state of development *(terminal differentiation),* is their ability to divide. Many structural changes occur within a cell during division. Membranes and the cytoskeleton undergo extensive reorganization. The cell is organized by a new structure, called the *spindle,* which functions to allow the distribution of chromosomes to daughter cells. These changes halt many of the former activities of the cell—gene expression, protein synthesis and secretion, and cell motility.[8]

The cell cycle, the period between the release of a newly formed cell as a progeny of a division and its own subsequent division into two daughter cells, consists of two parts.[9] Interphase, a relatively long period, represents the time during which the cell engages in its synthetic activities and reproduces its subcellular components. During interphase, the cell has a discrete nuclear compartment, containing a compact mass of chromatin. During mitosis, a relatively short period of time, the actual division into two daughter cells occurs. In cells in mitosis, the spindle replaces the internal organization of the cell, and individual chromosomes become apparent. The products of the series of mitotic divisions that generate the organism are called the *somatic cells.* During embryonic development, many or most of the somatic cells proceed through the cell cycle. In the adult organism, many cells are terminally differentiated and no longer divide. They remain in a stationary phase in which there is no DNA synthesis, equivalent to a perpetual interphase.

Mitosis recapitulates the chromosome constitution of the cell. Each daughter cell starts its life with two copies of each chromosome. These copies are called *homologues.* The total number of chromosomes is called the *diploid set* and has 2n members (see Chap. 8). During interphase, a growing cell duplicates its chromosomal material. At the beginning of mitosis, each chromosome appears to split longitudinally to generate two copies, called *sister chromatids.* The cell now contains 4n chromosomes, organized as 2n pairs of sister chromatids. The process of mitosis consists of four phases: prophase, metaphase, anaphase, and telophase, ending in cytokinesis, in which the cell divides and each daughter has the same complete set of chromosomes, one member of each pair derived from each parent (Fig. 7-2). Each phase consists of distinct movements of the centromere, the central, constriction region of the chromosome. These movements are essential to separation of the pairs of chromosomes into each daughter cell and completion of cell division.

Just before mitosis, double-stranded chromosomal breaks or other DNA damage is repaired by a series of cell cycle checkpoints.[10] Under normal conditions, cellular DNA is repaired and the cell completes mitosis. Cells in which DNA is not repaired undergo apoptosis, or programmed cell death.[11] This mechanism allows the perpetuation of cell division in which chromosomal DNA is intact. Carcinogenesis can result when cell division escapes checkpoint control, and cells with double-stranded DNA break or other forms of damaged DNA divide uncontrollably.

The essential proteins in cell cycle checkpoint control are the cyclins and the cyclin-dependent kinases (CDKs) (Fig. 7-3). The CDKs are holoenzyme complexes that contain cyclin regulatory subunits and CDK catalytic subunits. Four distinct phases of the cell cycle are regulated by cyclin-CDK complexes: Gap 1 or G1 phase, DNA replication or S phase, Gap 2 or G2 phase, and mitosis or M phase. Restriction point control in G1 phase is mediated by two CDKs, the cyclin D- and cyclin E-dependent kinases. The D-type cyclins (D1, D2, and D3) interact combinatorially with two catalytic partners, CDK4 and CDK6, early in G_1 to yield at least six holoenzymes expressed in tissue-specific patterns. Cyclin E enters into a complex with its catalytic partner CDK2 and collaborates with the cyclin D-dependent kinases to complete phosphorylation of the retinoblastoma tumor-suppressor protein (Rb) late in G1, which results in transit through the G1-S checkpoint into S phase.

Endogenous inhibitors of the cyclins-CDKs, termed the *cyclin-dependent kinase inhibitors* or CKIs, are expressed throughout G1 to inhibit phosphorylation and activation of cyclin-CDK complexes, resulting in G1 arrest. The CKIs function to prevent transition through the G1 checkpoint and inhibit mitosis, leading to growth arrest of cells. CKIs are classified into two families on the basis of their structures and CDK targets. The CIP/KIP proteins are broadly acting inhibitors that alter the activities of cyclin D, cyclin E-, and cyclin A-dependent kinases. This family includes p21(Cip1), p27(Kip1), and p57(Kip2). All three contain characteristic motifs in their amino-terminal regions that bind cyclin and CDK substrates. p21(Cip1) functions as a downstream effector of the transcription factor and tumor suppressor gene, p53, to cause DNA damage repair and/or promote apoptosis. p27(Kip1) is a potent inhibitor of cell proliferation in normal and diseased tissues and is a critical mediator in tissue injury, inflammation, and wound repair. The INK4 (*in*hibitor of CD*K4*) family of proteins consists of INK4A (p16), INK4B (p15), INK4C (p18), and INK4D (p19). These CKIs contain multiple ankyrin repeats, bind only to CDK4 and CDK6 and not to other CDKs, and specifically inhibit the catalytic subunits of CDK4 and CDK6. The INK proteins are important regulators of tumor growth and in developmental biology, but they play a lesser role in cardiovascular diseases.

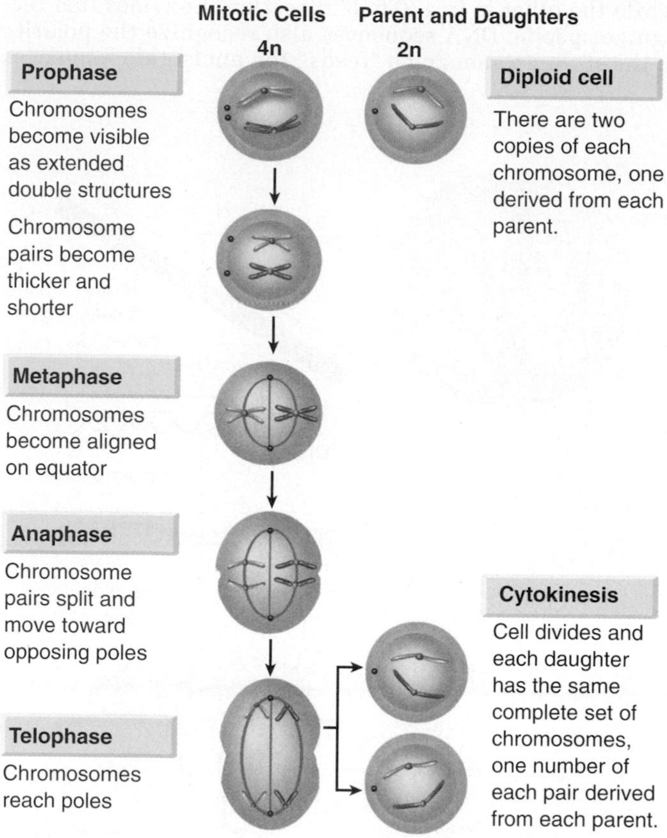

FIGURE 7–2 The process of mitosis in a mammalian cell in which the genetic material is duplicated and distributed during cell division (see text).

Injury to the heart or blood vessels leads to a remodeling process that is adaptive under normal conditions or maladaptive in conditions of disease pathophysiology (see Chaps. 22 and 38). In response to physiological stimuli, vascular smooth muscle cells (VSMCs) within the media proliferate and migrate into the intima to form a multilayered vascular wound or *neointima*. Normally, this is a self-limited process that results in a well-healed vascular wound and preservation of luminal blood flow. In certain vascular diseases, however, VSMC proliferation becomes excessive, leading to a pathological lesion in the blood vessel, which in turn produces clinical symptoms. These diseases are often characterized by systemic or local inflammation, which exacerbates the VSMC proliferative response. The CIP/KIP CKIs are important regulators of tissue remodeling in the vasculature.[12] p27(Kip1) is constitutively expressed in VSMCs and endothelial cells of arteries and is downregulated after vascular injury or exposure of VSMCs and endothelial cells to mitogens. After a proliferative burst, VSMCs synthesize and secrete extracellular matrix molecules, which signal to VSMCs and endothelial cells, leading to induction of p27(Kip1) and p21(Cip1) and suppression of cyclin E-CDK2. Expression of the CIP/KIP CKIs leads to cell cycle arrest and inhibition of cell division.[13] p27(Kip1) is also an important regulator of tissue inflammation through its effects on T-lymphocyte proliferation. In the vasculature, p27(Kip1) mediates vascular repair through its regulation of

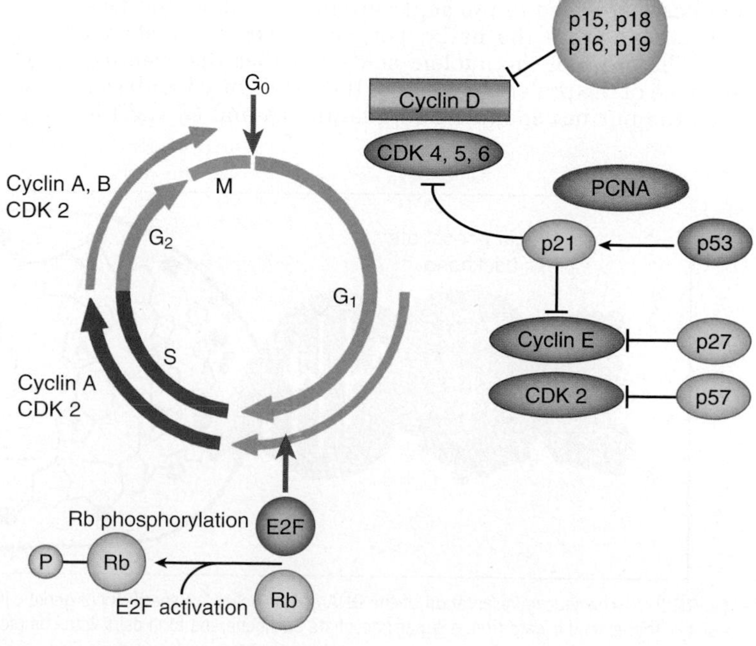

FIGURE 7–3 The mammalian cell cycle. The cyclins, cyclin-dependent kinases, and cyclin-dependent kinase inhibitors active in each phase are shown (see text for explanation and abbreviations).

proliferation, inflammation, and bone marrow progenitor cells. Genetic deletion of p27(Kip1) in mice results in a benign hyperplasia of epithelial and mesodermal cells in multiple organs including the heart and vasculature.

p21(Cip1) is required for growth and differentiation in the heart, bone, skin, and kidney, and it confers susceptibility to apoptosis.[14] This CKI functions in a p53-dependent and p53-independent manner. In the heart, p21(Cip1) is expressed independently of p53 in cardiac myocytes; overexpression of p21(Cip1) within myocytes leads to hypertrophy.

Most human cancer cells sustain mutations that alter the functions of p53 or Rb by direct mutation of gene sequences or by targeting genes that act epistatically to prevent their normal function. Rb limits cell proliferation by preventing entry into S phase. The mechanism is blockage of E2F transcription factors from activating genes required for DNA replication and nucleotide metabolism. p53 is mutated in more than 50 percent of human cancers. The protein accumulates in response to cellular stress from DNA damage, hypoxia, and oncogene activation. p53 initiates a transcriptional program that triggers cell cycle arrest or apoptosis.[15] When activated by p53, p21(Cip1) induces apoptosis in tumor and other cells.

The cell cycle functions as the major regulator of cell division. DNA replication and cytokinesis depend on normal functioning of the cell cycle. The cyclins, CDKs, and CKIs are, secondarily, important mediators of carcinogenesis, tissue inflammation, and wound repair.

THE GENETIC CODE: DNA, RNA, AND PROTEIN

DNA

DNA is the building block of human life (Fig. 7-4). Its double helical structure is deceptively simple, yet the rules encoded within this structure specify the form and function of all cells within an organism. DNA consists of two long strands of polydeoxyribonucleotides that twist around each other clockwise to form an unbroken double helix. Alternating deoxyribose-phosphate groups form the backbone of the helix, with the phosphate group making a 5′-3′ phosphodiester bond between the fifth carbon of one pentose ring and the third carbon of the next pentose ring (Fig. 7-5). Nucleic acid bases attached to the sugar groups of each strand face each other within the helix, perpendicular to the strand axis. The order of the nucleic acids specifies the eventual sequence of the protein product of the gene. Only four bases exist: the purines adenine and guanine (A and G) and the pyrimidines cytosine and thymine (C and T). During assembly of the double helix, a purine can pair only with a pyrimidine, and a pyrimidine with a purine. Each base pair (bp) forms one of the rungs in the twisted ladder of the DNA molecule, which can be millions of bases long. The two strands of DNA, which are held together by hydrogen bonds between complementary base pairs, have opposite chemical polarities. One strand is oriented in a 5′ to 3′ direction, while the other is in a 3′ to 5′ direction. Enzymes that recognize specific DNA sequences also recognize the polarity of the strand. An enzyme “reads” the nucleotide sequences

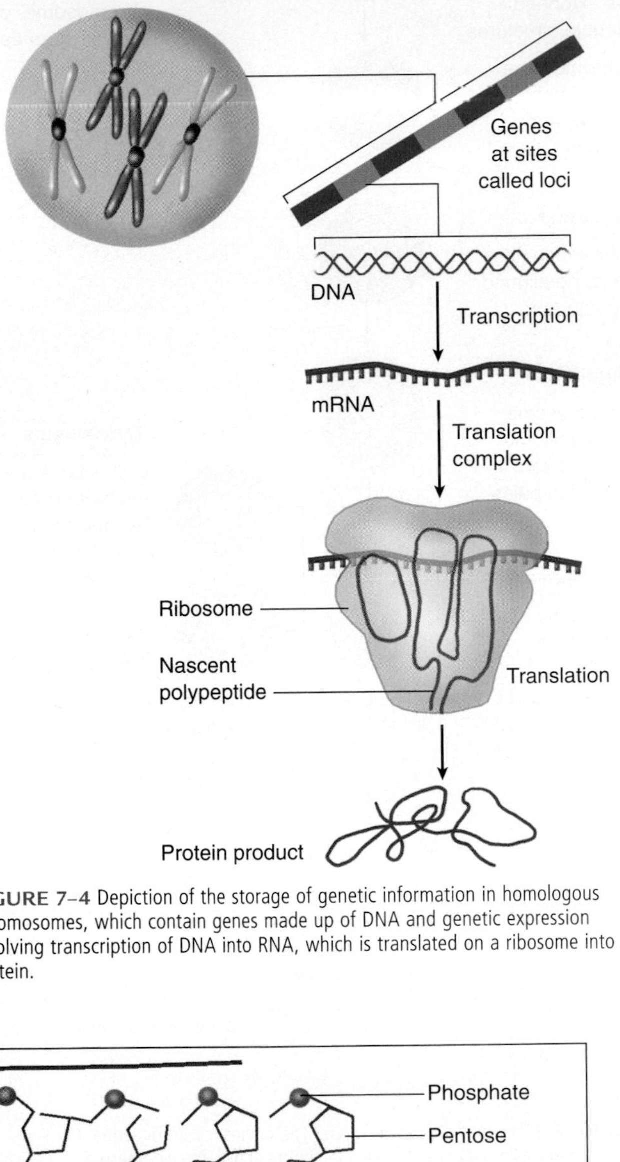

FIGURE 7–4 Depiction of the storage of genetic information in homologous chromosomes, which contain genes made up of DNA and genetic expression involving transcription of DNA into RNA, which is translated on a ribosome into protein.

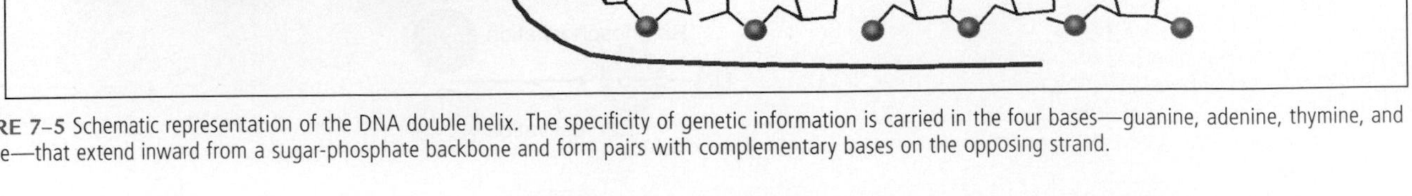

FIGURE 7–5 Schematic representation of the DNA double helix. The specificity of genetic information is carried in the four bases—guanine, adenine, thymine, and cytosine—that extend inward from a sugar-phosphate backbone and form pairs with complementary bases on the opposing strand.

on the two strands in opposite directions. Because the structure of the helical backbone is invariant, enzymes responsible for DNA copying, cleavage, and repairing strand breaks can act anywhere along the length of the DNA strand.

An important consequence of the A-T and G-C pairing is that the sequence of nucleotides on one strand of the double helix determines the sequence on the complementary strand. This base pairing rule is critical for the storage, retrieval, and transfer of genetic material, whether it be for duplication of DNA into a daughter cell, repair of a damaged DNA strand, or reading as a template for RNA transcription.

Chromosomes are long double helical strands of DNA tightly coiled into compacted, discrete lengths by nuclear proteins. Each chromosome varies in length and base pair composition. In human cells the nucleus contains 23 different pairs of chromosomes, each with a specific length and base pair sequence. The combined DNA sequences (approximately 3×10^9) on all the chromosomes within a cell comprise the genome.[16,17] The information carried within the genome is identical in all cells of an organism and varies little among members of a species. Indeed, the genome of humans, *Homo sapiens,* is approximately 99 percent identical among individuals.[18]

During cell division, enzymes called *polymerases* unwind the DNA helix in each chromosome and copy each of the two strands separately along their entire length. Each daughter cell, then, inherits a double-stranded DNA molecule containing one old and one new strand. Each of these strands can in turn generate a new strand that faithfully reproduces the original template. This fidelity of DNA replication is essential for accurate transfer of genetic information. Errors in this process are a common source of gene mutations, which are inherited in successive rounds of cell division.

A gene is a section of base sequences used as a template for the copying process of transcription and, therefore, is the fundamental unit of inherited DNA information. Genes comprise only a small fraction of all the DNA carried on a chromosome. Only 1 to 2 percent of its bases encode proteins, and the full complement of protein-coding sequences still remains to be established. The human genome contains an estimated 30,000 distinct genes.[16,17] The protein coding information contained within a single gene is not continuous but instead is encoded in multiple discontinuous packets called *exons.* Between these exons are variably sized stretches of DNA called *introns.* The function of these introns is not known. They probably contain the bulk of the regulatory information controlling the expression of the approximately 30,000 protein-coding genes, and myriad other functional elements such as non–protein-coding genes and the sequence determinants of chromosome dynamics. Even less is known about the function of the roughly half of the genome that consists of highly repetitive sequences or of the remaining noncoding, nonrepetitive DNA.

RNA

The first step in the expression of genetic information is transcription, which serves to carry the genetic information out of the nucleus into the cytoplasm, where the synthesis of proteins occurs. In this process, transcription of DNA to RNA requires the expression of a gene template called *messenger RNA* (mRNA) in the nucleus (Fig. 7-6). A specialized enzyme, RNA polymerase, copies one of the two DNA strands (the antisense strand), creating a complementary stretch of sequence that is an exact copy of the sense strand. RNA structure differs slightly from DNA. One of the RNA bases, uracil, replaces the DNA base thymine, and the RNA sugar phosphate component ribose replaces DNA deoxyribose. Ribose renders the RNA molecule much more susceptible to degradation than the more stable deoxyribose. This allows RNA to respond more rapidly to shifts in cellular signaling and move quickly to the cytoplasm for protein production.

From Genes to Proteins

The process of converting a gene to a protein involves two major steps: transcription of the DNA by RNA in the nucleus and translation of the RNA into protein in the cytoplasm. This is a complex and highly regulated process. Transcription begins in the nucleus by copying of the DNA sequence of the gene into mRNA (see Fig. 7-6). The single-stranded RNA is modified at both ends. At the 5′ end, a nucleotide structure called a *cap* is added to increase translation efficiency by allowing ribosomes to bind to RNA. At the 3′ end, a nucleotide recognizes an A/T rich sequence in a noncoding region and trims the transcript downstream by about 20 bp. An enzyme that adds a stretch of adenosine to form a polyA tail, which stabilizes the transcript, modifies the newly cleaved 3′ end. The transcript then undergoes splicing to remove intronic sequences. This is a highly regulated process because unspliced transcripts are highly unstable and are cleared rapidly from the cell. Splicing is an important control point in gene expression. It must be absolutely precise because the deletion or addition of a single nucleotide at the splice junction would throw out of frame the subsequent three-base codon translation of the RNA. The full significance of RNA splicing is not completely understood, but it must represent a critical point in the regulation of gene expression due to the large expanses of intron sequences and the inability of transcripts to leave the nucleus until their introns are removed.

Once in the cytoplasm, mRNA provides a template for translation or protein synthesis. Translation occurs on a macromolecular complex, like an assembly line, composed of *ribosomes.* The ribosomes read and translate the nucleotide sequence in mRNA into an amino acid sequence; that is, the four base mRNA code is translated into the 20 amino acid alphabet of proteins. This genetic code is remarkably simple and has been conserved in most organisms. Every three RNA nucleotides encode for a single amino acid; therefore the codon is a triplet of bases (Fig. 7-7). Permutations of the four RNA nucleotides result in 64 different triplets ($4 \times 4 \times 4$) so that any of the 20 amino acids can be specified by more than one codon. One of the triplets, AUG, specifies methionine, which is the amino acid that starts each protein. Three other triplets, UAA, UGA, and UAG, program the ribosome to end translation and are therefore called *stop codons.*

The conversion of a codon into an amino acid requires an adapter molecule, called *transfer RNA* (tRNA), to decode mRNA. Each tRNA uses a unique three-base sequence or anticodon to line up with the complementary codon in mRNA (see Fig. 7-6). Ribosomal enzymes link adjoining amino acids, which frees them from the tRNA adapters and adds them to the growing amino acid chain. The order of the amino acids is specified by the order of the codons on the corresponding mRNA template. Translation then completes the transfer of information from DNA in the nucleus to a unique protein structure.

Because the genetic code is preserved across species, human genetic sequences can be transferred into bacteria, yeast, or insect cells, where the sequences will be faithfully replicated and decoded into RNA and protein. This principle constitutes the basis of recombinant DNA technology, which is used to produce recombinant proteins for research and therapeutic purposes (e.g., tissue plasminogen activator).

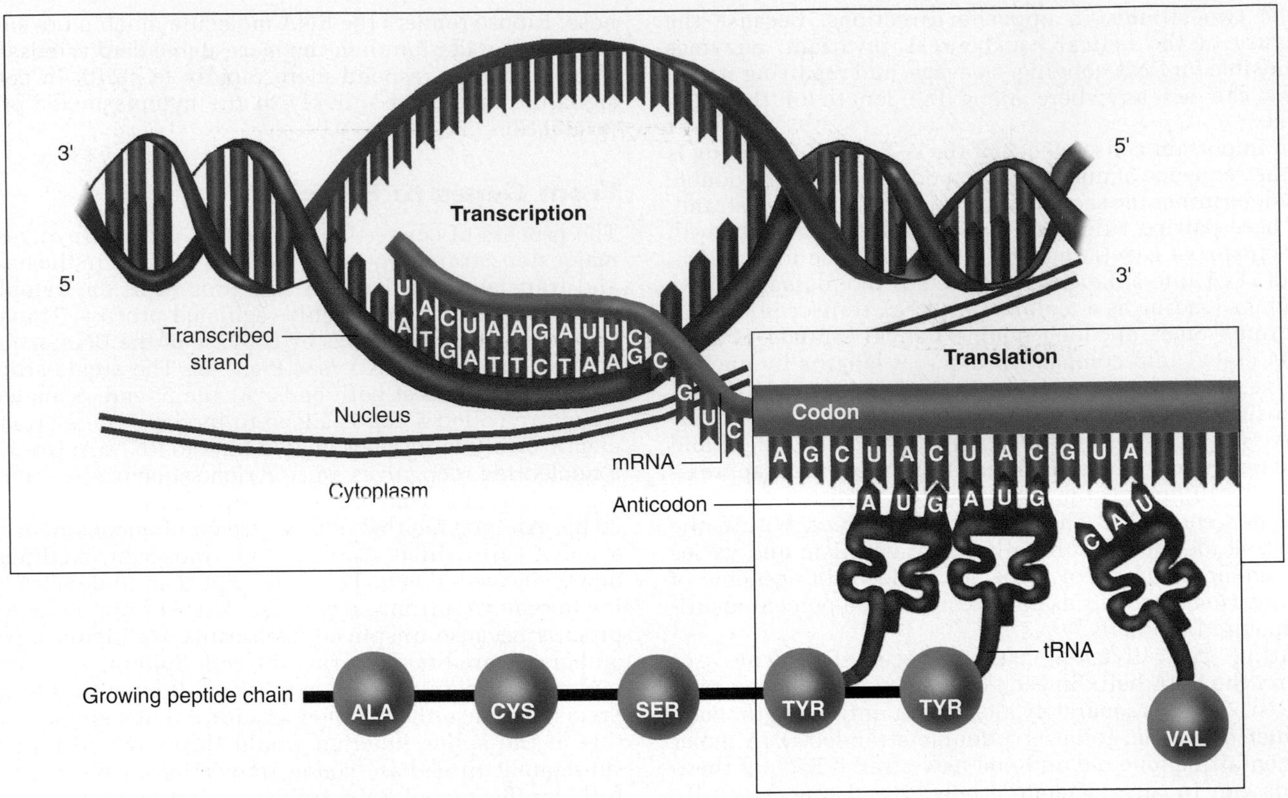

FIGURE 7–6 The flow of genetic information. Transcription in the nucleus creates a complementary ribonucleic acid copy from one of the DNA strands in the double helix. mRNA is transported into the cytoplasm, where it is translated into protein.

First Base	Second Base: U	Second Base: C	Second Base: A	Second Base: G
U	UUU, UUC } Phe UUA, UUG } Leu	UCU, UCC, UCA, UCG } Ser	UAU, UAC } Tyr UAA, UAG } TERM	UGU, UGC } Cys UGA TERM UGG Trp
C	CUU, CUC, CUA, CUG } Leu	CCU, CCC, CCA, CCG } Pro	CAU, CAC } His CAA, CAG } Gin	CGU, CGC, CGA, CGG } Arg
A	AUU, AUC, AUA } Ile AUG Met	ACU, ACC, ACA, ACG } Thr	AAU, AAC } Asn AAA, AAG } Lys	AGU, AGC } Ser AGA, AGG } Arg
G	GUU, GUC, GUA, GUG } Val	GCU, GCC, GCA, GCG } Ala	GAU, GAC } Asp GAA, GAG } Glu	GGU, GGC, GGA, GGG } Gly

FIGURE 7–7 The genetic code. The amino acids corresponding to each nucleotide triplet in the mRNA are shown. A single start codon (AUG) and three stop codons (UAG, UAA, UGA) are present.

The process of gene expression requires controlled and precise regulation at multiple steps. Only a small number of genes are expressed within a cell at a given time. One set of genes is constitutively expressed in most cells, referred to colloquially as "housekeeping genes." These genes are necessary for cell replication, energy generation, and survival functions. A second set of genes are expressed in a lineage-specific manner (i.e., within certain cells). These genes are required for cell-specific functions such as contractility. The precise regulation of lineage-specific genes determines the unique identity and function of a particular cell. Another set of genes is induced in response to environmental stimuli. These sets of controls are required to produce the complex and dynamic patterns of gene expression, which allow an organism to respond to internal and external signals.

PRINCIPLES AND TECHNIQUES OF MOLECULAR BIOLOGY

Recombinant DNA technologies developed in the 1970s as a response to the need for sufficient quantities of DNA for biochemical analysis. The method refers to the clipping of a segment out of surrounding DNA using sequence-specific endonucleases known as *restriction enzymes*. The segment can then be inserted at will into a vector that permits copying it millions of times (see later). The success of recombinant DNA techniques fueled most of the advances in molecular biology over the past 30 years. Many of these techniques are now commonplace in research laboratories. These approaches are used routinely for analysis of gene structure, expression, and organization; regulatory pathways by which cells control gene expression; and discovery of novel genes and therapeutics. These advances have changed the face of medical research. Genetic engineering in which an organism is modified to include new genes designed with desired characteristics is in routine practice in many research laboratories. Recombinant DNA technologies serve to mass-produce therapeutic proteins such as recombinant tissue plasminogen activator. The ability to manipulate the human genome has opened up new possibilities for the development of diagnostic tests and new therapies. Yet the techniques of molecular biology, like the structure of DNA itself, are surprisingly simple. The basic approaches are described here; the reader is guided to in-depth reviews for a primer on how to perform the techniques.[19]

Cloning DNA

Molecular cloning provides a means to produce millions of copies of a DNA sequence or gene within bacterial cells. A DNA fragment is first inserted into a cloning vector. The most commonly used vectors are small, circular DNA molecules called *plasmids* or bacterial viruses called *phage*. The vectors also contain genetic information that allows the bacterial cell to replicate the DNA sequence. After insertion of a DNA sequence, the plasmid or phage vector is introduced into a bacterial cell. The growing bacterial culture replicates the vector containing the DNA sequence in hundreds of copies per cell, yielding multiple identical clones of the original DNA sequence. The vectors are then harvested from the bacterial culture using the same restriction enzymes used to insert the DNA sequence into the vector.

The molecular biologist uses restriction endonucleases derived from bacteria as molecular scissors that cut DNA motifs at predictable sequences. Each restriction enzyme recognizes a specific nucleotide sequence. These recognition sites occur randomly along the DNA of any organism and consist of a short symmetric sequence motif called a *palindrome,* which is repeated in opposing orientation on both strands of the double helix DNA. For example, the enzyme EcoRI from the bacteria *Escherichia coli* recognizes and cuts the sequence GAATTC in double-strand DNA at GA and AG junctions. Most restriction enzymes cleave their palindromic sequence asymmetrically, leaving a single-stranded overhang on each end of the cut. These "sticky" ends have unique and complementary sequences that can be used to connect a fragment of human DNA with complementary ends of DNA from another source. An enzymatic reaction connects the continuous double-stranded DNA to form a smooth splice. These principles are used to construct various DNA rearrangements for multiple purposes such as gene cloning, generating knock-out mice, or constructing recombinant DNA therapies.

Blotting Techniques

Blotting is a tool that permits identification of DNA, RNA, or protein by its molecular size. Analysis of DNA is referred to as a Southern blot; RNA identification is a Northern blot; and protein isolation is a Western blot. The principles of blotting techniques are straightforward.[19] A mixture of molecules to be analyzed is subjected to gel electrophoresis, which separates different species according to size and/or electrical charge (Fig. 7-8). An agarose gel is used in which the molecules are loaded into wells at one end. The gel is submerged into a buffer and subjected to an electrical current. The molecules migrate across the electrical field. Because DNA and RNA are acids that carry a negative charge, they migrate toward the positive pole of the gel. The agarose matrix hinders the migration of larger molecules so

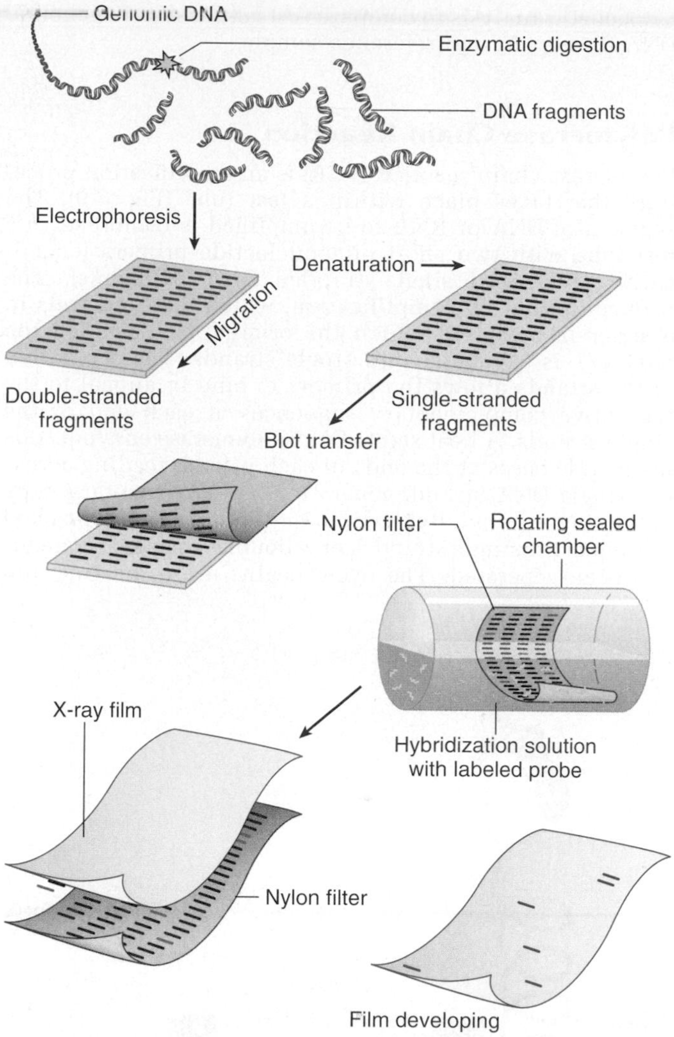

FIGURE 7–8 Blotting DNA. The process of Southern blotting to identify genomic DNA is shown.

that the molecules also separate by size. When the electrophoresis is completed, the gel is removed from the buffer, and a nylon filter and dry absorbent material are placed on top. The buffer from the gel is blotted into the absorbent material carrying with it the separated molecules, which remain on the nylon filter. The filter is treated to permanently fix the molecules on its surface, creating a mirror image of the original gel. The filter is then bathed with a tagged molecule (the probe) that recognizes (hybridizes to) the molecule of interest and washed to remove the unbound probe. For Southern (DNA) and Northern (RNA) blots, the probe is a small fragment of nucleic acid that carries a complementary sequence to the molecule being investigated. The nucleic acid is tagged with a radioactive element detectable by exposure to x-ray film or other techniques.

The position of the hybridized probe, which appears as a band, provides an estimate of the size of DNA or RNA segment. By running parallel lanes of molecular markers of known size, the precise size of the DNA or RNA element is determined. For protein identification (Western blot), the probe consists of a tagged antibody that recognizes the target protein. Size markers are also run in the gel to identify the size of the protein.

Blotting techniques are also used for other purposes including to map the position of restriction sites in a specific gene following restriction enzyme digestion and in cytogenetic analysis to compare restriction sites in genomic DNA from a test and reference sample.

Polymerase Chain Reaction

Polymerase chain reaction (PCR) is an amplification procedure that takes place within a test tube (Fig. 7-9). The segment of DNA or RNA to be amplified is combined in a test tube with two short oligonucleotide primers (chemically synthesized single-stranded DNA fragments). The primers initiate the amplification, which then proceeds in a series of cycles in which the original DNA, called the *template,* is separated into single strands. The separation of the strands allows the primers to bind or anneal to the respective complementary sequences at each end of the single strands. A heat-stable DNA polymerase enzyme adds nucleotide bases at the ends of each primer, reading across the single DNA strand, generating a complementary copy of the single strand. By the time the polymerase has reached the end of the single strand, a new double-stranded sequence has been generated. The cycle begins again, heating and separating the double strand, followed by the generation of a new strand by the primer and polymerase. Each round of PCR amplification doubles the number of DNA templates. Creating millions of copies of a DNA segment is possible in several hours by PCR, even when the starting material is a single copy of DNA. The entire amplification is carried out in a sealed test tube or well in a specially designed machine that can be programmed to automatically heat and cool the sample. PCR has now become a commonplace tool to generate a sufficient quantity of identical genetic material for analysis.

PRINCIPLES OF MOLECULAR GENETICS

Genotype and the Identification of Disease-Causing Genes

The discovery of the structure and function of DNA in 1953 laid the foundation for molecular genetics.[20] The completion of sequencing of the human genome has added considerably to this foundation.[16,17] Clinicians now have at hand the tools of molecular genetics with which they can pursue diagnoses and treatments. In this regard, three concepts prove particularly useful in cardiovascular genetics: genotype, genomics, and proteomics. Genotype is the composite of DNA sequences within an individual's set of genes, or the complete sequence of an individual's DNA on all 23 pairs of chromosomes. Genomics is the expression of gene sequences as RNA. The focus of genomics is "Which genes are expressed?" Proteomics is the study of proteins expressed within a cell or organism and seeks to understand the networks of protein–protein interactions.

Historically, the field of genetics focused on monogenic disorders, i.e., diseases caused by a single gene deletion or mutation (see Chap. 8). With the newer tools of genomics and proteomics, attention has turned to the evaluation of the genetic susceptibility to complex disease traits, such as coronary artery disease and diabetes. Understanding the genetic basis of complex diseases requires knowledge of gene sequences, the proteins encoded by the genes, and the functions of the proteins. However, it is becoming increasingly clear that

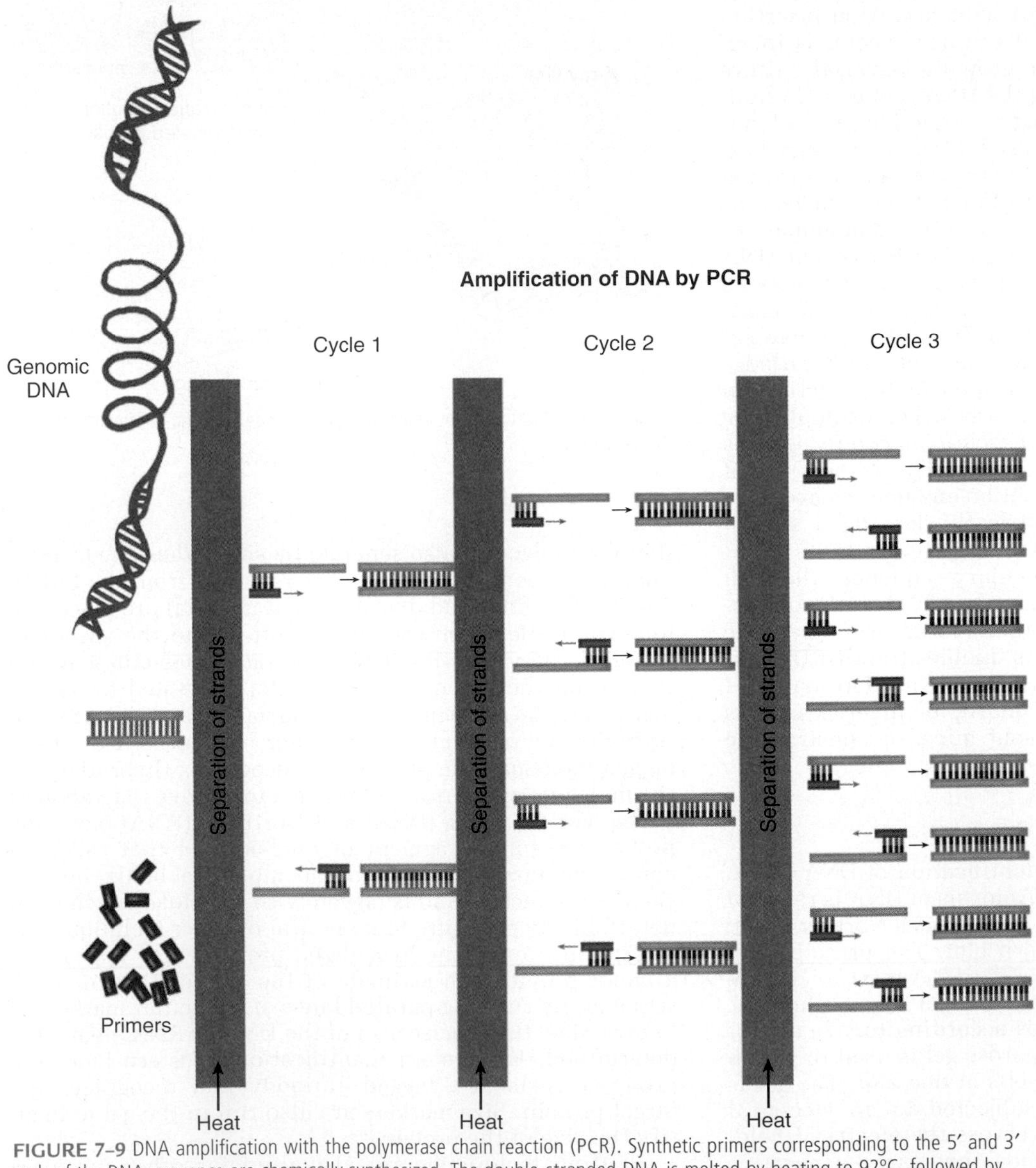

FIGURE 7–9 DNA amplification with the polymerase chain reaction (PCR). Synthetic primers corresponding to the 5′ and 3′ ends of the DNA sequence are chemically synthesized. The double-stranded DNA is melted by heating to 92°C, followed by cooling to 72°C to anneal the primers. A heat-stable DNA polymerase amplifies each strand of the target sequence, producing two copies of the DNA sequence. The process is repeated multiple times to achieve amplification of the target sequence.

complex cardiovascular problems will not be resolved solely by deriving the nucleotide sequence of the human genome or from unraveling the approximately 30,000 loci that encode the corresponding proteins or regulate other genes. Considerable work is required to define precisely the molecular mechanisms by which changes in an individual gene or set of genes specify or confer risk for a specific disease.

Monogenic Disorders

Medical genetics has classically focused on single gene or monogenic diseases, in which the cause of the disease is traced to a missing or mutated gene. Approximately 1000 disease-causing genes have been identified.[21] Monogenic disorders are rare and typically are inherited in a mendelian or autosomal manner. Interestingly, our understanding of the mechanism by which single genes cause disease, even though these mechanisms are uncommon, has led to an understanding of the pathogenesis of more common cardiovascular diseases.

Our current understanding of genetic factors in cardiovascular disease is reviewed in more detail elsewhere (see Chap. 8).[22] Briefly, each gene exists in two copies, known as *alleles.* An individual is homozygous at a given locus if the two alleles are identical, or heterozygous if the alleles are different. The specific alleles present at a given loci represent the genotype for those genes. Viewed more broadly, a genotype is a composite of the genetic factors responsible for creating a phenotype. A phenotype, in turn, is the visible or measurable properties resulting from a genotype, such as coronary artery disease or obesity. Phenotype can also be defined as the effect of gene action, whether due to a single gene or the entire genotype.

Differences in nucleotide sequences, either between two individuals or among all individuals within a population, constitute genetic *variation.* Differences that arise in nucleotide sequences and lead to a structural change in the proteins they encode are called *mutations.* A mutation is defined as occurring in less than 1 percent of a given population. Approximately 16,000 mutations in single-gene disorders have been identified.[21] Examples of mutations include missense, nonsense, frame shift, deletion, and insertion (Fig. 7-10). Missense mutations result from substitutions of one or more nucleotides in such a way as to change the primary sequence of the encoded protein. These missense mutations alter the function of the protein by changing its primary structure. A nonsense mutation introduces a premature stop codon into a gene, resulting in a truncated gene product that can display alterations in function and be unstable. Insertions or deletions of nucleotides add or subtract amino acids from the resulting proteins, if the nucleotide changes lead to an addition or deletion of a triplet. Frame-shift mutations occur when codons of a gene are read in the wrong reading frame. These mutations typically cause abnormal protein structure due to the introduction of out-of-frame termination codons, which lead to premature termination of proteins. Mutations in introns and exons cause splicing errors that also lead to alterations in protein structure or premature termination. Finally, mutations in the promoters or enhancers of genes can lead to alterations in the levels of expression of a protein, or the temporal or spatial patterns of gene expression of a protein.

A variety of mutations have been found in monogenic cardiovascular diseases (see Chap. 8). For example, although the primary defect in familial hypercholesterolemia is a deficit of low-density lipoprotein receptors (LDLRs), more than 600 mutations in the LDLR gene have been identified in patients with this disorder.[23] Likewise, hypertrophic cardiomyopathy, an autosomal dominant disease, is caused by mutations in the genes encoding proteins of the myocardial-contractile apparatus (see Chap. 10). Multiple causative

Wild-type Sequence							
...	AUG	GCC	TAC	GTT	CGA	CCC ...	
...	Met	Ala	Tyr	Val	Arg	Pro ...	
Missense							
	AUG	ACC	TAC	GTT	CGA	CCC	
	Met	Thr	Tyr	Val	Arg	Pro	
Nonsense							
	AUG	GCC	TAG	GTT	CGA	CCC	
	Met	Ala	Stop				
Frameshift							
	AUG	GCC	TAC	•TTC	CGA	CCC	
	Met	Ala	Tyr	Phe	Asp	...	
Deletion							
	AUG	GCC	TAC	GTT	...	CCC	
	Met	Ala	Tyr	Val	–	Pro	
OR							
	AUG	GCC	TA•	G	TT	CCC	
	Met	Ala	Stop ⟶				
Insertion							
	AUG	GCC	AAA	TAC	GTT	CGA	CCC
	Met	Ala	Lys	Tyr	Val	Arg	Pro
OR							
	AUG	GCC	ATA	CGT	TCG	ACC ...	
	Met	Ala	Ile	Arg	Ser	Thr ...	

FIGURE 7–10 Different types of mutations that alter the structure and expression of human genes.

mutations in at least 10 different sarcomeric proteins have been identified including cardiac beta-myosin heavy chain, cardiac myosin-binding protein, cardiac troponin T, cardiac troponin I, alpha-tropomyosin, essential and regulatory light chains, and cardiac actin.[24] Other monogenic cardiovascular disorders include familial long Q-T syndrome,[25] venous thrombosis due to factor V Leiden,[26] and inherited forms of hypertension.[27]

Complex Trait Analysis

Polymorphisms are common variations, defined as being present in more than 1 percent of the population. Single nucleotide polymorphisms (SNPs) are nucleotide substitutions that do not alter a protein structure (Fig. 7-11). SNPs are useful markers to map genes to chromosomal loci. An SNP may be a marker of disease susceptibility (i.e., it can associate with a disease due to either a direct effect of the SNP on the disease or linkage with a nearby susceptibility locus).[28] An estimated 1.4 million SNPs exist in the human genome.[29] Putative and confirmed SNPs are accessible through several public databases such as dbSNP, a database maintained by the National Center for Biotechnology Information.[30]

Wild-type Sequence							
...	AUG	GCC	TAC	GTT	CGA	CCC	...
...	Met	Ala	Tyr	Val	Arg	Pro	...
Polymorphism							
...	AUG	GCA	TAC	GTT	CGA	CCC	...
...	Met	Ala	Tyr	Val	Arg	Pro	...

FIGURE 7–11 A polymorphism is a nucleotide substitution that does not alter the primary amino acid structure of the resulting protein.

A haplotype is a set of SNPs grouped in a contiguous genetic region and inherited en bloc within a given population. Haplotypes may have a true association with a disease or may only appear to be associated due to confounding factors. If an SNP is associated with a disease, it is likely that the SNP is inherited as part of a haplotype in which other SNPs are also statistically associated with the disease. This nonrandom association of alleles is called *linkage disequilibrium.* Linkage disequilibrium exists when alleles at two distinct locations in the genome are inherited together more frequently than expected. Because an SNP may simply be a marker rather than cause of disease predisposition, proof of causality requires demonstration of altered gene function.

An international effort has identified all SNPs on all 22 somatic chromosomes in 300 individuals from diverse backgrounds in Asia, Africa, Europe, and the Americas. This project, called the Haplotype Map or HapMap, was initiated in 2002 to construct a genome-wide map of SNP clusters on the basis of DNA samples from different human populations, and the complete HapMap was published in 2005.[31] The HapMap provides an SNP roadmap for performing linkage analysis, association studies, and evaluation of SNP partners for contribution to a disease. SNPs, then, provide insight into the genetic basis for disease for several reasons: direct causal agents of altered gene function; markers of disease, regardless of causality; and genome-wide markers for genetic studies because of their presence at high density throughout the genome.

Linkage Analysis and Association Studies

Two types of genetic studies examine inheritance: linkage analysis and association studies. Linkage studies are performed in families to study coinheritance of two traits passed down from parent to child. SNP analyses are used because these markers can reveal co-inheritance of two traits or alleles that reside in close proximity to each other on a chromosomal locus. The genes encoding the two traits typically reside in close proximity to each other, and hence the alleles are linked. Linkage is determined by an LOD score, or the *l*ogarithm of the *od*ds that markers are linked at a particular distance, divided by the odds that they are linked at 50 percent co-inheritance (not linked at all). Linkage analysis is commonly used to identify and study Mendelian traits.[32,33] Allele-sharing methods are also used to compare similarity of alleles in closely affected individuals such as affected sibling pairs.

Population-based association studies are useful for investigations of common disorders without clear Mendelian inheritance.[34] Association studies often employ a case control approach in which experimental and reference groups are compared. Careful consideration of the most appropriate control population is necessary to draw valid conclusions and infer gene function from these studies. Case control studies should be sufficiently powered with a large enough sample size to achieve statistical significance. In this approach, known SNPs in candidate genes are investigated using the alleles of a given SNP as variables, which are then associated with the presence or absence of disease or a particular outcome. If SNPs in a candidate gene are not known, then the gene is directly sequenced in a subset of the study and in control populations to determine which SNPs are differentially represented in the two populations. Confirmation of SNPs is then performed in the remainder of the population using PCR-based techniques. Validation requires testing the association in an independent cohort. A limitation of the association approach is the bias inherent in selection of candidate genes. Only those genes known or of interest are often chosen for investigation. In contrast, identification of genes by positional cloning has frequently led to unanticipated discoveries.

Genome-Wide Scans

Genome-wide scans of SNPs are newer techniques performed on high-throughput platforms and assay for several hundred thousand SNPs simultaneously.[35-37] By taking advantage of the physical distribution of SNPs through the genome, chromosomal regions between SNPs can be associated with a disease using statistical methods. This is a powerful technique that assists the discovery of novel SNPs within or in close proximity to genes that cause or are associated with diseases, often complex cardiovascular diseases.[38,39] Genome-wide scans are also useful tools for hypothesis-driven research. This approach will likely receive considerable attention over the next 5 to 10 years as investigators study genetic susceptibility to complex cardiovascular diseases, genetic modifiers of diseases, and gene-environment interactions.

Genomics

Genomics is the study of gene function through the parallel measurements of genomes, most commonly using the techniques of microarrays and serial analysis of gene expression (SAGE). Microarray usage in drug discovery is expanding, and its applications include basic research and target discovery, biomarker determination, pharmacology, toxicogenomics, target selectivity, development of prognostic tests, and disease-subclass determination.

The basic technique involves extraction of RNA from biological samples in either normal or test states (Fig. 7-12).[40] The RNA is copied, while incorporating either fluorescent nucleotides or a tag that is later stained with fluorescence. The labeled RNA is then hybridized to a microarray, the excess is washed off, and the microarray is scanned under laser light. The end result is 4000 to 5000 measurements of gene expression per biological sample. Because a complete experiment might involve any number up to hundreds of microarrays, the resultant RNA-expression data sets can vary greatly in size.

cDNA Microarrays

cDNA (complementary DNA) microarrays are created from probe cDNA libraries (500 to 5000 bases) by spotting a cDNA corresponding to an individual gene or probe at a precise location on a microscope slide. Each microarray measures two samples and provides a relative measurement level for each RNA molecule. Target RNAs labeled with a fluorescent dye are hybridized to the cDNA microarray surface, along with a control sample. The two RNA samples compete for binding to each probe. RNA that matches the cDNA sequence hybridizes to the cDNA spot on the microscope slide. The fluorescent labels are laser activated, and the signal intensi-

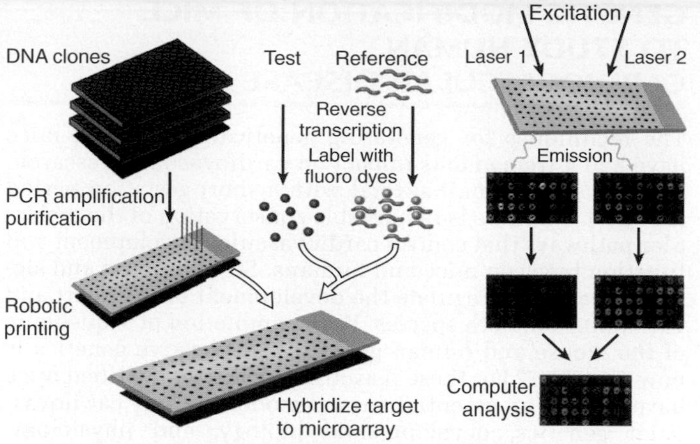

FIGURE 7–12 Detection of differential expression of mRNA from cells or tissues using gene expression profiling. After mRNA is isolated from cells or tissues, it is analyzed by hybridization to fluorescent-labeled cDNA clones imprinted onto a microscope slide. The fluorescent labels are laser activated, and the signal intensities from fluorescent probes binding cDNA spots are compared.

ties from fluorescent probes binding cDNA spots are compared. The comparison reflects the ratios of RNA abundance for each expressed gene. Normalization strategies that allow for standardization of inter-array comparisons are applied, followed by analytical methods, as described previously.

Oligonucleotide Arrays

Oligonucleotide arrays are created by attachment of synthetic nucleotide probes (12-80-mer oligonucleotides) representative of unique portions of genes to an array surface. cDNA is synthesized from the experimental mRNA sample, followed by an in vitro transcription step to create biotin-labeled cRNA, which hybridizes to the microarray target. The microarray is treated with a fluorescent dye tagged to avidin (a protein that binds tightly to biotin) and subjected to laser activation. With oligonucleotide arrays, each microarray measures a single sample and provides an absolute measurement level of each RNA molecule. Signal intensities are measured as a reflection of expression level for each gene.

SAGE

SAGE is a technique for characterization of gene expression based on direct sequencing of transcripts. Its major strength is determination and analysis of transcripts when the sequence is unknown. SAGE requires approximately 10-fold larger quantities of mRNA for analysis and hence is much more labor intensive than some array platforms, even with automated sequencers, because the simplest two-sample comparison requires sequencing of approximately 1.5×10^6 bases. This factor alone poses difficulties when RNA abundance is low, whereas a major advantage is its higher sensitivity for changes in expression level.[41,42]

After acquisition of data by image processing, data are analyzed in three steps: normalization, filtering, and computation. Normalization accounts for technical factors, such as array manufacturing, differences in dye incorporation, and irregularities in probe distribution during hybridization, and is performed to allow meaningful comparisons between individual arrays. Filtering of data refers to the selection of those data likely to represent significant findings. Typical criteria for filtering include assessment of signal quality and fold-change in gene expression level. Differential gene expression in microarray analysis is often defined by a 1.5- to 2-fold difference in relative gene expression level.

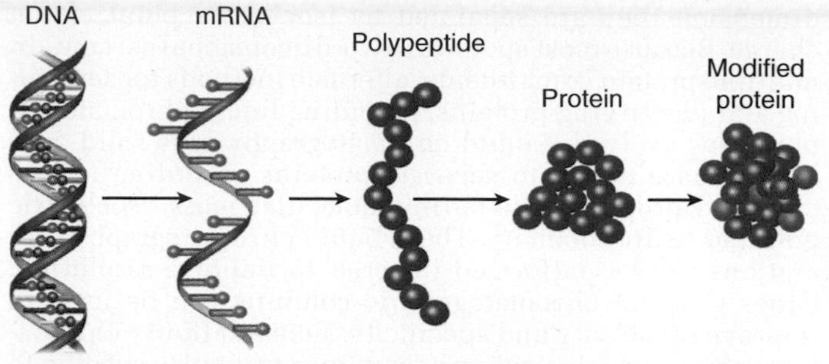

FIGURE 7–13 Relationship of the genome to the proteome. Examples of common posttranslational modifications include the addition to amino acids (blue balls) of sugars (glycosylation), phosphorylation, and prenylation depicted by the red and green balls.

Determination of similarity and dissimilarity is a critical component of the data analysis. Two general approaches are used: supervised and unsupervised. Supervised methods are employed for finding genes with expression levels that are significantly different among groups of samples and finding genes that accurately predict a characteristic of the sample. Two commonly used supervised techniques include "nearest neighbors" and "support vector machines." Users of unsupervised methods try to find internal structure or relationships in a data set instead of trying to determine how best to predict a correct answer. Four commonly used unsupervised techniques include hierarchical clustering, self-organizing maps, relevance networks, and principal-component analysis. These analytical methods are described in detail elsewhere.[43] These computational approaches are then followed by a statistical analysis. Before any microarray data are taken at face value, significant findings should be validated with independent testing of RNA expression levels using quantitative reverse transcription PCR or conventional Northern blotting techniques.

Proteomics

Proteomics is the study of proteins expressed by the genome. Genomics and proteomics should be viewed as complementary components of the genetic spectrum, beginning with DNA and ending with modified proteins (Fig. 7-13). Proteins are the final product of the human genome and ultimately define human biology. Proteins are responsible for biological form and function. Scientists have estimated that there are six to seven times as many proteins as genes (≈200,000) in humans because of splicing, exchange of structural cassettes among genes during transcription, and posttranslational modifications. The field of proteomics seeks to understand the complex interactions of all proteins expressed within a tissue or organism under normal or perturbed conditions. Indeed, human proteomics is in its infancy.[44]

The methods for proteome analysis are still under development and validation. However, there are five basic elements to any proteomic analysis: sample acquisition, protein extraction, protein separation, protein sequence determination, and sequence comparison to reference databases for protein identification.[45] Sample acquisition is straightforward, involving obtaining a tissue biopsy or a plasma sample from an individual (under informed consent). Protein extraction is generally performed by chemical methods, generally with methanol, to remove all DNA, RNA, carbohydrates, and lipids. Extracted proteins must be separated for identification, and this step has traditionally been performed by two-dimensional gel electrophoresis. In the first dimension proteins are separated by mass, and in the second dimension they are separated by isoelectric point or net charge. Because most spots on a two-dimensional gel contain multiple protein constituents, alternate methods for separating and identifying proteins, including liquid chromatography, have evolved. Liquid chromatography uses solid- and liquid-phase media to separate proteins according to biochemical properties including molecular mass, isoelectric point, or hydrophobicity. These liquid chromatography separations can be performed in series to improve resolution. Other types of chromatographic columns can be used to improve sensitivity and specificity, such as affinity chromatography in which a column contains antibodies specific to certain functions to achieve the desired separation. Following separation, the protein is identified, generally using some form of mass spectrometry (Fig. 7-14). Mass spectrometry converts proteins or peptides to charged species that can be separated on the basis of their mass-to-charge ratio. Several types of mass spectrometry ionization methods are in use including electrospray ionization and matrix-assisted laser desorption ionization (MALDI). Peptide sequences identified with these methods must next be analyzed by comparison with known database sequences to determine the unequivocal identity of the protein. Once proteins in a given proteome have been identified, their relative abundance levels are determined to compare relative abundance of proteins in a normal or diseased state. Finally, a thorough analysis of a proteome should include some measure of function, whether it is in cultured cells or in animal models. This approach is similar to functional genomic analysis, in which it is critical to gauge the importance of a gene or mutation through determination of gene function.

Proteomic analysis is currently limited by sensitivity, specificity, and throughput. However, this field and its methodologies are developing rapidly. The application of proteomics to cardiovascular disease holds great promise for understanding the function of the cardiovascular system in all its complexity.

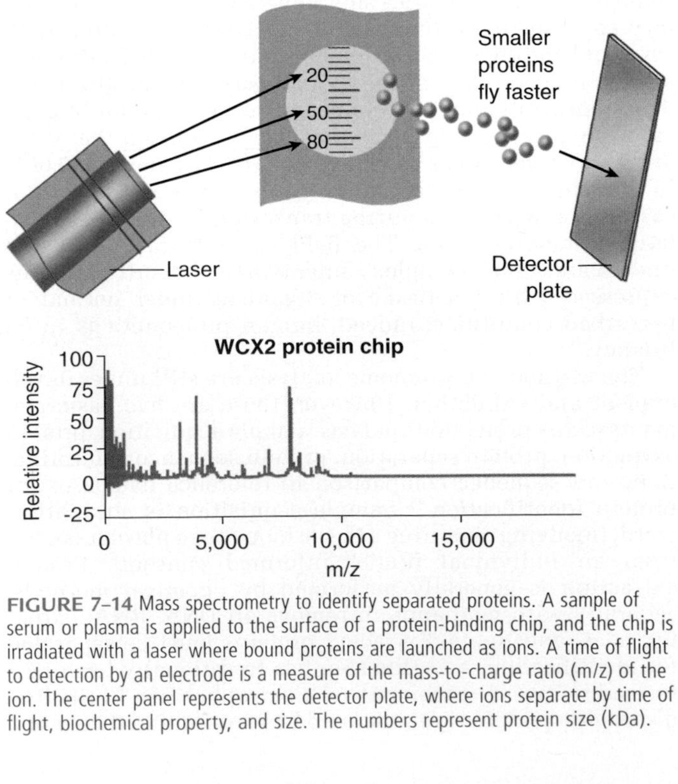

FIGURE 7–14 Mass spectrometry to identify separated proteins. A sample of serum or plasma is applied to the surface of a protein-binding chip, and the chip is irradiated with a laser where bound proteins are launched as ions. A time of flight to detection by an electrode is a measure of the mass-to-charge ratio (m/z) of the ion. The center panel represents the detector plate, where ions separate by time of flight, biochemical property, and size. The numbers represent protein size (kDa).

GENETIC MODIFICATION OF MICE TO STUDY HUMAN CARDIOVASCULAR DISEASE

The techniques for generating genetically modified mice have had a tremendous impact on cardiovascular research. The mouse is a small animal with a short gestation period (21 days). Yet there is remarkable conservation of the molecular pathways that control cardiovascular development and function between mice and humans. Similar genes and signaling pathways regulate the development of the heart and vasculature in both species. With completion of sequencing of the mouse and human genome, comparative genetics is now possible.[46] For these reasons, genetically modified mice have become an essential animal model to study cardiovascular genetics, developmental biology, and physiology. Limitations of mouse models to study human cardiovascular disease are evident, but due to the simplicity of genetic manipulation in the mouse, it has become a standard starting place for hypothesis testing before evaluation in a larger animal. This section briefly describes the principles of four approaches to genetic modification in the mouse: transgenics, gene deletion or "knockout," conditional knockout, and studying mouse physiology.

Transgenic Mice

Creation of a transgenic mouse involves four steps: cloning of the gene of interest; fusion of the gene to transcriptional regulatory sequences that program its expression in all tissues of the mouse or in specific tissues; injection of the purified transgene into the male pronucleus of a fertilized one-cell mouse embryo; and reimplantation of the injected embryo into a foster mother. The injected transgene randomly integrates into a chromosome of the fertilized embryo, resulting in a founder mouse that expresses the injected transgene and that passes the transgene to 50 percent of its progeny. Comparative studies can then be performed between the transgenic mouse and nontransgenic littermate mouse as a control. Production of a founder transgenic mouse is now routinely performed in many laboratories and is accomplished generally in less than a month. Similar techniques have been used to create transgenic rabbits, rats, and pigs.

Refinements of these techniques have assisted more sophisticated transgenic models. Cell-specific promoters program transgene expression exclusively in cardiomyocytes, endothelial cells, and vascular smooth muscle cells, creating a transgenic mouse with restricted expression in the cardiovascular system. Although overexpression of a transgene results in a gain-of-function, it is also possible to eliminate the function of a single gene by overexpressing a dominant-negative mutant of that gene, the encoded protein of which interferes with the function of the wild-type protein. Expression of a transgene can also be turned on or off by administration of a simple drug like tetracycline using a tet operon system. These mice allow precisely timed transgene expression as well as a comparison in the same animal of the phenotypes of transgene on and off states.

Gene Inactivation or Knockout Approaches

Gene deletion is a complementary approach to transgenesis for studying the role of a specific gene in mouse development and physiology (Fig. 7-15). In gene deletion studies, the expression of one or more genes is "knocked out" to produce a loss-of-function mutant mouse. The knockout approach involves the following steps: construction of a targeting vector containing the gene of interest with a deletion or nonsense mutation; transfection of a pluripotent mouse embryonic stem cell with the targeting vector; homologous recombination between the targeting construct and one copy of the endogenous gene, producing an embryonic stem cell with a homozygous deletion of the gene of interest; injection of the mutant embryonic stem cell into a fertilized mouse blastocyst; and implantation of the blastocyst into a foster mother. The resulting mouse pup is a chimera in which all tissues including the gonads are derived in part from the mutant embryonic stem cells and in part from the wild-type cells of the injected blastocysts. This chimeric animal is bred to a wild-type animal, and fertilization of a wild-type egg with a mutant sperm from the chimera produces a heterozygous knockout mouse in which one copy of the gene of interest in all cells is mutant and the other copy is wild-type. Heterozygous animals are then bred with each other to produce homozygous knockouts that have deletions of the gene of interest in all cells. The absence of the gene in the knockout animal produces a specific phenotype that reveals the direct function of the gene in development and normal and perturbed physiology. Creation of a knockout mouse is technically more challenging than transgenesis and often takes 9 to 12 months to complete.

Conditional Knockout Mice

Inactivation of important genes commonly results in early embryonic lethal phenotypes that are difficult to analyze and understand. As a result, methods have been developed to delete genes in a tissue-specific fashion and/or to inactivate genes at different times in development. In addition, it is often of interest to produce specific mutations of genes rather than to eliminate their expression completely. Homologous recombination is also used to introduce specific mutations into wild-type genes; the difference in technique is that these "knock-ins" use a targeting construct containing a mutant gene rather than a gene deletion. Other homologous recombination approaches permit introduction of a distinct or unrelated gene into a foreign genetic locus to regulate the new gene under the control of the promoter of the targeted locus.

Another approach to tissue-specific gene deletion is use of a bacterial phage recombination system called Cre-lox. A P1 bacteriophage encodes an enzyme called *Cre* that catalyzes recombination of DNA between two specific sequences (called loxP sites) that signal recombination. This system has been adapted in mice by producing a targeting construct in which the gene of interest is *f*lanked by *lox*P sites (a "floxed allele"). Mice homozygous for the floxed allele are bred with transgenic mice that express the Cre recombinase in a tissue-specific manner (e.g., endothelial cells, vascular smooth muscle cells, cardiomyocytes). The resulting mice have a deletion of the gene of interest only in the tissue expressing the Cre recombinase. By placing the Cre transgene under the control of a tetracycline responsive promoter, gene deletion is programmed only following tetracycline feeding.

Studies of Mouse Physiology

Realizing the advantage of the potential of mouse genetics requires technologies that can characterize the phenotype of mutant mice. The mouse is technically challenging because the heart and blood vessels are small in size, and the resting mouse heartbeat is greater than 500 beats/minute. Miniaturized instrumentation and microsurgical techniques have helped solve these problems. With these techniques, it is possible to take physiological measurements in anesthetized and intubated mice including aortic blood pressures, left ventricular pressure tracings, and cardiac hemodynamics before and after infusions of pharmacological agents, such as dobutamine or isoproterenol. Noninvasive imaging of the heart and vasculature has improved substantially, and two-dimensional echocardiograms are now routine in fetal and adult mice. Magnetic resonance imaging renders clear images of cardiac structure and function. These noninvasive techniques are used to measure end-systolic and end-diastolic left ventricular dimensions, left ventricular wall thickness and mass, and shortening fraction. Myocardial infarctions produced by coronary artery ligation, wire injuries to vessels that simulate angioplasty, and aortic banding to induce left ventricular hypertrophy are commonly performed in gene-modified mice. Exercise testing, 24-hour electrocardiogram recordings on conscious mice using implanted transducers, and electrophysiological studies to detect inducible cardiac arrhythmias are also standard techniques. With the availability of techniques to study cardiovascular physiology, genetically modified mice now provide an accurate and convenient way to evaluate the function of specific genes in cardiovascular disease.

GENE TRANSFER

Gene transfer is the introduction and expression of recombinant genes in mammalian cells. Gene transfer aims to introduce recombinant genes into target cells to study the mechanisms and consequences of gene expression. Genes are transfected into cells using vectors. The recombinant gene undergoes transcription into RNA and translation into protein by host enzymes, culminating in the expression of the recombinant protein. The recombinant protein remains intracellular or is secreted into the extracellular space or circulation. Gene expression is transient or stable, depending on whether integration into chromosomes occurs. The efficiency of DNA uptake and gene expression, often referred to as *transfection efficiency,* depends on many factors including delivery of DNA to the cell, uptake of DNA into the cytoplasm, degradation of DNA in endosomes, release of DNA from endosomes into the cytoplasm, transport to the nucleus, and persistence in the nucleus.

In vivo gene transfer is performed by cell-mediated or direct gene transfer methods. Cell-mediated or ex vivo gene transfer involves removing autologous cells from the host and transfecting the cells with the vector in vitro.[47] Genetically modified cells are reintroduced into the host by infusion or injection. Ex vivo gene transfer permits the introduction of recombinant genetic material into a specific cell—for example, endothelial or smooth muscle cells—and analysis of recombinant gene expression within that cell type.

In vivo gene transfer employs the direct introduction of recombinant genes into target cells and tissues.[48] Targeted gene transfer in the vasculature has been performed with cell-specific promoters to achieve gene expression within endothelial cells or smooth muscle cells. Both ex vivo and in vivo gene transfer approaches have been employed in the development of animal models of vascular disease and in clinical trials of gene transfer to the cardiovascular system.

Vectors

Transfection of appropriate target cells represents the critical first step in gene transfer. As a result, development of gene transfer methods has represented a significant area of research in the field. Both viral and nonviral vectors have been employed in vascular gene transfer studies. A common feature of these methods is the efficient delivery of genes

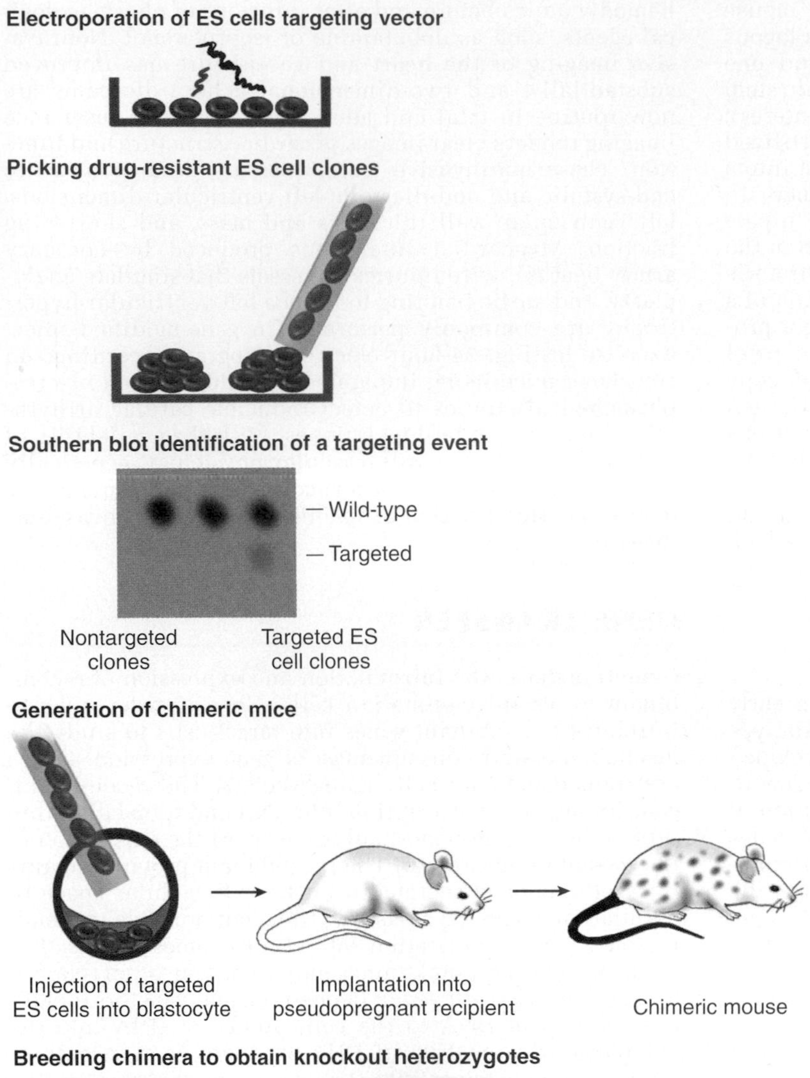

FIGURE 7–15 Scheme for generating heterozygous and homozygous gene knockout mice by homologous recombination in mouse embryonic stem cells.

into cells. Vectors differ, however, in the processing of foreign DNA and the frequency of integration into chromosomal DNA. In the case of retroviral and lentiviral vectors, the transferred sequences are stably integrated into the chromosomal DNA of the target cell. These vectors have been considered most often for ex vivo gene therapy. Other methods of gene transfer result primarily in the introduction of foreign DNA into target cell nuclei in an unintegrated form. These methods result in high, but transient, gene expression. These vectors including adenovirus, adeno-associated virus, and cationic liposomes have been employed predominantly for in vivo gene transfer studies.

RETROVIRUSES

Retroviruses were the first vectors employed in gene transfer studies, dating back to the 1980s. Initial interest in retroviruses as vectors arose from the observation that these vectors stably transduce nearly 100 percent of proliferating target cells in culture. Retroviral vectors were used initially in vascular gene transfer studies, primarily in ex vivo studies, but their use has been limited by low transfection efficiencies. Retroviral vectors have been used recently in clinical gene therapy studies for treatment of severe combined immune deficiency (SCID). Unfortunately, in one trial, two children experienced the complication of retroviral insertion into an oncogenic site of chromosome X, leading to leukemia.[49]

ADENOVIRUS

Adenovirus types 2 and 5 are the two serotypes used for vectors in cardiovascular gene transfer. The adenovirus genome is linear, double-stranded DNA, approximately 36 kb in length, which is divided into 100 map units, each of which is 360 base pairs in length. The DNA contains short inverted terminal repeats (ITRs) at the end of the genome that are required for viral DNA replication. The gene products are organized into early (E1-E4) and late (L1-L5) regions on the basis of expression before or after initiation of DNA replication. Adenoviruses have a lytic life cycle characterized by attachment to an adenoviral glycoprotein receptor on mammalian cells and entry into cells by receptor-mediated endocytosis. Adenoviral capsid proteins protect adenoviruses from lysosomal degradation, and viral DNA translocates to the nucleus. Expression of viral genes depends on cellular transcription factors and expression of the adenoviral E1 region, which encodes a transactivator of viral gene expression. During lytic infection, the viral genome replicates to several thousand copies per cell. The viral genome associates with core proteins and is packaged into capsids by self-assembling of major capsid proteins.

The adenovirus genome is rendered replication deficient to generate a vector. Vectors are constructed by homologous recombination in a cell line known as 293 cells by cotransfection of (1) a bacterial plasmid containing the cDNA of interest and a small region of adenoviral genome deleted from E1A and E1B regions (these regions regulate adenoviral transcription and are required for viral replication), and (2) an incomplete adenoviral genome. Homologous recombination between the two DNAs generates a recombinant genome in which the foreign gene replaces the E1 region. Viral stock is further propagated in 293 cells to high titer, generally 10^9 to 10^{10} plaque-forming units (pfu) per milliliter.

Adenoviral vectors have several additional advantages including efficient infection of mammalian cells and expression in nondividing cells in vitro and in vivo. These vectors are relatively stable and can be grown and concentrated to a high titer. Extrachromosomal replication of the vector greatly reduces the chance of mutation by random integration and dysregulation of host cellular genes. However, a number of shortcomings limit their use as gene transfer vectors. Gene expression in vascular and myocardial cells following adenoviral infection is short lived, persisting for only several weeks. Host immune response to adenoviral proteins presents a major limitation to their in vivo use. Although low levels of neutralizing antibodies do not appear to have adverse clinical effects, it remains to be determined whether host immune responses to the adenovirus will preclude repeated administrations of the same serotype of adenovirus. First-generation recombinant adenoviral vectors (deletion of E1A and E1B genes and partial deletion of E3 genes) have been used clinically in gene therapy studies, even though in animal models these vectors are often associated with tissue inflammation, particularly in the liver and lung. Direct exposure of diseased liver to high-titer adenoviral vectors is highly toxic and, in one case, unfortunately lethal.[50] Inactivation of the E2A gene prolongs gene expression and produces less inflammation in lung and liver. In arterial gene transfer studies employing adenoviral vectors, mononuclear inflammatory cell infiltrates have been observed in the adventitia of peripheral and pulmonary arteries, but no necrosis or vasculitis was observed.[51] Infection of pulmonary arteries with adenovirus was associated with mild degrees of perivascular inflammation; however, pulmonary arteries instilled with saline or liposomes also exhibited mild accumulation of perivascular mononuclear cells. Despite the limitations of immune responses to adenoviral capsid proteins, adenoviral vectors are attractive vehicles for in vivo gene transfer in animal models because of the efficiency of transfection. Whether adenoviral vectors will be used clinically remains to be seen.

ADENO-ASSOCIATED VIRUS

Adeno-associated virus (AAV) is a defective human parvovirus that has attractive features as a gene transfer vector. This viral vector is prepared at high titers, is not normally pathogenic in humans, and infects many cell types in vitro.[52] The AAV genome is a single-stranded, linear, 5 kb DNA molecule. The wild-type AAV integrates in a site-specific fashion into a single 7 kb region on human chromosome 19. The AAV genome is flanked by 145 base pair-inverted terminal repeats containing the sequences required for packaging, DNA replication, and integration. The coding region contains two open reading frames, which are deleted and replaced with one or more cDNAs plus transcriptional regulatory units during vector construction.[73] AAV vectors accept transgene cassettes of only 4 to 5 kb; this limits the types of transgenes that can be used. Propagation of AAV vectors requires complex packaging including AAV Rep and Cap proteins and five adenoviral proteins (E1A, E1B, E2A, E4, and VA). These complex packaging requirements have precluded construction of a helper cell line for AAV. Currently, vectors are constructed by cotransfection of cells with the AAV vector and a nonpackageable plasmid containing the AAV Rep and Cap proteins. This is followed by infection of the transfected cells with wild-type or mutant helper adenovirus. AAV is separated from contaminating adenovirus by heat treatment and equilibrium density gradation centrifugation. Protocols for constructing AAV vectors are described elsewhere.[52]

The AAV vectors infect multiple cell types in vitro, but their utility in vivo is uncertain. Transduction of vascular endothelial and smooth muscle cells remains unknown. Further limitations include a lack of packaging cell lines and a requirement for coinfection with adenovirus, making it difficult to prepare large quantities of pure AAV vectors. Deletion of viral genes during vector construction limits the ability of these vectors to integrate in a site-specific manner but does raise the possibility of insertional mutagenesis. AAV vectors have theoretic attractiveness, but considerable work is required before they can be employed clinically.

CATIONIC LIPOSOMES

Cationic lipids are preparations of positively charged lipids that spontaneously complex with negatively charged DNA to form DNA-lipid conjugates. The lipid component assists delivery of DNA to cells by fusion with plasmid membrane or with endosomal membranes after endocytosis. Following release from endosomes, plasmid DNA is maintained in an extrachromosomal form. Cationic liposomes have been employed in arterial gene transfer studies in many animal models including rats, rabbits, dogs, and pigs. Advantages of cationic liposomes include a favorable safety profile, a lack of viral coding sequences, and no cDNA size constraints. They have produced minimal biochemical, hemodynamic, or cardiac toxicity in animals or humans. These vectors are straightforward to prepare for experimental and clinical use. The limitations include a low transfection efficiency and short-term gene expression.

POLYMERS

Nucleic acids and drugs have been applied to polymer gels coated onto stents or balloons and directly applied to arteries. Many early polymers were associated with intense inflammatory reactions. Newer formulations have been successfully used in the development of drug-eluting stents.[53,54]

Animal Models

Gene transfer is a useful approach to introduce nucleic acids to somatic cells of an animal to define gene function, dissect disease pathophysiology, or achieve a therapeutic effect. Over the past decade, gene transfer has been employed in many animal models of cardiovascular disease. Gene- and cell-based approaches have been used including a recent interest in combining gene transfer with stem cell–based therapies.[55,56] Gene transfer as a tool to induce vascular growth is an illustrative example.

Vascular growth proceeds through the stages of angiogenesis, arteriogenesis, and lymphangiogenesis. Angiogenesis is the sprouting of new blood vessels from preexisting vessels. Arteriogenesis is the enlargement of muscular collateral blood vessels from preexisting arteriolar anastomoses and is often referred to as "collateralization." Lymphangiogenesis is the generation of new lymphatic vessels from preexisting ones. It has been widely used in preclinical and clinical studies. Two splice variants of vascular endothelial growth factor (VEGF A), $VEGF_{165}$ and $VEGF_{121}$, have angiogenic properties in animal models[57] and have been evaluated in clinical trials.[58] Placental growth factor (PlGF) also has angiogenic activity in animals. PlGF binds to VEGFR-1 and contributes to angiogenesis under pathological conditions. Interestingly, PlGF also promotes angiogenesis and arteriogenesis through mobilization of hematopoietic stem cells and endothelial progenitor cells from the bone marrow. The clinical relevance of VEGF, PlGF, and endothelial progenitor cells in the clinical treatment of ischemia remains undetermined, although there have been efforts at transducing stem cells with VEGF to enhance angiogenesis.[59,60] Other growth factors have been evaluated for their angiogenic properties in gene transfer models. Hypoxia-inducible transcription factor-1-alpha activates several angiogenic growth factors including VEGF-A, VEGFR-2, insulin-like growth factor-2, and erythropoietin. A leucine zipper transcription factor that activated VEGF transcription has also been recently described.[61]

The hypothesis that overexpression of growth factors will result in therapeutic vascular growth has been tested in several animal models of peripheral and myocardial ischemia including ex vivo transduction of stem cells and endothelial progenitor cells.[62] Adenoviral-mediated VEGF and fibroblast growth factor delivery and vascular growth has been demonstrated in the myocardium and skeletal muscle by the proliferation and enlargement of capillaries, although cessation of therapy (or extinction of the transgene) leads to regression of most of the vessels. Expression of VEGF for more than 4 weeks leads to sufficient vascular remodeling that new vessel growth persists for several months after VEGF treatment is withdrawn.[63] In animal models, hemodynamic factors and persistence of blood flow are important for stabilization of the newly formed vessels. Furthermore, the predictive value of a preclinical animal model is inversely related to the animal size. Many applications and vectors work well in smaller animals such as mice and rats, but scaling up to larger animals, such as pigs, dogs, and sheep, has proven difficult. Demonstration of efficacy in young, normal animals may not predict responses in older human patients with chronic diseases. Indeed, elderly and diabetic animals have impaired vascular growth.[64]

 Many of the beneficial biological effects reported in animals may not translate to humans, given the limitations of current vectors.

Clinical Trials

Cardiovascular gene therapy trials have had a checkered course. Many phase I trials have been completed, but few have proceeded to phase II studies. Concerns have been raised about the use of adenoviral vectors, even for cardiac or vascular applications, as well as low transfection efficiencies in vivo. The majority of studies have focused on stimulation of angiogenesis and arteriogenesis to improve perfusion of myocardial or skeletal muscle. Three phases of therapeutic angiogenesis trials have been conducted to date. Initial phase I trials employed plasmid DNA and adenoviruses to induce angiogenesis for peripheral or myocardial ischemia. These trials evaluated the safety of vectors and catheter or direct injection delivery in small numbers of patients. Consistent findings were evident: No serious adverse events were encountered attributable to the gene vector or delivery device. With this demonstration of safety, phase I/II trials evaluated larger numbers of patients with soft efficacy endpoints.[65,66] No major adverse events were reported, and although positive efficacy findings were reported, many of these trials were not controlled. Collectively, however, the following clinical insights accrued. Placebo effects are common in treated patients, perhaps due to altered hemodynamics or improved clinical care. Meaningful clinical endpoints were not always predefined and hence cast doubt on efficacy data. The absence of controlled, randomized studies also did not help the field move forward. A third phase of clinical trials has been initiated with placebo-controlled studies including larger numbers of patients and well-defined clinical endpoints.[67-74] Data from these phase III studies and long-term follow-up are essential in determining whether a gene therapy product will be approved by the Food and Drug Administration and clinically used to treat myocardial and/or peripheral ischemia. Improved understanding of the pharmacokinetics is essential.[75] Investigators must proceed with carefully conducted and evaluated trials.

FUTURE DIRECTIONS

Molecular and cellular biology have now joined the mainstream cardiovascular research. These approaches have advanced our understanding of the pathogenesis of cardiovascular diseases, have led to the development of extremely useful animal models, and have provided the basic principles for molecular therapies. Cardiovascular research is now turning to molecular genetics as the next scientific arena in which major advances will occur. To date, we have begun to understand the mechanisms by which single genes cause cardiovascular disease. These mechanisms have provided great insight into the pathophysiology of complex common cardiovascular disorders. The next major challenge in the field of molecular genetics is to understand with greater clarity genetic susceptibility to common cardiovascular diseases. Genotyping, genomics, and proteomics are approaches with promise and are in early stages of application. The information gleaned from these techniques will only be as good as the characterization of clinical phenotypes by thoughtful, observant physicians who detect unusual patterns of disease in their patients. Although many investigators remain hopeful, we do not know the role that genetic or cell-based therapies will play in the practice of clinical cardiology. The efforts of many physician-scientists and clinical investigators are required to conduct careful, well-considered studies. Only then can the promise of molecular genetics be realized and applied to the care of cardiovascular patients.

REFERENCES

Cell Biology and Signaling

1. Alberts B, Johnson A, Lewis J, et al: Molecular Biology of the Cell. New York, Garland Science, 2002.
2. Lewin B: Genes VII. Oxford, Oxford University Press, 2000.
3. Edidin M: Lipids on the frontier: A century of cell-membrane bilayers. Nat Rev Mol Cell Biol 4:414, 2003.
4. Shi Y, Massague J: Mechanisms of TGF-beta signaling from cell membrane to the nucleus. Cell 113:685, 2003.
5. Weis K: Regulating access to the genome: Nucleocytoplasmic transport throughout the cell cycle. Cell 112:441, 2003.
6. Bonifacino JS, Lippincott-Schwartz J: Coat proteins: Shaping membrane transport. Nat Rev Mol Cell Biol 1:409, 2003.
7. Williams RR, Fisher AG: Chromosomes, positions please! Nat Cell Biol 5:388, 2003.
8. Eichler EE, Sankoff D: Structural dynamics of eukaryotic chromosome evolution. Science 301:793, 2003.
9. Page SL, Hawley RS: Chromosome choreography: The meiotic ballet. Science 301:785, 2003.
10. Cline SD, Hanawalt PC: Who's on first in the cellular response to DNA damage? Nat Rev Mol Cell Biol 4:361, 2003.
11. Edinger AL, Thompson CB: Death by design: Apoptosis, necrosis and autophagy. Curr Opin Cell Biol 16:663, 2004.
12. Nabel EG: CDKs and CKIs: Molecular targets for tissue remodeling. Nat Rev Drug Discov 1:587, 2002.
13. Nabel EG, Boehm M, Akyurek LM, et at: Cell cycle signaling and cardiovascular disease. Cold Spring Harb Symp Quant Biol 67:163, 2002.
14. Gartel AL, Tyner AL: The role of the cyclin-dependent kinase inhibitor p21 in apoptosis. Mol Cancer Ther 1:639, 2002.

Molecular Basis of Genetics

15. Vogelstein B, Lane D, Levine AJ: Surfing the p53 network. Nature Nov 408:307, 2000.
16. Lander ES, Linton LM, Birren B, et al: Initial sequencing and analysis of the human genome. Nature 409:860, 2001.
17. Venter JC, Adams MD, Myers EW, et al: The sequence of the human genome. Science 291:1304, 2001.
18. Collins FS, Green ED, Guttmacher AE, et al: A vision for the future of genomics research. Nature 422:835, 2003.
19. Sambrook J, Russell DW: Molecular cloning: A laboratory manual. Cold Spring Harbor, Cold Spring Harbor Laboratory, 2001.
20. Watson JD, Crick FHC: Molecular structure of nucleic acids: A structure for deoxyribose nucleic acid. Nature 171:737, 1953.
21. NCBI:Online Mendelian Inheritance in Man. Available at: http://www.ncbi.nlm.nih.gov/omim
22. Nabel EG: Cardiovascular disease. N Engl J Med 349:60, 2003.
23. Cohen JC, Boerwinkle E, Mosley TH, et al: Sequence variations in PCSK9, low LDL, and protection against coronary heart disease. N Engl J Med 354:1264, 2006.
24. Seidman JG, Seidman C: The genetic basis for cardiomyopathy: From mutation identification to mechanistic paradigms. Cell 104:557, 2001.
25. Keating MT, Sanguinetti MC: Molecular and cellular mechanisms of cardiac arrhythmias. Cell 104:569, 2001.
26. Watkins H, Farrall M: Genetic susceptibility to coronary artery disease: From promise to progress. Nat Rev Genet 7:163, 2006.
27. Lifton RP, Gharavi AG, Geller DS: Molecular mechanisms of human hypertension. Cell 104:545, 2001.
28. Cargill M, Altshuler D, Ireland J, et al: Characterization of single-nucleotide polymorphisms in coding regions of human genes. Nat Genetics 22:231, 1999.
29. Sachidanandam R, Weissman D, Schmidt SC, et al: A map of human genome sequence variation containing 1.42 million single nucleotide polymorphisms. Nature 409:928, 2002.
30. National Center for Biotechnology Information: Single Nucleotide Polymorphism. NCBI (http://www.ncbi.nlm.nih.gov/SNP/).
31. The International HapMap Consortium. A haplotype map of the human genome. Nature 437:1299, 2005.
32. Zwick ME, Cutler DJ, Chakravarti A: Patterns of genetic variation in Mendelian and complex traits. Annu Rev Genomics Hum Genet 1:387, 2000.
33. Glazier AM, Nadeu JH, Altman TJ: Finding genes that underlie complex traits. Science 298:2345, 2002.
34. Lohmueller KE, Pearce CL, Pike M, et al: Meta-analysis of genetic association studies supports a contribution of common variants to susceptibility to common disease. Nat Genet 33:177, 2003.
35. Storey JD, Tibshirani R: Statistical significance for genomewide studies. Proc Natl Acad Sci 100:9440, 2003.
36. Kennedy GC, Matsuzaki H, Dong S, et al: Large-scale genotyping of complex DNA. Nat Biotechnol 21:1233, 2003.
37. Matsuzaki H, Loi H, Dong S, et al: Parallel genotyping of over 10,000 SNPs using a one-primer assay on a high-density oligonucleotide array. Genome Res 14:414, 2004.

38. Herbert A, Gerry NP, McQueen MB, et al: A common genetic variant is associated with adult and childhood obesity. Science 312:279, 2006.
39. Arking DE, Pfeufer A, Post W, et al: A common genetic variant in the NOS1 regulator NOS1AP modulates cardiac repolarization. Nat Genet 38:644, 2006.

Techniques for Molecular Investigations

40. Butte A: The use and analysis of microarray DNA. Nat Rev Drug Disc 1:951, 2002.
41. Velculescu VE, Vogelstein B, Kinzler KW: Analysing uncharted transcriptomes with SAGE. Trends Genet 16:423, 2000.
42. Patino WD, Mian OY, Hwang PM: Serial analysis of gene expression: Technical considerations and applications to cardiovascular biology. Circ Res 91:565, 2002.
43. Lockhart DJ, Winzeler EA: Genomics, gene expression and DNA arrays. Nature 405:827, 2000.
44. Loscalzo J: Proteomics in cardiovascular biology and medicine. Circulation 108:380, 2003.
45. Patterson SD, Aebersold RH: Proteomics: The first decade and beyond. Nat Genetics 33:311, 2003.
46. Mouse Genome Sequencing Consortium: Initial sequencing and comparative analysis of the mouse genome. Nature 420:520, 2002.

Molecular and Cellular Therapies

47. Nabel EG, Plautz G, Boyce FM, et al: Recombinant gene expression in vivo within endothelial cells of the arterial wall. Science 244:1342, 1989.
48. Nabel EG, Plautz G, Nabel GJ: Site-specific gene expression in vivo by direct gene transfer into the arterial wall. Science 249:1285, 1990.
49. Marshall E: Second child in French trial is found to have leukemia. Science 299:320, 2003.
50. Somia N, Verma IM: Gene therapy: Trials and tribulations. Nat Rev Genet 1:91, 2002.
51. Ohno T, Gordon D, San H, et al: Gene therapy for vascular smooth muscle cell proliferation after arterial injury. Science 265:781, 1994.
52. Tal J: Adeno-associated virus-based vectors in gene therapy. J Biomed Sci 7:279, 2000.
53. Sousa JE, Serruys PW, Costa MA: New frontiers in cardiology: Drug-eluting stents: Part I. Circulation 107:2274, 2003.
54. Sousa JE, Serruys PW, Costa MA: New frontiers in cardiology: Drug-eluting stents: Part II. Circulation 107:2383, 2003.
55. Mangi AA, Noiseux N, Kong D, et al: Mesenchymal stem cells modified with Akt prevent remodeling and restore performance of infarcted hearts. Nat Med 9:1195, 2003.
56. Hill JM, Dick AJ, Raman VK, et al: Serial cardiac magnetic resonance imaging of injected mesenchymal stem cells. Circulation 108:1009, 2003.
57. Isner JM: Myocardial gene therapy. Nature 415:234, 2002.
58. Yla-Herttuala S, Martin JF: Cardiovascular gene therapy. Lancet 355:213, 2000.
59. Iwaguro H, Yamaguchi J, Kalka C, et al: Endothelial progenitor cell vascular endothelial growth factor gene transfer for vascular regeneration. Circulation 105:672, 2002.
60. Nabel EG: Stem cells combined with gene transfer for therapeutic vasculogenesis. Circulation 105:672, 2002.
61. Rebar EJ, Huang Y, Hickey R, et al: Induction of angiogenesis in a mouse model using engineered transcription factors. Nat Med 8:1427, 2002.
62. Yla-Herttuala S, Alitalo K: Gene transfer as a tool to induce therapeutic vascular growth. Nat Med 9:694, 2003.
63. Dor Y, Djonov V, Abramovitch R, et al: Conditional switching of VEGF provides new insights into adult neovascularization and pro-angiogenic therapy. EMBO J 21:1939, 2002.
64. Schratzberger P, Walter DH, Rittig K, et al: Reversal of experimental diabetic neuropathy by VEGF gene transfer. J Clin Invest 107:1083, 2001.
65. Rajagopalan S, Shah M, Luciano A, et al: Adenovirus-mediated gene transfer of VEGF(121) improves lower-extremity endothelial function and flow reserve. Circulation 104:753, 2001.
66. Losordo DW, Vale PR, Hendel RC, et al: Phase 1/2 placebo-controlled, double-blind, dose-escalating trial of myocardial vascular endothelial growth factor 2 gene transfer by catheter delivery in patients with chronic myocardial ischemia. Circulation 105:2012, 2002.
67. Henry TD, Annex BH, McKendall GR, et al: The VIVA trial: Vascular endothelial growth factor in ischemia for vascular angiogenesis. Circulation 107:1359, 2003.
68. Simons M, Annex BH, Laham RJ, et al: Pharmacological treatment of coronary artery fibroblast growth factor-2: Double-blind, randomized, controlled clinical trial. Circulation 105:788, 2002.
69. Lederman RJ, Mendelsohn FO, Anderson RD, et al: TRAFFIC Investigators. Therapeutic angiogenesis with recombinant fibroblast growth factor-2 for intermittent claudication (the TRAFFIC study): A randomized trial. Lancet 359:2058, 2002.
70. Seiler C, Pohl T, Wustmann K, et al: Promotion of collateral growth by granulocyte-macrophage colony-stimulating factor in patients with coronary artery disease: A randomized, double-blind, placebo-controlled study. Circulation 104:2012, 2001.
71. Grines CL, Watkins MW, Helmer G, et al: Angiogenic Gene Therapy (AGENT) trial in patients with stable angina pectoris. Circulation 105:1291, 2002.
72. Hedman M, Hartikainen J, Syvanne M, et al: Safety and feasibility of catheter-based local intracoronary vascular endothelial growth factor gene transfer in the prevention of postangioplasty and in-stent restenosis and in the treatment of chronic myocardial ischemia: Phase II results of the Kuopio Angiogenesis Trial (KAT). Circulation 107:2677, 2003.
73. Stewart DJ, et al: A phase 2, randomized, multicenter, 26-week study to assess the efficacy and safety of BIOBYPASS (AdGVVEGF121) delivered through minimally invasive surgery versus maximum medical treatment in patients with severe angina, advanced coronary artery disease, and no options for revascularizations. Circulation 106:23, 2002.
74. Rajagopalan S, Mohler E 3rd, Lederman RJ, et al: Regional Angiogenesis with Vascular Endothelial Growth Factor Trial. Regional angiogenesis with vascular endothelial growth factor (VEGF) in peripheral arterial disease: Design of the RAVE trial. Am Heart J 145:1114, 2003.
75. Pislaru S, Janssens SP, Gersh BJ, Simari RD: Defining gene transfer before expecting gene therapy: Putting the horse before the cart. Circulation 106:631, 2002.

CHAPTER 8

General Principles of Genetic Factors in Cardiovascular Disease

Reed E. Pyeritz and Christine E. Seidman

GENETIC FACTORS IN DISEASE

Genes contribute to the cause and pathogenesis of virtually any abnormality of human physiology and behavior, including disorders of the heart and vascular system. This statement carries two messages in addition to the obvious one. First, disease associated with even the most "environmental" of causes, such as trauma, malnutrition, and drug abuse, depends on the human body's response to the insult. An individual's genotype defines to various but often poorly defined degrees the expression (phenotype) of the stress of the initial insult, and how the patient suffers and perhaps recovers. This concept is frequently overlooked. Some environmental insults, such as massive trauma or poisoning, are lethal to all, regardless of genotype. Nonetheless, as ongoing developments in fields such as pharmacogenetics and ecogenetics are defining genetic susceptibilities to human disease in better and simpler ways, physicians must become increasingly attuned to the importance of the genotype.[1]

Second, the introductory statement emphasizes that genetic factors have roles in both cause and process; causative factors and pathogenesis, although related, are conceptually distinct.[2] For example, a single mutant gene clearly causes sickle cell anemia, but whether a patient homozygous for this mutation expresses all, some, or none of the manifestations of the disease depends on many other genetic and nongenetic factors. Conversely, the cause of pneumococcal pneumonia is equally evident, but the severity and resolution of the disease depend on the patient's immune competence (which in turn depends on genetic and nongenetic factors) as much as on treatment with an antibiotic.

The genotype, therefore, can be detrimental in at least two distinct ways. First, mutant genes can so upset embryological and physiological processes that a clinical abnormality occurs. Whereas the phenotype of any particular mutation depends on a host of factors, including which homeostatic systems are available to modulate the action of the defect, the genotype has the principal role in causing the disease. This class of mutations is usually referred to as genetic diseases. Second, a mutation can facilitate the action of an extrinsic factor in producing disease. Inherited susceptibilities are part of the pathogenesis of disease and are one reason for taking a patient's family history. Until recently, clinicians could do little to pursue tantalizing findings, such as several relatives suffering myocardial infarction before the age of 50. The long-touted prospect of detecting a patient's inherited susceptibilities and intervening before irreversible clinical sequelae can occur is becoming reality.

Two caveats are important. There is a considerable gap between identifying an apparently inherited susceptibility and prescribing an intervention of proven benefit. For example, a parental history of sudden death identifies middle-aged men at increased risk of sudden death, independent of myocardial infarction.[3] However, effective clinical use of this association will require understanding the pathological factors and conducting outcome studies of potential interventions. Also, the risk of "genetic determinism" always remains. One study examined public perceptions of "a gene for heart disease"[4]; the concept was interpreted correctly by most of the sample, but an important minority thought in terms of an absolute risk that denoted inevitability.

Disorders Caused by Microscopic Alterations in Chromosomes (see Chap. 7)

The human genome contains about 35,000 genes. Two copies (termed *alleles*) of each gene are arrayed along 23 pairs of chromosomes. Twenty-two of the chromosomes are called autosomes (numbered 1 through 22), and the 23rd pair is the sex chromosomes, X and Y. Females have two X chromosomes and males have an X and a Y chromosome. Both autosomal alleles are potentially active in specifying RNA copies of their DNA sequences; whether a gene is active depends on the cell type, the developmental stage of the organism, and the regulatory molecules that interact with promoter and enhancer nucleotide sequences that control transcription of the gene. In cells with two X chromosomes (i.e., in all females, in persons with Klinefelter syndrome in which two Xs and one Y occur, and in persons with some other rare conditions), only one X is entirely active after early embryogenesis.

Human chromosomes can be examined by culturing cells capable of mitosis; T lymphocytes obtained from venous blood are the usual source, but fibroblasts, cells from chorionic villi, amniocytes, and leukocyte precursors present in bone marrow are also used clinically. Chromosomes are distinguished from one another by their size, shape (determined by the position of a constriction called the centromere, which functions as the attachment of the mitotic apparatus), and a characteristic banding pattern as revealed by any of several staining techniques. The chromosomes, from 1 through 22 and the sex chromosomes, are photographed, cut out, and arranged in pairs in a display called the karyotype. This display and its interpretation are the end results of a clinical study of a patient's chromosomes. The chromosome constitution of a cell is designated by first specifying the number of chromosomes present (46 being normal in diploid cells), then specifying the sex chromosomes, and finally describing any abnormalities. For example, a normal male is designated as 46,XY, and a female with an extra chromosome 21 is designated as 47,XX,+21.

ANEUPLOIDY. Chromosome aberrations, especially too many or too few chromosomes (aneuploidy), are extremely common in human embryos; more than half of all conceptuses are spontaneously aborted in early pregnancy, and at least half of them are aneuploid. Among live-born infants, about 0.5 percent have a chromosome aberration.

Gain or loss of chromosomes generally happens by nondisjunction, or the failure of a homologous pair of chromosomes to separate. Absence of one chromosome is termed *monosomy;* all autosomal monosomies are embryonic lethals, as is the presence of only a Y sex chromosome. The presence of three chromosomes is trisomy, and the presence of an entire extra set of chromosomes (for a total of 69) is triploidy. The most common autosomal aneuploidy, trisomy 21 associated with Down syndrome, and aneuploidy for sex chromosomes are compatible with survival into adulthood.

CHROMOSOME REARRANGEMENTS. A chromosome can break and rejoin within itself, potentially giving rise to an inversion of genetic material. Often, no apparent phenotypic effect occurs in people with an inversion, but because inversions can disrupt chromosome pairing during meiosis, their offspring may have more profound aberrations. Chromosomes can rearrange with each other, without apparent loss of material at the light microscopic level; these are called balanced rearrangements. However, 6 to 10 percent of people with an apparently balanced rearrangement have a clinical abnormality, suggesting that one gene, or perhaps two, was disrupted at the site of the translocation. In such situations, examining the chromosomes of the parents can shed light on the cause. If one parent has the same rearrangement but is phenotypically normal, then another cause of the offspring's disorder should be sought.

DELETIONS AND DUPLICATIONS. Just as their names imply, these aberrations are losses or gains of chromosomal material. Many clinical syndromes have been associated with aberrations of specific chromosome regions.[5] The smallest deletion detectable by light microscopy is associated with loss of considerable DNA, on the order of 1 million base pairs, so more than one gene is potentially disrupted or lost.

A number of conditions, each initially thought to be caused by a mutation in a single locus, are associated with small interstitial chromosome aberrations affecting a cluster of genes (Table 8-1). Rather than pleiotropic manifestations of one mutation, these conditions likely result from the effects of absences of several, and perhaps many, loci on one chromosome, and therefore are best thought of as genomic disorders. In the past, they were referred to as contiguous gene syndromes.[6] In the regions of the genome where these deletions occur, repetitive nucleotide sequences predispose to aberrant recombination, and this accounts for their surprising incidence.[7] In addition, such defects are potentially heritable, and the occurrence of the disorder in a family behaves as a mendelian dominant. Several interstitial deletions are relatively common and important causes of congenital heart disease. For example, deletion of the 22q11.2 region is the cause of the DiGeorge sequence, but also the cause of about half of all cases of interrupted aortic arch type B and of about 5 percent of cases of apparently isolated tetralogy of Fallot. The use of comparative genomic hybridization by means of molecular arrays has refined the search for deletions and duplications. The sensitivity outpaces the ability to associate genomic changes with phenotypes. As with chromosome rearrangements, if a molecular array abnormality is found in a patient, then the parents should be examined to determine whether the phenotype is linked.

Disorders Caused by Changes in Single Nuclear Genes

Mutations of genes located on the 22 pairs of autosomes and the two sex chromosomes produce phenotypes inherited according to the two principal tenets of Mendel—alleles segregate and nonalleles assort. The first principle refers to gametes receiving only one of the two alleles at a given locus as a result of meiosis. The second describes the results of recombination, the meiotic process of rearranging DNA between the two chromosomes of the pair (homologous chromosomes); if two loci are widely spaced along a chromosome, their chances of being separated by recombination are 50:50, and they are said to be unlinked.

The Human Genome Project, begun in 1990, had goals to map all expressed genes, create a physical map of overlapping pieces of DNA composing the entire genome, and sequence all 3.2 billion nucleotides in the haploid complement of human DNA. The project was completed well ahead of schedule, and about 99 percent of the entire sequence now exists in public databases.[8] More than 15,000 individual loci have been identified, either on the basis of the phenotype that mutations in single genes produce or through understanding the normal product or function of the gene.[9,10] The presumption of single-gene defects is based in most cases on the pattern of inheritance in families; segregation of the phenotype according to mendelian principles is the central piece of evidence. For an increasing number of loci, however, molecular genetic techniques have mapped the phenotype to a narrow chromosome region or to a single gene, or have even revealed the actual alteration in nucleotide sequence (see Chap. 7). The range of known mendelian variation in humans and information about gene mapping and molecular defects are routinely catalogued and updated and are available on-line.[11]

Of the many loci that have been clearly identified on the basis of an abnormal phenotype or a normal product, about 19 percent involve the heart and circulation.[11] Thousands of loci have been mapped to a specific region of the genome. Many of these loci, when mutated, cause mendelian disorders, and the genetic map of these loci represents the "morbid anatomy of the human genome." Knowledge of the molecular cause of the monogenic disorders, most of which are relatively rare, will undoubtedly lead to improved under-

TABLE 8–1 Genomic Disorders (Contiguous Gene Syndromes)

Syndrome	Acronym	Genetic Defect	Cardiovascular Abnormalities
With Cardiovascular Involvement			
Arteriohepatic dysplasia	AHD	del 20p11.23-p12.2	Peripheral pulmonic stenosis, hypoplasia
Cat-eye syndrome	CES	dup 22q11	Total anomalous pulmonary venous return
DiGeorge sequence	DGS	del 22q11	Truncus arteriosus, right aortic arch, TOF, PDA
Miller-Dieker syndrome	MDS	del 17p13	PDA, complex anomalies
Prader-Willi syndrome	PWS	del 15q12	Cor pulmonale (secondary to obesity and central apnea)
WAGR syndrome		del 11p13	Hypertension (secondary to Wilms tumor)
Without Frequent Cardiovascular Involvement			
Angelman syndrome	AS	del 15q12*	
Smith-Magenis syndrome	SMS	del 17p11.2	

*The deletion is often indistinguishable at the cytogenetic level from that of the Prader-Willi syndrome; genetic imprinting of locus *UBE3A* is thought to account in part for the phenotypic differences. In Prader-Willi syndrome, the deleted chromosome is always the chromosome 15 inherited from the father, whereas in Angelman syndrome, the deletion affects the maternal chromosome 15.

PDA = patent ductus arteriosus; TOF = tetralogy of Fallot; WAGR = ***W****ilms tumor,* ***a****niridia,* ***g****enitourinary, and* ***r****etardation.*

standing of the cause, pathogenesis, and treatment of more common conditions.[10,12]

Another product of the Human Genome Project is the identification and cataloguing of tens of thousands of single nucleotide polymorphisms (SNPs), nonpathological alterations in one nucleotide that occur in all humans at a prevalence of about 1 in 1100 nucleotides. Because many of these SNPs arose relatively recently in human evolution, those that are closely linked to one another will have the same genotype. Thus, identifying the genotype of one will specify many others in the region. This led to the HapMap (haplotype map) project, which has been completed.[8] Two types of genetic analyses can be performed using SNPs, linkage and association. Association analyses have been especially common in studies of common cardiovascular disease; however, most investigations of individual phenotypes, such as myocardial infarction, have produced conflicting results.[13] Improved precision will require larger numbers of subjects and careful attention to control populations, because the frequency and distribution of SNPs depend highly on ethnicity. Increasingly, studies of common conditions are melding large databases of medical history, genealogy, and genotypes based on SNPs.

Principles of Medical Genetics

Dominance and Recessiveness

The related concepts of dominance and recessiveness are characteristics of the phenotype, not of the gene. A phenotype is dominant when the patient is heterozygous for a mutation—when one copy of the mutant allele and one copy of the normal allele are present. This holds for genes on both autosomes and the X chromosome. A phenotype is recessive when the patient has two mutant alleles at the locus causing the condition. If the mutant alleles are identical, the patient is homozygous at that locus, a situation usually present when the allele is identical by descent through both parents (i.e., the parents had a common ancestor and are consanguineous) or when the mutant allele is common in the population (e.g., the most prevalent mutation for cystic fibrosis and the mutation for sickle cell anemia). Biochemical and molecular genetic assessment of mutant alleles has shown that most recessive phenotypes are caused by two distinct mutant alleles, a situation termed a *genetic compound,* indicative of the widespread heterogeneity in mutations at each locus. Males have only one X chromosome and each locus is therefore hemizygous; a mutant locus is always expressed in the phenotype of a male. Although virtually all X-linked traits are more severe in hemizygous males compared to heterozygous women, the vast majority of X-linked conditions are evident in females.

Whether a disorder is called dominant or recessive depends on how carefully the phenotype is assessed and how it is defined. For example, familial hypercholesterolemia is a relatively common hereditary disorder caused by defects in the receptor for low-density lipoprotein (LDL; see Chap. 42). The great majority of patients are heterozygous for a mutant allele at the *LDLR* locus on chromosome 19 and the disease is inherited as a mendelian dominant trait. However, if a man and a woman, each heterozygous for an LDLR mutation, produce a child, that child has a 25 percent risk of inheriting both mutant alleles and thereby is homozygous or has a genetic compound for mutations in *LDLR.* Such a child has a much more severe form of familial hypercholesterolemia that is inherited as a mendelian recessive trait. Similarly, homozygosity for the sickle hemoglobin mutation at the beta-globin locus on chromosome 11p15.5 produces the familiar autosomal recessive disease sickle cell anemia. However, heterozygosity for the same mutation rarely produces disease but rather sickling of erythrocytes when examined under conditions of low oxygen tension; this phenotype is transmitted as a dominant trait.

AUTOSOMAL RECESSIVE INHERITANCE. Almost all severe deficiencies of enzymatic activity—the classic inborn errors of metabolism first defined by Archibald Garrod in 1903—cause recessive phenotypes. Most homeostatic systems, which include all metabolic pathways, have sufficient flexibility to function well if one of the enzymatic steps functions at half-normal efficiency, as would occur in the case of heterozygosity for a mutant allele at a structural gene for an enzyme. However, homeostasis cannot cope if two mutant alleles cause a reduction in enzymatic activity to a few percent or less of normal activity. The characteristics of autosomal recessive inheritance, features common to such phenotypes, and a typical pedigree are shown in Figure 8-1.

AUTOSOMAL DOMINANT INHERITANCE. Only a few enzyme deficiencies, but many disorders of development and structure, are inherited as dominant traits. There are several reasons for this. One possibility is that developmental homeostasis has a limited repertoire of responses to stress and, when a structural or regulatory macromolecule is reduced to only half the normal amount, the system cannot cope. Another possibility, illustrated by mutations in procollagen molecules, pertains to gene products that must interact before becoming functional; an aberrant protein combined with a normal one would be a defective multimer, and the effect of being heterozygous for a mutation would be magnified, a dominant-negative effect.[2] The characteristics of autosomal dominant inheritance, features common to many such phenotypes, and a typical pedigree are shown in Figure 8-2.

Most human dominant traits are incomplete, because the heterozygote is less severely affected than the homozygote. Defects of *LDLR* are illustrative: the heterozygote has classic type IIa hyperlipidemia, whereas the homozygote has a quantitatively worse form of the same disease. It may well be that homozygosity for most alleles that cause dominant disorders is incompatible with life.

X-LINKED INHERITANCE. The characteristics of X-linked inheritance, features common to such phenotypes, and a typical pedigree are shown in Figure 8-3. Whereas virtually all diseases caused by mutations on the X chromosome are more severe in hemizygous males, women heterozygous for the same mutations often show some manifestations, albeit less severe and of later age of onset.

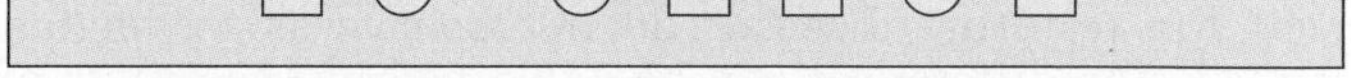

FIGURE 8–1 Characteristics of autosomal recessive inheritance: a single generation is affected; both genders are affected equally frequently; each parent is heterozygous (a carrier); each offspring of two carriers has a 25 percent chance of being affected, a 50 percent chance of being a carrier, and a 25 percent chance of inheriting neither mutant allele; two thirds of clinically normal offspring are carriers; the rarer the phenotype, the greater is the likelihood of consanguinity. Characteristics of autosomal recessive phenotypes: often caused by enzyme deficiencies; often more severe than dominant disorders; often early age of onset.

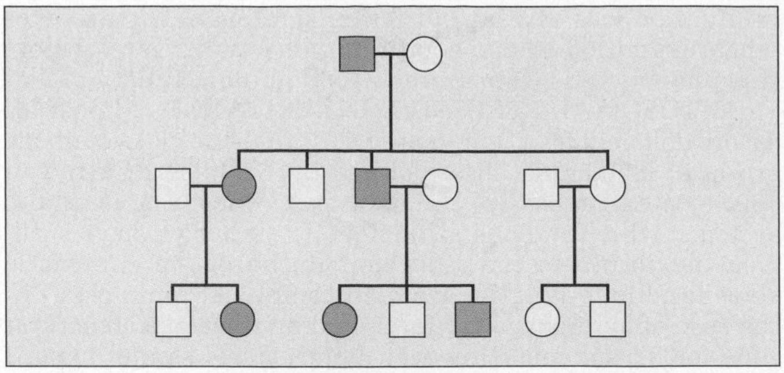

FIGURE 8–2 Characteristics of autosomal dominant inheritance: several generations are affected; both genders are affected equally frequently; in familial cases, only one parent need be affected; male-to-male transmission occurs; offspring of an affected parent has a 50 percent chance of being affected; the frequency of sporadic cases is higher, the more severe the condition; paternal age has an effect in sporadic cases. Characteristics of autosomal dominant phenotypes: often associated with malformations; often pleiotropic; usually variable; often age-dependent.

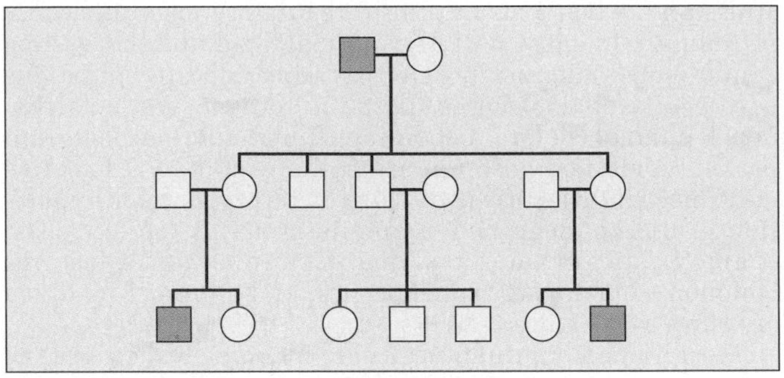

FIGURE 8–3 Characteristics of X-linked inheritance: no male-to-male transmission; all daughters of affected males are carriers; sons of a carrier mother have a 50 percent chance of being affected; daughters have a 50 percent chance of being carriers; some mothers of an affected male are not heterozygous in all cells of their body, but they may have more affected sons if germinal mosaicism is present. Characteristics of X-linked phenotypes: more severe in males; heterozygous females may be unaffected; variable, especially in females.

For example, most women carriers of alpha-galactosidase A deficiency (Fabry disease) eventually develop cerebrovascular disease or renal failure because of the accumulation of glycosphingolipids.[14]

MITOCHONDRIAL INHERITANCE. Energy generation through oxidative phosphorylation occurs in mitochondria in the cytoplasm of most cell types. Numerous mitochondria, each containing a single chromosome, exist in each cell. Some of the enzymes of oxidative phosphorylation are encoded by genes on the nuclear chromosomes and the proteins transported into the mitochondrion; the rest of the proteins are encoded by genes on the mitochondrial chromosome. Thus, genetic defects of oxidative phosphorylation can be caused by mutations of genes on the autosomes or the X chromosome, and the resulting diseases behave as mendelian recessive traits, or they can be caused by mutations of genes on the mitochondrial chromosome, in which case the resulting diseases do not behave as mendelian traits.[15] The differences can be explained by the events of conception. The spermatocyte contributes few, if any, mitochondria to the zygote, and the effective complement of mitochondria that will ever be present in the fetus is derived from the mitochondria already present in the cytoplasm of the oocyte. Thus, phenotypes caused by mutations of the mitochondrial chromosome show maternal inheritance (Fig. 8-4).

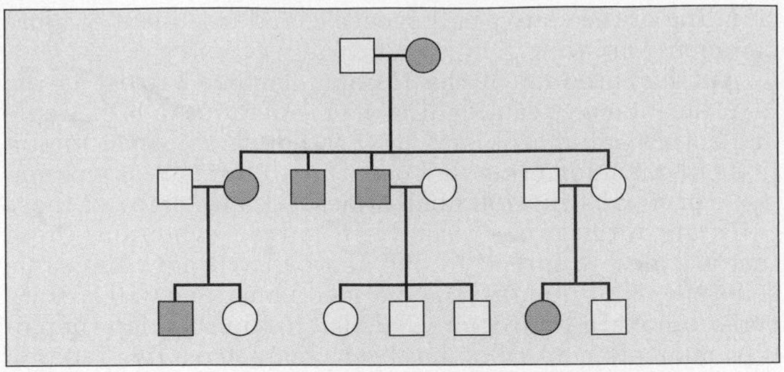

FIGURE 8–4 Characteristics of disorders caused by a mutation of the mitochondrial chromosome: both genders are equally frequently and severely affected; transmission is only through women; offspring of affected men are unaffected; all offspring of an affected woman may be affected; variability of expression can be extreme in a family, including apparent nonpenetrance; phenotypes may be age-dependent;

PLEIOTROPY. Most mutant alleles have effects on more than one organ system, and a mendelian phenotype frequently displays numerous, often diverse, manifestations. For example, Marfan syndrome is defined by abnormalities in the eye, skeleton, skin, dura mater, heart, and aorta and, until the recognition of a defect in extracellular microfibrils, the findings could not be linked by causative or pathogenetic factors.

VARIABILITY. The effects of the same mutant allele on phenotype can be different in people heterozygous (for dominant traits), homozygous (for autosomal recessive traits), or hemizygous (for X-linked traits) for the allele. Variability can be described in terms of the frequency of a particular pleiotropic manifestation in patients with the mutation, the severity of the phenotype, and the age of onset of manifestations. If a person has the mutant allele(s) but shows no phenotypic effect, the trait is called nonpenetrant. To an important degree, whether a clinical phenotype is called nonpenetrant depends on the sensitivity of the techniques used for detection. For example, two decades ago, based on bedside examination, cardiovascular abnormalities were thought to affect about 50 percent of people with Marfan syndrome; echocardiography now reveals aortic dilation in more than 90 percent. The term *incomplete penetrance* should not be used with reference to individuals but rather to indicate that prevalence of the phenotype is less than 100 percent in people known to carry the mutation. The Holt-Oram syndrome (see Chap. 61) is an instructive example. In this autosomal dominant syndrome of reduction anomalies of the upper limb and congenital heart defect, patients in the same family may have only arm anomalies, only a heart defect, or both. Moreover, the severity of the reduction defect varies widely, from a proximally placed thumb to almost total absence of the arm. The cardiac feature is incompletely penetrant because only about 50 percent of patients have it, but in any individual with the Holt-Oram allele, the heart is either structurally normal or not.

Numerous genetic and environmental factors can affect expression of a gene (Table 8-2), and it is often impossible to determine which factors are most important in a specific patient or particular disease. However, the pervasiveness of variable expression emphasizes that phenotypes determined by single genes are to some extent really multifactorial.

GENETIC HETEROGENEITY. Similar or even identical phenotypes can be caused by fundamentally distinct mutations, a phenomenon termed *genetic heterogeneity*. For example, Marfan syndrome and homocystinuria were long thought to be the same disorder, despite what now appear in retrospect to be obvious differences in inheritance pattern and intelligence.[16] As in the case of these two disorders, the

TABLE 8–2 Causes of Variability of Gene Expression
Genetic background
Age dependence
Sex influence
Sex limitation
Modifying loci—hypostasis and epistasis
Gene alteration
Somatic mutation
Somatic amplification
Transpositions and rearrangements
Mutations
Physiological rearrangements
Variation in X inactivation*
Endogenous complementation*
Maternal factors
Effects of mitochondrial genome
Intrauterine environment
Imprinting
Exogenous and ecological factors
Ecological factors—temperature, diet
Teratogens
Medical intervention
Chance

*Pertains to female heterozygotes for X-linked disorders.

causes may lie in two different genes whose products are functionally distinct. Osteogenesis imperfecta exemplifies a disorder in which mutations in two genes, alpha$_1$(I) and alpha$_2$(I) procollagen, can each produce the same phenotype because the two proteins interact to form type I collagen.[17] Genetic heterogeneity is pervasive at the intragenic level of analysis; except for sickle cell anemia, hemochromatosis, and achondroplasia, virtually all single-gene disorders are caused by a wide variety of mutations at a given locus.

Nonpathological Variation in the Cardiovascular System

CARDIAC STRUCTURE AND PHYSIOLOGY. The genome dictates all aspects of the ontogeny of the cardiovascular system. If, as seems most credible, few genes have a large effect and many have small contributions, any specific aspect of "normal" cardiovascular phenotype—size, shape, function—exhibits multifactorial inheritance. In other words, to the extent that any given phenotype can be quantified, it shows a normal distribution within the population, and near-relatives resemble each other more than distant relatives or the rest of the population. The twin method should demonstrate a higher concordance of the trait in monozygotic than dizygotic twins. However, surprisingly, few phenotypes have been examined.

Preliminary data on left ventricular dimensions measured echocardiographically have shown higher correlations between parent and child than between matched control subjects, suggesting a genetic contribution; however, as in many such studies, the effect of shared environment was not estimated. In an attempt to minimize environmental contributions, left ventricular sizes of twins who were not exercise-trained were compared; the mean intrapair differences in echocardiographic dimensions were less in the monozygotic than in the dizygotic twins and nontwin siblings. The caliber and branch geometry of coronary arteries show familial resemblance, and both parameters are much more similar in monozygotic twins than in other relatives.[18] Further support for the importance of genetic factors in normal development derives from studies that have demonstrated ethnic differences in structure. For example, the thickness of the intima and media of coronary arteries of children who died of noncardiovascular causes varied significantly with the ethnicity of the child.

Measures of cardiac electrophysiology have shown familial resemblance. Studies of both nuclear families and twins have suggested a genetic contribution to resting heart rate, conduction times, and repolarization time.[19] Polymorphic variation in the beta$_1$-adrenergic receptor is associated with resting heart rate.[20,21] Genetic control of normal cardiovascular function has been especially difficult to study because of the multitude of environmental (e.g., training, diet), stochastic (e.g., age), and clinical (e.g., subtle, unrecognized pathological condition) issues that confound comparisons of relatives and control subjects. The investigation of genetic factors that influence the capacity for physical conditioning is in its early stages. However, this area is sure to see considerable interest, especially as it relates to elite athletic performance.[20,22]

VASCULAR SYSTEM. All members of certain inbred animal strains show little variation in arterial anatomy, especially branch angles, and considerable variation with other strains of the same species. Except for the studies of coronary arterial anatomy already noted, similar studies of humans have not been reported.

One intriguing question of clinical importance is whether certain individuals are predisposed to arterial spasm and whether this susceptibility has a genetic basis. An examination of hereditary pathological and polymorphic variation in factors elaborated by endothelial cells, platelets, and leukocytes to maintain patency of blood vessels, such as prostacyclin, endothelium-derived relaxing factor (nitric oxide), or endothelin-1, may prove enlightening.[23,24] Similarly, is there a genetic contribution to arterial stiffness or its variation with age and conditioning?[25-27]

DISORDERS OF THE VASCULATURE

Some genetic conditions affect primarily arteries (and some of those primarily involve the aorta), whereas others affect veins and others lymphatics. Some involve the development of several types of vessels and their interconnections.

Disorders Primarily Affecting Arteries

Heritable Disorders of Connective Tissue

The two broad classes of connective tissue disorders are those caused by mutations in single genes that determine or somehow affect components of the extracellular matrix, and those caused by extrinsic factors affecting the extracellular matrix, such as rheumatoid arthritis and systemic lupus erythematosus. The former category includes many disorders that affect the cardiovascular system. Susceptibility to so-called acquired disorders of connective tissue is, in part, determined by genes (see Chap. 84).

MENDELIAN DISORDERS OF THE EXTRACELLULAR MATRIX

Almost 200 distinct phenotypes now make up this category, which was first defined about five decades ago with fewer

TABLE 8–3 Cardiovascular Manifestations of Heritable Disorders of Connective Tissue

Disorder	OMIM No.*	Cardiovascular Manifestations
Cutis laxa	219100, 123700	PS, PPS, CP MVP
Ehlers-Danlos syndrome		
Classic form	130000, 130010	MVP, occasional aortic root dilation
Hypermobile form	130020	MVP
Vascular form	130050	Arterial rupture, MVP, occasionally aortic dissection and arterial aneurysms, easy bruising
Ocular-scoliotic form	225400	MVP
Tenascin-X deficiency†	606408	MVP, easy bruising
Osteogenesis imperfecta		
I	166200	MVP, mild aortic root dilation
II	166210	CP, arterial calcification
III	259420	MVP
IV	166220	Aortic root dilation
Marfan syndrome	154700	MVP, aortic root dilation, aortic dissection
MASS phenotype	157700	MVP, mild aortic root dilation
Pseudoxanthoma elasticum	177850	Arteriolar sclerosis, claudication, myocardial infarction, endocardial fibroelastosis

CP = cor pulmonale; MASS = ***m***itral valve, ***a***orta, ***s***kin, and ***s***keletal abnormalities; MVP = mitral valve prolapse; OMIM = Online Mendelian Inheritance in Man; PPS = peripheral pulmonic stenosis; PS = valvular pulmonic stenosis.

*Data from Online Mendelian Inheritance in Man (http://www.ncbi.nlm.nih.gov/omim).

†Schalkwijk J, Zweers MC, Steijlen PM, et al: A recessive form of the Ehlers-Danlos syndrome caused by tenascin-X deficiency. N Engl J Med 345:1167, 2001.

than 10 disorders. Several reviews and textbooks have described the phenotypes, genetics, and causes of many of the conditions (Table 8-3).[25,26,28]

Several of these disorders cause arteriopathies of various types. Williams syndrome, which is a genomic disorder caused by deletion of genes at 7q11.23, including the one encoding tropoelastin, *ELN,* is covered elsewhere (see Chap. 61). Autosomal dominant supravalvular aortic stenosis, which has the same arteriopathy as Williams syndrome, is caused by mutations affecting only *ELN.* In some connective tissue disorders, the vascular problems seem to be caused by a weakening of the vessel wall, such as the arterial fragility seen in the vascular form of Ehlers-Danlos syndrome caused by mutations in the type III procollagen gene, *COL3A1.* The same sort of pathogenesis is probably true for the occasional aortic aneurysms and valve prolapse seen in the classic form of Ehlers-Danlos syndrome and osteogenesis imperfecta. However, the cardiovascular problems seen in Marfan syndrome, caused by mutations in the extracellular matrix glycoprotein, fibrillin-1, are not caused by "weak" connective tissue. Rather, most of the phenotypic features result from abnormal regulation of transforming growth factor-beta (TGF-β), which is ordinarily kept in check by binding to fibrillin.[29] Other mendelian arteriopathies have recently been shown to be caused by defects in TGF-β receptors.[30]

MARFAN SYNDROME

This autosomal dominant disorder is relatively frequent (2 to 3 per 10,000) and occurs in all races and ethnic groups.[25,26] Even with the discovery of the genetic and biochemical bases of the condition, the diagnosis of Marfan syndrome outside families with the classic phenotype remains largely clinical. Current criteria (Table 8-4) depend on the manifestations in the cardinal organ systems—eye, skeleton, heart, and aorta—and other systems, as well as the family history (Fig. 8-5).[31] The presence of manifestations more specific for Marfan syndrome, such as aortic dilation, aortic dissection in a nonhypertensive young person, ectopia lentis, and dural ectasia, clearly is more important diagnostically than features common in other connective tissue disorders and in the general population, such as scoliosis, joint hypermobility, myopia, and mitral valve prolapse (MVP).

TABLE 8–4 Diagnostic Criteria for Marfan Syndrome

Organ System	Phenotypic Manifestations*
Skeleton	Joint hypermobility, tall stature, pectus excavatum, reduced thoracic kyphosis, scoliosis, arachnodactyly, dolichostenomelia, pectus carinatum, erosion of the lumbosacral vertebrae from dural ectasia[d]
Eye	Myopia, retinal detachment, elongated globe, precocious cataracts, ectopia lentis[d]
Cardiovascular	Mitral valve prolapse, endocarditis, dysrhythmia, dilated mitral annulus, mitral regurgitation, tricuspid valve prolapse, aortic regurgitation, aortic dissection,[d] dilation of the aortic root[d]
Pulmonary	Apical blebs, spontaneous pneumothorax
Skin and integument	Inguinal hernias, incisional hernias, striae atrophicae
Central nervous system	Attention-deficit/hyperactivity disorder, verbal performance discrepancy, dural ectasia,[d] anterior pelvic meningocele[d]

*Manifestations are listed within each organ system in increasing specificity for Marfan syndrome, although none is completely specific; those indicated by superscript d are the most specific and constitute major criteria.

The most common cardiovascular features are MVP and dilation of the sinuses of Valsalva. Associated clinical problems of mitral regurgitation, aortic regurgitation, and aortic dissection, if untreated, account for most of the early mortality that results in an average age of death in the fourth and fifth decades of life.[32] Children tend to be more severely affected by mitral valve disease, whereas aortic problems are progressive and more likely in adolescence and beyond.

MITRAL VALVE INVOLVEMENT. MVP (see Chap. 62) is age-dependent and more common in women with Marfan syndrome. The incidence reaches 60 to 80 percent, and the valve leaflets generally have an elongated and redundant appearance. Progression of severity, as judged by the appearance or worsening of mitral regurgitation by clinical and echocardiographic criteria, occurs in at least 25 percent of patients, a much higher rate than in MVP found in the general population. The mitral annulus dilates and contributes to the regurgitation, as do stretching and occasional rupture of chordae. About 10 percent of patients with marked prolapse have calcification of the mitral annulus. Standard treatment for chronic mitral regurgitation is indicated, but coexistent aortic root dilation usually requires that increasing inotropy be avoided. When mitral regurgitation becomes severe enough to warrant surgical intervention, two considerations must be added to the balance:

1. Repair of the mitral apparatus is often successful and durable in patients with Marfan syndrome.[33] Repair is less easily accomplished when the cusps are extremely redundant, there is marked chordal damage, or the annulus is heavily calcified
2. The aorta may be enlarged enough to permit concomitant repair. With Marfan syndrome, as with virtually all of the heritable disorders of connective tissue, there is an increased susceptibility to dehiscence of prosthetic mitral valves, regardless of the care taken in placing them.

AORTIC ROOT INVOLVEMENT (see Chap. 56). The sinuses of Valsalva are often dilated at birth, and the rate of progression varies widely among patients in general and also among relatives (Fig. 8-6). Thus, predicting long-term risks of developing aortic regurgitation (which clearly associates positively with aortic root diameter), suffering aortic dissection (which is less clearly associated with diameter), or requiring aortic surgery is fraught with uncertainty.[34] Transthoracic echocardiography is sufficient for detecting and monitoring changes in diameter because, in the absence of dissection, dilation is limited to the proximal ascending aorta, and the rate of change is slow, measured in millimeters per year. Rare exceptions of primary dilation of the thoracic aorta can be monitored with transesophageal echocardiography or magnetic resonance imaging. Patients with dilation less than 1.5 times the mean diameter predicted for their body size can be observed annually; as the diameter increases, more frequent evaluation is necessary. Aortic regurgitation often appears in adults when the diameter is 50 mm. The risk of dissection increases with the size of the aorta and fortunately occurs infrequently below a diameter of 50 mm in the adult.

Many physicians have adopted the criterion of a 50-mm maximal aortic root dimension for performing elective surgery in adult patients with Marfan syndrome, even with minimal aortic regurgitation, although patients with a family history of aortic dissection should have surgery at smaller diameters.[32] The perioperative results of both elective and emergency repair of the aortic root have been excellent and a marked improvement from the precomposite graft era that ended in the mid-1970s. Long-term results of operation are limited by the problems of endocarditis and anticoagulation common to all prosthetic valves, but in the absence of chronic aortic dissection appear favorable for patients with Marfan syndrome.[35]

Several approaches to repairing the dilated or dissected aortic root while preserving the native aortic valve have been developed.[36] Findings at both short-term and now long-term follow-up of patients with Marfan syndrome who have undergone repair with the reimplantation technique have been favorable, and are superior to repair with the remodeling technique.[37,38] The operation must be performed before the root is widely dilated and the valve commissures and cusps markedly stretched or the cusps fenestrated. This approach is increasingly being taken in all patients when the maximal root dimension reaches 45 to 50 mm, and it is an

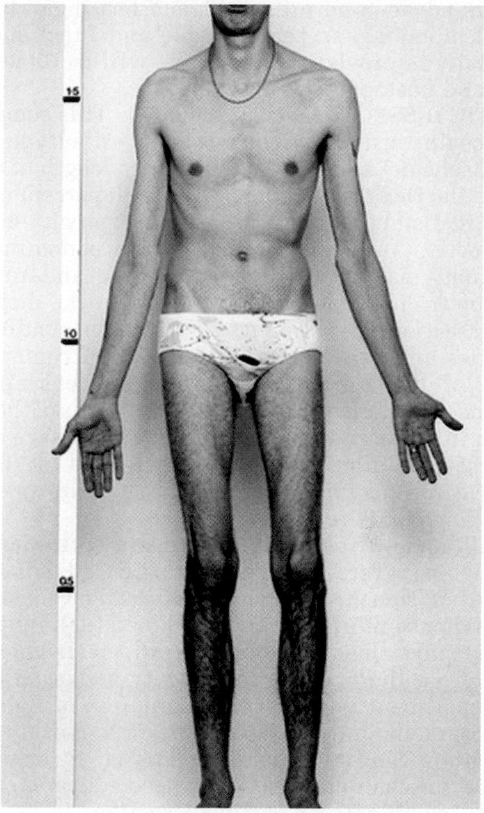

FIGURE 8–5 External phenotype of patients with Marfan syndrome, showing long extremities and digits, tall stature, and pectus carinatum. *(Used with permission from Mediscan, Medical-On-Line-Ltd, London.)*

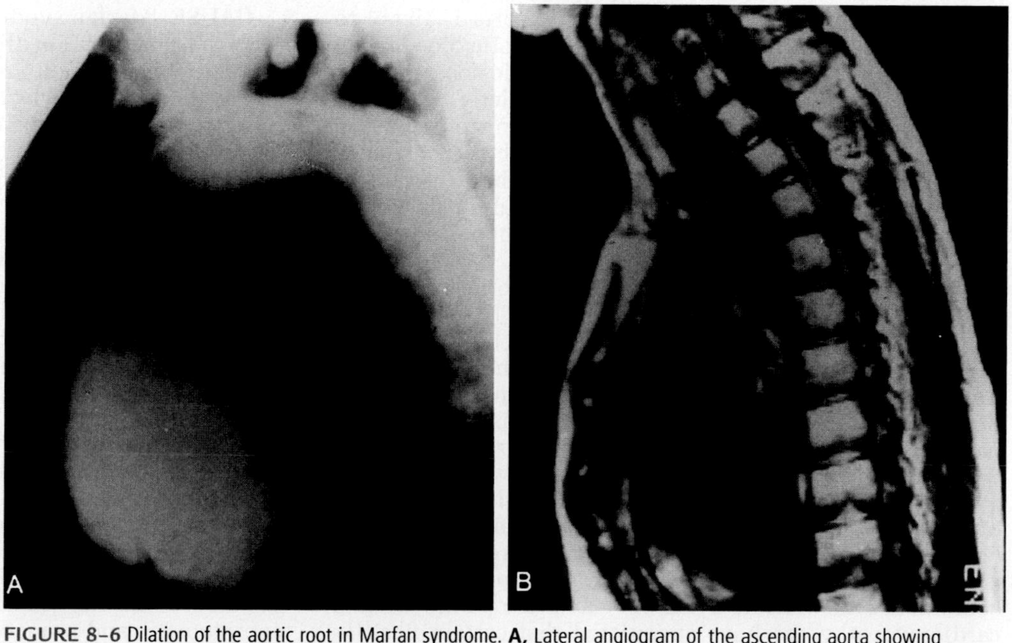

FIGURE 8–6 Dilation of the aortic root in Marfan syndrome. **A,** Lateral angiogram of the ascending aorta showing dilation of the sinuses of Valsalva and proximal ascending aorta and relatively normal caliber of the ascending aorta. **B,** Lateral magnetic resonance imaging scan of the same patient.

especially suitable procedure for women of childbearing age who want to consider pregnancy, as well as for all others in whom anticoagulation is contraindicated.

THORACIC ABNORMALITIES. Severe pectus excavatum can complicate cardiovascular surgery by hampering exposure of the heart by median sternotomy. For elective cardiovascular surgery, repair of the sternal deformity some months in advance permits sufficient healing of the costochondral junctions, so that a stable and functionally and cosmetically improved thoracic cage will facilitate further surgery and postoperative recovery.

AORTIC DISSECTION (see Chap. 56). This complication usually begins just above the coronary ostia (type A in the Stanford scheme) and extends the entire length of the aorta (type I in the DeBakey scheme). About 10 percent of dissections begin distal to the left subclavian artery (type B or III), but dissection rarely is limited to the abdominal aorta. Angiography, magnetic resonance imaging, and transesophageal echocardiography all have a role in the diagnosis of acute dissection in patients with Marfan syndrome; the capabilities and experience of the medical center and the stability of the patient are important determinants of the approach. Because many acute dissections of the ascending aorta in patients with Marfan syndrome have a stuttering course that culminates in death caused by rupture or hemopericardium, rapid transfer to a facility prepared to perform immediate repair is essential.

Not all acute dissections in patients with Marfan syndrome involve severe, tearing chest pain that radiates to the back; indeed, some extensive dissections have been occult. This experience reinforces the need for a high index of suspicion by physicians whenever a tall, nearsighted young person with a thoracic cage deformity arrives at an emergency department with vague complaints of lightheadedness, chest or abdominal discomfort, or a murmur of aortic regurgitation. Similarly, patients known to have Marfan syndrome and their close relatives need education about the signs and symptoms of aortic dissection. In general, the management of acute and chronic dissection in patients with Marfan syndrome follows standard practice, with several departures. First, all dissections of the ascending aorta should be repaired promptly. Second, regular evaluation with magnetic resonance imaging is important, because the diameter of any region of dissected aorta is likely to expand over time. Third, reduction of systolic blood pressure and administration of negative inotropic doses of beta-adrenergic blockers should be even more strictly adhered to than in dissections without a genetic connective tissue abnormality. In most cases, any region of the aorta should be repaired when complications of further dissection, branch vessel occlusion, or dilation beyond about 50 mm occur. A staged approach to total replacement of the Marfan aorta is now both feasible and successful.

DYSRHYTHMIAS. Some patients develop serious ventricular or supraventricular dysrhythmia.[39] The latter often accompanies chronic mitral regurgitation, but the former usually accompanies MVP, may be of high grade, and is difficult to suppress. The syndrome of autonomic dysfunction, atypical chest pain, and palpitations is seen in some patients with MVP unassociated with a flagrant connective tissue abnormality.

VENTRICULAR FUNCTION. Occasional patients with Marfan syndrome who have no clinically important valvular abnormalities develop moderate to severe left ventricular dysfunction. Although this could represent the unlikely coincidence of Marfan syndrome and idiopathic dilated cardiomyopathy, we have speculated that certain fibrillin mutations, directly or indirectly through TGF-β, could reduce myocardial function.[25,26] Evidence for and against this hypothesis has been found.[40,41] Further study is warranted.

MANAGEMENT (see Chap. 56). Routine cardiological management of Marfan syndrome is multifaceted: regular clinical and echocardiographic examinations, routine endocarditis prophylaxis for dental and other procedures; restriction of activity from heavy weight lifting, contact sports, and any exertion at maximal capacity; and long-term beta-adrenergic blocking agent therapy form the basic approach, with individual variation often appropriate. Support for the role of beta-adrenergic antagonists comes from several prospective studies that have shown a reduction in the rate of aortic dilation and the risk of aortic dissection in patients treated with negative inotropic doses of propranolol or atenolol.[42] Short-term administration of propranolol to patients with large sinus of Valsalva aneurysms, although reducing heart rate and peak systolic pressure, did not improve the impedance characteristics recorded in the ascending aorta. However, given studies that emphasize the importance of central pulse pressure to aortic dilation,[43] use of beta-adrenergic blocking agents seems warranted. In a mouse model of Marfan syndrome, the angiotensin receptor type 1 blocker losartan prevented the development of aortic wall abnormality when treatment was begun at birth and reversed the pathological findings, including dilation, when begun after 2 months of age.[44] A clinical trial in children and adolescents with substantial aortic root dilatation is underway.[45]

A woman with Marfan syndrome has two concerns about pregnancy. The first is the 50:50 risk that any child will inherit the condition; prenatal diagnosis can be attempted in certain cases. The second is the risk of dissection that the hemodynamic stresses of pregnancy place on the aorta. Several dozen case reports have attested to the heightened incidence of dissection during the third trimester, parturition, and the first months postpartum. However, serious aortic dilation was present in most cases. Prospective evaluation of 21 women through 45 pregnancies confirmed our earlier recommendation that the cardiovascular risks are relatively low if the aortic diameter does not exceed 40 mm and cardiac function is not compromised, a view shared by other investigators.[46] Obstetrical and fetal complications are increased in women with Marfan syndrome.[47]

CAUSE. Marfan syndrome is caused by mutations in the gene that encodes fibrillin-1 (*FBN1*), the major constituent of microfibrils, which are components of the extracellular matrix that are widely dispersed and perform numerous functions.[25,26] Microfibrils and tropoelastin form elastic fibers. Fragmentation and disorganization of elastic fibers in the aortic media have long been a histological marker (inappropriately called "cystic medial necrosis") of Marfan syndrome, although similar microscopic pathological lesions occur in familial aortic aneurysms and aging aortas in the normal population. Defects in microfibrils result in abnormal sequestration of the latent TGF-β–binding complex and increased TGF-β activity; this explains nearly all the pleiotropic manifestations of Marfan syndrome.[29,44,48,49]

Hundreds of distinct mutations in *FBN1* occur in different families, and only a few have emerged, by chance, in unrelated patients.[50] Because *FBN1* is such a large gene (approximately 9000 nucleotides in the mRNA, dispersed in 65 exons over 240 kb of chromosome 15q21.1), finding a mutation is still not simple or inexpensive.[51,52] Once the mutation is identified, diagnosis in that family is straightforward. In families with several living and cooperative affected members, linkage analysis can be used for presymptomatic and prenatal diagnosis. The use of molecular testing is confounded, however, by the discovery that autosomal dominant ectopia lentis, familial tall stature, MASS phenotype (denoting *m*itral valve, *a*orta, *s*kin, and *s*keletal abnormalities), and familial aortic aneurysm all are phenotypes caused by mutations in *FBN1* and are exactly the conditions clinicians are interested in excluding in their patients of questionable diagnosis.[25,26]

MITRAL VALVE PROLAPSE (see Chap. 62)

This trait is of heterogeneous cause and pathogenesis, although it has been called the most common abnormality of human heart valves. MVP is, equally clearly, not always an abnormality.[33,53] The heritable forms of MVP can be classified into three groups. The first is a familial form with minimal extracardiac involvement. The second is clinically variable, an autosomal dominant condition that merges at one end of its spectrum with Marfan syndrome; it could just as well be discussed as a heritable disorder of connective tissue. The third category is composed of the various mendelian syndromes that include MVP as a pleiotropic manifestation. In all these categories, prolapse of the tricuspid valve is a frequent accompaniment.

The first category, which some have called MVP syndrome or familial MVP, includes a condition centered on the mitral valve. The development of actual prolapse shows the age- and gender-dependent behavior characteristic of the idiopathic form. Formal genetic studies in most families have confirmed autosomal dominance with variable expression. This category has been partitioned into those patients with billowing of the mitral leaflets and those with excessive systolic mitral annular expansion; because this phenotype breeds relatively true, two distinct autosomal dominant forms may exist. The cause(s) of these entities is unknown. Moreover, when and how the phenotype of this condition can be distinguished from the sporadic cases of MVP and the cases with obvious evidence of a systemic disorder of connective tissue are unclear. The only consistent extracardiac manifestations are excessive arm span in women and relatively low body weight and systolic pressure. MVP has been mapped to three genetic loci; one of the genes has been identified to encode filamin A *(FMNA)*. The other two are autosomal loci, 11p15.4 and 16p11.2-p12.1.[54,55] Susceptibility to myxomatous degeneration of all cardiac valves can be inherited as an X-linked trait that maps to Xq28; the defect is in the gene encoding *FMNA*.[56]

Many clinical geneticists and cardiologists see patients referred with a suspicion of Marfan syndrome or Ehlers-Danlos syndrome. Some of these patients do not meet minimal diagnostic criteria for a recognized connective tissue disorder[31] but clearly have extracardiac features consistent with a defect of the extracellular matrix described later. MVP is commonly but not always present; when it is present and when evidence of a systemic abnormality of connective tissue is lacking, the patient should be considered to have *primary MVP*. The clinical spectrum of the patients with syndromic MVP includes abnormal striae atrophicae, excessive arm span and leg length, joint hypermobility, pectus excavatum, scoliosis, reduction in thoracic kyphosis ("straight back"), myopia, and mild aortic root dilation.[57] Aortic dilation beyond 3 SD above the mean for body surface area, aortic dissection, ectopia lentis, or a family history of any of these three features *removes* a patient from this category. For the remainder of patients, the MASS phenotype describes what certainly is a heterogeneous grouping of patients and families. The aorta is mentioned specifically because of the appropriate concern that progressive dilation and dissection will occur; in fact, neither has been the case, although prospective evaluation has been unsystematic. Many of the associations between MVP and deformity of the thoracic cage and spontaneous pneumothorax are explained by the MASS phenotype.

Finally, MVP frequently accompanies Marfan syndrome, several of the Ehlers-Danlos syndromes, and cutis laxa and occurs more often than expected in patients with osteogenesis imperfecta, Larsen syndrome, pseudoxanthoma elasticum, and other mendelian syndromes. In addition, occasional families with otherwise unclassified heritable disorders of connective tissue have prominent involvement of the mitral apparatus, with myxomatous deterioration, calcification, or both.

DISORDERS OF TRANSFORMING GROWTH FACTOR–BETA RECEPTORS

Several patients and families with some features of Marfan syndrome, but not meeting strict criteria for that diagnosis, were found to have mutations in the gene encoding TGF-β receptor-1 (*TGFBR1*).[58] Subsequently, families with only autosomal dominant aortic aneurysm have also been associated with mutations in this gene.[59] Loeys and colleagues found mutations in both *TGFBR1* and *TGFBR2* in patients with various phenotypes, including some who had been diagnosed as having incomplete Marfan syndrome for many years.[60] At the most severe end of the phenotypic spectrum are patients who have craniosynostosis, widely spaced eyes (hypertelorism), bifid uvula or cleft palate, club foot, arachnodactyly, dural ectasia, patent ductus arteriosus, dilation of the ascending aorta, tortuosity of the aorta, and a strong susceptibility to aortic dissection, even with minimal dilation. These patients do not develop ectopia lentis and are not tall. Molecular testing is important to confirm the diagnosis and to identify relatives who have inherited a mutation. Prophylactic aortic root repair is effective and should be considered at even smaller aortic root dimensions than in Marfan syndrome (i.e., less than 45 mm in the adult).[61] Neither the effectiveness of beta-adrenergic blockade nor angiotensin receptor blockade has been tested.

EHLERS-DANLOS SYNDROME

Ehlers-Danlos syndrome is a group of heterogeneous conditions linked by variable involvement of the skin and the joints, with hyperelasticity and fragility of the former occurring with hypermobility of the latter (Fig. 8-7).[62] Mitral valve prolapse is clearly increased in frequency in most clinical types, but the occurrence of aortic root dilation is controversial. One study found that 25 to 30 percent of patients with the classic and hypermobile forms of Ehlers-Danlos syndrome had mild dilation of the aortic root,[63] a finding counter to results of a previous survey.[64]

The most serious cardiovascular problems occur in patients with the vascular form of Ehlers-Danlos syndrome with spontaneous rupture of large- and medium-caliber arteries.[65] Various defects of type III collagen caused the phenotype in virtually all patients studied.[66] Analysis of collagen production by cultured skin fibroblasts should be used to confirm the diagnosis.[28] True aneurysms form infrequently; rather, a rupture without dissection usually occurs as a catastrophic event. Most prone are the abdominal aorta and its branches, the great vessels of the aortic arch, and the large arteries of the limbs. False aneurysms and fistulas may be one result in those patients who do not die of the initial rupture. Vascular surgery is difficult, because the normal-appearing vessels around the rent fail to hold sutures. As a consequence, elective surgery to repair vascular anomalies, such as false aneurysms, that are causing no immediate problem is contraindicated in most cases. The vascular form of Ehlers-Danlos syndrome is often sporadic but, when familial, is usually autosomal dominant.[67] Prenatal diagnosis is possible by examining collagen production in amniocytes. However, pregnancy is particularly hazardous to women with this condition because of vascular rupture, although some mutations may not be as dangerous.[65,68]

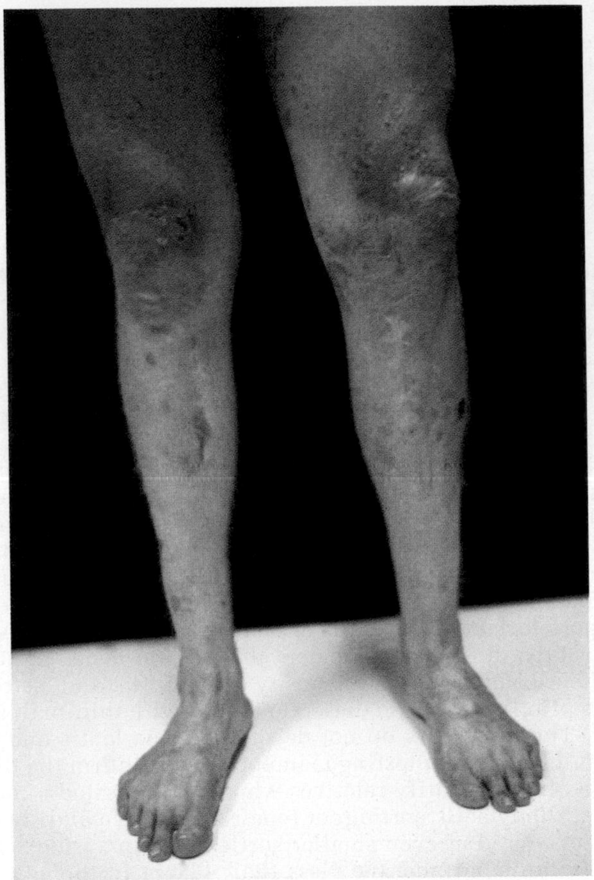

FIGURE 8–7 Legs of a patient with Ehlers-Danlos syndrome type IV who died of rupture of the subclavian artery. Note the mild joint hypermobility and the striking dermal abnormalities—elastosis perforans serpiginosa and thin, atrophic scars over areas of recurrent trauma.

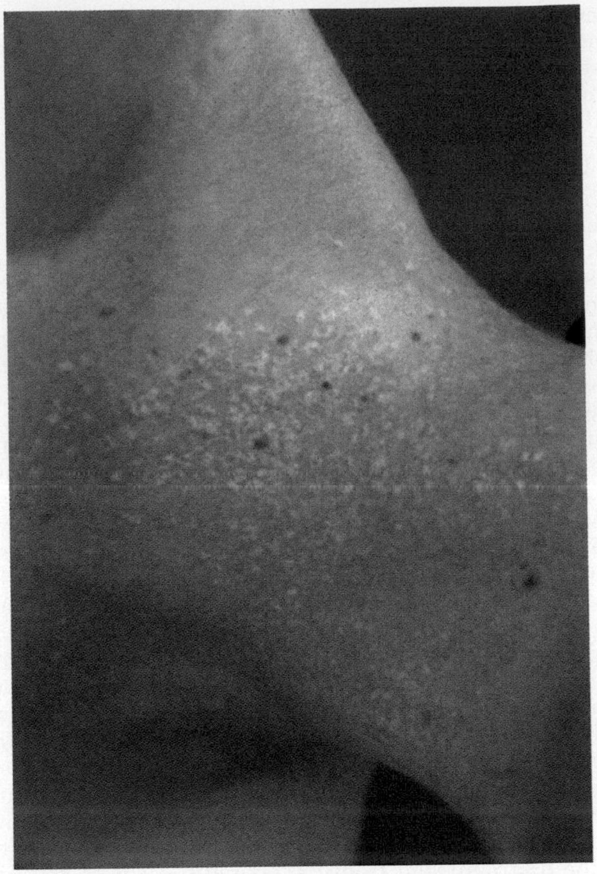

FIGURE 8–8 Skin of a young man with pseudoxanthoma elasticum. The neck is a typical location to notice the raised, yellowish papules from which the name of the condition derives.

PSEUDOXANTHOMA ELASTICUM

Pseudoxanthoma elasticum (PXE) is a clinically variable and genetically heterogeneous disorder caused by mutations in the gene *ABCC6,* which encodes a membrane protein of unclear function. Histopathological examination of affected tissues shows fragmentation and calcification of elastic fibers. The skin, eyes, gastrointestinal system, and cardiovascular system are the organs most severely affected.[69] The skin shows highly characteristic raised yellowish papules (pseudoxanthoma) overlying areas of flexural stress, such as the neck, cubital and popliteal fossae, and groin (Fig. 8-8). Breaks in the elastic lamella, Bruch membrane of the choroid, produce the funduscopic finding of angioid streaks. Gastrointestinal hemorrhage is common and potentially fatal; mucosal arterioles bleed, and because the calcified elastic fibers prevent effective vessel retraction, hemostasis is difficult. Selective arterial embolization was life-saving in one case. The heart is affected in a number of ways. Endocardial fibroelastosis is common, but because primarily the atria are involved, a restrictive cardiomyopathy is uncommon. One patient with marked endocardial fibroelastosis was helped by resection of calcified elastic bands within the left ventricle. Mitral valve prolapse may be increased in frequency but is rarely a clinical problem. Coronary artery disease with myocardial ischemia and infarction is a common cause of early death.

Elastic and muscular arteries, including the coronaries, develop a type of arteriosclerosis similar to Mönckeberg; progressive luminal narrowing occurs and can produce complete occlusion. This is initially most evident at the radial and ulnar arteries, where absence of pulses and a positive Allen test result are noted early in the course. Interestingly, carotid-femoral pulse wave velocity was not increased in patients with PXE, and radial artery stiffness was reduced in female patients.[70] Narrowing progresses slowly, so collateral arteries form, and peripheral ischemia is a late complication. Because the arterial stenoses tend to be diffuse, bypassing them often involves extensive surgery. Hypertension and all risk factors for atherosclerosis should be aggressively controlled.

OTHER RELATED DISORDERS

ADULT POLYCYSTIC KIDNEY DISEASE. Adult polycystic kidney disease (APKD) is a relatively common autosomal dominant disease that affects 0.5 million people and accounts for 8 to 10 percent of all long-term hemodialysis in the United States. Development of renal cysts is age-dependent, and presymptomatic detection of heterozygotes, even by ultrasonography, can be uncertain into adulthood. About half of patients are hypertensive, half have hepatic cysts, half eventually develop severe renal failure, and an unknown (but probably high) fraction have colonic diverticula. Elevated plasma renin levels contribute to hypertension long before renal failure occurs. The cardiovascular manifestations include MVP in 25 percent of cases, mild dilation of the aortic root, occasional thoracic and abdominal aneurysms, and a predisposition to regurgitation of the aortic, mitral, and tricuspid valves. The association of diverticula, organ cysts, and cardiovascular lesions reminiscent of, but milder than, that in Marfan syndrome suggests some involvement of the extracellular matrix.

The most serious vascular problem is typical berry aneurysms of the cerebral circulation that occur in about 10 percent of heterozygotes but may remain asymptomatic throughout life. Hypertension predisposes to subarachnoid hemorrhage. How to screen for and treat intracranial aneurysms in patients without neurological symptoms remain controversial. Cerebral angiography carries higher risks in patients with APKD because of dissection and heightened vascular reactivity. Magnetic resonance imaging detects most saccular aneurysms down to 2 to 3 mm in diameter. Whether to attempt prophylactic repair when a small aneurysm is detected has not been investigated systematically. Without question, aggressive blood pressure control is indicated in any patient with APKD.

At least three genes cause APKD. The greatest portion of cases is caused by mutations in a gene called *PBP* at the *PKD1* locus (16p13.3).[71] In most of the remaining families, the disease maps to *PKD2* in the region 4q23-q23. Families affected by mutations in *PKD2* tend to develop renal failure later and have a milder course.[72] In both *PKD1* and *PKD2* cases, the multiorgan cysts develop when a somatic mutation occurs in the normal allele at the respective mutant locus, analogous to the two-hit model familiar with tumorigenesis.[73] A French Canadian family was found to have disease typical of *PKD1* unlinked to either locus, indicating that a *PKD3* gene exists. Patients with mutations in *PKD1* and *PKD2* show marked intrafamilial variability. Discovering some of the factors that affect this variability could suggest novel approaches to modifying disease progression.[74]

ARTERIOHEPATIC DYSPLASIA. An autosomal dominant disorder of marked variability, Alagille syndrome causes neonatal jaundice caused by aplasia of intrahepatic bile ducts and congestive heart failure in the most severely affected infants, but may be asymptomatic in heterozygous relatives.[75] Cardiovascular findings include peripheral pulmonic and systemic arterial stenoses in most patients, occasionally associated with septal defects or patent ductus arteriosus.[76-78] A diffuse vasculopathy is present in some patients.[79] Renal disease can produce hypertension. The locus was initially mapped by studying chromosomes and finding in some patients that part or all of band 20p12 was missing (an interstitial deletion). Mutations in the gene that encodes the Notch receptor ligand Jagged 1 (*JAG1*), which mapped to this exact region, were then identified as the cause for most cases. Subsequently, mutations in *NOTCH2* were also identified in some families.[78]

FAMILIAL ARTERIAL ANEURYSM, ECTASIA, OR DISSECTION. Pedigrees abound in which dilation of the aortic root, aneurysm of the abdominal aorta, aortic dissection without dilation, or a combination of these problems occurs in an autosomal dominant pattern without evidence of a recognized heritable disorder of connective tissue.[80,81] Because of the variable presentation and natural history of the aortic disease, presymptomatic detection of presumed heterozygotes is uncertain, as is reassurance of relatives at risk who are of childbearing age and would prefer not to pass this condition to offspring.

The association of dissection of the ascending aorta with bicuspid aortic valve and aortic coarctation is well known, although the cause and pathogenesis remain unclear, except in rare families. In congenital bicuspid aortic valve, the proximal aortic wall shows abnormalities of elastic fibers and microfibrils.[82,83] A person with a congenital bicuspid aortic valve or aortic coarctation should be screened for dilation of the aortic root, and first-degree relatives should be screened for both lesions. This recommendation is based, in part, on the bicuspid aortic valve being a congenital heart defect of the left-sided flow category, with a relatively high recurrence risk in siblings and offspring. In several families, autosomal dominant inheritance of bicuspid aortic valve has been associated with mutations in *NOTCH1*.[84]

In two families with autosomal dominant transmission of arterial aneurysms and mildly increased skin fragility and bruisability, different mutations in the gene encoding type III procollagen occurred. Thus, depending on the mutation, deficiency of type III collagen can cause the vascular form of Ehlers-Danlos syndrome or a form of the much subtler but just as deadly syndrome, familial arterial rupture. For those families in which the mutations have been defined, reliable presymptomatic and prenatal diagnoses are available. However, suggestions that mutations in type III collagen would account for most aortic aneurysms, including abdominal aneurysms in the elderly, have proved unfounded.

Families with aneurysm, dissection, or both of the thoracic aorta have been studied extensively and the phenotypes have been linked to five loci: 3p25-p24.2, 5q13-q14, 9q33-q34, 11q23.3-q24, and 6p13.13-p13.12.[17,59,85-87] Mutations in the *TGFBR2* gene are responsible for disease in families linked to the 3p locus, whereas in one patient a mutation in *TGFBR1* (9q33-q34) was found.[88] Mutations in the myosin heavy chain 11 gene (*MYH11*) on 16p cause ascending aortic dissection associated with patent ductus arteriosus.[89] A predisposition to cervical arterial dissection in young people was found to be associated with diffuse lentiginosis in several families, with a suggestion of autosomal recessive inheritance. An association is also noted between cervical dissection and intracranial hemorrhage, which is increased when congenital cardiovascular defects are present, especially bicuspid aortic valve or aortic coarctation.

Formal genetic analysis of 91 families ascertained through a proband with abdominal aortic aneurysm has suggested that an autosomal recessive predisposition exists for late-onset aneurysms. This study and others[90] have provided a rationale for offering ultrasonographic screening to close relatives of patients with abdominal aortic dilation.

FAMILIAL ARTERIAL TORTUOSITY. This autosomal recessive condition is typically diagnosed in infants who have stroke-like episodes and are found to have very tortuous extracerebral and intracerebral arteries and peripheral pulmonic stenoses.[91,92] However, this disorder is not only found in young children.[93,94] Recently, a number of adults were diagnosed with marked tortuosity of various elastic and muscular arteries, often with minimal symptoms. The basic defect is a gene, *GLUT10*, that encodes a nuclear membrane glucose transporter.[30] The pathogenesis is proposed to be disordered regulation of extracellular matrix proteins that regulate expression of TGF-β. Thus, this syndrome bears some relationship to those associated with mutations in the TGF-β receptor genes.

FAMILIAL INTRACRANIAL HEMORRHAGE. Several genetic syndromes, including adult polycystic kidney disease, predispose to subarachnoid or cerebral hemorrhage. The cerebral arterial type of familial amyloidosis (type VI) is an autosomal dominant condition caused by a defect in the proteinase inhibitor cystatin O. This disease is rare outside Iceland and Holland. The walls of cerebral arteries are thickened by a material resembling amyloid, and the vessels become tortuous and fragile. Recurrent cerebral hemorrhage is common in the fifth and sixth decades of life.

Berry aneurysms without pleiotropic manifestations in other organs can occur as an autosomal dominant trait. Five loci have been mapped, but no gene has been identified.[95] How aggressively close relatives should be screened for intracranial aneurysms remains controversial because of the relatively low risk of hemorrhage compared with the morbidity and mortality of current surgical techniques for repairing defects.[96-98] A defect in type III collagen has been suggested by linkage analysis, but sequence analysis of the gene in 55 unrelated patients found no mutations. Familial hemangiomas have been reported infrequently to occur as an autosomal dominant condition. The brain and retina are the principal sites of vascular malformation, although cutaneous lesions occur in some pedigrees. The intracranial hemangioma can be large and the patient can present with varied neurological symptoms, including hemorrhage. A more benign familial disorder of primarily isolated cutaneous hemangiomas also exists.[99]

FAMILIAL ARTERIAL OCCLUSIVE DISEASES.[100] Fibromuscular dysplasia of the renal and other arteries occurs in neurofibromatosis type I and, along with pheochromocytoma, can be a cause of hypertension. Severe deficiency of alpha$_1$-antiprotease is another cause of fibromuscular dysplasia. The arterial lesion can occur by itself in families and produce stroke, myocardial infarction, intermittent claudication, and hypertension as early as childhood. Inheritance is most consistent with autosomal dominance.

Familial hypoplasia of the carotid arteries, familial arteriopathy caused by concentric thickening of systemic and pulmonic arteries, familial moyamoya disease (which has been mapped to 3p24.2-p26),[101] and generalized arterial calcification of infancy are rare, possibly mendelian, syndromes of unknown cause.

Cerebral autosomal dominant arteriopathy with subcortical infarcts and leukoencephalopathy (CADASIL) is caused by mutations in the *NOTCH3* gene.[102] Characteristic inclusions occur in vascular smooth muscle cells, and the deep, perforating cerebral arterioles develop occlusions that produce insidious onset of symptoms and transient ischemic attacks.

FAMILIAL HEMIPLEGIC MIGRAINE. Migraine complex is commonly familial. A severe form, associated with recurrent hemiplegia, is inherited as an autosomal dominant trait and is caused by mutations in a sodium channel gene.[103] However, some families with hemiplegic migraine and others with simple migraine are unlinked to this locus. In the same region of 19p is a locus causing autosomal dominant cerebral arteriopathy with subcortical infarcts. Whether the two conditions are related through allelism is unclear.

FAMILIAL PULMONARY HYPERTENSION (see Chap. 73). Primary pulmonary hypertension (PPH) is occasionally familial.[104] Inheritance is most consistent with an autosomal dominant predisposition, with a gender influence favoring expression in females.[105,106] Mutations in the *BMPR2* gene at 2q33 cause the disease in many families.[107] Mutations in *ALK1* can cause both hereditary hemorrhagic telangiectasia (see later) and PPH.[104] Pulmonary hypertension can occur in patients with neurofibromatosis caused by pulmonary fibrosis or as a primary vasculopathy.

GENETIC FACTORS PREDISPOSING TO ATHEROSCLEROSIS (see Chaps. 39 and 42)

Several issues impede investigations into the genetics of atherosclerosis. The first is the nature of the phenotype; the pathology in the artery is silent for years until a clinical event occurs. The age-dependency is caused by many factors, some of which are undoubtedly obscure at this time. Certainly, variable expression of genes of large and small effect and gene-environment interactions play a major role. People now tend to have small families and are having children later in life, which result in relatively few potential subjects in many families. Relying on historical information, especially death certificates, can be especially misleading. Many people who die suddenly without autopsy are said to have a heart attack when the cause of death may have been a dissection, ruptured abdominal aneurysm, or primary dysrhythmia. In studies that require unaffected controls, determining who is really unaffected presents challenges, because substantial atherosclerosis can be present, even when a coronary angiogram appears normal. Thus, studying atherosclerosis per se in humans is difficult. As a result, experimental animals, in which arteries can be examined pathologically at various stages, have proven useful. Imaging techniques that provide resolution sufficient to identify disease of human arteries in vivo hold considerable promise, but have not been widely applied. In addition, clinical surrogates of atherosclerosis pose a number of problems. Coronary artery disease (CAD) as manifest by angina or myocardial infarction, peripheral arterial disease as manifest by claudication, and cerebral vascular disease as manifest by transient ischemic attacks or stroke share frustrating features in that they are age-dependent, occasionally caused by conditions other than atherosclerosis, and often do not correlate with each other in the same individual or family. Furthermore, the event recorded in the medical record or death certificate, such as heart attack or stroke, is usually the result of some acute event that is unrelated to the pathogenesis of the chronic condition, atherosclerosis, such as plaque rupture and thrombosis.

Over more than 50 years, the full range of genetic techniques has been applied to the study of atherosclerosis. These approaches include twin and adoption studies,[108] segregation analyses in pedigrees, linkage analyses, association investigations involving candidate genes and whole genome marker sets in families or unrelated patient groups and controls[109,110] and, more recently, profiling of gene expression in pathological specimens.[111] A brief overview of the field is presented here; more complete reviews are available.[112]

Large investigations of CAD in populations, such as the Framingham study, have identified robust epidemiological risk factors (see Chap. 39). Most of them have important genetic determinants. In fact, the discovery of molecular defects in the LDL receptor, which cause familial hypercholesterolemia, has supported a reductionist model of the cause of atherosclerosis—find the genes of large effect that cause dysregulation of lipid metabolism, blood pressure, and glucose and most of the familial risk would be explained. However, although there are many mutations in many genes that predispose to atherosclerosis, most are rare and as a whole account for little of the overall genetic contribution. Some of these genes and their clinical implications are described in the chapters dealing with hypertension and lipids (see Chaps. 40 and 42). Thus, atherosclerosis and its clinical sequelae must be viewed as "complex disorders," meaning that multiple genes, each of small effect, interact with environmental factors to predispose to the pathology and disease.

One epidemiological risk factor for CAD that persists even when all others are considered is a positive family history of early angina and myocardial infarction, independent of all the other risk factors that clearly have genetic predispositions, such as hypercholesterolemia, hypertension, and diabetes mellitus. The definition of early varies considerably among studies, but typically means first occurrence at an age younger than 50 years for men and younger than 55 years for women. To determine which genes influence this independent risk, many linkage and association studies have been performed over the past decade. In some cases, candidate genes have been examined, with the choice of gene based on some real or potential role in the pathogenesis of atherosclerosis (e.g., mediators of inflammation) or the precipitant of the clinical phenotype (e.g., mediators of thrombosis). Most of the reported studies were underpowered in regard to detecting convincing relationships. Others have not been replicated in different ethnic groups. Some of the more enduring relationships are shown in Table 8-5.

Disorders Primarily Affecting Veins

VARICOSE VEINS. Although a familial susceptibility to varicosities of the lower extremities clearly exists and favors women in a ratio of 2:1, mendelian inheritance has not been confirmed. Marfan syndrome, various Ehlers-Danlos syndromes, and an autosomal recessive condition featuring distichiasis (a double row of eyelashes) predispose to varicose veins.

ATRETIC VEINS. Some patients with the Klippel-Trénaunay syndrome of cutaneous hemangioma and hemihypertrophy have atresia of the deep venous system. The concomitant superficial varicosities should not be stripped, lest the remaining venous drainage of the lower extremity be removed. This is a confusing syndrome that overlaps with several others; mendelian inheritance is uncertain.[113] Renal arterial aneurysm and hemangioma occurred in one patient.

CEREBRAL CAVERNOUS ANGIOMAS. Cavernous angiomas represent at least 15 percent of vascular malformations of the central nervous system, and familial occurrence is common. These are not arteriovenous malformations but primarily a tortuous collection of veins. Seizure is the most common presenting feature, followed by headache, stroke, and progressive neurological deficit. Magnetic resonance imaging (T2-weighted) is the procedure of choice because it is sensitive; arteriography is not likely to detect the venous malformation. In some families, hepatic angiomas are an important feature. Three genetic loci have been mapped to 7q, 7p, and 3q. Mutations in *KRIT1*, a gene on 7q of unclear function, account for about half of cases.[114-116] Many patients who are heterozygous for a *KRIT1* mutation are asymptomatic, even into the sixth decade; however, very few have no evidence of an angioma on magnetic resonance imaging.[48]

TABLE 8–5 Examples of Candidate Genes, Biomarkers, and Loci Linked to or Associated with Atherosclerotic Vascular Disease

Phenotype	Gene Symbol	OMIM No.*	Gene Map Locus
Disorders of Blood Pressure			
Hypertension, essential	*SAH*	145505	16p13.11
Hypertension, essential	*PNMT*	171190	17q21-q22
Hypertension, essential	*AGTR1*	106165	3q21-q25
Hypertension, essential	*GNB3*	139130	12p13
Hypertension, essential	*AGT*	106150	1q42-q43
Disorders of Coagulation and Thrombosis			
Dysfibrinogenemia, α type	*FGA*	134820	4q28
Factor VII level	*F7*	227500	13q34
Glycoprotein IIIa	*ITGB3*	173470	17q221.32
Plasminogen activator inhibitor deficiency	*PAI1*	173360	7q21.3-q22
Disorders of Lipid Metabolism			
Apolipoprotein A-I and apolipoprotein C-III deficiency	*APOA1*	107680	11q23
Apolipoprotein A-II deficiency	*APOA2*	107670	1q21-q23
Apolipoprotein B-100 ligand defect	*APOB*	107730	2p24
Cerebrotendinous xanthomatosis	*CYP27A1*	213700	2q33-qter
Combined familial hyperlipidemia	*LPL*	238600	8p22
3-Hydroxy-3-methylglutaryl coenzyme A synthetase-2 deficiency	*HMGCS2*	600234	1p13-p12
Hypercholesterolemia, familial	*LDLR*	143890	19p13.2-p13.1
Hypercholesterolemia, familial 3	*FH3*	603776	1p34.1-p32
Hypertriglyceridemia	*APOC3*	107720	11q23
Hypertriglyceridemia	*APOA1*	107680	11q23
Hypoalphalipoproteinemia	*APOA1*	107680	11q23
Hypobetalipoproteinemia	*APOB*	107730	2p24
Sitosterolemia	*STSL*	210250	2p21
Tangier disease	*HDLDT1*	205400	9q31
Metabolic Disorders with Secondary Effects in the Cardiovascular System			
Cerebral amyloid angiopathy	*CST3*	105150	20p11.2
Cerebrovascular disease, occlusive	*AACT*	107280	14q32.1
Coronary spasm, susceptibility to	*NOS3*	163729	7q36
Fabry disease	*GLA*	301500	Xq22
Homocystinuria	*CBS*	236200	21q22.3
Homocystinuria, MTHFR deficiency	*MTHFR*	236250	1p36.3
Mucopolysaccharidosis II	*IDS*	309900	Xq28
Progeria	*LMNA*	150330; 176670	1q21.1
Pseudoxanthoma elasticum	*PXE*	264800	16p13.1
Primary Disorders of Vasculature			
Fibromuscular dysplasia of arteries	*COL3A1*	120180	2q31
Components of (or Act on) the Vascular Wall			
Angiotensin-converting enzyme	*ACE*	106180	17q23
Endothelial nitric oxide synthase	*NOS3*	163729	7q36
MEF2A	*MEF2A*	600660	15q26
Phosphodiesterase 4D	*PDE4D*	600129	5q12
Mediators of Inflammation			
C-reactive protein	*CRP*	123260	1q21-q23
FLAP	*ALOX5AP*	603700	13q12
Intercellular adhesion molecule 1	*ICAM1*	147840	19p13.3-p13.2
Interleukin-6	*IL6*	147620	7p21
Membrane cofactor protein 1	*CCL*	158105	17q11.2-q12
P-selectin	*SELP*	173610	1q23-q25

FLAP = five-lipoxygenase–activating protein; MTHFR = methylenetetrahydrofolate reductase.

Disorders may have been mapped by the phenotype, gene, or both. The annotations p and q refer to band patterns in chromosomes detected cytochemically that mark specific regions.

*Refers to the entry for the locus in Online Mendelian Inheritance in Man (OMIM) (www.ncbi.nlm.nih.gov/omim).

Disorders Primarily Affecting Lymphatics

HEREDITARY LYMPHEDEMA. Several forms exist,[25,117] with the best studied inherited as autosomal dominant conditions. An early-onset form is called Nonne-Milroy lymphedema and can cause a protein-losing enteropathy and pleural effusion. A form called Meige lymphedema does not appear until about the time of puberty and is most severe in the legs, although one family with late-onset edema had involvement of the arms and face. Considerable intrafamilial variability in age of onset is noted, however, and whether two or more distinct conditions exist remains unclear. Mutations in one of the receptors for vascular endothelial growth factor, VEGFR3, have been found in some families.[118,119] Lymphedema associated with distichiasis is caused by mutations in *FOXC2,* which encodes a transcription factor, and hypotrichosis-lymphedema-telangiectasia syndrome is caused by mutations in another transcription factor gene, *SOX18.*[120]

Disorders Primarily Affecting Angiogenesis

HEREDITARY HEMORRHAGIC TELANGIECTASIA. Hereditary hemorrhagic telangiectasia (HHT),[121] an autosomal dominant condition previously called Osler-Rendu-Weber disease, is more common than is appreciated, in the range of 2 to 3 per 10,000. Because of marked intrafamilial and interfamilial variability, the condition can remain undiagnosed in affected patients for years, despite mild manifestations.[122,123] Mucocutaneous telangiectases, 0.5 to 3 mm in diameter, usually occur on the tongue, lips, trunk, and fingertips. Small and moderate-sized arteriovenous fistulas occur in the nose, leading to recurrent epistaxis; in the gastrointestinal system, where they cause recurrent bleeding and occult anemia; and in the lungs, resulting in hypoxemia, hemoptysis, polycythemia, clubbing, paradoxical embolization through the right-to-left shunt, and a hyperdynamic circulation. Less common sites of vascular malformations are the brain,[124] liver, and kidneys. Diffuse ectasia of the coronary arteries was noted in one patient, and hemorrhagic pericarditis with tamponade in another.[125]

Patients with HHT and their close relatives should be screened for pulmonary arteriovenous malformations (PAVMs) with contrast echocardiography.[126] Appearance of "bubbles" in the left atrium after 4 to 10 cardiac cycles is virtually pathognomonic of a shunt in the lung. A positive contrast echocardiogram should be followed by high-resolution computed tomographic angiography to document the number, size, and location of PAVMs. Therapeutic coil occlusion of any malformation with a feeding artery 1 mm or larger should be attempted to reverse hypoxemia and to prevent systemic embolization, especially to the brain.[127] In a few patients, epistaxis and gastrointestinal blood loss have been reduced by antifibrinolytic therapy with danazol or aminocaproic acid.[128] Controlled trials of various approaches to chronic management, taking into account clinical and genetic variables, are sorely needed. Cerebrovascular malformations in HHT occur in fewer than 25 percent of cases, are typically present by childhood, and usually do not progress in size. Thus, screening with magnetic resonance imaging should be performed as soon as the diagnosis of HHT is suspected and need not be repeated if neither malformations nor abscesses (caused by paradoxical embolization of septic clots) are detected and no new neurological symptoms or signs emerge. Vascular malformations of the spinal cord can occur but are infrequent.

At least six genes are capable of causing HHT; five have been mapped and three have been identified. The latter three involve the TGF-β and bone morphogenetic protein (BMP) signaling pathway. One locus, *ENG,* encodes a TGF-β–binding protein called endoglin, and various mutations segregate with HHT in different families. Another locus, *ALK1,* encodes an activin receptor-like kinase, which is a member of the serine-threonine kinase receptor family, expressed in endothelial cells. This suggests that defects in this gene might affect development or repair of vessels.[129] Hundreds of mutation in *ENG* and *ALK1* have been discovered in HHT, but occur in only about 65 to 75 percent of patients.[130] Patients with autosomal dominant juvenile polyposis of the gastrointestinal tract, caused by mutations in *SMAD4,* may show many features of HHT.[131] Thus, any person with juvenile polyps should be screened for manifestations of HHT. A fourth locus for HHT has been mapped to the short arm of chromosome 7, but the gene has not been identified.[132] It is likely that other uncommon loci remain to be discovered. However, by mutation detection or linkage analysis, presymptomatic and prenatal diagnoses are available to a large number of patients with a potentially life-threatening disorder.

The most common mendelian causes of arteriovenous malformations are the various forms of HHT. However, isolated arteriovenous malformations, especially of the brain, are relatively common findings,[133] and other genetic susceptibilities exist, such as the Parkes Weber syndrome.[113]

VON HIPPEL-LINDAU SYNDROME. The features of this autosomal dominant condition involve malformations and abnormal growth of small blood vessels. Retinal angioma, hemangioblastoma of the cerebellum, and hemangioma of the spinal cord occur in association with renal cell carcinoma, pancreatic and epididymal cystadenomas, and pheochromocytoma. Secondary hypertension caused by renal disease and pheochromocytoma, which is often bilateral, occurs and predisposes to subarachnoid hemorrhage. The cause is a tumor suppressor gene, *VHL,* at 3p26-p25. Patients inherit a germline mutation (and there is great diversity among families in the actual mutations) that is present in all cells. When a somatic mutation in the normal allele occurs in a susceptible cell, such as in the renal parenchyma or adrenal medulla, the cell becomes functionally homozygous for a lack of the gene product, and the cascade toward neoplasia is initiated.[134] How this gene product stimulates or permits angiomatous malformations is unclear.

REFERENCES

General

1. Childs B: Genetic Medicine: A Logic of Disease. Baltimore, Johns Hopkins University Press, 1999.
2. Murphy EA, Pyeritz RE: Pathogenetics. *In* Rimoin DL, Connor JM, Pyeritz RE, Korf BR (eds): Principles and Practice of Medical Genetics, 5th ed. Philadelphia, Churchill Livingstone, 2007, pp 319-332.
3. Jouven X, Desnos M, Guerot C, et al: Predicting sudden death in the population: The Paris Prospective Study I. Circulation 99:1978, 1999.
4. Bates BR, Templeton A, Achter PJ, et al: What does "a gene for heart disease" mean? A focus group study of public understandings of genetic risk factors. Am J Med Genet A 119:156, 2003.
5. Pai GS, Lewandowski RC Jr, Borgaonkar D: Handbook of Chromosomal Syndromes. New York, John Wiley & Sons, 2002.
6. Shaffer LG LD, Lupski JR: Molecular cytogenetics of contiguous gene syndromes: Mechanisms and consequences of gene dosage imbalance. *In* Scriver CR Beaudet AL, Sly WA, Valle D (eds): The Metabolic and Molecular Bases of Inherited Disease. New York, McGraw-Hill, 2001, pp 1291-326.
7. Bayes M, Magano LF, Rivera N, et al: Mutational mechanisms of Williams-Beuren syndrome deletions. Am J Hum Genet 73:1311, 2003.
8. Lander ES, Linton LM, Birren B, et al: Initial sequencing and analysis of the human genome. Nature 409:860, 2001.
9. Collins FS, Morgan M, Patrinos A: The Human Genome Project: Lessons from large-scale biology. Science 300:286, 2003.
10. Collins FS: 2005 William Allan Award address. No longer just looking under the lamppost. Am J Hum Genet 79:421, 2006.
11. Online Mendelian Inheritance in Man (http://www.ncbi.nlm.nih.gov/entrez/query. fcgi?db = OMIM).
12. Epstein JA, Rader DJ, Parmacek MS: Perspective: cardiovascular disease in the postgenomic era—lessons learned and challenges ahead. Endocrinology143:2045-50, 2002.
13. Hirschhorn JN, Lohmueller K, Byrne E, et al: A comprehensive review of genetic association studies. Genet Med 4:45, 2002.
14. Deegan PB, Baehner AF, Barba Romero MA, et al: Natural history of Fabry disease in females in the Fabry Outcome Survey. J Med Genet 43:347, 2006.
15. Wallace DC: Mitochondrial genetics. *In* Rimoin DL, Connor JM, Pyeritz RE, Korf BR (eds): Principles and Practice of Medical Genetics. 5th ed. Philadelphia, Churchill Livingstone, 2007, pp 194-298.
16. Pyeritz RE: Homocystinuria. *In* Beighton P (ed): McKusick's Heritable Disorders of Connective Tissue. 5th ed. St. Louis, CV Mosby, 1993, pp 137-178.
17. Guo D, Hasham S, Kuang SQ, et al: Familial thoracic aortic aneurysms and dissections: genetic heterogeneity with a major locus mapping to 5q13-14. Circulation 103:2461, 2001.
18. Herrington DM, Pearson TA: Clinical and angiographic similarities in twins with coronary artery disease. Am J Cardiol 59:366, 1987.
19. Friedlander Y, Lapidos T, Sinnreich R, et al: Genetic and environmental sources of QT interval variability in Israeli families: The kibbutz settlements family study. Clin Genet 56:200, 1999.
20. Macarthur DG, North KN: Genes and human elite athletic performance. Hum Genet 116:331, 2005.
21. Wilk JB, Myers RH, Pankow JS, et al: Adrenergic receptor polymorphisms associated with resting heart rate: The HyperGEN Study. Ann Hum Genet 70:566, 2006.
22. Brutsaert TD, Parra EJ: What makes a champion? Explaining variation in human athletic performance. Respir Physiol Neurobiol 151:109, 2006.
23. Rudic RD, Sessa WC: Nitric oxide in endothelial dysfunction and vascular remodeling: Clinical correlates and experimental links. Am J Hum Genet 64:673, 1999.
24. Wang XL, Mahaney MC, Sim AS, et al: Genetic contribution of the endothelial constitutive nitric oxide synthase gene to plasma nitric oxide levels. Arterioscler Thromb Vasc Biol 17:3147, 1997.

Marfan and Related Disorders

25. Ferrell RE, Pyeritz RE: Hereditary Disorders of the Lymphatic and Venous Systems. 5th ed. Philadelphia, Churchill Livingstone, 2007, pp 1214-1226.
26. Pyeritz RE: Marfan syndrome and related disorders. *In* Rimoin DL, Connor JM, Pyeritz RE, Korf BR (eds): Principles and Practice of Medical Genetics. 5th ed. Philadelphia, Churchill Livingstone, 2007, pp 3579-3624.
27. Rogers WJ, Hu YL, Coast D, et al: Age-associated changes in regional aortic pulse wave velocity. J Am Coll Cardiol 38:1123, 2001.

28. Byers PH: Disorders of collagen biosynthesis and structure. *In* Scriver CR, Beaudet AL, Sly WS, et al (eds): The Metabolic and Molecular Bases of Inherited Disease. 8th ed. New York, McGraw-Hill, 2001, pp 5241-86.
29. Kaartinen V, Warburton D: Fibrillin controls TGF-beta activation. Nat Genet 33:331, 2003.
30. Coucke PJ, Willaert A, Wessels MW, et al: Mutations in the facilitative glucose transporter GLUT10 alters angiogenesis and cause arterial tortuosity syndrome. Nat Genet 38:452, 2006.
31. De Paepe A, Devereux RB, Dietz HC, et al: Revised diagnostic criteria for the Marfan syndrome. Am J Med Genet 62:417, 1996.
32. Murdoch JL, Walker BA, Halpern BL, et al: Life expectancy and causes of death in the Marfan syndrome. N Engl J Med 286:804, 1972.
33. Bhudia SK, Troughton R, Lam BK, et al: Mitral valve surgery in the adult Marfan syndrome patient. Ann Thorac Surg 81:843, 2006.
34. van Karnebeek CD, Naeff MS, Mulder BJ, et al: Natural history of cardiovascular manifestations in Marfan syndrome. Arch Dis Child 84:129, 2001.
35. Gott VL, Greene PS, Alejo DE, et al: Replacement of the aortic root in patients with Marfan's syndrome. N Engl J Med340:1307-13, 1999.
36. de Oliveira NC, David TE, Ivanov J, et al: Results of surgery for aortic root aneurysm in patients with Marfan syndrome. J Thorac Cardiovasc Surg 125:7896, 2003.
37. Patel ND, Williams JA, Barreiro CJ, et al: Valve-sparing aortic root replacement: Early experience with the De Paulis Valsalva graft in 51 patients. Ann Thorac Surg 82:548, 2006.
38. Miller DC: Valve-sparing aortic root replacement in patients with the Marfan syndrome. J Thorac Cardiovasc Surg 125:773, 2003.
39. Yetman AT, Bornemeier RA, McCrindle BW: Long-term outcome in patients with Marfan syndrome: Is aortic dissection the only cause of sudden death? J Am Coll Cardiol 41:329, 2003.
40. Chatrath R, Beauchesne LM, Connolly HM, et al: Left ventricular function in the Marfan syndrome without significant valvular regurgitation. Am J Cardiol 91:914, 2003.
41. Porciani MC, Giurlani L, Chelucci A, et al: Diastolic subclinical primary alterations in Marfan syndrome and Marfan-related disorders. Clin Cardiol 25:416, 2002.
42. Shores J BK, Murphy EA, Additional A: Chronic -beta-adrenergic blockade protects the aorta in the Marfan syndrome: A prospective, randomized trial of propranolol. N Engl J Med 330:1335, 1994.
43. Jondeau G, Boutouyrie P, Lacolley P, et al: Central pulse pressure is a major determinant of ascending aorta dilation in Marfan syndrome. Circulation 99:2677, 1999.
44. Habashi JP, Judge DP, Holm TM, et al: Losartan, an AT1 antagonist, prevents aortic aneurysm in a mouse model of Marfan syndrome. Science 312:117, 2006.
45. Lacro RV, Dietz HC, Wruck L, et al: Rationale and design of a randomized clinical trial of beta-blocker therapy (atenolol) vs. angiotensin II receptor blocker therapy (losartan) in individuals with Marfan syndrome. J Clin Trials 2007 (in press).
46. Meijboom LJ, Vos FE, Timmermans J, et al: Pregnancy and aortic root growth in the Marfan syndrome: A prospective study. Eur Heart J 26:914, 2005.
47. Meijboom LJ, Drenthen W, Pieper PG, et al: Obstetric complications in Marfan syndrome. Int J Cardiol 110:53, 2006.
48. Denier C, Labauge P, Brunereau L, et al: Clinical features of cerebral cavernous malformations patients with KRIT1 mutations. Ann Neurol 55:213, 2004.
49. Neptune ER, Frischmeyer PA, Arking DE, et al: Dysregulation of TGF-beta activation contributes to pathogenesis in Marfan syndrome. Nat Genet 33:407, 2003.
50. Collod-Beroud G, Le Bourdelles S, Ades L, et al: Update of the UMD-FBN1 mutation database and creation of an FBN1 polymorphism database. Hum Mutat 22:199, 2003.
51. Summers KM, West JA, Peterson MM, et al: Challenges in the diagnosis of Marfan syndrome. Med J Aust 184:627, 2006.
52. Yuan B, Thomas JP, von Kodolitsch Y, et al: Comparison of heteroduplex analysis, direct sequencing, and enzyme mismatch cleavage for detecting mutations in a large gene, FBN1. Hum Mutat 14:440, 1999.
53. Nishimura RA, McGoon MD: Perspectives on mitral-valve prolapse. N Engl J Med 341:48, 1999.
54. Disse S, Abergel E, Berrebi A, et al: Mapping of a first locus for autosomal dominant myxomatous mitral-valve prolapse to chromosome 16p11.2-p12.1. Am J Hum Genet 65:1242, 1999.

Mitral Valve Prolapse

55. Freed LA, Acierno JS, Jr., Dai D, et al: A locus for autosomal dominant mitral valve prolapse on chromosome 11p15.4. Am J Hum Genet 72:1551-9, 2003.
56. Kyndt F, Schott JJ, Trochu JN, et al: Mapping of X-linked myxomatous valvular dystrophy to chromosome Xq28. Am J Hum Genet 62:627, 1998.
57. Glesby MJ, Pyeritz RE: Association of mitral valve prolapse and systemic abnormalities of connective tissue. A phenotypic continuum. JAMA 262:523, 1989.

Aneurysmal and Allied Disorders

58. Mizuguchi T, Collod-Beroud G, Akiyama T, et al: Heterozygous TGFBR2 mutations in Marfan syndrome. Nat Genet 36:855, 2004.
59. Pannu H, Fadulu VT, Chang J, et al: Mutations in transforming growth factor-beta receptor type II cause familial thoracic aortic aneurysms and dissections. Circulation 112:513, 2005.
60. Loeys BL, Chen J, Neptune ER, et al: A syndrome of altered cardiovascular, craniofacial, neurocognitive and skeletal development caused by mutations in TGFBR1 or TGFBR2. Nat Genet 37:275, 2005.
61. Williams JA, Loeys BL, Nwakanma LU, et al: Early surgical experience with Loeys-Dietz: A new syndrome of aggressive thoracic aortic aneurysm disease. Ann Thorac Surg 83:S757, 2007.
62. Beighton P, De Paepe A, Steinmann B, et al: Ehlers-Danlos syndromes: Revised nosology, Villefranche, 1997. Am J Med Genet 77:31, 1998.
63. Wenstrup RJ, Meyer RA, Lyle JS, et al: Prevalence of aortic root dilation in the Ehlers-Danlos syndrome. Genet Med 4:112, 2002.
64. Dolan AL, Mishra MB, Chambers JB, et al: Clinical and echocardiographic survey of the Ehlers-Danlos syndrome. Br J Rheumatol 36:459, 1997.
65. Pyeritz RE: Ehlers-Danlos syndrome. N Engl J Med 342:730, 2000.
66. Gilchrist D, Schwarze U, Shields K, et al: Large kindred with Ehlers-Danlos syndrome type IV caused by a point mutation (G571S) in the COL3A1 gene of type III procollagen: Low risk of pregnancy complications and unexpected longevity in some affected relatives. Am J Med Genet 82:305, 1999.
67. Pepin M, Schwarze U, Superti-Furga A, et al: Clinical and genetic features of Ehlers-Danlos syndrome type IV, the vascular type. N Engl J Med 342:673, 2000.
68. Lind J, Wallenburg HC; Pregnancy and the Ehlers-Danlos syndrome: A retrospective study in a Dutch population. Acta Obstet Gynecol Scand 81:293, 2002.
69. Uitto J, Ringpfeil F: Heritable disorders of elastic tissue: Cutis laxa, pseudoxanthoma elasticum and related disorders. *In* Rimoin DL, Connor JM, Pyeritz RE, Korf BR (eds): Principles and Practice of Medical Genetics. 5th ed. Philadelphia, Churchill Livingstone, 2007, pp 3647-3670.
70. Germain DP, Boutouyrie P, Laloux B, et al: Arterial remodeling and stiffness in patients with pseudoxanthoma elasticum. Arterioscler Thromb Vasc Biol 23:836, 2003.
71. Sutters M: The pathogenesis of autosomal dominant polycystic kidney disease. Nephron Exp Nephrol 103:e149, 2006.
72. Hateboer N, v Dijk MA, Bogdanova N, et al: Comparison of phenotypes of polycystic kidney disease types 1 and 2. European PKD1-PKD2 Study Group. Lancet 353:103, 1999.
73. Al-Bhalal L, Akhtar M: Molecular basis of autosomal dominant polycystic kidney disease. Adv Anat Pathol 12:126, 2005.
74. Peters DJ, Breuning MH; Autosomal dominant polycystic kidney disease: Modification of disease progression. Lancet 358:1439, 2001.
75. Piccoli DA, Spinner NB: Alagille syndrome and the Jagged1 gene. Semin Liver Dis 21:525, 2001.
76. Kamath BM, Spinner NB, Emerick KM, et al: Vascular anomalies in Alagille syndrome: A significant cause of morbidity and mortality. Circulation 109:1354, 2004.
77. Warthen DM, Moore EC, Kamath BM, et al: Jagged1 (JAG1) mutations in Alagille syndrome: Increasing the mutation detection rate. Hum Mutat 27:436, 2006.
78. McDaniell R, Warthen DM, Sanchez-Lara PA, et al: NOTCH2 mutations cause Alagille syndrome, a heterogeneous disorder of the notch signaling pathway. Am J Hum Genet 79:169, 2006.
79. McElhinney DB, Krantz ID, Bason L, et al: Analysis of cardiovascular phenotype and genotype-phenotype correlation in individuals with a JAG1 mutation and/or Alagille syndrome. Circulation 106:2567, 2002.
80. Biddinger A, Rocklin M, Coselli J, et al: Familial thoracic aortic dilatations and dissections: A case control study. J Vasc Surg 25:506, 1997.
81. Milewicz DM, Chen H, Park ES, et al: Reduced penetrance and variable expressivity of familial thoracic aortic aneurysms/dissections. Am J Cardiol 82:474, 1998.
82. Beroukhim RS, Kruzick TL, Taylor AL, et al: Progression of aortic dilation in children with a functionally normal bicuspid aortic valve. Am J Cardiol 98:828, 2006.
83. Homme JL, Aubry MC, Edwards WD, et al: Surgical pathology of the ascending aorta: A clinicopathologic study of 513 cases. Am J Surg Pathol 30:1159, 2006.
84. Garg V: Molecular genetics of aortic valve disease. Curr Opin Cardiol 21:180, 2006.
85. Tran-Fadulu V, Chen JH, Lemuth D, et al: Familial thoracic aortic aneurysms and dissections: Three families with early-onset ascending and descending aortic dissections in women. Am J Med Genet A 140:1196, 2006.
86. Hasham SN, Willing MC, Guo DC, et al: Mapping a locus for familial thoracic aortic aneurysms and dissections (TAAD2) to 3p24-25. Circulation 107:3184, 2003.
87. Vaughan CJ, Casey M, He J, et al: Identification of a chromosome 11q23.2-q24 locus for familial aortic aneurysm disease, a genetically heterogeneous disorder. Circulation 103:2469, 2001.
88. Matyas G, Arnold E, Carrel T, et al: Identification and in silico analyses of novel TGFBR1 and TGFBR2 mutations in Marfan syndrome-related disorders. Hum Mutat 27:760, 2006.
89. Zhu L, Vranckx R, Khau Van Kien P, et al: Mutations in myosin heavy chain 11 cause a syndrome associating thoracic aortic aneurysm/aortic dissection and patent ductus arteriosus. Nat Genet 38:343, 2006.
90. Multicentre Aneurysm Screening Study Group: Multicentre aneurysm screening study (MASS): Cost effectiveness analysis of screening for abdominal aortic aneurysms based on four year results from randomised controlled trial. BMJ 325:1135, 2002.
91. Franceschini P, Guala A, Licata D, et al: Arterial tortuosity syndrome. Am J Med Genet 91:141, 2000.
92. Hoop R, Steinmann B, Valsangiacomo Buechel ER: Cardiovascular findings in arterial tortuosity syndrome. Eur Heart J 27:2045, 2006.

CNS Vascular Diseases

93. Lan MY, Chang YY, Huang CC, et al: Segmental disruption of internal elastic lamina in spontaneous vertebral artery dissection combined with redundancy of multiple cervical arteries. J Clin Neurosci 13:367, 2006.
94. Cartwright MS, Hickling WH, Roach ES: Ischemic stroke in an adolescent with arterial tortuosity syndrome. Neurology 67:360, 2006.
95. Krischek B, Inoue I: The genetics of intracranial aneurysms. J Hum Genet 51:587, 2006.

96. Yanaka K, Nagase S, Asakawa H, et al: Management of unruptured cerebral aneurysms in patients with polycystic kidney disease. Surg Neurol 62:538; discussion, 45, 2004.
97. Magnetic Resonance Angiography in Relatives of Patients with Subarachnoid Hemorrhage Study Group: Risks and benefits of screening for intracranial aneurysms in first-degree relatives of patients with sporadic subarachnoid hemorrhage. N Engl J Med 341:1344, 1999.
98. Gaist D, Vaeth M, Tsiropoulos I, et al: Risk of subarachnoid haemorrhage in first-degree relatives of patients with subarachnoid haemorrhage: Follow-up study based on national registries in Denmark. BMJ 320:141, 2000.
99. Walter JW, Blei F, Anderson JL, et al: Genetic mapping of a novel familial form of infantile hemangioma. Am J Med Genet 82:77, 1999.
100. Wang MM: Genetics of ischemic stroke: Future clinical applications. Semin Neurol 26:523, 2006.
101. Sakurai K, Horiuchi Y, Ikeda H, et al: A novel susceptibility locus for moyamoya disease on chromosome 8q23. J Hum Genet 49:278, 2004.
102. Bianchi S, Dotti MT, Federico A: Physiology and pathology of notch signalling system. J Cell Physiol 207:3008, 2006.
103. Thomsen LL, Kirchmann M, Bjornsson A, et al: The genetic spectrum of a population-based sample of familial hemiplegic migraine. Brain 130:346, 2007.
104. Newman JH, Loyd JE, Phillips JA III: Primary pulmonary hypertension. *In* Rimoin DL, Connor JM, Pyeritz RE, Korf BR (eds): Principles and Practice of Medical Genetics. 5th ed. Philadelphia, Churchill Livingstone, 2007, pp 1187-1199.
105. Trembath RC, Harrison R: Insights into the genetic and molecular basis of primary pulmonary hypertension. Pediatr Res 53:883, 2003.
106. Runo JR, Loyd JE: Primary pulmonary hypertension. Lancet 361:1533, 2003.
107. Deng Z, Morse JH, Slager SL, et al: Familial primary pulmonary hypertension (gene PPH1) is caused by mutations in the bone morphogenetic protein receptor-II gene. Am J Hum Genet 67:737, 2000.
108. Holmes DR Jr, Kennel AJ, Smith HC, et al: Coronary artery disease in twins. Br Heart J 45:193, 1981.
109. Fan M, Kahonen M, Rontu R, et al: The p22phox C242T gene polymorphism is associated with a reduced risk of angiographically verified coronary artery disease in a high-risk Finnish Caucasian population. The Finnish Cardiovascular Study. Am Heart J 152:538, 2006.
110. Rhee EJ, Oh KW, Lee WY, et al: The differential effects of age on the association of KLOTHO gene polymorphisms with coronary artery disease. Metabolism 55:1344, 2006.
111. Chittenden TW, Sherman JA, Xiong F, et al: Transcriptional profiling in coronary artery disease: indications for novel markers of coronary collateralization. Circulation 114:1811, 2006.
112. Qasim A, Reilly MP: Genetic determinants of atherosclerotic disease. *In* Rimoin DL, Connor JM, Pyeritz RE, Korf B (eds): Principles and Practice of Medical Genetics. 5th ed. Philadelphia, Churchill Livingstone, 2007, pp 1329-1353.
113. Cohen MM Jr: Klippel-Trenaunay syndrome. Am J Med Genet 93:171, 2000.
114. Revencu N, Vikkula M: Cerebral cavernous malformation: New molecular and clinical insights. J Med Genet 43:716, 2006.
115. Cave-Riant F, Denier C, Labauge P, et al: Spectrum and expression analysis of KRIT1 mutations in 121 consecutive and unrelated patients with cerebral cavernous malformations. Eur J Hum Genet 10:733, 2002.
116. Liquori CL, Berg MJ, Squitieri F, et al: Low frequency of PDCD10 mutations in a panel of CCM3 probands: Potential for a fourth CCM locus. Hum Mutat 27:118, 2006.
117. Van Balkom ID, Alders M, Allanson J, et al: Lymphedema-lymphangiectasia-mental retardation (Hennekam) syndrome: A review. Am J Med Genet 112:412, 2002.
118. Wang QK: Update on the molecular genetics of vascular anomalies. Lymphat Res Biol 3:226, 2005.
119. Spiegel R, Ghalamkarpour A, Daniel-Spiegel E, et al: Wide clinical spectrum in a family with hereditary lymphedema type I caused by a novel missense mutation in VEGFR3. J Hum Genet 51:846, 2006.
120. Irrthum A, Devriendt K, Chitayat D, et al: Mutations in the transcription factor gene SOX18 underlie recessive and dominant forms of hypotrichosis-lymphedema-telangiectasia. Am J Hum Genet 72:1470, 2003.
121. Guttmacher A, Marchuk DA, Pyeritz RE: Hereditary hemorrhagic telangiectasia. *In* Rimoin DL, Connor JM, Pyeritz RE, Korf BR (eds): Principles and Practice of Medical Genetics. 5th ed. Philadelphia, Churchill Livingstone, 2007, pp 1200-1213.
122. Shovlin CL, Guttmacher AE, Buscarini E, et al: Diagnostic criteria for hereditary hemorrhagic telangiectasia (Rendu-Osler-Weber syndrome). Am J Med Genet 91:66, 2000.
123. McDonald JE, Miller FJ, Hallam SE, et al: Clinical manifestations in a large hereditary hemorrhagic telangiectasia (HHT) type 2 kindred. Am J Med Genet 93:320, 2000.
124. Folz BJ, Wollstein AC, Alfke H, et al: The value of screening for multiple arteriovenous malformations in hereditary hemorrhagic telangiectasia: A diagnostic study. Eur Arch Otorhinolaryngol 261:509, 2004.
125. Kopel L, Lage SG: Cardiac tamponade in hereditary hemorrhagic telangiectasia. Am J Med 105:252, 1998.
126. Lee WL, Graham AF, Pugash RA, et al: Contrast echocardiography remains positive after treatment of pulmonary arteriovenous malformations. Chest 123:351, 2003.
127. Pollak JS, Saluja S, Thabet A, et al: Clinical and anatomic outcomes after embolotherapy of pulmonary arteriovenous malformations. J Vasc Interv Radiol 17:35, 2006.
128. Longacre AV, Gross CP, Gallitelli M, et al: Diagnosis and management of gastrointestinal bleeding in patients with hereditary hemorhagic telangiectasia. Am J Gastroenterol 98:59, 2003.
129. Marchuk DA, Srinivasan S, Squire TL, et al: Vascular morphogenesis: Tales of two syndromes. Hum Mol Genet 12 Spec No 1:R97, 2003.
130. Bossler AD, Richards J, George C, et al: Novel mutations in ENG and ACVRL1 identified in a series of 200 individuals undergoing clinical genetic testing for hereditary hemorrhagic telangiectasia (HHT): Correlation of genotype with phenotype. Hum Mutat 27:667, 2006.
131. Gallione CJ, Repetto GM, Legius E, et al: A combined syndrome of juvenile polyposis and hereditary haemorrhagic telangiectasia associated with mutations in MADH4 (SMAD4). Lancet 363:852, 2004.
132. Bayrak-Toydemir P, Mcdonald J, Akarsu N, et al: A fourth locus for hereditary hemorrhagic telangiectasia maps to chromosome 7. Am J Med Genet A 140:2155, 2006.
133. Richling B, Killer M, Al-Schameri AR, et al: Therapy of brain arteriovenous malformations: Multimodality treatment from a balanced standpoint. Neurosurgery 59:S148, 2006.
134. Molino D, Sepe J, Anastasio P, et al: The history of von Hippel-Lindau disease. J Nephrol 19(Suppl 10):S119, 2006.

CHAPTER 9

Genetics of Cardiac Arrhythmias

Silvia G. Priori, Carlo Napolitano, and Peter J. Schwartz

Cardiac arrhythmias most often occur in the presence of an abnormal substrate that is responsible for derangement in impulse initiation and conduction. Although ischemic heart disease is the primary cause for the development of ventricular fibrillation, other structural heart diseases (such as hypertrophic and dilated cardiomyopathies, see Chaps. 64 and 65) account for most of the remaining cases. In several postmortem series of cardiac arrest victims, structural abnormalities were absent in approximately 5 to 8 percent[1] of cases, which, for many years, were referred to as cases of "idiopathic ventricular fibrillation" (IVF).[2] During the past 10 to 15 years, with the help of molecular biology, the substrate of IVF has been partially defined and substantial evidence now demonstrates that genetically determined abnormalities of proteins that control the electrical activity of the heart can cause cardiac arrest in the structurally intact heart. At least 14 genes (Table 9-1) have been associated with inherited arrhythmogenic diseases and are linked to sudden death in the apparently normal heart. Recent molecular evidence in large cohorts implicates cardiac channelopathies (mostly the long QT syndrome [LQTS]) in 35% of sudden unexplained deaths in the young and in 9% of cases of sudden infant death syndrome (SIDS).[3] In this chapter we review the clinical and genetic characteristics of the most common inherited arrhythmogenic diseases predisposing to arrhythmias and sudden death, the LQTS, Brugada syndrome, catecholaminergic polymorphic ventricular tachycardia and short QT syndrome (SQTS, see Chap. 35). In Table 9-1 we also report the most important clinical and genetic features of additional inherited arrhythmogenic disorders occurring in the structurally normal heart.

LONG QT SYNDROME

LQTS is an inherited arrhythmogenic disease characterized by susceptibility to life-threatening arrhythmias. Two major forms of LQTS have been identified, one transmitted as an autosomal dominant trait (Romano Ward syndrome), the second transmitted as an autosomal recessive disease in which the cardiac phenotype is associated with neurosensory deafness (Jervell and Lange-Nielsen syndrome). The electrocardiographic marker of LQTS consists of prolonged repolarization (i.e., prolonged QT interval), abnormal morphology of the T wave (Fig. 9-1), and of a characteristic polymorphic ventricular tachycardia called "torsades de pointes" that is usually induced by activation of the sympathetic nervous system but also by a sudden pause.[4]

Clinical Manifestations

Syncope and fainting, but also cardiac arrest and sudden death, are the typical manifestations of LQTS. Their occurrence is often precipitated by physical or emotional stress (e.g., fear, anger, loud noises, sudden awakening), but they may also occur at rest.[5] Onset of symptoms is typically in the first two decades of life including the neonatal period when LQTS can be misdiagnosed as SIDS,[6] and recent molecular evidence points to LQTS as a cause of approximately 10 percent of all SIDS cases.[7] However, the first symptoms may appear later in life, especially among females. The severity of the clinical manifestations of LQTS is highly variable, ranging from full-blown disease with markedly prolonged QT interval and recurrent syncope, to subclinical forms with borderline QT interval prolongation and no arrhythmias or syncopal events.[8]

Risk stratification, whenever possible aided by knowledge of the genotype, is important for clinical management.

GENETIC BASIS OF LONG QT SYNDROME

Following the identification, in 1995 and 1996, of the first three LQTS genes[9-11]—associated with the most frequently encountered variants (LQT1, LQT2, and LQT3)—there has been identification of other genes proven or thought to be associated with LQTS. This includes the genes for LQT4 through LQT10. Unfortunately, a terminology problem has developed because not all of these genes can be truly regarded as responsible for LQTS. Specifically, we consider that what have been called LQT4 and LQT7 (Andersen-Tawil syndrome) are complex clinical disorders in which a more or less modest prolongation of the QT interval—especially in the Andersen-Tawil syndrome—is only a secondary epiphenomenon and should not be regarded as part of LQTS. LQT5, LQT6, and LQT8, although rare, are certainly part of LQTS. For LQT9 and LQT10 there are only preliminary descriptions and at this time should be regarded as putative forms of LQTS.

From an epidemiological standpoint there is agreement that LQT1, LQT2, and LQT3 variants account for greater than 90 percent of all genotyped LQTS patients, whereas the remaining genes are responsible for a minority of cases. Another interesting observation is that the percentage of LQTS patients carrying more than one mutation (often defined as compound heterozygote) may be as high as 4 percent.[12]

TABLE 9–1 Genes Involved in Inherited Arrhythmogenic Disease

Disease	Variant	Gene	Protein	Effect of Mutations	Phenotype
Long QT Syndrome	LQT1	*KCNQ1*	I_{Ks} potassium channel alpha subunit (KvLQT1)	Loss of function—reduced K+ outward current	Prolonged QT interval
	LQT2	*KCNH2*	I_{Kr} potassium channel alpha subunit (HERG)	Loss of function—reduced K+ outward current	Prolonged QT interval
	LQT3	*SCN5A*	Cardiac sodium channel alpha subunit (Nav 1.5)	Gain of function—Increased inward Na+ current	Prolonged QT interval
	LQT4	*ANK2*	Ankyrin B, anchoring protein	Reduced membrane expression of Na+ and Ca2+ channels	Long QT, atrial fibrillation
	LQT5	*KCNE1*	I_{Ks} potassium channel beta subunit (MinK)	Loss of function—reduced K+ outward current	Prolonged QT interval
	LQT6	*KCNE2*	I_{Kr} potassium channel beta subunit (MiRP)	Loss of function—reduced K+ outward current	Prolonged QT interval
	LQT7, Andersen syndrome	*KCNJ2*	I_{K1} potassium channel (Kir2.1)	Loss of function—reduced outward K+ current	Long QT, Potassium sensitive periodic paralysis, low set hears, hypoplastic mandible
	LQT8, Timothy syndrome	*CACNA1c*	Voltage-gated calcium channel, CaV1.2	Gain of function—increased L-type Ca^{2+} current	Long QT, syndactyly, septal defect, patent foramen ovale, autism and developmental disorders
	LQT9	*CAV3*	Caveolin cardiac gene	Gain of function—increased INa current due to altered gating kinetic	Prolonged QT interval
	LQT10	*SCN4B*	Sodium channel beta-4 subunit	Reduced subunit expression causing increased sodium current (INa)	Prolonged QT interval
Brugada syndrome	BrS1	*SCN5A*	Cardiac sodium channel alpha subunit (Nav 1.5)	Loss of function—reduced outward Na+ current	ST segment elevation (V2-V3), right bundle branch block
	BrS2	*GPD1-L*	Glycerol-6-Phosphate-Dehydrogenase	Loss of function—reduced outward Na+ current	ST segment elevation (V2-V3), right bundle branch block
Catecholaminergic VT	CPVT1	*RyR2*	Cardiac Ryanodine receptor (RyR2)	Gain of function—diastolic Ca2+ release form SR	Adrenergically induced bidirectional or polymorphic VT, VF
	CPVT2	*CASQ2*	Cardiac Calsequestrin (CASQ2)	Loss of SR Ca2+ buffering capacity	Adrenergically induced bidirectional or polymorphic VT, VF
Short QT syndrome	SQTS1	*KCNH2*	I_{Kr} potassium channel alpha subunit (HERG)	Gain of function—increased outward K+ current	Short QT interval
	SQTS2	*KCNQ1*	I_{Ks} potassium channel alpha subunit (KvLQT1)	Gain of function—increased outward K+ current	Short QT interval
	SQTS3	*KCNJ2*	I_{K1} potassium channel (Kir2.1)	Gain of function—increased outward K+ current	Short QT interval
Cardiac conduction defect sick and sinus syndrome	PFHB1	*SCN5A*	Cardiac sodium channel alpha subunit (Nav 1.5)	Loss of function—reduced outward Na+ current	Atrioventricular and intraventricular conduction block
	SSS1	*SCN5A*	Cardiac sodium channel alpha subunit (Nav 1.5)	Loss of function—reduced outward Na+ current	Sinus bradycardia, sinus arrest, and/or sinoatrial block, atrial tachycardias
	SSS2	*HCN4*	Sinus node pacemaker current If	Loss of function—faster current deactivation	Bradycardia and sinus pauses
Atrial fibrillation	ATFIB1	*KCNQ1*	I_{Ks} potassium channel alpha subunit (KvLQT1)	Gain of function—increased K+ outward current	Lone atrial fibrillation
	ATFIB2	*KCNE2*	I_{Kr} potassium channel beta subunit (MiRP)	Gain of function—increased K+ outward current	Lone atrial fibrillation
	ATFIB3	*KCNJ2*	I_{K1} potassium channel (Kir 2.1)	Gain of function—increased K+ outward current	Lone atrial fibrillation

The main characteristic of all the LQTS genes identified so far is to encode cardiac ion channel subunits or, as in the case of the newly described CAV3, to modulate ionic currents: hence the use of the word "channelopathy" to indicate the group of diseases to which LQTS belongs. Table 9-1 summarizes the complete list of genes associated with QT prolongation and ventricular arrhythmias, the associated phenotypes (extracardiac), and the gene function.

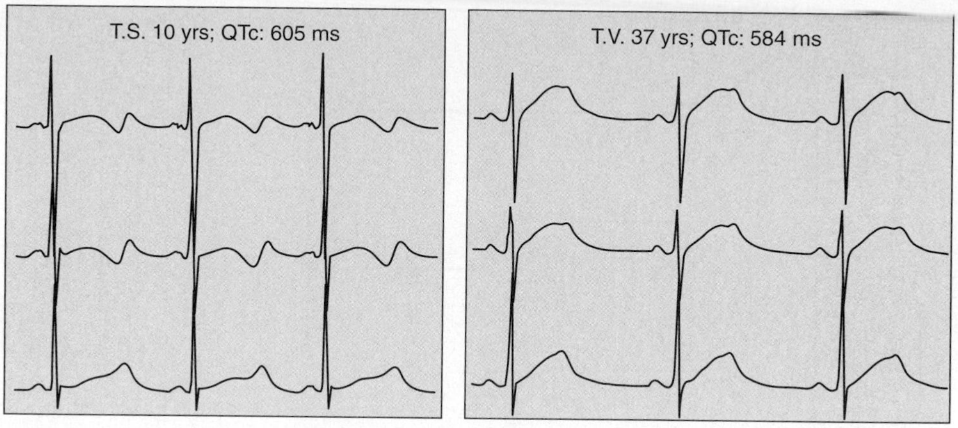

FIGURE 9–1 Typical electrocardiogram of two long QT syndrome patients showing QT interval prolongation and T wave morphological abnormalities.

Clinical Management of Long QT Syndrome

Recommendations for management of LQTS have been recently summarized in the joint ACC, ESC, AHA task force on ventricular arrhythmias (Table 9-2).[13]

Since the mid-1970s, the link between onset of cardiac events and increased sympathetic activity suggested the use of beta blockers in the treatment of the disease.[14] Recently, the efficacy of beta blockade in LQTS patients has been reassessed in large collaborative studies that showed an overall mortality below 2% over a mean follow-up exceeding 5 years.[15] Beta blockers are especially effective among LQT1 patients; in this group the combined incidence of resuscitated cardiac arrest (CA) and of sudden cardiac death (SCD) is only 1%.[16] This figure increases to almost 7 percent among LQT2 and to 14 percent among LQT3 patients (Fig. 9-2). Considering that the risk for CA/SCD among asymptomatic patients, untreated and younger than age 40, with a clearly prolonged QTc, is around 13 percent,[17] with few exceptions (mostly borderline QTc and LQT1 males older than age 25 to 30), all should be treated. All symptomatic patients should be treated as well. For the 20 to 30 percent of patients who may have a recurrence of syncope despite beta blockade, the main options are either left cardiac sympathetic denervation (LCSD)[18] or the prophylactic implantation of an implantable cardioverter defibrillator (ICD).

The analysis of cardiac events by genotype also showed that the presence of LQT2 or LQT3 genotypes, QTc intervals greater than 500 ms, and the occurrence of a first syncopal spell before age 7 years are independent predictors of failure of beta blockade. In these patients the use of ICD for primary prevention may be considered.[16]

Permanent pacemaker implantation is infrequently used today and only in selected LQTS patients with atrioventricular block or with bradycardia- or pause-dependent tachyarrhythmias, as an adjunct to beta blockade and after due consideration of an ICD.

On the basis of evidence that LQT3 is caused by an increased late I_{Na}, in 1995 the feasibility of this pharmacological intervention was tested in a few genotyped patients and, indeed, sodium channel blockade with mexiletine shortened the QT interval among LQT3 patients but not among LQT2 patients.[19] A growing number of anecdotal reports suggest the possible value, especially in LQT3 infants with major QT prolongation and storms of major arrhythmias, of mexiletine in combination with beta blockers.

Whereas for several years genotyping has been regarded primarily as a research tool, the existence of so many silent mutation carriers and the recognition of their arrhythmic risk should have a major impact on clinical management. Given the high probability (≈70 percent) of identifying the disease-causing mutation in the proband, this becomes an essential step in order to then rapidly screen the family members and implement protective strategies. Thus molecular screening should become part of the routine clinical management of LQTS. Genotyping is cost effective,[20] and strategies are available for a time- and cost-effective tiered approach to molecular screening for these patients.[12]

TABLE 9–2	Recommendations for Management of Long QT Syndrome (LQTS)
Class I	Lifestyle modification is recommended for patients with an LQTS diagnosis (clinical and/or molecular). *(Level of evidence: B)* Beta blockers are recommended for patients with an LQTS clinical diagnosis (i.e., in the presence of prolonged QT interval). *(Level of evidence: B)* Implantation of an ICD along with use of beta blockers is recommended for LQTS patients with previous cardiac arrest and who have reasonable expectation of survival with a good functional status for more than 1 year.
Class IIa	Beta blockers can be effective to reduce SCD in patients with a molecular LQTS analysis and normal QT interval. *(Level of evidence: B)* Implantation of an ICD with continued use of beta blockers can be effective to reduce SCD in LQTS patients experiencing syncope and/or ventricular tachycardia while receiving beta blockers and who have reasonable expectation of survival with a good functional status for more than 1 year. *(Level of evidence: B)*
Class IIb	Left cardiac sympathetic denervation may be considered for LQTS patients with syncope, torsades de pointes, or cardiac arrest while receiving beta blockers. *(Level of evidence: B)* Implantation of an ICD with use of beta blockers may be considered for prophylaxis of SCD for patients in categories possibly associated with higher risk of cardiac arrest (such as LQT2 and LQT3, QTc > 500 ms) and who have reasonable expectation of survival with a good functional status for more than 1 year. *(Level of evidence: B)*

ICD, implantable cardioverter defibrillator.

Genotype-Phenotype Correlation Studies

Recently, the distinguishing features of the three most common genetic variants of LQTS, namely LQT1, LQT2, and LQT3, have been outlined.[4,21] The analysis of the electrocardiographic patterns revealed a gene-specific morphology of the ST-T wave complex,[22] which may guide genotyping. The

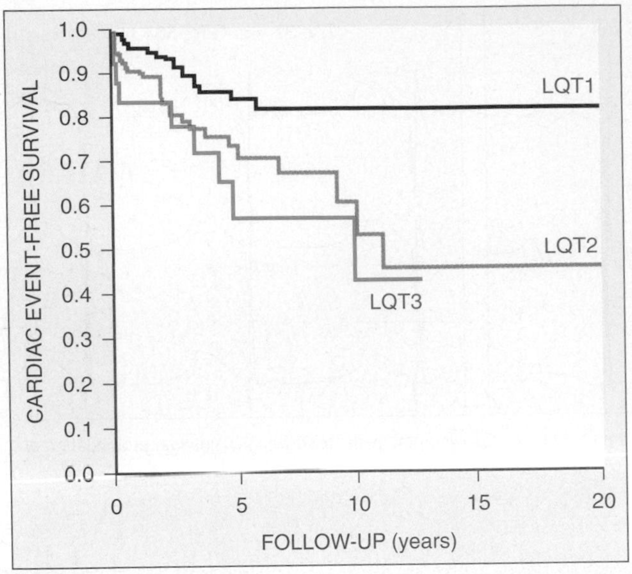

FIGURE 9–2 Kaplan-Meier analysis of cumulative cardiac event-free survival in genotyped long QT syndrome patients receiving beta blockers according to the genetic variant of the disease (log-rank $p < 0.001$). *(Modified and reproduced from Priori SG, Napolitano C, Schwartz PJ, et al: Association of long QT syndrome loci and cardiac events among patients treated with beta blockers. JAMA 292:1341, 2004.)*

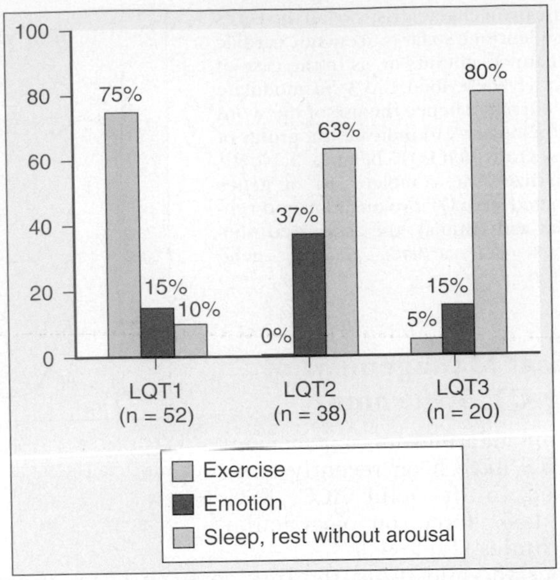

FIGURE 9–3 Fatal cardiac events classified according to the three main triggers in the three genotypes. *(Modified and reproduced from Schwartz PJ, Priori SG, Spazzolini C, et al: Genotype-phenotype correlation in the long-QT syndrome: Gene-specific triggers for life-threatening arrhythmias. Circulation 103:89, 2001.)*

overall penetrance of LQTS is 60 percent,[12,17] meaning that two out of five mutation carriers have a normal QT interval. Penetrance is variant specific, being LQT1 < LQT2 < LQT3. A clinically relevant concept is that the carriers with normal QT interval are at lower risk of spontaneous events but at high risk if treated with any of the many drugs containing an I_{Kr} blocker.

The triggers for cardiac events differ strikingly among the genetic variants of LQTS (Fig. 9-3).[5] LQT1 patients present an increased risk during physical or emotional stress: they experience 90% of lethal events under this setting as opposed to LQT3 patients who present most of their events (80 percent) at rest or while asleep and only 5 percent during exercise. LQT2 patients are at higher risk for lethal events during arousal or emotions (37 percent), but are also at risk during sleep and at rest (63%), and not at all during exercise. There are also triggers which appear as highly specific: indeed, 99% of cardiac events occurring while swimming involve LQT1 patients and 80% of events due to acoustic stimuli involve LQT2 patients.[23,24] These differences are also reflected in the differential response to beta blocker therapy discussed earlier and are consistent with the findings in a large group including only symptomatic patients: among them was a 4 percent incidence of CA/SCD for LQT1 and LQT2, to be contrasted with a 17 percent incidence for LQT3.[5]

Natural History and Risk Stratification

The increased availability of data collected among genotyped LQTS patients has allowed the development of risk stratification models on the basis of genetic substrate. Data from 647 LQTS patients from 193 genotyped families[17] show a lower cumulative event-free survival among LQT2 versus LQT1 patients, and a similar trend is present among LQT3 versus LQT1. Gender has no influence among LQT1 patients, whereas a higher risk is present for LQT2 females and LQT3 males. The percentage of genetically affected patients with a normal QT interval ("silent mutation carriers") differs strikingly among genotypes, being much more frequent ($p < 0.001$) in LQT1 patients (36 percent) than in LQT2 patients (19 percent) and especially so in LQT3 patients (10 percent). Quartiles of QTc distribution, determined within each genetic subgroup, allow recognition that among LQT1 and LQT2 patients, those with a QTc in the upper quartile have, respectively, a 5.3- and 8.4-fold risk increase compared with those in the first quartile. By contrast, QTc duration does not differentiate risk among LQT3 patients.

These data were incorporated in a risk quantification model by comparing the event-free survival in 12 categories including—for each genetic locus—the four combinations of gender and QTc below or above 500 ms. This provided the identification of a differential risk within these 12 categories (Fig. 9-4).

Risk stratification may be further refined by considering the location of a mutation. Mutations located in the carboxy terminus of the *KCNQ1* gene appear to be associated with a mild clinical phenotype and in LQT2 patients mutations in the pore region are associated with a greater risk for major cardiac events.[25] Even within the highly malignant Jervell and Lange-Nielsen syndrome,[26] the genotype allows risk stratification. The patients carrying the less common mutations on *KCNE1* have a better prognosis than those with mutations on *KCNQ1* (Fig. 9-5).

BRUGADA SYNDROME

Clinical Manifestations and Diagnosis

In 1992 Brugada and Brugada described patients presenting with ST segment elevation in the right precordial leads (V_1 to V_3) (in the absence of acute coronary syndrome), right bundle branch block, susceptibility to ventricular tachyarrhythmias, and structurally normal hearts. Familial distribution consistent with autosomal dominant inheritance was also reported, thus suggesting a genetic origin of the disease. This disease is now referred to as *Brugada syndrome* (BrS). Its prevalence is not known, but the disease seems to be more prevalent in the Far Eastern countries, possibly impacted by an Asian-specific genotype (see later).

The typical arrhythmia of BrS is a rapid polymorphic ventricular tachycardia that frequently degenerates into ventricular fibrillation. An increased propensity to atrial fibrillation has also been documented. Despite the fact that BrS is a genetically determined disease, clinical manifestations (syncope or cardiac arrest) are rare during pediatric age and exhibit increased severity in the third to fourth decades of life with a striking 8 : 1 male-to-female ratio in symptomatic individuals. The causes of such age- and gender-dependent risk are not yet understood. Cardiac events occur during sleep or at rest. Fever, tricyclic antidepressant usage, and cocaine assumption have been identified as specific triggers for events in some patients.

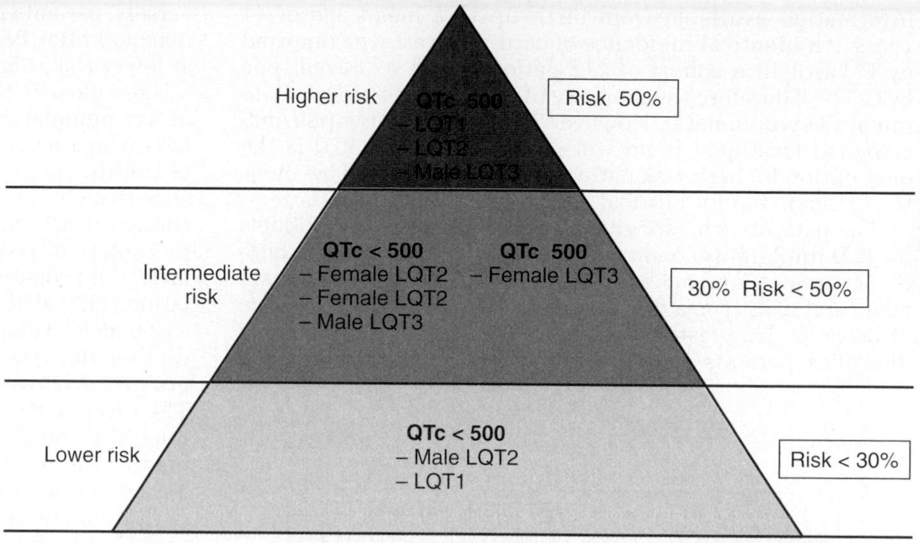

FIGURE 9–4 Risk stratification scheme in long QT syndrome patients according to genotype and gender. The risk groups have been defied on the basis of the probability of experiencing a first cardiac event (syncope, cardiac arrest, or sudden death) by age 40 years. Fifty percent or higher probability of events constitutes the higher-risk subgroup, a risk between 30 and 50 percent the intermediate risk group, and a risk less than 30 percent defines the lower-risk group.

The diagnosis of BrS is complicated by the intermittent nature of the electrocardiogram (ECG) pattern. Concealed forms may be unmasked only after performing provocative drug testing with selected class IC drugs: ajmaline (1 mg/kg), flecainide (2 mg/kg), or procainamide (15 mg/kg). Autonomic nervous system modulation can also modify the phenotype because intravenous administration of isoproterenol attenuates, whereas acetylcholine accentuates the ECG abnormalities in affected patients. This feature is consistent with the fact that cardiac events in BrS occur mostly at rest or during sleep. Diagnostic criteria for BrS have been refined over the years. Three ECG patterns have been identified, but only a "coved" ST or type I ECG (Fig. 9-6) segment elevation is presently considered diagnostic for the disease.[27] However, life-threatening cardiac events in patients with "saddle-back" ECG (type II, see Fig. 9-6) with genetically confirmed diagnosis can occur and challenge this concept, creating diagnostic uncertainty.

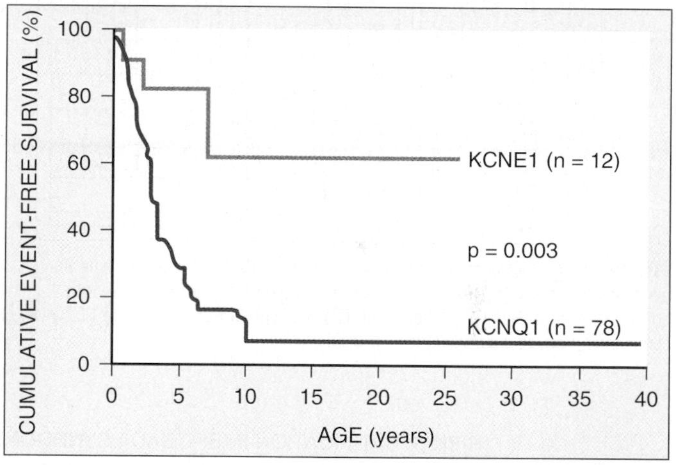

FIGURE 9–5 Kaplan-Meier curves of event-free survival and survival in Jervell and Lange-Nielsen syndrome patients. Numbers in parenthesis are number of patients for whom information on the time of the event are available *(From Priori SG, Napolitano C: Should patients with an asymptomatic Brugada electrocardiogram undergo pharmacological and electrophysiological testing? Circulation 112:279, 2005.)*

GENETIC BASIS OF BRUGADA SYNDROME

The first gene was identified in 1998 as being the cardiac sodium channel gene (*SCN5A*), the same gene responsible for the LQT3 variant of LQTS.[28] Therefore BrS and LQT3 are caused by mutations in the same gene but have opposite effects on cardiac sodium current: "loss of function" in BrS and "gain of function" in LQT3 (see Table 9-1). Interestingly, overlapping phenotypes between LQT3 and Brugada syndrome have been reported by independent groups[29,30] and they underscore the functional complexity of the cardiac "sodium channel disease." Interestingly, *SCN5A* mutations have been recently associated with dilated cardiomyopathy (CMD) (see Chap. 64),[31] thus suggesting that structural abnormalities can develop as a direct consequence of genetically impaired electrophysiological properties of cardiac cells.[31] This point is particularly relevant in BrS patients because the presence of structural abnormalities being part of the phenotype in some has been debated.[32] Recently it has been proposed that viral infection may be part of the trigger that accompanies the development of structural abnormalities in patients with BrS with or without SCN5A mutations.[33]

As a practical consequence for the clinical management of patients, it is safe to recommend a careful cardiac imaging evaluation in all patients with BrS.

Recently the second gene for BrS has been reported in a single large family harboring a mutation in the *GPD1-L* gene, encoding for a Glycerol-3-Phosphate-Dehydrogenase-one-like protein.[34] The function of this protein in the heart is not fully understood, but preliminary experimental evidence shows that the GPD1-L mutation causes a reduced expression of sodium current.

Unfortunately, *SCN5A* mutations account for only 20 to 25 percent of clinically confirmed Brugada syndrome cases[35] and preliminary evidence suggests that the *GPD1-L* gene accounts for approximately 1 percent of BrS cases (Priori SG, Napolitano C, personal communication).

Therefore the clinical impact of genetic testing in BrS is still limited, but, when available, this information is useful to identify silent carriers and for presymptomatic diagnosis of family members of a genotyped proband.

Prognostic Indicators and Management

Although initial data collected by Brugada and colleagues provided an alarming estimate of the lethality of the disease (close to 30 percent of deaths within 3 years from diagnosis), more recent analyses in larger cohorts have provided a more "reassuring" picture. Priori and colleagues[35] have reported an 11 percent incidence of cardiac arrest and 17 percent incidence of syncope among 200 patients with clinical information available from birth up to a mean age of 41 years. An identical incidence of cardiac arrest was reported by Eckardt in a cohort of 212 patients with a "coved-type ECG."[35,36] Therefore the majority of BrS patients are likely to remain asymptomatic. However, because effective pharmacological treatment is not yet available and the ICD is the only option for high-risk patients, risk stratification becomes the critical step for clinical management.

The patients who survived cardiac arrest are candidates for ICD implant (secondary prevention). Furthermore, there is agreement among investigators that a spontaneously abnormal ECG (i.e., a diagnostic pattern also in the absence of class IC drug test) associated with a history of syncope identifies patients in whom an ICD is indicated.[37,38] Conversely, patients in whom the diagnostic ECG (type I) is only detected after flecainide/ajmaline test are considered to be at lower risk (Fig. 9-7).

Less clear is the preferable strategy for the management of asymptomatic patients with a spontaneously abnormal ECG who are considered at "intermediate" risk (see Fig. 9-7) of life-threatening cardiac events. Registry data have consistently shown that neither a family history of juvenile sudden death nor the presence of late potentials are good predictors of risk of sudden death in these patients. Similarly, the prognostic value of programmed electrical stimulation (PES) still represents a matter of debate. Brugada and associates[38] suggested that PES is highly sensitive in predicting the risk of major cardiac events. However, other groups of investigators[35-37] did not confirm their findings. The disagreement is likely to be caused by the poor reproducibility of PES results in BrS either at short term[39] or medium term.[40] These results have been included in the Task Force on Sudden Cardiac Death of the European Society of Cardiology,[1] and the same recommendation has also been provided by joint ACC/AHA/ESC Guidelines[13] with a class IIb recommendation for PES in BrS. At present the use of PES for risk stratification is not definitely established.[37] Only the availability of ongoing prospective clinical trials will provide a clear answer to this issue.

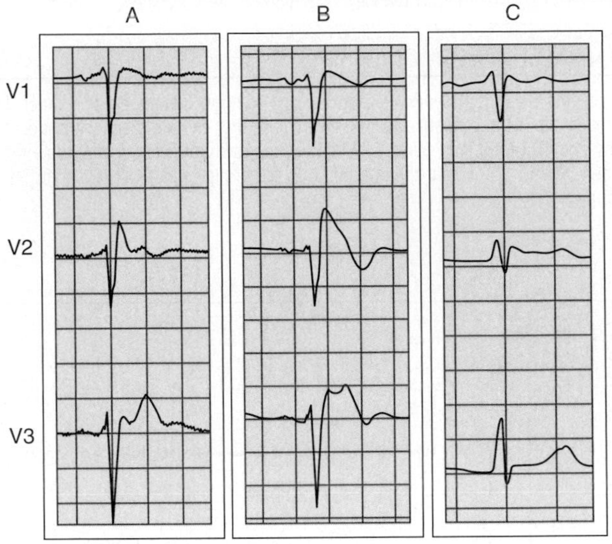

FIGURE 9–6 Electrocardiogram patterns in Brugada syndrome. **A,** Type II electrocardiogram (ECG) that is converted in a type I ECG after intravenous administration of 2 mg/kg of flecainide **(B)**. **C,** Type III ECG. Only type I ECG **(B)** is considered diagnostic for Brugada syndrome.

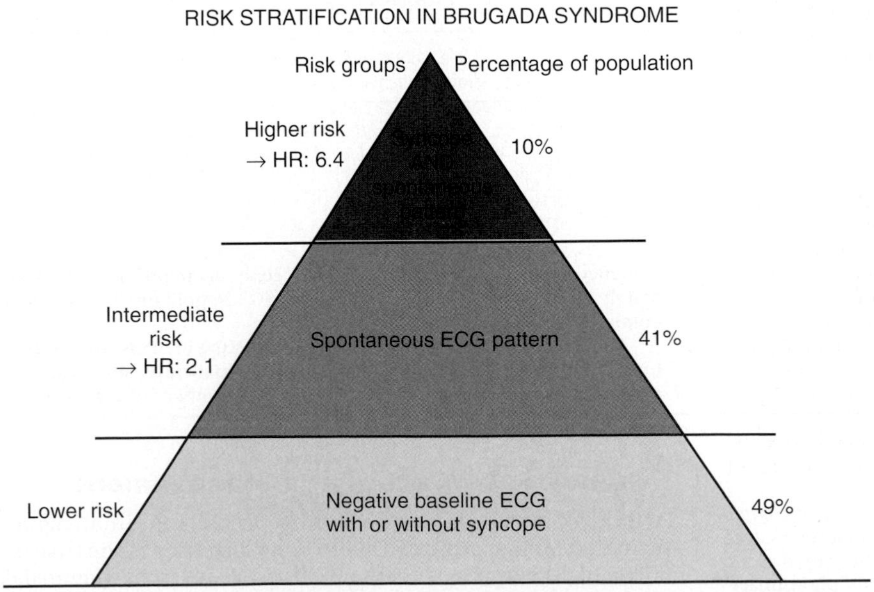

FIGURE 9–7 Risk stratification scheme in Brugada syndrome according to clinical presentation. Hazard ratios for cardiac arrest **(left)** are calculated keeping the lowest category (patients without spontaneously diagnostic electrocardiogram) as reference. Percentages **(right)** represent the relative frequency of patients in the three categories.

CATECHOLAMINERGIC POLYMORPHIC VENTRICULAR TACHYCARDIA

Catecholaminergic polymorphic ventricular tachycardia (CPVT) was originally described by Coumel and Leenhardt.[41,42] The disease is characterized by adrenergically induced ventricular tachycardia (VT), leading to syncope and sudden death in the absence of structural abnormalities of the heart. CPVT has now been recognized as a genetically determined arrhythmogenic disease, and its pathophysiological mechanisms are being progressively unveiled.

Clinical Manifestations

ELECTROCARDIOGRAPHIC CHARACTERISTICS. The resting ECG of patients with CPVT is unremarkable with the exception of a sinus bradycardia reported in some patients (Fig. 9-8). Physical activity and/or acute emotions are the specific triggers for arrhythmias. During graded exercise, CPVT patients typically and consistently develop ventricular ectopic beats at a "threshold" heart rate of 100 to 120 beats/min, followed by progressive worsening with increase in workload. If patients continue to exercise, the duration of nonsustained VT progressively increases and the arrhythmia can become sustained. A ventricular tachycardia with a 180-degree alternating QRS frontal plane axis on a beat-to-beat basis (i.e., the so-called *bidirectional VT*) is often the distinguishing presentation of CPVT (see Fig. 9-8), although some patients can also show irregular polymorphic VT. During exercise, several patients with CPVT also develop supraventricular arrhythmias such as runs of supraventricular tachycardia.

CARDIAC EVENTS AND CLINICAL MANIFESTATIONS. Syncope, triggered by exercise or acute emotion, is the typical symptom of CPVT. But sudden death or aborted cardiac arrest can be the first manifestation in approximately half of the patients. The mean age at the onset of symptoms is 12 years. Family history of juvenile (younger than 40 years of age) sudden death is reported in approximately 30 percent of cases. In 2002 we showed that CPVT is responsible for some unheralded cardiac arrests or sudden deaths occurring in subjects with apparently normal hearts and classified as idiopathic ventricular fibrillation (IVF), and other groups subsequently confirmed this finding.[43] Therefore the possibility of *RyR2* o r *CASQ2* mutations (see later) should be always considered among the causes of IVF occurring during exercise or in the setting of acute emotional stress (see Fig. 9-8). Untreated patients have a high risk of cardiac events (syncope or sudden death), as highlighted by natural history data showing that close to 80 percent of them experience at least one event before age 40 years.

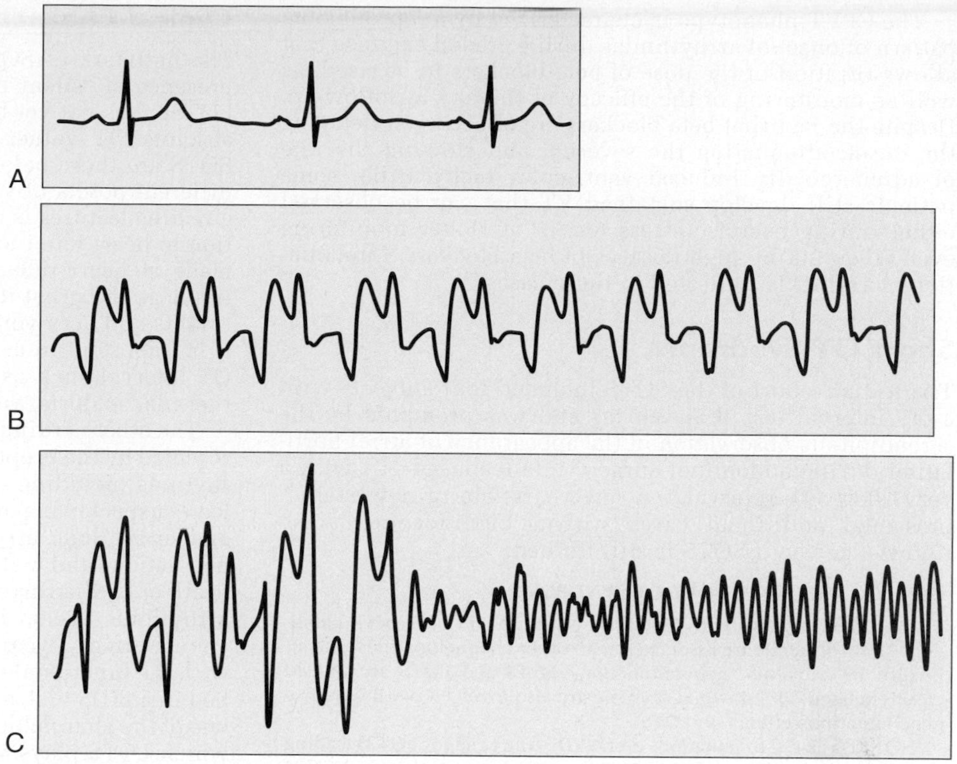

FIGURE 9–8 Electrocardiogram in catecholaminergic polymorphic ventricular tachycardia. **A,** Normal electrocardiogram at rest in a catecholaminergic polymorphic ventricular tachycardia patient. **B,** Example of a typical bidirectional ventricular tachycardia (VT) developing during exercise. **C,** Documentation of a bidirectional VT degeneration into VF in a patient resuscitated from cardiac arrest as the first manifestation of the disease.

GENETIC BASIS

Autosomal Dominant CPVT

Candidate gene screening based on a previous linkage mapping study[44] led Priori et al.[45] to the first identification of cardiac ryanodine receptor *(RyR2)* mutations in autosomal dominant CPVT.

RyR2 is a large tetrameric protein spanning sarcoplasmic reticulum membrane, in which it plays a major role in the regulation of intracellular calcium flux and excitation-contraction coupling. It is localized in close proximity with the L-type Ca2+ channels in the T-tubules, and it releases Ca^{2+} ions in response to Ca^{2+} entry through the L-type channels during phase 2 of the action potential. The identification of *RyR2* mutations in CPVT patients constitutes the first demonstration of the involvement of an intracellular ion channel in an inherited arrhythmia and points to the pivotal role of intracellular Ca^{2+} handling in arrhythmogenesis.[46] More than 60 *RyR2*-CPVT mutations have been reported in the literature, and several in vitro studies have shown that defective *RyR2* channels present uncontrolled Ca2+ leakage from SR to the cytosol that worsen on adrenergic activation.

Recently a CPVT transgenic mouse model harboring the R4496C mutation in the *RYR2* gene was developed. The knock-in mice present bidirectional VT on exposure to epinephrine and caffeine,[47] and myocytes isolated from their heart respond to beta adrenergic stimulation, developing delayed afterdepolarization (DADs) and triggered activity,[48] thus suggesting that this is likely to be the arrhythmogenic mechanism in CPVT patients.

Autosomal Recessive CPVT

In 2001 Lahat and associates[49] mapped an autosomal recessive CPVT trait in a 16-cM interval on chromosome 1p23-21. Subsequently, they identified *CASQ2* as the gene for this variant of CPVT. *CASQ2* encodes the cardiac isoform of calsequestrin. It serves as a major Ca^{2+} binding protein localized in the terminal cisternae of the sarcoplasmic reticulum, where it is physically and functionally bound to the *RyR2* channel. Few additional *CASQ2* mutations have been identified thereafter in patients of different ethnic backgrounds, suggesting that molecular screening of this gene is indicated when an autosomal recessive inheritance is compatible with the clinical presentation. *CASQ2* mutations disrupt sarcoplasmic reticulum Ca^{2+} storing and release functions via a reduced Ca^{2+} buffering capacity and a destabilization of the *CASQ2-RyR2* interaction at the level of the macromolecular complex formed by ryanodine receptor, calsequestrin, L-type Ca2+ channels and other regulatory proteins.[50,51]

Clinical Management

GENOTYPE-PHENOTYPE CORRELATION IN CATECHOLAMINERGIC POLYMORPHIC VENTRICULAR TACHYCARDIA. *RyR2* mutations are found in approximately 60 percent of CPVT patients, whereas *CASQ2* mutations are rare (1 to 2 percent). Thus the disease is genetically heterogeneous, and this lack of knowledge limits the definition of gene-specific therapeutic strategies and risk stratification schemes. Nonetheless, the high percentage of successfully genotyped patients makes worthwhile the genetic screening as a tool for presymptomatic diagnosis and primary prevention.

Some authors have suggested that the age of onset of the disease is delayed among patients not harboring *RyR2* genetic defects compared with *RyR2* mutation carriers and that resting heart rate is lower than normal in CPVT, particularly among *RyR2* mutation carriers.[43] Mild QT interval prolongation and the tendency to develop polymorphic instead of bidirectional VT among *CASQ2* mutation carriers has been suggested.

Therapy in Catecholaminergic Polymorphic Ventricular Tachycardia

Beta blockers are the drug of choice in all patients with clinical diagnosis of CPVT.[43] Furthermore, because sudden death may be the first manifestation of the disease, beta blockers are indicated in asymptomatic *RyR2* mutation carriers even in the absence of documented ventricular arrhythmias. Comparisons of effectiveness among different beta-blocking molecules are not available, but the experience reported in the published literature refers to patients treated with nadolol (1 to 3 mg/kg/day), propranolol (2 to 4 mg/kg/day) or metoprolol (1 to 3 mg/kg/day).

The CPVT phenotype is characterized by a reproducible pattern of onset of arrhythmias during graded exercise that allows titration of the dose of beta blockers to be used, as well as monitoring of the efficacy of therapy at follow-up. Despite the fact that beta blockers are effective in delaying the onset, attenuating the severity, and slowing the rate of adrenergically induced ventricular tachycardia, some patients still develop sustained VT that can be observed either during exercise stress test or at Holter monitoring even when taking high dosages of beta blockers. Implantation of an ICD is indicated in these cases.[43]

Short QT Syndrome

The initial report of the SQTS included four subjects with a QT interval less than 300 ms and was prompted by the serendipitous observation of the appearance of atrial fibrillation during abdominal surgery in a teenaged girl with a very short QT interval.[52] A few years later a new study[53] presented additional cases stirring significant interest. Knowledge about SQTS is still limited.

GENETIC BASIS OF SHORT QT SYNDROME

Three different genes with mutations causing SQTS have been identified. All three genes are associated with other channelopathies, and all involve K+ currents "gain-of-function." SQTS and LQTS are indeed closely related: all known SQTS gene are also involved, with opposite gene mutations effects, in LQTS.

SQT1 is related to mutations on *KCNH2* (the gene for LQT2) leading to increases in the IKr current.[54] SQT2 is related to mutations in *KCNQ1* (the gene for LQT1) leading to increases in the IKs current.[55] SQT3 is related to mutations in *KCNJ2* (the gene for the Andersen-Tawil syndrome) leading to increases in the IK1 current.[56]

Besides the apparently distinct shape of the T wave in SQT3,[56] characterized by an almost normal ascending phase and an impressively rapid terminal phase (Fig. 9-9), there are no distinctive features to suggest specific genotype-phenotype correlations in SQTS. However, this might just reflect the still scant existing knowledge.

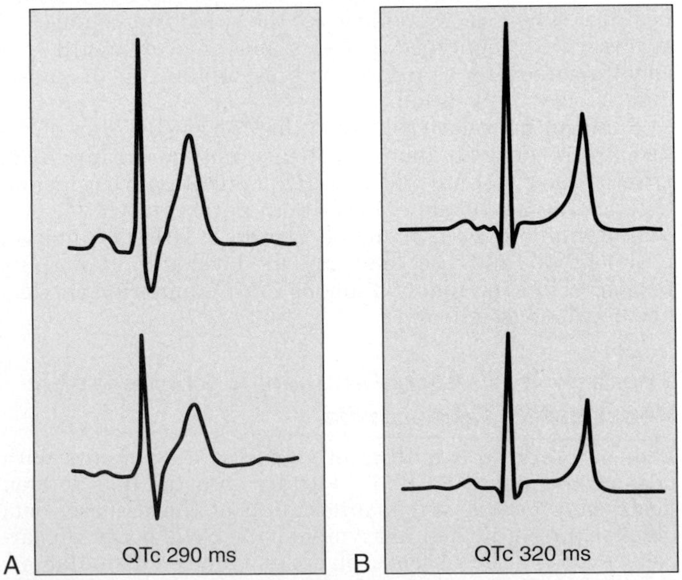

FIGURE 9–9 Electrocardiogram (ECG) in the short QT syndrome (SQTS). **A,** The ECG recorded in an SQTS patient with *KCNQ1* mutation (SQTS2). The "absence" of ST segment is evident. **B,** The peculiar T wave morphology of a patient with *KCNJ2* mutation *(SQTS3):* normal ST segment and extremely sharp descending limb of the T wave.

Clinical Characteristics

The hallmark of SQTS is a short QT interval. The likely presence of "silent mutation carriers," rather prevalent in LQTS6, has not yet been reported for SQTS. Currently, the absolute QT values considered as "strongly suggesting" SQTS are those below 300 to 320 ms, according to slightly different points of view.[57,58] However, as one of the distinguishing features is represented by an impaired QT adaptation to heart rate increases, these measurements should be made at heart rates below 80 beats/min.[58] An important implication is that it could be difficult to identify SQTS in infants and very young children. In the diagnostic process it is important to exclude the secondary causes of a short QT interval such as hypercalcemia, hyperkalemia, hyperthermia, acidosis, and digoxin therapy.

The other cardinal clinical manifestation of SQTS is represented by the propensity to both atrial and ventricular fast rhythms including fibrillation. Indeed, SQTS should be at least suspected in patients with a short QT interval (<350 ms) and either lone atrial fibrillation or primary ventricular fibrillation, and with a family history of sudden cardiac death or cardiac arrest or SIDS. Indeed, in addition to major arrhythmic events having been reported in three infants younger than 1 year of age,[53,59] recently a *KCNQ1* mutation with the functional effects typical for SQTS has been identified in a SIDS victim.[60] Thus SQTS should be considered as one of the channelopathies contributing to SIDS and among which LQTS plays a prominent role.[61] This concept is supported also by the recent identification of an infant with a *KCNQ1* mutation capable of shortening action potential duration, presenting with cardiac symptoms while still in utero and diagnosed as affected by SQTS after delivery by caesarean section.[62]

In the few patients who have undergone an electrophysiological study, the atrial and ventricular effective refractory periods were found to be short (mean between 140 and 150 ms). Moreover, almost all these patients had inducible ventricular fibrillation or flutter.

Clinical Management

Uncertainties still exist about the clinical management of SQTS, largely related to the small number of existing patients and to the limited follow-up.

Given the apparently high risk for sudden cardiac death and the lack of drugs with documented efficacy in preventing sudden cardiac death, the use of the ICD is recommended in secondary prevention of ventricular fibrillation. The ICD should be considered in selected patients for the primary prevention of ventricular fibrillation. The choice of when to use a prophylactic ICD remains a difficult one because there are no risk stratification parameters that allow identifying patients with increased risk of sudden death. Among the issues to be considered about deciding on the use of a prophylactic ICD is the concern generated by the report of inappropriate shocks due to T wave oversensing.[59]

The search for antiarrhythmic drug therapy, especially in infants and young children either as a bridge to the ICD or as an alternate modality of therapy, is progressing. Although sotalol, ibutilide, and flecainide all proved ineffective, quinidine has normalized the QT interval at resting heart rates in a small number of patients. These changes were accompanied by prolongation of the ventricular effective refractory periods.

REFERENCES

1. Priori SG, Aliot E, Blomstrom-Lundqvist C, et al: Update of the guidelines on sudden cardiac death of the European Society of Cardiology. Eur Heart J 24:13, 2003.

2. Survivors of out-of-hospital cardiac arrest with apparently normal heart. Need for definition and standardized clinical evaluation. Consensus Statement of the Joint Steering Committees of the Unexplained Cardiac Arrest Registry of Europe and of the Idiopathic Ventricular Fibrillation Registry of the United States. Circulation 95:265, 1997.
3. Schwartz PJ, Crotti L: Can a message from the dead save lives? J Am Coll Cardiol 49:247, 2007.

Long QT Syndrome

4. Schwartz PJ, Priori SG, Napolitano C: The Long QT Syndrome. *In* Zipes DP, Jalife J (eds): Cardiac Electrophysiology. From Cell to Bedside. 3rd ed. Philadelphia, WB Saunders, 2000, pp 597-615.
5. Schwartz PJ, Priori SG, Spazzolini C, et al: Genotype-phenotype correlation in the long-QT syndrome: Gene-specific triggers for life-threatening arrhythmias. Circulation 103:89-95, 2001.
6. Schwartz PJ, Priori SG, Bloise R, et al: Molecular diagnosis in a child with sudden infant death syndrome. Lancet 358:1342, 2001.
7. Arnestad M, Crotti L, Rognum TO, et al: Prevalence of long-QT syndrome gene variants in sudden infant death syndrome. Circulation 115:361, 2007.
8. Priori SG, Napolitano C, Schwartz PJ: Low penetrance in the long-QT syndrome: Clinical impact. Circulation 99:529, 1999.
9. Wang Q, Shen J, Splawski I, et al: SCN5A mutations associated with an inherited cardiac arrhythmia, long QT syndrome. Cell 80:805, 1995.
10. Curran ME, Splawski I, Timothy KW, et al: A molecular basis for cardiac arrhythmia: HERG mutations cause long QT syndrome. Cell 80:795, 1995.
11. Wang Q, Curran ME, Splawski I, et al: Positional cloning of a novel potassium channel gene: KVLQT1 mutations cause cardiac arrhythmias. Nat Genet 12:17, 1996.
12. Napolitano C, Priori SG, Schwartz PJ et al: Genetic testing in the long QT syndrome: Development and validation of an efficient approach to genotyping in clinical practice. JAMA 294:2975, 2005.
13. ACC/AHA/ESC 2006 Guidelines for the Management of Patients with Ventricular Arrhythmias and the Prevention of Sudden Cardiac Death. Europace 8:746, 2006.
14. Schwartz PJ, Periti M, Malliani A: The long Q-T syndrome. Am Heart J 89:378, 1975.
15. Moss AJ, Zareba W, Hall WJ, et al: Effectiveness and limitations of beta-blocker therapy in congenital long-QT syndrome. Circulation 101:616, 2000.
16. Priori SG, Napolitano C, Schwartz PJ, et al: Association of long QT syndrome loci and cardiac events among patients treated with beta-blockers. JAMA 292:1341, 2004.
17. Priori SG, Schwartz PJ, Napolitano C, et al: Risk stratification in the long-QT syndrome. N Engl J Med 348:1866, 2003.
18. Schwartz PJ, Priori SG, Cerrone M, et al: Left cardiac sympathetic denervation in the management of high-risk patients affected by the Long-QT syndrome. Circulation 109:1826, 2004.
19. Schwartz PJ, Priori SG, Locati EH, et al: Long QT syndrome patients with mutations of the SCN5A and HERG genes have differential responses to Na+ channel blockade and to increases in heart rate. Implications for gene-specific therapy. Circulation 92:3381, 1995.
20. Priori SG, Napolitano C: Role of genetic analyses in cardiology: Part I: Mendelian diseases: Cardiac channelopathies. Circulation 113:1130, 2006.
21. Schwartz PJ: The congenital long QT syndromes from genotype to phenotype: Clinical implications. J Interv Cardiol 259:39, 2006.
22. Zhang L, Timothy KW, Vincent GM et al: Spectrum of ST-T-wave patterns and repolarization parameters in congenital long-QT syndrome: ECG findings identify genotypes. Circulation 2000; 102:2849-2855.
23. Moss AJ, Robinson JL, Gessman L, et al. Comparison of clinical and genetic variables of cardiac events associated with loud noise versus swimming among subjects with the long QT syndrome. Am J Cardiol 84:876, 1999.
24. Schwartz PJ, Priori SG: Long QT syndrome—phenotype genotype considerations. *In* Zipes DP, Jalife J (eds): Cardiac Electrophysiology—4th ed. Philadelphia, Elsevier, 2004, pp 651-667.
25. Moss AJ, Zareba W, Kaufman ES, et al: Increased risk of arrhythmic events in long-QT syndrome with mutations in the pore region of the human ether-a-go-go-related gene potassium channel. Circulation 105:794, 2002.
26. Schwartz PJ, Spazzolini C, Crotti L, et al: The Jervell and Lange-Nielsen syndrome: Natural history, molecular basis, and clinical outcome. Circulation 113:783, 2006.

Brugada Syndrome

27. Antzelevitch C, Brugada P, Borggrefe M, et al: Brugada syndrome. Report of the Second Consensus Conference. Endorsed by the Heart Rhythm Society and the European Heart Rhythm Association. Circulation 111:659, 2005.
28. Chen Q, Kirsch GE, Zhang D, et al: Genetic basis and molecular mechanism for idiopathic ventricular fibrillation. Nature 392:293, 1998.
29. Bezzina C, Veldkamp MW, van Den Berg MP, et al: A single $Na^{(+)}$ channel mutation causing both long-QT and Brugada syndromes. Circ Res 85:1206, 1999.
30. Grant AO, Carboni MP, Neplioueva V, et al: Long QT syndrome, Brugada syndrome, and conduction system disease are linked to a single sodium channel mutation. J Clin Invest 110:1201, 2002.
31. Olson TM, Michels VV, Ballew JD, et al: Sodium channel mutations and susceptibility to heart failure and atrial fibrillation. JAMA 293:447, 2005.
32. Martini B, Nava A, Canciani B, et al: Right bundle branch block, persistent ST segment elevation and sudden cardiac death. J Am Coll Cardiol 22:633, 1993.
33. Frustaci A, Priori SG, Pieroni M, et al: Cardiac histological substrate in patients with clinical phenotype of Brugada syndrome. Circulation 112:3680, 2005.
34. London B, Shamarendra S, Michalec M, et al: A mutation in the glycerol-3-phosphate dehydrogenase 1-like gene (GPD1L) causes Brugada syndrome. Heart Rhythm 3 (abstr suppl): S32. 2006.
35. Priori SG, Napolitano C, Gasparini M, et al: Natural history of Brugada syndrome. Insights for risk stratification and management. Circulation 105:1342, 2002.
36. Eckardt L, Probst V, Smits JP, et al: Long-term prognosis of individuals with right precordial ST-segment-elevation Brugada syndrome. Circulation 111:257, 2005.
37. Priori SG, Napolitano C: Should patients with an asymptomatic Brugada electrocardiogram undergo pharmacological and electrophysiological testing? Circulation 112:279, 2005.
38. Brugada P, Brugada R, Brugada J, et al: Should patients with an asymptomatic Brugada electrocardiogram undergo pharmacological and electrophysiological testing? Circulation 112:279, 2005.
39. Eckardt L, Kirchhof P, Schulze-Bahr E, et al: Electrophysiologic investigation in Brugada syndrome; yield of programmed ventricular stimulation at two ventricular sites with up to three premature beats. Eur Heart J 23:1394, 2002.
40. Gasparini M, Priori SG, Mantica M, et al: Programmed electrical stimulation in Brugada syndrome: How reproducible are the results? J Cardiovasc Electrophysiol 13:880, 2002.

Catecholaminergic Polymorphic Ventricular Tachycardia

41. Coumel P, Fidelle J, Lucet V, et al: Catecholaminergic-induced severe ventricular arrhythmias with Adams-Stokes syndrome in children: Report of four cases. Br Heart J 40:28, 1978.
42. Leenhardt A, Lucet V, Denjoy I, et al: Catecholaminergic polymorphic ventricular tachycardia in children. A 7-year follow-up of 21 patients. Circulation 91:1512, 1995.
43. Priori SG, Napolitano C, Memmi M, et al: Clinical and molecular characterization of patients with catecholaminergic polymorphic ventricular tachycardia. Circulation 106:69, 2002.
44. Swan H, Piippo K, Viitasalo M, et al: Arrhythmic disorder mapped to chromosome 1q42-q43 causes malignant polymorphic ventricular tachycardia in structurally normal hearts. J Am Coll Cardiol 34:2035, 1999.
45. Priori SG, Napolitano C, Tiso N, et al: Mutations in the cardiac ryanodine receptor gene *(hRyR2)* underlie catecholaminergic polymorphic ventricular tachycardia. Circulation 103:196, 2001.
46. Priori SG, Napolitano C: Cardiac and skeletal muscle disorders caused by mutations in the intracellular Ca^{2+} release channels. J Clin Invest 115:2033, 2005.
47. Cerrone M, Colombi B, Santoro M, et al: Bidirectional ventricular tachycardia and fibrillation elicited in a knock-in mouse model carrier of a mutation in the cardiac ryanodine receptor *(RyR2)*. Circ Res 96:e77, 2005.
48. Liu N, Colombi B, Memmi M, et al: Arrhythmogenesis in catecholaminergic polymorphic ventricular tachycardia: Insights from a RyR2 R4496C knock-in mouse model. Circ Res 99:292, 2006.
49. Lahat H, Pras E, Olender T, et al: A missense mutation in a highly conserved region of CASQ2 is associated with autosomal recessive catecholamine-induced polymorphic ventricular tachycardia in Bedouin families from Israel. Am J Hum Genet 69:1378, 2001.
50. Viatchenko-Karpinski S, Terentyev D, Gyorke I, et al: Abnormal calcium signaling and sudden cardiac death associated with mutation of calsequestrin. Circ Res 94:471, 2004.
51. Terentyev D, Nori A, Santoro M, et al: Abnormal interactions of calsequestrin with the ryanodine receptor calcium release channel complex linked to exercise-induced sudden cardiac death. Circ Res 98:1151, 2006.

Short QT Syndrome

52. Gussak I, Brugada P, Brugada J, et al: Idiopathic short QT interval: A new clinical syndrome? Cardiology 94:99, 2000.
53. Gaita F, Giustetto C, Bianchi F, et al: Short QT syndrome: A familial cause of sudden death. Circulation 108:965, 2003.
54. Brugada R, Hong K, Dumaine R, et al: Sudden death associated with short-QT syndrome linked to mutations in HERG. Circulation 109:30, 2004.
55. Bellocq C, van Ginneken AC, Bezzina CR, et al: Mutation in the *KCNQ1* gene leading to the short QT-interval syndrome. Circulation 109:2394, 2004.
56. Priori SG, Pandit SV, Rivolta I, et al: A novel form of short QT syndrome (SQT3) is caused by a mutation in the *KCNJ2* gene. Circ Res 96:800, 2005.
57. Bjerregaard P, Gussak I: Short QT syndrome: Mechanisms, diagnosis and treatment. Nat Clin Pract 2:84, 2005.
58. Borggrefe M, Wolpert C, Antzelevitch C, et al: Short QT syndrome. Genotype-phenotype correlations. J Electrocardiol 38(4 suppl):75, 2005.
59. Schimpf R, Wolpert C, Gaita F, et al: Short QT syndrome. Cardiovasc Res 67:357, 2005.
60. Rhodes TE, Crotti L, Arnestad M, et al: Gain of function KCNQ1 mutation associated with sudden infant death syndrome. Heart Rhythm 3(abstr suppl):S2, 2006.
61. Schwartz PJ, Stramba-Badiale M: Prolonged repolarization and sudden infant death syndrome. *In* Zipes DP, Jalife J (eds): Cardiac Electrophysiology. From Cell to Bedside. 4th ed. Philadelphia, Saunders, 2004, pp 711-719.
62. Hong K, Bjerregaard P, Gussak I, et al: Short QT syndrome and atrial fibrillation caused by mutation in KCNH2. J Cardiovasc Electrophysiol 16:394, 2005.

CHAPTER 10

Genetic Factors in Myocardial Disease

Jonathan G. Seidman, Reed E. Pyeritz, and Christine E. Seidman

Application of molecular technologies to the study of myocardial diseases illustrates the considerable role for genetics in cardiac pathologies. Over the past 20 years, scores of genes and hundreds of mutations have been discovered that cause inherited and de novo (or sporadic) cardiomyopathies, primary cardiac arrhythmias, and congenital malformations. In addition to delineating causes for previously enigmatic cardiac diseases, molecular information provides novel insights about pathophysiology and suggests a rational and rigorous format for disease classification. In addition. genetic data can facilitate precise clinical diagnosis and preclinical recognition of disease risk. Beyond diagnosis, understanding the genetic diversity of heart diseases provides opportunities to consider whether natural history and clinical expressivity reflect, in part, differences in molecular cause. Of greater significance is the future promise that precise genetic knowledge can fuel development of novel and highly specific therapeutics to diminish or prevent cardiovascular genetic disease.

The opportunities for harnessing genetic insights to improve medical diagnosis, and to affect management and therapy, underpin the rationale for the establishment of molecular diagnostic laboratories. Although widely used in other medical fields, such as oncology, the potential for molecular genetics to help bring about advances in cardiovascular medicine is equally great. This chapter discusses major genetic advances in specific myocardial diseases, emphasizing contributions to adult cardiology, and outlines future expectations for this nascent field. See Chapter 8 for a review of the principles of human molecular genetics. See Chapter 10 Online Supplement on the website for additional detail regarding genetics of myocardial disease.

GENETIC CAUSES OF CARDIOMYOPATHY

Abnormal function triggers ventricular remodeling in response to various diverse stimuli, including gene mutations. Hypertrophic cardiomyopathy (HCM), dilated cardiomyopathy (DCM), and arrhythmogenic right ventricular dysplasia (ARVD), previously deemed idiopathic disorders, are now known to reflect human gene mutations that arise de novo and cause sporadic disease or inherited autosomal dominant disease. Similar to congenital heart disease gene defects, cardiomyopathy mutations are present at the time of conception, yet take years or even decades to evoke pathology. Age-related penetrance (the likelihood of clinical manifestations in gene carriers) of cardiomyopathy confounds early clinical recognition of individuals at risk for unexpected life-threatening arrhythmias and thromboembolic events that accompany these diseases. Discovery of a genetic cause overcomes this clinical conundrum. Identification of a molecular cause also provides a rigorous framework for classifying disorders with heterogeneous clinical manifestations and outcomes. Knowledge of the precise genetic cause of a cardiomyopathy can predict longitudinal course and foster strategies to prevent or diminish disease-related complications.

Gene mutations that cause adult-onset heart disease produce uniform clinical expression, unlike congenital heart disease genes. Whereas family members who share an identical cardiomyopathy mutation develop the same clinical phenotype, such as DCM, HCM, or ARVD, the same mutation in the cardiac transcription factor *NKX2-5* can cause a range of malformations, from ostium secundum defect to tetralogy of Fallot in mutation carriers. The diverse structural lesions produced by congenital heart disease genes may indicate that the encoded proteins function in global developmental processes. In contrast, cardiomyopathy gene mutations alter structural proteins with highly specialized functions in contraction, force transmission, or cell-cell communication. The degree to which a particular biophysical function is selectively altered by mutation may account for the extent of pathological remodeling that subsequently ensues. Although detailed consideration of the pathophysiology of cardiomyopathies appears in other chapters, the following sections examine molecular causes of cardiomyopathies and the relevance of genetics to diagnosis and management.

Cardiac Hypertrophy

Unexplained ventricular hypertrophy is estimated to occur in 1 in 500 individuals and is usually diagnosed by noninvasive imaging studies.[1] An echocardiographic finding of hypertrophy that occurs in the absence underlying hypertension or valvular heart disease can prompt diagnosis of HCM (see Chap. 65). However, the molecular causes of cardiac hypertrophy indicate that this clinical diagnosis can be parsed into two subtypes, reflecting mutations in genes encoding protein components of the sarcomere and genes encoding proteins that participate in myocyte metabolism. The distinct clinical manifestations, histopathology, and disease mechanisms[2] of these different classes of gene mutations that cause hypertrophy provides rationale for a molecular classification (Table 10-1).

Hypertrophic Cardiomyopathy: Sarcomere Mutations

Inherited as an autosomal dominant trait, HCM is caused by mutation in genes that encode proteins constituents of the cardiac sarcomere.[3] Over 300 mutations, which are often unique to individual HCM families, have been described (see http://cardiogenomics.med.harvard.edu).[4] Most mutations occur in genes that encode beta–cardiac myosin heavy chain (MHC;

TABLE 10–1 Gene Mutations in Cardiac Hypertrophy

Locus	Symbol	Name	Function
1q32	*TNNT2*	Cardiac troponin T	Sarcomere
2q31	*TTN*	Titin	Sarcomere
3p21	*MYL3*	Essential myosin light chain	Sarcomere
3p21-p14	*TNNC1*	Cardiac troponin C	Sarcomere
11p11.2	*MYBPC3*	Cardiac myosin binding protein C	Sarcomere
12q23-q24	*MYL2*	Regulatory myosin light chain	Sarcomere
14q12	*MYH7*	Beta-myosin heavy chain	Sarcomere
14q12	*MYH6*	Alpha-myosin heavy chain	Sarcomere
15q14	*ACTC*	Cardiac actin	Sarcomere
15q22	*TPM1*	Alpha-tropomyosin	Sarcomere
19p13.2	*TNNI3*	Cardiac troponin I	Sarcomere
7q36	*PRKAG2*	Protein kinase, AMP-activated, noncatalytic, gamma-2	Metabolism
Xq22	*GLA*	Alpha-galactosidase A	Lysosome, metabolism
Xq24	*LAMP2*	Lysosome-associated membrane protein B	Lysosome, metabolism

AMP = adenosine monophosphate.

MYH7), cardiac myosin binding protein C (*MYBPC3*), cardiac troponin I (*TNNI3*), or cardiac troponin T (*TNNT2*). Less commonly, HCM mutations occur in alpha-tropomyosin (*TPM1*), actin (*ACTC*), regulatory myosin light chain (*MYL2*), essential myosin light chain (*MYL3*), or titin (*TTN*). HCM mutations usually are missense mutations and result in the substitution of one amino acid for the normal residue. *MYBPC3* mutations can also be small deletions, insertions, or stop codons, or affect splice sites. HCM mutant proteins are incorporated into cardiac myofilaments and perturb biophysical functions that trigger hypertrophic remodeling. The impact of these mutations on sarcomere function[5-7] contributes in part to the clinical heterogeneity and affects the age of onset of hypertrophy, natural history, sudden death and, in rare cases, hypertrophic morphology.

First-degree family members of HCM patients have a substantial risk (50 percent) for inheriting the mutation and disease. Because HCM mutations cause latent or subtle disease in childhood and adolescence, at-risk individuals require longitudinal clinical assessment of disease status.[8] Discovery of molecular cause and the advent of Clinical Laboratory Improvement Amendment (CLIA)–approved gene-based HCM diagnosis provide efficient and accurate mutation status in individuals of any age (see www.genetests.org and www.hpcgg.org/LMM). Gene-based diagnosis typically reveals a single mutation in HCM patients, although two disease-causing mutations in the same or a different sarcomere protein gene are sometimes found in individuals with particularly severe disease. Genetic diagnosis of family members focuses clinical follow-up only in mutation carriers and alleviates the need for cardiac studies in individuals free of mutations.[9] Young mutation carriers who show no ventricular hypertrophy can demonstrate diastolic abnormalities by Doppler tissue imaging[10]; these results indicate that altered diastolic function is not a secondary consequence in HCM, but rather a primary and early manifestation of sarcomere dysfunction.

MUTATIONS IN THICK-FILAMENT PROTEINS. Missense mutations in beta–cardiac MHC (encoded by *MYH7* on chromosome 14) are prevalent causes of HCM and account for approximately 40 percent of cases.[4,11] Abundantly expressed in the adult heart, beta-MHC accounts for 70 percent of total ventricular myosin. A 200,000-kDa protein, beta-MHC contains an amino terminal globular head that interacts with actin to produce force, a carboxyl terminal rod, and a hinge region between these two domains. HCM mutations occur throughout the head domain and hinge region; HCM mutations in the rod are uncommon.

The alpha isoform of MHC (encoded by *MYH6* on chromosome 14) is expressed in the atria and ventricles during fetal development, but adult ventricular expression is markedly less than for the predominant beta isoform. Mutations in alpha-MHC (*MYH6*) are associated with sporadic cases of older onset HCH. Markedly lower expression of the alpha-MHC isoform in the adult ventricle may account for the delayed onset of hypertrophy.

Clinical manifestation of disease produced by beta-MHC mutations is generally overt, with substantial left ventricular hypertrophy (LVH) apparent by late adolescence. Although the clinical course associated with beta-MHC and other sarcomere protein gene mutations is heterogeneous, an increased risk of sudden death (Arg403Gln) and development of end-stage heart failure (Arg719Trp) is characteristic of particular defects. Rare individuals with homozygous *MYH7* mutations have particularly severe hypertrophy. *MYH7* mutations that result in a change in the charge of the substituted amino acid may cause more severe disease as a result of dramatic effects on protein structure and function. However, determinants of disease expression and prognosis are likely multifactorial and involve gene-gene and gene-environment interactions.[12]

Insights into the pathogenetic mechanisms of beta-MHC mutations have come from the study of animal models engineered to carry mutations.[13] Mice and rabbits with HCM mutations recapitulate the clinical features of human disease with cardiac hypertrophy, myocyte disarray, and diastolic dysfunction. Investigations of the biophysical properties of a mouse carrying HCM mutation Arg403Gln demonstrated unexpected enhanced myosin functions, including actin-activated ATPase activity, force generation and velocity of actin translocation along myosin. These data imply that human mutations produce a fundamental gain of myosin function, which generates a stimulus for hypertrophic remodeling.

Signal transduction pathways activated in mouse models have highlighted the important role of intracellular calcium in linking alterations of muscle contraction caused by myosin mutation with myocyte growth. Changes in calcium cycling by mutant sarcomeres occur early and in advance of histopathology as a result of diminished levels of calcium transport proteins such as calsequestrin and ryanodine receptors, with ultimate depletion of sarcoplasmic reticulum (SR) Ca^{2+} levels.[14] Treatment of mutant mice with diltiazem blunted this effect and restored normal calcium cycling between the sarcoplasmic reticulum and the cytoplasm, thereby interrupting the signals leading to hypertrophic remodeling. Fundamental dysregulation of calcium handling caused by myosin mutations may in part mediate the hypertrophic response of the myocyte, perhaps via the calcium–calmodulin-dependent kinase II (CaM kinase II) and histone deacetylase-4 (HDCA4) signaling pathway.[15]

Pharmacological studies have also been performed targeting pathways of myocardial fibrosis in HCM models.[16-18] Transgenic rabbits that express a beta-MHC mutation showed regression of hypertrophy and fibrosis and improved cardiac function when treated with the 3-hydroxy-3-methylglutaryl coenzyme A (HMG-CoA) reductase inhibitor, simvastatin or atorvastatin, effects attributable to the reduction of activation of the Ras- and mitogen-activated protein kinase (MAPK) pathway.

Mouse models of HCM have also been studied to assess factors that influence arrhythmia vulnerability in HCM. Myocardial disarray and fibrosis, characteristic pathological findings in HCM, have been suggested as factors that increase susceptibility to ventricular arrhythmias and sudden death risk. However, no correlation between disarray or fibrosis and arrhythmic vulnerability was found in analyses of a mouse model for HCM. In contrast, hypertrophy and increased contractility correlated with susceptibility to induced arrhythmias.[19] These results suggest that therapeutic approaches that mitigate myocyte growth in HCM may also attenuate the risk for cardiac arrhythmia.

Cardiac myosin binding protein-C (MyBPC), a 137-kDa protein encoded by *MYBPC3* on chromosome 11, provides structural support to the sarcomere by binding myosin heavy chain[20] and titin (see later) and modulates myosin ATPase activity and cardiac contractility in response to adrenergic stimulation. Missense, splice site, and deletion-insertion mutations in MyBPC collectively account for approximately 40 percent of cases of HCM.[4,11] Clinical expression of HCM is generally more mild and survival better with a MyBPC mutation than with a beta-MHC mutation. In significant subsets of individuals with MyBPC mutations, clinically apparent LVH is delayed until age 50 years or above. Consistent with this observation, there is an association between older onset HCM and mutations in MyBPC.

Mice engineered to express truncated MyBPC recapitulate human HCM,[13] with late-onset cardiac hypertrophy, myofibrillar disarray, and fibrosis. Mutant mice are not susceptible to arrhythmias, unlike HCM mice with myosin mutations, a result that underscores the importance of genotype in arrhythmic vulnerability. When truncated MyBPC protein is replaced in mice with MyBPC that cannot undergo phosphorylation in response to physiological signals, mice still develop HCM.[21] These data suggest that normal cardiac function requires MyBPC phosphorylation.

Mutations in the giant 3-kDa titin molecule, encoded by the *TTN* gene on chromosome 2, cause HCM.[22] Spanning the sarcomere from the Z-disc to the M-line, titin probably assembles contractile filaments and provides elasticity through serial spring-like elements. The considerable costs associated with genetic analyses of this huge gene have impeded comprehensive analyses in the HCM population. The few *TTN* mutations reported in HCM[23] have produced phenotypes indistinguishable from other sarcomere gene mutations.

The regulatory (encoded by *MYL2*) and essential (encoded by *MYL3*) myosin light chains belong to the EF hand superfamily of proteins with a helix-loop-helix motif that help determine the speed and force of actomyosin sliding by interacting with the head-rod junction of myosin heavy chains.[5] Mutations in myosin light chains are rarely genetic causes of HCM, accounting for less than 5 percent of cases of the disease.[24] One essential myosin light chain mutation (Met149Val) is associated with a distinctive HCM morphology, midcavitary hypertrophy associated with hemodynamic obstruction. Essential myosin light chain mutations may distort the stretch-activated response, an intrinsic property of muscle that results in oscillatory power and regional contraction properties of the heart that are particularly important for papillary muscle functions.

MUTATIONS IN THIN-FILAMENT PROTEIN. Approximately 5 percent of HCM is thought to be attributable to cardiac troponin T (cTnT) mutations.[11,25] Encoded by *TNNT2* on chromosome 1, cTnT is a 36- to 39-kDa amino acid peptide that links the troponin complex to alpha-tropomyosin and functions as a key regulator of contractile function. Several distinct isoforms are expressed in cardiac tissue via alternative splicing of 16 exons. Historically, the clinical phenotype of cTnT mutations has been characterized as modest hypertrophy,[12] but with increased risk of sudden death. Additional cTnT mutations are associated with better long-term survival. Rarely, homozygous cTnT mutations have been identified in consanguineous families. Doubling the dose of mutant cTnT peptide has markedly increased sudden death in children with homozygous mutations.

Transgenic mice that express HCM cTnT mutations[6] recapitulate human HCM phenotypes and provide evidence that like myosin mutations, these increase force and ATP consumption. Although cTnT mutant mice developed only modest hypertrophy, myocardial fibrosis, collagen and transforming growth factor-beta 1 (TGF-β1) and cardiac aldosterone expression is increased. Treatment with the angiotensin receptor-1 inhibitor losartan, the mineralocorticoid receptor antagonist spironolactone, or the antioxidant *N*-acetylcysteine reduced myocardial fibrosis. These results implicate the activation of multiple profibrotic molecules in HCM.

Cardiac troponin I (cTnI) missense mutations are increasingly recognized as causes of HCM.[26,27] The cardiac-specific isoform of troponin I (encoded by *TNNI3* on chromosome 19) is a 27- to 31-kDa protein that functions as the inhibitory subunit of the troponin complex, reducing actin-myosin interaction. Initial clinical findings reported with cTnI defects have suggested a greater predisposition for apical hypertrophy than occurs with other HCM genes. However, morphological manifestations associated with larger numbers of *TNNI3* mutations indicate a range of morphological phenotypes, although restrictive physiology may be particularly common.

Mutations in alpha-cardiac actin are rare causes of HCM. Encoded by the *ACTC* gene on chromosome 15, alpha-cardiac actin is a 41-kDa protein. Human mutations are clustered in proximity to a putative myosin binding site and may alter protein folding. The clinical phenotype of *ACTC* mutation is mild with respect to degree of hypertrophy and incidence of sudden death. Most *ACTC* mutations produce classic HCM morphologies, but a Glu101Lys missense mutation identified in multiple affected families uniformly caused apical hypertrophy.[24] Although the mechanisms for selective apical remodeling are unknown, *ACTC* Glu101Lys, like essential myosin light chain mutations, may particularly affect stretch activation responses.

Mutations in *TPM1* on chromosome 15 alter alpha-tropomyosin and account for a small proportion of HCM (less than 5 percent) in the general population.[11] These defects are prevalent in Finland because of a founding mutation.[28] Clinical phenotypes of HCM caused by *TPM1* mutations include variable degrees of hypertrophy and relatively good survival. Although alpha-tropomyosin protein is found in fast skeletal and cardiac muscle, disease is restricted to the heart. The lack of skeletal myopathy in *TPM1* mutations may indicate that HCM mutations occur in a domain of the molecule that interacts with the cardiac-specific isoform of cTnT. Alterations in calcium sensitivity may also play a role in the tissue specificity of *TPM1* mutations.

Cardiac Hypertrophy Caused by Metabolic Gene Mutations

Cardiac hypertrophy occurs from mutations in genes encoding metabolic proteins.[2] Prior to the elucidation of this distinct genetic cause, patients with these mutations were mistakenly classified as having HCM. Disarray and cardiac fibrosis are protean findings of sarcomeric protein gene mutations, but these findings are notably absent in metabolic cardiomyopathies. Histopathological studies of metabolic cardiomyopathies have shown myocyte-filled vacuoles that contain glycogen (*PRKAG2* mutations) or lysosomal remnants (*LAMP2* mutations[2]). With the distinct clinical course of metabolic cardiomyopathies and X-linked inheritance of *LAMP* mutations, accurate diagnosis of these disorders is imperative. Gene-based diagnosis is available in CLIA-approved molecular laboratories.

LYSOSOMAL PROTEIN MUTATIONS

Cardiac Fabry Disease. Mutation of the lysosomal hydrolase alpha-galactosidase A protein, encoded by *GLA* on chromosome X, causes Fabry disease. Although systemic manifestations include nephropathy, sensorineural deafness, skin lesions, and autonomic dysfunction, Fabry disease affects and can be limited to the heart.[29] Symptoms include angina, exercise intolerance, and palpitations. Concentric cardiac hypertrophy is found with progressive electrophysiological deficits. The duration (shortening) of the PR interval may indicate the severity of cardiac disease. Missense and splice site *GLA* mutations reduce enzymatic activities and increase cardiac globotriaosylceramide levels. Diagnosis should prompt enzyme replacement therapy with recombinant alpha-galactosidase A administration. Enzyme replacement is associated with reduction in cardiac hypertrophy and normalization of cardiac electrophysiology.

Cardiac Danon Disease. Mutation in the X-linked lysosome-associated membrane protein (*LAMP2*) causes Danon disease, a multisystem disorder with neurological, skeletal and heart muscle, and hepatic involvement or predominantly marked ventricular hypertrophy with mild systemic disease.[2,30] *LAMP2* mutations are clinically distinguished from HCM by male predominance and early onset, typically during childhood. The electrocardiogram shows markedly increased voltage with ventricular preexcitation, and echocardiograms demonstrate massive concentric hypertrophy. *LAMP2* cardiomyopathy is associated with frequent ventricular arrhythmias that can become refractory to medical management. Cardiac dysfunction is progressive and may prompt consideration of transplantation, albeit with thorough consideration of hepatic involvement. Arrhythmias and heart failure account for the shortened life expectancy in most patients. Affected males often die during the second decade of life; survival in females is better but may be complicated by heart failure.[2]

LAMP2 mutations produce a functionally null allele and resultant accumulation of autophagic vacuoles in the tissues of affected males.[31] Female carriers have half-normal *LAMP2* levels and do not exhibit systemic disease, although some increase in adult-onset heart failure has been reported. Rarely, massive cardiac hypertrophy occurs in females with *LAMP2* mutation, presumably because of the unfortunate inactivation of the normal X chromosome, with resultant *LAMP2* deficiency. The mechanisms by which deficiency in lysosomal proteins causes hypertrophy and electrophysiological dysfunction are incompletely understood, but the profound consequences of these mutations indicate critical roles for lysosomes in the heart.

GLYCOGEN STORAGE CARDIOMYOPATHY. Genetic studies of families and sporadic cases of unexplained LVH with conduction abnormalities (e.g., progressive atrioventricular block, atrial fibrillation, ventricular preexcitation–Wolff-Parkinson-White syndrome) have led to the identification of a glycogen cardiomyopathy caused by mutations in the $gamma_2$ regulatory subunit (*PRKAG2*) of adenosine monophosphate–activated protein kinase (AMPK).[32] In addition to cardiac hypertrophy, ventricular preexcitation typically occurs early and causes symptoms. Progressive conduction disease occurs with increasing age, necessitating permanent pacemaker implantation in 30 percent of affected individuals. Conduction system disease helps discriminate *PRKAG2* cardiomyopathy from HCM caused by sarcomere protein gene mutations. Severe clinical outcomes occur in some patients with *PRKAG2* mutations, including progression to end-stage heart failure or transplantation and sudden cardiac death.

AMPK is an energy sensor that is activated under conditions of energy depletion and alters substrate uptake, activation of glucose transport, stimulation of beta oxidation of fatty acids, inactivation of cholesterol synthesis, inhibition of creatine kinase, and transcriptional regulation of several genes.[33] *PRKAG2* mutations result in increased AMPK activity and glycogen accumulation. Hypertrophied myocytes contain vacuoles filled with glycogen and glycogen-protein complexes (amylopectin).[34] Because the $gamma_2$ subunit is expressed solely in the heart, *PRKAG2* mutations cause only a glycogen cardiomyopathy without the systemic manifestations found in *GAA* and *LAMP2* mutations.

Mouse models of *PRKAG2* mutations provide insight into the pathogenesis.[13] Transgenic expression of Asn488Ile mutation has demonstrated elevated AMPK activity, massive glycogen deposition in cardiac myocytes, approximately 30-fold above normal, marked left ventricular hypertrophy, ventricular preexcitation, and sinus node dysfunction. Aged Asn488Ile transgenic mice develop heart failure, similar to what is seen in human patients. Disruption of the annulus fibrosis by glycogen-filled myocytes was the anatomical substrate for preexcitation in *PRKAG2* mutant mice, which may account for electrophysiological defects in this and other human glycogen cardiomyopathies. Normalization of cardiac structure, function, and electrophysiology occurs in *PRKAG2* mutant mice that coexpress an inactivating mutation in the $alpha_2$ subunit of AMPK. Taken together, these data indicate that *PRKAG2* mutations produce a gain of function in the catalytic $alpha_2$ subunit of AMPK.

Cardiac Dilation

The prevalence of idiopathic dilated cardiomyopathy (DCM) is about double that of the hypertrophic form, or about 2 to 8 per 100,000. Approximately half of patients who are evaluated for unexplained DCM are left with the "idiopathic" designation. Clinical studies of first-degree relatives of patients with idiopathic DCM have suggested a familial component in 30 to 50 percent of cases. Most families (85 percent) show autosomal dominant inheritance, whereas others indicate recessive transmission and X-linked inheritance.[18]

Human DCM mutations affect proteins that participate in a wide range of myocyte functions, including force generation and transmission, metabolism, calcium homeostasis, and transcriptional regulation.[1] Although many disease genes are known, other human mutations are mapped to a chromosome region, but the causal gene remains undefined. This considerable genetic diversity of DCM limits the usefulness of selective gene-based diagnosis. Analysis of some DCM genes is available in CLIA-approved laboratories (see www.genetests.org and www.hpcgg.org/LMM); DNA studies are most informative when clinical manifestations implicate the involvement of particular genes. As with HCM mutations, identification of a DCM gene mutation in a family can predict disease development in at-risk relatives. Based on clinical manifestations of DCM gene mutations, these disorders fall into categories of isolated DCM and DCM that occurs with extracardiac manifestations (Table 10-2). Gene

TABLE 10–2 Gene Mutations and Loci in Cardiac Dilation

Locus	Symbol	Name	Additional Phenotype
1q32	*TNNT2*	Cardiac troponin T	None
1q42-q43	ACTN2	Alpha-actinin	
2q31	*TTN*	Titin	None
6q12-q16	*CMD1K*	Unknown	None
6q22.1	*PLN*	Phospholamban	None
9q13-q22	*CMD1B*	Unknown	None
9q22-q31	Unknown	Unknown	None
10 q 22.2-q23.3	*LDBD2*	Cipher ZASP	Left ventricular noncompaction
10q22.3-q23.2	*LDB3*		
11p11.2	*MYBPC3*	Cardiac myosin binding protein C	None
11p15.1	*CLP (CSRP3)*	Cardiac muscle LIM protein	None
12p12.1	ABCC9	ATP-sensitive K channel	None
14q12	*MYH7*	Beta-myosin heavy chain	None
15q14	*ACTC*	Cardiac actin	None
15q22	*TPM1*	Alpha-tropomyosin	None
16p11	*CTF1*	Cardiotrophin 1	None
1p1-q21	*LMNA*	Lamin A/C	Conduction disease, skeletal myopathy
2q14-q22	*CMD1H*	Unknown	Conduction disease
2q35	*DES*	Desmin	Skeletal myopathy
3p22-p25	Unknown	Unknown	Conduction disease
5q33	*SGCD*	Delta-sarcoglycan	Skeletal myopathy
6q23-q24	*EYA4*	Eyes absent 4	Skeletal myopathy, sensorineural hearing loss
10q22-q23	*MVCL*	Metavinculin	Mitral valve prolapse
17q12	*TCAP*	Telethonin	Limb-girdle muscular dystrophy
19q13.2	Unknown	Unknown	Conduction disease
Xp21.2	*DMD*	Dystrophin	Skeletal myopathy
Xq28	*TAZ*	Tafazzin	Skeletal myopathy
Xq28	EMD	Emerin	Skeletal myopathy

ATP = adenosine triphosphate.

mutations that cause isolated DCM further divide into those with or without conduction system disease.

Dilated Cardiac Myopathy without Conduction System Disease

Gene mutations that affect sarcomere proteins, calcium handling proteins, and other unidentified molecules cause DCM that is unaccompanied by extracardiac manifestations or conduction system diseases. Sarcomere mutations are most common,[18] and mutations have been identified in genes that encode actin (*ACTC*), beta–cardiac myosin heavy chain *MYH7*), cardiac troponin I (*TNNI3*), cardiac troponin T (*TNNT2*), alpha-tropomyosin (*TPM1*), titin (*TTN*), and cardiac troponin C (*TNNC1*). As in HCM, inheritance of sarcomere mutations in DCM is autosomal dominant. Disease onset is often earlier than with other DCM mutations, and both childhood presentation and rapid progression are recognized. In contrast, some adults with sarcomere mutations that cause DCM have normal cardiac function, indicating incomplete penetrance.

The histopathology of DCM caused by sarcomere mutations is notably different from HCM.[5,18] Degenerating myocytes and increased interstitial fibrosis occur without myocyte disarray, which serves to discriminate between primary DCM and the end-stage, burnt out phase of HCM. Types of sarcomere protein gene mutation found in DCM are comparable to those found in HCM patients; most encode missense amino acids or small deletion. Furthermore, the general location of the mutation within a gene does not predict its consequences (Fig. 10-1). Although the exact residue affected by a DCM or HCM mutation is distinct, the proximity of these to each other is remarkable. Biophysical analyses of mutant proteins and animal models have been used to explore the mechanisms by which sarcomere mutations cause DCM. These data indicate that sarcomere gene mutations cause DCM by affecting force production or force transmission.

Human DCM mutation, beta-MHC mutation Ser532Pro is located in the actin-binding domain (see Fig. 10-1), which is involved in initiating the power stroke of contraction.[35] Biophysical studies of this mutation have revealed reduced velocity of actin movement over mutant myosin, decreased ATPase activities, and slower rates of myocyte shortening.

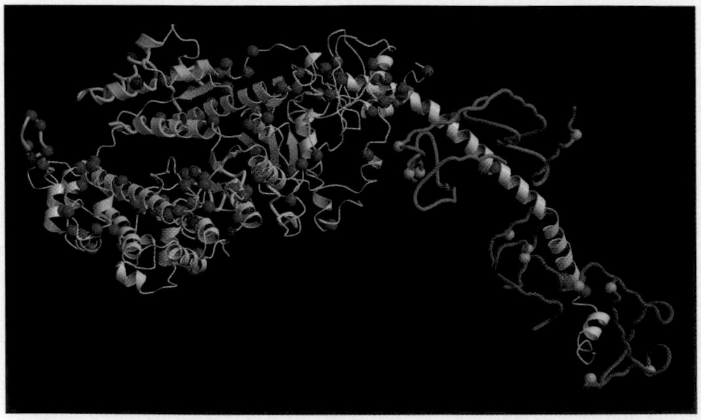

FIGURE 10–1. Computer reconstruction of the three-dimensional crystal structure of myosin, based on x-ray coordinates reported by Rayment and colleagues.[63] Protein backbone is shown as a gray ribbon. Binding sites for myosin (green) and adenosine triphosphate (yellow) are indicated. Essential and regulatory myosin light chains are shown in gold and purple, respectively. Blue spheres denote human hypertrophic cardiomyopathy (HCM) mutations in the myosin heavy chain (dark blue) and light chains (light blue). Red spheres denote human dilated cardiomyopathy (DCM) mutations. Note the close proximity of the HCM and DCM mutations.

These primary deficits in the motor functions of the mutant myosin in mice are contractile dysfunction with morphological and histopathological changes of DCM. Impaired contractile force is also the consequence of DCM mutations affecting thin-filament proteins. In vitro studies of mutations in troponin T, troponin C, and alpha-tropomyosin mutations have shown reduced activation in ATPase and motility assays, with decreased force generation. Depressed contractility, the net result of DCM mutations in sarcomere proteins, is an effect fundamentally opposite to that produced by HCM mutations.

Multiple human DCM mutations occur in specific domains of giant muscle protein titin that interact with sarcomere structures (see earlier).[22] DCM mutations localize within the cardiac-specific N2B domain that interacts with I-bands, the extensible thin filaments regions flanking Z-discs, and may cause deficits in force transmission. At the Z-disc, titin interacts with alpha-actinin, telethonin (encoded by *TCAP*), muscle LIM protein (encoded by *CLP*) and cipher ZASP (encoded by *LBD3*).[18] Mutations in these Z-disc interacting proteins are reported as causes of human DCM. Disease expression is incomplete in some mutation carriers from these families. Reported phenotypes associated with these mutations are limited to the heart, but elevations in serum enzyme levels may indicate a subclinical skeletal myopathy, a finding consistent with the shared roles for these Z-disc proteins in all striated muscles. Mutations in Z-disc proteins may either abolish titin interactions or make the titin–Z-disc complex unstable. As a consequence, normal detection and modulation of mechanical stress may be impaired and result in DCM.

To examine whether deficits in the transmission of force transmission between adjacent myocytes cause DCM, metavinculin, an isoform encoded by *VCL* on chromosome 10q22, was studied. Two mutations identified in DCM patients were also found in unaffected relatives, suggesting incomplete penetrance. *VCL* mutations are a rare cause of DCM.

Dominant mutations in phospholamban (*PLN,* encoded at 6q22) cause DCM by altering Ca^{2+} handling. Affected patients develop fulminant DCM and heart failure and require cardiac transplantation early in middle age. Phospholamban is the reversible inhibitor of the cardiac sarcoendoplasmic reticular Ca^{2+}-ATPase (SERCA) that regulates basal cardiac contractility. Phospholamban inhibition of SERCA is released following phosphorylation via beta-adrenergic stimulation of the heart. Dominant DCM mutations in the *PLN* mutation can prevent phosphorylation or cause superinhibition of SERCA; either change results in chronic delay in Ca^{2+} reuptake after sarcomere contraction.

Human DCM mutations in the regulatory SUR2A subunit (encoded by *ABCC9*) of KATP (ATP-sensitive potassium channels) may impair the ability of the heart to respond to stress.[36] KATP channels are multimeric proteins containing an inwardly rectifying potassium channel pore (Kir6.2), a regulatory SUR2A subunit, and an ATPase-harboring ATP-binding cassette protein. In the heart, these channels participate in decoding metabolic signals during stress adaptation. Human mutations render KATP channels insensitive to ADP-induced conformation changes, which alter channel opening and closure. Because hearts from KATP null mice are susceptible to calcium overload, some of the pathophysiology of human KATP mutations (DCM and arrhythmias) may reflect calcium increases triggered by myocyte stress.

Dilated Cardiac Myopathy with Conduction System Disease

Dominant mutations in the nuclear envelope protein lamin A/C (*LMNA* encoded at chromosome 1q) are the most common cause of DCM that occurs with progressive conduction system abnormalities.[37] Disease onset is usually in the third to fourth decade of life. Electrophysiological dysfunction usually precedes systolic dysfunction by many years, but because arrhythmias are often silent, conduction system disease may be undetected until heart failure symptoms prompt evaluation. The increased incidence of sudden death associated with *LMNA* mutations necessitates careful surveillance and appropriate intervention. Progressive cardiac dysfunction occurs despite progressive pacemaker implantation, indicating that *LMNA* mutations cause primary defects in all myocytes.

Ubiquitously expressed in all cells, lamin A/C participates in nuclear dissociation and reassembly during mitosis, but its function in terminally differentiated myocytes is unclear.[38] Analyses of myocytes and fibroblasts from mice deficient in lamin A/C have demonstrated deformities of the nucleus and the desmin cytoskeletal network, impaired mechanotransduction, diminished viability during periods of mechanical strain, and impaired activation of transcriptional programs in response to mechanical strain. Similar deformities of the nuclear architecture are present in skin fibroblasts of patients with *LMNA* mutations. Such *LMNA* mutations may impair normal adaptive mechanisms to mechanical strain; this is an appealing mechanism, but it fails to account for early-onset and progressive electrophysiological abnormalities.

LMNA mutations also cause familial partial lipodystrophy with insulin-resistant diabetes and skeletal muscular dystrophies.[38] The shared muscle and cardiac phenotypes in patients with lamin or emerin mutations (*EMD,* encoded by *EMD* on chromosome Xq28) likely relates to their common functions in supporting nuclear membrane integrity. Long-term survival in some patients with DCM *LMNA* mutations is associated with late-onset skeletal myopathy.

Dilated Cardiac Myopathy with Extracardiac Manifestations

Genetic causes of DCM can cause disease in other organ systems. The most common accompanying phenotype is a skeletal myopathy, presumably because of the many molecules common to all striated muscle cells. A broader array of manifestations is observed when the causal DCM gene also functions in processes vital to another organ system. These extracardiac manifestations can precede or follow the onset of DCM.

Mutations in several genes that cause DCM and skeletal myopathy encode protein components of dystrophin-associated complex, a protein scaffold that connects the nucleus to the extracellular matrix through the sarcolemma in all muscle cells.[39] Some mutations in muscle delta-sarcoglycan (*SGCD* encoded on chromosome 5q33), and dystrophin (*DMD* encoded on chromosome Xq33) cause predominantly cardiac disease, although subclinical skeletal myopathy may be coincident. A naturally occurring recessive DCM phenotype in Syrian hamsters is caused by homozygous delta-sarcoglycan mutation. Mice engineered to carry delta-sarcoglycan mutations exhibit coronary artery vasospasm with ischemia. Whether ischemia is also the mechanism by which human *SGCD* mutations cause skeletal and cardiac myopathy is unclear.

X-linked DCM can arise from rare mutations in the dystrophin gene. Unlike mutations in the protein coding sequences that cause classic Duchenne muscular dystrophy, some *DMD* mutations alter regulatory sequences that lead to more prominent involvement of the heart. A subclinical skeletal myopathy is often present[40] that may become overt with aging. DCM is also a prominent clinical feature in Duchenne muscular dystrophy.

A broader diversity of extracardiac manifestations occurs in DCM that accompanies Barth syndrome. Clinical manifestations include childhood onset of DCM and heart failure in the setting of skeletal myopathy, neutropenia, and growth retardation.[41] Mutations in tafazzin (*TAZ*), a molecule with putative enzyme functions involved in cardiolipin metabolism, are the cause of this X-linked syndrome. Cardiolipin levels, a mitochondrial phospholipid, are reduced in Barth syndrome patients; cardiolipin deficiency perturbs mitochondrial structure and causes suboptimal function of respiratory chain proteins.

EYA4, a transcriptional coactivator that may function as a nuclear phosphatase, causes DCM and sensorineural hearing loss.[7] Human mutations abolish *EYA4-SIX* protein interactions essential for translocation of the transcription coactivator into the nucleus. Target genes regulated by *EYA4* are unknown.

Dilated Cardiac Myopathy in Mitochondrial Syndromes

Mutations in genes that direct synthesis of ATP by oxidative phosphorylation can cause pleiomorphic diseases that frequently include DCM. Proteins involved in oxidative phosphorylation are primarily encoded in the nuclear genome, but 13 are encoded in the mitochondrial genome.[42,43] Unlike nuclear gene defects, mitochondrial mutations cause matrilineal inheritance (see Chap. 8). Because the mitochondrial chromosome is present in multiple copies and mutations are often heteroplasmic, not all copies are affected. These issues, coupled with the variable energy needs of different tissues, account for the considerable clinical diversity of mitochondrial gene mutations. Whereas most mitochondrial defects cause cardiomyopathy in the context of pleiomorphic syndromes such as Kearns-Sayre, ocular myopathy, MELAS (**m**itochondrial **e**ncephalomyopathy with **l**actic **a**cidosis, and **s**troke-like episodes), and MERRF (**m**yoclonus **e**pilepsy with **r**agged **r**ed **f**ibers), particular mitochondrial mutations may produce predominant or exclusive cardiac disease. In addition, an association between heteroplasmic mitochondrial mutations and DCM has been recognized. Deficits in energy may be a shared mechanism by which mutations in mitochondrial genes and tafazzin cause DCM.

Arrhythmogenic Right Ventricular Dysplasia

Arrhythmogenic right ventricular dysplasia (ARVD), a cardiomyopathy characterized by progressive fibrofatty degeneration of the myocardium with progressive dysfunction, electrical instability, and sudden death (see Chap. 35), is inherited as an autosomal dominant trait, with incomplete penetrance. Male gender may be associated with higher disease penetrance.[44] ARVD occurs as an isolated cardiomyopathy or in the context of two related disorders, Naxos or Carvajal syndromes, which have prominent skin (palmar-plantar keratosis), woolly hair, and either predominant right ventricular (RV; Naxos) or left ventricular (LV; Carvajal) manifestations. The higher prevalence of ARVD in some countries, particularly Italy, is not accounted for by founder mutations and may reflect surveillance and/or clinical awareness.

Recessive mutations in plakoglobin (*JUP*) cause Naxos and Carvajal syndromes. Cardiac disease in these disorders is comparable to that found in ARVD.[45] Dominant mutations in five genes cause isolated ARVD; the genes at other loci identified through linkage studies are unknown. Mutations occur in desmoplakin (*DSP*), plakophilin-2 (*PKP2*), desmogelin-2 (*DSG2*) and desmocolline-2 (*DSC2*), each of which encodes a protein component of desmosomes, highly organized cell membrane structures that maintain structural and functional contacts between adjacent cells (Table 10-3). Less common mutations occur in the cardiac ryanodine receptor (*RyR2*). Whether distinct mutations in these different genes are associated with clinical expression is unknown.

Two models have been proposed to account for how desmosome protein mutations cause ARVD. First, given the location and function of this organelle, mutations may render desmosomes inappropriately sensitive to mechanical stresses. An alternative model is based on analyses of signal transduction processes involving desmosome proteins. Cells engineered to express reduced levels of desmoplakin were found to have increased nuclear localization of plakoglobin that affected canonical Wnt/beta-catenin signaling and increased expression of an adipocyte and fibroblast gene program. These provocative results imply that the distinct histopathology of ARVD may reflect reprogramming of the cell biology of myocytes by ARVD mutations.

TABLE 10–3 Gene Mutations and Loci in Arrhythmogenic Right Ventricular Cardiomyopathy

Locus	Symbol	Name	Additional Phenotype
1q42-q43	*RYR2*	Ryanodine receptor	Catecholaminergic polymorphic ventricular tachycardia
2q32.1-q32.3	—	—	Left ventricular involvement
3p23	—	Unknown	—
6p24	*DSP*	Desmoplakin	—
10p12-p14	—	Unknown	Early onset, high penetrance
10q22	—	Unknown	Myofibrillar myopathy
12p11	*PKP2*	Plakophilin-2	—
14q12-q22	—	Unknown	—
14q23-q24	—	Unknown	—
17q21	*JUP*	Junctional plakoglobin	Naxos, Carvajal syndromes (recessive)
18q12	*DSG2*	Desmoglein	—
18q12.1	*DSC2*	Desmocollin 2	—

GENETIC CAUSES OF STRUCTURAL HEART DISEASE

Heart malformations are among the most common of all human congenital defects (for a fuller discussion of these abnormalities, consult the online version of this chapter) and occur in 5 to 7 per 1000 live births.[46] Higher rates (10 percent) are observed in stillbirths and in children with another congenital anomaly.[47] Teratogens, infectious agents, maternal environmental factors, and genetics all cause congenital heart defects. With major advances in surgical correction of heart defects over several decades, survival and reproductive fitness of congenital heart disease patients has improved. In concert with better detection of subtle lesions, an appreciation of the role of genetics in heart malformations has substantially increased.

Chromosomal aberrations provide overt evidence for the quintessential role played by genetics in congenital heart malformations. An extensive and varied array of structural heart disease is found in spontaneous abortuses and in children with major defects in chromosome number and structure. Although cytogenetic investigations have provided few clues about genetic causes, a clearer understanding has come from investigating mendelian forms of congenital heart defects. Dominant, recessive, and X-linked gene mutations can disrupt cardiac development and cause heart malformations. To date, dominant mutations have been defined, and strategies to identify recessive gene mutations in congenital heart defects are emerging. Given the observed increased incidence of structural heart defects recognized in children from consanguineous matings, discovery of recessive mutations may uncover other genes that contribute to the prevalence of congenital heart disease in the general population.

Discovery of gene defects that cause cardiac malformations has provided insights into the normal molecular signals and pathways that direct human cardiac morphogenesis, and clues as to why these processes sometimes fail. Three general principles have emerged from these discoveries. First, congenital heart disease genes encode transcription factors (*GATA4, TBX1, TBX5,* and *NKX2-5*), and signaling molecules (*PTPN11, KRAS, NOTCH1, JAG1*), proteins that direct and integrate temporal-spatial interactions of cells and tissues during cardiac development (Table 10-4). Unlike gene mutations that cause adult-onset disease (such as cardiomyopathies), remarkably few structural protein genes (*CRELD1, ELN, MYH6*) have been implicated in congenial heart malformations. With these data, researchers have capitalized on studies of model organisms, in which other key molecules that direct cardiac morphogenesis have been discovered. These provide a powerful collection of candidate genes for analyses of potential mutations in human patients. A second observation relates to the types of mutations in congenital heart disease genes; typically, these defects alter gene dosage and most often produce haploinsufficiency or loss of one functional copy (or allele) of the encoded molecule. That a change in gene dose causes congenital heart disease implies that expression levels of these molecules are critical for normal cardiac morphogenesis. A third observation relates to the expressivity of congenital heart disease mutations. Whereas some family members who share an identical gene defect may exhibit the preponderant malformation, others can have anatomically distinct malformations. Diversity of malformations triggered by one mutation also indicates the influence of other factors. These unknown factors likely include background genes and fetal environment, which affect phenotypic expression of gene defects. Furthermore, the clinical consequences of some mutations (*NKX2-5*) take years to emerge, which indicates that genes participating in cardiac morphogenesis also function in the adult myocardium. The considerable clinical heterogeneity of these human gene mutations supports the concept that various developmental pathways can be perturbed to cause congenital heart disease.

Most structural heart disease appears to be a sporadic occurrence. Uncovering the potential roles of genetics in isolated cases is an active research endeavor. Some sporadic cases may reflect de novo (or spontaneous) dominant mutations; other cases may reflect genetic recessive mutations or genetic variation in multiple genes that increase the risk for aberrant heart development. With the advent of technologies to assess genome-wide variation in populations, researchers now have opportunities to identify DNA variations that convey small increases in the risk for congenital heart disease throughout the general population. Undoubtedly, these discoveries will further advance our clinical recognition of the causes for these prevalent heart disorders and provide better understanding of the molecular basis for cardiac development and lifelong function.

Mendelian forms of congenital heart disease can be classified into three broad categories: isolated cardiovascular malformations, pleiotropic syndromes that frequently include congenital cardiovascular defects, and syndromes that only occasionally affect the cardiovascular system. Common examples of these first two categories, which are more likely to be seen by adult cardiologists, are considered here. A more complete presentation of additional disorders and syndromes is discussed in the Chapter 10 Online Supplement of this chapter and in Online Mendelian Inheritance in Man.[48]

Isolated Congenital Heart Disease

Atrial and Ventricular Septal Defects

Familial aggregation of isolated atrial and ventricular defects falls within two groups, those with and those without conduction system disease. Either group can be inherited as autosomal dominant traits that arise from mutation of cardiac transcription factor genes. Careful clinical evaluation and radiographic examination are important to exclude involvement of other organ systems. For example, the coexistence of upper limb malformations, even in a first-degree relative, should prompt consideration of hand-heart (e.g., Holt-Oram) syndromes.

Most isolated hereditary defects of cardiac septation involve the atria and result in familial ostium secundum defect. These are typically inherited as an autosomal dominant trait and, as such, the incidence of ASD in siblings and offspring of the affected patient greatly exceeds that in the general population.[49-51] Affected family members sometimes have other or additional structural defects, including atrial septal aneurysms, ventricular septal defect (VSD), atrioventricular canal, and/or aortic or pulmonary valve disease. Spontaneous closure of septation defects caused by gene mutation is uncommon; these usually require surgical correction.

Dominant mutations in three genes, *GATA4*,[52-54] *MYH6*,[55] and an unidentified gene on chromosome 5p, cause isolated familial atrial septal defects.[56] Loss of one gene copy (hemizygosity) of *GATA4* may also account for congenital heart disease in patients with interstitial deletions of 8p23, where the transcription factor is encoded. *GATA4* is a member of a zinc finger transcription factor gene family, which recognizes a consensus GATA: sequence motif in target gene promoters.[54,57] Although *GATA4* is also expressed in developing gut epithelium and gonads, the effects of human mutations in one gene copy appear limited to the heart. Model organisms engineered to lack *GATA4* are lethal to embryos because of failed cardiac development. Analyses of human mutations in model organisms have indicated that *GATA4* mutations disrupt interactions with cognate DNA sequences and reduce

TABLE 10–4 Gene Mutations and Loci in Congenital Heart Disease

Locus	Gene	Function	Malformations
1p31-p21	Unknown	—	AVCD
1q42	*LEFTY A*	Left-right axis	Heterotaxy
3p22	*CFC1*	Nodal-related signaling	Heterotaxy
3p25.3	*CRELD1*	Cell adhesion	ASD, VSD, AVC, heterotaxy
4p16	*EVC, EVC1*	Unknown	ASD, primum, Ellis-van Creveld
5p	*DNAH5*	Dynein, microtubule motor	Heterotaxy, Kartagener syndrome
5p	Unknown	—	ASD, aneurysm,
5q	*NKX2-5*	Transcription	ASD, VSD, TOF, conduction system
7p21	*DNAH11*	Dynein, microtubule motor	Heterotaxy, Kartagener syndrome
7q21	*SEMA3E*	Semaphorin, neural guidance	TOF, PDA, AVC, CHARGE syndrome
7q11.2	*ELN*	Vascular integrity	SVAS, PA stenosis
8q12	*CHD7*	Chromodomain helicase	TOF, PDA, AVC, CHARGE syndrome
8p23.1-p22	*GATA4*	Transcription	ASD
9p21	*DNAI1*	Dynein, microtubule motor	Heterotaxy, Kartagener syndrome
9q34.3	*NOTCH1*	Signaling	Bicuspid aortic valve
11p15.4	Unknown	—	MVP
12p12.1	*KRAS*	Signaling	PS, ASD, VSD, PDA, Noonan syndrome
12q24.1	*PTPN11*	Signaling	PS, ASD, VSD, PDA, Noonan syndrome
12q24.1	*TBX5*	Transcription	ASD, VSD, TOF, conduction system, Holt-Oram syndrome
12q24	Unknown	—	PDA
20q13	*SALL4*	Transcription	VSD, TOF, TA, Okihiro syndrome
20p12	*JAG1*	Signaling	PS, VSD, TOF, Alagille syndrome
14q12	*MYH6*	Alpha-myosin	ASD
16p11.2	Unknown	—	MVP
22q 11.2	*TBX1*	Transcription	TOF, TGA, DORV, DiGeorge syndrome
Xq26.2	*ZIC3*	—	Heterotaxy
Xq28	Unknown	—	MVP

ASD = atrial septal defect; AVC = atrioventricular conduction; AVCD = atrioventricular conduction disturbance; DORV = double outlet right ventricle; MVP = mitral valve prolapse; PA = pulmonary artery; PDA = patent ductus arteriosus; PS = pulmonic stenosis; SVAS = supraventricular arterial stenosis; TA = tricuspid atresia; TOF = tetralogy of Fallot; TGA = transposition of the great arteries; VSD = ventricular septal defect.

transcriptional activation of target genes.[52] *GATA4* may regulate genes critical for myocardial differentiation and function, including troponin C, alpha-myosin heavy chain,[58] and brain natriuretic peptide.[59]

A second gene implicated in septation defects is *MYH6*,[55] which encodes the structural protein alpha-myosin heavy chain. A single family with ostium secundum defects carried a *MYH6* missense mutation, which substitutes an asparagine for the normal isoleucine. The clinical expression of the mutation was incomplete, and some mutation carriers have structurally normal hearts. Expression of *MYH6* is regulated by two transcription factors, *TBX5* and *GATA4;* human mutations in each of these molecules also cause ASDs.

Inherited cardiac septation defects associated with postnatal onset of electrophysiological disease (Fig. 10-2) occur from a dominant mutation in *NKX2-5*.[53,54,60] Congenital malformations arising from *NKX2-5* mutations are more variable than those caused by *GATA4* mutations, and include secundum or cribriform type ASD, VSD (muscular type), tetralogy of Fallot, and double-orifice mitral valve. Adult-onset left ventricular hypertrophy caused by *NKX2-5* has been observed without demonstrable structural malformations.[60]

Electrophysiological defects produced by *NKX2-5* mutation include progressive atrioventricular conduction delay with Wenckebach-type second-degree heart block, sick sinus, and atrial fibrillation. In some individuals, electrophysiological manifestations occur without structural heart defects. Atrioventricular conduction delays evolve insidiously and necessitate permanent pacemaker implantation, even decades after diagnosis of the structural malformation (see Fig. 10-2B), thereby necessitating longitudinal evaluations of affected individuals. Electrocardiographic abnormalities in a patient with apparently sporadic atrial septal defect should prompt a detailed family history and evaluation of close relatives.

NKX2-5, the mammalian homologue of the *Drosophila tinman* gene (so-named because deletions abrogate development of the dorsal vessel, the insect's heart equivalent) is encoded on chromosome 5q34. *NKX2-5* is a member of the NK gene family of transcription factors that contain a homeobox sequence motif, and plays an essential role for the specification of cardiac progenitor cells from mesoderm tissue in mammalian and lower species.[61] Model organisms engineered to lack *NKX2-5* die early as a result of failed heart development. Among the target genes regulated by *NKX2-5* in the mouse, some have restricted expression in the atria and conduction system. Congenital heart mutations inactivate DNA binding by the *NKX2-5* protein,[62] reducing by half the physiological levels of this critical transcription factor.

Bicuspid Aortic Valve

Failure in the development of a trileaflet aortic valve is among the most common of congenital lesions, affecting 2 percent of live births. Although usually sporadic,

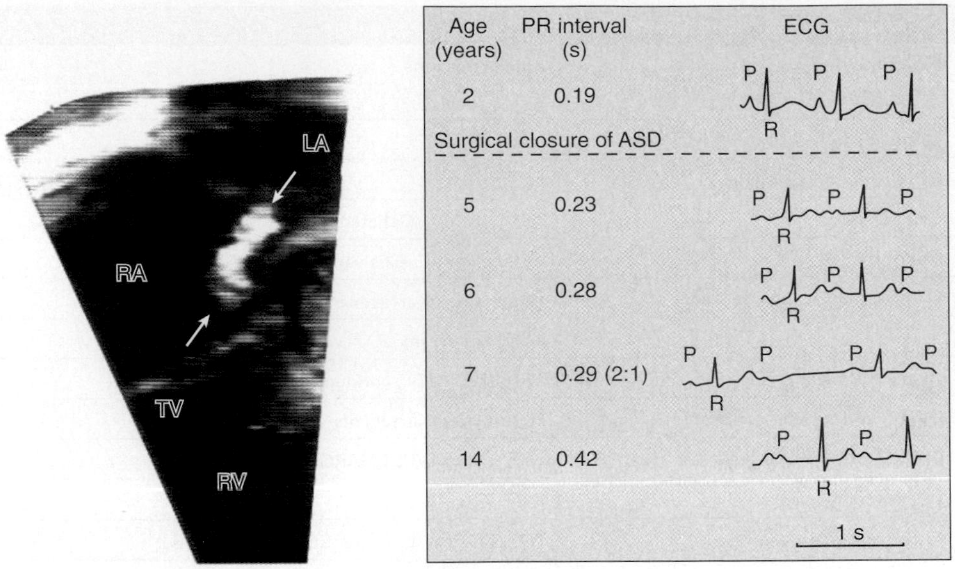

A B

FIGURE 10–2. Clinical manifestations of *NKX2-5* mutations. **A,** Doppler echocardiography detects atrial septal defect (ASD). **B,** Electrocardiogram (ECG) shows progressive atrioventricular delay through age 6. By age 7, 2:1 atrioventricular block is evident. A pacemaker was implanted at age 14. LA = left atrium; RA = right atrium; RV = right ventricle; TV = tricuspid valve. *(From Schott JJ, Benson DW, Basson CT, et al: Congenital heart disease caused by mutations in the transcription factor NKX2-5. Science 281:108, 1998.)*

familial inheritance of bicuspid aortic valve shows autosomal dominant transmission.[49] Mutations in the transcriptional regulator, *NOTCH1,* can produce bicuspid aortic valve; these are prone to progressive postnatal calcification. Clinical presentations of mutation carriers include aortic stenosis and aortic insufficiency. Less frequently, *NOTCH1* mutations cause hypoplastic left ventricle or tetralogy of Fallot.

NOTCH1 is a member of a gene family of transmembrane receptors with diverse roles in signaling cellular differentiation and cell fate. Activation of the receptor *NOTCH1* stimulates proteolytic cleavage and release of domains that translocate to the nucleus and participate in transcriptional activation. Human mutations in *NOTCH* receptors, *NOTCH* ligands, and *NOTCH* processing enzymes cause various diseases, with widely disparate phenotypes. *NOTCH1* mutations identified in familial bicuspid aortic valve development inactivate the receptor. Although the mechanism by which receptor inactivation affects valve development is unclear, late-onset calcium deposition in the misshaped valve may be caused by failed inhibition of *RUNX2,* a transcriptional regulator of osteoblast activity.

Mitral Valve Prolapse

Often called the most common abnormality of human heart valves, mitral valve prolapse (MVP) can arise alone or in the context of heritable disorder of connective tissue disorders (Marfan syndrome; see Chap. 8). Familial MVP that occurs without systemic disease shows age- and gender-dependent expression.[50] Familial occurrences can show distinct phenotypes (billowing of the mitral leaflets or excessive systolic mitral annular expansion) that breed relatively true. Genetic studies have indicated autosomal dominance with variable expression. Given the heritability of clinically distinct subtypes of MVP, genetic heterogeneity is expected. Two autosomal loci have been identified.[51] In addition, susceptibility to myxomatous degeneration of all cardiac valves can be inherited as an X-linked trait that maps to Xq28. The causal genes remain unknown.

Genetic Syndromes with Major Cardiovascular Defects

Holt-Oram Syndrome

The prototypic hand-heart disorder, Holt-Oram syndrome, is characterized by dysplasia of the upper limbs and cardiac septal defects.[48] Arm deformities are usually bilateral but often asymmetrical in severity, and range from subtle thumb abnormalities (distally placed and triphalangeal) to phocomelia. Hypoplastic thenar eminences, anomalies of the carpus, radial aplasia, and hypoplasia of the clavicles or shoulders may be present. Cardiac malformations are found in most (about 85 percent) of Holt-Oram syndrome patients. Secundum atrial septal defects are most common, but ventricular septal defects, patent ductus arteriosus (PDA), and a wide spectrum of complex heart and vascular malformations also occur. Patients can develop electrophysiological deficits beyond the atrioventricular node; conduction system disturbances can occur in the absence of structural heart disease. Patients with apparently "sporadic" atrial septal defect should be carefully examined for subtle limb malformations, because detection of Holt-Oram syndrome substantially increases the recurrence risk for offspring from 3 (empirical recurrence risk of an isolated septal defect) to 50 percent for this autosomal dominant condition.

Holt-Oram syndrome is caused by mutations in *TBX5,* a member of the T-box transcription factor gene family,[48] which shares conserved DNA-binding sequences, denoted as the T-box. Mutations typically inactivate one gene copy and reduce physiological levels by half, but clinical expression varies considerably among family members. Parental manifestations do not reliably predict the severity of malformations in offspring.

Deletion of one copy of the *TBX5* gene in mice recapitulates both hand and heart phenotypes of Holt-Oram syndrome.[48] Studies of the electrophysiological system in these mutant mice have revealed distinct morphological and functional defects in atrioventricular and bundle branch conduction systems. Anatomical absence of the right bundle branch has been observed, as well as right bundle branch block on electrocardiographic recordings, revealing a primary role for *TBX5* in the patterning of the cardiac conduction system. These results may account for the electrophysiological abnormalities found in Holt-Oram patients without structural heart defects.

Noonan Syndrome

This pleiotropic syndrome occurs with relatively high prevalence (1 in 1000 to 2500 live births) and frequent cardiovascular involvement.[48] An autosomal dominant disorder, features of Noonan syndrome include short stature, sometimes with an unusual pectus deformity, cubitus valgus, neck webbing, congenital lymphedema, and congenital heart defects. Mental retardation, hematopoietic abnormalities that can evolve into leukemia, and cryptorchidism also occur in those with Noonan syndrome. Lymphatic dysplasia, especially of the lower limbs, is common but causes clinical difficulties in less than 20 percent of cases. Chylothorax and a protein-losing enteropathy represent the severe end of the spectrum. Although phenotypically similar to Turner syndrome, Noonan syndrome affects both men and women. Because of the facial dysmorphism (hypertelorism, ptosis) and extensive cardiac involvement (occurring in 80 to 90 percent of patients), Noonan syndrome is often classified as a cardiofacial syndrome.

Valvular pulmonic stenosis is the most common defect in Noonan syndrome (found in approximately 40 percent of patients) and should always be considered in a patient with this lesion. Valve cusps are thickened and dysplastic, even in the absence of hemodynamic compromise. Pulmonary artery hypoplasia or infundibular subvalvular remodeling can occur and result in a cardiomyopathy that is hypertrophic, often asymmetrical, and predominant in either ventricle. ASD occurs in about one third of Noonan patients, usually in association with pulmonic stenosis. VSD and PDA each occur in about 10 percent of cases. Congenital anomalies of coronary arteries are found occasionally and unexpectedly during evaluation of more obvious defects.

Mutations in two genes, *PTPN11* and KRAS,[48] cause Noonan syndrome. Approximately 50 percent of Noonan patients have mutations in *PTPN11,* which encodes SHP-2, a tyrosine phosphatase, containing a Src homology 2 (SH2) domain that participates in signal transduction pathways involving RAS-mitogen activated protein kinase (MAPK).[122] Binding of guanosine diphosphate (GDP) and guanosine triphosphate (GTP) by RAS proteins regulates intracellular signals that control cell proliferation, differentiation, and survival. Human *PTPN11* mutations are clustered in sequences interacting with the SH2 domain and in domains involved in switching the protein between its active and inactive states; mutations result in excess SHP-2 activity and correlate with reduced transcriptional activation of NFAT (nuclear factor of activated T-cells).[48] Missense mutations in *KRAS,* which encodes two isoforms of the RAS family of proteins, account for only 2 percent of Noonan syndrome cases. Both *PTPN11* signaling via RAS-MAPK and *KRAS* mutations implicate other molecules in this pathway as gene candidates for Noonan syndrome mutations.

Trisomy 21 (Down Syndrome)

With an occurrence of 1 in 600 births, trisomy 21 is the most common defect of human chromosome dosage.[53] Clinical features of Down syndrome include characteristic morphological features with a typical facies, mental retardation, conductive hearing loss, and major congenital malformations, including structural heart defects (present in 40 to 50 percent of cases). Surviving patients have increased risk for hematological malignancy disease (10- to 20-fold above normal) and progressive dementia of the Alzheimer type, at a younger than expected age (fifth decade). Premature aging of the vasculature may also occur.

The prototypic cardiac anomaly of Down syndrome patients is atrioventricular canal defect and resultant pulmonary hypertension from increased blood flow.[54] Complex cardiac malformations occur in a third of patients, but transposition of the great arteries is extremely rare. Older patients develop MVP at a higher frequency than age- and gender-matched control subjects, and both aortic and pulmonary valve cusps are predisposed to fenestrations during adulthood in Down syndrome patients.

Most affected patients have three copies of chromosome 21 because of maternal errors in meiosis, events that exponentially increase with maternal age. Risk for trisomy 21 rises steeply after age 35, and reaches 4 percent in women older than 45. Critical regions within chromosome 21 for Down syndrome phenotypes have been identified and several genes that may be implicated in trisomy 21 heart disease are found in these regions. However, the gene responsible for the cardiac abnormalities associated with this condition has not been identified.

Turner Syndrome

About 1 in 2500 females have Turner syndrome.[55] Although classic morphological features include short stature, webbed neck, and bowed arms, clinical findings are variable and often mild. Diagnosis is sometimes prompted only during evaluation for short stature or amenorrhea.

Congenital cardiovascular defects occur in 20 to 50 percent of Turner syndrome patients.[56] Aortic coarctation, usually of the postductal type, is the most common defect and is found in 50 to 70 percent of Turner syndrome patients with heart disease. Other malformations occur alone or in combination with coarctation; these include bicuspid aortic valve, dilation of the ascending aorta, hypoplastic left heart, and partial anomalous pulmonary venous drainage without an accompanying ASD. Cardiac conduction system and repolarization abnormalities (notably QT prolongation) occur that may be intrinsic to the syndrome.[57] Hypertension is common in Turner patients, even without coarctation or following repair, and may reflect a high frequency of renal anomalies. Blood pressure elevation is strongly associated with dilation of the ascending aorta, so aggressive treatment is warranted. Treatment of children with human growth hormone to increase mature height has no apparent deleterious effect on cardiac performance.[58]

Turner syndrome is caused by complete or partial absence of the X chromosome, resulting in a 45,X karyotype. Mosaicism can also result in Turner syndrome with 46,XX or 46,XY karyotypes; these women are less likely to have cardiovascular defects.

CARDIAC TUMORS

Myxomas account for approximately 35 percent of all primary cardiac tumors.[59] Generally regarded as isolated benign tumors of the left atrium of middle-aged women, most cardiac myxomas are amenable to surgical resection and rarely recur, and therapy is important to prevent emboli and stroke. Almost 10 percent of cardiac myxomas occur as part of a dominant disorder, Carney complex.[60] Unlike sporadic myxomas, cardiac tumors in Carney complex affect men and women equally, arise commonly in the atria but also in the ventricles, may be multicentric and, despite complete surgical resection, frequently recur at distant cardiac sites. Extracardiac manifestations of Carney complex include myxomas, lentiginosis, hyperpigmentation, and endocrine dysfunction.[61] Clinical manifestations are variable, even among affected family members.

Carney complex is caused by mutations in the *PRKAR1α* gene that encodes the R1α regulatory subunit of cyclic adenosine monophosphate–dependent protein kinase A. All human mutations cause haploinsufficiency and reduce the normal kinase level by half. *PRKAR1α* may function as a tumor suppressor gene in the heart.[60] Unregulated myxomatous growth may reflect both a germline *PRKAR1α* mutation and an acquired mutation of another tumor suppressor gene, as occurs in *NF1* gene mutations in neurofibromatosis. Other Carney complex mutations affect perinatal myosin heavy chain and cause disease via uncertain mechanisms.[64]

FUTURE PERSPECTIVES

Mendelian disorders affecting the heart are prevalent causes of cardiovascular disease. Most cardiomyopathy disease genes encode structural proteins involved in critical contractile processes. Mutant structural proteins incorporated into functional complexes cause disease by their disruptive effects.

In contrast, congenital heart disease mutations affect transcription factors and signaling molecules that regulate cardiac development. These gene mutations usually reduce the levels of the encoded protein by half, implying that normal cardiac embryogenesis requires physiological doses of these genes. Congenital heart disease gene mutations have a wide range of clinical expression. Clinical gene-based diagnosis of cardiomyopathy and congenital heart disease is increasingly available to provide early, accurate diagnosis and evaluation of risk assessment in family members.

Therapies for cardiomyopathy and congenital heart disease remain limited. With gene discoveries and the development of animal models for these conditions, ongoing discoveries of pathways affected by mutant genes will increase and fuel the development of targeted therapies. Given the long latency of many cardiovascular genetic diseases such as cardiomyopathy, this knowledge can be expected to advance opportunities for intervention and disease prevention.

REFERENCES

Hypertrophic Cardiomyopathy

1. Morita H, Seidman J, Seidman CE: Genetic causes of human heart failure. J Clin Invest 115:518, 2005.
2. Arad M, Maron BJ, Gorham JM, et al: Glycogen storage diseases presenting as hypertrophic cardiomyopathy. N Engl J Med 352:362, 2005.
3. Seidman JG, Seidman C: The genetic basis for cardiomyopathy: From mutation identification to mechanistic paradigms. Cell 104:557, 2001.
4. Morita H, DePalma SR, Arad M, et al: Molecular epidemiology of hypertrophic cardiomyopathy. Cold Spring Harbor symposia on quantitative biology. 67:383, 2002.
5. LeWinter MM, VanBuren P: Sarcomeric proteins in hypertrophied and failing myocardium: An overview. Heart Fail Rev 10:173, 2005.
6. Tardiff JC: Sarcomeric proteins and familial hypertrophic cardiomyopathy: Linking mutations in structural proteins to complex cardiovascular phenotypes. Heart Fail Rev 10:237, 2005.
7. Ahmad F, Seidman JG, Seidman CE: The genetic basis for cardiac remodeling. Annu Rev Genomics Hum Genet 6:185, 2005.
8. Maron BJ, Seidman JG, Seidman CE: Proposal for contemporary screening strategies in families with hypertrophic cardiomyopathy. J Am Coll Cardiol 44:2125, 2004.
9. Havndrup O, Bundgaard H, Andersen PS, et al: Outcome of clinical versus genetic family screening in hypertrophic cardiomyopathy with focus on cardiac beta-myosin gene mutations. Cardiovasc Res 57:347, 2003.
10. Ho CY, Sweitzer NK, McDonough B, et al: Assessment of diastolic function with Doppler tissue imaging to predict genotype in preclinical hypertrophic cardiomyopathy. Circulation 105:2992, 2002.
11. Richard P, Charron P, Carrier L, et al: Hypertrophic cardiomyopathy: Distribution of disease genes, spectrum of mutations, and implications for a molecular diagnosis strategy. Circulation 107:2227, 2003.
12. Ho CY, Seidman CE: A contemporary approach to hypertrophic cardiomyopathy. Circulation 113:e858, 2006.
13. Tsoutsman T, Lam L, Semsarian C: Genes, calcium and modifying factors in hypertrophic cardiomyopathy. Clin Exp Pharmacol Physiol 33:139, 2006.
14. Semsarian C, Ahmad I, Giewat M, et al: The L-type calcium channel inhibitor diltiazem prevents cardiomyopathy in a mouse model. J Clini Invest 109:1013-20 2002.
15. Backs J, Song K, Bezprozvannaya S, et al: CaM kinase II selectively signals to histone deacetylase 4 during cardiomyocyte hypertrophy. J Clin Invest 116:1853, 2006.
16. Prestle J, Quinn FR, Smith GL: Ca(2+)-handling proteins and heart failure: Novel molecular targets? Curr Med Chem 10:967, 2003.
17. Takano H, Zou Y, Akazawa H, et al: Inhibitory molecules in signal transduction pathways of cardiac hypertrophy. Hypertens Res 25:491, 2002.
18. Chang AN, Potter JD: Sarcomeric protein mutations in dilated cardiomyopathy. Heart Fail Rev 10:225, 2005.
19. Wolf CM, Moskowitz IP, Arno S, et al: Somatic events modify hypertrophic cardiomyopathy pathology and link hypertrophy to arrhythmia. Proc Natl Acad Sci U S A 102:18123, 2005.
20. Flashman E, Watkins H, Redwood C: Localisation of the binding site of the C-terminal domain of cardiac myosin binding protein-C on the myosin rod. Biochem J 401:97, 2007.
21. Sadayappan S, Gulick J, Osinska H, et al: Cardiac myosin-binding protein-C phosphorylation and cardiac function. Circ Res 97:1156, 2005.
22. Hackman JP, Vihola AK, Udd AB: The role of titin in muscular disorders. Ann Med 35:434, 2003.
23. Bos JM, Poley RN, Ny M, et al: Genotype-phenotype relationships involving hypertrophic cardiomyopathy-associated mutations in titin, muscle LIM protein, and telethonin. Mol Genet Metab 88:78, 2006.
24. Arad M, Penas-Lado M, Monserrat L, et al: Gene mutations in apical hypertrophic cardiomyopathy. Circulation 112:2805, 2005.
25. Girolami F, Olivotto I, Passerini I, et al: A molecular screening strategy based on beta-myosin heavy chain, cardiac myosin binding protein C and troponin T genes in Italian patients with hypertrophic cardiomyopathy. J Cardiovasc Med (Hagerstown) 7:601, 2006.
26. Mogensen J, Murphy RT, Kubo T, et al: Frequency and clinical expression of cardiac troponin I mutations in 748 consecutive families with hypertrophic cardiomyopathy. J Am Coll Cardiol 44:2315, 2004.
27. Doolan A, Tebo M, Ingles J, et al: Cardiac troponin I mutations in Australian families with hypertrophic cardiomyopathy: clinical, genetic and functional consequences. J Mol Cell Cardiol 38:387, 2005.
28. Jaaskelainen P, Miettinen R, Karkkainen P, et al: Genetics of hypertrophic cardiomyopathy in eastern Finland: Few founder mutations with benign or intermediary phenotypes. Ann Med 36:23, 2004.
29. Pieroni M, Chimenti C, De Cobelli F, et al: Fabry's disease cardiomyopathy: Echocardiographic detection of endomyocardial glycosphingolipid compartmentalization. J Am Coll Cardiol 47:1663, 2006.
30. Yang Z, McMahon CJ, Smith LR, et al: Danon disease as an underrecognized cause of hypertrophic cardiomyopathy in children. Circulation 112:1612, 2005.
31. Eskelinen EL: Roles of LAMP-1 and LAMP-2 in lysosome biogenesis and autophagy. Mol Aspects Med 27:495, 2006.
32. Oliveira SM, Ehtisham J, Redwood CS, et al: Mutation analysis of AMP-activated protein kinase subunits in inherited cardiomyopathies: Implications for kinase function and disease pathogenesis. J Mol Cell Cardiol 35:1251, 2003.
33. Long YC, Zierath JR: AMP-activated protein kinase signaling in metabolic regulation. J Clin Invest 116:1776, 2006.
34. Burwinkel B, Scott JW, Buhrer C, et al: Fatal congenital heart glycogenosis caused by a recurrent activating R531Q mutation in the gamma 2-subunit of AMP-activated protein kinase (PRKAG2), not by phosphorylase kinase deficiency. Am J Hum Genet 76:1034, 2005.

Dilated Cardiomyopathy

35. Schmitt JP, Debold EP, Ahmad F, et al: Cardiac myosin missense mutations cause dilated cardiomyopathy in mouse models and depress molecular motor function. Proc Natl Acad Sci U S A 103:14525, 2006.
36. Kane GC, Liu XK, Yamada S, et al: Cardiac KATP channels in health and disease. J Mol Cell Cardiol 38:937, 2005.
37. Sylvius N, Tesson F: Lamin A/C and cardiac diseases. Curr Opin Cardiol 21:159, 2006.
38. Ben Yaou R, Muchir A, Arimura T, et al: Genetics of laminopathies. Novartis Found Symp 264:81; discussion, 90, 2005.
39. Wheeler MT, McNally EM: Sarcoglycans in vascular smooth and striated muscle. Trends Cardiovasc Med 13:238, 2003.
40. Feng J, Yan J, Buzin CH, et al: Mutations in the dystrophin gene are associated with sporadic dilated cardiomyopathy. Mol Genet Metab 77:119, 2002.
41. Barth PG, Valianpour F, Bowen VM, et al: X-linked cardioskeletal myopathy and neutropenia (Barth syndrome): An update. Am J Med Genet 126:349, 2004.
42. Dorn GW 2nd: Physiological growth and pathological genes in cardiac development and cardiomyopathy. Trends Cardiovasc Med 15:185, 2005.
43. Finsterer J: Mitochondriopathies. Eur J Neurol 11:163, 2004.
44. Corrado D, Thiene G: Arrhythmogenic right ventricular cardiomyopathy/dysplasia: Clinical impact of molecular genetic studies. Circulation 113:1634, 2006.
45. Antoniades L, Tsatsopoulou A, Anastasakis A, et al: Arrhythmogenic right ventricular cardiomyopathy caused by deletions in plakophilin-2 and plakoglobin (Naxos disease) in families from Greece and Cyprus: Genotype-phenotype relations, diagnostic features and prognosis. Eur Heart J 27:2208, 2006.

Structural Cardiovascular Disease

46. Thom T, Haase N, Rosamond W, et al: Heart disease and stroke statistics—2006 update: A report from the American Heart Association Statistics Committee and Stroke Statistics Subcommittee. Circulation 113:e85, 2006.
47. Wong SF, Chan FY, Cincotta RB, et al: Factors influencing the prenatal detection of structural congenital heart diseases. Ultrasound Obstet Gynecol 21:19, 2003.
48. McKusick V: Online Mendelian Inheritance in Man, 2006 (http://www.ncbi.nlm.nih.gov/omim).
49. McBride KL, Pignatelli R, Lewin M, et al: Inheritance analysis of congenital left ventricular outflow tract obstruction malformations: Segregation, multiplex relative risk, and heritability. Am J Med Genet 134:180, 2005.
50. Horne BD, Camp NJ, Muhlestein JB, et al: Evidence for a heritable component in death resulting from aortic and mitral valve diseases. Circulation 110:3143, 2004.
51. James PA, Aftimos S, Skinner JR: Familial mitral valve prolapse associated with short stature, characteristic face, and sudden death. Am J Med Genet 119:32, 2003.
52. Eroglu AG, Babaoglu K, Oztunc F, et al: Echocardiographic follow-up of children with supravalvular aortic stenosis. Pediatr Cardiol 27:707, 2006.
53. Antonarakis SE, Lyle R, Dermitzakis ET, et al: Chromosome 21 and down syndrome: From genomics to pathophysiology. Nat Rev Genet 5:725, 2004.
54. Vergara P, Digilio MC, Zorzi AD, et al: Genetic heterogeneity and phenotypic anomalies in children with atrioventricular canal defect and tetralogy of Fallot. Clin Dysmorphol 15:65, 2006.
55. Donaldson MD, Gault EJ, Tan KW, et al: Optimising management in Turner syndrome: From infancy to adult transfer. Arch Dis Child 91:513, 2006.
56. Doswell BH, Visootsak J, Brady AN, et al: Turner syndrome: An update and review for the primary pediatrician. Clin Pediatr (Phila) 45:301, 2006.

57. Bondy CA, Ceniceros I, Van PL, et al: Prolonged rate-corrected QT interval and other electrocardiogram abnormalities in girls with Turner syndrome. Pediatrics 118: e1220, 2006.
58. Gravholt CH, Hjerrild BE, Naeraa RW, et al: Effect of growth hormone and 17beta-oestradiol treatment on metabolism and body composition in girls with Turner syndrome. Clin Endocrinol (Oxf) 62:616, 2005.
59. Fieno DS, Saouaf R, Thomson LE, et al: Cardiovascular magnetic resonance of primary tumors of the heart: A review. J Cardiovasc Magn Reson 8:839, 2006.
60. Wilkes D, Charitakis K, Basson CT: Inherited disposition to cardiac myxoma development. Nat Rev Cancer 6:157, 2006.
61. Wilkes D, McDermott DA, Basson CT: Clinical phenotypes and molecular genetic mechanisms of Carney complex. Lancet Oncol 6:501, 2005.
62. Schott JJ, Benson DW, Basson CT, et al: Congenital heart disease caused by mutations in the transcription factor NKX2-5. Science 281:108, 1998.
63. Rayment I, Holden HM, Whittaker M, et al: Structure of the actin-myosin complex and its implications for muscle contraction. Science 261:58, 1993.
64. Veugelers M, Bressan M, McDermott DA, et al: Mutation of perinatal myosin heavy chain associated with a Carney complex variant. N Engl J Med 351:460, 2004.

PART III

Evaluation of the Patient

CHAPTER 11

The History and Physical Examination: An Evidence-Based Approach

James C. Fang and Patrick T. O'Gara

The approach to the patient with known or suspected cardiovascular disease begins with a directed history and targeted physical examination, the scope of which depends on the clinical context at time of presentation. Elective, ambulatory encounters allow comparatively more time for the development of a comprehensive assessment, whereas emergency department visits and urgent bedside consultations require a more focused strategy. The elicitation of the history, with its emphasis on major cardiovascular symptoms and their change over time, should not be delegated to a trainee or other health care provider. The history is an invaluable source of information and often will provide clues linking seemingly disparate aspects of the patient's presentation. It affords a unique opportunity to assess the patient's personal attitudes, his/her intelligence, comprehension, acceptance, denial, motivation, fear, and prejudices. The interview can reveal genetic influences and the impact of other medical conditions on the manifesting illness. Although time constraints have limited the emphasis on careful history taking in most clinical situations,[1] more recent concerns regarding the escalating costs of health care, driven to a large extent by the increasingly premature utilization of medical imaging, may slow or reverse this trend.

The past several years have witnessed a gradual decline in physical examination skills at every level, from student to faculty specialist, a development of great concern to clinicians and medical educators. On average, internal medicine and family practice residents recognize only 20 percent of classic cardiac findings.[2-4] Despite popular perception, performance does not predictably improve as a function of experience and the acquisition of new skills may become more difficult for the busy individual practitioner.[5] Both the time and expertise devoted to the mentored cardiovascular examination have suffered as a consequence of the growing number of expectations on physician performance and the need to allow adequate exposure to the rapidly expanding number of diagnostic and therapeutic innovations available for appropriate clinical application. This decline in bedside skills has spurred an increase in the utilization of noninvasive imaging studies to establish the presence and severity of cardiovascular disease, even when the clinical findings would suggest a low pretest probability of significant pathology. A growing experience with the use of handheld cardiac ultrasound devices does suggest that this technology can characterize chamber size, ventricular function, and valve performance more reliably than the physical examination.[6]

Nevertheless, an integrated approach to the patient, one that begins with an appropriate history and incorporates the findings from inspection, palpation, and auscultation, is both desirable and cost-effective. This method guides downstream testing and establishes the crucial bond between patient and doctor.[7] Educational techniques to improve diagnostic proficiency include repetition, patient-centered teaching conferences, and visual display feedback of auscultatory events and Doppler echocardiographic findings.[8-11]

The evidence base that justifies correlations between findings from the history and physical examination and cardiovascular disease severity and prognosis has been most rigorously established for heart failure, valvular heart disease, and coronary artery disease. For example, heart rate, blood pressure, signs of pulmonary congestion, and the presence of mitral regurgitation contribute importantly to bedside risk assessment in patients with acute coronary syndromes (ACS).[12,13] In this setting, observations from the physical examination inform clinical decision-making in real time and trigger application of specific therapies before results of biomarker testing are available. Accurate characterization of cardiac murmurs and any associated findings, a process that can be enhanced by digital recording and spectral display,[14] provides important insight into the natural history of many valvular heart lesions. This chapter will review the fundamental features of the cardiovascular history and physical examination and then apply what is known from correlative studies on the pathophysiology, natural history, and outcomes of specific diseases. The reader can consult earlier editions of the text for a more in-depth discussion of the specific elements of the cardiovascular history and physical examination.

THE HISTORY

The major symptoms associated with cardiac disease include chest discomfort, dyspnea, fatigue, edema, palpitations, and syncope. Cough, hemoptysis, and cyanosis are additional examples. Claudication, limb pain, edema, and skin discoloration usually indicate a vascular disorder. In most instances, the differential diagnosis of chest discomfort can be narrowed by careful attention to location, radiation, triggers, mode of onset, duration, alleviating factors, and associated symptoms (see also Chap. 49). Angina pectoris must be distinguished from the pain associated with pulmonary embolism, pericarditis, aortic dissection, esophageal reflux, and costochondritis. Although a history of chest discomfort alone does not suffice to render a diagnosis of an ACS, several aspects of the manifesting symptom increase or decrease the likelihood of ACS. For example, pain that is stabbing, pleuritic, positional, or reproducible with palpation is usually noncardiac (likelihood ratios [LRs] 0.2 to 0.3); whereas discomfort that radiates to one or both shoulders or is precipitated by exertion increases the likelihood of ACS (LRs 2.3 to 4.7).[15] Less typical symptoms ("anginal equivalents") such as indigestion, belching, and dyspnea should also command the clinician's attention when other features of the presentation suggest an ACS, even in the absence of chest discomfort. Less typical presentations are more common in women, the elderly, and patients with diabetes. Dyspnea may occur with exertion, recumbency (orthopnea), or even with standing (platypnea). Paroxysmal nocturnal dyspnea of cardiac origin usually occurs 2 to 4 hours after onset of sleep, compels the patient to sit upright or stand, and subsides gradually over several minutes. The patient's partner should be questioned about any signs of sleep disordered breathing, such as loud snoring and/or periods of apnea. Pulmonary embolism is often associated with dyspnea of sudden onset. Patients may use a variety of terms to describe their awareness of the heart beat (palpitations), such as "flutters," "skips," or "pounding." Cardiac syncope occurs suddenly and restoration of full consciousness occurs quickly. Patients with neurocardiogenic syncope may have an early warning (nausea, yawning), appear ashen and diaphoretic, and revive more slowly, albeit without signs of seizure or a prolonged postictal state. The complete history requires information pertaining to traditional cardiovascular risk factors, a general medical history, occupation, habits, family history, and systems review.

It is extremely important to obtain a semiquantitative assessment of symptom severity and to document any progressive change. The New York Heart Association (NYHA) and Canadian Cardiovascular Society (CCS) functional classification systems have served for decades and remain useful for both patient care and clinical research, despite their inherent limitations (Table 11-1).[16,17] Assignment of symptom severity, as approximated by these classification systems, contributes importantly to risk assessment, clinical decision-making, and patient outcomes. More quantitative classification systems, such as that based on activity-specific metabolic energy expenditures, have not gained widespread use.[18]

TABLE 11–1 A Comparison of Three Methods of Assessing Cardiovascular Disability

Class	New York Heart Association (NYHA) Functional Classification	Canadian Cardiovascular Society (CCS) Functional Classification	Specific Activity Scale
I	Patients with cardiac disease but without resulting limitations of physical activity. Ordinary physical activity does not cause undue fatigue, palpitation, dyspnea, or anginal pain.	Ordinary physical activity, such as walking and climbing stairs, does not cause angina. Angina with strenuous or rapid or prolonged exertion at work or recreation.	Patients can perform to completion any activity requiring >7 metabolic equivalents (e.g., can carry 24 lb up eight steps; carry objects that weigh 80 lb; do outdoor work [shovel snow, spade soil]; do recreational activities [skiing, basketball, squash, handball, jog/walk 5 mph]).
II	Patients with cardiac disease resulting in slight limitation of physical activity. They are comfortable at rest. Ordinary physical activity results in fatigue, palpitation, dyspnea, or anginal pain.	Slight limitation of ordinary activity. Walking or climbing stairs rapidly, walking uphill, walking or stair climbing after meals, in cold, in wind, or when under emotional stress, or only during the few hours after awakening. Walking more than two blocks on the level and climbing more than one flight of ordinary stairs at a normal pace and in normal conditions.	Patients can perform to completion any activity requiring >5 metabolic equivalents (e.g., have sexual intercourse without stopping, garden, rake, weed, roller skate, dance fox trot, walk at 4 mph on level ground), but cannot and do not perform to completion activities requiring ≥7 metabolic equivalents.
III	Patients with cardiac disease resulting in marked limitation of physical activity. They are comfortable at rest. Less than ordinary physical activity causes fatigue, palpitation, dyspnea, or anginal pain.	Marked limitation of ordinary physical activity. Walking one to two blocks on the level and climbing more than one flight in normal conditions.	Patients can perform to completion any activity requiring >2 metabolic equivalents (e.g., shower without stopping, strip and make bed, clean windows, walk 2.5 mph, bowl, play golf, dress without stopping), but cannot and do not perform to completion any activities requiring ≥5 metabolic equivalents.
IV	Patients with cardiac disease resulting in inability to carry on any physical activity without discomfort. Symptoms of cardiac insufficiency or of the anginal syndrome may be present even at rest. If any physical activity is undertaken, discomfort is increased.	Inability to carry on any physical activity without discomfort—anginal syndrome *may be* present at rest.	Patients cannot or do not perform to completion activities requiring ≥2 metabolic equivalents. *Cannot* carry out activities listed above (Specific Activity Scale, Class III).

From Goldman L, et al: Comparative reproducibility and validity of systems for assessing cardiovascular functional class: Advantages of a new specific activity scale. Circulation 64(6):1227-34, 1981.

THE GENERAL PHYSICAL EXAMINATION

The physical examination performed within the context of the history can help to establish a cardiovascular cause for a given symptom, assess disease severity and progression, and allow the clinician the opportunity to evaluate the impact of specific therapies over time. It can also identify the presence of early stage disease in patients without symptoms.

General Appearance

The examination begins with an appreciation of the general appearance of the patient, including his or her age, posture, demeanor, and general health status. Is the patient in pain, resting quietly, or visibly diaphoretic with a foreboding sense of doom? The autonomic response of diaphoresis is not volitional and implies serious disease. Does the patient choose to avoid certain positions to reduce or eliminate pain? The pain of acute pericarditis, for example, is often minimized by sitting up and breathing shallowly. The respiratory pattern is also important. Pursing of the lips, a breathy quality to the voice, and an increased anteroposterior chest diameter would favor a pulmonary rather than cardiovascular cause of dyspnea. Pallor suggests that anemia may contribute to exercise intolerance or dyspnea, independent of cardiovascular disease. Cyanosis and jaundice can be readily appreciated. Certain syndromes may be apparent from the patient's general appearance such as trisomy 21, Marfan syndrome, Holt-Oram syndrome, and Turner syndrome (see also Chaps. 8 and 10). The chronically ill–appearing, emaciated patient suggests long-standing heart failure or another systemic disorder (malignancy, infection), with or without secondary cardiovascular involvement. The vital signs, including height, weight, temperature, pulse rate, blood pressure (both arms), respiratory rate, and oxygen saturation, dictate the pace and scope of the evaluation and provide the initial clues as to the presence of a cardiovascular disorder. Mental status should be assessed continuously during the interview and examination. An impaired sensorium has multiple causes, of which reduced cerebral perfusion would be of concern in the appropriate context. The serendipitous observation of the respiratory pattern during sleep may reveal signs of disordered breathing (e.g., Cheyne Stokes, obstructive sleep apnea), a relatively common finding among patients with systolic heart failure, hypertension, obesity, and/or atrial fibrillation (AF).

The Skin

Central cyanosis is present with significant right to left shunting at the level of the heart or lungs, which allows deoxygenated blood to reach the systemic circulation. It is also a feature of hereditary methemoglobinemia. Peripheral or acrocyanosis of the fingers, toes, nose, and ears is characteristic of the reduced blood flow that accompanies small vessel constriction seen in severe heart failure, shock, or peripheral vascular disease. Differential cyanosis affecting the lower, but not the upper, extremities occurs with a patent ductus arteriosus and pulmonary artery (PA) hypertension with right to left shunting at the great vessel level. Hereditary telangiectases on the lips, tongue, and mucous membranes (Osler-Weber -Rendu syndrome) resemble spider nevi and, when present in the lungs, can be a source of right to left shunting and central cyanosis. Telangiectases are also seen in patients with scleroderma with or without pulmonary hypertension. Tanning or bronzing of the skin in unexposed areas can suggest iron overload and hemochromatosis. Jaundice may be first appreciated in the sclerae; it has a broad differential diagnosis. Ecchymoses are often present with either warfarin, aspirin, and/or thienopyridine use, whereas petechiae are a feature of thrombocytopenia, and purpuric skin lesions can be seen with endocarditis and other causes of leukocytoclastic vasculitis. Various lipid disorders can manifest with xanthomas, subcutaneously, along tendon sheaths, or over the extensor surfaces of the extremities. Xanthoma within the palmar creases are specific for type III hyperlipoproteinemia (pre-beta, intermediate density). The leathery, cobblestone, "plucked chicken" appearance of the skin in the axilla and skinfolds of a young person is highly characteristic for pseudoxanthoma elasticum, a disease with multiple cardiovascular manifestations. Extensive lentiginoses (freckle-like brown macules and café-au-lait spots over the trunk and neck) may be part of developmental delay—cardiovascular syndromes (LEOPARD, LAMB, and Carney) with multiple atrial myxomas, atrial septal defects, hypertrophic cardiomyopathy, and valvular stenoses (see Chap. 8). In a patient with heart failure or syncope, cardiovascular sarcoid should be suspected by the presence of lupus pernio, erythema nodosum, or granuloma annulare.

Head and Neck

The state of the dentition should be assessed in all patients, both as a source of infection as well as an index of general health and hygiene. A high-arched palate is a feature of Marfan syndrome. A large protruding tongue with parotid enlargement may suggest amyloid disease in the right setting. Ptosis and ophthalmoplegia suggest muscular dystrophies, and congenital heart disease is often accompanied by hypertelorism, low-set ears, micrognathia, and a webbed neck, as with Noonan, Turner, and Down syndromes. Proptosis, lid lag, and stare denote Grave's hyperthyroidism. Blue sclerae, mitral or aortic regurgitation (AR), and a history of recurrent nontraumatic skeletal fractures are observed in patients with osteogenesis imperfecta. Premature arcus senilis and prominent earlobe creases may be associated with hyperlipidemia and coronary artery disease, respectively, although the correlations are weak. The funduscopic examination is an important and underutilized feature of the evaluation of patients with hypertension, diabetes, endocarditis, neurological symptoms, or known carotid or aortic arch disease. Lacrimal hyperplasia may suggest sarcoidosis. The "mitral facies" of rheumatic mitral stenosis are characterized by pink, purplish patches with telangiectases over the malar eminences and can also be seen with other disorders associated with pulmonary hypertension and reduced cardiac output. Relapsing polychondritis is suggested by inflammation of the pinnae and nasal cartilage. The examiner should also palpate the thyroid gland and assess its size, symmetry, and consistency.

Extremities

The temperature of the extremities, presence of clubbing, arachnodactyly, and nail findings can be quickly surmised, often while talking to the patient. Clubbing implies the presence of central shunting, although it has also been described with endocarditis. The appearance of clubbing can range from cyanosis and softening of the root of the nail bed, to the classic loss of the normal angle between the base of the nail and skin ("drumsticking"), to the skeletal and periosteal bony changes of hypertrophic osteoarthropathy. The striking appearance of the unapposable "fingerized" thumb is a classic finding in the autosomal dominant Holt-Oram syndrome in which atrial septal defects and conduction abnormalities are found. Arachnodactyly ("spider fingers," Marfan syndrome) can be assessed using the "wrist" (overlapping of the thumb and little finger around the wrist) or "thumb" signs (protrusion of the thumb beyond the ulnar aspect of the hand when the fingers are clenched over the thumb in a fist). Janeway lesions (nontender, slightly raised hemorrhages on the palms and soles), Osler's nodes (tender, raised nodules on the pads of the fingers or toes), and splinter hemorrhages (linear petechiae in the mid-nailbed) may be seen in some patients with endocarditis.

Lower extremity or presacral edema with elevated jugular venous pressure occurs in many volume-overloaded states, including heart failure. Chronic venous insufficiency can be diagnosed when jugular venous pressure is normal and there are additional signs of venous disease, such as extensive varicosities, medial ulcers, or brownish pigmentation from hemosiderin deposition. Edema is also a common complication of dihydropyridine calcium channel blocker therapy. Anasarca is rare in heart failure unless longstanding, untreated, and accompanied by hypoalbuminemia. Asymmetrical swelling can reflect local or unilateral venous thrombosis, lymphatic obstruction, or the sequelae of previous vein graft harvesting. Muscular atrophy and the absence of hair in an extremity should suggest chronic arterial insufficiency or neuromuscular disorders.

Chest and Abdomen

Surprisingly, midline sternotomy or posterolateral thoracotomy scars, as well as palpable pacemaker and defibrillator generators, are often overlooked as obvious signs of heart disease, especially when patients may not volunteer such relevant history. Cutaneous venous collaterals over the anterior chest may suggest obstruction of the superior vena cava or subclavian vein, especially in the presence of indwelling catheters or leads. Thoracic cage abnormalities, such as pectus carinatum (pigeon chest) or pectus excavatum (funnel chest), may be seen in connective tissue disorders; the barrel chest of emphysema or advanced kyphoscoliosis may be associated with cor pulmonale. The characteristically severe kyphosis and compensatory lumbar, hip, and knee flexion of ankylosing spondylitis ("bamboo spine disease") should prompt careful auscultation for AR. The straight back syndrome (loss of normal kyphosis of the thoracic spine) can accompany mitral valve prolapse. Cyanotic congenital heart disease may result in asymmetry of the anterior chest wall, with the left hemithorax displaced anteriorly. A thrill may be present over well-developed intercostal arterial collaterals in patients with hypertension and severe aortic coarctation. The respiratory pattern should be noted during spontaneous breathing with attention to rate, depth, audible wheezing, and stridor. Palpation, percussion, and auscultation of the chest follow sequentially.

The cardiac impulse may be most readily felt in the epigastrium in patients with emphysema or substantial obesity. The liver is often enlarged and tender in heart failure; systolic hepatic pulsations signify severe tricuspid regurgitation. Patients with infective endocarditis of long duration may have splenomegaly. Ascites is a nonspecific finding and is present with advanced right heart failure, chronic constrictive pericarditis, or hepatic cirrhosis. This finding often leads to an erroneous pursuit of gastrointestinal pathology to explain abdominal pain, fullness, or nausea. The aorta may normally be palpated between the epigastrium and umbilicus in thin patients and children and its dimensions can be estimated (see also Chap. 56). The sensitivity of palpation for the detection of abdominal aortic aneurysm (AAA) disease increases as a function of aneurysm diameter. The positive predictive value of palpation for AAA (>3.0 cm) detection is 43 percent.[19] Palpation cannot reliably exclude AAA, especially in obese patients. Arterial bruits in the abdomen should be localized but are often diffuse and may be confused with murmurs radiating from the chest.

The Cardiovascular Examination

Jugular Venous Pressure and Wave Form

The jugular venous pressure is perhaps the single most important hemodynamic measurement to ascertain volume status at the bedside. The external (EJV) or internal (IJV) jugular vein may be used, although the IJV is preferred because the EJV is valved and not directly in line with the superior vena cava (SVC) and right atrium (RA). The EJV is easier to visualize when distended, and its appearance has been used to discriminate between a low and high central venous pressure when tested among a group of attending physicians, residents, and medical students.[20] An elevated left EJV pressure may also signify a persistent left-sided SVC or compression of the innominate vein from an intrathoracic structure such as a tortuous or aneurysmal aorta. If an elevated venous pressure is suspected but venous pulsations cannot be appreciated, the patient should be asked to sit with the feet dangling over the side of the bed. The pooling of blood in the lower extremities with this maneuver may suffice to make the venous pulsations appear. In contrast, in the hypotensive patient in whom hypovolemia is suspected, the patient may need to be lowered to a supine position to appreciate the waveform in the right supraclavicular fossa.

The venous waveform can sometimes be difficult to distinguish from the carotid artery pulse. The venous waveform has several characteristic features (Fig. 11-1, Table 11-2) and its several components can usually be identified. The *a* and *v* waves, and *x* and *y* descents, are defined by their temporal relation to electrocardiogram (ECG) events and heart sounds (S_1, S_2). The estimated height of the venous pressure is a surrogate measure of the central venous, or RA, pressure. There is wide variability among observers in the

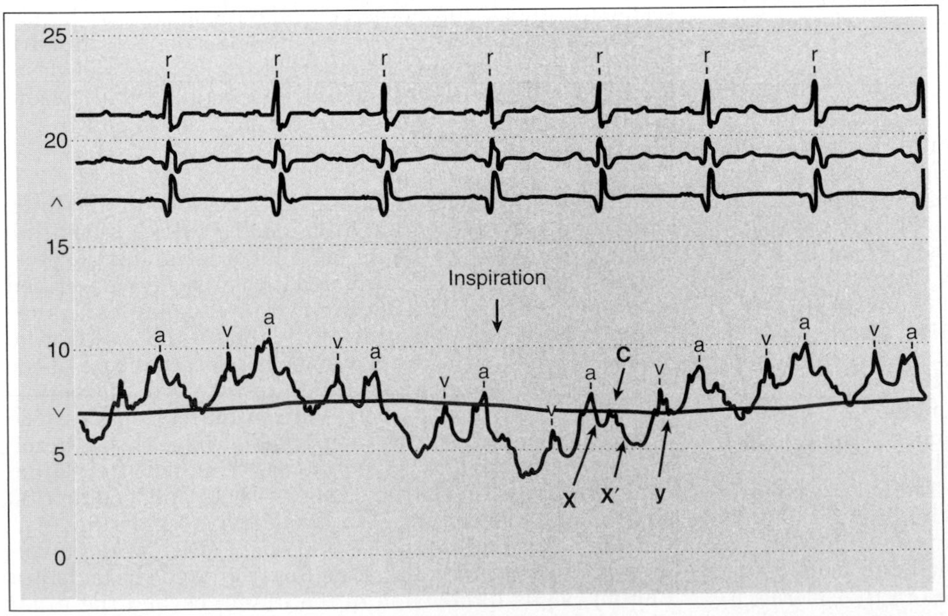

FIGURE 11–1 The normal jugular venous waveform recorded at cardiac catheterization. Note the inspiratory fall in pressure and the dominant X/X′ descent.

TABLE 11–2	Distinguishing the Jugular Venous Pulse from the Carotid Pulse	
Feature	**Internal Jugular Vein**	**Carotid Artery**
Appearance of pulse	Undulating two troughs and two peaks for every cardiac cycle (biphasic)	Single brisk upstroke (monophasic)
Response to inspiration	Height of column falls and troughs become more prominent	No respiratory change to contour
Palpability	Generally not palpable (except in severe TR)	Palpable
Effect of Pressure	Can be obliterated with gentle pressure at base of vein/clavicle	Cannot be obliterated

TR = tricuspid regurgitation.

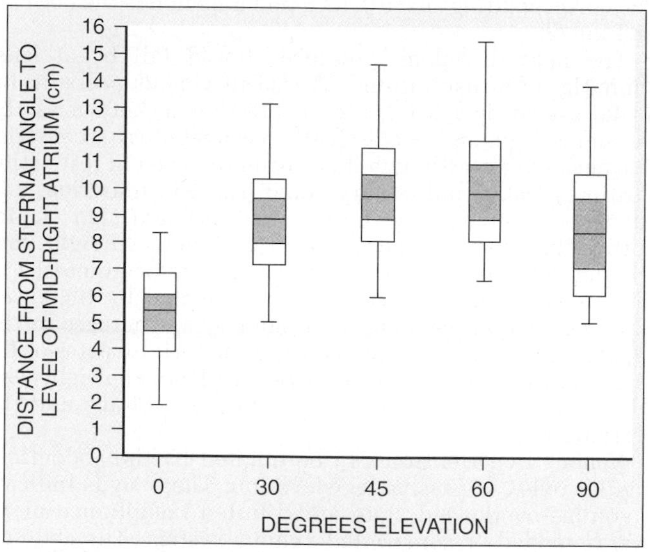

FIGURE 11–2 The distance between the angle of Louis and the mid-right atrium is highly variable among individual subjects and is a function of body position. Bars indicate minimum and maximum values. Box plots show 25th to 75th percentiles (gold) and 10th to 90th percentiles (white) and means. *(From Seth R, Magner P, Matziner F, vanWalraven C: How far is the sternal angle from the mid-right atrium? J Gen Intern Med 17[11]:852-6, 2002.)*

estimation of the central venous pressure.[21,22] In many instances, however, knowledge that the pressure is elevated, and not its specific value, will suffice for diagnosis and management.

The venous pressure is measured as the vertical distance between the top of the venous pulsation and the sternal inflection point, where the manubrium meets the sternum (angle of Louis). A distance of >3 cm is considered abnormal. Many have challenged this approach because the anatomical distance between the angle of Louis and mid-RA varies considerably, especially in obese patients.[23] In 160 consecutive patients receiving outpatient chest computed tomography (CT) scans, the median vertical distance ranged considerably by body position, with values of 8.0, 9.7, and 9.8 cm for body angles of 30, 45, and 60 degrees from supine, respectively. At 45 degrees, values ranged widely between patients, from 6 to 15 cm, and were independently correlated with smoking status, age, and anteroposterior chest dimension (Fig. 11-2).[24] In general, use of the sternal angle as a reference leads to systematic underestimation of venous pressure. In fact, some investigators recommend that this

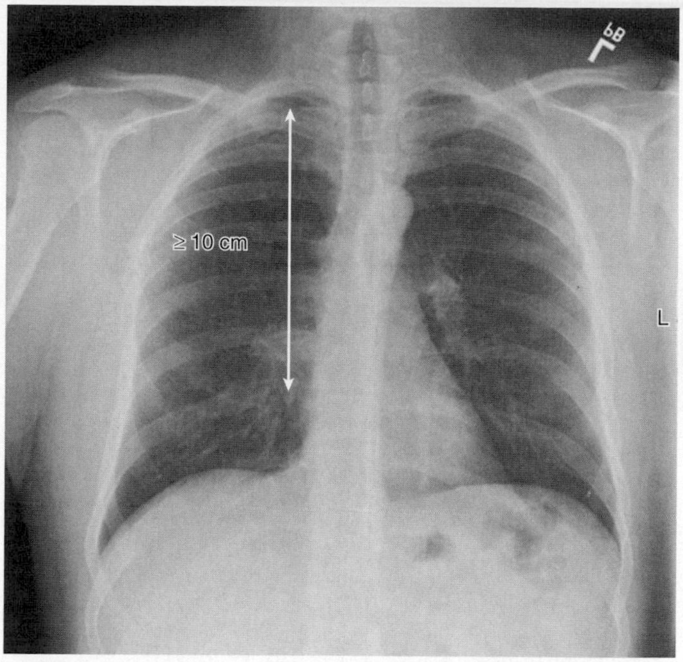

FIGURE 11–3 The clavicle can be used as a reference point to measure the jugular venous pressure in the upright position. The ability to see venous pulsations above the clavicle in the seated position is associated with an abnormally elevated venous pressure because, in most individuals, the clavicle is at least 10 cm above the right atrium.

method should not be used for quantification and that it can be used only to distinguish normal from abnormal central venous pressure.[22] The use of the mid-RA (estimated at the bedside using the mid-right chest) as the zero reference has also been challenged; other surface body points have been proposed on the basis of limited cadaveric studies or without specific rationale.[22] A point 5 cm below the fourth or 5th intercostal space at the left sternal border on the anterior chest wall may be the most accurate because it is the uppermost blood level in the left ventricular chamber in the supine position.[25] Practically, it is difficult to use even relatively simple landmarks. Critical care nurses varied by several centimeters in trying to locate an external reference point (the anterior axillary line at the 4th intercostal space) to measure the central venous pressure, despite a standardized approach.[26] Some clinicians choose to use the clavicle, especially with the patient in the seated position, as a constant reference. It is easily located and venous pulsations above that level are clearly abnormal, as the distance between the right atrium and the clavicle is at least 10 cm. (Fig. 11-3). The reliability of the bedside assessment of central venous pressure has been challenged and correlation with direct measurements has been only fair.[22] Differing reference standards, examiners, and variable definitions of normal values have limited previous studies. It is important to note that the measurements made at the bedside, which are in units of centimeters of blood or water, should be converted to millimeters of mercury (1.36 cm H_2O = 1.0 mm Hg), in order to correlate with accepted hemodynamic norms.

The venous waveforms are divided into several distinct peaks (*a*, *c*, and *v*; see Fig. 11-1). The *a* wave occurs with RA pre-systolic contraction, is coincident with the electrocardiographic P wave, and precedes the first heart sound (S_1). A prominent *a* wave is seen in patients with reduced right ventricular (RV) compliance from any cause. A cannon *a* wave occurs with A-V dissociation and RA contraction against a closed tricuspid valve (Fig. 11-4). The *a* wave is

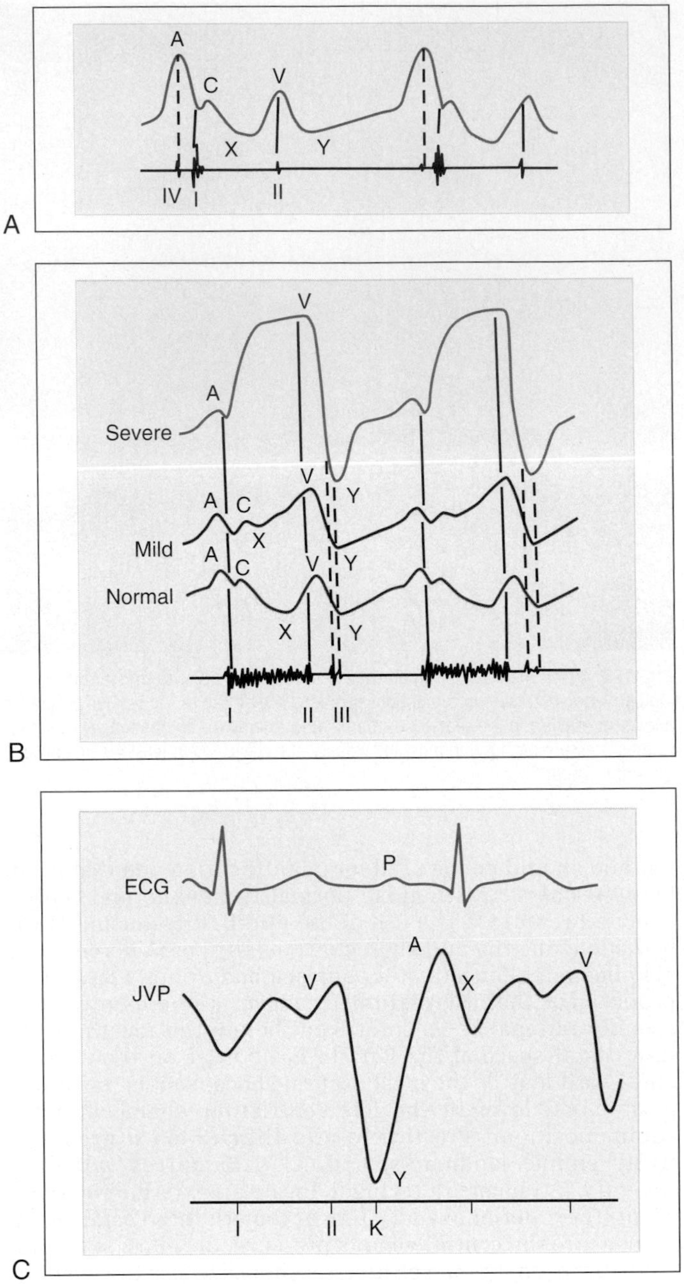

FIGURE 11–4 Abnormal jugular venous waveforms. **A,** Large *a* waves associated with reduced right ventricular (RV) compliance or elevated RV end-diastolic pressure. Phonocardiographic tracing **(below)** shows timing of the corresponding right-sided S4. **B,** Normal jugular venous waveform **(bottom),** mild tricuspid regurgitation (TR) **(middle)** and severe TR **(top),** with corresponding phonocardiogram. With severe TR, there is "ventricularization" of the jugular venous waveform, with a prominent V wave and rapid Y descent. The X descent is absent. **C,** Jugular venous waveform in constrictive pericarditis with a prominent Y descent. Note the timing of the pericardial knock (K) relative to S_2. The abrupt rise in pressure after the nadir of the Y descent is due to the rapid rise in venous pressure with ventricular filling. ECG = electrocardiogram; JVP = jugular venous pulse. *(From Abrams J: Synopsis of Cardiac Physical Diagnosis, 2nd ed. Boston, Butterworth Heinemann, 2001, pp 25-35.)*

absent with AF. The *x* descent defines the fall in RA pressure after the *a* wave peak. The *c* wave interrupts this descent as ventricular systole pushes the closed tricuspid valve into the right atrium, elevating its pressure. In the neck, the underlying carotid pulse may also be responsible for this wave. The *x′* descent follows and is the physiological consequence of atrial diastolic suction created by ventricular systole pulling the tricuspid valve and floor of the right atrium downward. In normal individuals, the *x′* descent is the predominant waveform in the jugular venous pulse. The *v* wave represents atrial filling, occurs at the end of ventricular systole, and follows just after S_2. Its height is determined by RA compliance and by the volume of blood returning to the RA—either antegrade from the vena cavae and/or retrograde through an incompetent tricuspid valve. The *v* wave is smaller than the *a* wave because of the normally compliant right atrium. In patients with atrial septal defect (ASD), the *a* and *v* waves may be of equal height; in tricuspid regurgitation (TR), the *v* wave is accentuated. With TR, the *v* wave will merge with the *c* wave because retrograde flow and antegrade right atrial filling will occur simultaneously (see Fig. 11-4). The *y* descent follows the *v* wave peak and reflects the fall in RA pressure after tricuspid valve opening. If there is resistance to ventricular filling in early diastole, the *y* descent will be blunted, as is the case with pericardial tamponade or tricuspid stenosis. The *y* descent will be steep when ventricular diastolic filling occurs early and rapidly, as with pericardial constriction. The corresponding auscultatory phenomenon is the pericardial knock.

The normal venous pressure should fall by at least 3 mm Hg with inspiration.[27] A rise in venous pressure (or its failure to decrease) with inspiration is known as the Kussmaul sign, and is classically associated with constrictive pericarditis, although it has been reported in restrictive cardiomyopathy, pulmonary embolism, RV infarction, and advanced systolic heart failure. A Kussmaul sign occurs with right-sided volume overload and reduced right ventricular compliance. Normally, the inspiratory increase in right-sided venous return is accommodated by increased right ventricular ejection, facilitated by an increase in the capacitance of the pulmonary vascular bed. In states of RV diastolic dysfunction and volume overload, the right ventricle cannot accommodate the enhanced volume and the pressure rises.

Venous hypertension can be elicited by the abdominojugular reflex or passive leg elevation. These signs indicate a volume-overloaded state and limited compliance of an overdistended or constricted venous system. The abdominojugular reflex is performed using firm and consistent pressure over the upper abdomen, preferably the right upper quadrant, for at least 10 seconds. A sustained rise of >3 cm in the venous pressure for at least 15 seconds after resumption of spontaneous respiration is a positive response. The patient should be coached to refrain from holding his or her breath or performing a Valsalva-like maneuver that can falsely elevate the venous pressure. The abdominojugular reflex is useful in predicting heart failure and a PA wedge pressure >15 mm Hg.[28]

Measuring the Blood Pressure

Auscultatory measurement of blood pressure (see also Chap. 40) based on the Korotkoff sounds yields lower systolic and higher diastolic values than direct intraarterial recording.[29] The measurement of blood pressure depends on body position, arm size, time of measurement, place of measurement, device, device size, technique, and examiner. For example, physician-recorded blood pressures are higher than nurse-recorded pressures by 6.3 mm Hg systolic and 7.9 mm Hg diastolic, respectively.[30] Nurse-recorded blood pressure is usually closer to the patient's average daytime blood pressure. Blood pressure should be measured in the seated position with the arm at the level of the heart using an appropriately sized cuff (Table 11-3). The patient should be relaxed for 5 to 10 minutes. In the supine position, the arm should be raised to bring it to the level of the mid-RA (i.e., elevated on a pillow). The length and width of the cuff's bladder should be 80 and 40 percent of the arm's circumfer-

TABLE 11–3	Important Aspects of Blood Pressure Measurement
· Seated comfortably, back supported, bared upper arm, legs uncrossed	
· Arm should be at heart level	
· Cuff length/width should be 80%/40% of arm circumference	
· Cuff should be deflated at <3 mm Hg per second	
· Column or dial should be read to nearest 2 mm Hg	
· First audible Korotkoff sound is systolic pressure; last sound is diastolic pressure	
· No talking between subject and observer	

ence, respectively (standard cuffs range from 12 to 16 cm × 22 to 36 cm). A common source of error in clinical practice is the use of an inappropriately small cuff, which results in overestimation of the true blood pressure and has particular relevance in obese patients. In one study from a hypertension referral clinic, 61 percent of patients had an arm circumference of >32 cm.[31] The blood pressure will be underestimated by a cuff that is too large for a smaller or thinner patient. The cuff should be placed 1 to 2 cm above the antecubital fossa to allow for placement of the stethoscope over the brachial artery. The cuff should be inflated to 30 mm Hg above the systolic pressure and the pressure should be released at 2 to 3 mm Hg per second. The first and fifth Korotkoff sounds mark the systolic and diastolic pressures, respectively. The sounds result from the turbulent blood flow and arterial wall oscillations in a partially occluded vessel.

On occasion, the Korotkoff sounds may disappear soon after the first sound, only to recur later before finally disappearing as phase 5. This phenomenon is known as the auscultatory gap and is attributed to venous engorgement of the upper extremity with poor antegrade arterial flow. It is more likely to occur in older, hypertensive patients with target end organ damage and may reflect intraarterial fluctuations in pressure.[32] The systolic pressure should be recorded at the first Korotkoff sound and not when the sound reappears. The gap can be eliminated by raising the arm for 30 seconds and clenching the fist several times before measuring the blood pressure. This finding should be distinguished from *pulsus paradoxus* (see later). Korotkoff sounds may be heard all the way down to 0 mm Hg with the cuff completely deflated in patients with chronic severe AR, children, pregnant patients, or in the presence of a large arteriovenous (AV) fistula. In these cases, both the phase 4 and 5 pressures should be noted.

The mercury sphygmomanometer is considered the most accurate device for measuring blood pressure, but it has fallen out of use because of concerns related to mercury toxicity. Aneroid sphygmomanometers are popular and use metal bellows and a system of levers to record the blood pressure. However, they require frequent calibration and there may be significant variability between manufacturers. Oscillometric devices are increasingly common in automated and hybrid sphygmomanometers and use empirically derived algorithms to obtain the systolic and diastolic pressures from mean pressure. The mean pressure is obtained using the point of maximal oscillations when a cuff is gradually deflated.

Blood pressure can be measured at the wrist. Systolic pressure increases and diastolic pressures decreases when measured in the more distal arteries, although there is little change in mean pressure from aorta to periphery. Blood pressure can also be measured without auscultation using the sphygmomanometer; palpation of a reestablished pulse distal to the cuff during deflation can be accurate to within 10 to 20 mm Hg of the systolic pressure. The diastolic pressure can be approximated when the character of the returned radial or brachial pulse changes to a brisk, normal rate of rise.

Blood pressure should be measured in both arms either in rapid succession or simultaneously; normally the measurements should differ by <10 mm Hg, independent of handedness. As many as 20 percent of normal subjects, however, have a >10 mm Hg arm blood pressure differential in the absence of symptoms or other examination findings, an observation of uncertain relevance.[33] A blood pressure differential of >10 mm Hg can be associated with subclavian artery disease (atherosclerotic or inflammatory), supravalvular aortic stenosis, aortic coarctation, or dissection. Systolic leg pressures may be as much as 20 mm Hg higher than arm pressures; greater leg-arm pressure differences are seen in patients with severe AR (Hill sign) and patients with extensive and calcified lower peripheral arterial disease (PAD).[34] Leg blood pressure should be measured using large thigh cuffs with auscultation at the popliteal artery or using a standard large arm cuff on the calf with simultaneous auscultation at the posterior tibial artery (Fig. 11-5). Measurement of lower extremity blood pressures forms the basis of the ankle brachial index (ABI), a powerful predictor of cardiovascular mortality (see later and Chaps. 57 and 59).

The blood pressure measured in the clinic may not accurately reflect the patient's mean blood pressure, as assessed by ambulatory or home-based recordings. Furthermore, isolated clinic measurements do not reflect other important aspects of blood pressure, including mean value, extent of normal diurnal fluctuation, and response to exercise. Consideration should be given to ambulatory blood pressure monitoring when uncertainty exists about the significance of recordings obtained in the clinic. This approach is especially useful for the patient with suspected "white coat" hypertension (more common in women and older men), defined by at least three separate clinic-based measurements of >140/90 mm Hg and at least two nonclinic-based measurements of <140/90 mm Hg, in the absence of end organ damage. Individuals with white coat hypertension may not benefit from drug therapy, but may be more likely to develop sustained hypertension over time. Masked hypertension (due to severe peripheral arterial disease) should be suspected when normal blood pressures are recorded and evidence of hypertensive end organ damage is present.

Orthostatic hypotension is defined by a fall in pressure of >20 mm Hg systolic and/or >10 mm Hg diastolic in response to moving from the supine to standing position within 3 minutes. There may be an additional lack of compensatory tachycardia, a response suggestive of autonomic insufficiency, as can be seen in patients with diabetes or Parkinson disease. The heart rate–blood pressure response to standing is also influenced by age, hydration, medications, food, conditioning, and ambient temperature.

Pseudohypertension is present when the sphygmomanometric pressure is greater than the intraarterial pressure and is usually due to stiff, calcified, noncompressible arteries. In this instance, decisions regarding the type and dosage of antihypertensive medications may be misguided. Osler maneuver is suggestive of pseudohypertension. The maneuver is positive when the radial pulse is still palpable despite an occlusive pressure over the more proximal brachial artery.[35] This sign is not specific; Osler maneuver is positive in as many as one third of unselected, elderly hospitalized patients.[36] Vascular stiffness can be quantified using other means. A wide pulse pressure (>50 mm Hg) in the absence of AR or other cause of diastolic run-off (e.g., an AV fistula) is due to the summation of the incident wave and the rapidly

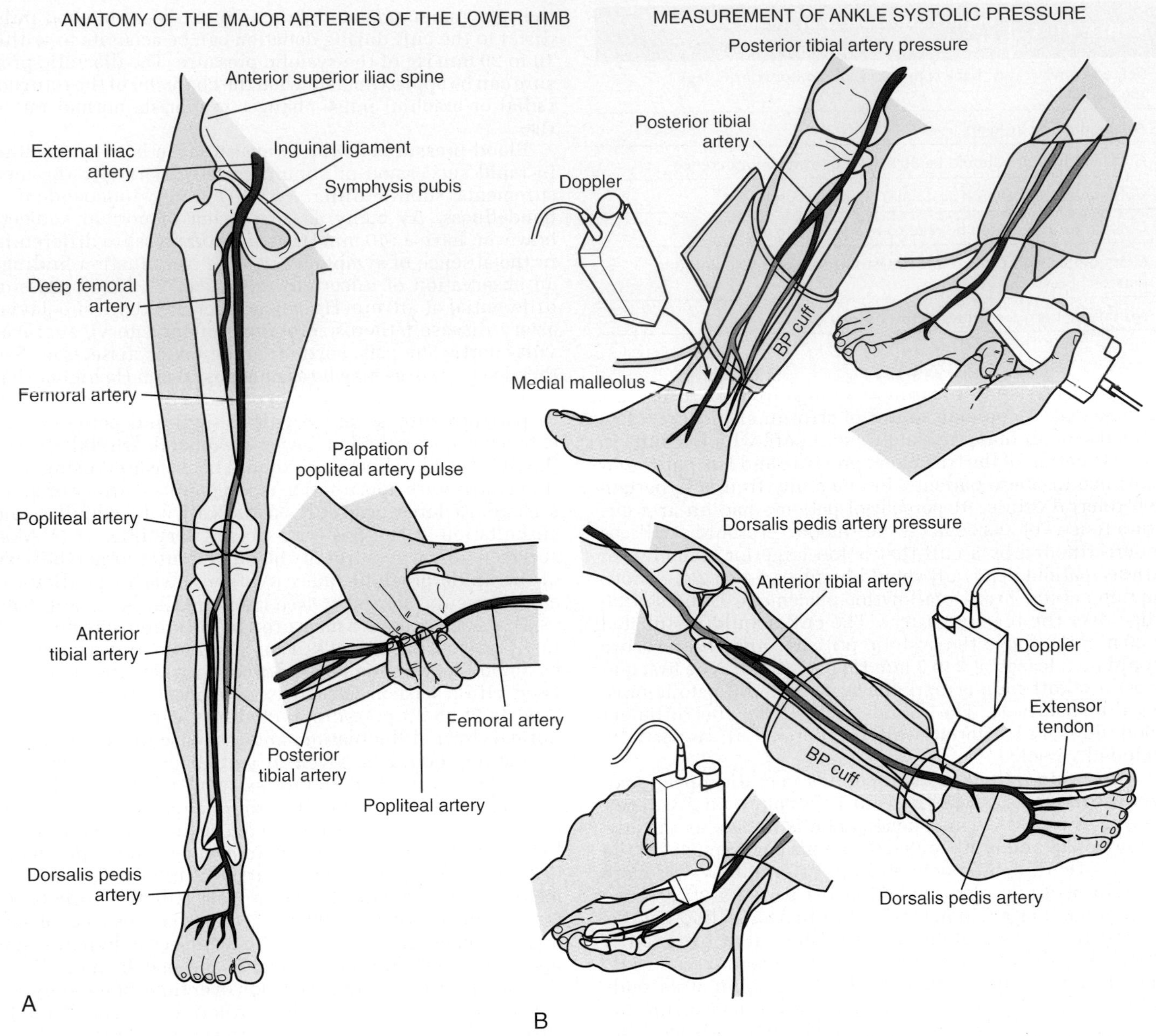

FIGURE 11–5 Measurement of the lower extremity blood pressures. *(From Khan NA, et al: Does the clinical examination predict lower extremity peripheral arterial disease? J Am Med Assoc 295:536-546, 2006.)*

reflected vascular pressure wave. The height of the systolic pressure and the nadir of the diastolic pressure are determined by the timing of the reflected wave as it sums with the primary forward stroke volume ejected into the vascular tree. An increase in pulse pressure in this circumstance represents increased vascular stiffness and is usually due to aging or atherosclerosis. The single best measure of vascular stiffness is unknown.[37] Peripheral indices may not correlate well with central aortic stiffness, which is a primary determinant of ventricular-vascular coupling. One measure, the augmentation index, is the percent increase in systolic pressure created by the premature return of the reflected wave during late systole. Such measurements can be obtained using peripheral tonometry and translated into central stiffness indices using mathematical transfer functions.[38]

Assessing the Pulses

The carotid artery pulse wave occurs within 40 msec of the ascending aortic pulse and reflects aortic valve and ascending aortic function. The aortic pulse is best appreciated in the epigastrium (abdominal aorta). The peripheral arterial pulses that should be assessed include the brachial, radial, ulnar, femoral, popliteal, dorsalis pedis, and posterior tibial. The temporal arteries can be easily palpated and should be examined in patients in whom the diagnosis of temporal arteritis or polymyalgia rheumatica has been raised. One of the two pedal pulses may not be palpable in a normal subject due to unusual anatomy (posterior tibial, <5 percent; dorsal pedis, <10 percent), but each pair should be symmetrical. True congenital absence of a pulse is rare (<2 percent) and in most cases pulses can be obtained with a handheld Doppler device when not palpable.[39] The integrity of the arcuate system of the hand can be assessed using the Allen test. All pulses should be examined for symmetry, volume, timing, contour, size, and strength. Simultaneous auscultation of the heart sounds will help to discern delays in upstroke. Concomitant palpation of the brachial or radial pulse with the femoral pulse should routinely be performed; a femoral delay in a patient with hypertension may be a clue for aortic coarctation. The carotid pulses should not be examined simultaneously or before auscultation for a bruit; light pressure should be used to avoid precipitation of carotid hypersensitivity syndrome in a susceptible individual.

The character and contour of the pulses depend on the stroke volume, ejection velocity, vascular capacity/compliance, and systemic resistance. These factors produce a palpable pulse that reflects the merging of both the antegrade pulsatile flow of blood and reflection of the propagated pulse returning from the peripheral arterial beds. These properties are most discernible in the more central arteries (i.e., the aorta and carotid pulses). The arterial pulse becomes more rapid and spiking as a function of its distance from the heart, reflecting the muscular status of the more peripheral arteries and the summation of incident and reflected waves. Normally, the incident (or percussion wave) begins with systolic ejection (just after S_1) and is the predominant monophasic pulse appreciated at the bedside (Fig. 11-6). The incisura or dicrotic notch signifies aortic valve closure. The modest rise in diastolic pressure after the incisura is not appreciated at the bedside and is discernible only with intraarterial pressure recordings. A bounding pulse indicates a large stroke volume with a rapid fall-off and may occur in hyperkinetic states such as fever, anemia, and thyrotoxicosis, or in pathological states such as severe bradycardia, AR, and arteriovenous fistula. A bifid pulse is created by two distinct pressure peaks. This phenomenon may occur with fever or after exercise in a normal individual and is consistent with increased vascular compliance. It is easily appreciated in patients on intraaortic balloon counterpulsation (with augmentation of diastolic pressure). With chronic severe AR, a large stroke volume ejected rapidly into a noncompliant arterial tree (as with hypertension or aging) produces a reflected wave of sufficient amplitude to be palpated during systole. Hypertrophic obstructive cardiomyopathy (HOCM) can rarely produce a bifid systolic pulse with percussion and tidal (or reflected) waves (see Fig. 11-6).

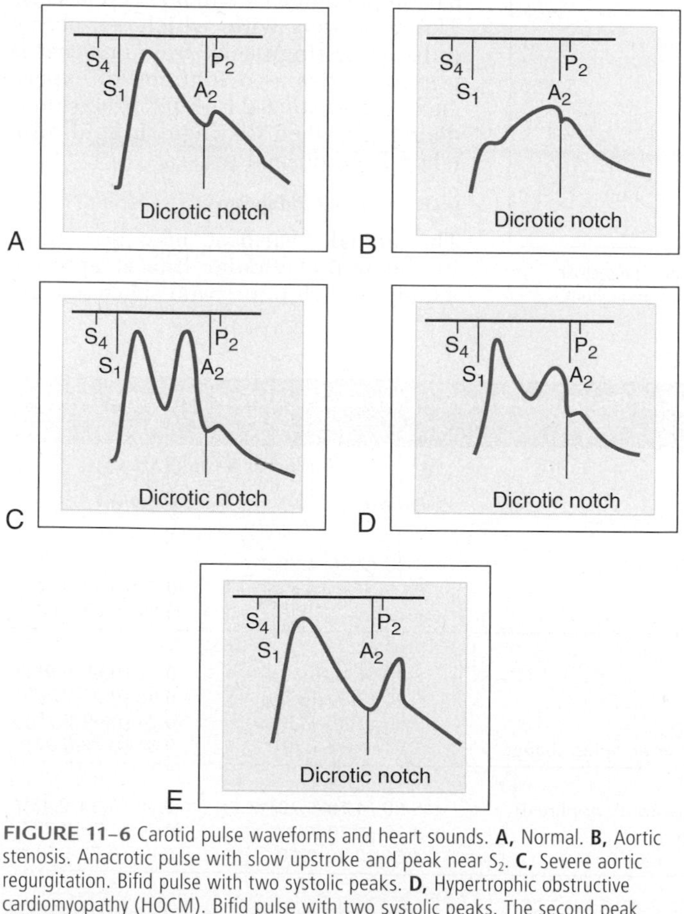

FIGURE 11–6 Carotid pulse waveforms and heart sounds. **A,** Normal. **B,** Aortic stenosis. Anacrotic pulse with slow upstroke and peak near S_2. **C,** Severe aortic regurgitation. Bifid pulse with two systolic peaks. **D,** Hypertrophic obstructive cardiomyopathy (HOCM). Bifid pulse with two systolic peaks. The second peak (tidal or reflected wave) is of lower amplitude than the initial percussion wave. **E,** Bifid pulse with systolic and diastolic peaks as may occur with sepsis or intraaortic balloon counterpulsation. A_2 = aortic component of S_2; P2 = pulmonic component of S_2; S_1 = first heart sound; S2 = second heart sound; S_4 = fourth heart sound. *(From Chatterjee K: Bedside evaluation of the heart: The physical examination.* In *Chatterjee K, Parmley W [eds]: Cardiology: An Illustrated Text/Reference. Philadelphia, JB Lippincott, 1991, pp 3.11-3.51; and Braunwald E: The clinical examination.* In *Braunwald E, Goldman L [eds]: Primary Cardiology, 2nd ed. Philadelphia, Elsevier, 2003, p 36.)*

A >10 mm Hg fall in systolic pressure with inspiration (*pulsus paradoxus*) is considered pathological and a sign of pulmonary or pericardial disease. It has also been described in obesity and pregnancy in the absence of clinical disease.[40] Pulsus paradoxus is measured by noting the difference between the systolic pressure at which the Korotkoff sounds are first heard (during expiration), and the systolic pressure at which the Korotkoff sounds are heard with each beat, independent of respiratory phase. Between these two pressures, the sounds are heard only intermittently (during exhalation). The cuff pressure must be decreased slowly to appreciate the finding. Tachycardia, AF, and tachypnea make its assessment very difficult. Pulsus paradoxus may be palpable when the pressure difference exceeds 20 mm Hg. The inspiratory fall in systolic pressure appears to be an exaggerated consequence of interventricular dependence. This phenomenon becomes amplified when ventricular volumes are fixed by an external constraint, as in the case of pericardial tamponade.[41] There is also a contribution from the inspiratory increase in transmural aortic wall pressure, which increases aortic impedance and LV afterload. Pulsus paradoxus is not specific for pericardial tamponade, and has been described with massive pulmonary embolus, hemorrhagic shock, severe obstructive lung disease, and tension pneumothorax.

Pulsus alternans is defined by the beat-to-beat variability of the pulse amplitude (Fig. 11-7). Pulsus alternans is present when only every other phase one Korotkoff sound is audible as the cuff pressure is slowly lowered, in a patient with a regular heart rhythm, independent of the respiratory cycle. It should be distinguished from the expected beat-to-beat variability of the pulse in a patient with bigeminy. Pulsus alternans is generally seen in severe heart failure and is exaggerated in severe AR, hypertension, and hypovolemic states. It is attributed to cyclic changes in intracellular calcium and action potential duration.[42] When associated with electrocardiographic T wave alternans, arrhythmic risk appears to be increased.[43]

Severe aortic stenosis may be suggested by a weak and delayed pulse, *pulsus parvus et tardus,* and best appreciated by careful palpation of the carotid arteries (see Fig. 11-6; see also Chap. 62). The delay is assessed during simultaneous auscultation of the heart sounds; the carotid upstroke should be coincident with S_1. This finding is less accurate in older, hypertensive patients with reduced vascular compliance and stiffer carotid arteries. A slow, notched, interrupted upstroke is known as an *anacrotic pulse;* a shudder or thrill may be appreciated with severe aortic stenosis. An abrupt carotid upstroke with rapid fall-off characterizes the pulse of AR (Corrigan or water-hammer pulse). The carotid upstroke is also rapid in elderly patients with isolated systolic hypertension and wide pulse pressures.

Ascending aortic aneurysms may rarely produce a systolic pulsation near the right sternoclavicular joint or in the upper right parasternal region. The abdominal aorta can be appreciated in the epigastric area (see earlier). Femoral and popliteal artery aneurysms should be sought in patients with AAA disease or underlying connective tissue disease.

Asymmetrical upper extremity systolic blood pressures, defined by a >10 mm Hg difference, may occur with left subclavian artery disease (atherosclerosis, inflammation, dissection). The site of obstruction in a patient with buttock or lower extremity claudication can be localized by the history and by appreciation of the level at which the pulse amplitude first decreases (see also Chap. 57). For example, a decreased femoral pulse suggests aortoiliac disease and a decreased popliteal pulse is consistent with femoral obstruction.

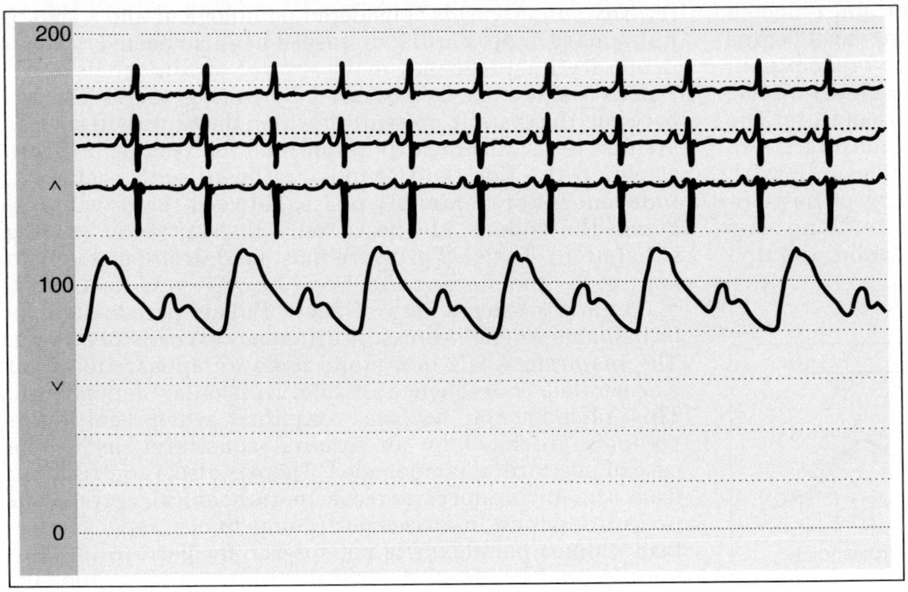

FIGURE 11–7 *Pulsus alternans* in a patient with severe left ventricular systolic dysfunction. The systolic pressure varies from beat-to-beat independently of the respiratory cycle. The rhythm is sinus throughout.

Arterial bruits are most commonly created by turbulent flow through narrowed arteries. The correlation between the presence of a bruit and the degree of vascular obstruction is weak.[44] A cervical bruit, for example, is a poor indicator of the degree of carotid artery narrowing, and the absence of a bruit does not rule out significant luminal compromise. If, however, the bruit extends into diastole, or a thrill is present, the obstruction is generally severe. Other causes of a bruit include AV fistulas and enhanced flow through normal arteries as, for example, in a young patient with fever.

The accuracy of the examination for the identification of lower extremity PAD can be improved by integrating the clinical history and presence of atherosclerotic risk factors with the observed findings.[39] The absence of claudication or the presence of normal pulses significantly decreases the likelihood of moderate to severe PAD. In an asymptomatic patient, the presence of a femoral bruit or any abnormality of the pulse increases the likelihood of PAD (LR 4.8, 95 percent CI 2.4 to 9.5 and 3.1, 95 percent CI 3.1 to 6.6, respectively). However, the likelihood of significant PAD increases when there are lower extremity symptoms and cool skin (LR 5.9, 95 percent CI 4.1 to 8.6), pulse abnormalities (LR 4.7, 95 percent CI 2.2 to 9.9), or any bruit (LR 5.6, 95 percent CI 4.7 to 6.7) (Table 11-4). The precision with which an absent pulse is distinguished from one that is present varies as a function of experience (K statistic 0.2 to 1.0).[45] Precision is decreased when distinguishing diminished from normal pulses.

Inspection and Palpation of the Heart

The apical heartbeat may be visible in the mid-clavicular line at approximately the 5th intercostal space in thin-

TABLE 11–4 Likelihood Ratios for Various Symptoms or Signs of Peripheral Arterial Disease, Stratified by Symptomatic or Screening Studies

Type of Study	Severity	Symptom or Sign	Likelihood Ratio (95% CI) Positive	Negative
Claudication				
Screening	Any disease	"Definite" or "Probable" claudication	3.30 (2.30-4.80)*	
	Moderate to severe	No claudication		0.57 (0.43-0.76)
	Any disease	No claudication		0.89 (0.78-1.00)
Skin Changes				
Symptomatic	Any disease	Cooler to touch	5.90 (4.10-8.60)	0.92 (0.89-0.95)
		Wounds or sores	5.90 (2.60-13.40)	0.98 (0.97-1.00)
		Discoloration	2.80 (2.40-3.30)	0.74 (0.69-0.79)
Screening	Moderate to severe	Hair, temperature, color, or atrophic change	1.50 (1.20-1.70)*	0.81 (0.72-0.92)*
Bruits				
Symptomatic	Any disease	At least one bruit (iliac, femoral, popliteal)	5.60 (4.70-6.70)*	0.39 (0.34-0.45)*
	Any disease	Femoral bruit	5.70 (4.70-7.00)	0.74 (0.70-0.78)
Screening	Any disease	Femoral bruit	4.80 (2.40-9.50)	0.83 (0.73-0.95)
Pulse Palpation				
Symptomatic	Any disease	Any palpable pulse abnormality	4.70 (2.20-9.90)	0.38 (0.23-0.64)
Screening	Moderate to severe	Any palpable pulse abnormality	3.00 (2.30-3.90)	0.44 (0.30-0.66)
	Any disease	Any palpable pulse abnormality	3.10 (1.40-6.60)	0.48 (0.22-1.04)
	Any disease	Absence of any palpable abnormality (in a lipid research clinic study)		0.27 (0.16-0.44)
	Any disease	Absence of any palpable abnormality (in high prevalence of diabetes)		0.87 (0.79-0.97)

*Results statistically homogeneous (all $P > 0.20$). Moderate to severe peripheral arterial disease defined by ankle-brachial index <0.50. Adapted from Khan NA, et al: JAMA 295:536-546, 2006.

chested adults. Visible pulsations anywhere other than the normally located ventricular apex beat are abnormal. The left anterior chest wall may heave in patients with enlarged and hyperdynamic left ventricles. Right upper parasternal and sternoclavicular pulsations suggest ascending aortic aneurysm disease. A left parasternal heave indicates RV pressure or volume overload. A proximal PA pulsation in the 3rd intercostal space to the left of the sternum indicates PA hypertension. In very thin, tall patients, or in patients with emphysema and flattened diaphragms, the RV impulse may be visible in the epigastrium and should be distinguished from a pulsatile liver edge.

Palpation of the heart should begin with the patient in the supine position at 30 degrees. If the heart is not palpable in this position, the patient should be examined either in the left lateral decubitus position with the left arm above the head or in the seated position, leaning forward. The point of maximal impulse is normally over the left ventricular apex beat and should be located in the mid-clavicular line at the 5th intercostal space. It is smaller than 2 cm in diameter, and moves quickly away from the fingers. It is best appreciated at end-expiration when the heart is closest to the chest wall. The apex beat is created by ventricular systole and counterclockwise rotation as the heart twists and shortens along its long axis. Rapid diastolic filling drops the apex beat away from the chest wall, producing a discrete, short, palpable impulse. The normal impulse may not be palpable in obese or muscular patients or in those with thoracic cage deformities. In such cases, the dominant pulse in the supine position may be in the epigastrium. The quality of the left ventricular apex beat can be appreciated by placing the patient in the left lateral decubitus position.

Left ventricular (LV) cavity enlargement, the most common cause of cardiomegaly, is manifested by leftward and downward displacement of an enlarged apex beat. A sustained apex beat is a sign of LV pressure overload (aortic stenosis, hypertension), but can be difficult to appreciate. A palpable, presystolic impulse corresponds to a fourth heart sound (S_4) and reflects the atrial contribution to late ventricular diastolic filling when LV compliance is reduced and diastolic pressure is increased. This presystolic impulse will feel like a "notching" of the sustained apex beat. A prominent, rapid early filling wave in patients with advanced systolic heart failure may result in a palpable third sound (S_3), which may be present when the gallop itself is not audible.[46] It can be visually exaggerated by the use of a pen or tongue depressor lightly pressed over the apex beat. The double or triple outward movements will be amplified at the distal tip of the pen or depressor and seen as two or three up and down excursions during a single cardiac cycle. In the presence of a large ventricular aneurysm, there may be a palpable and visible ectopic impulse, which is discrete from the apex beat. HOCM may rarely cause a triple cadence apex beat, with contributions from a palpable S_4 and the two components of the systolic pulse.

A parasternal lift occurs with RV pressure or volume overload. Signs of TR (jugular venous *cv* waves) and/or PA hypertension (loud or palpable P_2) should be sought. An enlarged RV impulse can extend across the precordium and obscure left-sided findings. Rarely, patients with severe mitral regurgitation (MR) will have a prominent left parasternal impulse because of systolic expansion of the left atrium (LA) and forward displacement of the heart within the thorax. The parasternal movement of an enlarged LA will begin and end after the LV apex beat; RV and LV impulses, on the other hand, occur simultaneously. Lateral retraction of the chest wall may also be present with isolated RV enlargement and is due to posterior displacement of the systolic LV impulse. Systolic and diastolic thrills signify turbulent, high velocity blood flow. Their locations help to identify the origins of heart murmurs.

Auscultation of the Heart

HEART SOUNDS

FIRST HEART SOUND (S_1). Ventricular systole is defined by the interval between the first and second heart sounds. The normal first heart sound (S_1) comprises mitral (M_1) and tricuspid (T_1) valve closure. The two components are usually best heard at the lower left sternal border in younger subjects. Splitting of S_1 is accentuated with complete right bundle branch block. The intensity of S_1 varies predominantly as a function of both the distance over which the anterior leaflet of the mitral valve must travel to return to its annular plane after onset of systole as well as its mobility. Intensity is increased in the early stages of rheumatic mitral stenosis when the valve leaflets are still pliable, in hyperkinetic states, and with short PR intervals (<160 msec). S_1 becomes softer in the late stages of mitral stenosis, when the leaflets are rigid and calcified, with contractile dysfunction, beta-adrenergic receptor blockers, and long PR intervals (>200 msec). Other factors that can decrease the intensity of the heart sounds and murmurs include mechanical ventilation, obstructive lung disease, obesity, pendulous breasts, pneumothorax, and pericardial effusion.

SECOND HEART SOUND (S_2). The second heart sound (S_2) comprises aortic (A_2) and pulmonic (P_2) valve closure. With normal, or physiological, splitting, the A_2-P_2 interval increases during inspiration and narrows with exhalation. The individual components are best heard at the second left interspace in the supine position. The A_2-P_2 interval widens with complete right bundle branch block because of delayed pulmonic valve closure and with severe mitral regurgitation because of premature aortic valve closure, although the normal directional variation with the respiratory cycle is maintained in both conditions. Unusually narrow but physiological splitting of S_2, with an increase in the intensity of P_2 relative to A_2, indicates PA hypertension. With fixed splitting, the A_2-P_2 interval is wide and remains unchanged during the respiratory cycle. Fixed splitting of S_2 is a feature of ostium secundum atrial septal defect. Reversed, or paradoxical, splitting occurs as a consequence of a pathological delay in aortic valve closure, as may occur with complete left bundle branch block, RV apical pacing, severe aortic stenosis, HOCM, and myocardial ischemia. A_2 is normally louder than P_2 and can be heard at most sites across the precordium. When both components can be heard at the lower left sternal border or apex, or when P_2 can be palpated at the second left interspace, pulmonary hypertension is present. The intensity of A_2 and P_2 decreases with aortic and pulmonic stenosis, respectively. A single S_2 may result.

SYSTOLIC SOUNDS. An ejection sound is a high-pitched, early systolic sound that coincides in timing to the upstroke of the carotid pulse and is usually associated with congenital bicuspid aortic or pulmonic valve disease. Ejection sounds are also audible in some patients with aortic or pulmonic root dilation and normal semilunar valves. The ejection sound that accompanies pulmonic valve disease decreases in intensity with inspiration, the only right-sided cardiac event to behave in this manner. Ejection sounds disappear as the culprit valve loses its pliability over time. Nonejection clicks, which occur after the upstroke of the carotid pulse, are related to mitral valve prolapse. A systolic murmur may or may not follow the click. With standing, ventricular preload decreases and the click and murmur move closer to S_1. With squatting, ventricular preload increases, the prolapsing mitral valve tenses later in systole, and the click and murmur move away from S_1 (Fig. 11-8).

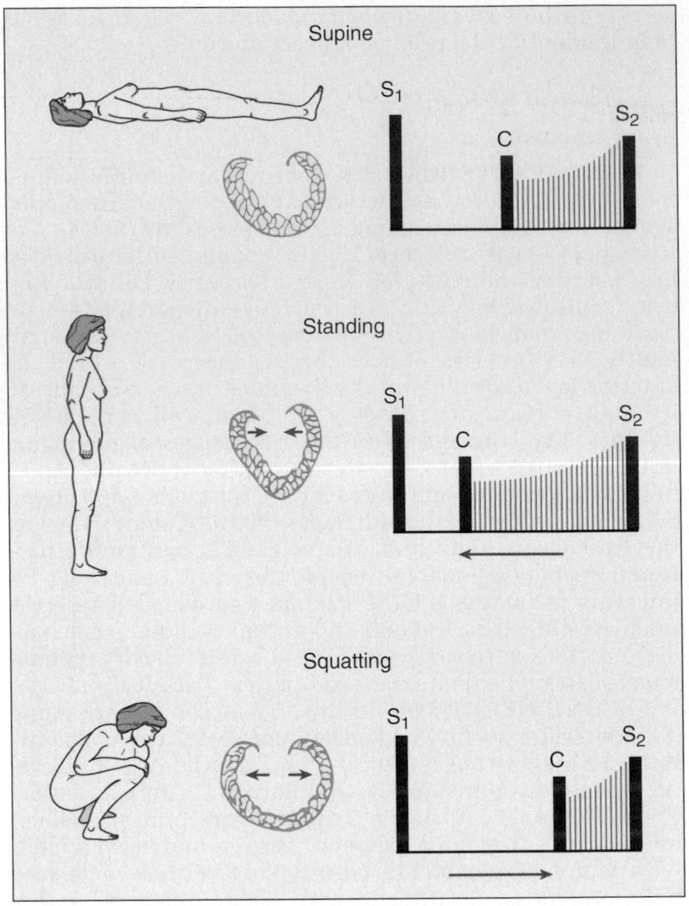

FIGURE 11–8 Behavior of the nonejection click (C) and systolic murmur of mitral valve prolapse. With standing, venous return decreases, the heart becomes smaller, and prolapse occurs earlier in systole. The click and murmur move closer to S_1. With squatting, venous return increases, causing an increase in left ventricular chamber size. The click and murmur occur later in systole and move away from S_1. *(From Shaver JA, Leonard JJ, Leon DF: Examination of the Heart. Part IV: Auscultation of the Heart. Dallas, American Heart Association, 1990, p 13. Copyright 1990, American Heart Association.)*

DIASTOLIC SOUNDS. Diastole is defined by the S_2-S_1 interval. The high-pitched opening snap (OS) of mitral stenosis occurs a short distance after S_2; the A_2-OS interval is inversely proportional to the height of the left atrium – LV diastolic pressure gradient. The intensity of both S_1 and the OS decreases with progressive calcification and rigidity of the anterior mitral leaflet. A pericardial knock is a high-pitched early diastolic sound, which corresponds in timing to the abrupt cessation of ventricular expansion after atrioventricular valve opening and with the prominent *y* descent seen in the jugular venous waveform in patients with constrictive pericarditis. A tumor plop is rarely heard with atrial myxoma; it is a low-pitched sound that may be appreciated only in certain positions and arises from the diastolic prolapse of the tumor across the mitral valve. A diastolic murmur may be present, although most myxomas cause no sound. A third heart sound (S_3) occurs during the rapid filling phase of ventricular diastole. An S_3 may be normally present in children, adolescents, and young adults, but it indicates systolic heart failure in older adults and carries important prognostic weight (see later). A left-sided S_3 is a low-pitched sound best heard over the LV apex in the left lateral decubitus position; whereas a right-sided S_3 is usually heard at the lower left sternal border or in the subxiphoid position with the patient supine and may become louder with inspiration. A fourth heart sound (S_4) occurs during the atrial filling phase of ventricular diastole and is felt to indicate presystolic ventricular expansion. An S_4 is especially common among patients who derive important benefit from the atrial contribution to ventricular filling, such as those with left ventricular hypertrophy or myocardial ischemia.

CARDIAC MURMURS (Table 11-5, Fig. 11-9)

Heart murmurs result from audible vibrations caused by increased turbulence and are defined by their timing within the cardiac cycle. Not all murmurs are indicative of valvular or structural heart disease. The accurate identification of a functional (benign) systolic murmur can obviate the need for echocardiography in many healthy subjects.[47] The magnitude, dynamic variability, and duration of the pressure difference between two cardiac chambers, or between the ventricles and their respective great arteries, dictate the duration, frequency, configuration, and intensity of the murmur. Intensity is graded on a scale of 1 to 6; a palpable thrill is present with murmurs of grade 4 or higher intensity. Other important attributes, which aid in identification, include location, radiation, and response to bedside maneuvers, including quiet respiration.

SYSTOLIC MURMURS. Systolic murmurs are early, mid-, late, or holo-systolic in timing. Acute severe MR results in a decrescendo, early systolic murmur, and is due to the progressive attenuation of the left ventricle – LA pressure gradient during systole because of the steep and rapid rise in pressure within the noncompliant LA (Fig. 11-10). Severe MR associated with posterior mitral leaflet abnormality radiates anteriorly and to the base; MR due to anterior leaflet involvement radiates posteriorly and to the axilla. With acute tricuspid regurgitation in patients with normal PA pressures, an early systolic murmur, which increases in intensity with inspiration, may be audible at the lower left sternal border, and regurgitant *cv* waves may be visible in the jugular venous pulse. Mid-systolic murmurs begin after S_1 and end before S_2; they are usually crescendo-decrescendo in configuration. Aortic stenosis (AS) is the most common cause of a mid-systolic murmur in an adult. Accurate characterization of the severity of the valve lesion at the bedside depends on cardiac output, the elasticity of the carotid arteries, and associated findings. There are several other causes of a mid-systolic heart murmur, including HOCM, pulmonic stenosis (PS), and increased pulmonary blood flow in patients with an ASD and a left-to-right shunt. An isolated grade 1 or 2 mid-systolic murmur in the absence of symptoms or other signs of heart disease is a benign finding that does not warrant further evaluation, including echocardiography.[48] A grade 1 or 2 mid-systolic murmur can often be heard at the left sternal border with pregnancy, hyperthyroidism, or anemia—physiological states that are associated with accelerated blood flow across normal semilunar valves. A murmur of this type is also commonly heard in healthy children and adolescents. A late, apical systolic murmur usually indicates mitral valve prolapse; one or more nonejection clicks may be present. A similar murmur may be heard transiently during an episode of acute myocardial ischemia. In this setting, the MR is due to apical tethering and mal-coaptation of the leaflets in response to structural and functional changes of the ventricle and mitral annulus. The intensity of the murmur will vary with left ventricular afterload. Holosystolic murmurs, which are in plateau configuration, derive from the continuous and wide pressure gradient between two cardiac chambers; the left ventricle and LA with chronic MR, the right ventricle and RA with chronic TR, and the left ventricle and right ventricle with a membranous ventricular septal defect (VSD) without pulmonary hypertension. In contrast to acute MR, in chronic MR, the LA is enlarged and its compliance

TABLE 11–5 Principal Causes of Heart Murmurs

Systolic Murmurs

- Early systolic
  - Mitral
    - Acute MR
  - VSD
    - Muscular
    - Nonrestrictive with pulmonary hypertension
  - Tricuspid
    - TR with normal pulmonary artery pressure
- Mid-systolic
  - Aortic
    - Obstructive
      - Supravalvular—supravalvular aortic stenosis, coarctation of the aorta
      - Valvular—AS and aortic sclerosis
      - Subvalvular—discrete, tunnel, or HOCM
    - Increased flow, hyperkinetic states, AR, complete heart block
    - Dilation of ascending aorta, atheroma, aortitis
  - Pulmonary
    - Obstructive
      - Supravalvular—pulmonary artery stenosis
      - Valvular—pulmonic valve stenosis
      - Subvalvular—infundibular stenosis (dynamic)
    - Increased flow, hyperkinetic states, left-to-right shunt (e.g., ASD)
    - Dilation of pulmonary artery
- Late systolic
  - Mitral
    - MVP, acute myocardial ischemia
  - Tricuspid
    - TVP
- Holosystolic
  - Atrioventricular valve regurgitation (MR, TR)
  - Left-to-right shunt at ventricular level (VSD)

Diastolic Murmurs

- Early diastolic
  - Aortic regurgitation
    - Valvular: congenital (bicuspid valve), rheumatic deformity, endocarditis, prolapse, trauma, postvalvulotomy
    - Dilation of valve ring: aorta dissection, annuloaortic ectasia, cystic medial degeneration, hypertension, ankylosing spondylitis
    - Widening of commissures: syphilis
  - Pulmonic regurgitation
    - Valvular: postvalvulotomy, endocarditis, rheumatic fever, carcinoid
    - Dilation of valve ring: pulmonary hypertension; Marfan syndrome
    - Congenital: isolated or associated with tetralogy of Fallot, VSD, pulmonic stenosis
- Mid-diastolic
  - Mitral
    - Mitral stenosis
    - Carey-Coombs murmur (mid-diastolic apical murmur in acute rheumatic fever)
    - Increased flow across nonstenotic mitral valve (e.g., MR, VSD, PDA, high-output states, and complete heart block)
  - Tricuspid
    - Tricuspid stenosis
    - Increased flow across nonstenotic tricuspid valve (e.g., TR, ASD, and anomalous pulmonary venous return)
  - Left and right atrial tumors (myxoma)
  - Severe or eccentric AR (Austin Flint murmur)
- Late-diastolic
  - Presystolic accentuation of mitral stenosis murmur
  - Austin Flint murmur of severe or eccentric AR

Continuous Murmurs

- PDA
- Coronary AV fistula
- Ruptured sinus of Valsalva aneurysm
- Aortic septal defect
- Cervical venous hum
- Anomalous left coronary artery
- Proximal coronary artery stenosis
- Mammary souffle of pregnancy
- Pulmonary artery branch stenosis
- Bronchial collateral circulation
- Small (restrictive) ASD with MS
- Intercostal AV fistula

AR = aortic regurgitation; AS = aortic stenosis; ASD = atrial septal defect; AV = arteriovenous; HOCM = hypertrophic obstructive cardiomyopathy; MR = mitral regurgitation; MS = mitral stenosis; MVP = mitral valve prolapse; PDA = patent ductus arteriosus; TR = tricuspid regurgitation; TVP = tricuspid valve prolapse; VSD = ventricular septal defect.

From Braunwald E, Perloff JK: *In* Zipes DP, Libby P, Bonow RO, Braunwald E (eds): Braunwald's Heart Disease, 7th ed. Philadelphia, Elsevier, 2005, pp 77-106; and Norton PJ, O'Rourke RA: Approach to the patient with a heart murmur. *In* Braunwald E, Goldman L (eds): Primary Cardiology, 2nd ed. Philadelphia, Elsevier, 2003, pp 151-168.

is normal or even increased, such that there is only a small increase in LA pressure from any increase in regurgitant volume. MR is best heard over the cardiac apex, TR at the lower left sternal border, and a VSD at the mid-left sternal border where a thrill is palpable in the majority of patients. Although there are several causes of primary TR, it most commonly occurs secondary to PA hypertension, right ventricle enlargement, annular dilation, papillary muscle displacement, and failure of leaflet coaptation.

DIASTOLIC MURMURS. Diastolic murmurs invariably signify cardiac abnormality. Chronic AR causes a high-pitched decrescendo early to mid-diastolic murmur. With primary aortic valve disease, the murmur is best heard along the left sternal border; whereas with root enlargement and secondary AR, the murmur tends to radiate along the right sternal border. A mid-systolic murmur due to augmented and accelerated forward flow is also present with moderate to severe AR, and need not signify valve or outflow tract obstruction.[49] The diastolic murmur is both softer and of shorter duration in acute AR, due to the rapid rise in LV diastolic pressure and the diminution of the aortic-LV diastolic pressure gradient. Additional features of acute AR include tachycardia, a soft first heart sound, and the absence of peripheral findings of significant diastolic run-off. The murmur of pulmonic regurgitation (PR) is heard along the left sternal border and is most often due to annular enlargement from chronic PA hypertension (Graham Steell murmur). Signs of RV pressure load are present. PR can also occur with a congenitally deformed valve and is invariably present after repair of tetralogy of Fallot. In these settings, the murmur is relatively softer and lower pitched; the severity of PR can be under-appreciated. Mitral stenosis is the classic cause of a mid- to late diastolic murmur. However, mitral stenosis may be "silent" and a murmur might be inaudible in patients with low cardiac output or large body habitus. The murmur is best heard over the apex in the left lateral decubitus position, is low-pitched (rumbling), and introduced by an OS in the early stages of the disease. Presystolic accentuation refers to an increase in the intensity of the murmur in late systole following atrial contraction in patients in sinus rhythm. Findings in patients with rheumatic tricuspid stenosis (TS) are usually obscured by

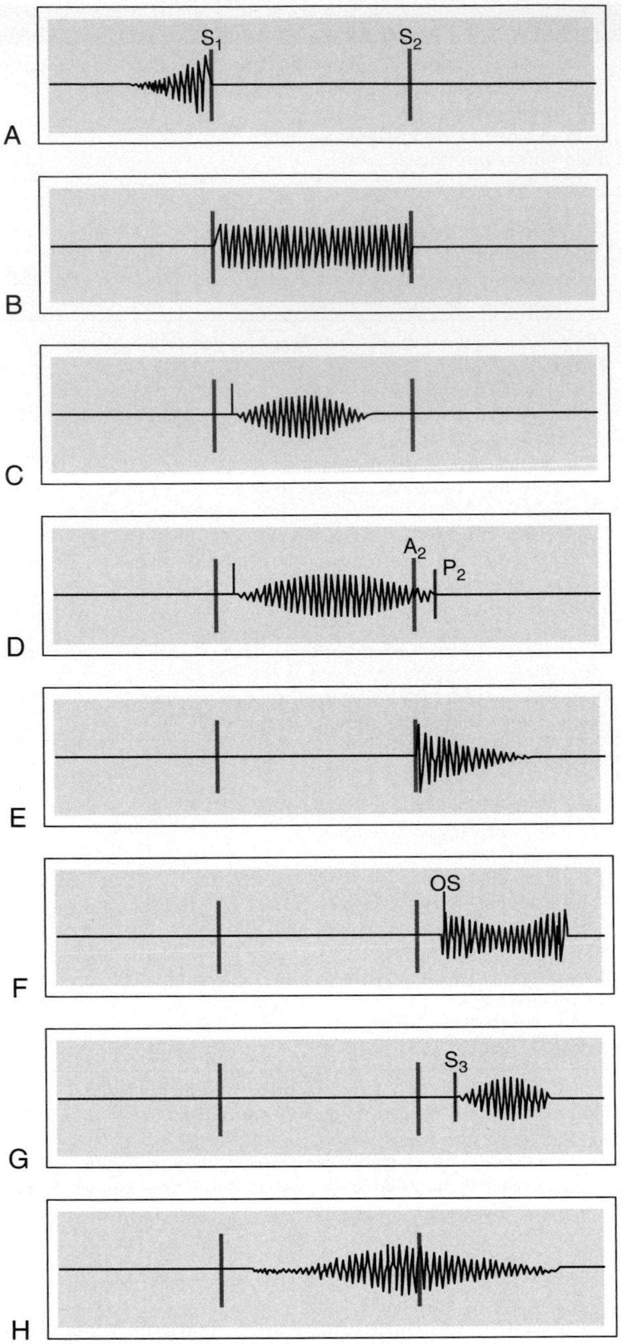

FIGURE 11–9 Diagram of principal heart murmurs. **A,** Presystolic accentuation of the murmur of mitral stenosis with sinus rhythm. **B,** Holosystolic murmur of chronic, severe mitral or tricuspid regurgitation, or ventricular septal defect without severe pulmonary hypertension. **C,** Ejection sound and crescendo-decrescendo murmur of bicuspid aortic stenosis. **D,** Ejection sound and crescendo-decrescendo murmur that extends to P_2 in bicuspid pulmonic stenosis. **E,** Early decrescendo diastolic murmur of aortic or pulmonic regurgitation. **F,** Opening snap and mid-diastolic rumble of mitral stenosis. **G,** Diastolic filling sound (S_3) and mid-diastolic murmur associated with severe mitral regurgitation, tricuspid regurgitation, or atrial septal defect with significant left to right shunt. **H,** Continuous murmur of patent ductus arteriosus that envelops S_2. OS = opening snap. *(Adapted from Wood P: Diseases of the Heart and Circulation. Philadelphia, Lippincott, 1968; and O'Rourke RA, Braunwald E: Physical examination of the cardiovascular system.* In *Kasper D, Braunwald E, Fauci A, Hauser S, Longo D, Jameson L [eds]: Harrison's Principles of Internal Medicine, 16th ed. New York, McGraw-Hill, 2005, p 1309.)*

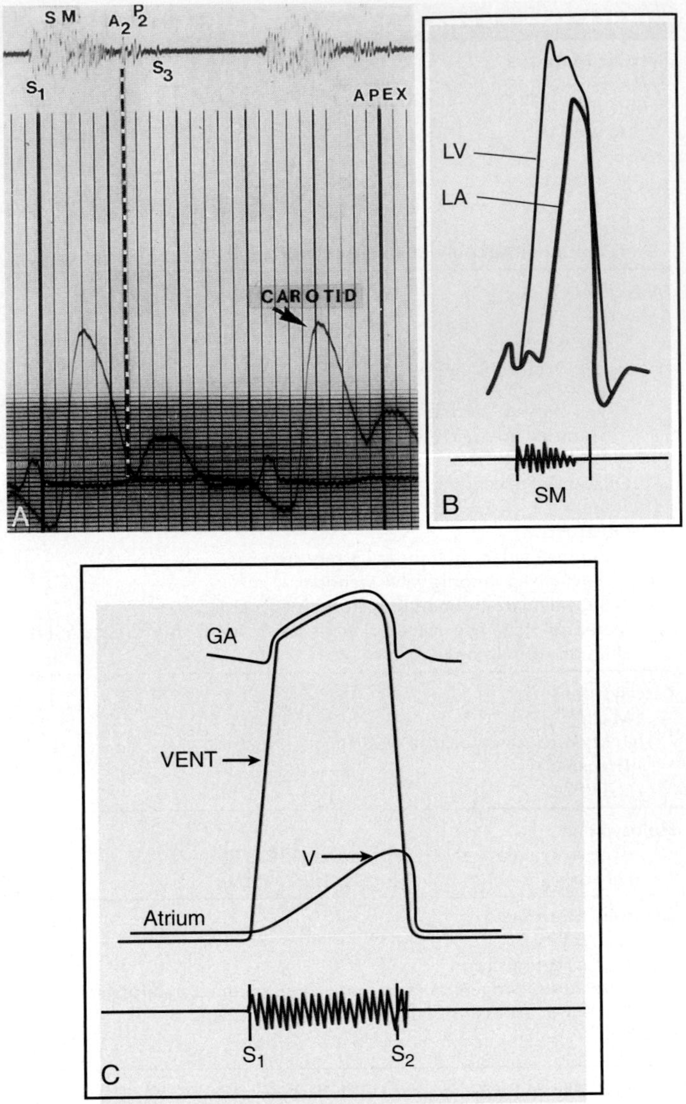

FIGURE 11–10 A, Phonocardiogram **(top)** of a patient with acute severe mitral regurgitation showing a decrescendo early systolic murmur and diastolic filling sound (S_3). **B,** left ventricle (LV) and left atrium (LA) pressure waveforms demonstrating the abrupt rise in LA pressure and attenuation of the LV-LA pressure gradient, resulting in the duration and configuration of the murmur. **C,** Phonocardiogram. Illustration of great artery (GA), ventricular (vent) and atrial pressures with resultant phonocardiogram in chronic mitral or tricuspid regurgitation. Note the holosystolic timing and plateau configuration of the murmur, both of which derive from the large ventricular-atrial pressure gradient throughout systole. SM = systolic murmur; V = v wave. *(From Braunwald E, Perloff JK: Physical examination of the heart and circulation.* In *Zipes D, Libby P, Bonow RO, Braunwald E [eds]: Braunwald's Heart Disease. A Textbook of Cardiovascular Medicine, 7th ed. Philadelphia, Elsevier, 2005, p 97.)*

left-sided events. Functional mitral stenosis or TS refers to mid-diastolic murmurs created by increased, accelerated transvalvular flow, without valvular obstruction, in the setting of severe MR, severe TR, or ASD with a large left to right shunt. The low-pitched mid- to late apical diastolic murmur associated with severe AR (Austin Flint murmur) can be distinguished from mitral stenosis on the basis of its response to vasodilators and the presence of associated findings. Less common causes of a mid-diastolic murmur include atrial myxoma, complete heart block, and acute rheumatic mitral valvulitis (Carey-Coombs murmur).

CONTINUOUS MURMURS. The presence of a continuous murmur implies a pressure gradient between two chambers or vessels during both systole and diastole. These murmurs begin in systole, peak near S_2, and then continue into diastole. They can be difficult to distinguish from systolic and diastolic murmurs in patients with mixed aortic or pulmonic valve disease. Examples include the murmurs associated with PDA, ruptured sinus of Valsalva aneurysm, and coronary, great vessel, or hemodialysis AV fistulas. The cervical venous hum and mammary souffle of pregnancy are two benign variants.

DYNAMIC AUSCULTATION

Simple bedside maneuvers can help identify heart murmurs and characterize their significance (Table 11-6). Right-sided events, save for the pulmonic ejection sound, increase with inspiration and decrease with exhalation; left-sided events behave oppositely (100 percent sensitivity, 88 percent specificity).[50] The intensity of the murmurs associated with MR, VSD, and AR will increase in response to maneuvers that increase LV afterload (handgrip, vasopressors) and decrease after exposure to vasodilating agents (amyl nitrite). Squatting is associated with an abrupt increase in ventricular preload and afterload; whereas rapid standing results in a sudden decrease in preload. In patients with mitral valve prolapse (MVP), the click and murmur will move away from S_1 with squatting, because of the delay in onset of leaflet prolapse at higher ventricular volumes. With rapid standing, the click and murmur move closer to S_1, as prolapse occurs earlier in systole at a smaller chamber dimension. The murmur of HOCM behaves in a directionally similar manner, becoming softer and shorter with squatting (95 percent sensitivity, 85 percent specificity) and longer and louder on rapid standing (95 percent sensitivity, 84 percent specificity).[50] The intensity of the murmur of HOCM also increases with the Valsalva maneuver (65 percent sensitivity, 95 percent specificity).[50] A change in the intensity of a systolic murmur in the first beat after a premature beat, or in the beat after a long cycle length in patients with AF, suggests AS rather than MR, particularly in an older patient in whom the murmur of AS is well transmitted to the apex (Gallavardin effect). Systolic murmurs due to LV outflow obstruction, including that due to AS, will increase in intensity in the beat following a premature beat because of the combined effects of enhanced LV filling and postextrasystolic potentiation of contractile function. Forward flow accelerates, causing an increase in the gradient and a louder murmur. The intensity of the murmur of MR does not change in the post-premature beat, as there is relatively little further increase in mitral valve flow or change in the left ventricle-LA gradient.

Indications for Echocardiography

Transthoracic echocardiography (TTE) can be deferred for patients with a mid-systolic murmur of grade 2 or less intensity, who lack symptoms and have no other signs of cardiovascular disease, and for patients with benign continuous murmurs (Fig. 11-11).[48] All other patients should undergo echocardiographic study to characterize cardiac structure and function and to estimate PA pressures. The findings from TTE, as well as those from the history and physical examination, verify the diagnosis and arrive at a treatment plan based on clinical risk assessment and knowledge of natural history.

TABLE 11–6 Interventions Used to Alter the Intensity of Cardiac Murmurs

Respiration	Right-sided murmurs generally increase with inspiration. Left-sided murmurs usually are louder during expiration.
Valsalva maneuver	Most murmurs decrease in length and intensity. Two exceptions are the systolic murmur of HOCM, which usually becomes much louder, and that of MVP, which becomes longer and often louder. After release of the Valsalva maneuver, right-sided murmurs tend to return to baseline intensity earlier than left-sided murmurs.
Exercise	Murmurs caused by blood flow across normal or obstructed valves (e.g., PS and MS) become louder with both isotonic and isometric (handgrip) exercise. Murmurs of MR, VSD, and AR also increase with handgrip exercise.
Positional changes	With standing, most murmurs diminish; two exceptions being the murmur of HOCM, which becomes louder, and that of MVP, which lengthens and often is intensified. With squatting, most murmurs become louder, but those of HCM and MVP usually soften and may disappear. Passive leg raising usually produces the same results as squatting.
Postventricular premature beat or AF	Murmurs originating at normal or stenotic semilunar valves increase in intensity during the cardiac cycle after a VPB or in the beat after a long cycle length in AF. By contrast, systolic murmurs due to atrioventricular valve regurgitation do not change, diminish (papillary muscle dysfunction), or become shorter after a premature beat (MVP).
Pharmacological interventions	During the initial relative hypotension after amyl nitrite inhalation, murmurs of MR, VSD, and AR decrease in intensity, whereas the murmur of AS increases in intensity because of increased stroke volume. During the later tachycardia phase, murmurs of MS and right-sided lesions also become louder. This intervention may help distinguish the murmur of the Austin-Flint phenomenon from that of MS. The response in MVP often is biphasic (softer and then louder than control).
Transient arterial occlusion	Transient external compression of both brachial arteries by bilateral cuff inflation to 20 mm Hg greater than peak systolic pressure augments the murmurs of MR, VSD, and AR, but not murmurs due to other causes.

AF = atrial fibrillation; AR = aortic regurgitation; AS = aortic stenosis; HOCM = hypertrophic obstructive cardiomyopathy; MR = mitral regurgitation; MS = mitral stenosis; MVP = mitral valve prolapse; PS = pulmonic stenosis; VPB = ventricular premature beat; VSD = ventricular septal defect.

Reprinted with permission from Bonow RO, et al. ACC/AHA 2006 guidelines for the management of patients with valvular heart disease: A report of the American College of Cardiology/American Heart Association Task Force on Practice Guidelines (writing Committee to Revise the 1998 guidelines for the management of patients with valvular heart disease) developed in collaboration with the Society of Cardiovascular Anesthesiologists endorsed by the Society for Cardiovascular Angiography and Interventions and the Society of Thoracic Surgeons. J Am Coll Cardiol 48(3):e1-148, 2006.

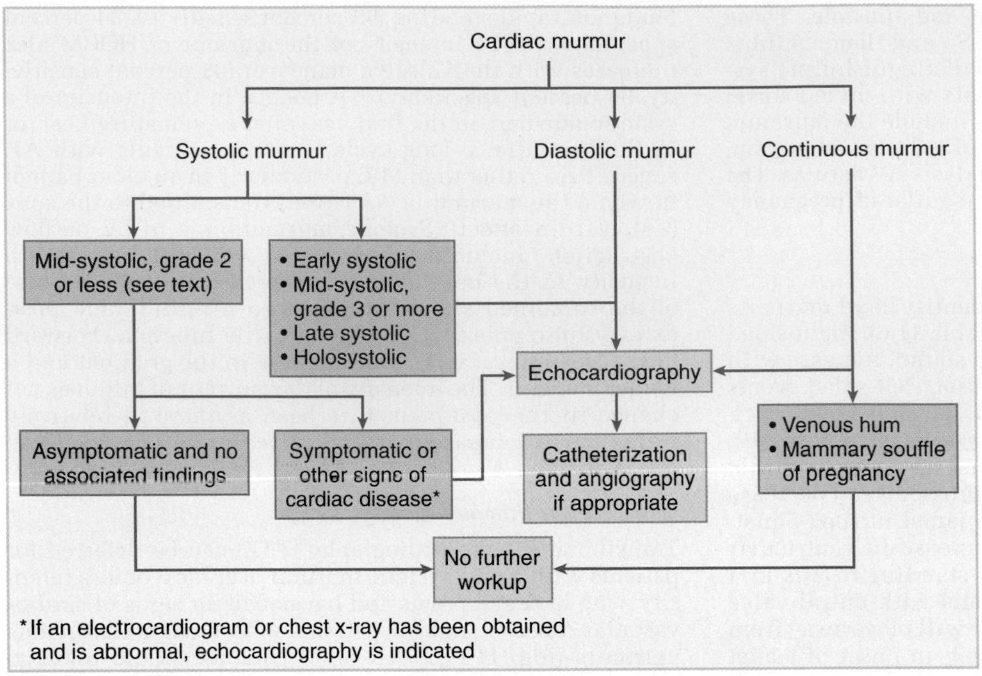

FIGURE 11–11 Strategy for the evaluation of heart murmurs. *(From Roldan CA, Shively BK, Crawford MH: Value of the cardiovascular physical examination for detecting valvular heart disease in asymptomatic subjects. Am J Cardiol 77[15]:1327-31, 1996.)*

INTEGRATED, EVIDENCE-BASED APPROACH

Heart Failure

History

Both exertional and resting symptoms should be explored. Common symptoms include dyspnea, fatigue, exercise limitation, orthopnea, and edema. Dyspnea, which is severe and sudden in onset, indicates acute pulmonary edema and typically is precipitated by ischemia, arrhythmia, sudden left-sided valvular regurgitation, or accelerated hypertension. It is important to exclude other causes such as pulmonary embolism and pneumothorax. The extent of limitation should also be defined because functional capacity, as assessed by NYHA class, strongly and independently predicts mortality for patients with heart failure. However, self-reported functional capacity and objectively measured cardiovascular performance can differ substantially.[51] Symptoms that occur at rest may have greater predictive value for the diagnosis of heart failure compared with symptoms that are exertional in nature.[52] Orthopnea is not specific for heart failure and can occur in patients with severe ascites or emphysema. Trepopnea, which is dyspnea or discomfort in the lateral decubitus position, may also be present. Patients with heart failure prefer sleeping on their right side, and trepopnea likely accounts for the predominance of right-sided pleural effusions in this population.[53] In a study of 75 heart failure patients with ejection fraction (EF) <0.45 and dyspnea, increased heart size, elevated PA wedge pressure, and lower cardiac output correlated with sleeping in the right rather than the left lateral decubitus position.[53] Paroxysmal nocturnal dyspnea is also common in heart failure. Cheyne-Stokes respirations may be apparent in the awake state. The prevalence of central sleep apnea or Cheyne-Stokes respirations ranges from 20 to 62 percent in various heart failure studies[54] and portends an increased mortality risk. Lower extremity edema is usually pitting and becomes more prominent as the day progresses for the ambulatory patient. Clinically evident edema likely indicates a volume excess at least 3 to 4 kilograms. In patients with advanced right heart failure, uncomfortable hepatomegaly and ascites may predominate. Patients with chronic heart failure often lack pulmonary rales or lower extremity edema.[55] In a study of 50 patients referred for heart transplantation, the combination of rales, edema, and an elevated jugular venous pressure were absent in 18 of 43 subjects with a measured PA wedge pressure >22 mm Hg; this combination of findings, however, had a sensitivity of 58 percent and specificity of 100 percent for the diagnosis of heart failure.[52]

Few studies have explored the predictive values of various symptoms of heart failure. Furthermore, symptoms often correlate poorly with objective evidence of cardiac dysfunction at rest.[51,56,57] For example, in Olmsted County, Minnesota, only 46 percent of a random sample of residents with severe diastolic dysfunction (as a marker of increased left ventricular filling pressure) had a validated heart failure diagnosis using the Framingham criteria (see Chap. 25, Table 25-4).[58] The available literature is also limited by small sample sizes, lack of proper controls, retrospective designs, variable interviewers and definitions, and referral bias. In a systematic review, orthopnea only modestly predicted increased filling pressures.[59] Dyspnea and edema were similarly useful but were most predictive when combined with physical examination findings (S_3, tachycardia, elevated jugular venous pressure, low pulse pressure, rales, abdominojugular reflux). When combined with other findings, a total of three or more symptoms or signs predicted a >90 percent likelihood of increased filling pressures if severe LV dysfunction was not known. In contrast, if one or no findings or symptoms were present, there was <10 percent likelihood of increased filling pressures.[59] Several studies have used this approach for the diagnosis of heart failure.[60-63] The European Society of Cardiology recommends that heart failure be defined by measurable cardiac dysfunction that accompanies symptoms.[64] The most commonly used system, the Framingham criteria, has only modest specificity (63 percent) and sensitivity (63 percent), when an EF of <0.40 is used to define heart failure.[57]

The distinction between systolic and nonsystolic heart failure can be made at the bedside with modest accuracy. For example, using multivariate analysis, Silver and others derived the following simple rule to predict an ejection fraction >0.40 after myocardial infarction (MI): (1) an interpretable electrocardiogram; (2) no previous Q wave MI; (3) no history of heart failure; and (4) an index infarction that is not a Q wave anterior infarction.[65] In both the derivation and validation sets, the positive predictive value of the rule was >98 percent.[64] In patients presenting with heart failure, systolic function is more likely to be preserved when there is significant hypertension (>160/100 mm Hg).[59] Systolic function is also more likely to be preserved when patients are female, elderly, and have an increased body mass index, but such findings lack adequate specificity or sensitivity to guide therapy.[66-69] Furthermore, diastolic dysfunction is not mutually exclusive of systolic dysfunction.[70] Clinical criteria for the diagnosis of nonsystolic heart failure have been developed but not validated.[64,71]

Physical Examination

The assessment of volume status is critical. Most patients with heart failure who require hospital admission will do so because of volume overload[72] and failure to relieve it has negative prognostic impact. Four signs are commonly used to predict elevated filling pressures: jugular venous distention/abdominojugular reflux, presence of an S_3 and/or S_4, rales, and pedal edema. In general, diagnostic accuracy is improved by using a combination of findings rather than relying on isolated clinical findings that have limited predictive value.[63,73]

Jugular Venous Pressure

The jugular venous pressure provides the readiest bedside assessment of left ventricular filling pressure. An abnormally elevated jugular venous pressure is generally defined as >8 to 10 cm H_2O or >3 to 5 cm H_2O above the angle of Louis. Although the jugular venous pressure estimates RV filling pressure, it has a predictable relationship with PA wedge pressure.[74] In 1000 consecutive patients with advanced heart failure undergoing right heart catheterization, Drazner and colleagues found that the RA pressure reliably predicted the PA wedge pressure (r = 0.64); the positive predictive value of an RA pressure >10 mm Hg for a PA wedge pressure >22 mm Hg was 88 percent. In addition, the PA systolic pressure could be estimated as twice the wedge pressure (r = 0.79).[74] As noted previously, agreement among observers that venous pressure is elevated is modest (K statistic 0.31 to 0.69)[21,59] and related in part to the experience of the observer as well as to the use of variable zero reference standards. The presence or absence of venous distention is more easily assessed than is the magnitude of venous pressure elevation.[22] In 52 patients with chronic heart failure, Butman and colleagues reported that an elevated jugular venous pressure had a predictive accuracy of 67 percent for a pulmonary capillary wedge pressure >18 mm Hg (positive predictive value 95 percent, negative predictive value 47 percent).[73] Unfortunately, studies are limited by small numbers of observations, bias by indication, and highly variable designs.

An elevated venous pressure has prognostic significance. Drazner and colleagues demonstrated that the presence of jugular venous distention at the time of enrollment in a large clinical heart failure trial (11 percent of the SOLVD treatment study participants), after adjusting for other markers of disease severity, predicted heart failure hospitalizations (RR 1.32, 95 percent CI 1.08 to 1.62), death from pump failure (RR 1.37, 95 percent CI 1.07 to 1.75), and death plus heart failure hospitalization (RR1.30, 95 percent CI 1.11 to 1.53)[74]; see Fig. 11-10). They extended these observations to asymptomatic individuals enrolled in the SOLVD prevention study in which jugular venous distention was less common (1.7 percent of study population).[75] These findings are especially noteworthy in that the presence of jugular venous distention was reported in a "yes or no" format by the multiple investigators who participated in the trial.

Inducible jugular venous distention (abdominojugular reflux) suggests excessive RV preload, which is most commonly related to elevated left ventricular filling pressures, but may also occur with other conditions (e.g., constrictive pericarditis, RV infarction). In patients presenting with dyspnea, the abdominojugular reflux is useful in predicting heart failure (LR + 6.0, 95 percent CI 0.8 to 51, LR −0.78, 95 percent CI 0.62 to 0.98) and is suggestive of a PA wedge pressure >15 mm Hg (LR +6.7, 95 percent CI 3.3 to 13.4, LR −0.08, 95 percent CI 0.01 to 0.52).[28] The presence of jugular venous distention, either at rest or inducible, had the best combination of sensitivity (81 percent), specificity (80 percent), and predictive accuracy (81 percent) for elevation of the PA wedge pressure (>18 mm Hg).[73]

THIRD AND FOURTH HEART SOUNDS. The third heart sound (S_3) predicts ejection fraction poorly because it reflects primarily diastolic rather than systolic performance. In patients with heart failure, S_3 is equally prevalent in those with or without LV systolic dysfunction (EF cut point 0.50).[67] The most rigorous contemporary assessment of the S_3 was conducted by Marcus and colleagues in 100 patients with a variety of cardiovascular conditions undergoing elective cardiac catheterization.[76,77] Cardiology fellows (n = 18, K statistic 0.37, $p < 0.001$) and faculty (n = 26, K statistic 0.29, $p = 0.003$) performed better than residents (n = 102, no significant agreement) for the identification of a phonocardiographically confirmed S_3. Furthermore, an S_3 heard by a cardiology fellow or faculty physician predicted an increase in both LV end-diastolic pressure (LVEDP) (>15 mm Hg) and B-type natriuretic peptide (>100 pg/ml), and depressed ventricular systolic function (EF < 0.50), though sensitivities were low (32 to 52 percent) (Fig. 11-12). An S_4 had comparable sensitivity (40 to 46 percent), but inferior specificity (72 to 80 percent for an S_4 versus 87 to 92 percent for an S_3) (Table 11-7). In several earlier studies of heart failure patients

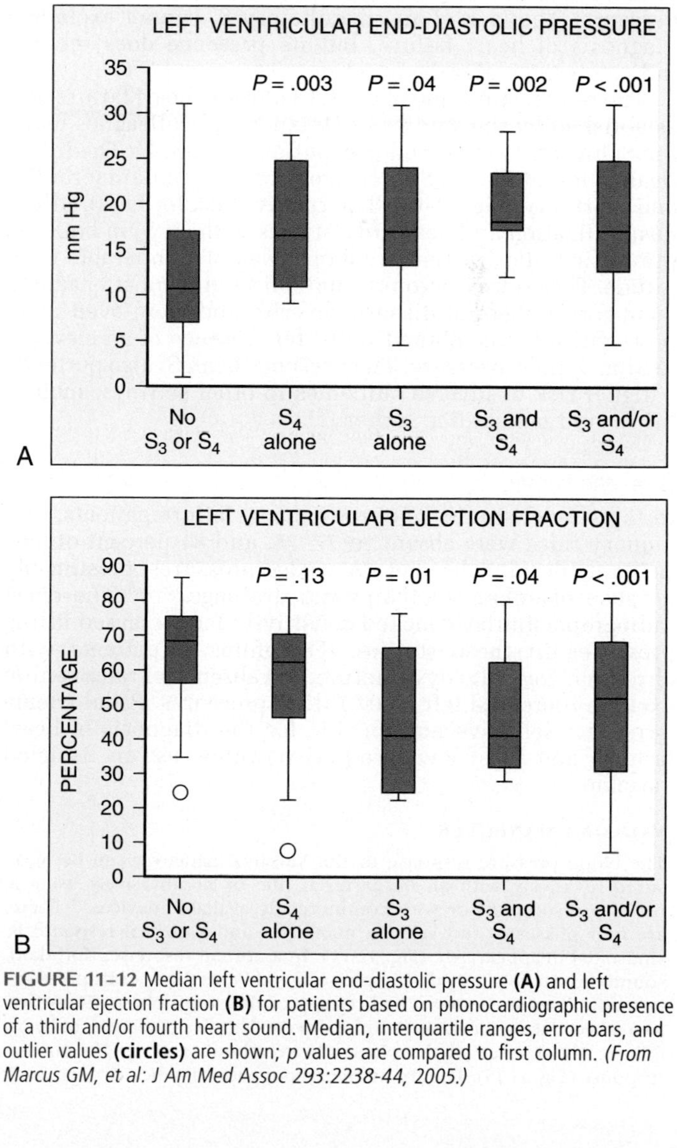

FIGURE 11–12 Median left ventricular end-diastolic pressure **(A)** and left ventricular ejection fraction **(B)** for patients based on phonocardiographic presence of a third and/or fourth heart sound. Median, interquartile ranges, error bars, and outlier values **(circles)** are shown; *p* values are compared to first column. *(From Marcus GM, et al: J Am Med Assoc 293:2238-44, 2005.)*

TABLE 11–7 Test Characteristics of Computerized Heart Sounds Detection

	LVEDP > 15 mm Hg	LVEF < 50%	BNP > 100 pg/ml
S_3			
Sensitivity	41 (26-58)	52 (31-73)	32 (20-46)
Specificity	92 (80-98)	87 (76-94)	92 (78-98)
Positive Predictive Value	81 (58-95)	57 (34-78)	85 (62-97)
Negative Predictive Value	65 (53-76)	84 (73-92)	48 (36-60)
Accuracy	69 (58-78)	78 (68-86)	56 (45-67)
S_4			
Sensitivity	46 (31-63)	43 (23-66)	40 (26-54)
Specificity	80 (66-90)	72 (59-82)	78 (61-90)
Positive Predictive Value	66 (46-82)	34 (18-54)	72 (52-87)
Negative Predictive Value	64 (51-76)	79 (66-88)	47 (34-60)
Accuracy	64 (54-74)	64 (54-74)	55 (44-66)
S_3 and/or S_4			
Sensitivity	68 (52-82)	74 (52-90)	57 (42-70)
Specificity	73 (59-85)	64 (52-76)	72 (55-86)
Positive Predictive Value	68 (52-82)	42 (26-58)	75 (59-87)
Negative Predictive Value	73 (59-85)	88 (75-95)	53 (38-67)
Accuracy	71 (61-80)	67 (56-76)	63 (52-73)

BNP = B-type natriuretic peptide; LVEDP = left ventricular end-diastolic pressure; LVEF = left ventricular ejection fraction. Data are presented as percentage (95% confidence intervals).

Adapted from Marcus GM, et al: JAMA 293:2238-2244, 2005.

referred for transplantation, a third heart sound was frequently heard but poorly predictive of elevated filling pressures.[52,73,78] The prevalence of an S_3 in a less ill cohort with systolic dysfunction (SOLVD prevention study) was 5.1 percent.[75] The lack of an auscultatory S_3 cannot exclude a diagnosis of heart failure, but its presence does reliably indicate ventricular dysfunction.

The prognostic value of an S_3 in chronic heart failure was established by the studies of Drazner and colleagues using the SOLVD treatment and prevention studies.[74,75] The investigators found that an S_3 predicted cardiovascular morbidity and mortality (Fig. 11-13). The relative risk for heart failure hospitalization and death in patients with an S_3 in both the prevention and treatment cohorts was of comparable magnitude. These observations remained significant after adjustment for markers of disease severity and were even more powerful when combined with the presence of an elevated jugular venous pressure. The presence of an S_3 also portends a higher risk of adverse outcomes in other settings, such as MI[79,80] and noncardiac surgery.[81]

Rales and Edema

In three older studies of chronic heart failure patients, pulmonary rales were absent in 77, 75, and 81 percent of participants despite elevated PA wedge pressures, presumably because of enhanced lymphatic drainage.[52,73,78] The chest radiograph similarly lacked sensitivity for increased filling pressures in these studies. Therefore, in patients with chronic LV systolic dysfunction, the absence of rales cannot exclude increased left heart filling pressures. Pedal edema is neither sensitive nor specific for the diagnosis of heart failure and has low predictive value as an isolated variable.

VALSALVA MANEUVER

The blood pressure response to the Valsalva maneuver can be measured invasively with an intraarterial line or noninvasively using a blood pressure cuff or with commercially available devices.[82] There are four phases in the Valsalva maneuver and a normal response is sinusoidal in appearance (Fig. 11-14). In a normal response, Korotkoff sounds are audible only during phases I and IV, as the systolic pressure normally rises at the onset and release of the strain phase. There are two recognized abnormal responses to the Valsalva maneuver in heart failure: (1) absence of the phase IV overshoot, and (2) the square response (Fig. 11-15). The absent overshoot pattern indicates decreased systolic function; the square wave response indicates elevated filling pressures and appears to be independent of ejection fraction.[83] The responses can be quantified using the pulse amplitude ratio if the pulse pressure is measured during the maneuver. This ratio compares the minimum pulse pressure at the end of the strain phase to the maximum pulse pressure at the onset of the strain phase; a greater ratio is consistent with a square wave response.

In a study of either stable patients undergoing catheterization or ill patients requiring a PA catheter in an intensive care unit (neither with a primary diagnosis of heart failure), McIntyre and others showed a strong correlation between the pulse amplitude ratio and the PA wedge pressure ($r = 0.80$ to 0.85) both at baseline and with changes in volume ($r = 0.79$).[84] The same group demonstrated similar findings in a chronic heart failure population with a sensitivity of 91 percent and a specificity of 100 percent for a wedge pressure >18 mm Hg. Using a noninvasive device, the Valsalva response was even better than the PA wedge pressure at estimating LVEDP.[82] The correlation with atrial and brain natriuretic peptide levels in heart failure patients is similarly robust.[85]

Other Findings

In the absence of hypertension, the pulse pressure is determined by the stroke volume and vascular stiffness and can be used to assess cardiac output. In a chronic heart failure cohort (EF 0.18 ± 0.06), the proportional pulse pressure ([systolic-diastolic]/systolic) correlated well with cardiac index ($r = 0.82$, $p < 0.001$), stroke volume index ($r = 0.78$, $p < 0.001$), and the inverse of systemic vascular resistance ($r = 0.65$, $p < 0.001$). Using a proportional pulse pressure of 25 percent, the cardiac index could be predicted: if the value was <25 percent, the cardiac index was <2.2 L/min/m^2 in 91 percent of patients; if >25 percent, the cardiac index was >2.2 L/min/m^2 in 83 percent of patients.[52] This prediction rule has not been reported in other patient groups, in larger cohorts, or in more contemporary studies. An increase in the intensity of the pulmonic component of the second heart sound (P_2) is strongly suggestive of PA hypertension. If P_2 can be heard at the apex, the systolic PA pressure is likely to be >50 mm Hg.[86]

Valvular Heart Disease (see also Chap. 62)

A careful history and physical examination can reveal much regarding lesion severity, natural history, indications for surgery, and outcomes in patients with valvular heart disease. Relevant symptoms that cannot be ascribed to a

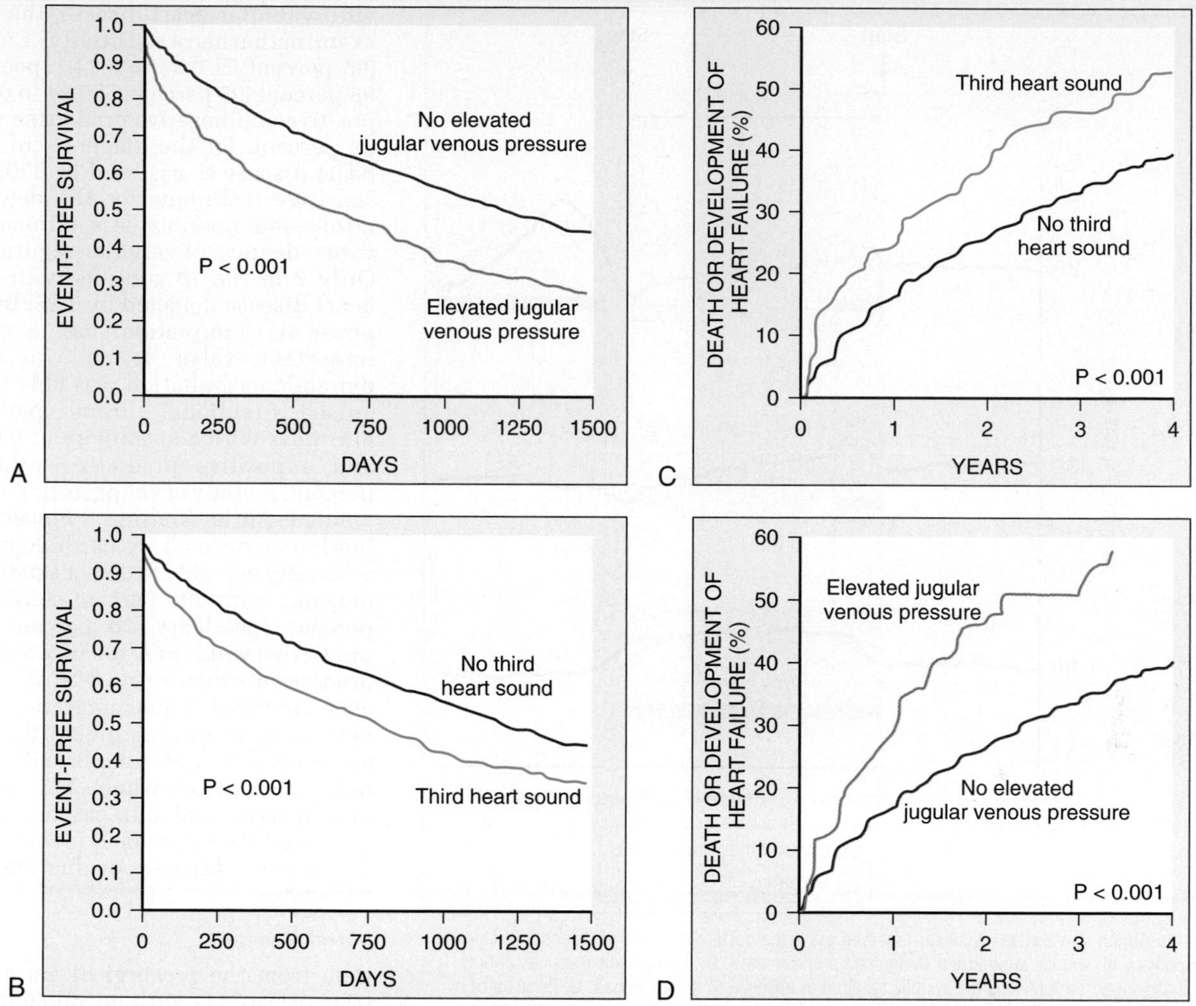

FIGURE 11–13 Kaplan-Meier plots demonstrating prognostic value of an elevated jugular venous pressure and third heart Sound (S_3) in symptomatic (**A** and **B**) and asymptomatic (**C** and **D**) heart failure patients with systolic dysfunction. *(**A** and **B**, from Drazner MH, et al: N Engl J Med 345:574, 2001; **C** and **D** from Drazner MH, et al: Am J Med 114:431, 2003.)*

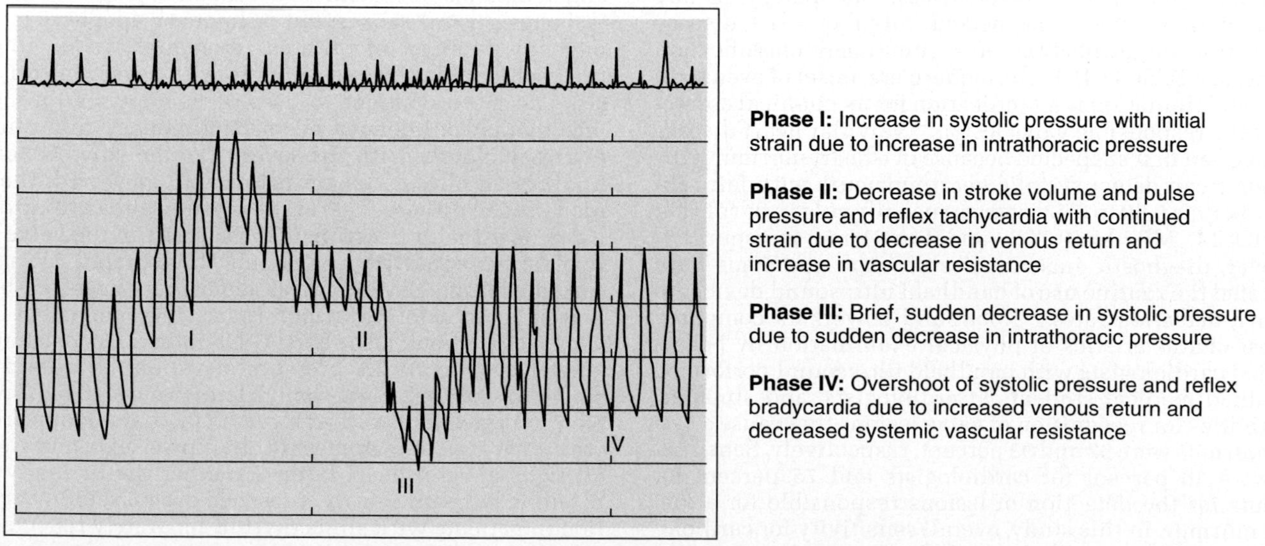

FIGURE 11–14 The normal Valsalva response. *(From Nishimura RA, Tajik AJ: Mayo Clin Proc 79:569-579, 2004.)*

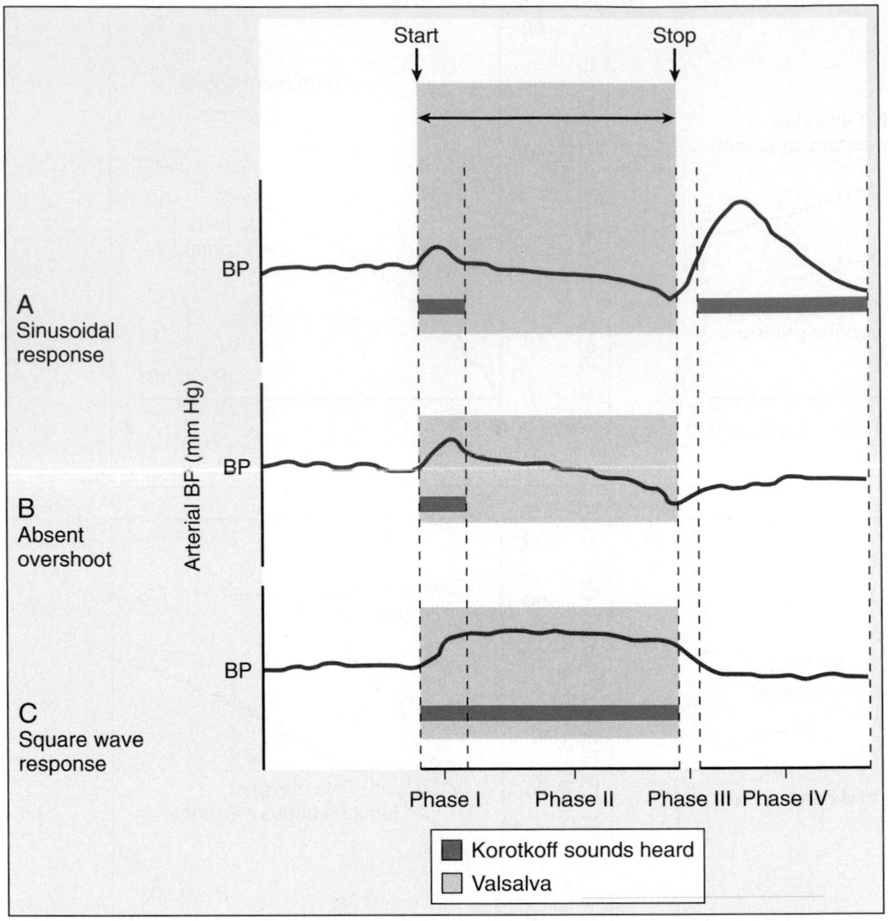

FIGURE 11–15 Abnormal Valsalva responses assessed using the pattern of Korotkoff sounds. **A,** Normal, sinusoidal response with sounds intermittent during strain and release. **B,** Briefly audible sounds during initial strain phase suggests only impaired systolic function in absence of fluid overload. **C,** Persistence of Korotkoff sounds throughout strain phase suggests elevated left ventricular filling pressures. BP = blood pressure. *(From Shamsham F, Mitchell J: Am Fam Physician 61[5]:1319-28, 2000.)*

noncardiac cause and signs of heart failure and/or pulmonary hypertension raise particular concern. The specificity of these findings decreases as a function of age and patient comorbidity. LV dysfunction from coronary artery disease is a common confounder. Nevertheless, the history in any patient with known or suspected valvular heart disease should rely on utilization of a functional classification scheme (see Table 11-1). In the modern era, onset of even mild functional limitation is an indication for mechanical correction of the responsible valve lesion.[48] Valvular heart disease is most often first suspected because of a heart murmur. Cardiologists can detect systolic heart murmurs with fair reliability (kappa 0.30 to 0.48) and can usually rule in or rule out AS, HOCM, MR, MVP, TR, and functional murmurs.[87,88] However, diagnostic inaccuracies do exist and some have advocated the routine use of handheld ultrasound devices to improve detection rates.[89] Kobal and coworkers compared the test characteristics of physical examination by board-certified cardiologists with handheld ultrasound performed by trained medical students.[6] Cardiologists' and students' sensitivities for recognition of valve lesions that cause a systolic murmur were 62 and 93 percent, respectively. Sensitivities were 16 percent for cardiologists and 75 percent for students for the detection of lesions responsible for a diastolic murmur. In this study, overall sensitivity for cardiologists for the detection of valvular heart disease was 50 versus 89 percent for the students using cardiac ultrasound ($p < 0.001$).[6] Spencer and coworkers had previously reported that cardiologists missed 59 percent of the cardiovascular findings on physical examination.[90] However, Roldan and colleagues have reported that among asymptomatic subjects with valvular heart disease, the physical examination had a sensitivity of 70 percent (95 percent CI 0.51 to 0.84), specificity of 98 percent (95 percent CI 0.94 to 0.99), and positive and negative predictive values of 92 percent, for the diagnosis of valvular heart disease as assessed by TEE, a more sensitive technique for the detection of mild—and possibly less clinically relevant—degrees of valvular regurgitation.[47] Only 2 of the 10 subjects with valvular heart disease detected by TEE, but not by physical examination, had a clinically important valve lesion. In addition, dynamic auscultation was able to distinguish functional from pathological murmurs with a specificity of 98 percent and a positive predictive value of 92 percent. A study of young military recruits yielded similar findings.[91] Physical examination performed by cardiology fellows or faculty was able to detect a pathological murmur with 100 percent sensitivity, 67 percent specificity, 30 percent positive predictive value, and 100 percent negative predictive value, using TTE as the reference standard. Thus, a careful and complete cardiac examination can first identify asymptomatic individuals with valvular heart disease for whom TTE, antibiotic prophylaxis, and clinical follow-up are indicated. It can similarly identify patients for whom further evaluation is not necessary.

Mitral Stenosis

Data from the presurgical era and registries of patients with mitral stenosis who refused intervention indicate that long-term survival declines following symptom onset and worsens with increasing degrees of functional limitation (NYHA Class) and as a function of the severity of pulmonary hypertension.[48] Prominent symptoms of mitral stenosis include dyspnea and fatigue. Palpitations, stroke, and symptoms of systemic embolization imply AF. Hemoptysis has several causes, but pulmonary apoplexy is attributed to rupture of dilated bronchial veins into the tracheobronchial tree in patients with severe mitral stenosis. The more common causes of hemoptysis (bronchitis, pneumonia, pulmonary edema, pulmonary infarction) do not track closely with the severity of the valve lesion. The findings on physical examination will vary with the chronicity of the disease, heart rate, rhythm, and cardiac output. It can be difficult to estimate the severity of the valve lesion in older patients with less pliable valves, rapid AF, and low cardiac output. Severe mitral stenosis is suggested by (1) a long or holodiastolic murmur, indicating a persistent LA-left ventricle gradient; (2) a short A_2-OS interval, consistent with greater degrees of LA pressure elevation; (3) a loud P_2 (or single S_2) and/or a right ventricle lift, suggestive of pulmonary hypertension; and (4) elevated jugular venous pressure with *cv* waves, hepatomegaly, and lower extremity edema, all signs of right heart failure. Neither the intensity of the diastolic murmur nor the presence of presystolic accentuation in patients with sinus rhythm accurately reflects lesion severity.

Mitral Regurgitation

The symptoms associated with mitral regurgitation (MR) depend on its severity and time course of development. The acute severe MR that occurs with papillary muscle rupture or endocarditis usually results in sudden and profound dyspnea from pulmonary edema. Examination findings may be misleading because the LV impulse is usually neither enlarged nor displaced and the systolic murmur is early in timing and decrescendo in configuration (see Fig. 11-10). It may also be best heard closer to the lower left sternal border or in the axilla rather than at the apex. A new systolic murmur early following MI may not be audible in a ventilated or obese patient and, thus, vigilance for MR requires a high clinical index of suspicion in this setting.

With chronic MR, symptoms reflect the severity of the regurgitant volume load and LV function and chamber geometry. They relate as well to the etiology of the MR. Fatigue (reduced forward output), dyspnea (increased LA and PA wedge pressures), and palpitations (AF from LA volume or pressure overload) are prominent. Chronic severe MR is suggested by (1) an enlarged, displaced, but dynamic LV apex beat; (2) an apical systolic thrill (murmur intensity grade 4 or greater); (3) a mid-diastolic filling complex comprising an S_3 and a short, low-pitched murmur, indicative of accelerated and enhanced diastolic mitral inflow; (4) wide but physiological splitting of S_2 due to early aortic valve closure; and (5) a loud P_2 or right ventricle lift. The examiner should strive to distinguish MR from other causes of a systolic heart murmur, based on location, radiation, timing, configuration, response to bedside maneuvers, and behavior following a premature beat, as reviewed earlier. The findings in patients with MVP can vary daily, depending on left ventricle loading conditions. The combination of a nonejection click and mid- to late-systolic murmur predicts MVP best as confirmed by TTE criteria (LR 2.43).[92]

Aortic Stenosis

The natural history of aortic stenosis (AS) is well known. Symptom onset indicates the need for valve replacement. The cardinal symptoms include exertional chest discomfort, often indistinguishable from angina, dyspnea, and lightheadedness. Syncope not attributable to another cause indicates severe AS. Warning symptoms may be more subtle in older, less active individuals and include fatigue, depression, and failure to thrive. A simple clinical prediction rule can establish moderate or severe AS (i.e., aortic valve area $<1.5\ cm^2$), based on the presence of a murmur in the 2nd right interspace and over the right clavicle, and several associated findings, including a slowly rising carotid upstroke (*pulsus tardus*), reduced carotid pulse amplitude (*pulsus parvus*), reduced intensity of A_2, and mid- to late-peaking of the systolic murmur.[87,93] The absence of a murmur over the right clavicle is associated with a negative LR of 0.10 (95 percent CI 0.01 to 0.44), whereas the presence of a systolic murmur in this location with 3 or 4 associated findings rules in AS (LR 40, 95 percent CI 6.6 to 240).[93] The intensity of the murmur depends on cardiac output and body size (peak momentum transfer[94] and does not reliably indicate stenosis severity. Munt and co-workers reported that no single physical examination finding had both a high sensitivity and specificity for the diagnosis of severe AS (valve area $<1.0\ cm^2$).[95] Univariate predictors of outcome (death, aortic valve replacement) included carotid upstroke delay and amplitude, systolic murmur grade and peak, and a single S_2. However, on multivariate Cox regression analysis, only carotid upstroke amplitude predicted outcome.[95] Clinical experience has established the difficulty in assessing carotid upstroke characteristics in the elderly, in patients with hypertension, and in low output states. It is also challenging to distinguish the murmur of AS from that due to mild or even moderate degrees of AS (Fig. 11-16). Aortic sclerosis is defined by focal calcification and thickening of the leaflets without restriction of motion and a peak transaortic velocity <2.5 msec. The murmur can be of grade 2 or 3 intensity, but it peaks in mid-systole. The carotid upstroke should be normal and A_2 preserved, and the ECG should lack evidence of left ventricular hypertrophy. Nevertheless, TTE is often necessary to clarify this distinction, especially in older patients with hypertension. The findings will affect decisions regarding prophylaxis for infective endocarditis and the frequency of clinical and TTE follow-up. Signal analysis of digitally captured cardiovascular sounds using spectral display can distinguish the murmur of aortic sclerosis from that due to hemodynamically significant AS.[14] The differential diagnosis of a systolic murmur related to LV outflow obstruction includes valvular AS, HOCM, discrete membranous subaortic stenosis (DMSS), and supravalvular aortic stenosis (SVAS). The presence of an ejection sound indicates a valvular etiology. HOCM can be distinguished on the basis of the response of the murmur to Valsalva and standing or squatting. The murmur intensifies during the strain phase of the Valsalva maneuver and after standing rapidly from a squatting position. It will decrease in intensity with squatting. Patients with DMSS will commonly have a diastolic murmur indicative of AR, but not an ejection sound, whereas in patients with SVAS, the right arm blood pressure is more than 10 mm Hg greater than the left arm blood pressure.

Aortic Regurgitation

Patients with acute severe aortic regurgitation (AR) present with pulmonary edema and symptoms and signs of low forward cardiac output. Tachycardia is invariably present; systolic blood pressure is not elevated, and the pulse pressure is not widened. S_1 is soft because of premature closure of the mitral valve. As noted, both the intensity and duration of the diastolic murmur are attenuated by the rapid rise in LV diastolic pressure and diminution of the aortic-LV diastolic pressure gradient. Interestingly, in patients with acute type A aortic dissection, the presence of a diastolic murmur (heard in nearly 30 percent of cases) does little to change the pretest probability of dissection (LR 1.4, 95 percent CI 1.0 to 2.0).[34,96] Acute severe AR is poorly tolerated and mandates surgical correction. Typical symptoms associated with chronic severe AR include dyspnea, fatigue, chest discomfort, and palpitations. As is the case for chronic MR, mild or moderate degrees of chronic AR are well tolerated and insufficient to cause symptoms, absent other cardiovascular abnormalities. The typical decrescendo diastolic blowing murmur suggests chronic AR. A mid-systolic murmur indicative of augmented LV outflow is invariably heard at the base. Aortic valve stenosis may coexist. The absence of the diastolic murmur significantly reduces the likelihood of moderate or greater AR (LR 0.1) and of mild or greater AR (LR 0.2 to 0.3). The presence of a typical diastolic murmur increases the likelihood of moderate or greater AR (LR 4.0 to 8.3) and of mild or greater AR (8.8 to 32.0).[34] In addition, in patients with chronic AR, the intensity of the murmur correlates with the severity of the lesion. A grade 3 diastolic murmur has an LR of 4.5 (95 percent CI 1.6 to 14.0) for distinguishing severe AR from mild or moderate AR. Data regarding the significance of an Austin Flint murmur (low-pitched, mid-to late apical diastolic murmur) are conflicting. Whereas Desjardins and colleagues reported that an Austin Flint murmur identified AR as moderate or greater (LR 25, 95 percent CI 2.8 to 243),[97] Rahko and colleagues attributed this murmur entirely to the direction of the regurgitant jet toward the anterior mitral leaflet and found no difference in the severity of AR between patients with and without an Austin Flint murmur.[98] Chronic severe AR will result in leftward and downward displacement of a vigorous LV apex beat. Little evidence supports the historical claims of the importance of nearly all the eponymous peripheral signs of chronic AR, of which there are at least a dozen.[99] The Hill sign (brachial-popliteal systolic blood pressure gradient >20 mm Hg) may be the single exception

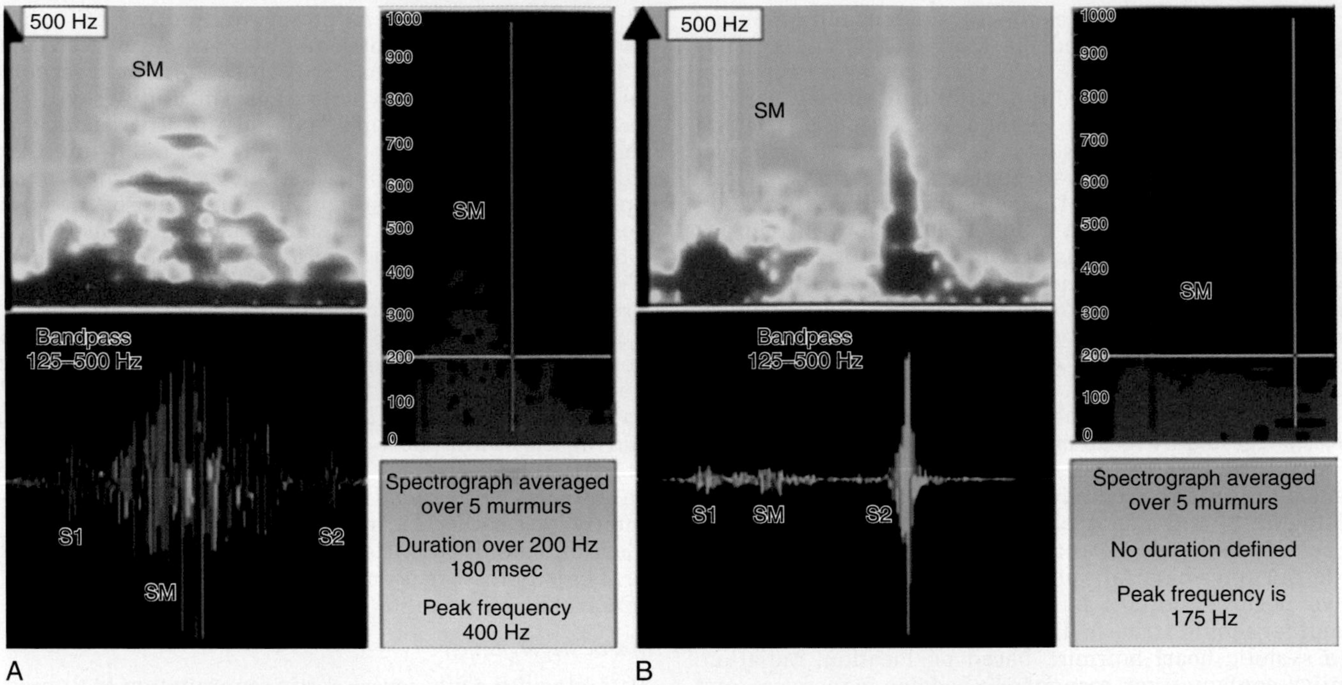

FIGURE 11–16 A, Example of a spectral display **(upper left panel)** recorded simultaneously with a waveform display **(lower left panel)** in a patient with severe aortic stenosis. A systolic murmur is noted that has a crescendo-decrescendo contour in the waveform display, whereas it also shows a crescendo-decrescendo frequency pattern in the spectral image. This latter image presents a colored plot in which the relative signal intensities correlate with the colors (i.e., greater intensity is shown in orange and lesser intensity is shown in yellow). Absence of sound is shown in green. The panel at the **right** shows a spectral average of murmurs derived from multiple cycles in this case. It is color-coded to demonstrate only more intense frequencies uniformly in red (i.e., after a given "cutoff" attenuation [−25 dB in this example], the red changes abruptly to black). Displayed in this way, this latter image shows a relatively high peak frequency of 400 Hz (vertical scale at the **left**). This display also allows for measurement of the time duration for the murmur to exceed any arbitrary frequency level, in this case 200 Hz. **B,** demonstrates a similar display for an individual with an innocent murmur, which appears primarily in early systole and does not reach a peak frequency of 200 Hz. SM = systolic murmur. *(Adapted from Tavel ME: Circulation 113:1255-1259, 2006.)*

(sensitivity 89 percent for moderate to severe AR), although its supporting evidence base is also weak.[99] Resurrection of these peripheral signs as indices of lesion severity awaits further research.

Tricuspid Valve Disease

The symptoms and signs of tricuspid stenosis (TS) are usually obscured by left-sided valve lesions, most notably, mitral stenosis. Fatigue (low output), palpitations (AF), increased abdominal girth, and lower extremity edema may develop. An elevated jugular venous pressure with a delayed *y* descent, abdominal ascites, and edema suggest severe TS. The auscultatory findings are difficult to appreciate but mimic those of mitral stenosis and may increase during inspiration. TR may be primary in origin (Ebstein's anomaly, prolapse, endocarditis, carcinoid syndrome), but occurs more often as a secondary complication of PA hypertension, RV enlargement, and annular dilation. The symptoms of TR resemble those of TS. Severe TR is manifested by elevated jugular venous pressure with prominent *cv* waves, a parasternal lift, pulsatile liver, ascites, and edema. The intensity of the holosystolic murmur of TR increases with inspiration (Carvallo sign). Murmur intensity does not accurately reflect the severity of the valve lesion.

Pulmonic Valve Disease

Progressive degrees of pulmonic stenosis (PS) may result in exertional fatigue, dyspnea, lightheadedness, and chest discomfort ("right ventricular angina"). Syncope denotes severe obstruction. The mid-systolic murmur of PS is best heard at the second left interspace. With severe PS, the interval between S_1 and the pulmonic ejection sound narrows, the murmur peaks in late systole and may extend beyond A_2, and P_2 becomes inaudible. Signs of significant RV pressure overload include a prominent jugular venous *a* wave and a parasternal lift. Pulmonic regurgitation (PR) occurs most commonly as a secondary manifestation of significant PA hypertension and annular dilation but may also reflect a primary valve disorder (congenital bicuspid valve) or develop as a complication of RV outflow tract surgery (e.g., for tetralogy of Fallot). Symptoms vary as a function of the severity of PA hypertension and the level of RV compensation. The diastolic murmur of secondary PR (Graham Steell) can be distinguished from that due to AR on the basis of its increase in intensity with inspiration, its later onset (after A_2 and with P_2), and its slightly lower pitch. When a typical murmur is audible, the likelihood of PR increases (LR 17), but the absence of a murmur does not exclude PR (LR 0.9).[34] With severe PA hypertension and PR, P_2 is usually palpable and there are signs of RV pressure and volume overload (parasternal lift, prominent jugular venous *a* wave). The intensity, pitch, and duration of the PR murmur may be misleadingly unimpressive in patients with severe degrees of PR following RV outflow tract surgery. The discrepancy is due to the associated rise in RV diastolic pressure and reduction in the PA-RV diastolic pressure gradient. The examiner should be alert to this phenomenon in the presence of other signs of RV volume overload (parasternal lift, elevated jugular venous pressure). TTE (or cardiac MR) is indicated for clarification.

Prosthetic Heart Valves

The differential diagnosis of recurrent functional limitation following valve replacement surgery includes prosthetic valve dysfunction, arrhythmia, and impairment of ventricular performance. Prosthetic valve dysfunction can occur as a result of thrombosis, pannus ingrowth, infection, and structural deterioration. Symptoms mimic those observed with native valve disease, and they may occur acutely or develop gradually over time. The first clue that prosthetic valve dysfunction may be present is often a *change* in the quality of the heart sounds or the appearance of a new murmur. The heart sounds with a bioprosthetic valve resemble those generated by native valves. A bioprosthesis in the mitral position is usually associated with a mid-systolic murmur (from turbulence created by systolic flow across the valve struts as they project into the LV outflow tract) and a soft, mid-diastolic murmur that occurs with normal LV filling. A high-pitched or holosystolic apical murmur signifies paravalvular or bioprosthetic regurgitation that requires TEE verification and careful follow-up. Depending on the magnitude of the regurgitant volume, a diastolic murmur may be more easily audible. Clinical deterioration can occur rapidly after first expression of bioprosthetic failure. A bioprosthesis in the aortic position is invariably associated with a grade 2 to 3 mid-systolic murmur at the base. A diastolic murmur of AR is abnormal and merits additional investigation. Bioprosthetic stenosis from pannus ingrowth in either the mitral or aortic position is relatively uncommon. A decrease in the intensity of either the opening or closing sounds of a mechanical prosthesis, depending on its type, is a worrisome finding. A high-pitched apical systolic murmur in patients with a mechanical mitral prosthesis, or a decrescendo diastolic murmur in patients with an aortic prosthesis, indicates prosthetic dysfunction (or dehiscence). Patients with prosthetic valve thrombosis may present with signs of shock, muffled heart sounds, and soft murmurs.

THE FUTURE

The history and physical examination will not lose their leading roles in the assessment of the patient with known or suspected cardiovascular disease. In fact, increasing concerns regarding the escalating costs of medical care, driven in large part by expenses related to imaging, may reinforce the value of these time-honored traditions. However, they will become more relevant only in relation to their proven value to provide incremental information regarding diagnosis, prognosis, and response to therapy. Additional studies are needed to establish the accuracy and performance characteristics of the history and examination, with the same rigor applied to treadmill exercise testing and biomarker use. Recognition of the need to reestablish the mentored patient evaluation as a dedicated component of physician training programs, along with mechanisms to allow practice, repetition, and provision of feedback, will be essential. The incorporation of either or both handheld Doppler echocardiography and spectral display of the heart sounds may improve clinician performance.

Acknowledgment

The authors wish to acknowledge the previous contributions of Drs. Eugene Braunwald, Joseph Perloff, Robert O'Rourke, and James A. Shaver, which have laid the foundation for this chapter.

REFERENCES

The General Physical Examination

1. Laukkanen A, Ikaheimo M, Luukinen H: Practices of clinical examination of heart failure patients in primary health care. Cent Eur J Public Health 14(2):86-9, 2006.
2. Paauw DS, Wenrich MD, Curtis JR, et al: Ability of primary care physicians to recognize physical findings associated with HIV infection. JAMA 274(17):1380-2, 1995.
3. Tavel M: Cardiac auscultation. A glorious past—but does it have a future? Circulation 93(6):1250-3, 1996.
4. Mangione S, Nieman LZ: Cardiac auscultatory skills of internal medicine and family practice trainees. A comparison of diagnostic proficiency. JAMA 278(9):717-22, 1997.
5. Vukanovic-Criley JM, Criley S, Warde CM, et al: Competency in cardiac examination skills in medical students, trainees, physicians, and faculty: A multicenter study. Arch Intern Med 166(6):610-6, 2006.
6. Kobal SL, Trento L, Baharami S, et al: Comparison of effectiveness of hand-carried ultrasound to bedside cardiovascular physical examination. Am J Cardiol 96(7):1002-6, 2005.
7. DeMaria AN: Wither the cardiac physical examination? J Am Coll Cardiol 48(10):2156-7, 2006.
8. Decara JM, Kirkpatrick JN, Spencer KT, Ward RP, et al: Use of hand-carried ultrasound devices to augment the accuracy of medical students' bedside cardiac diagnoses. J Am Soc Echocardiogr 18(3):257-63, 2005.
9. Hoyte H, Jensen T, Gjesdal K: Cardiac auscultation training of medical students: A comparison of electronic sensor-based and acoustic stethoscopes. BMC Med Educ 5(1):14, 2005.
10. Barrett MJ, Lacey CS, Sekara AE, et al: Mastering cardiac murmurs: The power of repetition. Chest 126(2):470-5, 2004.
11. March SK, Bedynek JL, Jr., Chizner MA: Teaching cardiac auscultation: Effectiveness of a patient-centered teaching conference on improving cardiac auscultatory skills. Mayo Clin Proc 80(11):1443-8, 2005.
12. Wiviott SD, Morrow DA, Frederick PD, et al: Performance of the thrombolysis in myocardial infarction risk index in the National Registry of Myocardial Infarction-3 and -4: A simple index that predicts mortality in ST-segment elevation myocardial infarction. J Am Coll Cardiol 44(4):783-9, 2004.
13. Wiviott SD, Morrow DA, Frederick PD, et al: Application of the thrombolysis in myocardial infarction risk index in non-ST-segment elevation myocardial infarction: Evaluation of patients in the National Registry of Myocardial Infarction. J Am Coll Cardiol 47(8):1553-8, 2006.
14. Tavel ME: Cardiac auscultation: A glorious past—and it does have a future! Circulation 113(9):1255-9, 2006.
15. Swap CJ, Nagurney JT: Value and limitations of chest pain history in the evaluation of patients with suspected acute coronary syndromes. JAMA 294(20):2623-9, 2005.
16. The Criteria Committee of the New York Heart Association: Nomenclature and Criteria for Diagnosis. 9th ed. Boston, Little Brown, 1994.
17. Campeau L: Grading of angina pectoris. Circulation 54:522, 1975.
18. Goldman L, Hashimoto B, Cook EF, Loscalzo A, et al: Comparative reproducibility and validity of systems for assessing cardiovascular functional class: Advantages of a new specific activity scale. Circulation 64(6):1227-34, 1981.
19. Lederle FA, Simel DL: The rational clinical examination. Does this patient have abdominal aortic aneurysm? JAMA 281(1):77-82, 1999.

Assessment of Venous Pressure

20. Vinayak AG, Levitt J, Gehbach B, et al: Usefulness of the external jugular vein examination in detecting abnormal central venous pressure in critically ill patients. Arch Intern Med 166(19):2132-7, 2006.
21. Cook DJ, Simel DL: The Rational Clinical Examination. Does this patient have abnormal central venous pressure? JAMA 275(8):630-4, 1996.
22. McGee SR: Physical examination of venous pressure: A critical review. Am Heart J 136(1):10-8, 1998.
23. Ramana RK, Senegala T, Lichtenberg R: A new angel on the Angel of Louis. Congest Heart Fail 12(4):196-9, 2006.
24. Seth R, Magner P, Matziner F, vanWalraven C: How far is the sternal angle from the mid-right atrium? J Gen Intern Med 17(11):852-6, 2002.
25. Courtois M, Fattal PG, Kovacs SJ, Jr., et al: Anatomically and physiologically based reference level for measurement of intracardiac pressures. Circulation 92(7):1994-2000, 1995.
26. Drake JJ: Locating the external reference point for central venous pressure determination. Nurs Res 23(6):475-82, 1974.
27. Hurrell DG, Nishimura RA, Higano ST, et al: Value of dynamic respiratory changes in left and right ventricular pressures for the diagnosis of constrictive pericarditis. Circulation 93(11):2007-13, 1996.
28. Wiese J: The abdominojugular reflux sign. Am J Med 109(1):59-61, 2000.

Assessment of Arterial Pressure

29. Pickering TG, Hall JE, Appel LJ, et al: Recommendations for blood pressure measurement in humans and experimental animals: Part 1: Blood pressure measurement in humans: A statement for professionals from the Subcommittee of Professional and Public Education of the American Heart Association Council on High Blood Pressure Research. Hypertension 45(1):142-61, 2005.
30. La Batide-Alanore A, Chatellier G, Bobrie G, et al: Comparison of nurse- and physician-determined clinic blood pressure levels in patients referred to a hypertension clinic: Implications for subsequent management. J Hypertens 18(4):391-8, 2000.
31. Graves JW: Prevalence of blood pressure cuff sizes in a referral practice of 430 consecutive adult hypertensives. Blood Press Monit 6(1):17-20, 2001.
32. Cavallini MC, Roman MJ, Blank SG, et al: Association of the auscultatory gap with vascular disease in hypertensive patients. Ann Intern Med 124(10):877-83, 1996.
33. Lane D, Beevers M, Barnes N, et al: Inter-arm differences in blood pressure: When are they clinically significant? J Hypertens 20(6):1089-95, 2002.

Assessment of Valvular Heart Disease

34. Choudhry NK, Etchells EE: The rational clinical examination. Does this patient have aortic regurgitation? JAMA 281(23):2231-8, 1999.
35. Messerli FH, Ventura HO, Amodeo C: Osler's maneuver and pseudohypertension. N Engl J Med 312(24):1548-51, 1985.
36. Belmin J, Visintin N, Salvatore R, et al: Osler's maneuver: Absence of usefulness for the detection of pseudohypertension in an elderly population. Am J Med 98(1):42-9, 1995.

37. Williams B, Lacy PS, Thom SM, et al: Differential impact of blood pressure-lowering drugs on central aortic pressure and clinical outcomes: Principal results of the Conduit Artery Function Evaluation (CAFE) study. Circulation 2006;113(9):1213-25, 2006.
38. Nichols WW, O'Rourke ME: McDonald's Blood Flow in Arteries: Theoretical, Experimental, and Clinical Principles, 5th ed. London, Edward Arnold, 1993.
39. Khan NA, Rahim SA, Anand SS, et al: Does the clinical examination predict lower extremity peripheral arterial disease? JAMA 295(5):536-46, 2006.
40. Lee JC, Atwood JE, Lee HJ, et al: Association of pulsus paradoxus with obesity in normal volunteers. J Am Coll Cardiol 47(9):1907-9, 2006.
41. Sagrista-Sauleda J, Angel J, Sambola A, et al: Low-pressure cardiac tamponade: Clinical and hemodynamic profile. Circulation 114(9):945-52, 2006.
42. Sipido KR: Understanding cardiac alternans: The answer lies in the $Ca2^+$ store. Circ Res 94(5):570-2, 2004.
43. Weiss JN, Karma A, Shiferaw Y, et al: From pulsus to pulseless: The saga of cardiac alternans. Circ Res 98(10):1244-53, 2006.
44. Magyar MT, Nam EM, Csiba L, et al: Carotid artery auscultation—anachronism or useful screening procedure? Neurol Res 24(7):705-8, 2002.
45. Lundin M, Wiksten JP, Perakyla T, et al: Distal pulse palpation: Is it reliable? World J Surg 1999;23(3):252-5, 1999.
46. Kono T, Rosman H, Alam M, et al: Hemodynamic correlates of the third heart sound during the evolution of chronic heart failure. J Am Coll Cardiol 21(2):419-23, 1993.
47. Roldan CA, Shively BK, Crawford MH: Value of the cardiovascular physical examination for detecting valvular heart disease in asymptomatic subjects. Am J Cardiol 77(15):1327-31, 1996.
48. Bonow RO, Bennett S, Casey DE, Jr.,et al: ACC/AHA 2006 guidelines for the management of patients with valvular heart disease: a report of the American College of Cardiology/American Heart Association Task Force on Practice Guidelines (writing Committee to Revise the 1998 guidelines for the management of patients with valvular heart disease) developed in collaboration with the Society of Cardiovascular Anesthesiologists endorsed by the Society for Cardiovascular Angiography and Interventions and the Society of Thoracic Surgeons. J Am Coll Cardiol 48(3):e1-148, 2006.
49. Heidenreich PA, Schnittger I, Hancock SL, et al: A systolic murmur is a common presentation of aortic regurgitation detected by echocardiography. Clin Cardiol 27(9):502-6, 2004.

CH 11

Assessment of Heart Failure

50. Lembo NJ, Dell'Italia LJ, Crawford MH, O'Rourke RA: Bedside diagnosis of systolic murmurs. N Engl J Med 318(24):1572-8, 1988.
51. Wilson JR, Rayes G, Yeoh TK, Gothard P: Dissociation between peak exercise oxygen consumption and hemodynamic dysfunction in potential heart transplant candidates. J Am Coll Cardiol 26(2):429-35, 1995.
52. Stevenson LW, Perloff JK: The limited reliability of physical signs for estimating hemodynamics in chronic heart failure. JAMA 261(6):884-8, 1989.
53. Leung RS, Bowman MF, Parker JD, et al: Avoidance of the left lateral decubitus position during sleep in patients with heart failure: Relationship to cardiac size and function. J Am Coll Cardiol 41(2):227-30, 2003.
54. Givertz MM, Fang JC: Diastolic Heart Failure. *In* Baughman KL, Baumgartner WA (eds): Treatment of Advanced Heart Disease. New York: Taylor and Francis; 2006, pp 227-246.
55. Hunt SA, Abraham WT, Chin MH, et al: ACC/AHA 2005 Guideline Update for the Diagnosis and Management of Chronic Heart Failure in the Adult: A report of the American College of Cardiology/American Heart Association Task Force on Practice Guidelines (Writing Committee to Update the 2001 Guidelines for the Evaluation and Management of Heart Failure): Developed in collaboration with the American College of Chest Physicians and the International Society for Heart and Lung Transplantation: Endorsed by the Heart Rhythm Society. Circulation 112(12):e154-235, 2005.
56. Franciosa JA, Park M, Levine TB: Lack of correlation between exercise capacity and indexes of resting left ventricular performance in heart failure. Am J Cardiol. 47(1):33-9, 1981.
57. Marantz PR, Tobin JN, Wassertheil-Smoller S, et al: The relationship between left ventricular systolic function and congestive heart failure diagnosed by clinical criteria. Circulation 77(3):607-12, 1988.
58. Redfield MM, Jacobsen SJ, Burnett JC Jr., et al: Burden of systolic and diastolic ventricular dysfunction in the community: Appreciating the scope of the heart failure epidemic. JAMA 289(2):194-202, 2003.
59. Badgett RG, Lucey CR, Mulrow CD: Can the clinical examination diagnose left-sided heart failure in adults? JAMA 277(21):1712-9, 1997.
60. McKee PA, Castelli WP, McNamara PM, Kannel WB: The natural history of congestive heart failure: The Framingham study. N Engl J Med 285(26):1441-6, 1971.
61. Harlan WR, Oberman A, Grim R, Rosati RA: Chronic congestive heart failure in coronary artery disease: Clinical criteria. Ann Intern Med 86(2):133-8, 1977.
62. Carlson KJ, Lee DC, Goroll AH, et al: An analysis of physicians' reasons for prescribing long-term digitalis therapy in outpatients. J Chronic Dis 38(9):733-9, 1985.
63. Rohde LE, Beck-da-Silva L, Goldraich L, et al: Reliability and prognostic value of traditional signs and symptoms in outpatients with congestive heart failure. Can J Cardiol 20(7):697-702, 2004.
64. How to diagnose diastolic heart failure. European Study Group on Diastolic Heart Failure. Eur Heart J 19(7):990-1003, 1988.
65. Silver MT, Rose GA, Paul SD, et al: A clinical rule to predict preserved left ventricular ejection fraction in patients after myocardial infarction. Ann Intern Med 121(10):750-6, 1994.
66. Ghali JK, Kadakia S, Cooper RS, Liao YL: Bedside diagnosis of preserved versus impaired left ventricular systolic function in heart failure. Am J Cardiol 67(11):1002-6, 1991.
67. Malki Q, Sharma ND, Afzal A, et al: Clinical presentation, hospital length of stay, and readmission rate in patients with heart failure with preserved and decreased left ventricular systolic function. Clin Cardiol 25(4):149-52, 2002.
68. Thomas JT, Kelly RF, Thomas SJ, et al: Utility of history, physical examination, electrocardiogram, and chest radiograph for differentiating normal from decreased systolic function in patients with heart failure. Am J Med 112(6):437-45, 2002.
69. Smith GL, Masoudi FA, Vaccarino V, et al: Outcomes in heart failure patients with preserved ejection fraction: Mortality, readmission, and functional decline. J Am Coll Cardiol 41(9):1510-8, 2003.
70. Yu CM, Lin H, Yang H, et al: Progression of systolic abnormalities in patients with "isolated" diastolic heart failure and diastolic dysfunction. Circulation 105(10):1195-201, 2002.
71. Vasan RS, Levy D: Defining diastolic heart failure: A call for standardized diagnostic criteria. Circulation 101(17):2118-21, 2000.
72. Fonarow GC, Adams KF, Jr., Abraham WT, et al: Risk stratification for in-hospital mortality in acutely decompensated heart failure: Classification and regression tree analysis. JAMA 293(5):572-80, 2005.
73. Butman SM, Ewy GA, Standen JR, et al: Bedside cardiovascular examination in patients with severe chronic heart failure: Importance of rest or inducible jugular venous distension. J Am Coll Cardiol 22(4):968-74, 1993.
74. Drazner MH, Hamilton MA, Fonarow G, et al: Relationship between right and left-sided filling pressures in 1000 patients with advanced heart failure. J Heart Lung Transplant 18(11):1126-32, 1999.
75. Drazner MH, Rame JE, Dries DL: Third heart sound and elevated jugular venous pressure as markers of the subsequent development of heart failure in patients with asymptomatic left ventricular dysfunction. Am J Med 114(6):431-7, 2003.
76. Marcus GM, Gerber IL, McKeown BH, et al: Association between phonocardiographic third and fourth heart sounds and objective measures of left ventricular function. JAMA 293(18):2238-44, 2005.
77. Marcus GM, Vessey J, Jordan MV, et al: Relationship between accurate auscultation of a clinically useful third heart sound and level of experience. Arch Intern Med 166(6):617-22, 2006.
78. Chakko S, Woska D, Martinez H, et al: Clinical, radiographic, and hemodynamic correlations in chronic congestive heart failure: Conflicting results may lead to inappropriate care. Am J Med 90(3):353-9, 1991.
79. Maisel AS, Gilpin E, Hoit B, et al: Survival after hospital discharge in matched populations with inferior or anterior myocardial infarction. J Am Coll Cardiol 6(4):731-6, 1985.
80. Ali AS, Rybicki BA, Alam W, et al: Clinical predictors of heart failure in patients with first acute myocardial infarction. Am Heart J 138(6 Pt 1):1133-9, 1999.
81. Goldman L, Caldera DL, Nussbaum SR, et al: Multifactorial index of cardiac risk in noncardiac surgical procedures. N Engl J Med 297(16):845-50, 1977.
82. Sharma GV, Woods PA, Lambrew CT, et al: Evaluation of a noninvasive system for determining left ventricular filling pressure. Arch Intern Med 162(18):2084-8, 2002.
83. Felker GM, Cuculich PS, Gheorghiade M: The Valsalva maneuver: A bedside "biomarker" for heart failure. Am J Med 119(2):117-22, 2006.
84. McIntyre KM, Vita JA, Lambrew CT, et al: A noninvasive method of predicting pulmonary-capillary wedge pressure. N Engl J Med 327(24):1715-20, 1992.
85. Brunner-La Rocca HP, Weilenmann D, Rickli H, et al: Is blood pressure response to the Valsalva maneuver related to neurohormones, exercise capacity, and clinical findings in heart failure? Chest 116(4):861-7, 1999.

The Value of the Physical Examination

86. Gaine SP, Rubin LJ: Primary pulmonary hypertension. Lancet 352(9129):719-25, 1998.
87. Etchells E, Bell C, Robb K: Does this patient have an abnormal systolic murmur? JAMA 277(7):564-71, 1997.
88. Attenhofer Jost CH, Turina J, Mayer K, et al: Echocardiography in the evaluation of systolic murmurs of unknown cause. Am J Med 108(8):614-20, 2000.
89. Vourvouri EC, Poldermans D, Deckers JW, et al: Evaluation of a hand carried cardiac ultrasound device in an outpatient cardiology clinic. Heart 91(2):171-6, 2005.
90. Spencer KT, Anderson AS, Bharqava A, et al: Physician-performed point-of-care echocardiography using a laptop platform compared with physical examination in the cardiovascular patient. J Am Coll Cardiol 37(8):2013-8, 2001.
91. Shry EA, Smithers MA, Mascette AM: Auscultation versus echocardiography in a healthy population with precordial murmur. Am J Cardiol 87(12):1428-30, 2001.
92. Olive KE, Grassman ED: Mitral valve prolapse: Comparison of diagnosis by physical examination and echocardiography. South Med J 83(11):1266-9, 1990.
93. Etchells E, Glenns V, Shadowitz S, et al: A bedside clinical prediction rule for detecting moderate or severe aortic stenosis. J Gen Intern Med 13(10):699-704, 1998.
94. Kuperstein R, Feinberg MS, Eldar M, Schwammenthal E: Physical determinants of systolic murmur intensity in aortic stenosis. Am J Cardiol 95(6):774-6, 2005.
95. Munt B, Legget ME, Kraft CD, et al: Physical examination in valvular aortic stenosis: Correlation with stenosis severity and prediction of clinical outcome. Am Heart J 137(2):298-306, 1999.
96. Klompas M: Does this patient have an acute thoracic aortic dissection? JAMA 287(17):2262-72, 2002.
97. Desjardins VA, Enriquez-Sarano M, Tajik AJ, et al: Intensity of murmurs correlates with severity of valvular regurgitation. Am J Med 100(2):149-56, 1996.
98. Rahko PS: Doppler and echocardiographic characteristics of patients having an Austin Flint murmur. Circulation 83(6):1940-50, 1991.
99. Babu AN, Kymes SM, Carpenter Fryer SM: Eponyms and the diagnosis of aortic regurgitation: What says the evidence? Ann Intern Med 138(9):736-42, 2003.

CHAPTER 12

Electrocardiography

David M. Mirvis and Ary L. Goldberger

The electrocardiogram (ECG) is the product of a series of technological and physiological advances pioneered over the past two centuries.[1,2] Early demonstrations of the heart's electrical activity reported during the last half of the 19th century were closely followed by direct recordings of cardiac potentials by Waller in 1887. The invention of the string galvanometer by Willem Einthoven in 1901 provided a reliable and direct method for registering electrical activity of the heart. By 1910, use of the string galvanometer had emerged from the research laboratory into the clinic.

Subsequent achievements built on the solid foundation supplied by the early electrocardiographers. The result has become a widely used and invaluable clinical tool for the detection, diagnosis, and treatment of virtually every type of heart disease. Recent advances have extended the importance of the ECG in determining the extent and severity of myocardial ischemia, localizing sites of origin and pathways of tachyarrhythmias, assessing therapeutic options for patients with heart failure, and identifying and evaluating patients with genetic diseases who are prone to arrhythmias.[2] As many as 20 million ECGs are performed in the United States each year, making the ECG the most commonly performed, as well as the oldest, cardiovascular laboratory procedure.

FUNDAMENTAL PRINCIPLES

The ECG is the final outcome of a complex series of physiological and technological processes[3] depicted in Figure 12-1. First, transmembrane ionic currents are generated by ion fluxes across cell membranes and between adjacent cells (see Chap. 31). These currents are synchronized by cardiac activation and recovery sequences to generate a cardiac electrical field in and around the heart that varies with time during the cardiac cycle. This electrical field passes through numerous other structures, including the lungs, blood, and skeletal muscle, that perturb the cardiac electrical field as it passes through them.

The currents reaching the skin are then detected by electrodes placed in specific locations on the extremities and torso that are configured to produce leads. The outputs of these leads are amplified, filtered, and displayed by various electronic devices to produce an electrocardiographic recording. Finally, diagnostic criteria are applied to these recordings to produce an interpretation. Each of these steps influences the final product, the clinical ECG, and are considered in detail in this chapter to provide a foundation for considering the common abnormalities found in clinical practice and as a basis for further learning.

Genesis of the Cardiac Electrical Field

IONIC CURRENTS AND CARDIAC ELECTRICAL FIELD GENERATION DURING ACTIVATION. Transmembrane ionic currents, discussed in detail in Chapter 31, are ultimately responsible for the cardiac potentials that are recorded as an ECG. Current may be modeled as being carried by positively charged or negatively charged ions. Through a purely arbitrary choice, electrophysiological currents are considered to be the movement of positive charge. A positive current moving in one direction is equivalent to a negative current of equal strength moving in the opposite direction.

The process of generating the cardiac electrical field during activation can be illustrated by considering the events depicted in Figure 12-2. A single cardiac fiber, 20 mm in length, is activated by a stimulus applied to its leftmost margin (see Fig. 12-2A). Transmembrane potentials (V_m) are recorded as the difference between intracellular and extracellular potentials (Φ_i and Φ_e, respectively). Figure 12-2B plots V_m along the length of the fiber at the instant (t_0) at which activation has reached the point designated as X_0. As each site is activated, it undergoes depolarization and the polarity of the transmembrane potential converts from negative to positive, as represented in the typical cardiac action potential. Thus, sites to the left of the point X_0 that have already undergone excitation have positive transmembrane potentials (i.e., the inside of the cell is positive relative to the outside of the cell), whereas those to the right of X_0 (which remain in a resting state) have negative transmembrane potentials. Near the site undergoing activation (site X_0), the potentials reverse polarity over a short distance.

Figure 12-2C displays the direction and magnitude of a transmembrane current (I_m) along the fiber at the instant (t_0) at which excitation has reached site X_0. Current flow is inwardly directed in fiber regions that have undergone activation (i.e., to the left of point X_0) and outwardly directed in neighboring zones still at rest (i.e., to the right of X_0). Sites of outward current flow are current sources and those with inward current flow are current sinks. As depicted in the figure, current flow is most intense in each direction near the site of activation X_0.

Because the border between inwardly and outwardly directed currents is relatively sharp, these currents can be visualized as though they were limited to the sites of maximal current flow, as depicted in Figure 12-2D, and separated by distance, d, which is usually 1.0 mm or less. As activation proceeds along the fiber, the source-sink pair

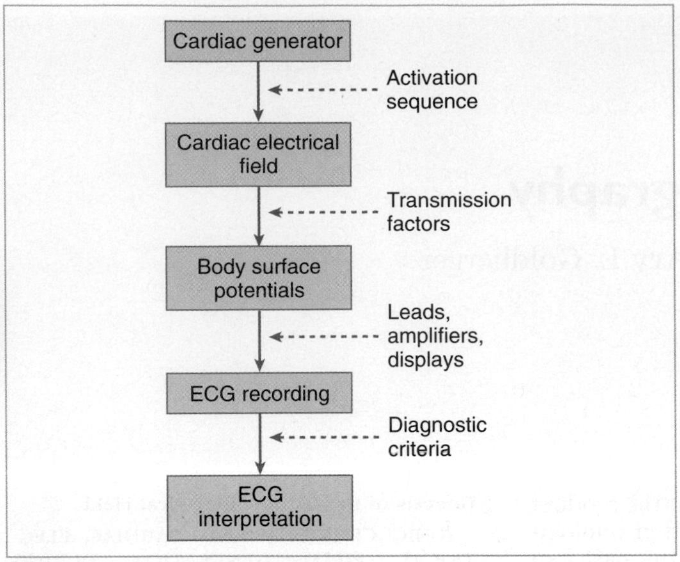

FIGURE 12–1 Schematic representation of the factors resulting in recording the electrocardiogram (ECG). The major paths leading to the ECG are marked by solid arrows and factors influencing or perturbing this path are shown with dashed arrows.

moves to the right at the speed of propagation for the particular type of fiber.

THE CARDIAC DIPOLE. Two point sources of equal strength but of opposite polarity located very near each other, such as the current source and the current sink illustrated in Figure 12-2D, can be represented as a current dipole. Thus, activation of a fiber can be modeled as a current dipole that moves in the direction of propagation of activation.

Such a dipole is fully characterized by three parameters: strength or dipole moment, location, and orientation. In this case, the location of the dipole is the site undergoing activation (point X_0), and its orientation is in the direction of activation (i.e., from left to right along the fiber). Dipole moment is proportional to the rate of change of intracellular potential—that is, action potential shape.

A current dipole produces a characteristic potential field with positive potentials projected ahead of it and negative potentials projected behind it. The actual potential recorded at any site within this field is directly proportional to the dipole moment, inversely proportional to the square of the distance from the dipole to the recording site, and directly proportional to the cosine of the angle between the axis of the dipole and a line drawn from the dipole to the recording site.

CARDIAC WAVE FRONTS. This example from one cardiac fiber can be generalized to the more realistic case, in which multiple adjacent fibers are activated in synchrony to produce an activation front. Activation of each fiber creates a dipole oriented in the direction of activation. The net effect of all the dipoles in this wave front is a single dipole with a strength and orientation equal to the (vector) sum of all the simultaneously active component dipoles. Thus, an activation front propagating through the heart can be represented by a single dipole that projects positive potentials ahead of it and negative potentials behind it.

This relationship between activation direction, orientation of the current dipole, and polarity of potentials is a critical concept in electrocardiography. It describes the fundamental relationship between the polarity of potentials sensed by an electrode and the direction of movement of an activation front—an electrode senses positive potentials when an activation front is moving toward it and negative potentials when the activation front is moving away from it.

The dipole model, although useful in describing cardiac fields and understanding clinical electrocardiography, has significant theoretical limitations. These limits result primarily from the inability of a single dipole to represent accurately more than one wave front that is propagating through the heart at any one instant. As will be discussed, during much of the time of ventricular excitation, more than one wave front is present.

THE SOLID ANGLE THEOREM. One important and commonly used method of estimating the potentials projected to some point away from an activation front is application of the solid angle theorem. A solid angle is a geometric measure of the size of a region when viewed

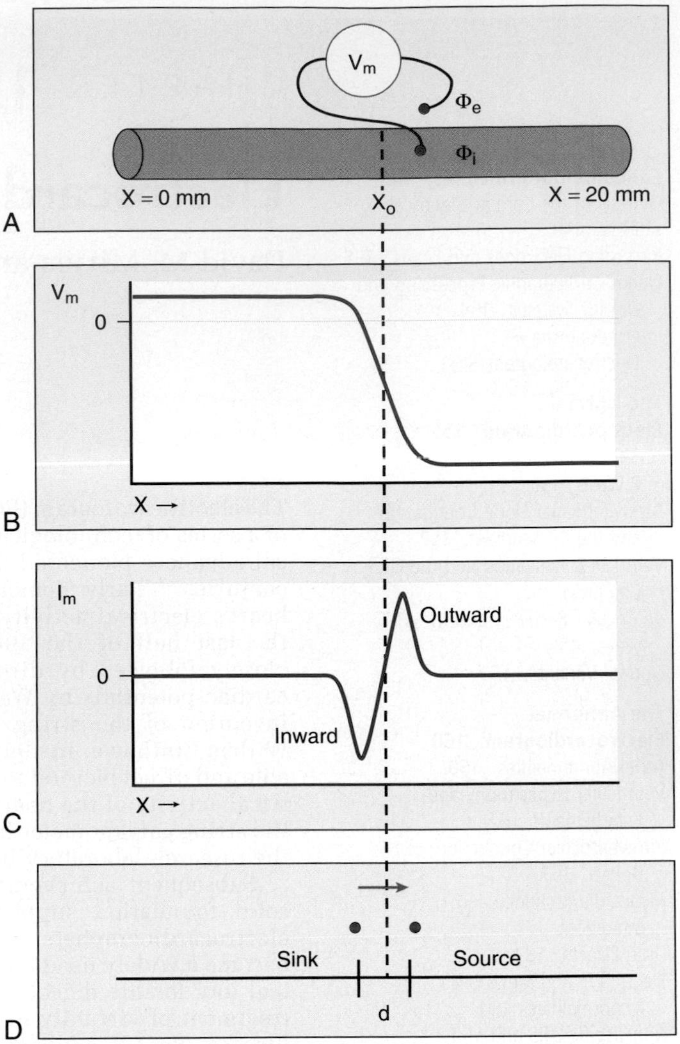

FIGURE 12–2 Example of potentials and currents generated by the activation of a single (e.g., ventricular) cardiac fiber. **A,** Intracellular (Φ_i) and extracellular (Φ_e) potentials are recorded with a voltmeter (V_m) from a fiber 20 mm in length. The fiber is stimulated at site X (0 mm), and propagation proceeds from left to right. **B,** Plot of transmembrane potential (V_m) at the instant in time at which activation reaches point X_0 as a function of the length of the fiber. Positive potentials are recorded from activated tissue to the left of site X_0, and negative ones are registered from not yet excited areas to the right of site X_0. **C,** Membrane current (I_m) flows along the length of the fiber at time t_0. The outward current is the depolarizing current that propagates ahead of activation site X_0, whereas an inward current flows behind site X_0. **D,** Representation of the sites of peak inward and outward current flow as two point sources, a sink (at the site of peak inward current flow) and a source (at the site of peak outward current flow) separated by distance d. The dipole produced by the source-sink pair is represented by the arrow. *(Modified from Barr RC: Genesis of the electrocardiogram.* In *MacFarlane PW, Lawrie TDV [eds]: Comprehensive Electrocardiography. New York, Pergamon Press, 1989, p 134.)*

from a distant site. It equals the area on the surface of a sphere of unit radius constructed around an electrode that is cut by lines drawn from the recording electrode to all points around the boundary of the region of interest. This region may be a wave front, a zone of infarction, or any other region in the heart.

The solid angle theorem states that the potential recorded by a remote electrode (Φ) is defined by the following equation:

$$\Phi = (\Omega/4p)(V_{m2} - V_{m1})K$$

where Ω is the solid angle, $V_{m2} - V_{m1}$ is the potential difference across the boundary under study, and K is a constant reflecting differences in intracellular conductivity.

This equation indicates that the recorded potential equals the product of two factors. First, the solid angle reflects spatial parameters, such as the size of the boundary of the region under study and the distance from the electrode to that boundary. The potential will rise as the boundary size increases and as the distance to the electrode shrinks. A second set of parameters includes nonspatial factors, such as the potential difference across the surface and intracellular and extracellular conductivities. Nonspatial effects include, as one example, myocardial ischemia, which changes transmembrane action potential shapes and alters conductivity.

THE CARDIAC ELECTRICAL FIELD GENERATION DURING VENTRICULAR RECOVERY. The cardiac electrical field during recovery (phases 1 through 3 of the action potential) is generated by forces analogous to those described during activation. However, recovery differs in several important ways from activation. First, intercellular potential differences and, hence, the directions of current flow during recovery are the opposite of those described for activation. As a cell undergoes recovery, its intracellular potential becomes progressively more negative. For two adjacent cells, the intracellular potential of the cell whose recovery has progressed further is more negative than that of an adjacent, less recovered cell. Intracellular currents then flow from the lesser toward the more recovered cell. An equivalent dipole can then be constructed for recovery, just as for activation. Its orientation, however, points from less to more recovered cells. Thus, the recovery dipole is oriented away from the direction of propagation of the activation front—that is, in the direction opposite that of the activation dipole.

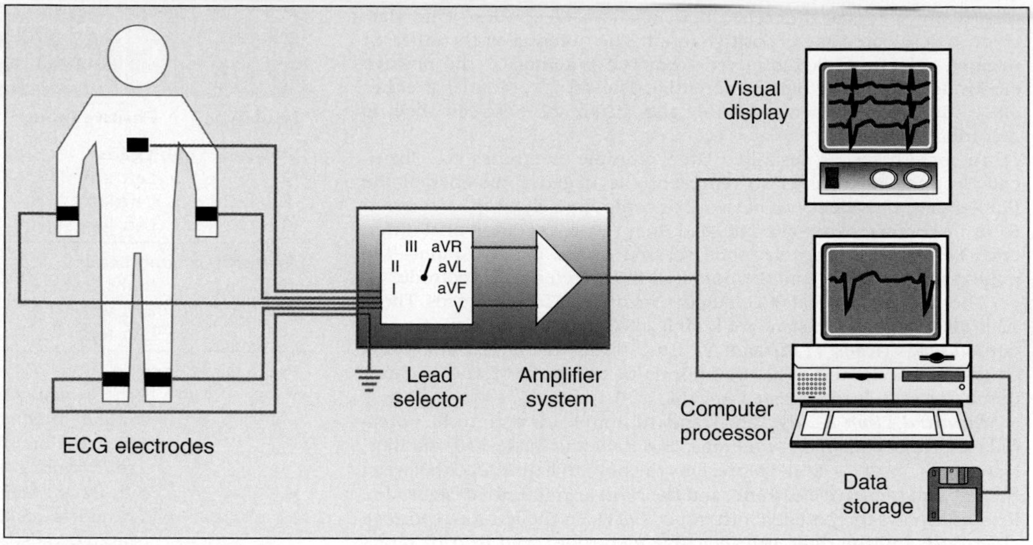

FIGURE 12–3 Components used in the recording and processing of an electrocardiogram. *(From Mirvis DM: Electrocardiography: A Physiologic Approach. St. Louis, Mosby-Year Book, 1993, p 83.)*

The moment, or strength, of the recovery dipole also differs from that of the activation dipole. The strength of the activation dipole is proportional to the rate of change in transmembrane potential. Rates of change in potential during the recovery phases of the action potential are considerably slower than during activation, so that the dipole moment at any one instant during recovery is less than during activation.

A third difference between activation and recovery is the rate of movement of the activation and recovery dipoles. Activation is rapid (as fast as 1 millisecond in duration) and occurs over only a small distance along the fiber. Recovery, in contrast, lasts 100 milliseconds or longer and occurs simultaneously over extensive portions of the fiber.

These features result in characteristic electrocardiographic differences between activation and recovery patterns. All other factors being equal (an assumption that is often not true, as described later), electrocardiographic waveforms generated during recovery of a linear fiber with uniform recovery properties may be expected to be of opposite polarity, lower amplitude, and longer duration than those caused by activation. As will be described, these features are explicitly demonstrated in the clinical ECG.

THE ROLE OF TRANSMISSION FACTORS. These activation and recovery fields exist within a complex three-dimensional physical environment (the volume conductor) that modifies the cardiac electrical field in significant ways. These contents of the volume conductor are called transmission factors to emphasize their effects on transmission of the cardiac electrical field throughout the body. They may be grouped into four broad categories: cellular factors, cardiac factors, extracardiac factors, and physical factors.

Cellular factors determine the intensity of current fluxes that result from local transmembrane potential gradients; they include intracellular and extracellular resistances and the concentrations of relevant ions, especially the sodium ion. Lower ion concentrations reduce the intensity of current flow and reduce extracellular potentials.

Cardiac factors affect the relationship of one cardiac cell to another. Two major factors are (1) anisotropy, the property of cardiac tissue that results in greater current flow and more rapid propagation along the length of a fiber than across its width, and (2) the presence of connective tissue between cardiac fibers, which disrupts effective electrical coupling of adjacent fibers. Recording electrodes oriented along the long axis of a cardiac fiber register larger potentials than electrodes oriented perpendicular to the long axis; waveforms recorded from fibers with little or no intervening connective tissue are narrow in width and smooth in contour, whereas those recorded from tissues with abnormal fibrosis are prolonged with prominent notching.

Extracardiac factors encompass all the tissues and structures that lie between the activation region and the body surface, including the ventricular walls, intracardiac and intrathoracic blood, pericardium, lungs, skeletal muscle, subcutaneous fat, and skin. These tissues alter the cardiac field because of differences in the electrical resistivity of adjacent tissues—that is, the presence of electrical inhomogeneities within the torso. For example, intracardiac blood has much lower resistivity (162 ohm-cm) than the lungs (2150 ohm-cm). When the cardiac field encounters the boundary between two tissues with differing resistivity, the field is altered.

Other transmission factors reflect basic laws of physics. First, changes in the distance between the heart and the recording electrode reduce potential magnitudes in proportion to the square of the distance. A related factor is the eccentricity of the heart within the chest; it lies closer to the anterior than to the posterior of the torso. The right ventricle and the anteroseptal aspect of the left ventricle are located closer to the anterior chest wall than other parts of the left ventricle and the atria. Therefore, electrocardiographic potentials will be higher anteriorly than posteriorly, and waveforms projected from the anterior left ventricle to the chest wall will be greater than those generated by posterior ventricular regions.

As a result of all these factors, body surface potentials have an amplitude of only 1 percent of the amplitude of transmembrane potentials and are smoothed in detail, so that surface potentials have only a general spatial relationship to the underlying cardiac events. Although changes in torso inhomogeneities within physiological ranges appear to have little impact on electrocardiographic potentials, pathological changes such as those produced by anasarca[4] may have a clinically relevant impact on the ECG.

Recording Electrodes and Leads

Potentials generated by the cardiac electrical generator and modified by transmission factors are sensed by electrodes placed on the torso that are configured to form various types of leads (Fig. 12-3).

ELECTRODE CHARACTERISTICS. The properties of the electrodes used to sense the cardiac electrical field are affected by the properties of the dermal and epidermal layers of the skin, the electrolytic paste applied to the skin, the electrode itself, and the mechanical contact between the electrode and skin. The net effect is a complex electrical circuit that includes resistances, capacitances, and voltages produced by these different components and the interfaces between them. Each of these factors modifies the cardiac potentials registered by the electrodes before they are displayed as an ECG.

ELECTROCARDIOGRAPHIC LEAD SYSTEMS. Electrodes are connected to form leads. Electrocardiographic leads are bipolar leads[3] that record the potential difference between two electrodes.* One electrode is designated as the positive input. The potential at the other, or negative, electrode is subtracted from the potential at the positive electrode to yield the bipolar potential. The actual potential at either electrode is not known, and only the difference between them is recorded.

In some cases, as described later, multiple electrodes are electrically connected together to represent the negative member of the bipolar pair. This electrode network or compound electrode is referred to as a reference electrode. The lead then records the potential difference between a single electrode serving as the positive input—the exploring electrode—and the potential in the reference electrode.

The standard clinical ECG includes recordings from 12 leads. These 12 leads include three standard limb leads (leads I, II, and III), six precordial leads (leads V_1 through V_6), and three augmented limb leads (leads aVR, aVL, and aVF). Definitions of the positive and negative inputs for each lead are listed in Table 12-1.

Standard Limb Leads. The standard limb leads record the potential differences between two limbs, as detailed in Table 12-1 and illustrated in Figure 12-4. Lead I represents the potential difference between the left arm (positive electrode) and the right arm (negative electrode), lead II displays the potential difference between the left foot (positive electrode) and the right arm (negative electrode), and lead III represents the potential difference between the left foot (positive electrode) and the left arm (negative electrode). The electrode on the right foot serves as a ground and is not included in these leads.

The electrical connections for these leads are such that the potential in lead II equals the sum of potentials sensed in leads I and III. That is,

$$I + III = II$$

This relationship is known as Einthoven's law, or Einthoven's equation.

Precordial Leads and the Wilson Central Terminal. The precordial leads register the potential at each of the six designated torso sites (see Fig. 12-4, bottom, left panel) in relation to a reference potential. To do so, an exploring electrode is placed on each precordial site and connected to the positive input of the recording system (see Fig. 12-4, bottom, right panel).

The negative, or reference, input is composed of a compound electrode known as the Wilson central terminal. This terminal is formed by combining the output of the left arm, right arm, and left leg electrodes through 5000-ohm resistances (see Fig. 12-4, bottom, right panel). The result is that each precordial lead registers the potential at a precordial site with reference to the average potential on three limbs.[5,6] The potential recorded by the Wilson central terminal remains relatively constant during the cardiac cycle, so the output of a precordial lead is determined predominantly by time-dependent changes in the potential at the precordial site.

Augmented Limb Leads. The three augmented limb leads are designated aVR, aVL, and aVF. The exploring electrode (Fig. 12-5) that forms the positive input is the right arm electrode for lead aVR, the left arm electrode for lead aVL, and the left foot electrode for aVF. The reference potential for the augmented limb leads is formed by connecting the two limb electrodes that are not used as the exploring electrode. For lead aVL, for example, the exploring electrode is on the left arm and the reference electrode is the combined output of the electrodes on the right arm and the left foot. Similarly, for lead aVF, the reference potential is the mean of the output of the two arm electrodes.

This modified reference system was designed to produce a larger amplitude signal than if the full Wilson central terminal were used as the reference electrode. When the Wilson central terminal was used, the output was small, in part because the same electrode potential was included in both the exploring and the reference potential input. Eliminating this duplication results in a theoretical increase in amplitude of 50 percent.

Other Lead Systems. Other lead systems can be used for specific purposes.[3] For example, additional right precordial leads can be used to assess right ventricular abnormalities, such as hypertrophy or infarction. Electrode locations posterior to V_6 (e.g., lead V_7 with the exploring electrode at the left posterior axillary line at the vertical level of V_6 and lead V_8 with the exploring electrode on the left midscapular line), can be used to help detect acute posterior-lateral infarctions (see Table 12-1). A vertical parasternal bipolar pair can facilitate detection of P waves for diagnosing arrhythmias.

Precordial and anteroposterior thoracic electrode arrays of 150 or more electrodes can be used to display the spatial distribution of body surface potentials as body surface isopotential maps. Other arrays have sought to reduce the number of electrodes and reconstruct the full 12-lead ECG. For example, lead sets requiring only five electrodes may reduce overall recording times in emergency situations.[7] Modified lead systems are also used in ambulatory electrocardiographic recording, exercise stress testing, and bedside cardiac monitoring, as described elsewhere.

Other lead systems that have had clinical use include those designed to record a vectorcardiogram (VCG). The VCG depicts the orientation and strength of a single cardiac dipole or vector at each instant during the cardiac cycle. Lead systems for recording the VCG are referred to as orthogonal systems because they record the three orthogonal or mutually perpendicular components of the dipole moment—the horizontal (x axis), frontal (y axis), and sagittal or anteroposterior (z axis) axes. An example of a normal VCG is shown in Figure 12-6. Clinical use of the VCG has waned in recent years, but the VCG can be useful in certain situations and, as described below, vectorial principles remain essential to understanding the origins of electrocardiographic waveforms.[8]

LEAD VECTORS AND HEART VECTORS. A lead can be represented as a vector (the lead vector). For simple bipolar leads, such as leads I, II, and III, the lead vectors are directed from the negative electrode toward the positive one (Fig. 12-7). For the augmented limb and precordial leads, the origin of the lead vector lies at the midpoint of the axis connecting the electrodes that make up the compound electrode. That is, for lead aVL, the vector points from the midpoint of the axis connecting the right arm and left leg electrodes toward the left arm (see Fig. 12-7, left). For the precordial leads, the lead vector points from the center of the triangle formed by the three standard limb leads to the precordial electrode site (see Fig. 12-7, right).

TABLE 12–1 Location of Electrodes and Lead Connections for Standard 12-Lead Electrocardiogram and Additional Leads

Lead Type	Positive Input	Negative Input
Standard Limb Leads		
I	Left arm	Right arm
II	Left leg	Right arm
III	Left leg	Left arm
Augmented Limb Leads		
aVR	Right arm	Left arm plus left leg
aVL	Left arm	Right arm plus left leg
aVF	Left leg	Left arm plus left arm
Precordial Leads*		
V_1	Right sternal margin, fourth intercostal space	Wilson central terminal
V_2	Left sternal margin, fourth intercostal space	Wilson central terminal
V_3	Midway between V_2 and V_4	Wilson central terminal
V_4	Left midclavicular line, fifth intercostal space	Wilson central terminal
V_5	Left anterior axillary line†	Wilson central terminal
V_6	Left midaxillary line†	Wilson central terminal
V_7	Posterior axillary line†	Wilson central terminal
V_8	Posterior scapular line†	Wilson central terminal
V_9	Left border of spine†	Wilson central terminal

*The right-sided precordial leads V_3R to V_6R are taken in mirror image positions on the right side of the chest.

†Leads V_5 to V_9 are taken in the same horizontal plane as V_4.

*Some electrodes used for the ECG, including the precordial electrodes and the augmented limb leads (see later), have been typically referred to as "unipolar" leads. Unipolar leads register the potential at one site in relation to an absolute zero potential. Referring to electrocardiographic leads as unipolar leads is based on the notion that the reference electrode—that is, the Wilson central terminal or the combination of two limb electrodes—represents a zero potential, so that the lead records the potential at a site in relation to a zero potential level, the definition of a unipolar lead. The choice of using the term *bipolar* for these leads reflects the recognition that the reference electrode is not exactly at zero potential but yields the average of the potentials sensed at the sites of the electrodes making up the compound electrode.[5,6]

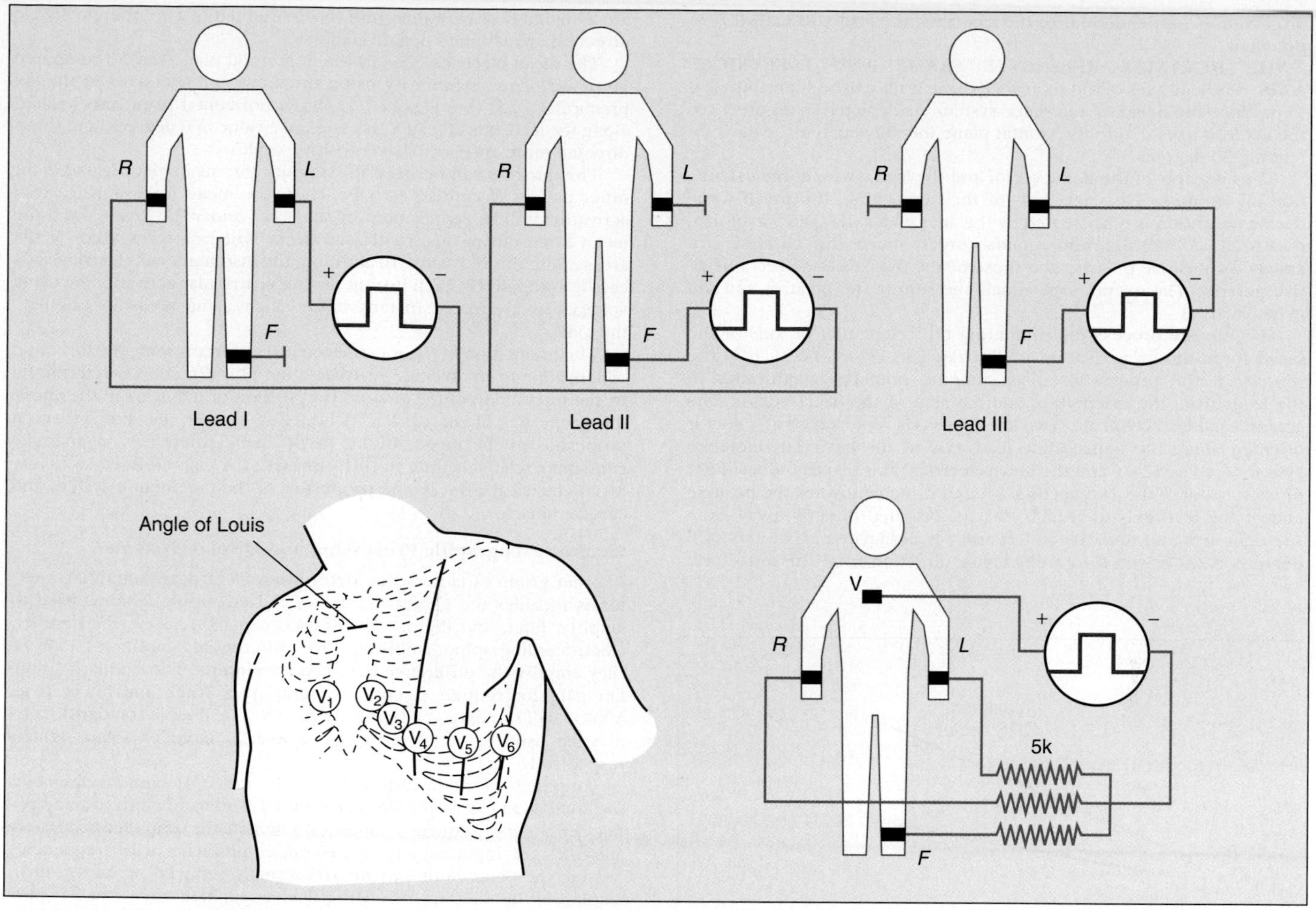

FIGURE 12–4 **Top,** Electrode connections for recording the three standard limb leads I, II, and III. *R, L,* and *F* indicate locations of electrodes on the right arm, the left arm, and the left foot, respectively. **Bottom,** Electrode locations and electrical connections for recording a precordial lead. **Left,** The positions of the exploring electrode (V) for the six precordial leads. **Right,** Connections to form the Wilson central terminal for recording a precordial (V) lead.

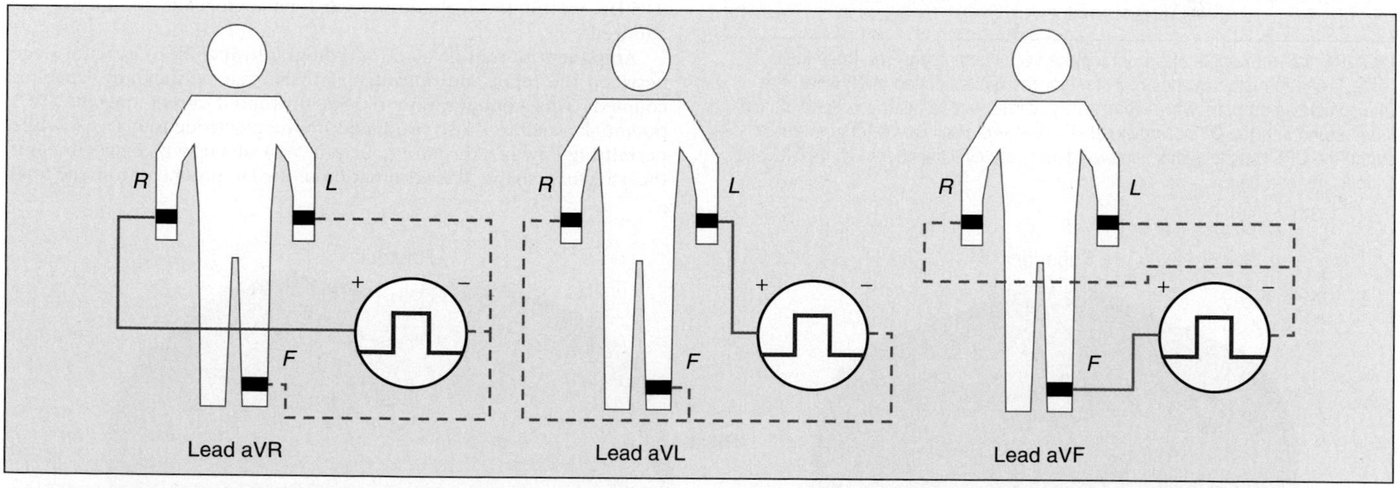

FIGURE 12–5 Electrode locations and electrical connections for recording the three augmented limb leads aVR, aVL, and aVF. Dashed lines indicate connections to generate the reference electrode potential.

As described earlier, instantaneous cardiac activity can also be approximated as a single dipole representing the vector sum of the various active wave fronts (the heart vector). Its location, orientation, and intensity vary from instant to instant because of the changing pattern of cardiac activation.

The amplitude and polarity of the potentials sensed in a lead equal the length of the projection of the heart vector on the lead vector multiplied by the length of the lead vector:

$$V_L = (H)(\cos \theta)(L)$$

where L and H are the length of the lead and heart vectors, respectively, as illustrated in Figure 12-8, and θ is the angle between the two vectors. Thus, if the projection of the heart vector on the lead vector points toward the positive pole of the lead axis, the lead will record a positive potential. If the projection is directed away from the positive pole of the lead axis, the potential will be negative. If the projection is perpendicular to the lead axis, the lead will record zero potential.

THE HEXAXIAL REFERENCE FRAME AND ELECTRICAL AXIS. The lead axes of the six frontal plane leads can be superimposed to produce the hexaxial reference system. As depicted in Figure 12-9, the six lead axes divide the frontal plane into 12 segments, each subtending 30 degrees.

The concepts of the heart vector and the lead vector allow calculation of the mean electrical axis of the heart. First, the mean force during activation is represented by the area under the QRS waveform, measured as millivolt-milliseconds. Areas above the baseline are assigned a positive polarity and those below the baseline have a negative polarity. The overall area equals the sum of the positive and the negative areas.

Second, the process for computing the orientation or axis of the mean force during activation is illustrated in Figure 12-10. It is the reverse of the process used to compute potential magnitudes in the leads from the orientation and moment of the heart vector. The area in each lead (typically, two are chosen) is represented as a vector oriented along the appropriate lead axis in the hexaxial reference system (see Fig. 12-9), and the mean electrical axis equals the resultant or vector sum of the two vectors. An axis directed toward the positive end of the lead axis of lead I—that is, oriented directly away from the right arm and toward the left arm—is designated as an axis of 0 degrees. Axes oriented in a clockwise direction from this zero level are assigned positive values and those oriented in a counterclockwise direction are assigned negative values.

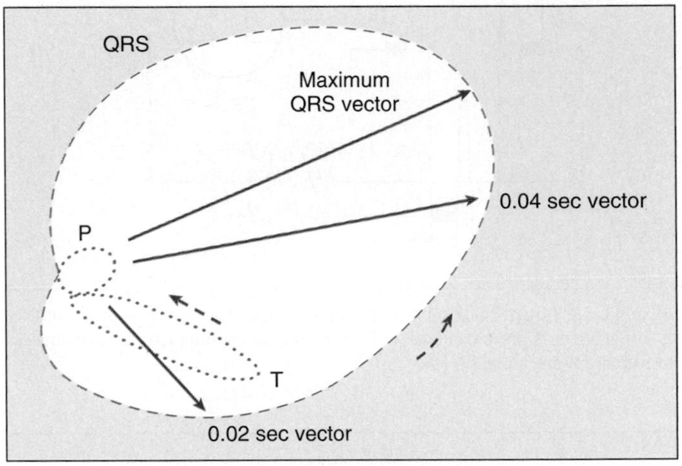

FIGURE 12–6 Example of a frontal plane vectorcardiogram. The three loops (QRS, T, and P) mark the ends of instantaneous vectors during the P wave, the QRS complex, and the T wave. Long arrows correspond to heart vectors 0.02 and 0.04 second into the QRS complex, at the instant of maximal vector strength during the QRS complex. Short arrows identify the direction in which the QRS and T loops are inscribed.

The mean electrical axis in the horizontal plane can be computed in an analogous manner by using the areas and lead axes of the six precordial leads (see Fig. 12-7, right). A horizontal plane axis located along the lead axis of lead V_6 is assigned a value of 0 degrees, and those directed more anteriorly have positive values.

This process can be used to compute the mean electrical axis for other phases of cardiac activity. Thus, the mean force during atrial activation will be represented by the areas under the P wave, and the mean force during ventricular recovery will be represented by the areas under the ST-T wave. In addition, the instantaneous electrical axis can be computed at each instant during ventricular activation by using voltages at a specific instant rather than using areas to calculate the axis.

The orientation of the mean electrical axis represents the direction of activation in an "average" cardiac fiber. This direction is determined by the interaction of the anatomical position of the heart in the chest, the properties of the cardiac conduction system, and the activation properties of the myocardium. In practice, differences in anatomy contribute relatively little to shifts in axis[9]; the major influences on the mean electrical axis are the properties of the conduction system and cardiac muscle.

Electrocardiographic Processing and Display Systems

Another group of factors that determines electrocardiographic waveforms includes the characteristics of the electronic systems used to amplify, filter, and digitize the sensed signals. As described earlier, electrocardiographic amplifiers are differential amplifiers—that is, they amplify the difference between two inputs. The standard amplifier gain for routine electrocardiography is 1000, and lower (e.g., 500 or half-standard) or higher (e.g., 2000 or double-standard) gains may be used to compensate for unusually large or small signals, respectively.

Amplifiers respond differently to the range of signal frequencies included in an electrophysiological signal. The bandwidth of an amplifier defines the frequency range over which the amplifier accurately amplifies the input signals. Waveform components with frequencies outside the bandwidth can be artifactually reduced or increased in amplitude. In addition, recording devices include high- and low-pass filters that intentionally reduce the amplitude of specific frequency ranges of the signal. Such reduction in amplitude may be intended—for example, to reduce the effect of body motion or line voltage frequencies (that is, 60-Hz interference). For routine electrocardiography, the standards of the American Heart Association require a bandwidth of 0.05 Hz to 150 Hz for adults, with an extension to 250 Hz for children.[3]

Amplifiers for routine electrocardiography include a capacitor stage between the input and output terminals; that is, they are capacitor coupled. This configuration blocks unwanted direct current (DC) potentials, such as those produced by the electrode interfaces, while permitting flow of alternating current (AC) signals which accounts for the waveform shape. The elimination of the DC potential from the final

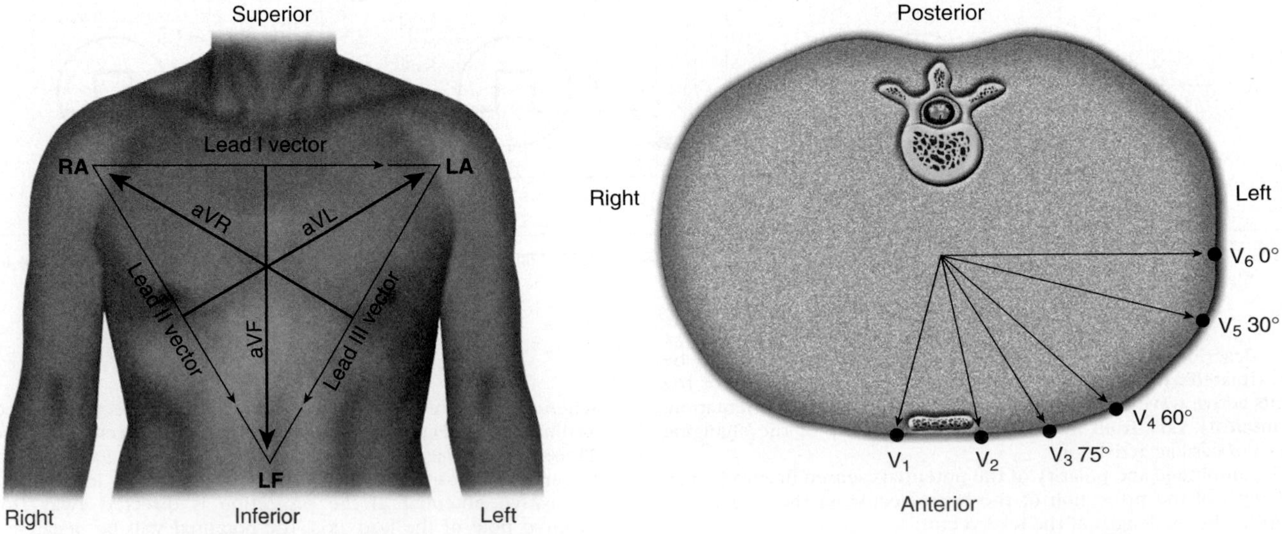

FIGURE 12–7 Lead vectors for the three standard limb leads, the three augmented limb leads **(left)**, and the six unipolar precordial leads **(right)**.

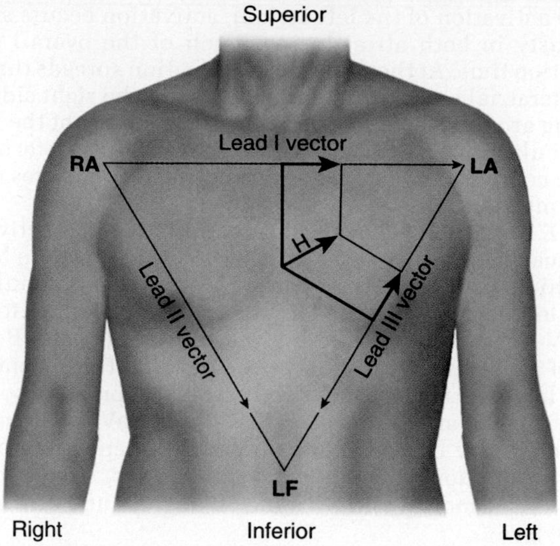

FIGURE 12–8 The heart vector H and its projections on the lead axes of leads I and III. Voltages recorded in lead I will be positive and potentials in lead III will be negative.

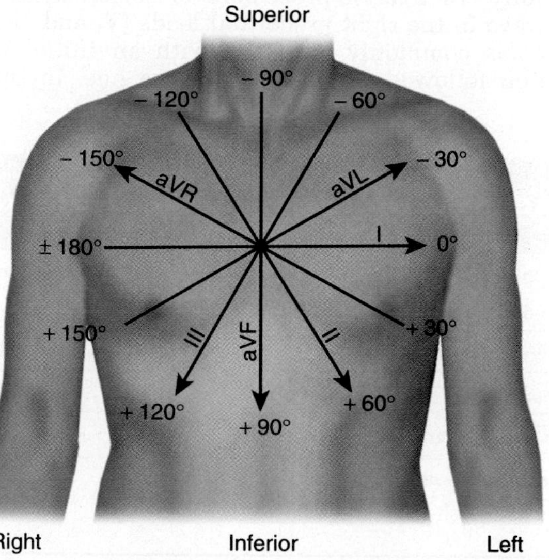

FIGURE 12–9 The hexaxial reference system composed of the lead axes of the six frontal plane leads. The lead axes of the six frontal plane leads have been rearranged so that their centers overlay one another. These axes divide the plane into 12 segments, each subtending 30 degrees. The positive ends of each axis are labeled with the name of the lead.

product means that electrocardiographic potentials are not calibrated against an external reference level (e.g., a ground potential). Rather, electrocardiographic potentials are measured in relation to another portion of the waveform that serves as a baseline. The TP segment, which begins at the end of the T wave of one cardiac cycle and ends with the onset of the P wave of the next cycle, is usually the most appropriate internal electrocardiographic baseline.

An additional issue is the sampling rate for computerized systems. Too low a sampling rate will miss brief signals, such as notches in QRS complexes or brief bipolar pacemaker spikes, and will reduce the precision and accuracy of waveform morphologies. Too fast a sampling rate may introduce artifacts, including high-frequency noise, and requires extensive digital storage capacity. In general, the sampling rate should be at least twice the frequency of the highest frequencies of interest in the signal being recorded. Standard electrocardiography is most commonly performed with a sampling rate of 1000 to 2000 Hz.

Cardiac potentials can be processed for display in numerous formats. The most common of these formats is the classic scalar ECG. Scalar recordings depict the potentials recorded from one lead as a function of time. For standard electrocardiography, amplitude is displayed on a scale of 1 mV to 10 mm vertical displacement and time as 400 msec/cm on the horizontal scale. Leads are generally displayed in

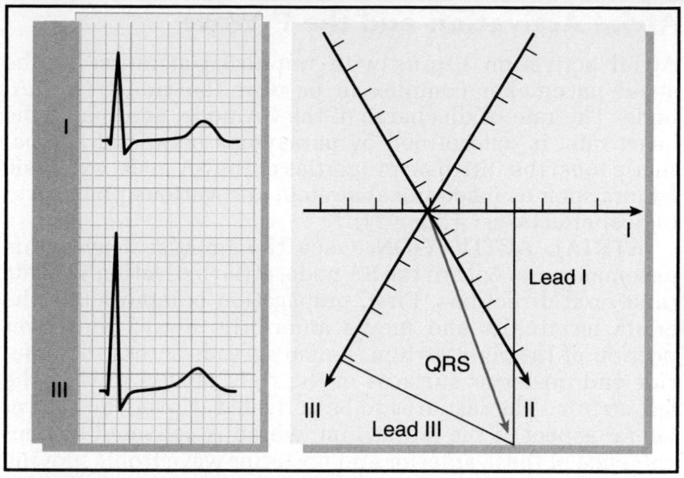

FIGURE 12–10 Calculation of the mean electrical axis during the QRS complex from the areas under the QRS complex in leads I and III. Magnitudes of the areas of the two leads are plotted as vectors on the appropriate lead axes, and the mean QRS axis is the sum of these two vectors. *(From Mirvis DM: Electrocardiography: A Physiologic Approach. St. Louis, Mosby-Year Book, 1993, p 147.)*

three groups—the three standard limb leads followed by the three augmented limb leads followed by the six precordial leads.

An alternative display format has been proposed,[10] in which the six limb leads are displayed in the sequence of the frontal plane reference frame (see Fig. 12-9). In addition, the polarity of lead aVR is reversed. That is, waveforms are displayed in this order: lead aVL, lead I, lead aVR (reversed in polarity), lead II, lead aVF, and lead III. Proposed advantages of this system include facilitating estimation of the electrical axis by the presenting the leads in the order in which they appear on the frontal plane reference frame and emphasizing the relevance of abnormalities in lead aVR by reversing its polarity.[11]

Interpreting the Electrocardiogram

The recorded or displayed electrocardiographic tracings are, finally, compared with various diagnostic criteria to identify specific abnormalities. In some cases, the electrocardiographic criteria are the sole basis for a diagnosis with no anatomical or physiological correlation. For example, the electrocardiographic findings of intraventricular conduction defects are diagnostic without reference to an anatomic standard.

For most electrocardiographic diagnoses, however, the criteria are based on statistical correlations between anatomical or physiological findings in large populations and electrocardiographic measurements. For example, the diagnostic criteria for ventricular hypertrophy depend on correlations between electrocardiographic patterns and an anatomical measure of chamber dimensions. These criteria are thus empirical rather than theoretical. The quantitative definition and the accuracy of the criteria depend on statistical analyses of electrocardiographic waveforms in large normal and abnormal populations rather than on a theoretical construct. As a result, many different criteria may exist for common abnormalities, such as left ventricular hypertrophy. The various criteria have different predictive accuracies so that the final diagnosis is usually not absolute but represents a statistical probability that the abnormality exists.

THE NORMAL ELECTROCARDIOGRAM

The heart is activated and recovers during each cardiac cycle in a characteristic manner determined by the anatomy and physiology of working cardiac muscle and the specialized cardiac conduction systems. The waveforms and intervals that make up the standard ECG are displayed in Figure 12-11, and a normal 12-lead ECG is shown in Figure 12-12. The P wave is generated by activation of the atria, the PR segment represents the duration of atrioventricular (AV) conduction, the QRS complex is produced by the activation of both ventricles, and the ST-T wave reflects ventricular recovery. Table 12-2 includes normal values for the various intervals and waveforms of the ECG.

Atrial Activation and the P Wave

Atrial activation begins with impulse generation in the atrial pacemaker complex in or near the sinoatrial (SA) node. The rate of discharge of the SA node, and hence the heart rate, is determined by parasympathetic and sympathetic tone, the intrinsic properties of the SA node, extrinsic factors such as mechanical stretch, and various pharmacological effects (see Chap. 31).

ATRIAL ACTIVATION. Once the impulse leaves this pacemaker site within the SA node, atrial activation spreads in several directions. First, propagation is rapid along the crista terminalis and moves anteriorly toward the lower portion of the right atrium. It also spreads across the anterior and posterior surfaces of the right atrium toward the left atrium. The last area to be activated is over the inferolateral aspect of the left atrium, which is activated by convergence of these anterior and posterior wave fronts moving from right to left. Although right atrial activation begins before activation of the left atrium, activation occurs simultaneously in both atria during much of the overall atrial activation time. At the same time, activation spreads through the interatrial septum, beginning high on the right side and moving around the fossa ovalis to reach the top of the interventricular septum. These patterns are largely determined by the complex anatomical and functional properties of the atrial musculature.

THE NORMAL P WAVE. The pattern of atrial activation noted earlier produces the normal P wave. Activation beginning high in the right atrium and proceeding simultaneously leftward toward the left atrium and inferiorly toward the AV node corresponds to a mean frontal plane P wave axis of approximately 60 degrees. Based on this orientation of the heart vector, normal atrial activation projects positive or upright P waves in leads I, II, aVL, and aVF. The pattern in lead III may be upright or downward, depending on the exact orientation of the mean axis—that is, upright if the mean axis is more positive than +30 degrees and downward otherwise.

P wave patterns in the precordial leads correspond to the direction of atrial activation wave fronts in the horizontal plane. Atrial activation early in the P wave is over the right atrium and is oriented primarily anteriorly; later, it shifts posteriorly as activation proceeds over the left atrium. Thus, the P wave in the right precordial leads (V_1 and, occasionally, V_2) is commonly biphasic, with an initial positive deflection followed by a later negative one. In the more

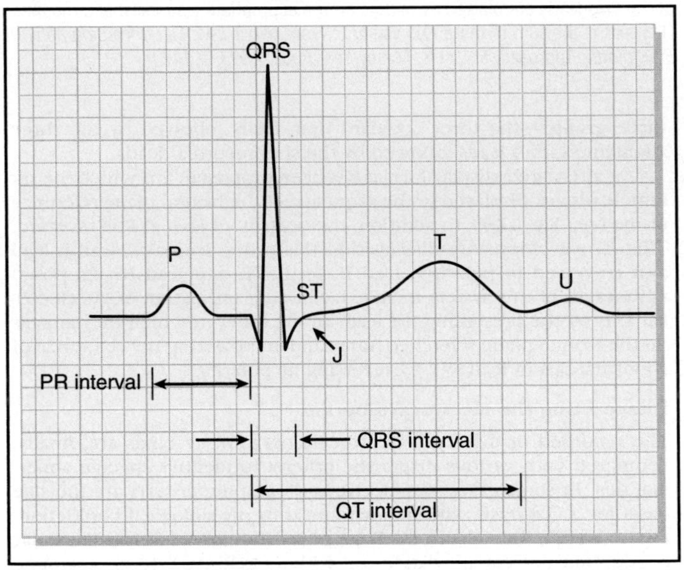

FIGURE 12–11 The waves and intervals of a normal electrocardiogram.

TABLE 12–2 Normal Values for Durations of Electrocardiographic Waves and Intervals in Adults

Wave, Interval	Duration (msec)
P wave duration	<120
PR interval	120-200
QRS duration	<110-120*
QT interval (corrected)	≤440-460*

*See text for further discussion.

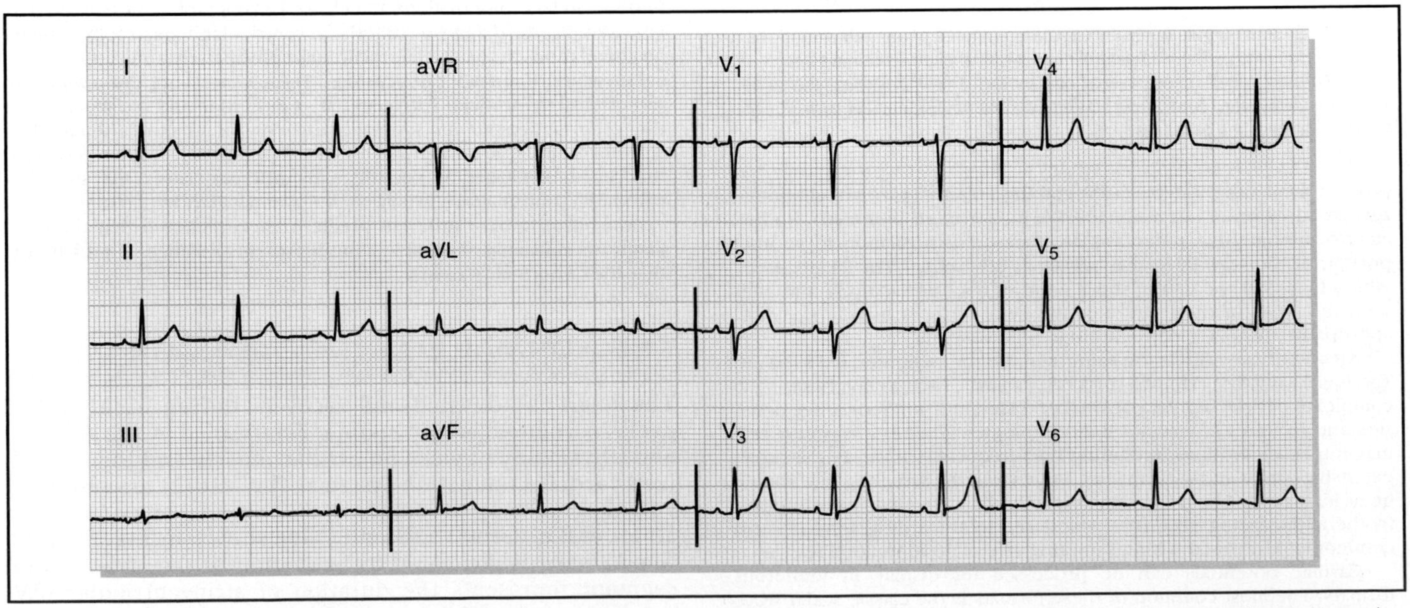

FIGURE 12–12 Normal electrocardiogram recorded from a 48-year-old woman. The vertical lines of the grid represent time, with lines spaced at 40-millisecond intervals. Horizontal lines represent voltage amplitude, with lines spaced at 0.1-mV intervals. Every fifth line in each direction is typically darkened. The heart rate is approximately 72 beats/min, the PR interval and QRS durations measure 140 and 84 milliseconds, respectively, the QT_c measures 400, and the mean QRS axis is approximately +35 degrees.

lateral leads, the P wave is upright and reflects right-to-left spread of the activation fronts.

P wave duration is normally less than 120 milliseconds, as measured in the lead with the widest P wave. The amplitude in the limb leads is normally less than 0.25 mV and the terminal negative deflection in the right precordial leads is normally less than 0.1 mV in depth.

ATRIAL REPOLARIZATION. Atrial depolarization is followed by atrial repolarization. The potentials generated by atrial repolarization are not usually seen on the surface ECG because of their low amplitude (usually less than 100 μV) and because they are superimposed on the much higher amplitude QRS complex. They may be observed as a low-amplitude wave with a polarity opposite that of the P wave (the T_a wave) during atrioventricular block and may have special significance in influencing electrocardiographic patterns during exercise testing (see Chap. 32). Deviation of the PR segment (corresponding to the atrial ST segment) is, as described later, also an important marker of acute pericarditis (see Chap. 70) and, more rarely, atrial infarction (see Chap. 50).

HEART RATE VARIABILITY. Ongoing attention continues to be directed to analysis of beat-to-beat changes in heart rate and related dynamics, termed *heart rate variability,* to gain insight into neuroautonomic control mechanisms (see Chap. 89) and their perturbations with aging, disease, and drug effects.[12] For example, high-frequency (0.15 to 0.5 Hz) fluctuations mediated by the vagus nerve occur phasically, with heart rate increasing during inspiration and decreasing during expiration. Attenuation of this respiratory sinus arrhythmia, and related short-term heart rate variability, is a consistent marker of physiological aging and also occurs with diabetes mellitus, congestive heart failure, and a wide range of other cardiac and noncardiac conditions that alter autonomic tone.[12,13] Relatively lower frequency (0.05 to 0.15 Hz) physiological oscillations in heart rate are associated with baroreflex activation and appear to be jointly regulated by sympathetic and parasympathetic interactions. Various complementary signal processing techniques are being developed to analyze heart rate variability. These methods include time domain statistics, frequency domain techniques based on spectral (Fourier) methods, and tools derived from nonlinear dynamics and complex systems. For further discussion, see Chapter 89.

Atrioventricular Node Conduction and the PR Segment

The PR segment is the isoelectric region beginning with the end of the P wave and ending with the onset of the QRS complex. It forms part of the PR interval, which extends from the onset of the P wave to the onset of the QRS complex. The overall PR interval is best determined from the lead with the shortest PR intervals (to avoid missing various preexcitation syndromes). The normal PR interval measures 120 to 200 milliseconds in duration.

The PR segment is the temporal bridge between atrial activation and ventricular activation. Most of the time during this segment is the result of slow conduction within the AV node. On exiting the AV node, the impulse rapidly traverses the bundle of His to enter the bundle branches and then finally travels through the specialized intraventricular conduction paths to activate ventricular myocardium.

The PR segment appears isoelectric because the potentials generated by these structures are too small to produce detectable voltages on the body surface at the normal amplifier gains used in clinical electrocardiography. Hence, the standard ECG detects only activation and recovery of working myocardium, not the specialized conduction system. Signals from elements of the conduction system may be recorded from the body surface by using very high gains (over 25,000) and signal-averaging techniques or from intracardiac recording electrodes placed against the base of the interventricular septum near the bundle of His, as described in Chapter 35.

Ventricular Activation and the QRS Complex

Normal ventricular activation is a complex event that is dependent on interactions between the physiology and the anatomy of the specialized ventricular conducting system and the ventricular myocardium. The net result is the multiphasic normal QRS complex.

VENTRICULAR ACTIVATION. Ventricular activation is the product of two temporally overlapping events, endocardial activation and transmural activation. Endocardial activation is guided by the anatomical distribution and physiology of the His-Purkinje system. The broadly dispersed ramifications of this tree-like (fractal) system and the rapid conduction within it result in the simultaneous activation of multiple endocardial sites and the depolarization of most of the endocardial surfaces of both ventricles within several milliseconds.

The sequence of ventricular endocardial activation[14] is depicted in Figure 12-13. Earliest activity begins in three sites: (1) the anterior paraseptal wall of the left ventricle; (2) the posterior paraseptal wall of the left ventricle; and (3) the center of the left side of the septum. These loci generally correspond to the sites of insertion of the three branches of the left bundle branch. Wave fronts spread from these sites in anterior and inferior and then superior directions to activate the anterior and lateral walls of the left ventricle. The posterobasal areas of the left ventricle are the last to be activated. Septal activation begins in the middle third of the left side and spreads across the septum from left to right and from apex to base.

Excitation of the right ventricle begins near the insertion point of the right bundle branch close to the base of the anterior papillary muscle and spreads to the free wall. The final areas to be involved are the pulmonary conus and the posterobasal areas. Thus, in both ventricles, the overall endocardial excitation pattern begins on septal surfaces and sweeps down and around the free walls to the posterior and basal regions in an apex to base direction.

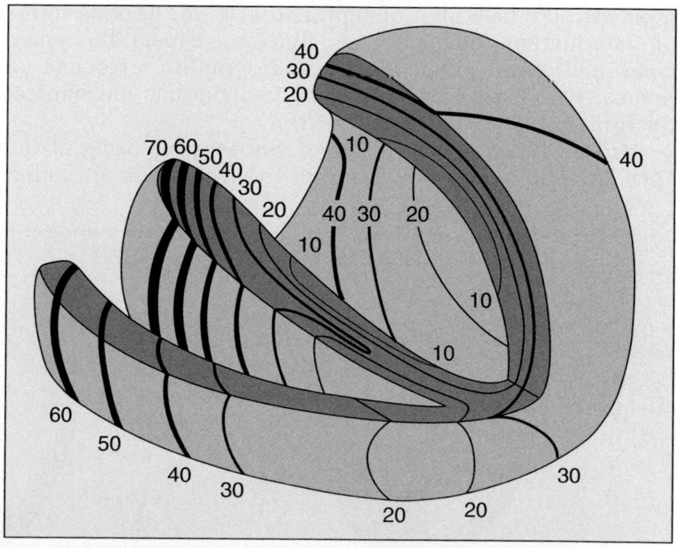

FIGURE 12–13 Activation sequence of the normal right and left ventricles. A portion of the left and right ventricles has been removed so that the endocardial surfaces of the ventricles and the interventricular septum can be seen. Isochrone lines connect sites that are activated at equal instants after the earliest evidence of ventricular activation. The numbers refer to isochrone lines in milliseconds during ventricular depolarization. *(From Durrer D: Electrical aspects of human cardiac activity: A clinical-physiological approach to excitation and stimulation. Cardiovasc Res 2:1, 1968.)*

The activation fronts then move from endocardium to epicardium. Excitation of the endocardium begins at sites of Purkinje–ventricular muscle junctions and proceeds by muscle cell to muscle cell conduction in an oblique direction toward the epicardium.

THE NORMAL QRS COMPLEX. The sequence of endocardial and transmural activation results in the characteristic waveforms of the QRS complex.

Terminology for the QRS Complex. QRS patterns are described by the sequence of waves constituting the complex. An initial negative deflection is called the Q wave, the first positive wave is the R wave, and the first negative wave after a positive wave is the S wave. A second upright wave following an S wave is an R′ wave. Tall waves are denoted by capital letters and smaller ones by lower case letters. A monophasic negative complex is referred to as a QS complex. Thus, for example, the overall QRS complex may be described as qRS if it consists of an initial small negative wave (the q wave) followed by a tall upright one (the R wave) and a deep negative one (an S wave). In an RSr′ complex, initial R and S waves are followed by a small positive wave (the r′ wave). In each case, the deflection must cross the baseline to be designated a discrete wave; changes in waveform direction that do not cross the baseline result in notches.

Early QRS Patterns. The complex pattern of activation described earlier can be simplified into two vectors, the first representing septal activation and the second representing left ventricular free wall activation (Fig. 12-14). Initial activation of the interventricular septum corresponds to a vector oriented from left to right in the frontal plane and anteriorly in the horizontal plane, corresponding to the anatomical position of the septum within the chest. This vector produces an initial positive wave in leads with axes directed to the right (lead aVR) or anteriorly (lead V_1). Leads with axes directed to the left (leads I, aVL, V_5, and V_6) will register initial negative waves (septal q waves). These initial forces are normally of low amplitude and are brief (less than 30 milliseconds).

The absence of these septal q waves is usually a normal variant and is not associated with any cardiac disease.[15] However, the absence or, particularly, recent loss of septal q waves may be a sign of septal infarction, various forms of conduction defects,[16] or fibrosis, especially when combined with other electrocardiographic evidence of myocardial infarction and left ventricular mechanical dysfunction.

Mid and Late QRS Patterns. Subsequent parts of the QRS complex reflect activation of the free walls of the left and right ventricles. Because right ventricular muscle mass is considerably smaller than that of the left ventricle, it contributes little to normal QRS complexes recorded in the standard ECG. Thus, the normal QRS can be considered to represent only left ventricular activity with relatively little oversimplification.

The complex interrelationships between cardiac position, conduction system function, and ventricular geometry result in a wide range of normal QRS patterns in the six limb leads. The QRS pattern in leads II, III, and aVF may be predominantly upright with qR complexes or these leads may show rS or RS patterns. Lead I may record an isoelectric RS pattern or a predominantly upright qR pattern.

This variability can be described in relation to the mean frontal plane QRS electrical axis, as described earlier in this chapter. The normal mean QRS axis in adults lies between −30 degrees and 90 degrees. The wide span of the normal axis corresponds to a wide range of QRS patterns, especially in the inferior leads, that can be understood by referring to the hexaxial reference system in Figure 12-9. If the mean axis is near 90 degrees, the QRS complex in leads II, III, and aVF will be predominantly upright with qR complexes; lead I will record an isoelectric RS pattern because the heart vector lies perpendicular to the lead axis. If the mean axis is nearer 0 degrees, the patterns will be reversed; lead I (and aVL) will register a predominantly upright qR pattern, and leads II, III, and aVF will show rS or RS patterns.

Mean QRS axes more positive than +90 to +100 degrees (usually with an rS pattern in lead I) represent right axis deviation, and those more negative than −30 degrees (with an rS pattern in lead aV_F) represent left axis deviation. Mean axes lying between −90 degrees and 180 degrees (or, equivalently, between +180 degrees and +270 degrees) are referred to as extreme axis deviations. The designation of indeterminate axis is applied when all six extremity leads show biphasic (QR or RS) patterns; this finding can occur as a normal variant or may be seen in various pathological conditions.

Normal QRS patterns in the precordial leads follow an orderly progression from right (V_1) to left (V_6). In the precordial leads V_1 and V_2, free wall activation generates S waves following the initial r waves generated by septal activation. These S waves are produced by the spread of activation in the free wall to the left and posteriorly, with generation of a heart vector directed away from the axes of these leads. Thus, these leads register rS patterns.

Patterns in the midprecordial leads V_3 and V_4 are more variable. Potentials sensed in these leads reflect the activation front in the ventricular free wall approaching the exploring electrode, followed by its moving leftward and posteriorly to more remote regions of the left ventricle. This front generates an R or r wave as it moves toward the electrode and later generates an S wave to produce rS or RS complexes as it moves away from the electrode. As the exploring electrode moves laterally to the left, however, the R wave becomes more dominant and the S wave becomes smaller (or is totally lost) because of the greater time period during which the activation front moves toward the positive end of the electrode. In the leftmost

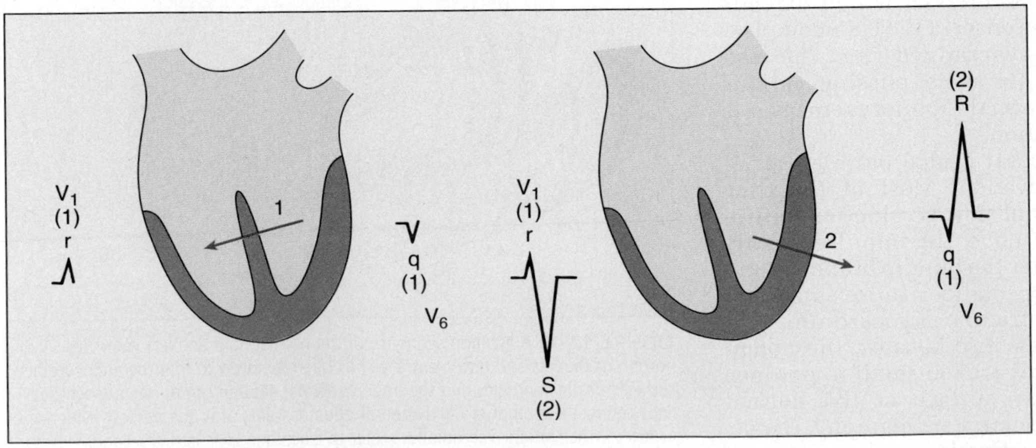

FIGURE 12–14 Schematic representation of ventricular depolarization as two sequential vectors representing septal **(left)** and left ventricular free wall **(right)** activation. QRS waveforms generated by each stage of activation in leads V_1 and V_6 are shown.

leads—that is, leads V_5 and V_6—the pattern also includes the septal q wave to produce a qRs or qR pattern.

Thus, in the precordial leads, the QRS complex is usually characterized by consistent progression from an rS complex in the right precordial leads to a qR pattern in the left precordial leads. The point during this transition at which the pattern changes from an rS to an Rs configuration—that is, the lead in which an isoelectric RS pattern is present—is known as the transition zone and normally occurs in leads V_3 or V_4. An example of a normal precordial QRS pattern is shown in Figure 12-12. Transition zones shifted to the right to lead V_2 are referred to as early transitions, and those shifted leftward to V_5 or V_6 are delayed transitions. (These variations in the horizontal plane axis were previously described as counterclockwise and clockwise rotations, respectively, of the heart, although these descriptors do not consistently correlate with cardiac anatomical findings.)

The amplitudes of the various parts of the QRS complex in normal people are similarly variable. Differences exist between genders, with higher amplitudes in men than in women, and among races, with higher amplitudes in African Americans[17] than in those of other races. Obese persons have lower amplitudes than thinner ones. These issues are considered later in this chapter when considering diagnostic criteria for ventricular hypertrophy.

QRS Duration. The upper normal value for QRS duration is traditionally given as shorter than 120 milliseconds (and often as shorter than 110 milliseconds) measured in the lead with the widest QRS duration. Women, on average, have somewhat smaller QRS durations than men (by about 5 to 8 milliseconds).

The Intrinsicoid Deflection. An additional feature of the QRS complex is the intrinsicoid deflection. An electrode overlying the ventricular free wall will record a rising R wave as transmural activation of the underlying ventricular free wall proceeds toward it. Once the activation front reaches the epicardium, the full thickness of the wall under the electrode will be in an active state. At that moment, the electrode will register negative potentials as activation proceeds in remote cardiac areas. The sudden reversal of potential with a sharp downslope is the intrinsicoid deflection and marks the timing of activation of the epicardium under the electrode.

Ventricular Recovery and the ST-T Wave

THE SEQUENCE OF VENTRICULAR RECOVERY. Recovery, like activation, occurs in a characteristic geometric pattern.[18,19] Differences in recovery timing occur both across the ventricular wall and between regions of the left ventricle. Transmural differences in recovery times are the net result of two effects, differences in action potential duration across the ventricular wall and the relatively slow spread of activation across the wall. As activation moves from endocardium to epicardium, sites further away from the endocardium are activated later and later in time. However, action potential durations are longest near the endocardium and shortest near the epicardium. Differences in action potential duration are greater than differences in activation times, so that recovery is completed near the epicardium before it is completed near the endocardium. For example, one endocardial site may be excited 10 milliseconds earlier than the overlying epicardium (i.e., transmural activation may require 10 milliseconds), and the action potential duration at the endocardium may be 22 milliseconds longer than on the epicardium. As a result, recovery will be completed 12 milliseconds earlier in the epicardium than in the endocardium.

The resulting recovery dipole will then be directed away from sites of less recovery (the endocardium) toward sites of greater recovery (near the epicardium). The orientation of this dipole is in the same direction as transmural activation dipoles, as described earlier.

This orientation is opposite to the expected direction described earlier in this chapter. If recovery times were uniform across the wall (or if differences in recovery times were less than differences in transmural activation times), the recovery dipole would have been directed toward the endocardium—that is, in the direction opposite the activation dipole. The result, in normal persons, is concordant QRS and ST-T wave patterns.

Regional differences in recovery properties similarly exist. Under normal conditions, it is the transmural gradients that predominantly determine ST patterns. These regional differences account for the discordant ST-T patterns observed with intraventricular conduction defects, as will be described.

THE NORMAL ST-T WAVE. The normal ST-T wave begins as a low-amplitude, slowly changing wave (the ST segment) that gradually leads to a larger wave, the T wave. The onset of the ST-T wave is the junction, or J point, and is normally at or near the isoelectric baseline of the ECG (see Figs. 12-11 and 12-12).

The polarity of the ST-T wave is generally the same as the net polarity of the preceding QRS complex. Thus, T waves are usually upright in leads I, II, aVL, aVF, and the lateral precordial leads. They are negative in lead aVR and variable in leads III and V_1 through V_2.

The amplitude of the normal S-T segment varies with gender and with age.[20] It is typically highest in lead V_2. In men ages 18 to 29 years, the normal S-T segment may reach 0.33 mV; maximal amplitudes fall thereafter to reach 0.24 mV by age 50. In women, the maximal normal amplitude is approximately 0.07 mV, regardless of age.

THE U WAVE. The T wave may be followed by an additional low-amplitude wave known as the U wave. This late repolarization wave, usually less than 0.1 mV in amplitude, normally has the same polarity as the preceding T wave and is largest in the midprecordial leads and at slow heart rates. Its basis in cardiac electrophysiology is uncertain; it may be caused by repolarization of the Purkinje fibers, by the long action potential of midmyocardial cells (M cells), or by delayed repolarization in areas of the ventricle that undergo late mechanical relaxation.[18,19]

THE QT INTERVAL. The QT interval is measured from the beginning of the QRS complex to the end of the T wave in the lead with the longest interval and without a prominent U wave. It includes the total duration of ventricular activation and recovery and, in a general sense, corresponds to the duration of the ventricular action potential.

When the T wave overlaps with the beginning of a U wave, the QT interval is sometimes referred to as the QT(U) interval; this designation is particularly appropriate when considering the electrocardiographic effects of certain metabolic abnormalities that alter the duration of repolarization and the amplitude of the U wave (see later).

The duration of the QT interval decreases as heart rate increases, as does the duration of the normal ventricular action potential duration. Thus, the normal range for the QT interval is rate dependent. Numerous formulas have been proposed to correct the measured QT interval for this rate effect. The most commonly used formula for relating QT interval duration to heart rate was developed by Bazett in 1920. The result is computation of a corrected QT interval, or QT_c, by using the following equation:

$$QT_c = QT/(RR)^{1/2}$$

where the QT and RR intervals are measured in seconds. The normal QT_c is generally accepted to be less than or equal to 440* and it is slightly longer, on average, in women. However, the precise upper limit for the QT_c is subject to discussion (see Chap. 35). Studies, based on the analysis of ECGs of family members of patients with genetic forms of long QT interval syndromes, have suggested that the upper limit should be set at 460 (see Chap. 9). Other epidemiological studies have suggested an upper limit of 450, with higher

*The QTc is traditionally reported in units of seconds or milliseconds. However, based on the formula, it is actually a ratio of seconds to the square root of seconds, which is equivalent to the square root of seconds ($sec^{1/2}$).

 values associated with increased mortality after adjustment for confounding variables.[22]

The Bazett formula, although widely used, has limited accuracy in predicting the effects of heart rate on the QT interval.[23,24] Large database studies have, for example, shown that the QT_c interval based on the Bazett formula remains significantly affected by heart rate and that as many as 30 percent of normal ECGs would be diagnosed as having a prolonged QT interval when this formula is used.[23]

Many other formulas and methods for correcting the QT interval for the effects of heart rate, including linear, logarithmic, hyperbolic, and exponential functions, have been developed and tested, but they also have limitations. The substantial variation in the relationship between QT interval duration and heart rate among individuals and patient groups reduces the accuracy of any single correction formula. In addition, these formulas do not account for the effects of autonomic tone on the QT interval independent of the effects on rate. They also do not account for the relatively slow adaptation of repolarization to changes in rate; for example, several minutes may be required for the QT interval to reach a new steady state after an abrupt change in heart rate.

QT Dispersion. A second property of the QT interval is that it varies from lead to lead. In normal persons, the QT interval varies between leads by up to 50 milliseconds and is longest in the midprecordial leads V_2 and V_3. This range of intervals, referred to as QT interval dispersion, has been related to electrical instability and the risk of ventricular arrhythmogenesis, as described later in more detail, although its practical clinical use appears limited.[25]

The QRST Angle. The concordance between the orientation of the normal QRS complex and the normal ST-T wave described earlier can be expressed vectorially. An angle can be visualized between the vector representing the mean QRS force and the vector representing the mean ST-T force, known as the QRST angle. This angle, in the frontal plane, is normally less than 60 degrees and usually less than 30 degrees. Abnormalities of the QRST angle reflect abnormal relationships between the properties of activation and recovery.

The Ventricular Gradient. If the two vectors representing mean activation and mean recovery forces are added, a third vector known as the ventricular gradient is created.[26] This third vector represents the net area under the QRST complex. The concept of the ventricular gradient was originally developed to assess differences in the properties of ventricular activation and recovery. According to this concept, the more variability that exists in regional repolarization properties, the greater will be the difference between the QRS and ST-T areas. In other words, the ventricular gradient correlates with the magnitude of regional differences in recovery properties. In addition, because changes in activation patterns produced, for example, by bundle branch block, cause corresponding changes in recovery patterns (see later), no change in the ventricular gradient typically results. The ventricular gradient should thus allow a measure of regional recovery properties that is independent of the activation pattern. This measurement has possible relevance to the genesis of reentrant arrhythmias that are caused, in part, by abnormal regional variations in refractory periods.

Normal Variants

These descriptions of the waveforms of the normal ECG represent patterns most often observed in normal adults. Understanding the limitations of assigning and interpreting the normal ranges of electrocardiographic measurements is important. Values for many of the intervals and amplitudes to be described vary widely within the population as a function of age, race, gender, and body habitus. Variation may also occur within an individual over time as a function of autonomic tone and activity level. Thus, what is normal in one condition may be abnormal in another. Some variations have already been described in this chapter including, for example, variations in rate, QRS axis, and QT intervals.

Normal variations that occur in the patterns of the ST segment and the T wave are also common. These variations are important to recognize because they may be mistaken for significant abnormalities. For example, as many as 40 percent of Olympic athletes have "abnormal" electrocardiograms and 15 percent have distinctly abnormal changes suggesting hypertrophic cardiomyopathy; however, fewer than 5 percent of these athletes have structural cardiac disease.[27] ST-T patterns are affected by maneuvers that change autonomic tone. For example, changing body position, hyperventilating, drinking cold water, and performing the Valsalva maneuver can produce modest ST segment depression and slight T wave inversion in as many as one third of subjects.

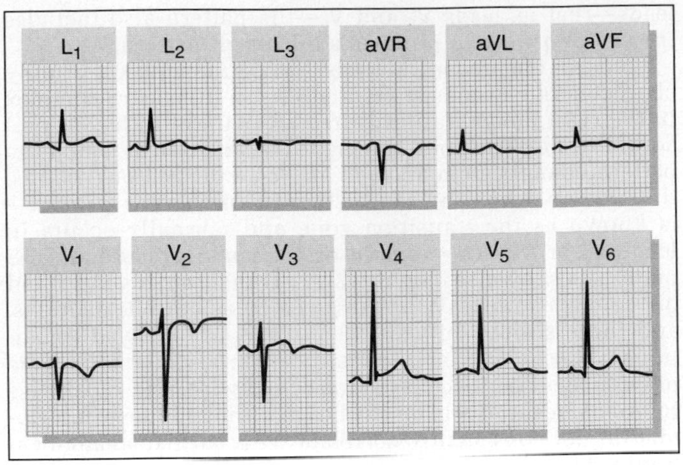

FIGURE 12–15 Normal tracing with a juvenile T wave inversion pattern in leads V_1, V_2, and V_3, as well as early repolarization patterns manifested by ST segment elevation in leads I, II, aVF, V_4, V_5, and V_6. *(Courtesy of Dr. C. Fisch.)*

T waves can be inverted in the right precordial leads in normal persons (Fig. 12-15).[28,29] T waves are commonly inverted in all precordial leads at birth but usually become upright as time passes. By the age of 10 years, T wave inversion is generally limited to leads V_1 and V_2, and only 1 to 3 percent of adults have inverted T waves in leads V_1 through V_3.[29] A persistent juvenile pattern with inverted T waves in leads to the left of V_1 may be more common in women than in men and in the African American population than in those in other racial or ethnic groups.

Second, the ST segment can be significantly elevated in normal persons, especially in the midprecordial leads (Fig. 12-16).[30] The elevation begins from an elevated J point, is usually concave in form, and is commonly associated with notching of the downstroke of the QRS complex. The magnitude of the ST segment elevation can reach 0.3 mV in amplitude. This pattern is more common at slow than at rapid heart rates and is most prevalent in young adults, especially African American men and those who are athletically active. The pattern is commonly referred to as early repolarization, and may be related to relative enhancement of vagal tone in healthy subjects.

THE ABNORMAL ELECTROCARDIOGRAM

Atrial Abnormalities

Various pathological and pathophysiological events alter the normal sequence of atrial activation and produce abnormal P wave patterns in the ECG. Three general categories of P wave changes are described here, reflecting abnormal sites or patterns of activation, left atrial abnormalities, and right atrial abnormalities.

Abnormal Atrial Activation and Conduction

Shifts in the site of initial activation within or away from the SA node to other ectopic sites can lead to major changes in the pattern of atrial activation and, hence, in the morphology of P waves. These shifts can occur either as escape rhythms if the normal SA nodal pacemaker fails or as accelerated ectopic rhythms if the automaticity of an ectopic site is enhanced (see Chap. 35). The resulting electrocardiographic abnormalities most commonly include negative P waves in the leads in which P waves are normally upright (leads I, II, aVF, and V_4 through V_6), with or without shortening of the PR interval.

P wave patterns can suggest the site of impulse formation based on simple vectorial principles. For example, a negative P wave in lead I suggests that the origin of activation is in the left atrium. Inverted P waves in the inferior leads normally correspond to a posterior atrial site. However, these correlations with location of origin are highly variable. Because of this, these patterns can, as a group, be referred to as ectopic atrial rhythms.

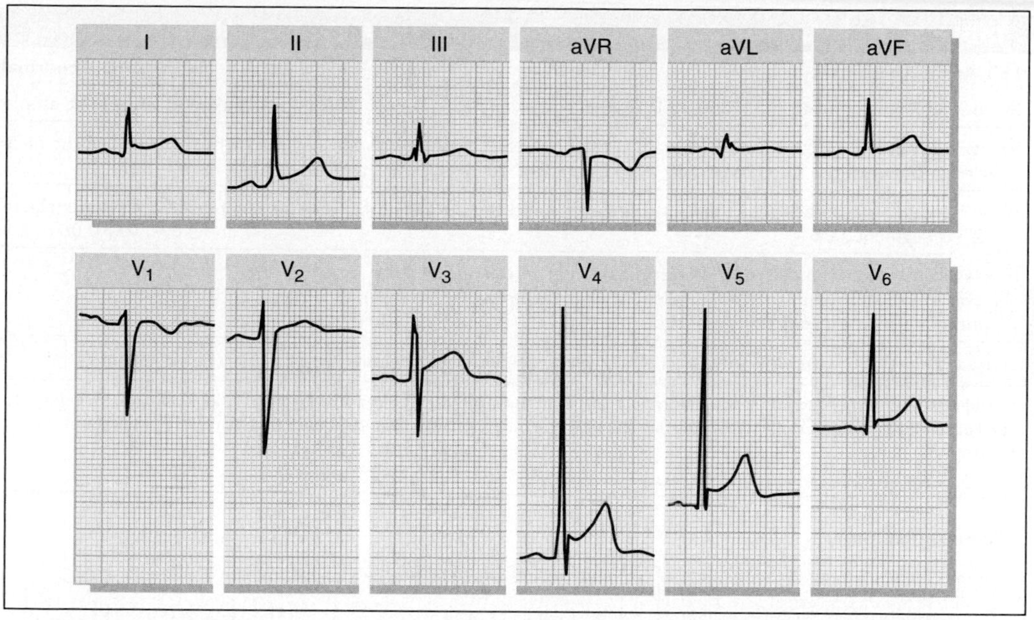

FIGURE 12–16 Normal variant pattern with functional ST elevations ("early repolarization" variant). These benign ST segment elevations are usually most marked in the midprecordial leads (here, V_4). Note the absence of reciprocal ST depression (except in lead aVR), as well as the absence of PR segment deviation, which may be helpful in the differential diagnosis of ischemia and pericarditis, respectively. Note also that lead II has a baseline recording shift. *(From Goldberger AL: Myocardial Infarction: Electrocardiographic Differential Diagnosis. 4th ed. St. Louis, Mosby-Year Book, 1991, p 201.)*

Conduction delays within the atria alter both the duration and pattern of P waves.[31] When conduction from the right to the left atrium within the Bachmann bundle is delayed, P wave duration is prolonged beyond 120 milliseconds and P waves appear to have two humps in lead II (P mitrale). With more advanced block, the sinus impulses reach the left atrium only after passing inferiorly near the AV junction and then superiorly through the left atrium. In this case, P waves are wide and biphasic in the inferior leads, with an initial positive wave reflecting inferior movement in the right atrium followed by a negative wave produced by superior movement within the left atrium. These conditions have been associated with atrial arrhythmias, including atrial fibrillation.

Left Atrial Abnormality

Anatomical or functional abnormalities of the left atrium alter the morphology, duration, and amplitude of the P waves in the clinical ECG. Specific abnormalities include increases in the amplitude and duration of the P wave in the limb leads, as well as an increase in the amplitude of the terminal negative portion of the P wave in lead V_1.

DIAGNOSTIC CRITERIA. Commonly used criteria for diagnosing left atrial abnormality are listed in Table 12-3. These features are illustrated in Figure 12-17.

MECHANISMS FOR ELECTROCARDIOGRAPHIC ABNORMALITIES. Increases in left atrial mass or chamber size cause increases in P wave amplitudes and durations. Because the left atrium is generally activated relatively late during P wave inscription, the increased electrical force accounts for the prolonged P wave duration and the increased P terminal force in the right precordial leads.

DIAGNOSTIC ACCURACY. Comparison of the various electrocardiographic abnormalities with echocardiographic criteria for left atrial enlargement demonstrates the limited sensitivity but high specificity for standard electrocardiographic criteria. For example, the presence of classic wide and notched P waves patterns has a sensitivity of only 20 percent but a specificity of over 90 percent for detecting echocardiographically enlarged left atria. Other studies have reported better correlations of these abnormalities with ventricular dysfunction (e.g., with reduced ventricular compliance) than with atrial pathology.

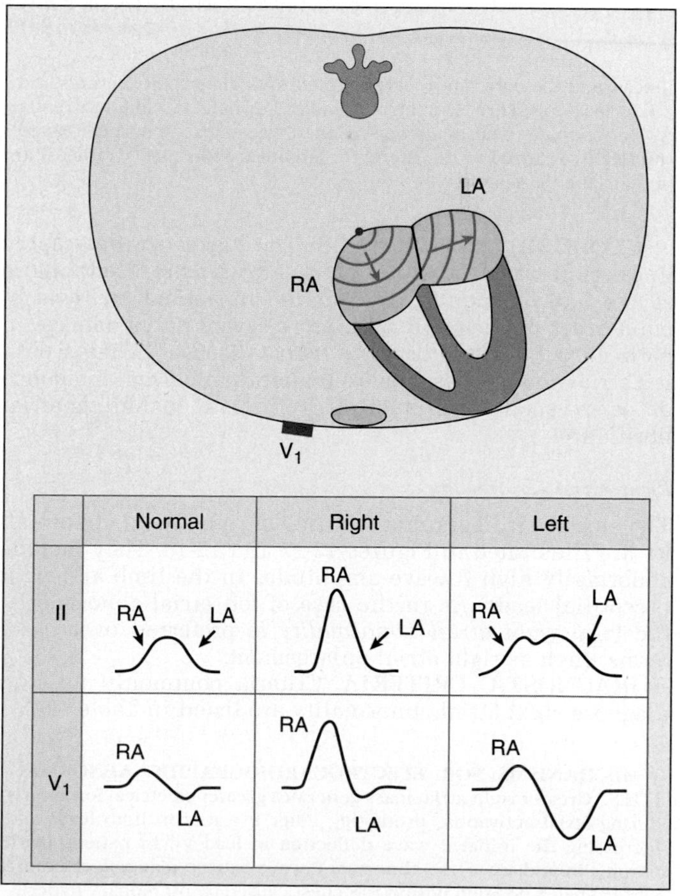

FIGURE 12–17 Schematic representation of atrial depolarization **(diagram)** and P wave patterns associated with normal atrial activation **(left panel)** and with right **(middle panel)** and left **(right panel)** atrial abnormalities. LA = left atrium; RA = right atrium. *(Modified from Park MK, Guntheroth WG: How to Read Pediatric ECGs. 3rd ed. St. Louis, Mosby-Year Book, 1993, p 51.)*

TABLE 12–3 Common Diagnostic Criteria for Left and Right Atrial Abnormalities*

Left Atrial Abnormality	Right Atrial Abnormality
Prolonged P wave duration >120 msec in lead II	Peaked P waves with amplitudes in lead II >0.25mV (P pulmonale)
Prominent notching of the P wave, usually most obvious in lead II, with an interval between the notches of >40 (P mitrale)	Rightward shift of the mean P wave axis to above +75 degrees
Ratio between the duration of the P wave in lead II and the duration of the PR segment >1.6	Increased area under the initial positive portion of the P wave in lead V_1 to >0.06 mm-sec
Increased duration and depth of the terminal negative portion of the P wave in lead V_1 (the P terminal force) so that the area subtended by it exceeds 0.04 mm-sec	
Leftward shift of the mean P wave axis to between −30 and −45 degrees	

*In addition to criteria based on P wave morphologies, right atrial abnormalities are suggested by QRS changes, including (1) Q waves (especially qR patterns) in the right precordial leads without evidence of myocardial infarction and (2) low-amplitude (under 600 μV) QRS complexes in lead V_1 with a threefold or greater increase in lead V_2.

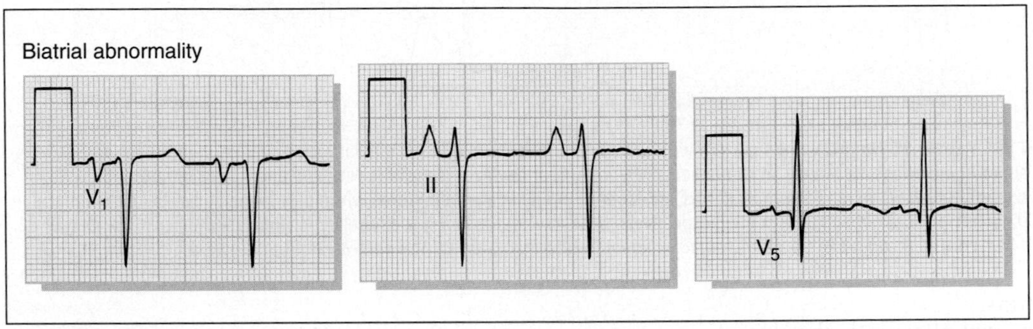

FIGURE 12–18 Biatrial abnormality, with tall P waves in lead II (right atrial abnormality) and an abnormally large terminal negative component of the P wave in lead V_1 (left atrial abnormality). The P wave is also notched in lead V_5.

Because of the correlation of these electrocardiographic features with high atrial pressure, intraatrial conduction defects, and ventricular dysfunction, as well as increased atrial size, these abnormalities are preferably referred to as criteria for left atrial abnormality rather than left atrial enlargement.

CLINICAL SIGNIFICANCE. The electrocardiographic findings of left atrial abnormality are associated with more severe left ventricular dysfunction in patients with ischemic heart disease and with more severe valve damage in patients with mitral or aortic valve disease. Patients with left atrial changes also have a higher than normal incidence of paroxysmal atrial tachyarrhythmias, including atrial fibrillation.

Right Atrial Abnormality

The electrocardiographic features of right atrial abnormality are illustrated in Figures 12-17 and 12-18. They include abnormally high P wave amplitudes in the limb and right precordial leads. As in the case of left atrial abnormality, the term *right atrial abnormality* is preferred over other terms, such as right atrial enlargement.

DIAGNOSTIC CRITERIA. Criteria commonly used to diagnose right atrial abnormality are listed in Table 12-3.

MECHANISMS FOR ELECTROCARDIOGRAPHIC ABNORMALITIES. Greater right atrial mass generates greater electrical force early during atrial activation, producing taller P waves in limb leads and increasing the initial P wave deflection in lead V_1. In patients with chronic lung disease, the abnormal P wave pattern may reflect a more vertical heart position within the chest caused by pulmonary hyperinflation rather than true cardiac damage. The QRS changes commonly associated with right atrial abnormalities correspond to the underlying pathological condition that is producing the right atrial hemodynamic changes (i.e., right ventricular hypertrophy [RVH]), which produces tall R waves in the right precordial leads, and a shift of the position of the heart within the chest by obstructive lung disease, which produces initial Q waves.

DIAGNOSTIC ACCURACY. Echocardiographic correlations have shown that the electrocardiographic findings of right atrial abnormality have limited sensitivity but high specificity for detecting right atrial enlargement.

CLINICAL SIGNIFICANCE. Patients with chronic obstructive pulmonary disease and this electrocardiographic pattern have more severe pulmonary dysfunction, as well as significantly reduced survival. However, comparison of electrocardiographic and hemodynamic parameters has not demonstrated a close correlation of P wave patterns and right atrial hypertension.

Other Atrial Abnormalities

Patients with abnormalities in both atria—that is, biatrial abnormality—can have electrocardiographic patterns reflecting each defect. Suggestive findings include large biphasic P waves in lead V_1 and tall and broad P waves in leads II, III, and aVF (see Fig. 12-18). P wave and PR segment changes can also be seen in patients with atrial infarction or pericarditis. The changes caused by these conditions are described later in this chapter.

Ventricular Hypertrophy and Enlargement

Left Ventricular Hypertrophy and Enlargement

Left ventricular hypertrophy (LVH) or enlargement produces changes in the QRS complex, the ST segment, and the T wave. The most characteristic finding is increased amplitude of the QRS complex. R waves in leads facing the left ventricle (i.e., leads I, aVL, V_5, and V_6) are taller than normal, whereas S waves in leads overlying the right ventricle (i.e., V_1 and V_2) are deeper than normal. These changes are illustrated in Figure 12-19.

ST-T wave patterns vary widely in patients with left ventricular enlargement and hypertrophy. ST segment and T wave amplitudes can be normal or increased in leads with tall R waves. In many patients, however, the ST segment is depressed and followed by an inverted T wave (Fig. 12-20). In most cases, the ST segment slopes downward from a depressed J point and the T wave is asymmetrically inverted (formerly called a "strain" pattern). These LVH-related repolarization changes usually occur in patients with QRS changes but can appear alone. Particularly prominent inverted T waves, or so-called giant negative T waves, are characteristic of hypertrophic cardiomyopathy with predominant apical thickening, especially in patients from the Pacific Rim (Yamaguchi syndrome; see Fig. 12-49).

Other QRS changes seen in cases of LVH include widening of the QRS complex beyond 110 milliseconds, a delay in the intrinsicoid deflection, and notching of the QRS complex. Other abnormalities may include prolongation of the QT interval and evidence of left atrial abnormality.

These electrocardiographic features are most typical of LVH induced by pressure overload of the left ventricle. Volume overload can produce a somewhat different pattern, including tall upright T waves and sometimes narrow (less than 30 milliseconds) but deep (0.2 mV or greater) Q waves in leads facing the left side of the septum (see Fig. 12-20). The diagnostic value of these changes in predicting the underlying hemodynamics is, however, very limited.

MECHANISMS FOR ELECTROCARDIOGRAPHIC ABNORMALITIES. Cardiac hypertrophy results in changes at the cellular, tissue, and volume conductor levels, all of which contribute to the electrocardiographic changes characteristic of left ventricular hypertrophy. These abnormalities may be compounded by changes caused by clinical conditions associated with hypertension, such as coronary artery disease and myocardial ischemia.

At the cellular level, hypertrophy is associated with a heterogeneous prolongation of action potential duration as well as an increase in action potential amplitude. These changes reflect a form of electrical remodeling cased by a downregulation of the transient outward potassium current I_{to} and the inward rectifier current I_{K1}, and reduced responsiveness to beta-adrenergic stimulation.[32]

These effects are augmented by an increase in the size of activation fronts moving across the thickened wall; these larger wave fronts subtend larger solid angles and result in higher body surface voltage. Prolonged transmural activation time required to activate the thickened wall, as well as delayed endocardial activation, contribute to the high voltage as well as QRS prolongation. Notching of the QRS complex can be produced by the fractionation of activation wave fronts by intramural scarring associated with wall thickening and damage.

In addition, changes in transmission factors can have an effect, although to a lesser degree. Left ventricular enlargement can shift the position of the heart so that the lateral free wall lies closer than normal to the chest wall, which increases body surface potentials in accordance with the inverse square law. Also, ventricular dilation increases the size of the highly conductive intraventricular blood pool that increases the potentials produced by transmural activation fronts, a phenomenon referred to as the Brody effect.

ST-T segment abnormalities may reflect a primary disorder of repolarization that accompanies the cellular processes of hypertrophy or they may reflect subendocardial ischemia. Patients with coronary artery disease have a higher prevalence of ST-T abnormalities with LVH than do those without coronary artery disease. Ischemia can be induced in the absence of coronary artery disease by the combination of high oxygen demand caused by high wall tension and limited blood flow to the subendocardium of the thickened wall.

DIAGNOSTIC CRITERIA. Many sets of diagnostic criteria for LVH have been developed on the basis

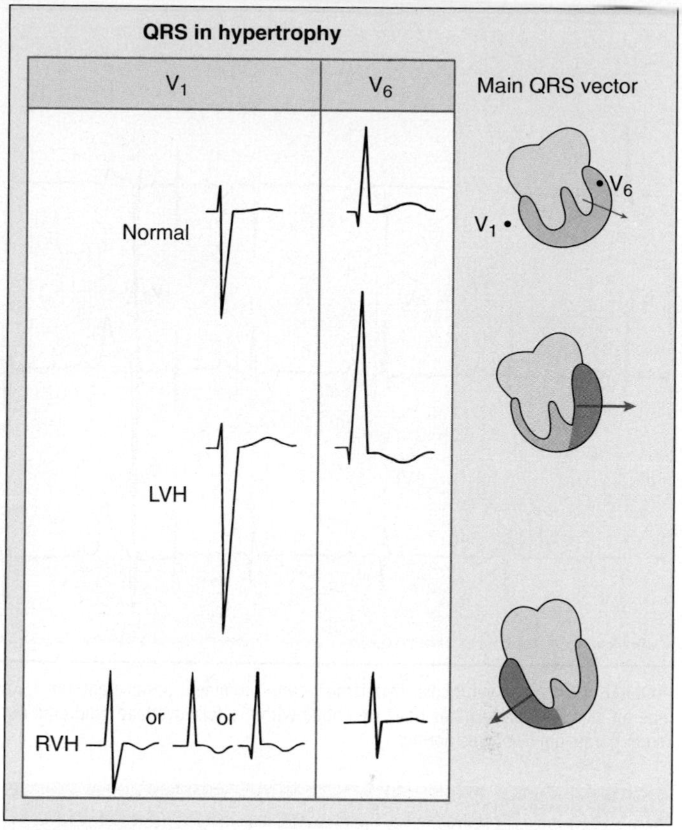

FIGURE 12–19 Left ventricular hypertrophy (LVH) increases the amplitude of electrical forces directed to the left and posteriorly. In addition, repolarization abnormalities can cause ST segment depression and T wave inversion in leads with a prominent R wave (formerly referred to as a "strain" pattern). Right ventricular hypertrophy (RVH) can shift the QRS vector to the right; this effect is usually associated with an R, RS, or qR complex in lead V_1, especially when caused by severe pressure overload. T wave inversions may be present in the right precordial leads. *(From Goldberger AL: Clinical Electrocardiography: A Simplified Approach. 7th ed. St. Louis, CV Mosby, 2006, p 64.)*

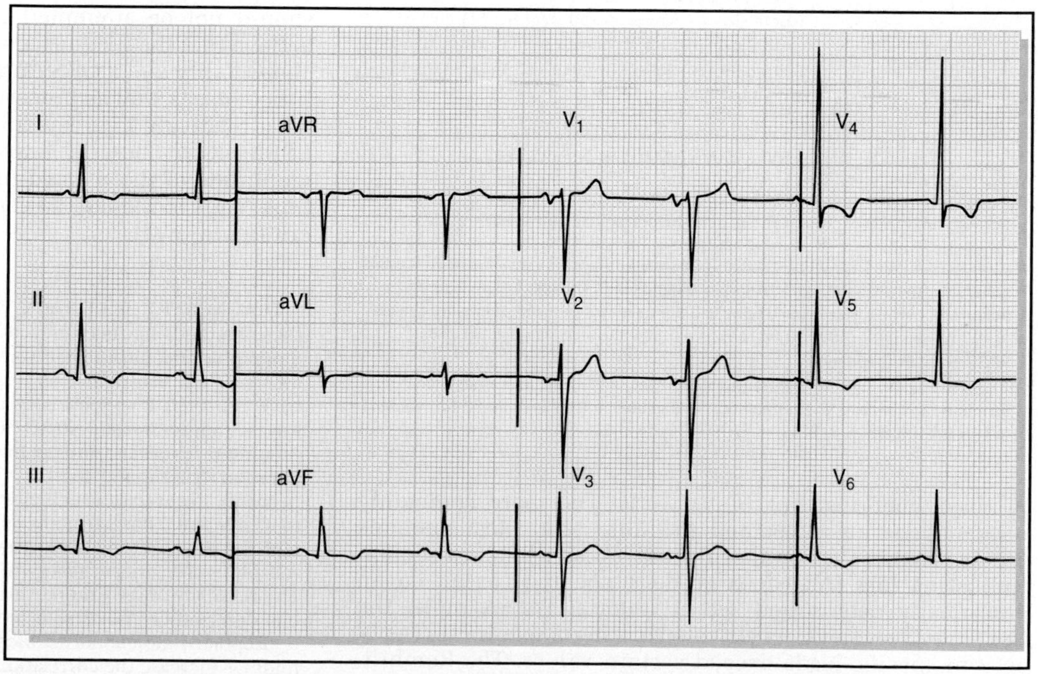

FIGURE 12–20 Marked left ventricular hypertrophy (LVH) pattern with prominent precordial lead QRS voltages. ST depression and T wave inversion can be seen with severe LVH in leads with a predominant R wave (compare with Fig. 12–21). Left atrial abnormality is also present.

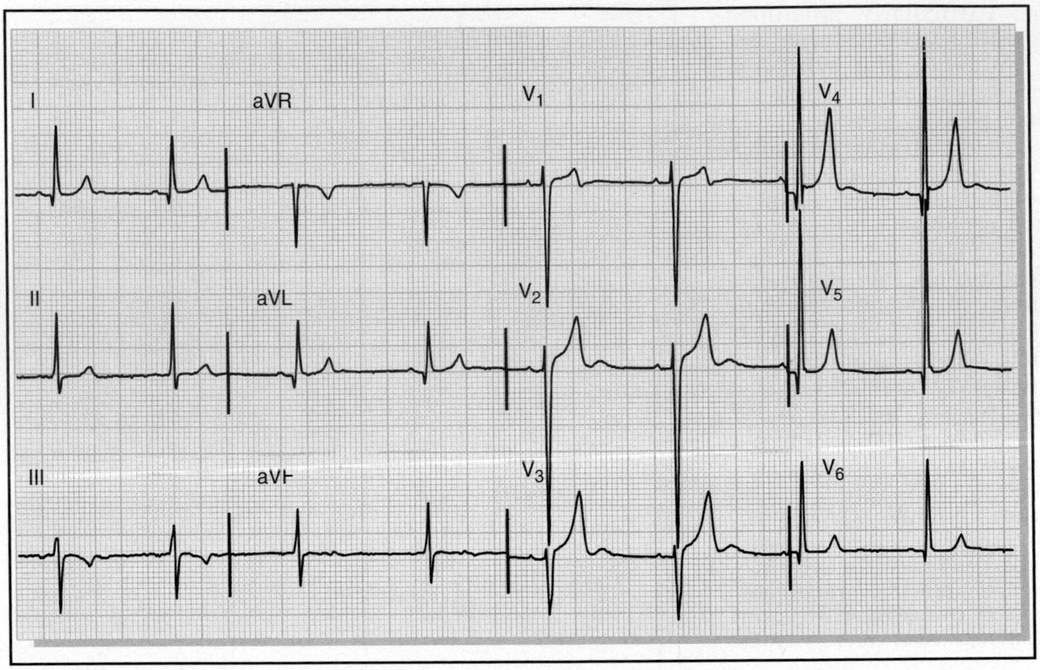

FIGURE 12–21 Left ventricular hypertrophy with prominent positive anterior T waves from a patient with severe aortic regurgitation. This pattern has been described with diastolic overload syndrome but has limited sensitivity and specificity. The serum potassium level was normal.

TABLE 12–4 Common Diagnostic Criteria for Left Ventricular Hypertrophy

Parameter	Criteria
Sokolow-Lyon index	$SV_1 + (RV_5 \text{ or } RV_6) > 3.5$ mV $RaVL > 1.1$ mV
Romhilt-Estes point score system (points)*	Any limb lead R wave or S wave ≥2.0 mV (3) *or* SV_1 or $SV_2 \geq 3.0$ mV (3) *or* RV_5 to $RV_6 \geq 3.0$ mV (3) ST-T wave abnormality (no digitalis therapy) (3) ST-T wave abnormality (digitalis therapy) (1) Left atrial abnormality (3) Left axis deviation ≤−30 degrees (2) QRS duration >90 msec (1) Intrinsicoid deflection in V_5 or $V_6 > 50$ msec (1)
Cornell voltage criteria	$SV_3 + SaVL \geq 2.8$ mV (for men) $SV_3 + SaVL \geq 2.0$ mV (for women)
Cornell voltage-duration measurement	QRS duration × Cornell voltage >2436 QRS duration × sum of voltages in all leads >17,472

*Probable left ventricular hypertrophy is diagnosed if 4 points are present and definite left ventricular hypertrophy is diagnosed if 5 or more points are present.

†Where $\exp = 4.558 - 0.092\ (RaVL + SV_3) - 0.306\ TV_1 - 0.212\ QRS - 0.278\ PTFV_1 - 0.859$ (gender).

Voltages are in mV, QRS is QRS duration in msec, PTF is the area under the P terminal force in lead V_1 (in mm-sec), and gender = 1 for men and 2 for women. LVH is present if $\exp < -1.55$.

of these abnormalities (Fig. 12-21). The more commonly used criteria are presented in Table 12-4. Most methods assess the presence or absence of LVH as a binary function indicating that LVH does or does not exist based on an empirically determined set of criteria. For example, the Sokolow-Lyon and Cornell voltage criteria require that voltages in specific leads exceed certain values. The Romhilt-Estes point score system assigns point values to amplitude and other criteria; definite LVH is diagnosed if 5 points are computed and probable LVH is diagnosed if 4 points are computed. The Cornell voltage-duration method includes measurement of QRS duration as well as amplitudes.

Other methods seek to quantify left ventricular mass as a continuum. Diagnosis of LVH can then be based on a computed mass that exceeds an independently determined threshold. One set of criteria applying this approach is the Cornell regression equation shown in the table.

Newer approaches include other variables in the diagnostic model. Some are based on multiple linear regression models[33] or include QT interval measurements[34] and QRS duration,[35] in addition to QRS amplitudes. Other criteria include nonelectrocardiographic variables, such as gender.

Concomitant abnormalities may interfere with the diagnosis of LVH. Because both LVH and conduction defects primarily alter QRS patterns, the existence of an intraventricular conduction defect may affect the accuracy of electrocardiographic criteria for LVH. In left anterior fascicular block, the larger R waves in leads I and aVL and smaller R waves but deeper S waves in leads V_5 and V_6 make criteria relying on R wave amplitude less valuable in this condition. In contrast, criteria that include the depth of the S wave in left precordial leads improve detection of LVH in the presence of left anterior fascicular block.

Left bundle branch block makes the diagnosis of LVH very difficult. Some have concluded that the diagnosis should not be attempted in this setting, whereas others believe that the diagnosis can be made. A left atrial P wave abnormality and a QRS duration longer than about 155 milliseconds, as well as precordial lead voltage criteria, tend to have relatively high specificity for LVH in the presence of LBBB. Right bundle branch block (RBBB) reduces the amplitude of the S wave in the right precordial leads and thus tends to reduce the sensitivity of electrocardiographic criteria for LVH.

DIAGNOSTIC ACCURACY. The relative diagnostic accuracy of these methods has been tested using autopsy, radiographic, echocardiographic and, most recently, magnetic resonance imaging[36] measurements of left ventricular size as standards. In general, these studies have reported low sensitivity and high specificity. Sensitivities are lowest (approximately 10 to 30 percent) for the Sokolow-Lyon and Romhilt-Estes criteria and are higher for the Cornell voltage and voltage duration criteria and for the Cornell regression methods (35 to 50 percent). In contrast, specificities for all measures vary from 85 percent to 95 percent. Thus, all methods are limited as screening tests in which high sensitivities (few false-negative results) are critical but have good reliability as diagnostic tests when few false-positive results are desired. The accuracy of the criteria varies from one trial to another so that no one criterion can be established as the preferred method.

Repolarization abnormalities associated with electrocardiographic findings increase the correlation with anatomical LVH. ST and T wave abnormalities are associated with a threefold greater prevalence of anatomical LVH in patients without coronary artery disease and a fivefold greater risk among patients with coronary disease.

The accuracy of the criteria also vary with the type of patient being evaluated. For example, precordial voltages are often higher in African Americans than in whites, which leads to a higher prevalence of false-positive electrocardiographic diagnoses of left ventricular hypertrophy in African Americans with hypertension. Body habitus, gender, and age also influence the accuracies of electrocardiographic criteria in complex ways that depend on the criterion being evaluated.

CLINICAL SIGNIFICANCE. An accurate electrocardiographic diagnosis of LVH is important to detect hypertrophy in association with overt cardiovascular disease (e.g., hypertension) or as an initial manifestation of various diseases, to assess prognosis, and to monitor progression or regression of hypertrophy during treatment.

The presence of electrocardiographic criteria for LVH identifies a subset of the general population with a significantly increased risk for cardiovascular morbidity and mortality. Among patients with hypertension, the Losartan Intervention for Endpoint Reduction in Hypertension (LIFE) study has reported that declines in measures such as the Cornell and Sokolow-Lyon voltages during antihypertensive therapy correlate with a fall in left ventricular mass and with lower likelihoods of cardiovascular mortality and morbidity independent of the extent of blood pressure lowering.[37]

Patients with repolarization abnormalities have, on average, more severe degrees of LVH and more commonly have symptoms of left ventricular dysfunction, in addition to a greater risk of cardiovascular events.[38,39] In the LIFE study referred to earlier, hypertensive patients with LVH-related ST-T wave abnormalities were 1.8 times as likely to develop congestive heart failure and 2.8 times as likely to experience heart failure-related death than were patients without such ST-T wave changes.[39]

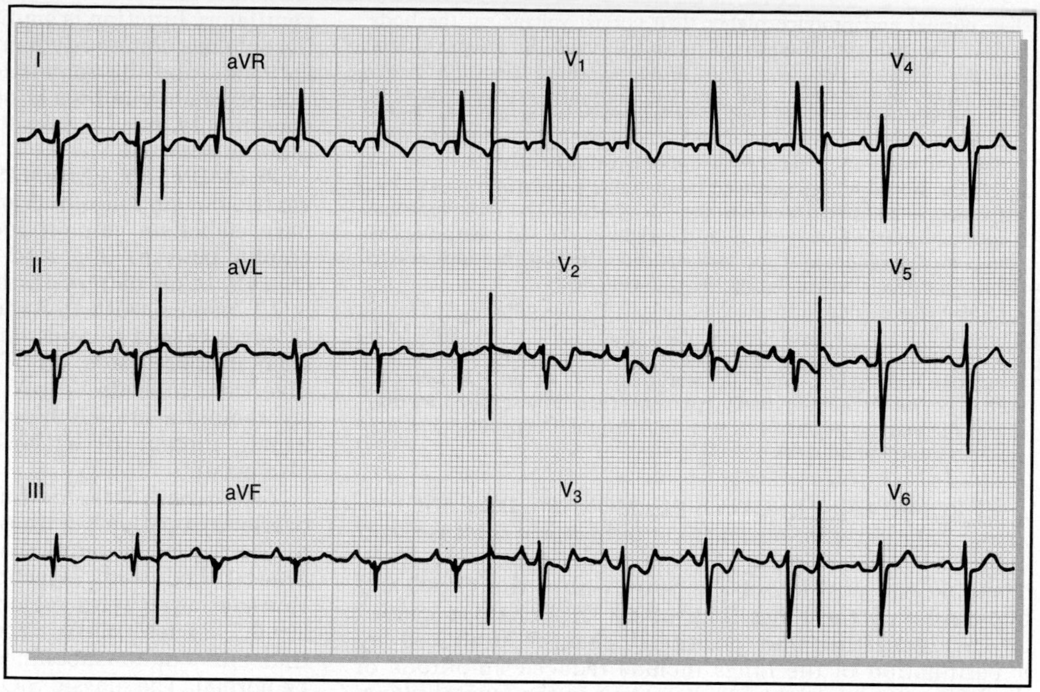

FIGURE 12–22 Right ventricular hypertrophy pattern most consistent with severe pressure overload. Note the combination of findings, including (1) a tall R wave in V_1 (as part of the qR complex), (2) right axis deviation, (3) T wave inversion in V_1 through V_3, (4) delayed precordial transition zone (rS in V_6), and (5) right atrial abnormality. An S_1Q_3 pattern is also present and can occur with acute or chronic right ventricular overload syndromes.

TABLE 12–5 Common Diagnostic Criteria for Right Ventricular Hypertrophy

Criterion	Sensitivity (%)	Specificity (%)
R in $V_1 \geq 0.7$ mV	<10	—
QR in V_1	<10	—
R/S in $V_1 > 1$ with R > 0.5 mV	<25	89
R/S in V_5 or $V_6 < 1$	<10	—
S in V_5 or $V_6 > 0.7$ mV	<17	93
R in V_5 or $V_6 \geq 0.4$ mV with S in $V_1 \geq 0.2$ mV	<10	—
Right axis deviation ≥ +90 degrees	<14	99
S_1Q_3 pattern	<11	93
S_1S_2S3 pattern	<10	—
P pulmonale	<11	97

From Murphy ML, Thenabadu PN, de Soyza N, et al: Reevaluation of electrocardiographic criteria for left, right and combined cardiac ventricular hypertrophy. Am J Cardiol 53:1140, 1984.

Right Ventricular Hypertrophy and Enlargement

The right ventricle is considerably smaller than the left ventricle and produces electrical forces that are largely concealed by those generated by the larger left ventricle. Thus, for RVH to be manifested on the ECG, it must be severe enough to overcome the concealing effects of the larger left ventricular forces. In addition, increasing dominance of the right ventricle changes the ECG in fundamental ways, whereas an enlarged left ventricle produces predominantly quantitative changes in underlying normal waveforms.

The electrocardiographic changes associated with moderate to severe concentric hypertrophy of the right ventricle include abnormally tall R waves in anteriorly and rightward-directed leads (leads aVR, V_1, and V_2), and deep S waves and abnormally small r waves in leftward-directed leads (I, aVL, and lateral precordial leads; Fig. 12-22). These changes result in a reversal of normal R wave progression in the precordial leads, a shift in the frontal plane QRS axis to the right, and the presence of S waves in leads I, II, and III (so-called $S_1S_2S_3$ pattern).

Less severe hypertrophy, especially when limited to the outflow tract of the right ventricle that is activated late during the QRS complex, produces less marked changes. Electrocardiographic abnormalities may be limited to an rSr′ pattern in V_1 and persistence of s (or S) waves in the left precordial leads. This pattern is typical of right ventricular volume overload as produced by an atrial septal defect.

DIAGNOSTIC CRITERIA. These abnormalities form the basis for the diagnostic criteria for RVH. The most commonly relied on criteria for the electrocardiographic diagnosis of RVH are listed in Table 12-5.

MECHANISMS FOR ELECTROCARDIOGRAPHIC ABNORMALITIES. These electrocardiographic patterns result from three effects of RVH. First, current fluxes between hypertrophied cells are stronger than normal and produce higher than normal voltage on the body surface. Second, activation fronts moving through the enlarged right ventricle are larger than normal and produce higher surface potentials, as predicted by the solid angle theorem. Third, the activation time of the right ventricle is prolonged. This last effect is particularly important in producing electrocardiographic changes; right ventricular activation now ends after the completion of left ventricular activation, so its effects are no longer canceled by the more powerful forces of the left ventricle and may emerge in the ECG. Because the right ventricle is located anteriorly as well as to the right of the left ventricle, the effects produce increased potentials in leads directed anteriorly and to the right, especially late during the QRS complex.

DIAGNOSTIC ACCURACY. The sensitivity and specificity of the individual electrocardiographic criteria are also shown in Table 12-5. The sensitivities of individual criteria are low and specificities are high. If any one feature is present, the sensitivity may be only 10 percent, with a specificity of more than 90 percent. These low sensitivities may reflect the marked degree of hypertrophy required to produce electrocardiographic abnormalities.

CHRONIC OBSTRUCTIVE PULMONARY DISEASE (see Chap. 73). Chronic obstructive pulmonary disease can induce electrocardiographic changes by producing RVH, changing the position of the heart within the chest, and hyperinflating the lungs (Fig. 12-23). QRS changes caused by the insulating and positional changes produced by hyperinflation of the lungs include reduced amplitude of the QRS complex, right axis deviation in the frontal plane, and delayed transition in the precordial leads (probably reflecting a vertical and caudal shift in heart position because of hyperinflation and a flattened diaphragm). Evidence of true RVH includes (1) marked right axis deviation (more positive than +110 degrees), (2) deep S waves in the lateral precordial leads, and (3) an $S_1Q_3T_3$ pattern, with an S wave in lead I (as an RS or rS complex), an abnormal Q wave in lead III, and an inverted T wave in the inferior leads.

The electrocardiographic evidence of RVH has limited value in assessing the severity of pulmonary hypertension or lung disease. QRS changes do not generally appear until ventilatory function is significantly depressed, with the earliest change commonly being a rightward shift in the mean QRS axis, and the correlation with either ventilatory function or hemodynamics is poor. The presence of right atrial abnormality, an $S_1S_2S_3$ pattern, or both is associated with reduced survival.

PULMONARY EMBOLISM (see Chap. 72). Acute right ventricular pressure overload such as produced by pulmonary embolism can produce characteristic electrocardiographic patterns (Fig. 12-24). These include the following: (1) a QR or qR pattern in the right ventricular leads; (2) an $S_1Q_3T_3$ pattern, with an S wave in lead I and new or increased Q waves in lead III and sometimes aVF, with T wave inversions in those leads; (3) ST segment deviation and T wave inversions in leads V_1 to V_3; and (4) incomplete or complete right bundle branch block (RBBB). Sinus tachycardia is usually present. Arrhythmias such as atrial fibrillation can also occur.

Electrocardiographic findings of acute right ventricular overload in patients with pulmonary embolism correspond to obstruction of more than 50 percent of the pulmonary arterial bed and significant pulmonary hypertension. However, even with major pulmonary artery obstruction, the ECG is notoriously deceptive and may show little more than minor or nonspecific waveform changes, or it may even be normal. The classic $S_1Q_3T_3$ pattern occurs in only about 10 percent of cases of acute pulmonary embolism (see Chap. 72). Furthermore, the specificity of this finding is limited, because it can occur acutely with other causes of pulmonary hypertension. A recent study of the ECGs of patients with right ventricular dilation due to acute pulmonary embolism reported positive predictive accuracies of 23 to 69 percent.[40]

Biventricular Enlargement

Enlargement or hypertrophy of both ventricles produces complex electrocardiographic patterns. In contrast to biatrial enlargement, the result is not the simple sum of the

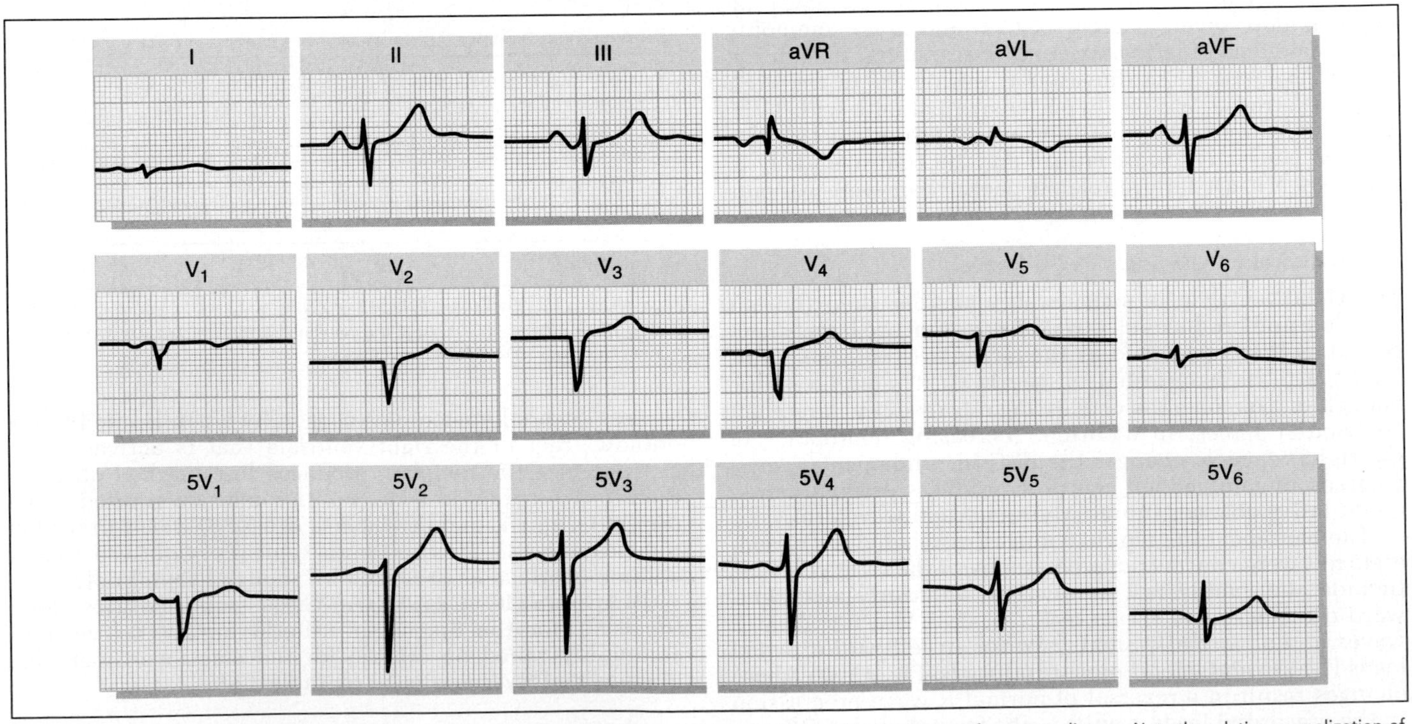

FIGURE 12–23 Pulmonary emphysema simulating anterior infarction in a 58-year-old man with no clinical evidence of coronary disease. Note the relative normalization of R wave progression with placement of the chest leads an interspace below their usual position ($5V_1$, $5V_2$, and so forth). *(From Chou TC: Pseudo-infarction (noninfarction Q waves). In Fisch C [ed]: Complex Electrocardiography. Vol 1. Philadelphia, FA Davis, 1973, p 203.)*

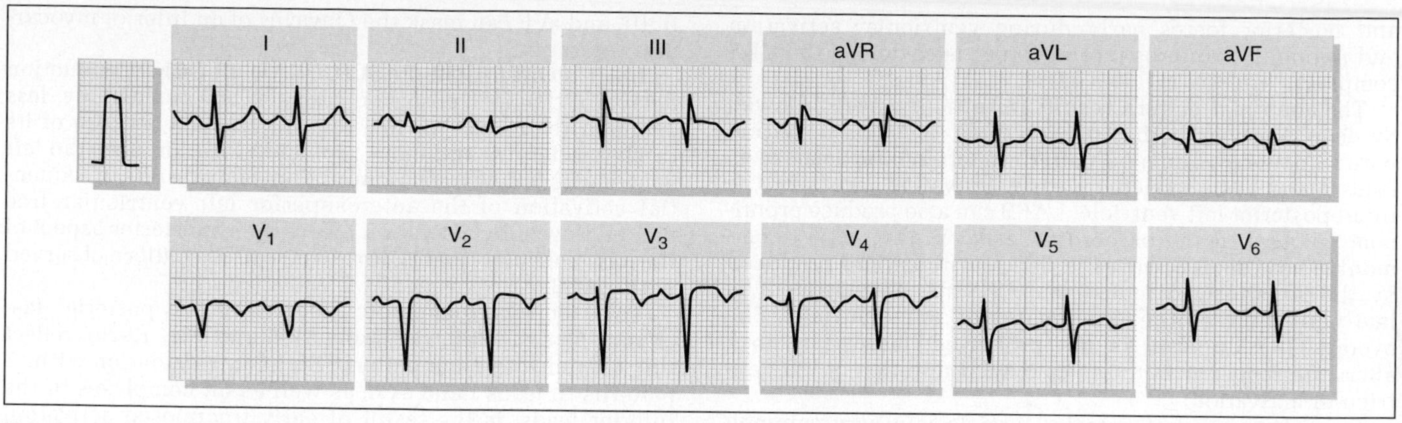

FIGURE 12–24 Acute cor pulmonale secondary to pulmonary embolism simulating inferior and anterior infarction. This tracing exemplifies the classic pseudoinfarct patterns sometimes seen: an $S_1Q_3T_3$, a QR in V_1 with poor R wave progression in the right precordial leads ("clockwise rotation"), and right precordial to midprecordial T wave inversion (V_1 to V_4). Sinus tachycardia is also present. The S_1Q_3 pattern is usually associated with a QR or QS complex, but not an rS, in aVR. Furthermore, acute cor pulmonale per se does not cause prominent Q waves in II (only in III and aVF).

two sets of abnormalities. The effects of enlargement of one chamber may cancel the effects of enlargement of the other. The greater left ventricular forces generated in LVH increase the degree of RVH needed to overcome the dominance of the left ventricle, and the anterior forces produced by RVH may cancel or be canceled by enhanced posterior forces generated by LVH.

Because of these factors, specific electrocardiographic criteria for RVH or LVH are seldom observed with biventricular enlargement. Rather, electrocardiographic patterns are usually a modification of the features of LVH and include the following: (1) tall R waves in both the right and left precordial leads; (2) vertical heart position or right axis deviation in the presence of criteria for LVH; (3) deep S waves in the left precordial leads in the presence of electrocardiographic criteria for LVH; and (4) a shift in the precordial transition zone to the left in the presence of LVH. The presence of prominent left atrial abnormality or atrial fibrillation with evidence of right ventricular or biventricular enlargement, especially LVH with a vertical or rightward QRS axis, should suggest chronic rheumatic valvular disease (Fig. 12-25; see Chaps. 62 and 83).

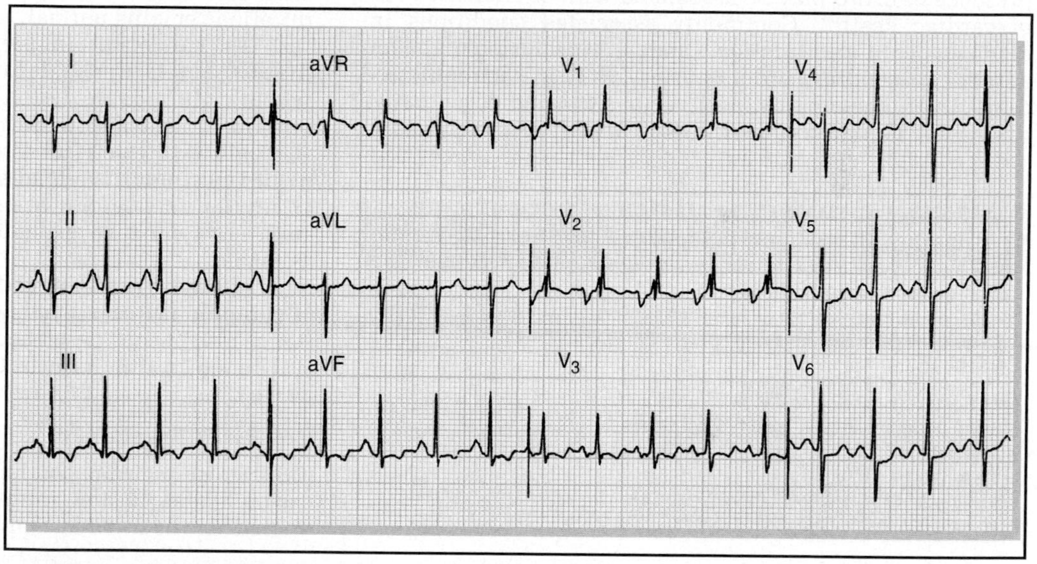

FIGURE 12–25 This electrocardiogram from a 45-year-old woman with severe mitral stenosis shows multiple abnormalities. The rhythm is sinus tachycardia. Right axis deviation and a tall R wave in lead V_1 are consistent with right ventricular hypertrophy. The very prominent biphasic P wave in lead V_1 indicates left atrial abnormality. The tall P waves in lead II suggest concomitant right atrial abnormality. Nonspecific ST-T changes and incomplete right bundle branch block are also present. The combination of right ventricular hypertrophy and marked left or biatrial abnormality is highly suggestive of mitral stenosis. *(From Goldberger AL: Clinical Electrocardiography: A Simplified Approach. 7th ed. St. Louis, CV Mosby, 2006, p 277.)*

Intraventricular Conduction Delays

The electrocardiographic patterns described in this section reflect abnormalities in the intraventricular conduction system (see Chaps. 32 and 35).

Fascicular Block

Under normal conditions, activation of the left ventricle begins simultaneously at the insertion points of the fascicles. Delayed conduction in a fascicle, referred to as fascicular block, results in activation of these sites sequentially rather than simultaneously. This produces an abnormal sequence of early left ventricular activation that, in turn, leads to characteristic electrocardiographic patterns. Even modest delays in conduction through the affected fascicle(s) may be enough to alter ventricular activation patterns sufficiently to produce characteristic electrocardiographic patterns; a complete block of conduction is not required.

LEFT ANTERIOR FASCICULAR BLOCK. The electrocardiographic features of left anterior fascicular block (LAFB) are listed in Table 12-6 and illustrated in Figure 12-26. The most characteristic finding is marked left axis deviation. However, LAFB is not synonymous with left axis deviation. Axis shifts to between −30 and −45 degrees commonly reflect other conditions, such as LVH, without conduction system damage and such patterns are best referred to as left axis deviation rather than as LAFB.

The left anterior fascicle normally activates the anterosuperior portion of the left ventricle early during the QRS complex. Left axis shift with LAFB is a result of delayed activation of this region. This causes unbalanced inferior and posterior forces early during ventricular activation and unopposed anterosuperior forces later during the QRS complex.

The abnormal pattern results in initial r waves followed by deep S waves in the inferior leads (left axis deviation with rS patterns) and a qR pattern in left-looking leads (e.g., leads I and aVL) caused by early activation forces in the inferoposterior left ventricle. LAFB can also produce prominent changes in the precordial leads; V_4 through V_6 commonly show deep S waves (a delayed transition) produced by the superiorly directed late QRS forces generated by late activation of the anterosuperior left ventricle. The overall QRS duration is not prolonged; fascicular block alters the sequence but not the overall duration of left ventricular activation.

Damage to the left anterior fascicle is a very common occurrence because of the delicate nature of the structure. Left anterior fascicular block is common in persons without overt cardiac disease, as well as in those with a wide range of diseases. In patients with coronary artery disease, the presence of LAFB may be associated with an increased risk of cardiac death.[41] Commonly associated conditions include myocardial infarction, especially occlusion of the left anterior descending coronary artery, LVH, hypertrophic and dilated cardiomyopathy, and various cardiac degenerative diseases. The development of LAFB with rS complexes in II, III, and aVF can mask the Q waves of an inferior myocardial infarction.

LEFT POSTERIOR FASCICULAR BLOCK. Conduction delay in the left posterior fascicle is considerably less common than delay in the anterior fascicle because of its thicker structure and more protected location near the left ventricular inflow tract. Conduction delay results in sequential activation of the anterosuperior left ventricular free wall, followed by activation of the inferoposterior aspect of the left ventricle—that is, the reverse of the pattern observed with LAFB.

The electrocardiographic features of left posterior fascicular block (LPFB; see Table 12-6 and Fig. 12-26), reflect this altered activation pattern. Right axis deviation with rS patterns in leads I and aVL, as well as qR complexes in the inferior leads, is the result of early unopposed activation forces from the anterosuperior aspect of the left ventricle (producing the initial q and r waves) and late unopposed forces from the inferoposterior free wall (generating the late S and R waves). As in the case of LAFB, the overall activation time of the ventricles is not prolonged and the QRS duration remains normal.

LPFB can occur in patients with almost any cardiac disease but is unusual in otherwise healthy persons in whom right axis deviation sometimes occurs as a normal variant. Other conditions that augment or appear to augment the rightward electrical forces in the frontal plane, such as right ventricular overload syndromes and extensive lateral infarction, can produce similar electrocardiographic patterns and must be excluded before a diagnosis of LPFB is made.

OTHER FORMS OF FASCICULAR BLOCK. Electrocardiographic patterns that suggest left septal fascicular block have also been described. The most common finding attributed to this form of block is the absence of septal q waves.[16]

TABLE 12–6 Common Diagnostic Criteria for Unifascicular Blocks

Left Anterior Fascicular Block
Frontal plane mean QRS axis of −45 to −90 degrees with rS patterns in leads II, III, and aVF and a qR pattern in lead aVL
QRS duration <120 msec
Left Posterior Fascicular Block
Frontal plane mean QRS axis >120 degrees
RS pattern in leads I and aVL with qR patterns in inferior leads
QRS duration <120 msec
Exclusion of other factors causing right axis deviation (e.g., right ventricular overload patterns, lateral infarction)

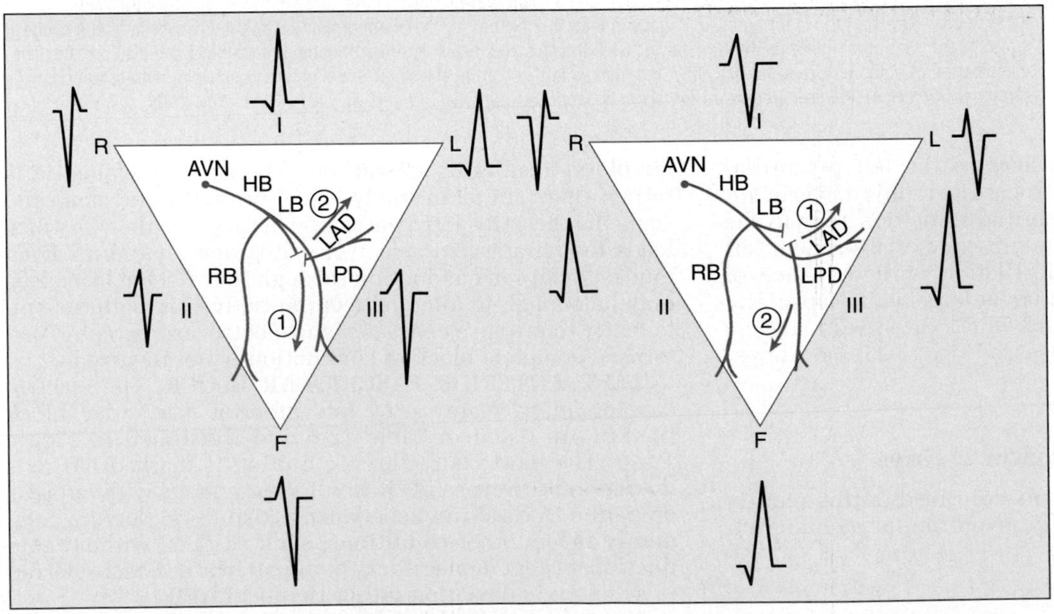

FIGURE 12–26 Diagrammatic representation of fascicular blocks in the left ventricle. **Left,** Interruption of the left anterior fascicle (LAF) results in an initial inferior (1) followed by a dominant superior (2) direction of activation. **Right,** Interruption of the left posterior fascicle (LPF) results in an initial superior (1) followed by a dominant inferior (2) direction of activation. AVN = atrioventricular node; HB = His bundle; LB = left bundle; RB = right bundle. *(Courtesy of Dr. C. Fisch.)*

Left Bundle Branch Block

LBBB results from conduction delay or block in any of several sites in the intraventricular conduction system, including the main left bundle branch, each of the two fascicles, the distal conduction system of the left ventricle or, less commonly, the fibers of the bundle of His that become the main left bundle branch. The result is extensive reorganization of the activation and recovery patterns of the left ventricle that produces extensive changes in the QRS complex and the ST-T wave.

ELECTROCARDIOGRAPHIC ABNORMALITIES. LBBB produces a prolonged QRS duration, abnormal QRS patterns, and ST-T wave abnormalities (Fig. 12-27). Commonly accepted diagnostic criteria for LBBB are listed in Table 12-7. Basic requirements include a prolonged QRS duration to 120 milliseconds or beyond; broad and commonly notched R waves in leads I, aVL, and

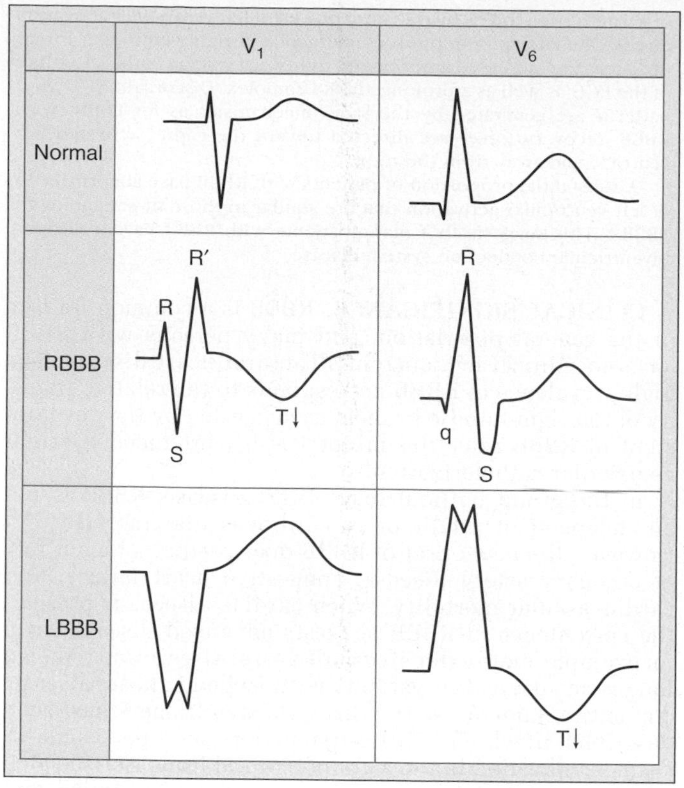

FIGURE 12–27 Comparison of typical QRS-T patterns in right bundle branch block (RBBB) and left bundle branch block (LBBB) with the normal pattern in leads V_1 and V_6. Note the secondary T wave inversions (arrows) in leads with an rSR′ complex with RBBB and in leads with a wide R wave with LBBB. *(From Goldberger AL: Clinical Electrocardiography: A Simplified Approach. 7th ed. St. Louis, CV Mosby, 2006, p 80.)*

TABLE 12–7 Common Diagnostic Criteria for Bundle Branch Blocks
Complete Left Bundle Branch Block
QRS duration ≥120 msec
Broad, notched R waves in lateral precordial leads (V_5 and V_6) and usually leads I and aVL
Small or absent initial r waves in right precordial leads (V_1 and V_2) followed by deep S waves
Absent septal q waves in left-sided leads
Prolonged intrinsicoid deflection (>60 msec) in V_5 and V_6*
Complete Right Bundle Branch Block
QRS duration ≥120 msec
Broad, notched R waves (rsr′, rsR′, or rSR′ patterns) in right precordial leads (V_1 and V_2)
Wide and deep S waves in left precordial leads (V_5 and V_6)

*Criterion required by some authors.

the left precordial leads; narrow r waves followed by deep S waves in the right precordial leads; and absent septal q waves. R waves are typically tall and S waves are deep. The mean QRS axis with LBBB is highly variable; it can be normal, deviated to the left or, less often, deviated to the right. In addition to these features, some electrocardiographers require a delayed intrinsicoid deflection (60 milliseconds or longer) to diagnose LBBB.

ST-T wave changes are prominent with LBBB. In most cases, the ST segment and T wave are discordant with the QRS complex. That is, the ST segment is depressed and the T wave is inverted in leads with positive QRS waves (e.g., leads I, aVL, V_5, and V_6), and the ST segment is elevated and the T wave is upright in leads with negative QRS complexes (e.g., leads V_1 and V_2).

An incomplete form of LBBB may result from lesser degrees of conduction delay in the left bundle branch system. Electrocardiographic features include (1) loss of septal q waves (reflecting reversal of the normal pattern of septal activation), (2) slurring and notching of the upstroke of R waves (because of the presence of competing activation fronts), and (3) modest prolongation of the QRS complex (between 100 and 120 milliseconds). An rSr′ morphology in lead V_1 (and sometimes V_2) with a narrow QRS duration (100 milliseconds) is a common physiological or positional variant.

MECHANISMS FOR THE ELECTROCARDIOGRAPHIC ABNORMALITIES. The electrocardiographic abnormalities of LBBB result from an almost completely reorganized pattern of left ventricular activation. Initial septal activation typically occurs on the right (rather than on the left) septal surface. This leads to right to left (rather than left to right) activation of the septum, resulting in the absence of normal septal q waves in the ECG. The site and timing of left septal activation has been shown to vary, suggesting differences in the pathophysiology of LBBB.[42,43] In some cases, earliest left septal activation occurs high along the septum, remote from the left side conduction system. This suggests transseptal activation. In other cases, earliest left septal activation occurs in the midseptal region in or just anterior to the left posterior fascicle. This suggests activation caused by slow conduction within the left bundle system rather than by transseptal spread. Approximately one third of patients with LBBB have near-normal left septal activation time, indicating a more peripheral site of block.[43]

After septal activation, free wall endocardial activation of the left ventricle may then require an additional 40 milliseconds, to more than 180 milliseconds, depending largely on the functional status of the distal left bundle and Purkinje systems. Thus, the overall QRS complex is prolonged and can be very wide, especially in patients with diffuse ventricular scarring from, for example, prior myocardial infarction.

Left ventricular free wall activation finally occurs near the end of the QRS complex.[44] Once left ventricular activation begins, it proceeds in a relatively simple and direct manner around the inferior free wall to the lateral wall and, finally, to the base of the heart.[43] This is in contrast to the multicentric overlapping patterns of activation seen under normal conditions. Spread predominantly through working muscle fibers rather than the specialized conduction system results in notching and slurring as a consequence of discontinuous anisotropy, as described earlier.

The discordant ST-T wave pattern is a result of the transventricular recovery gradients referred to earlier. With LBBB, the right ventricle is activated and recovers earlier than the left, so recovery vectors or dipoles are directed toward the right and away from the left. Hence, positive ST-T waves will be registered over the right ventricle and negatives ones over the left ventricle. These transventricular gradients play only a minor role during normal conduction because the simultaneous activation of multiple regions cancels the forces that they produce; with bundle branch block, activation is sequential and cancellation is reduced. Because the ST-T wave changes with LBBB are generated by abnormalities in conduction, they are called secondary ST-T wave abnormalities; as will be discussed later, ST-T wave changes produced by direct abnormalities of the recovery process are referred to as primary ST-T wave abnormalities.

CLINICAL SIGNIFICANCE. LBBB usually appears in patients with underlying heart disease, although as many as 12 percent of patients with LBBB have no demonstrable heart disease.[45] Even among persons without overt heart disease, LBBB is associated with a higher than normal risk of cardiovascular and all-cause mortality.[46] It is associated with substantially higher than expected risks of high-grade atrioventricular block and cardiac death, mostly as a result of sudden death outside the hospital setting.[47] Among patients with coronary artery disease, the presence of LBBB correlates with more extensive disease, more severe left ventricular dysfunction, and reduced survival rates.

Patients with associated left or right axis deviation have more severe clinical manifestations. Left axis deviation is associated with more severe conduction system disease that includes the fascicles as well as the main left bundle, whereas right axis deviation suggests dilated cardiomyopathy with biventricular enlargement.

In addition to the hemodynamic abnormalities produced by the underlying cardiovascular conditions, the abnormal ventricular activation pattern of LBBB itself induces hemodynamic changes. These include abnormal systolic function with dysfunctional contraction patterns, reduced ejection fraction and lower stroke volumes, and abnormal diastolic function,[44,48] which may represent a form of cardiomyopathy (see Chap. 34).[49] In addition, functional abnormalities in phasic coronary blood flow[50] often result in septal or anteroseptal defects on exercise perfusion scintigraphy in the absence of coronary artery disease.

A major impact of LBBB lies in obscuring or simulating other electrocardiographic patterns. The diagnosis of LVH is complicated by the increased QRS amplitude and axis shifts intrinsic to LBBB; in addition, the very high prevalence of anatomical LVH in combination with LBBB makes defining criteria with high specificity difficult. The diagnosis of myocardial infarction may be obscured; as will be described, the emergence of abnormal Q waves with infarction is dependent on a normal initial sequence of ventricular activation, which is absent with LBBB. In addition, electrocardiographic patterns of LBBB, including low R wave amplitude in the midprecordial leads and ST-T wave changes, can simulate anterior infarct patterns.

Right Bundle Branch Block

Right bundle branch block is a result of conduction delay in any portion of the right-sided intraventricular conduction system. The delay can occur in the main right bundle branch itself, in the bundle of His, or in the distal right ventricular conduction system. The latter is the common cause of RBBB after a right ventriculotomy is performed—for example, to correct the tetralogy of Fallot.[51]

ELECTROCARDIOGRAPHIC ABNORMALITIES. Major features of RBBB are illustrated in Figure 12-27 and commonly used diagnostic criteria are listed in Table 12-7. As with LBBB, the QRS complex duration exceeds 120 milliseconds. The right precordial leads show prominent and notched R waves with rsr′, rsR′, or rSR′ patterns, whereas leads I, aVL, and the left precordial leads demonstrate wide S waves that are longer in duration than the preceding R wave. The ST-T waves are, as in LBBB, discordant with the QRS complex, so that T waves are inverted in the right precordial leads (and other leads with a terminal R′ wave) and upright in the left precordial leads and in leads I and aVL.

The mean QRS axis is not altered by RBBB. Axis shifts can occur, however, as a result of the simultaneous occurrence of fascicular block along with RBBB, as described later. This combination of RBBB with either LAFB (producing left axis deviation) or LPFB (producing right axis deviation) is termed *bifascicular block.*

Features indicative of incomplete RBBB, produced by lesser delays in conduction in the right bundle branch system, are commonly seen. This finding is most frequently characterized by an rSr′ pattern in lead V_1, with a QRS duration between 100 and 120 milliseconds. Although these electrocardiographic changes of incomplete RBBB are commonly attributed to conduction defects, they can reflect RVH (especially with a rightward QRS axis) without intrinsic dysfunction of the conduction system.

MECHANISM FOR ELECTROCARDIOGRAPHIC ABNORMALITIES. With delay or block in the proximal right bundle branch system, activation of the right side of the septum is initiated only after slow transseptal spread of activation from the left septal surface.[50] The right ventricular anterior free wall is then excited slowly, followed by activation of the lateral right ventricular wall and, finally, the right ventricular outflow tract.

The result is delayed and slow activation of the right ventricle. Much or all of the right ventricle undergoes activation after depolarization of the left ventricle has been completed. This reduces the cancellation of RV activation forces by the more powerful left ventricular activation forces. The late and unopposed emergence of right ventricular forces produces the increased anterior and rightward voltage in the latter half of the ECG as well as a prolonged QRS complex. Discordant ST-T wave patterns are generated by the same mechanisms as for LBBB; with RBBB, recovery forces are directed toward the earlier activated left ventricle and away from the right.

A substantial proportion of patients with RBBB have abnormalities of left ventricular activation that are similar to those in patients with LBBB.[52] This suggests that many patients with RBBB have a diffuse, biventricular conduction system disease.

CLINICAL SIGNIFICANCE. RBBB is a common finding in the general population, and many persons with RBBB have no clinical evidence of structural heart disease. The high prevalence of RBBB corresponds to the relative fragility of the right bundle branch, as suggested by the development of RBBB after the minor trauma produced by right ventricular catheterization.

In the group without overt heart disease, RBBB is not an independent predictor of cardiovascular mortality.[44,47] However, the new onset of RBBB does predict a higher rate of coronary artery disease, congestive heart failure, and cardiovascular mortality. When cardiac disease is present, the coexistence of RBBB suggests advanced disease with, for example, more extensive multivessel disease and reduced long-term survival in patients with ischemic heart disease. An entity known as the Brugada syndrome[53] has been described, in which a RBBB-like pattern with persistent ST segment elevation in the right precordial leads is associated with susceptibility to ventricular tachyarrhythmias and sudden cardiac death (see Chaps. 9 and 35).

Right bundle branch block interferes with other electrocardiographic diagnoses, although to a lesser extent than LBBB. The diagnosis of RVH is more difficult to make with RBBB because of the accentuated positive potentials in lead V_1. RVH is suggested, although with limited accuracy, by the presence of an R wave in lead V_1 that exceeds 1.5 mV and a rightward shift of the mean QRS axis. The usual criteria for LVH can be applied but they have lower sensitivities than with normal conduction. The combination of left atrial abnormality or left axis deviation with RBBB also suggests underlying LVH.

Multifascicular Blocks

The term *multifascicular block* refers to conduction delay in more than one of the structural components of the specialized conduction system—that is, the left bundle branch, the left anterior and posterior fascicles of the left bundle branch, and the right bundle branch. Conduction delay in any two fascicles is called bifascicular block, and delay in all three fascicles is called trifascicular block. The term *bilateral bundle branch block* has been used to refer to concomitant conduction abnormalities in the left and right bundle branch systems.

Bifascicular block can have several forms. These include the following: (1) RBBB with LAFB, characterized by the electrocardiographic pattern of RBBB plus left axis deviation beyond −45 degrees (Fig. 12-28); (2) RBBB with LPFB, with an electrocardiographic pattern of RBBB and a mean QRS axis deviation to the right of +120 degrees (Fig. 12-29); and (3) LBBB alone that may be caused by delay in both the anterior and posterior fascicles. This form of LBBB represents one of the inadequacies of current electrocardiographic terminology and the simplification inherent in the trifascicular schema of the conduction system. The electrophysiological consequences of these abnormalities are discussed in Chapters 32 through 35.

Trifascicular block involves conduction delay in the right bundle branch plus delay in either the main left bundle branch or in both the left anterior and the left posterior fascicles. The resulting electrocardiographic pattern is dependent on (1) the relative degree of delay in the affected structures and (2) the shortest conduction time from the atria to the ventricles through any one part of the conducting system. Ventricular activation begins at the site of insertion of the branch with the fastest conduction time and spreads from there to the remainder of the ventricles. For example, if conduction in both the right and left bundle branches exists and the delay in the right bundle branch is less than the delay in the left bundle branch, activation will begin in the right ventricle and the QRS pattern will resemble that of LBBB. If the delay were greater in the right bundle branch than in the left bundle branch, the electrocardiographic pattern would be that of RBBB. The fascicle with the greatest delay can vary with, for example, the heart rate and lead to changing or alternating conduction patterns, as illustrated in Figure 12-30.

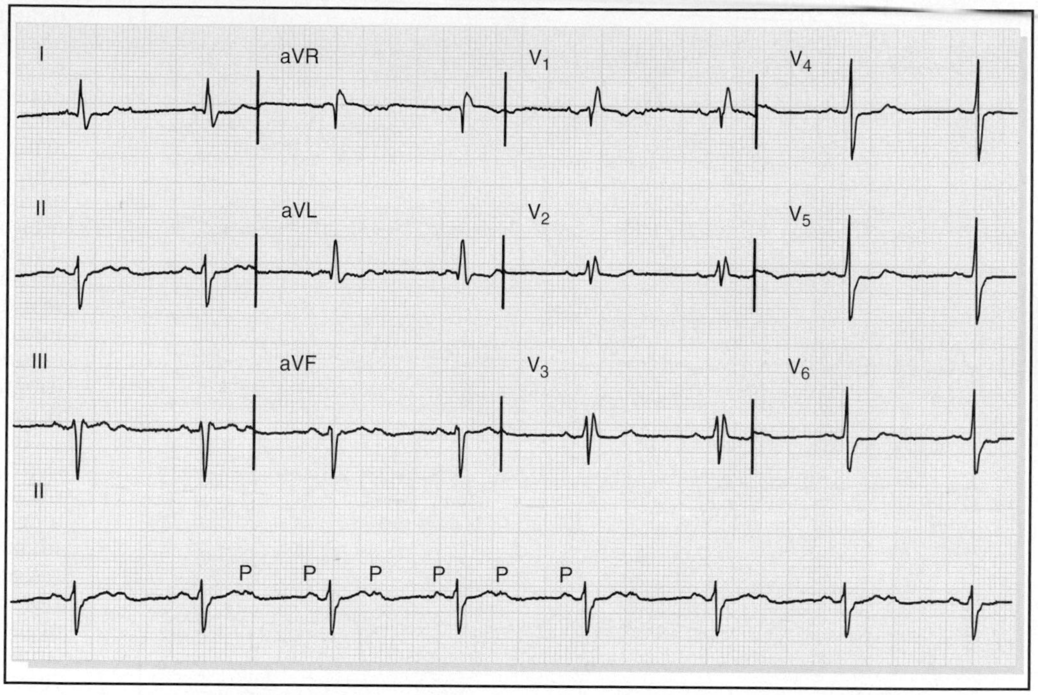

FIGURE 12–28 Sinus rhythm at 95 beats/min with 2:1 atrioventricular block. Conducted ventricular beats show a pattern consistent with bifascicular block with delay or block in the right bundle and left anterior fascicle. The patient underwent pacemaker implantation for presumed infrahisian block.

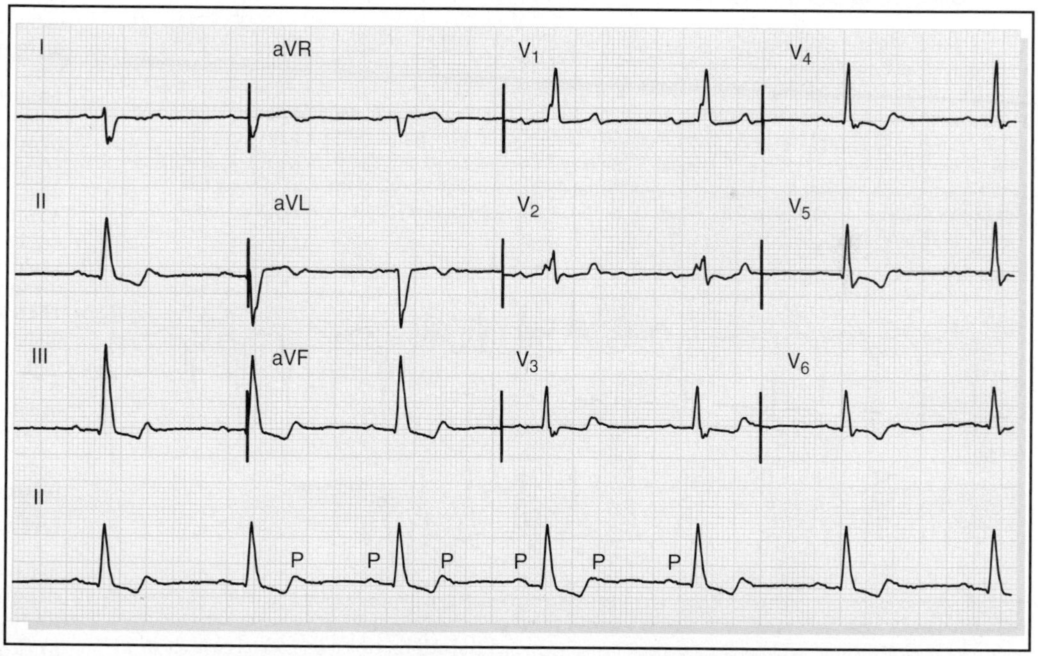

FIGURE 12–29 Sinus rhythm with a 2:1 atrioventricular block. QRS morphology in the conducted leads is consistent with bifascicular block with delay or block in the right bundle and left posterior fascicle. Subsequently, complete heart block was also noted. The patient underwent pacemaker implantation for presumed infrahisian block.

What distinguishes electrocardiographic patterns of trifascicular block from those of bifascicular block is an increase in the overall conduction time from the AV node to the ventricles. In bifascicular block, conduction time through the unaffected fascicle (and hence, overall conduction time) is normal in the absence of concomitant AV nodal conduction delay. In trifascicular block, however, the delay in conduction through even the least affected fascicle is abnormal and results in relative prolongation of the overall conduction time from the AV node to the ventricular myocardium. (Note that only delay, not block, of conduction is required. If block were present in all fascicles, conduction would fail and complete heart block would result. This situation is perhaps best illustrated by cases of alternating bundle branch block [see Fig. 12-30]; if the block were total in one bundle branch, development of block in the other would produce complete AV block rather than a change in bundle branch block patterns.) Thus, a diagnosis of trifascicular block requires an electrocardiographic pattern of bifascicular block *plus* evidence of prolonged conduction below the AV node.

This delay in conduction is most specifically observed as a prolongation of the His-ventricular (HV) time in intracardiac recordings. On the surface ECG, the delay in conduction delay may be manifested as a prolonged PR interval. However, the PR interval includes conduction time in the AV node as well as in the intraventricular conduction system. Prolonged intraventricular conduction may be insufficient to extend the PR interval beyond normal limits, whereas a prolonged PR interval can reflect delay in the AV node rather than in all three intraventricular fascicles. Thus, the finding of a prolonged PR interval in the presence of an electrocardiographic pattern of bifascicular block is not diagnostic of trifascicular block, whereas the presence of a normal PR interval does not exclude this finding (see Chap. 35).

The major clinical implication of a multifascicular block is its relation to advanced conduction system disease. It may be a marker for severe myocardial disease and may identify

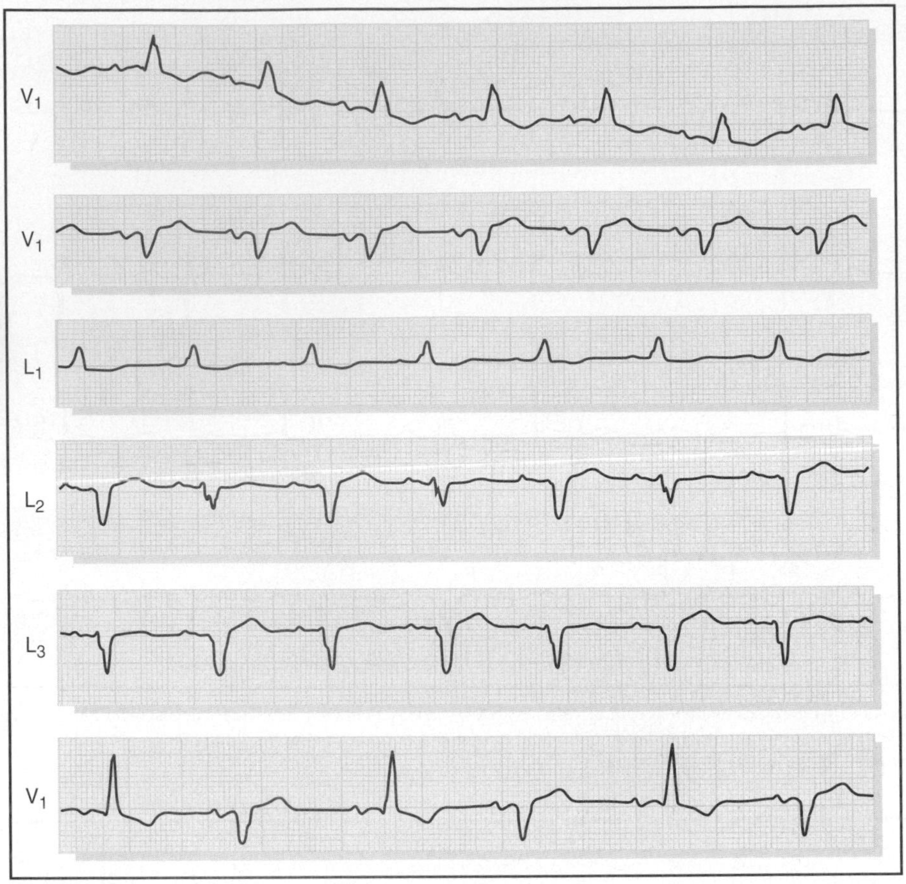

FIGURE 12–30 Multifascicular block manifested by alternating bundle branch blocks and PR intervals. **Top panel,** V_1 right bundle branch block (RBBB) with a PR interval of 280 milliseconds. **Middle panel,** V_1 left bundle branch block (LBBB) with a PR interval of 180 milliseconds. **Lower panel,** RBBB alternating with LBBB, along with alternation of the PR interval. The electrocardiographic records shown in leads I, II, and III (L_1 to L_3) exhibit left anterior fascicular block. An alternating bundle branch block of this type is consistent with trifascicular conduction delay. *(From Fisch C: Electrocardiography of Arrhythmias. Philadelphia, Lea & Febiger, 1990, p 433.)*

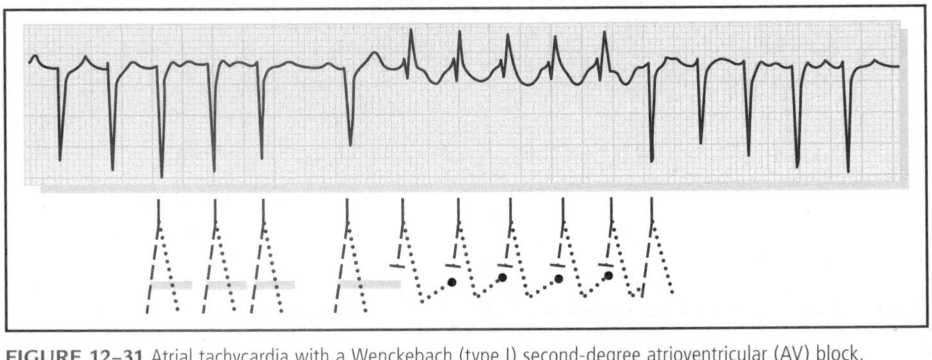

FIGURE 12–31 Atrial tachycardia with a Wenckebach (type I) second-degree atrioventricular (AV) block, ventricular aberration resulting from the Ashman phenomenon and probably concealed transseptal conduction. The long pause of the atrial tachycardia is followed by five QRS complexes with right bundle branch block (RBBB) morphology. The RBBB of the first QRS reflects the Ashman phenomenon. The aberration is perpetuated by concealed transseptal activation from the left bundle (LB) into the right bundle (RB), with block of anterograde conduction of the subsequent sinus impulse in the RB. Foreshortening of the R-R cycle, a manifestation of the Wenckebach structure, disturbs the relationship between transseptal and anterograde sinus conduction, and RB conduction is normalized. In the ladder diagram below the tracing, the solid lines represent the His bundle, the dashes represent the RB, the dots represent the LB, and the solid horizontal bars denote the refractory period. P waves and the AV node are not identified in the diagram. *(Courtesy of Dr. C. Fisch.)*

patients at risk for heart block (see Figs. 12-28 and 12-29), as discussed in Chapters 34 and 35.

Rate-Dependent Conduction Block (Aberration)

Intraventricular conduction delays can result from the effects of changes in the heart rate, as well as from fixed pathological lesions in the conduction system. Rate-dependent block or aberration can occur at relatively high or low heart rates. In acceleration (tachycardia)-dependent block, conduction delay occurs when the heart rate exceeds a critical value. At the cellular level, this aberration is the result of encroachment of the impulse on the relative refractory period (sometimes during phase 3 of the action potential) of the preceding impulse, which results in slower conduction. This form of rate-related block is relatively common and can have the electrocardiographic pattern of RBBB or LBBB (Figs. 12-31 and 12-32).

In deceleration (bradycardia)-dependent block, conduction delay occurs when the heart rate falls below a critical level. Although the mechanism is not clearly established, it may reflect abnormal phase 4 depolarization of cells, so that activation occurs at lower resting potentials. Deceleration-dependent block is less common than acceleration-dependent block and is usually seen only in patients with significant conduction system disease (Fig. 12-33).

Other mechanisms of ventricular aberration include concealed conduction (anterograde or retrograde) in the bundle branches (see Figs. 12-31 and 12-32; also see Chap. 35), premature excitation, depressed myocardial conduction as a result of drug effects or hyperkalemia (see Fig. 12-52, top), and the effect of changing cycle length on refractoriness (the Ashman phenomenon; see Chap. 32). The duration of the refractory period is a function of the immediately preceding cycle length: the longer the preceding cycle, the longer the subsequent refractory period. Therefore, abrupt prolongation of the immediately preceding cycle can result in aberration as part of a long cycle-short cycle sequence. These so-called Ashman beats usually have a RBBB morphology (see Fig. 12-31).

Myocardial Ischemia and Infarction

The ECG remains a key test in the diagnosis of acute and chronic coronary syndromes (see Chaps. 50, 53, and 54).[54-58] The findings vary considerably, depending importantly on four major factors: (1) the duration of the ischemic process (acute versus evolving or chronic); (2) its extent (large versus small); (3) its topography (anterior versus inferior-posterior and right ventricular); and (4) the presence of other underlying abnormalities (e.g., LBBB, Wolff-Parkinson-White pattern [see Chap. 35] or pacemaker patterns [see Chap. 34]) that can mask or alter the classic patterns.

Repolarization (ST-T Wave) Abnormalities

The earliest and most consistent electrocardiographic finding during acute ischemia is deviation of the ST segment

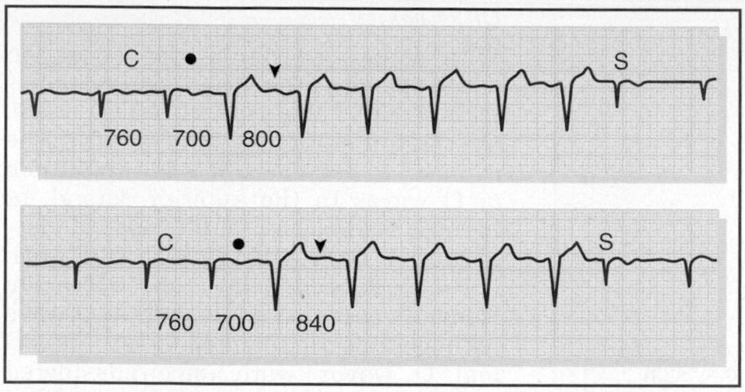

FIGURE 12–32 Acceleration-dependent QRS aberration with the paradox of persistence at a longer cycle and normalization at a shorter cycle than that which initiated the aberration. The duration of the basic cycle (C) is 760 milliseconds. Left bundle branch block (LBBB) appears at a cycle length of 700 milliseconds (dot) and is perpetuated at cycle lengths of 800 (arrowhead) and 840 (arrowhead) milliseconds; conduction normalizes after a cycle length of 600 milliseconds. Perpetuation of LBBB at a cycle length of 800 and 840 milliseconds is probably caused by transseptal concealment, similar to that described in Figure 12–31. Unexpected normalization of the QRS (S) following the atrial premature contraction is probably caused by equalization of conduction in the two bundles; however, supernormal conduction in the left bundle cannot be excluded. *(From Fisch C, Zipes DP, McHenry PL: Rate-dependent aberrancy. Circulation 48:714, 1973.)*

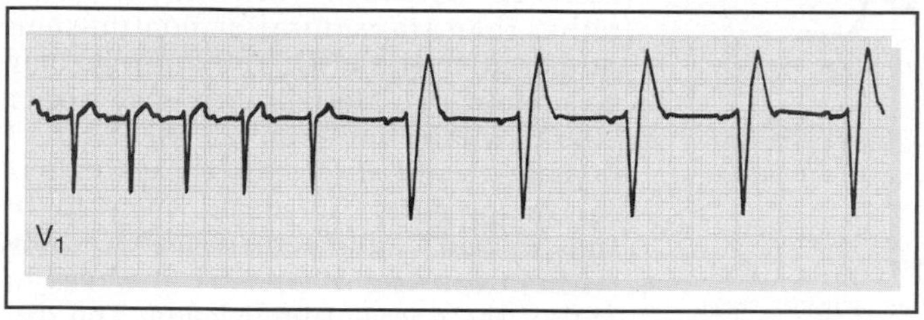

FIGURE 12–33 Deceleration-dependent aberration. The basic rhythm is sinus rhythm with a Wenckebach (type I) atrioventricular (AV) block. With 1:1 AV conduction, the QRS complexes are normal in duration; with a 2:1 AV block or after the longer pause of a Wenckebach sequence, left bundle branch block (LBBB) appears. Slow diastolic depolarization (phase 4) of the transmembrane action potential during the prolonged cycle is implicated as the cause of the LBBB. *(Courtesy of Dr. C. Fisch.)*

as a result of a current of injury mechanism. Under normal conditions, the ST segment is usually nearly isoelectric because virtually all healthy myocardial cells attain approximately the same potential during early repolarization—that is, during the plateau phase of the ventricular action potential.

Ischemia, however, has complex time-dependent effects on the electrical properties of myocardial cells. Severe acute ischemia can reduce the resting membrane potential, shorten the duration of the action potential in the ischemic area, and decrease the rate of rise and amplitude of phase 0 (Fig. 12-34). These changes cause a voltage gradient between normal and ischemic zones that leads to current flow between these regions. These currents of injury are represented on the surface ECG by deviation of the ST segment.

Both *diastolic* and *systolic injury currents* have been proposed to explain ischemic ST elevations (Fig. 12-35). According to the diastolic current of injury hypothesis, ischemic ST elevation is attributable to negative (downward) displacement of the electrical "diastolic" baseline (the TQ segment of the ECG). At least partly because of transmembrane leakage of intracellular potassium ions, ischemic cells may remain relatively depolarized during phase 4 of the ventricular action potential (i.e., lower membrane resting potential; see Fig. 12-34).[59] Depolarized muscle carries a negative extracellular charge relative to repolarized muscle. Therefore, during electrical diastole, current (the diastolic current of injury) will flow between the partly or completely depolarized ischemic myocardium and the neighboring, normally repolarized, uninjured myocardium. The injury current vector will be directed away from the more negative ischemic zone toward the more positive normal myocardium. As a result, leads overlying the ischemic zone will record a negative deflection during electrical diastole and produce depression of the TQ segment.

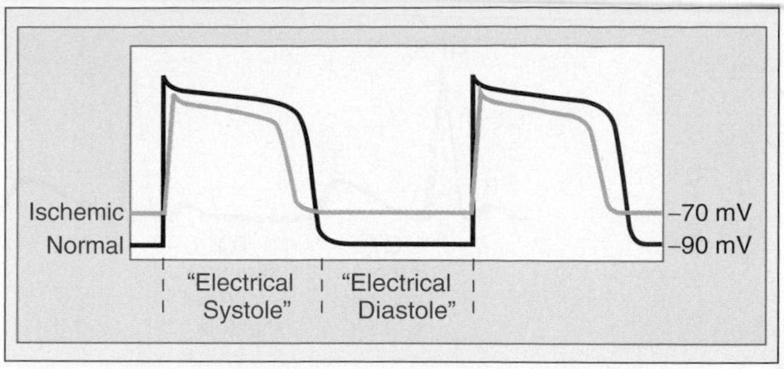

FIGURE 12–34 Acute ischemia may alter ventricular action potentials by inducing lower resting membrane potential, decreased amplitude and velocity of phase 0, and an abbreviated action potential duration (pathological early repolarization). These electrophysiological effects create a voltage gradient between ischemic and normal cells during different phases of the cardiac electrical cycle. The resulting currents of injury are reflected on the surface electrocardiogram by deviation of the ST segment (see Fig. 12-35).

TQ segment depression, in turn, appears as ST segment elevation because the electrocardiographic recorders in clinical practice use AC-coupled amplifiers that automatically "compensate" for any negative shift in the TQ segment. As a result of this electronic compensation, the ST segment will be proportionately elevated. Therefore, according to the diastolic current of injury theory, ST segment elevation represents an apparent shift. The true shift, observable only with DC-coupled electrocardiographic amplifiers, is the negative displacement of the TQ baseline.

Current evidence suggests that ischemic ST elevations (and hyperacute T waves) are also related to systolic injury currents. Three factors may make acutely ischemic myocardial cells relatively positive in comparison to normal cells with respect to their extracellular charge during electrical systole (QT interval): (1) pathological early repolarization (shortened action potential duration); (2) decreased action potential upstroke velocity; and (3) decreased action potential amplitude (see Fig. 12-34). The presence of one or more of these effects will establish a voltage gradient between normal and ischemic zones during the QT interval such that the current of injury vector will be directed toward the ischemic region. This systolic current of injury mechanism will result in primary ST elevation, sometimes with tall positive (hyperacute) T waves.

When acute ischemia is transmural (whether caused by diastolic or systolic injury currents, or both), the overall ST vector is usually shifted in the direction of the outer (epicardial) layers, and ST elevation and sometimes tall positive (hyperacute) T waves are produced over the ischemic zone (Fig. 12-36). Reciprocal ST depressions can appear in leads sensing the contralateral surface of the heart. Occasionally, the reciprocal changes can be more apparent than the primary ST elevations. When ischemia is confined primarily to the subendocardium, the overall ST vector typically shifts toward the inner ventricular layer and the ventricular cavity, such that the overlying (e.g., anterior precordial) leads show ST segment depression with ST elevation in lead aVR (see Fig. 12-36). This subendocardial ischemic pattern is the typical finding during spontaneous episodes of angina pectoris or during symptomatic or asymptomatic ("silent") ischemia induced by exercise or pharmacological stress tests (see Chap. 53).

Multiple factors can affect the amplitude of acute ischemic ST deviations. Profound ST elevation or depression in multiple leads usually indicates very severe ischemia. Conversely, prompt resolution of ST elevation following thrombolytic therapy or percutaneous coronary interventions[56,60]

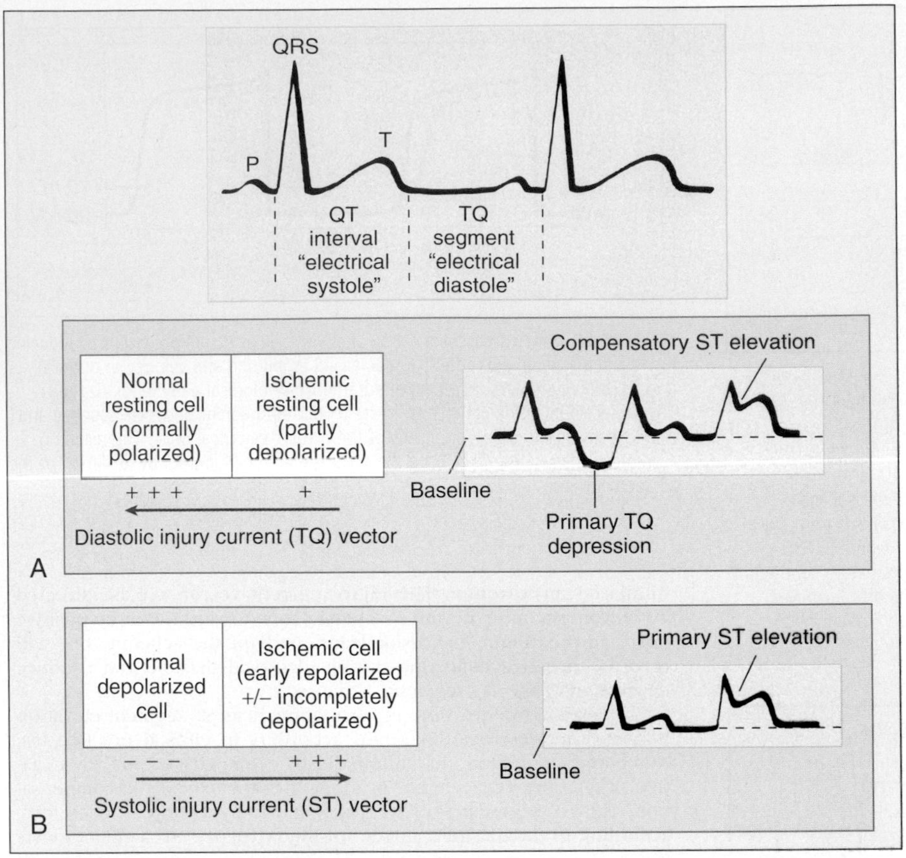

FIGURE 12–35 Pathophysiology of ischemic ST elevation. Two basic mechanisms have been advanced to explain the elevation seen with acute myocardial injury. **A,** Diastolic current of injury. In this case (first QRS-T complex), the ST vector will be directed away from the relatively negative, partly depolarized, ischemic region during electrical diastole (TQ interval), and the result will be primary TQ depression. Conventional alternating current electrocardiograms compensate for the baseline shift, and an apparent ST elevation (second QRS-T complex) results. **B,** Systolic current of injury. In this case, the ischemic zone will be relatively positive during electrical systole because the cells are repolarized early and the amplitude and upstroke velocity of their action potentials may be decreased. This injury current vector will be oriented toward the electropositive zone, and the result will be primary ST elevation. *(Modified from Goldberger AL: Myocardial Infarction: Electrocardiographic Differential Diagnosis. 4th ed. St. Louis, Mosby-Year Book, 1991, p 189.)*

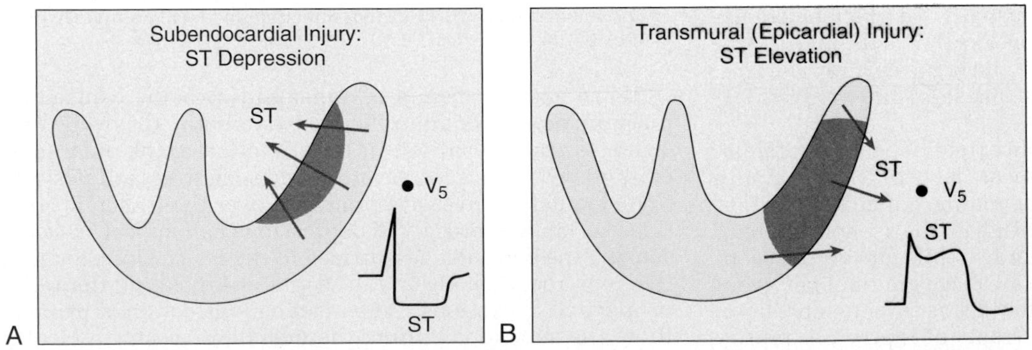

FIGURE 12–36 Current of injury patterns with acute ischemia. **A,** With predominant subendocardial ischemia the resultant ST vector is directed toward the inner layer of the affected ventricle and the ventricular cavity. Overlying leads therefore record ST depression. **B,** With ischemia involving the outer ventricular layer (transmural or epicardial injury), the ST vector is directed outward. Overlying leads record ST elevation. Reciprocal ST depression can appear in contralateral leads.

is a specific marker of successful reperfusion (see Chap. 55). These relationships are not universal, however, because severe ischemia or even infarction can occur with slight or even absent ST-T changes. Furthermore, a relative increase in T wave amplitude (hyperacute T waves) can accompany or precede the ST elevations as part of the injury current pattern attributable to ischemia with or without infarction (Fig. 12-37).

QRS Changes

With actual infarction, depolarization (QRS) changes often accompany repolarization (ST-T) abnormalities (Fig. 12-38). Necrosis of sufficient myocardial tissue can lead to decreased R wave amplitude or Q waves in the anterior, lateral, or inferior leads as a result of loss of electromotive forces in the infarcted area. Local conduction delays caused by acute ischemia can also contribute to Q wave pathogenesis in selected cases. Abnormal Q waves were once considered markers of transmural myocardial infarction, whereas subendocardial (nontransmural) infarcts were not thought to produce Q waves. However, careful experimental and clinical electrocardiographic-pathological correlative studies have indicated that transmural infarcts can occur without Q waves and that subendocardial infarcts can sometimes be associated with Q waves.[57,62] Accordingly, infarcts are better classified electrocardiographically as "Q wave" or "non-Q wave" rather than transmural or nontransmural based on the ECG. The findings may be somewhat different with posterior or lateral infarction (Fig. 12-39). Loss of depolarization forces in these regions can reciprocally increase R wave amplitude in lead V_1 and sometimes V_2, rarely without causing diagnostic Q waves in any of the conventional leads. The differential diagnosis of prominent right precordial R waves is given in Table 12-8.

Evolution of Electrocardiographic Changes

Ischemic ST elevation and hyperacute T wave changes occur as the earliest sign of acute infarction; these are typically followed within a period ranging from hours to days by evolving T wave inversion and sometimes Q waves in the same lead distribution (see Fig. 12-38). T wave inversion from evolving or chronic ischemia correlates with increased ventricular action potential duration, and these ischemic changes are often associated with QT prolongation. The T wave inversion can resolve after days or weeks or persist indefinitely. The extent of the infarct may be an important determinant of T wave evolution. In one series,[62] T waves that were persistently negative for more than 1 year in leads with Q waves were associated with a transmural infarction with fibrosis of the entire wall; in contrast, T waves that were positive in leads with Q waves correlated with nontransmural infarction with viable myocardium within the wall.

In the days to weeks or longer following infarction, the QRS changes can persist or begin to resolve.[63] Complete

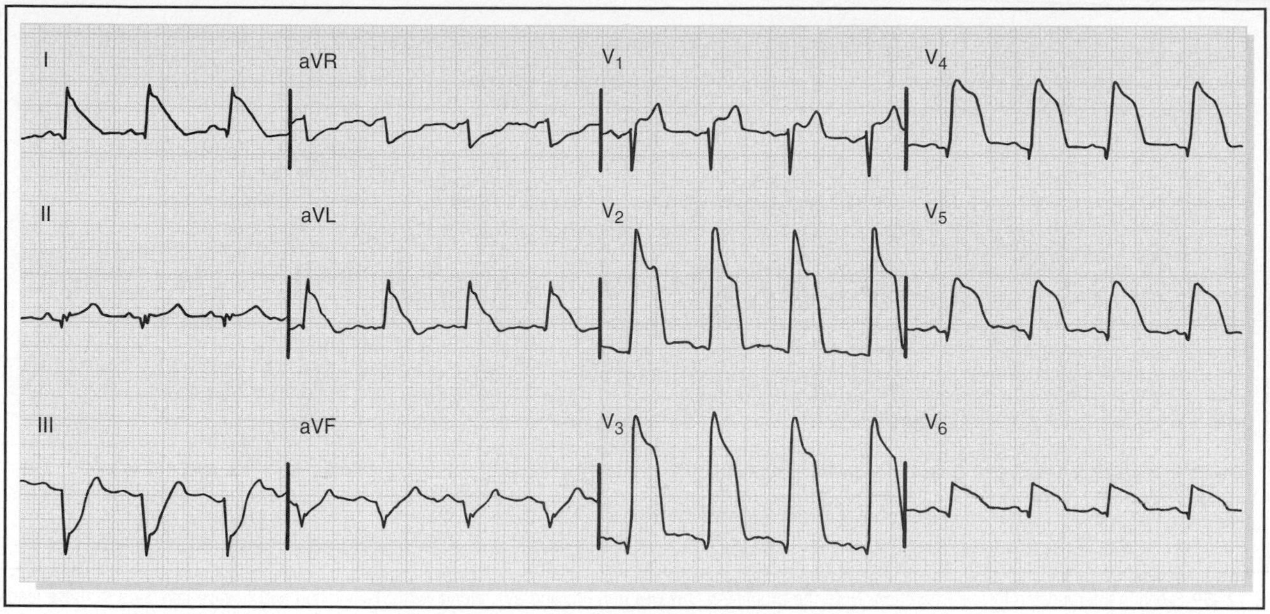

FIGURE 12–37 Hyperacute phase of extensive anterior-lateral myocardial infarction. Marked ST elevation melding with prominent T waves is present across the precordium, as well as in leads I and aVL. ST depression, consistent with a reciprocal change, is seen in leads III and aVF. Q waves are present in leads V_3 through V_6. Marked ST elevations with tall T waves caused by severe ischemia are sometimes referred to as a *monophasic* current of injury pattern. A paradoxical increase in R wave amplitude (V_2 and V_3) may accompany this pattern. This tracing also shows left axis deviation with small or absent inferior R waves, which raises the possibility of a prior inferior infarct.

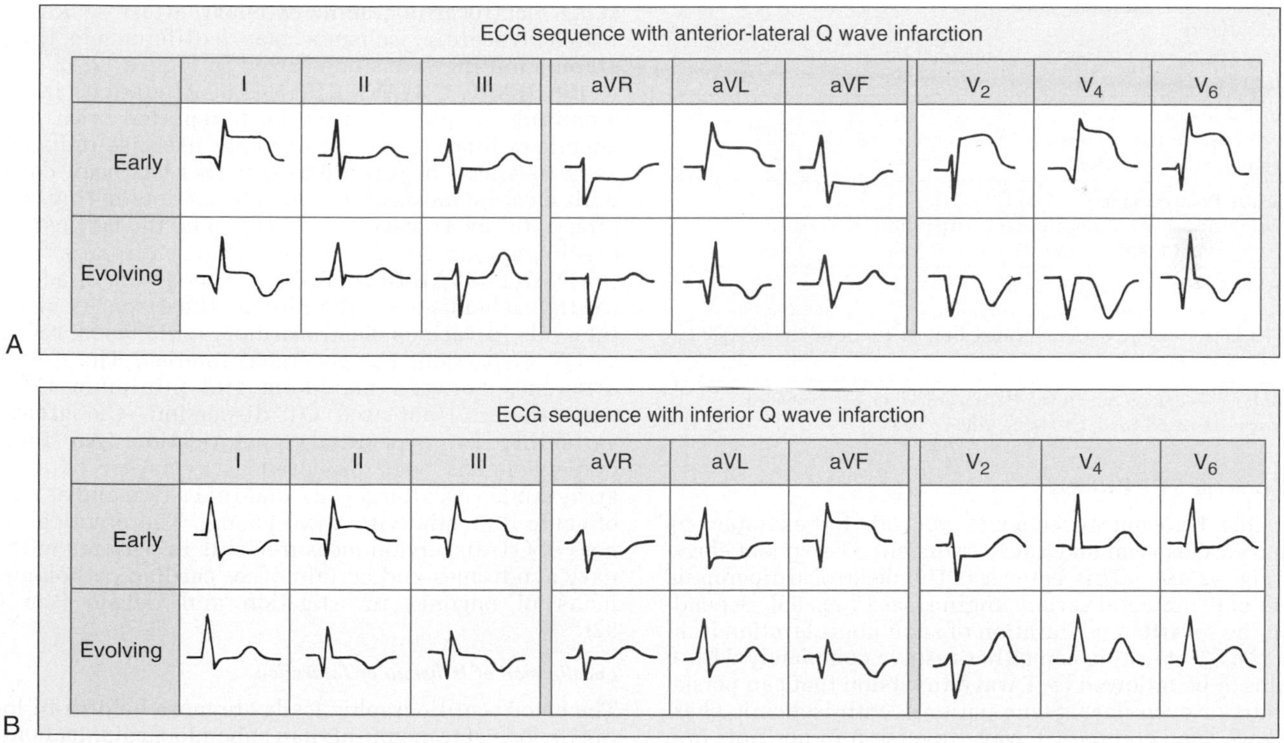

FIGURE 12–38 Sequence of depolarization and repolarization changes with **(A)** acute anterior-lateral and **(B)** acute inferior wall Q wave infarctions. With anterior-lateral infarcts, ST elevation in leads I, aV_l, and the precordial leads can be accompanied by reciprocal ST depression in leads II, III, and aV_f. Conversely, acute inferior (or posterior) infarcts can be associated with reciprocal ST depression in leads V_1 to V_3. *(Modified from Goldberger AL: Clinical Electrocardiography: A Simplified Approach. 7th ed. St. Louis, CV Mosby, 2006, p 90.)*

normalization of the ECG following Q wave infarction is uncommon but can occur, particularly with smaller infarcts and when the left ventricular ejection fraction and regional wall motion improve. This is usually associated with spontaneous recanalization or good collateral circulation and is a good prognostic sign. In contrast, persistent Q waves and ST elevation several weeks or more after an infarct correlate strongly with a severe underlying wall motion disorder (akinetic or dyskinetic zone), although not necessarily a frank ventricular aneurysm. The presence of an rSR′ or similar complex in the midleft chest leads or lead I is another reported marker of ventricular aneurysm.

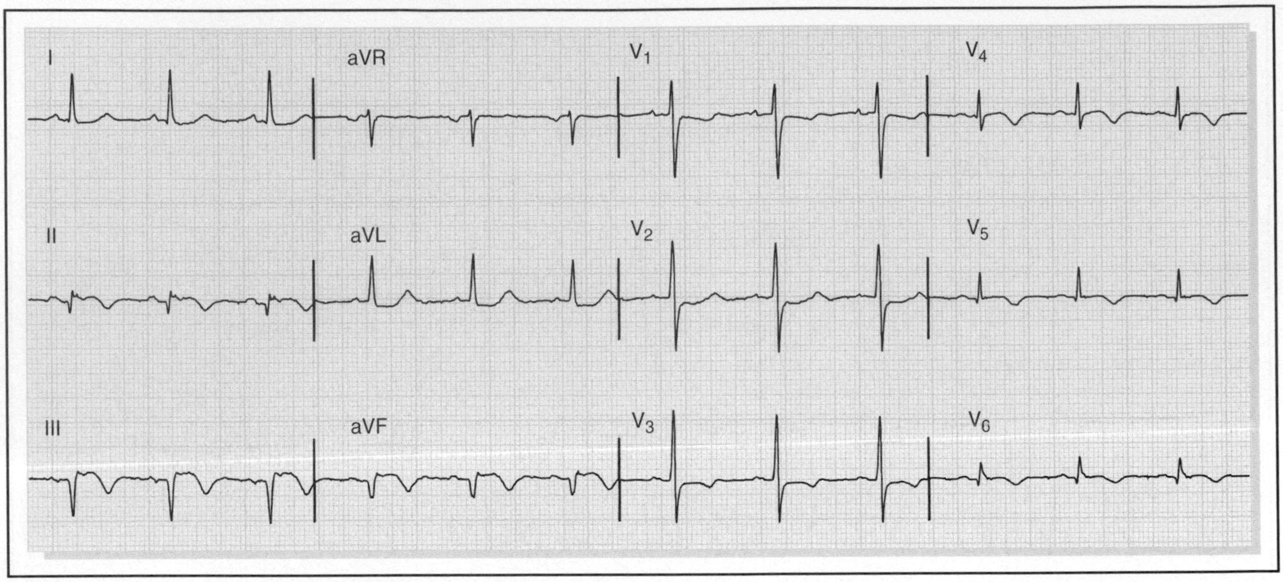

FIGURE 12–39 Evolving inferoposterolateral infarction. Note the prominent Q waves in II, III, and aVF, along with ST elevation and T wave inversion in these leads, as well as V_3 through V_6. ST depression in I, aVL, V_1, and V_2 is consistent with a reciprocal change. Relatively tall R waves are also present in V_1 and V_2.

TABLE 12–8	Differential Diagnosis of Tall R Waves in V_1/V_2
Physiological and Positional Factors Misplacement of chest leads Normal variants Displacement of heart toward right side of chest (dextroversion), congenital or acquired	
Myocardial Injury Posterior (and/or lateral) myocardial infarction (see Fig. 12-39) Duchenne muscular dystrophy	
Ventricular Enlargement Right ventricular hypertrophy (usually with right axis deviation) Hypertrophic cardiomyopathy	
Altered Ventricular Depolarization Right ventricular conduction abnormalities Wolff-Parkinson-White patterns (caused by posterior or lateral wall preexcitation)	

Modified from Goldberger AL: Clinical Electrocardiography: A Simplified Approach. 7th ed. St. Louis, CV Mosby, 2006, p 285.

Other Ischemic ST-T Patterns

Reversible transmural ischemia caused, for example, by coronary vasospasm may cause transient ST segment elevation (Fig. 12-40).[57] This pattern is the electrocardiographic marker of Prinzmetal variant angina (see Chap. 53). Depending on the severity and duration of such noninfarction ischemia, the ST elevation can either resolve completely within minutes or be followed by T wave inversion that can persist for hours or even days. Some patients with ischemic chest pain have deep coronary T wave inversion in multiple precordial leads (e.g., V_1 through V_4), with or without cardiac enzyme level elevations. This finding is typically caused by severe ischemia associated with a high-grade stenosis in the proximal left anterior descending (LAD) coronary artery system (LAD-T wave pattern). The T wave inversion can actually be preceded by a transient ST elevation that resolves by the time the patient arrives at the hospital. These T wave inversions, in the setting of unstable angina, can correlate with segmental hypokinesis of the anterior wall and suggest a "myocardial stunning" syndrome. The natural history of this syndrome is unfavorable, with a high incidence of recurrent angina and myocardial infarction. On the other hand, patients whose baseline ECG already shows abnormal T wave inversion can experience paradoxical T wave normalization (pseudonormalization) during episodes of acute transmural ischemia (Fig. 12-41). The four major classes of acute electrocardiographic-coronary artery syndromes in which myocardial ischemia leads to different electrocardiographic findings are summarized in Figure 12-42.

ISCHEMIC U WAVE CHANGES. Alterations in U wave amplitude or polarity have been reported with acute ischemia or infarction.[64] For example, exercise-induced transient inversion of precordial U waves has been correlated with severe stenosis of the left anterior descending coronary artery. Rarely, U wave inversion can be the earliest electrocardiographic sign of acute coronary syndromes.

QT INTERVAL DISPERSION. The effects of acute myocardial ischemia and infarction on the disparity among QT intervals in various electrocardiographic leads, referred to as QT dispersion, has generated interest. The greater the difference between maximum and minimum QT intervals—that is, increased QT dispersion—the greater the variability in myocardial repolarization. An increased dispersion has been proposed as a marker of increased arrhythmia risk after myocardial infarction and as a marker of acute ischemia with atrial pacing. The practical usefulness of QT dispersion measurements in patients with coronary syndromes and certain other cardiac pathologies is a focus of ongoing investigation and debate (see Chap. 32).[65-67]

Localization of Ischemia or Infarction

The electrocardiographic leads are more helpful in localizing regions of transmural than subendocardial ischemia. As examples, ST elevation and/or hyperacute T waves are seen in the following: (1) one or more of the precordial leads (V_1 through V_6) and in leads I and aVL with acute transmural anterior or anterolateral wall ischemia; (2) leads V_1 to V_3 with anteroseptal or apical[68] ischemia; (3) leads V_4 to V_6 with apical or lateral ischemia; (4) leads II, III, and aVF with inferior wall ischemia; and (5) right-sided precordial leads with right ventricular ischemia. Posterior wall infarction, which induces ST elevation in leads placed over the back of the heart such as leads V_7 to V_9,[5] can be induced by lesions in the right coronary artery or left circumflex artery. These lesions can produce both inferior and posterolateral injury, which may be indirectly recognized by reciprocal ST depression in leads V_1 to V_3. Similar ST changes can also be the primary electrocardiographic manifestation of anterior subendocardial ischemia. Posterior inferior wall infarction with reciprocal changes can be differentiated from primary anterior wall ischemia by the presence of ST segment elevations in posterior leads.

The ECG can also provide more specific information about the location of the occlusion within the coronary system (the culprit lesion).[58] In patients with an inferior wall myocardial infarction, the presence of ST segment elevation in lead III exceeding that in lead II, particularly when combined with ST elevation in V_1, is a useful predictor of occlusion in the proximal to midportion of the right coronary artery (Fig. 12-43). In contrast, the presence of ST segment elevation in lead II equal to or exceeding that in lead III, especially in concert with ST depression in leads V_1 to V_3 or ST elevation in leads I and aVL, strongly suggests occlusion of the left circumflex coronary artery or distal occlusion of a dominant right coronary artery. Right-sided ST elevation is indicative of acute right ventricular injury and usually indicates occlusion of the proximal right coronary artery. Of note is the finding that acute right ventricular infarction can project an injury current pattern in leads V_1 through V_3 or even V_4, thereby simulating anterior infarction. In other cases, simultaneous ST elevation in V_1 (V_2R) and ST depression in V_2 (V_1R) can occur (see Fig. 12-43). These and multiple other criteria proposed for localization of the site of coronary occlusion based on the initial ECG[58,69-72] require additional validation in test populations. Current and future criteria will always be subject to limitations and exceptions based on variations in coronary anatomy, the dynamic nature of acute electrocardiographic changes, the presence of multivessel involvement, and collateral flow.

For example, in some cases, ischemia can affect more than one region of the myocardium (e.g., inferolateral; see Fig. 12-38). Not uncommonly, the ECG will show the characteristic findings of

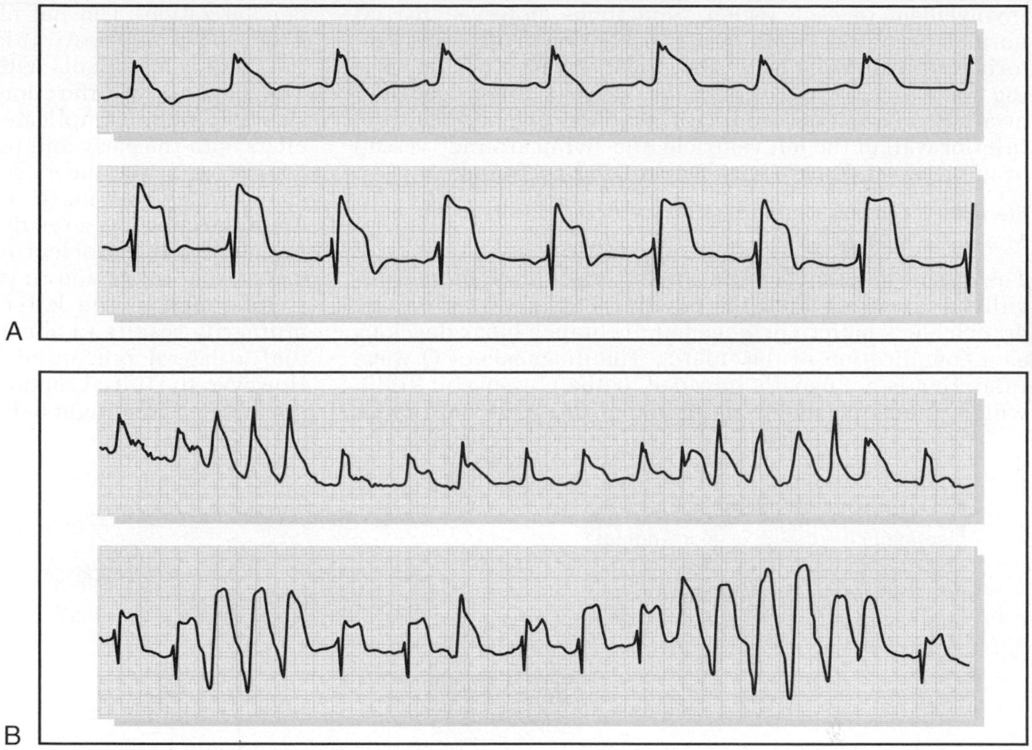

FIGURE 12–40 A, Prinzmetal angina with ST segment and T wave alternans. **B,** ST segment and T wave alternans associated with nonsustained ventricular tachycardia. *(Courtesy of Dr. C. Fisch.)*

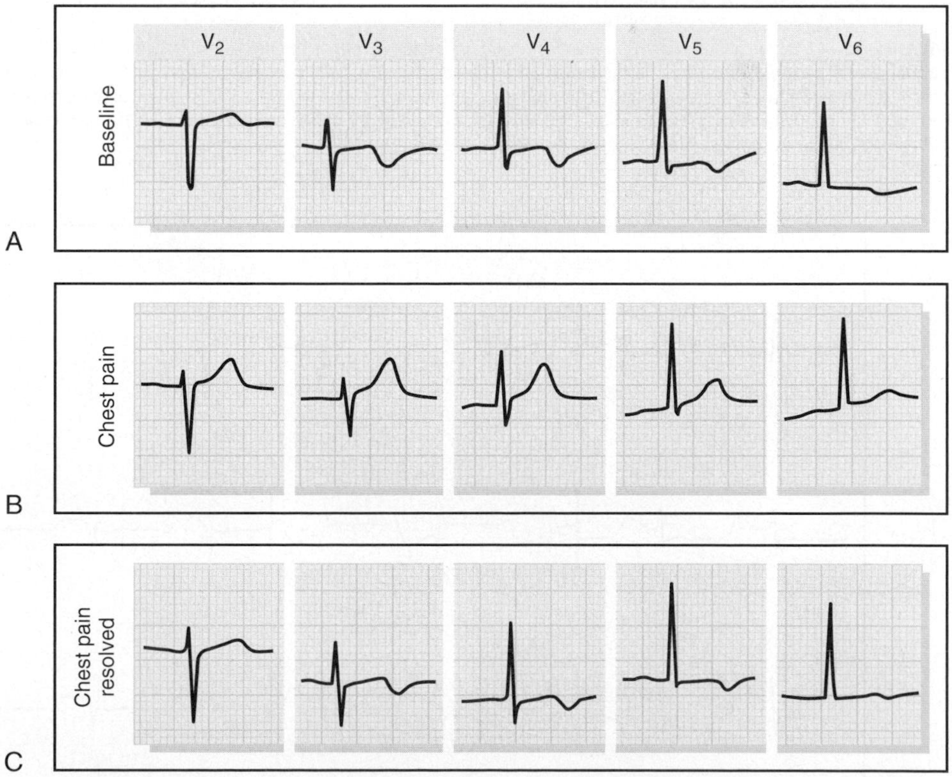

FIGURE 12–41 Pseudo (paradoxical) T wave normalization. **A,** The baseline electrocardiogram of a patient with coronary artery disease shows ischemic T wave inversion. **B,** T wave "normalization" during an episode of ischemic chest pain. **C,** Following resolution of the chest pain, the T waves have reverted to their baseline appearance. *(From Goldberger AL: Myocardial Infarction: Electrocardiographic Differential Diagnosis. 4th ed. St. Louis, Mosby-Year Book, 1991, p 330.)*

involvement in each region. Sometimes, however, partial normalization can result from cancellation of opposing vectorial forces. Inferior lead ST segment elevation accompanying acute anterior wall infarction suggests either occlusion of a left anterior descending artery that extends onto the inferior wall of the left ventricle (the "wrap around" vessel) or multivessel disease with jeopardized collaterals.

Electrocardiographic Diagnosis of Bundle Branch Blocks and Myocardial Infarction

The diagnosis of myocardial infarction is often more difficult in cases in which the baseline ECG shows a bundle branch block pattern or when bundle branch block develops as a complication of the infarct. The diagnosis of Q wave infarction is not usually impeded by the presence of RBBB, which affects primarily the terminal phase of ventricular depolarization. The net effect is that the criteria for the diagnosis of a Q wave infarct in a patient with RBBB are the same as in patients with normal conduction (Fig. 12-44). The diagnosis of infarction in the presence of LBBB is considerably more complicated and confusing, because LBBB alters both the early and late phases of ventricular depolarization and produces secondary ST-T changes. These changes may both mask and mimic the findings of myocardial infarction. As a result, considerable attention has been directed to the problem of diagnosing acute and chronic myocardial infarction in patients with LBBB (Fig. 12-45).[73]

Infarction of the left ventricular free (or lateral) wall ordinarily results in abnormal Q waves in the midprecordial to lateral precordial leads (and selected limb leads). However, the initial septal depolarization forces with LBBB are directed from right to left. These leftward forces produce an initial R wave in the midprecordial to lateral precordial leads, usually masking the loss of electrical potential (Q waves) caused by the infarction. Therefore, acute or chronic left ventricular free wall infarction by itself will not usually produce diagnostic Q waves in the presence of LBBB. Acute or chronic infarction involving both the free wall and the septum (or the septum itself) may produce abnormal Q waves (usually as part of QR-type complexes) in leads V_4 to V_6. These initial Q waves probably reflect posterior and superior forces from the spared basal portion of the septum (Fig. 12-46). Thus, a wide Q wave (40 milliseconds) in one or more of these leads

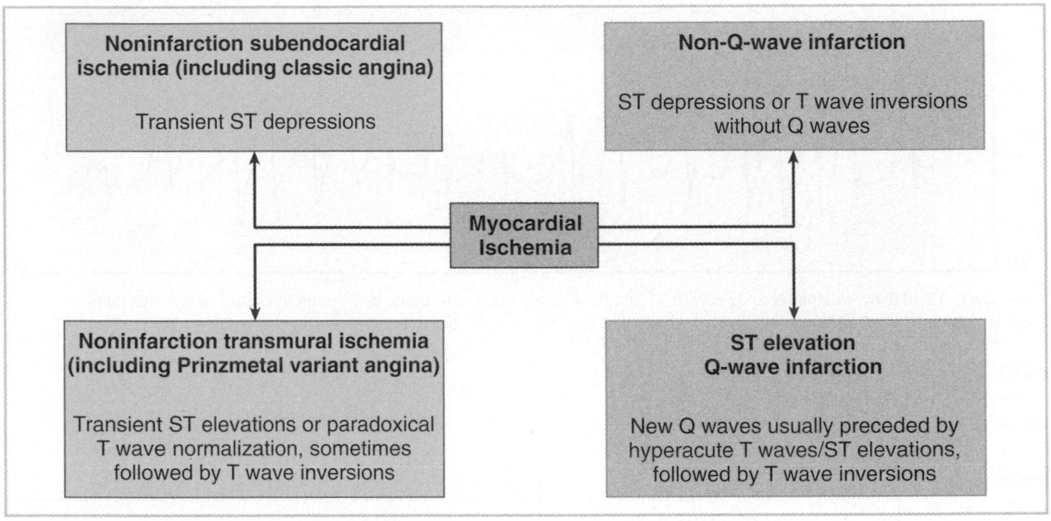

FIGURE 12–42 Variability of patterns in the electrocardiogram (ECG) with acute myocardial ischemia. The ECG may also be normal or nonspecifically abnormal. Furthermore, these categorizations are not mutually exclusive. For example, a non-Q-wave infarct can evolve into a Q wave infarct, ST elevation can be followed by a non-Q-wave infarct, or ST depression and T wave inversion can be followed by a Q wave infarct. *(Modified from Goldberger AL: Myocardial Infarction: Electrocardiographic Differential Diagnosis. 4th ed. St Louis, Mosby-Year Book, 1991, p 2.)*

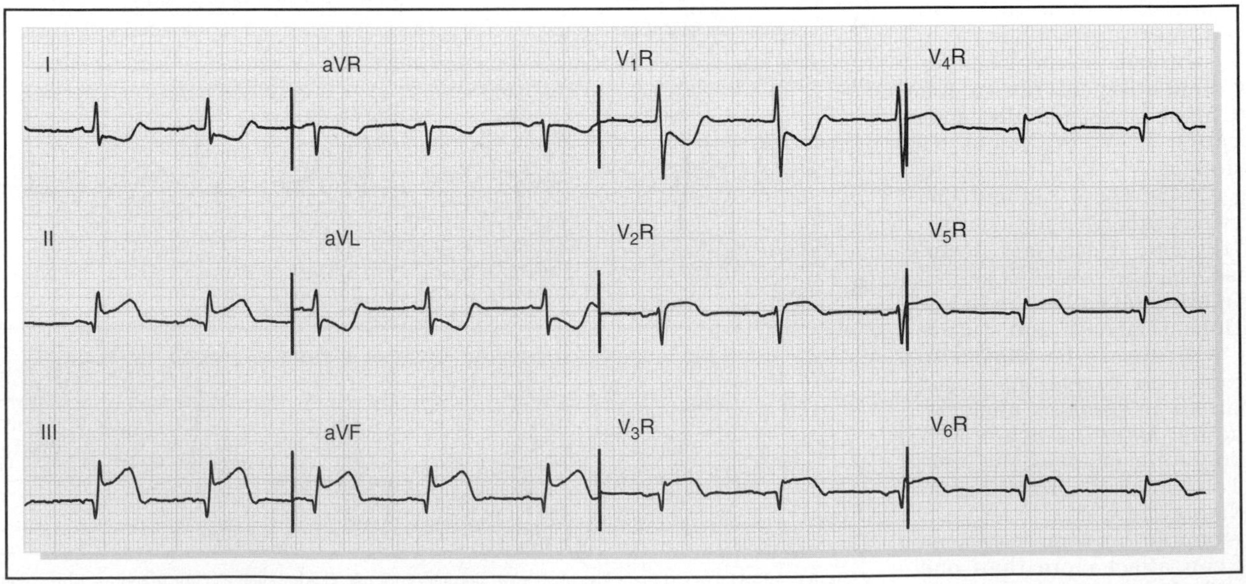

FIGURE 12–43 Acute right ventricular infarction with acute inferior wall infarction. Note the ST elevation in the right precordial leads, as well as in leads II, III, and aVF, with reciprocal change in I and aVL. ST elevation in lead III, greater than in lead II, and right precordial ST elevation are consistent with proximal to middle occlusion of the right coronary artery. The combination of ST elevation in conventional lead V_1 (lead V_2R here) and ST depression in lead V_2 (lead V_1R here) has also been reported with acute right ventricular ischemia or infarction.

is a reliable sign of underlying infarction. The sequence of repolarization is also altered in LBBB, with the ST segment and T wave vectors being directed opposite the QRS complex. These changes can mask or simulate the ST segment changes of actual ischemia.

The following points summarize the electrocardiographic signs of myocardial infarction in LBBB.

1. ST segment elevation with tall positive T waves are frequently seen in the right precordial leads with uncomplicated LBBB. Secondary T wave inversions are characteristically seen in the lateral precordial leads. However, the appearance of ST elevations in the lateral leads or ST depressions or deep T wave inversions in leads V_1 to V_3 strongly suggests underlying ischemia. More marked ST elevations (more than 0.5 mV) in leads with QS or rS waves may also be caused by acute ischemia, but false-positive findings occur, especially with large-amplitude negative QRS complexes.[6]
2. The presence of QR complexes in leads I, V_5, or V_6 or in II, III, and aVF with LBBB strongly suggests underlying infarction.
3. Chronic infarction is also suggested by notching of the ascending part of a wide S wave in the midprecordial leads (Cabrera sign) or the ascending limb of a wide R wave in I, aVL, V_5 or V_6 (Chapman sign). Similar principles can apply to the diagnosis of acute and chronic infarction in the presence of right ventricular pacing. Comparison between an ECG exhibiting the LBBB prior to the infarction and the present ECG is often helpful to show these changes.

The diagnosis of concomitant LAFB and inferior wall infarction can also pose challenges. This combination can result in loss of the small r waves in the inferior leads, so that leads II, III, and aVF show QS, not rS, complexes. LAFB, however, will occasionally hide the diagnosis of inferior wall infarction. The inferior orientation of the initial QRS forces caused by the fascicular block can mask inferior Q waves, with resultant rS complexes in leads II, III, and aVF. In other cases, the combination of LAFB and inferior wall infarction will produce qrS complexes in the inferior limb leads, with the initial q wave the result of the infarct and the minuscule r wave the result of the fascicular block.

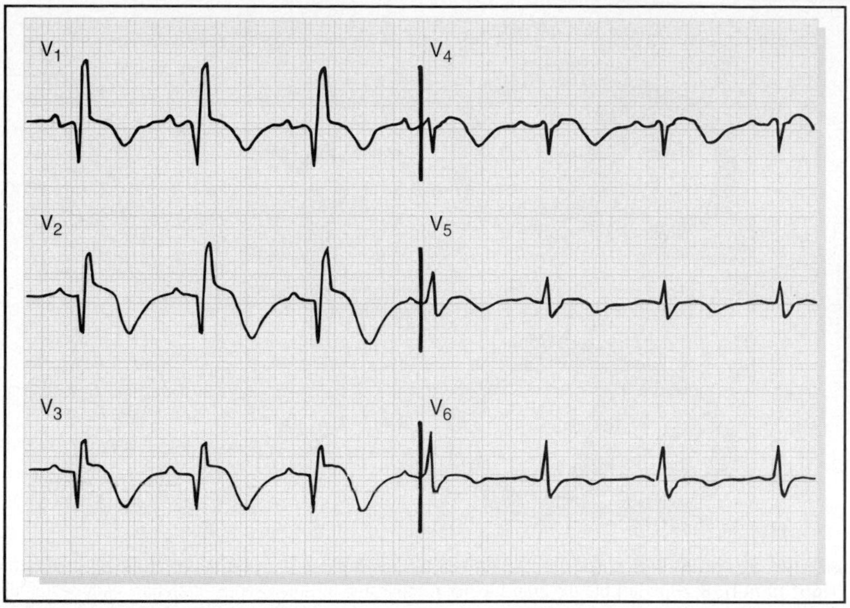

FIGURE 12–44 Right bundle branch block with acute anterior infarction. Loss of anterior depolarization forces results in QR-type complexes in the right precordial to midprecordial leads, with ST elevations and evolving T wave inversions (V_1 through V_6).

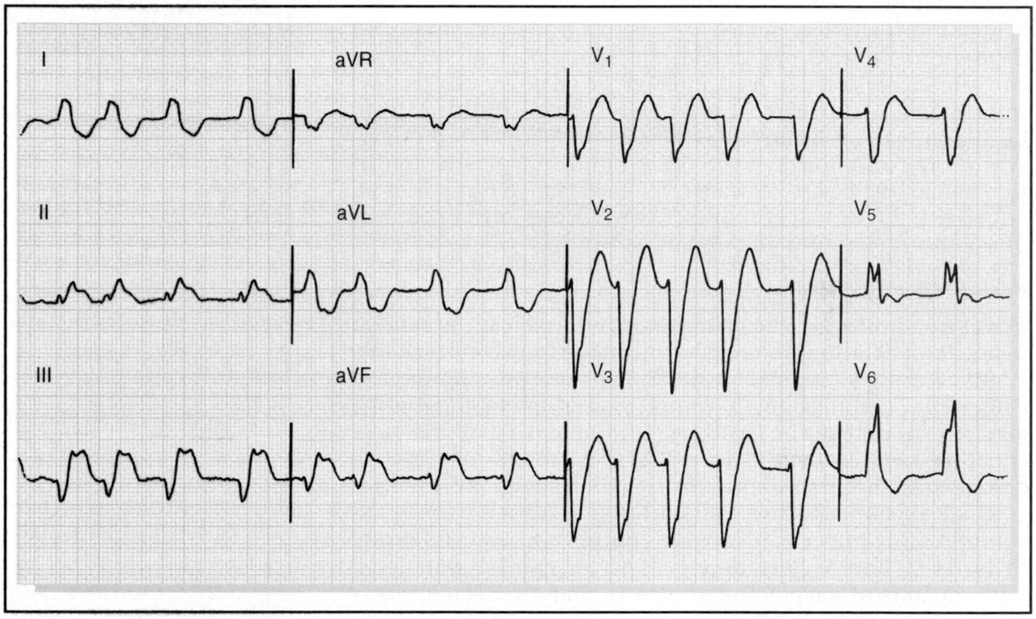

FIGURE 12–45 Complete left bundle branch block with acute inferior myocardial infarction. Note the prominent ST segment elevation in leads II, III, and aVF, with reciprocal ST segment depression in I and aVL superimposed on secondary ST-T changes. The underlying rhythm is atrial fibrillation.

Atrial Infarction

A number of electrocardiographic clues to the diagnosis of atrial infarction have been suggested, including localized deviations of the PR segment (e.g., PR elevation in V_5 or V_6 or the inferior leads[74,75]) changes in P wave morphology, and atrial arrhythmias. The sensitivity and specificity of these signs are limited, however. Diffuse PR segment changes, PR elevation in lead aVR with depression in the inferolateral leads with acute ventricular infarction usually indicate concomitant pericarditis (see later).

Electrocardiographic Differential Diagnosis of Ischemia and Infarction

The ECG has important limitations in both sensitivity and specificity in the diagnosis of coronary syndromes.[57] An initially normal ECG does not exclude ischemia or even acute infarction.[76] If the initial ECG is not diagnostic, but the patient remains symptomatic and there is high clinical suspicion for acute ischemia, it is recommended that the ECG be repeated at 5- to 10-minute intervals.[56] However, a normal ECG throughout the course of an alleged acute infarct is distinctly uncommon. As a result, prolonged chest pain without diagnostic electrocardiographic changes on repeat ECGs should always prompt a careful search for noncoronary causes of chest pain (see Chap. 49). Pathological Q

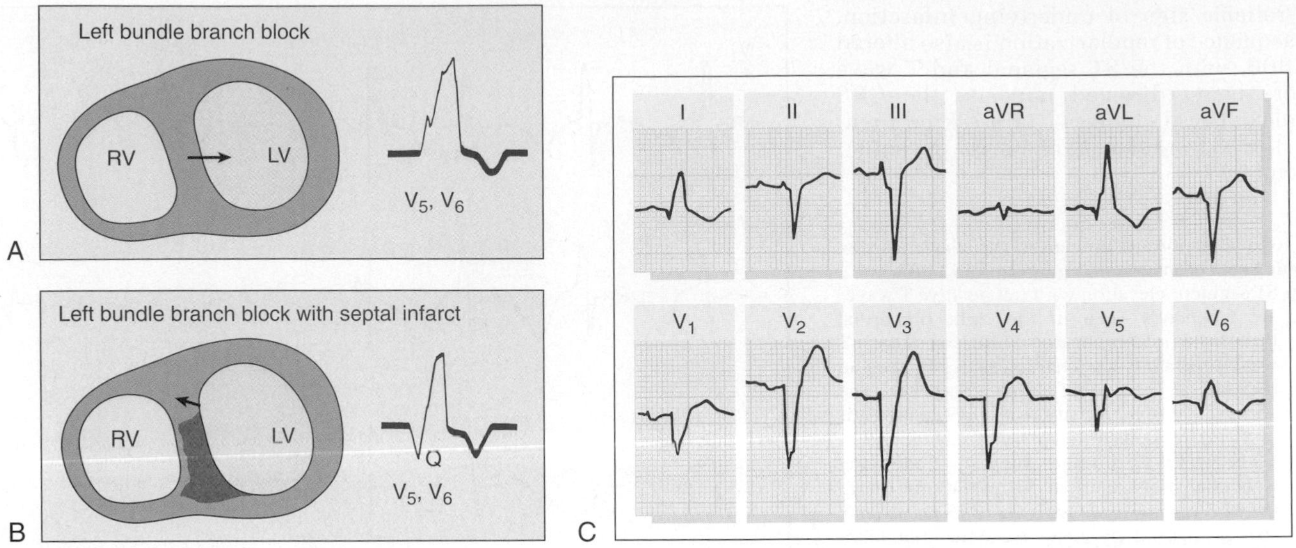

FIGURE 12–46 A, With uncomplicated left bundle branch block, early septal forces are directed to the left. Therefore, no Q waves will be seen in leads V_5 and V_6 **(right panel). B,** With left bundle branch block complicated by anteroseptal infarction, early septal forces can be directed posteriorly and rightward **(left panel).** Therefore, prominent Q waves may appear in V_5 and V_6 as a paradoxical marker of septal infarction **(right panel). C,** Anterior wall infarction (involving septum) with left bundle branch block. Note the presence of QR complexes in leads I, aVL, V_5, and V_6. ***(A and B** adapted from Dunn MI, Lipman BS: Lipman-Massie Clinical Electrocardiography. 8th ed. Chicago, Year Book, 1989, p 203.)*

waves can be absent even in patients with depressed left ventricular function caused by severe coronary disease and a previous infarct. As noted, the diagnosis of acute or chronic infarction can be completely masked by ventricular conduction disturbances, especially those resulting from LBBB, as well as ventricular pacing and Wolff-Parkinson-White preexcitation. On the other hand, diagnostic confusion can arise because Q waves, ST elevation, ST depression, tall positive T waves, and deep T wave inversion can be seen in a wide variety of noncoronary settings.

Noninfarction Q Waves

Q waves simulating coronary artery disease can be related to one (or a combination) of the following four factors (Table 12-9)[57]: (1) physiological or positional variants; (2) altered ventricular conduction; (3) ventricular enlargement; and (4) myocardial damage or replacement. Depending on the electrical axis, prominent Q waves (as part of QS- or QR-type complexes) can also appear in the limb leads (aVL with a vertical axis and III and aVF with a horizontal axis). A QS complex can appear in lead V_1 as a normal variant and rarely in leads V_1 and V_2. Prominent Q waves can be associated with various other positional factors that alter the orientation of the heart vis-à-vis a given lead axis. Poor R wave progression, sometimes with actual QS waves, can be the result solely of improper placement of chest electrodes above their usual position. In cases of dextrocardia, provided that no underlying structural abnormalities are present, normal R wave progression can be restored by recording leads V_2 to V_6 on the right side of the chest (with lead V_1 placed in the V_2 position; **see Chap. 61**). A rightward mediastinal shift in left pneumothorax can contribute to the apparent loss of left precordial R waves. Other positional factors associated with slow R wave progression include pectus excavatum, congenitally corrected transposition of the great vessels, and congenital absence of the left pericardium.

TABLE 12–9 Differential Diagnosis of Noninfarction Q Waves (with Selected Examples)

Physiological or Positional Factors
Normal variant "septal" Q waves
Normal variant Q waves in V_1 and V_2, III, and aVF
Left pneumothorax or dextrocardia: loss of lateral R wave progression
Myocardial Injury or Infiltration
Acute processes—myocardial ischemia without infarction, myocarditis, hyperkalemia (rare cause of transient Q waves)
Chronic myocardial processes—idiopathic cardiomyopathies, myocarditis, amyloid, tumor, sarcoid
Ventricular Hypertrophy/Enlargement
Left ventricular (slow R wave progression*)
Right ventricular (reversed R wave progression† or poor R wave progression, particularly with chronic obstructive lung disease)
Hypertrophic cardiomyopathy (can simulate anterior, inferior, posterior, or lateral infarcts; see Fig. 12-47)
Conduction Abnormalities
Left bundle branch block (slow R wave progression*)
Wolff-Parkinson-White patterns

*Small or absent R waves in the right precordial to midprecordial leads.

†Progressive decrease in R wave amplitude from V_1 to the midlateral precordial leads.

Modified from Goldberger AL: Clinical Electrocardiography: A Simplified Approach. 7th ed. St Louis, CV Mosby, 2006, p 285.

An intrinsic change in the sequence of ventricular depolarization can lead to pathological noninfarct Q waves. The two most important conduction disturbances associated with pseudoinfarct Q waves are LBBB and the Wolff-Parkinson-White (WPW) preexcitation patterns (see Chap. 35). With LBBB, QS complexes can appear in the right precordial to midprecordial leads and occasionally in one or more of leads II, III, and aVF. Depending on the location of the bypass tract, WPW preexcitation can mimic anteroseptal, lateral, or inferior-posterior infarction. LAFB is often cited as a cause of anteroseptal infarct patterns; however, LAFB usually has only minor effects on the QRS complex in horizontal plane leads. Probably the most common findings are relatively prominent S waves in leads V_5 and V_6. Slow R wave progression is not a consistent feature of LAFB, although minuscule q waves in leads V_1 to V_3 have been reported in this setting. These small q waves can become more apparent if the leads are recorded one interspace above their usual position and disappear in leads one interspace below their usual position. As a general clinical rule, however, prominent Q waves (as part of QS or QR complexes) in the right precordial to midprecordial leads should not be attributed to LAFB alone.

SLOW ("POOR") R WAVE PROGRESSION. In contrast, slow R wave progression, a nonspecific finding, is commonly observed with LVH and with acute or chronic right ventricular overload. Q waves in such settings can reflect various mechanisms, including a change in the balance of early ventricular depolarization forces and altered cardiac geometry and position. A marked loss of R wave voltage, sometimes with frank Q waves from V_1 to the lateral chest leads, can be seen with chronic obstructive pulmonary disease (see Fig. 12-23). The presence of low limb voltage and signs of right atrial abnormality ("P pulmonale") can serve as additional diagnostic clues. This loss of R wave progression may, in part, reflect right ventricular dilation. Furthermore, downward displacement of the heart in an emphysematous chest can play a major role in the genesis of poor R wave progression in this syndrome. Partial or complete normalization of R wave progression can be achieved in such cases simply by recording the chest leads an interspace lower than usual (see Fig. 12-23).

OTHER PSEUDOINFARCT PATTERNS IN VENTRICULAR OVERLOAD. Various pseudoinfarct patterns can occur with acute cor pulmonale caused by pulmonary embolism. Acute right ventricular overload in this setting can cause slow R wave progression and sometimes right precordial to midprecordial T wave inversion (formerly referred to as right ventricular "strain"), mimicking anterior ischemia or infarction. The classic $S_1Q_3T_3$ pattern can occur, but it is neither sensitive nor specific. A prominent Q wave (usually as part of a QR complex) can also occur in lead aVF along with this pattern (see Fig. 12-24). However, acute right overload by itself does not cause a pathological Q wave in lead II. Right heart overload, acute or chronic, may also be associated with a QR complex in lead V_1 and simulate anteroseptal infarction.

Pseudoinfarct patterns are an important finding in patients with hypertrophic cardiomyopathy, and the ECG can simulate anterior, inferior, posterior, or lateral infarction. The pathogenesis of depolarization abnormalities in this cardiomyopathy is not certain. Prominent inferolateral Q waves (II, III, aVF, and V_4 to V_6) and tall right precordial R waves are probably related to increased depolarization forces generated by the markedly hypertrophied septum (Fig. 12-47). Abnormal septal depolarization can also contribute to bizarre QRS complexes.

Q WAVE PATHOGENESIS WITH MYOCARDIAL DAMAGE. Loss of electromotive force associated with myocardial necrosis contributes to R wave loss and Q wave formation in cases of myocardial infarction. This mechanism of Q wave pathogenesis, however, is not specific for coronary artery disease with infarction. Any process, acute or chronic, that causes sufficient loss of regional electromotive potential can result in Q waves. For example, replacement of myocardial tissue by electrically inert material such as amyloid or tumor can cause noninfarction Q waves. Various dilated cardiomyopathies associated with extensive myocardial fibrosis can be characterized by pseudoinfarct patterns. Ventricular hypertrophy can also contribute to Q wave pathogenesis in this setting. Finally, Q waves caused by myocardial injury, whether ischemic or nonischemic in origin, can appear transiently and do not necessarily signify irreversible heart muscle damage. Severe ischemia can cause regional loss of electromotive potential without actual cell death ("electrical stunning" phenomenon). Transient conduction disturbances can also cause alterations in ventricular activation and result in noninfarctional Q waves. In some cases, transient Q waves may represent unmasking of a prior Q wave infarct. New but transient Q waves have been described in patients with severe hypotension from various causes, as well as with tachyarrhythmias, myocarditis, Prinzmetal angina, protracted hypoglycemia, phosphorus poisoning, and hyperkalemia.

FRAGMENTED QRS. Because Q waves are not always present and may regress or even disappear over time, alternative electrocardiographic markers of prior infarction are being evaluated, including a fragmented QRS complex (fQRS).[77] Regions of myocardial scar produce slow and disrupted activation; thus, the QRS morphology in leads overlying the scar may be altered, including the presence of RSR′-type waves or notching of the nadir of an S wave in two or more anatomically contiguous leads with QRS duration less than 120 milliseconds. Preliminary assessment in patients referred for evaluation of possible coronary artery disease has suggested that the visual detection of QRS fragmentation may enhance the sensitivity of conventional electrocardiographic criteria for prior myocardial infarction (MI) in selected groups, although the finding is not as specific as a pathological Q wave.[77] Further investigations in a wide range of populations are required both to confirm initially promising results of these findings and also to develop consistent, replicable definitions of QRS fragmentation.

ST-T Changes Simulating Ischemia

The differential diagnosis of ST segment elevation[54,57,78] includes acute pericarditis (see Chap. 70; Fig. 12-48), acute myocarditis (see Chap. 66), normal variant "early repolarization" (see Fig. 12-16), "Takotsubo" cardiomyopathy,[79] Brugada patterns[53] (see Chap. 9), and a number of other conditions listed in Table 12-10. Acute pericarditis, in contrast to acute myocardial infarction, typically induces diffuse ST segment elevation, usually in most of the chest leads and also in leads I, aVL, II, and aVF. Reciprocal ST depression is seen in lead aVR. An important clue to acute pericarditis, in addition to the diffuse nature of the ST elevation, is the frequent presence of PR segment elevation in lead aVR, with reciprocal PR segment depression in other leads, caused by a concomitant atrial current of injury (see Fig. 12-48). Abnormal Q waves do not occur with acute pericarditis, and the ST elevation may be followed by T wave inversion after a variable period. Acute myocarditis can, in some patients, exactly simulate the electrocardiographic pattern of acute myocardial infarction, including ST elevation and Q waves (see Chap. 66). These pseudoinfarct findings can be associated with a rapidly progressive course and increased mortality.

Takotsubo ("stress-induced") cardiomyopathy, also called transient left ventricular ballooning syndrome, is characterized by reversible wall motion abnormalities of the left ventricular apex and midventricle.[79] Patients, usually post-

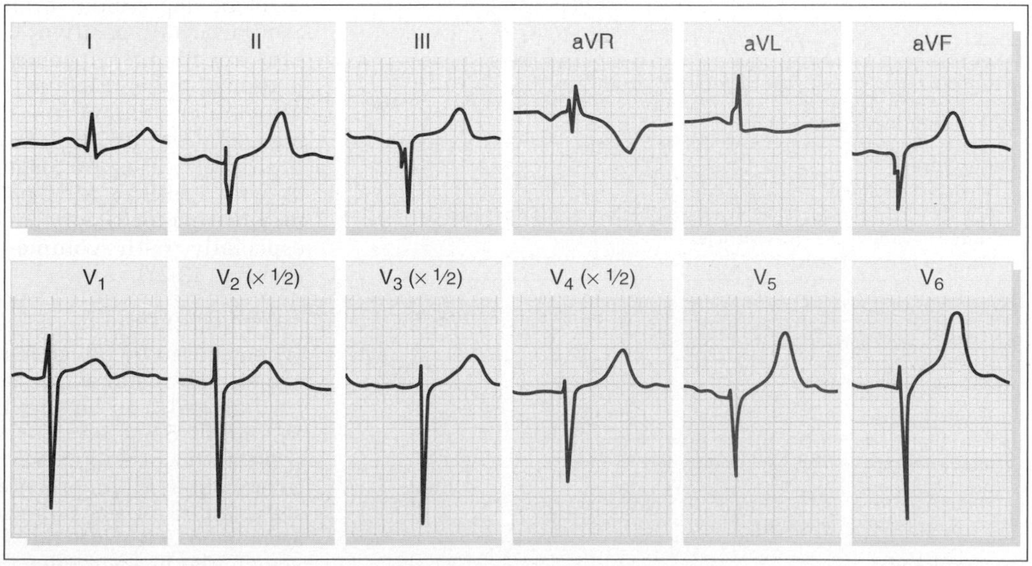

FIGURE 12–47 Hypertrophic cardiomyopathy simulating inferolateral infarction. This 11-year-old girl had a family history of hypertrophic cardiomyopathy. Note the W-shaped QS waves and the qrS complexes in the inferior and lateral precordial leads. *(From Goldberger AL: Myocardial Infarction: Electrocardiographic Differential Diagnosis. 4th ed. St. Louis, Mosby-Year Book, 1991, p 90.)*

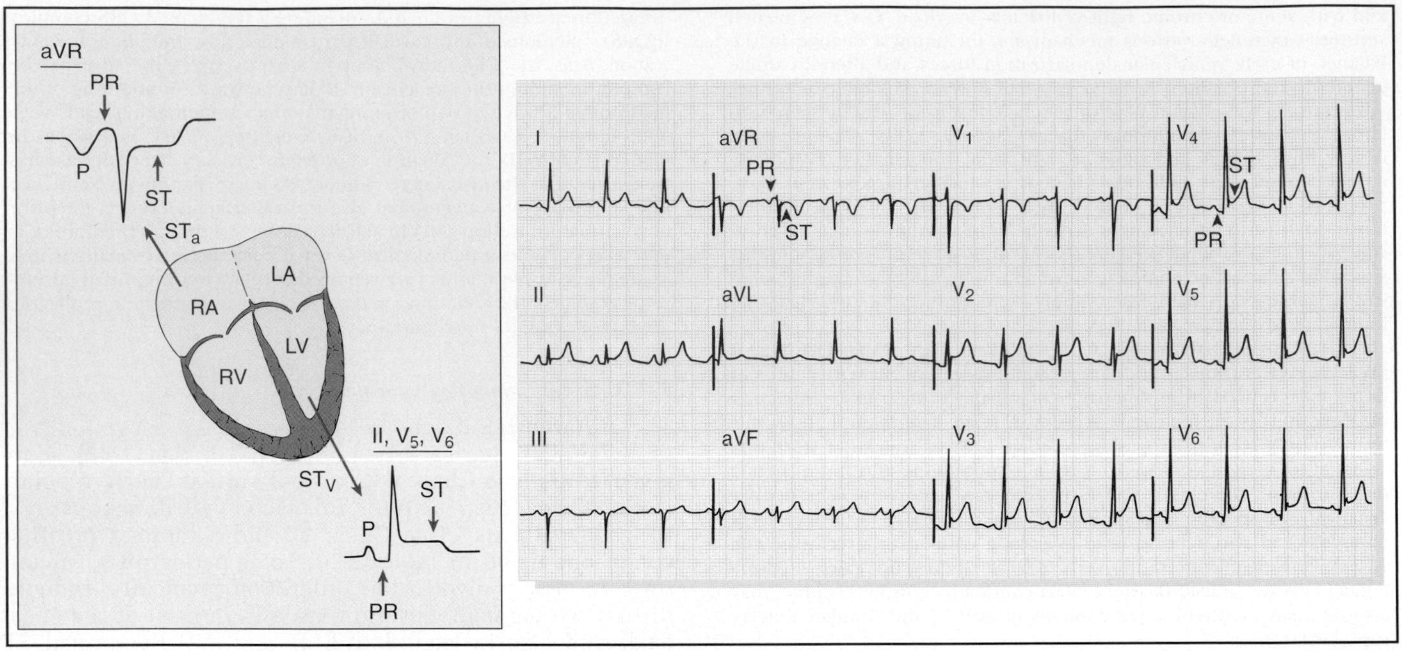

FIGURE 12–48 Acute pericarditis is often characterized by two apparent injury currents, one atrial, the other ventricular. The atrial injury current vector (ST_a) is usually directed upward and to the right and produces PR segment elevation in aVR with reciprocal PR depression in II, V_5, and V_6. The ventricular injury current (ST_V) is directed downward and to the left, associated with ST elevation in II, V_5, and V_6 with reciprocal ST depression in aVR. This characteristic PR-ST segment discordance is illustrated in the bottom-most tracing. Note the diffuse distribution of ST segment elevation in acute pericarditis (e.g., I, II, and V_2 through V_6, with reciprocal changes in aVR and perhaps minimally in V_1). Note the PR segment elevation in aV. LA = left atrium; LV = left ventricle; RA = right atrium; RV = right ventricle. *(From Goldberger AL: Myocardial Infarction: Electrocardiographic Differential Diagnosis. 4th ed. St. Louis, Mosby-Year Book, 1991.)*

TABLE 12–10	Differential Diagnosis of ST Segment Elevation
Myocardial ischemia or infarction	
Noninfarction, transmural ischemia (Prinzmetal angina pattern and possibly the Takotsubo syndrome; see Fig. 12-40)	
Acute myocardial infarction (see Fig. 12-37)	
Postmyocardial infarction (ventricular aneurysm pattern)	
Acute pericarditis (see Fig. 12-48)	
Normal variant ("early repolarization" pattern; see Fig. 12-16)	
LVH, LBBB (V_1-V_2 or V_3 only)	
Other (rarer) Myocardial injury Myocarditis (may look like myocardial infarction or pericarditis) Tumor invading the left ventricle Trauma to the ventricles	
Hypothermia (J wave, Osborn wave; see Fig. 12-53)	
After DC cardioversion	
Intracranial hemorrhage	
Hyperkalemia*	
Brugada pattern (RBBB-like pattern and ST elevations in right precordial leads)*	
Type 1C antiarrhythmic drugs*	
Hypercalcemia*	

*Usually most apparent in V_1 to V_2.

LBBB = left bundle branch block; LVH = left ventricular hypertrophy; RBBB = right bundle branch block.

Modified from Goldberger AL: Clinical Electrocardiography: A Simplified Approach. 7th ed. St Louis, CV Mosby, 2006, p 285.

menopausal women, present with chest pain, ST elevations, and elevated cardiac enzyme levels, exactly mimicking acute myocardial infarction. The syndrome is typically reported in the setting of emotional or physiological stress. Fixed epicardial coronary disease is absent. The exact pathophysiology is not known but may relate to coronary vasospasm or neurogenically mediated myocardial damage resulting in a transmural injury current pattern.

Various factors such as digitalis, ventricular hypertrophy, hypokalemia, and hyperventilation can cause ST segment depression mimicking subendocardial ischemia. Similarly, tall positive T waves do not invariably represent hyperacute ischemic changes but can reflect normal variants, hyperkalemia, cerebrovascular injury, and left ventricular volume loads resulting from mitral or aortic regurgitation, among other causes. ST elevation and tall positive T waves are also common findings in leads V_1 and V_2 with LBBB or LVH patterns. In addition, tall T waves may be seen occasionally in the left chest leads with LVH, especially with volume (diastolic) overload syndromes (see Fig. 12-21).

T Wave Inversion

When caused by physiological variants, T wave inversion is sometimes mistaken for ischemia. T waves in the right precordial leads can be slightly inverted, particularly in leads V_1 and V_2. Some adults show persistence of the juvenile T wave pattern (see Fig. 12-15), with more prominent T wave inversion in right precordial to midprecordial leads that show an rS or RS morphology. Such patterns, especially associated with left bundle branch block-type premature ventricular beats or relevant family history, also raise strong consideration of arrhythmogenic right ventricular dyplasia.[29,80] The other major normal variant that can be associated with notable T wave inversion is the early repolarization pattern (see Fig. 12-16). Some subjects with this variant have prominent, biphasic T wave inversion in association with the ST elevation. This pattern, which may simulate the initial stages of an evolving infarct, is most prevalent in young African American men and in athletes. These functional ST-T changes are probably caused by regional disparities in repolarization and can be normalized by exercise.

PRIMARY AND SECONDARY T WAVE INVERSIONS. Various pathological factors can alter repolarization and cause prominent T wave inversion (Fig. 12-49). As noted earlier, T wave alterations are usefully classified as primary or secondary. Primary T wave changes are caused by alterations in the duration or morphology of ventricular action potentials in the absence of changes in the activation sequence. Examples include ischemia, drug effects, and metabolic factors. Prominent primary T wave inversion (or, in some cases, tall positive T waves) is also a well-described feature of the ECG in cerebrovascular accidents, particularly with subarachnoid hemorrhage (see Chap. 58). The so-called cerebrovascular accident T wave pattern is characteristically diffuse, with a widely splayed appearance usually associated with marked QT prolongation (see Fig. 12-49). Some studies have implicated structural damage (myocytolysis) in the hearts of patients with such T wave changes, probably induced by excessive sympathetic stimulation mediated via the hypothalamus. A role for concomitant vagal activation in the pathogenesis of such T wave changes, which are usually associated with bradycardia, has also been postulated. Similar T wave changes have been reported after truncal vagotomy, radical neck dissection, and bilateral carotid endarterectomy. In addition, the massive diffuse T wave inversion seen in some patients after Stokes-Adams syncope may be related to a similar neurogenic mechanism. Patients with subarachnoid hemorrhage can also show transient ST elevation, as well as arrhythmias, including torsades de pointes. Ventricular dysfunction can even occur.

In contrast to these primary T wave abnormalities, secondary T wave changes are caused by altered ventricular activation, without changes in action potential characteristics. Examples include bundle branch block, Wolff-Parkinson-White preexcitation, and ventricular ectopic or paced beats. In addition, altered ventricular activation (associated with QRS interval prolongation) can induce persistent T wave changes that appear after normal ventricular depolarization has resumed. The term *cardiac memory T wave changes* has been used in this context to describe repolarization changes subsequent to depolarization changes caused by ventricular pacing, intermittent LBBB, intermittent Wolff-Parkinson-White preexcitation, and other alterations of ventricular activation (see Chap. 31).[81] Finally, the term *idiopathic global T wave inversion* has been used for cases in which no identifiable cause for often marked, diffuse repolarization abnormalities can be found. An unexplained female preponderance has been reported. Major causes of prominent T wave inversion are summarized in Table 12-11, with selected examples in Figure 12-49.

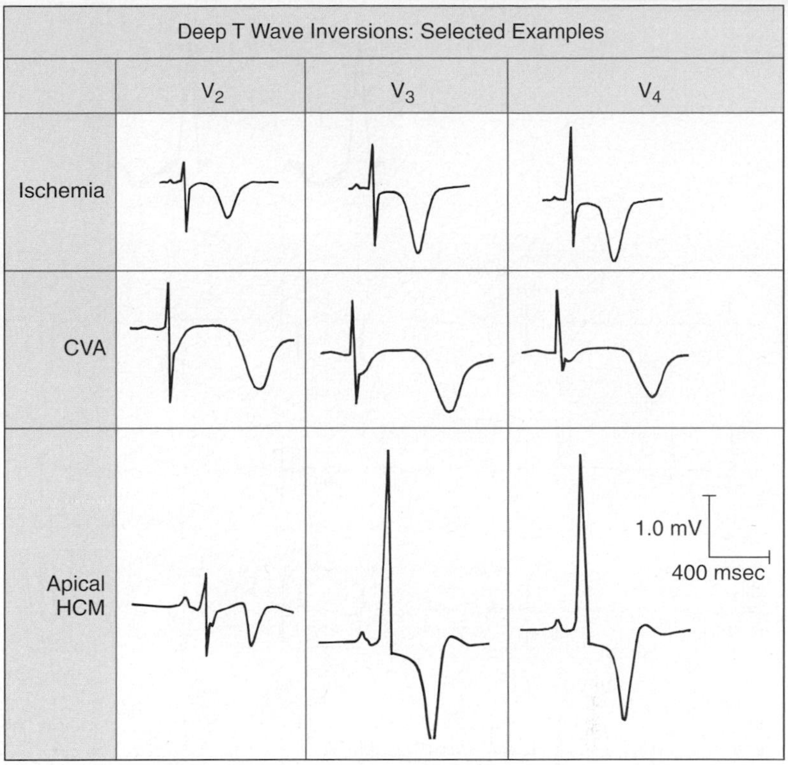

FIGURE 12–49 Deep T wave inversion can have various causes (see Table 12–11). Note the marked QT prolongation in conjunction with the cerebrovascular accident (CVA) T wave pattern caused here by subarachnoid hemorrhage. Apical hypertrophic cardiomyopathy (HCM) is another cause of deep T wave inversion that can be mistaken for coronary disease. *(From Goldberger AL: Deep T wave inversions. ACC Curr J Rev 5:28, 1996.)*

TABLE 12–11 Differential Diagnosis of Prominent T Wave Inversion

Normal variants Juvenile T wave pattern (see Fig. 12-15) Early repolarization variants (with ST elevation)
Myocardial ischemia or infarction (see Fig. 12-49)
Cardiomyopathies, including arrhythmogenic right ventricular dysplasia
Cerebrovascular accident (especially intracranial bleeding) and related neurogenic patterns (e.g., radical neck dissection, Stokes-Adams syndrome; see Fig. 12-49)
Left or right ventricular overload Classic left or right ventricular hypertrophy, enlargement repolarization abnormalities (formerly called "strain" patterns) Apical hypertrophic cardiomyopathy (Yamaguchi syndrome; see Fig. 12-49)
Post-tachycardia T wave pattern
Idiopathic global T wave inversion syndrome
Secondary T wave alterations—bundle branch blocks, Wolff-Parkinson-White patterns
Intermittent left bundle branch block, ventricular preexcitation, or ventricular pacing ("memory T waves")

Modified from Goldberger AL: Clinical Electrocardiography: A Simplified Approach. 7th ed. St Louis, CV Mosby, 2006, p 286.

Drug Effects

Numerous drugs can affect the ECG, often in association with nonspecific ST-T alterations.[54,55,81] More marked changes, as well as AV and intraventricular conduction disturbances, can occur with selected agents (see Chap. 33).

The digitalis effect[82] refers to the relatively distinctive "scooped" appearance of the ST-T complex and shortening of the QT interval, which correlates with abbreviation of the ventricular action potential duration (Fig. 12-50). Digitalis-related ST-T changes can be accentuated by an increased heart rate during exercise and result in false-positive stress test results (see Chap. 13). The digitalis effect can occur with therapeutic or toxic doses of the drug. The term *digitalis toxicity* refers specifically to systemic effects (e.g., nausea,

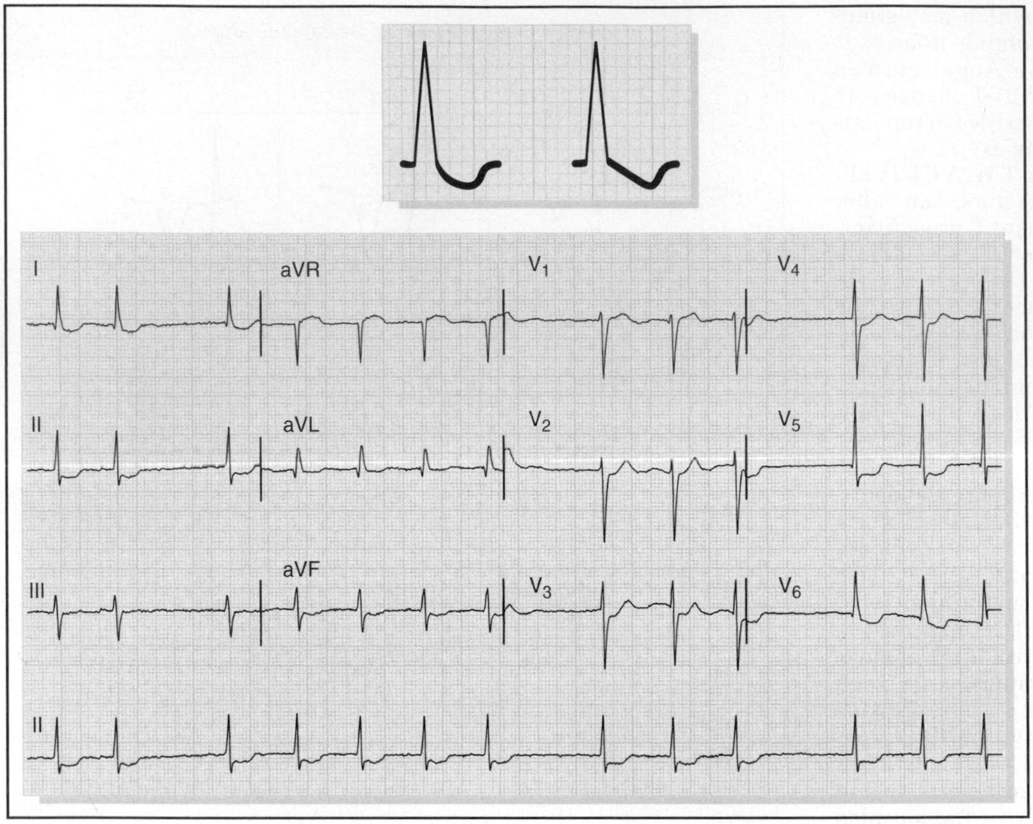

FIGURE 12–50 Top, Digitalis effect. Digitalis glycosides characteristically produce shortening of the QT interval with a "scooped" or downsloping ST-T complex. **Bottom,** Digitalis effect in combination with digitalis toxicity. The underlying rhythm is atrial fibrillation. A group-beating pattern of QRS complexes with shortening of the R-R intervals is consistent with nonparoxysmal junctional tachycardia with exit (atrioventricular Wenckebach) block. ST segment depression and scooping (V_6) are consistent with the digitalis effect, although ischemia or left ventricular hypertrophy cannot be excluded. Findings are strongly suggestive of digitalis excess; the serum digoxin level was greater than 3 ng/ml. Digitalis effect does not necessarily imply digitalis toxicity, however. *(Top from Goldberger AL: Clinical Electrocardiography: A Simplified Approach. 7th ed. St. Louis, CV Mosby, 2006, p 126.)*

anorexia) or conduction disturbances and arrhythmias caused by drug excess or increased sensitivity.

The electrocardiographic effects and toxicities of other cardioactive agents can be anticipated, in part, from ion channel effects (see Chap. 31). Inactivation of sodium channels by class 1 agents (e.g., quinidine, procainamide, disopyramide, flecainide) can cause QRS prolongation. Class 1A and 3 agents (e.g., amiodarone, dofetilide, ibutilide, sotalol) can induce an acquired long QT(U) syndrome (see Chap. 33). Psychotropic drugs (e.g., tricyclic antidepressants, phenothiazines), which have class 1A–like properties, can also lead to QRS and QT(U) prolongation. Toxicity can produce asystole or torsades de pointes. Right axis shift of the terminal 40-millisecond frontal plane QRS axis may be a helpful additional marker of tricyclic antidepressant overdose.

Electrolyte and Metabolic Abnormalities

In addition to the structural and functional cardiac conditions already discussed, numerous systemic metabolic aberrations affect the ECG, including electrolyte abnormalities, acid-base disorders, and systemic hypothermia.[54,55]

CALCIUM. Hypercalcemia and hypocalcemia predominantly alter the action potential duration. An increased extracellular calcium concentration shortens the ventricular action potential duration by shortening phase 2 of the action potential. In contrast, hypocalcemia prolongs phase 2 of the action potential. These cellular changes correlate with abbreviation and prolongation of the QT interval (ST segment portion) with hypercalcemia and hypocalcemia, respectively (Fig. 12-51). Severe hypercalcemia (e.g., serum Ca^{2+} concentration more than 15 mg/dl) can also be associated with decreased T wave amplitude, sometimes with T wave notching or inversion. Hypercalcemia sometimes produces a high takeoff of the ST segment in leads V_1 and V_2 and can thus simulate acute ischemia (see Table 12-10).

POTASSIUM. Hyperkalemia is associated with a distinctive sequence of electrocardiographic changes (Fig. 12-52A). The earliest effect is usually narrowing and peaking (tenting) of the T wave. The QT interval is shortened at this stage, associated with decreased action potential duration. Progressive extracellular hyperkalemia reduces atrial and ventricular resting membrane potentials, thereby inactivating sodium channels, which decreases V_{max} and conduction velocity. The QRS begins to widen and P wave amplitude decreases. PR interval prolongation can occur, followed sometimes by second- or third-degree AV block. Complete loss of P waves may be associated with a junctional escape rhythm or with a so-called sinoventricular rhythm. In the latter instance, sinus rhythm persists with conduction between the SA and AV nodes but occurs without producing an overt P wave. Moderate to severe hyperkalemia occasionally induces ST elevations in the right precordial leads (V_1 and V_2) and simulates an ischemic current of injury or Brugada-type patterns.[53] However, even severe hyperkalemia can be associated with atypical or nondiagnostic electrocardiographic findings. Very marked hyperkalemia leads to eventual asystole, sometimes preceded by a slow undulatory (sine wave) ventricular flutter-like pattern. The triad of (1) peaked T waves (from hyperkalemia), (2) QT prolongation (from hypocalcemia), and (3) LVH (from hypertension) is strongly suggestive of chronic renal failure (see Chap. 88).[53]

The electrophysiological changes associated with hypokalemia, in contrast, include hyperpolarization of myocardial cell membranes and increased action potential duration. The major electrocardiographic manifestations are ST depression with flattened T waves and increased U wave prominence (see Fig. 12-52B). The U waves can exceed the amplitude of T waves. Clinically, distinguishing T waves from U waves can be difficult or impossible from the surface ECG. Indeed, apparent U waves in hypokalemia and other pathological settings may actually be part of T waves whose morphology is altered by the effects of voltage gradients between M, or midmyocardial, cells and adjacent myocardial layers.[83] The prolongation of repolarization with hypokalemia, as part of an acquired long QT(U) syndrome, predisposes to torsades de pointes. Hypokalemia also predisposes to tachyarrhythmias from digitalis.

MAGNESIUM. Specific electrocardiographic effects of mild to moderate isolated abnormalities in magnesium ion concentration are not well characterized. Severe hypermagnesemia can cause AV and intraventricular conduction disturbances that may culminate in complete heart block and cardiac arrest (Mg^{2+} more than 15 mEq/liter). Hypomagnesemia is usually associated with hypocalcemia or hypokalemia. Hypomagnesemia can potentiate certain digitalis toxic arrhythmias. The role of magnesium deficiency in the pathogenesis and treatment of the acquired long QT(U) syndrome with torsades de pointes is discussed in Chapters 33 and 35.

OTHER FACTORS. Isolated hypernatremia or hyponatremia does not produce consistent effects on the ECG. Acidemia and alkalemia are often associated with hyperkalemia and hypokalemia, respectively. Systemic hypothermia may be associated with the appearance of a distinctive convex elevation at the junction (J point) of the ST segment and QRS complex (J wave or Osborn wave) (Fig. 12-53). The cellular mechanism of this type of pathological J wave appears to be related to an epicardial-endocardial voltage gradient associated with the localized appearance of a prominent epicardial action potential notch.

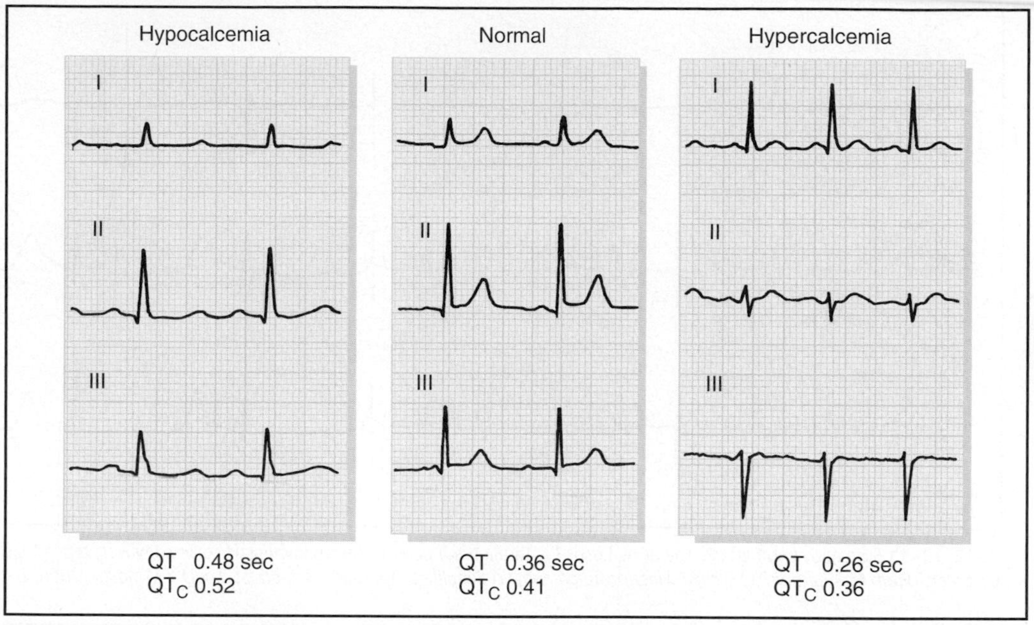

FIGURE 12–51 Prolongation of the QT interval (ST segment portion) is typical of hypocalcemia. Hypercalcemia may cause abbreviation of the ST segment and shortening of the QT interval. *(From Goldberger AL: Clinical Electrocardiography: A Simplified Approach. 7th ed. St. Louis, CV Mosby, 2006, p 133.)*

Nonspecific QRS and ST-T Changes

Low QRS voltage is said to be present when the total amplitude of the QRS complexes is 0.5 mV or less in each of the six extremity leads or 1.0 mV or less in leads V_1 through V_6. Low QRS voltage can relate to various mechanisms (Table 12-12), including the following: increased insulation of the heart by air (chronic obstructive pulmonary disease) or adipose tissue (obesity); replacement of myocardium—for example, by fibrous tissue (ischemic or nonischemic cardiomyopathy), amyloid, or tumor (see Chap. 69); or short-circuiting (shunting) effects caused by low resistance fluids (especially with pericardial or pleural effusions, or anasarca). The combination of relatively low limb voltage (QRS voltage less than 0.8 mV in each of the limb leads), relatively prominent QRS voltage in the chest leads (SV_1 or $SV_2 + RV_5$, or RV_6 more than 3.5 mV), and slow R wave progression (R wave less than the S wave in V_1 through V_4) has been reported as a relatively specific but not sensitive sign of dilated-type cardiomyopathies ("ECG–congestive heart failure triad").[54]

Many factors in addition to ischemia (e.g., postural changes, meals, drugs, hypertrophy, electrolyte and metabolic disorders, central nervous system lesions, infections, and pulmonary diseases) can affect the ECG. Ventricular repolarization is particularly sensitive to these effects, and can lead to various nonspecific ST-T changes. The term is usually applied to slight ST depression or T wave inversion, or to T wave flattening without evident cause. Care must be taken not to overinterpret such changes, especially in subjects with a low prior probability of heart disease. At the same time, subtle repolarization abnormalities can be markers of coronary or hypertensive heart disease or other types of structural heart disease and probably account for the association of relatively minor but persistent nonspecific

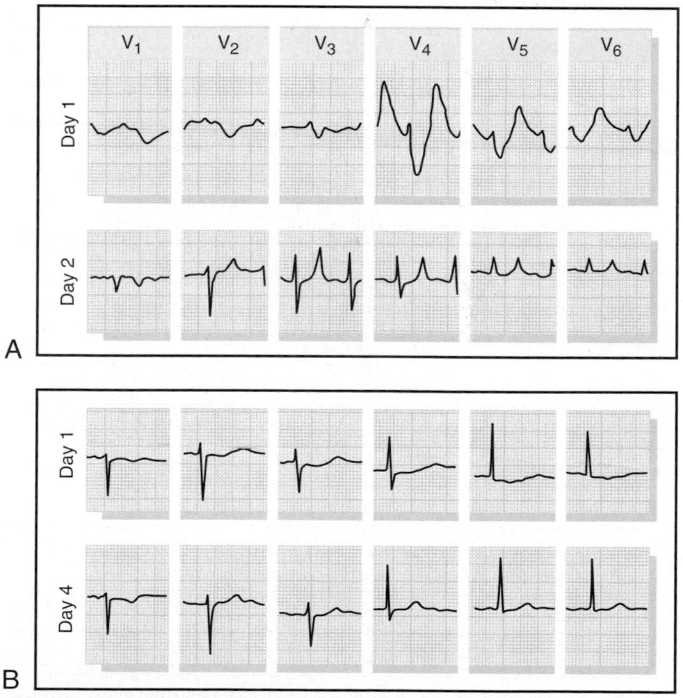

FIGURE 12–52 Electrocardiographic changes in hyperkalemia **(A)** and hypokalemia **(B)**. **A,** On day 1, at a K^+ level of 8.6 mEq/liter, the P wave is no longer recognizable and the QRS complex is diffusely prolonged. Initial and terminal QRS delay is characteristic of K^+-induced intraventricular conduction slowing and is best illustrated in leads V_2 and V_6. On day 2, at a K^+ level of 5.8 mEq/liter, the P wave is recognizable with a PR interval of 0.24 second, the duration of the QRS complex is approximately 0.10 second, and the T waves are characteristically tented. **B,** On day 1, at a K^+ level of 1.5 mEq/liter, the T and U waves are merged. The U wave is prominent and the QU interval is prolonged. On day 4, at a K^+ level of 3.7 mEq/liter, the tracing is normal. *(Courtesy of Dr. C. Fisch.)*

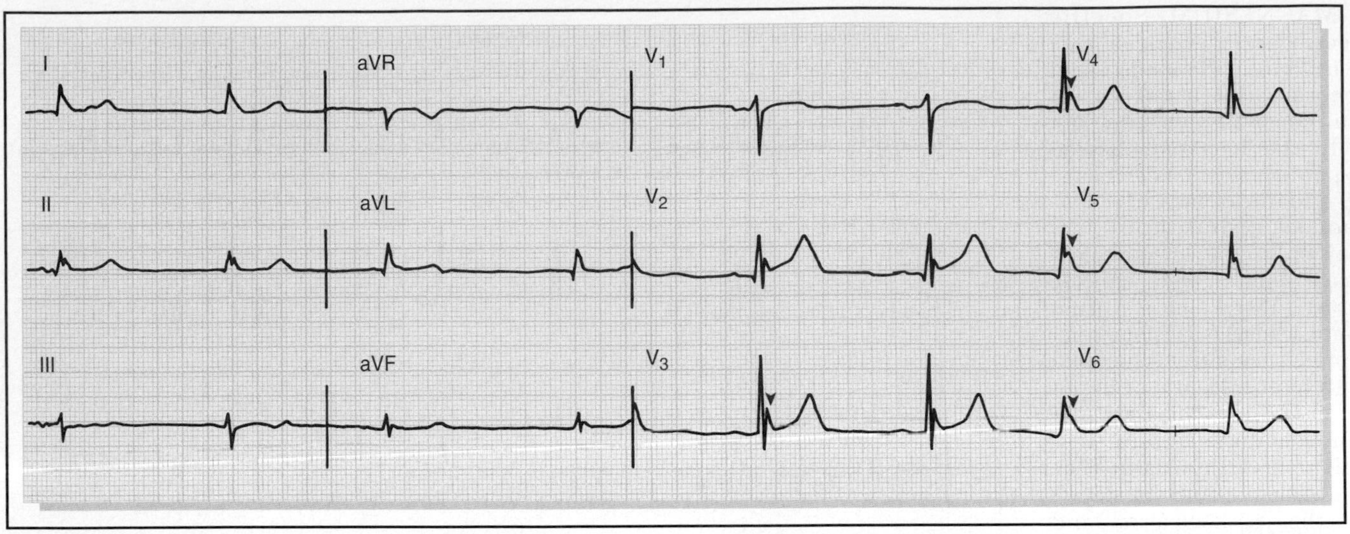

FIGURE 12–53 Systemic hypothermia. The arrowheads (V_3 through V_6) point to the characteristic convex J waves, termed *Osborn waves.* Prominent sinus bradycardia is also present. *(From Goldberger AL: Clinical Electrocardiography: A Simplified Approach. 7th ed. St. Louis, CV Mosby, 2006, p 133.)*

TABLE 12-12 Causes of Low-Voltage QRS Complexes
Artifactual or spurious—that is, unrecognized standardization of the electrocardiogram at half the usual gain (i.e., 5 mm/mV)
Adrenal insufficiency
Anasarca
Cardiac infiltration or replacement (e.g., amyloidosis, Chagas' disease, sarcoid, tumor)
Cardiac transplantation, especially with acute or chronic rejection
Cardiomyopathies, idiopathic or secondary*
Chronic obstructive pulmonary disease
Constrictive pericarditis
Hypothyroidism/myxedema (usually with sinus bradycardia)
Left pneumothorax (midleft chest leads)
Myocardial infarction, extensive
Myocarditis, acute or chronic
Normal variant
Obesity
Pericardial effusion or tamponade (latter usually with sinus tachycardia and sometimes with electrical alternans)
Pleural effusion
Postoperative (after cardiac surgery)

*Dilated cardiomyopathies can be associated with a combination of relatively low limb lead voltage and prominent precordial voltage.

ST-T changes with increased cardiovascular mortality in middle-aged men and women.[84]

Alternans Patterns

The term *alternans* applies to conditions characterized by the sudden appearance of a periodic beat-to-beat change in some aspect of cardiac electrical or mechanical behavior. These abrupt changes (AAAA pattern → ABAB pattern) are reminiscent of a generic class of subharmonic (period-doubling) bifurcation patterns observed in perturbed nonlinear control systems. Many different examples of electrical alternans have been described clinically (Table 12-13)[85,86]; a number of others have been reported in the laboratory. Most familiar is total electrical alternans with sinus tachycardia, a specific but not highly sensitive marker of pericardial effusion with tamponade physiology (Fig. 12-54) (see Chap. 70). This finding is associated with an abrupt transition

TABLE 12-13 Examples of Alternans Patterns in Electrocardiographic Diagnosis

Pattern	Comments
P wave alternans	Rare case reports; e.g., in pulmonary embolism
"Total" electrical alternans (P-QRS-T) with sinus tachycardia	Swinging-heart mechanism in pericardial effusion, tamponade* (see Fig. 12-54)
PR interval alternans	Dual AV nodal pathway pathophysiology; alternating bundle branch block (see Fig. 12-30)
ST segment alternans	Can precede ischemic ventricular tachyarrhythmias (see Fig. 12-40)
T wave (or ST-T) alternans	Can precede nonischemic or ischemic ventricular tachyarrhythmias
TU wave alternans	Can precede torsades de pointes in long QT(U) syndromes, congenital or acquired (see Fig. 12-55)
QRS alternans in supraventricular or ventricular tachycardias	Most common with AV reentrant tachycardias (concealed bypass tract mediated)
R-R (heart rate) alternans	With sinus rhythm, e.g., in congestive heart failure With non-sinus rhythm tachyarrhythmias (e.g.,in certain PSVTs)
Bidirectional tachycardias	Usually ventricular in origin; may be caused by digitalis excess
Intermittent bundle branch or fascicular blocks or Wolff-Parkinson-White patterns	Rarely occur on beat-to-beat basis; attributed to 2:1 block in part of conduction (see Fig. 12-31)

*Also rare report of QRS-T alternans with sinus tachycardia in acute pulmonary embolism.

AV = atrioventricular; PSVT = paroxysmal supraventricular tachycardia.

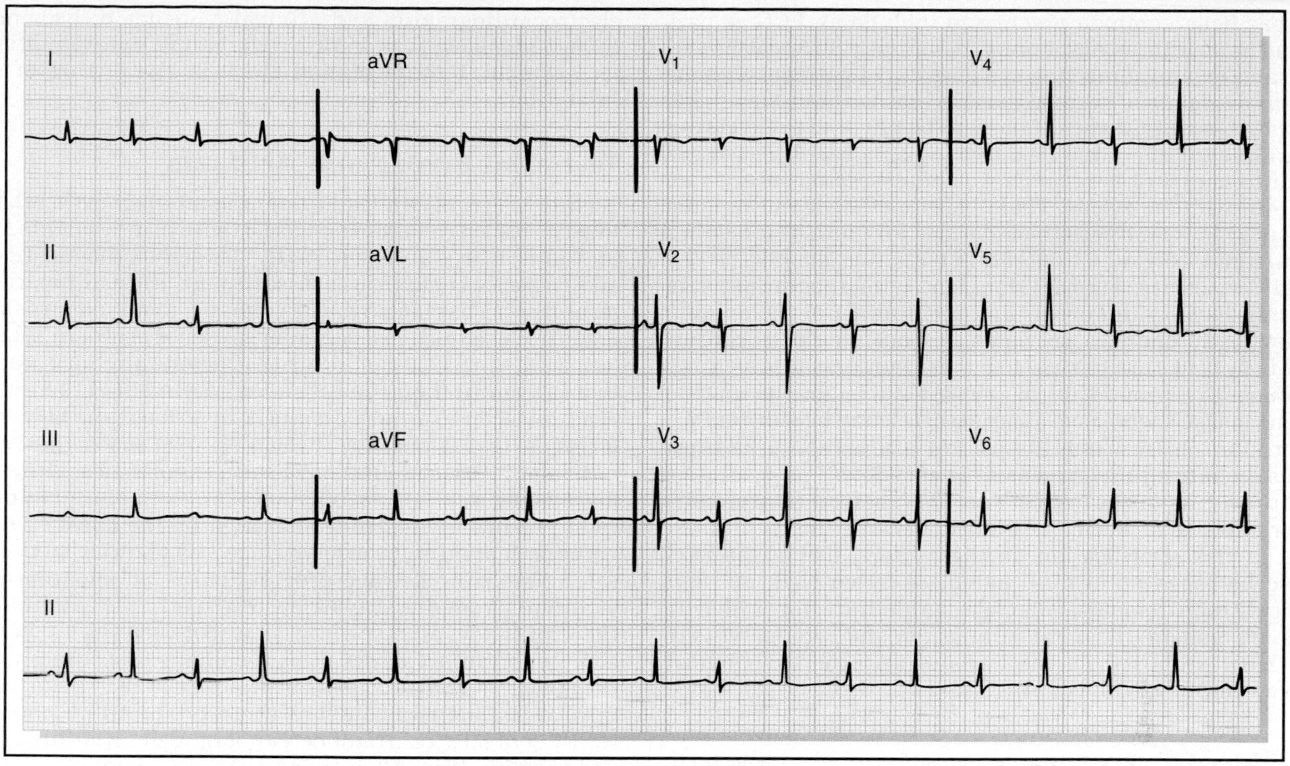

FIGURE 12–54 Total electrical alternans (P-QRS-T) caused by pericardial effusion with tamponade. This finding, particularly in concert with sinus tachycardia and relatively low voltage, is a highly specific, although not sensitive, marker of cardiac tamponade.

from a 1 : 1 to a 2 : 1 pattern in the "to-and-fro" swinging motion of the heart in the effusion. Other alternans patterns are the result of primary electrical rather than mechanical causes. ST-T alternans has long been recognized as a marker of electrical instability in cases of acute ischemia, where it may precede ventricular tachyarrhythmia (see Fig. 12-40). Considerable interest has recently been shown in the detection of microvolt T wave (or ST-T) alternans as a noninvasive marker of the risk of ventricular tachyarrhythmia in patients with chronic heart disease (see Chap. 32). Similarly, TU wave alternans (Fig. 12-55) may be a marker of imminent risk of a ventricular tachyarrhythmia, such as torsades de pointes in hereditary or acquired long QT syndromes.

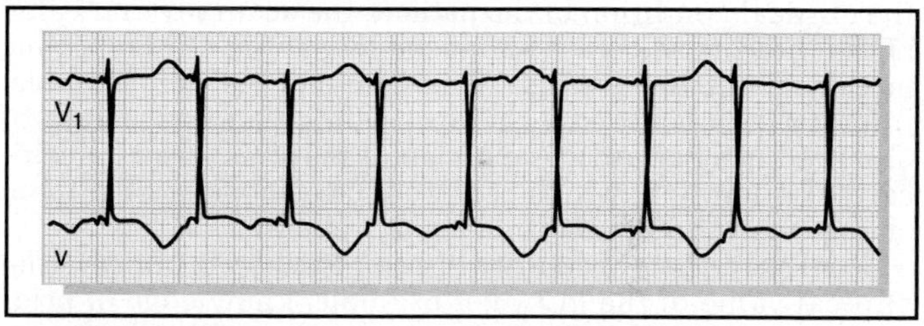

FIGURE 12–55 The QT(U) interval is prolonged (approximately 600 milliseconds) with TU wave alternans. The tracing was recorded in a patient with chronic renal disease shortly following dialysis. This type of repolarization alternans may be a precursor to torsades de pointes. *(Courtesy of Dr. C. Fisch.)*

CLINICAL ISSUES IN ELECTROCARDIOGRAPHIC INTERPRETATION

These principles and diagnostic electrocardiographic guidelines are, finally, subject to appropriate use in the clinical setting. The effectiveness of the ECG as a diagnostic tool depends on factors such as the indications for the procedure, the clinical context in which the ECG is used, proper technique, and the skills of the electrocardiographic reader.[96,97]

Indications for an Electrocardiogram

Limited attention has been paid to the indications for an ECG, probably because of its seeming simplicity, safety, and low cost. However, the cumulative expense of low-cost tests performed at high volume is significant, and the risk to the patient of a false diagnosis of cardiac disease can be damaging.

In patients with known cardiac disease, obtaining ECGs are warranted for the following: as part of a baseline examination; after initiating therapy known to produce electrocardiographic changes that correlate with therapeutic responses, progression of disease, or adverse effects; for intermittent follow-up with changes in signs or symptoms or relevant laboratory findings; or after significant intervals (usually 1 year or longer), even in the absence of clinical changes. In patients suspected of having cardiac disease or at high risk for cardiac disease, an ECG is appropriate as part of an initial evaluation in the presence of signs or symptoms suggesting cardiac disease; in patients with important risk factors such as cigarette abuse, diabetes mellitus, peripheral vascular disease, or family history of cardiac disease (including long-QT syndromes, arrhythmogenic right ventricular dysplasia, Brugada syndrome, and ventricular preexcitation); during therapy with cardioactive medications; and during follow-up if clinical events develop or at prolonged intervals (usually 1 year or more) if clinically stable. Preoperative tracings are appropriate for patients with known or suspected cardiac disease, although this application may also be questioned, especially if the cardiac condition is hemodynamically insignificant or the procedure is simple.

It has been common practice to include an ECG as part of routine health examinations, before any surgical procedure, and on any admission to a hospital of patients without current evidence of cardiac disease and without major risk factors. These ECGs are assumed to be of value in detecting any unknown abnormalities, serving as a baseline against which to compare later tracings, and assessing future risk of cardiovascular events. There is little evidence to support these practices, and recommendations for clinical screening by numerous organizations do not include an ECG.[87] The overall sensitivity of the ECG for identifying specific patients who will have future events and the number of therapeutic or diagnostic changes provoked by routine electrocardiographic findings are too low to warrant universal screening. Although the proportion of persons subjected to routine screening ECGs who have abnormalities may be substantial, the proportion in whom the electrocardiographic findings causes a change in management is very low.[88]

The routine recording of the ECG before noncomplex surgery has also been questioned because of its limited value in risk stratification. In these cases, use of the ECG should be based on clinical judgment rather than on rigid protocol requirements. Flexible guidelines for ordering ECGs on general hospital admission and preoperatively have been proposed on the basis of age, gender, medical history, and physical examination.

Knowledge of the Clinical Context and Prior Electrocardiographic Findings

Although most ECGs are read without a prior knowledge of the clinical condition of the patient, the accuracy and value of the interpretation are enhanced by having clinical information about the patient. This can include, for example, information about drug therapy, which can be a cause of observed electrocardiographic abnormalities, or prior myocardial infarction, which can produce electrocardiographic changes mimicking those of acute ischemia.

Similarly, the availability of prior ECGs can improve the clinical value of the ECG. For example, knowledge of prior electrocardiographic patterns can improve diagnostic accuracy and triage decisions for patients with current electrocardiographic and clinical evidence of ischemia or infarction, as well as improve the proper interpretation of, for example, bundle branch block in the setting of acute infarction.

Technical Errors and Artifacts

Technical errors can lead to significant diagnostic mistakes that can result in false diagnoses; these place patients at risk for unnecessary and potentially dangerous diagnostic tests and treatments that unnecessarily use limited health care resources. Misplacement of one or more electrocardiographic electrodes is a common cause for errors in interpretation of the ECG. Some misplacements produce patterns that can aid in their identification.[3] Reversal of the two arm electrodes, for example, results in inverted P and QRS waveforms in lead I but not in lead V_6, two leads that would normally be expected to have similar polarities. Other misplacements are not as obvious. For example, placing the right precordial electrodes too high on the chest can yield patterns that mimic those produced by anterior myocardial infarction (slow R wave progression) or an apparent intraventricular conduction delay (rSr′ patterns). Maintaining the constancy of recording sites between serial ECGs is also important to assess dynamic changes accurately, such as during episodes of myocardial ischemia.[89] Electrical or mechanical artifacts such as those produced by poor electrode contacts or tremors can simulate life-threatening arrhythmias (Fig. 12-56), and excessive body motion can cause excessive baseline wander that may simulate an ST segment shift of myocardial ischemia or injury.

Reading Errors

Errors in interpreting ECGs are common and may be increasing in frequency.[90,91] Studies assessing the accuracy of routine interpretations have demonstrated significant numbers of errors that can lead to clinical mismanagement, including failure to detect and triage patients with acute myocardial ischemia and other life-threatening situations appropriately. A review of the literature has documented that errors of "major proportions" may be identified in 4 to 32 percent of electrocardiographic interpretations.[90] Organizations such as the American College of Cardiology[92] and the American College of Physicians[90] have proposed minimal training and experience standards for electrocardiographers to help reduce these potentially serious errors, although there are little data to support specific recommendations.[90]

A final issue concerns overreliance on computerized interpretations. Computer systems have facilitated storage and retrieval of large numbers of ECGs and routine application of complex diagnostic algorithms[33] and, as diagnostic algorithms have become more accurate, have provided important adjuncts to the clinical interpretation of ECGs. However, measurements[93] and diagnoses[94] with current systems are not accurate enough, especially

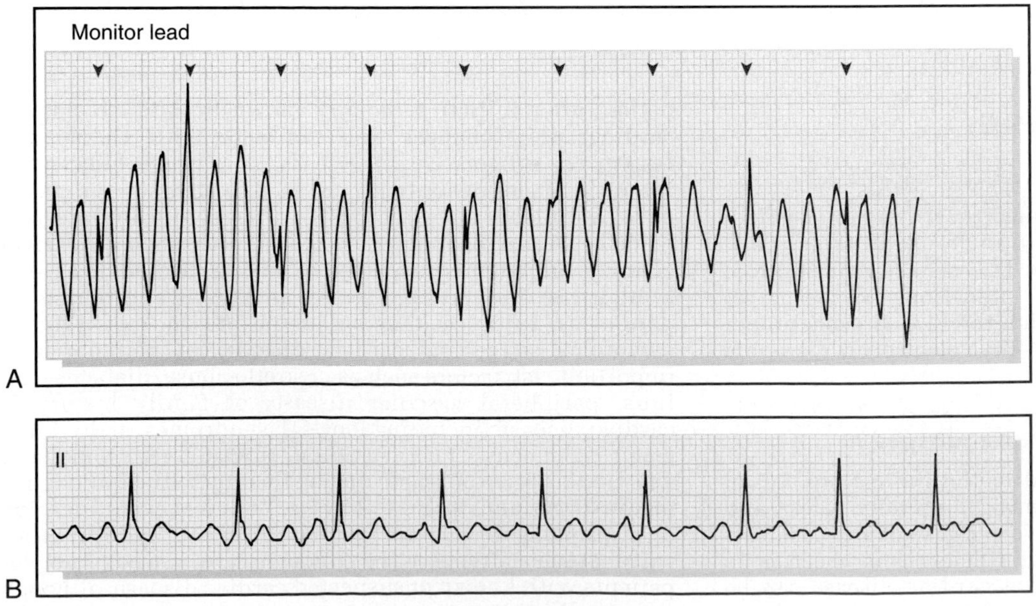

FIGURE 12–56 Artifacts simulating serious arrhythmias. **A,** Motion artifact mimicking ventricular tachyarrhythmia. Partly obscured normal QRS complexes (arrowheads) can be seen with a heart rate of about 100 beats/min. **B,** Parkinsonian tremor causing baseline oscillations mimicking atrial fibrillation. The regularity of QRS complexes may provide a clue to this artifact.

in the presence of complex abnormalities, to be relied on in critical clinical environments without expert review. New analysis techniques based on artificial intelligence concepts may lead to future improvements, and new hardware technology may result in expanded deployment of systems for prompt and expert interpretation.

Electrocardiograms for Self-Assessment

A number of websites feature ECGs for self-assessment and clinical instruction. For example, ECG Wave-Maven provides free access to more than 300 case studies of ECGs, with answers and multimedia adjuncts.[95]

REFERENCES

Introduction and Fundamental Principles

1. Kligfield P: The centennial of the Einthoven electrocardiogram. J Electrocardiol 35(Suppl):123, 2002.
2. Wellens HJJ, Gorgels AP: The electrocardiogram 102 years after Einthoven. Circulation 109:652, 2004.
3. Kligfield P, Gettes L, Bailey JJ, et al: Recommendations for the Standardization and Interpretation of the Electrocardiogram: Part I: The Electrocardiogram and its Technology: A Scientific Statement from the American Heart Association Electrocardiography and Arrhythmias Committee, Council on Clinical Cardiology; the American College of Cardiology Foundation; and the Heart Rhythm Society: endorsed by the International Society for Computerized Electrocardiology. Circulation 115:1306, 2007.
4. Madias J: Decrease/disappearance of pacemaker stimulus "spikes" due to anasarca: Further proof that the mechanism of attenuation of ECG voltage with anasarca is extracardiac in origin. Ann Noninvasive Electrocardiol 9:243, 2004.
5. Bacharova L, Selvester RH, Engblom H, Wagner GS: Where is the central terminal located? In search of understanding the use of the Wilson central terminal for production of 9 of the 12 electrocardiogram leads. J Electrocardiol 38:119, 2005.
6. Rautaharju PM: Elusive understanding of electrocardiographic lead networks. J Electrocardiol 38:128, 2005.
7. Rautaharju PM, Zhou SH, Hancock EW, et al: Comparability of 12-lead ECGs derived from EASI leads with standard 12-lead ECGS in the classification of acute myocardial ischemia and old myocardial infarction. J Electrocardiol 35(Suppl):35, 2002.
8. Hurst JW: Current status of clinical electrocardiography with suggestions for the improvement of the interpretive process. Am J Cardiol 92:1072, 2003.
9. Engblom H, Foster JE, Martin TN, et al: The relationship between electrical axis by 12-lead electrocardiogram and anatomical axis of the heart by cardiac magnetic resonance imaging in healthy subjects. Am Heart J 150:507, 2005.
10. Sgarbossa EB, Barold SS, Pinski SL, et al: Twelve-lead electrocardiogram: The advantages of an orderly frontal display including –aVr. J Electrocardiol 37:141, 2004.
11. Senaratne MP, Weerasinghe C, Smith G, Mooney D: Clinical utility of ST-segment depression in lead AVR in acute myocardial infarction. J Electrocardiol 36:11, 2003.

The Normal Electrocardiogram

12. Malik M, Camm AJ: Dynamic Electrocardiography. Elmsford, NY, Blackwell/Futura, 2004.
13. Mietus JE, Peng CK, Henry I, et al: The pNNx-files: Re-examining a widely-used heart rate variability measure. Heart 88:378, 2002.
14. Ramanathan C, Jia P, Ghanem R, et al: Activation and repolarization of the normal human heart under complete physiological condition. Proc Natl Acad Sci U S A 103:6309, 2006.
15. MacAlpin RN: Clinical significance of QS complexes in V_1 and V_2 without other electrocardiographic abnormality. Ann Noninvasive Electrocardiol 9:39, 2004.
16. MacAlpin RN: In search of left septal fascicular block. Am Heart J 144:948, 2002.
17. Okin PM, Wright JT, Nieminen MS, et al: Ethnic differences in electrocardiographic criteria for left ventricular hypertrophy: The LIFE study. Am J Hypertens 15:663, 2002.
18. Wu J, Wu J, Zipes DP: Early afterdepolarizations, U waves and torsades de pointes. Circulation 105:675, 2002.
19. Yan GX, Lankipalli RS, Burke JF, et al: Ventricular repolarization components on the electrocardiogram: cellular basis and clinical significance. J Am Coll Cardiol 42:401, 2003.
20. Macfarlane PW, Browne D, Devine B, et al: Modification of ACC/ESC criteria for acute myocardial infarction. J Electrocardiol 37(Suppl):98, 2004.
21. Miller MD, Porter CJ, Ackerman MJ: Diagnostic accuracy of screening electrocardiograms in long QT interval I. Pediatrics 108:8, 2001.
22. Robbins J, Nelson JC, Rautaharju PM, Gottdiener JS: The association between the length of the QT interval and mortality in the Cardiovascular Health Study. Am J Med 115:689, 2003.
23. Luo S, Michler K, Johnston P, Macfarlane PW: A comparison of commonly used QT correction formulae: The effect of heart rate on the QTc of normal ECGs. J Electrocardiol 37(Suppl):81, 2004.
24. Rautaharju PM, Prineas RJ, Kadish A, et al: Normal standards for QT and QT subintervals derived from a large ethnically diverse population of women aged 50 to 79 years (the Women's Health Initiative [WHI]). Am J Cardiol 97:730, 2006.
25. Shah BR, Yamazaki T, Engel G, et al: QT dispersion measurement and cardiovascular mortality in male veterans. Am J Cardiol 93:483, 2004.
26. Hurst JW: Thoughts about the ventricular gradient and its current clinical use. Clin Cardiol 28:175, 2005.
27. Pellicia A, DiPaolo FM, Maron BJ: The athlete's heart: Remodeling, electrocardiogram and preparticipation screening. Cardiol Rev 10:85, 2002.
28. Surawicz B, Parikh SR: Prevalence of male and female patterns of early repolarization in the normal ECG of males and females from childhood to old age. J Am Coll Cardiol 40:1870, 2002.
29. Marcus FI: Prevalence of T-wave inversion beyond V1 in young normal individuals and usefulness for the diagnosis of arrhythmogenic right ventricular cardiomyopathy/dysplasia. Am J Cardiol 95:1070, 2005.
30. Klatsky AL, Oehm R, Cooper RA, et al: The early repolarization normal variant electrocardiogram: correlates and consequences. Am J Med 115:171, 2003.

Atrial Abnormalities; Ventricular Hypertrophy and Enlargement

31. Ariyarajah V, Asad N, Tandar A, Spodick DH: Interatrial block. Pandemic prevalence, significance and diagnosis. Chest 128:970, 2005.
32. Perrier E, Kerfant BG, Lalevee N, et al: Mineralocorticoid receptor antagonism prevents the electrical remodeling that preceded cellular hypertrophy after myocardial infarction. Circulation 11:776, 2004.
33. Warner RA, Ariel Y, Gasperina MD, Okin PM: Improved electrocardiographic detection of left ventricular hypertrophy. J Electrocardiol 35(Suppl):111, 2002.
34. Salles G, Leocadio S, Bloch K, et al: Combined QT interval and voltage criteria improve left ventricular hypertrophy detection in resistant hypertension. Hypertension 46:1207, 2005.
35. Dhingra R, Ho Nam B, Benjamin EJ, et al: Cross-sectional relations of electrocardiogaphic QRS duration to left ventricular dimensions: The Framingham Heart Study. J Am Coll Cardiol 45:685, 2005.
36. Carlsson MB, Tragardh E, Engblom H, et al: Left ventricular mass by 12-lead electrocardiogram in healthy subjects: Comparison to cardiac magnetic resonance imaging. J Electrocardiol 39:67, 2006.
37. Okin PM, Devereux RB, Jern S, et al: Regression of electrocardiographic left ventricular hypertrophy during antihypertensive treatment and the prediction of major cardiovascular events. JAMA 292:2343, 2004.
38. Larsen CT, Blackburn H, Brown NE, et al: The ischemic electrocardiogram: A harbinger for ischemic heart disease independent of blood pressure level. The Copenhagen City Heart Study. Eur J Epidemiol 20:301, 2995.
39. Okin PM, Devereux RB, Nieminen MS, et al: Electrocardiographic strain pattern and prediction of new onset congestive heart failure in hypertensive patients: The Losartan Intervention for Endpoint Reduction in Hypertension (LIFE) study. Circulation 113:67, 2006.
40. Sukhija R, Aronow WS, Kakar P: Electrocardiographic abnormalities in patients with right ventricular dilatation due to acute pulmonary embolism. Cardiology 105:57, 2006.

Intraventricular Conduction Delays and Preexcitation

41. Biagini E, Elhendy A, Schinkel AF, et al: Prognostic significance of left anterior hemoblock in patients with suspected coronary artery disease. J Am Coll Cardiol 45:858, 2005.
42. Rodriguez LM, Timmermans C, Nabar A, et al: Variable patterns of septal activation with left bundle branch block and heart failure. J Cardiovasc Electrophysiol 14:135, 2003.
43. Auricchio A, Fantoni C, Regoli F, et al: Characterization of left ventricular activation in patients with heart failure and left bundle branch block. Circulation 109:133, 2004.
44. Turner MS, Bleasdale RA, Vinereanu D, et al: Electrical and mechanical components of dyssynchrony in heart failure patients with normal QRS duration and left bundle branch block. Circulation 109:2544, 2004.
45. Jain AC, Mehta MC: Etiologies of left bundle branch block and correlations to hemodynamic and angiographic findings. Am Heart J 91:1375, 2003..
46. Miller WL, Ballman KV, Hodge DO, et al: Risk factor implications of incidentally discovered uncomplicated bundle branch block. Mayo Clin Proc 80:1585, 2005.
47. Eriksson P, Wilhelmson L, Rosengren A: Bundle-branch block in middle-aged men: Risk of complications and death over 28 years. Eur Heart J 26:2300, 2005.
48. Breithardt OA, Stellbrink C, Herbots L, et al: Cardiac resynchronization therapy can reverse abnormal myocardial strain distribution in patients with heart failure and left bundle branch block. J Am Coll Cardiol 42:486, 2003.
49. Blanc JJ, Fatemi M, Bertault V, et al: Evaluation of left bundle branch block as a reversible cause of non-ischemic dilated cardiomyopathy with severe heart failure. Europace 7:604, 2005.
50. Youn HJ, Park CS, Cho EJ, et al: Left bundle branch block disturbs left anterior descending coronary blood flow: Study using transthoracic Doppler echocardiography. J Am Soc Echocardiogr 18:1093, 2005.
51. D'Andrea A, Caso P, Sarubbi B, et al: Right ventricular myocardial activation delay in adult patients with right bundle branch block late after repair of tetralogy of Fallot. Eur J Echocardiogr 5:123, 2004.
52. Fantoni C, Kawabata M, Massaro R, et al: Right and left ventricular activation sequence in patients with heart failure and right bundle branch block. J Cardiovasc Electrophysiol 16:112, 2005.
53. Antzelevitch C, Brugada P, Borggrefe M, et al: Brugada syndrome: Report of the second consensus conference. Heart Rhythm 2:429, 2005.

Myocardial Ischemia and Infarction

54. Goldberger AL. Clinical Electrocardiography: A Simplified Approach. 7th ed. St. Louis, Mosby/Elsevier, 2006.

55. Surawicz B, Knilans T: Chou's Electrocardiography in Clinical Practice: Adult and Pediatric. Philadelphia, WB Saunders, 2001.
56. Antman EM, Anbe DT, Armstrong PW, et al: ACC/AHA guidelines for the management of patients with ST-elevation myocardial infarction. A report of the American College of Cardiology/American Heart Association Task Force on Practice Guidelines. J Am Coll Cardiol 44:E1, 2004.
57. Goldberger AL: Myocardial Infarction: Electrocardiographic Differential Diagnosis. 4th ed. St. Louis, Mosby-Year Book, 1991.
58. Zimetbaum PJ, Josephson ME: Use of the electrocardiogram in acute myocardial infarction. N Engl J Med 348:933, 2003.
59. Kleber AG: ST-segment elevation in the electrocardiogram: A sign of myocardial ischemia. Cardiovasc Res 45:111, 2000.
60. Brodie BR, Stuckey TD, Hansen C, et al: Relation between electrocardiographic ST-segment resolution and early and late outcomes after primary percutaneous coronary intervention for acute myocardial infarction. Am J Cardiol 95;343, 2005.
61. Moon JC, De Arenaza DP, Elkington AG, et al: The pathologic basis of Q-wave and non-Q-wave myocardial infarction: A cardiovascular magnetic resonance study. J Am Coll Cardiol 44:554, 2004.
62. Bosimini E, Giannuzzi P, Temporelli PL, et al: Electrocardiographic evolutionary changes and left ventricular remodeling after acute myocardial infarction: Results of the GISSI-3 Echo substudy. J Am Coll Cardiol 35:127, 2000.
63. Voon WC, Chen YW, Hsu CC, et al: Q-wave regression after acute myocardial infarction assessed by Tl-201 myocardial perfusion SPECT. J Nucl Cardiol 11:165, 2004.
64. Correale E, Battista R, Ricciardiello V, et al: The negative U wave: A pathogenetic enigma but a useful, often overlooked bedside diagnostic and prognostic clue in ischemic heart disease. Clin Cardiol 27:674, 2004.
65. Chen A, Kusumoto FM: QT dispersion: much ado about something? Chest 125:1974, 2004.
66. Rautaharju PM: Why did QT dispersion die? Card Electrophysiol Rev 6:295, 2002.
67. Kligfield P, Okin PM, Lee KW, et al: Significance of QT dispersion. Am J Cardiol 91:1291, 2003.
68. Bogaty P, Boyer L, Rousseau L, Arsenault M: Is anteroseptal myocardial infarction an appropriate term? Am J Med 113:37, 2002.
69. Yamaji H, Iwasaki K, Kusachi S, et al: Prediction of acute left main coronary artery obstruction by 12-lead electrocardiography. ST segment elevation in lead aVR with less ST segment elevation in lead V1. J Am Coll Cardiol 38:1348, 2001.
70. Nikus KC, Sclarovsky S: ST elevation in lead aVR as a sign of left main disease—perpetuating an error? Am J Cardiol 94:542, 2004.
71. Kurum T, Birsin A, Ozbay G, et al: Differentiating the infarct-related artery on initial electrocardiogram in single or multi-vessel disease in acute inferior myocardial infarction and evaluating involvement of vessels using correspondence analysis. Angiology 56:385, 2005.
72. Fiol M, Carrillo A, Cygankiewicz I, et al: New criteria based on ST changes in 12-lead surface ECG to detect proximal versus distal right coronary artery occlusion in a case of acute inferoposterior myocardial infarction. Ann Noninvasive Electrocardiol 9:383, 2004.
73. Madias JE, Sinha A, Ashitani R, et al: A critique of the new ST-segment criteria for the diagnosis of acute myocardial infarction in patients with left bundle-branch block. Clin Cardiol 10:652, 2001.
74. Jim MH, Miu R, Siu CW: PR-segment elevation in inferior leads: An atypical electrocardiographic sign of atrial infarction. J Invasive Cardiol 16:219, 2004.
75. Neven K, Crijns H, Gorgels A: Atrial infarction: A neglected electrocardiographic sign with important clinical implications. J Cardiovasc Electrophysiol 14:306, 2003.
76. Welch RD, Zalenski RJ, Frederick PD, et al: Prognostic value of a normal or nonspecific initial electrocardiogram in acute myocardial infarction. JAMA 286:1977, 2001.
77. Das MK, Khan B, Jacob S, et al: Significance of a fragmented QRS complex versus a Q wave in patterns with coronary artery disease. Circulation 113:2495, 2006.
78. Wang K, Asinger RW, Marriott HJ: ST-segment elevation in conditions other than acute myocardial infarction. N Engl J Med 349:2128, 2003.
79. Bybee K, Rihal CS: Transient left ventricular apical ballooning. Ann Intern Med 142:678, 2005.
80. Nasir K, Bomma C, Tandri H, et al: Electrocardiographic features of arrhythmogenic right ventricular dysplasia/cardiomyopathy according to disease severity: A need to broaden diagnostic criteria. Circulation 21:1527, 2004.
81. Patberg KW, Shvilkin A, Plotnikov AN, et al: Cardiac memory: Mechanisms and clinical implications. Heart Rhythm 12:1376, 2005.

Drug Effects, Electrolyte and Metabolic Abnormalities; Nonspecific QRS and ST-T Abnormalities; Alternans Patterns

82. Sundqvist K, Jogestrand T, Nowak J: The effect of digoxin on the electrocardiogram of healthy middle-aged and elderly patients at rest and during exercise: A comparison with the ECG reaction induced by myocardial ischemia. J Electrocardiol 35:213, 2002.
83. Antzelevitch C, Shimizu W, Yan GX, et al: The M cell: Its contribution to the ECG and to normal and abnormal electrical function of the heart. J Cardiovasc Electrophysiol 10:1124, 1999.
84. Greenland P, Xie X, Liu K, et al: Impact of minor electrocardiographic ST-segment and/or T-wave abnormalities on cardiovascular mortality during long-term follow-up. Am J Cardiol 91:1068, 2003.
85. Maury P, Raczka F, Piot C, Davy JM: QRS and cycle length alternans during paroxysmal supraventricular tachycardia: What is the mechanism? J Cardiovasc Electrophysiol 13:92, 2002.
86. Pham Q, Quan KJ, Rosenbaum DS: T-wave alternans: Marker, mechanism, and methodology for predicting sudden cardiac death. J Electrocardiol 36(Suppl):75, 2003.

Clinical Issues in Electrocardiographic Interpretation

87. Stafford RS: Feedback intervention to reduce routine electrocardiogram use in primary care. Am Heart J 145:979, 2003.
88. Lesho G, Gey D, Forrester G, et al: The low impact of screening electrocardiograms in healthy individuals: a prospective study and review of the literature. Mil Med 168:15, 2003.
89. Madias JE: Serial ECG recordings via marked chest wall landmarks: An essential requirement for the diagnosis of myocardial infarction in the presence of left bundle branch lock. J Electrocardiol 35:299, 2002.
90. Salerno SM, Alguire PC, Waxman HS: Competency in interpretation of 12-lead electrocardiograms: A summary and appraisal of published evidence. Ann Intern Med 138:751, 2003.
91. Liebman J: Nonarrhythmia clinical electrocardiography—can it be returned to clinical utility? J Electrocardiol 35:293, 2002.
92. Kadish AH, Buxton AE, Kennedy HL, et al: ACC/AHA clinical competence statement on electrocardiography and ambulatory electrocardiography. Circulation 104:3169, 2001.
93. Eskola MJ, Nikus KC, Voipio-Pulkki LM, et al: Comparative accuracy of manual versus computerized electrocardiographic measurement of J-, ST- and T-wave deviations in patients with acute coronary syndromes. Am J Cardiol 96:1584, 2005.
94. Bogun F, Anh D, Kalahasty G, et al: Misdiagnosis of atrial fibrillation and its clinical consequence. Am J Med 117:636, 2004.
95. McClennen S, Nathanson LA, Safran C, Goldberger AL: ECG Wave-Maven: An Internet-based electrocardiography self-assessment program for students and clinicians. Med Educ Online 8:2, 2003 (http://www.med-ed-online.org/issue2.htm#v8).

Future Perspectives

96. Moss AJ: The electrocardiogram: From Einthoven to molecular genetics. Ann Noninvasive Electrocardiol 6:181, 2001.
97. Soffer A: Einthoven's machine, alive and well. Chest 128:487, 2005.

GUIDELINES *Thomas H. Lee*

Electrocardiography

Guidelines for the performance of electrocardiograms (ECGs) have evolved little in recent years. The most widely cited guidelines were published by the American College of Cardiology and American Heart Association (ACC/AHA) in 1992.[1] These guidelines make recommendations for the use of ECGs in patients with and without cardiovascular disease. Other guidelines were published by the AHA in 1987,[2] by a task force assembled by the Canadian government in 1991,[3] and by the U.S. Preventive Services Task Force (USPTF) in 1996.[4] An ACC/AHA task force published standards for clinical competence in 2001[5] and practice standards for electrocardiographic monitoring in hospitals in 2004.[6]

These guidelines use the older ACC/AHA convention of classifying indications according to one of three classes. Class I indications are conditions for which it is generally agreed that ECGs are useful. Class II indications are conditions for which opinions differ with respect to the usefulness of ECGs. Class III indications are conditions for which it is generally agreed that ECGs have little or no usefulness.

Patients with Known Cardiovascular Disease or Dysfunction

The ACC/AHA guidelines[1] endorse the use of ECGs in the baseline evaluation of all patients with known cardiovascular disease and for the evaluation of response to therapies likely to produce electrocardiographic changes (Table 12G-1). The ACC/AHA guidelines do not comment on the frequency of follow-up ECGs but do endorse the use of serial ECGs for patients with known cardiovascular disease whenever there are changes in symptoms, signs, or laboratory findings. Even in the absence of such changes, follow-up ECGs are considered appro-

TABLE 12G–1 ACC/AHA Guidelines for Electrocardiography in Patients with Known Cardiovascular Disease or Dysfunction

Indication	Class I (Indicated)	Class II (Equivocal)	Class III (Not Indicated)
Baseline or initial evaluation	All patients	None	None
Response to therapy	Patients in whom prescribed therapy is known to produce electrocardiographic changes that correlate with therapeutic responses or progression of disease Patients in whom prescribed therapy may produce adverse effects that may be predicted from or detected by electrocardiographic changes	None	Patients receiving pharmacological or nonpharmacological therapy not known to produce electrocardiographic changes or to affect conditions that may be associated with such changes
Follow-up	Patients with a change in symptoms, signs, or relevant laboratory findings Patients with an implanted pacemaker or antitachycardia device. Patients with symptoms such as the following conditions, even in the absence of new symptoms or signs, after an interval of time appropriate for the condition or disease: syncope and near-syncope; unexplained change in the usual pattern of angina pectoris; chest pain; new or worsening dyspnea Extreme and unexplained fatigue, weakness, and prostration; palpitation; new signs of congestive heart failure; new organic murmur or pericardial friction rub; new findings suggesting pulmonary hypertension; accelerating or poorly controlled systemic arterial hypertension; evidence of a recent cerebrovascular accident; unexplained fever in patients with known valvular disease; new onset of cardiac arrhythmia or inappropriate heart rate; chronic known congenital or acquired cardiovascular disease		Adult patients whose cardiovascular condition is usually benign and unlikely to progress (e.g., patients with asymptomatic mild mitral valve prolapse, mild hypertension, or premature contractions in the absence of organic heart disease) Adult patients with chronic stable heart disease seen at frequent intervals (e.g., 4 months) and who have no new or unexplained findings
Before surgery	All patients with known cardiovascular disease or dysfunction except as noted under Class II	Patients with hemodynamically insignificant congenital or acquired heart disease, mild systemic hypertension, or infrequent premature complexes in the absence of organic heart disease	None

ACC/AHA = American College of Cardiology/American Heart Association.

priate for patients with syndromes such as syncope, chest pain, and extreme fatigue. Follow-up ECGs are not considered appropriate for patients with mild chronic cardiovascular conditions that are not considered likely to progress (e.g., mild mitral valve prolapse). ECGs at each visit are considered inappropriate for patients with stable heart disease who are seen frequently (e.g., within 4 months) and have no evidence of clinical change.

Before surgical procedures, ECGs are considered appropriate for all patients with known cardiovascular disease or dysfunction, except those with insignificant or mild conditions such as mild systemic arterial hypertension.

Patients with Suspected Cardiovascular Disease or at High Risk for Cardiovascular Disease

The ACC/AHA guidelines make similar recommendations for patients with suspected cardiovascular disease and those who are at high risk for such conditions for the use of ECGs at baseline, for evaluation of the response to therapy, and before surgery (Table 12G-2). In the follow-up of patients at increased risk for heart disease, ECGs every 1 to 5 years are considered appropriate, but routine screening ECGs more frequently than yearly are not supported for patients who remain clinically stable, as long as they had not been previously demonstrated to have heart disease.

Patients without Known or Suspected Heart Disease

The various guidelines differ in their recommendations for the use of ECGs to screen for cardiovascular disease in healthy people. In the ACC/AHA guidelines, ECGs are considered appropriate screening tests in patients without apparent or suspected heart disease who are 40 years of age or older (Table 12G-3). Earlier guidelines from the AHA recommended that ECGs be obtained at ages 20, 40, and 60 years.[2] In contrast, the USPSTF and the task force assembled by the Canadian government did not find evidence to support the use of screening ECG.[3,4]

The ACC/AHA guidelines recommend ECGs for patients for whom drugs with a high incidence of cardiovascular effects (e.g., chemotherapy) or exercise testing is planned and for people of any age in occupations with high cardiovascular demands or whose cardiovascular status might affect the safety of many other people (e.g., airline pilots). ECGs are considered appropriate before surgery in patients 40 years of age or older and are equivocal in patients between the ages of 30 and 40 years in these guidelines. More recent guidelines from the ACC/AHA for perioperative evaluation[7] found good evidence for ECGs before noncardiac surgery in asymptomatic patients with diabetes (see Table 80G-1), but otherwise do not strongly endorse routine preoperative electrocardiographic testing in patients without cardiovascular symptoms.

TABLE 12G–2 ACC/AHA Guidelines for Electrocardiography in Patients Suspected of Having or Who Are at Increased Risk for Cardiovascular Disease or Dysfunction

Setting	Class I (Appropriate)	Class II (Equivocal)	Class III (Inappropriate)
Baseline or initial evaluation	All patients suspected of having or being at increased risk for cardiovascular disease Patients who may have used cocaine, amphetamines, or other illicit drugs known to have cardiac effects Patients who may have received an overdose of a drug known to have cardiac effects	None	None
Response to therapy	To assess therapy with cardioactive drugs in patients with suspected cardiac disease To assess response to the administration of any agent known to result in cardiac abnormalities or abnormalities on the ECG(e.g., antineoplastic drugs, lithium, antidepressant agents)	To assess the response to administration of any agent known to alter serum electrolyte concentrations	To assess the response to administration of agents known not to influence cardiac structure or function
Follow-up	Presence of any change in clinical status or laboratory findings suggesting interval development of cardiac disease or dysfunction Periodic follow-up (e.g., every 1 to 5 yr) of patients known to be at increased risk for cardiac disease Follow-up of patients after resolution of chest pain	None	Follow-up ECGs more often than once yearly not indicated for patients who remain clinically stable, not at increased risk for development of cardiac disease, and not demonstrated to have cardiac disease with previous studies
Before surgery	As part of the preoperative evaluation of any patient with suspected, or at increased risk of developing, cardiac disease or dysfunction	None	None

ACC/AHA = American College of Cardiology/American Heart Association; ECG = electrocardiogram.

TABLE 12G–3 ACC/AHA Guidelines for Electrocardiography in Patients with No Apparent or Suspected Heart Disease or Dysfunction

Setting	Class I (Appropriate)	Class II (Equivocal)	Class III (Inappropriate)
Baseline or initial evaluation	Persons aged 40 yr or older undergoing physical examination Before administration of pharmacological agents known to have a high incidence of cardiovascular effects (e.g., antineoplastic agents) Before exercise stress testing People of any age who are in special occupations that require very high cardiovascular performance (e.g., fire fighters, police officers) or whose cardiovascular performance is linked to public safety (e.g., pilots, air traffic controllers, critical process operators, bus or truck drivers, railroad engineers)	To evaluate competitive athletes	Routine screening or baseline ECG in asymptomatic persons younger than 40 yr with no risk factors
Response to therapy	To evaluate patients in whom prescribed therapy (e.g., doxorubicin) is known to produce cardiovascular effects	None	To assess treatment known not to produce any cardiovascular effects
Follow-up	To evaluate asymptomatic persons >40 yr of age	None	To evaluate asymptomatic adults who have had no interval change in symptoms, signs, or risk factors and who have had a normal ECG within the recent past
Before surgery	Patients >40 yr of age Patients being evaluated as donor for heart transplantation or as recipient of a noncardiopulmonary transplant	Patients 30-40 yr of age	Patients younger than 30 yr with no risk factors for coronary artery disease

ACC/AHA = American College of Cardiology/American Heart Association; ECG = electrocardiogram.

Clinical Competence

The ACC/AHA Clinical Competence Statement on electrocardiography[5] provides an overview for minimal standards for performance and interpretation of ECGs. In addition to making recommendations for the list of diagnoses with which ECG interpreters should be familiar, the statement asserts that computer interpretations must be reviewed by an experienced electrocardiographer. The USPSTF has recommended a minimum of 100 ECG interpretations/year to maintain competence.

Practice Standards for Electrocardiographic Monitoring in Hospital Settings

Electrocardiographic monitoring in hospital settings has expanded far beyond the original use of simple heart rate and basic rhythm determination. Despite significant advances in technology, human oversight is still needed in determining when electrocardiographic monitoring is needed and for interpreting data from the ECG. The AHA/ACC has developed best practices for hospital electrocardiographic monitoring

TABLE 12G-4 ACC/AHA Recommendations Regarding Best Practices for Electrocardiographic Monitoring in Hospital Settings

Setting	Class I	Class II	Class III
Cardiac arrhythmia monitoring	Patients resuscitated from a cardiac arrest Patients in the early phase of acute coronary syndromes Patients with unstable coronary syndromes and newly diagnosed high-risk coronary lesions Adults and children who have undergone cardiac surgery Patients who have undergone nonurgent percutaneous coronary intervention with complications Patients who have undergone implantation of an automatic defibrillator lead or pacemaker lead and are considered pacemaker-dependent Patients with a temporary pacemaker or transcutaneous pacing pads Patients with AV block Patients with arrhythmias complicating Wolff-Parkinson-White syndrome with rapid anterograde conduction over an accessory pathway Patients with long-QT syndrome and associated ventricular arrhythmias Patients receiving intraaortic balloon counterpulsation Patients with acute heart failure or pulmonary edema Patients with indications for intensive care Patients undergoing diagnostic or therapeutic procedures requiring conscious sedation or anesthesia Patients with any other hemodynamically unstable arrhythmia Diagnosis of arrhythmias in pediatric patients	Patients with post-acute MI Patients with chest pain syndromes Patients who have undergone uncomplicated, nonurgent, percutaneous coronary interventions Patients administered an antiarrhythmic drug or who require adjustment of drugs for rate control with chronic atrial tachyarrhythmias Patients who have undergone implantation of a pacemaker lead and are not pacemaker-dependent Patients who have undergone uncomplicated ablation of an arrhythmia Patients who have undergone routine coronary angiography Patients with subacute heart failure Patients being evaluated for syncope Patients with do-not-resuscitate orders with arrhythmias that cause discomfort	Postoperative patients at low risk for cardiac arrhythmias Obstetric patients, unless heart disease is present Patients with permanent, rate-controlled atrial fibrillation Patients undergoing hemodialysis (unless they have a Class I or II indication and undergo dialysis in the hospital, in which case monitoring of the ECG is recommended) Stable patients with chronic ventricular premature beats in the absence of major modulating factors such as acid-base imbalance, electrolyte abnormality, or myocardial ischemia
ST segment ischemia monitoring	Patients in the early phase of acute coronary syndromes Patients who present to the emergency department with chest pain or angina-equivalent symptoms Patients who have undergone nonurgent percutaneous coronary intervention with suboptimal angiographic results Patients with possible variant angina resulting from coronary vasospasm	Patients with post-acute MI Patients who have undergone nonurgent, uncomplicated, percutaneous coronary intervention Patients at high risk for ischemia after cardiac or noncardiac surgery Pediatric patients at risk of ischemia or infarction resulting from congenital or acquired conditions	Patients with left bundle branch block Patients with ventricular pacing rhythm Patients with other confounding arrhythmias that obscure the ST segment Patients who are agitated
QT interval and monitoring of the ECG for detection of proarrhythmia	Patients administered an antiarrhythmic drug known to cause torsades de pointes Patients who overdose from a potentially proarrhythmic agent Patients with new-onset bradyarrhythmias Patients with severe hypokalemia or hypomagnesemia	Patients who require treatment with antipsychotics or other drugs with possible risk of torsades de pointes Patients with acute neurological events	Healthy patients administered drugs that pose little risk for torsades de pointes

ACC/AHA = American College of Cardiology/American Heart Association; AV = atrioventricular; ECG = electrocardiogram; MI = myocardial infarction.

(Table 12G-4) based on expert opinion derived from clinical experience and related research in the field of electrocardiography, because randomized clinical trials in this area are almost nonexistent.

The AHA/ACC defines three categories for electrocardiographic monitoring:

Class I: Cardiac monitoring indicated in most, if not all, patients

Class II: Cardiac monitoring may be of benefit in some patients but is not considered essential for all

Class III: Cardiac monitoring is not indicated because the risk of a serious event is so low that monitoring has no therapeutic benefit

References

1. Schlant RC, Adolph RJ, DiMarco JP, et al: Guidelines for electrocardiography. A report of the American College of Cardiology/American Heart Association Task Force on Assessment of Diagnostic and Therapeutic Cardiovascular Procedures (Committee on Electrocardiography). J Am Coll Cardiol 19:473, 1992.
2. Grundy SM, Greenland P, Herd A, et al: Cardiovascular and risk factor evaluation of healthy American adults. A statement for physicians by an Ad Hoc Committee appointed by the Steering Committee, American Heart Association. Circulation 75:1340A, 1987.
3. Hayward RS, Steinberg EP, Ford DE, et al: Preventive care guidelines: 1991. American College of Physicians. Canadian Task Force on the Periodic Health Examination. United States Preventive Services Task Force. Ann Intern Med 114:758, 1991.
4. U.S. Preventive Services Task Force: Guide to Clinical Preventive Services. 2nd ed. Baltimore, Williams & Wilkins, 1996.
5. Kadish AH, Buxton AE, Kennedy HL, et al: ACC/AHA clinical competence statement on electrocardiography and ambulatory electrocardiography: A report of the ACC/AHA/ACP-ASIM task force on clinical competence (ACC/AHA Committee to develop a clinical competence statement on electrocardiography and ambulatory electrocardiography) endorsed by the International Society for Holter and noninvasive electrocardiology. Circulation 104:3169, 2001.
6. Drew BJ, Califf RM, Funk M, et al: Practice standards for electrocardiographic monitoring in hospital settings: An American Heart Association scientific statement from the Councils on Cardiovascular Nursing, Clinical Cardiology, and Cardiovascular Disease in the Young: endorsed by the International Society of Computerized Electrocardiology and the American Association of Critical-Care Nurses. Circulation 110:2721, 2004.
7. Eagle KA, Berger PB, Calkins H, et al: ACC/AHA guideline update for perioperative cardiovascular evaluation for noncardiac surgery—executive summary: A report of the American College of Cardiology/American Heart Association Task Force on Practice Guidelines (Committee to Update the 1996 Guidelines on Perioperative Cardiovascular Evaluation for Noncardiac Surgery). J Am Coll Cardiol 39:542, 2002.

CHAPTER 13

Exercise Stress Testing

Bernard R. Chaitman

Exercise is a common physiological stress used to elicit cardiovascular abnormalities not present at rest and to determine the adequacy of cardiac function.[1-11] Exercise electrocardiography is one of the most frequent noninvasive modalities used to assess patients with suspected or proven cardiovascular disease. The test is mainly used to estimate prognosis and to determine functional capacity, the likelihood and extent of coronary artery disease (CAD), and the effects of therapy. Hemodynamic and electrocardiographic measurements, combined with ancillary techniques such as metabolic gas analysis, radionuclide imaging, and echocardiography, enhance the information content of exercise testing in selected patients.[5]

EXERCISE PHYSIOLOGY

Anticipation of dynamic exercise results in an acceleration of ventricular rate caused by vagal withdrawal, increase in alveolar ventilation, and increased venous return, primarily as a result of sympathetic venoconstriction.[12] In normal persons, the net effect is to increase resting cardiac output before the start of exercise. The magnitude of hemodynamic response during exercise depends on the severity of the exercise and the amount of muscle mass involved. In the early phases of exercise in the upright position, cardiac output is increased by an augmentation in stroke volume mediated through the use of the Frank-Starling mechanism and heart rate; the increase in cardiac output in the latter phases of exercise is primarily caused by a sympathetic-mediated increase in ventricular rate. At fixed submaximal workloads below anaerobic threshold, steady-state conditions are usually reached after the second minute of exercise, following which heart rate, cardiac output, blood pressure, and pulmonary ventilation are maintained at reasonably constant levels. During strenuous exertion, sympathetic discharge is maximal and parasympathetic stimulation is withdrawn, resulting in vasoconstriction of most circulatory body systems, except for that in exercising muscle and in the cerebral and coronary circulations. Venous and arterial norepinephrine release from sympathetic postganglionic nerve endings, as well as plasma renin levels, are increased; the catecholamine release enhances ventricular contractility. As exercise progresses, skeletal muscle blood flow is increased, oxygen extraction increases by as much as threefold, total calculated peripheral resistance decreases, and systolic blood pressure, mean arterial pressure, and pulse pressure usually increase. Diastolic blood pressure does not change significantly. The pulmonary vascular bed can accommodate as much as a sixfold increase in cardiac output with only modest increases in pulmonary artery pressure, pulmonary capillary wedge pressure, and right atrial pressure; in normal individuals, this is not a limiting determinant of peak exercise capacity.

Cardiac output increases by four- to sixfold above basal levels during strenuous exertion in the upright position, depending on genetic endowment and level of training.[12] The maximum heart rate and cardiac output are decreased in older persons, partly because of decreased beta-adrenergic responsivity.[13,14] Maximum heart rate (HR) can be estimated from the following formula:

$$HR = 220 - \text{age (in years)}$$

with a standard deviation of 10 to 12 beats/min. The age-predicted maximum heart rate is a useful measurement for safety reasons. However, the wide standard deviation in the various regression equations used and the impact of drug therapy limit the usefulness of this parameter in estimating the exact age-predicted maximum for an individual patient.[8,15]

In the postexercise phase, hemodynamics returns to baseline within minutes of termination of exercise. Vagal reactivation is an important cardiac deceleration mechanism after exercise and is accelerated in well-trained athletes but blunted in patients with chronic heart failure (see later, "Nonelectrocardiographic Observations"). Intense physical work or significant cardiorespiratory impairment may interfere with achievement of a steady state, and an oxygen deficit occurs during exercise. The total oxygen uptake in excess of the resting oxygen uptake during the recovery period is the oxygen debt.[4,5]

Patient's Position

At rest, the cardiac output and stroke volume are higher when the person is in a supine position than when in an upright position. With exercise, in normal supine persons, the elevation of cardiac output results almost entirely from an increase in heart rate, with little augmentation of stroke volume. In the upright posture, the increase in cardiac output in normal individuals results from a combination of elevations in stroke volume and heart rate. A change from supine to upright posture causes a decrease in venous return, left ventricular end-diastolic volume and pressure, stroke volume, and cardiac index. Renin and norepinephrine levels are increased. End-systolic volume and ejection fraction are not significantly changed. In normal individuals, end-systolic volume decreases and ejection fraction increases to a similar extent from rest to exercise in the supine and upright positions. The magnitude and direction of change in end-diastolic volume from rest to maximum exercise in both positions are small and may vary according to the patient population studied. The net effect on exercise performance is an approximate 10 percent increase in exercise time, cardiac index, heart rate, and rate pressure product at peak exercise in the upright as compared with the supine position.

Cardiopulmonary Exercise Testing

Cardiopulmonary exercise testing involves measurements of respiratory oxygen uptake ($\dot{V}O_2$), carbon dioxide production ($\dot{V}CO_2$), and ventilatory parameters during a symptom-limited exercise test. The patient usually wears a nose clip and breathes through a nonrebreathing valve that separates expired air from room air. During testing, it is important that there be no air leaks in the system. Important measurements of expired gas are PO_2, PCO_2, and air flow. Ventilatory measurements include respiratory rate, tidal volume, and minute ventilation ($\dot{V}e$). PO_2 and PCO_2 are sampled breath by breath or by use of a mixing chamber. The $\dot{V}O_2$ and $\dot{V}CO_2$ can be computed from ventilatory volumes and differences between inspired and expired gases.[4,5] Under steady-state conditions, $\dot{V}O_2$ and $\dot{V}CO_2$ measured at the mouth are equivalent to total-body oxygen consumption and carbon dioxide production. The relationship between work output, oxygen consumption, heart rate, and cardiac output during exercise is linear (Fig. 13-1). The slope of the $\dot{V}O_2$-work relationship is a measure of the biochemical efficiency of exercise. $\dot{V}O_2$max is the product of maximal arteriovenous oxygen difference and cardiac output and represents the largest amount of oxygen a person can use while performing dynamic exercise involving a large part of total muscle mass. The $\dot{V}O_2$max decreases with age, is usually lower in women than in men, and can vary among individuals as a result of genetic factors.[4,5] $\dot{V}O_2$max is diminished by the degree of cardiovascular impairment and by physical inactivity. In untrained persons, the arterial-mixed venous oxygen difference at peak exercise is relatively constant (14 to 17 volume-percent), and $\dot{V}O_2$max is an approximation of maximum cardiac output. Measured $\dot{V}O_2$max can be compared with predicted values from empirically derived formulas based on age, gender, weight, and height.[3-5] Most clinical studies that use exercise as a stress to assess cardiac reserve report the peak $\dot{V}O_2$ (the highest $\dot{V}O_2$ attained during graded exercise testing) rather than $\dot{V}O_2$max. Peak exercise capacity is decreased when the ratio of measured to predicted $\dot{V}O_2$max is less than 85 to 90 percent. Oximetry, performed noninvasively, can be used to monitor arterial oxygen saturation, provided that a good signal pulse is obtained; the value normally does not decrease by more than 5 percent during exercise. In general, pulse oximeters are useful in monitoring trending phenomena, but may not be reliable in determining absolute magnitude of change. A significant desaturation should be confirmed with arterial blood gases.

ANAEROBIC THRESHOLD. Anaerobic threshold is a theoretical point during dynamic exercise when muscle tissue switches over to anaerobic metabolism as an additional energy source. All tissues do not shift simultaneously, and there is a brief interval during which exercise muscle tissue shifts from predominantly aerobic to anaerobic metabolism.[4,5] Lactic acid begins to accumulate when a healthy untrained subject reaches about 50 to 60 percent of the maximal capacity for aerobic metabolism. The increase in lactic acid becomes greater as exercise becomes more intense, resulting in metabolic acidosis. As lactate is formed, it is buffered in the serum by the bicarbonate system, resulting in increased carbon dioxide excretion, which causes reflex hyperventilation. The gas exchange anaerobic threshold is the point at which $\dot{V}e$ increases disproportionately relative to $\dot{V}O_2$ and work; it usually occurs at 40 to 60 percent of $\dot{V}O_2$max in normal untrained individuals, with a wide range of normal values between 35 and 80 percent. Below the anaerobic threshold, carbon dioxide production is proportional to oxygen consumption. Above the anaerobic threshold, carbon dioxide is produced in excess of oxygen consumption. The anaerobic threshold determination is influenced by age, modality (e.g., arm versus leg, ergometer versus treadmill), and exercise protocol. There are several methods to determine anaerobic threshold; these include the following: (1) the V-slope method, the point at which the rate of increase in $\dot{V}CO_2$ relative to $\dot{V}O_2$increases (see Fig. 13-1); (2) the point at which the $\dot{V}O_2$ and $\dot{V}CO_2$ slopes intersect; and (3) the point at which the ratio of $\dot{V}e/\dot{V}O_2$ and end-tidal oxygen tension begins to increase systematically, without an immediate increase in the $\dot{V}e/\dot{V}O_2$ (see Fig. 13-1). The anaerobic threshold is a useful parameter because work below this level encompasses most activities of daily living. Values below 40 percent of predicted $\dot{V}O_2$ may indicate significant cardiovascular disease, pulmonary disease, limited oxygen delivery to the tissues, or mitochondrial abnormalities. An increase in anaerobic threshold with training can enhance an individual's capacity to perform sustained submaximal activities, with consequent improvement in quality of life and daily living. Changes in anaerobic threshold and

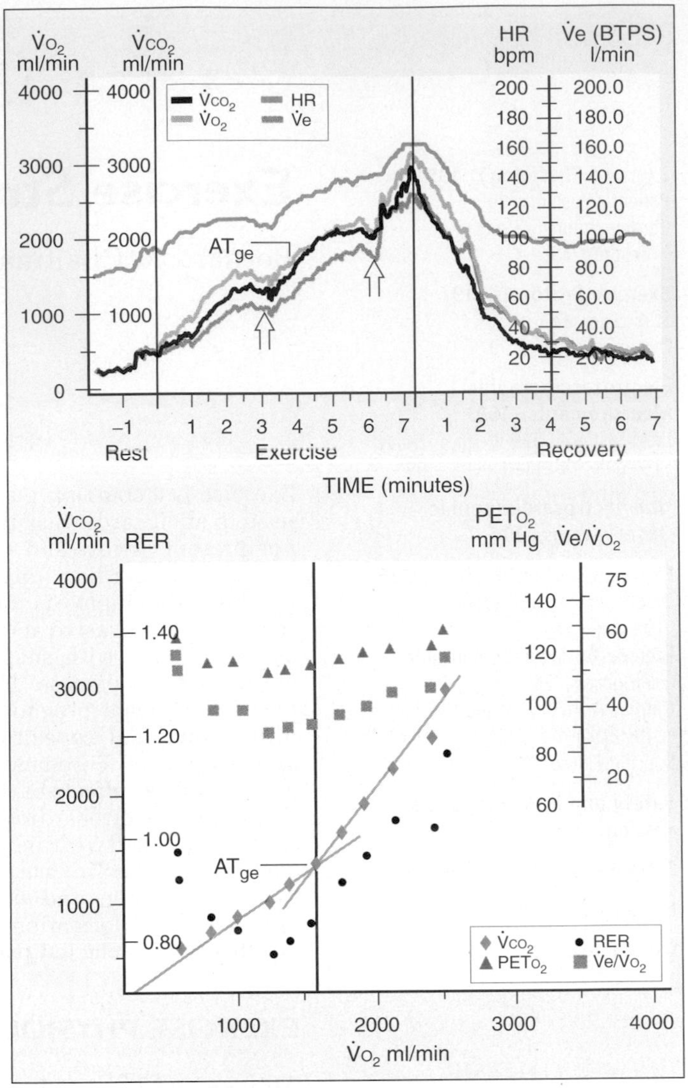

FIGURE 13–1 Cardiopulmonary exercise test in a healthy 53-year-old man using the Bruce protocol. The progressive linear increase in work output, heart rate (HR), and oxygen consumption $\dot{V}O_2$) is noted, with steady-state conditions reached after 2 minutes in each of the first two stages **(top).** Open arrows indicate the beginning of each new 3-minute stage. The subject completed 7 minutes and 10 seconds of exercise, and peak $\dot{V}O_2$ was 3.08 liters/min. The anaerobic threshold (AT_{ge}), determined by the V-slope method, is the point at which the slope of the relative rate of increase in $\dot{V}CO_2$ relative to $\dot{V}O_2$ changes; it occurred at a $\dot{V}O_2$ of 1.5 liters/min, or 49 percent of peak $\dot{V}O_2$, within predicted values for a normal sedentary population **(bottom).** The AT_{ge} determined by the point at which the $\dot{V}O_2$ and $\dot{V}CO_2$ slopes intersect (1.8 liters/min) **(top)** is slightly greater than the AT_{ge} determined by the V-slope method **(bottom).** The V-slope method usually provides a more reproducible estimate of AT_{ge}. $PETO_2$ = end-tidal pressure of oxygen; RER = respiratory exchange ratio; $\dot{V}e/\dot{V}O_2$ = ratio of ventilation to oxygen uptake.

peak $\dot{V}O_2$ with repeat testing can be used to assess disease progression, response to medical therapy, and improvement in cardiovascular fitness with training.

VENTILATORY PARAMETERS. In addition to peak $\dot{V}O_2$, minute ventilation and its relation to $\dot{V}CO_2$ and oxygen consumption are useful indices of cardiac and pulmonary function.[4,5] Exercise-induced changes in tidal minute ventilation ($\dot{V}e$), and breathing pattern (tidal volume, VT, and inspiratory frequency) are measured, along with assessment of ventilatory reserve. The ventilatory reserve determination corresponds to how close the peak minute ventilation achieved (ventilatory demand) during exercise ($\dot{V}e$ max) approaches maximum ventilatory capacity. The respiratory exchange ratio represents the amount of carbon dioxide produced divided by the amount of oxygen consumed. The respiratory exchange ratio ranges from 0.7 to 0.85 at rest and is partly dependent on the predominant fuel used for cellular metabolism (e.g., the respiratory exchange ratio for predominant carbohydrate use is 1.0, whereas the respiratory exchange ratio for predominant fatty acid use is 0.7). At high exercise levels, carbon dioxide production exceeds $\dot{V}O_2$, and a respiratory exchange ratio greater than 1.1 often indicates that the subject has performed at maximal effort.

METABOLIC EQUIVALENT. In current use, the term *metabolic equivalent* (MET) refers to a unit of oxygen uptake in a sitting, resting person; 1 MET is equivalent to 3.5 ml O_2/kg/min of body weight. Measured $\dot{V}O_2$ in ml O_2/kg/min divided by 3.5 ml O_2/kg/min determines the number of METs associated with activity. Work activities can be calculated in multiples of METs; this measurement is useful to determine exercise prescriptions, assess disability, and standardize the reporting of submaximal and peak exercise workloads when different protocols are used. An exercise workload of 3 to 5 METs is consistent with activities such as raking leaves, light carpentry, golf, and walking at 3 to 4 mph. Workloads of 5 to 7 METs are consistent with exterior carpentry, singles tennis, and light backpacking. Workloads in excess of 9 METs are compatible with heavy labor, handball, squash, and running at 6 to 7 mph. Estimating $\dot{V}O_2$ from work rate or treadmill time in individual patients may lead to misinterpretation of data if exercise equipment is not correctly calibrated, if the patient holds on to the front handrails, or if the patient fails to achieve steady state, is obese, or has peripheral vascular disease, pulmonary vascular disease, or cardiac impairment. $\dot{V}O_2$ does not increase linearly in some patients with cardiovascular or pulmonary disease as work rate is increased, and $\dot{V}O_2$ can thus be overestimated. The measurements obtained with cardiopulmonary exercise testing are useful in understanding an individual patient's response to exercise and can be useful in the diagnostic evaluation of a patient with unexplained dyspnea or exercise impairment, or in quantifying the degree of disability.[3-6,8]

EXERCISE PROTOCOLS

The main types of exercise are isotonic or dynamic exercise, isometric or static exercise, and resistive (combined isometric and isotonic) exercise. Dynamic protocols most frequently are used to assess cardiovascular reserve, and those suitable for clinical testing should include a low-intensity warm-up phase. In general, 6 to 12 minutes of continuous progressive exercise during which the myocardial oxygen demand is elevated to the patient's maximal level is optimal for diagnostic and prognostic purposes.[8] The protocol should include a suitable recovery or cool-down period. If the protocol is too strenuous for an individual patient, the test must be terminated early, and there is no opportunity to observe clinically important responses. If the exercise protocol is too easy for an individual patient, the prolonged procedure tests endurance and not aerobic capacity. Thus, exercise protocols should be individualized to accommodate a patient's limitations. Protocols may be set up at a fixed duration of exercise for a certain intensity to meet minimal qualifications for certain industrial tasks or sports programs.

Static Exercise

This form of isometric exercise generates force with little muscle shortening and produces a greater blood pressure response than dynamic exercise.[11] Cardiac output does not increase as much as with dynamic exercise, because increased resistance in active muscle groups limits blood flow. In a common form of static exercise, the patient's maximal force on a hand dynamometer is recorded. The patient then sustains 25 to 33 percent of maximal force for 3 to 5 minutes while the electrocardiogram (ECG) is obtained and blood pressure recorded. The increase in myocardial $\dot{V}O_2$ is often insufficient to initiate an ischemic response.

Dynamic Exercise

ARM ERGOMETRY. Arm crank ergometry protocols involve arm cranking at incremental workloads of 10 to 20 W for 2- or 3-minute stages. The heart rate and blood pressure responses to a given workload of arm exercise usually are greater than those for leg exercise. A bicycle ergometer with the axle placed at the level of the shoulders is used, and the subject sits or stands and cycles the peddles so that the arms are fully extended alternately. The most common frequency is 50 rpm. In normal individuals, maximal $\dot{V}O_2$ and $\dot{V}e$ for arm cycling approximates 50 to 70 percent of the same measures as leg cycling. Peak $\dot{V}O_2$ and peak heart rate are approximately 70 percent of the measures during leg testing. Arm ergometry exercise protocols for risk stratification of patients with suspected or documented coronary artery disease (CAD) before noncardiac surgery can be used as a stressor when leg exercise is not possible or insufficient to test cardiac reserve.

BICYCLE ERGOMETRY. Bicycle protocols involve incremental workloads calibrated in watts (W) or kilopond-meters per minute (kpm).[16] One watt is equivalent to approximately 6 kpm. Because exercise on a cycle ergometer is not weight-bearing, kilopond-meters per minute or watts can be converted to oxygen uptake in milliliters per minute. In mechanically braked bicycles, work is determined by force and distance and requires a constant pedaling rate of 60 to 80 rpm, according to the patient's preference. Electronically braked bicycles provide a constant workload despite changes in pedaling rate and are less dependent on a patient's cooperation. They are more costly than a mechanically braked bicycle but are preferred for diagnostic and prognostic assessment. Most protocols start with a power output of 10 or 25 W/min (150 kpm), usually followed by increases of 25 W every 2 or 3 minutes until endpoints are reached. Younger subjects can start at 50 W, with increases in 50-W increments every 2 minutes. A ramp protocol differs from the staged protocols in that the patient starts at 3 minutes of unloaded pedaling at a cycle speed of 60 rpm. Work rate is increased by a uniform amount each minute, ranging from 5- to 30-W increments, depending on a patient's expected performance. Exercise is terminated if the patient is unable to maintain a cycling frequency above 40 rpm. In the cardiac catheterization laboratory, hemodynamic measurements can be made during supine bicycle ergometry at rest and at one or two submaximal workloads. The bicycle ergometer is associated with a lower maximal $\dot{V}O_2$ and anaerobic threshold than the treadmill; maximal heart rate, maximal $\dot{V}e$, and maximal lactate values are often similar.

TREADMILL PROTOCOL. The treadmill protocol should be consistent with the patient's physical capacity and the purpose of the test. In healthy individuals, the standard Bruce protocol is popular, and a large diagnostic and prognostic data base has been published using this protocol.[1,2,7,8] The Bruce multistage maximal treadmill protocol has 3-minute periods to allow achievement of a steady state before workload is increased (Fig. 13-2; see Fig. 13-1). In older individuals or those whose exercise capacity is limited by cardiac disease, the protocol can be modified by two 3-minute warm-up stages at 1.7 mph and 0 percent grade and

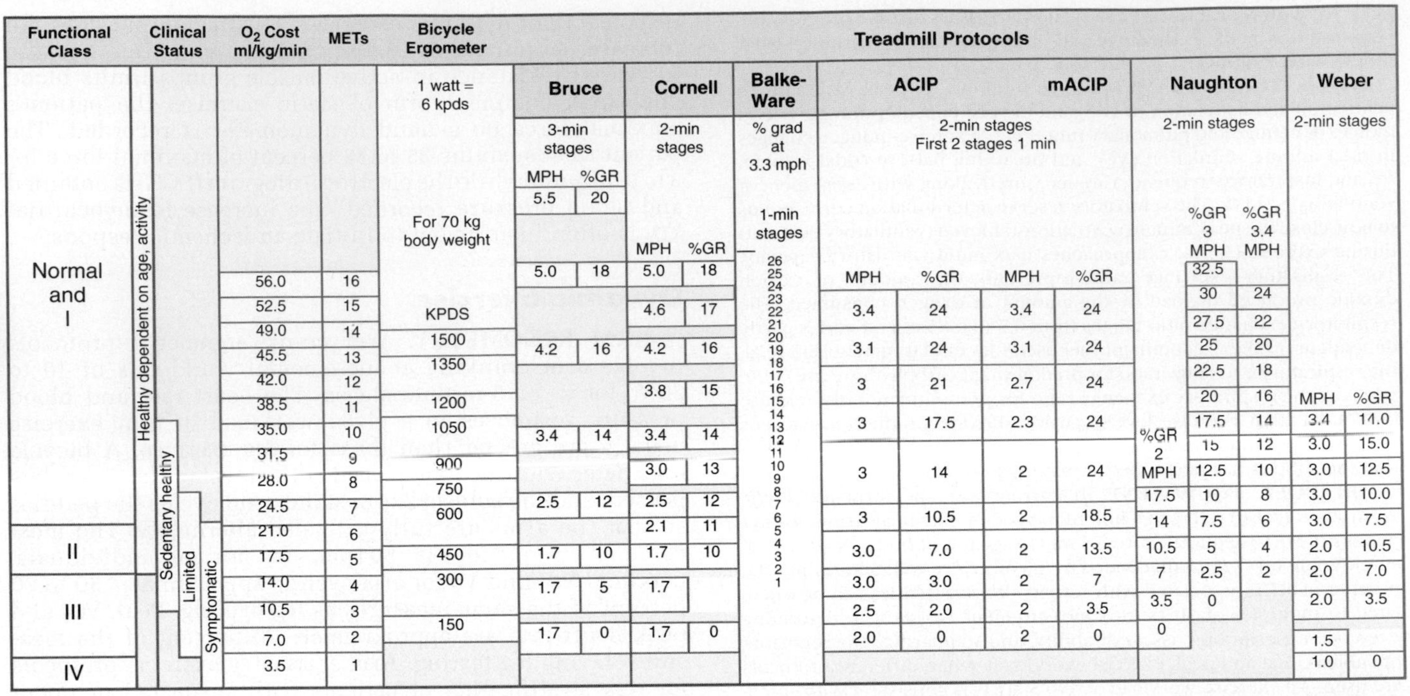

FIGURE 13–2 Estimated oxygen cost of bicycle ergometer and selected treadmill protocols. The standard Bruce protocol starts at 1.7 mph and 10 percent grade (5 METs), with a larger increment between stages than protocols such as the Naughton, ACIP, and Weber, which start at less than 2 METs at 2 mph and increase by 1- to 1.5-MET increments between stages. The Bruce protocol can be modified by two 3-minute warm-up stages at 1.7 mph and 0 percent grade and 1.7 mph and 5 percent grade. mACIP = modified ACIP; METs = metabolic equivalents. *(Adapted from Fletcher GF, Balady G, Amsterdam EA, et al: Exercise Standards for Testing and Training. A statement for healthcare professionals from the American Heart Association. Circulation 104:1694, 2001. © 2001 American Heart Association.)*

1.7 mph and 5 percent grade. A limitation of the Bruce protocol is the relatively large increase in $\dot{V}O_2$ between stages and the additional energy cost of running as compared with walking at stages in excess of Bruce's stage III. The Naughton and Weber protocols use 1- to 2-minute stages with 1-MET increments between stages; these protocols may be more suitable for patients with limited exercise tolerance, such as patients with compensated congestive heart failure. The Asymptomatic Cardiac Ischemia Pilot (ACIP) trial and modified ACIP (mACIP) protocols use 2-minute stages, with 1.5-MET increments between stages after two 1-minute warm-up stages with 1-MET increments. The ACIP protocols were developed to test patients with established CAD and result in a linear increase in heart rate and $\dot{V}O_2$, distributing the time to occurrence of ST segment depression over a wider range of heart rate and exercise time than protocols with more abrupt increments in workload between stages.[2] The mACIP protocol produces a similar aerobic demand as the standard ACIP protocol for each minute of exercise and is well suited for short or elderly individuals who cannot keep up with a walking speed of 3 mph (see Fig. 13-2).

Ramp protocols start the patient at a relatively slow treadmill speed, which is gradually increased until the patient has a good stride. The ramp angle of incline is progressively increased at fixed intervals (e.g., 10 to 60 seconds), starting at zero grade with the increase in grade calculated on the basis of the patient's estimated functional capacity so that the protocol will be complete at 6 to 12 minutes.[8] In this type of protocol, the rate of work increase is continuous and steady-state conditions are not reached. A limitation of ramp protocols is the need to estimate functional capacity from an activity scale; underestimation or overestimation of functional capacity occasionally results in an endurance test or premature cessation. One formula for estimating $\dot{V}O_2$ from treadmill speed and grade is as follows:

$$\dot{V}O_2(\text{ml } O_2 \times kg^{-1} \times min^{-1}) = (\text{mph} \times 2.68) + (1.8 \times 26.82 \times \text{mph} \times \text{grade} \div 100) + 3.5$$

The peak $\dot{V}O_2$ is usually the same regardless of treadmill protocol used; the difference is the rate of time at which the peak $\dot{V}O_2$ is achieved.

It is important to encourage patients not to grasp the handrails of the treadmill during exercise, particularly the front handrails. Functional capacity can be overestimated by as much as 20 percent in tests in which handrail support is permitted, and $\dot{V}O_2$ is decreased. Because the degree of handrail support is difficult to quantify from one test to another, more consistent results can be obtained during serial testing when handrail support is not permitted.

WALK TEST. A 6-minute walk test or a long-distance corridor walk test can be used to provide an estimate of functional capacity in patients who cannot perform bicycle or treadmill exercise, such as elderly patients or those with heart failure, claudication, or orthopedic limitations.[17,18] During a 6-minute walk test, patients are instructed to walk down a 100-foot corridor at their own pace, attempting to cover as much ground as possible in 6 minutes. At the end of the 6-minute interval, the total distance walked is determined and the symptoms experienced by the patient are recorded. During a long-distance corridor walk, patients are instructed to walk 400 meters in a hallway on a 20 meter/segment course for 10 laps (40 meters/lap) after a 2-minute warm-up. Performance of walk tests as a clinical measure of ambulatory function requires highly skilled personnel following a rigid protocol to elicit reproducible and reliable results.

Techniques. Patients should be instructed not to eat, drink caffeinated beverages, or smoke for 3 hours before testing and to wear comfortable shoes and loose-fitting clothes. Unusual physical exertion should be avoided before testing. A brief history and physical examination should be performed, and patients should be advised about the risks and benefits of the procedure. A written informed consent form is usually required. The indication for the test should be known. The supervising physician should be made aware of any recent deterioration in the patient's clinical status. The test should not be performed on subjects who are markedly hypertensive (e.g., blood pressure higher than 220/120 mm Hg) or who have unexplained hypotension (e.g., systolic blood pressure lower than 80 mm Hg) or other contraindications to exercise testing (see later, "Safety and Risks of Exercise Testing"). In many laboratories, the presence or absence of atherosclerotic risk factors is noted and cardioactive medication recorded. A standard 12-lead ECG is usually obtained, with the electrodes at the distal extremities. The timing of cardioactive medication ingestion before testing depends on the test indication.

After the standard 12-lead ECG is recorded, torso ECGs should be obtained with the patient in the supine position and in the sitting or standing position. Postural changes can elicit labile ST-T wave abnormalities. Hyperventilation is not recommended before exercise. If a false-positive test result is suspected, hyperventilation should be performed after the test, and the hyperventilation tracing compared with the maximal ST segment abnormalities observed. The ECG should be obtained and blood pressure recorded in both positions, and patients should be instructed on how to perform the test.

Adequate skin preparation is essential for high-quality recordings, and the superficial layer of skin needs to be removed to augment signal-to-noise ratio. The areas of electrode application are rubbed with an alcohol-saturated pad to remove oil and rubbed with free sandpaper or a rough material to reduce skin resistance to 5000 ohms or less. Silver chloride electrodes with a fluid column to avoid direct metal-to-skin contact produce high-quality tracings; these electrodes have the lowest offset voltage. The electrode fluid column can dry out over time and should be verified prior to application. This can be a cause of poor-quality tracings.

Cables connecting the electrodes and recorders should be light, flexible, and properly shielded. In a small minority of patients, a fishnet jersey may be required over the electrodes and cables to reduce motion artifact. The electrode-skin interface can be verified by tapping on the electrode and examining the monitor or by measuring skin impedance. Excessive noise indicates that the electrode needs to be replaced; replacement before the test rather than during exercise can save time. The electrocardiographic signal can be digitized systematically at the patient's end of the cable by some systems, reducing power line artifact. Cables, adapters, and the junction box have a finite life span and require periodic replacement to obtain the highest quality tracings. Exercise equipment should be calibrated regularly. Room temperature should be between 64° and 72°F (18° and 22°C) and humidity less than 60 percent.

Treadmill walking should be demonstrated to the patient. The heart rate, blood pressure, and ECG should be recorded at the end of each stage of exercise, immediately before and immediately after stopping exercise, at the onset of an ischemic response, and for each minute for at least 5 to 10 minutes in the recovery phase. A minimum of three leads should be displayed continuously on the monitor during the test. There is some controversy about optimal patient position in the recovery phase. In the sitting position, less space is required for a stretcher, and patients are more comfortable immediately after exertion. The supine position increases end-diastolic volume and has the potential to augment ST segment changes.[8]

ELECTROCARDIOGRAPHIC MEASUREMENTS

Lead Systems

The Mason-Likar modification of the standard 12-lead ECG requires that the extremity electrodes be moved to the torso to reduce motion artifact. The arm electrodes should be located in the most lateral aspects of the infraclavicular fossae, and the leg electrodes should be in a stable position above the anterior iliac crest and below the rib cage. The Mason-Likar modification results in a right axis shift and increased voltage in the inferior leads and may produce a loss of inferior Q waves and the development of new Q waves in lead aVL. Thus, the body torso limb lead positions cannot be used to interpret a diagnostic resting 12-lead ECG. The more cephalad the leg electrodes are placed, the greater is the degree of change and the greater is the augmentation of R wave amplitude.

Bipolar lead groups place the negative, or reference, electrode over the manubrium (CM_5), right scapula (CB_5), or RV_5 (CC_5), or on the forehead (CH_5), and the active electrode at V_5 or a proximate location to optimize R wave amplitude. Bipolar lead groups may provide additional diagnostic information and, in some medical centers, lead CM_5 is substituted for lead aVR in the Mason-Likar–modified lead system. Bipolar leads are frequently used when only a limited electrocardiographic set is required (e.g., in cardiac rehabilitation programs). The use of more elaborate lead set systems is usually reserved for research purposes.

ST Segment Displacement

Types of ST Segment Displacement

In normal persons, the PR, QRS, and QT intervals shorten as heart rate increases. P amplitude increases, and the PR segment becomes progressively more downsloping in the inferior leads. J point, or junctional, depression is a normal finding during exercise (Fig. 13-3). In patients with myocardial ischemia, however, the ST segment usually becomes more horizontal (flattens) as the severity of the ischemic response worsens. With progressive exercise, the depth of ST segment depression may increase, involving more ECG leads, and the patient may develop angina. In the immediate postrecovery phase, the ST segment displacement may persist, with downsloping ST segments and T wave inversion, gradually returning to baseline after 5 to 10 minutes (Figs. 13-4 and 13-5). Ischemic ST segment displacement may be seen only during exercise, emphasizing the importance of adequate skin preparation and electrode placement to capture high-quality recordings during maximum exertion (Fig. 13-6). In about 10 percent of patients, the ischemic response may appear only in the recovery phase.[19] This is a relevant finding, and the prevalence of reversible perfusion defects by single-photon emission computed tomography criteria (see Chap. 16) are comparable to those observed when the ischemic ST segment response occurs during and after exercise.[20-23] Patients should not leave the exercise laboratory area until the postexercise ECG has returned to

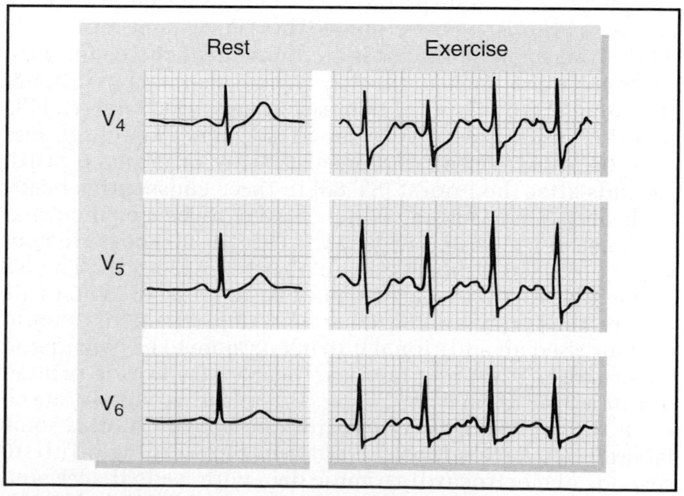

FIGURE 13-3 J point depression of 2 to 3 mm in leads V_4 to V_6 with rapid upsloping ST segments depressed approximately 1 mm 80 milliseconds after the J point. The ST segment slope in leads V_4 and V_5 is 3.0 mV/sec. This response should not be considered abnormal.

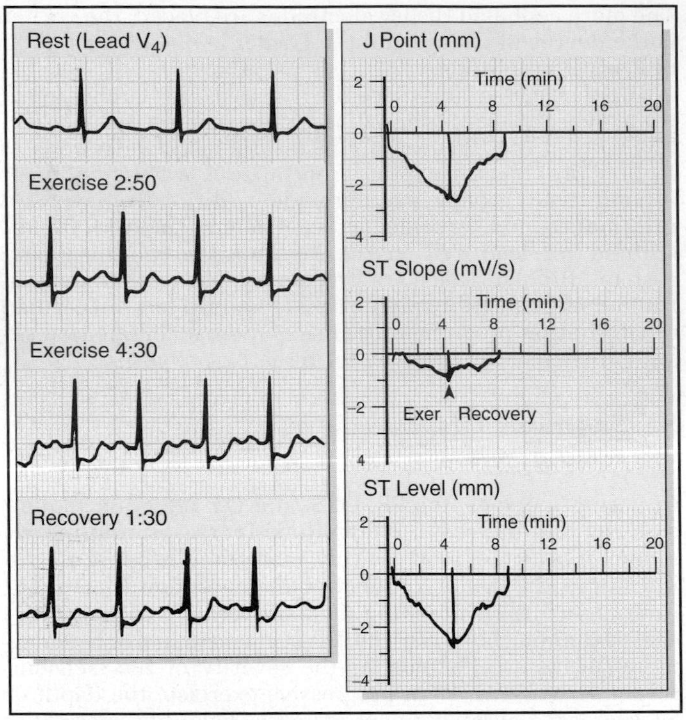

FIGURE 13–4 Bruce protocol. In lead V_4, the exercise electrocardiographic result is abnormal early in the test, reaching 0.3 mV (3 mm) of horizontal ST segment depression at the end of exercise. The ischemic changes persist for at least 1 minute and 30 seconds into the recovery phase. **Right panel,** Continuous plot of the J point, ST slope, and ST segment displacement at 80 milliseconds after the J point (ST level) during exercise and in the recovery phase. Exercise ends at the vertical line at 4.5 minutes (red arrow). The computer trends permit a more precise identification of initial onset and offset of ischemic ST segment depression. This type of electrocardiographic pattern, with early onset of ischemic ST segment depression, reaching more than 3 mm of horizontal ST segment displacement and persisting several minutes into the recovery phase, is consistent with a severe ischemic response.

baseline. Figure 13-7 illustrates eight different electrocardiographic patterns seen during exercise testing.

Measurement of ST Segment Displacement

For purposes of interpretation, the PQ junction is usually chosen as the isoelectric point. The TP segment represents a true isoelectric point but is an impractical choice for most routine clinical measurements. The development of 0.10 mV (1 mm) or more of J point depression measured from the PQ junction, with a relatively flat ST segment slope (e.g., less than 0.7 to 1 mV/sec), depressed 0.10 mV or more 80 milliseconds after the J point (ST 80) in three consecutive beats, with a stable baseline, is considered to be an abnormal response (Fig. 13-8). In general, the ST 60 measurement should be used at heart rates higher than 130/min. The ST segment at rest may occasionally be depressed. When this occurs, the J point and ST 60 or ST 80 measurements should be depressed an additional 0.10 mV or more to be considered abnormal. In most laboratories, the exercise ECG is printed out in a 3 × 4 format, or 2.5 sec/three-lead group. To maximize the opportunity of meeting the above criteria, some laboratories have adopted a strategy of recording a full 10 seconds of electrocardiographic data with leads II, aVF, and V_5 when the tracing starts to show abnormal beats below the ischemic threshold. This 10-second tracing increases the likelihood of capturing consecutive abnormal beats with a stable baseline.

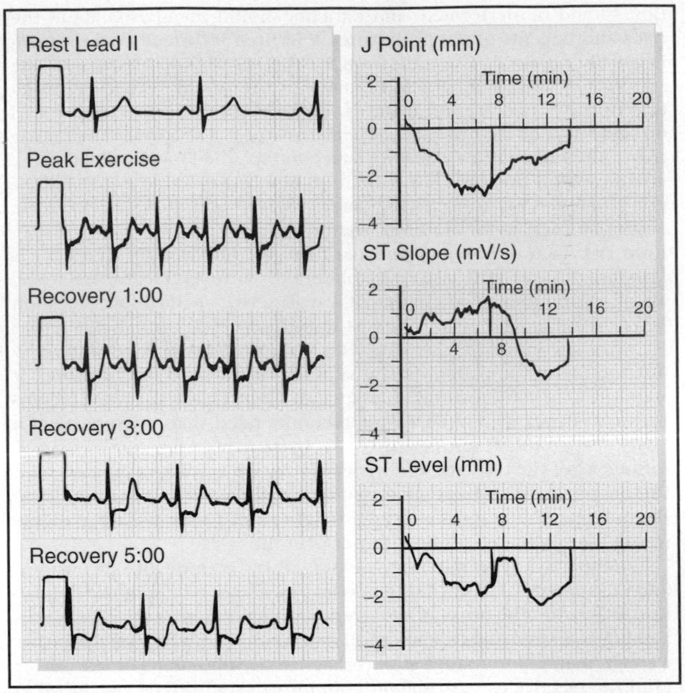

FIGURE 13–5 Bruce protocol. In this type of ischemic pattern, the J point at peak exertion is depressed 2.5 mm, the ST segment slope is 1.5 mV/sec, and the ST segment level is depressed 1.6 mm at 80 milliseconds after the J point. This "slow upsloping" ST segment at peak exercise indicates an ischemic pattern in patients with a high pretest prevalence of coronary disease. A typical ischemic pattern is seen at 3 minutes of the recovery phase when the ST segment is horizontal and 5 minutes after exertion when the ST segment is downsloping. **Right panels,** Exercise is discontinued at the vertical line at 7.5 minutes.

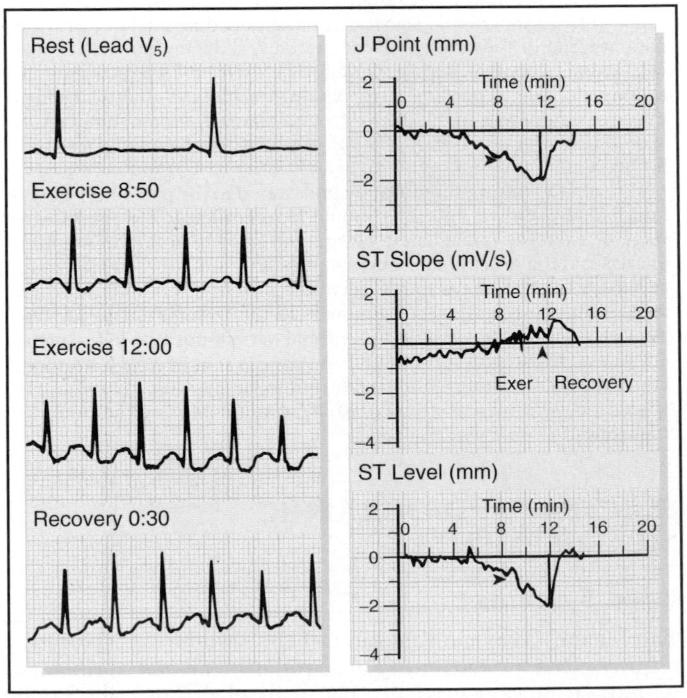

FIGURE 13–6 Bruce protocol. The exercise ECG result is not yet abnormal at 8:50 minutes but becomes abnormal at 9:30 minutes (horizontal arrows, **right**) of a 12-minute exercise test and resolves in the immediate recovery phase. This electrocardiographic pattern, in which the ST segment becomes abnormal only at high exercise workloads and returns to baseline in the immediate recovery phase, may indicate a false-positive result in an asymptomatic individual without atherosclerotic risk factors. Exercise myocardial imaging would provide more diagnostic and prognostic information if this were an older person with several atherosclerotic risk factors. Vertical arrow indicates termination of exercise.

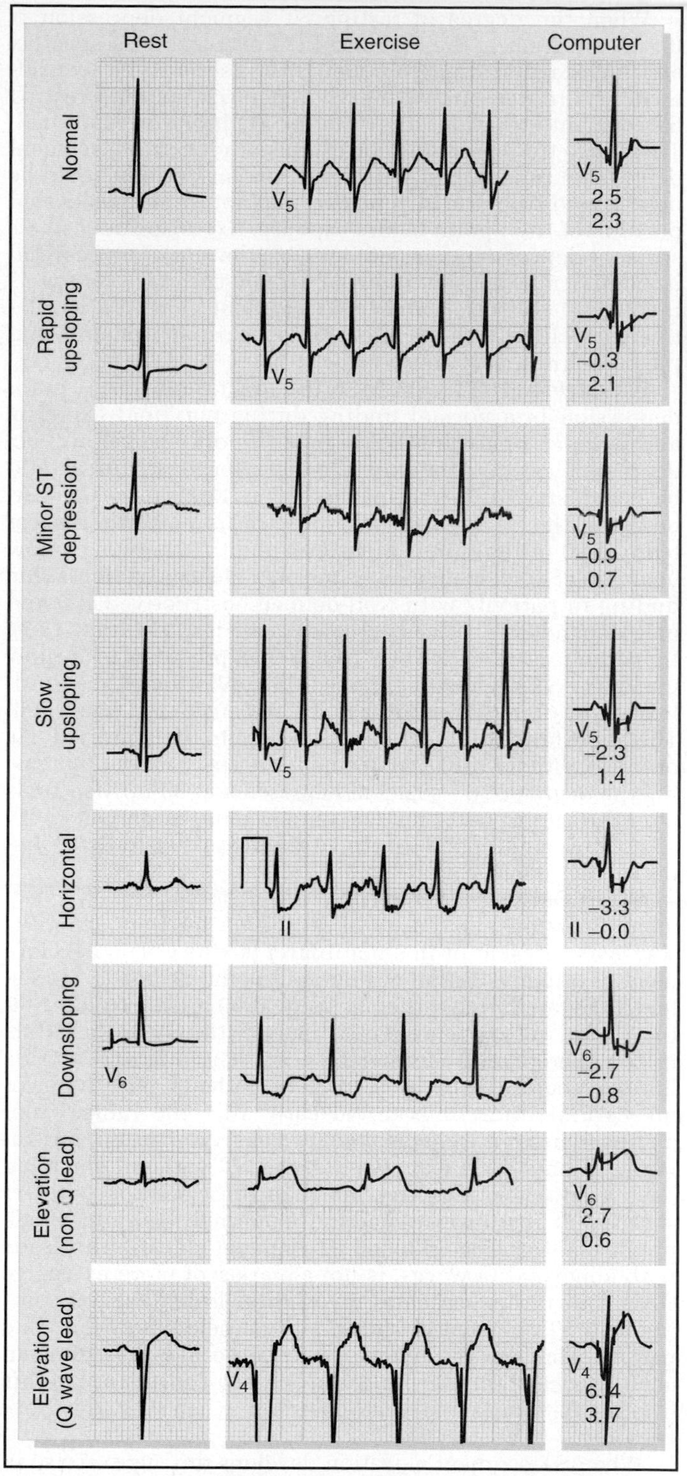

FIGURE 13–7 Eight typical exercise electrocardiographic patterns at rest and at peak exertion. The computer-processed incrementally averaged beat corresponds with the raw data taken at the same time point during exercise and is illustrated in the last column. The patterns represent worsening electrocardiographic responses during exercise. In the column of computer-averaged beats, ST 80 displacement (top number) indicates the magnitude of ST segment displacement 80 milliseconds after the J point relative to the PQ junction or E point. ST segment slope measurement (bottom number) indicates the ST segment slope at a fixed time point after the J point to the ST 80 measurement. At least three noncomputer average complexes with a stable baseline should meet criteria for abnormality before the exercise ECG result can be considered abnormal (see Fig. 13-9). The normal and rapid upsloping ST segment responses are normal responses to exercise. J point depression with rapid upsloping ST segments is a common response in an older, apparently healthy person. Minor ST depression can occur occasionally at submaximal workloads in patients with coronary disease; in this illustration, the ST segment is depressed 0.09 mV (0.9 mm) 80 milliseconds after the J point. The slow upsloping ST segment pattern often demonstrates an ischemic response in patients with known coronary disease or those with a high pretest clinical risk of coronary disease. Criteria for slow upsloping ST segment depression include J point and ST 80 depression of 0.15 mV or more and ST segment slope of more than 1.0 mV/sec. Classic criteria for myocardial ischemia include horizontal ST segment depression observed when both the J point and ST 80 depression are 0.1 mV or more and ST segment slope is within the range of 1.0 mV/sec. Downsloping ST segment depression occurs when the J point and ST 80 depression are 0.1 mV and the ST segment slope is −1.0 mV/sec. ST segment elevation in a non-Q-wave noninfarct lead occurs when the J point and ST 60 are 1.0 mV or higher and represents a severe ischemic response. ST segment elevation in an infarct territory (Q wave lead) indicates a severe wall motion abnormality and, in most cases, is not considered an ischemic response. *(From Chaitman BR: Exercise electrocardiographic stress testing. In Beller GA [ed]: Chronic Ischemic Heart Disease. In Braunwald E [series ed]: Atlas of Heart Diseases. Vol 5. Chronic Ischemic Heart Disease. Philadelphia, Current Medicine, 1995, pp 2.1-2.30.)*

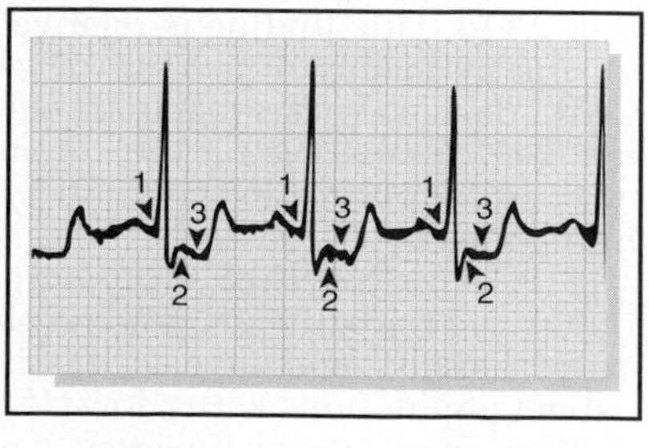

FIGURE 13–8 Magnified ischemic exercise-induced electrocardiographic pattern. Three consecutive complexes with a relatively stable baseline are selected. The PQ junction (1) and J point (2) are determined; the ST 80 (3) is determined at 80 milliseconds after the J point. In this example, average J point displacement is 0.2 mV (2 mm) and ST 80 is 0.24 mV (24 mm). The average slope measurement from the J point to ST 80 is −1.1 mV/sec.

When the degree of resting ST segment depression is 0.1 mV or greater, the exercise ECG becomes less specific, and myocardial imaging modalities should be considered.[1,2,8,24] In patients with early repolarization and resting ST segment elevation, return to the PQ junction is normal. Therefore, the magnitude of exercise-induced ST segment depression in a patient with early repolarization should be determined from the PQ junction and not from the elevated position of the J point before exercise. Exercise-induced ST segment depression does not localize the site of myocardial ischemia, nor does it indicate which coronary artery is involved.[25] Exercise-induced ST segment elevation is relatively specific for the territory of myocardial ischemia and the coronary artery involved.

UPSLOPING ST SEGMENTS. Junctional or J point depression is a normal finding during maximal exercise, and a rapid upsloping ST segment (more than 1 mV/sec) depressed less than 0.15 mV (1.5 mm) after the J point should be considered to be normal (see Fig. 13-3). Occasionally, however, the ST segment is depressed 0.15 mV (1.5 mm) or more at 80 milliseconds after the J point. This type of slow upsloping ST segment may be the only electrocardiographic finding in patients with well-defined obstructive CAD and may depend on the lead set used (see Figs. 13-5 and 13-7). In patient subsets with a high CAD prevalence, a slow upsloping ST segment depressed 0.15 mV or more at 80 milliseconds after the J point should be considered abnormal. The importance of this finding in asymptomatic individuals or those with a low CAD prevalence is less certain. Increasing the degree of ST segment depression at 80 milliseconds after the J point to 0.2 mV (2.0 mm) or more in patients with a slow upsloping ST segment increases specificity but decreases sensitivity.[1,2,7,8]

ST SEGMENT ELEVATION. Exercise-induced ST segment elevation may occur in an infarct territory where Q waves are present or in a noninfarct territory. The development of 0.10 mV (1 mm) or more of J point elevation, persistently elevated higher than 0.10 mV at 60 milliseconds after the J point in three consecutive beats with a stable baseline, is considered an abnormal response (see Fig. 13-7). This finding occurs more frequently in patients with anterior myocardial infarctions tested early after the index event and decreases in frequency by 6 weeks. As a group, postinfarct patients with exercise-induced ST segment elevation have a lower ejection fraction than those without, greater severity of resting wall motion abnormalities, and worse prognosis. Exercise-induced ST segment elevation in leads with abnormal Q waves, is not a marker of more extensive CAD, and rarely indicates myocardial ischemia. Exercise-induced ST segment elevation may occasionally occur in a patient who has regenerated embryonic R waves after an acute myocardial infarction; the clinical significance of this finding is similar to that observed when Q waves are present.

When ST segment elevation develops during exercise in a non-Q-wave lead in a patient without a previous myocardial infarction, the finding should be considered as likely evidence of transmural myocardial ischemia caused by coronary vasospasm or a high-grade coronary narrowing (Fig. 13-9). This finding is relatively uncommon, occurring in approximately 1 percent of patients with obstructive CAD. The electrocardiographic site of ST segment elevation is relatively specific for the coronary artery involved, and myocardial perfusion scintigraphy usually reveals a defect in the territory involved.

T WAVE CHANGES. The morphology of the T wave is influenced by body position, respiration, hyperventilation, drug therapy, and myocardial ischemia or necrosis. In patient populations with a low CAD prevalence, pseudonormalization of T waves (inverted at rest and becoming upright with exercise) is a nondiagnostic finding (Fig. 13-10). In rare cases, this finding may be a marker for myocardial ischemia in a patient with documented CAD, although it would need to be substantiated by an ancillary technique, such as the concomitant finding of a reversible myocardial perfusion defect.

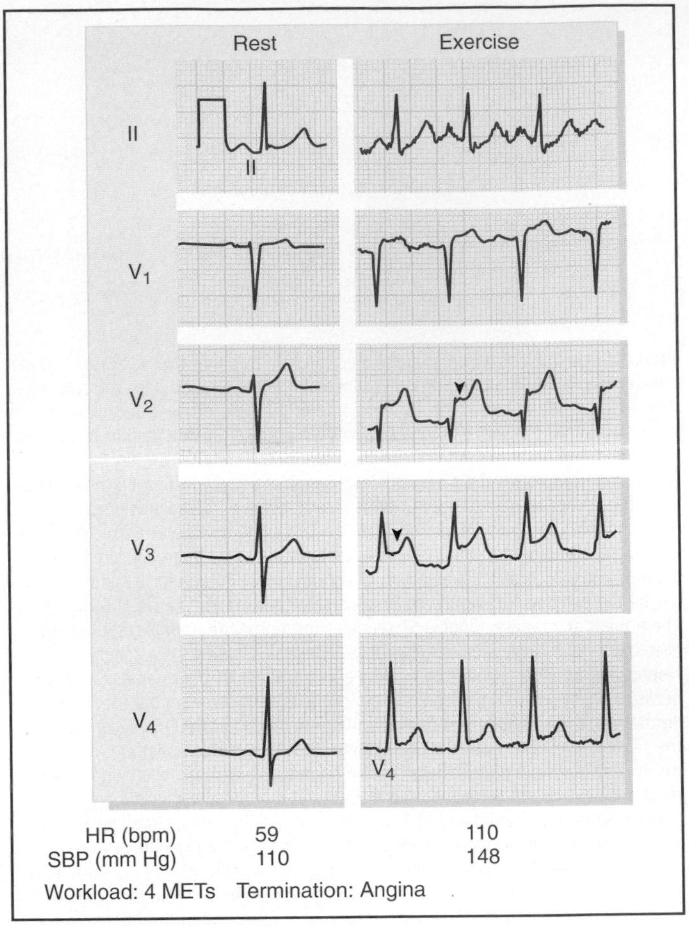

FIGURE 13–9 A 48-year-old man with several atherosclerotic risk factors and a normal resting ECG result developed marked ST segment elevation (4 mm [arrows]) in leads V_2 and V_3, with lesser degrees of ST segment elevation in leads V_1 and V_4 and J point depression with upsloping ST segments in lead II, associated with angina. This type of electrocardiographic pattern is usually associated with a full-thickness, reversible myocardial perfusion defect in the corresponding left ventricular myocardial segments and high-grade intraluminal narrowing at coronary angiography. Rarely, coronary vasospasm produces this result in the absence of significant intraluminal atherosclerotic narrowing. HR = heart rate; METs = metabolic equivalents; SBP = systolic blood pressure. *(From Chaitman BR: Exercise electrocardiographic stress testing.* In *Beller GA [ed]: Chronic Ischemic Heart Disease.* In *Braunwald E [series ed]: Atlas of Heart Diseases. Vol 5. Chronic Ischemic Heart Disease. Philadelphia, Current Medicine, 1995, pp 2.1-2.30.)*

OTHER ECG MARKERS. Changes in R wave amplitude during exercise are relatively nonspecific and are related to the level of exercise performed. When the R wave amplitude meets voltage criteria for left ventricular hypertrophy, the ST segment response cannot be used reliably to diagnose CAD, even in the absence of a left ventricular strain pattern. Loss of R wave amplitude, commonly seen after myocardial infarction, reduces the sensitivity of the ST segment response in that lead to diagnose obstructive CAD. Adjustment of the extent of ST segment depression by R wave height in individual leads has not been consistently shown to improve the diagnostic value of the exercise ECG for CAD. U wave inversion can occasionally be seen in the precordial leads at heart rates of 120 beats/min. Although this finding is relatively specific for CAD, it is relatively insensitive.

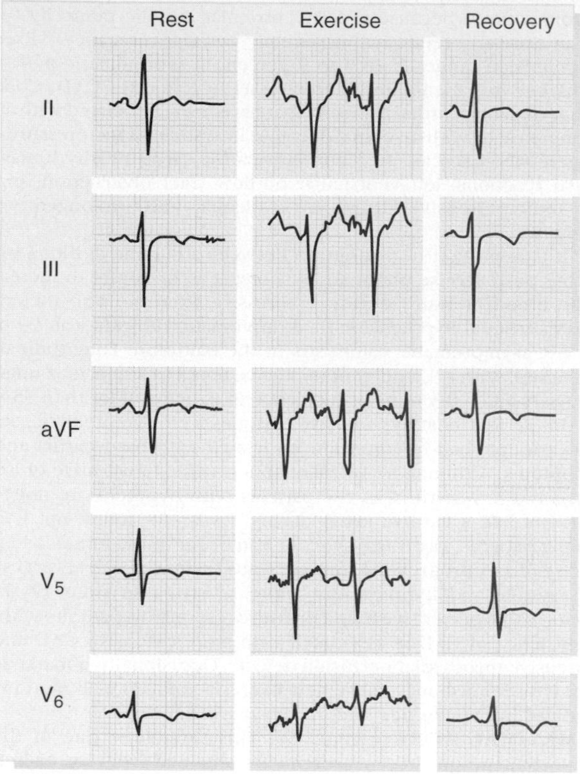

FIGURE 13–10 Pseudonormalization of T waves in a 49-year-old man referred for exercise testing. The patient had previously been seen for typical angina. The resting electrocardiogram in this patient with coronary artery disease shows inferior and anterolateral T wave inversion, an adverse long-term prognosticator. The patient exercised to 8 METs, reaching a peak heart rate of 142 beats/min and a peak systolic blood pressure of 248 mm Hg. At that point, the test was stopped because of hypertension. During exercise, pseudonormalization of T waves occurs, and it returns to baseline (inverted T wave) in the postexercise phase. The patient denied chest discomfort, and no arrhythmia or ST segment displacement was noted. Transient conversion of a negative T wave at rest to a positive T wave during exercise is a nonspecific finding in patients without prior myocardial infarction and does not enhance the diagnostic or prognostic content of the test; however, the ability to exercise to 8 METs without ischemic changes in the ST segment places this patient into a subset of lower risk. HR = heart rate; METs = metabolic equivalents; SBP = systolic blood pressure. *(From Chaitman BR: Exercise electrocardiographic stress testing.* In *Beller GA [ed]: Chronic Ischemic Heart Disease.* In *Braunwald E [series ed]: Atlas of Heart Diseases. Vol 5. Chronic Ischemic Heart Disease. Philadelphia, Current Medicine, 1995, pp 2.1-2.30.)*

Computer-Assisted Analysis

The use of computers has facilitated the routine analysis of and measurements required from the exercise ECG and can be performed online as well as off-line. When the raw ECG data are of high quality, the computer can filter and average or select median complexes from which the degree of J point displacement, ST segment slope, and ST displacement 60 to 80 milliseconds (ST 60 to 80) after the J point can be measured.[8] The selection of ST 60 or ST 80 depends on the heart rate response. At ventricular rates higher than 130 beats/min, the ST 80 measurement may fall on the upslope of the T wave, and the ST 60 measurement should be used instead. In some computerized systems, the PQ junction or isoelectric interval is detected by scanning before the R wave for the 10-millisecond interval with the least slope. J point, ST slope, and ST levels are determined (see Figs. 13-4, 13-5, and 13-6); the ST integral can be calculated from the area below the isoelectric line from the J point to ST 60 or ST 80. Computerized treatment of electrocardiographic complexes permits reduction of motion and myographic artifacts. However, the averaged or median beats may occasionally be erroneous because of electrocardiographic signal distortion caused by noise, baseline wander, or changes in conduction, and identification of the PQ junction and ST segment onset can be imperfect. Therefore, it is crucial to ensure that the computer-determined averages or median complexes reflect the raw electrocardiographic data; physicians should program the computer to print out raw data during exercise and inspect the raw data to be certain that the QRS template is accurately reproduced, and that the placement of the fiducial points are correctly placed at the PQ junction and J point before accepting the automatic measurements.

ST/HEART RATE SLOPE MEASUREMENTS. Heart rate adjustment of ST segment depression appears to improve the sensitivity of the exercise test, particularly the prediction of multivessel CAD.[26] The ST/heart rate slope depends on the type of exercise performed, number and location of monitoring electrodes, method of measuring ST segment depression, and clinical characteristics of the study population. Calculation of the maximal ST/heart rate slope in mV/beats/min is performed by linear regression analysis relating the measured amount of ST segment depression in individual leads to the heart rate at the end of each stage of exercise, starting at the end of exercise. An ST/heart rate slope of 2.4 mV/beats/min is considered abnormal, and values that exceed 6mV/beats/min are suggestive evidence of three-vessel CAD. The use of this measurement requires modification of the exercise protocol so that increments in heart rate are gradual, as in the Cornell protocol, as opposed to more abrupt increases in heart rate between stages, as in the Bruce or Ellestad protocols, which limit the ability to calculate valid ST segment/heart rate slopes statistically. The measurement does not provide an accurate estimate of prognosis in the early postinfarction phase. A modification of the ST segment/heart rate slope method is the ST segment/heart rate index calculation, which represents the average change of ST segment depression with heart rate throughout the course of the exercise test. The ST/heart rate index measurements are less than the ST/heart rate slope measurements, and an ST/heart rate index of 1.6 is defined as abnormal. A slight increase in the prognostic content of ST segment/heart rate slope measurements as compared with standard criteria was demonstrated in the Multiple Risk Factor Interventional Trial.[1,8]

Mechanism of ST Segment Displacement

PATHOPHYSIOLOGY OF THE MYOCARDIAL ISCHEMIC RESPONSE. Myocardial oxygen consumption (MO_2) is determined by heart rate, systolic blood pressure, left ventricular end-diastolic volume, wall thickness, and contractility (see Chap. 48).[1,2,7,8,12] The rate-pressure or double product (heart rate × systolic blood pressure) increases progressively with increasing work and can be used to estimate the myocardial perfusion requirement in normal persons and in many patients with coronary artery disease. The heart is an aerobic organ with little capacity to generate energy through anaerobic metabolism. Oxygen extraction in the coronary circulation is almost maximal at rest. The only significant mechanism available to the heart to increase oxygen consumption is to increase perfusion, and there is a direct linear relationship between MO_2 and coronary blood flow in normal individuals. The principal mechanism for increasing coronary blood flow during exercise is to decrease resistance at the coronary arteriolar level. In patients with progressive atherosclerotic narrowing of the epicardial vessels, an ischemic threshold occurs, and exercise beyond this threshold can produce abnormalities in diastolic and systolic ventricular function, electrocardiographic changes, and chest pain. The subendocardium is more susceptible to myocardial ischemia than the subepicardium because of increased wall tension, causing a relative increase in myocardial oxygen demand in the subendocardium. Dynamic changes in coronary artery tone at the site of an atherosclerotic plaque may result in diminished coronary flow during static or dynamic exercise instead of the expected increase that normally occurs from coronary vasodilation in a normal vessel; that is, perfusion pressure distal to the stenotic plaque actually falls as during exercise, resulting in reduced subendocardial blood flow.[27,28] Thus, regional left ventricular myocardial ischemia may result not only from an increase in myocardial oxygen demand during exercise but also from a limitation of coronary flow as a result of coronary vasoconstriction, or inability of vessels to vasodilate sufficiently as a result of diffuse atherosclerosis and abnormal endothelial function at or near the site of an obstructive atherosclerotic plaque.

Some patients with chronic angina have a warm-up phenomenon that can be demonstrated using sequential exercise testing.[29-31] Under these conditions, the time to angina and ischemic ST segment depression can be prolonged and can occur at a higher rate-pressure product on the second of two exercise tests performed within 10 to 30 minutes of each other. Improvement in performance on the second test is related to the magnitude of myocardial ischemia produced on the first test and usually myocardial ischemia of more than moderate intensity is required to produce the warm-up response.

In normal persons, the action potential duration of the endocardial region is longer than that of the epicardial region, and ventricular repolarization is from epicardium to endocardium. The action potential duration is shortened in the presence of myocardial ischemia and electrical gradients are created, resulting in ST segment depression or elevation, depending on the surface electrocardiographic leads. At the molecular level, activation of sarcolemmal ATP-sensitive potassium (K_{ATP}) channels by ischemic ATP depletion may play a role. Transgenic mice with homozygous knockout of the *Kir6.2* channel gene, which encodes the pore-forming subunit of cardiac surface K_{ATP} channels, lack the ability to generate an ST segment elevation response to acute coronary occlusion.[32] Increased myocardial oxygen demand associated with a failure to increase or with an actual decrease in regional coronary blood flow usually causes ST segment depression; ST segment elevation may occasionally occur in patients with more severe coronary flow reduction.

NONELECTROCARDIOGRAPHIC OBSERVATIONS

The ECG is only one part of the exercise response, and symptoms, abnormal hemodynamics or heart-rate response, and reduced functional capacity are even more important than ST segment shifts in determining long-term prognosis.

BLOOD PRESSURE. The normal exercise response is to increase systolic blood pressure progressively with increasing workloads to a peak response ranging from 160 to 200 mm Hg, with the higher range of the scale in older patients with less compliant vascular systems.[1,7,8,33] As a group, African American patients tend to have a higher systolic blood pressure response than white patients. At high exercise workloads, it is sometimes difficult to obtain a precise determination of systolic blood pressure by auscultation. In normal persons, the diastolic blood pressure does not usually change significantly. Failure to increase systolic blood pressure beyond 120 mm Hg, a sustained decrease greater than 10 mm Hg repeatable within 15 seconds, or a fall in systolic blood pressure below standing resting values during progressive exercise, when the blood pressure has otherwise been increasing appropriately, is abnormal and reflects inadequate elevation of cardiac output because of left ventricular systolic pump dysfunction or an excessive reduction in systemic vascular resistance.[36] Exertional hypotension ranges from 3 to 9 percent in symptomatic patients and is higher in patients with three-vessel or left main CAD. Conditions other than myocardial ischemia that have been associated with a failure to increase or with an actual decrease in systolic blood pressure during progressive exercise are cardiomyopathy, cardiac arrhythmias, vasovagal reactions, left ventricular outflow tract obstruction, ingestion of antihypertensive drugs, hypovolemia, and prolonged vigorous exercise.

It is important to distinguish between a decline in blood pressure in the postexercise phase and a decrease in or failure to increase systolic blood pressure during progressive exercise. The incidence of postexertional hypotension in asymptomatic subjects was 1.9 percent in 781 asymptomatic volunteers in the Baltimore Longitudinal Study on Aging, with a 3.1 percent incidence noted in subjects younger than 55 years and a 0.3 percent incidence in patients older than 55 years.[34] In this series, most hypotensive episodes were symptomatic, and only two patients had hypotension associated with bradycardia and vagal symptoms. Although ST segment abnormalities suggestive of ischemia occurred in one third of the patients with hypotension, none of the patients had a cardiac event during 4 years of follow-up. Rarely, in young patients, vasovagal syncope can occur in the immediate postexercise phase, progressing through sinus bradycardia to several seconds of asystole and hypotension before reverting to sinus rhythm. An abnormal hypertensive blood pressure response in patients with a high prevalence of CAD is associated with more extensive CAD and more extensive myocardial perfusion defects. Occasionally, a marked hypertensive response may cause new exercise-induced wall motion abnormalities in the absence of coronary disease.[35]

MAXIMAL WORK CAPACITY. This variable is one of the most important prognostic measurements obtained from an exercise test (Fig. 13-11).[1,2,7,8,10,36-41] Maximal work capacity in normal individuals is influenced by familiarization with the exercise test equipment, level of training, and environmental conditions at the time of testing. In patients with known or suspected CAD, a limited exercise capacity is associated with an increased risk of cardiac events and, in general, the more severe the limitation, the worse the CAD extent and prognosis. In estimating functional capacity, the amount of work performed (or exercise stage achieved) expressed in METs, not the number of minutes of exercise, should be the parameter measured. Estimates of peak functional capacity for age and gender have been well established for most of the exercise protocols in common use, subject to the limitations described in the section on cardiopulmonary testing. Comparison of an individual's performance against normal standards provides an estimate of the degree of exercise impairment. There is a rough correlation between observed peak functional capacity during exercise treadmill testing and estimates derived from clinical data and specific activity questionnaires.

Serial comparison of functional capacity in individual patients to assess significant interval change requires a careful examination of the exercise protocol used during both tests, drug therapy and time of ingestion, systemic blood pressure, and other conditions that might influence test performance. All these variables need to be considered before attributing changes in functional capacity to progression of CAD or worsening of left ventricular function. Major reductions in exercise capacity usually indicate significant worsening of cardiovascular status; modest changes may not.

SUBMAXIMAL EXERCISE. The interpretation of exercise test results for diagnostic and prognostic purposes requires consideration of maximal work capacity. When a patient is unable to complete moderate levels of exercise or reach at least 85 to 90 percent of age-predicted maximum, the level of exercise performed may be inadequate to test cardiac reserve. Thus, ischemic electrocardiographic, scintigraphic, or ventriculographic abnormalities may not be evoked and the test may be nondiagnostic. Nondiagnostic test results are more common in patients with peripheral vascular disease, orthopedic limitation, or neurological impairment and in patients with poor motivation. Pharmacological stress imaging studies should be considered in this setting.[1,2]

HEART RATE RESPONSE. The sinus rate increases progressively with exercise, mediated in part through sympathetic and parasympathetic innervation of the sinoatrial node and circulating catecholamines. In some patients who may be anxious about the exercise test, there may be an initial overreaction of heart rate and systolic blood pressure at the beginning of exercise, with stabilization after approximately 30 to 60 seconds. An inappropriate increase in heart rate at low exercise workloads may occur in patients who are in atrial fibrillation, physically deconditioned, hypovolemic, or anemic, or who have marginal left ventricular function; this increase may persist for several minutes in the recovery phase.

When the heart rate fails to increase appropriately with exercise, it is associated with an adverse prognosis.[1,8,42-44] Chronotropic incompetence is determined by decreased heart rate sensitivity to the normal increase in sympathetic tone during exercise and is defined as inability to increase heart rate to at least 85 percent of age-predicted maximum or as an abnormal heart rate reserve. Heart rate (HR) reserve is calculated as follows:

$$\%\text{HR reserve}_{used} = (\text{HR}_{peak} - \text{HR}_{rest})/(220 - \text{age} - \text{HR}_{rest})$$

The term *chronotropic index* refers to a heart rate increment per stage of exercise that is below normal or a peak heart rate below predicted at maximal workloads. It reflects an inability to use up all the heart rate reserve. This finding may indicate autonomic dysfunction, sinus node disease, drug therapy such as beta blockers, or a myocardial ischemic response. When the chronotropic index is 80 percent or less, long-term mortality is increased. Chronotropic incompetence should not be used to estimate prognosis in patients on beta blocker therapy.

HEART RATE RECOVERY. Abnormal heart rate recovery (HRR) refers to a relatively slow deceleration of heart rate following exercise cessation. This type of response reflects decreased vagal tone and is associated with increased mortality.[8,45-47]

$$\text{HRR} = \text{HR}_{peak} - \text{HR}_{1\ \text{minute later}}$$

When the postexercise phase includes an upright cool-down, a value 12 beats/min or less is abnormal. For patients undergoing stress echocardiography or otherwise assuming a supine position immediately after exercise, a value 18 beats/min or less is abnormal. When HRR is measured 2 minutes into recovery, a value 22 beats/min or less is abnormal. The prognostic value of abnormal HRR is independent of the exercise level attained, beta blocker usage, severity of coronary disease, left ventricular function, chronotropic incompetence, Duke treadmill score, and presence of exercise-induced angina or ischemic electrocardiographic abnormalities (Fig. 13-12). A submaximal heart rate response in a patient who is poorly motivated to complete the test or has a physical impairment that limits ability to perform sufficient exercise to test heart rate reserve (resulting in a nondiagnostic test, as described earlier) should be distinguished from a patient with chronotropic incompetence and an adequate test for prognostic estimates.

RATE-PRESSURE PRODUCT. The heart rate–systolic blood pressure product, an indirect measure of myocardial oxygen demand, increases progressively with exercise, and the peak rate-pressure product can be used to characterize cardiovascular performance. Most normal individuals develop a peak rate pressure product of 20 to 35 mm Hg × beats/min × 10^{-3}. In many patients with significant ischemic heart disease, rate-pressure products exceeding 25 mm Hg × beats/min × 10^{-3} are unusual. However, the cut point of 25 mm Hg × beats/min × 10^{-3} is not a useful diagnostic parameter; significant overlap exists between patients with disease and those without disease. Furthermore, cardioactive drug therapy significantly influences this measurement.

CHEST DISCOMFORT. Characterization of chest discomfort during exercise can be a useful diagnostic finding, particularly when the symptom complex is compatible with typical angina pectoris. In some patients, the exercise level during the test may exceed that which the patient exhibits in daily activities. Exercise-induced chest discomfort

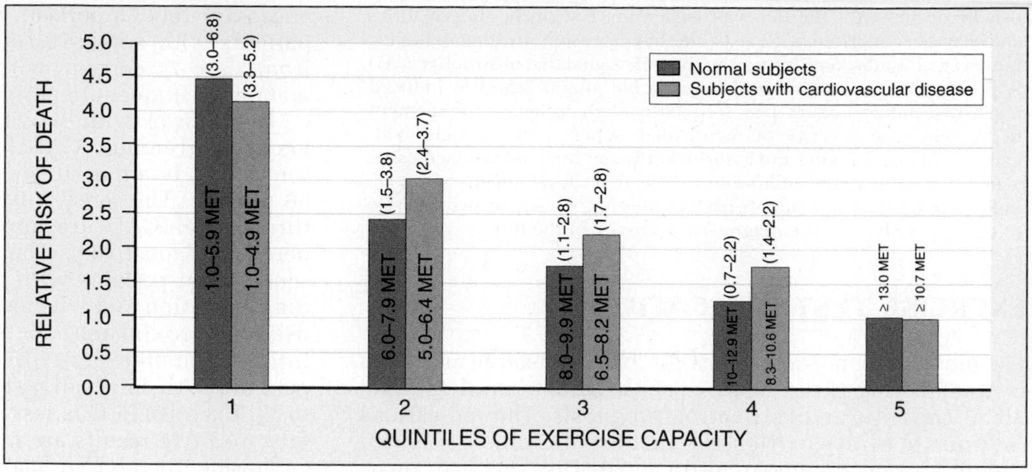

FIGURE 13–11 Age-adjusted relative risks of all-cause mortality by quintile of exercise capacity in 2534 subjects with a normal exercise test result and no history of cardiovascular disease and in 3679 subjects with an abnormal exercise test result or history of cardiovascular disease. The mean duration of follow-up was 6.2 ± 3.7 years. Quintile 5 was used as the reference category. For each 1-MET increase in exercise capacity, survival improved by 12 percent. *(From Myers J, Prakash M, Froelicher V, et al: Exercise capacity and mortality among men referred for exercise testing. N Engl J Med 346:793, 2002.)*

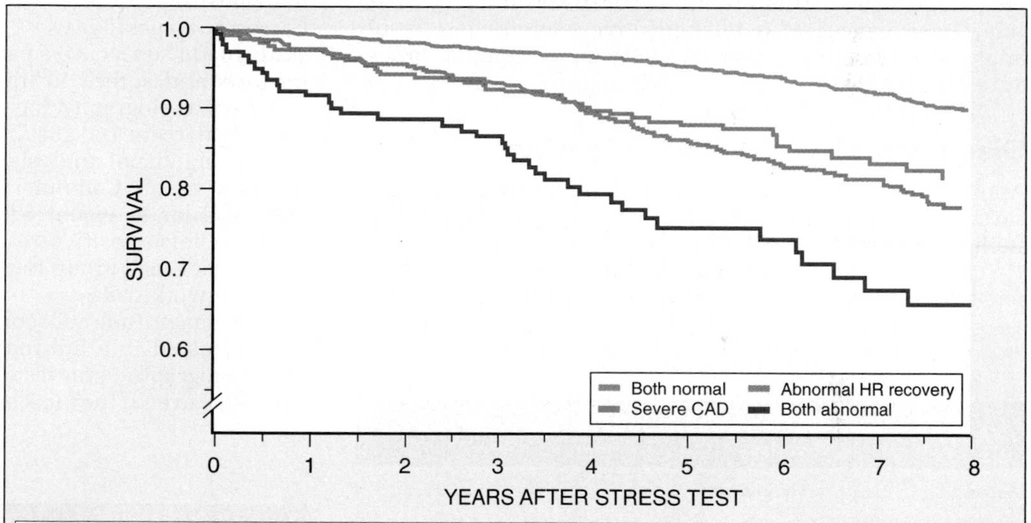

No. at risk	0	1	2	3	4	5	6	7	8
Both normal	1817	1802	1784	1666	1415	1170	868	706	475
Severe CAD	280	273	264	251	210	161	127	90	79
Abnl HR rec	697	678	665	614	508	395	299	243	143
Both abnormal	141	129	125	117	84	51	49	40	29

FIGURE 13–12 Six-year follow-up in 2935 patients who underwent an exercise test and coronary angiography. After adjustment for age, gender, standard risk factors, medications, exercise capacity, coronary disease extent, and left ventricular function, abnormal heart rate recovery (Abnl HR rec) was an independent predictor of mortality. The survival plot illustrates a mortality gradient, with the worst prognosis in patients with abnormal heart rate recovery and severe coronary artery disease (CAD). *(From Vivekananthan DP, Blackstone EH, Poithier CE, et al: Heart rate recovery after exercise is a predictor of mortality, independent of the angiographic severity of coronary disease. J Am Coll Cardiol 42:831, 2003.)*

usually occurs after the onset of ischemic ST segment abnormalities and may be associated with diastolic hypertension. In some patients, however, chest discomfort may be the only signal that obstructive CAD is present. In patients with chronic stable angina, exercise-induced chest discomfort occurs less frequently than ischemic ST segment depression. The severity of myocardial ischemia in a patient with exercise-induced angina and a normal ECG can often be assessed using a myocardial imaging technique.[1,2] The new development of an S_3, holosystolic apical murmur, or basilar rates in the early recovery phase of exercise enhances the diagnostic accuracy of the test.

EXERCISE TEST INDICATIONS

The most frequent indications for exercise testing are to aid in establishing the diagnosis of CAD, determining functional capacity, and estimating prognosis. The indications continue to evolve, with some that are uniformly accepted and others that are more controversial. The American Heart Association and American College of Cardiology Exercise Task Force have determined several categories of test indications drawn from a large body of published literature on exercise testing[1] (see later, "Guidelines"). Exercise testing should not be used to screen very low-risk asymptomatic individuals because the test has limited diagnostic and prognostic value in this situation, and the resultant undesirable consequences of a false-positive exercise test result might include unnecessary follow-up, additional procedures, anxiety, and exercise restrictions.[7,8]

Diagnostic Use of Exercise Testing

Appreciation of the noninvasive test literature to diagnose CAD requires an understanding of standard terminology such as *sensitivity, specificity,* and *test accuracy* (Table 13-1).[1,2,7,8] In patients selected for coronary angiography, the sensitivity of the exercise ECG in patients with CAD is approximately 68 percent, and specificity is 77 percent. In patients with single-vessel disease, the sensitivity ranges from 25 to 71 percent, with exercise-induced ST displacement most frequent in patients with left anterior descending CAD, followed by those with right CAD and those with isolated left circumflex CAD. In patients with multivessel CAD, sensitivity is approximately 81 percent and specificity is 66 percent. The sensitivity and specificity for left main or three-vessel CAD are approximately 86 percent and 53 percent, respectively. The exercise ECG tends to be less sensitive in patients with extensive anterior wall myocardial infarction and when a limited exercise ECG lead set is used. Approximately 75 to 80 percent of the diagnostic information on exercise-induced ST segment depression in patients with a normal resting ECG is contained in leads V_4 to V_6. Exercise ECG is less specific when patients in whom false-positive results are more common are included, such as those with valvular heart disease, left ventricular hypertrophy, marked resting ST segment depression, or digitalis therapy. Table 13-2 lists the more common causes of noncoronary exercise–induced ST segment depression.

Selective referral of patients with a positive test result for further study both decreases the rate of detection of true-negative test results and increases the rate of detection of false-positive results, thus increasing sensitivity and decreasing specificity.[1,2,7,8] Froelicher and colleagues, in a study of 814 consecutive patients who presented with angina pectoris and agreed to undergo both exercise testing and coronary angiography, have reported exercise ECG sensitivity of 45 percent and specificity of 85 percent for obstructive CAD using visual analysis in this population with reduced work-up bias.[48] Computerized ST segment measurements were similar to visual ST segment measurements in this study. A false-positive result is more common when only the inferior lead group (leads 2, 3, aVF) is abnormal at high exercise workloads.

The magnitude of coronary atherosclerosis is often undestimated in a luminal angiogram when intravascular ultrasonographic studies are performed, and may be quite extensive even if the most severe luminal narrowing appears

TABLE 13–1 Terms Useful in Evaluation of Test Results

Term	Definition
True positive (TP)	Abnormal test result in individual with disease
False positive (FP)	Abnormal test result in individual without disease
True negative (TN)	Normal test result in individual without disease
False negative (FN)	Normal test result in individual with disease
Sensitivity	Percentage of patients with CAD who have an abnormal result = TP/(TP + FN)
Specificity	Percentage of patients without CAD who have a normal result = TN/(TN + FP)
Predictive value of a positive test	Percentage of patients with an abnormal result who have CAD = TP/(TP + FN)
Predictive value of a negative test	Percentage of patients with a normal result who do not have CAD = TN/(TN + FN)
Test accuracy	Percentage of true test results = (TP + TN)/ total number tests performed
Likelihood ratio	Odds of a test result being true abnormal test result: sensitivity/(1 − specificity) normal test result: specificity/(1 − sensitivity)
Relative risk	Disease rate in persons with a positive test result/disease rate in persons with a negative test result

CAD = coronary artery disease.

TABLE 13–2 Noncoronary Causes of ST Segment Depression

Anemia
Cardiomyopathy
Digitalis use
Glucose load
Hyperventilation
Hypokalemia
Intraventricular conduction disturbance
Left ventricular hypertrophy
Mitral valve prolapse
Preexcitation syndrome
Severe aortic stenosis
Severe hypertension
Severe hypoxia
Severe volume overload (aortic, mitral regurgitation)
Sudden excessive exercise
Supraventricular tachyarrhythmias

less than 50%. A mildly abnormal coronary angiogram does not eliminate the possibility that a patient's symptoms may be ischemic in origin.

BAYES' THEOREM. The depth of exercise-induced ST-segment depression and the extent of the myocardial ischemic response can be thought of as continuous variables. Cut points such as 1 mm of horizontal or downsloping ST segment depression as compared with baseline cannot completely distinguish patients with disease from those without disease, and the requirement of more severe degrees of ST segment depression to improve specificity will decrease sensitivity. Sensitivity and specificity are inversely related, and false-negative and false-positive results are to be expected when electrocardiographic or angiographic cut points are selected to optimize the diagnostic accuracy of the test.

The use of Bayes' theorem incorporates the pretest risk of disease and the sensitivity and specificity of the test (likelihood ratio) to calculate the posttest probability of coronary disease. The patient's clinical information and exercise test results are used to make a final estimate about the probability of CAD. Atypical or probable angina in a 50-year-old man or a 60-year-old woman is associated with an approximately 50 percent probability for CAD before exercise testing is performed. The diagnostic power of the exercise test is maximal when the pretest probability of CAD is intermediate (30 to 70 percent).

MULTIVARIATE ANALYSIS. Multivariate analysis of noninvasive exercise tests to estimate posttest risk also can provide important diagnostic information. Multivariate analysis offers the potential advantage that it does not require that the tests be independent of each other or that sensitivity and specificity remain constant over a wide range of disease prevalence rates (see later, "Exercise Testing in Determining Prognosis"). However, the multivariate technique critically depends on how patients are selected to establish the reference data base.[49,50] Both bayesian and multivariate approaches are commonly used to provide diagnostic and prognostic estimates of patients with CAD.

SEVERITY OF ELECTROCARDIOGRAPHIC ISCHEMIC RESPONSE. The exercise ECG result is more likely to be abnormal in patients with more severe coronary arterial obstruction, with more extensive CAD, and after more strenuous levels of exercise. Early onset of angina, ischemic ST segment depression, and fall in blood pressure at low exercise workloads are the most important exercise parameters associated with an adverse prognosis and multivessel CAD.[1,2,7,8] Additional adverse markers include profound ST segment displacement, ischemic changes in five or more electrocardiographic leads, and persistence of the changes late in the recovery phase of exercise (Table 13-3).

TABLE 13–3 Exercise Parameters Associated with an Adverse Prognosis and Multivessel Coronary Artery Disease
Duration of symptom-limiting exercise <5 METs
Failure to increase systolic blood pressure ≥120 mm Hg, or a sustained decrease ≥10 mm Hg, or below rest levels, during progressive exercise
ST segment depression ≥2 mm, downsloping ST segment, starting at <5 METs, involving ≥5 leads, persisting ≥5 min into recovery
Exercise-induced ST segment elevation (aVR excluded)
Angina pectoris at low exercise workloads
Reproducible sustained (>30 sec) or symptomatic ventricular tachycardia

MET = metabolic equivalent.

Exercise Testing in Determining Prognosis

Exercise testing provides not only diagnostic information but also, more importantly, prognostic data.[1,2,7,8] The value of exercise testing to estimate prognosis must be considered in light of what is already known about a patient's risk status.[50-58] Left ventricular dysfunction, CAD extent, electrical instability, and noncoronary comorbid conditions must be taken into consideration when estimating long-term outcome.

ASYMPTOMATIC POPULATION. The prevalence of an abnormal exercise ECG result in middle-aged asymptomatic men ranges from 5 to 12 percent. Rywik and colleagues studied 1083 volunteers from the Baltimore Longitudinal Study of Aging to determine the prognostic value of different types of exercise ECG response for cardiac events defined as onset of angina, myocardial infarction, or cardiac death. After a 7.9-year follow-up, horizontal or downsloping ST segment depression 1 mm or more or intensification of minor preexercise ST segment depression to 1 mm or more independently predicted cardiac events.[51] In earlier studies from other institutions, the risk of developing a cardiac event such as angina, myocardial infarction, or death in men was approximately nine times greater when the test result was abnormal than when it was normal; however, over 5 years of follow-up, only one in four men suffered a cardiac event, and this was most commonly the development of angina. The data illustrate the difficulty in identifying asymptomatic subjects destined to develop abrupt changes in plaque morphology based on an abnormal exercise ECG. The future risk of cardiac events is greatest if the test result is strongly positive or if an asymptomatic subject has atherosclerotic risk factors such as diabetes, hypertension, hypercholesterolemia, smoking history, or familial history of premature coronary disease (Fig. 13-13).[51-57] Target extracardiac end-organ damage, such as peripheral vascular disease, proteinuria, or stroke, further escalates the risk in accordance with bayesian principles. Selection of asymptomatic subjects for an exercise test should be based on the atherosclerotic risk profile that can be used to provide a global risk estimate of the likelihood of death, myocardial infarction, or stroke. Appropriate asymptomatic subjects for exercise testing would be those with an estimated annual risk greater than 1 or 2 percent per year. In asymptomatic middle-aged or older men with several atherosclerotic risk factors, a markedly abnormal exercise response is associated with a significantly increased risk of subsequent cardiac events, particularly when there is additional supporting evidence for underlying CAD (e.g., coronary calcification, abnormal results of thallium scan). In one series of 710 asymptomatic men with a coronary artery calcium score higher than 100 by electron beam tomography, the age-adjusted hazard ratio for coronary heart disease events was 0.26 for men able to exercise more than 10 METS versus less than 10 METS after 3.5-year follow-up.[59] Several investigators have assessed prognostic risk by classifying asymptomatic subjects using the Framingham Risk Score and exercise testing.[52,53,55] Mora and associates[55] have reported that after adjustment for Framingham Risk Score, low peak METS achieved and low heart-rate recovery were significant predictors of cardiovascular death in 6126 men and women after 10- and 20-year follow-up (see Fig. 13-13). The exercise data added incremental prognostic information to the Framingham Risk Score in 50 percent of women with a Framingham Risk Score of 6 to 9 percent and 10 to 19 percent, and slightly less than 50 percent of men with a Framingham Risk Score of 10 to 19 percent. Blumenthal and colleagues[60] have studied 734 asymptomatic siblings of persons with documented

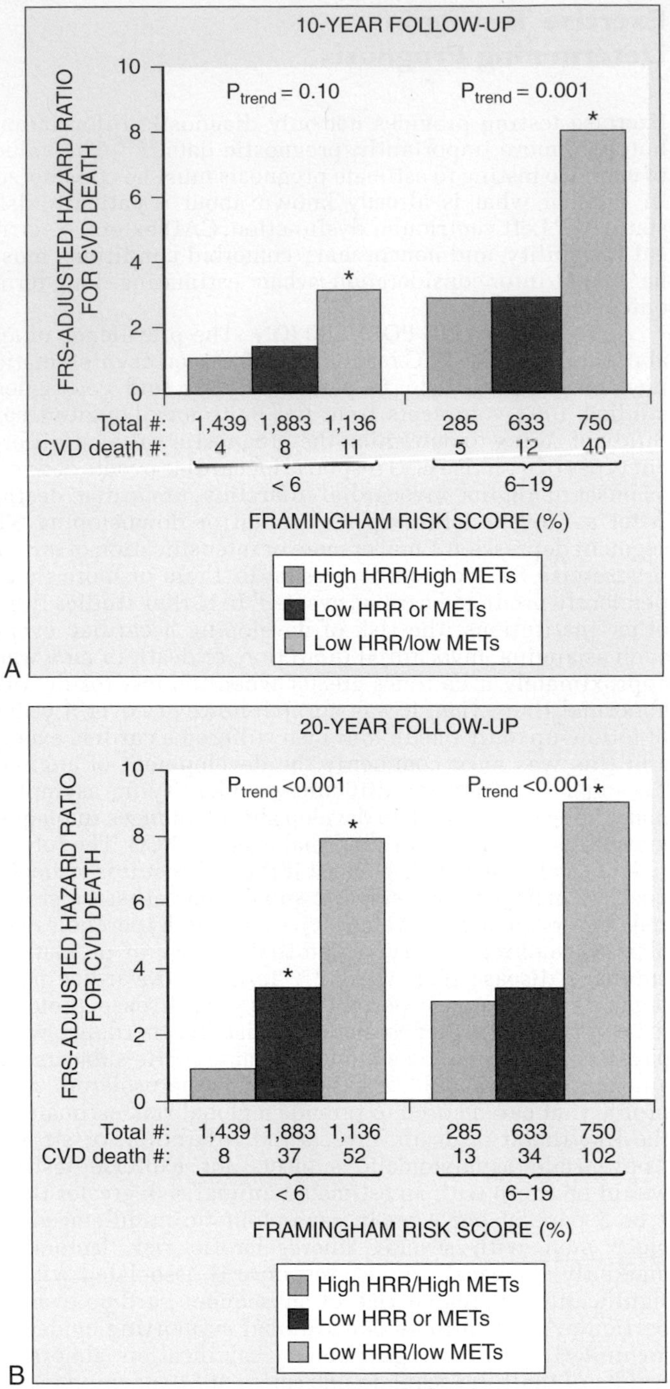

FIGURE 13–13 In 6126 asymptomatic subjects derived from the Lipid Research Clinics Prevalence Study, Framingham Risk Score (FRS)–adjusted hazard ratios for cardiovascular death are illustrated according to FRS categories for heart rate recovery (HRR)/METs groups at 10- **(A)** and 20-year **(B)** follow-up. P_{trend} values are for tests of significance for trend across the three HRR/METs groups in each FRS category. A low HRR/low METs finding was associated with significant increased risk of cardiovascular disease (CVD) death for FRS less than 6 percent and 6 to 19 percent. *(From Mora S, Redberg RF, Sharrett AR, et al: Enhanced risk assessment in asymptomatic individuals with exercise testing and Framingham risk scores. Circulation 112:1566, 2005).*

coronary disease and reported abnormal exercise perfusion results in 153 subjects, 95 percent of whom had mild to moderate atherosclerosis at angiography. Luminal narrowings higher than 50 percent were found in 70 percent of subjects with an abnormal exercise ECG and scan. Serial change of a negative exercise ECG result to a positive one in an asymptomatic person carries the same prognostic importance as an initially abnormal test result. However, the finding that an asymptomatic individual with an initially abnormal test result has significant worsening of electrocardiographic abnormalities at lower exercise workloads may indicate significant CAD progression; this warrants a more aggressive diagnostic work-up. The prevalence of an abnormal exercise ECG result in middle-aged asymptomatic women ranges from 20 to 30 percent.[1,2,7,8] In general, the prognostic value of an ST segment shift in women is less than in men (see later, "Specific Clinical Applications: Women").

SYMPTOMATIC PATIENTS. Exercise testing should be routinely performed (unless this is not feasible or unless there are contraindications) before coronary angiography in patients with chronic ischemic heart disease. Patients who have excellent exercise tolerance (e.g., more than 10 METs) and satisfactory management of their global atherosclerotic risk usually have an excellent prognosis, regardless of the anatomical extent of CAD.[1,2,36,38,39] The test provides an estimate of the functional significance of angiographically documented coronary artery stenoses. The impact of exercise testing in patients with proven or suspected CAD has been studied by Weiner and colleagues in 4083 medically treated patients in the CASS study.[61] A high-risk patient subset was identified (12 percent of the population), with an annual mortality rate of 5 percent when exercise workload was less than Bruce stage I (less than 4 METs) and the exercise ECG exhibited 0.1-mV (1-mm) ST segment depression or higher. A low-risk patient subset (34 percent of the population) who were able to exercise into Bruce stage III or higher and who had a normal exercise ECG result had an annual mortality rate of less than 1 percent over 4 years of follow-up. Similar electrocardiographic and workload parameters were useful in risk-stratifying patients with three-vessel CAD likely to benefit from coronary bypass grafting.

Mark and colleagues have developed a treadmill score based on 2842 consecutive patients with chest pain in the Duke data bank; these patients underwent treadmill testing using the Bruce protocol and cardiac catheterization.[62] Patients with left bundle branch block (LBBB) or those with exercise-induced ST elevation in a Q wave lead were excluded. The treadmill (TM) score is calculated as follows:

$$\text{TM score} = \text{exercise time} - (5 \times \text{ST deviation}) - (4 \times \text{TM angina index})$$

Angina index was assigned a value of 0 if angina was absent, 1 if typical angina occurred during exercise, and 2 if angina was why the patient stopped exercising. Exercise-induced ST deviation was defined as the largest net ST displacement in any lead. The 13 percent of patients with a TM score of −11 or less had a 5-year survival rate of 72 percent, as compared with a 97 percent survival rate among the 34 percent of patients at low risk, with a TM score of +5 or higher. The score added independent prognostic information to that provided by clinical data, coronary anatomy, and left ventricular ejection fraction. The stratified annual mortality rates predicted from the TM score were less in 613 outpatients referred for exercise testing from the same institution.[63] The score worked equally well in men and women, although women had a lower overall risk than men for similar scores. The Duke TM score is not as effective in estimating risk in subjects 75 years of age or older (see later, "Elderly Patients").[64,65] Exercise scoring systems can be used to identify prognostically intermediate- to high-risk patients in whom coronary angiography would be indicated to define coronary anatomy.[49,50,65] However, the decision to perform coronary revascularization should take into consideration the fact that in patients with less extensive CAD (e.g., one to two vessels narrowed and well-preserved left ventricular function), a similar degree of exercise-induced myocardial ischemia does not carry the same significant increased risk of cardiac events as in patients with more extensive disease (e.g., three vessels narrowed or impaired left ventricular function). When estimating prognosis in individual patients from the population-based data collected over the last 25 years or so, consideration should be given to the fact that actual survival rates currently are likely to be greater because of more aggressive treatment of atherosclerotic risk factors and the use of noninvasive testing to identify the highest risk subjects who would benefit from coronary revascularization.

SILENT MYOCARDIAL ISCHEMIA (see Chap. 54). In patients with documented CAD, the presence of exercise-induced ischemic ST segment depression confers an increased risk of subsequent cardiac events, regardless of whether angina occurs during the test.[66] The magnitude of the prognostic gradient in patients with an abnormal exercise ECG result with or without angina varies considerably in the published literature, most likely a feature of patient selection. In the CASS data bank, 7-year survival in patients with silent or symptomatic exercise-induced myocardial ischemia was similar in patients stratified by coronary anatomy and left ventricular function, with the worst survival in patients with the most extensive CAD.

ACUTE CORONARY SYNDROMES (see Chaps. 51 and 53). The prognostic risk assessment after an acute coronary syndrome should incorporate findings from the history, physical examination, resting 12-lead ECG, and level of serum markers to optimize mortality and morbidity estimates and to categorize patients into low-, intermediate-, and high-risk groups.[67,68] Exercise testing should be considered in the outpatient evaluation of low-risk patients with unstable angina (biomarker negative) who are free of active ischemic signs (e.g., electrocardiographic changes) or symptoms for a minimum of 8 to 12 hours, and in hospitalized low- to intermediate-risk ambulatory patients who are free of angina or heart failure symptoms for at least 48 hours.[68] In many intermediate- or high-risk patients, coronary angiography will have been performed during the acute phase of the illness; coronary disease extent, left ventricular function, and degree of coronary revascularization, if performed, should then be incorporated to determine the incremental value of the exercise test data to determine overall predischarge prognostic risk estimates. Patients who cannot perform or complete an exercise test for clinical reasons have a worse prognosis than those who can complete the protocol. Low functional capacity or abnormal hemodynamic responses to exercise are generally more predictive of an adverse prognosis than electrocardiographic measures of exercise-induced ischemia in patients with an acute coronary syndrome who have undergone partial or complete revascularization.

MYOCARDIAL INFARCTION. Exercise testing after myocardial infarction (both non-ST and ST elevation) is useful to determine (1) risk stratification and assessment of prognosis, (2) functional capacity for activity prescription after hospital discharge, and (3) assessment of adequacy of medical therapy and need to use supplemental diagnostic or treatment options.[1,2,7,8] The incidence of fatal or nonfatal cardiac events associated with exercise testing after myocardial infarction is low. The risk of events is approximately twofold greater for symptom-limited protocols compared with submaximal tests, although the overall fatal event rate is low with both types of exercise protocols. A low-level exercise test (achievement of 5 to 6 METs, or 70 to 80 percent of age-predicted maximum) is frequently performed before hospital discharge to establish the hemodynamic response and functional capacity.[1,2,67,68] The ability to complete 5 to 6 METs of exercise or 70 to 80 percent of age-predicted maximum in the absence of an abnormal ECG or blood pressure is associated with a 1-year mortality rate of 1 to 2 percent and may help guide the timing of early hospital discharge. Parameters associated with increased risk include inability to perform or complete the low-level predischarge exercise test, poor exercise capacity, inability to increase or a decrease in exercise systolic blood pressure, and angina or exercise-induced ST segment depression at low workloads. Many postinfarct patients referred for exercise testing have been prescribed beta-adrenergic blocking agents and angiotensin-converting enzyme inhibitors. Although beta-adrenergic blocking drugs may attenuate the ischemic response, they do not interfere with poor functional capacity as a marker of adverse prognosis and should be continued in patients referred for testing. The relative prognostic value of a 3- to 6-week postdischarge exercise test is minimal once clinical variables and the results of the low-level predischarge test are taken into consideration. For this reason, the timing of the exercise test after the infarct event favors predischarge exercise testing to allow implementation of a definitive treatment plan in patients in whom coronary anatomy is known, as well as risk stratification of patients in whom coronary anatomy has not yet been determined. In many medical centers, predischarge exercise testing is performed within 3 to 4 days in uncomplicated patients after acute myocardial infarction (e.g. absence of recurrent chest pain, heart failure, renal insufficiency, hemodynamic instability, or cardiac arrhythmias).[69,70] A 3- to 6-week test may be useful in clearing patients to return to work in occupations involving physical labor in which the MET expenditure is likely to be higher than that on a predischarge test.

The goals and basic principles of the predischarge evaluation have not been changed by the advent of reperfusion or direct percutaneous transluminal coronary angioplasty therapy for acute infarction. After undergoing intravenous thrombolytic therapy or direct coronary angioplasty, patients with uncomplicated myocardial infarction tend to exhibit exercise-induced angina and ST segment depression less frequently than consecutive postinfarct patients before these treatment strategies were widely applied. Exercise testing should be considered in the hospital or early after discharge in myocardial infarct patients not selected for cardiac catheterization and without high-risk features to assess the presence and extent of inducible ischemia.[68] In patients with baseline electrocardiographic abnormalities that compromise interpretation, myocardial imaging should be added to standard exercise testing.

RISK STRATIFICATION IN THE EMERGENCY DEPARTMENT. Patients who present to the emergency department are a heterogeneous population, with a large range of pretest risk for CAD. Clinical algorithms can identify lower risk persons who can safely be risk-stratified further using exercise testing.[71-73] In one series of 1000 symptomatic low-risk patients with chest pain, possibly of cardiac origin, who presented to the emergency department, Amsterdam and colleagues reported a positive, intermediate, and nondiagnostic exercise test result in 13, 64, and 23 percent, respectively.[73] There were no adverse effects of exercise testing. The cost-effectiveness of this approach has been demonstrated in both low- and intermediate-risk patients. The accuracy of exercise testing in the emergency department setting follows bayesian principles, with the greatest diagnostic and prognostic estimates in intermediate-risk clinical patient subsets. Exercise testing in the emergency department should not be performed when (1) new or evolving electrocardiographic abnormalities are noted on the rest tracing, (2) the levels of cardiac enzymes are abnormal, (3) the patient cannot adequately perform exercise, (4) the patient reports worsening or persistent chest pain symptoms, or (5) clinical risk profiling indicates that imminent coronary angiography is likely. Several series of clinically low-risk subjects reported 6-month cardiac event rates lower than 1 percent with a normal exercise test result.

PREOPERATIVE RISK STRATIFICATION BEFORE NONCARDIAC SURGERY (see Chap. 80). Exercise ECG before elective noncardiac surgery provides an objective measurement of functional capacity and the potential to identify the likelihood of perioperative myocardial ischemia in patients with a low ischemic threshold.[74] In patients with intermittent claudication and no prior history of cardiac disease, approximately 20 to 25 percent will have an abnormal exercise ECG result. In patients with a prior history of myocardial infarction or an abnormal resting ECG, 35 to 50 percent will have an abnormal exercise ECG result. The risks of perioperative cardiac events and adverse long-term outcome are significantly increased in patients with abnormal exercise ECG results at low workloads. Coronary angiography with revascularization, when feasible, should be considered in such patients before noncardiac operative interventions that are considered high risk, such as aortic and other major vascular surgery and anticipated prolonged procedures associated with large fluid shifts or blood loss.

CONGESTIVE HEART FAILURE (see Chap. 25). Cardiac and peripheral compensatory mechanisms are activated in patients with chronic congestive heart failure to restore impaired left ventricular performance partially or completely. Abnormal baroreflex function and increased norepinephrine spillover, sympathetic discharge, downregulation of beta-adrenergic receptors, depletion of myocardial sympathetic stores, and increased peripheral and central chemosensitivity with abnormally increased ventilatory response to exercise characterize the disease process resulting in the cardiopulmonary response to exercise.[75-85] There is a wide range of exercise capacity in patients who have a markedly reduced ejection fraction, with some patients having near-normal peak exercise capacity. The magnitude of exercise capacity impairment is a function of the relative inability to augment stroke volume and abnormalities in skeletal muscle metabolism, which may be the predominant cause of functional limitation in a significant proportion of patients with heart failure. Fatigue may be related to altered skeletal muscle metabolism secondary to chronic physical deconditioning, impaired perfusion, and chronic anemia. Symptoms in patients with congestive heart failure are related to an excessive increase in blood lactate during low exercise levels, reduction in quantity of oxygen consumed at peak exertion, and disproportionate increase in ventilation at submaximal and peak workloads. The increased ventilatory requirement assessed by the hyperventilatory response to exercise and increase in pulmonary dead space leads to rapid shallow breathing during exercise. Dyspnea and fatigue are the usual reasons for exercise termination. Arterial desaturation does not usually occur unless there is associated pulmonary disease.

Peak $\dot{V}O_2$ measurements in patients with compensated congestive heart failure are useful in risk-stratifying patients with congestive heart failure to determine the subsequent incidence of cardiac events (Fig. 13-14).[1,8,81,83] The ability to achieve a peak $\dot{V}O_2$ higher than 18 ml $O_2 \times kg^{-1} \times min^{-1}$ and anaerobic threshold higher than 14 ml $O_2 \times kg^{-1} \times min^{-1}$ is associated with a relatively good long-term prognosis and maximal cardiac output higher than 8 liters/min/m^2. Patients who are unable to achieve a peak $\dot{V}O_2$ of 10 ml $O_2 \times kg^{-1} \times min^{-1}$ and anaerobic threshold of 8 ml $O_2 \times kg^{-1} \times min^{-1}$ have a poor prognosis, and their maximal exercise cardiac output is usually less than 4 liters/min/m^2. When the peak $\dot{V}O_2$ ranges from 10 to 18 ml/kg/min, prognostic risk is moderate; in this setting, a $\dot{V}e/\dot{V}CO_2$ slope higher than 35 may help identify patients at increased risk.[8,83] The $\dot{V}e\dot{V}CO_2$ slope, usually expressed as the best-fit linear regression line relating $\dot{V}e$ and $\dot{V}CO_2$ below the ventilatory compensation point for exercise lactic acidosis, ranges between 20 and 30 in normal subjects. Values higher than 30 are common in patients with mild to moderate heart failure and values higher than 40 are often observed in those with more severe heart failure.

Patients with heart failure should be encouraged to exercise as closely as possible to a respiratory exchange ratio of 1.15 to determine motivation and to ensure that that the peak $\dot{V}O_2$ measurement is prognostically reliable. Failure of $\dot{V}O_2$ to decrease within 30 seconds after peak exertion, and accumulation of a large oxygen debt (recovery $\dot{V}O_2$ /work), is associated with more severe reductions in left ventricular ejection fraction and moderate to severe impairment of pulmonary gas exchange. Inability to increase oxygen pulse (milliliters of oxygen per beat) is related to a lack of or a minimal increase of stroke volume. A blunted heart rate response caused by postsynaptic desensitization of beta-adrenergic receptors is not uncommon in patients with congestive heart failure. Exercise protocols that limit exercise duration to 5 to 7 minutes are associated with the most reproducible peak $\dot{V}O_2$ measurements in patients with heart failure. In patients with heart failure with preserved systolic function (ejection fraction higher than 50%), impaired exercise ventilation appears to be a more robust predictor of mortality and subsequent hospitalization than peak $\dot{V}O_2$.[80] The interpretation of cardiopulmonary exercise test results in patients with heart failure can occasionally be difficult, because some patients hyperventilate during exercise, producing falsely low peak oxygen consumption, and it can be difficult to distinguish patients who are deconditioned from those who have impaired exercise performance and low peak $\dot{V}O_2$ caused by cardiac pathology. Randomized controlled trials of long-term moderate exercise training in patients with chronic heart failure have reported a 15 to 20 percent improvement in peak $\dot{V}O_2$ and prolonged onset of anaerobic metabolism.[88] Thus, clinical decisions such as listing a patient for cardiac transplantation based on peak $\dot{V}O_2$ measurements need to take into consideration interval training effects, as well as changes in pharmacological therapy, such as beta blockers.[76] Walk tests can also be used to evaluate functional capacity and to estimate prognosis in patients unable to exercise on a bicycle ergometer or treadmill. However, in patients with moderate to severe heart failure, peak $\dot{V}O_2$ measurements are more reliable than the walk test for clinical decisions.

Cardiac Arrhythmias and Conduction Disturbances

The genesis of cardiac arrhythmias includes reentry, triggered activity, and enhanced automaticity (see Chap. 31). Increased catecholamine levels during exercise accelerate impulse conduction velocity, shorten the myocardial refractory period, increase the amplitude of afterpotentials, and increase the slope of phase 4 spontaneous depolarization of the action potential. Other potentiators of cardiac rhythm disturbance include metabolic acidosis and exercise-induced myocardial ischemia. Ventricular premature complexes occur frequently during exercise testing and increase with age.[86-88] Repetitive forms occur in 0 to 5 percent of asymptomatic subjects without suspected cardiac disease and are not associated with an increased risk of cardiac death. Suppression of ventricular ectopic activity during

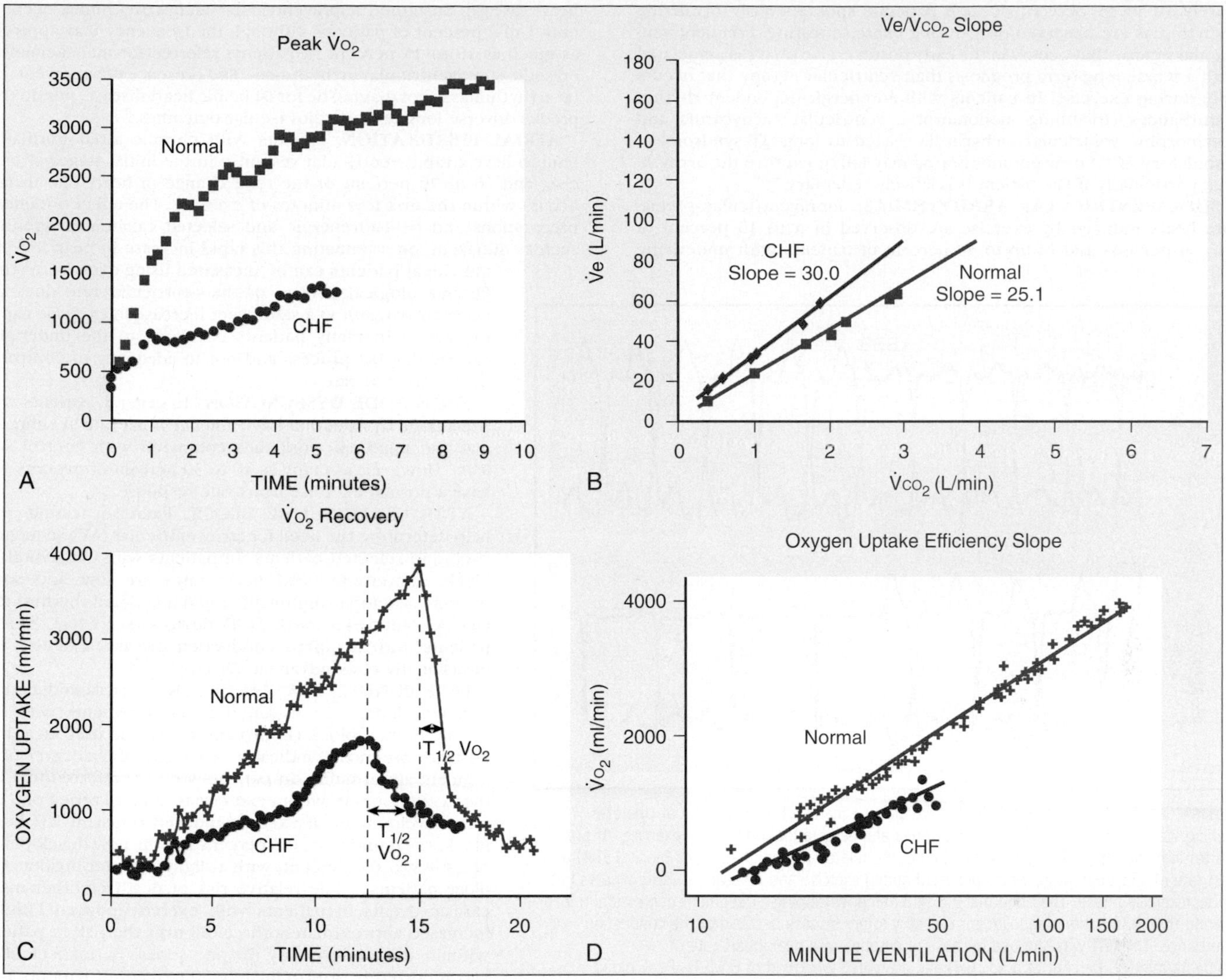

FIGURE 13–14 Examples of four different cardiopulmonary exercise test methods used to estimate prognosis in patients with cardiovascular disease. **A,** The peak $\dot{V}O_2$ responses are taken from a normal subject and a typical patient with chronic heart failure (CHF) of the same age. **B,** The $\dot{V}e\dot{V}CO_2$ slope is derived from the regression line between $\dot{V}e$ and $\dot{V}CO_2$, excluding points beyond the ventilatory threshold. **C,** $\dot{V}O_2$ in recovery shows a more graded recovery response in the heart failure patient (i.e., longer recovery time), despite the lower exercise capacity. T1/2 represents the time required for a 50 percent fall from the peak $\dot{V}O_2$ value. **D,** The oxygen uptake efficiency slope is derived by plotting $\dot{V}O_2$ against the log of $\dot{V}e$; a steeper slope reflects a lower $\dot{V}e$ for any given $\dot{V}O_2$—that is, more efficient ventilation. CHF = congestive heart failure. *(From Myers J: Applications of cardiopulmonary exercise testing in the management of a cardiovascular and pulmonary disease. (Int J Sports Med 26:S49, 2005).*

exercise is a nonspecific finding and may occur in patients with CAD, as well as in normal subjects. The prognostic importance of ventricular arrhythmias in patients with chronic ischemic heart disease after adjustment for baseline, clinical, and left ventricular function characteristics is low. Approximately 20 percent of patients with known heart disease and 50 to 75 percent of sudden cardiac death survivors have repetitive ventricular beats induced by exercise. In patients with a recent myocardial infarction, the presence of exercise-induced repetitive forms is associated with an increased risk of subsequent cardiac events. Beta-adrenergic blocking drugs may suppress exercise-induced ventricular arrhythmias. Exercise-induced ventricular arrhythmias tend to be more frequent in the recovery phase of exercise because peripheral plasma norepinephrine levels continue to increase for several minutes after cessation of exercise, and vagal tone is high in the immediate recovery phase. Five-year all-cause mortality rates are significantly higher in patients who have frequent ventricular ectopy or repetitive ventricular beats in the recovery phase of exercise as compared with those who have ventricular arrhythmias that occur only during exercise. The test is useful in evaluating the effects of antiarrhythmic drugs, detecting supraventricular arrhythmias, treating patients with chronic atrial fibrillation to test for ventricular rate control, and exposing possible drug toxicity in patients placed on antiarrhythmic drugs. Exercise testing is recommended in adult patients with ventricular arrhythmias who have an intermediate probability of coronary artery disease on the basis of age, gender, and symptoms, in patients with known or suspected exercise-induced ventricular arrhythmias, including catecholaminergic ventricular tachycardia, regardless of age, and in evaluating response to medical or ablation therapy in patients with known exercise-induced ventricular arrhythmias.

EVALUATION OF VENTRICULAR ARRHYTHMIAS. Exercise testing is useful in the assessment of patients with ventricular arrhythmias and has an important adjunctive role, along with ambulatory monitoring and electrophysiological studies.[1,2,7,8,86-88] Exercise testing provokes repetitive ventricular premature beats in most patients with a history of sustained ventricular tachyarrhythmia, and in approximately 10 to 15 percent of such patients, spontaneously occurring arrhythmias are observed only during exercise testing. Frequent ventricular ectopy that occurs in the early postexercise phase is associated with a worse long-term prognosis than ventricular ectopy that occurs only during exercise. In patients with adrenergic-dependent rhythm disturbances (including monomorphic ventricular tachycardia and polymorphic ventricular tachycardia related to long-QT syndromes), ambulatory ECG[3] or event monitoring may fail to capture the arrhythmia, particularly if the patient is relatively sedentary.[89,90]

SUPRAVENTRICULAR ARRHYTHMIAS. Supraventricular premature beats induced by exercise are observed in 4 to 10 percent of normal persons and in up to 40 percent of patients with underlying heart disease. Sustained supraventricular tachyarrhythmias occur in only 1 to 2 percent of patients, although the frequency may approach as much as 10 to 15 percent in patients referred for management of episodic supraventricular arrhythmias. The presence of supraventricular arrhythmias is not diagnostic for ischemic heart disease, nor do they predict adverse long-term cardiovascular outcomes.[91]

ATRIAL FIBRILLATION. Patients with chronic atrial fibrillation tend to have a rapid ventricular response in the initial stages of exercise, and 60 to 70 percent of the total change in heart rate usually occurs within the first few minutes of exercise. The effect of digitalis preparations and beta-adrenergic and selected calcium antagonists, such as diltiazem, on attenuating this rapid increase in heart rate for individual patients can be measured using exercise testing. Pharmacological control of the ventricular rate does not necessarily result in a significant increase in exercise capacity, which in many patients is related to the underlying cardiac disease process and not to adequacy of control of the ventricular rate.

SINUS NODE DYSFUNCTION. In general, patients with sinus node dysfunction have a lower heart rate at submaximal and maximal workloads compared with control subjects. However, as many as 40 to 50 percent of patients will have a normal exercise heart rate response.

ATRIOVENTRICULAR BLOCK. Exercise testing may help determine the need for atrioventricular (AV) sequential pacing in selected patients. In patients with congenital AV block, exercise-induced heart rates are low and some patients develop symptomatic rapid junctional rhythms that can be suppressed with DDD devices (see Chap. 34). In patients with acquired conduction disease, exercise can occasionally elicit advanced AV block.

LEFT BUNDLE BRANCH BLOCK. Exercise-induced ST segment depression is found in most patients with left bundle branch block (LBBB) and cannot be used as a diagnostic or prognostic indicator, regardless of the degree of ST segment abnormality. In patients who are referred to a tertiary center and in whom exercise testing is carried out, the new development of exercise-induced transient left hemiblock was found to be 0.3 percent and the new development of LBBB was 0.4 percent, with a slightly greater incidence in older patients.[92] The relative risk of death or other major cardiac events in patients with exercise-induced LBBB is increased approximately threefold over the risk in patients without this abnormality. In one series, permanent LBBB was reported in approximately 50 percent of patients who developed transient LBBB during exercise and who were monitored for an average of 6.6 years. High-grade AV block did not develop in any of the patients in this 15-patient series. The development of ischemic ST segment depression before the LBBB pattern appears or in the recovery phase after the LBBB has resolved does not attenuate the diagnostic yield of the ST segment shift. The ventricular rates at which the LBBB appears and disappears can be significantly different (Fig. 13-15).

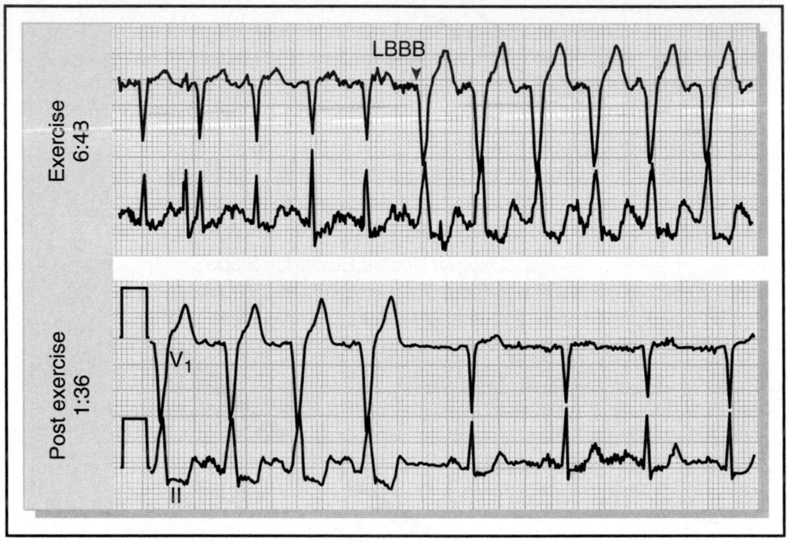

FIGURE 13–15 A 58-year-old hypertensive diabetic man with prior history of cigarette smoking was referred for evaluation of dyspnea and early fatigability during exercise. At 6:48 minutes into the test, the patient developed a rate-related left bundle branch block (LBBB) at a heart rate of 133 beats/min, which persisted during exercise and resolved at 1:36 minutes into the postexercise phase. The abnormal 2.5 to 3 mm downsloping ST segment depression in lead II during the LBBB is nondiagnostic for coronary artery disease because of the conduction disturbance. The test was stopped because of dyspnea at a peak heart rate of 138 beats/min (85 percent of predicted) and estimated workload of 6 METs. Peak blood pressure at the end of exercise was 174/94 mm Hg. Time to onset and offset of LBBB occurred at different ventricular rates related to fatigue in the left bundle, a common finding. METs = metabolic equivalents.

RIGHT BUNDLE BRANCH BLOCK. The resting ECG in patients with right bundle branch block (RBBB) is frequently associated with T wave and ST segment changes in the early anterior precordial leads (V_1 to V_3). Exercise-induced ST depression in leads V_1 to V_4 is a common finding in patients with RBBB and is nondiagnostic (Fig. 13-16). The new development of exercise-induced ST segment depression in leads V_5 and V_6 or leads 2 and aVF, reduced exercise capacity, and inability to increase systolic blood pressure adequately are useful in detecting patients who have CAD and a high clinical pretest risk of disease. The presence of RBBB decreases the sensitivity of the test. The new development of exercise-induced RBBB is relatively uncommon, occurring in approximately 0.1 percent of test results.

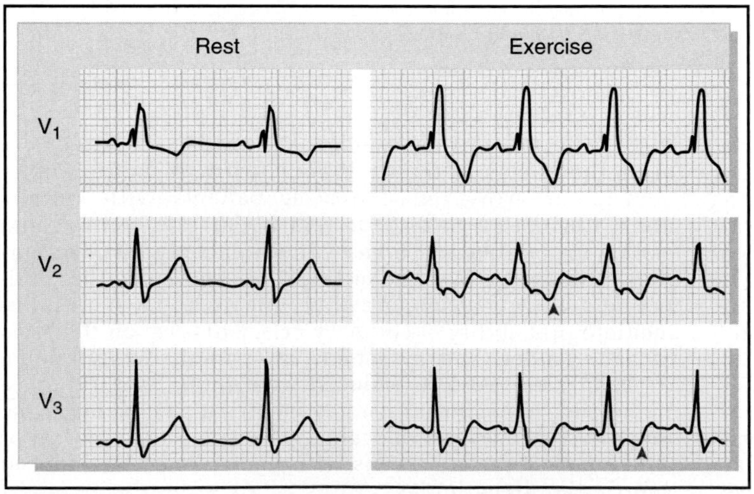

FIGURE 13–16 Exercise-induced ST segment depression is noted in leads V_2 to V_3 (arrows) in this patient with a resting right bundle branch block (RBBB) pattern. Exercise-induced horizontal or downsloping ST segment responses in the early anterior precordial leads (V_1 through V_4) are common in patients with RBBB and are secondary to the conduction disturbance. The presence of this finding in leads V_1 through V_4 is not diagnostic of obstructive coronary disease; however, if ischemic changes are seen in lead II or aVF, or in leads V_5 or V_6, the specificity for coronary disease is improved.

PREEXCITATION SYNDROME. The presence of Wolff-Parkinson-White syndrome invalidates the use of ST segment analysis as a diagnostic method for detecting CAD in preexcited as well as normally conducted beats; false-positive ischemic changes are frequently registered (Fig. 13-17).[93] In patients with persistent preexcitation, exercise may normalize the QRS complex, with disappearance of the delta wave in 20 to 50 percent of cases, depending on the series studied. Abrupt disappearance of the delta wave is presumptive evidence of a longer anterograde effective refractory period of the accessory pathway. Progressive disappearance of the delta wave is less reassuring and occurs when the improvement in AV node conduction is greater than in the accessory pathway; this finding does not preclude a possible significant or even critical shortening of the anterograde effective refractory period in the accessory pathway under the influence of sympathetic stimulation. Exercise-induced disappearance of the delta wave is more frequent with left-sided than right-sided accessory pathway positions. Although tachyarrhythmias appearing during an exercise test in patients with Wolff-Parkinson-White syndrome are rare, they provide an opportunity to evaluate AV conduction velocity when they do occur. The presence of Wolff-Parkinson-White syndrome does not cause a limitation of physical work capacity.

CARDIAC PACEMAKERS AND IMPLANTABLE CARDIOVERTER-DEFIBRILLATOR DEVICES. The exercise protocol used to assess chronotropic responsiveness in patients before and after cardiac pacemaker insertion should adjust for the fact that many patients with such devices are older persons and may not tolerate high exercise workloads or abrupt and relatively large increments in work between stages of exercise.[94,95] An optimal physiological cardiac pacemaker should normalize the heart rate response to exercise in proportion to oxygen uptake and should increase heart rate 2 to 4 beats/min for an increase in $\dot{V}O_2$ of 1 ml O_2/kg/min, with a slightly steeper slope for patients with severe left ventricular function impairment. The exercise test can be particularly useful in evaluating sensor-triggered rate-adaptive pacing, in terms of both maximum heart rate achieved and rate of increase in heart rate during progressive exercise. Exercise testing can also be used to assess performance following cardiac resynchronization therapy in patients with heart failure and ventricular conduction delay.

When testing patients with an implantable cardioverter-defibrillator (ICD), the program detection interval of the device should be known. If the ICD is implanted for ventricular fibrillation or fast ventricular tachycardia, the rate will normally exceed that attainable during sinus tachycardia and the test can be terminated as the heart rate approaches 10 beats/min below the detection interval of the device. In patients with slower programmed detection rates, the ICD can be reprogrammed to a faster rate to avoid accidental discharge during exercise testing or can be temporarily deactivated by a magnet. Exercise testing can be used to test the efficacy of tachycardic detection algorithms that apply criteria such as suddenness of onset and R-R variability.

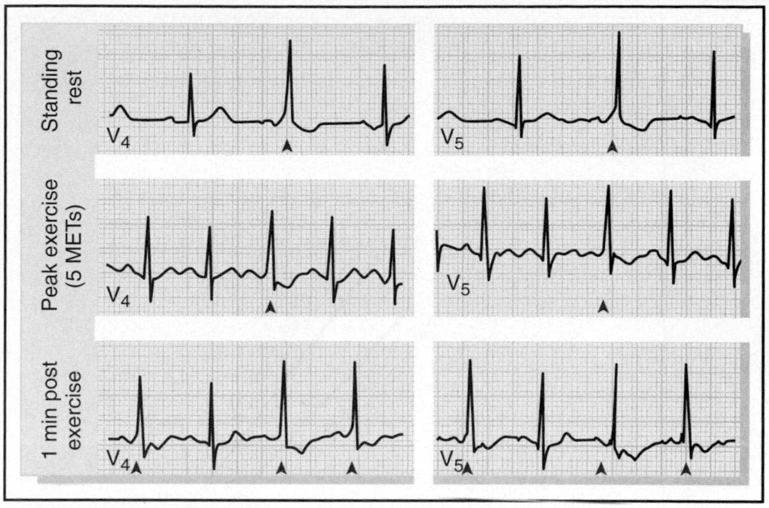

FIGURE 13–17 A 61-year-old man with atypical angina and a hiatal hernia was referred for diagnostic exercise testing. The test was stopped because of dyspnea. The standing resting ECG shows an intermittent Wolff-Parkinson-White pattern (arrows). In the nonpreexcited beats, ST segment depression does not occur at peak exercise or in the postexercise phase. However, in the preexcited beats (arrows), an additional 1.3 mm of downsloping ST segment depression is noted as compared with baseline during and after exertion. METs = metabolic equivalents.

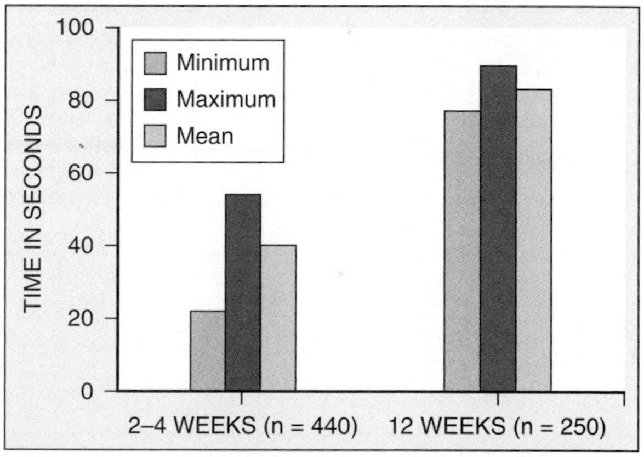

FIGURE 13–18 The average increase in total treadmill exercise duration with placebo in randomized trials of patients with chronic angina. After 2 to 4 weeks of placebo therapy, the average increase compared to baseline is 40 (minimum 25, maximum 55) seconds and, after 12 weeks of placebo therapy, it is 85 (75 to 90) seconds. *(From Chaitman BR: Efficacy and safety of a metabolic modulator drug in chronic angina: Review of evidence from clinical trials. J Cardiovasc Therapeut 9: S47, 2004).*

Specific Clinical Applications

INFLUENCE OF DRUGS AND OTHER FACTORS. Patients with CAD demonstrate individual variability in time to onset of exercise-induced angina, time to onset of exercise-induced ischemic ST segment depression of 0.1 mV or higher, and cardiovascular efficiency during exercise testing.[7,8] The average individual variability in time to onset of exercise-induced myocardial ischemia or peak anaerobic capacity approximates as much as 20 percent in placebo-controlled trials of antianginal drugs. Average increases in exercise duration approach 40 to 60 seconds after 2 to 4 weeks and as long as 90 seconds after 12 weeks of placebo therapy (Fig. 13-18).[96] Variability can be reduced by the patient's familiarization with the exercise protocol and equipment, controlling for antianginal drug therapy at the time of testing, and stable test performance conditions. When two or three exercise tests are conducted within weeks of each other, the greatest increase in exercise time usually occurs between the first test and the second test. The mechanisms of the attenuation response with reexercise may be the results of ischemic preconditioning, familiarization with the exercise protocol, and improved musculoskeletal efficiency but do not appear to be dependent on exercise protocol intensity or downregulation of myocardial contractility induced by the initial ischemic stimulus.[29-31] In cold-sensitive individuals, exercise testing in a cooler environment results in onset of ischemic ST segment depression earlier than under normal temperature-controlled conditions. Conditions that increase carbon monoxide levels, such as chronic cigarette smoking, lower the ischemic response threshold.

Digitalis glycosides can produce exertional ST segment depression even if the effect is not evident on the resting ECG and can accentuate ischemic exercise-induced ST segment changes, particularly in older individuals. Absence of ST segment deviation during an exercise test in a patient receiving a cardiac glycoside is considered a valid negative response. Hypokalemia in patients on long-term diuretic therapy can be associated with exercise-induced ST segment depression. Antiischemic drug therapy with nitrates, beta-blocking drugs, or calcium channel blocking drugs prolongs the time to onset of ischemic ST segment depression, increases exercise tolerance and, in a small minority of patients (10 to 15 percent), may normalize the exercise ECG

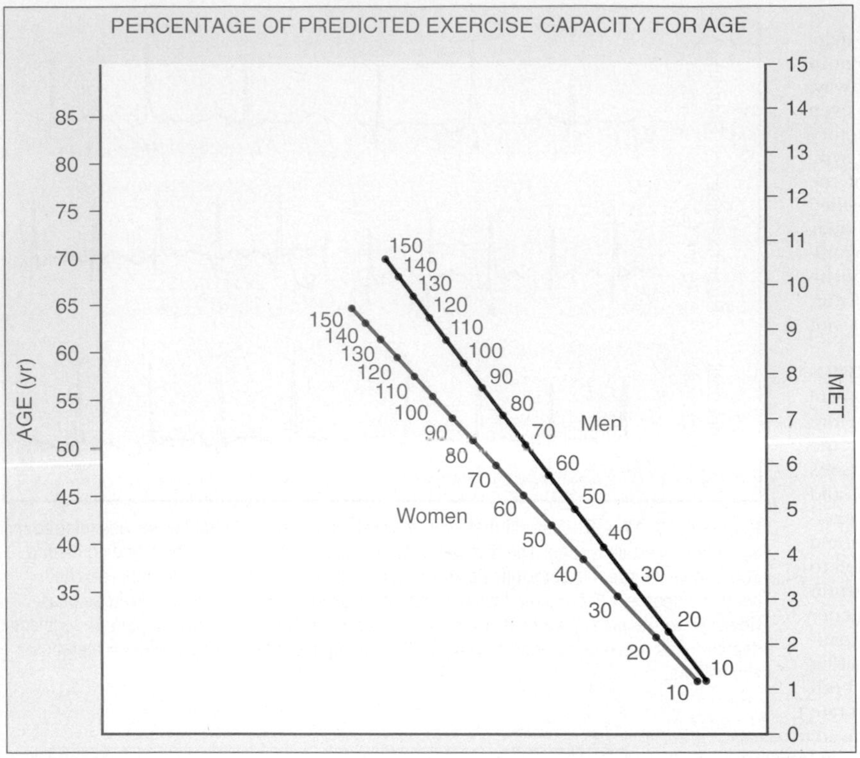

FIGURE 13–19 Nomogram of the percentage of predicted exercise capacity for age in asymptomatic men and women. A line drawn from the patient's age on the scale on the left to the MET value on the scale on the right crosses the percentage line at the point corresponding to the patient's percentage of predicted exercise capacity for age. The risk of death among asymptomatic and symptomatic women whose exercise capacity was less than 85 percent of that predicted for age is approximately twice that for women whose exercise capacity is more than 85 percent. MET = metabolic equivalent. *(From Gulati M, Black HR, Shaw LJ, et al: The prognostic value of a nomogram for exercise capacity in women. New Engl J Med 353:468, 2005.)*

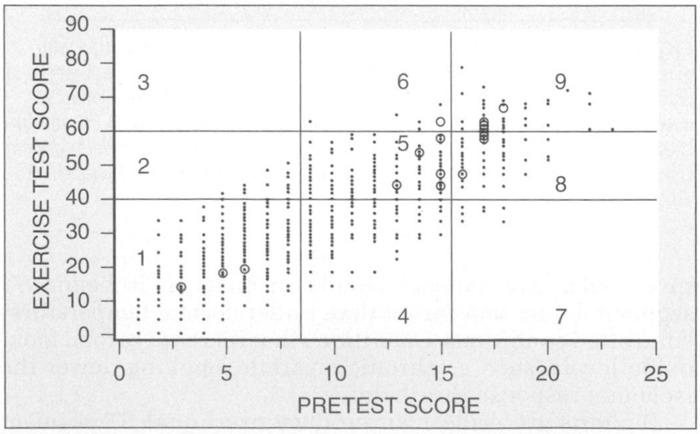

FIGURE 13–20 Scatter plot of exercise score as a function of pretest score for 1678 women referred for exercise testing. Points for those alive (closed circles) and dead (open circles) are shown. Heavy gridlines represent cut points for low-intermediate and intermediate-high risk groups for each score. Lowest risk patients (lowest pretest risk and lowest exercise score) are in sector 1 and highest risk patients (highest pretest risk and highest exercise score) are in sector 9. Mortality after a mean 2.6-year follow-up was highest in women with at least an intermediate pretest clinical score and exercise test score. Clinical variables include age, symptoms, diabetes, smoking, and estrogen status. Exercise ECG score variables include ST depression, peak heart rate, and Duke angina index. *(From Morise AP, Lauer MS, Froelicher VF: Development and validation of a simple exercise test score for use in women with symptoms of suspected heart disease. Am Heart J 144:818, 2002.)*

response in patients with documented CAD.[7,8] The time and dose of drug ingestion may affect exercise performance. In some laboratories, cardioactive drug therapy is withheld for three to five half-lives and digitalis for 1 to 2 weeks before diagnostic testing, but this is impractical in many cases.

WOMEN. The diagnostic accuracy of exercise-induced ST segment depression for obstructive CAD is less in women than in men. Populations of young and middle-aged women have less extensive coronary artery disease than men, resulting in a lower sensitivity to detect coronary disease using noninvasive tests such as exercise testing in this age group. Women tend to have a greater release of catecholamines during exercise, which could potentiate coronary vasoconstriction and augment the incidence of abnormal exercise ECG results, as well as a lower prevalence of coronary artery disease compared with men, and false-positive results have been reported to be more common during menses or preovulation, and in postmenopausal women on isolated estrogen replacement therapy.[97,98] The initial evaluation of women with suspected coronary artery disease and a normal resting ECG with adequate exercise capability should be an exercise ECG treadmill study. The exercise ECG data should be integrated with peak exercise capacity achieved, heart rate, and blood pressure changes to optimize prognostic accuracy.[99-104] In asymptomatic women, a low exercise capacity, low heart rate recovery, and failure to reach target heart rate are more important predictors of outcome than exercise-induced ECG changes (Fig. 13-19). Morise and colleagues have reported mortality rates ranging from 0.2 percent for a low-risk score to 7 percent for a high-risk score based on five clinical and three exercise test variables after an average 2.6-year follow-up in 442 symptomatic women referred for their first exercise test (Fig. 13-20).[49] In symptomatic women with an intermediate-high likelihood of coronary artery disease, imaging procedures should be considered as the initial test when the resting ECG is abnormal or exercise capacity is questionable.

HYPERTENSION. Exercise testing has been used in an attempt to identify patients who have an abnormal blood pressure response and are destined subsequently to develop hypertension. In asymptomatic normotensive individuals, an exaggerated exercise systolic and diastolic blood pressure response during exercise or an exaggerated peak systolic blood pressure response to 214 mm Hg or higher or an elevated systolic or diastolic blood pressure at the third minute of recovery is associated with significant increased long-term risk of hypertension (Fig. 13-21).[33,105,106] Severe systemic hypertension may interfere with subendocardial perfusion and cause exercise-induced ST segment depression in the absence of atherosclerosis, even when the resting ECG does not show significant ST or T wave changes. Beta- and calcium channel blocking drugs decrease submaximal and peak systolic blood pressure in many hypertensive patients.[106] Exercise tolerance is decreased in patients with poor blood pressure control.

ELDERLY PATIENTS. Maximal aerobic capacity $\dot{V}O_2$ max) declines 5 to 10 percent/decade in sedentary men and women, with an approximately 50 percent reduction in exercise capacity between the ages of 30 and 80 years, accel-

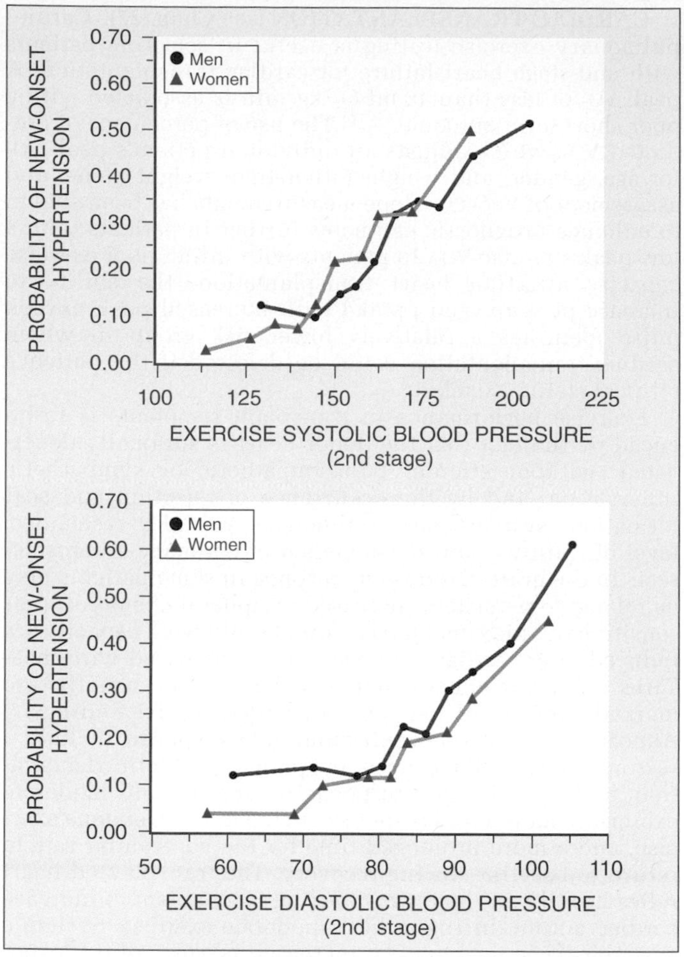

FIGURE 13–21 Probability of developing systemic hypertension within 8 years after exercise testing as a function of exercise-induced systolic **(top panel)** and diastolic **(bottom panel)** blood pressure responses in men and women. Crude probabilities of developing hypertension are displayed for mean systolic or diastolic blood pressure value for each exercise response during the second stage of treadmill testing. *(From Singh JP, Larson MG, Manolio TA, et al: Blood pressure response during treadmill testing is a risk factor for new onset hypertension. The Framingham Heart Study. Circulation 99:1831, 1999.)*

erating in the later decades of life.[1,2,14] The exercise protocol in elderly patients should be selected according to estimated aerobic capacity. In patients with limited exercise tolerance, the test should be started at the slowest speed, with a 0 percent grade, and adjusted according to the patient's ability. Older patients may need to grasp the handrails for support. The frequency of abnormal exercise ECG patterns is higher in older than in younger individuals, and the risk of cardiac events is significantly increased because of a concomitant increase in prevalence of more extensive CAD.[1,2,13,14,37,65,107,108]

The greater test sensitivity of the exercise ECG in elderly individuals is accompanied by a slight reduction in specificity. Cardiac arrhythmias, chronotropic incompetence, and hypertensive responses are more common in older individuals. The value of exercise testing to estimate prognosis in elderly subjects was evaluated in 3107 patients from Olmstead County, of whom 512 were 65 years of age or older. Workload expressed in METs was the only variable associated with all-cause mortality in subjects 65 years of age or older, whereas workload and exercise-induced angina were predictive of cardiac death or nonfatal myocardial infarction.[108] In elderly subjects 75 years of age or older, the Duke treadmill scoring system is less effective in estimating prognosis.[64] Most elderly patients tend to be categorized as intermediate risk, primarily because they cannot exercise long enough to be classified as low risk.

DIABETES MELLITUS. Coronary atherosclerosis and peripheral vascular disease are significantly increased in adult diabetic patients as compared with nondiabetic patients (see Chap. 60); the likelihood of atherosclerosis correlates closely with the duration of diabetes and the presence of microvascular disease, peripheral vascular disease, and autonomic neuropathy.[109] In patients with autonomic dysfunction and sensory neuropathy, anginal threshold may be increased, and abnormal exercise-induced heart rate and blood pressure responses are common. Once CAD is established, the incidence of exercise-induced electrocardiographic changes is similar to the incidence in nondiabetic persons. The probability of an adverse cardiac outcome in a diabetic person as compared with a nondiabetic person for a similar abnormal exercise test result is likely to be increased because of the increased risk of dyslipidemia, impaired fibrinolysis, and hypertension associated with the diabetic process. Patients with diabetes who wish to enroll in a moderate- to high-intensity exercise program are considered to have a class IIA indication for exercise testing.[1] Further research is required to determine optimal noninvasive test procedures to diagnose early endothelial dysfunction and the presence and extent of obstructive CAD in patients with diabetes.

VALVULAR HEART DISEASE AND HYPERTROPHIC CARDIOMYOPATHY. The hemodynamics of exercise provide an excellent opportunity to measure gradients across stenotic valves, assess ventricular function in patients with primary valvular regurgitation or mixed lesions, and assess pulmonary and systemic vascular resistance (see Chap. 62).[110-112] The use of echocardiographic Doppler techniques (see Chap. 14) is particularly valuable in evaluating patients whose symptoms are out of proportion to the degree of hemodynamic abnormalities observed at rest and in assessing the results of valvulotomy or valve replacement. Clinical and exercise noninvasive assessment of patients with valvular heart disease can provide useful information on the timing of operative intervention and help achieve a more precise estimate of a patient's degree of incapacitation than can assessment of symptoms alone. Studies of adults with moderate to severe aortic stenosis (e.g., valve area, 0.5 to 1.5 cm^2, and mean gradients, 18 to 64 mm Hg) have shown that exercise testing can be safely performed when appropriate exercise protocols and precautions are used.[110] Exercise testing is useful in evaluating aortic valve gradients during low-output flow states and, with Doppler echocardiography, provides important data on left ventricular functional reserve. Hypotension during exercise in asymptomatic patients with aortic stenosis may be a sufficient reason to consider valve replacement. In patients with mitral stenosis, excessive heart rate response to relatively low levels of exercise, reduction of cardiac output with exercise (manifested by exercise-induced hypotension), and chest pain (ischemia secondary to low output or pulmonary hypertension) are indicators that favor earlier valve repair. In patients with mitral valve prolapse without regurgitation at rest, exercise-induced mitral regurgitation has been associated with the subsequent development of progressive mitral regurgitation, heart failure symptoms, or syncope.

Peak $\dot{V}O_2$ and anaerobic threshold are reduced in symptomatic patients with hypertrophic cardiomyopathy as compared with sedentary subjects (see Chap. 65). Inability to increase blood pressure by 20 mm Hg during exercise may result from exercise-induced left ventricular systolic dysfunction and is associated with an adverse prognosis.[113] Abnormal blood pressure responses in patients with hypertrophic cardiomyopathy may normalize after transcoronary alcohol septal ablation, associated with only a slight increase in exercise time. Exercise testing is relatively safe in patients with hypertrophic cardiomyopathy and resting or inducible gradients.[114] Patients with high resting gradients (e.g., more than 4 meters/sec), NYHA Class III or IV symptoms, and a history of important ventricular arrhythmias are not generally tested.

CORONARY REVASCULARIZATION

Coronary Bypass Grafting (see Chap. 54). The degree of improvement in exercise-induced myocardial ischemia and aerobic capacity after coronary bypass grafting depends in part on the degree of revascularization achieved and on left ventricular function. Exercise-induced ischemic ST segment depression may persist when incomplete revascularization is achieved, albeit at higher exercise workloads. It also may persist in approximately 5 percent of patients in whom complete revascularization has been achieved. Stress imaging studies are likely to provide more useful information regarding the site and extent of myocardial ischemia after coronary revascularization procedures than the exercise electrocardiogram, and are the preferred modality when noninvasive testing is performed for management decisions. The diagnostic and prognostic usefulness of exercise testing late after coronary revascularization (e.g., 5 to 10 years) is much greater than early (less than 1 year) testing, because a late abnormal exercise response is more likely to indicate graft occlusion, stenosis, or progression of CAD, particularly in the presence of typical angina or conditions of accelerated atherosclerosis, such as diabetes mellitus, hemodialysis, or immunosuppressive therapy.[115] In selected patients with severe left ventricular dysfunction and symptomatic heart failure, coronary bypass surgery is associated with a significant increase in exercise capacity when a large amount of dysfunctional but viable myocardium (e.g., more than 25 percent of left ventricular mass) is revascularized.

Percutaneous Coronary Intervention (see Chap. 55). The risk of restenosis after percutaneous coronary intervention (PCI) is time dependent; stent restenosis usually occurs within the first 12 months after PCI, and is significantly reduced (less than 10 percent) with the use of drug-eluting stents. In the early post-PCI phase (less than 1 month), an abnormal exercise ECG result may be secondary to a suboptimal result, impaired coronary vascular reserve in a successfully dilated vessel, or incomplete revascularization.[30,116] Thus, exercise electrocardiography has a low diagnostic accuracy to detect restenosis or an incomplete dilation in the periprocedural phase. The optimal time to perform an exercise test after PCI depends in part on the success of the procedure and the degree of revascularization obtained. In an otherwise asymptomatic patient, a 6- to 12-month postprocedure test allows sufficient time to document restenosis should it occur and allows the dilated vessel an opportunity to heal. Serial conversion of an initially normal exercise test result after PCI to an abnormal result in the initial 6 months after the procedure, particularly when it occurs at a lower exercise workload, is usually associated with restenosis. The use of exercise myocardial imaging in selected patients enhances the diagnostic content of the test and can help localize the territory of myocardial ischemia and guide indications for repeat coronary angiography in patients who have undergone multivessel or multilesion PCI.

In general, routine periodic monitoring of asymptomatic patients after a coronary revascularization procedure (coronary artery bypass grafting or PCI) without a specific indication is not useful. The use of exercise testing without imaging to evaluate symptoms early after PCI is uncommon. Clinical stent thrombosis or access site complications were not increased in one randomized trial of exercise testing performed early after coronary stenting.[117]

CARDIAC TRANSPLANTATION (see Chap. 27). Cardiopulmonary exercise testing is useful in selecting patients with end-stage heart failure for cardiac transplantation. A peak $\dot{V}O_2$ of less than 10 ml O_2/kg/min is associated with a poor short-term outcome.[118-120] The use of percentage of predicted $\dot{V}O_2$, which adjusts an individual patient's peak $\dot{V}O_2$ for age, gender, and weight rather than weight alone, and assessment of $\dot{V}e/\dot{V}CO_2$ slope measurements has been shown to enhance prognostic estimates further in patients with a low peak exercise $\dot{V}O_2$. In patients with initial poor exercise capacity awaiting heart transplantation, the ability to increase peak oxygen uptake with increased peak oxygen pulse identifies a relatively lower risk group in whom cardiac transplantation could be deferred if the patient's clinical status is stable.

Exercise performance in transplant recipients is influenced by the fact that the donor heart is surgically denervated, without efferent parasympathetic or sympathetic innervation, and by the occurrence of rejection and scar formation, systemic and pulmonary vascular resistance, level of training, and development of coronary atherosclerosis in the graft. Exercise hyperpnea in some patients may be related to persistent increased peripheral chemoreceptor sensitivity.[118] Maximal oxygen uptake and work capacity are reduced after cardiac transplantation compared with measures in age-matched control subjects, but usually are markedly improved compared with preoperative findings.[119] Abnormalities of the ventricular rate response include a resting tachycardia caused by parasympathetic denervation, a slow heart rate response during mild to moderate exercise, a more rapid response during more strenuous exercise, and a more prolonged time for the ventricular rate to return to baseline during recovery. The transplanted heart relies heavily on the Frank-Starling mechanism to increase cardiac output during mild to moderate exercise. Systemic vascular resistance may be increased because of cyclosporine therapy. Sympathetic reinnervation of the sinus node may occur after cardiac transplantation and may partially restore a normal heart rate response to exercise, but in most patients will not return exercise capacity to normal. The exercise ECG is relatively insensitive in detecting coronary artery vasculopathy after cardiac transplantation. However, the new development of an abnormal exercise ECG result several years after cardiac transplantation may indicate focal intraluminal narrowing.

ADULT CONGENITAL HEART DISEASE. Exercise capacity is usually decreased in adults with congenital heart disease, even in the absence of symptoms.[121,122] Chronotropic response to exercise, pulmonary arterial hypertension, impaired pulmonary function, and underlying cardiac anatomy are important determinants of peak exercise capacity. Low peak $\dot{V}O_2$ measurements are associated with increased hospital admissions and survival (Fig. 13-22). Patients with simple noncyanotic lesions, with biventricular hearts without pulmonary arterial hypertension, have a significantly greater exercise capacity and better prognosis than patients with complex or cyanotic lesions and pulmonary arterial hypertension.

SAFETY AND RISKS OF EXERCISE TESTING

Exercise testing has an excellent safety record. The risk is determined by the clinical characteristics of the patient referred for the procedure. In nonselected patient populations, the mortality is less than 0.01 percent and morbidity is less than 0.05 percent.[123] The risk is greater when the test is performed soon after an acute ischemic event. In a survey of 151,941 tests conducted within 4 weeks of an acute myocardial infarction, mortality was 0.03 percent, and 0.09 percent of patients tested either had a nonfatal reinfarction or were resuscitated from cardiac arrest.[124] The relative risk of a major complication is about twice as great when a symptom-limited protocol is used as compared with a low-level protocol. Nevertheless, in the early postinfarction phase, the risk of a fatal complication during symptom-limited testing is only 0.03 percent. The risk is less for low-risk patients who are seen in the emergency department and who undergo exercise testing for risk stratification. Exercise testing can be safely performed in patients with compensated congestive heart failure, with no major complications reported in 1286 tests in which a bicycle ergometer was used.[125] The risk of exercise testing in patients referred for life-threatening ventricular arrhythmias was examined by Young and colleagues[126] in a series of 263 patients who underwent 1377 tests; 2.2 percent developed sustained ventricular tachyarrhythmias that required cardioversion, cardiopulmonary resuscitation, or antiarrhythmic drugs to restore sinus rhythm. The ventricular arrhythmias were more frequent in tests performed on patients who were receiving antiarrhythmic drug therapy as compared with the baseline drug-free state. In contrast to the high risk in the aforementioned patient subsets, the risk of complications in asymptomatic subjects is extremely low, with no fatalities reported in several series.[1,7,8]

The risk of incurring a major complication during exercise testing can be reduced by performing a careful history and physical examination before the test and observing patients closely during exercise with monitoring of the ECG, arterial pressure, and symptoms. The standard 12-lead ECG should be verified before the test for any acute or recent changes. The contraindications to exercise testing are well defined (Table 13-4). Patients with critical obstruction to left ventricular outflow are at increased risk of cardiac events during exercise. In selected patients, low-level exercise can be useful in determining the severity of the left ventricular outflow tract obstruction. The cool-down period should be prolonged to at least 2 minutes in patients with left ventricular outflow tract obstruction or stenotic valves to avoid sudden pressure-volume shifts, which occur in the immediate postexercise phase.

Uncontrolled systemic hypertension is a contraindication to exercise testing. Patients should continue antihypertensive drug therapy on the day of testing. Patients who present with systemic arterial pressure readings of 220/120 mm Hg or higher should rest for 15 to 20 minutes, and their blood pressure should be remeasured. If blood pressure remains at these levels, the test should be postponed until the hypertension is better controlled.

A resuscitation cart and defibrillator should be available in the room where the test procedure is carried out, and appropriate cardioactive medication should be available to treat cardiac arrhythmias, AV block, hypotension, and persistent chest pain. An intravenous line should be started in high-risk patients, such as those being tested for adequacy of control of life-threatening ventricular arrhythmias. The equipment and supplies in the cart should be checked on a regular basis. A previously specified routine for cardiac emergencies needs to be determined; this includes patient transfer and admission to a coronary care unit, if necessary.

Clinical judgment is required to determine which patients can be safely tested in an office as opposed to a hospital-based setting. The experience is acquired through training programs and maintenance of clinical competency.[127,128] High-risk patients, such as those with major left ventricular dysfunction, recent angina pectoris, cardiac syncope, or important ventricular ectopy on the pretest examination, should be tested in the hospital. Low-risk patients, such as asymptomatic individuals and those with a low pretest risk of disease, can be tested by specially trained nurses or physician assistants who have received advanced cardiac life support certification, with a physician in close proximity.

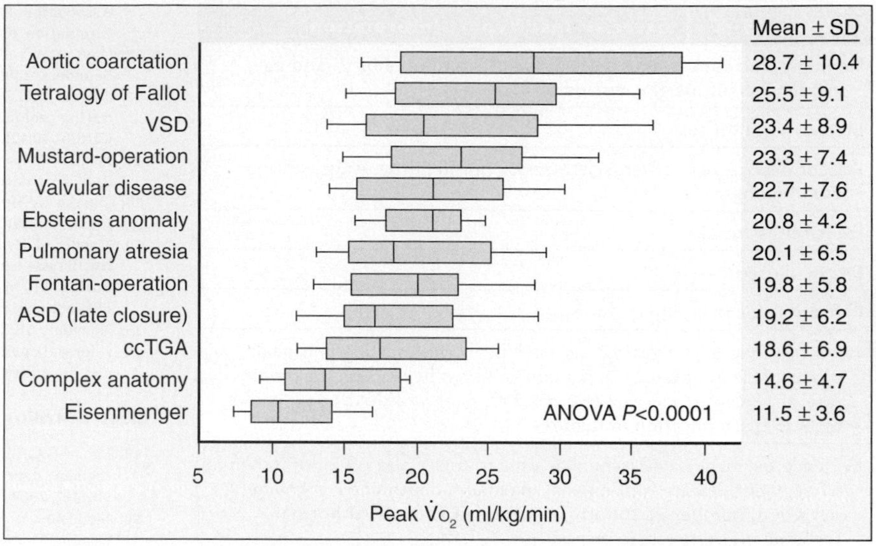

FIGURE 13–22 Distribution of peak V̇O_2 measurements in different diagnostic categories of a consecutive series of patients with adult congenital heart disease ($n = 335$) who underwent cardiopulmonary exercise testing. Peak V̇O_2 measurements were predictive of death and repeat hospital admissions over a median follow-up of 304 (range, 17 to 580) days. Cardiopulmonary exercise capacity (peak V̇O_2) was significantly worse in patients with cyanotic lesions, pulmonary hypertension, and complex pathology. ANOVA = analysis of variance between groups; ASD = atrial septal defect; ccTGA = congenitally corrected transposition of the great vessels; VSD = ventricular septal defect. *(From Diller GP, Dimopoulos K, Okonko D, et al: Exercise intolerance in adult congenital heart disease. Comparative severity, correlates, and prognostic implication. Circulation 112:828, 2005.)*

TABLE 13–4 Absolute Contraindications to Exercise Testing
Acute myocardial infarction (<2 d)
High-risk unstable angina
Decompensated heart failure
Uncontrolled cardiac arrhythmias with symptoms or hemodynamic compromise
Advanced atrioventricular block
Acute myocarditis or pericarditis
Severe symptomatic aortic stenosis
Severe hypertrophic obstructive cardiomyopathy
Uncontrolled hypertension
Acute systemic illness (pulmonary embolism, aortic dissection)

TERMINATION OF EXERCISE

The use of standard test indications to terminate an exercise test reduces risk (see Table 13G-2). Termination of exercise should be determined in part by the patient's recent activity level. The rate of perceived patient exertion can be estimated by the Borg scale. The scale is linear, with values of 9 for very light, 11 for fairly light, 13 for somewhat hard, 15 for hard, 17 for very hard, and 19 for very, very hard. Borg readings of 14 to 16 approximate anaerobic threshold, and readings of 18 or higher approximate a patient's maximum exercise capacity. It is helpful to grade exercise-induced chest discomfort on a 1 to 4 scale, with 1 indicating the initial onset of chest discomfort and 4 the most severe chest pain the patient has ever experienced. The exercise technician should note the onset of grade 1 chest discomfort on the work sheet, and the test should be stopped when the patient reports grade 3 chest pain. In the absence of symptoms, it is prudent to stop exercise when a patient demonstrates 0.3 mV (3 mm) or higher of ischemic ST segment depression or 0.1 mV (1 mm) or higher of ST segment elevation in a noninfarct lead without an abnormal Q wave. Significant worsening of ambient ventricular ectopy during

TABLE 13–5 Exercise Test Report Information
Demographic data—name, patient identifier, date of birth and age, gender, weight, height, test date
Indication(s) for test
Patient descriptors—atherosclerotic risk profile, drug usage, resting ECG findings
Exercise test results
Protocol used
Reason(s) for stopping exercise
Hemodynamic data—resting and peak heart rate, resting and peak blood pressure, percent maximum achieved heart rate, maximum rate of perceived exertion (Borg scale), peak workload, peak METs, total exercise duration in minutes
Evidence for myocardial ischemia—time to onset and offset of ischemic ST segment deviation or angina, maximum depth of ST segment deviation, number of abnormal exercise ECG leads, abnormal systemic blood pressure responses
General comments

ECG = electrocardiogram; METs = metabolic equivalents.

exercise or the unsuspected appearance of ventricular tachycardia is an indication to terminate exercise. A progressive, reproducible decrease in systolic blood pressure of 10 mm Hg or more may indicate transient left ventricular dysfunction or an inappropriate decrease in systemic vascular resistance, and is an indication to terminate exercise. The test should be stopped if the arterial blood pressure is 250 to 270/120 to 130 mm Hg or higher. Ataxia can indicate cerebral hypoxia.

The exercise test report should contain basic demographic data, the indication for testing, a brief description of the patient's profile, and exercise test results (Table 13-5).

REFERENCES

1. Gibbons RJ, Balady GJ, Bricker JT, et al: ACC/AHA 2002 guideline update for exercise testing. Summary article: A report of the ACC/AHA Task Force on Practice Guidelines (Committee to Update the 1997 Exercise Testing Guidelines). J Am Coll Cardiol 40:1531, 2002.
2. Fletcher GF, Balady GJ, Amsterdam EA, et al: Exercise standards for testing and training: A statement for healthcare professionals from the American Heart Association. Circulation 104:1694, 2001.
3. Whaley MH, Brubaker PH, Otto RM, Armstrong LE: ACSM's Guidelines for Exercise Testing and Prescription. 7th ed. Philadelphia, Lippincott Williams & Wilkins, 2006.
4. Wasserman K: Principles of Exercise Testing and Interpretation. 4th ed. Philadelphia, Lippincott Williams & Wilkins, 2005.
5. American Thoracic Society/American College of Chest Physicians: Statement on cardiopulmonary exercise testing. Am J Respir Crit Care Med 167:211, 2003.

Exercise Physiology

6. Skinner JS: Exercise Testing and Exercise Prescription for Special Cases: Theoretical Basis and Clinical Application. Philadelphia, Lippincott Williams & Wilkins, 2005.
7. Ellestad MH: Stress Testing: Principles and Practice. 5th ed. New York, Oxford University Press, 2003.
8. Froelicher, VF, Myers J: Exercise and the Heart. 5th ed. Philadelphia, WB Saunders, 2006.
9. Paridon SM, Alpert BS, Boas SR, et al: Clinical stress testing in the pediatric age group: A statement from the American Heart Association Council on Cardiovascular Disease in the Young, Committee on Atherosclerosis, Hypertension, and Obesity in Youth. Circulation 113:1905, 2006.
10. Fleg JL, Pina IL, Balady GJ, et al: Assessment of functional capacity in clinical and research applications: An advisory from the Committee on Exercise, Rehabilitation, and Prevention, Council on Clinical Cardiology, American Heart Association. Circulation 102:1591, 2000.
11. Pollock ML, Franklin BA, Balady GJ, et al: AHA Science Advisory. Resistance exercise in individuals with and without cardiovascular disease: Benefits, rationale, safety, and prescription. An advisory from the Committee on Exercise, Rehabilitation, and Prevention, Council on Clinical Cardiology, American Heart Association. Position paper endorsed by the American College of Sports Medicine. Circulation 101:828, 2000.
12. Guyton AC: Textbook of Medical Physiology. 11th ed. Philadelphia, Elsevier Saunders, 2006.
13. Correia LCL, Lakatta EG, O'Connor FC, et al: Attenuated cardiovascular reserve during prolonged submaximal cycle exercise in healthy older subjects. J Am Coll Cardiol 40:1290, 2002.
14. Fleg JL, Morrell CH, Bos AG, et al: Accelerated longitudinal decline of aerobic capacity in healthy older adults. Circulation 112:674, 2005.
15. Tanaka H, Monahan KD, Seals DR: Age-predicted maximal heart rate revisited. J Am Coll Cardiol 37:153, 2001.
16. Maeder M, Wolber T, Atefy R, et al: Impact of the exercise mode on exercise capacity. Bicycle testing revisited. Chest 128:2804, 2005.
17. Enright PL, McBurnie MA, Bittner V, et al: The 6-min walk test. A quick measure of functional status in elderly adults. Chest 123:387, 2003.
18. Newman AB, Simonsick EM, Naydeck BL, et al: Association of long-distance corridor walk performance with mortality, cardiovascular disease, mobility limitation and disability. JAMA 295:2018, 2006.

Electrocardiographic Measures

19. Lanza GA, Mustilli M, Sestito A, et al: Diagnostic and prognostic value of ST segment depression limited to the recovery phase of exercise stress test. Heart 90:1417, 2004.
20. Modesto KM, Rainbird A, Klarich KW: Comparison of supine bicycle exercise and treadmill exercise Doppler echocardiography in evaluation of patients with coronary artery disease. Am J Cardiol 91:1245, 2003.
21. Rywik TM, Zink RC, Gittings NS, et al: Independent prognostic significance of ischemic ST segment response limited to recovery from treadmill exercise in asymptomatic subjects. Circulation 97:2117, 1998.
22. Soto JR, Watson DD, Beller GA: Incidence and significance of ischemic ST-segment depression occurring solely during recovery after exercise testing. Am J Cardiol 88:670, 2001.
23. Akutsu Y, Shinozuka A, Nishimura H, et al: Significance of ST-segment morphology noted on electrocardiography during the recovery phase after exercise in patients with ischemic heart disease as analyzed with simultaneous dual-isotope single photon emission tomography. Am Heart J 144:335, 2002.
24. Fearon WF, Lee DP, Froelicher VF: The effect of resting ST segment depression on the diagnostic characteristics of exercise treadmill testing. J Am Coll Cardiol 35:1206, 2000.
25. Weinsaft JW, Wong FJ, Walden J, et al: Anatomic distribution of myocardial ischemia as a determinant of exercise-induced ST-segment depression. Am J Cardiol 96:1356, 2005.
26. Okin PM, Prineas RJ, Grandits G, et al: Heart rate adjustment of exercise-induced ST segment depression identifies men who benefit from a risk factor reduction program. Circulation 96:2899, 1997.
27. Julius BK, Vassalli G, Mandinov L, Hess OM: Alpha-adrenoreceptor blockade prevents exercise-induced vasoconstriction of stenotic coronary arteries. J Am Coll Cardiol 33:1499, 1999.
28. Maier W, Windecker S, Kung A, et al: Exercise-induced coronary artery vasodilation is not impaired by stent placement. Circulation 105:2373, 2002.
29. Kelion AD, Webb TP, Gardner MA, et al: The warm-up effect protects against ischemic left ventricular dysfunction in patients with angina. J Am Coll Cardiol 37:705, 2001.
30. Bogaty P, Poirier P, Boyer L, et al: What induces the warm-up ischemia/angina phenomenon: Exercise or myocardial ischemia? Circulation 107:1858, 2003.
31. Lambiase PD, Edwards RJ, Cusack MR, et al: Exercise-induced ischemia initiates the second window of protection in humans independent of collateral recruitment. J Am Coll Cardiol 41:1174, 2003.
32. Li RA, Leppo M, Miki T, et al: Molecular basis of electrocardiographic ST-segment elevation. Circ Res 87:837, 2000.

Nonelectrocardiographic Measures

33. Miyai N, Arita M, Miyashita K, et al: Blood pressure response to heart rate during exercise test and risk of future hypertension. Hypertension 39:761, 2002.
34. Fleg JL, Lakatta EG: Prevalence and significance of postexercise hypotension in apparently healthy subjects. Am J Cardiol 57:1380, 1986.
35. Ha JW, Juracan EM, Mahoney DW, et al: Hypertensive response to exercise: A potential cause for new wall motion abnormality in the absence of coronary artery disease. J Am Coll Cardiol 39:323, 2002.
36. Myers J, Prakash M, Froelicher V, et al: Exercise capacity and mortality among men referred for exercise testing. N Engl J Med 346:793, 2002.
37. Spin JM, Prakash M, Froelicher VF, et al: The prognostic value of exercise testing in elderly men. Am J Med 112:453, 2002.
38. Gulati M, Pandey DK, Arnsdorf MF, et al: Exercise capacity and the risk of death in women. The St. James Women Take Heart Project. Circulation 108:1554, 2003.
39. Mark DB, Lauer MS: Exercise capacity. The prognostic variable that doesn't get enough respect. Circulation 108:1534, 2003.
40. Lavie CJ, Kuruvanka T, Milani RV, et al: Exercise capacity in adult African-Americans referred for exercise stress testing. Is fitness affected by race? Chest 126:1962, 2004.
41. Falcone C, Buzzi MP, Klersy C, Schwartz PJ: Rapid heart rate increase at onset of exercise predicts adverse cardiac events in patients with coronary artery disease. Circulation 112:1959, 2005.
42. Elhendy A, Mahoney DW, Khandheria BK, et al: Prognostic significance of impairment of heart rate response to exercise: Impact of left ventricular function and myocardial ischemia. J Am Coll Cardiol 42:823, 2003.

43. Savonen KP, Lakka TA, Laukkanen JA, et al: Heart rate response during exercise test and cardiovascular mortality in middle-aged men. Eur Heart J 27:582, 2006.
44. Jouven X, Empana JP, Schwartz PJ, et al: Heart-rate profile during exercise as a predictor of sudden death. N Engl J Med 352:1951, 2005.
45. Chaitman BR: Abnormal heart rate responses to exercise predict increased long-term mortality regardless of coronary disease extent. The question is why? J Am Coll Cardiol 42:2049, 2003.
46. Morise AP: Heart rate recovery. Predictor of risk today and target of therapy tomorrow? Circulation 110:2778, 2004.
47. Vivekananthan DP, Blackstone EH, Pothier CE, Lauer MS: Heart rate recovery after exercise is a predictor of mortality, independent of the angiographic severity of coronary disease. J Am Coll Cardiol 42:831, 2003.

Diagnostic and Prognostic Applications

48. Froelicher VF, Lehmann KG, Thomas R, et al: The electrocardiographic exercise test in a population with reduced workup bias: Diagnostic performance, computerized interpretation and multivariable prediction. Veterans Affairs Cooperative Study in Health Services #016 (QUEXTA) Study Group. Quantitative Exercise Testing and Angiography. Ann Intern Med 128:965, 1998.
49. Morise AP, Lauer MS, Froelicher VF: Development and validation of a simple exercise test score for use in women with symptoms of suspected coronary artery disease. Am Heart J 144:818, 2002.
50. Morise AP, Jalisi F: Evaluation of pretest and exercise test scores to assess all-cause mortality in unselected patients presenting for exercise testing with symptoms of suspected coronary artery disease. J Am Coll Cardiol 42:842, 2003.
51. Rywik TM, O'Connor FC, Gittings NS, et al: Role of nondiagnostic exercise-induced ST-segment abnormalities in predicting future coronary events in asymptomatic volunteers. Circulation 106:2787, 2002.
52. Balady GJ, Larson MG, Vasan RS, et al: Usefulness of exercise testing in the prediction of coronary disease risk among asymptomatic persons as a function of the Framingham Risk Score. Circulation 110:1920, 2004.
53. Aktas MK, Ozduran V, Pothier CE, et al: Global risk scores and exercise testing for predicting all-cause mortality in a preventive medicine program. JAMA 292:1462, 2004.
54. Fowler-Brown A, Pignone M, Pletcher M, et al: Exercise tolerance testing to screen for coronary heart disease: A systematic review for the technical support for the U.S. Preventive Services Task Force. Ann Intern Med 140:W9, 2004.
55. Mora S, Redberg RF, Sharrett AR, Blumenthal RS: Enhanced risk assessment in asymptomatic individuals with exercise testing and Framingham Risk Scores. Circulation 112:1566, 2005.
56. Lauer M, Froelicher S, Williams M, Kligfield P: Exercise testing in asymptomatic adults. A statement for professionals from the American Heart Association on Clinical Cardiology, Subcommittee on Exercise, Cardiac Rehabilitation, and Prevention. Circulation 112:771, 2005.
57. Erikssen G, Bodegard J, Bjornholt JV, et al: Exercise testing of healthy men in a new perspective: From diagnosis to prognosis. Eur Heart J 25:978-986, 2004.
58. Shishehbor MH, Litaker D, Pothier CE, Lauer MS: Association of socioeconomic status with functional capacity, heart rate recovery, and all-cause mortality. JAMA 295:784, 2006.
59. LaMonte MJ, FitzGerald SJ, Levine BD, et al: Coronary artery calcium, exercise tolerance, and CHD events in asymptomatic men. Atherosclerosis 189:157, 2006.
60. Blumenthal RS, Becker DM, Yanek LR, et al: Detecting occult coronary disease in a high-risk asymptomatic population. Circulation 107:702, 2003.
61. Weiner DH, Ryan T, McCabe CH, et al: Prognostic importance of a clinical profile and exercise test in medically treated patients with coronary artery disease. J Am Coll Cardiol 3:772, 1984.
62. Mark DB, Hlatky MA, Harrell FE, et al: Exercise treadmill score for predicting prognosis in coronary heart disease. Ann Intern Med 106:793, 1987.
63. Mark DB, Shaw L, Harrell FE Jr, et al: Prognostic value of a treadmill exercise score in outpatients with suspected coronary artery disease. N Engl J Med 325:849, 1991.
64. Kwok JMF, Miller TD, Hodge DO, Gibbons RJ: Prognostic value of the Duke treadmill score in the elderly. J Am Coll Cardiol 39:1475, 2002.
65. Lai S, Kaykha A, Yamazaki T, et al: Treadmill scores in elderly men. J Am Coll Cardiol 43:606, 2004.
66. Valensi P, Paries J, Brulport-Cerisier V, et al: Predictive value of silent myocardial ischemia for cardiac events in diabetic patients: Influence of age in a French multicenter study. Diabetes Care 28:2722, 2005.
67. Braunwald E, Antman EM, Beasley JW, et al: ACC/AHA 2002 guideline update for the management of patients with unstable angina and non-ST-segment elevation myocardial infarction: A report of the American College of Cardiology/American Heart Association Task Force on Practice Guidelines (Committee on the Management of Patients With Unstable Angina), 2002 (http://www.acc.org/clinical/guidelines/unstable/unstable.pdf).
68. Antman E, Anbe DT, Green LA, et al: ACC/AHA guidelines for the management of patients with ST-elevation myocardial infarction—executive summary. J Am Coll Cardiol 44:671, 2004.
69. De Luca G, Suryapranata H, van't Hof AWJ, et al: Prognostic assessment of patients with acute myocardial infarction treated with primary angioplasty. Implications for early discharge. Circulation 109:2737, 2004.
70. Fernandez-Avilés F, Alonso JJ, Castro-Beiras A, et al: Routine invasive strategy within 24 hours of thrombolysis versus ischaemia-guided conservative approach for acute myocardial infarction with ST-segment elevation (GRACIA-1): A randomised controlled trial. Lancet 364:1045, 2004.
71. Stein RA, Chaitman BR, Balady GJ, et al: Safety and utility of exercise testing in emergency room chest pain centers: An advisory from the Committee on Exercise, Rehabilitation and Prevention, Council on Clinical Cardiology, American Heart Association. Circulation 102:1463, 2000.
72. de Filippi CR, Rosanio S, Tocchi M, et al: Randomized comparison of a strategy of predischarge coronary angiography versus exercise testing in low-risk patients in a chest pain unit: In-hospital and long-term outcomes. J Am Coll Cardiol 37:2050, 2001.
73. Amsterdam EA, Kirk JD, Diercks DB, et al: Immediate exercise testing to evaluate low-risk patients presenting to the emergency department with chest pain. J Am Coll Cardiol 40:251, 2002.
74. Eagle KA, Berger PB, Calkins H, et al: ACC/AHA guidelines for perioperative cardiovascular evaluation for noncardiac surgery update: Executive summary: A report of the American College of Cardiology/American Heart Association Task Force on Practice Guidelines (Committee to Update the 1996 Guidelines on Perioperative Cardiovascular Evaluation for Noncardiac Surgery). Circulation 105:1257, 2002.
75. Pina IL, Apstein CS, Balady GJ, et al: Exercise and heart failure: A statement from the American Heart Association Committee on Exercise, Rehabilitation, and Prevention. Circulation 107:1210, 2003.
76. O'Neill JO, Young JB, Pothier CE, Lauer MS: Peak oxygen consumption as a predictor of death in patients with heat failure receiving β-blockers. Circulation 111:2313, 2005.
77. Corra U, Mezzani A, Bosimini E, Giannuzzi P: Cardiopulmonary exercise testing and prognosis in chronic heart failure. A prognosticating algorithm for the individual patient. Chest 126:942, 2004.
78. Schalcher C, Rickli H, Brehm M, et al: Prolonged oxygen uptake kinetics during low-intensity exercise are related to poor prognosis in patients with mild-to-moderate congestive heart failure. Chest 124:580, 2003.
79. Mitchell SH, Steele NP, Leclerc KM, et al: Oxygen cost of exercise is increased in heart failure after accounting for recovery costs. Chest 124:572, 2003.
80. Guazzi M, Myers J, Arena R: Cardiopulmonary exercise testing in the clinical and prognostic assessment of diastolic heart failure. J Am Coll Cardiol 46:1883, 2005.
81. Lund LH, Aaronson KD, Mancini DM: Validation of peak exercise oxygen consumption and the heart failure survival score for serial risk stratification in advanced heart failure. Am J Cardiol 95:734, 2005.
82. Roveda F, Middlekauff HR, Rondon MU, et al: The effects of exercise training on sympathetic neural activation in advanced heart failure. J Am Coll Cardiol 42:854, 2003.
83. Rickli H, Kiowski W, Brehm M, et al: Combining low-intensity and maximal exercise test results improves prognostic prediction in chronic heart failure. J Am Coll Cardiol 42:116, 2003.
84. Gielen S, Adams V, Mobius-Winkler S, et al: Anti-inflammatory effects of exercise training in the skeletal muscle of patients with chronic heart failure. J Am Coll Cardiol 42:861, 2003.
85. Myers J: Applications of cardiopulmonary exercise testing in the management of cardiovascular and pulmonary disease. Int J Sports Med 26:S49, 2005.

Arrhythmias and Conduction Disturbances

86. Frolkis JP, Pothier CE, Blackstone EH, Lauer MS: Frequent ventricular ectopy after exercise as a predictor of death. N Engl J Med 348:781, 2003.
87. Morshedi-Meibodi A, Evans JC, Levy D, et al: Clinical correlates and prognostic significance of exercise-induced ventricular premature beats in the community. The Framingham Heart Study. Circulation 109:2417, 2004.
88. Partington S, Myers J, Cho S, et al: Prevalence and prognostic value of exercise-induced ventricular arrhythmias. Am Heart J 145:139, 2003.
89. Takenaka K, Ai T, Shimizu W: Exercise stress test amplifies genotype-phenotype correlation in the LQT1 and LQT2 forms of the long-QT syndrome. Circulation 107:838, 2003.
90. Dillenburg RF, Hamilton RM: Is exercise testing useful in identifying congenital long QT syndrome? Am J Cardiol 89:233, 2002.
91. Bunch TJ, Chandrasekaran K, Gersh BJ, et al: The prognostic significance of exercise-induced atrial arrhythmias. J Am Coll Cardiol 43:1236, 2004.
92. Grady TA, Chiu AC, Snader CE, et al: Prognostic significance of exercise-induced left bundle branch block. JAMA 279:153, 1998.
93. Shah PP, Nair M, Dhall A, et al: False-positive exercise stress electrocardiogram caused by accessory pathway in the absence of manifest preexcitation. Pacing Clin Electrophysiol 23:1051, 2000.
94. Tomczak CR, Wojcik W, Busse EFG, Haennel RG: Phase I and phase II oxygen uptake kinetics during atrioventricular dyssynchrony in chronotropically competent pacemaker patients. Chest 128:1782, 2005.
95. Auricchio A, Kloss M, Trautmann SI, et al: Exercise performance following cardiac resynchronization therapy in patients with heart failure and ventricular conduction delay. Am J Cardiol 89:198, 2002.

Specific Clinical Applications

96. Chaitman BR: Efficacy and safety of a metabolic modulator drug in chronic angina: Review of evidence from clinical trials. J Cardiovasc Pharmacol Therapeut 9:S47, 2004.
97. Bokhari S, Bergmann SR: The effect of estrogen compared to estrogen plus progesterone on the exercise electrocardiogram. J Am Coll Cardiol 40:1092, 2002.
98. Henzlova MJ, Croft LB, Diamond JA: Effect of hormone replacement therapy on the electrocardiographic response to exercise. J Nucl Cardiol 9:385, 2002.
99. Mieres JH, Shaw LJ, Arai A, et al: Role of noninvasive testing in the clinical evaluation of women with suspected coronary artery disease. Consensus Statement from the Cardiac Imaging Committee, Council on Clinical Cardiology, and the Cardiovascular Imaging and Intervention Committee, Council on Cardiovascular Radiology and Intervention, American Heart Association. Circulation 111:682, 2005.

100. Gulati M, Black HR, Shaw LJ, et al: The prognostic value of a nomogram for exercise capacity in women. N Engl J Med 353:468, 2005.
101. Mora S, Redberg RF, Cui Y, et al: Ability of exercise testing to predict cardiovascular and all-cause death in asymptomatic women. A 20-year follow-up of the Lipid Research Clinics Prevalence Study. JAMA 290:1600, 2003.
102. Nasir K, Redberg RF, Budoff MJ, et al: Utility of stress testing and coronary calcification measurement for detection of coronary artery disease in women. Arch Intern Med 164:1610, 2004.
103. Woo JS, Derleth C, Stratton JR, Levy WC: The influence of age, gender, and training on exercise efficiency. J Am Coll Cardiol 47:1049, 2006.
104. Kavanagh T, Mertens DJ, Hamm LF, et al: Peak oxygen intake and cardiac mortality in women referred for cardiac rehabilitation. J Am Coll Cardiol 42:2139, 2003.
105. Singh JP, Larson MG, Manolio TA, et al: Blood pressure response during treadmill testing as a risk factor for new-onset hypertension. The Framingham Study. Circulation 99:1831, 1999.
106. Kokkinos P, Chrysohoou C, Panagiotakos D, et al: Beta-blockade mitigates exercise blood pressure in hypertensive male patients. J Am Coll Cardiol 47:794, 2006.
107. Jeger RV, Zellweger MJ, Kaiser C, et al: Prognostic value of stress testing in patients over 75 years of age with chronic angina. Chest 125:1124, 2004.
108. Goraya TY, Jacobsen SJ, Pellikka PA, et al: Prognostic value of treadmill exercise testing in elderly persons. Ann Intern Med 132:862, 2000.
109. Albers AR, Krichavsky MZ, Balady GJ: Stress testing in patients with diabetes mellitus. Diagnostic and prognostic value. Circulation 113:583, 2006.
110. Bonow RO, Carabello B, Chatterjee K, et al: ACC/AHA 2006 guidelines for the management of patients with valvular heart disease: A report of the American College of Cardiology/American Heart Association Task Force on Practice Guidelines (Committee on Management of Patients with Valvular Heart Disease). J Am Coll Cardiol 48:589, 2006.
111. Lancellotti P, Lebrun F, Pierard LA: Determinants of exercise-induced changes in mitral regurgitation in patients with coronary artery disease and left ventricular dysfunction. J Am Coll Cardiol 42:1921, 2003.
112. Eichinger WB, Botzenhardt F, Keithahn A, et al: Exercise hemodynamics of bovine versus porcine bioprostheses: A prospective randomized comparison of the mosaic and perimount aortic valves. J Thorac Cardiovasc Surg 129:1056, 2005.
113. Ciampi Q, Betocchi S, Lombardi R, et al: Hemodynamic determinants of exercise-induced abnormal blood pressure response in hypertrophic cardiomyopathy. J Am Coll Cardiol 40:278, 2002.
114. Drinko JK, Nash PJ, Lever HM, Asher CR: Safety of stress testing in patients with hypertrophic cardiomyopathy. Am J Cardiol93:1443, 2004.
115. Krone RJ, Hardison RM, Chaitman BR, et al: Risk stratification after successful coronary revascularization: The lack of a role for routine exercise testing. J Am Coll Cardiol 38:136, 2001.
116. Garzon P, Sheppard R, Eisenberg MJ, et al: Comparison of event and procedure rates following percutaneous transluminal coronary angioplasty in patients with and without previous coronary artery bypass graft surgery (the Routine versus Selective Exercise Treadmill Testing after Angioplasty [ROSETTA] Registry). Am J Cardiol 89:251, 2002.
117. Roffi M, Wenaweser P, Windecker S, et al: Early exercise after coronary stenting is safe. J Am Coll Cardiol 42:1569, 2003.
118. Kavanagh T, Mertens DJ, Shephard RJ: Long-term cardiorespiratory results of exercise training following cardiac transplantation. Am J Cardiol 91:190, 2003.
119. Myers J, Geiran O, Simonsen S, et al: Clinical and exercise test determinants of survival after cardiac transplantation. Chest 124:2000, 2003.
120. Ciarka A, Cuylits N, Vachiery JL, et al: Increased peripheral chemoreceptors sensitivity and exercise ventilation in heart transplant recipients. Circulation 113:252, 2006.
121. Diller GP, Dimopoulos K, Okonko D, et al: Exercise intolerance in adult congenital heart disease. Comparative severity, correlates, and prognostic implication. Circulation112:828, 2005.
122. Glaser S, Opitz CF, Bauer U, et al: Assessment of symptoms and exercise capacity in cyanotic patients with congenital heart disease. Chest 125:368, 2004.

Safety and Risks of Exercise Testing

123. Stuart RJ, Ellestad MH: National survey of exercise stress testing facilities. Chest 77:94, 1980.
124. Hamm LF, Crow RS, Stull GA, Hannan P: Safety and characteristics of exercise testing early after acute myocardial infarction. Am J Cardiol 63:1193, 1989.
125. Tristani FE, Hughes CV, Archibald DG, et al: Safety of graded symptom-limited exercise testing in patients with congestive heart failure. Circulation 76:VI54, 1987.
126. Young DZ, Lampert S, Graboys TB, Lown B: Safety of maximal exercise testing in patients at high risk for ventricular arrhythmia. Circulation 70:184, 1984.
127. Beller GA, Bonow RO, Fuster V, et al: ACC revised recommendations for training in adult cardiovascular medicine core cardiology training II (COCATS 2) (Revision of the 1995 COCATS Training Statement). J Am Coll Cardiol 39:1242, 2002.
128. Rodgers GP, Ayanian JZ, Balady G, et al: American College of Cardiology/American Heart Association clinical competence statement on stress testing. A report of the American College of Cardiology/American Heart Association/American College of Physicians-American Society of Internal Medicine Task Force on Clinical Competence. J Am Coll Cardiol 36:1441, 2000.

GUIDELINES *Thomas H. Lee*

Exercise Stress Testing

Several sets of guidelines for the performance of exercise testing have been published by the American Heart Association and by committees commissioned jointly by the American College of Cardiology and the American Heart Association (ACC/AHA).[1-5] Use of exercise testing is addressed in guidelines for specific clinical syndromes, including acute myocardial infarction,[6] chronic stable angina,[7] valvular heart disease,[8] and congestive heart failure.[9] Recommendations for optimal use of treadmill exercise testing are also closely related to guidelines for the use of nuclear cardiology tests for detection of myocardial ischemia.[10]

Standards for Testing and Training

The AHA published standards for performance of exercise testing in 2001,[1] which defined absolute and relative contraindications to exercise testing; these recommendations were slightly modified in ACC/AHA guidelines published in 2002 (Table 13G-1). "Relative" contraindications are those that can be superseded if clinicians believe that the benefits of testing outweigh the risks of exercise. The AHA standards also provide recommendations for specific testing procedures, such as patient instructions for preparation for the procedure. This scientific statement does not offer explicit recommendations on when and whether beta blockers or other drugs (e.g., vasodilators, digitalis, diuretics) should be discontinued before testing.

Indications for termination of exercise testing from this scientific statement were updated in the most recent ACC/AHA guidelines on exercise testing[4] and are summarized in Table 13G-2. Again, relative indications for termination of testing are those that can be superseded when the clinician considers the benefits of continued exercise to exceed the risks.

Exercise testing should be performed under the supervision of a physician, who should be in the vicinity and immediately available during all exercise tests. However, the scientific statement indicates that a properly trained nonphysician (i.e., a nurse, physician assistant, or exercise physiologist or specialist) can perform the direct supervision for healthy younger persons and those with stable chest pain syndromes.[1] An ACC/AHA Clinical Competence Statement on exercise testing published in 2000 has described a "majority opinion" of its authors that supervising physicians should participate in at least 50 exercise test procedures during training and perform at least 25 exercise tests per year.[2] This statement also lists specific skills needed for competent test supervision and interpretation, and recommends that medical centers have a program of quality assurance to ensure systematic review and critique of a significant sample of exercise tests. Because computer processing can lead to an overestimation of ST depression, ACC/AHA guidelines recommend that the interpreting physician always be supplied with raw electrocardiographic tracings in addition to any computerized summaries.[4]

Clinical Indications for Exercise Testing

Guidelines published by the ACC/AHA in 1997[3] and updated in 2002[4] have assessed the appropriateness of exercise testing in specific clinical settings. The complete guidelines are available (www.americanheart.

TABLE 13G–1 ACC/AHA Guidelines: Absolute and Relative Contraindications to Exercise Testing

Absolute
Acute myocardial infarction (within 2 days)
High-risk unstable angina
Uncontrolled cardiac arrhythmias causing symptoms or hemodynamic compromise
Symptomatic severe aortic stenosis
Uncontrolled symptomatic heart failure
Acute pulmonary embolus or pulmonary infarction
Acute myocarditis or pericarditis
Acute aortic dissection
Relative
Left main coronary stenosis
Moderate stenotic valvular heart disease
Electrolyte abnormalities
Severe arterial hypertension (suggested definition—systolic blood pressure >200 mm Hg and/or diastolic blood pressure >100 mm Hg)
Tachyarrhythmias or bradyarrhythmias
Hypertrophic cardiomyopathy and other forms of outflow tract obstruction
Mental or physical impairment leading to inability to exercise adequately
High-degree atrioventricular block

ACC/AHA = American College of Cardiology/American Heart Association.

From Gibbons RJ, Balady GJ, Bricker JT, et al: ACC/AHA 2002 guideline update for exercise testing: Summary article. A report of the ACC/AHA Task Force on Practice Guidelines (Committee to Update the 1997 Exercise Testing Guidelines). Circulation 106:1883, 2002.

TABLE 13G–2 ACC/AHA Guidelines: Indications for Terminating Exercise Testing

Absolute
Drop in systolic blood pressure >10 mm Hg from baseline blood pressure despite an increase in workload, when accompanied by other evidence of ischemia
Moderate to severe angina
Increasing nervous system symptoms (e.g., ataxia, dizziness, or near-syncope)
Signs of poor perfusion (cyanosis or pallor)
Technical difficulties in monitoring electrocardiogram or systolic blood pressure
Subject's desire to stop
Sustained ventricular tachycardia
ST elevation (≥1.0 mm) in leads without diagnostic Q waves (other than V_1 or aVR)
Relative
Drop in systolic blood pressure >10 mm Hg from baseline blood pressure despite an increase in workload, in the absence of other evidence of ischemia
ST or QRS changes, such as excessive ST depression (>2 mm of horizontal or downsloping ST segment depression) or marked axis shift
Arrhythmias other than sustained ventricular tachycardia, including multifocal PVCs, triplets of PVCs, supraventricular tachycardia, heart block, or bradyarrhythmias
Fatigue, shortness of breath, wheezing, leg cramps, or claudication
Development of bundle-branch block or IVCD that cannot be distinguished from ventricular tachycardia
Increasing chest pain
Hypertensive response (suggested definition—systolic blood pressure >250 mm Hg and/or a diastolic blood pressure >115 mm Hg)

ACC/AHA = American College of Cardiology/American Heart Association; IVCD = intraventricular conduction delay; PVCs = premature ventricular contractions.

From Gibbons RJ, Balady GJ, Bricker JT, et al: ACC/AHA 2002 guideline update for exercise testing: Summary article. A report of the ACC/AHA Task Force on Practice Guidelines (Committee to Update the 1997 Exercise Testing Guidelines). Circulation 106:1883, 2002.

org or www.acc.org). As with other ACC/AHA guidelines, these recommendations have classified indications into one of three classes, including two levels of the intermediate group, as follows:

Class I: Conditions for which there is evidence and/or general agreement that exercise testing is useful and effective.

Class II: Conditions for which there is conflicting evidence and/or a divergence of opinion about the usefulness or efficacy of performing exercise testing.

Class IIa: Weight of evidence or opinion is in favor of usefulness or efficacy.

Class IIb: Usefulness or efficacy is less well established by evidence or opinion.

Class III: Conditions for which there is evidence and/or general agreement that exercise testing is not useful or effective and in some cases may be harmful.

Diagnosis of Obstructive Coronary Artery Disease

When the clinical question is whether obstructive coronary disease is present or absent in a patient (i.e., diagnosis), the ACC/AHA guidelines consider exercise testing most appropriate for patients with an "intermediate" pretest probability of coronary artery disease, such as patients with atypical or probable angina or younger patients with typical angina. Definitions of pretest risk status according to age, gender, and symptoms are summarized in Table 13G-3. Patients with high or low pretest probability of coronary disease are less likely to have their management altered by exercise testing; therefore, exercise testing is not strongly supported by these guidelines in these populations (Table 13G-4). Exercise electrocardiography is considered appropriate in patients with complete right bundle branch block and less than 1 mm of resting ST depression, but not in patients with electrocardiographic patterns more likely to lead to uninterpretable tracings. The 2002 ACC/AHA guidelines have lowered the threshold for using an imaging technology in patients with minor ST depression. The prior ACC/AHA guidelines considered exercise electrocardiography "the first test option" in such patients,[3] whereas the 2002 update has changed this phrase to "a reasonable first test option."

Risk Assessment and Prognosis in Patients with Coronary Disease

The ACC/AHA guidelines emphasize that exercise testing should be used to improve risk stratification as part of a process that begins with assessment of routinely available data from the clinical examination and other laboratory tests. The decision of whether to order an exercise test should reflect the chances that test results might alter management, and the interpretation of the results should be considered in the context of the patient's overall clinical status.

The recommendations endorse routine use of exercise testing for risk stratification of patients with suspected or known coronary disease (Table 13G-5), whether stable or after a change in clinical status. The guidelines emphasize the importance of consideration of multiple types of data from the exercise test (e.g., exercise duration) and encourage use of tools such as the Duke Treadmill Score[11] to integrate these data into a risk prediction.

For patients with unstable angina, the guidelines support exercise testing early (8 to 12 hours) after presentation in patients with a low clinical risk of complications (Table 13G-6) if they have been free of active ischemic or heart failure symptoms. A longer delay (2 to 3 days) is recommended for patients with an intermediate risk of complications, although the guidelines indicate that there is good supportive evidence for earlier exercise testing as part of chest pain management protocols for stable patients from this population if there is no evidence of active ischemia (class IIA indication). More detailed recommendations on exercise testing in chest pain centers have been provided

TABLE 13G–3 Pretest Probability of Coronary Artery Disease by Age, Gender and Symptoms

Age (yr)	Gender	Typical or Definite Angina Pectoris	Atypical or Probable Angina Pectoris	Nonanginal Chest Pain	Asymptomatic
30-39	Men	Intermediate	Intermediate	Low	Very low
	Women	Intermediate	Very low	Very low	Very low
40-49	Men	High	Intermediate	Intermediate	Low
	Women	Intermediate	Low	Very low	Very low
50-59	Men	High	Intermediate	Intermediate	Low
	Women	Intermediate	Intermediate	Low	Very low
60-69	Men	High	Intermediate	Intermediate	Low
	Women	High	Intermediate	Intermediate	Low

ACC/AHA = American College of Cardiology/American Heart Association.

From Gibbons RJ, Balady GJ, Bricker JT, et al: ACC/AHA 2002 guideline update for exercise testing: Summary article. A report of the ACC/AHA Task Force on Practice Guidelines (Committee to Update the 1997 Exercise Testing Guidelines). Circulation 106:1883, 2002.

TABLE 13G–4 ACC/AHA Guidelines for Exercise Testing to Diagnose Obstructive Coronary Artery Disease

Class	Indication
I (indicated)	Adult patients (including those with complete right bundle branch block or less than 1 mm of resting ST depression) with an intermediate pretest probability of CAD on the basis of gender, age, and symptoms (specific exceptions are noted under classes II and III, below)
IIA (good supportive evidence)	Patients with vasospastic angina
IIB (weak supportive evidence)	1. Patients with a high pretest probability of CAD by age, symptoms, and gender 2. Patients with a low pretest probability of CAD by age, symptoms, and gender 3. Patients with less than 1 mm of baseline ST depression and taking digoxin 4. Patients with electrocardiographic criteria for left ventricular hypertrophy and less than 1 mm of baseline ST depression
III (not indicated)	1. Patients with the following baseline ECG abnormalities: • Preexcitation (Wolff-Parkinson-White) syndrome • Electronically paced ventricular rhythm • More than 1 mm of resting ST depression • Complete left bundle branch block 2. Patients with a documented myocardial infarction or prior coronary angiography demonstrating significant disease who have an established diagnosis of CAD; however, ischemia and risk can be determined by testing.

ACC/AHA = American College of Cardiology/American Heart Association; CAD = coronary artery disease.

From Gibbons RJ, Balady GJ, Bricker JT, et al: ACC/AHA 2002 guideline update for exercise testing: Summary article. A report of the ACC/AHA Task Force on Practice Guidelines (Committee to Update the 1997 Exercise Testing Guidelines). Circulation 106:1883, 2002.

TABLE 13G–5 ACC/AHA Guidelines: Risk Assessment and Prognosis in Patients with Symptoms or a Prior History of Coronary Artery Disease

Class	Indication
I (indicated)	1. Patients undergoing initial evaluation with suspected or known CAD, including those with complete right bundle (indicated) branch block or less than 1 mm of resting ST depression (specific exceptions noted below in class IIB) 2. Patients with suspected or known CAD, previously evaluated, now presenting with significant change in clinical status 3. Low-risk unstable angina patients 8 to 12 hours after presentation who have been free of active ischemic or heart failure symptoms 4. Intermediate-risk unstable angina patients 2 to 3 days after presentation who have been free of active ischemic or heart failure symptoms
IIA (good supportive evidence)	Intermediate-risk unstable angina patients who have initial cardiac markers that are normal, a repeat ECG without significant change, and cardiac markers 6 to 12 hours after the onset of symptoms that are normal and no other evidence of ischemia during observation
IIB (weak supportive evidence)	1. Patients with the following resting ECG abnormalities: • Preexcitation (Wolff-Parkinson-White) syndrome • Electronically paced ventricular rhythm • 1 mm or more of resting ST depression • Complete left bundle branch block or any interventricular conduction defect with a QRS duration longer than 120 msec 2. Patients with a stable clinical course who undergo periodic monitoring to guide treatment.
III (not indicated)	1. Patients with severe comorbidity likely to limit life expectancy and/or candidacy for revascularization 2. High-risk unstable angina patients

ACC/AHA = American College of Cardiology/American Heart Association; CAD = coronary artery disease; ECG = electrocardiogram.

From Gibbons RJ, Balady GJ, Bricker JT, et al: ACC/AHA 2002 guideline update for exercise testing: Summary article. A report of the ACC/AHA Task Force on Practice Guidelines (Committee to Update the 1997 Exercise Testing Guidelines). Circulation 106:1883, 2002.

in a Science Advisory Statement from the American Heart Association in 2000.[5]

The guidelines discourage exercise testing for patients in whom the procedure would be dangerous (e.g., high-risk unstable angina patients), unlikely to add accurate information (e.g., patients with certain resting electrocardiogram [ECG] abnormalities), or unlikely to change management (e.g., patients with stable clinical courses or who were poor candidates for revascularization; see Table 13G-5).

After Acute Myocardial Infarction

Recommendations for the use of exercise testing after acute myocardial infarction (Table 13G-7) reflect an overall strategy for risk stratification and management described in the ACC/AHA guidelines on acute myocardial infarction.[6] In this approach (Fig. 13G-1), if the

TABLE 13G–6 ACC/AHA Classification System for Risk of Death or Nonfatal Myocardial Infarction in Patients with Unstable Angina

Feature	High Risk (at least one of the following features must be present)	Intermediate Risk (no high-risk feature but must have one of the following features)	Low Risk (no high-or intermediate-risk features, but may have any of the following features)
History		Prior MI, peripheral or cerebrovascular disease, or CABG, prior aspirin use	
Character of pain	Prolonged ongoing (>20 min) pain at rest	Prolonged (>20 min) resting angina, now resolved, with moderate or high likelihood of CAD Rest angina (<20 min) or relieved with rest or sublingual NTG	New-onset or progressive CCSC III or IV angina in the past 2 wk with moderate or high likelihood of CAD
Clinical findings	Pulmonary edema, most likely related to ischemia New or worsening MR murmur S_3 or new or worsening rales Hypotension, bradycardia, tachycardia Age older than 75 yr	Age older than 70 yr	
ECG findings	Angina at rest with transient ST changes ≥0.05 mV BBB, new or presumed new or sustained ventricular tachycardia	T-wave inversions greater than 0.2 mV, pathological Q waves	Normal or unchanged ECG during an episode of chest discomfort
Biochemical cardiac markers	Elevated (e.g., troponin T or T_1 level higher than 0.1 mg/ml)	Slightly elevated (e.g., troponin T > 0.01 but <0.1 mg/ml)	Normal

ACC/AHA = American College of Cardiology/American Heart Association; BBB = bundle branch block; CABG = coronary artery bypass graft; CAD = coronary artery disease; CCSC = Canadian Cardiovascular Society; ECG = electrocardiogram; MI = myocardial infarction; MR = mitral regurgitation; NTG = nitroglycerin.

From Gibbons RJ, Balady GJ, Bricker JT, et al: ACC/AHA 2002 guideline update for exercise testing: Summary article. A report of the ACC/AHA Task Force on Practice Guidelines (Committee to Update the 1997 Exercise Testing Guidelines). Circulation 106:1883, 2002.

TABLE 13G–7 ACC/AHA Guidelines for Exercise Testing after Acute Myocardial Infarction

Class	Indication
I (indicated)	1. Before discharge for prognostic assessment, activity prescription, evaluation of medical therapy (submaximal at about 4 to 76 days)* 2. Early after discharge for prognostic assessment, activity prescription, evaluation of medical therapy, and cardiac rehabilitation if the predischarge exercise test was not done (symptom-limited; about 14 to 21 days)* 3. Late after discharge for prognostic assessment, activity prescription, evaluation of medical therapy, and cardiac rehabilitation if the early exercise test was submaximal (symptom-limited; about 3 to 6 weeks)*
IIA (good supportive evidence)	After discharge for activity counseling and/or exercise training as part of cardiac rehabilitation in patients who have undergone coronary revascularization
IIB (weak supportive evidence)	1. Patients with the following electrocardiographic abnormalities: • Complete left bundle-branch block • Preexcitation syndrome • Left ventricular hypertrophy • Digoxin therapy • Greater than 1 mm of resting ST segment depression • Electronically paced ventricular rhythm 2. Periodic monitoring in patients who continue to participate in exercise training or cardiac rehabilitation
III (not indicated)	1. Severe comorbidity likely to limit life expectancy and/or candidacy for revascularization 2. At any time to evaluate patients with acute myocardial infarction who have uncompensated congestive heart failure, cardiac arrhythmia, or noncardiac conditions that severely limit their ability to exercise 3. Before discharge to evaluate patients who have already been selected for, or have undergone, cardiac catheterization; although stress test may be useful before or after catheterization to evaluate or identify ischemia in the distribution of a coronary lesion of borderline severity, stress imaging tests are recommended

*Exceptions are noted under classes IIB and III.

ACC/AHA = American College of Cardiology/American Heart Association.

From Ryan TJ, Antman EM, Brooks NH, et al: ACC/AHA guidelines for the management of patients with acute myocardial infarction: 1999 update. A report of the American College of Cardiology/American Heart Association Task Force on Practice Guidelines (Committee on Management of Acute Myocardial Infarction) (http://www.acc.org).

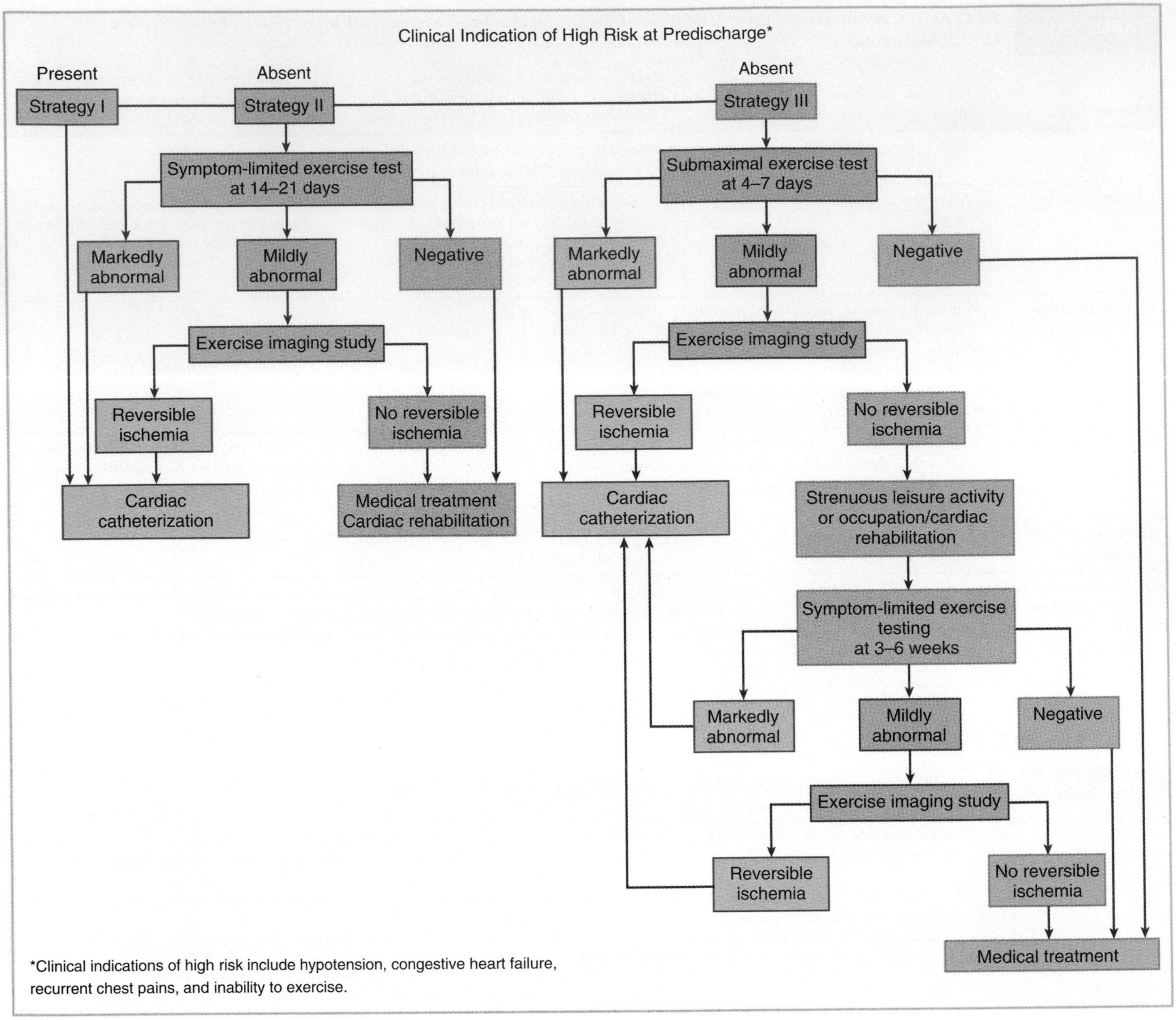

FIGURE 13G–1 Strategies for exercise test evaluation soon after myocardial infarction.

patient's clinical data suggest a high risk for complications, the patient should undergo invasive evaluation to determine whether he or she is a candidate for coronary revascularization procedures (strategy I). For patients with apparently low risk for complications, two strategies for performing exercise testing are endorsed. One uses a symptom-limited exercise test at 14 to 21 days (strategy II). An alternative strategy for low-risk patients (strategy III) is to perform a submaximal exercise test at 4 to 7 days after myocardial infarction or just before hospital discharge. If the exercise test result is negative, a second symptom-limited exercise test can be repeated at 3 to 6 weeks for patients undergoing vigorous activity during leisure time activities, at work, or exercise training as part of cardiac rehabilitation. Exercise imaging tests are reserved for patients with equivocal exercise electrocardiography tests or those with electrocardiographic findings that preclude interpretation of ST changes. The extent of ischemia on noninvasive studies helps determine whether patients should undergo cardiac catheterization.

Exercise Testing with Ventilatory Gas Analysis

Although measurement of maximal oxygen uptake is the best index of aerobic capacity, the ACC/AHA guidelines do not support ventilatory gas analysis as part of routine exercise testing or for routine measurement of exercise capacity (Table 13G-8). Ventilatory gas analysis is recommended when it is most likely to change management, such as in patients being considered for transplantation or those in whom clinical differentiation between pulmonary and cardiac causes of exercise limitation is difficult. Some support is provided for ventilatory gas exchange for patients in whom estimates of exercise capacity from other sources (e.g., exercise test time) are unreliable, but the guidelines discourage use of this technology for assessment of response to therapy or as a routine part of cardiac rehabilitation.

TABLE 13G-8 ACC/AHA Guidelines for Exercise Testing with Ventilatory Gas Analysis

Class	Indication
I (indicated)	1. Evaluation of exercise capacity and response to therapy in patients with heart failure who are being considered for heart transplantation 2. Assistance in the differentiation of cardiac versus pulmonary limitations as a cause of exercise-induced dyspnea or impaired exercise capacity when the cause is uncertain
IIA (good supportive evidence)	Evaluation of exercise capacity when indicated for medical reasons in patients in whom the estimates of exercise capacity from exercise test time or work rate are unreliable
IIB (weak supportive evidence)	1. Evaluation of the patient's response to specific therapeutic interventions in which improvement of exercise tolerance is an important goal or endpoint 2. Determination of the intensity for exercise training as part of comprehensive cardiac rehabilitation
III (not indicated)	Routine use to evaluate exercise capacity

ACC/AHA = American College of Cardiology/American Heart Association.
From Gibbons RJ, Balady GJ, Bricker JT, et al: ACC/AHA 2002 guideline update for exercise testing: Summary article. A report of the ACC/AHA Task Force on Practice Guidelines (Committee to Update the 1997 Exercise Testing Guidelines). Circulation 106:1883, 2002.

Special Populations

Exercise electrocardiography has poorer overall test performance in women compared with men, but the ACC/AHA guidelines recommend that exercise electrocardiography be the first-choice noninvasive test for coronary disease in women.[4] This recommendation reflects the fact that stress imaging technologies also have poorer sensitivity and higher false-positive rates in women, leading to the conclusion that there is insufficient evidence to recommend them as the initial diagnostic test in women.

The ACC/AHA guidelines discourage routine exercise testing for asymptomatic persons without known coronary artery disease (Table 13G-9) and conclude that only weak evidence is available to support its appropriateness for asymptomatic patients with multiple risk factors or patients about to embark on an exercise program. The guidelines are more supportive of exercise testing of patients with diabetes who are about to start vigorous exercise programs because of the high risk for atherosclerotic disease in this population.

Exercise testing is useful for assessing functional capacity in patients with valvular heart disease, particularly patients with regurgitant lesions (Table 13G-10). The guidelines note that exercise testing is usually not needed for symptomatic patients with stenotic valvular heart disease, and that severe aortic stenosis is classically considered to be a contraindication to exercise testing. However, the guidelines acknowledge that there are subsets of asymptomatic patients with stenotic valvular lesions in whom exercise testing may help assess functional capacity, such as determination of whether they are actually asymptomatic.

The ACC/AHA guidelines support the use of exercise testing as part of the evaluation of patients before revascularization with a coronary artery bypass graft (CABG) or percutaneous coronary interventions and for evaluation of recurrent symptoms or part of the rehabilitation process. However, the guidelines do not support routine periodic exercise testing of asymptomatic patients after revascularization (Table 13G-11).

The guidelines endorse exercise testing for patients with heart rhythm disorders when the test is intended to diagnose exercise-induced arrhythmias or evaluate therapy (e.g., settings for rate-adaptive pacemakers, or impact of therapy for patients with exercise-induced arrhythmias). However, there is little support for

TABLE 13G-9 ACC/AHA Guidelines for Exercise Testing in Asymptomatic Persons without Known Coronary Artery Disease (CAD)

Class	Indication
I (indicated)	None
IIA (good supportive evidence)	Evaluation of asymptomatic persons with diabetes mellitus who plan to start vigorous exercise
IIB (weak supportive evidence)	1. Evaluation of persons with multiple risk factors as a guide to risk reduction therapy* 2. Evaluation of asymptomatic men older than 45 yr and women older than 55 yr: • Who plan to start vigorous exercise (especially if sedentary) *or* • Who are involved in occupations in which impairment might impact public safety *or* • Who are at high risk for CAD because of other diseases (e.g., peripheral vascular disease and chronic renal failure)
III (not indicated)	Routine screening of asymptomatic men or women

*Multiple risk factors are defined as hypercholesterolemia (>240 mg/dl), hypertension (systolic blood pressure >140 mm Hg or diastolic blood pressure >90 mm Hg), smoking, diabetes, and family history of heart attack or sudden cardiac death in a first-degree relative younger than 60 years. An alternative approach might be to select patients with a Framingham Risk Score consistent with at least a moderate risk of serious cardiac events within 5 years.
ACC/AHA = American College of Cardiology/American Heart Association.
From Gibbons RJ, Balady GJ, Bricker JT, et al: ACC/AHA 2002 guideline update for exercise testing: Summary article. A report of the ACC/AHA Task Force on Practice Guidelines (Committee to Update the 1997 Exercise Testing Guidelines). Circulation 106:1883, 2002.

TABLE 13G-10 ACC/AHA Guidelines for Exercise Testing in Patients with Valvular Heart Disease

Class	Indication
I (indicated)	In chronic aortic regurgitation, assessment of functional capacity and symptomatic responses in patients with a history of equivocal symptoms
IIA (good supportive evidence)	1. In chronic aortic regurgitation, evaluation of symptoms and functional capacity before participation in athletic activities 2. In chronic aortic regurgitation, prognostic assessment before aortic valve replacement in asymptomatic or minimally symptomatic patients with left ventricular dysfunction
IIB (weak supportive evidence)	Evaluation of exercise capacity in patients with valvular heart disease
III (not indicated)	Diagnosis of coronary artery disease in patients with moderate to severe valvular disease or with the following baseline electrocardiographic abnormalities: • Preexcitation • Electronically paced ventricular rhythm • More than 1-mm ST depression • Complete left bundle branch block

ACC/AHA = American College of Cardiology/American Heart Association.
From Gibbons RJ, Balady GJ, Bricker JT, et al: ACC/AHA 2002 guideline update for exercise testing: Summary article. A report of the ACC/AHA Task Force on Practice Guidelines (Committee to Update the 1997 Exercise Testing Guidelines). Circulation 106:1883, 2002.

TABLE 13G–11 ACC/AHA Guidelines for Exercise Testing Before and After Revascularization

Class	Indication
I (indicated)	1. Demonstration of ischemia before revascularization 2. Evaluation of patients with recurrent symptoms that suggest ischemia after revascularization
IIA (good supportive evidence)	After discharge for activity counseling and/or exercise training as part of cardiac rehabilitation in patients who have undergone coronary revascularization
IIB (weak supportive evidence)	1. Detection of restenosis in selected, high-risk asymptomatic patients within the first 12 months after percutaneous coronary intervention 2. Periodic monitoring of selected, high-risk asymptomatic patients for restenosis, graft occlusion, incomplete coronary revascularization, or disease progression
III (not indicated)	1. Localization of ischemia for determining the site of intervention 2. Routine periodic monitoring of asymptomatic patients after percutaneous coronary intervention or coronary artery bypass grafting without specific indications

ACC/AHA = American College of Cardiology/American Heart Association.

From Gibbons RJ, Balady GJ, Bricker JT, et al: ACC/AHA 2002 guideline update for exercise testing: Summary article. A report of the ACC/AHA Task Force on Practice Guidelines (Committee to Update the 1997 Exercise Testing Guidelines). Circulation 106:1883, 2002.

TABLE 13G–12 ACC/AHA Guidelines for Exercise Testing for Investigation of Heart Rhythm Disorders

Class	Indication
I (indicated)	1. Identification of appropriate settings in patients with rate-adaptive pacemakers 2. Evaluation of congenital complete heart block in patients considering increased physical activity or participation in competitive sports
IIA (good supportive evidence)	1. Evaluation of patients with known or suspected exercise-induced arrhythmias 2. Evaluation of medical, surgical, or ablative therapy in patients with exercise-induced arrhythmias (including atrial fibrillation)
IIB (weak supportive evidence)	1. Investigation of isolated ventricular ectopic beats in middle-aged patients without other evidence of coronary artery disease 2. Investigation of prolonged first-degree atrioventricular block or type I second-degree Wenckebach block, left bundle branch block, right bundle branch block, or isolated ectopic beats in young patients considering participation in competitive sports
III (not indicated)	Routine investigation of isolated ectopic beats in young patients

ACC/AHA = American College of Cardiology/American Heart Association.

From Gibbons RJ, Balady GJ, Bricker JT, et al: ACC/AHA 2002 guideline update for exercise testing: Summary article. A report of the ACC/AHA Task Force on Practice Guidelines (Committee to Update the 1997 Exercise Testing Guidelines). Circulation 106:1883, 2002.

exercise testing for heart rhythm abnormalities that, in isolation, are not associated with a higher risk of cardiovascular complications, such as isolated ventricular or atrial premature beats (Table 13G-12).

References

1. Fletcher GF, Balady GJ, Amsterdam EA, et al: Exercise standards for testing and training: A statement for healthcare professionals from the American Heart Association. Circulation 104:1694, 2001.
2. Rodgers GP, Ayanian JZ, Balady G, et al: American College of Cardiology/American Heart Association clinical competence statement on stress testing. Circulation 102:1726, 2000.
3. Gibbons RJ, Balady GJ, Beasley JW, et al: ACC/AHA guidelines for exercise testing: A report of the American College of Cardiology/American Heart Association Task Force on Practice Guidelines (Committee on Exercise Testing). J Am Coll Cardiol 30:260, 1997.
4. Gibbons RJ, Balady GJ, Bricker JT, et al: ACC/AHA 2002 guideline update for exercise testing: Summary article. A report of the ACC/AHA Task Force on Practice Guidelines (Committee to Update the 1997 Exercise Testing Guidelines). Circulation 106:1883, 2002.
5. Stein RA, Chaitman BR, Balady GJ, et al: Safety and utility of exercise testing in emergency room chest pain centers. An advisory from the Committee on Exercise, Rehabilitation, and Prevention, Council on Clinical Cardiology, American Heart Association. Circulation 102:1463, 2000.
6. Ryan TJ, Antman EM, Brooks NH, et al: ACC/AHA guidelines for the management of patients with acute myocardial infarction: 1999 update. A report of the American College of Cardiology/American Heart Association Task Force on Practice Guidelines (Committee on Management of Acute Myocardial Infarction) (http://www.acc.org).
7. Gibbons RJ, Abrams J, Chatterjee K, et al: ACC/AHA 2002 guideline update for the management of patients with chronic stable angina: Summary article. A report of the American College of Cardiology/American Heart Association Task Force on Practice Guidelines (Committee on the Management of Patents With Chronic Stable Angina). Circulation 107:149, 2003.
8. Bonow RO, Carabello B, de Leon AC Jr, et al: ACC/AHA guidelines for the management of patients with valvular heart disease: Executive summary. A report of the American College of Cardiology/American Heart Association Task Force on Practice Guidelines (Committee on Management of Patients With Valvular Heart Disease). Circulation 98:1949, 1998.
9. Hunt SA, Baker DW, Chin MH, et al: ACC/AHA guidelines for the evaluation and management of chronic heart failure in the adult: A report of the American College of Cardiology/American Heart Association Task Force on Practice Guidelines (Committee to Revise the 1995 Guidelines for the Evaluation and Management of Heart Failure), 2001 (http://www.acc.org/clinical/guidelines/failure/hf_ index.htm).
10. Ritchie JL, Bateman TM, Bonow RO, et al: Guidelines for clinical use of cardiac radionuclide imaging. Report of the American College of Cardiology/American Heart Association Task Force on Assessment of Diagnostic and Therapeutic Cardiovascular Procedures (Committee on Radionuclide Imaging), developed in collaboration with the American Society of Nuclear Cardiology. J Am Coll Cardiol 25:521, 1995.
11. Mark DB, Shaw L, Harrell FE Jr, et al: Prognostic value of a treadmill exercise score in outpatients with suspected coronary artery disease. N Engl J Med 325:849, 1991.

CHAPTER 14

Echocardiography*

Heidi M. Connolly and Jae K. Oh

INTRODUCTION

Echocardiography is the most frequently used—and usually an initial—cardiac imaging test to evaluate all cardiovascular diseases related to a structural, functional, or hemodynamic abnormality of the heart or great vessels. Echocardiography began as a technique to display normal and abnormal structures in A (amplitude)-mode and M (motion)-mode. Ultrasound beams reflected by cardiovascular structures produce characteristic lines or shapes caused by normal or altered cardiac anatomy (Fig. 14-1). Subsequent advances in two-dimensional (2D) echocardiography have allowed visualization of cardiac structures in real time from multiple tomographic planes, and Doppler and color flow imaging have allowed a reliable assessment of cardiac hemodynamics and blood flow.[1] The creation of contrast agents that pass through the pulmonary circulation after intravenous administration has improved delineation of structures on the left side of the heart and made real-time myocardial perfusion imaging a clinical reality. Transesophageal echocardiography (TEE) has markedly improved resolution of 2D echocardiographic images, and tissue Doppler imaging (TDI) has enhanced the ability to assess systolic and diastolic function. Improvement in ultrasound transducer technology created the harmonic transducer, allowing real-time three-dimensional (3D) echocardiography.[2]

Reliable noninvasive hemodynamic evaluation and confident delineation of cardiovascular structures by echocardiography have markedly reduced the clinical necessity for hemodynamic cardiac catheterization. Increasingly, patients undergo valvular or congenital heart surgery on the basis of an echocardiographic diagnosis (see Chaps. 61 and 62). Echocardiographic units are also being miniaturized to become an extension of a clinician's physical examination. In our opinion, the appreciation of cardiac anatomy and hemodynamics by bedside echocardiography makes a physician's clinical evaluation, including physical examination, more relevant for the care of patients. For all physicians who care for patients with a cardiovascular problem, it is essential to know how echocardiographic images are obtained, what type of information echocardiography can provide, and how it should be used for patient management. Our intent is not to teach readers how to perform echocardiography but how to recognize abnormal cardiac structures, to evaluate cardiac function, to assess hemodynamics echocardiographically, and how to use echocardiographic information in clinical practice. This chapter first describes various echocardiographic modalities followed by specific diagnostic echocardiographic features and their clinical implications. The latter part of the chapter is best used in conjunction with other chapters in this book that describe the relevant clinical features of the same conditions.

M-MODE AND 2D/3D TRANSTHORACIC ECHOCARDIOGRAPHY

An echocardiographic examination begins with real-time 2D echocardiography, which produces high-resolution images of cardiac structures and their movements. These images are usually obtained from four standard transducer locations—parasternal, apical, subcostal, and suprasternal (Fig. 14-2A)—by manually rotating and angulating the transducer (Fig. 14-2B and C). Qualitative and quantitative measurements of cardiac dimensions, area, and volume are derived from 2D images or 2D-derived M-mode recordings.[3] Also, 2D echocardiography provides the framework for Doppler examination and color flow imaging. Newer matrix transducers with more than 3000 elements allow 3D or multidimensional images of the heart (Figs. 14-3 to 14-5). Different tomographic images can be obtained or derived from a full-volume 3D echocardiographic image. This shortens the examination time and minimizes variation in acquisition of cardiovascular images. With advances and clinical experience in 3D and multidimensional echocardiographic imaging, visualization and quantitation of cardiovascular structure, function, and hemodynamics will improve.

An M-mode recording is derived from 2D tomographic images and graphically represents the motion of cardiac structures. It is used primarily to measure cardiac chamber size and timing of cardiac events and to display subtle abnormalities of cardiac motion. Thus it is important to recognize the characteristic M-mode features to understand the pathophysiological mechanisms of cardiovascular disorders.

Measurement of cardiac dimensions from M-mode echocardiography has been standardized (Fig. 14-6). For these mea-

*Figures used with permission of Mayo Clinic.

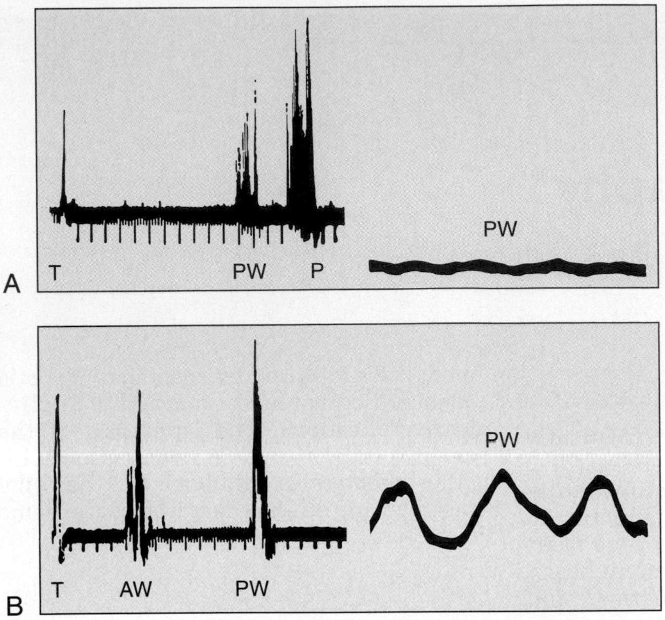

FIGURE 14–1 A-mode ultrasound recordings from a patient with cardiac tamponade and cardiomegaly seen on chest x-ray. **A,** Initial ultrasound recording showing two distinct signals in the vicinity of the posterior wall (PW). Signal to the right (P) failed to move with cardiac systole, and the signal on the left (PW) barely moved with cardiac motion (seen on the right). **B,** After surgical removal of the pericardium and 1 liter of pericardial fluid, the ultrasound examination showed only one signal in the vicinity of the posterior wall. This signal moved normally and was identified to originate from the unrestricted posterior wall of the heart. AW = anterior wall; T = transducer. *(From Feigenbaum H, Waldenhausen JA, Hyde LP: Ultrasound diagnosis of pericardial effusion. JAMA 191:711, 1965. Used with permission.)*

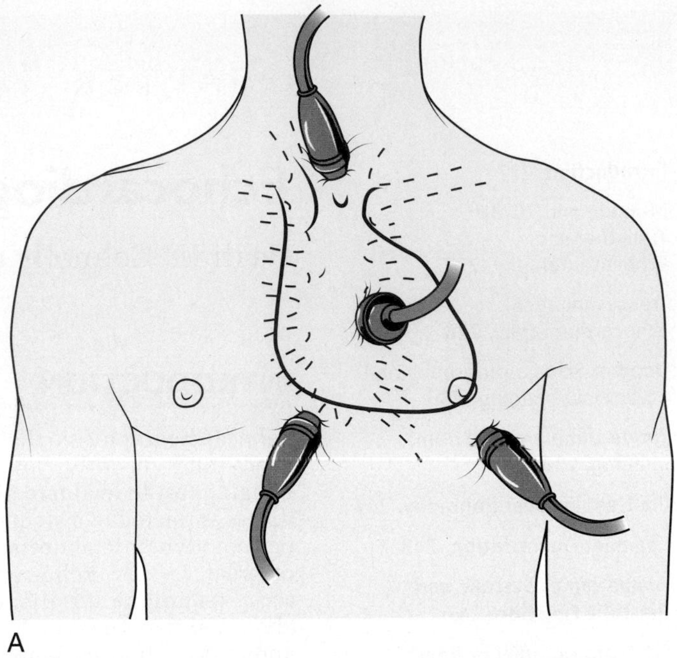

FIGURE 14–2 **A,** Four standard transducer positions: parasternal, apical, subcostal, and suprasternal, used to visualize the heart and great vessels.

surements, an M-mode cursor is drawn as a straight line from the transducer position in any direction in the sector to record the movement of the cardiac structure of interest. However, this traditional method of M-mode may overestimate the dimensions of the structure if the direction of the ultrasound beam is oblique to that structure. Anatomical M-mode allows the M-mode cursor to be positioned in any direction from anywhere in the heart; this allows a more reliable recording of cardiac structures. Figure 14-7 demonstrates the dynamic changes of cardiac structures documented with M-mode, 2D, and 3D echocardiography.

TRANSESOPHAGEAL ECHOCARDIOGRAPHY

With the proximity of the major cardiovascular structures (heart, aorta, and pulmonary arteries) to the esophagus, TEE provides excellent evaluation of cardiovascular anatomy, function, hemodynamics, and blood flow.

TEE is now considered essential in the evaluation of mitral valve lesions, the left atrium (LA) or LA appendage, an intracardiac mass, atrial septal defect, endocarditis and its complications, and thoracic aortic lesions such as aortic dissection (see Chaps. 56, 62, 63, 69).[4] Patients with atrial fibrillation undergo direct-current cardioversion without chronic anticoagulation if TEE does not show intracardiac thrombus, and with ablation procedures, atrial fibrillation has become one of the most common reasons for referral for TEE.[5] Another routine clinical use of TEE is in the operating room to assess the result of various valvular and repair procedures. During the 20-year clinical experience with TEE, it has been a low-risk procedure, with a complication rate less than 0.1 percent when transthoracic echocardiography is not diagnostic.[6]

The TEE probe is equipped with a multiplane transducer that rotates in a 180-degree arc, which produces a continuum of transverse and longitudinal image planes. These TEE images are identified by an icon that indicates the degree of transducer rotation (Fig. 14-8). The transverse plane, in the short axis of the body, is designated as 0 degree, and the longitudinal plane, in the long axis of the body, is designated as 90 degrees. Normally, from the midesophagus (35 to 40 cm from the teeth), the short axis of the heart is imaged at 45 to 60 degrees of rotation and the long axis at 120 to 135 degrees.

TEE tomographic views can be displayed similarly to those of TTE with the electronic transducer being at the bottom or, for the opposite orientation, with the transducer at the top of the screen (Fig. 14-9).

Primary Views

Four primary TEE views are obtained by rotating the transducer array from 0 to 135 degrees (see Fig. 14-9): (1) 0-degree (transverse plane)—the four-chamber view or an oblique view of the basal structures is obtained from this position; (2) 45 to 60 degrees—short-axis view of the aortic valve; this image is similar to the transthoracic parasternal short-axis view at the level of the aortic valve; (3) 75 to 90 degrees—longitudinal transducer orientation; this produces images oblique to the long axis of the heart; and (4) 120 to 135 degrees—the true long axis of the LA and left ventricle (LV) outflow tract (LVOT); this is analogous to the transthoracic parasternal long-axis view.

Secondary Longitudinal Views

With the transducer array at 75 to 90 degrees, the plane is sagittal to the body and oblique to the long axis of the heart. Sequential leftward (counterclockwise) and rightward (clockwise) rotations of the probe shaft develop a series of longitudinal TEE views[1] including the following: (a) counterclockwise rotation of the probe, producing a two-chamber view; (b) slight clockwise rotation of the scope from the neutral position, producing a long axis of the right ventricle (RV) outflow tract; (c) further rightward rotation, producing a long-axis view of the proximal ascending aorta; and (d) still further rightward clockwise rotation, producing a long-axis view of the venae cavae and atrial septum.

Transgastric Views

The short-axis view of the LV and RV is obtained with the transducer tip in the stomach (about 40 to 45 cm from the incisors) and the transducer array at 0 degree. Anteflexion of the transducer tip optimizes the basal short-axis view of the ventricles, and retroflexion of the tip results in a more apical short-axis view. The longitudinal two-chamber view of the LV is obtained with the transducer array at 75 to 90 degrees, and clockwise rotation shows both RV inflow and outflow areas. The LVOT and aortic valve can be imaged with the array at 110 to 135 degrees.

TEE View of the Aorta, Pulmonary Artery, and Pulmonary Veins

The ascending aorta is clearly visualized from the 120- to 135-degree transducer position. The arch and descending aorta are imaged by

Text continues on p. 236.

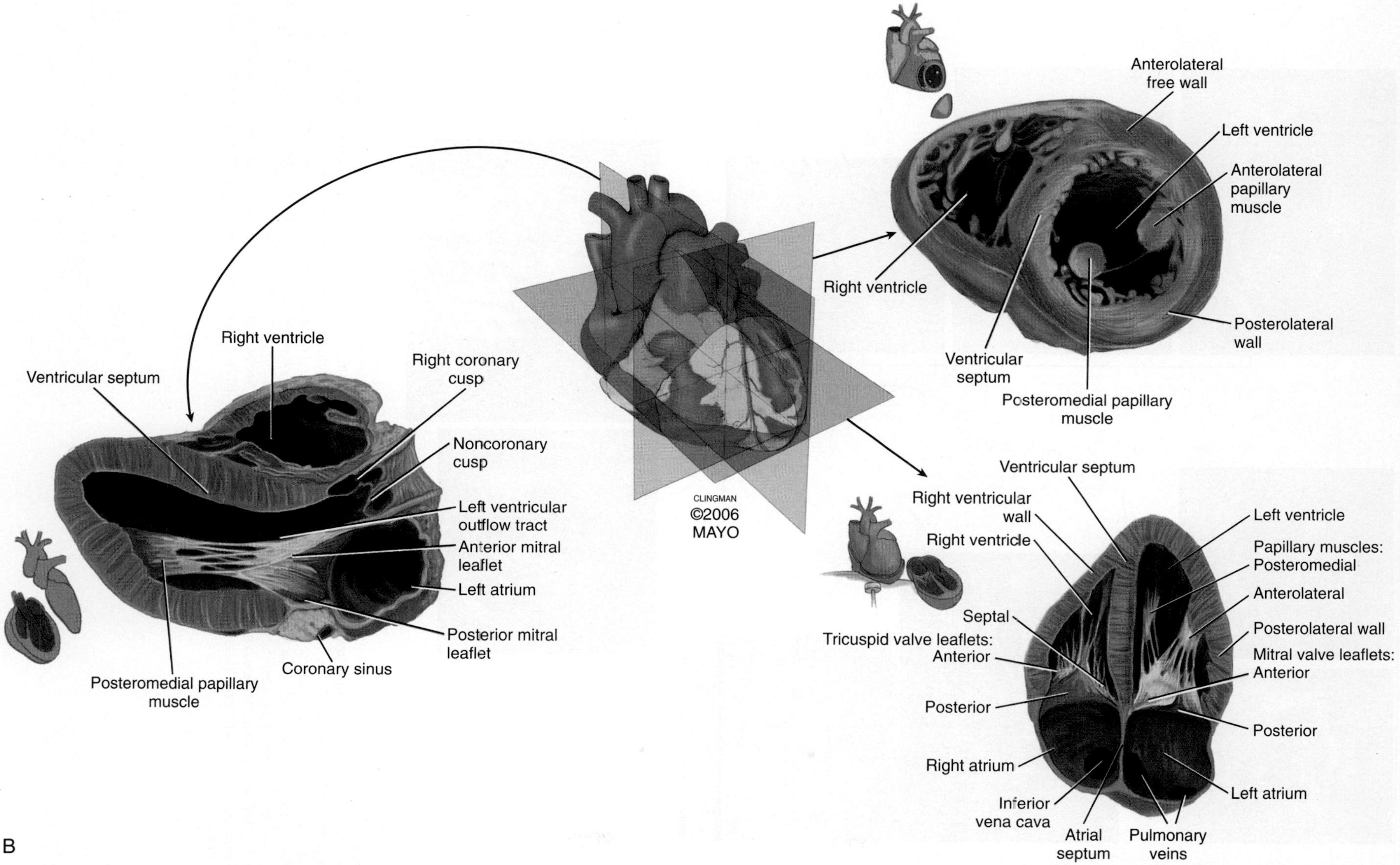

B

FIGURE 14–2, cont'd B, Diagram of cardiac structures from standard tomographic planes: parasternal long-axis view **(left)**, parasternal short-axis view **(upper right)**, and apical four-chamber view **(lower right)**.

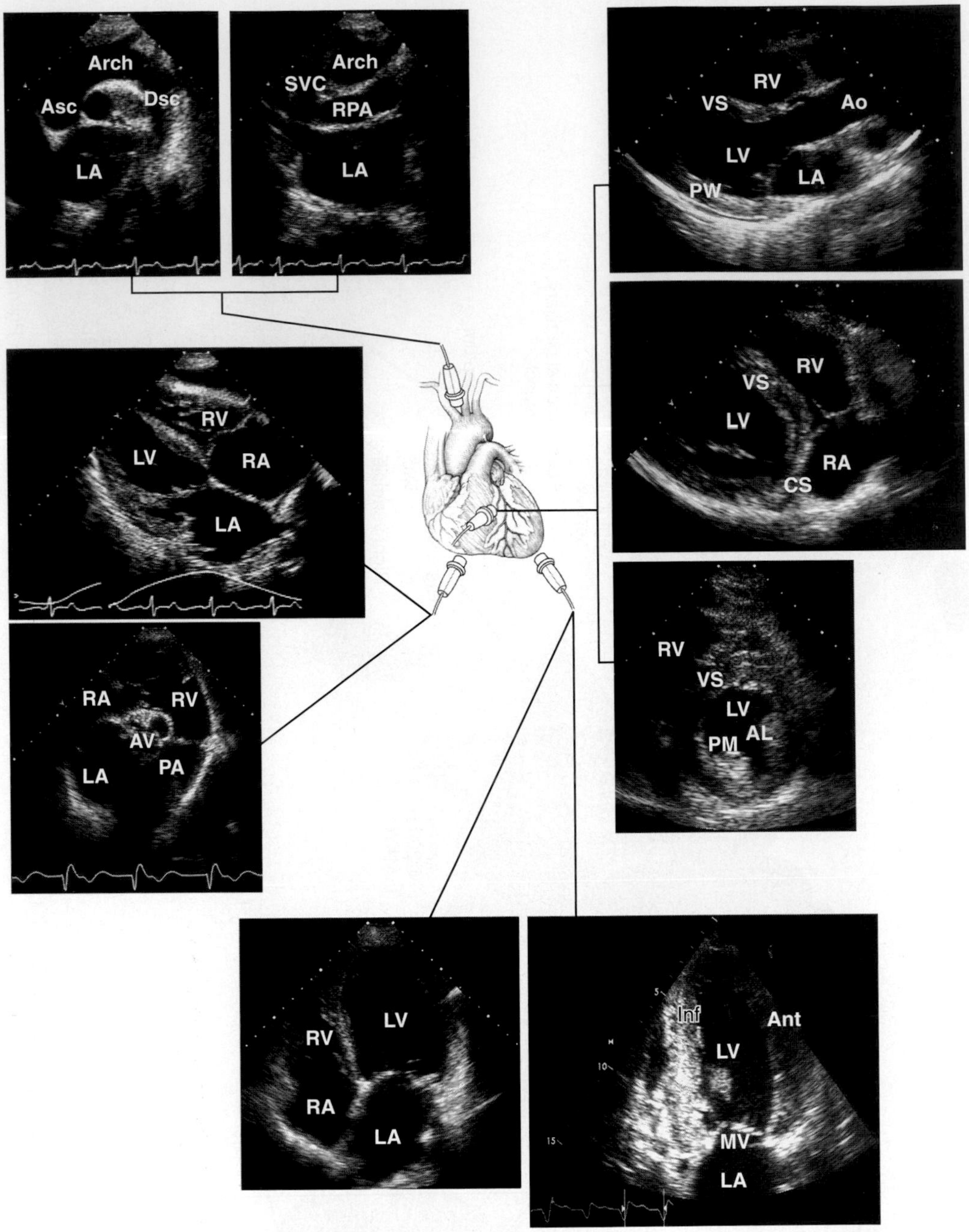

C

FIGURE 14–2, cont'd C, Still frame 2D echocardiographic images from various tomographic views: parasternal long-axis view **(right upper),** parasternal RV inflow view **(right middle),** parasternal short-axis view **(right lower),** apical four-chamber view **(left bottom),** apical two-chamber view **(right bottom),** subcostal four-chamber and short-axis views **(left middle and lower),** and suprasternal long- and short-axis views **(left upper).** These images are similar to the appearance of the diagram in **B.** AL = anterolateral; Ao = aorta; Asc = ascending aorta; CS = coronary sinus; Dsc = descending aorta; LA = left atrium; PM = papillary muscle; PW = posterior wall; RA = right atrium; RPA = right pulmonary artery; RV = right ventricle; SVC = superior vena cava; VS = ventricular septum. *(**A,** From Bansal RC, Tajik AJ, Seward JB, Offord KP: Feasibility of detailed two-dimensional echocardiographic examination in adults: Prospective study of 200 patients. Mayo Clin Proc 55:291, 1980. Used with permission of Mayo Foundation for Medical Education and Research. **B,** Modified from Tajik AJ, Seward JB, Hagler DJ, et al: Two-dimensional real-time ultrasonic imaging of the heart and great vessels: Technique, image orientation, structure identification, and validation. Mayo Clin Proc 53:271, 1978. Used with permission of Mayo Foundation for Medical Education and Research.)*

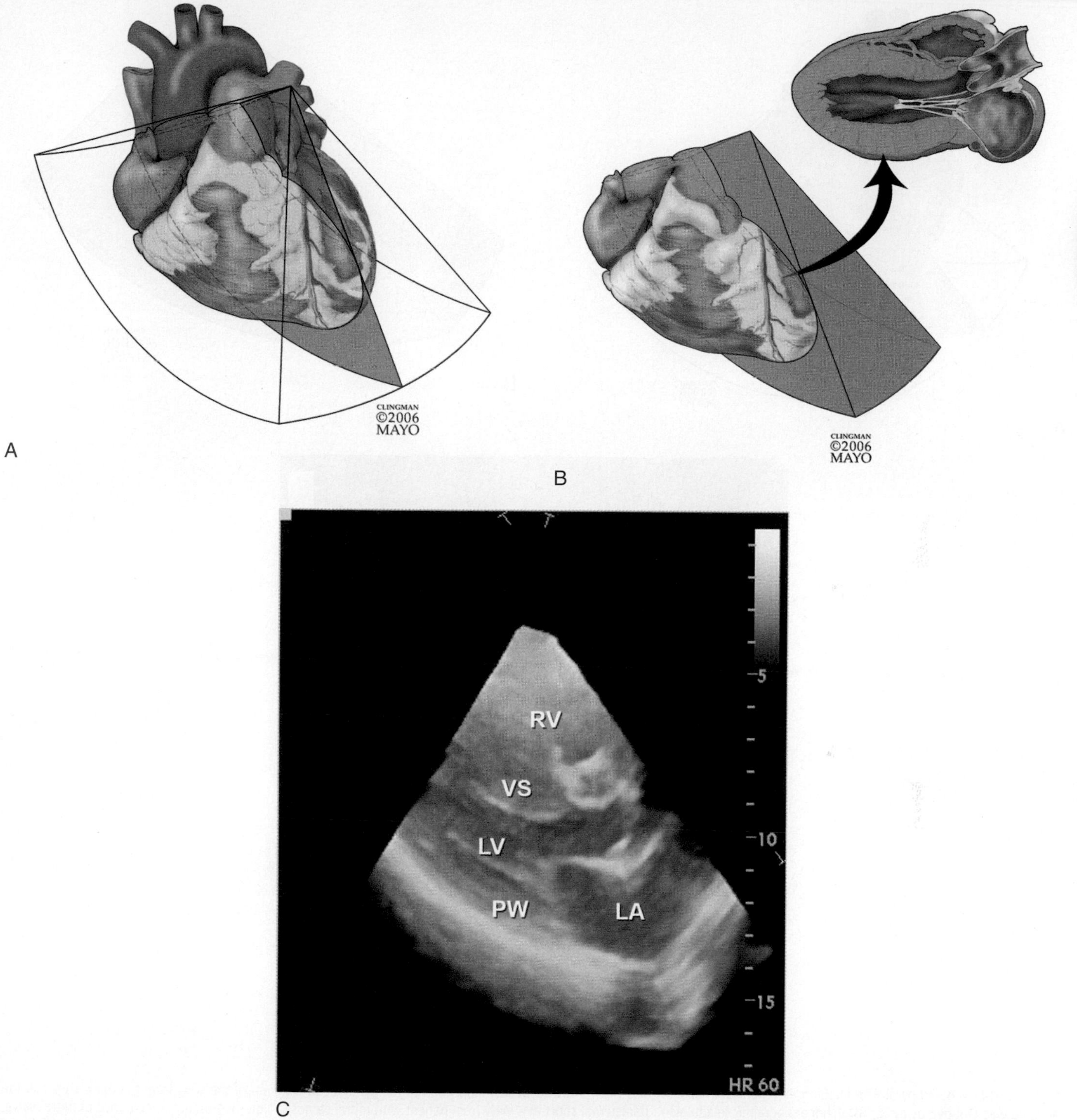

FIGURE 14–3 A, Parasternal long-axis view of 3D echocardiography pyramidal imaging. **Shaded area,** Center of pyramidal image along parasternal long-axis view. **B,** Removal of half the pyramidal image from left side of the heart produces a 3D image of the parasternal long-axis view. **C,** Still frame of real-time 3D imaging along parasternal long-axis view. The image can be rotated and tilted freely. This image was rotated clockwise to show better the mitral inflow area and left ventricular (LV) outflow tract area. LA = left atrium; PW = posterior wall; RV = right ventricle; VS = ventricular septum. *(From Oh JK, Seward JB, Tajik AJ: The Echo Manual. 3rd ed. Philadelphia, Lippincott Williams & Wilkins, 2006. Used with permission of Mayo Foundation for Medical Education and Research.)*

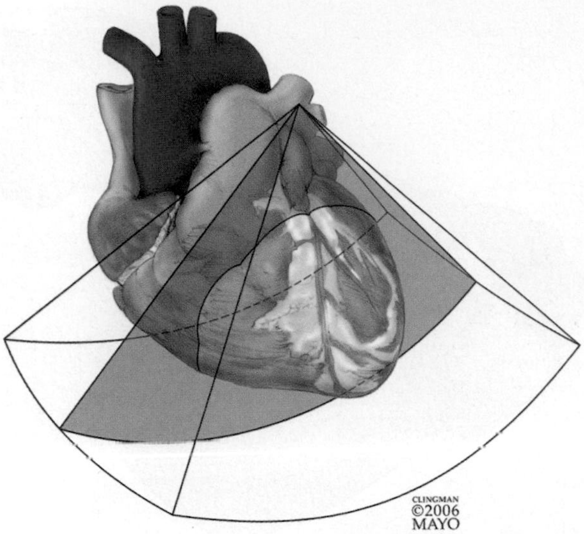

A

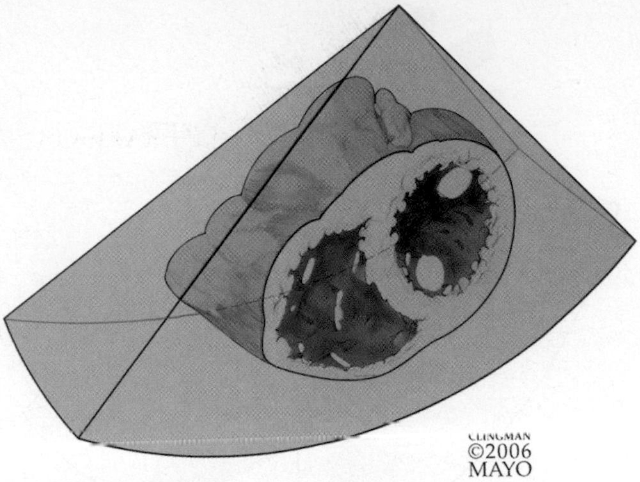

B

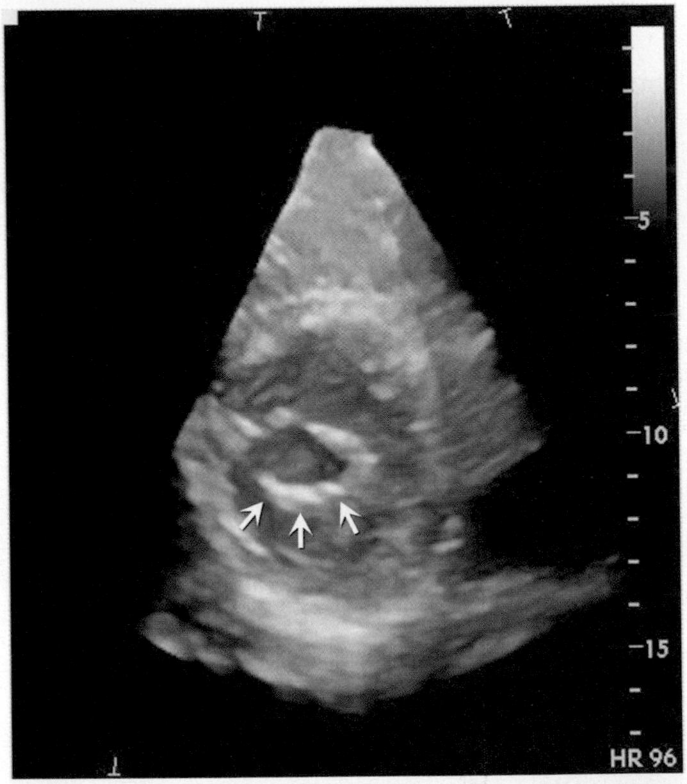

C

FIGURE 14–4 **A,** 3D pyramidal imaging along parasternal short-axis view. **Shaded area,** Midportion of the pyramid. **B,** Diagram of the view from the apex after half the pyramid was cropped away. **C,** 3D echocardiographic image along parasternal short-axis view from patient with mitral stenosis. Note fish-mouth appearance of mitral valve orifice (arrows). *(From Oh JK, Seward JB, Tajik AJ: The Echo Manual. 3rd ed. Philadelphia, Lippincott Williams & Wilkins, 2006. Used with permission of Mayo Foundation for Medical Education and Research.)*

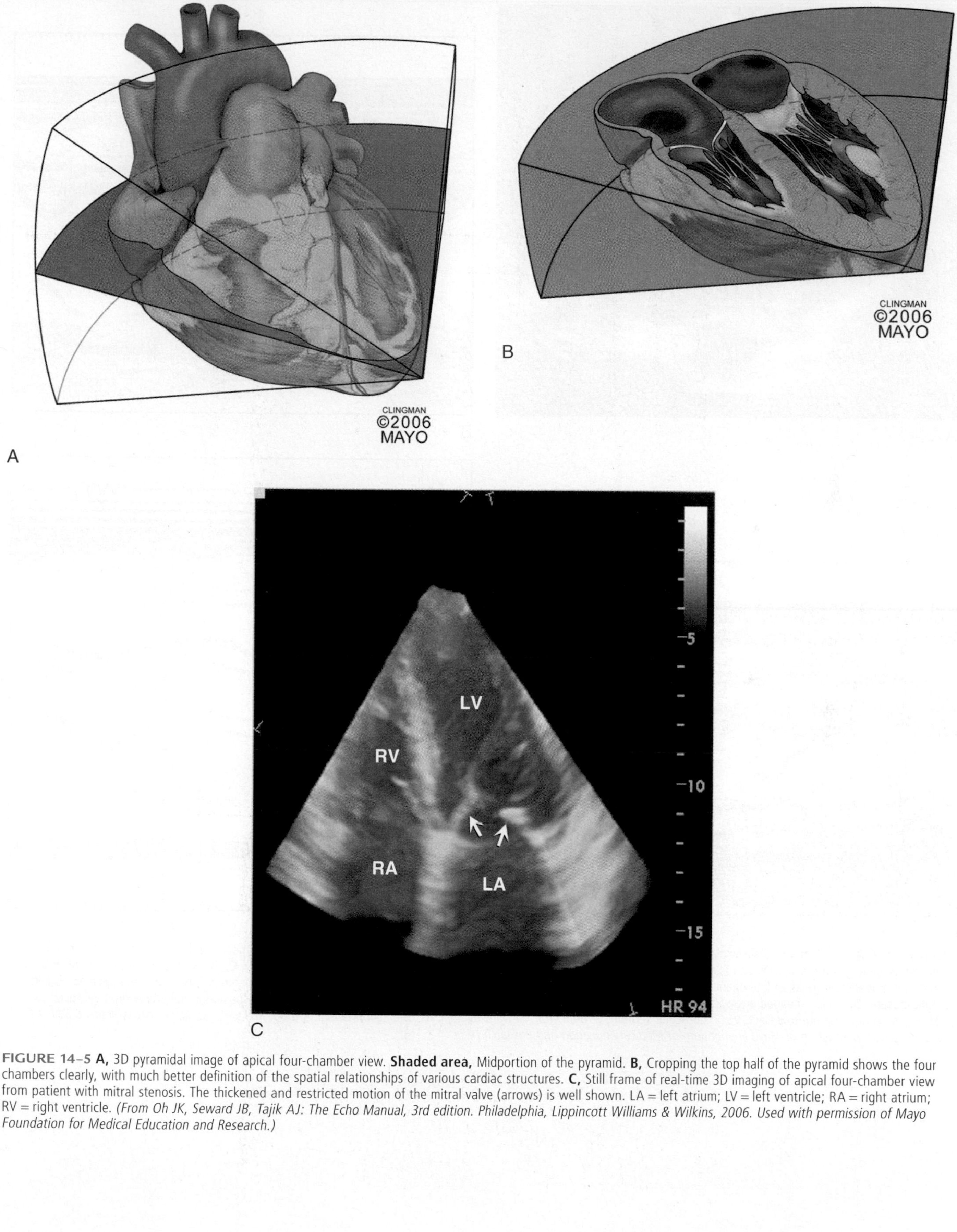

FIGURE 14–5 A, 3D pyramidal image of apical four-chamber view. **Shaded area,** Midportion of the pyramid. **B,** Cropping the top half of the pyramid shows the four chambers clearly, with much better definition of the spatial relationships of various cardiac structures. **C,** Still frame of real-time 3D imaging of apical four-chamber view from patient with mitral stenosis. The thickened and restricted motion of the mitral valve (arrows) is well shown. LA = left atrium; LV = left ventricle; RA = right atrium; RV = right ventricle. *(From Oh JK, Seward JB, Tajik AJ: The Echo Manual, 3rd edition. Philadelphia, Lippincott Williams & Wilkins, 2006. Used with permission of Mayo Foundation for Medical Education and Research.)*

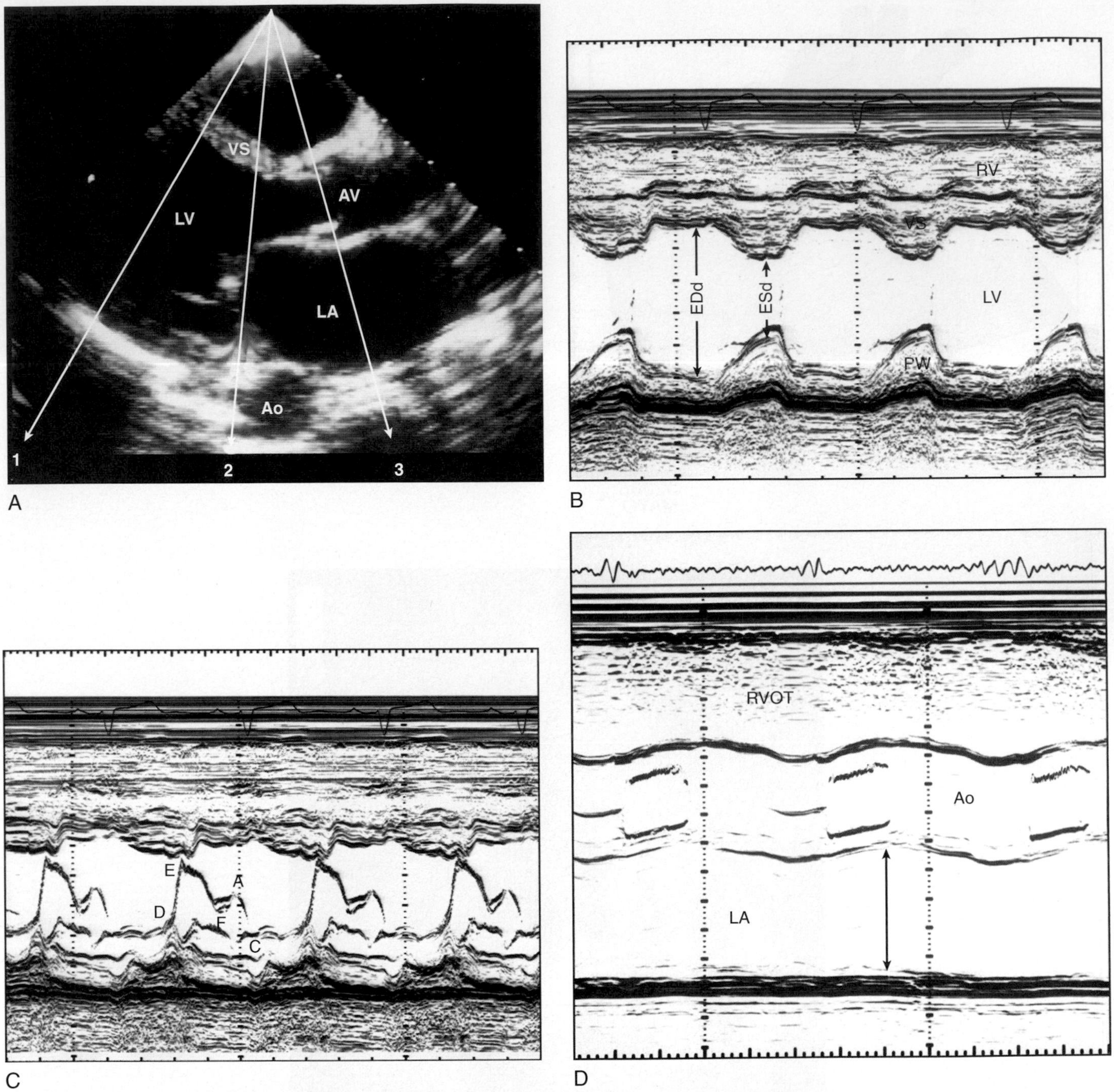

FIGURE 14–6 A, An M-mode cursor is placed along different levels (1, ventricular; 2, mitral valve; 3, aortic valve level) of the heart, with parasternal long-axis 2D echocardiographic guidance. **B,** EDd and ESd are end-diastolic and end-systolic dimensions, respectively, of the left ventricle (LV). **C,** M-mode echocardiogram of the anterior mitral leaflet: A, peak of late opening with atrial systole; C, closure of mitral valve; D, end-systole before mitral valve opening; E, peak of early opening; F, mid-diastolic closure. **D,** Double-headed arrow, dimension of the left atrium (LA) at end-systole. Ao = aorta; AV = aortic valve; PW = posterior wall; RV = right ventricle; RVOT = right ventricular outflow tract; VS = ventricular septum. *(From Oh JK, Seward JB, Tajik AJ: The Echo Manual. 3rd ed. Philadelphia, Lippincott Williams & Wilkins, 2006. Used with permission of Mayo Foundation for Medical Education and Research.)*

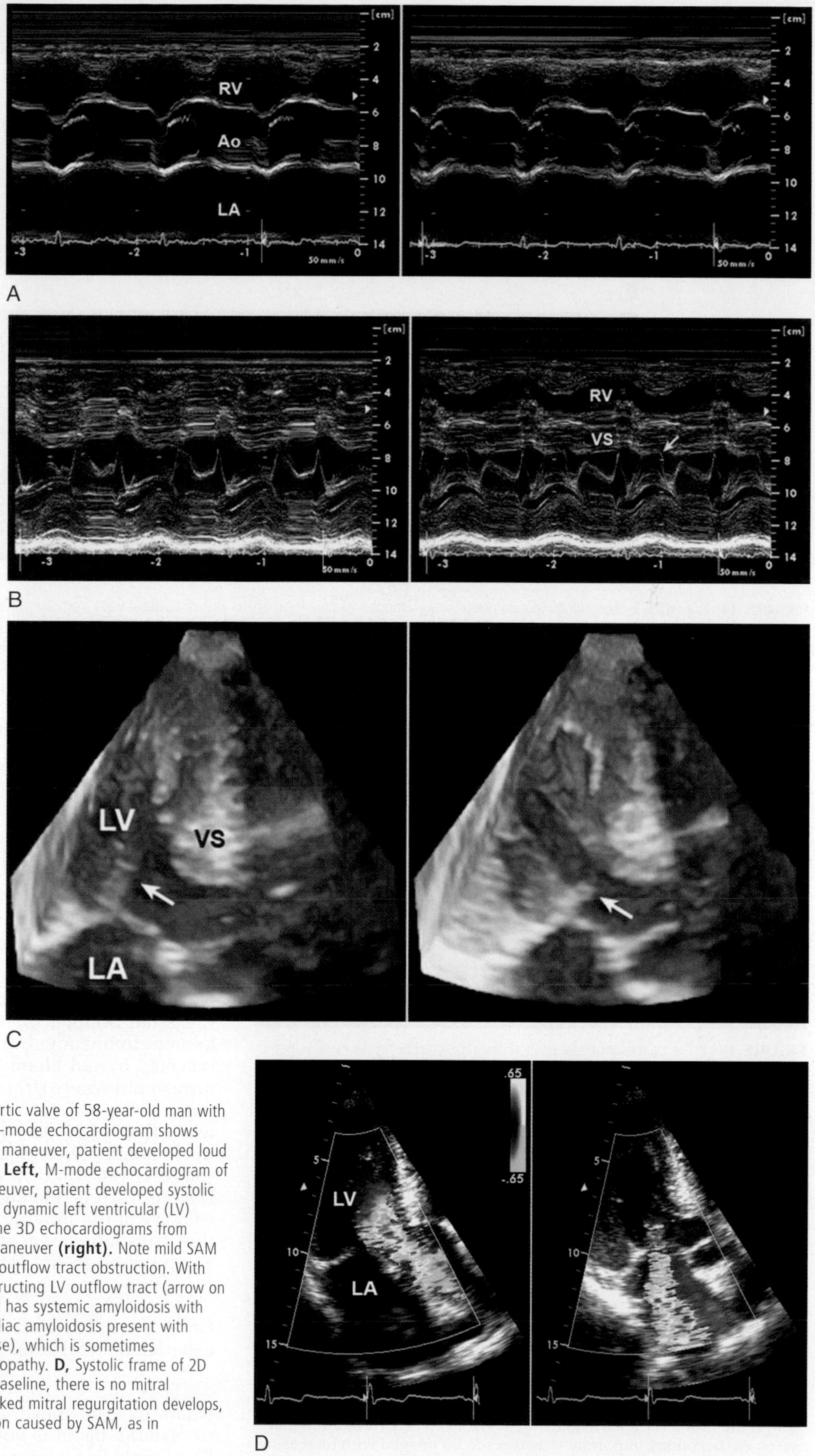

FIGURE 14–7 **A,** M-mode echocardiogram of aortic valve of 58-year-old man with heart failure and dysproteinemia. **Left,** Baseline M-mode echocardiogram shows normal aortic valve opening. **Right,** With Valsalva maneuver, patient developed loud murmur and mid-systolic closure of aortic valve. **B, Left,** M-mode echocardiogram of mitral valve at baseline. **Right,** With Valsalva maneuver, patient developed systolic anterior motion (SAM) of mitral valve (arrow) from dynamic left ventricular (LV) outflow tract obstruction. **C,** Still frames of real-time 3D echocardiograms from patient in **A** at baseline **(left)** and with Valsalva maneuver **(right).** Note mild SAM (arrow on left) at baseline without pronounced LV outflow tract obstruction. With Valsalva maneuver, SAM is more pronounced, obstructing LV outflow tract (arrow on right). Ventricular septum (VS) is thick. This patient has systemic amyloidosis with cardiac involvement. A subset of patients with cardiac amyloidosis present with dynamic LV outflow tract obstruction (as in this case), which is sometimes misdiagnosed as hypertrophic obstructive cardiomyopathy. **D,** Systolic frame of 2D and color flow imaging of same patient. **Left,** At baseline, there is no mitral regurgitation. **Right,** With Valsalva maneuver, marked mitral regurgitation develops, with a typical lateral direction of mitral regurgitation caused by SAM, as in hypertrophic cardiomyopathy.

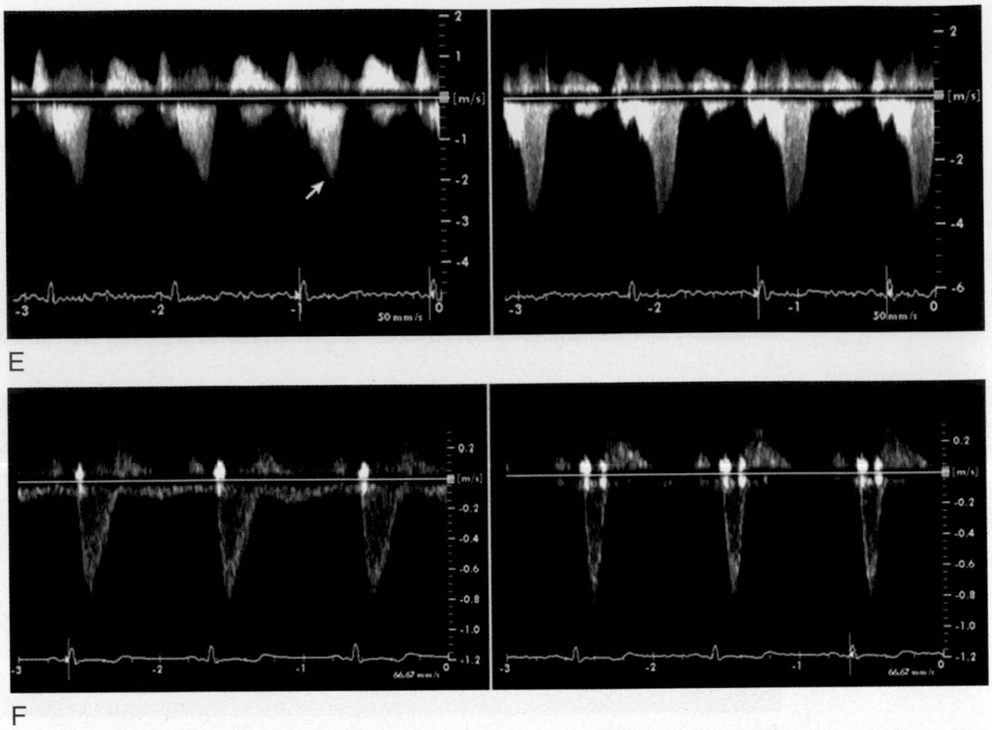

FIGURE 14–7, cont'd E, Recordings of continuous wave Doppler examination across the LV outflow tract from apical transducer position at baseline **(left)** and with Valsalva maneuver **(right)** show "dagger-shaped" systolic velocities below the baseline, characteristic for dynamic LV outflow tract gradient or obstruction. The peak velocity is 4 m/sec with Valsalva maneuver, which equals a 64-mm Hg gradient. **F,** Recordings of pulsed wave Doppler examination from suprasternal notch transducer position with sample volume in a proximal descending thoracic aorta at baseline **(left)** and with Valsalva maneuver **(right)** show marked reduction in flow duration and mid-systolic flow reversal with Valsalva maneuver. Ao = aorta; LA = left atrium; RV = right ventricle.

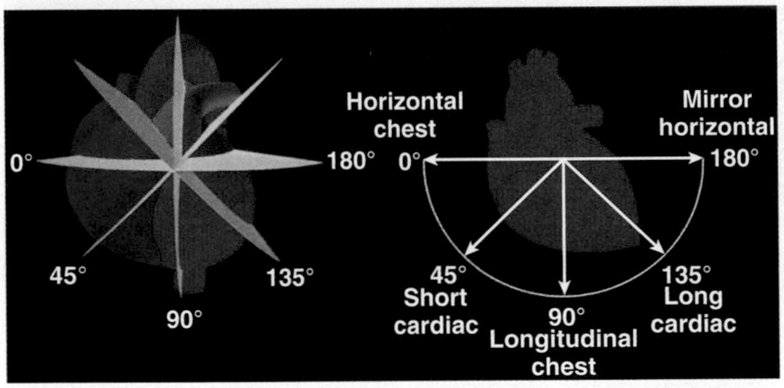

FIGURE 14–8 For transesophageal echocardiography, array rotations of selected degrees (0, 45, 90, 135, and 180 degrees) permit a logical sequence of standard transducer orientations and resultant images. Such a display helps the examiner acquire the desired views: 0-degree transverse orientation, which is horizontal to the chest at the midesophageal level; 45-degree short-axis orientation to the base of the heart from the midesophagus; 90-degree longitudinal orientation, which is in the sagittal plane of the body; 135-degree long-axis orientation to the heart from the midesophagus; and 180-degree rotation, which produces a mirror-image transverse plane. *(From Seward JB, Khandheria BK, Freeman WK, et al: Multiplane transesophageal echocardiography: Image orientation, examination technique, anatomic correlations, and clinical applications. Mayo Clin Proc 68:523, 1993. Used with permission of Mayo Foundation for Medical Education and Research.)*

directing the transducer to face posteriorly (Fig. 14-10). Aortic aneurysm, aortic dissection, and atheromatous plaques are reliably detected with TEE. The main, right, and proximal portion of the left pulmonary arteries are visualized from the 0-degree transverse transducer position if the probe is pulled slightly higher from the LA view. Pulmonary veins are becoming important structures to be imaged with increasing catheter-based or surgical procedures involving the structure. From the 60-degree short-axis view of the aortic valve, the probe is rotated clockwise to image the right pulmonary veins as a "Y" structure. Left pulmonary veins are best visualized by rotating the probe counterclockwise from the 130-degree long-axis view of the aorta. Pulmonary veins are also visualized from the 0-degree transverse view of the LA.

DOPPLER ECHOCARDIOGRAPHY AND COLOR FLOW IMAGING

Doppler Echocardiography

Doppler echocardiography measures blood flow velocities on the basis of the *Doppler effect,* which was described by Christian Doppler in 1842. When an ultrasound beam with known frequency (*fo*) is transmitted to the heart, it is reflected by red blood cells. The frequency of the reflected ultrasound waves (*fr*) increases when the red blood cells are moving toward the source of ultrasound and decreases when the red blood cells are moving away. The difference in frequency between transmitted sound and reflected sound is the *frequency,* or *Doppler, shift:* ($\Delta f = fr - fo$). The Doppler shift is related to the transmitted frequency (*fo*), the velocity of the moving target (*v*), and the angle (θ) between the ultrasound beam and the direction of the moving target, as expressed in the *Doppler equation* (Fig. 14-11):

$$\Delta f = 2\ fo \times v \times \cos\theta / c$$

Once Δf is calculated, the velocity of red blood cells can be calculated as follows:

$$V = \Delta f \times c / 2\ fo$$

where c is the speed of sound in blood (1540 m/sec). If the ultrasound beam is not parallel with the direction of blood flow, angle θ is greater than 0 degree. As angle θ increases, the corresponding cosine value becomes progressively less than 1, which results in underestimation of the Doppler shift (Δf) and, hence, peak velocity. Blood flow velocities

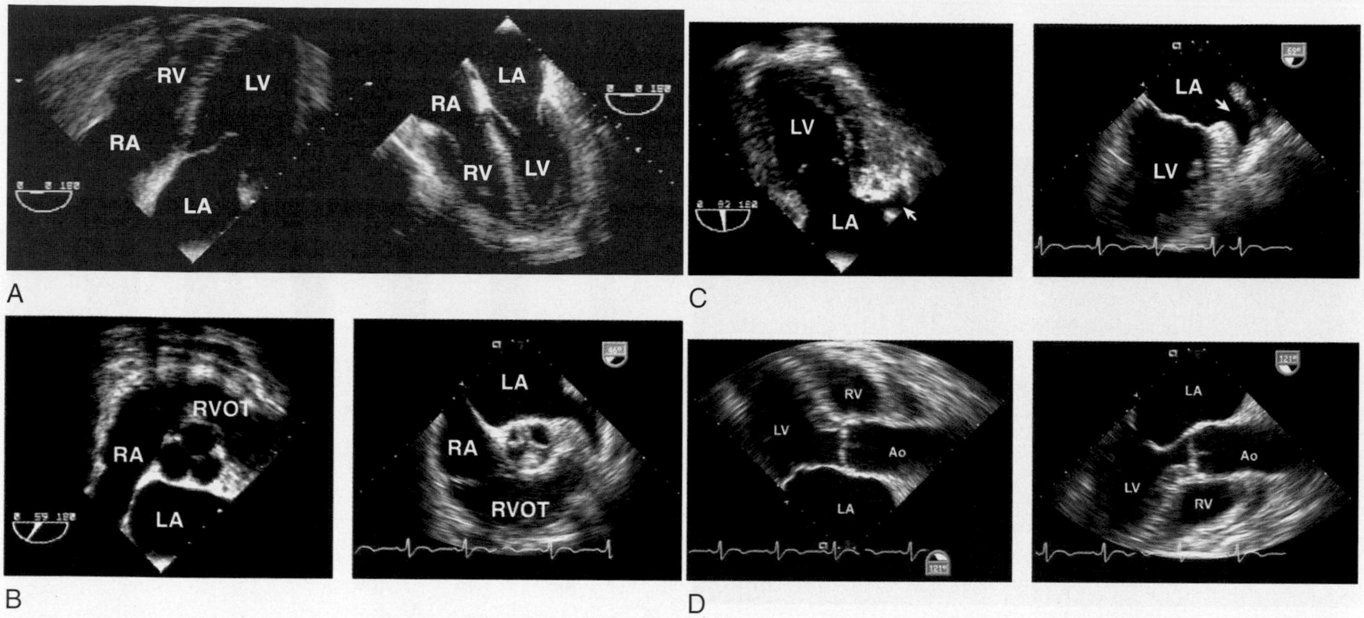

FIGURE 14–9 **A,** Four-chamber view (0 degrees with retroflexion of the transducer tip). Two different image orientations on the screen are shown: apex-up **(left)** and apex-down **(right)** views. **B,** Short-axis view (45 to 60 degrees) of the aortic valve in two different image displays. **Left,** Image display of left atrium (LA) at the bottom and right ventricular outflow tract (RVOT) at the top, similar to transthoracic parasternal short-axis view. **Right,** Image display of LA at the top and RVOT at the bottom. * = LA appendage. **C, Left** and **right,** Two-chamber view (65 to 100 degrees with leftward rotation of TEE shaft). Arrow, LA appendage in two different image displays. **D, Left** and **right,** Long-axis view (125 to 140 degrees) of the left ventricle (LV). Ao = aorta; RA = right atrium; RV = right ventricle. *(From Oh JK, Seward JB, Tajik AJ: The Echo Manual. 3rd ed. Philadelphia, Lippincott Williams & Wilkins, 2006. Used with permission of Mayo Foundation for Medical Education and Research.)*

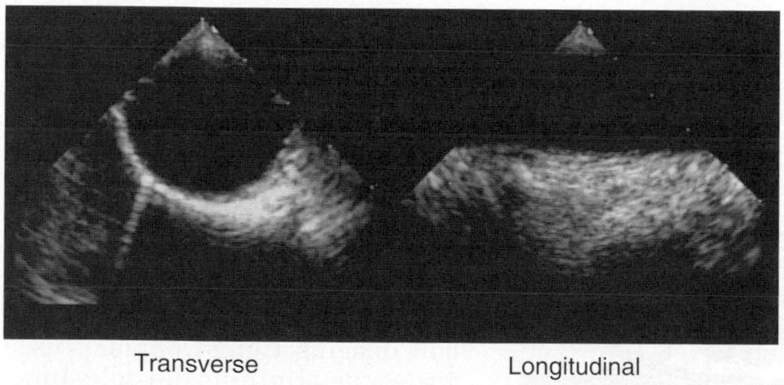

FIGURE 14–10 Transverse (0 degrees) and longitudinal (90 degrees) images of the normal descending thoracic aorta. *(From Oh JK, Seward JB, Tajik AJ: The Echo Manual. 3rd ed. Philadelphia, Lippincott Williams & Wilkins, 2006. Used with permission of Mayo Foundation for Medical Education and Research.)*

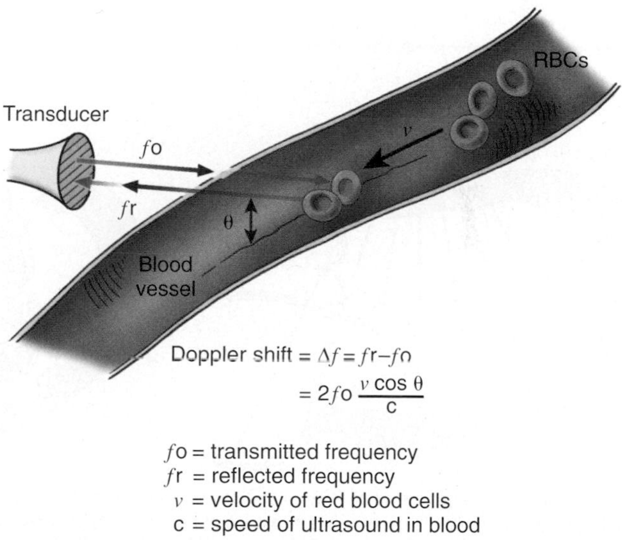

FIGURE 14–11 Diagram of the Doppler effect (see text for explanation). RBCs = red blood cells. *(From Oh JK, Seward JB, Tajik AJ: The Echo Manual. 3rd ed. Philadelphia, Lippincott Williams & Wilkins, 2006. Used with permission of Mayo Foundation for Medical Education and Research.)*

measured with Doppler echocardiography are used to derive various hemodynamic data.

Two forms of Doppler echocardiography exist: the *pulsed wave* and *continuous wave* forms (Fig. 14-12; see also Fig. 14-7). Pulsed wave Doppler is location specific. A single crystal sends a short burst of ultrasound at a pulse repetition frequency and receives sound beams reflected from moving red blood cells from a specified location that is determined by placement of a "sample volume." Thus the maximal frequency shift that pulsed wave Doppler can measure is one-half the pulse repetition frequency, called the *Nyquist frequency.* If the frequency shift is higher than the Nyquist frequency, *aliasing* occurs; that is, the frequency shift or the corresponding velocity higher than the Nyquist frequency is cut off at the Nyquist frequency, and the remaining frequency shift is recorded on the top or bottom of the opposite side of baseline. In continuous wave Doppler the transducer sends ultrasound waves and receives the reflected ultrasound waves continuously with the use of two separate crystals. Therefore the maximal frequency shift and velocity recorded with continuous wave Doppler are not limited by the pulse repetition frequency or Nyquist phenomenon. Unlike pulsed wave Doppler, continuous wave Doppler measures all frequency shifts (i.e., velocities) along its beam path; hence it is used to detect and record the highest flow velocity available.

Color Flow Imaging, or Color Doppler

Color flow imaging, or color Doppler, is a form of the pulsed wave Doppler that displays blood flow or myocardial velocities in various colors (usually red, blue, and green) or their combinations, depending on the velocity, direction, and turbulence. At each sampling site, the frequency shift is mea-

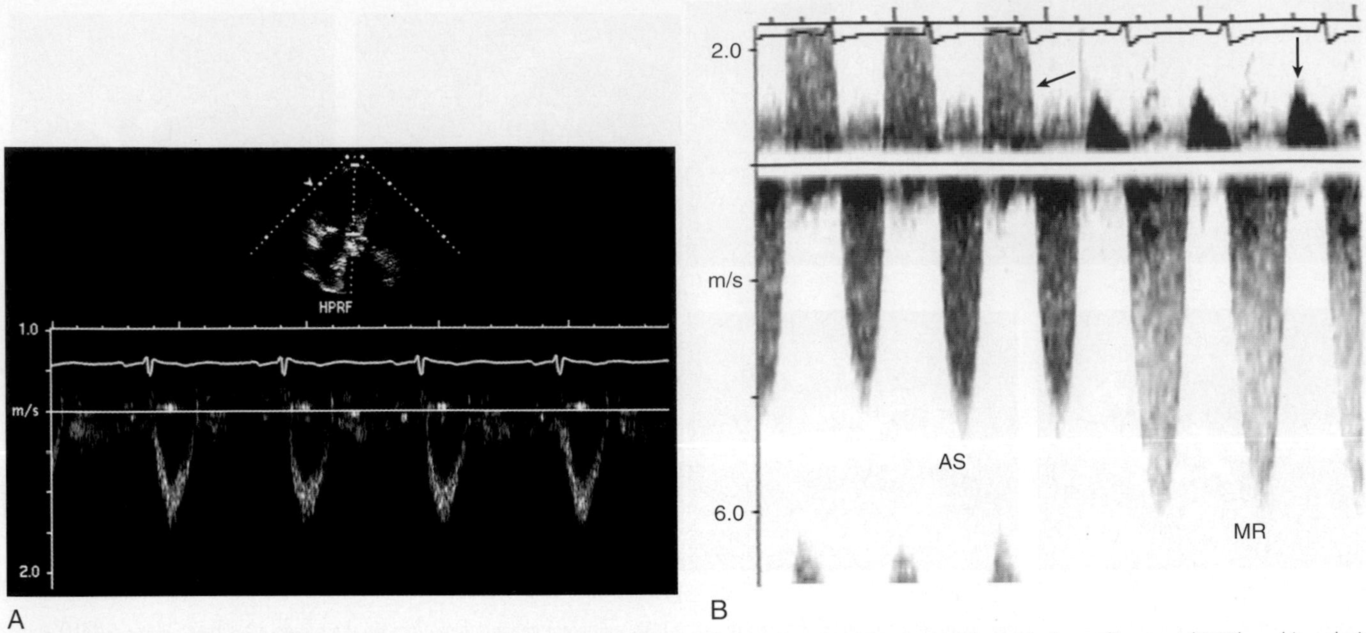

FIGURE 14–12 A, Pulsed wave Doppler records flow velocity from a specific location. The sample volume was in the left ventricular outflow tract (LVOT), and its velocity was 1.5 m/sec. **B,** Continuous wave Doppler records all velocities along the path of the ultrasound beam. Therefore a slight angulation of the transducer may record entirely different velocities. This continuous wave recording was obtained from the apical window with a pencil probe in a patient with severe aortic stenosis (AS) and moderate mitral regurgitation (MR). A slight change in the direction of the continuous wave Doppler probe recorded both AS and MR signals, as well as aortic regurgitation (left arrow) and mitral inflow (down arrow) during diastole. Note that the duration and peak velocity of AS are shorter and lower, respectively, than those of MR. *(**B,** From Oh JK, Seward JB, Tajik AJ: The Echo Manual. 3rd ed. Philadelphia, Lippincott Williams & Wilkins, 2006. Used with permission of Mayo Foundation for Medical Education and Research.)*

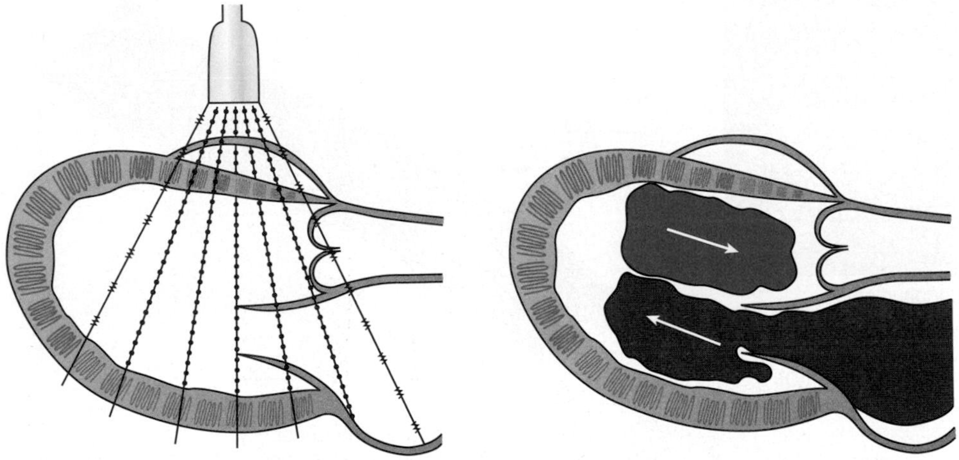

FIGURE 14–13 Drawing illustrating how color flow imaging is performed and displayed. The dots indicate multiple sampling sites (gates). The frequency shift measured at each gate is correlated automatically (autocorrelation) and converted to a preset color scheme (red for flow toward and blue for flow away from the transducer). *(From Oh JK, Seward JB, Tajik AJ: The Echo Manual. 3rd ed. Philadelphia, Lippincott Williams & Wilkins, 2006. Used with permission of Mayo Foundation for Medical Education and Research.)*

sured, converted to a digital format, automatically correlated (*autocorrelation*) with a preset color scheme, and displayed as color flow superimposed on 2D imaging (Fig. 14-13). For intracavitary flow, blood flow directed toward the transducer has a positive frequency shift and is color coded in shades of red. Blood flow directed away from the transducer has a negative frequency shift and is color coded in shades of blue. The lighter shades within each primary color are assigned to higher velocities within the Nyquist limit. When flow velocity is higher than the Nyquist frequency limit, color aliasing occurs and is depicted as a color reversal. *Turbulence* reflects the degree of the variance from the mean velocity of a region and is coded usually in a shade of green. Therefore abnormal blood flow is easily recognized by combinations of multiple colors according to the directions, velocities, and degrees of turbulence. The width and size of abnormal intracavitary blood flows are used to evaluate the degree of valvular regurgitation or cardiac shunt.

Almost all structural and hemodynamic abnormalities of the heart produce a disturbance in blood flow, hence, abnormality in color flow imaging. Color Doppler is used also for determining diastolic function and timing of intracardiac events (see Evaluation of Systolic and Diastolic Function later). Figure 14-7 demonstrates dynamic changes of valvular regurgitation and hemodynamics recorded with Doppler echocardiography and color flow imaging. Another important use of color display in echocardiography is parametric imaging, reflecting a predetermined characteristic of blood flow, or tissue Doppler velocities, including the timing of peak velocities.

TISSUE DOPPLER AND STRAIN IMAGING

Tissue Doppler imaging (TDI) records the motion of tissue or other structures with a velocity or frequency shift much lower than that of blood flow. Doppler echocardiography for blood flow measures the velocities of red blood cells (velocity usually higher than 20 cm/sec and up to 800 cm/sec in case of valvular disease). However, the velocities of myocardial tissue are much lower (<30 cm/sec), but with larger amplitudes than those produced by blood. Therefore pulsed wave Doppler was modified to record the low velocities of myocardial tissue and to reject the high velocities generated by blood flow. TDI can also be displayed in color mode (Fig. 14-14). A major limitation of tissue velocity recording is that tissue velocities measured by TDI may overestimate or underestimate the active component or function of the tissue because of translational motion or tethering, respectively. Strain (ε) and strain rate imaging can overcome this limitation by measuring the actual extent of stretching or contraction (see Fig. 14-14).[7,8]

Strain (ε) is the percentage change in length during myocardial contraction and relaxation and is expressed as "%." By convention, shortening is represented by negative values and lengthening by positive values for both strain and strain rate.

$$\varepsilon = \Delta L/L_0 = (L_1 - L_0)/L_0 = (V_a \times t - V_b \times t)/L_0 = (V_a - V_b) \times t/L_0$$

where L_0 is the original length, L_1 is final length, ΔL is change in length, $V_a - V_b$ is the instantaneous velocity difference at points a and b, and *t* is time interval.

Strain rate is the rate of instantaneous change in strain calculated as the difference between two velocities normalized to the distance (d) between them and expressed as "s^{-1}" (see Fig. 14-e1 on website).

$$\text{Strain rate} = (V_a - V_b)/d$$

Therefore strain (ε) is the sum of the instantaneous strain rate values over a time interval of deformation.

Tissue tracking or displacement is the integral of tissue velocity over a given time. It represents the distance a region of interest moves relative to its original location.

Tissue Doppler velocities, strain rate, displacement, and systolic strain of individual segments from healthy individuals are shown in Tables 14-1 to 14-3.

Speckle tracking is a method that uses 2D images to quantify myocardial motion in various planes.[9,10] Reflection, scattering, and interference of the ultrasound beam in the myocardial tissue produces formation of speckles. Myocardial regions with unique speckle patterns in the gray scale 2D image can be tracked frame to frame throughout the cardiac cycle. This allows LV rotational motion, often referred to as *torsion* or *twist,* to be assessed (Fig. 14-15). The spiral shape of LV myocardial fibers results in a complex 3D torsion mechanism for systolic contraction and untwisting for diastolic relaxation.[11,12] The degree of torsion or twisting appears to be related to aging and diastolic function, as well as systolic contraction. The LV myocardium consists of two layers: the subendocardial layer wraps around the LV cavity in a right-handed helical direction, and the subepicardial layer wraps around in a left-handed helical direction. Viewed from the LV apex, the apex rotates counterclockwise and the base rotates clockwise during systole.[13] As the two ends of the LV twist in opposite directions, the myocardium between the two thickens and shortens longitudinally. Speckle tracking is another method for measuring strain, using angle-independent 2D images instead of the angle-dependent tissue Doppler method described earlier. Hence the speckle tracking method can provide circumferential and radial strain, as well as longitudinal strain.

The clinical applications of TDI and strain imaging are increasing and provide incremental diagnostic and prognostic value over standard 2D and blood pool Doppler echocardiography. They have been used successfully in assessing regional and global systolic and diastolic function.[14-17] Myocardial strain becomes abnormal during the early stage of myocardial ischemia as well as in myopathies and appears to be more sensitive for identifying ischemic segments during stress echocardiography.[18,19] TDI has been used most commonly to evaluate diastolic function and to estimate diastolic filling pressures.[20,21] Both strain and tissue Doppler imaging allow reliable determination of cardiac timing

TABLE 14–1 Velocity of Individual Segments Determined with Tissue Doppler Echocardiography

	Septum	Lateral	Inferior	Anterior
S wave, cm/sec				
Basal	5.97±1.14	6.26±2.44	6.52±1.31	6.44±2.32
Mid	6.29±1.89	4.48±0.92	5.21±2.79	5.1±1.16
Apical	4.42±2.3	4.81±1.97	2.97±1.14	3.8±2.66
E wave, cm/sec				
Basal	7.91±2.16	8.54±2.77	9.01±2.44	8.09±2.48
Mid	8.39±2.5	6.85±1.86	6.82±3.16	7.22±2.04
Apical	6.03±2.95	6.74±2.58	4.76±1.94	4.52±2.95
A wave, cm/sec				
Basal	5.99±1.73	3.77±1.95	5.84±2.06	3.86±1.75
Mid	4.87±2.14	4.9±1.72	2.62±1.84	4.78±1.7
Apical	2.69±1.93	3.77±2.1	3.08±1.54	1.69±1.45

A=late diastolic velocity; E=early diastolic velocity; S=systolic velocity.
From Sun JP, Popovic ZB, Greenburg NL, et al: Noninvasive quantification of regional myocardial function using Doppler-derived velocity, displacement, strain rate, and strain in healthy volunteers: Effects of aging. J Am Soc Echocardiogr 17:132, 2004.

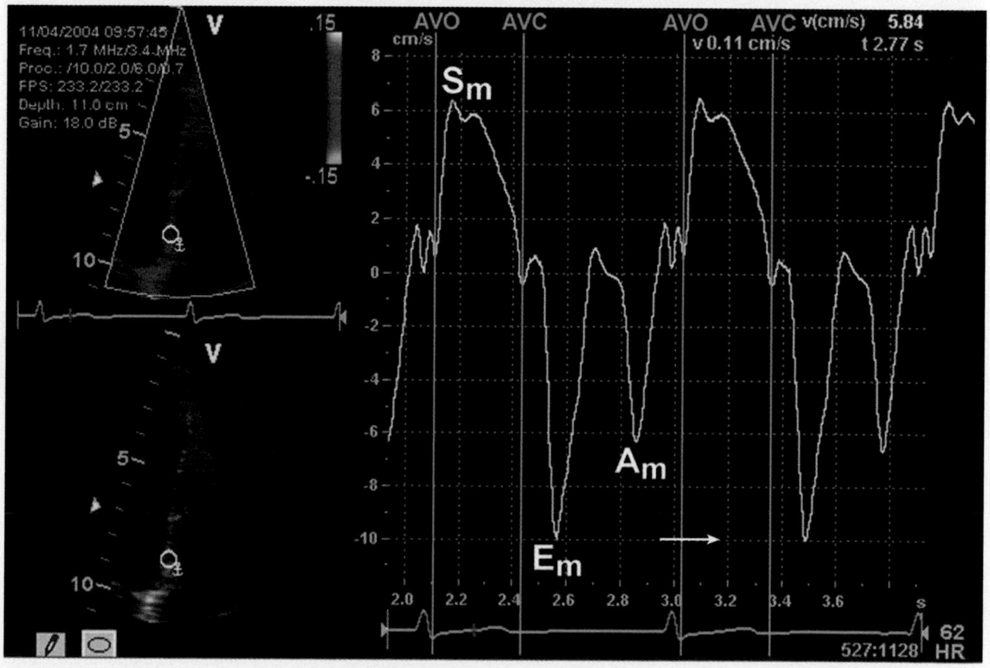

A

FIGURE 14–14 A, Recording of tissue velocity. The sample volume was placed at the basal portion of the inferior septum. Peak systolic velocity (Sm) was slightly more than 6 cm/sec, early diastolic velocity (Em) was 10 cm/sec, and late diastolic velocity (Am) was 6 cm/sec.

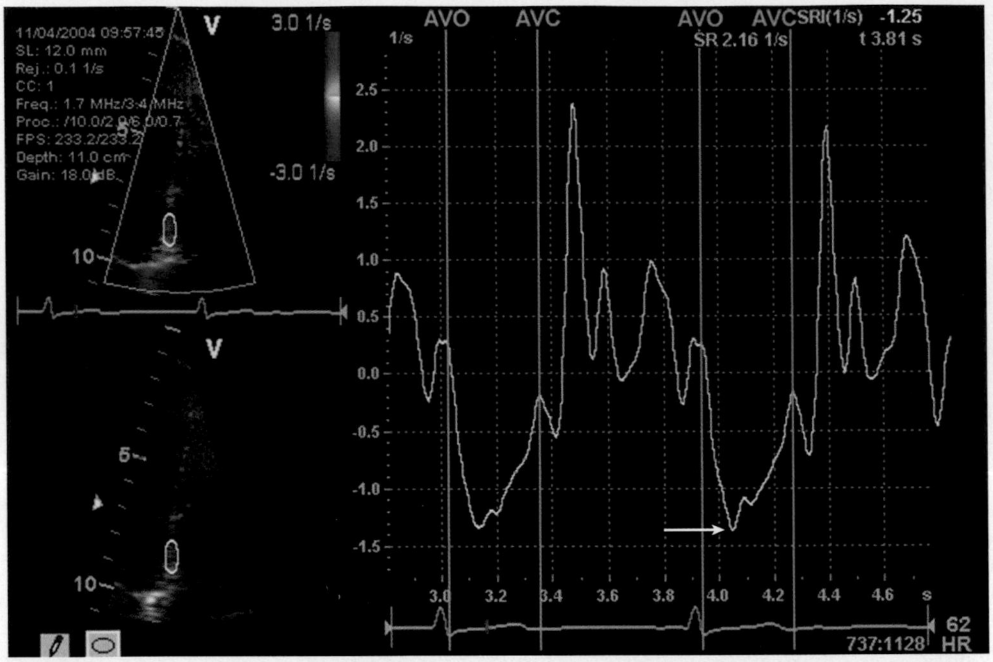

B

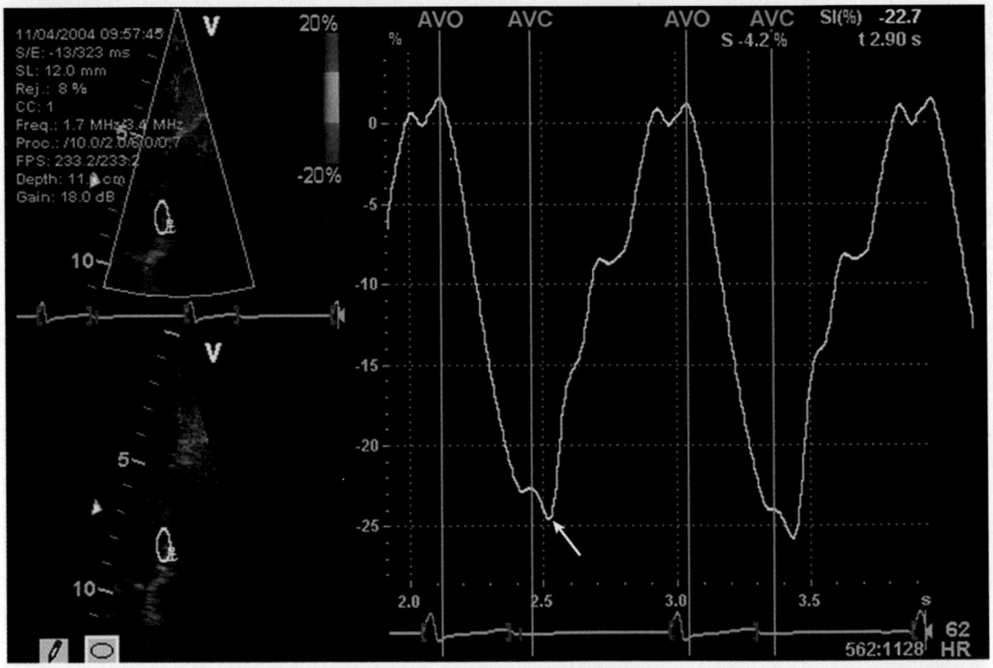

C

FIGURE 14–14, cont'd B, Recording of strain rate, which represents the rate of deformation; the peak negative strain rate (arrow) was −1.3/sec. **C,** Strain recording, which is the integration of the strain rates; the negative peak strain (arrow) occurred slightly after aortic valve closure (AVC). The normal strain value is usually more than −15 percent. AVO = aortic valve opening. *(From Oh JK, Seward JB, Tajik AJ: The Echo Manual. 3rd ed. Philadelphia, Lippincott Williams & Wilkins, 2006. Used with permission of Mayo Foundation for Medical Education and Research.)*

TABLE 14–2 Strain Rate of Individual Segments

	Septum	Lateral	Inferior	Anterior
Peak systolic wave, 1/s				
Basal	0.99±0.49	1.5±0.74	0.88±0.39	1.64±0.9
Mid	1.25±0.73	1.29±0.58	0.95±0.54	0.98±0.68
Apical	1.15±0.5	1.09±0.59	1.38±0.45	1.05±0.63
Early diastolic wave, 1/s				
Basal	1.95±0.89	1.92±1.11	1.85±0.89	2.03±0.99
Mid	1.94±0.97	1.71±0.66	1.92±1.2	1.7±0.82
Apical	1.91±0.66	1.81±0.87	2.29±0.88	1.76±0.98
Late diastolic wave, 1/s				
Basal	1.54±0.93	0.93±0.59	1.18±0.78	1.49±0.96
Mid	1.29±0.86	1.48±0.77	0.78±0.62	1.04±0.57
Apical	0.95±0.54	1.07±0.68	1.68±0.76	0.68±0.65

From Sun JP, Popovic ZB, Greenburg NL, et al: Noninvasive quantification of regional myocardial function using Doppler-derived velocity, displacement, strain rate, and strain in healthy volunteers: Effects of aging. J Am Soc Echocardiogr 17:132, 2004.

TABLE 14–3 Displacement and Systolic Strain of Individual Segments

	Septum	Lateral	Inferior	Anterior
Displacement, cm				
Basal	1.2±0.19	0.93±0.22	1.33±0.22	1.05±0.27
Mid	1.13±0.27	0.91±0.18	0.62±0.22	1.04±0.19
Apical	0.65±0.24	0.82±0.27	0.55±0.18	0.41±0.25
Systolic strain, %				
Basal	17.5±5.32	18.22±6.79	14.97±5.74	22.19±7.75
Mid	18.27±6.93	18.83±5.29	14.2±5.14	17.95±5.53
Apical	19.31±6.07	17.56±5.85	23.6±5.17	13.17±5.83

From Sun JP, Popovic ZB, Greenburg NL, et al: Noninvasive quantification of regional myocardial function using Doppler-derived velocity, displacement, strain rate, and strain in healthy volunteers: Effects of aging. J Am Soc Echocardiogr 17:132, 2004.

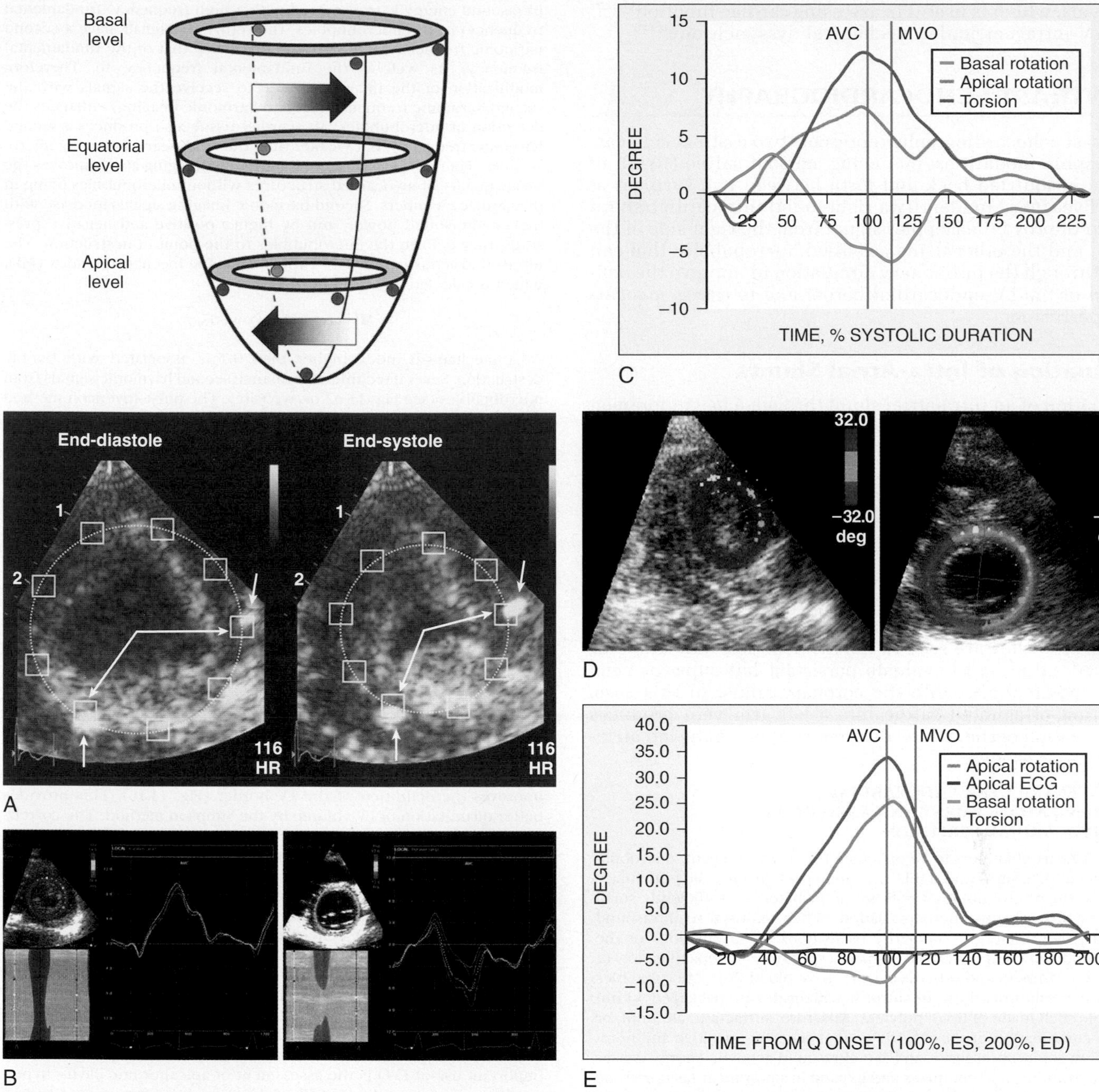

FIGURE 14–15 **A, Top,** Viewed from the apex, the apical rotation is counterclockwise (top thick arrow) and basal rotation is clockwise (bottom thick arrow). **Bottom,** Speckle tracking regions of interest are denoted by white boxes in the echocardiographic image of the animal model. Rotational changes are noted by the dotted white arrows during end-diastole and end-systole frames. **B,** Cardiac rotation in a normal person. The extent of rotation is colorized in these speckle tracking images. **Left,** Apical short-axis view with counterclockwise rotation colored blue. Maximal rotation occurred at end-systole, shown as the graph above the baseline. The extent of rotation of multiple segments is shown in different colors. The rectangle below the speckle image shows colorized rotation of different segments during one cardiac cycle, which is a color M-mode of left ventricular apical rotation. **Right,** The basal segment of the left ventricle, with clockwise rotation by color and graph. Because rotation is clockwise, the graph is recorded below the baseline. **C,** The mean apical rotation (7-degree counterclockwise) and basal rotation (5-degree clockwise rotation) at the time of aortic valve closing (AVC) are shown. They resulted in a net torsion of 12 degrees. Untwisting of the torsion starts the myocardial relaxation process. MVO = mitral valve opening. **D, Left,** Apical short-axis view with speckle imaging showing exaggerated counterclockwise rotation in a patient with abnormal myocardial relaxation. **Right,** Basal short-axis view showing clockwise rotation. **E,** Quantification of the extent of the rotation and resulting torsion is shown in this graph from the same patient as in **D.** Apical counterclockwise rotation is 25 degrees (above the baseline), and the peak basal rotation is clockwise (below the baseline) 9 degrees. Both apical and basal rotation is greater than that of a normal subject. Therefore torsion is higher than in a normal subject at 34 degrees. ED = end-diastole; ES = end-systole. *(**A,** From Helle-Valle T, Crosby J, Edvardsen T, et al: New noninvasive method for assessment of left ventricular rotation: speckle tracking echocardiography. Circulation 112:3149, 2005. Used with permission. **B-E,** Courtesy of C Miyazaki, MD.)*

 intervals, which is useful in assessing cardiac function[14,21,22] and LV intraventricular mechanical dyssynchrony.[23-26]

CONTRAST ECHOCARDIOGRAPHY

Contrast echocardiography represents two distinct echocardiographic modalities: one using agitated saline (10 mL of saline is squirted back and forth between two syringes at least five times) to identify a right-to-left intracardiac shunt and to improve the Doppler signal from the right side of the heart, and the other using gas-filled microbubbles that can pass through the pulmonary circulation to improve the definition of the LV endocardial border and to assess myocardial perfusion.

Evaluation of Intra-Atrial Shunts

Evaluation of an intra-atrial shunt through a patent foramen ovale (PFO) is the most frequent use of contrast echocardiography using agitated saline. Normally, when agitated saline is injected intravenously, the right atrium (RA) and RV become opacified by the contrast effect of the agitated saline and the left side of the heart remains contrast free. If there is an intra-atrial shunt via a PFO or atrial septal defect (see Chap. 61), the agitated saline appears in the LA immediately after the RA becomes opacified by bubbles from agitated saline. If a patient has an intrapulmonary shunt, the bubbles do not appear in the LA until several cardiac cycles after they are seen in the RA. Another indication for agitated saline is to evaluate persistent left superior vena cava, which drains into the coronary sinus. In this case, injection of agitated saline into a left arm vein produces opacification of the enlarged coronary sinus in the left atrioventricular groove.

LEFT VENTRICULAR ENDOCARDIAL BORDER ENHANCEMENT AND ASSESSMENT OF MYOCARDIAL PERFUSION

For left heart chambers to be opacified by a contrast agent, microbubbles need to be small and stable enough to pass through the pulmonary circulation. Microbubbles 4 to 5 μm in diameter are sufficiently small to pass through the microcirculation. When exposed to ultrasound signals, they undergo volumetric oscillations.[27,28] Oscillations of the microbubbles create acoustic signals responsible for opacification of cardiac chambers and other areas that have blood flow. Microbubbles (usually perfluorocarbons or sulfur hexafluoride) are packaged within a stable shell made of lipid, polymer, galactose, surfactant, albumin, or some combination of these.[27] Ultrasound generates positive and negative (sinusoidal) pressures, and the ultrasound acoustic energy causes the microbubbles to compress and expand in a nonlinear fashion if the acoustic pressure is at least as high as the resonant frequency of the microbubbles. Harmonic signals are generated by this nonlinear property of microbubbles when contacted by ultrasound energy. When ultrasound energy is transmitted with a high frequency (fundamental frequency) to the microbubbles, the returning signals have a second harmonic frequency, 2*fo* (a frequency twice that of the fundamental frequency), as well as the fundamental frequency, fo. Therefore modification of the imaging device to receive the signals with the second harmonic frequency (second harmonic imaging) enhances the detection of microbubbles. Myocardial tissue also produces a second harmonic frequency, but weaker than the nonlinearly behaving microbubbles. Therefore tissue second harmonic imaging also improves the image quality of myocardial structures without microbubbles being in the cardiac chambers. Second harmonic imaging signals increase with higher ultrasound power, and by higher positive and negative pressures, they deform the microbubbles to the point of destruction. The ultrasound acoustic power is expressed as the mechanical index (MI), which is calculated as follows:

$$\text{MI} = \text{Acoustic Power}/\sqrt{fo}$$

A mechanical index higher than 0.7 is associated with bubble destruction. Several techniques enhance second harmonic signals from microbubbles (see Fig. 14-e2 on website). The pulse-inversion method sends out two ultrasound pulses of inverted (or out of) phase to myocardial tissue and microbubbles. With its linear property, myocardial tissue produces two ultrasound signals of inverted phase at the fundamental frequency that are canceled by each other, but with their nonlinear property, microbubbles produce residual signals from two nonlinearly reflected signals. An alternative method is pulse modulation, which sends out two successive pulses, one signal with half the amplitude of the other signal. The returning signal of half-amplitude is doubled and subtracted from the other full signal. From myocardial tissue with a linear property, both signals are canceled, but from microbubbles with a nonlinear property, some signals remain to be imaged.

Because a high mechanical index may destroy the microbubbles, especially at the apex, low mechanical index (0.4 to 0.5) harmonic imaging is used to enhance the LV endocardial border definition between the blood pool and adjacent tissue or even mass. It is also important to use a sufficient amount of contrast agent to opacify the entire cavity.

Left ventricular opacification (LVO) obtained with microbubbles improves the definition of the LV border (Fig. 14-16). This provides better quantitation of LV volume by the Simpson method. The correlation between LV volume measured with cardiac magnetic resonance (CMR) and that measured with echocardiography is better with the use of LVO. Regional wall motion analysis can also be better with LVO. This is especially helpful during stress echocardiography. In critically ill patients in an intensive care unit, LVO is frequently necessary to assist in the echocardiographic evaluation of LV contractility and ejection fraction (LVEF). Also, LVO is helpful in the evaluation of intracardiac thrombus or mass and pseudoaneurysm. The presence or absence of vascularity of an intracardiac or paracardiac mass demonstrated with contrast echocardiographic pixel intensity measurements has been found to be useful in distinguishing between thrombus and tumor (see Chap. 69).[29] Another diagnostically important use of LVO is the assessment of apical or mid-cavity hypertrophic cardiomyopathy (see Chap. 65), which is often missed or mistaken for a dyskinetic apical segment because the epicardial motion of the hypertrophic apex appears to bulge outward unless the apical endocardium is clearly visualized, which is possible with the use of a contrast agent (Fig. 14-17).

After microbubbles are destroyed by a high mechanical index (>1.5) of ultrasound, myocardium with normal perfusion is replenished by microbubbles within 5 to 7 cardiac cycles (or 5 seconds), imaged as opacified myocardium (Fig. 14-18); however, myocardium with no or less than normal replenishment of microbubbles because of the lack of or decreased perfusion appears dark or patchy. The destruction and replenishment of microbubbles can be imaged in real time, providing a visual assessment of myocardial contractility, as well as myocardial perfusion.[27] A myocardial perfusion defect may be more sensitive

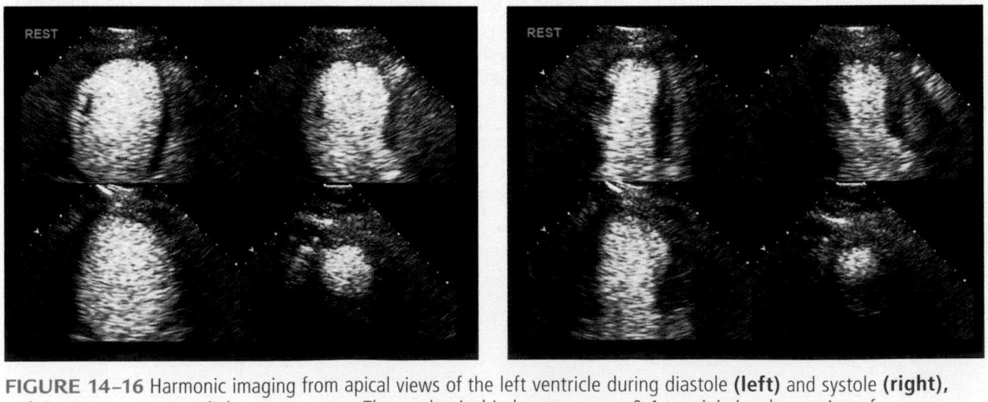

FIGURE 14–16 Harmonic imaging from apical views of the left ventricle during diastole **(left)** and systole **(right)**, with intravenous myocardial contrast agent. The mechanical index was set at 0.4 to minimize destruction of microbubbles. The definition of the left ventricular endocardial border is very clear with injection of contrast.

for the detection of myocardial ischemia than regional wall motion analysis in patients with chest pain syndrome.[30] Myocardial contrast perfusion imaging stress testing uses either dobutamine or a vasodilator such as dipyridamole or adenosine. Perfusion defects detected on myocardial contrast perfusion echocardiography with a vasodilator correlate well with perfusion defects seen on an exercise or dobutamine stress test, and perfusion defects demonstrated with myocardial contrast echocardiography correlate well with those seen on nuclear imaging (see Fig. 14-e3 on website) (see Chap. 16). No difference in sensitivity has been found between myocardial contrast echocardiography and SPECT for the detection of coronary artery disease (84 versus 82 percent, respectively).[31]

Theoretically, myocardial risk area, final infarct size, and amount of myocardial salvage by acute reperfusion therapy (a thrombolytic agent or percutaneous coronary intervention) can be measured with serial myocardial contrast perfusion echocardiography. In patients with acute myocardial infarction, the evaluation of myocardial viability soon after acute reperfusion therapy is possible with a myocardial contrast perfusion study.[32,33] After TIMI III coronary flow has been established with acute reperfusion therapy, almost one third of the patients may not recover myocardial function because of the "no reflow" phenomenon. TIMI III flow indicates the patency of the epicardial coronary artery but does not always indicate normal microvascular circulation. Myocardial perfusion imaging is a better way to assess the coronary microcirculation. We have performed contrast echocardiography with an intravenous contrast agent in patients who had revascularization (thrombolysis, percutaneous coronary intervention, or both) after acute myocardial infarction. Normal perfusion predicted functional recovery.[34] The accuracy of the technique was superior in myocardial segments supplied by the left anterior descending coronary artery, with a sensitivity of 80 percent and a specificity of 88 percent for detecting functional recovery. Therefore real-time intravenous myocardial contrast echocardiography is a helpful predictor of functional recovery of akinetic myocardium after myocardial infarction.

Myocardial contrast perfusion echocardiography has been an essential tool for alcohol ablation of the septal coronary artery in patients with obstructive hypertrophic cardiomyopathy (see Chap. 65).[35] Because the myocardial distribution of the septal perforator artery varies, knowledge about the amount of myocardium that would be damaged by the injection of alcohol into a septal perforator is critical before the procedure is performed.

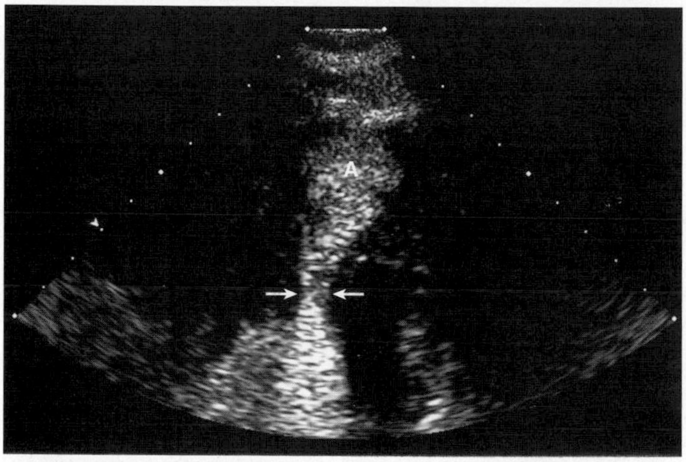

FIGURE 14–17 Apical view showing a mid cavity obstruction (arrows) that was not visualized clearly with 2D echocardiography without contrast injection. An apical pouch (A) is clearly seen. *(From Oh JK, Seward JB, Tajik AJ: The Echo Manual. 3rd ed. Philadelphia, Lippincott Williams & Wilkins, 2006. Used with permission of Mayo Foundation for Medical Education and Research.)*

CHAMBER QUANTITATION

The American Society of Echocardiography has published recommendations for chamber quantification with M-mode and 2D echocardiography.[3] It is critical that a method for chamber quantification be standardized because cardiac function is determined from the size of the chambers, which also frequently guides the strategy for patient management. It is recommended that the same range of normal values for chamber dimensions and volumes be used for both TEE and TTE (Tables 14-4 to 14-9).[3]

Left Ventricular Dimensions

Usually, LV dimensions are measured from 2D-guided M-mode echocardiograms of the LV at the level of mitral leaflet tips or the papillary muscle using the parasternal view (Fig. 14-19). If no significant regional wall motion abnormalities are present, the LV dimensions measured at the midventricular level can be used to calculate global LVEF (see later). The thicknesses of the ventricular posterior wall and the ventricular septum (from the leading edge to the trailing edge) are measured from the same M-mode echocardiogram. These values are used to calculate LV mass. The long-axis and short-axis dimensions of the ventricle can also be obtained directly from systolic and diastolic frames of the 2D parasternal long-axis view and apical view (Fig. 14-20). The LV end-diastolic and end-systolic dimensions are

TABLE 14–4 Reference Limits and Partition Values of Left Ventricular (LV) Size*

	Women				Men			
		Abnormal				Abnormal		
Measure	Reference Range	*Mildly*	*Moderately*	*Severely*	Reference Range	*Mildly*	*Moderately*	*Severely*
LV dimension								
Diastolic diameter	3.9-5.3	5.4-5.7	5.8-6.1	≥6.2	4.2-5.9	6.0-6.3	6.4-6.8	≥6.9
Diastolic diameter/BSA, cm/m²	2.4-3.2	3.3-3.4	3.5-3.7	≥3.8	2.2-3.1	3.2-3.4	3.5-3.6	≥3.7
Diastolic diameter/height, cm/m	2.5-3.2	3.3-3.4	3.5-3.6	≥3.7	2.4-3.3	3.4-3.5	3.6-3.7	≥3.8
LV volume								
Diastolic volume, mL	56-104	105-117	118-130	≥131	67-155	156-178	179-201	≥201
Diastolic volume/BSA, mL/m²	**35-75**	**76-86**	**87-96**	**≥97**	**35-75**	**76-86**	**87-96**	**≥97**
Systolic volume, mL	19-49	50-59	60-69	≥70	22-58	59-70	71-82	≥83
Systolic volume/BSA, mL/m²	**12-30**	**31-36**	**37-42**	**≥43**	**12-30**	**31-36**	**37-42**	**≥43**

*Boldface measures and volumes: recommended and best validated.

BSA = body surface area.

From Lang RM, Bierig M, Devereux RB, et al, Chamber Quantification Writing Group; American Society of Echocardiography's Guidelines and Standards Committee; European Association of Echocardiography: Recommendations for chamber quantification: A report from the American Society of Echocardiography's Guidelines and Standards Committee and the Chamber Quantification Writing Group, developed in conjunction with the European Association of Echocardiography, a branch of the European Society of Cardiology. J Am Soc Echocardiogr 18:1440, 2005.

TABLE 14–5 Reference Limits and Values and Partition Values of Left Ventricular Function*

Measure	Women				Men			
	Reference Range	Abnormal			Reference Range	Abnormal		
		Mildly	*Moderately*	*Severely*		*Mildly*	*Moderately*	*Severely*
Linear method								
Endocardial fraction shortening, %	27-45	22-26	17-21	≤16	25-43	20-24	15-19	≤14
Midwall fractional shortening, %	15-23	13-14	11-21	≤10	14-22	12-13	10-11	≤10
2D method								
Ejection fraction, %	**≥55**	**45-54**	**30-44**	**<30**	**≥55**	**45-54**	**30-44**	**<30**

*Boldface measures and values: recommended and best validated.
2D = two-dimensional.
From Lang RM, Bierig M, Devereux RB, et al, Chamber Quantification Writing Group; American Society of Echocardiography's Guidelines and Standards Committee; European Association of Echocardiography: Recommendations for chamber quantification: a report from the American Society of Echocardiography's Guidelines and Standards Committee and the Chamber Quantification Writing Group, developed in conjunction with the European Association of Echocardiography, a branch of the European Society of Cardiology. J Am Soc Echocardiogr 18:1440, 2005.

TABLE 14–6 Reference Limits and Partition Values of Left Ventricular (LV) Mass and Geometry*

Measure	Women				Men			
	Reference Range	Abnormal			Reference Range	Abnormal		
		Mildly	*Moderately*	*Severely*		*Mildly*	*Moderately*	*Severely*
Linear method								
LV mass, gm	67-162	163-186	187-210	≥211	88-224	225-258	259-292	≥293
LV mass/BSA, gm/m²	**43-95**	**96-108**	**109-121**	**≥122**	**49-115**	**116-131**	**132-148**	**≥149**
LV mass/height, gm/m	41-99	100-115	116-128	≥129	52-126	127-144	145-162	≥163
LV mass/height, gm/m	18-44	45-51	52-58	≥59	20-48	49-55	56-63	≥64
Relative wall thickness, cm	0.22-0.42	0.43-0.47	0.48-0.52	≥0.53	0.24-0.42	0.43-0.46	0.47-0.51	≥0.52
Septal thickness, cm	**0.6-0.9**	**1.0-1.2**	**1.3-1.5**	**≥1.6**	**0.6-1.0**	**1.1-1.3**	**1.4-1.6**	**≥1.7**
Posterior wall thickness, cm	**0.6-0.9**	**1.0-1.2**	**1.3-1.5**	**≥1.6**	**0.6-1.0**	**1.1-1.3**	**1.4-1.6**	**≥1.7**
2D method								
LV mass, gm	66-150	151-171	172-182	≥183	96-200	201-227	228-254	≥255
LV mass/BSA, gm/m²	**44-88**	**89-100**	**101-112**	**≥113**	**50-102**	**103-116**	**117-130**	**≥131**

*Boldface measures and values: recommended and best validated.
BSA = body surface area; 2D = two-dimensional.
From Lang RM, Bierig M, Devereux RB, et al, Chamber Quantification Writing Group; American Society of Echocardiography's Guidelines and Standards Committee; European Association of Echocardiography: Recommendations for chamber quantification: A report from the American Society of Echocardiography's Guidelines and Standards Committee and the Chamber Quantification Writing Group, developed in conjunction with the European Association of Echocardiography, a branch of the European Society of Cardiology. J Am Soc Echocardiogr 18:1440, 2005.

TABLE 14–7 Reference Limits and Partition Values of Right Ventricular (RV) and Pulmonary Artery (PA) Size

Dimension	Reference Range	Abnormal		
		Mildly	*Moderately*	*Severely*
RV dimension				
Basal RV diameter, cm	2.0-2.8	2.9-3.3	3.4-3.8	≥3.9
Mid RV diameter, cm	2.7-3.3	3.4-3.7	3.8-4.1	≥4.2
Base-to-apex length, cm	7.1-7.9	8.0-8.5	8.6-9.1	≥9.2
RVOT diameter				
Above aortic valve, cm	2.5-2.9	3.0-3.2	3.3-3.5	≥3.6
Above pulmonic valve, cm	1.7-2.3	2.4-2.7	2.8-3.1	≥3.2
PA diameter				
Below pulmonic valve, cm	1.5-2.1	2.2-2.5	2.6-2.9	≥3.0

From Lang RM, Bierig M, Devereux RB, et al, Chamber Quantification Writing Group; American Society of Echocardiography's Guidelines and Standards Committee; European Association of Echocardiography: Recommendations for chamber quantification: A report from the American Society of Echocardiography's Guidelines and Standards Committee and the Chamber Quantification Writing Group, developed in conjunction with the European Association of Echocardiography, a branch of the European Society of Cardiology. J Am Soc Echocardiogr 18:1440, 2005.

TABLE 14–8 Reference Limits and Partition Values of Right Ventricular (RV) Size and Function as Measured in the Apical Four-Chamber View

Measure	Reference Range	Abnormal		
		Mildly	*Moderately*	*Severely*
RV diastolic area, cm²	11-28	29-32	33-37	≥38
RV systolic area, cm²	7.5-16	17-19	20-22	≥23
RV fractional area change, %	32-60	25-31	18-24	≤17

From Lang RM, Bierig M, Devereux RB, et al, Chamber Quantification Writing Group; American Society of Echocardiography's Guidelines and Standards Committee; European Association of Echocardiography: Recommendations for chamber quantification: A report from the American Society of Echocardiography's Guidelines and Standards Committee and the Chamber Quantification Writing Group, developed in conjunction with the European Association of Echocardiography, a branch of the European Society of Cardiology. J Am Soc Echocardiogr 18:1440, 2005.

TABLE 14–9 Reference Limits and Partition Values for Atrial Dimensions and Volumes*

Measure	Women: Reference Range	Women: Abnormal Mildly	Women: Abnormal Moderately	Women: Abnormal Severely	Men: Reference Range	Men: Abnormal Mildly	Men: Abnormal Moderately	Men: Abnormal Severely
Atrial dimension								
LA diameter, cm	2.7-3.8	3.9-4.2	4.3-4.6	≥4.7	3.0-4.0	4.1-4.6	4.7-5.2	≥5.2
LA diameter/BSA, cm/m^2	1.5-2.3	2.4-2.6	2.7-2.9	≥3.0	1.5-2.3	2.4-2.6	2.7-2.9	≥3.0
RA minor axis dimension, cm	2.9-4.5	4.6-4.9	5.0-5.4	≥5.5	2.9-4.5	4.6-4.9	5.0-5.4	≥5.5
RA minor axis dimension/BSA, cm/m^2	1.7-2.5	2.6-2.8	2.9-3.1	≥3.2	1.7-2.5	2.6-2.8	2.9-3.1	≥3.2
Atrial area								
LA area, cm^2	<20	20-30	30-40	>40	<20	20-30	31-40	>40
Atrial volumes								
LA volume, mL	22-52	53-62	63-72	≥73	18-58	59-68	69-78	≥79
LA volume/BSA, mL/m^2	**22±6**	**29-33**	**34-39**	**≥40**	**22±6**	**29-33**	**34-39**	≥40

*Boldface measures and values: recommended and best validated.
BSA = body surface area; LA = left atrium; RA = right atrium.
From Lang RM, Bierig M, Devereux RB, et al, Chamber Quantification Writing Group; American Society of Echocardiography's Guidelines and Standards Committee; European Association of Echocardiography: Recommendations for chamber quantification: A report from the American Society of Echocardiography's Guidelines and Standards Committee and the Chamber Quantification Writing Group, developed in conjunction with the European Association of Echocardiography, a branch of the European Society of Cardiology. J Am Soc Echocardiogr 18:1440, 2005.

measured at the level of tips of the mitral leaflets as the largest and the smallest LV dimensions, respectively.

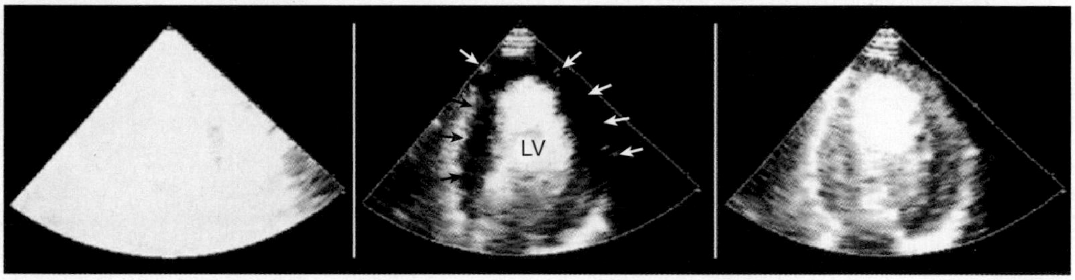

FIGURE 14–18 The process of performing real-time myocardial perfusion imaging. **A,** A high mechanical index of 1.7 is applied to the heart, destroying all microbubbles in the myocardium. **B,** Immediately after the destruction, no microbubbles are present (black areas indicated by arrows). **C,** Myocardium with normal perfusion is replenished with the microbubbles within five to seven cardiac cycles. LV = left ventricle. *(From Oh JK, Seward JB, Tajik AJ: The Echo Manual. 3rd ed. Philadelphia, Lippincott Williams & Wilkins, 2006. Used with permission of Mayo Foundation for Medical Education and Research. Courtesy of Namsik Chung, MD.)*

Right Ventricular Dimensions

Detection of RV dilatation may be the first clue to RV pressure or volume overload. Chronic RV pressure overload is accompanied by an increase in RV wall thickness in addition to dilatation, whereas in RV dysplasia, the RV wall is thin (see Chap. 64). The thickness of the RV wall is normally less than 5 mm and is measured best from the subcostal view at the peak of the R wave.[3] The size of the RV is measured best from the apical four-chamber view. An example of measuring the RV short axis and long axis is shown in Figure 14-21. The dimension of the LVOT is measured from the parasternal long-axis view, and the dimension of the RV outflow tract (RVOT) is measured from the parasternal short-axis view.

Left Atrial Size and Volume

Traditionally, LA dimension is determined from the parasternal long-axis view at end-systole. However, the size of the LA may be underestimated from the parasternal view because the chamber may enlarge longitudinally. Therefore LA size should also be measured from apical views (from the tip of the mitral valve to the posterior wall of the LA). However, LA volume is a better measure of LA size and provides better prognostic value. Four different methods are available for determining LA volume: (a) prolate ellipse, (b) biplane area-length, (c) biplane Simpson, and (d) 3D echocardiography.

The prolate ellipse method requires measuring LA dimensions from the parasternal long-axis view (D1) and apical four-chamber view (D2 and D3), from which LA volume is calculated as $D1 \times D2 \times D3 \times 0.523$. The biplane area-length method requires measurements of LA area from two orthogonal apical views (A1 and A2) and LA length (L), from which LA volume is calculated as $(0.85 \times A1 \times A2)/L$ (Fig. 14-22). When LA length is measured from two apical views, the shorter value is used to calculate LA volume. LA volume measured by the prolate ellipse method is usually 5 to 10 mL smaller than that measured by the biplane area-length method. Although LA volume can be measured by the biplane Simpson or 3D volumetric method, the biplane area-length method is currently the one recommended by the American Society of Echocardiography.[3] The influence of body surface area on LA volume is corrected by dividing LA volume by body surface area to calculate LA volume index. The normal value for all age groups for the LA volume index is 22 ± 6 mL/m^2. Left atrial size or volume is an important determinant of LA pressure, diastolic function, and prognosis.[36]

Left Ventricular Mass

Two methods are available for calculating LV mass from 2D echocardiography: the biplane area-length method and the truncated ellipsoid method. In both methods the LV wall volume is derived by subtracting intracavitary (endocardial) LV volume from the entire (epicardial) LV volume

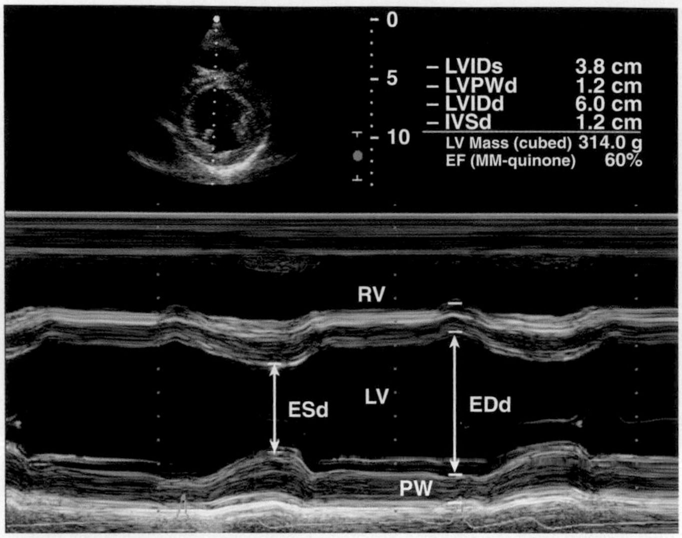

FIGURE 14–19 Two-dimensional-guided M-mode echocardiogram of left ventricle (LV) at the papillary muscle level. The LV end-diastolic internal dimension (EDd) measured at the onset of QRS is 60 mm, and the LV end-systolic internal dimension (ESd) is 38 mm. Therefore,

$$\text{LV ejection fraction (LVEF)} = \frac{60^2 - 38^2}{60^2} \times 100 = 60\% \text{ (uncorrected)}$$

If apical contractility is normal,

$$\begin{aligned} \text{Corrected LVEF} &= 60\% + [(100 - 60) \times 15\%] \\ &= 60\% + 6\% \\ &= 66\%. \end{aligned}$$

LV mass is also calculated from LV dimensions, posterior wall (PW) thickness, and ventricular septal (VS) thickness. RV = right ventricle. *(From Oh JK, Seward JB, Tajik AJ: The Echo Manual. 3rd ed. Philadelphia, Lippincott Williams & Wilkins, 2006. Used with permission of Mayo Foundation for Medical Education and Research.)*

including LV walls and ventricular septum. Myocardial mass is equal to the product of the volume and the specific gravity of the myocardium, 1.04 g/mL. LV mass can also be estimated from measurements of LV dimension and wall thicknesses on 2D or M-mode echocardiograms. Without measuring the major axis of the LV, LV mass is obtained from the LV short-axis dimension and a simple geometric cube formula. The following equation provides a reasonable determination of LV mass in grams:

$$1.04[(\text{LVID} + \text{PWT} + \text{IVST})^3 - \text{LVID}^3] \times 0.8 + 0.6$$

where LVID is the internal dimension, PWT is posterior wall thickness, IVST is interventricular septal thickness, 1.04 = specific gravity of the myocardium, and 0.8 is the correction factor. All measurements are made at end-diastole (at onset of the R wave) in centimeters.

Harmonic real-time 3D imaging has promised to be the most accurate echocardiographic measure for LV volume and mass. From a pyramidal volume data set, 3D echocardiography allows off-line selection of anatomically correct apical views without foreshortening. Tracing of endocardial and epicardial boundaries of anatomically correct, nonforeshortened apical views provides more accurate quantification of LV volume and mass. Compared with CMR, Mor-Avi and colleagues[37] showed that interobserver variability was 37 ± 19 percent of measured LV mass by 2D echocardiography and 7 ± 10 percent by real-time 3D echocardiography. Intraobserver variability was 19 ± 10 percent and 8 ± 5 percent, respectively.

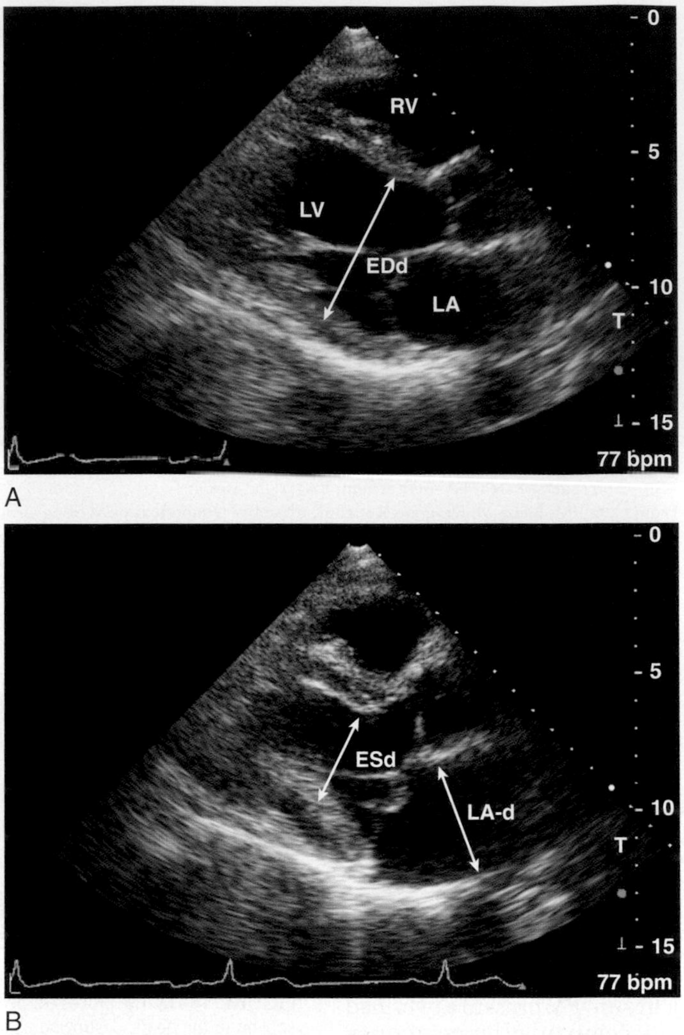

FIGURE 14–20 Measurement of LV dimensions from 2D echocardiography. Measurements of, **A,** diastolic dimensions and, **B,** systolic dimensions. Left ventricular (LV) end-diastolic dimension (EDd) and end-systolic dimension (ESd) are measured at the level of the mitral leaflet tips (at one-third the distance along the length of the long axis) from the parasternal long-axis view. The left atrial dimension (LA-d) is measured at end-systole, when it is largest. LA = left atrium; RV = right ventricle. *(From Oh JK, Seward JB, Tajik AJ: The Echo Manual. 3rd ed. Philadelphia, Lippincott Williams & Wilkins, 2006. Used with permission of Mayo Foundation for Medical Education and Research.)*

Left Ventricular Volume

With 2D echocardiography, LV volume is calculated best by the *modified Simpson method* or disk summation method (Fig. 14-23). The apical long axis is divided by the number of cylinders created within the LV, and the resulting distance (long-axis dimension ÷ number of cylinders) becomes the height of each cylinder. Therefore long-axis dimensions from two apical views should be similar to match the locations of each cylinder from two orthogonal views. In subjects with uniform contractility, the LV volume measured by single-plane disk summation is very close to that measured by the biplane Simpson method, which is preferred for LV volume measurements in patients with regional wall motion abnormalities. The endocardial borders of the LV can be traced manually or detected automatically with acoustic quantification or integrated backscatter information.[38] Reliable visualization of the LV endocardial blood-tissue border is a key for making reliable LV volume measurements with echocardiography. Contrast echocar-

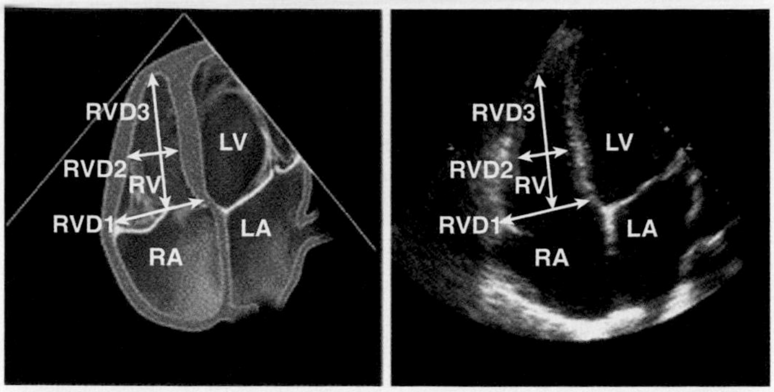

FIGURE 14–21 Measurements of right ventricular long-axis and short-axis dimensions (RVD1-RVD3) from apical four-chamber view. LA = left atrium; LV = left ventricle; RA = right atrium; RV = right ventricle. *(From Lang RM, Bierig M, Devereux RB, et al, Chamber Quantification Writing Group; American Society of Echocardiography's Guidelines and Standards Committee; European Association of Echocardiography: Recommendations for chamber quantification: A report from the American Society of Echocardiography's Guidelines and Standards Committee and the Chamber Quantification Writing Group, developed in conjunction with the European Association of Echocardiography, a branch of the European Society of Cardiology. J Am Soc Echocardiogr 18:1440, 2005. Used with permission.)*

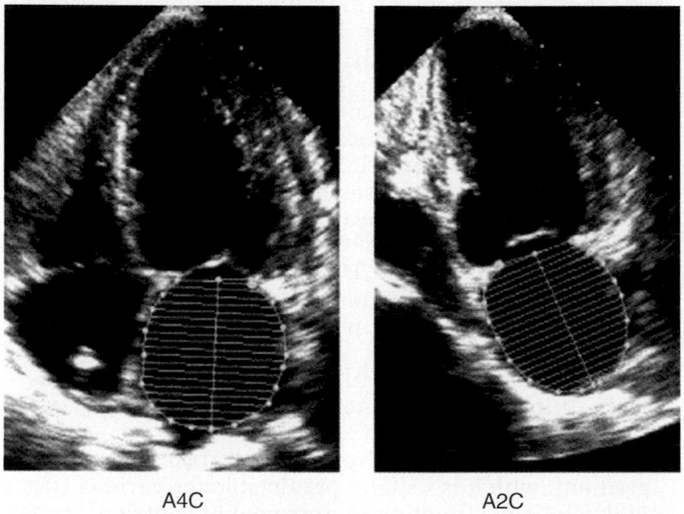

FIGURE 14–22 Left atrial volume measurement by biplane area-length method requires measurements of left atrial area from two orthogonal or apical views. A2C = apical 2-chamber view; A4C = apical 4-chamber view. *(From Lang RM, Bierig M, Devereux RB, et al, Chamber Quantification Writing Group; American Society of Echocardiography's Guidelines and Standards Committee; European Association of Echocardiography: Recommendations for chamber quantification: A report from the American Society of Echocardiography's Guidelines and Standards Committee and the Chamber Quantification Writing Group, developed in conjunction with the European Association of Echocardiography, a branch of the European Society of Cardiology. J Am Soc Echocardiogr 18:1440, 2005. Used with permission.)*

diography and harmonic imaging have improved definition of the endocardial border.

Early experience indicates that LV volume measurement is more reliable and accurate with real-time 3D echocardiography; this may well become the standard mode of measuring LV volume and LVEF in the future.[39] Comparison of real-time 3D echocardiography measurements of LV parameters with M-mode and 2D echocardiographic and CMR measurements showed that LV volume was underestimated by 2D echocardiography but much improved by real-time 3D echocardiography, with a mean difference of 4 ± 29 mL. However, the LVEF obtained with CMR was similar to that obtained with 2D and real-time 3D echocardiography. With 3D echocardiography, a real-time LV cast can be created

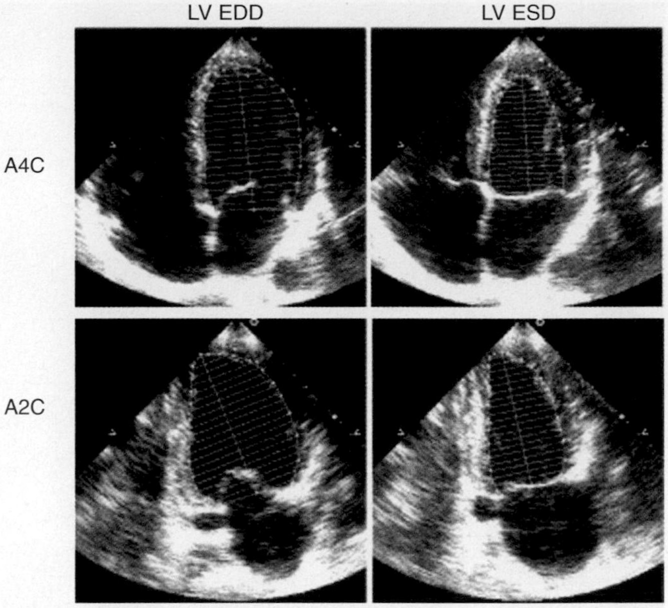

FIGURE 14–23 Left ventricular (LV) volume measurement by the biplane Simpson method requires two orthogonal apical views. LV is divided into 20 cylinders or disks, and their volumes are calculated and added to provide LV volume at end-diastole (LV EDD) and end-systole (LV ESD). A2C = apical 2-chamber view; A4C = apical 4-chamber view. *(From Lang RM, Bierig M, Devereux RB, et al, Chamber Quantification Writing Group; American Society of Echocardiography's Guidelines and Standards Committee; European Association of Echocardiography: Recommendations for chamber quantification: A report from the American Society of Echocardiography's Guidelines and Standards Committee and the Chamber Quantification Writing Group, developed in conjunction with the European Association of Echocardiography, a branch of the European Society of Cardiology. J Am Soc Echocardiogr 18:1440, 2005. Used with permission.)*

(Fig. 14-24) and regional volume changes can be displayed, which is useful for determining LV dyssynchrony.

EVALUATION OF SYSTOLIC AND DIASTOLIC FUNCTION

Systolic Functional Parameters

Echocardiography can measure several parameters as an expression of systolic function of the heart. These parameters are LVEF, fractional shortening, stroke volume and cardiac index, systolic tissue velocity of the mitral annulus and myocardium, strain, and regional wall motion analysis.

Left Ventricular Ejection Fraction

The most well-accepted expression of global LV function is LVEF. As the term indicates, it is a simple measure of how much end-diastolic volume is ejected from the LV with each contraction. Although it has many limitations, including load dependency, LVEF has been found to be a strong predictor of clinical outcome in almost all major cardiac conditions, and it is used to select optimal management strategies. In clinical practice, LVEF is frequently determined by "eye balling" 2D echocardiographic images of the LV. This visual assessment is reasonably reliable when performed by an experienced echocardiographer but varies widely among readers. Therefore LVEF should be measured more objectively whenever possible, using volumetric measurements as described by the following equation:

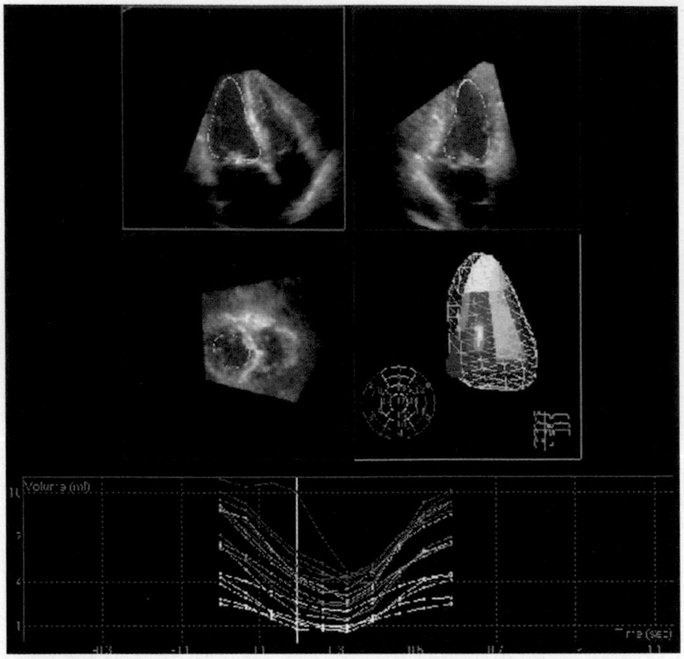

FIGURE 14–24 The left ventricular volume cast **(lower right)** was created from 3D echocardiography imaging. Regional left ventricular volume changes are shown in the plot at the bottom. The color of each line corresponds to the segment of the same color in the left ventricular cast. *(From Oh JK, Seward JB, Tajik AJ: The Echo Manual. 3rd ed. Philadelphia, Lippincott Williams & Wilkins, 2006. Used with permission of Mayo Foundation for Medical Education and Research.)*

$$LVEF = (LVEDV - LVESV)/LVEDV$$

where LVEDV and LVESV are LV end-diastolic volume and end-systolic volume, respectively.

LVEF can also be calculated from LV dimensions measured with M-mode or 2D echocardiography. M-mode or 2D echocardiographic measurement of LV dimensions from the mid ventricular level (see Fig. 14-19) is used to calculate LVEF as follows:

$$LVEF = (LVEDD^2 - LVESD^2)/LVEDD^2$$

where LVEDD and LVESD are end-diastolic dimension and end-systolic dimension, respectively. This equation is actually percentage change in LV area, or fractional shortening of the LV short axis, which equals LVEF if the apical long-axis dimension remains the same from diastolic phase to systolic contraction. Because the apical long axis normally shortens 10 to 15 percent with systole, an apical correction factor is added on the basis of the contractility of the apex; 5 to 7 percent for normal to hyperdynamic apical contraction, 3 percent for hypokinetic contraction, and 0 percent for akinetic apex.

Fractional Shortening

Fractional shortening (FS) is a percentage change in LV dimensions with each LV contraction:

$$FS = (LVEDD - LVESD)/LVEDD$$

This systolic function parameter is now rarely used for diagnosis or clinical decision making.

Stroke Volume

Stroke volume is the volume of blood ejected with each cardiac cycle as a final result of various factors affecting LV contraction. Stroke volume can be measured as the difference between LVEDV and LVESV obtained by the Simpson method or 3D echocardiography, as described. The difference should be equal to SV across the LVOT if there is no valvular regurgitation. If there is mitral regurgitation, regurgitant volume needs to be subtracted to obtain stroke volume across LVOT. LVOT stroke volume can also be obtained by the product of LVOT area and LVOT time velocity integral (TVI) (see "Hemodynamic Assessment").

Systolic Velocity of Myocardial Tissue or Mitral Annulus

The systolic component (S′) of the mitral annulus measured by TDI correlates well with LVEF and has been shown to be a good predictor of clinical outcome in various cardiovascular disorders.

Assessment of Diastolic Function

Assessment of diastolic function should be an integral part of an evaluation of cardiac function because about 50 percent of patients with heart failure have a preserved LVEF (see Chap. 26). Assessment of diastolic function requires an understanding of diastology and various means to evaluate diastolic function. Currently, echocardiography is the best noninvasive way to evaluate diastolic function and to estimate filling pressures. M-mode, 2D, and Doppler (blood flow, tissue, and color) echocardiography are all helpful in evaluating diastolic function. The following steps will ensure comprehensive assessment of diastolic function and the identification of heart failure related to diastolic dysfunction:

1. Look for M-mode and 2D echocardiographic evidence for diastolic dysfunction. Abnormal myocardial relaxation, an integral part of diastolic dysfunction, decreases the slope (in M-mode) and mitral annulus motion of early diastolic filling and increases LA size. LV wall thicknesses are usually, but not necessarily, increased.
2. Mitral inflow velocities reflect the transmitral pressure gradient, which is usually predictable for various stages of diastolic dysfunction. Assessment of ventricular compliance is possible from the configuration (velocities and flow duration) of mitral inflow velocities. Pulmonary vein flow velocities are also helpful.
3. Myocardial relaxation by tissue Doppler can be evaluated. Mitral annulus velocity (Ea) during early diastole correlates reasonably well with the status of myocardial relaxation (tau).
4. Mitral inflow velocities, Ea, mitral inflow propagation velocity, and their combination can estimate LV diastolic filling pressure at rest and with exercise.
5. Diagnosis of diastolic heart failure and separation of myocardial diastolic heart failure from pericardial diastolic heart failure (see "Pericardial Diseases" later) are possible from the above steps.

LV diastolic filling consists of a series of events that are affected by numerous factors including myocardial relaxation, compliance, cardiac rhythm, and pericardial compliance (see Chap. 21). Normal diastolic function ensures adequate filling of the ventricles during rest and exercise without an abnormal increase in diastolic pressure or pulmonary venous congestion. The initial diastolic event is myocardial relaxation,[40] an active energy-dependent process that causes LV pressure to decrease rapidly after the end of contraction. When LV pressure falls below LA pressure, the mitral valve opens, and rapid early diastolic filling begins. Under normal circumstances, a major determinant of the driving force of early diastolic filling is the elastic recoil caused by normal relaxation of the LV. Normally, 75 to 80 percent of LV filling occurs during this phase. During early diastolic filling, LV pressure continues to decrease until completion of myocardial relaxation (normally about 100 msec) before rising after reaching minimal pressure; this loss of positive driving force results in the deceleration of mitral inflow. Later, atrial contraction produces a positive transmitral pressure gradient and inflow, accounting for 20 to 25 percent of LV filling in normal subjects. The proportion of LV filling during the early and late diastolic phases depends on elastic recoil (suction), the rate of myocardial relaxation, chamber compliance, LA pressure, and heart rate. The LV filling pattern is the result of the transmitral pressure gradient produced by these various factors (Fig. 14-25).

The transmitral pressure gradient or the relationship between LA and LV pressures is accurately reflected by mitral inflow Doppler velocities.[20] Diastolic filling is usually classified initially on the basis of the peak mitral flow velocity of the early rapid filling wave (E), peak velocity of the late filling wave caused by atrial contraction (A), the E/A ratio, and deceleration time (DT), which is the time interval for the peak E velocity to reach zero baseline (see Fig. 14-25).

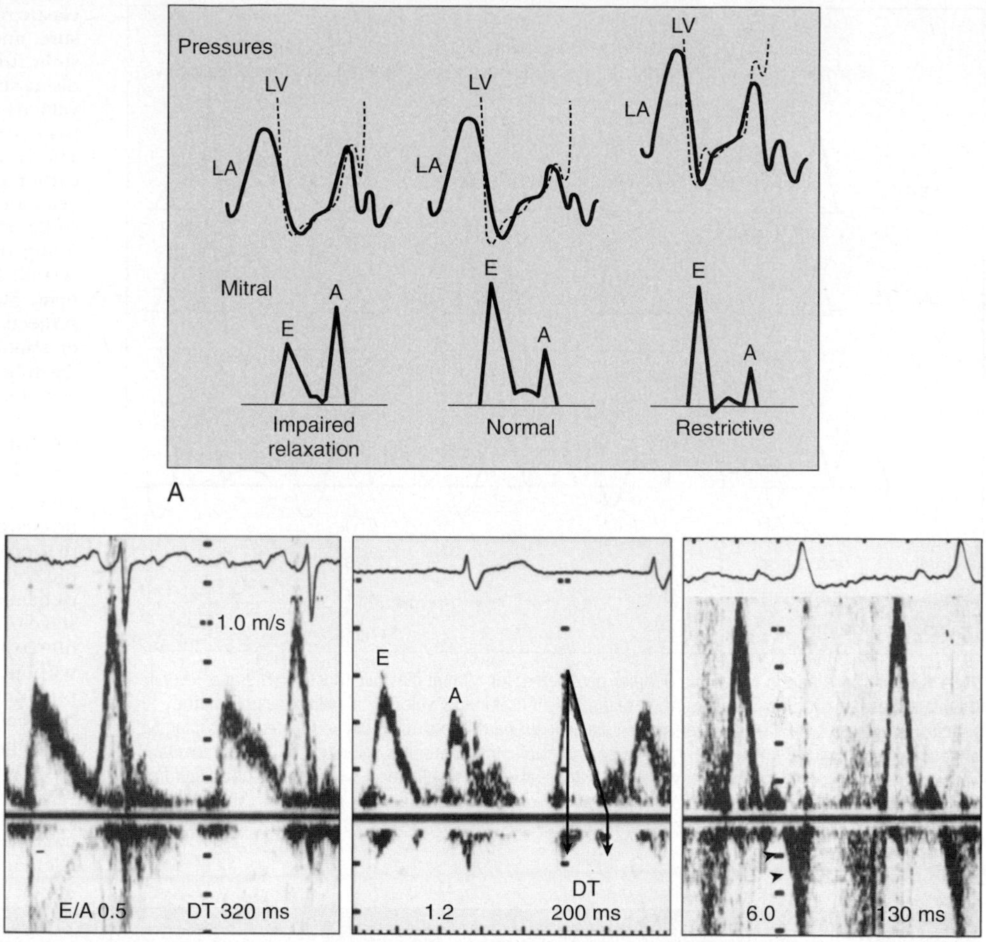

FIGURE 14–25 **A,** Left ventricular (LV) and left atrial (LA) pressure relationship and corresponding mitral inflow velocities in three different diastolic filling patterns: impaired relaxation, normal, and restrictive. **B,** Actual Doppler recordings of mitral inflow velocities, representing impaired relaxation **(left),** normal **(center),** and restrictive filling **(right)** patterns. Arrowheads indicate diastolic mitral regurgitation. A = late diastolic filling; DT = deceleration time; E = early diastolic filling. *(From Oh JK, Seward JB, Tajik AJ: The Echo Manual. 3rd ed. Philadelphia, Lippincott Williams & Wilkins, 2006. Used with permission of Mayo Foundation for Medical Education and Research.)*

With myocardial relaxation, the LV cavity elongates, expands laterally, and rotates. The longitudinal motion of the mitral annulus has been shown to correlate with the rate of myocardial relaxation. The velocity of the mitral annulus can be recorded by tissue Doppler imaging, which has become an essential part of evaluating diastolic function by echocardiography. Radial and circumferential function can also be assessed with speckle tracking strain imaging.[41,42]

Comprehensive assessment of diastolic filling and estimation of filling pressures by echocardiography require TDI, pulmonary vein Doppler, hepatic vein Doppler, and color M-mode of mitral inflow for propagation velocity (Vp)—sometimes with an alteration in a loading condition (Fig. 14-26). The Valsalva maneuver is used most frequently to decrease venous return by increasing intrathoracic pressure.[43]

GRADING OF DIASTOLIC DYSFUNCTION (OR DIASTOLIC FILLING PATTERN)

The grading of the diastolic filling pattern (or diastolic dysfunction) is based on several parameters (see Fig. 14-26).[20,44] In most (if not all) cardiac diseases, the initial diastolic abnormality is impaired relaxation. With further progression of disease and a mild-to-moderate increase in LA pressure, the mitral inflow velocity pattern appears similar to a normal filling pattern (pseudonormalized). With further decrease in LV compliance and increase in LA pressure, diastolic filling becomes restrictive. Most patients with restrictive filling are symptomatic and have a poor prognosis unless the restrictive filling can be reversed by treatment. However, restrictive filling may be irreversible and represent the end stage of diastolic heart failure. Therefore diastolic dysfunction can be graded according to the diastolic filling pattern[40]:

Grade 1 (mild dysfunction) = impaired relaxation with normal filling pressure

Grade 2 (moderate dysfunction) = pseudonormalized mitral inflow pattern

Grade 3 (severe reversible dysfunction) = reversible restrictive (high filling pressure)

Grade 4 (severe irreversible dysfunction) = irreversible restrictive (high filling pressure)

A grade 1 diastolic filling pattern usually implies a normal filling pressure despite a background of impaired myocardial relaxation. However, in patients with a marked relaxation abnormality, as in hypertrophic cardiomyopathy, the filling pressure can still be elevated with grade 1 mitral inflow velocity pattern (E/A < 1.0 and DT > 240 msec). This is classified as grade 1a (and hemodynamically should be similar to that for grade 2).

NORMAL DIASTOLIC FILLING PATTERN

In normal young subjects, LV elastic recoil is vigorous because of normal myocardial relaxation; therefore most filling is completed during early diastole. Thus E/A is usually ≥ 1.5, DT = 160-240 ms (septal), Ea ≥ 10 cm/s, E/Ea <8, and Vp ≥ 50 cm/s. Figure 14-27 shows mitral inflow, TDI, and color M-mode flow propagation in a young normal subject. This vigorous relaxation in normal subjects can also

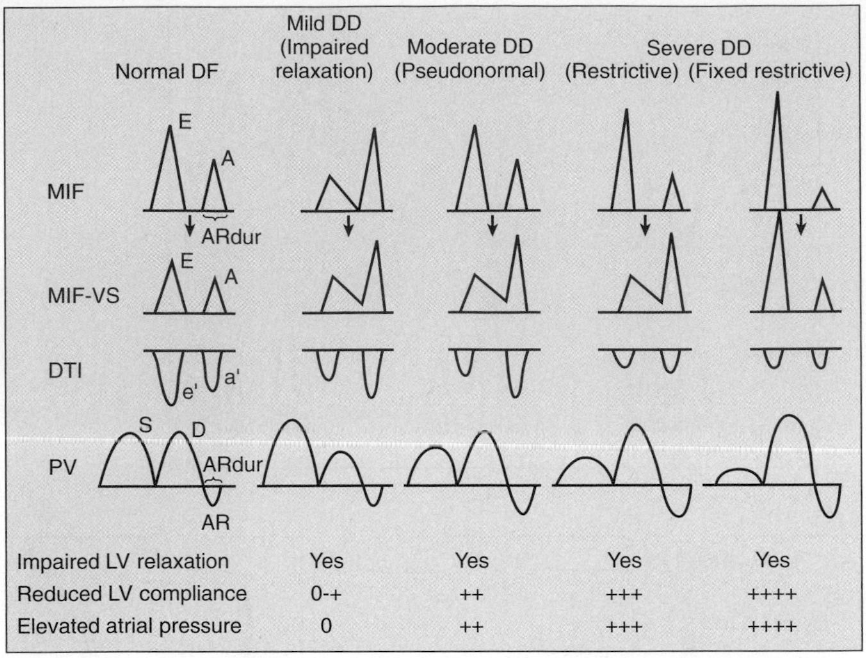

FIGURE 14–26 Diagram of various Doppler parameters for normal diastolic function (DF) and several stages of diastolic dysfunction (DD). A = late diastolic mitral inflow velocity; a′ = late diastolic mitral annulus velocity; AR = PV atrial reversal; D = diastolic forward PV velocity; DTI = Doppler tissue imaging; E = early diastolic mitral inflow velocity; e′ = early diastolic mitral annulus velocity; LV = left ventricular; MIF = mitral inflow; PV = pulmonary vein; S = systolic forward PV velocity; VS = Valsalva. *(Modified from Redfield MM, Jacobsen SJ, Burnett JC Jr, et al: Burden of systolic and diastolic ventricular dysfunction in the community: Appreciating the scope of the heart failure epidemic. JAMA 289:194-202, 2003. Used with permission.)*

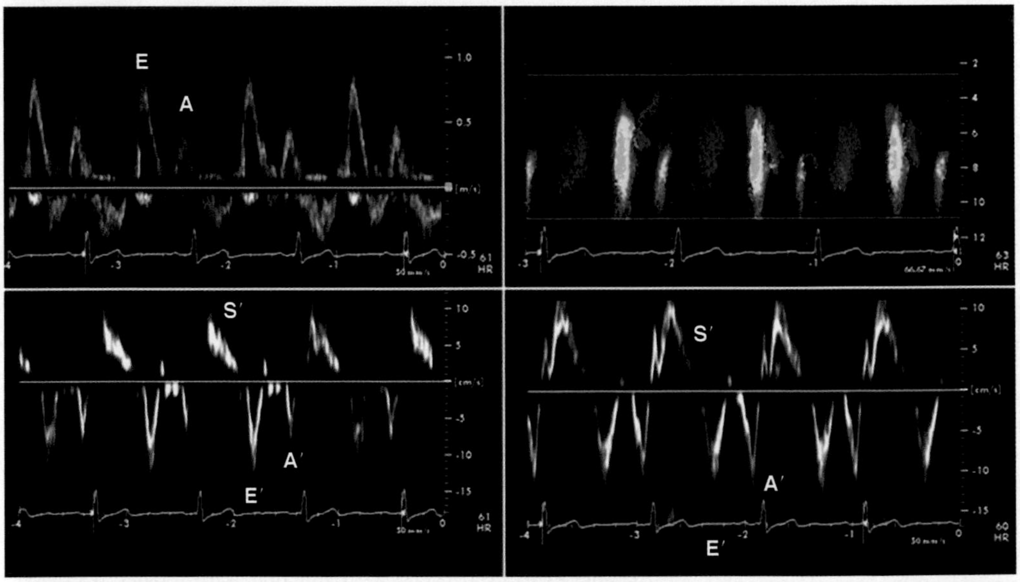

FIGURE 14–27 Mitral inflow, color M-mode, and tissue velocity of mitral annulus from a normal subject. Systolic velocity of the mitral annulus (S′) is normally >7 cm/sec. Early diastolic velocity (E′) of the mitral annulus is higher from the lateral annulus **(right lower)** than from the septal annulus **(left lower).** Color M-mode shows a rapid flow, with propagation velocity >50 cm/sec. A = late diastolic filling; A′ = late diastolic velocity; E = early diastolic filling.

be seen as active motion of the mitral annulus away from the apex during early diastole in parasternal long-axis and apical four-chamber views.

With normal myocardial relaxation, the longitudinal mitral annulus diastolic velocity pattern mirrors that of normal mitral inflow: early diastolic velocity (Ea) is higher than late diastolic velocity (Aa). Lateral annulus velocity is always higher (normal, >15 cm/sec) than septal Ea. Ea increases with exercise in healthy subjects so that E/Ea is similar at rest and with exercise (usually <8). With aging (see Chap. 75), there is a gradual decrease in the rate of myocardial relaxation, as well as in elastic recoil, resulting in slower decline of LV pressure, and filling becomes slower, producing a diastolic function pattern similar to grade 1 dysfunction discussed later. At roughly the age of 65 years, E velocity approaches A velocity, and in persons older than 70 years, the E/A ratio is usually less than 1.0.[45] The reversal of Ea/Aa occurs about 10 to 15 years earlier than that of E/A. Pulmonary venous flow velocities show similar changes with aging: Diastolic forward flow velocity decreases as more filling of the LV occurs at atrial contraction and systolic forward flow velocity becomes more prominent. Measurements of diastolic function in 1012 subjects without a history of cardiovascular disease or abnormal 2D echocardiograms showed that all diastolic function parameters are associated with age (Table 14-10).[45]

GRADE 1 DIASTOLIC DYSFUNCTION OR MILD DIASTOLIC DYSFUNCTION

An early abnormality of diastolic filling is abnormal myocardial relaxation. Typical cardiac conditions that produce abnormal relaxation are LV hypertrophy, hypertrophic cardiomyopathy, and myocardial ischemia or infarction, as well as aging. During this stage of diastolic dysfunction, an adequate diastolic filling period is critical to maintain normal filling without increasing filling pressure. As long as LA pressure remains normal, the pressure crossover between the LV and LA occurs late and the early transmitral pressure gradient is decreased. Consequently, the IVRT is prolonged. Mitral E velocity is decreased and A velocity is increased, producing an E/A ratio of less than 1, with prolonged DT. Pulmonary vein diastolic forward flow velocity (PVd) parallels mitral E velocity and is also decreased with compensatory increased flow in systole. The duration and velocity of pulmonary vein atrial flow reversal (PVa) are usually normal, but they may be increased if atrial compliance decreases or LV end-diastolic pressure is high. Ea and mitral flow propagation velocity are reduced, usually less than 7 cm/sec (at septal annulus) and less than 50 cm/sec, respectively. In most patients with the described mitral inflow velocity pattern, diastolic filling pressure is not increased and E/Ea is ≤ 8. In a subgroup of patients, E/Ea is greater than 15, with E/A less than 1. This pattern has been designated as grade 1a diastolic dysfunction to emphasize that filling pressure is increased while there is a typical grade 1 mitral inflow velocity pattern.

GRADE 2 DIASTOLIC DYSFUNCTION OR MODERATE DIASTOLIC DYSFUNCTION

This stage is also referred to as the *pseudonormalized mitral flow filling pattern,* and it represents a moderate stage of diastolic dysfunction.[20,44,45] As diastolic function worsens, the mitral inflow pattern goes through a phase resembling a normal diastolic filling pattern, that is, E/A ratio of 1 to 1.5 and normal DT (160 to 240 msec). This is the result of a moderately increased LA pressure superimposed on delayed myocardial relaxation. There are several means to differentiate the pseudonormal pattern from a true normal pattern in patients with grade 2 dysfunction:

1. Ea is usually less than 7 because myocardial relaxation is impaired.
2. Frequently, there is mid-diastolic flow because of marked impairment of myocardial relaxation (see Fig. 14-e4 on website).[46,47]

TABLE 14–10 Reference Ranges for Diastolic Function Parameters by Age*

	Age Groups, Yr					
Parameter	***45-49***	***50-54***	***55-59***	***60-64***	***65-69***	***≥70***
Mitral inflow						
E, m/sec	0.7 (0.5-0.9)	0.6 (0.5-0.9)	0.7 (0.5-0.9)	0.7 (0.5-0.9)	0.6 (0.4-0.8)	0.6 (0.4-1.0)
A, m/sec	0.5 (0.3-0.7)	0.5 (0.4-0.8)	0.6 (0.4-0.9)	0.6 (0.4-0.9)	0.7 (0.4-1.0)	0.8 (0.5-1.1)
E/A	1.3 (1.0-2.0)	1.2 (0.8-2.0)	1.2 (0.7-1.8)	1.0 (0.7-1.6)	1.0 (0.6-1.5)	0.8 (0.6-1.3)
E/(A-E at A)	1.50 (1.0-2.67)	1.40 (1.0-2.33)	1.29 (0.83-2.25)	1.20 (0.83-2.0)	1.00 (0.75-1.67)	1.00 (0.67-1.60)
DT, ms	208 (180-258)	217 (178-266)	210 (183-187)	222 (180-282)	227 (188-298)	242 (188-320)
A_{dur}, ms	140 (122-170)	147 (130-172)	147 (127-173)	147 (129-172)	150 (122-180)	150 (128-183)
Pulmonary vein flow						
P_S, m/sec	0.60 (0.40-0.80)	0.60 (0.40-0.80)	0.60 (0.40-0.80)	0.60 (0.40-0.80)	0.60 (0.50-0.80)	0.60 (0.40-0.80)
P_D, m/sec	0.40 (0.30-0.60)	0.40 (0.30-0.60)	0.40 (0.30-0.60)	0.40 (0.30-0.60)	0.40 (0.30-0.60)	0.40 (0.30-0.60)
P_S/P_D	1.25 (0.86-2.00)	1.40 (1.00-2.00)	1.40 (1.00-2.00)	1.50 (1.00-2.25)	1.60 (1.00-2.50)	1.67 (1.00-2.50)
$PVAR_{dur}$, ms	118 (100-140)	122 (103-142)	123 (105-157)	123 (103-160)	127 (110-152)	130 (112-170)
$PVAR_{dur}$-A_{dur}, ms	−25.0 (−53.3-0)	−25.0 (−51.7-0)	−21.6 (−50.0-11.7)	−23.3 (−51.7-13.4)	−21.7 (−55.0-12.5)	−22.3 (−51.7-31.6)
TDI-mitral annulus						
Septal						
E'_S, m/sec	0.10 (0.07-0.14)	0.09 (0.06-0.14)	0.09 (0.05-0.12)	0.09 (0.06-0.13)	0.08 (0.05-0.11)	0.07 (0.05-0.11)
A'_S, m/sec	0.10 (0.07-0.14)	0.10 (0.08-0.14)	0.11 (0.08-0.15)	0.11 (0.09-0.15)	0.11 (0.09-0.15)	0.11 (0.09-0.15)
E/E'_S	6.67 (4.62-11.25)	7.00 (4.55-11.67)	7.78 (4.62-13.33)	7.64 (5.0-12.0)	8.57 (5.45-13.33)	8.57 (4.55-16.67)
Lateral						
E'_L, m/sec	0.13 (0.09-0.17)	0.12 (0.08-0.16)	0.11 (0.07-0.15)	0.10 (0.07-0.15)	0.09 (0.07-0.12)	0.08 (0.05-0.11)
A'_L, m/sec	0.11 (0.07-0.16)	0.11 (0.07-0.15)	0.11 (0.08-0.16)	0.12 (0.08-0.17)	0.12 (0.09-0.16)	0.12 (0.08-0.18)
E/E'_L	5.38 (3.75-7.78)	5.45 (3.75-8.89)	6.0 (3.85-10.0)	6.67 (4.62-8.89)	7.0 (4.17-11.25)	7.78 (5.0-14.0)
Valsalva maneuver						
VS E/A	1.00 (0.60-1.33)	1.00 (0.57-1.33)	0.80 (0.44-1.25)	0.71 (0.43-1.20)	0.60 (0.40-1.00)	0.57 (0.30-1.00)
VS E/(A-E at A)	1.33 (0.80-2.50)	1.25 (0.67-3.00)	1.00 (0.60-2.50)	1.00 (0.50-2.00)	0.75 (0.50-1.67)	0.71 (0.33-1.50)
ΔE/A	0.37 (0-1.0)	0.40 (−0.05-1.0)	0.37 (0-1.0)	0.36 (−0.04-0.8)	0.31 (0-0.64)	0.29 (−0.04-0.70)
ΔE/(A-E at A)	0.0 (−1.3-1.0)	0.07 (−1.33-0.75)	0.17 (−1.0-0.77)	0.13 (−0.83-0.75)	0.17 (−0.58-0.57)	0.17 (−0.75-0.63)
Index of myocardial performance						
LIMP	0.30 (0.10-0.50)	0.30 (0.20-0.60)	0.30 (0.20-0.60)	0.40 (0.20-0.60)	0.40 (0.20-0.60)	0.40 (0.20-0.60)

*Data are median (5th and 95th percentile).

A=late diastolic mitral flow velocity; A_{dur}=duration of late mitral flow; A'_L=lateral mitral annulus velocity with atrial contraction; A'_S=late diastolic lateral annular velocity; DT=deceleration time of early diastolic mitral flow; E=early diastolic mitral flow velocity; E'_L=early diastolic lateral annular velocity; E'_S=early diastolic septal annular velocity; ΔE/A=change in E/A with Valsalva; ΔE/A-E=change in E/A-E at A with Valsalva; LIMP=left ventricular index of myocardial performance; P_D=pulmonary vein diastolic flow velocity; P_S=pulmonary vein systolic flow velocity; $PVAR_{dur}$=duration of pulmonary vein atrial flow reversal; TDI=tissue Doppler imaging; VS=peak Valsalva.

From Munagala VK, Jacobsen SJ, Mahoney DW, et al: Association of newer diastolic function parameters with age in healthy subjects: A population-based study. J Am Soc Echocardiogr 16:1049, 2003.

3. A decrease in preload, by having the patient sit or perform the Valsalva maneuver, may be able to unmask the underlying impaired relaxation of the LV, decreasing the E/A ratio by more than 0.5. If A velocity increases with the Valsalva maneuver, it is a positive sign.

4. Normal-appearing mitral inflow may occur in the setting of systolic dysfunction or increased wall thickness because impaired relaxation is expected as the baseline diastolic function without increased filling pressure in those situations, and a normal E/A ratio suggests that increased LA pressure is masking the abnormal relaxation.

5. Shortening of mitral A duration in the absence of a short PR interval and prolonged PVa exceeding mitral A duration.

6. Decreased rate of flow propagation (<45 cm/sec) by color M-mode of mitral inflow occurs. This is less reliable in patients with normal LV cavity size.

GRADE 3-4 DIASTOLIC DYSFUNCTION OR SEVERE DIASTOLIC DYSFUNCTION

Severe diastolic dysfunction is also termed *restrictive filling or physiology* and can be present in any cardiac abnormality or in a combination of abnormalities that produce decreased LV compliance and markedly increased LA pressure. Examples include decompensated congestive systolic heart failure, advanced restrictive cardiomyopathy, severe coronary artery disease, acute severe aortic regurgitation, and constrictive pericarditis. Early rapid diastolic filling into a less compliant LV causes a rapid increase in early LV diastolic pressure, with rapid equalization of LV and LA pressures producing a shortened DT. Atrial contraction increases LA pressure, but A velocity and duration are shortened because LV pressure increases even more rapidly. When LV diastolic pressure is markedly increased, there may be diastolic mitral regurgitation during mid-diastole or with atrial relaxation. Therefore restrictive filling with severe diastolic dysfunction is characterized by increased E velocity, decreased A velocity (<<E) with E/A ratio greater than 2, and shortened DT (<160 ms) and IVRT (<70 ms). Systolic forward flow velocity in the pulmonary vein is decreased because of increased LA pressure and decreased LA compliance (Fig. 14-28).

Because myocardial relaxation is impaired in patients with a restrictive filling pattern, mitral annulus Ea is reduced (<7 cm/sec). E/Ea is usually greater than 15. Flow propagation velocity may not be reduced in restrictive filling when the LV cavity is small and systolic function is well preserved. The Valsalva maneuver may reverse the restrictive filling pattern to a grade 1 to 2 pattern, indicating the reversibility of high filling pressure (grade 3 diastolic filling). However, even if the restrictive filling pattern does not change with the Valsalva maneuver, reversibility cannot be excluded because the Valsalva maneuver may not be adequate or filling pressure is too high to be altered by the Valsalva maneuver.

Evaluation of Cardiac Function by Cardiac Time Intervals[14]

Cardiac time intervals provide valuable mechanistic and diagnostic insight into systolic and diastolic function of the heart. In the 1960s the duration of isovolumic contraction (IVCT) and preejection period (PEP) were studied exten-

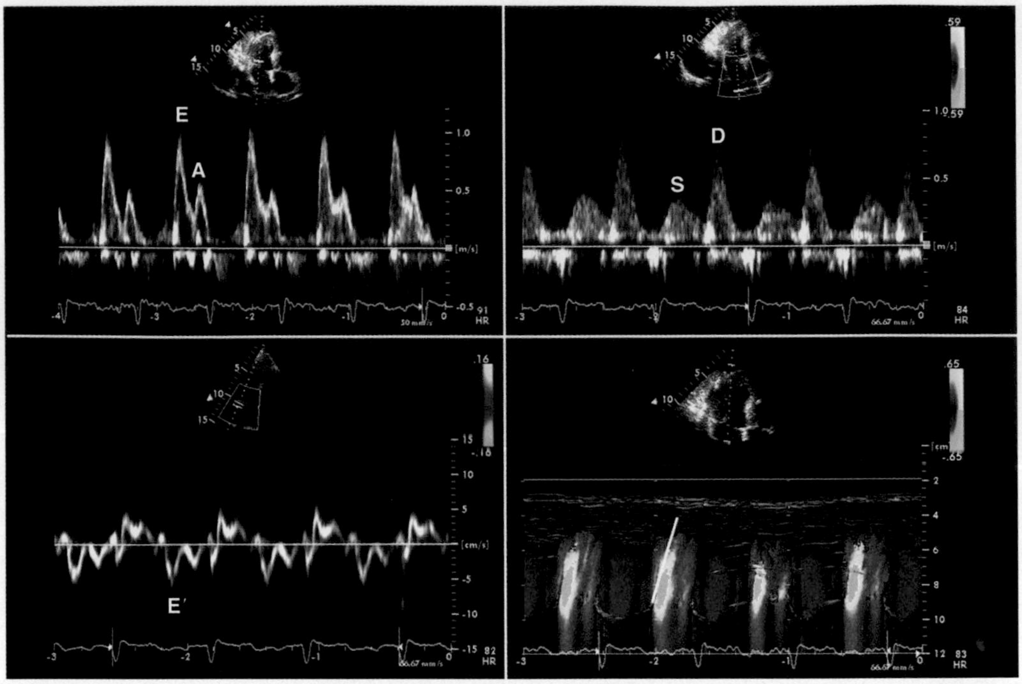

FIGURE 14–28 Mitral inflow **(upper left)**, pulmonary vein velocity **(upper right)**, septal mitral annular tissue Doppler **(lower left)**, and color M-mode **(lower right)** from a patient with restrictive diastolic dysfunction.

sively as a measure of cardiac systolic function, and LV ejection time (LVET) was used as a measure of LV stroke volume. Although myocardial dysfunction prolongs PEP and shortens LVET, these intervals are also influenced by many hemodynamic and electrical variables. Weissler and colleagues derived an index (PEP/LVET) called *systolic time interval,* which was less heart-rate dependent as a measure of LV systolic function. Since IVRT is also affected by LV function, Mancini and colleagues incorporated IVRT into an index called the *isovolumic index,* derived as (IVCT + IVRT)/LVET. The sum of IVCT and IVRT was measured by subtracting LVET from the peak of the R wave on the electrocardiogram (ECG) to the onset of mitral valve opening. The isovolumic index was considered more sensitive for cardiac dysfunction than the systolic time interval because it contains IVRT, as well as IVCT. However, the interval from the R wave peak to the onset of mitral valve opening contains an interval of electromechanical delay, which can be pronounced in patients with left bundle branch block. With the advent of Doppler echocardiography, it has become easier to determine cardiac time intervals more reliably. Tei and colleagues proposed a myocardial performance index (IMP or Tei index) that is independent of the electromechanical delay, (IVCT + IVRT)/LVET, with Doppler echocardiography used to identify the exact onset of isovolumic contraction.[48]

The time intervals necessary for calculating IMP are easily obtained with Doppler echocardiography and TDI,[22] as well as with M-mode echocardiography.[49] The normal value is 0.39 ± 0.05, and its mean value is 0.59 ± 0.10 in those with dilated cardiomyopathy. The index of myocardial performance was evaluated for the RV, especially in patients with pulmonary hypertension. This index was the single most powerful variable for differentiating patients with primary pulmonary hypertension from normal subjects (0.93 ± 0.34 versus 0.28 ± 0.04) (see Chap. 73). It may have an important role in assessing RV function. The Tei index has been well correlated with invasive measurements of ventricular function in an animal model.[50]

When myocardial relaxation is normal, the opening of the mitral valve is initiated by rapid suction of the LV; hence the onset of mitral valve opening is close to the onset of early diastolic movement (or velocity) of the mitral annulus.[15,21] However, if myocardial relaxation is delayed, the mitral valve opens by high LA pressure. Therefore the onset of diastolic motion of the mitral annulus follows the onset of mitral inflow. The time interval has been correlated with the degree of impairment in myocardial relaxation and LV filling pressure. With worsening of diastolic function, the time interval lengthens.[15,51]

Clinical Applications of Diastolic Function Assessment

Assessment of diastolic function echocardiographically has the following clinical applications and should be an integral part of an echocardiography examination:

1. Estimation of filling pressures at rest and with exercise—In patients with reduced LV systolic function (LVEF < 35 percent), mitral inflow E/A ratio ≥ 1.5 and DT ≤ 140 msec indicate increased filling pressures. However, these parameters do not have a good correlation with filling pressure in patients with normal LVEF and diastolic heart failure. For all degrees of LVEF, E/Ea is the best parameter to estimate filling pressure; pulmonary capillary wedge pressure (PCWP) is ≥ 20 mm Hg if E/Ea is ≥ 15 and PCWP is normal if E/Ea is < 8.[52] In case of 8 ≤ E/Ea < 15, pulmonary vein, flow duration, and the Valsalva maneuver can help estimate PCWP. In an important subset of patients with diastolic dysfunction, PCWP is normal at rest but increases only with exertion, causing exertional dyspnea. It is feasible and reliable to estimate PCWP with exercise by recording mitral inflow and annulus velocity.[53,54] In a normal population with normal diastolic function, filling pressure rarely increases with exercise.[53] Diastolic dysfunction (or impaired myocardial relaxation) is usually a prerequisite for developing exercise-induced high filling pressure. These patients increase cardiac output at the expense of increased filling pressure. In this situation, mitral E velocity increases while annulus Ea velocity does not increase as much or at all, resulting in an increase in E/Ea ratio. E/Ea correlates well with simultaneously measured PCWP with exercise, as well as during resting stage, and a ratio greater than 15 indicates PCWP greater than 20 mm Hg with exercise (see Fig. 14-e5 on website).[55]
2. Diagnosis of diastolic heart failure, cardiomyopathies, and constrictive pericarditis—Knowledge of the diastolic filling pattern and filling pressures allows the detection of cardiac diseases that are frequently missed or not suspected clinically, especially when the LVEF is normal. Patients with diastolic heart failure and normal LVEF have a large LA volume and evidence of impaired relaxation, as well as increased filling pressure. There are several reports that TDI of myocardial relaxation can diagnose the presence of various forms of cardiomyopathy (hypertrophic cardiomyopathy, Fabry disease, and amyloidosis) even before frank phenotypic manifestation.[56,57] The detection of constrictive pericarditis has been made much easier with the use of echocardiographic diastolic parameters and TDI (see Pericardial Diseases later).
3. Prognosis—Diastolic echocardiographic parameters, E, E/A, DT, E/Ea, and LA volume, have been found to be powerful prognostic indicators for various conditions.[58-62] Even in asymptomatic patients, the presence of diastolic dysfunction portends a poor clinical outcome.[44]

Although diastolic filling is affected by various factors, the direction of its change or progression is predictable in patients with known heart disease. Therefore assessment of the diastolic filling pattern allows LV filling pressures and LV compliance and relaxation to be estimated and understood so that optimal treatment strategies can be offered to symptomatic patients with diastolic dysfunction.

ECHOCARDIOGRAPHY IN HEART FAILURE (see Chap. 25)

Echocardiography is the single most useful test in the evaluation of patients with heart failure. It is important to demonstrate objective evidence of structural or functional abnormalities to explain a patient's symptoms of heart failure because the symptoms are not specific and more than one third of patients with a clinical diagnosis of heart failure may not actually have heart failure. Moreover, even when someone presents with symptoms typical of heart failure, a diagnostic test, most frequently echocardiography, is required to establish the underlying cause so that an optimal management strategy can be implemented. When a cardiac structural abnormality or systolic dysfunction is responsible for heart failure, it is usually obvious on 2D echocardiography. In systolic heart failure, however, echocardiography has many roles beyond the recognition of decreased LVEF because dilatation of the LV alters intracardiac geometry and hemodynamics, leading to increased morbidity and mortality. New medication strategies, devices, and surgical therapies are being developed to manage systolic heart failure. Echocardiography has been essential not only in identifying structural and hemodynamic abnormalities associated with systolic heart failure but also in monitoring responses to various therapies.

As well documented for the past 20 years, LV volume is one of the most important prognostic indicators in patients with ischemic or dilated cardiomyopathy. With LV remodeling and progressive dilatation of the heart—initially an adaptive response to myocardial damage—the LV becomes more spherical and the mitral annulus is dilated, with apical displacement of the mitral leaflets causing functional mitral valve regurgitation (see Chap. 62). The combination of LV dilatation and mitral valve regurgitation results in increased filling pressure, symptoms of heart failure, and death. It was demonstrated in the BEST trial that among various echocardiographic parameters, LV end-diastolic volume, DT of mitral E velocity, which is a surrogate for PCWP, and severity of mitral valve regurgitation were the strongest predictors of survival for patients with an LVEF less than or equal to 35 percent.[63] Because a smaller LV with less mitral regurgitation is associated with better functional capacity and survival, there are many management strategies for reducing LV volume and mitral regurgitation including surgical, pacing and other percutaneous devices, medications, and surgical revascularization. In heart failure trials, echocardiography is a valuable tool for measuring or assessing LV dimensions, volumes, sphericity index, severity of mitral regurgitation, diastolic filling parameters, and pulmonary artery systolic pressure.

Biventricular pacing improves functional status and survival of patients with reduced LVEF and ventricular conduction delay (see Chap. 25). Echocardiography has been used to assess the success of biventricular pacing by documenting a smaller LV volume, increased LVEF, increased dP/dT, and less mitral regurgitation, which are all signs of reverse remodeling. Another potentially critical role of echocardiography in biventricular pacing is to identify the patients who will benefit from the therapy because 30 to 50 percent of patients who receive biventricular pacing may not have improvement. Currently, mechanical dyssynchrony indexes obtained with TDI velocities are considered to be best for this (Fig. 14-29). Time intervals from the onset of QRS to the time of peak systolic velocity from 2 to 12 segments of the LV are used to determine the maximum or standard deviation interval.[64,65] The maximum interval of 100 msec or standard deviation interval of 34 msec was found to have the highest predictive power for identifying a positive responder. However, it has been discovered that such intervals identified with TDI are also present in normal subjects and patients without a decreased LVEF or conduction delay. Instead, time intervals from the QRS to the peak negative strain from 12 segments have been found to correlate better with LV remodeling parameters and hemodynamic improvement after cardiac resynchronization therapy.[66] Further clinical experience and simplification of current strain imaging procedure are required to use echocardiography routinely to identify positive responders to cardiac resynchronization therapy.

It has been well established that about 50 percent of patients with new onset of heart failure have a normal LVEF (see Chap. 26). This condition is often difficult to diagnose with 2D echocardiography alone, although this method can provide diagnostic clues. Compared with a normal heart, a heart with diastolic dysfunction has less vigorous mitral annulus motion during early diastole, corresponding to the period of active myocardial relaxation; the LV wall tends to be thicker than normal; and LA size is increased. These abnormalities suggest that the patient's diastolic function is abnormal and a more detailed Doppler assessment is required (as discussed in the previous section).

If mitral inflow velocity clearly demonstrates a restrictive filling pattern or high filling pressure at the resting stage, the diagnosis of diastolic heart failure or constrictive pericarditis is usually secure. TDI of the septal mitral annulus is helpful in differentiating pseudonormal from true normal mitral inflow velocities and differentiating constrictive pericarditis from myocardial diseases. It is more problematic when an evaluation of diastolic function shows relatively normal filling pressure or predominantly impaired myocardial relaxation at rest. In this situation, right heart failure, a pulmonary process, and a noncardiopulmonary process should be considered. Another important clinical condition that needs to be considered is exercise-induced increased filling pressure responsible for the symptoms of shortness of breath with exertion. Therefore filling pressure needs to be assessed with exercise, as well as at rest.

When plasma levels of brain natriuretic peptide (BNP) and mitral E/Ea ratio were correlated with PCWP, the correlation was better for the mitral E/Ea ratio than for BNP.[67] BNP has been shown to be helpful in triaging patients with dyspnea in the emergency department, but we should be mindful that the sensitivity and specificity of BNP for increased filling pressure is not optimal and probably lower than the echocardiographic estimation of filling pressure. Even when high filling pressure is detected with BNP in patients with heart failure, echocardiography is necessary to establish a cause and to provide optimal treatment. For patients with heart failure and normal LVEF, optimal therapy has not been established, although there are several large, ongoing clinical trials to identify the most efficacious management strategy in diastolic heart failure, and echocardiography is an integral part of these trials for identifying ideal patients and monitoring the response of various therapies.

CORONARY ARTERY DISEASE (see Chap. 54)

Evaluation of coronary artery disease is the most common use of echocardiography. From the diagnosis of coronary

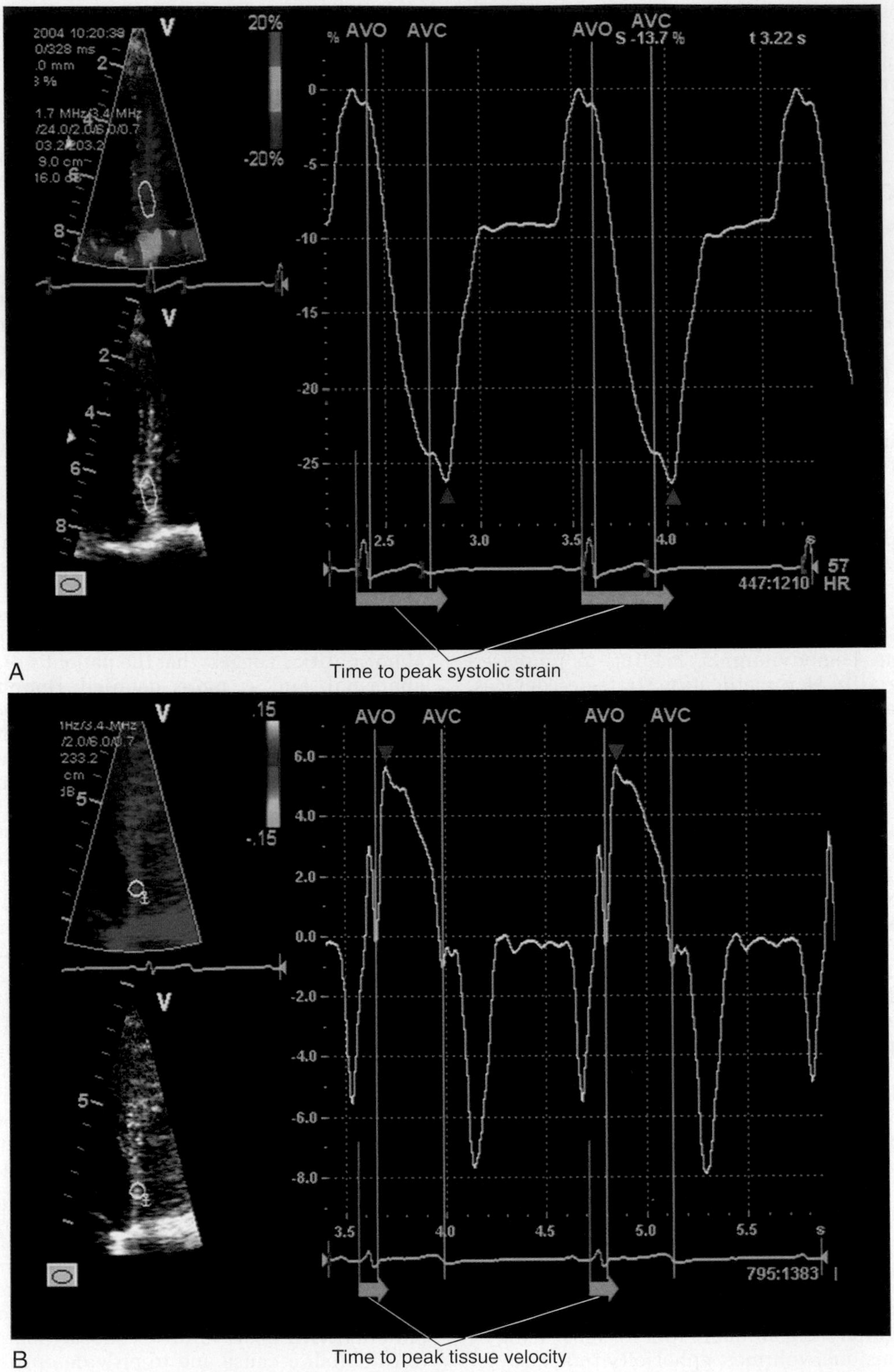

FIGURE 14–29 Measurement of intraventricular dyssynchrony by tissue velocity and strain imaging. **A,** Recording of strain from the basal segment of the ventricular septum from the apical four-chamber view. Time to peak systolic strain is measured from onset of QRS to the peak negative value including the postsystolic shortening. The timing of the peak negative strain is when shortening of the myocardium is maximum. **B,** Recording of tissue velocity from the basal segment of the ventricular septum. Peak systolic velocity is the positive wave during the ejection period. Time to peak tissue velocity is from onset of QRS to the positive peak velocity. The time interval is determined from 2 to 12 segments to measure intraventricular dyssynchrony. *(From Oh JK, Seward JB, Tajik AJ: The Echo Manual. 3rd ed. Philadelphia, Lippincott Williams & Wilkins, 2006. Used with permission of Mayo Foundation for Medical Education and Research.)*

artery disease with resting or stress echocardiography to the detection of a complication of acute myocardial infarction and prognostication using wall motion score, diastolic function, and stress-induced changes, echocardiography is helpful clinically. Myocardial perfusion, diastolic function, and contractility become abnormal immediately after the onset of ischemia, which can be detected readily with echocardiography,[68] even before other ischemic manifestations. Exercise or pharmacological stress echocardiography is valuable in evaluating myocardial viability and prognosis, as well as in detecting coronary artery disease.[69,70]

From the parasternal, apical, and sometimes subcostal imaging windows, 2D echocardiography can visualize all LV wall segments. For purposes of regional wall motion analysis, the American Society of Echocardiography has recommended a 16-segment model or, optionally, a 17-segment model[71] with an addition of the apical cap (Fig. 14-30). The following numerical score is assigned to each wall segment on the basis of its contractility as assessed visually: 1 = normal (>40 percent thickening with systole); 2 = hypokinesis (10 to 30 percent thickening); 3 = severe hypokinesis to akinesis (<10 percent thickening); 4 = dyskinesis; and 5 = aneurysm. On the basis of this wall motion analysis scheme, a wall motion score index (WMSI) is calculated to semiquantitate the extent of regional wall motion abnormalities:

$$\text{WMSI} = \frac{\text{Sum of wall motion scores}}{\text{Number of segments visualized}}$$

A normally contracting LV has a WMSI of 1, and the index increases as wall motion abnormalities become more severe. When 2D echocardiography was performed simultaneously with an injection of sestamibi in patients with acute STEMI (myocardial infarction with ST-segment elevation on the ECG), the overall correlation between the WMSI and the perfusion defect was good. Patients with a WMSI greater than 1.7 had a perfusion defect greater than 20 percent. The correlation was better for patients with an anterior wall myocardial infarction than for those with an inferior or lateral wall myocardial infarction with a smaller infarct size. A small area of subendocardial ischemia may not demonstrate wall motion abnormality, but contrast echocardiography can demonstrate a rim of subendocardial perfusion defect.

Moreover, the myocardium may remain akinetic for a period of time after successful coronary reperfusion in patients with acute myocardial infarction. Therefore knowledge of both myocardial contractility and perfusion is vital for the management of patients with coronary artery disease.

Echocardiography can be helpful in the evaluation of chest pain, especially during active chest pain. The absence of LV wall motion abnormalities during chest pain usually, but not always, excludes myocardial ischemia or infarction, and the presence of regional wall motion abnormalities has a high sensitivity for detecting myocardial ischemia or infarction, although it is not specific. Myocardial contrast imaging for perfusion provides incremental diagnostic value for patients with chest pain. When compared with gated single photon emission computed tomography (SPECT), myocardial contrast imaging was found to have a high concordance rate (77 to 84 percent).[30] Occasionally, echocardiography may be useful in detecting not an ischemic but another potentially life-threatening cause of chest pain syndrome, such as pulmonary embolism, aortic dissection, or cardiac tamponade (see later). However, a routine use of echocardiography in this setting requires availability of appropriately trained personnel to perform echocardiography and interpret its findings.

Echocardiography in Patients with Acute Myocardial Infarction (see Chaps. 51 and 52)

In patients with acute myocardial infarction, echocardiography has several important roles: (a) diagnosis and exclusion of acute myocardial infarction in patients with prolonged chest pain and nondiagnostic ECG findings, (b) estimation of the amount of myocardium at risk and final infarct size after reperfusion therapy, (c) evaluation of patients with unstable hemodynamics and detection of infarct complications, (d) evaluation of myocardial viability, and (e) risk stratification.

A 2D echocardiographic analysis of regional wall motion abnormalities is helpful even in patients with ST-elevation myocardial infarction (STEMI). When a patient presents with a STEMI, the affected myocardium is usually akinetic or dyskinetic. After the myocardium has been reperfused successfully within an appropriate time, it becomes more contractile. The improvement in regional myocardial contractility is evident within 24 to 48 hours and continues for several days to months. Therefore follow-up 2D echocardiographic imaging is useful in detecting reperfused myocardial segments or infarct expansion.

Persistent akinesis does not always indicate failed reperfusion. When the myocardium remains akinetic while being viable, low-dose dobutamine, contrast, or strain imaging echocardiography may be helpful to demonstrate its viability (see Chap. 48).[18,34,72,73]

In patients undergoing elective coronary angioplasty, systolic strain was reduced and postsystolic strain was increased, but delayed during transient ischemia.[74] Relaxation of ischemic myocardial segments is impaired and, as a consequence, the physiological early diastolic thinning and lengthening are replaced by ongoing postsystolic thickening and shortening.[75] Therefore regional strain or strain rate can be used as a marker of acute ischemia.

DETECTION OF MECHANICAL COMPLICATIONS OF ACUTE MYOCARDIAL INFARCTION

With effective acute reperfusion therapy during acute myocardial infarction, the incidence of mechanical complications from myocardial infarction has decreased; also, the timing of these events has changed. However, because these can be life threatening when they occur, reliable, timely identification of infarct-related complications is critical for optimal management. Two-dimensional and Doppler echocardiography with color flow imaging should be the first imaging modality to evaluate a clinical situation with a suspected mechanical complication or a patient with unstable hemodynamics. In this situation, TEE has become a very important imaging tool for obtaining diagnostic images under the most difficult clinical situations including in the critical care unit, in intubated patients and postoperative patients, and even during cardiopulmonary resuscitation, as well as in patients in whom precordial echocardiography is not possible for various reasons.[76] The presence of normal systolic function in a critically ill or hemodynamically unstable patient should lead immediately to the suspicion of a mechanical complication.

NEW SYSTOLIC MURMUR: VENTRICULAR SEPTAL RUPTURE, PAPILLARY MUSCLE RUPTURE, AND ACUTE LVOT OBSTRUCTION

The differential diagnosis of a new systolic murmur in patients with acute myocardial infarction includes infarct-related ventricular septal rupture, papillary muscle dysfunction or rupture, pericardial rub, and acute LVOT obstruction. After physical examination, echocardiography is the next logical noninvasive diagnostic procedure for all patients with a new murmur, especially for those who are hemodynamically unstable. Infarct-related ventricular septal defect is diagnosed by demonstration of a disrupted ventricular septum with a left-to-right shunt. The defect is always located in the region of the thinned myocardium with dyskinetic motion. The diagnosis usually can be established with a 2D TTE examination (Fig. 14-31). TEE may be necessary in a small subgroup of patients with a suboptimal precordial study (see Fig. 14-e6 on website). Peak flow velocity across the rupture measured with

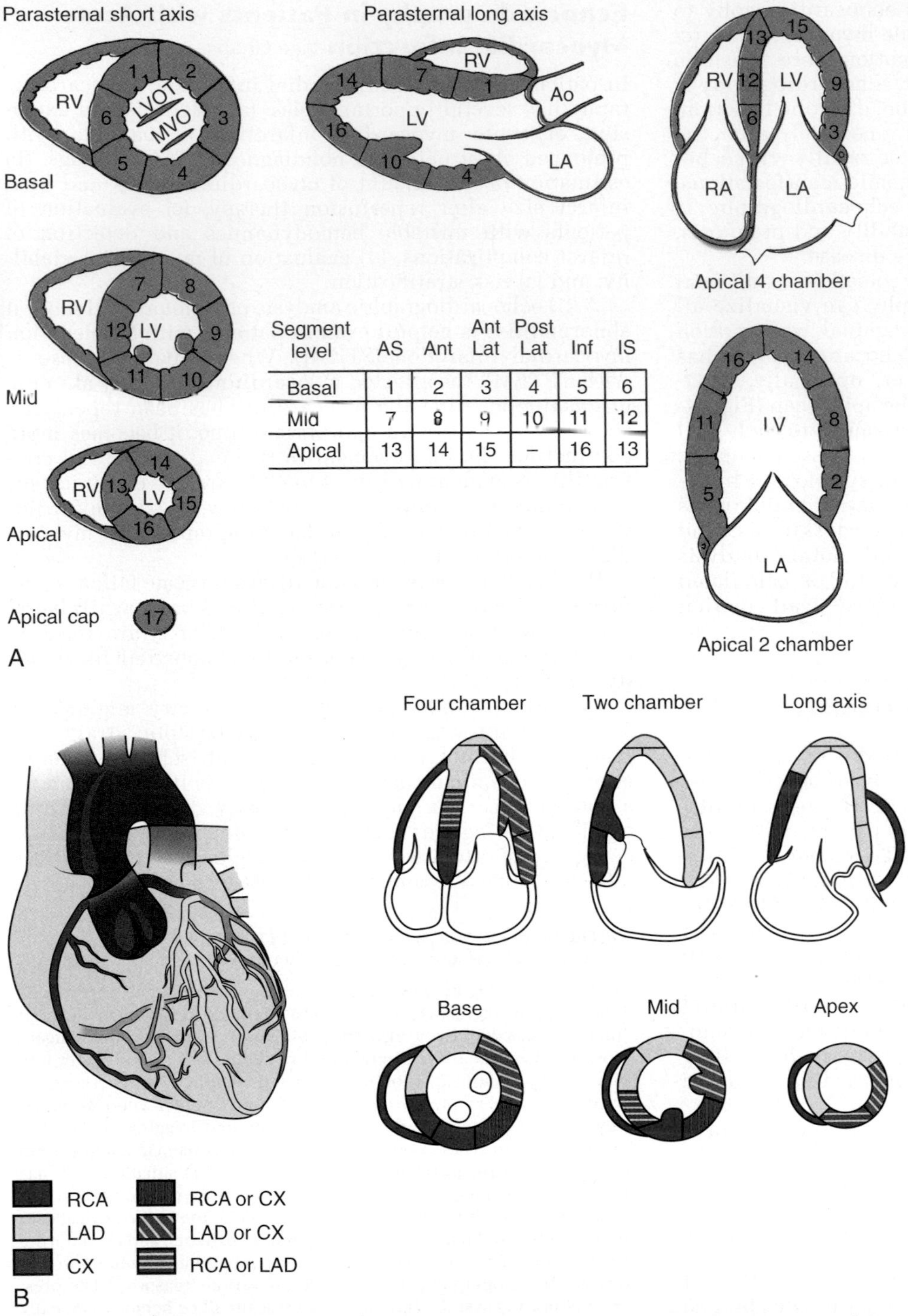

Segment level	AS	Ant	Ant Lat	Post Lat	Inf	IS
Basal	1	2	3	4	5	6
Mid	7	8	9	10	11	12
Apical	13	14	15	–	16	13

FIGURE 14–30 A, Diagrammatic cross sections of the left ventricle to show 17 segments for wall motion analysis. **B,** Left ventricular segments from three apical views and mid parasternal short-axis view with the corresponding coronary artery distribution. Cx = circumflex artery; LAD = left anterior descending artery; RCA = right coronary artery. *(**A,** From Oh JK, Seward JB, Tajik AJ: The Echo Manual. 3rd ed. Philadelphia, Lippincott Williams & Wilkins, 2006. Used with permission of Mayo Foundation for Medical Education and Research. **B,** Modified from Lang RM, Bierig M, Devereux RB, et al, Chamber Quantification Writing Group; American Society of Echocardiography's Guidelines and Standards Committee; European Association of Echocardiography: Recommendations for chamber quantification: A report from the American Society of Echocardiography's Guidelines and Standards Committee and the Chamber Quantification Writing Group, developed in conjunction with the European Association of Echocardiography, a branch of the European Society of Cardiology. J Am Soc Echocardiogr 18:1440, 2005. Used with permission.)*

continuous wave Doppler imaging can be used to estimate RV systolic pressure. When the rupture is located at the inferoseptum, the RV is usually involved by myocardial infarction, which portends a poor prognosis. An inferoseptal ventricular rupture can have a serpiginous septal tear, and an anteroapical ventricular septal rupture may be extended to an LV free wall rupture.

Acute mitral regurgitation is another important cause of systolic murmur. It is related to (a) LV global or regional remodeling, (b) papillary muscle dysfunction, (c) papillary muscle rupture (partial or complete), and (d) acute systolic anterior motion of the mitral valve. For optimal management, it is important to recognize the underlying cause of ischemic mitral regurgitation because papillary muscle rupture mandates urgent mitral valve replacement or repair, but mitral regurgitation caused by papillary muscle dysfunction or annulus dilatation may improve with afterload reduction or coronary revascularization (or both) (see Chap. 62). Mitral regurgitation caused by acute systolic anterior motion is managed by fluid, a beta blocker, or, occasionally, a pure alpha-agonist.

Hemodynamically, papillary muscle rupture is the most serious complication involving the mitral valve. The patients usually have a small infarct in the distribution of the right coronary or circumflex coronary artery. Because the posteromedial papillary muscle is supplied by a single coronary artery (as compared with the dual supply of the anterolateral papillary muscle), rupture of the posteromedial papillary muscle is more frequent. Echocardiography is the best way to diagnose papillary muscle dysfunction and rupture (Fig. 14-32; see also Fig. 14-e7 on website). Papillary muscle rupture can be partial (incomplete) or complete. The severity of mitral regurgitation is assessed with Doppler color flow imaging. Because patients with severe mitral regurgitation usually present with hemodynamic decompensation, TEE may be necessary to establish clearly the diagnosis and to assess the severity of mitral regurgitation. After papillary muscle rupture has been diagnosed, urgent mitral valve replacement with or without coronary revascularization is necessary for survival (see Chap. 62). Ischemic mitral regurgitation in the setting of chronic LV remodeling is discussed later.

A less known, but clinically important, entity resulting in new systolic murmur and an unstable hemodynamic condition is acute dynamic LVOT obstruction, which is related to the compensatory hyperdynamic motion of the posterior and inferolateral walls resulting in systolic anterior motion of the mitral leaflet, which causes mitral regurgitation, as well as the obstruction. It is more common after anterior wall myocardial infarction in elderly women who have basal septal hypertrophy caused by hypertension. It also has been noted in one third of patients with apical ballooning syndrome.[77] Patients with acute LVOT obstruction can develop severely unstable hemodynamics including shock and pulmonary edema. The most appropriate therapies are fluids, beta blockers, alpha-agonists, avoidance of vasodilators, and inotropics. This condition is not uncommon during the postoperative period in patients who receive inotropic support.

FREE WALL RUPTURE AND PSEUDOANEURYSM

Cardiac free wall rupture produces a sudden hemodynamic collapse caused by cardiac tamponade (from hemopericardium) and electromechanical dissociation. Alternatively, a patient may present

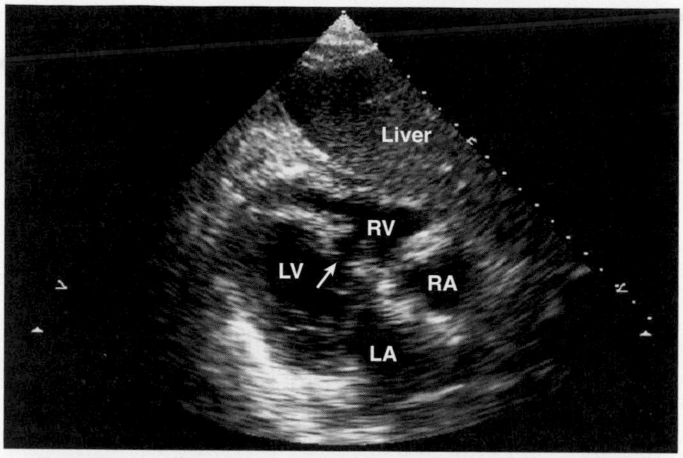

A

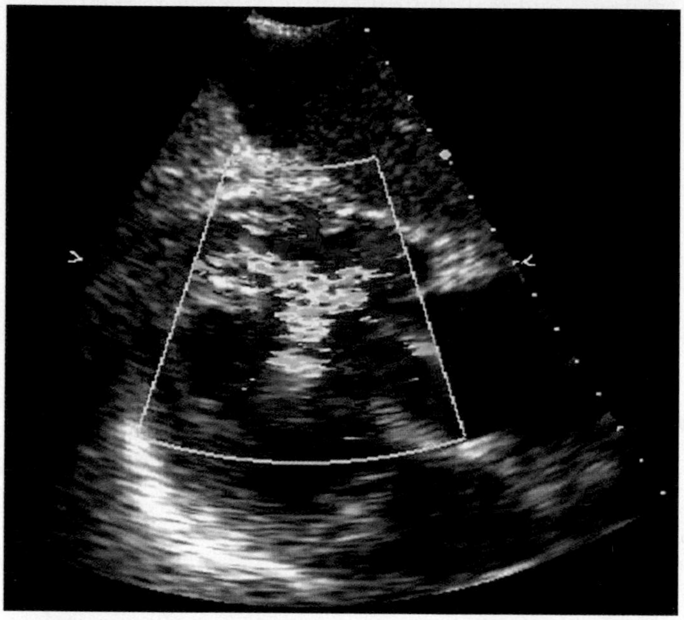

B

FIGURE 14–31 **A,** Transthoracic subcostal view showing a large inferoventricular septal defect (arrow). **B,** Color flow imaging showing a shunt from the left to right ventricle via the ventricular septal defect. LA = left atrium; LV = left ventricle; RA = right atrium; RV = right ventricle. *(From Oh JK, Seward JB, Tajik AJ: The Echo Manual. 3rd ed. Philadelphia, Lippincott Williams & Wilkins, 2006. Used with permission of Mayo Foundation for Medical Education and Research.)*

subacutely with syncope, hypotension, recurrent chest pain, or emesis (or some combination of these). Two-dimensional TTE may not be able to show the site of rupture but only demonstrate a pericardial effusion with or without Doppler characteristics of pericardial tamponade. The presence of pericardial effusion alone is not sufficient to diagnose a free wall rupture because pericardial effusion is common after acute myocardial infarction. Contrast echocardiography and/or color flow imaging may help in identifying the rupture site. Negative echocardiographic findings should not exclude myocardial rupture if clinical suspicion is high. In this case, another imaging technique such as CMR should be considered. In some cases, a pseudoaneurysm forms after a free wall rupture is contained within a limited portion of the pericardial space (most frequently in the posterior wall, followed by the lateral and apical walls). A pseudoaneurysm is traditionally characterized by a small neck communication between the LV and aneurysmal cavity (the ratio of the diameter of entry and the maximal diameter of the pseudoaneurysm is <0.5). However, it may have a wide neck communication (Fig. 14-33). There is always to-and-fro blood flow through the rupture site that can be documented with Doppler and color flow imaging. The clinical features of chronic pseudoaneurysm are nonspecific, and its detection is frequently incidental. Half of the patients have evidence of a mass on chest radiograph. Although there is concern that

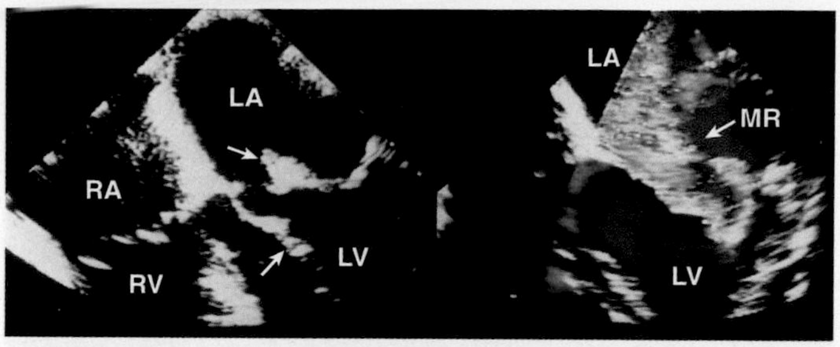

FIGURE 14–32 Transesophageal echocardiographic (TEE) images showing rupture and dysfunction of papillary muscle with severe mitral valve regurgitation. **Left,** This was the first complete rupture of papillary muscle diagnosed with TEE at Mayo Clinic. Transverse view (using monoplane) shows a ruptured papillary muscle prolapsing into the left atrium (LA) during diastole and attached to the posterior mitral leaflet (arrow in left atrium); arrow in left ventricle (LV) indicates the anterior mitral leaflet. **Right,** Color flow imaging shows severe mitral regurgitation with a broad mitral regurgitation (MR) jet. RA = right atrium; RV = right ventricle. *(From Patel AM, Miller FA Jr, Khandheria BK, et al: Role of transesophageal echocardiography in the diagnosis of papillary muscle rupture secondary to myocardial infarction. Am Heart J 118:1330, 1989. Used with permission.)*

pseudoaneurysms have a high incidence of rupture compared with true aneurysms, death caused by cardiac rupture is infrequent in patients with chronic pseudoaneurysm, even without surgical repair.[25]

Occasionally, a free wall rupture does not extend through the entire thickness of the wall and is contained by the epicardial layer (subepicardial aneurysm) (see Fig. 14-e8 on website).[78]

True LV Aneurysm and Thrombus

Compared with a pseudoaneurysm, a true aneurysm contains all layers of the myocardium and is characterized by myocardial thinning and bulging motion during systole. True aneurysm formation is related to transmural myocardial infarction and is found most frequently at the apex, followed by the inferobasal area. A ventricular aneurysm is the consequence of infarct expansion, which indicates a poor prognosis. Ventricular aneurysms frequently harbor a thrombus and can be the focus of malignant ventricular arrhythmias. Two-dimensional echocardiography has become the most practical and reliable imaging modality for detecting LV thrombus. It is important to differentiate thrombus from chordae or artifacts frequently seen at the apex. Characteristically, a thrombus has a nonhomogeneous echo density with a margin distinct from the underlying wall, which is akinetic to dyskinetic. Contrast echocardiography is also helpful in distinguishing LV thrombus from other structures.[29]

Evaluation of Left Ventricular Remodeling and Ischemic Mitral Regurgitation

LV remodeling represents progressive LV dilatation and systolic dysfunction after acute myocardial infarction. The LV becomes enlarged and has a more spherical shape, LVEF decreases, and mitral leaflets are pulled more apically, allowing an increasing amount of mitral regurgitation, all of which result in worsening of heart failure and death. Clinical trials have demonstrated lessening of the remodeling process or reverse remodeling with beta-blockade, angiotensin-converting enzyme inhibitors, and biventricular pacing. Large clinical trials are addressing the importance of surgical revascularization, surgical resection and reconstruction, passive constraint device, and mitral valve procedure in this patient population. Echocardiography is essential in identifying these patients and assisting clinical trials in LV remodeling by providing detailed information about LV size, LV volume, regional wall motion analysis,

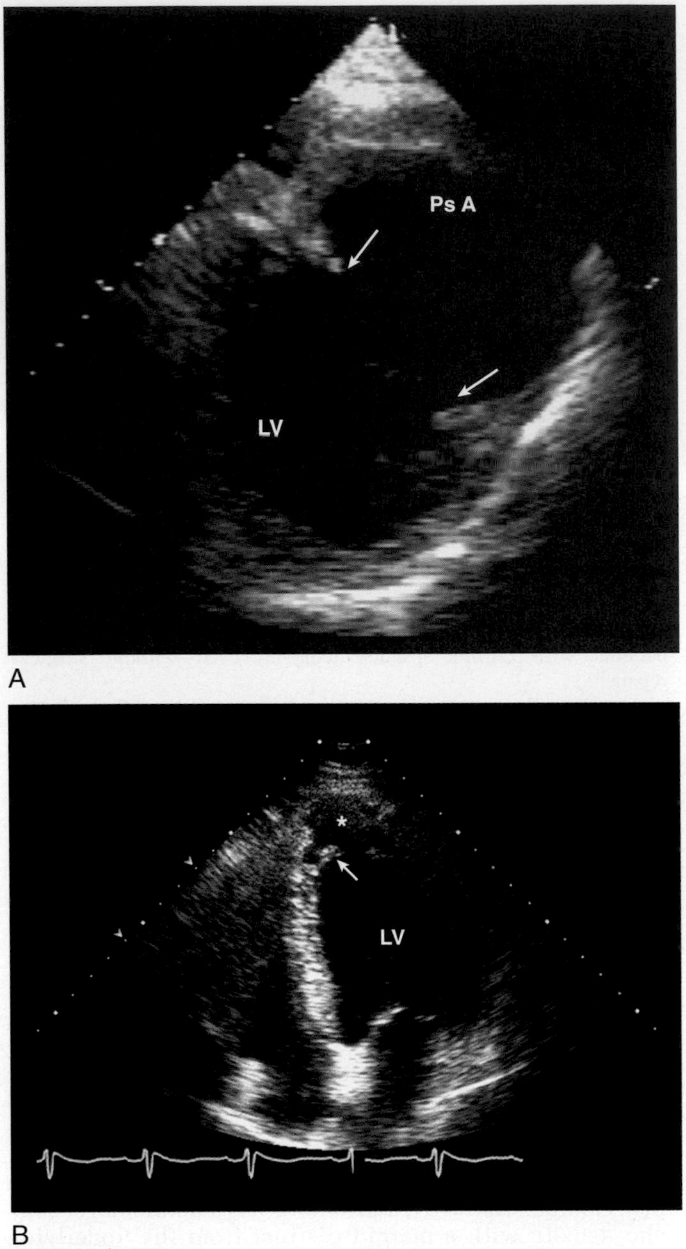

FIGURE 14–33 **A,** Parasternal short-axis view showing a tear or rupture of the anterolateral wall of the left ventricle (LV) communicating with a pseudoaneurysm (PsA) cavity. The space between the arrows is the mouth of the aneurysm cavity, which is relatively large. The myocardial rupture was repaired surgically. The rupture was found to be contained by the epicardial layer of the LV and pericardium. This entity has been termed *subepicardial aneurysm.* **B,** Apical four-chamber view in a 65-year-old man with atypical chest pain showing an apical pouch (*) with torn apical myocardium (arrow). Apical pseudoaneurysm was confirmed at the time of surgery. *(**A,** From Oh JK, Seward JB, Tajik AJ: The Echo Manual. 3rd ed. Philadelphia, Lippincott Williams & Wilkins, 2006. Used with permission of Mayo Foundation for Medical Education and Research.)*

myocardial viability, LV filling pressures, severity of mitral regurgitation, and pulmonary artery systolic pressure.[79]

Ischemic mitral regurgitation refers to chronic mitral regurgitation caused by LV remodeling due to coronary artery disease (see Chap. 62). As in the acute phase of myocardial infarction, chronic ischemic mitral regurgitation has been found to be an important prognostic indicator.[80] Even a mild degree of mitral regurgitation has been associated with increased mortality.[81] Whether reduction of mitral regurgitation by surgery or a percutaneous device procedure will improve a patient's quality of life or survival has not been determined by a clinical trial.[82] Determinants of functional mitral regurgitation are discussed further in the mitral regurgitation section in this chapter.

Right Ventricular Infarct

Mortality from a hemodynamically serious RV infarct is as high as one related to shock from LV infarct (see Chap. 50).[83] Echocardiographically, RV infarct is characterized by a dilated and hypokinetic to akinetic RV. The apical portion of the RV may be spared because it is supplied by the left anterior descending coronary artery, whereas the basal to mid-RV free walls are affected. The RA is also dilated, and tricuspid regurgitation develops as a result of tricuspid annulus dilatation. Because RV systolic pressure is not increased, peak tricuspid regurgitation velocity is low, usually less than 2 m/sec. TDI of the tricuspid valve annulus may be helpful in identifying depressed RV function in patients with inferior wall myocardial infarction. In patients with a PFO, an RV infarct creates an optimal clinical setting for a severe right-to-left shunt because of abnormal RV compliance and markedly increased RA pressure. If hypoxemia is a major problem after inferior wall myocardial infarction, an RV infarct and right-to-left shunt through a PFO should be considered. This diagnosis can be confirmed with contrast echocardiography (peripheral venous injection of agitated saline) or color flow imaging. Following opacification of the RA, the contrast medium enters the LA via the PFO. This situation is best assessed with TEE (see Fig. 14-e9 on website).

Apical Ballooning Syndrome or Takotsubo Cardiomyopathy

A subgroup of patients with acute myocardial infarction have no coronary artery stenosis on angiography. These patients may have typical ST-segment elevation, as well as elevation of troponin or creatine kinase with muscle subfraction (CK-MB). Echocardiography shows typical regional wall motion abnormalities, and these patients can also develop complications similar to those of patients with coronary artery disease. Clinical situations in which this scenario is found include coronary spasm, subarachnoid hemorrhage, pheochromocytoma, electroconvulsive treatment, and apical ballooning syndrome.[77,84,85] Usually the apical segment is involved more frequently, and acute LVOT obstruction has also occurred in this setting. Apical ballooning syndrome was initially described as "Takotsubo," or ampulla, cardiomyopathy by Satoh and colleagues.[86] Takotsubo is an octopus-catching device with a narrow neck, and the LV appears like a Takotsubo, with a ballooned apex and hyperdynamically contracting basal segment (Fig. 14-34). The Mayo Clinic experience showed the following interesting facts about apical ballooning syndrome:[77,84] (a) all patients were postmenopausal women (mean age, 71 years), (b) troponin T and CK-MB levels were mildly increased despite extensive apical akinesis to dyskinesis, with an initial LVEF of 39.5 percent, which returned to normal in a few days, (c) most patients had ST-segment elevation and a few developed LVOT obstruction, and (d) significant psychologic or physical stress was identified in almost all patients. These patients can have unstable hemodynamics and should be supported in the usual manner because almost all of them recover fully. Echocardiography is extremely helpful in this syndrome for monitoring the functional and hemodynamic response to treatment. A variant midventricular form of this syndrome has been described in which apical and basal segments are spared. Only the midportion of the LV was found to be akinetic on left ventriculography and echocardiography. Clinically, it is challenging to distinguish STEMI due to coronary occlusion from apical ballooning at presentation. Absence of coronary stenosis in STEMI patients may not always indicate apical ballooning syndrome because a subgroup of patients with STEMI may experience aborted myocardial infarction. When apical ballooning was compared with STEMI by echocardiography, the extent of wall motion abnormalities was greater in patients with apical ballooning, but the diastolic filling pattern was better, indicating less transmural involvement in apical ballooning.[87] Contrast echocardiography shows relatively normal perfusion in apical ballooning, indicating that wall motion abnormalities in apical ballooning are more demand related (such as increased catecholamine level) than supply related.

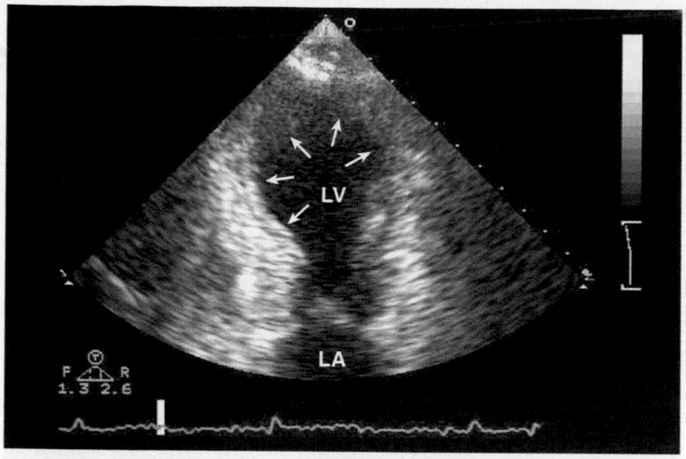

FIGURE 14–34 Apical four-chamber **(left)** and two-chamber **(right)** views demonstrating a dilated apical aneurysm or ballooning (arrows) in a 55-year-old woman with stress-induced apical ballooning syndrome. LA = left atrium; LV = left ventricle. *(From Oh JK, Seward JB, Tajik AJ: The Echo Manual. 3rd ed. Philadelphia, Lippincott Williams & Wilkins, 2006. Used with permission of Mayo Foundation for Medical Education and Research.)*

Risk Stratification by Echocardiography in Patients with Acute Myocardial Infarction

The most powerful prognostic indicators after myocardial infarction are the degree of systolic dysfunction, LV volume, the extent of coronary artery disease, mitral regurgitation, diastolic function, and the presence of heart failure (see Chap. 50). Therefore it is reasonable to predict that patients with a high WMSI have a greater chance of subsequently developing cardiac events. Most patients with Killip class II-IV heart failure after acute myocardial infarction had a WMSI of 1.7 or higher. In addition to the WMSI, restrictive Doppler filling variables derived from mitral inflow velocities correlate well with the incidence of postinfarct heart failure and LV filling pressures.[60] E/Ea, a reliable parameter to estimate PCWP, was found to be a strong predictor for long-term outcome after acute myocardial infarction.[62] Also, LA volume, a surrogate for chronic diastolic dysfunction and chronic elevation of LA pressure, was a strong predictor for outcome after acute myocardial infarction.[60] Stress echocardiography is sensitive in detecting residual ischemia, myocardial viability, and multivessel disease soon after myocardial infarction occurs. Usually, however, patients are unable to exercise adequately soon after an acute myocardial infarction. The myocardium remains akinetic for a time (days to weeks) after successful reperfusion of the occluded coronary artery. Demonstration of viability by augmentation of contractility (with dobutamine echocardiography) or demonstration of perfusion (with contrast echocardiography) predicts functional recovery. Both dobutamine and contrast echocardiography have a similar sensitivity and specificity for predicting fractional recovery, although myocardial perfusion echocardiography is better for evaluation of the anterior wall than the inferior or lateral wall.[88]

Stress Echocardiography

Maintaining a "reserve" capacity is mandatory for any system or organ to be able to perform satisfactorily under various conditions. Examination of a patient at resting condition may not be able to demonstrate the lack or reduction of reserve. Frequently, a patient's symptoms are precipitated or worsened by exercise or stress because of an abnormality in cardiovascular reserve. Increased demand cannot be met satisfactorily if the underlying pathologic condition (or diminished reserve) does not allow a normal or physiological increase in whatever is necessary to satisfy the demand (see Chap. 48). This can happen with coronary artery disease, valvular disease, and diastolic dysfunction. Stress echocardiography is an excellent method for comparing wall motion (regional contractility), myocardial perfusion, pressure gradient, pulmonary pressure, valvular regurgitation, or filling pressures before and after a stress to identify a pathological condition that is not apparent at rest. Stress echocardiography requires a comparison of echocardiographic data obtained at the time of or after stress with baseline resting data, and it is essential to review resting and stress images side-by-side using digital acquisition and display.[69,70] By allowing several successive cardiac cycles to be captured and stored in memory, digitized echocardiography enhances the capability of acquiring satisfactory comparative postexercise images. The most satisfactory postexercise image is selected and compared with the baseline image by side-by-side quad-screen display.

Stress echocardiography is performed with exercise or the administration of a pharmacological agent.[1] The exercise protocol includes a treadmill exercise test, with immediate postexercise echocardiographic images or upright or supine bicycle echocardiographic images obtained at peak exercise. Because exercise-induced regional wall motion abnormalities due to ischemia usually last for a few minutes after the termination of exercise, immediate postexercise images can be compared with the baseline preexercise images to detect exercise-induced regional wall motion abnormalities. The typical exercise echocardiography protocol is shown in Figure 14-35. Some centers favor a supine bike exercise protocol, which has an advantage of allowing echocardiographic images to be obtained at peak exercise. Supine bike exercise is a preferred form of stress test for evaluation of exercise-induced hemodynamics (for mitral stenosis or diastolic dysfunction).

When a patient cannot exercise, ischemia is induced pharmacologically with dobutamine, dipyridamole, or adenosine. Pharmacological stress is used most frequently for preoperative risk stratification, and dobutamine is the agent used most commonly in stress echocardiography (see Fig. 14-35). Contrast myocardial perfusion echocardiography can be used to identify ischemic myocardium.[89] To induce a perfusion defect, adenosine or dipyridamole is most frequently used. These vasodilating agents create a "coronary steal" so that myocardial segments subtended by a stenotic coronary artery show a decrease in myocardial perfusion (see Chaps. 16 and 48).

At our institution, the patient's medications usually are not discontinued before stress echocardiography; more than one third of our patients are taking a beta-blocker at the time of stress echocardiography. Atropine is used in 59 percent of dobutamine stress tests. Stress echocardiography is very safe, with no procedural mortality noted after more than 50,000 studies. Ventricular tachycardia occurred in 1.4 percent of exercise echocardiographic studies and in 4 percent of dobutamine stress echocardiographic studies. Ventricular fibrillation occurred in three patients (one with exercise and two with dobutamine studies). Supraventricular tachycardia and atrial fibrillation are more common.

Diagnostic Criteria for Stress Echocardiography

Normally with exercise, dobutamine, or pacing, LV wall motion becomes hyperdynamic (Fig. 14-36). Worsening of wall motion abnormalities or the development of new ones is the hallmark of stress-induced myocardial ischemia (Fig.

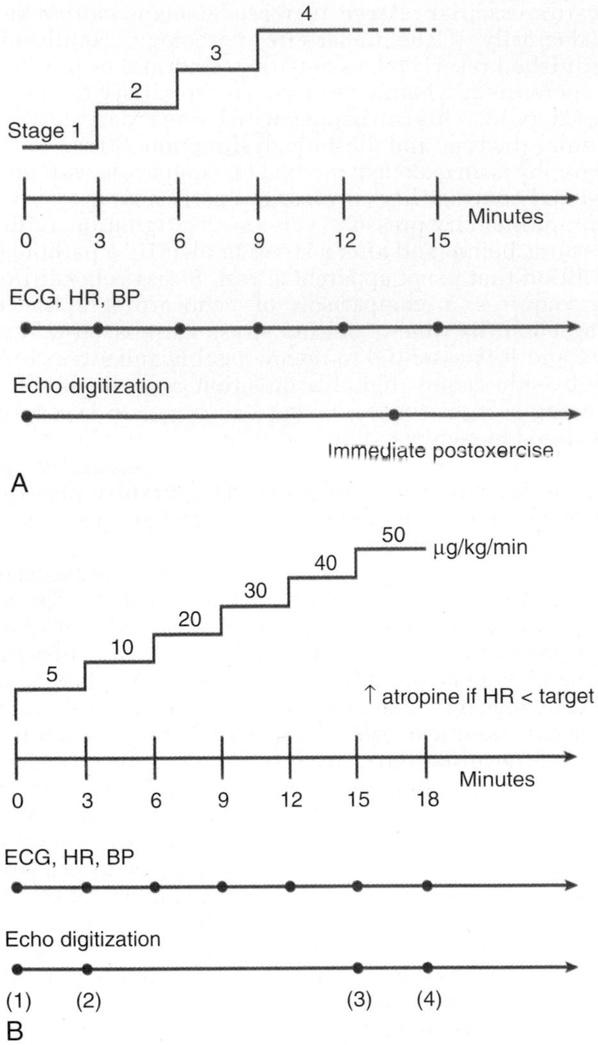

FIGURE 14–35 A, Typical exercise protocol. **B,** Protocol for pharmacological stress test. BP = blood pressure; ECG = electrocardiography; HR = heart rate. *(From Oh JK, Seward JB, Tajik AJ: The Echo Manual. 3rd ed. Philadelphia, Lippincott Williams & Wilkins, 2006. Used with permission of Mayo Foundation for Medical Education and Research.)*

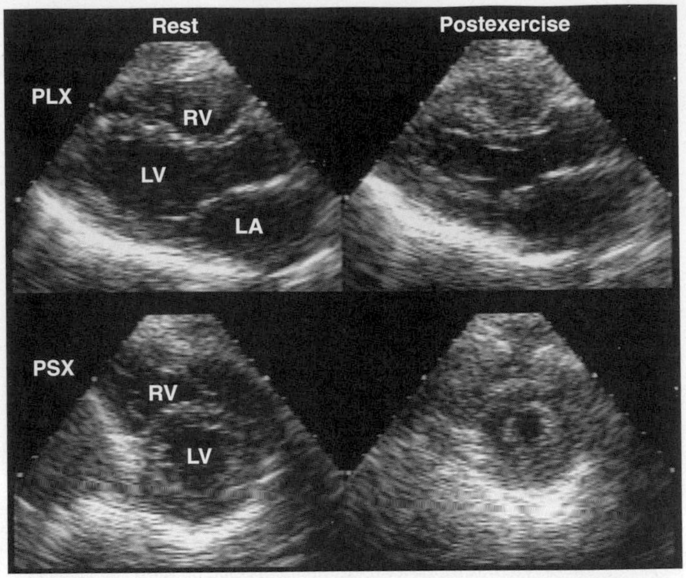

FIGURE 14–36 Still frame of end-systolic parasternal long-axis (PLX) and short-axis (PSX) views of normal exercise echocardiogram as shown in a quad-screen format. The left ventricular (LV) cavity is smaller and the walls are hyperdynamic in the postexercise period. LA = left atrium; RV = right ventricle. *(From Oh JK, Seward JB, Tajik AJ: The Echo Manual. 3rd ed. Philadelphia, Lippincott Williams & Wilkins, 2006. Used with permission of Mayo Foundation for Medical Education and Research.)*

14-37). The lack of hyperdynamic motion may indicate ischemia, but it is less specific. When the stress level is inadequate or the patient is taking a beta-blocker, however, the entire LV segment may contract normally without hyperdynamic motion. Not infrequently, an akinetic myocardial segment becomes dyskinetic during stress echocardiography. This change was not found to have any diagnostic or prognostic implication.[33]

Other adjunctive diagnostic criteria for a positive stress echocardiography test include LV cavity dilatation and a decrease in global systolic function. These adjunctive diagnostic criteria are more specific for detecting *severe* coronary artery disease. Also, it should be emphasized that the response to dobutamine is different from that due to exercise. Even in patients with severe coronary artery disease, including left main coronary artery disease, the LV cavity may not dilate and global systolic function may improve with dobutamine infusion despite new wall motion abnormalities due to severe coronary artery disease.

The use of TDI or strain imaging may be more sensitive for identifying ischemic segments.[74,90] Time from the QRS to the onset of regional relaxation has been found to be a good indication of ischemia.[18] Myocardial ischemia delays the onset and the rate of regional myocardial relaxation and the delay in relaxation can be quantified with TDI and strain rate imaging. Normally, it takes 350 to 400 msec from the QRS to the onset of regional myocardial relaxation, and the interval decreases by a mean of 34 ± 10 percent in normal myocardial segments with high-dose dobutamine, but the reduction in the interval is less (mean, 12 ± 18 percent) in ischemic segments.

It will be ideal if both myocardial contractility and perfusion data are available during stress echocardiography by real-time myocardial contrast perfusion study. A myocardial perfusion defect is usually seen as a dark area devoid of microbubbles in the subendocardium or the entire transmural myocardium area. Wall motion analysis is enhanced by LV opacification using contrast microbubbles. Currently, contrast is used for LV opacification in 25 percent of exercise and 50 percent of dobutamine echocardiography examinations in our laboratory. Biplane and 3D imaging may shorten the acquisition period of postexercise or peak-exercise images. This will improve the sensitivity of stress echocardiography, as well as minimize the technical strains imposed occasionally on sonographers or echocardiographers in obtaining challenging images.

DIAGNOSTIC ACCURACY

The sensitivity and specificity of stress echocardiography, with the use of wall motion criteria, are comparable with those of stress thallium or sestamibi SPECT (**see Chap. 16**).[69,70] In a large comparison study (112 patients), the overall sensitivity and specificity of exercise echocardiography were 85 percent and 88 percent, respectively, compared with 85 percent and 81 percent for exercise thallium imaging. The sensitivity of exercise echocardiography and exercise thallium imaging for coronary artery disease in patients with single-, double-, or triple-vessel involvement was also similar (58, 86, and 94 percent versus 61, 86, and 94 percent, respectively). However, according to our experience, the sensitivity of exercise echocardiography for predicting multivessel disease is about 70 percent. When a diagnostic test is used routinely, the diagnostic accuracy depends on the patient population, the expertise of the interpreter, and the quality of the image. Patients with seemingly normal wall motion but abnormal myocardial perfusion have been observed. Some stress-induced wall motion abnormalities resolve quickly before being documented by post-stress images. Another possibility is that our visual interpretation of regional wall

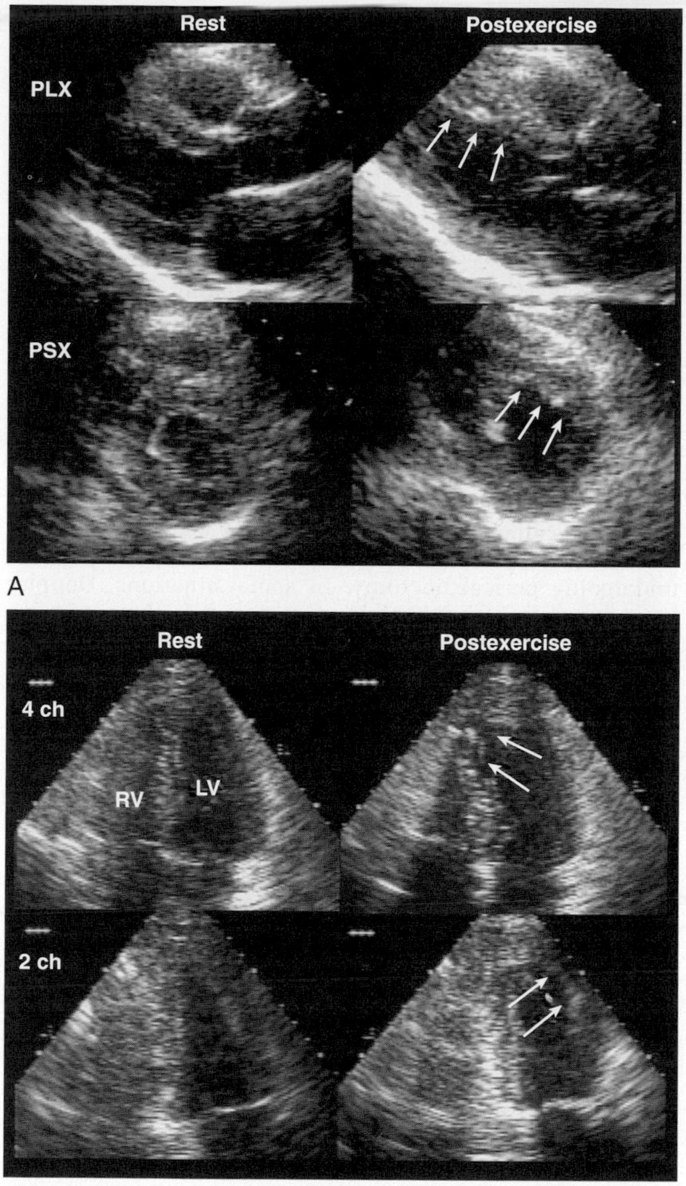

FIGURE 14–37 A, Still frame of end-systolic parasternal long-axis (PLX) and short-axis (PSX) views of an exercise echocardiogram positive for stress-induced myocardial ischemia. The anteroseptum and anterior wall became severely hypokinetic (arrows) with exercise. **B,** Still frame of end-systolic apical views of positive exercise echocardiogram. The apical septum and anteroapex became akinetic to dyskinetic (arrows). 2 ch = two-chamber view; 4 ch = four-chamber view; LV = left ventricle; RV = right ventricle. *(From OH JK, Seward JB, Tajik AJ: The Echo Manual. 3rd ed. Philadelphia, Lippincott Williams & Wilkins, 2006. Used with permission of Mayo Foundation for Medical Education and Research.)*

motion analysis is not always accurate. The ultimate technical goal of stress echocardiography for the evaluation of myocardial ischemia is to be able to assess regional contractility and myocardial perfusion at the same time. With further clinical experience, TDI, strain rate imaging, or color kinesis may be able to improve the accuracy of stress echocardiography.

STRESS ECHOCARDIOGRAPHY AS A PROGNOSTIC INDICATOR[1]

The likelihood of a cardiac event (cardiac death, nonfatal infarct, or coronary revascularization) occurring after normal stress echocardiography is extremely low. Among 1325 patients with normal findings on exercise echocardiography at Mayo Clinic, the event rate over 3 years of follow-up was less than 3 percent. The cardiac event rate per person-years of follow-up was 0.9 percent. Multivariate predictors of subsequent cardiac events were angina during a treadmill exercise test (TMET), low workload (<7 metabolic equivalents [METs] for men and <5 METs for women), LV hypertrophy, and advancing age. Therefore an interpretation of a normal exercise echocardiogram should consider the patient's symptoms and workload.

When the outcomes of 1874 patients who had good exercise capacity (≥5 METs for women and ≥7 METs for men) but an abnormal exercise echocardiogram were analyzed, the overall cardiac death or nonfatal myocardial infarction rate was 2 percent per person-year follow-up.[91] Diabetes mellitus, history of myocardial infarction, and an increase or no change in LV end-systolic size in response to exercise predicted a higher rate of a cardiac event, with risk ratio of 1.9, 2.4, and 1.6, respectively. When exercise capacity is reduced at the time of exercise echocardiography, an abnormal study is also a predictor[92] for a cardiac event, with a worse outcome for patients with a decreased LVEF and an increase or no change in LV size with exercise. Even within a group of patients with a high pretest probability of coronary artery disease, those with a normal exercise echocardiogram had a lower event rate than those with an abnormal exercise echocardiogram (2 versus 17 percent at 1 year and 4 versus 25 percent at 3 years).[93] The prognostic value of exercise echocardiography was also determined in 493 patients by Mazur and colleagues.[94] Independent predictors of cardiac events were WMSI with exercise, ST-segment depression greater than or equal to 1 mm, and treadmill time. The risk index (RI) was calculated as follows:

$$RI = 1.02\ (WMSI) + 1.04\ (\text{ST-segment change}) - 0.14\ (\text{treadmill time})$$

When the RI was in the upper quartile (+0.66 to +2.02), risk was highest (30 percent). The prognostic value of exercise echocardiography is comparable in women and men.

The most common indication for dobutamine stress echocardiography is preoperative cardiac evaluation. In 530 patients undergoing nonvascular surgery at Mayo Clinic, dobutamine stress echocardiography was a reliable predictor of postoperative events such as cardiac death and nonfatal myocardial infarction. An ischemic threshold <60 percent of age-predicted maximal heart rate identified a high-risk group (8 percent of patients), with 43 percent sustaining a postoperative event compared with 0 percent and 9 percent of patients with no ischemia or an ischemic threshold greater than or equal to 60 percent, respectively.

Assessment of Myocardial Viability

Generally, a myocardial segment of normal or near-normal thickness (≥6 mm) is considered viable, whereas a thinned and echodense (fibrotic) segment is considered scarred. More frequently than not, however, it is difficult to differentiate viable from nonviable myocardium by assessing just LV wall thickness.

It has been shown in animals that alpha-adrenergic stimulation improves contractility of a chronically ischemic or postischemic myocardium with regional wall motion abnormalities, but it does not improve contractility in infarcted myocardium. Several human studies have demonstrated that a low dose of dobutamine (5-20 μg/kg per minute) induces contractility in viable myocardium, whether stunned or hibernating. Dobutamine-responsive wall motion improvement predicts subsequent improvement in regional LV wall thickening after coronary revascularization (see Chap. 48).

It has been shown that, at least in hibernating myocardium, a biphasic response best predicts recovery of myocardial function after revascularization. During infusion of a low dose of dobutamine, coronary blood flow increases and recruitment of contractile reserve improves the wall motion of the dysfunctional myocardium. As the dobutamine dose is increased, coronary blood flow does not increase further and myocardial ischemia occurs because of stenosis of the coronary artery supplying the region, resulting in worsening of wall motion as compared with the previous lower dose of dobutamine. Most of the initial improvement in wall motion takes place with a low dose of dobutamine, between 10 and 20 μg/kg per minute, and worsening occurs at a higher dose, 30 to 40 μg/kg per minute, or with atropine.

Dobutamine is not as sensitive as thallium uptake or positron emission tomography (PET) for detecting myocardial viability (see Chap. 16). However, recovery of contractility of akinetic myocardium after revascularization is better predicted by increased contractility seen on dobutamine stress echocardiography than by SPECT or PET, which are more sensitive in detecting a small area of metabolically viable myocardium that may not be large enough to produce contractility. Showing perfusion in the myocardium with the use of contrast echocardiography is another way to demonstrate potential myocardial viability. Microbubbles from the contrast agent opacify the myocardium, indicating integrity of the microvascular circulation. The presence of microvascular integrity may not necessarily indicate the presence of sufficient myocardium to restore myocardial contractility. Therefore it appears that myocardial contrast echocardiography, like thallium perfusion, is less specific than dobutamine echocardiography in predicting functional recovery after revascularization. Dobutamine echocardiography may not demonstrate augmented contractility in a subset of myocardial segments in which myocardial contrast shows evidence of perfusion. Several studies including a multicenter dobutamine viability registry demonstrated that the outcome of patients with severe LV dysfunction and myocardial viability shown by dobutamine is better when they undergo revascularization.

Postsystolic shortening is an important feature of ischemic myocardium, and strain imaging is able to quantify postsystolic shortening. When postsystolic shortening is associated with systolic hypokinesis or akinesis, it indicates actively contracting and potentially viable myocardium. However, when combined with dyskinesis, postsystolic shortening appears to be a nonspecific marker of severe ischemia.[95] Strain imaging may be useful in assessing myocardial viability by quantifying postsystolic shortening but needs further clinical investigation.

DIASTOLIC STRESS TEST

Another important condition that needs to be evaluated is exercise-induced increased filling pressure, which is responsible for the symptoms of shortness of breath with exertion. Therefore, filling pressure needs to be assessed with exercise as well as at rest. The mitral annulus Ea velocity, which reflects the status of mitral relaxation, actually increases with exercise or increased preload when myocardial relaxation is normal, but Ea velocity does not augment as much with higher transmitral pressure gradient or with exercise when relaxation is impaired with increased tau. Therefore, in normal subjects, mitral inflow E velocity and mitral annulus Ea velocity increase proportionately so that E/Ea remains <15 at resting stage and exercise. However, in patients with diastolic dysfunction and exertional dyspnea, E velocity increases with exercise but Ea velocity remains less or increases less with exercise. Therefore, the E/Ea ratio increases with exercise compared with the resting stage in patients with diastolic dysfunction.

In normal subjects, mitral E velocity increases about 25 percent with exercise from baseline data, deceleration time decreases an average of 16 msec (from 192 to 176 msec), and Ea velocity increases about 25 percent. Therefore the E/Ea ratio remains the same (mean, 6.6) at baseline and with exercise in subjects with normal diastolic function.[53] However, in patients with diastolic dysfunction, the E/Ea ratio response to exercise varies. There are three groups of patients:[54] The first group has E/Ea greater than 15 (increased filling pressure) at rest, and the ratio remains elevated with exercise in all. The second group has relatively normal filling pressure and impaired myocardial relaxation pattern on mitral inflow velocity at rest, which changes to a restrictive filling pattern, with E/Ea greater than 15 with exercise. The third group has normal filling pressure and E/Ea less than 15 at rest and with exercise. Patients with increased filling pressure with exercise whether or not filling pressure is normal at rest (the first and second groups) have shorter exercise duration than patients (the third group) with normal filling pressure at rest and with exercise. Simultaneous cardiac catheterization and Doppler echocardiography has been performed in patients who were undergoing exercise testing in the cardiac catheterization laboratory for evaluation of exertional dyspnea. In this patient population, E/Ea correlated well with PCWP, not only at resting stage but also with exercise; specifically, an E/Ea ratio greater than 15 during exercise is associated with PCWP greater than 20 mm Hg.[96] Burgess and colleagues[55] have shown a similarly good correlation between E/Ea and PCWP at rest and exercise (see Fig. 14-e5 on website).

HEMODYNAMIC ASSESSMENT

Over the past 20 years, echocardiography has replaced cardiac catheterization for most hemodynamic assessments in our clinical practice. It is common practice that clinical decisions are based on an echocardiographic assessment of cardiac hemodynamics. Currently at our institution, less than 5 percent of patients undergo hemodynamic cardiac catheterization before aortic valve replacement for aortic stenosis. Even the most demanding hemodynamic assessment, such as evaluation of constrictive pericarditis, is performed reliably by echocardiography, and cardiac catheterization is performed in less than half of the patients undergoing pericardiectomy. In some situations, Doppler hemodynamic assessment is more accurate than invasive hemodynamic measurement, with the best example being the transmitral pressure gradient (see later). Therefore it is mandatory that all physicians who care for patients with cardiac disease be familiar with how echocardiography provides cardiac hemodynamics.

Transvalvular Gradients

Doppler echocardiography records blood flow velocities (in meters per second [m/sec]), and Doppler velocities are converted to pressure gradients (in millimeters of mercury [mm Hg]) according to the simplified Bernoulli equation (Fig. 14-38):

$$\text{Pressure gradient } (\Delta P) = 4 \times (v_2)^2 \text{ or } (2\ v_2)^2$$

When maximal Doppler velocity is converted to pressure gradient using the simplified Bernoulli equation, it represents the maximal instantaneous gradient. Mean gradient is an average of pressure gradients during the entire flow period. Maximal instantaneous or mean gradient obtained with Doppler echocardiography has been shown to correlate well with corresponding gradients simultaneously measured by cardiac catheterization (see Chap. 19). In some clinical situations, the Doppler-derived pressure gradient is more reliable than the catheter-derived gradient because the transmitral (normal, stenotic, native, or prosthetic valve) pressure gradient may be overestimated by cardiac catheterization if PCWP is used (instead of direct LA pressure) to calculate the pressure gradient.

Intracardiac Pressures

PULMONARY ARTERY PRESSURES. Flow velocities recorded with Doppler echocardiography are used to determine various intracardiac pressures. Tricuspid regurgitation velocity reflects the systolic pressure difference between the RV and the RA (see Fig. 14-38). Therefore RV systolic pressure can be obtained by adding the estimated RA pressure to the tricuspid regurgitation velocity$^2 \times 4$. If there is no RVOT obstruction, pulmonary artery systolic pressure is equal to the calculated RV systolic pressure. Pulmonary regurgitation velocity represents the diastolic pressure difference between the pulmonary artery and the RV. Hence pulmonary artery end-diastolic pressure (PAEDP) can be obtained by adding RV end-diastolic pressure (RVEDP) (which is equal to RA pressure) to (pulmonary regurgitation

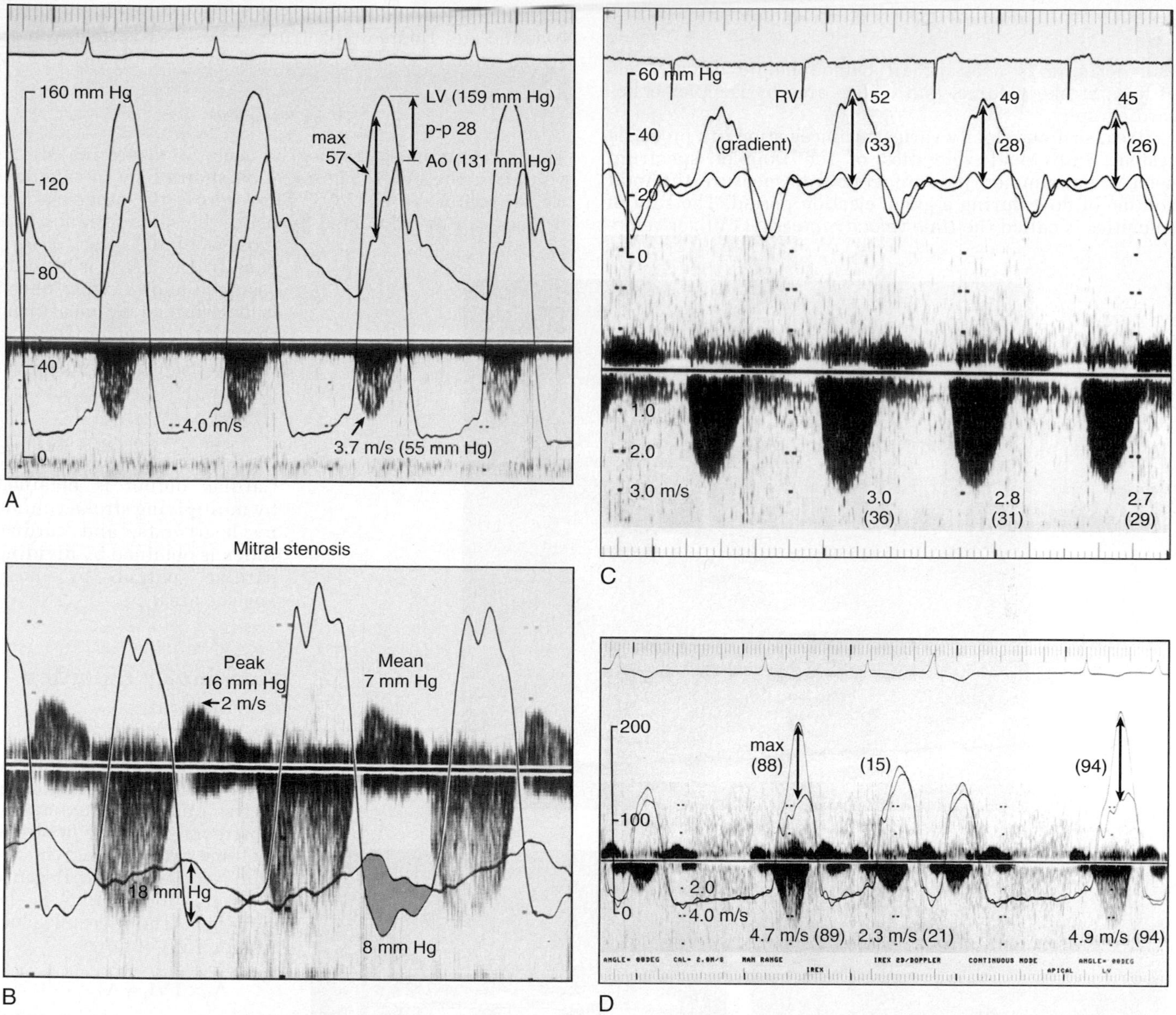

FIGURE 14–38 A, Simultaneous Doppler and cardiac pressure recordings show an excellent correlation between Doppler-derived and catheter-derived pressure gradients in aortic stenosis. Peak Doppler velocity (3.7 m/sec) from the third cardiac cycle is converted to a maximal instantaneous gradient (max) of 55 mm Hg, which corresponds well to the maximal gradient determined by catheter (57 mm Hg) but not to the peak-to-peak (p-p) gradient of 28 mm Hg. Ao = aorta; LV = left ventricle. **B,** Simultaneous left ventricular and left atrial pressure measurements and Doppler velocity recording of the mitral valve in mitral stenosis. Peak instantaneous and mean gradients correlate well. **C,** Simultaneous right ventricular (RV) and right atrial pressure tracings and tricuspid regurgitation velocity recording by continuous wave Doppler echocardiography. Pressure gradients (36, 31, and 29 mm Hg) derived from the peak Doppler velocities of the second, third, and fourth beats (3.0, 2.8, and 2.7 m/sec, respectively) are close to the catheter-derived RV and right atrial gradients (arrows, 33, 28, and 26 mm Hg). **D,** Simultaneous continuous wave Doppler and cardiac catheterization study. LV apex and outflow pressures are recorded to determine the severity of outflow obstruction. Doppler velocities are converted to pressure gradients with the simplified Bernoulli equation and correlate well with maximal (max) catheter-derived gradients. The resting gradient is 15 to 20 mm Hg, and it is markedly accentuated in the postextrasystolic contractions (second and fifth beats), with resultant gradients derived by catheter of 88 and 94 mm Hg and by Doppler of 89 and 94 mm Hg, respectively. Note that the LV pressure tracing has a late-peaking appearance corresponding to the late-peaking Doppler profile. *(**A,** From Currie PJ, Seward JB, Reeder GS, et al: Continuous wave Doppler echocardiographic assessment of severity of calcific aortic stenosis: A simultaneous Doppler-catheter correlative study in 100 adult patients. Circulation 71:1162, 1985. Used with permission. **B-D,** From Oh JK, Seward JB, Tajik AJ: The Echo Manual. 3rd ed. Philadelphia, Lippincott Williams & Wilkins, 2006. Used with permission of Mayo Foundation for Medical Education and Research.)*

end-diastolic velocity)$^2 \times 4$. The pulmonary artery mean pressure correlates well with the early diastolic pressure difference between the pulmonary artery and RV, hence (pulmonary regurgitation peak velocity)$^2 \times 4$.

LV END-DIASTOLIC PRESSURE. Aortic regurgitation (AR) velocity reflects the diastolic pressure difference between the aorta and the LV. Hence,

$$\text{LVEDP} = \text{DBP} - (\text{AR EDV})^2 \times 4$$

Where DBP is the diastolic blood pressure and EDV is end-diastolic velocity. LV end-diastolic pressure and LA pressure can also be estimated by various diastolic filling variables from mitral inflow, pulmonary venous flow velocities, tissue Doppler imaging, and color M-mode of mitral inflow[20] (see Diastolic Assessment later).

Stroke Volume and Cardiac Output

According to the hydraulic orifice formula, flow (rate) across a fixed orifice is equal to the product of the cross-sectional area (CSA) of the orifice and flow velocity:

$$\text{Flow rate} = \text{CSA} \times \text{flow velocity}$$

This formula is used in all hemodynamic calculations of flow, stroke volume, and orifice area by Doppler echocardiography.

Because flow velocity varies during ejection in a pulsatile system, individual velocities of the Doppler spectrum need to be summed (i.e., integrated) to measure the total volume of flow during a given ejection period. The sum of velocities is called the *time velocity integral* (TVI), or *velocity time integral* (VTI). It is equal to the area enclosed by the baseline and Doppler spectrum. After TVI is determined, stroke volume (SV) is calculated by multiplying TVI by CSA:

$$\text{SV} = \text{CSA} \times \text{TVI}$$

The location most frequently used to determine stroke volume is the LVOT. Figure 14-39 shows how to calculate stroke volume from LVOT. Flow across the other cardiac orifices can be calculated by using the same formula. The cross-sectional area of orifices in the heart is usually assumed to be a circle, and it is determined by measuring the orifice diameter (D):

$$\text{CSA} = (\text{D}/2)^2 \times \pi = \text{D}^2 \times 0.785$$

Hence,

$$\text{SV} = \text{D}^2 \times 0.785 \times \text{TVI}$$

Cardiac output is obtained by multiplying stroke volume by heart rate, and cardiac index is obtained by dividing cardiac output by body surface area.

Continuity Equation

(see Chap. 62)

Flow rate or stroke volume passing through a stenotic or regurgitant orifice is the same as the product of proximal (or upstream) flow rate or stroke volume across a known area and velocity (or TVI). Because flow rate (or volume) is the product of the area and velocity (or TVI) of flow:

$$A_1 \times \text{TVI}_1 = A_2 \times \text{TVI}_2$$

where A_1 is a known area at a location proximal to the unknown area, A_2. This is the continuity equation (Fig. 14-40), which is used to calculate the area of a stenotic[97] or regurgitant valve. Using the continuity equation, a stenotic or regurgitant orifice area is calculated from the following equation:

$$A_2 = A_1 \times \text{TVI}_1/\text{TVI}_2$$

In aortic stenosis, stroke volume across the aortic valve area (A_2) is the same as stroke volume across the LVOT (A_1). In mitral regurgitation, the flow rate across the regurgitant mitral valve orifice (A_2) is the same as that of a proximal isovelocity surface area known as *PISA* (A_1). It should be noted that the

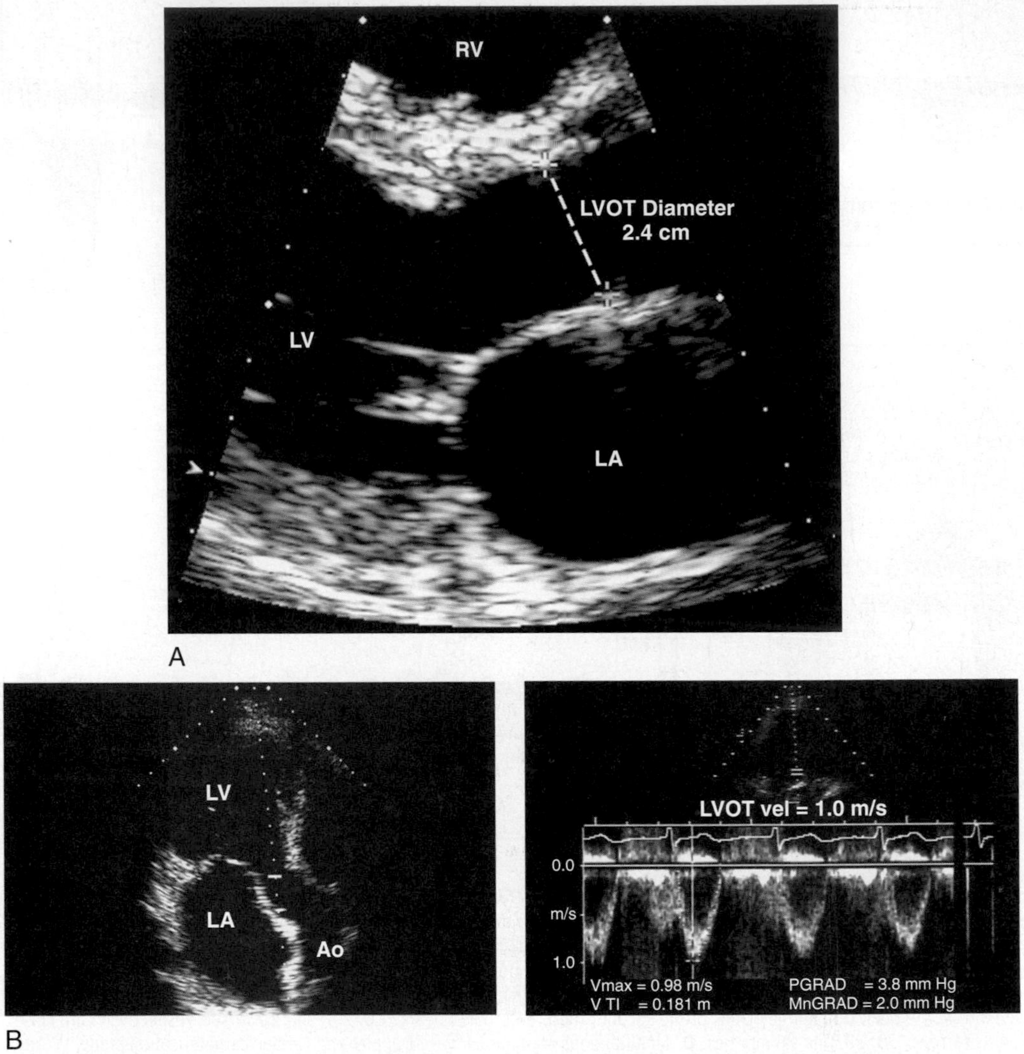

FIGURE 14–39 A, Step 1, Measurement of left ventricular outflow tract (LVOT) diameter from the expanded (zoom) parasternal long-axis view. The diameter is measured at the level of the aortic annulus during systole. The line is drawn from where the anterior aortic cusp meets the ventricular septum to where the posterior aortic cusp meets the anterior mitral leaflet and perpendicular to the anterior aortic wall. Distance (D) = 2.4 cm. Step 2, Calculation of LVOT area. Assuming a circular shape of LVOT,

$$\text{LVOT area (cm}^2) = \left(\frac{D}{2}\right)^2 \times \pi = D^2 \times 0.785$$

LVOT area = 4.5 cm^2 when D = 2.4 cm. LA = left atrium; LV = left ventricle; RV = right ventricle. **B, Left,** Step 3, Measurement of LVOT velocity (vel) and time velocity integral (TVI = VTI) from the apical long-axis view. A pulsed wave sample volume is placed at the center of the aortic annulus or 2 to 5 mm proximal to it. **Right,** TVI (cm) is the area under the velocity curve and is equal to the sum of velocities (cm/sec) during the ejection time (sec). TVI was measured to be 18 cm. Step 4, Calculation of stroke volume (SV) across the LVOT.

$$\begin{aligned}\text{SV (mL)} &= \text{Area (cm}^2) \times \text{TVI}\\ &= D^2 \times 0.785 \times \text{TVI}\\ &= 4.5\ \text{cm}^2 \times 18\ \text{cm} = 81\ \text{mL}\end{aligned}$$

Ao = aorta; MnGRAD = mean gradient; PGRAD = peak gradient. *(From Oh JK, Seward JB, Tajik AJ: The Echo Manual. 3rd ed. Philadelphia, Lippincott Williams & Wilkins, 2006. Used with permission of Mayo Foundation for Medical Education and Research.)*

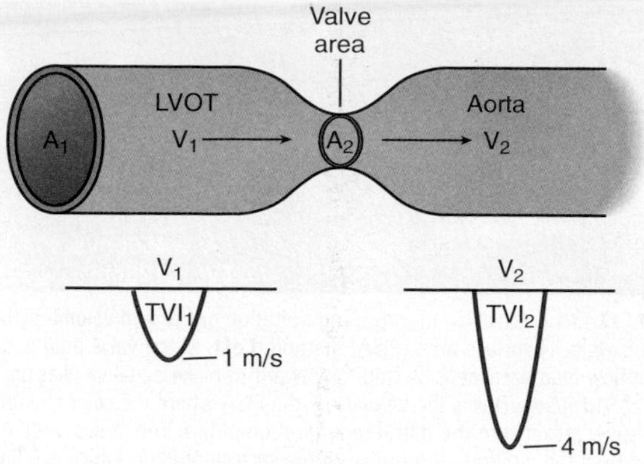

FIGURE 14–40 Diagram illustrating the continuity equation. $Area_1$ (A_1) is the known cross-sectional area. $Area_2$ (A_2) is the unknown cross-sectional area to be calculated:

$$SV_2 = SV_1$$
$$A_2 \times TVI_2 = A_1 \times TVI_1$$

LVOT = left ventricular outflow tract; SV = stroke volume; TVI = time velocity integral. *(From Oh JK, Seward JB, Tajik AJ: The Echo Manual. 3rd ed. Philadelphia, Lippincott Williams & Wilkins, 2006. Used with permission of Mayo Foundation for Medical Education and Research.)*

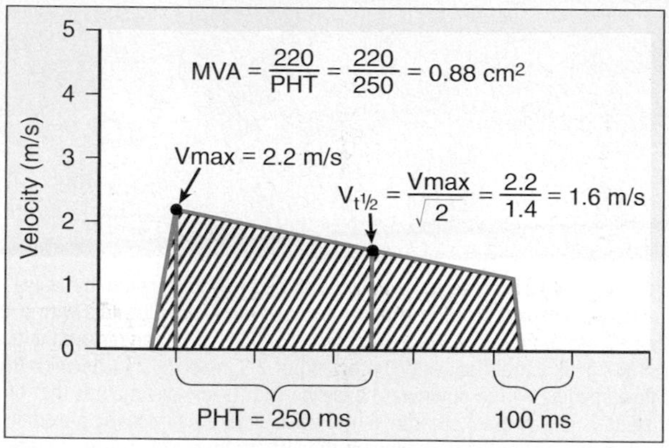

FIGURE 14–41 Diagram illustrating the calculation of pressure half-time (PHT). PHT is the time interval required for maximal pressure gradient (Pmax) to reach its half level ($P_{1/2}$). Hence,

$$P_{1/2} = 1/2\ Pmax$$
$$4 \times (V_{t1/2})^2 = 1/2(4 \times Vmax^2)$$

In this example, Vmax = 2.2 m/s; hence = 2.2/1.4 = 1.6 m/s. The time interval from Vmax (2.2 m/sec) to $V_{t1/2}$ (1.6 m/sec) is PHT (= 250 msec). In patients with native mitral valvular stenosis, mitral valve area (MVA) is estimated by dividing the constant, 220, by PHT. Vmax = maximal velocity; $V_{t1/2}$ = velocity at PHT. *(From Oh JK, Seward JB, Tajik AJ: The Echo Manual. 3rd ed. Philadelphia, Lippincott Williams & Wilkins, 2006. Used with permission of Mayo Foundation for Medical Education and Research.)*

ratio of the areas is inversely proportional to their TVI ratio:

$$A_2/A_1 = TVI_1/TVI_2$$

Pressure Half-time

Pressure half-time (PHT) is the time for the peak pressure gradient to reach its half level and is the same as the time for peak velocity to decrease to a velocity equal to the peak velocity divided by $\sqrt{2}$ (= 1.4) (Fig. 14-41). It is always proportionally related to deceleration time (DT):

$$PHT = 0.29 \times DT$$

Pressure half-time is used to estimate stenotic native mitral valve area (MVA) indirectly from an empirical formula:

$$MVA = 220/PHT$$

However, it overestimates the area of normal and prosthetic mitral valves. Another important clinical application of pressure half-time is to assess the severity of aortic regurgitation.

Regurgitant Volume, Fraction, and Orifice Area (see Chap. 62)

Regurgitant volume can be estimated two different ways with echocardiography: the *volumetric method,* and the *proximal isovelocity surface area* (PISA) *method.*[98]

Volumetric Method

Total forward volume across a regurgitant valve (Q total) is the sum of systemic stroke volume (Qs) and regurgitant volume. Hence, regurgitant volume can be obtained by calculating the difference between the total forward stroke volume and systemic stroke volume (Fig. 14-42):

$$\text{Regurgitant volume} = \text{Q total} - \text{Qs}$$

In mitral regurgitation, Q total is the mitral inflow volume, calculated as the product of mitral valve annulus area and mitral inflow TVI. Mitral inflow TVI is obtained by placing a sample volume at the center of the mitral annulus during diastole. Systemic stroke volume (Qs) is obtained from multiplying the LVOT area by LVOT TVI. Mitral valve regurgitant volume is calculated by subtracting the LVOT stroke volume from the mitral inflow volume. This calculation is not accurate (i.e., regurgitant volume is underestimated) if aortic regurgitation is pronounced. In aortic regurgitation, the aortic valve regurgitant volume is obtained by subtracting the mitral inflow stroke volume (Qs) from the LVOT forward stroke volume (Q total).

The *regurgitant fraction* is the percentage of regurgitant volume compared with the total forward flow across the regurgitant valve:

$$\text{Regurgitant fraction} = (\text{Regurgitant volume}/\text{Q total}) \times 100 \text{ percent}$$

Pisa Method

The regurgitant orifice area can be estimated using the concept of PISA. As blood flow converges toward the regurgitant orifice, blood flow velocity increases, with the formation of multiple shells of isovelocity of hemispheric shape. The flow rate at the surface of a hemispheric shell with the same flow velocity (isovelocity) should be equal to the flow rate across the regurgitant orifice (conservation of flow or modified form of the continuity equation). By adjusting the Nyquist limit of the color flow map, the flow velocity at a hemispheric surface proximal to the regurgitant orifice can be determined. In TTE, regurgitant flow travels away from the apical transducer position and toward the mitral regurgitation orifice. Hence the blood flow converging toward the mitral regurgitant orifice in the LV is color-coded blue until the velocity reaches the negative aliasing velocity of the selected color flow map, at which time the flow is color-coded light orange-red. If the negative aliasing velocity is decreased, the transition from blue to red-orange will occur farther from the regurgitant orifice, providing a larger hemispheric shell radius (r) (Fig. 14-43). An opposite color scheme occurs if TEE is used for quantification of mitral regurgitation by the PISA method. After a hemisphere of blood flow with known velocity (equal to negative aliasing velocity if TTE is used or positive aliasing velocity if TEE is used) is identified, the rate of flow through a hemispheric shell is equal to the area of the hemisphere multiplied by the flow velocity (which is the aliasing velocity). The area of hemisphere is calculated as $2\pi r^2$. Hence,

$$\text{Flow rate} = 6.28\ r^2 \times \text{Aliasing velocity}$$

This flow rate across PISA is equal to the flow rate across the effective regurgitant orifice (ERO):

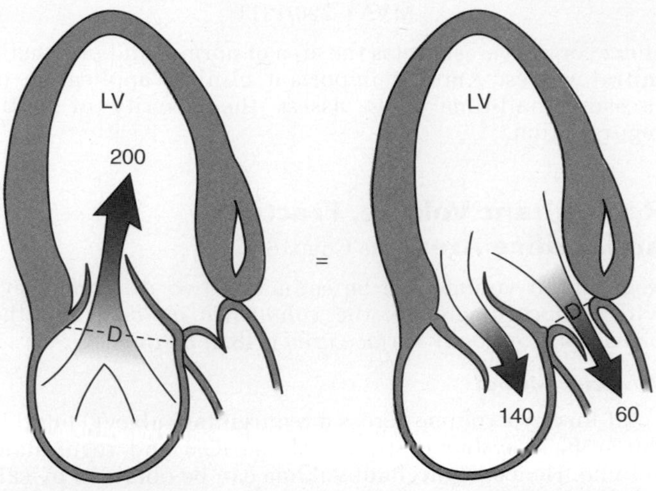

A

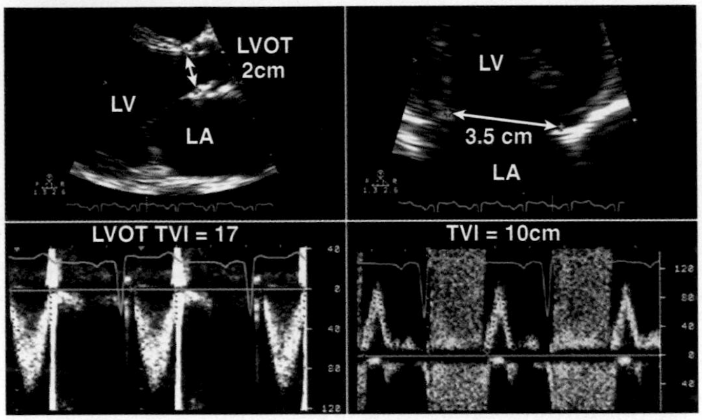

B

FIGURE 14–42 **A,** Estimation of regurgitant volume and regurgitant fraction using mitral regurgitation as an example. Assume that regurgitation is present only in the mitral valve. Therefore diastolic forward flow across the mitral valve (200 mL, **left**) is the sum of systolic flow across the left ventricular (LV) outflow tract (60 mL) and mitral regurgitant volume (140 mL); what goes into LV during diastole (mitral inflow) must come out of LV during systole (LV outflow tract [LVOT] flow + mitral regurgitant flow). The diagram shows a flail posterior mitral leaflet. Mitral inflow volume is the product of mitral annulus area and mitral flow time velocity integral (TVI) (flow = area × TVI). For this volumetric calculation, the sample volume is placed at the level of the mitral annulus:

$$\text{Mitral regurgitant volume} = \text{Mitral inflow} - \text{LVOT flow} = (D^2 \times 0.785 \times \text{TVI})\ \text{MV} - (D^2 \times 0.785 \times \text{TVI})\ \text{LVOT}$$

D = diameter. **B,** A representative case for calculating mitral regurgitation volume using the volumetric method. LVOT stroke volume is $(2)^2 \times 0.785 \times 17 = 53$ mL, and mitral inflow volume is $(3.5)^2 \times 0.785 \times 10 = 96$ mL. The difference, $96 - 53 = 43$ mL, is the mitral regurgitation volume. LA = left atrium. ***(A,** From Oh JK, Seward JB, Tajik AJ: The Echo Manual. 3rd ed. Philadelphia, Lippincott Williams & Wilkins, 2006. Used with permission of Mayo Foundation for Medical Education and Research.)*

$$\text{Flow rate} = \text{ERO} \times \text{Regurgitant velocity}$$

Therefore ERO can be obtained by dividing the flow rate by peak mitral regurgitant (MR) velocity across the regurgitant orifice:

$$\text{ERO} = \text{Flow rate/Peak MR velocity}$$

Regurgitant volume is equal to regurgitant orifice area multiplied by the mitral regurgitation TVI:

$$\text{Regurgitant volume} = \text{ERO} \times \text{MR TVI} = [6.28\ r^2 \times \text{Aliasing velocity/MR velocity}] \times \text{MR TVI}$$

The PISA method has several limitations, and its accuracy is based on reliable measurement of the PISA radius, which should be at midsystole. It is more accurate for a central mitral regurgitation jet. It is also important to have a correct aliasing velocity to produce a hemispheric PISA.

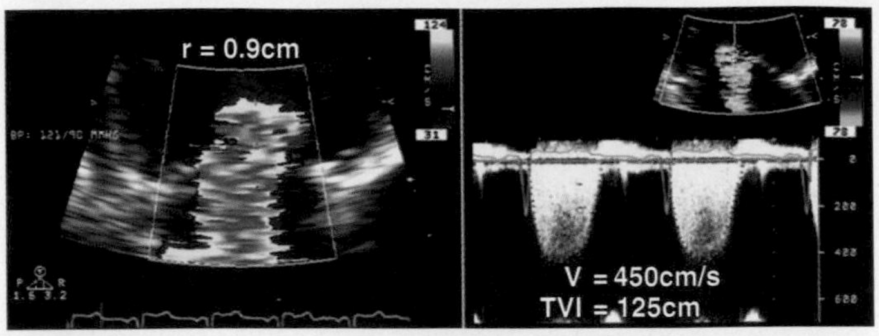

FIGURE 14–43 Calculation of mitral regurgitation orifice and volume by the proximal isovelocity surface area (PISA) method. **Left,** Mitral valve area is zoomed and color flow map baseline is shifted downward to make negative aliasing velocity of 31 cm/sec. This is the velocity of the PISA where the color changes from blue to yellow proximal to the mitral regurgitation orifice. The radius of PISA is measured from the regurgitation orifice to the surface of PISA, which is 0.9 cm. From these values, flow rate at PISA is calculated as follows: $6.28 \times (0.9)^2 \times 31 = 158$ cm/sec. To obtain effective regurgitant orifice (ERO), the flow rate is divided by the peak mitral regurgitation velocity shown on the right. **Right,** Continuous wave Doppler signal of mitral regurgitation shows the peak velocity of 4.5 m/sec or 450 cm/sec. ERO = 158/450 = 0.35 cm². Because volume is the product of ERO and time velocity integral (TVI) of mitral regurgitation, mitral regurgitant volume = 0.35 × 125 = 44 mL. These values are consistent with moderate degree of mitral regurgitation.

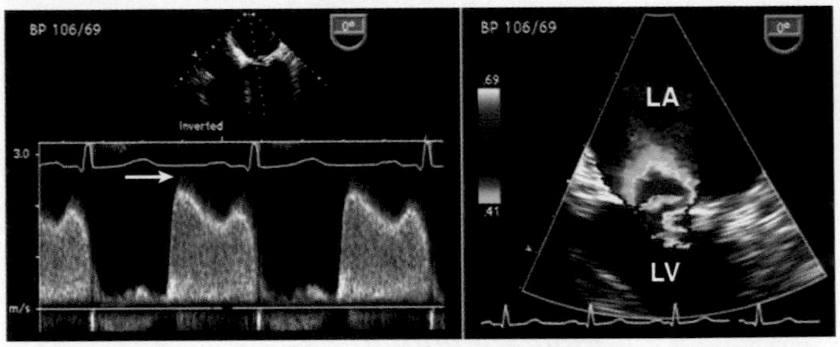

FIGURE 14–44 **Left,** A young woman with dyspnea following mitral valve repair. Transesophageal imaging shows narrowed mitral annulus area with a small soft tissue mass. Continuous wave Doppler recording across the repaired mitral valve shows peak mitral flow velocity (arrow) of 2.5 m/sec (= 250 cm/sec). **Right,** Color flow imaging with a downward baseline shift (same direction as that of mitral stenosis jet) across a stenotic mitral valve. A nice hemispheric proximal isovelocity surface area (PISA) is seen in the left atrium (LA) because of mitral stenosis. PISA radius is 1 cm. Hence, stenotic mitral valve area (MVA) is calculated as follows:

$$\text{MVA} = 6.28 \times (1)^2 \times 4/250 = 1.02\ \text{cm}^2$$

Because the surface of PISA is flat, no angle correction is necessary in this case. LV = left ventricle.

The concept of PISA can be applied for calculating the area of a stenotic orifice (Fig. 14-44). This method has been validated for mitral valve area in patients with mitral stenosis; however, it should be considered that PISA proximal to a stenotic mitral orifice may not be a complete hemisphere but rather a portion of a hemisphere because of the geometry of mitral leaflets on the atrial side. Therefore an angle correction factor may be necessary (but not in all cases):

$$\text{MVA} = [6.28\ r^2 \times \text{Aliasing velocity/Peak mitral stenosis velocity}] \times \alpha/180\ \text{degrees}$$

where α is the angle between two mitral leaflets on the atrial side.

Rate of Left Ventricular Pressure Change during Isovolumic Contraction (dP/dt)

The rate of LV pressure change during the isovolumic contraction period, *dP/dt*, is another index of LV contractility. During the isovolumic contraction, there is no significant change in LA pressure. Therefore mitral regurgitant velocity changes during this period reflect dP/dt. Usually, the

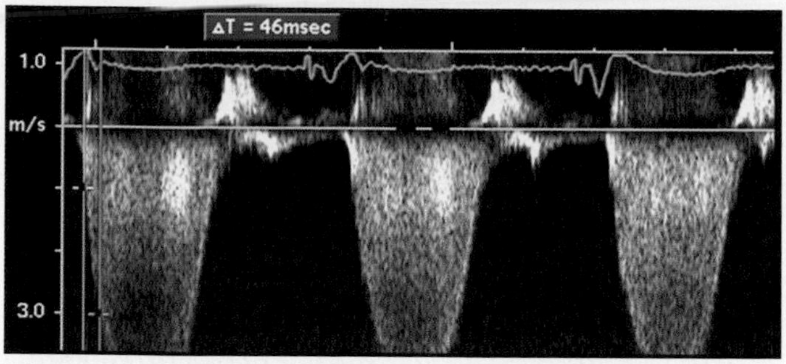

FIGURE 14-45 Continuous wave Doppler recording of mitral regurgitation. Time interval (ΔT) from 1 m/sec to 3 m/sec of the velocity is 46 msec. Therefore dP/dt = 32/0.046 = 696 mm Hg/sec.

interval between 1 m/sec and 3 m/sec on the mitral regurgitation velocity spectrum is measured (Fig. 14-45). For the Bernoulli equation, the pressure change from 1 m/sec to 3 m/sec is 32 mm Hg ($4 \times 3^2 - 4 \times 1^2$). The dP/dt (in mm Hg/sec) is calculated from the following formula: dP/dt = 32 mm Hg/time (seconds).

Several studies have demonstrated a good correlation between the noninvasive Doppler-derived and catheter-derived dP/dt. Normal dP/dt is greater than or equal to 1200 mm Hg/sec.

Resistance

Resistance is defined as a ratio of pressure (gradient) to flow. Because Doppler echocardiography is able to determine pressure (gradient) and flow, various resistances can be calculated noninvasively with 2D and Doppler echocardiographic measurements. Systemic vascular resistance (SVR) by echocardiography is determined as mitral regurgitant velocity/LVOT TVI. It correlates well with catheter-derived SVR (where SVR = [mean aortic pressure − RA pressure]/cardiac output). Mitral regurgitant velocity/LVOT TVI greater than 0.27 has been shown to have a 70 percent sensitivity and a 77 percent specificity for identifying SVR greater than 14 Wood units.[99]

Pulmonary vascular resistance is an important parameter to guide the management of patients with cardiopulmonary diseases (see Chap. 73). Because tricuspid regurgitant (TR) velocity provides pulmonary systolic pressure and TVI of the RVOT provides pulmonary flow, the TR velocity/RVOT TVI ratio has been correlated with invasively determined pulmonary vascular resistance (PVR). The following regression formula was found to be reliable in estimating PVR by TR velocity/RVOT TVI.[100]

$$PVR = (TR\ velocity/RVOT\ TVI) \times 10 + 0.16$$

VALVULAR HEART DISEASE (see Chap. 62)

Echocardiography provides a comprehensive and reliable hemodynamic assessment of patients with valvular heart disease including determination of pressure gradients, stenotic and regurgitant valve orifice area, regurgitant volume, and pulmonary artery pressures. TEE complements TTE by allowing improved delineation of valvular morphology, and 3D echocardiography may enhance its applications in valvular heart diseases because it can provide better delineation of valvular structures. On the basis of a comprehensive echocardiography examination, which outlines structure, function, and hemodynamic information, physicians can decide optimal treatment strategy including the timing of surgical intervention for patients with valvular heart disease.

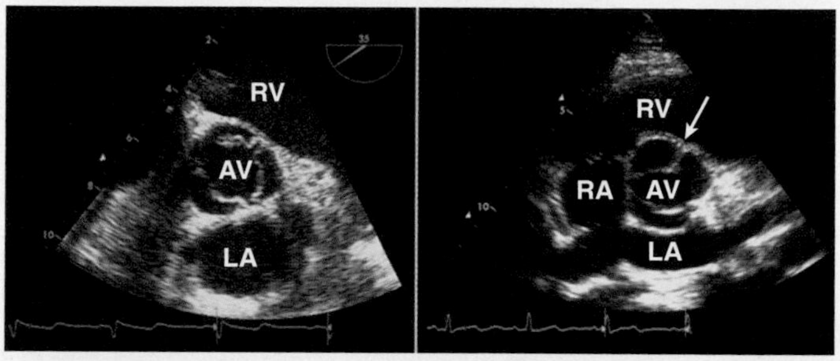

A

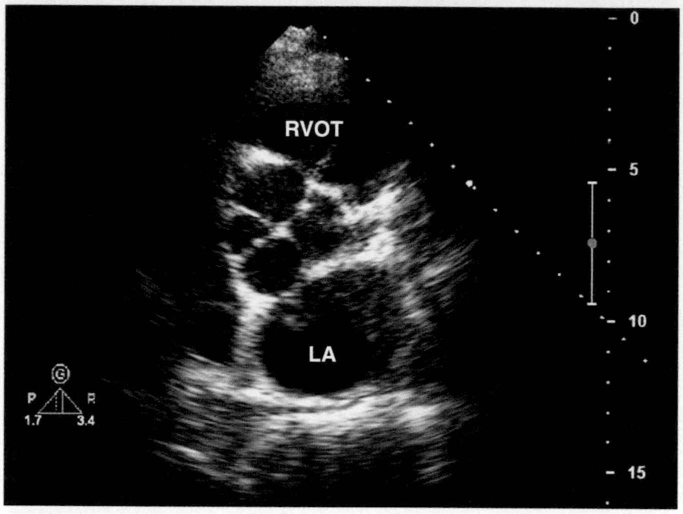

B

FIGURE 14-46 **A, Left,** Transesophageal echocardiographic image of tricuspid aortic valve (AV) from short-axis view. **Right,** Transthoracic image of a typical bicuspid aortic valve with fusion of the right and left cusps forming a raphe (arrow) and commissures at the 4 and 9 o'clock positions. **B,** Transthoracic image of quadracuspid aortic valve. LA = left atrium; RA = right atrium; RV = right ventricle; RVOT = RV outflow tract.

Aortic Stenosis

Most commonly, aortic stenosis is caused by degenerative valvular calcification. Thickened and calcified cusps cause reduced systolic opening. The aortic valve is reliably visualized with 2D echocardiography, which differentiates noncalcific (doming of aortic cusps in bicuspid aortic valve) from calcific aortic stenosis. The 2D TTE parasternal short-axis view at the level of the aortic valve is used to visualize the number of aortic cusps. Additional delineation of cusp anatomy can be obtained by TEE and 3D echocardiography (Fig. 14-46). Important ancillary information in patients with aortic stenosis readily obtained with echocardiography includes the degree of valvular calcification, aortic annulus and supravalvular ascending aorta size, degree of LV hypertrophy and the presence and degree of subvalvular obstruction, and aortic valve regurgitation.

The echocardiographic assessment of aortic stenosis severity relies on acquiring the following hemodynamic Doppler parameters: peak aortic valve velocity (v), mean pressure gradient (Fig. 14-47), aortic valve area, and the ratio of the LVOT to the aortic valve velocity or TVI. As aortic stenosis severity increases, the valve area becomes smaller and flow velocity and pressure gradients increase. The modified Bernoulli equation (pressure gradient = $4 \times v^2$ or $[2 \times v]^2$) is used to reliably measure the pressure gradient across the aortic valve. There may be a small difference between aortic valve pressure gradients obtained by Doppler and catheter methods because of the pressure recovery phenomenon. The pressure gradient depends on stroke volume; thus aortic valve area is a better measure to determine the severity of aortic stenosis, especially when stroke volume and cardiac output are decreased. Aortic valve area (AVA) is calculated from the continuity equation (see previous section on hemodynamics) (Fig. 14-48):

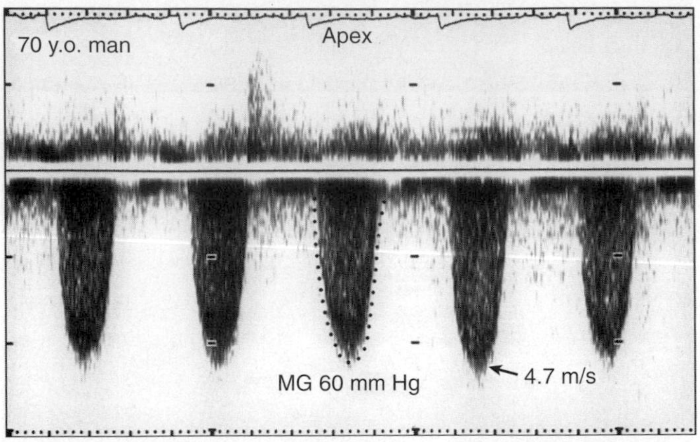

FIGURE 14–47 Continuous wave Doppler spectra from a patient with severe aortic stenosis. The velocity was obtained from the apical window. The peak velocity is 4.7 m/sec, and the mean pressure gradient (MG) is 60 mm Hg. *(From Oh JK, Seward JB, Tajik AJ: The Echo Manual. 3rd ed. Philadelphia, Lippincott Williams & Wilkins, 2006. Used with permission of Mayo Foundation for Medical Education and Research.)*

$$AVA = (LVOT\ area \times LVOT\ TVI)/AV\ TVI$$

LVOT area, LVOT TVI, and aortic valve (AV) TVI are reliably measured with 2D and Doppler echocardiography. All available transducer positions should be used to record the highest velocity from the aortic valve. When there is marked calcification of the aortic valve and annulus, it may be difficult to measure LVOT diameter and area. The continuity equation can be rearranged as:

$$AVA/LVOT\ area = LVOT\ TVI/AV\ TVI$$

The LVOT TVI and AV TVI ratio is inversely proportional to AVA and LVOT area ratio. Hence LVOT TVI/AV TVI of 0.25 indicates that AVA is 25 percent of the LVOT area. Because the LVOT area is usually 3 to 3.5 cm^2, a ratio of less than 0.25 indicates AVA of 0.8 cm^2 or less, consistent with severe aortic stenosis.

SEVERE AORTIC STENOSIS BY ECHOCARDIOGRAPHY

Aortic stenosis is usually severe when patients with normal LV systolic function and cardiac output demonstrate the following echo-Doppler hemodynamics: (a) peak aortic valve velocity is greater than or equal to 4.5 m/sec, (b) the mean pressure gradient is greater than or equal to 50 mm Hg, (c) LVOT/AV TVI less than or equal to 0.25, or (d) the aortic valve area is less than or equal to 0.75 cm^2. ACC/AHA Guidelines recommendations (see Chap. 62) selected a lower degree of stenosis with which to consider aortic valve replacement in patients with symptoms, LV dysfunction, or need for coronary artery bypass surgery.[101] These criteria include a peak velocity of greater than 4.0 m/sec, a mean pressure gradient greater than 40 mm Hg, and an aortic valve area less than 1.0 cm^2. The peak velocity threshold of 4 m/sec was selected

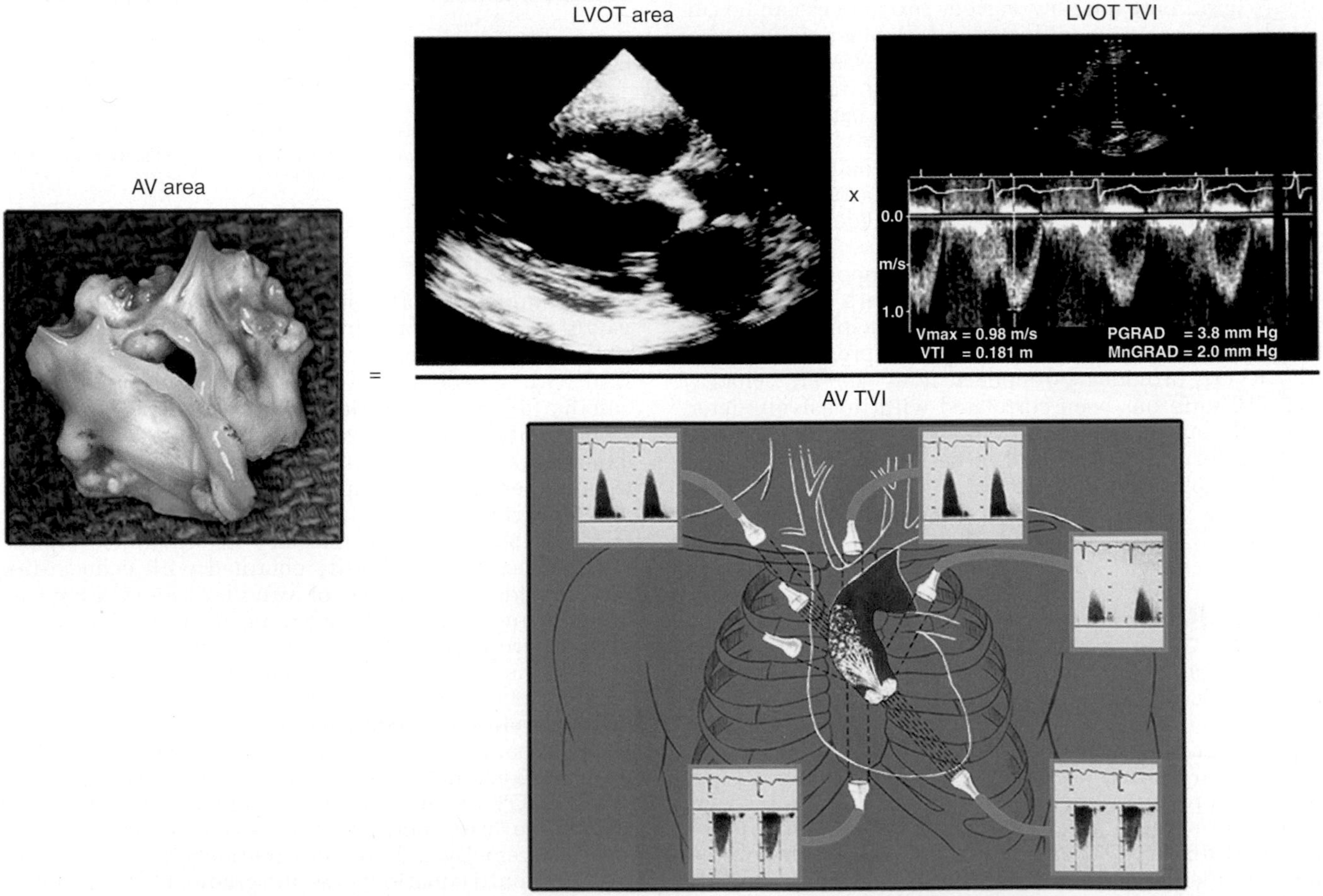

FIGURE 14–48 Continuity equation to calculate aortic valve (AV) area: AV area = LVOT $D^2 \times 0.785 \times TVI_{LVOT}/TVI_{AV}$. LVOT = left ventricular outflow tract; TVI = time velocity integral. Diagram of multiple transducer positions used to obtain aortic stenosis jet velocity. The maximal velocity is obtained most commonly (85 percent of the time) from the apical transducer position. The second most commonly successful position is the right parasternum. However, all transducer positions should be used to ensure securing the maximal velocity. *(From Oh JK, Seward JB, Tajik AJ: The Echo Manual. 3rd ed. Philadelphia, Lippincott Williams & Wilkins, 2006. Used with permission of Mayo Foundation for Medical Education and Research.)*

because of natural history data[102] indicating a high likelihood of symptoms or other indications for surgery at this degree of stenosis (see Chap. 62).

The Doppler-derived aortic pressure gradient is generally higher, and the Doppler-derived aortic valve area is smaller than the catheter-derived aortic pressure gradient and aortic valve area. Thus the American Heart Association/American College of Cardiology recommendation[101] that aortic valve area less than or equal to 1 cm^2 is severe aortic stenosis overestimates the severity of aortic stenosis when aortic valve area is calculated with 2D Doppler echocardiography.

Determination of aortic valve hemodynamics depends on LV systolic function and cardiac output. The peak aortic velocity and mean aortic pressure gradient may be less than 4.5 m/sec and less than 50 mm Hg, respectively, in patients with severe aortic stenosis when LV function and stroke volume decrease. Conversely, aortic stenosis may not be severe even when the peak velocity is greater than or equal to 4.5 m/sec and the mean gradient is greater than or equal to 50 mm Hg when cardiac output is increased, as in aortic regurgitation or anemia. In these situations, the LVOT/aortic valve TVI (or velocity) ratio and aortic valve area are more helpful in determining the severity of aortic stenosis because of proportional change in velocities.

SEVERE AORTIC STENOSIS WITH LOW AORTIC PRESSURE GRADIENT

In patients with LV systolic dysfunction and reduced cardiac output, a small aortic valve area may represent true anatomically severe aortic stenosis or functionally severe aortic stenosis because the aortic valve with moderate stenosis may not open fully because of low stroke volume. Aortic stenosis is likely severe if (a) the aortic valve area by the continuity equation is less than or equal to 0.75 cm^2, and (b) the LVOT/AV TVI (or velocity) ratio is less than or equal to 0.25. A dobutamine infusion is often used to increase stroke volume and may be helpful in differentiating morphologically severe aortic stenosis from pseudosevere aortic stenosis.[103,104] In true anatomically severe aortic stenosis, aortic valve area remains less than 1 cm^2 and the mean gradient increases proportional to an increase in stroke volume with dobutamine infusion (Fig. 14-49). Dobutamine infusion in patients with low-gradient aortic stenosis also assesses contractile reserve, defined as an increase in stroke volume of greater than 20 percent with dobutamine. Contractile reserve affects perioperative outcome; when it is absent, perioperative mortality for aortic valve replacement in a multicenter study was 50 versus 7 percent when present.[103,104] Based on these data, when dobutamine infusion increases stroke volume (or LVOT TVI) by greater than or equal to 20 percent and the aortic valve area remains less than or equal to 1 cm^2, aortic valve replacement can be performed with relatively low risk.[104,105]

NATURAL PROGRESSION OF ASYMPTOMATIC AORTIC STENOSIS

Understanding the natural progression of the severity of aortic stenosis is helpful in timing follow-up and surgical intervention. In asymptomatic patients with valvular aortic stenosis, the aortic jet velocity increases by 0.32 ± 0.34 m/sec per year, mean gradient by 7 ± 7 mm Hg per year, and valve area decreases by 0.12 ± 0.19 cm^2 per year (see Chap. 62). When peak aortic velocity is greater than 4 m/sec, the likelihood of the patient remaining alive without valve replacement at 2 years is only 21 ± 18 percent. Pellikka and colleagues[102] reported on more than 600 patients with isolated, asymptomatic aortic stenosis and peak systolic velocity greater than or equal to 4 m/sec by Doppler echocardiography who were not referred for surgery at the initial evaluation. During follow-up, most patients with asymptomatic, hemodynamically significant aortic stenosis developed symptoms within 5 years. Sudden death occurred in approximately 1 percent per year. Patients with peak velocity greater than or equal to 4.5 m/sec had a higher likelihood of developing symptoms or having surgery or cardiac death.

Mitral Stenosis

Valvular mitral stenosis is usually caused by rheumatic disease. Uncommon causes of mitral stenosis include congenital, degenerative calcification, radiation, hypereosinophilia, medication toxicity, and vegetation. The typical M-mode and 2D echocardiographic features of rheumatic mitral stenosis are shown in Figure 14-50. The parasternal short-axis view is used to measure mitral valve area using

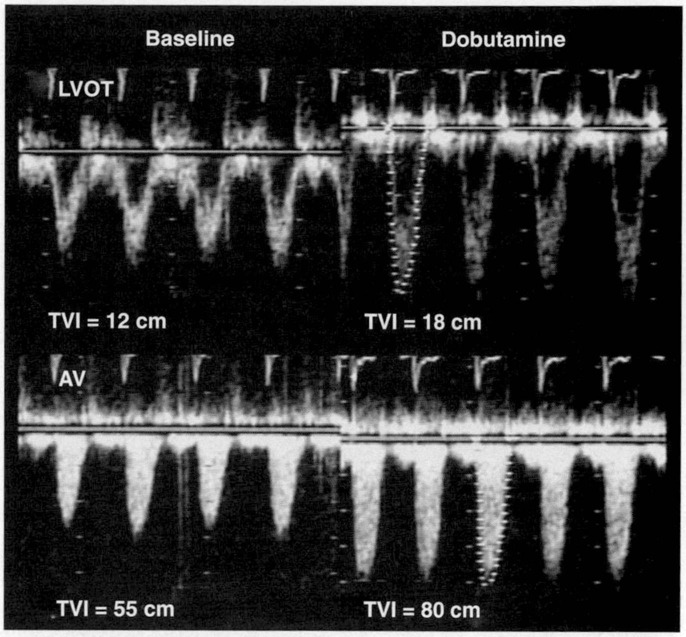

FIGURE 14–49 Example of dobutamine Doppler hemodynamic measurement in a patient with severe aortic stenosis and a low gradient. At baseline, LVOT TVI was low (12 cm), indicating a low stroke volume, and aortic valve (AV) peak velocity was 3 m/sec, with TVI of 55 cm. TVI ratio between LVOT and AV was 0.22. With infusion of dobutamine (up to 20 μg/kg/min), LVOT TVI increased to 18 cm, which is a 50 percent increase in stroke volume, and AV TVI increased a similar degree to 80 cm. TVI ratio was 0.23, similar to the baseline ratio. This result indicates that the aortic valve is truly stenotic, with a low gradient. The patient successfully underwent aortic valve replacement. LVOT, left ventricular outflow tract; TVI = time velocity integral. *(From Oh JK, Seward JB, Tajik AJ: The Echo Manual. 3rd ed. Philadelphia, Lippincott Williams & Wilkins, 2006. Used with permission of Mayo Foundation for Medical Education and Research.)*

planimetry. Three-dimensional echocardiography may provide a better determination of the stenotic mitral valve area (see Fig. 14-4C) in patients with calcified valves or prior commissurotomy.

Mitral balloon valvuloplasty is a successful form of intervention for many patients with mitral stenosis (see Chap. 62). An echocardiographic score based on valve thickness, calcification, mobility, and subvalvular thickening can be used to predict the outcome of the procedure (Table 14-11). Patients with an echocardiographic score of 8 or less generally have a more favorable result from mitral balloon valvuloplasty than those with a score higher than 8. Commissural calcification or fusion is an additional important determinant of outcome after percutaneous valvuloplasty or valvotomy.

Calculation of mitral valve area is the most reliable means of determining the severity of mitral stenosis, and several methods in addition to planimetry of the mitral valve are available.[106,107] The comprehensive echo-Doppler evaluation of mitral stenosis should include determination of:

1. Peak mitral diastolic velocity by continuous wave Doppler echocardiography
2. Mean pressure gradient and TVI by tracing mitral velocity (Fig. 14-51B)
3. Mitral valve area (MVA) by the pressure half-time (PHT) method: MVA = 220/PHT
4. MVA by the continuity equation and by the PISA method (see Fig. 14-44)

The PHT method is easiest to use, but is less reliable immediately after balloon valvuloplasty or in patients with severe aortic regurgitation or high filling pressure. This method underestimates the severity of mitral stenosis in

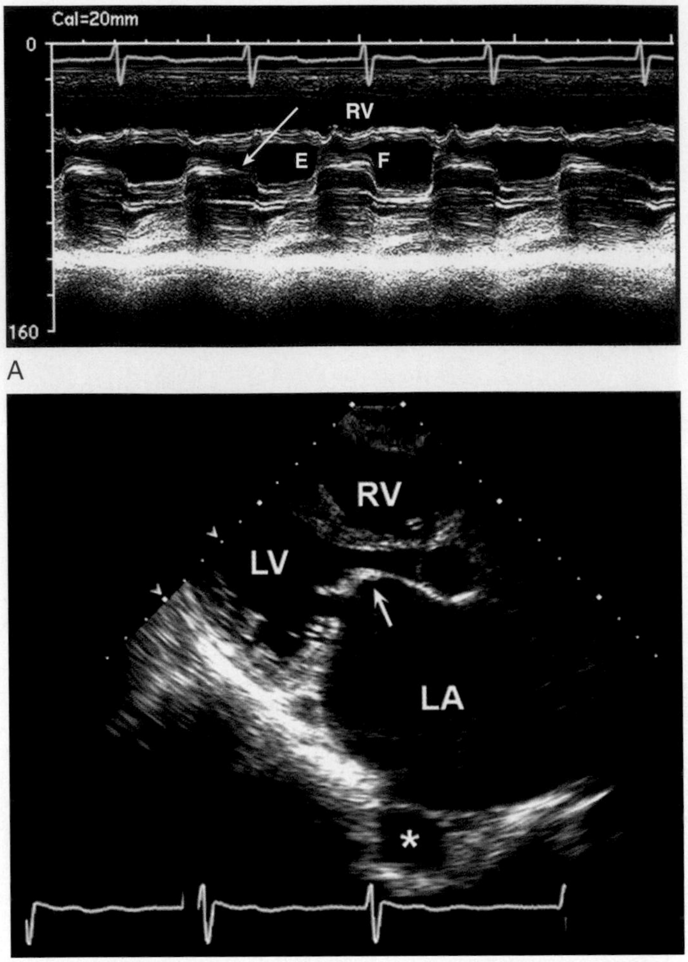

FIGURE 14–50 **A,** M-mode echocardiogram of a patient with mitral stenosis. Note the abnormal motion of the anterior mitral valve leaflet as demonstrated by the E-F slope (arrow). **B,** 2D echocardiogram of parasternal long-axis view during diastole of a patient with mitral stenosis. The mitral valve leaflets are thickened and have the typical "hockey-stick" appearance (arrow). Left atrium (LA) is enlarged. LV = left ventricle; RV = right ventricle; * = descending thoracic aorta.

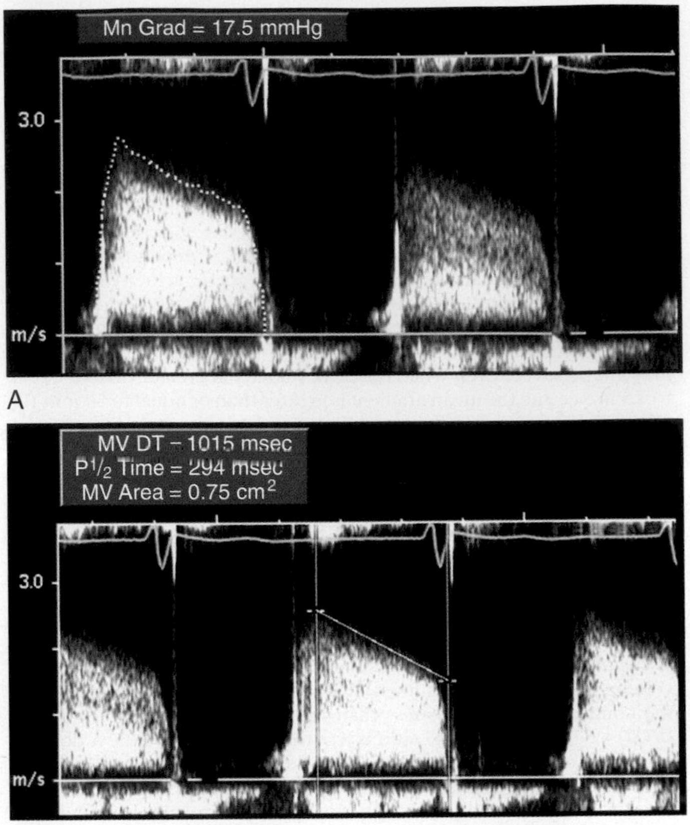

FIGURE 14–51 **A,** Continuous wave Doppler velocity measurement from the apex. The mean gradient (Mn Grad) is 17.5 mm Hg. **B,** Pressure half time (P1/2) is drawn from peak velocity and is 294 msec. Mitral valve area is calculated as 220/294 = 0.75 cm^2.

these situations because PHT becomes shortened. The continuity equation cannot be used if there is significant aortic or mitral regurgitation. The PISA method is not affected by other valvular lesions. Severe mitral stenosis by echocardiography is defined as follows:

1. Resting mean pressure gradient is greater than or equal to 10 mm Hg
2. Mitral valve area is less than or equal to 1 cm^2
3. Pressure half-time is greater than or equal to 220 ms

It may be helpful to perform a Doppler hemodynamic assessment during bicycle exercise, after treadmill exercise, or during dobutamine infusion for symptomatic patients who do not clearly show severe mitral stenosis. A marked increase in the transmitral gradient, LA pressure, and pulmonary artery pressure occurs with the exercise-related increase in cardiac output and heart rate. A mean gradient greater than 15 mm Hg with exercise is considered severe mitral stenosis. A dobutamine-induced mean mitral pressure gradient greater than or equal to 18 mm Hg predicted clinical events with 90 percent accuracy.[95] In patients with mitral stenosis, symptoms have been shown to correlate best with the degree of pulmonary hypertension. In this setting, patients may be treated with a beta blocker to decrease heart rate response to exercise or with mitral valvotomy.

TEE is used for patients with mitral stenosis primarily to exclude LA or LA appendage thrombus after an embolic event or before mitral balloon valvuloplasty. Occasionally, TEE or intracardiac echocardiography is performed during mitral balloon valvuloplasty to guide transseptal puncture or the position of the balloon.

TRICUSPID STENOSIS

Tricuspid stenosis is caused primarily by rheumatic fever (see Chap. 62). Uncommon causes are congenital, tumor, vegetation, carcinoid heart disease, and valvular damage from catheter or pacemaker leads. Tricuspid valve morphology is assessed with 2D echocardiography. The severity of tricuspid stenosis is determined by Doppler echocardiography, similar to the method described for mitral stenosis. Tricuspid stenosis is considered severe when the mean gradient is greater than or equal to 7 mm Hg and pressure half-time is greater than or equal to 190 msec (constant of 190 was proposed for the pressure half-time method).

PULMONARY STENOSIS

Pulmonary stenosis is usually an isolated congenital cardiac lesion but may be part of a more complex congenital cardiac disorder. It may also be an acquired valve disease caused by carcinoid heart disease or vegetation. Occasionally, an intracardiac or extracardiac mass obstructs or compresses the pulmonary outflow tract. Subvalvular pulmonary stenosis can occur with congenital heart disease or as a result of right-sided hypertrophic cardiomyopathy. The morphologic features of each of these lesions are easily identified on 2D and Doppler echocardiography

Aortic Regurgitation

Aortic regurgitation may be caused by an abnormal aortic valve such as a congenitally abnormal valve, endocarditis, drug-related valvulopathy, or degenerative calcific aortic

TABLE 14–11 Echocardiographic Score Used to Predict Outcome of Mitral Balloon Valvuloplasty*

Grade	Mobility	Subvalvular Thickening	Thickening	Calcification
1	Highly mobile valve with only leaflet tips restricted	Minimal thickening just below the mitral leaflets	Leaflets near normal in thickness (4-5 mm)	A single area of increased echo brightness
2	Leaflet mid and base portions have normal mobility	Thickening of chordal structures extending up to one third of the chordal length	Midleaflets normal, considerable thickening of margins (5-8 mm)	Scattered areas of brightness confined to leaflet margins
3	Valve continues to move forward in diastole, mainly from the base	Thickening extending to the distal third of the chords	Thickening extending through the entire leaflet (5-8 mm)	Brightness extending into the midportion of the leaflets
4	No or minimal forward movement of the leaflets in diastole	Extensive thickening and shortening of all chordal structures extending down to the papillary muscles	Considerable thickening of all leaflet tissue (>8-10 mm)	Extensive brightness throughout much of the leaflet tissue

*The total echocardiographic score was derived from an analysis of mitral leaflet mobility, valvular and subvalvular thickening, and calcification, which were graded from 0 (normal) to 4 according to the above criteria. This gave a total score of 0 to 16.

From Oh JK, Seward JB, Tajik AJ: The Echo Manual. 3rd ed. Philadelphia, Lippincott Williams & Wilkins, 2006. Used with permission of Mayo Foundation for Medical Education and Research.

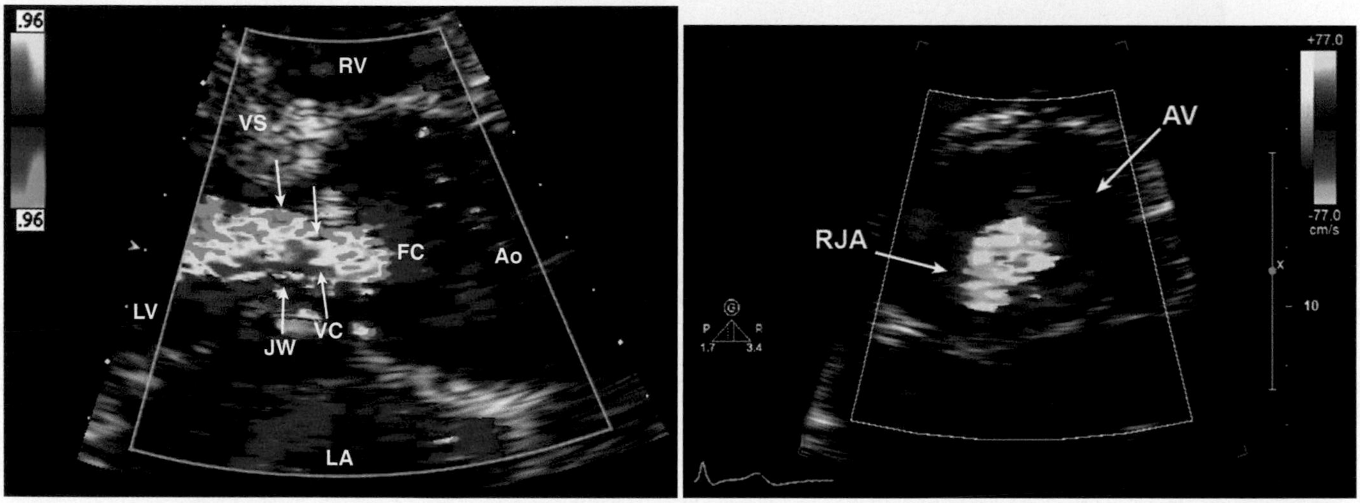

A B

FIGURE 14–52 A, Color flow imaging to estimate severity of aortic regurgitation. Parasternal long-axis view showing aortic regurgitation by color flow imaging. Left ventricular (LV) outflow height and jet width (JW) are determined from the parasternal long-axis view. Vena contracta (VC) is the smallest region below the aortic valve and flow convergence (FC). The jet spreads out into the LV outflow tract. Aortic JW is about two thirds of the LV outflow tract diameter, consistent with severe aortic regurgitation. VS = ventricular septum. **B,** Regurgitant jet area (RJA) is measured from the parasternal short-axis view at the aortic valve (AV) level. Ao = aorta; LA = left atrium; RV = right ventricle; VS = ventricular septum. ***(A,** From Oh JK, Seward JB, Tajik AJ: The Echo Manual. 3rd ed. Philadelphia, Lippincott Williams & Wilkins, 2006. Used with permission of Mayo Foundation for Medical Education and Research.)*

valve. Ascending aorta causes of aortic regurgitation include a dilated aortic root and aortic dissection. Structural abnormalities causing aortic regurgitation are usually detected on 2D echocardiography. In patients with chronic severe aortic valve regurgitation, the LV is dilated and pulsation of the aorta is evident.

Echo-Doppler methods of assessing aortic regurgitation include the following[107]: (a) The aortic regurgitant jet area is assessed from the parasternal short-axis view relative to the short-axis area of the LVOT at the level of the aortic annulus (Fig. 14-52). The width of the regurgitant jet at its origin relative to the dimension of the LVOT is also a good predictor of the severity of aortic regurgitation (see Fig. 14-52). (b) Pressure half-time measures the continuous wave Doppler signal, which corresponds to the pressure difference between the aorta and the LV (Fig. 14-53A). The pressure half-time of aortic regurgitation becomes significantly shorter with severe aortic regurgitation because of a rapid increase in LV diastolic pressure and decrease in aortic pressure. However, this velocity may also be shortened by increased LV diastolic pressure from other causes. (c) Holo-diastolic retrograde flow can be demonstrated in the descending thoracic aorta (see Fig. 14-53B) and in the abdominal aorta in severe aortic valve regurgitation. (d) In case of acute severe aortic regurgitation, LV diastolic pressure increases rapidly, resulting in a restrictive diastolic filling pattern in mitral inflow. (e) Regurgitant volume and orifice area can be quantified with the volumetric or PISA method. (f) The vena contracta is the smallest neck of the color flow region at the level of the aortic valve, immediately below the flow convergence region (see Fig. 14-52). The vena contracta is usually measured from the parasternal long-axis view, and a vena contracta greater than 6 mm is specific for severe aortic regurgitation.[107] Severe aortic regurgitation by echocardiography:

1. Regurgitant jet width/LVOT diameter ratio greater than or equal to 60 percent
2. Vena contracta greater than 6 mm
3. Regurgitant jet area/LVOT area ratio greater than or equal to 60 percent

4. Aortic regurgitation pressure half-time less than or equal to 250 ms
5. Restrictive mitral flow pattern (usually in acute setting)
6. Holodiastolic flow reversal in the descending thoracic or abdominal aorta
7. Effective regurgitant orifice greater than or equal to 0.30 cm^2
8. Regurgitant volume greater than or equal to 60 mL
9. Regurgitant fraction greater than or equal to 50 percent

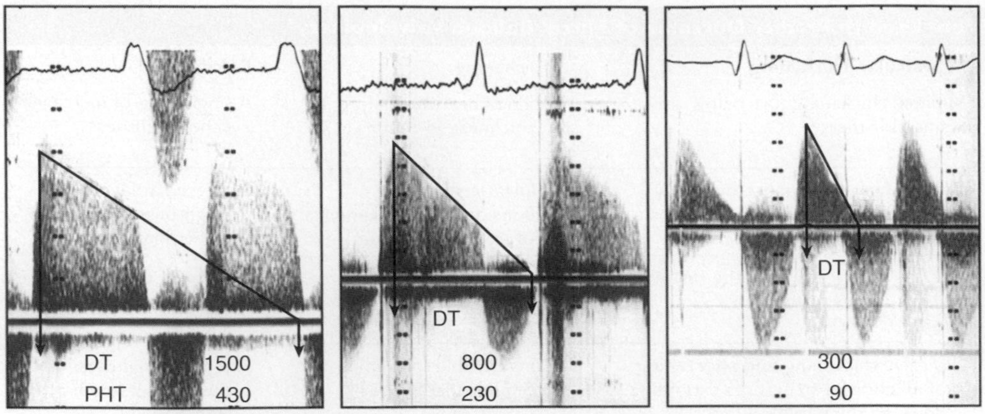

A

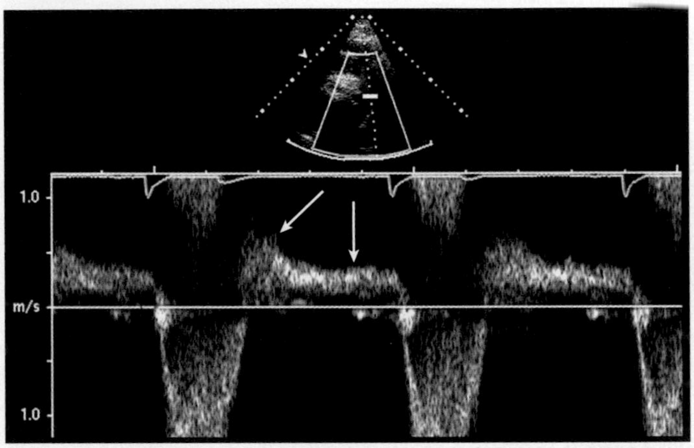

B

FIGURE 14–53 **A,** Continuous wave Doppler spectra of aortic regurgitation from three patients illustrating decreased deceleration time (DT) and pressure half-time (PHT) with more severe aortic regurgitation. **Left,** Mild regurgitation, with a PHT of 430 msec; **right,** severe regurgitation, with a PHT of 90 msec; and **middle,** moderately severe regurgitation. **B,** Holodiastolic reversal flow (arrows) in the descending aorta indicates severe aortic regurgitation. Similar diastolic reversal can be seen in a descending thoracic aneurysm or shunt into the aorta during diastole (as in Blalock-Taussig shunt). The sample volume is usually located just distal to the takeoff of the left subclavian artery. *(From Oh JK, Seward JB, Tajik AJ: The Echo Manual. 3rd ed. Philadelphia, Lippincott Williams & Wilkins, 2006. Used with permission of Mayo Foundation for Medical Education and Research.)*

Mitral Regurgitation

Comprehensive echocardiography identifies the underlying cause of mitral regurgitation (see Chap. 62), which may be related to a cleft or other congenital mitral valve abnormality, mitral valve prolapse, mitral annulus calcification or dilatation, papillary muscle dysfunction or rupture, rheumatic valve involvement, drug-induced valvulopathy, endocarditis, or perforation.

Echo-Doppler methods of assessing mitral regurgitation include the following[107]: (a) qualitative assessment using color flow imaging—the area of the regurgitant jet relative to the size of the LA has been shown to correlate well with regurgitant severity determined with angiography when the jet is not eccentric (Fig. 14-54). However, color flow imaging of valvular regurgitation depends on technical machine settings, loading conditions, and jet geometry. A flow jet directed against the atrial wall appears smaller than a free jet of the same regurgitant volume (Coanda effect). (b) Antegrade flow (*mitral inflow*) velocity increases with severe regurgitation. (c) The continuous wave Doppler spectrum may have a characteristic configuration (due to the V wave) with increased intensity (see Fig. 14-e10 on website) and reduced systolic velocity as the increase in LA pressure reduces the transmitral systolic gradient (see Fig. 14-e10 on website). (d) In severe mitral regurgitation, there may be systolic flow reversal in the pulmonary vein (see Fig. 14-e11 on website). (e) The vena contracta is the narrowest portion of the mitral regurgitation jet downstream from the orifice (Fig. 14-55).[107] It represents the physiological or effective orifice area of the regurgitant jet as opposed to the actual anatomical orifice area,[108] and the vena contracta width correlates well with other quantitative measures of mitral regurgitation severity.[107,108] (f) Regurgitant volume, fraction, and orifice area can be calculated with the volumetric or PISA method to assess the severity of mitral regurgitation (Fig. 14-56). It should be emphasized that the determination of regurgitation severity should incorporate LV volume, which should increase with severe degrees of chronic aortic or mitral regurgitation. A normal LV volume is not consistent with severe chronic aortic or mitral regurgitation.

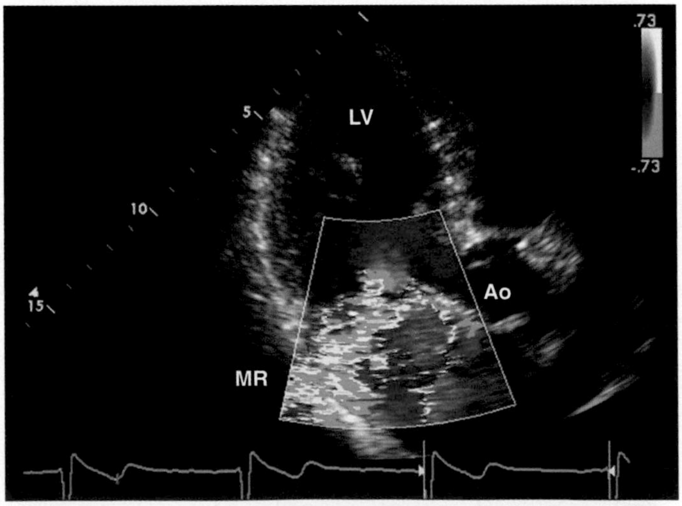

FIGURE 14–54 Standard color flow imaging of mitral regurgitation (MR) from apical long-axis view. Ao = aorta; LV = left ventricle. *(From Oh JK, Seward JB, Tajik AJ: The Echo Manual. 3rd ed. Philadelphia, Lippincott Williams & Wilkins, 2006. Used with permission of Mayo Foundation for Medical Education and Research.)*

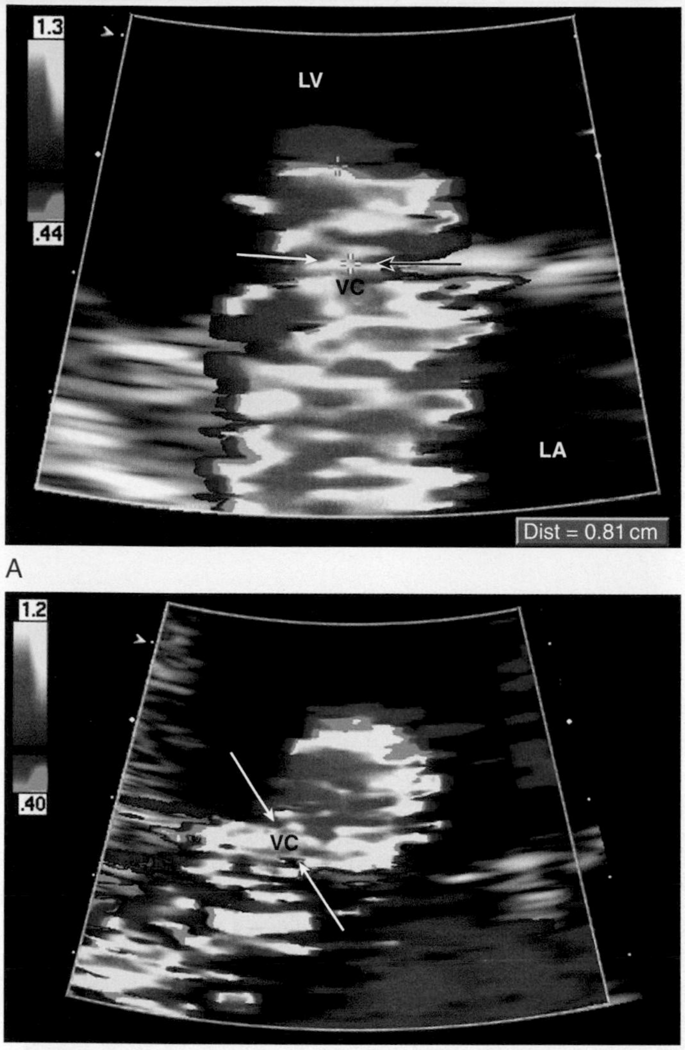

FIGURE 14–55 Measurement of the vena contracta (VC between arrows) in two different patients. **A,** With a central mitral regurgitation jet and, **B,** with an eccentric mitral regurgitation jet (note change in color flow baseline). LA = left atrium; LV = left ventricle. *(From Oh JK, Seward JB, Tajik AJ: The Echo Manual. 3rd ed. Philadelphia, Lippincott Williams & Wilkins, 2006. Used with permission of Mayo Foundation for Medical Education and Research.)*

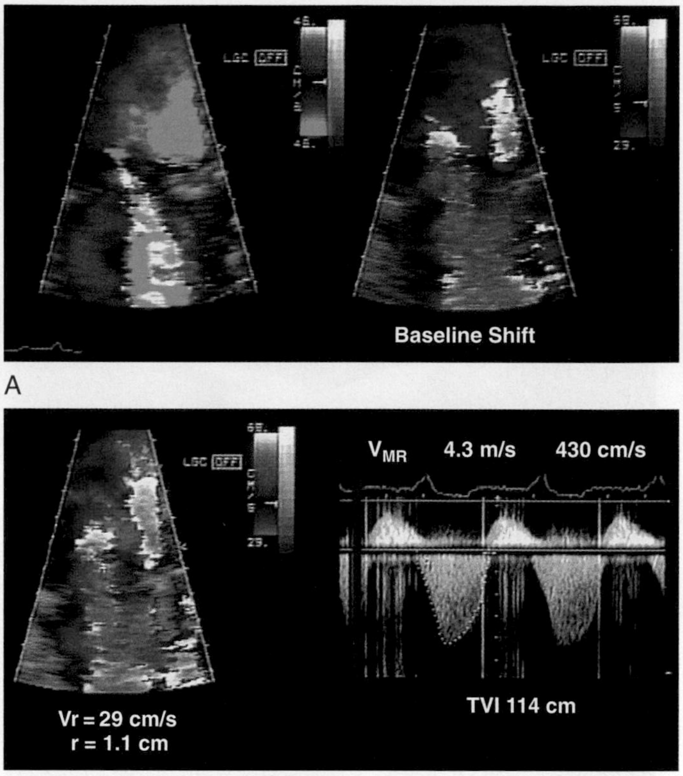

FIGURE 14–56 **A,** Apical four-chamber view and color flow imaging of mitral regurgitation, with mitral regurgitation jet zoomed. **Left,** Aliasing velocity is 46 cm/sec in either direction. The baseline for the color flow map has not been shifted. **Right,** Color flow map baseline is shifted downward so that negative aliasing velocity was reduced from 46 cm/sec to 29 cm/sec. The downward baseline shift makes the change of color flow farther from the mitral regurgitant orifice because blood flow converging toward the mitral regurgitant orifice has a lower velocity farther away from the regurgitant orifice. Therefore a downward baseline shift makes the radius of the identified proximal isovelocity surface area (PISA) larger. **B,** The measured radius (r) was 1.1 cm, with an aliasing velocity (Vr) of 29 cm/s. Mitral regurgitation velocity (V_{MR}) was obtained with continuous wave Doppler from the apex, and the peak velocity was 4.3 m/sec (430 cm/sec), with a time velocity integral (TVI) of 114 cm. From the data of PISA radius, color flow map aliasing velocity, mitral regurgitation peak velocity, and mitral regurgitation TVI, the mitral regurgitation effective regurgitant orifice and regurgitant volume can be calculated. *(From Oh JK, Seward JB, Tajik AJ: The Echo Manual. 3rd ed. Philadelphia, Lippincott Williams & Wilkins, 2006. Used with permission of Mayo Foundation for Medical Education and Research.)*

MITRAL VALVE PROLAPSE

The echocardiographic diagnosis of mitral valve prolapse is primarily based on the parasternal long-axis view (see Chap. 62). Mitral valve prolapse is defined as systolic displacement (>2 mm) of one or both mitral leaflets into the LA, below the plane of the mitral annulus (Fig. 14-57A and B). The mitral leaflets are often thickened (>5 mm) or myxomatous. If a strict definition is used, the prevalence of mitral valve prolapse is 1.7 to 2.4 percent. The calculation of mitral regurgitant volume is more accurate than a visual assessment of its severity in mitral valve prolapse because the duration of mitral regurgitation is shorter (see Fig. 14-57). Severe mitral regurgitation by echocardiography:

1. Two-dimensional echocardiographic evidence of disruption of the mitral valve apparatus (papillary muscle rupture, flail mitral leaflet)
2. Effective regurgitant orifice is greater than or equal to 0.40 cm^2
3. Mitral regurgitation volume is greater than or equal to 60 mL
4. Regurgitation fraction is greater than or equal to 50 percent
5. Vena contracta width is greater than or equal to 7 mm
6. Mitral regurgitation color flow jet reaching the posterior wall of the LA (with a high aliasing velocity of the color map)
7. Pulmonary vein systolic flow reversals

Mitral regurgitation can be dynamic, related to afterload and ischemia. Occasionally, assessment of clinically important mitral regurgitation requires change in loading conditions or exercise. For example, the severity of mitral regurgitation in the operating room is usually less than that of the preoperative evaluation. Mitral regurgitation needs to be assessed after an increase in afterload with an isoproterenol infusion. In patients with ischemia, mitral regurgitation, and LV dysfunction, the effective regurgitant orifice and mitral regurgitant volume may increase with exercise.[103] In patients with exercise-induced systolic anterior motion of the mitral valve, mitral regurgitation may be evident only with exercise, Valsalva maneuver, or in a standing position.

FUNCTIONAL MITRAL REGURGITATION

Functional mitral regurgitation is regurgitation caused by regional or global LV remodeling in ischemic or dilated cardiomyopathy without structural valve abnormalities (see Chap. 62). The functional mitral regurgitation jet is usually central in origin, and color flow imaging tends to overestimate its severity. After 5 years, total mortality and cardiac mortality for patients with at least moderate degree (effective regurgitant orifice ≥20 mm^2 and regurgitant volume ≥30 mL) ischemic mitral regurgitation (62 ± 5 and 50 ± 6 percent, respectively) were

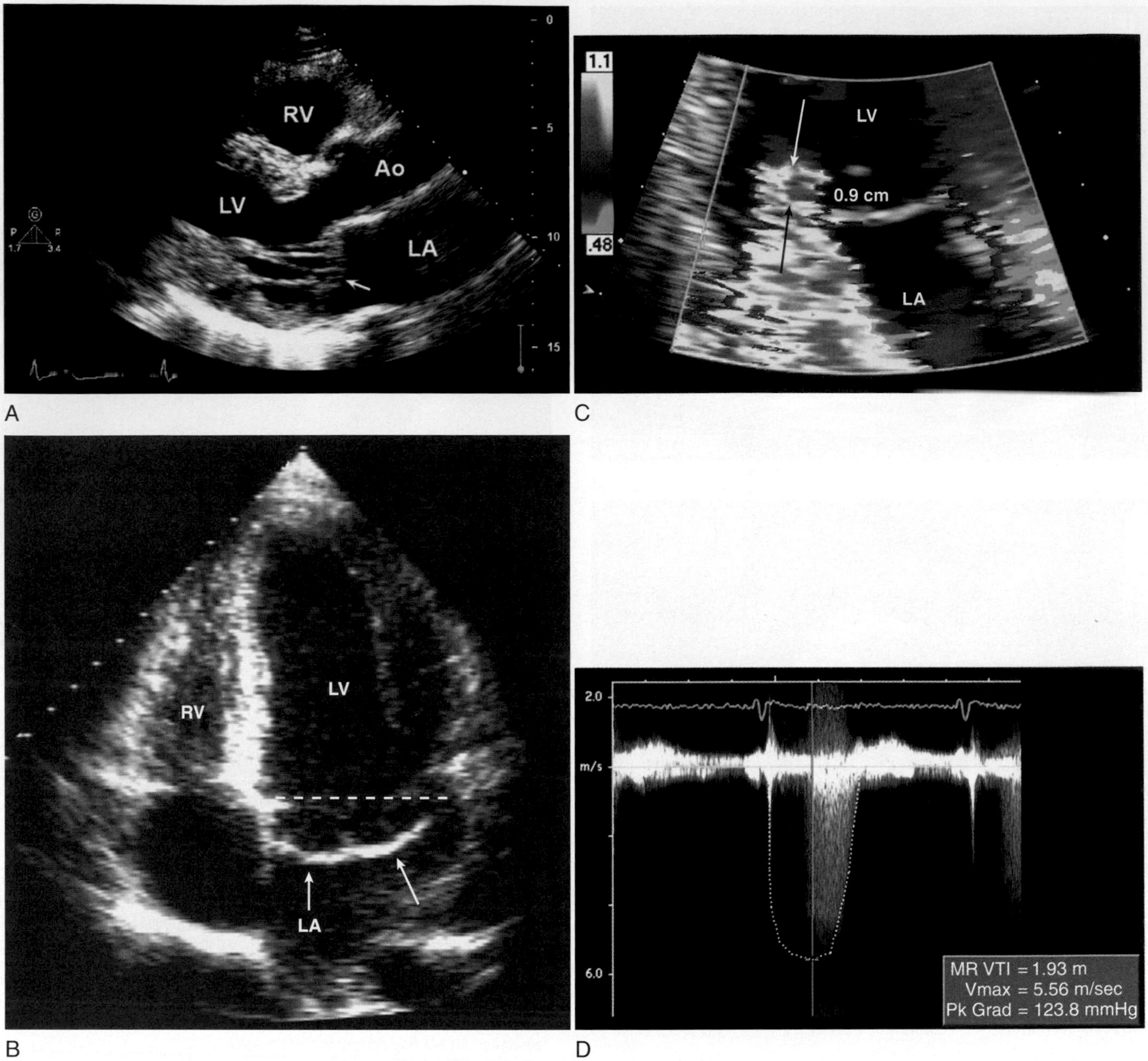

FIGURE 14–57 A, From the parasternal long-axis view, there is systolic displacement of the anterior mitral leaflet (arrow) into the left atrium (LA) beyond the plane of the mitral annulus. **B,** Apical four-chamber view showing prolapse of both mitral leaflets (arrows). Dotted line, plane of the mitral annulus. Generally, the apical view should not be used to make the diagnosis of mitral valve prolapse. **C,** Quantification of mitral regurgitation (MR) in mitral valve prolapse. Proximal isovelocity surface area (PISA) of MR caused by mitral valve prolapse with color flow aliasing velocity of 48 cm/sec. PISA radius is 0.9 cm, which usually indicates severe MR. **D,** Continuous wave Doppler recording of MR velocity shows mid to late systolic MR. Peak MR velocity is 556 cm/sec, hence:

$$\text{Effective regurgitant orifice (ERO)} = 6.28 \times (0.9)^2 \times 48/556 = 0.44\ \text{cm}^2$$

consistent with severe MR. MR time velocity integral (TVI) is 193 cm if the entire systolic interval is included, which provides the following calculation of MR volume:

$$\text{MR volume} = \text{ERO} \times \text{TVI} = 0.44 \times 193 = 85\ \text{mL}$$

MR volume also indicates severe MR. However, the actual TVI is about half because MR starts at mid-systole, which estimates MR volume to be about 40 mL (more consistent with moderate MR). Ao = aorta; LV = left ventricle; RV = right ventricle. *(**B-D,** From Oh JK, Seward JB, Tajik AJ: The Echo Manual. 3rd ed. Philadelphia, Lippincott Williams & Wilkins, 2006. Used with permission of Mayo Foundation for Medical Education and Research.)*

higher than for those without ischemic mitral regurgitation (39 ± 6 and 30 ± 5 percent, respectively). The major determinant of the effective regurgitant orifice is mitral deformation (i.e., systolic mitral valvular tenting area) (Fig. 14-58).[33] The tenting area is determined by apical and posterior displacement of the papillary muscles and by the wall motion score index (WMSI) of the segments supporting the papillary muscles. A tenting area greater than or equal to 6 cm^2 usually indicates grade 3 or higher mitral regurgitation.

Transesophageal Echocardiography

TEE visualizes the mitral valve apparatus clearly including the identification of the flail mitral leaflet scallops (Fig. 14-59) and can be used in conjunction with TTE to determine the cause and severity of mitral regurgitation. TEE often provides invaluable clinical and anatomical information in

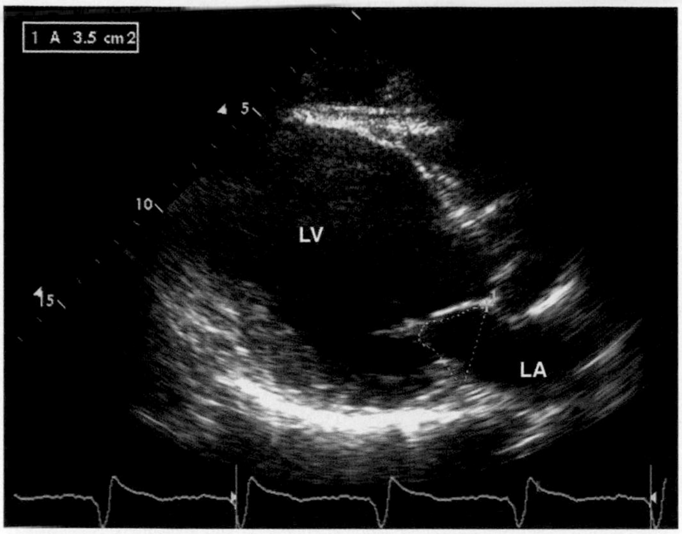

FIGURE 14–58 Parasternal long-axis view of dilated cardiomyopathy. Mitral tenting (dotted area) is caused by the markedly dilated left ventricular (LV) cavity. The tenting area (A), is 3.5 cm^2. LA = left atrium.

the setting of severe acute mitral regurgitation and is routinely used in the operating room to assess the mitral valve before and after operative intervention.

Tricuspid Regurgitation

A mild degree of tricuspid regurgitation is common, and its velocity is routinely used to estimate RV systolic pressure. However, a more-than-moderate tricuspid regurgitation has been found to adversely affect survival.[109] A flail tricuspid valve leaflet is associated with excess mortality, especially when associated with severe enlargement of right-sided chambers.[110]

Tricuspid regurgitation may be caused by primary valve disease, such as Ebstein anomaly, rheumatic valve, prolapse, carcinoid, rupture, or injury from trauma or a pacemaker or defibrillator wire.[111] Alternatively, tricuspid regurgitation may be secondary to annular dilatation, RV infarct, or pulmonary hypertension.[112]

Echocardiographic methods used to assess tricuspid regurgitation severity are similar to those used to assess mitral regurgitation and include (Fig. 14-60) (a) assessment

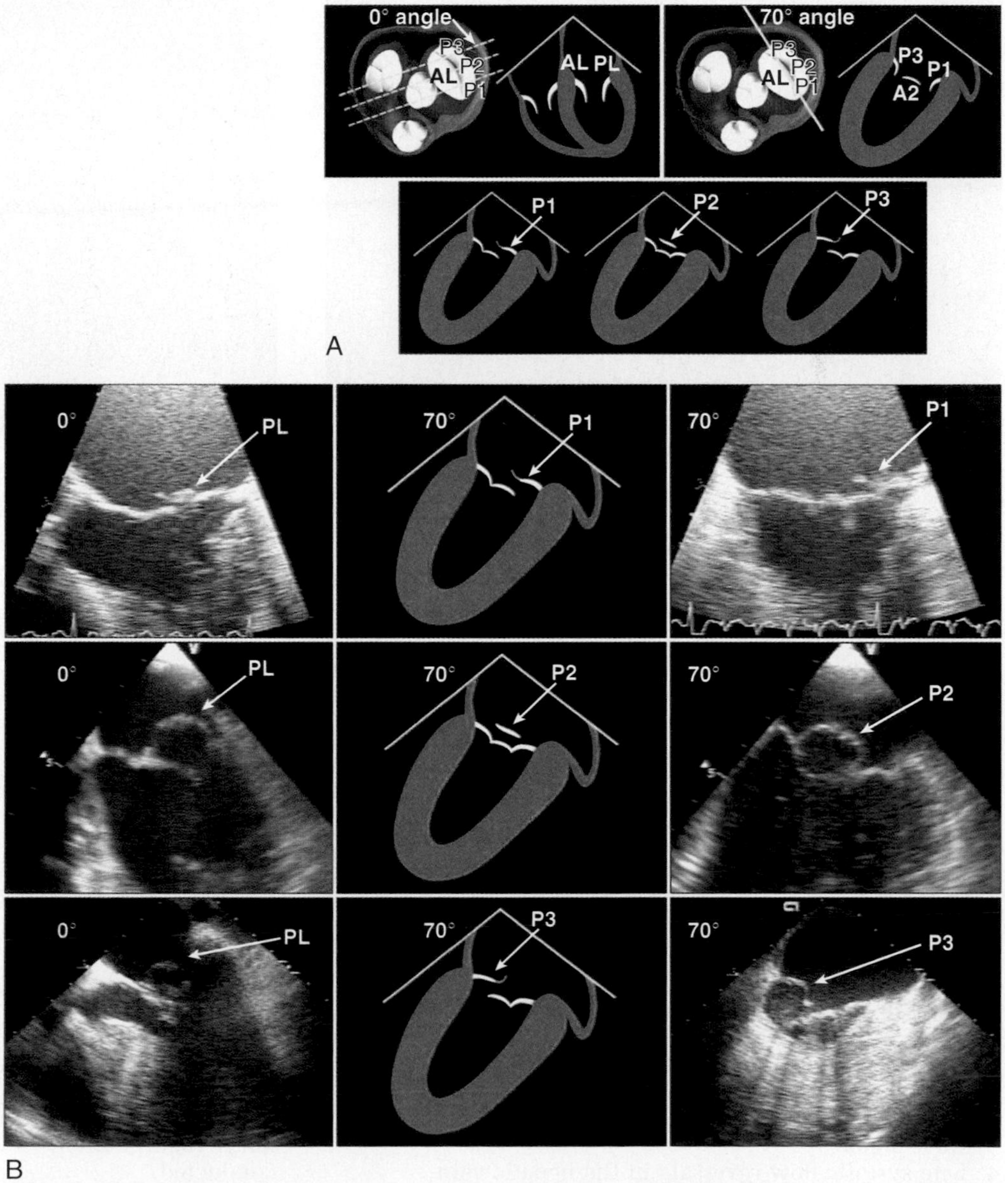

FIGURE 14–59 **A,** TEE identification of mitral valve scallops. **Upper left,** First view at 0 degrees to determine if anterior or posterior (AL = anterior leaflet; PL = posterior leaflet). **Upper right,** Next, the probe is rotated to about 70 degrees, cutting across the valve medial to lateral to identify the individual scallops (P3, medial posterior scallop; P2, middle scallop; P1, lateral scallop; A2, middle portion of the anterior leaflet). P2 is across from A2 and seen when flail. **Lower panels,** Examples of the three posterior leaflet flail views. **B,** Examples of flail mitral valve scallops. **Left column,** Transesophageal images at 0 degrees. The scallop location cannot be adequately assessed at 0 degrees. **Middle column,** Drawings of the lateral (P1), middle (P2), and medial (P3) flail scallops. **Right column,** The corresponding transesophageal echocardiographic images at 70 degrees. *(From Oh JK, Seward JB, Tajik AJ: The Echo Manual. 3rd ed. Philadelphia, Lippincott Williams & Wilkins, 2006. Used with permission of Mayo Foundation for Medical Education and Research.)*

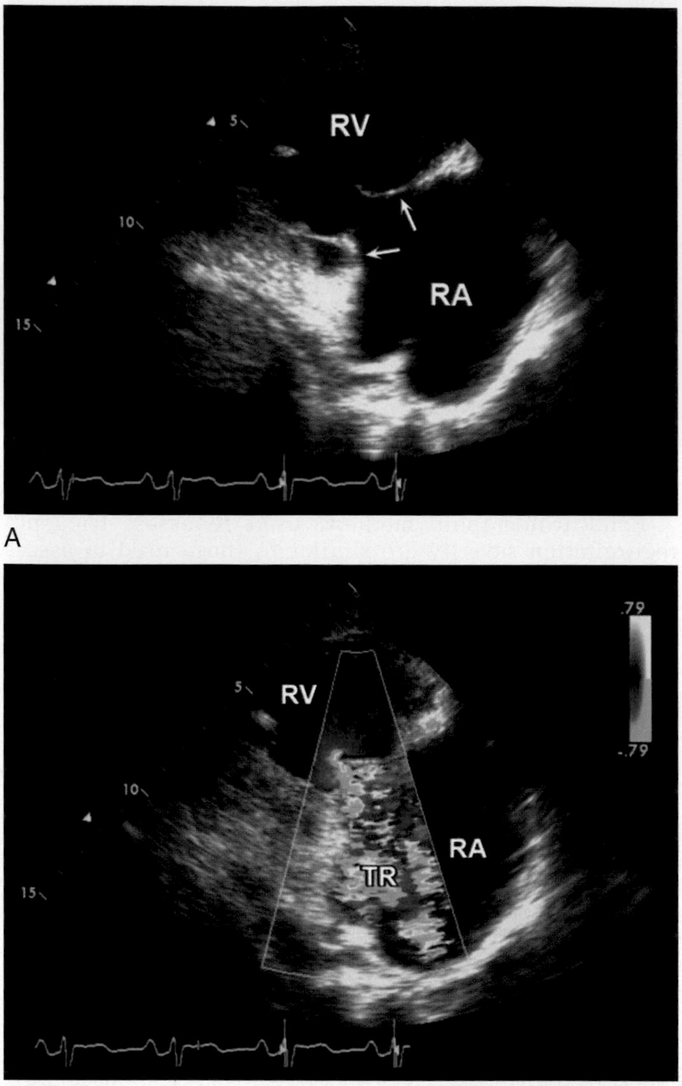

FIGURE 14–60 **A,** 2D systolic frame of right ventricular (RV) inflow view showing carcinoid involvement of the tricuspid valve. Anterior and septal tricuspid leaflets (arrows) do not coapt because of retraction and thickening, which results in severe tricuspid regurgitation. **B,** Color flow imaging shows severe tricuspid regurgitation (TR). RA = right atrium.

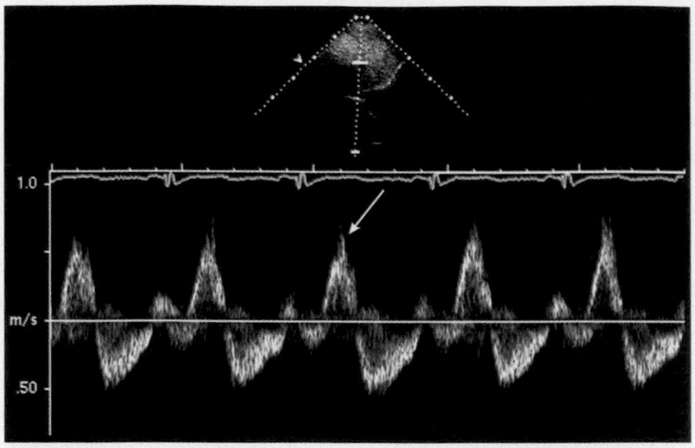

FIGURE 14–61 Pulsed wave Doppler recording showing late systolic flow reversal (arrow) in the hepatic vein. *(From Oh JK, Seward JB, Tajik AJ: The Echo Manual. 3rd ed. Philadelphia, Lippincott Williams & Wilkins, 2006. Used with permission of Mayo Foundation for Medical Education and Research.)*

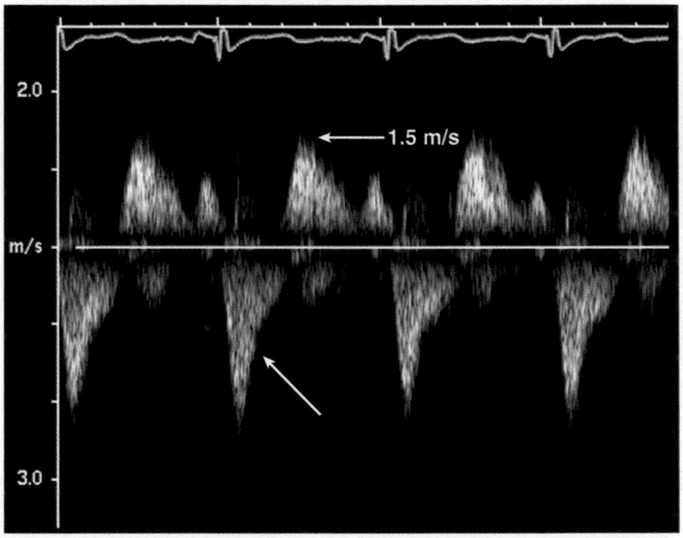

FIGURE 14–62 Continuous wave Doppler recording of tricuspid flow in a patient with severe tricuspid regurgitation. Because of the large amount of tricuspid regurgitation, there is an indentation (arrow) in tricuspid regurgitation velocity spectrum during mid-late systole (i.e., V wave). Diastolic velocity is also increased (1.5 m/sec) from increased flow across the tricuspid valve. *(From Oh JK, Seward JB, Tajik AJ: The Echo Manual. 3rd ed. Philadelphia, Lippincott Williams & Wilkins, 2006. Used with permission of Mayo Foundation for Medical Education and Research.)*

of regurgitant jet area with color flow imaging, (b) identification of late-peaking systolic flow reversal in the hepatic veins (Fig. 14-61) (this should not be confused with early-peaking systolic flow reversals caused by RV dysfunction or increased RA pressure), (c) demonstration of continuous wave Doppler signal with increased forward flow velocity, relatively decreased tricuspid regurgitation velocity, and concave late systolic configuration of tricuspid regurgitation due to a large RA V wave (Fig. 14-62), (d) use of the vena contracta width to quantify the severity of tricuspid regurgitation (see Fig 62-42),[107] and (e) calculation of the effective regurgitant orifice and regurgitant volume with the PISA method, as for the mitral valve. Severe tricuspid regurgitation by echocardiography:

1. Color flow regurgitant jet area is greater than or equal to 30 percent of RA area
2. Annulus dilatation (≥4 cm) or inadequate cusp coaptation
3. Late systolic concave configuration of the continuous wave signal
4. Late systolic flow reversals in the hepatic vein
5. Effective regurgitant orifice is greater than or equal to 0.4 cm^2
6. Regurgitant volume is greater than or equal to 45 mL
7. Width of vena contracta is greater than or equal to 6.5 mm

Pulmonary Regurgitation

Mild degrees of pulmonary regurgitation have been reported in 40 to 78 percent of patients with normal pulmonary valves and no structural heart disease. Pulmonary regurgitation is often related to pulmonary hypertension; previous operative intervention for congenital pulmonary stenosis; and, less commonly, carcinoid or rheumatic or other acquired valve disease. Because of difficulties imaging the pulmonary valve and the low prevalence of severe pulmonary regurgitation, few validation studies have been conducted.

Evaluation of the pulmonary valve is usually possible with 2D echocardiography. Identification of valve anatomy including bicuspid valve, prolapse, dysplasia, or absence of the pulmonary valve may help define the mechanism of regurgitation (see Fig. 14-e12A on website). Color Doppler imaging shows a diastolic jet in the RVOT, beginning at the region of the pulmonary valve (see Fig. 14-e12B on website). Planimetered jet areas, indexed for body surface area, have been shown to correlate well with the severity of pulmonary regurgitation determined angiographically. The continuous wave Doppler profile demonstrates rapid deceleration of the regurgitation jet to baseline (Fig. 14-63; see also Fig. 62-44). The vena contracta width may be used to evaluate the severity of pulmonary regurgitation with color Doppler imaging; however, this technique has not been validated for the pulmonary valve.

Drug-Induced Valvular Heart Disease

Several drugs have been associated with regurgitant or stenotic valvular heart disease, including ergot preparations, appetite suppressants, and pergolide. These drugs induce valvular abnormalities similar in echocardiographic appearance to carcinoid heart disease or rheumatic valve disease (Fig. 14-64).[113]

Summary

An integrated comprehensive echocardiographic approach should provide a complete assessment of valvular heart disease in most patients. Discrepancies between a clinical assessment and measures of severity should be explained, and additional diagnostic imaging considered if discrepancies persist. When surgical intervention is necessary, hemodynamic evaluation by cardiac catheterization is necessary only when comprehensive echocardiography is not adequate (<5 percent).

Prosthetic Valve Evaluation (see Chap. 62)

The echocardiographic evaluation of prosthetic valves requires a thorough knowledge of the normal structure and hemodynamic profiles, as well as the surgical techniques used for different prostheses. Identification of prosthetic valve structural abnormalities requires an understanding of the echocardiographic characteristics including reflectance of the prosthetic material, attenuation of the ultrasound beam, and ultrasound reverberations from the prosthesis. All these factors may cause difficulties in echocardiographic interpretation. Structural abnormalities of a prosthesis, such as dehiscence, vegetation, thrombus, and tissue prosthesis degeneration, can be assessed with 2D TTE, complemented by TEE when needed because of the challenges in visualizing structures around and behind the cardiac prosthesis.

Doppler echocardiography is used to determine pressure gradients across prosthetic valves with the use of the modified Bernoulli equation. Invasive dual-catheter pressure measurements made simultaneously across various prosthetic valves (Fig. 14-65) have demonstrated an excellent correlation with Doppler-derived gradients. However, because of the *pressure recovery phenomenon,* it has been shown in vitro that the aortic prosthetic gradients determined with Doppler velocities are overestimated compared

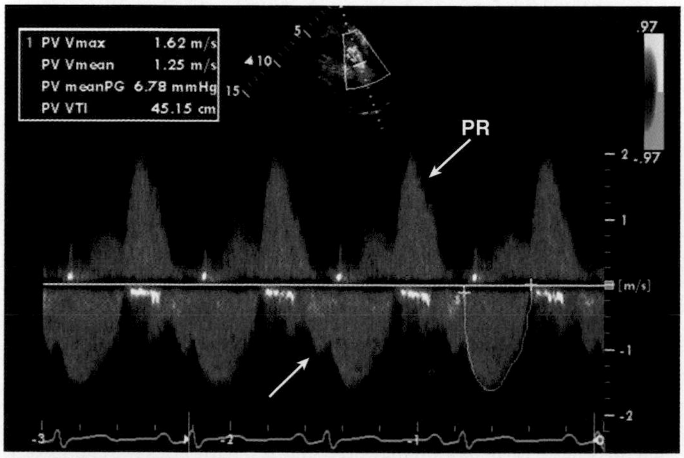

FIGURE 14–63 Continuous wave Doppler signal showing a pulmonary regurgitant (PR) signal with a short deceleration time because of rapid equalization (downward arrow) of the right ventricular and pulmonary artery diastolic pressures before the onset of QRS. There is also diastolic flow (upward arrow) across the pulmonary valve caused by a rapid increase in right ventricular diastolic pressure.

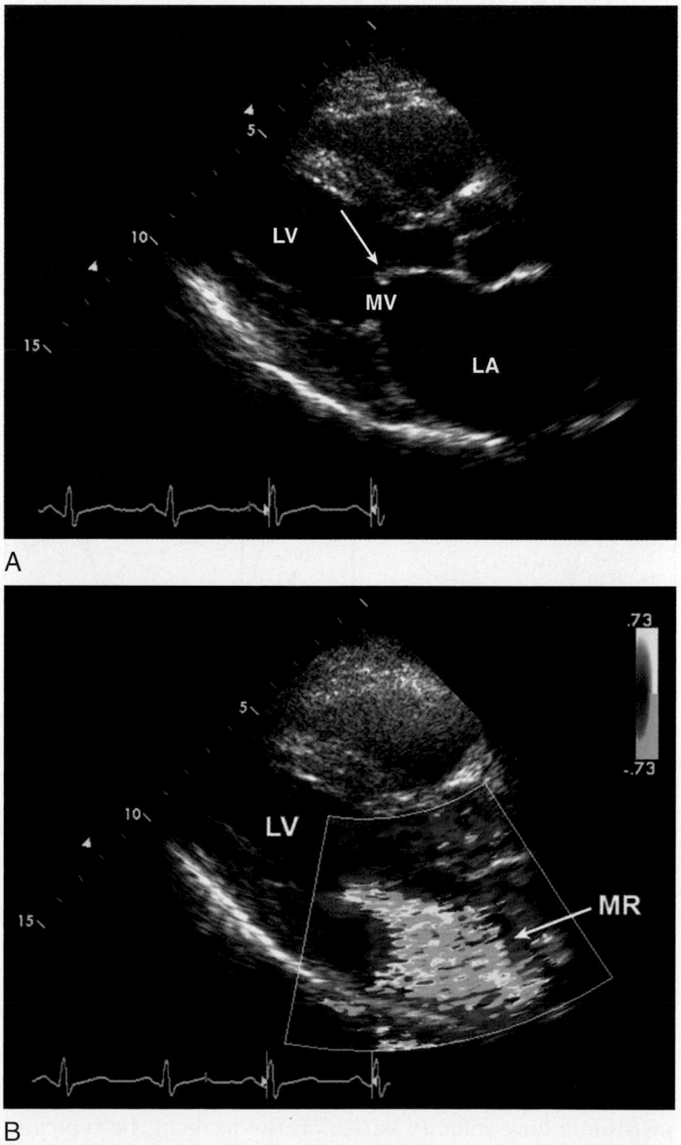

FIGURE 14–64 A, Typical echocardiographic features of mitral valve associated with fenfluramine treatment. The mitral valve (MV) is thickened. The anterior mitral leaflet (arrow) has doming during diastole, resembling a rheumatic MV. **B,** Color flow imaging shows severe mitral regurgitation (MR). LA = left atrium; LV = left ventricle.

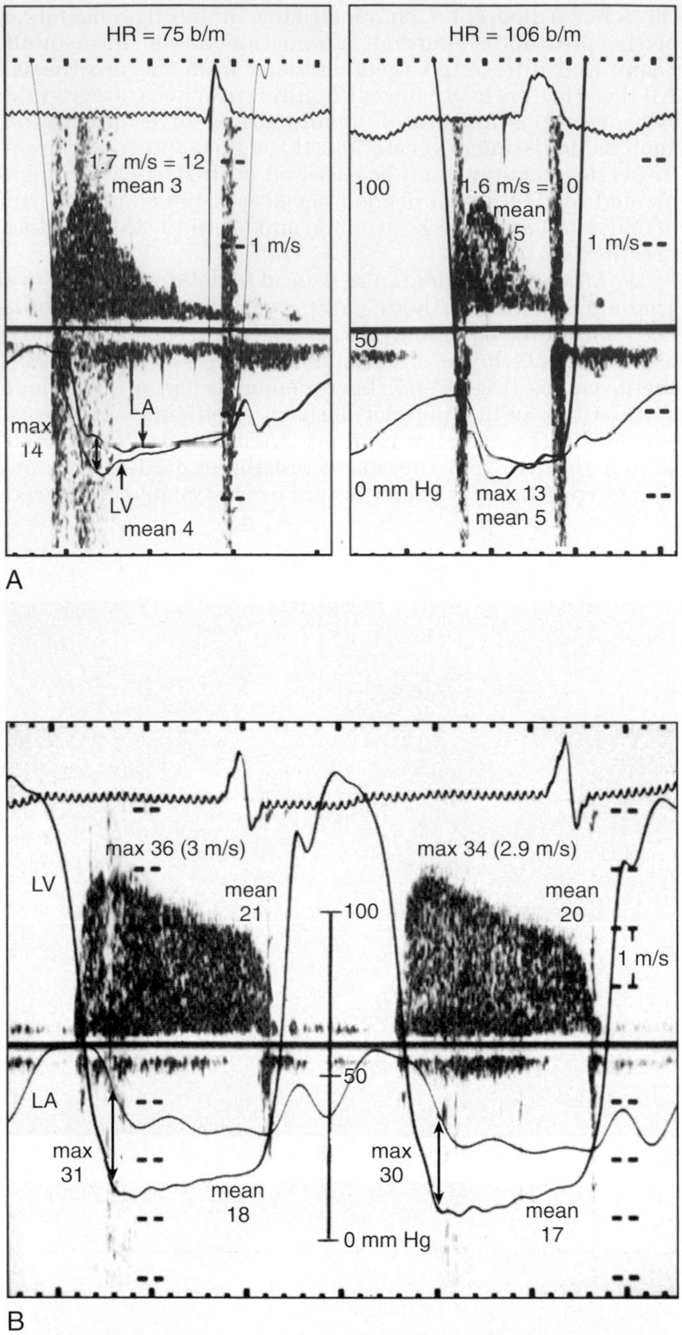

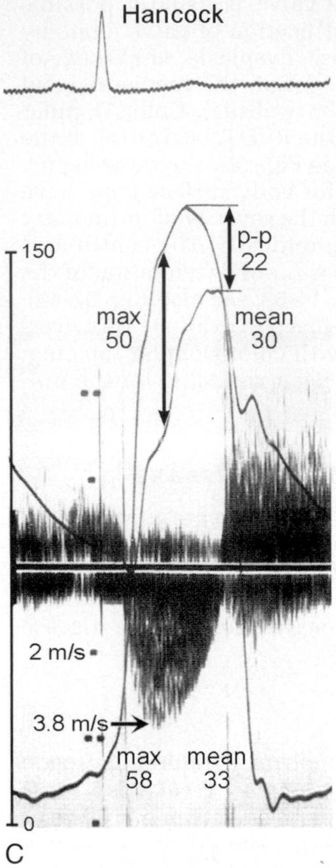

FIGURE 14–65 **A,** Simultaneous Doppler and catheterization study of a normal mechanical mitral prosthesis. The correlation between the two techniques at different heart rates (HR) is good. b/m = beats per minute; LA = left atrium; LV = left ventricle. **B,** Simultaneous continuous wave Doppler and catheter pressure measurements in a patient with an obstructed Hancock mitral prosthesis. The maximal (36 versus 31 mm Hg) and mean (21 versus 18 mm Hg by Doppler and catheter, respectively) gradients derived from these two techniques correlate well. **C,** Simultaneous Doppler and catheterization study in a patient with a Hancock aortic prosthesis. The correlation between Doppler-derived and catheter-derived maximal (58 versus 50 mm Hg) and mean (33 versus 30 mm Hg) pressure gradients is good. A good correlation was also noted for the mechanical aortic prosthesis. Note that the peak-to-peak (p-p) gradient, which is a nonphysiological assessment, underestimates the severity of obstruction (p-p gradient, 22 mm Hg; catheter-derived mean gradient, 30 mm Hg). *(**A,** From Oh JK, Seward JB, Tajik AJ: The Echo Manual. 3rd ed. Philadelphia, Lippincott Williams & Wilkins, 2006. Used with permission of Mayo Foundation for Medical Education and Research. **B** and **C,** From Burstow D, Nishimura R, Bailey K, et al: Continuous wave Doppler echocardiographic measurement of prosthetic valve gradients: A simultaneous Doppler-catheter correlative study. Circulation 80:504, 1989. Used with permission.)*

with catheter-derived gradients. In pressure recovery, part of the kinetic energy, which is lost during flow passage through a small orifice, is recovered. Therefore this pressure recovery results in a higher absolute pressure in the ascending aorta away from the stenotic aortic valve, accounting for the pressure gradient being lower than the Doppler-derived pressure gradient, which measures the highest value. Pressure recovery is smaller when the aorta is dilated.[114] The discrepancy is minor in a large mechanical prosthesis and in tissue prostheses.

The prosthetic valve is inherently stenotic, and normal prosthetic flow velocity varies on the basis of the type and size of the prosthesis, the location, and the cardiac output. Normal Doppler values for each type of aortic, mitral, tricuspid, and pulmonary prosthesis in a large number of patients has been reported (Tables 14-12 to 14-15). Not only is it important to know the normal values for each prosthesis but also to have an early postoperative baseline Doppler study that can be used as an individual reference baseline for comparison with later studies. Increased flow velocities across a prosthetic valve may be caused by regurgitation from increased flow across the prosthesis or obstruction indicating a smaller orifice.

Thrombus is the most common cause of mitral mechanical prosthesis obstruction (Fig. 14-66), whereas pannus formation is usually the cause of aortic mechanical prosthesis obstruction. The reduced motion of the disk, ball, or leaflets in an obstructed prosthetic valve may be difficult to visualize and quantify with TTE, whereas normal and abnormal prosthetic valve motion may be visualized with TEE (see Fig. 14-e13 on website). Doppler echocardiography is the most accurate method for detecting and quantifying the degree of prosthetic obstruction; however, increased flow velocities may be related to a high-output state or severe prosthetic regurgitation and should be excluded. The maximal and mean pressure gradients and the effective valve area can be calcu-

TABLE 14–12	Hemodynamic Profiles of 609 Normal Aortic Valve Prostheses			
Type of Prosthesis	No. of Prostheses	Peak Velocity, m/sec	Mean Gradient, mm Hg	LVOT TVI/ AV TVI
Heterograft	214	2.4±0.5	13.3±6.1	0.44±0.21
Ball-cage	160	3.2±0.6	23.0±8.8	0.32±0.09
Björk-Shiley	141	2.5±0.6	13.9±7.0	0.40±0.10
St. Jude Medical	44	2.5±0.6	14.4±7.7	0.41±0.12
Homograft	30	1.9±0.4	7.7±2.7	0.56±0.10
Medtronic-Hall	20	2.4±0.2	13.6±3.3	0.39±0.09
Total	609	2.6±0.7	15.8±8.3	0.40±0.16

AV=aortic valve; LVOT=left ventricular outflow tract; TVI=time velocity integral.
From Miller F Jr, Callahan J, Taylor C, et al. Normal aortic valve prosthesis hemodynamics: 609 prospective Doppler examinations [abstract]. Circulation 80(Suppl 2):II-169, 1989.

TABLE 14–13	Doppler Hemodynamic Profiles of 456 Normal Mitral Valve Prostheses			
Type of Prosthesis	No. of Prostheses	Peak Velocity, m/sec	Mean Gradient, mm Hg	Effective Area, cm^2
Heterograft	150	1.6±0.3	4.1±1.5	2.3±0.7
Ball-cage	161	1.8±0.3	4.9±1.8	2.4±0.7
Björk-Shiley	79	1.7±0.3	4.1±1.6	2.6±0.6
St. Jude Medical	66	1.6±0.4	4.0±1.8	3.0±0.8

From Lengyel M, Miller F Jr, Taylor C, et al: Doppler hemodynamic profiles in 456 clinically and echo-normal mitral valve prostheses [abstract]. Circulation 82(Suppl 3):III-43, 1990.

lated using the same formulas and equations described for the native valve (see Fig. 14-e14 on website). In patients with an obstructed mitral or tricuspid valve prosthesis, flow velocities increase and the pressure half-time is prolonged. When the velocity across the mitral or tricuspid prosthesis is increased because of severe regurgitation, the pressure half-time is normal or shortened and LVOT velocity is decreased because forward flow is decreased.

The increase in flow velocity across the obstructed aortic prosthesis is not accompanied by increased LVOT velocity, but it is with severe regurgitation. The LVOT and aortic prosthesis velocity or TVI ratio are helpful in differentiating increased flow velocity across an aortic prosthesis due to a prosthetic obstruction (ratio, ≤0.20) from increased velocity due to regurgitation (normal ratio, ≥0.3).

The pressure half-time constant, 220, was derived for native mitral valve stenosis and not for calculating the effective orifice area of a mitral prosthesis. Thus, the pressure half-time method overestimates the area of a mitral prosthesis. The continuity equation is the preferred method for estimating the functional orifice area of prosthetic aortic and mitral valves when there is no pronounced aortic or mitral regurgitation.

A small amount of leakage volume regurgitation is detected in about 30 percent of normal mechanical prostheses examined with TTE and in up to 44 and 95 percent for aortic and mitral prostheses, respectively, examined with TEE. The size and type of mechanical prosthesis also have an effect on the degree of regurgitation. Pathological prosthetic valve regurgitation can be distinguished from the normal regurgitation by examining the morphology of the valve and the number and location of regurgitant jets.

TABLE 14–14	Doppler Hemodynamic Profiles of Normal Tricuspid Valve Prostheses			
Type of Prosthesis	No. of Prostheses	Peak Velocity, m/sec	Mean Gradient, mm Hg	Pressure Half-Time, m/sec
Heterograft	41	1.3±0.2	3.2±1.1	146±39
Ball-cage	33	1.3±0.2	3.1±0.8	144±46
St. Jude Medical	7	1.2±0.3	2.7±1.1	108±32
Björk-Shiley	1	1.3	2.2	144
Total	82	1.3±0.2	3.1±1.0	142±42

Modified from Connolly HM, Miller FA Jr, Taylor CL, et al: Doppler hemodynamic profiles of eighty-six normal tricuspid valve prostheses (abstract). J Am Coll Cardiol 17:69A, 1991.

TABLE 14–15	Doppler Echocardiographic Data for Pulmonary Prostheses				
Type of Prosthesis	No.	Size, mm	Peak Velocity, m/sec	Mean Gradient, mm Hg	Trivial/Mild Regurgitation, No.
Carpentier-Edwards	24	26.5±1.8	2.4±0.5	12.1±5.3	7
Pulmonary homograft	17	24.2±1.8	1.8±0.6*	8.4±4.8	15
Aortic homograft	3	22.3±1.2	2.5±0.4	14.4±3.4	3
Hancock	3	26.0±3.0	2.4±0.5	14.0±5.7	1
Ionescu-Shiley	2	25.0±0.0	2.4±0.4	12.5±3.5	2
St. Jude Medical	1	25	2.6	12.0	1
Björk-Shiley	1	25	2.0	7.0	1

*Compared with all heterografts combined, $p=0.002$.
From Novaro GM, Connolly HM, Miller FA Jr: Doppler hemodynamics of 51 clinically and echocardiographically normal pulmonary valve prostheses. Mayo Clin Proc 76:155, 2001. Copyright Mayo Foundation for Medical Education and Research.

Color flow imaging is the principal technique used to detect prosthetic valvular regurgitation. Semiquantification of prosthetic valvular and perivalvular regurgitation is possible by using the same criteria as for native valvular regurgitation. TEE is often necessary when assessing mitral or tricuspid prostheses for regurgitation because of the inability to visualize the atria adequately that is related to attenuation of the ultrasound beam. Aortic prosthetic regurgitation often requires combined TTE and TEE assessments to determine location and severity. Transverse imaging of the prosthesis sewing ring and transgastric imaging may help delineate periprosthetic aortic regurgitation.

TEE complements the echocardiographic assessment of patients with prosthetic valves and is commonly used in conjunction with comprehensive hemodynamic assessment by TTE to assess patients with possible endocarditis, abscess, dehiscence, and intracardiac masses or thrombi. With TEE, filamentous prosthetic valve strands related to fibroblasts and collagen are often noted,[115] but their role in cardioembolic events is uncertain.

Prosthesis-Patient Mismatch

A subset of patients with prosthetic aortic valves have a prosthesis that is too small in relation to body size, resulting

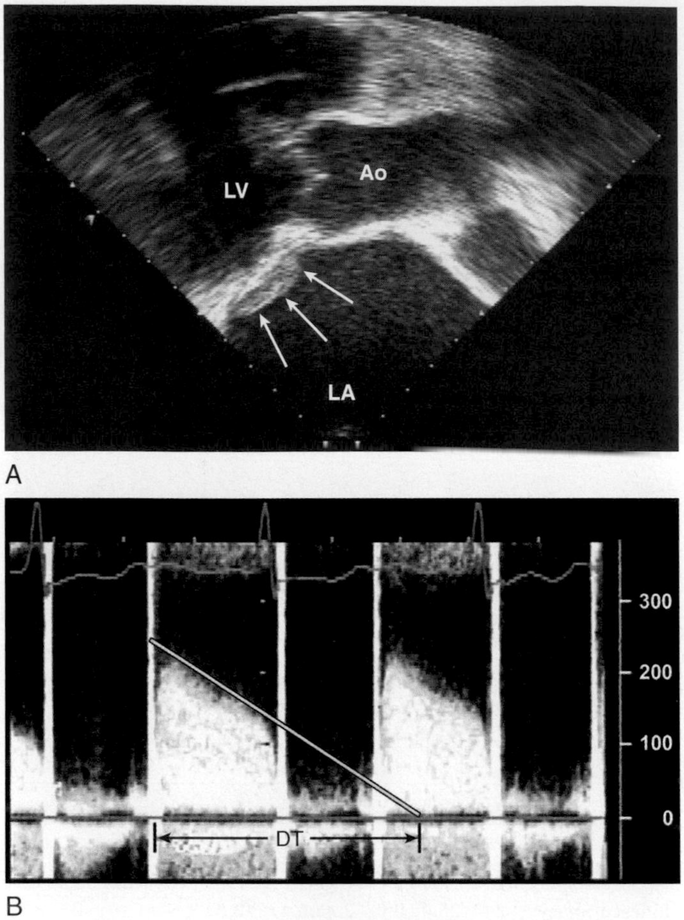

FIGURE 14–66 A, Transesophageal echocardiography examination showing a large thrombus (arrows) attached to the atrial surface of a mitral mechanical prosthesis, causing an obstruction. Ao = aorta; LA = left atrium; LV = left ventricle. **B,** Continuous wave Doppler recording across the obstructive mitral prosthesis. Peak mitral prosthesis velocity is higher than 2 m/sec and pressure half-time and deceleration time (DT) are prolonged. *(From Oh JK, Seward JB, Tajik AJ: The Echo Manual. 3rd ed. Philadelphia, Lippincott Williams & Wilkins, 2006. Used with permission of Mayo Foundation for Medical Education and Research.)*

in an increased transvalvular gradient and cardiovascular disability (see Chap. 62). Subsequent studies have defined prosthesis-patient mismatch as:

1. Mild—indexed effective orifice area greater than 0.85 cm^2/m^2
2. Moderate—effective orifice area less than or equal to 0.85 cm^2/m^2 and greater than 0.65 cm^2/m^2
3. Severe—effective orifice area less than or equal to 0.65 cm^2/m^2

More than a moderate degree of prosthesis-patient mismatch is associated with increased mortality, especially in patients with LVEF less than 40 percent.[116]

INFECTIVE ENDOCARDITIS

The diagnosis of infective endocarditis is frequently suggested on the basis of echocardiography, which is the diagnostic procedure of choice for detecting valvular vegetations (see Chap. 63). Identification of a vegetation is one of two major diagnostic criteria for infective endocarditis.

The echocardiographic features typical for infective endocarditis are (a) an oscillating intracardiac mass on a valve or supporting structure or in the path of a regurgitation jet or on a device, (b) abscesses, (c) new partial dehiscence of a prosthetic valve, or (d) new valvular regurgitation.

TABLE 14–16	Complications of Endocarditis
Structural Cusp or leaflet rupture/flail	
Perforation	
Abscess	
Aneurysm	
Fistula	
Dehiscence of prosthetic valve	
Pericardial effusion (more frequent with abscess)	
Hemodynamic compromise Valvular regurgitation Acute mitral regurgitation Acute aortic regurgitation Premature mitral valve closure Restrictive mitral inflow pattern Valvular stenosis Shunt Congestive heart failure	
Embolization Systemic Cerebral Pulmonary	

From Oh JK, Seward JB, Tajik AJ: The Echo Manual. 3rd ed. Philadelphia, Lippincott Williams & Wilkins, 2006. Copyright Mayo Foundation for Medical Education and Research.

The initial attachment site of a vegetation is usually on the ventricular surface of the semilunar valves and on the atrial surface of the atrioventricular valves (Fig. 14-67). Vegetations frequently show high-frequency flutter or oscillations and can be linear, round, irregular, or shaggy.[117]

The sensitivity for detecting vegetation with 2D TTE is 65 to 80 percent and 95 percent with TEE but depends on vegetation size, location, and the echocardiographic window. The yield of TTE is poor in patients with prosthetic valve endocarditis, but the sensitivity for TEE is 90 percent. A baseline TTE examination is often recommended for patients with suspected endocarditis (see Chap. 63). Serial studies are dictated by the patient's clinical and hemodynamic status. Right-sided valvular vegetations are often larger than left-sided ones, and TEE rarely improves the diagnostic accuracy of TTE in detecting vegetations (Fig. 14-68). After successful medical treatment of endocarditis, vegetations frequently persist but are not associated with late complications.

By identifying and characterizing vegetations, echocardiography is useful in predicting complications related to endocarditis (Fig. 14-69) including embolization, destruction of valvular or intracardiac structures, abscess, and hemodynamic deterioration (Table 14-16). In left-sided valve endocarditis, mobility, extent, consistency, and size of the vegetation affect the frequency of complications. More than 50 percent of patients developed at least one complication when vegetations were greater than 10 mm. In another series, vegetations greater than or equal to 10 mm in size had a higher incidence of embolism when the microorganism was *Staphylococcus* and the mitral valve was infected.[118] Tricuspid valve endocarditis causes pulmonary embolism in 69 percent of cases.

TRANSESOPHAGEAL ECHOCARDIOGRAPHY IN ENDOCARDITIS

The sensitivity of TEE for detecting vegetations or complications of endocarditis is much higher than that of TTE.[119] Thus TEE should be performed in all patients who have nondiagnostic TTE findings, per-

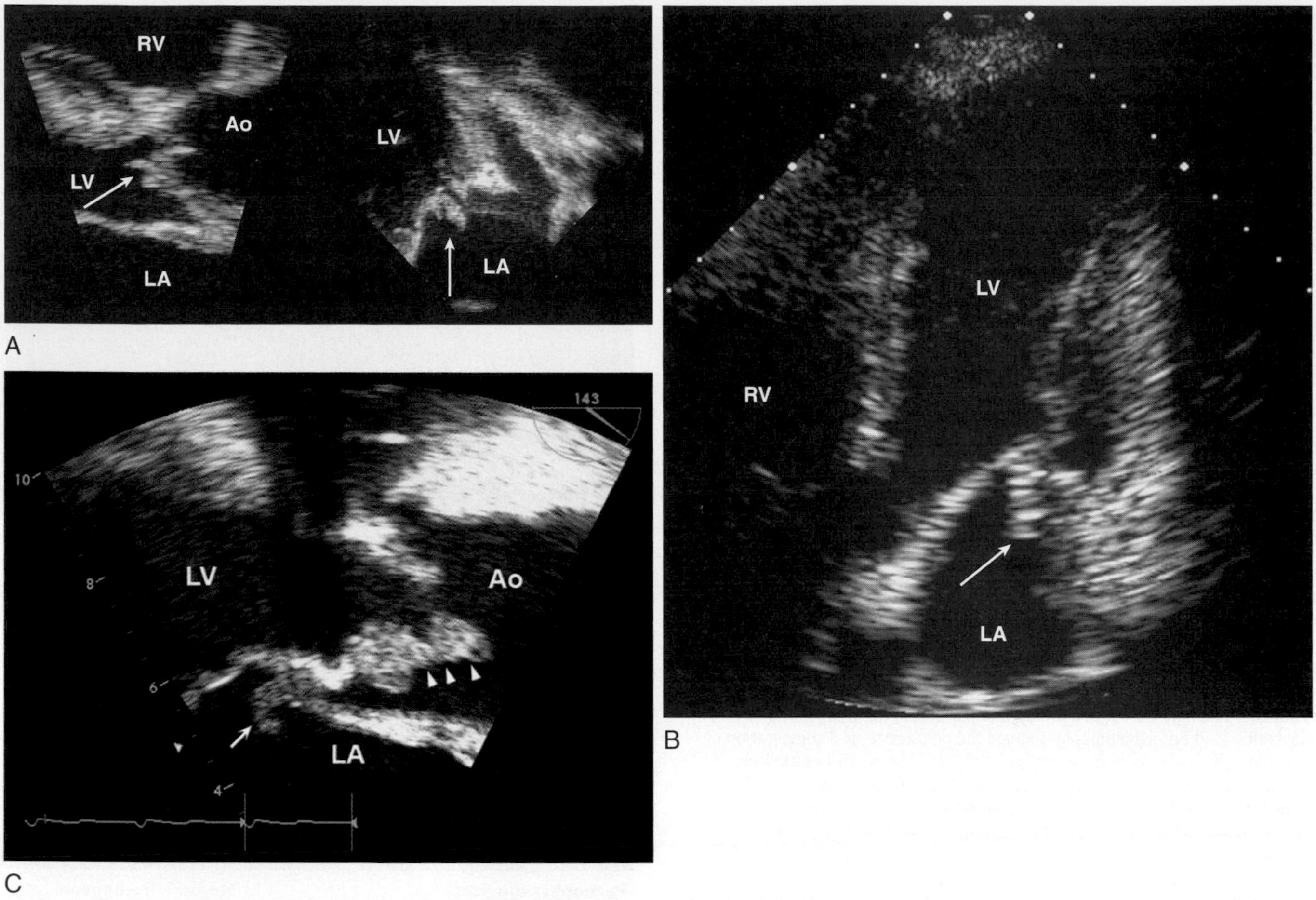

FIGURE 14–67 **A,** Transesophageal echocardiograms of aortic valve (left) and mitral valve (right) showing the typical attachment site for vegetation. The initial attachment site to the aortic valve is usually on the ventricular surface (left arrow), and, for the mitral and tricuspid valves, it is on the atrial side (right arrow). It results from the high velocity blood jet from the high-pressure chamber to the low-pressure chamber. When the regurgitation jet is eccentric, as in mitral valve prolapse, satellite vegetation lesions can develop along the direction of the mitral regurgitation jet. **B,** Transthoracic apical view showing a mobile mass attached to the atrial surface (arrow) of the mitral valve. **C,** Vegetation (arrowheads) attached to the aortic bioprosthesis comes through (arrow) the intervalvular fibrosa into the left atrium (LA). Ao = aorta; LV = left ventricle; RV = right ventricle. *(**A** and **B,** From Oh JK, Seward JB, Tajik AJ: The Echo Manual. 3rd ed. Philadelphia, Lippincott Williams & Wilkins, 2006. Used with permission of Mayo Foundation for Medical Education and Research.)*

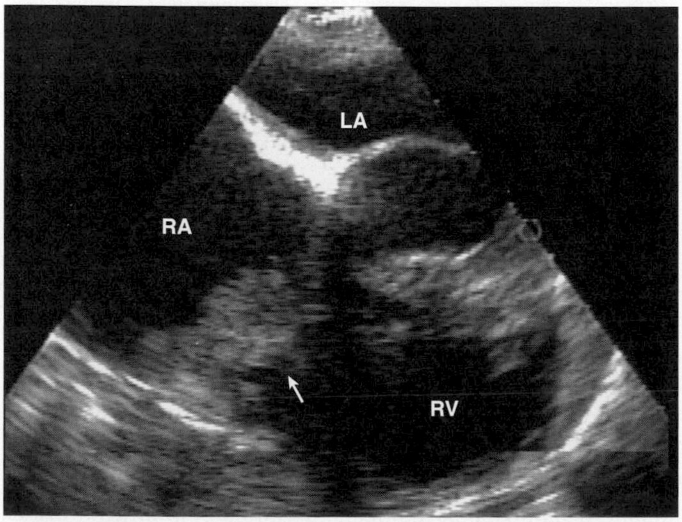

FIGURE 14–68 Transesophageal view of abnormal tricuspid valve due to *Staphylococcus aureus* endocarditis (arrow). LA = left atrium; RA = right atrium; RV = right ventricle. *(From Oh JK, Seward JB, Tajik AJ: The Echo Manual. 3rd ed. Philadelphia, Lippincott Williams & Wilkins, 2006. Used with permission of Mayo Foundation for Medical Education and Research.)*

sistent fever, persistent positive blood cultures, or heart failure without a demonstrable cause (see Chap. 63). Currently, TEE is the diagnostic procedure of choice for excluding vegetation and for detecting complications of infective endocarditis. The effect of TEE in patients with aortic valve endocarditis was demonstrated when consecutive patients were examined with TEE and anatomical complications were identified more frequently than expected. Forty-four percent of patients with aortic valve endocarditis had involvement of subaortic structures: mitral-aortic intervalvular fibrosa aneurysm (see Fig. 14-69),[120] perforation with communication into the LA, aortic annular abscess, or perforation of the mitral leaflet. TTE suggested complications in only one-half of these patients. In pediatric patients TTE has a higher sensitivity for detecting vegetation and TEE may be used less frequently.[121]

Nonbacterial Thrombotic Endocarditis

In 1924 Libman and Sacks described four cases of valvular and mural lesions of verrucous appearance designated as *atypical verrucous.* Antiphospholipid antibody syndrome is a cause of nonbacterial thrombotic endocarditis. Patients often present with cerebral embolic events; thus echocardiography is performed to identify a potential cardiac source. The mitral valve is usually involved (Fig. 14-70), causing regurgitation. The aortic valve is involved less frequently. A surgical pathology study found that all vegeta-

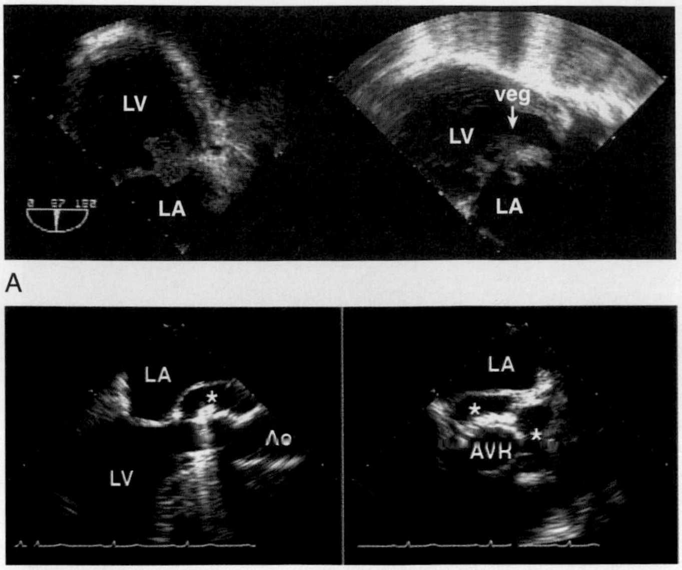

FIGURE 14–69 A, Transesophageal echocardiogram of a patient with *Staphylococcus aureus* endocarditis. **Right,** Vegetation (veg) is attached to the mitral valve, specifically the anterior leaflet of the mitral valve. As a complication, the anterior leaflet of the mitral valve with vegetation had a dehiscence from the mitral annulus, causing severe mitral valve regurgitation. The patient suddenly developed pulmonary edema and a loud murmur during the treatment of endocarditis, and echocardiography showed the dehiscence as a complication of endocarditis. **B,** Transesophageal long-axis (left) and short-axis (right) views showing an abscess cavity (*) at the aortic and mitral valve intervalvular fibrosa in a patient with prosthetic aortic valve endocarditis. The increased echodensity in the region posterior to the aortic valve is consistent with an infectious process. Ao = aorta; AVR = aortic valve prosthesis; LA = left atrium; LV = left ventricle. *(**A,** From Oh JK, Seward JB, Tajik AJ: The Echo Manual. 3rd ed. Philadelphia, Lippincott Williams & Wilkins, 2006. Used with permission of Mayo Foundation for Medical Education and Research.)*

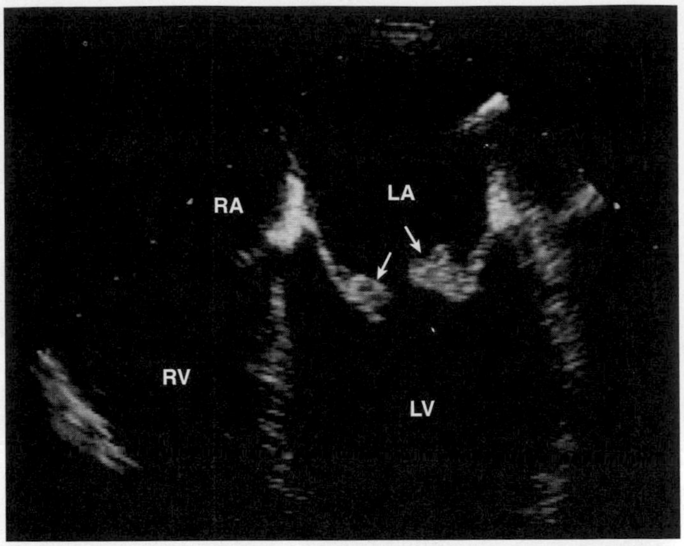

FIGURE 14–70 Transesophageal echocardiographic view of round masses attached to the tip of the mitral leaflet (arrows) of a patient with systemic lupus erythematosus and no clinical evidence of bacterial endocarditis. Diastolic frame of the horizontal transesophageal echocardiographic view of the mitral valve shows large verrucous vegetations (arrows). LA = left atrium; LV = left ventricle; RA = right atrium; RV = right ventricle. *(From Oh JK, Seward JB, Tajik AJ: The Echo Manual. 3rd ed. Philadelphia, Lippincott Williams & Wilkins, 2006. Used with permission of Mayo Foundation for Medical Education and Research.)*

tions in nonbacterial thrombotic endocarditis consist primarily of platelets and fibrin and may respond to warfarin therapy. Patients with advanced adenocarcinoma may develop a similar vegetation, which was termed a *marantic vegetation.*

CARDIOMYOPATHIES

The World Health Organization/International Society and Federation of Cardiology Task Force recommended that cardiomyopathies be classified by the dominant pathophysiological mechanism or etiologic/pathogenic factor (Table 14-17), thus the following classification: (a) *dilated cardiomyopathy,* (b) *hypertrophic cardiomyopathy,* (c) *restrictive cardiomyopathy,* and (d) *arrhythmogenic right ventricular dysplasia* or *cardiomyopathy.* Noncompaction of the ventricular myocardium is another form of cardiomyopathy that has been described more recently[122,123] and has not yet been classified as a distinct entity by the World Health Organization. Each class of cardiomyopathy has distinctive morphological and functional characteristics, with salient echocardiographic features.[1]

TABLE 14–17 Classification of Cardiomyopathies According to Pathophysiological and Etiological/Pathogenic Factors

Pathophysiological	Etiological/Pathogenic
Dilated cardiomyopathy	Ischemic cardiomyopathy
Hypertrophic cardiomyopathy	Valvular cardiomyopathy
Restrictive cardiomyopathy	Hypertensive cardiomyopathy
Arrhythmogenic right ventricular cardiomyopathy	Inflammatory cardiomyopathy
Unclassified cardiomyopathies	Metabolic cardiomyopathy General systemic disease Muscular dystrophy Neuromuscular disorders Sensitivity and toxic reaction Peripartum cardiomyopathy

From Richardson P, McKenna W, Bristow M, et al: Report of the 1995 World Health Organization/International Society and Federation of Cardiology Task Force on the definition and classification of cardiomyopathies. Circulation 93:841, 1996.

Dilated Cardiomyopathy (see Chap. 64)

In dilated cardiomyopathy, the LV cavity is enlarged and global systolic function is decreased (Fig. 14-71). End-diastolic and end-systolic dimensions and volumes are increased, and systolic function is decreased. With gradual dilatation, the LV cavity becomes more spherical, with a sphericity index (long-axis dimension/short-axis dimension) nearing the value of 1 (normally, ≥1.5). LV mass is uniformly increased (eccentric hypertrophy), and wall thickness is typically within normal limits. Ventricular contractility usually is globally reduced, but regional wall motion abnormalities can be present. Similar echocardiographic findings occur in patients with cardiomyopathy related to ischemia, myocarditis, alcohol abuse, hemochromatosis, sarcoidosis, acute catecholamine crisis, acquired immunodeficiency syndrome, severe sepsis, or doxorubicin (Adriamycin) toxicity and in peripartum cardiomyopathy.

Secondary features may be identified by echocardiography in patients with dilated cardiomyopathy and include

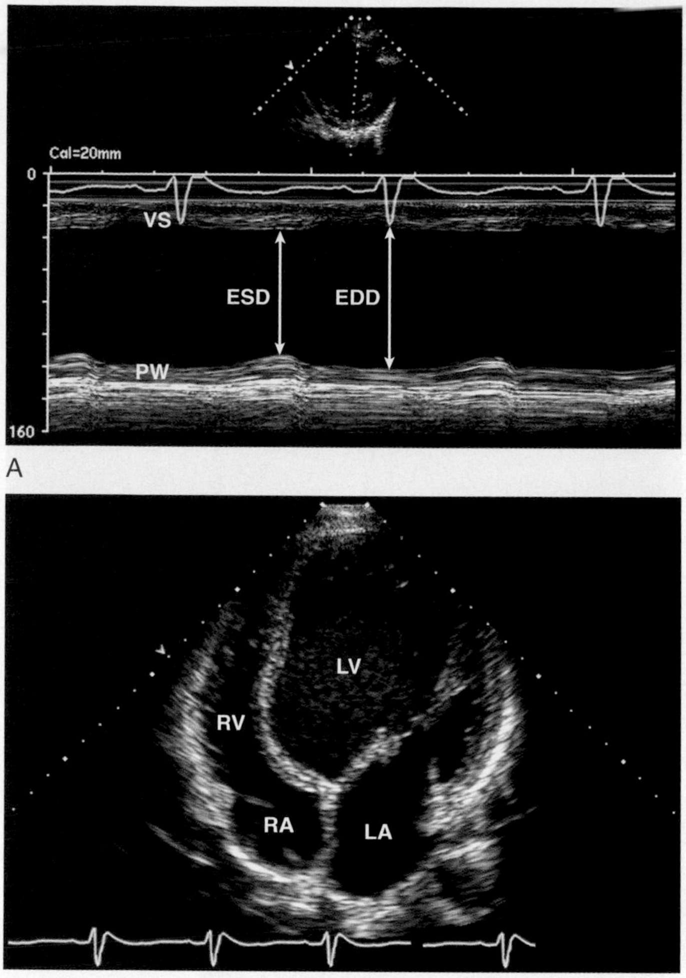

FIGURE 14–71 A, 2D echocardiography-guided M-mode echocardiogram in dilated cardiomyopathy. End-diastolic dimension (EDD = 86 mm) and end-systolic dimension (ESD = 76 mm) were markedly dilated. Contractility is globally reduced, although it is better in the posterior wall (PW) than in the ventricular septum (VS). According to the simplified Quinones method, left ventricular ejection fraction is calculated as:

$$EF = \frac{(86)^2 - (76)^2}{(86)^2} \times 100 = 22\%$$

B, End-diastolic frame of apical four-chamber view in dilated cardiomyopathy (from the same patient as in **A**). The left ventricle (LV) is markedly dilated, and systolic function is reduced in real time. This is typical end-stage dilated cardiomyopathy, with a more spherical shape caused by more dilatation of the short axis (86 mm) than the long axis (100 mm). LA = left atrium; RA = right atrium; RV = right ventricle. *(From Oh JK, Seward JB, Tajik AJ: The Echo Manual. 3rd ed. Philadelphia, Lippincott Williams & Wilkins, 2006. Used with permission of Mayo Foundation for Medical Education and Research.)*

(a) dilated mitral annulus with incomplete mitral leaflet coaptation causing functional mitral regurgitation; (b) evidence of low cardiac output (decreased excursion of mitral leaflets); (c) enlarged atrial cavities; (d) RV enlargement; and, occasionally (e) apical mural thrombus. Intraventricular mechanical dyssynchrony caused by left or right bundle branch block is common and contributes to further cardiac dysfunction.[124,125] In view of the incidence (20 to 50 percent) of familial dilated cardiomyopathy, echocardiographic screening of immediate family members is recommended.[126] Appropriate medical therapy for patients with dilated cardiomyopathy may normalize LV size and function, producing reverse remodeling.

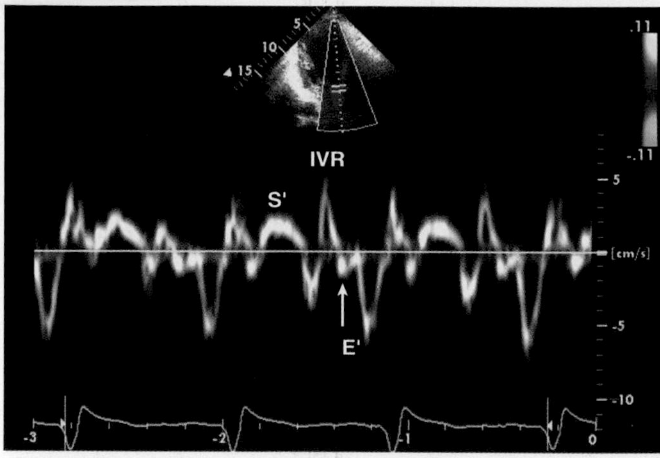

FIGURE 14–72 Tissue Doppler recording of the septal mitral annulus showing decreased systolic velocity (*S'*), early diastolic velocity (*E'*), and prominent bidirectional velocities during isovolumic relaxation (*IVR*).

Doppler echocardiography is useful for determining hemodynamics in patients with dilated cardiomyopathy. Important hemodynamic data routinely obtained include (a) cardiac output and (b) LV filling pressures and diastolic function using mitral inflow filling patterns, TDI, and color M-mode (Fig. 14-72). Both mitral annulus systolic (S′) and early diastolic (E′) velocities are reduced in dilated cardiomyopathy.[15]

Diastolic function analysis correlates well with PCWP and has incremental prognostic power over what LVEF can provide in dilated cardiomyopathy.[127] Patients who are compensated with near-normal stroke volume and cardiac output have an impaired relaxation pattern (grade 1 diastolic dysfunction) (Fig. 14-73A). Patients who are decompensated have decreased stroke volume and a restrictive diastolic filling pattern (see Fig. 14-73B) because of decreased compliance and increased LV filling pressures. Patients with reversible restrictive filling have a high probability of improvement with medical therapy and excellent survival. The persistence of the restrictive filling pattern after therapy is associated with high mortality and transplantation rates. Doppler-derived pulmonary artery pressure measurement also has prognostic significance in dilated cardiomyopathy. Patients with a tricuspid regurgitation velocity greater than or equal to 3 m/sec have a higher mortality rate, a higher incidence of heart failure, a restrictive diastolic filling pattern, and more frequent hospitalizations than those with a velocity less than 3 m/sec. Therefore a restrictive diastolic filling pattern and a high tricuspid regurgitation velocity identify patients who are at increased risk for death and heart failure. Mitral regurgitation is common in dilated cardiomyopathy and is related to the LV remodeling process (see Fig. 14-58) (see Chap. 62). Treatment directed toward reverse remodeling improves mitral regurgitation, as well as LV systolic function.

Echocardiography in Management of Dilated Cardiomyopathy

Increasingly, LV filling parameters have been recognized to have an important effect on LV filling. The PR interval affects diastolic LV filling and has been demonstrated to have an important effect on optimizing cardiac output. If the PR interval becomes prolonged (>200 msec), atrial contraction may occur before early diastolic filling is completed. If the PR interval is too short (60 to 100 msec), the atrium may contract at the same time the ventricle contracts. The PR interval can be optimized with the guidance of Doppler imaging in patients with pacemakers; this may increase cardiac output and improve symptoms.

TDI and other modified techniques are able to quantify the degree of intraventricular dyssynchrony (Fig. 14-73C). Initial data suggest that patients with greater dyssynchrony receive more benefit from cardiac resynchronization therapy (see Chap. 25).[128,129] Deciding which echocardiographic

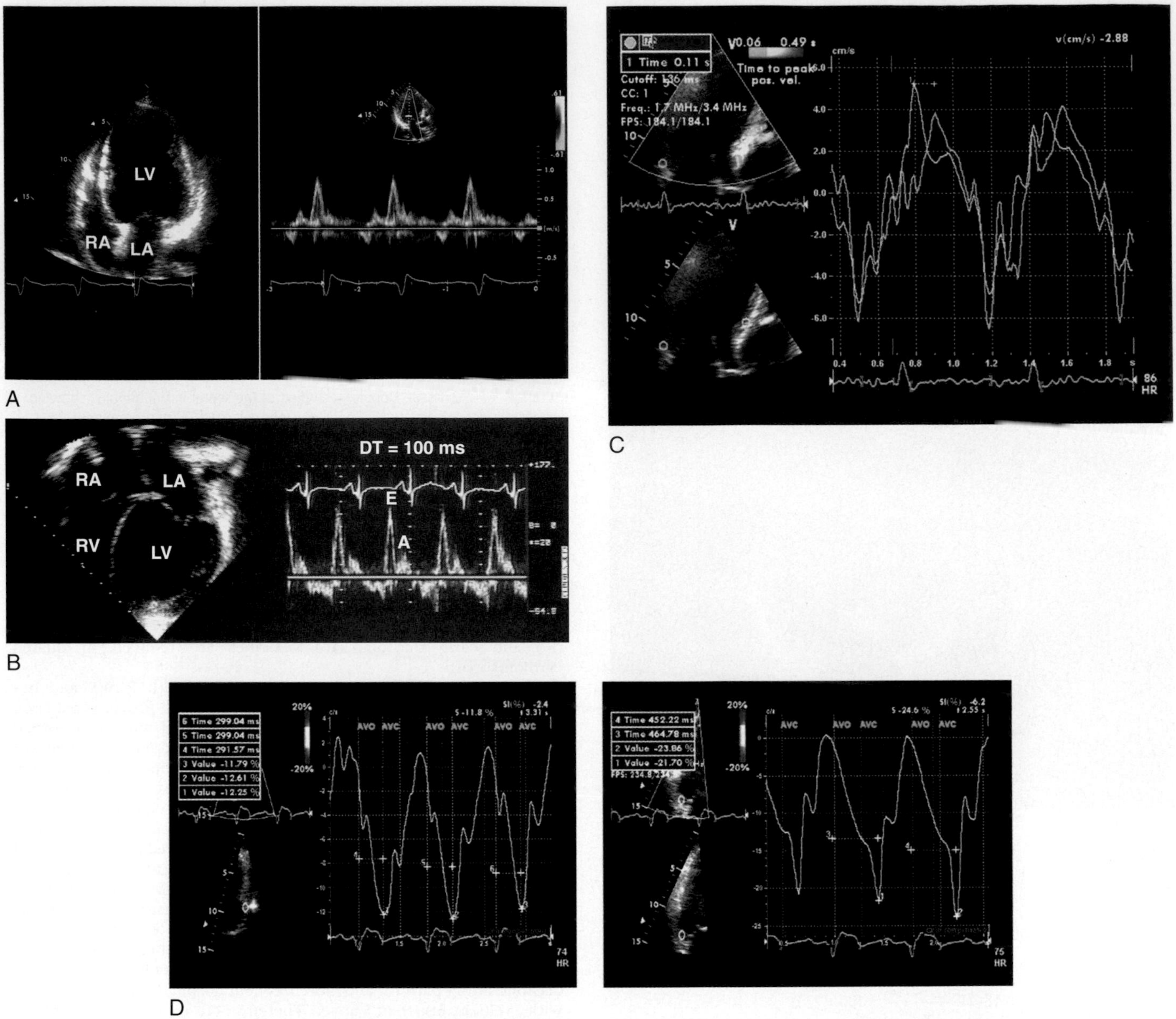

FIGURE 14–73 **A,** Apical four-chamber view **(left)** and pulsed wave Doppler velocity recording of mitral valve inflow **(right)** in a patient with dilated ischemic cardiomyopathy showing a relaxation abnormality pattern with increased A velocity. Patients with this type of diastolic filling pattern usually have minimal to mild symptoms, despite severe left ventricular (LV) systolic dysfunction. **B,** In this patient with dilated cardiomyopathy, the MV inflow velocity pattern shows restrictive physiology, with a markedly decreased A velocity and an increased E/A ratio. Deceleration time (DT) of mitral E velocity is shortened. Patients with this type of diastolic filling have increased filling pressure and symptomatic congestive heart failure. **C,** Tissue Doppler velocity recordings from the basal septal **(yellow)** and basal lateral **(blue)** walls. Septal peak velocity occurs first, then lateral peak velocity. The timing difference (+----+) is 110 msec, indicating dyssynchronous contraction. **D,** Intraventricular dyssynchrony can be measured with strain imaging, which we prefer. **Left,** Strain recording from the basal septal wall. The time from the onset of QRS to peak negative strain (when the maximum contraction occurs) is measured from three cardiac cycles. The time intervals measured for the three cycles are 299, 299, and 291 msec. **Right,** Strain recording from the basal lateral wall. The peak strain occurs after aortic valve closure (AVC), which is termed *postsystolic shortening.* The time interval measured from the onset of QRS to peak negative is 452 and 464 msec, much later than that of the septal wall. The timing difference between the septal and lateral segments is more than 150 msec, indicating marked dyssynchrony. AVO = aortic valve opening; LA = left atrium; RA, right atrium; RV, right ventricle. *(**B,** From Oh JK, Seward JB, Tajik AJ: The Echo Manual. 3rd ed. Philadelphia, Lippincott Williams & Wilkins, 2006. Used with permission of Mayo Foundation for Medical Education and Research.)*

parameters are most helpful in predicting a positive response to cardiac resynchronization requires further clinical experience.[1]

Hypertrophic Cardiomyopathy (see Chap. 65)

Hypertrophic cardiomyopathy is a genetic disorder caused by a missense mutation in 1 of at least 10 genes that encode the proteins of the cardiac sarcomere.[130] Mutations associated with hypertrophic cardiomyopathy are scattered throughout sarcomeric genes, with mutations in the gene encoding the beta-myosin heavy chain representing one of the most common genetic causes of this condition.[131] The phenotypic expression of hypertrophic cardiomyopathy, which occurs in 1 of every 500 adults, includes abnormal LV hypertrophy. Although asymmetrical septal hypertrophy is the most common type of morphological pattern, hypertrophic cardiomyopathy can present with concentric, apical, or free wall LV hypertrophy.[130] The basal septal hypertrophy causes narrowing of the LVOT and provides a substrate for dynamic obstruction. The blood flow velocity across the narrowed LVOT produces the *Venturi effect.* Con-

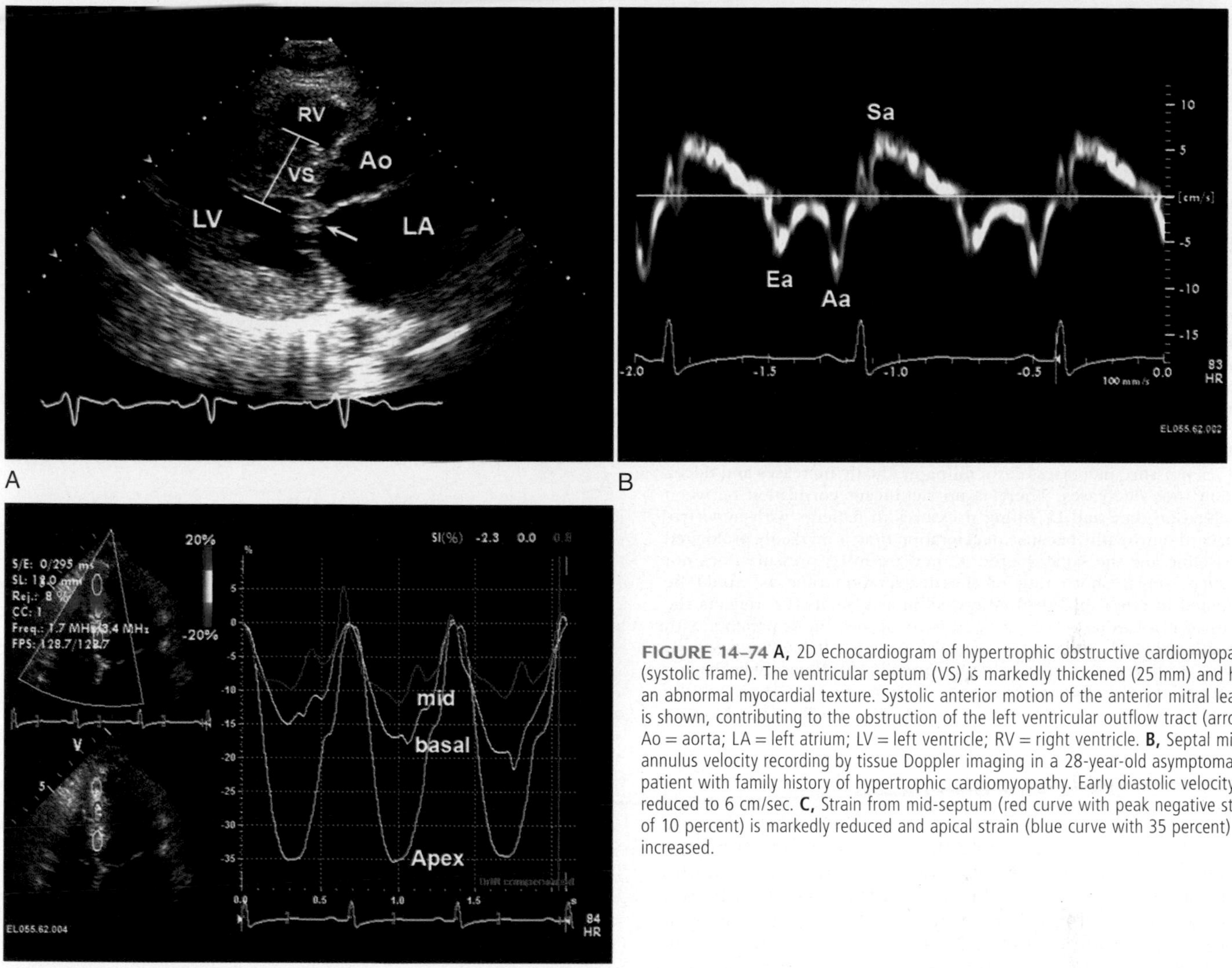

A B C

FIGURE 14–74 **A,** 2D echocardiogram of hypertrophic obstructive cardiomyopathy (systolic frame). The ventricular septum (VS) is markedly thickened (25 mm) and has an abnormal myocardial texture. Systolic anterior motion of the anterior mitral leaflet is shown, contributing to the obstruction of the left ventricular outflow tract (arrow). Ao = aorta; LA = left atrium; LV = left ventricle; RV = right ventricle. **B,** Septal mitral annulus velocity recording by tissue Doppler imaging in a 28-year-old asymptomatic patient with family history of hypertrophic cardiomyopathy. Early diastolic velocity is reduced to 6 cm/sec. **C,** Strain from mid-septum (red curve with peak negative strain of 10 percent) is markedly reduced and apical strain (blue curve with 35 percent) is increased.

sequently, the mitral leaflets and support apparatus are drawn toward the septum (i.e., systolic anterior motion), contributing to the LVOT obstruction (Fig. 14-74A) and causing variable mitral regurgitation. Obstruction in hypertrophic cardiomyopathy is often dynamic and varies with the loading conditions, LV size, and contractility.

Currently, 2D echocardiography is the diagnostic method of choice for hypertrophic cardiomyopathy. Three-dimensional echocardiography may provide additional anatomical delineation (see Fig. 14-e15 on website). Diffuse hypertrophy of the ventricular septum and anterolateral free wall is the most common variety of hypertrophic cardiomyopathy in the West (70 to 75 percent), followed by basal septal hypertrophy (10 to 15 percent), concentric hypertrophy (5 percent), apical hypertrophy (<5 percent), and hypertrophy of the lateral wall (1 to 2 percent). The magnitude of hypertrophy is related to the risk of sudden death. In one study, the cumulative risk for sudden death was about zero for wall thickness less than or equal to 19 mm and 40 percent for greater than or equal to 30 mm.[132] In some patients with hypertrophic cardiomyopathy, the RV wall is also markedly hypertrophied, which may obstruct the RVOT.

The degree of LV obstruction is readily assessed with continuous wave Doppler echocardiography. The continuous wave Doppler spectrum has a characteristic late-peaking *dagger-shaped* appearance (Fig. 14-75). With the simplified

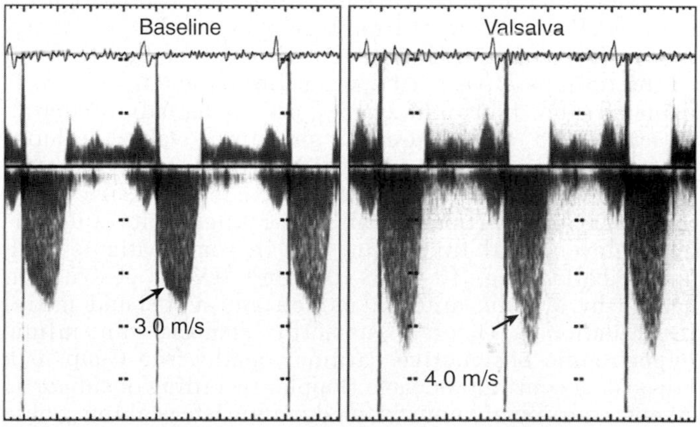

FIGURE 14–75 Continuous wave Doppler spectra obtained from the apex showing dynamic left ventricular outflow tract obstruction. Note the typical late-peaking configuration resembling a dagger or ski slope (arrow). The baseline **(left)** velocity is 2.8 m/sec, corresponding to the peak left ventricular outflow tract gradient of 31 mm Hg (= 4×2.8^2). With the Valsalva maneuver **(right),** the velocity increased to 3.5 m/sec, corresponding to the gradient of 50 mm Hg. *(From Oh JK, Seward JB, Tajik AJ: The Echo Manual. 3rd ed. Philadelphia, Lippincott Williams & Wilkins, 2006. Used with permission of Mayo Foundation for Medical Education and Research.)*

Bernoulli equation, the peak velocity can be converted to the peak pressure gradient across the LVOT. The correlation between Doppler-derived and catheter-derived pressure gradients is good. The dynamic nature of LVOT obstruction can be documented with continuous wave Doppler imaging during the Valsalva maneuver, positional change (from supine to standing), or amyl nitrite inhalation (see Fig. 14-75).[1] Mitral regurgitation frequently accompanies the obstructive form of hypertrophic cardiomyopathy and is related to systolic anterior motion of the mitral valve.

DIASTOLIC FILLING PATTERN AND TISSUE DOPPLER IMAGING

Markedly impaired myocardial relaxation is the predominant diastolic abnormality in hypertrophic cardiomyopathy; this is caused by the hypertrophied myocardium. Atrial contraction makes an important contribution to LV filling, and when atrial contraction is compromised because of tachycardia or atrial fibrillation, cardiac output decreases and pulmonary venous congestion occurs. As compliance decreases and LA pressure increases, early filling gradually increases and deceleration time decreases. There is no significant correlation between deceleration time and LV filling pressures in patients with hypertrophic cardiomyopathy because deceleration time is markedly prolonged at baseline and the same degree of increase in LA pressure does not produce similar shortening of the deceleration time as would be expected in other disorders. Mitral annulus velocity, Ea, reflects the status of myocardial relaxation and is reduced in most patients with hypertrophic cardiomyopathy (see Fig. 14-74B). It has been shown that Ea is decreased in patients with preclinical disease who have a genotype positive for hypertrophic cardiomyopathy.[1] Strain of the myocardium is also altered in hypertrophic cardiomyopathy (see Fig. 14-74C).

Dynamic LVOT Obstruction in Other Diseases

Not all dynamic LVOT obstruction is caused by hypertrophic cardiomyopathy. Hyperdynamic LV systolic function, caused by medication or other factors, can cause dynamic LVOT obstruction hemodynamically indistinguishable from hypertrophic cardiomyopathy in patients with basal septal hypertrophy. Elderly patients with hypertension treated with vasodilators, diuretics, or digoxin may develop dynamic obstruction and associated symptoms of dyspnea, chest pain, or hypotension exacerbated by treatment. This has been called *hypertensive hypertrophic cardiomyopathy,* but it is clearly different from true hypertrophic cardiomyopathy. Dynamic LVOT obstruction is also commonly noted in the postoperative period when intravascular volume is depleted and inotropic agents are being administered. Patients with aortic stenosis or mitral valve prolapse are especially vulnerable to LVOT obstruction after aortic valve replacement or mitral valve repair, respectively. Acute LVOT obstruction can occur after acute anterior-apical myocardial infarction, and in some patients with apical ballooning, there is dynamic LVOT obstruction caused by systolic anterior motion and associated mitral regurgitation.[133] Discrete subaortic stenosis can mimic hypertrophic obstructive cardiomyopathy (see Chap. 61); however, a continuous wave Doppler recording of subaortic stenosis does not demonstrate a dynamic late peaking profile but resembles that of valvular aortic stenosis. Dynamic LVOT obstruction may also be an initial presentation of cardiac amyloidosis.

Apical Hypertrophic Cardiomyopathy

Apical hypertrophic cardiomyopathy may be missed by parasternal 2D echocardiography because the hypertrophy is usually confined to the cardiac apex (Fig. 14-76). Apical hypertrophic cardiomyopathy is best visualized from apical short-axis and four-chamber views with good endocardial definition; echocardiography of patients with this condition shows thickened apical walls and obliteration of the apical cavity during systole. Because of massive apical hypertrophy, epicardial motion may suggest a dyskinetic apex. Apical hypertrophy should be differentiated from obliteration of the apical cavity caused by hypereosinophilic syndrome or abnormal apical trabeculation in noncompaction. Intravenous administration of a contrast agent is extremely helpful in delineating the small apical cavity with a configuration of the "ace of spades," typical of apical hypertrophic cardiomyopathy (Fig. 14-77). This condition is associated typically with giant T-wave inversion in the precordial leads.[134]

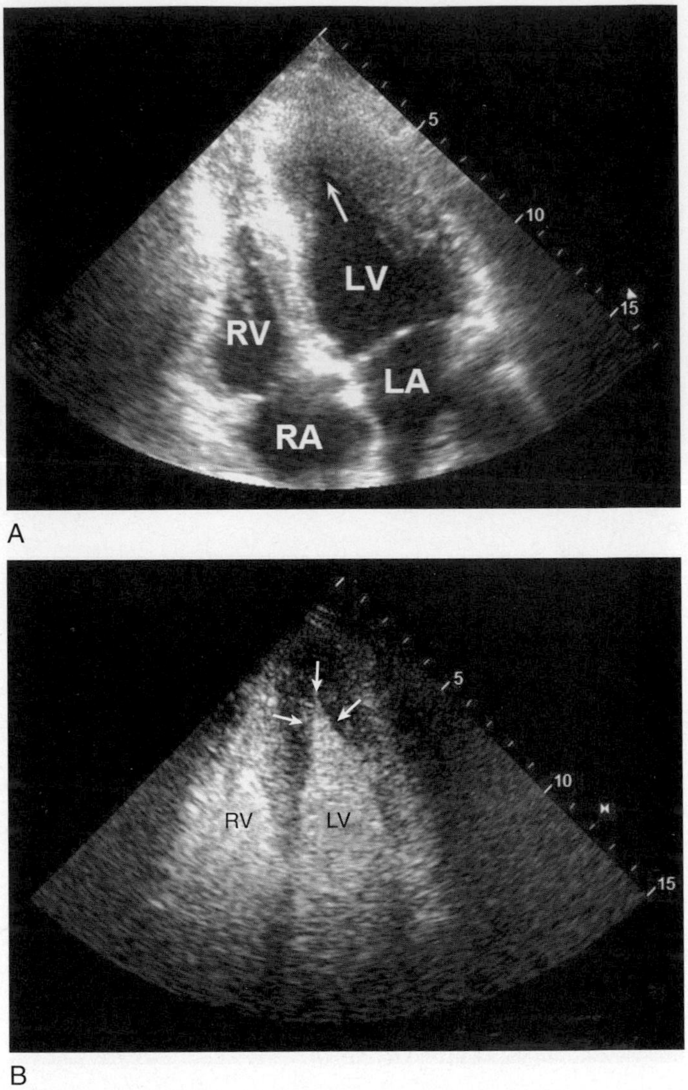

FIGURE 14–76 A, 2D apical four-chamber view during diastole in a patient with apical hypertrophic cardiomyopathy. The apical wall thickness during diastole is markedly increased (arrow), and the apical cavity is nearly obliterated except for a small slit during diastole. **B,** 2D apical four-chamber view with contrast shows apical hypertrophy and obliteration of the apical cavity (arrows). LA = left atrium; LV = left ventricle; RA = right atrium; RV = right ventricle.

Management of Hypertrophic Obstructive Cardiomyopathy

When medical therapy fails to provide relief from symptoms or obstruction, septal reduction by surgical myectomy or alcohol ablation should be considered (see Chap. 65).[135] Echocardiography can outline the extent and location of

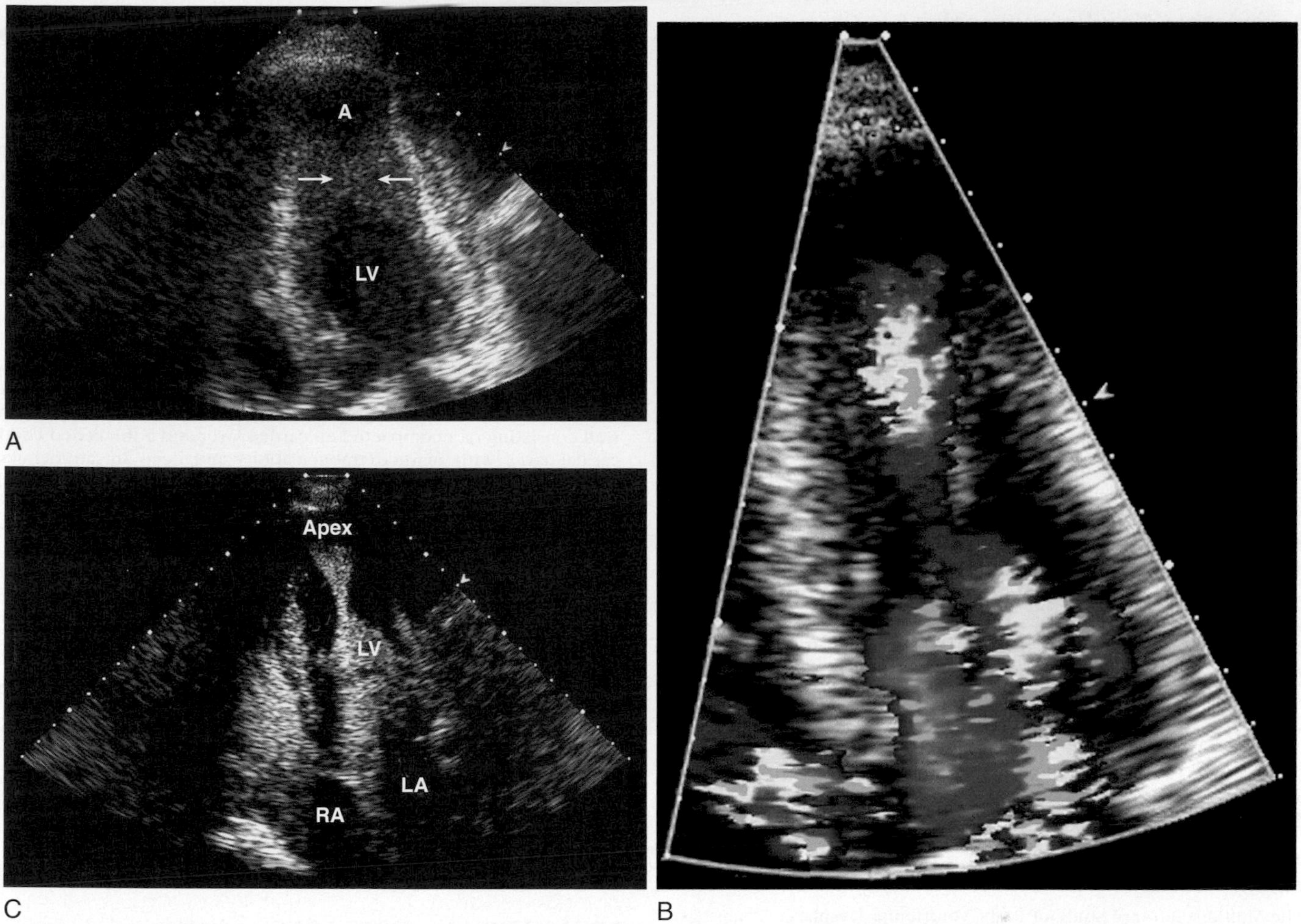

FIGURE 14–77 Apical view with color flow imaging and intravenous administration of a contrast agent showing an apical pouch characteristic of mid-cavitary obstruction. **A,** 2D echocardiography shows increased left ventricular (LV) wall thickness and systolic obstruction (arrows) at mid ventricle. The apical portion (A) is not well seen. **B,** Color flow imaging shows increased flow velocity at the obstructed mid cavity. **C,** Contrast echocardiography for LV opacification shows the apical cavity best. LA = left atrium; RA = right atrium. *(From Oh JK, Seward JB, Tajik AJ: The Echo Manual. 3rd ed. Philadelphia, Lippincott Williams & Wilkins, 2006. Used with permission of Mayo Foundation for Medical Education and Research.)*

hypertrophy and help guide intervention. Alcohol septal ablation is an effective method for reducing LVOT obstruction in selected patients. It creates infarction of the basal septum, which widens the LVOT area. Because the myocardial area supplied by the septal perforator varies, it is critical to visualize the area to be infarcted by septal ablation before the procedure. Myocardial contrast echocardiography is well suited for this purpose. The basal septum becomes atrophied from alcohol-induced myocardial damage (see Fig. 14-e16 on website), decreasing the LVOT gradient, which is accurately assessed with continuous wave Doppler echocardiography.[136] Surgical myectomy remains the gold standard for relief of LVOT obstruction. It is the preferred method of management in the setting of diffuse septal hypertrophy or anomalous papillary muscle contributing to obstruction and in patients who have another indication for cardiac surgery.[135]

Other Conditions Can Mimic Hypertrophic Cardiomyopathy

Although echocardiography is the diagnostic procedure of choice in hypertrophic cardiomyopathy, many other disorders have similar echocardiographic features including chronic hypertension, RV hypertrophy, cardiac amyloidosis (see Fig. 14-7), athlete's heart, pheochromocytoma, long-term hemodialysis, Fabry disease, and Friedreich ataxia. Therefore the echocardiographic finding of increased LV wall thickness and dynamic LVOT obstruction should be interpreted in its clinical context. Apical hypertrophy should be differentiated from apical cavity obliteration caused by hyper-eosinophilic syndrome or noncompaction. Contrast echocardiography is helpful in differentiating apical hypertrophic cardiomyopathy from other entities.[137]

Athlete's Heart versus Hypertrophic Cardiomyopathy

LV hypertrophy occurs after years of intense athletic training, and the 2D echocardiographic findings of athlete's heart are similar to those of hypertrophic cardiomyopathy. The following characteristics of athlete's heart can differentiate it from hypertrophic cardiomyopathy[138]:

1. Symmetrical hypertrophy
2. Hypertrophy is rarely greater than 17 mm
3. LV cavity dimension is increased, whereas it is decreased in hypertrophic cardiomyopathy
4. Diastolic function is normal (Ea > 7 cm/sec)
5. Tissue Doppler velocities and strain values are normal

Restrictive Cardiomyopathy (see Chap. 64)

Primary restrictive cardiomyopathy is characterized by limited ventricular filling resulting from an idiopathic nonhypertrophied myocardial abnormality (fibrosis or decreased compliance or both).[1] Early in the disease, ventricular systolic function is usually preserved, but diastolic function is abnormal, which causes increased atrial pressures and marked biatrial enlargement. The characteristic features of primary restrictive cardiomyopathy on 2D echocardiography include normal ventricular cavity size, wall thicknesses, and usually preserved global systolic function, with biatrial enlargement (Fig. 14-78). Restrictive cardiomyopathy is accompanied by restrictive diastolic filling, but restrictive diastolic filling pattern can also be present in other cardiac diseases. The typical ventricular diastolic pressure tracing in restrictive cardiomyopathy is the dip-and-plateau, or square root configuration, which corresponds to shortened deceleration time of the mitral inflow E velocity. The increase in LA pressure causes (a) the mitral valve to open at a higher pressure, resulting in a decrease in IVRT, (b) increased transmitral pressure gradient with associated increased mitral E velocity, and (c) a decrease in pulmonary venous flow velocity during systole and an increase during diastole (Fig. 14-79). With high end-diastolic ventricular pressure, atrial contribution to ventricular filling is minimal, and A velocity is usually decreased (see Fig. 14-79), causing the E/A ratio to increase markedly (>2). In contrast to constrictive pericarditis, hepatic vein diastolic flow reversal is greater during inspiration (Fig. 14-80). Myocardial relaxation is universally impaired so that mitral annulus E′ velocity obtained from the septal annulus is usually less than 7 cm/sec.[139]

ARRHYTHMOGENIC RIGHT VENTRICULAR DYSPLASIA/ CARDIOMYOPATHY (see Chap. 64)

The Multidisciplinary Study of Right Ventricular Dysplasia Group has reported 2D echocardiographic findings of arrhythmogenic RV dysplasia (ARVD) from 29 patients.[140] The systolic and diastolic RVOT and RV inflow tract dimensions are increased, with diastolic RVOT enlargement being most common (RVOT diameter was >25 mm in all patients). An RVOT dimension greater than 30 mm from the parasternal long-axis view had the highest sensitivity (89 percent) and specificity (86 percent) for the diagnosis of ARVD. RV function was abnormal in 62 percent, and RV regional wall motion abnormalities were frequent, most commonly affecting the apex and anterior wall. Morphologically, RV trabecular derangements, hyperreflective moderator band, and sacculations were present in 54, 34, and 17 percent, respectively (Fig. 14-81). In some patients LV dilatation and dysfunction also occur. The tricuspid regurgitation velocity is usually less than 2 m/sec, suggesting an RV systolic pressure in the low-normal range. Contrast echocardiography is useful in delineating RV morphology and contractility. CMR or computed tomography (CT) for fat in the RV myocardium has been helpful in some patients. A multidisciplinary study for patients with ARVD/C (cardiomyopathy) is obtaining data regarding risk stratification and proper treatment of this interesting but potentially fatal condition.[141]

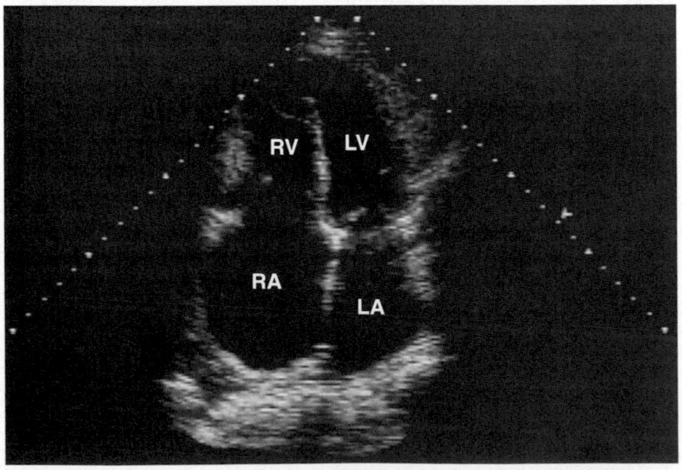

FIGURE 14–78 Apical four-chamber view of typical restrictive cardiomyopathy with normal left ventricular (LV) cavity size, normal systolic function, and marked biatrial enlargement. LA = left atrium; RA = right atrium; RV = right ventricle. *(From Oh JK, Seward JB, Tajik AJ: The Echo Manual. 3rd ed. Philadelphia, Lippincott Williams & Wilkins, 2006. Used with permission of Mayo Foundation for Medical Education and Research.)*

NONCOMPACTION CARDIOMYOPATHY (ISOLATED VENTRICULAR NONCOMPACTION)

Isolated ventricular noncompaction (IVNC) occurs from embryonic arrest of compaction, previously described as persistent intramyocardial sinusoids. It is characterized by segmental thickening of the LV wall consisting of a compacted epicardial layer and a thickened endocardial layer with marked trabeculations and deep intratrabecular recesses (Fig. 14-82). The following major complications in patients with noncompaction cardiomyopathy have been reported from a referral center series: heart failure (53 percent), thromboembolic events (24 percent), ventricular tachycardia (41 percent), and sudden death.

The following echocardiographic criteria for IVNC have been reported by Jenni et al:

1. The absence of any coexisting cardiac anomalies
2. The characteristic appearance of numerous, excessively prominent trabeculations and deep intertrabecular recesses
3. Intertrabecular spaces filled by direct blood flow from the ventricular cavity, as visualized on color flow imaging
4. An end-systolic ratio of noncompacted-to-compacted layers greater than 2

The ratio of noncompacted-to-compacted layers can be determined better with contrast enhancement (see Fig. 14-82). Predominant areas of the trabeculations in IVNC are midlateral, midinferior, and apical segments.[142]

PERICARDIAL DISEASES (see Chap. 70)

Detection of pericardial effusion was one of the first clinical applications of echocardiography (see Fig. 14-1), and echocardiography continues to be invaluable in the evaluation and management of various pericardial diseases. Pericardial effusion, tamponade, pericardial cyst, and absence of pericardium are readily recognized on 2D echocardiography. The unique echocardiographic features of constrictive pericarditis and the use of tissue Doppler imaging have added reliability and confidence to the noninvasive diagnosis of constrictive pericarditis and for differentiating it from restrictive myocardial disease. Pericardiocentesis can be performed most safely under the guidance of 2D echocardiography.[143]

Congenitally Absent Pericardium

Congenital absence of the pericardium is usually partial and involves the left side of the pericardium. The defect is more frequent in males, and it occasionally causes symptoms such as chest pain, dyspnea, or syncope. With the defect in the pericardium, cardiac motion, especially the posterior wall of the LV, is exaggerated. Congenital absence of the pericardium demonstrates typical 2D echocardiographic features, which include (a) the appearance of RV cavity enlargement from the standard parasternal windows, mimicking the RV volume overload pattern on echocardiography (see Fig. 14-e17 on website) (this finding is caused by the entire cardiac structure being shifted to the left), (b) displacement of the apical imaging window into the axilla (with the patient on the left side), and (c) the appearance of compressed atria. The diagnosis can be confirmed with CT or CMR.[144]

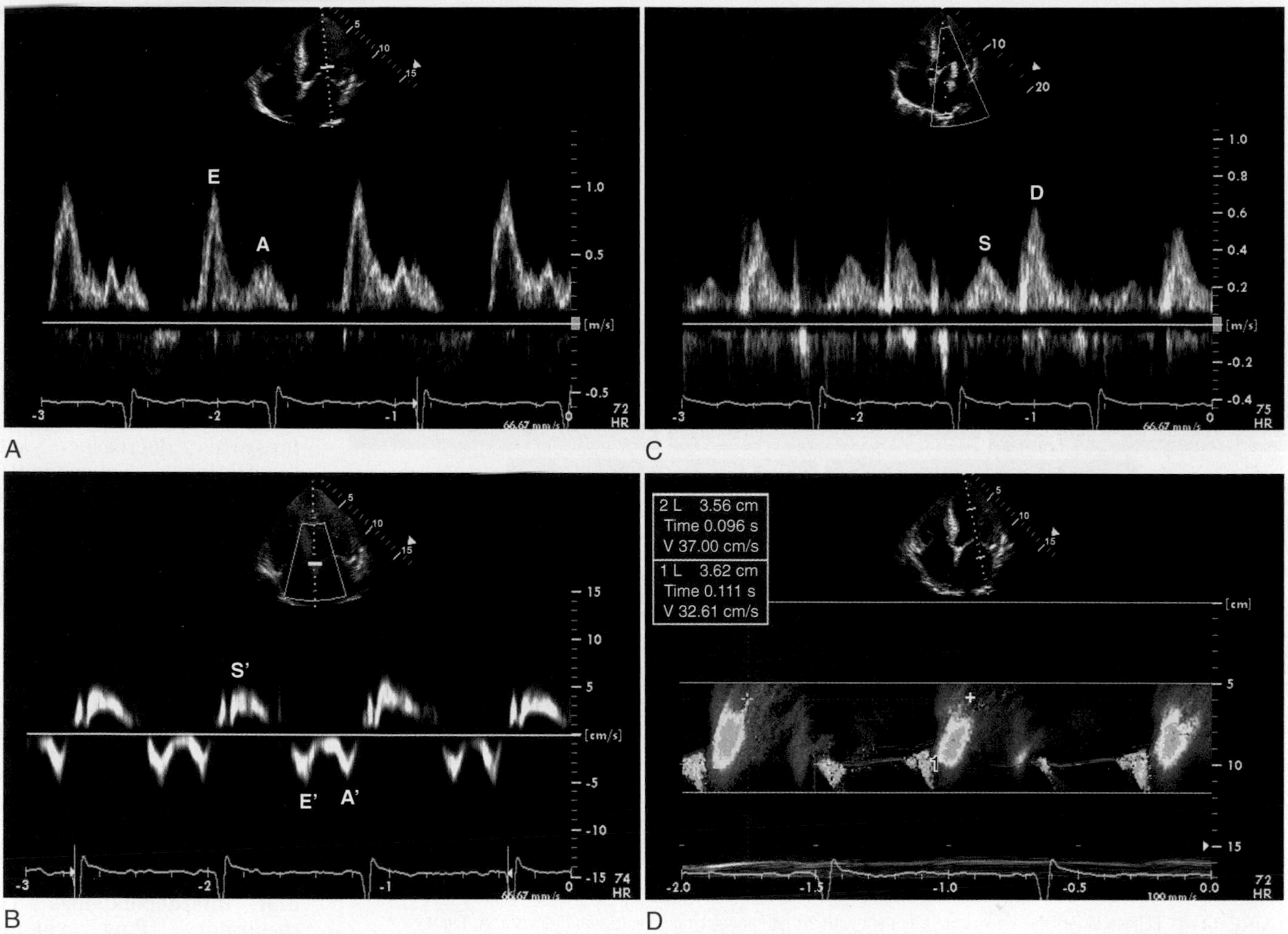

FIGURE 14–79 **A,** Mitral inflow; **B,** tissue Doppler septal mitral annulus; **C,** pulmonary vein; and **D,** color M-mode of mitral inflow velocity in a patient with restrictive cardiomyopathy. **A,** E/A ratio is greater than 2, and deceleration time is short. **B,** E′ is decreased because of abnormal relaxation; S′ is also decreased. **C,** Pulmonary vein systolic velocity (S) is reduced and diastolic velocity (D) deceleration time is shortened. **D,** Mitral inflow color propagation velocity (V) is reduced to 32-37 cm/sec. A = late diastolic mitral flow velocity; A′ = late diastolic mitral annulus velocity; E = early diastolic mitral flow velocity; E′ = early diastolic mitral annulus velocity; S′ = systolic velocity of mitral annulus.

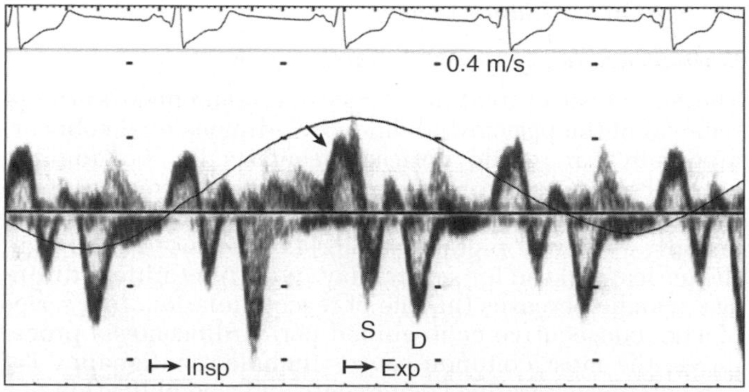

FIGURE 14–80 Hepatic vein pulsed wave Doppler recording together with respirometer recording from a patient with restrictive physiology. Note the higher diastolic velocity (D) than systolic velocity (S) and greater reversal of diastolic flow during inspiration (Insp) (arrow). Exp = expiration. *(From Oh JK, Seward JB, Tajik AJ: The Echo Manual. 3rd ed. Philadelphia, Lippincott Williams & Wilkins, 2006. Used with permission of Mayo Foundation for Medical Education and Research.)*

Pericardial Cyst

A pericardial cyst is a benign fluid-filled abnormality of the pericardium that is usually detected as a mass lesion on chest radiography or as a cystic echo-free structure on 2D echocardiography. Pericardial cysts are usually located on the right side (Fig. 14-83), but they also are found in the left costophrenic angle, hilum, and superior mediastinum. They should be differentiated from tumors, cardiac chamber enlargement, and diaphragmatic hernia. Pericardial cysts also have a characteristic appearance on CT and CMR (see Fig. 14-83B).

Pericardial Effusion/Tamponade

Pericardial effusion is detected as an echo-free space. In a large pericardial effusion, the heart may have a "swinging" motion in the pericardial cavity that causes the typical electrocardiographic manifestation of cardiac tamponade, *electrical alternans* (Fig. 14-84). Cardiac tamponade usually occurs with a large pericardial effusion but can occur with a small amount of fluid if the fluid accumulation occurs rapidly (see Chap. 70).[145] M-mode and 2D echocardiographic features caused by the characteristic hemodynamics of tam-

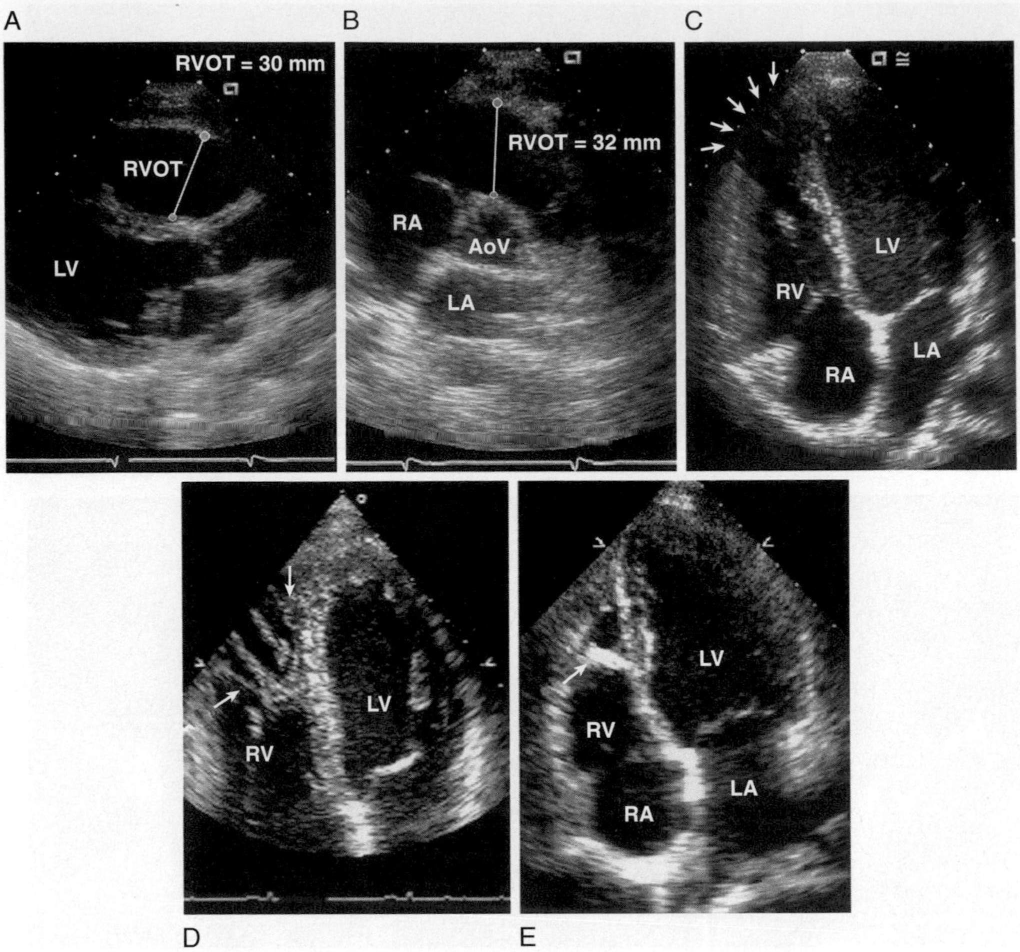

FIGURE 14–81 Echocardiographic views from a patient with arrhythmogenic right ventricular dysplasia. **A,** Right ventricular outflow tract (RVOT) enlargement from the parasternal long-axis view. **B,** RVOT enlargement from the parasternal short-axis view. Apical four-chamber views showing, **C,** a focal right ventricular (RV) apical aneurysm (arrows), **D,** excessive trabeculations (arrows), and, **E,** a hyperreflective moderator band (arrow). AoV = aortic valve; LA = left atrium; LV = left ventricle; RA = right atrium. *(From Yoerger DM, Marcus F, Sherrill D, et al, Multidisciplinary Study of Right Ventricular Dysplasia Investigators: Echocardiographic findings in patients meeting task force criteria for arrhythmogenic right ventricular dysplasia: New insights from the multidisciplinary study of right ventricular dysplasia. J Am Coll Cardiol 45:860, 2005. Used with permission.)*

ponade include (a) early diastolic collapse of the RV and late diastolic RA inversion related to intrapericardial pressure increasing above the intracardiac pressures (diastolic collapse of the right heart may not occur if right-heart pressure is elevated), (b) abnormal ventricular septal motion related to respiratory variation in ventricular filling, (c) respiratory variation in ventricle chamber size, and (d) plethora of the inferior vena cava with blunted respiratory changes. Clotted blood, or hemopericardium, may be seen in the pericardial sac of patients with myocardial rupture or proximal aortic dissection (Fig. 14-85). Pneumopericardium, or air in the pericardial sac as a result of esophageal perforation, causes inadequate TTE and TEE imaging because ultrasound does not penetrate air well.

Pericardial and pleural effusions may be difficult to differentiate from each other. In the parasternal long axis view, pericardial effusion is located anterior to the descending thoracic aorta, whereas a pleural effusion is posterior to the aorta (see Fig. 14-e18 on website). The presence of only an anterior echo-free space suggests an epicardial fat pad rather than pericardial effusion; a pericardial effusion is usually circumferential.

Doppler echocardiographic features of pericardial tamponade are more sensitive than the 2D echocardiographic features. The Doppler findings of cardiac tamponade are based on the characteristic respiratory variations in intrathoracic and intracardiac hemodynamics (see Chap. 70).[1] Normally, intrapericardial pressure (hence LA and LV diastolic pressures) and intrathoracic pressure (hence PCWP) decrease the same degree during inspiration, but in cardiac tamponade, intrapericardial (and intracardiac) pressure falls substantially less than intrathoracic pressure. Therefore the LV filling pressure gradient from PCWP to LV diastolic pressure decreases with inspiration. Consequently, mitral E velocity is reduced with inspiration. LV filling and mitral E velocity increase with expiration. In cardiac tamponade the degree of ventricular filling depends on the other ventricle because of the relatively fixed combined cardiac volume (ventricular interdependence); thus reciprocal changes occur in the right-heart chambers (Fig. 14-86). Increased venous return to the right-heart chambers with inspiration also contributes to the increased ventricular interdependence. The respiratory flow velocity changes across the mitral and tricuspid valves are also reflected in the pulmonary and hepatic venous flow velocities, respectively: inspiratory decrease and expiratory increase in pulmonary vein diastolic forward flow and expiratory decrease in hepatic vein forward flow and increase in expiratory reversal flow.[1]

Echocardiographically Guided Pericardiocentesis

The most effective treatment for cardiac tamponade is prompt removal of the pericardial fluid. Two-dimensional echocardiography can guide pericardiocentesis by locating the optimal site of puncture and by monitoring the results of the pericardiocentesis. Under most circumstances, a catheter (usually a 5F or 6F pigtail catheter) is introduced and left in the pericardial sac for several days with intermittent drainage, which decreases the rate of reaccumulation. In a series of 1127 consecutive echo-guided pericardiocentesis procedures, the most common causes included malignancy (34 percent), postoperative (25 percent), and a complication of a catheter-based procedure (10 percent). The procedure was successful in 97 percent of cases, and complications occurred in 4.4 percent. Major complications were death (1 patient), cardiac laceration (5), vessel laceration (1), pneumothorax (5), infection (1), and sustained ventricular tachycardia (1).

Constrictive Pericarditis

Constrictive pericarditis is caused by abnormally thickened, adherent, inflamed, or calcific pericardium limiting

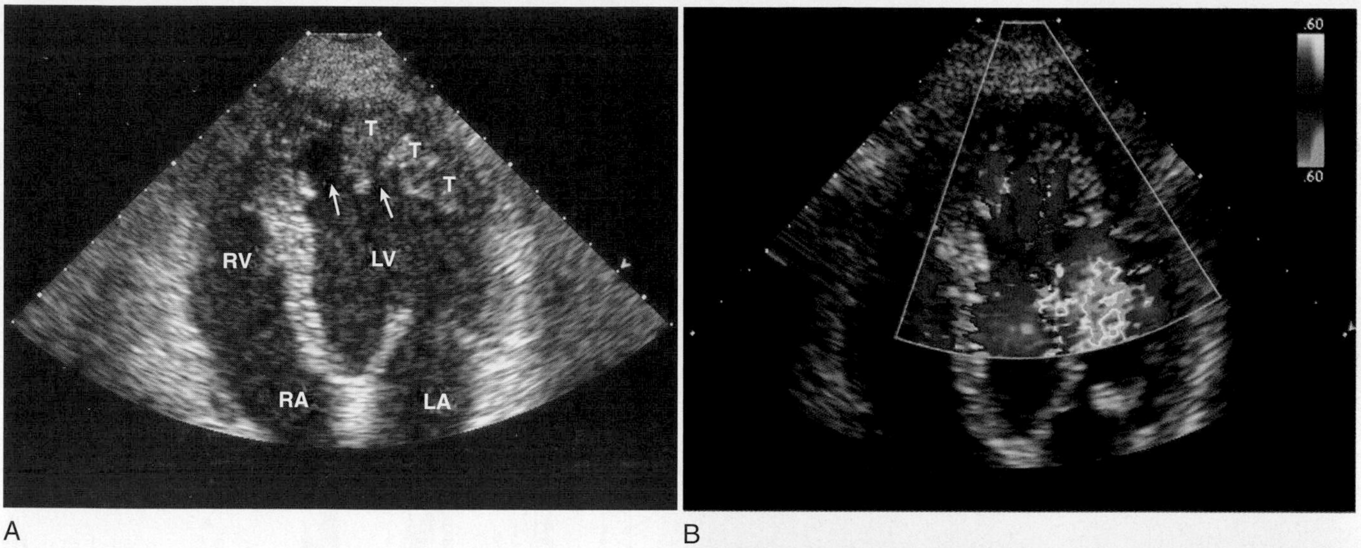

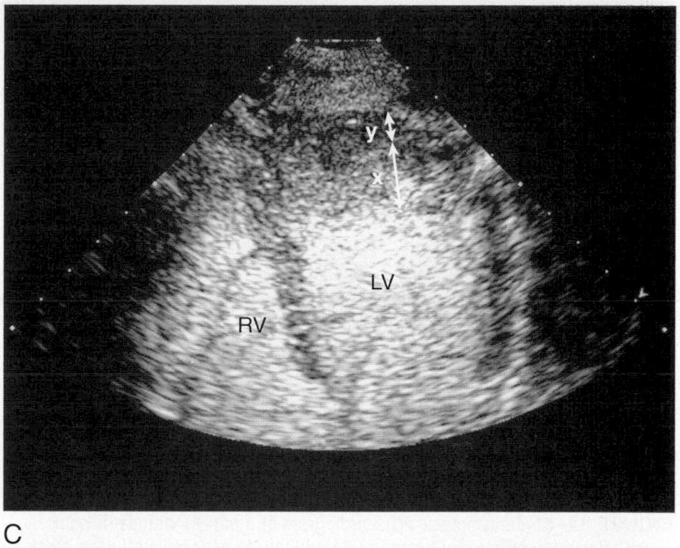

FIGURE 14–82 A, Apical four-chamber 2D echocardiographic view showing characteristic increase in trabeculations (T) and deep recesses (arrows) in noncompaction cardiomyopathy. **B,** Color flow imaging showing flow into the intratrabecular recesses. **C,** Contrast administration shows trabeculations at the apex; the appearance is different from that of apical hypertrophic cardiomyopathy. With contrast enhancement, the ratio of noncompacted layer (x) to compacted layer (y) can be calculated. In this patient, x = 1.8 cm, y = 0.8 cm, with x/y = 2.3. LA = left atrium; LV = left ventricle; RA = right atrium; RV = right ventricle. *(From Oh JK, Seward JB, Tajik AJ: The Echo Manual. 3rd ed. Philadelphia, Lippincott Williams & Wilkins, 2006. Used with permission of Mayo Foundation for Medical Education and Research.)*

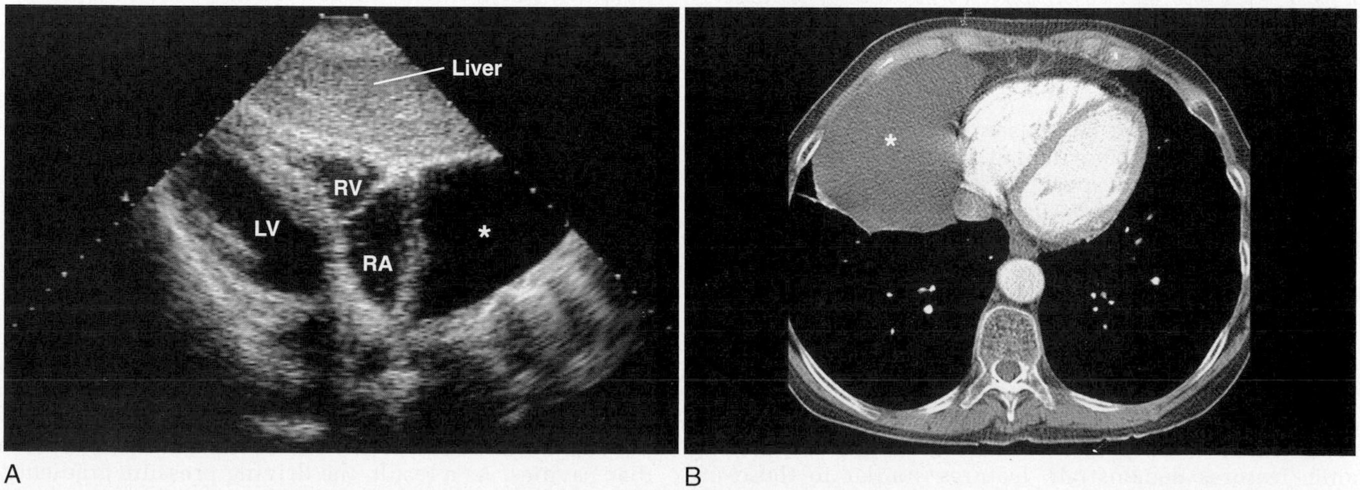

FIGURE 14–83 A, 2D still frame obtained from the normal subcostal position in a patient with a pericardial cyst (*). **B,** Computed tomographic image of the chest showing a large fluid-filled space adjacent to the heart on the right side, consistent with a pericardial cyst (*). LV = left ventricle; RA = right atrium; RV = right ventricle. *(From Oh JK, Seward JB, Tajik AJ: The Echo Manual. 3rd ed. Philadelphia, Lippincott Williams & Wilkins, 2006. Used with permission of Mayo Foundation for Medical Education and Research.)*

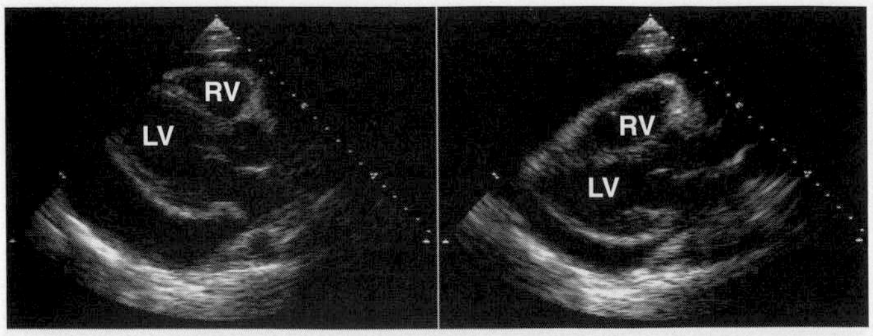

FIGURE 14–84 With a large amount of pericardial effusion, the heart has a swinging motion, which is an ominous sign of cardiac tamponade. When the left ventricular (LV) cavity is close to the surface **(left),** the QRS voltage increases on the electrocardiogram, but it decreases when the LV swings away from the surface **(right),** producing electrical alternans. RV = right ventricle. *(From Oh JK, Seward JB, Tajik AJ: The Echo Manual. 3rd ed. Philadelphia, Lippincott Williams & Wilkins, 2006. Used with permission of Mayo Foundation for Medical Education and Research.)*

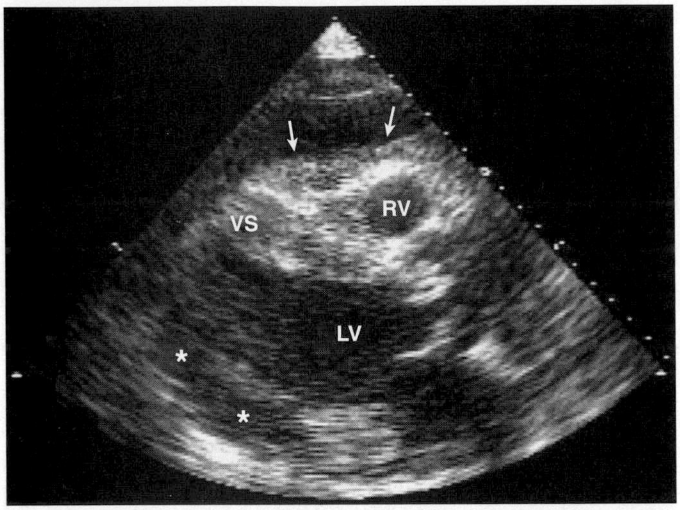

FIGURE 14–85 Transthoracic echocardiogram of a patient with cardiogenic shock after acute myocardial infarction. In addition to pericardial effusion, there is an echo-dense structure posteriorly (*) and anteriorly (arrows) that indicate clot formation. LV = left ventricle; RV = right ventricle; VS = ventricular septum. *(From Oh JK, Seward JB, Tajik AJ: The Echo Manual. 3rd ed. Philadelphia, Lippincott Williams & Wilkins, 2006. Used with permission of Mayo Foundation for Medical Education and Research.)*

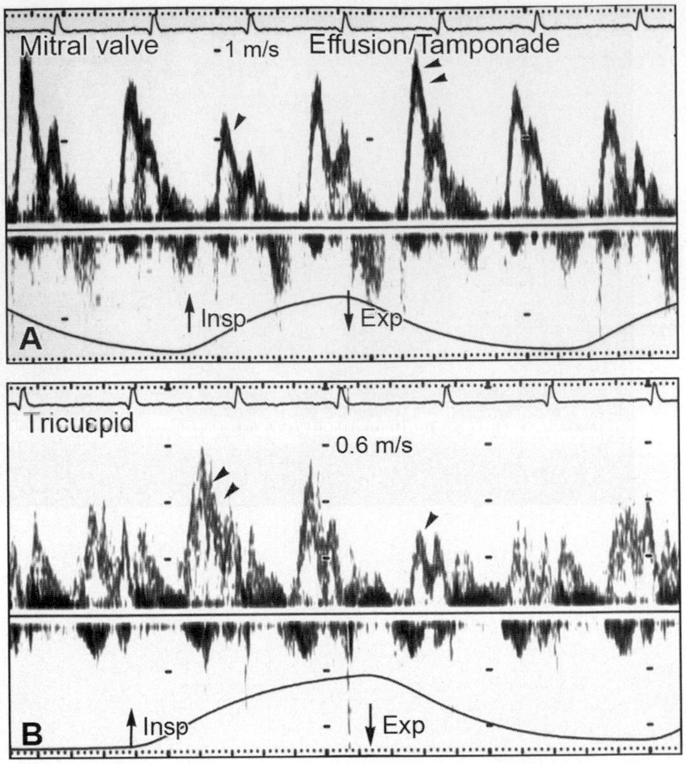

FIGURE 14–86 Typical pulsed wave Doppler pattern of tamponade recorded with a nasal respirometer. **A,** Mitral inflow velocity decreases (single arrowhead) after inspiration (Insp) and increases (double arrowheads) after expiration (Exp). **B,** Tricuspid inflow velocity has the opposite changes. E velocity increases (double arrowheads) after inspiration and decreases (single arrowhead) after expiration. *(From Oh JK, Hatle LK, Mulvagh SL, Tajik AJ: Transient constrictive pericarditis: diagnosis by two-dimensional Doppler echocardiography. Mayo Clin Proc 68:1158, 1993. Used with permission of Mayo Foundation for Medical Education and Research.)*

diastolic filling of the heart (see Chap. 70). Constrictive pericarditis is a curable cause of severe heart failure and should be considered, especially when systolic function is normal and/or there is a predisposing factor. Previous cardiac surgery is now the most common cause of constriction in the United States,[146] followed by viral pericarditis, radiation to the chest, and collagen vascular disease. In one fourth of patients, the cause of constriction cannot be found. In areas where tuberculosis is endemic, it is the most frequent cause of constriction.

The pericardium is usually thickened in patients with constrictive pericarditis, but pericardial thickness may be normal in up to 20 percent of cases.[147] Invasive hemodynamic features demonstrate features similar to those of restrictive cardiomyopathy and other myocardial diseases. Improved understanding of the mechanism of constrictive pericarditis has allowed development of specific echo-Doppler diagnostic criteria for constriction.[148] The M-mode and 2D echocardiographic features of constrictive pericarditis include (a) thickened pericardium, (b) abnormal ventricular septal motion reflecting ventricular interdependence, (c) flattening of the LV posterior wall during diastole, (d) respiratory variation in ventricular size, and (e) a dilated inferior vena cava (Fig. 14-87), but these findings are not sensitive or specific for constriction. The hemodynamic events of constriction in regard to respiratory variation in LV and RV filling are similar to the findings in cardiac tamponade, although the underlying pathological mechanism is different. To establish the diagnosis of constrictive pericarditis, two hemodynamic characteristics need to be demonstrated either with 2D/Doppler echocardiography or with cardiac catheterization: (a) disassociation between intrathoracic and intracardiac pressures and (b) exaggerated ventricular interdependence.[1]

A thickened pericardium prevents full transmission of the intrathoracic pressure changes that occur with respiration to the intracardiac cavities, creating respiratory variations in the pressure difference between the pulmonary vein and LA. With inspiration, intrathoracic pressure decreases (normally 3 to 5 mm Hg) and the pressure in the pulmonary veins and capillaries decreases to a similar degree. In constriction, this inspiratory pressure change is not fully transmitted to the intrapericardial and intracardiac cavities. As a result, the driving pressure gradient for LV filling decreases immediately after inspiration and increases with expiration. This characteristic hemodynamic pattern is best illustrated with simultaneous pressure recordings from the LV and the PCWP together with mitral inflow velocities (Fig. 14-88).[1]

Within the noncompliant, adherent pericardium, the combined ventricular volume is relatively fixed; thus the

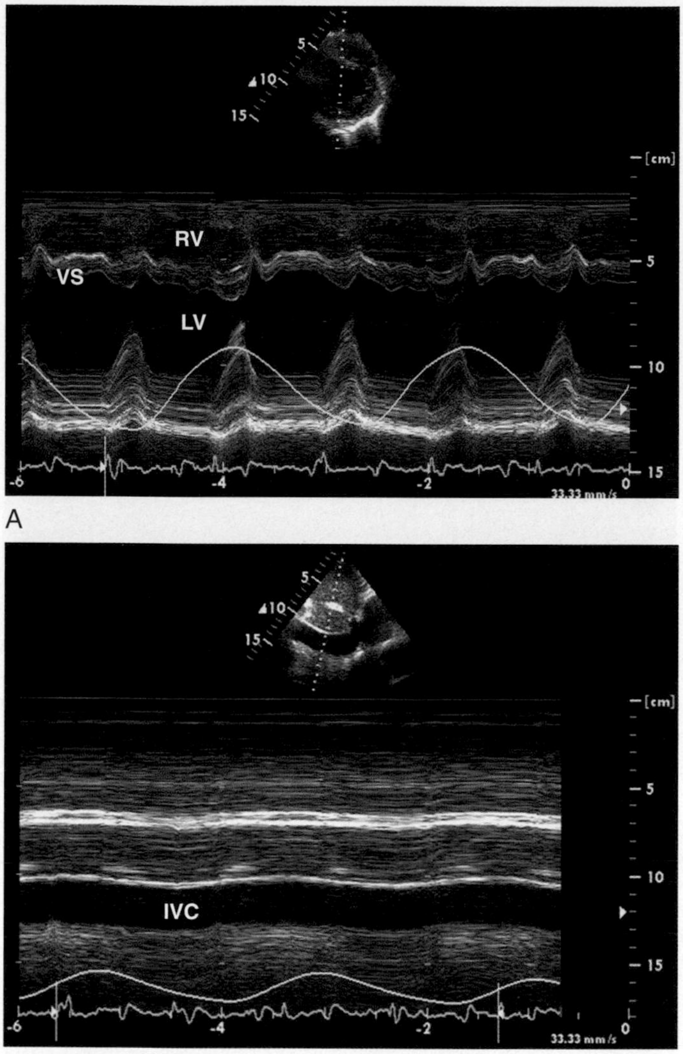

FIGURE 14–87 **A,** M-mode echocardiogram from the parasternal window of a patient with constrictive pericarditis recorded simultaneously with the respirometer tracing. An upward deflection of the respirometer recording indicates onset of inspiration, and downward deflection indicates onset of expiration. Typical features of constrictive pericarditis include thickened pericardium, abnormal ventricular septal (VS) motion with septal shift toward the left ventricle (LV) on inspiration and toward the right ventricle (RV) on expiration (resulting in the respiratory variation in ventricular size), and flattening of the LV posterior wall because of limited diastolic filling. **B,** M-mode from subcostal view of the inferior vena cava (IVC), which is plethoric and does not collapse with inspiration in constrictive pericarditis.

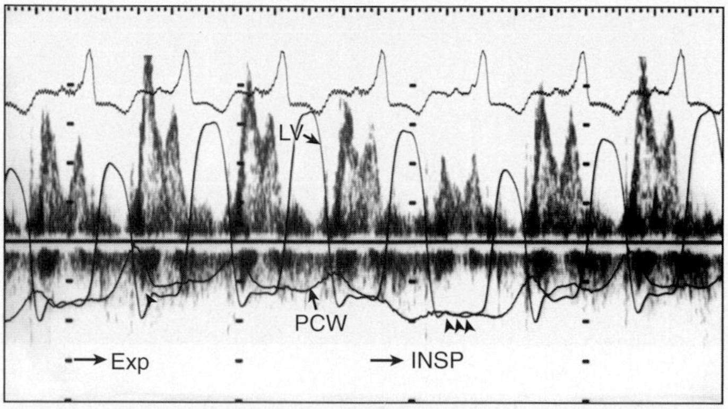

FIGURE 14–88 Diagrams of left ventricular (LV) and pulmonary capillary wedge (PCW) pressure tracings to demonstrate dissociation between intrathoracic (or PCW) and intracardiac (or LV) pressure change with respiration (see text). EXP = expiration (single arrowhead); INSP = inspiration (triple arrowheads); PCW = pulmonary capillary wedge. *(From Oh JK, Seward JB, Tajik AJ: The Echo Manual. 3rd ed. Philadelphia, Lippincott Williams & Wilkins, 2006. Used with permission of Mayo Foundation for Medical Education and Research.)*

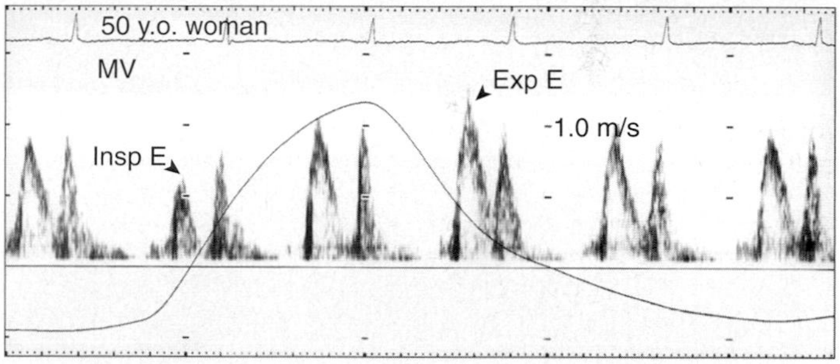

FIGURE 14–89 Typical mitral inflow pulsed wave Doppler recordings in constrictive pericarditis along with simultaneous recording of respiration (onset of inspiration at upward deflection and onset at expiration at downward deflection). The first mitral inflow is at the onset of inspiration, and the fourth mitral inflow is soon after the onset of expiration. Mitral inflow E velocity is decreased with inspiration (1st and 6th beat). MV = mitral valve. *(From Oh JK, Seward JB, Tajik AJ: The Echo Manual. 3rd ed. Philadelphia, Lippincott Williams & Wilkins, 2006. Used with permission of Mayo Foundation for Medical Education and Research.)*

diastolic filling of each ventricular chamber relies on the other, accounting for reciprocal respiratory changes in the filling of the ventricles in constrictive pericarditis (see Chap. 70). With inspiration, LV filling decreases and the ventricular septum shifts to the left, which allows increased RV filling. Consequently, tricuspid inflow E velocity and hepatic vein diastolic forward flow velocity increase. With expiration, LV filling increases, causing the ventricular septum to shift to the right, which limits RV filling. Tricuspid inflow decreases and hepatic vein diastolic forward flow decreases, with significant flow reversals during diastole. When the Doppler features for constrictive pericarditis were described initially, respiratory variation of greater than or equal to 25 percent in the mitral inflow E velocity and increased hepatic vein diastolic flow reversal with expiration were proposed as diagnostic criteria for constrictive pericarditis (Fig. 14-89). However, it is now recognized that up to 50 percent of patients with constrictive pericarditis have less than 25 percent respiratory variation in mitral E velocity.[139,148] Because LA pressure is markedly elevated, the respiratory variation in mitral E velocity becomes more blunted. Therefore the lack of respiratory variation in mitral inflow velocities should not exclude the diagnosis of constrictive pericarditis. Hepatic vein flow reversal at the beginning of expiration continues to be a reliable diagnostic feature, even in atrial fibrillation (Fig. 14-90). Mitral annulus velocity recorded with TDI has become a valuable Doppler parameter in establishing the diagnosis of constriction[139,148] and in differentiating it from myocardial disease or restrictive cardiomyopathy (Fig. 14-91A and B). Myocardial relaxation is relatively well preserved in constriction unless the myocardium is also involved, as in radiation heart injury. The longitudinal motion, hence, mitral septal annulus velocity, is well preserved in constriction (Ea > 7 cm/sec) and increases further as the constriction becomes worse with higher filling pressure, paradoxical to its change in myocardial disease. This phenomenon has been termed *annulus paradoxus.*[1]

Acute dilatation of the heart, pulmonary embolism, RV infarct, pleural effusion, and chronic obstructive lung disease can produce similar respiratory Doppler changes as constrictive pericarditis, and most can be differentiated on the basis of clinical features. However, patients

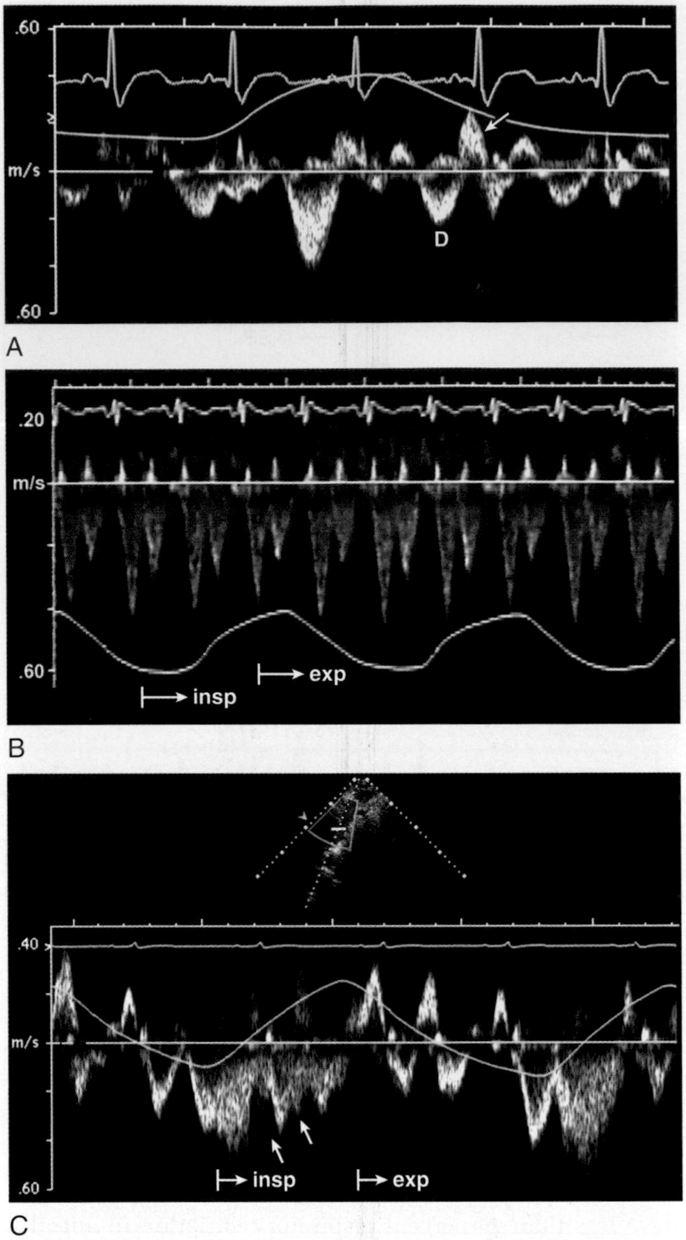

FIGURE 14–90 **A,** Pulsed-wave Doppler recording from the hepatic vein of a patient with advanced constrictive pericarditis. The hepatic vein has flow reversal after the onset of expiration (arrow), with decreased forward flow during diastole (D) as compared with the flow velocities on inspiration. **B,** Superior vena cava velocity in constriction. There is no notable difference in systolic velocity with respiration. **C,** Superior vena cava velocity in chronic obstructive lung disease. There is marked increase in flow velocities (arrows) with inspiration (insp), then decrease with expiration (exp).

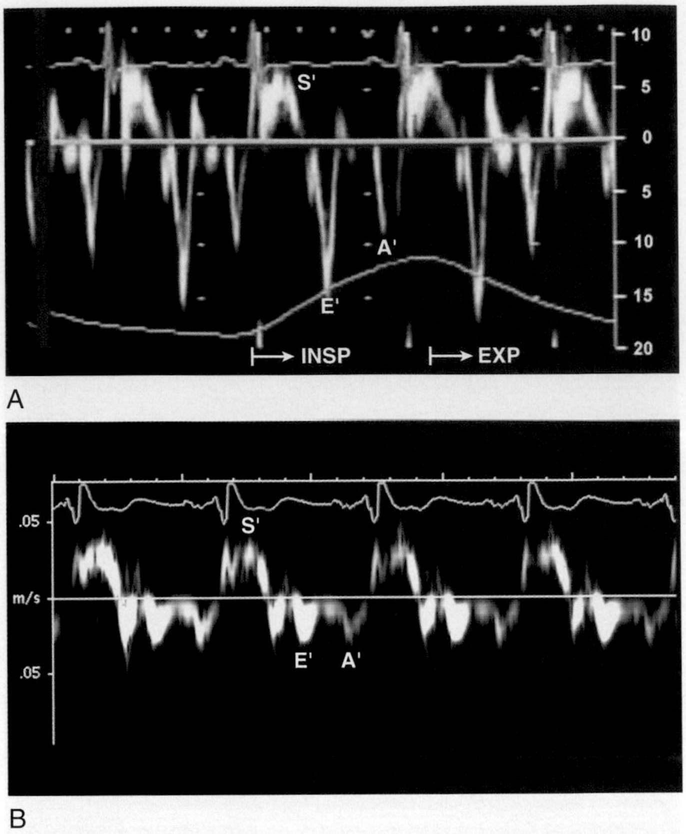

FIGURE 14–91 Tissue Doppler imaging of the septal mitral annulus in constriction **(A)** and restriction **(B)**. **A,** Early diastolic septal mitral annulus velocity (E′) is 12 cm/sec, indicating relatively normal or even greater than normal longitudinal motion of the mitral annulus. In patients with heart failure and increased jugular venous pressure, E′ velocity greater than or equal to 8 cm/sec should be equated with constrictive pericarditis until proven otherwise. **B,** E′ is markedly decreased in this patient with myocardial disease and heart failure. Decreased E′ correlates with abnormality in myocardial relaxation, which is reduced in almost all forms of cardiomyopathies. A′ = late diastolic septal mitral annulus velocity; Exp = expiration; Insp = inspiration; S′ = longitudinal systolic velocity. *(From Oh JK, Seward JB, Tajik AJ: The Echo Manual. 3rd ed. Philadelphia, Lippincott Williams & Wilkins, 2006. Used with permission of Mayo Foundation for Medical Education and Research.)*

with chronic obstructive lung disease may have symptoms of right-sided heart failure similar to those of constrictive pericarditis and may be difficult to differentiate from those who have constrictive pericarditis. Respiratory variation in ventricular filling in chronic obstructive lung disease is related to increased respiratory effort causing marked reduction in intrathoracic pressure with inspiration. This is also manifested as a marked increase in forward flow velocity in the superior vena cava that is not present in patients with constrictive pericarditis (see Fig. 14-90). Atrial fibrillation makes the interpretation of respiratory variation in Doppler velocities difficult. Patients with constrictive pericarditis and atrial fibrillation still have typical 2D echocardiographic features and require longer observation of Doppler velocities to detect velocity variation with respiration, regardless of underlying cardiac cycle length. Hepatic vein diastolic flow reversal with expiration is an important Doppler finding that suggests constrictive pericarditis, even when mitral inflow velocity pattern is not diagnostic.[1] Occasionally, a temporary pacemaker is used to regularize the patient's rhythm in an attempt to evaluate the respiratory variation of Doppler velocities. Strain imaging may be able to add more diagnostic features useful in distinguishing pericardial from myocardial diastolic heart failure. Preliminary data suggest normal strain of the ventricular septum in constriction but decreased strain in myocardial diseases, especially at the basal septum. Doppler echocardiographic features of constrictive pericarditis are summarized by the following: (a) a restrictive mitral inflow velocity pattern with or without respiratory variation, (b) increased hepatic vein diastolic flow reversals with expiration, (c) mitral annulus septal Ea greater than 7 cm/sec, (d) less than 20 cm/sec respiratory variation in superior vena cava systolic velocity, and (e) normal strain imaging of the ventricular septum.

A subset of patients with constrictive pericarditis presents with pericardial effusion. Patients usually present with clinical or hemodynamic evidence of increased filling pressures caused by a pericardial effusion and/or tamponade.[149,150] However, constrictive hemodynamics persist even after removal or the resolution of pericardial effusion and after intrapericardial pressure has normalized. This condition is called *effusive-constrictive pericarditis* (see Chap. 70). Most of these patients have inflammation of the pericardium that causes constriction; the constrictive hemodynamics resolve spontaneously or after treatment with antiinflammatory agents. The latter condition has been termed *transient constrictive pericarditis*.[151] Occasionally, the underlying constrictive pericarditis requires pericardiectomy.

Transient Constrictive Pericarditis

About 7 to 10 percent of patients with acute pericarditis have a transient constrictive phase. These patients usually have a moderate amount of pericardial fluid, and as the pericardial effusion disappears, the pericardium remains inflamed, thickened, and noncompliant, resulting in constrictive hemodynamics. The patient presents with features of chronic constrictive pericarditis including dyspnea, peripheral edema, increased jugular venous pressure, and sometimes ascites. This transient constrictive phase may last 2 to 3 months before it gradually resolves either spontaneously or with antiinflammatory therapy. When hemodynamics and findings typical of constriction develop in patients with acute pericarditis, initial treatment is indomethacin and/or colchicine for 4 to 6 weeks and, if there is no response, corticosteroids for 1 to 2 months (60 mg daily for 1 week, then tapered over 6 to 8 weeks) after ensuring that the pericarditis is not caused by bacterial infection. The thickened pericardium usually returns to normal thickness, and constrictive hemodynamics resolve. All causes of chronic constrictive pericarditis except radiation treatment have been identified to cause transient constrictive pericarditis.[151] It is possible that constrictive pericardium is curable during the initial phase of the disease, and it may be worthwhile treating patients with antiinflammatory agents (nonsteroidal and/or steroidal) if the onset of constriction is recent. There appears to be an increased response to medical therapy by patients with thickened pericardium and markers of inflammation. Inflammation of the pericardium is best assessed by CMR with delayed enhancement, using gadolinium (see Chap. 17).

TEE in Pericardial Diseases

If TTE does not provide adequate imaging of the pericardium and hemodynamic assessment of ventricular filling, TEE should be considered. A loculated pericardial effusion may be difficult to detect on TTE, and TEE has been especially helpful in postoperative patients with loculated hemopericardium as a cause of tamponade. TEE also provides useful pulmonary venous flow pulsed-wave Doppler velocities with simultaneous respirometer recording, which may be helpful in the evaluation of constrictive pericarditis. Furthermore, TEE is helpful in measuring the thickness of the pericardium.

CARDIAC DISEASES CAUSED BY SYSTEMIC ILLNESS

Multiple systemic disorders, genetic diseases, chemicals, acute illnesses such as sepsis, and medications can cause morphological, functional, and hemodynamic abnormalities of the heart. Cardiac abnormalities include secondary cardiomyopathies (dilated, infiltrative, or restrictive), valvular diseases, pericardial diseases, intracardiac mass, and marantic or nonbacterial thrombotic (Libman-Sacks) endocarditis. Frequently, echocardiographic detection of a cardiac abnormality may be the first diagnostic clue to a systemic disease (e.g., the typical tricuspid and pulmonary valve involvement and appearance in carcinoid or increased ventricular wall thickness and granular appearance in cardiac amyloidosis). Table 14-18 lists various cardiac manifestations of systemic illnesses frequently seen in the echocardiography laboratory.

Amyloidosis (see Chap. 64)

Myocardial infiltration is primarily interstitial in amyloidosis, and an increase in myocardial wall thickness without dilatation of the LV cavity is the predominant morphological feature. However, normal wall thickness does not exclude the diagnosis. Amyloid deposits can affect most cardiac structures, such as the valves, thus causing multivalvular regurgitation. Amyloid deposition in the myocardium causes a characteristic sparkling appearance on 2D echocardiography (Fig. 14-92). Importantly, the sparkling appearance alone is not diagnostic of cardiac amyloidosis, but occurs commonly with harmonic imaging or in other

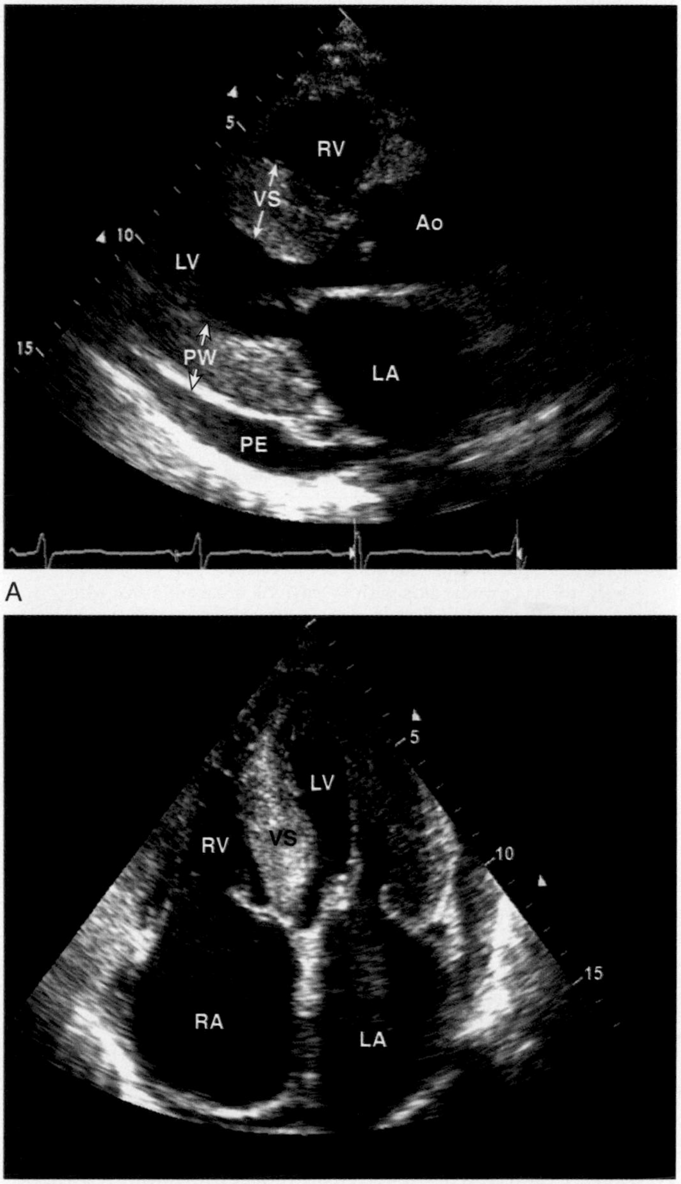

FIGURE 14–92 A, Parasternal long-axis view showing typical findings in cardiac amyloidosis: concentric increase in left ventricular (LV) wall thickness, sparkling granular appearance of the myocardium, and thickened valve leaflets. Arrows, 23-mm-thick ventricular septum (VS) and 19-mm-thick posterior wall (PW). There is a small pericardial effusion (PE). **B,** Apical four-chamber view showing marked increase in VS wall thickness and marked dilatation of both atria. Ao = aorta; LA = left atrium; RA = right atrium; RV = right ventricle. *(From Oh JK, Seward JB, Tajik AJ: The Echo Manual. 3rd ed. Philadelphia, Lippincott Williams & Wilkins, 2006. Used with permission of Mayo Foundation for Medical Education and Research.)*

TABLE 14–18 Echocardiographic Features of Cardiac Manifestations of Systemic Illnesses

Amyloidosis	Increased LV and RV wall thickness (moderate to marked) Normal LV cavity size Gradual deterioration of ventricular systolic function Granular appearance of myocardium (abnormal texture) Pericardial effusion Spectrum of diastolic dysfunction Thickening of the valves and multivalvular regurgitation
Ankylosing spondylitis	Dilatation of the aortic annulus Dilatation of sinuses of Valsalva Thickened aortic valve with aortic regurgitation
Carcinoid	Thickening and retraction of tricuspid valve with severe tricuspid regurgitation Tricuspid stenosis, usually mild Pulmonary valve thickening and retraction with pulmonic stenosis RV volume overload Thickening of valves on left side (<15%)
Friedreich ataxia	LV hypertrophy, usually concentric (68%), resembling hypertrophic cardiomyopathy Dilated LV with systolic dysfunction (7%)
Hemochromatosis	Appearance of dilated cardiomyopathy, dilated LV with decreased systolic function Normal ventricular wall thickness Restrictive diastolic filling characteristic at advanced stage
HIV infection or AIDS	Pericardial effusion Dilated cardiomyopathy Pulmonary hypertension
Hypereosinophilic syndrome	Posterior mitral leaflet thickening and tethering Ventricular apical thrombus with cavity obliteration Rarely, diffuse myocarditis with LV cavity increased in size with systolic dysfunction Hyperthyroidism or hypothyroidism Pericardial effusion LV systolic dysfunction
Marfan syndrome	Dilatation of the ascending aorta Dilatation of the aortic annulus and the sinus of Valsalva Aortic dissection Mitral valve prolapse
Muscular dystrophy (Duchenne)	Posterior basal and lateral wall fibrosis
Pheochromocytoma	Concentric LV hypertrophy (20%) Myocarditis (acute) with catecholamine crisis
Rheumatoid arthritis	Pericardial effusion Constrictive pericarditis Cardiac granuloma
Sarcoidosis	Regional wall motion abnormalities Thinning of the basal and posterolateral walls Posterobasal aneurysm Restrictive morphology
Scleroderma	Pericardial effusion Pulmonary hypertension Valvular sclerosis
Systemic lupus erythematosus	Pericarditis Tamponade Myocarditis Endocarditis, Libman-Sacks
Tuberous sclerosis	Rhabdomyoma Cardiomyopathy

AIDS=acquired immunodeficiency syndrome; HIV=human immunodeficiency virus; LV=left ventricle; RV=right ventricle.

From Oh JK, Seward JB, Tajik AJ: The Echo Manual. 3rd ed. Philadelphia, Lippincott Williams & Wilkins, 2006. Used with permission of Mayo Foundation for Medical Education and Research.

conditions such as hypertensive disease (especially in patients with renal failure), glycogen storage disease, and hypertrophic cardiomyopathy. Patients with cardiac amyloidosis usually have low QRS voltage or a pseudoinfarct pattern on the electrocardiogram, whereas increased QRS voltage is noted in those with LV hypertrophy, hypertrophic cardiomyopathy, or glycogen storage disease.

During an early stage of cardiac amyloidosis, systolic function can be hyperdynamic, and systolic anterior motion of the mitral valve with intracavitary obstruction may be present, similar to hypertrophic cardiomyopathy. The initial diastolic abnormality in cardiac amyloidosis is abnormal relaxation (grade 1 diastolic dysfunction) resulting from increased ventricular wall thickness. As amyloid infiltration progresses, systolic function gradually deteriorates and the diastolic filling pattern becomes restrictive (grade 3-4 diastolic dysfunction), decreasing LV compliance and increasing LA pressure. Diastolic function is an important prognostic variable in cardiac amyloidosis (Fig. 14-93). The shorter the deceleration time, the poorer the prognosis: the average survival for patients with a deceleration time of less than or equal to 150 msec is less than 1 year, compared with 3 years if deceleration time is greater than 150 msec. TDI demonstrates decreased systolic and early diastolic velocities of the mitral annulus (usually <6 cm/sec) in cardiac amyloidosis (see Fig. 14-93C). Color M-mode imaging of mitral inflow may not show delayed propagation despite marked abnormality in myocardial relaxation because of the small LV cavity. However, the longitudinal myocardial velocity gradient ([myocardial velocity at the base − myocardial velocity at mid LV]/[distance between two sample sites]) appears to identify patients with heart failure.[152]

Carcinoid Disease (see Chaps. 62 and 64)

Carcinoid tumors arise from enterochromaffin cells typically located in the gastrointestinal tract. Cardiac involvement occurs primarily with hepatic metastases, except in patients with ovarian carcinoid. Valve disease is caused by hormonally active substances released from the primary tumor and metastases, such as serotonin. Cardiac involvement predominantly affects the endocardium and valves on the right side of the heart because the tumor substances are inactivated by the lung. Left-sided valve disease is noted in 7 percent of cases and is usually related to a PFO, which allows the tumor substances to pass from the RA to the LA or, less commonly, to high circulating levels of serotonin or to pulmonary metastasis. The characteristic tricuspid and pulmonary valve thickening causes restricted motion of the valves and secondary severe tricuspid valve regurgitation

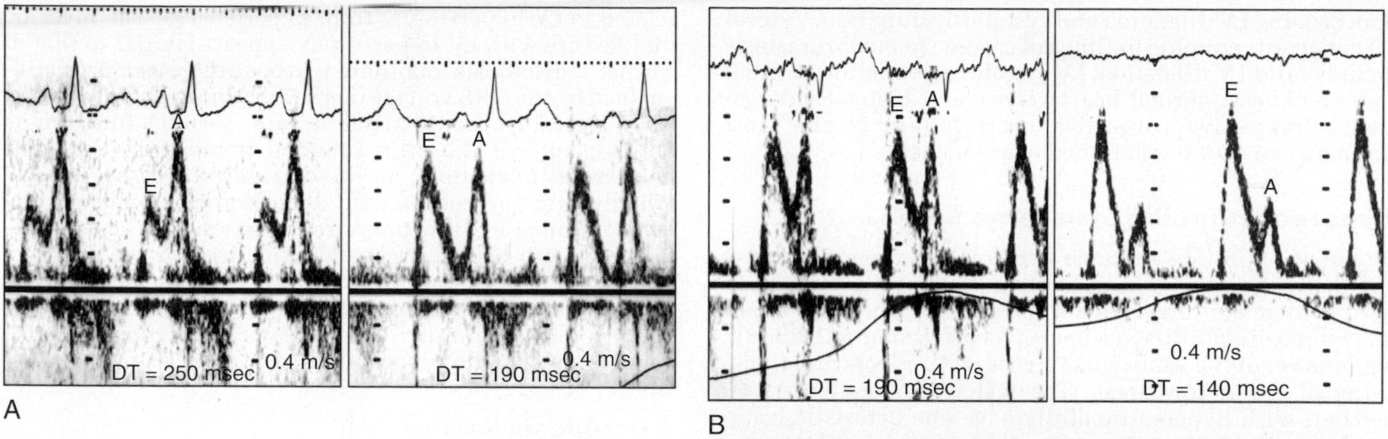

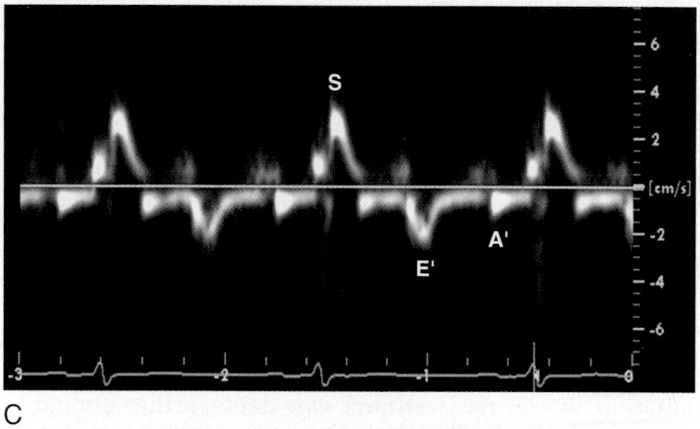

FIGURE 14–93 Serial mitral inflow Doppler velocities from two patients with cardiac amyloidosis. **A,** The initial Doppler study **(left)** showed a relaxation abnormality, with decreased E, increased A, and prolonged deceleration time (DT). Six months later **(right),** it had become pseudonormalized, with progressive cardiac amyloidosis. **B,** In another patient, the initial study **(left)** showed a DT of 190 msec, with normal E and A. Seven months later **(right),** the mitral inflow became typical of a restrictive pattern (increased E, decreased A, and decreased DT), indicating that the initial Doppler pattern was of "pseudonormalized" inflow. **C,** Tissue Doppler imaging of mitral annulus in a patient with cardiac amyloidosis. Longitudinal systolic (S) and diastolic (E′ and A′) velocities are decreased: S′ = 3.4 m/sec, E′ = 2.5 cm/sec, and A′ = 1 cm/sec. *(**A** and **B**, From Klein AL, Hatle LK, Taliercio CP, et al: Serial Doppler echocardiographic follow-up of left ventricular diastolic function in cardiac amyloidosis. J Am Coll Cardiol 16:1135, 1990. Used with permission. **C**, From Oh JK, Seward JB, Tajik AJ: The Echo Manual. 3rd ed. Philadelphia, Lippincott Williams & Wilkins, 2006. Used with permission of Mayo Foundation for Medical Education and Research.)*

(see Fig. 14-60; see also Fig. 62-40), minimal tricuspid stenosis, and various degrees of pulmonic stenosis and regurgitation. Surgical pathology examination of 75 cases at Mayo Clinic showed that all valve dysfunction was related to carcinoid plaques that caused thickening and retraction.[153] Thickening was the result of both cellular proliferation (myofibroblasts) and deposition of extracellular matrix (collagen, myxoid, and elastin).

Characteristic 2D echocardiographic features demonstrate tricuspid valve thickening and retraction, with limited mobility. Coaptation is incomplete, resulting in severe tricuspid regurgitation that produces an RV volume overload pattern. The pulmonary valve thickening and retraction result in mixed pulmonic stenosis and regurgitation; the pulmonary valve is characteristically difficult to image with TTE (see Fig. 14-63); however, Doppler and color flow imaging readily outlines hemodynamic features. Doppler recordings from the tricuspid and pulmonic valves demonstrate severe valve regurgitation and rapid rise in RV diastolic pressure. Liver metastasis and hepatic vein Doppler systolic flow reversal from severe tricuspid regurgitation are important features noted on subcostal imaging. Carcinoid also may produce a metastatic tumor embedded in the myocardium (see Fig. 14-e19 on website).[154] The 2D echocardiographic features of carcinoid heart disease are distinctive and readily distinguishable from other lesions producing right-sided heart failure. Rarely, cardiac valvular lesions resembling carcinoid involvement may develop with excessive use of ergot, pergolide, or a diet pill combination (fenphen). Progression of carcinoid heart disease has been correlated to high peak urinary levels of 5-hydroxyindoleacetic acid and previous chemotherapy.[155] Operative risk is higher for patients with carcinoid than for patients undergoing operation for other types of valve disease; however, operative intervention improves survival of patients with carcinoid disease.[156]

Drug-Induced Cardiac Diseases

Drugs have been identified as responsible agents for myocardial, valvular, and pericardial abnormalities. The chemotherapy agent doxorubicin (Adriamycin) causes LV dilatation and systolic dysfunc-tion that usually occurs after a dose of more than 450 gm/m^2 and may not be reversible (see Chap. 85). Cardiac toxicity is dose related and potentiated by concurrent or previous radiotherapy. Daunorubicin (>600 mg/m^2) and cyclophosphamide (>6.2 gm/m^2) cause a similar cardiomyopathy. Pericardial effusion or tamponade may also develop after cyclophosphamide treatment. LV systolic dysfunction has been reported in bulimic patients who ingested ipecac. Emetine, the principal component of ipecac, causes mitochondrial damage by inhibiting oxidative phosphorylation. High-dose corticosteroid therapy, phenothiazine, and tricyclic antidepressants may also cause LV systolic dysfunction.

Long-term use of chloroquine may result in a reversible infiltrative cardiomyopathy similar to Fabry disease, with increased LV and, occasionally, RV wall thickness, biatrial enlargement, restrictive diastolic filling, and valvular regurgitation. Chloroquine is taken up by lysosomes, and abnormal lysosomal enzymatic activity results in the accumulation of glycogen and phospholipids. Light microscopy findings include vacuolated cytoplasm of myocytes preferentially found in the ventricular septum, which may explain the conduction abnormality in this disorder.[157]

Cardiac valves may be affected by drug toxicity. Ergot alkaloids, appetite suppressants (see Fig. 14-64), and pergolide may produce valvular lesions similar to those of rheumatic or carcinoid valve disease.[113] The 2D echocardiographic findings are similar to those of rheumatic valve disease, but microscopic examination shows fibrous plaque stuck on relatively normal valve tissue.

Hemochromatosis (see Chap. 64)

Hemochromatosis is characterized by large deposits of iron in various organs including the heart, liver, testes, and pancreas. Cardiac involvement occurs in advanced disease, and the severity of myocardial dysfunction is proportional to the amount of iron deposited in the myocardium. Excessive myocardial iron interferes with myocardial cellular function, causing LV dilatation and systolic dysfunction. Typical 2D echocardiographic findings of cardiac hemochromatosis include mild LV dilatation, LV systolic dysfunction, normal wall thickness, normal heart valves, and biatrial enlargement. Progressive congestive heart failure is the most common cause of death in hemochromatosis.

Hypereosinophilic Syndrome (see Chap. 64)

Hypereosinophilic syndrome is defined as a persistent (>6 months) eosinophilia of more than 1500 eosinophils/mm^3 with evidence of organ involvement. Cardiac involvement in hypereosinophilic syndrome involves thrombotic-fibrotic obliteration of the ventricular apices and endocardial thickening of the inflow areas. The majority of patients (>50 percent) with hypereosinophilia have characteristic echocardiographic findings including limited motion of the posterior mitral leaflet resulting in mitral regurgitation, thickening of the inferobasal LV wall, endocardial thrombotic-fibrotic lesion, and biventricular apical obliteration by thrombus. Myocardial contrast imaging confirms apical thrombus (Fig. 14-94).[157] Ventricular compliance is reduced, and ventricular diastolic filling is limited by apical cavity obliteration and eosinophilic endocardial involvement. Acute hypereosinophilic crisis produces diffuse myocarditis, with ventricular cavity dilatation and marked decrease in systolic function.

Radiation-Induced Cardiac Disease (see Chap. 64)

Radiation to the mediastinum can damage the coronary arteries and cause pericardial effusion, constrictive pericarditis, regurgitant or stenotic valve disease, restrictive cardiomyopathy, or a combination of these. Radiation-induced valve damage causes thickening and regurgitation of any valve, most frequently the tricuspid valve. Constrictive pericarditis or restrictive cardiomyopathy (or both) cause severe symptoms, and radiation-induced constriction has a poor prognosis, even after pericardiectomy.

Renal Failure (see Chap. 88)

The predominant echocardiographic finding in patients with chronic renal failure is increased LV wall thickness related to LV hypertrophy from hypertension. The myocardial texture with LV hypertrophy appears similar to that of cardiac amyloidosis, but these two conditions can be distinguished by the QRS voltage on the electrocardiogram. In the early stage of chronic renal failure, systolic function is normal, but not diastolic function because of decreased myocardial relaxation. As the disease progresses, LV systolic dysfunction occurs with decreased compliance of the myocardium, LV filling pressure increases, and the diastolic filling pattern becomes pseudonormalized or even restrictive. Small pericardial effusions are common, especially in patients undergoing chronic hemodialysis. Valvular sclerosis and mitral annulus and leaflet calcification are also common in chronic renal failure.

Sarcoidosis (see Chap. 64)

Sarcoidosis is a multiorgan granulomatous disease of unknown cause. Pulmonary involvement, resulting in diffuse pulmonary fibrosis, right-sided heart failure, and pulmonary hypertension, is the most common cause of cardiovascular disease. The 2D echocardiographic features of myocardial involvement with sarcoidosis occur in less than 20 percent of sarcoid patients and include a dilated LV with regional wall motion abnormalities, especially at the mid and basal levels of the LV. Characteristically, the wall motion abnormalities do not correspond to a defined coronary distribution.

Sepsis

LV dilatation and decreased LVEF are common in patients with sepsis and septic shock.[158] The cause of myocardial dysfunction may be related to a circulating myocardial depressant, such as an endotoxin, tumor necrosis factor, or interleukin, but this is not completely understood.[159] Echocardiography frequently shows a dilated LV and decreased LVEF. Stroke volume may be maintained (normal LVOT TVI and velocity) or reduced. In patients who survive sepsis, LV dilatation and systolic dysfunction are reversible. Certain infections result in characteristic cardiac and echocardiographic abnormalities: pericarditis in viral, bacterial, or tuberculosis infection; an intracardiac mass in echinococcosis or tuberculosis; and ventricular aneurysm in Chagas disease.

Systemic Lupus Erythematosus (see Chap. 84)

Lupus is a systemic disease that produces immune complexes, which cause inflammation of various organs. Pericarditis is the most common cardiac manifestation and is found in more than two thirds of patients. Thus one of the diagnostic criteria for systemic lupus erythematosus is the detection of pericardial effusion. The myocardium may be involved by vasculitis, resulting in myocarditis, but significant LV diastolic dysfunction is rare. Another characteristic cardiac lesion is that of Libman-Sacks endocarditis.

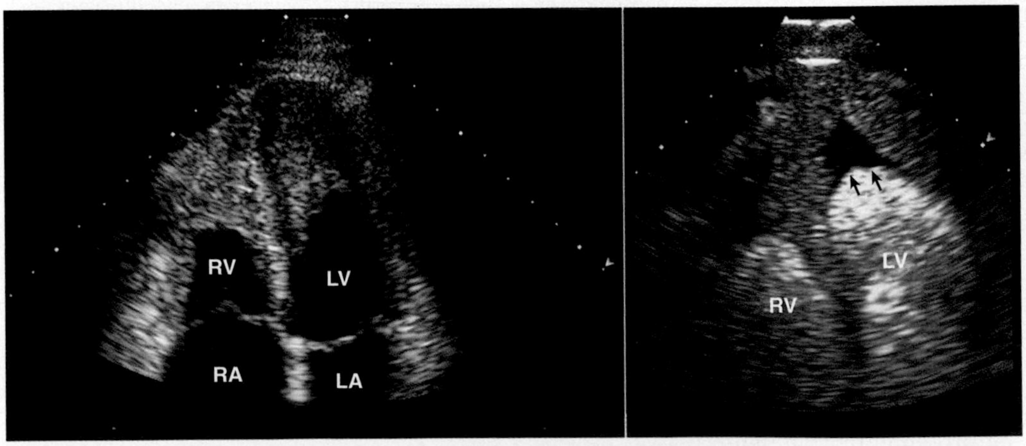

FIGURE 14–94 Apical four-chamber views in a patient with hypereosinophilic syndrome showing apical (both left [LV] and right [RV] ventricular) obliteration caused by deposits of thrombus and eosinophils. **Left,** Obliterative thrombus material is shown only in the apex of the LV. This condition should be differentiated from apical hypertrophic cardiomyopathy, in which the apical cavity is obliterated by hypertrophied myocardium but still with a slitlike cavity inside the hyperdynamic myocardium. **Right,** Myocardial contrast shows black wedge-shaped thrombus (arrows) in the LV apex, which has good perfusion. It is very different from apical hypertrophic cardiomyopathy. LA = left atrium; RA = right atrium. *(From Oh JK, Seward JB, Tajik AJ: The Echo Manual. 3rd ed. Philadelphia, Lippincott Williams & Wilkins, 2006. Used with permission of Mayo Foundation for Medical Education and Research.)*

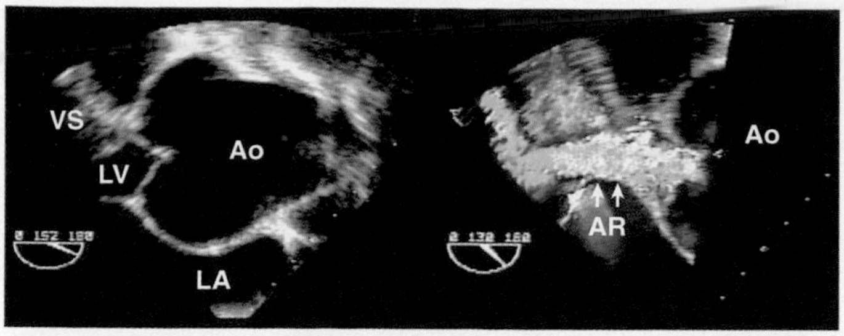

FIGURE 14–95 Multiplane transesophageal view of the aorta in a patient with Marfan syndrome. **Left,** Long-axis view of the aorta (Ao) with a transducer at 130 to 150 degrees showing the dilated sinus of Valsalva. **Right,** Color-flow imaging of severe aortic regurgitation (AR) (arrows). LA = left atrium; LV = left ventricle; VS = ventricular septum. *(From Oh JK, Seward JB, Tajik AJ: The Echo Manual. 3rd ed. Philadelphia, Lippincott Williams & Wilkins, 2006. Used with permission of Mayo Foundation for Medical Education and Research.)*

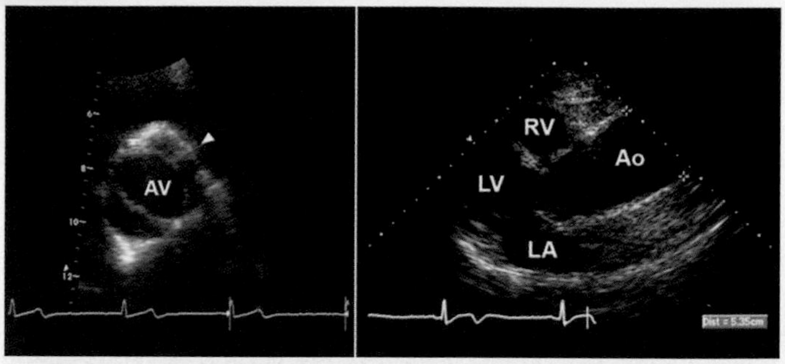

FIGURE 14–96 **Left,** Parasternal short-axis view showing a bicuspid aortic valve with fusion of the left and right cusps (arrowhead). The valve was functionally normal. **Right,** Parasternal long-axis view of marked enlargement of the mid ascending aorta (5.4 cm) in patient with bicuspid aortic valve.

DISEASES OF THE AORTA (see Chap. 56)

Aortic Aneurysm

Aortic aneurysms occur frequently and, in the elderly population, are usually related to hypertension or atherosclerosis. Aneurysms also are found in patients with congenital aortic valve disease, Marfan syndrome, familial aortic aneurysmal disease, or annuloaortic ectasia. Generally, aortic dilatation is easily detected with TTE and TEE. When the ascending aneurysm reaches a diameter greater than 5 cm, there is increased risk of rupture, and replacement is generally indicated.[160,161] Smaller aneurysms require serial follow-up studies to measure the aorta at specific locations.

Marfan syndrome is the most common inherited connective tissue disease, and cardiovascular complications occur in the majority of patients. Aortic root dilatation, aortic regurgitation (Fig. 14-95), and aortic dissection are the most common cardiovascular findings, and the ones of most concern. Prophylactic beta-blockade has been demonstrated to be effective in slowing the rate of aortic dilatation and reducing the development of aortic complications. A recent study demonstrated that the angiotensin receptor blocker losartan has an important effect on vascular development in the mouse model of Marfan syndrome.[162] These data have not been confirmed in humans who have Marfan syndrome or other aortic disorders but are being evaluated.

BICUSPID AORTIC VALVE AND AORTOPATHY (see Chap. 62)

More than 50 percent of young patients with normally functioning bicuspid aortic valve disease have echocardiographic evidence of aortic root dilation. A bicuspid aortic valve is an independent risk factor for progressive aortic dilation, aneurysm formation, and dissection. The vascular complications of bicuspid aortic valve disease are not secondary to valvular dysfunction and may be noted in young adults without pronounced aortic valve disease or in patients in whom the native bicuspid aortic valve was replaced by a prosthesis. Bicuspid aortic valve is associated with accelerated degeneration of the aortic media, indicating that the disease is an ongoing pathological process rather than a discrete developmental event. These lesions are similar to those of the aorta in patients with Marfan syndrome. Aortic dilation should be monitored carefully with echocardiography. The region of maximal dilatation usually involves the mid ascending aorta (Fig. 14-96) but may also involve the aortic sinuses. Comprehensive evaluation and monitoring with TTE is feasible in most patients. If these images are limited, alternative imaging should include TEE, CT, or CMR. Aortic root replacement is recommended for patients with a bicuspid aortic valve whose aortic root size is greater than or equal to 5 cm. Aortic valve preservation with a supracoronary graft or repair in combination with a valve-sparing root replacement can be performed successfully in young patients who have normally functioning bicuspid valves or aortic valve regurgitation and aortic dilation, respectively.[163] The benefit of beta blockers or losartan to prevent aortic dilation in bicuspid aortic valve patients is not clear; however, hypertension should be monitored carefully and controlled.

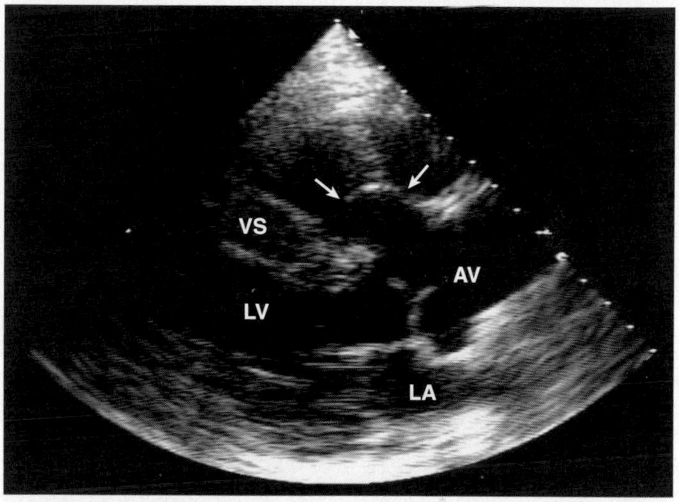

FIGURE 14–97 Transthoracic parasternal long-axis view of aneurysm (arrows) of the sinus of Valsalva. AV = aortic valve; LA = left atrium; LV = left ventricle; VS = ventricular septum. *(From Meier JH, Seward JB, Miller FA Jr, et al: Aneurysms in the left ventricular outflow tract: Clinical presentation, causes, and echocardiographic features. J Am Soc Echocardiogr 11:729, 1998. Used with permission.)*

ANEURYSM OF THE SINUS OF VALSALVA

The localized absence of the media in the aortic wall results in aneurysm of the sinus of Valsalva. It may be an incidental finding. The aneurysm can rupture into the adjacent cardiac chambers, most commonly the RA or RV, or into the ventricular septum (Fig. 14-97) or compress adjacent structures.[164] The parasternal and apical long-axis views are helpful in distinguishing this from an aneurysm of a membranous ventricular septum. A sinus of Valsalva aneurysm is located on the aortic side of the aortic valve, whereas an aneurysm of the membranous septum is located on the ventricular side of the aortic valve. These aneurysms can be distinguished confidently with comprehensive TTE and TEE examinations.[164] The natural history of sinus of Valsalva aneurysm has not been fully delineated, but it has been associated with an increased incidence of endocarditis, potentially fatal rupture, embolic events, and fistulous communication with a cardiac chamber. Surgical repair is recommended when the aneurysm is associated with rupture because of the recognized complication associated with the chronic left-to-right shunt. Repair of an unruptured sinus of Valsalva aneurysm is individualized.[164]

Atherosclerosis and Aortic Debris

On a routine TEE examination, atherosclerotic plaques and debris are common findings in elderly patients. Aortic plaques usually are irregularly shaped and frequently mobile (Fig. 14-98). As part of the Stroke Prevention Assessment of Risk in a Community (SPARC) study, TEE was performed in an asymptomatic population.[165] In this study, age,

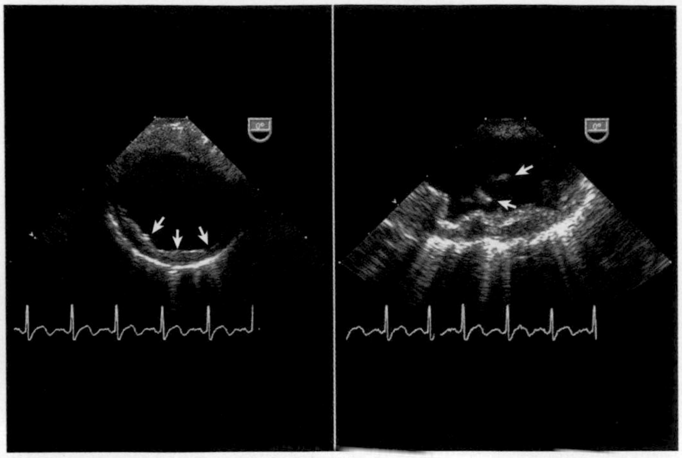

FIGURE 14–98 Transesophageal short-axis image of aortic debris in the descending thoracic aorta (**left,** arrows) and arch **(right)** with mobile irregular masses (in real time) (arrows). This appearance is typical of an atherosclerotic plaque in the aorta.

smoking history, and systolic blood pressure were independently associated with aortic atherosclerosis and aortic debris was common in patients who had had an embolic event. Ulcerated plaques in the aortic arch were studied in patients who had a stroke, and they were present in 26 percent of 239 patients who had a cerebrovascular accident but in only 5 percent of the 261 patients without neurological disease. Preliminary data suggest that chronic anticoagulation with warfarin may be beneficial in patients with atheromatous plaque to decrease embolic events, and surgical removal is indicated if embolism recurs during anticoagulation.

AORTIC DISSECTION, INTRAMURAL HEMATOMA, AND AORTIC ULCER

Although most patients with aortic dissection have a dilated aorta on 2D echocardiography, an intimal flap is often difficult to see on TTE (Fig. 14-99). Another limitation of TTE is the inability to visualize the descending thoracic aorta. Therefore TTE is a rapid screening tool for aortic dissection, but negative findings or a suboptimal examination requires further diagnostic evaluation.

A good initial imaging modality for visualizing proximal aortic dissection is TEE. With TEE, the entire thoracic aorta can be visualized because of the intimate anatomic relation between the esophagus and thoracic aorta. In a horizontal transesophageal view, the distal portion of the ascending aorta and the proximal portion of the transverse aorta may not be well visualized because of the interposed trachea. However, this blind area on the horizontal plane can be visualized with the longitudinal view. With a clearer and more complete view of the entire aorta, TEE has changed the role of echocardiography in the diagnosis

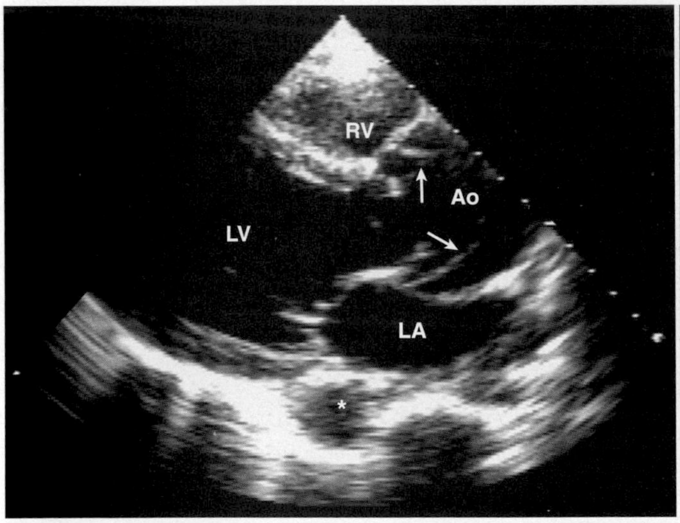

A

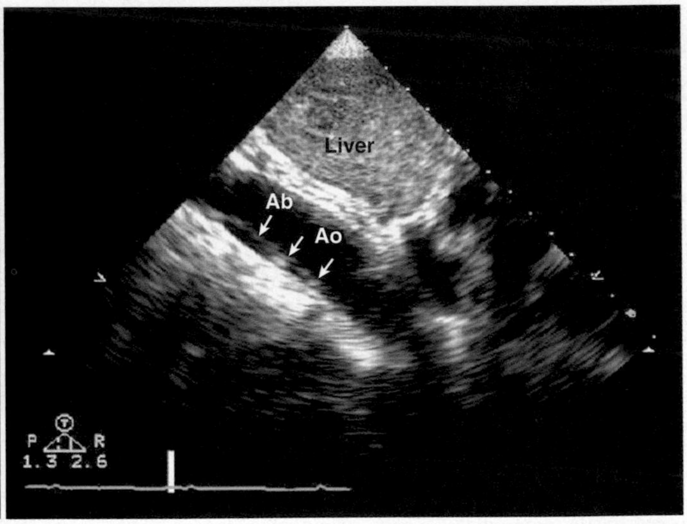

C

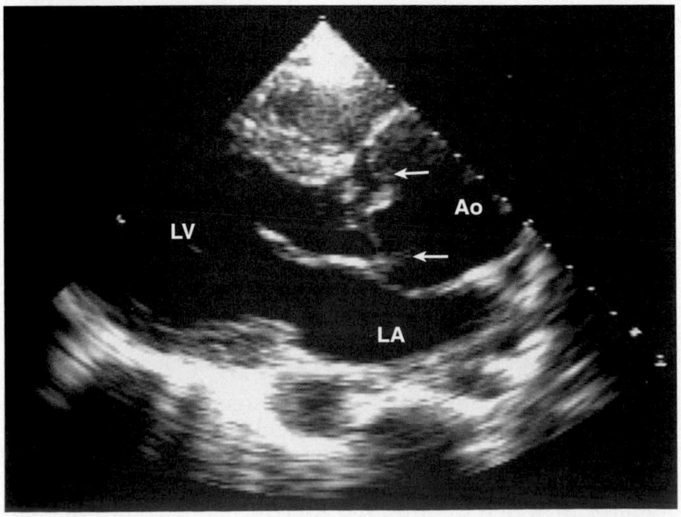

B

FIGURE 14–99 **A,** Transthoracic parasternal long-axis view showing a dilated ascending aorta and an undulating intimal flap in proximal aortic dissection. Systolic frame shows an intimal flap (arrows) in the aorta (Ao), which is dilated. * = Descending thoracic aorta, which is not dilated. **B,** Diastolic frame shows movement of the flap (arrows) toward the aortic valve. **C,** Abdominal aorta (Ab Ao) from the subcostal view also shows an intimal flap (arrows). LA = left atrium; LV = left ventricle; RV = right ventricle. *(From Oh JK, Seward JB, Tajik AJ: The Echo Manual. 3rd ed. Philadelphia, Lippincott Williams & Wilkins, 2006. Used with permission of Mayo Foundation for Medical Education and Research.)*

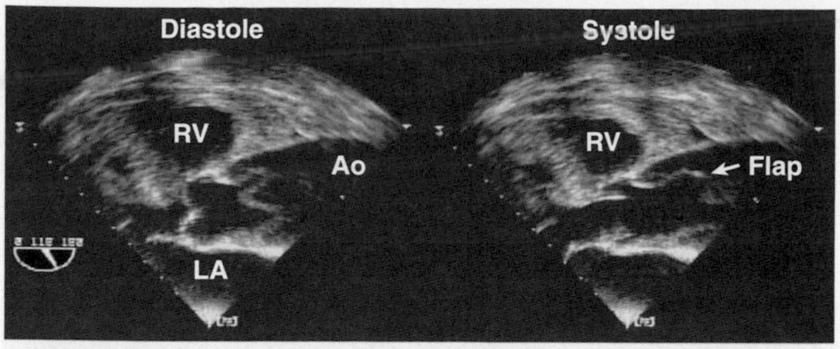

FIGURE 14–100 Transesophageal echocardiography was performed because of bloody pericardial effusion. Long-axis diastolic (left) and systolic (right) views of the ascending aorta (Ao) (141 degrees) shows dilated ascending aorta with an intimal flap. LA = left atrium; RV = right ventricle. *(From Oh JK, Seward JB, Tajik AJ: The Echo Manual. 3rd ed. Philadelphia, Lippincott Williams & Wilkins, 2006. Used with permission of Mayo Foundation for Medical Education and Research.)*

and management of aortic dissection (Fig. 14-100) (see Chap. 56).[1] The International Registry of Acute Aortic Dissection (IRAD) has reported imaging modalities used for diagnosis of aortic dissection. From an initial 13 international medical centers, 628 patients with acute aortic dissection were reviewed.[166] CT and TEE were the most common initial imaging tests for the diagnosis of aortic dissection.

The multicenter European Cooperative Study Group of Echocardiography was the first to demonstrate that TEE was equal to or even superior to CT and aortography for the diagnosis of aortic dissection (sensitivity, 99 percent). Subsequent studies validated the highly accurate diagnostic capability of TEE in aortic dissection. As TEE became more widespread in clinical use, its diagnostic sensitivity became slightly less (88 percent) in the IRAD, compared with the 93 percent sensitivity of CT.[166] Currently, TEE or CT with contrast agent is the initial diagnostic procedure of choice for suspected aortic dissection. Although the diagnostic accuracy of CMR was reported by a small number of studies to be excellent, its clinical role is limited by the longer examination time, difficulties with monitoring patients during the procedure, and the remote location of the imaging facility from the emergency department.[166]

Intramural hematoma is a precursor of aortic dissection. It is often associated with hypertension and advanced age. From 15 to 20 percent of patients with aortic dissection may present with intramural hematoma. It has been found to progress to aortic dissection or rupture in up to 45 percent.[167] Intramural hematoma has been reported to regress completely in 34 percent of patients, progress to aortic dissection in 12 percent, aneurysm in 20 percent, and evolve to pseudoaneurysm in 24 percent.[168] Intramural hematoma, best visualized on TEE, appears as increased echodensity along the wall of the aorta, corresponding to thrombus formation between the intima and the adventitia (Fig. 14-101). This should be differentiated from atheromatous plaque in the aorta, or aortitis. Intramural hematoma is also easily identified on CT and CMR. Aortography is the least valuable diagnostic modality for detecting intramural hematoma.

Penetrating atherosclerotic aortic ulcer describes the condition in which ulceration of an aortic atherosclerotic lesion penetrates the internal elastic lamina into the media. This lesion may result in intramural hematoma, aortic dissection, or aortic rupture and should be suspected in a hypertensive patient presenting with chest or back pain similar to that of aortic dissection. The ulcer is usually located in the descending aorta. With TEE, the penetrating aortic ulcer has a crater-like or focal outpouching appearance in an atherosclerotic aortic wall.

Aortic Rupture and Pseudoaneurysm

(see Chap. 71)

Aortic rupture is a complication of deceleration injury caused by a motor vehicle accident, and survival depends on prompt diagnosis and surgical treatment. Because TEE is able to visualize the entire thoracic aorta, it is an excellent diagnostic procedure for patients with suspected rupture of the thoracic aorta. Aortography, CT, or CMR may also be used to diagnose aortic rupture.

Pseudoaneurysm results from a tear in the aortic wall, with leakage of blood from the aorta into a contained aneurysmal cavity. This can be caused by trauma, previous operation, or infection. Pseudoaneurysm has a different appearance from true aneurysm, with a sharply demarcated rupture site where communication occurs between the aorta and the pseudoaneurysm (see Fig. e20 on website). Repair is usually recommended because of the risk of rupture.

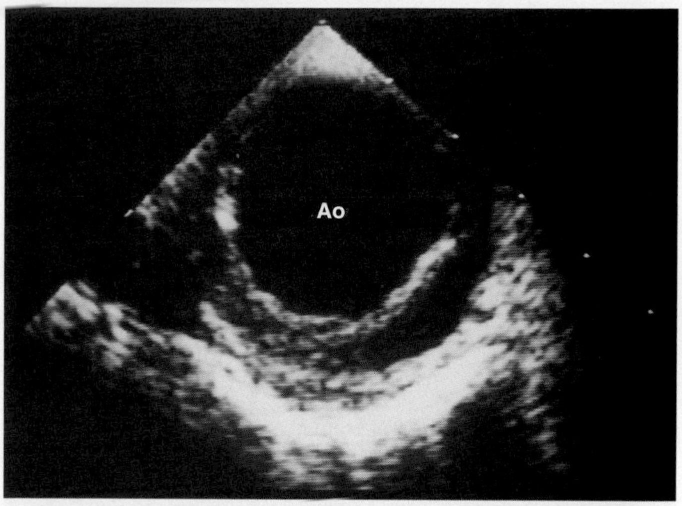

A

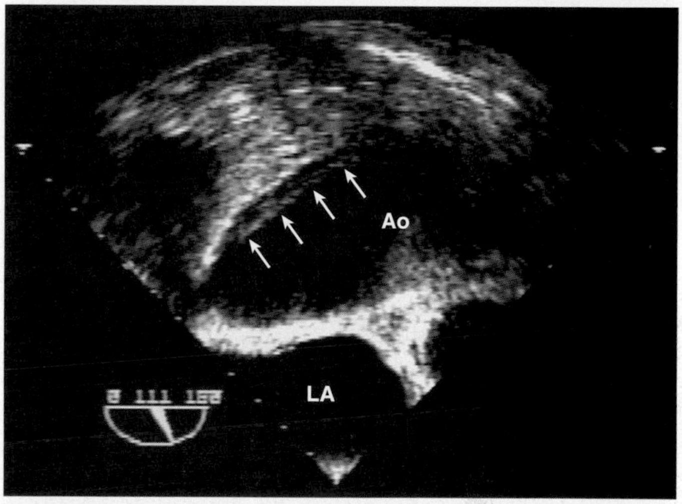

B

FIGURE 14–101 A, Transverse transesophageal view of the descending thoracic aorta (Ao) showing an intramural hematoma in a patient with hypertension and severe back pain. The soft-tissue mass with a smooth surface appears different from aortic debris. During the next 6 months, the intramural hematoma disappeared while the patient was taking antihypertensive medications, including a beta blocker. **B,** Long-axis transesophageal view showing intramural hematoma in the ascending aorta (arrows). LA = left atrium. *(From Oh JK, Seward JB, Tajik AJ: The Echo Manual. 3rd ed. Philadelphia, Lippincott Williams & Wilkins, 2006. Used with permission of Mayo Foundation for Medical Education and Research.)*

Aortitis (see Chap. 84)

Aortitis is an inflammation of the aortic wall caused by infection (syphilitic or mycotic), giant cell arteritis, Takayasu disease, ankylosing spondylitis, rheumatoid arthritis, or relapsing polychondritis. Aortic involvement is usually an expression of the systemic nature of the underlying disease. Aortic wall thickness is increased, making it difficult to differentiate the TEE findings from those of intramural hematoma (Fig. 14-102). Thoracic or abdominal aortic narrowing with obstruction may occur in patients with Takayasu disease. Syphilitic aortitis is uncommon but characteristically affects the ascending aorta.

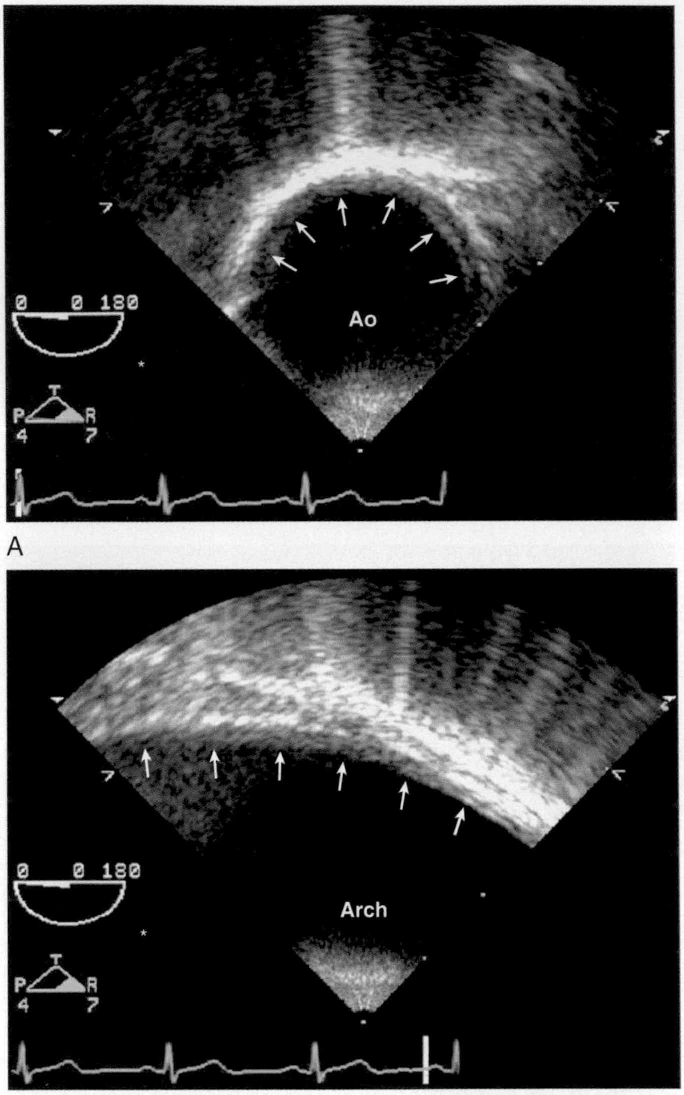

FIGURE 14–102 Transesophageal images from a patient with giant cell arteritis who presented with fever of unknown origin, erythrocyte sedimentation rate of 102 mm/1 hr, and jaw claudication. Descending thoracic aorta (Ao) **(A)** and arch **(B)** view showed increased thickness of the intima (arrows), which has an appearance similar to that of intramural hematoma. *(From Oh JK, Seward JB, Tajik AJ: The Echo Manual. 3rd ed. Philadelphia, Lippincott Williams & Wilkins, 2006. Used with permission of Mayo Foundation for Medical Education and Research.)*

Ankylosing spondylitis is characterized by aortic root thickening and dilatation. Aortic valve nodularity and aortic root enlargement cause progressive aortic valve regurgitation that may require valve replacement. Aortic regurgitation with dilatation of the aorta is also seen in patients with Reiter syndrome, psoriatic arthritis, and Behçet syndrome.[169]

CARDIAC TUMORS AND MASSES
(see Chap. 69)

Cardiac masses can be caused by tumor, thrombus, vegetation, iatrogenic material, normal variant, or extracardiac structure. The size, shape, location, mobility, and attachment site of a cardiac mass, as well as the clinical presentation, usually help in diagnostic differentiation. Accurate diagnosis is crucial and misinterpretation may result in incorrect management, including an unnecessary surgical procedure.

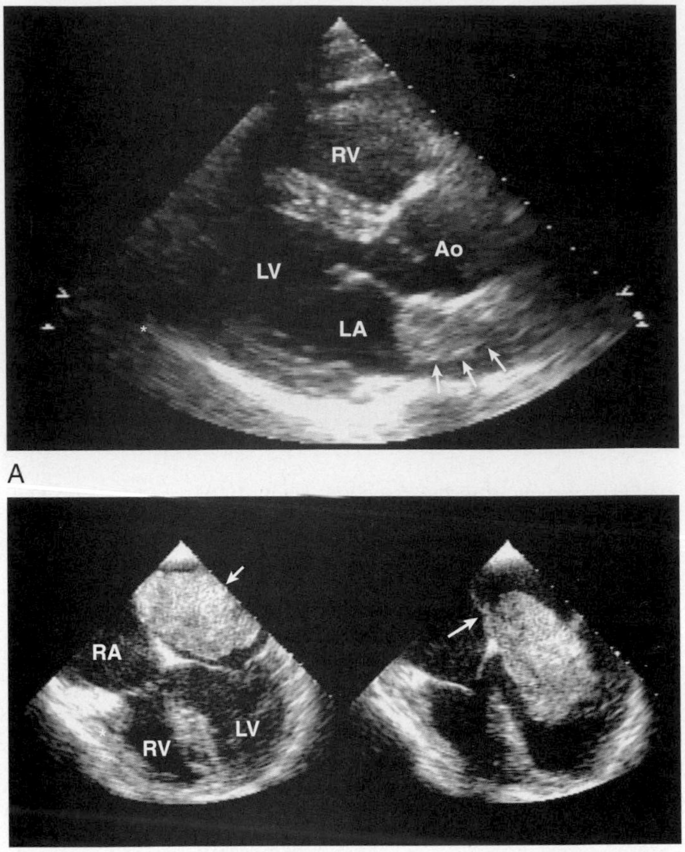

FIGURE 14–103 **A,** Left atrial (LA) myxoma (arrows) recorded from the parasternal long-axis position. The myxoma appears attached to the posterior wall of the aorta (Ao), although its attachment site is actually atrial septum. **B,** Systolic **(left)** and diastolic **(right)** frames of transesophageal view of a large LA myxoma (left arrow) attached to the atrial septum (right arrow). LV = left ventricle; RA = right atrium; RV = right ventricle. *(From Oh JK, Seward JB, Tajik AJ: The Echo Manual. 3rd ed. Philadelphia, Lippincott Williams & Wilkins, 2006. Used with permission of Mayo Foundation for Medical Education and Research.)*

Myxoma

Myxomas originate from multipotential mesenchymal cells of the endocardium. Cardiac myxomas are the most common primary cardiac tumor in adults, representing up to 83 percent of all primary tumors of the heart. Myxomas usually occur between the third and sixth decades of life and show a 2 : 1 female predominance. The majority of myxomas occur in the LA, with attachment to the atrial septum (83 to 88 percent), but they have been identified in all other chambers and also attached to cardiac valves. Myxomas usually have a typical echocardiographic appearance characterized by a gelatinous and friable mass and, occasionally, central necrosis (Fig. 14-103). Up to 7 percent of myxoma cases are familial, with the most notable condition being Carney syndrome, an autosomal dominant complex of cutaneous findings including lentigines, ephelides, and blue nevi; cardiac myxomas, classically occurring at age younger than 40 years, with an atypical location, and often multiple; and endocrine abnormalities. This syndrome is caused by a gene defect on the long arm of chromosome 17. Although sporadic atrial myxomas usually are highly amenable to curative surgical resection, familial lesions frequently recur, often at locations distant from the initial site of resection.

Complications associated with myxoma include embolic events occurring primarily with small myxomas; obstruc-

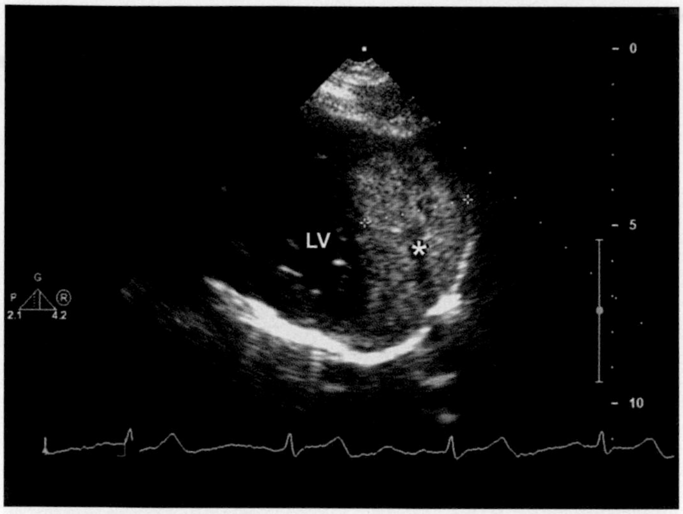

FIGURE 14-104 Parasternal short-axis view of a left ventricular (LV) fibroma (*). It is large and well circumscribed in the posterior free wall. It may cause ventricular arrhythmia but does not produce any hemodynamic abnormality. Surgical removal was successful despite tumor size.

tion to inflow or outflow; systemic illness; and, rarely, metastases.

Fibroma

Fibromas are usually located in the LV free wall, the ventricular septum, or at the apex. It is well demarcated from the surrounding myocardium by multiple calcifications (Fig. 14-104). Fibromas can grow into the LV cavity and interfere with ventricular filling or cause malignant arrhythmias. Also, fibromas can cause congestive heart failure. When located at the apex, a fibroma may be misinterpreted by other imaging modalities as apical hypertrophic cardiomyopathy.

Rhabdomyoma

Rhabdomyoma is the most common cardiac tumor in children, particularly in those with tuberous sclerosis, and can be diagnosed before birth with fetal echocardiography. Rhabdomyomas are often multiple and present in the RV, RVOT, or the pulmonary artery (see Fig. 14-e21 on website), but they often regress spontaneously after birth.

Papillary Fibroelastoma

Papillary fibroelastoma, or papilloma, is a benign intracardiac tumor with a characteristic appearance on echocardiograms. It is usually small (average size, <15 mm) and has a characteristic stippled edge, with a shimmering appearance at the tumor-blood interface. There are fingerlike projections consistent with the fronds that are described pathologically as a "sea anemone." The most frequent location is the aortic valve on either the aortic or ventricular surface (Fig. 14-105), followed by either the atrial or ventricular surface of the mitral valve. Papillomas can be found in any chamber or on any surface and are usually single, but multiple tumors occur in approximately 10 percent of patients. Papillary fibroelastoma can cause embolus and is a potential cause of stroke when located in the left cardiac chambers.[170]

Pheochromocytoma

Primary cardiac pheochromocytomas are rare. They are usually located along the atrioventricular groove, are well circumscribed and ovoid, and range from 1.5 to 5 cm in diameter.[171] Both TTE and TEE demonstrate this tumor well (Fig. 14-106).

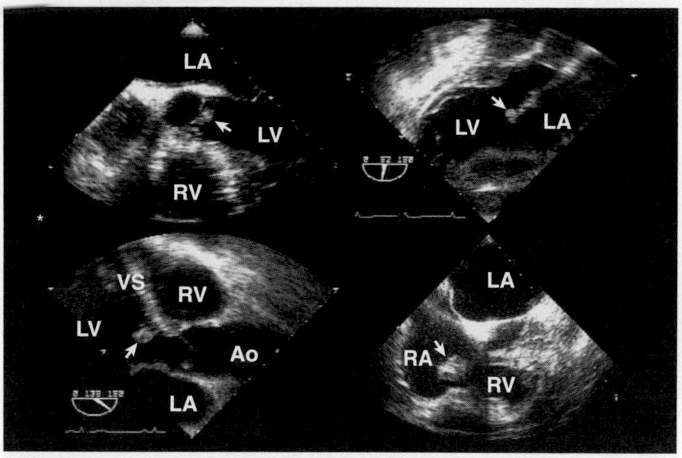

FIGURE 14-105 Transesophageal echocardiographic examples of aortic valve **(upper left)**, mitral valve **(upper right)**, left ventricular outflow tract **(lower left)**, and tricuspid valve **(lower right)** papillary fibroelastomas (arrows). These tumors were not detected with transthoracic echocardiography. Ao = aorta; LA = left atrium; LV = left ventricle; RA = right atrium; RV = right ventricle; VS = ventricular septum. *(From Oh JK, Seward JB, Tajik AJ: The Echo Manual. 3rd ed. Philadelphia, Lippincott Williams & Wilkins, 2006. Used with permission.)*

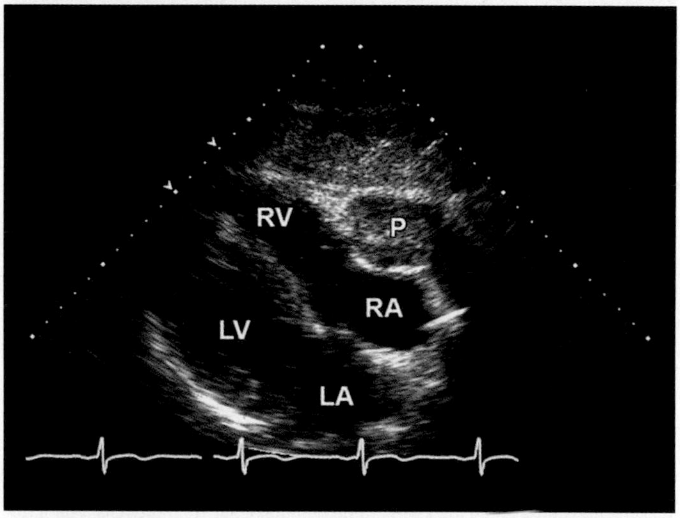

FIGURE 14-106 Subcostal transthoracic image of a tumor (P) in the right atrioventricular groove. The patient had a history of severe hypertension, and laboratory findings were consistent with pheochromocytoma. Pathology study confirmed cardiac pheochromocytoma. LA = left atrium; LV = left ventricle; RA = right atrium; RV = right ventricle.

Malignant Tumors of the Heart

Malignant primary cardiac tumors are uncommon and generally have a poor prognosis. These tumors are angiosarcoma, rhabdomyosarcoma, myxosarcoma, osteosarcoma, fibrosarcoma, and synovial sarcoma. Angiosarcoma usually occurs in the RA and is commonly associated with pericardial effusion. Rhabdomyosarcoma and fibrosarcoma can occur anywhere in the heart. Synovial sarcoma is rare and usually occurs in the RA.

Metastatic malignant tumors are more common than primary tumors to the heart. Most frequently, they are from the lung, breast, kidney, liver, lymphoma, melanoma, and osteogenic sarcoma. Whenever an RA mass is detected, the inferior vena cava should be carefully scanned because

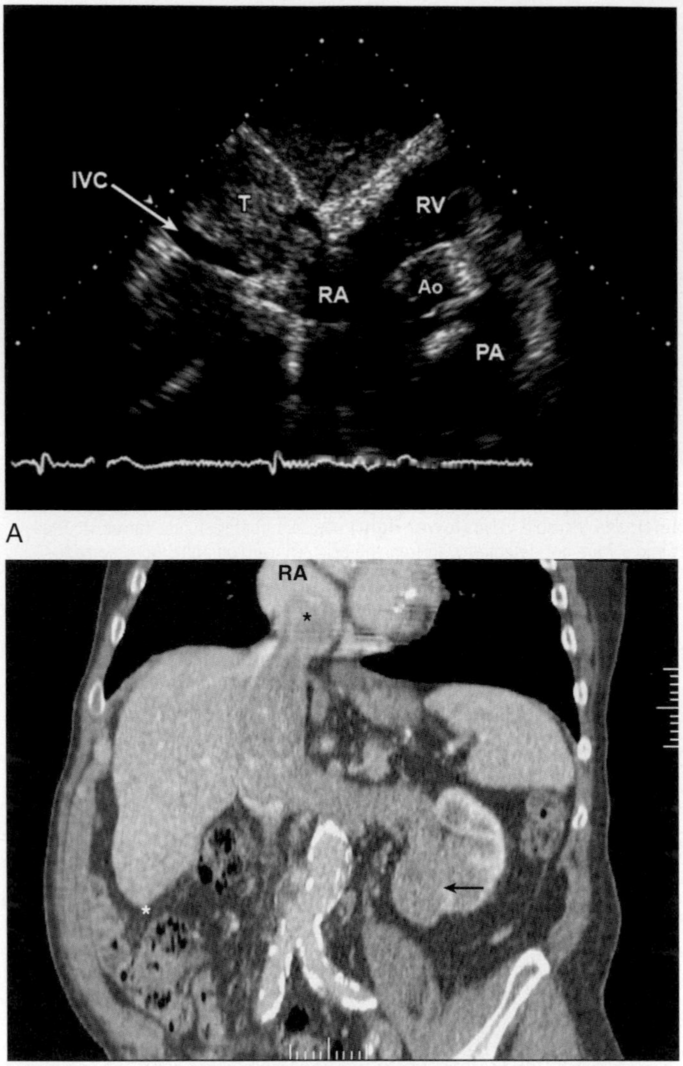

FIGURE 14–107 **A,** Subcostal transthoracic image of a tumor (T) in the inferior vena cava (IVC) extending to the level of the right atrium (RA). Ao = aorta; PA = pulmonary artery; RV = right ventricle. **B,** Computed tomography confirmed that the mass arises from the kidney (arrow) and extends from the renal vein into the inferior vena cava and presents as a mass in the right atrium (RA)(*). The tumor is a hypernephroma. The patient underwent nephrectomy and removal of the mass from the inferior vena cava and RA.

hypernephroma, hepatoma, and intravenous leiomyomatosis from the uterus tend to metastasize to the inferior vena cava and RA (Fig. 14-107).

OTHER MASSES

Lipomatous atrial septal hypertrophy can be misinterpreted as a cardiac tumor (Fig. 14-108). The RA often harbors structures that appear as a mass on 2D echocardiography; these include the eustachian valve, pacemaker wire or central-line catheter infection, cyst, and thrombus. Infection and abscess in the heart can present as a mass. Echinococcal cyst, tuberculoma, or vegetations attached to the ventricular free wall or intracardiac catheter are also examples. Thrombi from the deep veins must go through the RA and RV to cause pulmonary embolism. They are mobile, have a characteristic snakelike appearance, and usually are associated with pulmonary embolism (Fig. 14-109). Occasionally, an RA thrombus is identified passing through a patent foramen ovale, and this may cause a paradoxical embolus (see Fig. 14-109). A similar mobile structure may be seen in patients with intravenous leiomyomatosis.[172]

Left atrial thrombus is most common in patients with atrial fibrillation or mitral stenosis. TEE should be used when thrombus is suspected in the LA or LA appendage (Fig. 14-110). Ventricular thrombus is differentiated from a tumor because the former is associated with abnormal regional wall motion, except apical thrombus noted in hypereosinophilic syndrome and, occasionally, in lymphoma. Contrast echocardiography can be helpful in differentiating an apical mass or thrombus. Thrombus is visualized as a dark structure on contrast echocardiography because it is not vascular.

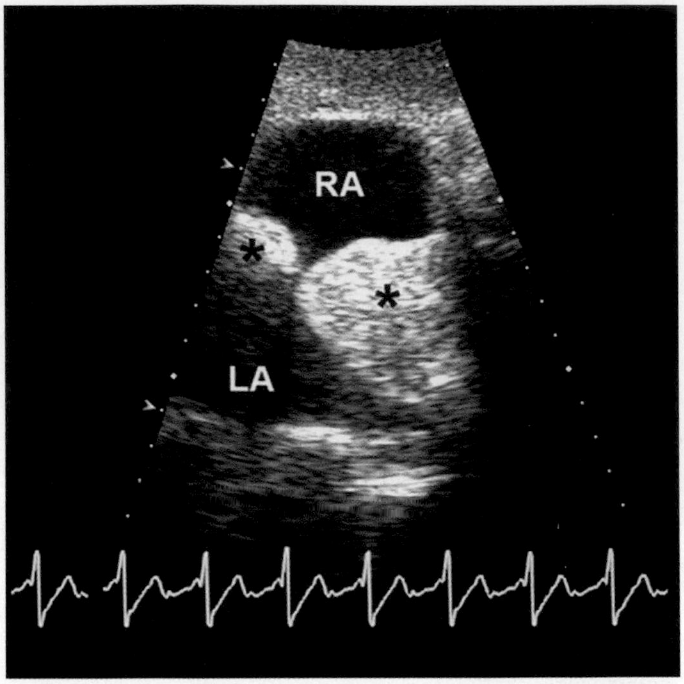

FIGURE 14–108 Subcostal long-axis view showing lipomatous hypertrophy (*) involving the atrial septum. This is occasionally misinterpreted as a tumor or indeterminate mass. The characteristic features include sparing of the fossa ovalis membrane, resulting in a so-called dumbbell appearance. LA = left atrium; RA = right atrium.

ECHOCARDIOGRAPHY IN ATRIAL FIBRILLATION (see Chap. 35)

Atrial fibrillation is the most common sustained cardiac rhythm disturbance, and it is increasing in frequency. It causes substantial cardiovascular morbidity and mortality. Echocardiography has an important role in the evaluation of patients with atrial fibrillation and in making management decisions. During the initial evaluation, TTE is usually performed to screen for occult cardiovascular disease that may precipitate atrial fibrillation, and it provides information that will alter the approach to therapy. Systemic thromboembolism is a potentially catastrophic complication of atrial fibrillation. The risk of thromboembolism is substantially reduced by anticoagulation, but because of the potential hazards of anticoagulation, risk-stratifying patients to determine who will benefit most from anticoagulation is appropriate. Information acquired with TTE can assist with the decision about anticoagulation in patients with atrial fibrillation.

Prospective data from large population-based studies have established a relationship between LA diameter and the risk of developing atrial fibrillation. Recently, it was reported that LA volume is a superior measure to LA diameter for predicting outcomes including atrial fibrillation[173] and provided prognostic information that was incremental to clinical risk factors.

TEE is frequently performed in patients with atrial fibrillation (see Chap. 35). The primary purpose of TEE is to detect LA appendage thrombi (see Fig. 14-110) and to iden-

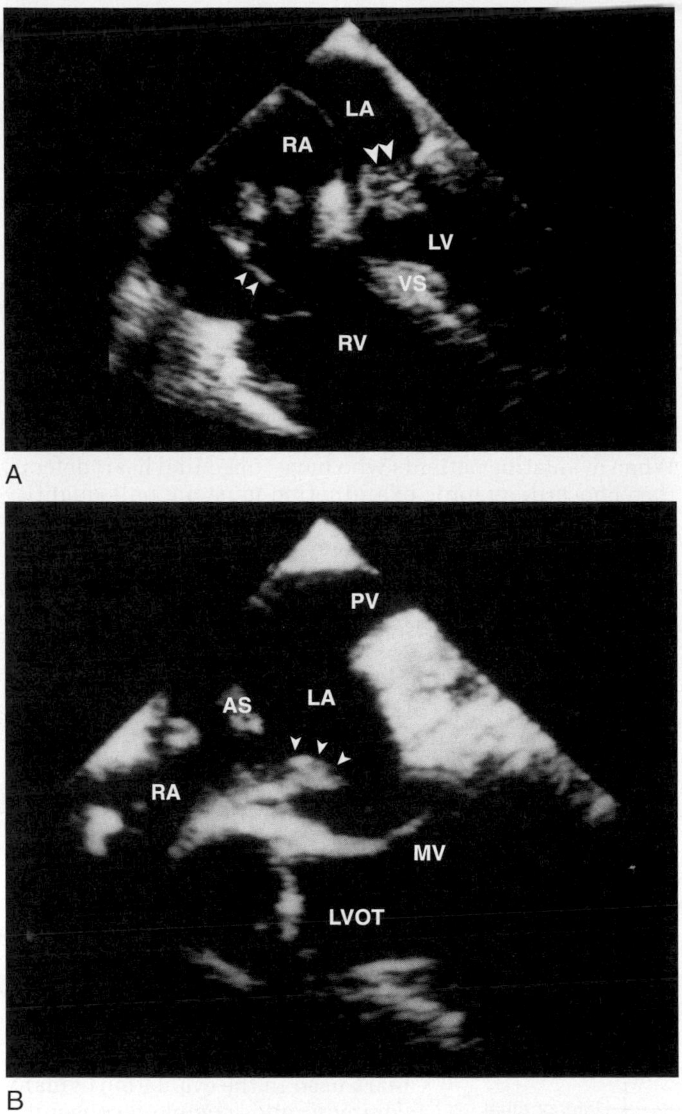

FIGURE 14–109 **A,** Transverse transesophageal view showing biatrial thrombi (large arrowheads) in a patient with dyspnea and cold left foot caused by a peripheral embolic event. Small arrowheads, a pacemaker wire. The atrial septum bulges toward the left atrium (LA) because of increased right atrial (RA) pressure caused by pulmonary embolism. The RA and right ventricle (RV) are dilated. LV = left ventricle; VS = ventricular septum. **B,** Basal transverse transesophageal view in the same patient showing thrombus (arrowheads) traversing the patent foramen ovale. This is a typical example of paradoxical embolism. This patient had undergone hip surgery 1 month before this echocardiography examination, and deep venous thrombosis, pulmonary embolism, and paradoxical embolism developed. AS = atrial septum; LVOT = LV outflow tract; MV = mitral valve; PV = pulmonary vein. *(From Oh JK, Seward JB, Tajik AJ: The Echo Manual. 3rd ed. Philadelphia, Lippincott Williams & Wilkins, 2006. Used with permission of Mayo Foundation for Medical Education and Research.)*

tify patients at increased risk for cardiogenic embolism. Patients at moderate risk for both stroke and hemorrhagic complications with anticoagulation may benefit from risk stratification with TEE. Compared with TTE, TEE provides a superior assessment of the LA appendage in most patients. The LA appendage is a multilobed muscular extension of the LA, and meticulous imaging in several planes is essential because of the complexity of the structure and its anatomical variability. Common artifacts include prominent trabeculations, duplication artifacts, and adipose tissue within the transverse sinus. It is also important to image the RA appendage in patients with atrial fibrillation.

In sinus rhythm the LA appendage is protected from thrombus formation by high-velocity blood flow. Function

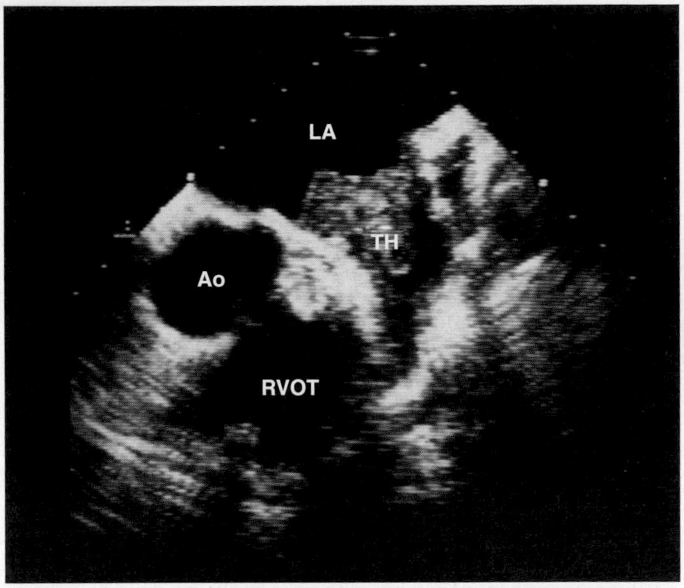

FIGURE 14–110 Transverse transesophageal view of the left atrium (LA) and its appendage with thrombus (TH) in a patient with atrial fibrillation. Ao = aorta; RVOT = right ventricular outflow tract. *(From Oh JK, Seward JB, Tajik AJ: The Echo Manual. 3rd ed. Philadelphia, Lippincott Williams & Wilkins, 2006. Used with permission of Mayo Foundation for Medical Education and Research.)*

of the LA appendage can be assessed with pulsed wave Doppler interrogation of the chamber (see Fig. 14-e22 on website) during TEE. In patients in sinus rhythm, the appendage contracts once per cardiac cycle, and flow velocities have a biphasic pattern, with peak velocities generally exceeding 40 cm/sec. Patients with atrial fibrillation have lower flow velocities. An LA appendage peak flow velocity <20 cm/sec is independently associated with increased risk of thromboembolic events.

Spontaneous echo contrast is commonly identified with TEE in patients with atrial fibrillation. The smoke-like echo reflections are likely produced by backscatter from red cell aggregates at low flow rates, and they are a marker of stasis and a prothrombotic environment. Variables that have been associated with the presence of spontaneous echo contrast include age, fibrinogen levels, hematocrit, LA appendage velocity, and atherosclerotic aortic plaque. In retrospective studies, dense spontaneous echo contrast has been associated with increased thromboembolic risk.

TRANSESOPHAGEAL ECHOCARDIOGRAPHY-GUIDED CARDIOVERSION

A strategy of TEE to exclude LA thrombus, followed immediately by cardioversion, has been shown to be an efficient means of restoring sinus rhythm without requiring long-term precardioversion anticoagulation (see Chap. 35). Although TEE-guided cardioversion has been found to be a safe alternative to the standard approach of 3 to 4 weeks of anticoagulation followed by cardioversion, it has not been shown to result in a higher success rate for either initial conversion to sinus rhythm or maintenance of sinus rhythm at 1 year. Evidence suggests that the risk of stroke might be reduced by incorporating TEE into the treatment algorithm, compared with standard anticoagulation management. In an observational study, thrombus was discovered in 7.7 percent of patients and dense spontaneous echo contrast was observed in 10 percent despite therapeutic anticoagulation levels before TEE.[174] All patients should receive anticoagulation after cardioversion for 6 weeks to 6 months because of atrial stunning and the likelihood of new thrombus formation. Stunning appears to occur regardless of the method used for cardioversion. Echocardiographic studies have demonstrated that the timing of this recovery appears to depend on the duration of atrial fibrillation before cardioversion and may take as long as 1 month.

TEE-facilitated cardioversion has several theoretical advantages over the conventional strategy. First, in patients with no thrombus identified on TEE, the total duration of anticoagulation can be reduced. In addition, accelerated cardioversion with a TEE-guided approach may prevent the remodeling that is believed to perpetuate atrial fibrillation. Second, a TEE-based strategy could lower total costs by limiting laboratory tests, reducing preprocedural bleeding events, and improving clinical outcomes. Third, adherence to the traditional guidelines can often be difficult for patient and physician.

The TEE study, ACUTE, a multicenter prospective randomized study, showed that TEE-guided cardioversion is a safe alternative to conventional anticoagulant therapy in patients with atrial fibrillation. However, controversy persists about whether TEE-guided therapy is superior to the conventional strategy, and there is concern that accelerated cardioversion might be harmful, with increased mortality. The incidence of spontaneous cardioversion in the conservative arm was double that in the TEE-facilitated group. With use of either strategy, extremely low stroke rates make it difficult to justify extending the TEE-guided strategy to all patients with planned cardioversion. In the majority of patients with atrial fibrillation, long-term anticoagulant therapy may be recommended, regardless of rhythm status, based on the results of the AFFIRM trial. Thus the minimal reduction in bleeding events provided by the TEE-guided algorithm may become insignificant.[175] Still, TEE-guided cardioversion should be strongly considered in certain subgroups of patients with atrial fibrillation, including those with hemodynamic compromise caused by poor rate control, those with persistent symptoms, and those at high risk of hemorrhage with outpatient anticoagulation therapy, keeping in mind that postcardioversion anticoagulation is still necessary.

Various catheter-based and surgical procedures are performed for atrial fibrillation including ablation and catheter obliteration of the LA appendage (see Chap. 35). Preprocedural TEE is routinely requested to exclude the presence of atrial thrombus and, for catheter ablation, to assess pulmonary vein anatomy. During either procedure, TEE or intracardiac echocardiography is usually performed to help guide therapy. Postprocedural TEE imaging is often performed to reassess the pulmonary veins for stenosis related to the catheter-based procedure. Intraoperative TEE and postoperative TTE are commonly performed in patients who have had the surgical Maze procedure.

CONGENITAL HEART DISEASE (see Chap. 61)

Echocardiography has markedly changed the evaluation, diagnosis, and management of patients with congenital heart disease. Congenital heart defects are the most common birth defects, occurring in about 1 percent of live births. Today, most infants born with cardiac defects are expected to live into adulthood, and the number of adults with a congenital heart defect now exceeds the number of children. A complete echocardiographic examination can establish management, reduce the need for confirmatory cardiac catheterization, and provide serial evaluation of residua and sequelae of congenital heart disease.

Systematic Tomographic Approach to Imaging in Congenital Heart Disease

When evaluating patients who have congenital heart defects, the echocardiographic examination must not only quantify function but also define any anatomical and physiological deviations from normal that may be present. The systematic approach can be applied to all cardiac anomalies and conforms to the recommendations of the American Society of Echocardiography (ASE) and the Society of Pediatric Echocardiography (SOPE).

For a congenital TTE examination, it is easiest to begin with the examination of the upper abdomen to establish the position of the viscera and heart. The location of the heart and the base-to-apex orientation are established to determine levocardia (cardiac apex in the left side of the chest), mesocardia (cardiac apex in the midline), or dextrocardia (cardiac apex in the right side of the chest). When imaging congenital anomalies, apex-down is used because it orients cardiac structures in a manner most closely resembling classic anatomical dissections and surgical approaches to the heart. Thus four-chamber views orient the heart as though looking at the patient from the front.

The internal cardiac crux is an important echocardiographic landmark used in the evaluation of many common and complex congenital cardiac anomalies (Fig. 14-111). In the four-chamber plane, the components of the internal crux include the atrial septum, ventricular septum, and septal portions of the mitral and tricuspid valves. The tricuspid valve originates from the crest of the ventricular septum, whereas the septal portion of the mitral valve inserts at a higher level off the lower atrial septum. The portion of the ventricular septum between the two valves represents the atrioventricular septum (i.e., a potential communication between the LV and RA). The anatomy of the internal cardiac crux can be used to diagnose both ventricular and atrioventricular valve morphology and abnormalities. The higher inserting morphologic mitral valve is predictably committed to the morphological LV, and the lower inserting morphological tricuspid valve to the morphologic RV. The anatomy of the crux is best imaged from a precordial apical, subcostal, or transesophageal four-chamber view.

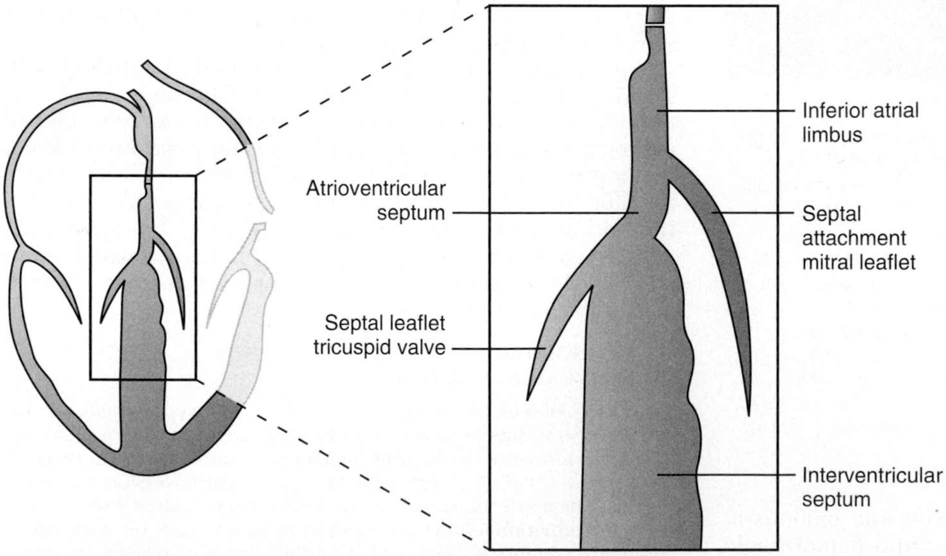

FIGURE 14–111 Diagram of the internal cardiac crux: the joining of the inflow atrial and ventricular septa and respective leaflets of the mitral and tricuspid valves form a crosslike configuration within the heart. This view is predictably obtained with an apical four-chamber view. The normal internal cardiac crux (i.e., cross) is characterized by a lower insertion of the septal leaflet of the morphological tricuspid valve. In fact, this characteristic relationship of crux attachment of the atrioventricular valves can predict the morphology of these valves (i.e., tricuspid and mitral) and ventricular morphology. This also allows for potential communication between left ventricle and right atrium through the atrioventricular septum. The morphologic tricuspid valve is always committed to the morphologic right ventricle and the mitral valve to the morphologic left ventricle. Note that with partial (i.e., primum atrial septal defect) and complete (primum atrial septal defect and inflow ventricular septal defect) congenital canal defects, the mitral valve is characteristically displaced downward. This downward displacement and loss of the atrioventricular septum (i.e., potential communication from the left ventricle directly into the right atrium) results in a deficiency of the mitral leaflet (i.e., a cleft). A large number of congenital anomalies are characterized by diagnostic alterations of the internal cardiac crux.

Many complex anomalies of the heart are diagnosed most confidently by their alteration of the crux anatomy, such as Ebstein anomaly, congenitally corrected transposition, double-inlet ventricle, and others (Fig. 14-112).

Transesophageal Echocardiography

Because of the superb visualization of cardiovascular structures, TEE is increasingly being used in the diagnosis of congenital heart disease. TEE is particularly useful in the operating room or during interventional procedures. However, intracardiac echocardiographic imaging is increasingly used for monitoring during percutaneous procedures. TEE is used routinely intraoperatively[176] and to complement TTE. Currently, a comprehensive 2D and Doppler echocardiography examination is considered the primary means of diagnosing and characterizing most congenital cardiac anomalies and the primary method for evaluating anatomy and hemodynamics during follow-up.

Fetal Congenital Heart Disease

High-resolution echocardiography can now be used to confidently diagnose congenital heart disease in a fetus. Fetal echocardiography is used most effectively to anticipate fetal or neonatal problems, allow prenatal counseling, plan pregnancy, delivery, neonatal care, and treatment strategies.

Atrial Septal Defect

Atrial septal defects comprise approximately 10 percent of congenital heart disease (see Chap. 61). The four distinct types of atrial septal defect are (1) secundum (Fig. 14-113), (2) primum or partial atrioventricular canal (Fig. 14-114), (3) sinus venosus (Fig. 14-115), and (4) coronary sinus atrial septal defect (Fig. 14-116). A complete TTE examination can detect most primum and secundum atrial septal defects, but sinus venosus defect is visualized in only about 70 percent of patients. However, TEE is exquisitely sensitive for the identification of all types of atrial septal defect, as well as associated anomalous pulmonary venous connections.

Each form of atrial septal defect is normally associated with a left-to-right shunt, which eventually results in RA and RV volume overload. It is not necessary or recommended to quantify shunt volume by Doppler measurements. These assessments are often inaccurate because of the number of component measurements involved in the calculation of multiple stroke volumes. The TTE finding of an atrial septal defect with associated right-heart enlargement is enough to warrant closure of the defect in the absence of pulmonary hypertension. Pulmonary hypertension of a magnitude that would preclude surgical or device closure is rare and can be recognized on 2D and Doppler echocardiography studies. Confirmation of fixed pulmonary hypertension requires

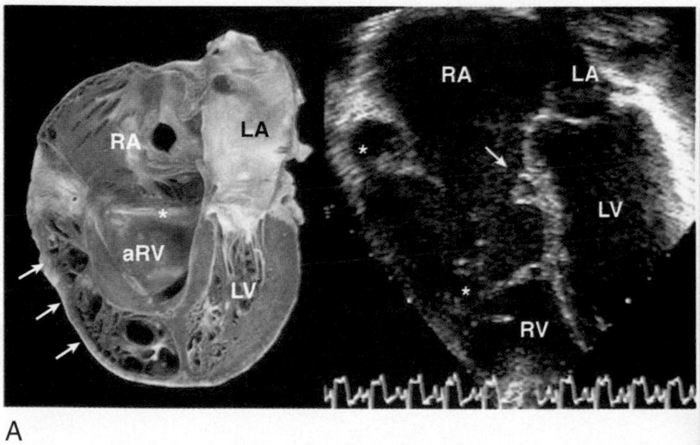

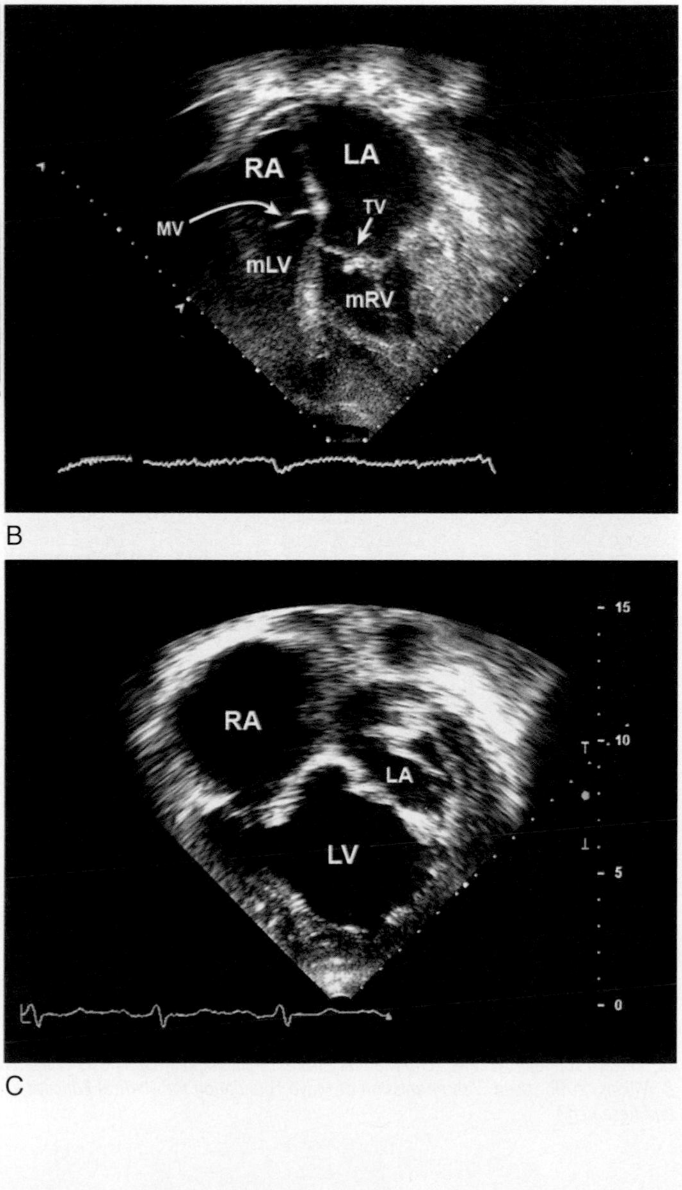

FIGURE 14–112 **A,** Ebstein anomaly. **Left,** Pathology specimen shows right atrial (RA) and right ventricular (RV) enlargement with a large atrialized portion of the RA (aRV). The anterior tricuspid valve leaflets are tethered to the lateral wall of the RV (arrows). The left atrium (LA) and left ventricle (LV) are small. * = Anatomical tricuspid annulus. **Right,** Apical four-chamber view. The septal leaflet of the tricuspid valve (arrow) inserts lower than the septal attachment of the mitral valve. The portion of the RV below the tricuspid valve annulus and the downwardly displaced septal tricuspid valve leaflet (arrow) is an atrialized RV. The anterior leaflet is inserted directly into the papillary muscle (*), which impairs mobility. Note that the heart cavities on the right side (RA and RV) become enlarged because of associated tricuspid regurgitation and an atrial septal defect that is usually present (not shown in this example). **B,** Congenitally corrected transposition of the great arteries. The right atrium (RA) communicates with a right-sided morphologically left ventricle (mLV), which connects to the pulmonary artery. The left atrium (LA) communicates with a left-sided morphologically right ventricle (mRV), which connects to the aorta. Four-chamber echocardiogram showing the reversed relationship of the cardiac crux (i.e., the right-sided mitral valve [MV] inserts higher than the left-sided tricuspid valve [TV]). The mLV is to the left below the RA and the mRV is below the LA. The RV is trabeculated. **C,** Double-inlet LV. Systole. The left-sided and right-sided atrioventricular valves are committed to the LV. Both atrioventricular valves can be committed to a single ventricular chamber. This is referred to as *double-inlet ventricle*. *(**A,** From Oh JK, Seward JB, Tajik AJ: The Echo Manual. 3rd ed. Philadelphia, Lippincott Williams & Wilkins, 2006. Used with permission of Mayo Foundation for Medical Education and Research.)*

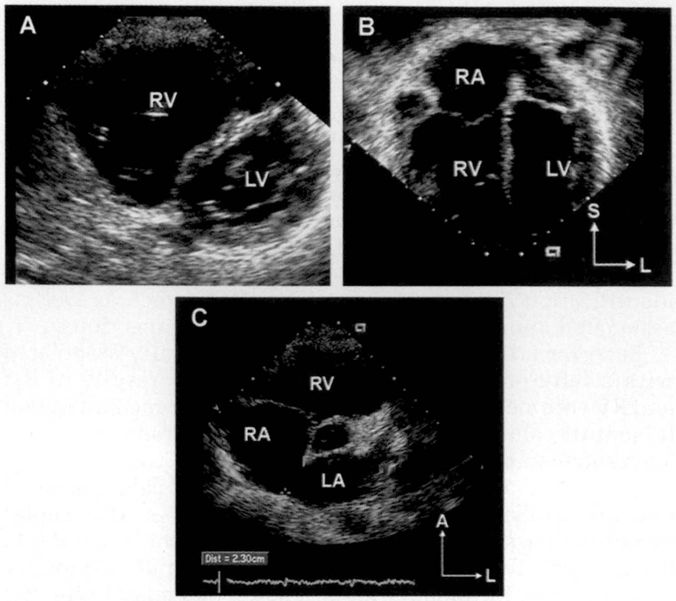

FIGURE 14–113 2D Echocardiographic features of atrial septal defect. Short-axis imaging **(A)** shows right ventricular (RV) enlargement from RV volume overload. **B,** Apical four-chamber image shows right atrial (RA) and RV enlargement and drop out in the atrial septum from the secundum atrial septal defect. **C,** Basal short-axis view of RA and RV enlargement and the secundum atrial septal defect (2.3 cm). LA = left atrium; LV = left ventricle. A = anterior; L = left; S = superior. *(From Oh JK, Seward JB, Tajik AJ: The Echo Manual. 3rd ed. Philadelphia, Lippincott Williams & Wilkins, 2006. Used with permission of Mayo Foundation for Medical Education and Research.)*

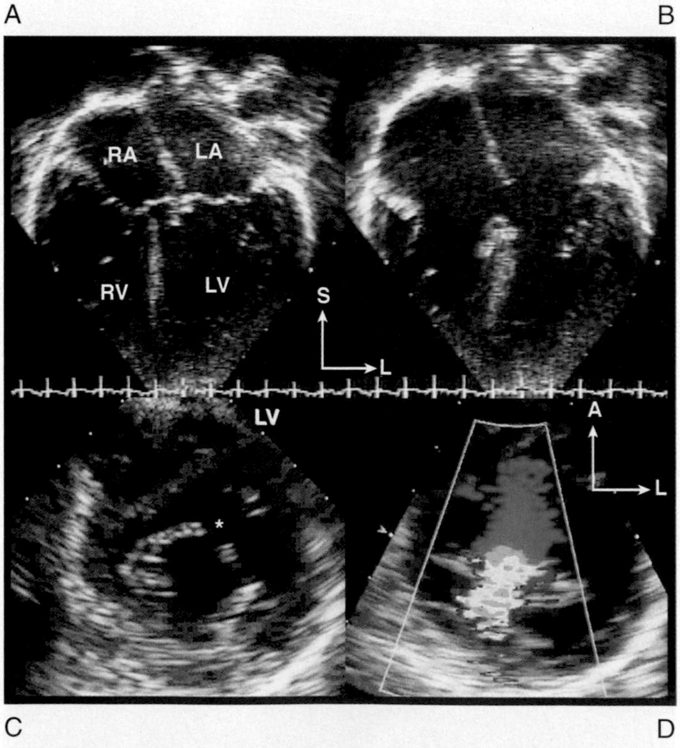

FIGURE 14–114 Primum atrial septal defect is characterized by a defect in the lower atrial septum and downward displacement of the atrioventricular valves, as seen with apical four-chamber imaging during systole **(A)** and diastole **(B)**. Short-axis 2D imaging **(C)** shows a mitral valve cleft (*) and **(D)** color-flow imaging shows mitral regurgitation through the cleft. LA = left atrium; LV = left ventricle; RA = right atrium; RV = right ventricle. Orientation: A = anterior; L = left. *(From Oh JK, Seward JB, Tajik AJ: The Echo Manual. 3rd ed. Philadelphia, Lippincott Williams & Wilkins, 2006. Used with permission of Mayo Foundation for Medical Education and Research.)*

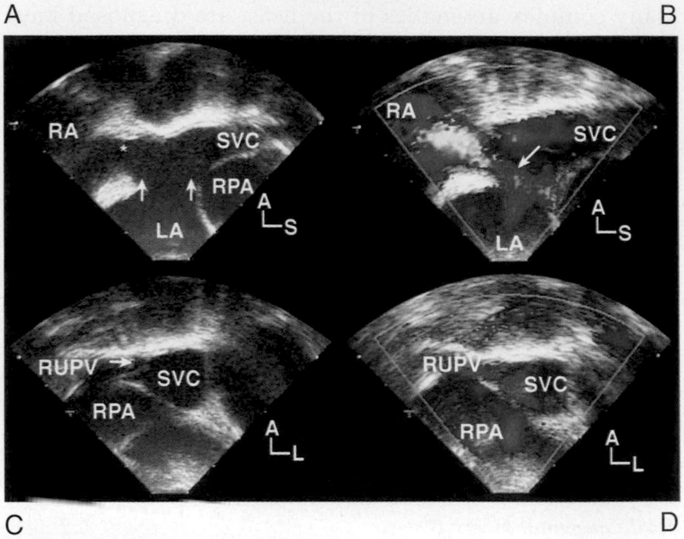

FIGURE 14–115 Sinus venosus atrial septal defect (ASD). **A,** Long-axis transesophageal examination aligned with the superior vena cava (SVC). Note the large atrial septal defect (arrows) just beneath the SVC, where this vessel enters (*) the right atrium (RA). Note the volume-enlarged right pulmonary artery (RPA) and that no atrial septal tissues are attached to the wall adjacent to the RPA (absence of the superior limbus of the atrial septum). These features are pathognomonic of sinus venosus ASD. Note the intact membranous portion of the fossa ovalis. **B,** Color flow Doppler shows left-to-right shunt flow across the sinus venosus ASD. Also visualized is blood entering the SVC from the anomalously connecting right pulmonary vein (arrow). **C,** Transesophageal short-axis view at the level of the RPA, which is displayed in its long axis. Normally, SVC is circular, but in this example, it has a teardrop shape because an anomalous connecting pulmonary vein (RUPV) (arrow) enters the lateral wall of the SVC. **D,** On color flow Doppler study, note blood flow from the anomalously connecting RUPV into the SVC. A sinus venosus ASD is commonly associated with anomalous connection of the right middle and upper pulmonary veins, which enter either the RA or SVC. LA = left atrium. Orientation: A = anterior; L = left; S = superior. *(From Oh JK, Seward JB, Tajik AJ: The Echo Manual. 3rd ed. Philadelphia, Lippincott Williams & Wilkins, 2006. Used with permission of Mayo Foundation for Medical Education and Research.)*

cardiac catheterization and hemodynamic assessment. Routine cardiac catheterization is not required to establish the diagnosis of atrial septal defect.

Ventricular Septal Defect

Ventricular septal defects are common, occurring in approximately 20 to 25 percent of patients with congenital heart disease (see Chap. 61). Often, they are small, isolated defects that cause no symptoms, but multiple ventricular septal defects may occur in the same patient. Large ventricular septal defects cause a large left-to-right shunt and pulmonary hypertension. Left-heart volume overload and RV hypertrophy are features that should suggest the presence of a large ventricular septal defect. If unrepaired, large defects may cause irreversible pulmonary vascular obstructive disease, even in young children. These defects can occur in various locations in the ventricular septum. There are four major categories of ventricular septal defect. The most common type in adults is the membranous type (Fig. 14-117). These are located at the junction of the muscular, atrioventricular, and outlet portions of the septum. They are adjacent to the aortic and tricuspid valves, which may eventually cause aortic or tricuspid valve regurgitation; thus, prolonged echocardiographic surveillance is recommended.

The most common ventricular septal defect in children is the muscular type (Fig. 14-118). They are most often located in the apical two thirds of the ventricular septum. Remote from any cardiac valve, they are not associated with progressive valve dysfunction. Most of these defects

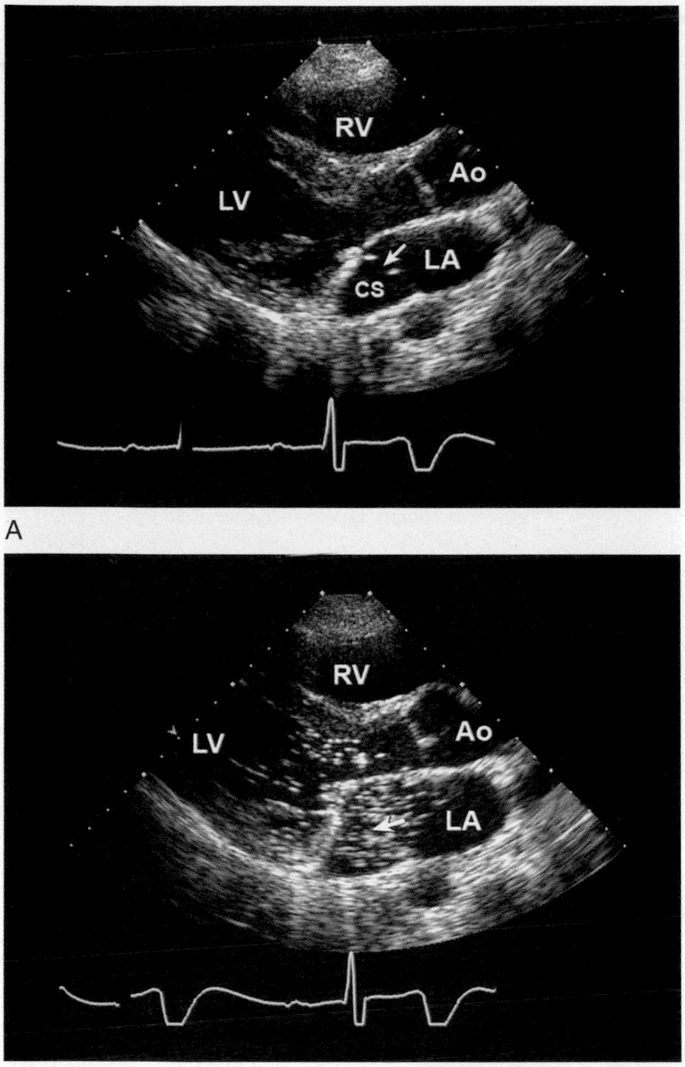

FIGURE 14–116 Coronary sinus atrial septal defect (ASD), the most rare ASD, is characterized by the absence of the roof of the coronary sinus, which is located in the floor of the left atrium (LA). **A,** Parasternal long-axis image of dilated coronary sinus (CS) and a defect in the wall (arrow) between CS and LA. Ao = aorta; LV = left ventricle; RV = right ventricle. **B,** Left upper extremity agitated saline injection shows prompt filling of the CS and LA (arrow). Thus LA blood can enter the unroofed coronary sinus and cross its orifice into the right atrium (i.e., "coronary sinus ASD"). Ao = aorta; LV = left ventricle; RV = right ventricle.

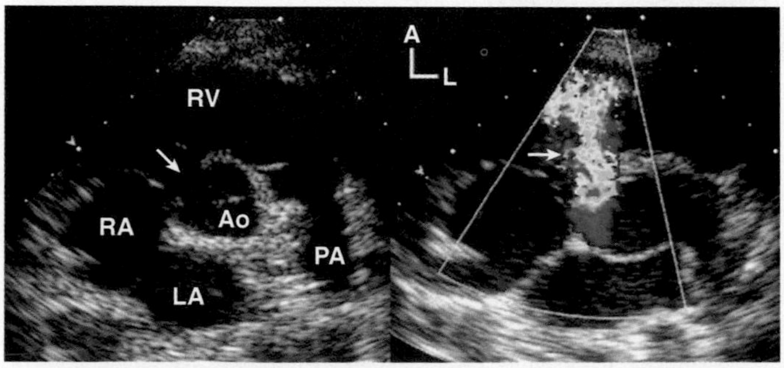

FIGURE 14–117 Membranous ventricular septal defect. **Left,** Parasternal short-axis view. The ventricular septal defect (arrow) is located on the medial aspect of the left ventricle outflow. **Right,** Color flow imaging shows left-to-right shunt from across the membranous VSD (arrow). Ao = aorta; LA = left atrium; PA = pulmonary artery; RA = right atrium; RV = right ventricle. Orientation: A = anterior; L = left. *(From Oh JK, Seward JB, Tajik AJ: The Echo Manual. 3rd ed. Philadelphia, Lippincott Williams & Wilkins, 2006. Used with permission of Mayo Foundation for Medical Education and Research.)*

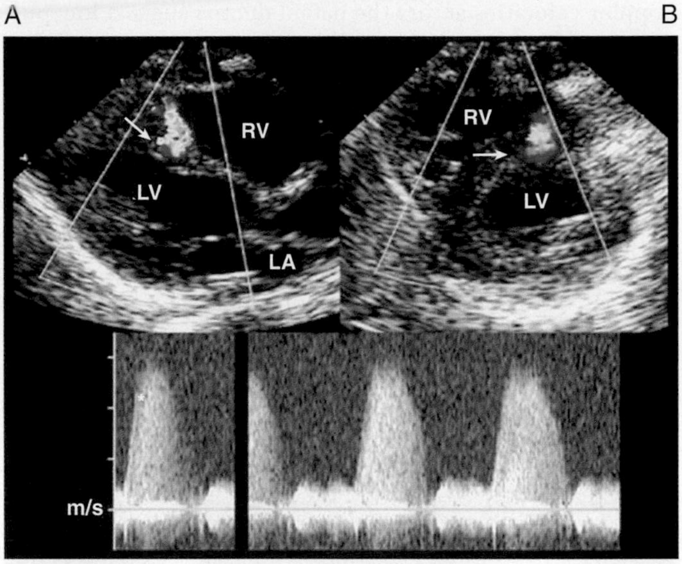

FIGURE 14–118 Muscular ventricular septal defect (VSD). **A,** Parasternal long-axis image with color flow Doppler of a muscular VSD (arrow) shows flow from left ventricle (LV) to right ventricle (RV). LA = left atrium. **B,** Short-axis imaging with color flow Doppler of a muscular VSD (arrow) shows flow from LV to RV. **C,** Continuous wave Doppler signal from the VSD demonstrates left-to-right high-velocity flow. *(From Oh JK, Seward JB, Tajik AJ: The Echo Manual. 3rd ed. Philadelphia, Lippincott Williams & Wilkins, 2006. Used with permission of Mayo Foundation for Medical Education and Research.)*

are small and close spontaneously early in life. A large muscular ventricular septal defect can cause a large left-to-right shunt, with eventual pulmonary hypertension.

The third most frequent type of ventricular septal defect is the one seen with complete atrioventricular septal defects. This type usually occurs as part of a complete atrioventricular canal defect, but occasionally it may be seen in isolation.

The supracristal, or subarterial, ventricular septal defect is rare. It is located in the outlet septum, immediately adjacent to both the aortic and pulmonary valve annulus at the base of the heart. As a result, the right aortic cusp may be unsupported and prolapse into the ventricular septal defect (Fig. 14-119). Aortic cusp prolapse restricts the functional size of the defect but distorts the aortic valve and is associated with aortic valve regurgitation. Elective repair of this ventricular septal defect is usually recommended to prevent progressive aortic cusp prolapse and regurgitation.

A comprehensive TTE examination can identify a ventricular septal defect in more than 90 percent of cases. Continuous wave Doppler echocardiography can measure the blood flow velocity and gradient across the defect. A large ventricular septal defect will have a smaller pressure difference between the ventricles; conversely, a small defect would have a large gradient (i.e., velocity). Rarely, TEE is used to improve imaging in patients with a known or suspected ventricular septal defect.

Patent Ductus Arteriosus

Patent ductus arteriosus is an arterial communication between the upper descending aorta and the distal main pulmonary artery, near the origin of the left pulmonary artery (see Chap. 61). Echocardiographic diagnosis is based on demonstrating a persistent anatomical connection and flow between the descending thoracic aorta and the pulmonary artery (Fig. 14-120). The best imaging views include the high left parasternal long-axis scan of the RVOT and main pulmonary artery and the suprasternal view. A patent ductus arteriosus associated with pulmonary hypertension may be difficult to visualize with TTE or TEE because of equalization of pressures between the two vessels. High

 Doppler velocities across the patent ductus suggest low pulmonary artery pressure.

Coarctation of the Aorta

Aortic coarctation usually occurs as a discrete posterior infolding of the aortic media, causing a narrowing in the upper descending thoracic aorta (see Chaps. 56 and 61). This narrowing can be seen just distal to the left subclavian artery in the region opposite the origin or remnant of the ductus arteriosus, so-called *juxtaductal coarctation.* Coarctation of the aorta occurs in 6 to 8 percent of patients with congenital heart disease. The physiology of the coarctation varies depending on age at presentation, severity and location of the stenosis, and associated lesions. Clinical presentation can range from severe heart failure and shock in a young infant to asymptomatic systemic hypertension with diminished femoral pulses or a murmur in an older child or adult.

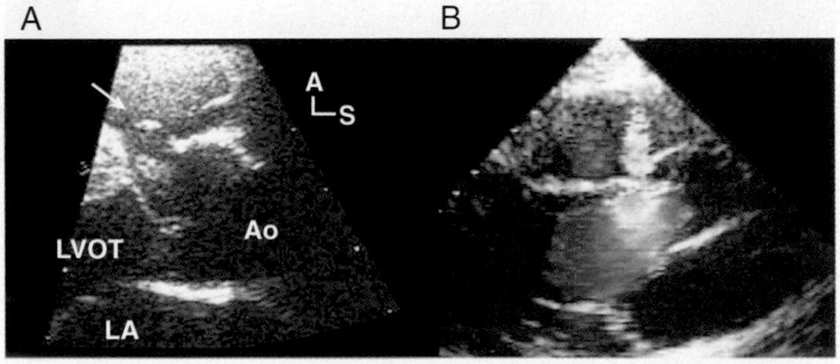

FIGURE 14–119 Supracristal ventricular septal defect (VSD). **A,** Parasternal long-axis image shows dilatation of the right aortic sinus and a ventricular septal defect (arrow). Ao = aorta; LA = left atrium; LVOT = left ventricular outflow tract. **B,** Color flow image shows left-to-right shunt through the VSD. *(From Oh JK, Seward JB, Tajik AJ: The Echo Manual. 3rd ed. Philadelphia, Lippincott Williams & Wilkins, 2006. Used with permission of Mayo Foundation for Medical Education and Research.)*

With TTE, the area of aortic narrowing can often be seen from the suprasternal or high left parasternal transducer position; however, continuous wave Doppler echocardiography is the best method for quantifying the magnitude of obstruction. Doppler recordings of hemodynamically sig-

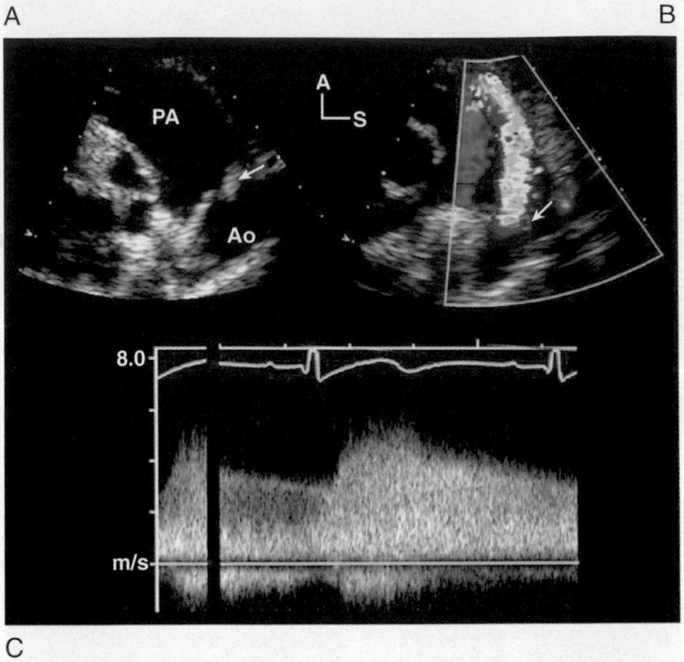

FIGURE 14–120 Patent ductus arteriosus. **A,** Parasternal short-axis image shows communication between the aorta (Ao) and pulmonary artery (PA) (arrow) by 2D echocardiography, which is confirmed on color flow imaging **(B). C,** Continuous wave Doppler signal shows high systolic velocity and persistent flow through diastole. Orientation: A = anterior; S = superior. *(From Oh JK, Seward JB, Tajik AJ: The Echo Manual. 3rd ed. Philadelphia, Lippincott Williams & Wilkins, 2006. Used with permission of Mayo Foundation for Medical Education and Research.)*

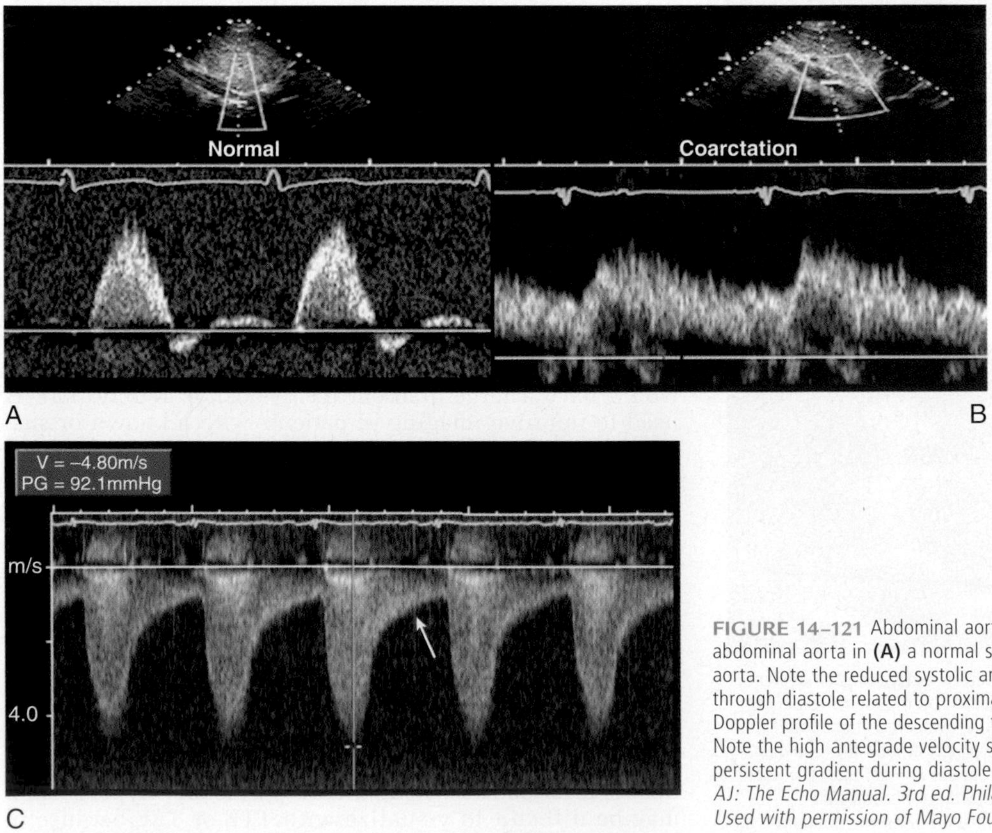

FIGURE 14–121 Abdominal aorta in coarctation. Pulsed wave Doppler study of abdominal aorta in **(A)** a normal subject and **(B)** a patient with coarctation of the aorta. Note the reduced systolic antegrade velocity, late rise, and persistent flow through diastole related to proximal obstruction of the aorta. **C,** Continuous wave Doppler profile of the descending thoracic aorta in a patient with severe coarctation. Note the high antegrade velocity suggesting severe systolic obstruction and the persistent gradient during diastole (arrow). *(**A** and **B**, From Oh JK, Seward JB, Tajik AJ: The Echo Manual. 3rd ed. Philadelphia, Lippincott Williams & Wilkins, 2006. Used with permission of Mayo Foundation for Medical Education and Research.)*

nificant coarctation are characterized by an increased flow velocity in the descending thoracic aorta that extends into diastole. The systolic gradient in severe coarctation may underestimate the severity of obstruction when there is an extensive collateral network. Thus ancillary data are obtained; in severe coarctation, a pulsed wave examination of the abdominal aorta shows distorted flow velocity, with decreased systolic amplitude, and persistent flow in diastole (Fig. 14-121). Abnormal abdominal flow is helpful in recognizing (re)coarctation in adults. In older patients and any patient with a repaired coarctation, CMR or CT has replaced angiography for definitive diagnosis and overall vascular assessment of coarctation or recoarctation.

REFERENCES

Transthoracic, Transesophageal, and Doppler Echocardiography

1. Oh JK, Seward JB, Tajik AJ: The Echo Manual. 3rd ed. Philadelphia, Lippincott Williams & Wilkins, 2006.
2. Zamorano J, Cordeiro P, Sugeng L, et al: Real-time three-dimensional echocardiography for rheumatic mitral valve stenosis evaluation: An accurate and novel approach. J Am Coll Cardiol 43:2091, 2004.
3. Lang RM, Bierig M, Devereux RB, et al: Chamber Quantification Writing Group; American Society of Echocardiography's Guidelines and Standards Committee; European Association of Echocardiography: Recommendations for chamber quantification: A report from the American Society of Echocardiography's Guidelines and Standards Committee and the Chamber Quantification Writing Group, developed in conjunction with the European Association of Echocardiography, a branch of the European Society of Cardiology. J Am Soc Echocardiogr 18:1440, 2005.
4. Kuhl HP, Hanrath P: The impact of transesophageal echocardiography on daily clinical practice. Eur J Echocardiogr 5:455, 2004.
5. Klein AL, Murray RD, Becker ER, et al: ACUTE Investigators: Economic analysis of a transesophageal echocardiography-guided approach to cardioversion of patients with atrial fibrillation: The ACUTE economic data at eight weeks. J Am Coll Cardiol 43:1217, 2004.
6. Min JK, Spencer KT, Furlong KT, et al: Clinical features of complications from transesophageal echocardiography: A single-center case series of 10,000 consecutive examinations. J Am Soc Echocardiogr 18:925, 2005.

Tissue Doppler and Strain Imaging

7. Sutherland GR, Di Salvo G, Claus P, et al: Strain and strain rate imaging: a new clinical approach to quantifying regional myocardial function. J Am Soc Echocardiogr 17:788, 2004.
8. Yip G, Abraham T, Belohlavek M, Khandheria BK: Clinical applications of strain rate imaging. J Am Soc Echocardiogr 16:1334, 2003.
9. Notomi Y, Setser RM, Shiota T, et al: Assessment of left ventricular torsional deformation by Doppler tissue imaging: validation study with tagged magnetic resonance imaging. Circulation 111:1141, 2005.
10. Helle-Valle T, Crosby J, Edvardsen T, et al: New noninvasive method for assessment of left ventricular rotation: Speckle tracking echocardiography. Circulation 112:3149, 2005.
11. Notomi Y, Martin-Miklovic MG, Oryszak SJ, et al: Enhanced ventricular untwisting during exercise: a mechanistic manifestation of elastic recoil described by Doppler tissue imaging. Circulation 113:2524, 2006.
12. Foster E, Lease KE: New untwist on diastole: what goes around comes back. Circulation 113:2477, 2006.
13. Sengupta PP, Khandheria BK, Korinek J, et al: Apex-to-base dispersion in regional timing of left ventricular shortening and lengthening. J Am Coll Cardiol 47:163, 2006.
14. Oh JK, Tajik AJ: The return of cardiac time intervals: The phoenix is rising. J Am Coll Cardiol 42:1471, 2003.
15. Hasegawa H, Little WC, Ohno M, et al: Diastolic mitral annular velocity during the development of heart failure. J Am Coll Cardiol 41:1590, 2003.
16. Derumeaux G, Mulder P, Richard V, et al: Tissue Doppler imaging differentiates physiological from pathological pressure-overload left ventricular hypertrophy in rats. Circulation 105:1602, 2002.
17. Wang M, Yip GW, Wang AY, et al: Tissue Doppler imaging provides incremental prognostic value in patients with systemic hypertension and left ventricular hypertrophy. J Hypertens 23:183, 2005.
18. Abraham TP, Belohlavek M, Thomson HL, et al: Time to onset of regional relaxation: Feasibility, variability and utility of a novel index of regional myocardial function by strain rate imaging. J Am Coll Cardiol 39:1531, 2002.
19. Rambaldi R, Bax JJ, Rizzello V, et al: Post-systolic shortening during dobutamine stress echocardiography predicts cardiac survival in patients with severe left ventricular dysfunction. Coron Artery Dis 16:141, 2005.
20. Oh JK, Hatle L, Tajik AJ, Little WC: Diastolic heart failure can be diagnosed by comprehensive two-dimensional and Doppler echocardiography. J Am Coll Cardiol 47:500, 2006.
21. Diwan A, McCulloch M, Lawrie GM, et al: Doppler estimation of left ventricular filling pressures in patients with mitral valve disease. Circulation 111:3281, 2005. Erratum in: Circulation 112:e76, 2005.
22. Kjaergaard J, Hassager C, Oh JK, et al: Measurement of cardiac time intervals by Doppler tissue M-mode imaging of the anterior mitral leaflet. J Am Soc Echocardiogr 18:1058, 2005.
23. Yu CM, Zhang Q, Fung JW, et al: A novel tool to assess systolic asynchrony and identify responders of cardiac resynchronization therapy by tissue synchronization imaging. J Am Coll Cardiol 45:677, 2005.
24. Gorcsan J III, Kanzaki H, Bazaz R, et al: Usefulness of echocardiographic tissue synchronization imaging to predict acute response to cardiac resynchronization therapy. Am J Cardiol 93:1178, 2004.
25. Mele D, Pasanisi G, Capasso F, et al: Left intraventricular myocardial deformation dyssynchrony identifies responders to cardiac resynchronization therapy in patients with heart failure. Eur Heart J 27:1070, 2006.
26. Miyazaki C, Espinosa RE, Hayes DL, et al: Baseline dyssynchrony derived by strain imaging correlates with the effect of cardiac resynchronization therapy at 1-month follow-up [abstract]. J Am Coll Cardiol 47(4 Suppl A):102A, 2006.

Contrast Echocardiography

27. Lepper W, Belcik T, Wei K, et al: Myocardial contrast echocardiography. Circulation 109:3132, 2004.
28. Kaul S, Ito H: Microvasculature in acute myocardial ischemia: Part I: Evolving concepts in pathophysiology, diagnosis, and treatment. Circulation 109:146, 2004.
29. Kirkpatrick JN, Wong T, Bednarz JE, et al: Differential diagnosis of cardiac masses using contrast echocardiographic perfusion imaging. J Am Coll Cardiol 43:1412, 2004.
30. Kaul S, Senior R, Firschke C, et al: Incremental value of cardiac imaging in patients presenting to the emergency department with chest pain and without ST-segment elevation: A multicenter study. Am Heart J 148:129, 2004.
31. Jeetley P, Hickman M, Kamp O, et al: Myocardial contrast echocardiography for the detection of coronary artery stenosis: A prospective multicenter study in comparison with single-photon emission computed tomography. J Am Coll Cardiol 47:141, 2006.
32. Main ML, Magalski A, Morris BA, et al: Combined assessment of microvascular integrity and contractile reserve improves differentiation of stunning and necrosis after acute anterior wall myocardial infarction. J Am Coll Cardiol 40:1079, 2002.
33. Kaul S, Ito H: Microvasculature in acute myocardial ischemia: Part II: Evolving concepts in pathophysiology, diagnosis, and treatment. Circulation 109:310, 2004.
34. Hillis GS, Mulvagh SL, Gunda M, et al: Contrast echocardiography using intravenous octafluoropropane and real-time perfusion imaging predicts functional recovery after acute myocardial infarction. J Am Soc Echocardiogr 16:638, 2003.
35. Holmes DR Jr, Valeti US, Nishimura RA: Alcohol septal ablation for hypertrophic cardiomyopathy: indications and technique. Catheter Cardiovasc Interv 66:375, 2005.

Cardiac Chamber Size and Function

36. Abhayaratna WP, Seward JB, Appleton CP, et al: Left atrial size: physiologic determinants and clinical applications. J Am Coll Cardiol 47:2357, 2006.
37. Mor-Avi V, Sugeng L, Weinert L, et al: Fast measurement of left ventricular mass with real-time three-dimensional echocardiography: comparison with magnetic resonance imaging. Circulation 110:1814, 2004.
38. Mor-Avi V, Korcarz CE, Collins KA, et al: Simultaneous real-time echocardiographic imaging of myocardial perfusion and regional function using color-encoded, contrast-enhanced power modulation. J Am Soc Echocardiogr 16:1258, 2003.
39. Caiani EG, Corsi C, Zamorano J, et al: Improved semiautomated quantification of left ventricular volumes and ejection fraction using 3-dimensional echocardiography with a full matrix-array transducer: Comparison with magnetic resonance imaging. J Am Soc Echocardiogr 18:779, 2005.
40. Zile MR, Baicu CF, Gaasch WH: Diastolic heart failure: abnormalities in active relaxation and passive stiffness of the left ventricle. N Engl J Med 350:1953, 2004.
41. Amundsen BH, Helle-Valle T, Edvardsen T, et al: Noninvasive myocardial strain measurement by speckle tracking echocardiography: Validation against sonomicrometry and tagged magnetic resonance imaging. J Am Coll Cardiol 47:789, 2006.
42. Langeland S, D'hooge J, Wouters PF, et al: Experimental validation of a new ultrasound method for the simultaneous assessment of radial and longitudinal myocardial deformation independent of insonation angle. Circulation 112:2157, 2005.
43. Nishimura RA, Tajik AJ: The Valsalva maneuver: 3 centuries later. Mayo Clin Proc 79:577, 2004.
44. Redfield MM, Jacobsen SJ, Burnett JC Jr, et al: Burden of systolic and diastolic ventricular dysfunction in the community: Appreciating the scope of the heart failure epidemic. JAMA 289:194, 2003.
45. Munagala VK, Jacobsen SJ, Mahoney DW, et al: Association of newer diastolic function parameters with age in healthy subjects: A population-based study. J Am Soc Echocardiogr 16:1049, 2003.
46. Frommelt PC, Pelech AN, Frommelt MA: Diastolic dysfunction in an unusual case of cardiomyopathy in a child: Insights from Doppler and Doppler tissue imaging analysis. J Am Soc Echocardiogr 16:176, 2003.
47. Lam CS, Han L, Ha JW, et al: The mitral L wave: a marker of pseudonormal filling and predictor of heart failure in patients with left ventricular hypertrophy. J Am Soc Echocardiogr 18:336, 2005.
48. Spencer KT, Kirkpatrick JN, Mor-Avi V, et al: Age dependency of the Tei index of myocardial performance. J Am Soc Echocardiogr 17:350, 2004.

49. Tham EB, Silverman NH: Measurement of the Tei index: A comparison of M-mode and pulse Doppler methods. J Am Soc Echocardiogr 17:1259, 2004.
50. LaCorte JC, Cabreriza SE, Rabkin DG, et al: Correlation of the Tei index with invasive measurements of ventricular function in a porcine model. J Am Soc Echocardiogr 16:442, 2003.
51. Rivas-Gotz C, Khoury DS, Manolios M, et al: Time interval between onset of mitral inflow and onset of early diastolic velocity by tissue Doppler: A novel index of left ventricular relaxation: experimental studies and clinical application. J Am Coll Cardiol 42:1463, 2003.
52. Gonzalez-Vilchez F, Ayuela J, Ares M, et al: Comparison of Doppler echocardiography, color M-mode Doppler, and Doppler tissue imaging for the estimation of pulmonary capillary wedge pressure. J Am Soc Echocardiogr 15:1245, 2002.
53. Ha JW, Lulic F, Bailey KR, et al: Effects of treadmill exercise on mitral inflow and annular velocities in healthy adults. Am J Cardiol 91:114, 2003.
54. Ha JW, Oh JK, Pellikka PA, et al: Diastolic stress echocardiography: A novel noninvasive diagnostic test for diastolic dysfunction using supine bicycle exercise Doppler echocardiography. J Am Soc Echocardiogr 18:63, 2005.
55. Burgess MI, Jenkins C, Sharman JE, Marwick TH: Diastolic stress echocardiography: hemodynamic validation and clinical significance of estimation of ventricular filling pressure with exercise. J Am Coll Cardiol 47:1891, 2006.
56. Nagueh SF, Bachinski LL, Meyer D, et al: Tissue Doppler imaging consistently detects myocardial abnormalities in patients with hypertrophic cardiomyopathy and provides a novel means for an early diagnosis before and independently of hypertrophy. Circulation 104:128, 2001.
57. Pieroni M, Chimenti C, Ricci R, et al: Early detection of Fabry cardiomyopathy by tissue Doppler imaging. Circulation 107:1978, 2003.
58. Zile MR, Brutsaert DL: New concepts in diastolic dysfunction and diastolic heart failure: Part I: diagnosis, prognosis, and measurements of diastolic function. Circulation 105:1387, 2002.
59. Tsang TS, Barnes ME, Gersh BJ, et al: Risks for atrial fibrillation and congestive heart failure in patients ≥65 years of age with abnormal left ventricular diastolic relaxation. Am J Cardiol 93:54, 2004.
60. Temporelli PL, Giannuzzi P, Nicolosi GL, et al: GISSI-3 Echo Substudy Investigators: Doppler-derived mitral deceleration time as a strong prognostic marker of left ventricular remodeling and survival after acute myocardial infarction: Results of the GISSI-3 echo substudy. J Am Coll Cardiol 43:1646, 2004.
61. Schillaci G, Pasqualini L, Verdecchia P, et al: Prognostic significance of left ventricular diastolic dysfunction in essential hypertension. J Am Coll Cardiol 39:2005, 2002.
62. Hillis GS, Moller JE, Pellikka PA, et al: Noninvasive estimation of left ventricular filling pressure by E/e' is a powerful predictor of survival after acute myocardial infarction. J Am Coll Cardiol 43:360, 2004.

Heart Failure

63. Grayburn PA, Appleton CP, DeMaria AN, et al: BEST Trial Echocardiographic Substudy Investigators: Echocardiographic predictors of morbidity and mortality in patients with advanced heart failure: the Beta-blocker Evaluation of Survival Trial (BEST): J Am Coll Cardiol 45:1064, 2005.
64. Bax JJ, Bleeker GB, Marwick TH, et al: Left ventricular dyssynchrony predicts response and prognosis after cardiac resynchronization therapy. J Am Coll Cardiol 44:1834, 2004.
65. Yu CM, Fung JW, Zhang Q, et al: Tissue Doppler imaging is superior to strain rate imaging and postsystolic shortening on the prediction of reverse remodeling in both ischemic and nonischemic heart failure after cardiac resynchronization therapy. Circulation 110:66, 2004.
66. Miyazaki C, Cha Y-M, Espinosa RE, et al: Correlation between acute effect of cardiac resynchronization therapy and mechanical dyssynchrony measured by tissue velocity and strain parameters [abstract]. J Am Coll Cardiol 47(4 Suppl A):95A, 2006.
67. Dokainish H, Zoghbi WA, Lakkis NM, et al: Optimal noninvasive assessment of left ventricular filling pressures: A comparison of tissue Doppler echocardiography and B-type natriuretic peptide in patients with pulmonary artery catheters. Circulation 109:2432, 2004.

Coronary Artery Disease

68. Tsutsui JM, Kusler M, Porter TR: Intravenous myocardial contrast echocardiography for the diagnosis of coronary artery disease. Curr Opin Cardiol 20:381, 2005.
69. Pellikka PA: Stress echocardiography for the diagnosis of coronary artery disease: Progress towards quantification. Curr Opin Cardiol 20:395, 2005.
70. Armstrong WF, Zoghbi WA: Stress echocardiography: Current methodology and clinical applications. J Am Coll Cardiol 45:1739, 2005.
71. Cerqueira MD, Weissman NJ, Dilsizian V, et al: American Heart Association Writing Group on Myocardial Segmentation and Registration for Cardiac Imaging: Standardized myocardial segmentation and nomenclature for tomographic imaging of the heart: A statement for healthcare professionals from the Cardiac Imaging Committee of the Council on Clinical Cardiology of the American Heart Association. Circulation 105:539, 2002.
72. Senior R, Monaghan M, Becher H, et al: British Society of Echocardiography: Stress echocardiography for the diagnosis and risk stratification of patients with suspected or known coronary artery disease: A critical appraisal. Supported by the British Society of Echocardiography. Heart 91:427, 2005.
73. Smiseth OA, Stoylen A, Ihlen H: Tissue Doppler imaging for the diagnosis of coronary artery disease. Curr Opin Cardiol 19:421, 2004.
74. Marwick TH: Measurement of strain and strain rate by echocardiography: Ready for prime time? J Am Coll Cardiol 47:1313, 2006.
75. Voigt JU, Lindenmeier G, Exner B, et al: Incidence and characteristics of segmental postsystolic longitudinal shortening in normal, acutely ischemic, and scarred myocardium. J Am Soc Echocardiogr 16:415, 2003.
76. Vignon P: Hemodynamic assessment of critically ill patients using echocardiography Doppler. Curr Opin Crit Care 11:227, 2005.
77. Bybee KA, Kara T, Prasad A, et al: Systematic review: transient left ventricular apical ballooning: A syndrome that mimics ST-segment elevation myocardial infarction. Ann Intern Med 141:858, 2004.
78. Bunch TJ, Oh JK, Click RL: Subepicardial aneurysm of the left ventricle. J Am Soc Echocardiogr 16:1318, 2003.
79. Anand IS, Florea VG, Solomon SD, et al: Noninvasive assessment of left ventricular remodeling: concepts, techniques, and implications for clinical trials. J Card Fail 8(Suppl 6):S452, 2002.
80. Bursi F, Enriquez-Sarano M, Jacobsen SJ, Roger VL: Mitral regurgitation after myocardial infarction: A review. Am J Med 119:103, 2006.
81. Bursi F, Enriquez-Sarano M, Nkomo VT, et al: Heart failure and death after myocardial infarction in the community: The emerging role of mitral regurgitation. Circulation 111:295, 2005.
82. Wu AH, Aaronson KD, Bolling SF, et al: Impact of mitral valve annuloplasty on mortality risk in patients with mitral regurgitation and left ventricular systolic dysfunction. J Am Coll Cardiol 45:381, 2005.
83. Jacobs AK, Leopold JA, Bates E, et al: Cardiogenic shock caused by right ventricular infarction: A report from the SHOCK registry. J Am Coll Cardiol 41:1273, 2003.
84. Bybee KA, Prasad A, Barsness GW, et al: Clinical characteristics and thrombolysis in myocardial infarction frame counts in women with transient left ventricular apical ballooning syndrome. Am J Cardiol 94:343, 2004.
85. McCully RB, Karon BL, Rummans TA, et al: Frequency of left ventricular dysfunction after electroconvulsive therapy. Am J Cardiol 91:1147, 2003.
86. Satoh H, Tateishi H, Uchida T: Takotsubo-type cardiomyopathy due to multivessel spasm. In Kodama K, Haze K, Hon M (eds): Clinical Aspect of Myocardial Injury: From Ischemia to Heart Failure [Japanese]. Tokyo, Kagakuhyouronysa, 1990, pp 56-64.
87. Reynolds HR, Anand SK, Fox JM, et al: Restrictive physiology in cardiogenic shock: Observations from echocardiography. Am Heart J 151:890.e9, 2006.
88. Moller JE, Hillis GS, Oh JK, et al: Left atrial volume: A powerful predictor of survival after acute myocardial infarction. Circulation 107:2207, 2003.
89. Hillis GS, Mulvagh SL, Pellikka PA, et al: Comparison of intravenous myocardial contrast echocardiography and low-dose dobutamine echocardiography for predicting left ventricular functional recovery following acute myocardial infarction. Am J Cardiol 92:504, 2003.
90. Hillis GS, Oh JK, Mahoney DW, et al: Akinesia becoming dyskinesia after exercise testing: Prevalence and relationship to clinical outcome. J Am Coll Cardiol 43:599, 2004.
91. Hanekom L, Jenkins C, Jeffries L, et al: Incremental value of strain rate analysis as an adjunct to wall-motion scoring for assessment of myocardial viability by dobutamine echocardiography: A follow-up study after revascularization. Circulation 112:3892, 2005.
92. McCully RB, Roger VL, Mahoney DW, et al: Outcome after abnormal exercise echocardiography for patients with good exercise capacity: prognostic importance of the extent and severity of exercise-related left ventricular dysfunction. J Am Coll Cardiol 39:1345, 2002.
93. Elhendy A, Mahoney DW, Burger KN, et al: Prognostic value of exercise echocardiography in patients with classic angina pectoris. Am J Cardiol 94:559, 2004.
94. Mazur W, Rivera JM, Khoury AF, et al: Prognostic value of exercise echocardiography: Validation of a new risk index combining echocardiographic, treadmill, and exercise electrocardiographic parameters. J Am Soc Echocardiogr 16:318, 2003.
95. Skulstad H, Edvardsen T, Urheim S, et al: Postsystolic shortening in ischemic myocardium: Active contraction or passive recoil? Circulation 106:718, 2002.
96. Talreja DR, Nishimura RA, Oh JK: Estimation of left ventricular filling pressure with exercise by Doppler echocardiography in patients with normal systolic function: A simultaneous echocardiographic-cardiac catheterization study. J Am Soc Echocardiogr 2007 (in press).

Valvular Heart Disease

97. Otto CM: Valvular aortic stenosis: disease severity and timing of intervention. J Am Coll Cardiol 47:2141, 2006.
98. Enriquez-Sarano M, Avierinos JF, Messika-Zeitoun D, et al: Quantitative determinants of the outcome of asymptomatic mitral regurgitation. N Engl J Med 352:875, 2005.
99. Abbas AE, Fortuin FD, Patel B, et al: Noninvasive measurement of systemic vascular resistance using Doppler echocardiography. J Am Soc Echocardiogr 17:834, 2004.
100. Abbas AE, Fortuin FD, Schiller NB, et al: A simple method for noninvasive estimation of pulmonary vascular resistance. J Am Coll Cardiol 41:1021, 2003.
101. Bonow RO, Carabello Ba, Kanu C, et al: American College of Cardiology/American Heart Association Task Force on Practice Guidelines, Society of Cardiovascular Anesthesiologists, Society for Cardiovascular Angiography and Interventions, Society of Thoracic Surgeons: ACC/AHA 2006 guidelines for the management of patients with valvular heart disease: A report of the American College of Cardiology/American Heart Association Task Force on Practice Guidelines (writing committee to revise the 1998 Guidelines for the management of patients with valvular heart disease): Developed in collaboration with the Society of Cardiovascular Anesthesiologists: Endorsed by the Society for Cardiovascular angiography and Interventions and the Society of Thoracic Surgeons. Circulation 114:e84, 2006.
102. Pellikka PA, Sarano ME, Nishimura RA, et al: Outcome of 622 adults with asymptomatic, hemodynamically significant aortic stenosis during prolonged follow-up. Circulation 111:3290, 2005.

103. Lancellotti P, Troisfontaines P, Toussaint AC, Pierard LA: Prognostic importance of exercise-induced changes in mitral regurgitation in patients with chronic ischemic left ventricular dysfunction. Circulation 108:1713, 2003.
104. Monin JL, Quere JP, Monchi M, et al: Low-gradient aortic stenosis: Operative risk stratification and predictors for long-term outcome: A multicenter study using dobutamine stress hemodynamics. Circulation 108:319, 2003.
105. Pereira JJ, Lauer MS, Bashir M, et al: Survival after aortic valve replacement for severe aortic stenosis with low transvalvular gradients and severe left ventricular dysfunction. J Am Coll Cardiol 39:1356, 2002.
106. Mohan JC, Patel AR, Passey R, et al: Is the mitral valve area flow-dependent in mitral stenosis? A dobutamine stress echocardiographic study. J Am Coll Cardiol 40:1809, 2002.
107. Zoghbi WA, Enriquez-Sarano M, Foster E, et al: American Society of Echocardiography: Recommendations for evaluation of the severity of native valvular regurgitation with two-dimensional and Doppler echocardiography. J Am Soc Echocardiogr 16:777, 2003.
108. Roberts BJ, Grayburn PA: Color flow imaging of the vena contracta in mitral regurgitation: Technical considerations. J Am Soc Echocardiogr 16:1002, 2003.
109. Nath J, Foster E, Heidenreich PA: Impact of tricuspid regurgitation on long-term survival. J Am Coll Cardiol 43:405, 2004.
110. Messika-Zeitoun D, Aubry MC, Detaint D, et al: Evaluation and clinical implications of aortic valve calcification measured by electron-beam computed tomography. Circulation 110:356, 2004.
111. Lin G, Nishimura RA, Connolly HM, et al: Severe symptomatic tricuspid valve regurgitation due to permanent pacemaker or implantable cardioverter-defibrillator leads. J Am Coll Cardiol 45:1672, 2005.
112. Sadeghi HM, Kimura BJ, Raisinghani A, et al: Does lowering pulmonary arterial pressure eliminate severe functional tricuspid regurgitation? Insights from pulmonary thromboendarterectomy. J Am Coll Cardiol 44:126, 2004.
113. Pritchett AM, Morrison JF, Edwards WD, et al: Valvular heart disease in patients taking pergolide. Mayo Clin Proc 77:1280, 2002.
114. Garcia D, Dumesnil JG, Durand LG, et al: Discrepancies between catheter and Doppler estimates of valve effective orifice area can be predicted from the pressure recovery phenomenon: practical implications with regard to quantification of aortic stenosis severity. J Am Coll Cardiol 41:435, 2003.
115. Rozich JD, Edwards WD, Hanna RD, et al: Mechanical prosthetic valve-associated strands: pathologic correlates to transesophageal echocardiography. J Am Soc Echocardiogr 16:97, 2003.
116. Blais C, Dumesnil JG, Baillot R, et al: Impact of valve prosthesis-patient mismatch on short-term mortality after aortic valve replacement. Circulation 108:983, 2003.

Infective Endocarditis

117. Baddour LM, Wilson WR, Bayer AS, et al: Committee on Rheumatic Fever, Endocarditis, and Kawasaki Disease, Council on Cardiovascular Disease in the Young, Councils on Clinical Cardiology, Stroke, and Cardiovascular Surgery and Anesthesia, American Heart Association, Infectious Diseases Society of America: Infective endocarditis: diagnosis, antimicrobial therapy, and management of complications: A statement for healthcare professionals from the Committee on Rheumatic Fever, Endocarditis, and Kawasaki Disease, Council on Cardiovascular Disease in the Young, and the Councils on Clinical Cardiology, Stroke, and Cardiovascular Surgery and Anesthesia, American Heart Association: Endorsed by the Infectious Diseases Society of America. Circulation 111:e394, 2005. Erratum in: Circulation 112:2373, 2005.
118. Vilacosta I, Graupner C, San Roman JA, et al: Risk of embolization after institution of antibiotic therapy for infective endocarditis. J Am Coll Cardiol 39:1489, 2002.
119. Jacob S, Tong AT: Role of echocardiography in the diagnosis and management of infective endocarditis. Curr Opin Cardiol 17:478, 2002.
120. Graupner C, Vilacosta I, SanRoman J, et al: Periannular extension of infective endocarditis. J Am Coll Cardiol 39:1204, 2002.
121. Humpl T, McCrindle BW, Smallhorn JF: The relative roles of transthoracic compared with transesophageal echocardiography in children with suspected infective endocarditis. J Am Coll Cardiol 41:2068, 2003.

Cardiomyopathies

122. Ali SK, Omran AS, Najm H, Godman MJ: Noncompaction of the ventricular myocardium associated with mitral regurgitation and preserved ventricular systolic function. J Am Soc Echocardiogr 17:87, 2004.
123. Oechslin E, Jenni R: Isolated left ventricular non-compaction: Increasing recognition of this distinct, yet "unclassified" cardiomyopathy. Eur J Echocardiogr 3:250, 2002.
124. Sutton TM, Stewart RA, Gerber IL, et al: Plasma natriuretic peptide levels increase with symptoms and severity of mitral regurgitation. J Am Coll Cardiol 41:2280, 2003.
125. Leclercq C, Hare JM: Ventricular resynchronization: Current state of the art. Circulation 109:296, 2004.
126. Burkett EL, Hershberger RE: Clinical and genetic issues in familial dilated cardiomyopathy. J Am Coll Cardiol 45:969, 2005.
127. Troughton RW, Prior DL, Pereira JJ, et al: Plasma B-type natriuretic peptide levels in systolic heart failure: Importance of left ventricular diastolic function and right ventricular systolic function. J Am Coll Cardiol 43:416, 2004.
128. Sogaard P, Egeblad H, Kim WY, et al: Tissue Doppler imaging predicts improved systolic performance and reversed left ventricular remodeling during long-term cardiac resynchronization therapy. J Am Coll Cardiol 40:723, 2002.
129. Yu CM, Chau E, Sanderson JE, et al: Tissue Doppler echocardiographic evidence of reverse remodeling and improved synchronicity by simultaneously delaying regional contraction after biventricular pacing therapy in heart failure. Circulation 105:438, 2002.
130. Nishimura RA, Holmes DR Jr: Clinical practice: hypertrophic obstructive cardiomyopathy. N Engl J Med 350:1320, 2004. Erratum in: N Engl J Med 351:1038, 2004.
131. Van Driest SL, Jaeger MA, Ommen SR, et al: Comprehensive analysis of the beta-myosin heavy chain gene in 389 unrelated patients with hypertrophic cardiomyopathy. J Am Coll Cardiol 44:602, 2004.
132. Maron MS, Olivotto I, Betocchi S, et al: Effect of left ventricular outflow tract obstruction on clinical outcome in hypertrophic cardiomyopathy. N Engl J Med 348:295, 2003.
133. Abe Y, Kondo M, Matsuoka R, et al: Assessment of clinical features in transient left ventricular apical ballooning. J Am Coll Cardiol 41:737, 2003.
134. Moukarbel GV, Alam SE, Abchee AB: Contrast-enhanced echocardiography for the diagnosis of apical hypertrophic cardiomyopathy. Echocardiography 22:831, 2005.
135. Ommen SR, Maron BJ, Olivotto I, et al: Long-term effects of surgical septal myectomy on survival in patients with obstructive hypertrophic cardiomyopathy. J Am Coll Cardiol 46:470, 2005.
136. Jassal DS, Neilan TG, Fifer MA, et al: Sustained improvement in left ventricular diastolic function after alcohol septal ablation for hypertrophic obstructive cardiomyopathy. Eur Heart J 27:1805, 2006.
137. Ward RP, Weinert L, Spencer KT, et al: Quantitative diagnosis of apical cardiomyopathy using contrast echocardiography. J Am Soc Echocardiogr 15:316, 2002.
138. Pelliccia A, Maron BJ, De Luca R, et al: Remodeling of left ventricular hypertrophy in elite athletes after long-term deconditioning. Circulation 105:944, 2002.
139. Ha JW, Ommen SR, Tajik AJ, et al: Differentiation of constrictive pericarditis from restrictive cardiomyopathy using mitral annular velocity by tissue Doppler echocardiography. Am J Cardiol 94:316, 2004.
140. Yoerger DM, Marcus F, Sherrill D, et al: Multidisciplinary Study of Right Ventricular Dysplasia Investigators: Echocardiographic findings in patients meeting task force criteria for arrhythmogenic right ventricular dysplasia: New insights from the multidisciplinary study of right ventricular dysplasia. J Am Coll Cardiol 45:860, 2005.
141. Hulot JS, Jouven X, Empana JP, et al: Natural history and risk stratification of arrhythmogenic right ventricular dysplasia/cardiomyopathy. Circulation 110:1879, 2004.
142. de Groot-de Laat LE, Krenning BJ, ten Cate FJ, Roelandt JR: Usefulness of contrast echocardiography for diagnosis of left ventricular noncompaction. Am J Cardiol 95:1131, 2005.

Pericardial Diseases

143. Tsang TS, Enriquez-Sarano M, Freeman WK, et al: Consecutive 1127 therapeutic echocardiographically guided pericardiocenteses: clinical profile, practice patterns, and outcomes spanning 21 years. Mayo Clin Proc 77:429, 2002.
144. Abbas AE, Appleton CP, Liu PT, Sweeney JP: Congenital absence of the pericardium: Case presentation and review of literature. Int J Cardiol 98:21, 2005.
145. Spodick DH: Acute pericarditis: current concepts and practice. JAMA 289:1150, 2003.
146. Bertog SC, Thambidorai SK, Parakh K, et al: Constrictive pericarditis: etiology and cause-specific survival after pericardiectomy. J Am Coll Cardiol 43:1445, 2004.
147. Talreja DR, Edwards WD, Danielson GK, et al: Constrictive pericarditis in 26 patients with histologically normal pericardial thickness. Circulation 108:1852, 2003.
148. Ha JW, Oh JK, Ommen SR, et al: Diagnostic value of mitral annular velocity for constrictive pericarditis in the absence of respiratory variation in mitral inflow velocity. J Am Soc Echocardiogr 15:1468, 2002.
149. Sagrista-Sauleda J, Angel J, Sanchez A, et al: Effusive-constrictive pericarditis. N Engl J Med 350:469, 2004.
150. Sohn DW, Kim YJ, Kim HS, et al: Unique features of early diastolic mitral annulus velocity in constrictive pericarditis. J Am Soc Echocardiogr 17:222, 2004.
151. Haley JH, Tajik AJ, Danielson GK, et al: Transient constrictive pericarditis: causes and natural history. J Am Coll Cardiol 43:271, 2004.

Systemic Diseases Affecting the Heart

152. Koyama J, Davidoff R, Falk RH: Longitudinal myocardial velocity gradient derived from pulsed Doppler tissue imaging in AL amyloidosis: A sensitive indicator of systolic and diastolic dysfunction. J Am Soc Echocardiogr 17:36, 2004.
153. Simula DV, Edwards WD, Tazelaar HD, et al: Surgical pathology of carcinoid heart disease: A study of 139 valves from 75 patients spanning 20 years. Mayo Clin Proc 77:139, 2002.
154. Pandya UH, Pellikka PA, Enriquez-Sarano M, et al: Metastatic carcinoid tumor to the heart: echocardiographic-pathologic study of 11 patients. J Am Coll Cardiol 40:1328, 2002.
155. Moller JE, Connolly HM, Rubin J, et al: Factors associated with progression of carcinoid heart disease. N Engl J Med 348:1005, 2003.
156. Moller JE, Pellikka PA, Bernheim AM, et al: Prognosis of carcinoid heart disease: Analysis of 200 cases over two decades. Circulation 112:3320, 2005.
157. Naqvi TZ, Luthringer D, Marchevsky A, et al: Chloroquine-induced cardiomyopathy-echocardiographic features. J Am Soc Echocardiogr 18:383, 2005.
158. Hotchkiss RS, Karl IE: The pathophysiology and treatment of sepsis. N Engl J Med 348:138, 2003.
159. Lancel S, Joulin O, Favory R, et al: Ventricular myocyte caspases are directly responsible for endotoxin-induced cardiac dysfunction. Circulation 111:2596, 2005.

160. Milewicz DM, Dietz HC, Miller DC: Treatment of aortic disease in patients with Marfan syndrome. Circulation 111:e150, 2005.
161. Elefteriades JA: Natural history of thoracic aortic aneurysms: Indications for surgery, and surgical versus nonsurgical risks. Ann Thorac Surg 74:S1877, 2002.
162. Habashi JP, Judge DP, Holm TM, et al: Losartan, an AT1 antagonist, prevents aortic aneurysm in a mouse model of Marfan syndrome. Science 312:117, 2006.
163. Veldtman GR, Connolly HM, Orszulak TA, et al: Fate of bicuspid aortic valves in patients undergoing aortic root repair or replacement for aortic root enlargement. Mayo Clin Proc 81:322, 2006.
164. Banerjee S, Jagasia DH: Unruptured sinus of Valsalva aneurysm in an asymptomatic patient. J Am Soc Echocardiogr 15:668, 2002.
165. Agmon Y, Khandheria BK, Meissner I, et al: Is aortic dilatation an atherosclerosis-related process? Clinical, laboratory, and transesophageal echocardiographic correlates of thoracic aortic dimensions in the population with implications for thoracic aortic aneurysm formation. J Am Coll Cardiol 42:1076, 2003.
166. Moore AG, Eagle KA, Bruckman D, et al: Choice of computed tomography, transesophageal echocardiography, magnetic resonance imaging, and aortography in acute aortic dissection: International Registry of Acute Aortic Dissection (IRAD). Am J Cardiol 89:1235, 2002.
167. von Kodolitsch Y, Csosz SK, Koschyk DH, et al: Intramural hematoma of the aorta: predictors of progression to dissection and rupture. Circulation 107:1158, 2003.
168. Evangelista A, Dominguez R, Sebastia C, et al: Long-term follow-up of aortic intramural hematoma: Predictors of outcome. Circulation 108:583, 2003.
169. Tsui KL, Lee KW, Chan WK, et al: Behcet's aortitis and aortic regurgitation: A report of two cases. J Am Soc Echocardiogr 17:83, 2004.

Cardiac Tumors

170. Ngaage DL, Mullany CJ, Daly RC, et al: Surgical treatment of cardiac papillary fibroelastoma: A single center experience with eighty-eight patients. Ann Thorac Surg 80:1712, 2005.
171. Osranek M, Bursi F, Gura GM, et al: Echocardiographic features of pheochromocytoma of the heart. Am J Cardiol 91:640, 2003. Erratum in: Am J Cardiol 92:772, 2003.
172. Mahilmaran A, Seshadri M, Nayar PG, et al: Familial cardiac myxoma: Carney's complex. Tex Heart Inst J 30:80, 2003.

Atrial Fibrillation

173. Tsang TS, Abhayaratna WP, Barnes ME, et al: Prediction of cardiovascular outcomes with left atrial size: Is volume superior to area or diameter? J Am Coll Cardiol 47:1018, 2006.
174. Seidl K, Rameken M, Drogemuller A, et al: Embolic events in patients with atrial fibrillation and effective anticoagulation: Value of transesophageal echocardiography to guide direct-current cardioversion. Final results of the Ludwigshafen Observational Cardioversion Study. J Am Coll Cardiol 39:1436, 2002.
175. Wyse DG, Waldo AL, DiMarco JP, et al: Atrial Fibrillation Follow-up Investigation of Rhythm Management (AFFIRM) Investigators: A comparison of rate control and rhythm control in patients with atrial fibrillation. N Engl J Med 347:1825, 2002.

Congenital Heart Disease

176. Randolph GR, Hagler DJ, Connolly HM, et al: Intraoperative transesophageal echocardiography during surgery for congenital heart defects. J Thorac Cardiovasc Surg 124:1176, 2002.

GUIDELINES *Thomas H. Lee*

Use of Echocardiography

The American College of Cardiology and the American Heart Association (ACC/AHA) published their first joint set of guidelines for the use of echocardiography in 1997.[1] These were updated in 2003,[2] the same year the ACC/AHA, in collaboration with several other professional societies, issued recommendations regarding standards of clinical competence.[3] Recommendations regarding the use of echocardiography are also included in guidelines for specific clinical syndromes, such as management of valvular heart disease (see Chap. 62) and suspected endocarditis (see Chap. 63).

The ACC/AHA guidelines provide recommendations for the use of echocardiography in various clinical settings in which this tool is considered likely or unlikely to contribute information that improves the management of patients. The guidelines include a new section on the use of intraoperative transesophageal echocardiography (TEE) to update guidelines published by the American Society of Anesthesiologists and the Society of Cardiovascular Anesthesiologists.[4] They also make recommendations for the frequency with which Doppler echocardiography should be repeated for some clinical issues. In general, the guidelines urge restraint in the use of echocardiography for patients whose initial evaluations indicated minimal or mild abnormalities, unless there is a change in clinical status. They do not recommend the use of echocardiography for screening purposes, because of the cost and the very real possibility of generating false-positive results that could lead to further testing or inappropriate therapy.

In these guidelines, the term *echocardiography* refers to Doppler analysis, M-mode echocardiography, two-dimensional transthoracic echocardiography (TTE) and, when indicated, TEE.

As with other ACC/AHA guidelines, these use the standard ACC/AHA classification system for indications:

Class I: Conditions for which there is evidence and/or general agreement that the test is useful and effective
Class II: Conditions for which there is conflicting evidence and/or a divergence of opinion about the usefulness/efficacy of performing the test
Class IIa: Weight of evidence or opinion is in favor of usefulness/efficacy
Class IIb: Usefulness or efficacy is less well established by evidence or opinion.
Class III: Conditions for which there is evidence and/or general agreement that the test is not useful or effective and in some cases may be harmful

Three levels are used to rate the evidence on which recommendations have been based. Level A recommendations are derived from data from multiple randomized clinical trials, level B recommendations are derived from a single randomized trial or nonrandomized studies, and level C recommendations are based on the consensus opinion of experts.

Murmurs and Valvular Heart Disease

The ACC/AHA guidelines for the use of echocardiography in patients with known or suspected valvular heart disease reflect the critical role of this test in assessing cardiac structure and function (Table 14G-1). Accordingly, echocardiography is considered appropriate in any patient with cardiorespiratory symptoms and a heart murmur, and any asymptomatic patient with a murmur in whom there is a reasonable probability of structural heart disease. However, the guidelines also emphasize that echocardiography is not a substitute for a careful clinical evaluation. The guidelines repeatedly state that this test is not appropriate for patients with murmurs or other clinical findings that an experienced observer identifies as functional or innocent. Serial or follow-up testing is discouraged in the absence of any change in symptoms or signs. These recommendations are reiterated in the 2006 ACC/AHA guidelines on the management of patients with valvular heart disease.[5]

For patients with known or suspected valvular stenosis, the guidelines support the use of echocardiography for assessing the severity of valvular stenosis and ventricular dysfunction. Reevaluation with echocardiography is considered appropriate with changing symptoms or signs, and also for patients with severe valvular stenosis, even if asymptomatic. Pregnancy in a patient with valvular stenosis is considered a sufficient change in clinical status to justify echocardiographic evaluation.

Doppler echocardiography is the test of choice to evaluate valvular regurgitation and assess the need for surgical intervention. Because left ventricular dysfunction is such a critical issue in the management of many patients, serial use of echocardiography is appropriate for asymptomatic patients with severe regurgitation or with left ventricular dilation, as well as for those with changes in symptoms or signs or who have become pregnant. The guidelines are less supportive of

TABLE 14G-1 ACC/AHA Guidelines for Use of Echocardiography in the Evaluation of Patients with Murmurs or Valvular Heart Disease

Indication	Class I (Indicated)	Class IIa (Good Supportive Evidence)	Class IIb (Weak Supportive Evidence)	Class III (Not Indicated)
Evaluation of heart murmurs	Patients with a murmur and cardiorespiratory symptoms Asymptomatic patients with a murmur and clinical features indicating at least a moderate probability that the murmur reflects structural heart disease	Asymptomatic patients with a murmur and a low probability of heart disease but in whom the diagnosis of heart disease cannot be reasonably excluded by the standard cardiovascular clinical evaluation		Asymptomatic adults with a heart murmur that has been identified by an experienced observer as functional or innocent
Valvular stenosis	Diagnosis; assessment of hemodynamic severity LV and RV size, function, and/or hemodynamics Reevaluation of known valvular stenosis with changing symptoms or signs Assessment of changes in hemodynamic severity and ventricular compensation in patients with known valvular stenosis during pregnancy Reevaluation of asymptomatic patients with severe stenosis	Assessment of the hemodynamic significance of mild to moderate valvular stenosis by stress Doppler echocardiography Reevaluation of patients with mild to moderate aortic stenosis with LV dysfunction or hypertrophy, even without clinical symptoms	Reevaluation of patients with mild to moderate aortic valvular stenosis with stable signs and symptoms Dobutamine echocardiography for the evaluation of patients with low-gradient aortic stenosis and ventricular dysfunction	Routine reevaluation of asymptomatic adult patients with mild aortic stenosis, stable physical signs, and normal LV size and function Routine reevaluation of asymptomatic patients with mild to moderate mitral stenosis and stable physical signs
Native valvular regurgitation	Diagnosis; assessment of hemodynamic severity Initial assessment and reevaluation (when indicated) of LV and RV size, function, and/or hemodynamics Reevaluation of patients with mild to moderate valvular regurgitation with changing symptoms Reevaluation of asymptomatic patients with severe regurgitation Assessment of changes in hemodynamic severity and ventricular compensation in patients with known valvular regurgitation during pregnancy Reevaluation of patients with mild to moderate regurgitation with ventricular dilation without clinical symptoms Assessment of the effects of medical therapy on the severity of regurgitation and ventricular compensation and function when it might change medical management Assessment of valvular morphology and regurgitation in patients with a history of anorectic drug use, or the use of any drug or agent known to be associated with valvular heart disease, who are symptomatic, have cardiac murmurs, or have a technically inadequate auscultatory examination		Reevaluation of patients with mild to moderate mitral regurgitation without chamber dilation and without clinical symptoms Reevaluation of patients with moderate aortic regurgitation without chamber dilation and without clinical symptoms	Routine reevaluation in asymptomatic patients with mild valvular regurgitation with stable physical signs, normal LV size and function Routine repetition of echocardiography in past users of anorectic drugs with normal studies or known trivial valvular abnormalities
Mitral valve prolapse (MVP)	Diagnosis; assessment of hemodynamic severity, leaflet morphology, and/or ventricular compensation in patients with physical signs of MVP	To exclude MVP in patients who have been diagnosed but without clinical evidence to support the diagnosis To exclude MVP in patients with first-degree relatives with known myxomatous valve disease Risk stratification in patients with physical signs of MVP or known MVP		Exclusion of MVP in patients with ill-defined symptoms in the absence of a constellation of clinical symptoms or physical findings suggestive of MVP or a positive family history Routine repetition of echocardiography in patients with MVP with no or mild regurgitation and no changes in clinical signs or symptoms

Continues

TABLE 14G–1 ACC/AHA Guidelines for Use of Echocardiography in the Evaluation of Patients with Murmurs or Valvular Heart Disease—cont'd

Indication	Class I (Indicated)	Class IIa (Good Supportive Evidence)	Class IIb (Weak Supportive Evidence)	Class III (Not Indicated)
Infective endocarditis—native valves	Detection and characterization of valvular lesions, their hemodynamic severity, and/or ventricular compensation* Detection of vegetations and characterizations of lesions in patients with congenital heart disease suspected of having infective endocarditis Detection of associated abnormalities (e.g., abscesses, shunts)* Reevaluation studies in complex endocarditis (e.g., virulent organism, severe hemodynamic lesion, aortic valve involvement, persistent fever or bacteremia, clinical change, or symptomatic deterioration) Evaluation of patients with high clinical suspicion of culture-negative endocarditis* If TTE is equivocal, TEE evaluation of bacteremia, especially staphylococcal bacteremia and fungemia without a known source	Evaluation of persistent nonstaphylococcal bacteremia without a known source* Risk stratification in established endocarditis*	Routine reevaluation in uncomplicated endocarditis during antibiotic therapy	Evaluation of transient fever without evidence of bacteremia or new murmur
Infective endocarditis—prosthetic valves	Detection and characterization of valvular lesions, their hemodynamic severity, and/or ventricular compensation* Detection of associated abnormalities (e.g., abscesses, shunts)* Reevaluation in complex endocarditis (e.g., virulent organism, severe hemodynamic lesion, aortic valve involvement, persistent fever or bacteremia, clinical change, or symptomatic deterioration)* Evaluation of suspected endocarditis and negative cultures* Evaluation of bacteremia without known source*	Evaluation of persistent fever without evidence of bacteremia or new murmur	Routine reevaluation in uncomplicated endocarditis during antibiotic therapy	Evaluation of transient fever without evidence of bacteremia or new murmur
Interventions for valvular heart disease and prosthetic valves	Assessment of the timing of valvular intervention based on ventricular compensation, function, and/or severity of primary and secondary lesions Selection of alternative therapies for mitral valve disease (e.g., balloon valvuloplasty, operative valve repair, valve replacement)* Use of echocardiography (especially TEE) in guiding the performance of interventional techniques and surgery (e.g., balloon valvotomy and valve repair) for valvular disease Postintervention baseline studies for valve function (early) and ventricular remodeling (late) Reevaluation of patients with valve replacement with changing clinical signs and symptoms; suspected prosthetic dysfunction (stenosis, regurgitation) or thrombosis*	Routine reevaluation study after baseline studies of patients with valve replacements with mild to moderate ventricular dysfunction, without changing clinical signs or symptoms	Routine reevaluation at the time of increased failure rate of a bioprosthesis without clinical evidence of prosthetic dysfunction	Routine reevaluation of patients with valve replacements without suspicion of valvular dysfunction and with unchanged clinical signs and symptoms Patients whose clinical status precludes therapeutic interventions

*TEE may provide incremental value in addition to information obtained by TTE.

ACC/AHA = American College of Cardiology/American Heart Association; ECG = electrocardiogram; LV = left ventricular; RV = right ventricular; TEE = transesophageal echocardiography; TTE = transthoracic echocardiography.

routine serial echocardiography for patients with mild to moderate valvular regurgitation without chamber dilation or clinical symptoms, and discourage its use in patients with mild regurgitation who have stable physical signs and normal left ventricular size and function.

The guidelines emphasize that diagnosis of mitral valve prolapse should be made on the basis of the physical examination, in part because of the high rates of false-positive results with echocardiography. Specifically discouraged is the use of echocardiography to exclude mitral valve prolapse in patients with ill-defined symptoms but no other clinical evidence for this condition and the use of serial echocardiography in patients with mild mitral valve prolapse and little or no regurgitation.

Echocardiography is strongly supported in virtually all patients with known or suspected infective endocarditis. (ACC/AHA guidelines on the use of echocardiography in this setting are discussed in the Guidelines in Chap. 63.) Similarly, the guidelines support the use of echocardiography before and after operative interventions for valvular heart disease. The incremental value of transesophageal echocardiography over transthoracic echocardiography is acknowledged for several clinical issues related to patients for whom procedures are contemplated or have been performed. Specific recommendations about the ideal interval for repeat evaluations in patients without changes in symptoms or signs are not made.

Endocarditis of prosthetic valves is more difficult to diagnose than endocarditis of native valves using the transthoracic technique. In these cases, TEE may provide diagnostic value over and above that of TTE.

For the evaluation of prosthetic valves, which is a challenging task, the guidelines recommend obtaining baseline postoperative studies for future comparison and assessment of changes in hemodynamics and ventricular function following surgery. The use of routine reevaluation in patients with unchanged clinical signs and symptoms remains controversial.

Chest Pain and Ischemic Heart Disease

Ischemic heart disease and other cardiac conditions (e.g., pericarditis and acute aortic dissection) are major diagnostic considerations in the evaluation of acute chest pain. Accordingly, the ACC/AHA guidelines support the use of echocardiography when routinely available clinical data, including the electrocardiogram, are not diagnostic in patients with suspected aortic dissection, acute myocardial ischemia, or severe hemodynamic instability (Table 14G-2). This test is not considered necessary for routine use in patients with a high likelihood of myocardial ischemia or infarction or when a noncardiac cause is apparent.

For patients with suspected acute myocardial ischemic syndromes, echocardiography is considered an appropriate tool for detection of ischemia or injury when other data are not conclusive; for evaluations of left and right ventricular function; and for detection of mechanical complications, such as ruptured papillary muscles or a mural thrombus. Once the diagnosis of acute ischemic heart disease is established, the ACC/AHA guidelines support the use of echocardiography to assess the extent of myocardial injury and assess ventricular function, to help assess prognosis as part of pharmacological or exercise stress testing, and to assess myocardial viability in candidates for coronary revascularization. The guidelines are less certain but generally supportive of the use of echocardiography for in-hospital or early post-discharge assessment of inducible ischemia, guidance of therapy during recovery, and assessment of left ventricular function after revascularization (Class IIa).

For patients with chronic ischemic heart disease, the guidelines support echocardiography as appropriate for the diagnosis of myocardial ischemia in symptomatic and other selected patients (see Table 14G-2), assessment of ventricular function, and assessment of myocardial viability and jeopardy through exercise or pharmacological stress testing. However, the guidelines explicitly state that echocardiography should not be routinely substituted "for treadmill exercise

TABLE 14G–2 ACC/AHA Guidelines for Use of Echocardiography in the Evaluation of Patients with Chest Pain and Known or Suspected Ischemic Heart Disease

Indication	Class I (Indicated)	Class IIa (Strong Supportive Evidence)	Class IIb (Weak Supportive Evidence)	Class III (Not Indicated)
Patients with chest pain	Diagnosis of underlying cardiac disease in patients with chest pain and clinical evidence of valvular, pericardial, or primary myocardial disease Evaluation of chest pain in patients with suspected acute myocardial ischemia, when baseline ECG and other laboratory markers are nondiagnostic and when study can be obtained during pain or within minutes after its abatement Evaluation of chest pain in patients with suspected aortic dissection Evaluation of patients with chest pain and hemodynamic instability unresponsive to simple therapeutic measures			Evaluation of chest pain for which a noncardiac cause is apparent Diagnosis of chest pain in a patient with electrocardiographic changes diagnostic of myocardial ischemia or infarction
Diagnosis of acute myocardial ischemic syndromes	Diagnosis of suspected acute ischemia or infarction not evident by standard means Measurement of baseline LV function Evaluation of patients with inferior myocardial infarction and clinical evidence suggesting possible RV infarction Assessment of mechanical complications and mural thrombus*	Identification of location and severity of disease in patients with ongoing ischemia		Diagnosis of acute myocardial infarction already evident by standard means

Continues

TABLE 14G–2 ACC/AHA Guidelines for Use of Echocardiography in the Evaluation of Patients with Chest Pain and Known or Suspected Ischemic Heart Disease—cont'd

Indication	Class I (Indicated)	Class IIa (Strong Supportive Evidence)	Class IIb (Weak Supportive Evidence)	Class III (Not Indicated)
Risk assessment, prognosis, and assessment of therapy in acute myocardial ischemic syndromes	Assessment of infarct size and/or extent of jeopardized myocardium In-hospital assessment of ventricular function when the results are used to guide therapy In-hospital or early postdischarge assessment of the presence and extent of inducible ischemia whenever baseline abnormalities are expected to compromise electrocardiographic interpretation† Assessment of myocardial viability when required to define potential efficacy of revascularization†‡	In-hospital or early postdischarge assessment of the presence and extent of inducible ischemia in the absence of baseline abnormalities expected to compromise electrocardiographic interpretation* Reevaluation of ventricular function during recovery when results are used to guide therapy Assessment of ventricular function after revascularization	Assessment of late prognosis (2 yr or more after acute myocardial infarction)	Routine reevaluation in the absence of any change in clinical status
Diagnosis and prognosis of chronic ischemic heart disease	Diagnosis of myocardial ischemia in symptomatic individuals† Exercise echocardiography for diagnosis of myocardial ischemia in selected patients (those in whom electrocardiographic assessment is less reliable because of digoxin use, LVH or with more than 1 mm ST depression at rest on the baseline ECG, those with pre-excitation (Wolff-Parkinson-White) syndrome, complete left bundle branch block with an intermediate pretest likelihood of CAD Assessment of global ventricular function at rest Assessment of myocardial viability (hibernating myocardium) for planning revascularization‡ Assessment of functional significance of coronary lesions (if not already known) in planning percutaneous transluminal coronary angioplasty†	Prognosis of myocardial ischemia in selected patients (those in whom electrocardiographic assessment is less reliable) with the following abnormalities on the ECG: preexcitation (Wolff-Parkinson-White) syndrome, electronically paced ventricular rhythm, more than 1 mm of ST depression at rest, complete left bundle branch block† Detection of coronary arteriopathy in patients who have undergone cardiac transplantation‡ Detection of myocardial ischemia in women with an intermediate pretest likelihood of CAD†	Assessment of an asymptomatic patient with positive results from a screening treadmill test† Assessment of global ventricular function with exercise†	Screening of asymptomatic persons with a low likelihood of CAD Routine periodic reassessment of stable patients for whom no change in therapy is contemplated Routine substitution for treadmill exercise testing in patients for whom electrocardiographic analysis is expected to suffice†
Assessment of interventions in chronic ischemic heart disease	Assessment of LV function when needed to guide institution and modification of drug therapy in patients with known or suspected LV dysfunction Assessment for restenosis after revascularization in patients with atypical recurrent symptoms†	Assessment for restenosis after revascularization in patients with typical recurrent symptoms† Assessment of LV function in patients with previous myocardial infarction when needed to guide possible implantation of implantable cardioverter-defibrillator (ICD) in patients with known or suspected LV dysfunction		Routine assessment of asymptomatic patients after revascularization

*TEE is indicated when TTE studies are not diagnostic.
†Exercise or pharmacological stress echocardiogram.
‡Dobutamine stress echocardiogram.
ACC/AHA = American College of Cardiology/American Heart Association; CAD = coronary artery disease; ECG = electrocardiogram; LV = left ventricular; LVH = left ventricular hypertrophy; RV = right ventricular; TEE = transesophageal echocardiography; TTE = transthoracic echocardiography.

testing in patients for whom electrocardiographic analysis is expected to suffice."

Cardiomyopathy and Assessment of Left Ventricular Function

Echocardiography is the ideal first test for assessment of global and regional left ventricular function because current techniques enable a comprehensive assessment of left ventricular size and function. It is thus the preferred first-line test for patients with symptoms or signs consistent with impaired left ventricular function (Table 14G-3). TEE is recommended when TTE is not diagnostic. The 2005 ACC/AHA guidelines on diagnosis and management of heart failure recommend performing two-dimensional echocardiography with Doppler during the initial evaluation of patients presenting with heart failure to assess left ventricular ejection fraction, left ventricular size, wall thickness, and valve function.[6] Echocardiography is also recommended for assessment of patients with edema or dyspnea and a high suspicion of clinical heart disease. It provides important insight into the cause of heart failure, and is recommended for patients with suspected hypertrophic cardiomyopathy. restrictive cardiomyopathy, and diastolic dysfunction. Use of the test is discouraged for routine evaluation of clinically stable patients in whom no change in management is contemplated and in patients with edema but normal venous pressures and no evidence of heart disease.

PERICARDIAL DISEASE

Echocardiography remains the test of choice for detection of pericardial effusion, and is an appropriate test for the diagnosis of other pericardial diseases (see Table 14G-3). The guidelines discourage the use of echocardiography for routine follow-up of clinically stable patients with pericardial effusion and when findings are unlikely to change management. They also note that pericardial friction rubs are common after acute myocardial infarction and early after cardiac surgery, and echocardiography is not routinely needed in such settings. Echocardiographic assessment of pericardial thickness to assess the diagnosis of constrictive pericarditis is not supported by these guidelines, which note that other technologies (computed tomography or magnetic resonance imaging) provide more accurate data.

TABLE 14G–3 ACC/AHA Guidelines for Use of Echocardiography in the Evaluation of Left Ventricular Function and Other Cardiac Anatomy

Indication	Class I (Indicated)	Class IIa (Strong Supportive Evidence)	Class IIB (Weak Supportive Evidence)	Class III (Not Indicated)
Patients with dyspnea, edema, or cardiomyopathy	Assessment of LV size and function in patients with suspected cardiomyopathy or clinical diagnosis of heart failure† Edema with clinical signs of elevated central venous pressure when a potential cardiac cause is suspected or when central venous pressure cannot be estimated with confidence and clinical suspicion of heart disease is high† Dyspnea with clinical signs of heart disease Patients with unexplained hypotension, especially in the intensive care unit† Patients exposed to cardiotoxic agents, to determine the advisability of additional or increased dosages Reevaluation of LV function in patients with established cardiomyopathy when there has been a documented change in clinical status or to guide medical therapy Suspicion of hypertrophic cardiomyopathy based on abnormal physical examination, ECG, or family history Contrast echocardiographic assessment of myocardial infarct zone during interventional septal alcohol ablation studies		Reevaluation of patients with established cardiomyopathy when there is no change in clinical status but where the results might change management Reevaluation of patients with edema when a potential cardiac cause has already been demonstrated	Evaluation of LV ejection fraction in patients with recent (contrast or radionuclide) angiographic determination of ejection fraction Routine reevaluation in clinically stable patients in whom no change in management is contemplated and for whom the results would not change management In patients with edema, normal venous pressure, and no evidence of heart disease
Pericardial disease	Patients with suspected pericardial disease, including effusion, constriction, or effusive-constrictive process Patients with suspected bleeding in the pericardial space (e.g., trauma, perforation) Follow-up study to evaluate recurrence of effusion or to diagnose early constriction; repeat studies may be goal-directed to answer a specific clinical question Pericardial friction rub developing in acute myocardial infarction accompanied by symptoms such as persistent pain, hypotension, and nausea	Follow-up studies to detect early signs of tamponade in the presence of large or rapidly accumulating effusions; a goal-directed study may be appropriate Echocardiographic guidance and monitoring of pericardiocentesis	Postsurgical pericardial disease, including postpericardiotomy syndrome, with potential for hemodynamic impairment In the presence of strong clinical suspicion and nondiagnostic TTE, TEE assessment of pericardial thickness to support a diagnosis of constrictive pericarditis	Routine follow-up of small pericardial effusion in clinically stable patients Follow-up studies in patients with cancer or other terminal illness for whom management would not be influenced by echocardiographic findings Assessment of pericardial thickness in patients without clinical evidence of constrictive pericarditis Pericardial friction rub in early uncomplicated myocardial infarction or in the early postoperative period after cardiac surgery

Continues

TABLE 14G–3 ACC/AHA Guidelines for Use of Echocardiography in the Evaluation of Left Ventricular Function and Other Cardiac Anatomy—cont'd

Indication	Class I (Indicated)	Class IIa (Strong Supportive Evidence)	Class IIB (Weak Supportive Evidence)	Class III (Not Indicated)
Patients with cardiac masses and tumors	Evaluation of patients with clinical syndromes and events that suggest an underlying cardiac mass Evaluation of patients with underlying cardiac disease known to predispose to mass formation for whom a therapeutic decision regarding surgery or anticoagulation will depend on the results of echocardiography Follow-up or surveillance studies after surgical removal of masses known to have a high likelihood of recurrence (e.g., myxoma) Patients with known primary malignancies when echocardiographic surveillance for cardiac involvement is part of the disease staging process			Screening persons with disease states likely to result in mass formation but for whom no clinical evidence for the mass exists Patients for whom the results of echocardiography will have no impact on diagnosis or clinical decision-making
Suspected thoracic aortic disease*	Aortic dissection, diagnosis, location, and extent Aortic aneurysm‡ Aortic intramural hematoma Aortic rupture Aortic root dilation in Marfan syndrome or other connective tissue syndromes‡ Degenerative or traumatic aortic disease with clinical atheroembolism Follow-up of aortic dissection, especially when complication or progression is suspected First-degree relative of a patient with Marfan syndrome or other connective tissue disorder for whom TTE is recommended‡	Follow-up of a patient with surgically repaired aortic dissection†		

*TEE is the technique indicated for examination of the entire aorta, especially in emergency situations.
†TEE is indicated when TTE studies are not diagnostic.
‡TTE should be the first choice in these situations, and TEE should only be used if the examination is incomplete or more information is needed.
ACC/AHA = American College of Cardiology/American Heart Association; ECG = electrocardiogram; LV = left ventricular; RV = right ventricular; TEE = transesophageal echocardiography; TTE = transthoracic echocardiography.

CH 14

Cardiac Masses and Tumors

Echocardiography is also the first-line test for detection of cardiac masses and tumors and is therefore considered appropriate in patients with syndromes suggestive of such abnormalities (e.g., patients with arterial emboli of unknown origin or patients with auscultatory findings suggesting intermittent obstruction of intracardiac flow; see Table 14G-3). Other candidates include patients with malignancies with a high incidence of cardiovascular involvement, such as hypernephroma, metastatic melanoma, or malignancies of intrathoracic organs.

Diseases of the Great Vessels

Transthoracic echocardiography is often adequate for detection of abnormalities of the aortic root and proximal pulmonary vasculature, but TEE is a far more sensitive tool for evaluation of most conditions affecting the great vessels. Therefore, TEE is the procedure of choice for evaluation of possible aortic dissection or rupture (see Table 14G-3). Because TTE is a less invasive and expensive procedure than TEE, it is recommended for follow-up of patients after repair of aortic dissection who do not have suspicion of complications or progression and of first-degree relatives of patients with Marfan syndrome or other connective tissue disorders.

Primary Pulmonary and Pulmonary Vascular Disease

Primary pulmonary disease often compromises the quality of TTE, but echocardiography can be an appropriate test for evaluation of the right ventricle and right-sided heart pressures that may be abnormal in patients with conditions such as pulmonary hypertension and pulmonary emboli (Table 14G-4). The guidelines recommend echocardiography for diagnosis of suspected pulmonary hypertension and, when other clinical data are not diagnostic, consider echocardiography to be appropriate for attempts to distinguish cardiac and noncardiac causes of dyspnea. There is somewhat less support for the use of echocardiography for detecting pulmonary emboli and measurement of exercise pulmonary artery pressure. Echocardiography is not considered necessary for routine evaluation of patients with pulmonary disease or patients with pulmonary disease without changes in clinical status.

Systemic Hypertension

Use of echocardiography in patients with hypertension is supported by ACC/AHA guidelines when the assessment of left ventricular function or hypertrophy is likely to influence management. An example of

TABLE 14G–4 ACC/AHA Guidelines for the Use of Echocardiography in the Evaluation of Other Clinical Syndromes

Indications	Class I (Indicated)	Class IIa (Strong Supportive Evidence)	Class IIb (Weak Supportive Evidence)	Class III (Not indicated)
Pulmonary and pulmonary vascular disease	Suspected pulmonary hypertension For distinguishing cardiac versus noncardiac cause of dyspnea in patients in whom all clinical and laboratory clues are ambiguous* Follow-up of pulmonary artery pressures in patients with pulmonary hypertension to evaluate response to treatment Lung disease with clinical suspicion of cardiac involvement (suspected cor pulmonale)	Pulmonary emboli and suspected clots in the right atrium or ventricle or main pulmonary artery branches* Measurement of exercise pulmonary artery pressure Patients being considered for lung transplantation or other surgical procedure for advanced lung disease*		Lung disease without any clinical suspicion of cardiac involvement Reevaluation studies of RV function in patients with chronic obstructive lung disease without a change in clinical status
Hypertension	When assessment of resting LV function, hypertrophy, or concentric remodeling is important in clinical decision-making (see LV function) Detection and assessment of functional significance of concomitant CAD by stress echocardiography (see coronary) Follow-up assessment of LV size and function in patients with LV dysfunction when there has been a documented change in clinical status or to guide medical therapy	Identification of LV diastolic filling abnormalities with or without systolic abnormalities Assessment of LV hypertrophy in a patient with borderline hypertension without LV hypertrophy on ECG to guide decision-making regarding initiation of therapy; limited goal-directed echocardiogram may be indicated for this purpose	Risk stratification for prognosis by determination of LV performance	Reevaluation to guide antihypertensive therapy based on LV mass regression Reevaluation in asymptomatic patients to assess LV function
Neurological events or other vascular occlusive events	Patients of any age with abrupt occlusion of a major peripheral or visceral artery Younger patients (typically younger than 45 yr) with cerebrovascular events Older patients (typically older than 45 yr) with neurological events without evidence of cerebrovascular disease or other obvious cause Patients for whom a clinical therapeutic decision (e.g., anticoagulation) will depend on results of echocardiography	Patients with suspicion of embolic disease and with cerebrovascular disease of questionable significance	Patients with a neurological event and intrinsic cerebrovascular disease of a nature sufficient to cause the clinical event	Patients for whom the results of echocardiography will not affect a decision to institute anticoagulant therapy or otherwise alter the approach to diagnosis or treatment
Arrhythmias and palpitations	Arrhythmias with clinical suspicion of structural heart disease Arrhythmia in a patient with a family history of a genetically transmitted cardiac lesion associated with arrhythmia such as tuberous sclerosis, rhabdomyoma, or hypertrophic cardiomyopathy Evaluation of patients as a component of the workup before electrophysiological ablative procedures	Arrhythmia requiring treatment TEE or intracardiac ultrasound guidance of radiofrequency ablative procedures	Arrhythmias commonly associated with, but without clinical evidence of, heart disease Evaluation of patients who have undergone radiofrequency ablation in the absence of complications (in centers with established ablation programs, a postprocedural echocardiogram may not be necessary) Postoperative evaluation of patients undergoing maze procedure to monitor atrial function	Palpitation without corresponding arrhythmia or other cardiac signs or symptoms Isolated premature ventricular contractions for which there is no clinical suspicion of heart disease

Continues

TABLE 14G-4 ACC/AHA Guidelines for the Use of Echocardiography in the Evaluation of Other Clinical Syndromes—cont'd

Indications	Class I (Indicated)	Class IIa (Strong Supportive Evidence)	Class IIb (Weak Supportive Evidence)	Class III (Not indicated)
Before cardioversion	Patients requiring urgent (not emergent) cardioversion for whom extended precardioversion anticoagulation is not desirable* Patients who have had prior cardioembolic events thought to be related to intra-atrial thrombus* Patients for whom anticoagulation is contraindicated and for whom a decision about cardioversion will be influenced by TEE results* Patients for whom intraatrial thrombus has been demonstrated in previous TEE* Evaluation of patients for whom a decision concerning cardioversion will be affected by knowledge of prognostic factors (such as LV function or coexistent mitral valve disease)	Patients with atrial fibrillation of less than 48-hr duration and other heart disease*	Patients with atrial fibrillation of less than 48-hr duration and no other heart disease* Patients with mitral valve disease or hypertrophic cardiomyopathy who have been on long-term anticoagulation at therapeutic levels before cardioversion, unless there are other reasons for anticoagulation (e.g., prior embolus or known thrombus on previous TEE)* Patients undergoing cardioversion from atrial flutter*	Patients requiring emergent cardioversion Patients who have been on long-term anticoagulation at therapeutic levels and who do not have mitral valve disease or hypertrophic cardiomyopathy before cardioversion unless there are other reasons for anticoagulation (e.g., prior embolus or known thrombus on previous TEE)* Precardioversion evaluation of patients who have undergone previous TEE and with no clinical suspicion of a significant interval change
Syncope	Syncope in a patient with clinically suspected heart disease Periexertional syncope	Syncope in a patient in a high-risk occupation (e.g., pilot)	Syncope of occult cause with no findings of heart disease on history or physical examination	Recurrent syncope in a patient in whom previous echocardiographic or other testing demonstrated a cause of syncope Syncope in a patient for whom there is no clinical suspicion of heart disease Classic neurogenic syncope
Screening	Patients with a family history of genetically transmitted cardiovascular disease Potential donors for cardiac transplantation Patients with phenotypic features of Marfan syndrome or related connective tissue diseases Baseline and reevaluations of patients undergoing chemotherapy with cardiotoxic agents First-degree relatives (parents, siblings, children) of patients with unexplained dilated cardiomyopathy in whom no cause has been identified		Patients with systemic disease that may affect the heart	General population Routine screening echocardiogram for participation in competitive sports in patients with normal cardiovascular history, ECG, and examination
Critically ill patients	Hemodynamically unstable patient Suspected aortic dissection (TEE)			Hemodynamically stable patient not expected to have cardiac disease Reevaluation follow-up studies on hemodynamically stable patients

TABLE 14G–4 ACC/AHA Guidelines for the Use of Echocardiography in the Evaluation of Other Clinical Syndromes—cont'd

Indications	Class I (Indicated)	Class IIa (Strong Supportive Evidence)	Class IIb (Weak Supportive Evidence)	Class III (Not indicated)
Critically injured patients	Serious blunt or penetrating chest trauma (suspected pericardial effusion or tamponade) Mechanically ventilated multiple-trauma or chest trauma patient Suspected preexisting valvular or myocardial disease in the trauma patient Hemodynamically unstable multiple-injury patient without obvious chest trauma but with mechanism of injury suggesting potential cardiac or aortic injury (deceleration or crush) Widening of the mediastinum, postinjury suspected aortic injury (TEE) Potential catheter, guidewire, pacer electrode, or pericardiocentesis needle injury with or without signs of tamponade	Evaluation of hemodynamics in multiple-trauma or chest trauma patients with pulmonary artery catheter monitoring and data disparate with clinical situation Follow-up study on victims of serious blunt or penetrating trauma		Suspected myocardial contusion in the hemodynamically stable patient with a normal ECG who has no abnormal cardiac or thoracic physical findings and/or lacks a mechanism of injury suggesting cardiovascular contusion
Adult patients with congenital heart disease	Patients with clinically suspected congenital heart disease, as evidenced by signs and symptoms such as a murmur, cyanosis, or unexplained arterial desaturation, and an abnormal ECG or radiograph suggesting congenital heart disease Patients with known congenital heart disease on follow-up when there is a change in clinical findings Patients with known congenital heart disease for whom there is uncertainty about the original diagnosis or when the precise nature of the structural abnormalities or hemodynamics is unclear Periodic echocardiograms in patients with known congenital heart lesions and for whom ventricular function and atrioventricular valve regurgitation must be followed (e.g., patients with a functional single ventricle after Fontan procedure, transposition of the great vessels after Mustard procedure, L-transposition and ventricular inversion, and palliative shunts) Patients with known congenital heart disease for whom following pulmonary artery pressure is important (e.g., patients with hemodynamically important, moderate, or large ventricular septal defects, atrial septal defects, single ventricle, or any of the above with an additional risk factor for pulmonary hypertension) Periodic echocardiography in patients with repaired (or palliated) congenital heart disease with the following: change in clinical condition or clinical suspicion of residual defects, obstruction of conduits and baffles, LV or RV function that must be followed, or a possibility of hemodynamic progression or a history of pulmonary hypertension		Follow-up echocardiographic study, annually or once every 2 years, in patients with known hemodynamically significant congenital heart disease without evident change in clinical condition	Multiple repeat echocardiography in patients with repaired patent ductus arteriosus, atrial septal defect, ventricular septal defect, coarctation of the aorta, or bicuspid aortic valve without change in clinical condition Repeat echocardiography in patients with known hemodynamically insignificant congenital heart lesions (e.g., small atrial septal defect, small ventricular septal defect) without a change in clinical condition

Continues

TABLE 14G-4 ACC/AHA Guidelines for the Use of Echocardiography in the Evaluation of Other Clinical Syndromes—cont'd

Indications	Class I (Indicated)	Class IIa (Strong Supportive Evidence)	Class IIb (Weak Supportive Evidence)	Class III (Not indicated)
	To direct interventional catheter valvotomy, radiofrequency ablation, and interventions in the presence of complex cardiac anatomy Identification of site of origin and initial course of coronary arteries (TEE may be indicated for some patients)*			

*TEE is indicated when TTE studies are not diagnostic.

ACC/AHA = American College of Cardiology/American Heart Association; CAD = coronary artery disease; ECG = electrocardiogram; LV = left ventricular; RV = right ventricular; TEE = transesophageal echocardiography; TTE = transthoracic echocardiography.

such a case would be a patient with mild hypertension in whom the detection of left ventricular hypertrophy would lead to initiation of drug therapy. The guidelines explicitly state that not every patient with hypertension should have a left ventricular function assessment and discourage serial echocardiography to assess changes in left ventricular mass as patients are treated.

Neurological Disease and Other Cardioembolic Disease

The ACC/AHA guidelines support the use of echocardiography for the evaluation of patients with embolic events affecting any major peripheral or visceral artery (see Table 14G-4). Echocardiography is considered clearly appropriate in younger patients with cerebrovascular events, older patients with neurological events who have no evidence of cerebrovascular disease, and patients for whom echocardiography can guide clinical decision-making, such as the appropriateness of anticoagulation. Echocardiography is discouraged when results will not influence management.

Arrhythmias and Palpitations

Because arrhythmias can be a manifestation of underlying structural heart disease, the ACC/AHA guidelines consider echocardiography appropriate in several subsets of patient with arrhythmias and palpitations, as well as part of the workup for electrophysiological ablative procedures (see Table 14G-4). There is less support for its use to assess arrhythmias commonly associated with heart disease in the absence of clinical heart disease or to evaluate patients who have undergone radiofrequency or surgical ablative procedures (Class IIb). The use of echocardiography is discouraged in most patients with palpitations or isolated ventricular premature complexes if they have no other evidence for structural or arrhythmic cardiac disease.

Echocardiography can be used to help identify patients most likely to be successfully cardioverted and maintain sinus rhythm, as well to assess the risk of thromboembolic events in patients under atrial fibrillation if the need to proceed to cardioversion is urgent and an extended course of anticoagulation is not desirable (see Table 14G-4). There is also support for this strategy in patients with other heart disease whose duration of atrial fibrillation is less than 48 hours; the guidelines are less bullish on this strategy in patients without other heart disease whose duration of atrial fibrillation is less than 48 hours.

The ACC/AHA guidelines discourage the routine use of echocardiography for the evaluation of classic neurogenic syncope or for patients in whom there is no suspicion of cardiac disease (see Table 14G-4). ACC/AHA guidelines on the evaluation of syncope published in 2006[7] somewhat broaden the use of echocardiography, indicating that it is a helpful screening test when the history, physical examination, and electrocardiogram (ECG) do not provide a diagnosis. Echocardiography is considered appropriate for patients with clinical evidence of cardiac disease or periexertional syncope, and there is limited support for its use in patients with syncope in high-risk professions, such as airline pilots (Class IIa).

Screening

The ACC/AHA guidelines do not support using echocardiography to screen for heart disease in the general population or asymptomatic athletes (see Table 14G-4). Examples of settings in which screening echocardiography may be appropriate include those involving patients with a family history of genetically transmitted cardiovascular diseases, potential donors for heart transplantation, patients with phenotypic features of Marfan syndrome or related connective tissue diseases, first-degree relatives of patients with unexplained dilated cardiomyopathy, and serial evaluation of patients receiving potentially cardiotoxic chemotherapy.

Critically Ill and Injured Patients

Echocardiography is often useful for establishing the diagnosis in hemodynamically unstable, critically ill, and injured patients (see Table 14G-4). TEE is particularly useful in several situations, including:

- The hemodynamically unstable patient with suboptimal TTE images
- The hemodynamically unstable patient on a ventilator
- Major trauma or postoperative patients who cannot be positioned for adequate TTE
- Suspected aortic dissection
- Suspected aortic injury

Adult Patients with Congenital Heart Disease

Echocardiography is useful for diagnosis of congenital heart disease in adults and for follow-up of manifestations of disease, such as ventricular function and hemodynamically significant shunts. The guidelines discourage the overuse of serial echocardiography in patients without changes in clinical status, particularly if they are known to have lesions of minor hemodynamic significance, such as small atrial or ventricular septal defects.

Intraoperative Echocardiography

The use of echocardiography during various adult and pediatric cardiac surgeries has been expanding over the past two decades. Echocardiography is now indicated in the evaluation of serious hemodynamic disturbances with uncertain ventricular function, repair of valvular lesions, hypertrophic obstructive cardiomyopathy, and aortic dissection, evaluation of complex valve replacements, and placement of most intracardiac devices (Table 14G-5). Echocardiography is not

TABLE 14G-5 ACC/AHA Guidelines for Use of Intraoperative Echocardiography

Level of Evidence	Indication
Class I (indicated)	Evaluation of acute, persistent, and life-threatening hemodynamic disturbances in which ventricular function and its determinants are uncertain and have not responded to treatment Surgical repair of valvular lesions, hypertrophic obstructive cardiomyopathy, and aortic dissection with possible aortic valve involvement Evaluation of complex valve replacements requiring homografts or coronary reimplantation, such as the Ross procedure Surgical repair of most congenital heart lesions that require cardiopulmonary bypass Surgical intervention for endocarditis when preoperative testing was inadequate or extension to perivalvular tissue is suspected Placement of intracardiac devices and monitoring of their position during port access and other cardiac surgical interventions Evaluation of pericardial window procedures in patients with posterior or loculated pericardial effusions.
Class IIa (strong supportive evidence)	Surgical procedures in patients at increased risk of myocardial ischemia, myocardial infarction, or hemodynamic disturbances Evaluation of valve replacement, aortic atheromatous disease, maze procedure, cardiac aneurysm repair, removal of cardiac tumors, intracardiac thrombectomy, and pulmonary embolectomy Detection of air emboli during cardiotomy, heart transplant operations, and upright neurosurgical procedures
Class IIb (weak supportive evidence)	Evaluation of suspected cardiac trauma, repair of acute thoracic aortic dissection without valvular involvement, and anastomotic sites during heart and/or lung transplantation Evaluation of regional myocardial function during and after off-pump coronary artery bypass grafting Evaluation of pericardiectomy, pericardial effusions, and pericardial surgery Evaluation of myocardial perfusion, coronary anatomy, or graft patency Dobutamine stress testing to detect inducible demand ischemia or to predict functional changes after myocardial revascularization Assessment of residual duct flow after interruption of patent ductus arteriosus
Class III (not indicated)	Surgical repair of uncomplicated secundum atrial septal defect

ACC/AHA = American College of Cardiology/American Heart Association.

indicated for repair of uncomplicated secundum atrial septal defect, and the benefits and risks of its use in other situations are under investigation.

Standards for Clinical Competence

A joint statement on standards for Clinical Competency was issued in 2003 by the ACC/AHA and other professional societies.[3] It described three levels of expertise and standards for the duration and depth of training. Level I training (3 months, 75 examinations performed, 150 examinations interpreted) constitutes the minimum amount of training that must be achieved by all trainees in adult cardiovascular medicine. Level II training (6 months, 150 cases performed, 300 cases interpreted) is the minimum training for physicians who perform and interpret echocardiograms independently. Level III training (12 months, 300 cases performed, 750 cases interpreted) is appropriate for physicians who direct echocardiography laboratories and supervise quality control systems for interpretation of tests. Different criteria are recommended for experienced echocardiographers who completed training before these guidelines were established.

For competence in TEE, trainees in cardiovascular medicine should perform at least 25 esophageal intubations with an echocardiographic probe and perform approximately 50 TEEs under the supervision of a level III-trained echocardiographer. To maintain competence in TEE, the task force recommends a minimum of 25 to 50 cases/year.

References

1. Cheitlin MD, Alpert JS, Armstrong WF, et al: ACC/AHA Guidelines for the Clinical Application of Echocardiography. A report of the American College of Cardiology/American Heart Association Task Force on Practice Guidelines (Committee on Clinical Application of Echocardiography). Developed in collaboration with the American Society of Echocardiography. Circulation 95:1686, 1997.
2. Cheitlin MD, Armstrong WF, Aurigemma GP, et al: ACC/AHA/ASE 2003 guideline update for the clinical application of echocardiography—summary article: A report of the American College of Cardiology/American Heart Association Task Force on Practice Guidelines (ACC/AHA/ASE Committee to Update the 1997 Guidelines for the Clinical Application of Echocardiography). J Am Coll Cardiol 42:954, 2003.
3. Quinones MA, Douglas PS, Foster E, et al: American College of Cardiology/American Heart Association clinical competence statement on echocardiography: A report of the American College of Cardiology/American Heart Association/American College of Physicians—American Society of Internal Medicine Task Force on Clinical Competence. Circulation 107:1068, 2003.
4. Practice guidelines for perioperative transesophageal echocardiography. A report by the American Society of Anesthesiologists and the Society of Cardiovascular Anesthesiologists Task Force on Transesophageal Echocardiography. Anesthesiology 84:986, 1996.
5. Bonow RO, Carabello BA, Kanu C, et al: ACC/AHA 2006 guidelines for the management of patients with valvular heart disease: A report of the American College of Cardiology/American Heart Association Task Force on Practice Guidelines (writing committee to revise the 1998 Guidelines for the Management of Patients With Valvular Heart Disease): Developed in collaboration with the Society of Cardiovascular Anesthesiologists: endorsed by the Society for Cardiovascular Angiography and Interventions and the Society of Thoracic Surgeons. Circulation 114:e84, 2006.
6. Hunt SA, Abraham WT, Chin MH, et al: ACC/AHA 2005 Guideline Update for the Diagnosis and Management of Chronic Heart Failure in the Adult: A report of the American College of Cardiology/American Heart Association Task Force on Practice Guidelines (Writing Committee to Update the 2001 Guidelines for the Evaluation and Management of Heart Failure): Developed in collaboration with the American College of Chest Physicians and the International Society for Heart and Lung Transplantation: endorsed by the Heart Rhythm Society. Circulation 112:e154, 2005.
7. Strickberger SA, Benson DW, Biaggioni I, et al: AHA/ACCF scientific statement on the evaluation of syncope: from the American Heart Association Councils on Clinical Cardiology, Cardiovascular Nursing, Cardiovascular Disease in the Young, and Stroke, and the Quality of Care and Outcomes Research Interdisciplinary Working Group; and the American College of Cardiology Foundation In Collaboration With the Heart Rhythm Society. J Am Coll Cardiol 47:473, 2006.

CHAPTER 15

The Chest Radiograph in Cardiovascular Disease

Michael A. Bettmann

The chest radiograph was one of the first clinical studies to use the then-new technology of diagnostic x-ray.[1] The major variables that determine the diagnostic value of the chest x-ray include the specific technical factors involved in producing the radiographs, patient-specific factors (e.g., body habitus, age, physiological status, ability to stand and to take and hold a deep breath), and training, experience, and focus of the interpreter. This chapter aims to review how chest radiographs are obtained, to present a basic approach on how to interpret them, and to discuss and illustrate common and characteristic findings relevant to cardiovascular disease in adults.

TECHNICAL CONSIDERATIONS

The usual chest radiograph consists of a frontal and a lateral view. The frontal view is a posteroanterior (PA) view, with the patient standing with the chest toward the film or other recording medium and the back to the x-ray tube. The lateral is also taken with the patient standing, with the left side toward the film. For both, the x-ray tube is kept at a distance of 6 feet from the film. The rationale for these conventions is based on simple physics. X-rays are created by first inducing a high current across a diode, thereby generating electrons. These electrons are aimed at a metal target. When the electrons interact with the target, x-ray photons are produced. To prevent overheating and destruction of the target, it is made to rotate at a high speed, so that over a brief period of time, the x-rays are produced from different portions of this rotating anode. The anode has an angled edge, so the x-rays emerge at essentially a right angle to the incoming electron beam. The x-rays are allowed to emerge from the tube housing only through a small opening, the focal spot. The smaller the focal spot, the higher must be the energy applied to deliver a given number of photons. Also, the smaller the focal spot, the narrower the x-ray beam, leading to improved imaging geometry. The ability of the x-rays to penetrate structures is determined by the combination of the kilovoltage, milliamperage, and time used to produce them—in other words, by the characteristics of the electron beam directed at the target that result in the production of the x-ray photons. These factors are also the major (but not sole) determinants of the exposure that the patient receives.[2,3]

In theory, x-rays emerge from the x-ray tube as a point source, remain parallel, and do not diverge from each other; there is no geometrical distortion of structures as they pass through the body and are recorded on film. In reality, however, the x-rays form a cone-shaped beam, diverging from the focal spot and becoming less parallel as the distance from the focal spot increases. When the incident x-rays interact with film or other recording medium, there is geometrical distortion as a function of the distance from the midline of the x-ray beam and the distance of the structure from the film. If one imagines a wide-diameter structure, such as the thorax, that is perpendicular to the center of the x-ray beam, the farther an object is from the tube, the more parallel are the x-rays that penetrate it (Fig. 15-1). Conversely, the closer the object and the film are to the X-ray tube, the more the incident x-rays must diverge to cover the edges of the object. Thus, the farther an object is from the source, the less geometrical distortion is encountered. The greater the distance from the source, however, the more energy must be applied to penetrate the object to be imaged and to expose the x-ray film. In simple terms, resolution is improved by increasing the source-image distance (SID) but tube energy and thus exposure to the patient must also be increased as the SID is increased. To balance these opposing concerns, a standard convention has been developed—routine standing chest radiographs are obtained with an SID of 6 feet.

X-rays are blocked from the film or other recording medium to varying degrees by various structures, leading to shades of gray that allow discrimination between the heart, which is fluid filled and is relatively impervious to x-rays, and the air-filled lung parenchyma, which blocks few x-rays. The exposure the patient receives is a function of the strength and duration of the current applied to the x-ray tube (or, more accurately, of the strength and duration of the x-ray photons produced), size of the focal spot, length of the exposure, distance from the tube to the patient, and degree to which the x-rays are blocked within the patient. Most patient exposure is caused not by the x-rays that penetrate but rather by those that interact with tissues, are slowed and changed, and in the process deposit residual energy in tissue. This process is what is broadly referred to as scatter. As the amount of tissue that attenuates photons increases, the amount of energy deposition within the patient will increase. Patients who are very thin require an inherently lower x-ray dose to achieve diagnostically satisfactory deposition of x-ray photons on an imaging medium, and have less energy deposition within the body. In patients who are obese, a higher x-ray dose is necessary to penetrate the patient and produce a diagnostic exposure. Such patients also cause more dispersion of the x-ray beam and will receive a higher dose.

Scatter not only leads to deposition of energy in the patient, but also deposits energy on surrounding structures. This

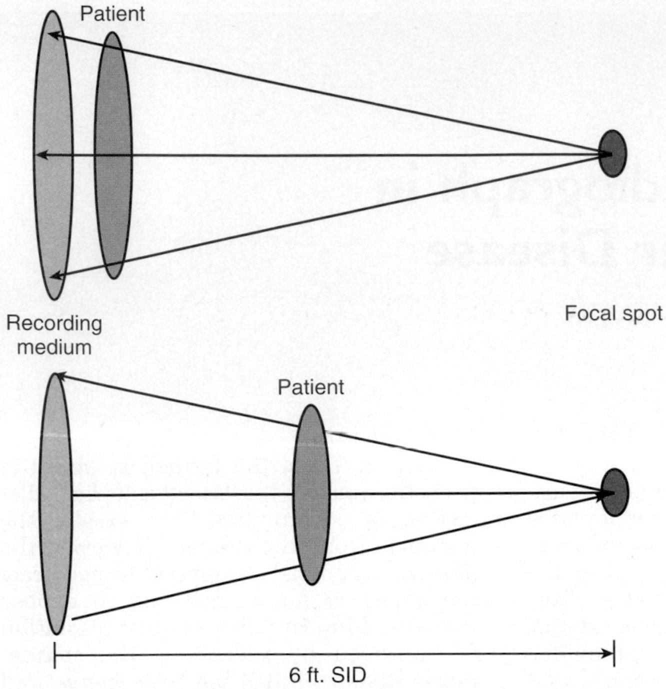

FIGURE 15–1 Position of the patient in relation to the source-image distance (SID) between x-ray source (focal spot) and recording medium. The closer the patient is to the source, the greater the x-ray divergence and the resulting geometric distortion.

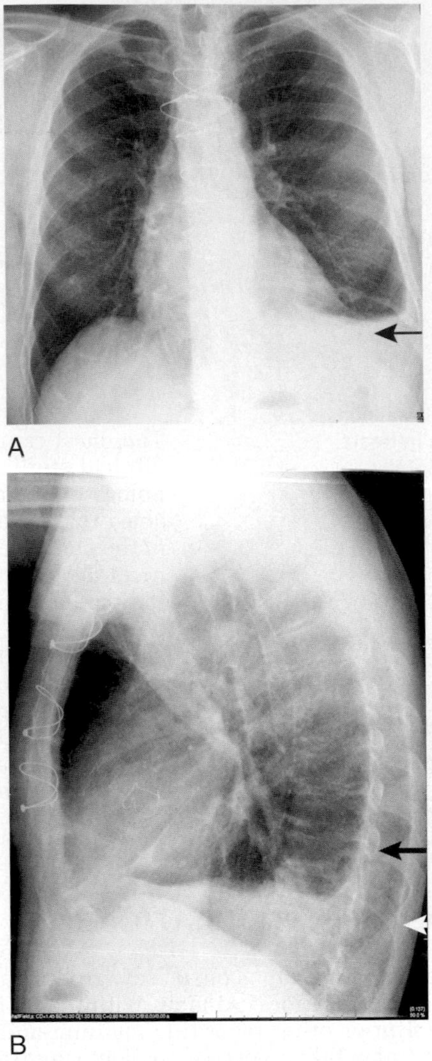

FIGURE 15–2 Standard upright chest radiographs of a 74-year-old man who has undergone aortic valve replacement. **A,** Posteroanterior (PA) view shows median sternotomy wires, a left pleural effusion (arrow), and normal pulmonary vascular pattern. **B,** Lateral view. Note that the right ribs (white arrow) are magnified compared with the left (black arrow), and the effusion can be localized to the left. Also, note that the gastric air bubble is displaced inferiorly (PA) and anteroinferiorly (lateral), indicating an enlarged left ventricle.

includes personnel, if they are close to the patient (as with fluoroscopy), and also the recording medium. That is, the film or other recording medium is altered by incident x-rays to produce an image but is also altered by scatter, which does not reflect anatomical structures but will detract from the resolution of these structures. The more scatter deposited on the recording medium, the more the image quality is denigrated and the worse the resolution. This is in part why the resolution of chest radiographs is lower in heavier than in thinner patients when all other factors remain constant.

Several additional practical observations can be made based on the physics of chest radiographs. The standard chest radiograph is obtained with deep inspiration and the patient facing the film. If patients are unable to stand, chest radiographs are generally obtained with their chest toward the tube and their back toward the film (i.e., in the anteroposterior [AP] position). With the standard PA (posteroanterior) view, the heart appears smaller and its size and contour are more accurately depicted than on an AP view. With AP views, which are standard for portable films, there is a resultant greater divergence of x-rays because the heart lies relatively anteriorly (and thus farther from the film) and the SID is short. Similarly, on a standard lateral film, the right ribs appear larger than the left (Fig. 15-2). In both cases, this effect occurs because a structure is further from the film. As a result, there is increased divergence of the x-rays from the midline point source, and relative magnification. The side of an effusion, therefore, can generally be delineated on a lateral radiograph by determining whether the effusion is associated with the side on which the ribs appear larger or appear smaller (see Fig. 15-2).

There are several inherent practical limitations to portable chest radiographs. Most are obtained with patients positioned supine or semisupine. The degree of inspiration is therefore likely to be substantially less than with an erect film, making the heart appear relatively larger and providing less optimal visualization of the lungs, because they are not optimally expanded. Furthermore, portable radiographs are invariably taken as AP views and the SID is less than 6 feet, of necessity, because of the nature of the portable x-ray machine and the usual position of the patient, sitting or lying in a bed. Most portable x-ray units are not able to generate sufficient energy to penetrate a patient adequately and to expose the film from 6 feet. Space constraints and the patient's position are additional disadvantages. Also, because exposure time must usually be longer than with fixed units, cardiac and respiratory motion are more likely to interfere, and edge definition is compromised. For all these reasons, the inherent resolution is poorer with portable radiographs, and the accuracy is limited. Because of the lower available kilovoltage with portable x-ray units and the longer exposure time necessary, radiation exposure to the patient is also higher than with a standard PA film. Portable films are most useful for answering relatively simple questions, such as whether the pacemaker or implantable cardioverter-defibrillator (ICD) is properly positioned, the endotracheal tube is in the correct location, and the mediastinum is in the midline (Fig. 15-3).[2,4]

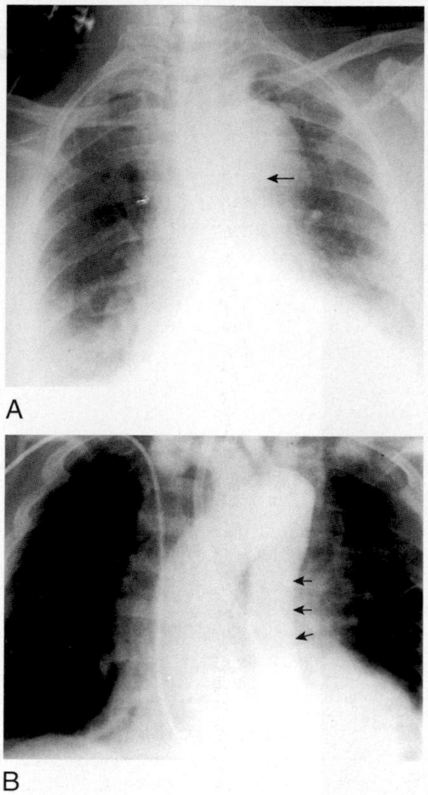

FIGURE 15–3 **A,** Portable chest radiograph of a 70-year-old man with spontaneous dissection of the thoracic aorta. The portable frontal view cannot accurately demonstrate heart size or pulmonary vascularity but shows a double density (arrow) at the level of the descending aorta. Note also the widened superior mediastinum, with the nasogastric tube deviated toward the right. **B,** Levo phase of a right-heart angiogram shows an evident Stanford type B dissection, with a flap (arrows) beginning at the level of the left subclavian artery, and filling of the true (but not the false) lumen of the descending aorta.

Image Recording

Chest radiographs have generally been recorded on high-resolution x-ray film. With optimal technique and a cooperative patient who can hold a deep inspiration, the result is a study that clearly and accurately depicts very small structures, such as the contour of small pulmonary arteries. With x-ray film, the incident x-rays (and scattered photons) alter silver iodide crystals in an emulsion. When the film is developed, these alterations produce an image reflecting the extent to which x-rays have interacted with specific areas of the film. There is inherently very high resolution of structures because of the small size of the silver iodide crystals and their sensitivity to incident x-ray photons.

Increasingly, chest radiographs are being stored on digital media. There are two principal ways to do this. The first, less expensive approach, has been called computed radiography (CR). It is essentially a digital conversion of conventionally obtained chest radiographs. With this method, x-rays are recorded on a reusable imaging screen, much like a fluoroscopic screen but with the ability to provide better resolution, and the image is converted to a digital format in which it is postprocessed, reviewed, and stored. The second method, DR, a filmless form of radiography, is the direct recording of images by digital means, without conversion of analog to digital information. There is an inherent difference, with the elimination of added noise and lost information that occurs with this conversion. True DR can be carried out by various means. The most promising is flat plate technology because of better resolution, usefulness, and, over the long term, cost. It involves the use of an image-sensing plate that directly converts the incident photons into a digital signal rather than producing a transient conversion, as with an image intensifier, a reusable CR plate, or alteration of a silver iodide crystal in a film emulsion. DR is truly filmless and CR can be either; the classic chest radiograph relies on film that is exposed and developed.[5-13]

Resolution with DR may be marginally decreased because the pixel size is larger than that of the silver iodide crystals in the emulsion on x-ray film, although this is a function of the specific system used as well as of the exposure factors.[3,6,13] If there is a decrease, it is generally below the ability of the eye to detect and does not worsen the diagnostic usefulness of the resultant image.[5,6,9] Currently, DR equipment is more costly than standard radiographic or CR rooms.

Both DR and CR have significant advantages for several reasons. First, with the widespread adoption of picture archiving and communication systems (PACS), films that are obtained digitally or directly converted to digital format are immediately available for review at any location at which there is a PACS-enabled workstation. This system obviates the problem of lost films (all films are digitally archived) and the need to go to a remote location to review a film.[14,15] Also, each film is available for review immediately after it is obtained and stored. The dose to an individual patient may or may not be lower; this is a function of patient factors and the specific imaging system.[3,10,11] The overall exposure to patients, however, is decreased because the need to repeat films because of inadequate positioning or exposure is substantially eliminated. This occurs because digital radiography provides the ability to manipulate the image after it is obtained; the relative density (window and level), magnification, and even area included can be altered without re-exposing the patient, which adds substantial information to the examination (Fig. 15-4). Storage of conventional x-ray films is relatively straightforward, although time- and space-intensive. Storage of digital images is clearly more complex, but eliminates many of the major problems encountered with storage of standard x-ray films. Most PACS, rather than using stand-alone systems, now use large-volume local storage devices and the Internet for gaining access to images, further simplifying availability. Integration with hospital-wide information systems allows improved access and use compared with what was available even a decade ago.[16]

THE NORMAL CHEST RADIOGRAPH

Interpreting standard PA and lateral chest radiographs is a daunting task. The amount of information is huge, and there are countless relevant variables. It is imperative to have a systematic and standardized approach, based on an assessment first of anatomy and then of physiology. Any approach must, of course, be based on an understanding of what is normal.[17,18]

In the standard PA chest study, the overall heart diameter is normally less than 50 percent of the transverse diameter of the thorax (Fig. 15-5). The heart overlies the thoracic spine, roughly three fourths to the left of the spine and one fourth to the right. The mediastinum is narrow superiorly and, normally, the descending aorta can be defined from the arch to the dome of the diaphragm, on the left. Below the aortic arch, the pulmonary hila are seen, slightly higher on the left than the right. On the lateral film (Fig. 15-6), the left main pulmonary artery can be seen coursing superiorly and posteriorly compared with the right. On both frontal and lateral views, the ascending aorta (aortic root) is normally obscured by the main pulmonary artery and both atria. The location of the pulmonary outflow tract is usually clear on the lateral film.

Cardiac Chambers and Aorta

On the PA view, the right contour of the mediastinum contains the right atrium but also the ascending aorta and the superior vena cava. The right ventricle is located partially overlying the left ventricle on

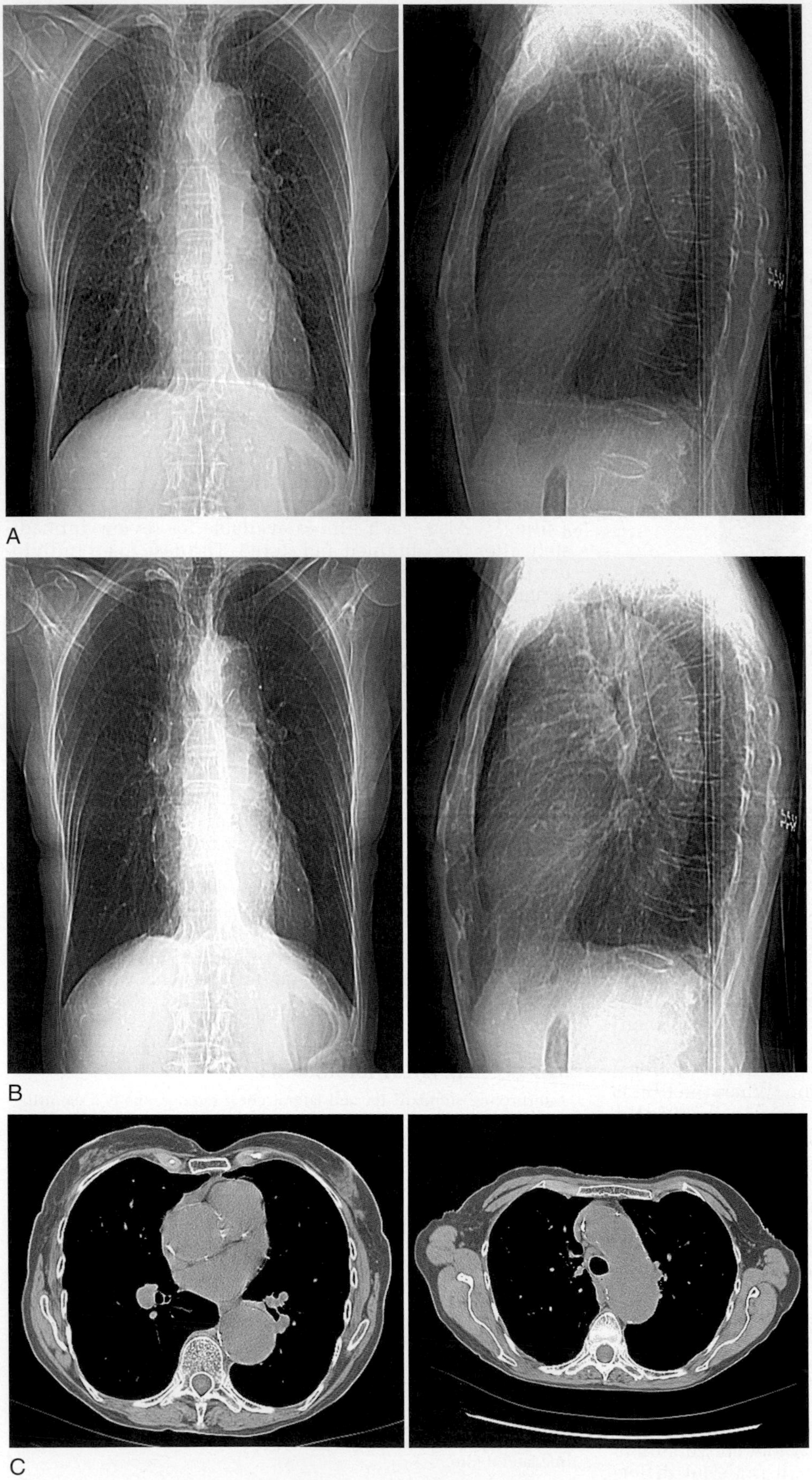

FIGURE 15–4 A and **B,** Posteroanterior and lateral digital chest radiographs with different window and leveling. **A,** With pulmonary window and level, the lung fields, including the pulmonary vascularity, are well visualized, but the mediastinal structures are not well defined. **B,** Rewindowed, the mediastinal structures are now well visualized, showing a dilated, calcified aortic root and descending thoracic aorta. The pulmonary vascularity cannot be defined in these images. **C,** Computed tomography scans at the level of the aortic root (left) and arch (right) confirm marked ectasia of the entire thoracic aorta.

both frontal and lateral views.[19] The left atrium is located just inferior to the left pulmonary hilum. In normal individuals, there is a concavity at this level, which is the location of the left atrial appendage. The atrium constitutes the upper portion of the posterior contour of the heart on the lateral film but cannot normally be differentiated from the left ventricle. The left ventricle constitutes the prominent rounded apex of the heart on the frontal view, as well as the sloping inferior portion of the mediastinum on the lateral (see Figs. 15-5 and 15-6).

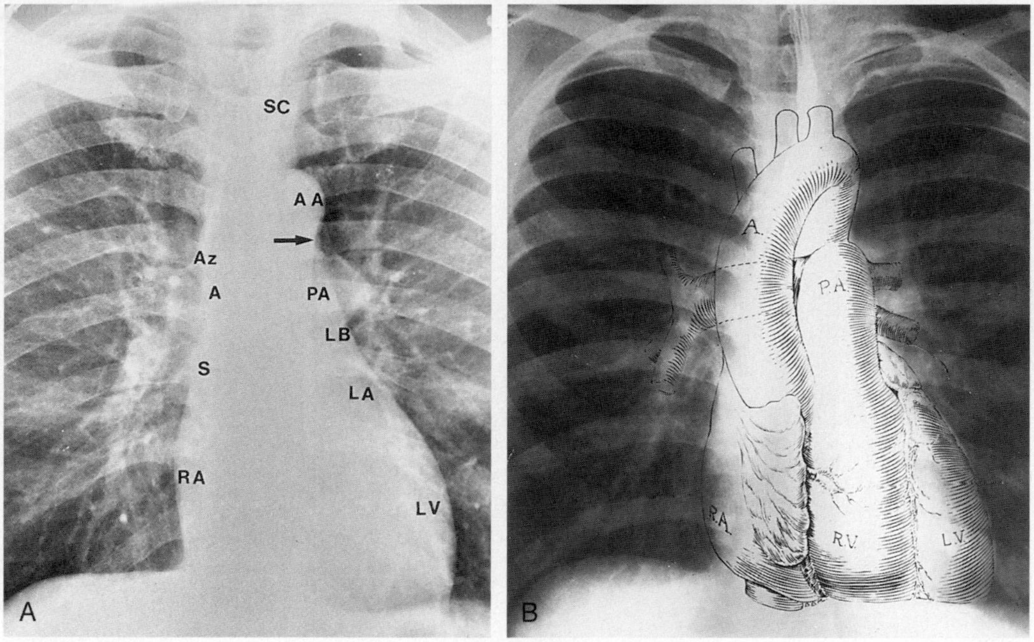

FIGURE 15–5 Frontal projection of the heart and great vessels. **A,** Left and right heart borders in the frontal projection. **B,** Line drawing in the frontal projection demonstrates the relationship of the cardiac valves, rings, and sulci to the mediastinal borders. A = ascending aorta; AA = aortic arch; Az = azygous vein; LA = left atrial appendage; LB = left lower border of pulmonary artery; LV = left ventricle; PA = main pulmonary artery; RA = right atrium; S = superior vena cava; SC = subclavian artery.

The apex is often not clearly delineated for a reason related to x-ray attenuation. A fat pad of varying thickness surrounds the apex of the heart (Figs. 15-7 and 15-8). Fat has a density greater than that of air and marginally less than that of blood. As it covers the ventricular apex, the fat pad is relatively thick and dense. As it thins out toward the left lateral chest wall, it is progressively less dense—hence the hazy, poorly marginated appearance of the apex. Similarly, a fat pad may be seen on the lateral chest film as a wedge-shaped density overlying the anterior aspect of the left ventricle. The pericardial sac cannot normally be defined (Fig. 15-9). Normally, the borders of the cardiac silhouette are moderately but not completely sharp in contour. Even though the exposure time for a chest x-ray is very short (less than 100 milliseconds), there is usually sufficient cardiac motion to cause minor haziness of the silhouette. If a portion of the heart border does not move, as in the case of a left ventricular aneurysm, the border may be unusually sharp (Fig. 15-10). The aortic arch, however, is usually visible, because the aorta courses posteriorly and is surrounded by air. Most of the descending aorta is also visible. The position and the size of each can be easily evaluated (see Fig. 15-4) using the frontal and lateral views.

The contour that the inferior vena cava (IVC) makes with the heart is clearly seen on the lateral film (see Fig. 15-2B). Its relationship to the cardiac contour varies markedly, depending on minor degrees of rotation of the patient. That is, the IVC lies on the right of the mediastinum and posterior to the contour of the heart. This contour is made up of the left atrium and ventricle, which lie toward the left side of the thorax. If the patient is placed laterally, with the left side against the film, the right is relatively slightly magnified compared with the left (see Fig. 15-2B). If the patient rotates minimally anterior or posterior to true lateral, the relationship between the IVC and the left-sided contours changes substantially. This anatomical relationship is important to understand, because in the past a formula was used to determine left ventricular enlargement as a function of its relationship to the IVC (referred to as the Rigler sign).[20] This sign, although sometimes still used, is not accurate and should not be relied on.[21,22]

Lungs and Pulmonary Vasculature

Lung size varies as a function of inspiratory effort, age, body habitus, water content, and intrinsic pathological processes. For example, because lung distensibility decreases with age, with normal aging the lungs appear subtly but progressively smaller, even with maximal inspiratory effort. As lung expansion decreases with age, the heart appears relatively slightly larger, even though it may not actually change in size. However, the heart does not exceed half the transverse diameter of the chest in a good-quality PA film unless there is true cardiomegaly. Conversely, left ventricular dysfunction may lead to interstitial fluid in the lungs and decreased lung compliance, and therefore expansion as seen on a chest x-ray decreases. In chronic obstructive pulmonary disease, with or without bulla formation, the lungs appear both larger and blacker, the diaphragm may appear flattened, and the heart often appears small or normal in size, even in the presence of cardiac dysfunction.

In normal subjects, pulmonary vascularity has a predictable pattern.[23] Pulmonary arteries are usually easily visible centrally in the hila and progressively less so more peripherally. The central main right and left pulmonary arteries are usually not individually identifiable, because they lie within the mediastinum (see Figs. 15-5 and 15-6). If the lung is considered in three zones, the major arteries are central, the clearly distinguishable midsized pulmonary arteries (third or fourth order branches) are in the middle zone, and the small arteries and arterioles, which are normally below the limit of resolution, are in the outer zone. The visible small and midsized arteries have sharp, clearly definable margins because of the sharp border between water density and air density structures. In the standard, standing PA chest film, the arteries in the lower zone are larger than those in the upper zone and are at an equal distance from the hila, related to the effect of gravity on the normal, low-pressure lung circulation. This effect of gravity on the distribution of normal intravascular lung volume is reflected in a normal perfusion lung scan; because the radionuclide is generally administered with the patient supine, there is a greater concentration posteriorly than anteriorly, as confirmed in the count rates. If the patient is sitting or standing when the radionuclide is injected, the count rate is higher at the lung base than at the apices.

The angles that the lungs make with the diaphragm are normally very sharp and can be delineated bilaterally on frontal and lateral views. The pleura is usually tightly applied and is not separated from the ribs on the PA or lateral view.

Normal Variations

Anatomical variables and aging present challenges in the evaluation of chest radiographs, in addition to those posed by decreased lung compliance. The aorta and great vessels normally dilate and become more tortuous and prominent with increasing age, leading to widening of the superior mediastinum. As noted, the heart appears larger because of decreasing lung compliance. Patients who are obese are likely to have a degree of inhibition of maximal lung expansion that may make a normal heart appear slightly larger. Patients with pectus excavatum have a narrowed AP diameter of the chest, increasing the transverse diameter. Consequently, the heart may appear enlarged on the frontal view but the narrow AP diameter seen on the lateral view explains this. There may also be lack of definition of the right heart border on the frontal view because of compression by the sternum. Marked

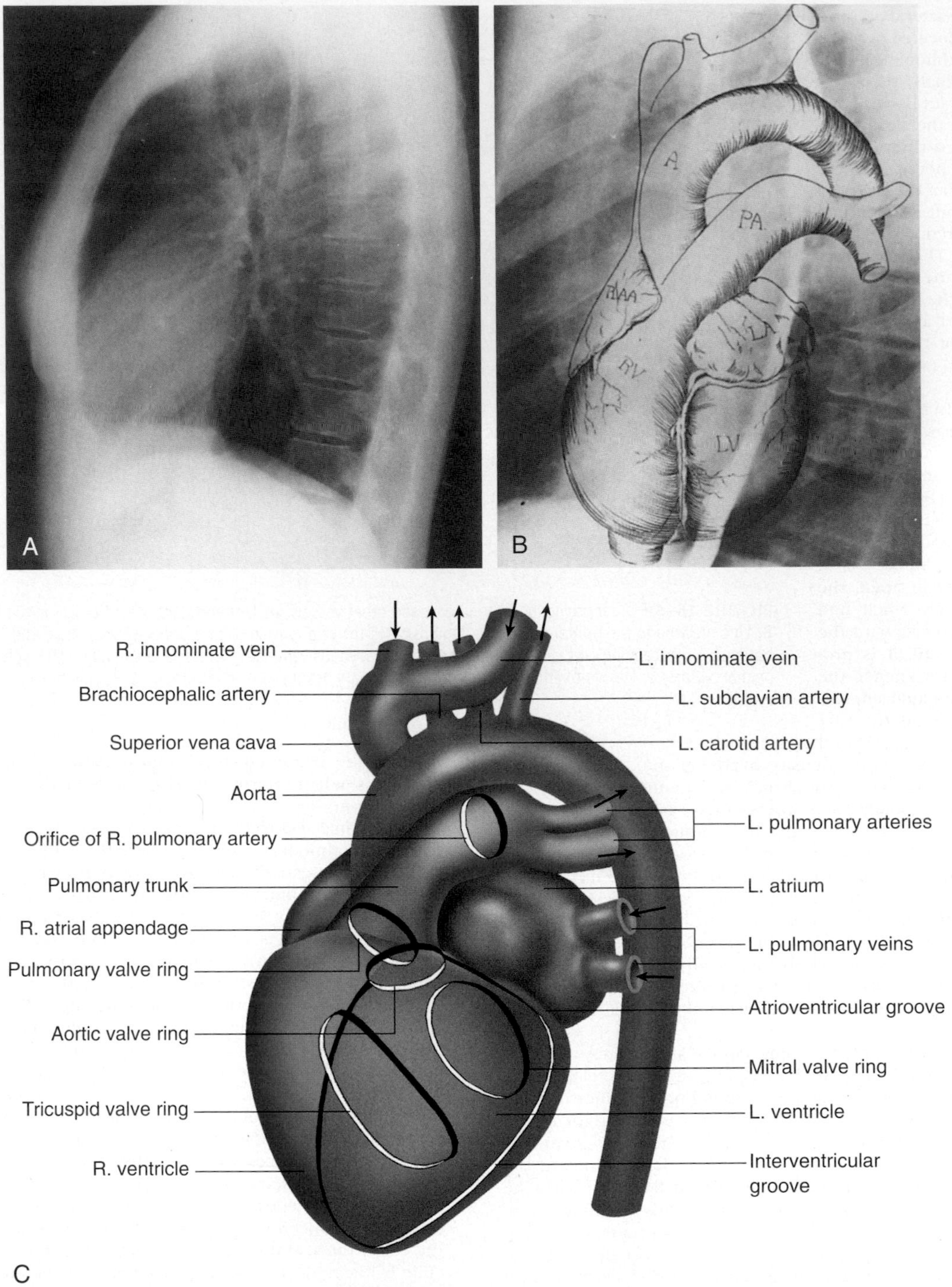

FIGURE 15–6 A, Lateral chest radiograph. **B,** Superimposed anatomical drawing of the cardiac chambers and great vessels. **C,** Diagram of the lateral projection of the heart showing the position of the cardiac chambers, valve rings, and sulci. Arrows indicate direction of blood flow.

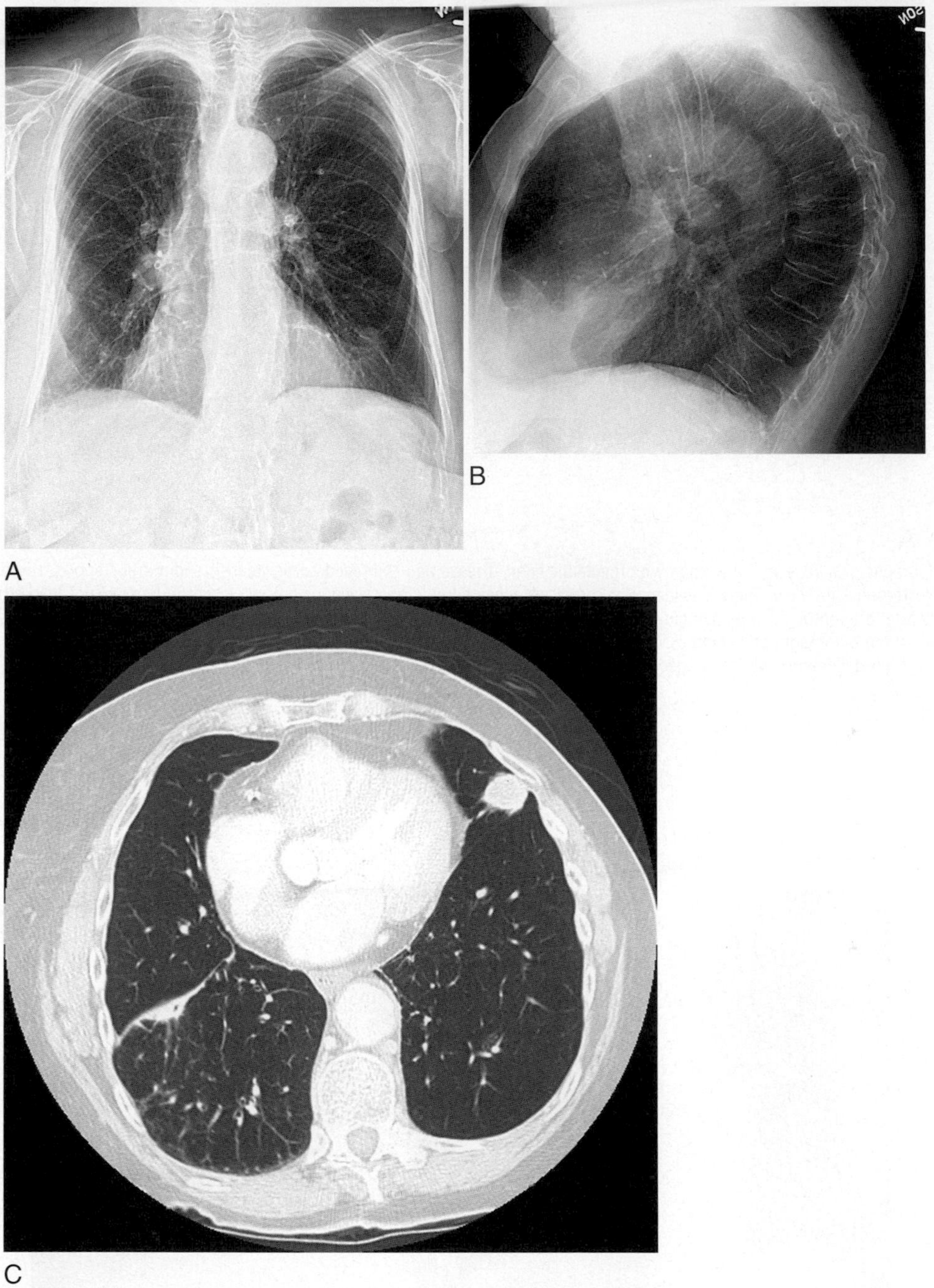

FIGURE 15–7 Posteroanterior (PA) **(A)** and lateral **(B)** chest radiographs show prominent apical fat pad, with suggestion of rounded density seen on PA but not lateral view. Fat pad is manifest in the gradual decrease in density over the left ventricular apex on the frontal view and the triangle-shaped density overlying the anterior aspect of the left ventricular contour on the lateral view. **C,** Computed tomography scan shows fat surrounding much of the cardiac silhouette, as well as a mass in the left lung and thickening of the major fissure in the right lung.

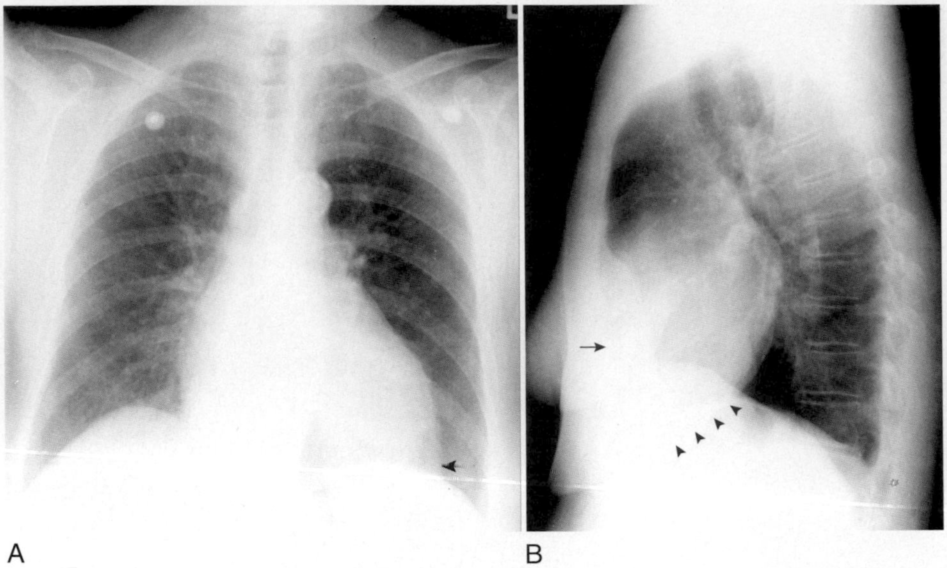

FIGURE 15–8 Chest radiographs of a 70-year-old woman with rheumatic heart disease and combined aortic stenosis and mitral stenosis. Her pulmonary capillary wedge pressure is 30 mm Hg. **A,** Posteroanterior view. There is evidence of chronically elevated pulmonary venous pressures with moderate (not marked) pulmonary vascular redistribution. There is moderate left ventricular enlargement and prominence of the left atrial appendage. **B,** Lateral view. Note enlargement of the left ventricle (arrowheads), extending below the diaphragm and compressing the gastric bubble. Also note the apical fat pad, seen as the hazy density on the frontal view (**A,** arrow), and the anterior, retrosternal, well-delineated, wedge-shaped density on the lateral view (**B,** arrow).

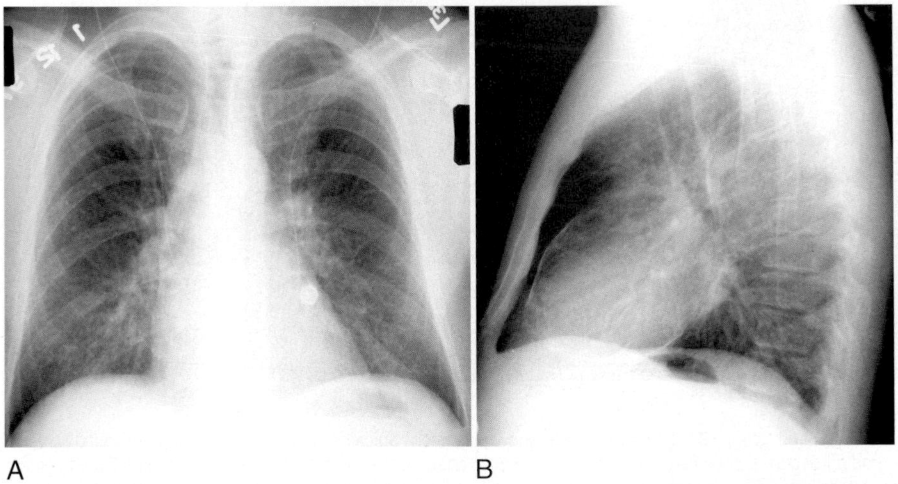

FIGURE 15–9 Chest radiographs of a 45-year-old man with calcific pericarditis. **A,** Posteroanterior view is essentially normal. **B,** Lateral view demonstrates thin, irregular calcification of pericardium around the left ventricular contour.

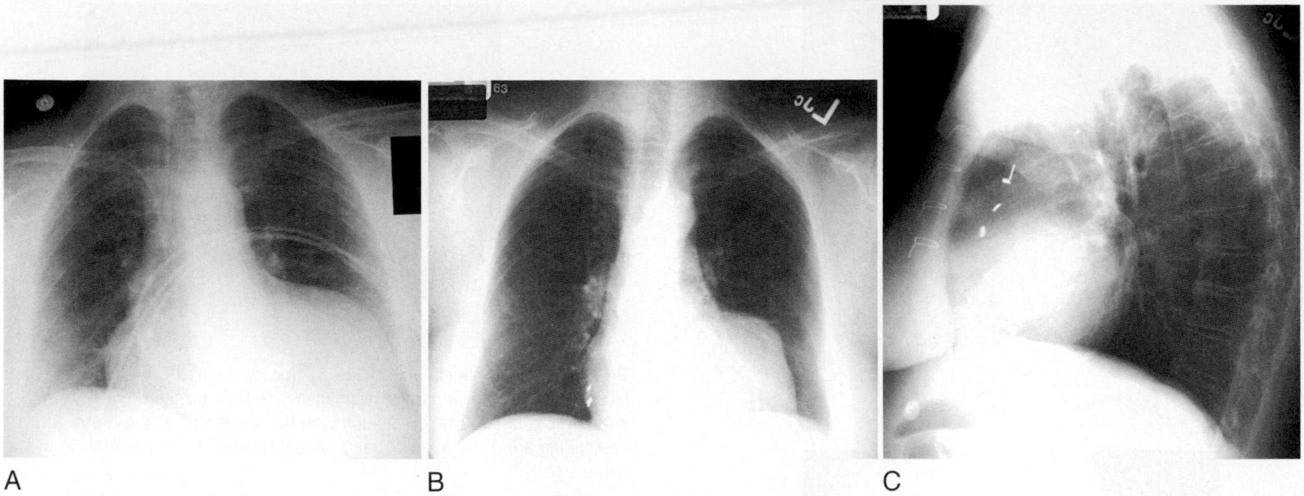

FIGURE 15-10 Chest radiographs of a 53-year-old woman with coronary artery disease and heart failure following a large anterolateral myocardial infarction. **A,** Frontal portable view suggests cardiomegaly and heart failure. Sharp horizontal contour of the left ventricle is suggestive of anterior wall aneurysm. Posteroanterior **(B)** and lateral **(C)** views after revascularization and aneurysmectomy demonstrate persistence of an abnormal contour of the left ventricle, consistent with recurrent aneurysm, and clips on side branches of the saphenous vein graft to the right coronary artery.

kyphosis or scoliosis can also cause the heart or mediastinum to look abnormal. It is thus important to evaluate the spine and other bone structures systematically when looking at a chest radiograph. Delineation of all anatomical abnormalities is beyond the scope of this chapter. For an in-depth discussion, *Fraser and Pare's Diagnosis of Diseases of the Chest*[24] remains a useful reference.

EVALUATING THE CHEST RADIOGRAPH IN HEART DISEASE

There is no single best way to read a chest film, but a systematic approach to the evaluation of a chest radiograph is imperative to distinguish normal from abnormal and to define the underlying pathology and pathophysiology. The first step is to decide what type of film is being evaluated—PA and lateral, PA alone, or AP (either portable or one obtained in the AP view because the patient is unable to stand). The next step is to determine whether prior films are available for comparison,[25] because many abnormalities can be put into appropriate perspective by determining whether or not they are new. Common examples are a prominent aortic arch, a visible major fissure related to prior inflammatory process, or a widened superior mediastinum related to aortic ectasia (see Fig. 15-4) or a substernal thyroid.

Any system should incorporate a routine that includes a deliberate attempt to observe areas that are easily ignored. These include the thoracic spine, neck (for masses and tracheal position), costophrenic angles, lung apices, retrocardiac space, and retrosternal space. Looking at these areas allows definition of the mediastinal position and cardiac and aortic situs and the presence of pleural effusions, scarring, or diaphragmatic elevation. Next, the lung fields are evaluated. This evaluation should involve a careful search for infiltrates or masses, even when examining a chest radiograph for cardiovascular abnormalities, keeping in mind that many with coronary artery disease have a history of tobacco abuse and are, therefore, at increased risk for lung malignancies (see Fig. 15-7).

The overall size of the cardiac silhouette, its position, and the location of the ascending and descending aorta must be specifically evaluated. Dextrocardia and a right descending aorta are rare, particularly in adults, but are easy to find. They are important to recognize because of their association with congenital cardiac and abdominal situs abnormalities. It is also important to look at the site and position of the stomach, which can help differentiate between a high diaphragm and a pleural effusion (see Fig. 15-2). Overall cardiomegaly can be judged with reasonable accuracy on the PA view by noting whether or not the diameter of the heart exceeds half the diameter of the thorax. Cardiomegaly is a common but nonspecific finding (Fig. 15-11).[26-30]

Lungs and Pulmonary Vasculature

Evaluation of the pulmonary vascular pattern is difficult and imprecise, but very important. As noted earlier, it varies with the patient's position (erect versus supine) and is altered substantially by underlying pulmonary disease. It is best to define pulmonary vascularity by looking at the middle zone of the lungs (i.e., the third of the lungs between the hilar region and the peripheral region laterally) and comparing a region in the upper lung field with a region in the lower lung field at equal distances from the hilum.[20] Vessels should be larger in the lower lung but sharply marginated in both the upper and lower zones. In normal persons, the vessels taper and bifurcate and are difficult to define in the outer third of the lung. They normally cannot be seen near the pleura.

Two distinct patterns of abnormality are recognizable. When pulmonary arterial flow is increased, as in patients with a high-output state (e.g., pregnancy, severe anemia, hyperthyroidism) or left-to-right shunt, the pulmonary vessels are seen more prominently than usual in the periphery of the lung (Fig. 15-12). They are uniformly enlarged and can be traced almost to the pleura, but their margins remain clear. With elevated pulmonary artery pressure, in contrast, the vessel borders become hazy, the lower zone vessels constrict, and the upper zone vessels enlarge, and vessels become visible farther toward the pleura, in the outer third of the lungs (see Fig. 15-11). With increasing left ventricular end-diastolic pressure (LVEDP) or left atrial pressure, interstitial edema occurs, and ultimately pulmonary edema develops. There is a reasonably good correlation between the pulmonary vascular pattern and pulmonary capillary wedge pressure (PCWP). At a PCWP less than 8 mm Hg, the vascular pattern is normal. As the PCWP increases to 10 to 12 mm Hg, the lower zone vessels appear equal in diameter to or smaller than the upper zone vessels. At pressures of

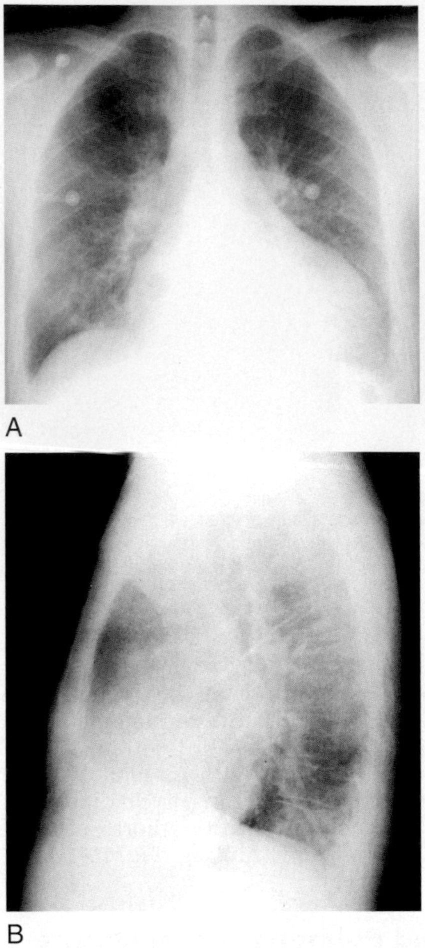

FIGURE 15–11 Chest radiographs of a 53-year-old man with severe ischemic cardiomyopathy and marked cardiomegaly. Frontal **(A)** and lateral **(B)** views show markedly enlarged cardiac silhouette, without clear enlargement of individual chambers, and marked pulmonary vascular redistribution.

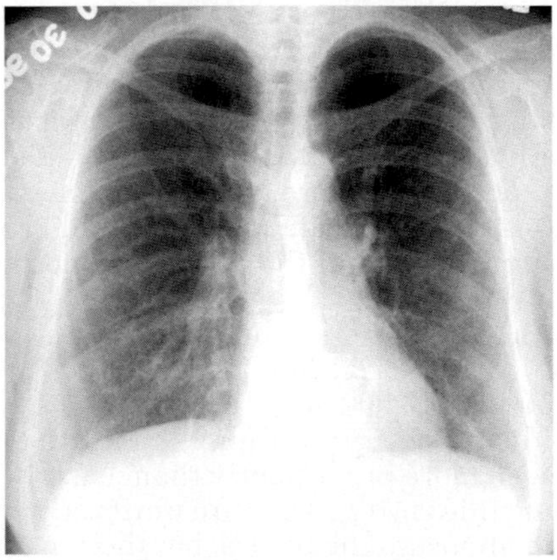

FIGURE 15–12 Chest radiograph of a 47-year-old asymptomatic woman with an atrial septal defect. The posteroanterior view shows a normal cardiac contour, with mild pulmonary vascular plethora at the periphery of the lung fields.

12 to 18 mm Hg, the vessel borders become progressively hazier because of increasing extravasation of fluid into the interstitium. This effect is sometimes evident as Kerley B lines, which are horizontal, pleura-based, peripheral linear densities. As PCWP increases acutely above 18 to 20 mm Hg pulmonary edema occurs, with interstitial fluid present in sufficient amounts to cause a perihilar bat wing appearance (Fig. 15-13).

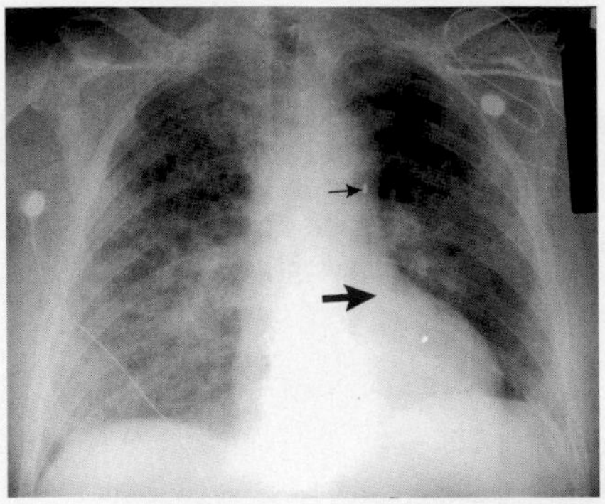

FIGURE 15–13 Patient with acute pulmonary edema. Note engorged hila bilaterally, with typical pattern of pulmonary edema on the right. Also, note intraaortic counterpulsation balloon with radiopaque tip at the top of the descending aorta (small arrow) and the balloon expanded in the aorta below it (large arrow).

Again, these typical appearances may be altered for various reasons. In patients with extensive pulmonary fibrosis or multiple bullae, the vascular pattern is abnormal at baseline and, as the PCWP increases, it does not change in predictable ways. In patients with chronic heart failure, there are chronic changes in the pulmonary vascular pattern that do not correlate with the changes that occur in patients with normal left ventricular pressure at baseline.[20,31] For example, a patient with a chronic elevation of LVEDP to 25 to 30 mm Hg may have a normal pulmonary vascular pattern or only moderate rather than marked redistribution (see Fig. 15-8 and compare with Fig. 15-13). In general, heart size increases over time with increasing pulmonary vascular redistribution. If pulmonary edema is independent of left ventricular dysfunction, however, as may occur at high altitude or following cerebral trauma, the heart size may remain normal. A more frequently encountered disparity is that in the setting of an acute, large transmural myocardial infarction, the heart is usually minimally or mildly enlarged, despite a marked increase in LVEDP (see Fig. 15-13).

Cardiac Chambers and Great Vessels

Evaluation of the heart must also be done systematically. After assessing overall size and pulmonary vascular pattern, as a reflection of left-heart physiological status, the individual chambers should be examined. It is not possible to define individual chambers clearly in a normal chest radiograph (see Figs. 15-5 and 15-6). Furthermore, when the cardiac silhouette is enlarged, it is often related to biventricular failure, and individual chamber enlargement is not discernible (see Fig. 15-11). In acquired valvular disease and in many types of congenital heart disease, however, individual chamber enlargement develops and is crucial to plain film (and often clinical) diagnosis.[17,26,31] This information is now readily available with other, more expensive imaging modalities, namely echocardiography, cardiac magnetic resonance (CMR), and computed tomography (CT) (see also Chaps. 14, 17, and 18).[32] Nonetheless, plain films remain important, because they allow fairly straightforward and inexpensive assessment of current status as well as changes over time and are routinely and readily available.[33-37]

RIGHT ATRIUM. Right atrial enlargement is essentially never isolated except in the presence of congenital tricuspid atresia or the Ebstein anomaly (see Chap. 61). In adults, the right atrium may dilate in the presence of pulmonary hypertension or tricuspid regurgitation, but right ventricular dilation usually predominates and prevents definition of the atrium. The right atrial contour blends with that of the superior vena cava, right main pulmonary artery, and right ventricle.

RIGHT VENTRICLE. The classic signs of right ventricular enlargement are a boot-shaped heart and filling in of the retrosternal airspace.[19] The former is caused by transverse displacement of the apex of the right ventricle as it dilates (Fig. 15-14A). In adults, it is unusual for the right ventricle to dilate without left ventricular dilation, so this boot shape is not often obvious. It is most commonly seen as an isolated finding in congenital heart disease, classically in tetralogy of Fallot (see Chap. 61). As the right ventricle dilates, it expands superiorly as well as laterally and posteriorly, filling in the retrosternal airspace (see Fig. 15-14B). The classic teaching is that the soft tissue density is confined to less than one third of the distance from the suprasternal notch to the tip of the xyphoid in a normal lateral chest radiograph. If the soft tissue fills in more than a third, in the absence of other explanations, it is a reliable indication of right ventricular enlargement. There are, however, other causes of increased soft tissue density in this region that usually are readily definable. Common causes that are generally easy to distinguish from right ventricular enlargement include retrosternal adenopathy, midmediastinal mass (e.g., lymphoma or thymoma), marked dilation of the main pulmonary artery (Fig. 15-15), and marked aortic root dilation (see Fig. 15-4). The most common cause of increased retrosternal soft tissue is prior median sternotomy, with resultant scarring and haziness of this region (see Fig. 15-10C). Right ventricular enlargement is most often seen in mitral valve disease, secondary to pulmonary hypertension (Fig. 15-16; see also Fig. 15-14). Less commonly, it is the result of primary pulmonary hypertension (see Chap. 73).

LEFT ATRIUM. Several classic signs define left atrial enlargement.[17,37] First is dilation of the left atrial appendage, which appears as a focal convexity where there is normally a concavity between the left main pulmonary artery and the left border of the left ventricle on the frontal view (Fig. 15-17; see also Fig. 15-16A). Second, because of its location, as the left atrium enlarges, it elevates the left main stem bronchus. In so doing, it widens the angle of the carina (see Figs. 15-16A and 15-17A).[38] Third, as the left atrium enlarges posteriorly, it may cause focal bowing of the middle to low thoracic aorta toward the left. This bowing is distinguishable from the tortuosity seen with progressive atherosclerosis, which involves the descending thoracic aorta either in its upper portion or diffusely. Fourth, with marked left atrial enlargement, a double density can be seen on the frontal view, because the left atrium projects laterally toward the right as well as posteriorly, and the discrete outline of the blood-filled left atrium is surrounded by air-filled lung (see Figs. 15-16A and 15-17A). Finally, on the lateral film, left atrial enlargement appears as a focal, posteriorly directed bulge (see Fig. 15-16B).

Isolated left atrial enlargement in the adult develops in mitral stenosis (see Fig. 15-17), and definable left atrial enlargement is the hallmark of mitral valve disease (see Chap. 62). In mitral stenosis, there is evidence of pulmonary vascular redistribution (often with Kerley B lines) and ultimately enlargement of the right ventricle as the disease progresses. The left ventricle remains normal in size (see Fig. 15-17). In contrast, in mitral regurgitation, with increased volume in the left atrium and ventricle, both enlarge over time (Fig. 15-18). The pattern of pulmo-

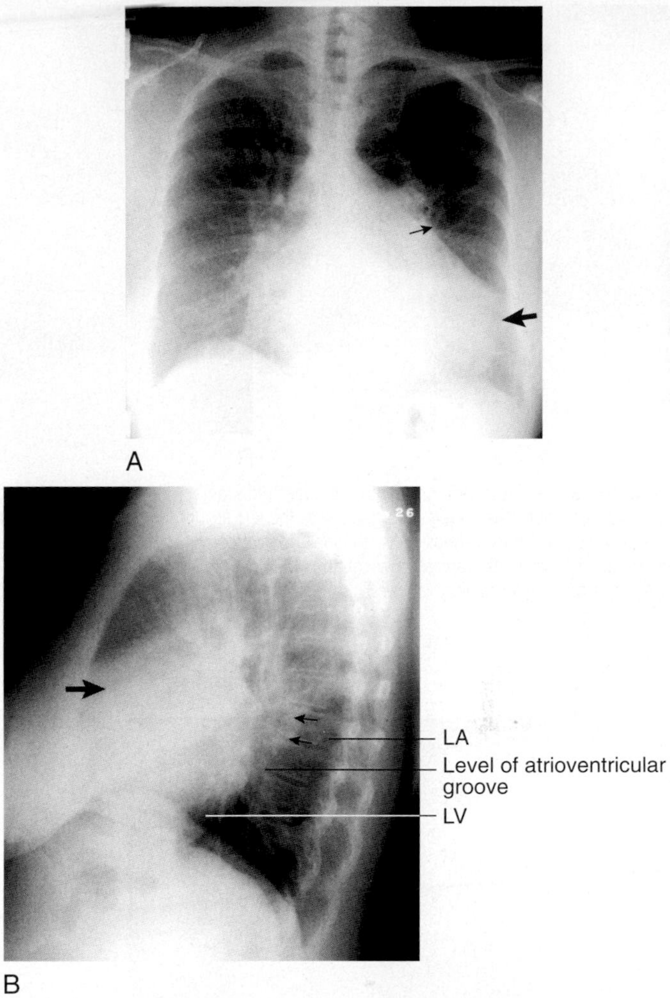

FIGURE 15–14 Chest radiographs of a 59-year-old woman with history of rheumatic heart disease and mitral stenosis. **A,** Posteroanterior view demonstrates enlarged cardiac silhouette, with suggestion of a double density seen through the heart (left atrial enlargement), prominent convexity of the left atrial appendage (small arrow), and slightly elevated cardiac apex (large arrow), suggestive of right ventricular (rather than left ventricular) enlargement. There is significant elevation of the pulmonary venous pressures. **B,** The lateral view confirms marked right ventricular (large arrow) and left atrial (small arrows) enlargement. Note filling in of the retrosternal airspace. LA = left atrium; LV = left ventricle.

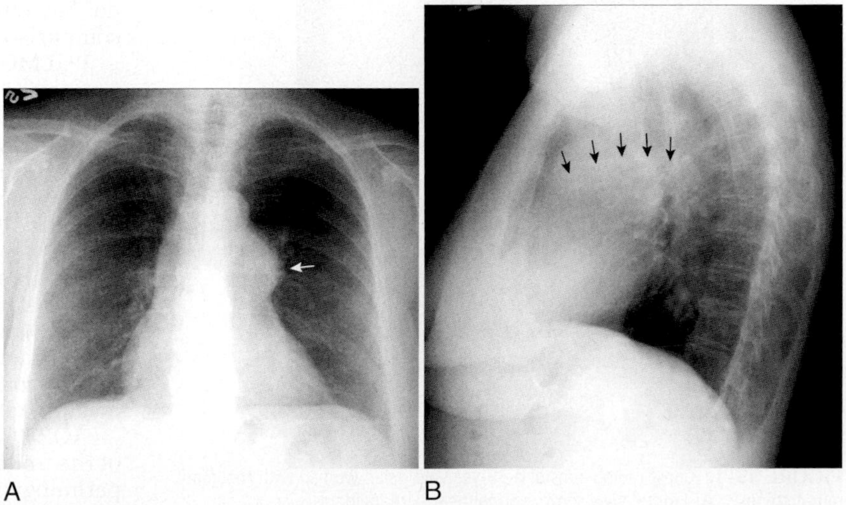

FIGURE 15–15 Chest radiographs of a 56-year-old asymptomatic woman with incidentally discovered pulmonic stenosis. **A,** Posteroanterior view shows marked enlargement of the main pulmonary trunk extending into the left main pulmonary artery (arrow). **B,** Lateral view confirms prominence of the pulmonary outflow tract and main and left pulmonary arteries (arrows).

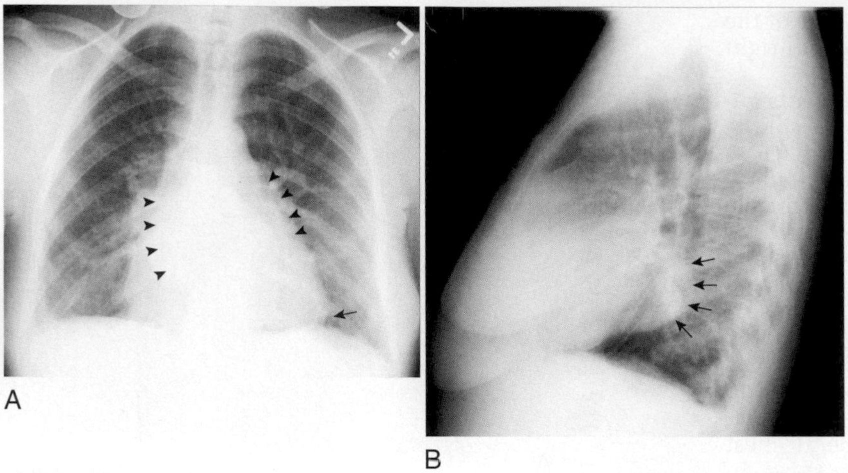

FIGURE 15–16 Chest radiographs of a 60-year-old woman with severe mitral stenosis. **A,** Posteroanterior view shows enlargement of the left atrium (arrowheads), prominence of the hilar vessels, and pulmonary venous redistribution. Transverse angle of the apex suggests right ventricular enlargement (arrow). **B,** Lateral view confirms this, with filling in of the retrosternal airspace. Note also severe left atrial enlargement (arrows).

nary vascular redistribution is more variable in mitral regurgitation than in mitral stenosis, as is right ventricular dilation. It is also important to note mitral annulus calcification. This common finding does not have a strong association with valvular dysfunction but does have an association with premature coronary artery disease (Fig. 15-19).[39]

LEFT VENTRICLE. Left ventricular enlargement is characterized by a prominent, downwardly directed contour of the apex, as distinguished from the transverse displacement seen with right ventricular enlargement. On the PA film, the overall cardiac contour is also usually enlarged, although this is a nonspecific finding. On the lateral film, left ventricular enlargement appears as a posterior bulge below the level of the mitral annulus (Fig. 15-20). It may also be seen inferiorly, pushing the gastric bubble (see Fig. 15-8B). Such left ventricular enlargement is an illustration of findings that lie outside the usual confines of the chest and is another example of the value of looking at the entire chest radiograph.

Focal left ventricular enlargement in adults occurs commonly with aortic insufficiency, often with associated aortic root dilation (see Fig. 15-20), whereas mitral regurgitation also manifests left atrial dilation (see Fig. 15-18). In contrast, aortic stenosis is characterized by left ventricular hypertrophy rather than dilation, and the left ventricle dilates only when aortic stenosis is accompanied by heart failure.[21-23,31,40]

In most patients with an acute myocardial infarction, the cardiac silhouette is not enlarged but there is pulmonary vascular redistribution, consistent with an acute increase in LVEDP. This condition is most easily defined when the chest radiograph is compared with a prior or subsequent one. After infarction, various alterations can occur. Left ventricular aneurysms, either true (generally in the distribution of the left anterior descending artery; see Fig. 15-10) or false (usually involving the base or the posterior wall) are uncommon. Although the location generally differs, the appearance of both is similar—there is focal prominence (of the anterolateral cardiac contour with true aneurysms), there may be linear myocardial calcification, and the margin is unusually sharp because the area of the aneurysm does not have normal cardiac motion. Again, this is best seen in comparison with prior chest radiographs.

PULMONARY ARTERIES. The main pulmonary arteries are abnormal in many clinical settings. In patients with pulmonic stenosis, the main pulmonary artery and the left pulmonary artery dilate (see Fig. 15-15), a finding thought to be caused by the jet effect through the stenotic valve. The main pulmonary artery continues straight into the left main pulmonary artery, but the right comes off at a fairly sharp angle and is not generally affected by the jet from the stenotic valve. This enlargement can be seen with a prominent left hilum on the frontal view and a prominent pulmonary outflow tract on the lateral. It is important to remember that the pulmonic valve lies higher and more peripherally in the outflow tract than the aortic valve (see Fig. 15-6). It is also located anterior to the aortic valve on the lateral view.

AORTA. The aorta dilates in different ways as a function of the underlying pathology. It is often possible to define the pathology not only by the pattern of aortic dilation but also by associated cardiac abnormalities.[41] On the frontal chest radiograph, aortic dilation is seen as a prominence to the right of the middle mediastinum (see Fig. 15-20A). There is also a prominence in the anterior mediastinum on the lateral

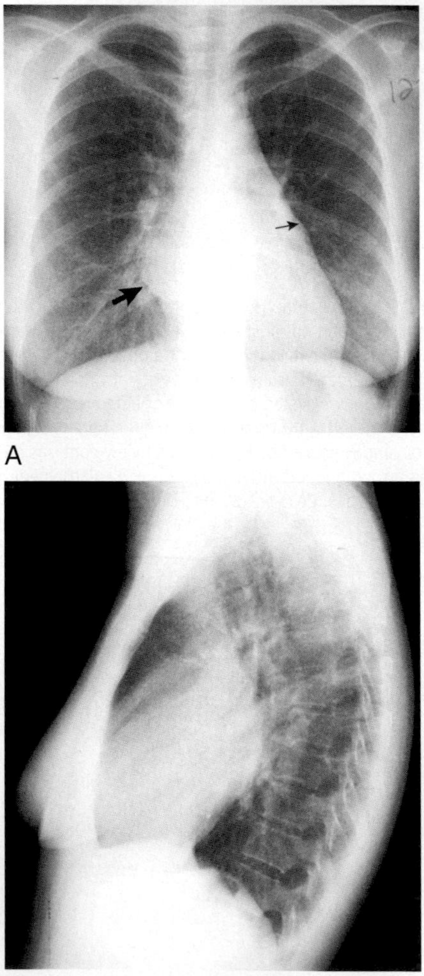

FIGURE 15–17 Chest radiographs of a 39-year-old Asian woman with rheumatic mitral stenosis. **A,** Frontal view shows normal heart size, mild vascular redistribution, and marked focal enlargement of the left atrium (small arrow), which extends to the right of the midline (large arrow). There is elevation of the left main stem bronchus. **B,** Lateral view shows dilated right ventricle, with filling in of the retrosternal airspace. The left ventricle is normal in size and contour.

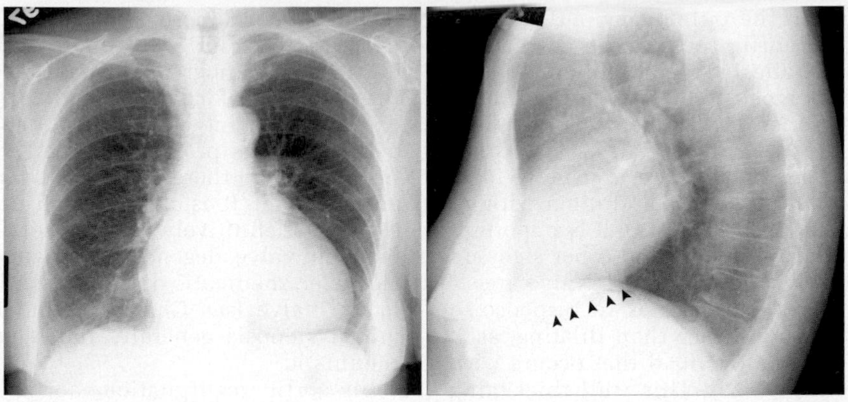

FIGURE 15–18 Chest films of a 78-year-old woman with pure mitral regurgitation and atrial fibrillation. **A,** Posteroanterior view shows enlargement of the left atrium and left ventricle with mild pulmonary vascular redistribution. **B,** Lateral view confirms these findings. Arrowheads indicate prominent left ventricular contour.

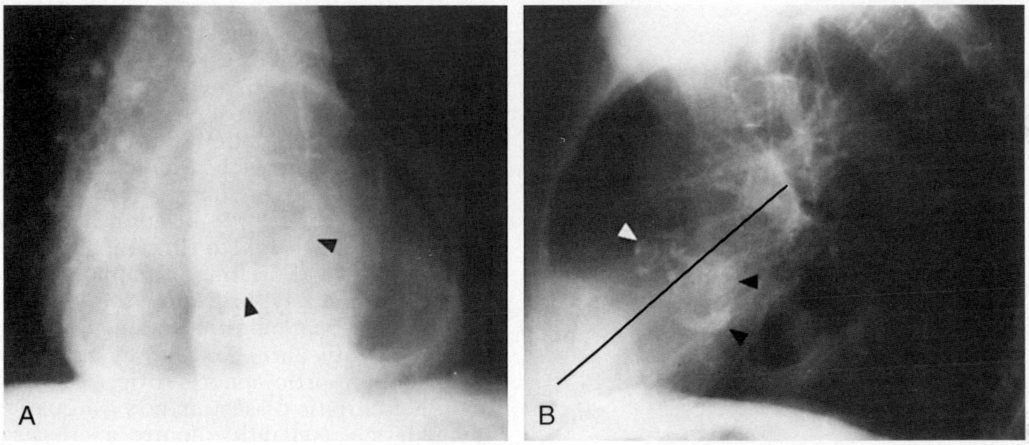

FIGURE 15–19 Mitral annulus calcification in posteroanterior **(A)** and lateral **(B)** projections. This calcification (black arrowheads) lies below the line drawn from the left main bronchus to the anterior costophrenic sulcus, which localizes it to the mitral valve. The calcified aortic valve in this patient lies more anteriorly and above this line (white arrowhead).

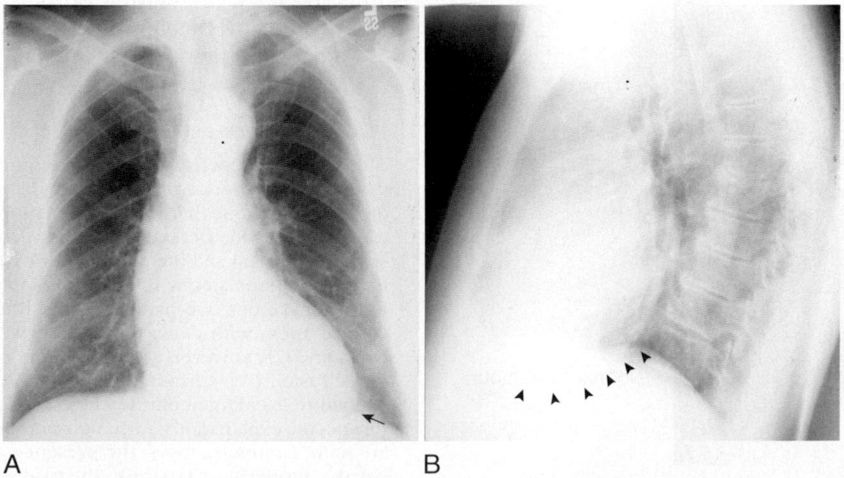

FIGURE 15–20 Chest radiographs of a 63-year-old man with chronic aortic regurgitation. **A,** Posteroanterior view shows downward displacement of the apex (arrow), suggestive of left ventricular enlargement. There is prominence and enlargement of the ascending aorta, creating a convex right border of the mediastinum. **B,** Lateral view shows prominent left ventricular enlargement (arrowheads). The aortic root is m arkedly enlarged in the retrosternal airspace but is separate from the sternum (in contrast to findings in right ventricular enlargement; see Figs. 15-16B and 15-17B).

view, behind and superior to the pulmonary outflow tract (Fig. 15-21). Dilation of the aortic root occurs with aortic valve disease (both stenosis and regurgitation) but is more frequent in other settings, most commonly longstanding systemic hypertension or generalized atherosclerosis with ectasia.

In aortic stenosis (see Chap. 62), there is usually focal dilation of the aortic root, often subtle, and often without left ventricular enlargement (see Fig. 15-21). It is important to look for this, because there are often no other signs on the chest radiograph, even with a very small valve area.[40] The left ventricle generally hypertrophies in response to increased resistance to outflow rather than dilating, as it does in response to the volume overload that occurs with aortic regurgitation (see Fig. 15-20). This wall thickening with hypertrophy is seen with echocardiography, CT, or CMR, but the ventricle may appear entirely normal on the chest radiograph despite severe aortic stenosis. Aortic valve calcification (see Fig. 15-21B) is usually difficult to see on a chest radiograph because of the overlying soft tissue densities and the minimal blurring caused by cardiac motion, even with a very stenotic valve. If calcification is present, it is much more easily seen with fluoroscopy. Despite the decreased resolution of fluoroscopy compared with standard chest radiography, real-time visualization facilitates the detection of calcification.[42-44]

It is important to remember that a subset of patients with aortic stenosis present with left ventricular decompensation, in whom there is both left ventricular and aortic root enlargement. It is not possible on a chest radiograph to establish definitively whether aortic stenosis is caused by a bicuspid valve, degenerative changes, or rheumatic disease. However, rheumatic disease essentially always involves the mitral valve (see Chap. 62), and the absence of signs of mitral stenosis generally indicates that the cause is not rheumatic.

In aortic regurgitation, aortic involvement is usually more diffuse than in aortic stenosis and more easily seen (see Chap. 62). In pure aortic regurgitation, the left atrium is generally not enlarged. Over time, however, dilation of the mitral annulus may occur secondary to the left ventricular dilation, with resultant mitral regurgitation and left atrial dilation. Although aortic regurgitation most often develops from intrinsic diseases of the valve, such as congenital defects, degenerative valve disease, or rheumatic heart disease (with associated mitral valve involvement), it may also be caused by diseases of the aortic root, including cystic medial necrosis, with or without Marfan syndrome. In cystic medial necrosis, the involvement is diffuse, and there is generally dilation of the aorta from the level of the valve at least through the arch, with a gradual transition to normal diameter (see Chaps. 8 and 56). Aortic regurgitation may occur secondary to dilation of the valve or to aortic dissection into the valve ring. Bicuspid aortic valves are a common cause of dilation of the aortic root and ascending aorta. In tertiary syphilis, now rarely seen, the characteristic finding is marked dilation of the aorta from the root to the arch, with abrupt return to normal diameter at this level. Other aortic abnormalities, such as acute (see Fig. 15-3B) or chronic dissection and traumatic rupture or pseudoaneurysm, generally require a cross-sectional imaging modality for clear delineation (see Chap. 56). Chest radiography may delay appropriate diagnosis and intervention in acute trauma, such as in the case of suspected aortic rupture. The findings on the chest films are generally nonspecific and indirect, such as the presence of mediastinal widening, blood at the left lung apex, a large left pleural effusion (presumably blood), deviation of the trachea to the right, or rib fractures. Multislice or even helical CT can provide a rapid and accurate diagnosis (see Chap. 18).

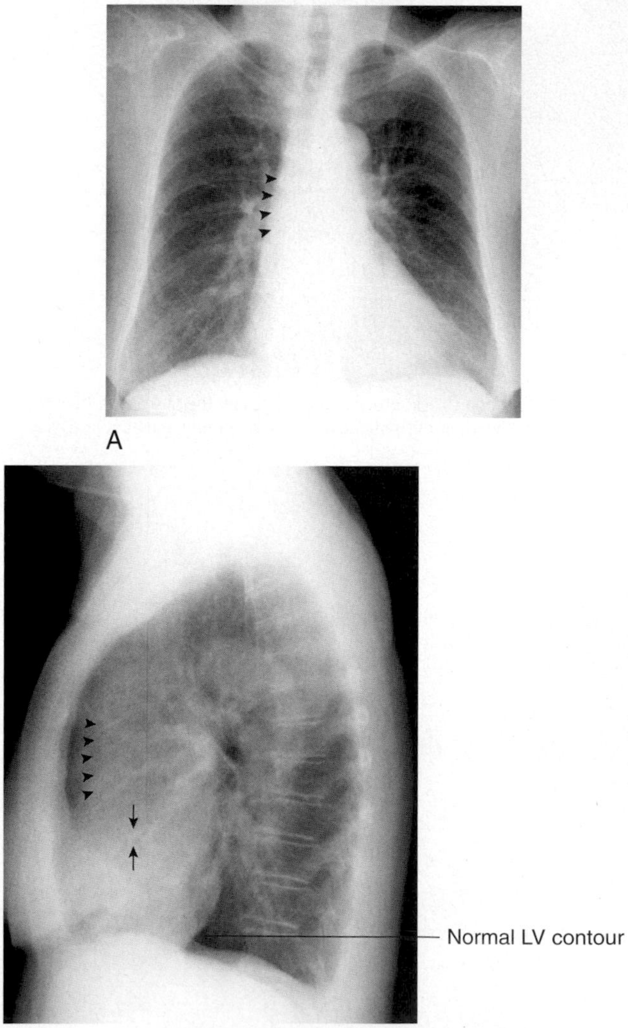

FIGURE 15–21 Chest radiographs of a 65-year-old woman with severe aortic stenosis. **A,** Frontal view shows prominent aortic root to the right of the midline (arrowheads). Note absence of cardiomegaly and presence of normal pulmonary vascular pattern. **B,** Lateral view demonstrates calcification of the aortic valve leaflets (arrows), suggestive of a bicuspid valve. There is a prominent, mildly dilated aortic root (arrowheads).

Pleura and Pericardium

The pleura and pericardium also require systematic evaluation (see Chap. 70). The pericardium is rarely distinctly definable on plain films of the chest,[45] but there are two situations in which it can be seen: effusion and constriction. In the presence of a large pericardial effusion, the visceral and the parietal pericardium separate. Because there is a fat pad associated with each, it is sometimes possible on the lateral film to make out two parallel lucent lines, usually in the area of the cardiac apex, with density (fluid) between them. Echocardiography, CMR, and CT, however, are all far more reliable for defining a pericardial effusion (see Chaps. 14, 17, and 18). Nonetheless, if the cardiac silhouette is enlarged on the chest radiograph, it is important to look for specific explanations. Although cardiac dilation and valvular disease are more common causes, the presence of an unsuspected effusion is worth considering. Classically, the cardiac silhouette has a water bottle shape in the presence of a pericardial effusion, but such a shape is not in itself diagnostic.

Both pleural and pericardial calcification can occur (see Fig. 15-9), but they are often not obvious. Pericardial calcification is associated with a history of pericarditis, with tuberculosis and various viruses the most common causes. Such calcification is usually thin and linear and follows the contour of the pericardium. Because the calcification is thin, it is often seen only on one view (see Fig. 15-9). Myocardial calcification secondary to a large myocardial infarction with transmural necrosis is rare but can generally be distinguished from pericardial calcification. It tends to appear thicker, more focal, and less consistent with the outer contour of the heart. Pleural calcification is essentially pathognomonic for asbestos exposure, associated with a high risk of malignant mesothelioma. Usually, it is easily distinguished from pericardial calcification by its location.

IMPLANTABLE DEVICES

A final important and broad area concerns the chest radiograph following surgery or other procedures. In these situations, it is crucial to recognize devices that have been implanted and changes that may occur. Among the most common are various percutaneous septal closure devices,[46] valve prostheses,[47] pacemakers (Fig. 15-22),[48] and implantable cardiac defibrillators (ICDs; Fig. 15-23), and intraaortic counter pulsation balloons (see Fig. 15-13). There are also clear changes that occur after surgery, such as the presence of clips on the side branches of saphenous veins used for coronary artery bypass grafting (see Fig. 15-10B and C) and retrosternal blurring (see Fig. 15-22) and effusions (see Fig. 15-2).[49] Some of these findings may be temporary, such as lines and tubes associated with surgery and effusions.

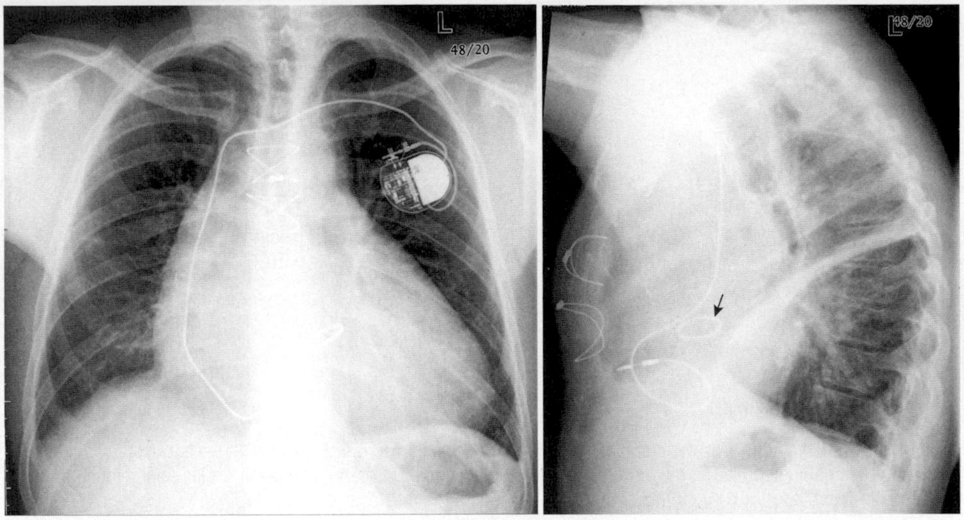

A B

FIGURE 15–22 Chest radiographs of a 28-year-old man who has undergone aortic valve replacement with a porcine bioprosthesis. **A,** Posteroanterior view. There is marked left ventricular (LV) enlargement, with a downwardly displaced apex. Note pacemaker wire with tip in the right ventricular (RV) apex. **B,** Lateral view confirms primary LV dilation, with the valve ring indicating the position of the aortic valve (arrow). This and the location of the pacing wire tip in the RV apex confirms LV versus RV dilation.

Pacemakers and ICDs present specific questions (see Chap. 34). The first is whether or not the leads are intact,[50,51] and the second is the position of the tip. Although course and tip position are generally confirmed fluoroscopically at the time of placement, malposition can occur. If there are two leads, the tips should generally be in the anterolateral wall of the right atrium and the apex of the right ventricle. If the leads are not positioned in this way, the reasons should be carefully determined (Fig. 15-24). That is, are they positioned because of error or because of anatomical variants, such as a persistent left superior vena cava that empties into the coronary sinus and then the right atrium (see Fig. 15-23)?[52] Additionally, the position of the wires and of valve prostheses can help in the definition of specific chamber enlargement (see Figs. 15-22 and 15-24).

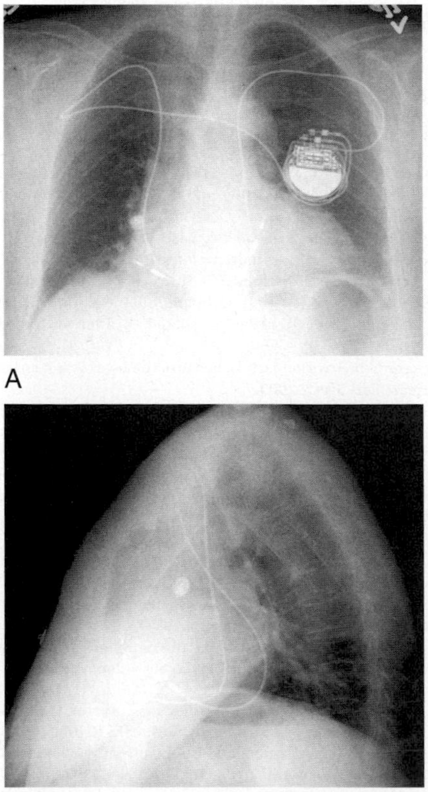

A

B

FIGURE 15–23 Chest radiographs of a 62-year-old woman with two pacemakers, with left-sided pacemaker implanted because of failure of the right. As seen on frontal **(A)** and lateral **(B)** views, the right-sided wire traverses the right superior vena cava and right atrium and its tip lies superiorly and anteriorly in the pulmonary outflow tract. The left-sided wire traverses a persistent left superior vena cava (a normal anatomical variant) and coronary sinus and its tip, the lower of the two, is in the right atrium.

CONCLUSION

Chest radiographs provide a wealth of physiological and anatomical information. As such, they play a central role in the evaluation and management of patients with a wide variety of cardiovascular and other disorders. Portable chest films should be used as infrequently as possible, because the information they provide is limited and may even be misleading (e.g., in defining cardiomegaly or in ruling out a pneumothorax or effusion). Standard 6-foot frontal and lateral chest films, on the other hand, are almost always useful. If they are evaluated carefully, using a systematic approach and compared with prior chest radiographs (when possible), whether recorded conventionally or digitally, it is hard to overstate their importance.

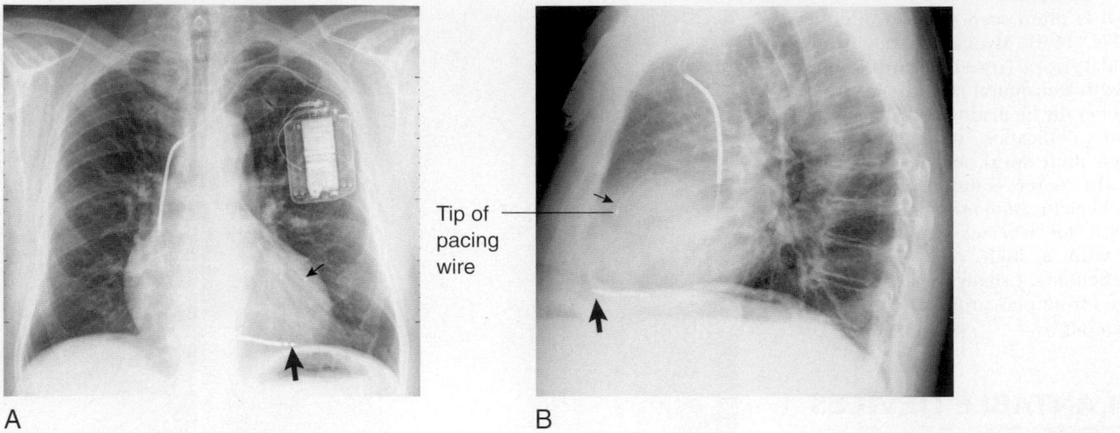

FIGURE 15–24 A and **B,** Chest radiographs of a 78-year-old man after aortic valve replacement. Note wire position (arrow), through the coronary sinus into the great coronary vein (running parallel to the left anterior descending coronary artery), and biventricular enlargement. Also, note the position of the separate implantable cardioverter-defibrillator (ICD) tip in right ventricular apex (large arrow).

REFERENCES

1. Williams FH: A method for more fully determining the outline of the heart by means of a fluoroscope together with other uses of the instrument in medicine. Boston Med Surg J 135:335, 1896.

Technical Considerations

2. Hintenlang KM, Williams JL, Hintenlang DE: A survey of radiation dose associated with pediatric plain-film chest X-ray examinations. Pediatr Radiol 32:771, 2002.
3. Volk M, Hamer OW, Feuerbach S, Strotzer M: Dose reduction in skeletal and chest radiography using a large-area flat-panel detector based on amorphous silicon and thallium-doped cesium iodide: Technical background, basic image quality parameters, and review of the literature. Eur Radiol 14:827, 2004.
4. Krivopal M, Shlobin OA, Schwartzstein RM: Utility of daily routine portable chest radiographs in mechanically ventilated patients in the medical ICU. Chest 123:1607, 2003.
5. Rong XJ, Shaw CC, Liu X, et al: Comparison of an amorphous silicon/cesium iodide flat-panel digital chest radiography system with screen/film and computed radiography systems: A contrast-detail phantom study. Med Phys 28:2328, 2000.
6. Garmer M, Hennigs SP, Jäger HJ, et al: Digital radiography versus conventional radiography in chest imaging: Diagnostic performance of a large area flat-panel detector in a clinical CT-controlled study. AJR Am J Roentgenol 174:75, 2000.
7. Chotas HG, Dobbins JT, Ravin CE: Principles of digital radiography with large-area electronically readable detectors: A review of the basics. Radiology 210:595, 1999.
8. Bacher K, Smeets P, Bonnarens K, et al: Dose reduction in patients undergoing chest imaging: Digital amorphous silicon flat-panel detector radiography versus conventional film-screen radiography and phosphor-based computed radiography. AJR 181:923, 2003.
9. Konen E, Greenberg I, Rozenman J: Visibility of normal thoracic anatomic landmarks on storage phosphor digital radiography versus conventional radiography. Isr Med Assoc J 7:495, 2005.
10. Pascoal A, Lawinski CP, Mackenzie A, et al: Chest radiography: A comparison of image quality and effective dose using four digital systems. Radiat Prot Dosimetry 114:273, 2005.
11. Eisenhuber E, Stadler A, Prokop M, et al: Detection of monitoring materials on bedside chest radiographs with the most recent generation of storage phosphor plates: Dose increase does not improve detection performance. Radiology 227:216, 2003.
12. Prato A, Ropolo R, Fava C: Digital chest radiography system with amorphous selenium flat-panel detectors: Qualitative and dosimetric comparison with a dedicated film-screen system. Radiol Med (Torino) 110:561, 2005.
13. Kroft LJ, Veldkamp WJ, Mertens BJ, et al: Comparison of eight different digital chest radiography systems: Variation in detection of simulated chest disease. AJR Am J Roentgenol 185:339, 2005.
14. Ganten M, Radeleff B, Kampschulte A, et al: Comparing image quality of flat-panel chest radiography with storage phosphor radiography and film-screen radiography. AJR Am J Roentgenol 181:171, 2003.
15. Weatherburn GC, Ridout D, Strickland NH, et al: A comparison of conventional film, CR hard copy and PACS soft copy images of the chest: Analyses of ROC curves and inter-observer agreement. Eur J Radiol 47:206, 2003.
16. Honeyman-Buck J: PACS adoption. Semin Roentgenol 38:256, 2003.

The Normal Chest Radiograph

17. Baron MG: The cardiac silhouette. J Thorac Imaging 15:230, 2000.
18. Ohye RG, Kulik TA: Images in cardiovascular medicine. Normal chest x-ray. Circulation 105:2455, 2002.
19. Boxt LM: Radiology of the right ventricle. Radiol Clin North Am 37:379, 1999.
20. Hoffman RB, Rigler LG: Evaluation of left ventricular enlargement in the lateral projection of the chest. Radiology 85:93, 1965.
21. Freeman V, Mutatiri C, Pretorius M, et al: Evaluation of left ventricular enlargement in the lateral position of the chest using the Hoffman and Rigler sign. Cardiovasc J S Afr 14:134, 2003.
22. Jung G, Landwehr P, Schanzenbacher G, et al: Value of thoracic radiography in the assessment of cardiac size. A comparison with left ventricular cardiography. Rofo Fortschr Geb Rontgenstr Neuen Bildgeb Verfahr 162:368, 1995.
23. Sharma S, Bhargave A, Krishnakumar R, et al: Can pulmonary venous hypertension be graded by the chest radiograph? Clin Radiol 53:899, 1998.
24. Fraser RS, Muller NL, Colman N, et al (eds): Fraser and Pare's Diagnosis of Diseases of the Chest. 4th ed. Philadelphia, WB Saunders, 1999.

Evaluating the Chest Radiograph in Heart Disease

25. Berbaum KS, Smith WL: Use of reports of previous radiologic studies. Acad Radiol 5:111, 1998.
26. Satou GM, Lacro RV, Chung T, et al: Heart size on chest x-ray as a predictor of cardiac enlargement by echocardiography in children. Pediatr Cardiol 22:218, 2001.
27. Thomas JT, Kelly RF, Thomas SJ, et al: Utility of history, physical examination, electrocardiogram, and chest radiograph for differentiating normal from decreased systolic function in patients with heart failure. Am J Med 112:437, 2002.
28. Ernst ER, Shub C, Bailey KR, et al: Radiographic measurements of cardiac size as predictors of outcome in patients with dilated cardiomyopathy. J Card Fail 7:13, 2001.
29. Petrie MC: It cannot be cardiac failure because the heart is not enlarged on the chest X-ray. Eur J Heart Fail 5:117, 2003.
30. Perez AA, Ribeiro AL, Barros MV, et al: Value of the radiological study of the thorax for diagnosing left ventricular dysfunction in Chagas' disease. Arq Bras Cardiol 80:208, 2003.
31. Hoilund-Carlsen PF, Gadsboll N, Hein E, et al: Assessment of left ventricular systolic function by the chest x-ray: Comparison with radionuclide ventriculography. J Card Fail 11:299, 2005.
32. Schmermund A, Rensing BJ, Sheedy PF, et al: Reproducibility of right and left ventricular volume measurements by electron-beam CT in patients with congestive heart failure. Int J Card Imaging 14:201, 1998.
33. Ferri C, Emdin M, Nielsen H, et al: Assessment of heart involvement. Clin Exp Rheumatol 21:S24, 2003.
34. Rothrock SG, Green SM, Costanzo KA, et al: High-yield criteria for obtaining non-trauma chest radiography in the adult emergency department population. J Emerg Med 23:117, 2002.
35. Oeppen RS, Fairhurst JJ, Argent JD: Diagnostic value of the chest radiograph in asymptomatic neonates with a cardiac murmur. Clin Radiol 57:736, 2002.
36. Gardiner S: Are routine chest x ray and ECG examinations helpful in the evaluation of asymptomatic heart murmurs? Arch Dis Child 88:638, 2003.
37. Laya BF, Goske MJ, Morrison S, et al: The accuracy of chest radiographs in the detection of congenital heart disease and in the diagnosis of specific congenital cardiac lesions. Pediatr Radiol 36:677, 2006.
38. Murray JG, Brown AL, Anagnostou EA, et al: Widening of the tracheal bifurcation on chest radiographs: Value as a sign of left atrial enlargement. AJR Am J Roentgenol 164:1089, 1995.
39. Atar S, Jeon DS, Luo H, et al: Mitral annular calcification: A marker of severe coronary artery disease in patients under 65 years old. Heart 89:161, 2003.
40. Rodan BA, Chen JT, Halber MD, et al: Chest roentgenographic evaluation of the severity of aortic stenosis. Invest Radiol 17:453, 1982.

41. Yamamoto H, Shavelle D, Takasu J, et al: Valvular and thoracic aortic calcium as a marker of the extent and severity of angiographic coronary artery disease. Am Heart J 146:153, 2003.
42. Cook C, Styles C, Hopkins R: Calcification on the chest X-ray: A pictorial review. Hosp Med 62:210, 2001.
43. Li J, Galvin HK, Johnson SC, et al: Aortic calcification on plain chest radiography increases risk for coronary artery disease. Chest 121:1468, 2002.
44. Kiryu S, Raptopoulos V, Baptista J, et al: Increased prevalence of coronary artery calcification in patients with suspected pulmonary embolism. Acad Radiol 10:840, 2003.
45. Wang ZJ, Reddy GP, Gotway MB, et al: CT and MR imaging of pericardial disease. Radiographics 23:S167, 2003.
46. Kim JH, Siegel MJ, Goldstein JA, et al: Radiologic findings of two commonly used cardiac septal occluders with clinical correlation. J Thorac Imaging 18:183, 2003.
47. Bordlee RP: Cardiac valve reconstruction and replacement: A brief review. Radiographics 12:659, 1992.
48. Bejvan SM, Ephron JH, Takasugi JE, et al: Imaging of cardiac pacemakers. AJR Am J Roentgenol 169:1371, 1997.
49. Kurihara Y, Yakushiji YK, Nakajima Y, et al: The vertical displacement sign: A technique for differentiating between left and right ribs on the lateral chest radiograph. Clin Radiol 54:367, 1999.
50. Morishima I, Sone T, Tsuboi H, et al: Follow-up X rays play a key role in detecting implantable cardioverter defibrillator lead fracture: A case of incessant inappropriate shocks due to lead fracture. Pacing Clin Electrophysiol 26:911, 2003.
51. Drucker EA, Brooks R, Garan H, et al: Malfunction of implantable cardioverter defibrillators placed by a nonthoracotomy approach: Frequency of malfunction and value of chest radiography in determining cause. AJR Am J Roentgenol 165:275, 1995.
52. Schummer W, Schummer C, Frober R: Persistent left superior vena cava and central venous catheter position: Clinical impact illustrated by four cases. Surg Radiol Anat 25:315, 2003.

CHAPTER 16

Nuclear Cardiology

James E. Udelson, Vasken Dilsizian, and Robert O. Bonow

The era of noninvasive radionuclide cardiac imaging in humans began in the early 1970s, with the first reports of noninvasive evaluation of resting myocardial blood flow. Since that time, there have been major advances in the technical ability to image cardiac physiology and pathophysiology, including that of myocardial blood flow, myocardial metabolism, and ventricular function. Just as important has been a major growth in the understanding of how to apply the image information to care of patients and the effect of that information on clinical decision-making. Ultimately, the role of information derived from any imaging procedure is to enhance the clinician's decision-making process to improve symptoms or clinical outcomes, or both.

TECHNICAL ASPECTS OF IMAGE ACQUISITION, DISPLAY, AND INTERPRETATION

SPECT Imaging of Perfusion and Function

The most commonly performed imaging procedure in nuclear cardiology is single-photon emission computed tomography (SPECT) imaging of myocardial perfusion. Following injection of the chosen radiotracer, the isotope is extracted from the blood by viable myocytes and retained within the myocyte for some period of time. Photons are emitted from the myocardium in proportion to the magnitude of tracer uptake, in turn, related to perfusion. The standard camera used in nuclear cardiology studies, a gamma camera, captures the gamma ray photons, and converts the information into digital data representing the *magnitude of uptake* and the *location of the emission.* The photoemissions collide along their flight path with a detector crystal. There, the gamma photons are absorbed and converted into visible light events (a "scintillation event"). Emitted gamma rays are selected for capture and quantitation by a *collimator* attached to the face of the camera-detector system. Most often, parallel hole collimators are used so that only photon emissions coursing perpendicular to the camera head and parallel to the collimation holes are accepted (Fig. 16-1). This arrangement allows better appropriate *localization of the source* of the emitted gamma rays. Photomultiplier tubes, the final major component in the gamma camera, sense the light-scintillation events and convert the events into an electrical signal to be further processed (see Fig. 16-1). The final result of SPECT imaging is the creation of multiple tomograms, or slices, of the organ of interest, comprising a digital display representing radiotracer distribution throughout the organ.[1] With SPECT myocardial perfusion imaging (MPI), the display represents the distribution of perfusion throughout the myocardium.

SPECT IMAGE ACQUISITION

To construct the three-dimensional model of the heart from which tomograms are created, the myocardial perfusion data must be sampled from multiple angles over 180 or 360 degrees around the patient. Multiple images, each comprising 20 to 25 seconds of emission data, are collected. Each one of the separate "projection" images constitutes a two-dimensional snapshot of myocardial perfusion from the angle at which the projection was acquired. Then, the imaging information from each of the angles is *back projected* onto an imaging matrix, creating a reconstruction of the organ of interest. The reader is referred to detailed reviews for more extensive information on the technical aspects of SPECT imaging and image reconstruction.[1]

SPECT IMAGE DISPLAY

From the three-dimensional reconstruction of the heart, computer processing techniques are used to identify the long axis of the left ventricle, and standardized tomographic images in three standard planes are derived. *Short-axis* images, representing "doughnut-like" slices of the heart cut perpendicular to the long axis of the heart, are displayed beginning toward the apex and moving toward the base. This tomographic orientation is similar to the short-axis view in two-dimensional echocardiography, although shifted counterclockwise (Fig. 16-2A). Tomographic slices cut parallel to the long axis of the heart and also parallel to the long axis of the body are termed *vertical long-axis* tomograms (see Fig. 16-2B), and slices also cut parallel to the long axis of the heart but perpendicular to the vertical long axis slices are known as *horizontal long-axis* tomograms (see Fig. 16-2C). From all of these tomographic planes, the entire three-dimensional myocardium is sampled and displayed, minimizing overlap of structures.

Basics of Quality Control

The quality of SPECT MPI and the "accuracy" of the representation of regional myocardial perfusion are dependent on multiple quality control issues. These issues include the stability of the tracer distribution in the organ of interest during the acquisition interval, the absence of motion of the patient or organ of interest, or both, during the acquisition, and the absence of overlying structures that would attenuate the photon emissions from one region relative to another region across the different projection images. Those issues are related to the patient and the organ being imaged, and other quality control issues involve the camera and detector system, including the unifor-

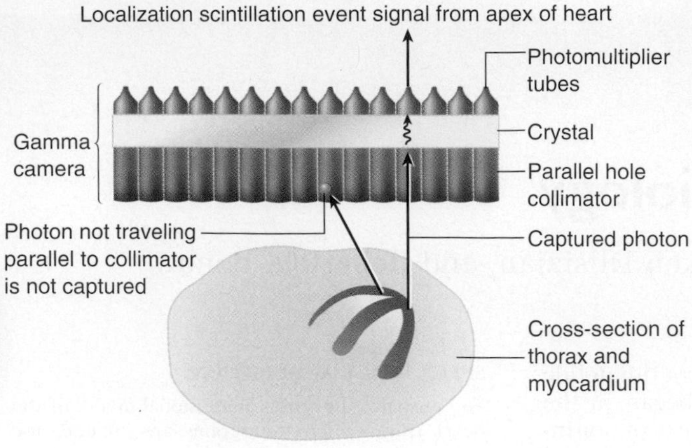

FIGURE 16–1 Capture of emitted photons by a gamma camera. Emissions are captured by a parallel hole collimator, allowing photons to interact with a detector crystal, and are recorded as scintillation events. The event is localized on the basis of where the photon interacts with the crystal.

mity of photon detection efficiency across the camera face as well as the stability of the camera across the entire orbit of acquisition.[2]

It is important when interpreting SPECT images to be aware of possible sources of image artifacts. Discrete motion of the patient (and thus motion of the heart outside its original field) causes an abnormality in the final images that may be corrected with motion correction software. Imaging artifacts commonly occur because of the effects of overlying structures that attenuate photon emissions. These include breast attenuation in women and attenuation of the inferobasal wall related to the diaphragm, most commonly seen in men. Strategies to overcome quality problems such as attenuation are described subsequently.

SPECT Perfusion Tracers and Protocols

THALLIUM-201. Thallium-201 was introduced in the 1970s and propelled the clinical application of myocardial perfusion imaging (MPI) as an adjunct to exercise treadmill testing. Thallium-201 is a monovalent cation with biological properties similar to those of potassium. Because potassium is the major intracellular cation in muscle and is virtually absent in scar tissue, thallium-201 is a well-suited radionuclide for differentiating normal and ischemic from scarred myocardium.[3] Thallium-201 emits 80 keV of photon energy and has a physical half-life of 73 hours. The initial myocardial uptake early after intravenous injection of thallium is proportional to regional blood flow. First-pass extraction fraction (the proportion of tracer extracted from the blood as it passes through the myocardium) is high—in the range of 85 percent. It is transported across the myocyte cell membrane by the Na^+,K^+-adenosine triphosphatase (ATPase) transport system and by facilitative diffusion. Peak myocardial concentration of thallium occurs within 5 minutes of injection, with rapid clearance from the intravascular compartment. Although the initial uptake and distribution of thallium are primarily a function of blood flow, the subsequent *redistribution* of thallium, which begins within 10 to 15 minutes after injection, is unrelated to flow but is related to the rate of thallium clearance from myocardium, linked to the concentration gradient between myocytes and the blood levels of thallium (Fig. 16-3A). Thallium clearance is more rapid from normal myocardium with high thallium activity compared with myocardium with reduced thallium activity (ischemic myocardium), a process termed "differential washout" (see Fig. 16-3B).

Thallium studies can be divided into protocols in which thallium-201 is administered during stress or at rest.[3] Following stress, the reversal of a thallium defect from the initial peak stress to delayed 3- to 4-hour or 24-hour redistribution images is a marker of reversibly ischemic, viable myocardium. When thallium is injected at *rest,* the extent of thallium defect reversibility from the initial rest images to delayed redistribution images (at 3 to 4 hours) reflects viable myocardium with resting hypoperfusion. When scarred myocardium is present, the initial rest or stress thallium defect persists over time, termed an "irreversible" or "fixed" defect. However, in some patients with coronary artery disease (CAD), the initial uptake of thallium during stress may be severely decreased, and tracer accumulation from the recirculating thallium in the blood during the redistribution phase may be slow or even absent because of rapid decline of thallium levels in the blood. The result is that some severely ischemic but viable regions may show no redistribution on either early (3- to 4-hour) or late (24-hour) imaging, *even if viable myocardium is present.* Viable myocardium in this situation can be revealed by raising blood levels of thallium by reinjecting a small dose (1 mCi) of thallium at rest. Thus, in some patients, thallium reinjection is necessary to identify viable myocardium when there are irreversible defects on stress-redistribution images.

TECHNETIUM 99m-LABELED TRACERS. Tc 99m-labeled myocardial perfusion tracers were introduced in the clinical arena in the 1990s.[3] Technetium 99m emits 140 keV of photon energy and has a physical half-life of 6 hours. Despite the excellent myocardial extraction and flow kinetics properties of thallium, its energy spectrum of 80 keV is suboptimal for conventional gamma cameras (ideal photopeak in the 140-keV range). In addition, thallium's long physical half-life (73 hours) limits the amount of thallium that may be administered to stay within acceptable radiation exposure parameters. Thus, Tc 99m-labeled tracers improve on these two limitations of thallium. Although three Tc 99m-labeled tracers (sestamibi, teboroxime, and tetrofosmin) have received U.S. Food and Drug Administration (FDA) approval for detection of CAD, only sestamibi and tetrofosmin are available for clinical use at present.

Sestamibi and tetrofosmin are lipid-soluble cationic compounds with first-pass extraction fraction in the range of 60 percent. Myocardial uptake and clearance kinetics of both tracers are similar. They cross sarcolemmal and mitochondrial membranes of myocytes by passive distribution, driven by the transmembrane electrochemical gradient, and they are retained within the mitochondria.[3] There is minimal redistribution of these tracers compared with thallium. Thus, myocardial perfusion studies with Tc 99m-labeled tracers require *two separate injections, one at peak stress and the second at rest.*

There are three basic protocols[2] with Tc 99m-labeled tracers: (1) a single-day study, in which myocardial blood flow is interrogated at rest and at peak stress, or in the reverse order, as long as the first injected dose is low (8 to 10 mCi) and the second injected dose is high (22 to 30 mCi); (2) a 2-day study (commonly performed in patients with large body habitus) in which higher doses of the tracer are injected (20 to 30 mCi) both at rest and at peak stress to optimize myocardial count rate; and (3) a dual-isotope technique, which combines injection of thallium at rest followed by injection of a Tc 99m tracer at peak stress. The last approach takes advantage of the favorable properties of each of the two tracers, including high-quality gated SPECT images from Tc 99m and the potential of acquiring redistribution images from thallium (either at 4 hours prior to the stress study or at 24 hours after the Tc 99m activity has decayed). A comparison of the properties of the available isotopes for perfusion imaging is shown in Table 16-1.

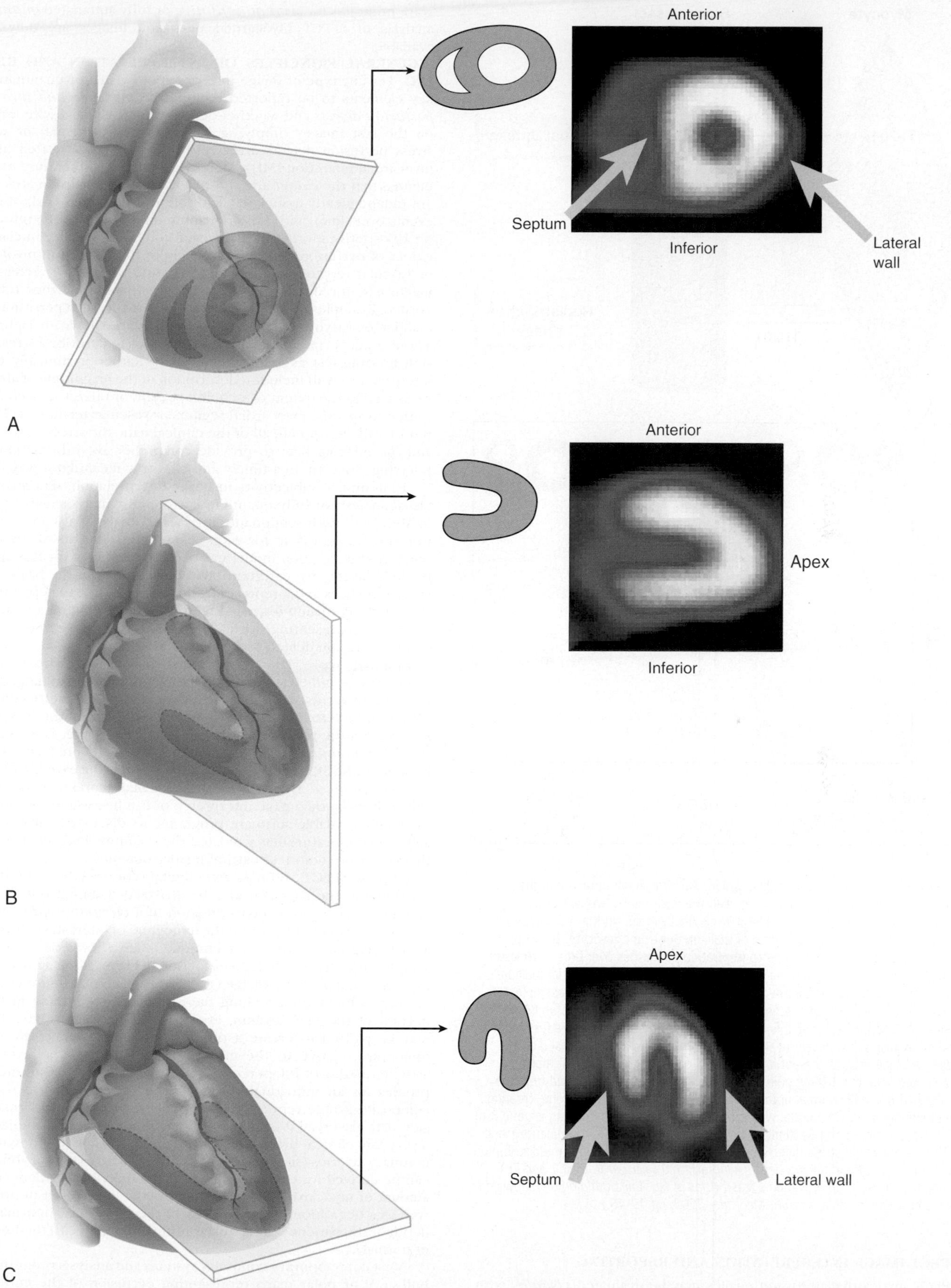

FIGURE 16–2 Standard single-photon emission computed tomography imaging display. **A,** The short-axis images each represent a portion of the anterior, lateral, inferior, and septal walls. **B,** Vertical long-axis images represent the anterior wall, apex, and inferior wall. **C,** Horizontal long-axis images represent the septum, apex, and lateral walls.

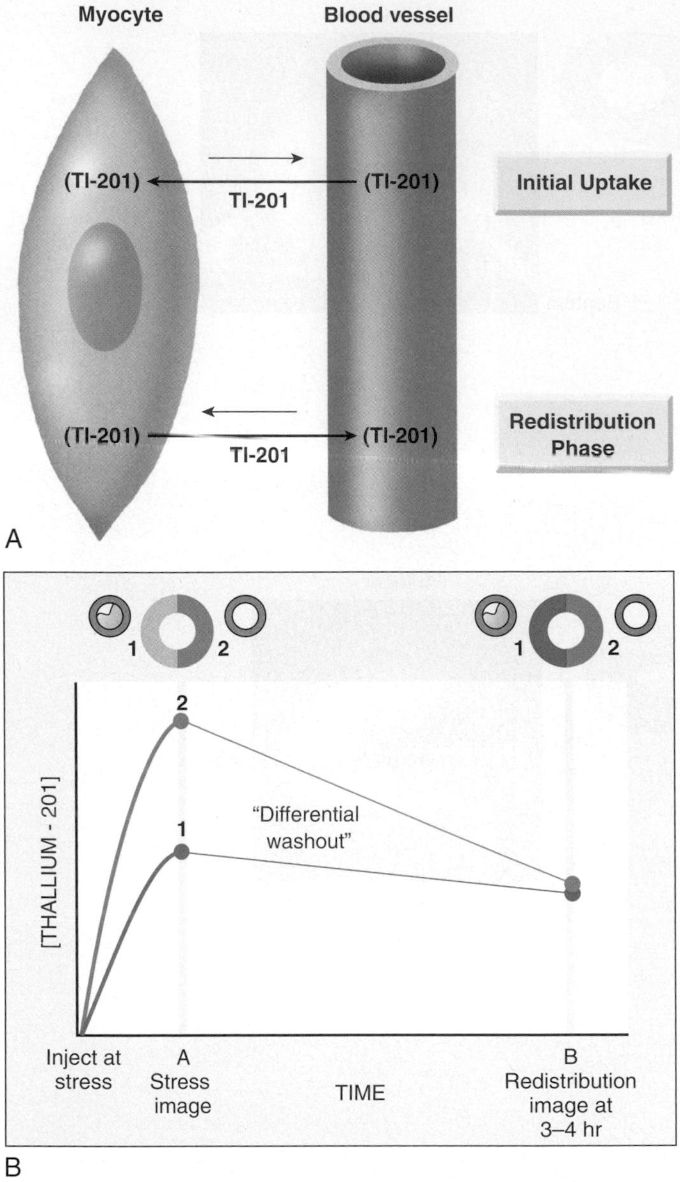

FIGURE 16–3 Thallium-201 redistribution. **A,** After initial uptake into the myocyte, an equilibrium is created between the intracellular and extracellular concentrations of thallium. After blood levels diminish during the redistribution phase, the equilibrium favors egress of thallium out of the myocyte. **B,** On the basis of that equilibrium, thallium concentration diminishes over time in zones of normal uptake, while diminishing more slowly in zones with less initial thallium uptake, i.e., those with diminished flow reserve or ischemia. In this example, segment 1 of the myocardial schematic is supplied by an artery with an 80 percent stenosis and segment 2 is supplied by a normal artery. During peak stress, normal blood flow reserve is present in segment 2; blunted flow reserve, based on the presence of stenosis, is present in segment 1, and there is less initial thallium uptake into segment 1 (time point A). Thallium washout is more rapid from the territory with initially normal uptake and slower from the ischemic zone, creating the phenomenon of differential washout. When redistribution imaging is done 3 to 4 hours later (time point B), thallium concentrations are equal in segments 1 and 2. Thus, a reversible stress defect is seen in segment 1, based on the redistribution properties and differential washout. *(Adapted from Dilsizian V: SPECT and PET techniques.* In *Dilsizian V, Narula J [eds]: Atlas of Nuclear Cardiology. Braunwald E [series ed]. Philadelphia, Current Medicine, 2003, pp 19-46.)*

SPECT IMAGE INTERPRETATION AND REPORTING

SPECT myocardial perfusion images may be evaluated *visually,* with the interpreter describing the perfusion pattern findings on stress, and then visually interpreting whether defects observed on the stress images are, or are not, reversible. Because the imaging data are digital, computer-aided quantitative analysis may also be used. Validated software programs for *semi-quantitative* or fully automated *quantitative* analysis of SPECT myocardial perfusion images are now widely available.

GENERAL PRINCIPLES OF INTERPRETATION AND REPORTING. For any type of image interpretation, visual or quantitative, the key elements to be reported include the *presence and location of perfusion defects* and whether defects on stress images are *reversible* on the rest images (implying stress-induced ischemia) or whether stress perfusion defects are *irreversible or "fixed"* (often implying myocardial infarction [MI]). Moreover, substantial literature has documented that the *extent* and the *severity* of the perfusion abnormality are independently associated with clinical outcomes (risk of adverse events over time), and thus contribute importantly to the information on risk-stratification to be conveyed to the ordering clinician.[4] The *extent* of perfusion abnormality refers to the amount of myocardium or vascular territory that is abnormal, and the *severity* refers to the magnitude of reduction in tracer uptake in abnormal zone relative to normal. Examples of stress and rest SPECT myocardial perfusion abnormalities of varying extents and severities are shown in Figure 16-4. These concepts imply that it is not sufficient to describe a stress perfusion imaging test as simply "abnormal." Rather, a clinically relevant interpretation will include a description of the magnitude of abnormality as well as the extent of ischemia, extent of infarct, as well as localization to specific myocardial regions or vascular territories. The final report will incorporate all of the clinical data, the stress testing result, and the imaging data to provide comprehensive information to the referring clinician, in a timely and clinically meaningful way.

To minimize subjectivity in image interpretation, semiquantitative visual analysis or fully quantitative computer analysis may be applied to MPI data.[5] With semiquantitative visual analysis, a score is assigned to represent perfusion for each of multiple segments of the myocardium. A segmentation model has been standardized for this approach by dividing the myocardium into 17 segments[6] on the basis of three short-axis slices and a representative long-axis slice to depict the apex (Fig. 16-5). Perfusion is graded within each segment on a scale of 0 to 4, with 0 representing normal perfusion and 4 representing a very severe perfusion defect. Scores for all 17 segments are added to create a "summed" score. The sum of the segmental scores from the stress images (the summed stress score, SSS) represents the extent and severity of stress perfusion abnormality, the magnitude of perfusion defects related to *both ischemia and infarction.* The sum of the 17 segmental scores from the rest images (the summed rest score, SRS) represents the *extent of infarction.* The summed difference score (SDS) is derived by subtracting SRS from the SSS, and represents the extent and severity of *stress-induced ischemia.* The segmental scores can be assigned subjectively by the image interpreter, or can be assigned automatically by widely available software programs. As discussed subsequently, a substantial literature has validated these summed scores, particularly the SSS, as predictors of natural history outcomes.

Because SPECT MPI data are a digital representation of radiotracer distribution, the data can also be analyzed quantitatively. The most common technique involves creation of a *circumferential profile* of relative tracer activity around the tomogram of interest, such as a short-axis tomogram. With this technique, each short-axis tomogram is sampled at every 3 to 6 degrees for 360 degrees, along a ray extending from the center of the image (Fig. 16-6A). The maximum counts at a picture element (pixel) along the ray, usually occurring in the midportion of the myocardium, are recorded for each angle. The data may be plotted to create a profile of the perfusion pattern of that tomogram relative to the most "normal" area of uptake, which is assigned a value of 100 percent uptake (see Fig. 16-6B). Circumferential profiles for an individual patient can be compared directly with a composite profile representing normal perfusion. The normal perfusion data are created from studies performed in normal subjects with a very low clinical probability of CAD or in those with known normal coronary arteries (see Fig. 16-6B). A quantitative extent of abnormality can be derived for each tomogram of the individual patient (the total amount of myocardium that falls below the lower limit of normal) as well as a derivation of the severity of the perfusion abnormality (the depth of the patient's perfusion abnormality relative to the lower limit of normal).

Most contemporary computer systems and analysis programs create bull's-eye or polar maps representing perfusion of the entire three-dimensional myocardium in a two-dimensional plot (see Fig. 16-6C and D). Quantitative data may be derived on the extent of global perfusion abnormality, abnormality within vascular territories, as well as the extent of reversible and fixed defects (see Fig. 16-6D). These are often

TABLE 16–1 Properties of SPECT Tracers

Tracer	Physical Half-Life (hr)	Uptake	Myocardial Clearance	"Differential Washout"	Maximum Extraction Fraction
Thallium-201	73	Active	~50% at 6 hr	Yes	~0.70
Tc 99m sestamibi	6	Passive	Minimal	Minimal	0.39
Tc 99m tetrofosmin	6	Passive	Minimal	Minimal	0.24
Tc 99m teboroxime	6	Passive	~50% at 10 min	Yes	0.72

SPECT = single-photon emission computed tomography.

From Gerson MC, McGoron A, Roszell N, et al: Myocardial perfusion imaging: Radiopharmaceuticals and tracer kinetics. *In* Gerson MC (ed): Cardiac Nuclear Medicine. New York, McGraw Hill, 1997, pp 3-27.

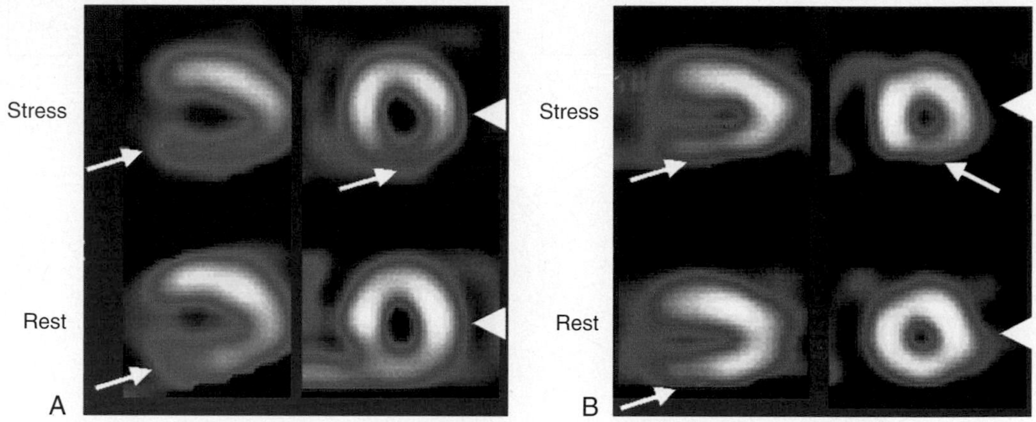

FIGURE 16–4 Abnormal single-photon emission computed tomography images of different extent and severity. **A,** A large, moderately severe, reversible inferior wall defect (arrows) reflecting a severe flow reserve abnormality. **B,** A milder reversible inferior wall defect (arrows) reflecting a less severe stenosis or a more severe stenosis with well-developed collaterals minimizing the defect severity. In both patients, there is also a mild lateral wall reversible defect (arrowheads). Note how the lateral wall brightens relative to the septum on the rest images compared with the stress images.

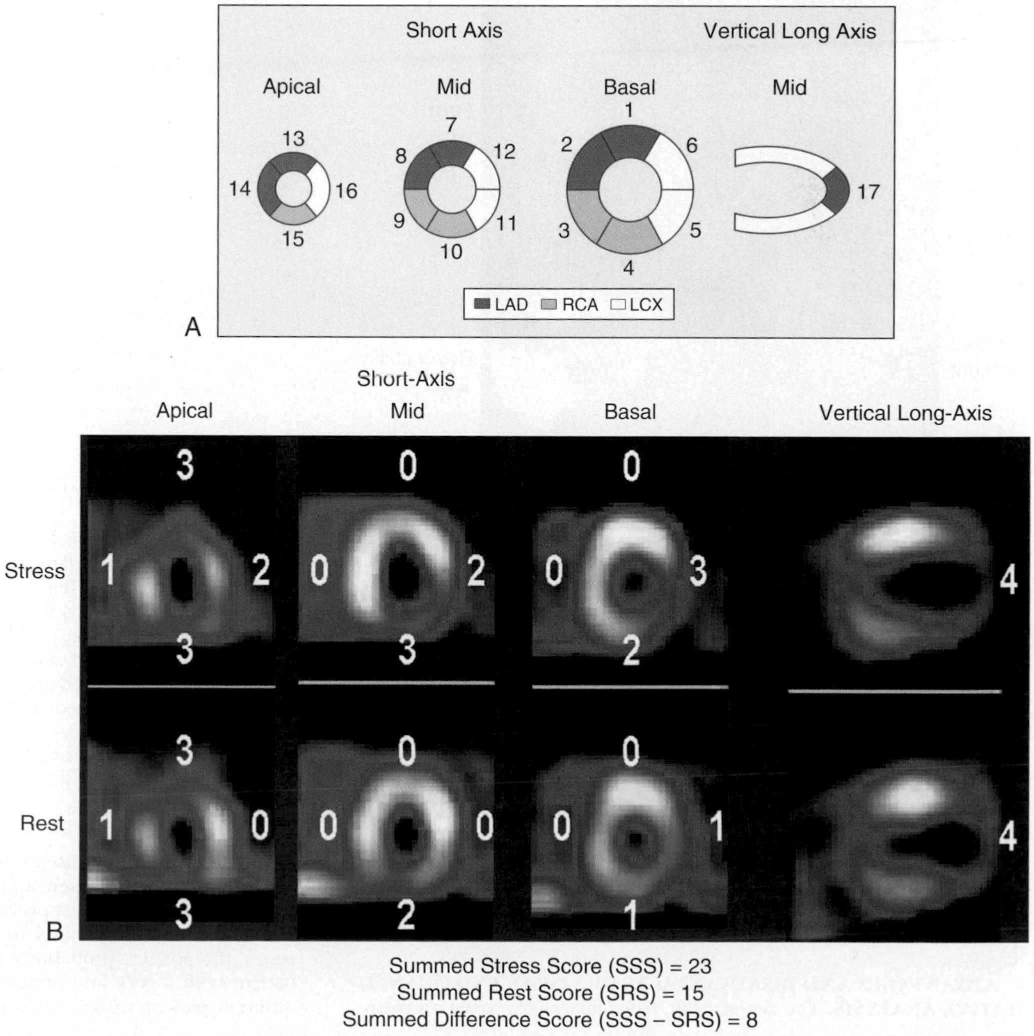

FIGURE 16–5 A, Standard segmental myocardial display for semiquantitative visual analysis in a 17-segment model, with corresponding vascular territory schematic. **B,** Segmental scoring of a patient whose stress and rest single-photon emission computed tomography perfusion images show a severe apical fixed defect (in the vertical long axis), extending into the inferoapical and anteroapical walls (in the apical short axis), with evidence of reversible defects in the inferior and lateral walls (in the mid and basal short axis). The summed stress score (SSS = 23) represents extensive perfusion abnormality at stress (reflecting ischemia and infarct); the summed rest score (SRS = 15) represents the extent of infarct; and the summed difference score (SDS = SSS – SRS = 8) represents the extent of ischemia. LAD = left anterior descending (artery); LCX = left circumflex (coronary artery); RCA = right coronary artery.

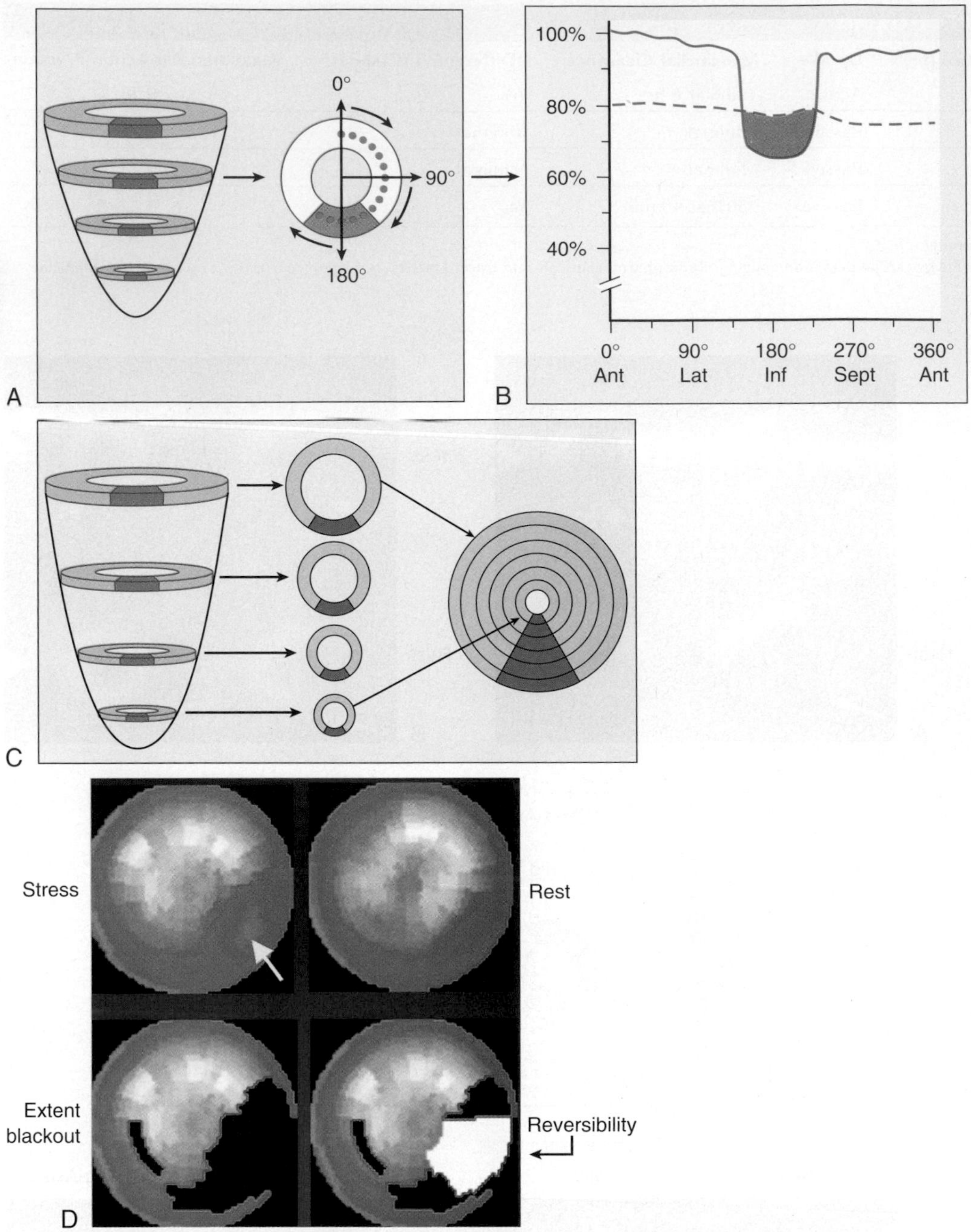

FIGURE 16–6 Quantitative analysis of single-photon emission computed tomography imaging. **A,** Circumferential profile analysis of tracer uptake along rays emanating from the center of the short-axis tomogram. From this procedure, a circumferential profile of tracer uptake around the myocardium is developed for each short-axis tomogram. In this example, there is a perfusion defect in the inferior wall (darker purple area). **B,** The data are plotted relative to location around the myocardium (*x*-axis) and "normalized" to the point of peak uptake, which is assigned a value of 100 percent (*y*-axis). The patient's data (solid line) are compared with lower limits of normal (dashed line) derived from a group of subjects without coronary artery disease of the same gender. From this comparison, the quantitative extent and severity of the perfusion abnormality can be derived (orange area). **C,** Data from all of the individual short-axis tomograms can be combined to create a bull's-eye polar plot, representing a two-dimensional compilation of all of the three-dimensional short-axis perfusion data. The extent of the inferior wall perfusion defect (gray area on individual profiles and polar plot) is seen on the two-dimensional map. **D,** Example of a bull's-eye polar plot for a patient with a reversible defect of the inferolateral wall (yellow arrow on the stress bull's-eye plot, upper left). The "blackout" area (on the extent blackout plot, lower left) represents the myocardium that falls below the lower limits of normal, and in the reversibility plot (lower right) the white area represents the extent of that abnormality that is reversible (ischemic) on rest imaging. *(Images courtesy of Ernest Garcia, PhD.)*

displayed as "blackout" maps, in which any pixel values falling below a set number of standard deviations below the normal limits is assigned the color black, and the extent of that abnormality is expressed as a percent of the presumed vascular territory and as a percent of the left ventricle.

ADVANTAGES AND DISADVANTAGES OF VISUAL AND QUANTITATIVE ANALYSIS. The accuracy of visual analysis is based on many factors, which include the experience and training of the reader, as well as the quality of the imaging study. The well-trained reader will incorporate information from the raw data (such as the presence of apparent breast attenuation, or an elevated diaphragm potentially attenuating the inferior wall) and adjust their threshold for interpreting an abnormality to optimize accuracy. Visual analysis is inherently subjective, however, and subject to variability, both between readers as well as within an individual reader. The quantitative programs and comparisons to normal databases can perform with little or no human interaction. Thus, the results are highly reproducible. This approach attempts to account for potential artifacts such as breast or diaphragm attenuation by the comparison of patient image data to image data from normal, gender-matched subjects (in which, for example, the lower limits of normal for the anterolateral wall of a woman would be lower than that of a man because of the presence of breast tissue). Nonetheless, artifacts that are not accounted for by the normal data comparison, such as those introduced by motion or other suboptimal quality issues that the trained reader may recognize as likely artifactual, may often be called abnormal by quantitation. Thus, in practice, many readers will interpret MPI studies using both visual analysis as well as incorporating the quantitative data to arrive at a final conclusion. The more objective and reproducible nature of the quantitative analysis is a strength with regard to its use in clinical trials that interrogate the effect of therapies on serial changes in myocardial perfusion.

INCORPORATING BAYESIAN PRINCIPLES INTO IMAGE INTERPRETATION. Although it is possible to interpret MPI data in isolation and report only on what the images demonstrate, a more accepted interpretive methodological principle is that the final interpretation should take into account the entirety of the data at hand—the image data built on the already known clinical and stress test data—when interpreting MPI data. An understanding of Bayesian probability principles is useful in this regard. Bayes' theorem posits that the posttest probability of disease (or risk of an event) after a test is influenced not only by the sensitivity and specificity of the test, but also importantly by the pretest probability of disease (see Chaps. 4 and 13). This principle is illustrated in Figure 16-7. For a given positive test result, the posttest probability of disease may be distinctly lower in a patient with a very low pretest probability of disease compared to a different patient with a much higher pretest probability (see Fig. 16-

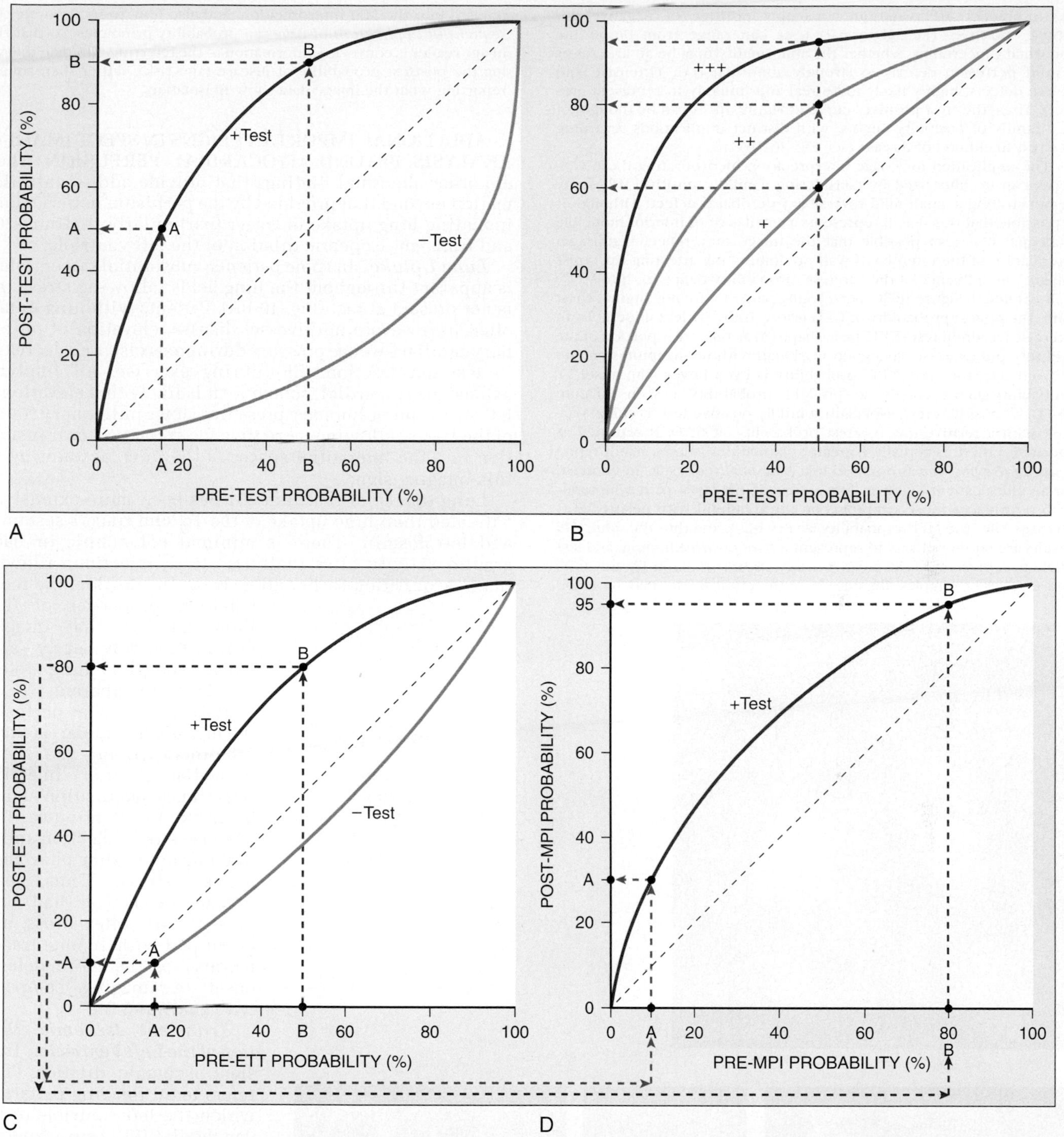

FIGURE 16–7 The influence of the "pretest" probability on posttest interpretation and application of Bayes' theorem. **A,** For a patient with a low pretest probability of disease (point A at 15 percent on the *x*-axis) with a positive test result, the posttest probability of disease (point A at 50 percent on the *y*-axis) is lower compared to a different patient with a higher pretest probability with the same positive test result (point B at 50 percent pretest probability on the *x*-axis, 90 percent posttest probability on the *y*-axis). **B,** The "test positive" curve can be thought of as a family of curves influenced by how strongly positive the images might be. For a given pretest probability, the posttest probability becomes progressively higher as the image becomes more strongly abnormal. For a borderline abnormal study ("+" curve), the posttest probability may be only slightly higher then the pretest value. For a strongly positive study ("+++" curve), the posttest probability is very high no matter what the pretest probability. **C** and **D,** Sequential application of Bayes' theorem. For a young patient with nonanginal chest pain, the pretest probability of CAD is low (~15 percent, point A on *x*-axis of **C**). If the patient with the 15% pretest probability undergoes an exercise treadmill test (ETT) and exercises to a good workload with no symptoms and no ECG change, the "post-ETT" probability is even lower (10 percent on *y*-axis in **C**). The post-ETT probability then becomes the "pre-MPI" probability, as seen in **D** (point A on *x*-axis). A "positive" MPI test is still associated with a relative low posttest probability of CAD (point A at 30 percent probability on *y*-axis). If reported as "positive," there is actually a greater chance that such a result represents a *false-positive result* (70 percent) as opposed to a *true-positive* result (30 percent). For an older patient with chest pain (higher pretest probability, point B on *x*-axis of **C**), who reproduces those symptoms on the treadmill with positive ECG changes, the "post-ETT" probability rises (point B on *y*-axis of **C**), and that becomes the high "pre-MPI" probability (point B on *x*-axis of **D**). Thus the same MPI results are far more likely to represent a *true positive* finding (point B on *y*-axis of **D,** 95 percent), and less likely to represent a false-positive study (5 percent).

7A). In practice, MPI results are not simply "positive" or "negative" but rather, "positive" (i.e., abnormal) tests can range from borderline abnormal (uncertainty whether the abnormality may be an artifact or a mild perfusion defect) to strongly abnormal (i.e., extensive and severe defects, highly likely to be real and unlikely to represent artifact). Thus, the "test positive" curve in Figure 16-7A can be thought of as a family of positivity curves, with distinct implications regarding posttest likelihood of disease (see Fig. 16-7B).

The implication for image interpretation incorporating these concepts can be illustrated by considering a mildly positive MPI study demonstrating a small mild reversible inferobasal defect. Although it is possible that this defect represents a small area of inferior inducible ischemia, it is also possible that the image may reflect diaphragm attenuation of the inferobasal wall predominantly affecting the stress image. The influence of the "pretest" probability data (i.e., "pre-MPI") is illustrated in Figure 16-7C. For a young patient with nonanginal chest pain, the pretest probability of CAD is low. If the patient undergoes an exercise treadmill test (ETT) (see Chap. 13) as the stress portion of the MPI test and exercises to a good workload with no symptoms and no ECG change, the "post-ETT" probability is even lower. The post-ETT probability then becomes the "pre-MPI" probability, as seen in Figure 16-7D. A "positive" test, especially a mildly positive test, is still associated with a relative low posttest probability of CAD. If reported as "positive," there is actually a greater chance that such a result represents a *false-positive* as opposed to a *true-positive* result. In contrast, for an older patient being evaluated for anginal chest pain symptoms, who reproduces those symptoms on the treadmill with positive ECG changes, the "pre-MPI" probability is very high, and thus the same MPI results are far more likely to represent a *true positive* finding, and less likely to represent a false-positive study, as illustrated in Figure 16-7C and D. These examples illustrate how the clinical data may be incorporated into the MPI interpretation, and also how to incorporate the *sequential application* of Bayesian probability principles, so that the image reader is conveying information to the referring clinician reflecting the posttest probability of disease (and risk), rather than simply reporting what the image data show in isolation.

ADDITIONAL IMPORTANT SIGNS IN SPECT IMAGING ANALYSIS BEYOND MYOCARDIAL PERFUSION. There are other abnormal findings that provide additional information beyond that provided by the perfusion pattern alone, including lung uptake of tracer (particularly thallium-201) and transient ischemic dilation of the left ventricle.

Lung Uptake. In some patients, substantial tracer uptake is apparent throughout the lung fields following stress that is not present at rest (Fig. 16-8A). Patients with lung uptake often have severe multivessel disease, elevation of pulmonary capillary wedge pressure during exercise, and decreases in ejection fraction (EF) during exercise, all implying extensive myocardial ischemia.[3] It is likely that elevation in left atrial and pulmonary pressures slows pulmonary transit of the tracer, allowing more time for extraction or transudation into the interstitial spaces of the lung, accounting for this imaging sign.

Lung uptake of thallium-201 has been more extensively validated than lung uptake of the Tc 99m tracers sestamibi and tetrofosmin. There is minimal splanchnic or background activity after thallium stress injection, allowing image acquisition earlier after stress. In addition, the redistribution properties of thallium mandate that imaging begin relatively early after stress, and thus lung uptake may be more apparent.

With the Tc 99m perfusion tracers, liver uptake is more prominent than the heart immediately after injection; thus, image acquisition should begin 15 to 30 minutes after exercise stress injection and 30 to 60 minutes after pharmacological stress. Thus, lung uptake, even if it had been present early after stress, may be missed with Tc 99m tracers because of the more delayed onset of imaging compared with thallium.

Transient Ischemic Dilation of the Left Ventricle. Transient ischemic dilation (TID) refers to an imaging pattern in which the left ventricle or left ventricular (LV) cavity appears larger on the stress images than at rest (see Fig. 16-8B).[7] For patients in whom the entire left ventricle appears larger during stress, the pathophysiology is probably related to extensive ischemia and prolonged postischemic systolic dysfunction, resulting in a dilated, dysfunctional left ventricle during the stress acquisition relative to the rest acquisition. In other patients, the epicardial silhouette appears similar at stress and rest, but there is apparent dila-

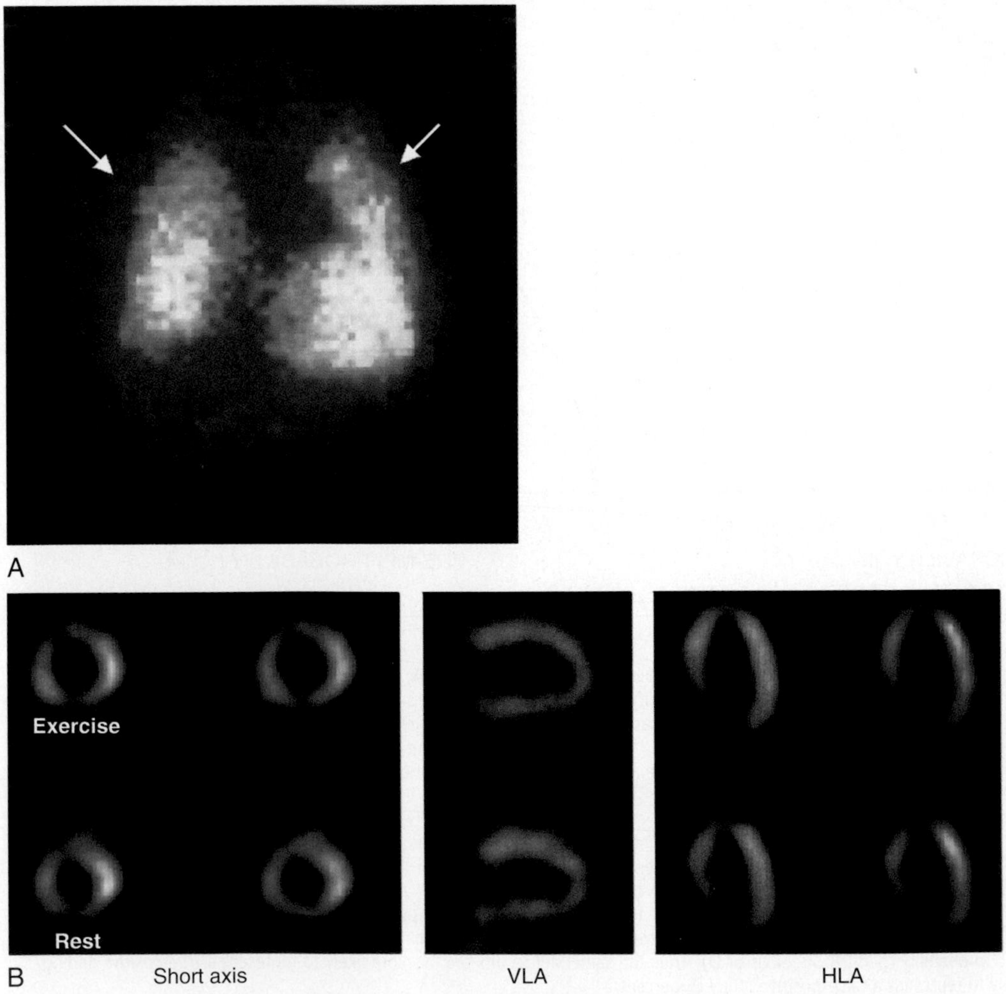

FIGURE 16–8 A, Increased lung uptake of thallium-201, imaged in the anterior projection. Lung uptake such as this is associated with extensive coronary artery disease and an adverse prognosis. **B,** Transient ischemic dilation of the left ventricle after stress. In the exercise stress images (top row), the apparent size of the left ventricular cavity is larger compared with the rest images (bottom row), i.e., transiently dilated. HLA = horizontal long axis; VLA = vertical long axis.

tion in the LV cavity. This probably represents diffuse subendocardial ischemia (relatively less tracer uptake in the subendocardium creating the appearance of an enlarged LV cavity) and is also associated with severe and extensive CAD. Contemporary processing systems can automatically quantify TID.

Both lung uptake and TID provide clues to more extensive CAD than may have been suspected from the perfusion pattern alone. Both signs have been associated with angiographically extensive and severe CAD and with unfavorable long-term outcomes and thus are considered "high-risk" findings.

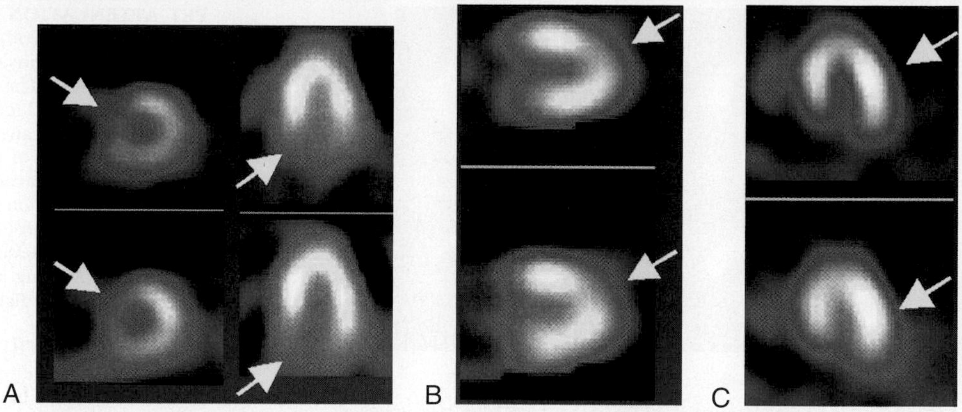

FIGURE 16–9 Normal variations in single-photon emission computed tomography perfusion imaging. **A,** Normal "dropout" of the basal septum (arrows). **B,** Normal apical thinning. **C,** The lateral wall is often slightly "hotter" than the septum, another normal variation.

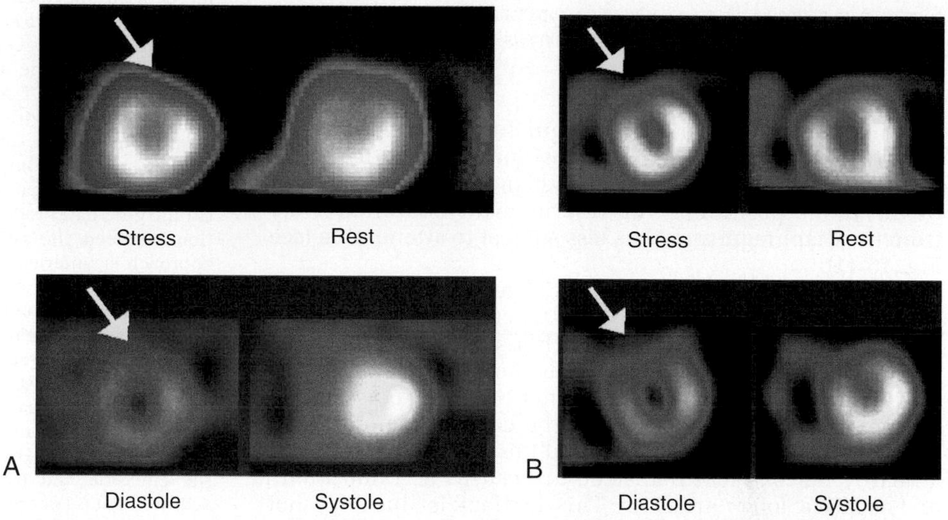

FIGURE 16–10 Breast attenuation artifact. **A,** Top row: a mild fixed anterior defect related to a possible breast attenuation artifact. In the bottom row, diastolic and systolic frames from an electrocardiographic-gated single-photon emission computed tomography (SPECT) acquisition demonstrating preserved wall thickening in the territory of the mild anterior fixed defect. The preserved wall thickening supports the conclusion that the mild defect is an attenuation artifact. **B,** A more severe anterior fixed defect is unlikely to represent an artifact on the basis of the severity and is more likely to represent myocardial infarction. In the bottom row, diastolic and systolic frames from the gated SPECT acquisition demonstrate abnormal thickening, supporting the interpretation of infarct rather than artifact.

Common Normal Variations in SPECT Imaging

Normal variations in perfusion images can be falsely interpreted as a defect. These perturbations from a completely homogeneous tracer pattern throughout the myocardium are related to structural variations of the myocardium as well as technical factors associated with image acquisition.

One example is the "dropout" of the upper septum because of the muscular septum merging with the membranous septum (Fig. 16-9A). Apical thinning is another variation of normal that can be mistaken for a perfusion defect (see Fig. 16-9B). The apex is anatomically thinner than other myocardial regions, creating this appearance. In normal SPECT images, the lateral wall may often appear brighter than the contralateral septum (see Fig. 16-9C). This is not due to a difference in lateral versus septal wall myocardial blood flow. Rather, during a SPECT acquisition, the camera is physically closer to the lateral myocardial wall (in close proximity to the lateral chest wall) than to the septum, thus subject to less soft tissue attenuation and associated with more efficient count capture. A careful review of a series of normal volunteers or subjects with a low probability of CAD with one's own equipment is an important step in minimizing the influence of these normal variations on the sensitivity and specificity for detecting CAD.

Technical Artifacts Affecting Image Interpretation

BREAST ATTENUATION. In patients with large or dense breasts, significant attenuation may create artifacts varying considerably in their appearance and location (Fig. 16-10A and B). A review of the cine display of the raw projection images may reveal the presence of potential breast attenuation.[4] Gender-matched quantitative data bases have had a favorable, although modest, impact on this issue, as such data bases generally consist of subjects who are of average body and breast size.

Several approaches toward minimizing the impact of breast tissue have been taken to improve specificity (lowering the false-positive rate) in women. Most well documented is the use of Tc 99m-based agents with SPECT imaging with ECG gating. In the setting of a mild to moderately severe fixed defect, most often of the anterior or anterolateral wall, that may represent breast attenuation artifact versus nontransmural MI, the *presence of preserved wall motion suggests the absence of infarct* and supports the interpretation of attenuation artifact (see Fig. 16-10A, bottom). Specificity for ruling out CAD in women has been improved significantly with this technique,[4] as discussed subsequently.

INFERIOR WALL ATTENUATION. Inferior wall attenuation artifacts are commonly encountered in SPECT imaging. This artifact may be caused by extracardiac structures such as the diaphragm overlapping the inferior wall (Fig. 16-11). In addition, during a SPECT acquisition, the longer distance from the inferior wall to the camera means that photons must traverse a greater degree of tissue before reaching the detectors, which may increase the degree of scatter and attenuation.

As with breast attenuation artifact detection, the demonstration of preserved wall thickening by gated SPECT

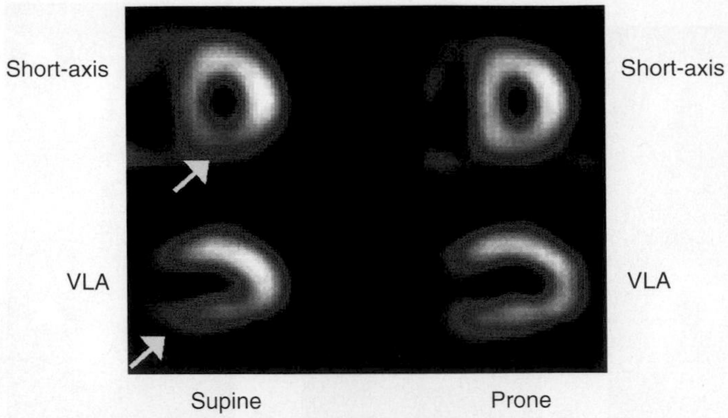

FIGURE 16–11 Left, Attenuation of the inferior basal wall (yellow arrows) possibly related to attenuation by overlying left hemidiaphragm. Most commonly, this appears as a tapering of the inferior wall seen best on the vertical long-axis (VLA) image. **Right,** One solution to the problem of inferior wall attenuation is reimaging the patient in the prone position. In this position, the inferior wall is pulled somewhat away from the diaphragm. In this example, the inferior wall appears more normal in the prone acquisition, suggesting that the apparent reduction in counts in the usual supine acquisition represented attenuation artifact.

imaging may be helpful in distinguishing attenuation artifact from infarct. The patient's positioning may also minimize the degree of attenuation. When patients are imaged in the *prone* position,[2,4] the inferior wall is shifted away from the diaphragm and thus less subject to attenuation (see Fig. 16-11).

ARTIFACTS RELATED TO EXTRACARDIAC TRACER UPTAKE. Tracer in extracardiac structures can cause artifacts in SPECT images. When such a structure is near the heart, increased counts may reach the detector. This may falsely elevate the number of counts the system assigns to the nearby cardiac wall, so that the cardiac region is displayed as falsely "hotter." A second possibility occurs when a nearby hot extracardiac structure causes a "ramp filter" or "negative lobe" artifact.[2] This artifact is due to a hot extracardiac structure "stealing" counts from the heart during the calculation of the summed SPECT images. The adjacent myocardium appears falsely "cool." If substantial extracardiac uptake is noted, image acquisition may be repeated after waiting a longer period of time before imaging. Having the patient drink cold water may enhance clearance of tracer from visceral organs, particularly bowel.

ATTENUATION CORRECTION METHODS

Attenuation of photons refers to undetected events in the heart due to interaction of atoms with the intervening soft tissue, breast, or diaphragm. Attenuation of photons can produce artifactual defects in both positron emission tomography (PET) and SPECT cardiac imaging that mimic true myocardial perfusion defects, and thus reduce specificity (increase false-positive findings). The 511 keV photons emitted by positron emitting radiotracers in PET imaging are attenuated less per centimeter of soft tissue than are the lower energy 80-140 keV photons typically emitted by SPECT radiotracers. In SPECT imaging, a single photon needs to travel from the heart to the camera, whereas in PET imaging two coincident photons (i.e., emitted simultaneously) need to travel across the entire body to reach their respective detectors. Although the total attenuation may actually be greater for PET than for SPECT, an important distinction in the case of PET is that the attenuation is the same along a projection line (the path the pair of photons traverse) independent of how deep in the body the annihilation took place. Thus, in PET, only the total attenuation through the whole body along a specific direction must be known. On the other hand, in SPECT, the exact depth along a projection line where the radioactive decay took place is necessary to correct for attenuation. Thus, attenuation correction for SPECT is theoretically more challenging. In recent years, several approaches to correct for attenuation in both PET and SPECT imaging have emerged—with the goal of "correcting" attenuation artifacts to minimize false positive defects and improve specificity.

PET ATTENUATION CORRECTION. To measure the attenuation correction factor, a rod that rotates about the patient is filled with a relatively long-lived positron emitter germanium-68 or a single photon emitter cesium-137. The rod is first made to rotate at a fixed speed in the gantry and total coincident counts are measured without the patient (the blank scan) and repeated with the patient (the transmission scan). The ratio of coincident counts of blank scan and transmission scan yields the array of attenuation correction factors needed to correct each projection line. Once each projection line has been corrected for attenuation (and scatter), the emission data may be reconstructed into an attenuation-corrected emission image for clinical interpretation. As long as the patient does not move during the scanning procedure, cardiac PET images will be free from attenuation artifacts.

SPECT ATTENUATION CORRECTION. Similar approaches to those in PET have been attempted to correct attenuation artifacts in SPECT, but these have not been widely adopted, because the problem of attenuation correction is fundamentally more challenging in SPECT than in PET. There are a number of commercially available SPECT gamma cameras that have the ability to acquire transmission data and perform attenuation correction. Several published studies suggest that incorporating attenuation correction into SPECT interpretation may increase the specificity of CAD diagnosis. However, the increased cost of SPECT attenuation correction systems and the additional time required to quality control, acquire, and process studies are factors that have slowed the widespread deployment of this technology.

TYPES OF SPECT ATTENUATION CORRECTION. Accurate attenuation correction with SPECT requires both emission and transmission acquisitions from a single study, and there are a number of potential approaches to accomplish this. The first is a sequential attenuation correction, which can be done with the emission acquisition (the clinical imaging data) following the transmission scan. However, registration between the two acquisitions can be challenging. A second approach is "interleaved" attenuation correction, where emission and transmission scans are acquired sequentially, at each stop. While this reduces the emission-transmission misalignment, the acquisition time is significantly longer. The third approach is simultaneous attenuation correction, which reduces the length of the study as well as emission-transmission misalignment. Whether a two-headed (90 degree) or three-headed gamma camera is used, one of the heads can be dedicated to acquire the transmission data and the other head (or two) to acquire the emission data. However, crosstalk by scattered photons between the emission and transmission photons unavoidably degrades the acquired data. For three-headed SPECT cameras, a line source can be added at one of the gaps between the three camera heads. In this approach, the opposing camera head with a fan beam collimator is then used to detect the transmitted photons. Because the fan beam collimator focuses down to a line in about 50 cm, it is possible that a portion of the patient's body will not intersect the fan beam and thus be out of the camera's field of view. This can lead to loss of data, termed truncation artifacts, when reconstructing the attenuation image. Although a number of schemes have been proposed to account for the truncation artifact, none has proved to be clinically robust. Clinical validation has been performed for several, but not all, of the commercially available systems just described. Despite these technical challenges, the application of attenuation correction in multicenter clinical trials, with different hardware and software approaches, has been shown to add to the diagnostic accuracy of stress myocardial perfusion SPECT, predominantly by improving specificity (Fig. 16-12). As a result, the American Society of Nuclear Cardiology and the Society of Nuclear Medicine have published a joint statement with the recommendation that the weight of current evidence is in favor of applying attenuation correction in addition to ECG-gating with SPECT MPI to optimize diagnostic accuracy.[8] This recommendation, however, presumes that personnel highly knowledgeable about the technique and its stringent quality control apply the attenuation correction methodology.

Combined PET/CT and SPECT/CT Scanners

Combined PET/CT and SPECT/CT scanners provide a tool for obtaining complementary anatomical and functional information in a single imaging session. CT angiography provides information on the presence and extent of luminal narrowing of epicardial coronary arteries with high sensitivity and specificity (see Chap. 18), whereas PET and SPECT provide information on the downstream functional consequences of anatomical lesions. Cardiac CT angiography is suited to determine whether an "obstructive" coronary artery stenosis is present, although the ability to accurately determine stenosis severity is limited with current generation CT angiography systems. PET and SPECT, on the other hand, are more suited to determine if such a stenosis is physiologically significant regarding limitation of flow reserve. With the advent of hybrid PET/CT or SPECT/CT systems, such complementary information of anatomy and physiology can be realized immediately, at the same imaging session. The combination of these anatomical and functional modalities is particularly relevant in patients who have an intermediate finding on either SPECT/PET or CT angiography. The advantage of the combined scanner is that the corresponding images are *spatially aligned,* and can be acquired during a single imaging session (Fig. 16-13).

CT ATTENUATION CORRECTION FOR PET AND SPECT. A subsidiary benefit of hybrid PET/CT and SPECT/CT imaging systems is in the potential to use the CT image to compute the attenuation map for the MPI data. This approach has allowed the replacement of germanium-68 or cesium-137 transmission scans with faster CT scans, reducing the overall duration of the PET procedure. One potential problem of using fast CT scans for attenuation correction, however, is the motion of the organs during respiration. The CT scanner "freezes" the heart, lungs, and liver at one point in the respiratory cycle, while the PET emission data are averaged over many respiratory cycles. Methods using respiratory gating to correct this problem are currently under investigation.

Gated SPECT Display, Interpretation, and Quantitation

An important advance in the use and application of SPECT MPI has been the incorporation of ECG-gated SPECT perfusion imaging for *simultaneous assessment of LV function as well as perfusion.* Prior to the use of gated SPECT, comprehensive information on both perfusion and function required separate testing modalities, such as SPECT MPI and a separate radionuclide ventriculogram (RVG) or echocardiogram.

Electrocardiographically Gated Radionuclide Techniques to Assess the Physiology of Ventricular Function

To assess parameters of cardiac function with echocardiography, LV endocardial borders are drawn over several beats to derive parameters such as EF. With contrast left ventriculography, endocardial borders are drawn for either one beat or an average of several beats to calculate EF. In contrast, the commonly used radionuclide techniques to assess ventricular function create *one cardiac cycle for analysis that represents an average of several hundred beats* acquired over a period of 8 to 15 minutes, using a technique known as ECG gating (Fig. 16-14).

During an ECG-gated image acquisition, the patient's ECG is monitored simultaneously with the image. As the peak of an R wave is detected, the gate opens and a set number of milliseconds of imaging information is stored in a frame. For a typical gated SPECT acquisition, each R-R interval is divided into eight frames. For example, if the patient's resting heart rate is 60 beats/min (1000 milliseconds per beat), an eight-frame acquisition across the cardiac cycle comprises 125 milliseconds per frame. After the first 125 milliseconds of imaging data have been recorded in frame 1, the gate closes and then instantly reopens, allowing the second 125 milliseconds of information to be recorded in frame 2 (see Fig. 16-14A). This sequence continues through the prespecified number of frames throughout the cardiac cycle. When the R wave of the next beat is detected by the ECG-gated system, the sequence is repeated for each beat that occurs throughout the image acquisition.

The number of counts recorded during any individual cardiac cycle is insufficient to create an interpretable image. When several hundred beats have been recorded, an average cardiac cycle representing all the recorded beats can be reconstructed by redisplaying the frames sequentially in a cine or movie format.[9] The first few frames represent systolic events, and the latter frames represent diastolic events (see Fig. 16-14A).

High-quality ECG-gated images require that included cardiac cycles have reasonably homogeneous beat lengths. This is usually accomplished by "beat-length windowing,"

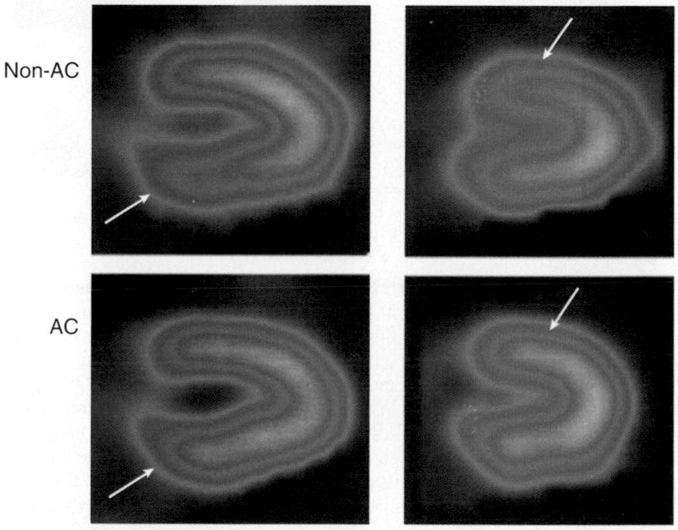

FIGURE 16–12 Impact of attenuation correction (AC). In the non-AC images (top row) there are examples of an inferior defect (left column) and an anterior defect (right column), which may represent diaphragmatic and breast attenuation, respectively, or may represent a true perfusion abnormality. With the application of AC (bottom row), both images become normal, suggesting that the abnormalities in the non-AC images were highly likely to represent artifact. *(Courtesy of Ernest Garcia, PhD.)*

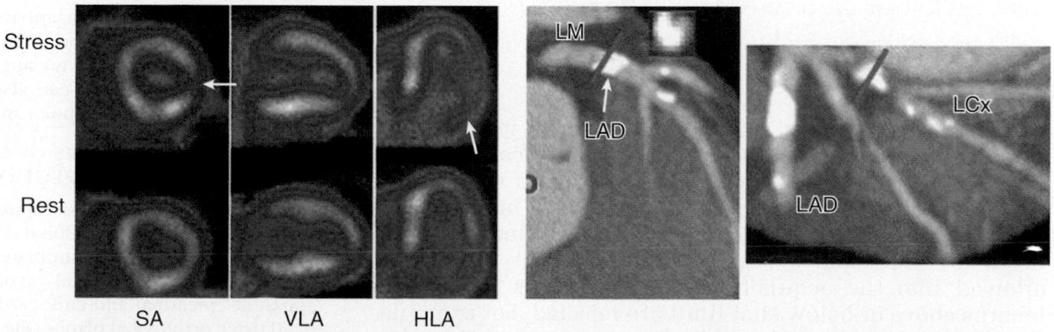

FIGURE 16–13 Combined positron emission tomographic (PET) images of stress and rest perfusion (left) and cardiac computed tomographic (CT) angiography and calcium imaging (right). The PET images demonstrate a lateral wall reversible defect consistent with ischemia (arrows in the short-axis [SA] and horizontal long-axis [HLA] images). However the CT images demonstrate more extensive calcification and stenosis of the left main (LM), left anterior descending (LAD) and left circumflex (LCx) vessels. The combined information suggests that although the physiological ischemia predominantly involves the lateral wall/LCx territory, more extensive CAD is present. VLA = vertical long-axis.

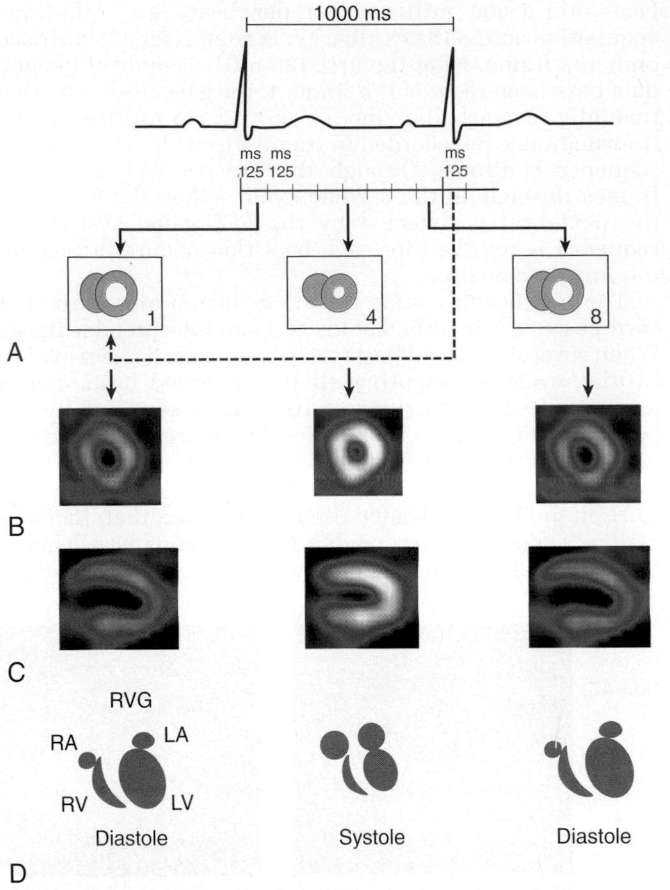

FIGURE 16–14 Basis for the technique of electrocardiographic (ECG) gating. **A,** The scintigraphic acquisition data are collected in conjunction with the electrocardiogram. The R-R interval is divided into a prespecified number of frames (in this example eight frames). At a heart rate of 60 beats/min (1000 msec/beat), each of the eight frames would comprise 125 milliseconds. For the first 125 milliseconds after the peak of the initial R wave, all imaging data are recorded in frame 1; the second 125 milliseconds are recorded in frame 2 and so on until the peak of the next R wave is detected, and this is repeated for each beat in the acquisition. Frame 1 thus represents the end-diastolic events, and one of the frames in the middle of the acquisition (frame 4 in this example) represents end-systolic events. **B,** Examples of gated single-photon emission computed tomography perfusion imaging. Short-axis images are seen at end diastole and at end systole. **C,** Similar timing with images displayed from the vertical long-axis orientation. Visually, wall thickening and brightening are seen across the course of systole. These events represent regional wall thickening and changes in global function across the cardiac cycle. **D,** ECG-gated equilibrium radionuclide ventriculographic (RVG) schematic images are shown at diastole and at end systole. LA = left atrium; LV = left ventricle; RA = right atrium; RV = right ventricle. *(Adapted from Germano G, Berman DS: Acquisition and processing for gated SPECT: Technical aspects.* In *Germano G, Berman DS [eds]: Clinical gated cardiac SPECT. Armonk, NY, Futura Publishing, 1999, pp 93-114.)*

whereby the computer acquisition system is programmed to accept beats into the acquisition of only certain cycle lengths. Typically, cycles with the beat length represented by the average heart rate of the patient (1000 milliseconds in the preceding example), along with cycles fluctuating up to 10 to 15 percent around the average beat length, are allowed into the acquisition. Cardiac cycles with cycle lengths above or below that limit are rejected. For example, the short cardiac cycle from the R wave of a normal beat to the R wave of a premature ventricular contraction (PVC) would not be allowed into the acquisition, nor would the long cycle representing the post-PVC pause. This makes physiological sense; the short pre-PVC beat and the more prolonged post-PVC beat have distinctly different systolic and diastolic characteristics than the beats during normal sinus rhythm.

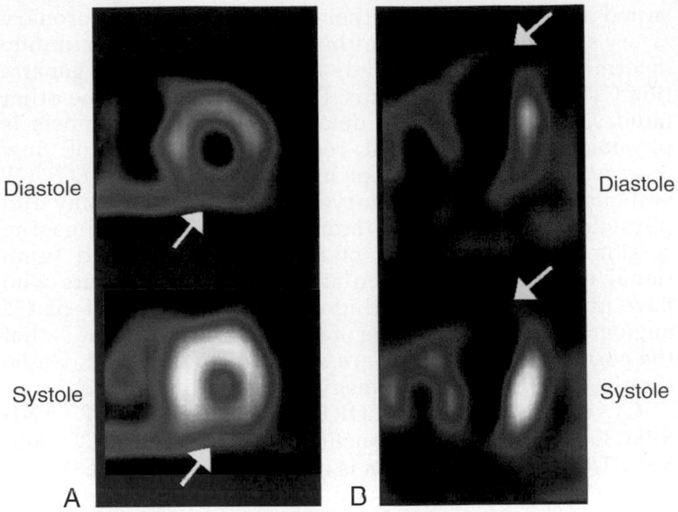

FIGURE 16–15 Examples of regional dysfunction detected by ECG-gated single-photon emission computed tomography perfusion imaging. **A,** The *severely hypokinetic* inferior region appears to brighten less (arrows) than the other regions from diastole to systole. The lateral wall also brightens less than the normal septum, and thus would be interpreted as *hypokinetic.* **B,** The *akinetic* apex in the horizontal long axis (arrows) appears to have no change from diastole to systole, in contrast to the normally thickening (brightening) lateral wall.

ECG-GATED SPECT IMAGING. The clinical technique most commonly used to assess ventricular function is ECG-gated SPECT imaging.[9] Normal regional systolic function is depicted as brightening of the wall during systole (see Fig. 16-14B). The wall appears to thicken, and there is apparent endocardial excursion. Assessment of regional LV function by gated SPECT imaging is based on an effect known in imaging physics as the *partial volume effect,* sometimes referred to as the *recovery coefficient* effect. When objects being imaged fall below a certain thickness threshold, count (or photon) recovery from the object is related not only to the tracer concentration within that object but also to the thickness of the object.[9] For SPECT imaging, usually all myocardial wall thicknesses fall below that threshold. Although tracer concentration within the myocardium is constant during a gated SPECT image acquisition, the recovery of counts (and thus the brightness of the object being imaged) is related to wall thickness. Hence, during systolic wall thickening, it appears that the LV wall becomes brighter and thicker, even though the isotope concentration per gram of myocardial tissue is actually unchanged. This principle forms the basis for gated SPECT imaging.

Regional myocardial function is usually assessed visually, in a manner similar to the analysis performed in echocardiography. Regions that brighten normally have normal regional systolic performance, and those with diminished but apparent brightening are labeled hypokinetic. Regions with slight brightening are interpreted as severely hypokinetic and regions with no apparent brightening as akinetic (Fig. 16-15). Regional function can also be analyzed by quantitative techniques and displayed in a polar map format.

QUANTITATIVE ANALYSIS OF GLOBAL LEFT VENTRICULAR FUNCTION BY GATED SPECT IMAGING

All contemporary camera-computer systems have software capable of quantitative analysis of global LV function. These computer-based methodologies are fully automated and thus extremely reproducible. The most common method involves automated interrogation of the apparent epicardial and endocardial borders of all of the tomograms in all three orthogonal planes (Fig. 16-16A). These multiple two-dimensional contours are then reconstructed to create a surface-rendered three-dimensional display representing global LV function across a typical cardiac cycle (see Fig. 16-16B) that can be viewed from any direction by simple maneuvering of the computer display screen or cursor.[9] The three-dimensional display is accompanied by automated calculation of EF and LV volumes.

EF measurements from automated analysis of ECG-gated SPECT MPI have been extensively validated against other quantitative techniques assessing LV function, such as equilibrium RVG, angiographic contrast left ventriculography, and cardiac magnetic resonance imaging (see Chaps. 17 and 19).[9] Across a wide range of LV function, and even in the setting of severe perfusion defects, ECG-gated SPECT imaging provides robust, highly reproducible estimates of LVEF.

The incorporation of ECG-gated SPECT imaging into a SPECT acquisition is now routine in MPI and is recommended as standard by contemporary guidelines.[2] As discussed subsequently, the addition of LV function data to the perfusion information provides incremental and independent prognostic information in addition to its practical importance in management decisions. Gated SPECT imaging has also been an important advance in helping to differentiate attenuation artifacts from infarct, as regions with persistent low counts that show normal motion and thickening represent soft tissue artifacts rather than scar. Thus, gated SPECT has improved the specificity of perfusion imaging for ruling out CAD, particularly in women.[10]

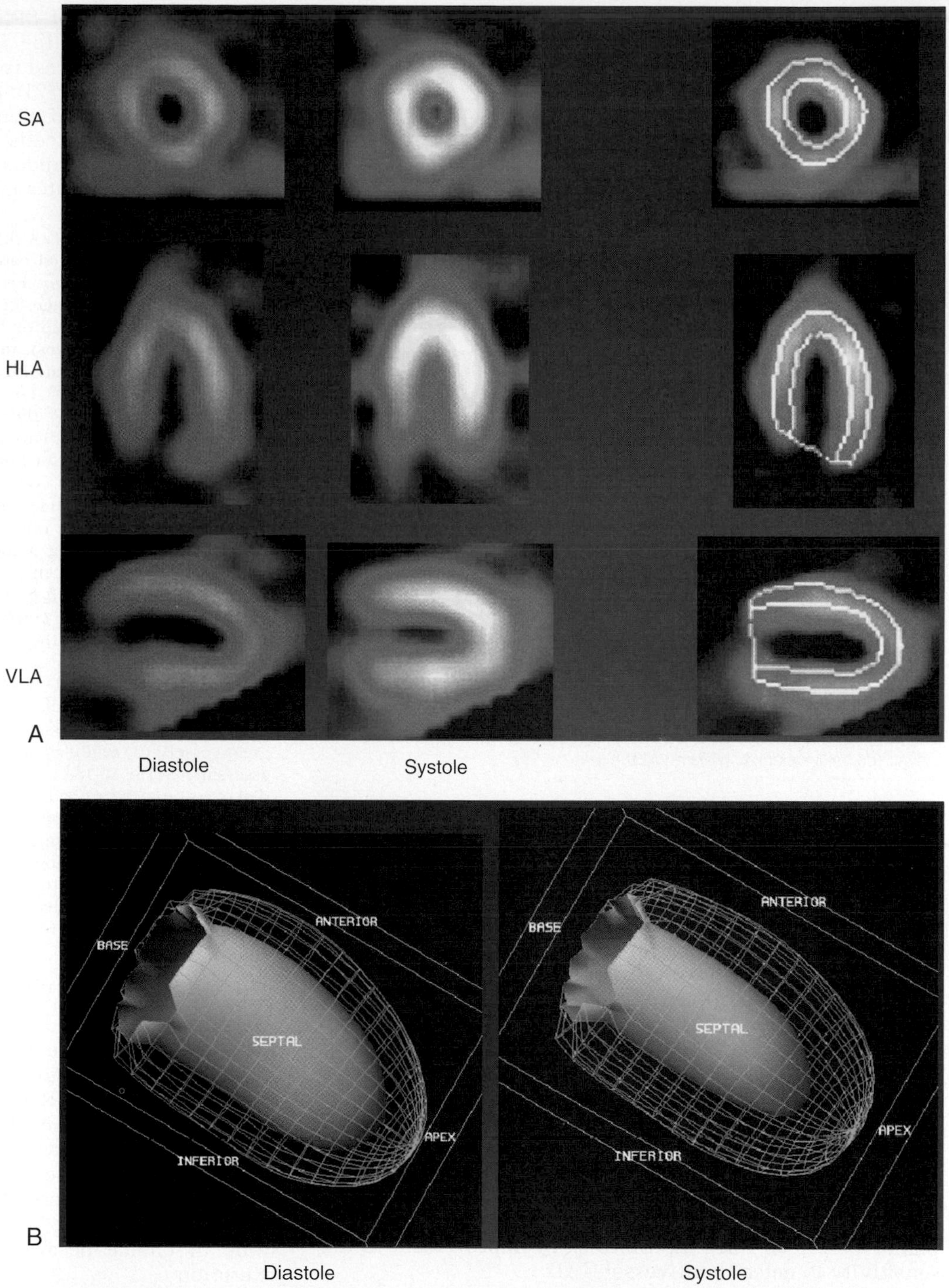

FIGURE 16–16 **A,** ECG-gated single-photon emission computed tomography (SPECT) perfusion images in short axis (SA), vertical long axis (VLA), and horizontal long axis (HLA), shown frozen at diastole (left column) and at end systole (middle column). Endocardial and epicardial borders are shown on the diastolic frames as automatically assigned by the software analysis program (right column). **B,** From the contours that are created from all of the two-dimensional tomograms, a three-dimensionally surface-rendered image of the left ventricle can be created and displayed in multiple orientations here frozen at end diastole (left) and end systole (right). The green "mesh" represents the epicardium, and the gray surface represents the endocardium. Ejection fraction is quantitated from the volume change. During image interpretation, gated SPECT images are displayed in the cine format, as an endless loop movie rather than as the still frames depicted here.

Planar Myocardial Perfusion Imaging

Prior to the widespread application of tomographic (SPECT) perfusion imaging techniques, planar imaging was the standard acquisition and display methodology. In planar imaging, three separate two-dimensional images are obtained with the gamma camera following radiotracer injection and uptake into the myocardium.[2] The three standard views are an anterior, a left anterior oblique, and a more lateral view (Fig. 16-17).

Using planar imaging, the imaging views are standard and the reader must account for the different orientations of the heart in assigning regional abnormalities. In contrast, because the tomographic SPECT slices are constructed perpendicular and parallel to an assigned long axis, SPECT images are oriented in a uniform manner for display and interpretation without influence by the individual patient's cardiac orientation.

An advantage of planar imaging over SPECT imaging is its simplicity. Each of the three views can be acquired over 5 to 8 minutes with patients lying on a table with their arms by their side. Planar imaging is less affected by patient motion than is SPECT imaging. With planar imaging, there is no extensive image processing as with SPECT, which creates many more sources of potential error and artifact. However, given the two-dimensional nature of planar imaging, in each of the standard views there is substantial overlap of myocardial regions and less ability to differentiate smaller and particularly milder perfusion abnormalities. The more standard orientation of SPECT imaging lends

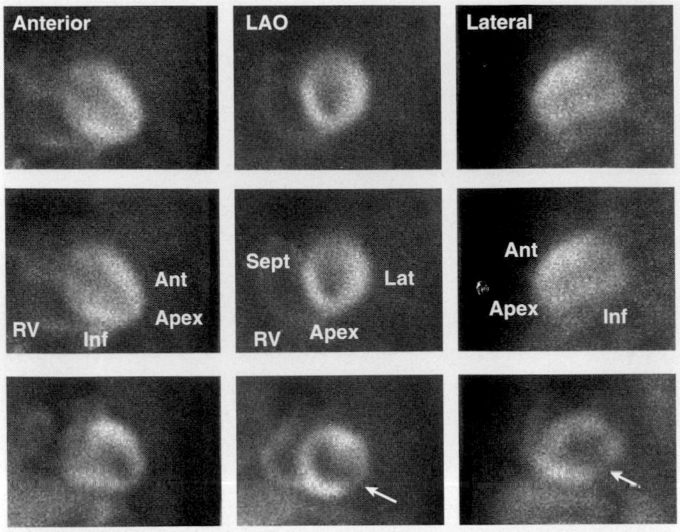

FIGURE 16–17 Examples of planar myocardial perfusion imaging. **Top row:** A normal stress planar perfusion study in the anterior, shallow left anterior oblique (LAO), and more lateral views. Tracer uptake is uniform throughout the myocardial walls. **Middle row:** The same normal planar stress perfusion images are shown, with the myocardial walls that are seen in each view labeled. The anterior wall (ant), apex, and inferior (inf) walls are seen in the anterior view as well as the right ventricle (RV). The septum (sept), apex, and lateral walls (lat) and the RV are seen in the shallow LAO view, and the anterior wall, apex, and inferior walls are seen in the lateral view. **Bottom row:** Example of an abnormal planar study showing a lateral wall stress perfusion defect in the shallow LAO view (arrow), extending into the inferior wall in the lateral view (arrow). Rest images are not shown. *(Courtesy of Kim A. Williams, M.D.)*

itself to easier understanding of the localization of perfusion abnormalities.

The original data on the sensitivity and specificity of perfusion imaging for CAD, as well as the prognostic value of perfusion imaging, were developed using planar imaging and later revalidated using SPECT imaging. In contemporary practice, planar imaging may be used for patients who do not tolerate the position that must be maintained during a SPECT acquisition, those who have difficulty coping with the larger SPECT camera being so close to the body, or those with large body habitus that surpasses the weight and size limits of SPECT systems.[4]

Quantitative analytical techniques such as the circumferential profile technique were originally developed using planar perfusion imaging. A substantial literature has documented that when quantitative analysis is applied to planar perfusion imaging, there is an improvement in the sensitivity to detect multivessel CAD.

Radionuclide Angiography or Ventriculography

RVG, also known as radionuclide angiography (RNA) or blood pool imaging, may be performed by *first-pass* or by *equilibrium gated* techniques.[10] The equilibrium technique is often referred to as multiple-gated acquisition (MUGA) scanning. Although the two techniques use distinct tracers and data recording, they provide similar results for global EF and chamber volumes. Both techniques provide a highly reproducible means to quantify global LV and right ventricular (RV) EF.

Equilibrium Radionuclide Angiography or Ventriculography (Gated Blood Pool Imaging)

In *equilibrium* RVG studies, data are recorded in a computer system synchronized with the R wave of the patient's ECG, similar to ECG-gated SPECT (see Fig. 16-14). Most commonly, Tc 99m labeling is applied to red blood cells or albumin. Image contrast is usually better with ^{99m}Tc-labeled red blood cells, but ^{99m}Tc-labeled albumin is preferable in patients in whom red blood cell labeling may be difficult. Labeling of red blood cells with ^{99m}Tc pertechnetate requires a reducing agent, stannous pyrophosphate, which is administered 15 to 30 minutes prior to pertechnetate injection.

IMAGE ACQUISITION. Although relatively few counts are recorded during a *single* ECG-gated cardiac cycle, the *summation of counts from 800 to 1000 cardiac cycles* produces an average cardiac cycle with high resolution. Images of the heart are usually acquired in three standard projections: anterior, left anterior oblique (best separation of the left and right ventricles), and left lateral (or left posterior oblique). The minimum framing rate for a resting RVG study is 16 frames/cycle (about 50 msec/frame).[10] For quantitative assessment of diastolic indices and regional EF, the framing rate should be increased to 32 frames/cycle (about 25 msec/frame). For adequate counting statistics, images are acquired for a preset count of at least 250,000 per frame or count density of 300 counts per pixel, which corresponds to an acquisition time of 5 to 10 minutes per projection. For exercise studies, adequate counts can be obtained in the best septal view with a 2-minute acquisition using a high-sensitivity collimator. Arrhythmias such as multiple PVCs can adversely affect the study if these beats account for more than 10 percent of the total. In patients with atrial fibrillation, there may be considerable beat-to-beat variability, and the mean EF obtained over the period of acquisition may underestimate the actual LVEF.[10]

IMAGE DISPLAY AND ANALYSIS. Qualitative inspection of equilibrium studies as an endless cinematic loop of the cardiac cycle (see Fig. 16-14D) allows assessment of (1) the size of heart chambers and great vessels; (2) regional wall motion; (3) global function (qualitative assessment) (Fig. 16-18A and B); (4) ventricular wall thickness, pericardial effusion, pericardial fat pad or paracardiac mass; and (5) extracardiac uptake (such as splenomegaly). Quantification of systolic and diastolic indices and volumes is derived from the ventricular time-activity curve,[10] which is analogous to the angiographic time-volume curve (Fig. 16-19). In addition to the time-activity curve, functional images, such as amplitude and phase images, can be produced that have been useful in characterizing regional asynergy and asynchrony.

First-Pass Radionuclide Angiography or Ventriculography

In *first-pass* RVG studies, the bolus of radioactivity passes initially through the right chambers of the heart, then through the lungs, and finally through the left-sided chambers of the heart. Radiopharmaceuticals used for this purpose must produce adequate counts in a short period of time at an acceptably low radiation dose to the patient.[10] Although both ^{99m}Tc-diethylenetriaminepentaacetic acid (DTPA) and ^{99m}Tc pertechnetate have short intravascular residence time, ^{99m}Tc-DTPA is the recommended radionuclide of choice because the DTPA salt enhances renal excretion.

IMAGE ACQUISITION. Images are acquired very rapidly as the tracer passes through the heart chambers. Separation of the right and left ventricles is achieved because of the temporal separation of the bolus. Image quality is related to the injection technique, which should be rapid (more than 2 to 3 seconds) in order to achieve an uninterrupted bolus (Fig. 16-20). Images are acquired in the supine position following the rapid injection of 25 mCi of tracer through an 18-gauge or larger intravenous catheter placed in the medial antecubital or external jugular vein. The shallow (20 to 30 degree) right anterior oblique projection is used to optimize separation of the atria and great vessels from the ventricles and to view the ventricles parallel to their long axes. Although the right anterior oblique view maximizes overlap of the right and left ventricles, this is not a problem in most patients because the timing of tracer appearance reliably identifies each chamber sequentially. A 1-mCi tracer dose may be used to ensure proper positioning so that the right and left ventricles are in the field of view.

IMAGE ANALYSIS. To identify the RV and LV phases, regions of interest are drawn around the right and left ventricles at end diastole.[10]

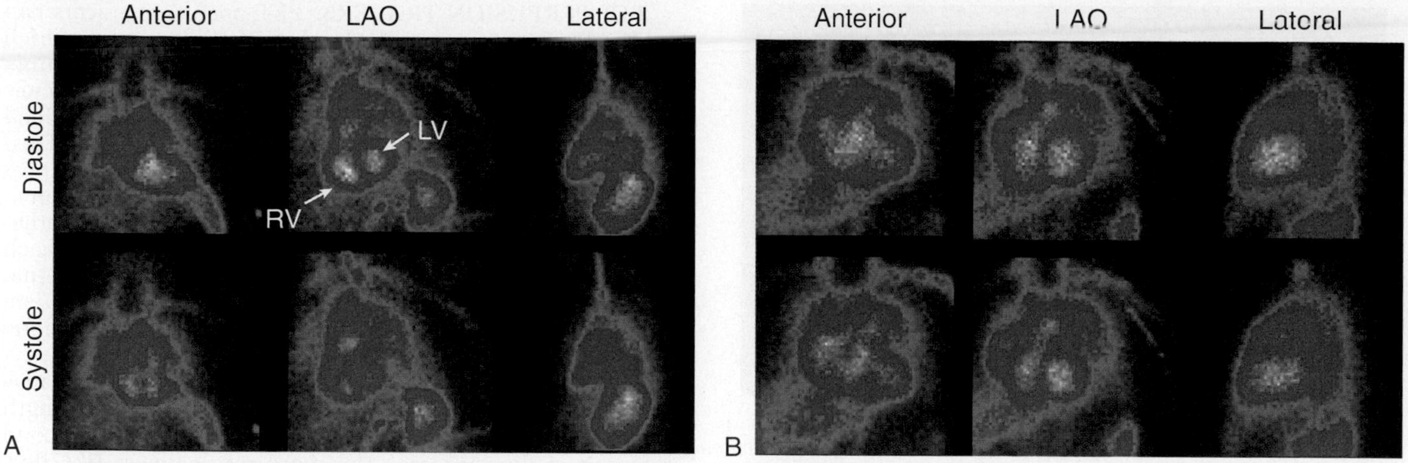

FIGURE 16–18 Equilibrium radionuclide ventriculography (RVG). The isotope (Tc99m) is labeled to red blood cells, and hence the images represent the blood "pools" in the left ventricle (LV), the right ventricle (RV), the other cardiac chambers and the great vessels, as well as the spleen. Typically, three views are obtained, as shown. **A,** Normal left ventricular function, with end-diastolic images in the top row and end-systolic images in the bottom row. LV and RV volumes diminish from diastole to systole. **B,** Images obtained in a patient with LV dysfunction. There is significant LV and RV dilatation at both end diastole (top) and end systole (bottom), and severely diminished LV systolic function (i.e., much less volume change from end diastole to end systole compared to the study in panel A). LAO = left anterior oblique projection.

Time-activity curves are generated, and cycles around and including the peak time-activity curve are used to calculate EFs. In general, two to five cardiac cycles are summed for the RV phase, and five to seven cycles are summed for the LV phase. From these data, quantitative analysis of LV and RV EF is performed.

COMPARISON OF EQUILIBRIUM AND FIRST-PASS TECHNIQUES. Advantages of the first-pass technique are the high target-to-background ratio, more distinct temporal separation of the cardiac chambers, and rapidity of imaging. RV EF may be more readily assessed using the first-pass technique because of the more distinct separation of this structure from the other chambers with that technique. Advantages of equilibrium technique are the potential for repeated assessment of cardiac function during rapidly varying physiological conditions, high count density, and acquisition of images in multiple projections. In contemporary practice, the equilibrium technique is performed more commonly.[2,4]

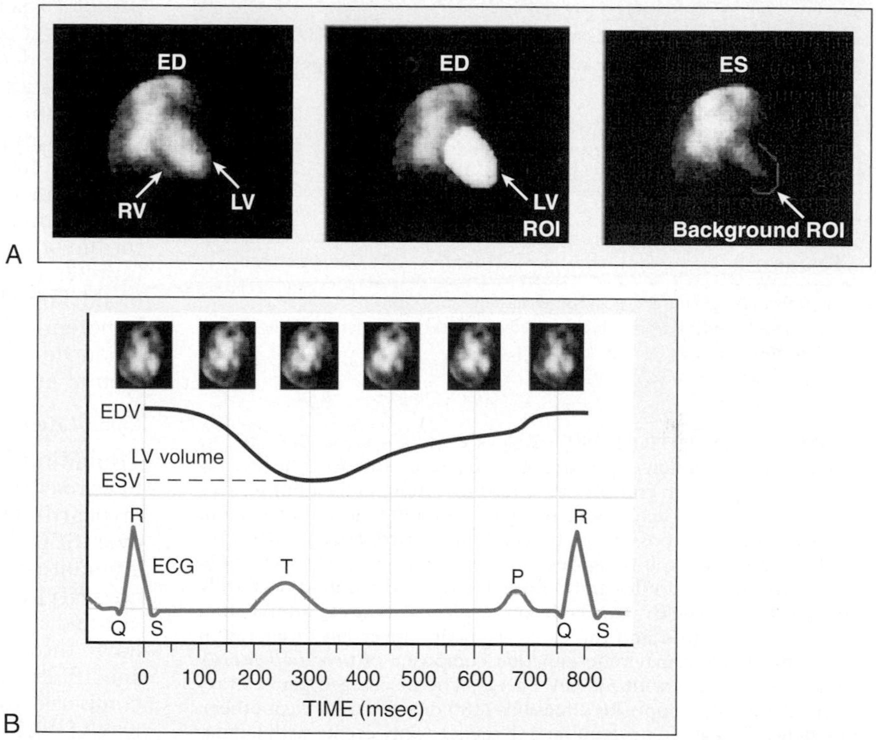

FIGURE 16–19 Quantitative analysis of equilibrium ECG-gated radionuclide ventriculography. **A,** The left anterior oblique view of the left ventricle (LV) and right ventricle (RV) is shown at end diastole (ED) **(left),** with a region of interest (ROI) identifying the LV contour at end diastole **(middle)** and a "background" ROI drawn at end systole (ES) **(right),** used to correct for count activity in front of and behind the LV. In **B,** a time-activity curve is demonstrated that illustrates the change in counts within the regions of interest shown in A across a cardiac cycle. Because count activity is related to LV chamber volume, the time-activity curve represents the relative volume change of the LV chamber across a cardiac cycle, from end diastole to end systole and back to end diastole. EDV = end-diastolic volume; ESV = end-systolic volume. *(From Green MV, Bacharach SL, Douglas MA, et al: The measurement of left ventricular function and the detection of wall motion abnormalities with high temporal resolution ECG-gated scintigraphic angiocardiography. IEEE Trans Nucl Sci NS-23, 1976.)*

Positron-Emission Tomography

Because of the quantitative capabilities of PET, measurement of myocardial perfusion and metabolism can be obtained with PET in *absolute quantitative terms,* a potential advantage compared with SPECT imaging. The radiotracers used in PET are labeled with positron-emitting isotopes that have chemical and physical properties identical to those of naturally occurring elements, such as carbon, oxygen, nitrogen, and fluorine. *Incorporating such elements allows interrogation of physiologically relevant processes in normal and diseased states.*[11] Although most positron-emitting radiotracers are cyclotron produced with short half-lives, the development of *generator-produced* positron-emitting isotopes, such as rubidium-82, makes it feasible for laboratories to perform cardiac PET studies without an on-site cyclotron.

Clinically available cardiac PET radiotracers fall within two broad categories: those that evaluate myocardial perfusion and those that evaluate myocardial metabolism (Table 16-2).[4] The perfusion tracers, rubidium-82 and [^{13}N]ammonia, and the myocardial metabolic tracer 2-[^{18}F]fluoro-2-deoxyglucose (FDG), have received FDA approval.

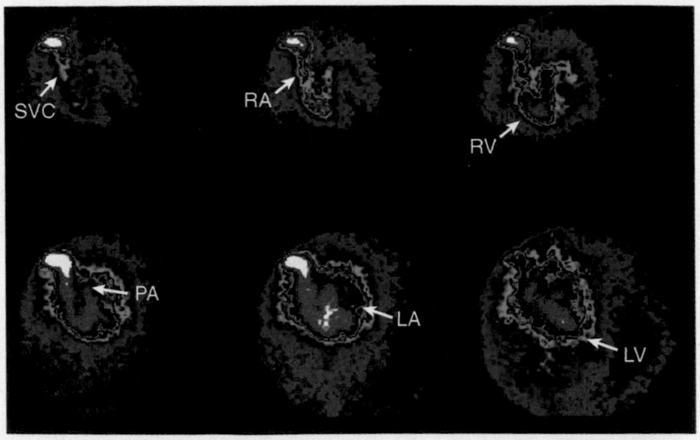

FIGURE 16–20 First-pass radionuclide ventriculography. Individual frames from a first-pass acquisition, illustrating the path of the bolus isotope through the superior vena cava (SVC), the right atrium (RA), the right ventricle (RV), the pulmonary outflow tract and lungs (pulmonary artery, PA), the left atrium (LA), and the left ventricular (LV) phase, from which the isotope bolus is then distributed systemically.

TABLE 16–2 Properties of Selected Positron-Emission Tomography Tracers

Tracer	Produced	Half-Life	Compound
Perfusion			
Oxygen-15	Cyclotron	2.1 min	H_2O
Nitrogen-13	Cyclotron	10 min	NH_3
Rubidium-82	Generator	76 sec	RbCl
Metabolism			
Carbon-11	Cyclotron	20.4 min	Acetate palmitate
Fluorine-18	Cyclotron	110 min	Deoxyglucose

Adapted from Bergmann SR: Positron-emission tomography of the heart. *In* Gerson MC (ed): Cardiac Nuclear Medicine. New York, McGraw-Hill, 1997, pp 267-300.

IMAGE ACQUISITION. PET employs camera systems designed to optimize the detection of positron-emitting radioisotopes. The process by which a positron-emitting radionuclide attempts to stabilize over time is termed beta decay, which occurs when the nucleus of an atom emits a positron, a positively charged beta particle (Fig. 16-21). After a high-energy positron is emitted from a nucleus, it travels a few millimeters in tissue and ultimately collides with an electron (a negatively charged beta particle). This collision results in complete annihilation of both the positron and the electron, with conversion to energy in the form of electromagnetic radiation composed of *two high-energy gamma rays,* each with 511-keV energy. The discharged gamma rays travel in perfectly opposite directions (180 degrees from each other). PET detectors can be programmed to register only events with temporal *coincidence* of photons that strike at directly opposing detectors. The outcome of such selective *coincidence detection* is an improvement in spatial and temporal resolution of PET compared with SPECT imaging.[12] Unlike the procedure in SPECT, in which an extrinsic collimator is used to limit the direction at which photons enter the detector, the coincidence detection with PET provides intrinsic collimation and improves the sensitivity of the camera.

In addition, an important distinction between PET and SPECT is in the ease of labeling primary substrates for energy metabolism and membrane receptor subtypes in the heart, allowing the interrogation of such physiological pathways in vivo. Moreover, dynamic mode PET scanning allows potential analysis of the *change in tracer content* in a specific region of interest in the heart with time, allowing potential interrogation of the rate of change of a physiological process.

IMAGE ANALYSIS. Emission data are displayed as tomograms in the horizontal and vertical long-axis and short-axis views.[12] If the data are acquired in dynamic mode, with appropriate mathematical modeling, myocardial perfusion and metabolic data can be displayed in absolute terms: in milliliters per gram per minute for blood flow and moles per gram per minute for metabolism.

PET PERFUSION TRACERS. PET perfusion tracers can be divided into two types (1) freely diffusible tracers, which accumulate and wash out from myocardial tissue as a function of blood flow; and (2) nondiffusible tracers, characterized by retention in myocardial tissue as a function of blood flow.[11] The rapid physiological washout of the freely diffusible tracers, such as [^{15}O]water, makes it possible to repeat studies in rapid sequence. The images of the distribution of such tracers are usually not visually meaningful; mathematical modeling is done to arrive at flow values at each pixel. An advantage of freely diffusible tracers is that they do not depend on a metabolic trapping mechanism that might change as a function of a changing metabolic environment.

The nondiffusible flow tracers are easier to image because the tracer is retained in myocardium for a reasonable length of time. Rubidium-82 and [^{13}N]ammonia fall into this second category of flow tracers—the more microsphere-like flow tracers. Rubidium-82 is a cation, with biological properties similar to those of potassium and thallium, and uptake across the sarcolemmal membrane reflects active transport by the Na^+,K^+-ATPase pump. In experimental studies, its extraction fraction does not change significantly over a wide range of metabolic conditions. However, the very short half-life of 75 seconds for ^{82}rubidium means that any trapped ^{82}rubidium quickly disappears from the myocardium by physical decay. Despite its short half-life, ^{82}rubidium is easily obtained as it is generator produced, and it can be used clinically without the need for an on-site cyclotron.

[^{13}N]Ammonia is an extractable perfusion tracer, with a physical half-life of 10 minutes. Its transport across cell membranes may occur by passive diffusion or by the active Na-K transport mechanism. Retention of [^{13}N]ammonia in the myocyte involves metabolic trapping. As with rubidium-82, myocardial uptake of ammonia reflects absolute blood flows up to 2 to 3 ml/gm/min and plateaus at more hyperemic flows. The use of this tracer to assess myocardial blood flow has been extensively validated in both experimental and clinical studies.[12]

Clinical Application of PET Perfusion Imaging

^{82}Rubidium and [^{13}N]ammonia are the two PET tracers that have received FDA approval for clinical application to assess myocardial perfusion. Advantages of PET perfusion imaging over SPECT include higher spatial resolution, improved attenuation and scatter correction, and the potential for quantifying regional blood flow. As a result, a number of clinical studies with either ^{82}rubidium or [^{13}N]ammonia PET have shown an improvement in either the sensitivity or specificity (as high as 95 percent) for detection of CAD when compared to SPECT (Fig. 16-22). However, the widespread use of PET myocardial perfusion studies in the clinical setting has been hampered by the requirement of an onsite cyclotron for ^{13}N-ammonia and the high cost of monthly generator replacement for ^{82}rubidium. Moreover, the relatively short half lives of both ^{82}rubidium and [^{13}N]ammonia limit the utility of PET perfusion studies to patients undergoing pharmacological stress only. As the exercise component of MPI studies has independent prognostic and diagnostic value, this represents an important limitation. On the other hand, the potential for quantifying myocardial blood flow in absolute terms is highly desirable, with potential clinical applications. Patients with multivessel CAD may have a uniform decrease in flow reserve, and the relative perfusion data from SPECT may fail to detect this balanced ischemia. On the other extreme, detection of mild abnormalities in myocardial blood flow reserve with PET potentially allows early identification of CAD, characterized by endothelial dysfunction in asymptomatic patients with elevated cholesterol, smoking, hypertension, and insulin

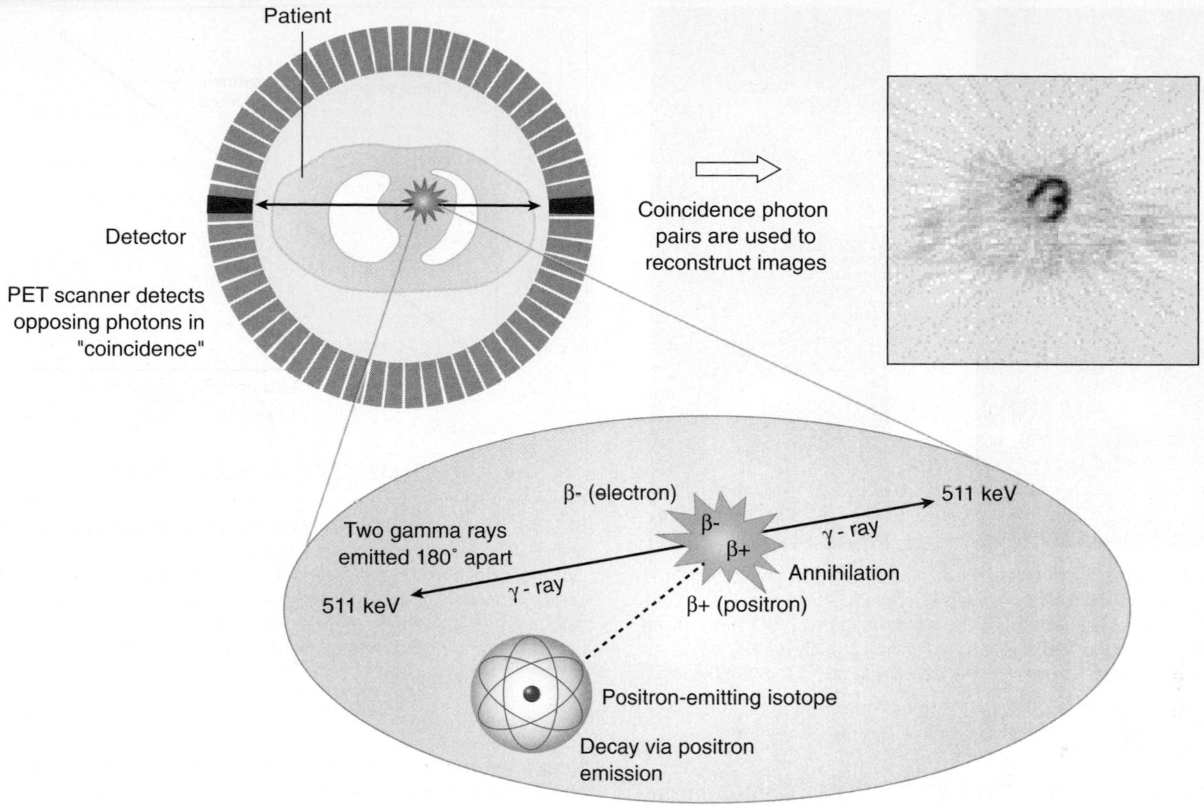

FIGURE 16–21 Schematic of positron and electron beta particle emission, with detection by a coincidence camera, as the basis of positron-emission tomography (PET) imaging.

resistance. Recent studies have also shown that abnormal blood flow reserve by PET may be predictive of future cardiovascular outcomes among patients with cardiomyopathies in the absence of CAD,[13] such as patients with idiopathic dilated cardiomyopathy[14] and hypertrophic cardiomyopathy.[15]

ASSESSMENT OF THE PHYSIOLOGY AND PATHOPHYSIOLOGY OF MYOCARDIAL BLOOD FLOW, MYOCARDIAL METABOLISM, AND VENTRICULAR FUNCTION

Assessment of Myocardial Blood Flow by Radionuclide Imaging

Resting Myocardial Blood Flow

Myocardial blood flow at rest is tightly regulated to provide nutritive perfusion to viable, contractile myocytes (see Chap. 48). Although SPECT tracers to image myocardial blood flow are commonly referred to as "perfusion tracers," they require viable myocyte cell membranes for uptake and retention.[3] Thus, the uptake and retention of these tracers do reflect regional flow differences, but myocyte cell membrane integrity is also a prerequisite. Although visualization of myocardial regions suggests the presence of working, viable cell membranes, lack of visualization of myocardium does not necessarily indicate the absence of viable cells. Decreased regional myocardial tracer uptake at rest could reflect either lack of cell membrane integrity in an area of infarcted myocardium or reduced blood flow secondary to hibernating but viable myocardium. A severe reduction in tracer activity usually signifies infarction, but a more moderate reduction in regional activity of a blood flow tracer *alone* cannot always differentiate hibernating from partially scarred myocardium in patients with ischemic LV dysfunction. In that setting, techniques that assess intact cellular metabolic processes (e.g., FDG, or the myocardial potassium space, e.g., thallium-201 redistribution) may be used as an adjunct to resting myocardial blood flow.[3]

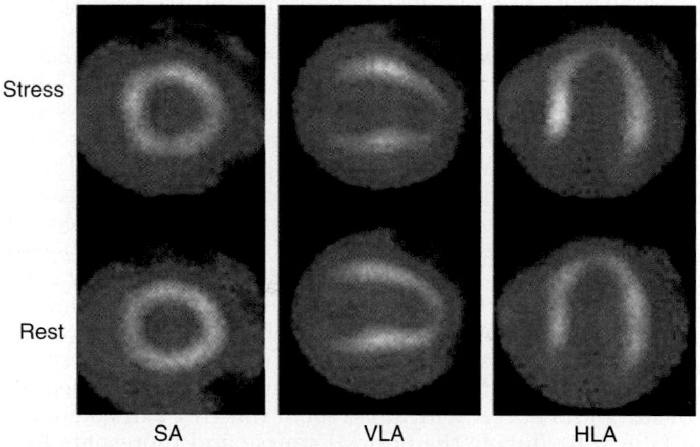

FIGURE 16–22 Example of high quality stress and rest PET perfusion images, using ^{82}rubidium as the perfusion tracer, in the short-axis (SA), vertical long-axis (VLA), and horizontal long-axis (HLA).

IMAGING MYOCARDIAL INFARCTION. In patients with prior MI, blood flow to the infarcted region is usually diminished, often severely, and there are few viable myocytes within the scarred territory.[4] Thus, severely reduced uptake of a radionuclide perfusion tracer in a resting study is a good marker of presence, location, and extent of MI (Fig. 16-23).

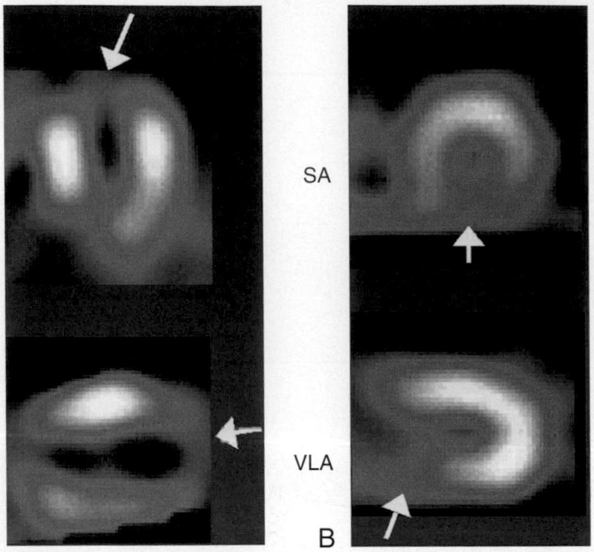

FIGURE 16–23 Single-photon emission computed tomography perfusion images demonstrating myocardial infarction in different locations. **A,** An apical infarction (arrow) in the horizontal long-axis (HLA) and vertical long-axis (VLA) views. **B,** An inferior infarction in the short-axis (SA) and VLA views. In both studies, the *severity* of the defect suggests minimal myocyte viability within those territories.

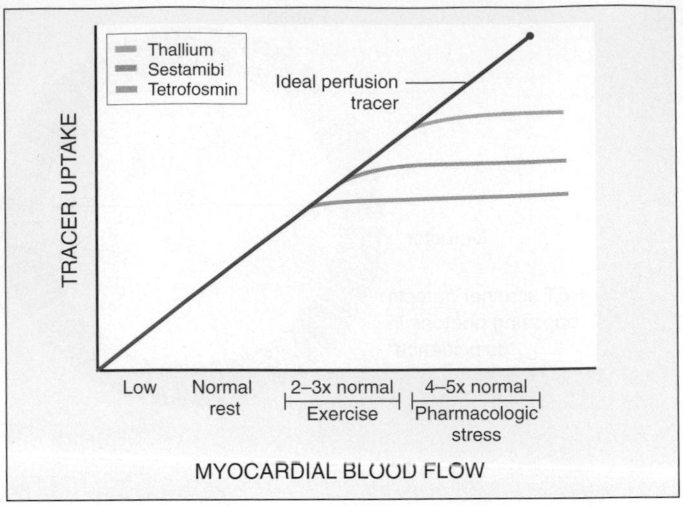

FIGURE 16–24 The relation between myocardial blood flow and perfusion tracer uptake. The ideal perfusion tracer would track myocardial blood flow across the entire range of physiologically relevant flows (red line). However, the available perfusion tracers "roll off" at higher levels of flow. The different tracers begin to reach a plateau at different levels of myocardial blood flow, as demonstrated in this schematic example based on multiple studies in animal models.

ASSESSMENT OF INFARCT SIZE. Contemporary studies have used ^{99m}Tc sestamibi to provide an assessment of infarct size.[16] Because there is minimal clearance from the myocardium following initial uptake of this tracer, images acquired even hours after initial injection represent a "snapshot" of blood flow conditions and tracer uptake at the time of injection.

Infarct size as assessed by quantitative analysis of resting sestamibi uptake has been validated against many other measures of infarct size.[16] Moreover, a significant association between SPECT infarct size and mortality over long-term follow-up has been demonstrated. Many clinical trials now use "final infarct size" by sestamibi SPECT imaging as an early post-MI surrogate endpoint to assess new agents to reduce infarct size.

When a tracer such as sestamibi is injected *during acute infarction* in the setting of an occluded infarct-related artery *before reperfusion therapy,* the resulting defect, even when imaged hours later after successful reperfusion, represents the *area-at-risk* of the occluded artery.[16] A second injection of sestamibi at rest with subsequent imaging can be done at a later time during the post-MI course and represents *final infarct size.* The change in defect size between the initial image acquired in the acute stage and the later image represents the *magnitude of salvaged myocardium from reperfusion.* Hence, SPECT imaging at rest in the early postinfarct period can provide important information regarding final infarct size and infarct zone viability.

Assessment of Myocardial Perfusion During Stress

Coronary blood flow must respond rapidly to changing metabolic conditions and oxygen demand to meet the nutrient needs of myocytes being called on to contract more quickly and with more force. Oxygen extraction by the myocardium is near maximum at rest; thus, any increase in oxygen demand can be met only through increasing coronary blood flow to deliver more oxygen per unit time (see Chap. 48). The major determinants of coronary blood flow include the perfusion pressure at the head of the system (principally aortic diastolic pressure) and the downstream resistance, residing predominantly in the coronary *arteriolar* bed. Because aortic diastolic pressure during exercise varies little from the resting value, the major mechanism responsible for increasing coronary blood flow during stress involves a reduction in coronary vascular resistance. During *exercise* stress, coronary blood flow can increase approximately two to three times over resting levels. During *pharmacological* stress to minimize coronary arteriolar resistance, with intravenous coronary arteriolar vasodilator agents such as dipyridamole or adenosine (discussed later), coronary blood flow can increase up to four to five times over resting levels. The magnitude of blood flow increase secondary to any stress relative to resting flow values is termed *coronary blood flow reserve.*[17]

PERFUSION TRACERS AND CORONARY BLOOD FLOW RESERVE. The ideal perfusion tracer should track myocardial blood flow across the entire physiologically relevant range of blood flow achievable in animal models and in humans (Fig. 16-24). It should be extracted rapidly (from the blood into the myocyte) because the hemodynamic conditions during peak stress are not maintained for long periods of time. The ideal tracer should also be extracted as completely as possible out of the bloodstream, and it should be retained in myocardium for a sufficient period to be imaged. Moreover, perturbations in metabolic conditions, such as ischemia or commonly used cardioactive drugs, should neither influence nor interfere with uptake so that the resulting regional tracer concentrations primarily reflect myocardial perfusion.[3]

Despite its excellent first-pass myocardial extraction (85 percent), the energy spectrum of thallium is lower (69 to 80 keV) than optimum for current gamma cameras. The 140-keV energy spectrum of ^{99m}Tc perfusion tracers results in less scatter and soft tissue attenuation, with improved spatial resolution compared with thallium.[3] However, the first-pass myocardial extraction of both sestamibi and tetrofosmin is only in the 60 percent range with nonlinear extraction at high flows. Thus, none of the clinically available SPECT perfusion tracers have all of the properties of an ideal perfusion tracer (see Fig. 16-24). Regional differences in myocardial tracer uptake during exercise or pharmacological stress have provided important diagnostic, as well as prognostic, information.[4]

The PET perfusion tracer [^{13}N]ammonia displays an extraction fraction exceeding 90 percent; rubidium-82 has a lower extraction fraction and reaches a plateau more rapidly at hyperemic range of flow. In the clinical setting, the evaluation of regional myocardial blood flow and flow reserve with [^{13}N]ammonia and rubidium-82 have been validated for detecting and localizing CAD.[11] As noted earlier, most PET studies evaluating coronary flow reserve use pharmacological rather than exercise stress.

EFFECT OF A CORONARY STENOSIS ON CORONARY BLOOD FLOW RESERVE. (See Chap. 48.) In animal models wherein discrete coronary stenoses of varying degrees are induced, *resting* coronary blood flow is maintained by autoregulatory dilation of the downstream arteriolar resistance vessels until a stenosis between 80 and 90 percent diameter was reached (Fig. 16-25). As stenosis severity increases further, the arteriolar vasodilatory capacity to maintain resting flow is exhausted—at which point resting coronary blood flow diminishes.[17]

In contrast, *maximum coronary blood flow reserve* begins to decrease when the upstream coronary stenosis reaches 50 percent diameter. There are three levels of resistance that influence coronary blood flow: that provided by the large conductance epicardial vessels (R1), the coronary arteriolar resistance (R2), and the resistance in the subendocardium by wall tension from the ventricular chamber (R3) (see Fig. 16-25). Under normal conditions, most of the resistance at rest is provided by R2, and most of the increase in coronary flow during heightened demand occurs through reduction of resistance at this level, potentially increasing flow as much as four times as demand increases. Normal epicardial vessels dilate slightly (R1 decreases slightly) in response to increased coronary flow as a consequence of normal endothelial cell function. Depending on the type of exercise that is performed, the R3 component may remain unchanged or may increase, with an increase in chamber radius and wall tension. Achieving maximal flow is predominantly dependent on the vasodilatory capacity of the downstream resistance vessels.[17] With a coronary stenosis, in which some vasodilatory reserve has been used to maintain resting flow, less vasodilatory reserve is available to minimize resistance during stress. Thus, in a vessel with a moderate stenosis, *coronary blood flow reserve* is blunted and detectable by a perfusion tracer (see Fig. 16-25).

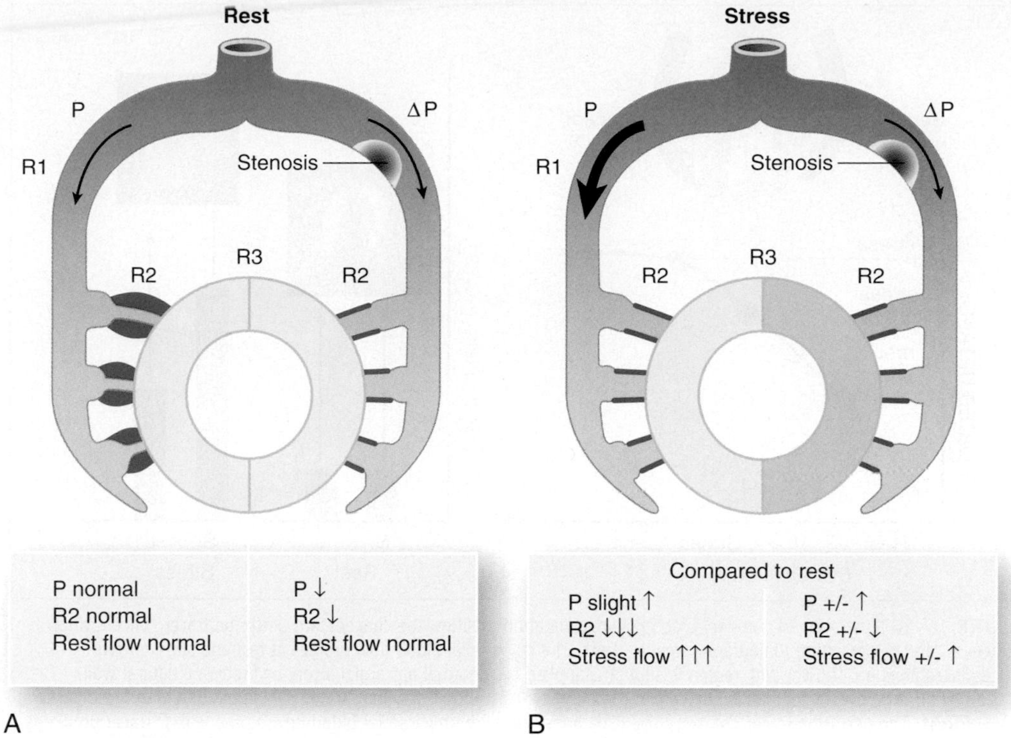

FIGURE 16–25 Effect of coronary resistance on coronary blood flow reserve. **A,** At rest, flow is driven by the pressure head (P) at the proximal end of the system. R1 refers to resistance offered by the large epicardial conductance vessels. R2 represents the coronary arteriolar resistance, which predominantly regulates coronary blood flow. R3 represents the resistance provided by wall tension in the subendocardium. At rest in the normal vessel (left vessel), some vasoconstrictor resistance is present. In the setting of an epicardial coronary stenosis (right vessel), blood flow at rest can be maintained, as coronary resistance can be lowered downstream (R2 decreased) by autoregulatory dilation of the arterioles. Thus, with lower resistance, resting flow may be maintained despite the lower pressure head at the distal end of the stenosis. **B,** With a demand stress or with the administration of a coronary arteriolar vasodilator such as dipyridamole or adenosine, perfusion increases substantially in the area supplied by the normal epicardial artery (left vessel) as resistance (R2) becomes minimal. However, there is *blunted flow reserve* in the area supplied by the stenosis (right vessel) because most vasodilator reserve at the R2 level has been used to maintain resting flow. Thus, heterogeneity of flow is established (based on the presence of the upstream stenosis), and can be imaged with a perfusion tracer as a defect in the territory supplied by the stenotic vessel. *(Adapted from Follansbee WP: Alternatives to leg exercise in the evaluation of patients with coronary artery disease: Functional and pharmacological stress modalities.* In *Gerson MC [ed]: Cardiac Nuclear Medicine. New York, McGraw-Hill, 1997, pp 193-236.)*

In contrast to animal models, human CAD is more complex. Stenoses may not be discrete, the length and complexity of the stenosis may affect the coronary reserve, and impaired endothelial function plays a role.[18] In subjects with preserved endothelial function, the increased coronary flow during stress leads to coronary arterial and arteriolar vasodilation, contributing to maximal coronary flow reserve. Endothelial function is often abnormal with early atherosclerosis, or risk factors for atherosclerosis, contributing to the blunting of coronary flow reserve. The development of collaterals to the distal perfusion bed of a myocardial territory with a severe upstream coronary stenosis also influences blood flow at rest and during stress.[19]

With SPECT imaging, *relative* regional differences of tracer uptake can be detected and quantified (Fig. 16-26), whereas with PET imaging, *absolute* regional coronary blood flow at rest and during stress (in milliliters per gram per minute) can be quantified.[11,12]

DETECTING STRESS-INDUCED ISCHEMIA VERSUS INFARCT WITH MYOCARDIAL PERFUSION IMAGING

In standard practice, stress and rest myocardial perfusion images are compared to determine the presence, extent, and severity of stress-induced perfusion defects and to determine whether such defects represent regions of myocardial ischemia or infarction.[2,4] ***Regions with stress-induced perfusion abnormalities, which have normal perfusion at rest, are termed reversible perfusion defects and represent viable regions with blunted coronary blood flow reserve*** (Fig. 16-27A). Strictly speaking, SPECT MPI is demonstrating stress-induced reversible abnormalities in perfusion reserve, although these findings are often referred to as "ischemia." Regional myocardial *tissue ischemia* per se is not being demonstrated, although it is indeed often present, based on a mismatch between oxygen supply and demand. Perfusion abnormalities at stress that are *irreversible,* or *fixed,* as seen on resting images (unchanged from stress to rest) most often represent infarction, particularly if the defect is severe (see Fig. 16-27B). When both viable myocardium and scarred myocardium are present, thallium redistribution or technetium 99m tracer reversibility is incomplete, giving the appearance of partial reversibility on the delayed thallium or rest technetium 99m images.

Exercise Stress to Induce Coronary Hyperemia

SPECT MPI is commonly performed with exercise stress to induce coronary hyperemia and is particularly suitable for patients with exertional symptoms because this provides the opportunity to link the *symptoms* induced during exercise to the location, extent, and severity of abnormal perfusion patterns.[4] Performing exercise stress in conjunction

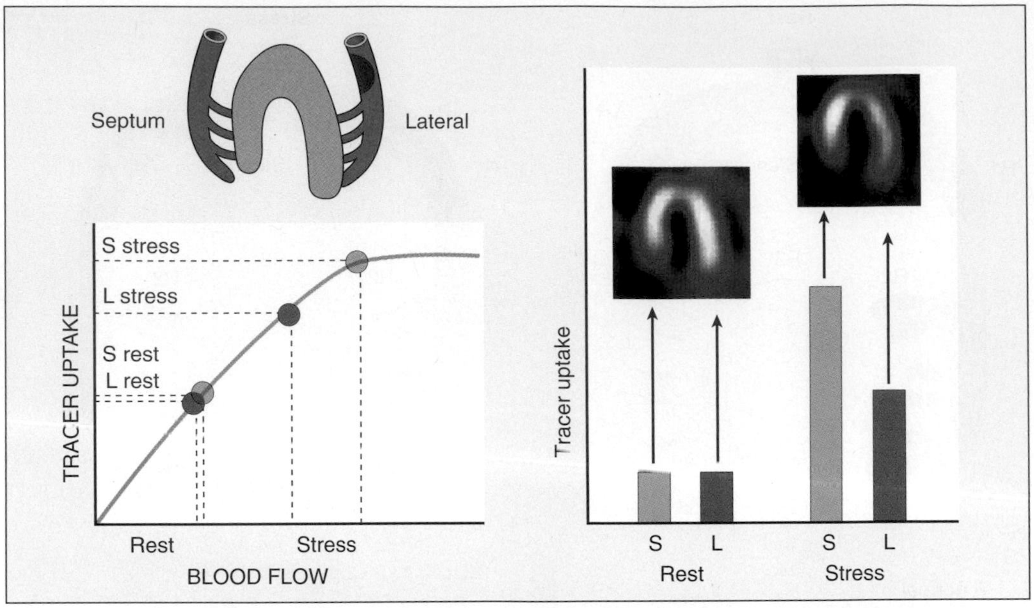

FIGURE 16–26 Illustration of coronary blood flow reserve abnormalities, the concomitant perfusion tracer concentration differences, and the resulting tomographic images. **Left,** The myocardial blood flow profiles at rest and stress of two myocardial regions are shown, with region S (septum) supplied by a normal epicardial artery and region L (lateral wall) supplied by an artery with a significant epicardial coronary stenosis. Blood flow at stress is diminished in region L compared with S. **Right,** The perfusion tracer uptake profile is demonstrated with myocardial blood flow on the *y*-axis. Tracer uptake is diminished in region L relative to S during stress. In the resulting perfusion images, a relative "defect" of tracer uptake is seen in the lateral wall compared with the septum, whereas at rest both regions demonstrate similar tracer uptake. The lateral wall thus demonstrates a reversible perfusion defect, reflecting the blunted coronary blood flow reserve and indirectly reflecting the presence of the coronary stenosis.

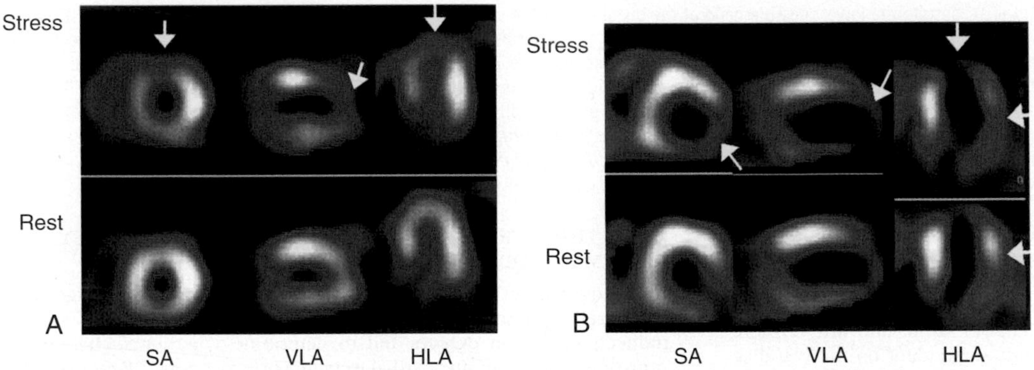

FIGURE 16–27 A, Example of single-photon emission computed tomography anterior and apical reversible perfusion defects (arrows), representing inducible regional myocardial ischemia in the short axis (SA), vertical long axis (VLA), and horizontal long axis (HLA). **B,** Example of irreversible or fixed defects of the inferolateral wall in the SA and of the apex in the VLA image (arrows), representing predominant myocardial infarction. There is also evidence of a reversible lateral wall defect (arrowhead) in the HLA image representing lateral wall ischemia.

with MPI allows the opportunity to incorporate additional information on functional capacity, stress-induced ECG changes or arrhythmias, and utilization of heart rate reserve and heart rate recovery in the assessment of CAD probability or prognosis.[20]

Pharmacological Stress to Induce Coronary Hyperemia

Exercise stress is the preferred modality for inducing coronary hyperemia as it allows a correlation between exertional symptoms and the perfusion pattern and provides information on exercise duration, workload achieved, and the presence and extent of ischemic ECG changes—all of which provide important diagnostic and prognostic information.[4] However, a substantial proportion of patients are incapable of attaining a sufficient level of exercise. Patients with exertional symptoms may not exercise adequately to reproduce these symptoms, and patients may not achieve more than 85 percent of the maximum predicted heart rate for age (see Chap. 13), considered the optimal level of exertion to achieve coronary hyperemic responses.[4,20] As the population ages and comorbid disease states such as peripheral vascular disease and diabetes in-crease, the proportion of patients referrod for stress testing who are unable to achieve adequate levels of exercise will increase.

In such patients, *pharmacological stress testing* can be used to induce coronary hyperemia. The most widely used agents for pharmacological stress testing can be divided into those that act as coronary arteriolar vasodilators, adenosine and dipyridamole, and adrenergic agents such as dobutamine.[2,4]

MECHANISM OF CORONARY ARTERIOLAR VASODILATOR PHARMACOLOGICAL STRESS

Stimulation of adenosine A_{2a} receptors on the smooth muscle cells leads to enhanced production of adenylate cyclase, increased intracellular cyclic adenosine monophosphate, and other effects that produce vasorelaxation. With maximal arteriolar vasodilation (maximal decrease in coronary resistance), coronary blood flow increases.

Adenosine is a powerful, endogenous molecule that acts as a regulator of blood flow in many organ beds, including the coronary circulation (see Chap. 48). It has many other effects mediated by different receptor subtypes (Fig. 16-28). Adenosine A_1 receptors are present in the sinus node and atrioventricular (AV) node and mediate diminished heart rate and AV nodal conduction. Adenosine A_{2b} receptors are present in bronchioles and the peripheral vasculature, and stimulation may result in bronchial constriction and peripheral vasodilation.

Initial studies of adenosine demonstrated that a dose of 140 μg/kg/min induced maximal coronary hyperemia, with no further increase in maximum coronary blood flow at higher doses.[21] Following the onset of intravenous adenosine infusion, maximum coronary flow occurs at an average of 84 seconds with a range of up to 125 seconds. Dipyridamole blocks the intracellular retransport of adenosine and inhibits adenosine deaminase, responsible for the intracellular breakdown of adenosine.[21] Thus, dipyridamole acts as an indirect coronary arteriolar vasodilator, increasing intracellular and interstitial concentrations of adenosine (see Fig. 16-28).

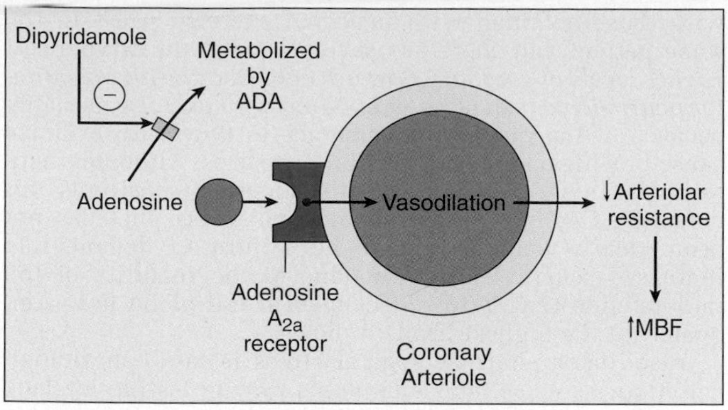

FIGURE 16–28 Schematic of the mechanism of action of dipyridamole and adenosine. Exogenously administered adenosine acts directly on its receptor to result in coronary arteriolar vasodilation and thus an increase in myocardial blood flow (MBF) as resistance is minimized. The adenosine A_{2a} receptor mediates coronary arteriolar vasodilation, which is the basis for pharmacological stress testing. Dipyridamole blocks the intracellular retransport of adenosine and also inhibits adenosine deaminase (ADA), resulting in increased intracellular and interstitial concentrations of adenosine, which then interacts with its receptor. *(Adapted from Follansbee WP: Alternatives to leg exercise in the evaluation of patients with coronary artery disease: Functional and pharmacological stress modalities. In Gerson MC [ed]: Cardiac Nuclear Medicine. New York, McGraw-Hill, 1997, pp 193-236.)*

HETEROGENEITY OF CORONARY HYPEREMIA WITH PHARMACOLOGICAL STRESS

With the administration of dipyridamole or adenosine, the resistance vessels in the area subtended by a normal epicardial vessel dilate, diminishing coronary resistance and resulting in an increment in coronary blood flow four to five times above normal. Coronary resistance in a bed supplied by a stenotic epicardial vessel is diminished at rest (i.e., coronary vasodilator reserve has been utilized), and only minor or no further reductions can take place. Thus, myocardial blood flow in that territory does not change or may even decrease slightly because of the peripheral vasodilation and drop in diastolic blood pressure characteristic of pharmacological stress. The net result of these changes is heterogeneity in myocardial blood flow (increased in the normal territory and relatively unchanged in the territory supplied by the stenotic epicardial vessel). Perfusion tracer administration in this setting demonstrates a defect in the area supplied by the stenotic vessel (see Fig. 16-25).[21]

During exercise stress, the increase in myocardial oxygen demand and limitation of oxygen supply create a supply-demand mismatch often resulting in cellular ischemia. With pharmacological stress, the perfusion defect may represent merely the heterogeneity in coronary flow reserve. "Demand" may change little during pharmacological stress; there is often a reduction in blood pressure accompanied by a reflex although modest increase in heart rate. Therefore, double product, reflecting oxygen demand, changes little during the vasodilator "stress." Thus, a supply-demand mismatch may not occur and cellular ischemia may not be present despite vasodilator-induced perfusion defects.[21]

Under certain conditions, true myocardial ischemia may be present, related to development of a *coronary steal.* This phenomenon appears to occur when the myocardial perfusion bed supplied by a severe epicardial stenosis is also dependent on collateral vessels from remote coronary arteries. Blood flow through coronary collaterals is dependent on perfusion pressure, particularly if the collaterals are jeopardized; that is, their parent blood vessel is compromised by a moderate coronary stenosis. In this setting, administration of a vasodilator stress agent diminishes the perfusion pressure supplying the collaterals, and collateral flow diminishes. Flow to the bed supplied by a severe epicardial stenosis may then *decrease* compared with resting flow, and the diminished supply may create supply-demand mismatch and true myocardial ischemia.

HEMODYNAMIC EFFECTS OF VASODILATOR PHARMACOLOGICAL STRESS. Dipyridamole and adenosine result in adenosine receptor-mediated systemic as well as coronary vasodilation, causing an average 8 to 10 mm Hg reduction in systolic and diastolic blood pressure, often accompanied by a reflex increase in heart rate.[21] The magnitude of the heart rate increase is variable, usually between 10 and 20 beats/min. A blunted heart rate response may be observed in patients who are taking beta blockers or in diabetic patients with underlying autonomic insufficiency.

SIDE EFFECTS ASSOCIATED WITH VASODILATOR PHARMACOLOGICAL STRESS. The side effects associated with pharmacological vasodilator stress are the result of stimulation of the adenosine A_1, A_{2b}, and A_3 receptors and are common.[21,22] Following dipyridamole stress, approximately 50 percent of patients experience some side effect. In a large registry study, more than 80 percent of patients undergoing adenosine stress experienced untoward side effects, most commonly flushing, chest pain, or shortness of breath.[2,21,22]

As a result of adenosine's effect on the conduction system, AV block may develop during adenosine administration. Approximately 10 percent of patients manifest first-degree AV block, with 5 percent developing either second- or third-degree AV block. AV block is more common in patients who are studied while taking beta blockers or heart rate–lowering calcium channel blockers. Patients with baseline evidence of second- or third-degree AV block in the absence of a pacemaker should not receive adenosine. However, patients with first-degree AV block or left bundle branch block (LBBB) appear to tolerate adenosine infusion well, without an exacerbation of conduction abnormalities.[2,4]

Ischemic ST depression is observed in 10 to 15 percent of patients undergoing pharmacological vasodilator stress, probably representing the physiological consequence of induction of a coronary steal and regional myocardial ischemia. Such patients often have extensive and severe perfusion defects on imaging and more often have collateralized multivessel disease on angiography.

Chest pain, even typical angina pectoris, develops commonly during pharmacological vasodilator stress testing. Although it may reflect regional myocardial ischemia based on a coronary steal, chest pain may also occur in patients with no ischemic ECG changes and with normal perfusion studies because of involvement of adenosine A_1 receptors in the nociceptive pathway influencing the sensation of chest pain.[21,22] Thus, chest pain by itself is a nonspecific finding during vasodilator pharmacological stress.

In early reports of dipyridamole testing, infrequent but severe episodes of bronchospasm occurred, possibly related to a nonspecific adenosine receptor-mediated mechanism. Thus, patients with a significant history of reactive airways disease should not undergo vasodilator stress testing.[4,10] However, patients with obstructive lung disease without a reactive airways component generally tolerate the procedure well.

New vasodilator pharmacological stress agents are under development that are more specific agonists at the adenosine A_{2a} receptor. Early studies suggest that the results of imaging are similar to the effects of adenosine, although side effects are fewer and less severe, consistent with greater A_{2a} receptor specificity.[22]

REVERSING THE EFFECTS OF VASODILATOR PHARMACOLOGICAL STRESS. Methylxanthine compounds such as theophylline and caffeine act as competitive antagonists of adenosine at the receptor level, and infusion of intravenous aminophylline antagonizes the effects of dipyridamole or adenosine.[2,4] Because adenosine has a very short half-life (~20 to 30 seconds), administration of aminophylline is rarely required during adenosine testing; simply stopping the infusion results in cessation of symptoms within 20 to 30 seconds. Following intravenous dipyridamole, infusion of aminophylline at approximately 1 to 2 mg/kg, given over 30 seconds, reverses side effects (as well as the coronary vasodilator effects), usually within 1 to 2 minutes. Because the coronary vasodilator effects are reversed as well, reversal of the dipyridamole effect should be delayed until at least 1 to 2 minutes after radionuclide administration if clinically safe, otherwise the true stress perfusion pattern may not be manifest. Generally, side effects from vasodilator pharmacological stress, although common, may be tolerated for this period of time. However, with more severe side effects such as severe shortness of breath or bronchospasm or with more dramatic ST segment abnormalities, reversal of the dipyridamole effect more quickly is prudent. Because caffeine is a methylxanthine compound and antagonizes the effect of adenosine at its receptor, it is critical that patients be instructed to withhold caffeine, ideally for 24 hours prior to vasodilator pharmacological stress testing.

In some patients, myocardial ischemia provoked during vasodilator stress testing triggers a cascade of events that maintains ischemia even after reversal of the vasodilator effect with aminophylline. The sensation of chest pain may drive a heightened sympathetic response, with an elevation of heart rate and blood pressure. In that setting, when aminophylline has been given to reverse the effects of the vasodilator, it is safe to administer sublingual nitroglycerin or other measures to relieve myocardial ischemia. It is *not safe* to give sublingual nitroglycerin *prior to* aminophylline to treat signs of myocardial ischemia. Because systemic vasodilation is present during vasodilator stress testing, administration of nitroglycerin prior to aminophylline may result in substantial systemic hypotension.

In contemporary practice, a small number of patients may be encountered who are taking oral dipyridamole preparations for their antiplatelet effects. As dipyridamole is an adenosine deaminase inhibitor and prevents the usual rapid breakdown of adenosine, infusion of intravenous adenosine in patients receiving oral dipyridamole may be accompanied by a far more prolonged adenosine effect than usual. Thus, for adenosine testing, oral dipyridamole compounds must be stopped at an appropriate period of time before testing. Oral dipyridamole as background therapy does not complicate the performance of intravenous dipyridamole testing.

PROTOCOLS FOR PHARMACOLOGICAL STRESS TESTING. The accepted protocols for performing vasodilator pharmacological stress testing are listed in Table 16-3.[2,4] Since the original descriptions of these protocols, iterations have been studied, with the goal of shortening the test procedure or minimizing side effects, or both,[23] by shortening the duration of the adenosine infusion or adding low-level exercise.

Handgrip exercise may be used in order to raise peripheral blood pressure and thus coronary perfusion pressure. Reports are mixed on whether image quality is improved. This approach may be useful in patients with borderline low blood pressure prior to the test to avoid significant hypotension.

Low-level treadmill exercise has been increasingly applied in combination with vasodilator stress testing. Although no clear advantage in diagnostic performance has been demonstrated, a reduction in side effects of pharmacological stress testing has been demonstrated, as well as a reduction in extracardiac tracer uptake that improves image quality.[23]

Initial reports of intravenous adenosine testing described a protocol in which the dose was progressively increased. More commonly, adenosine is given now as an infusion starting with the maximum dose. This allows a shortened total infusion period of 4 minutes rather than 6 minutes, with radionuclide injected at 3 minutes into the 4-minute infusion. Published data suggest that diagnostic sensitivity is maintained while decreasing the overall time of testing.[21]

DIFFERENCES BETWEEN VASODILATOR AND EXERCISE STRESS. The perfusion images obtained using vasodilator pharmacological stress are generally concordant with those obtained with maximal exercise stress in the same patient, but there are several important differences. *Higher levels of coronary flow are achieved during vasodilator pharmacological stress compared with exercise,* possibly because of the increased resistance to flow with exercise caused by higher subendocardial pressures. Although theoretically this should result in increased sensitivity for detecting CAD with pharmacological stress, that has not been clearly demonstrated. The failure to demonstrate increased sensitivity may be due to the inability of the radionuclide tracers to reflect myocardial blood flow adequately at the highest levels of flow.[3]

Vasodilator pharmacological stress is less "physiological" than exercise, and symptoms during testing (or lack thereof) cannot be as clearly linked to the perfusion pattern. Optimal diagnostic performance of MPI during exercise is often dependent on the patient achieving a maximal level of stress, which does not always occur. In contrast, vasodilator pharmacological stress affords generally predictable coronary flow responses.[3,21]

Antiischemic medications may significantly affect the results of MPI during exercise.[4] Reports have now suggested that the extent and severity of myocardial perfusion defects may be affected in an important way by background medication during pharmacological stress.[24,25] Thus, antianginal medications should be withheld, if possible, prior to the study.

TABLE 16–3 Pharmacological Stress Protocols

	Dose (μg/kg/min)	Duration	Isotope Injection
Dipyridamole	142	4 min by hand infusion or pump	3 min after completion of infusion
Adenosine	140	6 min infusion by pump	At 3 min into infusion

Dobutamine Stress to Induce Coronary Hyperemia

In some patients, vasodilator pharmacological stress is contraindicated because of reactive bronchospastic airways disease or background methylxanthines. In such situations, intravenous dobutamine hydrochloride may be used to induce coronary hyperemia.[2,4] Dobutamine has a relatively rapid onset of action, with a half-life of approximately 2 minutes. This agent is given starting at a dose of 5 μg/kg/min and increased in a stepwise fashion by 5 μg/kg/min every 3 minutes, to a maximum dose of 40 μg/kg/min. Dobutamine is a broad adrenergic receptor agonist, at varying doses stimulating the $beta_1$, $beta_2$, and $alpha_1$ receptors. At relatively low doses, the predominant effect is an increase in contractility through adrenergic receptors. As the dose is increased beyond 10 μg/kg/min, heart rate rises steadily, and the increase in oxygen demand stimulates an increase in myocardial blood flow.

The hemodynamic response to dobutamine generally involves a modest increase in systolic blood pressure with a modest decrease in diastolic blood pressure through doses up to 20 μg/kg/min, with only small further changes after that point. As the increase in myocardial blood flow is dependent on the increase in oxygen demand, optimal sensitivity for MPI based on optimizing heterogeneity of flow is dependent on achieving a high dose of dobutamine.

The increment in myocardial blood flow during maximal doses of dobutamine appears to be less than that achieved during vasodilator pharmacological stress; hence, the degree of heterogeneity of coronary flow with a coronary stenosis is also less. Thus, vasodilator stress is the preferred pharmacological modality for MPI in patients who cannot exercise adequately. Dobutamine stress is reserved for cases in which vasodilator stress is contraindicated or cannot be performed because of background medications.[2,4]

Side effects during dobutamine are frequent and can be bothersome.[2] The most common side effects include palpitations and chest pain, and arrhythmias including PVCs and nonsustained ventricular tachycardia may be encountered. Hypotension occurs in approximately 10 percent of patients, possibly as a result of myocardial mechanoreceptor stimulation during increased contractility with resulting withdrawal of peripheral constrictor tone. Hypotension during dobutamine stress does not have the same prognostic implications as exercise-induced hypotension. Because of the relatively short half-life, side effects generally resolve within a few minutes of stopping the infusion and can be aborted more quickly with intravenous beta blockade.[2,4]

Assessment of Myocardial Cellular Metabolism and Physiology by Radionuclide Imaging

Myocardial Ischemia and Viability (see Chap. 48)

PROGRAMMED CELL SURVIVAL. Imbalance between oxygen supply and demand results in myocardial ischemia. If the imbalance is transient (i.e., triggered by exertion), it represents reversible ischemia. However, if supply-demand imbalance is prolonged, high-energy phosphates are depleted, and regional contractile function progressively deteriorates. If the supply-demand balance is sufficiently prolonged, cell membrane rupture with cell death follows.

The myocardium has several mechanisms of acute and chronic adaptation to a temporary or sustained reduction in coronary blood flow (Fig. 16-29), known as stunning, hibernation, and ischemic preconditioning (see Chap. 48). These responses to ischemia preserve sufficient energy to protect the structural and functional integrity of the cardiac myocyte. In contrast to programmed cell death, or apoptosis, the term "programmed cell survival" has been used to describe the commonality between myocardial stunning, hibernation, and ischemic preconditioning despite their distinct pathophysiology.[26]

STUNNED AND HIBERNATING MYOCARDIUM. In stunned and hibernating myocardium, *myocardial function is depressed at rest but myocytes remain viable.* Although LV dysfunction may be reversible in both stunning and hibernation, these states differ in the relation between myocardial perfusion and function. *Stunned myocardium* is most commonly observed after a *transient period of ischemia followed by reperfusion* (depressed function at rest but preserved perfusion). The ischemic episodes can be single or multiple, brief or prolonged, but never severe enough to result in injury. *Hibernating myocardium* refers to adaptive responses of the myocardium to *repetitive episodes of ischemia resulting in myocardial hypoperfusion at rest*[27] (depressed function and perfusion at rest). Clinically, it is likely that the adaptive responses of hibernation and stunning coexist (see Chap. 48).

MYOCARDIAL VIABILITY. Requirements for cellular viability include (1) sufficient myocardial blood flow, (2) cell membrane integrity, and (3) preserved metabolic activity. Myocardial blood flow has to be adequate to deliver substrate to the myocyte for metabolic processes and to remove the end products of metabolism. If blood flow is severely reduced, metabolites accumulate, causing inhibition of the enzymes of the metabolic pathway, depletion of high-energy phosphates, cell membrane disruption, and cell death. Thus, with severe reduction in blood flow, perfusion tracers alone provide information regarding myocardial viability.[4] However, in regions in which the reduction in blood flow is less severe, perfusion information alone may be an insufficient signal to identify clinically relevant viability—additional data, such as metabolic indices, would be important.[4]

Because cell membrane integrity, another requisite for cell survival, is dependent on preserved intracellular metabolic activity to generate high-energy phosphates, tracers that reflect cation flux (thallium-201), electrochemical gradients (sestamibi or tetrofosmin), or metabolic processes (FDG) provide insight into myocardial viability (Fig. 16-30).[3,26]

Major Myocardial Fuels and Energetics in Normal and Ischemic Myocardium

High-energy phosphates, such as adenosine triphosphate (ATP), provide the fuel that powers the myocyte contractile proteins (see Chap. 21). ATP is generated in the myocardium by two different but integrated metabolic processes: *oxidative phosphorylation* and *glycolysis.*[12] Fatty acids, glucose, and lactate are the major sources of energy in the heart, and depending on the arterial concentration of each and the physiological condition, any one of these three can be the principal substrate (see Fig. 16-30B). Increased uptake and utilization of one substrate leads to a decreased contribution by the others.

In the fasting state, long-chain free fatty acids are the preferred source of energy in the heart, with glucose accounting for only 15 to 20 percent of the total energy supply. When the oxygen supply is *normal,* high levels of ATP and tissue citrate formed by breakdown of fatty acids suppress the oxidation of glucose. When the oxygen supply is *decreased,* ATP and citrate levels fall, and the rate of glycolysis is accelerated. Anaerobic glycolysis can be maintained only if lactate and hydrogen ion (the byproducts of glycolysis) are removed and do not accumulate. In the setting of *severe* hypoperfusion, these end products of the glycolytic pathway accumulate, causing inhibition of the glycolytic enzymes and depletion of high-energy phosphates, resulting in cell membrane disruption and cell death.[26] Thus, even to maintain anaerobic glycolysis, minimally sufficient blood flow is necessary.

IMAGING ALTERATIONS IN MYOCARDIAL METABOLISM

Imaging Fatty Acid Metabolism

[^{11}C]PALMITATE. Because fatty acids are the primary source of myocardial energy production in the fasting state, early PET studies focused on characterizing the kinetics of long-chain fatty acids, such as [^{11}C]palmitate.[28] Measurement by dynamic PET imaging allows determination of tracer inflow (by regional perfusion), peak accumulation, and release within a region of interest. Once the tracer is in the cell, it either (1) enters the endogenous lipid pool or (2) moves to the mitochondria, where rapid degradation by beta-oxidation results in the generation of carbon dioxide. Depending on demand, about 80 percent of extracted [^{11}C]palmitate is activated for transport from the lipid pool into the mitochondria for breakdown by beta-oxidation. Because of its complicated kinetic modeling and numerous confounding effects, [^{11}C]palmitate imaging has not gained wide clinical acceptance.

[^{123}I]BMIPP. Fatty acid imaging with radioiodine-labeled fatty acid analogs such as iodine-123-beta-methyliodopentadecanoic acid (BMIPP) using SPECT is an investigational area for the assessment of *ischemic memory.*[29] After an ischemic episode, fatty acid metabolism may be suppressed for a prolonged time, and BMIPP imaging can demonstrate a regional metabolic defect even if perfusion has returned to normal. This metabolic signal of recent ischemia has been termed "ischemic memory" and may be clinically useful, for example, in patients who report to an emergency department (ED) with chest pain that resolved hours earlier. Although BMIPP is approved for clinical use in Japan, it has not yet received approval by the FDA.

Imaging Glucose Metabolism

Whereas fatty acids are the primary source of fuel in the *fasting state,* increased arterial glucose concentration in the *fed state* results in an increase in insulin levels, stimulating glucose metabolism while inhibiting lipolysis.[11,12] The result is a switch in myocardial metabolism from predominantly fatty acid utilization to glucose utilization.

The principle of using a metabolic tracer that tracks glycolysis is based on the concept that glucose utilization may be preserved or increased relative to flow in hypoperfused but viable (hibernating) myocardium, termed *metabolism-perfusion mismatch.*[11,12,30] Myocardial glucose utilization is absent in scarred or fibrotic tissue, represented by *metabolism-perfusion match* (Fig. 16-31). Although the amount of energy produced by glycolysis may be adequate to maintain myocyte viability and preserve the electrochemical gradient across the cell membrane, it may not be sufficient to sustain contractile function.[26]

2-[^{18}F]FLUORO-2-DEOXYGLUCOSE. FDG is a glucose analog for imaging myocardial glucose utilization with PET.[11,12,26] Following injec-

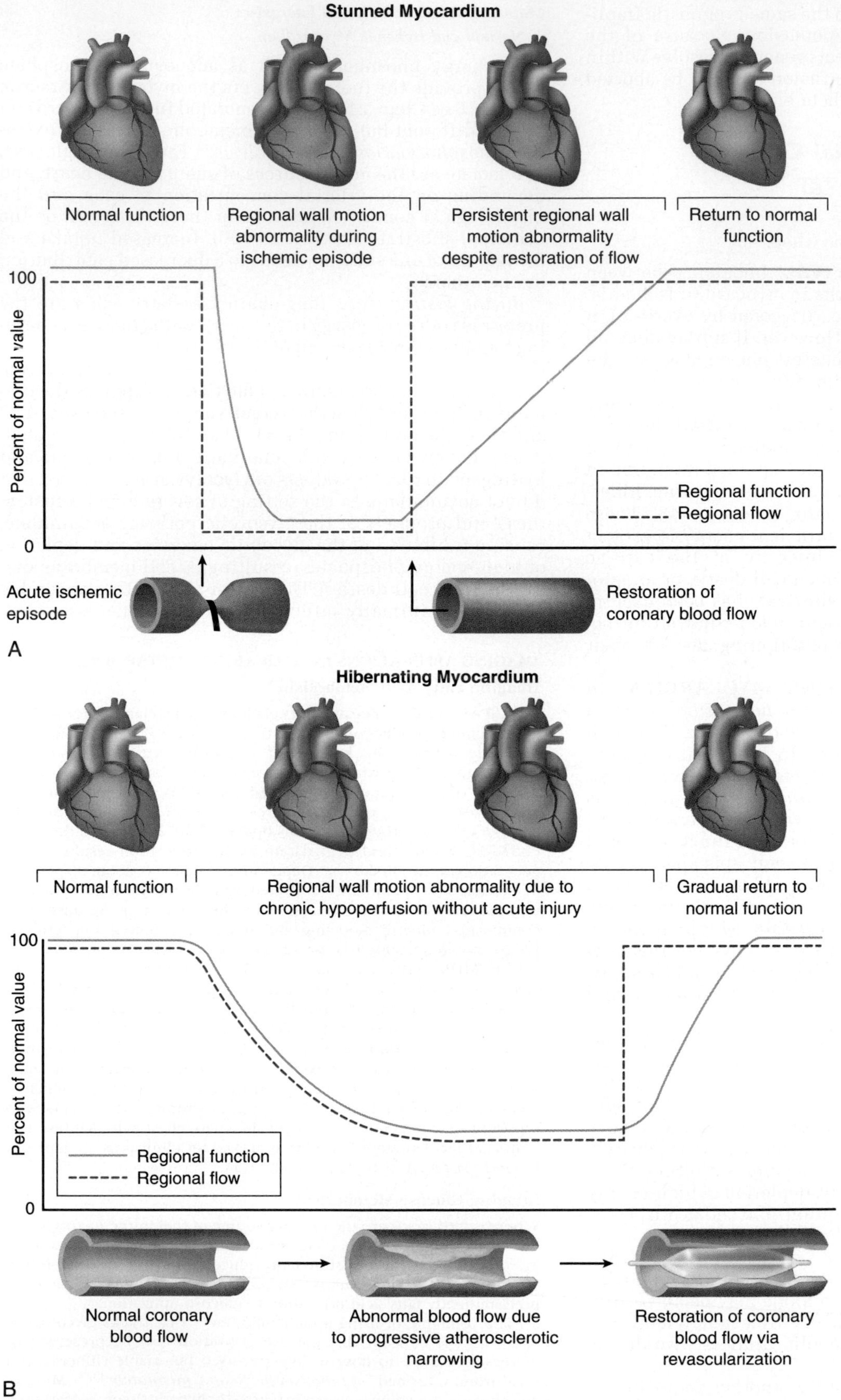

FIGURE 16–29 Pathophysiology of stunning and hibernation, representing different mechanisms of acute and chronic reversible left ventricular dysfunction. *(Adapted from Dilsizian V: Myocardial viability: Reversible left ventricular dysfunction.* In *Dilsizian V, Narula J, Braunwald E [eds]: Atlas of Nuclear Cardiology. Philadelphia, Current Medicine, 2006.)*

tion of 5 to 10 mCi, FDG rapidly exchanges across the capillary and cellular membranes. It is phosphorylated by hexokinase to FDG-6-phosphate (see Fig. 16-30B) and not metabolized further or used in glycogen synthesis. Because the dephosphorylation rate of FDG is slow, it becomes trapped in the myocardium, permitting PET or SPECT imaging of regional glucose utilization. FDG uptake may be increased in hibernating but viable myocardium, and FDG uptake in asynergic myocardial regions with reduced blood flow at rest has become a scintigraphic marker of hibernation.

Diagnostic quality of FDG imaging is critically dependent on hormonal milieu and substrate availability. Most clinical FDG studies are performed after 50 to 75 g of glucose loading in the form of oral dextrose approximately 1 to 2 hours before the FDG injection to increase glucose metabolism, increase FDG uptake, and improve image quality.[11,12] Although 90 percent of FDG images are of diagnostic quality in nondiabetic patients, the quality of FDG images after glucose loading alone is less certain in patients with clinical or subclinical diabetes because the increase in plasma insulin levels may be attenuated, tissue lipolysis may not be inhibited, and free fatty acid levels may remain high. Standardization schemes to optimize FDG image quality in diabetic patients include[11,12] (1) intravenous insulin injections after glucose loading; (2) hyperinsulinemic-euglycemic clamping; and (3) use of nicotinic acid derivative.

Imaging Oxidative Metabolism and Mitochondrial Function

[^{11}C]ACETATE. All oxidative fuels are metabolized in the tricarboxylic acid (TCA) cycle after conversion to acetyl coenzyme A (CoA). [^{11}C] Acetate is avidly extracted by the myocardium and metabolized predominantly by conversion to [^{11}C]acetyl-CoA in the cytosol and oxidation by the TCA cycle in the mitochondria to [^{11}C]carbon dioxide and water. Hence, the rapid myocardial turnover and clearance of [^{11}C]acetate in the form of [^{11}C]carbon dioxide may reflect myocardial oxidative metabolism and provide insight into mitochondrial function. In patients with recent MI and chronic stable angina, clearance rates of [^{11}C]acetate predict myocardial viability and functional recovery after revascularization. Despite encouraging data in the literature, [^{11}C]acetate remains an investigational tracer.

Assessment of Ventricular Function by Radionuclide Imaging

Assessing the Physiology of Ventricular Function

The EF as an index of global systolic LV performance is influenced by many factors, including the intrinsic state of contractility, preload, and afterload as well as neurohormonal and inotropic influences. Despite its load dependence, EF has proved clinically quite useful as a marker of ventricular performance. In the aftermath of acute MI, the postinfarction EF is among the most powerful indices predictive of subsequent mortality.[4,31] The radionuclide techniques used to image ventricular function, RVG, and gated SPECT imaging have provided substantial insight into the physiology of LV function and the response to disease states.

ASSESSING THE LEFT VENTRICULAR RESPONSE TO EXERCISE. Equilibrium-gated RVG and first-pass RVG are among the few noninvasive imaging techniques that can evaluate ventricular performance *during exercise.*[10] Most often, this is accomplished by imaging the patient during bicycle exercise, supine or semisupine for equilibrium RVG, and upright for first-pass RVG. EF measurements during exertion can then be compared with the resting EF.[10]

This technique has been used to study the response of LV function and volumes to exercise. For example, in younger normal subjects, the normal increase in EF and cardiac output is accomplished by decreasing end-systolic volume. In contrast, among older normal subjects, the increase in EF and cardiac output during exercise is accomplished by increasing end-diastolic volume (utilizing preload reserve). In healthy subjects, the normal EF response to exercise is an increase of more than five EF units. The underlying physiology of this increase changes as normal subjects age.[10]

The relative ease by which the EF response to exercise may be studied with RVG techniques led to many reports in the late 1970s and throughout the 1980s. However, evaluation of LV function during exercise by RVG has now been largely replaced by exercise echocardiography (see Chap. 14).

EVALUATION OF LEFT VENTRICULAR VOLUMES. With the RVG technique, the counts detected from the LV region of interest are proportional to ventricular volume.

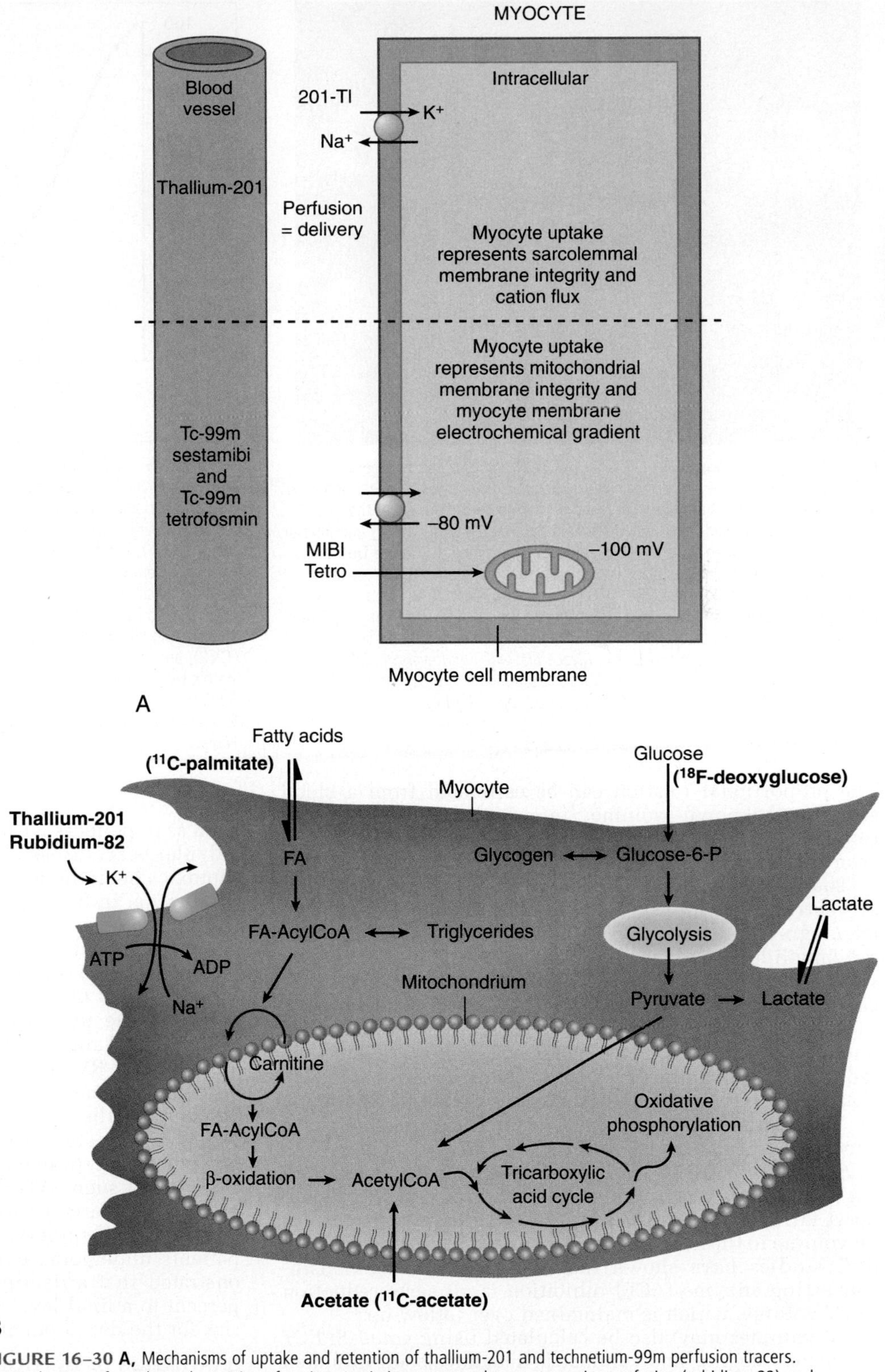

FIGURE 16–30 **A,** Mechanisms of uptake and retention of thallium-201 and technetium-99m perfusion tracers. **B,** Mechanism of uptake and retention of positron emission tomography agents tracing perfusion (rubidium-82) and oxidative and anaerobic metabolism (^{11}C-acetate, ^{11}C-palmitate, and ^{18}F-deoxyglucose). ADP = adenosine diphosphate; ATP = adenosine triphosphate; CoA = coenzyme A; FA = fatty acid. (***B** adapted from Dilsizian V: SPECT and PET techniques.* In *Dilsizian V, Narula J, Braunwald E [eds]: Atlas of Nuclear Cardiology. Philadelphia, Current Medicine, 2006.)*

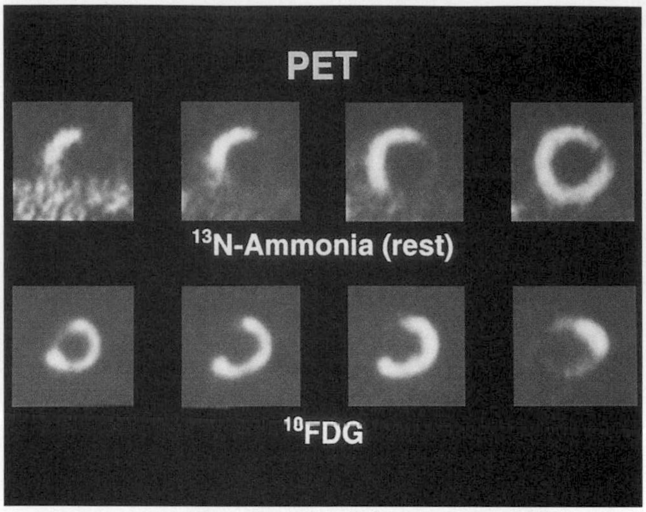

FIGURE 16–31 Assessment of viability by PET imaging. In the **top row,** ^{13}N-ammonia is used as a tracer of myocardial blood flow at rest in these short-axis images starting toward the apex (left) and moving toward the base of the heart (right). There is reduced resting blood flow in the anterolateral, lateral, and inferior walls (defects best seen on the first three images from the left). In the **bottom row,** ^{18}F-fluorodeoxyglucose (FDG) is used as a tracer of myocardial glucose metabolism. There is *enhanced* FDG uptake relative to blood flow in the anterolateral, lateral, and inferior walls, referred to as the "PET mismatch" pattern, indicative of viable myocardium in areas with diminished resting flow, or hibernation. *(Adapted from Dilsizian V: Myocardial viability: Reversible left ventricular dysfunction.* In *Dilsizian V, Narula J, Braunwald E [eds]: Atlas of Nuclear Cardiology. Philadelphia, Current Medicine, 2003, pp 131-145.)*

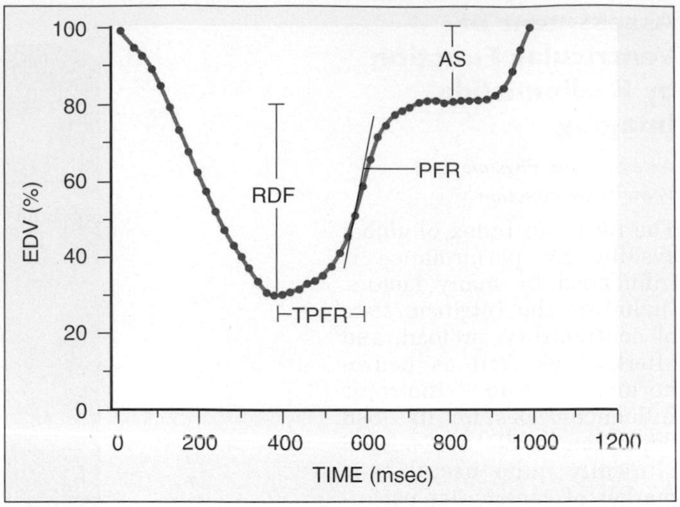

FIGURE 16–32 Quantitative analysis of systolic and diastolic events by radionuclide ventriculography. The *x*-axis represents time across one average cardiac cycle, and the *y*-axis represents count activity within the left ventricular region of interest, which is expressed as a percentage of end-diastolic volume (percent EDV). The time-activity curve represents the relative change in volume within the ventricle during the cardiac cycle. In this high-temporal-resolution example, each point represents 20 milliseconds. Indices of diastolic function may be computed from analysis of the filling portion of the curve, including the peak rate of rapid filling (PFR), the time from end systole at which peak filling occurs (TPFR), and the relative contribution of rapid diastolic filling (RDF) and of atrial systole (AS) to total stroke volume. *(Adapted from Udelson JE, Bonow RO: Radionuclide ventriculography in left ventricular diastolic dysfunction.* In *Gaasch WH, LeWinter M [eds]: Heart Failure and Diastolic Dysfunction. Philadelphia, Lea & Febiger, 1994, pp 167-191.)*

The proportional relation can be estimated from a blood sample of known volume, in which the quantitative relation between counts and volume can be determined after correction for attenuation.[2,4,10]

The major advantage of the RVG technique for evaluation of ventricular volumes (and function) over contrast ventriculographic and echocardiographic methods is that the radionuclide techniques *do not require assumptions about ventricular geometry.* Using RVG techniques, volumes are calculated from count rates over a region of interest involving the left or right ventricle, or both, and are based on photon emissions from the region of interest.[10] Thus, the radionuclide techniques are *not dependent on any assumption of ventricular geometry* and are suitable for the study of ventricular volumes when ventricular geometry is abnormal.

Serial studies of LV volumes have been useful in evaluating the process of LV remodeling after MI and in chronic heart failure,[32] in which there is a progressive increase in LV volume in the absence of neurohormonal blockade. Serial RVG studies have shown that the effect of angiotensin-converting enzyme (ACE) inhibition is an early reduction in LV volume, which is maintained over follow-up.[32]

LV volumes may also be calculated using *gated SPECT perfusion imaging,* and volumetric data have been validated against other quantitative techniques.[33] At this time, there is less experience using gated SPECT perfusion imaging for serial evaluation of LV volumes compared with equilibrium RVG volumetric techniques. The ability to evaluate simultaneously LV function, perfusion, and volumes demonstrates the clinical versatility of gated SPECT MPI.

SERIAL EVALUATION OF LEFT VENTRICULAR FUNCTION. The quantitative nature of radionuclide analysis of ventricular function and the high reproducibility of the measurement make ECG-gated RVG or ECG-gated SPECT imaging well suited for serial follow-up of changes in LV systolic performance. There are many clinical situations in which serial changes in LV function are clinically relevant, such as in patients with heart failure,[34] those observed with valvular heart disease,[35,36] and those being treated with cardiotoxic chemotherapy.[37] Serial RVG studies demonstrating diminution in EF suggesting the early onset of myocardial dysfunction can herald the onset of a higher risk clinical course thereby directing clinical management decisions.

The accuracy and reproducibility of the RVG technique for assessment of LV function make this technique particularly suitable for serial follow-up assessment of patients with regurgitant valvular heart disease. As an example, studies using RVGs have shown that patients being followed with asymptomatic chronic severe aortic regurgitation who demonstrate the onset of LV dysfunction, even when remaining asymptomatic, are at higher risk for adverse clinical outcomes than those with preserved LV performance.[35,36] On the basis of such RVG data, the onset of LV dysfunction in an asymptomatic patient with aortic regurgitation is an indication for surgery. Similarly, serial RVG follow-up of patients undergoing cardiotoxic chemotherapy[37] has demonstrated that a decline in EF as detected by RVG of 10 percent to a final level less than 50 percent indicates high risk for the development of subsequent heart failure.

EVALUATION OF DIASTOLIC FUNCTION WITH RADIONUCLIDE TECHNIQUES

Although the most important quantitative variable derived from RVG evaluation of LV function in the majority of cardiac diseases is the EF, numerous other quantitative variables, including indices describing LV diastolic performance, may also be derived.

LEFT VENTRICULAR DIASTOLIC FILLING. Radionuclide assessment of LV filling properties is based on analysis of the LV time-activity curve, usually obtained using equilibrium RVG techniques,[2] which represents relative volume changes throughout the cardiac cycle (Fig. 16-32). With appropriate data acquisition methods and attention to technical considerations, several parameters of diastolic function may be computed from the time-activity curve, including the peak rate of rapid diastolic filling, the time to peak filling rate, and the relative contributions of the rapid filling period and of atrial systole to total LV

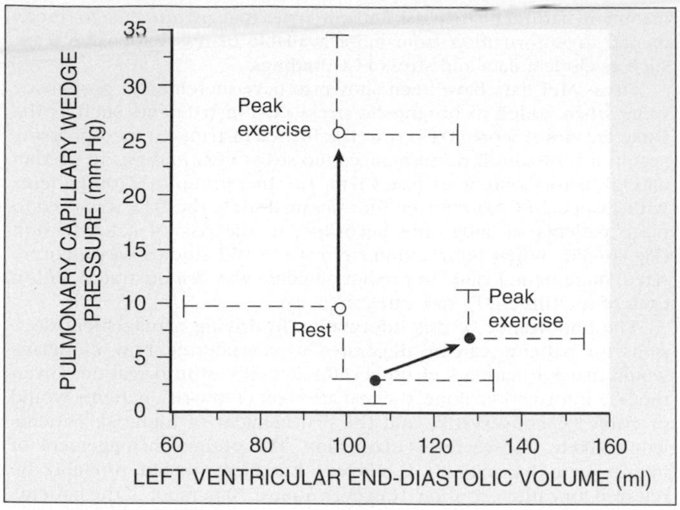

FIGURE 16–33 Use of radionuclide ventriculography to evaluate changes in end-diastolic volume (EDV) during exercise. In normal subjects (closed symbols), there is an increase in EDV during exercise (recruitment of preload reserve) with only minor change in pulmonary capillary wedge (PCW) pressure. In contrast, patients with heart failure and preserved systolic function (open symbols) manifest no change in EDV during exercise despite substantial increase in PCW pressure, to levels that would be associated with symptoms such as shortness of breath. *(Adapted from Kitzman DW, Higginbotham MB, Cobb FR, et al: Exercise intolerance in patients with heart failure and preserved left ventricular systolic function: Failure of the Frank-Starling mechanism. J Am Coll Cardiol 17:1065, 1991.)*

stroke volume. Several studies have shown good correlation between various radionuclide and Doppler echocardiographic measures of filling, as both techniques assess physiological events during the filling period.[2,4]

Evaluation of Diastolic Filling by Equilibrium Radionuclide Ventriculography Techniques in Disease States

HYPERTROPHIC CARDIOMYOPATHY. Abnormal diastolic properties of the hypertrophied ventricle are a characteristic feature of hypertrophic cardiomyopathy (HCM), contributing notably to clinical manifestations.[38] Studies using RVG evaluation of diastolic filling have demonstrated that the rate and extent of rapid filling are reduced in HCM, that the time to peak filling rate is prolonged, and that the contribution of atrial systole to total LV stroke volume is increased.[38]

HEART FAILURE. Radionuclide studies have provided evidence of an abnormal end-diastolic volume response to exercise in patients with heart failure and *preserved* systolic performance, supporting the concept of diastolic dysfunction as an underlying cause for symptoms. Patients with heart failure but preserved systolic performance do not increase end-diastolic volume during exercise associated with a substantial increase in wedge pressure (Fig. 16-33). In contrast, normal subjects demonstrate an increase in end-diastolic volume associated with no change in wedge pressure, recruiting preload despite no change in left atrial driving pressure. Patients with heart failure and normal systolic performance require higher filling pressures to maintain stroke volume, at the cost of an increased pulmonary wedge pressure, resulting in shortness of breath. Thus, abnormal diastolic performance, manifested by an *impaired ability to recruit end-diastolic volume (preload reserve),* as demonstrated by equilibrium RVG techniques, results in physiological abnormalities leading to heart failure in these patients with normal systolic function.

DISEASE DETECTION, RISK STRATIFICATION, AND CLINICAL DECISION-MAKING

Stable Chest Pain Syndromes

Application of Radionuclide Imaging: Answering the Clinical Questions

For patients with stable symptoms of suspected CAD who are referred for noninvasive testing, the two major goals of testing are (1) determination of whether CAD is present or absent (the "diagnostic" construct); and (2) determination of the longer term prognosis or risk of an adverse outcome over time (the "prognostic" construct). These goals of testing are linked to the two main treatment goals for any patients with suspected or known CAD: (1) amelioration of symptoms in everyday life; and (2) improvement in natural history.

Establishing the presence of or ruling out of CAD is an important goal of testing. The performance characteristics of radionuclide imaging for this purpose are often based on an angiographic definition of stenosis greater than or equal to 50 or 70 percent stenosis in an individual epicardial vessel. This definition of CAD is, in part, based on seminal studies in animal models showing that a 50 percent stenosis begins to blunt coronary flow reserve. However, over time, a view has emerged that CAD is a more complex process than can be simply defined dichotomously by a 50 percent or even a 70 percent luminal stenosis. Throughout the progression of plaque growth, there is a risk of transformation from a stable plaque to an unstable plaque, with the potential for an acute coronary syndrome (ACS) that abruptly alters the natural history of the patient (see Chaps. 38 and 50).[39] Plaque encroachment of the lumen occurs later in the process but has a potentially important impact on the patient's everyday quality of life by causing symptoms related to exertional ischemia.

PATIENT-RELATED OUTCOMES AS A GOLD STANDARD. The evolution of preventive therapies (see Chap. 45), such as 3-hydroxy-3-methylglutaryl (HMG) CoA reductase inhibitors, to reduce cardiovascular risk has focused attention on the ability of global risk scores or noninvasive testing to *assess risk of future events* to best target strategies to reduce risk.[40,41] Thus, from the perspective of improving natural history, knowledge of whether or not a greater than 50 percent stenosis is present in a patient with stable anginal symptoms becomes less important than *knowledge of the patient's risk of a cardiovascular event* (i.e., cardiac death or nonfatal MI). After initial investigations of the performance of radionuclide imaging to detect or rule out CAD (sensitivity and specificity), the trajectory of the literature has been toward gaining more understanding of how noninvasive imaging results assess prognosis and stratify the risk of future cardiac events.[4] This has occurred in parallel with similar directions in primary prevention efforts, such as the use of a Framingham risk score, with a goal of life-style and treatment interventions to lower that risk.[40] In much the same way, risk stratification and assessment of prognosis by noninvasive imaging will influence clinical management decisions geared toward reducing risk of MI and cardiac death, and optimizing the selection of patients for revascularization and medical therapies.

Risk Stratification in Stable Chest Pain Syndromes

DEFINITIONS FOR UNDERSTANDING THE LITERATURE. For prognostic assessment, an important goal is to detect patients at risk for "hard" cardiac events. This definition includes *nonfatal MI* as well as *cardiac death* or *all-cause mortality,* irreversible events important to prevent.[42] "Soft" cardiac events include revascularization and hospital admission for unstable angina or heart failure. Such events occur more often than the hard cardiac events and contribute to a larger number of endpoints for data analysis. However, these events are not as important in terms of natural history and may be driven by subjective changes in symptoms and, in the case of revascularization, by the results of the imaging tests themselves.

Risk categories as described in the American College of Cardiology/American Heart Association (ACC/AHA) stable angina guidelines include (1) low risk, defined as a less than 1 percent per year risk of hard event; (2) intermediate risk, defined as a 1 to 3 percent per year risk, and (3) high risk, defined as a greater than 3 percent per year risk of hard cardiac events.[43] These definitions are conceptually linked to implied treatment strategies. Patients with greater than 3 percent per year risk would be most likely to benefit from a revascularization strategy, whereas those at low risk would be least likely to benefit from revascularization, in terms of natural history, and thus could be treated medically—with treatment directed against symptoms as well as risk factor modification.

THE RELATION BETWEEN THE EXTENT OF PERFUSION DEFECT AND NATURAL HISTORY OUTCOMES. Seminal studies in the 1980s demonstrated that the *extent of perfusion abnormality* by stress MPI has an important relation with the *subsequent likelihood of an adverse natural history outcome* (cardiac death or nonfatal MI). Among patients presenting with chest pain and *suspected* CAD (without any known CAD history, such as an MI or revascularization), the risk of cardiac death or MI increased as the number of reversible perfusion defects (i.e., the extent of inducible ischemia) increased (Fig. 16-34).

This concept has been confirmed many times by investigators around the world. This robust concept not only applies to *exercise* stress MPI but also extends across the spectrum of procedural variation in nuclear cardiology, including different stressors (vasodilator pharmacological stress, dobutamine stress), isotopes (thallium-201 and ^{99m}Tc agents), and imaging protocols (including dual-isotope imaging).[4] An example of data on risk stratification implying therapeutic management strategies is demonstrated by the images shown in Figure 16-34A and B. In two older men with typical exertional angina, it would be predicted that the probability of CAD is very high, according to established guidelines. However, what is *not* established from that clinical information is the *natural history risk*. These examples demonstrate that patients presenting with similar symptoms might be identified as having distinct natural histories on the basis of perfusion imaging data, with distinct implications for subsequent management.

THE INCREMENTAL VALUE OF PERFUSION IMAGING. The term "incremental value" implies that perfusion imaging data provide information on natural history risk and outcomes that are *additive to* (incremental to) information from more available or less expensive tests, such as clinical data and stress ECG findings.

Stress MPI data have been shown to have incremental prognostic value when added to prognostic stress ECG instruments such as the Duke Treadmill Score (DTS), a well-validated instrument incorporating symptoms, treadmill performance, and stress ECG findings to predict natural history outcomes (see Chap. 13). In a group of 2200 patients with suspected CAD referred for nuclear testing, the DTS was used to place patients in subgroups according to the risk of a hard event (Fig. 16-35). When information from stress MPI studies was incorporated, incremental value to predict outcome was demonstrated within each of the three DTS risk categories.

The importance of this information in driving management decisions for patients can be illustrated by considering how clinicians would manage patients given certain amounts of information. Given the DTS information alone, the management of low-risk patients would probably be conservative and the management of high-risk patients would likely involve revascularization. The optimal management of intermediate-risk patients is unclear, but many would probably be referred for catheterization. However, almost 70 percent of the patients in the intermediate DTS category had a *normal* stress perfusion study (see Fig. 16-35A), associated with a very low-risk natural history, implying that conservative management would be a safe and effective strategy.

Another method used to demonstrate the incremental value of MPI data over clinical, stress, and even angiographic data involves the creation of a multivariable model to measure the strength of association of individual factors with the natural history outcomes.[44] This is often illustrated by assessing the incremental chi-square value measuring the strength of the association of the factor with subsequent cardiac death and nonfatal MI (see Fig. 16-35B).

IDENTIFICATION OF TREATMENT BENEFIT FOLLOWING RISK STRATIFICATION. Although numerous studies intimate that the extent and severity of perfusion abnormality are related to subsequent natural history risk, few studies have documented *reduction* in that risk associated with a particular therapy. Current information suggests that more extensive ischemia determined by MPI identifies patients in whom revascularization may lead to an improvement in outcome. In a group of more than 10,000 patients with suspected CAD studied by stress MPI, the extent of ischemic myocardium predicted reduction in the risk of death with revascularization compared with medical therapy (Fig. 16-36), beginning at just over 10 percent of ischemic myocardium.[45] As the percentage of ischemic myocardium increased, the magnitude of benefit of revascularization increased as well. Thus, MPI data can predict the magnitude of a potential treatment benefit from revascularization, helping to guide management decisions.

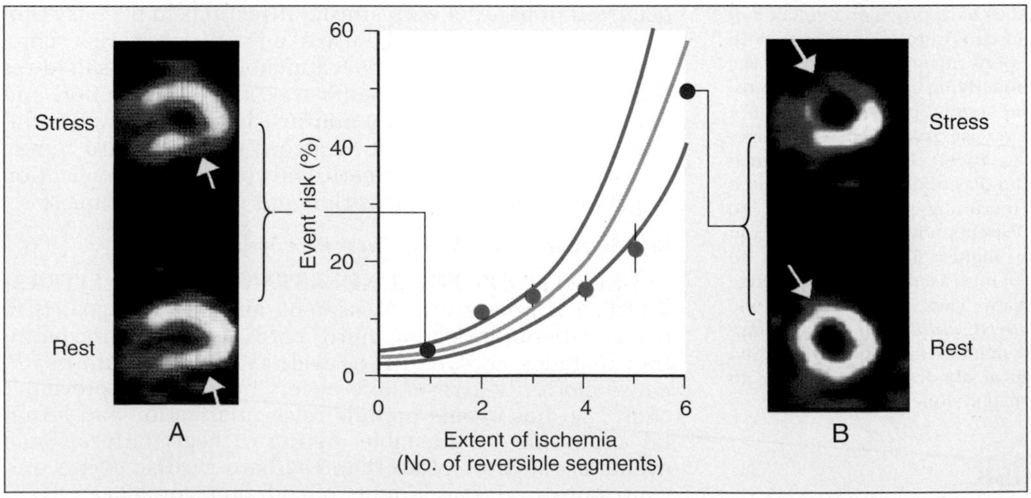

FIGURE 16-34 Prognostic implications of myocardial perfusion imaging. The graph in the middle panel depicts the cardiac event rate (risk of cardiac death or myocardial infarction) on the y-axis as a function of the extent of inducible ischemia on the x-axis. There is an exponential relationship between the extent of ischemia and risk of cardiac events. **A** and **B,** Single-photon emission computed tomography perfusion images in two patients with stable anginal symptoms. **A,** Small area of inferoapical ischemia (arrows). When this extent of ischemia is plotted on the graph (line to red circle), the patient is placed in a low-risk category. **B,** In contrast, the large, severe area of anterior and septal ischemia in this patient (yellow arrows) places him in a high-risk group (line to red circle). *(Graph adapted from Ladenheim ML, Pollock BH, Rozanski A, et al: Extent and severity of myocardial hyperfusion as predictors of prognosis in patients with suspected coronary artery disease. J Am Coll Cardiol 7:464, 1986.)*

THE PROGNOSTIC VALUE OF NORMAL MYOCARDIAL PERFUSION IMAGING. A consistent finding in studies assessing prognosis has been the benign outcome associated with a normal stress MPI study. As summarized in the ACC/AHA/American Society for Nuclear Cardiology (ASNC) Radionuclide Imaging Guidelines,[4] data on outcomes associated with a normal stress SPECT MPI study now involve almost 21,000 patients. In patients with a normal study, the hard event rate (i.e., rate of cardiac death or nonfatal MI) occurring over an average follow-up of 2 years is 0.7 percent per year. This concept applies across a broad spectrum of isotopes, protocols, and stressors.[4,46] The prediction of low-risk outcome following a normal MPI extends approximately 2 years after testing (i.e., the "warranty period").[47] Patients who at baseline represent higher risk subsets (i.e., those with diabetes) have a slightly higher risk of an adverse outcome after a normal stress MPI,[48] consistent with Bayes' theorem; that is, given a certain MPI finding, the posttest probability (outcome risk) is related in part to the pretest risk.

Even when angiographic CAD is present with a stable symptom complex, a normal stress MPI study is associated with a low-risk outcome (~0.9 percent per year).[4] The mechanism for a normal MPI despite established CAD has not been conclusively demonstrated but may involve preserved endothelial function, allowing appropriate flow-mediated vasodilation during stress, reducing the impact of an angiographic stenosis on downstream myocardial perfusion. If this is true, such preserved endothelial function may identify a patient less susceptible to plaque fissuring or rupture and more likely to have a stable clinical course.

DYNAMIC ASSESSMENT OF PROGNOSIS BY SERIAL SCINTIGRAPHIC STUDIES: A NEW PARADIGM? Although there is an important correlation between the extent of ischemia and subsequent outcome, the specificity of such determinations is low. That is, among patients with high-risk scintigraphic signs, only a minority suffer an important cardiac event during follow-up and the majority of "high-risk" patients remain event-free. As most of these high-risk patients undergo catheterization and intervention, many patients who will not have an event are receiving interventions to prevent these events in the minority. Clinicians accept this trade-off, but evolving data suggest that the response of scintigraphic ischemia to

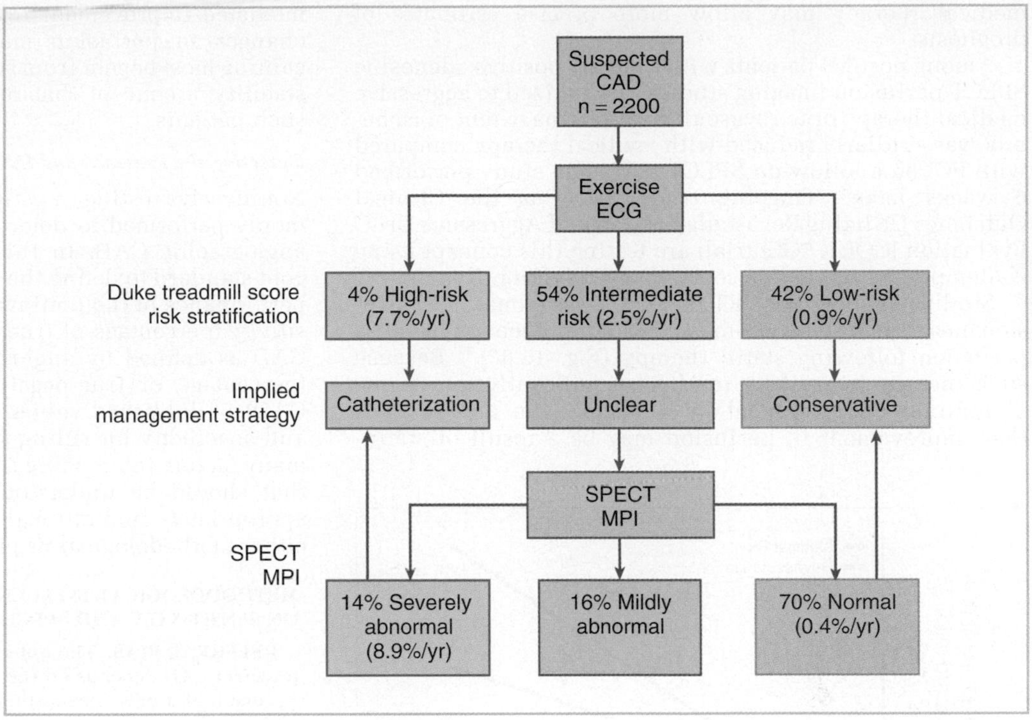

A

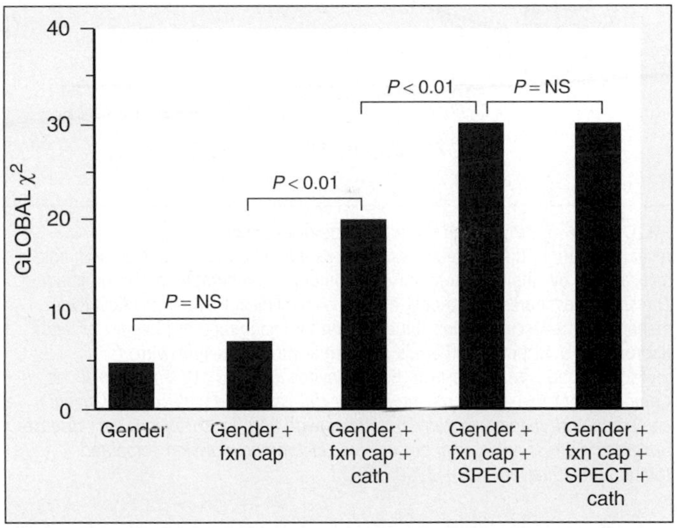

B

FIGURE 16–35 Incremental value of single-photon emission computed tomography (SPECT) perfusion imaging. **A,** Comparison with the Duke Treadmill Score (DTS). A large group of patients with suspected coronary artery disease (CAD) was initially risk stratified by the well-validated DTS. Figures in parentheses are the observed annual event rates. The majority of the population is classified as "intermediate risk" by DTS, and management strategy is not clear. High-risk patients may be managed aggressively, and low-risk patients may be managed conservatively. Among patients originally categorized as intermediate risk by the DTS, almost 70 percent had a normal SPECT perfusion study, associated with a very low event rate. Following SPECT myocardial perfusion imaging (MPI), more patients are classified at the "extremes" of risk (low or high), where management is more clearly implied by the risk prediction. Thus, the imaging data allowed further stratification and had incremental value over the DTS information. **B,** The incremental value of imaging data may be expressed as the incremental chi-square value, a statistical measure of the strength of the association of clinical, demographic, stress, or imaging factors to risk stratification. Among patients with known CAD who had undergone catheterization (cath), clinical information is added on the *x*-axis, with the global chi-square value associated with the information depicted on the *y*-axis. The larger the chi-square value, the stronger the relation between the combination of factors on the *x*-axis and the natural history outcome of cardiac death or myocardial infarction. Even when anatomical information is available, the physiological information provided by SPECT MPI adds significantly to risk prediction ability. fxn cap = functional capacity. *(**A,** Adapted from Hachamovitch R, Berman DS, Kiat H, et al: Exercise myocardial perfusion SPECT in patients without known coronary artery disease: Incremental prognostic value and use in risk stratification. Circulation 93:905, 1996;* ***B,*** *Adapted from Beller GA: First annual Mario S. Verani, MD, Memorial Lecture: Clinical value of myocardial perfusion imaging in coronary artery disease. J Nucl Cardiol 10:529, 2003.)*

medical therapy may allow more precise estimates of prognosis.

Among post-MI patients with strongly positive adenosine SPECT perfusion imaging studies randomized to aggressive medical therapy or to revascularization, the extent of ischemia was similarly reduced with medical therapy compared with PCI on a follow-up SPECT perfusion study performed 6 weeks later.[24] Ongoing trials (such as the Clinical Outcomes Utilizing Revascularization and Aggressive DruG Evaluation [COURAGE] trial) are testing this concept using contemporary aggressive secondary prevention therapies.[49]

Studies using either PET or SPECT assessment of perfusion have concordantly demonstrated improvement in stress perfusion following statin therapy (Fig. 16-37).[50] Because such therapy is unlikely to affect significantly the degree of luminal encroachment by a plaque, the data suggest that improvement in perfusion may be a result of statin-mediated improvement in endothelial function. Favorable changes in perfusion may identify cohorts of patients gaining most benefit from statin therapy in terms of vascular stability, a concept that requires longer term follow-up of such patients.

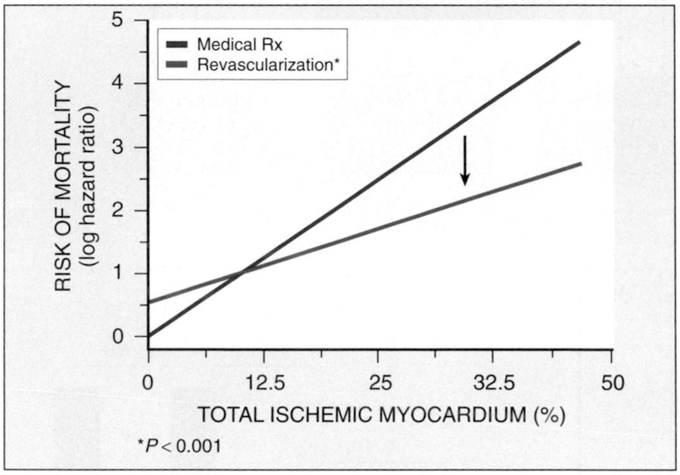

FIGURE 16–36 Predicting the magnitude of treatment benefit by revascularization. Risk of death is plotted as a function of the percent ischemic myocardium by single-photon emission computed tomography perfusion imaging. The solid lines represent patients treated with medical therapy (medical Rx, magenta) or revascularization (blue). When the magnitude of ischemia exceeds approximately 12 percent, there is a potential survival benefit with revascularization. *(Adapted from Hachamovitch R, Hayes SW, Friedman JD, et al: Comparison of the short-term survival benefit associated with revascularization compared with medical therapy in patients with no prior coronary artery disease undergoing stress myocardial perfusion single photon emission computed tomography. Circulation 107:2900, 2003.)*

Detecting the Presence and Extent of Coronary Artery Disease

Noninvasive testing in patients with suspected CAD is commonly performed to determine the presence or absence of angiographic CAD. In this paradigm, angiography is the gold standard to define the presence or absence of CAD, and performance of the noninvasive test is measured by its *sensitivity* (percentage of true-positive tests among those with CAD as defined by angiography) as well as its *specificity* (percentage of true-negative tests among those without CAD).[4,51] Published values of sensitivity for detecting CAD and specificity for ruling out CAD vary widely.[4] There are many factors influencing these performance characteristics that should be understood to incorporate imaging data appropriately into clinical decision-making. These include either methodological or physiological factors.

METHODOLOGICAL INFLUENCES ON SENSITIVITY AND SPECIFICITY

REFERRAL BIAS. The *apparent* accuracy of any noninvasive test to detect CAD depends on the indications for coronary angiography. Accuracy of a new diagnostic test is usually determined initially in patients who are undergoing coronary angiography. As the test becomes implemented in routine diagnostic strategies, its results determine which patients are to be referred for coronary angiography (Fig. 16-38). For example, patients with abnormal MPI are more likely to undergo coronary angiography than those with normal MPI. This results in a phenomenon termed "posttest referral bias," in which the specificity of a diagnostic test declines over time as it is accepted into clinical practice and plays a gatekeeper role in determining which patients undergo angiography.[4] In its extreme form, in which only patients with an abnormal test are referred for angiography (as in Figure 16-38), posttest referral bias drives the specificity to zero (all patients with normal coronary arteriograms have false-positive MPI results and there are no true-negatives). The same phenomenon artificially increases the sensitivity of the test and in its extreme drives the sensitivity to 100 percent (all patients with abnormal coronary arteriograms have true-positive MPI, with no false-negatives). This concept holds not only for MPI but also for any diagnostic test that might determine the indications for angiography.

The concept of "normalcy rate" has been developed in an attempt to compensate for this referral bias.[4] Normalcy is calculated in the same manner as specificity but includes only the imaging test results of patients with a clinically low or very low pretest likelihood of CAD, whether or not they are referred for cardiac catheterization. Normalcy rates tend to be greater than specificity rates.

ANGIOGRAPHY AS THE GOLD STANDARD. In humans, coronary atherosclerosis is a complex disease most often involving the coronary arteries diffusely and not merely focally. Moreover, whether a given discrete stenosis, imaged at rest during coronary angiography, results in a perfusion abnormality during stress is dependent on a number of factors besides the percent of stenosis. These factors include the dilatory or constrictor response of the vessel during stress (mediated by endothelial function) and the presence or absence of collaterals.[51] For example, a vessel with 70 percent stenosis but with preserved endothelial function and a well-developed collateral supply may *not* be associated with an abnor-

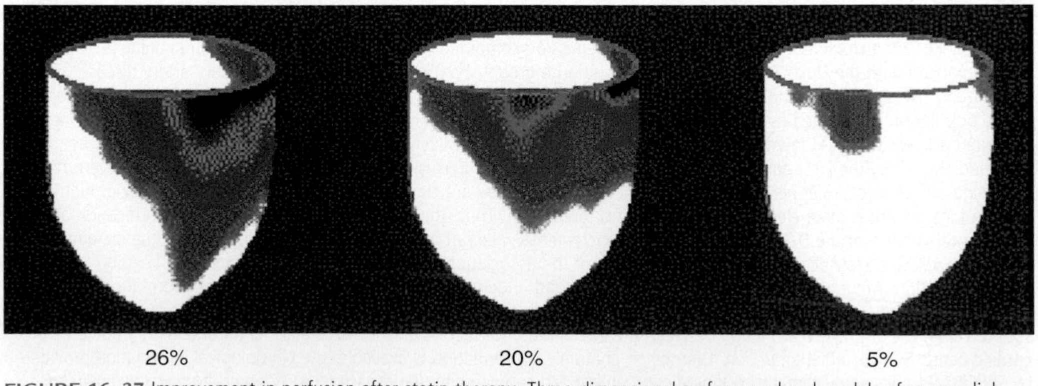

FIGURE 16–37 Improvement in perfusion after statin therapy. Three-dimensional surface-rendered models of myocardial perfusion before statin therapy **(left)** and after 6 weeks **(middle)** and 6 months **(right)** of therapy, viewed from the inferior surface of the heart. White areas represent normal perfusion, with red, blue, and black representing increasingly severe degrees of ischemia. The extent of ischemia is below each image, expressed as a percentage of total myocardium. There is a substantial improvement in the degree of inferior wall ischemia over the course of statin therapy. *(Adapted from Schwartz RG, Pearson TA, Kalaria VG, et al: Prospective serial evaluation of myocardial perfusion and lipids during the first six months of pravastatin therapy: Coronary artery disease regression single photon emission computed tomography monitoring trial. J Am Coll Cardiol 42:600, 2003.)*

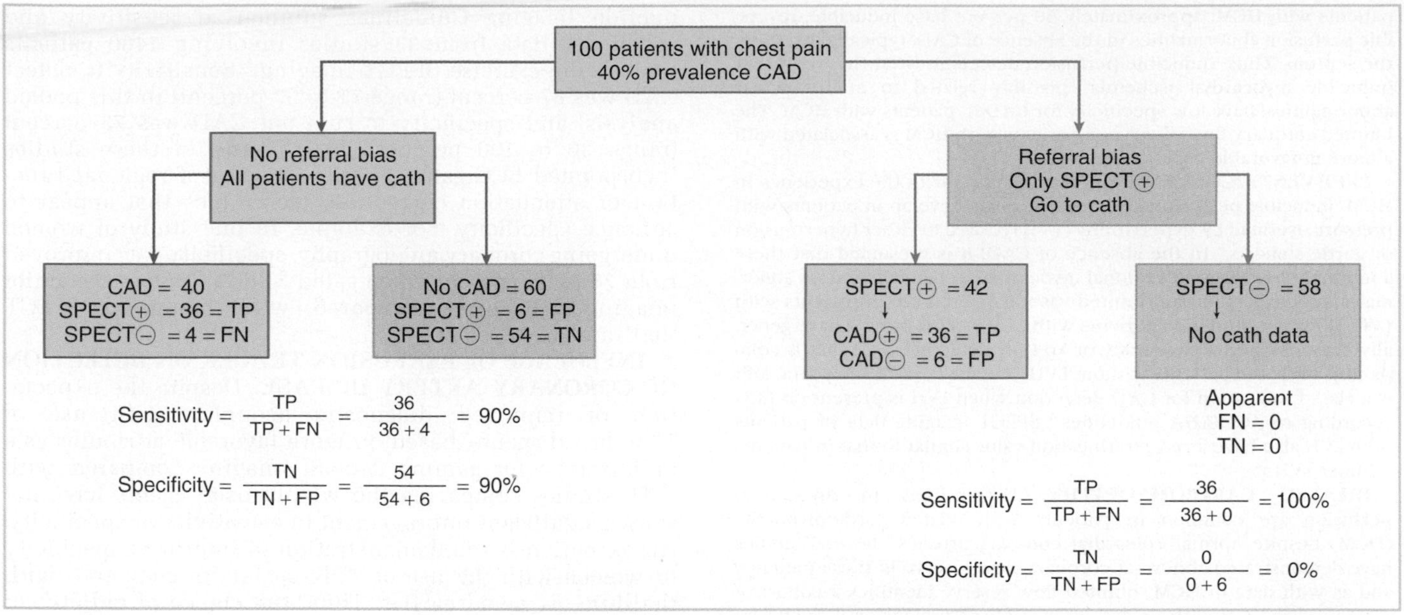

FIGURE 16–38 The effect of referral bias on specificity calculation. If the test being evaluated is used as the gatekeeper to coronary angiography, many patients who are true negatives (i.e., have a normal test and do not have coronary disease) will not undergo angiography and thus will not be included in the specificity calculations **(right).** This has an effect of artificially reducing the apparent specificity of the noninvasive test in question. CAD = coronary artery disease; FN = false negative; FP = false positive; TN = true negative; TP = true positive. *(Adapted from Rozanski A, Diamond GA, Berman D, et al: The declining specificity of exercise radionuclide ventriculography. N Engl J Med 309:518, 1983.)*

mality on stress MPI. In a diagnostic construct, such a result would be categorized as a false-negative finding, reducing MPI sensitivity. However, the MPI data may be providing the *correct physiological information* regarding the functional significance of the angiographic finding, demonstrating that collateral flow during exercise or normal endothelial function, or both, were associated with preserved coronary blood flow reserve despite the coronary stenosis. This example illustrates the limitation of using angiography as a gold standard in evaluating a physiological modality.

Many published studies define CAD as greater than or equal to 50 percent stenosis, whereas others use a threshold of greater than or equal to 70 percent stenosis.[2,4] Using the former would decrease sensitivity (as some 50 to 70 percent stenoses are not hemodynamically significant) and increase specificity. In contrast, using the latter threshold would increase sensitivity, as more such stenoses are likely to be associated with perfusion abnormality, but decrease specificity, as any positive scan result with 50 to 70 percent stenosis would be considered false-positive.

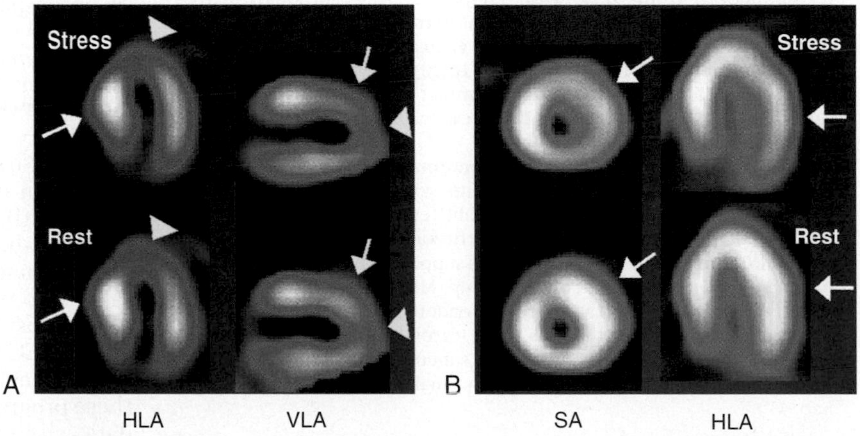

FIGURE 16–39 Single-photon emission computed tomography perfusion imaging in hypertrophic cardiomyopathy (HCM) in young asymptomatic patients with normal coronary arteries. **A,** Fixed perfusion defect of the apex consistent with infarction, indicated by yellow arrowheads in the horizontal (HLA) and vertical (VLA) long-axis images, with a reversible defect of the anterior wall (yellow arrows in the VLA images). The hypertrophied septum is evident (white arrows in the HLA images). **B,** Extensive inducible silent ischemia in the anterior, lateral, and inferior walls (white arrows). Transient ischemic cavity dilation is also present, possibly related to subendocardial ischemia. *(Based on data from O'Gara PT, Bonow RO, Maron BJ, et al: Myocardial perfusion abnormalities in patients with hypertrophic cardiomyopathy: Assessment with thallium-201 emission computed tomography. Circulation 76:1214, 1987; and Udelson JE, Bonow RO, O'Gara PT, et al: Verapamil prevents silent myocardial perfusion abnormalities during exercise in asymptomatic patients with hypertrophic cardiomyopathy. Circulation 79:1052, 1989.)*

PHYSIOLOGICAL INFLUENCES ON SENSITIVITY AND SPECIFICITY

A number of disease processes involving the coronary vasculature or the myocardium may result in abnormalities in myocardial perfusion in the *absence of a discrete coronary stenosis.* In a diagnostic construct for CAD, such abnormalities would be labeled false-positive, reducing specificity (i.e., the test is positive in the absence of epicardial CAD). However, MPI may actually be providing correct information regarding perfusion physiology.

LEFT BUNDLE BRANCH BLOCK. Isolated reversible perfusion defects of the septum in patients with left bundle branch block (LBBB) may be seen in the absence of stenosis of the left anterior descending (LAD) coronary artery.[2,4] This phenomenon may represent true heterogeneity of flow between the LAD and left circumflex territories, related to delayed relaxation of the septum in LBBB leading to reduced coronary flow reserve in early diastole, or reduced oxygen demand as a result of late septal contraction when wall stress is decreasing. The specificity and predictive value of a septal perfusion defect with LBBB are thus low. However, apical or anterior involvement in septal perfusion defects increases the specificity for CAD.[4] Because a septal defect in LBBB is most commonly seen at high heart rates, pharmacological stress improves specificity, and vasodilator stress is recommended in the setting of LBBB.[4]

HYPERTROPHIC CARDIOMYOPATHY. The asymmetrical septal hypertrophy in many patients with HCM can lead to the appearance of a greater amount of tracer uptake in the hypertrophied septum relative to the lateral wall, creating the impression of a mild lateral wall perfusion defect, especially when polar maps are employed.

Many reports have demonstrated myocardial perfusion abnormalities in patients with HCM in the absence of epicardial CAD.[15] Such findings have important pathophysiological relevance: patients with fixed perfusion defects are likely to have thinned akinetic walls on echocardiography and diminished EF (Fig. 16-39). Of asymptomatic patients with HCM, approximately 50 percent have inducible, reversible perfusion abnormalities in the absence of CAD, typically involving the septum. Thus, inducible perfusion defects in HCM that represent inducible myocardial ischemia, possibly related to microvascular abnormalities, have low specificity for CAD in patients with HCM. The blunted coronary flow reserve in patients with HCM is associated with a more unfavorable natural history.[15]

LEFT VENTRICULAR HYPERTROPHY. As with the experience in HCM, inducible perfusion abnormalities may develop in patients with pressure overload LV hypertrophy (LVH) related to either hypertension or aortic stenosis.[4] In the absence of CAD, it is presumed that these abnormalities represent regional myocardial ischemia based on abnormal microcirculation and limited vasodilator reserve in patients with LVH. However, studies in patients with LVH by ECG criteria have generally demonstrated an accuracy of MPI for detecting CAD that is comparable to that in patients without LVH.[4] On the basis of such data, MPI is a class I indication for CAD detection when LVH is present on ECG according to ACC/AHA guidelines.[4] SPECT imaging data in patients with LVH also have a risk stratification value similar to that in patients without LVH.[52]

DILATED CARDIOMYOPATHY. Abnormalities in myocardial perfusion are common in patients with dilated cardiomyopathy (DCM) despite normal epicardial coronary arteries.[4] Several studies have demonstrated abnormal coronary flow reserve in these patients, and as with data in HCM, blunted flow reserve identifies a cohort of patients with DCM with a more unfavorable natural history.[14] Such data support the relevance of the perfusion abnormalities rather than simply classifying them as false-positive if epicardial CAD is not present.

An important diagnostic consideration in patients with LV systolic dysfunction involves distinguishing those whose cardiomyopathy may be primarily due to CAD (many of whom have potentially reversible LV dysfunction) from those with idiopathic DCM. Although many patients with DCM may have perfusion abnormalities detected on MPI, the *absence* of perfusion abnormalities virtually excludes CAD as the etiology of the cardiomyopathy (Fig. 16-40).[53] *Extensive* perfusion abnormalities in the setting of LV dysfunction are virtually always associated with CAD rather than DCM, especially when the perfusion defects are segmental.

ENDOTHELIAL DYSFUNCTION. Abnormalities in myocardial perfusion detected by SPECT MPI in patients with coronary endothelial dysfunction, in the absence of "significant" epicardial vessel stenosis, have been demonstrated. That these perfusion findings represent true abnormalities in coronary flow reserve is supported by studies showing *improvement* in perfusion on follow-up MPI after treatment with medical therapies directed at improving endothelial function.[54] Further support for this concept comes from cardiac magnetic resonance imaging studies demonstrating blunted subendocardial coronary flow reserve in patients with angina and normal coronary arteries (see Chap. 17).[55]

SENSITIVITY AND SPECIFICITY OF MYOCARDIAL PERFUSION IMAGING. The 2003 ACC/AHA/ASNC Radionuclide Imaging Guidelines summarize sensitivity and specificity data from 33 studies involving 4480 patients undergoing exercise SPECT imaging.[4] Sensitivity to detect CAD was 87 percent (range 71 to 97 percent) in this pooled analysis, and specificity to rule out CAD was 73 percent (range 36 to 100 percent). Few if any of these studies incorporated ECG-gated SPECT imaging of regional function or attenuation correction, techniques that appear to enhance specificity. For example, in one study of women undergoing coronary angiography, specificity was improved from 76 to 96 percent when gated SPECT Tc 99m sestamibi imaging was used compared with non-gated SPECT thallium-201.[4]

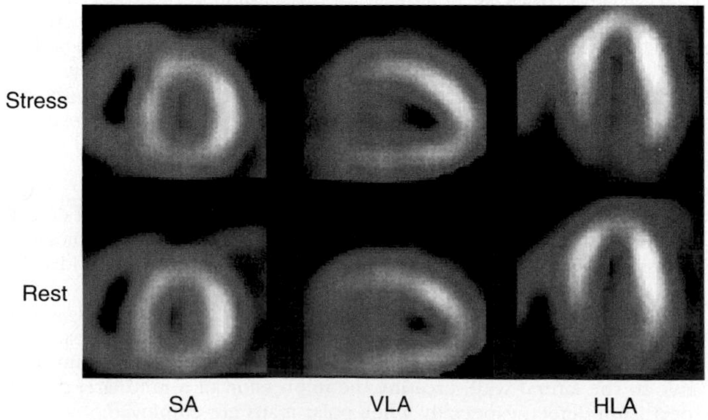

FIGURE 16-40 Single-photon emission computed tomography perfusion images at stress and rest from a patient with heart failure. The images depict a dilated left ventricle but with normal perfusion patterns, suggesting a low likelihood that coronary artery disease is the etiology of heart failure. HLA = horizontal long axis; SA = short axis; VLA = vertical long axis.

INFLUENCE OF PERFUSION TRACER ON DETECTION OF CORONARY ARTERY DISEASE. Despite the expectation of improved diagnostic accuracy with use of ^{99m}Tc-based agents, based on more favorable attributes as a radioisotope for gamma camera imaging compared with ^{201}Tl, studies comparing the widely used agents have not shown significant improvement in sensitivity or specificity. An exception is the demonstration of improved specificity in women with the use of ^{99m}Tc sestamibi compared with thallium, as noted earlier. Thus, the choice of radiotracer for MPI does not notably affect the discrimination between the presence or absence of CAD. It is important to recognize that published studies often involve subjects who may not fully represent those who are most challenging to image. It would be expected that the ^{99m}Tc-based agents, with their greater photon energy, would offer improved performance in obese patients and those with large breasts as well as allow the option of higher quality gated images.

Influence of Automated Quantitation of Myocardial Perfusion Images in Detection of Coronary Artery Disease. There may be significant intra- and interobserver variability in the visual analysis of myocardial perfusion images. Several methods of quantitative analysis of MPI have been developed[1,4] to reduce the variability in reading by objectifying image analysis, by comparing regional uptake values with a normal data base.

Automated quantitative analysis systems are incorporated into most SPECT camera-computer equipment. Some of the most common are Emory Toolbox, Cedars QPS,[56] and 4D MSPECT (Fig. 16-41). Although published data do not clearly demonstrate improved sensitivity or specificity of these programs over visual analysis for CAD detection, such data arise from expert centers, often where the quantitative software was developed, and the visual analysis data are derived from experienced readers in laboratories with excellent quality control. In practice, the use of contemporary quantitative programs can improve image acquisition quality as well as interpretation. Some programs incorporate motion-sensing algorithms that interrogate the raw data and alert the technologist that motion correction may be needed.

PHARMACOLOGICAL STRESS TESTING FOR DETECTION OF CORONARY ARTERY DISEASE. Reports examining the sensitivity and specificity of vasodilator pharmacological stress combined with MPI for the detection of CAD have achieved results similar to those reported with exercise stress. A pooled analysis from the 2003 ACC/AHA/ASNC Radionuclide Imaging Guidelines involving 2465 catheterized patients in 17 studies[4] demonstrated sensitivity of 89 percent and specificity of 75 percent, similar to values from exercise SPECT MPI studies.

The more powerful hyperemic stress response achieved with vasodilator stress compared with exercise might be expected to result in improved sensitivity to detect CAD, particularly more moderate stenoses. This has not been demonstrated, possibly because of the "roll off" property of the common perfusion tracers, caused by diffusion limitation at hyperemic blood flow levels.[3] Thus, the more favorable hyperemic stress achieved with pharmacological stress is offset by the lack of linear tracer uptake in the areas with the highest flow.

The diagnostic ability of dobutamine stress imaging appears to be generally similar to that of other pharmacological and exercise stress modalities for the detection of CAD.[4] One study demonstrated that there is an increase in false-negative scans when patients with known positive dobutamine MPI are retested after receiving intravenous propranolol.[2,10] On the basis of these considerations, dobutamine is used only when adenosine or dipyridamole is contraindicated, such as in a patient with reactive airways disease.

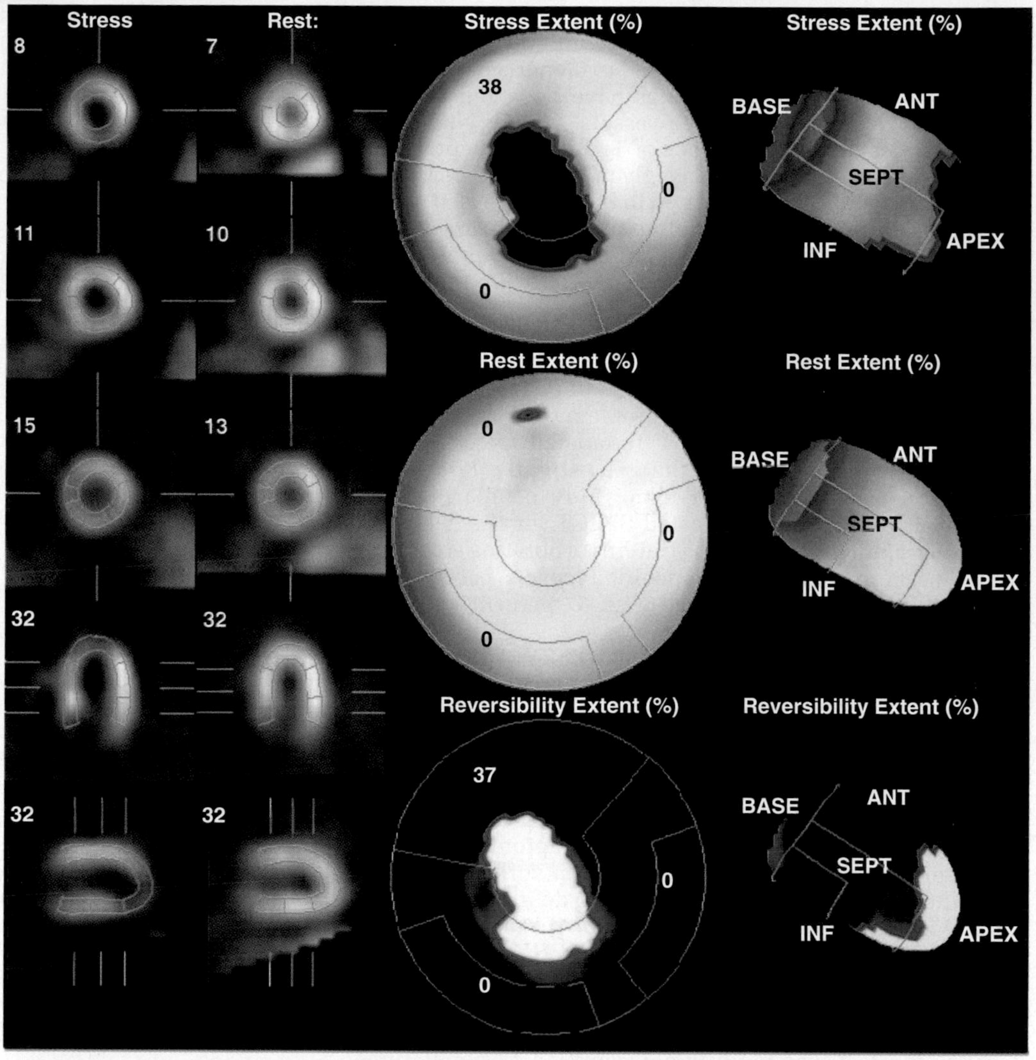

FIGURE 16–41 Automated quantitative analysis software. Selected short- and long-axis tomograms from stress and rest studies **(two left columns)** are automatically segmented and scored. Bull's-eye plots are created **(third column)** representing the stress **(top)** and rest **(middle)** data and demonstrate a large apical reversible defect. The bottom bull's-eye plot displays the extent of ischemic myocardium (white area), which measures 23 percent of the total myocardium. The bull's-eye information is also displayed in a three-dimensional format (**right column, top, middle, and bottom,** respectively). *(Images courtesy of Guido Germano, PhD.)*

EFFECT OF SUBMAXIMAL EXERCISE PERFORMANCE ON CORONARY ARTERY DISEASE DETECTION. The sensitivity of MPI to detect CAD is optimized by achieving the highest possible level of oxygen demand to stimulate the greatest increment in coronary flow reserve. In exercise ECG testing, sensitivity to detect CAD falls significantly if greater than 85 percent of maximum predicted heart rate for age is not achieved (see Chap. 13).[57] Because perfusion heterogeneity usually develops at a lower degree of supply-demand mismatch than ECG changes, the sensitivity of MPI to detect CAD is maintained at somewhat lower workloads. In one study, patients with CAD were stressed with MPI at a maximal workload and then again at a less than maximal workload.[4,10] There was no difference in sensitivity between the maximal and the submaximal tests. However, the extent and severity of reversible perfusion defects are diminished at submaximal compared with maximal workloads, which may affect the prognostic value of the test.

The selection of a stress protocol can be summarized as follows[2,4]: exercise is the preferred stressor because it allows the optimal potential association of symptoms with perfusion abnormalities. The use of exercise also allows incorporation of validated stress test criteria such as the DTS, heart rate reserve, or heart rate recovery with the MPI data.[20] For patients who cannot exercise adequately, vasodilator stress with adenosine or dipyridamole is the procedure of choice, with dobutamine used for patients with a contraindication to the vasodilators.[2,4] For patients who begin exercise but do not reach 85 percent of maximum predicted heart rate for age *or* who do not reach an appropriate symptomatic endpoint, isotope injection can be withheld, the exercise portion of the test terminated, and vasodilator stress performed to optimize diagnostic and risk stratification information.

DETECTING AND DEFINING THE EXTENT OF CORONARY ARTERY DISEASE. In formulating a management strategy for patients, it is important to determine the *extent* of disease rather than just the *presence or absence* of disease. The term "extensive CAD" refers to angiographic patterns of CAD that have prognostic significance and suggest treatment benefit from revascularization, such as left main or severe three-vessel CAD involving the proximal LAD artery.

SPECT MPI is limited by the relative nature of the perfusion information; if all areas are hypoperfused in the presence of three-vessel CAD, the least hypoperfused area appears normal and the true extent of CAD may be underestimated. However, incorporation of other findings, including regional functional abnormalities, can be used to estimate more correctly the probability of disease extent.

Wall motion abnormalities on poststress gated SPECT imaging may be of benefit in the detection of extensive CAD. In one study,[58] incorporating the finding of poststress wall motion abnormality on gated SPECT imaging along with the degree of perfusion abnormality allowed improved sensitivity (85 to 91 percent) for detecting proximal 90 percent LAD lesions or multivessel disease related to 90 percent or greater proximal lesions. Similar findings have been reported for improving detection of three-vessel CAD.[59] Numerous reports suggest that the presence of TID raises the probability of multivessel CAD for any given extent of perfusion abnormality.[2,4] Findings unrelated to imaging are also useful in enhancing the diagnosis of left main or three-vessel CAD. The development of greater than 2 mm of ST depression or hypotension on ECG treadmill testing increases the likelihood of left main or three-vessel CAD.[57]

DETECTION OF CORONARY ARTERY DISEASE IN WOMEN. The detection of CAD using exercise ECG testing is problematic in women.[43,57] The use of ^{201}Tl for detecting CAD in women is limited by problems associated with breast attenuation. The use of ^{99m}Tc-labeled tracers should improve specificity because there is slightly less tissue attenuation, as demonstrated in a study comparing ^{201}Tl SPECT with ^{99m}Tc sestamibi gated SPECT for the detection of angiographic CAD.[4] With the incorporation of gated SPECT sestamibi imaging, a specificity of 92 percent was achieved in one study compared with 67 percent with ^{201}Tl (see Fig. 16-10).

DETECTION OF CORONARY ARTERY DISEASE IN VALVULAR HEART DISEASE. Several studies have evaluated the use of MPI in the assessment of the possible copresence of CAD in patients with valvular heart disease; most of the published studies involved patients with aortic stenosis. Sensitivity of MPI has ranged from 61 to 100 percent, with specificity 64 to 77 percent.[4] Although it is potentially useful in selected cases to assist in symptom evaluation, these performance characteristics are not sufficient to preclude the use of coronary angiography to define the presence of CAD in patients being considered for surgery.[36]

RADIONUCLIDE VENTRICULOGRAPHY FOR DETECTION OF CORONARY ARTERY DISEASE. Early reports of exercise RVG to detect CAD included predominantly patients with extensive CAD, resulting in high sensitivity. Because the test was more widely applied to populations with less extensive disease, sensitivity values were lower. However, although the EF response to exercise may be a relatively insensitive marker of CAD, it is a powerful prognostic marker.[4]

As the LVEF response to exercise may be normal in many patients with less extensive CAD, a regional wall motion abnormality during exercise may be more sensitive for identifying CAD. RVG data during exercise are usually acquired in only one view, the left anterior oblique "best septal" view.[10] Thus, the view of the inferior wall is limited, and regional wall motion abnormalities are insensitive for disease of the right coronary artery.

The normal range for an exercise EF response was initially defined by a group of young normal volunteers, a population that differs from those with chest pain and normal coronary arteriograms. Posttest referral bias has also been invoked to explain the decline in specificity in exercise RVG. However, as with a normal MPI study, a preserved ventricular response to exercise is associated with a good prognosis,[10] despite the presence of CAD.

In contrast to studies of MPI demonstrating little change in the ability to detect CAD at slightly submaximal workloads, the sensitivity for detecting CAD by exercise RVG is impaired at submaximal workloads.[10] A similar problem would be expected with stress echocardiographic studies of inducible regional wall motion abnormalities. Although exercise RVG is rarely used in contemporary practice, the EF response to exercise or the absolute value of the exercise EF is a powerful prognostic indicator in suspected or known CAD, and these data have informed the contemporary use of post-stress ECG-gated SPECT imaging as well as stress echocardiography (see Chap. 14).

Imaging in Patients with Established Coronary Artery Disease

There are several potential roles for SPECT MPI in patients who are known to have established CAD. Clinical questions may remain after angiography regarding the physiological significance of stenoses. The results of stress-rest SPECT MPI correlate generally with invasive measures of coronary flow reserve. Moreover, improvement of SPECT evidence of ischemia has been commonly documented after successful PCI, suggesting that SPECT MPI can identify the culprit ischemic lesion.[4]

IMAGING AFTER CORONARY ARTERY BYPASS SURGERY. Studies of patients who develop recurrent symptoms after coronary artery bypass graft (CABG) surgery have demonstrated that SPECT MPI can accurately detect the presence and location of graft stenoses, even if the symptoms are atypical for ischemia.

A number of studies have concordantly demonstrated the risk stratification value of SPECT MPI in patients after CABG, especially late after CABG, even if symptoms are not present.[4] The extent of perfusion abnormality is related to the subsequent risk of cardiac death and nonfatal MI, and SPECT information has incremental predictive value over clinical and stress data. As the outcome risk is generally low in the early years after CABG, *routine* assessment for the presence and extent of ischemia in an asymptomatic patient is not recommended by current guidelines. Still, in a study of almost 900 asymptomatic patients studied with SPECT MPI after CABG,[4] perfusion defects were common and were associated with significantly increased relative risk of death or major events (as was impaired exercise capacity), even when controlling for time after CABG. In *symptomatic* post-CABG patients, such information can guide the need for catheterization and intervention. In *asymptomatic* patients, in whom aggressive secondary prevention strategies should be in place, the implications for clinical decision-making are less clear. In this situation, the *extent* of SPECT abnormality is important, as a more extensive perfusion abnormality is associated with a progressively higher risk of subsequent cardiac death or MI[60] and at some threshold may justify an invasive approach.

IMAGING AFTER PERCUTANEOUS CORONARY INTERVENTION. Exercise MPI is superior in detecting the presence and location of restenosis after PCI compared with exercise ECG, and current guidelines recommend stress imaging in symptomatic post-PCI patients.[4] The extent of SPECT MPI abnormality in patients studied after PCI is correlated with the subsequent risk of cardiac death or MI on long-term follow-up, even late after PCI, and this appears to hold true in patients even in the absence of symptoms.[61] Thus, although *routine* assessment of asymptomatic patients after PCI with SPECT MPI is not currently recommended, important information may be gleaned by imaging of symptomatic patients to guide decisions regarding reintervention and in selected high-risk asymptomatic patients late after PCI, to assess subsequent risk.[4] Reports have suggested that very early after PCI, SPECT MPI may demonstrate a mild reversible defect in the territory of the treated vessel (although less severe than before PCI).[4] This may be due to delayed return of full coronary flow reserve after PCI, thus representing a true physiological phenomenon.

LEFT VENTRICULAR FUNCTION DURING EXERCISE IN PATIENTS WITH KNOWN CORONARY ARTERY DISEASE. The EF response to exercise (as determined by exercise RVG) can be considered a reflection of the impact of regional ischemia on global LV performance. Even among patients with three-vessel disease by angiography, the EF response to exercise may be maintained. This finding may be due to the possibility that only small areas of the left ventricle become ischemic if some of the stenoses are not physiologically significant or if distal vessels are well collateralized. Patients with three-vessel disease who have an abnormal exercise EF response are at high risk for adverse events over follow-up and thus are more likely to benefit from revascularization.[10] In contrast, patients who manifest a more normal EF response to exercise have a more favorable natural history and thus are less likely to benefit from revascularization in terms of natural history.

Detection of Preclinical Coronary Artery Disease and Risk Stratification in Asymptomatic Subjects

As sudden cardiac death is too often the first manifestation of CAD, there is interest in screening populations for CAD or for CAD risk. On the basis of Bayesian principles, the low prevalence of CAD in the general asymptomatic population results in low predictive value of a positive test, although negative predictive value is high. Current guidelines do not recommend routine stress MPI in asymptomatic populations.[4]

There may be circumstances, however, in which the baseline risk of a specific asymptomatic population may warrant testing with MPI. In a study of asymptomatic siblings of patients with known CAD, an abnormal SPECT MPI was associated with a fivefold increase in risk for cardiac events, with higher relative risk if both stress MPI and ECG were abnormal.[62] A key question in considering the use of testing such as SPECT MPI in asymptomatic populations is how the information will be used to manage or reduce risk. Current guidelines suggest aggressive risk factor reduction in those at high clinical risk for the development of vascular disease.[63] Whether further intensification of risk factor reduction in the setting of an abnormal imaging test or diminished aggressiveness of risk factor reduction in the setting of a normal MPI study results in improved outcomes is unproved and worthy of study.

Patients with diabetes are at significant risk for CAD development and cardiac events. An emerging body of literature suggests that a substantial proportion of *asymptomatic* diabetic patients have abnormal SPECT MPI studies and that such patients may be at even higher risk for events over time. Studies have suggested that 20 to 40 percent of asymptomatic diabetic patients have abnormal SPECT MPI studies, often with evidence of inducible, silent ischemia.[64-66] SPECT MPI has substantial risk stratification value in patients with diabetes, with risk being higher for any given perfusion abnormality than in nondiabetic patients. Similar risk stratification value has been demonstrated for diabetic patients who are *asymptomatic and without known CAD.*[66] Although guidelines at present do not suggest routine screening of asymptomatic diabetic patients with stress SPECT MPI, ongoing studies of prognosis and randomized trials in asymptomatic diabetic patients should clarify the role of SPECT MPI in diabetes.

Myocardial Perfusion Imaging Following Computed Tomographic Coronary Calcium Imaging or Computed Tomographic Angiography

With the growing availability and use of non-invasive computed tomographic (CT) cardiac imaging (see Chap. 18), clinicians are now commonly faced with a patient with substantial coronary calcium, raising the possibility of multivessel CAD, or with apparent moderate or even severe stenoses seen on CT coronary angiography, raising questions regarding physiological significance and risk stratification.

SPECT MPI AND CORONARY CALCIUM IMAGING. Although extensive coronary artery calcium (CAC) and a high coronary calcium score is indicative of atherosclerosis, studies to date have suggested that even extensive CAC is associated with important myocardial perfusion abnormalities only in a *minority* of patients. In one study of over 1000 patients (approximately 50 percent of whom were asymptomatic), among those with the highest coronary calcium scores (>400), only approximately 10 percent had abnormal perfusion on stress SPECT MPI, and only 5 percent had high-risk SPECT MPI perfusion patterns,[67] suggesting potential benefit from revascularization (Fig. 16-42A). Thus, the presence of even extensive CAC on CT imaging, although well validated for representing *atherosclerosis deserving of aggressive risk-factor modification,* does not always represent *obstructive* stenoses resulting in stress-induced perfusion abnormalities. Based on this concept, stress SPECT MPI is an appropriate test to perform to evaluate the need and potential benefit of catheterization and potential revascularization after CT imaging demonstration of CAC.[68]

REFINING RISK STRATIFICATION BY INCORPORATING BOTH CT CALCIUM IMAGING AND SPECT MPI. Substantial literature now documents that patients with CAC, especially if extensive, are at higher risk of cardiac events over time compared to those with no CAC. Yet among those with extensive calcification, many will have normal stress perfusion on MPI, a finding that extensive published data suggest is associated with low risk. How can these seemingly contradictory bodies of literature be reconciled? It is important to understand that "high risk" is a relative term (i.e., patients with extensive CAC are at higher risk *than those without CAC*) but among those with extensive CAC, most will still not have events. Investigators have suggested that combining data from CT assessment of CAC and information from SPECT MPI may allow a refinement of risk stratification.[69] Conceptually, those patients with no CAC and normal SPECT MPI should have the lowest risk, and those patients with evidence of *both* CAC and an abnormal SPECT MPI should have the highest risk. Patients with

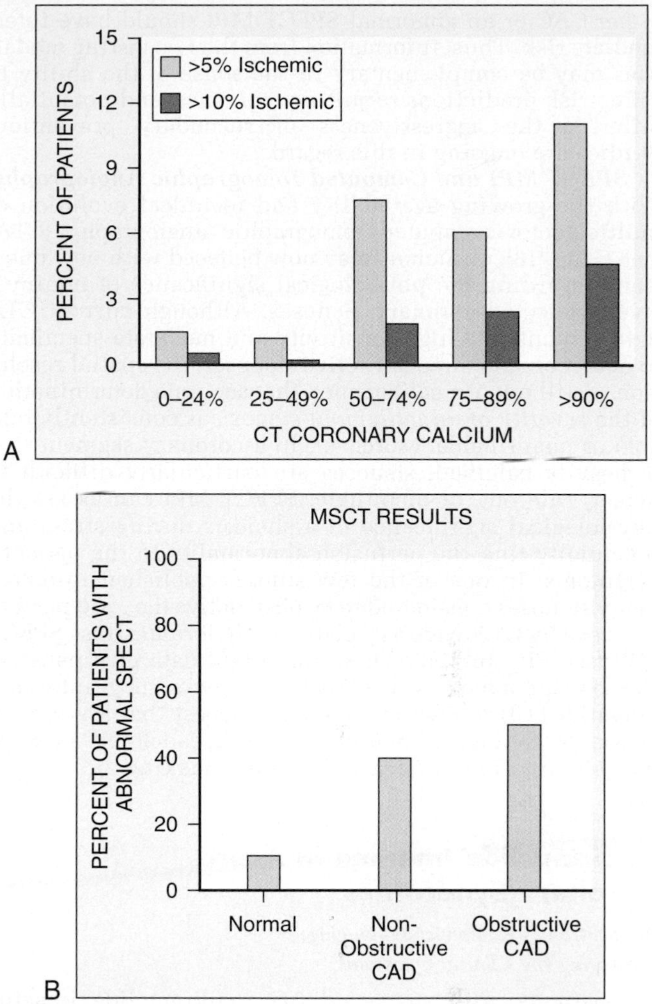

FIGURE 16–42 A, In a study of 1195 patients without known coronary artery disease (CAD) who underwent both single-photon emission computed tomography (SPECT) perfusion imaging and assessment of coronary calcium by computed tomography (CT), the *x*-axis categorizes patients by the age-corrected percentile of coronary calcium. Even when coronary calcium is at a level >90 percent or age is present, only 11 percent of patients had ischemia involving >5 percent of the left ventricle on SPECT, and only ~5 percent of such patients had ischemia >10 percent of the left ventricle. **B,** Prevalence of an abnormal SPECT perfusion study based on results of multislice computed tomographic (MSCT) angiography. Even when "obstructive" CAD (stenosis >50 percent) is present by CT angiography, abnormal perfusion is present in only ~50 percent of patients. *(**A,** Adapted from Berman DS, Wong ND, Gransar H, et al: Relationship between stress-induced myocardial ischemia and atherosclerosis measured by coronary calcium tomography. J Am Coll Cardiol 44[4]:923-930, 2004; **B,** Adapted from Schuijf JD, Wijns W, Jukema JW, et al: Relationship between noninvasive coronary angiography with multi-slice computed tomography and myocardial perfusion imaging. J Am Coll Cardiol 48:2508-2514, 2006.)*

either CAC or an abnormal SPECT MPI should have intermediate risk. Thus, information from the two testing modalities may be complementary in the sense of the ability to refine risk predictions regarding outcomes, and potentially tailoring the aggressiveness of secondary prevention. Studies are ongoing in this regard.

SPECT MPI and Computed Tomographic Angiography. With the growing availability and technical evolution of multidetector computed tomographic angiography (CTA) (see Chap. 18), clinicians may now be faced with new questions regarding the physiological significance of noninvasively detected coronary stenoses. Although current CTA data demonstrate high sensitivity and moderate specificity to detect or rule out obstructive stenoses, the spatial resolution is still not of a caliber such that accurate determination of the *severity of an individual stenosis* is consistently reliable or quantifiable. Moreover, in a coronary segment that is heavily calcified, stenoses are particularly difficult to detect, rule out, or quantitate. SPECT MPI can assess the physiological significance of a stenosis during stress and potentially link the perfusion abnormality to the patient's symptoms. In one of the few studies published to date,[70] many stenoses considered to be obstructive (i.e., >50 percent stenosis) by CTA were associated with *normal* stress SPECT MPI (see Fig. 16-42B). These important data give pause to the concept of moving directly to invasive angiography (and potential PCI) following CTA, and suggest that assessment of the physiological significance of CTA-defined stenoses may be important for clinical decision-making.

Radionuclide Imaging in Acute Coronary Syndromes

Application of Radionuclide Imaging: Answering the Clinical Questions

For patients with *suspected* ACS, radionuclide imaging techniques can play both a diagnostic role (is the clinical syndrome due to ischemia and CAD?) and provide prognostic information. Among patients who present with an ACS and ST segment depression or elevation, the typical role for imaging is in the stabilized patient, to provide risk stratification information to drive management strategies aimed at improving natural history.

SUSPECTED ACUTE CORONARY SYNDROMES IN THE EMERGENCY DEPARTMENT

Many patients presenting to EDs with symptoms suggestive of ACS but with nondiagnostic initial ECG and biomarker findings are admitted to an observation unit for serial biomarker studies and possible stress testing. ^{99m}Tc-based perfusion agents may be administered to a patient in the ED at rest, with images acquired 45 to 60 minutes later,[71] and because there is minimal redistribution, images reflect myocardial blood flow *at the time of injection*.

In this setting, negative predictive value for ruling out MI is high in all observational series.[71] Patients with positive MPI have a higher risk of cardiac events during the index hospitalization as well as during follow-up (Fig. 16-43). Thus, rest SPECT MPI can provide information to assist triage decisions (admit or not admit) in the ED.

One study[71] reported that SPECT sestamibi imaging performed in the ED was 92 percent sensitive for detecting acute MI, whereas *initial* troponin I values in samples drawn at the same time had a sensitivity of only 39 percent. The maximum troponin I over the first 24 hours had a sensitivity similar to that of rest sestamibi imaging but at a distinctly later time point. Thus, acute MPI has the potential to identify ACS *earlier* than biomarkers. SPECT perfusion imaging data have been shown to provide incremental risk stratification value over clinical data for predicting unfavorable cardiac events.[4] One small randomized study[72] of 46 ED patients with ongoing chest pain and a nondiagnostic ECG reported that an MPI-guided strategy incurred lower costs and resulted in shorter lengths of stay.

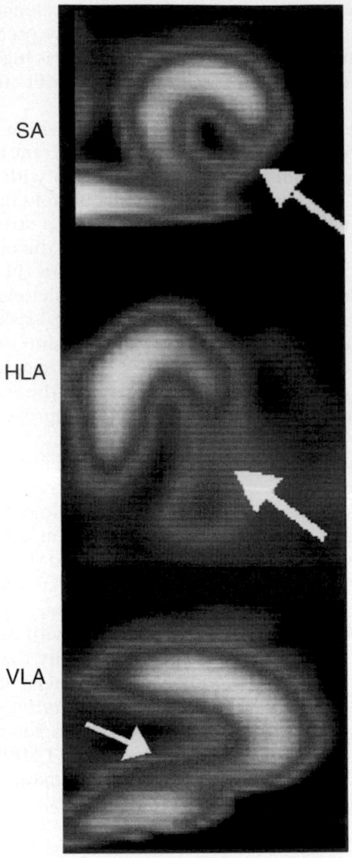

FIGURE 16–43 Example of resting single-photon emission computed tomography (SPECT) images in a patient evaluated in the emergency department with chest pain and nondiagnostic initial electrocardiographic findings. A severe inferolateral resting perfusion defect is seen (arrows), suggestive of resting ischemia or infarction in that territory. Subsequent emergent angiography demonstrated an occluded left circumflex artery.

The Emergency Room Assessment of Sestamibi for Evaluation of (ERASE) Chest Pain Trial[73] of 2475 patients with symptoms suggestive of ACS reported a significant 20 percent relative reduction in unnecessary admissions of patients ultimately found *not to have* ACS for those randomly assigned to incorporate MPI into the ED evaluation strategy. The imaging data were among the most powerful factors associated with the decision to discharge the patient appropriately from the ED.

Thus, evidence from controlled, randomized trials suggests that incorporating SPECT MPI in ED patients with suspected ACS but no definitive ECG changes can improve triage decisions. The ACC/AHA/ASNC Radionuclide Imaging Guidelines classify MPI in this setting as a class I, level A indication.[4]

Non-ST Segment Elevation Myocardial Infarction and Unstable Angina

Guidelines suggest that patients with high-risk clinical characteristics in the setting of unstable angina (UA) should undergo direct catheterization.[42] Contemporary clinical trials suggest that patients with positive biomarkers, or those with a high-risk Thrombolysis in Myocardial Infarction (TIMI) score, benefit in terms of outcomes from an "invasive" strategy.[74] For patients with intermediate or low clinical risk (i.e., with "medically stabilized" UA) stress MPI has been shown to have substantial risk stratification value.[4] Patients without ischemia or infarct, especially in the presence of preserved LV function, have a low-risk outcome, suggesting that such patients can be managed conservatively without catheterization (Fig. 16-44), whereas patients with significant inducible ischemia are at high-risk and are selected for intervention. The ACC/AHA/ASNC Radionuclide Imaging Guidelines[4] classify the use of stress

MPI for detecting residual ischemia and as a class I indication.

Although the results of randomized clinical trials such as Treat Angina with Aggrastat and determine Cost of Therapy with an Invasive or Conservative Strategy (TACTICS)-TIMI 18 and others suggest slight superiority of an invasive approach in patients with UA or non-ST segment elevation MI (NSTEMI), subgroup analyses suggest that an important proportion of patients may be well managed by the conservative strategy of risk stratification by MPI followed by more selective catheterization and intervention. Moreover, a recent large randomized trial of patients with ACS and positive troponin T found no difference in outcomes between an invasive strategy and a selectively invasive strategy in which patients were examined for the presence of ischemia prior to selection for catheterization while on contemporary aggressive medical therapy.[75] In TACTICS-TIMI 18, the troponin-positive subgroup, composing 60 percent of the total population, had a larger reduction in death or MI with the early invasive strategy, whereas there was no difference in outcomes in those patients with negative troponins.[74] Therefore, TACTICS type patients without elevation of troponin or high TIMI risk score[76] may be optimally managed by a more conservative approach with risk stratification by using imaging techniques.

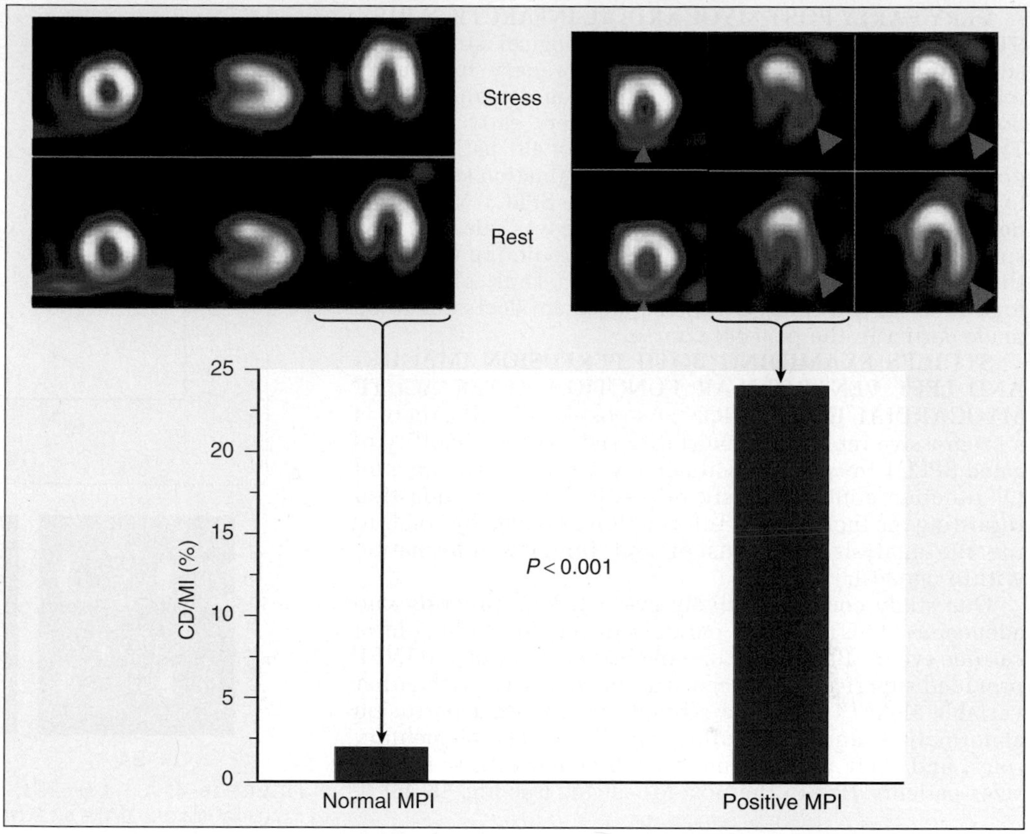

FIGURE 16–44 Single-photon emission computed tomography (SPECT) perfusion imaging in patients after medical stabilization of unstable angina. **Upper left,** Normal study, associated with a low risk of cardiac events during follow-up, suggesting that such a patient can be managed conservatively without catheterization, but with aggressive secondary preventive strategies. The bottom graph is a summary of predictive values of SPECT imaging in the aftermath of unstable angina from multiple studies. Similar to the concepts in populations with stable chest pain, the presence of abnormal perfusion imaging after unstable angina is associated with a substantial increase in the risk of cardiac death or myocardial infarction (CD/MI) during follow-up. **Upper right,** An example of a high-risk stress-rest SPECT myocardial perfusion imaging (MPI) study in the aftermath of unstable angina. Despite the stabilization of symptoms, extensive reversible perfusion abnormalities in the inferior and lateral walls suggest high risk of cardiac death or myocardial infarction, or both, during follow-up. Thus, this patient would be managed more aggressively with catheterization and intervention. *(Adapted in part from Brown KA: Management of unstable angina: The role of noninvasive risk stratification. J Nucl Cardiol 4:S164, 1997.)*

ST Segment Elevation Myocardial Infarction

Clinical variables such as recurrent ischemia, heart failure, and nonacute arrhythmias during hospitalization for acute ST segment elevation MI (STEMI) identify a subgroup of patients at high risk in whom early catheterization and intervention are indicated.[77] However, patients surviving the initial acute period may have a relatively stable course, and current guidelines suggest that noninvasive risk stratification prior to hospital discharge is appropriate.[4,77]

ASSESSMENT OF INDUCIBLE ISCHEMIA AFTER ACUTE MYOCARDIAL INFARCTION. Three major determinants of natural history risk following an acute MI include residual resting LV function; the extent of ischemic, jeopardized myocardium; and the susceptibility to ventricular arrhythmias. Gated SPECT MPI, on the basis of the comprehensive ability to provide much of this information, has the potential to be the single most important test in the stable patient following STEMI.

In one of the earliest studies to examine the relation of MPI data to outcomes in stable patients following MI, thallium-201 scintigraphic data contained the most robust information on stratifying post-MI risk. A "low-risk" thallium-201 image (no reversible defects and no lung uptake) was associated with a low-risk natural history outcome after MI.[44]

An important proportion of patients following uncomplicated MI are not able to exercise, even to a submaximal workload. Using pharmacological stress MPI in the post-MI setting, the presence of reversible defects has been reported as the only significant predictor of cardiac events on multivariable analysis,[44] whereas the absence of reversible defects identified a low-risk cohort.

Studies in the reperfusion era have reported generally similar results regarding the relation of stress-induced ischemia to post-MI outcomes. In a study of 134 consecutive patients within 14 days of an uncomplicated MI, the extent of ischemia on the SPECT MPI was the only significant correlate of a future cardiac event on Cox regression analysis (Fig. 16-45). The extent of SPECT ischemia remained a strong correlate of a cardiac event in those who received thrombolytic therapy. The *quantitated* extent of ischemia on adenosine SPECT MPI has also been shown to be an important predictor of cardiac events in post-MI risk stratification. Post-MI patients with extensive inducible ischemia are at high risk for future cardiac events, and interventional management is likely to result in improved outcome.

VERY EARLY POST-MYOCARDIAL INFARCTION RISK STRATIFICATION. Because pharmacological stress with adenosine or dipyridamole induces coronary hyperemia with only minimal increments in oxygen demand, it may potentially be performed safely even very early after MI. This concept was examined in a study of 451 patients randomly assigned to a standard post-MI evaluation strategy or to a strategy incorporating dipyridamole SPECT MPI 2 to 3 days after uncomplicated MI. The testing was safe, and MPI supplied better risk-stratification data-predicting outcomes than the submaximal stress MPI data.[21] Thus, pharmacological stress can safely allow management decisions to be made earlier in the post-MI course.

STUDIES EXAMINING BOTH PERFUSION IMAGING AND LEFT VENTRICULAR FUNCTION AFTER ACUTE MYOCARDIAL INFARCTION. As post-MI EF falls, there is a progressive increase in mortality risk. The availability of gated SPECT imaging to evaluate myocardial perfusion and LV function simultaneously raises an important question regarding the incremental information provided by combining the analysis of perfusion and function information within one test.

One study comprehensively evaluated LV function and adenosine SPECT MPI in patients in relation to long-term cardiac events. Both the extent of perfusion defect and LVEF provided superior risk categorization compared with either variable alone. These data strongly suggest that perfusion abnormalities and LVEF following MI have complementary roles, and their measurement together powerfully categorizes patients' risk in the post-MI setting (see Fig. 16-45).

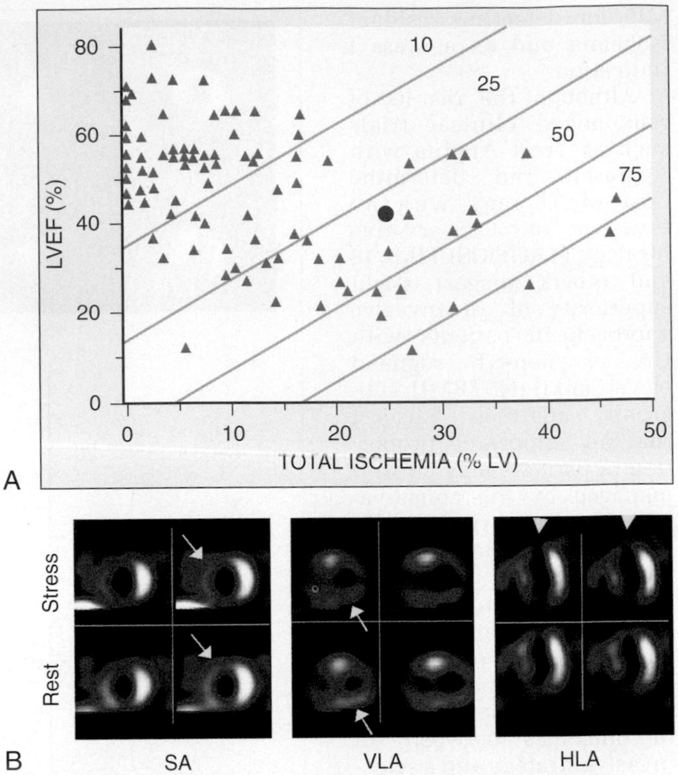

FIGURE 16–45 A, Risk of cardiac event during long-term follow-up after myocardial infarction (MI) is predicted by the combination of infarct size (represented by left ventricular ejection fraction [LVEF]) and the extent of reversible ischemia. As the extent of inducible ischemia increases (*x*-axis), and the LVEF decreases (*y*-axis), the outcome risk increases. The blue lines represent isobars of 10, 25, 50, and 75 percent risk of an adverse event during post-MI follow-up. The large red symbol corresponds to the images in **B,** which is an example of a patient studied several days after acute ST segment elevation MI and medical stabilization. Besides the fixed defect representing the MI in the anterior wall and apex (arrowheads), there is extensive inducible ischemia both within and remote from the infarct territory (septum and inferior walls, arrows), involving 25 percent of the ventricle. Gated single-photon emission computed tomography EF was 38 percent. On the basis of the data in A, there is an approximately 25 percent risk of post-MI adverse event (large red circle in A). HLA = horizontal long axis; SA = short axis; VLA = vertical long axis. *(Adapted from Mahmarian JJ, Mahmarian AC, Marks GF, et al: Role of adenosine thallium-201 tomography for defining long-term risk in patients after acute myocardial infarction. J Am Coll Cardiol 25:1333, 1995.)*

Radionuclide Imaging for Acute Coronary Syndromes: Research Directions

IMAGING ISCHEMIC MEMORY. A possible future approach to risk stratification in patients with *suspected* ACS involves the imaging of fatty acid metabolism. As noted earlier, following a regional ischemic insult, abnormalities in fatty acid metabolism may persist long after perfusion has returned to normal, a finding termed ischemic memory. Imaging fatty acid metabolism may, therefore, allow assessment of *recent* ischemia. Uptake of the radiolabeled fatty acid analog BMIPP has been imaged with SPECT 1 to 5 days after presentation in patients with suspected ACS. The BMIPP images showed greater sensitivity than did rest MPI in identifying the presence and site of the culprit coronary stenosis (Fig. 16-46).[78] Future studies will determine whether such techniques can help guide management decisions.

IMAGING OF POTENTIALLY UNSTABLE ATHEROSCLEROTIC PLAQUES AND PLATELET ACTIVATION. Plaque rupture exposes the lipid core to platelet activation. ^{125}I-labeled low-density lipoprotein has been used to image atherosclerotic disease in carotid arteries. A radionuclide target for macrophages, ^{131}I-labeled monocyte chemoattractant protein-1, has been shown to accumulate in lipid-rich, macrophage-rich regions in animal models of atherosclerosis.[79,80] Whether these favorable results in animals can be translated to the clinical setting of patients with potentially unstable atherosclerosis is a subject of ongoing study.

Assessment of Heart Failure with Radionuclide Imaging

Is Coronary Artery Disease the Etiology of Heart Failure?

Determining whether LV dysfunction is due predominantly to the consequences of CAD or to one of the many other etiologies included in the term "nonischemic" cardiomyopathy is a critical early step in the management of patients with heart failure. Because CAD is the most common cause of heart failure in developed countries,[81] noninvasive assessment of myocardial ischemia and viability would identify the subgroup of patients with heart failure who have a potentially *reversible* degree of LV dysfunction and may benefit from revascularization. Therapeutic interventions that improve dysfunctional but viable myocardium may significantly affect global LVEF, LV remodeling, and survival. The identification of CAD in patients with heart failure also has implications in secondary prevention strategies because recurrent MI is a common mechanism of death in patients with heart failure.

A *normal* stress MPI scan in a patient with heart failure and LV dysfunction is highly predictive for the *absence* of CAD. Studies of MPI for detecting CAD in patients with LV dysfunction have shown high sensitivity but modest specificity (Fig. 16-47; see Fig. 16-40).[53] The modest specificity of MPI to rule out CAD is explained, in part, by pathological as well as cardiac magnetic resonance imaging studies[82] demonstrating that patients with "nonischemic" cardiomyopathy may have patchy or larger confluent territories of fibrosis or scarring (see Chap. 17), manifest as fixed defects on SPECT MPI. Invasive studies, as well as PET imaging, have demonstrated attenuated coronary blood flow at rest and during hyperemic stress in nonischemic cardiomyopathy,[14,83] which could be manifest as reversible defects.

Although the presence of *any* perfusion abnormality is not specific for ruling out CAD, the *pattern* of perfusion abnormality may assist in the differentiation between CAD and "nonischemic" etiology of heart failure. *More exten-*

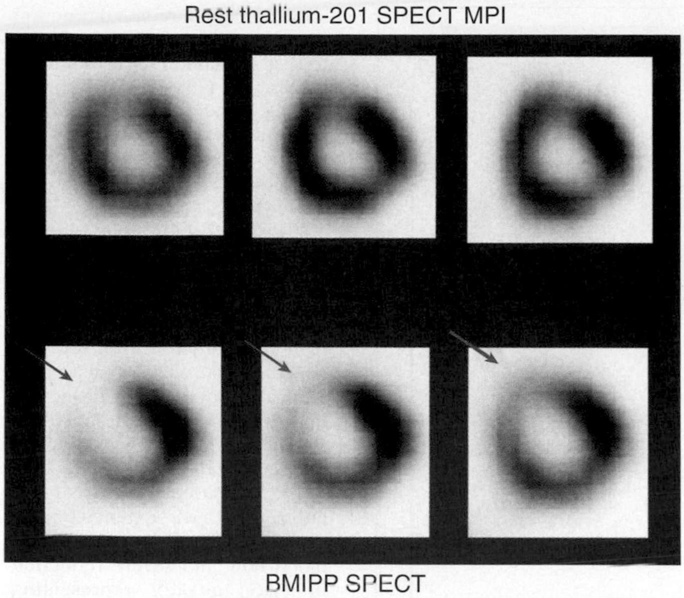

FIGURE 16–46 Iodine-123-beta-methyliodopentadecanoic acid (BMIPP) imaging of ischemic memory. In the **top row,** multiple short-axis tomograms of thallium-201 uptake at rest demonstrate near-homogeneous resting perfusion in a patient who presented to an emergency department and whose symptoms of chest pain had resolved many hours earlier. The BMIPP images in the same short-axis tomographic planes demonstrate a significant anteroseptal defect (arrows), suggesting prolonged postischemic suppression of fatty acid metabolism, referred to as "ischemic memory." MPI = myocardial perfusion imaging; SPECT = single-photon emission computed tomography. *(Adapted from Kawai Y, Tsukamoto E, Nozaki Y, et al: Significance of reduced uptake of iodinated fatty acid analogues for the evaluation of patients with acute chest pain. J Am Coll Cardiol 38: 1888, 2001.)*

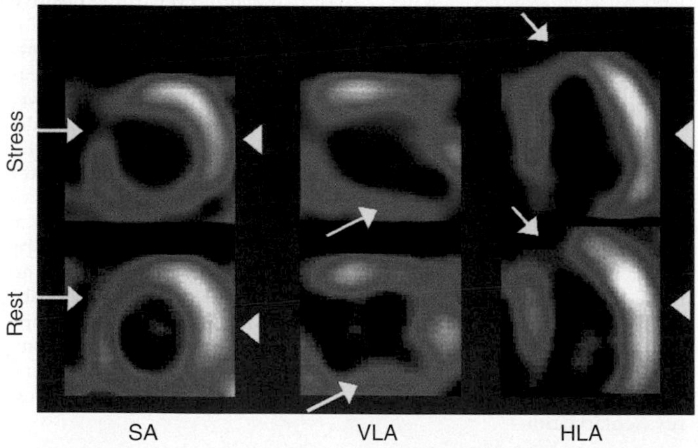

FIGURE 16–47 Single-photon emission computed tomography perfusion imaging demonstrating extensive severe fixed defects of the septum, apex, and inferior wall (arrows) suggestive of extensive prior myocardial infarction, as well as extensive inducible ischemia of the lateral wall (arrowheads). This strongly suggests that coronary artery disease is the etiology of the heart failure syndrome in this patient. HLA = horizontal long axis; SA = short axis; VLA = vertical long axis.

sive or *more severe* perfusion defects, or both, are more likely to represent CAD, whereas smaller and milder defects are more likely in patients with nonischemic cardiomyopathy.[4,53]

Assessment of Myocardial Viability and the Potential Benefit of Revascularization

The goal of assessing viability is to optimize selection of patients with heart failure whose symptoms and natural history may improve following revascularization. Data suggest that hibernation and stress-induced ischemia are common in patients with stable heart failure, even in the

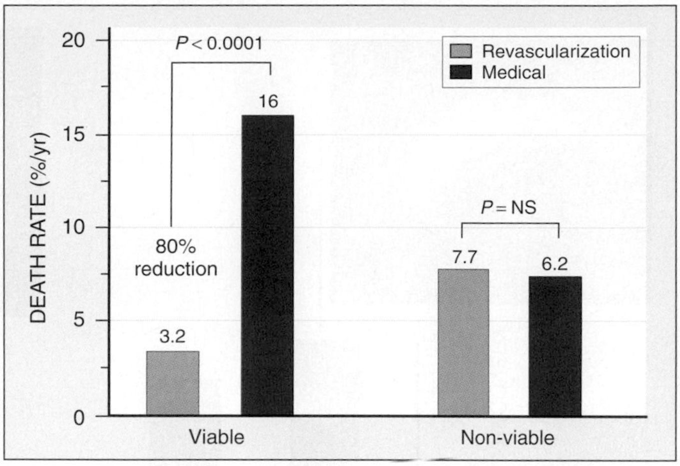

FIGURE 16–48 Outcome of patients with ischemic left ventricular dysfunction after viability testing. Among patients determined to have predominantly viable myocardium, treatment with medical therapy is associated with a 16 percent annual risk of cardiac death. Similar patients treated with revascularization have only a 3.2 percent annual risk of cardiac death, representing an 80 percent reduction in risk with revascularization. In contrast, patients with predominantly nonviable myocardium have no difference in outcome whether they are treated with medical therapy or revascularization. These data suggest that noninvasive interrogation of myocardial viability can identify treatment strategies associated with more favorable long-term outcomes. *(Adapted from Allman K, Shaw L, Hachamovitch R, Udelson JE: Myocardial viability testing and impact of revascularization on prognosis in patients with coronary artery disease and left ventricular dysfunction: A meta-analysis. J Am Coll Cardiol 39:1151, 2002.)*

absence of angina.[84] In a clinical trial of stable community-based patients with heart failure of whom only a minority had angina, hibernation or stress-induced ischemia, or both, were demonstrated by SPECT imaging in approximately 70 percent of patients, suggesting that an important subpopulation of patients with heart failure may benefit from a noninvasive search for viability and ischemia.

Studies have demonstrated that the *potential for improved heart failure symptoms* following revascularization correlates with the magnitude of the PET "mismatch" pattern (i.e., enhanced FDG uptake relative to perfusion).[4] In a meta-analysis of outcome studies after viability imaging, patients with evidence of preserved myocardial viability[85] who underwent revascularization had a substantial reduction in the *risk of cardiac death* during long-term follow-up (Fig. 16-48). Revascularization conferred no natural history advantage in patients without substantial myocardial viability. These data suggest that noninvasive imaging of viability and ischemia can play an important role in selecting patients for revascularization, with the expectation of improving symptoms and natural history.

PRINCIPLES OF ASSESSING MYOCARDIAL VIABILITY BY RADIONUCLIDE TECHNIQUES

The radionuclide tracers and techniques most often used to assess viability have been evaluated for their relation to preserved tissue viability directly by correlating tracer uptake with histologically confirmed extent of tissue viability. Quantitative analysis of tracer uptake correlates directly with the magnitude of preservation of tissue viability, and tracer uptake represents a *continuous variable*—the magnitude of tracer uptake directly reflects the magnitude of preserved tissue viability.[86] For a dysfunctional segment or territory, the probability of functional recovery after revascularization is related to the magnitude of tracer uptake, representing the degree of preserved myocardial viability (extent of hibernation or stunning) within that territory. A dysfunctional territory with normal or only mildly reduced tracer uptake has a high likelihood of improved function after revascularization. In contrast, a territory with a severe reduction in tracer uptake would represent predominant infarction, and the likelihood of improved function after revascularization would be low (Fig. 16-49). The magnitude of potential improvement of *global LV function* after

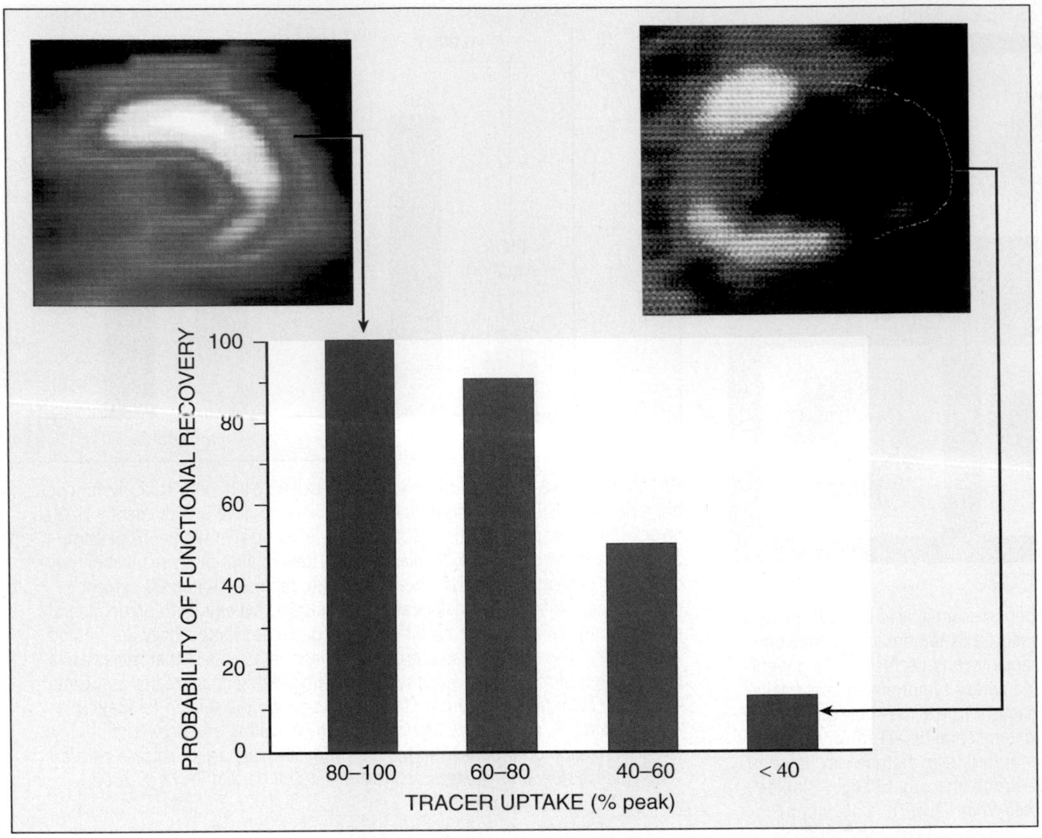

FIGURE 16–49 Relation between tracer uptake in a dysfunctional territory and the subsequent probability of functional recovery after revascularization. The probability of improved regional left ventricular function after revascularization is significantly related to the quantitative degree of tracer uptake. **Upper right,** A patient with a large, severe defect in the anterior and apical walls. The severity of the defect suggests that significant functional recovery would not be expected with revascularization. **Upper left,** Extensive myocardial viability in a patient with left ventricular dysfunction (ejection fraction 30 percent) and severe three-vessel coronary disease. There is substantial tracer uptake throughout the anterior wall and apex (arrow), territories with significant regional dysfunction. The retained degree of tracer uptake suggests extensive myocardial (myocyte) viability and high probability of functional recovery after revascularization. *(Adapted from Bonow RO: Assessment of myocardial viability with thallium-201.* In *Zaret BL, Beller GA [eds]: Nuclear Cardiology: State of the Art and Future Directions. St. Louis, Mosby, 1999, pp 503-512; and Udelson JE: Assessment of myocardial viability with technetium-99m-labeled agents.* In *Zaret BL, Beller GA [eds]: Nuclear Cardiology: State of the Art and Future Directions. St. Louis, Mosby, 1999, pp 513-533.)*

revascularization is, in turn, determined by the extent of viable dysfunctional myocardium.

Imaging Protocols for Assessing Myocardial Viability

THALLIUM-201. The presence of thallium-201 after redistribution implies preserved myocyte cellular viability. However, because the *absence* of thallium-201 uptake on the redistribution images is not a sufficient sign of the *absence* of regional viability, iterations of the standard thallium-201 protocol have been investigated[6] to optimize the assessment of regional viability (Fig. 16-50). After thallium-201 *reinjection,* approximately 50 percent of regions with "fixed" defects on stress-redistribution imaging show significant enhancement of thallium-201 uptake, predictive of improvement in regional LV function. The presence of a severe thallium-201 defect after reinjection identifies areas with a very low probability of improvement in function.

Late redistribution imaging, 24 to 48 hours after the initial stress thallium-201 injection, allows more time for redistribution to occur and has good positive predictive value for improvement in function. The negative predictive value is suboptimal because redistribution does not take place in some patients even after a prolonged time, and image quality may be suboptimal.[3,4]

With *rest-redistribution thallium-201 imaging,* images are obtained 15 to 20 minutes after tracer injection at rest, reflecting resting regional blood flow, and images obtained 3 to 4 hours following redistribution reflect preserved viability. The finding of a *reversible resting defect* may identify areas of myocardial hibernation (see Fig. 16-50). This finding appears to be an insensitive, although specific, sign of potential improvement in regional function.[4]

TECHNETIUM 99M SESTAMIBI AND TETROFOSMIN. Studies have demonstrated that the performance of these agents for predicting improvement in regional function after revascularization is similar to that of thallium-201.[4] Administration of nitrates to improve resting blood flow prior to injection of sestamibi appears to improve slightly the ability of these tracers to detect myocardial viability.[3,4]

POSITRON-EMISSION TOMOGRAPHY. The extent of the PET mismatch pattern (enhanced FDG uptake relative to blood flow) correlates with improvement in LV function after revascularization as well as with the clinical course, magnitude of improvement in heart failure symptoms, and survival after revascularization (see Fig. 16-29).[4,11,12] Patients with heart failure and an extensive PET match pattern (diminished blood flow and severe reduction in FDG uptake), representing predominant infarction, are unlikely to benefit clinically from revascularization.

COMPARISON OF IMAGING TECHNIQUES FOR VIABILITY ASSESSMENT. On the basis of a meta-analysis evaluating the ability of the various radionuclide techniques to predict improvements in regional function, all the radionuclide techniques (as well as low-dose dobutamine echocardiography) perform in a relatively similar manner regarding positive and negative predictive values for improvements in regional function.[87] SPECT techniques appear to be slightly more sensitive, dobutamine echocardiography slightly more specific, and PET techniques appear to have better accuracy. A randomized trial of patients with moderate LV dysfunction being considered for revascularization randomly allocated to have viability information supplied by either PET imaging or SPECT stress-rest sestamibi imaging found no difference in outcomes over long-term follow-up.[88] As noted previously, a meta-analysis of observational outcome studies related to myocardial viability demonstrated no difference between the techniques commonly used to assess viability (PET versus SPECT versus dobutamine echocardiography) with regard to reduction of mortality after revascularization.[85]

Selection of Patients with Heart Failure for Viability Assessment

Guidelines suggest that patients with heart failure *and* active angina benefit in terms of natural history from revascularization and should be referred directly for angiography.[89] In some situations, subsequent noninvasive definition of regional viability and ischemia may be important for planning the revascularization strategy when the anatomy is known.

For patients with heart failure and *no angina,* recommendations are less clear. Studies suggest that ischemia and viability may be present in a significant proportion of such patients, who have potential benefit from revascularization,[84] and for most patients with heart failure, a search for underlying ischemia and viability would be an appropriate clinical strategy at some point in their evaluation. If substantial ischemia or viability of dysfunctional territories is found in the setting of vessels technically amenable to revascularization, the literature would suggest a *clinical benefit* from revascularization.[4] In the *absence* of substantial ischemia or viability, such a benefit is less likely. The imaging data can be used in decision-making to help balance the *risks and benefits* of revascularization in a patient with heart failure and LV dysfunction, by supplying information on potential *benefit* of a revascularization strategy.

Assessment of Left Ventricular Function in Heart Failure

For patients with the clinical syndrome of heart failure, the distinction between those patients with preserved and those with impaired systolic function has important clinical relevance. Clinical trials evaluating the use of such therapies as ACE inhibitors, angiotensin receptor blockers, and beta blockers have focused on the subpopulation of heart failure patients with impaired systolic function.[89] Thus, accurate determination of LV function in a patient with heart failure defines the evidence-based therapeutic approach that should be undertaken.

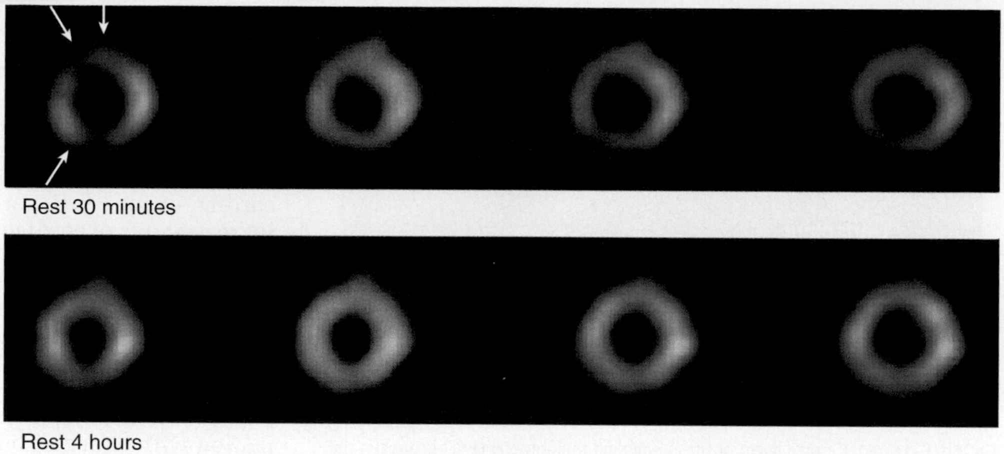

FIGURE 16–50 Myocardial viability imaging with single-photon emission computed tomography. Rest-redistribution thallium imaging, demonstrating redistribution in regions with initial reductions in thallium uptake, particularly the anterior wall, septum, and inferior walls (arrows), indicating resting hypoperfusion.

On the basis of the quantitative and reproducible nature of the EF results, equilibrium RVG techniques have been used in large clinical trials to identify systolic dysfunction.[4,89] In contemporary practice, the ECG-gated SPECT technique is often used for determination of systolic function. The *simultaneous* assessment of LV systolic function as well as stress and rest perfusion by gated SPECT imaging can provide a range of information relevant to the care and clinical decision-making for patients with heart failure, including the state of LV function, the probability of CAD as the etiology of heart failure, and the presence and extent of viability and ischemia.

Imaging in Inflammatory and Infiltrative Cardiomyopathies

MYOCARDITIS. Inflammatory injury to the myocardium by infective agents, postinfective immune processes (i.e., Chagas disease, rheumatic carditis), hypersensitivity, and autoimmune conditions can cause myocardial dysfunction (see Chap. 66). The clinical manifestation of such an inflammatory process is acute myocarditis and cardiac allograft rejection. As myocyte necrosis is an obligatory component of myocarditis (cellular infiltrates, predominantly lymphocytes and macrophages, clustered around necrotic myocytes), ^{111}In-labeled antimyosin antibody, which specifically targets myosin heavy chain, has been used for the detection of necrosis associated with myocarditis and heart transplant rejection. In patients with biopsy-positive myocarditis, the sensitivity of an antimyosin scan is approximately 95 percent, with a negative predictive value of approximately 95 percent. However, the specificity and positive predictive value of antimyosin imaging are modest—in the 50 percent range.[90] In cardiac allograft recipients, there is a general relation between the severity of transplant rejection by biopsy and the magnitude of antimyosin uptake by scintigraphy. However, the highly variable antimyosin uptake across the severity range of rejection precludes antimyosin imaging as a sufficiently reliable noninvasive test for detection of transplant rejection.[91] Observational studies with myocardial perfusion, gated blood pool, and ^{123}I metaiodobenzylguanidine (MIBG) imaging have reported regional perfusion defects, wall motion abnormalities, and sympathetic denervation in patients who present with myocarditis, in the absence of significant CAD.[4]

SARCOID HEART DISEASE. Cardiac involvement occurs in about 20 percent of patients with sarcoidosis (see Chap. 64). In patients presenting with advanced AV block, myocardial perfusion SPECT or gallium-67 imaging (a nonspecific indicator of inflammation) along with magnetic resonance imaging or chest computed tomography can localize myocardial involvement of sarcoidosis.[4] Focal fibromuscular dysplasia found in the small coronary arteries may provide an explanation for focal ischemic injuries and reversible defects described on myocardial perfusion SPECT. Perfusion defects involving the left ventricle have been associated with AV block and heart failure, and defects involving the right ventricle on SPECT have been associated with ventricular tachycardia of right ventricular origin.[92]

CARDIAC AMYLOIDOSIS. Cardiac involvement of amyloidosis involves the deposition of light chain amino acids into the myofibrils, which leads to impaired relaxation (see Chap. 64). Patients with amyloidosis may demonstrate abnormally prolonged LV diastolic filling and an increased atrial contribution to the total diastolic filling. ^{99m}Tc pyrophosphate scintigraphy may be useful in identifying patients with cardiac amyloidosis—demonstrating diffuse uptake throughout the myocardium.[4] ^{123}I MIBG imaging has shown marked cardiac sympathetic denervation, providing insight into the pathogenesis of cardiac conduction disturbances in amyloidosis.[93]

Radionuclide Imaging in Heart Failure and Left Ventricular Dysfunction: Research Directions

ASSESSMENT OF CARDIAC SYMPATHETIC INNERVATION. An emerging area of risk stratification involves the use of ^{123}I MIBG imaging of cardiac sympathetic innervation. In the post-MI setting, the territory of abnormal MIBG uptake (corresponding to sympathetic *denervation*) often exceeds the final infarct size, and such patients are at higher risk for subsequent ventricular arrhythmias.[53,94,95] Should this finding prove prognostic for outcomes in patients with LV dysfunction, as suggested by earlier studies, MIBG imaging may have a role in selecting post-MI patients who may optimally benefit from defibrillators.[95]

IMAGING OF APOPTOSIS. Another potential approach to evaluating patients with LV dysfunction after MI is the visualization of apoptosis, or programmed cell death, in humans using ^{99m}Tc-labeled annexin V, which localizes to apoptotic cells.[96] In one study, positive uptake of this agent was seen in six of seven post-MI patients, localized to areas of resting perfusion defects.[97] This agent may herald the onset of the ability to track this process noninvasively in syndromes such as heart failure and to study approaches to attenuate the unfavorable pathophysiology of apoptosis.

RADIONUCLIDE IMAGING OF CELL- OR GENE-BASED REGENERATIVE THERAPY. Local targeted gene delivery or implantation of autologous skeletal myoblasts, bone marrow stromal cells, or hematopoietic stem cells may functionally revitalize scarred, noncontractile myocardial regions. Noninvasive assessment of the fate of myogenic cell grafts and therapeutic genes in vivo may provide insight into the mechanism by which they improve cardiac function or prevent remod-

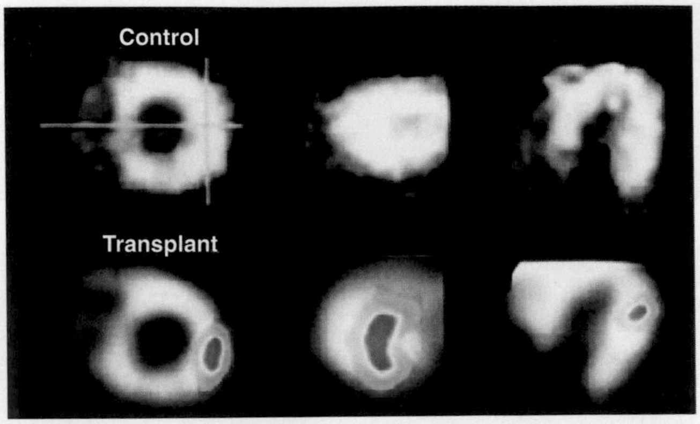

FIGURE 16–51 Cardiac micro positron emission tomography (PET) images in the short-axis (SA), vertical long-axis (VLA), and horizontal long-axis (HLA) views of a rat heart transplanted with cardiomyoblasts expressing a PET reporter gene. The gray/white uptake represents homogeneous perfusion by $^{13}N\text{-}NH_3$, and the color uptake in the lateral wall represents the viable transplanted cardiomyoblasts studied in vivo **(bottom row).** There is no uptake in the control heart, with normal perfusion **(top row).** *(Adapted from Wu JC, Chen IY, Sundaresan G, et al: Molecular imaging of cardiac cell transplantation in living animals using optical bioluminescence and positron emission tomography. Circulation 108:1302, 2003.)*

eling. In animal studies, transplanted cardiomyoblasts expressing a PET reporter gene have been imaged longitudinally to gain insight into the pattern of cell survival.[98] Using cardiac micro-PET imaging, detailed tomographic locations of transplanted cells were obtained (Fig. 16-51). This may become an important method to study regenerative therapies in human studies.

IMAGING THE TISSUE ANGIOTENSIN-CONVERTING ENZYME RECEPTOR SYSTEM. Radionuclide imaging has been used in experimental systems to study the tissue ACE receptor system directly. Using the radiotracer [^{18}F]fluorobenzyl-lisinopril,[99] observations have shown a relation between ACE and collagen replacement, as ACE was absent in the collagen-stained areas and was increased in the juxtaposed areas of replacement fibrosis.[100] These data suggest that increased ACE may be a stimulus for collagen replacement and remodeling. In the future, noninvasive imaging with PET in patients with heart failure may allow monitoring of changes in ACE patterns in vivo, possibly reflecting progression of disease and the effect of therapies before collagen replacement ensues.

Imaging to Assess Cardiac Risk Prior to Noncardiac Surgery

The clinical role of MPI for evaluating patients prior to elective noncardiac surgery has grown, as CAD represents an important perioperative and long-term risk in such patients (see Chap. 80). The ischemic burden from the stress of surgery and postoperative recovery can result in MI or cardiovascular death. Prospective identification of such patients has important prognostic and preventive implications.

Initial cardiac assessment of patients undergoing noncardiac surgery should be based on (1) the prevalence of CAD in a given surgical population; (2) the type of the surgical procedure and the institutional event rate; (3) cardiac history and risk factors; and (4) functional capacity.[101] Surgical procedures can be classified as high-risk procedures (cardiac risk greater than 5 percent), such as major vascular surgery. If the institutional event rate for an elective operation is less than 2 to 3 percent, most screening studies are inefficient with regard to lowering the cardiac event rate in the perioperative period.

Clinical parameters of increased risk include advanced age (older than 70 years), diabetes, history of angina or recent ACS, heart failure, and ventricular arrhythmias. Patients with known prior CAD may be considered to have a low perioperative cardiac risk on the basis of their functional capacity and symptoms. Asymptomatic patients with known CAD who have had revascularization within the past 5 years generally require no further evaluation.[101] Patients with intermediate risk on the basis of clinical predictors, functional capacity, and type of surgery are op-timal candidates for further stratification by imaging procedures.

Studies of MPI using pharmacological stress have uniformly shown that a normal MPI study predicts a low likelihood (~1 percent) for perioperative or longer term postoperative cardiac events.[101] Reversible perfusion defects predict an increased risk of cardiac events, and the magnitude of risk is related to the extent of ischemia. Although fixed perfusion defects (infarct) portend a lower risk for perioperative cardiac events than ischemia, the risk is higher than that with a normal scan, and patients with infarct or LV dysfunction are at higher *long-term* risk for death or heart failure.[101]

In clinical practice, most patients in whom extensive ischemia is demonstrated preoperatively undergo catheterization with expectation of revascularization. Clinical trial evidence supporting this point provides conflicting evidence,[102-105] and the threshold of ischemia extent above which revascularization might *reduce* short- or long-term cardiac risk is not known.

Future Perspectives

Over the next few years, the advances in the field of nuclear cardiology are likely to involve further refinement of quantitative methods to model and deliver imaging information and results, further development of metabolic imaging and greater accessibility of positron emission tomography for perfusion imaging, and continuing advances in the area of molecular imaging.

Data bases linking imaging results and outcomes are now published that are on the scale of major epidemiological studies, some involving more than 10,000 patients. This has allowed sophisticated modeling of the relation between the imaging results and outcomes, and has permitted the prediction of not only outcomes, but outcomes based on a management strategy, as depicted in Figure 16-36. In the future, incorporation of information on the *risks* of revascularization (including factors such as age, renal function, and so on) could potentially provide clinicians with a robust support tool for clinical decision-making in complex patients. It is likely that greater accessibility of PET instrumentation will fuel growth in PET perfusion imaging, with potential improved diagnostic ability in previously challenging patients. With greater use of CT angiography, the need to carefully assess the physiological significance of imaged anatomical stenoses will also likely grow.

Molecular imaging exploits the targeting of expressed cell surface molecules, intracellular processes, and gene expression. The growth of molecular imaging has been further heightened by the availability of transgenic disease models and multiple technological advances including microSPECT, microPET, and hybrid devices with CT. Radionuclide tracers by their nature reflect physiological processes at the cellular level. Targeting intracellular metabolic processes for imaging, for example, should expand our ability to diagnose and treat subclinical or progressive cardiovascular disorders that often remain elusive with traditional imaging techniques. Hence, nuclear cardiology is uniquely primed to provide insight into the molecular basis of cardiovascular disease and foster the development and growth of novel therapeutic interventions in the future.

REFERENCES

Technical Aspects of Image Acquisition, Display, and Interpretation

1. Garcia EV, Galt JR, Faber TL, Chen J: Principles of nuclear cardiology imaging. *In* Dilsizian V, Narula J, Braunwald E: Atlas of Nuclear Cardiology, 2nd ed. Current Medicine. Philadelphia, 2006

2. DePuey EG, Corbett JR, Friedman JD, et al: American Society of Nuclear Cardiology. Imaging guidelines for nuclear cardiology procedures. J Nucl Cardiol 13:888, 2006.
3. Dilsizian V: SPECT and PET Imaging: Tracers and Techniques. *In* Dilsizian V, Narula J, Braunwald E: Atlas of Nuclear Cardiology, 2nd ed. Current Medicine. Philadelphia, 2006
4. Klocke FJ, Baird MG, Bateman TM, et al: ACC/AHA/ASNC guidelines for the clinical use of cardiac radionuclide imaging: A report of the American College of Cardiology/American Heart Association Task Force on Practice Guidelines (ACC/AHA/ASNC Committee to Revise the 1995 Guidelines for the Clinical Use of Radionuclide Imaging). 2003. American College of Cardiology Web Site. Available at: http://www.acc.org/clinical/guidelines/radio/rni_fulltext.pdf.
5. Berman DS, Hachamovitch R, Germano G: Risk stratification and patient management. *In* Dilsizian V, Narula J, Braunwald E: Atlas of Nuclear Cardiology, 2nd ed. Current Medicine. Philadelphia, 2006.
6. Cerqueira MD, Weissman NJ, Dilsizian V, et al: Standardized myocardial segmentation and nomenclature for tomographic imaging of the heart: A statement for healthcare professionals from the cardiac imaging committee of the council on clinical cardiology of the American Heart Association. Circulation 105:539, 2002.
7. McLaughlin MG, Danias PG: Transient ischemic dilation: A powerful diagnostic and prognostic finding of stress myocardial perfusion imaging. J Nucl Cardiol 9:663, 2002.
8. Hendel RC, Corbett JR, Cullom SJ, et al: The value and practice of attenuation correction for myocardial perfusion SPECT imaging: A joint position statement from the American Society of Nuclear Cardiology and the Society of Nuclear Medicine. J Nucl Cardiol 9:135, 2002.
9. Germano G, Berman DS: Acquisition and processing for gated SPECT: Technical aspects. *In* Germano G, Berman DS (eds): Clinical Gated Cardiac SPECT. Armonk, NY, Blackwell-Futura Publishing, 2006.
10. Germano G, Borer JS, Berman DS: Myocardial function assessment by nuclear techniques. *In* Dilsizian V, Narula J, Braunwald E: Atlas of Nuclear Cardiology, 2nd ed. Current Medicine. Philadelphia, 2006.
11. Dilsizian V: SPECT and PET techniques. *In* Dilsizian V, Narula J, Braunwald E (eds): Atlas of Nuclear Cardiology. Philadelphia, Current Medicine, 2003, pp 131-146.
12. Bacharach SL, Bax JJ, Case J, et al: PET myocardial glucose metabolism and perfusion imaging: Part I—Guidelines for patient preparation and data acquisition. J Nucl Cardiol 10:543, 2003.
13. Yoshinaga K, Chow BJ, William K, et al What is the prognostic value of myocardial perfusion imaging using rubidium-82 positron emission tomography? J Am Coll Cardiol 48:1029, 2006.
14. Neglia D, Michelassi C, Trivieri MG, et al: Prognostic role of myocardial blood flow impairment in idiopathic left ventricular dysfunction. Circulation 105:186-193, 2002.
15. Cecchi F, Olivotto I, Gistri R, et al: Coronary microvascular dysfunction and prognosis in hypertrophic cardiomyopathy, N Engl J Med 349:1027, 2003.

Assessment of the Physiology and Pathophysiology of Myocardial Blood Flow, Myocardial Metabolism, and Ventricular Function

16. Gibbons RJ, Miller TD, Christian TF: Infarct size measured by single photon emission computed tomographic imaging with ^{99m}Tc-sestamibi: A measure of the efficacy of therapy in acute myocardial infarction. Circulation 101:101, 2000.
17. Kern MJ, Meier B: Evaluation of the culprit plaque and the physiological significance of coronary atherosclerotic narrowings. Circulation 103:3142, 2001.
18. Gould KL, Nakagawa Y, Nakagawa K, et al: Frequency and clinical implications of fluid dynamically significant diffuse coronary artery disease manifest as graded, longitudinal, base-to-apex myocardial perfusion abnormalities by noninvasive positron emission tomography. Circulation 101:1931, 2000.
19. He Z, Mahmarian JJ, Verani MS: Myocardial perfusion in patients with total occlusion of a single coronary artery with and without collateral circulation. J Nucl Cardiol 8:452, 2001.
20. Mark DB, Lauer MS: Exercise capacity: The prognostic variable that doesn't get enough respect. Circulation 108:1534, 2003.
21. Miller DD: Pharmacologic stressors in coronary artery disease. *In* Dilsizian V, Narula J, Braunwald E (eds): Atlas of Nuclear Cardiology. Philadelphia, Current Medicine, 2003, pp 47-62.
22. Udelson JE, Heller GV, Wackers FJ, et al: A randomized, controlled dose-ranging study of the selective adenosine A_{2A} receptor agonist binodenoson for pharmacologic stress as an adjunct to myocardial perfusion imaging. Circulation 109:457, 2004.
23. Thomas GS, Prill NV, Majmundar H, et al: Treadmill exercise during adenosine infusion is safe, results in fewer adverse reactions, and improves myocardial perfusion imaging quality. J Nucl Cardiol 7:439, 2000.
24. Mahmarian JJ, Dakik HA, Filipchuk NG, et al. An Initial Strategy of Intensive Medical Therapy Is Comparable to That of Coronary Revascularization for Suppression of Scintigraphic Ischemia in High-Risk But Stable Survivors of Acute Myocardial Infarction. J Am Coll Cardiol 48:2458, 2006.
25. Taillefer R, Ahlberg AW, Masood Y, et al: Acute beta-blockade reduces the extent and severity of myocardial perfusion defects with dipyridamole Tc-99m sestamibi SPECT imaging. J Am Coll Cardiol 42:1475, 2003.
26. Taegtmeyer H: Modulation of responses to myocardial ischemia: Metabolic features of myocardial stunning, hibernation, and ischemic preconditioning. *In* Dilsizian V (ed): Myocardial Viability: A Clinical and Scientific Treatise. Armonk, NY, Futura Publishing, 2000, pp 25-36.
27. Selvanayagam JB, Jerosch-Herold M, Porto I, et al. Resting myocardial blood flow is impaired in hibernating myocardium: A magnetic resonance study of quantitative perfusion assessment. Circulation 112:3289, 2005.
28. Feinendegen LE: Myocardial imaging of lipid metabolism with labeled fatty acids. *In* Dilsizian V (ed): Myocardial Viability: A Clinical and Scientific Treatise. Armonk, NY, Futura Publishing Company, 2000, pp 349-389.
29. Dilsizian V, Bateman TB, Bergmann SR, et al. Metabolic imaging with ß-Methyl-*p*-[^{123}I]-iodophenyl-pentadecanoic acid identifies ischemic memory after demand ischemia. Circulation 112:2169, 2005.
30. Dilsizian V, Bacharach SL, Maung KM, Smith MF: Fluorine-18-deoxyglucose SPECT and coincidence imaging for myocardial viability: Clinical and technological issues. J Nucl Cardiol 8:75, 2001.
31. Jafary F, Udelson JE: Assessment of myocardial perfusion and left ventricular function in acute coronary syndromes: Implications for gated SPECT imaging. *In* Germano G, Berman DS (eds): Clinical Gated Cardiac SPECT. Armonk, NY, Blackwell-Futura Publishing, 2006.
32. Anand IS, Florea VG, Solomon SD, et al: Noninvasive assessment of left ventricular remodeling: Concepts, techniques, and implications for clinical trials. J Card Fail 8:S452, 2002.
33. Germano G, Berman DS: Quantitative gated perfusion SPECT. *In* Germano G, Berman DS (eds): Clinical Gated Cardiac SPECT. Armonk, NY, Blackwell-Futura Publishing, 2006.
34. Metra M, Giubbini R, Nodari S, et al: Differential effects of ß-blockers in patients with heart failure: A prospective, randomized, double-blind comparison of the long-term effects of metoprolol versus carvedilol. Circulation 102:546, 2000.
35. Borer JS, Bonow RO; Contemporary approach to aortic and mitral regurgitation. Circulation 108:2432, 2003.
36. Bonow RO, Carabello B, Chatterjee K, et al: ACC/AHA 2006 guidelines for the management of patients with valvular heart disease: A report of the American College of Cardiology/American Heart Association Task Force on Practice Guidelines (Committee on Management of Patients with Valvular Heart Disease). J Am Coll Cardiol 48:589, 2006.
37. Imitani I, Jain D, Joska TM, et al: Doxorubicin cardiotoxicity: Prevention of congestive heart failure with serial cardiac function monitoring with equilibrium radionuclide angiocardiography in the current era. J Nucl Cardiol 10:132, 2003.
38. Maron BJ: Hypertrophic cardiomyopathy: A systematic review. JAMA 287:1308, 2002.

Stable Chest Pain Syndromes

39. Libby P, Ridker PM, Maseri A: Inflammation and atherosclerosis Circulation 105:1135, 2002.
40. Expert Panel on Detection, Evaluation, and Treatment of High Blood Cholesterol in Adults: Executive Summary of the Third Report of the National Cholesterol Education Program (NCEP) Expert Panel on Detection, Evaluation and Treatment of High Blood Cholesterol in Adults (Adult Treatment Panel III). JAMA 285:2486, 2001.
41. Fletcher GF, Balady GJ, Vogel RA: Preventive cardiology: How can we do better? 33rd Bethesda Conference. J Am Coll Cardiol 40:579, 2002.
42. Braunwald E, Antman EM, Beasley JW, et al: ACC/AHA 2002 guideline update for the management of patients with unstable angina and non-ST-segment elevation myocardial infarction: A report of the American College of Cardiology/American Heart Association Task Force on Practice Guidelines (Committee on the Management of Patients with Unstable Angina). 2002. Available at: http://www.acc.org/clinical/guidelines/unstable/incorporated/index.htm.
43. Gibbons RJ, Abrams J, Chatterjee K, et al: ACC/AHA 2002 guideline update for the management of patients with chronic stable angina-Summary article: A report of the American College of Cardiology/American Heart Association Task Force on Practice Guidelines (Committee on the Management of Patients with Chronic Stable Angina). Circulation 107:149, 2003.
44. Beller GA: First Annual Mario S. Verani, MD, Memorial Lecture: Clinical value of myocardial perfusion imaging in coronary artery disease. J Nucl Cardiol 10:529, 2003.
45. Hachamovitch R, Hayes SW, Friedman JD, et al: Comparison of the short-term survival benefit associated with revascularization compared with medical therapy in patients with no prior coronary artery disease undergoing stress myocardial perfusion single photon emission computed tomography. Circulation 107:2900, 2003.
46. Shaw LJ, Hendel R, Borges-Neto S, et al, for the Myoview Multicenter Registry: Prognostic value of normal exercise and adenosine 99mTc-tetrofosmin SPECT imaging: Results from the multicenter registry of 4728 patients. J Nucl Med 44:134, 2003.
47. Hachamovitch R, Hayes S, Friedman JD, et al: Determinants of risk and its temporal variation in patients with normal stress myocardial perfusion scans. What is the warranty period of a normal scan? J Am Coll Cardiol 41:1329, 2003.
48. Giri S, Shaw LJ, Murthy DR, et al: Impact of diabetes on the risk stratification using stress single-photon emission computed tomography myocardial perfusion imaging in patients with symptoms suggestive of coronary artery disease. Circulation 105:32, 2002.
49. Boden WE, O'Rourke RA, Teo KK, et al. Optimal medical therapy with or without PCI for stable coronary disease. N Engl J Med 356:1503, 2007.
50. Schwartz RG, Pearson TA, Kalaria VG, et al: Prospective serial evaluation of myocardial perfusion and lipids during the first six months of pravastatin therapy: Coronary artery disease regression single photon emission computed tomography monitoring trial. J Am Coll Cardiol 42:600, 2003.
51. Beller GA, Zaret BL: Contributions of nuclear cardiology to diagnosis and prognosis of patients with coronary artery disease. Circulation 101:1465, 2000.
52. Amanullah AM, Berman DS, Kang X, et al: Enhanced prognostic stratification of patients with left ventricular hypertrophy with the use of single-photon emission computed tomography. Am Heart J 140:3456, 2000.
53. Udelson JE, Shafer CD, Carrio I: Radionuclide imaging in heart failure: Assessing etiology and outcomes and implications for management. J Nucl Cardiol 9:S40, 2002.

54. Masoli O, Perez Baliño N, Sabaté D, et al: Effect of endothelial dysfunction on regional perfusion in myocardial territories supplied by normal and diseased vessels in patients with coronary artery disease. J Nucl Cardiol 7:199, 2000.
55. Panting JR, Gatehouse PD, Yang GZ, et al: Abnormal subendocardial perfusion in cardiac syndrome X detected by cardiovascular magnetic resonance imaging. N Engl J Med 346:1948, 2002.
56. Germano G, Berman DS: Quantitative gated SPECT. J Nucl Med 42:528, 2001.
57. Gibbons RJ, Balady GJ, Timothy B, et al: ACC/AHA 2002 guideline update for exercise testing: Summary article. A report of the American College of Cardiology/American Heart Association Task Force on Practice Guidelines (Committee to Update the 1997 Exercise Testing Guidelines). J Am Coll Cardiol 40:1531, 2002.
58. Sharir T, Bacher-Stier C, Dhar S, et al: Identification of severe and extensive coronary artery disease by postexercise regional wall motion abnormalities in Tc-99m sestamibi gated single-photon emission computed tomography. Am J Cardiol 86:1171, 2000.
59. Lima RSL, Watson DD, Goode AR, et al: Incremental value of combined perfusion and function over perfusion alone by gated SPECT myocardial perfusion imaging for detection of severe three-vessel coronary artery disease. J Am Coll Cardiol 42:64, 2003.
60. Zellweger M, Lewin H, Shenghan L, et al: When to stress patients after coronary artery bypass surgery? Risk stratification in patients early and late post-CABG using stress myocardial perfusion SPECT: Implications of appropriate clinical strategies. J Am Coll Cardiol 37:144, 2001.
61. Acampa W, Petretta M, Florimonte L, et al: Prognostic value of exercise cardiac tomography performed late after percutaneous coronary intervention in symptomatic and symptom-free patients. Am J Cardiol 9:259, 2003.
62. Blumenthal RS. Becker DM, Yanek LR, et al: Comparison of coronary calcium and stress myocardial perfusion imaging in apparently healthy siblings of individuals with premature coronary artery disease. Am J Cardiol 97(3):328, 2006.
63. Smith SC, Greenland P, Grundy SM: Prevention Conference V: Beyond secondary prevention: Identifying the high-risk patient for primary prevention: Executive summary. Circulation 101:111, 2000.
64. Wackers FJ, Young LH, Inzucchi SE, et al: Detection of Ischemia in Asymptomatic Diabetics Investigators. Detection of silent myocardial ischemia in asymptomatic diabetic subjects: the DIAD study. Diabetes Care 27:1954, 2004.
65. Scholte AJ,Bax JJ,Wackers FJ: Screening of asymptomatic patients with type 2 diabetes mellitus for silent coronary artery disease: Combined use of stress myocardial perfusion imaging and coronary calcium scoring. J Nucl Cardiol 13(1):11-18, 2006.
66. De Lorenzo A, Lima RS, Siqueira-Filho AG, Pantoja MR: Prevalence and prognostic value of perfusion defects detected by stress technetium-99m sestamibi myocardial perfusion single-photon emission computed tomography in asymptomatic patients with diabetes mellitus and no known coronary artery disease. Am J Cardiol 90:827, 2002.
67. Berman DS, Wong ND, Gransar H, et al: Relationship between stress-induced myocardial ischemia and atherosclerosis measured by coronary calcium tomography. J Am Coll Cardiol 44:923, 2004.
68. Brindis RG, Douglas PS, Hendel RC, et al: ACCF/ASNC appropriateness criteria for single-photon emission computed tomography myocardial perfusion imaging (SPECT MPI): A report of the American College of Cardiology Foundation Quality Strategic Directions Committee Appropriateness Criteria Working Group and the American Society of Nuclear Cardiology endorsed by the American Heart Association. J Am Coll Cardiol 46:1587, 2005.
69. Berman DS, Hachamovitch R, Shaw LJ, Friedman JD, et al: Roles of nuclear cardiology, cardiac computed tomography, and cardiac magnetic resonance: Noninvasive risk stratification and a conceptual framework for the selection of noninvasive imaging tests in patients with known or suspected coronary artery disease. J Nucl Med 47:1107, 2006.
70. Schuijf JD, Wijns W, Jukema JW, et al: Relationship between noninvasive coronary angiography with multi-slice computed tomography and myocardial perfusion imaging. J Am Coll Cardiol 48:2508, 2006.

Acute Coronary Syndromes

71. Wackers FJ, Brown KA, Heller GV, et al: American Society of Nuclear Cardiology position statement on radionuclide imaging in patients with suspected acute ischemic syndromes in the emergency department or chest pain center. J Nucl Cardiol 9:246, 2002.
72. Stowers SA, Eisenstein EL, Wackers FJ, et al: An economic analysis of an aggressive diagnostic strategy with single photon emission computed tomography myocardial perfusion imaging and early exercise stress testing in emergency department patients who present with chest pain but non diagnostic electrocardiograms: Results from a randomized trial. Ann Emerg Med 35:17, 2000.
73. Udelson JE, Beshansky JR, Ballin DS, et al: Myocardial perfusion imaging for evaluation and triage of patients with suspected acute cardiac ischemia: A randomized controlled trial. JAMA 288:2693, 2002.
74. Cannon CP, Weintraub WS, Demopoulos LA, et al: Comparison of early invasive and conservative strategies in patients with unstable coronary syndromes treated with the glycoprotein IIb/IIIa inhibitor tirofiban. N Engl J Med 344:1879, 2001.
75. de Winter RJ, Windhausen F, Cornel JH, et al: Early invasive versus selectively invasive management for acute coronary syndromes. N Engl J Med 353:1095, 2005.
76. Antman EM, Cohen M, Bernink PJ, et al: The TIMI risk score for unstable angina/non-ST elevation MI: A method for prognostication and therapeutic decision making. JAMA 284:835, 2000.
77. Antman EM, Anbe DT, Armstrong PW, et al: ACC/AHA guidelines for the management of patients with ST-elevation myocardial infarction-executive summary: A report of the American College of Cardiology/American Heart Association Task Force on practice guidelines (writing committee to revise the 1999 guidelines for the management of patients with acute myocardial infarction) J Am Coll Cardiol 44:671, 2004.
78. Kawai Y, Tsukamoto E, Nozaki Y, et al: Significance of reduced uptake of iodinated fatty acid analogues for the evaluation of patients with acute chest pain. J Am Coll Cardiol 38:1888, 2001.
79. Narula J, Virmani R, Zaret BL: Radionuclide imaging of atherosclerotic lesions. *In* Dilsizian V, Narula J, Braunwald E (eds): Atlas of Nuclear Cardiology. Philadelphia, Current Medicine, 2003, pp 217-236.
80. Ohtsuki K, Hayase M, Akashi K, et al: Detection of monocyte chemoattractant protein-1 receptor expression in experimental atherosclerotic lesions: An autoradiographic study. Circulation 104:203, 2001.

Heart Failure

81. Gheorghiade M, Sopko G, De Luca L, et al. Navigating the crossroads of coronary artery disease and heart failure. Circulation 114:1202, 2006.
82. McCrohon JA, Moon JCC, Prasad SK, et al: Differentiation of heart failure related to dilated cardiomyopathy and coronary artery disease using gadolinium-enhanced cardiovascular magnetic resonance. Circulation 108:54, 2003.
83. Bennett SK, Smith MF, Gottlieb SS, et al: Effect of metoprolol on absolute myocardial blood flow in patients with heart failure secondary to ischemic or nonischemic cardiomyopathy. Am J Cardiol 89:1431, 2002.
84. Cleland JG, Pennell DJ, Ray SG, et al: Myocardial viability as a determinant of the ejection fraction response to carvedilol in patients with heart failure (CHRISTMAS trial): Randomised controlled trial. Lancet 362:14, 2003.
85. Allman K, Shaw L, Hachamovitch R, UdelsonJE: Myocardial viability testing and impact of revascularization on prognosis in patients with coronary artery disease and left ventricular dysfunction: A meta-analysis. J Am Coll Cardiol 39:1151, 2002.
86. Bonow RO: Myocardial viability and prognosis in patients with ischemic left ventricular dysfunction. J Am Coll Cardiol 39:1159, 2002.
87. Bax JJ, Poldermans D, Elhendy A, et al: Assessment of myocardial viability by nuclear imaging techniques. Curr Cardiol Rep 7:124, 2005.
88. Siebelink HM, Blanksma P, Crijns H, et al: No difference in cardiac event-free survival between positron emission tomography and single-photon emission computed tomography-guided patient management. J Am Coll Cardiol 37:81, 2001.
89. Hunt SA, Abraham WT, Chin MH, et al. ACC/AHA 2005 Guideline Update for the Diagnosis and Management of Chronic Heart Failure in the Adult: A Report of the American College of Cardiology/American Heart Association Task Force on Practice Guidelines (Writing Committee to Update the 2001 Guidelines for the Evaluation and Management of Heart Failure). J Am Coll Cardiol 46:e1, 2005.
90. Margazi ZJ, Anastasiou-Nana MI, Terrovitis J, et al: Indium-111 monoclonal antimyosin cardiac scintigraphy in suspected acute myocarditis: Evolution and diagnostic impact. Int J Cardiol 90:239, 2003.
91. Puig M, Ballester M, Matias-Guiu X, et al: Burden of myocardial damage in cardiac allograft rejection: Scintigraphic evidence of myocardial injury and histologic evidence of myocyte necrosis and apoptosis. J Nucl Cardiol 7:132-139, 2000.
92. Eguchi M, Tsuchihashi K, Hotta D, et al: Technetium-99m sestamibi/tetrofosmin myocardial perfusion scanning in cardiac and noncardiac sarcoidosis. Cardiology 94:193, 2000.
93. Hongo M, Urushibata K, Kai R, et al: Iodine-123 metaiodobenzylguanidine scintigraphic analysis of myocardial sympathetic innervation in patients with AL (primary) amyloidosis. Am Heart J 144:122, 2002.
94. Carrio I: Cardiac neurotransmission imaging. J Nucl Med 42:1062, 2001.
95. Arora R, Ferrick KJ, Nakata T, et al: 123-metaiodobenzylguanidine (MIBG) imaging and heart rate variability analysis to predict the need for an implantable cardioverter defibrillator. J Nucl Cardiol 10:121, 2003.
96. Narula J, Kietselaer B, Hofstra L: Role of molecular imaging in defining and denying death. J Nucl Cardiol 11:349, 2004.
97. Hofstra L, Liem IH, Dumont EA, et al: Visualization of cell death in vivo in patients with acute myocardial infarction. Lancet 356:209, 2000.
98. Wu JC, Chen IY, Sundaresan G, et al: Molecular imaging of cardiac cell transplantation in living animals using optical bioluminescence and positron emission tomography. Circulation 108:1302, 2003.
99. Lee YHC, Kiesewetter DO, Lang L, et al: Synthesis of 4-[^{18}F]fluorobenzoyllisinopril: A radioligand for angiotensin converting enzyme (ACE) imaging with positron emission tomography. J Labelled Cpd Radiopharm 44:S268, 2001.
100. Dilsizian V, Eckelman WC, Loredo ML, et al. Evidence for tissue angiotensin converting enzyme in explanted hearts of ischemic cardiomyopathy patients using targeted radiotracer technique. J Nucl Med 48:1-6, 2007.

Risk Assessment for Noncardiac Surgery

101. Eagle KA, Berger PB, Calkins H, et al: ACC/AHA guideline update for perioperative cardiovascular evaluation for noncardiac surgery: Executive summary: A report of the American College of Cardiology/American Heart Association Task Force on Practice Guidelines (Committee to Update the 1996 Guidelines on Perioperative Cardiovascular Evaluation for Noncardiac Surgery). Circulation 105:1257, 2002.
102. Cohen MC, Eagle KA: Preoperative risk stratification: An overview. *In* Zaret BL, Beller GA (eds): Nuclear Cardiology: State of the Art and Future Directions. St. Louis, Mosby, 1999, pp 346-367.
103. Poldermans D, Boersma E, Bax JJ, et al: The effect of bisoprolol on perioperative mortality and myocardial infarction in high-risk patients undergoing vascular surgery. N Engl J Med 341:1789, 1999.
104. Landesberg G, Mosseri M, Wolf YG, et al. Preoperative thallium scanning, selective coronary revascularization and long-term survival after major vascular surgery. Circulation 108:177, 2003.
105. McFalls EO, Ward HB, Moritz TE, et al. Coronary-artery revascularization before elective major vascular surgery. N Engl J Med 351:2795, 2004.

Nuclear Cardiology

Guidelines for the use of cardiac radionuclide imaging were published by the American Heart Association (AHA), the American College of Cardiology (ACC), and the American Society of Nuclear Cardiology (ASNC) in 2003.[1] Other recent commentaries on the role of nuclear cardiology tests are included under guidelines for exercise testing published in 2002[2] and for the management of acute myocardial infarction in 1999.[3] These guidelines reaffirm the fundamental theme and recommendations of the 1995 ACC/AHA radionuclide imaging guidelines.[4] The consistent message is that radionuclide imaging should be used in situations in which the history, electrocardiographic changes, and other laboratory measurements do not provide reliable information to guide management.

As with most ACC/AHA guidelines, the indications for use of nuclear cardiology tests are classified into one of three classes:

Class I: Conditions for which there is evidence and/or general agreement that testing is useful and effective.

Class II: Conditions for which there is conflicting evidence and/or a divergence of opinion about the usefulness/efficacy of performing testing.

Class IIa: Weight of evidence/opinion is in favor of usefulness/efficacy.

Class IIb: Usefulness/efficacy is less well established by evidence/opinion.

Class III: Conditions for which there is evidence and/or general agreement that testing is not useful/effective and in some cases may be harmful.

Acute ST Segment Elevation Myocardial Infarction

The ACC/AHA/ASNC guidelines indicate that radionuclide imaging should have a limited role in the diagnosis of acute myocardial infarction. These technologies are not appropriate for routine diagnosis and should be used only when information from the history, electrocardiogram, and laboratory tests is not sufficient. The task force considered evidence to be supportive of the use of radionuclide imaging for the assessment of infarct size, for the diagnosis of right ventricular infarction, or for cases in which the diagnosis of myocardial infarction was unclear and the patient presented late (more than 24 hours and less than 7 days) after the onset of symptoms (Table 16G-1).

For evaluation of prognosis after acute myocardial infarction, stress myocardial perfusion imaging was considered appropriate to assess the presence and extent of stress-induced ischemia. The guidelines do not address settings in which radionuclide imaging is preferable to exercise electrocardiography, but the 1999 guidelines on care of acute myocardial infarction indicate that exercise electrocardiography should be the first test used for risk stratification after acute myocardial infarction; imaging studies should be reserved for cases in which the electrocardiogram is likely to be uninterpretable or when the exercise electrocardiograph is equivocal.[3] Radionuclide angiography was considered useful for assessment of ventricular function after acute myocardial infarction, but echocardiography is cited as a low-cost, convenient, widely accessible alternative technology for this purpose.[3]

Unstable Angina/Non-ST Segment Elevation Myocardial Infarction

The ACC/AHA/ASNC guidelines consider radionuclide imaging to be potentially useful for diagnosis and assessment of severity of ischemia in patients with unstable angina and for assessment of left ventricular function when angina is satisfactorily stabilized with medical therapy. Myocardial perfusion imaging was also considered potentially useful (class IIa) for patients with ongoing ischemia who undergo imaging at rest. For patients presenting to emergency departments with a possible acute coronary syndrome but with nondiagnostic initial ECG and biomarkers, the guidelines recommend perfusion imaging at rest as a class I indication, based, in part, on a randomized controlled trial that found that sestamibi imaging can improve emergency department triage decision-making for patients with suspected acute cardiac ischemia.[5]

Chronic Ischemic Heart Disease

The ACC/AHA/ASNC guidelines consider exercise or pharmacological myocardial perfusion imaging to be appropriate (class I) for evaluation of the extent and severity of coronary artery disease in patients with chronic ischemic heart disease. The guidelines consider thallium-201 and technetium-99m to be sufficiently similar to be used interchangeably in this population. Review of data on the three most commonly used agents in pharmacological perfusion imaging (dipyridamole, adenosine, and dobutamine) led the task force to conclude that adenosine or dipyridamole is preferred for patients who cannot exercise adequately. The ACC/AHA guidelines on exercise testing continue to assert that exercise electrocardiography remains the first-choice test for women as well as men, and the imaging technologies should be used when patients cannot exercise or when the electrocardiogram is likely to be uninterpretable.[2]

Asymptomatic Patients

The ACC/AHA/ASNC guidelines do not consider cardiac radionuclide imaging an appropriate routine test for diagnosis of coronary artery disease in patients who are not symptomatic. However, radionuclide imaging is considered potentially useful for determining the need for coronary angiography in patients with positive exercise electrocardiography tests.

Before Noncardiac Surgery

Most studies of the radionuclide imaging in patients undergoing noncardiac surgery have been performed in patients undergoing major vascular procedures. Such testing was considered appropriate (class I) in patients with chronic ischemic heart disease (see Table 16G-1). However, the guidelines discourage use of radionuclide imaging before noncardiac surgery in most patients undergoing nonvascular surgery because of the lower cardiac risk of these procedures.

Before and After Revascularization Procedures

Myocardial perfusion imaging is appropriate for planning for coronary revascularization procedures and for detection of ischemia in patients who are symptomatic after these procedures (see Table 16G-1). However, the guidelines discourage routine assessment of patients who are asymptomatic after revascularization because of lack of data supporting interventions in such patients. These conclusions are consistent with recent guidelines for exercise testing.[2]

Heart Failure

The ACC/AHA/ASNC guidelines consider radionuclide assessment of left and right ventricular function to be useful in the initial work-up for heart failure, although echocardiography provides additional information on valvular disease. The noninvasive assessment of the copresence of coronary artery disease (CAD) by myocardial perfusion imaging in patients with heart failure without angina is considered a class IIa indication. The guidelines recommend radionuclide assess-

TABLE 16G–1 American College of Cardiology/American Heart Association/American Society of Nuclear Cardiology Guidelines for the Clinical Use of Cardiac Radionuclide Imaging*

Indication	Class I (Indicated)	Class IIa (Good Supportive Evidence)	Class IIb (Weak Supportive Evidence)	Class III (Not Indicated)
Diagnosis of STE acute myocardial infarction		Right ventricular infarction Infarction not diagnosed by standard means—late presentation		Routine diagnosis with ischemia/necrosis already documented clinically
Risk assessment, prognosis, and assessment of therapy after STE acute myocardial infarction	Rest RV/LV function Presence/extent of stress-induced ischemia Detection of infarct size and residual viable myocardium			
Diagnosis, prognosis, and assessment of therapy in patients with unstable angina/NSTEMI	Identificationof ischemia in the distribution of the culprit lesion or in remote areas Measurement of baseline LV function Identification of the severity/extent of disease in patients whose angina is satisfactorily stabilized with medical therapy	Identification of the severity/extent of disease in patients with ongoing ischemia but nondiagnostic ECG	Diagnosis of myocardial ischemia in patients when the combination of history and ECG changes is unreliable	
Suspected ACS in the emergency department with nondiagnostic ECG and initial biomarkers	Assessment of risk with rest MPI Stress MPI for diagnosis of CAD after negative biomarkers or normal rest MPI			
Diagnosis of chronic ischemic heart disease	Diagnosis of symptomatic and selected patients with asymptomatic myocardial ischemia Assessment of ventricular performance (rest or exercise) Planning PTCA—identifying lesions causing myocardial ischemia, if not otherwise known Risk stratification before noncardiac surgery in select patients			Screening of asymptomatic patients with low likelihood of disease
Assessment of severity/prognosis/risk stratification of chronic ischemic heart disease	Assessment of LV performance Identification of extent and severity of ischemia and localization of ischemia† Risk stratification in patients with an intermediate risk Duke Treadmill Score Assessment of functional significance of intermediate coronary stenosis	MPI as the initial test in patients with diabetes or with >20% 10-yr CHD risk	Redefining risk 1-3 yr after initial MPI in patients with stable symptoms	
Assessment of interventions in chronic ischemic heart disease	Assessment for restenosis after PCI (symptomatic) Assessment of ischemia in symptomatic patients after CABG	Assessment 3-5 yr after CABG or PCI in select, high-risk asymptomatic patients	Assessment of drug therapy for myocardial perfusion	Routine assessment of asymptomatic patients after PTCA or CABG
Heart failure	Determination of initial LV and RV performance in heart failure Initial evaluation of LV function in patients receiving chemotherapy with doxorubicin Assessment of myocardial viability in patients with CAD and LV dysfunction without angina	Assessment of the co-presence of CAD in patients without angina	Routine serial assessment of LV and RV function Detection of myocarditis Diagnosis of CAD in hypertrophic cardiomyopathy	
After cardiac transplantation	Assessment of ventricular performance		Detection and assessment of coronary angiopathy	
Valvular heart disease	Initial and serial assessment of LV and RV function		Detection and assessment of function significance of concomitant coronary artery disease	

*Table represents a compilation of recommendations from the 1995 and 2003 guidelines.

†Exercise MPI in patients with baseline ECG abnormalities, vasodilator pharmacological stress MPI in patients who cannot exercise adequately or who have LBBB or paced rhythm.

ACS = acute coronary syndrome; CABG = coronary artery bypass graft; CAD = coronary artery disease; CHD = coronary heart disease; ECG = electrocardiographic; LBBB = left bundle branch block; LV = left ventricular; MPI = myocardial perfusion imaging; NSTEMI = non-ST segment elevation myocardial infarction; PCI = percutaneous coronary intervention; PTCA = percutaneous transluminal coronary angioplasty; RV = right ventricular; STE = ST segment elevation.

ment of myocardial viability as a class I indication for consideration of revascularization in patients with known CAD and left ventricular systolic dysfunction who do not have active angina.

Other Conditions

Radionuclide angiography is considered to be useful for assessment of ventricular function in patients who have undergone cardiac transplantation or who have valvular heart disease. It is also considered to be useful for baseline and serial monitoring of left ventricular function during therapy with cardiotoxic drugs.

Appropriateness Criteria

Recently, the American College of Cardiology Foundation and the American Society of Nuclear Cardiology published "Appropriateness Criteria" for SPECT imaging,[6] as a guide for clinicians as to the appropriateness of ordering a SPECT procedure in various clinical scenarios. These criteria are meant to complement and incorporate Guideline recommendations as much as possible, while acknowledging that many clinical scenarios faced by clinicians do not fit neatly into the evidence base from the published literature on which more formal Guidelines are built. As an example, for stable outpatients with chest pain syndromes, patients with an intermediate- or high pretest likelihood of CAD are thought to be appropriate for nuclear imaging along with stress testing, whereas those with a low pretest likelihood who can exercise are not. Patients within 1 year of successful PCI who had pre-PCI symptoms and remain asymptomatic post-PCI are felt to be inappropriate candidates for SPECT (i.e., routine "surveillance"). It is likely that payors will use these criteria as a basis for reimbursement decisions at some point in the future.

References

1. Klocke FJ, Baird MG, Bateman TM, et al: ACC/AHA/ASNC Guidelines for the Clinical Use of Cardiac Radionuclide Imaging: A Report of the American College of Cardiology/American Heart Association Task Force on Practice Guidelines, 2003. (http://www.acc.org/clinical/guidelines/radio/index.pdf)
2. Gibbons RJ, Balady GJ, Bricker JT, et al: ACC/AHA 2002 guideline update for exercise testing: Summary article: A report of the ACC/AHA Task Force on Practice Guidelines (Committee to Update the 1997 Exercise Testing Guidelines). Circulation 106:1883, 2002.
3. Ryan TJ, Antman EM, Brooks NH, et al: ACC/AHA guidelines for the management of patients with acute myocardial infarction: 1999 Update: A report of the American College of Cardiology/American Heart Association Task Force on Practice Guidelines (Committee on Management of Acute Myocardial Infarction). (http:www.acc.org)
4. Guidelines for Clinical Use of Cardiac Radionuclide Imaging. A Report of the American College of Cardiology/American Heart Association Task Force on the Assessment of Cardiovascular Procedures (Committee on Nuclear Imaging). J Am Coll Cardiol 25:521, 1995.
5. Udelson JE, Beshansky JR, Ballis DS, et al: Myocardial perfusion imaging for evaluation and triage of patients with suspected acute cardiac ischemia: A randomized controlled trial. JAMA 288:2693, 2002.
6. Brindis RG, Douglas PS, Hendel RC, et al: ACCF/ASNC appropriateness criteria for single photon emission computed tomographic myocardial perfusion imaging (SPECT MPI): A report of the American College of Cardiology Foundation Quality Strategy Directions Committee Appropriateness Criteria Working Group and the American Society of Nuclear Cardiology. J Am Coll Cardiol 46:1587-1605, 2005.

CHAPTER 17

Cardiovascular Magnetic Resonance

Dudley Pennell

Cardiovascular magnetic resonance (CMR), as it is called by the international scientific community, has grown considerably in recent years and is now firmly established in clinical and research cardiovascular medicine in the larger centers.[1] This growth and acceptance stems from a number of factors, including technical advancements (e.g., speed, reliability, ease of use, new applications), superb image quality and field of view, and the reporting of CMR-derived new insights in regard to entrenched problem areas in cardiology. In addition, a recognition of the excellent reproducibility of CMR images has encouraged widespread adoption of its use by those in academic medicine and the pharmaceutical industry. Research trials can be completed with noteworthy findings and substantially reduced sample sizes, which hasten the process and lower costs. It is also worth noting that in the modern climate of safety priority, radiowave and ultrasound technology have an inescapable advantage over x-ray and gamma ray modalities, suggesting that these nonionizing technologies may be preferable in the future. Further strengthening this perspective is the appreciation that echocardiography is the faster and more portable modality, but CMR typically provides superior image quality at a higher entry price. Thus, echocardiography and CMR are powerful and complementary partners.

FUNDAMENTAL PRINCIPLES OF MAGNETIC RESONANCE

The abbreviated physics background of MR is presented here to facilitate understanding the technical terms used throughout this chapter; greater detail can be found in more specialized texts.[2] The physical interaction required for MR is at the level of the atomic nucleus, as first described in 1946. It was also found at that time that the frequency of radiowave absorption depends on the strength of the external magnetic field. These two key findings form the basis for modern clinical MR imaging. Because MR does not therefore interfere with electrons in the outer atomic shell that are responsible for chemical binding, it is fundamentally safe, unlike ionizing radiation, such as x-rays, which may interact with electron binding, damaging molecules such as DNA. Magnetic resonance only occurs in atomic nuclei with unpaired spin (nucleons). In clinical practice, this means hydrogen-1, which is abundant in water and fat. Because hydrogen is abundant in the human body, and has good sensitivity to the phenomenon of magnetic resonance, high signal-to-noise images can be obtained. Other important elements are useful for investigation in the laboratory to characterize biochemical processes (^{13}C, ^{17}O, ^{19}F, ^{23}Na, ^{39}K) but these are not used clinically. Human spectroscopy usually makes use of the phosphorus-31 nucleus; this is important because it occurs in compounds involved in energy metabolism, such as adenosine triphosphate (ATP) and phosphocreatine (PCr). MR spectra are rarely used to construct images, however, and the data generally are used to quantify metabolite concentrations.

Hydrogen nuclei behave like magnets and align to an external magnetic field. At baseline, the nuclei precess randomly about a 1.5-T magnetic field at a resonant frequency of 63 MHz, which is in the radiowave range. A body region can be excited by a pulse of radiowaves at this frequency, which has the effect of causing all the excited hydrogen nuclei to rotate away from the direction of the main magnetic field axis (the flip angle) and precess in a coordinated manner, which causes a net magnetization. After the excitation pulse is finished, the net magnetization decays to its former position (relaxation), and energy is transmitted as a radio signal. Typically, this signal is formed into a radiowave echo by the scanner, such that it can be used to form an image by a receiver antenna. The contrast between different tissues in the image depends on the delay between excitation and the signal readout (TE, echo time) and the time between repetitive radiowave excitations (TR, repeat time). The different forms of contrast are derived from two principal relaxation processes that affect the net magnetization, decay in the longitudinal axis (T1) and the transverse plane (T2). Additional magnetic fields (gradient fields) are required, which can be rapidly switched on and off to localize the radiowaves coming from the body. An MR image therefore represents a spatially resolved map of radio signals.

The Cardiovascular Magnetic Resonance Scanner

A modern CMR scanner consists of major hardware components. The superconducting magnet produces the static magnetic field, which is highly homogeneous, stable over time, and large enough for chest examinations. Currently, CMR is usually performed at 1.5 T, but some centers are exploring the use of 3-T magnets, which offers greater signal but at the cost of increased artifacts and inability to use some sequences because of radiofrequency heating problems. The gradient fields are generated by gradient amplifiers with ultrafast capability, which rapidly drive large currents at high voltages through the resistive gradient coils within the bore of the magnet. The radiofrequency amplifier generates the excitation pulses and a radiofrequency antenna receives the radio signals coming from the patient. A computer controls all the scanner components with complex software. It is also used to perform the Fourier transformation and other complex mathematical processes on the raw radio signal data matrix (known as k-space), which ultimately generates the images. Of growing importance are the receiver coils that gather the radiowave signals from the body. New technology using multiple coil arrays allows improved image quality and/or accelerated imaging by acquiring multiple lines of signal simultaneously. This has been particularly important for acquisitions that are stretched for signal and speed, such as perfusion imaging, which has greatly improved clinical usefulness.

Cardiovascular Magnetic Resonance Sequences

A CMR scanner can only generate useful images if the various component pieces of hardware are intricately coordinated. The timing and magnitude of radiowave and magnetic field pulses, along with data collection, form MR sequences, which are controlled by the scanner computer. Sequences have various components, such as preparation pulses (used to alter contrast between tissues), excitation pulses (shape and location of the area of the body to be excited by radiowaves), gradient and magnetic field pulses (formation of a radiowave echo to generate a useful signal for image formation), and signal readout (filling of the raw data matrix, or k-space). There are a large variety of sequences; this can appear daunting at first. Fundamentally, however, it is a knowledge of the properties of the sequences rather than their exact nature that is required for medical interpretation.

For CMR, most images are obtained using two basic sequences, spin-echo and gradient-echo. Spin-echo sequences are also known as "black blood" and gradient-echo as "white blood," although this is a simplification. Spin-echo sequences are routinely used for multislice anatomical imaging, whereas gradient-echo sequences are used for physiological assessment of function through cine acquisitions. The most common prepulse is known as inversion recovery—this gives strong T1 weighting, which is valuable for infarct and viability imaging. Alternatively, T2 preparations are used for coronary imaging. The readout of the signal can be achieved in many ways, leading to sequences with other names. Usually, the readout is modified for CMR so that it is as fast as possible. Images or cines can be acquired within single breath-holds; the faster schemes include fast low-angle shot (FLASH), steady state with free precession (SSFP, also known as FISP and FIESTA), spiral imaging, and echoplanar imaging (EPI). These fast sequences yield images during a 4- to 20-second breath-hold, which substantially reduces artifact from respiratory motion and also allows three-dimensional acquisitions.

Some other sequences are also very useful in examination of the cardiovascular system. Velocity mapping displays each pixel in the image as a pixel velocity rather than as a signal magnitude. This is derived from encoding of the phase of the radio signal by using modified gradient profiles. Higher pixel velocities cause a higher phase shift and this information can be recovered during Fourier transformation of the signal readout. This is invaluable for measurement of peak velocities through stenotic values and true flow for shunt assessment, which is calculated from the integral over time throughout the cardiac cycle of the product of the mean velocity and area of a vessel. For coronary CMR, some high-resolution acquisitions cannot be completed within a breath-hold, and a specialized sequence called a navigator echo is used to reduce respiratory motion significantly. The diaphragm movement is monitored in real time and the scanning computer calculates the coronary position corrected for the position in the breathing cycle. A sequence called tagging is being used to study myocardial contraction. In this sequence, a grid of dark lines is laid across the image in diastole. The lines of altered magnetization persist and deform throughout the cardiac cycle. Using computer analysis, the intersections of the lines can be used to calculate myocardial strain, which is a quantitative and observer-independent measure of myocardial contractility. CMR angiography is a rapidly growing technique in which three- or four-dimensional visualization of a vessel lumen is achieved, usually after intravenous injection of a gadolinium-based MR contrast agent.

Cardiovascular Magnetic Resonance Contrast Agents

There are a number of classes of contrast agents used for MR but, for the cardiovascular system, only the gadolinium agents are currently in clinical use. Gadolinium has seven unpaired electrons in its outer shell, which allows it to couple efficiently with excited water spins, so that their relaxation is hastened. This predominantly results in a shortening of T1, which increases the signal on T1-weighted images. Gadolinium is a toxic element and is therefore chelated to other molecules for clinical use. The properties of the chelator determine the distribution of the gadolinium, and all currently used gadolinium contrast agents remain in the extracellular compartment. These agents have proved invaluable for arterial angiography and viability imaging. Many other MR contrast agents exist; some are based on other elements such as iron, manganese, or dysprosium, which have powerful effects on shortening T2, thereby reducing the MR signal. Iron-based contrast agents have been evaluated in humans for angiography and perfusion and for showing macrophage activity in atherosclerotic plaque. Finally, a class of targeted contrast agents has been described; in this group, large numbers of gadolinium atoms are linked through an intermediary compound to antibody fragments, which in principle allows any biological epitope to be selectively imaged. This has been demonstrated for thrombus, and may become a powerful CMR tool of the future.

Cardiovascular Magnetic Resonance Gating and Safety

All cardiac and many vascular CMR sequences rely on cardiac gating to prevent artifact from appearing in the periodic cardiac contraction cycle. In almost all current scanners, this is achieved through gating to the R wave of the electrocardiogram (ECG). In some CMR scanners, gating is linked to the vector ECG (two-dimensional electrical activation over time), which may have advantages of reliability, more consistent timing to the R wave peak, and more effective arrhythmia rejection. Older scanners also used gating to the peripheral pulse, but this is now largely abandoned. Most recently, cardiac gating has been achieved without the ECG by gating the CMR acquisition to bulk cardiac motion detected directly during imaging.[3]

The safety of CMR is well described and, in comparison with x-ray based techniques, there are obvious advantages. However, two main problems with CMR must be considered. The first is the issue of flying projectiles in the magnet room, which have the potential to strike the patient. The problem items are iron-based, with ferromagnetic properties. These include scissors, electrical items with power transformers such as injection pumps, and oxygen cylinders. Strict adherence to protocols restricting access to the magnet room by only fully trained staff is essential. The second major issue is that of metallic implants or implanted electronic devices. Most metallic implants are CMR-compatible, including all prosthetic cardiac valves, vascular stents, and orthopedic implants. Although some stent manufacturers have suggested abstinence from CMR for a period after implantation, there are no published data to support this, and several reports have concurred with clinical experience—CMR images may be obtained at any time after implantation with the absence at 1.5 T of magnetic attraction, heating, or adverse clinical risk.[4] Conventional cardiac stents cause localized signal loss on CMR, but some new stent designs are artifact-free.[5] There remain problems with some neurological devices such as cerebrovascular clips, and specialized neurological advice is required for these patients. Electronic implants are more problematic for MR and, hypothetically, the high magnetic field of MR will interfere with the electronics and programming of such devices. For CMR, the main implants in question are pacemakers and implantable cardioverter-defibrillators; their presence is a strong relative contraindication for CMR. The main reason for caution is that the wires can couple to the radiofrequency waves and heat significantly. However, some studies have shown that there are strategies that will allow CMR in these patients, in particular if the device can be turned off for the duration of the scan[6,7] but, until further evidence is available, this can only be considered in patients for whom benefit clearly exceeds risk.

CLINICAL APPLICATIONS

Coronary Artery Disease

ASSESSMENT OF VENTRICULAR VOLUMES, MASS, AND FUNCTION. CMR is well validated for quantifying the volumes and mass of the ventricles and has become the clinical gold standard against which other techniques are measured because of its three-dimensional nature, which does not rely on geometric assumptions. Comparisons with other techniques show wide variability in individual patients and are not greatly instructive, other than illustrating the difficulties in comparing clinical techniques.[8] The accuracy and reproducibility of the measurements make CMR useful for the longitudinal follow-up of patients and for hemodynamic and remodeling research studies using small sample sizes.

The accuracy of CMR for measurement of global left ventricular (LV) volume is well established,[9] initially by comparing CMR images of ex vivo ventricles with the water displacement volume of casts of the ventricles. In vivo, volume validation is more difficult to achieve but the grounds for asserting accuracy depend on comparing LV stroke volume (SV) with right ventricular (RV) stroke volume or with aortic flow measured using velocity mapping, and showing their equivalence in normal human subjects. RV volumes have also been validated against water displacement of casts and by comparing RV SV with pulmonary artery flow. LV mass measurements have been validated against human autopsy hearts and in animals.[10] RV mass measurements have been validated against ex vivo animal hearts. More recently, LV volumes and systolic and diastolic function have been comprehensively described with normalization to gender, body surface area, and age.[11]

An important feature of CMR is the excellent interstudy reproducibility of volume and mass measurements. Other forms of reproducibility are often quoted for functional techniques (interobserver, intraobserver), but they have little statistical import, whereas interstudy reproducibility can be used directly to quantify sample sizes in research studies, with minimal clinical difference observable, and this represents a true clinical change. Interstudy reproducibility is measured as the standard deviation (SD) of the differences in two measurements of a parameter over a reasonable period during which no clinical change is expected, but no substantial recollection is expected by the operator of patient positioning and other procedural factors. SD is often expressed as a coefficient of variability by division into the parameter mean value. Sample sizes for trials are easily calculated from the technique interstudy SD, and low SDs are important, because a reduction between techniques leads to a squared reduction in sample size (i.e., half the SD equals one quarter of the sample size). The interstudy SD for volumes and mass by CMR is excellent for both LV[12] and RV studies,[13] and considerably superior to that of two-dimensional echocardiography.[12] Many drug trials have now used CMR as a primary or major endpoint.[14-16]

CMR is valuable for the assessment of regional contractile function. This is usually achieved clinically by visual inspection of cines in standard imaging planes. Quantification of wall motion and thickening using conventional techniques is possible for both the left and right ventricles, but is not widely used. A preferable CMR technique is tagging, which directly assesses myocardial strain and other deformations as a measure of contractility. Tagging CMR has been validated using sonomicrometer studies and can be applied for full three-dimensional myocardial analysis by collective modeling of the numerous small individual myocardial elements.[17] Advanced tagging CMR acquisitions have now greatly increased spatial and temporal resolution and considerably simplified post processing. Clinical applications are just starting to emerge.

ASSESSMENT OF MYOCARDIAL INFARCTION AND VIABILITY. Myocardial infarction (MI) can be detected with high resolution using a protocol known as late gadolinium enhancement CMR. Gadolinium is given intravenously and CMR is performed after a delay, using an inversion recovery sequence. Little gadolinium enters areas of normal myocardium, because there is uniform tightly packed muscle, and gadolinium is an extracellular contrast agent. However, the extracellular compartment is expanded in areas of MI because of cellular rupture, and therefore differential distribution occurs. The kinetics of entry of gadolinium into the MI territory is delayed and the optimal time for imaging of the distribution of gadolinium is after 10 to 15 minutes. By nulling (forcing to near-zero) the normal myocardial signal with adjustment of the inversion time, the area of infarction can be demonstrated with extremely high contrast relative to the black normal myocardium. A simple mnemonic is that "bright is abnormal." The transmural distribution of MI can be visualized in vivo for the first time using this technique because of its high resolution. Animal models have validated this (Fig. 17-1).[18] In humans, late gadolinium enhancement CMR detects Q wave and non-Q-wave MI accurately[19] and with such high sensitivity that small MIs can be demonstrated that are usually not apparent using gated perfusion single-photon emission computed tomography (SPECT; Fig. 17-2A)[20]; also, microinfarcts can be shown after percutaneous coronary intervention.[21] In the acute setting, the extent of late gadolinium enhancement is related to the magnitude of cardiac enzyme release and the functional outcome after recovery. Late gadolinium enhancement CMR reveals a permanent record of MI (both acute and chronic) and is proving very useful clinically for the diagnosis of MI in cases of doubt, or when other techniques are inconclusive. The technique has clarified the pathological significance of Q waves after MI.[22] It has good interstudy reproducibility,[23] suggesting a useful role in studies of therapies for limiting MI in the acute setting. In the setting of acute MI, data have shown that the area at risk from coronary occlusion can be determined from T2-weighted imaging because the severely ischemic but noninfarcted myocardium becomes edematous; this significantly lengthens T2, which increases the signal.[24] The increase in T2 signal persists for many days, allowing edema to be imaged well after the acute event. The area at risk (T2 scan) is larger than the final infarction (late gadolinium enhancement scan) when myocardial salvage has occurred with physical or pharmacological intervention. This makes the combination of these two scans very attractive for studies of techniques to improve salvage and thence prognosis.[25] Late gadolinium enhancement has been shown to be a major predictor of cardiac events in patients without a history of infarction, but in whom infarction is nonetheless present (see Fig. 17-2B).[26]

Further work has shown that CMR can differentiate between the densely bright infarct core and the adjacent periinfarct zone, which appears with lower signal intensity because of the admixture of infarct and viable tissue. The greater the extent of the periinfarct zone, the greater the likelihood of future cardiac death and events.[27]

In the assessment of myocardial viability to determine the likely benefit from coronary bypass surgery, both con-

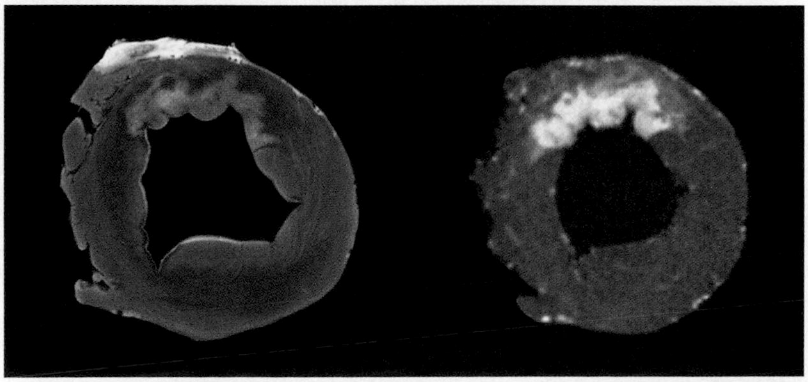

FIGURE 17–1 Validation of late gadolinium-enhanced cardiovascular magnetic resonance (CMR). A subendocardial infarct has been produced by ligation of a coronary artery in a dog, and gadolinium was injected shortly before sacrifice. **Left,** TTC-negative area indicates the extent and shape of the infarct, which is closely matched by the ex vivo CMR scan **(right).** Studies such as this have shown increased gadolinium concentration within the infarct zone and close correlation between the total infarct size by histology and CMR. Note the transmural resolution of the CMR scan and the similarity in shape of the infarctions. Gd = gadolinium; TTC = triphenyltetrazolium chloride. *(Courtesy of Dr. R. J. Kim and Dr. R. M. Judd.)*

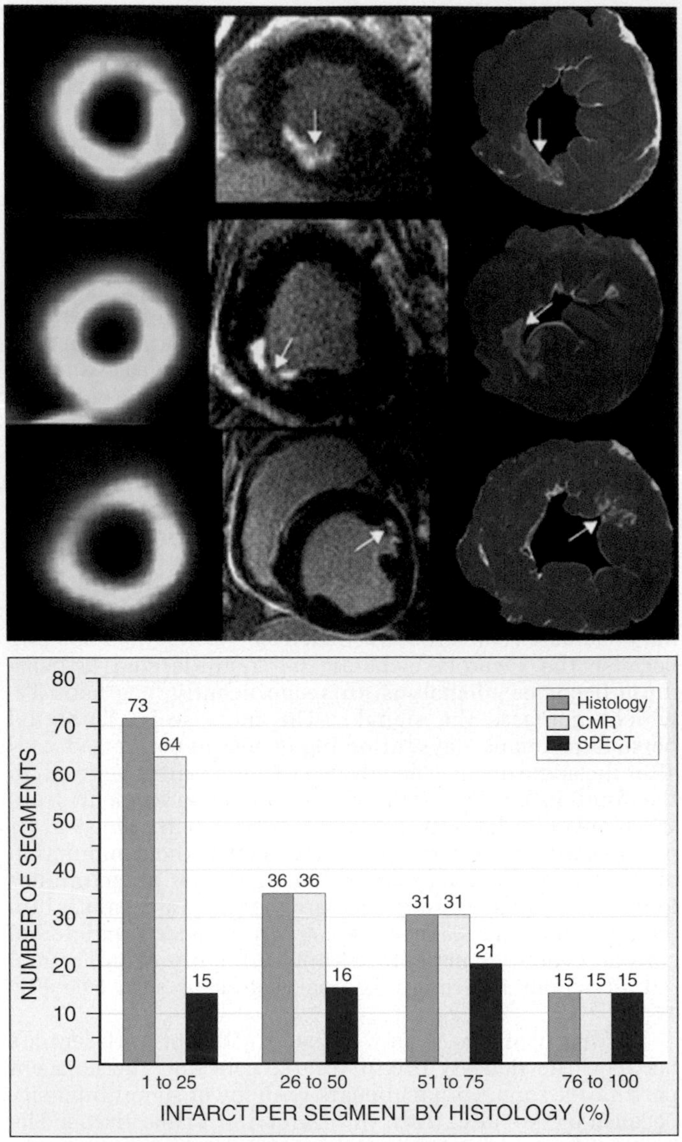

A

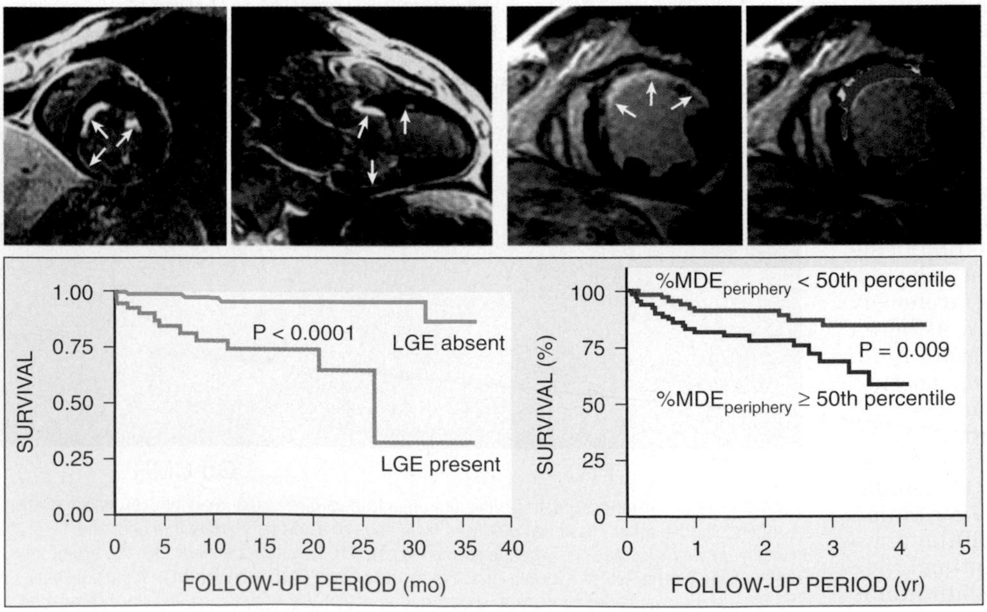

B

FIGURE 17–2 A, Comparison of cardiovascular magnetic resonance (CMR), Tc-99m sestamibi single-photon emission computed tomography (SPECT), and histological findings in subendocardial infarction. **Top panel,** Findings from SPECT **(left),** late gadolinium-enhanced CMR **(middle),** and triphenyltetrazolium chloride histology **(right)** are compared in three different dogs with experimentally induced subendocardial infarction. There is close similarity between histology and CMR but, in all three cases, SPECT fails to demonstrate the infarction because of inadequate resolution. **Bottom panel,** These findings are summarized in this graph, which shows excellent agreement between histology and CMR in regard to the number of segments with infarction categorized by the percentage of infarction per segment. The agreement with SPECT, however, is only satisfactory in segments with more than 75 percent infarction per segment. This indicates that CMR is significantly more accurate in identifying small infarctions and the extent of infarction than SPECT. **B,** The importance of high-resolution detection and assessment of infarction is demonstrated. **Top left panels,** Small infarctions (arrows) are seen in a patient with no history of infarction (unrecognized infarction). Although small, these have profound prognostic impact, as shown in the difference between the Kaplan-Meier cardiac mortality curves over 3 years **(bottom left panel). Top right panels,** An infarction analyzed with semiautomatic software that divides the infarct zone (white arrows) into the densely bright infarct core (shown in red), and the adjacent gray zone periinfarction region (shown in yellow), to quantify the percentage of the infarct that can be classified as periinfarct, and potentially therefore at risk of further damage or arrhythmia generation. **Bottom right panel,** The extent of the periinfarct region (percent $MDE_{periphery}$) was a powerful predictor of outcome, as shown by the divergence of the all-cause mortality curves over 4 years, stratified by values above or below the median. This predictive power was incremental to end-systolic volume and ejection fraction. *(**A** from Wagner A, Mahrholdt H, Holly TA, et al: Contrast-enhanced MRI and routine single photon emission computed tomography (SPECT) perfusion imaging for detection of subendocardial myocardial infarcts: An imaging study. Lancet 361:374, 2003; **B** from Kwong RY, Chan AK, Brown KA, et al: Impact of unrecognized myocardial scar detected by cardiac magnetic resonance imaging on event-free survival in patients presenting with signs or symptoms of coronary artery disease. Circulation 113:2733, 2006, and Yan AT, Shayne AJ, Brown KA, et al: Characterization of the periinfarct zone by contrast-enhanced cardiac magnetic resonance imaging is a powerful predictor of post-myocardial infarction mortality. Circulation 114:32, 2006.)*

ventional and late gadolinium enhancement CMR are useful. One conventional approach is to measure myocardial wall thickness in areas of chronic transmural MI, using the premise from pathological studies that preserved thickness (more than 5 mm) indicates preserved viability. This simple criterion shows good correlation in chronic MI with fluorodeoxyglucose (FDG) positron emission tomography (PET).[28] In dysfunctional myocardium, improved thickening shown by low-dose dobutamine CMR is also in good agreement with FDG-PET. However, there are problems with this simple measure, because recovery of function of very thinned myocardium has been recently described.[29] This suggests that there are mechanisms of reverse remodeling that are currently not understood. The morphological measure of the transmural extent of late gadolinium enhancement by CMR has been shown to be highly predictive of viability, with high likelihood of recovery when the transmural extent of infarction is less than 50 percent (Fig. 17-3).[30] Unlike wall thickness measurements, however, which can only be applied in chronic MI, late gadolinium enhancement is also useful for prediction of functional recovery in acute MI.[31] There is high concordance of late gadolinium enhancement CMR with PET,[32] and superior results have been shown in comparison with thallium-201 SPECT.[33]

EVALUATION OF ACUTE CORONARY SYNDROMES. CMR has been used for the assessment of acute chest pain.[34] CMR showed a sensitivity and specificity of 84 and 85 percent, respectively, was the strongest predictor of an acute coronary syndrome, and added diagnostic value over the usual clinical parameters, including the electrocardiogram, troponin level, and Thrombolysis in Myocardial Infarction (TIMI) risk score. CMR also can be used to identify microvascular obstruction in acute MI.[35] This is demonstrated approximately 1 to 2 minutes after intravenous injection of gadolinium during the vascular distribution phase of the contrast agent and well before late gadolinium enhancement CMR is performed. Areas within the MI that have severely compromised perfusion appear black, indicating microvascular collapse. Microvascular obstruction detected by CMR is associated with ventricular remodeling and an increased likelihood of cardiovascular events, which is independent of the size of the MI. The use of CMR to assess myocardial salvage and prognosis has been mentioned previously.[24,52]

A

B

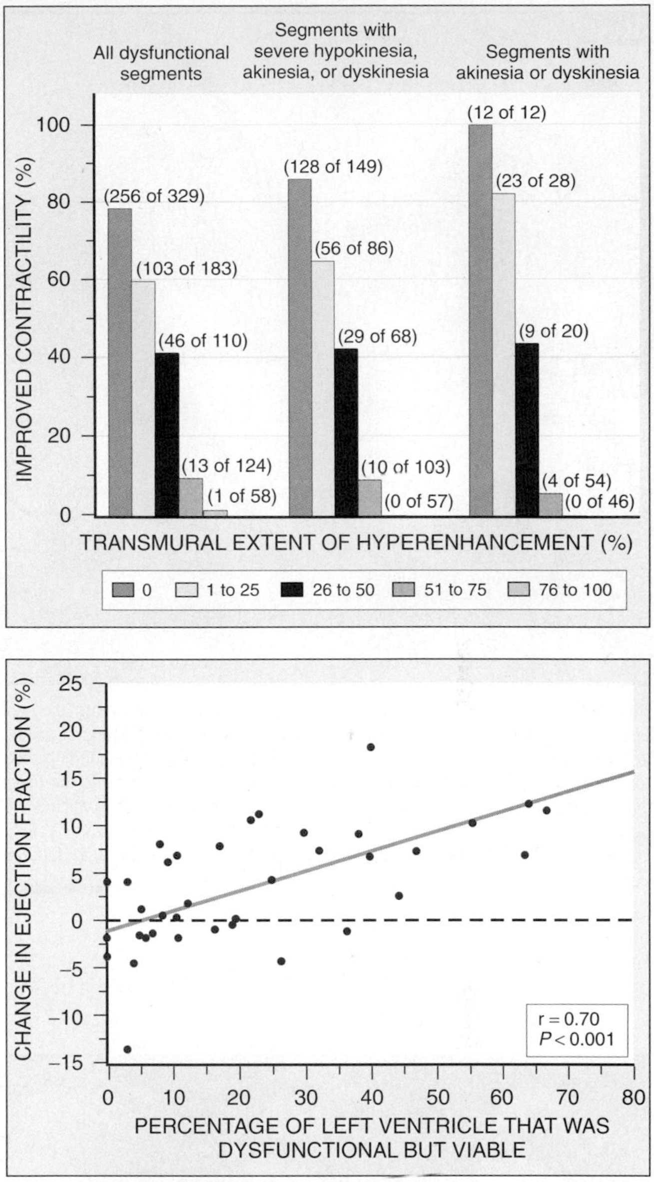

FIGURE 17–3 Assessment of myocardial hibernation by late gadolinium-enhanced cardiovascular magnetic resonance (CMR). There is a significant relationship between the likelihood of improvement of contraction in a segment that is dysfunctional, and the preoperative transmural extent of late gadolinium enhancement. **A,** Relationship for all dysfunctional segments, those with at least severe hypokinesis, and those with at least akinesis. The discrimination is greatest for the most dysfunctional segments. **B,** The change in left ventricular ejection fraction was directly related to the percentage of the left ventricle which was dysfunctional but viable using the late gadolinium enhancement technique. *(From Kim RJ, Wu E, Rafael A, et al: The use of contrast-enhanced magnetic resonance imaging to identify reversible myocardial dysfunction. N Engl J Med 16:1445, 2000.)*

STRESS VENTRICULOGRAPHY. Stress CMR using dobutamine is now clinically established for diagnosing obstructive coronary artery disease (CAD) through the induction of new wall motion abnormalities (Fig. 17-4). Pharmacological stress is preferred to dynamic exercise within the magnet to prevent motion artifacts. Stress CMR is superior to dobutamine stress echocardiography, which is a function of higher image quality. Stress CMR is effective in the diagnosis of CAD in patients who are unsuitable for dobutamine echocardiography (see Chap. 14). Stress CMR has been shown to be very reproducible.[36,37] Outcome studies following normal stress CMR have been limited, but have shown a low event rate.[38,39] CMR has been used for preoperative risk assessment, and higher risk has been shown with demonstration of ischemia.[38] Real-time stress CMR may hasten the acquisition and make the study easier for the patient by eliminating the need for breath-holding.[40]

A valuable adjunct to stress CMR would be the quantification of wall motion assessment, which would reduce the observer variability encountered with dobutamine echocardiography. This has been approached in several ways with early results. A center line method for assessing wall thickening while using dobutamine, with comparison with normal ranges, has improved the accuracy for detection of CAD in patients with single-vessel disease. Tagging CMR has also been applied, and this is expected to be more useful because of the independence of intrinsic strain measurements from endocardial motion. Increased sensitivity with tagging has been shown,[39] but larger clinical trials and improved postprocessing techniques are needed to demonstrate clinical applicability. Other work in quantification has included assessment of stress diastolic function and stress global LV function measured with velocity mapping of aortic flow. Further work is required to determine the clinical role of these modalities.

MYOCARDIAL PERFUSION. Myocardial perfusion CMR is a well-validated technique[41] and is used in clinical practice in early adoption centers. This has the potential for significant impact because of the combination of greatly enhanced resolution with no ionizing radiation. Full ventricular segmental coverage is achieved by using multiple contiguous short-axis slices or mixed short- and long-axis planes. The number of slices achievable in each cardiac cycle has increased through the use of parallel imaging,[42] and the resulting improvement in temporal resolution has decreased endocardial artifacts,[43] which has boosted clinical robustness significantly. Improved contrast with perfusion

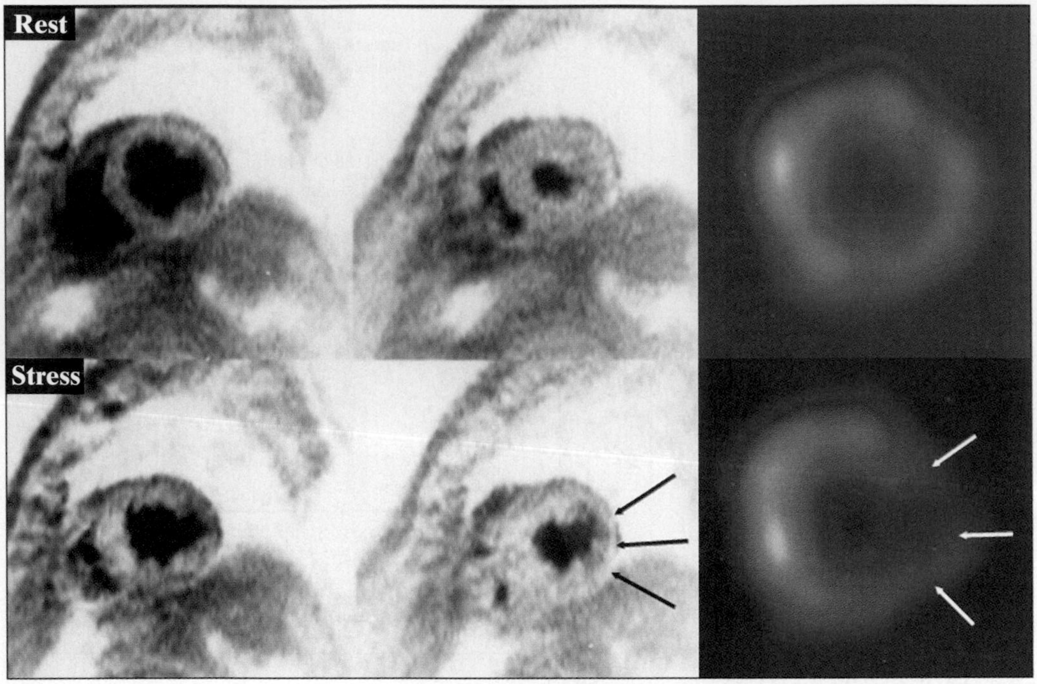

FIGURE 17–4 Cardiovascular magnetic resonance (CMR) stress ventriculography in a patient with left circumflex stenosis. **Left** and **middle panels** show end-diastolic and end-systolic frames, respectively, from CMR cines (the video scale is inverted, and blood therefore appears black). **Right panel,** Corresponding slice by thallium single-photon emission computed tomography (SPECT). The **upper row** shows images taken at rest and the **lower row** shows images taken during dobutamine stress. There is stress-induced wall motion abnormality, which is well shown in the end-systolic stress image (arrows) which is similar in location and extent to the ischemia shown on the stress thallium scan (arrows). *(From Pennell DJ, Underwood SR, Manzara CC, et al: Magnetic resonance imaging during dobutamine stress in coronary artery disease. Am J Cardiol 70:34, 1992.)*

imaging at 3 T has also been reported.[44] A fast intravenous bolus (typically, 5 to 7 ml/sec) of gadolinium contrast agent is given using a power injector, and the myocardial signal changes during the first pass are measured. Ideally, each slice is imaged with each cardiac cycle to maximize the quality of the analysis, although imaging on alternate cycles has been performed with good results. Low signal areas representing reduced perfusion can be visualized directly. Alternatively, computer quantification of parameters, such as the signal upslope, can be used to generate parametric relative perfusion maps (Fig. 17-5) or measures of perfusion index at rest and stress.[45] More complex analyses for quantification of myocardial perfusion or perfusion reserve include preprocessing to remove respiratory motion and deconvolution of the myocardial signal curve with the input function taken from the LV blood pool. Perfusion CMR has been validated using microspheres in animal models[46] and using PET in humans.

For clinical application, several perfusion CMR protocols are being tested using adenosine as a pharmacological stress agent. One approach is to assess stress

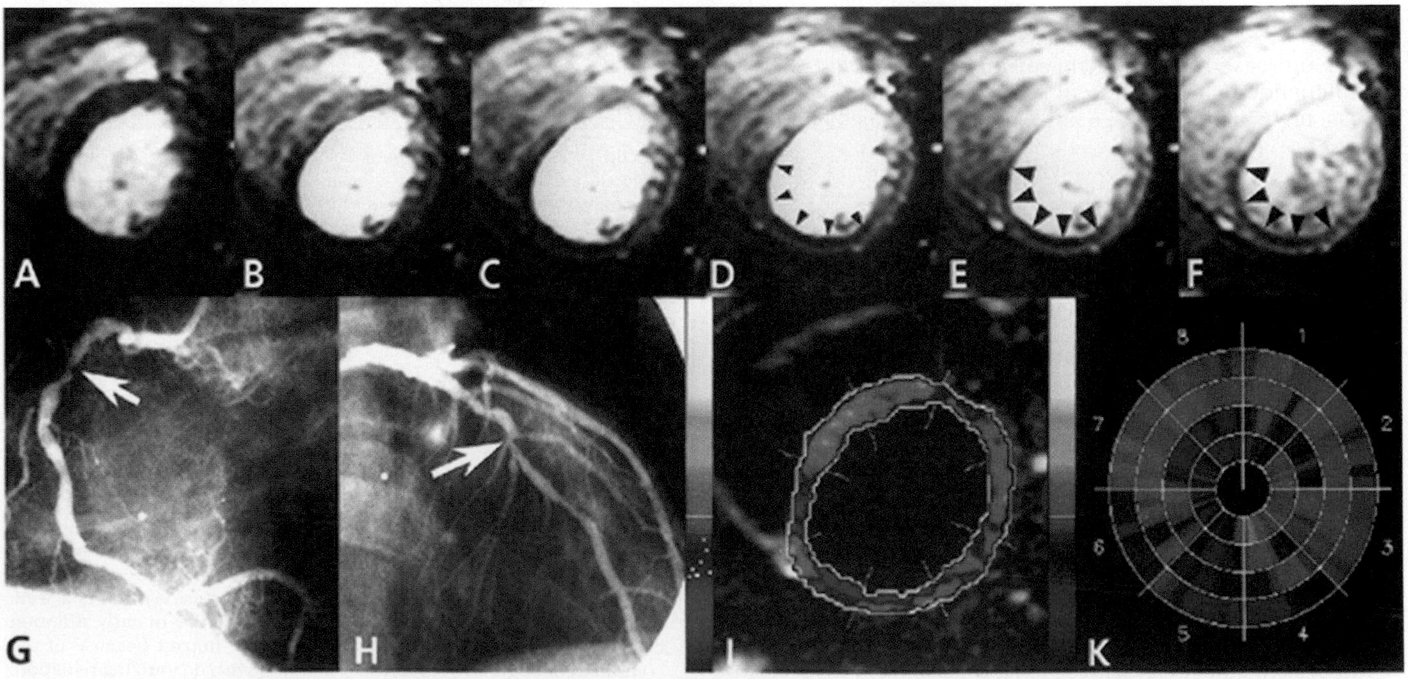

FIGURE 17–5 Perfusion cardiovascular magnetic resonance (CMR) and parametric maps in a patient with stenosis of the right coronary and left anterior descending arteries (arrows in **G** and **H**). A single slice shown in **A** through **F** shows delayed wash in the inferior wall of gadolinium during first pass (arrowheads). The parametric map in **I** shows this abnormality in blue. The polar map shown in **K** indicates areas of abnormal perfusion in blue and both the inferoseptal and the anteroseptal abnormal areas are seen, corresponding to right coronary and left anterior descending artery stenoses, respectively. *(From Schwitter J, Nanz D, Kneifel S, et al: Assessment of myocardial perfusion in coronary artery disease by magnetic resonance: A comparison with positron emission tomography and coronary angiography. Circulation 103:2230-2235, 2001.)*

myocardial perfusion only and to define areas of nonviability using late gadolinium enhancement. A more conventional approach is to perform both stress and rest myocardial perfusion CMR. This has some advantage in identifying artifacts and enables perfusion reserve measurements. If stress and rest studies are performed, the stress images are typically obtained first, because these are the most important. The second series has residual gadolinium from the first injection, which has the potential to interfere with interpretation. The optimal perfusion CMR sequence is not fully resolved. Superior coverage and reduced artifact are obtained with a hybrid gradient-echo-EPI sequence but higher signal is possible with SSFP, and FLASH yields intermediate results.[47] All sequences yield good results with experience, and all are improved with parallel imaging. There is general consensus that fast gadolinium injection is desirable for quantification, although for purely qualitative analysis this is not necessary. There is little difference among gadolinium contrast agents for perfusion CMR; all currently distribute into the extracellular space, although those with lower viscosity can be injected at lower pressures, which has some patient safety advantages. A technique that does not require ultrafast imaging or gadolinium contrast has also been described, called T2* blood oxygen level-dependent (BOLD),[48] but the sensitivity of T2* to perfusion change may be low and currently there is no clinical role.

Myocardial perfusion CMR has shown very good results for the detection of CAD versus PET and SPECT (see Chap. 16).[49] Multicenter trials have shown good performance of CMR compared with coronary angiography,[50,51] and prognostic studies using adenosine CMR are consonant with established literature for SPECT in predicting cardiac events.[52] Improvements in myocardial perfusion reserve have been shown after coronary angioplasty. The excellent resolution of perfusion CMR has also allowed visualization of nonepicardial coronary artery-related perfusion abnormality in other conditions, such as cardiac syndrome X (Fig. 17-6),[45] which agrees with results of CMR spectroscopy. Perfusion CMR is likely to improve our understanding of the pathophysiology of these types of conditions and of perfusion heterogeneity in the normal heart.[53]

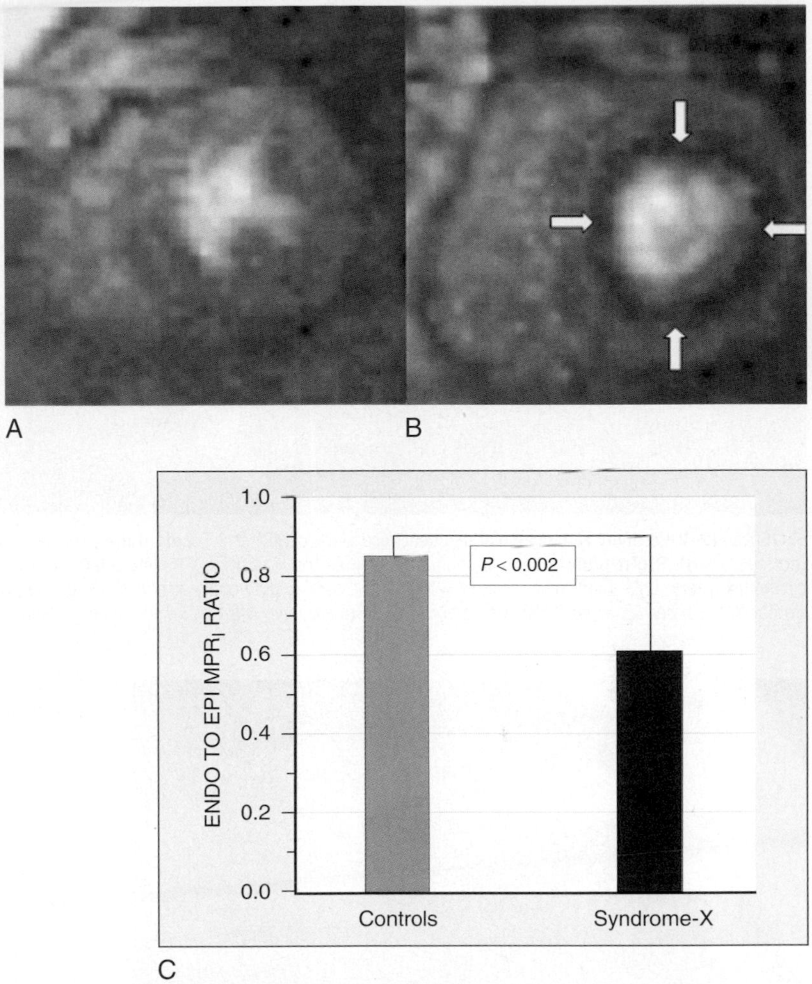

FIGURE 17–6 Perfusion cardiovascular magnetic resonance (CMR) in syndrome X. The high resolution of CMR allows the in vivo visualization of subendocardial perfusion defects for the first time. A perfusion CMR study at rest **(A)** and during adenosine stress **(B)** is shown in a patient with syndrome X (typical angina, greater than 2-mm ST segment depression during exercise electrocardiography, and normal coronary arteries). The two CMR images are from peak enhancement during the first pass of gadolinium, and the image at baseline is normal but the image during adenosine shows subendocardial hypoperfusion. **C,** The graph depicts the myocardial perfusion reserve ratio between the endocardium and epicardium in a group of syndrome X patients and controls. The ratio is significantly lower in syndrome X, indicating reduced endocardial perfusion reserve. *(With permission from Panting JR, Gatehouse PD, Yang GZ, et al: Abnormal subendocardial perfusion in cardiac syndrome-X detected by cardiovascular magnetic resonance imaging. N Engl J Med 346:1948, 2002.)*

CORONARY ANGIOGRAPHY AND FLOW. Coronary CMR angiography is technically challenging for determining both the presence and severity of coronary stenosis because of small arterial size, tortuosity, complex anatomy, and cardiac and respiratory motion. Using highly optimized three-dimensional acquisitions, there has been gradual improvement in resolution and clinical robustness using both breath-holding and navigator techniques.[54] The most significant clinical study, with multicenter participation, has shown good results for the exclusion of multivessel proximal CAD requiring operative intervention.[55] However, current limitations of spatial resolution and rapid coronary motion during the acquisition allow for only broad categorization of diameter stenosis, and distal runoff assessment is difficult for surgical planning.

These limitations of lumen stenosis imaging are not problematic for the assessment of the course of anomalous coronary arteries, where CMR plays a significant clinical role. The malignant course of some coronary arteries between the aorta and pulmonary artery is significantly better depicted by CMR than by x-ray coronary angiography because of the three-dimensional CMR tomograms in comparison with two-dimensional x-ray projections, with overlapping structures. Coronary CMR sequences can image coronary artery bypass grafts. Black and white blood approaches are approximately 90 percent accurate for identifying graft patency. This may prove useful in postoperative chest pain syndromes, but vein graft stenoses and distal anastomoses cannot be assessed directly by luminal assessment. Although coronary imaging for luminal stenosis remains suboptimal, some technical advances may prove valuable. These include high magnetic field scanners (Fig. 17-7), intravascular contrast agents, novel sequences for correction for heart rate variability,[56] and correction of all three dimensions of chest movement during breathing.

Assessment of coronary function can also be achieved by measuring coronary flow velocities using CMR. Adenosine stress coronary flow has been reported in animals and in humans, and the coronary flow reserve has been used to identify stenosis of the left anterior descending artery and in-stent restenosis.[57] It has also been shown that reduced baseline flow and flow reserve in vein grafts is useful for identifying significant stenosis.[58]

ARTERIAL WALL FUNCTION AND STRUCTURE. The arterial wall offers opportunities for assessment of atherosclerosis by CMR that could yield important additional information compared with luminal imaging, from endothelial dysfunction to arterial mechanical properties, total

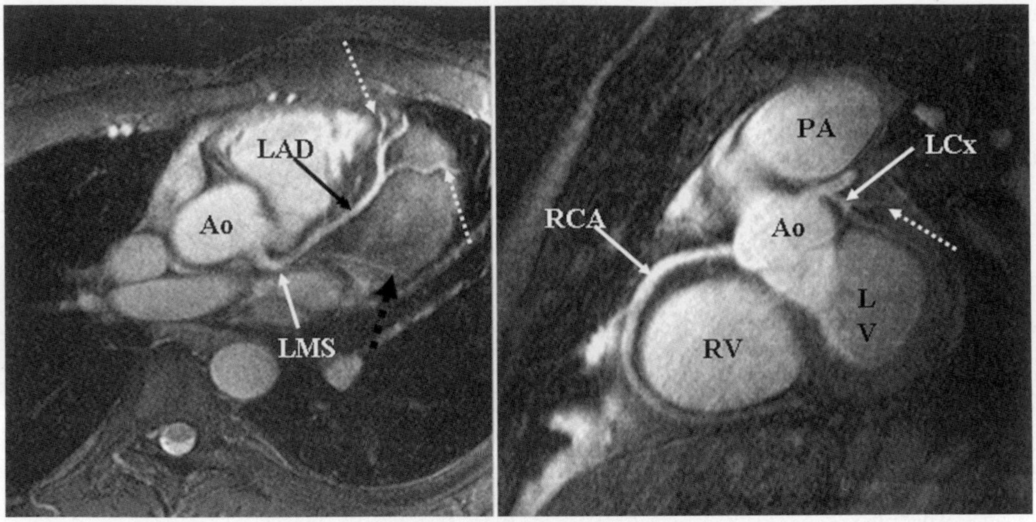

FIGURE 17–7 Coronary cardiovascular magnetic resonance (CMR) at 3 T. **Left panel,** Left coronary artery and branches (dotted arrows). **Right panel,** Right coronary artery (RCA). Ao = aorta; LAD = left anterior descending artery; LCx = left circumflex artery; LMS = left main stem; LV = left ventricle; PA = pulmonary artery; RV = right ventricle. *(From Stuber M, Botnar RM, Fischer SE, et al: Preliminary report on in vivo coronary MRA at 3 T in humans. Magn Reson Med 48:425, 2002.)*

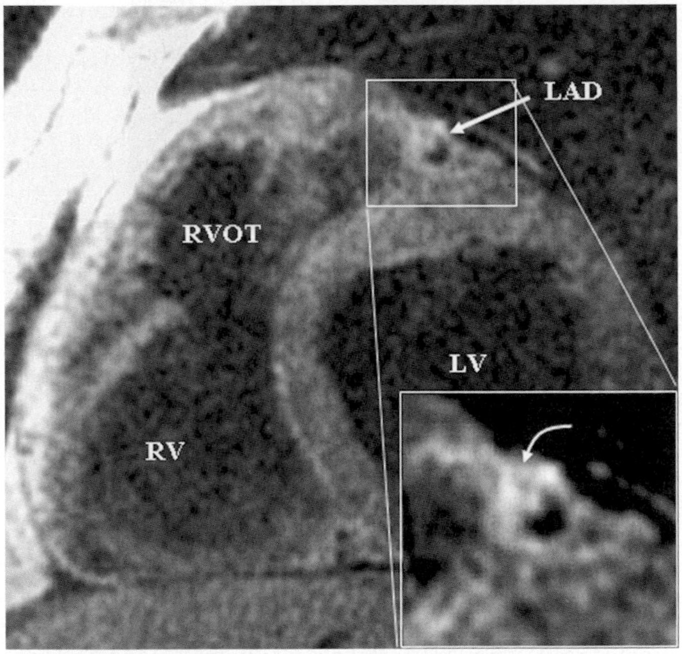

FIGURE 17–8 Coronary wall cardiovascular magnetic resonance (CMR). Short-axis cut of the ventricles at the base of the heart, with the left anterior descending artery (LAD) lying in the interventricular groove. This is enlarged in the **inset,** in which a substantial eccentric plaque is identified (curved arrow). The lumen is still widely patent. LV = left ventricle; RV = right ventricle; RVOT = right ventricular outflow tract. *(From Fayad ZA, Fuster V, Fallon JT, et al: Noninvasive in vivo human coronary artery lumen and wall imaging using black-blood magnetic resonance imaging. Circulation 102:506, 2000.)*

plaque burden, and plaque characterization, including vulnerability. Most CMR data have been derived from work on the aorta and carotid and brachial arteries, but more coronary wall studies have been published (Fig. 17-8).

Endothelial function is considered one of the earliest triggers of atherosclerosis. As with ultrasound, this can be examined noninvasively by CMR using stimuli that cause arterial vasodilation, such as flow-mediated dilation (endothelium dependent) and direct-acting drugs such as glyceryl trinitrate (endothelium independent). Flow-mediated dilation is assessed by forearm cuff occlusion for a standard time period followed by release, which induces increased endothelial shear, the release of nitric oxide, and arterial dilation. This technique has been performed using CMR on the brachial artery but, unlike ultrasound, which measures arterial diameter, CMR measures arterial area and thus has significant advantages.[59] These include improved determination that the imaging is perpendicular to the vessel, greater immunity to arterial shape changes with transducer application and patient movement during the procedure, and increased sensitivity. Validation studies have been performed in humans using invasive techniques, and repeated measurements by CMR appear to have greater reproducibility than the use of ultrasound, suggesting smaller sample sizes for trials using CMR.[59] An additional advantage of CMR is that flow changes can also be measured directly in response to standard stimuli. Arterial dilation measurements have also been performed by CMR in the proximal coronaries.[60]

The mechanical properties of the arterial wall are significantly affected by sclerosis and, in the aorta, this increases pulse pressure, afterload, and cardiac workload, resulting in reduced organ perfusion. Sclerosis of the vessel wall can be assessed in a number of ways, but CMR has usually been used to measure compliance in the ascending aorta (change of aortic sectional volume normalized to pulse pressure, in μl/mm Hg) and pulse wave velocity around the aortic arch (rate of propagation of the flow wave in early systole, in m/sec). These measures have an age-dependent normal range, are abnormal in early atherosclerosis, and have been shown to be predictive of cardiac events.[61]

Arterial wall CMR can also be used to identify total plaque burden within an imaging volume. Plaque burden is usually assessed on T1-weighted images with double or triple inversion to suppress blood signal in the lumen. Quantification of the vessel wall volume over the imaging stack is achieved by planimetry summation of the difference between the outer and inner vessel boundaries in each image. This total vessel volume includes the normal vessel wall and atherosclerotic burden, which is dominant in disease and dynamic for longitudinal studies of natural history and treatment. CMR studies have shown sufficient sensitivity to measure the effectiveness of antiatheroma therapy such as statin treatment over 12 months, showing a reduction in total wall volume.[62] The technique has been extended to the coronary arteries, and wall thickening has been identified.[63] Studies at 3 T are promising in this regard.[64]

Plaque constituents can be assessed using a combination of T1-, T2-, and proton density–weighted images, which allows assessment of plaque vulnerability.[65] Cholesterol pools are identified from low signal on T1 and T2 images,[66] and the fibrous cap can be identified overlying this.[67] Thin or disrupted caps on CMR have been strongly linked with cerebrovascular events.[68] Contrast agents have been used to characterize plaque further and show inflammation,[69] neovasculature,[70] and the fibrous cap.[71] Early results of molecular imaging to identify plaque constituents have shown promise.[72] Longitudinal study by CMR has followed changes in the lipid pool.[73] Coronary plaque constituents have also been identified, but improved resolution is needed to improve assessment in these small vessels.[63]

Cardiomyopathy

DILATED CARDIOMYOPATHY (see Chap. 64). CMR demonstrates the functional abnormalities in dilated cardiomyopathy (DCM), and ventricular volumetric analysis is useful for follow-up. The right ventricle is usually involved in DCM, which may be a useful diagnostic marker. The quantitative effects of therapy can be assessed.[14,15] A key clinical question in the diagnosis of DCM is its differentiation from heart failure resulting from CAD. In many centers, coronary angiography is routinely performed for this. In those patients with unobstructed coronary arteries and no other causative factor, the diagnosis of DCM is usually made. This differentiation is important clinically for several reasons in patients with CAD: they have a worse prognosis; they may benefit from revascularization and/or aneurysmectomy; and secondary preventive pharmacotherapy with statins and aspirin are indicated. Conversely, in DCM patients, secondary causes, such as excess ethanol ingestion or myocardial iron overload,[74] need to be excluded and, as genetic studies of DCM begin to identify inherited abnormalities, accurate phenotyping and family screening are important for early diagnosis. Late gadolinium enhancement CMR has been shown to be very useful in this respect. In a study of heart failure patients with the clinical diagnosis of DCM following normal coronary angiography, 59 percent showed no gadolinium enhancement, 28 percent showed patchy or longitudinal striae of midwall enhancement, which is clearly different than that of the distribution in CAD patients, and 13 percent showed gadolinium enhancement indistinguishable from patients with CAD (Fig. 17-9).[75] These data suggest that using the coronary angiogram as the arbiter for the presence of LV dysfunction resulting from CAD could have led to an incorrect assignment of DCM cause, possibly because of postinfarction coronary recanalization. The midwall myocardial enhancement in DCM patients correlates with fibrosis found at autopsy, has not been visualized in vivo with other techniques, and predicts an adverse outcome.[76] CMR is useful therefore in the diagnostic workup of DCM by allowing direct and highly sensitive assessment of the myocardial substrate for CAD, rather than relying on the coronary angiogram, which yields problems with false-positive results (e.g., incidental coronary disease in DCM that has not caused myocardial infarction[77,78]) and false-negative results (e.g., normal coronaries despite previous myocardial damage, caused by arterial recanalization). Such accurate phenotyping is particularly useful for genotyping and providing family counseling. CMR spectroscopy can also be used to assess prognosis in DCM, in which adverse outcomes are predicted by a low PCr/ATP ratio.

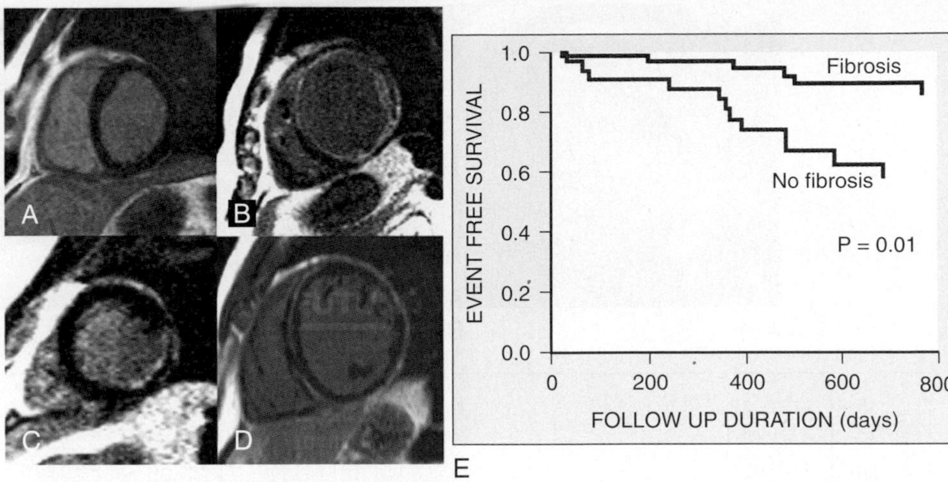

FIGURE 17–9 A-D, Images relating to late gadolinium-enhanced cardiovascular magnetic resonance (CMR) in dilated cardiomyopathy (DCM). **A,** Patient with DCM and no gadolinium enhancement. **B,** Patient with known previous myocardial infarction resulting in heart failure. Late gadolinium enhancement is seen throughout the subendocardium, causing thinning particularly in the septum and inferolateral wall. **C,** Patient with the presumed clinical diagnosis of DCM because of the presence of a dilated heart with symptoms of heart failure but with normal coronary arteries by coronary angiography. This late gadolinium-enhanced CMR image clearly shows an inferolateral infarction despite the normal coronary arteries, and it is likely that this patient's heart failure relates to coronary disease and not DCM. **D,** Patient with DCM who has late gadolinium enhancement of the midwall of the septum in the ventricular circumferential fibers. This pattern of fibrosis is recognized by pathologists, but has not been previously visualized in vivo. **E,** Kaplan-Meier survival curves of the occurrence of major cardiac events in patients with proven DCM according to the presence of intramural fibrosis. Fibrosis was a powerful predictor of outcome which was incremental to cardiac volumes and ejection fraction. *(**A-D** from McCrohon JA, Moon JC, Prasad SK, et al: Differentiation of heart failure related to dilated cardiomyopathy and coronary artery disease using gadolinium-enhanced cardiovascular magnetic resonance. Circulation 108:54, 2003; **E** from Assomull RG, Prasad SK, Lyne J, et al: Cardiovascular magnetic resonance, fibrosis, and prognosis in dilated cardiomyopathy. J Am Coll Cardiol 48:1977, 2006.)*

HYPERTROPHIC CARDIOMYOPATHY (see Chap. 65). CMR is very useful in the diagnosis and assessment of hypertrophic cardiomyopathy (HCM), with comprehensive coverage of both ventricles for localization of hypertrophy. CMR may be used as a first-line test because of superior identification of regional hypertrophy, particularly in the basal anteroseptal wall[79] and apex.[80] Cines oriented in the plane of the LV outflow tract show obstruction, and velocity mapping can be used to assess peak velocities. Systolic anterior motion of the mitral valve is also clearly seen. Improvement in obstruction after septal ablation or resection can be demonstrated, as well as the location and size of the associated infarction with late gadolinium enhancement, which is helpful for planning repeat procedures. CMR myocardial tagging identifies abnormal patterns of strain, shear, and torsion in HCM, demonstrating significant dysfunction in hypertrophic areas. CMR spectroscopy shows bioenergetic defects in HCM patients with varying genetic mutations, which supports the hypothesis that the underlying substrate for HCM might be inefficient energy uptake.[81] The accuracy of the phenotypic determination of HCM by CMR is helpful for family screening, and genetic linkage studies for causative mutations have been improved. Late gadolinium enhancement occurs in HCM, which represents myocardial fibrosis.[82] Most patients have no gadolinium enhancement, and a common benign pattern is two stripes running along the junction of the RV insertion into the left ventricle. Enhancement is more commonly seen in hypertrophic areas than elsewhere. More extensive gadolinium enhancement can be dense and plaque-like or diffuse. The greater the gadolinium enhancement, the higher the risk of heart failure or sudden death, presumably because of reentrant tachycardias and systolic failure from myocyte replacement (Fig. 17-10).[83] More work needs to be done in this promising area. CMR has also proved useful in differentiating causes of hypertrophy, which can mimic HCM. This

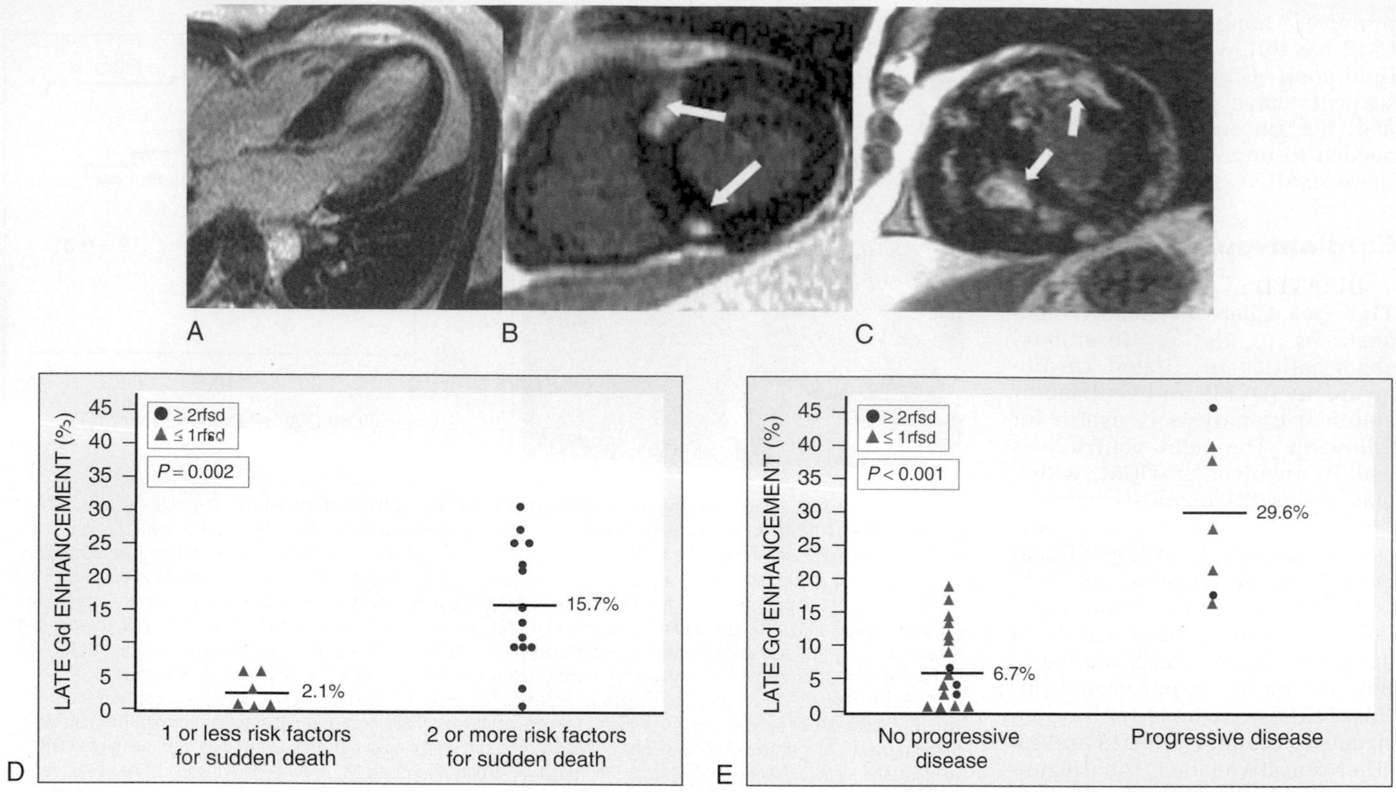

FIGURE 17–10 Late gadolinium enhancement and risk assessment in hypertrophic cardiomyopathy (HCM). **A,** HCM patient with no gadolinium enhancement. **B,** HCM patient with longitudinal striae of late gadolinium enhancement at the insertion points of the right ventricle into the left ventricle (arrows), **C,** HCM patient with extensive plaque-like fibrosis (arrows). The relationship between the extent of late gadolinium enhancement and the number of risk factors for sudden death (rfsd) is shown in **D** and documented progression of ventricular dilation toward heart failure is shown in **E.** In both cases, extensive gadolinium enhancement indicated a poor prognosis. *(From Moon JCC, McKenna WJ, McCrohon JA, et al: Toward clinical risk assessment in hypertrophic cardiomyopathy with gadolinium cardiovascular magnetic resonance. J Am Coll Cardiol 41:1561, 2003.)*

includes Fabry disease (α-galactoside deficiency) which occurs in 4 percent of HCM populations. It is an X-linked genetic disorder causing accumulation of glycosphingolipid in myocytes and endothelium, in which CMR shows unusual lateral wall gadolinium enhancement.[84] Other differential diagnoses, including amyloidosis[85] and athletic heart,[86] can be distinguished by CMR.

IRON OVERLOAD CARDIOMYOPATHY (see Chap. 64). Iron overload, or siderotic cardiomyopathy, occurs in patients with severe inherited anemia who require regular blood transfusions. The iron load of the transfusions may be exacerbated by increased intestinal iron absorption in anemia. This leads to tissue iron deposition because the body has no mechanism for iron excretion. The iron is toxic and causes oxidative cellular damage and organ dysfunction. The most important of these conditions is beta-thalassemia major, in which 71 percent die from heart failure at a young age. This is a substantial worldwide health problem, with 60,000 affected children born annually who require long-term treatment. It has not been possible so far to measure cardiac iron levels except by myocardial biopsy, which is highly problematic. This has led to usual clinical management based on blood ferritin and liver iron levels, but this is patently unsuccessful in identifying those at risk of heart failure. Recently, CMR has been introduced with measurement of myocardial T2*, which is a relaxation parameter that is directly related to tissue iron.[87] A low myocardial T2*, below 20 milliseconds, indicates iron overload,[74] and this correlates with LV dysfunction and increased ventricular volumes and mass, providing clinical validation of the technique (Fig. 17-11). Myocardial T2* increases as iron is cleared from the heart with iron chelation, and this is associated with LV function recovery.[88] CMR has demonstrated differential effects of different chelators on myocardial iron,[89] which has improved management of cardiac siderosis[90] and has been linked with improved mortality.[91] The T2* CMR sequence can be completed in a single breath-hold and should prove cost-effective in areas with large numbers of affected people, such as in Asia and the Mediterranean.

ARRHYTHMOGENIC RIGHT VENTRICULAR CARDIOMYOPATHY (see Chaps. 35 and 64). CMR is widely used in specialized centers for the investigation of arrhythmogenic right ventricular dysplasia (ARVD) because of good depiction of the structural and functional abnormalities of the right ventricle, with no limitation from the retrosternal location. The diagnostic criteria of ARVD are well defined, and the genetic understanding of this disease as a desmosomopathy is advanced.[92] CMR is helpful in ascertaining whether there are RV regional wall motion abnormalities, increased volumes, morphological abnormalities, and fibrous or fatty infiltration. Follow-up of the quantitative parameters over time can also be clinically useful. Problems occur if the CMR images are overinterpreted, because the right ventricle has substantial normal variation, including reduced regional wall motion in the region of the moderator band insertion, highly variable trabeculation, and substantial fat around the coronary vessels and epicardium. Therefore, sufficient experience in recognizing the normal variants is important. In addition, it is important to recognize the limitations of CMR, because poor-quality breath-holds with fast spin-echo images may lead to the misinterpretation of artifacts as wall thinning, not distinguishing epicardial fat clearly from RV myocardium, and artifacts giving rise to increased wall RV signal that mimics that of fat. Fatty infiltration is not considered a definitive sign of the disease in any case, because it may occur in other circumstances. Late gadolinium enhancement has been used in ARVD, and preliminary results have suggested that RV fibrosis can be identified.[93] Left ventricular forms (so-called arrhythmogenic left ventricular dysplasia, ALVD) have also been reported, in which CMR is very helpful.[94] It is also clear that crossover variants exist that can mimic DCM. An abnormal CMR scan has been linked to an adverse prognosis,[95] but more work needs to be done in this area.

MYOCARDIAL SARCOIDOSIS (see Chap. 64). Myocardial sarcoidosis is uncommon, but sudden death may be its initial clinical presentation. Standard imaging techniques suffer from low diagnostic accuracy, and the clinical diagnosis is difficult. CMR is valuable, with gadolinium enhancement occurring in presumed areas of fibrosis.[96,97] Enhancement may decrease after steroid treatment and is therefore a potential

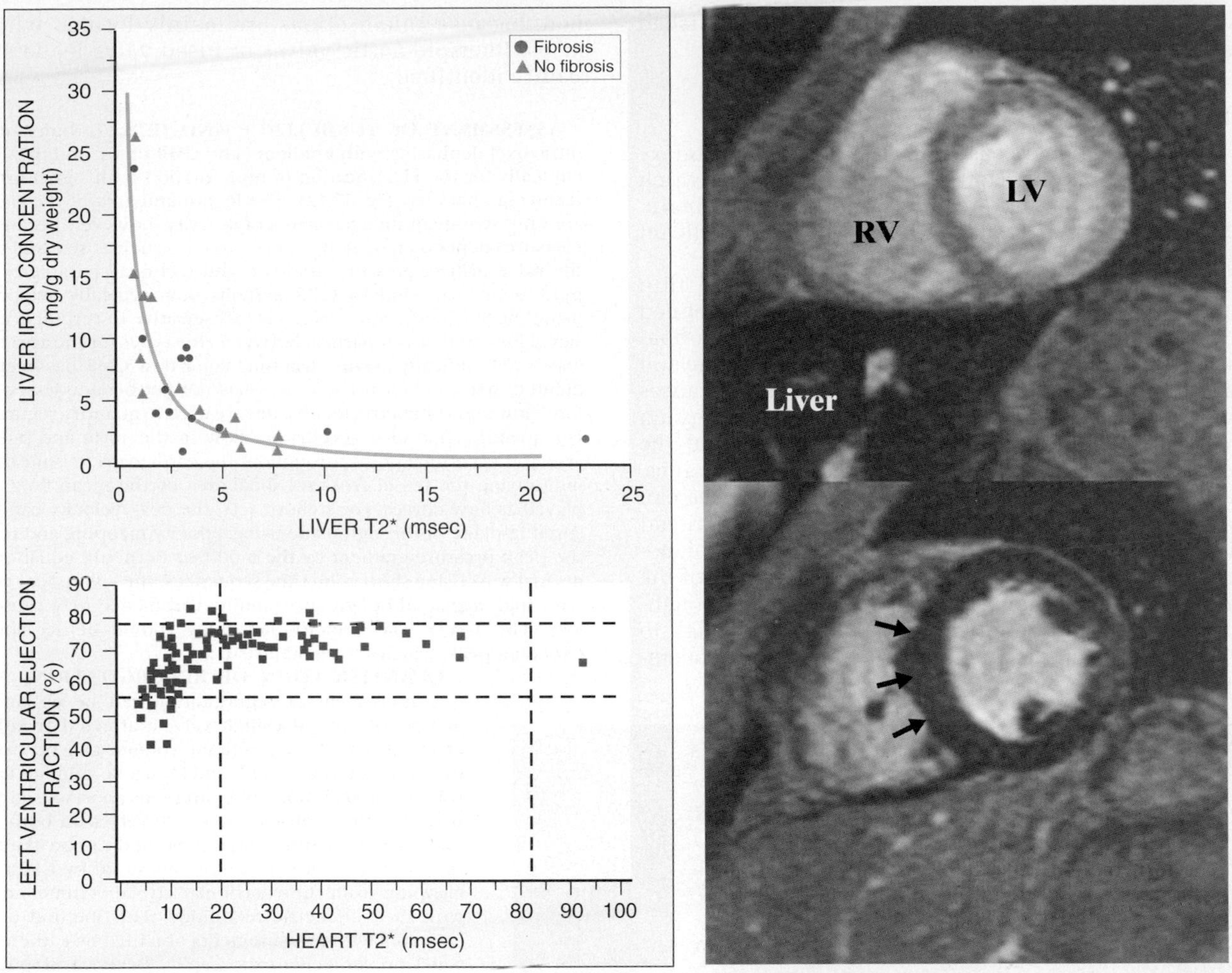

FIGURE 17–11 T2* cardiovascular magnetic resonance (CMR) in patients with iron overload cardiomyopathy. **Left,** Tissue calibration between T2* of the liver and liver biopsy is shown in the **upper graph.** The fit is best for the nonfibrotic liver samples, as expected. The curvilinear relationship is transformed into a linear relationship with a log-log plot. **Lower graph,** Relationship between myocardial T2* and the left ventricular ejection fraction. Normal values for heart T2* are greater than 20 milliseconds and, in this range, the ejection fraction is normal. Below this range, there is a marked fall in ejection fraction related to iron toxicity. The two CMR scans **(right panel)** are short-axis cuts showing both the ventricular myocardium and the liver. **Top,** Iron-loaded liver (dark) but normal heart appearance. If there were concern about this patient's heart iron status, liver biopsy would suggest iron loading, which could lead to an increase in chelation therapy with desferrioxamine and the risk of significant side effects. **Bottom,** The opposite scenario is shown, in which the liver has a normal signal but the heart is iron-loaded (dark, arrows). Should this patient have a liver biopsy, the result would be falsely reassuring; chelation therapy would not be increased, and the patient would be at risk of death from heart failure and arrhythmias. These disparities in iron between the heart and liver help explain why heart failure is the greatest cause of mortality in thalassemia patients. LV = left ventricle; RV = right ventricle. *(From Anderson LJ, Holden S, Davies B, et al: Cardiovascular T2* magnetic resonance for the early diagnosis of myocardial iron overload. Eur Heart J 22:2171, 2001.)*

therapeutic marker of myocardial activity.[98] The use of T2-weighted sequences is helpful in identifying active myocardial inflammation.[98]

MYOCARDIAL AMYLOIDOSIS. CMR is useful in amyloidosis, which can be recognized by morphofunctional features such as diastolic dysfunction, ventricular hypertrophy, and interatrial septum thickening. In addition, typical late gadolinium enhancement is widespread and greatest in the subendocardium.[85] The myocardial amyloid load leads to substantial myocardial gadolinium uptake, and this lowers the global myocardial T1. In principle, therefore, myocardial T1 can be used to monitor myocardial amyloid burden,[85] which is not otherwise possible.

MYOCARDITIS (see Chap. 66). The diagnosis and investigation of myocarditis using conventional techniques have been difficult. CMR has transformed this situation, allowing a confident diagnosis and differentiation from other acute conditions. CMR shows patchy increases of myocardial signal in acute myocarditis using late gadolinium enhancement CMR, which is typically subepicardial and involves the inferolateral wall.[99] Involvement of the septum may also occur, and there is evidence that different viruses affect different myocardial locations. Interestingly, detecting virus using LV myocardial biopsy is improved when guided by prior CMR. Relative myocardial T1 enhancement compared with skeletal muscle also occurs, and edema is identified by T2-weighted CMR.[100] Normalization of late gadolinium enhancement often occurs with healing, because patchy dead cell resorption leaves microscars, which are beyond the resolution of CMR. Residual midwall striae such as those found in DCM have also been reported. Anthracycline toxicity has also been shown to increase relative myocardial T1 enhancement, presumably through inflammatory mechanisms.

Heart Transplantation

Acute rejection results in an increase in myocardial mass, reduction in ventricular function, high myocardial signal intensity, and increased T2, which occur with myocardial edema or cellular infiltration. These changes are not reliable indicators of acute rejection, particularly in the early stages. In early rejection, decreased PCr/ATP ratios are evident by

CMR spectroscopy, although this has to be distinguished from ischemia.

Valvular Heart Disease (see Chap. 62)

CMR is useful in valve disease but often plays a secondary role to echocardiography. However, in situations in which adequate echocardiographic results are difficult to obtain, particularly in valvular regurgitation, CMR has significant clinical usefulness.[101]

VALVE MORPHOLOGY. Normal heart valves are thin and rapidly moving, and the leaflets become well defined on CMR on a routine basis only with the use of breath-hold sequences. Abnormal valves are thicker and less mobile and are thus more easily visualized, but calcification causes local signal loss, which may obscure valve pathology on black-blood images. Valve leaflet function throughout the cardiac cycle is well assessed using gradient echo cines, especially with the latest SSFP techniques. Valve area can be assessed by direct planimetry using a cross-sectional plane immediately downstream from the valve, and plane-following techniques can be used to ensure tracking of the valve movement throughout the cycle to eliminate through-plane motion errors. Calcification has the potential to increase valve area on direct planimetry but this is uncommon, because calcifications are mainly located within the cusps. Bicuspid aortic valves or fused valve leaflets can be readily identified.

ASSESSMENT OF TURBULENCE AND JETS. Turbulence causes intravoxel dephasing with gradient echo CMR cines, and this is useful clinically for the identification of regurgitation with signal loss in the receiving chamber (Fig. 17-12). The length and area of the signal loss are only semiquantitive measures of severity, however, because these measures depend on hemodynamic variables such as size and shape of the valve orifice, pressure gradient, and technical parameters of the pulse sequence. Modern CMR systems now typically acquire cines using the SSFP technique, which is less sensitive to turbulence-related signal loss, so that comparison between cine types for the area of signal loss is not clinically useful. Real-time color flow CMR has been implemented, but its clinical usefulness has not yet been assessed. Therefore, flow and volumetric techniques are used to quantify regurgitation. For quantification of regurgitation, flow in the aorta and pulmonary artery at each time point throughout the cardiac cycle is measured by multiplying the vessel cross-sectional area by the mean flow and displayed as flow curves. For stenotic jets, the peak velocity can be measured in-plane or through-plane using velocity mapping and related to the peak pressure gradient by the modified Bernoulli equation in the normal way. Using short echo time sequences, the jets appear coherent with high signal, although surrounding turbulence may cause signal loss (Fig. 17-13). The velocity sensitivity should be set above the expected peak velocity to avoid aliasing.

QUANTIFICATION OF REGURGITATION. Quantitative assessment of regurgitation can be obtained in a number of ways. If a single valve is affected on either side of the heart, the regurgitant volume can be calculated from the difference of RV and LV stroke volumes using the volumetric technique of contiguous short-axis cine slices spanning the ventricles. If single valves on both sides of the heart are regurgitant, the method can be extended by subtracting great vessel flow measured by CMR velocity mapping from the ventricular stroke volumes measured with the volumetric technique. This method compares favorably with measurements obtained by catheterization and Doppler echocardiography. Reversal of pulmonary vein flow indicates severe mitral regurgitation, as with echocardiography. Direct methods for measuring systolic regurgitant flow and ventricular inflow at the mitral annulus level are less satisfactory because of annulus motion and jet eccentricity. An alternative technique for measurement of pulmonary or aortic regurgitation is the direct assessment of regurgitation using flow mapping immediately downstream of the valve by measuring the retrograde volume flow after valve closure (see Fig. 62-44). The diastolic backflow is divided into the systolic forward flow to derive a regurgitant fraction. This simple

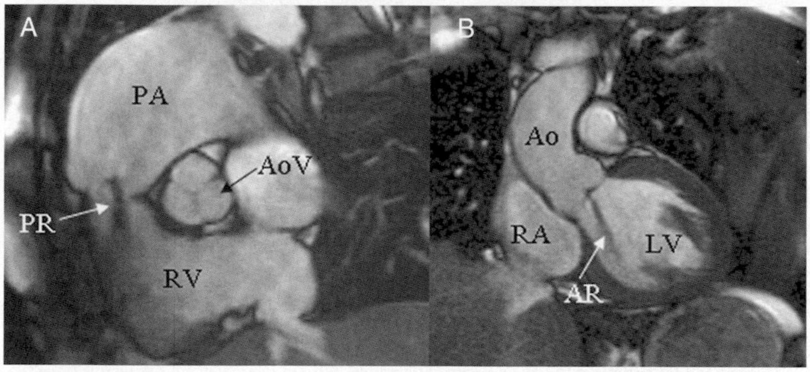

FIGURE 17–12 Cardiovascular magnetic resonance (CMR) of valvular regurgitation. **A,** Patient with pulmonary hypertension with a dilated pulmonary artery. The images are from a steady state with free precession (SSFP) cine in diastole, and the aortic valve (AoV) is seen to be closed. A jet of pulmonary regurgitation (PR) can be seen entering the right ventricle. **B,** Patient with aortic regurgitation (AR) in the coronal plane (arrow). Ao = aorta; LV = left ventricle; PA = pulmonary artery; RA = right atrium; RV = right ventricle.

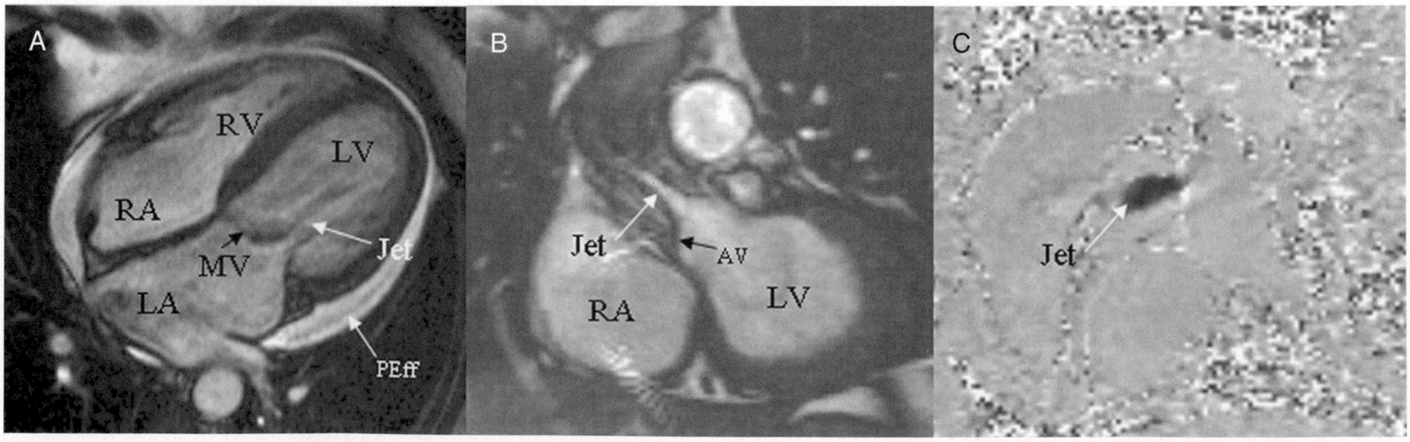

FIGURE 17–13 Cardiovascular magnetic resonance (CMR) of valvular stenosis. **A,** Diastolic frame from a four-chamber steady state with free precession (SSFP) cine. The mitral valve (MV) is thickened and there is poor opening, with jet formation and surrounding signal loss from turbulence (Jet). The left atrium (LA) is enlarged and there is pericardial effusion (PEff). **B,** Aortic stenosis, with central bright jet formation and surrounding signal loss from turbulence. **C,** Velocity map taken through the aortic stenotic jet, with a measured velocity of 4.3 m/sec equal to a calculated pressure drop of 74 mm Hg. AV = aortic valve; LA = left atrium; LV = left ventricle; PA = pulmonary artery; RA = right atrium; RV = right ventricle.

technique has been used to assess responses to treatment. It has good interstudy reproducibility, suggesting that it may be valuable for longitudinal follow-up of regurgitation severity over time.

QUANTIFICATION OF STENOSIS. To quantify the velocity of a jet through a valve stenosis, it is necessary to adjust the imaging parameters so that signal is present in the jet core. For higher velocities, this requires a very short TE to prevent signal loss or other artifacts that would interfere with the measurement. Turbulence around the jet core is usual, appears dark on the cine, and does not interfere with measurements within the jet. There is good agreement between CMR and other techniques for evaluating mitral and aortic valve stenosis.[102] The valve area can also be measured by direct planimetry in aortic stenosis.[103] Because echocardiography is usually the first-line clinical test to investigate valve stenosis (see Chap. 14), CMR is used when acoustic windows are poor or when discordant imaging and invasive results occur. Improved LV and microvascular function and reduced hypertrophy,[104] as well as improved myocardial metabolism and diastolic function, have been shown by CMR after valve replacement for aortic stenosis. Comparisons of the results of different bioprosthetic valves on LV function have also been performed using CMR.[105]

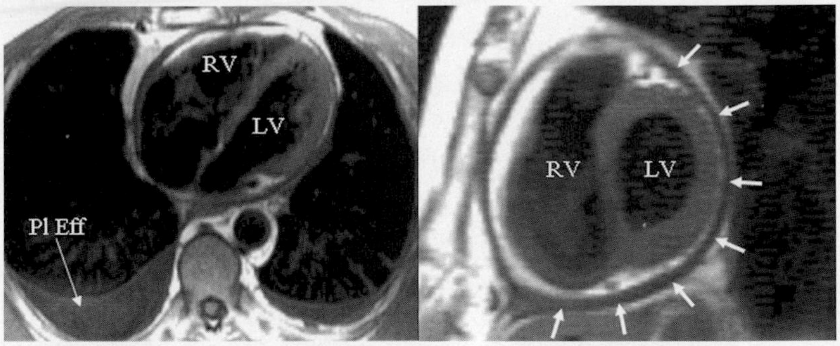

FIGURE 17–14 Cardiovascular magnetic resonance (CMR) of constrictive pericarditis. **Right panel,** Basal short-axis view of the ventricles, showing a thickened pericardium encasing the heart (arrows). **Left panel,** Transaxial view, again showing the thickened pericardium, particularly over the right heart, but also a pleural effusion (Pl Eff). LV = left ventricle; RV = right ventricle.

PROSTHETIC VALVES. CMR of all prosthetic heart valves at 1.5 T is safe, because there is no substantial magnetic interaction and heating is negligible. However, metallic valve components produce artifacts and signal loss, which are mild on spin-echo images but more apparent on gradient-echo cines. Small paravalvular jets may be obscured by the artifact but velocity profiles close to aortic valve prostheses have been measured using valve tracking techniques.

Diseases of the Pericardium (see Chap. 70)

CMR is well suited to define functional and anatomical abnormalities associated with the pericardium,[106] but is mainly used when echocardiography yields incomplete information. CMR is very sensitive in detection of pericardial effusion, which has high signal intensity with SSFP cine imaging and has clinical value when the effusion is loculated or complex. Signal from effusion is usually low on spin-echo images. Pericardial constriction is usually but not invariably associated with pericardial thickening, and this is well depicted with both spin-echo and gradient-echo imaging (Fig. 17-14). The signal of the normal pericardium is low, and appears as a thin dark line between fat outside the visceral and parietal layers. The thickness in normal subjects is 1 to 2 mm, but the upper range of normal for CMR is usually taken as 4 mm, which allows for chemical shift signal cancellation effects at the fat-pericardium border. Pericardial thickening is often inhomogeneous in acute and chronic pericardial disease, and the signal characteristics can be variable. Acute inflammation may give rise to a pericardium with increased signal on spin-echo images that enhances early after gadolinium. It is important to distinguish pericardial thickening from pericardial effusion, because both may appear dark on spin-echo images, and this is achieved by using cine sequences. Calcium is not seen directly by CMR but appears dark, and computed tomography (CT) should be used if this information is clinically required. Other pericardial abnormalities can also be identified by CMR. Cysts have characteristic signal intensity, with low signal on T1-weighted spin-echo images, but high signal with T2 weighting. Complete absence of the pericardium is indicated by a leftward shift of the long axis of the heart, and partial absence is seen as a protrusion of a portion of the heart.

Cardiac Tumors (see Chap. 69)

Cardiac tumors are usually first diagnosed or suspected following transthoracic echocardiography, often as an incidental finding. Information can be obtained by echocardiography about tumor localization, origin, extent, and resectability but characterization may well be incomplete. CMR may then be very helpful.[107] The wide field of view of CMR significantly improves the delineation of the relationship of the tumor to adjacent structures for surgical planning, as well as for identifying infiltration into the pericardium. CMR also offers a number of means of tumor characterization, which may have important clinical value. The most obvious example is that of a well-circumscribed high signal intensity lesion that shows complete signal suppression using fat saturation techniques, which is diagnostic of lipoma (Fig. 17-15). A variant of this diagnosis that is also very well demonstrated by CMR is atrial lipomatous hypertrophy. Alternatively, an irregular tumor that shows signal increase during the first-pass bolus of gadolinium (perfusion), significant early tissue enhancement (increased vascularity), and significant late enhancement (fibrosis or necrosis) is typically an angiosarcoma (Fig. 17-16). Other useful signal characteristics include a high T1-weighted signal in recent hemorrhage (caused by the paramagnetic effects of the breakdown of hemoglobin), cysts with high protein content, and melanoma. In contrast, there is a low T1-weighted signal in cysts with low protein content, calcified lesions, or air. There is a high T2-weighted signal in cysts. With gadolinium-enhanced imaging, there is a high signal during the first pass of the contrast agent in hemangioma (noninvasive) and angiosarcoma (invasive), necrotic areas highlighted against surrounding enhancement in malignant tumors 1 to 2 minutes after intravenous gadolinium, absence of early gadolinium enhancement in most benign tumors with the exclusion of hemangioma and myxoma, and late gadolinium enhancement in fibrosis and its absence in cysts. The clinical setting and location of the tumor also yield important diagnostic information.

Finally, CMR is excellent at identifying thrombus. Thrombus is usually hypointense on SSFP cines. On spin-echo images, thrombus is usually visible against the black blood pool and, in the subacute phase, may have areas of high signal intensity resulting from the paramagnetic effect of hemoglobin breakdown products. Thrombus is also identified with high accuracy using an inversion recovery technique, with a long inversion time 2 minutes after gadolinium injection. The thrombus has low vascularity and appears as a dark area surrounded by intense blood and myocardial signal.

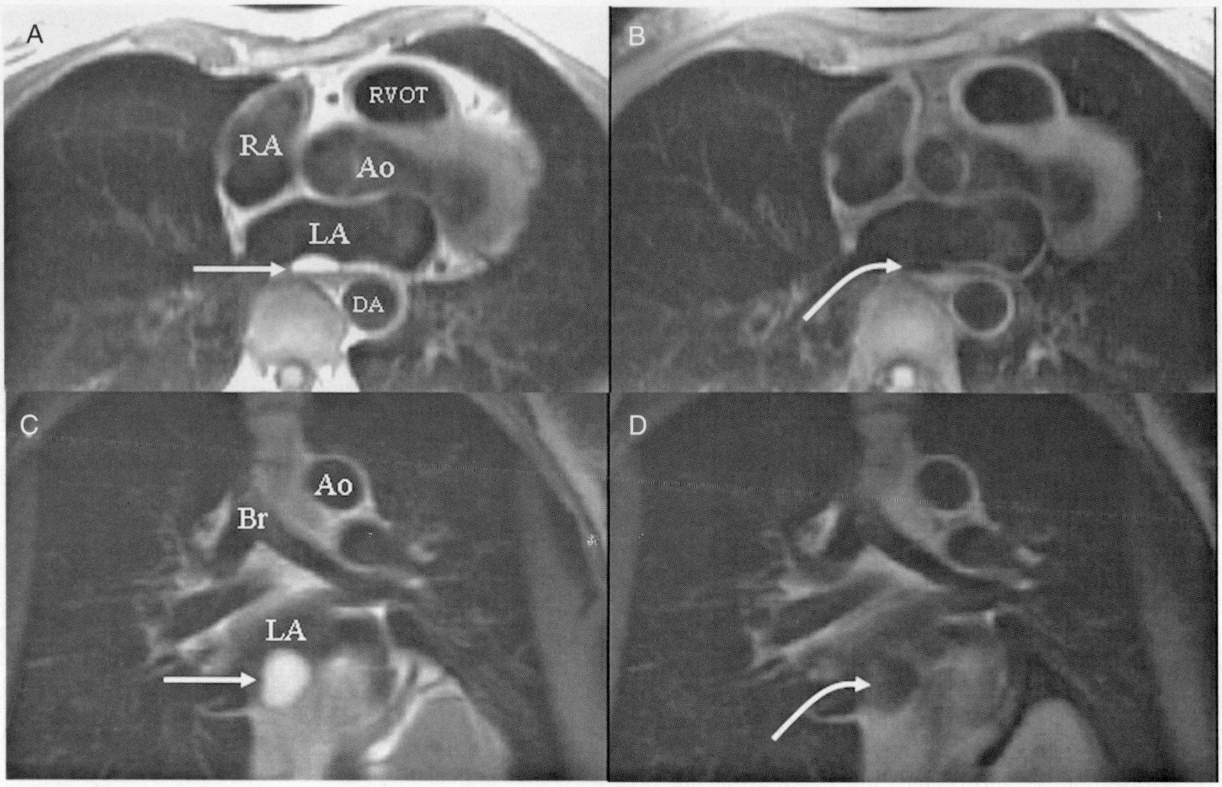

FIGURE 17–15 Cardiovascular magnetic resonance (CMR) images of retroatrial lipoma. **A, B,** Transaxial cuts through the heart. **C, D,** Coronal cuts posteriorly. A tumor is present posterior to the left atrium (straight arrow). **B, D,** Equivalent images with fat suppression turned on and abolition of signal within the tumor (curved arrow), therefore confirming the diagnosis of lipoma. Ao = aorta; Br = bronchus; DA = descending aorta; LA = left atrium; LV = left ventricle; RA = right atrium; RVOT = right ventricular outflow tract.

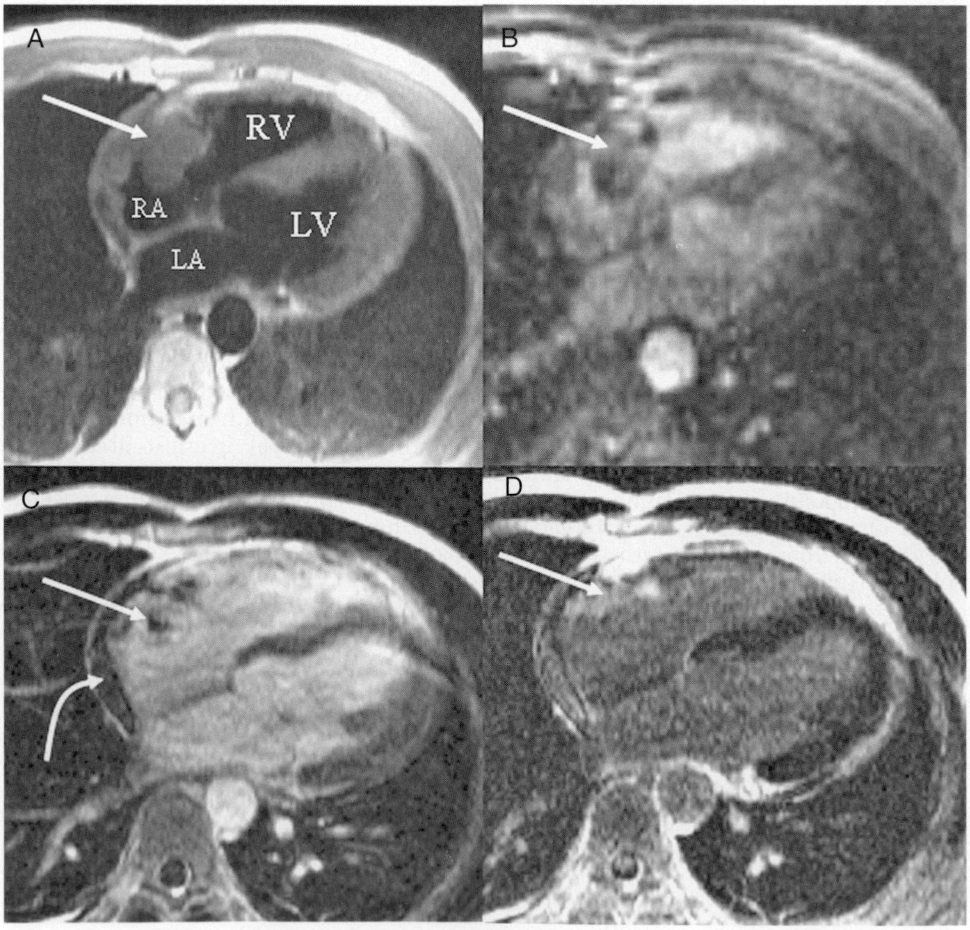

FIGURE 17–16 Cardiovascular magnetic resonance (CMR) images of right atrial angiosarcoma. All images are in the transaxial plane at the same level. **A,** T1-weighted spin-echo image showing a tumor (straight arrow) in the right atrial wall. For characterization, gadolinium was given intravenously as a bolus. **B,** Image taken during the first pass of gadolinium. There is considerable signal within the tumor, indicating high vascularity (arrow). **C,** Inversion recovery image taken 1 to 2 minutes after injection, showing areas of absent signal within the tumor compatible with microvascular obstruction (straight arrow). There is also a pericardial effusion best seen in this image (curved arrow). **D,** Late gadolinium enhancement. The tumor has a high signal, indicating fibrosis. All these features taken together indicate a likely diagnosis of angiosarcoma, and this was confirmed at operation. LA = left atrium; LV = left ventricle; RA = right atrium; RV = right ventricle.

Congenital Heart Disease (see Chap. 61)

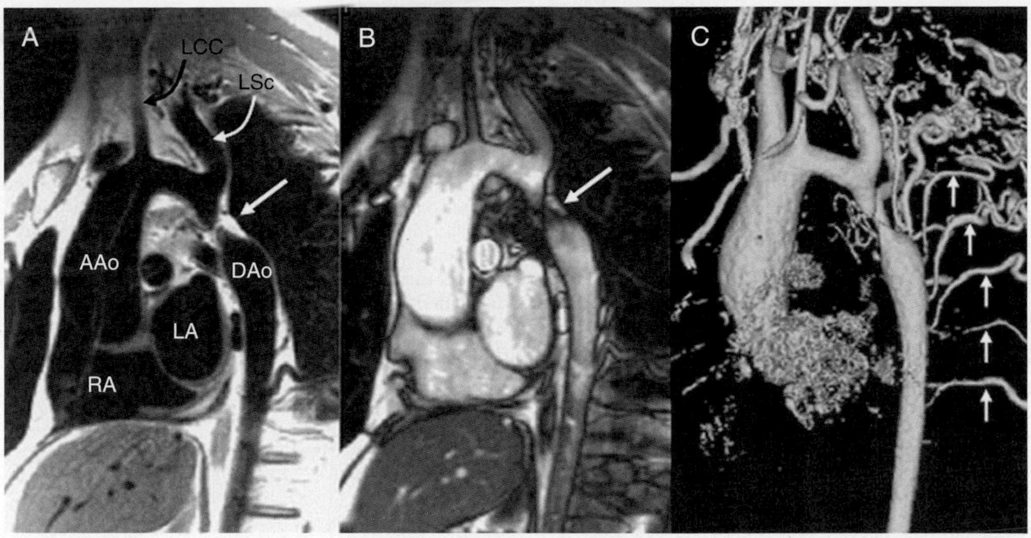

FIGURE 17–17 Cardiovascular magnetic resonance (CMR) images of aortic coarctation. **A,** Oblique sagittal view showing the ascending aorta (AAo), which is dilated, giving rise to dilated left common carotid (LCC) and left subclavian (LSc) arteries. Immediately distal to the left subclavian is the coarctation (straight arrow), after which the descending aorta (DAo) is formed. Similar findings are seen in **B,** which shows one frame from a steady state with free precession (SSFP) cine. **C,** Projection from a three-dimensional CMR angiogram, which shows multiple intercostal collateral arteries joining the descending aorta (small arrows); these can be responsible for rib notching on the chest x-ray. LA = left atrium; RA = right atrium. *(With permission from Babu-Narayan SV, Kilner PJ, Gatzoulis MA: When to order cardiovascular magnetic resonance in adults with congenital heart disease. Curr Cardiol Rep 5:324, 2003.)*

CMR is ideally suited for the evaluation of congenital heart disease (CHD) for several reasons. Three-dimensional contiguous data sets are very effective for the complete depiction of anatomy, functional assessments are readily combined with the anatomical data, and CMR is less operator-dependent than echocardiography.[108,109] In addition, long-term follow-up is greatly facilitated by good reproducibility, noninvasiveness, access to relatively unrestricted fields of view, and freedom from ionizing radiation. The combination of CMR with transesophageal echocardiography has been particularly effective in patient evaluation, because the two investigations often yield complementary information. Hence, the need for invasive catheterization has diminished in recent years. However, the ease of use and value of CMR depend on the age and clinical condition of the patient. For small children, anesthesia or sedation is required for CMR and monitoring may be demanding; echocardiography is usually adequate. The contributions of CMR tend to increase in older children and adults. CMR is also relatively more effective in evaluating patients with more complex anatomy and in the many patients now surviving after surgery, because scar tissue and limitations of acoustic access are increasing problems for echocardiography. CMR is thus the preferred technique for the serial evaluation of RV volumes, mass, and function,[13] valvular regurgitation, the pulmonary arteries, and extracardiac conduits. Expertise in CMR is highly recommended in centers specialized in the care of patients with congenital heart disease.

GREAT VESSEL ABNORMALITIES. Coarctation usually occurs in the proximal descending aorta opposite the ductus arteriosus, just distal to the left subclavian artery. CMR is the optimal technique for assessment of coarctation (Fig. 17-17), especially in adults and after operative repair. CMR identifies the coarctation site and extent, any involvement of arch vessels, and poststenotic dilation. Velocity mapping of the coarctation jet yields a pressure gradient in most cases, and the jet duration into diastole is a useful index of severity. Usually, CMR angiography is performed to assess the size of collateral vessels, but flow mapping of upper and lower sites in the descending aorta may also be used to assess the volume of collateral flow. Long-term follow-up is advised for these patients because of the complications of restenosis and repair site aneurysms. Tortuosity of the isthmal region without significant obstruction (pseudocoarctation) occurs with no significant narrowing or jet formation and no collateral flow.

CMR displays vascular rings in detail, including the relationship between aortic arch anomalies and other structures. A double aortic arch may cause compression from encirclement of the trachea and esophagus. A vascular sling is also well demonstrated by CMR, in which an anomalous left pulmonary artery arises from the right pulmonary artery and courses between the trachea and esophagus and back to the left lung, which can result in airway compression. In infants, patent ductus arteriosus is usually well visualized by echocardiography, but CMR has a role in older patients. CMR is also useful in depicting the aortopulmonary window. CMR is valuable in anomalous pulmonary venous drainage, in which some or all of the pulmonary veins do not enter the left atrium. Anomalous pulmonary veins may be missed with conventional cardiological investigation, but the anatomy is easily visualized with standard CMR sequences or, more commonly, CMR angiography.[110] CMR correctly identifies anomalies of the systemic venous system (e.g., bilateral superior cava, interrupted inferior cava), including connection to the left heart in patients with occult arterial desaturation. Finally, the pulmonary arteries are well depicted by CMR, including their presence, size, confluence, and relationship to other structures. Main and branch vessel stenosis can be detected, the pressure gradient assessed, and differential pulmonary flow measured. CMR angiography is very effective for demonstrating systemic to pulmonary collateral vessels.[111]

ATRIAL AND VENTRICULAR MORPHOLOGY. The morphological right atrium has a broad-based triangular appendage, whereas the morphological left atrium has a narrow entrance to the appendage, with a tubular configuration. The right atrium is also connected to the inferior vena cava in almost all cases. Furthermore, atrial situs is nearly always concordant with the visceral situs, and therefore the morphological right atrium is on the side of the short main bronchus and liver. The morphological left atrium similarly is on the side of the long main bronchus and the aorta, spleen, and stomach. The morphological right ventricle is characterized by a prominent moderator band, a more apical insertion point of the tricuspid valve into the ventricular septum, and an infundibulum or conus separating the tricuspid and pulmonary valves. The morphological left ventricle is more smoothly contoured toward the apex, lacks a muscular infundibulum, and therefore has a fibrous continuity between the mitral and aortic valves. In situs solitus, the normal atrial arrangement applies; the left pulmonary artery passes over the left main bronchus and the right pulmonary artery runs anterior and slightly inferior to the right bronchus. The atrial arrangement is reversed in situs inversus. In atrial isomerism, both atria are alike and develop sidedness according to the thoracic and abdominal viscera. Left-sided isomerism is associated with polysplenia and right-sided isomerism with asplenia. Because CMR provides anatomical data that can be easily related to the surrounding structures of the body, reliable diagnosis of situs is possible, even in difficult cases.

ATRIOVENTRICULAR CONNECTION ABNORMALITIES. Because of its excellent ability to define the atrial and ventricular morphology, CMR demonstrates atrioventricular discordance well. Atrioventricular discordance is present in congenitally corrected transposition (combined with ventriculoarterial discordance), in which the left atrium drains into the right ventricle, which supplies the systemic arterial circulation. Other abnormalities of atrial connection include atrioventricular valve atresia, connection of both atria to a single ventricle, and connection of one valve to both ventricles. CMR also provides excellent visualization of crisscrossed atrioventricular connections, conditions in which ventricular positions are rotated with respect to the atrium, with connections being concordant or discordant.

VENTRICULOARTERIAL CONNECTION ABNORMALITIES. CMR well demonstrates the anatomy of transposition of the great arteries (discordant ventriculoarterial connections), with the connections between the ventricles and great vessels showing an anterior aorta arising from the morphological right ventricle and the posterior pulmonary artery arising from the morphological left ventricle. CMR is effective for assessing intraatrial baffles after atrial repair of transposition of the great arteries (Fig. 17-18). After arterial switch repair, which has now become the operation of choice, CMR provides good views of the right ventricular outflow tract and pulmonary arteries, which may be stenosed. A double-outlet right ventricle is defined as an abnormal ventriculoarterial connection in which more than half of both the aorta and pulmonary artery arise from the morphological right ventricle. This typically presents with the aorta to the right of the pulmonary artery at the semilunar valve level. An additional feature is a complete muscle rim separating both semilunar valves from the anterior leaflet of the mitral valve. Truncus arteriosus is a failure of the embryonic truncus to separate into an individual aorta and pulmonary artery. A single large artery arises above a ventricular septal defect from which the aorta and pulmonary, and coronary arteries arise, and this is well shown by CMR. Because of the problem with graft degeneration, CMR is valuable for assessing long-term postoperative conduit patency and stenosis, regurgitation, or aneurysm formation. Echocardiography can be limited in evaluating conduits because of their retrosternal position and calcification.

SEPTAL DEFECTS. The anatomy of atrial and ventricular septal defects is usually well delineated by CMR, especially using SSFP sequences. The defect location and size can be determined directly and the systemic-to-pulmonary flow ratio measured, all of which are useful for planning of intervention. The effects on RV function can also be quantified. CMR is relatively more valuable than echocardiography in patients with more complex anatomy, especially those with additional abnormalities. In addition, CMR is valuable for excluding shunting from other sources, such as anomalous pulmonary venous drainage, in which echocardiography is problematic (Fig. 17-19).[112] This is important, because partial

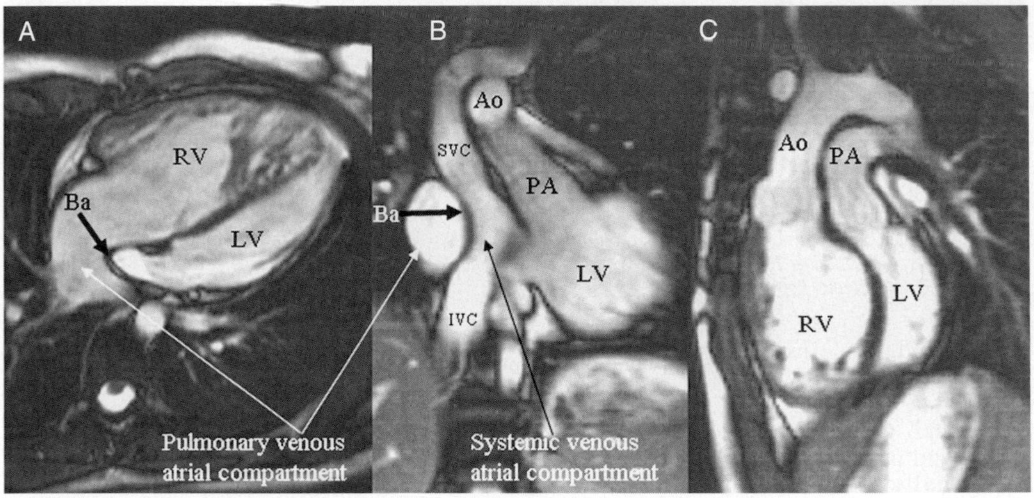

FIGURE 17–18 Cardiovascular magnetic resonance (CMR) of transposition of the great arteries following Senning procedure, with insertion of atrial baffle. **A, B, and C,** Single frames from steady state with free precession (SSFP) cines. **A,** Oblique transaxial plane. **B,** Oblique coronal plane. **C,** Oblique sagittal plane. The atrial baffle (Ba) is seen in **A** and **B.** The pulmonary venous atrial compartment is unobstructed, as seen in **A** and **B,** and the systemic venous atrial compartment is similarly unobstructed, as seen in **B. C,** Aorta arising from the right ventricle and the pulmonary artery arising from the left ventricle. This is a good late postoperative result. Ao = aorta; IVC = inferior vena cava; LV = left ventricle; PA = pulmonary artery; RV = right ventricle; SVC = superior vena cava.

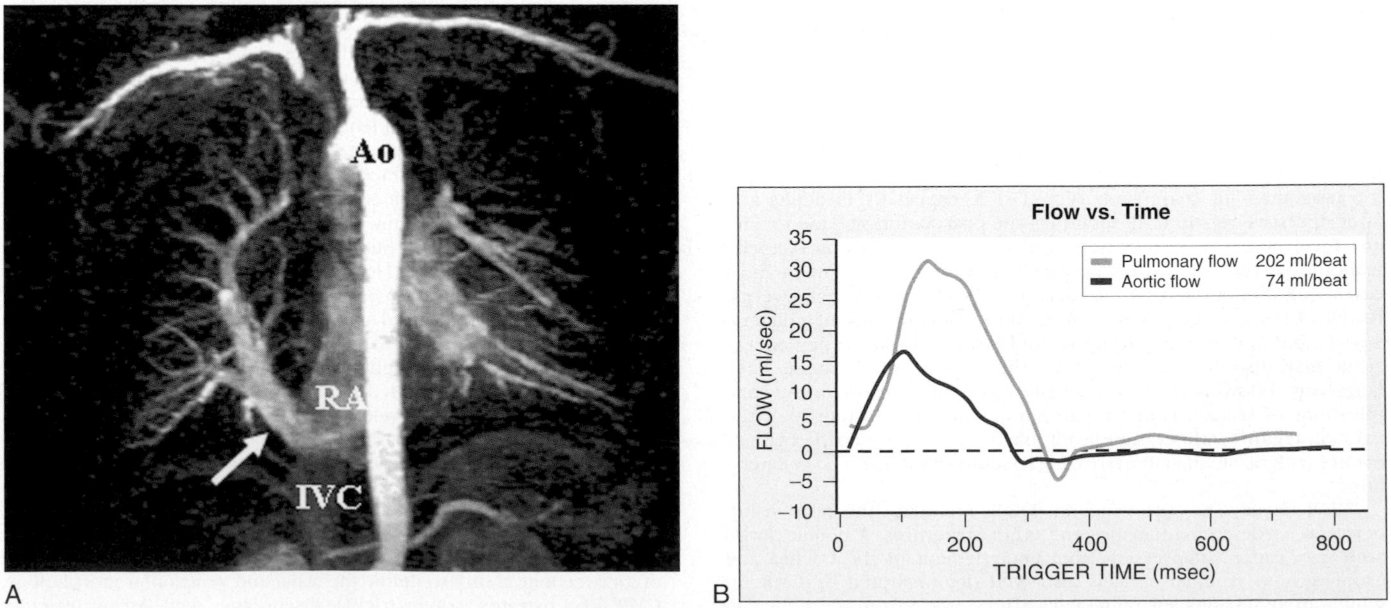

FIGURE 17–19 Cardiovascular magnetic resonance (CMR) angiography of anomalous pulmonary venous drainage. **A,** The pulmonary venous angiogram shows the right upper and lower pulmonary veins draining into a common trunk (arrow) and into the inferior vena cava (IVC) and right atrium (RA). **B,** Direct flow measurements of the pulmonary artery and aorta are shown in this graph, which yielded a Qp/Qs ratio of 2.7. Ao = aorta. *(With permission from Tan RS, Behr ER, McKenna WJ, Mohiaddin RH: Images in cardiovascular medicine. Occult anomalous pulmonary venous drainage: The clinical value of cardiac magnetic resonance imaging. Circulation 105:E27, 2002.)*

anomalous venous return may coexist with atrial septal defect.

VALVULAR ABNORMALITIES. Simple (e.g., mitral stenosis) and complex (e.g., Ebstein anomaly of the tricuspid valve) congenital valve abnormalities can be assessed by CMR, but echocardiography has the significant primary role. CMR is particularly helpful in the assessment of valve regurgitation and the effects of valve pathology on the volumes and function of the associated ventricle. This has proved particularly useful for assessment of pulmonary regurgitation in tetralogy of Fallot and surgical RV to pulmonary artery conduits.

TETRALOGY OF FALLOT. This condition is well assessed by CMR both before intervention and in long-term follow-up. The full tetralogy includes an overriding aorta with membranous ventricular septal defect, infundibular or pulmonary stenosis, and RV hypertrophy, but additional features are common, such as stenosis of the pulmonary arteries and, in severe cases, aortopulmonary collaterals. As adults, most patients will have undergone corrective surgery, and CMR is ideal for monitoring RV volumes and function as well as pulmonary regurgitation, which is common after correction. RV arrhythmias and failure are the most important causes of mortality.

SINGLE VENTRICLE. CMR is useful in determining the anatomical features of this condition, including the ventricular morphology, atrioventricular and ventriculoarterial connections, situs, and presence of associated anomalies. Compared to the dominant ventricle, a rudimentary right ventricle is usually anterosuperior and a rudimentary left ventricle usually is posteroinferior. In adults, a dominant left ventricle is most common. Some single ventricles have no characteristic morphological features and are termed *indeterminate.*

CORONARY ARTERY ANOMALIES. CMR is useful in defining congenital or inflammatory changes of the coronary arteries, as in Kawasaki disease.[113] In adults, the course of congenitally anomalous coronary arteries can be reliably depicted by CMR in patients with otherwise normal anatomy and in those with other types of congenital heart disease, where the prevalence reaches 30 percent. CMR has significant advantages over x-ray angiography in clarifying the spatial relationship of these arteries, most importantly whether the proximal portion runs between the aorta and pulmonary artery, which is associated with sudden death. In other forms of congenital heart disease, the course and location of the coronary arteries can be important for surgical planning.

Acquired Disease of the Major Arteries

CMR angiography of the major central arteries has advanced rapidly and, in experienced centers, is replacing invasive x-ray techniques.[114] Substantial diagnostic information can often be gained in the larger vessels from conventional CMR, but gadolinium-enhanced three-dimensional CMR angiography can now be completed in a few seconds and is routinely used for large and small vessels. The older non–gadolinium CMR angiographic techniques, such as time-of-flight angiography, are not used commonly in the central circulation but do have application elsewhere.

GREAT VESSELS (see Chap. 56). CMR is an ideal technique for assessing the aorta because of its large field of view and ability of CMR angiography to image obliquely and in three dimensions. CMR accurately depicts aortic aneurysms showing cross-sectional diameter and the relationship to branch vessels and associated thrombus. Additional CMR angiography shows associated branch vessel occlusive disease and is useful to define the relationship of the aneurysm to smaller vessels. Inflammatory abdominal aortic aneurysms show enhancement with gadolinium. CMR may be used for stent planning and follow-up. Aortic dissection is a well-established indication for CMR, and the diagnosis can be made rapidly (Fig. 17-20). The associated complications of dissection, such as extent, aortic regurgitation, pericardial effusion, and branch vessel involvement, are all readily assessed by CMR. Other techniques, however, may be used in the acute setting, which mainly reflects availability. In the chronic follow-up setting, CMR is the technique of choice. CMR is also useful for depiction of intramural hematoma and penetrating ulcer. CMR is ideal for the assessment and long-term follow-up of patients with Marfan syndrome. CMR angiography is also useful for assessment of the pulmonary arteries. Reasonable results have been obtained in pulmonary embolism using three-dimensional contrast-enhanced CMR angiography,[115] but CT remains the study of choice because of superior spatial resolution and a shorter breath-hold requirement (see Chap. 18). Pulmonary artery aneurysms and dissections are well evaluated by CMR.

ARTERIAL BRANCHES OF THE AORTA. CMR angiography of the internal carotid artery has proved valuable and both three-dimensional time-of-flight and gadolinium-enhanced techniques have similar accuracy to invasive x-ray techniques, although the gadolinium technique is faster, with improved coverage in the superior-inferior direction. Gadolinium CMR angiography is used for renal (Fig. 17-21) and mesenteric vessels. The lower spatial resolution of CMR compared with x-ray angiography limits quantitative assessment of the degree of stenosis and evaluation of accessory or branch vessels. For the arteries to the leg, three-dimensional gadolinium CMR angiography is very useful diagnostically, and has been used for interventional planning of limb-threatening ischemia. For the arms, there is less clinical experience, but gadolinium CMR angiography has been used with good results.

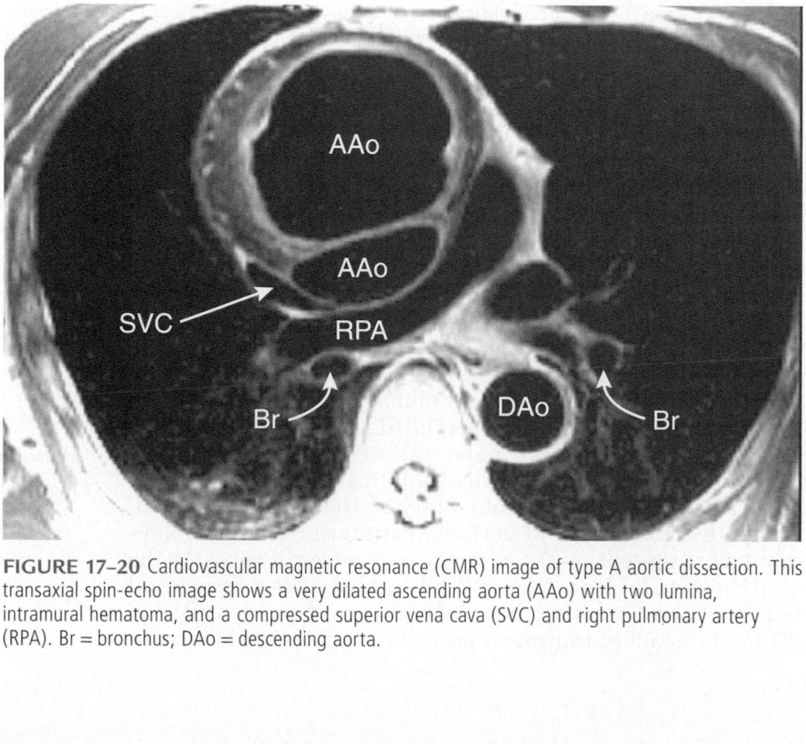

FIGURE 17–20 Cardiovascular magnetic resonance (CMR) image of type A aortic dissection. This transaxial spin-echo image shows a very dilated ascending aorta (AAo) with two lumina, intramural hematoma, and a compressed superior vena cava (SVC) and right pulmonary artery (RPA). Br = bronchus; DAo = descending aorta.

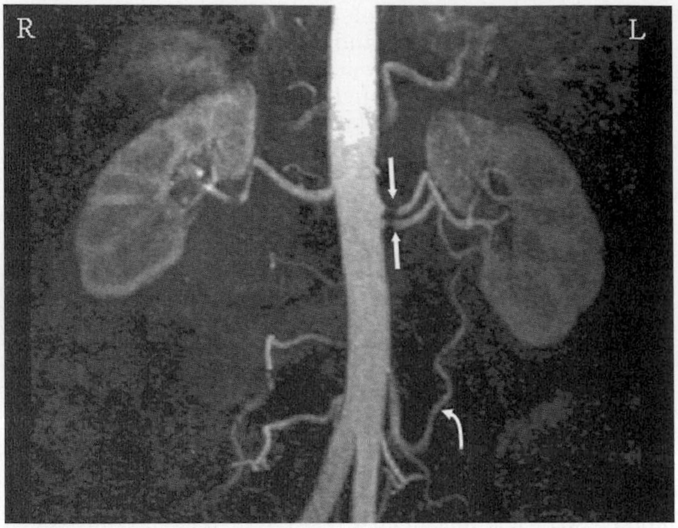

FIGURE 17–21 Cardiovascular magnetic resonance (CMR) renal angiography. Shown is a projection of a three-dimensional CMR angiogram of both kidneys, from the thoracic aorta to beyond the bifurcation into the iliac arteries. The right kidney and renal artery are normal. Three renal arteries supply the left kidney. The upper pair, which are opposite the right renal artery, are both stenosed (straight arrows). Shortly before the bifurcation of the aorta, an accessory renal artery is seen, which is not stenosed (curved arrow).

Intravascular and Interventional Cardiovascular Magnetic Resonance

There is active research into the use of CMR for intravascular and interventional applications because of its whole-body imaging capability in any plane without exposure to x-rays.[116] This requires the combination of a number of techniques, including real-time image acquisition and reconstruction, angiography, and image guidance. In addition, the instruments required must be safe to use in the MR environment, and magnet designs must allow sufficient patient access for the operator. For the cardiovascular system, a key component is the tracking of the catheter and guidewire. This can be achieved by incorporating a small receive-only coil in the tip of the device. The coil generates a signal that can be rapidly localized in three dimensions and shown on a previously acquired MR image, and different coils and receivers can be used for multiple devices. Such technical advances are still being investigated. Results have been reported for renal angiography, femoral angioplasty, wall imaging, placement of stents, coronary angiography, and assessment of radiofrequency ablation procedures. Stem cell therapy is another application under investigation, with significant promise.[117] Dual x-ray–CMR facilities have been proposed for more efficient diagnostic and interventional procedures during a single anesthesia session.[118] The future of this technology is uncertain at present, but there is considerable interest in its development.

FUTURE PERSPECTIVES

CMR has developed into a mainstream investigative tool in clinical cardiology and will continue to improve understanding of pathophysiology through multifaceted tissue characterization at high resolution. Sequence development, such as late gadolinium enhancement, has recently energized this, and hardware advances in MR technology, such as parallel imaging and improved magnet design, have also given ultrafast imaging a robust clinical platform, allowing myocardial perfusion to enter the clinical arena. In the immediate future, the clinical application of established CMR procedures will therefore rely on the results of cardiomyopathy, viability, and perfusion studies. Future development of interventional CMR holds great promise, and the challenge will be to take full advantage of the speed and tissue characterization now available and to identify the clinical impact of improved procedures, such as ablation in electrophysiology and delivery and monitoring of stem cells for myocardial regeneration.

CLASSIC REFERENCES

Anderson LJ, Holden S, Davis B, et al: Cardiovascular T2-star (T2*) magnetic resonance for the early diagnosis of myocardial iron overload. Eur Heart J 22:2174, 2001.

Kim RJ, Wu E, Rafael A, et al: The use of contrast-enhanced magnetic resonance imaging to identify reversible myocardial dysfunction. N Engl J Med 343:1445-1453, 2000.

Neubauer S, Horn M, Cramer M, et al: Myocardial phosphocreatine-to-ATP ratio is a predictor of mortality in patients with dilated cardiomyopathy. Circulation 96:2190-2196, 1997.

Schwitter J, Nanz D, Kneifel S, et al: Assessment of myocardial perfusion in coronary artery disease by magnetic resonance: A comparison with positron emission tomography and coronary angiography. Circulation 103:2230-2235, 2001.

Wu KC, Zerhouni EA, Judd RM, et al: Prognostic significance of microvascular obstruction by magnetic resonance imaging in patients with acute myocardial infarction. Circulation 97:765-772, 1998.

REFERENCES

Principles of Magnetic Resonance

1. Pennell DJ, Sechtem UP, Higgins CB, et al: European Society of Cardiology; Society for Cardiovascular Magnetic Resonance: Clinical indications for cardiovascular magnetic resonance (CMR): Consensus Panel report. J Cardiovasc Magn Reson 6:727, 2004.
2. Manning WJ, Pennell DJ: Cardiovascular Magnetic Resonance. Philadelphia, Churchill Livingstone, 2002.
3. Larson AC, White RD, Laub G, et al: Self-gated cardiac cine MRI. Magn Reson Med 51:93, 2004.
4. Gerber TC, Fasseas P, Lennon RJ, et al: Clinical safety of magnetic resonance imaging early after coronary artery stent placement. J Am Coll Cardiol 42:1295, 2003.
5. Spuentrup E, Ruebben A, Mahnken A, et al: Artifact-free coronary magnetic resonance angiography and coronary vessel wall imaging in the presence of a new, metallic, coronary magnetic resonance imaging stent. Circulation 111:1019, 2005.
6. Martin ET, Coman JA, Shellock FG, et al: Magnetic resonance imaging and cardiac pacemaker safety at 1.5-tesla. J Am Coll Cardiol 43:1315, 2004.
7. Roguin A, Zviman MM, Meininger GR, et al: Modern pacemaker and implantable cardioverter/defibrillator systems can be magnetic resonance imaging safe:in vitro and in vivo assessment of safety and function at 1.5 T. Circulation 110:475, 2004.

Ventricular Volumes, Mass, and Function

8. Bellenger NG, Burgess M, Ray SG, et al: Comparison of left ventricular ejection fraction and volumes in heart failure by two-dimensional echocardiography, radionuclide ventriculography and cardiovascular magnetic resonance: Are they interchangeable? Eur Heart J 21:1387, 2000.
9. Bellenger NG, Pennell DJ: Ventricular function. *In* Manning WJ, Pennell DJ (eds): Cardiovascular Magnetic Resonance. New York, Churchill Livingstone, 2002, pp 99-111.
10. Myerson SG, Bellenger NG, Pennell DJ: Assessment of left ventricular mass by cardiovascular magnetic resonance. Hypertension 39:750, 2002.
11. Maceira AM, Prasad SK, Khan M, Pennell DJ: Normalized left ventricular systolic and diastolic function by steady state free precession cardiovascular magnetic resonance. J Cardiovasc Magn Reson 8:417, 2006.
12. Grothues F, Smith GC, Moon JCC, et al: Comparison of interstudy reproducibility of cardiovascular magnetic resonance with two-dimensional echocardiography in normal subjects and in patients with heart failure or left ventricular hypertrophy. Am J Cardiol 90:29, 2002.
13. Grothues F, Moon JC, Bellenger NG, et al: Interstudy reproducibility of right ventricular volumes, function, and mass with cardiovascular magnetic resonance. Am Heart J 147:218, 2004.
14. Bellenger NG, Rajappan K, Rahman SL, et al: Effects of carvedilol on left ventricular remodelling in chronic stable heart failure:a cardiovascular magnetic resonance study. Heart 90:760, 2004.
15. Prasad SK, Dargie HJ, Smith GC, et al: Comparison of the dual receptor endothelin antagonist enrasentan with enalapril in asymptomatic left ventricular systolic dysfunction:a cardiovascular magnetic resonance study. Heart 92:798, 2006.
16. Pennell DJ, Berdoukas V, Karagiorga M, et al: Randomized controlled trial of deferiprone or deferoxamine in beta-thalassemia major patients with asymptomatic myocardial siderosis. Blood 107:3738, 2006.
17. Pai VM, Axel L: Advances in MRI tagging techniques for determining regional myocardial strain. Curr Cardiol Rep 8:53, 2006.

Myocardial Infarction and Viability

18. Elliott MD, Kim RJ: Late gadolinium cardiovascular magnetic resonance in the assessment of myocardial viability. Coron Artery Dis 16:365, 2005.
19. Wu E, Judd RM, Vargas JD, et al: Visualisation of presence, location and transmural extent of healed Q-wave and non-Q-wave myocardial infarction. Lancet 357:21, 2001.
20. Wagner A, Mahrholdt H, Holly TA, et al: Contrast-enhanced MRI and routine single photon emission computed tomography (SPECT) perfusion imaging for detection of subendocardial myocardial infarcts: An imaging study. Lancet 361:374, 2003.

21. Selvanayagam JB, Porto I, Channon K, et al: Troponin elevation after percutaneous coronary intervention directly represents the extent of irreversible myocardial injury: Insights from cardiovascular magnetic resonance imaging. Circulation 111:1027, 2005.
22. Moon JC, De Arenaza DP, Elkington AG, et al: The pathologic basis of Q-wave and non-Q-wave myocardial infarction: A cardiovascular magnetic resonance study. J Am Coll Cardiol 44:554, 2004.
23. Mahrholdt H, Wagner A, Holly TA, et al: Reproducibility of chronic infarct size measurement by contrast-enhanced magnetic resonance imaging. Circulation 106:2322, 2002.
24. Aletras AH, Tilak GS, Natanzon A, et al: Retrospective determination of the area at risk for reperfused acute myocardial infarction with T2-weighted cardiac magnetic resonance imaging: Histopathological and displacement encoding with stimulated echoes (DENSE) functional validations. Circulation 113:1865, 2006.
25. Pennell D: Myocardial salvage: Retrospection, resolution, and radio waves. Circulation 113:1821, 2006.
26. Kwong RY, Chan AK, Brown KA, et al: Impact of unrecognized myocardial scar detected by cardiac magnetic resonance imaging on event-free survival in patients presenting with signs or symptoms of coronary artery disease. Circulation 113:2733, 2006.
27. Yan AT, Shayne AJ, Brown KA, et al: Characterization of the periinfarct zone by contrast-enhanced cardiac magnetic resonance imaging is a powerful predictor of post-myocardial infarction mortality. Circulation 114:32, 2006.
28. Mahrholdt H, Wagner A, Judd RM, Sechtem U: Assessment of myocardial viability by cardiovascular magnetic resonance imaging. Eur Heart J 23:602, 2002.
29. John AS, Dreyfus GD, Pennell DJ: Images in cardiovascular medicine. Reversible wall thinning in hibernation predicted by cardiovascular magnetic resonance. Circulation 111:e24, 2005.
30. Selvanayagam JB, Kardos A, Francis JM, et al: Value of delayed-enhancement cardiovascular magnetic resonance imaging in predicting myocardial viability after surgical revascularization. Circulation 110:1535, 2004.
31. Gerber BL, Garot J, Bluemke DA, et al: Accuracy of contrast-enhanced magnetic resonance imaging in predicting improvement of regional myocardial function in patients after acute myocardial infarction. Circulation 106:1083, 2002.
32. Klein C, Nekolla SG, Bengel FM, et al: Assessment of myocardial viability with contrast-enhanced magnetic resonance imaging:comparison with positron emission tomography. Circulation 105:162, 2002.
33. Kitagawa K, Sakuma H, Hirano T, et al: Acute myocardial infarction:Myocardial viability assessment in patients early thereafter—comparison of contrast enhanced MR imaging with resting 201-Tl SPECT. Radiology 226:138, 2003.
34. Kwong RY, Schussheim AE, Rekhraj S, et al: Detecting acute coronary syndrome in the emergency department with cardiac magnetic resonance imaging. Circulation 107:531, 2003.
35. Wu KC, Lima JA: Noninvasive imaging of myocardial viability: Current techniques and future developments. Circ Res 93:1146, 2003.

Stress Ventriculography and Myocardial Perfusion

36. Syed MA, Paterson DI, Ingkanisorn WP, et al: Reproducibility and inter-observer variability of dobutamine stress CMR in patients with severe coronary disease: implications for clinical research. J Cardiovasc Magn Reson 7:763, 2005.
37. Paetsch I, Jahnke C, Ferrari VA, et al: Determination of interobserver variability for identifying inducible left ventricular wall motion abnormalities during dobutamine stress magnetic resonance imaging. Eur Heart J 27:1459, 2006.
38. Hundley WG, Morgan TM, Neagle CM, et al: Magnetic resonance imaging determination of cardiac prognosis. Circulation 106:2328, 2002.
39. Kuijpers D, Ho KY, van Dijkman PR, et al: Dobutamine cardiovascular magnetic resonance for the detection of myocardial ischemia with the use of myocardial tagging. Circulation 107:1592, 2003.
40. Schalla S, Klein C, Paetsch I, et al: Real-time MR image acquisition during high-dose dobutamine hydrochloride stress for detecting left ventricular wall-motion abnormalities in patients with coronary arterial disease. Radiology 224:845, 2002.
41. Jerosch-Herold M, Muehling O, Wilke N: MRI of myocardial perfusion. Semin Ultrasound CT MR 27:2, 2006.
42. Kellman P, Derbyshire JA, Agyeman KO, et al: Extended coverage first-pass perfusion imaging using slice-interleaved TSENSE. Magn Reson Med 51:200, 2004.
43. Di Bella EV, Parker DL, Sinusas AJ: On the dark rim artifact in dynamic contrast-enhanced MRI myocardial perfusion studies. Magn Reson Med 54:1295, 2005.
44. Araoz PA, Glockner JF, McGee KP, et al: 3 TMR imaging provides improved contrast in first-pass myocardial perfusion imaging over a range of gadolinium doses. J Cardiovasc Magn Reson 7:559, 2005.
45. Panting JR, Gatehouse PD, Yang GZ, et al: Abnormal subendocardial perfusion in cardiac syndrome-X detected by cardiovascular magnetic resonance imaging. N Engl J Med 346:1948, 2002.
46. Epstein FH, London JF, Peters DC, et al: Multislice first pass cardiac perfusion MRI: Validation in a model of myocardial infarction. Magn Reson Med 47:482, 2002.
47. Lyne JC, Gatehouse PD, Assomull RG, et al: Direct comparison of myocardial perfusion cardiovascular magnetic resonance sequences with parallel acquisition. J Magn Reson Imaging 2007 (in press).
48. Wacker CM, Hartlep AW, Pfleger S, et al: Susceptibility-sensitive magnetic resonance imaging detects human myocardium supplied by a stenotic coronary artery without a contrast agent. J Am Coll Cardiol 41:834, 2003.
49. Sakuma H, Suzawa N, Ichikawa Y, et al: Diagnostic accuracy of stress first-pass contrast-enhanced myocardial perfusion MRI compared with stress myocardial perfusion scintigraphy. Am J Roentgenol 185:95, 2005.
50. Wolff SD, Schwitter J, Coulden R, et al: Myocardial first-pass perfusion magnetic resonance imaging: A multicenter dose-ranging study. Circulation 110:732, 2004.
51. Giang TH, Nanz D, Coulden R, et al: Detection of coronary artery disease by magnetic resonance myocardial perfusion imaging with various contrast medium doses: First European multi-centre experience. Eur Heart J 25:1657, 2004.
52. Ingkanisorn WP, Kwong RY, Bohme NS, et al: Prognosis of negative adenosine stress magnetic resonance in patients presenting to an emergency department with chest pain. J Am Coll Cardiol 47:1427, 2006.
53. Muehling OM, Jerosch-Herold M, Panse P, et al: Regional heterogeneity of myocardial perfusion in healthy human myocardium: Assessment with magnetic resonance perfusion imaging. J Cardiovasc Magn Reson 6:499, 2004.

Imaging the Coronary Arteries

54. Appelbaum E, Botnar RM, Yeon SB, Manning WJ: Coronary magnetic resonance imaging: Current state-of-the-art. Coron Artery Dis 16:345, 2005.
55. Kim WY, Danias PG, Stuber M, et al: Coronary magnetic resonance angiography for the detection of coronary stenosis. N Engl J Med 345:1863, 2001.
56. Leiner T, Katsimaglis G, Yeh EN, et al: Correction for heart rate variability improves coronary magnetic resonance angiography. J Magn Reson Imaging 22:577, 2005.
57. Nagel E, Thouet T, Klein C, et al: Noninvasive determination of coronary blood flow velocity with cardiovascular magnetic resonance in patients after stent deployment. Circulation 107:1738, 2003.
58. Langerak SE, Vliegen HW, Jukema JW, et al: Value of magnetic resonance imaging for the noninvasive detection of stenosis in coronary artery bypass grafts and recipient coronary arteries. Circulation 107:1502, 2003.
59. Sorenson MB, Collins P, Ong PJL, et al: Long-term use of contraceptive depot medroxyprogesterone acetate in young women impairs arterial endothelial function assessed by cardiovascular magnetic resonance. Circulation 106:1646, 2002.
60. Terashima M, Meyer CH, Keeffe BG, et al: Noninvasive assessment of coronary vasodilation using magnetic resonance angiography. J Am Coll Cardiol 45:104, 2005.
61. Mohiaddin RH: Assessment of the biophysical mechanical properties of the arterial wall. *In* Manning WJ, Pennell DJ (eds): Cardiovascular Magnetic Resonance. New York, Churchill Livingstone, 2002, pp 272-280.
62. Corti R, Fuster V, Fayad ZA, et al: Lipid lowering by simvastatin induces regression of human atherosclerotic lesions: Two years' follow-up by high-resolution noninvasive magnetic resonance imaging. Circulation 106:2884, 2002.
63. Fayad ZA, Choudhury RP, Fuster V: Magnetic resonance imaging of coronary atherosclerosis. Curr Atheroscler Rep 5:411, 2003.
64. Botnar RM, Stuber M, Lamerichs R, et al: Initial experiences with in vivo right coronary artery human MR vessel wall imaging at 3 tesla. J Cardiovasc Magn Reson 5:589, 2003.
65. Cai JM, Hatsukami TS, Ferguson MS, et al: Classification of human carotid atherosclerotic lesions with in vivo multicontrast magnetic resonance imaging. Circulation 106:1368, 2002.
66. Yuan C, Mitsumori LM, Ferguson MS, et al: In vivo accuracy of multispectral magnetic resonance imaging for identifying lipid-rich necrotic cores and intraplaque hemorrhage in advanced human carotid plaques. Circulation 104:2051, 2001.
67. Mitsumori LM, Hatsukami TS, Ferguson MS, et al: In vivo accuracy of multisequence MR imaging for identifying unstable fibrous caps in advanced human carotid plaques. J Magn Reson Imaging 17:410, 2003.
68. Yuan C, Zhang SX, Polissar NL, et al: Identification of fibrous cap rupture with magnetic resonance imaging is highly associated with recent transient ischemic attack or stroke. Circulation 105:181, 2002.
69. Ruehm SG, Corot C, Vogt P, et al: Magnetic resonance imaging of atherosclerotic plaque with ultrasmall superparamagnetic particles of iron oxide in hyperlipidemic rabbits. Circulation 103:415, 2001.
70. Kerwin W, Hooker A, Spilker M, et al: Quantitative magnetic resonance imaging analysis of neovasculature volume in carotid atherosclerotic plaque. Circulation 107:851, 2003.
71. Wasserman BA, Smith WI, Trout HH 3rd, et al: Carotid artery atherosclerosis:in vivo morphologic characterization with gadolinium-enhanced double-oblique MR imaging initial results. Radiology 223:566, 2002.
72. Winter PM, Caruthers SD, Wickline SA, Lanza GM: Molecular imaging by MRI. Curr Cardiol Rep 8:65, 2006.
73. Zhao XQ, Yuan C, Hatsukami TS, et al: Effects of prolonged intensive lipid-lowering therapy on the characteristics of carotid atherosclerotic plaques in vivo by MRI: A case-control study. Arterioscler Thromb Vasc Biol 21:1623, 2001.

Cardiomyopathy

74. Pennell DJ: T2* magnetic resonance and myocardial iron in thalassemia. Ann N Y Acad Sci 1054:373, 2005.
75. McCrohon JA, Moon JC, Prasad SK, et al: Differentiation of heart failure related to dilated cardiomyopathy and coronary artery disease using gadolinium-enhanced cardiovascular magnetic resonance. Circulation 108:54, 2003.
76. Assomull RG, Prasad SK, Lyne J, et al: Cardiovascular magnetic resonance, fibrosis, and prognosis in dilated cardiomyopathy. J Am Coll Cardiol 48:1977, 2006.
77. Felker GM, Shaw LK, O'Connor CM: A standardized definition of ischemic cardiomyopathy for use in clinical research. J Am Coll Cardiol 39:210, 2002.
78. Repetto A, Dal Bello B, Pasotti M, et al: Coronary atherosclerosis in end-stage idiopathic dilated cardiomyopathy: An innocent bystander? Eur Heart J 26:1519, 2005.
79. Rickers C, Wilke NM, Jerosch-Herold M, et al: Utility of cardiac magnetic resonance imaging in the diagnosis of hypertrophic cardiomyopathy. Circulation 112:855, 2005.

80. Moon JC, Fisher NG, McKenna WJ, Pennell DJ: Detection of apical hypertrophic cardiomyopathy by cardiovascular magnetic resonance in patients with non-diagnostic echocardiography. Heart 90:645, 2004.
81. Crilley JG, Boehm EA, Blair E, et al: Hypertrophic cardiomyopathy due to sarcomeric gene mutations is characterized by impaired energy metabolism irrespective of the degree of hypertrophy. J Am Coll Cardiol 41:1776, 2003.
82. Moon JC, Reed E, Sheppard MN, et al: The histologic basis of late gadolinium enhancement cardiovascular magnetic resonance in hypertrophic cardiomyopathy. J Am Coll Cardiol 43:2260, 2004.
83. Moon JC, McKenna WJ, McCrohon JA, et al: Toward clinical risk assessment in hypertrophic cardiomyopathy with gadolinium cardiovascular magnetic resonance. J Am Coll Cardiol 41:1561, 2003.
84. Moon JC, Sachdev B, Elkington AG, et al: Gadolinium-enhanced cardiovascular magnetic resonance in Anderson-Fabry disease. Evidence for a disease specific abnormality of the myocardial interstitium. Eur Heart J 24:2151, 2003.
85. Maceira AM, Joshi J, Prasad SK, et al: Cardiovascular magnetic resonance in cardiac amyloidosis. Circulation 111:186, 2005.
86. Petersen SE, Selvanayagam JB, Francis JM, et al: Differentiation of athlete's heart from pathological forms of cardiac hypertrophy by means of geometric indices derived from cardiovascular magnetic resonance. J Cardiovasc Magn Reson 7:551, 2005.
87. Wood JC, Otto-Duessel M, Aguilar M, et al: Cardiac iron determines cardiac T2*, T2, and T1 in the gerbil model of iron cardiomyopathy. Circulation 112:535, 2005.
88. Anderson LJ, Westwood MA, Holden S, et al: Myocardial iron clearance during reversal of siderotic cardiomyopathy with intravenous desferrioxamine: A prospective study using T2* cardiovascular magnetic resonance. Br J Haematol 127:348, 2004.
89. Anderson LJ, Wonke B, Prescott E, et al: Comparison of effects of oral deferiprone and subcutaneous desferrioxamine on myocardial iron levels and ventricular function in beta thalassemia. Lancet 360:516, 2002.
90. Pennell DJ, Berdoukas V, Karagiorga M, et al: Randomized controlled trial of deferiprone or deferoxamine in beta-thalassemia major patients with asymptomatic myocardial siderosis. Blood 107:3738, 2006.
91. Borgna-Pignatti C, Cappellini MD, De Stefano P, et al: Cardiac morbidity and mortality in deferoxamine- or deferiprone-treated patients with thalassemia major. Blood 107:3733, 2006.
92. Macrae CA, Birchmeier W, Thierfelder L: Arrhythmogenic right ventricular cardiomyopathy: Moving toward mechanism. J Clin Invest 116:1825, 2006.
93. Tandri H, Saranathan M, Rodriguez ER, et al: Noninvasive detection of myocardial fibrosis in arrhythmogenic right ventricular cardiomyopathy using delayed-enhancement magnetic resonance imaging. J Am Coll Cardiol 45:98, 2005.
94. Norman M, Simpson M, Mogensen J, et al: Novel mutation in desmoplakin causes arrhythmogenic left ventricular cardiomyopathy. Circulation 112:636, 2005.
95. Keller DI, Osswald S, Bremerich J, et al: Arrhythmogenic right ventricular cardiomyopathy: Diagnostic and prognostic value of the cardiac MRI in relation to arrhythmia-free survival. Int J Cardiovasc Imaging 19:537, 2003.
96. Smedema JP, Snoep G, van Kroonenburgh MP, et al: Evaluation of the accuracy of gadolinium-enhanced cardiovascular magnetic resonance in the diagnosis of cardiac sarcoidosis. J Am Coll Cardiol 45:1683, 2005.
97. Smedema JP, Snoep G, van Kroonenburgh MP, et al: The additional value of gadolinium-enhanced MRI to standard assessment for cardiac involvement in patients with pulmonary sarcoidosis. Chest 128:1629, 2005.
98. Stauder NI, Bader B, Fenchel M, et al: Images in cardiovascular medicine. Follow-up of cardiac sarcoidosis by magnetic resonance imaging. Circulation 111:e158, 2005.
99. Mahrholdt H, Goedecke C, Wagner A, et al: Cardiovascular magnetic resonance assessment of human myocarditis: A comparison to histology and molecular pathology. Circulation 109:1250, 2004.
100. Abdel-Aty H, Boye P, Zagrosek A, et al: Diagnostic performance of cardiovascular magnetic resonance in patients with suspected acute myocarditis: Comparison of different approaches. J Am Coll Cardiol 45:1815, 2005.

Valvular Heart Disease and Pericardial Disease

101. Mohiaddin RH, Kilner PJ: Valvular heart disease. *In* Manning WJ, Pennell DJ (eds): Cardiovascular Magnetic Resonance. Philadelphia, Churchill Livingstone, 2002, pp 355-363.
102. Lin SJ, Brown PA, Watkins MP, et al: Quantification of stenotic mitral valve area with magnetic resonance imaging and comparison with Doppler ultrasound. J Am Coll Cardiol 44:133, 2004.
103. Caruthers SD, Lin SJ, Brown P, et al: Practical value of cardiac magnetic resonance imaging for clinical quantification of aortic valve stenosis: Comparison with echocardiography. Circulation 108:2236, 2003.
104. Rajappan K, Rimoldi OE, Camici PG, et al: Functional changes in coronary microcirculatory function after valve replacement in patients with aortic stenosis. Circulation 107:3170, 2003.
105. Perez de Arenaza D, Lees B, Flather M, et al: ASSERT (Aortic Stentless versus Stented valve assessed by Echocardiography Randomized Trial) Investigators: Randomized comparison of stentless versus stented valves for aortic stenosis: Effects on left ventricular mass. Circulation 112:2696, 2005.
106. Vick GW, Rokey R: CMR evaluation of the pericardium in health and disease. *In* Manning WJ, Pennell DJ (eds): Cardiovascular Magnetic Resonance. Philadelphia, Churchill Livingstone, Philadelphia, 2002, pp 355-363.
107. Frank H: Cardiac masses. *In* Manning WJ, Pennell DJ (eds): Cardiovascular Magnetic Resonance. Philadelphia, Churchill Livingstone, 2002, pp 342-354.

Congenital Heart Disease

108. Wyttenbach R, Bremerich J, Higgins CB: Cardiovascular magnetic resonance of complex congenital heart disease in the adult. *In* Manning WJ, Pennell DJ (eds): Cardiovascular Magnetic Resonance. New York, Churchill Livingstone, 2002, pp 311-323.
109. Kilner PJ: Adult congenital heart disease. *In* Higgins CB, de Roos A (eds): Cardiovascular MRI and MRA. Philadelphia, Lippincott, Williams & Wilkins, 2003, pp 353-366.
110. Prasad SK, Soukias N, Hornung T, et al: Role of magnetic resonance angiography in the diagnosis of major aortopulmonary collateral arteries and partial anomalous pulmonary venous drainage. Circulation 109:207, 2004.
111. Geva T, Greil GF, Marshall AC, et al: Gadolinium-enhanced three-dimensional magnetic resonance angiography of pulmonary blood supply in patients with complex pulmonary stenosis or atresia: Comparison with x-ray angiography. Circulation 106:473, 2002.
112. Prasad SK, Soukias N, Hornung T, et al: Role of magnetic resonance angiography in the diagnosis of major aortopulmonary collateral arteries and partial anomalous pulmonary venous drainage. Circulation 109:207, 2004.
113. Greil GF, Stuber M, Botnar RM, et al: Coronary magnetic resonance angiography in adolescents and young adults with Kawasaki disease. Circulation 105:908, 2002.

Diseases of the Major Arteries

114. Prince MR, Meaney JF: Expanding role of MR angiography in clinical practice. Eur Radiol 16(Suppl 2):B3, 2006.
115. Oudkerk M, van Beek EJ, Wielopolski P, et al: Comparison of contrast-enhanced magnetic resonance angiography and conventional pulmonary angiography for the diagnosis of pulmonary embolism: A prospective study. Lancet 359:1643, 2002.

Interventional CMR

116. Henk CB, Higgins CB, Saeed M: Endovascular interventional MRI. J Magn Reson Imaging 22:451, 2005.
117. Rickers C, Kraitchman D, Fischer G, et al: Cardiovascular interventional MR imaging: A new road for therapy and repair in the heart. Magn Reson Imaging Clin N Am 13:465, 2005.
118. Kuehne T, Saeed M, Higgins CB, et al: Endovascular stents in pulmonary valve and artery in swine: Feasibility study of MR imaging-guided deployment and post-interventional assessment. Radiology 226:475, 2003.

GUIDELINES *Thomas H. Lee*

Appropriateness Guidelines: Cardiovascular Magnetic Resonance

The explosive growth in cardiovascular imaging has sometimes outpaced the evidence on which use of new technologies should be based. In an effort to guide rational use of these technologies, eight scientific organizations—American College of Cardiology Foundation, American College of Radiology, Society of Cardiovascular Computed Tomography, Society for Cardiovascular Magnetic Resonance, American Society of Nuclear Cardiology, North American Society for Cardiac Imaging, Society for Cardiovascular Angiography and Interventions, and Society of Interventional Radiology—have embarked on a process to determine the appropriateness of selected indications for cardiovascular imaging procedures.

Panelists rated 33 indications for cardiovascular magnetic resonance (CMR) imaging as appropriate (7 to 9 points), uncertain (4 to 6 points), and inappropriate (1 to 3 points), based on the following definition of appropriateness[1]:

An appropriate imaging study is one in which the expected incremental information, combined with clinical judgment, exceeds the expected negative consequences by a sufficiently wide margin for a specific indication that the procedure is generally considered acceptable care and a reasonable approach for the indication. (Negative consequences include the risks of the procedure [i.e., radiation or contrast exposure] and the downstream impact of poor test

TABLE 17G–1 Joint Professional Society* Evaluation of Appropriate Indications for Cardiac Magnetic Resonance

Indication	Appropriateness (Median Score)
DETECTION OF CAD: SYMPTOMATIC	
Evaluation of Chest Pain Syndrome (Use of Vasodilator Perfusion CMR or Dobutamine Stress Function CMR) Intermediate pretest probability of CAD ECG uninterpretable *or* unable to exercise	A (7)
High pretest probability of CAD	U (5)
Intermediate pretest probability of CAD ECG interpretable *and* able to exercise	U (4)
Low pretest probability of CAD ECG interpretable *and* able to exercise	I (2)
Evaluation of Chest Pain Syndrome (Use of MR Coronary Angiography) Intermediate pretest probability of CAD ECG interpretable *and* able to exercise	I (2)
Intermediate pretest probability of CAD ECG uninterpretable OR unable to exercise	I (2)
High pretest probability of CAD	I (1)
Evaluation of Intracardiac Structures (Use of MR Coronary Angiography) Evaluation of suspected coronary anomalies	A (8)
Acute Chest Pain (Use of Vasodilator Perfusion CMR or Dobutamine Stress Function CMR) Intermediate pretest probability of CAD No changes on the ECG and serial cardiac enzymes negative	U (6)
High pretest probability of CAD ECG—ST segment elevation and/or positive cardiac enzymes	I (1)
RISK ASSESSMENT WITH PRIOR TEST RESULTS (Use of Vasodilator Perfusion CMR or Dobutamine Stress Function CMR)	
Coronary angiography (catheterization or CT) Stenosis of unclear significance	A (7)
Equivocal stress test (exercise, stress SPECT, or stress echo) Intermediate CHD risk (Framingham)	U (6)
Normal prior stress test (exercise, nuclear, echo, MRI) High CHD risk (Framingham) Within 1 year of prior stress test	I (2)
RISK ASSESSMENT: PREOPERATIVE EVALUATION FOR NONCARDIAC SURGERY	
Low-Risk Surgery (Use of Vasodilator Perfusion CMR or Dobutamine Stress Function CMR) Intermediate perioperative risk predictor	I (2)
Intermediate- or High-Risk Surgery (Use of Vasodilator Perfusion CMR or Dobutamine Stress Function CMR) Intermediate perioperative risk predictor	U (6)
DETECTION OF CAD: POSTREVASCULARIZATION (PCI OR CABG)	
Evaluation of Chest Pain Syndrome (Use of MR Coronary Angiography) Evaluation of bypass grafts	I (2)
History of percutaneous revascularization with stents	I (1)
STRUCTURE AND FUNCTION	
Evaluation of Ventricular and Valvular Function[†] Assessment of complex congenital heart disease, including anomalies of coronary circulation, great vessels, and cardiac chambers and valves Procedures may include LV-RV mass and volumes, MR angiography, quantification of valvular disease, and contrast enhancement	A (9)
Evaluation for arrhythmogenic right ventricular cardiomyopathy (ARVC) Patients presenting with syncope or ventricular arrhythmia	A (9)
Evaluation of LV function following myocardial infarction *or* in heart failure patients Patients with technically limited images from echocardiogram	A (8)
Quantification of LV function Discordant information that is clinically significant from prior tests	A (8)
Evaluation of specific cardiomyopathies (infiltrative [amyloid, sarcoid], HCM, or caused by cardiotoxic therapies) Use of delayed enhancement	A (8)

TABLE 17G–1 Joint Professional Society* Evaluation of Appropriate Indications for Cardiac Magnetic Resonance—cont'd

Indication	Appropriateness (Median Score)
Characterization of native and prosthetic cardiac valves, including planimetry of stenotic disease and quantification of regurgitant disease Patients with technically limited images from echocardiogram or TEE	A (8)
Evaluation of myocarditis or myocardial infarction with normal coronary arteries Positive cardiac enzymes without obstructive atherosclerosis on angiography	A (8)
Evaluation of LV function following myocardial infarction *or* in heart failure patients	U (6)
Evaluation of Intra- and Extracardiac Structures Evaluation of cardiac mass (suspected tumor or thrombus) Use of contrast for perfusion and enhancement	A (9)
Evaluation of pericardial conditions (pericardial mass, constrictive pericarditis)	A (8)
Evaluation for aortic dissection	A (8)
Evaluation of pulmonary veins prior to radiofrequency ablation for atrial fibrillation Left atrial and pulmonary venous anatomy, including dimensions of veins for mapping purposes	A (8)
DETECTION OF MYOCARDIAL SCAR AND VIABILITY	
Evaluation of Myocardial Scar (Use of Late Gadolinium Enhancement) To determine viability prior to revascularization Viability assessment by SPECT or dobutamine echo has provided "equivocal" or "indeterminate" results	A (9)
To determine viability prior to revascularization To establish likelihood of recovery of function with revascularization (PCI or CABG) or medical therapy	A (9)
To determine the location and extent of myocardial necrosis, including no-reflow regions Post-acute myocardial infarction	A (7)
To detect post PCI myocardial necrosis	U (4)

*American College of Cardiology Foundation, American College of Radiology, Society of Cardiovascular Computed Tomography, Society for Cardiovascular Magnetic Resonance, American Society of Nuclear Cardiology, North American Society for Cardiac Imaging, Society for Cardiovascular Angiography and Interventions, and Society of Interventional Radiology.

†Procedures may include LV/RV mass and volumes, MR angiography, quantification of valvular disease, and delayed contrast enhancement.

CABG = coronary artery bypass grafting; CAD = coronary artery disease; CHD = congenital heart disease; CMR = cardiovascular magnetic resonance; CT = computed tomography; ECG = electrocardiogram; HCM = hypertrophic cardiomyopathy; LV = left ventricular; MRI = magnetic resonance imaging; PCI = percutaneous coronary intervention; RV = right ventricular; SPECT = single-photon emission computed tomography; TEE = transesophageal echocardiography.

performance such as delay in diagnosis [false negatives] or inappropriate diagnosis [false positives].)

Of the 33 cardiac computed tomography indications, 17 were deemed appropriate, 7 were uncertain, and 9 were rated as inappropriate (Table 17G-1).

The panel stressed that appropriateness criteria are not substitutes for sound clinical judgment and practice experience. Medical reasons may preclude applying the appropriateness criteria to specific patients, and clinician judgment should be used at all times in applying the criteria. For example, the rating of an indication as inappropriate should not dissuade a provider from performing CMR imaging when patient- and condition-specific data support that decision, and not performing a study rated as appropriate may be the correct decision in light of unique patient, clinical, and other relevant information.

Reference

1. Hendel RC, Patel MR, Kramer CM, et al; American College of Cardiology Foundation Quality Strategic Directions Committee Appropriateness Criteria Working Group; American College of Radiology; Society of Cardiovascular Computed Tomography; Society for Cardiovascular Magnetic Resonance; American Society of Nuclear Cardiology; North American Society for Cardiac Imaging; Society for Cardiovascular Angiography and Interventions; Society of Interventional Radiology: ACCF/ACR/SCCT/SCMR/ASNC/NASCI/SCAI/SIR 2006 appropriateness criteria for cardiac computed tomography and cardiac magnetic resonance imaging: A report of the American College of Cardiology Foundation Quality Strategic Directions Committee Appropriateness Criteria Working Group, American College of Radiology, Society of Cardiovascular Computed Tomography, Society for Cardiovascular Magnetic Resonance, American Society of Nuclear Cardiology, North American Society for Cardiac Imaging, Society for Cardiovascular Angiography and Interventions, and Society of Interventional Radiology. J Am Coll Cardiol 48:1475, 2006 (http://www.acc.org/qualityandscience/clinical/pdfs/ CCT.CMR.pdf).

CHAPTER 18

Computed Tomography of the Heart

Stephan Achenbach and Werner G. Daniel

PRINCIPLES OF COMPUTED TOMOGRAPHY

Computed tomography (CT) imaging was introduced in 1972. The ability to obtain cross-sectional images of the body revolutionized medicine and, for the development of computer-assisted tomography, Sir Geoffrey N. Hounsfield and Allan M. Cormack were awarded the Nobel Prize in Medicine in 1979. CT is an x-ray–based technique. An x-ray source that rotates on a circular path around the patient emits a fan-shaped beam of x-rays that passes through the body. Collimators are used to confine the x-ray beam to the slice that shall be imaged; its thickness can vary from less than one to several millimeters. Opposite the x-ray source, extremely sensitive detectors record the intensity of x-rays that have passed through the body. Based on the x-ray attenuations obtained from a multitude of angles, a cross-sectional image of the body can be calculated. Each pixel of the reconstructed image is assigned an x-ray attenuation value (also called CT number), which is expressed in Hounsfield units (HU). The Hounsfield scale is calibrated in a way that yields 0 HU for water and –1000 HU for air. CT numbers within one cross section of the body can thus range from close to –1000 HU (e.g., the lungs) to several thousand HU (e.g., bone or metal; Table 18-1). Because the human eye cannot distinguish a gray scale over such a wide range, adjustments (window width and window level or center) are made when displaying the reconstructed images. The width value represents the range of CT numbers, which are displayed on a gray scale. Each value below that range will be displayed in black, and each value exceeding the range will be displayed in white. The level or center value determines the CT number around which the window is centered (e.g., in an image displayed with a center of 500 HU and width of 400 HU, each pixel with a density of less than 300 HU will displayed in black and each pixel with a density greater than 700 HU will be displayed in white). By convention, body images obtained by CT are displayed as if looking upward from the patient's feet (Fig. 18-1).

Special Considerations for Cardiac Imaging

Because of technical limitations, the clinical value of CT for imaging of the heart has, for a long time, been very limited. Cardiac imaging requires a very high temporal resolution, because the heart is in constant, rapid motion. Conventional CT imaging, on the other hand, is an imaging modality with low temporal resolution: the heavy x-ray tube and the detector array must be moved very accurately in a circular pattern around the body, so that centrifugal forces and the need to keep the geometry of source and detectors exactly aligned limit the rotation speed. Therefore, dedicated scanner designs needed to be developed to increase acquisition speed.

Cardiac CT imaging requires one further prerequisite—to provide contiguous cross-sectional images of the heart, every displayed image must be of the same cardiac phase. Otherwise, gaps may occur if adjacent images depict the heart in different phases of the cardiac cycle. Data acquisition must therefore be triggered by the patient's electrocardiogram (ECG) or, in case of continuous acquisition of x-ray data, image reconstruction must be synchronized to a function correlated to cardiac motion, such as the simultaneously recorded ECG (retrospective ECG gating).

Lastly, the heart is subjected not only to intrinsic motion because of cardiac contraction, but also to motion caused by breathing. To avoid artifacts, CT imaging of the complete heart has to be performed within one single breath-hold and CT scanners have to provide for sufficiently fast volume coverage. In practice, image acquisition times of up to 35 seconds can be tolerated by a cooperative patient.

Electron Beam Tomography

The electron beam tomography (EBT) scanner was the first commercially available CT scanner that could be applied to imaging of the heart. It had been developed specifically for cardiac imaging, initially with the purpose of analyzing left ventricular function. In contrast to conventional (mechanical) CT scanners, the EBT scanner does not use a mechanically moving x-ray tube. Instead, a stationary high-voltage electron gun produces a beam of electrons (Fig. 18-2). A system of electromagnetic deflection coils focuses and steers the electron beam to sweep over tungsten targets, which constitute the anode and are arranged in a semicircular array under the patient table. Where the electron beam hits the anode, a fan of x-rays is created that penetrates the patient. Stationary detector arrays are mounted opposite the targets. Because of this design, cross-sectional images can be acquired without the constraints of mechanical motion, and image acquisition times as short as 33 msec/image are possible. In addition, image acquisition by EBT can be prospectively triggered to the patient's ECG. X-rays are emitted only at one or several predefined time points in the cardiac cycle. The EBT scanner had its main application in the assessment of coronary artery

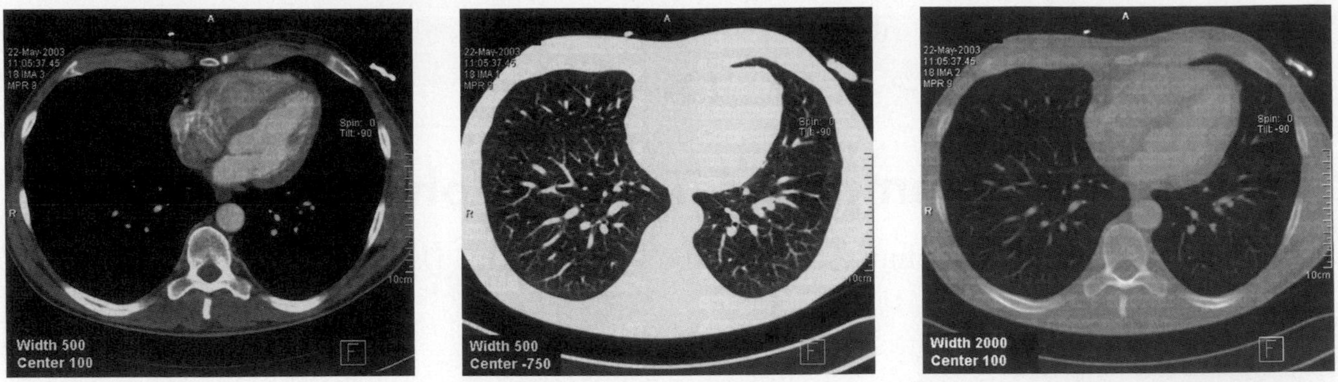

A B C

FIGURE 18–1 The same contrast enhanced cross-sectional computed tomography (CT) images of the chest are displayed in three different window and level settings. **A,** Window width of 500 HU and center of 100 HU provides good soft tissue contrast. Lungs (low CT attenuation) are displayed in black, and bones (high attenuation) are displayed in white. **B,** Same image, displayed with a window width of 500 HU and center of −750 HU. All structures with a CT number of −500 HU or more are now displayed in white, and low-density structures (e.g., the lungs) are displayed with good contrast. **C,** Window width of 2000 HU and center of 100 HU. The image has low contrast but displays all structures from very low (lungs) to high density (bones). In CT, by convention, images are displayed as if looking up from the patient's feet.

TABLE 18–1 Typical Attenuation Values in Noncontrast Computed Tomography

Tissue Type	Attenuation (HU)
Air	−1000
Lungs	−900-750
Fat	−120-50
Water	0-10
Muscle	20-70
Fresh thrombus	20-90
Blood	35-65
Bone	800-3000

HU = Hounsfield units.

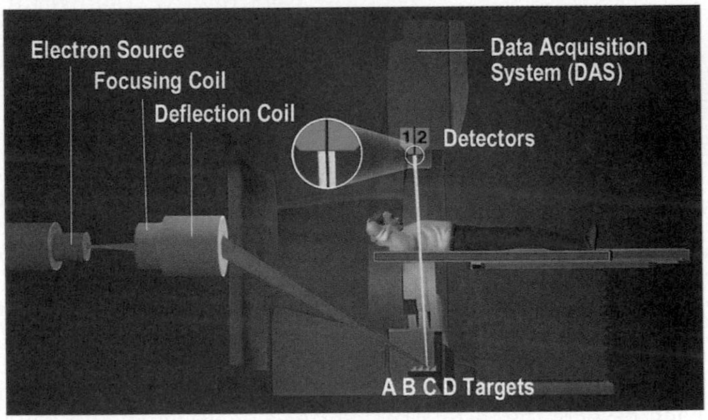

FIGURE 18–2 Principle of electron beam tomography (EBT). An electron beam is created by a high-voltage electron gun. In a large vacuum chamber, the electron beam is focused and deflected by electromagnetic coils to sweep over anode rings arranged in a semicircular fashion below the patient. Where the electron beam hits the anode, x-rays are created. They penetrate the patient and are received by an array of detectors arranged on the opposite side. To create one image, the electron beam needs to perform a 210-degree sweep over the anodes, which requires 33 to 100 milliseconds.

calcifications. Limited spatial resolution, high cost, and limited applicability for non–cardiac imaging prevented more widespread use of the EBT scanner and it is no longer manufactured.

Mechanical Computed Tomography

Substantially improved temporal resolution of conventional (mechanical) CT scanners, the ability to obtain images in defined phases of the cardiac cycle by correlation to the patient's ECG, and growing spatial resolution have continuously increased the applicability of mechanical CT scanners for visualization of the heart and the clinical use of cardiac CT imaging in recent years. In modern multidetector computed tomography (MDCT) scanners, the time for one 360-degree tube rotation has been decreased to 500 milliseconds or less. The scanners can be operated in sequential (step and shoot) mode or in spiral (or helical) mode and permit simultaneous image acquisition in four or more parallel cross sections, with collimation as low as 0.5 mm/slice. Currently, the ability to acquire data in at least 16 slices simultaneously is considered a prerequisite for high-resolution imaging of the heart and coronary arteries, and 64-slice systems are the current state of the art for cardiac CT.

Sequential and Spiral Scan Modes

In sequential mode, images are acquired at one level and, after enough data have been collected for image reconstruction, the table is advanced so that data can be acquired at another level (usually in the next cardiac cycle; Fig. 18-3). Spiral mode offers faster coverage of large volumes. While the gantry is rotating and data are acquired continuously, the table is advanced at a constant speed. After the x-ray data set has been collected, images can retrospectively be reconstructed at any desired level. To reconstruct an image at a given level, a set of projections from numerous angles has to be obtained at that very plane. Because the tube does not perform a full rotation in any given plane, x-ray data for every projection angle are interpolated from the preceding and following tube rotation (see Fig. 18-3).

Partial Scan Reconstruction

One of the major prerequisites for cardiac imaging is high temporal resolution (short image acquisition times). Modern scanners have gantry rotation times of 500 milliseconds or less, but because of the

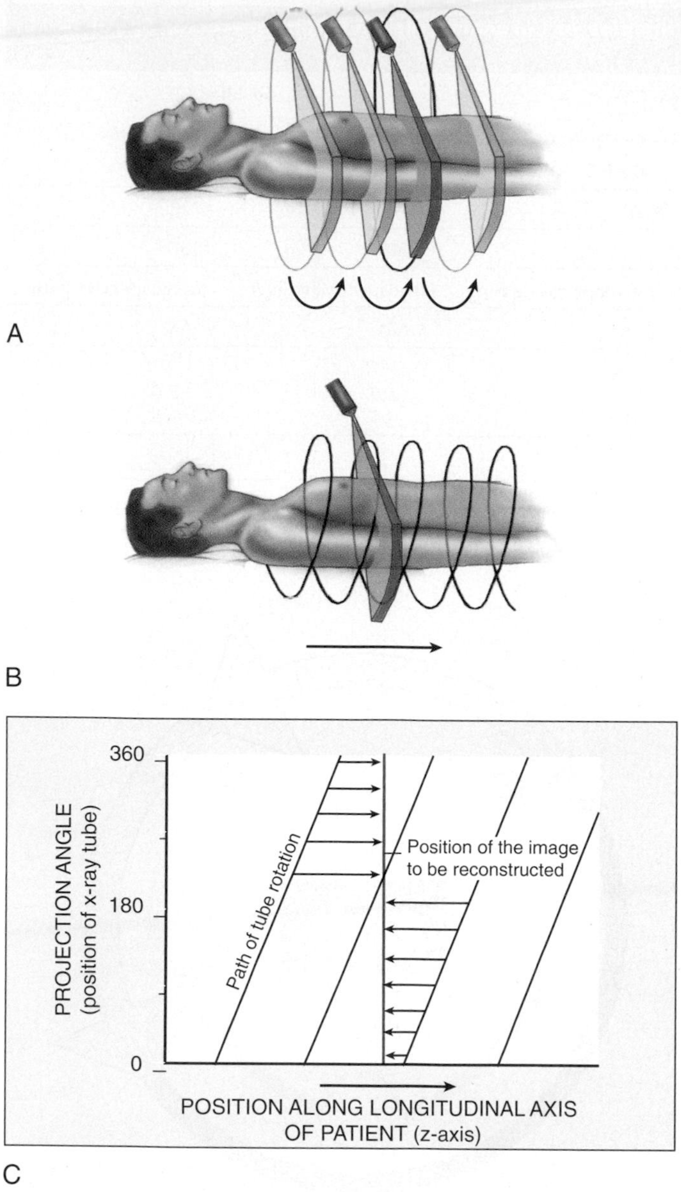

FIGURE 18–3 Principle of sequential and spiral scan modes. **A,** Sequential scanning. X-ray data are acquired at one table position, with the x-ray source and detectors on a circular path. After enough data have been collected for image reconstruction, the x-ray tube is switched off and the table is advanced so that data can be acquired in another level. With multidetector computed tomography (CT), several (4 to 16) image slices can be acquired at each table position. Usually, table movement and image acquisition are triggered to the electrocardiogram so that every acquisition will be performed at the same instant in the cardiac cycle. **B,** Spiral scanning. X-ray data are continuously acquired, with the x-ray tube and detectors in constant circular motion. Simultaneously, the patient table is advanced at a constant speed. The x-ray tube and detectors thus move on a spiral (or helical) path relative to the patient. **C,** Image reconstruction in spiral CT. To reconstruct an image at a given level, a set of projections from numerous angles has to be obtained at that very plane. Because the tube does not perform a full rotation at any given imaging plane, x-ray data for every projection angle are interpolated from the preceding and following tube rotation.

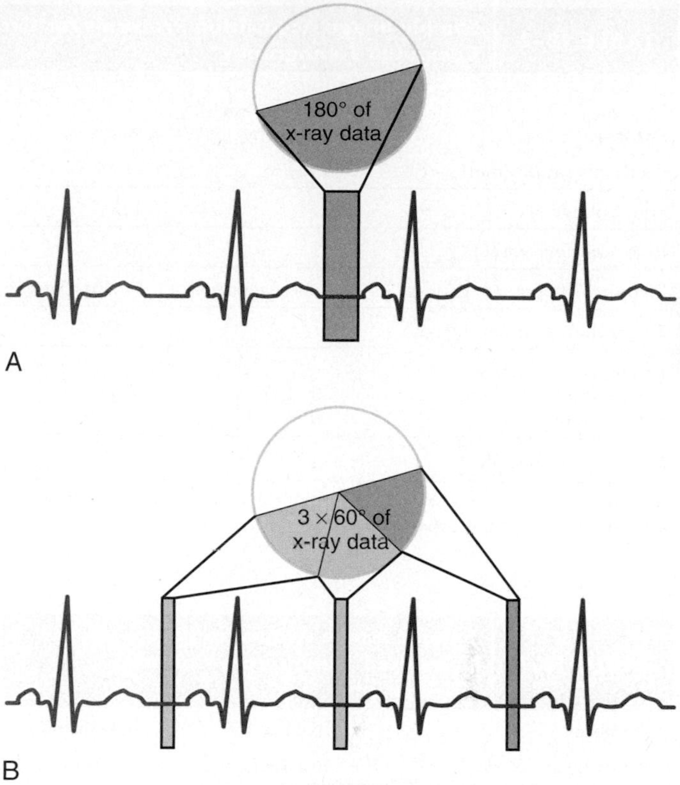

FIGURE 18–4 Half-scan and multisegment reconstruction algorithms. To reconstruct one tomographic image, x-ray data have to be available in projections over approximately 180 degrees. In cardiac computed tomography (CT), the data used for image reconstruction are synchronized to the patient's electrocardiogram (ECG) to ascertain that they all correspond to the same phase of the cardiac cycle. **A,** In half-scan reconstruction algorithms, the data for one tomographic image are collected during one single 180-degree sweep of the x-ray tube so that the temporal resolution corresponds to half of the gantry rotation time. **B,** Multisegment reconstruction algorithms use data collected over several heartbeats (in this case, three heart beats) to fill the 180 degrees of projections for reconstruction of a cross-sectional image at a given level. Temporal resolution (width of the time window used for image reconstruction in each cardiac cycle) can be substantially shorter than in half-scan reconstruction, but is dependent on the relationship between rotation speed, speed of table movement, and heart rate. The obtained image contains data from several consecutive cardiac cycles.

rapid cardiac motion, even reconstructing images with an acquisition window of 500 milliseconds will not be fast enough to suppress cardiac motion artifacts reliably. However, it is not necessary to use x-ray data from a full rotation (360 degrees) to reconstruct one image. Parts of the data are redundant (e.g., attenuation will be the same when an x-ray beam passes through the body from back to front or from front to back). To reconstruct one complete cross-sectional image, it is only necessary to use data from projections over 180 degrees plus the width of the fan angle emitted by the x-ray tube (approximately 50 degrees for most manufacturers). Image reconstruction algorithms that use projections covering less than 360 degrees are called partial scan reconstruction algorithms. The most commonly used algorithms for cardiac imaging use x-ray data from a single sweep over 180 degrees (plus the fan angle) and are usually referred to as half-scan reconstruction algorithms. With this reconstruction technique, a temporal resolution of half the gantry rotation time can be achieved in the center of the scan field.

For multidetector systems, more advanced partial scan reconstruction algorithms are available that make use of less than 180 degrees of tube rotation (so-called multisegment reconstruction algorithms). To fill gaps and provide missing projection angles for reconstruction of an image at a given level, data are used that are acquired during a later heartbeat by another detector and assigned to the correct heart phase by means of the simultaneously recorded ECG (Fig. 18-4). Even though, theoretically, a better temporal resolution can be achieved by confining image reconstruction to shorter segments of the cardiac cycle, the necessity to combine data from several successive heartbeats constitutes a disadvantage of this approach. Because the heart may not return to exactly the same position from heartbeat to heartbeat, this may reduce image quality. A clear advantage of these techniques over half-scan reconstruction has so far not been shown.

Electrocardiographic Gating

Another prerequisite for cardiac imaging by CT is the ability to synchronize the obtained images to the cardiac cycle. To achieve this, image acquisition can be triggered by the patient's ECG in sequential scan modes. In spiral scan mode, x-ray data are continuously acquired,

TABLE 18–2 Sample Image Acquisition Protocols for Cardiac Imaging of Coronary Calcium by Multidetector Spiral Computed Tomography*

Parameter	Electron Beam Tomography	16-Slice CT *Prospective*	16-Slice CT *Retrospective*	64-Slice CT *Prospective*	64-Slice CT *Retrospective*
Slice collimation (mm)	2×3.0	16×1.5	16×1.5	64×1.2	64×1.2
Tube voltage (kV)	130	120	120	120	120
Rotation time (msec)	—	375	375	330	330
Electrocardiographic gating	Prospective trigger	Prospective trigger	Retrospective gating	Prospective trigger	Retrospective gating
Temporal resolution (msec)	50	188*	188*	165*	165*
Image reconstruction Slice thickness (mm) Increment (mm)	 3.0 3.0	 3.0 1.5	 3.0 1.5	 3.0 1.5	 3.0 1.5
Contrast enhancement	—	—	—	—	—

*Temporal resolution in the center of the scan field, for a half-scan reconstruction algorithm.
Scan protocols will vary depending on scanner type.

TABLE 18–3 Sample Image Acquisition Protocols for Computed Tomography Coronary Angiography

Parameter	16-Slice CT	64-Slice CT
Slice collimation (mm)	16×0.75	64×0.6
Tube voltage (kV)	120	120
Rotation time (msec)	375	330
Electrocardiographic gating	Retrospective gating	Retrospective gating
Temporal resolution (msec)	188*	165*
Image reconstruction Slice thickness (mm) Increment (mm)	 1.0 0.7	 0.75 0.5
Scan duration (sec)	~18	~10
Contrast enhancement	Intravenous iodinated contrast (~100 ml)	Intravenous iodinated contrast (~65 ml)

*Temporal resolution in the center of the scan field, for a half-scan reconstruction algorithm.
Scan protocols will vary depending on scanner type.

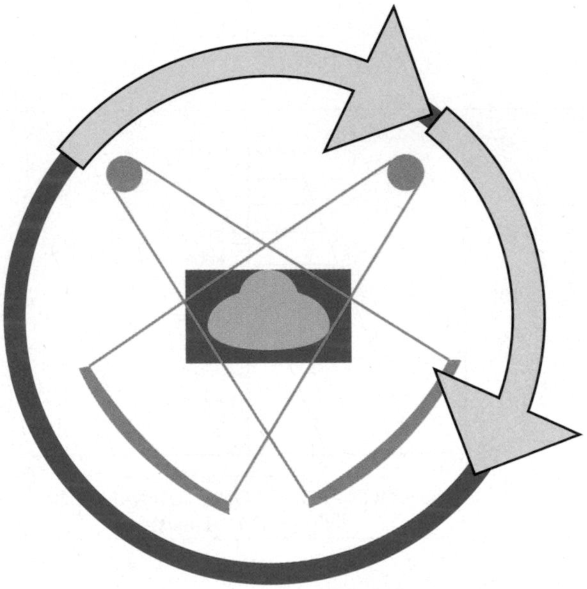

FIGURE 18–5 Design principle of the dual-source computed tomography (DSCT) scanner. Two arrays of tubes and detectors are mounted orthogonally in a single gantry. To acquire x-ray data over 180 degrees of projections, a quarter-rotation is sufficient. At a gantry rotation speed of 330 milliseconds, temporal resolution is 83 milliseconds in the center of the scan field.

and modern CT systems permit simultaneous recording of the patient's ECG with the x-ray data. Using the partial scan reconstruction methods described earlier, it is therefore possible to reconstruct cross-sectional images at any given instant in the cardiac cycle. This technique can be used to minimize motion artifacts (by retrospectively selecting the cardiac phase with the fewest artifacts) or to provide data sets during systole and diastole, which permits dynamic analysis of cardiac function. Although the availability of data throughout the cardiac cycle represents an advantage of continuous data acquisition and retrospective electrocardiographic gating, this scanning mode is associated with a higher radiation dose than sequential scan modes.[1-3] Tables 18-2 and 18-3 list typical scan parameters for EBT and multidetector spiral CT of the heart; Table 18-4 lists typical values for radiation exposure.[1-5]

Future Developments of Computed Tomography Technology

Technology of cardiac CT continues to develop rapidly and much of the development of new CT technology is driven by cardiac imaging applications. As this book goes to print, two new CT scanner designs are being introduced. One concept is to expand the number of detectors from 64 to 256. With a detector width of 0.5 mm, this will yield a coverage of approximately 120 mm that can be obtained in one rotation. Thus, it is possible to visualize the entire volume of the heart in a single rotation, which can be performed during one heartbeat.[6] As opposed to previous scanner generations, this will decrease the length of the necessary breath-hold, decrease the amount of contrast agent necessary to achieve intravascular enhancement during the scan, and may be useful in patients with an inconstant heart rate or arrhythmias. Another new approach is the dual-source CT (DSCT) scanner.[7,8] Two arrays of tubes and detectors are mounted orthogonally in a single gantry (Fig. 18-5). It is therefore possible to obtain x-ray data in 180-degree projections by performing only a quarter-rotation of the gantry. Temporal resolution is thus substantially higher than with previous scanners. It corresponds to one quarter of the rotation time (83 milliseconds temporal resolution at 330 milliseconds gantry rotation time) using a half-scan reconstruction algorithm, without the need to average data over several heartbeats. A further recent development is the combination of positron emission tomography (PET)–CT scanners. Further scientific and clinical assessments are necessary to define the role of these combined scanners in clinical cardiology.

TABLE 18–4 Radiation Exposure Estimates for Cardiac Computed Tomography

Study	Scan	Scanner	Scan Mode	Effective Dose (mSv)	Dose Compared with Invasive Coronary Angiography (mSv)
Morin et al[1]	Calcium	EBT	Sequential	0.7	
	Calcium	4-Slice MDCT	Sequential	1.0	
	Calcium	4-Slice MDCT	Spiral	4.1	
	CTA	4-Slice MDCT	Spiral	9.3	
Hunold et al[2]	Calcium	EBT	Sequential	1.0-1.3	
	Calcium	4-Slice MDCT	Sequential	1.5-1.8	
	Calcium	4-Slice MDCT	Spiral	3.0-6.2	
	CTA	4-Slice MDCT	Spiral	6.7-9.2	2.1-2.5
Trabold et al[3]	Calcium	16-Slice CT	Spiral	2.9-3.6	
	Calcium	16-Slice CT	Spiral	1.6-2.0*	
	CTA	16-Slice CT	Spiral	8.1-10.9	
	CTA	16-Slice CT	Spiral	4.3-5.6*	
Coles et al[4]	CTA	16-Slice CT	Spiral	14.2-15.3	5.4-5.8
Hausleiter et al[5]	CTA	16-Slice CT	Spiral	10.6	
	CTA	16-Slice CT	Spiral	5.0-6.4*	–
	CTA	64-Slice CT	Spiral	14.8	
	CTA	64-Slice CT	Spiral	5.4-9.4*	

*Dose estimates obtained for protocols that incorporated electrocardiogram-correlated modulation of tube current (reduction of tube current in systole).
CT = computed tomography; CTA = CT coronary angiography; EBT = electron beam tomography; MDCT = multidetector CT.

VISUALIZATION OF THE HEART IN COMPUTED TOMOGRAPHY

Nonenhanced Imaging

CT imaging of the heart can be performed with and without injection of a contrast agent. The x-ray attenuation of soft tissue (e.g., myocardium) and blood is almost identical. In cardiac images obtained without injection of contrast agent, it is therefore not possible to discern structures within the heart (Fig. 18-6). Epicardial fat has a lower CT attenuation value, so that the proximal coronary arteries, which are frequently surrounded by fat, can often be recognized (see Fig. 18-6). Nonenhanced CT studies of the heart are almost exclusively performed to assess calcified structures within the heart, most notably coronary artery calcification.

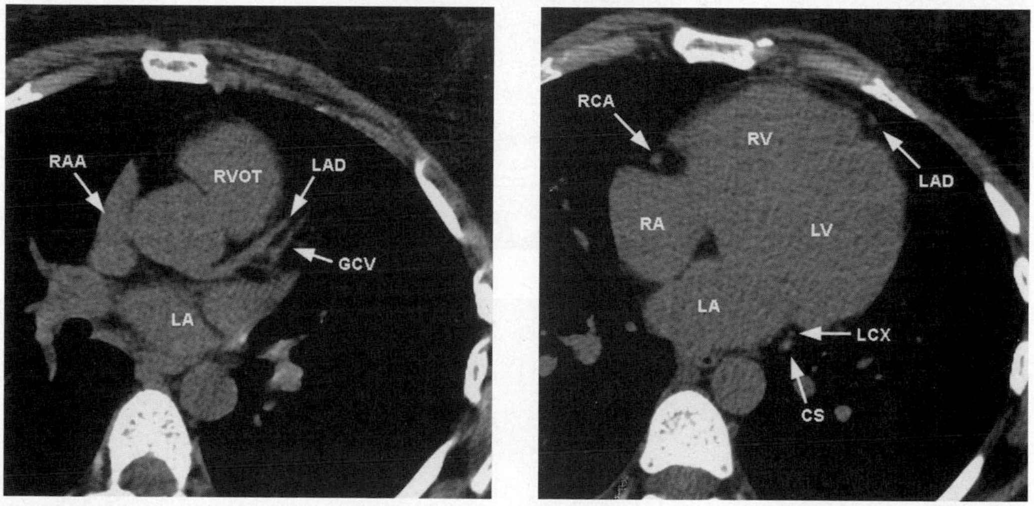

A B

FIGURE 18–6 Normal cardiac anatomy as depicted by nonenhanced computed tomography (CT). Images are in the axial (transverse) plane and displayed as if looking up from the patient's feet. Blood has a similar CT attenuation as connective tissue (e.g., the myocardium). It is therefore not possible to delineate the ventricular cavities or other structures within the heart. **A,** Level of the left coronary artery ostium from the aortic root. **B,** Level of the mid–right coronary artery (RCA). CS = coronary sinus; GCV = great cardiac vein; LA = left atrium; LAD = left anterior descending coronary artery; LCX = left circumflex coronary artery; LV = left ventricle; RA = right atrium; RAA = right atrial appendage; RV = right ventricle; RVOT = right ventricular outflow tract.

Contrast-Enhanced Imaging

To increase the CT attenuation of the blood pool, an iodinated contrast agent can be injected. During the time of CT data acquisition (approximately to 6 to 20 seconds for a high-resolution MDCT scan, depending on scanner type and scan parameters), maximum enhancement of the blood pool should be maintained. To limit the amount of contrast agent that needs to be injected and to achieve good contrast, the correct timing of the actual CT scan relative to contrast injection is important. The CT scan should start when the contrast agent arrives in the ascending aorta, which is usually 15 to 25 seconds after the start of contrast injection into a peripheral vein. Individual determination of the contrast agent transit time is recommended for each patient. If only arterial structures (left ventricle, coronary arteries) are to be investigated, the duration of contrast injection should be approximately the same as the duration of the scan. If structures of the right heart and pulmonary circulation are also to be analyzed, contrast injection must be longer to maintain enhancement in the right heart until the end of the scan.

Contrast-enhanced CT studies permit delineation of the cardiac chambers, valves, great cardiac vessels and, under the prerequisite of sufficient spatial resolution and successful suppression of motion artifacts, the coronary artery lumen (Fig. 18-7). Contrast enhancement in the right atrium can be inhomogeneous because blood saturated with con-

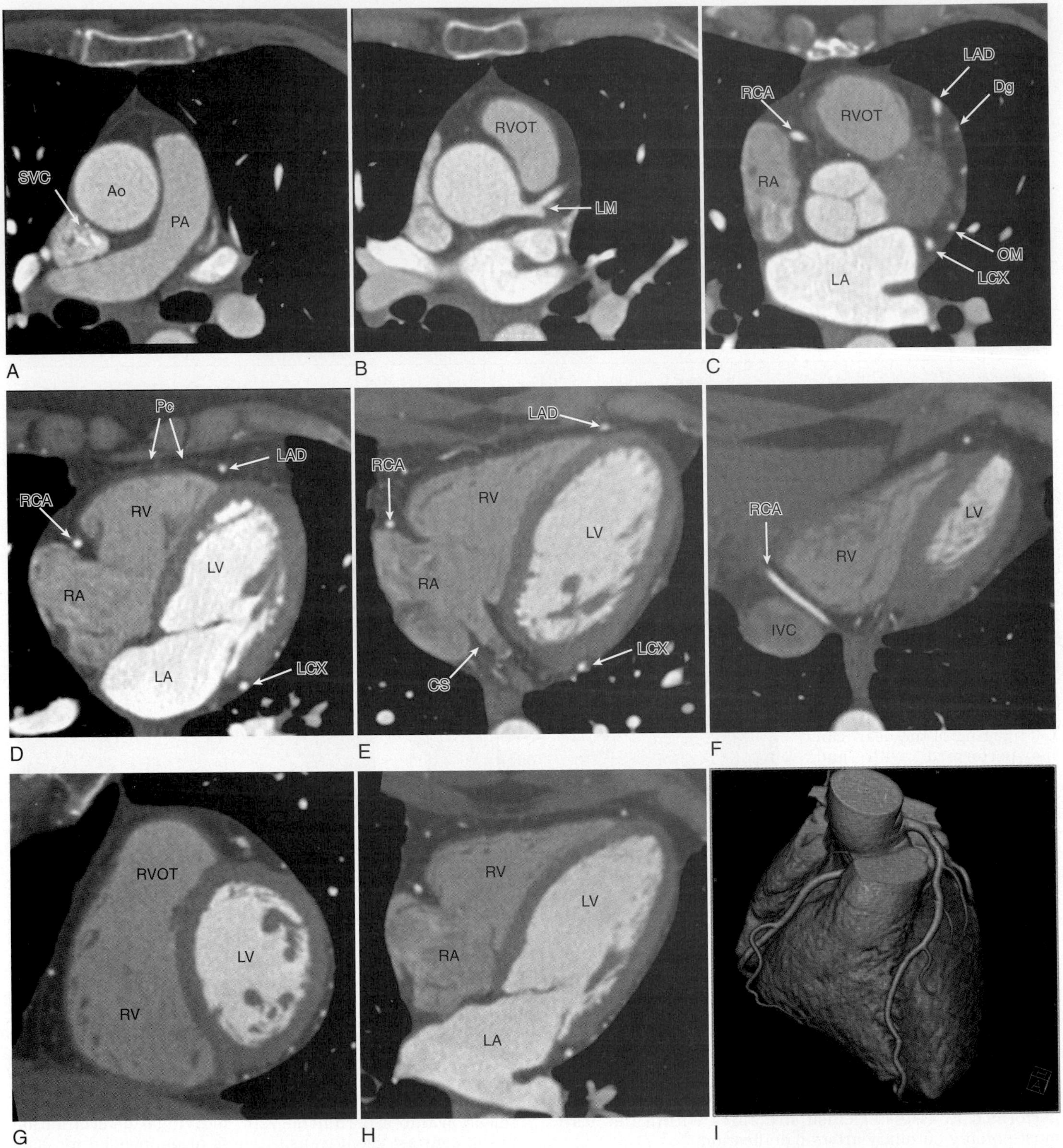

FIGURE 18–7 Normal cardiac anatomy as depicted by contrast-enhanced multidetector computed tomography (MDCT). **A** to **G,** Axial (transverse) cross sections acquired with 165 milliseconds temporal resolution. A craniocaudal sequence of noncontiguous cross sections is shown. **A,** Level of the ascending aorta (Ao) and pulmonary artery, usually the topmost level of a cardiac CT image data set. **B,** Level of the left main coronary artery (LM), which can be seen originating from the aortic root and dividing into the left anterior descending coronary artery and left circumflex coronary artery (arrow). **C,** Level of the proximal right coronary artery (RCA). **D,** Midventricular level. **E,** Level of the caudal right atrium. The drainage of the coronary sinus into the right atrium (RA) can be seen. **F,** Level of the distal right coronary artery. **G,** Multiplanar reconstruction to create a short axis view. **H,** Multiplanar reconstruction to create a four-chamber view. **I,** Three-dimensional surface reconstruction, shown from an anterior view. The coronary arteries can be recognized on the surface of the heart. CS = coronary sinus; Dg = diagonal branch; IVC = inferior vena cava; LA = left atrium; LAA = left atrial appendage; LAD = left anterior descending coronary artery; LCX = left circumflex coronary artery; LV = left ventricle, OM = obtuse marginal branch; Pc = pericardium; PA = pulmonary artery; RA = right atrium; RV = right ventricle; RVOT = right ventricular outflow tract; SVC = superior vena cava.

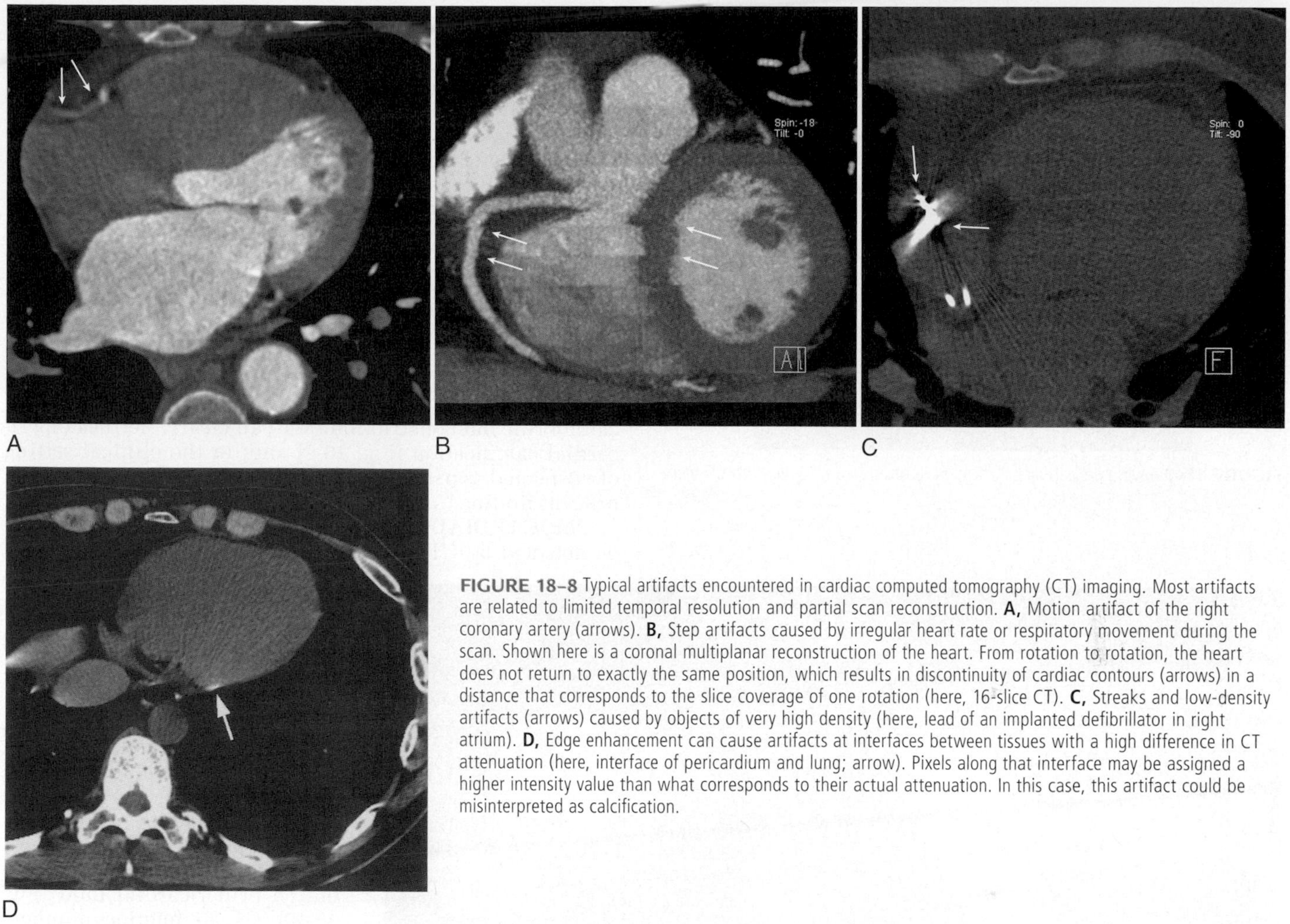

FIGURE 18–8 Typical artifacts encountered in cardiac computed tomography (CT) imaging. Most artifacts are related to limited temporal resolution and partial scan reconstruction. **A,** Motion artifact of the right coronary artery (arrows). **B,** Step artifacts caused by irregular heart rate or respiratory movement during the scan. Shown here is a coronal multiplanar reconstruction of the heart. From rotation to rotation, the heart does not return to exactly the same position, which results in discontinuity of cardiac contours (arrows) in a distance that corresponds to the slice coverage of one rotation (here, 16-slice CT). **C,** Streaks and low-density artifacts (arrows) caused by objects of very high density (here, lead of an implanted defibrillator in right atrium). **D,** Edge enhancement can cause artifacts at interfaces between tissues with a high difference in CT attenuation (here, interface of pericardium and lung; arrow). Pixels along that interface may be assigned a higher intensity value than what corresponds to their actual attenuation. In this case, this artifact could be misinterpreted as calcification.

trast material from the superior vena cava mixes with nonenhanced blood from the inferior vena cava. The resulting artifacts can impair visualization of structures in the right atrium, the interatrial septum, and the tricuspid valve.

Typical Artifacts

CT imaging of the heart is prone to artifacts, because it stretches the temporal and spatial resolution of CT scanners to their limits and additional artifacts can be introduced by the partial scan reconstruction algorithms. It is important to recognize typical artifacts to avoid misinterpretation. Motion artifacts will typically blur the contours of the heart, especially of the coronary arteries (Fig. 18-8). Inconsistent triggering or arrhythmias may cause misalignment of adjacent slices (see Fig. 18-8). In combination with motion, partial scan reconstruction can cause streaks and low-density artifacts adjacent to regions of very high CT density (e.g., metal or calcium). Edge-enhancing reconstruction filters can lead to artifacts along borders between areas of very low and high density (e.g., the interface between lung and cardiac tissue) by assigning artificially high CT numbers to pixels along that border (see Fig. 18-8). Finally, the partial volume effect is a general phenomenon in CT imaging: if an image pixel is only partially filled by a structure of very high attenuation (e.g., metal or bone), a very high CT number will be assigned to the complete pixel, which will thus appear bright on the image. This may lead to overestimation of the dimensions of high-intensity objects (e.g., calcifications within coronary arteries) and may cause difficulties in image interpretation.

CLINICAL APPLICATIONS

Cardiac Morphology

Computed tomography imaging has a relatively high spatial resolution, and a high contrast between the blood pool and other tissues can be achieved after injection of contrast agent. CT imaging therefore has the ability to provide high-resolution morphologic imaging of the heart. Clinically, however, CT imaging does not play a very prominent role in evaluating cardiac morphology, because echocardiography or cardiac magnetic resonancec (CMR) can provide all relevant information in most clinical situations (see Chaps. 14 and 17). Because echocardiography and CMR neither expose the patient to radiation nor require the injection of potentially nephrotoxic contrast agents, echocardiography, possibly followed by CMR, will usually be the preferred approach to imaging for assessment of cardiac morphology. However, cardiac CT imaging can be clinically helpful in various situations, including the need for cross-sectional imaging after echocardiography in patients with pacemakers or other devices that preclude CMR. Also, CT techniques have an extremely high accuracy for the depiction of calcified structures. Finally, cardiac CT imaging is increasingly applicable for coronary artery visualization.

Pericardial Disease (see Chap. 70)

Because the pericardium is usually embedded in epicardial and pericardial fat, it can, in most cases, be delineated in CT images. It usually appears as a thin line (see Fig. 18-7) and is best delineated on the anterior face of the heart. Con-

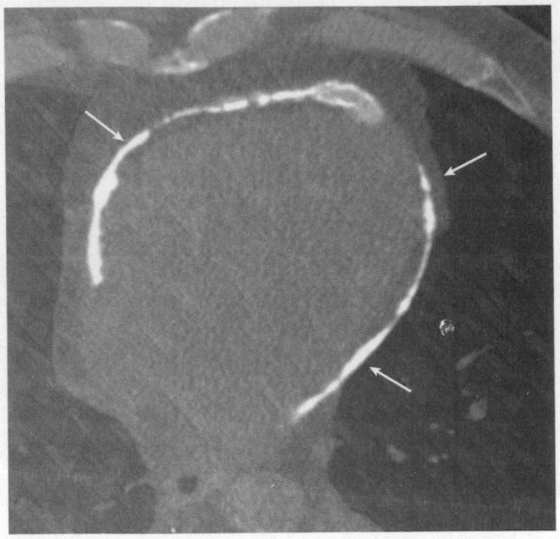

FIGURE 18–9 Severe pericardial calcification (arrows) in a nonenhanced CT scan.

genital absence of the pericardium can be complete or partial. This condition is infrequent, and patients are usually asymptomatic. A CT scan can be helpful in establishing the absence or presence of a segment of pericardium, but lack of visualization, especially on the posterior surface, is not a sufficient criterion for making the diagnosis.[9] Studies have found the normal thickness of pericardium on high-resolution scans to range between 1 and 2 mm.[10,11] Pericardial thickening of more than 4 to 6 mm, even if only localized, can be a helpful finding in cases of suspected constriction, but it does not prove any hemodynamic relevance.[10,11] Thickened pericardium can be found in many situations, including the early postoperative period, uremia, rheumatic heart disease, and sarcoidosis or as a consequence of radiation therapy, and does not constitute proof of constriction per se. Similarly, a normal pericardial thickness cannot rule out constriction.[9] CT can clearly delineate pericardial calcification (Fig. 18-9) and, in the clinical setting of suspected constriction, this should be considered a significant finding.[9]

PERICARDIAL FLUID. Pericardial fluid can reliably be detected by CT, and small amounts of fluid in pericardial recesses can frequently be observed in healthy individuals.[12] Although echocardiography has an excellent sensitivity to detect relevant pericardial effusion in most clinical situations (see Chap. 14), its application can be limited in postoperative patients, and some localized effusions may be outside the echocardiographic acoustic windows. CT can clearly delineate the anatomical distribution of pericardial fluid (Fig. 18-10). CT attenuation numbers measured in the pericardial fluid may give some indication as to the genesis of the effusion. Densities higher than water (above approximately 10 HU) suggest high protein content (e.g., blood).[10]

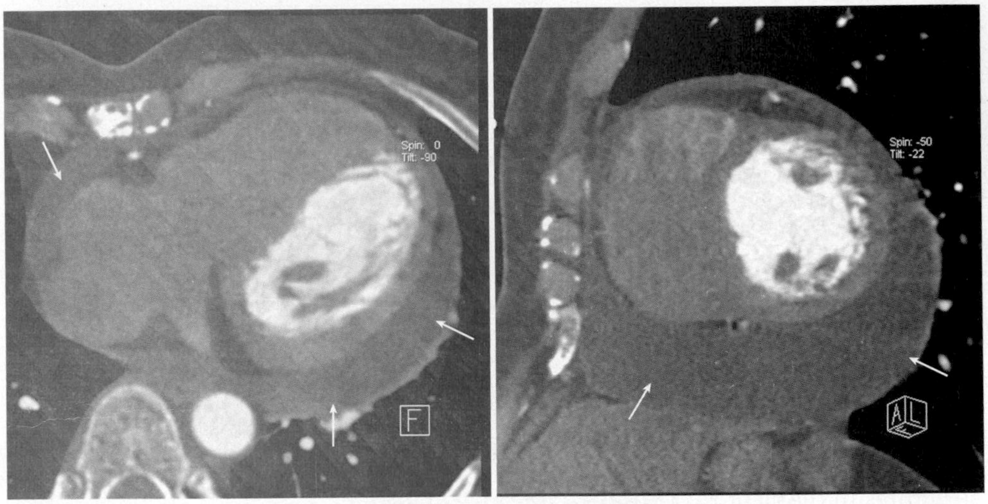

A B

FIGURE 18–10 Pericardial effusion. **A,** Large circumferential pericardial effusion (arrows) in transaxial orientation. **B,** Same patient as in **A**; short-axis orientation.

PERICARDIAL CYSTS AND NEOPLASMS. Pericardial cysts appear on CT images as paracardiac masses, typically in the right cardiophrenic angle. The cysts have a thin capsule that is not always visualized but may occasionally be calcified. The cysts are usually filled with fluid of water-equivalent density (Fig. 18-11). Bronchiogenic cysts or teratomas may mimic pericardial cysts in location and appearance. Primary neoplasms of the pericardium are infrequent but can be the reason for thickened pericardium on CT scans. Both primary neoplasms and secondary involvement of the pericardium can be accompanied by hemorrhagic pericardial effusions.[13]

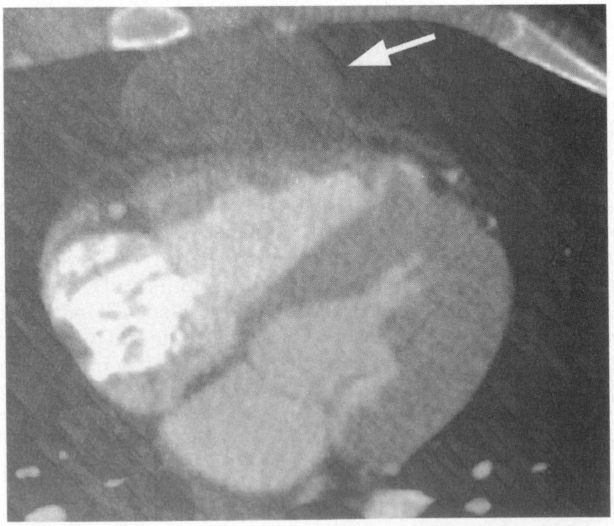

FIGURE 18–11 Pericardial cyst located anterior to the right ventricle in a contrast-enhanced electron beam CT scan (arrow).

Myocardial Disease (see Chaps. 64 and 65)

The role of CT in the assessment of myocardial disease is limited. Even though CT can clearly show left ventricular geometry, wall thickness,[14] and also function, the diagnosis of dilated or hypertrophic cardiomyopathy does not require cross-sectional imaging. Except for occasional case reports, little is known about the value of CT in assessing infiltrative myocardial disease. CT imaging can be useful in the assessment of arrhythmogenic right ventricular dysplasia. Typical findings that can be obtained by CT include dilation of the right ventricle and infiltration of the myocardium with fatty tissue of low CT attenuation (less than

0 HU), as well as aneurysms and local bulging of the right ventricular free wall (Fig. 18-12).[15,16] CT may be especially useful when the diagnosis of arrhythmogenic right ventricular dysplasia is suspected or needs to be confirmed in patients who already have implanted devices, or if intermittent arrhythmias or claustrophobia prevent cardiac MRI.

Valvular Disease (see Chap. 62)

Visualization of the tricuspid and pulmonary valves by CT is inconsistent, but the mitral and aortic valves can reliably be depicted in contrast-enhanced cardiac CT scans (Fig. 18-13). Although CT is unable to provide measurements of transvalvular flow and pressure gradients, dynamic imaging of the open and closed valve is possible (Fig. 18-14). Initial work has demonstrated that CT can quantify the regurgitant orifice area in mitral regurgitation.[17] For the normal and stenotic aortic valve, several recent studies have demonstrated the ability of MDCT to measure the orifice area, with close correlation to transesophageal echocardiography and invasive assessment of the aortic orifice area.[18-21] However, in the setting of severely calcified stenosis, measurements of the opening area by CT may become unreliable. Nonenhanced CT can be used to quantify aortic valve calcium. Accuracy and reproducibility are high and the progression of aortic valve calcification can be assessed.[22,23] This may develop into clinically relevant applications with respect to the prognostic relevance of aortic valve sclerosis,[24] as well as the problem of bioprosthesis calcification. The movement of metallic valve prostheses can be accurately visualized (Fig. 18-15).

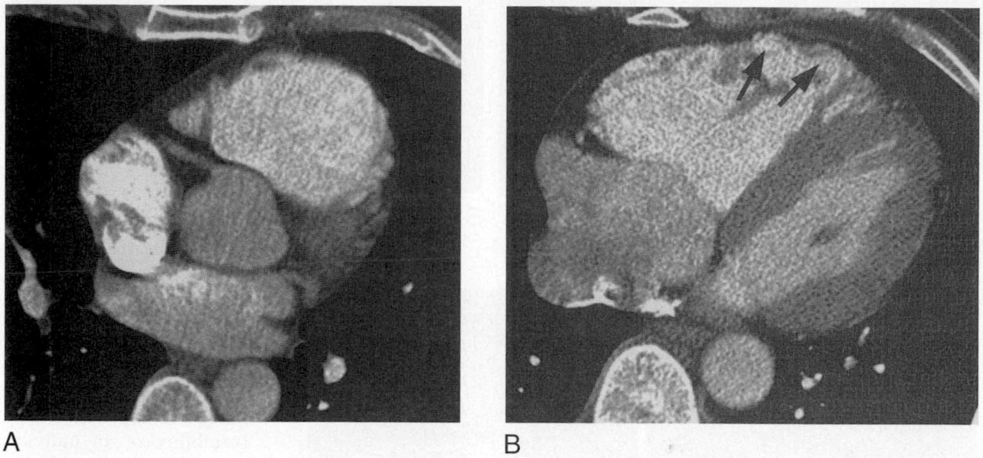

FIGURE 18-12 A and **B,** Dilated right ventricle and aneurysmal bulging of the right ventricular free wall (arrows) in a patient with arrhythmogenic right ventricular dysplasia. *(Courtesy of Dr. J. F. Breen, Mayo Clinic, Rochester, Minn.)*

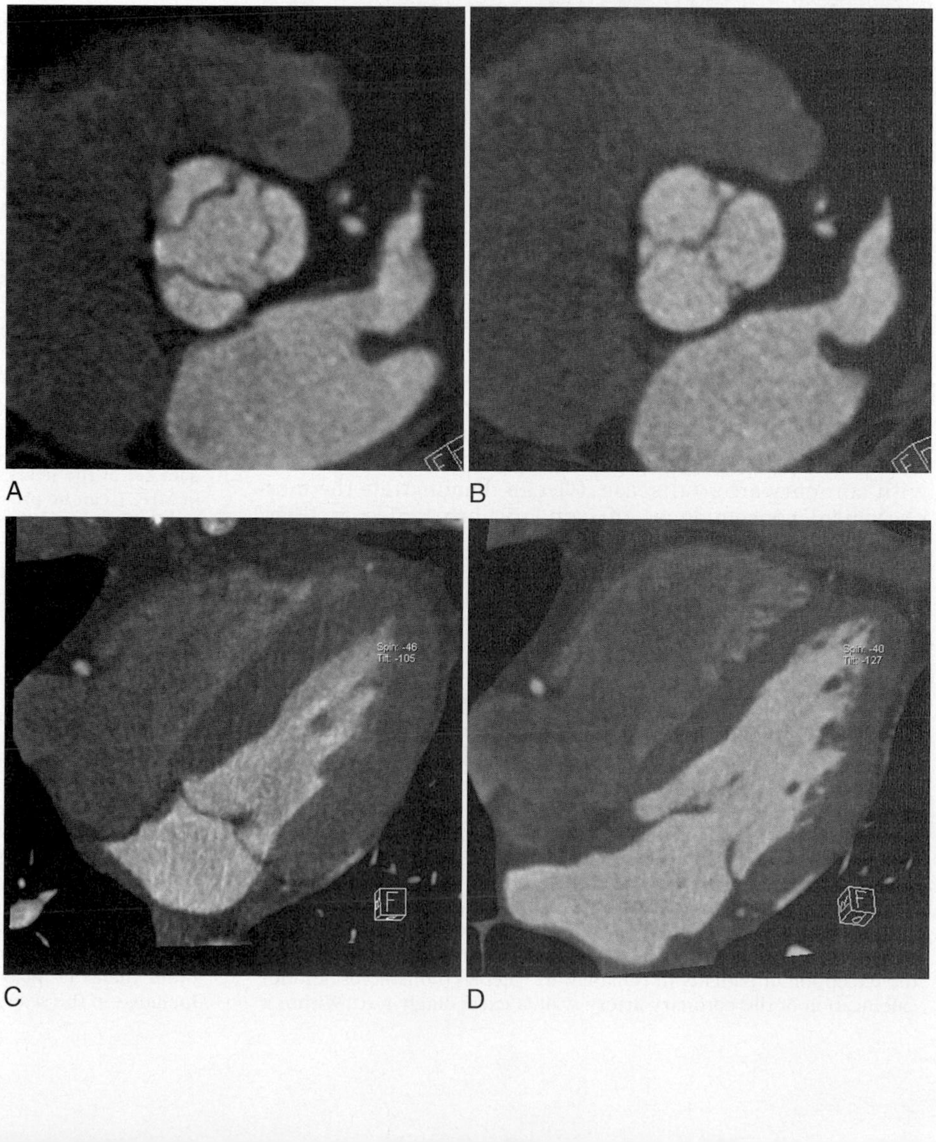

FIGURE 18-13 Visualization of cardiac valves by computed tomography. Visualization of a normal aortic valve in open **(A)** and closed **(B)** positions by multidetector computed tomography. Visualization of a normal mitral valve in closed **(C)** and open **(D)** positions.

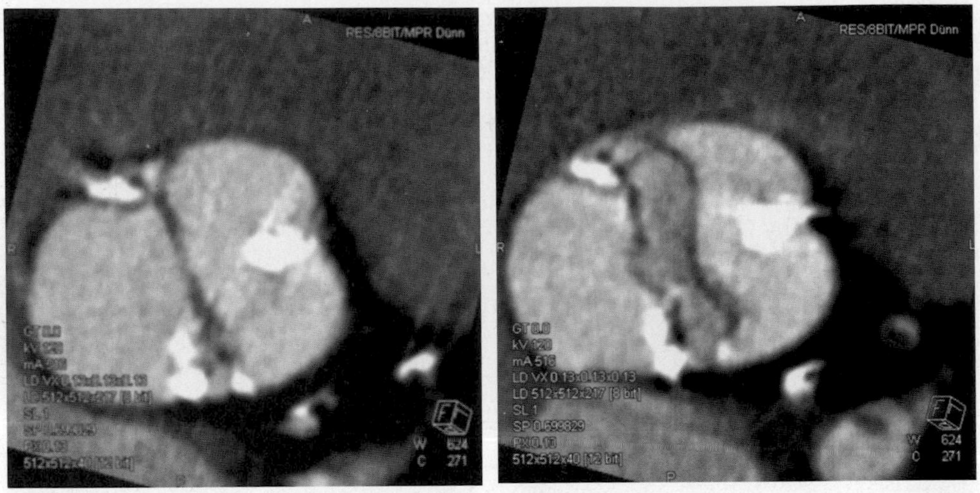

A B

FIGURE 18-14 Bicuspid aortic valve with calcification and impaired opening visualized in diastole **(A)** and systole **(B)** by multidetector computed tomography after intravenous injection of contrast agent.

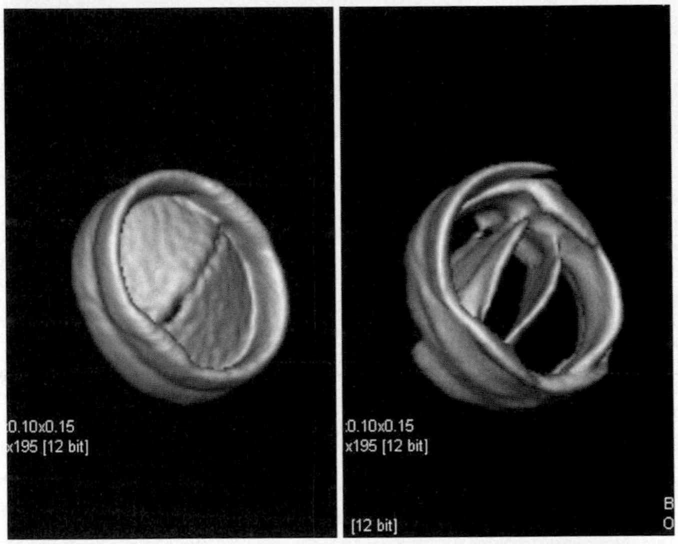

FIGURE 18-15 In vivo visualization of function of a prosthetic bileaflet aortic valve. This three-dimensional reconstruction shows normal opening (right) and closure (left) of the two leaflets.

Coronary Artery Disease (see Chap. 54)

Cardiac CT has several potential applications for patients with coronary artery disease. CT can demonstrate the morphological consequences of ischemic heart disease (Figs. 18-16 and 18-17) and assess ventricular function and perfusion, and has been applied with increasing success to visualize coronary arteries. In addition, the assessment of coronary artery calcification has received considerable attention with respect to its potential role in the early detection of subclinical atherosclerosis. In the diagnostic workup of coronary artery disease, the emerging abilities of CT imaging compete with many other well-established and readily available diagnostic modalities. In this context, the most appropriate clinical use of CT is made when limiting its application to situations in which clinical evidence shows advantages over other modalities.

Coronary Artery Calcification

PATHOLOGY. Coronary calcium is a surrogate marker for coronary atherosclerotic plaque. In the coronary arteries, calcifications occur almost exclusively in the context of atherosclerotic changes.[25,26] With the exception of patients in renal failure, medial (nonatherosclerotic) calcification of the coronary artery wall is exceedingly rare. Within a coronary vessel or larger segment of the vessel, the amount of coronary calcium correlates moderately closely with the extent of atherosclerotic plaque burden.[25,26] On the other hand, not every atherosclerotic coronary plaque is calcified. The presence or absence of calcium is not closely associated with the propensity of an individual atherosclerotic plaque to rupture, and calcification is neither a sign of stability nor instability of an individual plaque.[25] Plaques with healed ruptures almost invariably contain calcium, whereas plaque erosions are frequently not calcified. In the vast majority of patients with acute coronary syndromes, coronary calcium can be detected, and the amount of calcium in these patients is substantially greater than in matched control subjects without coronary artery disease.[27-29]

Although there is a strong quantitative relationship between coronary calcification and coronary plaque burden, there is only a weak nonlinear correlation between the amount of coronary calcium and the angiographic severity of obstructive coronary artery disease.[26] The complete absence of coronary calcium makes the presence of significant coronary luminal obstruction highly unlikely, however.[26]

In patients with end-stage renal disease, the prevalence and extent of coronary calcification are high. However, the relationship of coronary calcium to coronary atherosclerosis is less well established in this patient group.[25]

DETECTION OF CORONARY CALCIUM. Although mechanical CT without ECG gating is unsuitable for the reliable detection of coronary artery calcium,[30] EBT and ECG-gated spiral CT with subsecond rotation permit detection and quantification of coronary artery calcium with equal accuracy.[31] The vast majority of existing data concerning histopathological validation and clinical evaluation of coronary calcium assessment has been obtained using EBT.

The usual protocol to detect and quantify coronary calcification by CT consists of the acquisition of a high-resolution axial cross-sectional data set of the heart without contrast enhancement. Data acquisition in MDCT can be prospectively triggered to the ECG or retrospectively gated; the latter provides for higher quality data sets, albeit at the expense of higher radiation dose. By convention, images are reconstructed with a slice thickness of 3.0 mm. Although no overlap is used in EBT data sets, MDCT data sets generally use an overlap of 1.5 mm to improve the spatial resolution of the data set.

The presence of calcifications is assumed if contiguous pixels with a density exceeding 130 HU are found within the coronary artery system (Fig. 18-18).[26] The Agatston score has most frequently been used to quantify the amount of coronary calcium in CT. The Agatston score is derived by measuring the area of each calcified coronary lesion and multiplying it by a coefficient of 1 to 4, depending on the maximum CT attenuation within the lesion. The sum of all lesions represents the Agatston score for the patient. Several large reference data sets are available that describe the distribution of Agatston scores found in the respective (usually self-referred) population, stratified by age and gender.[28,32-34] Other means of quantifying the amount of coronary calcification, such as the calcified mass or volume, have been proposed and often display a slightly better reproducibility than the Agatston score. Because there is a lack of large reference data sets for scores other than the Agatston score, it is recommended that all scores be included in the scan report.

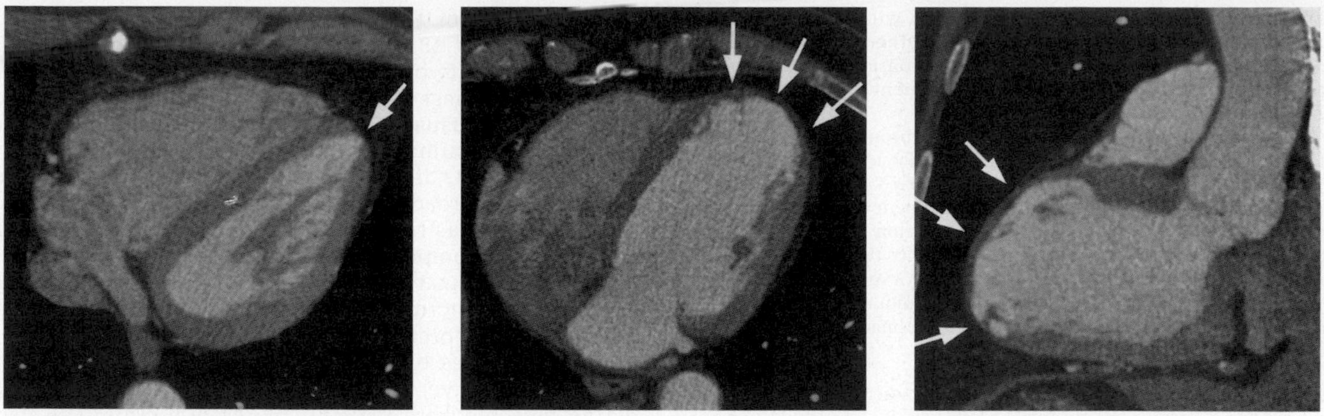

A B C

FIGURE 18-16 Computed tomography (CT) clearly depicts regional wall thinning as a consequence of myocardial infarction. It is important to note that in healthy subjects, the left ventricular wall in the very apical region can be paper thin, which constitutes a frequent normal finding.[14] **A,** Normal tapering of the left ventricular apex as frequently observed in high-resolution CT scans (arrow). Infarction of the anterior wall (arrows) in an axial cross section **(B)** and multiplanar reformat **(C)**.

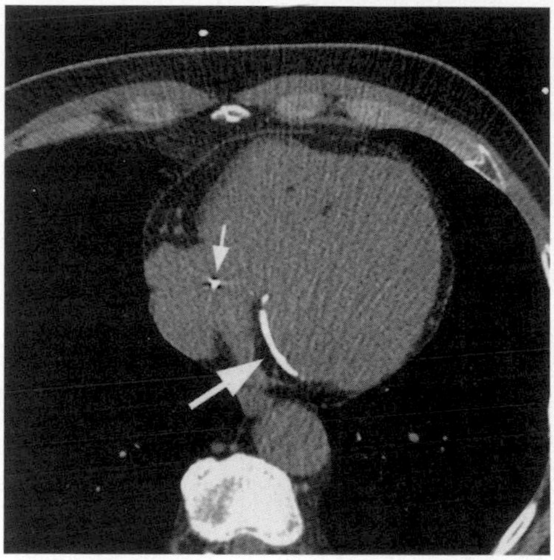

FIGURE 18-17 Calcified left ventricular aneurysm (large arrow) as a consequence of posterior myocardial infarction in a nonenhanced multidetector CT scan (small arrow = pacemaker lead).

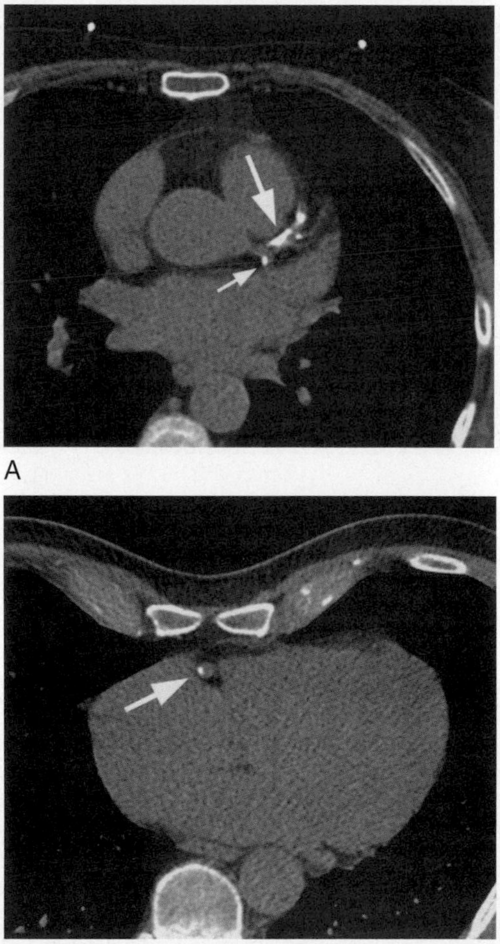

A

B

FIGURE 18-18 Examples of coronary calcification. **A,** Calcification of the left anterior descending coronary artery (large arrow) and left circumflex coronary artery (small arrow). **B,** Calcification of the right coronary artery (arrow).

The analysis of coronary calcification in coronary CT images is usually straightforward. Difficulties in interpretation can arise in the presence of motion artifacts (Fig. 18-19). The close proximity of the left circumflex coronary artery to the mitral valve and annulus can sometimes lead to misinterpreting mitral calcification as coronary calcium (see Fig. 18-19). Interscan variability for calcium quantification can be high for patients with small amounts of calcium, but is lower for higher calcium scores. One recent study has found an average variability of 20 percent for the Agatston score and 18 percent for the calcified volume in a population sample.[31]

CLINICAL SIGNIFICANCE OF CORONARY CALCIUM. Coronary calcium correlates with the presence and extent of coronary atherosclerosis. The absence of coronary calcium thus rules out the presence of significant coronary artery stenoses, with high predictive value.[26] However, because even pronounced coronary atherosclerotic plaque burden is not necessarily associated with hemodynamically relevant luminal narrowings, even the detection of large amounts of calcium does not imply the presence of significant stenoses. Thus, the finding of pronounced calcifications by itself does not necessitate invasive coronary angiography.

Several cohort studies have shown that the presence of coronary calcium demonstrated by computed tomography in asymptomatic individuals is a prognostic parameter with high predictive power regarding the development of hard cardiac events during the following 3 to 5 years.[28,35-43] A meta-analysis has demonstrated that a calcium score higher than the median is associated with an unadjusted odds ratio of 4.2 (95 percent confidence interval [CI], 1.6 to 11.3) for myocardial infarction or death.[44] Whereas the predictive value of coronary calcium in asymptomatic individuals is widely accepted,[26,45] it is less clear which patients or individuals will profit from having a coronary calcium scan performed. It is currently assumed that individuals who seem to be at intermediate risk for coronary events (1.0 to 2.0 percent annual risk), based on traditional risk factor analysis, will be most likely to profit from noninvasive testing for subclinical atherosclerosis, and the use of coronary calcification measurement is considered "reasonable" in this situation.[26] Unselected screening or patient self-referral is uniformly not recommended.[26,46]

Coronary calcification has been found to be progressive over time.[47] Initial studies have observed a higher coronary artery disease event rate in patients with more rapid progression of coronary artery calcium.[48] Studies that have assessed the influence of lipid-lowering therapy on the progression of coronary calcium report conflicting results.[49-54] The lack of data that would support the use of repeated calcium scans to guide the intensity of risk factor modification and the measurement variability, especially for small amounts of calcification, currently do not allow recommendations to be made for repeat coronary calcium scanning.[46]

Visualization of the Coronary Artery Lumen (see Chap. 20)

Computed tomography can be applied for visualization of the coronary artery lumen after intravenous injection of a contrast agent (coronary CT angiography). Based on axial cross sections of the heart, a two- or three-dimensional reconstruction of the coronary arteries can be rendered (Figs. 18-20 and 18-21). Concerning the detection of coronary stenoses, two-dimensional forms of reconstruction provide the highest diagnostic accuracy. Three-dimensional reconstruction usually adds no further information but may be useful to document findings.

Because of its higher spatial resolution, faster volume coverage, and broader availability, MDCT with 16 or more detector rows has replaced EBT for coronary CT angiography. However, temporal resolution is still the major limiting factor for visualization of the coronary arteries by MDCT. It has been convincingly demonstrated that regular and low heart rates are a prerequisite for reliable visualization of the coronary arteries by 16- to 64-slice MDCT.[55] Hence, most investigators have proposed the administration of short-acting beta blockers prior to the MDCT scan. The use of sublingual nitroglycerin is also recommended to achieve coronary vasodilation and maximize image quality.

Numerous studies have compared the accuracy of coronary artery stenosis detection by MDCT with invasive coronary angiography (see Figs. 18-20 and 18-21). Results depend on several factors, such as the technology used, the patient group studied (e.g., prevalence of disease), scan protocols (e.g., systematic lowering of heart rate), criteria used to define a significant coronary stenosis, and the basis for evaluation (per coronary segment, per coronary artery, or per patient). Table 18-5 compares the accuracy for the detection of coronary artery stenoses on a per-segment basis in studies performed with recent generations of 16- to 64-slice CT in comparison with invasive coronary angiography. Table 18-6 lists studies that have performed a per-patient analysis, which, in clinical terms, may be even more rel-

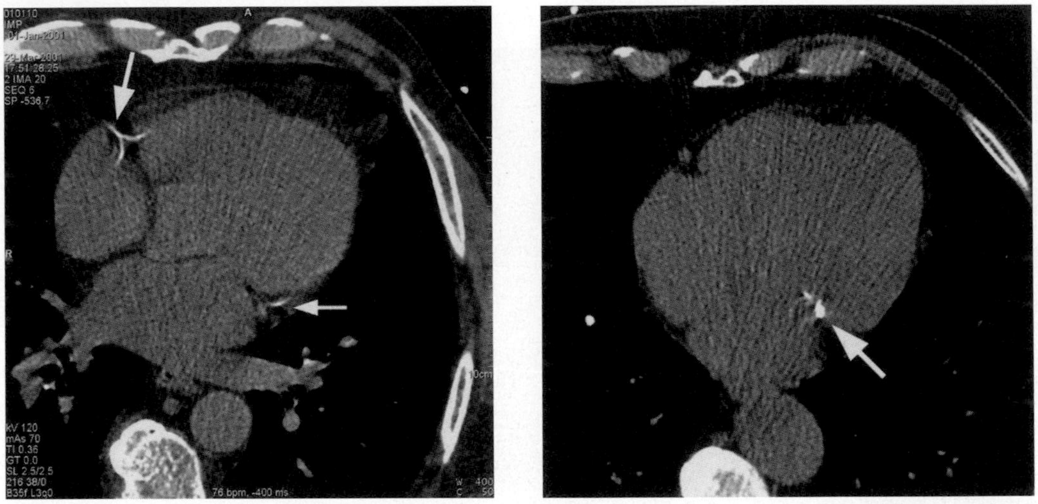

A B

FIGURE 18-19 Interpretation problems in coronary calcium scans. **A,** Motion artifacts of the right coronary artery (large arrow) and, to a lesser extent, of the left circumflex coronary artery (small arrow) in prospective electrocardiographically triggered sequential multidetector computed tomography (four-slice scanner, 500-millisecond rotation, patient with a heart rate of 75/min). **B,** Calcification of the mitral annulus (arrow). Because of the proximity of the course of the left circumflex coronary artery, mitral calcification can be misinterpreted as calcium in the left circumflex coronary artery.

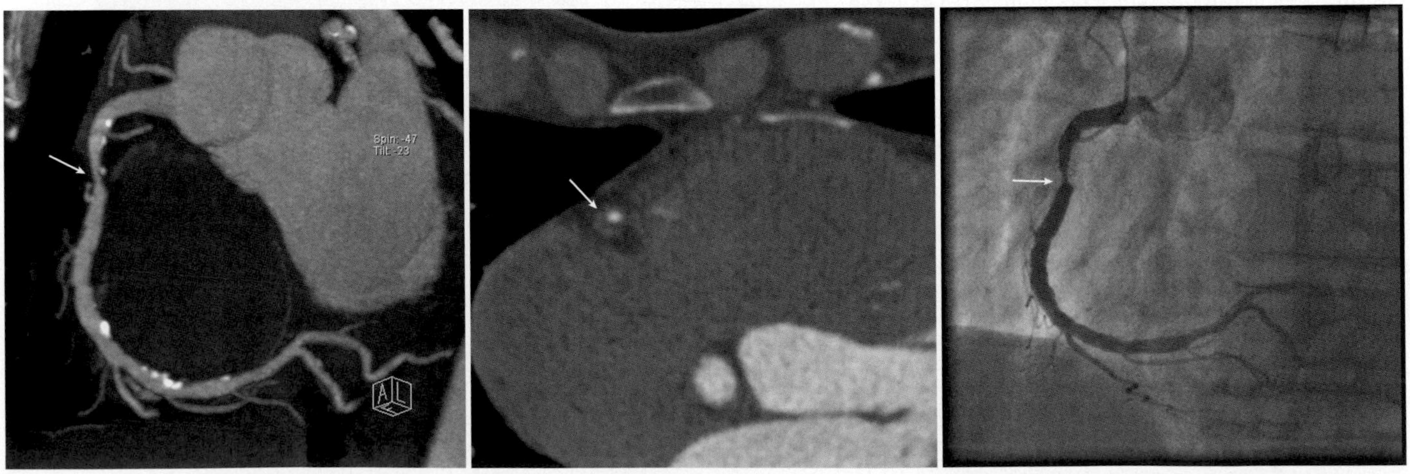

A B C

FIGURE 18-20 Noninvasive coronary angiography by multidetector computed tomography. This patient had a high-grade right coronary artery stenosis (arrows). **A,** Two-dimensional reconstruction (maximum intensity projection). **B,** Transaxial cross section at the level of right coronary artery stenosis, showing substantial narrowing of the contrast-enhanced lumen caused by noncalcified plaque. **C,** Corresponding invasive coronary angiogram.

TABLE 18–5 Accuracy of 16-Slice CT with Recent Technology and 64-Slice CT for the Detection of Coronary Artery Stenoses*

Study	No. of Patients	Rotation (msec)	Sensitivity (%)	Specificity (%)	NPV (%)	PPV (%)	Unevaluable
16-Slice CT							
Kuettner et al[56]	124	375	85	98	96	87	7
Mollet et al[57]	51	375	95	98	99	79	—
Morgan-Hughes et al[58]	58	500	83	97	97	80	2
Hoffmann et al[55]	103	420	95	98	99	87	6
Achenbach et al[59]	50	375	94	96	99	69	4
Garcia et al[60]	187	420	85	91	99	36	29
64-Slice CT							
Leschka et al[61]	53	370	94	97	99	87	—
Raff et al[62]	70	330	86	95	98	66	12
Leber et al[63]	59	330	88†	97	99	—	—
Mollet et al[64]	52	330	99	95	99	76	2
Ropers et al[65]	82	330	95	93	99	56	4
Fine et al[66]	66	330	95	96	95	97	6
Nikolaou et al[67]	72	330	86	95	97	72	10

*On a per-segment or per-artery basis in comparison with invasive, catheter-based coronary angiography.
†Mid and proximal segments.
CT = computed tomography; NPV = negative predictive value; PPV = positive predictive value.

TABLE 18–6 Accuracy of Coronary CT Angiography to Identify Patients with at Least One Coronary Artery Stenosis*

Study	No. of Patients	Collimation/Rotation (msec)	Sensitivity (%)	Specificity (%)	NPV (%)	PPV (%)
Mollet[57]	51	16 × 0.75/375	100	100	100	100
Hoffmann[55]	103	16 × 0.75/420	95	97	94	98
Achenbach[59]	50	16 × 0.75/375	100	83	100	86
Garcia et al[60]	187	16 × 0.75/420	98	54	99	50
Leschka[61]	53	64 × 0.6/375	100	100	100	100
Raff[62]	70	64 × 0.6/330	95	90	93	93
Leber[63]	59	64 × 0.6/330	94	—	—	—
Mollet[64]	52	64 × 0.6/330	100	92	100	97
Ropers[65]	82	64 × 0.6/330	96	91	98	83
Nikolaou[67]	72	64 × 0.6/330	97	72	95	83

*In comparison with invasive, catheter-based coronary angiography.
CT = computed tomography; NPV = negative predictive value; PPV = positive predictive value.

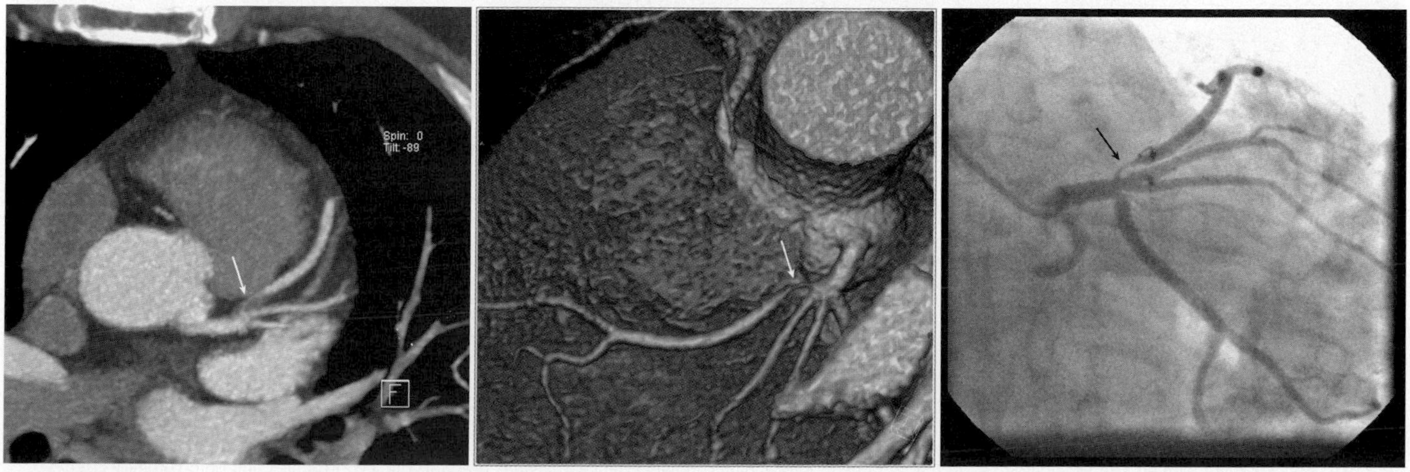

A B C

FIGURE 18-21 Patient with a high-grade ostial stenosis of the left anterior descending coronary artery (arrows). **A,** Two-dimensional reconstruction (maximum intensity projection) obtained by multidetector computed tomography. **B,** Three-dimensional reconstruction. **C,** Corresponding invasive coronary angiogram.

evant to identify *patients* with or without significant coronary artery stenosis. It is remarkable that in both types of evaluation, the negative predictive value was uniformly found to be high, ranging from 93 to 100 percent. Even though this may partly be influenced by a rather low prevalence of coronary artery stenoses in most patient groups studied, it does indicate the method's ability to rule out the presence of coronary artery stenoses reliably if the MDCT scan is expertly acquired and evaluated, has sufficient image quality, and fails to demonstrate coronary artery stenoses. The positive predictive value has usually been found to be lower, ranging from 50 to 100 percent on a per-patient basis and from 36 to 97 percent on a per-segment basis.[56-67] MDCT, therefore, does tend to overestimate disease severity in comparison with invasive coronary angiography. Accurate grading of the severity of a coronary lesion (percentage of stenosis) is currently not possible on a routine basis and, even in optimally prepared patients, pronounced coronary calcifications, trigger artifacts caused by arrhythmias, or high image noise can prevent analysis of coronary segments in regard to the presence of stenoses.

While CT coronary angiography presently cannot be considered a routine replacement for invasive coronary angiography, clinical application, especially to rule out coronary stenoses in patients who do not have a high pretest likelihood of disease, is conceivable. This pertains to patients with stable symptoms but potentially also to patients with acute chest pain.[68] A recently published consensus document lists several indications for coronary CT angiography as "appropriate," including symptomatic patients with intermediate likelihood of disease but in whom stress testing is not possible or the result of stress testing is equivocal or uninterpretable, as well as patients with acute chest pain and intermediate likelihood of disease but absence of ECG changes and normal mycoardial enzyme levels.[69]

Imaging of coronary stents has been demonstrated (Fig. 18-22), but partial volume effects and artifacts caused by metal frequently prevent adequate visualization of the coronary lumen inside stents. Stent size substantially influences the ability to analyze the stent lumen by CT. In a small study investigating left main coronary artery stents with a mean diameter of 3.9 mm, good results for stenosis detection were found.[70] However, visualization of the stent lumen is currently not reliably possible in unselected patients and therefore does not constitute an indication for clinical application of CT coronary angiography.

In contrast-enhanced MDCT, patency and occlusion of bypass grafts can be established with very high accuracy (Fig. 18-23),[71-77] but limitations exist concerning the detection of stenoses at the site of the anastomosis to the coronary artery and in the peripheral run-off vessels. Clinical situations that might benefit from noninvasive assessment of bypass patency by CT are therefore currently limited.

Because of the three-dimensional nature of the tomographic data set, CT coronary angiography is an excellent tool to investigate patients with known or suspected congenital coronary artery anomalies (Fig. 18-24). MDCT can classify both the origin and the often complex course of anomalous coronary vessels.[78-81] Although the necessity for contrast agent injection and radiation exposure are certain drawbacks of CT as compared with MRI, which has also been suggested as a diagnostic tool in coronary artery anomalies, the ease of data acquisition, and the predictability with which a high-resolution data set with optimal image quality for evaluation can be expected, make cardiac CT a valid first choice for the work-up of known or suspected anomalous coronary anatomy.

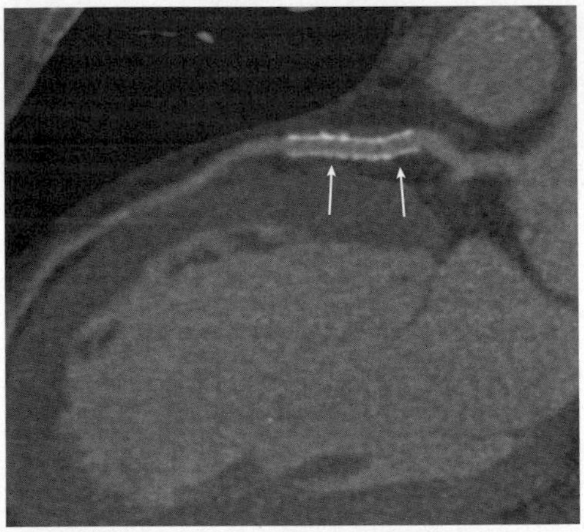

FIGURE 18-22 Visualization of a patent stent (arrows) in the proximal left anterior descending coronary artery (stent diameter, 3.5 mm).

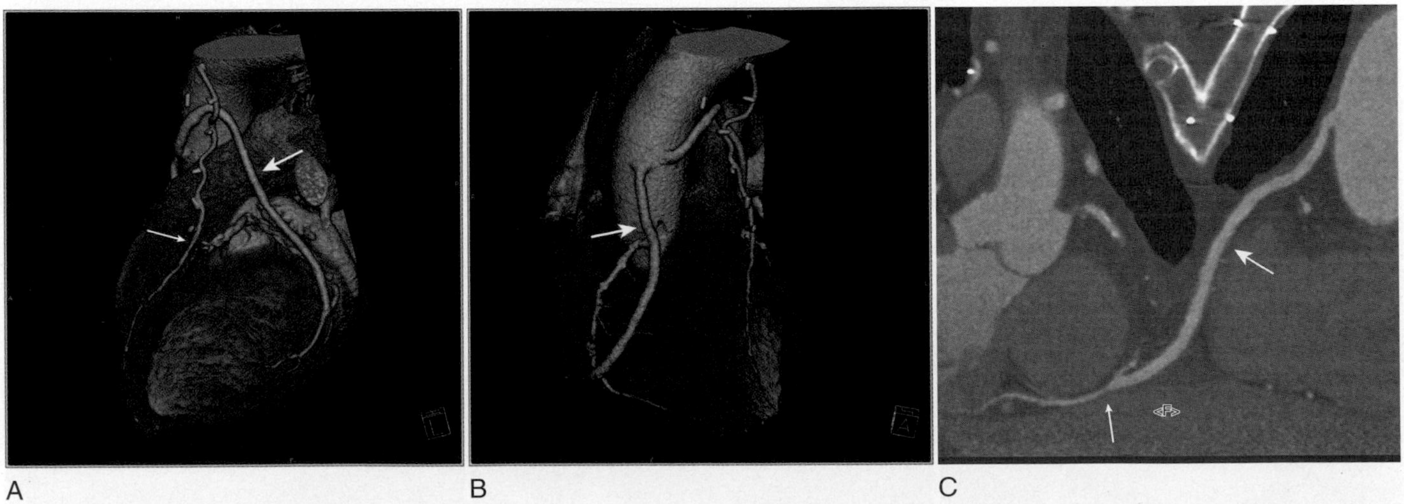

FIGURE 18-23 Patient with an arterial bypass graft to the left anterior descending coronary artery and venous grafts to the left circumflex and right coronary arteries. **A** and **B,** Three-dimensional reconstructions showing the arterial graft to the left anterior descending coronary artery (small arrow) and the venous grafts to the left circumflex and right coronary artery (large arrows). **C,** Curved multiplanar reconstruction showing the right coronary artery bypass graft (large arrow) as well as the anastomosis to the distal right coronary artery (small arrow).

The image quality of noninvasive coronary and bypass angiography by CT has been rapidly improving. Technical innovations and the development of faster scanners with higher resolution are ongoing. With increasing image quality, it can be anticipated that the accuracy and clinical applicability of noninvasive coronary angiography by MDCT will continue to improve.

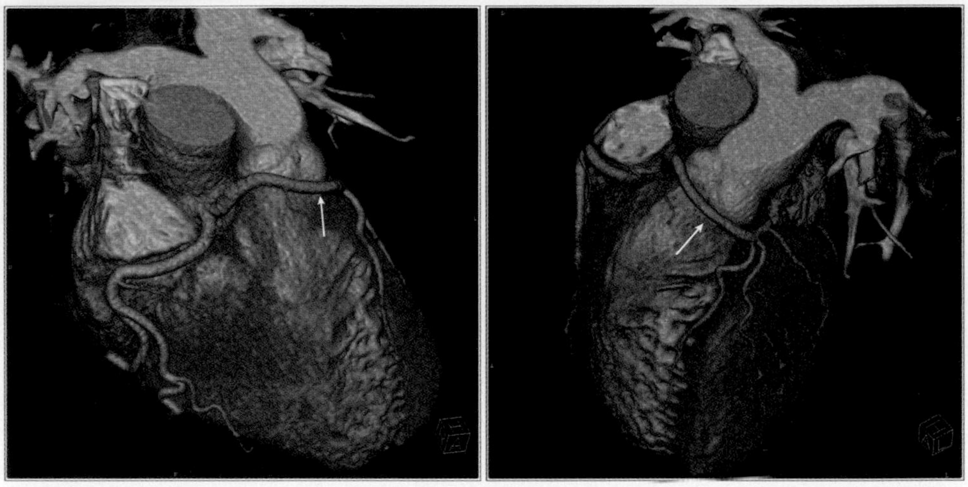

FIGURE 18-24 **A** and **B**, Patient with a coronary anomaly. The left coronary artery arises from the right coronary ostium and courses anterior to the right ventricular outflow tract and pulmonary artery (arrows).

Visualization of Noncalcified Coronary Artery Plaque

Contrast-enhanced high-resolution CT scans of the coronary arteries allow the visualization not only of coronary artery stenoses, but also of noncalcified atherosclerotic plaque in lesions that are not associated with a significant stenosis. Detection, quantification, and characterization of coronary plaque by CT are currently the subjects of intense evaluation, because potential applications in risk stratification are assumed (Fig. 18-25). Several validation studies against intravascular ultrasound have reported sensitivities of 53 to 83 percent for the detection of noncalcified plaque by 16- and 64-slice CT.[82-84] However, the ability to quantify plaque volumes by CT is limited and suffers from high interobserver variability.[84] CT measurements can potentially contribute to the further characterization of noncalcified plaque, because lipid-rich plaque is, on average, associated with lower CT Hounsfield attenuation numbers than fibrous plaques (14 to 72 HU for fibrous plaques and 90 to 121 HU for lipid-rich plaques).[83,85-88] However, in clinical CT scans, the variability of these measurements is high and does not allow accurate classification of a single plaque.[88] In addition, whereas coronary calcification can be reliably detected by CT at a relatively low radiation dose, and coronary calcium has clearly been shown to be associated with an increased risk of future coronary artery disease events in asymptomatic individuals, available clinical data are scarce for the detection of noncalcified plaque by contrast-enhanced CT. In several smaller trials, patients with acute coronary syndromes were found to have a higher prevalence of noncalcified as compared with calcified plaque than patients with stable coronary artery disease,[89-91] which suggests a potential advantage of noncalcified plaque assessment over mere detection of calcium for risk stratification. Current data, however, do not justify the addi-tional expense in radiation exposure and contrast agent for noncalcified plaque detection as compared with the assessment of coronary calcium. Thus, the clinical implications of the intriguing observation that CT may be able to visualize and characterize noncalcified plaque are currently unclear.

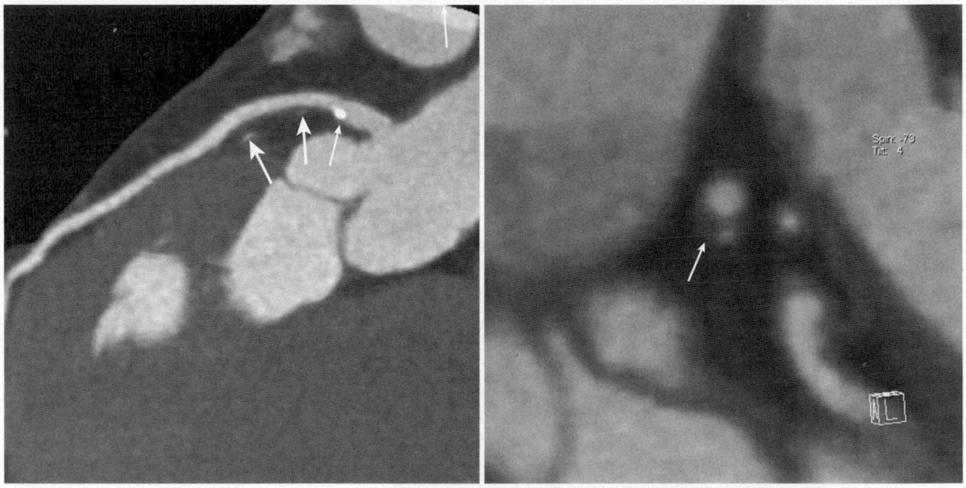

FIGURE 18-25 Visualization of a nonstenotic atherosclerotic plaque in the proximal left anterior descending coronary artery. The plaque has a small calcification (small arrows) but is largely noncalcified (large arrows). **A**, Curved multiplanar reconstruction yields a longitudinal view of the proximal left anterior descending coronary artery. **B**, Cross-sectional view of the proximal left anterior descending coronary artery (arrow).

Cardiac Masses (see Chap. 69)

Although echocardiography is the first-line diagnostic tool for cardiac masses, CT can provide helpful additional information because of its high resolution and ability to visualize cardiac morphology clearly without the restriction of acoustic windows. CT provides less information concerning the tissue type than CMR but may provide limited insight into the nature of a mass through measurement of the x-ray attenuation (CT numbers).[92] Lipomas have low CT numbers (typically less than 50 HU), whereas cysts have water-like density (0 to 10 HU). CT numbers of intracardiac thrombi usually range from 20 to 90 HU,[93] but their density values may overlap with those of myocardium, and correct delineation of the extent of mural thrombi must be done with great care (Fig. 18-26). As they age, hematomas may develop calcifications or even take up contrast agent. CT can identify thrombi in the left atrial appendage, but because of poor enhancement of the left atrial appendage, scans can yield false-positive results for left atrial thrombi.

Atrial myxomas are the most frequent primary intracardiac tumor. They have an average CT number of approxi-

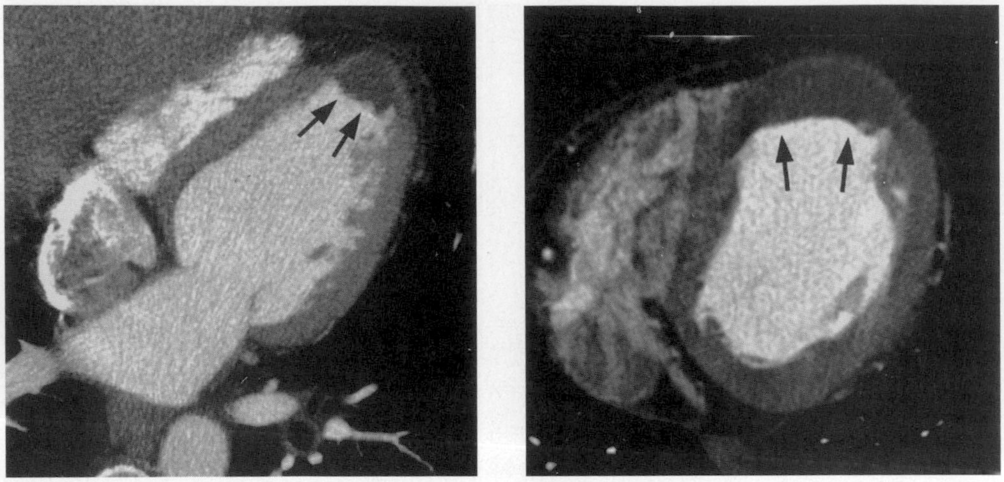

FIGURE 18-26 Left ventricular thrombi in contrast-enhanced computed tomography (CT) images. **A,** Spherical apical thrombus after myocardial infarction (arrows). **B,** Large mural thrombus (arrows) in a patient with a large anterior infarction. The attenuation of the thrombus in the CT scan is only a little less than the density of the adjacent myocardium.

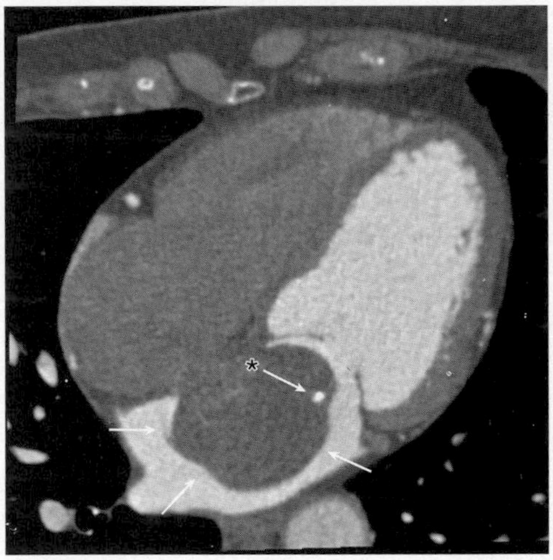

FIGURE 18-27 Large left atrial myxoma (arrows) in a typical position, with attachment to the interatrial septum. The myxoma contains a small calcification (asterisk).

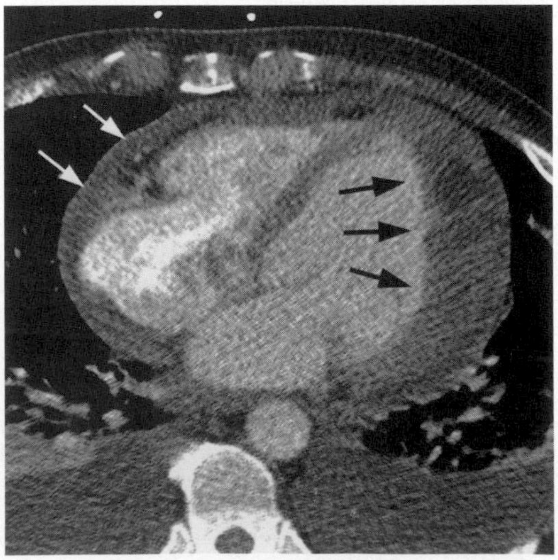

FIGURE 18-28 Primary cardiac lymphoma in a patient who presented with ventricular arrhythmias. Inhomogeneous thickening of the lateral left ventricular wall (black arrows) is caused by infiltrative growth of the lymphoma. Pericardial effusion (white arrows) and bilateral pleural effusion are present.

mately 30 HU and may also contain calcification (Fig. 18-27).[94] Neoplasms can have an attenuation close to that of myocardium and, if displaying a diffusely infiltrative pattern of growth, such as cardiac lymphoma, may be difficult to outline in CT images (Fig. 18-28). In primary cardiac neoplasms and with metastatic cardiac or pericardial involvement, pericardial effusion (often with above-water CT numbers) may be the only finding in CT.[13,92]

Congenital Heart Disease

(see Chap. 61)

Although echocardiography constitutes the first-line diagnostic modality for patients with congenital heart disease, cross-sectional imaging may be warranted to delineate cardiac morphology, especially the anatomy of the great arteries, pulmonary veins, and anomalous coronary arteries (Figs. 18-29 and 18-30). Newer generation CT scanners can cover a large imaging volume within one breath-hold and can acquire thin transaxial cross sections that permit reformatting in any desired plane. This has substantially increased the diagnostic value of CT in the setting of congenital heart disease. Limitations in obtaining information about flow or shunts and the necessity for contrast injection and radiation exposure constitute disadvantages of CT over CMR (see Chap. 17). However, CT provides morphological analysis with very high resolution and is not limited by the presence of implanted devices such as pacemakers or ICDs, which are encountered with increasing frequency in adults with congenital heart disease (Fig. 18-31). The systematic use of EBT and MDCT imaging has been described, especially for the analysis of great vessels and pulmonary venous return[95] and for the exact delineation of the course of anomalous coronary arteries. The fact that detailed information about the dimensions and function of both ventricles can be obtained by CT may be important in the follow-up of adults with surgically corrected disease, because right ventricular assessment may be especially problematic using echocardiography.

Function, Perfusion, and Viability

Computed tomography permits detailed and accurate analysis of left and right ventricular function. Using retrospective electrocardiographic gating, spiral CT data sets can be reconstructed at any desired phase of the cardiac cycle. EBT provides the option of prospectively acquiring high-resolution data sets at several predefined points in the cardiac cycle. The high contrast between the ventricular cavity and myocardium in contrast-enhanced scans permits accurate measurements of ventricular volumes at systole and diastole, thus enabling exact analysis of global function and regional wall motion (Fig. 18-32; see corresponding video clips on the companion website).[96,97] Thus, information about ventricular function can be obtained as a byproduct of contrast-enhanced data sets acquired for other reasons, such as coronary artery visualization or cardiac morphology in cases of congenital heart disease. In clinical reality, however, it is seldom necessary to resort to CT imaging to obtain information about global or regional wall motion.

EBT is well suited to analyze myocardial perfusion after bolus injection of contrast agent with high resolution.[98] Studies can be performed at rest and during exercise. In fact, wall motion and perfusion analysis can be combined into one single scan. Because of the ready availability of alternative imaging modalities (see Chap. 16), however, clinical applications have so far been limited.

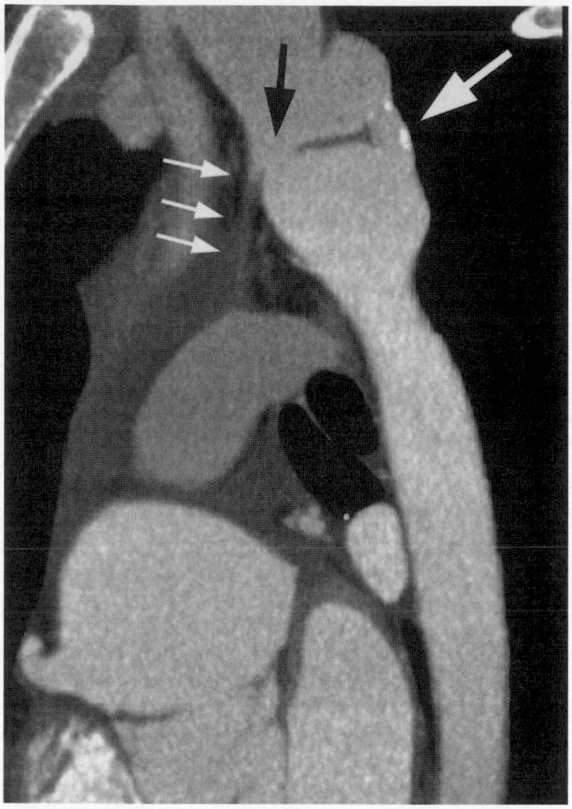

FIGURE 18-29 A 31-year-old patient with aortic coarctation. A sagittally reformatted multidetector computed tomography scan shows the descending aorta (black arrow = coarctation). A partly calcified, patent bypass conduit that was implanted at the age of 9 years can be seen (large white arrow). Note the obliterated ductus arteriosus (small white arrows).

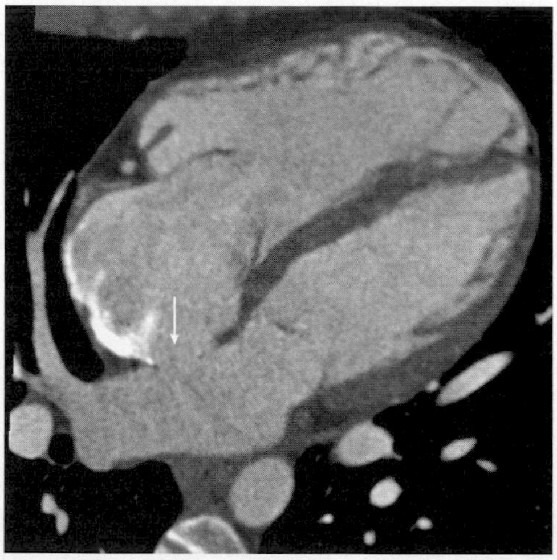

FIGURE 18-30 Atrial septal defect (arrow) visualized by multidetector computed tomography after intravenous injection of contrast agent.

Because iodinated contrast agents accumulate in infarcted myocardium, it is possible to visualize chronic myocardial infarction by computed tomography in a fashion similar to the delayed enhancement method of CMR (Fig. 18-33).[99,100] CT acquisitions are performed approximately 10 minutes after injection of contrast agent and relatively thick tomographic slices (e.g., 10 mm) are reconstructed to improve the signal-to-noise ratio. Because the signal of noninfarcted myocardium cannot be suppressed, the signal of the infarcted myocardium is not as clear as with CMR (see Chap. 17). Also, it currently seems that the amount of contrast agent necessary may be substantially higher than for visualization of the coronary arteries, so that delayed enhancement

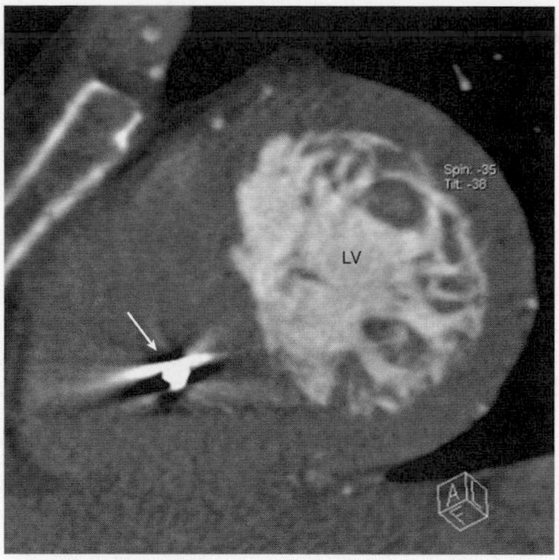

FIGURE 18-31 Computed tomography scan in a patient with left ventricular noncompaction (note increased trabecularization in the left ventricle, LV). The right ventricular lead (arrow) of an implanted defibrillator causes some artifacts, but these do not impair the evaluability of the data set.

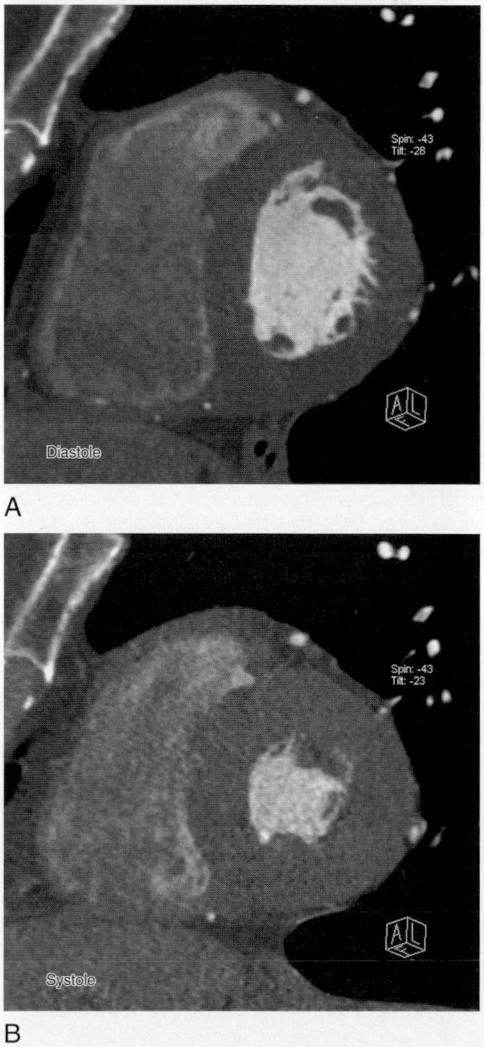

FIGURE 18-32 Analysis of left ventricular function by computed tomography. A, Multiplanar reconstruction of the heart in short-axis orientation during diastole. B, Multiplanar reconstruction in the same plane during systole. (See the corresponding video clips on the companion website, which show a dynamic analysis of left ventricular function in short-axis and two-chamber views.)

information cannot be obtained as a simple by-product of the coronary computed tomography angiography (CTA) investigation. Rather, it requires additional expense in regard to contrast agent and radiation.

Great Vessels

Thoracic Aorta

Computed tomography is extremely accurate for the diagnosis of aortic disease, including aneurysms, dissection, and intramural hematoma. Demonstration of the intimal flap (low CT attenuation within contrast-enhanced aortic lumen) is required for the diagnosis of aortic dissection (Fig. 18-34). Differentiation between true and false lumina is important, especially in the context of endovascular repair. The true lumen tends to be smaller than the false, and thrombus formation and aortic cobwebs are pathognomonic for the false lumen.[101] A dissection with complete thrombosis of the false lumen may be difficult to differentiate from an aortic aneurysm with mural thrombus; a delayed second scan after recontrast injection may be helpful. Also, inward displacement of calcium toward the aortic lumen may help indicate dissection in this case. Higher temporal resolution and the availability of electrocardiographic triggering have substantially reduced pulsation artifacts that could misdiagnose dissection, especially in the ascending aorta, and the accuracy of CT for establishing the diagnosis of dissection, assuming optimal technology, is close to 100 percent.[102,103] The individual clinical situation must dictate whether transesophageal echocardiography, CMR, or CT constitutes the optimal approach in a given patient (see Chaps. 14 and 17). Speed of acquisition, detailed visualization of the aorta and branch vessels, and ready availability represent the advantages of CT, whereas the need for contrast injection is a drawback. The ability of CT to depict the lumen of metallic stents in the aorta and to detect leaks by demonstrating extravasation of contrast agent makes it a useful follow-up tool after interventional treatment of aortic aneurysms.[103]

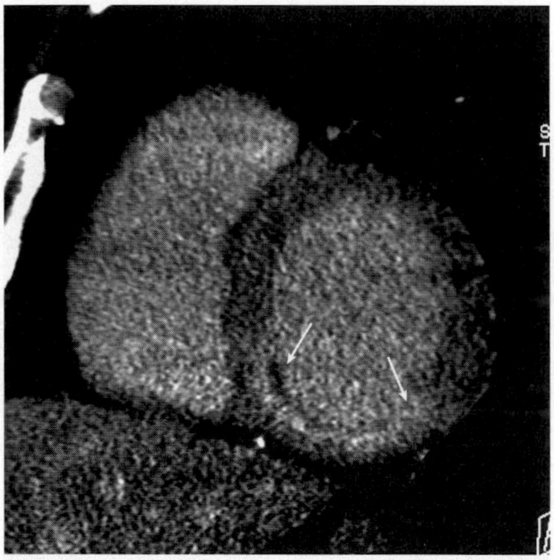

FIGURE 18-33 Example of delayed enhancement by computed tomography (CT) in an acquisition obtained 10 minutes after injection of an iodinated contrast agent. The arrows indicate an area of increased CT attenuation in the posterior wall, corresponding to a chronic myocardial infarction. *(Courtesy of Dr. R. Cury, Department of Radiology, Massachusetts General Hospital, Boston.)*

Pulmonary Veins

In the context of electrophysiological interventions (e.g., to isolate the pulmonary veins electrically for prevention of atrial fibrillation, visualization of the exact anatomy of pulmonary veins, and detection of supernumerary veins) are of clinical importance. Suitable imaging information can reduce the duration of the interventional procedure. In addition, pulmonary vein stenosis is a possible consequence of ablation and difficult to assess with echocardiography. Similar to CMR, CT can provide two-dimensional and three-dimensional images that show the exact anatomy of pulmonary veins (Figs. 18-35 and 18-36).[104] Image quality may be degraded if the CT examination is performed during atrial fibrillation but usually remains sufficiently high. Anomalous pulmonary venous return can be present in congenital heart disease and is also clearly depicted by CT.

Pulmonary Embolism (see Chap. 72)

EBT[105] and MDCT[106,107] have been demonstrated to provide high diagnostic accuracy for the detection of pulmonary embolism. In contrast-enhanced scans, the thrombi appear as filling defects in the pulmonary arteries (Fig. 18-37). There is consensus that a thin-collimation CT scan of the thorax with 1- to 2-mm image reconstruction can be used for the diagnostic evaluation of patients with suspected pulmonary embolism[108-110] and that a normal CT scan, possibly in combination with ultrasonography or CT venography of the lower extremity veins or other clinical findings,

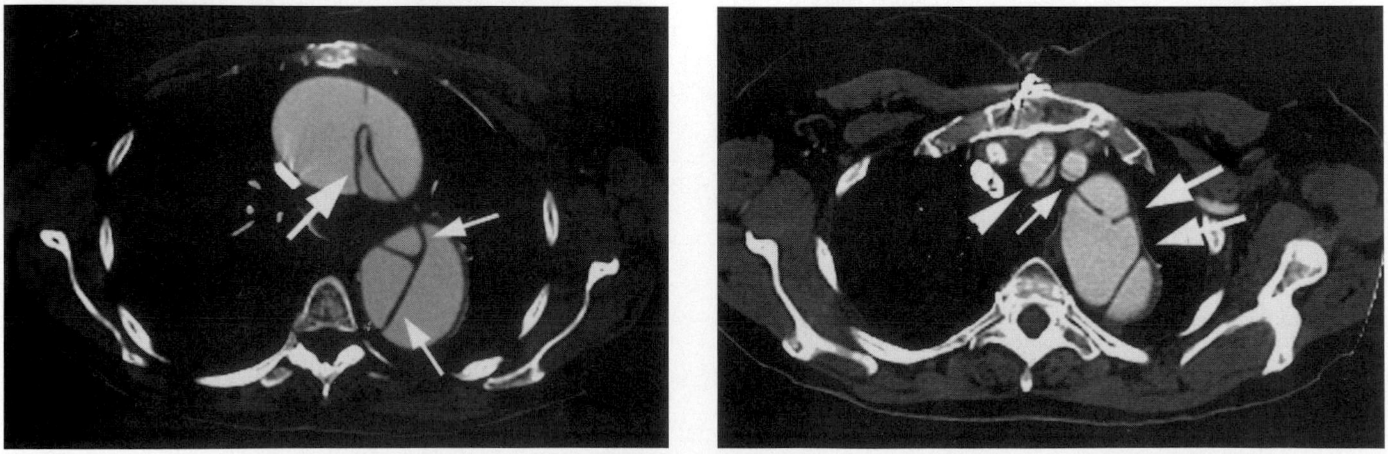

A B

FIGURE 18-34 Aortic dissection. **A,** Dissection membranes clearly visualized in the ascending aorta (large arrow) and descending aorta (small arrows). **B,** Same patient as in A. Shown is the dissection membrane, partially fenestrated, in the aortic arch (large arrows). The dissection extends into the left common carotid artery (small arrow) and innominate artery (arrowhead). *(Courtesy of Dr. R. C. Gilkeson, Case Western Reserve University, Cleveland.)*

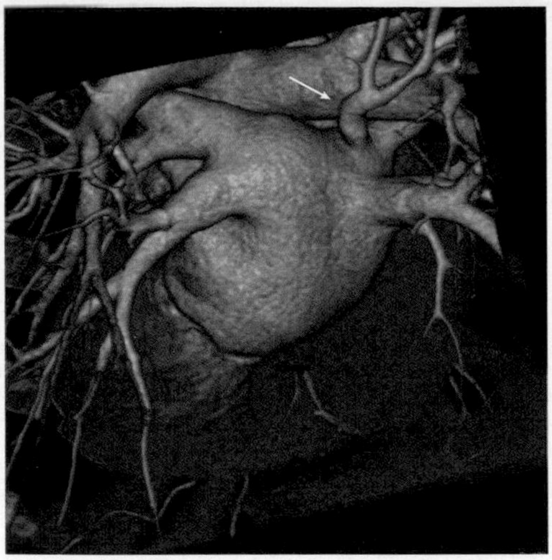

FIGURE 18-35 Three-dimensional visualization of pulmonary vein anatomy by computed tomography. In a posterior view, an accessory pulmonary vein is visible (arrow).

is sufficient to withhold anticoagulation therapy. Guidelines have incorporated MDCT as the first-line imaging test in stable patients with suspected pulmonary embolism, with no further diagnostic work-up or treatment to follow if CT is negative.[111] In patients with suspected massive pulmonary embolism, the individual clinical situation will drive the decision toward appropriate initial testing, and echocardiography will usually be sufficient to reach a treatment decision (see Chap. 14).

FUTURE PERSPECTIVES

The technology of cardiac computed tomography will continue to progress. Whereas radiation exposure sets a limit to increases in spatial resolution, temporal resolution will most likely be increased considerably, which will reduce artifact, especially in the context of coronary artery visualization. Careful clinical studies of appropriate size and design will be needed to clarify the role of coronary CT angiography, especially in the context of stable and acute chest pain. Most likely, CT angiography will prove a benefi-

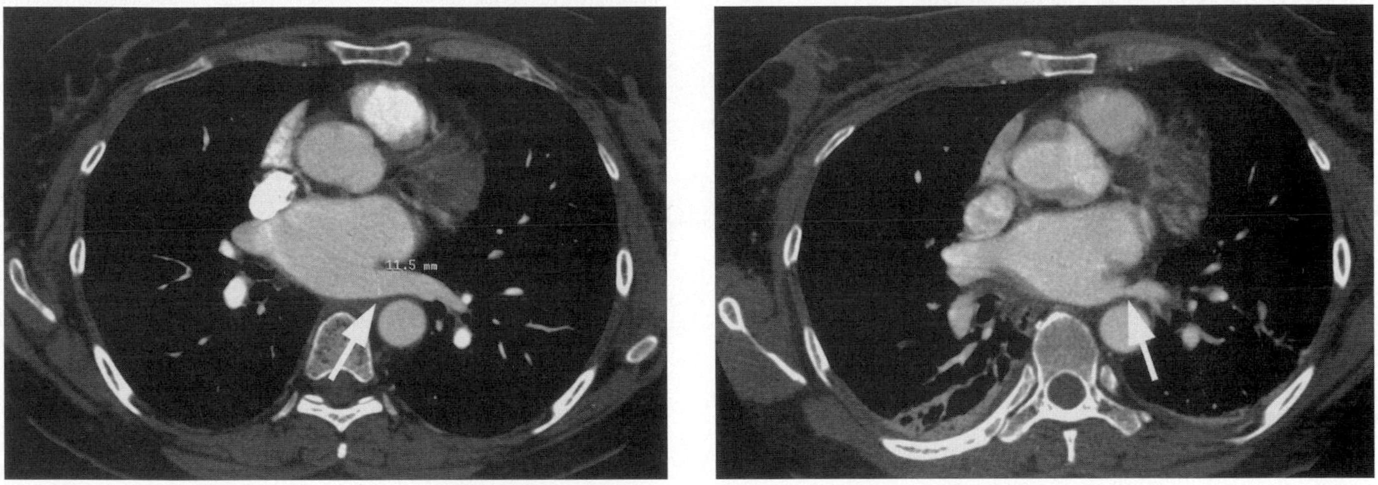

A B

FIGURE 18-36 Visualization of pulmonary veins before and after ablation of the pulmonary vein ostium for atrial fibrillation. **A,** Transaxial cross section at the ostium of the left inferior pulmonary vein (arrow). Normal anatomy prior to ablation. **B,** Same patient 6 weeks after ablation. Severe stenosis can be seen at the ostium of the pulmonary vein (arrow). *(Courtesy of Dr. J. F. Breen, Mayo Clinic, Rochester, Minn.)*

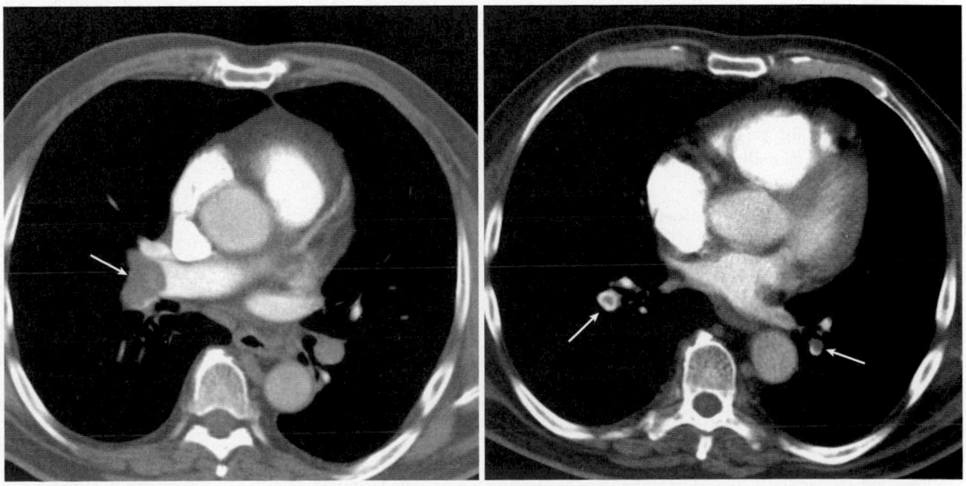

A B

FIGURE 18-37 Visualization of pulmonary embolism by contrast-enhanced computed tomography in central pulmonary arteries after injection of contrast agent. **A,** Central embolism in the bifurcation of the right pulmonary artery (arrow). **B,** Embolism in peripheral arteries (arrows).

 cial application in selected subgroups of these patients, as will general CT imaging of cardiac morphology for some disease entities that cannot be sufficiently evaluated by echocardiography or CMR.

REFERENCES

Technical Principles

1. Morin RL, Gerber TC, McCollough CH: Radiation dose in computed tomography of the heart. Circulation 107:917, 2003.
2. Hunold P, Vogt FM, Schmermund A, et al: Radiation exposure during cardiac CT: Effective doses at multi-detector-row CT and electron beam CT. Radiology 226:145, 2003.
3. Trabold T, Buchgeister M, Küttner A, et al: Estimation of radiation exposure in 16-detector row computed tomography of the heart with retrospective ECG-gating. Rofo Fortschr Geb Rontgenstr Bildgeb Verf 175:1051, 2003.
4. Coles DR, Smail MA, Negus IS, et al: Comparison of radiation dose from multislice computed tomography and conventional diagnostic coronary angiography. J Am Coll Cardiol 47:1840, 2006.
5. Hausleiter J, Meyer T, Hadamitzky M, et al: Radiation dose estimates from cardiac multislice computed tomography in daily practice. Circulation 113:1305, 2006.
6. Mori S, Endo M, Tsunoo T, et al: Physical performance evaluation of a 256-slice CT-scanner for four-dimensional imaging. Med Phys 31:1348, 2004.
7. Flohr TG, McCollough CH, Bruder H, et al: First performance of a dual-source CT (DSCT) system. Eur Radiol 16:256, 2006.
8. Achenbach S, Ropers D, Kuettner A, et al: Contrast-enhanced coronary artery visualization by dual-source computed tomography—initial experience. Eur J Radiol 57:331, 2006.

Diseases of the Pericardium and Myocardium

9. Breen JF: Imaging of the pericardium. J Thorac Imaging 16:47, 2001.
10. Wang ZJ, Reddy GP, Gotway MB, et al: CT and MR imaging of pericardial disease. Radiographics 23:167, 2003.
11. Ayama N, Oyama M, Komuro K, et al: Computed tomography and magnetic resonance imaging of the pericardium: Anatomy and pathology. Magn Reson Med Sci 3:145, 2004.
12. Broderick LS, Brooks GN, Kuhlman JE: Anatomic pitfalls of the heart and pericardium. Radiographics 25:441, 2005.
13. Chiles C, Woodard P, Gutierrez FR, et al: Metastatic involvement of the heart and pericardium: CT and MR imaging. Radiographics 21:439, 2001.
14. Ferencik M, Abbara S, Hoffmann U, et al: Left ventricular thin point detection using multi-detector spiral computed tomography. Am J Cardiol 93:949, 2004.
15. Kimura F, Sakai F, Sakomura Y, et al: Helical CT features of arrhythmogenic right ventricular cardiomyopathy. Radiographics 22:1111, 2002.
16. Tandri H, Bomma C, Calkins H, Bluemke DA: Magnetic resonance and computed tomography imaging of arrhythmogenic right ventricular dysplasia. J Magn Reson Imaging 19:848, 2004.

Valvular Heart Disease

17. Alkadhi H, Wildermuth S, Bettex DA, et al: Mitral regurgitation: Quantification with 16-detector-row CT—initial experience. Radiology 238:454, 2006.
18. Alkadhi H, Wildemuth S, Plass A, et al: Aortic stenosis: Comparative evaluation of 16-detector row CT and echocardiography. Radiology 240:47-55, 2006.
19. Abbara S, Pena AJ, Maurovich-Horvat P, et al: Feasibility and optimization of aortic valve planimetry with MDCT. Am J Roentgenol 188:356, 2007.
20. Feuchtner GM, Dichtl W, Friedrich GJ, et al: Multislice computed tomography for detection of patients with aortic valve stenosis and quantification of severity. J Am Coll Cardiol 47:1410, 2006.
21. Gilkeson RC, Markowitz AH, Balgude A, Sachs PB: MDCT evaluation of aortic valvular disease. AJR Am J Radiol 186:350, 2006.
22. Willmann JK, Weishaupt D, Lachat M, et al: Electrocardiographically gated multidetector row CT for assessment of valvular morphology and calcification in aortic stenosis. Radiology 225:120, 2002.
23. Pohle K, Maffert R, Ropers D, et al: Progression of aortic valve calcification: Association with coronary atherosclerosis and cardiovascular risk factors. Circulation 104:1927, 2001.
24. Otto CM, Lind BK, Kitzman DW, et al: Association of aortic-valve sclerosis with cardiovascular mortality and morbidity in the elderly. N Engl J Med 341:142, 1999.

Coronary Artery Calcification

25. Burke AP, Virmani R, Galis Z, et al: 34th Bethesda Conference: Task Force #2—What is the pathologic basis for new atherosclerosis imaging techniques? J Am Coll Cardiol 41:1874, 2003.
26. Greenland P, Bonow RO, Brundage BH, et al: ACCF/AHA 2007 Clinical expert consensus document on coronary artery calcium scoring by computed tomography in global cardiovascular risk assessment and in evaluation of patients with chest pain. Circulation 115:402, 2006.
27. Pohle K, Ropers D, Mäffert R, et al: Coronary calcifications in young patients with first, unheralded myocardial infarction: A risk factor–matched analysis by electron beam tomography. Heart 89:625, 2003.
28. Raggi P, Callister TQ, Cooil B, et al: Identification of patients at increased risk of first unheralded acute myocardial infarction by electron-beam computed tomography. Circulation 101:850, 2000.
29. Schmermund A, Schwartz RS, Adamzik M, et al: Coronary atherosclerosis in unheralded sudden coronary death under age fifty: Histopathologic comparison with “healthy” subjects dying out of hospital. Atherosclerosis 155:499, 2001.
30. Goldin JG, Yoon HC, Greaser LE 3rd, et al: Spiral versus electron-beam CT for coronary artery calcium scoring. Radiology 221:213, 2001.
31. Detrano RC, Anderson M, Nelson J, et al: Coronary calcium measurements: Effect of CT scanner type and calcium measure on rescan reproducibility—MESA study. Radiology 236:477, 2005.
32. Hoff JA, Chomka EV, Krainik AJ, et al: Age and gender distribution of coronary artery calcium detected by electron beam tomography in 35246 adults. Am J Cardiol 87:1335, 2001.
33. McClelland RL, Chung H, Detrano R, et al: Distribution of coronary artery calcium by race, gender, and age. Results from the Multi-Ethnic Study of Atherosclerosis (MESA). Circulation 113:30, 2006.
34. Schmermund A, Mohlenkamp S, Berenbein S, et al: Population-based assesment of subclinical coronary atherosclerosis using electron-beam computed tomography. Atherosclerosis 185:117, 2006.
35. Arad Y, Spadaro LA, Goodman K, et al: Prediction of coronary events with electron beam computed tomography. J Am Coll Cardiol 36:1253, 2000.
36. Park R, Detrano R, Xiang M, et al: Combined use of computed tomography coronary calcium scores and C-reactive protein levels in predicting cardiovascular events in nondiabetic individuals. Circulation 106:2073, 2002.
37. Vliegenthart R, Oudkerk M, Song B, et al: Coronary calcification detected by electron-beam computed tomography and myocardial infarction. The Rotterdam Coronary Calcification Study. Eur Heart J 23:1596, 2002.
38. Wong ND, Hsu JC, Detrano RC, et al: Coronary artery calcium evaluation by electron beam computed tomography and its relation to new cardiovascular events. Am J Cardiol 86:495, 2000.
39. Kondos GT, Hoff JA, Sevrukov A, et al: Electron-beam tomography coronary artery calcium and coronary events: A 37-month follow-up of 5635 initially asymptomatic low- to intermediate-risk adults. Circulation 107:2571, 2003.
40. Church TS, Levine BD, McGuire DK, et al: Coronary artery calcium score, risk factors, and incident coronary heart disease events. Atherosclerosis 190:224, 2007.
41. Taylor AJ, Bindeman J, Feuerstein I, et al: Coronary calcium independently predicts incident premature coronary heart disease over measured cardiovascular risk factors: Mean three-year outcomes in the Prospective Army Coronary Calcium (PACC) project. J Am Coll Cardiol 46:807, 2005.
42. Greenland P, LaBree L, Azen SP, et al: Coronary artery calcium score combined with Framingham score for risk prediction in asymptomatic individuals. JAMA 291:210, 2004.
43. Arad Y, Goodman KJ, Roth M, et al: Coronary calcification, coronary disease risk factors, C-reactive protein, and atherosclerotic cardiovascular disease events: The St. Francis Heart Study. J Am Coll Cardiol 46:158, 2005.
44. O´Malley PG, Taylor AJ, Jackson JL, et al: Prognostic value of coronary electron-beam computed tomography for coronary heart disease events in asymptomatic patients. Am J Cardiol 85:945, 2000.
45. De Backer G, Ambrosioni E, Borch-Johnsen K, et al: European guidelines on cardiovascular disease prevention in clinical practice. Third Joint Task Force of European and Other Societies on Cardiovascular Disease Prevention in Clinical Practice. Eur Heart J 24:1601, 2003.
46. Taylor AJ, Bairey Merz CN, Udelson JE: 34th Bethesda Conference: Executive summary—Can atherosclerosis imaging techniques improve the detection of patients at risk for ischemic heart disease? J Am Coll Cardiol 41:1860, 2003.
47. Schmermund A, Baumgart D, Möhlenkamp S, et al: Natural history and topographic pattern of progression of coronary calcification in symptomatic patients. Arterioscler Thromb Vasc Biol 21:421, 2001.
48. Raggi P, Callister TQ, Shaw LJ: Progression of coronary artery calcium and risk of first myocardial infarction in patients receiving cholesterol-lowering therapy. Arterioscler Thromb Vasc Biol 24:1272, 2004.
49. Callister TQ, Raggi P, Cooil B, et al: Effect of HMG-CoA reductase inhibitors on coronary artery disease as assessed by electron-beam computed tomography. N Engl J Med 339:1972, 1998.
50. Achenbach S, Ropers D, Pohle K, et al: Influence of lipid-lowering therapy on the progression of coronary artery calcification: a prospective evaluation. Circulation 106:1077, 2002.
51. Budoff MJ, Lane KL, Bakhsheshi H, et al: Rates of progression of coronary calcium by electron beam tomography. Am J Cardiol 86:8, 2000.
52. Raggi P, Davidson M, Callister TQ, et al: Aggressive versus moderate lipid-lowering therapy in hypercholesterolemic postmenopausal women: Beyond Endorsed Lipid Lowering with EBT Scanning (BELLES). Circulation 112:563, 2005.
53. Schmermund A, Achenbach S, Budde T, et al: Effect of intensive versus standard lipid-lowering treatment with atorvastatin on the progression of calcified coronary atherosclerosis over 12 months: A multicenter, randomized, double-blind trial. Circulation 113:427, 2006.
54. Arad Y, Spadaro LA, Roth M, et al: Treatment of asymptomatic adults with elevated coronary calcium scores with atorvastatin, vitamin C, and vitamin E: The St. Francis Heart Study randomized clinical trial. J Am Coll Cardiol 46:166, 2005.

Visualization of the Coronary Artery Lumen

55. Hoffmann MH, Shi H, Schmitz BL, et al: Noninvasive coronary angiography with multislice computed tomography. JAMA 293:2471, 2005.
56. Kuettner A, Beck T, Drosch T, et al: Image quality and diagnostic accuracy of noninvasive coronary imaging with 16-detector slice spiral computed tomography with 188 ms temporal resolution. Heart 91:938, 2005.
57. Mollet NR, Cademartiri F, Krestin GP, et al: Improved diagnostic accuracy with 16-row multi-slice computed tomography coronary angiography. J Am Coll Cardiol 45:128, 2005.

58. Morgan-Hughes GJ, Roobottom CA, Owens PE, Marshall AJ: Highly accurate coronary angiography with submillimetre, 16 slice computed tomography. Heart 91:308, 2005.
59. Achenbach S, Ropers D, Pohle FK, et al: Detection of coronary artery stenoses using multi-detector CT with 16 × 0.75 mm collimation and 375 ms rotation. Eur Heart J 26:1978, 2005.
60. Garcia MJ, Lessick J, Hoffmann MH: CATSCAN Study Investigators: Accuracy of 16-row multidetector computed tomography for the assessment of coronary artery stenosis. JAMA 296:403, 2006.
61. Leschka S, Alkadhi H, Plass A, et al: Accuracy of MSCT coronary angiography with 64-slice technology: First experience. Eur Heart J 26:1482, 2005.
62. Raff GJ, Gallagher MJ, O'Neill WW, Goldstein JA: Diagnostic accuracy of noninvasive angiography using 64-slice spiral computed tomography. J Am Coll Cardiol 46:552, 2005.
63. Leber AW, Knez A, von Ziegler F, et al: Quantification of obstructive and nonobstructive coronary lesions by 64-slice computed tomography. A comparative study with quantitative coronary angiography and intravascular ultrasound. J Am Coll Cardiol 46:147, 2005.
64. Mollet NR, Cademartiri F, van Mieghem CA, et al: High-resolution spiral computed tomography coronary angiography in patients referred for diagnostic conventional coronary angiography. Circulation 112:2318, 2005.
65. Ropers D, Rixe J, Anders K, et al: Usefulness of multidetector row computed tomography with 64 × 0.6 mm collimation and 330-ms rotation for the noninvasive detection of significant coronary artery stenoses. Am J Cardiol 97:343, 2006.
66. Fine JJ, Hopkins CB, Ruff N, Newton FC: Comparison of accuracy of 64-slice cardiovascular computed tomography with coronary angiography in patients with suspected coronary artery disease. Am J Cardiol 97:173, 2006.
67. Nikolaou K, Knez A, Rist C, et al: Accuracy of 64-MDCT in the diagnosis of ischemic heart disease. Am J Radiol 187:111, 2006.
68. Hoffmann U, Nagurney JT, Moselewski F, et al: Coronary multidetector computed tomography in the assessment of patients with acute chest pain. Circulation 114:2251, 2006.
69. Hendel RC, Patel MR, Kramer CM, et al: ACCF/ACR/SCCT/SCMR/ASNC/NASCI/SCAI/SIR 2006 appropriateness criteria for cardiac computed tomography and cardiac magnetic resonance imaging. J Am Coll Cardio 48:1475, 2006.
70. Gilard M, Cornily JC, Rioufol G, et al: Noninvasive assessment of left main coronary stent patency with 16-slice computed tomography. Am J Cardiol 95:110, 2005.
71. Martuscelli E, Romagnoli A, D'Eliseo A, et al: Evaluation of venous and arterial conduit patency by 16-slice spiral computed tomography. Circulation 110:3234, 2004.
72. Schlosser T, Konorza T, Hunold P, et al: Noninvasive visualization of coronary artery bypass grafts using 16-detector row computed tomography. J Am Coll Cardiol 44:1224, 2004.
73. Chiurlia E, Menozzi M, Ratti C, et al: Follow-up of coronary artery bypass graft patency by multislice computed tomography. Am J Cardiol 95:1094, 2005.
74. Moore RKG, Sampson C, Mac Donald S, et al: Coronary artery bypass graft imaging using ECG-gated multislice computed tomography: Comparison with catheter angiography. Clin Radiol 60:990, 2005.
75. Burgstahler C, Beck T, Kuettner A, et al: Non-invasive evaluation of coronary artery bypass grafts using 16-row multi-slice computed tomography with 188 ms temporal resolution. Int J Cardiol 106:244, 2006.
76. Salm LP, Bax JJ, Jukema JW, et al: Comprehensive assessment of patients after coronary artery bypass grafting by 16-detector-row computed tomography. Am Heart J 150:775, 2005.
77. Anders K, Baum U, Schmid M, et al: Coronary artery bypass graft (CABG) patency: Assessment with high-resolution submillimeter 16-slice multidetector-row computed tomography (MDCT) versus coronary angiography. Eur J Radiol 57:336, 2006.
78. Ropers D, Moshage W, Daniel WG, et al: Visualization of coronary artery anomalies and their course by contrast-enhanced electron beam tomography and three-dimensional reconstruction. Am J Cardiol 87:193, 2001.
79. Deibler AR, Kuzo RS, Vohringer M, et al: Imaging of congenital coronary anomalies with multislice computed tomography. Mayo Clin Proc 79:1017, 2004.
80. Datta J, White CS, Gilkeson RC, et al: Anomalous coronary arteries in adults: Depiction at multi-detector row CT angiography. Radiology 235:812, 2005.
81. Schmid M, Achenbach S, Ludwig J, et al: Visualization of coronary artery anomalies by contrast-enhanced multi-detector row spiral computed tomography. Int J Cardiol 111:430, 2006.

Imaging of Coronary Artery Plaque

82. Achenbach S, Moselewski F, Ropers D, et al: Detection of calcified and noncalcified coronary atherosclerotic plaque by contrast-enhanced, submillimeter multidetector spiral computed tomography: A segment-based comparison with intravascular ultrasound. Circulation 109:14, 2004.
83. Leber AW, Knez A, Becker A, et al: Accuracy of multidetector spiral computed tomography in identifying and differenitating the composition of coronary atherosclerotic plaques: A comparative study with intracoronary ultrasound. J Am Coll Cardiol 43:1241, 2004.
84. Leber AW, Becker CR, Knez A, et al: Accuracy of 64-slice computed tomography to classify and quantify plaque volumes in the proximal coronary system: A comparative study using intravascular ultrasound. J Am Coll Cardiol 47:672, 2006.
85. Schroeder S, Kopp AF, Baumbach A, et al: Noninvasive detection and evaluation of atherosclerotic coronary plaques with multislice computed tomography. J Am Coll Cardiol 37:1430, 2001.
86. Becker CR, Nikolaou K, Muders M, et al: Ex vivo coronary atherosclerotic plaque characterization with multi-detector-row CT. Eur Radiol 13:2094, 2003.
87. Carrascosa PM, Capunay CM, Garcia-Merletti P, et al: Characterization of coronary atherosclerotic plaques by multidetector computed tomography. Am J Cardiol 97:598, 2006.
88. Pohle K, Achenbach S, MacNeill B, et al: Characterization of non-calcified coronary atherosclerotic plaque by multi-detector row CT: Comparison to IVUS. Atherosclerosis 190:174, 2007.
89. Hoffmann U, Moselewski F, Nieman K, et al: Noninvasive assessment of plaque morphology and composition in culprit and stable lesions in acute coronary syndrome and stable lesions in stable angina by multidetector computed tomography. J Am Coll Cardiol 47:1655, 2006.
90. Inoue F, Sato Y, Matsumoto N, et al: Evaluation of plaque texture by means of multislice computed tomography in patients with acute coronary syndrome and stable angina. Circ J 68:840, 2004.
91. Leber AW, Knez A, White CR, et al: Composition of coronary atherosclerotic plaque in patients with acute myocardial infarction and stable angina pectoris determined by contrast-enhanced multislice computed tomography. Am J Cardiol 91:714, 2003.

Other Cardiac Applications

92. Araoz PA, Eklund HE, Welch TJ, et al: CT and MR imaging of primary cardiac malignancies. Radiographics 19:1421, 1999.
93. Kirchhof K, Welzel T, Mecke C, et al: Differentiation of white, mixed, and red thrombi: Value of CT in estimation of the prognosis of thrombolysis—phantom study. Radiology 228:126, 2003.
94. Grebenc ML, Rosado-de-Christenson ML, Green CE, et al: Cardiac myxoma: Imaging features in 83 patients. Radiographics 22:673, 2002.
95. Gilkeson RC, Ciancibello L, Zahka K: Multidetector CT evaluation of congenital heart disease in pediatric and adult patients. AJR Am J Roentgenol 180:973, 2003.
96. Halliburton SS, Petersilka M, Schvartzman PR, et al: Evaluation of left ventricular dysfunction using multiphasic reconstructions of coronary multi-slice computed tomography data in patients with chronic ischemic heart disease: Validation against cine magnetic resonance imaging. Int J Cardiovasc Imaging 19:73, 2003.
97. Juergens KU, Grude M, Maintz D, et al: Multi-detector row CT of left ventricular function with dedicated analysis software versus MR imaging: Initial experience. Radiology 230:403, 2004.
98. Mohlenkamp S, Lerman LO, Lerman A, et al: Minimally invasive evaluation of coronary microvascular function by electron beam computed tomography. Circulation 102:2411, 2000.
99. Lardo AC, Cordeiro MA, Silva C, et al: Contrast-enhanced multidetector computed tomography viability imaging after myocardial infarction: Characterization of myocyte death, microvascular obstruction, and chronic scar. Circulation 223:394, 2006.
100. Gerber BL, Belge B, Legros GJ, et al: Characterization of acute and chronic myocardial infarcts by multidetector computed tomography: Comparison with contrast-enhanced magnetic resonance. Circulation 113:823, 2006.

Great Vessels and the Pulmonary Circulation

101. Manghat NE, Morgan-Hughes GJ, Roobottom CA: Multi-detector row computed tomography: Imaging in acute aortic syndrome. Clin Radiol 60:1256, 2005.
102. Hartnell GG: Imaging of aortic aneurysms and dissection: CT and MRI. J Thorac Imaging 16:35, 2001.
103. Erbel R, Alfonso F, Boileau C, et al: Diagnosis and management of aortic dissection. Recommendations of the Task Force on Aortic Dissection, European Society of Cardiology. Eur Heart J 22:1642, 2001.
104. Schwartzman D, Lacomis J, Wigginton WG: Characterization of left atrium and distal pulmonary vein morphology using multidimensional computed tomography. J Am Coll Cardiol 41:1349, 2003.
105. Teigen CL, Maus TP, Sheedy PF, et al: Pulmonary embolism: Diagnosis with contrast-enhanced electron beam CT and comparison with pulmonary angiography. Radiology 194:313, 1995.
106. Quiroz R, Kucher N, Zou KH, et al: Clinical validity of a negative computed tomography scan in patients with suspected pulmonary embolism: A systematic review. JAMA 293:2012, 2005.
107. Stein PD, Fowler WE, Goodman LR, et al: Multidetector computed tomography for acute pulmonary embolism, N Engl J Med 354:2317, 2006.
108. Donato AA, Scheirer JJ, Atwell MS, et al: Clinical outcomes in patients with suspected acute pulmonary embolism and negative helical computed tomographic results in whom anticoagulation was withheld. Arch Intern Med 163:2033, 2003.
109. American College of Emergency Physicians Clinical Policies Committee; Clinical Policies Committee Subcommittee on Suspected Pulmonary Embolism: Clinical policy: Critical issues in the evaluation and management of adults presenting with suspected pulmonary embolism. Ann Emerg Med 41:257, 2003.
110. Kruip MJ, Leclercq MG, Heul CV, et al: Diagnostic strategies for excluding pulmonary embolism in clinical outcome studies: A systematic review. Ann Intern Med 138:941, 2003.
111. British Thoracic Society Standards of Care Committee Pulmonary Embolism Guideline Development Group: British Thoracic Society guidelines for the management of suspected acute pulmonary embolism. Thorax 58:470, 2003.

Appropriateness Guidelines: Cardiac Computed Tomography

The explosive growth in cardiovascular imaging has sometimes outpaced the evidence on which use of new technologies should be based. In an effort to guide rational use of these technologies, eight scientific organizations—American College of Cardiology Foundation, American College of Radiology, Society of Cardiovascular Computed Tomography, Society for Cardiovascular Magnetic Resonance, American Society of Nuclear Cardiology, North American Society for Cardiac Imaging, Society for Cardiovascular Angiography and Interventions, and Society of Interventional Radiology—have embarked on a process to determine the appropriateness of selected indications for cardiovascular imaging procedures.

Panelists rated 39 indications for cardiac computed tomography (CCT) as appropriate (7 to 9 points), uncertain (4 to 6 points), and inappropriate (1 to 3 points) based on the following definition of appropriateness[1]:

An appropriate imaging study is one in which the expected incremental information, combined with clinical judgment, exceeds the expected negative consequences by a sufficiently wide margin for a specific indication that the procedure is generally considered acceptable care and a reasonable approach for the indication. (Negative consequences include the risks of the procedure [i.e., radiation or contrast exposure] and the downstream impact of poor test performance such as delay in diagnosis [false negatives] or inappropriate diagnosis [false positives].)

Thirteen of the 39 CCT indications were deemed appropriate, 12 were uncertain, and 14 were rated as inappropriate (Table 18G-1).

The panel stressed that appropriateness criteria are not substitutes for sound clinical judgment and practice experience. Medical reasons may preclude applying the appropriateness criteria to specific patients, and clinician judgment should be used at all times in applying the criteria. For example, the rating of an indication as inappropriate should not dissuade a provider from performing a CCT procedure when patient- and condition-specific data support that decision, and not performing a study rated as appropriate may be the correct decision in light of unique patient, clinical, and other relevant information.

References

1. Hendel RC, Patel MR, Kramer CM, et al; American College of Cardiology Foundation Quality Strategic Directions Committee Appropriateness Criteria Working Group; American College of Radiology; Society of Cardiovascular Computed Tomography; Society for Cardiovascular Magnetic Resonance; American Society of Nuclear Cardiology; North American Society for Cardiac Imaging; Society for Cardiovascular Angiography and Interventions; Society of Interventional Radiology: ACCF/ACR/SCCT/SCMR/ASNC/NASCI/SCAI/SIR 2006 appropriateness criteria for cardiac computed tomography and cardiac magnetic resonance imaging: A report of the American College of Cardiology Foundation Quality Strategic Directions Committee Appropriateness Criteria Working Group, American College of Radiology, Society of Cardiovascular Computed Tomography, Society for Cardiovascular Magnetic Resonance, American Society of Nuclear Cardiology, North American Society for Cardiac Imaging, Society for Cardiovascular Angiography and Interventions, and Society of Interventional Radiology. J Am Coll Cardiol 48:1475, 2006 (http://www.acc.org/qualityandscience/clinical/pdfs/ CCT.CMR.pdf).

TABLE 18G–1 Joint Professional Society Evaluation* of Appropriate Indications for Cardiac Computed Tomography

Indication	Appropriateness† (Median Score)
DETECTION OF SYMPTOMATIC CAD	
Evaluation of Chest Pain Syndrome (Use of CT Angiogram) Intermediate pretest probability of CAD ECG uninterpretable *or* unable to exercise	A (7)
Intermediate pretest probability of CAD ECG interpretable *and* able to exercise	U (5)
High pretest probability of CAD	I (2)
Evaluation of Intracardiac Structures (Use of CT Angiogram) Evaluation of suspected coronary anomalies	A (9)
Acute Chest Pain (Use of CT Angiogram) Intermediate pretest probability of CAD No electrocardiographic changes and serial enzymes negative	A (7)
High pretest probability of CAD No electrocardiographic changes and serial enzymes negative	U (6)
Low pretest probability of CAD No electrocardiographic changes and serial enzymes negative	U (5)
Triple rule out—exclude obstructive CAD, aortic dissection, and pulmonary embolism Intermediate pretest probability for one of the above ECG—no ST segment elevation and initial enzymes negative	U (4)
High pretest probability of CAD ECG—ST segment elevation and/or positive cardiac enzymes	I (1)
DETECTION OF CAD: ASYMPTOMATIC (without Chest Pain Syndrome)	
Asymptomatic (Use of CT Angiogram) High CHD risk (Framingham)	U (4)
Moderate CHD risk (Framingham)	I (2)
Low CHD risk (Framingham risk)	I (1)
RISK ASSESSMENT: GENERAL POPULATION	
Asymptomatic (Calcium Scoring) Moderate CHD risk (Framingham)	U (6)
High CHD risk (Framingham)	U (5)
Low CHD risk (Framingham)	I (1)
DETECTION OF CAD WITH PRIOR TEST RESULTS	
Evaluation of Chest Pain Syndrome (Use of CT Angiogram) Uninterpretable or equivocal stress test (exercise, perfusion, or stress echocardiography)	A (8)
Evidence of moderate to severe ischemia on stress test (exercise, perfusion, or stress echocardiography)	I (2)
RISK ASSESSMENT WITH PRIOR TEST RESULTS	
Asymptomatic (Calcium Scoring) Prior calcium score within previous 5 years	I (1)
Asymptomatic (Use of CT Angiogram) High CHD risk (Framingham) Prior calcium score ≥400	I (3)
High CHD risk (Framingham) Within 2 years, prior cardiac CT angiogram or invasive angiogram without significant obstructive disease	I (2)
RISK ASSESSMENT: PREOPERATIVE EVALUATION FOR NONCARDIAC SURGERY	
Low-Risk Surgery (Use of CT Angiogram) Intermediate perioperative risk	I (1)
Intermediate- or High-Risk Surgery (Use of CT Angiogram) Intermediate perioperative risk	U (4)
DETECTION OF CAD: POSTREVASCULARIZATION (PCI or CABG)	
Evaluation of Chest Pain Syndrome (Use of CT Angiogram) Evaluation of bypass grafts and coronary anatomy	U (6)
History of percutaneous revascularization with stents	U (5)

TABLE 18G–1 Joint Professional Society Evaluation* of Appropriate Indications for Cardiac Computed Tomography—cont'd

Indication	Appropriateness† (Median Score)
Asymptomatic (Use of CT Angiogram) Evaluation of bypass grafts and coronary anatomy ≥5 years after CABG	I (3)
Evaluation of bypass grafts and coronary anatomy <5 years after CABG	I (2)
Evaluation for in-stent restenosis and coronary anatomy after PCI	I (2)
STRUCTURE AND FUNCTION	
Morphology (Use of CT Angiogram) Assessment of complex congenital heart disease, including anomalies of coronary circulation, great vessels, and cardiac chambers and valves	A (7)
Evaluation of coronary arteries in patients with new-onset heart failure to assess cause	A (7)
Evaluation of Ventricular and Valvular Function (Use of CT Angiogram) Evaluation of LV function following myocardial infarction *or* in heart failure patients Patients with technically limited images from echocardiography	U (5)
Characterization of native and prosthetic cardiac valves Patients with technically limited images from echocardiography, MRI, or TEE	U (5)
Evaluation of left ventricular function following myocardial infarction *or* in heart failure patients	I (3)
Evaluation of Intra- and Extracardiac Structures (Use of Cardiac CT) Evaluation of cardiac mass (suspected tumor or thrombus) Patients with technically limited images from echocardiography, MRI, or TEE	A (8)
Evaluation of pericardial conditions (pericardial mass, constrictive pericarditis, or complications of cardiac surgery) Patients with technically limited images from echocardiography, MRI, or TEE	A (8)
Evaluation of pulmonary vein anatomy prior to invasive radiofrequency ablation for atrial fibrillation	A (8)
Noninvasive coronary vein mapping prior to placement of biventricular pacemaker	A (8)
Noninvasive coronary arterial mapping, including internal mammary artery prior to repeat cardiac surgical revascularization	A (8)
Evaluation of Aortic and Pulmonary Disease (Use of CT Angiogram‡) Evaluation of suspected aortic dissection or thoracic aortic aneurysm	A (9)
Evaluation of suspected pulmonary embolism	A (9)

*American College of Cardiology Foundation, American College of Radiology, Society of Cardiovascular Computed Tomography, Society for Cardiovascular Magnetic Resonance, American Society of Nuclear Cardiology, North American Society for Cardiac Imaging, Society for Cardiovascular Angiography and Interventions, and Society of Interventional Radiology.

†A = appropriate; U = uncertain; I = inappropriate.

‡Nongated CT angiogram, which has a sufficiently large field of view for these applications.

CABG = coronary artery bypass grafting; CAD = coronary artery disease; CT = computed tomography; ECG = electrocardiogram; MRI = magnetic resonance imaging; PCI = percutaneous coronary intervention; TEE = transesophageal echocardiography.

CHAPTER 19

Cardiac Catheterization

Charles J. Davidson and Robert O. Bonow

INDICATIONS FOR DIAGNOSTIC CARDIAC CATHETERIZATION

As with any procedure, the decision to recommend cardiac catheterization is based on an appropriate risk-benefit ratio. In general, diagnostic cardiac catheterization is recommended whenever it is clinically important to define the presence or severity of a suspected cardiac lesion that cannot be adequately evaluated by noninvasive techniques. Because the risk of major complication from cardiac catheterization is less than 2 percent, with mortality of less than 0.08 percent, there are few patients who cannot be studied safely in an active laboratory. Intracardiac pressure measurements and coronary arteriography are procedures that can be performed with reproducible accuracy only by invasive catheterization. Noninvasive estimation of intracardiac pressures can be obtained with echocardiography (see Chap. 14). Coronary computed tomography (CT) angiography shows promise for assessment of coronary anatomy (see Chap. 18). However, current limitations of spatial resolution, heart rate variability, patient cooperation, and radiation dosing make coronary CT angiography useful only as a preliminary screening technique in most patients.

To understand the various indications for diagnostic cardiac catheterization, integration of knowledge from a number of American College of Cardiology/American Heart Association (ACC/AHA) guidelines are necessary. In addition to the diagnostic coronary angiography guidelines,[1] other groups have addressed cardiac catheterization indications, including the guidelines for management of patients with valvular heart disease,[2] chronic heart failure,[3] acute myocardial infarction,[4] percutaneous coronary intervention (PCI),[5] and coronary artery bypass surgery.[6]

Expansion of traditional indications for cardiac catheterization has been in two divergent directions. At one extreme, many critically ill and hemodynamically unstable patients are evaluated during acute myocardial ischemia, severe heart failure, or cardiogenic shock. At the other end of the spectrum, an increasing number of procedures are being performed in an outpatient setting, including hospitals with or without cardiac surgery capability and freestanding or mobile laboratories.[7]

Cardiac catheterization should be considered as a diagnostic test to be used in combination with complementary noninvasive tests. For example, cardiac catheterization in patients with valvular or congenital heart disease is best done with full noninvasive imaging and functional information. The catheterization can be directed and simplified without obtaining redundant anatomical information that is reliably available using echocardiography, cardiac magnetic resonance (CMR), or CT.

Identification of coronary artery disease (CAD), with assessment of its extent and severity, are the most common indications for cardiac catheterization in adults (see Chap. 54). The information obtained by catheterization is crucial to assess the severity of CAD to optimize the mechanical and/or medical therapy of patients with various chest pain syndromes. In addition, the presence of dynamic coronary vascular lesions, such as spasm, myocardial bridging, or thrombosis, can be identified. The consequences of coronary heart disease, such as ischemic mitral regurgitation or left ventricular dysfunction, can be defined. During PCI for acute coronary syndromes, patients are studied during evolving acute myocardial infarction or unstable angina, or in the early period after acute myocardial injury (see Chap. 52). The approach of individual centers in evaluating such patients often depends on local facilities, off-hour capabilities, and treatment philosophies, as well as the availability of surgical support.

In patients with myocardial disease and left ventricular dysfunction, cardiac catheterization provides critical information (see Chaps. 23 and 64). It can evaluate whether CAD is the cause of symptoms, quantify left ventricular dysfunction, and measure right heart pressures and cardiac outputs in patients with cardiomyopathy. In patients with angina and impaired ventricular function, noninvasive testing is of limited value and clinicians should proceed directly to coronary angiography.[37] Cardiac catheterization also permits quantification of the severity of both diastolic and systolic dysfunction, differentiation of myocardial restriction from pericardial constriction, assessment of the extent of valvular regurgitation, and assessment of the cardiovascular response to acute pharmacological intervention.

In patients with valvular heart disease, cardiac catheterization provides confirmatory and complementary data with noninvasive echocardiography, CMR, and nuclear studies (see Chap. 62). Cardiac catheterization can define the severity of valvular stenosis or regurgitation, particularly when noninvasive studies are inconclusive or disparate with clinical findings. Knowledge of the presence or absence of CAD is critical in most adults older than 35 years when valve surgery is planned.[2] However, catheterization may be unnecessary in some preoperative situations, such as patients with an atrial myxoma or younger patients (younger than 35 years) with endocarditis or acute valvular regurgitation. Identification of anomalies, quantification of the hemodynamic consequences of the valvular lesions (such as pulmonary hypertension), and occasionally the acute hemodynamic response to pharmacological therapy all provide useful preoperative information that defines the operative risk, predicts response to surgery, and permits a more directed surgical approach.[2]

The current role of cardiac catheterization in certain congenital disease states is not as clear (see Chap. 61). Echocardiography with Doppler and CMR often provide adequate information. Because gross cardiac anatomy can generally be well defined by these methods, catheterization is required only if certain hemodynamic information (e.g., shunt size or pulmonary vascular resistance) is important in determining the indications for surgical procedures or if percutaneous interventional methods are being used.

There is no true absolute contradiction to cardiac catheterization other than refusal by the competent patient. The procedure can be successfully performed even in the most critically ill patient with a relatively low risk. The relative contradictions of cardiac catheterization are summarized in Table 19-1.

TECHNICAL ASPECTS OF CARDIAC CATHETERIZATION

CATHETERIZATION LABORATORY FACILITIES

Cardiac catheterization facilities have several venues, including traditional hospital-based laboratories with in-house cardiothoracic surgical programs, hospital-based laboratories without on-site surgical programs, free-standing laboratories, and mobile laboratories. At present, about 75 percent of cardiac catheterization laboratories have on-site surgical back-up. The goals of freestanding and mobile cardiac catheterization facilities are to reduce cost while offering services in a convenient location for low-risk patients. The safety of mobile catheterization in properly selected low-risk patients has been well established and appears comparable with that of other settings.

As a result of the documented safety and cost-effectiveness of diagnostic cardiac catheterization in the outpatient setting, there has been increasing use of this approach. Currently, about 50 percent of most hospital-based procedures are done on an outpatient basis. In general, patients who require preprocedural hospitalization for diagnostic catheterization are uncommon, such as those with severe congestive heart failure or renal insufficiency requiring prehydration. The need for hospitalization to change from warfarin to heparin is no longer a requirement. Unfractionated or low-molecular-weight heparin may be used as an outpatient bridge for anticoagulation.[2]

TABLE 19–1	Relative Contraindications to Diagnostic Cardiac Catheterization
Acute gastrointestinal bleeding	
Electrolyte imbalance, especially hypokalemia	
Medication toxicity including digitalis	
Anticoagulation, with international normalized ratio >1.8 or severe coagulopathy	
Anaphylactoid reaction to contrast medium	
Acute stroke	
Acute renal failure or severe chronic nondialysis-dependent kidney disease	
Unexplained fever or untreated active infection	
Severe anemia	
Uncooperative patient	

Noninvasive testing can identify patients who would be more appropriately evaluated in a setting in which cardiac surgery is available, such as patients with severe ischemia discovered during stress testing, ischemia at rest, known or highly suspected severe left main or proximal three-vessel disease, critical aortic stenosis, and severe comorbid disease. Most patients can be discharged on the same day within 2 to 6 hours postprocedure.

The most common complication requiring postprocedural hospitalization is hematoma formation necessitating additional bed rest and observation. Also, diagnosis from the procedure may require hospitalization, such as the finding of left main or severe three-vessel disease. Other considerations for postprocedure hospitalization include uncompensated heart failure, unstable ischemic symptoms, severe aortic stenosis with left ventricular dysfunction, renal insufficiency requiring further hydration, and the need for continuous anticoagulation.[7]

PERSONNEL

Personnel in the catheterization laboratory include the medical director, physicians, nurses, cardiology trainees (fellows), physician extenders, including nurse practitioners and physician assistants, and radiological technologists. All members should be trained in cardiopulmonary resuscitation and preferably in advanced cardiac life support. For full-service laboratories, it is highly desirable for facilities to be associated with a cardiothoracic surgical program. High-risk diagnostic studies and all elective percutaneous interventions should be performed in laboratories with on-site surgical facilities.[5]

LABORATORY CASELOAD

To maintain proficiency, laboratories for adult studies should perform a minimum of 300 procedures/year. According to Accreditation Council for Graduate Medical Education (ACGME) guidelines for diagnostic catheterization, physicians in training must perform a total of 8 months and handle more than 300 cases, including more than 200 as a primary operator, to be credentialed for level II diagnostic cardiac catheterization procedures in practice. However, the minimum caseload for established physicians in practice has not been established.[7,8] Regular evaluation with quality indicator assessment of laboratory, physician, nurse, and technologist performance and outcomes are mandatory. The laboratory director should possess at least 5 years of catheterization experience. In a laboratory performing PCI, the director should be board-certified in interventional cardiology. The director is responsible for credentialing of physicians, reviewing laboratory, physician, and ancillary personnel performance, and providing necessary training. Other responsibilities involve establishing and maintaining quality control of staff and equipment, patient outcome monitoring, and budget analysis.

EQUIPMENT

Necessary equipment for cardiac catheterization includes the radiographic system, physiological data monitoring, including recording and acquisition instrumentation, sterile supplies, and an emergency cart. Also necessary is support equipment, consisting of a power injector, image processing (preferably with digital archiving capabilities), adequate viewing equipment, and a uniform method of report generation.

RADIOGRAPHIC EQUIPMENT. High-resolution x-ray imaging is required for optimal performance of catheterization procedures. Necessary equipment includes a generator, x-ray tube, image intensifier, video system, and either digital archiving or a cine camera (Fig. 19-1).[9] Newer x-ray systems use a flat panel detector rather than an image intensifier, and therefore do not use video cameras. The flat panel detector produces a video image directly without the intermediate visible light stage, thus improving image quality.

Almost all facilities have transitioned from traditional film-based cineangiography to digital angiography, thus becoming "cinefilm-less" laboratories. There are many advantages of digital acquisition and archiving, including immediate on-line review, elimination of film development, quantitative computer analysis, image manipulation capabilities, road maps, flicker-free images at low frame rates, and minimization of radiation exposure. Using these technologies, transfer of images among cardiac catheterization laboratories, hospitals, and physician offices can be accomplished using a common network. The development of digital imaging and communication (DICOM) standards for cardiac angiography has allowed compatibility among different systems. Digital image quality is superior to cinefilm and allows for a telemedicine approach to cardiac catheterization. Increased computer storage capabilities allow storage and remote access to thousands of cases.

PHYSIOLOGICAL MONITORS. Continuous monitoring of blood pressure and the electrocardiogram (ECG) is required during cardiac catheterization. Systemic, pulmonary, and intracardiac pressures are generally recorded using fluid-filled catheters connected to strain-gauge pressure transducers and then transmitted to a monitor. Equipment for determination of thermodilution, Fick cardiac output, and blood gas levels, as well as that for a standard 12-lead ECG, are necessary.

RADIATION SAFETY

Radiation effects can be classified as deterministic or stochastic effects. Both have a delay between radiation and effect, which may be hours to weeks. Deterministic effects are dose-related in that below a certain dose, there is no effect. However, when exceeding a threshold, the severity increases with dose. Examples of deterministic effects include skin erythema, desquamation, cataracts, hair loss, and skin necrosis. Stochastic effects are related to probability and are not related to dose, although the likelihood of an effect is related to dose. Examples of this effect include neoplasms and genetic defects. The estimated dose range for cardiac catheterization is 1 to 10 millisieverts (mSv), which is the equivalent of 2 to 3 years of natural background radiation.[9]

The basic principles of minimizing radiation exposure include minimizing fluoroscopic beam time, using beam collimation, positioning the x-ray source and image reception optimally, using the least magnification possible, changing radiographic projection in long procedures to minimize entrance port skin exposure, recording the estimated patient dose, and selecting equipment with dose-reduction features.

For laboratory personnel, the most important factors are maximizing distance from the source of x-rays and using appropriate shielding, including lead aprons, thyroid collars, lead eyeglasses, and movable leaded barriers. Severely angulated views, especially the left anterior oblique view, substantially increase the radiation exposure of the operator.

A method for measuring radiation exposure for personnel is required. It is recommended that two film badges be worn, one on the outside of the apron at the neck and another under the apron at the waist. The latter monitors the effectiveness of the lead apron. The maximum allowable whole-body radiation dose/year for those working with radiation is 5 rem (roentgen-equivalents-man), or a maximum of 50 rem in a lifetime.[7]

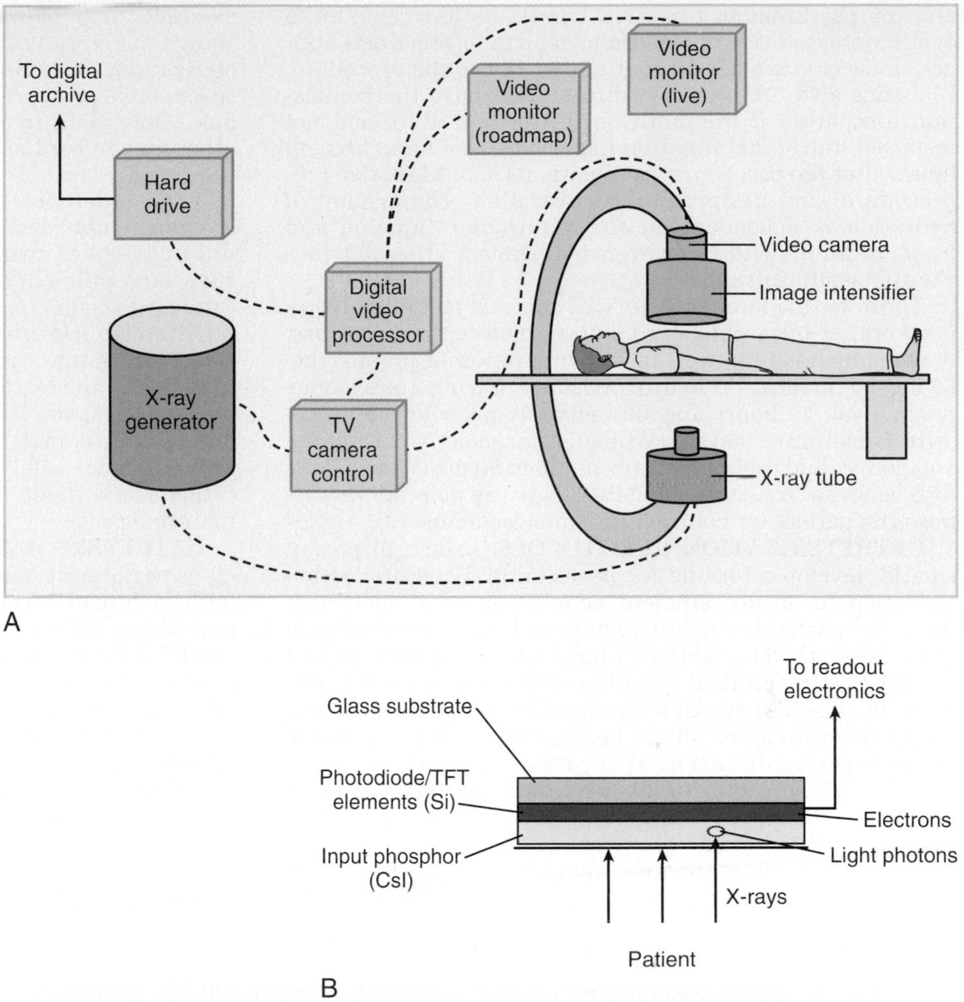

FIGURE 19–1 A, Block diagrams of a filmless x-ray cinefluorographic unit. The unit consists of a patient positioning system, x-ray source, x-ray image detector and digital video image processor, recorder, and display system. X-rays are produced in the x-ray tube from highly controlled electrical power that is applied by the x-ray generator. X-rays that penetrate the patient form an image that is detected and converted to a visible light image by the image intensifier. The visible light image is detected by the video camera and converted to a digital video signal, which is processed and displayed as a visible light image on video monitors. Feedback circuitry from the digital video processor communicates with the x-ray generator. This enables modulation of x-ray output to achieve appropriate subject penetration by the x-ray beam and, accordingly, proper image brightness. X-ray systems that have flat panel detectors rather than image intensifiers do not have video cameras, because the flat-panel detector produces a digital video image directly without the intermediate visible light stage. **B,** Flat panel detector. TFT = thin film transistor. *(Modified from Hirshfeld JW Jr, Balter S, Brinker JA, et al: ACCF/AHA/HRS/SCAI clinical competence statement of physician knowledge to optimize patient safety and image quality in fluoroscopically guided invasive cardiovascular procedures. J Am Coll 44: 2259, 2004.)*

Catheterization Laboratory Protocol

PREPARATION OF THE PATIENT. Before arrival in the catheterization laboratory, the cardiologist responsible for the procedure should explain the procedure fully, including the risk and benefits, and answer questions from the patient and/or family. Precatheterization evaluation includes obtaining the patient's history, physical examination, and ECG. Routine laboratory studies include complete blood count with platelets, serum electrolyte levels, with creatinine and glucose, prothrombin time with international normalized ratio (INR), and partial thromboplastin time (in patients receiving heparin). Important components of the history that need to be addressed include diabetes mellitus (insulin or non–insulin requiring), kidney disease, anticoagulation status, and peripheral vascular disease, as well as previous contrast medium or latex allergy. Full knowledge of any prior procedures, including cardiac catheterizations, PCI procedures, peripheral arterial interventions or surgery, and cardiac surgery, is necessary.

Patients should be fasting at least 6 hours, and an intravenous line should be established. Oral or intravenous sedation is usually administered (e.g., benzodiazepine). Pulse oximetry should be used to monitor respiratory status when these agents are used. Some laboratories routinely premedicate patients with antihistamines such as diphenhydramine (25 IV push) for its antiallergic properties and prolongation of sedation. Oral anticoagulants should be discontinued and the prothrombin time INR should be less than 1.8 to avoid increased risk of bleeding. Aspirin or other oral antiplatelet agents are not discontinued prior to the procedure. Diabetics also taking metformin should have the medication discontinued the morning of the procedure and not restarted until renal function has been stable for at least 48 hours after the procedure.[10] All patients should receive preprocedural and postprocedural hydration. The amount of hydration is dependent on the ventricular function and baseline fluid status. However, if tolerated, at least 1 liter should be administered.

Those with a known history of contrast medium allergy need oral or intravenous prophylaxis before the procedure. A recommended regimen is administration of prednisone, 60 mg by mouth, or hydrocortisone, 100 mg intravenous push, given 12 hours and immediately prior to the procedure. Cimetidine, 300 mg IV push, a nonselective histamine antagonist, and diphenhydramine, 25 to 50 mg IV push, may also be given. A history of shellfish allergy does not predispose the patient for contrast medium reactions.

CATHETERIZATION PROTOCOLS. Each physician should develop a routine for performing diagnostic catheterization to ensure efficient acquisition of all pertinent data. The particular technical approach and necessary procedures should be established individually for each patient so that specific clinical questions can be addressed (Table 19-2). In general, hemodynamic measurements and cardiac output determination should be done before angiography to reflect basal conditions most accurately and to guide angiography. When angiography is performed, the vessel or chamber with most clinical importance should be visualized first in case an adverse event occurs.

Right-heart catheterization should not be performed in all patients undergoing routine coronary angiography. An example of a balloon flotation catheter (Swan-Ganz) is shown in Figure 19-2. Despite limited risks, right-heart catheterization, including screening oximetric analysis, measurement of pressures, and determination of cardiac output, has a low yield in patients with suspected CAD without other known cardiac disease. Right-heart catheterization is indicated when the clinical question cannot be answered by isolated left-heart catheterization or when a patient has left ventricular dysfunction, congestive heart failure, complicated acute myocardial infarction, valvular disease, suspected pulmonary hypertension, a congenital anomaly, intracardiac shunts, or pericardial disease.

Although the use of a temporary pacemaker is not indicated for routine cardiac catheterization, operators should understand the techniques for proper insertion and setting of the pacemaker, if needed. Even in patients with isolated left bundle branch block, right-heart catheterization can generally be safely performed with balloon flotation catheters without causing any additional conduction disturbance.

CATHETERS AND ASSOCIATED EQUIPMENT. Physicians performing cardiac catheterization should be familiar with technical aspects of the equipment used during the procedure. Catheters used for cardiac catheterization are available in various lengths, sizes, and shapes. Typical catheter lengths vary between 50 and 125 cm, with 100 cm being the most commonly used length for adult left-heart catheterization by the femoral approach. The outer diameter of the catheter is specified using French units; 1 French unit (F) = 0.33 mm. The inner diameter of the catheter is smaller than the outside diameter because of the thickness of the catheter material. Guidewires used during the procedure must be small enough to pass through the inner diameters of the introducer needle and catheter. Guidewires are

TABLE 19-2 Catheterization Protocol

Clinical Issue	LHC	RHC	CORO	LV	AO	RV	PA	BX	PROVO	IABP
Known or suspected coronary artery disease										
Stable angina	✓		✓	✓						
Positive stress-test result	✓		✓	✓						
Preoperative evaluation	✓		✓	✓						
Atypical chest pain	✓		✓	✓					±	
Unstable or new-onset angina	✓		✓	✓						
Acute myocardial infarction	✓	±	✓	±						±
Failed thrombolysis	✓	±	✓	±						±
Postinfarction angina	✓		✓	±						±
Cardiogenic shock	✓	✓	✓	±						✓
Mechanical complications	✓	✓	✓	✓	±					✓
Sudden cardiac death	✓	✓	✓	✓						
Valvular heart disease	✓	✓	✓	✓	±					
Myocardial disease	✓	✓	✓	✓	±			±		
Pericardial disease	✓	✓	✓	✓						
Congenital heart disease	✓	✓	✓	✓	±	±	±			
Aortic dissection	✓	±	✓	±	✓					
Pulmonary disease	✓	✓	✓	✓		±	±			

AO = aortography; BX = biopsy; CORO = coronary angiography; IABP = intraaortic balloon pump; LHC = left-heart catheterization, including measurement of left ventricular end-diastolic pressure and aortic valve gradient; LV = left ventriculography; PA = pulmonary angiography or wedge pulmonary angiography; PROVO = provocative challenge (e.g., ergot alkaloids, acetylcholine); RHC = right-heart catheterization, including pressure measurement, determination of cardiac output, oximetric analysis; RV = right ventriculography; ✓ = appropriate; ± = may be appropriate in certain clinical circumstances.

described by their length in centimeters, diameter in inches, and tip conformation. A commonly used wire is a 150-cm, 0.035-inch, J-tip wire. The introducer sheaths are specified by the French number of the largest catheter that passes freely through the inner diameter of the sheath, rather than its outer diameter. Therefore, a 7F introducer sheath accepts a 7F catheter but has an outer diameter of more than 7F, or 2.31 mm.

The choice of the catheter size to be used is made by balancing the need to opacify the coronary arteries and cardiac chambers adequately, have adequate catheter manipulation, limit vascular complications, and permit early ambulation. Although the larger catheters (7 and 8F) allow greater catheter manipulation and excellent visualization, the more commonly used smaller catheters (4 to 6F) permit earlier ambulation after catheterization. Catheter technology has advanced so that 4 to 6F systems are used for routine angiography without significant compromise of angiographic quality. The smaller catheters require greater technical skill of manipulation and have lower flow rates. Thus, their use in tortuous anatomy or in patients with large body habitus may be limited. The relationship between sheath size and vascular complications is not clear. Rather, the arterial puncture technique, anticoagulation status, including use of thienopyridines, glycoprotein IIb/IIIa receptor inhibitors, and bleeding disorders are more important factors related to vascular complications.[11]

BALLOON FLOTATION CATHETERS. Balloon flotation catheters are the simplest and most widely used. If thermodilution cardiac outputs must be determined, catheters that contain thermistors, such as Swan-Ganz catheters, are used (see Fig. 19-2). Determining intracardiac pressure and oxygen saturation to evaluate intracardiac shunts can also be done. These catheters are flexible and flow-directed but, when the femoral approach is used, fluoroscopic guidance is almost always necessary to cannulate the pulmonary artery and to determine pulmonary capillary wedge position. Right-heart catheters have a J-shaped curvature distally to facilitate passage from the SVC to the pulmonary

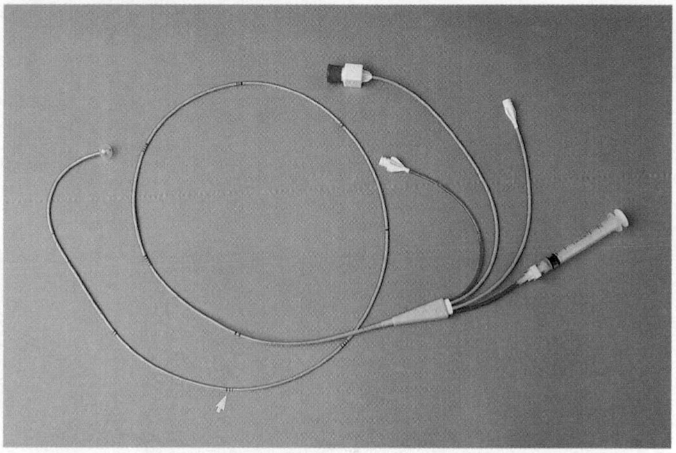

FIGURE 19–2 Typical Swan-Ganz catheter. Proximal ports, left to right, are proximal injection hub, thermistor connector, distal lumen hub, and balloon inflation valve with syringe. The distal end of the catheter has a balloon and a distal end-hole. The proximal injectate port exits 30 cm from the distal lumen (arrow). The thermistor lies just proximal to the balloon.

Techniques

Right-Heart Catheterization

Right-heart catheterization allows measurement and analysis of right atrial, right ventricular, pulmonary artery, and pulmonary capillary wedge pressures; measurement of cardiac output by thermodilution; and screening for intracardiac shunts. Screening blood samples for oximetry should be obtained from the superior vena cava (SVC) and pulmonary artery. Right-heart catheterization is performed antegrade through the inferior vena cava (IVC) or SVC. Percutaneous entry is achieved through the femoral, subclavian, jugular, or antecubital vein. The anatomy of the major arteries and veins used for cardiac catheterization is shown in Figures 19-3 and 19-4.

When left-heart catheterization is performed via the Judkins technique, the femoral venous access approach is used most often. However, when the catheter is left indwelling following the procedure, the internal jugular approach may be preferable. This approach allows the patient to sit up in bed rather than lying flat. The internal jugular approach is preferred to the subclavian to lessen the risk of pneumothorax. A micropuncture kit using a 21-gauge needle and introducer can minimize potential trauma caused by inadvertent puncture of the carotid artery. When the jugular vein has been entered, the micropuncture assembly can be exchanged for a larger sheath (e.g., 7F) necessary for the right-heart catheterization. Also, the adjunctive use of portable vascular ultrasound probes can help locate and establish the patency of the jugular vein in difficult cases, such as patients with short thick necks or following multiple previous catheterizations.

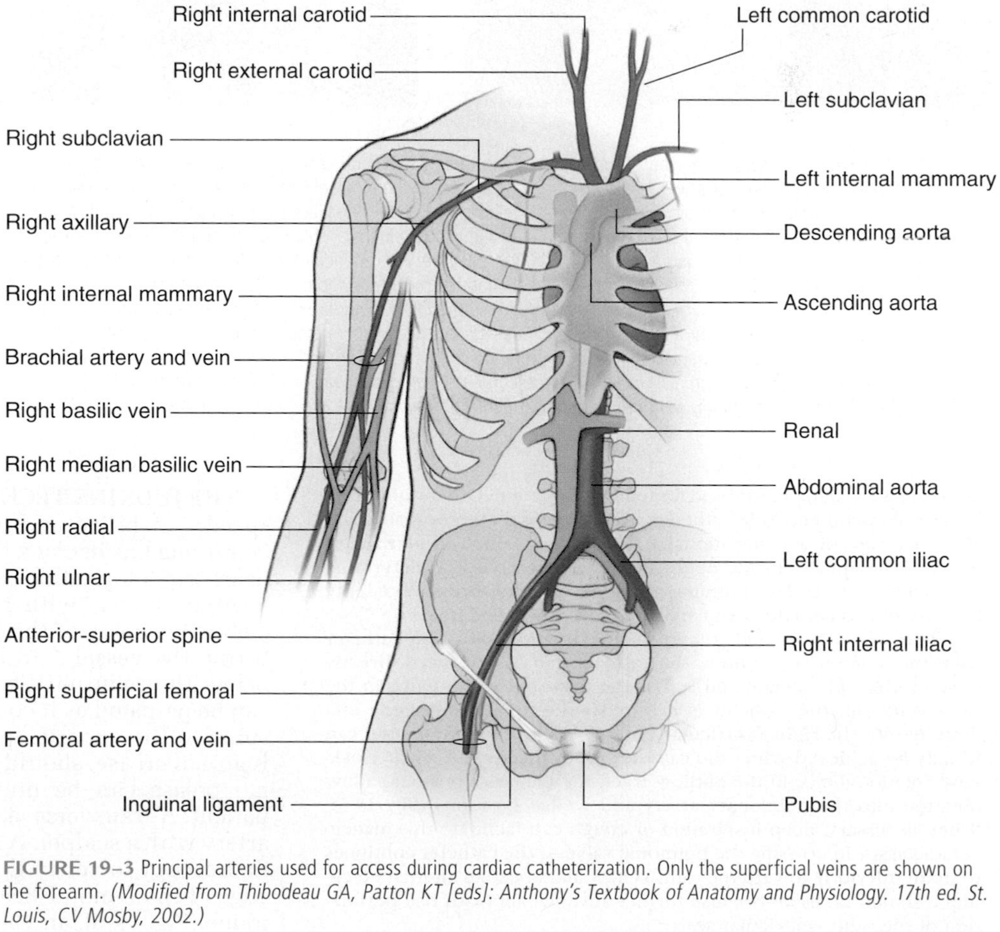

FIGURE 19–3 Principal arteries used for access during cardiac catheterization. Only the superficial veins are shown on the forearm. *(Modified from Thibodeau GA, Patton KT [eds]: Anthony's Textbook of Anatomy and Physiology. 17th ed. St. Louis, CV Mosby, 2002.)*

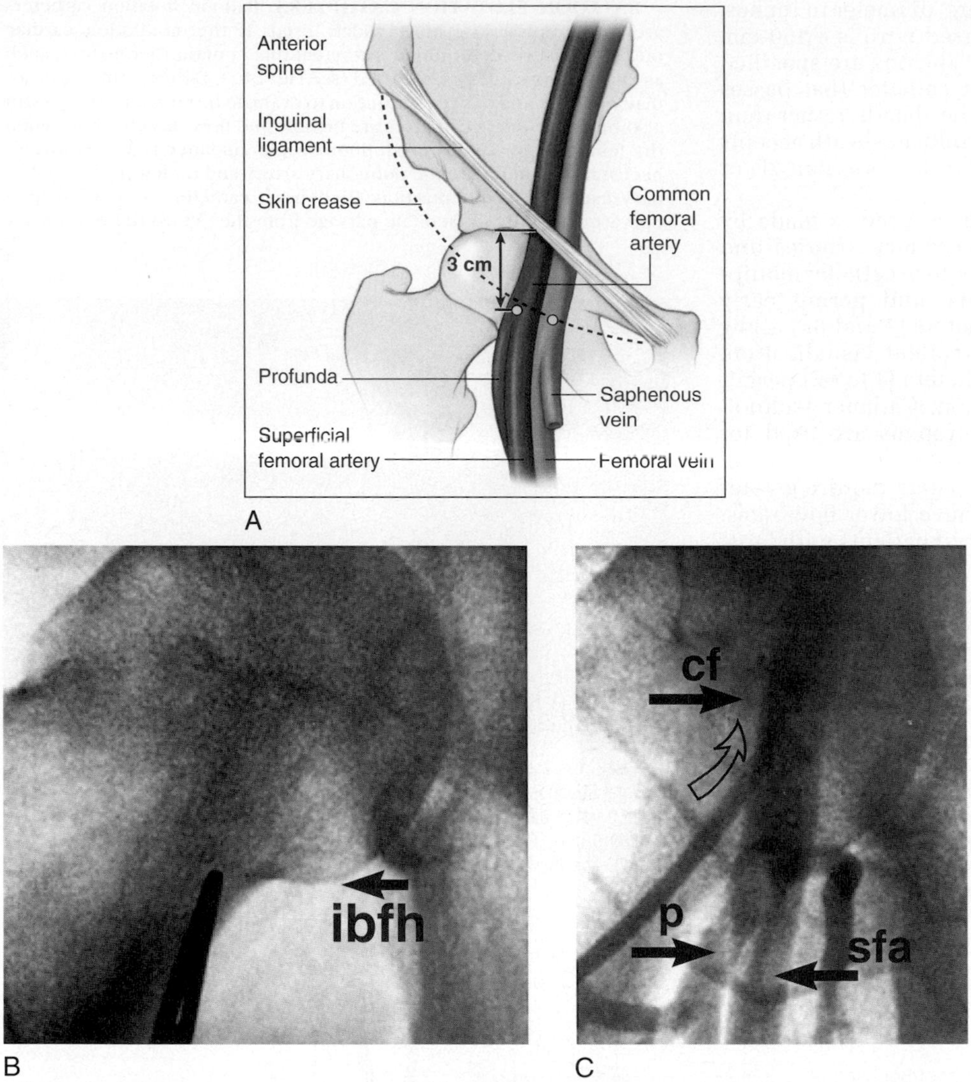

FIGURE 19–4 Regional anatomy relevant to percutaneous femoral arterial and venous catheterization. **A,** Schematic diagram showing the right femoral artery and vein coursing underneath the inguinal ligament, which runs from the anterior superior iliac spine to the pubic tubercle. The arterial skin nick should be placed approximately 3 cm below the ligament and directly over the femoral arterial pulsation, and the venous skin nick should be placed at the same level but approximately one fingerbreadth more medially. Although this level corresponds roughly to the skin crease in most patients, the anatomical localization relative to the inguinal ligament provides a more constant landmark.
B, Fluoroscopic localization of skin nick (marked by clamp tip) to the inferior border of the femoral head (ibfh).
C, Catheter (open arrow) inserted through this skin nick has entered the common femoral artery (cf), above its bifurcation into the superficial femoral artery (sfa) and profunda (p) branches (arrows). (See also Fig. 20-1) *(From Baim DS, Grossman W: Percutaneous approach, including transseptal and apical puncture. In Baim DS, Grossman W [eds]: Cardiac Catheterization, Angiography, and Intervention. 7th ed. Philadelphia, Lea & Febiger, 2006, p 81.)*

artery, or an S-shaped distal end for femoral insertion. Other right-heart balloon flotation end-hole catheters are more rigid and torquable and allow passage of a conventional 0.035- or 0.038-inch guidewire to improve manipulation. Although these lack the ability to determine thermodilution cardiac outputs, they yield better pressure fidelity because of less catheter whip artifact and a larger end hole.

There are two methods for advancing a balloon flotation catheter from the femoral vein. Often, the catheter can be advanced directly through the right atrium and across the tricuspid valve. Once in the right ventricle, the catheter is manipulated to point superiorly and directly into the right ventricular outflow tract. This orientation can usually be achieved while the catheter is advanced with slight clockwise rotation. Once in the outflow tract, the balloon tip should allow flotation into the pulmonary artery and wedge positions (Fig. 19-5). When necessary, deep inspiration or cough can facilitate this maneuver and assist in crossing the pulmonic valve. If the catheter continues to point inferiorly toward the right ventricular apex, an alternate technique should be used, because further advancement can risk perforation of the right ventricular apex.

Another technique for performing right-heart catheterization with a balloon flotation catheter is shown in Figure 19-5. A loop is formed in the right atrium, with the catheter tip directed laterally. The loop can be created by hooking the catheter tip on the hepatic vein or by advancing the catheter while it is directed laterally in the right atrium. Once the loop is formed, the catheter should be advanced further, which directs the tip inferiorly and then medially across the tricuspid valve. Antegrade blood flow should then direct the catheter into the pulmonary artery. After the catheter is placed into the wedge position, the redundant loop can be removed by slow withdrawal.

NONFLOTATION CATHETERS. When an end-hole catheter (e.g., Cournand or multipurpose) that does not have a balloon tip is used, the technique for cannulating the pulmonary artery is markedly different. Manipulation and torquing of the nonflotation catheter are necessary to advance into the pulmonary artery. The catheter should be directed inferiorly across the tricuspid valve and then superiorly into the right ventricular outflow tract. It is generally recommended that one attempt be made to form a loop in the right atrium before advancement into the right ventricle to lessen the risk of perforation.

A probe-patent foramen ovale is present in 20 to 30 percent of adult patients, which allows access to the left atrium. It can be entered using a multipurpose catheter with the tip directed medially and slightly posteriorly. The catheter is withdrawn slowly from the SVC or high right atrium until a slight forward and medial motion is observed. The catheter then prolapses into the left atrium with mild pressure against the interatrial septum in patients with a probe-patent foramen ovale. Left atrial position can be verified by the pressure waveform, blood samples demonstrating arterial saturation, or manual contrast medium injection. If left atrial access is necessary and cannot be obtained with this technique, a transseptal catheterization should be undertaken (see later, "Transseptal Catheterization").

Left-Heart Catheterization and Coronary Arteriography

THE JUDKINS TECHNIQUE. Because of its relative ease, speed, reliability, and low complication rate,[1,7] the Judkins technique has become the most widely used method of left-heart catheterization and coronary arteriography. After local anesthesia with 1 percent lidocaine (Xylocaine), percutaneous entry of the femoral artery is achieved by puncturing the vessel 1 to 3 cm (or one to two fingerbreadths) below the inguinal ligament (see Fig. 19-4). The ligament can be palpated as it courses from the anterior superior iliac spine to the superior pubic ramus. This ligament, not the inguinal crease, should be used as the landmark. The inguinal crease can be misleading, particularly in the obese patient. A transverse skin incision is made over the femoral artery with a scalpel. A hemostatic clamp can be used under fluoroscopy to verify that the nick is made over the inferior edge of the femoral head. Using a modified Seldinger technique (Fig. 19-6), an 18-gauge thin-walled needle (Fig. 19-7)

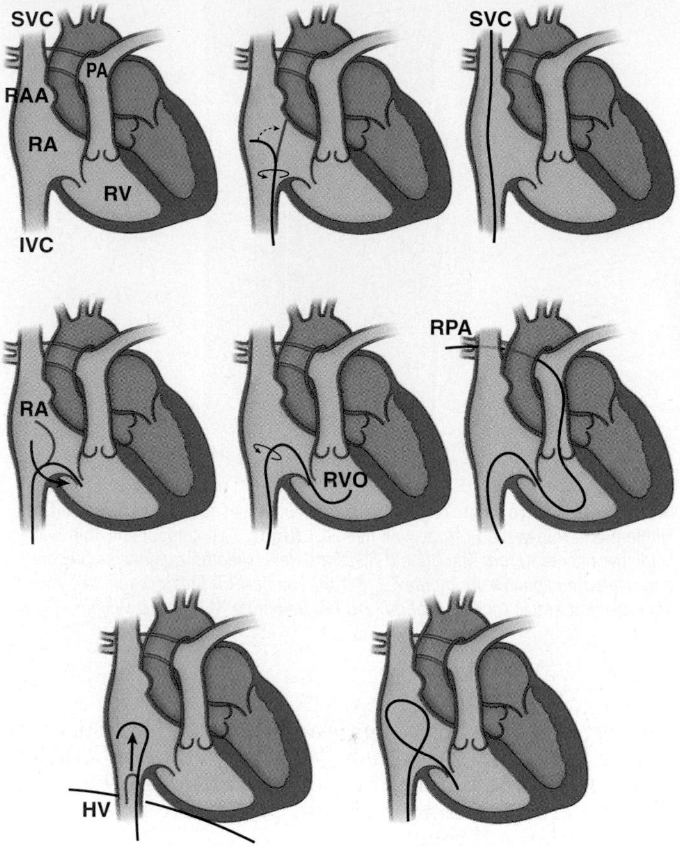

FIGURE 19–5 Right-heart catheterization from the femoral vein, shown in cartoon form. **Top row,** The right-heart catheter is initially placed in the right atrium (RA) aimed at the lateral atrial wall. Counterclockwise rotation aims the catheter posteriorly and allows advancement into the superior vena cava (SVC). Although not evident in the figure, clockwise catheter rotation into an anterior orientation would lead to advancement into the right atrial appendage (RAA), precluding SVC catheterization. **Center row,** The catheter is then withdrawn back into the right atrium and aimed laterally. Clockwise rotation causes the catheter tip to sweep anteromedially and cross the tricuspid valve. With the catheter tip in a horizontal orientation just beyond the spine, it is positioned below the right ventricular outflow (RVO) tract. Additional clockwise rotation causes the catheter to point straight up, allowing advancement into the main pulmonary artery and from there into the right pulmonary artery (RPA). **Bottom row,** Two maneuvers useful in catheterization of a dilated right heart. A larger loop with a downward-directed tip may be required to reach the tricuspid valve and can be formed by catching the catheter tip in the hepatic vein (HV) and advancing the catheter quickly into the right atrium. The reverse loop technique (bottom right) gives the catheter tip an upward direction, aimed toward the outflow tract. IVC = inferior vena cava; PA = pulmonary artery; RV = right ventricle. *(From Baim DS, Grossman W: Percutaneous approach, including transseptal and apical puncture. In Baim DS, Grossman W [eds]: Cardiac Catheterization, Angiography, and Intervention. 7th ed. Philadelphia, Lea & Febiger, 2006, p 86.)*

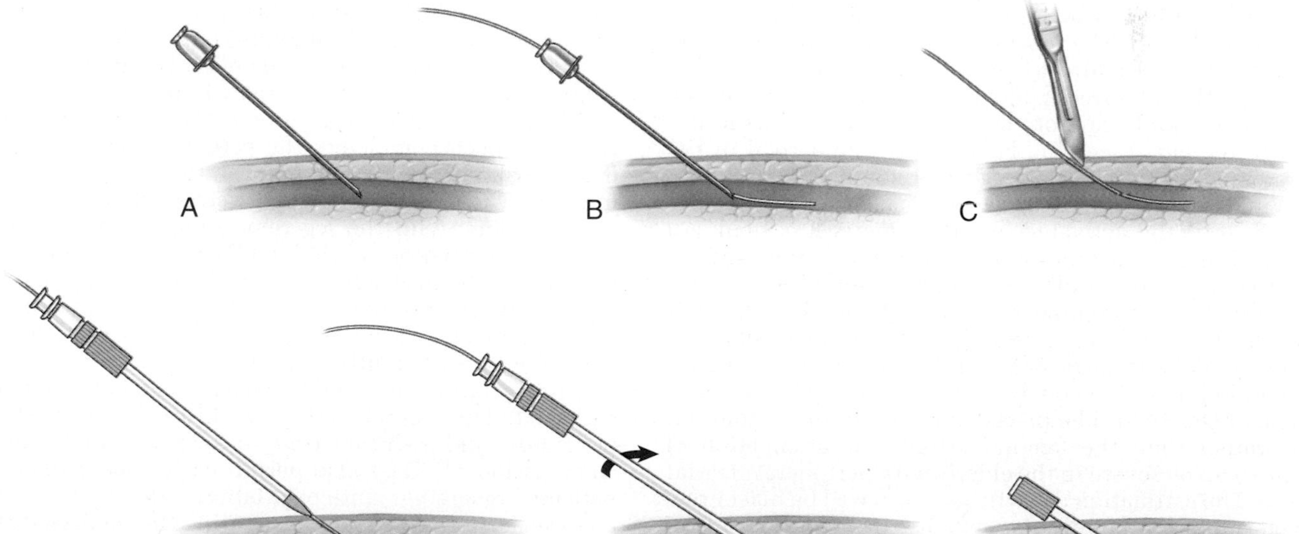

FIGURE 19–6 Modified Seldinger technique for percutaneous catheter sheath introduction. **A,** Vessel punctured by needle. **B,** Flexible guidewire placed into the vessel through the needle. **C,** Needle removed, guidewire left in place, and the hole in the skin around the wire enlarged with a scalpel. **D,** Sheath and dilator placed over the guidewire. **E,** Sheath and dilator advanced over the guidewire and into the vessel. **F,** Dilator and guidewire removed while the sheath remains in the vessel. *(From Hill JA, Lambert CR, Vlietstra RE, Pepine CJ: Review of general catheterization techniques. In Pepine CJ, Hill JA, Lambert CR [eds]: Diagnostic and Therapeutic Cardiac Catheterization. 3rd ed. Baltimore, Williams & Wilkins, 1998, p 107.)*

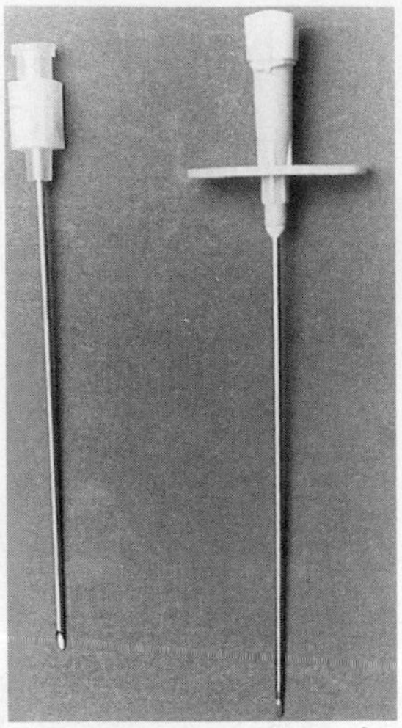

FIGURE 19–7 Two most commonly used needle types for vascular access. **Left,** Single-piece, thin-walled "front-wall needle." **Right,** Two-component, thin-walled Seldinger needle. *(From MacDonald RG: Catheters, sheaths, guidewires, needles, and related equipment.* In *Pepine CJ, Hill JA, Lambert CR [eds]: Diagnostic and Therapeutic Cardiac Catheterization. 3rd ed. Baltimore, Williams & Wilkins, 1998, p 130.)*

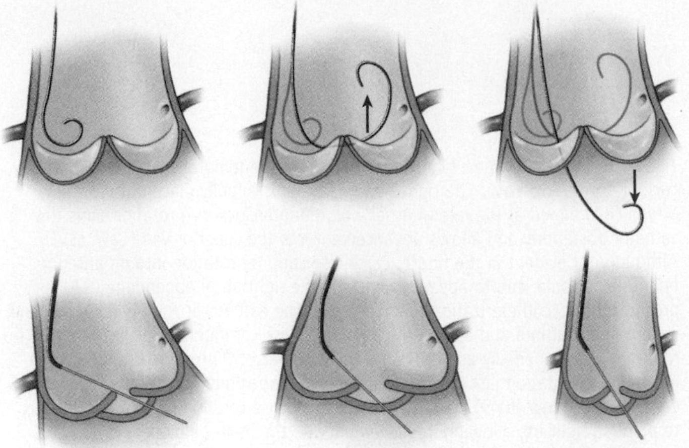

FIGURE 19–8 Technique for retrograde crossing of an aortic valve using a pigtail catheter. **Top row,** Technique for crossing a normal aortic valve. **Bottom row,** Use of a straight guidewire and pigtail catheter in combination. Increasing the length of protruding guidewire straightens the catheter curve and causes the wire to point more toward the right coronary ostium; reducing the length of protruding wire restores the pigtail contour and deflects the guidewire tip toward the left coronary artery. When the correct length of wire and the correct rotational orientation of the catheter have been found, repeated advancement and withdrawal of catheter and guidewire together allow retrograde passage across the valve. In a dilated aortic root, the angled pigtail catheter is preferable. In a small aortic root (bottom row, right), a right coronary Judkins catheter may have advantages. In patients with bicuspid valves, an Amplatz left catheter is often used, because it directs the wire more superiorly. *(From Baim DS, Grossman W: Percutaneous approach including transseptal and apical puncture.* In *Baim DS, Grossman W [eds]: Cardiac Catheterization, Angiography, and Intervention. 6th ed. Philadelphia, Lea & Febiger, 2006, p 93.)*

is inserted at a 30- to 45-degree angle into the femoral artery, and a 0.035- or 0.038-inch J-tip polytetrafluoroethylene (Teflon)–coated guidewire is advanced through the needle into the artery. The wire should pass freely up the aorta, like a hot knife through butter.

After arterial access is obtained, a sheath at least equal in size to the coronary catheter is usually inserted into the femoral artery. The routine use of heparin for diagnostic cardiac catheterization has not been established. However, in prolonged procedures, such as patients with bypass grafts or stenotic valve disease, it may be administered at 2000 to 3000 units IV push. The routine administrator of protamine following the procedure to reverse heparin is not recommended. Although rare, hypotensive reactions to protamine can be severe and are more common in patients with diabetes. In patients receiving heparin prior to arrival in the laboratory, an activated clotting time should be determined following access. Sheath removal is usually not recommended until the activated clotting time is less than 170 seconds, unless a vascular closure device is being used.

Left ventricular systolic and end-diastolic pressures can be obtained by advancing a pigtail catheter into the left ventricle (Fig. 19-8). In assessing valvular aortic stenosis, left ventricular and aortic or femoral artery pressures should be recorded simultaneously with two transducers. The aortic catheter should be placed at least into the abdominal aorta, rather than the femoral artery. The attenuation of pressure can be severe in the elderly with peripheral arterial disease. The estimation of aortic pressure will be inaccurate for determination of valvular severity. In suspected mitral stenosis, left ventricular and wedge or left atrial pressures should be determined simultaneously. Left ventriculography is performed in the 30-degree right anterior oblique and 45- to 50-degree left anterior oblique views. A pigtail catheter is most commonly used for this purpose. A power injection of contrast medium into the ventricle, 30 to 40 ml at 12 to 15 ml/sec, is used to assess left ventricular function and the severity of mitral regurgitation. After ventriculography, left ventricular systolic and end-diastolic pressure measurements may be repeated and the systolic pressure recorded as the catheter is withdrawn from the left ventricle into the aorta. If an aortic transvalvular gradient is present, recording these pressures can detect it. For measurement of suspected intraventricular gradients, a multipurpose catheter with an end hole is desirable to localize the gradient in the left ventricle. Pigtail catheters contain side holes, which obscure the capacity to define whether the gradient is intraventricular, subvalvular, or transvalvular.

After coronary arteriography and left-heart catheterization have been completed, the catheters are removed and firm pressure is applied by hand to the femoral area for 10 minutes. The patient should be instructed to lie in bed for several hours, with the leg remaining straight to prevent hematoma formation. With 4 to 6F catheters, 2 hours of bed rest is usually sufficient, whereas use of a catheter larger than 6F usually requires at least 3 to 4 hours of bed rest.

Alternatively, vascular closure devices may be used. Four types are currently available—collagen plugs, suture closure, metallic clips, and hemostatic patches. Each allows early ambulation of the patient, within 1 to 2 hours after the procedure, and a shorter time to hemostasis than manual compression.[12,13] They also permit early sheath removal in patients receiving anticoagulation. However, a meta-analysis has raised concern regarding the increased risk of pseudoaneurysm and hematoma with arterial puncture closure devices.[14] The ultimate success of any means of achieving hemostasis relies on a single front wall puncture of the common femoral artery.

The main advantage of the Judkins technique is speed and ease of selective catheterization. These attributes do not, however, preclude the importance of extensive operator experience to ensure quality studies with an acceptable degree of safety. The main disadvantage of this technique is its use in patients with severe iliofemoral atherosclerotic disease, in whom retrograde passage of catheters through areas of extreme narrowing or tortuosity may be difficult or impossible. However, with careful technique, passage through synthetic aortofemoral grafts can be achieved with low complication rates.

BRACHIAL ARTERY TECHNIQUE—SONES TECHNIQUE. Sones and colleagues introduced the first technique for coronary artery catheterization by means of a brachial artery cutdown. The technically demanding Sones technique is still popular in some centers and is described in Chapter 20.

PERCUTANEOUS BRACHIAL ARTERY TECHNIQUE. A modification of the Sones technique is the percutaneous brachial artery technique using preformed Judkins catheters. This technique uses the Seldinger method of percutaneous brachial artery entry. A 4 to 6F sheath is placed into the brachial artery, and 3000 to 5000 U of heparin is infused into the side port. A guidewire is then advanced to the ascending aorta under fluoroscopic control. Judkins left, right, and pigtail catheters are passed over the guidewire for routine arteriography and ventriculography. The guidewire may occasionally be necessary to direct the left coronary catheter into the left sinus of Valsalva and the ostium of the left main coronary artery. Alternatively, an Amplatz left or multipurpose catheter is used to intubate the coronary ostium. Following removal of the sheath, the arm should be maintained straight with an arm board for 4 to 6 hours, with observation of radial and brachial pulses.

The main advantage of the percutaneous brachial technique is that it avoids a brachial artery cutdown and repair. The main disadvantage is that manipulation of catheters can be difficult. Compared with the femoral technique, patient's comfort, hemostasis time, and time to ambulation favor the brachial technique, whereas procedural efficiency, time of radiation exposure, and diagnostic image quality are more favorable with the femoral approach. The complication rates appear similar.

PERCUTANEOUS RADIAL ARTERY TECHNIQUE. Left-heart catheterization by the radial artery approach was developed as an alternative to the percutaneous transbrachial approach in an attempt to limit vascular complications. The inherent advantages of the transradial approach are that the hand has a dual arterial supply connected through the palmar arches and that there are no nerves or veins at the site of puncture. In addition, bed rest is unnecessary after the procedure, allowing more efficient outpatient angiography.

The procedure requires a normal Allen test result. After manual compression of both the radial and ulnar arteries during fist clenching, the hand is blanched. Normal color returns to the opened hand within 10 seconds after releasing pressure over the ulnar artery, and significant reactive hyperemia is absent on releasing pressure over the radial artery.

The arm is abducted and the wrist hyperextended over a gauze roll. Routine skin anesthesia is used, a small incision is made just proximal to the styloid process of the radius, and the subcutaneous tissue is tunneled using forceps. An 18-gauge needle is introduced at a 45-degree angle and an exchange length 0.035- or 0.038-inch J-tip guidewire is inserted. A 23-cm-long 4 or 5F sheath is then introduced. Heparin, 5000 U, is administered through the side arm of the sheath. Coronary catheters are then advanced over the exchange wire into the ascending aorta. The left and right coronary arteries are intubated in a manner similar to that for the brachial approach. Hemostasis is obtained at the end of the procedure after sheath removal, using direct pressure. It is recommended that the arterial puncture site be allowed to bleed for several beats before maintaining direct pressure. The radial pulse should be monitored regularly for several hours after the procedure.

The potential limitations of this procedure include the inability to cannulate the radial artery because of its smaller size and propensity to develop spasm, poor visualization of the coronary arteries resulting from use of small-caliber catheters with limited manipulation potential, and risk of radial arterial occlusion caused by dissection or thrombus formation. In addition, when right-heart catheterization is required, additional approaches are necessary. If intervention is contemplated, device selection may be limited by guide catheter size. Although there is little debate that the femoral approach is the simplest and probably the safest technique for left-heart catheterization, the transradial approach for left-heart catheterization has gained in popularity in some centers.[15]

TRANSSEPTAL CATHETERIZATION. Transseptal left-heart catheterization has received renewed interest with the advent of percutaneous balloon mitral commissurotomy as a viable option to surgical commissurotomy (see Chap. 62), with electrophysiological procedures requiring access to pulmonary veins (see Chap. 35), with the early development of percutaneous valve replacement and repair, and with use of disc-type prosthetic valves in the aortic position. This type of mechanical prosthetic valve cannot be crossed safely and prohibits retrograde left-heart catheterization. When performed by experienced operators, the technique has a low complication rate, less than 1 percent.[16,17]

The transseptal catheter is a short curved catheter with a tapered tip (Fig. 19-9). Alternatively, an 8F Mullins sheath and dilator combination is used. The Brockenbrough needle is an 18-gauge needle that tapers to 21 gauge at the distal tip. One commonly used approach is to place a 0.032-inch guidewire through the femoral vein, through the right atrium, and into the SVC. The Mullins transseptal sheath and dilator are then advanced over the wire into the SVC. The guidewire is removed and replaced with a Brockenbrough needle, and the distal port is connected to a pressure manifold. With the needle tip just proximal to the Mullins sheath tip, the entire catheter system is withdrawn. The catheter is simultaneously rotated from a 12 to a 5 o'clock position. The operator observes two abrupt rightward movements. The first occurs as the catheter descends from the SVC to the right atrium. The second occurs as the Mullins

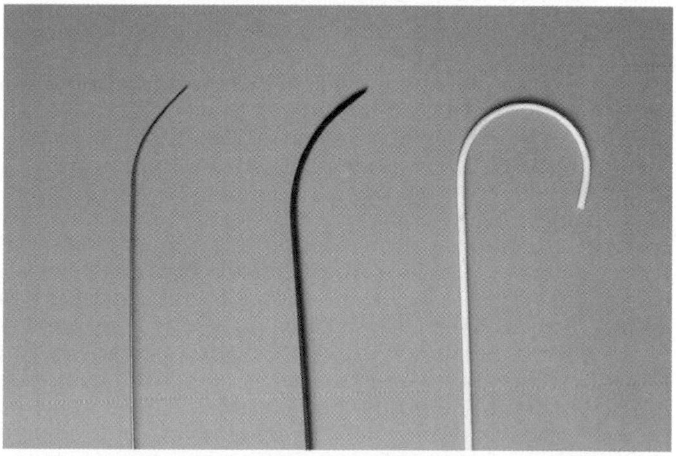
A

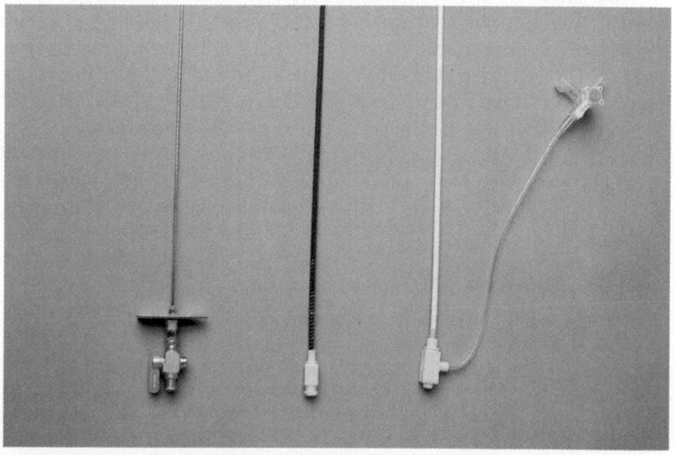
B

FIGURE 19–9 Transseptal catheters. **A,** Distal catheters. **B,** Proximal catheters. **A** and **B,** Mullins transseptal sheath (left), introducer (dilator) placed inside sheath to add stiffness to the catheter (middle), Brockenbrough transseptal needle placed inside the sheath and used to penetrate the septum (right).

dilator tip passes over the limbic edge into the fossa ovalis. The curve of the sheath and needle should be oriented slightly anteriorly. The dilator and needle can then be advanced gently as a unit. Steady gentle pressure is often adequate to advance the system through the fossa ovalis into the left atrium. If not, the needle should be advanced across the interatrial septum while holding the Mullins sheath in place. In patients in whom transseptal puncture is technically difficult because of a large right atrium, postsurgical condition, or anatomical variant, intracardiac echocardiography can be useful to localize the fossa ovalis and interatrial septum.[18]

Left atrial position can be confirmed by the overall increase in pressure with left atrial a and v waveforms, hand injection of contrast medium, or measurement of arterial oxygen saturation. When the position is confirmed, the catheter should be rotated toward 3 o'clock and the dilator and sheath safely advanced 2 to 3 cm into the left atrium. The sheath is held firmly, and the dilator and needle are removed. Left atrial pressure measurements should then be repeated. If measurement of left ventricular pressure, left ventriculography, or both is necessary, the catheter can usually be advanced easily into the left ventricle after slight counterclockwise rotation. The major risk of transseptal catheterization lies in inadvertent puncture of atrial structures, such as the atrial free wall, left atrial appendage, or coronary sinus, or entry into the aortic root or pulmonary artery.

Direct Transthoracic Left Ventricular Puncture

The sole indication for direct left ventricular puncture is to measure left ventricular pressure and to perform ventriculography in patients with mechanical prosthetic valves in both the mitral and aortic positions, preventing retrograde arterial and transseptal catheterization. Crossing tilting-disc valves with catheters should be avoided because it may result in catheter entrapment, occlusion of the valve, or possible dislodgment of the disc with embolization.

The procedure is performed after localizing the left ventricular apex by palpation or, preferably, by using echocardiography.[19,20] After local anesthesia is administered, an 18- or 21-gauge 6-inch Teflon catheter system is inserted at the upper rib margin and directed slightly posteriorly and toward the right second intercostal space until the impulse is encountered. The needle and sheath are advanced into the left ventricle. The stylet and needle are removed, and the sheath is connected for pressure measurement.

The risks of this procedure include cardiac tamponade, hemothorax, pneumothorax, laceration of the left anterior descending coronary artery, embolism of left ventricular thrombus, vagal reactions, and ventricular arrhythmias. The risk of pericardial tamponade, however, is limited in patients who have undergone prior cardiac surgery because mediastinal fibrosis is present. However, with current noninvasive imaging techniques, including transesophageal echocardiography, this procedure is infrequently indicated.

Endomyocardial Biopsy

Endomyocardial biopsy is performed most commonly using a disposable or, less frequently, a reusable bioptome. The most popular devices used for the internal jugular vein approach include preshaped 50-cm bioptomes. Right ventricular biopsy may be performed using the internal jugular vein (see "Right-heart Catheterization" for internal jugular technique), subclavian vein, or femoral vein. Left ventricular biopsy is usually performed using the femoral arterial approach.

When performing right ventricular biopsy through the right internal jugular vein, a 7 to 9F short straight sheath is introduced by the usual Seldinger technique. A 7 to 8F bioptome is advanced under fluoroscopic guidance to the lateral wall of the right atrium. Using counterclockwise rotation, the device is advanced across the tricuspid valve and toward the interventricular septum. Position of the bioptome against the interventricular septum is confirmed using 30-degree right anterior oblique and 60-degree left anterior oblique fluoroscopic projections. Alternatively, two-dimensional echocardiography rather than fluoroscopy has been used to guide the position of the bioptome. Contact with the myocardium is confirmed by the presence of premature ventricular contractions, resistance to further advancement, and transmission of the ventricular impulse to the operator. The bioptome is then slightly withdrawn from the septum, the forceps jaws are opened, the bioptome is readvanced to make contact with the myocardium, and the forceps closed. A slight tug is felt on removal of the device. Another technique uses a preshaped sheath with a flexible straight bioptome. The configurations are shorter replicates of those sheaths used in the femoral venous approach. Approximately four to six samples of myocardium are required for adequate pathological analysis. Preprocedural consultation with a pathologist should be obtained to ensure appropriate specimen collection and processing.

Right ventricular biopsy from the femoral vein requires insertion of a long 6 or 7F sheath directed toward the portion of the ventricle to be sampled. Various configurations of sheaths are used for right ventricular biopsy. The conventional sheath has a 45-degree angle on its distal end to allow access to the right ventricle. However, newer sheaths have dual curves. These catheters possess the usual 180-degree curve and an additional distal perpendicular septal plane curve of 90 degrees, which allows improved manipulation and positioning toward the interventricular septum.

The bioptome is advanced through the sheath, and should be visualized in both the 30-degree right anterior oblique and 40-degree left anterior oblique views. The right anterior oblique view ensures that the catheter is in the midventricle, away from the apex. The left anterior oblique view verifies that the sheath tip is oriented toward the interventricular septum. Contrast medium infusion through the side port of the sheath can be confirmatory. Samples of myocardium are taken in a manner similar to that described earlier.

If left ventricular biopsy is to be performed, the biopsy sheath is generally inserted through the femoral artery and positioned over a multipurpose or pigtail catheter that has been placed in the ventricle. The sheath is advanced below the mitral apparatus and away from the posterobasal wall. The catheter is then withdrawn, and a long left ventricular bioptome is inserted. Care must be taken when left ventricular biopsy is performed to prevent air embolism while introducing the bioptome into the sheath. A constant infusion of flush solution through the sheath minimizes the risk of air or thrombus embolism.

Complications of endomyocardial biopsy include cardiac perforation with cardiac tamponade, emboli (air, tissue embolus, or thromboembolus), arrhythmias, electrical conduction disturbances, injury to heart valves, vasovagal reactions, and pneumothorax. The overall complication rate is between 1 and 2 percent, with the risk of cardiac perforation with tamponade generally reported as less than 0.05 percent.[21] Systemic embolization and ventricular arrhythmias are more common with left ventricular biopsy. Left ventricular biopsy should generally be avoided in patients with right bundle branch block because of the potential for developing complete atrioventricular block, as well as in patients with known left ventricular thrombus.

The indications for endomyocardial biopsy remain controversial.[3] It is generally agreed that endomyocardial biopsy is indicated to monitor cardiac allograft rejection and that it may also be useful to monitor for anthracycline cardiotoxicity. However, considerable persistent controversy surrounds the use of endomyocardial biopsy to evaluate the cause of dilated cardiomopathy.[3] Other possible indications for endomyocardial biopsy include differentiation between restrictive and constrictive myopathies,[22] determination of whether myocarditis is the cause of ventricular arrhythmias, and assessment of patients with left ventricular dysfunction associated with human immunodeficiency virus infection.[23]

Percutaneous Intraaortic Balloon Pump Insertion

Intraaortic balloon counterpulsation devices are positioned in the descending thoracic aorta. They have a balloon volume of 30 to 50 ml, use helium as the inflation gas, and are timed to inflate during diastole and deflate during systole. Balloon size is based on the patient's height. The device is inserted through the femoral artery using the standard Seldinger technique, so that the tip is 2 to 3 cm below the level of the left subclavian artery. Both 8 and 9.5F systems are used.[24] Optimal positioning requires fluoroscopic guidance. Timing of the balloon is adjusted during 1 : 2 pumping (one inflation for each two beats), so that inflation of the balloon occurs at the aortic dicrotic notch and deflation occurs immediately before systole. This timing ensures maximal augmentation of diastolic flow and maximal systolic unloading. Figure 19-10 displays the optimal timing of an intraaortic balloon pump (IABP).[25]

Favorable hemodynamic effects include reduction in left ventricular afterload and improvement in myocardial oxygenation.[26] IABP insertion is indicated for patients with angina refractory to medical therapy, cardiogenic shock, or mechanical complications of myocardial infarction (e.g., severe mitral regurgitation, ventricular septal defect) or for those who have severe left main coronary artery stenosis. IABP may also be valuable in patients undergoing high-risk PCI or after primary angioplasty in the setting of acute myocardial infarction.[27,28] IABP insertion is contraindicated in patients with moderate or severe aortic regurgitation, aortic dissection, aortic aneurysm, patent ductus arteriosus, severe peripheral vascular disease, bleeding disorders, or sepsis.

Complications of IABP insertion include limb ischemia requiring early balloon removal or vascular surgery, balloon rupture, balloon entrapment, hematomas, and sepsis.[25,27] The incidence of vascular complications ranges from 12 to more than 40 percent.[25,27] Most patients in whom limb ischemia develops after insertion of a balloon pump device have resolution of the ischemia on balloon removal and do not require surgical intervention (e.g., thrombectomy, vascular repair, fasciotomy, amputation). The risk of limb ischemia is heightened in patients with diabetes or peripheral vascular disease, in women, and in patients with a postinsertion ankle-brachial index lower than 0.8. However, with the development of smaller catheters (8 to 9.5F) and the advent of sheathless insertion techniques, vascular complications have been reduced.[25-28]

HEMODYNAMIC DATA

The hemodynamic component of the cardiac catheterization procedure focuses on pressure measurements, the measurement of flow (e.g., cardiac output, shunt flows, flow across a stenotic orifice, regurgitant flows, and coronary blood flow), and the determination of vascular resistances. Simply stated, flow through a blood vessel (Q) is determined by the pressure (P) difference within the vessel and the vascular resistance (R), as described by Ohm's law:

$$Q = \Delta P/R$$

Pressure Measurements

Accurate recording of pressure waveforms and correct interpretation of physiological data derived from these waveforms are major goals of cardiac catheterization. A pressure wave is the cyclical force generated by cardiac muscle contraction, and its amplitude and duration are influenced by various mechanical and physiological parameters. The pressure waveform from a particular cardiac chamber is influenced by the force of the contracting chamber and its surrounding structures, including the contiguous chambers of the heart, pericardium, lungs, and vasculature. Physiological variables of heart rate and the respiratory cycle also influence the pressure waveform. An understanding of the components of the cardiac cycle is essential to the correct interpretation of hemodynamic data obtained in the catheterization laboratory.

FLUID-FILLED SYSTEMS. Intravascular pressures are typically measured using a fluid-filled catheter attached to a pressure transducer. The pressure wave is transmitted from the catheter tip to the transducer by the fluid column within the catheter. Most pressure transducers used currently are disposable electrical strain gauges. The pressure wave distorts the diaphragm or wire within the transducer. This energy is then converted to an electrical signal proportional to the pressure being applied, using the principle of the Wheatstone bridge. This signal is then amplified and recorded as an analog signal.[29]

There are a number of sources of error when pressures are measured using a fluid-filled catheter-transducer system. Distortion of the output signal occurs as a result of the frequency response characteristics and damping characteristics of the system. The frequency response of the system is the ratio of the output amplitude to input amplitude over a range of frequencies of the input pressure wave. The natural frequency is the frequency at which the system oscillates when it is shock-excited in the absence of friction. Dissipation of the energy of the system, such as by friction, is called damping. To ensure a high-frequency response range, the pressure measurement system should have the highest possible natural frequency and optimal damping. With optimal damping the energy is dissipated gradually, thus maintaining the frequency response curve as close as possible to an output-to-input ratio of 1 as it approaches the system's natural frequency. Optimal damping is achieved by using a short, wide-bore, noncompliant catheter tubing system that is directly connected to the transducer using a low-density liquid from which all air bubbles have been removed.[29]

The pressure transducer must be calibrated against a known pressure, and the establishment of a zero reference must be undertaken at the start of the catheterization procedure. To "zero" the transducer, the transducer is placed at the level of the atria, which is approximately midchest. If the transducer is attached to the manifold and is therefore at variable positions during the procedure, a second fluid-filled catheter system should be attached to the transducer and positioned at the level of the midchest. All transducers being used during the procedure should be zeroed and calibrated simultaneously. Because of possible variable drift during the procedure, all transducers should be rebalanced immediately prior to obtaining simultaneous recordings for transvalvular gradient or simultaneous pressure determinations.

Potential sources of error include catheter whip artifact (motion of the tip of the catheter within the measured chamber), end-pressure artifact (an end-hole catheter measures an artificially elevated pressure because of streaming or high velocity of the pressure wave), catheter impact artifact (when the catheter is struck by the walls or valves of the cardiac chambers), and catheter tip obstruction within small vessels or valvular orifices occurring because of the size of the catheter itself. The operator must be aware of the many sources of potential error and, when there is a discrepancy between the observed data and the clinical scenario, the system should be examined for errors or artifacts.

MICROMANOMETER CATHETERS. The use of these catheters, which have the pressure transducer mounted at their tip, greatly reduces many of the errors inherent in fluid-filled systems. However, their usefulness is limited by the additional cost and time needed for properly calibrating and using the system. These catheters have higher natural frequencies and more optimal damping characteristics because the interposing fluid column is eliminated. In

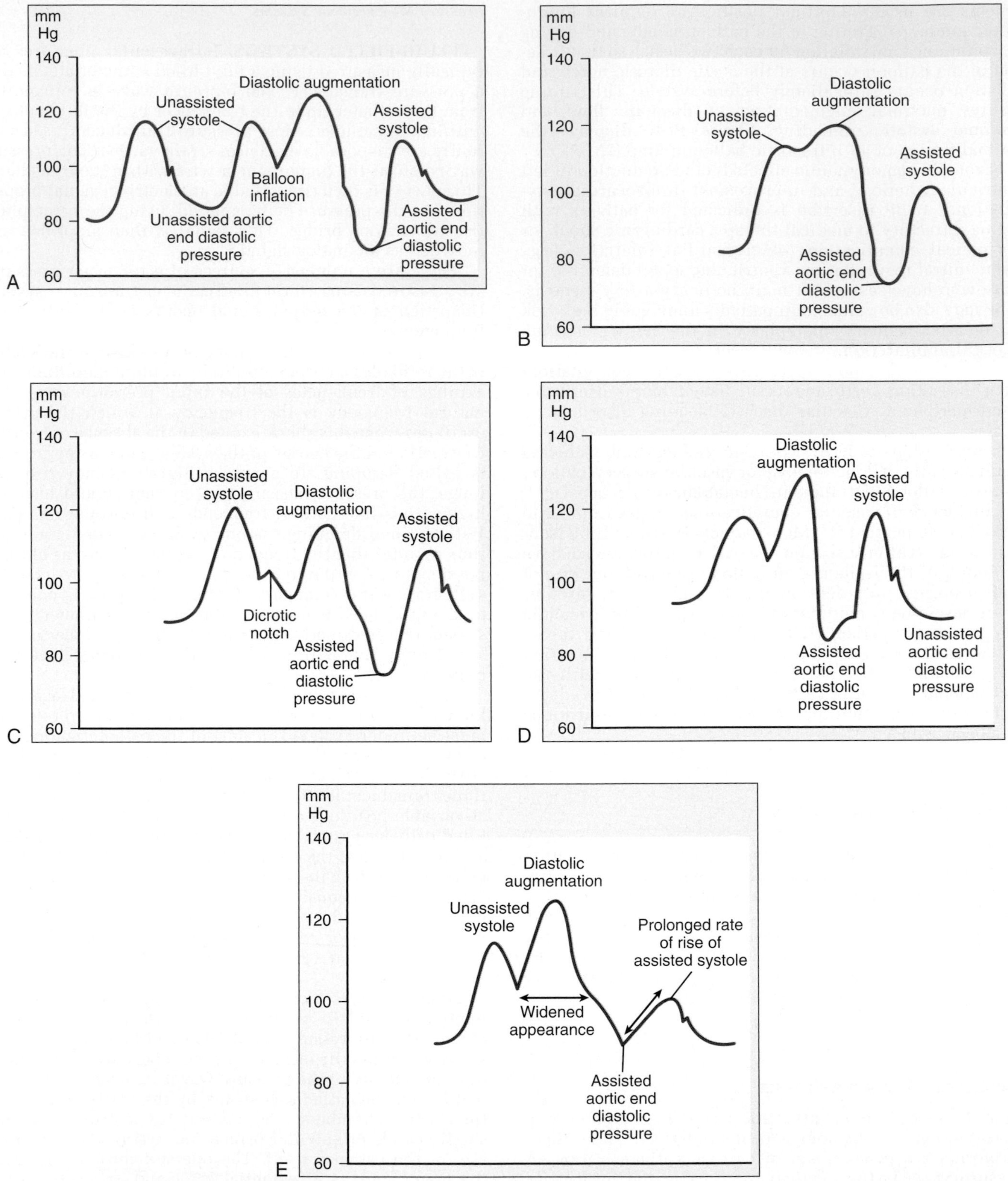

FIGURE 19–10 Optimal timing and arterial waveforms with intraaortic balloon pump (IABP). **A,** Systemic arterial pressure waveform from a patient with a normally functioning IABP device in whom the IABP device is programmed to inflate during every other cardiac cycle (commonly referred to as 1 : 2 inflation for every two cardiac cycles). With the first beat, aortic systolic and end-diastolic pressures are shown without IABP support and are therefore unassisted. With the second beat, the balloon inflates with the appearance of the dicrotic notch, and peak-augmented diastolic pressure is inscribed. With balloon deflation, assisted end-diastolic pressure and assisted systolic pressure are observed. To confirm that IABP is producing maximal hemodynamic benefit, the peak diastolic augmentation should be higher than the unassisted systolic pressure, and the assisted systolic and diastolic pressures should be less than the unassisted values. **B,** Systemic arterial pressure waveform from a subject in whom balloon inflation occurs too early, before aortic valve closure. Consequently, the left ventricle is forced to empty against an inflated balloon; the corresponding increase in afterload may increase myocardial oxygen demands and worsen systolic function. **C,** Systemic arterial pressure waveform from a patient in whom balloon inflation occurs too late, well after the beginning of diastole, thereby minimizing diastolic pressure augmentation. **D,** Systemic arterial pressure waveform from a patient in whom balloon deflation occurs too early, before the end of diastole. This may shorten the period of diastolic pressure augmentation. A corresponding transient decrease in aortic pressure may promote retrograde arterial flow from the carotid or coronary arteries, possibly inducing cerebral or myocardial ischemia. **E,** Systemic arterial pressure waveform from a subject in whom balloon inflation occurs too late, after the end of diastole, thereby producing the same deleterious consequences as early balloon inflation (increased LV afterload, with a resultant increase in myocardial oxygen demands and a worsening of systolic function). *(From Trost JC, Hillis LD: Intra-aortic balloon counterpulsation, Am J Cardiol 97:1391, 2006).*

addition, there is a decrease in catheter whip artifact. The pressure waveform is less distorted and is without the 30- to 40-millisecond delay seen in the fluid-filled catheter-transducer system. Commercially available high-fidelity micromanometer systems have both an end hole and side holes to allow over-the-wire insertion into the circulation while also permitting angiography. Catheters that have two transducers separated by a short distance are useful for accurate measurement of gradients across valvular structures and within ventricular chambers. The micromanometer system has been used for research purposes to assess the rate of ventricular pressure rise (dP/dt), wall stress, the rate of ventricular pressure decay (−dP/dt), the time constant of relaxation (tau), and ventricular pressure-volume relationships (see Chap. 23).

Micromanometer catheter systems have several disadvantages, including their expense, fragility, and added procedural time. In addition, the zero level of these systems can drift after the pressure is zeroed to the fluid-filled lumen within the catheter.

NORMAL PRESSURE WAVEFORMS

An understanding of the normal pressure waveform morphologies is necessary for comprehending the abnormalities that characterize certain pathological conditions. Normal pressures in the cardiac chambers and great vessels are listed in Table 19-3. Simply stated, whenever fluid is added to a chamber or compressed within a chamber, the pressure usually rises; conversely, whenever fluid exits from a chamber or the chamber relaxes, the pressure usually falls. One exception to this rule is in the early phase of ventricular diastolic filling, when ventricular volume increases after mitral valve opening but ventricular pressure continues to decrease because of active relaxation. Examples of normal-pressure waveforms are shown in Figure 19-11.

ATRIAL PRESSURE. The right atrial pressure waveform has three positive deflections, the a, c, and v waves. The a wave occurs as a result of atrial systole and follows the P wave of the ECG. The height of the a wave depends on atrial contractility and the resistance to right ventricular filling. The *x* descent follows the a wave and represents relaxation of the atrium and downward pulling of the tricuspid annulus by right ventricular contraction. The *x* descent is interrupted by the c wave, which is a small positive deflection caused by protrusion of the closed tricuspid valve into the right atrium. Pressure in the atrium rises after the *x* descent because of passive atrial filling. The atrial pressure then peaks as the v wave, which represents right ventricular systole. The height of the v wave is related to atrial compliance and the amount of blood returning to the atrium from the periphery. The right atrial v wave is generally smaller than the a wave. The *y* descent occurs after the v wave and reflects tricuspid valve opening and right atrial emptying into the right ventricle. During spontaneous respiration, right atrial pressure declines during inhalation as intrathoracic pressure falls. Right atrial pressure rises during exhalation as intrathoracic pressures increase. The opposite effect is seen when patients are mechanically ventilated.

The left atrial pressure waveform is similar to that of the right atrium, although normal left atrial pressure is higher, reflecting the high-pressure system of the left side of the heart. In the left atrium, as opposed to the right atrium, the v wave is generally higher than the a wave. This difference occurs because the left atrium is constrained posteriorly by the pulmonary veins, whereas the right atrium can easily decompress throughout the IVC and SVC. The height of the left atrial v wave most accurately reflects left atrial compliance.

PULMONARY CAPILLARY WEDGE PRESSURE. The pulmonary capillary wedge pressure waveform is similar to the left atrial pressure waveform but is slightly damped and delayed as a result of transmission through the lungs. The a and v waves with both *x* and *y* descents are visible, but c waves may not be seen. In the normal state, the pulmonary artery diastolic pressure is similar to the mean pulmonary capillary wedge pressure because the pulmonary circulation has low resistance. In certain disease states associated with elevated pulmonary vascular resistance (e.g., hypoxemia, pulmonary embolism, chronic pulmonary hypertension), and occasionally after mitral valve surgery, the pulmonary capillary wedge pressure may overestimate true left atrial pressure. In this circumstance, accurate measurement of the mitral valve gradient may require obtaining direct left atrial pressure.[30]

VENTRICULAR PRESSURE. Right and left ventricular waveforms are similar in morphology. They differ mainly with respect to their magnitudes. The durations of systole and isovolumic contraction and relaxation are longer and the ejection period shorter in the left than in the right ventricle. There may be a small (5-mm Hg) systolic gradient between the right ventricle and the pulmonary artery. Ventricular diastolic pressure is characterized by an early rapid filling wave during which most of the ventricle fills, a slow filling phase, and the a wave denoting atrial systolic activity. End-diastolic pressure is generally measured at the C point, which is the rise in ventricular pressure at the onset of isovolumic contraction. When the C point is not well seen, a line is drawn from the R wave on the simultaneous ECG to the ventricular pressure waveform, and this is used as the end-diastolic pressure.

GREAT VESSEL PRESSURES. The contour of the central aortic and pulmonary artery pressure tracing consists of a systolic wave, the incisura (indicating closure of the semilunar valves), and a gradual decline in pressure until the following systole. The pulse pressure reflects the stroke volume and compliance of the arterial system. The mean aortic pressure more accurately reflects peripheral resistance. As the systemic pressure wave is transmitted through the length of the aorta, the systolic wave increases in amplitude and becomes more triangular, and the diastolic wave decreases until it reaches the midthoracic aorta and then increases. The mean aortic pressures, however, are usually similar, with the mean peripheral arterial pressure typically equal to or less than 5 mm Hg lower than the mean central aortic pressure. The difference in systolic pressures between the central aorta and the peripheral arteries (femoral, brachial, or radial arteries) is highest in younger patients because of their increased vascular compliance. These potential differences between proximal aorta and peripheral artery must be considered to measure and interpret the peak systolic pressure gradient between the left ventricle and systemic arterial system in patients with suspected aortic stenosis. When a transvalvular gradient is present, the most accurate measure of the aortic pressure is obtained at the level of the coronary arteries. This measurement avoids the effect of pressure recovery, which is defined as the variable increase in lateral pressure downstream from a stenotic orifice (see Chap. 62). This approach can become clinically important in cases of mild to moderate aortic stenosis, particularly when the aorta is small.[31,32] There will be an underestimation of the transvalve gradient because of higher pressure in the femoral artery. This can be accomplished with a dual-lumen pigtail catheter, which measures pressure in the left ventricle and ascending aorta simultaneously.

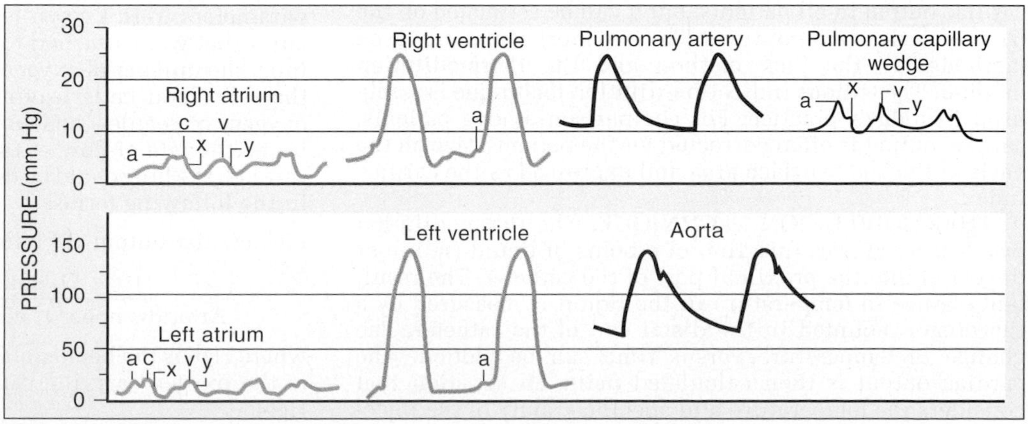

FIGURE 19–11 Normal right- and left-heart pressures recorded from fluid-filled catheter systems in a human. *(From Pepine C, Hill JA, Lambert CR [eds]: Diagnostic and Therapeutic Cardiac Catheterization. 3rd ed. Baltimore, Williams & Wilkins, 1998, p 451.)*

TABLE 19–3 Normal Pressures and Vascular Resistances

Pressures	Average (mm Hg)	Range (mm Hg)
Right atrium		
a wave	6	2-7
v wave	5	2-7
Mean	3	1-5
Right ventricle		
Peak systolic	25	15-30
End-diastolic	4	1-7
Pulmonary artery		
Peak systolic	25	15-30
End-diastolic	9	4-12
Mean	15	9-19
Pulmonary capillary		
Wedge		
Mean	9	4-12
Left atrium		
a wave	10	4-16
v wave	12	6-21
Mean	8	2-12
Left ventricle		
Peak systolic	130	90-140
End-diastolic	8	5-12
Central aorta		
Peak systolic	130	90-140
End-diastolic	70	60-90
Mean	85	70-105
Vascular Resistance	**Mean (dyne-sec · cm^{-5})**	**Range (dyne-sec · cm^{-5})**
Systemic vascular resistance	1100	700-1600
Total pulmonary resistance	200	100-300
Pulmonary vascular resistance	70	20-130

Abnormal Pressure Characteristics

Abnormal pressure waveforms may be diagnostic of specific pathological conditions. Table 19-4 summarizes the more commonly encountered waveforms.

Cardiac Output Measurements

There is no completely accurate method of measuring cardiac output in all patients, but it can be estimated on the basis of various assumptions. The two most commonly used methods are the Fick method and the thermodilution method. The tedious indication-dilution technique is rarely used in today's practice. For comparison among patients, cardiac output is often corrected for the patient's size on the basis of the body surface area and expressed as the cardiac index.

THERMODILUTION TECHNIQUE. The thermodilution procedure requires injection of a bolus of liquid (saline or dextrose) into the proximal port of the catheter. The resultant change in temperature in the liquid is measured by a thermistor mounted in the distal end of the catheter. The change in temperature versus time can be plotted. The cardiac output is then calculated using an equation that considers the temperature and specific gravity of the injectate and the temperature and specific gravity of the blood, along with the injectate volume. A calibration factor is also used. The cardiac output is inversely related to the area under a thermodilution curve, plotted as a function of temperature versus time, with a smaller area indicative of a higher cardiac output. Temperature fluctuation in the circuit can affect accuracy,[33] but the use of two thermistors can significantly improve the accuracy of this technique.[34]

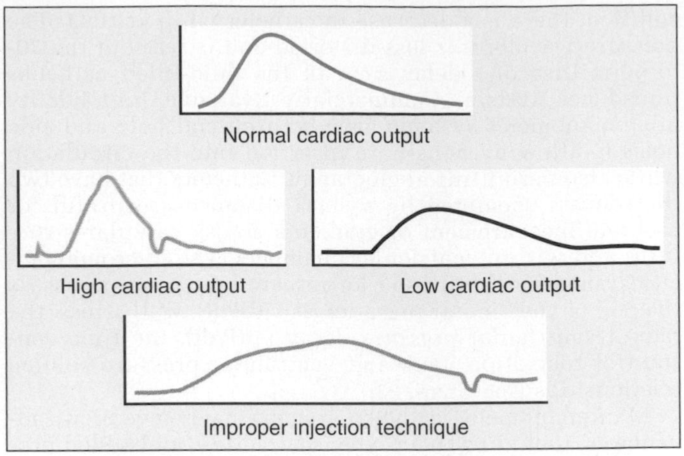

FIGURE 19–12 Thermodilution cardiac output curves. A normal curve has a sharp upstroke following an injection of saline. A smooth curve with a mildly prolonged downslope occurs until it returns to baseline. The area under the curve is inversely related to the cardiac output. At low cardiac output, a prolonged period is required to return to baseline. Therefore, there is a larger area under the curve. In a high cardiac output state, the cooler saline injectate moves faster through the right side of the heart and temperature returns to baseline more quickly. The area under the curve is smaller and the output is higher.

The thermodilution method has several advantages. It obviates the need for withdrawal of blood from an arterial site and is less affected by recirculation. Perhaps its greatest advantage is the rapid display of results using computerized methods (Fig. 19-12). However, a significant error occurs in patients with severe tricuspid regurgitation. Also, in patients with low outputs (especially less than 2.5 liter/min), thermodilution tends to overestimate the cardiac output.

FICK METHOD. The Fick principle assumes that the rate at which oxygen is consumed is a function of the rate of blood flow times the rate of oxygen pick-up by the red blood cells. The basic assumption is that the flow of blood in a given period of time is equal to the amount of substance entering the stream of flow in the same period of time, divided by the difference between the concentrations of the substance in the blood upstream and downstream from its point of entry into the circulation (Fig. 19-13). The same number of red blood cells that enter the lung must leave the lung if no intracardiac shunt is present. Thus, if certain parameters were known (e.g., the number of oxygen molecules that were attached to the red blood cells entering the lung, the number of oxygen molecules that were attached to the red blood cells leaving the lung, and the number of oxygen molecules consumed during travel through the lung), the rate of flow of these red blood cells as they pass through the lung could be determined. This can be expressed in the following terms:

$$\text{Fick cardiac output (L/min)} = \frac{O_2 \text{ consumption (ml/min)}}{\text{Arteriovenous } O_2 \text{ difference (vol\%)} \times 1.36 \times \text{Hgb} \times 10}$$

where Hgb is the hemoglobin concentration (mg/dl) and 1.36 is the oxygen-carrying capacity of hemoglobin (ml O_2/gm Hgb).

Measurements must be made in the steady state. Automated methods can accurately determine the oxygen content of the blood samples. Thus, the greatest source of

TABLE 19–4 Pathological Waveforms

- I. Right atrial pressure waveforms
  - A. Low mean atrial pressure
    1. Hypovolemia
    2. Improper zeroing of the transducer
  - B. Elevated mean atrial pressure
    1. Intravascular volume overload states
    2. Right ventricular failure caused by valvular disease (tricuspid or pulmonic stenosis or regurgitation)
    3. Right ventricular failure caused by myocardial disease (right ventricular ischemia, cardiomyopathy)
    4. Right ventricular failure caused by left-sided heart failure (mitral stenosis/regurgitation, aortic stenosis/regurgitation, cardiomyopathy, ischemia)
    5. Right ventricular failure caused by increased pulmonary vascular resistance (pulmonary embolism, chronic obstructive pulmonary disease, primary pulmonary hypertension)
    6. Pericardial effusion with tamponade physiology
    7. Obstructive atrial myxoma
  - C. Elevated a wave (any increase to ventricular filling)
    1. Tricuspid stenosis
    2. Decreased ventricular compliance caused by ventricular failure, pulmonic valve stenosis, or pulmonary hypertension
  - D. Cannon a wave
    1. Atrial-ventricular asynchrony (atria contract against a closed tricuspid valve, as during complete heart block, following premature ventricular contraction, during ventricular tachycardia, with ventricular pacemaker)
  - E. Absent a wave
    1. Atrial fibrillation or atrial standstill
    2. Atrial flutter
  - F. Elevated v wave
    1. Tricuspid regurgitation
    2. Right ventricular heart failure
    3. Reduced atrial compliance (restrictive myopathy)
  - G. a wave equal to v wave
    1. Tamponade
    2. Constrictive pericardial disease
    3. Hypervolemia
  - H. Prominent *x* descent
    1. Tamponade
    2. Subacute constriction and possibly chronic constriction
    3. Right ventricular ischemia with preservation of atrial contractility
  - I. Prominent *y* descent
    1. Constrictive pericarditis
    2. Restrictive myopathies
    3. Tricuspid regurgitation
  - J. Blunted *x* descent
    1. Atrial fibrillation
    2. Right atrial ischemia
  - K. Blunted *y* descent
    1. Tamponade
    2. Right ventricular ischemia
    3. Tricuspid stenosis
  - L. Miscellaneous abnormalities
    1. Kussmaul sign (aspiratory rise or lack of decline in right atrial pressure)—constrictive pericarditis, right ventricular ischemia
    2. Equalization (≤5 mm Hg) of mean right atrial ventricular diastolic, pulmonary artery diastolic, pulmonary capillary wedge, and pericardial pressures in tamponade
    3. M or W patterns—right ventricular ischemia, pericardial constriction, congestive heart failure
    4. Ventricularization of the right atrial pressure: severe tricuspid regurgitation
    5. Sawtooth pattern—atrial flutter
    6. Dissociation between pressure recording and intracardiac electrocardiogram—Ebstein anomaly
- II. Left atrial pressure–pulmonary capillary wedge pressure waveforms
  - A. Low mean pressure
    1. Hypovolemia
    2. Improper zeroing of the transducer
  - B. Elevated mean pressure
    1. Intravascular volume overload states
    2. Left ventricular failure caused by valvular disease (mitral or aortic stenosis or regurgitation)
    3. Left ventricular failure caused by myocardial disease (ischemia or cardiomyopathy)
    4. Left ventricular failure caused by systemic hypertension
    5. Pericardial effusion with tamponade physiology
    6. Obstructive atrial myxoma
  - C. Elevated a wave (any increase to ventricular filling)
    1. Mitral stenosis
    2. Decreased ventricular compliance caused by ventricular failure, aortic valve stenosis, or systemic hypertension
  - D. Cannon a wave
    1. Atrial-ventricular asynchrony (atria contract against a closed mitral valve, as during complete heart block, following premature ventricular contraction, during ventricular tachycardia, or with ventricular pacemaker)
  - E. Absent a wave
    1. Atrial fibrillation or atrial standstill
    2. Atrial flutter
  - F. Elevated v wave
    1. Mitral regurgitation
    2. Left ventricular heart failure
    3. Ventricular septal defect
  - G. a wave equal to v wave
    1. Tamponade
    2. Constrictive pericardial disease
    3. Hypervolemia
  - H. Prominent *x* descent
    1. Tamponade
    2. Subacute constriction and possibly chronic constriction
  - I. Prominent *y* descent
    1. Constrictive pericarditis
    2. Restrictive myopathies
    3. Mitral regurgitation
  - J. Blunted *x* descent
    1. Atrial fibrillation
    2. Atrial ischemia
  - K. Blunted *y* descent
    1. Tamponade
    2. Ventricular ischemia
    3. Mitral stenosis
  - L. Pulmonary capillary wedge pressure not equal to left ventricular end-diastolic pressure
    1. Mitral stenosis
    2. Left atrial myxoma
    3. Cor triatriatum
    4. Pulmonary venous obstruction
    5. Decreased ventricular compliance
    6. Increased pleural pressure
    7. Placement of catheter in a nondependent zone of the lung
- III. Pulmonary artery pressure waveforms
  - A. Elevated systolic pressure
    1. Primary pulmonary hypertension
    2. Mitral stenosis or regurgitation
    3. Congestive heart failure
    4. Restrictive myopathies
    5. Significant left-to-right shunt
    6. Pulmonary disease (pulmonary embolism, hypoxemia, chronic obstructive pulmonary disease)
  - B. Reduced systolic pressure
    1. Hypovolemia
    2. Pulmonary artery stenosis
    3. Subvalvular or supravalvular stenosis
    4. Ebstein anomaly
    5. Tricuspid stenosis
    6. Tricuspid atresia
  - C. Reduced pulse pressure
    1. Right-heart ischemia
    2. Right ventricular infarction
    3. Pulmonary embolism
    4. Tamponade

Table continues

TABLE 19–4 Pathological Waveforms—cont'd

D. Bifid pulmonary artery waveform
  1. Large left atrial v wave transmitted backward (e.g., mitral regurgitation)

E. Pulmonary artery diastolic pressure higher than pulmonary capillary wedge pressure
  1. Pulmonary disease
  2. Pulmonary embolus
  3. Tachycardia

IV. Ventricular pressure waveforms
  A. Systolic pressure elevated
    1. Pulmonary or systemic hypertension
    2. Pulmonary valve or aortic stenosis
    3. Ventricular outflow tract obstruction
    4. Supravalvular obstruction
    5. Right ventricular pressure elevation with significant:
      a. Atrial septal defect
      b. Ventricular septal defect
    6. Right ventricular pressure elevation caused by factors that increase pulmonary vascular resistance (see factors that increase right atrial pressure)
  B. Systolic pressure reduced
    1. Hypovolemia
    2. Cardiogenic shock
    3. Tamponade
  C. End-diastolic pressure elevated
    1. Hypervolemia
    2. Congestive heart failure
    3. Diminished compliance
    4. Hypertrophy
    5. Tamponade
    6. Regurgitant valvular disease
    7. Pericardial constriction
  D. End-diastolic pressure reduced
    1. Hypovolemia
    2. Tricuspid or mitral stenosis
  E. Diminished or absent a wave
    1. Atrial fibrillation or flutter
    2. Tricuspid or mitral stenosis
    3. Tricuspid or mitral regurgitation when ventricular compliance is increased
  F. Dip and plateau in diastolic pressure wave
    1. Constrictive pericarditis
    2. Restrictive myopathies
    3. Right ventricular ischemia
    4. Acute dilation associated with:
      a. Tricuspid regurgitation
      b. Mitral regurgitation
  G. Left ventricular end-diastolic pressure>right ventricular end-diastolic pressure
    1. Restrictive myopathies

V. Aortic pressure waveforms
  A. Systolic pressure elevated
    1. Systemic hypertension
    2. Arteriosclerosis
    3. Aortic insufficiency
  B. Systolic pressure reduced
    1. Aortic stenosis
    2. Heart failure
    3. Hypovolemia
  C. Widened pulse pressure
    1. Systemic hypertension
    2. Aortic insufficiency
    3. Significant patent ductus arteriosus
    4. Significant ruptures of sinus of Valsalva aneurysm
  D. Reduced pulse pressure
    1. Tamponade
    2. Congestive heart failure
    3. Cardiogenic shock
    4. Aortic stenosis
  E. Pulsus bisferiens
    1. Aortic insufficiency
    2. Obstructive hypertrophic cardiomyopathy
  F. Pulsus paradoxus
    1. Tamponade
    2. Chronic obstructive airway disease
    3. Pulmonary embolism
  G. Pulsus alternans
    1. Congestive heart failure
    2. Cardiomyopathy
  H. Pulsus parvus et tardus
    1. Aortic stenosis
  I. Spike and dome configuration
    1. Obstructive hypertrophic cardiomyopathy

CH 19

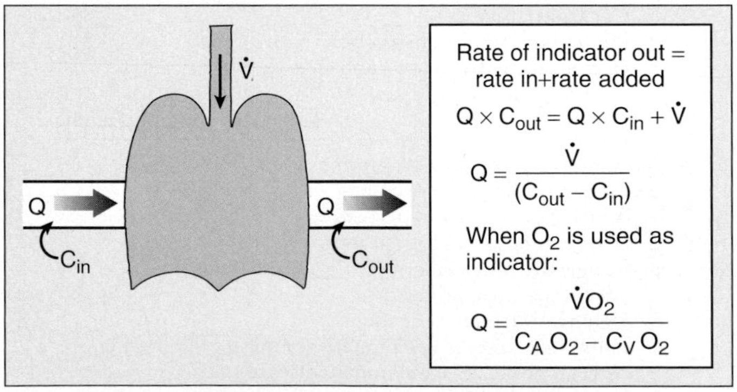

FIGURE 19–13 Schematic illustration of flow measurement using the Fick principle. Fluid containing a known concentration of an indicator (C_{in}) enters a system at flow rate Q. As the fluid passes through the system, indicator is continuously added at rate $\dot{V}$, raising the concentration in the outflow to C_{out}. In a steady state, the rate of indicator leaving the system (QC_{out}) must equal the rate at which it enters (QC_{in}), plus the rate at which it is added ($\dot{V}$). When oxygen is used as the indicator, cardiac output can be determined by measuring oxygen consumption ($\dot{V}O_2$), arterial oxygen content (C_AO_2), and mixed venous oxygen content (C_VO_2). *(From Winniford MD, Kern MJ, Lambert CR: Blood flow measurement. In Pepine CJ, Hill JA, Lambert CR [eds]: Diagnostic and Therapeutic Cardiac Catheterization. 3rd ed. Baltimore, Williams & Wilkins, 1998, p 400.)*

measurement variability is the oxygen consumption. In the original Fick determinations, expiratory gas samples were collected in a large bag over a specified period. By measuring the expiratory oxygen concentration and by knowing the concentration of oxygen in room air, the quantity of oxygen consumed over time could be determined. Techniques that allow measurement of the expired oxygen concentration are quantified by using a polarograph. This device can be connected to the patient by use of a plastic hood or by a mouthpiece and tubing.

The advantage of the Fick method is that it is the most accurate method in patients with low cardiac output and thus is preferred over the thermodilution method in these circumstances. It is also independent of the factors that affect curve shape and cause errors in thermodilution cardiac output. The Fick method suffers primarily from the difficulty in measuring oxygen consumption accurately and the inability to obtain a steady state under certain conditions. Because the method assumes mean flow over a period of time, it is not suitable during rapid changes in flow. Also, the patient must be breathing room air during blood sample collection.

Many laboratories use an "assumed" Fick method, in which the oxygen consumption index is assumed on the basis of the patient's age, gender, and body surface area or an estimate is made on the basis of body surface area (125 ml/m²). However, when assumed oxygen consumption, rather than measured oxygen consumption is used, large errors can occur.[35]

ANGIOGRAPHIC CARDIAC OUTPUT. Angiographic stroke volume can be calculated by tracing the end-diastolic and end-systolic images. Stroke volume is the quantity of blood ejected with each beat. End-diastolic volume is the maximum left ventricular volume and occurs immediately before the onset of systole. It occurs immediately after atrial contraction in patients in sinus rhythm. End-systolic volume is the minimum volume during the cardiac cycle. Calibration of the images with grids or ventricular phantoms is necessary to obtain accurate ventricular volumes. Angiographic cardiac output and stroke volume are derived from the following equations:

$$\text{Stroke volume} = \text{EDV} - \text{ESV}$$

$$\text{Cardiac output} = (\text{EDV} - \text{ESV}) \times \text{heart rate}$$

where EDV = end-diastolic volume and ESV = end-systolic volume. The inherent inaccuracies of calibrating angiographic volumes often make this method of measurement unreliable. In cases of valvular regurgitation or atrial fibrillation, angiographic cardiac output does not accurately measure true systemic outputs. However, the angiographic or thermodilution cardiac output is preferred over the Fick or thermodilution output for calculation of stenotic valve areas in patients with significant aortic or mitral regurgitation.

Determination of Vascular Resistance

Vascular resistance calculations are based on hydraulic principles of fluid flow, in which resistance is defined as the ratio of the decrease in pressure between two points in a vascular segment and the blood flow through the segment. Although this straightforward analogy to Ohm's law represents an oversimplification of the complex behavior of pulsatile flow in dynamic and diverse vascular beds, the calculation of vascular resistance based on these principles has proven to be of value in a number of clinical settings.

Determination of the resistance in a vascular bed requires measurement of the mean pressure of the proximal and distal ends of the vascular bed and accurate measurement of cardiac output. Vascular resistance (R) is usually defined in absolute units (dyne-sec·cm^{-5}):

$$R = [\text{mean pressure gradient (dyne/cm}^2)]/[\text{mean flow (cm}^3/\text{sec})]$$

Hybrid units (Wood units) are less often used.[36]

Systemic vascular resistance in absolute units is calculated using the following equation:

$$\text{SVR} = [80(\text{Ao}_m - \text{RA}_m)]/Q_s$$

where Ao_m and RA_m are the mean pressures (in mm Hg) in the aorta and right atrium, respectively, and Q_s is the systemic cardiac output (in liters/min). The constant 80 is used to convert units from mm Hg/liter/min (Wood units) to the absolute resistance units (dyne-sec·cm^{-5}). If the right atrial pressure is not known, the term RA_m can be dropped, and the resulting value is called the total peripheral resistance (TPR):

$$\text{TPR} = 80(\text{Ao}_m)/Q_s$$

Similarly, the pulmonary vascular resistance (PVR) is derived from the following equation:

$$\text{PVR} = [80(\text{PA}_m - \text{LA}_m)]/Q_p$$

where PA_m and LA_m are the pulmonary artery and left atrial pressures, respectively, and Q_p is the pulmonary blood flow. Mean pulmonary capillary wedge pressure is commonly substituted for mean left atrial pressure if the latter has not been measured directly, although errors can occur because of this substitution. In the absence of an intracardiac shunt, Q_p is equal to the systemic cardiac output. Normal values are listed in Table 19-3.

Elevated resistances in the systemic and pulmonary circuits may represent reversible abnormalities or may be fixed because of irreversible anatomical changes. In several clinical situations, such as congestive heart failure, valvular heart disease, primary pulmonary hypertension, and congenital heart disease with intracardiac shunting, determination of whether elevated systemic or pulmonary vascular resistance can be lowered transiently in the catheterization laboratory may provide important insights into potential management strategies. Interventions that can be used in the laboratory for this purpose include the administration of vasodilating drugs (e.g., sodium nitroprusside), exercise and, in patients with pulmonary hypertension, oxygen or nitric oxide inhalation or intravenous epoprostenol, a pulmonary and systemic vasodilator (see Chap. 73).

Vascular impedance measurements account for blood viscosity, pulsatile flow, reflected waves, and arterial compliance. Hence, vascular impedance has the potential to describe the dynamic relation between pressure and flow more comprehensively than would be possible using the simpler calculations of vascular resistance. Because the simultaneous pressure and flow data required for the calculation of impedance are complex and difficult to obtain, however, the concept of impedance has failed to gain widespread acceptance, and vascular impedance has not been adopted as a routine clinical index.

Evaluation of Valvular Stenosis (see Chap. 62)

Determining the severity of valvular stenosis on the basis of the pressure gradient and flow across the valve is one of the most important aspects of the evaluation of patients with valvular heart disease. In many patients, the magnitude of the pressure gradient alone is sufficient to distinguish clinically significant from insignificant valvular stenosis.

Determination of Pressure Gradients

In patients with aortic stenosis, the transvalvular pressure gradient is best measured with a catheter in the left ventricle and another in the proximal aorta. Although it is convenient to measure the gradient between the left ventricle and the femoral artery, downstream augmentation of the pressure signal and delay in pressure transmission between the proximal aorta and femoral artery may alter the pressure waveform substantially and introduce errors into the measured gradient.[31,32]

Left ventricular–femoral artery pressure gradients may suffice in many patients as an estimate of the severity of aortic stenosis to confirm the presence of a severely stenotic valve. If the side port of the arterial introducing sheath is used to monitor femoral pressure, the inner diameter of the sheath should be at least 1F size larger than the outer diameter of the left ventricular catheter.

The operator should obtain simultaneous ascending aortic and femoral artery pressures to verify similarity between the two sites. The left ventricular–femoral artery pressure gradient may not always be relied on in the calculation of valve orifice area in patients with moderate valve gradients. A careful single-catheter pull-back from left ventricle to aorta is often preferable to simultaneous measurement of left ventricular and femoral artery pressures. Alternatively, a single catheter with distal and proximal lumina or a micromanometer catheter with distal and proximal transducers may be used for simultaneous measurement of left ventricular and central aortic pressures. Another method is to place two arterial catheters, one in the aorta and the second in the left ventricle. However, this requires puncture of two arteries and is rarely used.

In patients with very severe aortic stenosis, the left ventricular catheter itself may reduce the effective orifice area, resulting in an artifactual increase in the measured pressure gradient. However, this overestimation of the severity of aortic stenosis is rarely an important clinical issue, because the diagnosis of severe aortic stenosis is already apparent in such patients.

The mean pressure gradient across the aortic valve is determined by planimetry of the area separating the left ventricular and aortic pressures using multiple beats (Fig. 19-14); it is this gradient that is applied when calculating the valve orifice area. The peak-to-peak gradient, measured as the difference between peak left ventricular pressure and

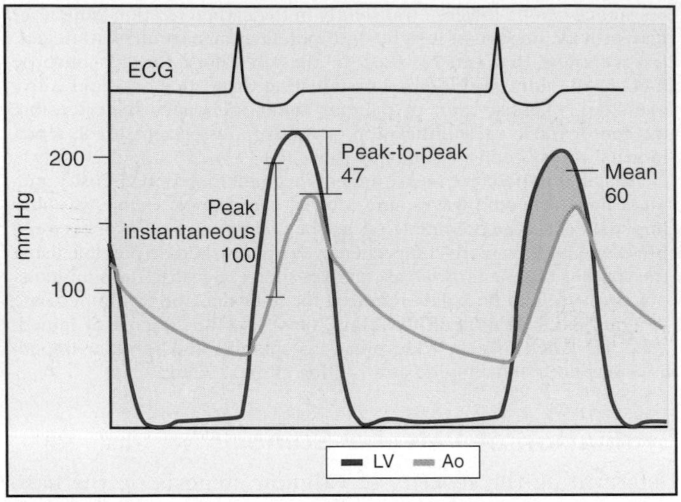

FIGURE 19–14 Various methods of describing an aortic transvalvular gradient. The peak-to-peak gradient (47 mm Hg) is the difference between the maximal pressure in the aorta (Ao) and the maximal left ventricle (LV) pressure. The peak instantaneous gradient (100 mm Hg) is the maximal pressure difference between the Ao and LV when the pressures are measured in the same moment (usually during early systole). The mean gradient (green shaded area) is the integral of the pressure difference between the LV and Ao during systole (60 mm Hg). ECG = electrocardiogram. *(From Bashore TM: Invasive Cardiology: Principles and Techniques. Philadelphia, BC Decker, 1990, p 258.)*

peak aortic pressure, is commonly used to quantify the valve gradient, because this measurement is rapidly determined and can be estimated visually. However, there is no physiological basis for the peak-to-peak gradient because the maximum left ventricular and aortic pressures rarely occur simultaneously. The peak-to-peak gradient measured in the catheterization laboratory is generally lower than the peak instantaneous gradient measured in the echocardiography laboratory (see Chap. 14). It is lower because the peak instantaneous gradient represents the maximum pressure difference between the left ventricle and aorta when measured simultaneously. This maximum pressure difference occurs on the upslope of the aortic pressure tracing (see Fig. 19-14). The mean aortic transvalvular gradient and aortic valve area are well correlated with both techniques.[37]

In patients with mitral stenosis, the most accurate means of determining the mitral valve gradient is measurement of the left atrial pressure using the transseptal technique, with simultaneous measurement of left ventricular pressure and planimetry of the area bounded by the left ventricular and left atrial pressures in diastole using several cardiac cycles (Fig. 19-15). In most laboratories, the pulmonary capillary wedge pressure is substituted for the left atrial pressure, because the pulmonary wedge pressure is more readily determined. The pulmonary wedge pressure tracing must be realigned with the left ventricular tracing for accurate mean gradient determination. Although it has been generally accepted that pulmonary capillary wedge pressure is a satisfactory estimate of left atrial pressure, some studies have indicated that the pulmonary wedge pressure may systematically overestimate the left atrial pressure by 2 to 3 mm Hg, thereby increasing the measured mitral valve gradient.[30] In addition, accurate wedge tracings may be difficult to obtain in patients with mitral stenosis because of pulmonary hypertension or dilated right-sided heart chambers. Improperly wedged catheters, resulting in damped pulmonary artery pressure recordings, further overestimate the severity of mitral stenosis. If there is doubt about accurate positioning of the catheter in the wedge position, the position can be confirmed by slow withdrawal of blood for oximetric analysis. An oxygen

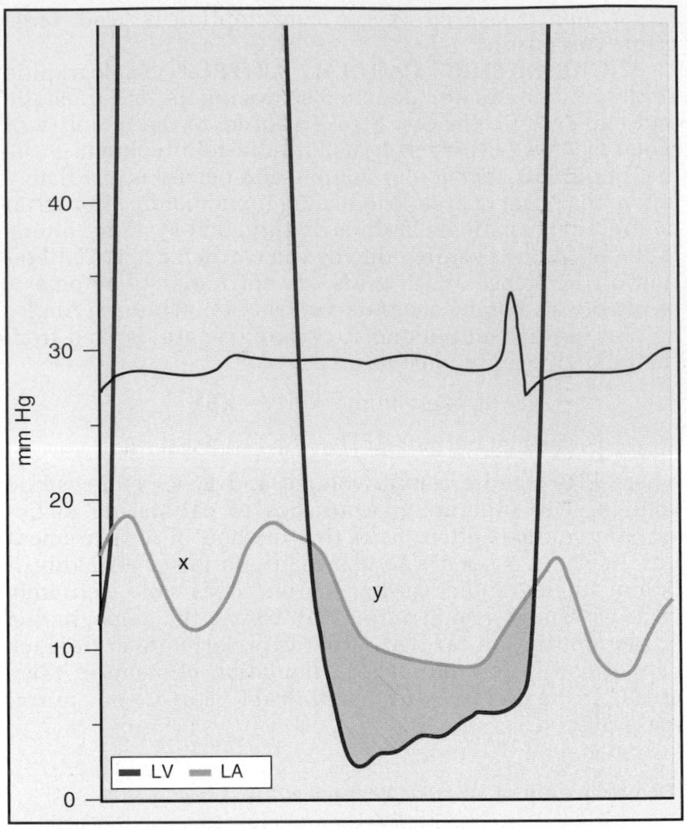

FIGURE 19–15 Pressure gradient in a patient with mitral stenosis. The pressure in the left atrium (LA) exceeds the pressure in the left ventricle (LV) during diastole, producing a diastolic pressure gradient (green shaded area). *(From Bashore TM: Invasive Cardiology: Principles and Techniques. Philadelphia, BC Decker, 1990, p 264.)*

saturation equal to that of the systemic circulation confirms the wedge position.

In pulmonic stenosis, the valve gradient is usually obtained by a catheter pull-back from the pulmonary artery to the right ventricle or by placing separate catheters in the right ventricle and pulmonary artery. Multilumen catheters are also available for simultaneous pressure recordings. Tricuspid valve gradients should be assessed, with simultaneous recording of right atrial and right ventricular pressures.

CALCULATION OF STENOTIC VALVE ORIFICE AREAS. The stenotic orifice area is determined from the pressure gradient and cardiac output using the formula developed by Gorlin and Gorlin from the fundamental hydraulic relationships linking the area of an orifice to the flow and pressure drop across the orifice. Flow (F) and orifice area (A) are related by the following fundamental equation:

$$F = cAV$$

where V is velocity of flow and c is a constant accounting for central streaming of fluid through an orifice, which tends to reduce the effective orifice size. Hence,

$$A = F/cV$$

Velocity is related to the pressure gradient through the relation $V = k\sqrt{(2g\Delta P)}$, where k is a constant accounting for frictional energy loss, g is the acceleration because of gravity (980 cm/sec^2), and ΔP is the mean pressure gradient (mm Hg). Substituting for V in the orifice area equation, and combining c and k into one constant, C, yields the following equation:

$$A = F44.3C\sqrt{\Delta P}$$

Gorlin and Gorlin have determined the value of the constant C by comparing the calculated valve area with the actual valve area measured at autopsy or at surgery in 11 mitral valves. The maximal discrepancy between the actual mitral valve area and calculated values was only 0.2 cm^2 when the constant 0.85 was used. No data were obtained for aortic valves, a limitation noted by the Gorlins, and a constant of 1.0 was assumed. Because flow across the aortic valve occurs only in systole, the flow value for calculating aortic valve area (cm^2) is the cardiac output in milliliters per minute divided by the systolic ejection period (SEP) in seconds per beat multiplied by the heart rate (HR) in beats per minute. The systolic ejection period is defined from aortic valve opening to closure. Hence, the aortic valve area (AVA) is calculated from the Gorlin formula using the following equation:

$$\text{AVA}\left(\text{cm}^2\right) = \frac{\text{cardiac output}\left(\text{liters/min}\right) \times 1000}{(44.3)(\text{HR})(\text{SEP})\sqrt{\text{mean gradient}}}$$

where the mean gradient is in mm Hg.

Similarly, because mitral flow occurs only in diastole, the cardiac output is corrected for the diastolic filling period (DFP) in seconds per beat in the equation for mitral valve area, where the diastolic filling period is defined from mitral valve opening to mitral valve closure:

$$\text{Mitral valve area}\left(\text{cm}^2\right) = \frac{\text{cardiac output}\left(\text{liters/min}\right) \times 1000}{(37.7)(\text{HR})(\text{DFP})\sqrt{\text{mean gradient}}}$$

The normal aortic valve area is 2.6 to 3.5 cm^2 in adults. Valve areas smaller than 1.0 cm^2 represent severe aortic stenosis. The normal mitral valve area is 4 to 6 cm^2, and severe mitral stenosis is present with valve areas smaller than 1.0 cm^2.

The calculated valve area is often crucial in management decisions for patients with aortic stenosis or mitral stenosis. Hence, it is essential that accurate and simultaneous pressure gradient and cardiac output determinations be made, especially in patients with borderline or low pressure gradients.

There are limitations of the orifice area. Because the square root of the mean gradient is used in the Gorlin formula, the valve area calculation is more strongly influenced by the cardiac output than the pressure gradient. Thus, errors in measuring cardiac output may have profound effects on the calculated valve area, particularly in patients with low cardiac outputs, in whom the calculated valve area is often of greatest importance.

As noted earlier, the thermodilution technique may provide inaccurate cardiac output data when cardiac output is reduced or when concomitant aortic, mitral, or tricuspid regurgitation is present. Thus, the Fick method of determining cardiac output is the most accurate for assessing cardiac output, especially in low-output states. In patients with mixed valvular disease (stenosis and regurgitation) of the same valve, the use of forward flow as determined by the Fick method or the thermodilution technique overestimates the severity of the valvular stenosis. This overestimation occurs because the Gorlin formula depends on total forward flow across the stenotic valve, not net forward flow. If valvular regurgitation is present, the angiographic cardiac output is the most appropriate measure of flow. If both aortic and mitral regurgitation are present, flow across a single valve cannot be determined and neither aortic valve area nor mitral valve area can be assessed accurately.

Other potential errors and limitations are inherent in the use of the Gorlin formula, related both to inaccuracies in measurement of valve gradients and to more fundamental issues regarding the validity of the assumptions underlying the formula. In low-output states, the Gorlin formula may systematically predict smaller valve areas than are actually present. Several lines of evidence indicate that the aortic valve area from the Gorlin formula increases with increases in cardiac output. Although this may represent an actual greater opening of stenotic valves by the higher proximal opening pressures that result from increases in transvalvular flow, the flow dependence of the calculated valve area may also reflect inherent errors in the assumptions underlying the Gorlin formula, particularly with respect to the aortic valve. Tricuspid aortic valve stenosis determinations appear particularly influenced by flow.[38]

A study has been performed to compare simultaneous aortic valve area determinations by transesophageal echocardiographic planimetry and the Gorlin formula.[39] The study demonstrated that with increases in transvalvular flow, the Gorlin valve area also increases. This finding was not associated with alterations in direct planimetry of the aortic valve area. The results suggest that flow-related variation in the Gorlin aortic valve area occurs because of disproportional flow dependence of the formula and not a true change in the valve area.

An alternative simplified formula for determining valve areas has been proposed. The effects of the systolic ejection period and the diastolic filling period are relatively constant at normal heart rates, and these terms can be eliminated from the equation. This assumes that $\text{HR} \times \text{SEP} \times 44.3 \cong 1000$ in most circumstances. In this modified approach, the aortic valve area can be quickly estimated from the following formula:

$$\text{AVA}\left(\text{cm}^2\right) = \frac{\text{cardiac output}\left(\text{liters/min}\right)}{\sqrt{\text{peak-to-peak or mean gradient}\left(\text{in mm Hg}\right)}}$$

Use of either the mean aortic transvalvular gradient or peak-to-peak gradient produces similar correlation with the Gorlin formula.

One approach to patients with a low aortic transvalvular gradient and low cardiac output is to calculate the aortic valve resistance. However, the clinical usefulness is unproven. Patients with low-output, low-gradient aortic stenosis remain a challenge for accurate determination of valve area either by cardiac catheterization or echocardiography. Whether afterload mismatch or intrinsic contractile dysfunction is the primary problem in ventricular impairment can be difficult to ascertain. Thus, the use of pharmacological stress with low-dose dobutamine infusion has been advocated to distinguish moderate from severe aortic stenosis.[40,41] The concept is that patients without true anatomical, severe AS will have an increase in valve areas with little change in transvalvular gradient.[2] If dobutamine increases the AVA more than 0.2 cm^2, with no change in gradient, it is likely that the baseline evaluation overestimated the severity of aortic stenosis.[2] It has also been shown that patients who increase stroke volume by less than 20 percent lack contractile reserve and have a poor prognosis with medical or surgical therapy.[41]

Despite theoretical limitations, the Gorlin formula has proved to be a reliable clinical determination for evaluating patients with suspected aortic stenosis.

Measurement of Intraventricular Pressure Gradients (see Chap. 65)

The demonstration of an intracavitary pressure gradient is among the most interesting yet challenging aspects of diagnostic catheterization. Simultaneous pressure measurements are usually obtained in either the central aorta or femoral artery and from within the ventricular cavity. Pullback of the catheter from the ventricular apex to a posterior position, just beneath the aortic valve, demonstrates an intracavitary gradient. An erroneous intracavitary gradient may be seen if the catheter becomes entrapped by the hypertrophic myocardium.

The intracavitary gradient is distinguished from aortic valvular stenosis by the loss of the aortic–left ventricular gradient when the catheter is still in the left ventricle yet proximal to the myocardial obstruction. In addition, careful analysis of the upstroke of the aortic pressure waveform distinguishes a valvular from a subvalvular stenosis, because the aortic pressure waveform demonstrates a slow upstroke in aortic stenosis. Other methods for localizing intracavitary gradients include the use of a dual-lumen catheter, a double-sensor micromanometer catheter, and placement of an end-hole catheter in the left ventricular outflow tract while a transseptal catheter is advanced into the left ventricle, with pressure measured simultaneously. An intracavitary gradient may be increased by various provocative maneuvers, including the Valsalva maneuver, inhalation of amyl nitrate, introduction of a premature ventricular beat, and isoproterenol infusion (see "Physiological and Pharmacological Maneuvers").

Assessment of Valvular Regurgitation (see Chap. 62)

The severity of valvular regurgitation is generally graded by visual assessment, although calculation of the regurgitant fraction is used occasionally. According to ACC/AHA guidelines, hemodynamic evaluation of either aortic or mitral regurgitant lesions is recommended as a class I indication when pulmonary artery pressure is disproportionate to the severity of regurgitation assessed noninvasively, or when there is a discrepancy between clinical and noninvasive findings.[2] Exercise with hemodynamic assessment may also provide useful information.

VISUAL ASSESSMENT OF REGURGITATION. Valvular regurgitation may be assessed visually by determining the relative amount of radiographic contrast medium that opacifies the chamber proximal to its injection. The estimation of regurgitation depends on the regurgitant volume as well as the size and contractility of the proximal chamber. The original classification scheme, devised by Sellers and colleagues, remains the standard in most catheterization laboratories:

- \+ Minimal regurgitant jet seen. Clears rapidly from proximal chamber with each beat.
- ++ Moderate opacification of proximal chamber, clearing with subsequent beats.
- +++ Intense opacification of proximal chamber, becoming equal to that of the distal chamber.
- ++++ Intense opacification of proximal chamber, becoming more dense than that of the distal chamber. Opacification often persists over the entire series of images obtained.

REGURGITANT FRACTION. A gross estimate of the degree of valvular regurgitation may be obtained by determining the regurgitant fraction (RF). The difference between the angiographic stroke volume and the forward stroke volume can be defined as the regurgitant stroke volume. The RF is that portion of the angiographic stroke volume that does not contribute to the net cardiac output:

$$\text{Regurgitant stroke volume} = \text{angiographic stroke volume} - \text{forward stroke volume}$$

Forward stroke volume is the cardiac output determined by the Fick or thermodilution method divided by the heart rate. Thermodilution cardiac output cannot be used if there is significant concomitant tricuspid regurgitation.

As detected visually, 1+ regurgitation is roughly equivalent to an RF less than or equal to 20 percent, 2+ regurgitation to an RF of 21 to 40 percent, 3+ to an RF of 41 to 60 percent, and 4+ to an RF of more than 60 percent.

The assumption underlying the determination of RF is that the angiographic and forward cardiac outputs are accurate and comparable, a state requiring similar heart rates, stable hemodynamic states between measurements, and only a single regurgitant valve. Given these conditions, the equation yields only a gross approximation of regurgitant flow.

Shunt Determinations (see Chap. 61)

Normally, pulmonary blood flow and systemic blood flow are equal. With an abnormal communication between intracardiac chambers or great vessels, blood flow is shunted from the systemic circulation to the pulmonary circulation (left-to-right shunt), from the pulmonary circulation to the systemic circulation (right-to-left shunt), or in both directions (bidirectional shunt). Although many shunts are suspected before cardiac catheterization, physicians performing the procedure should be vigilant in determining the cause of unexpected findings. For example, an unexplained pulmonary artery oxygen saturation exceeding 80 percent should raise the operator's suspicion of a left-to-right shunt, whereas unexplained arterial desaturation (less than 93 percent) may indicate a right-to-left shunt.[42] Arterial desaturation commonly results from alveolar hypoventilation and associated "physiological shunting," the causes of which include oversedation from premedication, pulmonary disease, pulmonary venous congestion, pulmonary edema, and cardiogenic shock. If arterial desaturation persists after the patient takes several deep breaths or coughs, or after administration of 100 percent oxygen, a right-to-left shunt must be highly suspected.

Several noninvasive and invasive methods are available for the detection of intracardiac shunts. Noninvasive methods include echocardiographic, radionuclide, and magnetic resonance imaging techniques. The most commonly used method in the cardiac catheterization laboratory is the oximetric method.

OXIMETRIC METHOD. The oximetric method is based on blood sampling from various cardiac chambers for the determination of oxygen saturation. A left-to-right shunt is detected when a significant increase in blood oxygen saturation is found between two right-sided vessels or chambers.

A screening oxygen saturation measurement for any left-to-right shunt is often performed with right-heart catheterization by sampling blood in the SVC and the pulmonary artery. If the difference in oxygen saturation between these samples is 8 percent or more, a left-to-right shunt may be present, and an oximetry run should be carried out. This run includes obtaining blood samples from all right-sided locations, including the SVC, IVC, right atrium, right ventricle, and pulmonary artery. In cases of interatrial or interventricular shunts, it is recommended to obtain multiple samples from the high, middle, and low right atrium or the right ventricular inflow tract, apex, and outflow tract to localize the level of the shunt. One may miss a small left-to-right shunt using the right atrium for screening purposes rather than the SVC because of incomplete mixing of blood in the right atrium, which receives blood from the IVC, SVC, and coronary sinus. Oxygen saturation in the IVC is higher than in the SVC because the kidneys use less oxygen relative to their blood flow than other organs, whereas coronary sinus blood has very low oxygen saturation. Mixed venous saturation is most accurately measured in the pulmonary artery after complete mixing has occurred.

A full saturation run involves obtaining samples from the high and low IVC, high and low SVC, high, middle, and low right atrium, right ventricular inflow and outflow tracts and midcavity, main pulmonary artery, left or right pulmonary artery, pulmonary vein and left atrium, if possible, left ventricle, and distal aorta. When a right-to-left shunt must be localized, oxygen saturation samples must be taken from the pulmonary veins, left atrium, left ventricle, and aorta. Although the major weakness of the oxygen step-up method is its lack of sensitivity, clinically significant shunts are generally detected by this technique. Obtaining multiple samples from each chamber can improve sampling error and variability. Most instruments analyze samples with a measurement error ranging from 2.5 to 1 percent saturation or better.[43] Another method of oximetric determination of intracardiac shunts uses a balloon-tipped fiberoptic catheter; this allows continuous registration of oxygen saturation as it is withdrawn from the pulmonary artery through the right-heart chambers into the SVC and IVC.

Shunt Quantification. The principles used to determine Fick cardiac output are also used to quantify intracardiac shunts. To determine the size of a left-to-right shunt, pulmonary blood flow (PBF) and systemic blood flow (SBF) determinations are required. PBF is simply oxygen consumption divided by the difference in oxygen content across the pulmonary bed, whereas SBF is oxygen consumption divided by the difference in oxygen content across the systemic bed. The effective blood flow (EBF) is the fraction of mixed venous return received by the lungs without contamination by the shunt flow. In the absence of a shunt, PBF, SBF, and EBF all are equal. These equations are as follows:

$$\text{PBF} = \frac{O_2 \text{ consumption (ml/min)}}{(P\bar{v}O_2 - PaO_2)}$$

$$\text{SBF} = \frac{O_2 \text{ consumption (ml/min)}}{(SaO_2 - M\bar{v}O_2)}$$

$$\text{EPF} = \frac{O_2 \text{ consumption (ml/min)}}{(P\bar{v}O_2 - M\bar{v}O_2)}$$

where $P\bar{v}O_2$, PaO_2, SaO_2, and $M\bar{v}O_2$ are the oxygen contents (in ml O_2/liter of blood) of pulmonary venous, pulmonary arterial, systemic arterial, and mixed venous bloods, respectively. The oxygen content is determined as outlined in the section on Fick cardiac output.

If a pulmonary vein is not sampled, systemic arterial oxygen content may be substituted, assuming that the systemic arterial saturation is 95 percent or more. As discussed earlier, if systemic arterial saturation is less than 95 percent, a right-to-left shunt may be present. If arterial desaturation is present but not secondary to a right-to-left shunt, systemic arterial oxygen content is used. If a right-to-left shunt is present, pulmonary venous oxygen content is calculated as 98 percent of the oxygen capacity.

The mixed venous oxygen content is the average oxygen content of the blood in the chamber proximal to the shunt. When assessing a left-to-right shunt at the level of the right atrium, one must calculate mixed venous oxygen content on the basis of the contributing blood flow from the IVC, SVC, and coronary sinus. The most common method used is the Flamm formula:

$$M\bar{V}O_2 = \frac{3(\text{SVC } O_2 \text{ content}) + 1(\text{IVC } O_2 \text{ content})}{4}$$

Assuming conservation of mass, the size of a left-to-right shunt, when there is no associated right-to-left shunt, is simply

$$L \rightarrow R \text{ shunt} = PBF - SBF$$

When there is evidence of a right-to-left shunt in addition to a left-to-right shunt, the approximate left-to-right shunt size is

$$L \rightarrow R \text{ shunt} = PBF - EBF$$

and the approximate right-to-left shunt size is

$$R \rightarrow L \text{ shunt} = SBF - EBF$$

The flow ratio PBF/SBF (or Q_p/Q_s) is used clinically to determine the significance of the shunt. A ratio of less than 1.5 indicates a small left-to-right shunt, and a ratio of 1.5 to 2.0 indicates a moderate-sized shunt. A ratio of 2.0 or more indicates a large left-to-right shunt and generally requires percutaneous or surgical repair to prevent future pulmonary or right ventricular complications, or both. A flow ratio of less than 1.0 indicates a net right-to-left shunt. If oxygen consumption is not measured, the pulmonic-to-systemic blood flow ratio may be calculated as follows:

$$PBF/SBF = \frac{(SaO_2 - M\bar{V}O_2)}{(P\bar{V}O_2 - PaO_2)}$$

where SaO_2, $M\bar{V}O_2$, $P\bar{V}O_2$, and PaO_2 are systemic arterial, mixed venous, pulmonary venous, and pulmonary arterial blood oxygen saturations, respectively.

INDICATOR-DILUTION METHOD. Although the indicator-dilution method is more sensitive than the oximetric method for detection of small shunts, it cannot be used to localize the level of a left-to-right shunt. An indicator such as indocyanine green dye is injected into a proximal chamber while a sample is taken from a distal chamber using a densitometer, and the density of dye is displayed over time. To detect a left-to-right shunt, dye is injected into the pulmonary artery and sampling is performed in a systemic artery. Presence of a shunt is indicated by early recirculation of the dye on the downslope of the curve. Although shunts may also be quantified using this technique, it is uncommonly used in clinical practice.

PHYSIOLOGICAL AND PHARMACOLOGICAL MANEUVERS

Potentially significant cardiac abnormalities might be absent in the resting condition but may be unmasked by stress. Therefore, if the physician performing a cardiac catheterization procedure cannot elucidate the cause of a patient's symptoms at rest, various physiological and pharmacological maneuvers can be considered.

Physiological Maneuvers

DYNAMIC EXERCISE. Dynamic exercise in the catheterization laboratory is most commonly performed using supine bicycle ergometry, although straight leg raises or arm or upright bicycle exercise may be used. Upright treadmill exercise may also be performed outside the catheterization laboratory using a balloon flotation catheter inserted through an antecubital vein to measure pulmonary artery and wedge pressures and cardiac output. The associated changes in heart rate, cardiac output, oxygen consumption, and intracardiac pressures are monitored at a steady state during progressive stages of exercise. Normally, the increased oxygen requirements of exercise are met by an increase in cardiac output and an increase in oxygen extraction from arterial blood. Patients with cardiac dysfunction are unable to increase their cardiac output appropriately in response to exercise and must meet the demands of the exercising muscle groups by increasing the extraction of oxygen from arterial blood, thereby increasing the arteriovenous oxygen difference.

The relationship between cardiac output and oxygen consumption is linear, and a regression formula can be used to calculate the predicted cardiac index at a given level of oxygen consumption. The actual cardiac index divided by the predicted cardiac index is defined as the exercise index. A value of 0.8 or higher indicates a normal cardiac output response to exercise. The exercise factor is another method of describing the same relationship between the cardiac output and oxygen consumption. The exercise factor is the increase in cardiac output divided by the increase in oxygen consumption. Normally, for every 100-ml/min increase in oxygen consumption with exercise, the cardiac output should increase by at least 600 ml/min. Therefore, a normal exercise factor should be 0.6 or higher.[44]

Supine exercise normally causes a rise in mean arterial and pulmonary pressures. There is a proportionately greater decrease in systemic vascular resistance compared with pulmonary vascular resistance and an increase in heart rate. Myocardial contractility increases because of increased sympathetic tone and increased heart rate. Left ventricular ejection fraction rises. During early levels of exercise, increased venous return augments left ventricular end-diastolic volume, leading to an increase in stroke volume. At progressively higher levels of exercise, left ventricular end-systolic and end-diastolic volumes decrease, leading to a negligible rise in stroke volume. Thus, the augmentation in cardiac output during peak supine exercise in the catheterization laboratory is generally caused by an increase in heart rate (see Chap. 13). For this reason, all agents that could impair the chronotropic response should be discontinued before catheterization if exercise is contemplated during the procedure.

Exercise may provoke symptoms in a patient who had been found to have valvular disease of borderline significance in the resting state (see Chap. 62). Exercise increases the gradient across the mitral valve and pulmonary artery pressures in mitral stenosis and may provoke symptoms not experienced at rest. The hemodynamic response to exercise is also useful in evaluating regurgitant valvular lesions. Clinically important valvular regurgitation exists if an increase occurs in left ventricular end-diastolic pressure, pulmonary capillary wedge pressure, and systemic vascular resistance, in conjunction with a reduced exercise index (less than 0.8) and abnormal exercise factor (less than 0.6). Simultaneous echocardiographic data may also be useful in equivocal cases. Patients with myocardial disease, ischemic or otherwise, may have pronounced increases in left ventricular end-diastolic pressure with exercise.

ISOMETRIC EXERCISE. Isometric handgrip exercise causes an increase in heart rate, mean arterial pressure, and cardiac output. Because the systemic vascular resistance does not increase, the elevation in arterial pressure is because of the rise in cardiac output rather than a vasoconstrictor response. Patients with left ventricular dysfunction respond abnormally to isometric exercise (i.e., significant increase in left ventricular end-diastolic pressure, a failure to increase stroke work appropriately, and a blunted rise in left ventricular peak dP/dT).[44]

PACING TACHYCARDIA. Rapid atrial or ventricular pacing increases myocardial oxygen consumption and myocardial blood flow. With pacing, in contradistinction to dynamic or isometric exercise, left ventricular end-diastolic volume decreases and there is little change in cardiac output. This method may be used to determine the significance of coronary artery disease or valvular abnormalities. For example, the gradient across the mitral valve increases with rapid atrial pacing because of the increase in heart rate. Pacing has the advantage of allowing greater control and rapid termination of the induced stress.

PHYSIOLOGICAL STRESS. Various physiological stresses alter the severity of obstruction in hypertrophic cardiomyopathy (see Chap. 65). The Valsalva maneuver (forcible expiration against a closed glottis) increases the systolic subaortic pressure gradient in the strain phase, during which there is a decrease in venous return and decreased left ventricular volume. This maneuver is also abnormal in patients with congestive heart failure. The Müller maneuver (forced inspiration against a closed glottis) has the opposite effect. Another useful maneuver in patients with hypertrophic obstructive cardiomyopathy is the introduction of a premature ventricular beat (Brockenbrough maneuver). Premature ventricular contractions normally increase the pulse pressure of the subsequent ventricular beat. In obstructive hypertrophic cardiomyopathy, the outflow gradient is increased during the postpremature beat, with a decrease in the pulse pressure of the aortic contour. A premature ventricular beat may also accentuate the spike and dome configuration of the aortic pressure waveform.

Rapid volume loading may reveal occult pericardial constriction (see Chap. 70) when atrial and ventricular filling pressures are relatively normal under baseline conditions because of hypovolemia, and can help distinguish pericardial constriction from myocardial restriction. The Kussmaul sign occurs in pericardial constriction. With inspiration, it is demonstrated when right atrial pressure fails to decrease or actually increases in relation to impaired right ventricular filling.[45]

Pharmacological Maneuvers

Dobutamine infusion during cardiac catheterization is indicated in patients with low-flow, low-gradient aortic stenosis[2] (see Chap. 62). In patients with a mean gradient lower than 30 mm Hg and a low cardiac output, the Gorlin formula may not reflect the true valve area. Provocation with dobutamine infusion can assist in distinguishing intrinsic contractile dysfunction versus afterload mismatch from valvular stenosis.

Resting hemodynamic measurements, including transvalvular gradient, cardiac output, and aortic valve area, should be obtained. Dobutamine is infused at 5 μg/kg/min and increased by 3 to 10 μg/kg/min every 5 minutes, with a maximum of 40 μg/kg/min, mean gradient higher than 40 mm Hg, 50 percent increase in the cardiac output, or heart rate more than 140 beats/min. Patients with a final aortic valve area smaller than 1.2 cm^2 and mean gradient higher than 30 mm Hg are considered to have severe aortic stenosis.[40]

Nitric oxide (NO) is an endothelium-derived vasodilator with selective pulmonary vasodilator proportions. Inhaled NO is rapidly inactivated in contrast to an intravenous vasodilator, which can cause severe systemic hypotension.[46] It has been well established that lowering of pulmonary artery pressure with vasodilators predicts a favorable clinical outcome in patients with pulmonary hypertension (see Chap. 73).

It has been shown that inhaled NO can safely and effectively assess the capacity of a patient for pulmonary vasodilator response without causing systemic hypotension. It can predict a response to subsequent medical therapy accurately.[47] Doses of 10, 20, and 40 parts/million can be tested over 5- to 10-minute intervals with several samplings of mean pulmonary artery pressure and calculation of the pulmonary vascular resistance. A significant response is noted with a decrease in either parameter of more than 20 percent.[47]

Isoproterenol infusion may be used to simulate supine dynamic exercise, although untoward side effects limit its applicability. This drug's positive inotropic and chronotropic effects can increase the gradient in obstructive hypertrophic cardiomyopathy and mitral stenosis. Nitroglycerin and amyl nitrate decrease preload and accentuate the systolic gradient in patients with obstructive hypertrophic cardiomyopathy (see Chap. 65). Amyl nitrate is generally inhaled, and its onset and offset of action are very rapid. Agents that increase systemic vascular resistance, such as phenylephrine, reduce the gradient in obstructive hypertrophic cardiomyopathy. Use of an intravenous inotropic agent such as dobutamine may clarify the precise severity of aortic stenosis in patients with a low cardiac output and low transvalvular gradient.[2,40,41] Infusion of sodium nitroprusside may improve the cardiac output and filling pressures in patients with dilated cardiomyopathies and in those with mitral regurgitation by lowering systemic and pulmonary vascular resistances. A favorable response to sodium nitroprusside infusion may predict a good clinical outcome.

Methylergonovine maleate has replaced ergonovine as a safer and more specific provocation test for coronary artery spasm caused by endothelial dysfunction. Small intracoronary increments of 5 to 10 μg are given. The total dose should not exceed 50 μg. Intracoronary acetylcholine, although not as sensitive, appears safer than methylergonovine and has largely replaced it in clinical practice.[48]

ADJUNCTIVE DIAGNOSTIC TECHNIQUES

Coronary Pressure and Blood Flow Determinations

Five methods are available for measuring human coronary blood flow in the cardiac catheterization laboratory—thermodilution, digital subtraction angiography, electromagnetic flowmeters, Doppler velocity probes, and pressure wires.[49] Although most current methods measure relative changes in coronary blood flow, useful information about the physiological significance of stenosis, cardiac hypertrophy, and pharmacological interventions can be obtained. Doppler flow wires and translesional gradients are the most commonly used clinical techniques (see Chap. 48).

Left Ventricular Electromechanical Mapping

Advances in catheter design and navigational technology have resulted in catheter-based three-dimensional mapping systems for evaluating regional and global left ventricular function. The system provides simultaneous electrical, mechanical, and anatomic information.[50] An ability of the electromechanical left ventricular maps to distinguish viable from nonviable myocardium and ischemic from nonischemic myocardium has been suggested.

The clinical experience with this system is limited. However, preliminary data indicate that the mapping system has promise in predicting recovery of function following revascularization.[51] This technique holds promise for guiding delivery of myocardial regeneration therapies, such as local stem cell injection.[52]

Intracardiac Echocardiography

Intracardiac echocardiography (ICE) has become available for transvenous imaging within the cardiac chambers. It consists of an 8 or 10F, 90-cm-long device that permits two planes of bidirectional steering in the anterior-posterior and left-right directions. The transducers have variable frequencies of 5 to 10 MHz with multiple phased array features, including two-dimensional imaging and color and spectral Doppler.

ICE can provide imaging of interatrial or interventricular septum and left-heart structures from the right atrium or ventricle, with penetration up to 15 cm. Current applications include guidance of percutaneous atrial septal defect and patent foramen ovale closures (see Chap. 61), thus mitigating the need for transesophageal echocardiography and anesthesia (Fig. 19-16). In patients requiring transseptal puncture, ICE can facilitate localization of the fossa ovalis. ICE can also be used to guide electrophysiological procedures, with identification of anatomical structures difficult to view by fluoroscopy (e.g., pulmonary veins or fossa ovalis for transseptal puncture).[18]

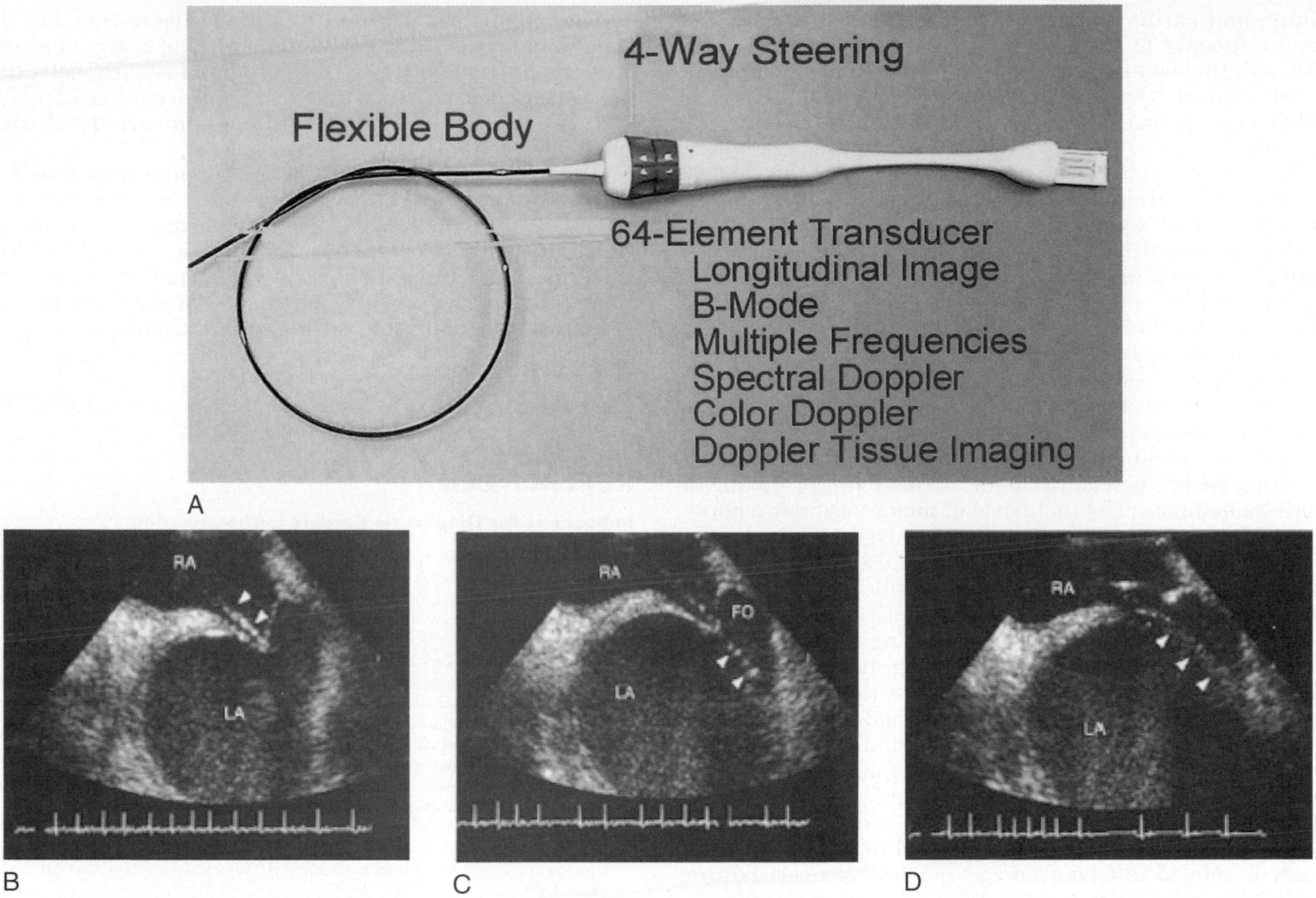

FIGURE 19–16 A, Intracardiac echo disposable transducer (Siemens Medical, Malvern, PA). The steering apparatus is on the proximal end, the body is flexible, with a transducer on the distal tip of the catheter. **B,** Tenting of the membranous fossa by the dilator-needle assembly. The transseptal needle assembly (arrowheads) is advanced to indent the fossa membrane. **C,** Advancement of the transseptal needle across the membranous fossa. Here, the needle (arrowheads) is seen near the posterosuperior left atrial wall. The membrane remains tented because the dilator has not yet crossed the septum. **D,** Dilator and sheath passage across the interatrial septum (arrowheads). The dilator and sheath assembly has now advanced into the left atrium, releasing the tenting of the membranous fossa. FO = fossa ovalis; LA = left atrium; RA = right atrium. *(From Johnson SB, Seward JB, Packer DL: Phased-array intracardiac echocardiography for guiding transseptal catheter placement: Utility and learning curve. Pacing Clin Electrophysiol 25:402, 2002.)*

COMPLICATIONS ASSOCIATED WITH CARDIAC CATHETERIZATION (Table 19-5)

Cardiac catheterization is a relatively safe procedure but has a well-defined risk of morbidity and mortality. The potential risk of major complications during cardiac catheterization may be difficult to ascertain because of the confounding aspects of comorbid disease and disparities in methods used to collect complication data. The use of low-osmolar and isosmolar contrast media, lower profile diagnostic catheters, reduced anticoagulation, and extensive operator experience all serve to reduce the incidence of complications further. Several large studies have provided insight into the incidence of major events and delineated cohorts of patients that are at increased risk.[1,53,54]

Death related to diagnostic cardiac catheterization occurs in 0.08 to 0.75 percent of patients, depending on the population studied. Data from the Society for Cardiac Angiography have identified subsets of patients with an increased mortality rate.[54] In an analysis of 58,332 patients, multivariate predictors of significant complications were moribund status, advanced New York Heart Association functional class, hypotension, shock, aortic valve disease, renal insufficiency, unstable angina, mitral valve disease, acute myocardial infarction within 24 hours, congestive heart

TABLE 19–5 Risk of Cardiac Catheterization and Coronary Angiography*

Complication	Risk (%)
Mortality	0.11
Myocardial infarction	0.05
Cerebrovascular accident	0.07
Arrhythmia	0.38
Vascular complications	0.43
Contrast reaction	0.37
Hemodynamic complications	0.26
Perforation of heart chamber	0.03
Other complications	0.28
Total of major complications	1.70

*No. of patients = 59,792.

From Scanlon PJ, Faxon DP, Audet AM, et al: ACC/AHA guidelines for coronary angiography: A report of the American College of Cardiology/American Heart Association Task Force on Practice Guidelines (Committee on Coronary Angiography). J Am Coll Cardiol 33:1760, 1999.

failure, and cardiomyopathy. The risk of cardiac catheterization appears to be further increased in octogenarians. Although the overall mortality is approximately 0.8 percent in this cohort, the risk of nonfatal major complications, which are primarily peripheral vascular, is about 5 percent.

The risk of myocardial infarction varies from 0.03 to 0.06 percent, of neurological complications from 0.03 to 0.2 percent, and of significant bradyarrhythmias or tachyarrhythmias from 0.56 to 1.3 percent.[54] One study using serial cranial magnetic resonance imaging has demonstrated a 22 percent incidence of focal acute cerebral embolic events following retrograde crossing of stenotic aortic valves. Three percent of patients demonstrated clinically apparent neurological deficits.[55] However, the results of this study were in contradistinction to previously published large clinical series and require additional validation.

The most common complication is arterial access site bleeding, which is usually manifested by minor oozing or small hematomas. The incidence of major vascular complications has varied, with most series suggesting a slightly higher frequency when the Sones brachial approach is used. The incidence of major vascular complications has been reported as approximately 0.40 percent.[54] Major vascular complications include occlusion requiring arterial repair or thrombectomy, retroperitoneal bleeding, hematoma formation, pseudoaneurysm, arteriovenous fistula formation, and infection. In a patient with unexplained hypotension or back pain, retroperitoneal hematoma should be suspected. Evaluation should include serial complete blood count determinations, evaluation of anticoagulation status, and CT or ultrasound evaluation of the groin, pelvis, and abdomen. The risk of requiring surgical repair for vascular injury is related to advanced age, congestive heart failure, and larger body surface area. With ultrasound guidance, many pseudoaneurysms can be successfully treated percutaneously with directed infusion of thrombin, and surgical repair can often be avoided.

The proper management of the arterial sheath is important in avoiding complications. Because dwell times correlate with hematoma formation, all sheaths should be removed as soon as possible, with an activated clotting time (ACT) less than 170 seconds. Frequent blood pressure and pulse monitoring is essential.

Systemic complications can vary from mild vasovagal responses to severe vagal reactions that lead to prolonged hypotension. Minor complications occur in approximately 4 percent of patients undergoing routine cardiac catheterization.[56] The most common untoward effects are transient hypotension and brief episodes of angina lasting less than 10 minutes.

Hives can occur but are less commonly observed with low-osmolar contrast and with intraarterial administration. They are readily treated with intravenous corticosteroids and diphenhydramine. Rarely, anaphylactoid complications are observed.

The most common complications of right-heart catheterization are nonsustained atrial and ventricular arrhythmias. Major complications associated with right-heart catheterization are infrequent. These include pulmonary infarction, pulmonary artery or right ventricular perforation, and infection.

FUTURE PERSPECTIVES

In many ways, diagnostic cardiac catheterization is at a crossroads. The development of high-resolution coronary CT angiography will likely mitigate the need for cardiac catheterization in low-risk patients in whom coronary artery disease can be excluded with noninvasive testing. On the other hand, the widespread availability of many noninvasive imaging modalities will likely provide early detection of coronary heart disease that will require cardiac catheterization to precisely define the extent and severity of coronary, vascular and valvular disease.

The expansion of modalities for percutaneous repair of coronary, valvular, and structural heart disease will also stimulate the growth of cardiac catheterization in conjunction with the percutaneous therapeutic procedure. The safety of the technique has been well established and continues to improve with experience, standardized quality assurance programs, and advances in technology.

Acknowledgment

The authors would like to thank Robert Fishman, MD, for his contribution to a previous edition of this chapter.

REFERENCES

Indications for Diagnostic Cardiac Catheterization

1. Scanlon PJ, Faxon DP, Audet AM, et al: ACC/AHA guidelines for coronary angiography: A report of the American College of Cardiology/American Heart Association Task Force on Practice Guidelines (Committee on Coronary Angiography). Developed in collaboration with the Society for Cardiac Angiography and Interventions. J Am Coll Cardiol 33:1756, 1999.
2. American College of Cardiology; American Heart Association Task Force on Practice Guidelines (Writing Committee to revise the 1998 guidelines for the management of patients with valvular heart disease); Society of Cardiovascular Anesthesiologists; Society for Cardiovascular Angiography and Interventions; Society of Thoracic Surgeons; Bonow RO, Carabello BA, Chatterjee K, et al: ACC/AHA 2006 guidelines for the management of patients with valvular heart disease: a report of the American College of Cardiology/American Heart Association Task Force on Practice Guidelines (Writing Committee to Revise the 1998 guidelines for the management of patients with valvular heart disease) developed in collaboration with the Society of Cardiovascular Anesthesiologists endorsed by the Society for Cardiovascular Angiography and Interventions and the Society of Thoracic Surgeons. J Am Coll Cardiol 48:e1, 2006.
3. Hunt SA, Abraham WT, Chin MH, et al; American Heart Association Task Force on Practice Guidelines; American College of Chest Physicians; International Society for Heart and Lung Transplantation; Heart Rhythm Society; American College of Cardiology: ACC/AHA 2005 Guideline Update for the Diagnosis and Management of Chronic Heart Failure in the Adult: A report of the American College of Cardiology/American Heart Association Task Force on Practice Guidelines (Writing Committee to Update the 2001 Guidelines for the Evaluation and Management of Heart Failure): developed in collaboration with the American College of Chest Physicians and the International Society for Heart and Lung Transplantation: endorsed by the Heart Rhythm Society. Circulation 112:e154, 2005.
4. Antman EM, Anbe DT, Armstrong PW, et al; American College of Cardiology; American Heart Association Task Force on Practice Guidelines; Canadian Cardiovascular Society: ACC/AHA guidelines for the management of patients with ST-elevation myocardial infarction: A report of the American College of Cardiology/American Heart Association Task Force on Practice Guidelines (Committee to Revise the 1999 Guidelines for the Management of Patients with Acute Myocardial Infarction). Circulation 110:e82, 2004.
5. Smith SC Jr, Feldman TE, Hirshfeld JW Jr, et al; American College of Cardiology/American Heart Association Task Force on Practice Guidelines; ACC/AHA/SCAI Writing Committee to Update 2001 Guidelines for Percutaneous Coronary Intervention: ACC/AHA/SCAI 2005 guideline update for percutaneous coronary intervention: A report of the American College of Cardiology/American Heart Association Task Force on Practice Guidelines (ACC/AHA/SCAI Writing Committee to Update 2001 Guidelines for Percutaneous Coronary Intervention. Circulation 113:e166, 2006.
6. Eagle KA, Guyton RA, Davidoff R, et al; American College of Cardiology; American Heart Association: ACC/AHA 2004 guideline update for coronary artery bypass graft surgery: A report of the American College of Cardiology/American Heart Association Task Force on Practice Guidelines (Committee to Update the 1999 Guidelines for Coronary Artery Bypass Graft Surgery). Circulation 110:e340, 2004.
7. Bashore TM, Bates ER, Berger PB, et al: ACC/SCAI Clinical expert consensus document on cardiac catheterization laboratory standards. J Am Coll Cardiol 37:2170, 2001.

Technical Aspects

8. Jacobs AK, Faxon DP, Hirshfeld JW, Holmes DR: Task force 3: Training in diagnostic cardiac catheterization and interventional cardiology. Revision of the 1995 COCATS training statement. J Am Coll Cardiol 39:1242, 2002.
9. Hirshfeld JW Jr, Balter S, Brinker JA, et al: ACCF/AHA/HRS/SCAI Clinical competence statement of physician knowledge to optimize patient safety and image quality in fluoroscopically guided invasive cardiovascular procedures. J Am Coll Cardiol 44:2259, 2004.
10. Heupler FA Jr: Guidelines for performing angiography in patients taking metformin. Members of the Laboratory Performance Standards Committee of the Society for Cardiac Angiography and Interventions. Cathet Cardiovasc Diagn 43:121, 1998.

11. Piper WD, Malenka DJ, Ryan TR Jr: Predicting vascular complications in percutaneous coronary interventions. Am Heart J 145:1022, 2003.
12. Kussmaul WG, Buchbinder M, Whitlow P, et al: Rapid arterial hemostasis after cardiac catheterization and percutaneous transluminal angioplasty—results of a randomized trial of a novel hemostatic device. J Am Coll Cardiol 25:1685, 1995.
13. Baim DS, Knopf WDD, Hinohara T, et al: Suture-mediated closure of the femoral access site after cardiac catheterization. Am J Cardiol 85:864, 2000.
14. Koreny M, Riedmuller E, Nikfardjam M, et al: Arterial puncture closing devices compared with standard manual compression after cardiac catheterization. JAMA 291:350, 2004.
15. Archbold RA, Robinson NM, Schilling RJ: Radial artery access for coronary angiography and percutaneous coronary intervention. BMJ 329:443, 2004.
16. Baim DS: Percutaneous approach, including transseptal and apical puncture. *In* Baim DS, Grossman W (eds): Cardiac Catheterization, Angiography, and Intervention, 7th ed. Philadelphia, Lippincott Williams & Wilkins, 2006, pp 79-106.
17. DePonti R, Cappato R, Curnis A, et al: Trans-septal catheterization in the electrophysiology laboratory. Data from a multicenter survey spanning 12 years. J Am Coll Cardiol 47:1037, 2006.
18. Jongbloed MRM, Schalij MJ, Zeppenfeld K, et al: Clinical applications of intracardiac echocardiography in interventional procedures. Heart 91:981, 2005.
19. Zuguchi M, Shindoh C, Chida K, et al: Safety and clinical benefits of transsubxiphoidal left ventricular puncture. Catheter Cardiovascular Int 55:58, 2001.
20. Walters DL, Sanchez PL, Rodriquez-Alemparte M, et al: Transthoracic left ventricular puncture for the assessment of patients with aortic and mitral valve prosthesis. The Massachusetts General experience 1989-2000. Cathet Cardiovasc Interv 58:539, 2003.
21. Wu LA, Lapeyre AC 3rd, Cooper LT: Current role of endomyocardial biopsy in the management of dilated cardiomyopathy and myocarditis. Mayo Clin Proc 76:1030, 2001.
22. Mehta A, Mehta M, Jain AC: Constrictive pericarditis. Clin Cardiol 22:334, 1999.
23. Barbaro G, DiLorenzo G, Grisorio B, et al: Incidence of dilated cardiomyopathy and detection of HIV in myocardial cells in HIV-positive patients. N Engl J Med 339:1093, 1998.
24. Cohen M, Ferguson JJ 3rd, Freedman RJ Jr, et al: Comparison of outcomes after 8 vs. 9.5 French size intra-aortic balloon counterpulsation catheters based on 9,332 patients in the prospective Benchmark registry. Cathet Cardiovasc Interv 56:200, 2002.
25. Trost JC, Hillis LD: Intra-aortic balloon counterpulsation. Am J Cardiol 97:1391, 2006.
26. O'Rourke MF: Augmentation of coronary blood flow with intra-aortic balloon pump counter-pulsation. Circulation 103:e129, 2001.
27. Ferguson JJ, Cohen M, Freedman RJ: The current practice of intra-aortic balloon counterpulsation: Results from the Benchmark registry. J Am Coll Cardiol 38:1456, 2001.
28. Stone GW, Ohman EM, Miller MF: Contemporary utilization and outcomes of intra-aortic balloon counterpulsation in acute myocardial infarction: The Benchmark registry. J Am Coll Cardiol 41:1940, 2003.

Hemodynamic Data

29. Grossman W: Pressure measurement. *In* Grossman W, Baim DS (eds): Cardiac Catheterization, Angiography, and Intervention. 7th ed. Philadelphia, Lea & Febiger, 2006, pp 13-35.
30. Hildick-Smith DJ, Walsh JT, Shapiro LM: Pulmonary capillary wedge pressure in mitral stenosis accurately reflects mean left atrial pressure but overestimates transmitral gradient. Am J Cardiol 85:512, 2000.
31. Schobel WA, Voelker W, Haase KK: Extent, determinants and clinical importance of pressure recovery in patients with aortic valve stenosis. Eur Heart J 20:1355, 1999.
32. Niederberger J, Schima H, Maurer G, Baumgartner H: Importance of pressure recovery for the assessment of aortic stenosis by Doppler ultrasound. Circulation 94:1934, 1996.
33. Moise SF, Sinclair CJ, Scott DHT: Pulmonary artery blood temperature and the measurement of cardiac output by thermodilution. Anaesthesia 57:562, 2002.
34. Lehmann KG, Platt MS: Improved accuracy and precision of thermodilution cardiac output measurement using a dual thermistor catheter system. J Am Coll Cardiol 33:883, 1999.
35. Fakler U, Pauli C, Hennig M, et al: Assumed oxygen consumption frequently results in large errors in the determination of cardiac output. J Thoracic Cardiovascular Surgery 130:272, 2005.
36. Nichols WW, O'Rourke MF (eds): McDonald's Blood Flow in Arteries. 4th ed. New York, Oxford University Press, 1998.
37. Otto CM: Cardiac catheterization and angiography. *In* Otto CM (ed): Valvular Heart Disease. 2nd ed. Philadelphia, WB Saunders, 2004, pp 93-108.
38. Shively BK, Charlton GA, Crawford MH, Chaney RK: Flow dependence of valve area in aortic stenosis: Relation to valve morphology. J Am Coll Cardiol 31:654, 1998.
39. Tardif JC, Rodrigues AG, Hardey JF, et al: Simultaneous determination of aortic valve area by the Gorlin formula and by transesophageal echocardiography under different transvalvular flow conditions. J Am Coll Cardiol 29:1296, 1997.
40. Nishimura RA, Grantham JA, Connolly HM, et al: Low-output, low-gradient aortic stenosis in patients with depressed left ventricular systolic function: The clinical utility of the dobutamine challenge in the catheterization laboratory. Circulation 106:809, 2002.
41. Monin JL, Quere JP, Monchi M, et al: Low-gradient aortic stenosis: Operative risk stratification and predictors for long-term outcome: A multicenter study using dobutamine stress hemodynamics. Circulation 108:319, 2003.
42. Grossman W: Shunt detection and quantification. *In* Grossman W, Baim DS (eds): Cardiac Catheterization, Angiography, and Intervention. 7th ed. Philadelphia, Lea & Febiger, 2006, pp 163-172.
43. Shepherd AP, McMahon CA: Role of oximeter error in the diagnosis of shunts. Cathet Cardiovasc Diagn 37:435, 1996.
44. Grossman W: Stress testing during cardiac catheterization: Exercise and pacing tachycardia. *In* Grossman W, Baim DS (eds): Cardiac Catheterization, Angiography, and Intervention. 7th ed. Philadelphia, Lea & Febiger, 2006, pp 283-303.
45. Higano ST, Azrak E, Tahirkheli NK, Kern MJ: Hemodynamic rounds series II: Hemodynamics of constrictive physiology: Influence of respiratory dynamics on ventricular pressures. Cathet Cardiovasc Interv 46:473, 1999.
46. Ichinose F, Roberts JD, Zapol WM: Inhaled nitric oxide: A selective pulmonary vasodilator: Current uses and therapeutic potential. Circulation 109:3106, 2004.
47. Krasuski RA, Warner JJ, Wang A, et al: Inhaled nitric oxide selectively dilates pulmonary vasculature in adult patients with pulmonary hypertension, irrespective of etiology. J Am Coll Cardiol 36:2204, 2000.
48. Konidala S, Gutterman DD: Coronary vasospasm and the regulation of coronary blood flow. Prog Cardiovasc Dis 46:349, 2004.

Adjunctive Diagnostic Techniques

49. Kern MJ: Curriculum in interventional cardiology: Coronary pressure and flow measurements in the cardiac catheterization laboratory. Cathet Cardiovasc Interv 54:378, 2001.
50. Underwood SR, Bax JJ, Vom Dahl J, et al: Imaging techniques for the assessment of myocardial hibernation. Report of a study group of the European Society of Cardiology. Eur Heart J 25:815, 2004.
51. Koch KC, Wenderdel M, Stellbrink C, et al: Electromechanical assessment of left ventricular function following successful percutaneous coronary revascularization. Cathet Cardiovasc Interv 54:466, 2001.
52. Vale PR, Losordo DW, Milliken CE, et al: Left ventricular electromechanical mapping to assess efficacy of phVEGF(165) gene transfer for therapeutic angiogenesis in chronic myocardial ischemia. Circulation 102:965, 2000.

Complications Associated with Cardiac Catheterization

53. Davidson CJ, Mark DB, Pieper KS, et al: Thrombotic and cardiovascular complications related to nonionic contrast media during cardiac catheterization. Analysis of 8517 patients. Am J Cardiol 65:1481, 1990.
54. Laskey W, Boyle J, Johnson LW: Multivariable model for prediction of risk of significant complication during diagnostic cardiac catheterization. The Registry Committee of the Society for Cardiac Angiography and Interventions. Cathet Cardiovasc Diagn 30:185, 1993.
55. Omran H, Schmidt H, Hackenbroch M, et al: Silent and apparent cerebral embolism after retrograde catheterisation of the aortic valve in valvular stenosis: A prospective, randomised study. Lancet 361:1241, 2003.
56. Davidson CJ, Hlatky M, Morris GG, et al: Cardiovascular and renal toxicity of a nonionic radiographic contrast agent after cardiac catheterization. Ann Intern Med 110:119, 1989.

CHAPTER 20

Coronary Arteriography and Intravascular Imaging

Jeffrey J. Popma

Coronary arteriography remains the standard for identifying the presence or absence of arterial narrowings related to atherosclerotic coronary artery disease (CAD) and provides the most reliable anatomical information for determining the appropriateness of medical therapy, percutaneous coronary intervention (PCI), or coronary artery bypass graft (CABG) surgery in patients with ischemic CAD. First performed by Sones in 1959, coronary arteriography has subsequently become one of the most widely used invasive procedures in cardiovascular medicine. It is performed by directly injecting radiopaque contrast material into the coronary arteries and recording radiographic images on 35-mm cinefilm or digital recordings. More than 2 million patients will undergo coronary arteriography in the United States this year alone, and coronary arteriography is now available in 25% of acute care hospitals in this country.

The methods used to perform coronary arteriography have improved substantially since 1959. Smaller (5 to 6 French [5 to 6F]), high-flow injection catheters have replaced larger (8F), thick-walled catheters, and the reduced sheath size has allowed same-day coronary arteriography, ambulation, and discharge. Complication rates associated with coronary arteriography have fallen due to a better understanding of the periprocedural management of patients undergoing cardiac catheterization. "Filmless" digital, and, more recently, flat-panel laboratories now permit high-quality image acquisition, electronic (rather than 35-mm cinefilm) storage, and rapid image transfer and dissemination.[1] Adjunctive invasive imaging modalities, such as intravascular ultrasonography (IVUS), optical coherence tomography, and intracoronary temperature measurements, can now provide the clinician with more precise characterization of the vessel wall and extent of atherosclerotic risk than is available with conventional angiography.

This chapter reviews the indications for and techniques of coronary arteriography, the normal coronary anatomy and pathological coronary variants, the qualitative and quantitative angiographic methods for assessing severity of stenoses, and the advantages and limitations of invasive imaging for characterizing atherosclerotic plaque.

INDICATIONS FOR CORONARY ARTERIOGRAPHY

(See also later, "Guidelines: Coronary Arteriography.")

Coronary arteriography establishes the presence or absence of coronary stenoses, defines therapeutic options, and determines the prognosis of patients with symptoms or signs of ischemic CAD.[2] Coronary arteriography can also be used as a research tool to evaluate serial changes that occur after PCI or pharmacological therapy. The American College of Cardiology/American Heart Association (ACC/AHA) Task Force established indications for coronary arteriography in patients with known or suspected CAD (Table 20-1).[2]

Patients with suspected CAD who have severe stable angina (Canadian Cardiovascular Society [CCS] class III or IV) or those who have less severe symptoms or are asymptomatic but demonstrate "high-risk" criteria for an adverse outcome on noninvasive testing should undergo coronary arteriography. High-risk features include resting or exercise-induced left ventricular dysfunction (left ventricular ejection fraction [LVEF] <35 percent) or a standard exercise treadmill test demonstrating hypotension or 1 to 2 mm or more ST segment depression associated with decreased exercise capacity.[2] Stress imaging that demonstrates a moderate or large perfusion defect (particularly in the anterior wall), multiple defects, a large fixed perfusion defect with left ventricular dilation or increased lung uptake (see Chapter 16), or extensive stress or dobutamine-induced wall motion abnormalities (see Chapter 14) also indicate high risk for an adverse outcome. Patients resuscitated from sudden cardiac death, particularly those with residual ventricular arrhythmias, are also candidates for coronary arteriography, given the favorable outcomes associated with revascularization in these patients. In the absence of symptoms and signs of ischemia, the presence of coronary calcification on fluoroscopy and a high calcium score by ultrafast computed tomographic scanning are not indications for coronary arteriography.

Patients with unstable angina (see Chapter 53) who develop recurrent symptoms despite medical therapy or who are at intermediate or high risk for subsequent death or myocardial infarction (MI) are also candidates for coronary arteriography.[2,3] High-risk features include prolonged ongoing (>20 minutes) chest pain, pulmonary edema, worsening mitral regurgitation, dynamic ST segment depression of 1 mm or more, and hypotension.[2] Intermediate-risk features include angina at rest (>20 minutes) relieved with rest or sublingual nitroglycerin, angina associated with dynamic electrocardiographic

TABLE 20–1 Indications for Coronary Arteriography

Class I	Class IIa	Class IIb	Class III
Asymptomatic or Stable Angina			
CCS class III and IV on medical therapy High-risk criteria on noninvasive testing irrespective of angina Successfully resuscitated from sudden cardiac death with sustained monomorphic VT or nonsustained polymorphic VT	CCS class III or IV that improves to class I or II with medical therapy Worsening noninvasive testing Patients with angina and severe illness that precludes risk stratification CCS class I or II angina with intolerance to medical therapy Individuals whose occupation affects the safety of others	CCS class I or II angina with demonstrable ischemia but no high-risk criteria on noninvasive testing Asymptomatic men or postmenopausal women with >two major clinical risks with low-risk noninvasive testing and no prior CAD Asymptomatic patients with prior MI, normal LV function, and no high-risk noninvasive testing	Angina in patients who prefer to avoid revascularization Angina in patients who are not candidates for revascularization or in whom it will not improve QOL As a screening test for CAD After CABG when there is no evidence of ischemia on noninvasive testing Coronary calcification on fluoroscopy or EBCT
Unstable Angina			
High or intermediate risk for adverse outcome in patients refractory to medical therapy High or intermediate risk that stabilizes after initial treatment Initially low short-term risk that is high risk on noninvasive testing Suspected Prinzmetal variant angina	None	Low short-term risk unstable angina without high-risk criteria on noninvasive testing	Recurrent chest discomfort suggestive of unstable angina but without objective signs of ischemia and with a normal coronary angiogram within the past 5 years Unstable angina in patients who are not candidates for revascularization
Postrevascularization Ischemia			
Suspected abrupt closure or subacute stent thrombosis after PCI Recurrent angina and high-risk criteria on noninvasive evaluation within 9 months of PCI	Recurrent symptomatic ischemia within 12 months of CABG Noninvasive evidence of high-risk criteria occurring anytime after CABG Recurrent angina inadequately controlled by medications	Asymptomatic post-PCI patient suspected of having re-stenosis within the first months after PCI because of an abnormal but not high-risk noninvasive test Recurrent angina without high-risk criteria on noninvasive testing occurring 1 year postoperatively Asymptomatic post-CABG patient in whom a deteriorating noninvasive test is found	Symptoms in a post-CABG patient who is not a candidate for revasascularization Routine angiography after PCI or CABG unless part of an approved research protocol
After QWMI or NQWMI			
Spontaneous myocardial ischemia or ischemia provoked with minimal exertion Before surgical therapy for acute MR, VSD, true or pseudoaneurysm Persistent hemodynamic instability	Suspected MI due to coronary embolism, arteritis, trauma, certain metabolic diseases, or coronary spasm Survivors of acute MI with LVEF <0.40, CHF, prior PCI or CABG, or malignant ventricular arrhythmias	For a suspected persistent occlusion of the IRA to perform delayed PCI Coronary arteriography performed without risk stratification to identify the presence of left main or three-vessel CAD All patients after NQWMI Recurrent ventricular tachycardia despite antiarrhyhtmic therapy without ongoing ischemia	Patients who are not a candidate for or refuse revascularization
Nonspecific Chest Pain			
High-risk features on noninvasive testing	None	Patients with recurrent hospitalizations for chest pain who have abnormal or equivocal findings on noninvasive testing	All other patients with nonspecific chest pain

Class I: conditions for which there is agreement that the procedure is useful and effective; Class IIa: weight of the evidence is in favor of usefulness and efficacy; Class IIb: weight of the evidence is less well established by evidence and opinion; Class III: conditions for which there is general agreement that the procedure is not useful and effective and in some cases may be harmful.

CABG = coronary artery bypass graft surgery; CAD = coronary artery disease; CCS = Canadian Cardiovascular Society; CHF = congestive heart failure; EBCT = electron beam computed tomography; IRA = infarct-related artery; LV = left ventricular; MI = myocardial infarction; MR = mitral regurgitation; NQWMI = non-Q-wave MI; PCI = percutaneous coronary intervention; QOL = quality of life; QWMI = Q-wave MI; VSD = ventricular septal defect; VT = ventricular tachycardia.

From Scanlon P, Faxon D, Audet A, et al: ACC/AHA guidelines for coronary angiography. J Am Coll Cardiol 33:1756, 1999.

changes, recent-onset angina with a high likelihood of CAD, pathological Q waves or ST segment depression less than 1 mm in multiple leads, and age older than 65 years.[2]

Patients with an ST segment elevation myocardial infarction (STEMI), a non-ST segment elevation myocardial infarction (NSTEMI), or unstable angina who develop spontaneous ischemia; or with ischemia at a minimal workload; or who have MI complicated by congestive heart failure (CHF), hemodynamic instability, cardiac arrest, mitral regurgitation, or ventricular septal rupture should undergo coronary arteriography. Patients with angina or provocable ischemia after MI should also undergo coronary arteriography because revascularization may reduce the high risk of reinfarction in these patients.

Patients who present with chest pain of unclear etiology, particularly those who have high-risk criteria on noninvasive testing, may benefit from coronary arteriography to diagnose or exclude the presence of significant CAD.[2] Patients who have undergone prior revascularization should undergo coronary arteriography if there is suspicion of abrupt vessel closure or when recurrent angina develops that meets high-risk noninvasive criteria.

Coronary arteriography should be performed in patients scheduled to undergo noncardiac surgery who demonstrate high-risk criteria on noninvasive testing, have angina unresponsive to medical therapy, develop unstable angina, or have equivocal noninvasive test results and are scheduled to undergo high-risk surgery (see also Chap. 80 and its Guidelines). Coronary arteriography is also recommended for patients scheduled to undergo surgery for valvular heart disease or congenital heart disease, particularly those with multiple cardiac risk factors and those with infective endocarditis and evidence of coronary embolization.[2]

Coronary arteriography should be performed annually in patients after cardiac transplantation in the absence of clinical symptoms because of the characteristically diffuse and often asymptomatic nature of graft atherosclerosis (see Chaps. 27 and 38). Coronary arteriography is useful in potential donors for cardiac transplantation whose age or cardiac risk profile increases the likelihood of CAD. The arteriogram often provides important diagnostic information about the presence of CAD in patients with intractable arrhythmias before electrophysiological testing or in patients who present with a dilated cardiomyopathy of unknown etiology.

CONTRAINDICATIONS. Although there are no absolute contraindications for coronary arteriography, relative contraindications include unexplained fever, untreated infection, severe anemia with hemoglobin less than 8 mg/dl, severe electrolyte imbalance, severe active bleeding, uncontrolled systemic hypertension, digitalis toxicity, previous contrast reaction but no pretreatment with corticosteroids, and ongoing stroke.[2] Other disease states that are relative contraindications to coronary arteriography include acute renal failure; decompensated CHF; severe intrinsic or iatrogenic coagulopathy (International Normalized Ratio [INR] greater than 2.0); and active endocarditis.[2] Risk factors for significant complications after catheterization include advanced age as well as several general medical, vascular, and cardiac characteristics (Table 20-2).

Given that the majority of these conditions are self-limited, deferral of coronary arteriography until important comorbidities have been stabilized is generally preferred unless there is evidence of ongoing myocardial necrosis. It is recognized that coronary arteriography performed under emergency conditions is associated with a higher risk of procedural complication. The risks and benefits of the procedure and its alternatives should be carefully reviewed with the patient and family in all circumstances before undertaking coronary arteriography in the presence of relative contraindications.

TABLE 20–2 Patients at Increased Risk for Complications after Coronary Arteriography

Increased General Medical Risk
Age >70 years
Complex congenital heart disease
Morbid obesity
General debility or cachexia
Uncontrolled glucose intolerance
Arterial oxygen desaturation
Severe chronic obstructive lung disease
Renal insufficiency with creatinine greater than 1.5 mg/dl
Increased Cardiac Risk
Three-vessel coronary artery disease
Left main coronary artery disease
Functional class IV
Significant mitral or aortic valve disease or mechanical prosthesis
Ejection fraction less than 35%
High-risk exercise treadmill testing (hypotension or severe ischemia)
Pulmonary hypertension
Pulmonary artery wedge pressure greater than 25 mm Hg
Increased Vascular Risk
Anticoagulation or bleeding diathesis
Uncontrolled systemic hypertension
Severe peripheral vascular disease
Recent stroke
Severe aortic insufficiency

Adapted from Scanlon P, Faxon D, Audet A, et al: ACC/AHA guidelines for coronary angiography. J Am Coll Cardiol 33:1756, 1999.

TABLE 20–3 Risk of Cardiac Catheterization

Complication	SCAI Registry (%)
Mortality	0.11
Myocardial infarction	0.05
Cerebrovascular accident	0.07
Arrhythmias	0.38
Vascular complications	0.43
Contrast reaction	0.37
Hemodynamic complications	0.26
Perforation of heart chamber	0.03
Other complications	0.28
Total of major complications	1.70

SCAI = Society for Cardiac Angiography and Intervention.

Adapted from Scanlon P, Faxon D, Audet A, et al: ACC/AHA guidelines for coronary angiography. J Am Coll Cardiol 33:1756, 1999.

COMPLICATIONS OF CORONARY ARTERIOGRAPHY

Major complications are uncommon (<1 percent) after coronary arteriography (Table 20-3)[4,5] and include death (0.10 to 0.14 percent), MI (0.06 to 0.07 percent), contrast agent reactions (0.23 percent), stroke (0.07 to 0.14 percent), and local vascular complications (0.24 to 0.1 percent).[6] The incidence of death during coronary arteriography is higher in the presence of left main coronary artery (LMCA) disease (0.55 percent), with LVEF less than 30 percent (0.30 percent), and with New York Heart Association functional Class IV disease (0.29 percent). Stroke may develop due to embolization of atherosclerotic debris into the cerebral circulation or embolization of clot that formed on the injection catheters, particularly in patients with prior CABG who have a diseased ascending aorta. More recently, acute stroke complicating diagnostic catheterization has been amenable to neurovascular intervention.[7] Recent series have shown no increase, and in one study a decline[5] in the major complication rates associated with coronary arteriography, despite increased morbidity of patients and higher lesion complexity.[4]

Minor complications are also uncommon (<2 percent) after coronary arteriography. Air embolus is rare (0.1 percent) during diagnostic coronary arteriography and is generally preventable with meticulous flushing and elimination of air within the manifold. If an air embolus and air lock do occur, 100 percent oxygen should be administered, which allows resorption of smaller amounts of air within 2 to 4 minutes. Ventricular arrhythmias associated with air embolus can be treated with lidocaine and direct-current cardioversion. Cholesterol embolization is also uncommon, but may occur with catheter manipulation in a diffusely diseased abdominal aortic aneurysm (see also Chaps. 56 and 57).[8] Nerve pain after diagnostic catheterization is infrequent and generally resolves spotaneously.[9] Although lactic acidosis may develop after coronary angiography in diabetic patients taking metformin, this complication has been minimized with metformin discontinuation after coronary arteriography until renal function has recovered.

With the expanded use of complex PCI (see Chap. 55), patients may now return for multiple procedures over their lifetime that may subject them to the risk of cumulative radiation injury.[10] An average PCI procedure imparts 150 times the radiation exposure received with a single chest x-ray and 6 times the annual radiation received by background environmental radiation.[10] Reports of radiodermatitis related to prolonged x-ray exposure have led to the recommendation that patients who receive fluoroscopy for more than 60 minutes be counseled about the delayed effects of radiation injury to the skin, although proportionately more radiation is received with digital cineangiography than fluoroscopy alone. Radiation-induced lesions are generally identified by their location in the region of the x-ray tube and are manifest by an acute erythema, delayed pigmented telangiectasia, and indurated or ulcerated plaques in the upper back or below the axilla.

TECHNIQUE OF CORONARY ARTERIOGRAPHY

PREPARATION OF THE PATIENT. Elective coronary arteriography should be performed alone or in conjunction with right-heart catheterization or contrast left ventriculography when comorbid conditions, such as CHF, diabetes mellitus, or renal insufficiency, are stable. A baseline ECG, electrolyte and renal function tests, complete blood cell count, and coagulation panel should be reviewed before coronary arteriography. Patients who may undergo PCI should receive aspirin, 162 to 325 mg, at least 2 hours before the procedure if PCI is planned. Warfarin should be discontinued 2 days before elective coronary arteriography, and the INR should be less than 2.0 before arterial puncture. Patients at increased risk for systemic thromboembolism on withdrawal of warfarin, such as those with atrial fibrillation, mitral valve disease, or a prior history of systemic thromboembolism, may be treated with intravenous unfractionated heparin or subcutaneous low-molecular-weight heparin in the periprocedural period.

VASCULAR ACCESS. A variety of vascular approaches are available for coronary arteriography. The selection of the vascular access depends on the operator and patient preferences, anticoagulation status, and presence of peripheral vascular disease.

Femoral Artery Approach. The right or left femoral arteries are the most commonly used access sites for coronary arteriography. The common femoral artery courses medially to the femoral head and the bifurcation of the common femoral artery into its branches is generally distal to the middle third of the femoral head, which can be localized by fluoroscopy before arterial puncture (Fig. 20-1A). The anterior wall of the common femoral artery should be punctured several centimeters below the inguinal ligament but proximal to the bifurcation of the superficial femoral and profunda arterial branches (see Fig. 20-1B). If the puncture site is proximal to the inguinal ligament, hemostasis after the procedure may be difficult with manual compression, leading to an increased risk of retroperitoneal hemorrhage. If the puncture site is at or distal to the femoral bifurcation, there is a higher risk of pseudoaneurysm formation after sheath removal. Ipsilateral cannulation of the femoral artery and femoral vein also increases the risk of arteriovenous fistula formation.

Radial and Brachial Artery Approaches. Although Sones first introduced the cutdown approach to the brachial artery for coronary arteriography, access to the brachial and radial arteries is now most often obtained percutaneously. These approaches are preferred to the femoral approach in the presence of severe peripheral vascular disease and morbid

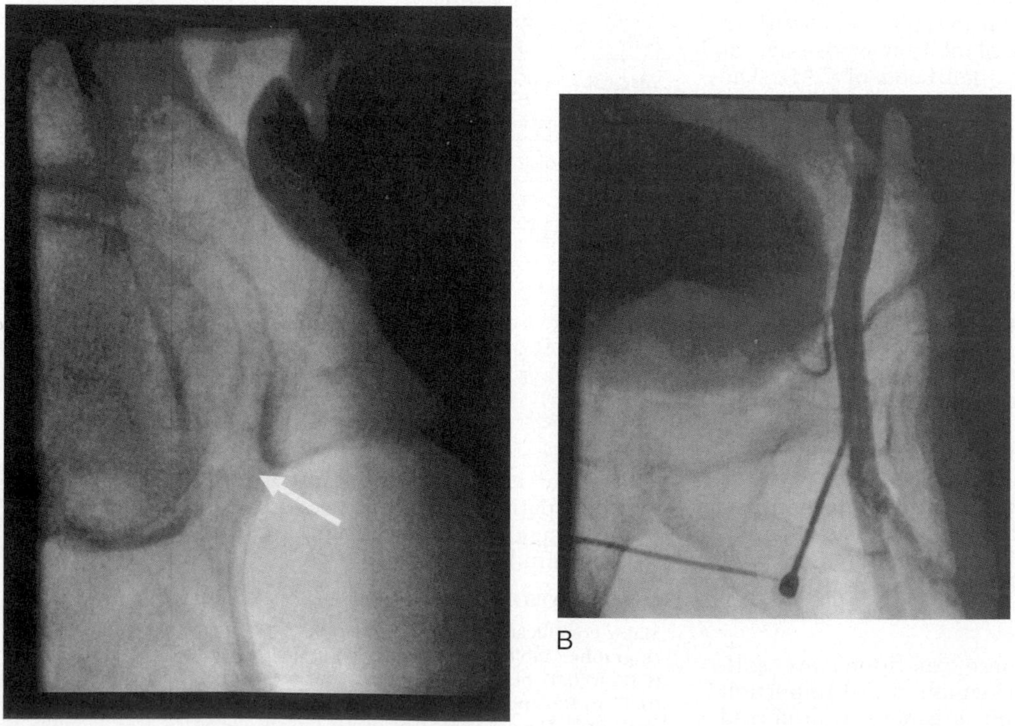

A

B

FIGURE 20–1 Radiographic landmarks can be used to identify the course of the common femoral artery. **A,** The middle third of the right femoral head identifies the usual course of the common femoral artery (arrow). **B,** The arterial sheath is shown placed proximally to the bifurcation of the femoris superficial femoral artery and the profunda femoris.

obesity,[11,12] and radial artery access is generally preferred to brachial catheterization due to its ease of catheter entry and removal.[13] The brachial artery easily accommodates an 8F (1F = 0.33 mm in diameter) sheath, whereas the radial artery is smaller and generally limited to 5 to 7F catheters. Before radial artery access is attempted, an Allen test should be carried out to ensure that the ulnar artery is patent in the event of radial artery occlusion.[14] Systemic anticoagulation with intravenous heparin or bivalirudin is used for both approaches to prevent catheter thrombosis. Use of a hydrophilic sheath[15] and administration of intraarterial verapamil and nitroglycerin reduce the occurrence of radial artery spasm, although rare episodes of radial artery trauma and avulsion have been reported.[16]

The radial artery approach allows immediate ambulation after coronary arteriography with lower cost (compared with femoral closure devices) and improved coronary visualization (compared with smaller 4F diameter femoral catheters).[17] Saphenous vein grafts (SVGs) can be engaged using either brachial or radial artery, but cannulation of the internal mammary artery (IMA) is best performed from the left brachial or radial artery. Engagement of the left IMA from the right brachial or radial artery is technically challenging but may be performed using a "headhunter" or another shaped catheter for selective entry into the left subclavian artery. A 0.035-inch angled hydrophilic guidewire is the most useful support wire for access to the subclavian artery.

CATHETERS

Diagnostic catheters developed for coronary arteriography are generally constructed from polyethylene or polyurethane with a fine wire braid within the wall to allow advancement and directional control (torque) and to prevent kinking. The outer diameter size of the catheters ranges from 4 to 8F, but 5 and 6F catheters are used most commonly for diagnostic arteriography.

JUDKINS CATHETERS. The Judkins left catheter is preshaped to allow entry into the left coronary ostium from the femoral approach with minimal catheter manipulation (Figs. 20-2 and 20-3). A preformed Judkins left catheter can also be used from the left brachial or radial artery, but a catheter with 0.5 cm less curvature than required for the femoral approach is generally better suited for coronary cannulation.

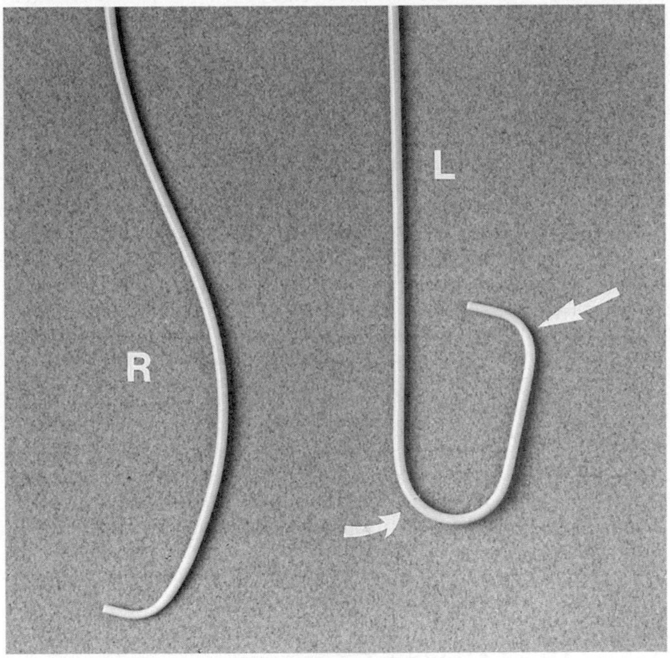

FIGURE 20–2 Right (R) and left (L) Judkins catheters. The primary (straight arrow) and secondary (curved arrow) curves of the Judkins left catheter are shown. (*Courtesy of Cordis Corporation.*)

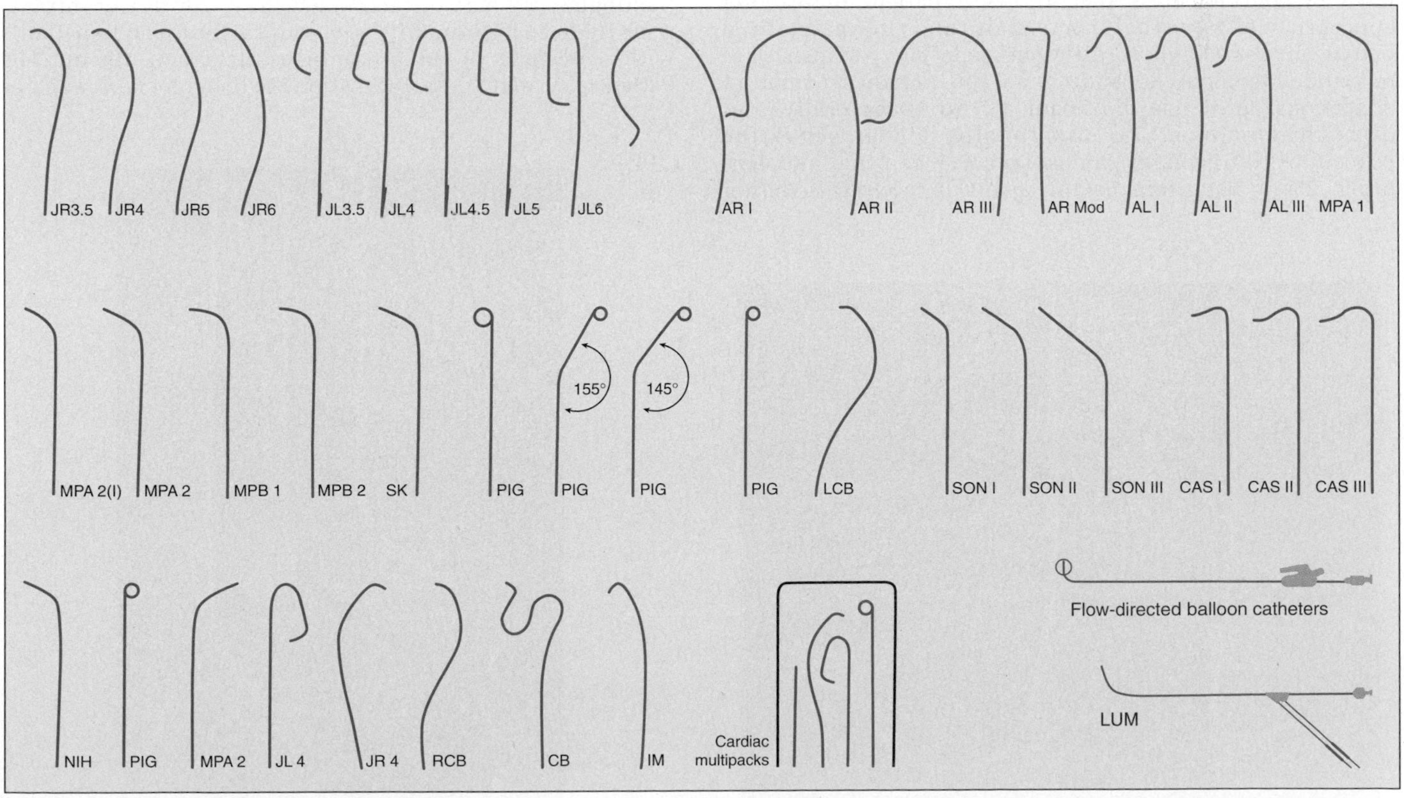

FIGURE 20–3 Tip configurations for several catheters useful in coronary arteriography. AL = Amplatz left; AR = Amplatz right; CAS = Castillo; CB = coronary bypass catheter; IM = internal mammary; JL = Judkins left; JR = Judkins right; LCB = left coronary bypass graft; LUM = lumen; Mod = modified; MP = multipurpose; NIH = National Institutes of Health; PIG = pigtail; RCB = right coronary bypass graft; SON = Sones. (*Courtesy of Cordis Corporation.*)

The Judkins right catheter is shaped to permit entry into the right coronary artery (RCA) with a small amount of rotational (clockwise) catheter manipulation from any vascular approach.

Selection of Judkins catheter shape is based on the body habitus of the patient and size of the aortic root. The left coronary artery (LCA) is easily engaged with the Judkins left 4.0 catheter from the femoral approach in most patients, whereas patients with a dilated ascending aorta (e.g., in the setting of congenital aortic stenosis and poststenotic dilation) may require the use of a Judkins left 5.0 or 6.0 catheter. Patients with large ascending aortic aneurysms may require arteriography with heat-modified catheters to achieve Judkins left 7.0 to 10.0 shapes. Use of a Judkins shape that is too small for the ascending aorta often leads to folding of the catheter within the aortic root. The best technique for removing a folded Judkins left catheter from the body involves withdrawing the folded catheter into the descending aorta and advancing a guidewire anterograde in the contralateral common iliac artery. On withdrawal of the catheter and guidewire together, the catheter straightens and can be removed safely from the body without disrupting the arterial access site.

AMPLATZ CATHETERS. Amplatz catheters can be used for the femoral or brachial approach to coronary arteriography (Fig. 20-4). The Amplatz catheters are an excellent alternative in cases in which the Judkins catheter is not appropriately shaped to enter the coronary arteries. The Amplatz L-1 or L-2 catheter may be used for coronary angiography from the right brachial or radial approach. A modified Amplatz right catheter (AR-1 or AR-2) can be used for engagement of a horizontal or upward takeoff RCA or SVG.

OTHER CATHETERS. Other catheters used for coronary arteriography include the IMA left catheter with an angulated tip that allows engagement of the IMA or an upward takeoff RCA. Catheter shapes that permit engagement of SVGs include the multipurpose catheter (Fig. 20-5), Judkins right, modified Amplatz right, and hockey stick catheters. Specially designed catheters for engagement of the coronary arteries from the radial artery have also been developed.

Drugs Used During Coronary Arteriography

ANALGESICS. The goal of analgesic use is to achieve a state of conscious sedation, defined by a minimally depressed level of consciousness that allows a patient to respond appropriately to verbal commands and to maintain a patent airway. Several different sedation regimens are recommended, but depending on the patient's comorbid conditions, most use diazepam, 2.5 to 10 mg orally, and diphenhydramine, 25 to 50 mg orally, 1 hour before the procedure. Intravenous midazolam, 0.5 to 2 mg, and fentanyl, 25 to 50 µg, are useful agents to provide sedation during the procedure. Patients undergoing conscious sedation should have continuous hemodynamic, electrocardiographic, and oximetry monitoring as well as access to oxygen and suction ports and a resuscitation cart.

ANTICOAGULANTS. Intravenous unfractionated heparin is no longer required during routine coronary arteriography. Patients at increased risk for thromboembolic complications, including those with severe aortic stenosis, critical peripheral arterial disease, or arterial atheroembolic disease or those undergoing procedures in which there is a need for prolonged (>1 to 2 minutes) use of guidewires in the central circulation may be given intravenous unfractionated heparin, 2000 to 5000 units. Patients undergoing brachial or radial artery catheterization should also receive systemic anticoagulation with unfractionated heparin or bivalirudin. Frequent flushing of all diagnostic and guiding catheters with heparinized saline prevents the formation of microthrombi within the catheter tip. A continuous flush through the arterial access sheath may also lower the occurrence of distal thromboembolism.

The anticoagulant effect of unfractionated heparin can be reversed with protamine, 1 mg for every 100 units of heparin. Protamine causes anaphylaxis or serious hypotensive episodes in approximately 2 percent of patients, and protamine should not be administered to patients with prior exposure to NPH insulin, to those with a history of unstable angina or high-risk coronary anatomy, or to patients who have undergone coronary arteriography by means of the brachial or radial arteries. Femoral sheaths can be removed after the anticoagulant effect of unfractionated heparin has dissipated, as assessed by an activated clotting time less than 150 to 180 seconds.

TREATMENT OF PERIPROCEDURAL ISCHEMIA. Patients may develop angina during coronary arteriography because of ischemia induced by tachycardia, hypertension, contrast agents, microembolization, coronary spasm or enhanced vasomotor tone, or dynamic platelet aggregation. Sublingual (0.3 mg), intracoronary (50 to 200 µg), or intravenous (10 to 25 µg/min) nitroglycerin can be given to patients with a systolic blood pressure greater than 100 mm Hg. Patients without contraindications to beta blockers, such as

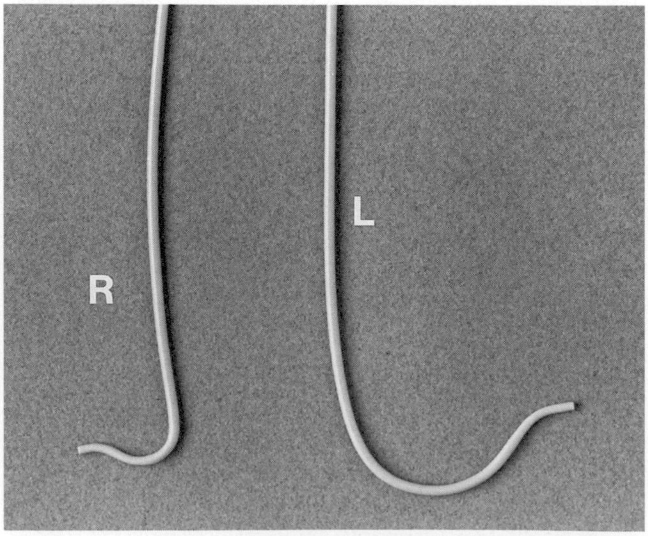

FIGURE 20–4 Amplatz right (R) and left (L) catheters. (*Courtesy of Cordis Corporation.*)

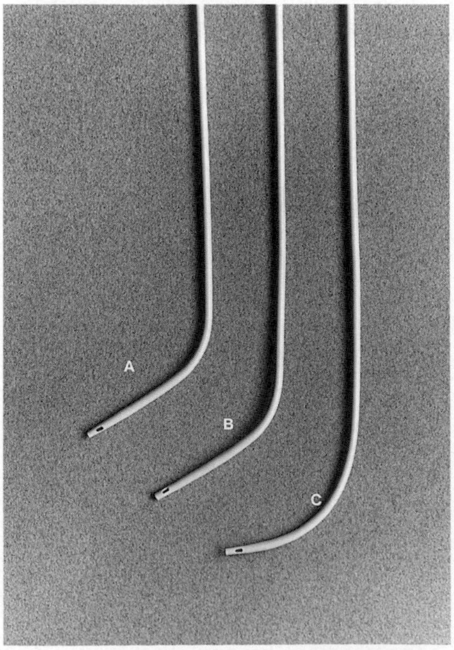

FIGURE 20–5 Multipurpose A, B, and C type catheters. (*Courtesy of Cordis Corporation.*)

TABLE 20–4 Characteristics of Radiocontrast Agents

Compound	Brand Name	Osmolality (mOsm/kg H_2O)	Viscosity at 37°C	Iodine (mg/ml)	Sodium (mEq/liter)	Additives	Side Effects Profile
High Osmolar Ionic Agents							
Sodium diatrizoate	Hypaque	1690	9.0	37.0	160	Calcium disodium EDTA	Electophysiologic (++++) Hemodynamic (++++) Anticoagulant (++++) Nephrotoxicity (+++) Allergic (+++)
Sodium meglumine diatrizoate	Renografin	1940	8.4	370	160	Sodium citrate, disodium EDTA	
Nonionic or Low Osmolar Agents							
Ioxaglate	Hexabrix	600	7.5	320	150	Calcium disodium EDTA	Electophysiologic (+) Hemodynamic (+) Anticoagulant (+) Nephrotoxicity (+) Allergic (+)
Iohexol	Omnipaque	844	10.4	350	5	Tromethamine calcium disodium EDTA	
Iopamidol	Isovue	790	9.4	370	2	Tromethamine calcium disodium EDTA	
Ioversol	Optiray	702	5.8	320	2	Tromethamine calcium disodium EDTA	
Iodixanol	Visipaque	290	11.8	320	19	Tromethamine calcium disodium EDTA + 0.15 mEq/liter calcium	

++++ = common; +++ = occasional; ++ = infrequent; + = rare; EDTA = ethylene diaminetetraacetic acid (a divalent cation chelating agent).

Modified from Hill J, Lambert C, Pepine C: Radiographic contrast agents. *In* Pepine C, Hill J, Lambert C (eds): Diagnostic and Therapeutic Cardiac Catheterization. Baltimore, Williams & Wilkins, 1994, pp 182-194.

bradycardia, bronchospasm, or left ventricular dysfunction, can be given intravenous metoprolol, 2.5 to 5.0 mg, or propranolol, 1 to 4 mg. Intraaortic balloon counterpulsation is also a useful adjunct in patients with coronary ischemia and left main CAD, cardiogenic shock, or refractory pulmonary edema.

Contrast Agents

All radiographic contrast agents contain iodine, which effectively absorbs x-rays in the energy range of the angiographic imaging system. Radiographic contrast agents currently used for coronary arteriography may also produce a number of adverse hemodynamic, electrophysiological, and renal effects. The frequency of these side effects varies among the different radiocontrast agents because of differences in their ionic content, osmolality, and viscosity (Table 20-4).

IONIC CONTRAST AGENTS. The monomeric ionic contrast agents initially used for coronary arteriography were the high-osmolar meglumine and sodium salts of diatrizoic acid. These substances dissociated into cations and iodine-containing anions that have a higher serum osmolality (>1500 mOsm) than human plasma (300 mOsm). The hypertonicity of these compounds produced sinus bradycardia, heart block, QT interval and QRS prolongation, ST segment depression, giant T wave inversion, decreased left ventricular contractility, decreased systolic pressure, and increased left ventricular end-diastolic pressure, owing, in part, to the calcium-chelating properties of these agents. Ventricular tachycardia and fibrillation occurred in 0.5 percent of cases and developed more often when ionic contrast agents were injected into a damped (ventricularized) coronary catheter, were given too rapidly, or were administered in too great a volume. Because of the availability of other, less toxic contrast agents, ionic contrast agents are now rarely used for coronary arteriography. When ionic agents are selected, additional precautions are needed to avoid complications. Patients should be counseled about coughing, which helps clear contrast material from within the coronary artery, before the first selective coronary arteriogram is performed and the minimal amount of contrast agent needed to fill the entire coronary artery should be given.

NONIONIC AND LOW-OSMOLAR CONTRAST AGENTS. Nonionic agents do not ionize in solution and provide more iodine-containing particles per milliliter of contrast material than ionic agents. Their osmolality is substantially reduced (<850 mOsm) because these agents exist in solution as single neutral molecules and do not chelate calcium, potentially leading to fewer side effects.

Side Effects. Unwanted reactions may also occur after use of nonionic radiocontrast agents, related in part to the hyperosmolality of these agents. These reactions include hot flushing, nausea, vomiting, and arrhythmia. Hypotension after contrast medium administration may be due to an anaphylactoid reaction, a direct toxic effect, or a vasovagal reaction. Ionic radiocontrast agents may inhibit clot formation when mixed with blood. Although nonionic agents exhibit less of an anticoagulant effect, potentially leading to clots within the manifold where low-osmolar and nonionic contrast agents and blood are in direct contact with one another, the clinical effects of this finding related to embolization of thrombus into the coronary arteries are not known. The low-osmolality ionic dimer methylglucamine-sodium ioxaglate retains most of the anticoagulant properties of diatrizoate sodium but has more complications than the isosmolar, nonionic dimer contrast agent iodixanol. Iodixanol may also be the preferred contrast agent in diabetic patients with underlying renal insufficiency.[18]

CONTRAST-INDUCED NEPHROPATHY. Worsening of renal function may occur after contrast agent administration in 13 to 20 percent of patients, particularly in those with prior renal insufficiency, diabetes mellitus, dehydration before the procedure, CHF, larger volumes of contrast material, and recent (<48 hours) contrast exposure (see also Chap. 88). Fluid administration (with sodium bicarbonate),[19] preprocedural use of *N*-acetylcysteine, and use of the isosmolar contrast agent iodixanol in diabetic patients with underlying renal insufficiency are recommended to prevent this complication.[20]

CONTRAST REACTION PROPHYLAXIS. Reactions to radiocontrast agents are classified as mild (grade I: single episode of emesis, nausea, sneezing, or vertigo), moderate (grade II: hives, multiple episodes of emesis, fevers, or chills), or severe (grade III: clinical shock, bronchospasm, laryngospasm or edema, loss of consciousness, hypotension, hypertension, cardiac arrhythmias, angioedema, or pulmonary edema) (Table 20-5). Although mild or moderate reactions occur in approximately 9.0 percent of patients, severe reactions are uncommon (0.2 to 1.6 percent).[21,22] Contrast reactions may be more difficult to manage in patients receiving beta blocker therapy. Recurrence rates may approach 50 percent on reexposure to contrast agents, and prophylactic use of H_1 and H_2 histamine blocking agents and aspirin therapy has been advocated. In a meta-analysis of nine trials addressing the value of premedication in patients with a history of contrast reactions, there was a 70% reduction in the occurrence of grade III reactions associated with the pretreatment with corticosteroids (from 0.9 to 0.2 percent in premedicated patients; odds ratio = 0.28; 95 percent confidence intervals: 0.13 to 0.60). Although these reductions appear clinically relevant, 100 to 150 patients would require pretreatment to prevent a single contrast-related event, which has led to the recommendations by one group that premedication is not routinely needed.[21] Nevertheless, patients with a suspected severe prior contrast reaction should receive two doses of prednisone, 60 mg (or its equivalent) the night before and again at 2 hours before the procedure. Diphenhydramine, 50 mg, and cimetidine, 300 mg, may also be given before the procedure.

TABLE 20–5	Toxicities Associated with Radiocontrast Agents
Allergic (anaphylactoid) reactions	
Grade I: Single episode of emesis, nausea, sneezing, or vertigo	
Grade II: Hives, multiple episodes of emesis, fevers, or chills	
Grade III: Clinical shock, bronchospasm, laryngospasm or edema, loss of consciousness, hypotension, hypertension, cardiac arrhythmia, angioedema, or pulmonary edema	
Cardiovascular toxicity	
Electrophysiologic	
Bradycardia (asystole, heart block)	
Tachycardia (sinus, ventricular)	
Ventricular fibrillation	
Hemodynamic	
Hypotension (cardiac depression, vasodilation)	
Heart failure (cardiac depression, increased intravascular volume)	
Nephrotoxicity	
Discomfort	
Nausea, vomiting	
Heat and flushing	
Hyperthyroidism	

Anatomy and Variations of the Coronary Arteries

The basic principle of radiographic coronary imaging is that radiation produced by the x-ray tube is attenuated as it passes through the body and detected by the image intensifier (Fig. 20-6). Iodinated contrast medium injected into the coronary arteries enhances the absorption of x-rays and produces a sharp contrast with the surrounding cardiac tissues. The x-ray shadow is then converted into a visible light image by an image intensifier, displayed on fluoroscopic monitors, and stored on 35-mm cinefilm or a digital storage system. Although 35-mm cinefilm has better image resolution (4 line pairs/mm) than digital imaging (2.5 line pairs/mm) archived in a standard DICOM3 512 × 512 × 8 bit pixel matrix format, digital imaging has largely replaced 35-mm cinefilm for coronary angiography because of its versatility with respect to image transfer, low-cost acquisition and storage, and capability for image enhancement after image acquisition. More recently, direct digital imaging systems, termed *flat-panel catheterization laboratories,* have eliminated the analog to digital converters of the conventional image intensifiers without compromise of the image integrity.[23] This has resulted in reduced radiation exposure and enhanced image quality.[1,24]

The major epicardial branches and their second- and third-order branches can be visualized using coronary arteriography. The network of smaller intramyocardial branches generally are not seen because of their size, cardiac motion, and limitations in resolution of cineangiographic systems. These fourth-order and higher "resistance" vessels play a major role in autoregulation of coronary blood flow (see Chap. 48), may limit myocardial perfusion during stress, and contribute to ischemia in patients with left ventricular hypertrophy or systemic hypertension. Coronary perfusion in these smaller branch vessels can be quantitatively assessed using the myocardial blush score which has important prognostic significance in patients with ST segment elevation MI and those undergoing percutaneous coronary intervention.[25]

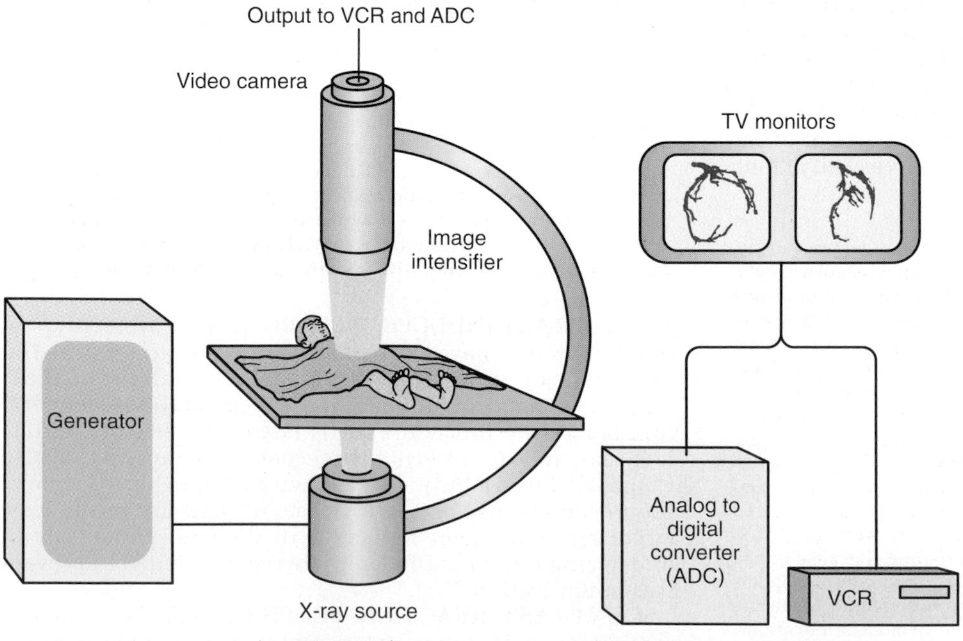

FIGURE 20–6 Cineangiographic equipment. The major components include a generator, x-ray tube, image intensifier attached to a positioner such as a C-arm, optical system, video camera, videocassette recorder (VCR), analog to digital converter (ADC), and television monitors. The x-ray tube is the source of the x-ray beam, which passes superiorly through the patient.

ARTERIAL NOMENCLATURE AND EXTENT OF DISEASE. The Coronary Artery Surgery Study (CASS) investigators established the nomenclature most commonly used to describe the coronary anatomy, defining 27 segments in three major coronary arteries (Table 20-6). The Bypass Angioplasty Revascularization Investigators (BARI) modified these criteria by addition of two segments for the ramus intermedius and the third diagonal branch. In this system, the three

TABLE 20–6 Classification System for Coronary Segments

Number	Map Location	Number	Map Location	Number	Map Location
Right Coronary Artery		**Left Main Coronary Artery**		**Left Circumflex Artery**	
1	Proximal RCA	11	Left main coronary artery	18	Proximal LCx artery
2	Mid RCA	**Left Anterior Descending Artery**		19	Distal LCx artery
3	Distal RCA	12	Proximal LADA	20	1st obtuse marginal
4	Right posterior descending branch	13	Mid LADA	21	2nd obtuse marginal
5	Right posterior atrioventricular	14	Distal LADA	22	Third obtuse marginal
6	First right posterolateral	15	1st diagonal	23	LCx atrioventricular groove
7	Second right posterolateral	16	2nd diagonal	24	1st left posterolateral branch
8	Third right posterolateral	17	LADA septal perforators	25	2nd left posterolateral branch
9	Posterior descending septals	29	3rd diagonal	26	3rd left posterolateral branch
10	Acute marginal segment	27	Left posterior descending branch		
		28	Ramus intermedium branch		

LADA = left anterior descending artery; LCx = left circumflex artery; RCA = right coronary artery.

From CASS Principal Investigators and their Associates: Coronary Artery Surgery Study (CASS): A randomized trial of coronary artery surgery: Survival data. Circulation 68:939, 1983.

major coronary arteries include the left anterior descending (LAD) artery, left circumflex (LCx) artery, and RCA with a right-dominant, balanced, or left-dominant circulation (see later). CAD is defined as a more than 50 percent diameter stenosis in one or more of these vessels, although it is clear that stenoses of less than 50 percent have major prognostic implications because these lesions most commonly lead to plaque rupture and acute MI. Subcritical stenoses of less than 50 percent are best characterized as nonobstructive CAD; obstructive CAD is classified as one-, two-, or three-vessel disease.

A number of "jeopardy scores" were developed to quantitate plaque burden, predict patient-based clinical outcomes, and identify risk factors for the presence of atherosclerosis and its progression.[26] The Califf scoring system divided the coronary circulation into six segments with two points allotted for each coronary stenosis of 75 percent or more (score range: 0 to 12). The Gensini scoring system used an ordinal ranking based on stenosis severity in 11 coronary segments (score range: 0 to 72). The Candell-Riera scoring system used an ordinal ranking (from 1 to 5) of 13 coronary segments (score range: 0 to 65). Differences between these scoring systems were primarily related to definitions rather than to their ability to provide unique prognostic information, as one comparative study found that 80 percent of the prognostic information in one jeopardy index was obtained with other indices using subtly different methodologies. In CASS, the major determinants of 6-year outcome included the number of diseased vessels, the number of diseased proximal segments, and the global left ventricular function; these three factors accounted for 80 percent of the prognostic information.

ANGIOGRAPHIC PROJECTIONS. The major coronary arteries traverse the interventricular and atrioventricular grooves, aligned with the long and short axes of the heart, respectively. Because the heart is oriented obliquely in the thoracic cavity, the coronary circulation is generally visualized in the right anterior oblique (RAO) and left anterior oblique (LAO) projections to furnish true posteroanterior and lateral views of the heart, but these views are limited by vessel foreshortening and superimposition of branches. Simultaneous rotation of the x-ray beam in the sagittal plane provides a better view of the major coronary arteries and their branches. A simple nomenclature has evolved for the description of these sagittal views, which characterizes the relationship between the image intensifier and the patient. Assuming that the x-ray tube is under the patient's table and the image intensifier is over the patient's table, the projection is referred to as the "cranial" view if the image intensifier is tilted toward the head of the patient (Figs. 20-7 and 20-8). The projection is referred to as the "caudal" view if the image intensifier is tilted down toward the feet of the patient.

It is difficult to predict which angulated views will be most useful for any particular patient because the "optimal" angiographic projection depends largely on body habitus, variation in the coronary anatomy, and location of the lesion. It is recommended that the coronary arteries be visualized in both the LAO and RAO projections using both cranial and caudal angulation.

Left Coronary Artery

CANNULATION. The Judkins left 4.0 coronary catheter is used most often to engage the LCA (Fig. 20-9). If the Judkins left catheter begins to turn out of profile (so that one or both curves of the catheter are no longer visualized en face), it can be rotated clockwise very slightly and advanced slowly to enter the left sinus of Valsalva, permitting the catheter tip to engage the ostium of the LCA. When the ascending aorta is dilated or the aortic arch is unfolded, advancement of the Judkins left 4.0 coronary catheter may result in the formation of an acute secondary angle of the catheter, pointing the tip of the catheter upward, away from the left coronary ostium. Further advancement of the Judkins left catheter in this position should be avoided because the catheter then prolapses on itself and becomes folded in the ascending aortic arch. In the event this occurs, a guidewire can be temporarily reinserted into the catheter to straighten the secondary bend and permit the catheter to be advanced to the left sinus of Valsalva. If the ascending aorta is significantly dilated, the Judkins left 4.0 catheter should be exchanged for a larger size (e.g., Judkins left 5.0 or 6.0). If the tip of the Judkins left catheter advances beyond the ostium of the LCA without engagement, the primary bend of the catheter can be reshaped within the patient's body by further careful advancement and prompt withdrawal of the catheter, allowing the tip to "pop into" the ostium of the LCA. This maneuver, along with gentle clock-

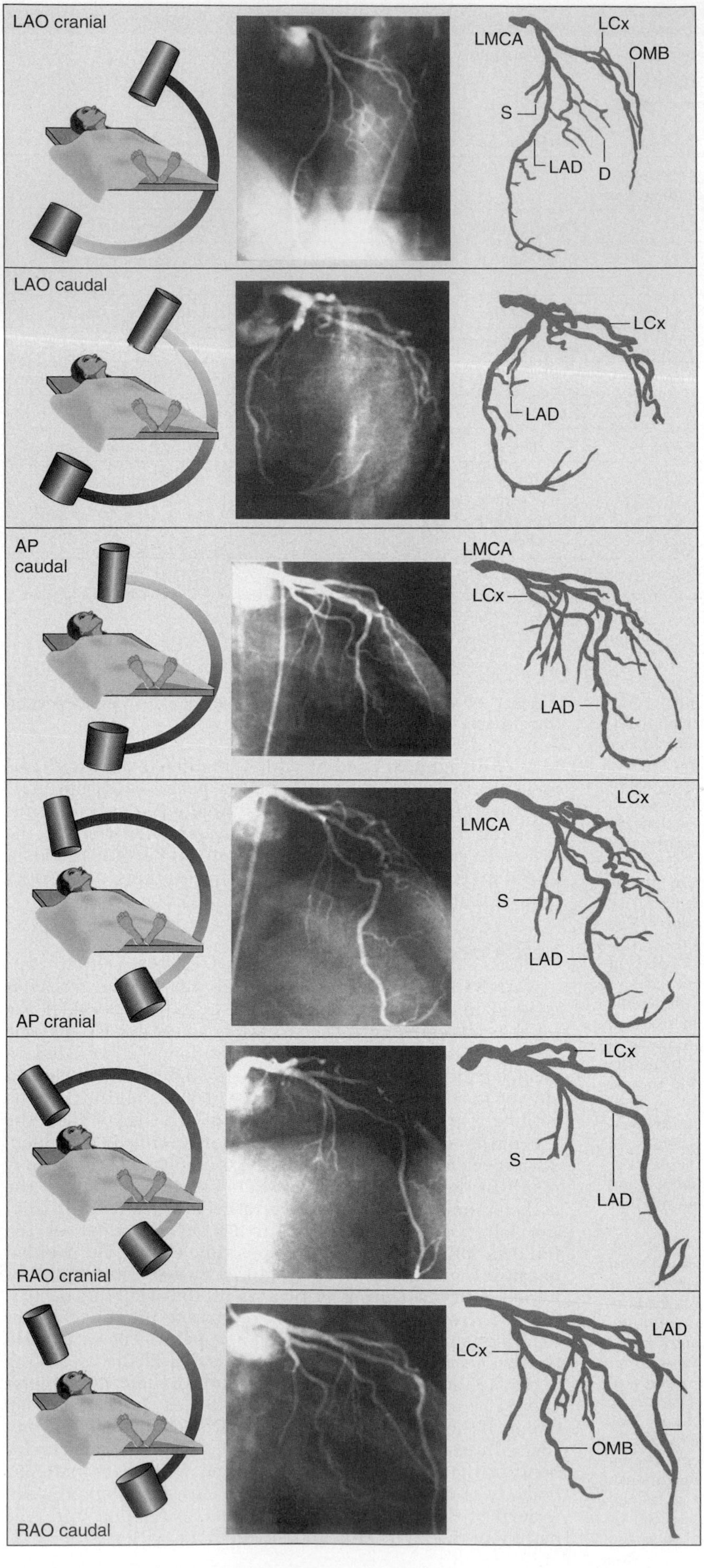

FIGURE 20–7 Angiographic views of the left coronary artery. The approximate positions of the x-ray tube and image intensifier are shown for each of the commonly used angiographic views. The 60-degree left anterior oblique (LAO) view with 20 degrees of cranial angulation (LAO cranial) shows the ostium and distal portion of the left main coronary artery (LMCA), the middle and distal portions of the left anterior descending (LAD) artery, septal perforators (S), diagonal branches (D), and the proximal left circumflex (LCx) and superior obtuse marginal branch (OMB). The 60-degree left anterior oblique view with 25 degrees of caudal angulation (LAO caudal) shows the proximal LMCA and the proximal segments of the LAD and LCx arteries. The anteroposterior (AP) projection with 20 degrees of caudal angulation (AP caudal) shows the distal LMCA and proximal segments of the LAD and LCx arteries. The anteroposterior (AP) projection with 20 degrees of cranial angulation (AP cranial) also shows the mid-portion of the LAD artery and its septal (S) branches. The 30-degree right anterior oblique (RAO) projection with 20 degrees of cranial angulation (RAO cranial) shows the course of the LAD artery and its septal (S) and diagonal branches. The 30-degree right anterior oblique projection with 25 degrees of caudal angulation (RAO caudal) shows the LCx and obtuse marginal branches (OMB).

wise or counterclockwise rotation, frequently permits selective engagement of the LCA when the initial attempt has failed. If the catheter tip is located below the origin of the LCA, as in the case of a smaller aortic root, a shorter Judkins left 3.5 catheter can be used to allow coaxial engagement of the LCA.

Use of the Amplatz left catheters to cannulate the LCA requires more catheter manipulation than with the standard Judkins left catheter. In this circumstance, the broad secondary curve of the Amplatz left 1 or 2 catheter is positioned so that it rests on the right aortic cusp with its tip pointing toward the left aortic cusp. Alternating advancement and retraction of the catheter with slight clockwise rotation allows the catheter tip to advance slowly and superiorly along the left sinus of Valsalva to enter the left coronary ostium. When the tip enters the ostium, the position of the catheter can usually be stabilized with slight retraction of the catheter. After the left coronary ostium has been cannulated, the pressure at the tip of the catheter should be checked immediately to ensure that there is no damping or ventricularization of the pressure contour. If a damped or ventricularized pressure tracing is obtained, the catheter should be removed immediately from the LCA, and an attempt at repositioning should be made. If abnormal pressure recording persists, the catheter should be withdrawn from the coronary artery and a nonselective injection of contrast medium into the LCA should be performed in the anteroposterior (AP) view to evaluate the LMCA. If the pressure measured at the catheter tip is normal and a test injection of contrast agent suggests the absence of LMCA disease, left coronary arteriography is then performed using standard techniques. To remove the Amplatz left catheter from the coronary artery, the catheter should be advanced forward in the body to disengage the catheter tip superiorly from the coronary ostium. Simply withdrawing the Amplatz left catheter results in deep seating of the catheter tip within the coronary artery, potentially resulting in catheter-induced arterial dissection.

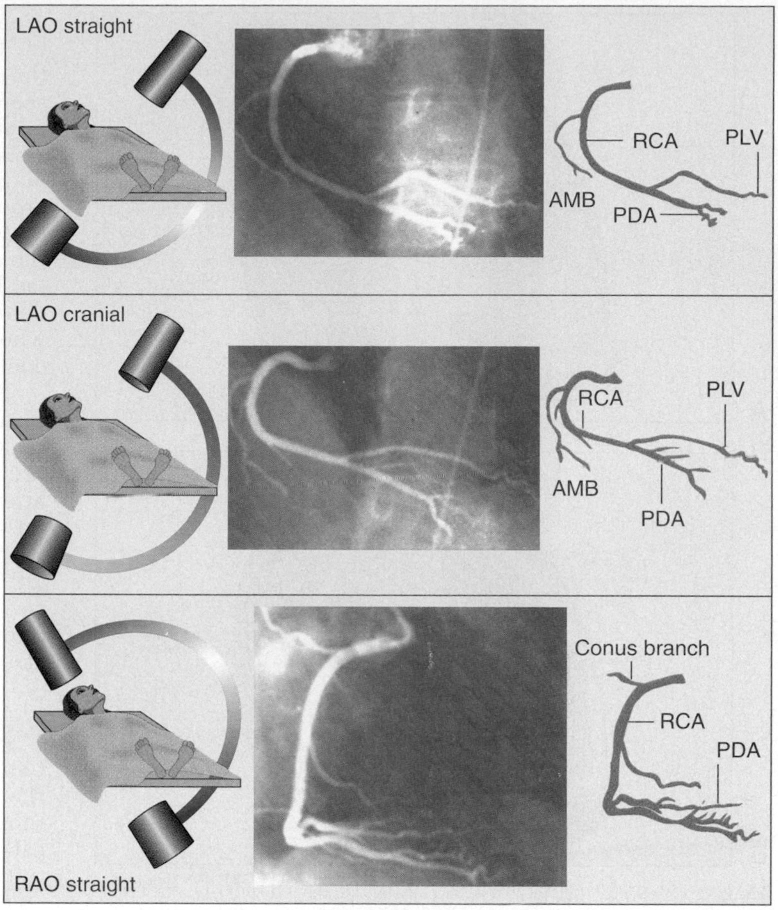

FIGURE 20–8 Angiographic views of the right coronary artery (RCA). The approximate positions of the x-ray tube and image intensifier are shown for each of the commonly used angiographic views. The 60-degree left anterior oblique view (LAO straight) shows the proximal and mid-portions of the RCA as well as the acute marginal branches (AMB) and termination of the RCA in the posterior left ventricular branches (PLV). The 60-degree left anterior oblique view with 25 degrees of cranial angulation (LAO cranial) shows the mid-portion of the RCA and the origin and course of the posterior descending artery (PDA). The 30-degree right anterior oblique view (RAO) shows the mid-portion of the RCA, the conus branch, and the course of the PDA.

LEFT MAIN CORONARY ARTERY. The LMCA arises from the superior portion of the left aortic sinus, just below the sinotubular ridge of the aorta, which defines the border separating the left sinus of Valsalva from the smooth (tubular) portion of the aorta. The LMCA ranges from 3 to 6 mm in diameter and may be up to 10 to 15 mm in length. The LMCA courses behind the right ventricular outflow tract and usually bifurcates into the LAD artery and LCx branches. Rarely, the LMCA is absent, and there are separate ostia of the LAD and LCx arteries. The LMCA is best visualized in the AP projection with slight (0 to 20 degrees) caudal angulation, but it should be viewed in several projections with the vessel off the spine to exclude LMCA stenosis (Figs. 20-10 and 20-11).

LEFT ANTERIOR DESCENDING ARTERY. The LAD courses along the epicardial surface of the anterior interventricular groove toward the cardiac apex. In the RAO projection, it extends along the anterior aspect of the heart; in the LAO projection, it passes down the cardiac midline, between the right and left ventricles (see Fig. 20-7).

The major branches of the LAD are the septal and diagonal branches. The septal branches arise from the LAD at approximately 90-degree angles and pass into the interventricular septum, varying in size, number, and distribution. In some cases there is a large first septal branch that is vertically oriented and divides into a number of secondary "pitch forking" branches that ramify throughout the septum. In other cases, a more horizontally oriented, large first septal branch is present that passes parallel to the LAD itself within the myocardium. In still other cases, a number of septal arteries are roughly comparable in size. These septal branches interconnect with similar septal branches passing upward from the posterior descending branch of the RCA to produce a network of potential collateral channels. The interventricular septum is the most densely vascularized area of the heart.

The diagonal branches of the LAD pass over the anterolateral aspect of the heart. Although virtually all patients have a single LAD in the anterior interventricular groove, there is wide variability in the number and size of diagonal branches. Most patients (90 percent) have one to three diagonal branches, and acquired atherosclerotic occlusion of the diagonal branches should be suspected if no diagonal branches are seen, particularly if there are unexplained contraction abnormalities of the anterolateral left ventricle. Visualization of the origin of the diagonal branches often requires very steep (50 to 60 degrees) LAO and angulated cranial (20 to 40 degrees) skews.

In some patients, the LMCA trifurcates into the LAD, LCx, and ramus intermedius. When present, the ramus intermedius arises between the LAD and LCx arteries. This vessel is analogous to either a diagonal branch or an obtuse marginal branch, depending on its anterior or posterior course along the lateral aspect of the left ventricle. In most patients (80 percent), the LAD courses around the left ventricular apex and terminates along the diaphragmatic aspect of the left ventricle. In the remaining patients, the LAD fails to reach the diaphragmatic surface, terminating instead either at or before the cardiac apex. In this circumstance, the posterior descending branch (PDA) of

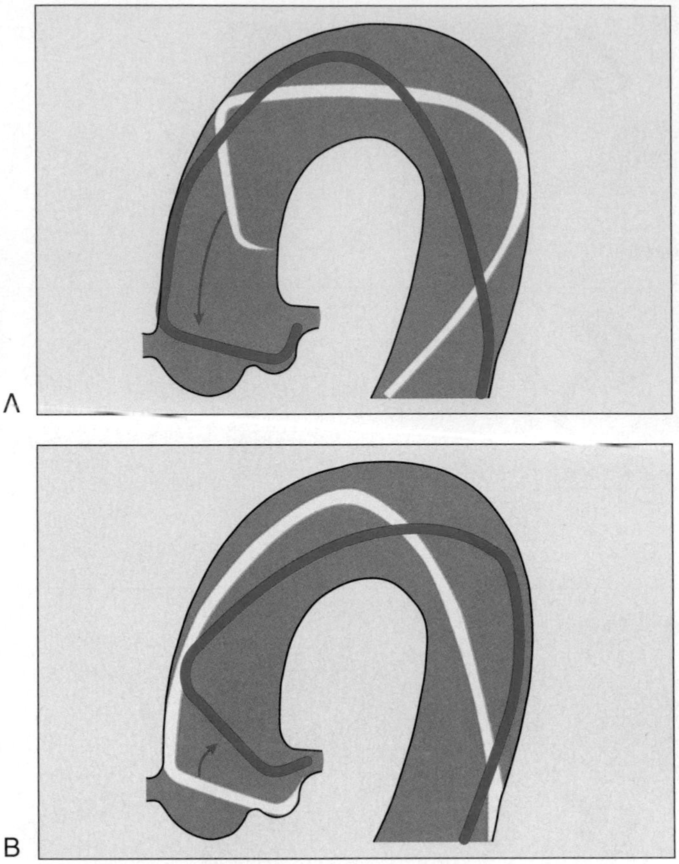

FIGURE 20–9 Push-pull technique for catheterizing the left coronary artery with the Judkins left catheter. In the left anterior oblique view, the coronary catheter is positioned in the ascending aorta over a guidewire and the guidewire is removed. The catheter is advanced so that the tip enters the left sinus of Valsalva. If the catheter does not selectively engage the ostium of the left coronary artery, further slow advancement into the left sinus of Valsalva imparts a temporary acute angle at the catheter. Prompt withdrawal of the catheter allows easy entry into the left coronary artery.

the RCA or LCx is larger and longer than usual and supplies the apical portion of the ventricle.

The best angiographic projections for viewing the course of the LAD are the cranially angulated LAO, AP, and RAO views. The LAO cranial view displays the mid-portion of the LAD and separates the diagonal and septal branches. The RAO cranial view displays the proximal, middle, and distal segment of the LAD and allows separation of the diagonal branches superiorly and the septal branches inferiorly. The AP view requiring cranial (20 to 40 degrees) skew often projects the mid-portion of the LAD, separating the vessel from its diagonal and septal branches. The LAO caudal view also displays the origin of the LAD in a horizontally oriented heart, and the AP caudal or shallow RAO caudal view visualizes the proximal LAD as it arises from the LMCA. The RAO caudal projection is also useful for visualizing the distal LAD and its apical termination.

In some patients with no LMCA but separate ostia for the LAD and LCx, the LAD generally has a more anterior origin than the LCx. The LAD can be engaged with the Judkins left catheter in this setting with paradoxical counterclockwise rotation, which rotates the secondary bend of the catheter to a posterior position in the aorta and turns the primary bend and tip of the catheter to an anterior position. The opposite maneuver may be used to engage the LCx selectively in the setting of separate LAD and LCx ostia. A Judkins catheter, such as a Judkins left 5.0 with a larger curve, selectively engages the downward coursing LCx, and a catheter with shorter curve, such as a Judkins left 3.5, tends to engage selectively the more anterior and superior LAD.

LEFT CIRCUMFLEX ARTERY. The LCx artery originates from the LMCA and courses within the posterior (left) atrioventricular groove toward the inferior interventricular groove (see Fig. 20-7). The LCx artery is the dominant vessel in 15 percent of patients, supplying the left PDA from the distal continuation of the LCx. In the remaining vessels, the distal LCx varies in size and length, depending on the number of posterolateral branches supplied by the distal RCA. The LCx usually gives off one to three large obtuse marginal branches as it passes down the atrioventricular groove. These are the principal branches of the LCx because they supply the lateral free wall of the left ventricle. Beyond the origins of the obtuse marginal branches, the distal LCx tends to be small. The actual position of the LCx can be determined on the late phase of a left coronary injection when the coronary sinus becomes opacified with diluted contrast material.

The RAO caudal and LAO caudal projections are best for visualizing the proximal and middle LCx and obtuse marginal branches. The AP (or 5- to 15-degree RAO) caudal projections also show the origins of the obtuse marginal branches. More severe rightward angulation often superimposes the origins of the obtuse marginal branches on the LCx. If the LCA is dominant, the optimal projection for the left PDA is the LAO cranial view. The LCx artery also gives rise to one or two left atrial circumflex branches. These branches supply the lateral and posterior aspects of the left atrium.

Right Coronary Artery

Cannulation of the origin of the RCA is also performed in the LAO position but requires different maneuvers than those for cannulation of the LCA. Whereas the Judkins left catheter naturally seeks the ostium of the LCA, the Judkins right or modified Amplatz catheters must be rotated to engage the vessel. This is usually accomplished by first passing the catheter to a point just superior to the aortic valve in the left sinus of Valsalva with the tip of the catheter facing rightward and then rotating the catheter clockwise while withdrawing the catheter slightly, which forces the tip to move anteriorly from the left sinus of Valsalva to the right sinus of Valsalva along the sinotubular ridge (Fig. 20-12). Sudden rightward and downward movement of the catheter tip signifies the entry into the right coronary ostium. If the ostium of the RCA is not easily located, the most common reason is that the ostium has a more superior and anterior origin than anticipated. Repeated attempts to engage the RCA should be made at a level slightly more distal to the aortic valve. Nonselective contrast agent injections in the right sinus of Valsalva may reveal the site of the origin of the RCA. Positioning an Amplatz left catheter in the ostium of the RCA requires a technique similar to that used with the Judkins right catheter. If a gentle attempt to withdraw the Amplatz catheter results in paradoxical deep entry into the coronary artery, removal of the catheter can be achieved by clockwise or counterclockwise rotation and advancement to prolapse the catheter into the aortic sinus.

An abnormal pressure tracing showing damping or ventricularization may suggest the presence of an ostial stenosis or spasm, selective engagement of the conus branch, or deep intubation of the RCA. If an abnormal pressure tracing has been encountered, the catheter tip should be gently rotated counterclockwise and withdrawn slightly in an effort to free the tip of the catheter. If persistent damping occurs, a very small amount of contrast medium (<1 ml) can be injected carefully and the catheter immediately withdrawn in a "shoot-and-run" maneuver, which may allow the cause of damping to be identified. The frequency of ventricular fibrillation and iatrogenic coronary dissection are higher when the RCA is injected in the presence of a damped pressure tracing. If the pressure tracing is normal on entry into the RCA, the vessel should be imaged in at least two

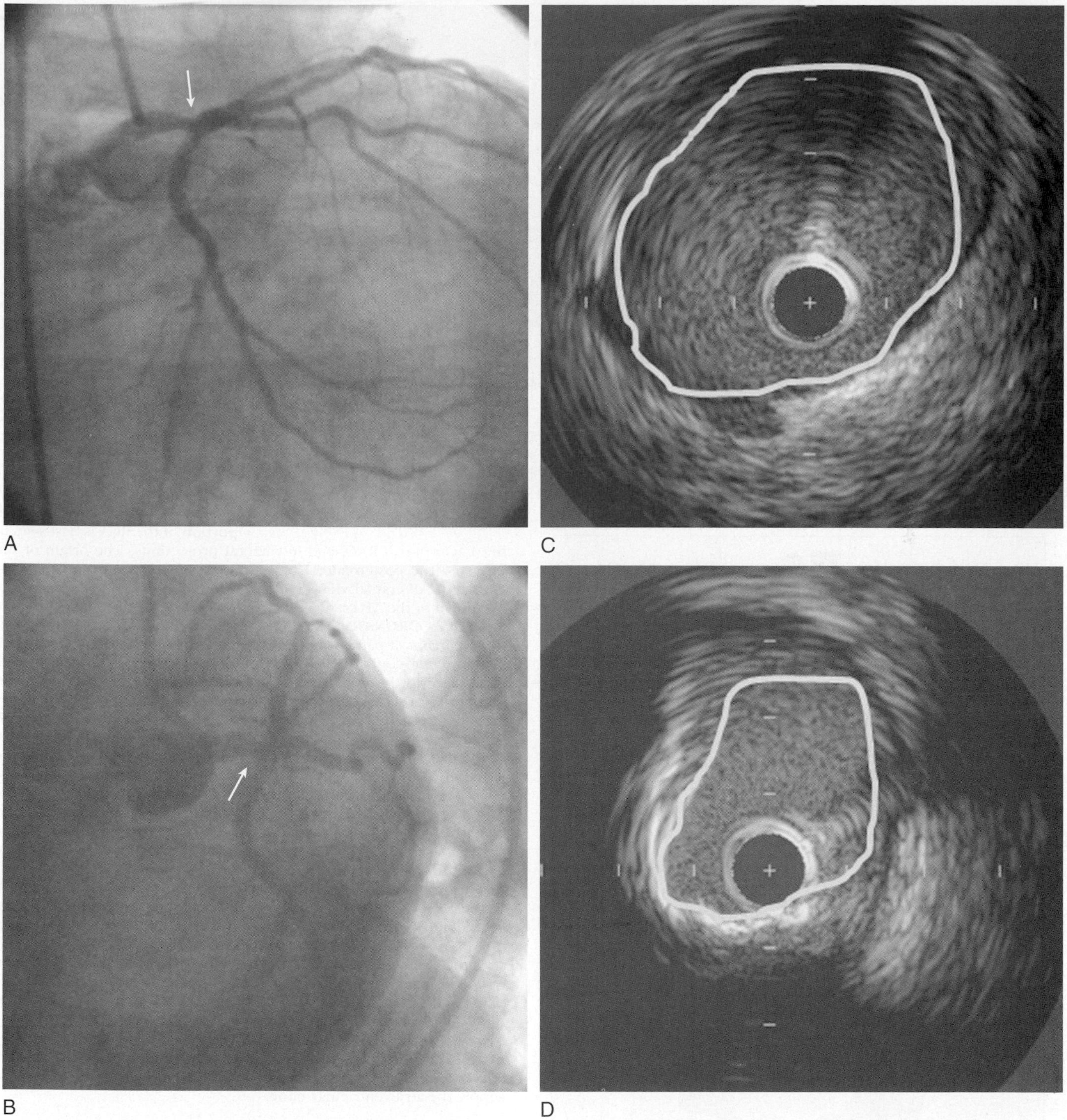

FIGURE 20–10 Intermediate left main coronary artery (LMCA) stenosis evaluated with intravascular ultrasound (IVUS). **A,** Left coronary arteriography in the standard right anterior oblique projection with caudal angulation (arrow indicates distal left main coronary artery). **B,** The left anterior oblique projection with caudal angulation shows a tapered stenosis of the LMCA (arrow). **C,** IVUS of the proximal LMCA shows a minimal cross-sectional area 16 mm^2 (white circle). **D,** IVUS of the distal LMCA shows an LMCA stenosis with a lumenal cross-sectional area = 6.5 mm^2 (white outline), which is consistent with a hemodynamically significant LMCA stenosis.

projections. The initial injection should be gentle because of the possibility that forceful injection through a catheter whose tip is immediately adjacent to the vessel wall may also lead to dissection. Coronary spasm of the RCA ostium may also occur as a result of catheter intubation. When an ostial stenosis of the RCA is seen, intracoronary nitroglycerin or calcium channel antagonists may be useful in excluding catheter-induced spasm as a cause of the coronary artery narrowing.

The RCA originates from the right anterior aortic sinus somewhat inferior to the origin of the LCA (see Fig. 20-8). It passes along the right atrioventricular groove toward the crux (a point on the diaphragmatic surface of the heart where the anterior atrioventricular groove, the posterior atrioventricular groove, and the inferior interventricular groove coalesce. The first branch of the RCA is generally the conus artery, which arises at the right coronary ostium or within the first few millimeters of the RCA in about 50 percent of patients. In the remaining patients, the conus artery arises from a separate ostium in the right aortic sinus just above the right coronary ostium. The second branch

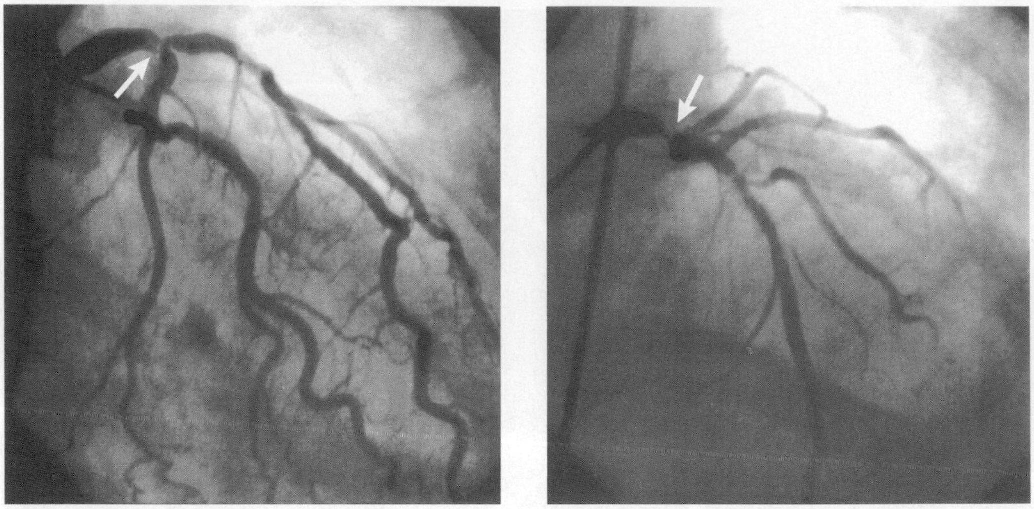

A B

FIGURE 20–11 Severe stenosis of the distal left main coronary artery. **A,** Right anterior oblique projection with caudal angulation demonstrates a severe ulcerated stenosis in the distal portion of the left main coronary artery (arrow). **B,** An anteroposterior view with cranial angulation demonstrates this stenosis in a second view. Limited coronary arteriography should be performed when severe left main coronary artery stenosis (arrow) has been demonstrated.

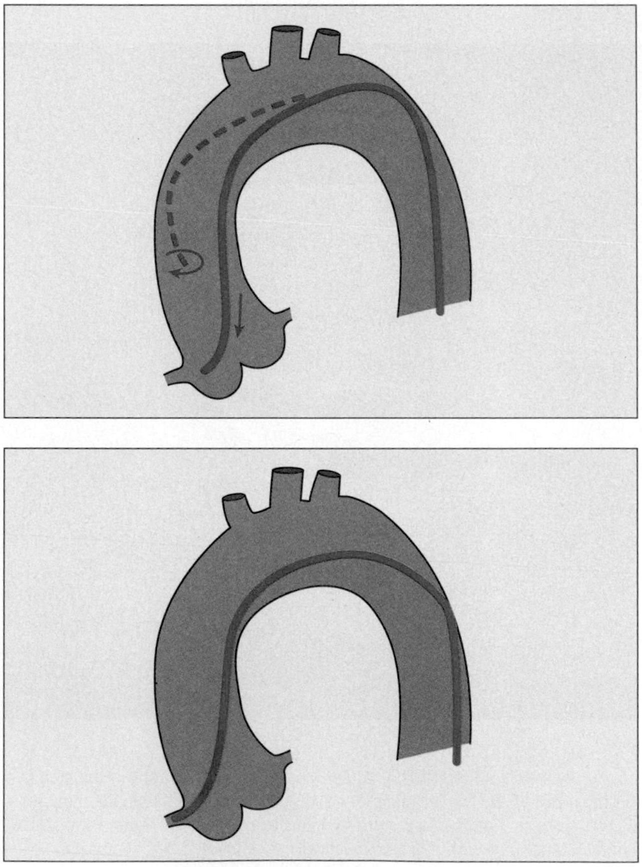

A B

FIGURE 20–12 Cannulation of the right coronary artery using the Judkins right catheter. **A,** The catheter is advanced to a point just superior to the aortic valve in the left sinus of Valsalva with the tip of the catheter facing rightward, and then the catheter is rotated clockwise while withdrawing the catheter slightly. **B,** Sudden rightward and downward movement of the catheter tip signifies the entry into the right coronary ostium.

of the RCA is usually the sinoatrial node artery. It has been found that this vessel arises from the RCA in just under 60 percent of patients, from the LCx artery in just under 40 percent, and from both arteries with a dual blood supply in the remaining cases. The mid-portion of the RCA usually gives rise to one or several medium-sized acute marginal branches. These branches supply the anterior wall of the right ventricle and may provide collateral circulation in patients with LAD occlusion. The RCA terminates in a PDA and one or more right posterolateral branches.

Because the RCA traverses both the atrioventricular and the interventricular grooves, multiple angiographic projections are needed to visualize each segment of the RCA. The ostium of the RCA is best evaluated in the LAO views, with or without cranial or caudal angulation. The left lateral view is also useful for visualizing the ostium of the RCA in difficult cases. The ostium is identified by the reflux of contrast material from the RCA that also delineates the aortic root with swirling of contrast in the region of the ostium. The proximal RCA is generally evaluated in the LAO cranial or LAO caudal projections but is markedly foreshortened in the RAO projections. The mid-portion of the RCA is best seen in the LAO cranial, RAO, and left lateral projections. The origin of the PDA and the posterolateral branches are best evaluated in the LAO cranial or AP cranial views, whereas the mid-portion of the PDA can be shown in the AP cranial or RAO projection.

RIGHT CORONARY ARTERY DOMINANCE. The RCA is dominant in 85 percent of patients, supplying the PDA and at least one posterolateral branch (right dominant) (Figs. 20-13 to 20-15). The PDA courses in the inferior interventricular groove and gives rise to a number of small inferior septal branches, which pass upward to supply the lower portion of the interventricular septum and interdigitate with superior septal branches passing down from the LAD artery. After giving rise to the PDA, the dominant RCA continues beyond the crux cordis (the junction of the atrioventricular and interventricular grooves) as the right posterior atrioventricular branch along the distal portion of the posterior (left) atrioventricular groove, terminating in one or several posterolateral branches that supply the diaphragmatic surface of the left ventricle. The RCA is nondominant in 15 percent of patients. One half of these patients have a left PDA and left posterolateral branches that are provided by the distal LCx artery (left dominant circulation). In these cases, the RCA is very small, terminates before reaching the crux, and does not supply any blood to the left ventricular myocardium. The remaining patients have an RCA that gives rise to the PDA with the LCx artery providing all the posterolateral branches (balanced or codominant circulation). In about 25 percent of patients with RCA dominance, there are significant anatomical variations in the origin of the PDA. These variations include partial supply of the PDA territory by acute marginal branches, double PDA, and early origin of the PDA proximal to the crux. At or near the crux, the dominant artery gives rise to a small atrioventricular node artery, which passes upward to supply the atrioventricular node.

CORONARY BYPASS GRAFTS. Selective cannulation of bypass grafts may be more challenging than cannulation of the native coronary arteries because the locations of graft ostia are more variable, even when surgical clips or ostia markers are used. Knowledge of the number, course, and type of bypass grafts obtained from the operative report is invaluable for the identification of the location of the bypass grafts during arteriography.

SAPHENOUS VEIN GRAFTS. SVGs from the aorta to the distal RCA or PDA originate from the right anterolateral aspect of the aorta approximately 5 cm superior to the sinotubular ridge. SVGs to the LAD artery (or diagonal branches) originate from the anterior portion of the aorta about 7 cm superior to the sinotubular ridge. SVGs to the obtuse marginal branches arise from the left anterolateral aspect of the aorta 9 to 10 cm superior to the sinotubular ridge. In most

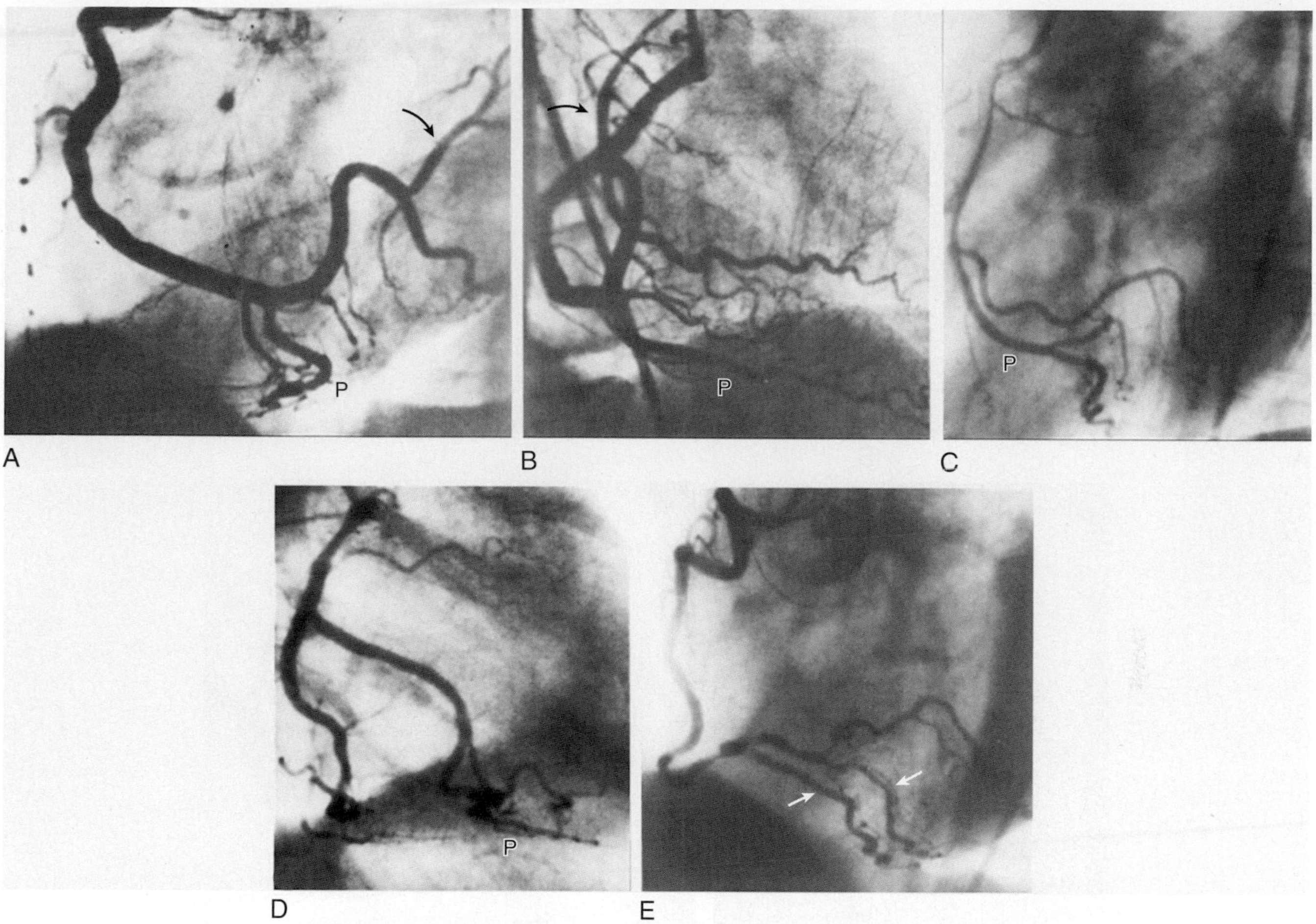

FIGURE 20–13 Strongly dominant right coronary artery (RCA). **A** and **B,** Left anterior oblique and right anterior oblique views of the RCA show that the distal segment (arrows) extends to the left atrioventricular groove. After giving rise to the posterior descending artery, the RCA gives rise to multiple posterior left ventricular branches. **C,** A variation in the origin of the posterior descending artery, which originates early from the RCA, runs parallel to it, and enters the posterior interventricular groove. **D,** Right anterior oblique right coronary arteriogram showing the posterior descending artery (P) arising from a right ventricular branch of the RCA. **E,** Left anterior oblique right coronary arteriogram showing duplicated posterior descending arteries (arrows). *(From Levin DC, Baltaxe HA: Angiographic demonstration of important anatomic variations of the posterior descending artery. AJR 116:41, 1972.)*

patients, all SVGs can be engaged with a single catheter, such as a Judkins right 4.0 or a modified Amplatz right 1 or 2. Other catheters useful for engaging SVGs include the right and left bypass graft catheters. Amplatz left 1 to 2 catheters are useful for superiorly oriented SVGs (see Fig. 20-4). A multipurpose catheter may also be useful for the cannulation of the downward takeoff SVG to the RCA or PDA.

Viewed in the LAO projection, the Judkins right 4 or Amplatz right 2 catheters rotate anteriorly from the leftward position as the catheter is rotated in a clockwise direction. The relation between the movement of catheter shaft at the femoral artery and the response of catheter tip on fluoroscopy immediately indicates whether the catheter tip is anteriorly positioned in the aorta and likely to enter an SVG ostium or posteriorly positioned and unlikely to engage an SVG. Steady advancement and withdrawal of the catheter tip proximal and distal in the ascending aorta, 5 to 10 cm above the sinotubular ridge, with varying degrees of rotation, usually result in entry into the SVG. Entry into the SVG is associated with abrupt outward motion of the tip of the catheter. When this occurs, a small test injection of contrast material verifies that the catheter is in the SVG. A well-circumscribed "stump" is almost always present if the SVG is occluded. Each SVG or stump must be viewed in nearly orthogonal views. The relation between the origin of the SVGs and surgical clips confirms whether all targeted SVGs have been visualized. If neither a patent SVG nor a stump can be located, it may be necessary to perform an ascending aortogram (preferably in biplane) in an attempt to visualize all SVGs and their course to the coronary arteries.

The goal of SVG angiography is to assess the ostium of the SVG, its entire course, and the distal insertion ("touchdown") site at the anastomosis between the bypass SVG and the native coronary vessel. The ostium of a SVG must be evaluated by achieving a coaxial engagement of the catheter tip and the origin of the SVG. The mid-portion (body) of the SVG must be evaluated with complete contrast filling of the SVG because inadequate opacification produces an angiographic artifact suggestive of friable filling defects. It is critical to assess the SVG insertion or anastomotic site in full profile without any overlap of the distal SVG or the native vessel. Angiographic assessment of the native vessels beyond SVG anastomotic sites requires views that are conventionally used for the native segments themselves. Sequential grafts are those that supply two different epicardial branches in a side-to-side fashion (for the more proximal epicardial artery) and terminating in an end-to-side anastomosis (for the more distal epicardial artery). A "Y" graft is one in which there is a proximal anastomosis in an end-to-side fashion to another saphenous vein or arterial graft with two distal end-to-side anatomoses to the two epicardial grafts from these two grafts.

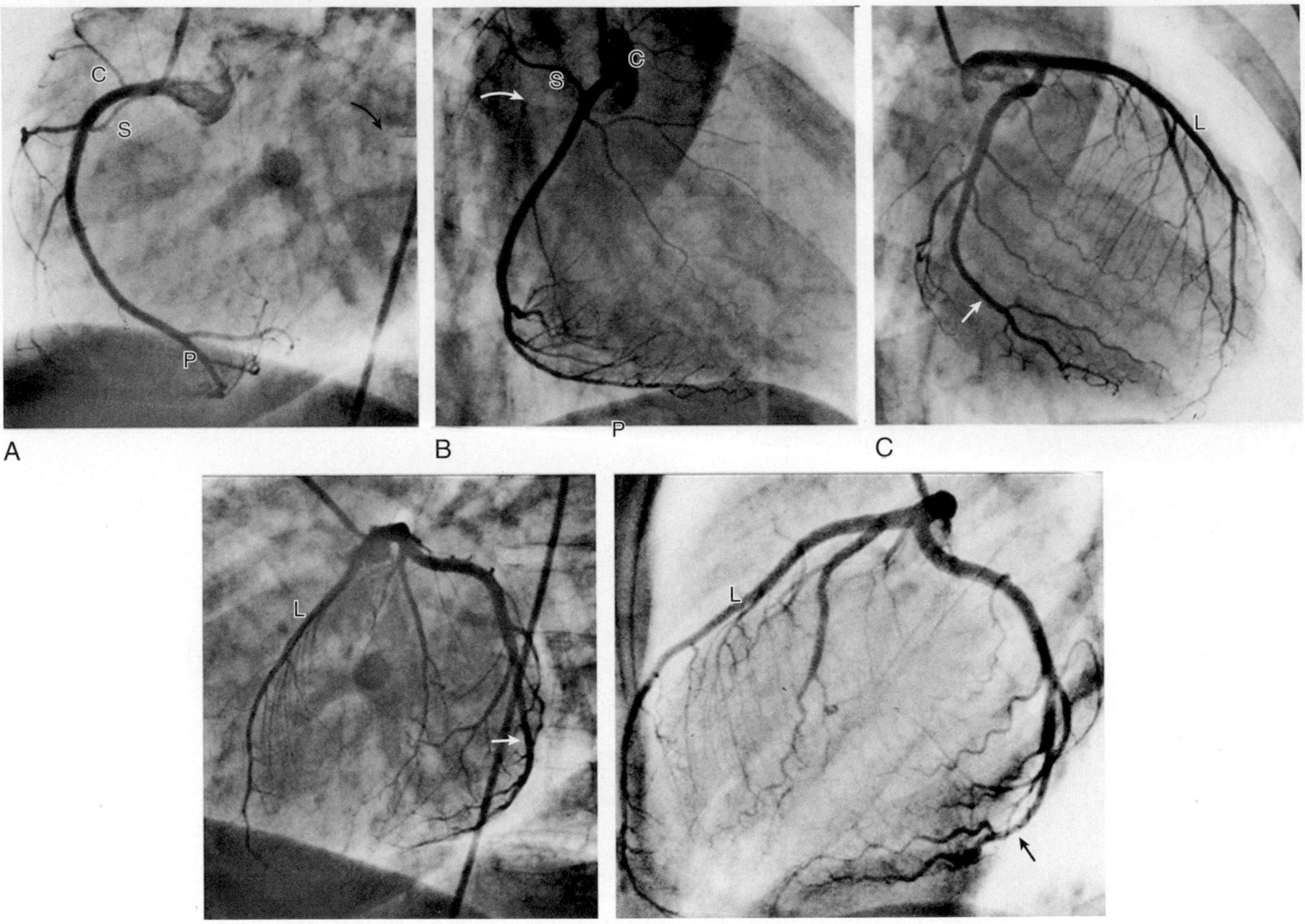

A B C D E

FIGURE 20–14 Weakly dominant right coronary artery (RCA). **A** and **B,** Left anterior oblique and right anterior oblique views of the RCA. Both the conus and sinoatrial node artery arise from the RCA. The distal portion of the RCA beyond the origin of the posterior descending artery is short and gives rise to a single small posterior left ventricular branch (arrow indicates left atrium). **C** to **E,** Left coronary artery in the right anterior oblique, left anterior oblique, and left lateral projections. Note that the circumflex artery gives rise to four obtuse marginal branches, the most distal of which (arrow) supplies some of the diaphragmatic surface of the left ventricle. The left anterior descending artery gives rise to two small and one medium-sized diagonal branches. C = conus branch; L = left anterior descending artery; P = posterior descending artery; S = sinoatrial nodal artery.

INTERNAL MAMMARY ARTERY. The left IMA arises inferiorly from the left subclavian artery approximately 10 cm from its origin. Catheterization of the left IMA is performed with a specially designed J-tip IMA catheter (see Fig. 20-3, bottom row). The catheter is advanced into the aortic arch distal to the origin of the left subclavian artery in the LAO projection and then rotated counterclockwise and is gently withdrawn with the tip pointing in a cranial direction, allowing entry into the left subclavian artery (Fig. 20-16). A 0.035 J or angled Terumo guidewire is advanced to the left subclavian artery under fluoroscopy, and the catheter is advanced into the subclavian artery. The RAO or AP projections then can be used to cannulate the IMA selectively by withdrawing and slightly rotating the catheter anteriorly (counterclockwise) with the tip down. The right IMA can also be cannulated with the IMA catheter. The innominate artery is entered in the LAO projection, and the guidewire is advanced cautiously to avoid entry into the right common carotid artery. When the guidewire is positioned in the distal right subclavian artery, the IMA catheter is advanced to a point distal to the expected origin of the right IMA. The catheter is withdrawn in the LAO view and rotated to cannulate the right IMA.

The IMA itself is rarely affected by atherosclerosis. Angiographic studies of the IMAs should assess not only the patency of the graft itself but also the distal anastomosis, where most IMA graft compromise occurs. Although the LAO cranial view may be limited in its ability to demonstrate the anastomosis of the IMA and the LAD because of vessel overlap, the left lateral or AP cranial projection usually provides adequate visualization of the left LIMA-LAD anastomotic site. The risk of catheter-induced dissection of the origin of the IMA can be reduced by careful manipulation of the catheter tip and avoidance of forceful advancement without the protection of the guidewire. If the IMA cannot be selectively engaged because of tortuosity of the subclavian artery, nonselective arteriography can be enhanced by placing a blood pressure cuff on the ipsilateral arm and inflating it to a pressure above systolic arterial pressure. Alternatively, the ipsilateral brachial or radial artery may be used to facilitate coaxial IMA engagement. IMA spasm can be treated with 50 to 200 μg of intraarterial nitroglycerin or 50 to 100 μg of intraarterial verapamil. The patient may feel chest warmth or discomfort with contrast injection due to injection into small IMA branches supplying the chest wall.

GASTROEPIPLOIC ARTERY. The right gastroepiploic artery (GEA) is the largest terminal artery of the gastroduodenal artery and was briefly used as an alternative in situ arterial conduit to the PDA in patients undergoing CABG. The gastroduodenal artery arises from the common hepatic artery in 75 percent of cases, but it may also arise from the

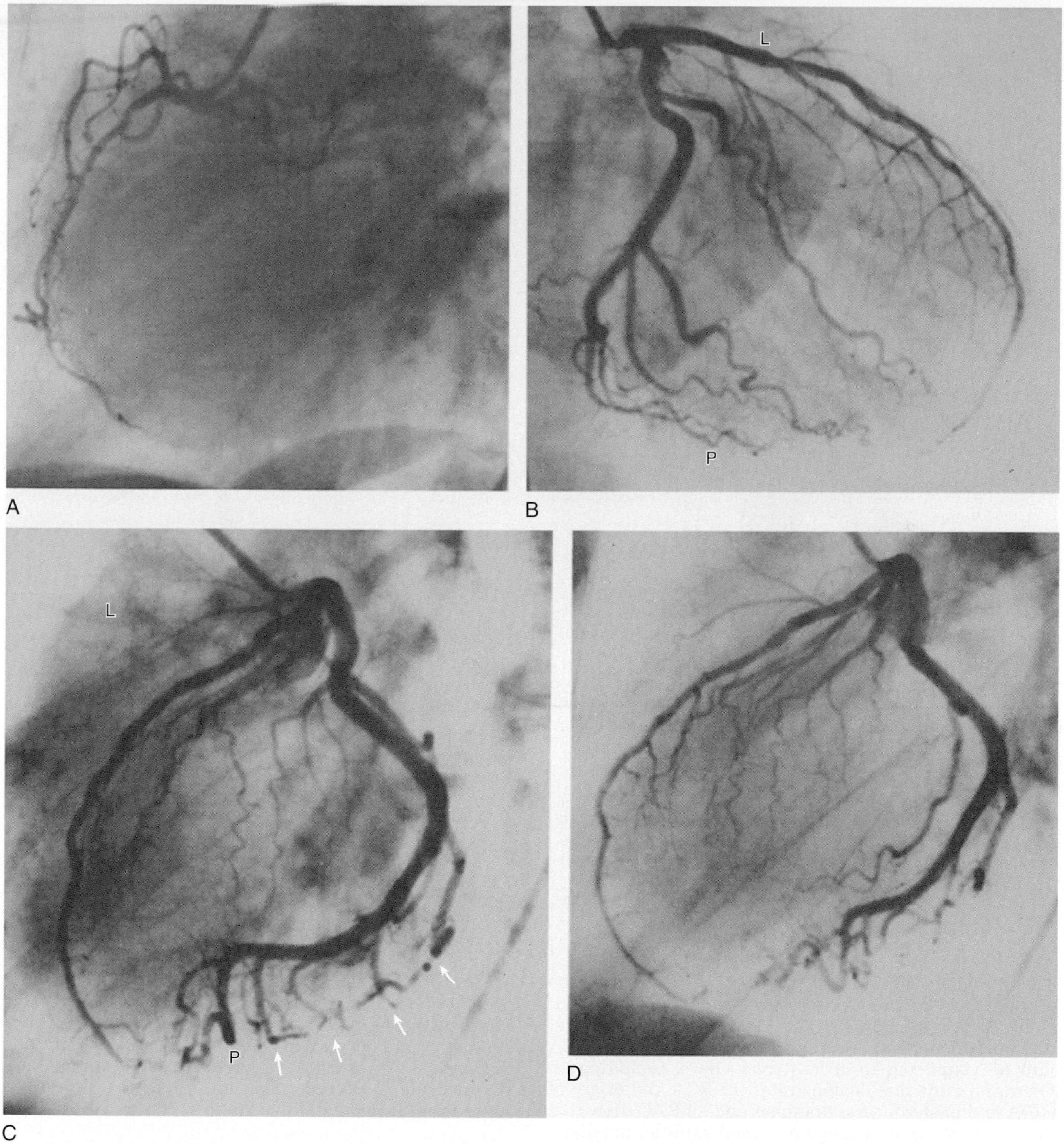

FIGURE 20–15 Dominant left coronary system. **A,** The left anterior oblique projection shows that the right coronary artery is small and terminates before reaching the crux. **B** to **D,** The right anterior oblique, left anterior oblique, and left lateral projections show that the left circumflex artery is large and gives rise to the posterior descending artery at the crux of the heart and to several posterior descending arteries. Arrows indicate posterolateral branches. L = left anterior descending coronary artery; P = posterior descending artery.

right or left hepatic artery or the celiac trunk. Catheterization of the right GEA is carried out by first entering the common hepatic artery with a cobra catheter (Fig. 20-17). A torquable, hydrophilic-coated guidewire is advanced to the gastroduodenal artery and then to the right GEA. The cobra catheter is then exchanged for a multipurpose or Judkins right coronary catheter, which then permits selective arteriography of the right GEA.

STANDARDIZED PROJECTION ACQUISITION. Although general recommendations can be made for sequences of angiographic image acquisition that are applicable to most patients, tailored views may be needed to accommodate individual variations in anatomy. As a general rule, each coronary artery should be visualized with a number of different projections that minimize vessel foreshortening and overlap (Fig. 20-18). An AP view with shallow caudal angulation is often performed first to evaluate the possibility of LMCA disease. Other important views include[1] the LAO cranial view used to evaluate the middle and distal LAD, which should have sufficient leftward positioning of the image intensifier to allow separation of the LAD, diagonal, and septal branches[2]; the LAO caudal view to evaluate

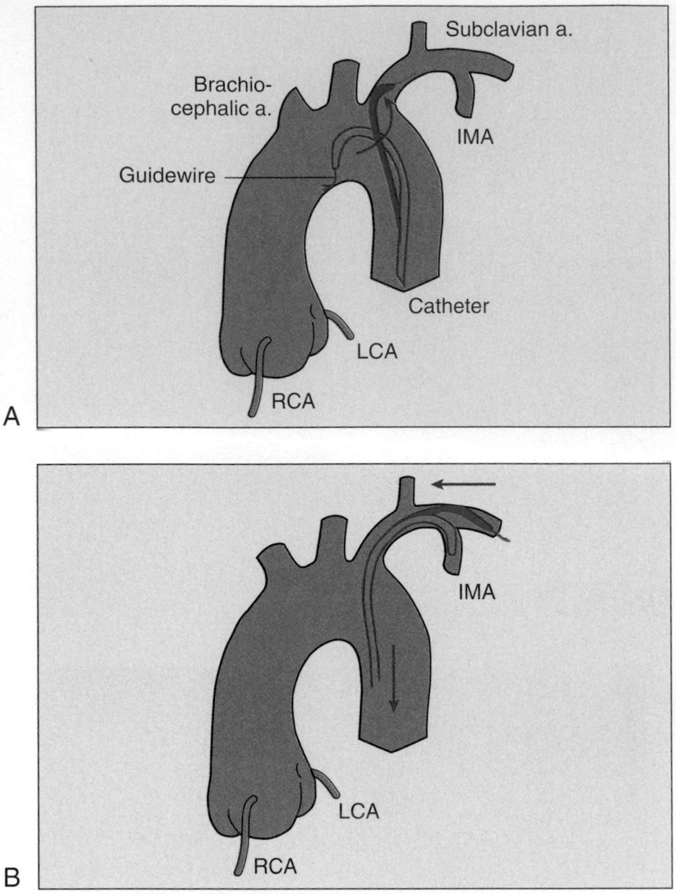

FIGURE 20–16 Catheterization of the left internal mammary artery (IMA). The IMA is positioned in the aortic arch and visualized in the left anterior oblique position. The catheter tip is rotated so that it engages the origin of the left subclavian artery immediately subjacent to the head of the clavicle **(A).** This is followed by gentle advancement of the guidewire into the left subclavian artery to a point distal to the origin of the left IMA. After the guidewire is removed, the left subclavian artery is visualized in the right anterior oblique projection, the catheter is withdrawn, and the catheter tip engages the ostium of the left IMA selectively **(B).** LCA = left coronary artery; RCA = right coronary artery. *(From Judkins MW: Coronary arteriography.* In *Douglas JS Jr, King SB III [eds]: Coronary Arteriography and Intervention. New York, McGraw-Hill, 1985, p 231.)*

the LMCA, origin of the LAD, and proximal segment of the LCx[3]; the RAO caudal view to assess the LCx and marginal branches; and[4] a shallow RAO or AP cranial view to evaluate the mid-portion and distal portion of the LAD. The RCA should be visualized in at least two views, including an LAO cranial view that demonstrates the RCA and origin of the PDA and posterolateral branches and an RAO view that demonstrates the mid-RCA and proximal, middle, and distal termination of the PDA. An AP cranial projection may also be useful for the demonstration of the distal termination of the RCA, and a left lateral view is useful to visualize the ostium of the RCA and mid-portion of the RCA with separation of the RCA and its right ventricular branches.

Congenital Anomalies of the Coronary Circulation

Coronary anomalies are defined as those angiographic findings in which the number, origin, course, and termination of the arteries are rarely encountered in the general population. Coronary anomalies may occur in 1 to 5 percent of patients undergoing coronary arteriography, depending on the threshold for defining an anatomical variant (Table 20-7).[27,28]

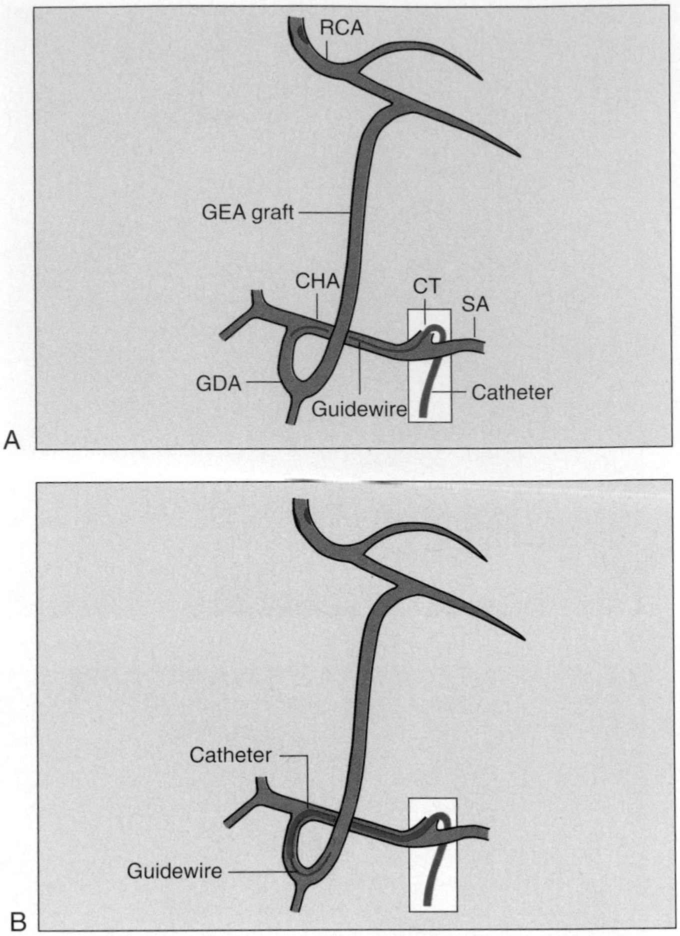

FIGURE 20–17 Catheterization of the right gastroepiploic artery (GEA) graft. The celiac trunk (CT) is selectively engaged with a cobra catheter, and a guidewire is gently advanced to the gastroduodenal artery (GDA) and the GEA. The catheter is advanced over the guidewire for selective arteriography of the GEA graft. CHA = common hepatic artery; RCA = right coronary artery; SA = splenic artery.

The major reason for appropriately identifying and classifying coronary anomalies is to determine their propensity to develop fixed or dynamic myocardial ischemia and sudden cardiac death, particularly in young and otherwise healthy individuals.[29] Documentation of precise ischemia risk for some of these anomalies using conventional exercise stress testing or intravascular Doppler flow studies is poorly predictive and may fail to detect significant anatomic abnormalities.[28,30,31] Accordingly, coronary artery anomalies are divided into those that cause and those that do not cause myocardial ischemia (Table 20-8).[28]

ANOMALOUS PULMONARY ORIGIN OF THE CORONARY ARTERIES (APOCA). This syndrome is characterized by the origin of the coronary artery arising from the pulmonary artery. The most common variant is an anomalous origin of the LCA from the pulmonary artery (ALCAPA), although single vessel origins of the RCA, LCx coronary artery, or LAD artery from the pulmonary artery have also been reported.[31] Untreated, and in the absence of an adequate collateral network, most (95%) infants with APOCA die within the first year. In the presence of an extensive collateral network, patients may survive into adulthood. Aortography typically shows a large RCA with absence of a left coronary ostium in the left aortic sinus. During the late phase of the aortogram, patulous LAD and LCx branches fill by means of collateral circulation from RCA branches. Still later in the filming sequence, retrograde flow from the LAD and LCx arteries opacifies the LMCA and its origin from the main pulmonary artery (Fig. 20-19).[31] Once detected, coronary artery bypass surgery is recommended because of the high incidence of sudden death, cardiomyopathy, and arrhythmias associated with APOCA.[31]

ANOMALOUS CORONARY ARTERY FROM THE OPPOSITE SINUS (ACAOS). Origin of the LCA from the proximal RCA or the right aortic sinus with subsequent passage between the aorta and the right ventricular outflow tract has been associated with sudden death during or shortly after exercise in young persons (Figs. 20-20 to Fig. 20-22).[31,32] The increased risk of sudden death may be due to a slit-like ostium, a bend with acute takeoff angles of the aberrant coronary arteries, or arterial compression between the pulmonary trunk and aorta when there is increased blood flow through these vessels with exercise and stress.[33] Origin of the RCA from the LCA or left aortic sinus with passage between the aorta and the right ventricular outflow tract is also associated with myocardial ischemia and sudden death.[34,35] In rare cases of anomalous origin of the LCA from the right sinus, myocardial ischemia may occur even if the LCA passes anterior to the right ventricular outflow tract or posterior to the aorta (i.e., not through a tunnel between the two great vessels). Although coronary bypass surgery has been the traditional revascularization approach in patients with

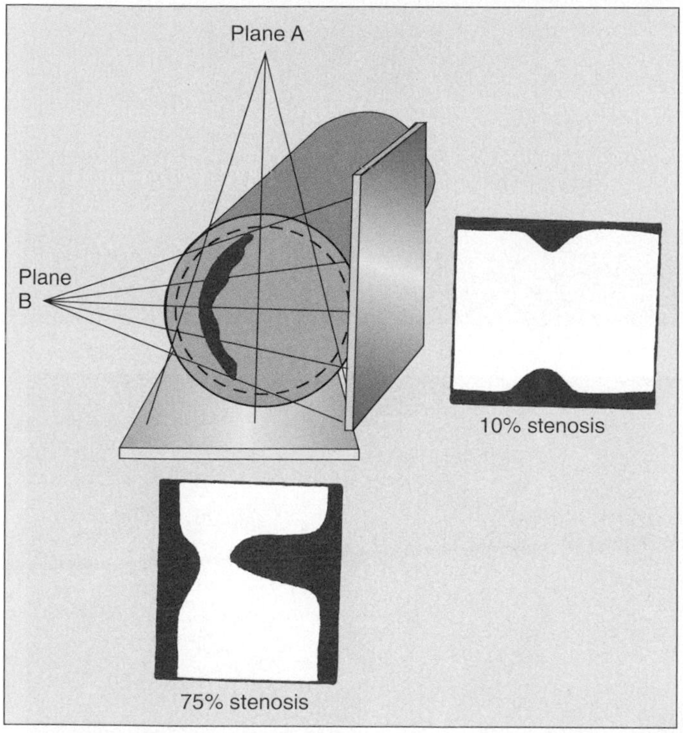

FIGURE 20–18 Importance of orthogonal projections. Each vascular segment of the coronary artery must be recorded in two orthogonal or nearly orthogonal views to avoid missing important diagnostic information about eccentric stenoses. In plane A the image is associated with 75 percent stenosis, but in plane B the image results in 10 percent stenosis.

TABLE 20–7 Incidence of Coronary Anomalies among 1950 Angiograms

Variable	Number	Percent
Coronary anomalies	110	5.64
Split RCA	24	1.23
Ectopic RCA (right cusp)	22	1.13
Ectopic RCA (left cusp)	18	0.92
Fistulas	17	0.87
Absent left main coronary artery	13	0.67
LCx artery arising from right cusp	13	0.67
LCA arising from right cusp	3	0.15
Low origin of RCA	2	0.1
Other anomalies	3	0.15

LCx = left circumflex; RCA = right coronary artery.
From Angelini P (ed): Coronary Artery Anomalies: A Comprehensive Approach. Philadelphia, Lippincott Williams and Wilkins, 1999, p 42.

TABLE 20–8 Ischemia Occurring in Coronary Anomalies

Type of Ischemia	Coronary Anomaly
Absence of ischemia	Majority of anomalies (split RCA, ectopic RCA from right cusp, ectopic RCA from left cusp)
Episodic ischemia	Anomalous origin of a coronary artery from the opposite sinus (ACAOS); coronary artery fistulas; myocardial bridge
Obligatory ischemia	Anomalous left coronary artery from the pulmonary artery (ALCAPA); coronary ostial atresia or severe stenosis

RCA = right coronary artery.
Modified from Angelini P (ed): Coronary Artery Anomalies: A Comprehensive Approach. Philadelphia, Lippincott Williams & Wilkins, 1999, p 42.

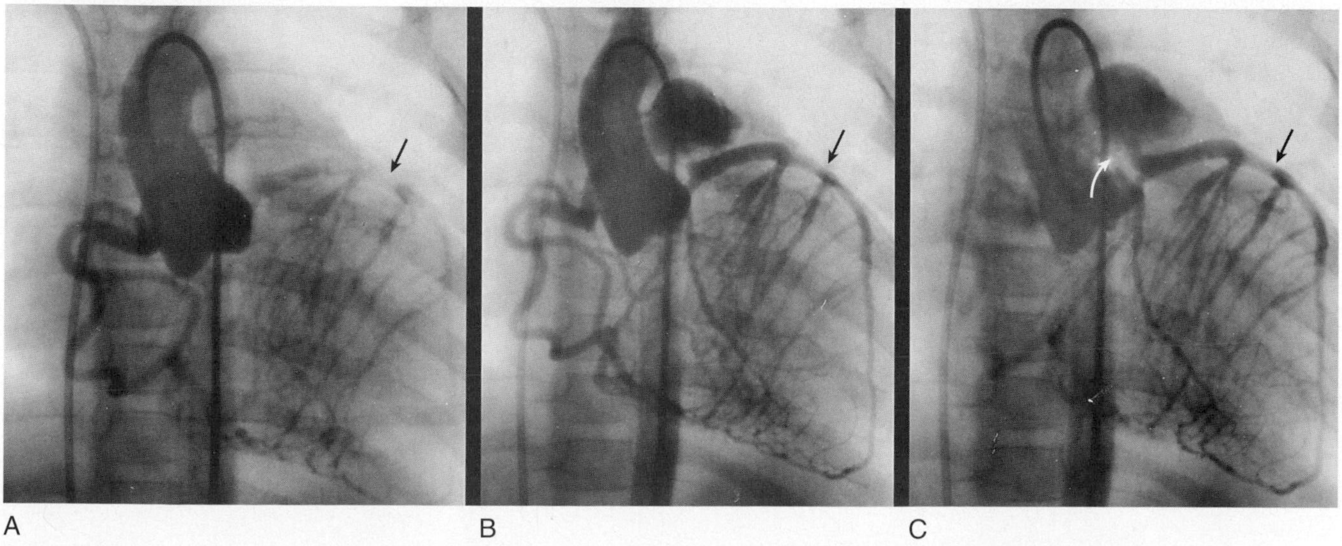

FIGURE 20–19 Anomalous origin of the left coronary artery (LCA) from the pulmonary artery. **A** to **C,** The thoracic aortogram shows a large right coronary artery (RCA) and no antegrade filling of the LCA. The LCA fills primarily through extensive collaterals from the RCA to the LADA (straight arrows). The anomalous origin of the LCA from the pulmonary artery is demonstrated in late phases of the aortogram (**C,** curved arrow).

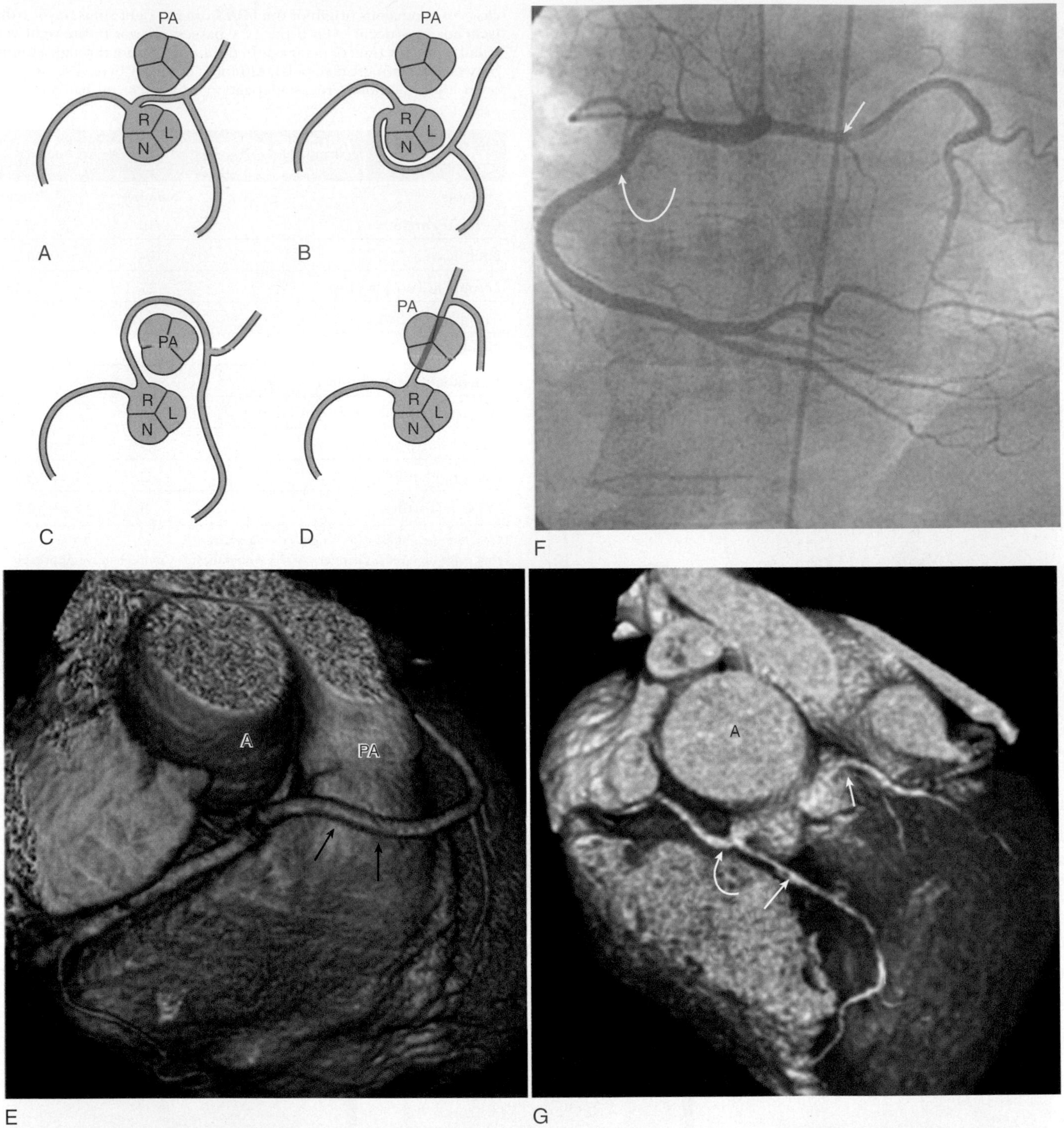

FIGURE 20–20 Four possible pathways of the anomalous left coronary artery arising from the right coronary sinus (R): **A,** Interarterial (between the aorta and the pulmonary artery [PA]); **B,** retroaortic; **C,** prepulmonic; and **D,** septal (beneath the right ventricular outflow tract). L = left coronary sinus, N = non-coronary sinus. **E,** Computed tomographic (CT) angiography showing the left coronary artery taking a prepulmonic course, passing anterior to the pulmonary artery (PA) (arrows). A = aorta. **F,** The left anterior descending artery arising from the right coronary sinus and taking a septal (subpulmonic) course. The right coronary artery has a normal origin from the right coronary sinus (curved arrow) but the left anterior descending artery arises from the right coronary cusp and courses beneath the pulmonary artery (straight arrow). **G,** CT angiography showing the left circumflex coronary artery (short straight arrow) arising from its normal location in the left coronary sinus. A (aorta). The curved arrow represents the right coronary artery arising from the right coronary sinus. The aberrant left anterior descending artery arises from the right coronary sinus and takes a subpulmonic course (large straight arrow). *(Reproduced from Kim SY, Seo JB, Do KH, et al: Coronary artery anomalies: Classification and ECG-gated multi-detector row CT findings with angiographic correlation. Radiographics 26:317-333; discussion 333-334, 2006.)*

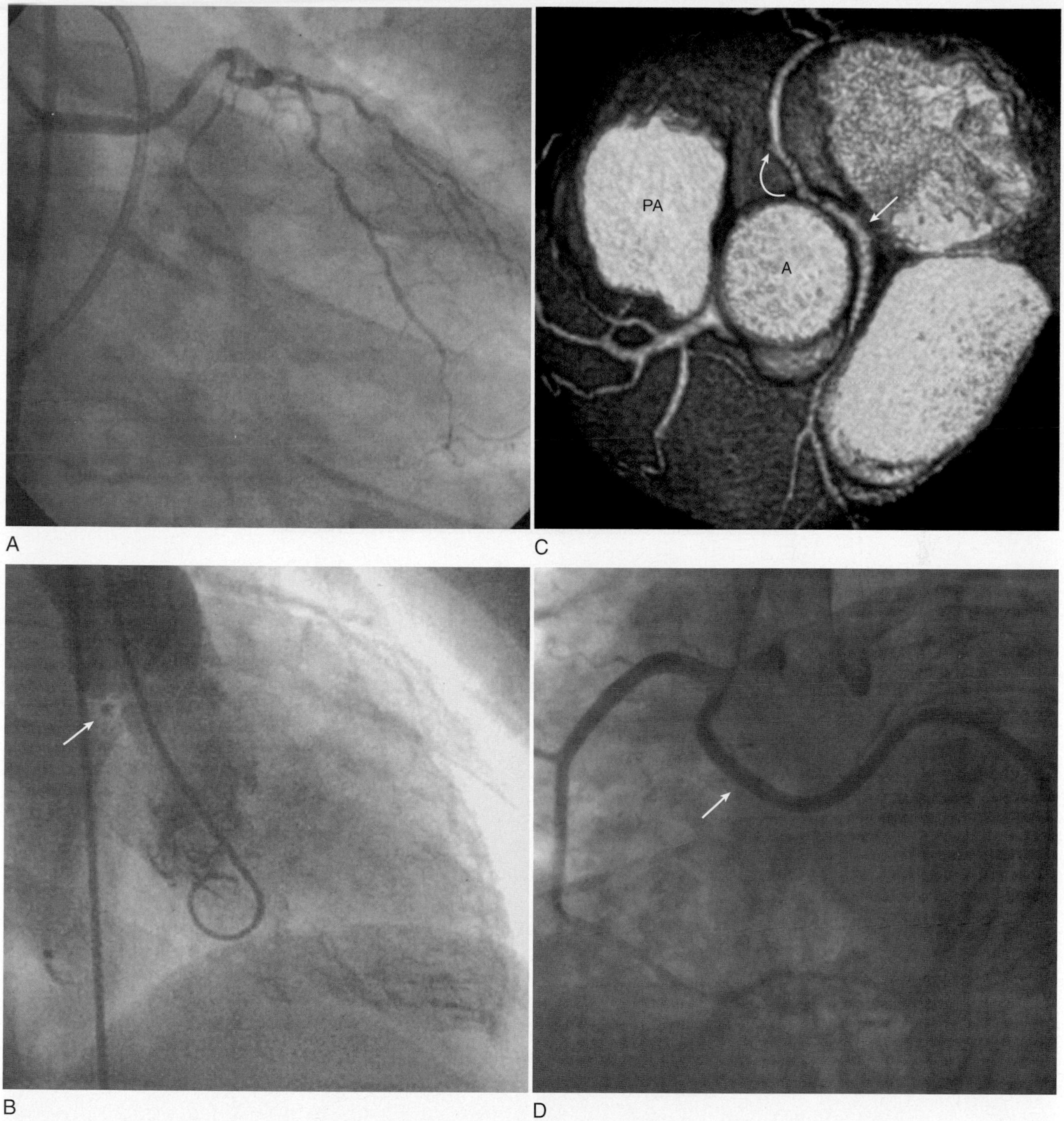

FIGURE 20–21 Anomalous origin of the left circumflex coronary artery from the right coronary sinus. **A,** The left anterior descending artery arises from the left coronary sinus in usual location but there is absence of the left circumflex artery. **B,** A left ventriculogram in the right anterior oblique projection shows the "button sign" (arrow) of the anomalous left circumflex artery coursing behind the aorta. **C,** Computed tomographic angiography shows the origin of the left circumflex artery from the right coronary sinus and passing behind the aorta (A) (arrow). Angiographic demonstration of the anomalous left circumflex artery (arrows) from the right coronary sinus shown in the left anterior oblique projection **(D)** and the right anterior oblique projection **(E).** PA = pulmonary artery. *Figure continues on next page.*

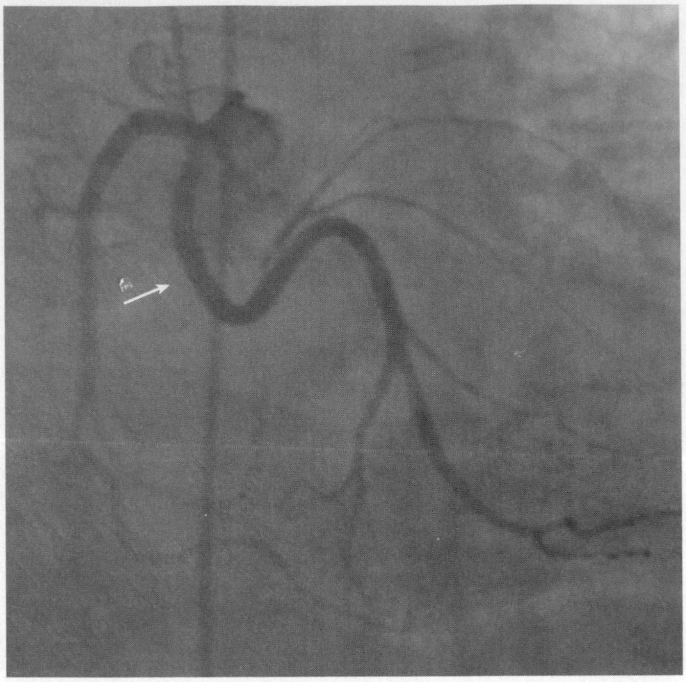

E

FIGURE 20–21, cont'd

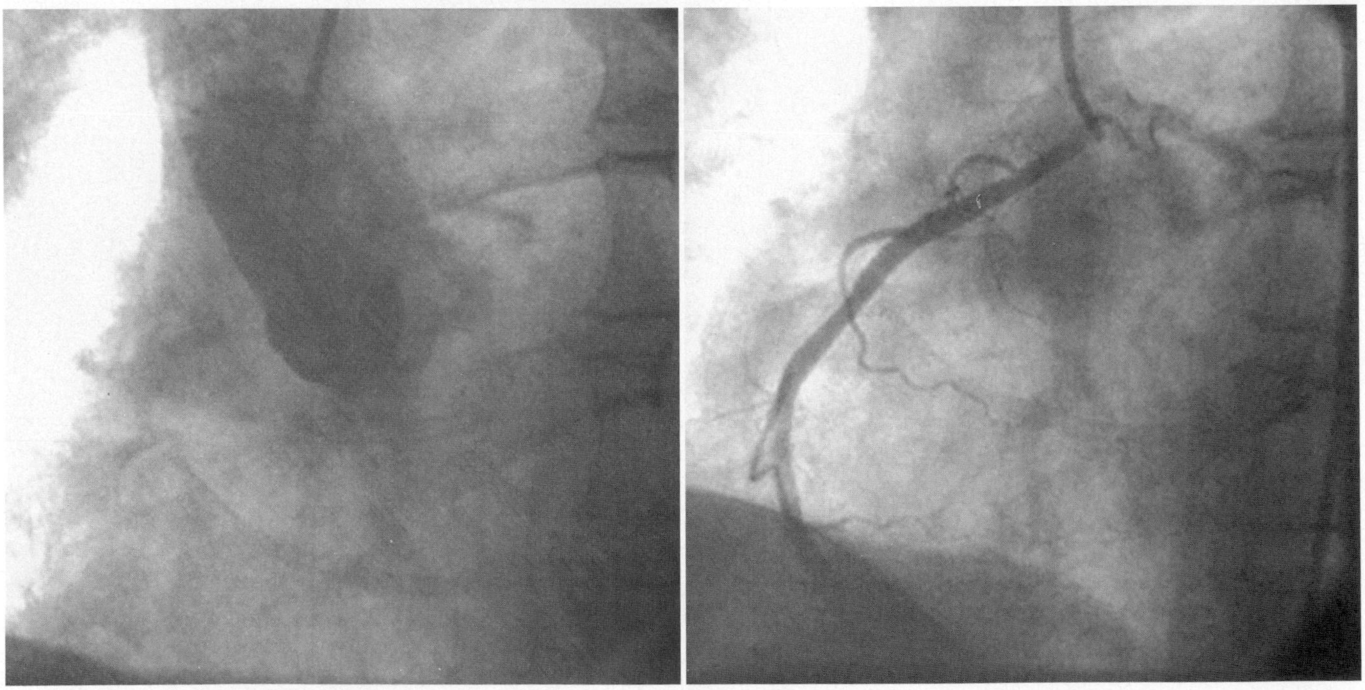

A B

FIGURE 20–22 Anomalous origin of the right coronary artery from the left coronary sinus. **A,** An aortogram in left oblique projection shows the absence of the right coronary artery from the right coronary sinus. **B,** Selective injection of the right coronary artery from the left coronary sinus. *Figure continues opposite.*

ACAOS, coronary stenting has also been reported with acceptable medium-term success.[36]

The course of the anomalous coronary arteries is easily assessed by angiography in the RAO view. The four common courses for the anomalous LCA arising from the right sinus of Valsalva include a septal, anterior, interarterial, or posterior course.[37] The posterior course of the anomalous LCA arising from the right sinus of Valsalva is similar to the course of the anomalous LCx artery arising from the right sinus of Valsalva (see Fig. 20-21), whereas the common interarterial course of the anomalous RCA from the left sinus of Valsalva is similar to the interarterial course of the anomalous LCA arising from the right sinus of Valsalva.

When either the LCA or the LAD arises anomalously from the right sinus, another angiographic method to identify the course of the anomalous vessel is to pass a catheter into the main pulmonary artery and then perform an arteriogram of the aberrant coronary artery in the steep AP caudal projection. This places the aberrant coronary artery, the rightward and anterior pulmonary valve, and the leftward and posterior aortic valve all in one plane. From this "laid-back" aortogram, which can be used even in mapping the course of anomalous coronary arteries in transposition of the great vessels, it is usually possible to confirm whether the course of the aberrant coronary artery is between the great vessels. Although angiography is useful for establishing the presence of anomalous coronary arteries, computed tomographic (CT) angiography may also be an important adjunctive diagnostic tool for establishing the course of the vessels (see Chap. 18).[38,39]

CORONARY ARTERY FISTULAS. Coronary artery fistulas are defined as abnormal communications between a coronary artery and a cardiac chamber or major vessel, such as the vena cava, right or left ventricle, pulmonary vein, or pulmonary artery.[40,41] Fistulas arise from the RCA or its branches in about one half of the cases, and drainage generally occurs into the right ventricular, right atrium, and pulmonary arteries; coronary artery fistulas terminating in the left ventricle are uncommon (3%)[40] (Figs. 20-23 to Fig. 20-25). Coronary arteriography is the best method for demonstrating the origin of these fistulas.

The clinical presentation associated with coronary artery fistulas is dependent on the type of fistula, shunt volume, site of the shunt, and presence of other cardiac conditions, although patients (50%) often remain asymptomatic.[40] Dyspnea on exertion, fatigue, congestive heart failure, pulmonary hypertension, bacterial endocarditis, and arrhythmias are common presentations in symptomatic patients. Myocardial ischemia may also occur, but the mechanism remains speculative.[40] Symptomatic patients or those with severe shunts may be treated with surgical closure, although percutaneous closure with coil embolization may also be tried.

CONGENITAL CORONARY STENOSIS OR ATRESIA. Congenital stenosis or atresia of a coronary artery can occur as an isolated lesion or in association with other congenital diseases, such as calcific coronary sclerosis, supravalvular aortic stenosis, homocystinuria, Friedreich ataxia, Hurler syndrome, progeria, and rubella syndrome. In these cases, the atretic vessel usually fills by means of collateral circulation from the contralateral side.

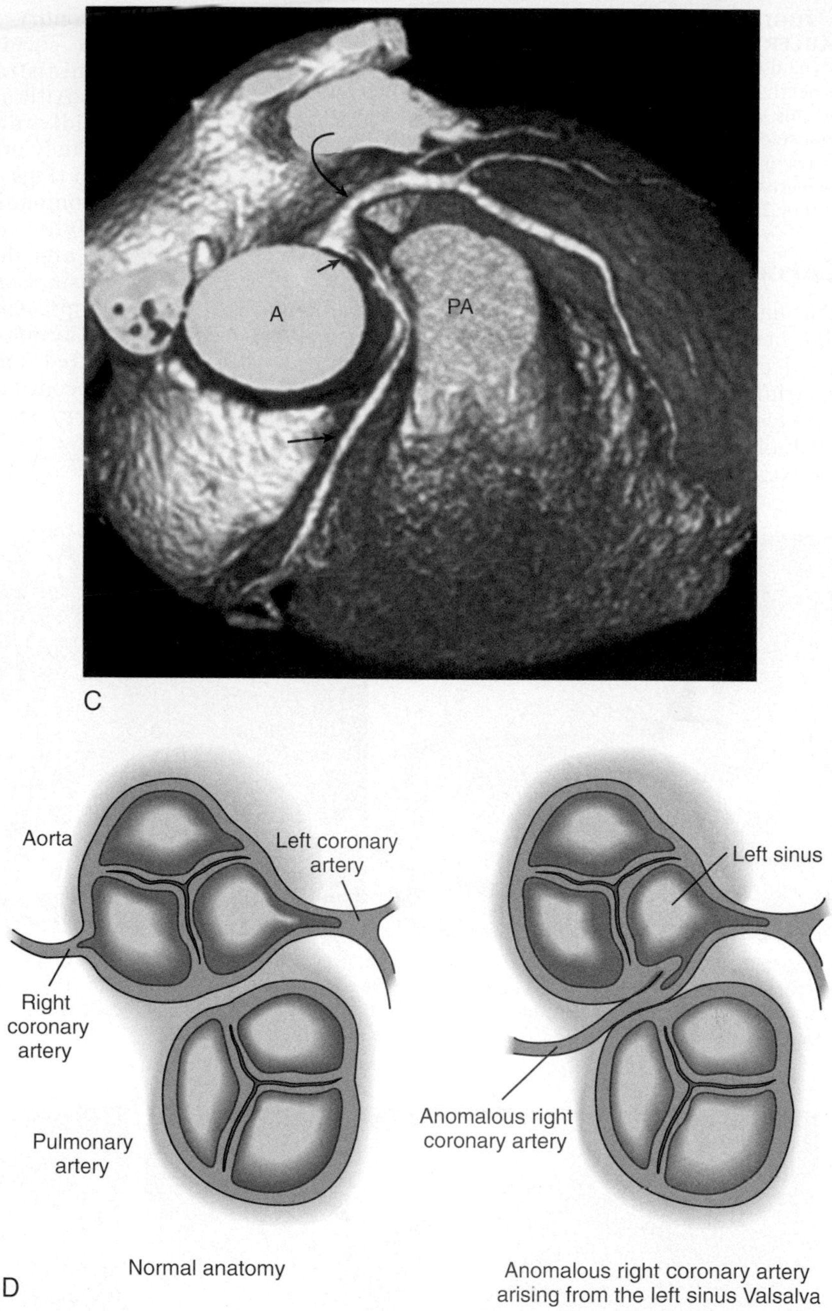

FIGURE 20–22, cont'd C, Computed tomographic angiography shows the slit-like origin of the right coronary artery (straight arrow) from the left coronary sinus and normal origin of the left coronary artery (curved arrow). The right coronary artery courses between the aorta (A) and pulmonary artery (PA). **D,** The normal anatomy of the right and left coronary arteries is shown in the left plane, and the anomalous origin of the right coronary artery is shown coursing between the aorta and pulmonary artery. *(Reproduced from Kim SY, Seo JB, Do KH, et al: Coronary artery anomalies: Classification and ECG-gated multi-detector row CT findings with angiographic correlation. Radiographics 26:317-33; discussion 333-4, 2006; and Qayyum U, Leya F, Steen L, Sochanski M, Grassman E, Cho L, et al: New catheter design for cannulation of the anomalous right coronary artery arising from the left sinus of Valsalva. Catheter Cardiovasc Interv 60:382-388, 2003.)*

MYOCARDIAL BRIDGING. The three major coronary arteries generally course along the epicardial surface of the heart. On occasion, however, short coronary artery segments descend into the myocardium for a variable distance. This abnormality, termed myocardial bridging, occurs in 5 to 12 percent of patients, and is usually confined to the LAD (Fig. 20-26).[42] Because a "bridge" of myocardial fibers passes over the involved segment of the LAD, each systolic contraction of these fibers can cause narrowing of the artery. Myocardial bridging has a characteristic appearance on angiography with the bridged segment of normal caliber during diastole and abruptly narrows with each systole. Although bridging is not thought to have any hemodynamic significance in most cases, myocardial bridging has been associated with angina, arrhythmia, depressed left ventricular function, myocardial stunning, early death after cardiac transplantation, and sudden death.[42] Intracoronary Doppler studies have shown that diastolic flow abnormalities may be present in patients with myocardial bridging.[42] Medical treatment generally includes beta blockers, although nitrates should be avoided because they may worsen symptoms.[42] Intracoronary stents and surgery have been attempted in selected patients, but the results have been mixed.[42]

HIGH ANTERIOR ORIGIN OF THE RIGHT CORONARY ARTERY. This anomaly is commonly encountered but is of no hemodynamic significance. The inability to engage the ostium of the RCA selectively by conventional catheter manipulation raises the question of this superior origin of the RCA above the sinotubular ridge. Forceful, nonselective injection of contrast medium into the right sinus of Valsalva may reveal the anomalous takeoff of the RCA, which can then be selectively engaged with a Judkins right 5.0 catheter or an Amplatz left 1.0 or 2.0 catheter.

Coronary Artery Spasm

Coronary artery spasm is defined as a dynamic and reversible occlusion of an epicardial coronary artery caused by focal constriction of the smooth muscle cells within the arterial wall. Initially described by Prinzmetal and colleagues ("Prinzmetal" or "variant" angina) in 1959, this form of angina was not provoked by the usual factors, such as exercise, emotional upset, cold, or ingestion of a meal. Coronary artery spasm can be invoked by cigarette smoking, cocaine use, alcohol, intracoronary radiation, and administration of catecholamines during general anesthesia. Although the ST segment elevation is often striking, it rapidly reverts to normal when the pain disappears spontaneously or is terminated by the administration of nitroglycerin (Figs. 20-27 and 20-28). Coronary artery spasm may be accompanied by atrioventricular block, ventricular ectopic activity, ventricular tachycardia, or ventricular fibrillation. MI and death are rare manifestations of coronary artery spasm. Coronary artery spasm can also be superimposed on the presence of an intramyocardial bridge.[43]

Coronary arteriography is useful in patients with suspected coronary artery spasm to exclude the presence of concomitant CAD and to document an episode of coronary artery spasm using provocative intravenous medications. Three provocative tests can be performed to detect the presence of coronary artery spasm. Intravenous ergonovine maleate can elicit two types of responses. A diffuse coronary vasoconstriction that occurs in all the epicardial arteries is a physiological response to ergonovine not diagnostic of coronary artery spasm. The second response to ergonovine is a focal, occlusive spasm of the epicardial artery that is associated with chest pain and ST segment elevation. Nitroglycerin should be administered directly into the coronary artery to relieve the coronary spasm. A second provocative test is the use of intravenous acetylcholine. Although it is more sensitive than ergonovine, it may be less specific because of the positive response in patients with atherosclerotic

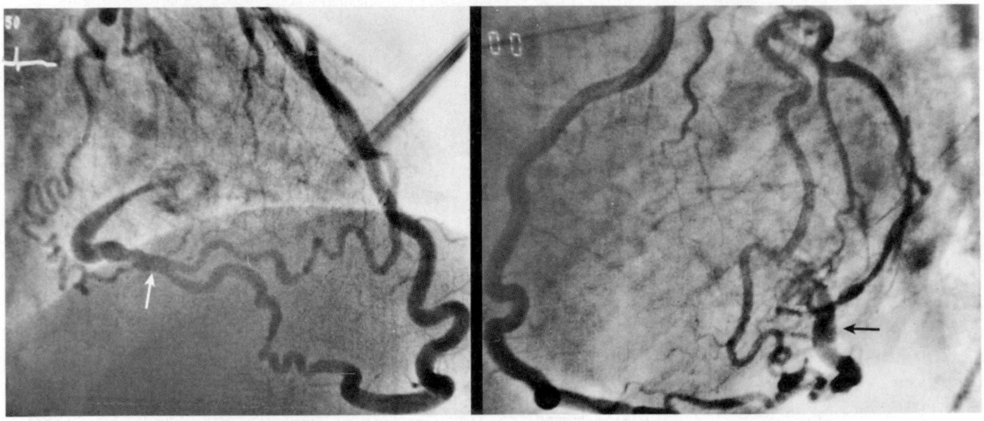

FIGURE 20–23 Congenital fistula to the left ventricle. **A,** Right anterior oblique cranial view of the left coronary arteriogram shows a congenital fistula (arrow) arising from branches of both the left anterior descending and left circumflex arteries and draining into the left ventricle. **B,** Left anterior oblique view of the left coronary arteriogram shows the fistula (arrow).

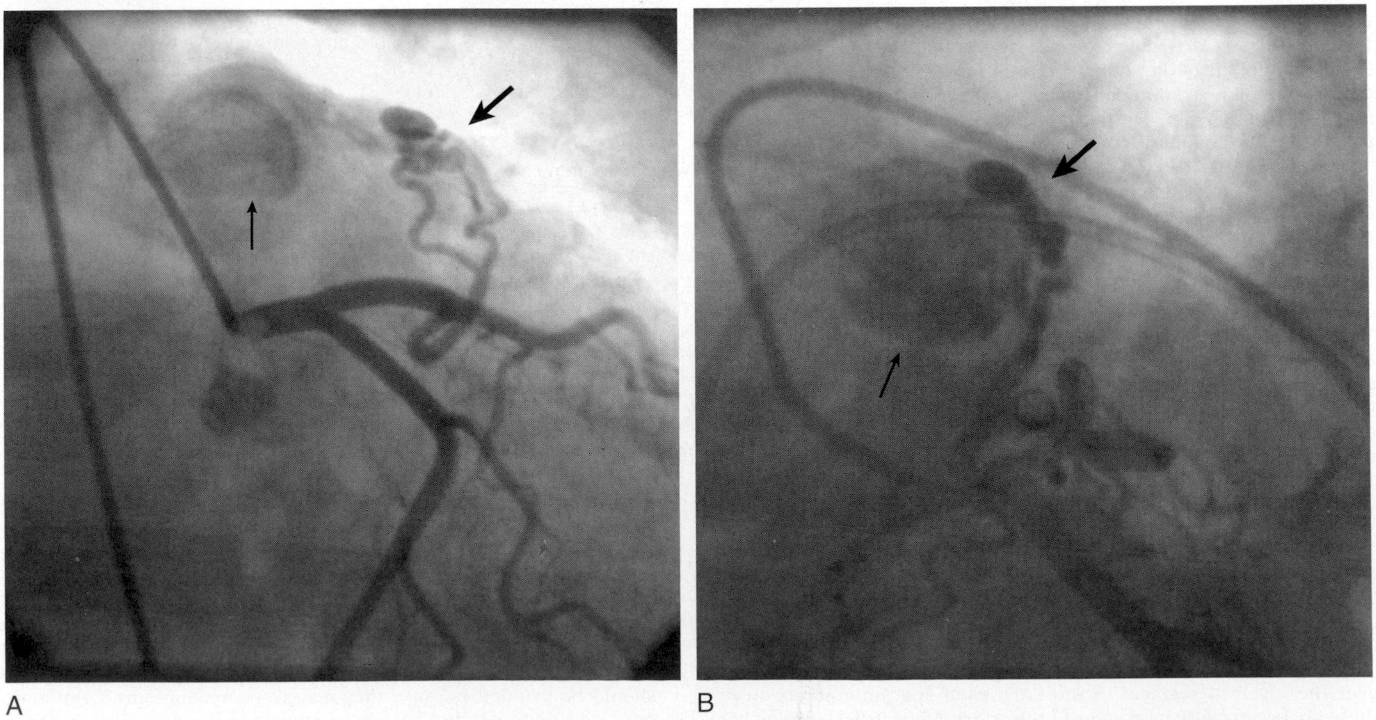

FIGURE 20–24 Congenital fistula to the pulmonary artery. The left coronary arteriogram shows a congenital fistula arising from the left anterior descending (large arrow) and terminating (small arrow) in the pulmonary artery demonstrated in the right anterior oblique **(A)** and left anterior oblique with caudal angulation **(B)**.

CAD. The final provocative test is hyperventilation during coronary arteriography, which is less sensitive but highly specific for the presence of coronary artery spasm.

In the absence of a positive stimulation test, the diagnosis of coronary artery spasm must rely instead on clinical features and response to treatment with nitrates and calcium channel blockers. Sole therapy with beta blockers should be avoided because it can worsen the occurrence of coronary artery spasm. Coronary artery spasm that is refractory to conventional therapy with long-acting calcium channel blockers and nitrates can be treated with coronary stenting.

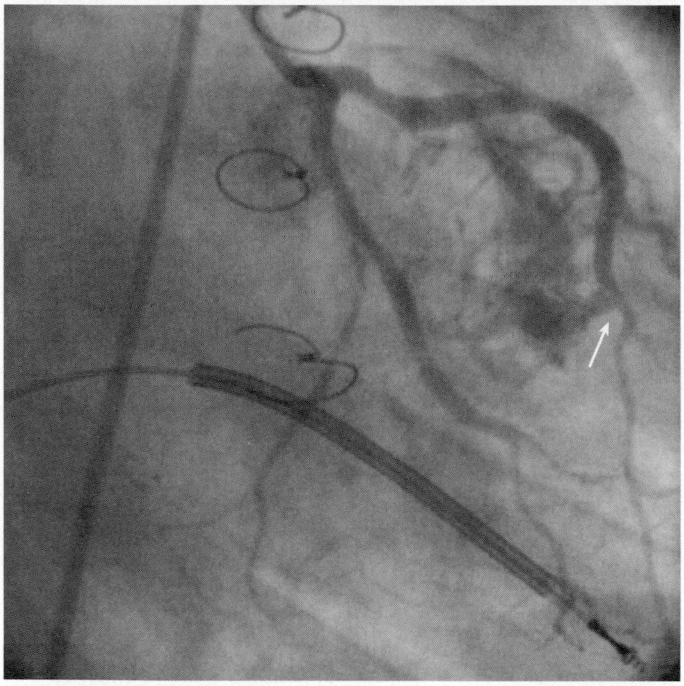

FIGURE 20–25 Iatrogenic fistula of the left anterior descending artery. This patient had undergone prior cardiac transplantation and developed a fistula between the left anterior descending artery and the right ventricle following right ventricular biopsy (arrow).

Lesion Complexity

Heterogeneity of the composition, distribution, and location of atherosclerotic plaque within the native coronary artery results in unique patterns of stenosis morphology in patients with CAD. These patterns have been used to identify risk factors for procedural outcome and complications after PCI and to assess the risk for recurrent events in patients who present with an acute coronary syndrome.[44] Criteria established by a joint ACC/AHA task force suggested that procedure success and complication rates were related to a number of different lesion characteristics (Table 20-9). Over the decade following the publication of these criteria, despite substantial improvements in the techniques used for coronary intervention, the most complex lesion morphologies (i.e., "type C" lesions) remain associated with reduced procedural success in patients with ischemic CAD (Table 20-10).

The predictive value of two other risk scores has been compared to the ACC/AHA lesion complexity score.[45,46] The Society for Cardiac Angiography and Interventions (SCAI) risk score used an ordinal ranking of two composite criteria (vessel patency and complex morphology) to classify lesions into four groups: non-type C–patent, type C–patent, non-type C–occluded, and Type C–occluded.[45] For correctly classifying lesion success, the ACC/AHA classification had a C-statistic of 0.69; the modified ACC/AHA system had a C-statistic of 0.71; and the SCAI classification had a C-statistic of 0.75. The Mayo Clinic Risk Score added the integer scores for the presence of eight morphological variables and provided a better risk stratification than the ACC/AHA lesion classification for the predicting cardiovascular complications, whereas the ACC/AHA lesion classification was a better system for identifying angiographic success.[46]

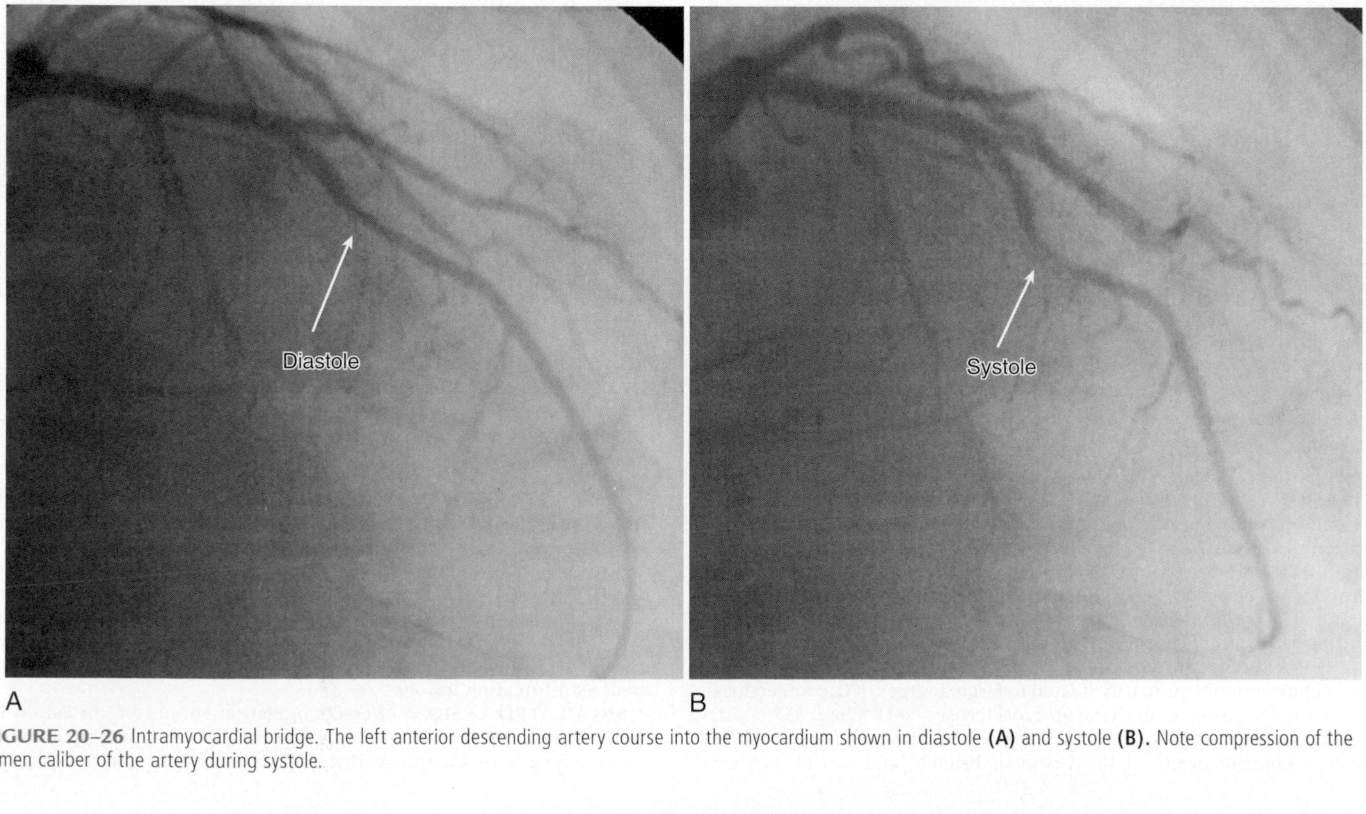

FIGURE 20–26 Intramyocardial bridge. The left anterior descending artery course into the myocardium shown in diastole **(A)** and systole **(B)**. Note compression of the lumen caliber of the artery during systole.

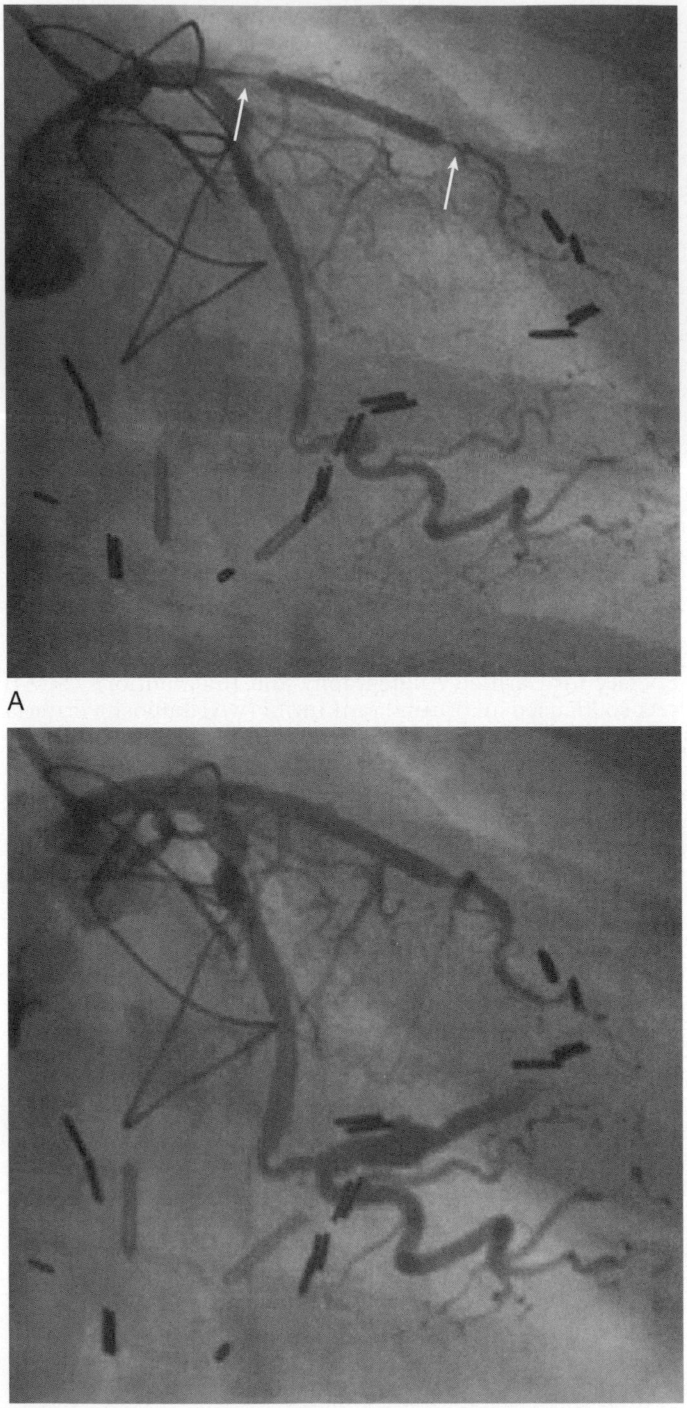

FIGURE 20–27 Coronary artery spasm. **A,** Proximal and distal coronary artery spasm was found after stent placement in the left anterior descending coronary artery (arrows) that was relieved with intracoronary nitroglycerin **(B).**

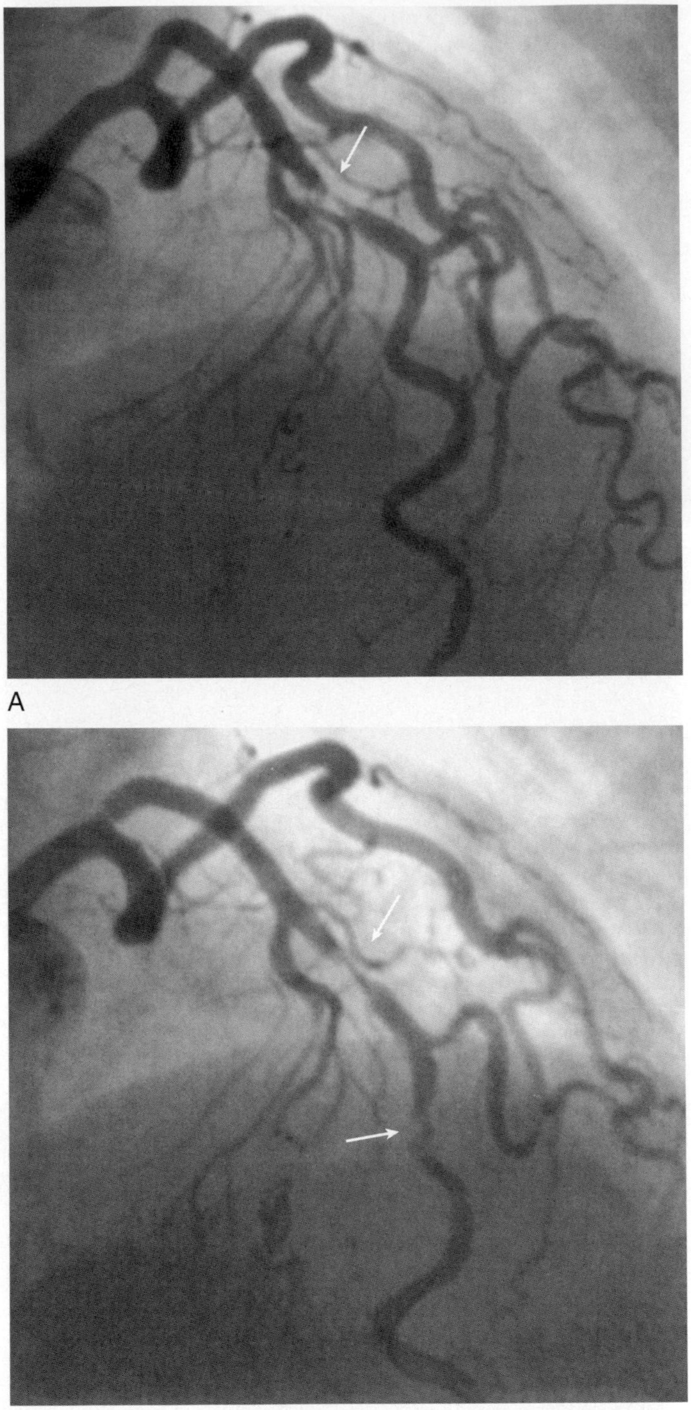

FIGURE 20–28 "Wire pleating." **A,** A focal stenosis (top arrow) is shown in the left anterior descending artery. **B,** A 0.014 inch coronary guidewire was advanced across the stenosis but straightened the vessel, resulting in downstream wire pleating mimicking a coronary stenosis or dissection (bottom arrow). *Figure continues opposite.*

LESION LENGTH. Lesion length may be measured using a number of methods, including measurement of the "shoulder-to-shoulder" extent of atherosclerosis narrowed by more than 20 percent, quantifying the lesion length more than 50 percent narrowed, and estimating the distance between the proximal and distal angiographically "normal" segment; the last method is used most commonly in clinical practice and provides a longer length than more quantitative methods. Diffuse (>20 mm) lesions are associated with reduced procedural success with drug-eluting stents, primarily related to large degrees of late lumen loss and more extensive underlying atherosclerosis[47] (see Chap. 55).

OSTIAL LOCATION. Ostial lesions are defined as those arising within 3 mm of origin of the vessel or branch, and can be further characterized into aorto-ostial and non–aorto-ostial. Aorto-ostial lesions are often fibrocalcific and rigid, requiring additional ablative devices, such as rotational atherectomy in the presence of extensive calcification, in order to obtain adequate stent expansion. Positioning of the proximal portion of the stent in the aorto-ostial location so that no more than 1 mm of stent extends into the aorta requires meticulous care. Ostial stenoses that do not involve the aorta may also be more elastic than non-ostial lesion and require the same principles for treatment as bifurcation lesions.

ANGULATED LESIONS. Vessel angulation should be measured in the most unforeshortened projection at the site of maximum stenosis using a length of curvature that approximates the balloon length.

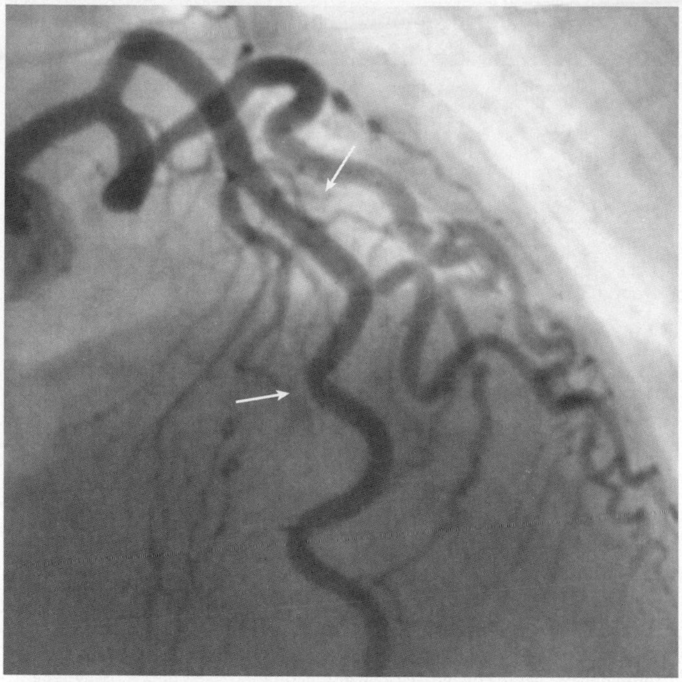

C

FIGURE 20–28, cont'd C. After a stent was placed in the proximal left anterior descending artery (top arrow), the pseudostenosis was no longer present (bottom arrow).

TABLE 20–9 Characteristics of Type A, B, and C Coronary Lesions

Type A Lesions (high success, >85%; low risk)	
Discrete (<10 mm)	Little or no calcium
Concentric	Less than totally occlusive
Readily accessible	Not ostial in locations
Nonangulated segment, <45 degrees	No major side branch involvement
Smooth contour	Absence of thrombus
Type B Lesions (moderate success, 60-85%; moderate risk)	
Tubular (10 to 20 mm length)	Moderate to heavy calcification
Eccentric	Total occlusions <3 mo old
Moderate tortuosity of proximal segment	Ostial in location
Moderately angulated segment, ≥45 degrees, <90 degrees	Bifurcation lesion requiring double guidewire
Irregular contour	Some thrombus present
Type C Lesions (low success, <60%; high risk)	
Diffuse (>2 cm length)	Total occlusion >3 mo old
Excessive tortuosity of proximal segment	Inability to protect major side branches
Extremely angulated segments, ≥90 degrees	Degenerated vein grafts with friable lesions

From Ryan TJ, Bauman WB, Kennedy JW, et al: Guidelines for percutaneous coronary angioplasty. A report of the American Heart Association/American College of Cardiology Task Force on Assessment of Diagnostic and Therapeutic Cardiovascular Procedures (Subcommittee on Percutaneous Transluminal Coronary Angioplasty). Circulation 88:2987, 1993.

TABLE 20–10 Definitions of Preprocedural Lesion Morphology

Feature	Frequency (%)	Definition
Eccentricity	48.0	Stenosis that is noted to have one of its luminal edges in the outer one quarter of the apparent normal lumen
Irregularity	17.9	Characterized by lesion ulceration, intimal flap, aneurysm, or saw-toothed pattern
Ulceration	12.1	Lesions with a small crater consisting of a discrete luminal widening in the area of the stenosis
Intimal flap	3.22	A mobile, radiolucent extension of the vessel wall into the arterial lumen
Aneurysm	5.49	Segment of arterial dilation larger than the dimensions of the normal arterial segment
Saw-toothed pattern	0.84	Multiple, sequential stenosis irregularities
Length		Measured "shoulder to shoulder" in an unforeshortened view
Discrete	55.0	Lesion length <10 mm
Tubular	34.8	Lesion length 10-20 mm
Diffuse	10.2	Lesion length >20 mm
Ostial location	10.0	Origin of the lesion within 3 mm of the vessel origin
Angulation		Vessel angle formed by the center line through the lumen proximal and distal to the stenosis
Moderate	15.3	Lesion angulation ≥45 degrees
Severe	0.93	Lesion angulation ≥90 degrees
Bifurcation stenosis	6.05	Stenosis involving the parent and daughter branch if a medium or large branch (>1.5 mm) originates within the stenosis and if the side branch is completely surrounded by stenotic portions of the lesion to be dilated
Proximal tortuosity		
Moderate	15.3	Lesion is distal to two bends >75 degrees
Severe	NR	Lesion is distal to three bends >75 degrees
Degenerated SVG	7.1	Graft characterized by luminal irregularities or ectasia constituting >50% of the graft length
Calcification	34.3	Readily apparent densities noted within the apparent vascular wall at the site of the stenosis
Total occlusion	6.4	TIMI 0 or 1 flow
Thrombus	3.4	Discrete, intraluminal filling defect is noted with defined borders and is largely separated from the adjacent wall. Contrast staining may or may not be present.

NR = not reported; SVG = saphenous vein graft; TIMI = thrombolysis in myocardial infarction.
Data obtained from 846 lesions undergoing qualitative angiographic analysis at the Washington Hospital Center Angiographic Core Laboratory.

Balloon angioplasty of angulated lesions increased the risk for dissections, although with the advent of coronary stenting, the inability to deliver the stent and subsequent straightening of the vessel that may predispose to late stent fracture are the largest challenges of highly angulated lesions.

BIFURCATION LESIONS. The optimal strategic approach for bifurcation lesions remains controversial, and the risk for side branch occlusion during PCI relates to the relative size of the parent and branch vessel, the location of the disease in the parent vessel, and the stenosis severity in the origin of the side branch. In general, placement of one stent is preferable to stent placement in both the parent vessel and side branch. (See Chap. 55.)

DEGENERATED SAPHENOUS VEIN GRAFTS. A serial angiographic study in patients undergoing coronary bypass surgery showed that 25% of SVGs occlude within the first year after coronary bypass surgery.[48] Although a drug-eluting stent may reduce the recurrence rate due to restenosis,[49] only embolic protection devices have reduced procedural complications. A study that evaluated the extent of graft degeneration and estimated volume of plaque in the target lesion found that the independent correlates of increased 30-day major adverse cardiac event rates were more extensive vein graft degeneration ($p = 0.0001$) and bulkier lesions (larger estimated plaque volume, $p = 0.0005$).[50]

LESION CALCIFICATION. Coronary artery calcium is an important marker for coronary atherosclerosis. Conventional angiography is moderately sensitive for the detection of extensive lesion calcification, but is less sensitive for detecting the presence of milder degrees of lesion calcification. Severely calcified lesions tend to be more rigid and undilatable than noncalcified lesions, and rotational atherectomy may be useful before stenting to ensure stent delivery and complete stent expansion.

THROMBUS. Although conventional angiography is a relatively insensitive method for detecting coronary thrombus, its presence is associated with a higher risk of procedural complications, primarily relating to embolization of thrombotic debris into the distal circulation. Large, intracoronary thrombi may be treated with a combination of pharmacological agents (e.g., glycoprotein IIb/IIIa inhibitors) and mechanical devices (e.g., rheolytic thrombectomy) (see Chap. 55).

TOTAL OCCLUSION. Total coronary occlusion is identified as an abrupt termination of the epicardial vessel; anterograde and retrograde collaterals may be present and are helpful in quantifying the length of the totally occluded segment. Success in passage of a coronary guidewire across the occlusion depends on the occlusion duration and on certain lesion morphological features, such as bridging collaterals, occlusion length greater than 15 mm, and the absence of a "nipple" to guidewire advancement. Newer guidewires and improved operator experience have improved procedural success rates, although the presence of a total occlusion remains one of the major reasons for referring patients for coronary bypass surgery.

CORONARY PERFUSION. Perfusion distal to a coronary stenosis can occur anterograde by means of the native vessel, retrograde through collaterals, or through a coronary bypass graft. The rate of anterograde coronary flow is influenced by both the severity and complexity of the stenosis and the status of the microvasculature. The Thrombolysis in Myocardial Infarction (TIMI) study group established criteria to assess the degree of anterograde coronary reperfusion in patients with acute MI and found that complete restoration of anterograde perfusion by TIMI 3 flow was associated with the lowest mortality rate (Table 20-11). TIMI frame count and the TIMI myocardial perfusion grade permit further quantification of anterograde flow and assessment of distal microvascular perfusion.

Coronary Collateral Circulation

Networks of small anastomotic branches interconnect the major coronary arteries and serve as precursors for the collateral circulation that maintains myocardial perfusion despite the development of severe proximal atherosclerotic narrowings.[51] Collateral channels may not be seen in patients with normal or mildly diseased coronary arteries because of their small (<200 μm) caliber, but as CAD progresses and becomes more severe (>90 percent stenosis), a pressure gradient is generated between the anastomotic channels and the distal vessel that is hypoperfused.[52] The trans-stenosis pressure gradient facilitates blood flow through the anastomotic channels, which progressively dilate and eventually become visible as collateral vessels (Fig. 20-29).

TABLE 20–11 Thrombolysis in Myocardial Infarction (TIMI) Flow

Grade 3 (complete reperfusion)	Anterograde flow into the terminal coronary artery segment through a stenosis is as prompt as anterograde flow into a comparable segment proximal to the stenosis. Contrast material clears as rapidly from the distal segment as from an uninvolved, more proximal segment.
Grade 2 (partial reperfusion)	Contrast material flows through the stenosis to opacify the terminal artery segment. However, contrast material enters the terminal segment perceptibly more slowly than more proximal segments. Alternatively, contrast material clears from a segment distal to a stenosis noticeably more slowly than from a comparable segment not preceded by a significant stenosis.
Grade 1 (penetration with minimal artery perfusion)	A small amount of contrast material flows through the stenosis but fails to opacify fully the epicardial vessel.
Grade 0 (no perfusion)	No contrast flow through the stenosis.

Modified from Sheehan F, Braunwald E, Canner P, et al: The effect of intravenous thrombolytic therapy on left ventricular function: A report on the tissue-type plasminogen activator and streptokinase from the Thrombolysis in Myocardial Infarction (TIMI) phase 1 trial. Circulation 72:817, 1989.

The visible collateral channels arise either from the contralateral coronary artery, from the ipsilateral coronary artery through intracoronary collateral channels, or through "bridging" channels that have a serpiginous course from the proximal coronary artery to the coronary artery distal to the occlusion. These collaterals may provide up to 50 percent of anterograde coronary flow in chronic total occlusions, and may allow the development of a "protected" region of myocardial perfusion that does not develop ischemia during enhanced myocardial oxygen demands. Recruitment of collateral channels may occur quickly in patients who develop an acute ST segment elevation MI caused by a sudden thrombotic occlusion. Other factors that affect collateral development are patency of the arteries supplying the collateral and the size and vascular resistance of the segment distal to the stenosis. Grading of flow of collaterals can be classified using the Rentrop criteria, including Rentrop grade 0 (no filling), Rentrop grade 1 (small side branches filled), Rentrop grade 2 (partial epicardial filling of the occluded artery), or Rentrop grade 3 (complete epicardial filling of the occluded artery).[52]

Quantitative Angiography

Although visual estimations of coronary stenosis severity are used by virtually all clinicians to guide clinical practice, "eyeball" estimates of percent diameter stenosis are limited by substantial observer variability and bias. More reliable and objective "on-line" quantitative coronary measurements have had limited clinical use, however, being largely supplanted by more physiological measures of stenosis severity, such as direct measurements of fractional

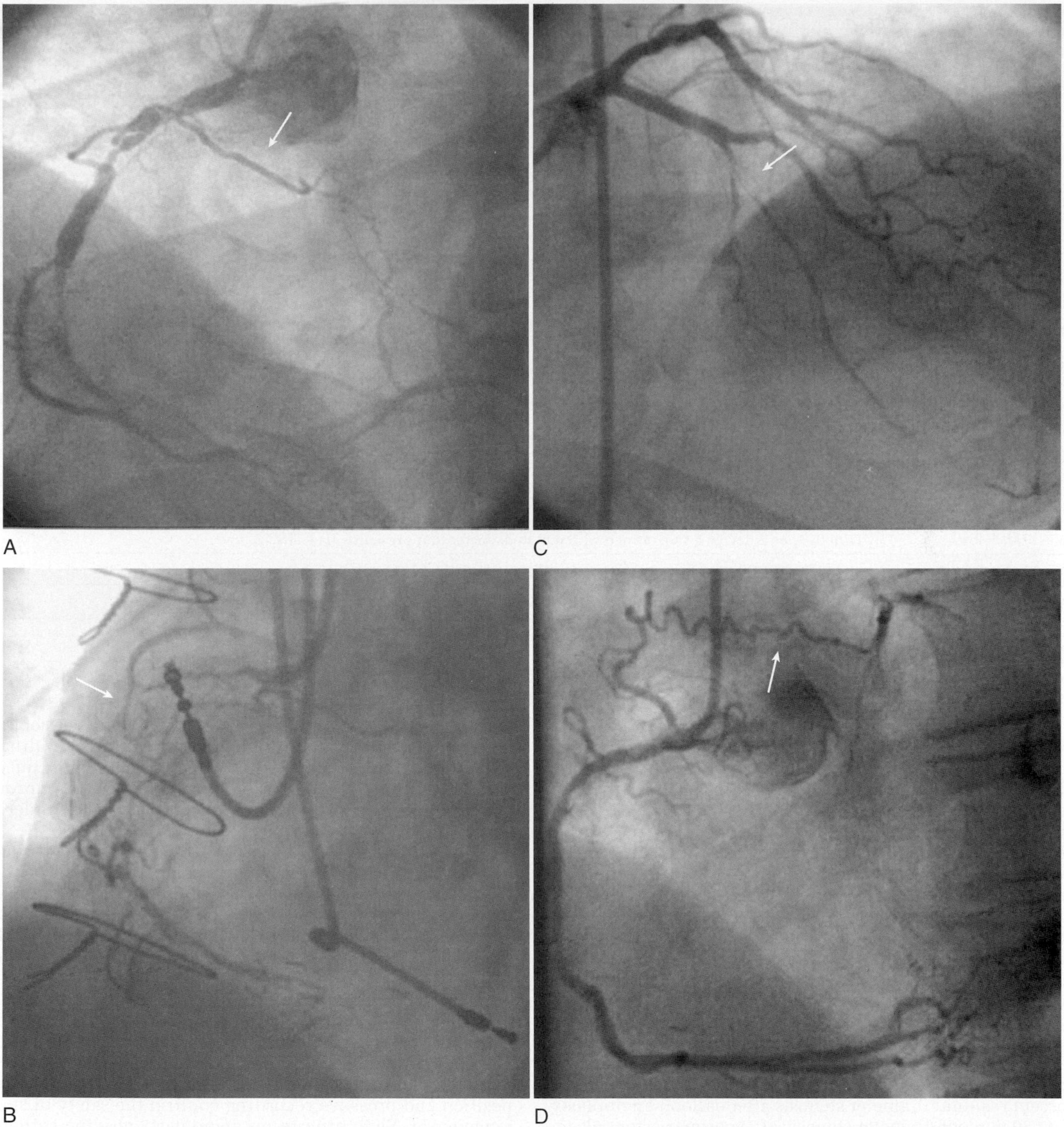

FIGURE 20–29 Coronary collaterals. **A,** Kugel's branch arises from the proximal right coronary artery and extends to the distal posterior descending branch of the right coronary artery (arrow). **B,** "Bridging" collaterals (arrow) connecting the proximal and distal right coronary artery. **C,** A "microchannel" in the mid-left anterior descending artery. **D,** A Viessen collateral extends from the proximal right coronary artery to the left anterior descending artery (arrow).

and coronary flow reserve in regions of intermediate (40 to 70 percent) stenosis severity. Nevertheless, a number of angiographic measures have been developed to more quantitatively assess early and late procedural outcome after PCI for research protocols and registry reports (Table 20-12); these methods have been used to determine the value of new devices and drugs for the treatment of patients with ischemic CAD.

Quantitative coronary angiography was initially performed by Greg Brown and colleagues at the University of Washington nearly 30 years ago. Using hand-drawn arterial contours that corrected for pincushion distortion and reconstructed a three-dimensional representation of the arterial contour, reference vessel and minimal lumen diameters were measured and were used to evaluate the effect of pharmacological intervention for a number of angiographic plaque regression studies. These initial quantitative angiographic methods were time consuming and cumbersome, and have now been largely replaced with computer-assisted methods for automated arterial contour detection that have utilized improved microprocessor speed and storage capacity.

TABLE 20–12 Standardized Criteria for Postprocedural Lesion Morphology

Feature	Definition
Abrupt closure	Obstruction of contrast flow (TIMI 0 or 1) in a dilated segment with previously documented anterograde flow
Ectasia	A lesion diameter greater than the reference diameter in one or more areas
Luminal irregularities	Arterial contour that has a saw-toothed pattern consisting of opacification but not fulfilling the criteria for dissection or intracoronary thrombus
Intimal flap	A discrete filling defect in apparent continuity with the arterial wall
Thrombus dissection*	Discrete, mobile angiographic filling defect with or without contrast staining
A	Small radiolucent area within the lumen of the vessel
B	Linear, nonpersisting extravasation of contrast material
C	Extraluminal, persisting extravasation of contrast material
D	Spiral-shaped filling defect
E	Persistent lumen defect with delayed anterograde flow
F	Filling defect accompanied by total coronary occlusion
Dissection, length (mm)	Measure end to end for type B through F dissections
Dissection, staining	Persistence of contrast within the dissection after washout of contrast material from the remaining portion of the vessel
Perforation	
Localized	Extravasation of contrast material confined to the pericardial space immediately surrounding the artery and not associated with clinical tamponade
Nonlocalized	Extravasation of contrast material with a jet not localized to the pericardial space, potentially associated with clinical tamponade
Side branch loss	TIMI 0, 1, or 2 flow in a side branch >1.5 mm in diameter that previously had TIMI 3 flow
Distal embolization	Migration of a filling defect or thrombus to distally occlude the target vessel or one of its branches
Coronary spasm	Transient or permanent narrowing >50% when a <25% stenosis has been previously noted

*National Heart, Lung and Blood Institute classification system for coronary dissection.
TIMI: thrombolysis in myocardial infarction.

Quantitative angiographic analysis is divided into several distinct processes, including film digitization (when needed), image calibration, and arterial contour detection. The contrast-filled diagnostic or guiding catheter can be used as a scaling device for determining absolute vessel dimensions, yielding a calibration factor in millimeters per pixel. Catheter and arterial contours are obtained by drawing a center line through the segment of interest. Linear density profiles are then constructed perpendicular to the center line, and a weighted average of the first and second derivative function is used to define the catheter or arterial edges. Individual edge points are then connected using an automated algorithm, and outliers are discarded and the edges are smoothed. The automated algorithm is then applied to a selected arterial segment, and absolute coronary dimensions and percent diameter stenosis are obtained.

The measures obtained using quantitative angiography are used to document angiographic success, defined as a <50 percent residual diameter stenosis after balloon angioplasty or a <20 percent diameter stenosis after coronary stent placement. Long-term results following stent placement, and, more recently, drug-eluting stent placement, are described using binary angiographic restenosis, defined as a 50 percent or greater follow-up diameter stenosis, and late lumen loss, defined as the loss in lumen diameter during the intermediate (6 to 9 month) period of follow-up. Both the follow-up percent diameter stenosis and late lumen loss has been correlated with clinical restenosis, manifest by ischemia-driven target lesion revascularization.

PITFALLS OF CORONARY ARTERIOGRAPHY

Errors in image acquisition and interpretation can have a profound impact on management strategies in patients with ischemic CAD, particularly when there is disagreement between angiographic, physiological, and clinical findings. Attention to those factors that affect angiographic image quality at the time of image acquisition will improve the ultimate course selected for patients who undergo arteriography.

INADEQUATE VESSEL OPACIFICATION. Inadequate filling of the coronary artery with contrast medium results in incomplete vessel opacification or "streaming," which may misrepresent the degree of ostial and side branch disease and overestimate the amount of thrombus within the vessel. The causes of contrast streaming include competition from increased native coronary blood flow in the setting of left ventricular hypertrophy associated with aortic insufficiency or anemia or inadequate placement of the diagnostic catheter that is not coaxial (or "in line") with the coronary ostium. Contrast streaming can be overcome by a more forceful contrast agent injection as long as catheter tip position and pressure recording confirm the safety of such a maneuver. Switching to an angioplasty-guiding catheter with a soft, short tip and a larger lumen than a diagnostic catheter may allow more complete opacification of the target coronary artery or bypass graft. Superselective injection of contrast medium into the LCx artery (or LAD) through a short LMCA may give the impression of total occlusion of the LAD (or LCx).

ECCENTRIC STENOSES. By its nature, coronary atherosclerosis is a ubiquitous process that leads to asymmetrical plaque distribution within the coronary artery. Although most segments of the artery wall are involved in the atherosclerotic process, eccentric or slit-like lesions may be seen by angiography in regions of more focal plaque accumulation. The hemodynamic significance of eccentric lesions is dependent on the percent area stenosis rather then the "worst" percent diameter stenosis. A related problem is that of the hazy band-like or membranous stenosis, which may be exceedingly difficult to characterize using standard angiographic views. These unique lesions may simply represent atherosclerosis or they may be caused by congenital membranous bands. Because of the difficulty in ascertaining the hemodynamic significance of these eccentric and band-like lesions, measurement of a fractional flow reserve using a micromanometer-tip guidewire across the region of abnormality during intravenous adenosine administration may be useful in identifying those patients with hemodynamically significant narrowings.

SUPERIMPOSITION OF BRANCHES. Superimposition of major branches of the left and right arteries can result in failure to detect significant stenoses or total occlusions of these branches. Although this problem most commonly affects the LAD artery and parallel diagonal branches, side branch overlap may also occur with the ostium of the obtuse marginal branch lesion of the left circumflex and the origin of the right ventricular branch of the right coronary artery. Moreover, when the LAD is occluded beyond the origin of the first septal branch, this branch often becomes quite enlarged in an attempt to provide collateral circulation to the vascular bed of the distal LAD. It is important to obtain sufficient angulation for these views to identify the exact anatomy at the origin of the side branch, such as cranial projections for the LAD artery, caudal projections for the left circumflex, and left lateral projection for the RCA.

MICROCHANNEL RECANALIZATION. It is sometimes difficult to differentiate very severe (>90 percent) coronary stenoses (with an anterograde lumen) from total occlusions (with no anterograde lumen) that have been recanalized with microchannels and bridging collaterals. Pathological studies suggest that approximately one third of totally occluded coronary arteries ultimately recanalize, resulting in the development of multiple tortuous channels that are quite small and close to one another, and creating the impression on angiography of a single, slightly irregular channel. As angiography lacks sufficient spatial resolution to demonstrate this degree of detail in most patients with recanalized total occlusions, wire crossing may not be possible in some cases unless advanced wire techniques are used.

Intravascular Ultrasonography and Related Invasive Imaging Methods

Contrast coronary arteriography is limited in its ability to quantify the extent or distribution of atherosclerosis or to identify changes within the vessel wall over time. Intravascular ultrasound (IVUS) is a safe, accurate, and reproducible method of detecting vessel wall structure and disease and it lends insight into the dynamic changes before, after, and late after PCI (see also Chap. 55). The two-dimensional tomographic images provided by IVUS also permit 360-degree characterization of arterial lumen dimensions in regions that are difficult to assess using conventional angiography, such as the LMCA and the ostia of the LAD, LCx artery, and RCA. When a mechanized pull-back of the IVUS ca-theter is performed at a fixed rate, a three-dimensional reconstruction of the arterial wall and its lumen can be obtained.

TECHNICAL ISSUES. IVUS has evolved substantially since the early 1990s, resulting in the commercial availability of rapid exchange, mechanical, or dynamic-array imaging catheters—ranging in size from 2.6 to 3.2F—compatible with 6 to 7F guiding catheters, and yielding a 30 to 40 MHz imaging frequency for enhanced tissue characterization. Longitudinal or three-dimensional display of the arterial wall is best performed using an automated pull-back device, which uses side branches and other anatomical landmarks to ascertain the plaque location along the axial length of the vessel.

VESSEL WALL COMPOSITION. In nondiseased arteries, IVUS differentiates the vessel wall into three components[1]: the intima, which is composed of endothelial cells, subjacent smooth muscle cells, and extracellular matrix, is 150 to 200 μm in diameter and partitioned from the media by the internal elastic lamina[2]; the media, which is composed of smooth muscle cells, elastin, and collagen, is 100 to 350 μm in diameter and encircled by the external elastic membrane (EEM); and the adventitia,[3] which contains fibrous tissue, is 300 to 500 μm in diameter and encased by perivascular stroma and epicardial fat. Differences in acoustic impedance between the cell layers generally account for the "three-layer" appearance seen in the normal vessel wall of most patients by IVUS. A "two-layer" coronary artery is seen in some patients, depending on the IVUS transducer frequency (<30 MHz), intimal thickness (<160 μm), and collagen content of the media.

In diseased arteries, the differentiation between vessel wall components becomes more obscure and, depending on the cellular composition of the atherosclerotic plaque, at least three plaque types can be described. Hypoechoic, or soft, plaques are echolucent compared with the EEM and indicate a high lipid content (Fig. 20-30). IVUS has also been used to assess the changes in plaque volume after lipid-lowering therapy[53,54] and has demonstrated that multiple plaques may develop simultaneous rupture in patients with acute MI.[55]

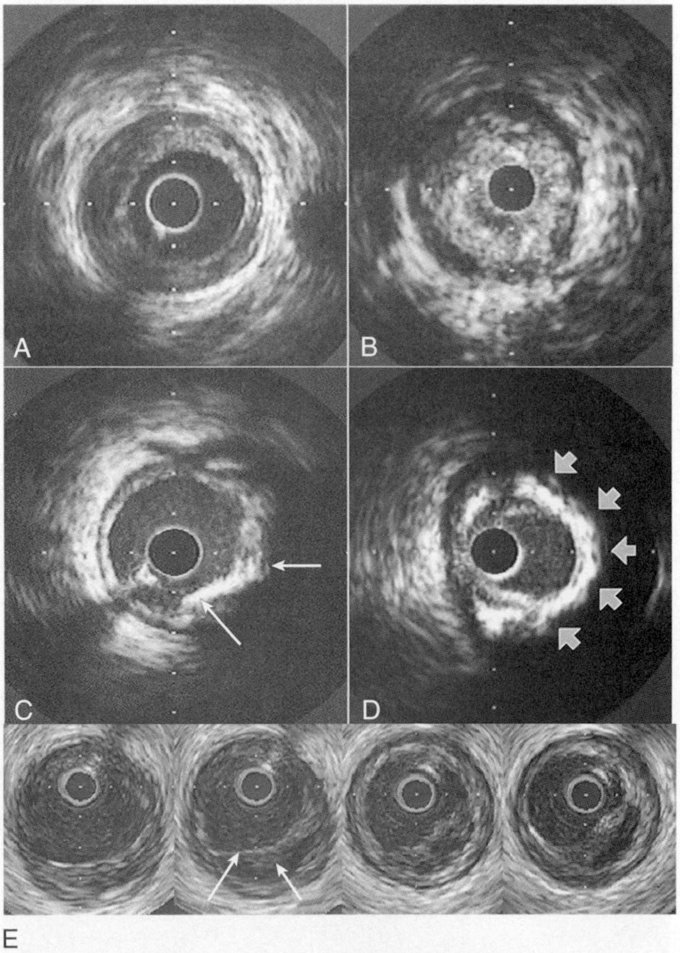

FIGURE 20-30 Intravascular ultrasound (IVUS) characterization of plaque morphology. **A,** A concentric "soft" plaque with concentric vessel wall involvement is less echogenic than a fibrous plaque that presumably contains more collagenous components. **B,** Calcification within the vessel is characterized by a bright leading edge with echo dropout (acoustic shadowing) behind the calcification, and may be focal **(C)** (arrows) or extensive **(D)** (arrows). (*Courtesy of Steven Nissen, MD.*) **E,** Adjacent IVUS cross sections of a "vulnerable" plaque show a thin fibrous cap (long arrow) and a large lipid core (short arrow). (*Courtesy of Gary Mintz, MD.*)

Thrombus within the vessel lumen often can be mistaken for soft plaque, but it can be distinguished from soft plaque by its mobility, lobular edges, and movement away from the vessel wall during the cardiac cycle. Fibrous plaques have brightness similar to that of the adventitia and consistent with a higher content of collagen and elastin. Calcified plaques are identified by their bright, echogenic components with acoustic shadowing of the underlying vascular structures. A calcified plaque may be characterized as superficial or deep and quantified by its circumferential extent (from 0 to 360 degrees) and by its axial length (in millimeters).

IVUS studies in patients undergoing PCI have also demonstrated that coronary atherosclerosis is more diffuse than appreciated using conventional angiography (Fig. 20-31). In an IVUS series of 884 angiographically "normal" reference segments, only 6.8 percent were free of atherosclerosis, with an average 51 percent cross-sectional plaque area found proximal or distal to the target lesion. IVUS studies have also confirmed an earlier pathological finding of Glagov and colleagues, suggesting that the coronary artery undergoes "adaptive" remodeling, or vessel expansion, in most patients in the early stages of atherosclerosis, maintaining a nonobstructive coronary lumen diameter (Figs. 20-32 and 20-33; see also Chap. 38). Once the EEM has expanded by 40 percent, further accumulation of plaque encroaches on the arterial lumen. Arterial constriction does occur in some patients, particularly diabetic patients because of "negative" arterial remodeling.

USE OF INTRAVASCULAR ULTRASONOGRAPHY DURING PERCUTANEOUS CORONARY INTERVENTION. IVUS may be used for several purposes during PCI:[1] to characterize baseline plaque composition, vessel size, and lesion accessibility to select the best single device or combination of devices for PCI[2]; to confirm (or refute) angiographic estimates of stenosis severity, particularly in regions difficult to visualize using conventional methods; and to assess anatomical results and detect complications, including dissections and residual minimal cross-sectional area, after PCI. In general, a minimal cross-sectional area <4.0 mm^2 in a native coronary artery and <7.0 mm^2 in the left main coronary artery suggest the presence of functionally significant native vessel lesions.

VESSEL WALL CHANGES AFTER PERCUTANEOUS CORONARY INTERVENTION. IVUS provides unique insight into the dynamic changes that occur within the vessel wall after PCI. Sequential IVUS studies show that lumen renarrowing after balloon angioplasty and atherectomy is related to both arterial remodeling and, to a lesser extent, intimal hyperplasia. In contrast to these findings, IVUS studies have also shown that lumen renarrowing after stent implantation is primarily due to intimal hyperplasia within the axial length of the stent or its border. (See Chap. 55.)

USE OF INTRAVASCULAR ULTRASOUND AFTER DRUG-ELUTING STENTS. IVUS has been a critical tool in assessing the initial procedural results[56] and in quantifying the degree of reduction of late (9-month) intimal hyperplasia in patients undergoing treatment with drug-eluting

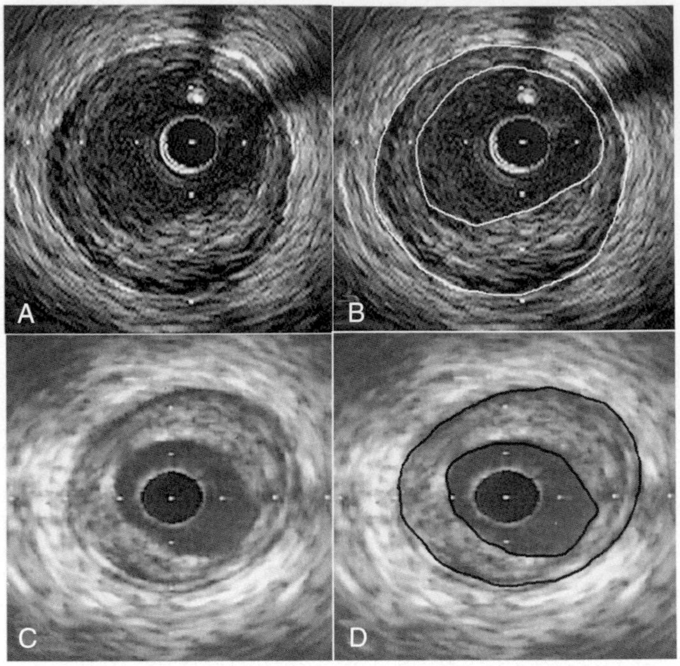

FIGURE 20–32 Quantitative intravascular ultrasound (IVUS) measurements. **A,** IVUS image obtained using a mechanical imaging transducer. **B,** The external elastic membrane is identified by the outer circle and the lumen cross-sectional area is demonstrated by the inner circle. (*Courtesy of Gary Mintz, MD.*) **C,** IVUS cross-sectional image obtained using a phased-array catheter. **D,** The external elastic membrane is identified by the outer circle and the lumen cross-sectional area is demonstrated by the inner circle. (*Courtesy of Steven Nissen, MD.*)

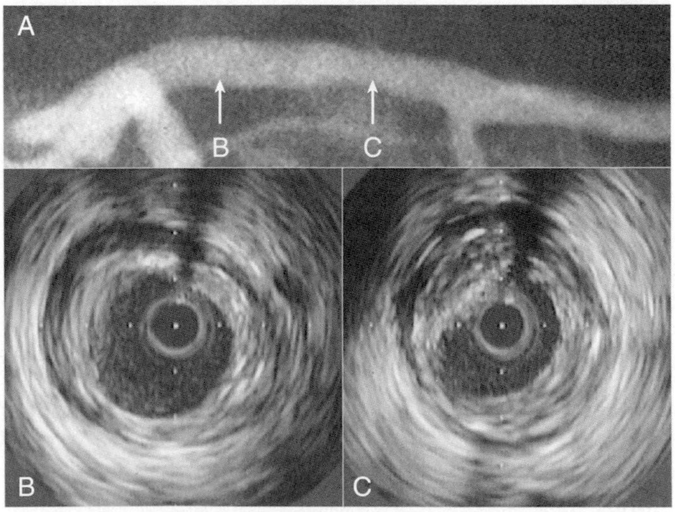

FIGURE 20–31 Discordance between angiographic and intravascular ultrasound (IVUS) findings. **A,** Angiographic imaging of the mid-portion of the LADA shows only minor lumen irregularities within the vessel. The arrows show the sites imaged in cross section by IVUS below. IVUS imaging of the angiographically normal site **(B)** and the most normal aspect **(C)** of the LADA. Note the substantial atherosclerotic plaque within the wall of the coronary artery that is not appreciated by angiography. (*Courtesy of Steven Nissen, MD.*)

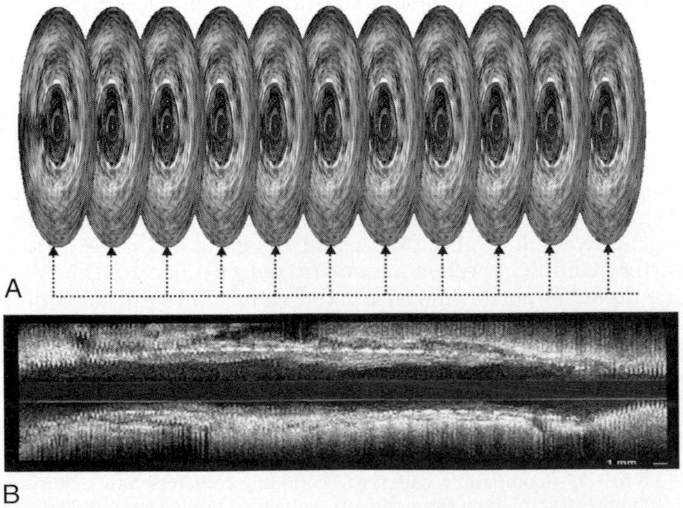

FIGURE 20–33 Longitudinal intravascular ultrasound (IVUS) imaging. Motorized "pull-back" IVUS allows reconstruction of the individual two-dimensional cross-sectional images **(A)** into a longitudinal display that characterizes the coronary artery in three dimensions **(B).** (*Courtesy of Peter Fitzgerald, MD.*)

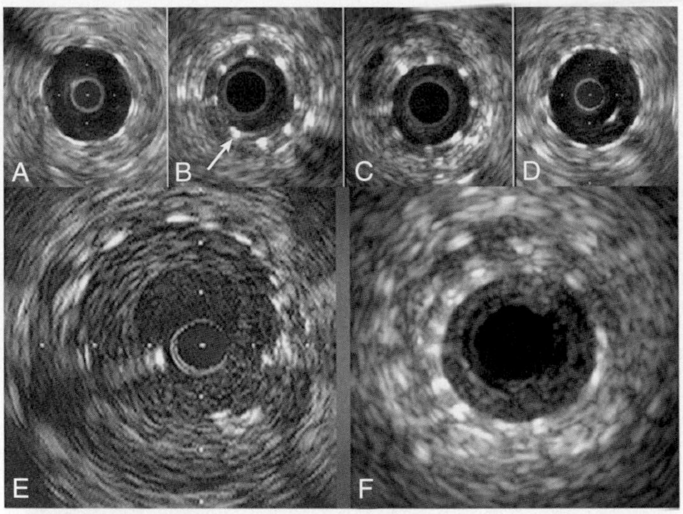

FIGURE 20–34 Stent deployment and in-stent restenosis assessed by intravascular ultrasound (IVUS). **A–D,** Coronary stent apposed against the vessel wall (**B,** arrow). **E,** IVUS Obtained in a patient who developed in-stent restenosis, as assessed by the soft-shadowed intimal hyperplasia that obstructs the lumen. **F,** Complete catheter entrapment with the soft intimal hyperplasia that results in stent restenosis. (*Courtesy of Gary Mintz, MD, and Neil Weissman, MD.*)

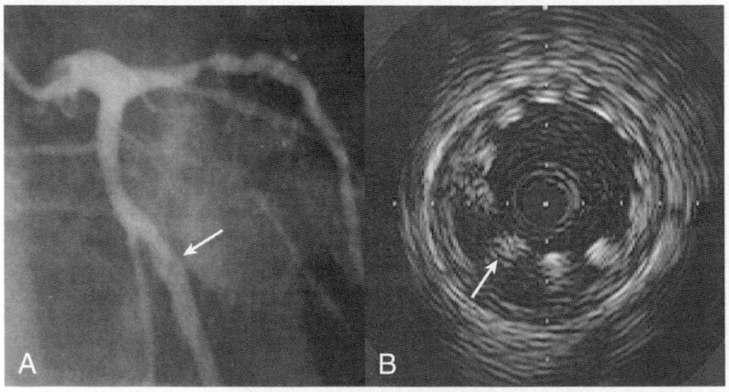

FIGURE 20–35 Incomplete stent apposition. Intravascular ultrasound (IVUS) imaging after coronary stent deployment. **A,** Excellent angiographic result after stent deployment (arrow). **B,** Despite this initial angiographic result, the stent struts are not completely apposed against the vessel wall (arrow). (*Courtesy of Peter Fitzgerald, MD.*)

stents[57] (Fig. 20-34). Nine-month percent intimal hyperplasia volume was reduced from 33.4% in patients treated with bare metal stents to 3.1% in patients treated with sirolimus-eluting stents ($P < 0.001$),[58] and from 23.3% in patients treated with bare metal stents to 7.8% in patients treated with paclitaxel-eluting stents.[59] Suppression of intimal hyperplasia is generally uniform across the length of the drug-eluting stent. Some have suggested that complete stent expansion is less critical in patients treated with drug-eluting stents due to the profound reduction in intimal hyperplasia.[60]

A unique finding in patients undergoing drug-eluting stent placement is the finding of late stent malapposition, in which stent struts are no longer adjacent to the vessel wall late following stent implantation (Fig. 20-35).[57,61] Although the clinical implications of this finding are not known,[62] some cases of very late drug-eluting stent thrombosis have been attributed to abnormal vessel wall healing and late stent malapposition, and extended follow-up studies are ongoing.

LIMITATIONS OF INTRAVASCULAR ULTRASONOGRAPHY. A number of factors have limited the widespread use of IVUS during PCI, including its cost, its cumbersome setup for occasional IVUS users, the steep "learning curve" for "on-line" IVUS interpretation, and the improved outcomes associated with routine use of stents. Current catheter-based IVUS systems are also limited by their inability to assess lumen diameters less than 1.0 mm because of the catheter size and "ring-down" artifact, and the limited spatial resolution of a 30-MHz imaging transducer (theoretical spatial resolution, 80 μm; usual spatial resolution, 120 to 150 μm) makes IVUS detection of a "vulnerable" plaque somewhat problematic. Nevertheless, IVUS will remain useful for lesions difficult to assess using conventional angiography as these limitations are addressed with newer IVUS designs. IVUS provides a powerful research tool for clinical trials, taking advantage of its ability to visualize the vessel wall as well as the lumen. Insights into the efficacy of therapeutic interventions have already emerged from application of this tool to clinical trials.

Novel Invasive Imaging Modalities

OPTICAL COHERENCE TOMOGRAPHY. Optical coherence tomography (OCT) is a novel catheter-based imaging modality that provides cross-sectional imaging of coronary arteries at a high resolution (4 to 10 microns),[63,64] permitting plaque characterization[65,66] and identification of the thickness of the fibrous cap (Fig. 20-36; Table 20-13).[67,68] More recently, OCT has been used to assess early and late results in patients undergoing coronary intervention.[69] Advantages of OCT include its high data acquisition rate, small (0.014 inch) guidewires and catheters, and ability to be combined with adjuvant optical techniques.[70,71] OCT also provides higher resolution of plaque compared with IVUS.[72] Its disadvantages are the need to eliminate blood from the imaging field and the long time required to acquire the image.[73] Although OCT images may give an indication of the overall composition of large homogeneous signal-poor regions, such as lipids or calcified areas, they could be unreliable in differentiating areas with heterogeneous composition.[73]

INTEGRATED BACKSCATTER ANALYSIS ("VIRTUAL HISTOLOGY"). This technology converts radiofrequency backscatter signals provided by IVUS into color-coded regions to characterize calcified, fibrofatty, calcified necrotic, and lipid-rich plaque (Fig. 20-37).[74-76] Although some have shown that the percentage of lipid core was significantly higher in patients with acute coronary syndromes and that the percentage of fibrotic content was higher in patients with stable angina,[77] others have found opposite findings using this technique.[78] These disparities underscore the need for careful prospective studies and analysis to correlate findings with virtual histology and late clinical outcome.

INTRACORONARY THERMOGRAPHY. Inflamed atherosclerotic plaques have higher surface temperatures that correlate with the pathological studies that find increased numbers of macrophages and decreased fibrous-cap thickness. Several coronary temperature-mapping catheters have been developed and correlated with the risk for late cardiac events[79] as well as therapeutic responsiveness to lipid-lowering therapy.[80]

PALPOGRAPHY. Intraarterial palpography assesses the local mechanical properties of tissue using the deformation caused by the intraluminal pressure and may permit the differentiation of fibrous and fatty tissue (see Fig. 20-37).[81,82] High-strain region can be determined using palpography and shows higher strain values in fatty than in fibrous plaques, and is highly predictive for the presence of macrophages within the artery. In contrast, calcified plaque showed low-strain values. Using this technique, patients with MI or unstable angina may be identified by more high-strain spots in their coronary arteries than patients with stable angina.[81,83]

COMPUTATIONAL FLOW DYNAMICS. Variations in shear stress elicit markedly different metabolic responses in patients with CAD.[84] Areas of low shear stress may promote atherosclerosis, whereas areas of high shear stress prevent atherosclerosis but predispose to plaque

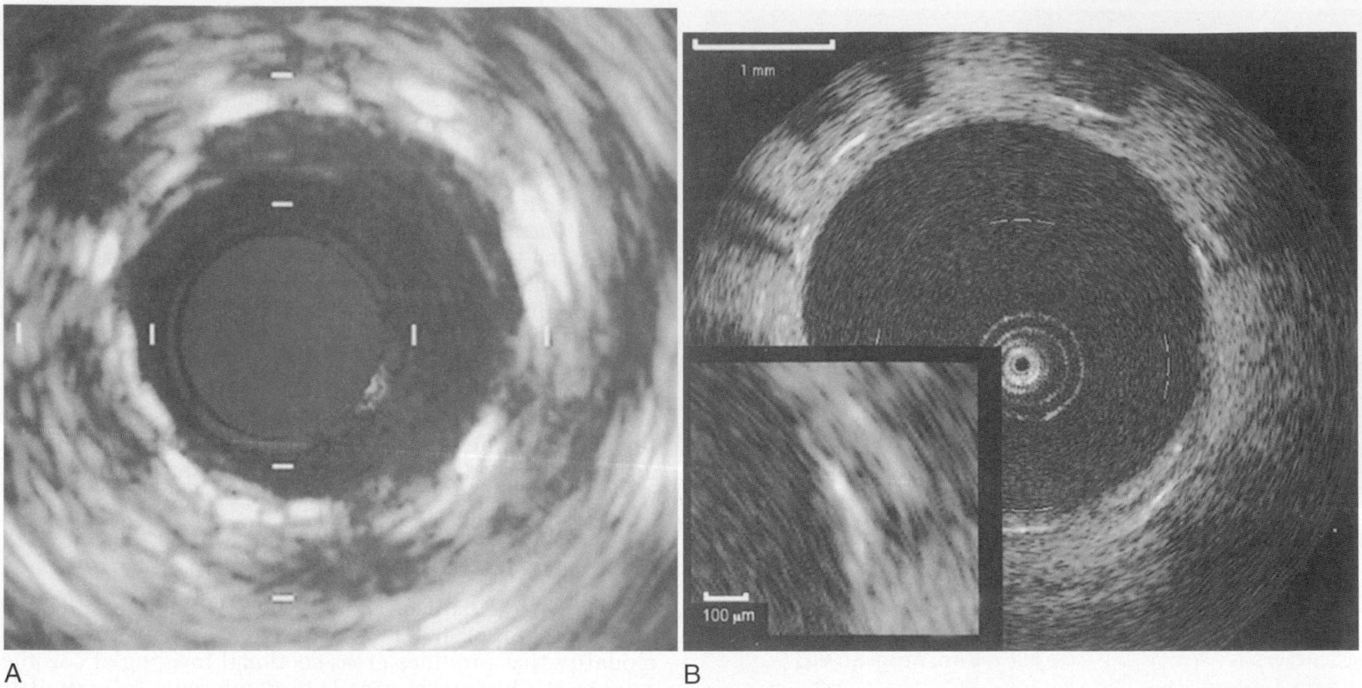

FIGURE 20–36 Invasive imaging using optical coherence tomography (OCT). **A,** IVUS imaging of a stented region. This image shows a typical visualization of the luminal border, vessel layers, and bright presentation of stent struts without precise detection of neointimal proliferation. **B,** OCT imaging of a stented region. Focusing on the inner vessel layer, OCT illustrates a very thin neointimal area at follow-up, as well as the doubled stenting markedly discriminating each stent strut. Segment magnification demonstrating the high resolution of OCT (insert). *(Reproduced from Grube E, Gerckens U, Buellesfeld L, Fitzgerald PJ: Images in cardiovascular medicine. Intracoronary imaging with optical coherence tomography: A new high-resolution technology providing striking visualization in the coronary artery. Circulation 106:2409-2410, 2002.)*

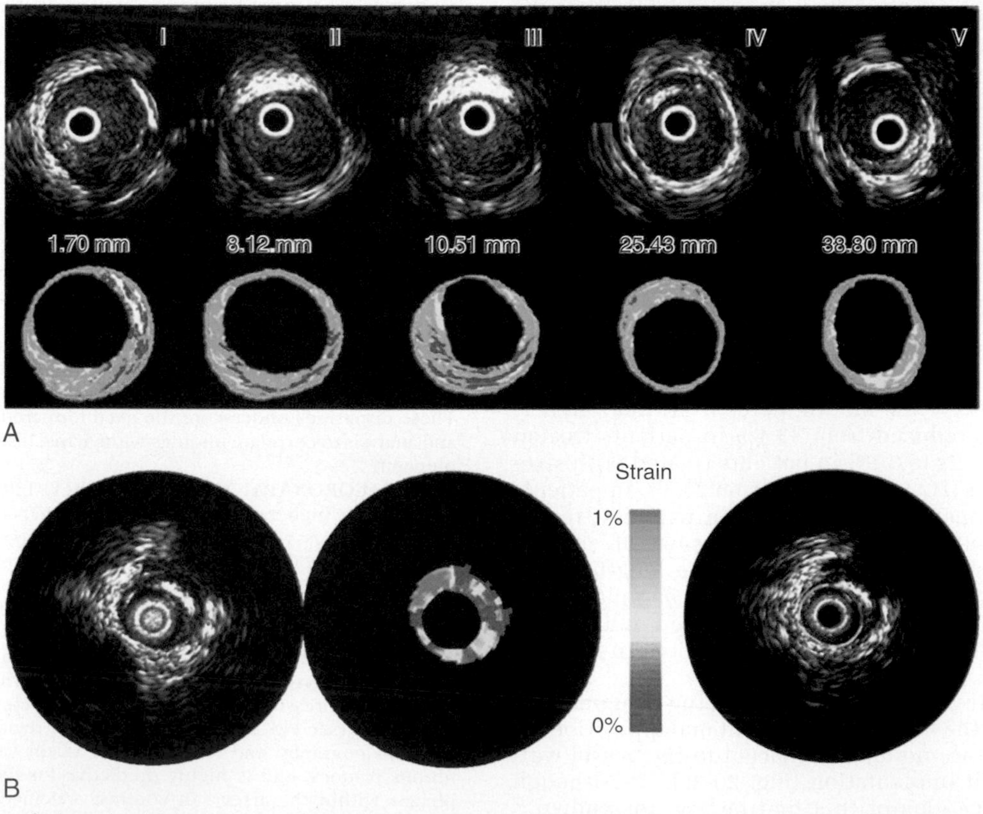

FIGURE 20–37 Detection of atherosclerotic plaque characteristics using alternative invasive imaging modalities. **A,** Intravascular ultrasound with virtual histology (IVUS-VH) along a coronary vessel. IVUS-VH cross-sectional areas in a representative patient showing the change in plaque composition (calcium: white; fibrous: green; fibrolipidic: greenish-yellow; and lipid core: red) along the longitudinal axis of the vessel. The distance between the cross-sectional area and the ostium of the vessel is reported in millimeters (mm). **B.** In vivo echogram (left panel), elastogram (center) and palpogram (right panel) of a cross section in the left anterior descending artery of a patient. The echogram reveals calcified material between noon and 3 o'clock. In this region, a very low strain value was assessed on both the elastogram and the palpogram (color-coded in red). *(**A,** Reproduced from Valgimigli M, Malagutti P, Rodriguez-Granillo G, et al: J Am Coll Cardiol 47[8]:1530-1537, 2006; **B,** Modified from Carlier SG, et al: Imaging of atherosclerosis. Elastography. J Cardiovasc Risk 9:237-245, 2002.)*

TABLE 20–13 Comparison of Noninvasive and Invasive Imaging Modalities for Detection of Individual Characteristics of Vulnerable Plaque

Imaging Modality	Resolution	Penetration	Fibrous Cap	Lipid Core	Inflammation	Calcium	Thrombus	Current Status
IVUS	100 μm	Good	+	++	–	+++	+	CS/CA
Angioscopy	UK	Poor	+	++	–	–	+++	CS/CA*
OCT	10 μm	Poor	+++	+++	+	+++	+	CS
Thermography	0.5 mm	Poor	–	–	+++	–	–	CS
Spectroscopy	NA	Poor	+	++	++	++	–	PCS
Intravascular MRI	160 μm	Good	+	++	++	++	+	PCS

*Clinically approved for commercial use in Japan.
CA = clinically approved for commercial use; CS = clinical studies; PCS = preclinical studies; IVUS = intravascular ultrasound, OCT = optical coherence tomography; MRI = magnetic resonance imaging; NA = not applicable; UK = unknown. +++ >90% sensitivity; ++80-90% sensitivity; + = 50-80% sensitivity; – <50%.
Adapted from MacNeill BD, Lowe HC, Takano M, et al: Intravascular modalities for detection of vulnerable plaque: Current status. Arterioscler Thromb Vasc Biol 23:1333-1342, 2003.

rupture. A novel integrated, but reproducible, technique of assessing endothelial shear stress using a combination of intracoronary ultrasound and biplane coronary angiography has been developed.[84] Using computational fluid dynamics, flow reversals, significant swirling, and large variations of local velocity and shear stress can be measured within the artery.[84] Long-term outcome studies assessing the clinical significance of these measurements are ongoing.[85]

Acknowledgment

The author acknowledges the contributions of Dr. Alexandra Almonacid for her assistance in the preparation of this chapter and Dr. John Bittl for his contribution to prior versions of this chapter.

REFERENCES

1. Holmes DR, Laskey WK, Wondrow MA, Cusma JT: Flat-panel detectors in the cardiac catheterization laboratory: Revolution or evolution—what are the issues? Catheter Cardiovasc Interv 63:324-30, 2004.

Indications for Coronary Arteriography

2. Scanlon P, Faxon D, Audet A, et al: ACC/AHA Guidelines for coronary angiography. J Am Coll Cardiol 33:1756-1824, 1999.
3. Braunwald E, Antman E, Beasley J, et al: ACC/AHA 2002 guideline update for the management of patients with unstable angina and non-ST-segment elevation myocardial infarction—summary article: A report of the American College of Cardiology/American Heart Association task force on practice guidelines (Committee on the Management of Patients With Unstable Angina). J Am Coll Cardiol 40(7):1366-74, 2002.

Complications of Coronary Arteriography

4. Ammann P, Brunner-La RH, Angehrn W, et al: Procedural complications following diagnostic coronary angiography are related to the operator's experience and the catheter size. Catheter Cardiovasc Interv 59(1):13-8, 2003.
5. West R, Ellis G, Brooks N: Complications of diagnostic cardiac catheterisation: Results from a confidential inquiry into cardiac catheter complications. Heart (England) 92:810-4, 2006.
6. Samal A, White C: Percutaneous management of access site complications. Catheter Cardiovasc Interv 57(1):12-23, 2002.
7. Khatri P, Kasner SE: Ischemic strokes after cardiac catheterization: Opportune thrombolysis candidates? Arch Neurol 63:817-21, 2006.
8. Fukumoto Y, Tsutsui H, Tsuchihashi M, et al: The incidence and risk factors of cholesterol embolization syndrome, a complication of cardiac catheterization: A prospective study. J Am Coll Cardiol 42(2):211-6, 2003.
9. Butler R, Webster M: Meralgia paresthetica: An unusual complication of cardiac catheterization via the femoral artery. Catheter Cardiovasc Interv 56(1):69-71, 2002.
10. Efstathopoulos EP, Karvouni E, Kottou S, et al: Patient dosimetry during coronary interventions: A comprehensive analysis. Am Heart J 147:468-75, 2004.

Technique of Coronary Arteriography

11. McNulty P, Ettinger S, Field J, et al: Cardiac catheterization in morbidly obese patients. Catheter Cardiovasc Interv 56(2):174-7, 2002.
12. Cox N, Resnic FS, Popma JJ, et al: Comparison of the risk of vascular complications associated with femoral and radial access coronary catheterization procedures in obese versus nonobese patients. Am J Cardiol 94:1174-7, 2004.
13. Agostoni P, Biondi-Zoccai GG, deBenedictus ML, et al: Radial versus femoral approach for percutaneous coronary diagnostic and interventional procedures: Systematic overview and meta-analysis of randomized trials. J Am Coll Cardiol 44:349-56, 2004.
14. Greenwood MJ, Della-Siega AJ, Fretz EB, et al: Vascular communications of the hand in patients being considered for transradial coronary angiography: Is the Allen's test accurate? J Am Coll Cardiol 46:2013-7, 2005.
15. Kiemeneij F, Fraser D, Slagboom T, et al: Hydrophilic coating aids radial sheath withdrawal and reduces patient discomfort following transradial coronary intervention: A randomized double-blind comparison of coated and uncoated sheaths. Catheter Cardiovasc Interv 59:161-4, 2003.
16. Abu-Ful A, Benharroch D, Henkin Y: Extraction of the radial artery during transradial coronary angiography: An unusual complication. J Invasive Cardiol 15:351-2, 2003.
17. Reddy BK, Brewster PS, Walsh T, et al: Randomized comparison of rapid ambulation using radial, 4 French femoral access, or femoral access with AngioSeal closure. Catheter Cardiovasc Interv 62:143-9, 2004.
18. Aspelin P, Aubry P, Fransson S, et al: Nephrotoxic effects in high-risk patients undergoing angiography. N Engl J Med 348(6):491-9, 2003.
19. Merten GJ, Burgess WP, Gray LV, et al: Prevention of contrast-induced nephropathy with sodium bicarbonate: A randomized controlled trial. JAMA 291:2328-34, 2004.
20. Pannu N, Wiebe N, Tonelli M: Prophylaxis strategies for contrast-induced nephropathy. JAMA 295:2765-79, 2006.
21. Tramer MR, von Elm E, Loubeyre P, Hauser C: Pharmacological prevention of serious anaphylactic reactions due to iodinated contrast media: systematic review. BMJ 333:675, 2006.
22. Thomsen HS, Morcos SK: Management of acute adverse reactions to contrast media. Eur Radiol 14:476-81, 2004.

Anatomy and Variations of the Coronary Arteries

23. Van Herck PL, Gavit L, Gorissen P, et al: Quantitative coronary arteriography on digital flat-panel system. Catheter Cardiovasc Interv 63:192-200, 2004.
24. Tsapaki V, Kottou S, Kollaros N, et al: Comparison of a conventional and a flat-panel digital system in interventional cardiology procedures. Br J Radiol (England) 77:562-7, 2004.
25. Gibson CM, Morrow DA, Murphy SA, et al: A randomized trial to evaluate the relative protection against post-percutaneous coronary intervention microvascular dysfunction, ischemia, and inflammation among antiplatelet and antithrombotic agents: The PROTECT-TIMI-30 trial. J Am Coll Cardiol 47:2364-73, 2006.
26. Graham MM, Faris PD, Ghali WA, et al: Validation of three myocardial jeopardy scores in a population-based cardiac catheterization cohort. Am Heart J 142:254-61, 2001.

Congenital Anomalies of the Coronary Circulations

27. Angelini P, Velasco JA, Flamm S: Coronary anomalies: Incidence, pathophysiology, and clinical relevance. Circulation 105:2449-54, 2002.
28. Angelini P: Coronary artery anomalies—current clinical issues: Definitions, classification, incidence, clinical relevance, and treatment guidelines. Tex Heart Inst J 29(4):271-8, 2002.
29. Eckart RE, Jones SO, Shry EA, et al:. Sudden death associated with anomalous coronary origin and obstructive coronary disease in the young. Cardiol Rev 14:161-3, 2006.
30. Basso C, Maron BJ, Corrado D, Thiene G: Clinical profile of congenital coronary artery anomalies with origin from the wrong aortic sinus leading to sudden death in young competitive athletes. J Am Coll Cardiol 35:1493-501, 2000.
31. von Kodolitsch Y, Franzen O, Lund GK, et al: Coronary artery anomalies Part II: Recent insights from clinical investigations. Z Kardiol (Germany) 94:1-13, 2005.
32. Porto I, MacDonald ST, Selvanayagam JB, Banning AP: Intravascular ultrasound to guide stenting of an anomalous right coronary artery coursing between the aorta and pulmonary artery. J Invasive Cardiol 17:E33-6, 2005.
33. Qayyum U, Leya F, Steen L, et al: New catheter design for cannulation of the anomalous right coronary artery arising from the left sinus of Valsalva. Catheter Cardiovasc Interv 60:382-8, 2003.

34. Cohen M, Tolleson T, Peter R, et al: Successful percutaneous coronary intervention with stent implantation in anomalous right coronary arteries arising from the left sinus of Valsalva: A report of two cases. Catheter Cardiovasc Interv 55(1):105-8, 2002.
35. Garcia-Rinaldi R: Right coronary arteries that course between aorta and pulmonary artery. Ann Thorac Surg 74(3):973-4, 2002.
36. Doorey AJ, Pasquale MJ, Lally JF, et al: Six-month success of intracoronary stenting for anomalous coronary arteries associated with myocardial ischemia. Am J Cardiol 86:580-2, A10, 2000.
37. Rentoukas E, Alpert M, Deftereos S, et al: Anomalous left coronary artery arising from the right sinus of Valsalva in a man with unstable angina pectoris and right coronary artery stenosis. Am J Med Sci 323(4):223-6, 2002.
38. Kim SY, Seo JB, Do KH, et al: Coronary artery anomalies: Classification and ECG-gated multi-detector row CT findings with angiographic correlation. Radiographics 26:317-33; discussion 333-4, 2006.
39. Sevrukov A, Aker N, Sullivan C, et al: Identifying the course of an anomalous left coronary artery using contrast-enhanced electron beam tomography and three-dimensional reconstruction. Catheter Cardiovasc Interv 57:532-6, 2002.

40. Luo L, Kebede S, Wu S, Stouffer GA: Coronary artery fistulae. Am J Med Sci (United States) 332:79-84, 2006.
41. Burma O, Rahman A, Ilkay E: Coronary arteriovenous fistulas from both coronary arteries to pulmonary artery. Eur J Cardiothorac Surg 21(1):86, 2002.
42. Alegria JR, Herrmann J, Holmes DR, et al: Myocardial bridging. Eur Heart J 26:1159-68, 2005.
43. Rozenberg V, Nepomnyashchikh L: Pathomorphology of myocardial bridges and their role in the pathogenesis of coronary disease. Bull Exp Biol Med 134(6):593-6, 2002.

Lesion Complexity

44. Smith S, Feldman T, Hirshfeld J, et al: ACC/AHA/SCAI 2005 Guideline Update for Percutaneous Coronary Intervention—summary article: A report of the American College of Cardiology/American Heart Association Task Force on Practice Guidelines (ACC/AHA/SCAI Writing Committee to Update the 2001 Guidelines for Percutaneous Coronary Intervention). Circulation 113(1):156-75, 2006.
45. Krone R, Shaw R, Klein L, et al: Evaluation of the American College of Cardiology/American Heart Association and the Society for Coronary Angiography and Interventions lesion classification system in the current "stent era" of coronary interventions (from the ACC-National Cardiovascular Data Registry). Am J Cardiol 92(4):389-94, 2003.
46. Singh M, Rihal CS, Lennon RJ, et al: Comparison of Mayo Clinic risk score and American College of Cardiology/American Heart Association lesion classification in the prediction of adverse cardiovascular outcome following percutaneous coronary interventions. J Am Coll Cardiol 44:357-61, 2004.
47. Popma J, Leon M, Moses J, et al: Quantitative assessment of angiographic restenosis after sirolimus-eluting stent implantation in native coronary arteries. Circulation 110(25):3773-80, 2004.
48. Alexander JH, Hafley G, Harrington RA, et al: Efficacy and safety of edifoligide, an E2F transcription factor decoy, for prevention of vein graft failure following coronary artery bypass graft surgery: PREVENT IV: A randomized controlled trial. JAMA 294:2446-54, 2005.
49. Hoye A, Lemos PA, Arampatzis CA, et al: Effectiveness of the sirolimus-eluting stent in the treatment of saphenous vein graft disease. J Invasive Cardiol 16:230-3, 2004.
50. Giugliano GR, Kuntz RE, Popma JJ, et al: Determinants of 30-day adverse events following saphenous vein graft intervention with and without a distal occlusion embolic protection device. Am J Cardiol 95:173-7, 2005.
51. Koerselman J, van der Graaf Y, de Jaegere PP, Grobbee DE: Coronary collaterals: An important and underexposed aspect of coronary artery disease. Circulation 107(19):2507-2511, 2003.
52. Werner GS, Ferrari M, Heinke S, et al: Angiographic assessment of collateral connections in comparison with invasively determined collateral function in chronic coronary occlusions. Circulation 107(15):1972-1977, 2003.

Intravascular Ultrasonography and Related Invasive Imaging Methods

53. Nicholls SJ, Sipahi I, Schoenhagen P, et al: Application of intravascular ultrasound in anti-atherosclerotic drug development. Nat Rev Drug Discov 5:485-92, 2006.
54. Schoenhagen P, Tuzcu EM, Apperson-Hansen C, et al: Determinants of arterial wall remodeling during lipid-lowering therapy: Serial intravascular ultrasound observations from the Reversal of Atherosclerosis with Aggressive Lipid Lowering Therapy (REVERSAL) trial. Circulation 113:2826-34, 2006.
55. Mintz G, Maehara A, Bui A, Weissman N: Multiple versus single coronary plaque ruptures detected by intravascular ultrasound in stable and unstable angina pectoris and in acute myocardial infarction. Am J Cardiol 91(11):1333-5, 2003.
56. Futamatsu H, Sabate M, Angiolillo DJ, et al: Characterization of plaque prolapse after drug-eluting stent implantation in diabetic patients: A three-dimensional volumetric intravascular ultrasound outcome study. J Am Coll Cardiol 48:1139-45, 2006.
57. Mintz GS, Weissman NJ: Intravascular ultrasound in the drug-eluting stent era. J Am Coll Cardiol 48:421-9, 2006.
58. Moses J, Leon M, Popma J, Fitzgerald P, et al: Sirolimus-eluting stents versus standard stents in patients with stenosis in a native coronary artery. N Engl J Med 349(14):1315-23, 2003.
59. Colombo A, Drzewiecki J, Banning A, et al: Randomized study to assess the effectiveness of slow- and moderate-release polymer-based Paclitaxel-eluting stents for coronary artery lesions Circulation 108(7):788-94, 2003.
60. Cheneau E, Pichard AD, Satler LF, et al: Intravascular ultrasound stent area of sirolimus-eluting stents and its impact on late outcome. Am J Cardiol 95:1240-2, 2005.
61. Costa MA, Sabate M, Angiolillo DJ, et al: Intravascular ultrasound characterization of the "black hole" phenomenon after drug-eluting stent implantation. Am J Cardiol 97:203-6, 2006.
62. Kimura M, Mintz GS, Carlier S, et al: Outcome after acute incomplete sirolimus-eluting stent apposition as assessed by serial intravascular ultrasound. Am J Cardiol 98:436-42, 2006.
63. Jang IK, Bouma BE, Kang DH, et al: Visualization of coronary atherosclerotic plaques in patients using optical coherence tomography: Comparison with intravascular ultrasound. J Am Coll Cardiol 39:604-9, 2002.
64. Jang IK, Tearney GJ, MacNeill B, et al: In vivo characterization of coronary atherosclerotic plaque by use of optical coherence tomography. Circulation 111:1551-5, 2005.
65. Stamper D, Weissman NJ, Brezinski M: Plaque characterization with optical coherence tomography. J Am Coll Cardiol 47:C69-79, 2006.
66. Rieber J, Meissner O, Babaryka G, et al: Diagnostic accuracy of optical coherence tomography and intravascular ultrasound for the detection and characterization of atherosclerotic plaque composition in ex-vivo coronary specimens: A comparison with histology. Coron Artery Dis 17:125-30, 2006.
67. Kume T, Akasaka T, Kawamoto T, et al: Measurement of the thickness of the fibrous cap by optical coherence tomography. Am Heart J 152:755.e1-4, 2006.
68. Grube E, Gerckens U, Buellesfeld L, Fitzgerald PJ: Images in cardiovascular medicine. Intracoronary imaging with optical coherence tomography: A new high-resolution technology providing striking visualization in the coronary artery. Circulation 106:2409-10, 2002.
69. Diaz-Sandoval LJ, Bouma BE, Tearney GJ, Jang IK. Optical coherence tomography as a tool for percutaneous coronary interventions. Catheter Cardiovasc Interv 65:492-6, 2005.
70. Brezinski M: Characterizing arterial plaque with optical coherence tomography. Curr Opin Cardiol 17:648-55, 2002.
71. MacNeill BD, Lowe HC, Takano M, et al: Intravascular modalities for detection of vulnerable plaque: Current status. Arterioscler Thromb Vasc Biol 23:1333-42, 2003.
72. Kawasaki M, Bouma BE, Bressner J, et al: Diagnostic accuracy of optical coherence tomography and integrated backscatter intravascular ultrasound images for tissue characterization of human coronary plaques. J Am Coll Cardiol 48:81-8, 2006.
73. Manfrini O, Mont E, Leone O, et al: Sources of error and interpretation of plaque morphology by optical coherence tomography. Am J Cardiol 98:156-9, 2006.
74. De Maria AN, Narula J, Mahmud E, Tsimikas S: Imaging vulnerable plaque by ultrasound. J Am Coll Cardiol 47:C32-9, 2006.
75. Sano K, Kawasaki M, Ishihara Y, et al: Assessment of vulnerable plaques causing acute coronary syndrome using integrated backscatter intravascular ultrasound. J Am Coll Cardiol 47:734-41, 2006.
76. Valgimigli M, Malagutti P, Rodriguez-Granillo G, et al: Distal left main coronary disease is a major predictor of outcome in patients undergoing percutaneous intervention in the drug-eluting stent era: An integrated clinical and angiographic analysis based on the Rapamycin-Eluting Stent Evaluated At Rotterdam Cardiology Hospital (RESEARCH) and Taxus-Stent Evaluated At Rotterdam Cardiology Hospital (T-SEARCH) registries. J Am Coll Cardiol 47(8):1530-7, 2006.
77. Rodriguez-Granillo GA, McFadden EP, Valgimigli M, et al: Coronary plaque composition of nonculprit lesions, assessed by in vivo intracoronary ultrasound radio frequency data analysis, is related to clinical presentation. Am Heart J 151:1020-24, 2006.
78. Surmely JF, Nasu K, Fujita H, et al: Coronary plaque composition of culprit/target lesions according to the clinical presentation: A virtual histology intravascular ultrasound. Eur Heart J 27:2939-44, 2006.
79. Madjid M, Willerson JT, Casscells SW: Intracoronary thermography for detection of high-risk vulnerable plaques. J Am Coll Cardiol 47:C80-5, 2006.
80. Toutouzas K, Drakopoulou M, Mitropoulos J, et al: Elevated plaque temperature in non-culprit de novo atheromatous lesions of patients with acute coronary syndromes. J Am Coll Cardiol 47:301-6, 2006.
81. Schaar JA, van der Steen AF, Mastik F, et al: Intravascular palpography for vulnerable plaque assessment. J Am Coll Cardiol 47:C86-91, 2006.
82. Carlier SG, de Korte CL, Brusseau E, et al: Imaging of atherosclerosis. Elastography. J Cardiovasc Risk 9:237-45, 2002.
83. Schaar JA, Regar E, Mastik F, et al: Incidence of high-strain patterns in human coronary arteries: Assessment with three-dimensional intravascular palpography and correlation with clinical presentation. Circulation 109:2716-9, 2004.
84. Feldman CL, Ilegbusi OJ, Hu Z, et al: Determination of in vivo velocity and endothelial shear stress patterns with phasic flow in human coronary arteries: A methodology to predict progression of coronary atherosclerosis. Am Heart J 143:931-9, 2002.
85. Stone PH, Coskun AU, Kinlay S, et al: Effect of endothelial shear stress on the progression of coronary artery disease, vascular remodeling, and in-stent restenosis in humans: In vivo 6-month follow-up study. Circulation 108:438-44, 2003.

Coronary Arteriography

The American College of Cardiology (ACC) and the American Heart Association (AHA) first published guidelines for coronary angiography in 1987.[1] These were updated in 1999, in collaboration with the Society for Cardiac Angiography and Intervention.[2] Although these guidelines have not been revised since then, recommendations for the use of coronary angiography are included in several more recent practice guidelines, including those for stable angina,[3] unstable angina and non-ST-elevation myocardial infarction,[4] acute ST-elevation myocardial infarction,[5] noncardiac surgery,[6] heart failure,[7] and valvular disease.[8] The text and tables that follow present an amalgam of recommendations from the 1999 ACC/AHA coronary angiography guidelines and from more recent condition-specific guidelines.

As with other ACC/AHA guidelines, these use the standard ACC/AHA classification system for indications:

Class I: Conditions for which there is evidence and/or general agreement that the test is useful and effective

Class II: Conditions for which there is conflicting evidence and/or a divergence of opinion about the usefulness or efficacy of performing the test

Class IIa: Weight of evidence or opinion is in favor of usefulness or efficacy.

Class IIb: Usefulness or efficacy is less well established by evidence or opinion.

Class III: Conditions for which there is evidence and/or general agreement that the test is not useful or effective and in some cases may be harmful.

Three levels are used to rate the evidence on which recommendations have been based. Level A recommendations are derived from data from multiple randomized clinical trials, level B recommendations are derived from a single randomized trial or nonrandomized studies, and level C recommendations are based on the consensus opinion of experts.

Coronary Arteriography in Asymptomatic Patients or Those with Stable Angina

The 1999 ACC/AHA guidelines do not support routine use of coronary angiography as a first-line test for asymptomatic patients, but consider angiography possibly appropriate (Class IIa) in patients with high-risk criteria suggestive of ischemia on noninvasive testing (Table 20G-1). Angiography is clearly indicated (Class I) for patients with chest pain who have survived a sudden cardiac arrest, and for patients with known chronic coronary disease who have disabling symptoms, high-risk criteria on noninvasive testing, and/or clinical evidence of heart failure (see Table 20G-1).

Coronary Arteriography in Patients with ST-Elevation Myocardial Infarction

The ACC/AHA guidelines on coronary angiography[3] and ST-elevation myocardial infarction (STEMI)[5] do not recommend coronary angiography as a routine diagnostic tool for STEMI. However, coronary angiography is strongly supported for patients eligible for primary or rescue percutaneous coronary intervention (PCI), as well as those with cardiogenic shock or other structural cardiac injury (e.g., ventricular septal rupture or severe mitral regurgitation) or other major complications (Table 20G-2).

Coronary Arteriography in Patients with Unstable Angina/Non-ST-Elevation Myocardial Infarction

Coronary angiography is not generally recommended as part of the routine evaluation for unstable angina/non-ST-elevation myocardial infarction (UA/NSTEMI), but a low threshold for angiography is endorsed as part of an early invasive strategy for patients with high-risk indicators, such as recurrent symptoms of ischemia despite adequate medical therapy, high-risk noninvasive test results, depressed left ventricular (LV) systolic function, severe arrhythmia, and prior revascularization (Table 20G-3).

Coronary Arteriography in Patients with Nonspecific Chest Pain

The 1999 ACC/AHA guidelines on coronary angiography,[2] as well as the 2002 guidelines on UA/NSTEMI, discourage use of coronary angiography for patients with nonspecific chest pain unless they have high-risk findings on noninvasive testing. The guidelines do support angiography for patients with chest pain after cocaine use if ST segments remain elevated after medical therapy (Table 20G-4). Coronary angiography is also endorsed for patients with clinical evidence of coronary spasm.

Coronary Arteriography for Patient Follow-Up

Coronary angiography is not supported as part of routine follow-up of patients who have no change in clinical status (Table 20G-5), but it is supported for patients with marked limitations of functional status despite maximal medical therapy, or who have evidence of ongoing ischemia after revascularization procedures.

Coronary Arteriography for the Evaluation and Assessment of Heart Failure

The 2005 ACC/AHA guidelines on heart failure[7] recommend that clinicians proceed directly to coronary angiography in patients who have heart failure or impaired LV function and clinical evidence of ischemia given the benefits of revascularization in this high-risk population (Table 20G-6). There is weaker support for the use of angiography for patients with heart failure in the absence of clear-cut cardiac chest pain, because revascularization has not been shown to improve clinical outcomes in patients without angina.

Coronary Arteriography in Patients with Valvular Disease

Coronary angiography for patients with valvular heart disease is generally used as a prelude to surgery to provide insight into whether the patient has coexisting coronary disease that might warrant concomitant revascularization (Table 20G-7). Cardiac catheterization is occasionally needed to obtain hemodynamic data, but advances in noninvasive testing have greatly reduced the role of catheterization for that purpose. The ACC/AHA guidelines on valvular heart disease recommend preoperative coronary angiography in men older than 35 years, premenopausal women older than 35 years with coronary risk

TABLE 20G–1 ACC/AHA Recommendations for Coronary Arteriography in Asymptomatic Patients or Those with Stable Angina

Indication	Class I (Indicated)	Class IIa (Strong Supportive Evidence)	Class IIb (Weak Supportive Evidence)	Class III (Not Indicated)
Establishing a diagnosis in patients with suspected angina or a significant change in anginal symptoms	Patients with known or possible angina pectoris who have survived sudden cardiac death (B)	Patients with an uncertain diagnosis after noninvasive testing in whom the benefit of a more certain diagnosis outweighs the risk and cost of coronary angiography (C) Patients who cannot undergo noninvasive testing because of disability, illness, or morbid obesity (C) Patients with an occupational requirement for a definitive diagnosis (C) Patients who by virtue of young age at onset of symptoms, noninvasive imaging, or other clinical parameters are suspected of having a nonatherosclerotic cause for myocardial ischemia (e.g., coronary artery anomaly, Kawasaki disease, primary coronary artery dissection, radiation-induced vasculopathy) (C) Patients in whom coronary artery spasm is suspected and provocative testing may be necessary (C) Patients with a high pretest probability of left main or three-vessel CAD (C)	Patients with recurrent hospitalization for chest pain in whom a definite diagnosis is judged necessary (C) Patients with an overriding desire for a definitive diagnosis and a greater than low probability of CAD (C)	Patients with significant comorbidity in whom the risk of coronary arteriography outweighs the benefit of the procedure (C) Patients with an overriding personal desire for a definitive diagnosis and a low probability of CAD (C)
Risk stratification in patients with chronic stable angina	Patients with disabling (Canadian (CCS classes III and IV) chronic stable angina, despite medical therapy (B) Patients with high-risk criteria on noninvasive testing regardless of anginal severity (B) Patients with angina who have survived sudden cardiac death or serious ventricular arrhythmia (B) Patients with angina and symptoms and signs of HF (C) Patients with clinical characteristics that indicate a high likelihood of severe CAD (C)	Patients with significant left ventricular dysfunction (ejection fraction less than 45%), CCS class I or II angina, and demonstrable ischemia but less than high-risk criteria on noninvasive testing (C) Patients with inadequate prognostic information after noninvasive testing (C)	Patients with CCS class I or II angina, preserved LV function (ejection fraction more than 45%), and less than high-risk criteria on noninvasive testing (C) Patients with CCS class III or IV angina, which improves with medical therapy to class I or II (C) Patients with CCS class I or II angina but intolerance (unacceptable side effects) to adequate medical therapy (C)	Patients with CCS class I or II angina who respond to medical therapy and who have no evidence of ischemia on noninvasive testing (C) Patients who prefer to avoid revascularization (C)
Risk stratification in asymptomatic patients		Patients with high- risk criteria suggesting ischemia on noninvasive testing (C)	Patients with inadequate prognostic information after noninvasive testing (C) Patients with clinical characteristics that indicate a high likelihood of severe CAD (C)	Patients who prefer to avoid revascularization (C)
Monitoring of symptoms and antianginal therapy	Coronary angiography in patients with marked limitation of ordinary activity (CCS class III), despite maximal medical therapy (C)			

ACC = American College of Cardiology; AHA = American Heart Association; CAD = coronary artery disease; CCS = Canadian Cardiovascular Society; HF = heart failure.
From Gibbons RJ, Abrams J, Chatterjee K, et al: ACC/AHA 2002 guideline update for the management of patients with chronic stable angina: A report of the American College of Cardiology/American Heart Association Task Force on practice guidelines (Committee on the Management of Patients With Chronic Stable Angina). J Am Coll Cardiol 41:159, 2003.

TABLE 20G–2 ACC/AHA Recommendations for Coronary Arteriography in Patients with ST-Elevation Myocardial Infarction

Indication	Class I (Indicated)	Class IIa (Strong Supportive Evidence)	Class IIb (Weak Supportive Evidence)	Class III (Not Indicated)
Diagnosis of STEMI	Diagnostic coronary angiography should be performed: a. In candidates for primary or rescue percutaneous coronary intervention (A) b. In patients with cardiogenic shock who are candidates for revascularization (A) c. In candidates for surgical repair of VSR or severe mitral regurgitation (B) d. In patients with persistent hemodynamic and/or electrical instability (C)			Coronary angiography should not be performed in patients with extensive comorbidities in whom risks of revascularization likely to outweigh benefits (C)
Treatment of STEMI	(see "Guidelines," Chap. 52)			
Hospital management of STEMI	Coronary arteriography should be performed in patients with spontaneous episodes of myocardial ischemia or episodes of myocardial ischemia provoked by minimal exertion during recovery from STEMI (A) Coronary arteriography should be performed for intermediate- or high-risk findings on noninvasive testing after STEMI (B) Coronary arteriography should be performed if the patient is sufficiently stable before definitive therapy of a mechanical complication of STEMI, such as acute mitral regurgitation, VSR, pseudoaneurysm, or LV aneurysm (B) Coronary arteriography should be performed in patients with persistent hemodynamic instability (B) Coronary arteriography should be performed in survivors of STEMI who had clinical heart failure during the acute episode but subsequently demonstrated well-preserved LV function (C)	Reasonable to perform coronary arteriography when STEMI is suspected to have occurred by mechanism other than thrombotic occlusion of an atherosclerotic plaque, including coronary embolism, certain metabolic or hematological diseases, or coronary artery spasm (C) Coronary arteriography is reasonable in STEMI patients with any of the following: diabetes mellitus, LV ejection fraction less than 0.40, congestive heart failure, prior revascularization, or life-threatening ventricular arrhythmias (C)	Catheterization and revascularization may be considered as part of strategy of routine coronary arteriography for risk assessment after fibrinolytic therapy (B)	Coronary arteriography should not be performed in survivors of STEMI thought not to be candidates for coronary revascularization (A)

ACC = American College of Cardiology; AHA = American Heart Association; CAD = coronary artery disease; CCS = Canadian Cardiovascular Society; HF = heart failure; LV = left ventricular; STEMI = ST-elevation myocardial infarction; VSR = ventricular septal rupture.

From Antman EM, Anbe DT, Armstrong PW, et al: ACC/AHA guidelines for the management of patients with ST-elevation myocardial infarction: A report of the American College of Cardiology/American Heart Association Task Force on Practice Guidelines (Committee to Revise the 1999 Guidelines for the Management of Patients with Acute Myocardial Infarction). Circulation 110:e82, 2004.

TABLE 20G–3 ACC/AHA Recommendations for Coronary Arteriography in Patients with Non-ST-Elevation Myocardial Infarction

Indication	Class I (Indicated)	Class IIa (Strong Supportive Evidence)	Class IIb (Weak Supportive Evidence)	Class III (Not Indicated)
Management of UA/NSTEMI	An early invasive strategy in patients with UA/NSTEMI and any of the following high-risk indicators (A): a. Recurrent angina or ischemia at rest or with low-level activities despite intensive anti-ischemic therapy b. Elevated TnT or TnI level c. New or presumably new ST segment depression d. Recurrent angina/ischemia with CHF symptoms, an S_3 gallop, pulmonary edema, worsening rales, or new or worsening MR e. High-risk findings on noninvasive stress testing f. Depressed LV systolic function (e.g., EF less than 0.40 on noninvasive study)	An early invasive strategy in patients with repeated presentations for ACS despite therapy and without evidence for ongoing ischemia or high risk (C)		Coronary angiography in patients with extensive comorbidities (e.g., liver or pulmonary failure, cancer), in whom the risks of revascularization are not likely to outweigh the benefits (C) Coronary angiography in patients with acute chest pain and a low likelihood of ACS (C)

Continues

TABLE 20G–3 ACC/AHA Recommendations for Coronary Arteriography in Patients with Non-ST-Elevation Myocardial Infarction—cont'd

Indication	Class I (Indicated)	Class IIa (Strong Supportive Evidence)	Class IIb (Weak Supportive Evidence)	Class III (Not Indicated)
	g. Hemodynamic instability h. Sustained ventricular tachycardia i. PCI within 6 months j. Prior CABG In the absence of these findings, either an early conservative or an early invasive strategy in hospitalized patients without contraindications for revascularization (B)			Coronary angiography in patients who will not consent to revascularization, regardless of the findings (C)
Postdischarge follow-up	Patients managed initially with a conservative strategy who experience recurrent unstable angina or severe (CCS class III) chronic stable angina despite medical management who are suitable for revascularization (B)			

ACC = American College of Cardiology; ACS = acute coronary syndrome; AHA = American Heart Association; CABG = coronary artery bypass grafting; CAD = coronary artery disease; CCS = Canadian Cardiovascular Society; CHF = congestive heart failure; EF = ejection fraction; MR = mitral regurgitation; LV = left ventricular; PCI = percutaneous coronary intervention; TnI = troponin I; TnT = troponin T; UA/NSTEMI = unstable angina/non-ST-elevation myocardial infarction.

From Braunwald E, Antman EM, Beasley JW, et al: ACC/AHA guidelines for the management of patients with unstable angina and non-ST-segment elevation myocardial infarction. A report of the American College of Cardiology/American Heart Association Task Force on Practice Guidelines (Committee on the Management of Patients With Unstable Angina). J Am Coll Cardiol 36:970, 2000.

TABLE 20G–4 ACC/AHA Recommendations for Coronary Arteriography in Patients with Nonspecific Chest Pain

Indication	Class I (Indicated)	Class IIa (Strong Supportive Evidence)	Class IIb (Weak Supportive Evidence)	Class III (Not Indicated)
General*	High-risk findings on noninvasive testing (B)		Patients with recurrent hospitalizations for chest pain who have abnormal (but not high-risk) or equivocal findings on noninvasive testing (B)	All other patients with nonspecific chest pain (C)
Chest pain after cocaine use†	Immediate coronary arteriography, if possible, when ST segments remain elevated after nitroglycerin and calcium antagonists; thrombolysis (with or without PCI) if thrombus is detected (C)	Coronary arteriography, if available in patients with ST segment depression or isolated T wave changes not known to be old and who are unresponsive to nitroglycerin and calcium antagonists (C)		Coronary arteriography in patients with chest pain without ST-T wave changes (C)
Variant (Prinzmetal) angina†	Coronary arteriography in patients with episodic chest pain and ST segment elevation that resolves with nitroglycerin and/or calcium antagonists (B)	Provocative testing in patients with a nonobstructive lesion on coronary arteriography, clinical picture of coronary spasm, and transient ST segment elevation (B)	Provocative testing without coronary arteriography (C) In the absence of significant CAD on coronary arteriography, provocative testing with methylergonovine, acetylcholine, or methacholine when coronary spasm is suspected but there is no evidence on the ECG of transient ST segment elevation (C)	Provocative testing in patients with high-grade obstructive lesions on coronary arteriography (B)
Cardiac syndrome X, coronary microvascular disease†	If ECGs are not available during chest pain and coronary spasm cannot be ruled out, coronary arteriography and provocative testing with methylergonovine, acetylcholine, or methacholine (C)			

*From Scanlon PJ, Faxon DP, Audet AM, et al: ACC/AHA guidelines for coronary angiography: executive summary and recommendations. A report of the American College of Cardiology/American Heart Association Task Force on Practice Guidelines (Committee on Coronary Angiography) developed in collaboration with the Society for Cardiac Angiography and Interventions. Circulation 99:2345, 1999.

†From Braunwald E, Antman EM, Beasley JW, et al: ACC/AHA 2002 guideline update for the management of patients with unstable angina and non-ST-segment elevation myocardial infarction—summary article: A report of the American College of Cardiology/American Heart Association task force on practice guidelines (Committee on the Management of Patients With Unstable Angina). J Am Coll Cardiol 40:1366, 2002.

ACC = American College of Cardiology; AHA = American Heart Association; CAD = coronary artery disease; ECG = electrocardiogram; PCI = percutaneous coronary intervention.

TABLE 20G–5 ACC/AHA Recommendations for Coronary Arteriography for Patient Follow-Up

Indication	Class I (Indicated)	Class IIa (Strong Supportive Evidence)	Class IIb (Weak Supportive Evidence)	Class III (Not Indicated)
Monitoring of symptoms and antianginal therapy*	Coronary angiography in patients with marked limitation of ordinary activity (CCS class III) despite maximal medical therapy (C)			Repeat coronary angiography in patients with no change in clinical status, no change on repeat exercise testing or stress imaging, and insignificant coronary artery disease on initial evaluation (C)
After coronary artery bypass grafting (CABG) in patients with UA/NSTEMI†	Maintain a low threshold for angiography, given the many anatomical possibilities that might be responsible for recurrent ischemia (B) Patients managed initially with a conservative strategy who experience recurrent unstable angina or severe (CCS class III) chronic stable angina, despite medical management, who are suitable for revascularization should undergo coronary arteriography (B)			
Postrevascularization ischemia‡	Suspected abrupt closure or subacute stent thrombosis after percutaneous revascularization (B) Recurrent angina or high-risk criteria on noninvasive evaluation (see Table 20-G1) within 9 months of percutaneous revascularization (C)	Recurrent symptomatic ischemia within 12 months of coronary artery bypass graft (B) Noninvasive evidence of high-risk criteria at any time postoperatively (B) Recurrent angina inadequately controlled by medical means after revascularization (C) For patients undergoing PCI for unprotected left main coronary obstructions, coronary angiography follow-up between 2 and 6 months after PCI is reasonable (C)§	Asymptomatic post-PTCA patient suspected of having restenosis within the first months after angioplasty because of an abnormal noninvasive test result but without noninvasive high-risk criteria (B) Recurrent angina without high-risk criteria on noninvasive testing occurring >1 yr postoperatively (C) Asymptomatic postbypass patient in whom a deterioration in serial noninvasive testing has been documented but who is not at high risk on noninvasive testing (C)	Symptoms in a postbypass patient who is not a candidate for repeat revascularization (C) Routine angiography in asymptomatic patients after PTCA or other surgery, unless as part of an approved research protocol (C)

*From Gibbons RJ, Abrams J, Chatterjee K, et al: ACC/AHA 2002 guideline update for the management of patients with chronic stable angina–summary article: A report of the American College of Cardiology/American Heart Association Task Force on practice guidelines (Committee on the Management of Patients With Chronic Stable Angina). J Am Coll Cardiol 41:159, 2003.

†From Braunwald E, Antman EM, Beasley JW, et al: ACC/AHA 2002 guideline update for the management of patients with unstable angina and non-ST-segment elevation myocardial infarction–summary article: A report of the American College of Cardiology/American Heart Association task force on practice guidelines (Committee on the Management of Patients With Unstable Angina). J Am Coll Cardiol 40:1366, 2002.

‡From Scanlon PJ, Faxon DP, Audet AM, et al: ACC/AHA guidelines for coronary angiography: executive summary and recommendations. A report of the American College of Cardiology/American Heart Association Task Force on Practice Guidelines (Committee on Coronary Angiography) developed in collaboration with the Society for Cardiac Angiography and Interventions. Circulation 99:2345, 1999.

§From Smith SC, Jr., Feldman TE, Hirshfeld JW Jr, et al: ACC/AHA/SCAI 2005 guideline update for percutaneous coronary intervention: A report of the American College of Cardiology/American Heart Association Task Force on Practice Guidelines (ACC/AHA/SCAI Writing Committee to Update the 2001 Guidelines for Percutaneous Coronary Intervention). J Am Coll Cardiol 47:e1, 2006.

ACC = American College of Cardiology; AHA = American Heart Association; CCS = Canadian Cardiovascular Society; ECG = electrocardiogram; PCI = percutaneous coronary intervention; PTCA = percutaneous transluminal coronary angioplasty; UA/NSTEMI = unstable angina/non-ST-elevation myocardial infarction.

factors, and postmenopausal women who have symptoms of coronary artery disease (CAD) and/or LV dysfunction. Routine coronary angiography is not indicated in younger patients (younger than 45) undergoing surgery for mitral regurgitation caused by mitral valve degeneration in the absence of symptoms and without risk factors.

Coronary Arteriography before and after Noncardiac Surgery

In general, indications for preoperative coronary angiography are similar to those identified for the nonoperative setting. The ACC/AHA guidelines on perioperative cardiovascular evaluation for noncardiac surgery[6] indicate that coronary angiography is an appropriate intervention for patients with high-risk criteria on noninvasive testing, as well as those with angina symptoms that would warrant consideration of revascularization, even if they were not candidates for noncardiac surgery (Table 20G-8).

Coronary Arteriography in Patients with Congenital Heart Disease

In patients with congenital heart disease, there are two main indications for coronary angiography: assessment of the hemodynamic

TABLE 20G–6 ACC/AHA Recommendations for Initial and Serial Clinical Assessment of Patients Presenting with Heart Failure

Class	Indication	Level of Evidence
Class I (indicated)	Coronary arteriography should be performed in patients presenting with HF who have angina or significant ischemia unless the patient is not eligible for revascularization of any kind.	B
Class IIa (weak supportive evidence)	Coronary arteriography is reasonable for patients presenting with HF who have chest pain that may or may not be of cardiac origin who have not had evaluation of their coronary anatomy and who have no contraindications to coronary revascularization.	C
	Coronary arteriography is reasonable for patients presenting with HF who have known or suspected coronary artery disease but who do not have angina unless the patient is not eligible for revascularization of any kind.	C

ACC = American College of Cardiology; AHA = American Heart Association; HF = heart failure.

From Hunt SA, Abraham WT, Chin MH, et al: ACC/AHA 2005 guideline update for the diagnosis and management of chronic heart failure in the adult. Circulation 112: e154, 2005.

TABLE 20G–7 ACC/AHA Recommendations for Coronary Arteriography in Patients with Valvular Disease

Indication	Class I (Indicated) [Level of Evidence]	Class IIa (Strong Supportive Evidence) [Level of Evidence]	Class IIb (Weak Supportive Evidence) [Level of Evidence]	Class III (Not Indicated) [Level of Evidence]
Aortic stenosis (AS)	Coronary angiography recommended before AVR for patients with AS at risk for CAD [B] Cardiac catheterization for hemodynamic measurements recommended for assessment of severity of AS for symptomatic patients when noninvasive tests are inconclusive or when there is discrepancy between noninvasive tests and clinical findings regarding severity of AS [C] Coronary angiography recommended before AVR for patients with AS for whom a pulmonary autograft (Ross procedure) is contemplated and if origin of coronary arteries was not identified by noninvasive technique [C]			Cardiac catheterization for hemodynamic measurements not recommended for assessment of severity of AS before AVR when noninvasive tests are adequate and concordant with clinical findings [C] Cardiac catheterization for hemodynamic measurements not recommended for assessment of LV function and severity of AS in asymptomatic patients [C]
Aortic regurgitation (AR)	Cardiac catheterization with aortic root angiography and measurement of LV pressure indicated for assessment of severity of regurgitation, LV function, or aortic root size when noninvasive tests are inconclusive or discordant with clinical findings in patients with AR [B] Coronary angiography indicated before AVR for patients at risk for CAD [C]			Cardiac catheterization with aortic root angiography and measurement of LV pressure not indicated for assessment of LV function, aortic root size, or severity of regurgitation before AVR when noninvasive tests are adequate and concordant with clinical findings and coronary angiography is not needed [C] Cardiac catheterization with aortic root angiography and measurement of LV pressure not indicated for assessment of LV function and severity of regurgitation for asymptomatic patients when noninvasive tests are adequate [C]

TABLE 20G-7 ACC/AHA Recommendations for Coronary Arteriography in Patients with Valvular Disease—cont'd

Indication	Class I (Indicated) [Level of Evidence]	Class IIa (Strong Supportive Evidence) [Level of Evidence]	Class IIb (Weak Supportive Evidence) [Level of Evidence]	Class III (Not Indicated) [Level of Evidence]
Mitral regurgitation (MR)	Left ventriculography and hemodynamic measurements indicated when noninvasive tests are inconclusive regarding severity of MR, LV function, or need for surgery [C] Hemodynamic measurements indicated when pulmonary artery pressure is out of proportion to severity of MR as assessed by noninvasive testing [C] Left ventriculography and hemodynamic measurements indicated when there is a discrepancy between clinical and noninvasive findings regarding severity of MR [C] Coronary angiography indicated before mitral valve repair or mitral valve replacement for patients at risk for CAD [C]			Left ventriculography and hemodynamic measurements not indicated for patients with MR in whom valve surgery is not contemplated [C]
Diagnosis of concurrent coronary artery disease	Coronary angiography indicated before valve surgery (including infective endocarditis) or mitral balloon commissurotomy for patients with chest pain, other objective evidence of ischemia, decreased LV systolic function, history of CAD, or coronary risk factors (including age). Patients undergoing mitral balloon valvotomy need not undergo coronary angiography solely on basis of coronary risk factors [C] Coronary angiography indicated for patients with apparently mild to moderate valvular heart disease but with progressive angina (Canadian Heart Association functional class II or greater), objective evidence of ischemia, decreased LV systolic function, or overt congestive heart failure [C] Coronary angiography should be performed before valve surgery in men 35 yr or older, premenopausal women 35 yr or older who have coronary risk factors, and postmenopausal women [C]	Surgery without coronary angiography reasonable for patients having emergency valve surgery for acute valve regurgitation, aortic root disease, or infective endocarditis [C]	Coronary angiography may be considered for patients undergoing catheterization to confirm severity of valve lesions before valve surgery without preexisting evidence of CAD, multiple coronary risk factors, or advanced age [C]	Coronary angiography not indicated for young patients undergoing nonemergency valve surgery when no further hemodynamic assessment by catheterization is deemed necessary and there are no coronary risk factors, no history of CAD, and no evidence of ischemia [C] Patients should not undergo coronary angiography before valve surgery if severely hemodynamically unstable [C]

ACC = American College of Cardiology; AHA = American Heart Association; AVR = aortic valve replacement; CAD = coronary artery disease; HF = heart failure; LV = left ventricular.

From Bonow RO, Carabello BA, Kanu C, et al: ACC/AHA 2006 guidelines for the management of patients with valvular heart disease: a report of the American College of Cardiology/American Heart Association Task Force on Practice Guidelines (writing committee to revise the 1998 Guidelines for the Management of Patients With Valvular Heart Disease): Developed in collaboration with the Society of Cardiovascular Anesthesiologists: endorsed by the Society for Cardiovascular Angiography and Interventions and the Society of Thoracic Surgeons. Circulation 114:e84, 2006.

TABLE 20G-8 ACC/AHA Recommendations for Coronary Arteriography before and after Noncardiac Surgery

Class I (Indicated)	Class IIa (Strong Supportive Evidence)	Class IIb (Weak Supportive Evidence)	Class III (Not Indicated)
Evidence for high risk of adverse outcome based on noninvasive test results Angina unresponsive to adequate medical therapy Unstable angina, particularly when facing intermediate- or high-risk noncardiac surgery Equivocal noninvasive test results in patients at high clinical risk undergoing high-risk surgery	Multiple markers of intermediate clinical risk and planned vascular surgery (noninvasive testing should be considered first) Moderate to large region of ischemia on noninvasive testing but without high-risk features and without lower LVEF Nondiagnostic, noninvasive test results in patients of intermediate clinical risk undergoing high-risk noncardiac surgery Urgent noncardiac surgery while convalescing from acute MI	Medically stabilized class III or IV angina and planned low-risk or minor surgery	Low-risk noncardiac surgery with known CAD and no high-risk results on noninvasive testing Asymptomatic after coronary revascularization with excellent exercise capacity (≥7 METs) Mild stable angina with good left ventricular function and no high-risk noninvasive test results Noncandidate for coronary revascularization because of concomitant medical illness, severe left ventricular dysfunction (e.g., LVEF less than 0.20), or refusal to consider revascularization Candidate for liver, lung, or renal transplantation older than 40 yr, as part of evaluation for transplantation, unless noninvasive testing reveals high risk for adverse outcome

ACC = American College of Cardiology; AHA = American Heart Association; CAD = coronary artery disease; LVEF = left ventricular ejection fraction; METs = metabolic equivalents; MI = myocardial infarction.

From Eagle KA, Berger PB, Calkins H, et al: ACC/AHA guideline update for perioperative cardiovascular evaluation for noncardiac surgery–executive summary: A report of the American College of Cardiology/American Heart Association Task Force on Practice Guidelines (Committee to Update the 1996 Guidelines on Perioperative Cardiovascular Evaluation for Noncardiac Surgery). J Am Coll Cardiol 39:542, 2002.

TABLE 20G-9 ACC/AHA Recommendations for Coronary Arteriography in Patients with Congenital Heart Disease

Class I (indicated)	Class IIa (Strong Supportive Evidence)	Class IIb (Weak Supportive Evidence)	Class III (Not Indicated)
Before surgical correction of congenital heart disease when chest discomfort or noninvasive evidence suggests associated CAD (C) Before surgical correction of suspected congenital anomalies such as congenital coronary artery stenosis, coronary arteriovenous fistula, and anomalous origin of left coronary artery (C) Forms of congenital heart disease frequently associated with coronary artery anomalies that may complicate surgical management (C) Unexplained cardiac arrest in a young patient [B]	Before corrective open heart surgery for congenital heart disease in an adult whose risk profile increases the likelihood of coexisting coronary disease (C)	During left-heart catheterization for hemodynamic assessment of congenital heart disease in an adult in whom the risk of coronary disease is not high (C)	In routine evaluation of congenital heart disease in asymptomatic patients for whom heart surgery is not planned (C)

ACC = American College of Cardiology; AHA = American Heart Association; CAD = coronary artery disease.
From Scanlon PJ, Faxon DP, Audet AM, et al: ACC/AHA guidelines for coronary angiography: executive summary and recommendations. A report of the American College of Cardiology/American Heart Association Task Force on Practice Guidelines (Committee on Coronary Angiography) developed in collaboration with the Society for Cardiac Angiography and Interventions. Circulation 99:2345, 1999.

TABLE 20G-10 ACC/AHA Recommendations for Other Uses of Coronary Arteriography

Class I (Indicated)
Diseases affecting the aorta when knowledge of the presence or extent of coronary artery involvement is necessary for management (e.g., aortic dissection or aneurysm with known CAD) (B)
Hypertrophic cardiomyopathy with angina, despite medical therapy, when knowledge of coronary anatomy might affect therapy (C)
Hypertrophic cardiomyopathy with angina when heart surgery is planned (B)
Class IIa (Strong Supportive Evidence)
High risk for coronary disease when other cardiac surgical procedures are planned (e.g., pericardiectomy or removal of chronic pulmonary emboli) (C)
Prospective immediate cardiac transplant donors whose risk profile increases the likelihood of coronary disease.(B)
Asymptomatic patients with Kawasaki disease who have coronary artery aneurysms on echocardiography (B)
Before surgery for aortic aneurysm/dissection in patients without known coronary disease
Recent blunt chest trauma and suspicion of acute myocardial infarction, without evidence of preexisting CAD (C)

ACC = American College of Cardiology; AHA = American Heart Association; CAD = coronary artery disease.
From Scanlon PJ, Faxon DP, Audet AM, et al: ACC/AHA guidelines for coronary angiography: executive summary and recommendations. A report of the American College of Cardiology/American Heart Association Task Force on Practice Guidelines (Committee on Coronary Angiography) developed in collaboration with the Society for Cardiac Angiography and Interventions. Circulation 99:2345, 1999.

impact of congenital coronary lesions and assessment of the presence of coronary anomalies that potentially could compromise the heart during correction of other congenital heart lesions (Table 20G-9). The ACC/AHA guidelines indicate that it is prudent to perform coronary angiography in patients being considered for repair of congenital heart disease if angina, ischemia on noninvasive testing, or multiple coronary risk factors are present.

Other Uses of Coronary Arteriography

The ACC/AHA guidelines[2] recommend coronary angiography for patients with aortic aneurysm, hypertrophic cardiomyopathy, and other conditions when knowledge of coronary artery involvement or the presence of CAD is necessary (Table 20G-10).

References

1. Guidelines for coronary angiography. A report of the American College of Cardiology/American Heart Association Task Force on Assessment of diagnostic and therapeutic cardiovascular procedures (subcommittee on coronary angiography). J Am Coll Cardiol 10:935, 1987.
2. Scanlon PJ, Faxon DP, Audet AM, et al: ACC/AHA guidelines for coronary angiography: executive summary and recommendations. A report of the American College of Cardiology/American Heart Association Task Force on Practice Guidelines (Committee on Coronary Angiography) developed in collaboration with the Society for Cardiac Angiography and Interventions. Circulation 99:2345, 1999.
3. Gibbons RJ, Abrams J, Chatterjee K, et al: ACC/AHA 2002 guideline update for the management of patients with chronic stable angina—summary article: A report of the American College of Cardiology/American Heart Association Task Force on practice guidelines (Committee on the Management of Patients With Chronic Stable Angina). J Am Coll Cardiol 41:159, 2003.
4. Braunwald E, Antman EM, Beasley JW, et al: ACC/AHA 2002 guideline update for the management of patients with unstable angina and non-ST-segment elevation myocardial infarction—summary article: A report of the American College of Cardiology/American Heart Association task force on practice guidelines (Committee on the Management of Patients With Unstable Angina). J Am Coll Cardiol 40:1366, 2002.
5. Antman EM, Anbe DT, Armstrong PW, et al: ACC/AHA guidelines for the management of patients with ST-elevation myocardial infarction: A report of the American College of Cardiology/American Heart Association Task Force on Practice Guidelines (Committee to Revise the 1999 Guidelines for the Management of Patients with Acute Myocardial Infarction). Circulation 110:e82, 2004.
6. Eagle KA, Berger PB, Calkins H, et al: ACC/AHA guideline update for perioperative cardiovascular evaluation for noncardiac surgery—executive summary: A report of the American College of Cardiology/American Heart Association Task Force on Practice Guidelines (Committee to Update the 1996 Guidelines on Perioperative Cardiovascular Evaluation for Noncardiac Surgery). J Am Coll Cardiol 39:542, 2002.
7. Hunt SA, Abraham WT, Chin MH, et al: ACC/AHA 2005 guideline update for the diagnosis and management of chronic heart failure in the adult. Circulation 112:e154, 2005.
8. Bonow RO, Carabello BA, Chatterjee K, et al: ACC/AHA 2006 guidelines for the management of patients with valvular heart disease: A report of the American College of Cardiology/American Heart Association Task Force on Practice Guidelines (writing Committee to Revise the 1998 guidelines for the management of patients with valvular heart disease) developed in collaboration with the Society of Cardiovascular Anesthesiologists endorsed by the Society for Cardiovascular Angiography and Interventions and the Society of Thoracic Surgeons. J Am Coll Cardiol 48:e1, 2006.
9. Smith SC Jr, Feldman TE, Hirshfeld JW Jr, et al: ACC/AHA/SCAI 2005 guideline update for percutaneous coronary intervention: A report of the American College of Cardiology/American Heart Association Task Force on Practice Guidelines (ACC/AHA/SCAI Writing Committee to Update the 2001 Guidelines for Percutaneous Coronary Intervention). J Am Coll Cardiol 47:e1, 2006.

PART IV

Heart Failure

CHAPTER 21

Mechanisms of Cardiac Contraction and Relaxation

Lionel H. Opie

MICROANATOMY OF CONTRACTILE CELLS AND PROTEINS

Ultrastructure of Contractile Cells

The major function of myocardial muscle cells (cardiomyocytes or myocytes) is to execute the cardiac contraction-relaxation cycle. The contractile proteins of the heart lie within these myocytes, which constitute about 75% of the total volume of the myocardium, although only about one third in number of all the cells. About half of each ventricular cell is occupied by myofibers and about one quarter to one third by mitochondria (Table 21-1). A myofiber is a group of myocytes (Fig. 21-1) held together by surrounding collagen connective tissue, the latter being the major component of the extracellular matrix. Further strands of collagen connect myofibers to each other. Excess collagen, one cause of left ventricular (LV) diastolic dysfunction, accumulates as part of the growth response to LV pressure overload.

The individual contractile myocytes that account for more than half of the heart's weight are roughly cylindrical in shape (Fig. 21-2). Those in the atrium are quite small, being less than 10 μm in diameter and about 20 μm in length. Relative to atrial cells, human ventricular myocytes are large, measuring about 17 to 25 μm in diameter and 60 to 140 μm in length (see Table 21-1).

When examined under the light microscope, the atrial and ventricular myocytes have cross striations and are branched. Each myocyte is bounded by a complex cell membrane, the sarcolemma (*sarco*, flesh; *lemma*, thin husk), and is filled with rod-like bundles of myofibrils (see Fig. 21-1). The latter are the contractile elements. The sarcolemma of the myocyte invaginates to form an extensive tubular network (the T tubules) that extends the extracellular space into the interior of the cell (see Figs. 21-1 and 21-2). The nucleus, which contains almost all the cell's genetic information, is often centrally located. Some myocytes have several nuclei. Interspersed between the myofibrils and immediately beneath the sarcolemma are many mitochondria, the main function of which is to generate the energy in the form of adenosine triphosphate (ATP) needed to maintain the heart's contractile function and the associated ion gradients. Of the other organelles, the sarcoplasmic reticulum (SR) is most important (see Fig. 21-1). When the wave of electrical excitation reaches the closely approximated T tubules, the tubular calcium channels open to a relatively small amount of calcium to trigger the release of much more calcium from the calcium release channels of the SR. This is the calcium that initiates myocardial contraction. When the calcium is once again taken up into the SR, relaxation ensues.

Anatomically, the SR is a fine network spreading throughout the myocytes, demarcated by its lipid bilayer, which is rather similar to that of the sarcolemma. The calcium release channels (also called the ryanodine receptors) are found in the expanded parts of the SR that lie in very close apposition to the T tubules. These are called subsarcolemmal cisternae (Latin,

TABLE 21–1 Characteristics of Cardiac Cells, Organelles, and Contractile Proteins

	Microanatomy of Heart Cells		
Characteristic	***Ventricular Myocyte***	***Atrial Myocyte***	***Purkinje Cells***
Shape	Long and narrow	Elliptical	Long and broad
Length, μm	60-140	About 20	150-200
Diameter, μm	About 20	5-6	35-40
Volume, cubic μm	15,000-45,000	About 500	135,000-250,000
T tubules	Plentiful	Rare or none	Absent
Intercalated disc	Prominent end-to-end transmission	Side-to-side as well as end-to-end transmission	Very prominent, abundant gap junctions; fast; end-to-end transmission
General appearance	Mitochondria and sarcomeres very abundant; rectangular branching bundles with little interstitial collagen	Bundles of atrial tissue separated by wide areas of collagen	Fewer sarcomeres, paler

	Composition and Function of Ventricular Cells	
Organelle	***% of Cell Volume***	***Function***
Myofibril	About 50-60	Interaction of thick and thin filaments during contraction cycle
Mitochondria	16 in neonate; 33 in adult rat; 23 in adult human	Provide ATP chiefly for contraction
T system	About 1	Transmission of electrical signal from sarcolemma to cell interior
Sarcoplasmic reticulum (SR)	33 in neonate; 2 in adult	Takes up and releases Ca^{2+} during contraction cycle
Terminal cisternae of SR	0.33 in adult	Site of calcium storage and release
Rest of network of SR	Rest of volume	Site of calcium uptake en route to cisternae
Sarcolemma	Very low	Control of ionic gradients; channels for ions (action potential); maintenance of cell integrity; receptors for drugs and hormones
Nucleus	About 5	Protein synthesis
Lysosomes	Very low	Intracellular digestion and proteolysis
Sarcoplasm (cytoplasm) (plus nuclei and other structures)	About 12 in adult rat; 18 in humans	Provides cytosol in which increase and decrease of ionized calcium occurs; contains other ions and small molecules

boxes or baskets), or the junctional SR. The second part of the SR, the longitudinal or network SR, consists of ramifying tubules (see Fig. 21-1) and is involved with the uptake of calcium that initiates relaxation. This uptake is achieved by the ATP-requiring calcium pump, also called SERCA (***s***arco***e***ndoplasmic ***r***eticulum ***C***a^{2+}-***A***TPase), which increases its activity in response to beta-adrenergic stimulation. Calcium taken up into the SR is then stored at high concentration in a number of storage proteins, including calsequestrin, before being released again in response to the next wave of depolarization.

The cytoplasm is the intracellular fluid and proteins therein, contained within the sarcolemma but excluding the contents of organelles such as mitochondria and the SR. The fluid component of the cytoplasm, minus the proteins, is called the cytosol. It is in the cytosol that the concentrations of calcium ions rise and fall to cause cardiac contraction and relaxation. The proteins of the sarcoplasm include myriads of specialized molecules, enzymes, which accelerate the conversion of one chemical form to another, thereby stimulating crucial metabolic or signaling pathways and thereby eventually promoting energy production.

SUBCELLULAR MICROARCHITECTURE. The molecular signal systems that convey messages from surface receptors to intracellular organelles may be directed to specific sites by molecules that anchor components of the internal messenger chain to specific organelles, as when the beta-adrenergic chain must link up with the calcium pump of the sarcoplasmic reticulum (see later). Scaffolding proteins bring interacting molecules closely together, as in the case of the signaling chain leading to myocyte growth. An example of physiological subcellular compartmentalization is the local unloading of ATP where it is needed by the exact location of the enzyme, creatine kinase, which converts creatine phosphate to ATP.

Contractile Proteins

The major molecules involved in the contraction-relaxation cycle are the two chief contractile proteins, the thin actin filament and the thick myosin filament (see Fig. 21-1). Calcium ions initiate the contraction cycle by interacting with troponin C to relieve the inhibition otherwise exerted by troponin I (Fig. 21-3). Titin is a large elastic molecule that supports myosin (Fig. 21-4). During contraction, the filaments slide over each other, without the individual molecules of actin or myosin actually shortening. As they slide, they pull together the two ends of the fundamental contractile unit called the sarcomere. On electron microscopy, the sarcomere is limited on either side by the Z-line (from German *Zuckung*, contraction) to which the actin filaments are attached (see Fig. 21-2). Conversely, the myosin filaments extend from the center of the sarcomere in either direction toward but not actually reaching the Z-lines.

The interaction of the myosin heads with actin filaments, when sufficient calcium arrives from the sarcoplasmic reticulum (see Fig. 21-1), is called cross-bridge cycling. As the actin filaments move inward toward the center of the sarcomere, they draw the Z-lines closer together, so that the sarcomere shortens. The energy for this shortening is provided by the breakdown of ATP, chiefly made in the mitochondria.

TITIN AND LENGTH SENSING. Titin is a giant molecule, the largest protein yet described. It is an extraordinarily long, flexible, and slender myofibrillar protein (see Fig. 21-4). Titin acts as a third filament to provide elasticity. The titin molecule is between 0.6 and 1.2 μm in length and extends from the Z-line, stopping just short of the M-line (see Fig. 21-1). It has two distinct segments, an inextensible anchoring segment and an extensible elastic segment that stretches as sarcomere length increases. Titin has multiple functions. First, it indirectly tethers the myosin molecule to the Z-line, thereby stabilizing the contractile proteins. Second, as it stretches and relaxes, its elasticity explains the stress-strain relation of cardiac and skeletal muscles. At short sarcomere lengths, the elastic domain is folded on itself to generate restoring forces (see Fig. 21-4). These changes in titin help to explain the series elastic element; this postulates that there is elasticity in series between the contractile elements and the ends of the muscle. Third, increased diastolic stretch of titin, as the sarcomere length of cardiac muscle is increased, causes the enfolded part of the titin molecule to straighten. This stretched molecular spring then contracts more vigorously in systole.[1] Such enhanced systolic contraction helps explain the Frank-Starling mechanism (see later). Fourth, titin may transduce mechanical stretch into growth signals. In sustained diastolic stretch, as in volume overload, the elastic segment of titin is constantly under strain and transmits this mechanical signal to the muscle LIM protein (MLP) attached to the terminal part of titin, which forms part of the Z-disc complex.[2] The MLP protein has been proposed as the stretch sensor that transmits the signals that result in the myocyte growth pattern characteristic of volume overload.[2] This signal system may be defective in a subset of human dilated cardiomyopathy.[2]

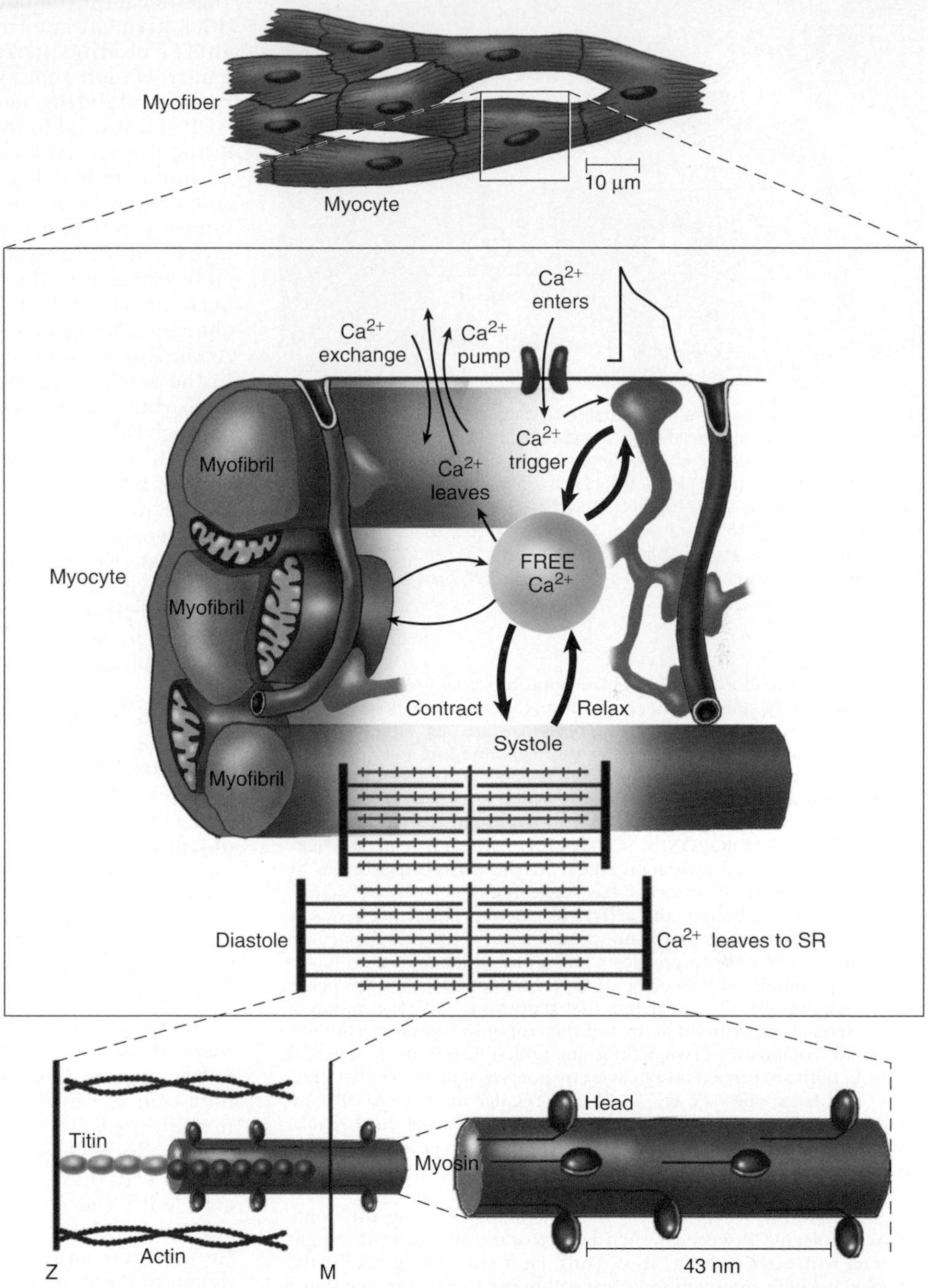

FIGURE 21–1 The crux of the contractile process lies in the changing concentrations of Ca^{2+} ions in the myocardial cytosol. **Upper panel,** Difference between the myocardial cell or myocyte, and the myofiber, composed of many myocytes. **Middle and lower panels,** Ca^{2+} ions are schematically shown as entering via the calcium channel that opens in response to the wave of depolarization that travels along the sarcolemma. These Ca^{2+} ions trigger the release of more calcium from the sarcoplasmic reticulum (SR) and thereby initiate a contraction-relaxation cycle. Eventually, the small amount of calcium that has entered the cell will leave predominantly by a Na^+/Ca^{2+} exchanger, with a lesser role for the sarcolemmal calcium pump. The varying actin-myosin overlap is shown for systole, when calcium ions arrive, and diastole, when calcium ions leave. The myosin heads, attached to the thick filaments, interact with the thin actin filaments, as shown in Figure 21-5. For the role of titin, see Figure 21-4. *(Middle and bottom panels, from Opie LH: Heart Physiology: From Cell to Circulation. Philadelphia, Lippincott Williams & Wilkins, 2004. © LH Opie, 2004. Upper panel from Braunwald E, Ross J, Sonnenblick EH, et al: Mechanisms of Contraction of the Normal and Failing Heart. 2nd ed. Little Brown, Boston, 1976.)*

STRONG AND WEAK BINDING STATES. Although, at a molecular level, the events underlying the cross-bridge cycle are exceedingly complex, one simple current hypothesis is that the cross bridges exist in a strong or weak binding state (Fig. 21-5). The arrival of calcium ions at the contractile proteins is a crucial link in the series of events known as excitation-contraction coupling. The ensuing interaction of calcium with troponin C and the deinhibition of troponin I puts the cross bridges in the strong binding state. As long as enough calcium ions are present, the strong binding state potentially dominates (see Fig. 21-5). If, however, the strong binding state were continuously present, then the contractile proteins could never relax. Thus, it has been hypothesized that the binding of ATP to the myosin head puts the cross bridges into a weak binding state, even when the calcium level is high. Conversely, when ATP is hydrolyzed to ADP (adenosine diphosphate) and P_i (inorganic phosphate), the strong binding state again predominates (see Fig. 21-5). The ATP-induced changes in the molecular configuration of the

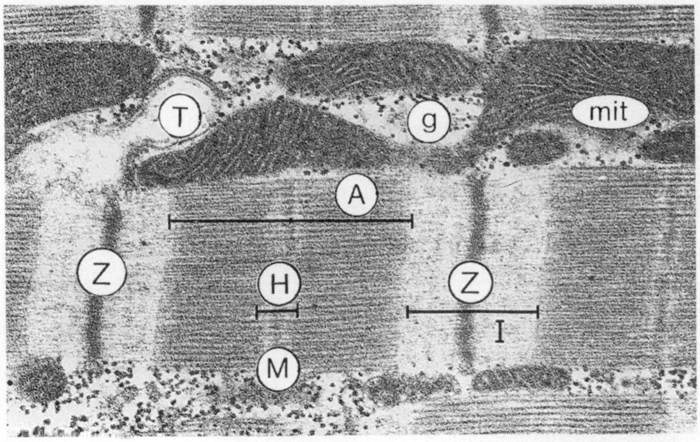

FIGURE 21–2 The sarcomere is the distance between the two Z-lines. Note the presence of numerous mitochondria (mit) sandwiched between the myofibrils, and the presence of T tubules (T), which penetrate into the muscle at the level of the Z-lines. This two-dimensional picture should not disguise the fact that the Z-line is really a Z-disc, as is the M-line (M), also shown in Figure 21-1. A = band of actin-myosin overlap; g = glycogen granules; H = central clear zone containing only myosin filament bodies and the M-line; I = band of actin filaments, titin, and Z-line. (×32,000, rat papillary muscle.) *(Courtesy of Dr. J Moravec, Dijon, France.)*

myosin head therefore result in corresponding variations in the physical properties (a similar concept as in metabolic regulation). Length activation also promotes the strong binding state (see later, "Length-Dependent Activation"). Conversely, the weak binding state predominates when cytosolic calcium levels fall at the start of diastole. As the calcium ions leave troponin C, a master switch is turned off and tropomyosin again assumes the inhibitory configuration.

ACTIN AND TROPONIN COMPLEX. Although calcium ions provide the essential switch-on signal to the cross-bridge cycle by binding to troponin C, evidence has suggested more than an "on-off" signaling process. Rather, the arrival of calcium initiates a series of interactions between the troponin components of the thin filament to allow movement of the tropomyosin molecule, which in turn promotes the strong binding state (see Fig. 21-5) so that contraction takes place. Understanding the role of calcium first requires a brief description of the molecular structure of actin and the troponin complex. Thin filaments are composed of two actin units, which intertwine in a helical pattern; both are carried on a heavier tropomyosin molecule that functions as a backbone (see Fig. 21-5A). At regular intervals of 38.5 nm along this twisting structure is a closely bound group of three regulatory proteins called the troponin complex. Of these proteins, it is troponin C that responds to the calcium ions that are released in large amounts from the SR to start the cross-bridge cycle.

Schematically, when the cytosolic calcium level is low, the tropomyosin molecule is twisted in such a way that the myosin heads cannot interact with actin (see Fig. 21-3). Thus, most cross bridges are in the blocked position, although some are still in the weakly binding state.[1] As calcium ions increasingly arrive at the start of the contractile cycle and interact with troponin C, the activated troponin C binds tightly to the inhibitory molecule, troponin I. The latter moves to a new position on the thin filament, thereby weakening the interaction between troponin T and tropomyosin (see Fig. 21-3). Ultimately, tropomyosin is repositioned on the thin filament,[1] thereby removing most of the inhibition exerted by tropomyosin on the actin-myosin interaction. Thus, weakly bound or blocked cross bridges enter the strongly bound state and the cross-bridge cycle is initiated. As the strong cross bridges form, they activate close neighbors and thereby spread the activation process.[1] They also promote further tropomyosin movement to cause more forceful cross-bridge interaction.

MYOSIN AND MOLECULAR BASIS OF MUSCULAR CONTRACTION. Each myosin head is the terminal part of a heavy chain. The bodies of two of these chains intertwine and each terminates in a short neck, which carries the elongated myosin head (see Fig. 21-3). According to the Rayment model, it is the base of the head, also sometimes called the neck, that changes configuration in the contractile cycle.[3] Together with the bodies of all the other heads, the myosin thick filament is formed. Each lobe of the bilobed head has an ATP binding pocket (also called a nucleotide pocket) and a narrow cleft that extends from the base of this pocket to the actin-binding face.[3] ATP and its breakdown products ADP and P_i bind to the nucleotide pocket in close proximity to the myosin ATPase activity, which breaks down ATP to its products (see Fig. 21-3). Currently, there is controversy about the role in the contractile cycle of the narrow actin-binding cleft that splits the central 50-kDa segment of the myosin head. According to the revised Rayment model,[1] this cleft responds to the binding of ATP or its breakdown products to the nucleotide pocket so that the conformational changes necessary for movement of the head are produced. According to Dominguez and associates,[1] the cleft is closed in the weakly attached states before the power stroke (Fig. 21-6), but opens when inorganic phosphate is released through the cleft, whereon the myosin head attaches strongly to actin to induce the power stroke (see Fig. 21-5D and E).

Starting with the rigor state (see Fig. 21-5A), the binding of ATP to its pocket changes the molecular configuration of the myosin head so that the head detaches from actin to terminate the rigor state (see Fig. 21-5B). Next, the ATPase activity of the myosin head splits ATP into ADP and P_i and the head flexes (see Fig. 21-5C). As ATP is hydrolyzed, the myosin head binds to an adjacent actin unit. P_i is then released from the head through the cleft, and there is strong binding of the myosin head to actin (see Fig. 21-5D). Next, the head extends—that is, it straightens. A power stroke takes place, the actin molecule moves by about 10 nm,[1] and the myosin head is now in the rigor state. The pocket then releases ADP, ready to accept ATP, and the cycle repeats. The Rayment model[3] has postulated that straightening and not flexion of the light chain region of the head (i.e., the neck) produces the power stroke. The lever-arm model[1] is more applicable to many cells and organelles that depend on movement of myosin rather than of actin—for example, for intracellular transport. By contrast, in contracting cardiomyocytes, myosin is fixed and tethered by titin and myosin-binding protein C. The lever-arm model proposes that movements of the neck, which is the lever arm, produce large displacements that translate into movement of the entire myosin molecule. This model provides evolutionary data that reinforce the crucial nature of movements of the myosin neck (shown as the flexible domain in Fig. 21-5C).

Myosin ATPase activity normally responds to calcium in such a way that increases in calcium concentration, associated with the contraction cycle in the heart, result in a several-fold increase in the myosin ATPase activity in addition to increasing calcium binding to troponin C and force development (see Fig. 21-6).[1]

Myosin heavy chain (MHC) isoforms help regulate myosin ATPase activity. Each myosin filament consists of two heavy chains, the bodies of which are intertwined, with each ending in one head, and four light chains, two in apposition to each head. The heavy chains, containing the myosin ATPase activity on the heads, occur in two isoforms, beta and alpha, of the same molecular weight but with substantially different ATPase activities. The beta-heavy chain (beta-MHC) isoform has lower ATPase activity and is the predominant form in the adult human. In small animals, the faster alpha-MHC form changes to a predominantly beta-MHC pattern in heart failure.[1]

MYOSIN HEADS: TWO ARE BETTER THAN ONE. The double-headed structure is required to produce the full displacement of actin, about 10 nm, versus only 6 nm with single-headed myosin.[1] The myosin neck is chiefly formed by a long alpha helix (see Fig. 21-3B), surrounded by two light chains (four per bilobed head) that act as a cervical collar. The light chain that is more proximal to the myosin head, the essential myosin light chain (MLC-1), may inhibit the contractile process by interaction with actin. The other regulatory light chain (MLC-2) is a potential site for phosphorylation (e.g., in response to beta-adrenergic stimulation). Such phosphorylation (the gaining of a phosphate grouping) may promote cross-bridge cycling by increasing the affinity of myosin for actin.[1] Mutation of this light chain in one type of human cardiomyopathy impairs the contractile response to tachycardia.[1] In vascular smooth muscle, the phosphorylation that occurs under the influence of the enzyme myosin light chain kinase (MLCK) is an obligatory step in the initiation of the contractile process.

Myosin-binding protein C runs at approximately a right angle to the myosin molecules to tether myosin molecules by linking the structures that lie around subfragments of the myosin heads. This binding protein, which stabilizes the myosin head, itself flexes and extends at the level of the light chains. Defects in binding protein C may be involved in some types of hypertrophic cardiomyopathy.

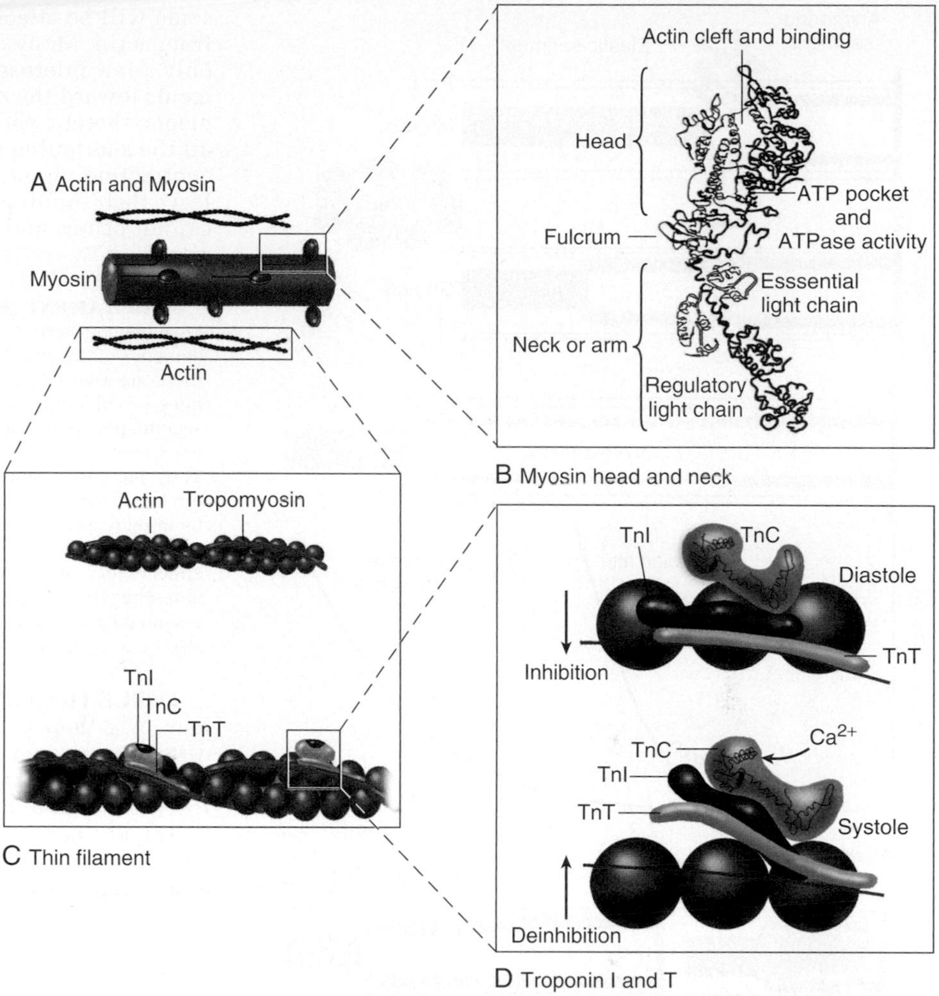

FIGURE 21–3 Major molecules of the contractile system. The thin actin filament **(A)** interacts with the myosin head **(B)** when Ca^{2+} ions arrive at troponin C, TnC **(C)**. A complex interaction between TnC and the other troponins moves tropomyosin to uncover an actin site to which a myosin head can attach (see Fig. 21-7). The molecular aspects are as follows. **A,** The thin actin filament contains TnC and its Ca^{2+} binding sites. When TnC is not activated by Ca^{2+}, then troponin I (TnI) inhibits the actin-myosin interaction. Troponin T (TnT) is an elongated protein that interacts with all the other components of the thin filament,[7] thereby participating in the activation cycle **(D)**. **B,** Myosin head molecular structure (based on work by Rayment and associates[3]) is composed of heavy and light chains. The heavy head chain in turn has two major domains, one of 70 kDa (70,000 molecular weight) that interacts with actin at the actin cleft and has an ATP-binding pocket. The neck domain of 20 kDa, also called the lever, is an elongated alpha helix that extends and bends and has two light chains surrounding it as a collar. The essential light chain is part of the structure. The other regulatory light chain may respond to phosphorylation to influence the extent of the actin-myosin interaction. **C,** Troponin C with sites in the regulatory domain for activation by calcium and for interaction with troponin I. **D,** Calcium binding to TnC induces a conformational change in TnC that elongates (compare systole with diastole). TnI closes up to TnC, and the normal inhibition of TnI on actin-tropomyosin is lessened. There is a strengthening of the interaction between TnC and TnT. These changes allow repositioning of tropomyosin in relation to actin, with lessening of its normal inhibitory effects, as shown in the bottom panel. Now the contractile cycle can start. *(**A-C** modified from Opie LH: Heart Physiology: From Cell to Circulation. Philadelphia, Lippincott Williams & Wilkins, 2004. © LH Opie, 2004; **D** modified from Solaro RJ, Van Eyk J: Altered interactions among thin filament proteins modulate cardiac function, J Mol Cell Cardiol 28:217, 1999.)*

GRADED EFFECTS OF INCREASED CYTOSOLIC CALCIUM LEVELS ON CROSS-BRIDGE CYCLE. Calcium ions play a crucial role in linking external neurohumoral control of the heart to stimulation of the contractile process by acting at multiple control sites.[1] Calcium interaction with troponin C is essential for cross-bridge cycling. Does calcium act as an on-off switch to regulate the total number of cycling cross bridges? According to this hypothesis, the enhanced force development in response to a greater calcium ion concentration must be caused by the recruitment of additional cross bridges. Alternatively, to explain the graded model, the following mechanisms might be applicable: (1) a graded response of troponin C to calcium ions, including altered rates of calcium binding and release; (2) a graded response of myosin ATPase to calcium; (3) near-neighbor self-activation, whereby actin-myosin interaction activates additional cross bridges, even in the absence of increased binding of calcium to the troponin C of those cross bridges[1]; and (4) alterations in the extent of myosin light chain phosphorylation.[1] Of specific interest is the proposal that tightly bound cross bridges act to spread activation on the thin filament to near-neighbor units to achieve full activation.[1] By such mechanisms, one calcium-troponin complex could activate as many as 14 actin molecules.

LENGTH-DEPENDENT ACTIVATION. In addition to the cytosolic calcium concentration, the other major factor influencing the strength of contraction is the length of the muscle fiber at the end of diastole, just before the onset of systole. Starling has observed that the greater the volume of the heart in diastole, the more forceful the contraction.[1] The increased heart volume translates into an increased muscle length, which acts by a length-sensing mechanism (see Fig. 21-6). Previously, this relation was ascribed to a more optimal overlap between actin and myosin. The current view is that an increased sarcomere length leads to greater sensitivity of the contractile apparatus to the prevailing cytosolic calcium ion concentration.[1] A plausible mechanism for this regulatory change may reside in the decreasing interfilament spacing as the heart muscle is stretched. This rather satisfactory lattice-dependent explanation for the Frank-Starling relationship has been dealt a setback by careful x-ray diffraction studies.[1] Reducing sarcomere lattice spacing by osmotic compression fails to influence calcium

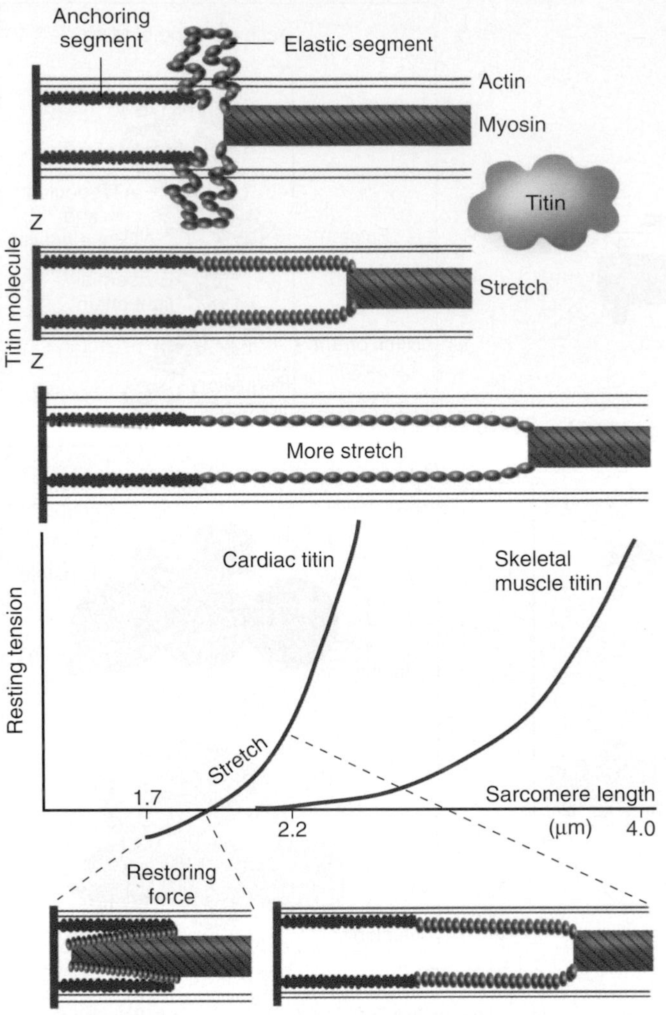

FIGURE 21–4 Titin, a very large elongated protein with elasticity, binds myosin to the Z-line. It may act as a bi-directional spring that develops passive forces in stretched sarcomeres, and resting forces in shortened sarcomeres. As the sarcomere is stretched to its maximum physiological diastolic length of 2.2 µm (see Fig. 21-20), titin first undergoes straightening (up to 2 µm) and then elongation, with the latter rapidly increasing the passive forces generated. At low sarcomere lengths, when sarcomeres are slack at about the diastolic limit of 1.85 µm (see Fig. 21-20), the mechanically active elastic domain is folded on top of itself. At even shorter lengths, which may not be physiological in the intact heart, there are substantial restoring forces generated. *(Modified from Trombitas K, Jian-Ping J, Granzier H: The mechanically active domain of titin in cardiac muscle. Circ Res 77:856, 1995; and Helmes M, Trombitas K, Granzier H: Titin develops restoring force in rat cardiac myocytes. Circ Res 79:619, 1996.)*

sensitivity. Alternatively, sarcomere stretch increases the passive forces built up by titin, which could in turn hypothetically influence the position of myosin heads. Another proposal, that troponin C is the length sensor, is currently less favored.[1] Several mechanisms are probably at work.

CROSS-BRIDGE CYCLING DIFFERS FROM CARDIAC CONTRACTION-RELAXATION CYCLE. The cardiac cycle of Wiggers (see later) must be distinguished from the cross-bridge cycle. The former reflects the overall pressure changes in the left ventricle, whereas the latter is the repetitive interaction between myosin heads and actin. According to the Rayment model,[3] the binding of ATP or ADP regulates in part whether the cross bridges are weak or strong in nature (see Fig. 21-5). As long as enough calcium ions are bound to troponin C, many repetitive cycles of this type occur. Thus, at any given moment, some myosin heads will be flexing or flexed, some will be extending or extended, some will be attached to actin, and some will be detached from actin. Many of these cross-bridge cycles, each lasting only a few microseconds, actively move the thin actin filaments toward the central bare area of the thick myosin filaments, thereby shortening the sarcomere. The sum total of all the shortening sarcomeres leads to systole, which is the contraction phase of the cardiac cycle. When calcium ions leave their binding sites on troponin C, cross-bridge cycling cannot occur, and the diastolic phase of the cardiac cycle sets in.

MYOFILAMENT RESPONSE TO HEMODYNAMIC DEMANDS. Myofilament activity is coupled to the prevailing hemodynamic demands of the circulation. In addition to length-dependent activation, there are two other chief mechanisms. First, there may be variable rates of calcium binding and release from troponin C (see earlier). Second, phosphorylation and dephosphorylation of the contractile proteins may help control the extent of activation of the myofilaments. Thus, increased beta-adrenergic dependent phosphorylation of troponin I reduces the myofilament sensitivity to calcium and thereby leads to an increased rate of relaxation during beta-adrenergic stimulation.[1] Hypothetically, this mechanism enhances the relaxant (lusitropic) effect of increased uptake rates of calcium into the sarcoplasmic reticulum. The effects of phosphorylation of other proteins, such the myosin essential light chains and C protein, still imperfectly understood, may also be important.[1]

FORCE TRANSMISSION. Volume and pressure overload may owe their different effects on myocardial growth to different patterns of force transmission. Whereas increased diastolic forces are transmitted longitudinally via titin to reach the postulated sensor, the MLP protein (see earlier, "Titin and Length Sensing"), increased systolic forces may be transmitted laterally (i.e., at right angles) via the Z-disk and cytoplasmic actin to reach the proteins of the cell-matrix junctions, such as the focal adhesion complex. How these mechanical forces become translated into signals that activate the growth pathways, such as those leading to MAP (mitogen-activated protein) kinase, still remains to be elucidated.

Current proposals for the onward transmission of mechanical forces from sarcomere[4] show different patterns for systole and diastole, which could explain why greater end-systolic stress leads to thicker myocytes and greater end-diastolic stress to longer myocytes. During systole, the sarcomere shortens as a result of myosin head flexion and movement of actin filaments towards the M-line. Increased horizontal force is exerted on the Z-line, which in turn transmits lateral forces to the sarcolemma by the thin and intermediate filaments, cytoplasmic actin and desmin. Further transmission is to the integrins of the costameres and associated cytoskeletal proteins that connect the stress generated in the Z-lines of the sarcomeres to the extracellular matrix, from where the intracellular hypertrophy program is activated.[4]

During diastole, as the sarcomere stretches, the elastic segment of titin expands and transmits force via MLP, which acts as a mechanical sensor (see Fig. 21-4).[2] When of long duration, as in sustained volume overload, MLP-induced stimuli may induce myocyte lengthening, as in the dilated failing heart. Further signaling is not clear. Pressure and volume overload may induce distinctly different signal transduction paths; pressure overload rapidly activates Akt and the expected downstream kinases, whereas volume overloading results in delayed Akt activation that does not involve the same downstream signals.[5] This rather clear separation between the molecular mechanisms, whereby pressure and volume loading induce different patterns of hypertrophy, is marred by the observation that MLP colocalizes with calcineurin and nuclear factor of activated T cells (NFAT), both of which are associated with transverse rather than longitudinal myocyte growth.[6] Thus, the MLP sensor could participate in the response to both volume and pressure loading.

CONTRACTILE PROTEINS AND CARDIOMYOPATHY. It has been postulated that genetic-based hypertrophic and dilated cardiomyopathies not only produce hearts that look and behave very differently, but have diverse molecular causes. Hypertrophic cardiomyopathy is generally linked to mutant genes that cause abnormalities in the force-generating system, such as the beta-myosin heavy chain. Less commonly, there may be defects in the genes encoding troponin T, myosin light chain isoforms, troponin I and C isoforms, myosin-binding protein C, and alpha-tropomyosin (see Chaps. 8 and 65). The current hypothesis is that these mutations increase the contractile performance and/or the energy demand, but how such defects translate into hypertrophic cardiomyopathy is still obscure.[7] In contrast, dilated cardiomyopathy can be related to mutations in non–force-generating cytoskeletal proteins, such as dystrophin, nuclear lamin, cytoplasmic actin, and titin, as well as defects in the enzymes that control the integrity of the matrix (see Chaps. 8 and 22).[8] This distinction between the two types of cardiomyopathy remains useful but is oversimplified, with several examples of overlapping mechanisms.[9]

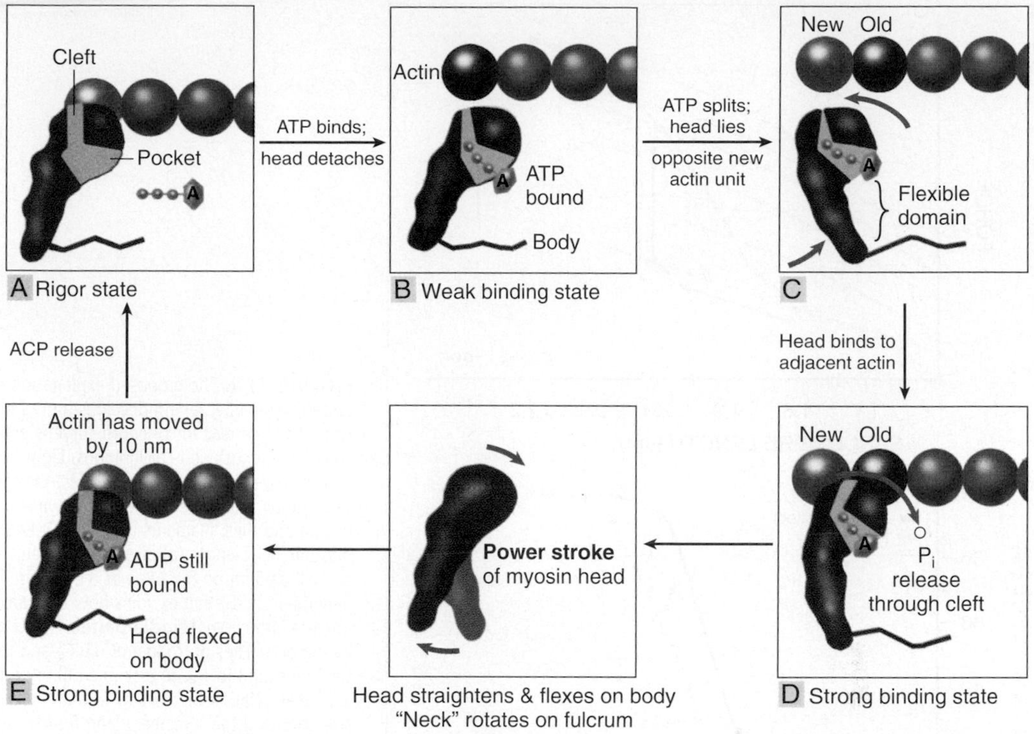

FIGURE 21–5 Cross-bridge cycling molecular model (updated from the original Rayment five-step model for interaction between the myosin head and the actin filament[3]), taking into account other models. The cross bridge (only one myosin head depicted) is pear-shaped and consists of the catalytic motor domain that interacts with the actin molecule and an extended alpha helical neck region acting as a lever arm. The nucleotide pocket receiving and binding ATP is a depression near the center of the catalytic domain. The actin-binding cleft bisects the catalytic motor domain. During the cross-bridge cycle, the width of the actin-binding cleft changes in size, although details remain controversial. Starting with the rigor state **(A)**, the binding of ATP to the pocket **(B)** is followed by ATP hydrolysis **(C)**, which partly closes the actin-binding cleft. The cleft opens when phosphate is released (through the cleft rather than through the pocket) and the myosin head strongly attaches to actin to induce the power stroke **(D, E)**. During the power stroke, the latter rotates about a fulcrum in the region where the helix terminates in the catalytic motor domain. As the head flexes, the actin filament is displaced by about 10 nm (**E**). In the process, ADP is also released so that the binding pocket becomes vacant. Finally, the rigor state is reached **(A)** and the myosin head is again ready to receive ATP to reinitiate the cross-bridge cycle. P_i = inorganic phosphate; spheres = actin monomer with which the myosin head is interacting. *(Professor Caspar Rüegg, Heidelberg University, Germany, gave valuable advice. For references to Cooke and colleagues, see Opie.[1])*

CALCIUM ION FLUXES IN CARDIAC CONTRACTION-RELAXATION CYCLE

Calcium Movements and Excitation-Contraction Coupling

Calcium has a crucial role in regulating the contraction and relaxation phases of the cardiac cycle. The details of the associated calcium ion fluxes that link contraction to the wave of excitation (excitation-contraction coupling) have now been reasonably well delineated.[1] The generally accepted hypothesis is based on the crucial role of calcium-induced calcium release from the SR. Relatively small amounts of calcium ions, the trigger calcium ions, actually enter and leave the cardiomyocyte during each cardiac cycle, whereas much larger amounts move in and out of the SR (Fig. 21-7). The basic proposal is that each wave of depolarization traveling down the T tubules opens the L-type calcium channels, which are physically closely approximated to that part of the SR lying close to the T tubule, to activate the calcium release channels, collectively called the ryanodine receptors. Thereby, depolarization releases relatively large amounts of calcium ions into the cytosol in response to the much smaller amounts entering the cardiomyocyte.[1] This process greatly elevates (by about tenfold) the concentration of calcium ions in the cytosol, resulting in the increasing interaction of calcium ions with troponin C to trigger the contractile process. This theory has received strong support from several studies: (1) the tight proximity of the ryanodine receptors on the SR to the L-type calcium channels of the T tubules; (2) the molecular characterization of the calcium-releasing ryanodine receptor on the SR (Fig. 21-8); (3) proof of the control of this receptor not only by calcium ions but by beta-adrenergic–mediated phosphorylation and by binding proteins of the FKBP (FK-506 binding protein) family[10]; and (4) electrophysiological evidence closely linking the duration of the action potential with the extent of Ca^{2+} release.[1]

Calcium Release and Uptake by the Sarcoplasmic Reticulum

RYANODINE RECEPTORS. Each L-type calcium channel of the sarcolemma controls a cluster of possibly 6 to 20 SR release channels because of close anatomical proximity of the calcium channels on the T tubules to the calcium release channels situated on the SR. The calcium release channel is part of the complex structure known as the ryanodine receptor, so called because it coincidentally binds the potent insecticide ryanodine (often abbreviated as RyR2 to indicate the cardiac isoform). Ryanodine receptors have a dual function, both containing the calcium release channels of the SR and acting as scaffolding proteins that localize numerous key regulatory proteins to the junctional complexes.[1]

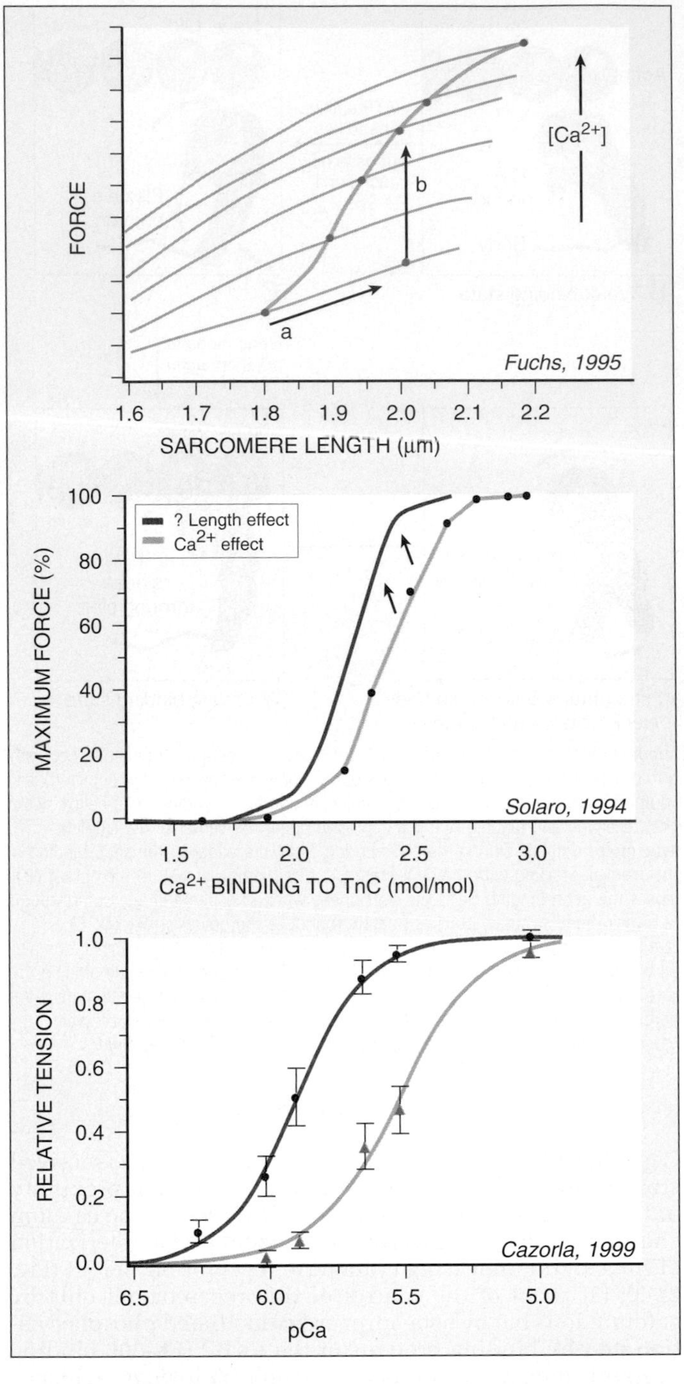

FIGURE 21–6 The proposed explanation for the Starling effect, whereby a greater end-diastolic fiber length develops a greater force. **Top panel,** The steep ascending limb of the cardiac force-length curve is explained by an interaction between sarcomere length and calcium ions. Light lines show a family of hypothetical force-length curves for increasing free Ca^{2+} concentrations, with each drawn on the assumption that the shape of the curve is determined solely by the degree of overlap of thin and thick filaments (see Fig. 21-1). It is postulated that an increase in end-diastolic fiber length (a) at any given free Ca^{2+} concentration would increase force by a small amount on the basis of the change in filament overlap. In addition, length-dependent activation explains how the sarcomere can upgrade itself (b) to a higher force-length curve. **Middle panel,** The effects of Ca^{2+} and length can be explained by the properties of troponin C (TnC) and the binding of calcium to TnC. As more Ca^{2+} ions bind to TnC in a skinned fiber preparation, more force is developed. There is a steep relationship, similar to that shown in the top panel. When the fiber is stretched and the sarcomere length increased, it is postulated that for any given number of Ca^{2+} ions binding to TnC, there is a greater force development. **Bottom panel,** Ca^{2+} concentration influences the development of tension at long (red circles) and shorter (blue triangles) sarcomere lengths. *(Top panel modified from Fuchs F: Mechanical modulation of the Ca^{2+} regulatory protein complex in cardiac muscle. News Physiol Sci 10:6, 1995; middle panel modified from Solaro RJ, Wolska BM, Westfall M: Regulatory proteins and diastolic relaxation. In Lorell BH, Grossman W [eds]: Diastolic Relaxation of the Heart. Norwell, Mass, Kluwer, 1994, pp 43-53; right panel modified from Cazorla O, Vassort G, Garnier D, LeGuennec J-Y: Length modulation of active force in rat cardiac myocytes: Is titin the sensor? J Mol Cell Cardiol 31:1215, 1995.)*

These proteins include the important stabilizing protein (technically known as FKBP-12.6) that responds to phosphorylation to coordinate the opening of neighboring ryanodine calcium channels by the process of coupled gating. Phosphatases (see Fig. 21-8) work in the opposite direction. The anatomical basis of the scaffolding function is that part of the ryanodine receptor extends from the membrane of the SR toward the T tubule, constituting the junctional calcium release complex, which bridges the gap between the SR and the T tubule. Here, the ryanodine receptors are packed in large organized arrays of perhaps 50 to 300 per junction. The ryanodine receptor is very large, and four of these link to form a megacomplex containing one calcium release channel (see Fig. 21-8). In addition to this are all the proteins adhering to the complex via their binding sites, so that the total megacomplex has a molecular weight approximating that of titin. After the wave of depolarization has reached the T tubule and opened the voltage-operated L-type calcium channels, the trigger calcium ions enter the cardiomyocyte to reach the junctional regions of the SR with their ryanodine receptors. The result is a change in the molecular configuration of the ryanodine receptor that opens the calcium release channel of the SR to discharge calcium ions into the subsarcolemmal space between the foot and the T tubule, and from there into the cytosol.

PHYSIOLOGICAL IMPLICATIONS: FIGHT OR FLIGHT VERSUS HEART RATE–INDUCED CALCIUM RELEASE. An interesting proposal is that there are different sites of phosphorylation for the catecholamine-mediated fight-or-flight reaction versus the heart rate–induced increase in contraction. During fight or flight, protein kinase A (PKA), linked to its anchoring protein, AKAP (see Fig. 21-8), targets the stabilizing protein FKBP-12.6 (which binds FK-506, also called calstabin 2) at a specific site, serine 2809. The proposed result

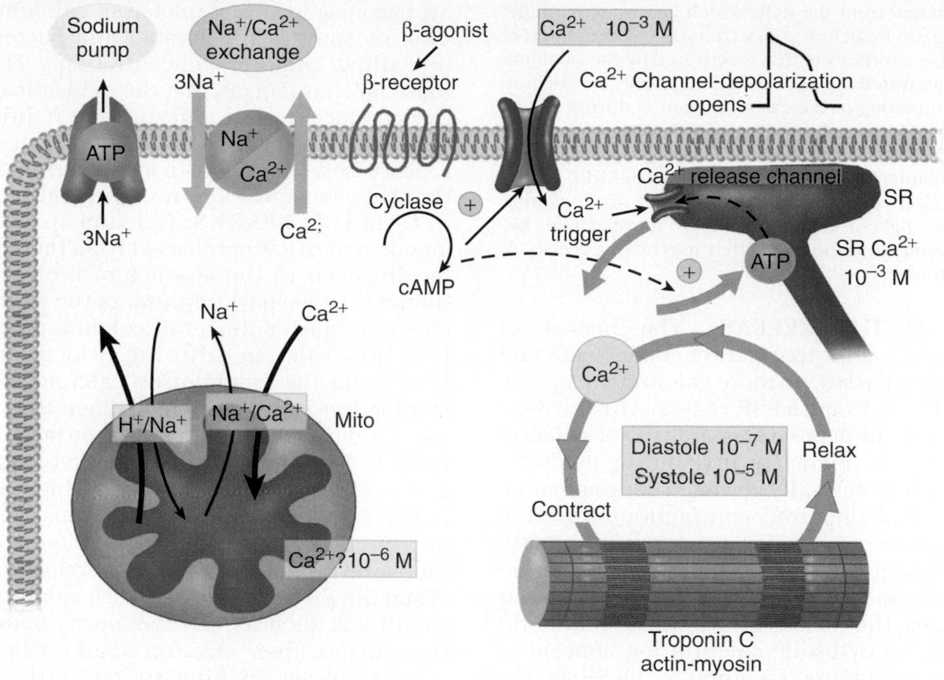

FIGURE 21–7 Calcium fluxes in the myocardium. Crucial features are (1) entry of Ca^{2+} ions via the voltage-sensitive L-type Ca^{2+} channels, acting as a trigger to the release of Ca^{2+} ions from the sarcoplasmic reticulum (SR); (2) the effect of alpha-adrenergic stimulation with adenylyl cyclase forming cyclic AMP, the latter both helping to open the Ca^{2+} channel and to increase the rate of uptake of Ca^{2+} into the SR; and (3) exit of Ca^{2+} ions, chiefly via the Na^+/Ca^{2+} exchange, with the sodium pump thereafter extruding the Na^+ ions gained in this process, which requires ATP. Note the much higher extracellular (10^{-3} M) than intracellular cytosolic Ca^{2+} concentration, with much higher calcium levels in the SR because of its storage function, and a hypothetical mitochondrial value of about 10^{-6} M. The mitochondria can act as a buffer against excessive changes in the free cytosolic calcium concentration. Mito = mitochondria. *(From Opie LH: Heart Physiology: From Cell to Circulation. Philadelphia, Lippincott Williams & Wilkins, 2004. © LH Opie, 2004.)*

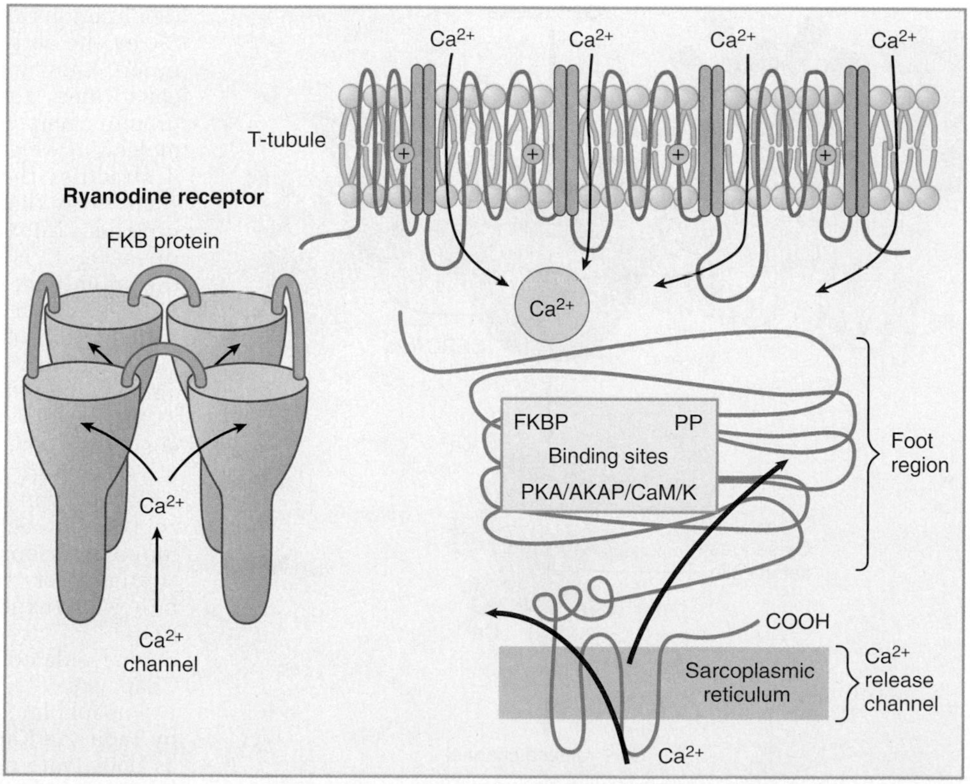

FIGURE 21–8 Role of ryanodine receptor (RyR) in calcium-induced calcium release. The RyR protein forms a link between the T tubule and the sarcoplasmic reticulum and is a scaffolding protein, which binds other proteins, such as kinases and phosphatases. This makes a macromolecular complex, also called the "foot" region. One high-affinity RyR is composed of four RyR monomer proteins. The molecular model of one RyR is schematically shown at the right. The four RyR proteins make a single calcium release channel, in a manner similar to the formation of some other ion channels (schematic, left). Depolarization stimulates the L-type calcium channel of the T tubule to allow calcium ion entry. The incoming calcium binds to the RyR to cause molecular conformational changes that result in opening of the calcium release channel, and calcium release from the SR. FKBP = FKBP-12.6 channel stabilizing subunit; PKA = protein kinase A; AKAP = anchoring protein for PKA; CaM/K = calmodulin/calmodulin kinase; PP = protein phosphatases. *(From Opie LH: Heart Physiology: From Cell to Circulation. Philadelphia, Lippincott Williams & Wilkins, 2004. © LH Opie, 2004.)*

is that FKBP-12.6 is detached from the RyR, which is now temporally destabilized to allow a greater calcium efflux from the SR through the RyR channel.[11] By contrast, another site that is activated by the calcium-dependent enzyme is activated by the greater amount of calcium brought in by repetitive opening of the calcium channel during tachycardia. This enzyme is Ca^{2+}/calmodulin-dependent protein kinase II (CaMKII); it phosphorylates at serine 2815 to cause a larger opening of the calcium release channel without any dissociation of FKBP-12.6.[11] Thus, if both PKA and CaMKII stimuli were applied at once, as in a genuine life-threatening fight-or-flight response, there could be maximal release of calcium from the SR, with a maximal increase in the cardiac contractile force.

TURN-OFF OF CALCIUM RELEASE. The increase of cytosolic calcium that triggers contraction comes to an end as the wave of excitation passes, no more calcium ions enter, and the release of calcium from the SR ceases. This turn-off of release is not as well understood as control of calcium release from the SR, but is important in avoiding cytosolic calcium overload with potentially serious consequences, such as arrhythmias and impaired contraction-relaxation cycles. Several proposals have been put forth to explain turn-off: (1) the increasing cytosolic calcium ion concentration inhibits the release process; (2) when the tubular calcium channel closes, the release of calcium from the SR ceases; (3) the increasing cytosolic calcium ion concentration can activate the calcium uptake pump of the SR; (4) the SR becomes locally depleted of calcium; and (5) the ryanodine receptor is inactivated and becomes resistant to the prevailing calcium concentration.[1] The overall effect of these mechanisms is that the cytosolic calcium ion concentration starts to fall and diastole is initiated. As the cytosolic calcium level decreases, calcium binding to troponin C decreases, tropomyosin again starts to inhibit the interaction between actin and myosin, and relaxation proceeds.

CALCIUM SPARKS. Calcium sparks are the very small amounts of calcium released from the SR spontaneously and locally, even in the absence of L channel opening. Hypothetically, the spark represents the spontaneous opening of one or at most a cluster of calcium release channels. There is so little calcium diffusing away from a spark that it fails to activate the neighboring calcium release channels and contraction is not initiated. When the calcium channels of the T tubules open, several thousand calcium sparks can unite to become a subsarcolemmal calcium wave that triggers excitation-contraction coupling.[12] This model predicts that the graded response in calcium release can be explained by the increased number of channels opened and the increased amount of calcium released by each channel. When the SR is overloaded with calcium, as in pathological conditions such as catecholamine toxicity or during early reperfusion, then calcium sparks can lead to propagated calcium waves, risking serious arrhythmias or impaired contractile activity.

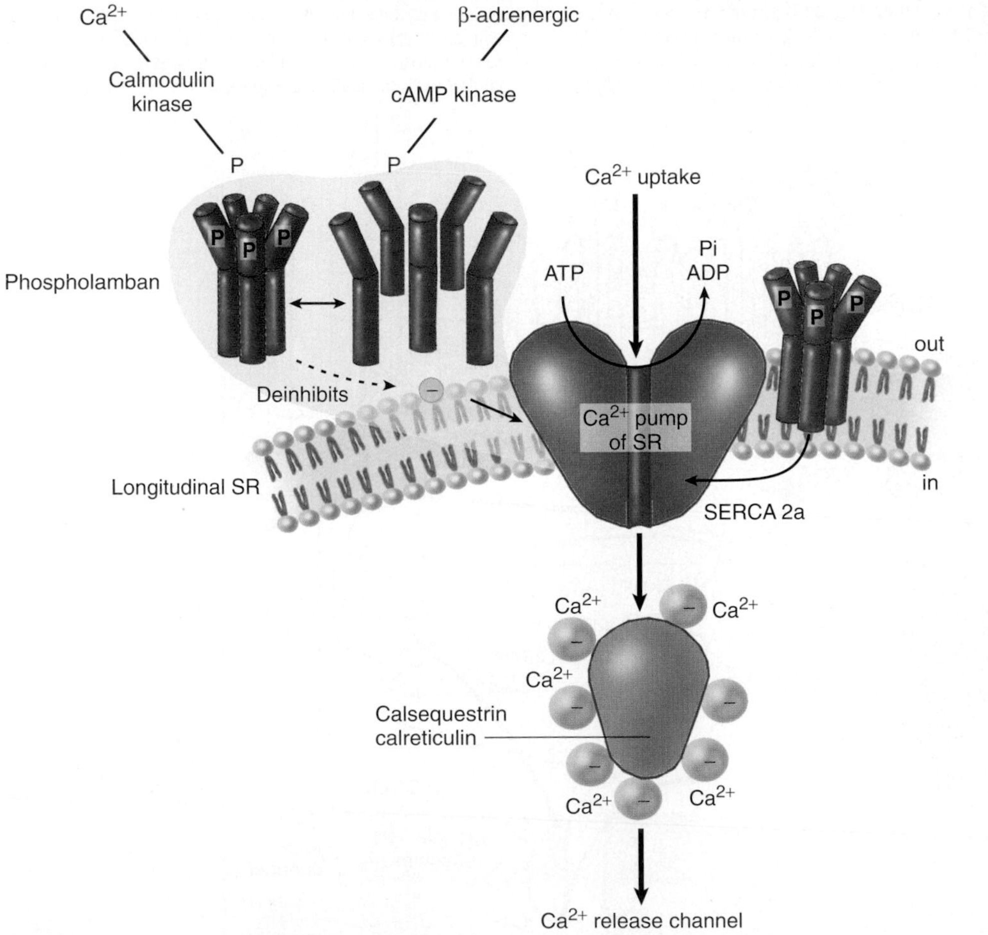

FIGURE 21–9 Lusitropic mechanism of calcium uptake into the sarcoplasmic reticulum (SR) by the energy-requiring calcium pump, SERCA 2a. Phospholamban can be phosphorylated (P) to remove the inhibition exerted by its dephosphorylated form (positive charges) on the calcium pump. Thereby, calcium uptake is increased, either in response to an enhanced cytosolic calcium or in response to alpha-adrenergic stimulation. Thus, there are two phosphorylations activating phospholamban at two distinct sites and their effects are additive. An increased rate of uptake of calcium into the SR enhances the rate of relaxation (lusitropic effect). ADP = adenosine diphosphate; ATP = adenosine triphosphate; cAMP = cyclic adenosine monophosphate; Pi = inorganic phosphate. *(Modified from Opie LH: Heart Physiology: From Cell to Circulation. Philadelphia, Lippincott Williams & Wilkins, 2004. © LH Opie, 2004.)*

Calcium Uptake by SERCA into the Sarcoplasmic Reticulum

Calcium ions are taken up into the SR by the activity of the calcium pump known as SERCA, which constitutes almost 90% of the protein component of the SR. Its molecular weight is about 115 kDa; it straddles the SR membrane in such a way that part of it actually protrudes into the cytosol. It exists in several isoforms, of which the dominant cardiac form is SERCA 2a. For each mole of ATP hydrolyzed by this enzyme, two calcium ions are taken up and accumulate in the SR (Fig. 21-9). Part of the source of the energy is from cytosolic generation of ATP via glycolysis.[12] Important links between SERCA and cardiac contractile activity have been found in various animal and human studies. For example, in heart failure, the expression and/or functional activity of SERCA 2a is downregulated (see Fig. 21-27 and Chap. 22).

Phospholamban was so named by Tada and Katz; it can be defined as *phosphate receiver*.[13] The activity of phospholamban is governed by a state of phosphorylation, a process that alters the molecular configuration of SERCA to promote its activity (see Fig. 21-9). Two major protein kinases are involved at two different phosphorylation sites[1]; one is activated by PKA in response to beta-adrenergic stimulation and cyclic AMP and the other is activated by calcium ions and calmodulin. When phospholamban responds to beta-adrenergic stimulation of the cardiomyocyte by enhancing the uptake of calcium by SERCA into the SR, thus increasing the rate of relaxation, the major activation is phosphorylation of the PKA site. It has also been postulated that the enhanced store of calcium in the SR correspondingly increases the amount of calcium released by the ryanodine receptor in response to subsequent waves of depolarization to give an increased rate and force of contraction.[1] This sequence is strongly supported by a transgenic mouse model, totally deficient in phospholamban, with hyperdynamic hearts, in which rates of contraction and relaxation are maximal and with attenuated responses to added beta-adrenergic stimulation by isoproterenol. Conversely, in hearts overexpressing phospholamban, cardiac function is depressed.[1]

Calcium, taken up into the SR by the calcium uptake pump, is stored within the SR prior to further release. The highly charged storage protein, calsequestrin, is found in that part of the SR that lies near the T tubules. Calcium stored with calsequestrin becomes available for the release process as calsequestrin discharges Ca^{2+} into the inner mouth of the calcium release channel. This process replaces the calcium ions liberated from the outer mouth into the cytosol. Calreticulin is another Ca^{2+}-storing protein, very similar in structure to calsequestrin and probably similar in function. Hypothetically, calsequestrin and two other proteins located in the SR membrane (junctin and triadin) may help regulate the properties of the ryanodine receptor.[1]

Sarcolemmal Control of Calcium and Sodium Ions

Calcium Channels

Models of excitation-contraction coupling ascribe a crucial role to the voltage-induced opening of the sarcolemmal L-type calcium channels in the initiation of the contractile process. Channels are pore-forming macromolecular proteins that span the sarcolemmal lipid bilayer to allow a highly selective pathway for ion transfer into the heart cell when the channel changes from a closed to an open state. Ion channels have two major properties, gating and permeation. Guarding each channel are two or more hypothetical gates that control its opening. Ions can permeate through the channel only when both gates are open. In the case of the sodium and calcium channels, which are best understood, the activation gate is shut at the normal resting membrane potential and the inactivation gate is open, so that the channels are voltage-gated. Depolarization opens the activation gate.

MOLECULAR STRUCTURE OF L-TYPE CALCIUM CHANNELS. There is a superfamily of voltage-gated ion channels that includes the sodium and calcium channels and some of the potassium channels. The potassium channels have the simpler structure, from which it is thought that the more complex sodium and calcium channels evolved. Both sodium and calcium channels contain a major alpha subunit with four transmembrane subunits or domains, very similar to each other in structure.[12] In addition, both sodium and calcium channels include in their overall structure a number of other subunits whose function is less well understood, such as the alpha subunit. Each of the four transmembrane domains of the alpha subunit is made up of six helices and is folded in on itself, so that the four S5-S6 spans structurally combine to form the single functioning pore of each calcium channel.[12] Activation is now understood in molecular terms as the change in charge on the fourth transmembrane segment, S4, called the voltage sensor, of each of the four subunits of the sodium or calcium channel.[12] Inactivation is the process whereby the current initially elicited by depolarization decreases with time, despite continuation of the original stimulus. The alpha subunit acts to enhance the calcium current flow through the alpha subunit pores. Channels are not simply open or closed. Rather, the open state is the last of a sequence of many molecular states, varying from a fully closed to a fully open configuration. Therefore, it is more correct to speak of the probability of channel opening.

CURRENT ACTIVATION AND DEACTIVATION. Having been activated by depolarization, the L-type calcium current is inactivated by the increasing voltage during depolarization, at a more positive potential than for activation, and by the increasing internal calcium ion concentration. In particular, the calcium flowing from the ryanodine receptor pushes up the subsarcolemmal internal calcium ion concentration near the mouth of the L channels of the T tubules to terminate current flow.[12]

T- AND L-TYPE CALCIUM CHANNELS. There are two major subpopulations of sarcolemmal calcium channels relevant to the cardiovascular system, the T and L channels. The T (transient) channels open at a more negative voltage, have short bursts of opening, and do not interact with conventional calcium antagonist drugs.[12] T channels presumably account for the earlier phase of the opening of the calcium channel, which may also give them a special role in the early electrical depolarization of the sinoatrial node, and hence of initiation of the heart beat. Although T channels are found in atrial cells, their existence in normal ventricular cells is controversial. T channels are not found in T tubules.[1]

The sarcolemmal L (long-lasting) channels are the standard calcium channels found in the myocardium and T tubules, which are involved in calcium-induced calcium release, and are inhibited by calcium channel blockers such as verapamil, diltiazem, and the dihydropyridines. During beta-adrenergic stimulation, the cyclic AMP level increases within the cell and phosphate groups are transferred from ATP to the $alpha_1$ subunit.[12] The electrical charges near the inner mouth of the nearby pores are thereby altered to induce changes in the molecular conformation of the pores, so that there is an increased probability of opening of the L-type calcium channels. The L channels are also part of the cellular cardiac protective pathway leading from insulin-like growth factor-1 (IGF-1) via phosphatidylinositol 3-kinase (PI3K) and Akt to physiological hypertrophy and protection from ischemia-reperfusion injury (see later, Fig. 21-27).[14]

Ion Exchangers and Pumps

To balance the small amount of calcium ions entering the heart cell with each depolarization, a similar quantity must leave the cell by one of two processes. First, calcium can be exchanged for sodium ions entering by the Na^+/Ca^{2+} exchange, and second, an ATP-consuming sarcolemmal calcium pump can transfer calcium into the extracellular space against a concentration gradient.

SODIUM-CALCIUM EXCHANGER. During relaxation, the sarcoplasmic calcium uptake pump and the Na^+/Ca^{2+} exchanger compete for the removal of cytosolic calcium, with the SR pump normally being dominant.[1] Restitution of calcium balance takes place by the activity of a series of transsarcolemmal exchangers, the chief of which is the Na^+/Ca^{2+} exchanger. The direction of ion exchange is responsive to the membrane potential and to the concentrations of sodium and calcium ions on either side of the sarcolemma. Because sodium and calcium ions can exchange inwardly or outwardly in response to the membrane potential, there must be a specific membrane potential, called the reversal or equilibrium potential, at which the ions are distributed so that they can move as easily in one direction as the other. The reversal potential may lie about halfway between the resting membrane potential and the potential of the fully depolarized state.

The major factor influencing the activity of the exchanger is the concentration of sodium and calcium ions on either side of the sarcolemma. Thus, of the calcium entering the cardiomyocyte with each depolarization-induced opening of the calcium channel, normally about 25 percent is extruded by this exchanger (see Fig. 21-7). In this case, the exchanger is operating in the forward mode (Na^+ in, Ca^{2+} out). However, changing the membrane potential from the resting value of perhaps −85 to +20 mV in the phase of rapid depolarization of the action potential and entry of sodium ions will therefore briefly reverse the direction of Na^+/Ca^{2+} exchange. Thus, the sodium ions that have just entered during the opening of the sodium channel will tend to leave and calcium ions will tend to enter. This process is known as reverse mode exchange. Such transsarcolemmal calcium entry may participate in calcium-induced calcium release.[1] There is evidence that enhanced reversed exchange contributes to the slow decline of the Ca^{2+} transient,[12] which may help explain delayed diastolic relaxation. Prolongation of the action potential duration also provokes reverse mode exchange, with risk of ventricular arrhythmias.[1] Also relevant is the influence of phospholemman, a newly discovered sarcolemmal protein that when phosphorylated by PKA, such as during the excess beta-adrenergic stimulation of heart failure (Fig. 21-10), limits the exchanger.[15] Such inhibition of normal forward exchange could potentially retain calcium within the myocyte and exaggerate diastolic calcium overload of heart failure.

Heart Rate and Na^+/Ca^{2+} Exchanger. This exchanger may participate in the force-frequency relationship (Treppe or Bowditch phenomenon). According to the sodium pump lag hypothesis, the rapid accumulation of calcium ions during fast stimulation of the myocardium outstrips the ability of the Na^+/Ca^{2+} exchanger and the sodium pump to return to ionic normality. The result is an accumulation of calcium ions in the SR and an increased force of contraction.

SODIUM PUMP (Na^+/K^+-ATPase). The sarcolemma becomes highly permeable to Na^+ only during the opening of the Na^+ channel during early depolarization, and Na^+ will also enter during the exit of Ca^{2+} by Na^+/Ca^{2+} exchange. Most of this influx of Na^+ across the sarcolemma must be corrected by the activity of the Na^+/K^+ pump, also called the Na^+/K^+-ATPase or simply the Na^+ pump. The pump is activated by internal Na^+ or external K^+.[1] One ATP molecule is used per transport cycle. The ions are first secluded within the pump protein and then extruded to either side. Although there has been some dispute about the exact ratio of Na^+ to K^+ ions that are pumped, a generally accepted model is that for each three Na^+ exported, two K^+ are imported. During this process, one positive charge must leave the cell. Hence, the pump is electrogenic and is also called the electrogenic Na^+ pump.[1] The current induced by sustained activity of the pump may contribute about −10 mV to the resting membrane potential.[12] Because the pump must extrude Na^+ ions entering by either Na^+/Ca^{2+} exchange or the Na^+ channel, its sustained activity is essential for the maintenance of normal ion balance.

BETA-ADRENERGIC SIGNAL SYSTEMS

During the sympathetic adrenergic response, norepinephrine is released into the synaptic cleft from small swellings, the terminal varicosities, lying on minute end branches of the neurons of the adrenergic nervous system (see Fig. 21-10). Norepinephrine is synthesized in the varicosities by two compounds, dopa and dopamine, and ultimately from the amino acid tyrosine, which is taken up from the circulation. The norepinephrine thus synthesized is stored in the terminals in storage granules (or vesicles) to be released on stimulation by an adrenergic nervous impulse. Thus, when central stimulation increases during excitement or exercise, an increased number of adrenergic impulses liberate an increased amount of norepinephrine from the terminals. Most of the released norepinephrine is taken up again by the nerve terminal varicosities to re-enter the storage vesicles or to be metabolized. The norepinephrine remaining in the synaptic cleft interacts with the postsynaptic beta-adrenergic receptors in the heart and alpha-adrenergic receptors in the arterioles. From these receptors, the messages are passed on by a series of messengers, with two major physiological end results. Whereas increased beta-adrenergic activity causes the heart to beat faster, with stronger contractions, increased alpha-adrenergic activity causes arteriolar constriction to increase the blood pressure.

Neuromodulation is the process whereby the release of norepinephrine from the terminal neurons is increased or decreased. The most powerful positive neuromodulator stimulating the release of norepinephrine is angiotensin II. Negative neuromodulators, which decrease the release of

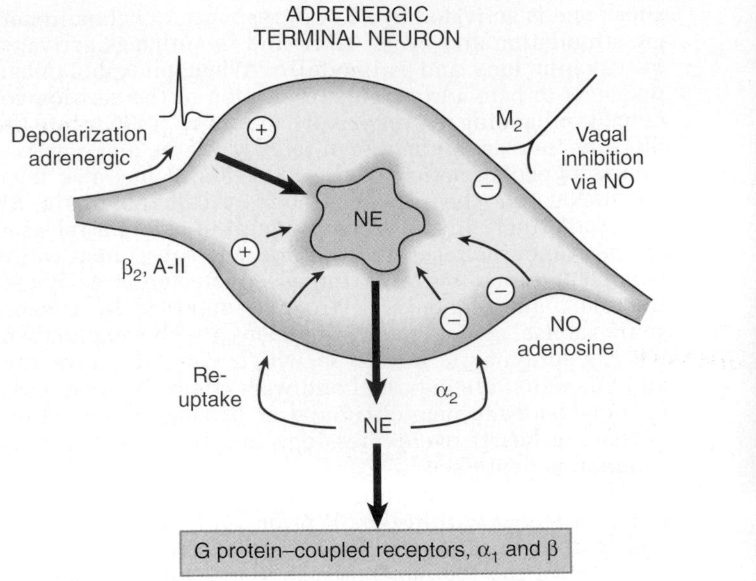

FIGURE 21–10 Control of release of norepinephrine (NE) from terminal neuron. NE is released from the storage granules of the terminal sympathetic neurons into the narrow cleft that separates the terminals from the G protein–coupled receptors (GPCRs), located in the sarcolemma of the myocytes of the heart or arterial wall. In cardiomyocytes, alpha-adrenergic receptors dominate, so that their stimulation increases heart rate and contractile force. In arterioles, NE has predominantly vasoconstrictive effects, acting via postsynaptic $alpha_1$-receptors (see Fig. 21-17). In addition, NE stimulates presynaptic $alpha_2$-receptors to invoke feedback inhibition of its own release, thereby modulating excess release of NE. Parasympathetic cholinergic stimulation, acting via nitric oxide (NO; see Fig. 21-16), inhibits the release of NE and thereby indirectly reduces the heart rate or causes vasodilation. Circulating epinephrine (E) stimulates vascular vasodilatory $alpha_2$-receptors but also presynaptic receptors on the nerve terminal that promote release of NE. Angiotensin II is also powerfully vasoconstrictive, acting both by inhibition of NE release (presynaptic receptors, schematically shown to the left of the terminal neuron) and also directly on arteriolar receptors. E = epinephrine; A-II = angiotensin II; M_2 = muscarinic receptor, subtype two. *(Modified from Opie LH: Heart Physiology: From Cell to Circulation. Philadelphia, Lippincott Williams & Wilkins, 2004. © LH Opie, 2004.)*

norepinephrine, include the local messengers adenosine and nitric oxide formed during exercise. Norepinephrine release is also lessened when there is increased cholinergic activity, as at night, when the muscarinic presynaptic receptors on the terminal neurons are stimulated (see Fig. 21-10).

Beta-Adrenergic Receptor Subtypes

Cardiac beta-adrenergic receptors are chiefly the beta$_1$ subtype, whereas most noncardiac receptors are beta$_2$. There are also beta$_2$ receptors in the human heart, about 20 percent of the total beta receptor population in the left ventricle and about twice as many as in the atria. Whereas the beta$_1$ receptors are linked to the stimulatory G protein, G_s, a component of the G protein–adenylyl cyclase system, beta$_2$ receptors are linked to both G_s and to the inhibitory G_i, so that their signaling pathway bifurcates at the very first postreceptor step, which has been a matter of controversy.[1] Hypothetically, beta$_2$ receptors are normally more strongly coupled to G_s but, in heart failure, this coupling is weakened and that to G_i is strengthened.[1] The beta-adrenergic receptor site is highly stereospecific, the best fit among catecholamines being obtained with the synthetic agent isoproterenol (ISO) rather than with the naturally occurring catecholamines, norepinephrine (NE) and epinephrine (E). In the case of beta$_1$ receptors, the order of agonist activity is ISO > E = NE, whereas in the case of beta$_2$ receptors, the order is ISO > E > NE. Human beta$_1$ and beta$_2$ receptors have now both been cloned.[1] The transmembrane domains are believed to be the site of agonist and antagonist binding, whereas the cytoplasmic domains interact with G proteins.

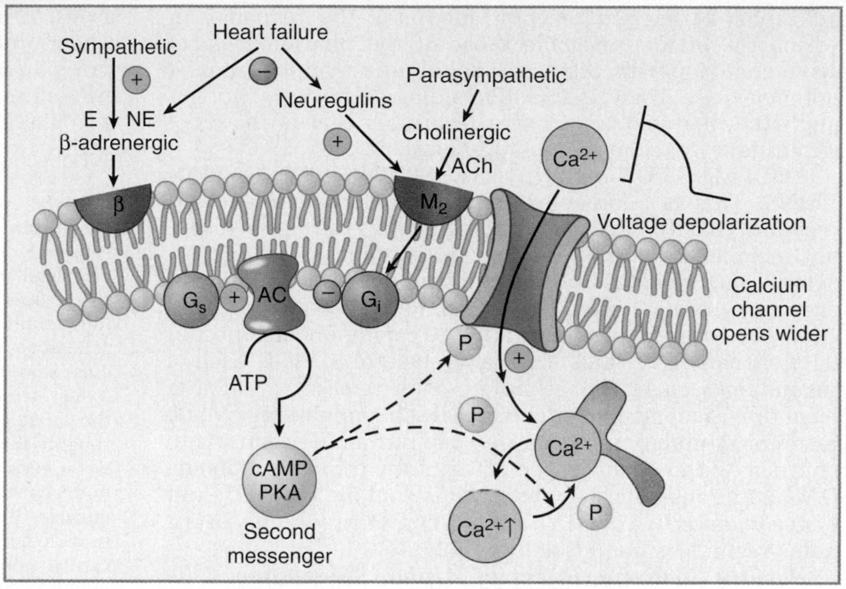

FIGURE 21–11 Interaction between sympathetic and parasympathetic systems could best be explained by countervailing influences on the second messenger, cyclic AMP (cAMP), mediated respectively by the stimulatory or inhibitory G proteins, G_s and G_i. In response to M_2 receptor stimulation, note the formation of G_i, with inhibitory effects on the formation of cyclic AMP. M_2 = muscarinic receptor, subtype 2; E = epinephrine; NE = norepinephrine; AC = adenylyl cyclase; PKA = protein kinase A; ACh = acetylcholine; P = phosphate group. *(From Opie LH: Heart Physiology: From Cell to Circulation. Philadelphia, Lippincott Williams & Wilkins, 2004. © LH Opie, 2004.)*

G Proteins

STIMULATORY G PROTEIN, G_s. G proteins are a superfamily of proteins that bind guanine triphosphate (GTP) and other guanine nucleotides. G proteins are crucial in carrying the signal from the first messenger and its receptor to the membrane-bound enzyme system, which produces the second messenger (Fig. 21-11).[1] The triple combination of the beta receptor, the G protein complex, and adenylyl cyclase is termed the beta-adrenergic system. The G protein itself is a heterotrimer composed of G_α, G_β, and G_γ, which on receptor stimulation splits into the alpha subunit, which is bound to GTP, and the beta-gamma subunit. Either of these subunits may regulate differing effectors, such as adenylyl cyclase, phospholipase C, and ion channels. The activity of adenylyl cyclase is controlled by two different G-protein complexes, namely G_s, which stimulates, and G_i, which inhibits. The alpha subunit of G_s (alpha$_s$) combines with GTP and then separates from the other two subunits to enhance activity of adenylyl cyclase. The beta and gamma subunits (beta-gamma) appear to be linked structurally and functionally.

INHIBITORY G PROTEIN, G_i. In contrast, a second trimeric GTP-binding protein, G_i, is responsible for inhibition of adenylyl cyclase.[1] During cholinergic signaling, the muscarinic receptor is stimulated and GTP binds to the inhibitory alpha subunit, alpha$_i$. The latter then dissociates from the other two components of the G protein complex, which are, as in the case of G_s, the combined beta-gamma subunits. The beta-gamma subunits act as follows. By stimulating the enzyme GTPase, they break down the active alpha$_s$-subunit (alpha$_s$-GTP), so that the activation of adenylyl cyclase in response to alpha stimulation becomes less. Furthermore, the beta-gamma subunit activates the K_{ACh} channel, which, in turn, can inhibit the sinoatrial node to contribute to the bradycardiac effect of cholinergic stimulation. The alpha$_i$ subunit activates another potassium channel (K_{ATP}) whose physiological function in the myocardium is still unclear. Pathophysiologically, preconditioning may link to this channel (see Chap. 48).

THIRD G PROTEIN, G_q. G_q links a group of heptahelical (*hepta*, seven) myocardial receptors, including the alpha-adrenergic receptor and those for angiotensin II and endothelin, to another membrane-associated enzyme, phospholipase C, and thence to protein kinase C (see later). G_q has at least four isoforms, of which two have been found in the heart. This G protein, unlike G_i, is not susceptible to inhibition by the pertussis toxin. Overexpression of Gq in mice induces a dilated cardiomyopathy,[1] which is of interest because angiotensin II and endothelin, which act through G_q, are overactive in human heart failure. Conversely, when the activity of G_q is genetically inhibited, the hypertrophic response to pressure overload attenuates and wall stress increases, but cardiac function is relatively well maintained (see later, Fig. 21-27).

Alpha-Adrenergic Receptor Subtypes

There are two types of alpha-adrenergic receptors. Those situated on the sarcolemma are called postsynaptic or postjunctional receptors, whereas those situated on the terminal varicosities are called the presynaptic or prejunctional receptors (see Fig. 21-10). Norepinephrine can inhibit its own release from the terminal neurons, acting on the presynaptic alpha$_2$-adrenergic receptors, whereas the postsynaptic alpha$_1$-adrenergic receptors act on the arteriolar sarcolemma to regulate arterial tone.[12] Pharmacologically, an alpha$_1$-adrenergic receptor mediates the response in which the effects resemble those of the pharmacological agent phenylephrine. Among catecholamines, alpha$_1$-agonist potencies are NE > E > ISO. Physiologically, it is norepinephrine liberated from nerve terminals that is the chief stimulus to vascular alpha$_1$-adrenergic activity.

COUPLING OF ALPHA$_1$ RECEPTORS BY G PROTEINS. This is another example of a G protein–coupled receptor (GPCR). When an agonist occupies the alpha$_1$ receptor, members of the G protein family, such as G_h and G_q, couple the receptor to the activity of the sarcolemmal enzyme system, phospholipase C, to form phosphatidyl inositol. The latter in turn is split into two components, inositol triphosphate (IP_3) and 1,2-diacylglycerol (DAG), each a second messenger. IP_3 stimulates the release of calcium from the sarcoplasmic reticulum, which explains why alpha receptor stimulation can cause vascular smooth muscle to contract without any entry of calcium from the outside. DAG is the messenger that activates protein kinase C, and hence eventually the MAP kinase complex, which in turn helps regulate growth (see Fig. 21-26).

Positive Inotropic Effect of Alpha$_1$-Stimulation. This effect is not thought to be of major importance in the normal myocardium, when the prime regulation of contraction is through the beta-adrenergic system. Nonetheless, the small positive inotropic effect associated with the formation of IP_3 could be active in heart failure as a supportive positive inotropic mechanism.

CYCLIC ADENOSINE MONOPHOSPHATE AND PROTEIN KINASE A

Adenylyl Cyclase. This is a transmembrane enzyme system, also called adenylate or adenyl cyclase, that responds to input from G proteins. When stimulated by G_s, adenylyl cyclase produces the second messenger, cyclic adenosine monophosphate (cAMP), which then acts through a further series of intracellular signals—specifically the third messenger protein kinase A—to increase cytosolic calcium transients. In contrast, cholinergic stimulation exerts inhibitory influences, largely on the heart rate, but also on contraction, acting at least in part by decreasing the rate of formation of cAMP.

Adenylyl cyclase is the only enzyme system producing cyclic AMP; it specifically requires low concentrations of ATP (and magnesium) as substrate. Surprisingly, the proposed molecular structure resembles certain channel proteins, such as that of the calcium channel. Most of the protein is located on the cytoplasmic side, the presumed site of interaction with the G protein. Another cyclic nucleotide, cyclic GMP, acts as a second messenger for some aspects of vagal activity. In vascular smooth muscle, cyclic GMP is the second messenger of the nitric oxide messenger system. These messenger chemicals are present in the heart cell in minute concentrations, that of cyclic AMP being roughly about 10^{-9} M and that of cyclic GMP about 10^{-11} M. Cyclic AMP has a very rapid turnover as a result of a constant dynamic balance between its formation by adenylyl cyclase and removal by another enzyme, phosphodiesterase. In general, directional changes in the tissue content of cyclic AMP can be related to directional changes in cardiac contractile activity. For example, beta-adrenergic stimulation increases both, whereas beta blockade inhibits the increases induced by beta agonists. Forskolin, a direct stimulator of adenylyl cyclase, increases cyclic AMP and contractile activity. Adenosine, acting through A_1 receptors, inhibits adenylyl cyclase, decreases cyclic AMP, and lessens contractile activity. A number of hormones or peptides can couple to myocardial adenylyl cyclase independently of the beta-adrenergic receptor. These are glucagon, thyroid hormone, prostacyclin (PGI_2), and the calcitonin gene-related peptide.

INHIBITION OF ADENYLYL CYCLASE. The major physiological stimulus to G_i is thought to be vagal muscarinic receptor stimulation. In addition, adenosine, by interaction with alpha$_1$ receptors, couples to G_i to inhibit contraction and heart rate. The adenosine A_2 receptor paradoxically increases cyclic AMP. The latter effect, only of ancillary significance in the myocardium, is of major importance in vascular smooth muscle, where it induces vasorelaxation. Pathologically, inhibitory G_i is increased in experimental postinfarct heart failure and in donor hearts prior to cardiac transplantation.[1]

CYCLIC AMP-DEPENDENT PROTEIN KINASES. It is now clear that most, if not all, the effects of cyclic AMP are ultimately mediated by protein kinase A, which phosphorylates various key proteins and enzymes (Fig. 21-12).[1] Phosphorylation is the donation of a phosphate group to the enzyme concerned, acting as a fundamental metabolic switch that can amplify the signal extensively.

Each protein kinase is composed of two subunits, regulatory (R) and catalytic (C). When cyclic AMP interacts with the inactive protein kinase, it binds to the R subunit to liberate the active kinase, which is the C subunit:

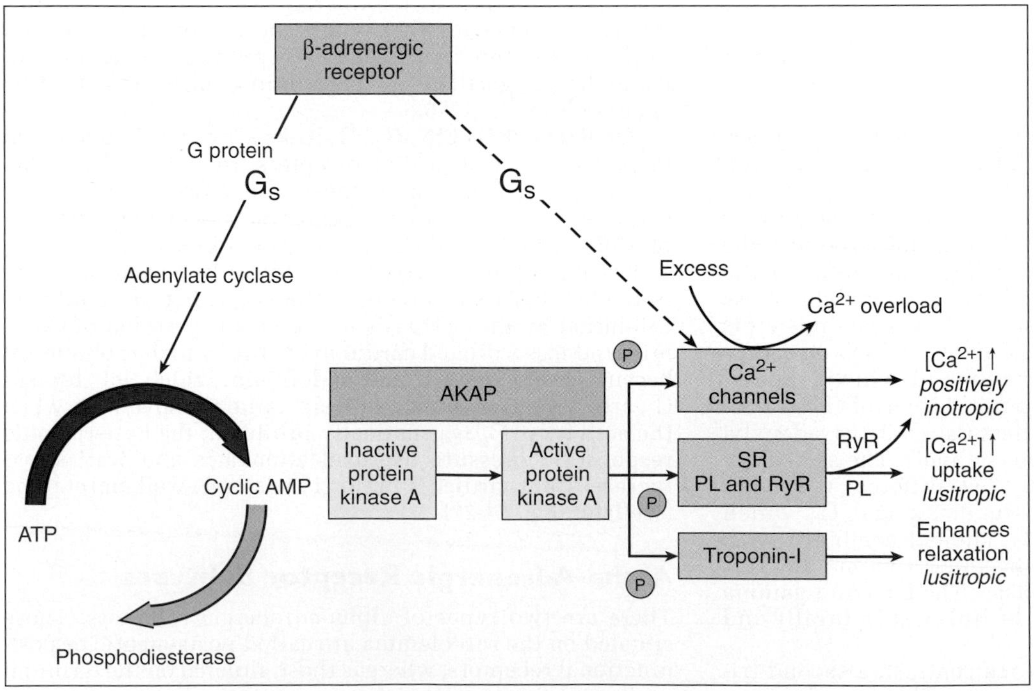

FIGURE 21–12 Key role of protein kinase A in the alpha-adrenergic response. The major intracellular effects of beta agonist catecholamines are by formation of cyclic AMP, which increases the activity of the cAMP-dependent protein kinase A (PKA). The latter achieves its optimal intracellular site by localizing to the scaffolding protein, A-kinase anchoring protein (AKAP), whereupon PKA phosphorylates various proteins involved in contraction and relaxation. SR = sarcoplasmic reticulum; PL = phospholamban; RyR = ryanodine receptor. For inotropic and lusitropic mechanisms, see Figure 21-13. *(From Opie LH: Heart Physiology: From Cell to Circulation. Philadelphia, Lippincott Williams & Wilkins, 2004. © LH Opie, 2004.)*

$$(R_2 + C_2) + 2cAMP \rightarrow 2RcAMP + 2C$$

At a molecular level, this active kinase catalyzes the transfer of the terminal phosphate of ATP to serine and threonine residues of the protein substrates, leading to phosphorylation and modification of the properties of the proteins concerned, thereby promoting further key reactions. PKA occurs in different cells in two isoforms; PKA-II predominates in cardiac cells. The proposed anchorage of this kinase by its anchoring proteins (AKAPs) to specific organelles, such as the SR, explains the phenomenon of cyclic AMP compartmentalization,[1] because anchored PKA requires focal elevation of cyclic AMP, even at an unchanged cytosolic concentration. In addition, the G protein system may not be evenly spread throughout the sarcolemma but localized to certain focal areas. Thus, it is very likely that there is only a specific subcompartment of cyclic AMP available to increase contractile activity.

COMPARTMENTALIZATION OF CYCLIC AMP AND PROTEIN KINASE A. These second and third messengers are not simply evenly distributed thoughout the cytosol. Rather, there is increasing evidence for subcellular compartmentalization of cyclic AMP and its further messenger PKA, in which the scaffolding or anchoring protein, AKAP, plays an important role (see Figs. 21-12 and 21-13), so that PKA is colocalized with its target.[16] Thus, during beta-adrenergic stimulation, there is subsarcolemmal formation of cyclic AMP with a multimolecular signaling complex involving PKA, PKA-anchoring proteins, and the phosphodiesterase-4 (PDE-4) isoform, the latter breaking down PKA.[17] Furthermore, this sequence of events is linked to activation of the cardiac L-type calcium channels and by inference also to phosphorylation of the RyR receptor.

PHYSIOLOGICAL BETA$_1$-ADRENERGIC EFFECTS. The probable sequence of events describing the positive inotropic effects of catecholamines is as follows (see Fig. 21-11):

Catecholamine stimulation → beta receptor → molecular changes → binding of GTP to alpha$_s$-subunit of G protein → GTP-alpha$_s$ subunit stimulates adenylyl cyclase → formation of cyclic AMP from ATP → activation of cyclic AMP-dependent PKA, locally bound by an A-kinase anchoring protein (AKAP) → phosphorylation of a sarcolemmal protein p27 → increased entry of calcium ion through increased opening of the voltage-dependent L-type calcium channels → greater calcium-induced calcium release via ryanodine receptor of sarcoplasmic reticulum, coupled with phosphorylation of the ryanodine receptor → greater and more rapid rise of intracellular free calcium ion concentration → increased calcium–troponin C interaction, with deinhibition of tropomyosin effect on actin-myosin interaction → increased rate and number of cross bridges interacting with increased myosin ATPase activity → increased rate and peak of force development.

The increased lusitropic (relaxant) effect is the consequence of increased PKA-mediated phosphorylation of phospholamban. Also, increased phosphorylation of troponin I may help desensitize the contractile apparatus to calcium ions (Fig. 21-13).

Physiological Switch Off, Beta-Agonist Receptor Kinase, and Arrestin

There is a potent feedback mechanism whereby the degree of postreceptor response to a given degree of beta-adrenergic receptor stimulation can be muted (Fig. 21-14). Sustained beta agonist stimulation rapidly induces the activity of the beta agonist receptor kinase (βARK), also called G protein–coupled receptor kinase (GRK2) that is involved in the transfer of the phosphate group to the phosphorylation site on the terminal COOH tail of the receptor, a process that of itself does not markedly affect the signaling properties. Rather, βARK increases the affinity of the beta receptor for another protein family, the arrestins, which cause the uncoupling. Beta-arrestin is a scaffolding protein that links to one of the cytoplasmic loops of the G protein–coupled beta-adrenergic receptor,[1] thus uncoupling receptor occupancy from G_s and lessening activation of adenylyl cyclase, thereby inhibiting the functioning of this receptor. Furthermore, beta-arrestin switches the agonist coupling from G_s to G_i.[18] Resensitization of the receptor occurs if the phosphate group is split off by a phosphatase; the receptor may then more readily be linked to G_s.

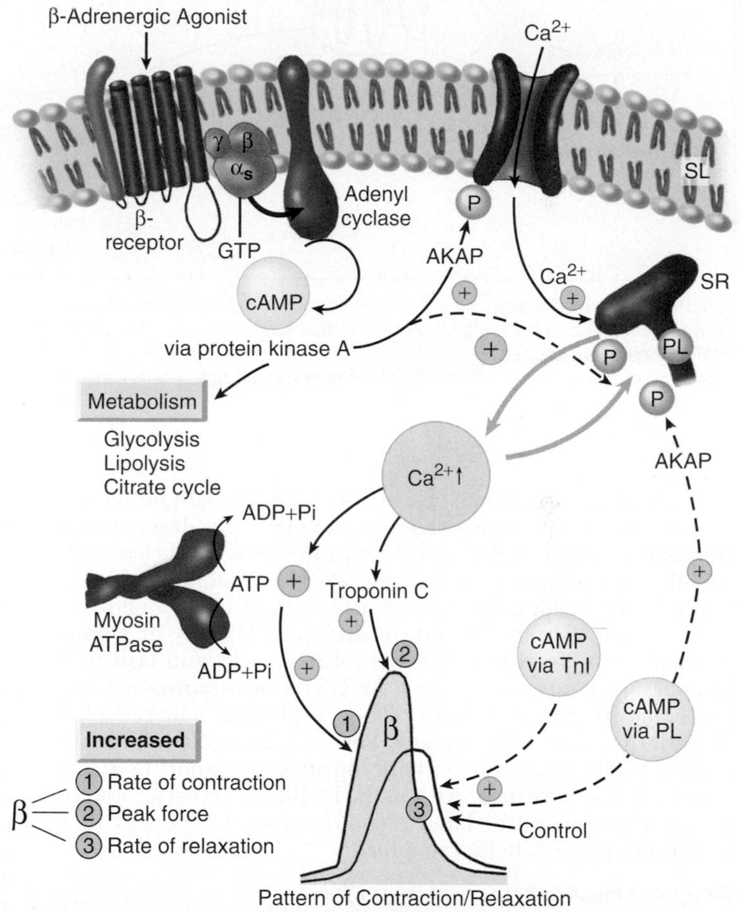

FIGURE 21–13 Signal systems involved in positive inotropic and lusitropic (enhanced relaxation) effects of alpha-adrenergic stimulation. When the alpha-adrenergic agonist interacts with the alpha receptor, a series of G-protein–mediated changes (see Fig. 21-11) leads to activation of adenylyl cyclase and formation of cyclic AMP (cAMP). The latter acts via protein kinase A to stimulate metabolism (on the left) and to phosphorylate the calcium channel protein. The result is an enhanced opening probability of the calcium channel, thereby increasing the inward movement of Ca^{2+} ions through the sarcolemma (SL) of the T tubule. These Ca^{2+} ions release more calcium from the sarcoplasmic reticulum (SR; see Fig. 21-7) to increase cytosolic calcium and to activate troponin C. Calcium ions also increase the rate of breakdown of ATP to ADP and inorganic phosphate (P_i). Enhanced myosin ATPase activity explains the increased rate of contraction, with increased activation of troponin C explaining increased peak force development. An increased rate of relaxation is explained because cyclic AMP also activates the protein phospholamban, situated on the membrane of the SR, that controls the rate of uptake of calcium into the SR (see Fig. 21-9). The latter effect explains enhanced relaxation (lusitropic effect). P = phosphorylation; PL = phospholamban; SL = sarcolemma; SR = sarcoplasmic reticulum. AKAP = A-kinase anchoring proteins. *(From Opie LH: Heart Physiology: From Cell to Circulation. Philadelphia, Lippincott Williams & Wilkins, 2004. © LH Opie, 2004.)*

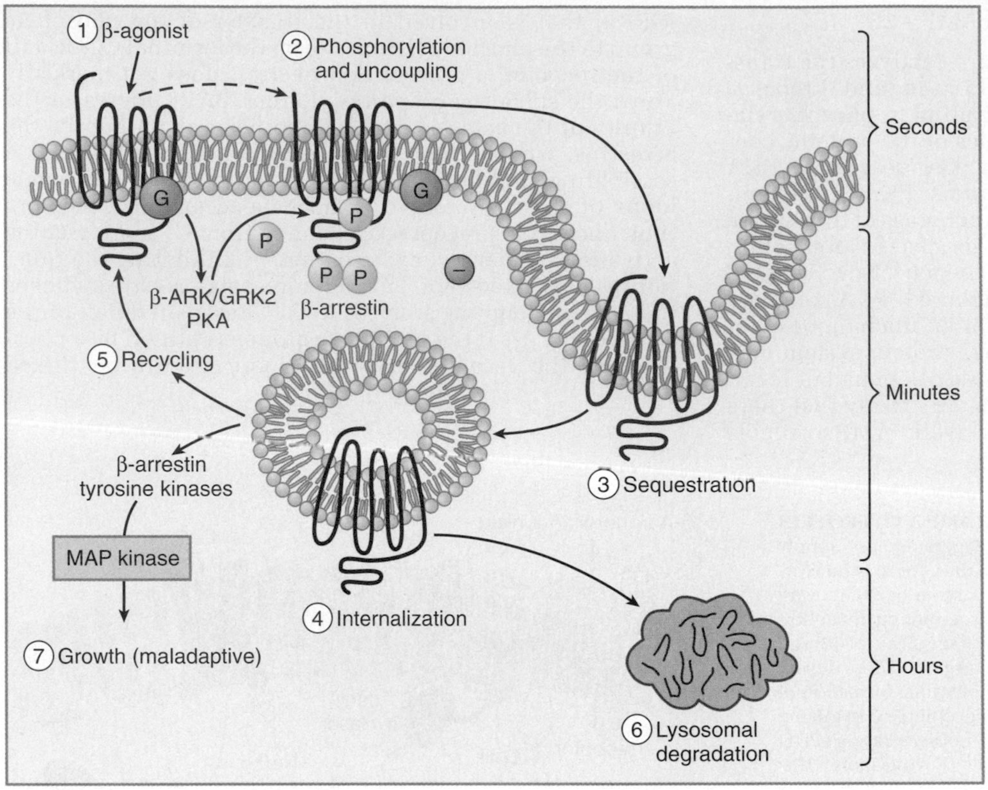

FIGURE 21–14 Mechanisms of alpha-adrenergic receptor desensitization and internalization. Note links between the internalized receptor complex with growth stimulation via mitogen-activated protein (MAP) kinase. β-ARK = beta-agonist receptor kinase or G-coupled receptor kinase (GRK2); PKA = protein kinase A. *(Modified from Hein L, Kobilka BK: Adrenergic receptors. From molecular structures to in vivo function. Trends Cardiovasc Med 7:137, 1997.)*

Physiologically, the βARK-arrestin mechanism helps terminate the beta receptor signal by a very rapid desensitization of the beta receptor, within minutes to seconds (see Fig. 21-14). As discussed in Chapter 22, this mechanism also plays a role in long-term desensitization of the beta-adrenergic receptor in heart failure and participates in signal transduction, leading to hypertrophic growth and failure.[19] Conversely, transgenic mice with GRK2 overexpression are protected from heart failure.[19] Thus, prolonged beta receptor stimulation may have adverse end results, both impairing contractile function and enhancing adverse signaling in the course of heart failure. Although the βARK-arrestin effects are best described for $beta_2$ receptors, they also occur to a lesser extent with $beta_1$ receptors.[1]

Beta₂- and Possible Beta₃-Adrenergic Effects

In the normal ventricle, about 20 percent of the receptors are $beta_2$ in nature; however, in heart failure, this figure can double because of $beta_1$ receptor downregulation (See Chap. 22). The $beta_2$ postreceptor signaling involves both the stimulatory and the inhibitory G proteins.[1] In humans, the positive inotropic response to $beta_2$ stimulation by salbutamol occurs, at least in part, through $beta_2$ receptors on the terminal neurons of the cardiac sympathetic nerves, thereby releasing norepinephrine, which in turn exerts dominant $beta_1$ effects.[1] Indirect evidence suggests that the G_i inhibitory path is relatively augmented in heart failure, whereas the strength of the stimulatory G_s path is lessened because of uncoupling of G_s from the $beta_2$ receptor.

Regarding $beta_3$-adrenergic receptors, some studies have proposed a negative inotropic effect through nitric oxide and formation of inhibitory cyclic guanosine monophosphate (cyclic GMP).[20] By contrast, in more recent studies, these receptors are associated with the formation of cyclic AMP, with negative modulation by cyclic GMP.[21] Thus, the physiological role of the $beta_3$-receptors remains in doubt.

CHOLINERGIC AND NITRIC OXIDE SIGNALING

Cholinergic Signaling

Parasympathetic stimulation reduces heart rate and is negatively inotropic. The key features of its signaling system are similar to those of the $beta_1$-adrenergic system. Again, there is an extracellular first messenger (acetylcholine), a receptor system (the cholinergic muscarinic receptor), a sarcolemmal signaling system (the G protein system, specifically the inhibitory G_i), and a second messenger (cyclic GMP). The myocardial muscarinic receptor (M_2) is associated specifically with the activity of the vagal nerve endings. Receptor stimulation produces a negative chronotropic response that is inhibited by atropine. Nitric oxide (NO) facilitates cholinergic signaling at two levels, the nerve terminal and the activity of the enzyme system that produces cyclic GMP. Neuroregulins are growth factors that maintain the activity of the muscarinic receptor, thereby indirectly helping balance the normal parasympathetic modulation of excess beta-adrenergic stimulation.[22]

MECHANISMS OF VAGAL HEART RATE LOWERING. Cyclic GMP acts as a second messenger to vagal stimulation, just as cyclic AMP does to beta-adrenergic stimulation. Of note, cell-permeable analogues of cyclic GMP have antiadrenergic effects. Cholinergic stimulation of the M_2 receptor activates guanylyl (= guanylate = guanyl) cyclase to form cyclic GMP, with consequent stimulation of protein kinase G (PKG), which results in inhibitory cardiac effects, such as a decreased heart rate and negative inotropic response.[23] These effects are largely achieved by modulation of calcium ion entry through the L calcium channel and through inhibition of internal calcium cycling.[24] In addition, muscarinic M_2 stimulation acts via G_i to lessen the G_s activation that results from beta receptor occupation. Thus, the vagus has a dual effect on second messengers, inhibiting the formation of cyclic AMP and increasing that of cyclic GMP, thereby providing one of several explanations for sympathetic-parasympathetic interaction. In the sinus node, formation of cyclic GMP may occur not only by guanylyl cyclase (Fig. 21-15) but also by a muscarinic-mediated formation of nitric oxide.

COMPARTMENTALIZATION OF CYCLIC GMP. To date, two compartments of cyclic GMP have been localized, the particulate, or subsarcolemmal, pool and the soluble, or cytosolic, pool.[17] Particulate cGMP is activated by the natriuretic peptides, such as brain natriuretic peptide (BNP), whereas the soluble pool is activated by nitric oxide and cholinergic stimulation (see Fig. 21-15). Cyclic GMP is broken

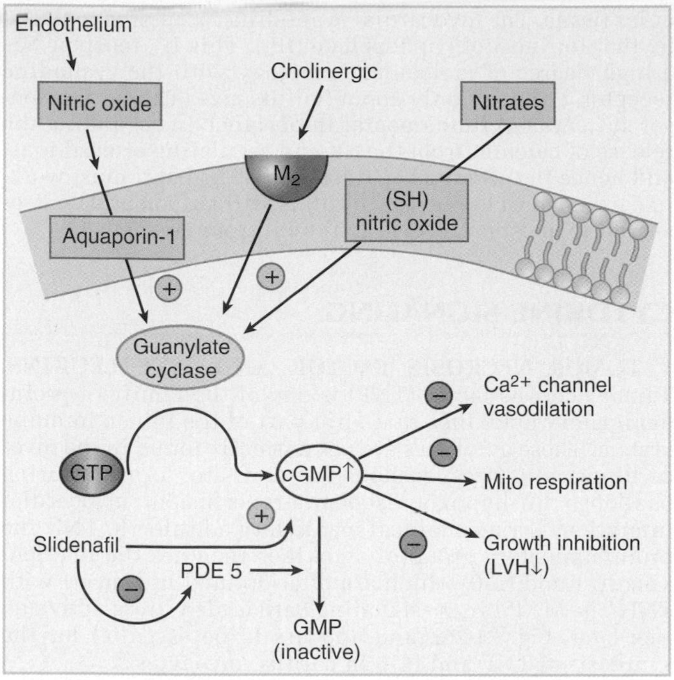

FIGURE 21–15 Nitric oxide messenger system. Illustrated is the proposed role of nitric oxide in stimulating soluble guanylyl cyclase to form cyclic guanosine monophosphate (cGMP) to cause vasodilation and a negative inotropic effect. In the myocardium, there is inhibition of maladaptive growth. Antianginal nitrates also cause coronary vasodilation by this mechanism. Cholinergic stimulation, by acting on the muscarinic receptors (M_2), also increases vascular and myocardial cGMP. Mito = mitochondrial; PDE = phosphodiesterase; LVH = left ventricular hypertrophy. *(From Opie LH: Heart Physiology: From Cell to Circulation. Philadelphia, Lippincott Williams & Wilkins, 2004. © LH Opie, 2004.)*

down by phosphodiesterase 5 (PDE 5), which has achieved prominence as a result of its inhibition by sildenafil and related compounds that all enhance penile vasodilation. Emerging data show wider therapeutic potential. Thus, sildenafil, by accumulation of cyclic GMP, combats harmful excessive adrenergic stimulation of contractile function.[25] Furthermore, sildenafil via cyclic GMP can inhibit excess LV growth in response to aortic constriction.[26] The next messenger of cyclic GMP, protein kinase G (PKG), like its counterpart PKA, colocalizes with its targets to control substrate phosphorylation.[16] The anchoring protein for PKG may be the same AKAP as for cyclic AMP, allowing tight subcellular colocalization and regulation of the counterpoised activities of cyclic AMP and cyclic GMP, and hence of the balance between adrenergic and cholinergic regulation.

Regarding the negative inotropic effect of vagal stimulation (see Fig. 21-15), the mechanisms include the following: (1) heart rate slowing (negative Treppe phenomenon); (2) inhibition of the formation of cyclic AMP; and (3) direct negative inotropic effect mediated by cyclic GMP. It has been controversial whether ventricular tissue is as responsive to muscarinic agonists as atrial tissue, although the receptor populations are similar in density. However, using pressure-volume loops and the slope of the pressure-volume relationship (see Fig, 21-24, line Es) as an index of contractile function, vagal stimulation in humans markedly decreases this load-independent measure.[1]

The sympathetic terminal neurons are another site of parasympathetic-sympathetic interaction. Here, the presynaptic muscarinic M_2 receptor inhibits the release of norepinephrine. Additionally, adrenergic and cholinergic stimuli exert important and often opposing effects on ion channels and cardiac function (Table 21-2). The presence of such mechanisms involved in the inhibitory effects of vagal stimulation on the heart rate, inotropic state, and arrhythmogenicity, suggest that "braking" of beta-adrenergic stimulation is desirable. Otherwise, the risk may be that intense beta-adrenergic stimulation would increase the heart rate or inotropic state excessively or provoke potentially fatal arrhythmias.

TABLE 21–2 Comparative Cardiovascular Effects of Alpha- and Beta-Adrenergic Receptor Stimulation

Parameter	Alpha$_1$-Mediated	Beta-Mediated
Electrophysiological effects	±	++ Conduction; pacemaker; heart rate
Myocardial mechanics	±	++ Contractility; stroke volume; cardiac output
Myocardial metabolism	±; glycolysis	++ O_2 uptake ↑; ATP
Signal systems	GPCR coupled, can activate MAP kinase	GPCR coupled, can activate MAP kinase
Coronary arterioles	++ Constriction	+ Direct dilation +++ Indirect dilation (metabolic)
Peripheral arterioles	+++ Constriction SVR↑ SBP↑	+ Dilation SVR↓ SBP↓

± = variable effect; + = clear effect, positive; ++ = increasing effect, positive; +++ = maximal effect, positive.

SVR = systemic vascular resistance; SBP = systolic blood pressure; GPCR = G protein–coupled receptor.

Modified from Opie LH: Heart Physiology: From Cell to Circulation. 4th ed. Philadelphia, Lippincott Williams & Wilkins, 2004, Table 7-4.

Nitric Oxide Signaling

Nitric oxide (NO), the focus of the Nobel Prize in 1998, is a unique messenger; it is formed in so many tissues, is a gas, and is a physiological free radical. It should more correctly be written as ˙NO (Fig. 21-16; also see Fig. 21-15), but the standard abbreviation is NO. Although usually thought to be freely diffusible through cell membranes, it has recently been discovered that an integral membrane protein, aquaporin-1, facilitates and may regulate diffusion of NO into cells.[27] NO is generated in the heart by one of three isoenzymes.[24] Vasodilatory NO is generated in the vascular endothelium by endothelial nitric oxide synthase (eNOS; also called NOS-3) in response to increased blood flow, increased cardiac load, or bradykinin. Excess NO is generated in cardiomyocytes in disease states such as cardiogenic or septic shock by the inducible enzyme iNOS (also called NOS-2). Generation of NO by neuronal NOS (nNOS; also called NOS-1), the form of the synthase found in vagal nerve terminals, enhances the release of acetylcholine.[28] The enhanced vagal activity of exercise training depends on increased expression of nNOS.[28] Exercise also acts peripherally to enhance the expression of vasodilatory eNOS in humans with coronary disease.[29] Because the activity of guanylyl cyclase, promoted by cholinergic stimulation, is sensitive to and enhanced by NO,[23] previous concepts have been revised. NO is now seen as augmenting parasympathetic stimulation both upstream and downstream from acetylcholine. Furthermore, the increase in cyclic GMP induced by eNOS-derived NO potentially adds to that of cholinergic stimulation (see Fig. 21-15). Such increases of cyclic GMP are potentially protective from adverse excess adrenergic stimulation.[25] Whereas physiological amounts of NO are cardio-

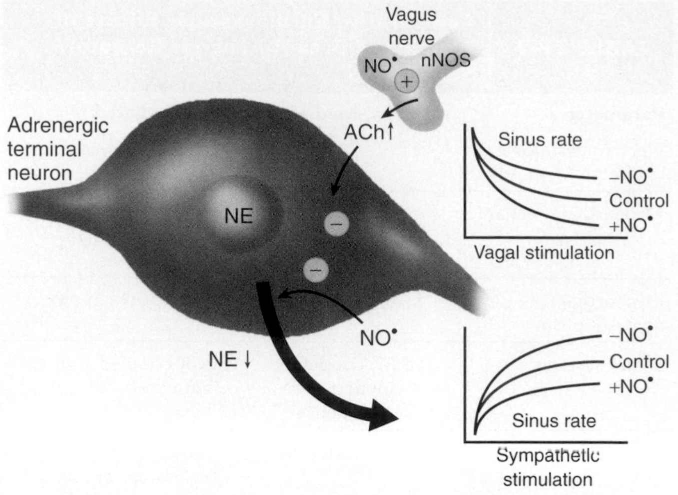

FIGURE 21–16 Nitric oxide (NO) mediates the release of acetylcholine (ACh) from vagal nerve terminals. NO, produced in the terminal vagal nerve endings, increases the release of acetylcholine (ACh) and decreases that of norepinephrine (NE). Thus, the sinus rate response to vagal or sympathetic stimulation is changed accordingly. nNOS = neuronal nitric oxide synthase. *(From Opie LH: Heart Physiology: From Cell to Circulation. Philadelphia, Lippincott Williams & Wilkins, 2004. © LH Opie, 2004.)*

protective (see Chap. 22), excessive levels of nitric oxide are harmful.

REACTIVE OXYGEN SPECIES AS SIGNALING MOLECULES. Although excess reactive oxygen species (ROS) production is linked to many cardiovascular diseases, it is often forgotten that ROS probably have important physiological roles. Many pathways for formation are present, as are the endogenous antioxidants and antioxidant enzymes (see Chap. 22).[30] Thus, ROS are part of protective oxygen-sensing mechanisms, allowing cells to adapt to hypoxia.[30] Increased contraction frequency of cardiomyocytes also gives rise to ROS of unknown physiological function.[30] As discussed in Chapter 22, excessive ROS production in the heart has numerous consequences.

OTHER INHIBITORY SIGNAL SYSTEMS. Adenosine, in addition to being a physiological vasodilator, acts on myocardial A_1 receptors that are coupled to adenylyl cyclase by the inhibitory G protein (α_i subunit). Opioids released in the central nervous system are known to participate in cardiovascular regulation by inhibiting sympathetic and promoting parasympathetic outflow. In the heart, the delta receptors inhibit the adrenergic system by coupling to G_i, thereby inhibiting the activation of adenylyl cyclase by alpha-adrenergic stimulation and stimulating the PKC pathway (see later).[31]

VASOCONSTRICTIVE SIGNALING

VASCULAR G PROTEIN–COUPLED RECEPTORS. Agonists with vasoconstriction as their major physiological role include alpha$_1$-adrenergic catecholamines, angiotensin II, and endothelin (Fig. 21-17). By regulating the degree of vasoconstriction, the peripheral vascular resistance can be tuned to the needs of the circulation—for example, with vasoconstriction occurring in response to alpha$_1$-adrenergic stimulation during the stress of blood loss. Each of these agonists is coupled to its appropriate seven-transmembrane spanning receptor, linked via the G protein G_q to different effectors from those of adrenergic and cholinergic signaling. Specifically, a different calcium release signal system is involved to achieve vasoconstrictive calcium release in vascular tissue. The myocardial ryanodine receptor is replaced by that for inositol triphosphate (IP_3). This IP_3 receptor has a high degree of molecular homology with the ryanodine receptor, although only about half its size. The IP_3 messenger system is of fundamental importance in regulating the release of calcium from the SR and regulating arterial tone, and hence the afterload against which the heart must work. In cardiac muscle, the role of IP_3 is still sufficiently controversial to question its role in the inotropic response.

CYTOKINE SIGNALING

TUMOR NECROSIS FACTOR AND INTERLEUKINS. Tumor necrosis factor (TNF) is one of the family of proinflammatory cytokines that form part of the innate immune system. These cytokines are not normally found in the myocardium, are stress-responsive, and are formed during challenge by hypoxia, ischemia-reperfusion, myocardial infarction,[32] or mechanical loading. In addition to TNF, the proinflammatory group of cytokines includes the interleukins IL-1 and IL-6, which are often formed in concert with TNF. The MAP-kinase signaling path is also stress-activated (see later, Fig. 21-26), and appears to be essential for the synthesis of TNF and IL-6 in cardiac myocytes.[33]

Such cytokines mediate local events and are distinct from circulating neurotransmitters or hormones. TNF stimulation has bifunctional effects, mediating both protective signals as a component of preconditioning[34] and adverse cardiodepressant signaling in response to diffuse myocardial ischemia, as in embolization.[1] The signaling paths involved are complex, starting with two surface receptors for TNF proceeding via sphingolipids to apparently bifurcating paths. One path is adaptive and sends further signals via nuclear factor kappa B to the nucleus for the manufacture of protective molecules. The other maladaptive path leads to apoptosis via the activation of caspases. These paths are neither simple nor well-understood. For example, nitric oxide can act upstream and downstream from TNF.[1] Currently, it is not known why the intracellular signaling paths activated by TNF sometimes lead to beneficial effects, such as preconditioning and cell survival, and at other times lead to depressed myocardial function and apoptosis. It has been proposed first, that there are short-term adaptive and long-term maladaptive effects of TNF and, second, that low concentrations are adaptive and high concentrations are maladaptive.[35]

CARDIOTROPHIN. This member of the IL-6 family of cytokines is briskly released from the perfused heart in response to ventricular stretch.[36] It interacts with the gp130 receptor, which in turn can activate cellular signaling pathways linked to physiological hypertrophy (see later, Fig. 21-26). However, because of possible cross talk, interaction with maladaptive paths is also possible.

CONTRACTILE PERFORMANCE OF THE INTACT HEART

There are three main determinants of myocardial mechanical performance—loading conditions (preload and afterload; Frank-Starling mechanism), contractile state, and heart rate. This section describes the cardiac cycle and the determinants of LV function.

The Cardiac Cycle

The cardiac cycle, fully delineated by Lewis[37] but first conceived by Wiggers,[38] yields important information on the temporal sequence of events in the cardiac cycle. The three basic events are (1) LV contraction, (2) LV relaxation, and (3) LV filling (Table 21-3). Although similar mechanical events occur in the right side of the heart, the focus here is those on the left side.

LEFT VENTRICULAR CONTRACTION. LV pressure starts to build up when the arrival of calcium ions at the contractile proteins starts to trigger actin-myosin interaction. On the electrocardiogram (ECG), the advance of the wave of depolarization is indicated by the peak of the R wave (Fig. 21-18). Soon after, LV pressure in the early contraction phase builds up and exceeds that in the left atrium (normally, 10 to 15 mm Hg) followed about 20 milliseconds later by M_1, the mitral component of the first heart sound. The exact relationship of M_1 to mitral valve closure is controversial. Although mitral valve closure is often thought to coincide with the crossover point at which the LV pressure starts to exceed the left atrial pressure,[1] in reality mitral valve closure is delayed because the valve is kept open by the inertia of the blood flow. Shortly thereafter, pressure changes in the right ventricle, similar in pattern but lesser in magnitude to those in the left ventricle, cause the tricuspid valve to close, thereby creating T_1, the second component of the first heart sound. During this phase of contraction between mitral valve and aortic valve opening, the LV volume is fixed (isovolumic contraction) because aortic and mitral valves are shut. As more and more myofibers enter the contracted state, pressure development in the left ventricle proceeds. The interaction of actin and myosin increases and cross-bridge cycling rises. When the pressure in the left ventricle exceeds that in the aorta, the aortic valve opens, usually a clinically silent event. Opening of the aortic valve is followed by the phase of rapid ejection. The rate of ejection is determined not only by the pressure gradient across the aortic valve, but also by the elastic properties of the aorta and the arterial tree, which undergoes systolic expansion. LV pressure rises to a peak and then starts to fall.

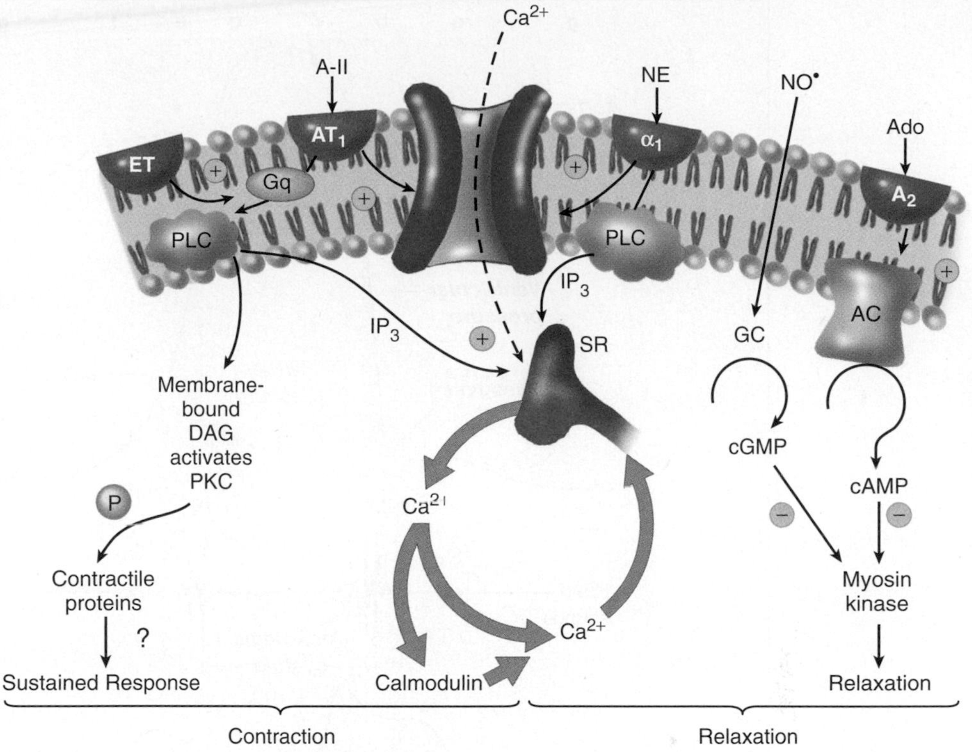

FIGURE 21–17 Patterns of contraction and relaxation in vascular smooth muscle. Thus, the angiotensin-II (A-II) signaling system is coupled via a G-protein to phospholipase C (PLC), which breaks down membrane-bound phosphatidylinositol to 1,2-diacylglycerol (DAG) and IP_3 (inositol triphosphate). DAG translocates protein kinase C (PKC) from cytosol to the sarcolemma, thereby activating PKC. Signals beyond PKC are not clear. It may phosphorylate ion channels to give the sustained vasoconstrictive response. IP_3 releases calcium from the sarcoplasmic reticulum to initiate vascular smooth muscle contraction. Other vasoconstrictors such as endothelin (ET receptor) act by the same signal system. In response to norepinephrine (NE), an $alpha_1$ agonist, a similar sequence of events occurs to promote contraction. Relaxation is achieved by inhibition of myosin kinase, when cyclic GMP or cyclic AMP is formed in response, respectively, to nitric oxide (NO) or adenosine (Ado). AC = adenylyl cyclase; GC = guanylyl cyclase. *(From Opie LH: Heart Physiology: From Cell to Circulation. Lippincott Williams & Wilkins, Philadelphia, 2004. © LH Opie, 2004.)*

TABLE 21–3	The Cardiac Cycle
LV Contraction	
Isovolumic contraction (b)	
Maximal ejection (c)	
LV Relaxation	
Start of relaxation and reduced ejection (d)	
Isovolumic relaxation (e)	
LV Filling	
LV filling, rapid phase (f)	
Slow LV filling (diastasis) (g)	
Atrial systole or booster (a)	

The letters a-g refer to the phases of the cardiac cycle shown in Figure 21-18. These letters are arbitrarily allocated so that atrial systole (a) coincides with the A wave and (c) with the C wave of the jugular venous pressure.

LEFT VENTRICULAR RELAXATION. As the cytosolic calcium ion concentration starts to decline because of uptake of calcium into the SR under the influence of activated phospholamban, more and more myofibers enter the state of relaxation and the rate of ejection of blood from the left ventricle into the aorta falls (phase of reduced ejection). During this phase, blood flow from the left ventricle to the aorta rapidly diminishes but is maintained by aortic recoil—the Windkessel effect. The pressure in the aorta exceeds the falling pressure in the left ventricle. The aortic valve closes, creating the first component of the second sound, A_2 (the second component, P_2, results from closure of the pulmonary valve as the pulmonary artery pressure exceeds that in the right ventricle). Thereafter, the ventricle continues to relax. Because the mitral valve is closed during this phase, the LV volume cannot change (isovolumic relaxation). When the LV pressure falls to below that in the left atrium, the mitral valve opens (normally silent) and the filling phase of the cardiac cycle restarts (see Fig. 21-18).

LEFT VENTRICULAR FILLING PHASES. As LV pressure drops below that in the left atrium, just after mitral valve opening, the phase of rapid or early filling occurs, which accounts for most of the ventricular filling.[1] Active diastolic relaxation of the ventricle may also contribute to early filling (see later, "Ventricular Suction During

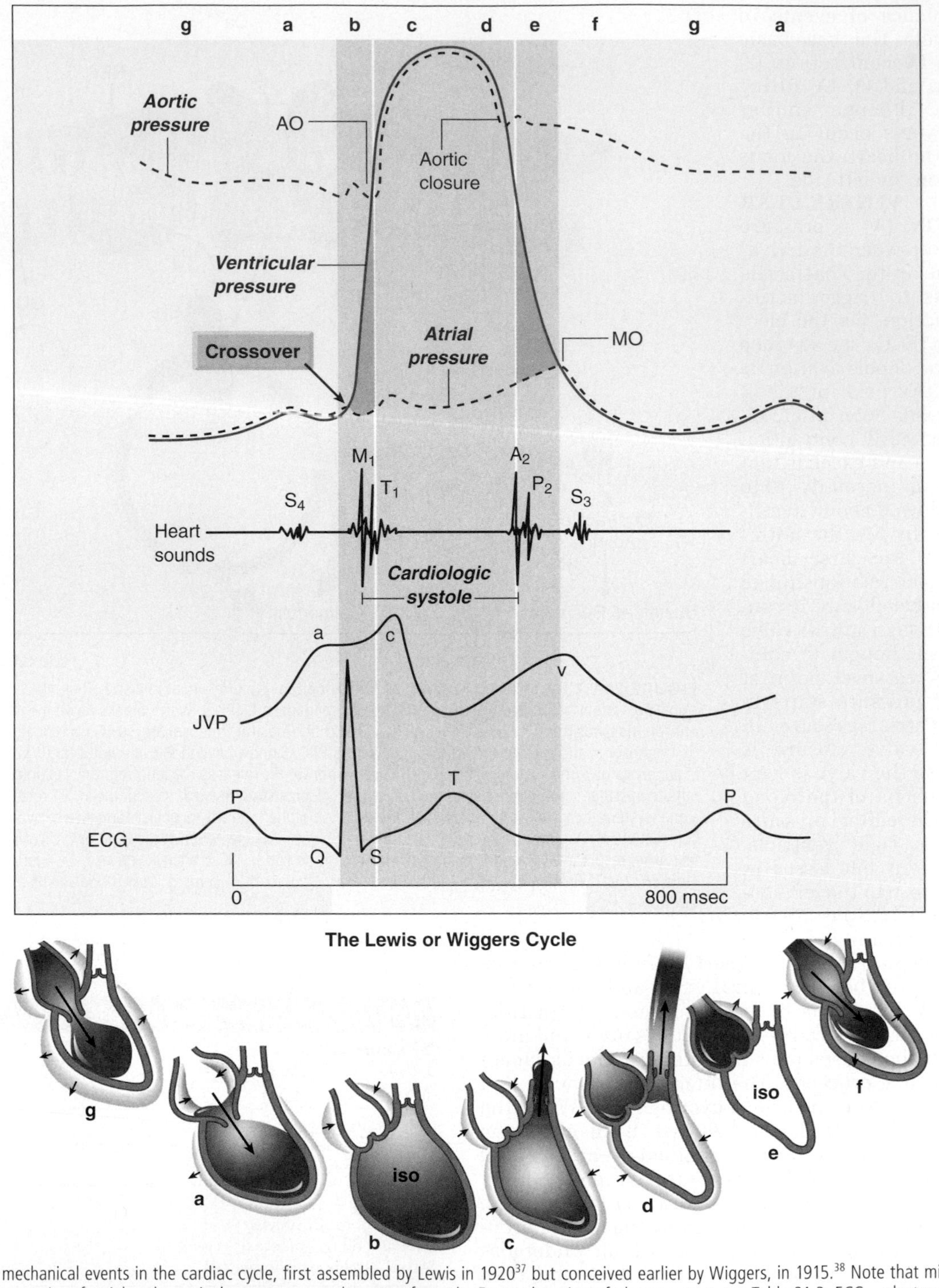

FIGURE 21–18 The mechanical events in the cardiac cycle, first assembled by Lewis in 1920[37] but conceived earlier by Wiggers, in 1915.[38] Note that mitral valve closure occurs *after* the crossover point of atrial and ventricular pressures at the start of systole. For explanation of phases a to g, see Table 21-3. ECG = electrocardiogram; JVP = jugular venous pressure; M_1 = mitral component of first sound at time of mitral valve closure; T_1 = tricuspid valve closure, second component of first heart sound; AO = aortic valve opening, normally inaudible; A_2 = aortic valve closure, aortic component of second sound; P_2 = pulmonary component of second sound, pulmonary valve closure; MO = mitral valve opening, may be audible in mitral stenosis as the opening snap; S_3 = third heart sound; S_4 = fourth heart sound; a = wave produced by right atrial contraction; c = carotid wave artifact during rapid LV ejection phase; v = venous return wave, which causes pressure to rise while tricuspid valve is closed. Cycle length of 800 milliseconds for 75 beats/min. *(Top panel from Opie LH: Heart Physiology: From Cell to Circulation. Lippincott Williams & Wilkins, Philadelphia, 2004. © LH Opie, 2004; bottom panel modified from Shepherd JT, Vanhoutte PM: The Human Cardiovascular System. New York, Raven Press, 1979, p 68.)*

Diastole"). Such rapid filling may cause the physiological third heart sound (S_3), particularly when there is a hyperkinetic circulation.[1] As pressures in the atrium and ventricle equalize, LV filling virtually stops (diastasis, separation). Renewed filling requires that the pressure gradient from the atrium to the ventricle increase. This is achieved by atrial systole (or the left atrial booster), which is especially important when a high cardiac output is required, as during exercise, or when the LV fails to relax normally, as in left ventricular hypertrophy.[1]

Definitions of Systole and Diastole

In Greek, *systole* means contraction and *diastole* means to send apart. The start of systole can be regarded as (1) the beginning of isovolumic contraction, when LV pressure exceeds the atrial pressure, or as (2) mitral valve closure (M_1). These correspond reasonably well, because mitral valve closure actually occurs only about 20 milliseconds after the crossover point of the pressures. Thus, in practice, the term *isovolumic contraction* often also includes this brief period of early systolic contraction, even before the mitral valve shuts, when the heart volume does not change substantially. Physiological systole lasts from the start of isovolumic contraction (when LV pressure crosses over atrial pressure; see Fig. 21-18) to the peak of the ejection phase, so that physiological diastole commences as LV pressure starts to fall (Table 21-4). This concept fits well with the standard pressure-volume curve. Physiological diastole commences as calcium ions are taken up into the sarcoplasmic reticulum, so that myocyte relaxation dominates over contraction and the LV pressure starts to fall, as shown on the pressure-volume curve. In contrast, *cardiological systole* is demarcated by the interval between the first and second heart sounds, lasting from the first heart sound (M_1) to the closure of the aortic valve (A_2). The remainder of the cardiac cycle automatically becomes cardiological diastole. Thus, cardiological systole, demarcated by heart sounds rather than by physiological events, starts fractionally later than physiological systole and ends significantly later. For the cardiologist, protodiastole is the early phase of rapid filling, when the third heart sound (S_3) can be heard. This sound probably reflects ventricular wall vibrations during rapid filling and becomes audible with an increase in LV diastolic pressure, wall stiffness, or rate of filling.

Contractile Function versus Loading Conditions

CONTRACTILE FUNCTION (see Chap. 23). Contractile function is the inherent capacity of the myocardium to contract independently of changes in the preload or afterload. It is a key word in cardiological language. At a molecular level, an increased inotropic state can be explained by enhanced interaction between calcium ions and contractile proteins. Increased contractile function means a greater rate of contraction to reach a greater peak force. Often, increased contractile function is associated with enhanced rates of relaxation, called the lusitropic effect. Alternate names for contractile function are the inotropic state (*ino*, fiber; *tropos*, to move) or the contractile state. Contractile function is an important regulator of the myocardial oxygen uptake. Factors that increase contractile function include exercise, adrenergic stimulation, digitalis, and other inotropic agents.

PRELOAD AND AFTERLOAD. It is important to stress that any change in the contractile state should be independent of the loading conditions. The preload is the load present before contraction has started, at the end of diastole (the afterload is discussed later). The preload reflects the venous filling pressure that fills the left atrium, which in turn fills the left ventricle during diastole. When the preload increases, the left ventricle distends during diastole, and the stroke volume rises according to Starling's law (see later, next section). The heart rate also increases by stimulation of the atrial mechanoreceptors, which enhances the rate of discharge of the sinoatrial node. Thus, the cardiac output (stroke volume times heart rate) rises.

TABLE 21–4 Physiological Versus Cardiological Systole and Diastole

	Physiological	Cardiological
Systole	Isovolumic contraction Maximal ejection	From M_1 to A_2, including: Major part of isovolumic contraction* Maximal ejection Reduced ejection
Diastole	Reduced ejection Isovolumic relaxation Filling phases	A_2-M_1 interval (filling phases included)

*Note that M_1 occurs with a definite although short delay after the start of LV contraction.

Starling's Law of the Heart

VENOUS FILLING PRESSURE AND HEART VOLUME. Starling, in 1918, related the venous pressure in the right atrium to the heart volume in the dog heart-lung preparation.[12] He proposed that within physiological limits, the larger the volume of the heart, the greater the energy of its contraction and the amount of chemical change at each contraction. Starling did not, however, measure sarcomere length but could only relate LV volume to cardiac output. This holds true in normal, compliant hearts. One modern version of Starling's law is that stroke volume is related to the end-diastolic volume.

The LV volume can now be directly measured with two-dimensional echocardiography. However, the value determined depends on a number of simplifying assumptions, such as a spherical LV shape, and neglects the confounding influence of the complex anatomy of the left ventricle. From the investigational point of view, real-time three-dimensional echocardiographic recordings can now indicate global LV volume and endocardial function.[39] In practice, LV volume is not often measured, but instead uses various surrogate measures, such as LV end-diastolic pressure and pulmonary capillary wedge pressure. The relationship between LV end-diastolic volume and LV end-diastolic pressure is curvilinear, depending on LV compliance.

The left ventricular diastolic filling pressure, the difference between the left atrial pressure and the left ventricular diastolic pressure, is easier to measure and, in diseased noncompliant hearts, may be used as a surrogate for heart volume. The venous filling pressure can indirectly be measured in humans by the technique of Swan-Ganz catheterization, as can the stroke volume. The left ventricular pressure and volume are, however, not linearly related because of variations in the compliance of the myocardium. Therefore, a jump from pressure to volume is required to apply the Starling concept to the hemodynamic management of those critically ill who are undergoing Swan-Ganz catheterization.

FRANK AND ISOVOLUMIC CONTRACTION. If a larger heart volume increases the initial length of the muscle fiber to increase the stroke volume and hence the cardiac output, then diastolic stretch of the LV actually increases contractile function. Frank, in 1895, had already reported that the greater the initial LV volume, the more rapid the rate of rise, the greater the peak pressure reached, and the faster the rate of relaxation.[12] He described both a positive inotropic effect and an increased lusitropic effect. These complementary findings of Frank and Starling are often combined into the Frank-Starling law, which can account for two of the mechanisms underlying the increased stroke volume of exercise—

namely, increased diastolic filling (Starling's law) and increased inotropic state (Frank's findings).

AFTERLOAD. This is the systolic load on the left ventricle after it has started to contract. In the nonfailing heart, the left ventricle can overcome any physiological acute increase in load. Chronically, however, the LV must hypertrophy to overcome sustained arterial hypertension or significant aortic stenosis. In clinical practice, the arterial blood pressure is often taken to be synonymous with the afterload while ignoring the aortic compliance—the extent to which the aorta can yield during systole. A stiff aorta, as in isolated systolic hypertension of the elderly, increases the afterload.

INTERLINKED PRELOAD AND AFTERLOAD. These distinctions between preload and afterload do not allow for those situations when the two change concurrently. By the Frank-Starling law, an increased LV volume leads to increased contractile function, which in turn will increase the systolic blood pressure and hence the afterload. Nonetheless, in general, the preload is related to the degree to which the myocardial fibers are stretched at the end of diastole, and the afterload is related to the wall stress generated by those fibers during systole.

FORCE-LENGTH RELATIONSHIPS AND CALCIUM TRANSIENTS. Evidence that there is no increase in the calcium transient as the sarcomere length increases has been provided by direct measurements (Fig. 21-19). The favored explanation for the steep length-tension relationship of cardiac muscles is length-dependent activation, whereby an increase in calcium sensitivity is the major factor explaining the steep increase of force development as the initial sarcomere length increases. This change may be explained by stretch of the titin molecule (see Fig. 21-4). Is the degree of overlap of actin and myosin also involved? Whereas the overlap theory explains the force-length relationship in skeletal muscle, the situation is different for cardiac muscle . In cardiac muscle, even at 80 percent of the maximal length, only 10 percent or less of the maximal force is developed. Thus, it can be predicted that cardiac sarcomeres must function near the upper limit of their maximal length (L_{max}). Rodriguez and colleagues[40] have tested this prediction by relating sarcomere length changes to volume changes of the intact heart. By implanting small radiopaque beads in only about 1 cm^3 of the LV free wall and using biplane cineradiography, the motion of the markers could be tracked through various cardiac cycles, with allowances made for local myocardial deformation. Thus, the change in sarcomere length from approximately 85 percent of L_{max} to L_{max} itself can result in physiological LV volume changes (Fig. 21-20). This estimate is remarkably close to the normal fiber shortening of 15 percent in the human heart in situ.[1]

ANREP EFFECT: ABRUPT INCREASE IN AFTERLOAD. When the aortic pressure is elevated abruptly, a positive inotropic effect follows within 1 or 2 minutes. This was formerly called homeometric autoregulation (*homeo,* the same; *metric,* length), because it was apparently independent of muscle length and, by definition, a true inotropic effect. A reasonable speculation would be that increased LV wall tension could act on myocardial stretch receptors to increase the cytosolic sodium level and then, by Na^+/Ca^{2+} exchange, the cytosolic calcium level. Thus, this effect would be different from that of an increase in preload, which acts by length activation.

Wall Stress

A more exact definition of the afterload is the wall stress during LV ejection. Technically, wall stress develops when tension is applied to a cross-sectional area, and the units are force per unit area. According to the Laplace law (Fig. 21-21):

$$\text{Wall stress} = (\text{pressure} \times \text{radius})/(2 \times \text{wall thickness})$$

This equation, although an oversimplification, emphasizes two points. First, the larger the left ventricle and the greater its radius, the greater is the wall stress. Second, at any given

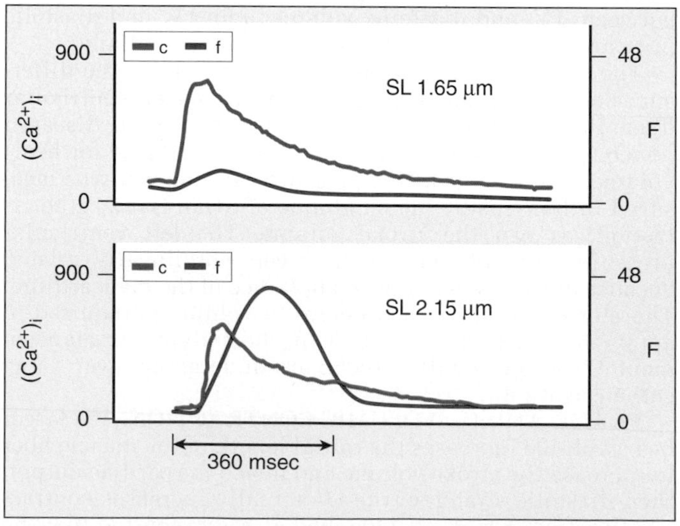

FIGURE 21–19 Length sensitization of the sarcomere. **Top panel,** Sarcomere length (SL) is 1.65 μm, which gives very little force (f) development (see Fig. 21-20). **Bottom panel,** At near-maximum sarcomere length (see Fig. 21-20), the same Ca^{2+} transient (c) with the same peak value and overall pattern causes a much greater force development. Therefore, there has been length-induced calcium sensitization. *(Modified from Backx PH, ter Keurs HEDJ: Fluorescent properties of rat cardiac trabeculae microinjected with fura-2 salt. Am J Physiol 264:H1098, 1993.)*

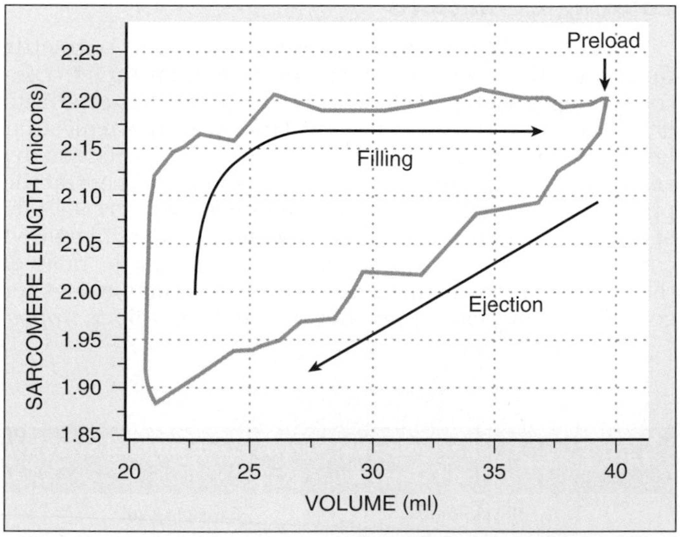

FIGURE 21–20 Changes in sarcomere length during a typical cardiac contraction-relaxation cycle. During diastole the sarcomere length is 2.2 μm, reducing to 1.90 μm during systole in the intact dog heart. Starting at the top right, the *preload* is the maximum sarcomere length just before the onset of contraction. As ejection decreases the left ventricular volume, by somewhat more than half, the sarcomere length decreases from 2.20 to 1.90 μm. Then, during the rapid phase of filling (see Fig. 21-18), the sarcomere length increases from 1.90 to 2.15 μm and is followed by the phase of constant sarcomere length (diastasis). (Modified from Rodriguez EK, Hunter WC, Royce MJ, et al: A method to reconstruct sarcomere lengths and orientations to transmural sites in beating canine hearts. Am J Physiol 263:H293, 1992.).

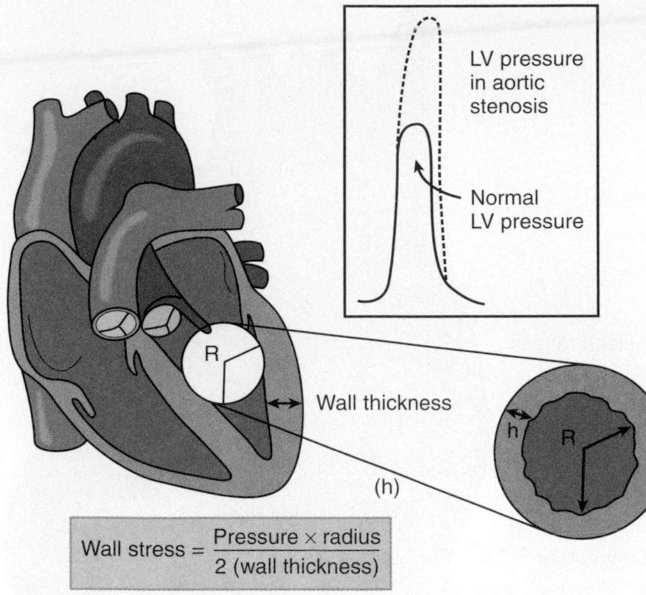

FIGURE 21–21 Wall stress increases as the afterload increases. The formula shown is derived from the Laplace law. The increased left ventricular (LV) pressure in aortic stenosis is compensated for by LV wall hypertrophy, which decreases the denominator on the right side of the equation. R = radius. *(From Opie LH: Heart Physiology: From Cell to Circulation. Philadelphia, Lippincott Williams & Wilkins, 2004. © LH Opie, 2004.)*

radius (LV size), the greater the pressure developed by the left ventricle, the greater the wall stress. An increase in wall stress achieved by either of these two mechanisms (LV size or intraventricular pressure) will increase myocardial oxygen uptake. This is because a greater rate of ATP use is required as the myofibrils develop greater tension. (For more details and formulas for circumferential and meridional wall stress, see Chap. 23.)

In cardiac hypertrophy, the Laplace law explains the effects of changes in wall thickness on wall stress (see Fig. 21-21). The increased wall thickness caused by hypertrophy balances the increased pressure, and the wall stress remains unchanged during the phase of compensatory hypertrophy. This change, previously regarded as compensatory and beneficial, has been seriously challenged by a mouse model, in which the process of hypertrophy was genetically inhibited so that wall stress increased in response to a pressure load; however, these mice had better cardiac mechanical function than the wild type mice, which developed compensatory hypertrophy.[1] Despite this "mighty mouse" challenge, it is difficult to see how a patient with significant aortic stenosis could develop the required intraventricular pressure to eject blood through the stenosed valve without the development of LV hypertrophy.

Another clinically useful concept is that in congestive heart failure, the heart dilates so that the increased radius elevates wall stress. Furthermore, because ejection of blood is inadequate, the radius stays too large throughout the contractile cycle, and end-diastolic and end-systolic tensions are higher. Compensation for the LV enlargement may be that myocytes need to contract less to maintain stroke volume. Overall reduction of heart size decreases wall stress and improves LV function.

WALL STRESS, PRELOAD, AND AFTERLOAD. These definitions take both the volume and the fiber length that define the radius into consideration. Preload can now be defined more exactly as the wall stress at the end of diastole and therefore at the maximal resting length of the sarcomere (see Fig. 21-20). Measurement of wall stress in vivo is difficult because the radius of the left ventricle (see preceding sections) neglects the confounding influence of the complex anatomy of the left ventricle. Surrogate measurements of the indices of preload include LV end-diastolic pressure or dimensions; the latter includes the major and minor axes of the heart in a two-dimensional echocardiographic view. The afterload, being the load on the contracting myocardium, is also the wall stress during LV ejection. Increased afterload means that an increased intraventricular pressure has to be generated first to open the aortic valve and then generated during the ejection phase. These increases will translate themselves into an increased myocardial wall stress, which can be measured either as an average value or at end-systole. Peak systolic wall stress reflects the three major components of the afterload–peripheral resistance, arterial compliance, and peak intraventricular pressure. Decreased arterial compliance and increased afterload can be anticipated when there is aortic dilation, as in severe systemic hypertension or in the elderly. Generally, in clinical practice, it is a sufficient approximation to take the systolic blood pressure as an indirect measure of the afterload (reflecting both peripheral resistance and peak intraventricular pressure), provided that there is neither significant aortic stenosis nor a change in arterial compliance.

AORTIC IMPEDANCE. Aortic impedance (arterial input impedance) represents another accurate measure of the afterload. The aortic impedance is the aortic pressure divided by the aortic flow at that point, so that this index of the afterload varies at each stage of the contraction cycle. Factors reducing aortic flow, such as a high arterial blood pressure, aortic stenosis, or loss of aortic compliance, will increase impedance and therefore the afterload. During systole, when the aortic valve is open, an increased afterload will communicate itself to the ventricles by increasing wall stress. In LV failure, aortic impedance is augmented not only by peripheral vasoconstriction but by decreases in aortic compliance. The problem with the clinical measurement of aortic impedance is that invasive instrumentation is required. An approximation can be obtained by using transesophageal echocardiography to determine aortic blood flow at, for example, the time of maximal increase of aortic flow, just after aortic valve opening.

Heart Rate and Force-Frequency Relationship

TREPPE OR BOWDITCH EFFECT. An increased heart rate progressively enhances the force of ventricular contraction, even in an isolated papillary muscle preparation (Bowditch staircase phenomenon). Alternative names are the *treppe* (German, steps) phenomenon, positive inotropic effect of activation, or force-frequency relationship (Fig. 21-22). Conversely, a decreased heart rate has a negative staircase effect. When stimulation becomes too rapid, force decreases. It has been hypothesized that during rapid stimulation, more sodium and calcium ions enter the myocardial cell than can be handled by the sodium pump, and the mechanisms for calcium control are overwhelmed. Opposing the force-frequency effect is the negative contractile influence of the decreased duration of ventricular filling at high heart rates. The longer the filling interval, the better the ventricular filling and the stronger the subsequent contraction. This phenomenon can be shown in patients with atrial fibrillation with a variable filling interval. In heart failure, the phenomenon is muted or lost.

Postextrasystolic potentiation and the inotropic effect of paired pacing can be explained by the same model, again assuming an enhanced contractile state after the prolonged interval between beats. Nonetheless, the exact cellular mechanism remains to be clarified.

FORCE-FREQUENCY RELATIONSHIP AND OPTIMAL HEART RATE. Normally, peak contractile force at a fixed muscle length (isometric contraction) increases and a peak

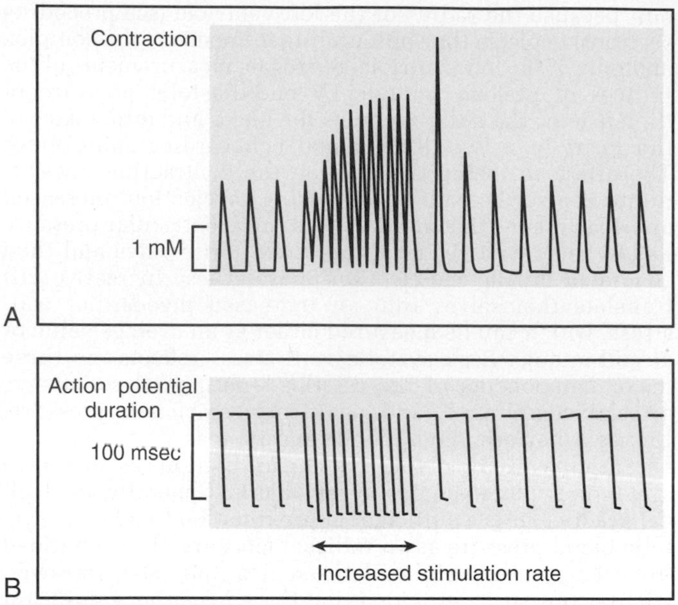

FIGURE 21–22 Bowditch, or treppe, phenomenon. A faster stimulation rate (bottom panel) increases the force of contraction (top panel). The stimulus rate is shown as the action potential duration (milliseconds) on an analog analyzer. The tension developed by papillary muscle contraction is shown in mN (millinewtons) in the top panel. On cessation of rapid stimulation, the contraction force gradually declines. Hypothetically, the explanation for the increased contraction during the increased stimulation is repetitive Ca^{2+} entry with each depolarization and, hence, an accumulation of cytosolic calcium. *(From Noble MIM: Excitation-contraction coupling. In Drake-Holland AJ, Noble MIM [eds]: Cardiac Metabolism. Chichester, UK, John Wiley, 1983, pp 49-71.)*

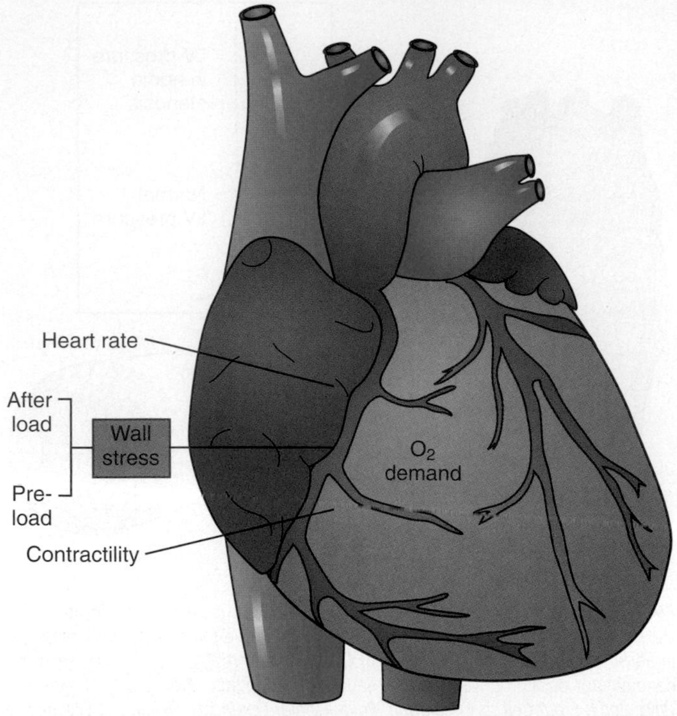

FIGURE 21–23 Major determinants of the oxygen (O_2) demand of the normal heart—heart rate, wall stress, and contractile function. For use of pressure-volume area as index of oxygen uptake, see Figure 21-24. *(Modified from Opie LH: Heart Physiology: From Cell to Circulation. Philadelphia, Lippincott Williams & Wilkins, 2004. © LH Opie, 2004.)*

is reached at about 150 to 180 stimuli/min.[1] This is the human counterpart of the treppe phenomenon. In situ, the optimal heart rate is not only the rate that would give maximal mechanical performance of an isolated muscle strip, but is also determined by the need for adequate time for diastolic filling. In normal humans, it is not possible to attach exact values to the heart rate required to decrease rather than increase cardiac output or to keep it steady. Pacing rates of up to 150 beats/min can be tolerated, whereas higher rates cannot because of the development of AV block. In contrast, during exercise, indices of LV function still increase up to a maximum heart rate of about 170 beats/min, presumably because of enhanced contractile function and peripheral vasodilation.[1] In patients with severe left ventricular hypertrophy, the critical heart rate is between 100 and 130 beats/min, with a decrease in LV function at higher rates.[12]

Myocardial Oxygen Uptake

The myocardial oxygen demand can be increased by heart rate, preload, or afterload (Fig. 21-23), factors that can all precipitate myocardial ischemia in those with coronary artery disease. The oxygen uptake can also be augmented by increased contractile function, as during beta-adrenergic stimulation. Because myocardial oxygen uptake ultimately reflects the rate of mitochondrial metabolism and of ATP production, any increase in ATP requirement will be reflected by an increased oxygen uptake. In general, factors increasing wall stress will increase the oxygen uptake. An increased afterload causes an increased systolic wall stress, which needs a greater oxygen uptake. An increased diastolic wall stress, resulting from an increased preload, will also require more oxygen, because the greater stroke volume must be ejected against the afterload. In states of enhanced contractile function, the rate of change of wall stress is increased. Thus, thinking in terms of wall stress provides a comprehensive approach to the problem of myocardial oxygen uptake. Because the systolic blood pressure is an important determinant of the afterload, a practical index of the oxygen uptake is systolic blood pressure multiplied by heart rate, the double product. In addition, there may be a metabolic component to the oxygen uptake that is usually small but may be prominent in certain special conditions, such as the oxygen wastage found during periods of abnormally high circulating free fatty acid levels. The concept of wall stress in relation to oxygen uptake also explains why heart size is such an important determinant of the myocardial oxygen uptake, because the larger radius increases wall stress.

WORK OF THE HEART. External work is done when, for example, a mass is lifted a certain distance. In terms of the heart, the cardiac output is the mass moved, and the resistance against which it is moved is the blood pressure. Because volume work needs less oxygen than pressure work, it might be supposed that external work is not an important determinant of the myocardial oxygen uptake. However, three determinants of the myocardial oxygen uptake are involved—preload (because this helps determine the stroke volume), the afterload (in part determined by the blood pressure), and heart rate, as can be seen in the following formula:

$$\text{Minute work} = \text{SBP} \times \text{SV} \times \text{heart rate}$$

where SBP = systolic blood pressure and SV = stroke volume. Thus, it is not surprising that heart work is related to oxygen uptake. The pressure-work index takes into account both the double product (SBP × heart rate) and the heart rate × SV (i.e. cardiac output). The pressure-volume area is another index of myocardial oxygen uptake, requiring invasive monitoring for accurate measurements. External cardiac work can account for up to 40 percent of the total myocardial oxygen uptake.

Internal Work (Potential Energy). The total oxygen consumption is related to the total work of the heart (area abcd in Fig. 21-24), meaning both the external work (the area abce) and the volume-pressure triangle joining the end-systolic volume-pressure point to the origin (the area cde; marked PE).[41] Although this area has been called internal work, more precisely it should be called potential energy, which is generated within each contraction cycle but not converted to external work. Such potential energy at the end of systole (point c) may be compared with the potential energy of a compressed spring.

Kinetic Work. Strictly speaking, the work performed (power production) needs to take into account not only pressure but kinetic components. It is the pressure work that has been discussed (product of cardiac output and peak systolic pressure). The kinetic work is the component required to move the blood against the afterload. Normally, kinetic work is less than 1 percent of the total. In aortic stenosis, kinetic work increases sharply as the cross-sectional area of the aortic valve narrows, whereas pressure work increases as the gradient across the aortic valve rises. Noninvasive measures of peak power production have been assessed as indices of cardiac contractile function.

Efficiency of work is the relationship between the work performed and the myocardial oxygen uptake. Exercise increases the efficiency of external work, an improvement that offsets any metabolic cost of the increased contractile function. Metabolically, efficiency is increased by promotion of glucose rather than fatty acids as major myocardial fuel. Conversely, heart failure decreases the efficiency of work, possibly by beta-adrenergic–promoted fatty acid metabolism.[1] The subcellular basis for changes in efficiency of work is not fully understood. Because as little as 12 to 14 percent of the oxygen uptake may be converted to external work, it is probably the internal work that becomes less demanding. Internal ion fluxes ($Na^+/K^+/Ca^{2+}$) account for about 20 to 30 percent of the ATP requirement of the heart, so that most ATP is spent on actin-myosin interaction, and much of that on generation of heat rather than on external work. An increased initial muscle length sensitizes the contractile apparatus to calcium (see Fig. 21-19), thereby theoretically increasing the efficiency of contraction by diminishing the amount of calcium flux required.

Measurements of Contractile Function

FORCE-VELOCITY RELATIONSHIP AND MAXIMUM CONTRACTILE FUNCTION IN MUSCLE MODELS. If the concept of contractile function is truly independent of the load and the heart rate, then unloaded heart muscle stimulated at a fixed rate should have a maximum value of contractile function for any given magnitude of the cytosolic calcium transient. This value, the V_{max} of muscle contraction, is defined as the maximal velocity of contraction when there is no load on the isolated muscle or no afterload to prevent maximal rates of cardiac ejection. Beta-adrenergic stimulation increases V_{max}, and converse changes are found in the failing myocardium. V_{max} is also referred to as V_0, the maximum velocity at zero load. The problem with this relatively simple concept is that V_{max} cannot be measured directly but is extrapolated from the peak rates of shortening in unloaded muscle obtained from the intercept on the velocity axis. In another extreme condition, there is no muscle shortening at all (zero shortening), and all the energy goes into the development of pressure (P_0) or force (F_0). This situation is an example of isometric shortening (*iso,* the same; *metric,* length). Because the peak velocity is obtained at zero load, when there is no external force development, the relationship is usually termed the *force-velocity relationship.*

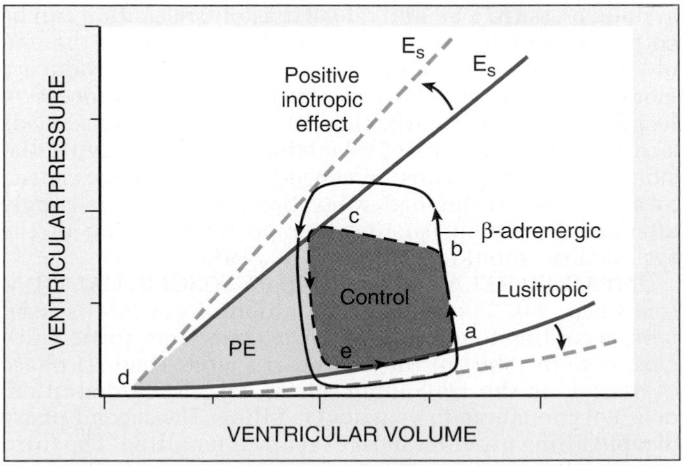

FIGURE 21–24 Pressure-volume loop of left ventricle. Note the effects of alpha-adrenergic catecholamines with both positive inotropic (increased slope of line E_s) and increased lusitropic (relaxant) effects. The total pressure-volume area (for control area, see abcd) is closely related to the myocardial oxygen uptake. The area cde is that component of work spent in generating potential energy (PE). E_s = slope of pressure-volume relationship. *(Modified from Opie LH: Heart Physiology: From Cell to Circulation. Philadelphia, Lippincott Williams & Wilkins, 2004. © LH Opie, 2004.)*

V_{max}. The concept of V_{max} has been subject to much debate over many years, chiefly because of the technical difficulties in obtaining truly unloaded conditions. Braunwald and associates[42] used cat papillary muscle to define a hyperbolic force-velocity curve, with V_{max} relatively independent of the initial muscle length, but increased by the addition of norepinephrine. Another preparation used to examine force-velocity relations uses single cardiac myocytes isolated by enzymatic digestion of the rat myocardium and then permeabilized with a staphylococcal toxin. Again, the force-velocity relationship is hyperbolic, suggesting the existence of intracellular passive elastic elements, such as those generated by titin (see Fig. 21-4) that contribute to the load on the isolated myocyte.

MECHANISM OF ALPHA-ADRENERGIC EFFECTS ON FORCE-VELOCITY RELATIONSHIP. The data on papillary muscles showing that norepinephrine can increase V_{max} could be explained by an effect of beta-adrenergic stimulation on enhancing calcium ion entry, a direct effect on the contractile proteins, or both. The overall concept would be that beta-adrenergic stimulation mediates the major component of its inotropic effect through increasing the cytosolic calcium transient and the factors controlling it, such as the rate of entry of calcium ions through the sarcolemmal L-type channels, the rate of calcium uptake under the influence of phospholamban into the SR, and the rate of calcium release from the ryanodine receptor in response to calcium entry in association with depolarization.

ISOMETRIC VERSUS ISOTONIC CONTRACTION. Despite the similarities in the force-velocity patterns between the data obtained from studies of papillary muscle and isolated myocytes, it should be considered that a number of different types of muscular contraction may be involved. For example, data for P_0 are obtained under isometric conditions (length unchanged). When muscle is allowed to shorten against a steady load, the conditions are isotonic (*iso,* same; *tonic,* contractile force). Thus, the force-velocity curve may be a combination of initial isometric conditions followed by isotonic contraction and then followed by the abrupt and total unloading to measure V_{max}. Although isometric conditions can be found in the whole heart as an approximation during isovolumic contraction, isotonic conditions cannot prevail, because the load is constantly changing during the ejection period and complete unloading is impossible. Therefore, the application of force-velocity relations to the heart in vivo is limited.

PRESSURE-VOLUME LOOPS (see Chap. 23). Measurements of pressure-volume loops are among the best of the current approaches to the assessment of the contractile performance of the intact heart (see Fig. 21-24). A crucial measurement in pressure volume loops is the relationship between end-systolic pressure and end-systolic volume (E_s, or end-systolic pressure-volume relationship, ESPVR). When the loading conditions are changed, changes in the slope of this line joining the different values for E_s is considered to represent a reliable load-independent index of the contractile performance of the heart (see Chap. 23). In clinical practice, the need to change the loading conditions and the requirement for invasive monitoring, required for the full pressure-volume loop, lessen the usefulness of this index. Measuring LV volume adequately and continuously throughout the cardiac cycle is difficult. During a positive inotropic intervention, the pressure-volume loop reflects a smaller end-systolic volume and a higher end-systolic pressure, so that the slope of E_s has moved upward and to the left (see Fig. 21-24). When the positive inotropic intervention is by beta-adrenergic stimulation, then enhanced relaxation (lusitropic effect) results in a lower pressure-volume curve during ventricular filling than in controls.

POWER PRODUCTION AND CONTRACTILE FUNCTION. Power production is the basis of another approach to assess contractile function. Power is defined as work per unit time, where F equals force:

$$\text{Power} = \text{work/time} = (\text{F} \times \text{cm})/\text{time}$$

Power is composed of kinetic and pressure components.[12] The peak power index is the maximal power divided by the end-diastolic volume, which is proposed as a load-independent index of contractile function.[25] Maximum power in turn is approximated by peak aortic flow and systolic pressure, which in practice can be measured invasively as the maximal instantaneous product of pressure and flow.[25]

DEFECTS IN THE CONTRACTILE FUNCTION CONCEPT. Despite all the procedures discussed earlier, which can be modified in an attempt to measure true contractile function, the concept has at least two serious defects: (1) the absence of any potential index that can be measured in situ and is free of significant criticism and, in particular, the absence of any acceptable noninvasive index; and (2) the impossibility of separating the cellular mechanisms of contractile function changes from those of load or heart rate. Therefore, an increased heart rate through the sodium pump lag mechanism gives rise to an increased cytosolic calcium level, which is thought to explain the treppe phenomenon. An increased preload involves increased fiber stretch, which in turn causes length activation, explicable by sensitization of the contractile proteins to the prevailing cytosolic calcium concentration. An increased afterload may increase cytosolic calcium through stretch-sensitive channels. *Thus, there is a clear overlap between contractile function, which should be independent of load or heart rate, and the effects of load and heart rate on the cellular mechanisms.* The traditional separation of inotropic state from load and heart rate effects as two independent regulators of cardiac muscle performance is no longer a simple concept now that the underlying cellular mechanisms have been uncovered. An example of this dilemma is in patients with atrial fibrillation and a constantly varying force-frequency relationship. Contractile function, as measured in situ by pressure-volume loops, constantly changes from beat to beat, and the explanation could be either a true change in contractile function or the operation of the Frank-Starling mechanism resulting from varying diastolic filling times.[1]

CONTRACTILE FUNCTION: ESSENTIAL CONCEPT, CONTINUING INVESTIGATION. Whatever the defects of the concept and the problems of measuring it, contractile function remains an essential cardiac concept to separate the effects of a primary change in loading conditions or heart rate from an intrinsic change in the force of contraction. An analogy could be that the rate at which a truck travels is determined not only by external loading factors, such as the weight of the products carried on the back and by the slope of the road, but also by internal factors, such as the horsepower of the engine and the gear used. Consequently, the quest for the perfect index of contractile function continues. Currently, myocardial acceleration during isovolumic contraction, as measured by tissue Doppler imaging, is being assessed as an index of contractile function.[43]

Ventricular Relaxation and Diastolic Dysfunction

The fact that diastolic dysfunction and diastolic heart failure can occur in the presence of normal or relatively normal systolic function (now often referred to as a preserved or normal ejection fraction) is now widely accepted (see Chap. 26). Indeed, approximately 40 to 50 percent of patients with heart failure will have a normal ejection fraction. Among the many complex physiological and pathological factors influencing relaxation, four are of major concern:

1. The cytosolic calcium level must fall to cause the relaxation phase, a process requiring ATP and phosphorylation of phospholamban for uptake of calcium into the SR.
2. The inherent viscoelastic properties of the myocardium are of importance. In the hypertrophied heart with increased fibrosis, relaxation occurs more slowly. Particularly in the early stages of the hypertrophied heart, during hypertension and aortic stenosis, a situation arises in which systolic function is relatively well preserved but diastolic relaxation is impaired. The probable explanation is that hypertrophy is accompanied by increasing fibrosis.[44]
3. Increased phosphorylation of troponin I enhances the rate of relaxation.[1]
4. Relaxation is influenced by the systolic load.[1]

Thus, the history of contraction affects cross-bridge relaxation. Within limits, the greater the systolic load, the faster the rate of relaxation. This complex relationship has been explored in detail by Brutsaert's group[45] but could perhaps be simplified as follows. When the workload is high, peak cytosolic calcium is also high. Thus, the rate of decrease of the calcium level is also greater, provided that the diastolic uptake mechanisms function effectively. In this way, the systolic pressure load and rate of diastolic relaxation can be correlated. Furthermore, a larger muscle length at the end of systole, when the workload is high, should produce a more rapid rate of relaxation by the opposite process to length-dependent sensitization. When the afterload exceeds a certain limit, the rate of relaxation is delayed,[12] with diastolic dysfunction. Thus, in congestive heart failure caused by an excess systolic load, relaxation becomes increasingly afterload-dependent, so that therapeutic reduction of the systolic load should improve LV relaxation.

IMPAIRED RELAXATION AND CYTOSOLIC CALCIUM (see Chap. 26). The clinical definition of diastole is used here, according to which diastole extends from aortic valve closure to the start of the first heart sound. The first phase of diastole is the isovolumic phase, which, by definition, does not contribute to ventricular filling. The second phase of rapid filling provides most of ventricular filling. The third phase of slow filling, or diastasis, accounts for only 5 percent of the total filling. The final atrial booster phase accounts for the remaining 15 percent.

Isovolumic relaxation is energy-dependent, requiring ATP for the uptake of calcium ions by the SR (Fig. 21-25), which is an active and not a passive process. Impaired relaxation is an early event in angina pectoris. A proposed metabolic explanation is that there is impaired

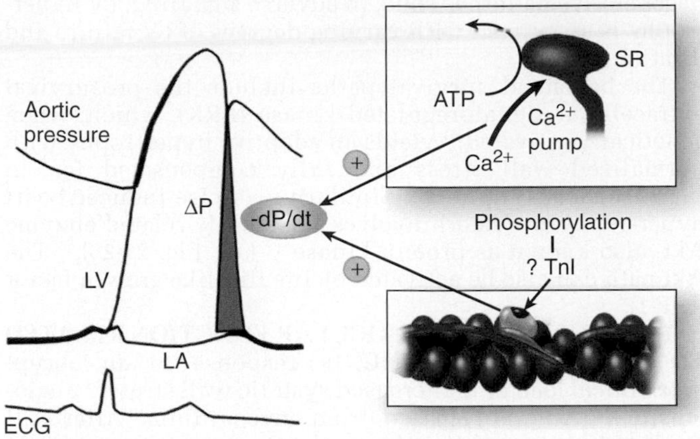

FIGURE 21–25 Factors governing the isovolumic relaxation phase of the cardiac cycle. This period of the cycle extends from the aortic second sound (A_2) to the crossover point between the left ventricular and left atrial pressures (see Fig 21-18). The maximum negative rate of pressure development ($-dP/dt_{max}$), which gives the isovolumic relaxation rate, is measured either invasively or by a continuous-wave Doppler velocity spectrum in aortic regurgitation. Isovolumic relaxation is increased (+ sign) when the rate of calcium uptake into the sarcoplasmic reticulum (SR) is enhanced—for example, during alpha-adrenergic stimulation (see Fig. 21-11). Isovolumic relaxation may also be enhanced when phosphorylation of troponin I (TnI), as in response to alpha-adrenergic stimulation, may decrease the affinity of the contractile system for calcium (see Fig. 21-3). *(From Opie LH: Heart Physiology: From Cell to Circulation. Philadelphia, Lippincott Williams & Wilkins, 2004. © LH Opie, 2004.)*

generation of energy, which diminishes the supply of ATP required for the early diastolic uptake of calcium by the SR. The result is that the cytosolic calcium level, at a peak in systole, delays its return to normal in the early diastolic period. In other conditions as well there is a relationship between the rate of diastolic decay of the calcium transient and diastolic relaxation, with a correlation to impaired function of the SR.[12] Also, regional nonuniformity of contraction may impair isovolumic relaxation. When the rate of relaxation is prolonged by hypothyroidism, the rate of return of the systolic calcium elevation is likewise delayed, whereas opposite changes occur in hyperthyroidism. In congestive heart failure, diastolic relaxation also is delayed and irregular, as is the rate of decay of the cytosolic calcium elevation. Most patients with coronary artery disease have various abnormalities of diastolic filling, probably related to those also found in angina pectoris. Theoretically, such abnormalities of relaxation are potentially reversible because they depend on changes in patterns of calcium ion movement.

MEASUREMENT OF ISOVOLUMIC RELAXATION. The rate of isovolumic relaxation is best measured by negative dP/dt_{max} at invasive catheterization. Tau, the time constant of relaxation, describes the rate of fall of LV pressure during isovolumic relaxation and also requires invasive techniques for precise determination. Tau is increased as the systolic LV pressure rises. Other indices of isovolumic relaxation can be obtained echocardiographically or from tissue Doppler measurements to monitor the peak rate of wall thinning.

VENTRICULAR SUCTION DURING EARLY DIASTOLE. The idea that LV suction by active relaxation could increase the pressure gradient from the left atrium to the left ventricle during the early filling phase has now been substantiated.[46] The suction effect can be found by carefully comparing LV and left atrial pressures; it occurs especially during the early diastolic phase of rapid filling as a result of the LV elastic recoil. During catecholamine stimulation, the rate of relaxation increases to enhance the sucking effect and prolong the period of filling. In mitral stenosis, the mitral valve does not respond as it otherwise should in response to diastolic suction, thereby impairing diastolic filling. In dilated cardiomyopathy, there is a double defect. The impaired LV elastic recoil lessens the diastolic suction, whereas the pattern of blood flow from the mitral valve to the apex is abnormal, deviating from the longitudinal axis of the ventricle, with the formation of vortices.[46] The proposed molecular mechanism of sucking is that in early diastole, myosin is pulled into the space between the two anchoring segments of titin to lower the intraventricular pressure to below that in the atrium.[1] Ventricular suction, by propagating a dominant backward pressure wave, is also responsible for diastolic coronary filling and is attenuated in LV hypertrophy.[47]

ATRIAL FUNCTION

The left atrium has five main functions.[1,48] The best-known function is that of a blood-receiving reservoir chamber. Second, it also is a contractile chamber, which, by presystolic contraction and its atrial booster function, helps complete LV filling. Third, it functions as a conduit that empties its contents into the LV down a pressure gradient after the mitral valve opens. Fourth, it is the volume sensor of the heart, releasing atrial natriuretic peptide (ANP) in response to intermittent stretch, so that an ANP-induced diuresis can help restore blood volume to normal. Fifth, the atrium contains receptors for the afferent arms of various reflexes, including mechanoreceptors that increase sinus discharge rate, thereby contributing to the tachycardia of exercise as the venous return increases (Bainbridge reflex). The atrial pressure-volume loop is very different in shape from that of the ventricles, resembling a figure-of-8. During atrial pacing, the preload is increased and the atria are distended, so that the volume part of the loop is small and the pressure part of the loop is much enlarged.[49] The atria have a number of differences in structure and function from the ventricles, including smaller myocytes and a shorter action potential duration, as well as a more fetal type of myosin (both in heavy and light chains). The more rapid atrial repolarization is thought to be caused by increased outward potassium ionic currents, such as I_{to} and $I_{K.ACh}$. In general, these histological and physiological changes can be related to the decreased need for the atria to generate high intrachamber pressures; instead, they are sensitive to volume changes while retaining enough contractile action to help with LV filling and to respond to inotropic stimuli. Atrial remodeling refers to various ionic, structural, contractile, and metabolic changes induced by insults such as chronic atrial tachyarrhythmias, including atrial fibrillation,[49] or by left atrial stretch and enlargement. Cellular mechanisms include decreased L-type calcium channel activity,[49] increased abnormal collagen,[50] and probably adverse stretch-induced signaling. The results include poor contractile performance and an increased initiation and perpetuation of atrial fibrillation.

CONTRACTILE PATTERNS IN PHYSIOLOGICAL AND PATHOLOGICAL HYPERTROPHY

Effects of Mechanical Load on Contraction and Relaxation

WALL STRESS AND COMPENSATED LEFT VENTRICULAR HYPERTROPHY. Meerson, in 1962, studied the cardiac hypertrophic response to experimental constriction of the aorta.[51] He described the prolonged protective state of "compensatory hyperfunction" of the heart. Thereafter, if the pressure load were continued, the left ventricle developed fibrosis with a transition to the decompensated state, with failure and dilation. To explain the mechanism of the LV hypertrophy, Grossman, in 1975,[51] proposed that the hypertrophic response was evoked by increased wall stress, the result of an increased intraventricular LV pressure (see Fig. 21-27). According to his systolic stress correction hypothesis, pressure overload causes myocytes to grow wider and to thicken (see Figs. 21-21 and 21-27). Then, according to the Laplace law, the increased wall thickness would decrease and even normalize the increased wall stress.[51] This hypothesis has been challenged by studies on transgenic mice, but the compensated hypertrophic state is often cited as a clinical entity.[44] An examination of the signaling paths involved in LV hypertrophy can explain such apparent contradictions.

LEFT VENTRICULAR RESPONSE TO MECHANICAL STRESS. There are two basic patterns of response to a sustained LV pressure load, hypothetically associated with adaptive and maladaptive signals (Fig. 21-26). According to the signaling stimulus invoked by the load, the myocyte can either survive, leading to beneficial hypertrophy, or undergo adverse patterns of signaling that lead to hypertrophy-associated apoptosis (programmed cell death) and related degenerative patterns. Thus, in adverse signaling, LV hypertrophy is associated with varying degrees of LV failure and dilation.[51]

The beneficial survival paths include the prosurvival extracellular signal–regulated kinase (ERK), which, when genetically activated,[51] yields an adaptive hypertrophy with normalized wall stress and fully compensated for an increased load (Fig. 21-27). Similarly, exercise-induced heart hypertrophy (see later) involves the closely related enzyme Akt, also known as protein kinase B (see Fig. 21-26).[52] The Akt path can also be activated by insulin-like growth factor (IGF-1).

IMPAIRED LEFT VENTRICULAR FUNCTION RELATED TO ADVERSE SIGNALING. In response to an abrupt mechanical load or to increased systolic wall stress,[51] angiotensin II (A-II) is released from myocardium. After A-II binds to its receptor, it activates the G protein, G_q, to initiate a signaling complex signaling sequence that leads to the enzyme complex mitogen-activated protein (MAP)–kinase (see Fig. 21-26). Some of the MAP-kinase components, such as ERK, promote prosurvival signaling, whereas others, such as JNK, stimulate apoptosis and decrease myocyte survival.[51] Other maladaptive paths include those that act through calcium-calmodulin, calcineurin, and the nuclear factor NFAT,[53] while yet others promote fibrosis in response to A-II, aldosterone, and transforming growth factor-beta (TGF-β). Cytokines such as tumor necrosis factor-alpha (TNF-α) appear to have bidirectional effects, with transient low levels being protective and sustained high levels being maladaptive.[35]

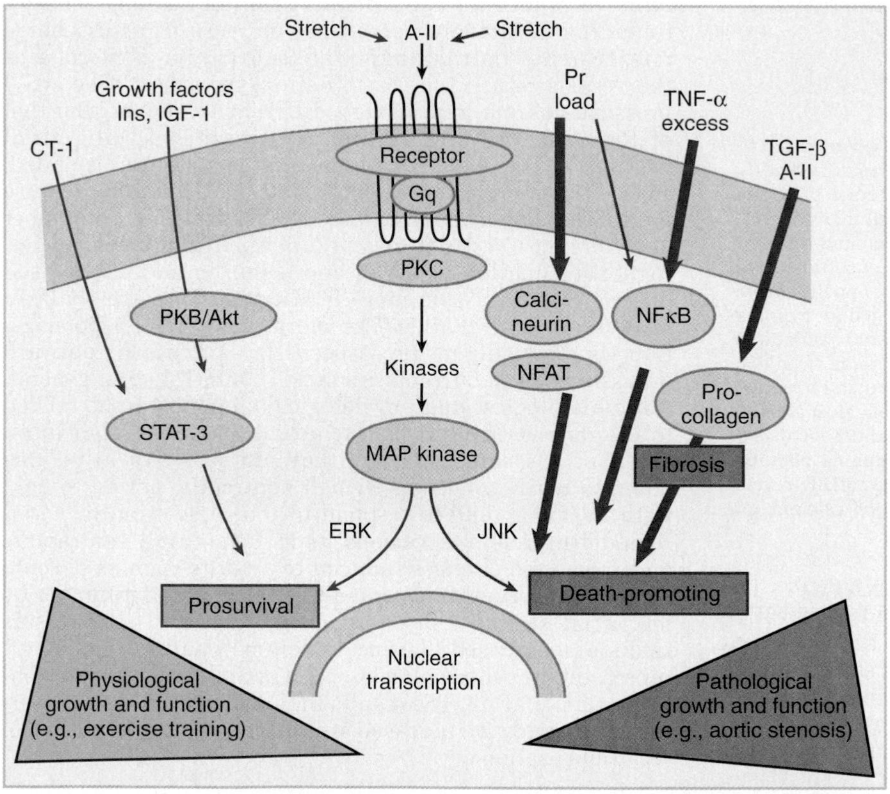

FIGURE 21–26 Consequences of physiological versus pathological signaling for mechanical function. Pathways on the left half of the figure lead predominantly to myocyte survival and adaptive hypertrophy, with enhanced contraction-relaxation function, whereas those in the right half lead to death-promoting fibrosis and apoptosis. Angiotensin II (A-II), released from myocardial cells by biomechanical stress such as prolonged stretch or pressure, leads to both prosurvival (on the left) and death-promoting pathways (on the right), the former via ERK (extracellular signal-regulated kinase) and the later via JNK (Jun N-terminal kinase). Tumor necrosis factor-alpha (TNF-α) acting physiologically, as in the left panel, is prosurvival, but in excess probably acts adversely via NFκB (nuclear factor kappa B), which is also where prolonged pressure loading acts. Transforming growth factor-beta (TGF-β) promotes the conversion of procollagen to fibrosis. Thus, depending on the nature of the biomechanical stress, the myocardium can adapt in such a way that mechanical function is either enhanced (left side of figure) or depressed (right side of figure). A similar two-way potential is envisaged for the effects of reactive oxygen species. IGF-1 = insulin-like growth factor; Ins = insulin; PKB/Akt = protein kinase B/Akt; PKC = protein kinase C; MAP = mitogen-activated protein. *(From Opie LH: Heart Physiology: From Cell to Circulation. Philadelphia, Lippincott Williams & Wilkins, 2004. © LH Opie, 2004.)*

Thus, if pressure-induced A-II stimulation leads to more maladaptive than adaptive growth, and more apoptosis, then genetic interruption of the A-II path would lessen hypertrophy but still protect the myocardium. In a mouse model in which part of the A-II receptor–related signaling system was transgenically inactivated by elimination of the G protein, G_q, pressure loading gave less than predicted hypertrophy with decreased correction of wall stress.[54] However, contractile function was better than in the wild type, which had more LVH (see Fig. 21-27). This finding shows that the wall stress model is not infallible, depending on the signaling path that promotes the hypertrophy.

LEFT VENTRICULAR HYPERTROPHY AND DIASTOLIC DYSFUNCTION (see Chap. 26). In hearts with concentric hypertrophy, as in chronic hypertension or severe aortic stenosis, abnormalities of diastole are common and may precede systolic failure. Morphologically and functionally, there are clear differences between human hypertrophic hearts with diastolic failure when compared with hearts in systolic failure.[55,56] There is increased cardiomyocyte stiffness, relieved by the addition of protein kinase A, possibly acting by phosphorylation of titin and its conversion to a less stiff isoform.[56] Regarding the signaling paths involved in aortic stenosis with LV hypertrophy, there is strong evidence for growth signals such as A-II and TGF-β being associated not only with myocyte growth, but also with maladaptive fibrosis, myocyte degeneration, and eventual myocyte loss.[44] Overall, taking both experimental and limited patient data into account, a sustained pressure load, as in aortic stenosis, is a mixed stimulus that produces both beneficial adaptive and adverse maladaptive remodeling. The latter could explain why the wall stress correction hypothesis does not always apply, and why in patients with aortic stenosis, increased LV mass predicts systolic dysfunction and heart failure.[57]

LEFT VENTRICULAR VOLUME LOADING AND THE SIGNALS INVOLVED. Volume differs from pressure loading in several important ways (see Fig. 22-11). From the signaling point of view, volume-induced mechanical stress with progressively greater LV volumes releases increasing amounts of TNF from the normal myocardium. Passive stretch of ventricular muscle promotes TNF mRNA synthesis. Low-level TNF stimulation interlinks with other cytokines such as cardiotrophin-1 acting on the gp130 receptor to promote prosurvival pathways (see Fig 21-26) so that the sarcomere units form in series to result in eccentric hypertrophy.[51] Remodeling in early volume overload may be related to stretch-induced signaling via adaptive signals such as cardiotrophin-1, low-level TNF-α, cyclic GMP, and IGF-1. In one of the few direct comparisons with pressure loading mechanisms, pressure but not volume overload increased the potentially adverse signal JNK,[58] compatible with the scheme in Figure 21-26.

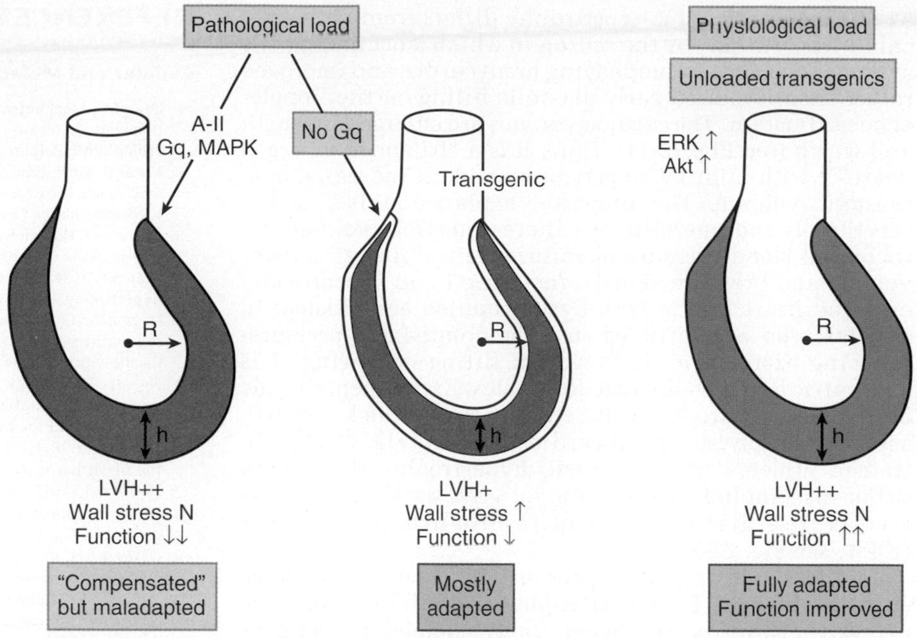

FIGURE 21–27 Compensated hypertrophy functions poorly compared with transgenic models and athlete's heart. **Left panel,** Left ventricular hypertrophy (LVH) in which wall stress, the relationship between the radius of the LV chamber and the thickness of the LV wall (h), is normalized (N) in response to sustained pressure load acting via angiotensin II (A-II). Contrary to the wall stress correction hypothesis, LV mechanical function is reduced and not maintained. The impaired mechanical function is the direct result of increased fibrosis and apoptosis intermixed with growth signaling. **Middle panel,** Lesser hypertrophic response to pressure load in transgenic mice with inhibited G_q signaling, so that angiotensin II that leads to maladaptive signaling (see Fig. 21-26) cannot operate. Although the transgenic wall stress has increased, as shown by the lower ratio of wall thickness, h, to the radius, R, mechanical function is less reduced than in the "compensated" heart of the wild type. **Right panel,** Adaptive growth patterns if ERK kinase is transgenically overexpressed or in the athlete's heart through Akt activation, when the truly compensated well-adapted state is reached. N = normal; MAPK = mitogen-activated protein kinase; ERK = extracellular signal–regulated kinase; Akt = protein kinase B. *(Modified from Opie LH: Heart Physiology: From Cell to Circulation. Philadelphia, Lippincott Williams & Wilkins, 2004. © LH Opie, 2004.)*

DOES THE STRESS CORRECTION HYPOTHESIS HOLD FOR A VOLUME LOAD? Experimentally, following 3 months of severe mitral regurgitation in dogs, LV mass increased with cardiomyocyte lengthening, whereas end-diastolic volume and wall stress (both diastolic and systolic) increased substantially.[59] Overall, the data are compatible with the Grossman concept of increased diastolic wall stress as the initiator of longitudinal myocyte growth in response to a chronic volume load.[51] However, in severe experimental mitral regurgitation, end-diastolic wall stress is much higher (by about fourfold), so that stress correction has not occurred. This problem could be predicted because as myocyte length increases, so does the radius, thus increasing rather than decreasing wall stress. Furthermore, volume-induced ventricular enlargement may be self-perpetuating by promotion of increasing mitral regurgitation and increasing ventricular sphericity.[51] At this late stage, it is likely that the growth paths stimulated are chiefly those with maladaptive patterns (see Fig. 21-26)—for example, in response to excess TNF.

Contractile Patterns in Physiological Hypertrophy: Athlete's Heart

In the endurance-trained athlete's heart, true physiological hypertrophy occurs[60] and must be distinguished from pathologic hypertrophy, as in hypertrophic cardiomyopathy, which can cause sudden death in young athletes (Table

TABLE 21–5 Contractile Patterns in Physiological Versus Pathological Hypertrophy

	Physiological	Pathological
Signaling pattern	Prosurvival	Proapoptotic, profibrotic
Key signals	IGF-1; PI3K/Akt (also inhibits pathological growth); STAT-3	p38 MAP kinase; JNK; TGF-β; angio-II
Fetal gene program	No	Yes
Interstitial fibrosis	No	Yes
Myocyte apoptosis	No	Yes
Systolic contraction	Normal or increased	Decreased
Diastolic relaxation	Normal or increased	Decreased
Doppler LV filling	Normal	Impaired

IGF = insulin-like growth factor; PI3K = phosphatidylinositol 3-phosphate kinase; Akt = another term for protein kinase B; STAT-3 = signal transducer and activator of transcription; LV = left ventricular; MAP kinase = mitogen-activated protein kinase; JNK = Jun *N*-terminal kinase; TGF-β = transforming growth factor-beta; angio-II = angiotensin II.

From Opie LH, Commerford PJ, Gersh BJ, Pfeffer MA: Controversies in ventricular remodelling. Lancet 367:356, 2006; Walsh K: Akt signaling and growth of the heart. Circulation 113:2032, 2006; and Derumeaux G, Mulder P, Richard V, et al: Tissue Doppler imaging differentiates physiological from pathological pressure-overload left ventricular hypertrophy in rats. Circulation 105:1602, 2002.

21-5). Physiological LV hypertrophy differs from pathological LV hypertrophy by the setting in which it occurs, signals systems involved, accompanying bradycardia, and improved rather than impaired early diastolic filling on the Doppler echocardiogram. The cardiomyocytes are enlarged in length and width (see Fig. 22-11). Thus, it is a "balanced enlarged heart,"[60] with both LV hypertrophy and an increased end-diastolic volume. The proposed explanation is that the repetitively and intermittently increased stroke volume and increased blood pressure of endurance training stimulates volume and pressure signals, resulting in an eccentrically enlarged heart that is both hypertrophied and dilated. In athletes who are involved in a predominantly pressure-inducing exercise, such as weight lifting or rowing, it is concentric hypertrophy that dominates. Experimentally, the beneficial hypertrophic paths involve Akt as the key signal, essential for physiological cardiac growth (Fig. 21-27).[52] In trained athletes with eccentric hypertrophy, the growth paths also include stimulation of Akt, as shown by the increased cardiac formation of insulin-like growth factor (IGF-1; see Fig. 21-27).[61]

In those with repeated pressure-induced hypertrophy, such as rowers, LV hypertrophy and dilation may be excessive. However, the hypertrophy completely regresses when the training stops, whereas some dilation persists.[62] It has been speculated that excess pressure stimulation can evoke some pathological changes and growth patterns similar to those found in patients with severe aortic stenosis.[44]

FUTURE PERSPECTIVES

In the future, there will be an increasing focus on the abnormalities of contraction and relaxation and regulation of calcium cycles, especially in relation to ventricular dysfunction. I speculate that calcium ion movements will be more clearly understood in terms of microdomains, with increasing subsubcellular compartmentalization. Lipid rafts will hold together molecules that regulate signaling sequences. Key intracellular regulators, such as cyclic AMP and GMP, will be found to be "snuggling up" to their molecular partners in a very localized way.

It has been proposed that "The most attractive, though somewhat speculative concept. . . . is that it matters through which adenylyl cyclase isoform cyclic AMP is formed and through which phosphodiesterase isoform it is degraded, and that its subcellular localization and its accordingly different targets matter."[63] Similar arguments hold for subcellular affinity domains for cyclic GMP and possibly for other messengers, such as protein kinases and their scaffolding proteins, and the relevant paths for synthesis and degradation. These findings may lead to consideration of different agonists and inhibitors acting on a single microdomain, perhaps involving protein kinase A generation or molecular disorders of the proteins associated with ryanodine receptors. In the therapy of heart failure, clinically applicable stabilizers of the ryanodine receptor may soon be developed.[10] The advent of drugs selectively regulating these calcium microdomains will make the administration of beta blockers and L-type calcium channel blockers, although still remaining useful, seem clumsy and unfocused.

Acknowledgments

Professor Gerd Heusch is thanked for critical review of this chapter. Additional useful references can be found in the previous edition of this text.[1]

REFERENCES

Cellular and Molecular Mechanisms

1. Opie LH: Mechanisms of cardiac contraction and relaxation. *In* Zipes DP, Libby P, Bonow R, Braunwald E (eds): Heart Disease. A Textbook of Cardiovascular Medicine. 7th ed. Philadelphia, Elsevier Saunders, 2005, pp 457-489.
2. Knoll R, Hoshijima M, Hoffman HM, et al: The cardiac mechanical stretch sensor machinery involves a Z disc complex that is defective in a subset of human dilated cardiomyopathy. Cell 111:943, 2002.
3. Rayment I, Holden HM, Whittaker M: Structure of the actin-myosin complex and its implications for muscle contraction. Science 261:58, 1993.
4. Brancaccio M, Hirsch E, Notte A, et al: Integrin signalling: The tug-of-war in heart hypertrophy. Cardiovasc Res 70:422, 2006.
5. Miyamoto T, Takeishi Y, Takahashi H, et al: Activation of distinct signal transduction pathways in hypertrophied hearts by pressure and volume overload. Basic Res Cardiol 99:328, 2004.
6. Heineke J, Ruetten H, Willenbockel C, et al: Attenuation of cardiac remodeling after myocardial infarction by muscle LIM protein-calcineurin signaling at the sarcomeric Z-disc. Proc Natl Acad Sci U S A 102:1655, 2005.
7. Ertz-Berger BR, He H, Dowell C, et al: Changes in the chemical and dynamic properties of cardiac troponin T cause discrete cardiomyopathies in transgenic mice. Proc Natl Acad Sci U S A 102:18219, 2005.
8. Fedak PW, Smookler DS, Kassiri Z, et al: TIMP-3 deficiency leads to dilated cardiomyopathy. Circulation 110:2401, 2004.
9. Chien KR: Genotype, phenotype: Upstairs, downstairs in the family of cardiomyopathies. [commentary]. J Clin Invest 111:175, 2003.
10. Wehrens XH, Lehnart SE, Reiken S, et al: Enhancing calstabin binding to ryanodine receptors improves cardiac and skeletal muscle function in heart failure. Proc Natl Acad Sci U S A 102:9607, 2005.
11. Wehrens XH, Lehnart SE, Reiken SR, Marks AR: Ca^{2+}/calmodulin-dependent protein kinase II phosphorylation regulates the cardiac ryanodine receptor. Circ Res 94:e61, 2004.
12. Opie LH: Heart Physiology: From Cell to Circulation. 4th ed. Philadelphia, Lippincott Williams & Wilkins, 2004.
13. Tada M, Katz AM: Phosphorylation of the sarcoplasmic reticulum and sarcolemma. Annu Rev Physiol 44:401, 1982.
14. Kamp TJ, Chiamvimonvat N: Mission impossible: IGF-1 and PTEN specifically "Akt"ing on cardiac L-type Ca^{2+} channels. Circ Res 98:1349, 2006.
15. Zhang XQ, Ahlers BA, Tucker AL, et al: Phospholemman inhibition of the cardiac Na^+/Ca^{2+} exchanger. Role of phosphorylation. J Biol Chem 281:7784, 2006.

Cell Signaling

16. Dodge-Kafka KL, Langeberg L, Scott JD: Compartmentalization of cyclic nucleotide signaling in the heart: The role of A-kinase anchoring proteins. Circ Res 98:993, 2006.
17. Castro LR, Verde I, Cooper DM, Fischmeister R: Cyclic guanosine monophosphate compartmentalization in rat cardiac myocytes. Circulation 113:2221, 2006.
18. Baillie GS, Sood A, McPhee I, et al: Beta-arrestin-mediated PDE4 cAMP phosphodiesterase recruitment regulates beta-adrenoceptor switching from Gs to Gi. Proc Natl Acad Sci U S A 100:940, 2003.
19. Penela P, Murga C, Ribas C, et al: Mechanisms of regulation of G protein-coupled receptor kinases (GRKs) and cardiovascular disease. Cardiovasc Res 69:46, 2006.
20. Apstein CS, Opie LH: A challenge to the metabolic approach to myocardial ischaemia. Eur Heart J 26:956, 2005.
21. Sterin-Borda L, Bernabeo G, Ganzinelli S, et al: Role of nitric oxide/cyclic GMP and cyclic AMP in beta3 adrenoceptor-chronotropic response. J Mol Cell Cardiol 40:580, 2006.
22. Okoshi K, Nakayama M, Yan X, et al: Neuregulins regulate cardiac parasympathetic activity: Muscarinic modulation of beta-adrenergic activity in myocytes from mice with neuregulin-1 gene deletion. Circulation 110:713, 2004.
23. Friebe A, Koesling D: Regulation of nitric oxide-sensitive guanylyl cyclase. Circ Res 93:96, 2003.
24. Ziolo MT, Bers DM: The real estate of NOS signaling. Location, location, location. Circ Res 92:1279, 2003.
25. Borlaug BA, Melenovsky V, Marhin T, et al: Sildenafil inhibits beta-adrenergic-stimulated cardiac contractility in humans. Circulation 112:2642, 2005.
26. Takimoto E, Champion HC, Li M, et al: Chronic inhibition of cyclic GMP phosphodiesterase 5A prevents and reverses cardiac hypertrophy. Nat Med 11:214, 2005.
27. Kone BC: NO break-ins at water gate. Hypertension 48:29, 2006.
28. Danson EJ, Paterson DJ: Enhanced neuronal nitric oxide synthase expression is central to cardiac vagal phenotype in exercise-trained mice. J Physiol 546:225, 2003.
29. Hambrecht R, Adams V, Erbs S, et al: Regular physical activity improves endothelial function in patients with coronary artery disease by increasing phosphorylation of endothelial nitric oxide synthase. Circulation 107:3152, 2003.
30. Shah AM, Sauer H: Transmitting biological information using oxygen: Reactive oxygen species as signalling molecules in cardiovascular pathophysiology. Cardiovasc Res 71:191, 2006.
31. Gross GJ: Role of opioids in acute and delayed preconditioning. J Mol Cell Cardiol 35:709, 2003.
32. Valgimigli M, Ceconi C, Malagutti P, et al: Tumor necrosis factor-alpha receptor 1 is a major predictor of mortality and new-onset heart failure in patients with acute myocardial infarction: The Cytokine-Activation and Long-Term Prognosis in Myocardial Infarction (C-ALPHA) study. Circulation 111:863, 2005.

33. Li M, Georgakopoulos D, Lu G, et al: p38 MAP kinase mediates inflammatory cytokine induction in cardiomyocytes and extracellular matrix remodeling in heart. Circulation 111:2494, 2005.
34. Lecour S, Smith RM, Woodward B, et al: Identification of a novel role for sphingolipid signalling in TNF-α and ischemic preconditioning mediated protection. J Mol Cell Cardiol 34:509, 2002.
35. Mann DL: Stress-activated cytokines and the heart: From adaptation to maladaptation. Annu Rev Physiol 65:81, 2003.
36. Pemberton CJ, Raudsepp SD, Yandle TG, et al: Plasma cardiotrophin-1 is elevated in human hypertension and stimulated by ventricular stretch. Cardiovasc Res 68:109, 2005.

Contractile Performance of the Heart

37. Lewis T: The Mechanism and Graphic Registration of the Heart Beat. London, Shaw and Sons, 1920.
38. Wiggers CJ: Modern Aspects of Circulation in Health and Disease. Philadelphia, Lea and Febiger, 1915.
39. Corsi C, Lang RM, Veronesi F, et al: Volumetric quantification of global and regional left ventricular function from real-time three-dimensional echocardiographic images. Circulation 112:1161, 2005.
40. Rodriguez EK, Hunter WC, Royce MJ: A method to reconstruct myocardial sarcomere lengths and orientations at transmural sites in beating canine hearts. Am J Physiol 263:H293, 1992.
41. Suga H, Hisano R, Hirata S, Hayashi T, Ninomiya I. Mechanism of higher oxygen consumption rate: Pressure-loaded vs volume-loaded heart. Am J Physiol 242:H942, 1982.
42. Braunwald E, Sonnenblick EH, Ross J: Normal and abnormal circulatory function. *In* Braunwald E (ed): Heart Disease. A Textbook of Cardiovascular Medicine. 4th ed. Philadelphia, WB Saunders, 1992, pp 351-392.
43. Lyseggen E, Rabben SI, Skulstad H, et al: Myocardial acceleration during isovolumic contraction: Relationship to contractility. Circulation 111:1362, 2005.
44. Hein S, Amon E, Kostin S, et al: Progression from compensated hypertrophy to failure in the pressure-overloaded human heart. Structural deterioration and compensatory mechanisms. Circulation 107:984, 2003.
45. Zile MR, Brutsaert DL: New concepts in diastolic dysfunction and diastolic heart failure: Part 1. Circulation 105:1387, 2002.
46. Little WC: Diastolic dysfunction beyond distensibility: Adverse effects of ventricular dilatation. Circulation 112:2888, 2005.
47. Davies JE, Whinnett ZI, Francis DP, et al: Evidence of a dominant backward-propagating "suction" wave responsible for diastolic coronary filling in humans, attenuated in left ventricular hypertrophy. Circulation 113:1768, 2006.
48. Pagel PS, Kehl F, Gare M, et al: Mechanical function of the left atrium: new insights based on analysis of pressure-volume relations and Doppler echocardiography. Anesthesiology 98:975, 2003.
49. Schotten U, Duytschaever M, Ausma J, et al: Electrical and contractile remodeling during the first days of atrial fibrillation go hand in hand. Circulation 107:1433, 2003.
50. Xu J, Cui G, Esmailian F, et al: Atrial extracellular matrix remodeling and the maintenance of atrial fibrillation. Circulation 109:363, 2004.
51. Opie LH, Commerford PJ, Gersh BJ, Pfeffer MA: Controversies in ventricular remodelling. Lancet 367:356, 2006.
52. Walsh K: Akt signaling and growth of the heart. Circulation 113:2032, 2006.
53. Dorn GW, 2nd, Force T: Protein kinase cascades in the regulation of cardiac hypertrophy. J Clin Invest 115:527, 2005.
54. Esposito G, Rapacciuolo A, Prasad SVN, et al: Genetic alterations that inhibit in vivo pressure-overload hypertrophy prevent cardiac dysfunction despite increased wall stress. Circulation 105:85, 2002.
55. Aurigemma GP, Zile MR, Gaasch WH: Contractile behavior of the left ventricle in diastolic heart failure: With emphasis on regional systolic function. Circulation 113:296, 2006.
56. van Heerebeek L, Borbely A, Niessen HW, et al: Myocardial structure and function differ in systolic and diastolic heart failure. Circulation 113:1966, 2006.
57. Kupari M, Turto H, Lommi J: Left ventricular hypertrophy in aortic valve stenosis: Preventive or promotive of systolic dysfunction and heart failure? Eur Heart J 26:1790, 2005.
58. Sopontammarak S, Aliharoob A, Ocampo C, et al: Mitogen-activated protein kinases (p38 and c-Jun NH2-terminal kinase) are differentially regulated during cardiac volume and pressure overload hypertrophy. Cell Biochem Biophys 43:61, 2005.
59. Perry GJ, Wei CC, Hankes GH, et al: Angiotensin II receptor blockade does not improve left ventricular function and remodeling in subacute mitral regurgitation in the dog. J Am Coll Cardiol 39:1374, 2002.
60. Scharhag J, Schneider G, Urhausen A, et al: Athlete's heart. Right and left ventricular mass and function in male endurance athletes and untrained individuals determined by magnetic resonance imaging. J Am Coll Cardiol 40:1856, 2006.
61. Neri Serneri GG, Boddi M, Modesti PA, et al: Increased cardiac sympathetic activity and insulin-like growth factor-I formation are associated with physiological hypertrophy in athletes. Circ Res 89:977, 2001.
62. Pelliccia A, Maron BJ, De Luca R, et al: Remodeling of left ventricular hypertrophy in elite athletes after long-term deconditioning. Circulation 105:944, 2002.
63. Leineweber K, Böhm M, Heusch G: Cyclic AMP in acute myocardial infarction with heart failure—slayer or savior? Circulation 114:365, 2006.
64. Derumeaux G, Mulder P, Richard V, et al: Tissue Doppler imaging differentiates physiological from pathological pressure-overload left ventricular hypertrophy in rats. Circulation 105:1602, 2002.

CHAPTER 22

Pathophysiology of Heart Failure

Douglas L. Mann

OVERVIEW

Despite repeated attempts to develop a unifying hypothesis that describes the clinical syndrome of heart failure (HF), no single conceptual paradigm has withstood the test of time. Thus it is not surprising that clinicians and investigators have used a variety of increasingly complex model systems in an attempt to describe the syndrome of HF. Although clinicians initially viewed HF as a problem of excessive salt and water retention that was caused by abnormalities of renal blood flow (the "cardiorenal model"[1]), as they began to perform careful hemodynamic measurements, it also became apparent that HF was associated with a reduced cardiac output and excessive peripheral vasoconstriction. This latter realization led to the development of the "cardiocirculatory" or "hemodynamic" model for HF,[1] wherein HF was thought to arise largely as a result of abnormalities of the pumping capacity of the heart and excessive peripheral vasoconstriction. However, although both the cardiorenal and cardiocirculatory models for HF explained the excessive salt and water retention that HF patients experience, neither of these models explained the relentless "disease progression" that occurs in this syndrome. Indeed, although the cardiorenal models provided the rational basis for the use of diuretics to control the volume status of patients with HF, and the cardiocirculatory model provided the rational basis for the use of inotropes and intravenous vasodilators to augment cardiac output, these therapeutic strategies have not prevented HF from progressing, nor have they led to prolonged life for patients with moderate to severe HF.

On the basis of these arguments, it has become increasingly apparent that HF can no longer be defined in simple hemodynamic terms. Accordingly, in this chapter we focus on the molecular and cellular changes that underlie HF with depressed systolic function, with an emphasis on the role of neurohormonal activation and left ventricular (LV) remodeling as the primary determinants for disease progression in HF. The hemodynamic, contractile, and wall motion disorders in systolic HF are discussed in the chapters on echocardiography (see Chap. 14), cardiac catheterization (see Chap. 19), radionuclide imaging (see Chap. 16), and the clinical assessment of the patients with HF (see Chap. 23). The pathogenesis of HF with a normal ejection fraction is discussed elsewhere (see Chap. 26).

PATHOGENESIS

As shown in Figure 22-1, HF may be viewed as a progressive disorder that is initiated after an "index event" either damages the heart muscle, with a resultant loss of functioning cardiac myocytes, or alternatively disrupts the ability of the myocardium to generate force, thereby preventing the heart from contracting normally. This index event may have an abrupt onset, as in the case of a myocardial infarction (MI); it may have a gradual or insidious onset, as in the case of hemodynamic pressure or volume overloading; or it may be hereditary, as in the case of many of the genetic cardiomyopathies. Regardless of the nature of the inciting event, what is common to each of these index events is that they all, in some manner, produce a decline in pumping capacity of the heart. In most instances patients will remain asymptomatic or minimally symptomatic following the initial decline in pumping capacity of the heart, or will develop symptoms only after the dysfunction has been present for some time. Although the precise reasons why patients with LV dysfunction remain asymptomatic are not certain, one potential explanation is that a number of compensatory mechanisms become activated in the setting of cardiac injury or depressed cardiac output and appear to modulate LV function within a physiological/homeostatic range, such that the functional capacity of the patient is preserved or is depressed only minimally. However, as patients transition to symptomatic HF, the sustained activation of neurohormonal and cytokine systems leads to a series of end-organ changes within the myocardium, referred to collectively as "LV remodeling." As discussed later, LV remodeling is sufficient to lead to disease progression in HF independent of the neurohormonal status of the patient.

HEART FAILURE AS A PROGRESSIVE MODEL

Neurohormonal Mechanisms

Some experts have suggested that HF should be viewed as a neurohormonal model, in which HF progresses as a result of the overexpression of biologically active molecules that are capable of exerting deleterious effects on the heart and circulation.[1] The compensatory mechanisms that have been described thus far include activation of the adrenergic nervous systemic and renin angiotensin system (RAS), which are responsible for maintaining cardiac output through increased retention of salt and water, peripheral arterial vasconstriction and increased contractility, and activation of inflammatory mediators that are responsible for cardiac repair and remodeling. It bears emphasis that the terminology "neurohormone" is largely a historical

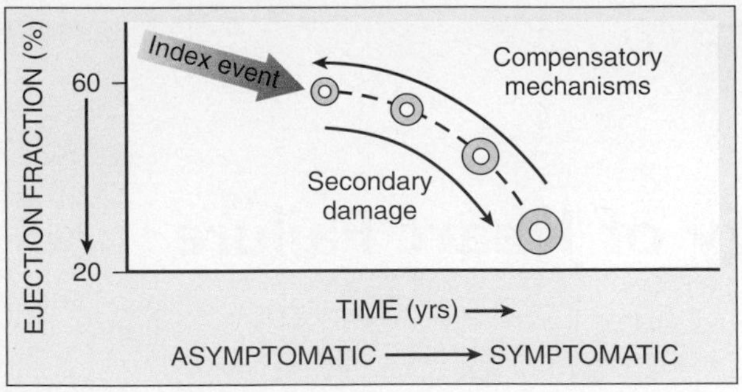

FIGURE 22–1 Pathogenesis of heart failure (HF). HF begins after an "index event" produces an initial decline in pumping capacity of the heart. Following this initial decline in pumping capacity of the heart, a variety of compensatory mechanisms are activated including the adrenergic nervous system, the renin angiotensin system, and the cytokine systems. In the short term these systems can restore cardiovascular function to a normal homeostatic range with the result that the patient remains asymptomatic. However, with time the sustained activation of these systems can lead to secondary end-organ damage within the ventricle, with worsening LV remodeling and subsequent cardiac decompensation. As a result of this worsening LV remodeling and cardiac decompensation, patients undergo the transition from asymptomatic to symptomatic HF. *(From Mann DL: Mechanisms and models in HF: A combinatorial approach. Circulation 100:99, 1999.)*

term, reflecting the original observation that many of the molecules that were elaborated in HF were produced by the neuroendocrine system and thus acted on the heart in an endocrine manner. However, it has since become apparent that many of the so-called classical neurohormones such as norepinephrine (NE) and angiotensin II are synthesized directly within the myocardium and thus act in autocrine and paracrine manner. Nonetheless, the important unifying concept that arises from the neurohormonal model is that the overexpression of portfolios of biologically active molecules contributes to disease progression by virtue of the deleterious effects these molecules exert on the heart and circulation.

ACTIVATION OF THE SYMPATHETIC NERVOUS SYSTEM. The decrease in cardiac output in HF activates a series of compensatory adaptations that are intended to maintain cardiovascular homeostasis. One of the most important adaptations is activation of the sympathetic (adrenergic) nervous system, which occurs early in the course of HF. As shown in Figure 22-2, activation of the sympathetic nervous system in HF is accompanied by a concomitant withdrawal of parasympathetic tone. Although these disturbances in autonomic control were initially attributed to loss of the inhibitory input from arterial or cardiopulmonary baroreceptor reflexes, there is increasing evidence that excitatory reflexes may also participate in the autonomic imbalance that occurs in HF.[2] Under normal conditions inhibitory inputs from "high pressure" carotid sinus and aortic arch baroreceptors and the "low pressure" cardiopulmonary mechanoreceptors are the principal inhibitors of sympathetic outflow, whereas discharge from the nonbaroreflex peripheral chemoreceptors and muscle "metaboreceptors" are the major excitatory inputs to sympathetic outflow. The vagal limb of the baroreceptor heart rate reflex is also responsive to arterial baroreceptor afferent inhibitory input. Healthy individuals display low sympathetic discharge at rest and have a high heart rate variability. However, in HF patients inhibitory input from baroreceptors and mechanoreceptors decreases and excitatory input increases, with the net result that there is a generalized increase in sympathetic nerve traffic and blunted parasympathetic nerve traffic, with a resultant loss of heart rate variability and increased peripheral vascular resistance.[2]

As a result of the increase in sympathetic tone, there is an increase in circulating levels of NE, a potent adrenergic neurotransmitter. The elevated levels of circulating NE result from a combination of increased release of NE from adrenergic nerve endings and its consequent "spillover" into the plasma, as well as reduced uptake of NE by adrenergic nerve endings. In patients with advanced HF, the circulating levels of NE in resting patients are two to three times those found in normal subjects. Indeed, plasma levels of NE predict mortality in patients with HF. Whereas the normal heart usually extracts NE from the arterial blood, in patients with moderate HF the coronary sinus NE concentration exceeds the arterial concentration, indicating increased adrenergic stimulation of the heart. However, as HF progresses there is a significant decrease in the myocardial concentration of NE. The mechanism responsible for cardiac NE depletion in severe HF is not clear and may relate to an "exhaustion" phenomenon resulting from the prolonged adrenergic activation of the cardiac adrenergic nerves in HF. In addition, there is decreased activity of myocardial tyrosine hydroxylase, which is the rate-limiting enzyme in the synthesis of NE. In patients with cardiomyopathy, iodine-131-labeled metaiodobenzylguanidine (MIBG), a radiopharmaceutical that is taken up by adrenergic nerve endings, is not taken up normally, suggesting that NE reuptake is also impaired in HF.

Increased sympathetic activation of the beta$_1$-adrenergic receptor results in increased heart rate and force of myocardial contraction, with a resultant increase in cardiac output (see Chap. 21). In addition, the heightened activity of the adrenergic nervous system leads to stimulation of myocardial alpha$_1$-adrenergic receptors, which elicits a modest positive inotropic effect, as well as peripheral arterial vasoconstriction. Although NE enhances both contraction and relaxation and maintains blood pressure, myocardial energy requirements are augmented, which can intensify ischemia when myocardial O_2 delivery is restricted. The augmented adrenergic outflow from the central nervous system may also trigger ventricular tachycardia or even sudden cardiac death, particularly in the presence of myocardial ischemia. Thus activation of the sympathetic nervous system provides short-term support that has the potential to become maladaptive in the long term.

ACTIVATION OF THE RENIN-ANGIOTENSIN SYSTEM. In contrast to the sympathetic nervous system, the components of the renin-angiotensin system (RAS) are activated comparatively later in HF. The presumptive mechanisms for RAS activation in HF include renal hypoperfusion; decreased filtered sodium reaching the macula densa in the distal tubule; and increased sympathetic stimulation of the kidney, leading to increased renin release from a juxtaglomerular apparatus. As shown in Figure 22-3, renin cleaves four amino acids from circulating angiotensinogen, which is synthesized in the liver, to form the biologically inactive decapeptide angiotensin I. Angiotensin-converting enzyme (ACE) cleaves two amino acids from angiotensin I to form the biologically active octapeptide (1-8) angiotensin II. The majority (≈90%) of ACE activity in the body is found in tissues; the remaining 10 percent of ACE activity is found in a soluble (non–membrane bound) form in the interstitium of the heart and vessel wall. The importance of tissue ACE activity in HF is suggested by the observation that ACE mRNA, ACE binding sites, and ACE activity are increased in explanted human hearts.[3] Angiotensin II can also be synthesized through renin-independent pathways, through the enzymatic conversion of angiotensinogen to angiotensin I by kallikrein and cathepsin G (Fig. 22-4). The tissue production of angiotensin II may also occur through ACE independent pathways, through the activation of chymase. This latter pathway may be of major importance in the myocardium, particularly when the levels of renin and angiotensin I are increased by the use of ACE inhibitors. Angiotensin II itself can undergo further proteolysis to generate three biologically active fragments—angiotensin III (2-8) and angiotensin IV (3-8), which promote vasconstriction,[4] as well as angiotensin (1-7), which may act to counteract the deleterious effects of angiotensin II on endothelial function.

Angiotensin II exerts its effects by binding to two G-protein coupled receptors termed *angiotensin type 1* (AT_1) and *angiotensin type 2* (AT_2). The predominant angiotensin receptor in the vasculature is the AT_1 receptor. Although both the AT_1 and AT_2 receptor subtypes are present in human myocardium, the AT_2 receptor predominates in a 2 : 1 molar ratio. Cellular localization of the AT_1 receptor in the heart is most abundant in nerves distributed in the myocardium, whereas the AT_2 receptor is localized more highly in fibroblasts and the interstitium. Activation of the AT_1 receptor leads to vasoconstriction, cell growth, aldosterone secretion, and catecholamine release, whereas activation of the AT_2 receptor leads to vasodilation, inhibition of cell growth, natriuresis, and bradykinin release. Studies have shown that the AT_1 receptor and mRNA levels are downregulated in failing human hearts, whereas AT_2 receptor density is increased or unchanged, with the result that the ratio of AT_1 to AT_2 receptors decreases.[3]

Angiotensin II has several important actions that are critical to maintaining short-term circulatory homeostasis (see later). However, the sustained expression of angiotensin II is maladaptive and leads to fibrosis of the heart, kidneys, and other organs. Angiotensin II can also lead to worsening neurohormonal activation by enhancing the release of NE from sympathetic nerve endings, as well as stimulating the zona glomerulosa of the adrenal cortex to produce aldosterone. Analogous to angiotensin II, aldosterone provides short-term support to the circulation by promoting the reabsorption of sodium in exchange for potassium, in the distal segments of the nephron. However, the sustained expression of aldosterone may exert harmful effects by provoking hypertrophy and fibrosis within the vasculature and the myocardium, thus contributing to reduced vascular compliance and increased ventricular stiffness. In addition, aldosterone provokes endothelial cell dysfunction, baroreceptor

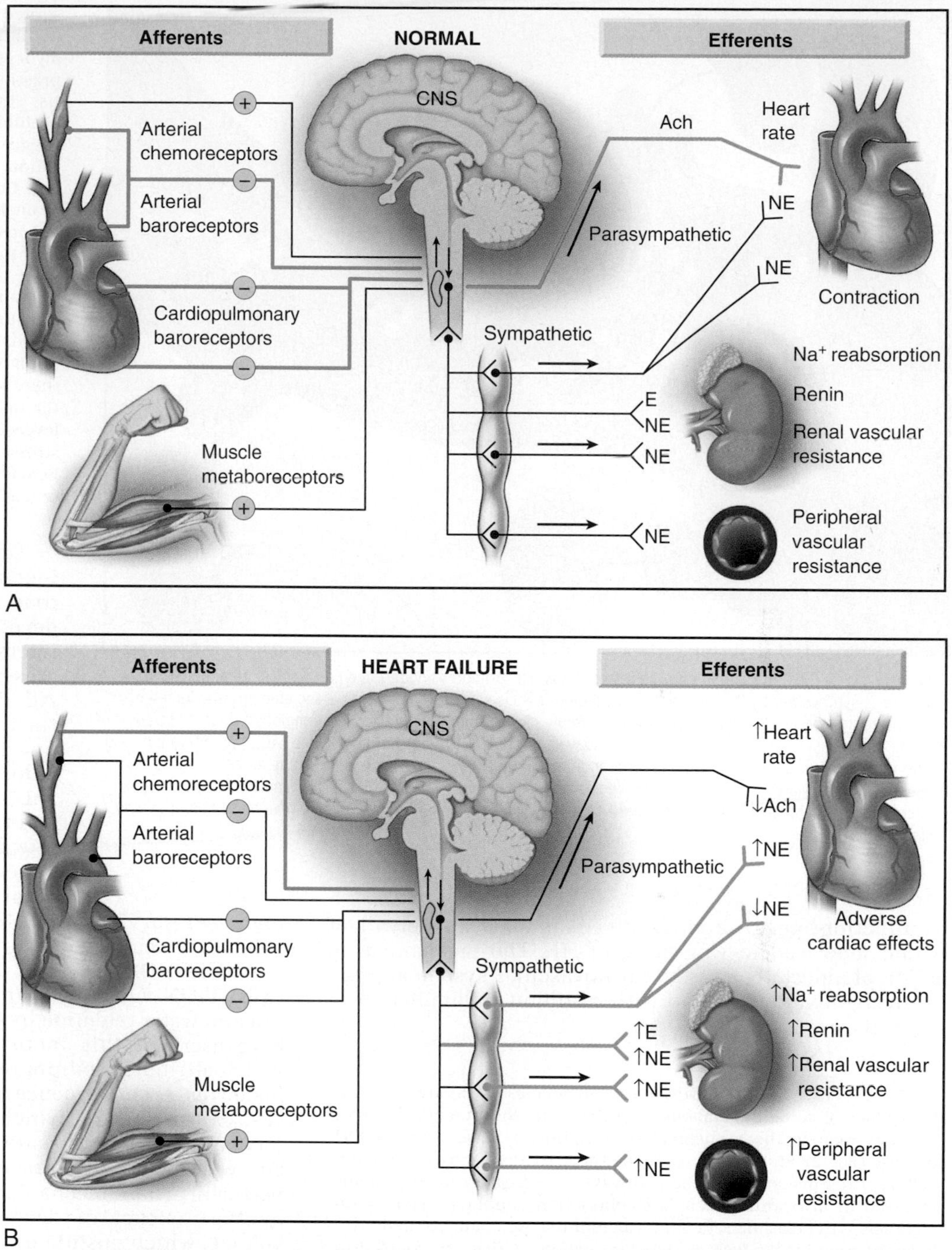

FIGURE 22–2 Mechanisms for generalized sympathetic activation and parasympathetic withdrawal in HF. **A,** Under normal conditions, inhibitory (–) inputs from arterial and cardiopulmonary baroreceptor afferent nerves are the principal influence on sympathetic outflow. Parasympathetic control of heart rate is also under potent arterial baroreflex control. Efferent sympathetic traffic and arterial catecholamines are low, and heart rate variability is high. **B,** As HF progresses, inhibitory input from arterial and cardiopulmonary receptors decreases and excitatory (+) input increases. The net response to this altered balance includes a generalized increase in sympathetic nerve traffic, blunted parasympathetic and sympathetic control of heart rate, and impairment of the reflex sympathetic regulation of vascular resistance. Anterior wall ischemia has additional excitatory effects on efferent sympathetic nerve traffic. See text for details. Ach = acetylcholine; CNS = central nervous system; E = epinephrine; Na^+ = sodium; NE = norepinephrine. *(From Floras JS: Alterations in the sympathetic and parasympathetic nervous system in HF. In Mann DL [ed]: Heart Failure: A Companion to Braunwald's Heart Disease. Philadelphia, Elsevier, 2004, pp 247-278.)*

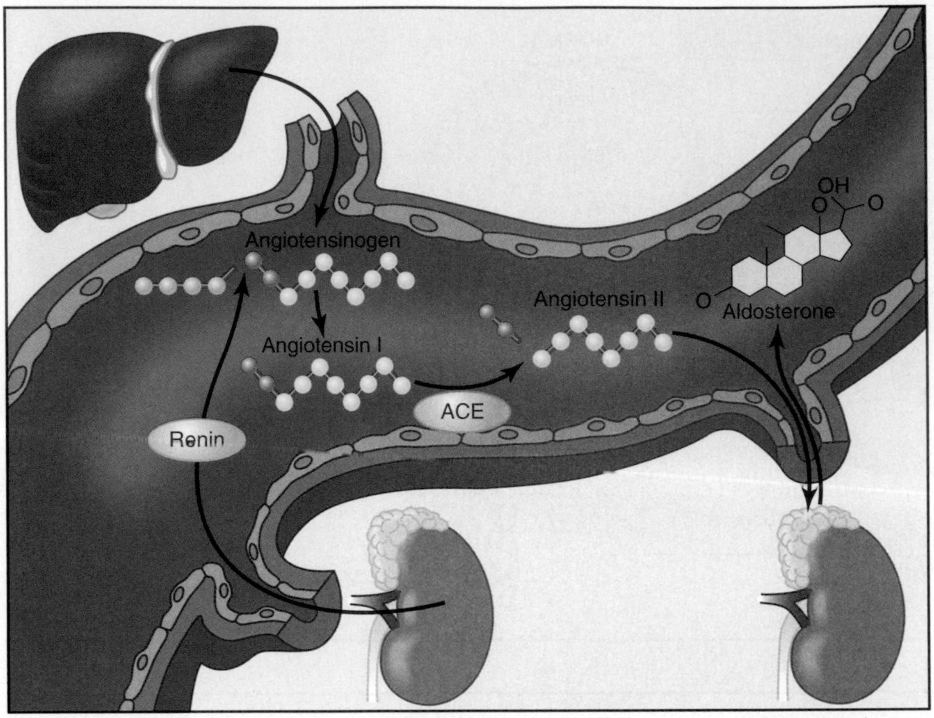

FIGURE 22–3 The renin-angiotensin-aldosterone system. Angiotensinogen, the precursor of all angiotensin peptides, is synthesized by the liver. In the circulation it is cleaved by renin, which is secreted into the lumen of renal afferent arterioles by juxtaglomerular cells. Renin cleaves four amino acids from angiotensinogen, thereby forming angiotensin I. In turn, angiotensin I is cleaved by angiotensin-converting enzyme (ACE), an enzyme bound to the membrane of endothelial cells, to form angiotensin II. In the zona glomerulosa of the adrenal cortex, angiotensin II stimulates the production of aldosterone. Aldosterone production is also stimulated by potassium, corticotropin, catecholamines (e.g., NE), and ET. *(From Weber KT: Aldosterone in congestive heart failure. N Engl J Med 345:1689, 2001.)*

dysfunction, and inhibition of NE uptake, any or all of which may lead to worsening of HF. The mechanism of action of aldosterone in the cardiovascular system appears to involve oxidative stress with resultant inflammation in target tissues.

OXIDATIVE STRESS. Reactive oxygen species (ROS) are a normal byproduct of aerobic metabolism. In the heart the potential sources for ROS include the mitochondria, xanthine oxidase, and NADPH oxidase (Fig. 22-5). ROS can modulate the activity of a variety of intracellular proteins and signaling pathways including essential proteins involved in myocardial excitation-contraction coupling, such as ion channels, sarcoplasmic reticulum calcium release channels, and myofilament proteins, as well as signaling pathways that are coupled to myocyte growth (see Fig. 22-e1 on website).[5] "Oxidative stress" occurs when the production of ROS exceeds the buffering capacity of antioxidant defense systems, leading to an excess of ROS within the cell. In the heart the mitochondrial enzymes manganese superoxide dismutase (MnSOD) and glutathione peroxidase appear to be the most important antioxidant systems for controlling myocardial levels of superoxide and hydrogen peroxide. Indeed, MnSOD knockout mice developed a dilated cardiomyopathy and died at a young age.[6] Substantial evidence indicates that the level of oxidative stress is increased both systemically and in the myocardium of HF patients. Oxidative stress in the heart may be due to reduced antioxidant capacity and/or the increased production of ROS, which may arise secondary to mechanical strain of the myocardium, neurohormonal stimulation (angiotensin II, aldosterone, alpha-adrenergic agonists, endothelin-1 [ET-1]), and/or inflammatory cytokines (tumor necrosis factor [TNF], interleukin-1 [IL-1]). Excessive mitochondrial-derived ROS in cardiac myocytes have been demonstrated in experimental models of HF and may contribute to contractile dysfunction in advanced HF. Increased xanthine oxidase expression and activity have been reported in canine rapid pacing–induced HF and patients with end-stage HF. Moreover, increased expression and activity of myocardial NADPH oxidases have recently been demonstrated in both experimental and human HF.[5] In cultured cardiac myocytes ROS stimulate myocyte hypertrophy (see Fig. 22-5), reexpression of fetal gene programs, and apoptosis. ROS can also modulate fibroblast proliferation and collagen synthesis and can trigger increased MMP abundance and activation. ROS affects the peripheral vasculature in HF by decreasing the bioavailability of nitric oxide (NO). These and other observations have led to the suggestion that strategies to reduce ROS may be of therapeutic value in HF. The OPT-CHF (Oxypurinol Therapy in Congestive Heart Failure) with oxypurinol (a xanthine oxidase inhibitor) failed to alter the primary composite endpoint of hospitalization or CV death, although there was a trend toward improvement for the subgroup of patients with the highest levels of uric acid (a biomarker for oxidative stress), suggesting that this therapy may benefit patients with the highest degree of oxidative stress.

Transgenic mice with a selective increase in activation of the aldosterone receptors in cardiac myocytes develop myocardial hypertrophy and interstitial fibrosis, leading to progressive LV dilation, HF, and death. All of these events can be blocked by treatment with an aldosterone receptor antagonist. The importance of aldosterone, independent of angiotensin II, has been demonstrated by clinical trials (see Chap. 25) showing that low doses of spironolactone, an aldosterone antagonist, increased the survival of patients with systolic HF[7] and improved survival after MI,[8] independent of changes in volume or electrolyte status.

NEUROHORMONAL ALTERATIONS OF RENAL FUNCTION. One signature of advancing HF is increased salt and water retention by the kidneys. Traditional theories have ascribed this increase to either "forward" failure, which attributes sodium retention to inadequate renal perfusion as a consequence of impaired cardiac output, or "backward" failure, which emphasizes the importance of increased venous pressure in favoring transudation of salt and water from the intravascular to the extracellular compartment. These mechanisms have largely been supplanted by the concept of decreased "effective arterial" blood volume, which postulates that despite blood volume expansion in HF, inadequate cardiac output sensed by baroreceptors in the vascular tree leads to a series of compensatory neurohormonal adaptations that resemble the homeostatic response to acute blood loss.[9] As illustrated in Figure 22-6, a falling cardiac output and/or redistribution of the circulating blood volume is sensed by baroreceptors in the left ventricle, aortic arch, carotid sinus, and renal afferent arterioles. The loss of inhibitory input from arterial or cardiopulmonary baroreceptor reflexes leads to sustained activation of the sympathetic nervous and the renin-angiotensin systems.

There is little evidence to suggest that a primary renal abnormality is responsible for excessive sodium retention in HF. Rather, it is likely secondary to a functional derangement of renal physiology in response to several factors, all of which have the potential to cause increased sodium reabsorption including activation of the sympathetic nervous system, activation of RAS, reduced renal perfusion pressures, and blunting of renal responsiveness to natriuretic

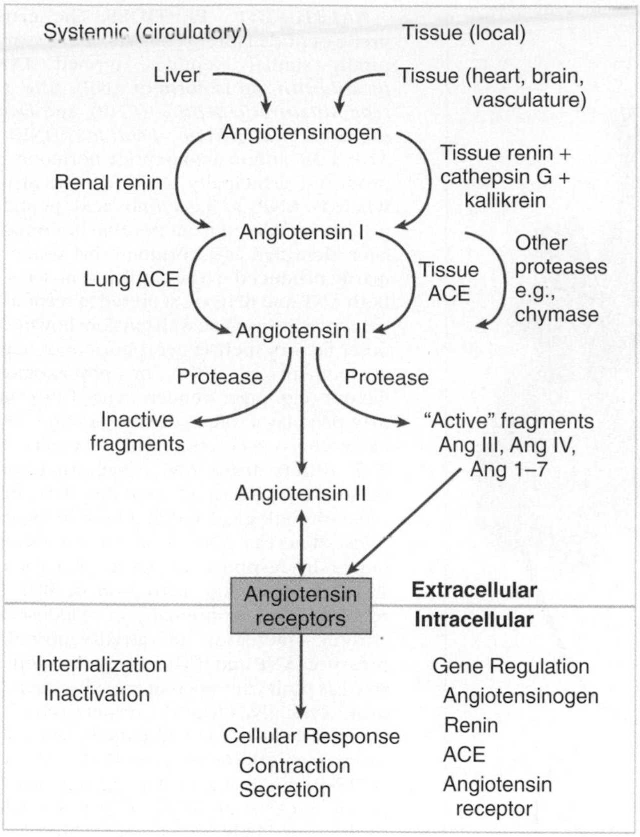

FIGURE 22–4 The systemic and tissue components of the renin-angiotensin system. Several tissues including myocardium, vasculature, kidney, and brain have the capacity to generate angiotensin II independent of the circulating renin-angiotensin system. Angiotensin II produced at the tissue level may play an important role in the pathophysiology of HF. ACE = angiotensin-converting enzyme. *(Modified from Timmermans PB, Wong PC, Chiu AT, et al: Angiotensin II receptors and angiotensin II receptor antagonists. Pharmacol Rev 45:205, 1993.)*

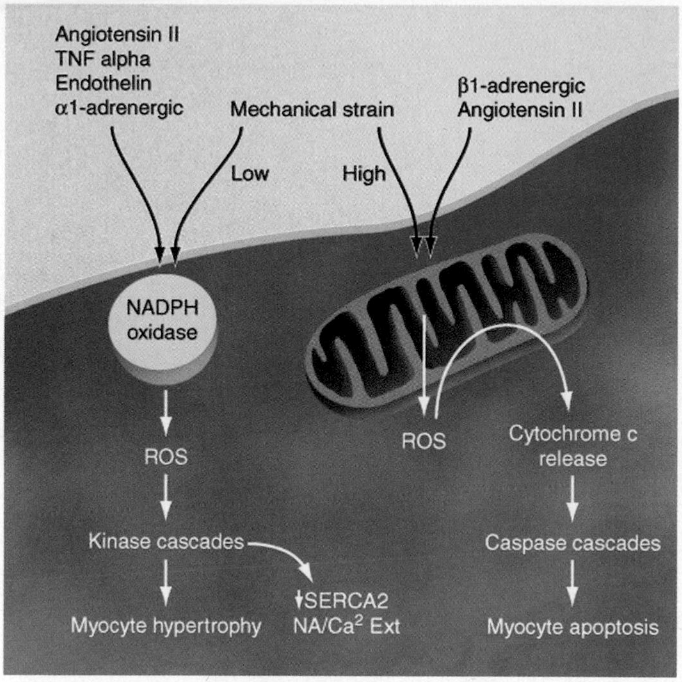

FIGURE 22–5 Effects of reactive oxygen species (ROS) on cardiac myocyte phenotype. Through activation of kinase cascades such as mitogen-activated protein kinase (MAPK), ROS can induce myocyte hypertrophy. ROS can also alter the activity and expression of Ca^{2+}-handling proteins including SERCA2A and the Na^+/Ca^{2+} exchanger to alter myocardial contractility. Mitochondrial ROS may be particularly prone to induce apoptosis by stimulating the mitochondrial release of cytochrome c, which is necessary for the activation of caspase cascades. NADPH = reduced nicotinamide adenine dinucleotide phosphate; TNF = tumor necrosis factor. *(From Mann DL [ed]: Heart Failure: A Companion to Braunwald's Heart Disease. Philadelphia, Elsevier, 2004. Modified from Sawyer DB, Siwik DA, Xiao L, et al: Role of oxidative stress in myocardial hypertrophy and failure. J Mol Cell Cardiol 34:379, 2002.)*

peptides. Increased renal sympathetic nerve–mediated vasconstriction leads to decreased renal blood flow, as well as increased renal tubular sodium and water reabsorption throughout the nephron. Renal sympathetic stimulation can also lead to the nonosmotic release of arginine vasopressin (AVP) from the posterior pituitary, which reduces the excretion of free water and contributes to worsening peripheral vasoconstriction, as well as increased ET production.[9]

ARGININE VASOPRESSIN. Arginine vasopressin (AVP) is a pituitary hormone that plays a central role in the regulation of free water clearance and plasma osmolality (see Fig. 22-6). Under normal circumstances AVP is released in response to an increase in plasma osmolality, leading to increased retention of water from the proximal duct. Of note, circulating AVP is elevated in many patients with HF, even after correction for plasma osmolality (i.e., nonosmotic release),[10] and may contribute to the hyponatremia that occurs in HF. The cellular effects of AVP are mediated mainly by interactions with three types of receptors: V_{1a}, V_{1b}, and V2. The V_{1a} receptor is the most widespread subtype and is found primarily in vascular smooth muscle cells. The V_{1b} receptor has a more limited distribution and is located mainly in the central nervous system. The V2 receptors are found primarily in the epithelial cells in the renal collecting duct and the thick ascending limb. AVP receptors are members of the G protein–coupled receptors. The V_{1a} receptors mediate vasoconstriction, platelet aggregation, and stimulation of myocardial growth factors, whereas V_{1b} modulates ACTH secretion from the anterior pituitary and the V2 receptor mediates antidiuretic effects by stimulating adenylyl cyclase to increase the rate of insertion of vesicles containing water channels into the apical membrane. Because these vesicles contain preformed functional water channels, termed *aquaporins,* their localization in the apical membranes in response to V2 stimulation increases the water permeability of the apical membrane, leading to water retention. In dogs with pacing-induced HF, the selective inhibition of V1 receptors increased cardiac output without affecting electrolytes or hormone levels. In contrast, inhibition of V2 receptors increased serum sodium concentration, plasma renin activity, and plasma AVP levels but did not affect hemodynamics. When the two inhibitors were combined, the hemodynamic effects were potentiated.[11] The "vaptans," vasopressin receptor antagonists with V_{1a} (relcovaptan) or V2 (tolvaptan, lixivaptan) selectivity or nonselective V_{1a}/V2 activity (conivaptan), are currently being evaluated in clinical trials (see also Chap. 25).

Increased renal sympathetic activity leads to increased renin production of renin by the kidneys, with a resultant sustained activation of RAS, despite an expanded extracellular volume. Angiotensin II assists retention of sodium and water by multiple renal mechanisms including a direct proximal tubular effect and through activation of aldosterone, which leads to increased sodium resorption in the distal tubule. Angiotensin II also stimulates the thirst center of the brain and provokes the release of AVP and aldosterone, which can both lead to further dysregulation of salt and water homeostasis.

A number of counterregulatory neurohormonal systems become activated in HF in order to offset the deleterious effects of the vasoconstricting neurohormones (see Table 22-e1 on website). Metabolites of vasodilatory prostaglandins including prostaglandin E_2 (PGE_2) and prostacyclin (PGI_2), are elevated in patients with HF. In addition to being a vasodilator, PGE_2 enhances renal sodium excretion and

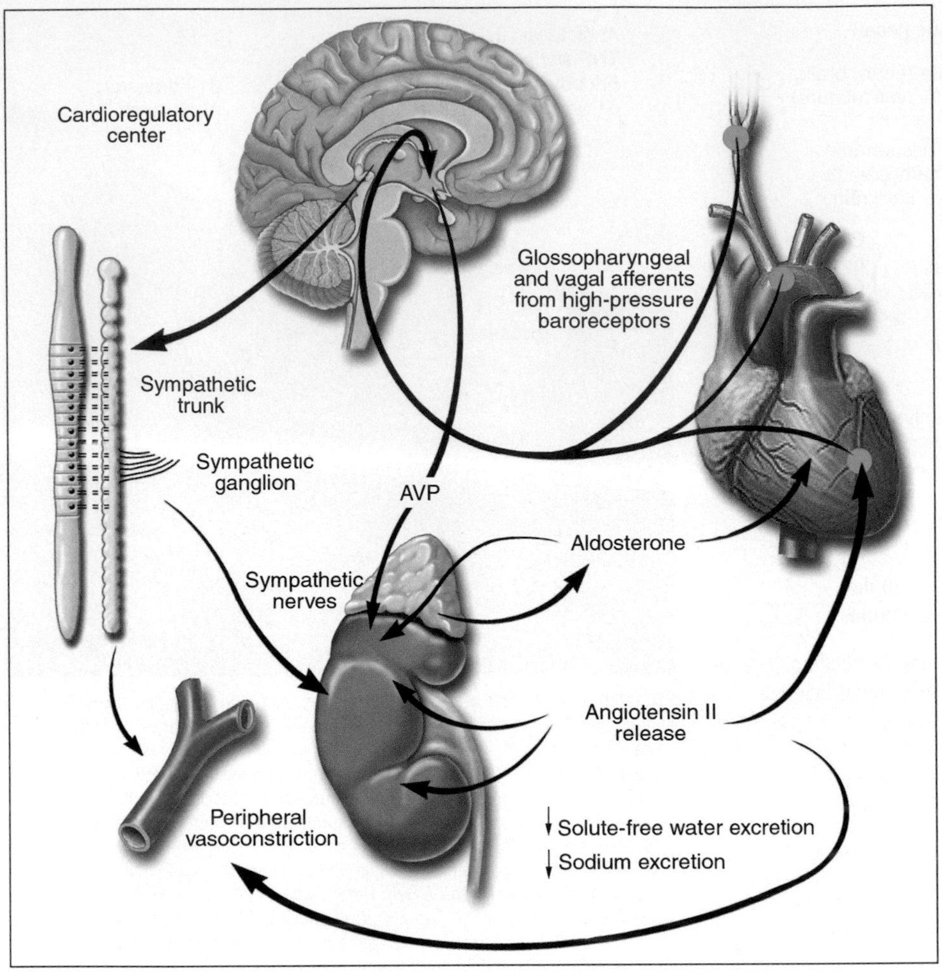

FIGURE 22–6 Unloading of high-pressure baroceptors (circles) in the left ventricle, carotid sinus, and aortic arch generates afferent signals that stimulate cardioregulatory centers in the brain, resulting in the activation of efferent pathways in the sympathetic nervous system. The sympathetic nervous system appears to be the primary integrator of the neurohumoral vasoconstrictor response to arterial underfilling. Activation of renal sympathetic nerves stimulates the release of arginine vasopressin (AVP). Sympathetic activation also causes peripheral and renal vasoconstriction, as does angiotensin II. Angiotensin II constricts blood vessels and stimulates the release of aldosterone from the adrenal gland, and it also increases tubular sodium reabsorption and causes remodeling of cardiac myocytes. Aldosterone may also have direct cardiac effects, in addition to increasing the reabsorption of sodium and the secretion of potassium and hydrogen ions in the collecting duct. The lines designate circulating hormones. (See also Chaps. 40 and 88). *(Modified from Schrier RW, Abraham WT: Hormones and hemodynamics in heart failure. N Engl J Med 341:577, 1999.)*

modulates the antidiuretic action of AVP. Among the most important counterregulatory neurohormonal systems that become activated in HF are the natriuretic peptides including atrial natriuretic peptide (ANP) and brain type natriuretic peptide (BNP). Under physiological conditions, ANP and BNP function as natriuretic hormones that are released in response to increases to atrial and/or myocardial stretch, often secondary to excessive sodium intake. Once released, these cardiac peptides act on the kidney and peripheral circulation to unload the heart, through increased excretion of sodium and water, while inhibiting the release of renin and aldosterone. In the setting of RAS activation the release of ANP and BNP may serve as an important counterregulatory mechanism that maintains sodium and water homeostasis. However, for reasons that are not entirely clear, the renal effects of the natriuretic peptides appear to become blunted with advancing HF, leaving the effects of RAS unopposed (see Fig. 22-e2 on website).[12] Potential reasons for this blunting include low renal perfusion pressure, relative deficiency or altered molecular forms of the natriuretic peptides, or decreased levels of natriuretic peptide receptors.

NATRIURETIC PEPTIDES. The natriuretic peptide system consists of five structurally similar peptides, termed *ANP, urodilantin* (an isoform of ANP), *BNP, C-type natriuretic peptide* (CNP), and *Dendroaspis natriuretic peptide* (DNP).[13] ANP, a 28–amino acid peptide hormone, is produced principally in the cardiac atria, whereas BNP, a 32–amino acid peptide originally isolated from porcine brain, was later identified as a hormone that was primarily produced in the cardiac ventricles.[14] Both ANP and BNP are secreted in response to increasing cardiac wall tension; however, other factors such as neurohormones (e.g., angiotensin II, ET-1) or physiological factors (e.g., age, gender, renal function) may also play a role in their regulation. The biosynthesis, secretion, and clearance of BNP differs from ANP, suggesting that these two natriuretic peptides have discrete physiological and pathophysiological roles. Whereas ANP is secreted in short bursts in response to acute changes in atrial pressure, the activation of BNP is regulated transcriptionally in response to chronic increases in atrial/ventricular pressure. ANP and BNP are initially synthesized as prohormones that are subsequently proteolytically cleaved, respectively, by corin and furin, to yield large biologically inactive N-terminal fragments (NT-ANP or NT-BNP) and smaller biologically active peptides (ANP or BNP). ANP has a relatively short half-life of approximately 3 minutes, whereas BNP has a plasma half-life of approximately 20 minutes. CNP, which is located primarily in the vasculature, is also released as a prohormone that is cleaved into a biologically inactive form (NT-CNP) and a 22–amino acid biologically active form (CNP).

Figure 22-7 illustrates the signaling pathway of the natriuretic peptide system. The natriuretic peptides stimulate the production of the intracellular second messenger cGMP via binding to the natriuretic peptide A receptor (NPR-A), which preferentially binds ANP and BNP, and the natriuretic peptide B receptor (NPR-B), which preferentially binds CNP. Both NPR-A and NPR-B receptors are coupled to particulate guanylate cyclase. Activation of NPR-A and NPR-B results in natriuresis, vasorelaxation, inhibition of renin and aldosterone, inhibition, inhibition of fibrosis, and increased lusitropy. The natriuretic peptide C receptor (NPR-C) is not linked to cGMP and serves as a clearance receptor for the natriuretic peptides. Natriuretic peptides are degraded by neutral endopeptidase 24.11 (NEP), which is widely expressed in multiple tissues, where it is often colocalized with ACE. Inhibition of NEP may further potentiate the renal actions of ANP and BNP. The infusion of the endopeptidase inhibitor candoxatrilat into patients with HF resulted in a reduction in left- and right-sided filling pressures that was associated with suppression of plasma NE levels and a transient reduction in plasma vasopressin.[15] Vasopeptidase inhibitors such as omapatrilat, which inhibit both neutral endopeptidase and ACE, were developed with the intent of inhibiting RAS while concurrently elevating natriuretic peptide levels. Although some early trials suggested that neutral endopeptidase inhibition would have a greater benefit than ACE inhibition, more recent trials have found the two classes of drug to exert similar effects on survival.[16]

The biological importance of the natriuretic peptides in renal sodium handling has been demonstrated in multiple studies employing natriuretic peptide receptor antagonists, as well as overexpression of ANP or BNP.[12] In experimental HF models, either acute blockade of the natriuretic A and B receptors or chronic genetic disruption of the natriuretic peptide A receptor, blunts the renal natriuretic response to acute volume expansion, demonstrating the renal protective action of natriuretic peptide activation.[17] The infusion of a recombinant human (rh) BNP exerts beneficial hemodynamic effects that are characterized by decreases in arterial and venous pressures, an increase in cardiac output, and suppression of neurohormonal activation. Indeed, the unique properties of the natriuretic peptides have resulted in their clinical development as therapeutic agents for human HF. Recombinant human (rh) BNP has been approved by the U.S. Food and Drug Administration for use in acute decompensated HF (see Chap. 24). In addition to their important biological role, the natriuretic peptides have provided important diagnostic and prognostic information in HF (see Chap. 23).

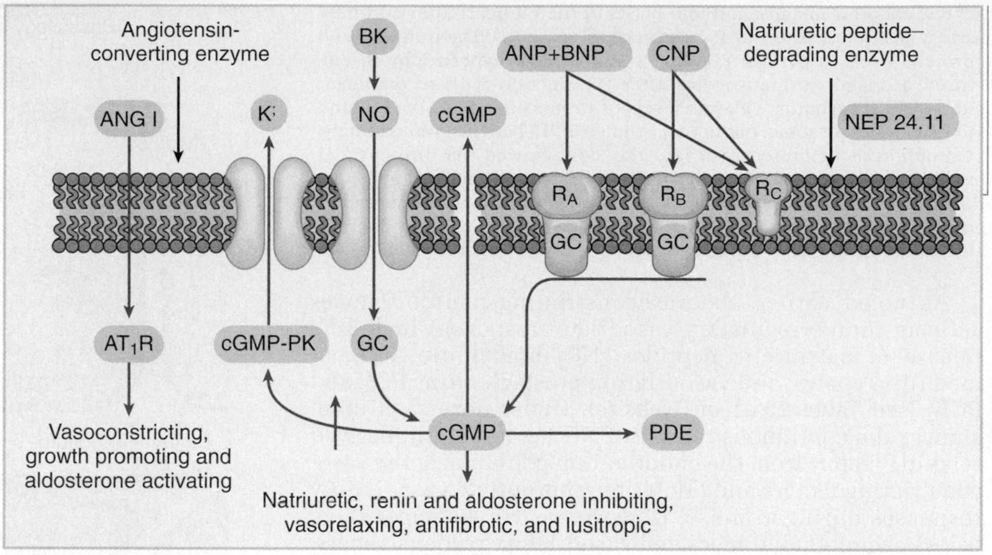

FIGURE 22–7 Cellular actions in signaling of the natriuretic peptide system. Ang 1 = angiotensin I; ANP = atrial natriuretic peptide; AT_1R = angiotensin type 1 receptor; BK = bradykinin; BNP = brain natriuretic peptide; cGMP = cyclic guanosine monophosphate; CNP = C-type natriuretic peptide; GC = guanylate cyclase; NEP = neutral endopeptidase; PDE = phosphodiesterase; PK = phosphokinase; R_A = particulate guanylate cyclase A receptor; Rc = particulate guanylate cyclase C receptor; R_s = particulate guanylate cyclase S receptor. *(From Burnett JC, Costello-Boerrigter L, Boerrigter G: Alterations in the kidney in heart failure: The cardiorenal axis in the regulation of sodium homeostasis.* In *Mann DL [ed]: Heart Failure: A Companion to Braunwald's Heart Disease. Philadelphia, Elsevier, 2004, pp 279-289.)*

NEUROHORMONAL ALTERATIONS IN THE PERIPHERAL VASCULATURE. In patients with HF the complex interactions between the autonomic nervous system and local autoregulatory mechanisms tend to preserve circulation to the brain and heart while decreasing blood flow to the skin, skeletal muscles, splanchnic organs, and kidneys. This intense visceral vasoconstriction during exercise helps to divert the limited cardiac output to exercising muscle but contributes to hypoperfusion of the gut and kidneys. The most powerful stimulus for peripheral vasoconstriction is sympathetic activation, which releases the potent vasoconstrictor NE. Other vasoconstrictors that contribute to maintaining circulatory homeostasis include angiotensin II, ET, neuropeptide Y, urotensin II, thromboxane A_2, and AVP (see Table 22-e1 on website). The increased sympathetic adrenergic stimulation of the peripheral arteries and the increased concentrations of circulating vasoconstrictors contribute to the arteriolar vasoconstriction and to the maintenance of arterial pressure, while the sympathetic stimulation of the veins contributes to an increase in venous tone, which helps to maintain venous return and ventricular filling and support cardiac performance by Starling's law of the heart (see Chap 23).

ENDOTHELIN. All three endothelin peptides (ET-1, ET-2, and ET-3) are potent vasoconstrictors. Although primarily released by endothelial cells, ET can also be synthesized and released by a variety of other cell types such as cardiac myocytes. ET-1 is the predominant isoform of the ET peptide family and is ubiquitously expressed. ET-1 is synthesized as a protein precursor termed *preproET-1.* Preproendothelin-1 is processed by multiple proteases in a process that involves the proteolytic release of proendothelin-1 ("big endothelin"), followed by C-terminal trimming by a carboxypeptidase and further processing by endothelin-converting enzyme (ECE) to generate the biologically active 21-amino acid ET-1 peptide. However, studies in ECE knockout mice show that significant levels of mature ET-1 exist, suggesting that there may be alternative ECE-independent (e.g., chymase, non-ECE metalloproteinases) pathways for generation of ET-1. At least two subtypes of ET receptors (types A and B) have been identified in human myocardium. Endothelin ET(A) receptors mediate vasoconstriction, cell proliferation, pathological hypertrophy, fibrosis, and increased contractility, whereas ET(B) receptors are involved in the clearance of ET-1 and the release of NO and prostacyclin. The release of ET from endothelial cells in vitro can be enhanced by several vasoactive agents (e.g., NE, angiotensin II, thrombin) and cytokines (e.g., TGF-beta, TNF, and IL-1). Several reports have documented an increase in circulating levels of ET-1 in patients with HF and have shown that ET levels correlate with patient outcomes. Further, plasma ET concentrations correlate directly with pulmonary artery pressure, pulmonary vascular resistance, and pulmonary vascular resistance. On the basis of the biological properties of ET, ET receptor antagonists were developed for the treatment of patients with HF. Although early experimental studies showed that ET(A) receptor antagonists inhibited myocardial hypertrophy in rats with pressure overload–induced hypertrophy caused by aortic banding and prevented cardiac remodeling in rats with MI,[18] and although early clinical studies confirmed the ability of these new agents to improve hemodynamics, the effects of chronic ET receptor antagonism have not been beneficial in clinical HF trials and have led to worsening outcomes in some settings.[19] This statement notwithstanding, ET receptor antagonists have been shown to be beneficial in the setting of pulmonary hypertension and are currently approved by the U.S. Food and Drug Administration for the treatment of pulmonary artery hypertension in patients with moderate disability (functional class III).

NEUROPEPTIDE Y. Neuropeptide Y (NPY) is a vasconstricting peptide that is released together with NE from sympathetic nerve endings. NPY is abundant in cerebral cortex, hippocampus, thalamus, hypothalamus, and brainstem. Of note, the inhibitory effects of NPY on NE release in the paraventricular nucleus are blunted in animals with HF following an acute infarction, leading to an increase in sympathetic nerve activity and peripheral NE levels. NPY elicits peripheral vasoconstriction by interacting with Y1 receptors, which are located postjunctionally at the sympathetic neuroeffector junction in blood vessels. In addition, NPY potentiates the vasoconstrictor effects of other extracellular messengers including alpha-adrenergic agonists and angiotensin II, and inhibits acetylcholine release from parasympathetic nerve endings in the heart. Although the role of NPY in HF is not known, circulating concentrations of NPY-like immunoreactivity are significantly increased in moderate to severe forms of HF and correlated with circulating levels of NE.[20]

UROTENSIN II. Mammalian U-II is the most potent endogenous cardiostimulatory peptide identified thus far, with an 8- to 110-fold greater potency than ET-1. The effects of urotensin II are mediated by binding to the urotensin receptor. Urotensin II mediates vascular tone and increased contractile force in human atrium and ventricle. Analogous to ET-1, urotensin II provokes trophic and/or mitogenic actions in vascular smooth muscle cells, cardiac myocytes, and cardiac fibroblasts. However, unlike ET-1, which uniformly constricts most blood vessels, the vasoactive effects of U-II are both species and vascular bed dependent. Urotensin receptor expression is increased in cardiac myocytes, endothelial cells, and fibroblasts in the rat heart after coronary artery ligation. Urotensin II treatment increased collagen mRNA and protein levels in cardiac fibroblasts and cardiac hypertrophy in cultured neonatal cardiomyocytes after transfection with recombinant urotensin II receptor.[21] Plasma levels of urotensin II have been found to be elevated in some, but not all, studies in HF patients. Interestingly, iontophoresis of urotensin II into the skin showed that urotensin II mediated a dose-dependent vasodilator response in normal subjects, whereas urotensin II mediated a dose-dependent vasoconstrictor response in patients with HF, suggesting that urotensin II may contribute to the increased peripheral vascular tone that occurs in HF.[22]

As noted earlier, the vasoconstricting neurohormones activate counterregulatory vasodilator responses including release of natriuretic peptides, NO, bradykinin, adrenomedullin, apelin, and vasodilating prostaglandins PGI_2 and PGE_2 (see Table 22-e1 on website). Under normal circumstances the continuous release of NO (endothelium-derived relaxing factor) from the endothelium counteracts the vasoconstricting factors and allows for appropriate vasodilatory responses during exercise. However, as HF advances there is loss of endothelial-mediated vasodilatory responsiveness, which contributes to the excessive peripheral arterial vasoconstriction that is emblematic of advanced HF. Of interest, the vasodilator response can be restored by the administration of L-arginine, a precursor of endothelium-derived NO.[23]

NITRIC OXIDE. The free radical gas NO is produced by three isoforms of nitric oxide synthase (NOS). All three isoforms are present in the heart including NOS1 (nNOS, "neuronal" NOS); NOS2 (iNOS or "inducible" NOS); and NOS3 (eNOS, "endothelial-constitutive" NOS). NOS1 has been detected in cardiac conduction tissue, intracardiac neurons, and the sarcoplasmic reticulum of cardiac myocytes; NOS2 is an inducible isoform that is not normally expressed in the myocardium but is synthesized de novo in virtually all cells in the heart in response to inflammatory cytokines, whereas NOS3 is expressed in coronary endothelium, endocardium, and in the sarcolemma and T-tubule membranes of cardiac myocytes. NOS1 and NOS3 can be activated by calcium or calmodulin, whereas the induction of NOS2 is calcium independent. NO activates soluble guanylate cyclase (Fig. 22-8). This activation leads to the production of cGMP, which in turn activates protein kinase G and a cascade of different signaling events. In normal subjects NO released by endothelial cells mediates vasodilation in the peripheral vasculature through cGMP-mediated relaxation of vascular smooth muscle (see Fig. 22-7). In patients with HF, endothelium-dependent NO-mediated dilation of the peripheral vasculature is blunted, which has been attributed to decreased NOS3 expression and activity. The actions of NO on the myocardium are complex and include both short-term alterations in function and energetics and longer-term effects on structure. NO modulates the activity of several key calcium channels involved in excitation contraction coupling, as well as mitochondrial respiratory complexes. This type of regulation is accomplished by spatial localization of different NOS isoforms in distinct cellular microdomains involved in excitation-contraction coupling. Specifically, NOS1 localizes to the sarcoplasmic reticulum in proximity to the ryanodine receptor and the SR Ca^{2+} ATPase (SERCA2a), and NOS3 is found in sarcolemmal caveolae compartmentalized with cell-surface receptors and the L-type Ca^{2+} channel.

Evidence indicates that the subcellular location of NO becomes disrupted in HF. In HF NOS3 relocalizes from the SR to the cell membrane, resulting in reduced localization with the ryanodine receptor and increased amounts of NOS3 localized to caveolin-3 in the cell membrane, in close proximity to the L-type Ca^{2+} channel. Consequently, NO can participate in abnormal excitation-contraction coupling by

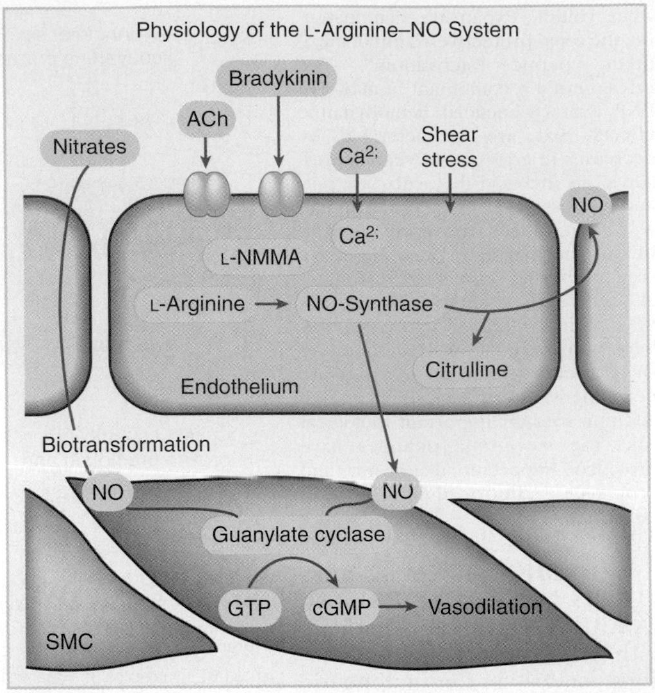

FIGURE 22–8 Physiology of the L-arginine-nitric oxide (NO) system. NO is synthesized in the endothelial cell from the amino-acid L-arginine by the endothelial NO synthase (NOS3). Following uptake into the vascular smooth muscle cell (SMC), NO stimulates guanylate cyclase to form cyclic guanosine monophosphate (cGMP), resulting in vasodilation. ACh = acetylcholine; GTP = guanosine triphosphate; L-NMMA = N^G-monomethyl-L-arginine. (See also Chap. 48.) *(From Drexler H, Hornig B: Role of the peripheral circulation and endothelial cell dysfunction.* In *Mann DL [ed]: Heart Failure: A Companion to Braunwald's Heart Disease. Philadelphia, Elsevier, 2004, pp 109-122.)*

increasing its inhibition of membrane voltage-dependent L-type Ca^{2+} channel, while reducing its favorable modulatory effects on calcium cycling in the SR (Fig. 22-9).[24] NO also participates in mitochondrial respiration, the process that fuels excitation-contraction coupling. The different NOS isoforms may also participate in the process of cardiac remodeling. LV remodeling was ameliorated and survival improved after MI in transgenic mice deficient in NOS2.[25] In contrast, overexpression of NOS3 resulted in improved remodeling after MI. These contrasting effects of NOS2 and NOS3 may reflect the differences in amount of NO produced, which is much higher with NOS2.

BRADYKININ. Kinins are vasodilators that are released from inactive protein precursors (kininogens) through the action of proteolytic enzymes termed ***kallikreins***. The biological actions of the kinins are mediated by binding to B_1 and B_2 receptors. Most cardiovascular actions are initiated by the B_2 receptor, which is distributed widely in tissues, where it binds bradykinin and kallidin. The B_1 receptor binds the metabolites of bradykinin and kallidin. Stimulation of the B_2 receptor leads to vasodilation, which is mediated by the activation of NOS3, phospholipase A2, and adenylyl cyclase. Studies suggest that bradykinin plays an important role in the regulation of vascular tone in HF.[26] The breakdown of bradykinin is catalyzed by ACE, so this enzyme not only leads to the formation of a potent vasoconstrictor (angiotensin II) but also mediates the breakdown of a vasodilator (bradykinin). The augmentation of bradykinin levels likely contributes to the beneficial actions of ACE inhibitors (see Chap. 25).

ADRENOMEDULLIN. Adrenomedullin is a 52-amino acid vasodilatory peptide that was originally discovered in human pheochromocytoma tissue. Subsequently, high levels of adrenomedullin immunoreactivity were detected in cardiac atrium and adrenal and pituitary glands, with lower levels detected in the ventricle, kidney, and vasculature.[27] Adrenomedullin binds to a number of G protein–coupled receptors including the calcitonin receptor-like receptor and one specific for the adrenomedullin peptide. Adrenomedullin receptors are present in multiple tissue beds, as well as both endothelial and vascular smooth muscle cells. Circulating concentrations of adrenomedullin are elevated in cardiovascular disease and HF in proportion to the severity of cardiac and hemodynamic impairment. There is increasing evidence that adrenomedullin may play a compensatory role in HF by offsetting the deleterious effects of excessive peripheral vasoconstriction. Administration of adrenomedullin in experimental and human HF leads to a decrease in blood pressure and cardiac filling pressures, improves cardiac output, and leads to improved renal function and suppression of plasma aldosterone.[27]

APELIN. Apelin is a recently discovered (1993) vasoactive peptide that is an endogenous ligand for the G protein–coupled receptor APJ. In the cardiovascular system, apelin elicits endothelium-dependent, NO-mediated vasorelaxation and reduces arterial blood pressure. In addition, apelin demonstrates potent inotropic activity without stimulating concomitant cardiac myocyte hypertrophy. Apelin also produces diuresis by inhibition of arginine vasopressin activity. In experimental animals, apelin concentrations are significantly lower in failing hearts and are increased following treatment with an angiotensin receptor blocker. Further, apelin levels are significantly reduced in HF patients when compared with controls and are significantly increased following cardiac resynchronization.

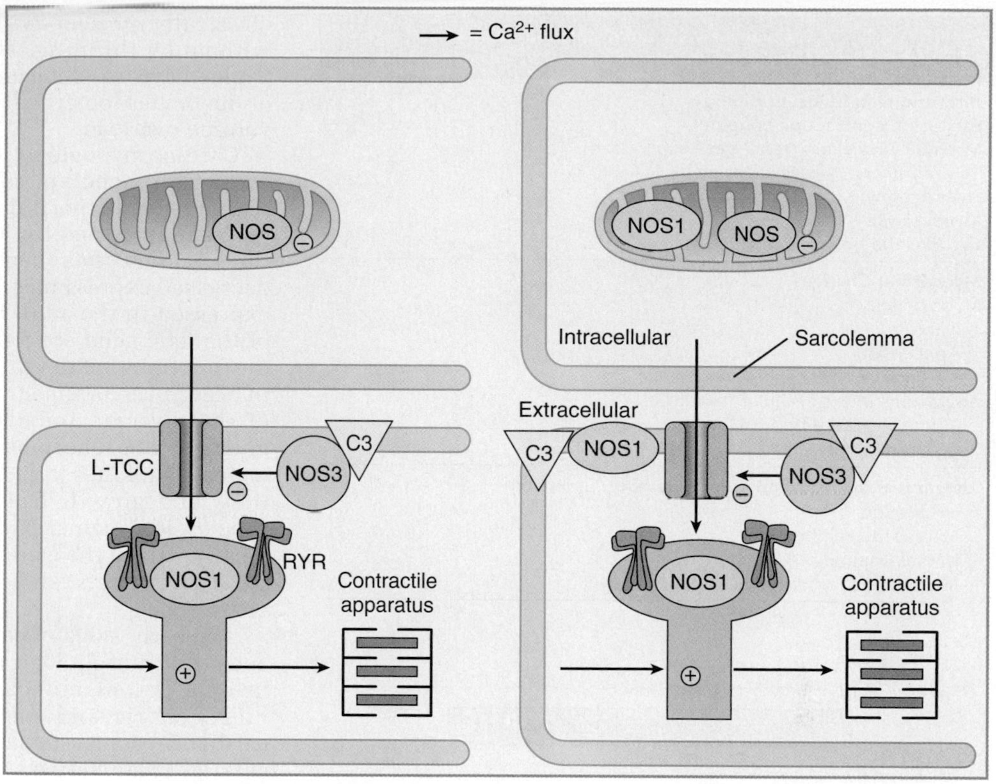

FIGURE 22–9 Potential mechanisms for NOS involvement in abnormal cardiac function in HF. **Left,** NOS1 is normally found in sarcoplasmic reticulum and NOS3 at cell membrane, bound to caveolin-3 (C3). **Right,** In HF, subcellular localization of NOS isoforms becomes disrupted. NOS1 translocates from sarcoplasmic reticulum to cell membrane, resulting in reduced amount bound to ryanodine receptor (RYR, also known as sarcoplasmic-reticulum Ca^{2+}-release channel) but increased amount associated with caveolin-3. Consequently, nitric oxide can participate in abnormal excitation-contraction coupling by increasing its inhibition of membrane voltage-dependent L-type Ca^{2+} channel (L-TCC) while reducing its favorable modulatory effects on calcium cycling in sarcoplasmic reticulum. If NOS1 were also to translocate to mitochondria, inhibition of energy production could contribute to reduced cardiac function. Plus or minus signs show direction of physiological effects of nitric oxide in each subcellular location. *(From Hare JM: Spatial confinement of isoforms of cardiac nitric-oxide synthase: Unravelling the complexities of nitric oxide's cardiobiology. Lancet 363:1338, 2004.)*

Is the neurohormonal model adequate to explain the progression of heart failure? Despite the many strengths of the neurohormonal model in terms of explaining disease progression and the many insights that neurohormonal models have provided in terms of drug development for HF, increasing clinical evidence suggests that our current neurohormonal models fail to completely explain disease progression in HF. That is, our current medical therapies for HF will stabilize HF, and in some cases reverse certain aspects of the disease process. However, in the overwhelming majority of patients HF will progress, albeit at a slower rate. Moreover, as HF progresses, many patients will be refractory and/or intolerant to conventional medical therapy and often require withdrawal of conventional medical therapies. In addition, many types of neurohormonal inhibition have been shown to be ineffective or even harmful in HF patients.[28] Although the precise mechanism(s) for this attenuation or loss of effectiveness of neurohormonal antagonism is not known, there is increasing evidence that progressive LV remodeling may lead to worsening HF, independent of the neurohormonal status of the patient.

Left Ventricular Remodeling

Natural history studies have shown that progressive LV remodeling is directly related to future deterioration in LV performance and a less favorable clinical course in patients with HF.[29] Although the complex changes that occur in the heart during LV remodeling have canonically been described in anatomical terms, the process of LV remodeling has an important effect on the biology of the cardiac myocyte, on changes in the volume of myocyte and nonmyocyte components of the myocardium, and on the geometry and architecture of the LV chamber (Table 22-1).

ALTERATIONS IN THE BIOLOGY OF THE CARDIAC MYOCYTE. Numerous studies have suggested that failing human cardiac myocytes undergo a number of important changes that might be expected to lead to a progressive loss of contractile function including decreased alpha-myosin heavy chain gene expression with a concomitant increase in beta-myosin heavy chain expression, progressive loss of myofilaments in cardiac myocytes, alterations in cytoskeletal proteins, alterations in excitation-contraction coupling, as well as desensitization of beta-adrenergic signaling (see Table 22-1).

CARDIAC MYOCYTE HYPERTROPHY. Two basic patterns of cardiac hypertrophy occur in response to hemodynamic overload (Fig. 22-10). In pressure overload hypertrophy (e.g., with aortic stenosis or hypertension), the increase in systolic wall leads to the addition of sarcomeres in parallel, an increase in myocyte cross-sectional area (Fig. 22-11), and increased LV wall thickening. This pattern of remodeling has been referred to as "concentric" hypertrophy (see Fig. 22-10). In contrast, in volume overload hypertrophy (e.g., with aortic and mitral regurgitation), increased diastolic

TABLE 22–1 Overview of Left Ventricular (LV) Remodeling
Alterations in Myocyte Biology
Excitation contraction coupling
Myosin heavy chain (fetal) gene expression
Beta-adrenergic desensitization
Hypertrophy
Myocytolysis
Cytoskeletal proteins
Myocardial Changes
Myocyte loss
Necrosis
Apoptosis
Autophagy
Alterations in extracellular matrix
Matrix degradation
Myocardial fibrosis
Alterations in Left Ventricular Chamber Geometry
LV dilation
Increased LV sphericity
LV wall thinning
Mitral valve incompetence

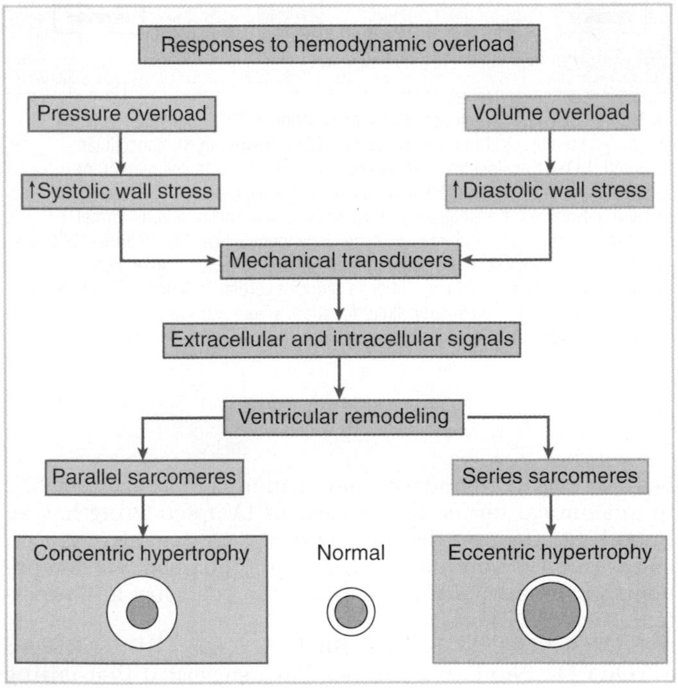

FIGURE 22–10 The pattern of cardiac remodeling that occurs in response to hemodynamic overloading depends on the nature of the inciting stimulus. When the overload is predominantly due to an increase in pressure (e.g., with systemic hypertension or aortic stenosis), the increase in systolic wall stress leads to the parallel addition of sarcomeres and widening of the cardiac myocytes, resulting in concentric cardiac hypertrophy. When the overload is predominantly due to an increase in ventricular volume, the increase in diastolic wall stress leads to the series addition of sarcomeres, lengthening of cardiac myocytes, and LV dilation, which is referred to as *eccentric chamber hypertrophy. (From Colucci WS [ed]: Heart Failure: Cardiac Function and Dysfunction. 2nd ed. Philadelphia, Current Medicine, 1999, p 4.2.)*

wall stress leads to an increase in myocyte length with the addition of sarcomeres in series (see Fig. 22-11), thereby engendering increased LV dilation (see Fig. 22-10). This pattern of remodeling has been referred to as "eccentric hypertrophy" (so named because of the position of the heart in the chest), or a "dilated" phenotype. Patients with HF classically present with a dilated left ventricle with or without LV thinning. The myocytes from these failing ventricles have an elongated appearance that is characteristic of myocytes obtained from hearts subjected to chronic volume overload.

Cardiac myocyte hypertrophy also leads to change in the biological phenotype of the myocyte that are secondary to reactivation of portfolios of genes that are normally not expressed postnatally. The reactivation of these fetal genes, the so-called "fetal gene program," is also accompanied by decreased expression of a number of genes that are normally expressed in the adult heart. As discussed later, activation of the fetal gene program may contribute to the contractile dysfunction that develops in the failing myocyte. As shown in Figure 21-26, the stimuli for the genetic reprogramming of the myocyte include mechanical stretch/strain of the myocyte, neurohormones (e.g., NE, angiotensin II), inflammatory cytokines (e.g., TNF, interleukin-6 [IL-6]), other peptides and growth factors (e.g., ET), and reactive oxygen species (e.g., superoxide, NO). These stimuli occur both locally within the myocardium, where they exert autocrine/paracrine effects, and systemically where they exert endocrine effects.

The early stage of cardiac myocyte hypertrophy is characterized morphologically by increases in the number of myofibrils and mitochondria, as well as enlargement of mitochondria and nuclei (Fig. 22-12). At this stage the cardiac myocytes are larger than normal and have preserved cellular organization. As hypertrophy continues, there is an increase in the number of mitochondria, as well as the addition of new contractile elements in localized areas of the cell. Cells subjected to longstanding hypertrophy show more obvious disruptions in cellular organization, such as markedly enlarged nuclei with highly lobulated membranes, accompanied by the displacement of adjacent myofibrils with loss of the normal registration of the Z-bands. The late stage of hypertrophy is characterized by loss of contractile elements (myocytolysis) with marked disruption of Z bands and severe disruption of the normal parallel arrangement of the sarcomeres, accompanied by dilation and increased tortuosity of T tubules (see Fig. 22-12).

ALTERATIONS IN EXCITATION-CONTRACTION COUPLING. As discussed in Chapter 21, excitation-contraction (EC) coupling refers to the cascade of biological events that begins with the cardiac action potential and ends with myocyte contraction and relaxation. Classic studies from explanted failing hearts have shown that patients with end-stage HF exhibit abnormal prolongation of the action potential, as well as depressed developed force and impaired relaxation.[30] The intracellular Ca^{2+} transient, as assessed by the fluorescent indicator fura-2, demonstrates a blunted rise following depolarization, reflecting slower delivery of Ca^{2+} to the contractile apparatus (causing slower activation), followed by a slowed rate of fall during repolarization (causing slowed relaxation). Changes in the abundance and/or phosphorylation state of critical Ca^{2+} regulatory proteins likely play an important role in the contractile dysfunction of failing cardiac myocytes.

SARCOPLASMIC RETICULUM IN THE FAILING HEART. The normal function of the sarcoplasmic reticulum (SR) is described in detail in Chapter 21. As shown in Table 22-2, a number of alterations in SR proteins/function occur in the failing heart. Given the central role for SERCA2A (sarcoendoplasmic reticulum Ca^{2+}) in excitation-contraction coupling, it has been suggested that the reduced activity of SERCA2A may play an important role in the pathogenesis of HF. Indeed, several (but not all) studies have reported that the levels of SERCA2A mRNA and protein are reduced in animal models of HF, as well as in myocardium samples obtained from patients with end-stage HF. The downregulation in SERCA2A expression was associated with a corresponding reduction in SR Ca^{2+} reuptake in some (but not all) in myo-

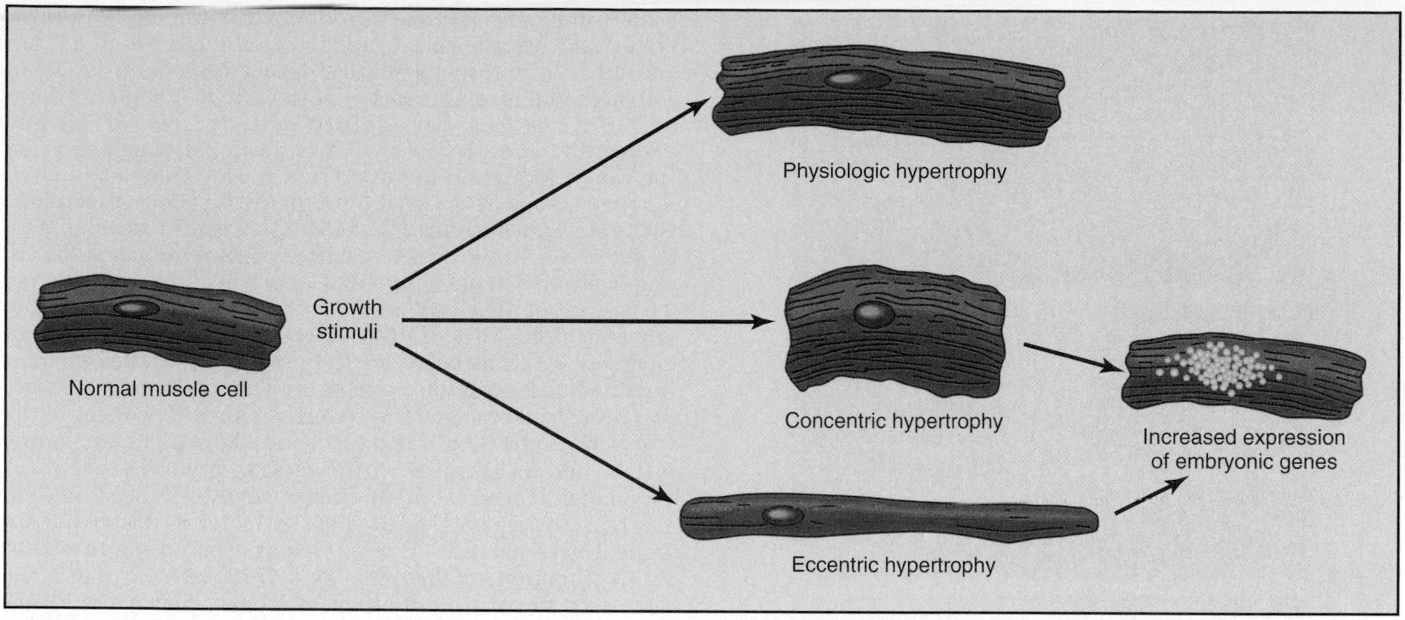

FIGURE 22–11 Morphology of cardiac myocytes in response to hemodynamic pressure and volume overloading. Phenotypically distinct changes occur in the morphology of myocyte in response to the type of hemodynamic overload that is superimposed. When the overload is predominantly due to an increase in pressure, the increase in systolic wall stress leads to the parallel addition of sarcomeres and widening of the cardiac myocytes. When the overload is predominantly due to an increase in ventricular volume, the increase in diastolic wall stress leads to the series addition of sarcomeres and thus lengthening of cardiac myocytes. The expression of maladaptive embryonic genes (see Table 22-2) is increased in both eccentric and concentric hypertrophy, but not in physiological myocyte hypertrophy that occurs with exercise. *(Modified from Hunter JJ, Chien KR: Signaling pathways for cardiac hypertrophy and failure. N Engl J Med 341:1276, 1999.)*

TABLE 22–2 Changes in the Biology of the Failing Myocyte

Protein	Change in Human Heart Failure
Plasma Membrane	
L-type calcium channels	Decreased*†
Sodium/calcium exchanger	Increased*†
Sodium pump	Reexpression of fetal isoforms
$Beta_1$-adrenergic receptor	Decreased*†
$Beta_2$-adrenergic receptor	Increased*
$Alpha_1$-adrenergic receptor	Increased*
Contractile Proteins	
Myosin heavy chain	Reversion to fetal isoform
Myosin light chain	Reversion to fetal isoform
Actin	Normal*
Troponin I	Normal*
Troponin T	Reversion to fetal isoform
Troponin C	Normal*
Tropomyosin	Normal*
Sarcoplasmic Reticulum	
SERCA2A	Normal or decreased*†
Phospholamban	Decreased*†
Ryanodine receptor	Decreased*†
Calsequestrin	Normal*
Calreticulin	Normal*

*Protein level.
†Functional activity.
Modified from Katz AM: Physiology of the Heart. Philadelphia, Lippincott Williams & Wilkins, 2001.

cardial samples obtained from patients with severe failure. This reduction in the abundance and/or functional activity of SERCA2A could explain the slow decay of the Ca^{2+} transient and the reduced SR Ca^{2+} storage and release that have been observed in failing myocytes.[30] Importantly, overexpression of SERCA2A improves myocardial performance in the senescent heart, prevents the development of HF following aortic banding, and improves the contractile performance of human cardiac myocytes taken from the explanted hearts of HF patients. However, SERCA2A abundance (or Ca^{2+} uptake rate) has also been reported to be normal in some failing hearts with depressed contractility, suggesting that there may also be functional abnormalities in other molecules that regulate SR function. For example, decreases in phospholamban phosphorylation and/or activity in the failing human heart could disrupt normal SR function or, alternatively, could exacerbate the effect of decreased SERCA abundance. As a case in point, studies in transgenic mice with a defect in muscle LIM protein ($MLP^{-/-}$), a structural protein involved in muscle development, develop a dilated cardiomyopathy that can be completely repaired by knocking out phospholamban.[31] Another mechanism that has been proposed relates to the "leakage" of the ryanodine receptor, which is closed during diastole and thus allows Ca^{2+} that is transported into the SR to accumulate until activation by the L-type Ca^{2+} leads to SR Ca^{2+} release. Studies in experimental models of HF and failing human myocardium suggest that ryanodine receptor is "hyperphosphorylated" by protein kinase A (PKA) and that this hyperphosphorylation increases the open probability of the ryanodine receptor, causing a persistent leak of Ca^{2+} from the SR.[32]

L-TYPE CALCIUM CHANNEL. The L-type calcium channel opens when the membrane depolarizes during the upstroke of the cardiac action potential. The subsequent Ca^{2+} influx helps to produce the plateau phase of the action potential and elevates $[Ca^{2+}]$ in the cytosol. Studies have shown that there is a reduction in the mRNA and protein levels and an increased level of phosphorylation of the L-type Ca^{2+} channels in HF.[30] Both of these abnormalities would reduce both the magnitude and homogeneity of the inward Ca^{2+} current and thus adversely affect SR Ca^{2+} release.

Na^+/Ca^{2+} EXCHANGER. Under normal conditions, Ca^{2+} enters myocytes from the extracellular space down a large electrochemical gradient. At a normal resting potential of −80 mV and with normal intracellular Na^+ levels, energy in the Na^+ electrochemical gradient is sufficient to remove approximately 20 percent of the Ca^{2+} from the cytoplasm via the Na^+/Ca^{2+} exchanger (forward mode conductance [see Chap. 21]). In HF mRNA, protein levels and activity levels of the Na^+/Ca^{2+} exchanger have been reported to be increased.[33] It has been suggested that the increased expression of the Na^+/Ca^{2+} exchanger compensates for decreased Ca^{2+} uptake because of the reduction in SERCA2A activity in HF. However, this seems unlikely to be the case in human HF, insofar as SERCA2A Ca^{2+} uptake occurs when forward mode conductance is minimal. Recently, it has been suggested that Ca^{2+} entry via reverse-mode Na^+/Ca^{2+} exchanger activity contributes to abnormal Ca^{2+} handling in HF.[33]

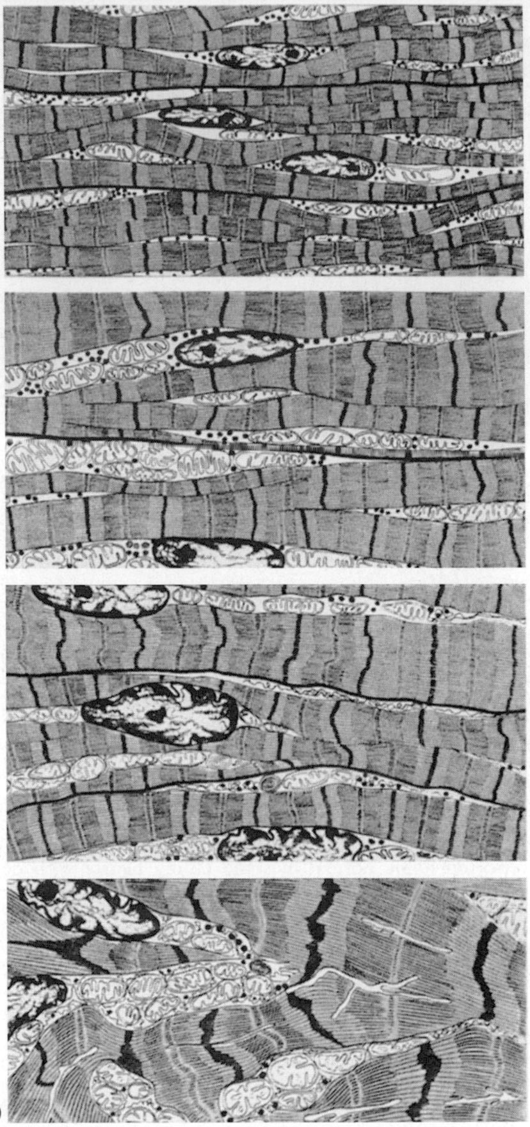

FIGURE 22–12 The early stage of cardiac hypertrophy **(A)** is characterized morphologically by increases in the number of myofibrils and mitochondria, as well as enlargement of mitochondria and nuclei. Muscle cells are larger than normal, but cellular organization is largely preserved. At a more advanced stage of hypertrophy **(B),** preferential increases in the size or number of specific organelles such as mitochondria, as well as irregular addition of new contractile elements in localized areas of the cell, result in subtle abnormalities of cellular organization and contour. Adjacent cells may vary in their degree of enlargement. Cells subjected to longstanding hypertrophy **(C)** show more obvious disruptions in cellular organization such as markedly enlarged nuclei with highly lobulated membranes, which displace adjacent myofibrils and cause breakdown of normal Z-band registration. The early preferential increase in mitochondria is supplanted by a predominance (by volume) of myofibrils. The late stage of hypertrophy **(D)** is characterized by loss of contractile elements with marked disruption of Z bands, severe disruption of the normal parallel arrangement of the sarcomeres, deposition of fibrous tissue, and dilation and increased tortuosity of T tubules. *(From Ferrans VJ: Morphology of the heart in hypertrophy. Hosp Pract 18:69, 1983. Copyright 1983, McGraw-Hill Companies, Inc.)*

ABNORMALITIES IN CONTRACTILE AND REGULATORY PROTEINS (see Table 22-2). Early studies showed that the activity of myofibrillar ATPase was reduced in the hearts of patients who died of HF. Furthermore, reductions in the activities of myofibrillar ATPase, actomyosin ATPase, or myosin ATPase have been demonstrated in several animal models of HF. Subsequent studies showed that these abnormalities in ATPase activity could be explained by a shift to the fetal isoform of myosin heavy chain (MHC) in cardiac hypertrophy and failure. In rodents the predominant MHC is the "fast" V1 isoform (alpha-MHC), which has high ATPase activity. With pressure-induced hypertrophy or after MI in rodents there is re-expression of the "slow" V3 fetal isoform of MHC that has low ATPase activity (beta-MHC) and decreased expression of the V1 isoform. Although translating this information to human HF proved to be more challenging, insofar as the predominant MHC isoform in humans is the slower V3 isoform (beta-MHC), with the development of the polymerase chain reaction, it has been possible to demonstrate that the alpha-MHC accounts for approximately 33 percent of MHC mRNA in normal human myocardium, whereas alpha-MHC mRNA abundance decreases to about 2 percent in failing heart. Further, in human studies wherein myocardial biopsies were obtained in patients who were receiving beta-blockers there were reciprocal changes in the levels of alpha-MHC (increase) and beta-MHC (decrease) mRNA and an increase in the ratio of alpha/beta-MHC in the patients who had an improvement in LV function, whereas these changes in myosin isoform shifts did not occur in HF patients in whom there was no improvement in LV function on beta-blockers (Fig. 22-13).[34] Thus the decreased expression of alpha-MHC may play a significant role in the pathophysiology of dilated cardiomyopathy. Another important modification of contractile proteins that contributes to contractile dysfunction is proteolysis of the myofilaments themselves (myocytolysis). Myocardial biopsy samples from patients with advanced LV dysfunction show a significant reduction in the volume of myofibrils per cell, which may contribute to the development of cardiac decompensation.

Alterations in the expression or activity, or both, of myofilament regulatory proteins has also been proposed as a potential mechanism for the decrease in cardiac contractile function in HF (see Table 22-2) including changes in the myosin light chains and the troponin-tropomyosin complex in HF. Changes in myosin light chain isoforms have been observed in the atria and ventricles of patients whose hearts have been subjected to mechanical overload. Although changes in the abundance and/or isoforms of TnI and TnC (see also Chap. 21) have not been reported in HF, isoform shifts have been reported in TnT. In normal adult myocardium, troponin T is expressed as a single isoform (cTnT3). However, in myocardium samples from patients with end-stage HF, both the fetal cTnT1 and the cTnT4 isoforms are expressed at increased levels, which might be expected to lead to a decrease in maximal active tension.[35]

ABNORMALITIES IN CYTOSKELETAL PROTEINS. The cytoskeleton of cardiac myocytes consists of actin, the intermediate filament desmin, the sarcomeric protein titin (see Chap. 21), and alpha- and beta-tubulin that form the microtubules by polymerization. Vinculin, talin, dystrophin, and spectrin represent a separate group of membrane-associated proteins. In numerous experimental studies the role of cytoskeletal and/or membrane-associated proteins has been implicated in the pathogenesis of HF. In patients with dilated cardiomyopathy, titin is downregulated, whereas the cytoskeletal proteins desmin and membrane-associated proteins such as vinculin and dystrophin are upregulated. Recently, proteolytic digestion of the dystrophin molecule was identified as a possible reversible cause of HF.[36] Loss of integrity of the cytoskeleton and its linkage of the sarcomere to the sarcolemma and extracellular matrix would be expected to lead to contractile dysfunction at the myocyte level, as well as at the myocardial level.

BETA-ADRENERGIC DESENSITIZATION (see Fig. 21-14). Ventricles obtained from HF patients demonstrate a marked reduction in beta-adrenergic receptor density, isoproterenol-mediated adenylyl cyclase stimulation, and the contractile response to beta-adrenergic agonists.[37] The downregulation of beta-adrenergic receptors is likely mediated by increased levels of NE in the vicinity of the receptor. In patients with dilated cardiomyopathy, this reduction in receptor density involves primarily the beta$_1$-receptor protein and mRNA, and is proportional to the severity of HF. In contrast, the level of beta$_2$-adrenergic receptor protein and mRNA are unchanged. In addition, there are increases in the expression of beta-adrenergic receptor kinase 1 (βARK1 [also called G protein–coupled receptor kinase 2]), a member of the family of G protein–coupled receptor kinases, in failing human hearts. As noted in Chapter 21, βARK phosphorylates the cytoplasmic loops of both beta$_1$- and beta$_2$-adrenergic receptors and increases the affinity of these receptors for a scaffolding protein termed *beta-arrestin* (see Fig. 21-14). The binding of beta-arrestins to the cytoplasmic tail of the beta-receptor not only uncouples the receptor from heterotrimeric G proteins but also targets the receptor for internalization in clathrin-coated vesicles. Although this internalization fosters receptor dephosphorylation and serves as a prelude to recycling the beta-receptor to the surface for reactivation, at some point receptor entry via endocytosis is not followed by recycling but rather leads to receptor trafficking to lysosomes and receptor degradation. Increased βARK activity may therefore contribute to the desensitization of both beta$_1$- and beta$_2$-adrenergic receptors in patients with HF. Desensitization of the beta-receptors can be both beneficial and deleterious in HF. By reducing LV contractility, desensitization may be deleterious; however, by reducing energy expenditure of the energy-starved myocardium and protecting the myocyte from the deleterious effects of sustained adrenergic stimulation, this adaptive response is beneficial. Of interest, transgenic mice that overexpress βARK are protected from developing HF.[38]

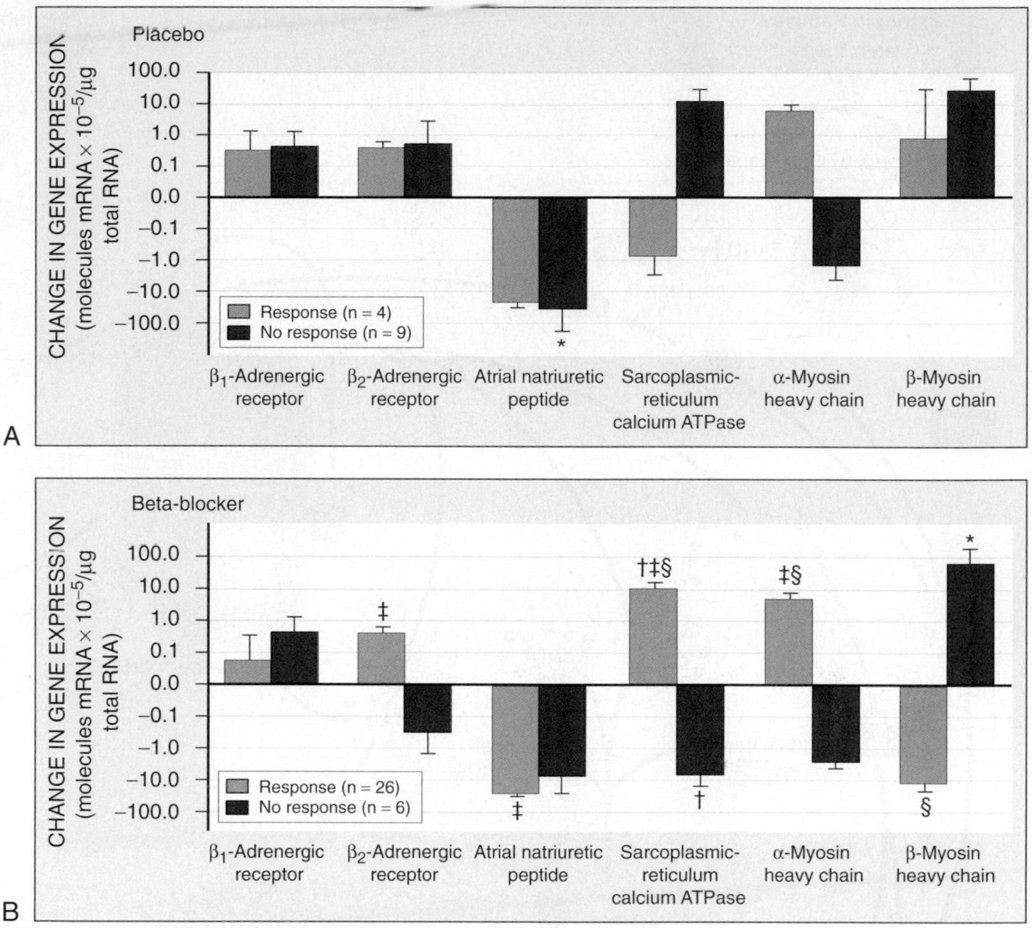

FIGURE 22–13 Changes in myocardial messenger RNA (mRNA) expression and beta-adrenergic receptor protein levels. **A** and **B,** Changes between baseline and the end of the 6-month study in the abundance of myocardial mRNA for six contractility-regulating or hypertrophy-regulating proteins in patients who received a placebo or beta blocker. The changes in patients who had an improvement in left ventricular ejection fraction (a "response," defined as an increase by at least five ejection fraction [EF] units) were compared with the changes in patients who did not have such a response. Gene expression is shown as molecules of mRNA per microgram of total RNA on a logarithmic scale. The asterisk indicates $p < 0.10$ for the change between the baseline value and the value measured at 6 months by the paired t-test, the daggers $p < 0.05$ for the comparison with the placebo group by the test for interaction, the double daggers $p < 0.05$ for the change between the baseline value and the value measured at 6 months by the paired t-test, and the section marks $p < 0.05$ for the comparison with patients who did not have a response. Each panel shows results for patients with complete data for the indicated mRNA and receptor protein measurements. *(From Lowes BD, Gilbert EM, Abraham WT, et al: Myocardial gene expression in dilated cardiomyopathy treated with beta blocking agents. N Engl J Med 346:1357, 2002.)*

ALTERATIONS IN THE MYOCARDIUM IN HEART FAILURE. The alterations that occur in failing myocardium may be categorized broadly into those that occur in the volume of cardiac myocytes and those that occur in the volume and composition of the extracellular matrix. With respect to the changes that occur in the cardiac myocyte component of the myocardium, increasing evidence suggests that progressive myocyte loss, through necrotic, apoptotic, or autophagic cell death pathways, may contribute to progressive cardiac dysfunction and LV remodeling.

NECROSIS. Necrosis is an "accidental" form of cell death that occurs following extreme myocyte injury. The hallmark of necrosis is cell rupture, which is generally preceded by distention of various cellular organelles, clumping, and random degradation of nuclear DNA and cell swelling, culminating in disruption of the plasma membrane barrier. In the heart, increased plasma membrane permeability allows calcium to leak into the cell, exposing the contractile proteins to high concentrations of this activator, which in turn initiates extreme interactions among the myofilaments (contraction-bands), further contributing to disruption of the cellular membrane. Necrotic myocyte death occurs in ischemic heart disease, myocardial injury, toxin exposure (e.g., daunorubicin [see Chap. 85]), infection, and inflammation. Neurohormonal activation can also lead to necrotic cell death. For example, concentrations of NE that are available within myocardial tissue, as well as in circulating levels in patients with advanced HF, are sufficient to provoke myocyte necrosis in experimental model systems. Moreover, excessive stimulation with either angiotensin II or ET has been shown to provoke myocyte necrosis in experimental models. Myocyte necrosis was sevenfold greater than apoptosis in explanted hearts from male and female HF patients. Interesting, necrotic cell death was twofold higher in men than in women.[39] Additional evidence for the existence of ongoing myonecrosis in patients with HF is suggested by studies showing that levels of circulating troponin I and T are increased significantly in patients with advanced HF. In contrast to apoptosis (see later), the rupture of cell membranes with cell necrosis releases intra-

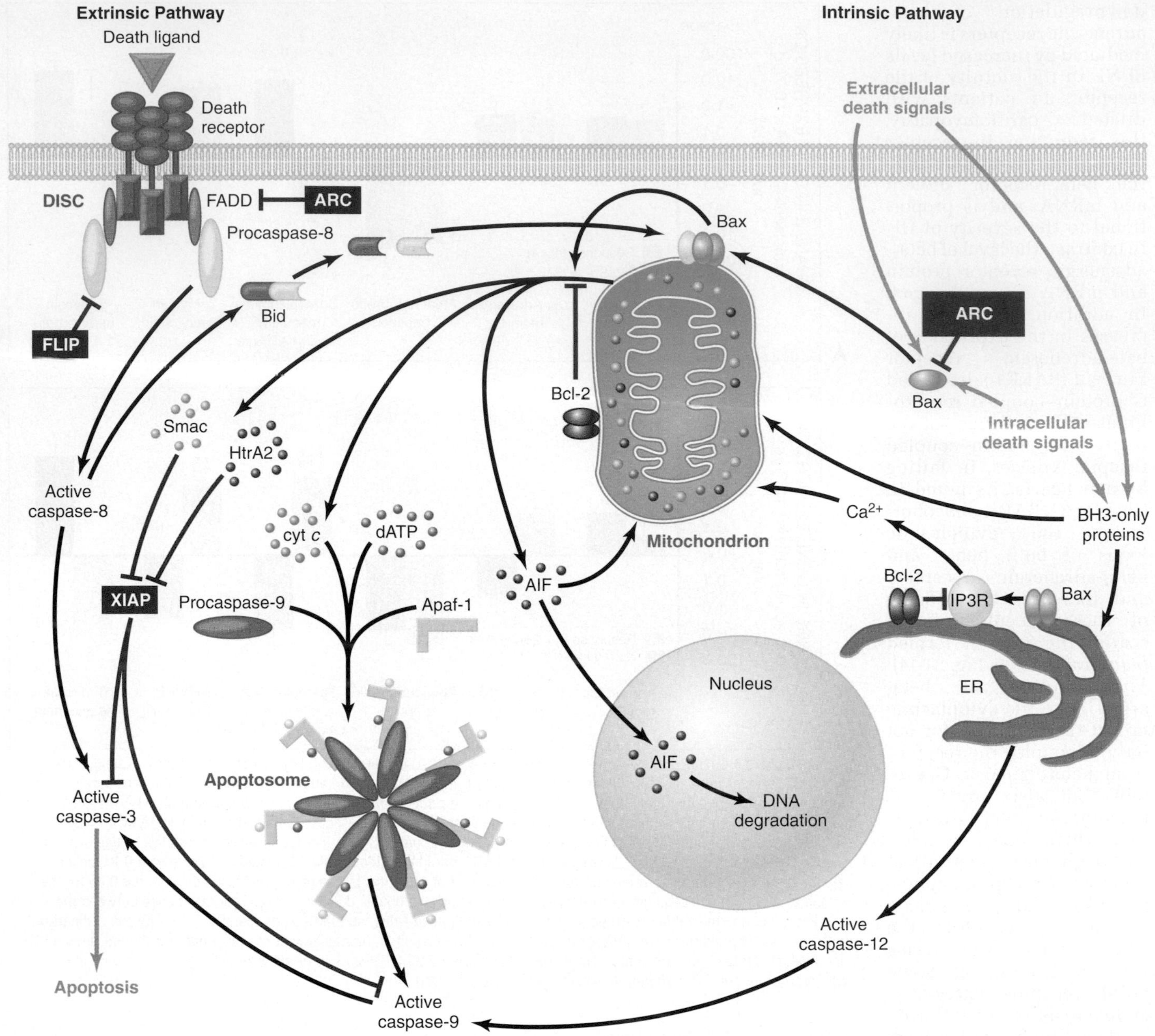

FIGURE 22–14 Intrinsic and extrinsic cell death pathways in cardiac myocytes. In the extrinsic pathway, ligand binding induces death receptors to recruit FADD, which recruits procaspase-8. Within this complex (DISC), procaspase-8 dimerizes and activates. Caspase-8 proteolytically activates procaspase-3, which cleaves cellular proteins causing cell death. In the intrinsic pathway, extracellular and intracellular stimuli signal to the mitochondria through a variety of BH3-only proteins (e.g., Bid) and through Bax, which translocates to and inserts into the outer mitochondrial membrane. Bax and Bak (not shown) stimulate the release of cytochrome c (cyt c) and other apoptogens. Once released, cytochrome c binds Apaf-1 along with dATP. This triggers oligomerization of Apaf-1 and recruitment of procaspase-9. Within this complex (apoptosome), procaspase-9 dimerizes and activates. Caspase-9 proteolytically activates procaspase-3. Caspase-8 also cleaves Bid, and its C-terminal fragment translocates to the mitochondria, where it activates Bax and Bak stimulating apoptogen release. Activation of the extrinsic pathway is prevented by the antiapoptotic proteins c-FLIP and ARC, whereas activation of the intrinsic pathway is prevented by the antiapoptotic proteins ARC, Bcl-2 or Bcl-X_L (not shown). The X-linked inhibitor of apoptosis (XIAP) blocks the activation of caspase 3. AIF translocates to the nucleus and, in conjunction with a presumed endonuclease, mediates large-scale DNA fragmentation in a caspase-independent manner. *(Modified from Foo RS, Mani K, Kitsis RN: Death begets failure in the heart. J Clin Invest 115:565, 2005.)*

cellular contents that evoke an intense inflammatory reaction, leading to the influx of granulocytes, macrophages, as well as collagen secreting fibroblasts into the area of injury. The final result is a fibrotic scar, which may alter the structural and functional properties of the myocardium (see later).

APOPTOSIS (Fig. 22-14). Apoptosis, or programmed cell death, is an evolutionarily conserved process that allows multicellular organisms to selectively remove cells through a highly orchestrated program of cell suicide. The ensemble of proteins that are responsible for activating apoptosis is preprogrammed into the genetic code of the cells that are destined to die. However, under pathological circumstances such as acute ischemia and/or in dilated cardiomyopathy, the apoptotic program can be triggered inappropriately, resulting in inadvertent cell death. Apoptosis requires energy and activation of specific biochemical steps that are involved in triggering and executing cell death through activation of "intrinsic" (mitochondrial) and "extrinsic" (death receptor mediated) pathways that lead to the activation of executioner caspases (see Fig. 22-14). In contrast to the cell swelling that characterizes necrosis, during apoptosis the cell shrinks and eventually breaks up into small, membrane-surrounded fragments. The latter often contain bits of condensed chromatin, referred to as apoptotic bodies. Maintenance of plasma membrane integrity until late in the apoptotic process allows the dying cell to be engulfed by macrophages, which prevents the release of the reactive intracellular contents, thereby preventing an inflammatory reaction. An important distinction between necrosis and apoptosis is the manner in which DNA is degraded. In necrosis, DNA is broken down into randomly sized fragments, whereas the endonuclease-mediated breakdown of DNA in apoptosis leads to the generation of multiples of 180 to 200 base pair fragments that resemble a ladder ("DNA laddering") when they are run out on electrophoretic gels. Another characteristic feature of apoptosis is that the type of DNA cleavage that occurs has a characteristic single 3′ overhang, which can be detected readily by a number of molecular probes (see later).

The gold standard for identification of apoptotic cells is ultrastructural evidence of chromatin condensation, the earliest characteristic morphological feature. However, although ultrastructural evidence of chromatin condensation is highly reliable, the routine use of electron microscopy to detect chromatin condensation is impractical because it is labor intensive and costly. The terminal deoxynucleotidyl transferase (TUNEL) method is the most widely used technique because the microscopic evaluation of myocardial samples is relatively easy and inexpensive (see Fig. 22-e3 on website). The TUNEL method uses a molecular probe that anneals to DNA with double-strand breaks characteristic of apoptosis (i.e., with 3′ overhangs). The Taq polymerase method follows a similar principle.[40] However, the TUNEL technique not only labels apoptotic nuclei but also necrotic and oncotic nuclei, as well as nuclei undergoing DNA repair. Similar limitations apply to the Taq polymerase method, albeit to a lesser extent.

Cardiac myocyte apoptosis has been shown to occur in failing human hearts.[41] Indeed, many factors that have been implicated in the pathogenesis of HF including catecholamines acting through $beta_1$-adrenergic receptor, angiotensin II, reactive oxygen species, NO, inflammatory cytokines, and mechanical strain, have been shown to trigger apoptosis in vitro. Moreover, activation of either the extrinsic[42] or intrinsic[43] cell death pathways provokes progressive LV dilation and decompensation in transgenic mice. Nonetheless, the exact physiological significance and consequence(s) of apoptosis in human HF have been difficult to determine because of the tremendous uncertainty with respect to the actual rate of cardiac myocyte apoptosis in the failing human heart (reviewed in reference 40). This statement notwithstanding, the aggregate clinical and experimental data suggest that apoptosis is likely to play an important role in HF.

AUTOPHAGY. Autophagy refers to the homeostatic cellular process of sequestering organelles and long-lived proteins in a double-membrane vesicle inside the cell (autophagosome), where the contents are subsequently delivered to the lysosome for degradation. When autophagy involves the total destruction of the cell, it is referred to as autophagic cell death. Recent studies have demonstrated the existence of autophagic cell death in hypertrophied, failing, and hibernating myocardium.[44] Approximately 0.3 percent of the cardiac myocytes in explanted hearts from patients with HF exhibited autophagic cell death,[45] whereas the predominant form of cell death in pressure-overloaded human hearts was mainly by autophagy and oncosis.[46]

The distinction between necrosis and apoptosis is obvious in certain circumstances, whereas the dividing line between these two conditions is often less clear in the failing heart. And indeed, similar mechanisms can operate in both types of cell death. For example, cell death that begins as apoptosis can also lead to necrosis if the decline in adenosine triphosphate (ATP) content results in cell rupture (secondary necrosis) before the cell can be engulfed by macrophages. Moreover, cardiac myocytes can undergo either necrotic or apoptotic cell death in response to different stimuli (e.g., NE). Ultimately, what determines cell fate in the failing heart is the intensity and/or rapidity of the injury, the expression levels of the downstream proapoptotic and antiapoptotic proteins, as well as the extent of the calcium overload and the intracellular ATP levels. Thus instead of the existence of distinct types of cell death in HF, there is likely a continuum of cell death responses that contribute to progressive myocyte loss and disease progression.

Changes within the extracellular matrix (ECM) constitute the second important myocardial adaptation that occurs during cardiac remodeling. The myocardial ECM consists of a basement membrane, a fibrillar collagen network that surrounds the myocytes, proteoglycans and glycosaminoglycans, and biologically active signaling molecules. The major fibrillar collagens in the heart are types I and III, with the ratio of type I to type III of approximately 1.3 : 1 to 1.9 : 1. The organization of myocardial fibrillar types I and III collagen ensures the structural integrity of adjoining myocytes and is essential for maintaining alignment of myofibrils within the myocyte through the interaction of collagen, integrins, and the cytoskeleton (Fig. 22-15). During cardiac remodeling, important changes in the ECM include changes in fibrillar collagen synthesis and degradation (Fig. 22-16), changes in the degree of collagen cross-linking, as well as loss of collagen struts that connect the individual cardiac myocytes.[47] Markers of collagen turnover have been shown to be increased in patients with dilated cardiomyopathy compared with age-matched control subjects.[47] In patients with idiopathic or ischemic dilated cardiomyopathy, serum N-terminal type III collagen peptide (PIIINP) levels have

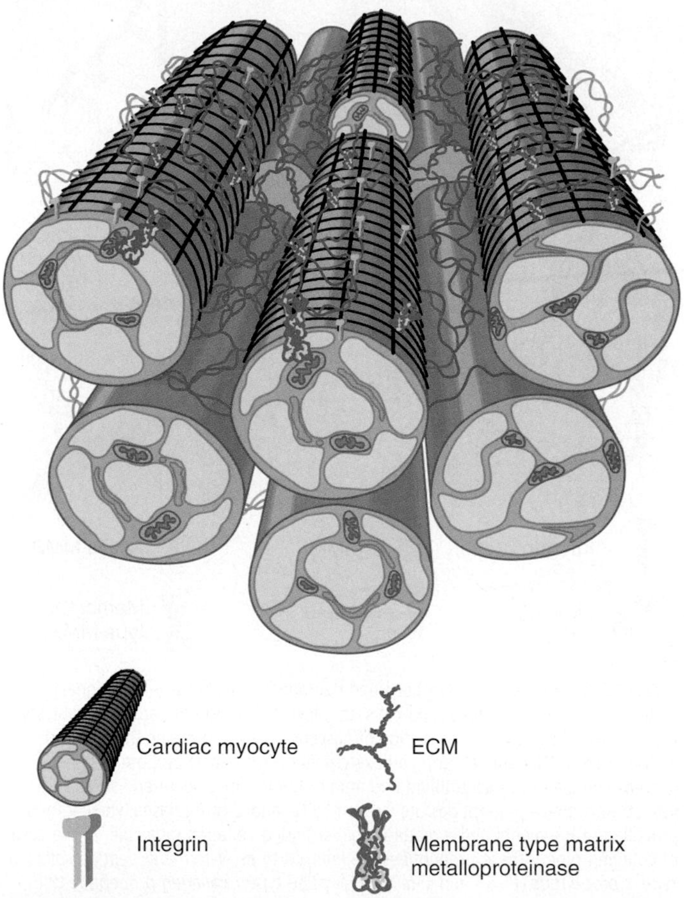

FIGURE 22–15 Relationship between the fibrillar collagen extracellular matrix and cardiac myocytes. The myocytes are interconnected by a complex of fibrillar collagen weave and extracellular matrix proteins, such as fibronectin. As shown, the myocyte adheres to the ECM through a family of transmembrane proteins referred to as integrins. Integrins are comprised of alpha and beta subunits that each contain a single transmembrane domain. The engagement of the integrins allows for the transduction of sarcomere shortening into myocyte shortening, which in turn facilitates muscle fiber shortening. In addition, the integrins form an important intracellular signaling role by activation of intracellular signaling pathways. The membrane type MMP (MT-MMP) is an important proteolytic enzyme that is responsible for ECM degradation/remodeling. As shown, MT-MMPs may colocalize with the integrins. The activation of the MT-MMPs may cause local ECM degradation and in turn alter the degree of integrin engagement and ultimately intracellular signaling pathways. *(Modified from Deschamps AM, Spinale FG: Extracellular matrix. In Walsh RA [ed]: Molecular Mechanisms of Cardiac Hypertrophy and Failure. Boca Raton, Fla., Taylor & Francis, 2005, pp 101-116.)*

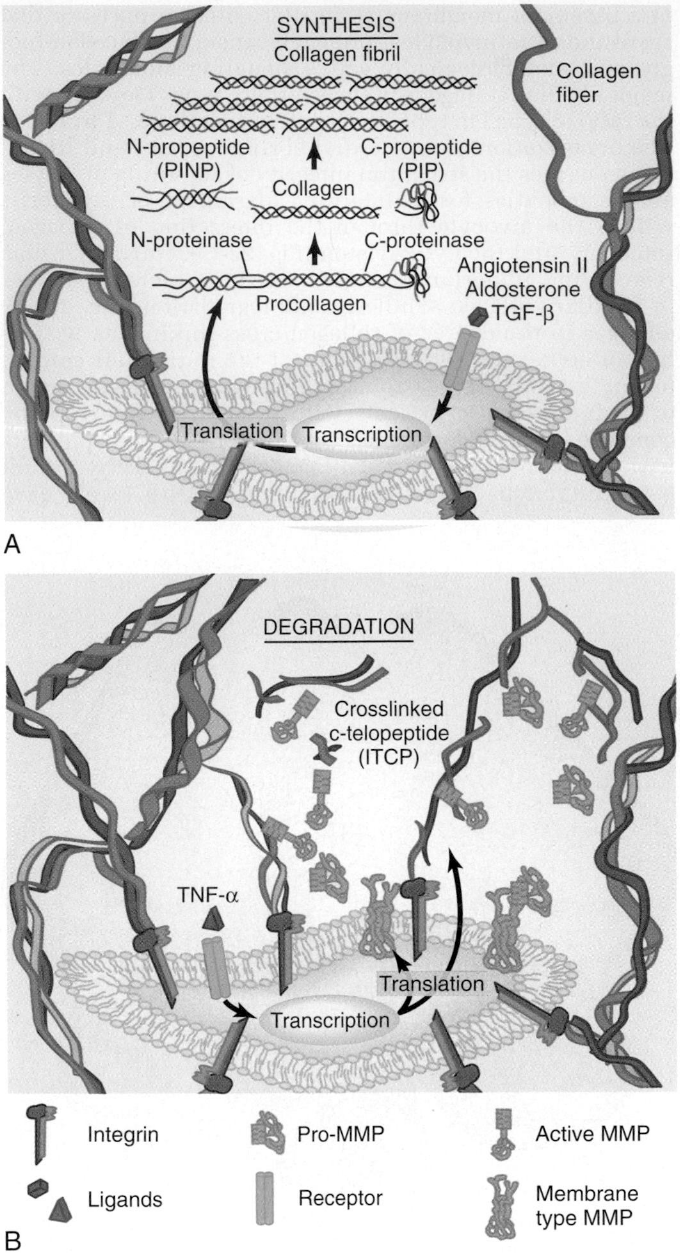

FIGURE 22–16 Collagen synthesis and degradation. **A,** Intracellular signals generated by neurohormonal and/or mechanical stimulation of cardiac fibroblasts result in transcription and translation of nascent collagen proteins that contain aminoterminal (N-terminal) and carboxyterminal (C-terminal) propeptides that prevent collagen from assembling into mature fibrils. Once secreted into the interstitium, these propeptides are cleaved by N- and C-proteinases, yielding two procollagen fragments and a mature triple-stranded collagen molecule. In the case of collagen type I, these propeptides are referred to as *N-terminal peptide collagen type 1 propeptide* (PINP) and *C-terminal peptide type I collagen propeptide* (PIP). Removal of the propeptide sequences allows the secreted collagen molecule to integrate into growing collagen fibrils, which can then further assemble into collagen fibers. After the collagen fibrils form in the extracellular space, their tensile strength is greatly strengthened by the formation of covalent cross-links between the lysine residues on the collagen molecules. **B,** The degradation of the collagen matrix within the myocardium involves a number of biochemical events involving a number of protease systems. Degradation of collagen fibrils occurs through catalytic cleavage of the 3 collagen alpha-chains at a single locus by interstitial collagenase, yielding 36-kDa and 12-kDa collagen telopeptides that maintain their helical structure and hence are resistant to further proteolytic degradation. The big 36-kDa telopeptide spontaneously denatures into nonhelical gelatin derivatives, which in turn are completely degraded by interstitial gelatinases. The small 12-kDa pyridinoline cross-linked C-terminal telopeptide resulting from the cleavage of collagen type I (ICTP) is found intact in blood, where it appears to be derived from tissues with a stoichiometric ratio of 1 : 1 between the number of collagen type I molecules degraded and that of ITCP released. *(From Deschamps AM, Spinale FG: Extracellular matrix.* In *Walsh RA [ed]: Molecular Mechanisms of Cardiac Hypertrophy and Failure. Boca Raton, Fla., Taylor & Francis, 2005, pp 101-116.)*

been shown to be independent predictors of mortality.[48] In the RALES trial (see Chap. 25), serum PIP and PIIINP were assessed at baseline and at 6 months. At 6 months both PIIINP and PINP were decreased in the spironolactone-treated patients, whereas they were increased or unchanged in the placebo group, suggesting that aldosterone may play an important role in ECM synthesis.

CARDIAC FIBROBLASTS AND MAST CELLS. The cardiac fibroblast, which comprises the vast majority (>90 percent) of nonmyocyte cells in the heart, is the primary cell type that is responsible for the secretion of the majority of ECM components in the heart such as collagens I, III, and IV; laminin; and fibronectin. In response to mechanical stress and/or neurohormonal activation, a subset of fibroblasts undergo phenotypic conversion to myofibroblasts that are characterized by increased expression of alpha smooth muscle actin and enhanced secretory activity. Myofibroblasts migrate into the area surrounding tissue injury, where they are responsible for the collagen secretion and contraction/realignment of the nascent collagen fibors and thus play an important role in the final scar formation at the site of injury. Increasing evidence indicates that mast cells, which are bone marrow–derived cells that "home" to and reside in the myocardium, also play an important role in remodeling of the ECM. Myocardial mast cells are located mainly around blood vessels and among myocytes, where they are capable of releasing profibrotic cytokines and growth factors that influence ECM remodeling. Experimental studies have shown that mast cell proliferation and degradation contribute to the remodeling process.[49]

As noted earlier, one of the histological signatures of advancing HF is the progressive increase in collagen content of the heart (myocardial fibrosis). Studies in failing human myocardium have shown that there is a quantitative increase in collagens I, III, VI, and IV; fibronectin; laminin; and vimentin and that the ratio of type I to type III collagen is decreased in patients with ischemic cardiomyopathy. Moreover, clinical studies suggest that there is a progressive loss of cross-linking of collagen in the failing heart, as well as loss of connectivity of the collagen network with individual myocytes, which would be expected to result in profound alterations in LV structure and function. Further, loss of cross-linking of the fibrillar collagen has been associated with progressive LV dilation following myocardial injury. The accumulation of collagen can occur on a "reactive" basis around intramural coronary arteries and arterioles (perivascular fibrosis) or in the interstitial space (interstitial fibrosis), and does not require myocyte cell death (Fig. 22-17). Alternatively, collagen accumulation can occur as a result of microscopic scarring (replacement fibrosis) that develops in response to cardiac myocyte cell necrosis. This scarring or "replacement fibrosis" is an adaptation to the loss of parenchyma and is therefore critical to preserve the structural integrity of the heart. The increased fibrous tissue would be expected to lead to increased myocardial stiffness, which would presumably result in decreased myocardial shortening for a given degree of afterload. In addition, myocardial fibrosis may provide the structural substrate for atrial and ventricular arrhythmias, thus potentially contributing to sudden death (see Chap. 31). Although the full complement of molecules that are responsible for fibroblast activation are not known, many of the classical neurohormones (e.g., angiotensin II, aldosterone) and cytokines (ET, transforming growth factor-beta [TGF-beta], cardiotrophin-1) that are expressed in HF are sufficient to provoke fibroblast activation. And indeed, the use of ACE inhibitors, beta-blockers, and aldosterone receptor antagonists has been associated with a decrease in myocardial fibrosis in experimental HF models.[1]

Although the fibrillar collagen matrix was initially considered to form a relatively static complex, it is now recognized that these structural proteins can undergo rapid turnover. One of the more exciting developments with respect to understanding the pathogenesis of cardiac remodeling has been the discovery that a family of collagenolytic enzymes, collectively referred to as *matrix metalloproteinases* (MMPs), are activated within the failing myocardium. Conceptually, disruption of the extracellular matrix would be expected to lead to LV dilation and wall thinning as a result of mural realignment ("slippage") of myocyte bundles and/or individual myocytes within the left ventricular wall (see Fig. 22-e4 on website), as well as LV dysfunction as a result of dyssynchronous contraction of the left ventricle. While the precise biochemical triggers that are responsible for activation of MMPs are not known, it bears emphasis that TNF, as well as other cytokines and peptide growth factors that are expressed within the failing myocardium are capable of activating MMPs. However, the biology of matrix remodeling in HF is likely to be much more complex than the simple presence or absence of MMP activation, insofar as degradation of the matrix is also controlled by glycoproteins termed "tissue inhibitors of matrix metalloproteinases" (TIMPs), that are capable of regulating the activation of MMPs by binding to and preventing these enzymes from degrading the collagen matrix of the heart. The TIMP family presently consists of four distinct members, known as TIMP-1, -2, -3 and -4, each of which is constitutively expressed in the heart by fibroblasts, as well as myocytes. TIMPs-1, -2, - 3, -4 are secreted proteins that act as the natural inhibitors of active forms of all MMPs, although the efficiency of MMP inhibition varies among the different members.

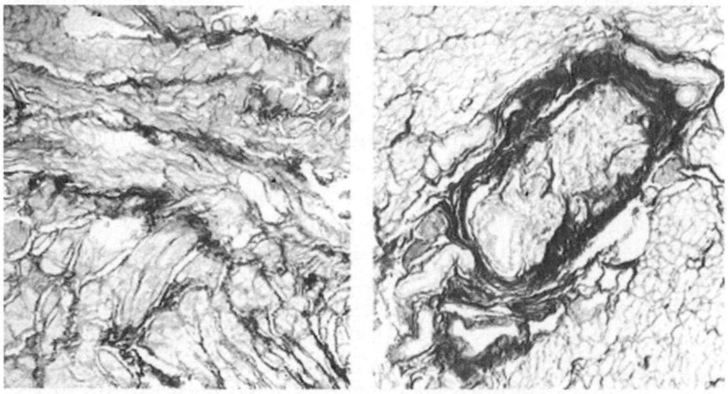

FIGURE 22–17 Myocardial fibrosis. Histological section of a human myocardial biopsy specimen showing **(A)** interstitial and **(B)** perivascular fibrosis using picrosirius red staining. *(Modified from Lopez B, Gonzales A, Varo N, et al: Biochemical assessment of myocardial fibrosis in hypertensive heart disease. Hypertension 38:1222, 2001.)*

MATRIX METALLOPROTEINASES. The matrix metalloproteinases (MMPs) represent a family of zinc-dependent proteases that play an important role in normal tissue remodeling, as well as in pathological processes such as inflammation, tumor invasion, and metastasis. The MMPs are secreted as inactive zymogens that must be activated by cleavage of the N-terminal sequence of the propeptide domain, which allows the Zn^{2+} binding site of the catalytic domain to become exposed. The exception is membrane-type 1 MMP (MT1-MMP), which is cell-surface bound and processed before cell-surface localization by a furin-dependent mechanism. The MMPs can be classified into subgroups on the basis of substrate specificity or structure, or both (Table 22-3). This classification includes the collagenases (e.g., MMP-1 and MMP-13), the stromelysins (e.g., MMP-3), the gelatinases (e.g., MMP-9 and MMP-2), and the membrane-type MMPs (MT-MMPs). Once activated, the MMPs are capable of degrading all of the ECM components.[50] Myocardial MMP abundance and activation have been assessed in end-stage human HF (see Table 22-3).[50] Although the majority of MMP species are increased in HF (see Table 22-3), the abundance of MMP-1 is significantly reduced in HF patients.[50] Furthermore, different levels of MMP-2 abundance and activity have been observed in CHF myocardium of ischemic or nonischemic origin. Loss of TIMP-mediated inhibitory control has been suggested as a reason for enhanced MMP activity in patients with dilated cardiomyopathy, in whom a reduction in relative myocardial levels of TIMP-1 and TIMP-3 and/or alterations in MMP/TIMP binding have been reported. This disparity between MMP and TIMP levels favors a persistent MMP activation, enhanced ECM proteolysis, and progressive LV dilation.[50] The role of MMP inhibition in the postinfarction setting was examined in humans in the PREMIER (Prevention of Myocardial Infarction Early Remodeling) trial, in which 253 patients with ST-segment elevation MI and an EF between 15 and 40 percent were randomized in a 1 : 1 ratio to placebo or an MMP inhibitor (PG-116800) with high affinity for MMP-1, -3, -8, -9, -13 and -14. In this small study MMP inhibition failed to reduce LV remodeling or improve clinical outcomes after MI. The failure to show a benefit may have been related to inadequate dosing of the MMP inhibitor.[51]

ALTERATIONS IN THE LEFT VENTRICULAR STRUCTURE IN HEART FAILURE. The aforementioned changes in the biology of the failing myocyte, as well as in the failing myocardium, are largely responsible for the progressive LV dilation and LV dysfunction that occur during cardiac remodeling. As discussed later, many of the structural changes in LV remodeling may contribute to worsening HF (see Table 22-e2 on website). Indeed, one of the first observa-

TABLE 22–3 Classes of Matrix Metalloproteinases (MMPs) That Have Been Identified in Human Myocardium

Name	Number	Substrate/Function	Abundance/Activity in Heart Failure
Collagenase		Collagens I, II, III, VII; and basement membrane components	
Interstitial collagenases	MMP-1		Decreased
Collagenase 3	MMP-13	Collagens I, II, III	Increased
Neutrophil collagenase	MMP-8	Collagens I, II, III; and basement membrane components	
Gelatinase			
Gelatinase A	MMP-2	Gelatins; collagens I, IV, V, VII and basement membrane components	Increased/unchanged
Gelatinase B	MMP-9	Gelatins; collagens IV, V, XIV; and basement membrane components	Increased
Stromelysin			
Stromelysin 1	MMP-3	Fibronectin; laminin; collagens III, IV, IX; and MMP activation	Increased
Membrane-type MMP			
MT1-MMP	MMP-14	Collagens I, II, III; fibronectin; laminin-1; activates pro-MMP-2 and pro-MMP-13	Increased

Modified from Deschamps AM, Spinale FG: Extracellular matrix. *In* Walsh RA (ed): Molecular Mechanisms of Cardiac Hypertrophy and Failure. Boca Raton, Fla., Taylor & Francis, 2005, pp 101-116.

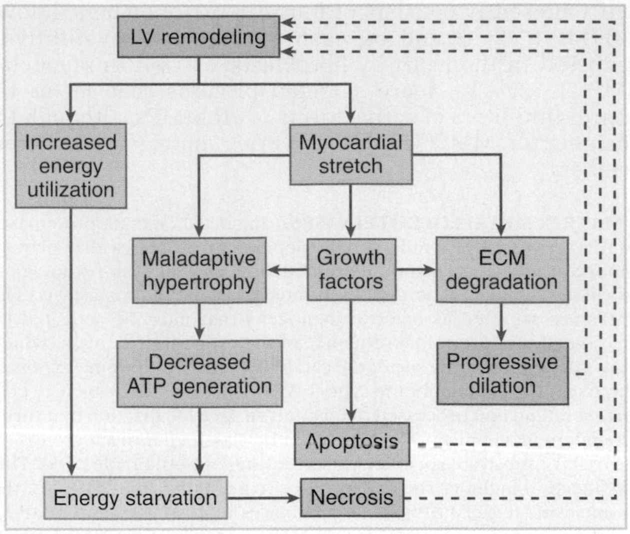

FIGURE 22–18 Self-amplifying nature of left ventricular (LV) remodeling. LV remodeling results in increased afterload on the heart, which increases energy utilization and further stimulates cardiac growth through stretch-mediated activation of growth factors. The former contributes directly to a state of energy starvation, whereas the latter contributes to further cardiac remodeling including increased myocyte hypertrophy and further matrix remodeling. The sustained activation of growth stimuli also promotes apoptosis and myocardial fibrosis, which contribute to LV dysfunction and LV remodeling. ATP = adenosine triphosphate; ECM = extracellular matrix. *(Modified from Katz AM: Heart Failure. Philadelphia, Lippincott Williams & Wilkins, 2000.)*

tions with respect to the abnormal geometry of remodeled ventricle was the consistent finding that the remodeled heart was not only larger but also more spherical in shape.[29] Of note is the change in LV shape from a prolate ellipse to a more spherical shape that results in an increase in meridional wall stress of the left ventricle, thereby creating a de novo energetic burden for the failing heart (see Fig. 22-e5 on website). Inasmuch as the load on the ventricle at end diastole contributes importantly to the afterload that the ventricle faces at the onset of systole, it follows that LV dilation itself will increase mechanical energy expenditure of the ventricle, which exacerbates the underlying problems with energy utilization in the failing ventricle (Fig. 22-18).

CARDIAC ENERGETICS. Studies of myocardial ATP concentrations in humans with end-stage cardiomyopathy have shown that the total adenine nucleotide pool (ATP, AMP, and AMP), creatine kinase (CK) activity (required for synthesis of ATP), the concentrations of creatine phosphate (CrP), and the CPr/ATP ratio are all decreased. In addition, decreased levels of creatine phosphokinase have been reported, which would slow phosphocreatine shuttle and thereby further exacerbate energy utilization in the failing heart. Although several mechanisms have been proposed to explain the fall in ATP content in HF, the one that has received the most recent attention relates to changes in substrate utilization in HF. Under normal conditions, the adult heart derives most of its energy through oxidation of fatty acids in mitochondria. The genes involved in this key energy metabolic pathway are transcriptionally regulated by members of the nuclear receptor superfamily, specifically the fatty acid–activated peroxisome proliferator activated receptors (PPARs) and the nuclear receptor coactivator, PPARgamma coactivator-1alpha (PGC-1alpha). In experimental HF models there is an initial decrease in the oxidation of fatty acids secondary to downregulation of fatty acid metabolizing genes, as well as decreased glucose metabolism, with an overall shift toward glycolytic metabolism.[52] Of interest, the use of partial fatty acid oxidase inhibitors (PFox) has led to an improvement in patient functional class, exercise capacity, quality of life, and ejection fraction when compared with standard HF therapy alone, suggesting that the shift to glycolytic metabolism may be beneficial in HF (see also Chap. 29).[53] In addition to loss of substrate, ATP generation may be impaired in the failing heart secondary to decreased capillary density, which can lead to hypoxia because of the increased diffusion distance of oxygen to reach the core fibers in muscle. Reduced coronary artery flow reserve can also contribute to the imbalance between energy production and consumption, especially in underperfused subendocardial regions of the ventricle. Finally, it has been suggested that a decrease in the free energy of ATP hydrolysis and a reduction in the allosteric effects of high ATP concentrations are also likely to be important in the energy starvation of the failing heart. That is, in addition to providing energy for contraction, ATP exerts important regulatory effects that accelerate ion pumps and ion exchangers and inhibit interactions between the actin and myosin filaments. These allosteric effects of ATP occur at higher concentrations than those at which it serves as a substrate, so modest declines in AT levels observed in the failing heart may be of pathophysiological significance.

In addition to the increase in LV end-diastolic volume, LV wall thinning also occurs as the ventricle begins to remodel. The increase in wall thinning, along with the increase in afterload created by LV dilation, leads to a functional "afterload mismatch" that may further contribute to a decrease in forward cardiac output. Increased LV wall stress can also lead to sustained expression of stretch-activated genes (angiotensin II, ET, and TNF) and/or stretch activation of hypertrophic signaling pathways. Moreover, the high end-diastolic wall stress might be expected to lead to episodic hypoperfusion of the subendocardium with resultant worsening of LV function, as well as increased oxidative stress, with the resultant activation of families of genes that are sensitive to free radical generation (e.g., TNF and IL-1beta). Another important mechanical problem that results from progressive LV dilation is that the papillary muscles are pulled apart, resulting in incompetence of the mitral valve and development of functional mitral regurgitation. Apart from the more obvious problem of loss of forward blood flow, mitral regurgitation results in further hemodynamic volume overloading of the ventricle. Taken together, the mechanical burdens engendered by LV remodeling might be expected to lead to increased LV dilation, decreased forward cardiac output, and increased hemodynamic overloading (see Fig. 22-18), any or all of which are sufficient to contribute to worsening LV function independently of the neurohormonal status of the patient.

INFLAMMATORY MEDIATORS. One of the recent conceptual advances with respect to our understanding of the pathogenesis of HF has been the insight that proinflammatory cytokines, such as TNF and IL-1, may contribute to the progressive cardiac remodeling that occurs in HF. Proinflammatory cytokines have traditionally been thought to be produced by the immune system, but it is now recognized that these molecules are produced locally within the myocardium by cells that reside within the myocardium including cardiac myocytes in direct response to one or more different forms of cardiac injury. Although the primary role for these molecules is to initiate repair of the injured myocardium, when expressed for protracted periods of time and/or when expressed at high levels, these molecules are sufficient to recapitulate virtually all aspects of the HF phenotype, by provoking deleterious changes in cardiac myocytes and nonmyocytes, as well as changes in the myocardial extracellular matrix (Table 22-4).[54] Moreover, in experimental models there is substantial cross-talk between proinflammatory cytokines and RAS, such that angiotensin II upregulates the expression of TNF through an NF-κB dependent pathway, and the expression of inflammatory mediators leads to upregulation of RAS through increased activation of myocardial ACE and chymase. Circulating levels of proinflammatory cytokines including TNF and interleukin-6 are increased in patients with HF and correlate with adverse patient outcomes.[55] Conversely, the plasma concentrations of antiinflammatory cytokines such as IL-10 are reduced in patients with HF and are decreased more in

TABLE 22–4	Effects of Inflammatory Mediators on Left Ventricular Remodeling
Alterations in the Biology of the Myocyte	
Myocyte hypertrophy	
Fetal gene expression	
Negative inotropic effects	
Increased oxidative stress	
Alterations in the Biology of the Nonmyocytes	
Conversion of fibroblasts to myofibroblasts	
Upregulation of AT_1 receptors on fibroblasts	
Increased matrix metalloproteinase secretion by fibroblasts	
Alterations in the extracellular matrix	
Degradation of the matrix	
Myocardial fibrosis	
Progressive Myocyte Loss	
Necrosis	
Apoptosis	

patients with severe HF, suggesting that the imbalance between proinflammatory and antiinflammatory cytokine expression may contribute to progressive HF.

Reversibility of Left Ventricular Remodeling (Myocardial Recovery)

Clinical studies have shown that currently approved medical and device therapies for HF have favorable effects on cardiac remodeling, inasmuch as they result in a stabilization and/or reversal of LV chamber mass and LV chamber dilation. For want of a better term, this process of myocardial recovery, which encompasses a myriad of changes at the molecular, cellular, tissue, and organ levels, has been referred to as "reverse remodeling." Although the precise cellular and molecular mechanisms that are responsible for the remarkable return toward normal LV size and shape are not fully known, there is a fairly consistent theme with respect to the parameters that return toward baseline following pharmacological or device therapy (Table 22-5). For example, recent studies in patients who have been treated with beta blockers showed that patients who had an improvement in ejection fraction also had an increase in SERC2A mRNA and alpha-myosin heavy chain mRNA and a decrease in beta-myosin heavy chain mRNA, thus demonstrating that the improvement in ventricular function following treatment with beta blockers is associated with favorable changes in myocardial gene expression (see Fig. 22-13).[34] Similar findings have been obtained when examining myocardial recovery following pharmacological support with ACE inhibitors, LVADs, or cardiac support devices, suggesting that there may be specific gene programs that accompany myocardial recovery. Indeed, in patients with dilated cardiomyopathy who were supported with an LVAD, a specific pharmacological regimen consisting of an ACE inhibitor, an angiotensin receptor blocker, an aldosterone antagonist, and a beta blocker, followed by treatment with a $beta_2$-adrenergic-receptor agonist (clenbuterol), resulted in sufficient myocardial recovery to allow for explantation of the LVAD, and an improvement in quality of life and freedom from recurrent heart failure for 1 to 4 years following LVAD explantation.[56] However, although many of the individual elements of recovery have been identified, it is still not clear how the decrease in LV chamber mass and LV chamber dilation are coordinated during the process of myocardial recovery. Moreover, it is also clear from clinical studies that there are limits to the amount of myocardial recovery that can occur with current pharmacological and device support.

FUTURE DIRECTIONS

In this chapter we have described the clinical syndrome of HF in terms of several different clinical model systems including a cardiorenal model, a hemodynamic model, and a neurohormonal model. As noted, each model has strengths and weaknesses in terms of understanding the mechanisms responsible for HF, as well as developing effective new therapies for HF. Nonetheless, as noted earlier, our current models for understanding the mechanisms for HF are inadequate and do not adequately describe disease progression in HF. Moreover, they do not provide an adequate scaffold for understanding newer device therapies that appear to work through neurohormonal independent mechanisms. For this reason we have emphasized the importance of cardiac remodeling as a neurohormonal independent mechanism that fosters worsening LV function and disease progression in HF. Viewed together, these observations suggest that HF can be viewed as a *biomechanical model* in which HF develops and progresses as a result of the deleterious changes in cardiac function and cardiac remodeling that occur as the result of sustained neurohormonal activation.[1] Although this point of view does not obviate the importance of neurohormonal activation in the setting of HF, it suggests that future therapies will likely be focused on reversing and/or stabilizing the downstream biological consequences

TABLE 22–5 Cellular and Molecular Determinants of Myocardial Recovery

	ACE Inhibitor	Beta Blocker	LVAD	CSD
Myocyte Defects				
Hypertrophy	Decreased	Decreased	Decreased	Decreased
Myocytolysis	ND	Decreased	Decreased	ND
E-C coupling	Increased	Increased	Increased	Increased
Fetal gene expression	Decreased	Decreased	Decreased	Decreased
Beta-adrenergic desensitization	Decreased	Decreased	Decreased	Decreased
Cytoskeletal proteins	ND	ND	Increased	ND
Myocyte contractility	ND	Increased	Increased	Increased
Myocardial Defects				
Myocyte necrosis	Decreased	Decreased	Decreased	ND
Myocyte apoptosis	Decreased	Decreased	Decreased	Decreased
MMP activation	Decreased	Decreased	Decreased	Decreased
Fibrosis	Decreased	Decreased	Decreased	Decreased
LV Dilation	Stabilized	Decreased	Decreased	Decreased

ACE = angiotensin-converting enzyme; CSD = cardiac support device, LVAD = left ventricular assist device; MMP = matrix metalloproteinase; ND = not done.

 of neurohormonal activation, rather than on neurohormonal activation per se.

REFERENCES

Neurohormonal Mechanisms

1. Mann DL, Bristow MR: Mechanisms and models in heart failure: The biomechanical model and beyond. Circulation 111:2837, 2005.
2. Floras JS: Sympathetic activation in human heart failure: Diverse mechanisms, therapeutic opportunities. Acta Physiol Scand 177:391, 2003.
3. Dell'Italia L, Sabri A: Activation of the renin-angiotensin system in hypertrophy and heart failure. *In* Mann DL (ed): Heart Failure: A Companion to Braunwald's Heart Disease, Saunders, Philadelphia, 2004, pp 129-143.
4. Haulica I, Petrescu G, Slatineanu SM, et al: New bioactive angiotensins formation pathways and functional involvements. Rom J Intern Med 42:27, 2004.
5. Grieve DJ, Shah AM: Oxidative stress in heart failure. More than just damage. Eur Heart J 24:2161, 2003.
6. Sawyer DB, Siwik DA, Xiao L, et al: Role of oxidative stress in myocardial hypertrophy and failure. J Mol Cell Cardiol 34:379, 2002.
7. Pitt B, Zannad F, Remme WJ, et al: The effect of spironolactone on morbidity and mortality in patients with severe heart failure. Randomized Aldactone Evaluation Study Investigators. N Engl J Med 341:709, 1999.
8. Pitt B, Remme W, Zannad F: Eplerenone, a selective aldosterone blocker, in patients with left ventricular dysfunction after myocardial infarction. N Engl J Med 348:1309, 2003.
9. Schrier RW, Abraham WT: Hormones and hemodynamics in heart failure. N Engl J Med 341:577, 1999.
10. Tang WH, Bhavnani S, Francis GS: Vasopressin receptor antagonists in the management of acute heart failure. Expert Opin Investig Drugs 14:593, 2005.
11. Naitoh M, Suzuki H, Murakami M, et al: Effects of oral AVP receptor antagonists OPC-21268 and OPC-31260 on congestive heart failure in conscious dogs. Am J Physiol 267:H2245-H2254, 1994.
12. Burnett JC Jr, Costello-Boerrigter L, Boerriger G: Alterations in the kidney in heart failure: The cardiorenal axis in the regulation of sodium homeostasis. *In* Mann DL (ed): Heart Failure: A Companion to Braunwald's Heart Disease. Philadelphia, Saunders, 2003, pp 279-289.
13. Cea LB: Natriuretic peptide family: New aspects. Curr Med Chem Cardiovasc Hematol Agents 3:87, 2005.
14. Rademaker MT, Richards AM: Cardiac natriuretic peptides for cardiac health. Clin Sci (Lond) 108:23, 2005.
15. Munzel T, Kurz S, Holtz J, et al: Neurohormonal inhibition and hemodynamic unloading during prolonged inhibition of ANF degradation in patients with severe chronic heart failure. Circulation 86:1089, 1992.
16. Packer M, Califf RM, Konstam MA, et al: Comparison of omapatrilat and enalapril in patients with chronic heart failure: The Omapatrilat Versus Enalapril Randomized Trial of Utility in Reducing Events (OVERTURE). Circulation 106:920, 2002.
17. Cataliotti A, Burnett JC Jr: Natriuretic peptides: Novel therapeutic targets in heart failure. J Investig Med 53:378, 2005.
18. Podesser BK, Siwik DA, Eberli FR, et al: ET(A)-receptor blockade prevents matrix metalloproteinase activation late postmyocardial infarction in the rat. Am J Physiol Heart Circ Physiol 280:H984, 2001.
19. Teerlink JR: Recent heart failure trials of neurohormonal modulation (OVERTURE and ENABLE): Approaching the asymptote of efficacy? J Card Fail 8:124, 2002.
20. Feng QP, Hedner T, Andersson B, et al: Cardiac neuropeptide Y and noradrenaline balance in patients with congestive heart failure. Br Heart J 71:261, 1994.
21. Onan D, Pipolo L, Yang, E, et al: Urotensin II promotes hypertrophy of cardiac myocytes via mitogen-activated protein kinases. Mol Endocrinol 18:2344, 2004.
22. Lim M, Honisett S, Sparkes CD, et al: Differential effect of urotensin II on vascular tone in normal subjects and patients with chronic heart failure. Circulation 109:1212, 2004.
23. Scherrer-Crosbie M, Ullrich R, Bloch KD, et al: Endothelial nitric oxide synthase limits left ventricular remodeling after myocardial infarction in mice. Circulation 104:1286, 2001.
24. Damy T, Ratajczak P, Shah AM, et al: Increased neuronal nitric oxide synthase-derived NO production in the failing human heart. Lancet 363:1365, 2004.
25. Sam F, Sawyer DB, Xie Z, et al: Mice lacking inducible nitric oxide synthase have improved left ventricular contractile function and reduced apoptotic cell death late after myocardial infarction. Circ Res 89:351, 2001.
26. Sharma JN, Sharma J: Cardiovascular properties of the kallikrein-kinin system. Curr Med Res Opin 18:10, 2002.
27. Rademaker MT, Cameron VA, Charles CJ, et al: Adrenomedullin and heart failure. Regul Pept 112:51, 2003.
28. Mann DL, Deswal A, Bozkurt B, et al: New therapeutics for chronic heart failure. Annu Rev Med 53:59, 2002.

Left Ventricular Remodeling

29. Mann DL: Left ventricular size and shape: determinants of mechanical signal transduction pathways. Heart Fail Rev 10:95, 2005.
30. Houser SR, Margulies KB: Is depressed myocyte contractility centrally involved in heart failure? Circ Res 92:350, 2003.
31. Minamisawa S, Hoshijima M, Chu G, et al: Chronic phospholamban-sarcoplasmic reticulum calcium ATPase interaction is the critical calcium cycling defect in dilated cardiomyopathy. Cell 99:313, 1999.
32. Reiken S, Wehrens XH, Vest JA, et al: Beta-blockers restore calcium release channel function and improve cardiac muscle performance in human heart failure. Circulation 107:2459, 2003.
33. Margulies K, House SR: Myocyte abnormalities in human heart failure. *In* Mann DL (ed): Heart Failure: A Companion to Braunwald's Heart Disease. Philadelphia, Saunders, 2003, pp 41-56.
34. Lowes BD, Gilbert EM, Abraham WT, et al: Myocardial gene expression in dilated cardiomyopathy treated with beta- blocking agents. N Engl J Med 346:1357, 2002.
35. Nassar R, Malouf NN, Mao L, et al: cTnT1, a cardiac troponin T isoform, decreases myofilament tension and affects the left ventricular pressure waveform. Am J Physiol Heart Circ Physiol 288:H1147, 2005.
36. Vatta M, Stetson SJ, Perez-Verdia A, et al: Molecular remodeling of dystrophin in patients with end-stage cardiomyopathies and reversal in patients on assistance-device therapy. Lancet 359:936, 2002.
37. Bristow MR: Beta-adrenergic receptor blockade in chronic heart failure. Circulation 101:558, 2000.
38. Penela P, Murga C, Ribas C, et al: Mechanisms of regulation of G protein–coupled receptor kinases (GRKs) and cardiovascular disease. Cardiovasc Res 69:46, 2006.
39. Guerra S, Leri A, Wang X, et al: Myocyte death in the failing human heart is gender dependent. Circ Res 85:856, 1999.
40. Rodriguez M, Schaper J: Apoptosis: Measurement and technical issues. J Mol Cell Cardiol 38:15, 2005.
41. Garg S, Narula J, Chandrashekhar Y: Apoptosis and heart failure: Clinical relevance and therapeutic target. J Mol Cell Cardiol 38:73, 2005.
42. Wencker D, Chandra M, Nguyen K, et al: A mechanistic role for cardiac myocyte apoptosis in heart failure. J Clin Invest 111:1497, 2003.
43. Yussman MG, Toyokawa T, Odley A, et al: Mitochondrial death protein Nix is induced in cardiac hypertrophy and triggers apoptotic cardiomyopathy. Nat Med 8:725, 2002.
44. Kostin S, Pool L, Elsasser A, et al: Myocytes die by multiple mechanisms in failing human hearts. Circ Res 92:715, 2003.
45. Knaapen MW, Davies MJ, De Bie M, et al: Apoptotic versus autophagic cell death in heart failure. Cardiovasc Res 51:304, 2001.
46. Hein S, Arnon E, Kostin S, et al: Progression from compensated hypertrophy to failure in the pressure-overloaded human heart: Structural deterioration and compensatory mechanisms. Circulation 107:984, 2003.
47. Deschamps AM, Spinale FG: Matrix modulation and heart failure: New concepts question old beliefs. Curr Opin Cardiol 20:211, 2005.
48. Zannad F, Dousset B, Alla F: Treatment of congestive heart failure: Interfering the aldosterone-cardiac extracellular matrix relationship. Hypertension 38:1227, 2001.
49. Shiota N, Rysa J, Kovanen PT, et al: A role for cardiac mast cells in the pathogenesis of hypertensive heart disease. J Hypertens 21:1935, 2003.
50. Spinale FG: Matrix metalloproteinases: Regulation and dysregulation in the failing heart. Circ Res 90:520, 2002.
51. Hudson MP, Armstrong PW, Ruzyllo W, et al: Effects of selective matrix metalloproteinase inhibitor (PG-116800) to prevent ventricular remodeling after myocardial infarction: Results of the PREMIER (Prevention of Myocardial Infarction Early Remodeling) trial. J Am Coll Cardiol 48:15, 2006.
52. Huss JM, Kelly DP: Nuclear receptor signaling and cardiac energetics. Circ Res 95:568, 2004.
53. Fragasso G, Palloshi A, Puccetti P, et al: A randomized clinical trial of trimetazidine, a partial free fatty acid oxidation inhibitor, in patients with heart failure. J Am Coll Cardiol 48:992, 2006.
54. Mann DL: Inflammatory mediators and the failing heart: Past, present, and the foreseeable future. Circ Res 91:988, 2002.
55. Deswal A, Petersen NJ, Feldman, AM, et al: Cytokines and cytokine receptors in advanced heart failure: An analysis of the cytokine database from the Vesnarinone Trial (VEST). Circulation 103:2055, 2001.
56. Birks EJ, Tansley PD, Hardy J, et al: Left ventricular assist device and drug therapy for the reversal of heart failure. N Engl J Med 355:1873, 2006.

CHAPTER 23

Clinical Assessment of Heart Failure

Otto M. Hess and John D. Carroll

Heart failure is a complex clinical syndrome that arises secondary to abnormalities of cardiac structure and/or function (inherited or acquired) that impair the ability of the left ventricle to fill or eject blood. The cardinal manifestations of heart failure are dyspnea and fatigue. These abnormalities may impair the functional capacity and quality of life of affected individuals; however, they do not necessarily dominate the clinical picture concurrently.[1] Furthermore, many of the typical signs and symptoms of heart failure are not directly attributable to the cardiac abnormalities that occur in the failing heart, but rather arise secondarily to abnormalities that occur in remote organs (e.g., kidney) or tissues (e.g., skeletal muscle). The dysfunction that occurs in these organs and tissues cannot be explained solely by decreased perfusion pressure, suggesting that other systemic processes (e.g., neurohormonal activation; see Chap. 22) must contribute to the syndrome of heart failure. Although heart failure was once thought to arise primarily in the setting of depressed left ventricular (LV) ejection fraction (EF), epidemiological studies have shown that approximately 50 percent of patients who develop heart failure have a normal or preserved EF (see Chap. 26). Accordingly, patients may be broadly categorized as having heart failure with depressed EF (commonly referred to as systolic failure), or having heart failure with a normal EF or heart failure with a preserved EF (sometimes referred to as "diastolic failure"). Epidemiological studies have also shown that patients may have significant abnormalities of LV contraction and relaxation and yet have no symptoms, in which case these patients are referred to as having asymptomatic heart failure. When a patient with chronic heart failure deteriorates, the patient is referred to as having decompensated or, alternatively, acute decompensated heart failure if the symptoms arise abruptly. Congestive heart failure is largely an outdated term that reflects the original clinical observation that patients with heart failure were frequently edematous or volume-overloaded. However, with current medical and device therapy, most patients with heart failure remain euvolemic, and are therefore referred to simply as having heart failure. Cardiomyopathy and LV dysfunction are more general terms that describe abnormalities of cardiac structure or function, or both, which may lead to heart failure.[2] Circulatory failure is not synonymous with heart failure because various noncardiac conditions (e.g., hemorrhagic shock) can lead to circulatory collapse while cardiac function is preserved. The terms *backward failure* and *forward failure* are largely historical terms that do not take into account the full spectrum of pathophysiological changes that contribute to ventricular remodeling and disease progression in patients with chronic heart failure, and thus have largely been abandoned.

APPROACH TO THE PATIENT

Cardiac History

The clinical examination of heart failure patients begins with a history and physical examination, which remain the cornerstone of the clinical assessment in heart failure. The principles and techniques for obtaining a detailed and objective cardiovascular history for patients with heart failure are summarized here and are intended to complement the principles of the general cardiovascular history and physical examination described in Chapter 11.

Symptoms

The cardinal symptoms of heart failure are dyspnea, exercise intolerance, and fatigue (Table 23-1). Although the fatigue has been traditionally ascribed to a low cardiac output in heart failure, abnormalities of skeletal muscles and other noncardiac comorbidities such as anemia are also likely to contribute to this symptom. In early heart failure, dyspnea is observed only during exertion; however, as heart failure advances, dyspnea occurs with progressively less strenuous activity and ultimately is present even at rest. The origin of dyspnea is likely multifactorial. The most important mechanism is pulmonary congestion, with accumulation of interstitial or intraalveolar fluid in the alveolus, which activates juxtacapillary J receptors and stimulates the rapid, shallow breathing characteristic of cardiac dyspnea. Other factors that contribute to dyspnea on exertion include abnormalities in pulmonary compliance, increased airway resistance, respiratory muscle and/or diaphragm fatigue, and anemia. Dyspnea may become less frequent with the onset of right ventricular failure and tricuspid regurgitation.

ORTHOPNEA AND PAROXYSMAL NOCTURNAL DYSPNEA. Orthopnea is defined as dyspnea that occurs in the recumbent position and is usually a later manifestation of heart failure than exertional dyspnea. Orthopnea is generally relieved by sitting upright or by sleeping with additional pillows. It results from the redistribution of fluid from the splanchnic circulation and lower extremities into the central circulation during recumbency, with a resultant increase in pulmonary capillary pressures. Nocturnal cough is a frequent manifestation of this process, and is a frequently overlooked symptom of heart failure. Although orthopnea is a relatively specific symptom of heart failure, it

TABLE 23–1 Symptoms in Heart Failure	
Major Symptoms	**Minor Symptoms**
Dyspnea	Weight loss
Orthopnea	Cough
Paroxysmal nocturnal dyspnea	Nocturia
Ankle edema	Palpitations
Pulmonary edema	Peripheral cyanosis
Fatigue	Depression
Exercise intolerance	
Cachexia	

TABLE 23–2 Physical Findings in Heart Failure	
Major Symptoms	**Minor Symptoms**
Tachycardia	Mitral regurgitation
Elevated venous pressure	Cardiomegaly
Positive hepatojugular reflux	Splenomegaly
Pulmonary rales	Hypotension
Tachypnea	Pulsus alternans
Third heart sound	Extrasystoles
Hepatomegaly	Atrial fibrillation
Ankle edema	Weight loss
Ascites	
Pleural effusion	

may occur in pulmonary patients with abdominal obesity or ascites, and in pulmonary patients whose lung mechanics favor an upright posture. Paroxysmal nocturnal dyspnea (PND) refers to acute episodes of severe shortness of breath and coughing that generally occur at night and awaken the patient from sleep, usually 1 to 3 hours after the patient retires. PND may be manifest by coughing or wheezing, possibly because of increased pressure in the bronchial arteries leading to airway compression, along with interstitial pulmonary edema leading to airway resistance. Whereas orthopnea may be relieved by sitting upright at the side of the bed with the legs dependent, in the patient with paroxysmal nocturnal dyspnea, coughing and wheezing often persist, even in this position.[2] PND is a relatively specific symptom of heart failure. Cardiac asthma is closely related to paroxysmal nocturnal dyspnea, is characterized by wheezing secondary to bronchospasm, and must be differentiated from primary asthma and pulmonary causes of wheezing.

ACUTE PULMONARY EDEMA. This results from transudation of fluid into the alveolar spaces as a result of an acute rise in capillary hydrostatic pressure secondary to depressed cardiac function or an increase in intravascular volume (see Chap. 24). Pulmonary edema may manifest as cough or progressive dyspnea. In its most severe form, pulmonary edema is associated with extreme shortness of breath and the expectoration of blood-tinged fluid. If not treated promptly, acute pulmonary edema may be fatal.

CHEYNE-STOKES RESPIRATION. This is also referred to as periodic respiration or cyclic respiration, is common in advanced heart failure, and is usually associated with low cardiac output. Cheyne-Stokes respiration is caused by a diminished sensitivity of the respiratory center to arterial P_{CO_2} (see Chap. 25). There is an apneic phase, during which the arterial P_{O_2} falls and the arterial P_{CO_2} rises. These changes in the arterial blood stimulate the depressed respiratory center, resulting in hyperventilation and hypocapnia, followed in turn by the recurrence of apnea. Cheyne-Stokes respiration may be perceived by the patient or the patient's family as severe dyspnea or as a transient cessation of breathing.

OTHER SYMPTOMS. Patients with heart failure may also present with gastrointestinal symptoms. Anorexia, nausea, and early satiety associated with abdominal pain and fullness are frequent complaints and may be related to edema of the bowel wall and/or a congested liver. Congestion of the liver and stretching of its capsule may lead to right upper quadrant pain. Cerebral symptoms such as confusion, disorientation, and sleep and mood disturbances may be observed in patients with severe heart failure, particularly elderly patients with cerebral arteriosclerosis and reduced cerebral perfusion. Nocturia is common in heart failure and may contribute to insomnia.

Physical Examination (see Chap. 11)

A careful physical examination is always warranted in the evaluation of patients with heart failure. The purpose of the examination is to help determine the cause of heart failure, as well as to assess the severity of the syndrome.[3] Obtaining additional information about the hemodynamic profile, the response to therapy, and determination of the prognosis are important additional goals of the physical examination (Table 23-2).

GENERAL APPEARANCE AND VITAL SIGNS. In mild or moderately severe heart failure, the patient appears in no distress at rest, except for feeling uncomfortable when lying flat for more than a few minutes. In more severe heart failure, the patient may have labored breathing and may not be able to finish a sentence because of shortness of breath. Systolic blood pressure may be normal or high, but is generally reduced in advanced heart failure because of severe LV dysfunction. The pulse pressure may be diminished, reflecting a reduction in stroke volume, and the diastolic arterial pressure may be elevated as a consequence of generalized vasoconstriction. Sinus tachycardia is a nonspecific sign caused by increased sympathetic activity. Peripheral vasoconstriction leading to cool peripheral extremities and cyanosis of the lips and nailbeds is also caused by excessive sympathetic activity.

JUGULAR VEINS AND EXAMINATION OF THE NECK. Examination of the jugular veins provides an estimation of right atrial pressure and, by inference, left atrial pressure. The jugular venous pressure is best appreciated with the patient lying recumbent, with the head tilted at 45 degrees. The jugular venous pressure should be quantified in centimeters of water (normal, less than 8 cm) by estimating the height of the venous column of blood above the sternal angle in centimeters and then adding 5 cm (in any posture). In the early stages of heart failure, the venous pressure may be normal at rest but may become abnormally elevated, with sustained pressure on the abdomen (positive hepatojugular reflux). Giant V waves indicate the presence of tricuspid valve incompetence.

PULMONARY EXAMINATION. Pulmonary crackles (rales or crepitations) result from the transudation of fluid from the intravascular space into the alveoli. In patients with pulmonary edema, rales may be heard widely over both lung fields and may be accompanied by expiratory wheezing (cardiac asthma). When present in patients without concomitant lung disease, rales are specific for heart failure. However, it bears emphasis that rales are frequently absent in most patients with chronic heart failure, even when the pulmonary capillary wedge pressure is more than 20 mm Hg, because of increased lymphatic drainage of alveolar fluid. Pleural effusions result from the elevation of pleural capillary pressure and the resultant transudation of fluid into the pleural cavities. Because the pleural veins drain into both the systemic and pulmonary veins, pleural effusion occurs most commonly with biventricular failure. Although pleural effusions are usually bilateral, they occur more frequently in the right pleural space than in the left.

CARDIAC EXAMINATION. Examination of the heart, although essential, frequently does not provide useful information about the severity of heart failure. If cardiomegaly is present, the point of maximal impulse is usually displaced below the fifth intercostal space and/or lateral to the midclavicular line, and the impulse is palpable over two interspaces. Severe LV hypertrophy leads to a sustained precordial impulse. Examination of the precordial pulsation is inadequate to assess the degree of LV dysfunction. In some patients, a third heart sound is audible and palpable at the apex. Patients with enlarged or hypertrophied right ventricles may have a sustained and prolonged left parasternal impulse extending throughout systole. A third heart sound (or gallop rhythm) is most commonly present in patients with volume overload who have tachycardia and tachypnea, and often signifies severe hemodynamic compromise.[4] A fourth heart sound is not a specific indicator of heart failure, but it is usually present in patients with diastolic dysfunction. The murmurs of mitral and tricuspid regurgitation are frequently present in patients with advanced heart failure.

EXAMINATION OF ABDOMEN AND EXTREMITIES. Hepatomegaly is an important but uncommon sign in patients with heart failure. When present, the enlarged liver is frequently tender and may pulsate during systole if tricuspid valve regurgitation is present. Ascites also occurs as a consequence of transudation and results from increased pressure in the hepatic veins and the veins draining the peritoneum. Jaundice is also a late finding in heart failure and is associated with elevations of both direct and indirect bilirubin levels. It results from impairment of hepatic function secondary to hepatic congestion and hepatocellular hypoxia. Peripheral edema is a cardinal manifestation of heart failure, but is nonspecific and is usually absent in patients who have been adequately treated with diuretics. Peripheral edema is usually symmetrical and dependent in heart failure, and occurs predominantly in the ankles and pretibial region in ambulatory patients. In bedridden patients, edema may be found in the sacrum and scrotum. Long-standing edema may be associated with indurated and pigmented skin.

CARDIAC CACHEXIA. With severe chronic heart failure, there may be marked weight loss and cachexia. Although the mechanism of cachexia is not entirely understood, it is likely multifactorial and includes elevation of the resting metabolic rate, anorexia, nausea, and vomiting caused by congestive hepatomegaly and abdominal fullness, elevation of circulating concentrations of inflammatory cytokines, and impairment of intestinal absorption resulting from congestion of the intestinal veins. When present, cachexia augurs a poor overall prognosis.

Diagnostic Laboratory Tests

As shown in Table 23-3, the diagnostic sensitivity and specificity of the clinical history and physical examination for diagnosing patients with heart failure is relatively poor. For this reason, laboratory testing has assumed a progressively greater role in establishing the diagnosis of heart failure. The goal of diagnostic laboratory testing is threefold: (1) to determine that there is some abnormality of cardiac structure or function that explains the patient's symptoms; (2) to identify abnormalities that may lead to specific interventions; and (3) to determine the severity and prognosis of the heart failure.[5] In the classic sense, routine laboratory testing relates to blood and urine tests; however, as shown in Table 23-4, echocardiography, computed tomography (CT) scanning, radionuclide angiography, and magnetic resonance imaging (MRI) have assumed a major role in the clinical

TABLE 23–3 Sensitivity, Specificity, and Predictive Accuracy of Symptoms and Signs for Diagnosing Heart Failure

Symptoms or Signs	Sensitivity (%)	Specificity (%)	Predictive Accuracy (%)
Exertional dyspnea	66	52	23
Orthopnea	21	81	2
Paroxysmal	33	76	26
History of edema	23	80	22
Resting heart rate	7	99	6
Rales	13	91	21
Third heart sound	31	95	61
Jugular venous distention	10	97	2
Edema (on examination)	10	93	3

Modified from Harlan WR, Oberman A, Grimm R, et al: Chronic congestive heart failure in coronary artery disease: Clinical criteria. Ann Intern Med 86:133, 1977.

TABLE 23–4 Evaluation of Patients with Heart Failure

Modality	Examples; Indicated?
Routine laboratory testing	Blood count, CRP, BNP, creatinine, electrolytes, CK, troponin, liver function tests, TSH, urine analysis
Chest x-ray	Yes
Electrocardiography	Yes
Echocardiography	Yes
Holter monitoring	No, unless symptoms of an arrhythmia
Exercise testing	Yes† ($V\text{O}_2$max)
Radionuclide angiography	No, unless EF during exercise indicated
Computed tomography scanning	No; special indication (coronary calcifications, coronary anatomy)
Magnetic resonance imaging	No; special indication (late enhancement, myocardial perfusion, myocardial tagging)
Coronary angiography*	Selected patients with suspected CAD
Follow-up	Clinical examination, electrolyte and BNP levels; electrocardiography and echocardiography, when indicated

CAD = coronary artery disease; CRP = C-reactive protein, BNP = brain natriuretic peptide, CK = creatine kinase, TSH = thyroid-stimulating hormone, EF = ejection fraction; $V\text{O}_2$max = maximal oxygen uptake during exercise.[11]

*Catheter-based pressure and flow measurements in selected patients in whom noninvasive measurements may be inadequate (i.e., for assessment of pulmonary hypertension).

†Not routinely recommended for all patients with heart failure, but useful in the assessment of cardiac transplantation patients.

 noninvasive assessment of heart failure. In many patients, invasive laboratory testing may still be necessary to determine the correct diagnosis, assess severity, and provide catheter-based measurements when noninvasive testing results are indeterminate or limited by the quality of the data.

ROUTINE LABORATORY TESTS. Routine blood tests are mandatory in patients with heart failure for several reasons: (1) to detect anemia, (2) to identify electrolyte disorders (hypokalemia and/or hyponatremia), (3) to assess renal and liver function, and (4) to measure brain natriuretic peptide (severity of hemodynamic impairment). Serum electrolyte levels are usually normal in mild to moderate heart failure but may become abnormal in severe heart failure when drug therapy is increased. The serum potassium level is usually normal but prolonged use of kaliuretic diuretics such as thiazides or loop diuretics may lead to hypokalemia. The degree of hyponatremia is a marker for the severity of heart failure, insofar as the level of serum sodium indirectly reflects the degree of activation of the renin angiotensin system (see Chap. 22). In addition, sodium restriction together with intensive diuretic therapy may lead to hyponatremia. Other electrolyte disturbances include hypophosphatemia, hypomagnesemia and hyperuricemia. Anemia may aggravate heart failure caused by its increase in cardiac output which is associated with an increase in myocardial volume overload (see Chap. 25). It has been shown[6] that approximately 25 percent of all severely limited heart failure patients have anemia with a hemoglobin value of less than 12 gm/dL. It is strongly recommended to determine brain natriuretic peptide (BNP) levels in all patients to assess the extent of hemodynamic impairment and to evaluate clinical outcome (see later). Renal function plays a key role in the progression of ventricular dysfunction and heart failure. Decreases in renal function, specifically glomerular filtration rate, predict cardiac mortality more powerfully than functional classification, according to the New York Heart Association (NYHA).

Liver function is often abnormal in heart failure as a result of the accompanying hepatomegaly. Aspartate aminotransferase (AST) and alanine aminotransferase (ALT) levels are increased, whereas prothrombin time may be prolonged. In rare cases, hyperbilirubinemia may occur. Urinalysis should be done in all patients with heart failure to search for bacterial infections, microalbuminuria, and microhematuria. Specific attention should be paid to urine concentration and excretion volume in patients with renal impairment and diuretic therapy.[7]

BIOMARKERS. Biomarkers are becoming increasingly useful in terms of providing important diagnostic and prognostic information about patients with heart failure. Myocardial biomarkers such as natriuretic peptides have emerged as useful adjunctive tools in the diagnosis of patients with heart failure. As noted in Chapter 22, both atrial natriuretic peptide (ANP) and BNP are secreted in response to increasing cardiac wall tension and/or circulating neurohormones. ANP and BNP are initially synthesized as prohormones that are subsequently cleaved proteolytically to yield large, biologically inactive N-terminal fragments (NT-ANP or NT-BNP) and smaller biologically active peptides (ANP or BNP).

Because ANP has a short half-life, only NT-ANP is clinically useful. For BNP, both N-terminal pro-BNP and BNP have been shown to be clinically useful. Circulating levels of ANP and BNP are increased in patients with systolic dysfunction and are also elevated, albeit to a lesser extent, in patients with heart failure with a normal ejection fraction. In systolic heart failure, BNP levels have been shown[8] to be directly related to wall stress, ejection fraction, and functional classification (Fig. 23-1).

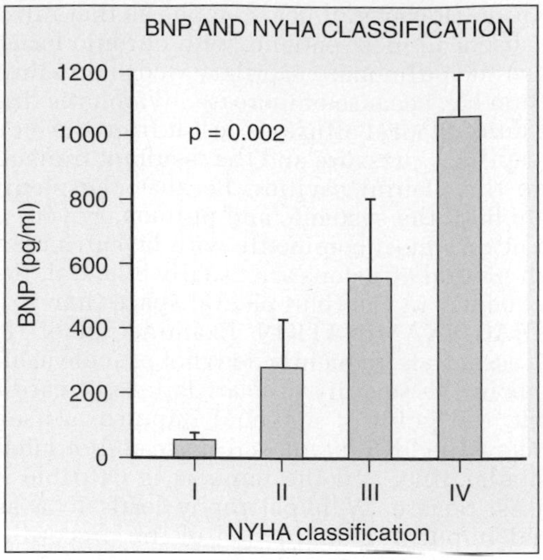

FIGURE 23–1 Brain natriuretic peptide (BNP) values in patients with systolic, diastolic, or combined dysfunction in patients with heart failure. The highest values are observed in those patients with combined failure and lowest in normals. Patients with diastolic dysfunction show slightly lower values than those with pure systolic failure.[11] *(With permission from Maisel A, Koon J, Krishnaswamy P, et al: Am Heart J 141:367, 2001.)*

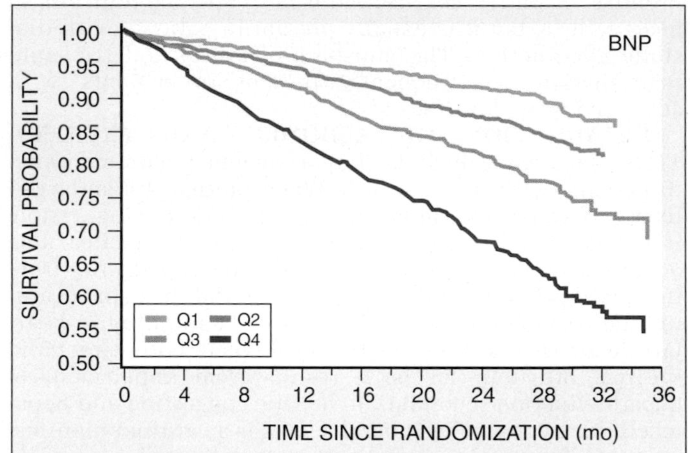

	Q1	Q2	Q3	Q4
BNP (pg/ml)	<41	41–<97	97–<238	≥238
Mortality (%)	9.7	14.3	20.7	32.4

FIGURE 23–2 Plasma brain natriuretic peptide (BNP) was measured before randomization and during follow-up in approximately 4300 patients in the Valsartan Heart Failure Trial. The baseline values for BNP in quartiles were less than 41, 41 to less than 97, 97 to less than 238, and greater than or equal to 238 pg/ml. Kaplan-Meier curves show a significant quartile-dependent increase in mortality and first morbid events. *(From Anand IS, Fisher LD, Chiang YT, et al: Changes in brain natriuretic peptide and norepinephrine over time and mortality and morbidity in the Valsartan Heart Failure Trial (Val-HeFT). Circulation 107:1278, 2003.)*

The plasma BNP level has been shown to be useful in distinguishing cardiac from noncardiac causes of dyspnea, and provides prognostic information in patients with chronic heart failure and/or acute coronary syndromes (Fig. 23-2). Recently, changes in the level of NT-BNP have been shown to predict response to treatment in heart failure. Moreover, elevated BNP levels are a more powerful predictor of LV systolic dysfunction and diastolic dysfunction than elevated levels of NT-ANP. Although population screening using BNP levels is not currently recommended, in patients at risk for heart failure, BNP levels may facilitate earlier identification of those who would benefit from initiation of therapy to prevent or delay progression to overt heart failure. Natriuretic peptide levels increase with age and renal impairment, are more elevated in women, and can be elevated in right heart failure from any cause.[9] The explanation for the higher BNP values in women is not known, but may be caused by the higher wall stress in the smaller female heart. Levels can be falsely low in obese patients and may normalize in some patients following appropriate treatment. A normal serum BNP level has a high negative predictive value of 95 percent to exclude the diagnosis of heart failure.[10] Other common cardiac abnormalities that may cause elevated natriuretic peptide levels include left ventricular hypertrophy, valvular heart disease, acute or chronic ischemia, hypertension, cor pulmonale, and pulmonary embolism.

Other biomarkers, such as C-reactive protein, tumor necrosis factor receptor, and uric acid levels, are elevated in heart failure, and may provide important prognostic information (see Chap. 25). Creatine kinase (CK) and troponin (I or T) may be modestly elevated in severe heart failure when wall stress is high and/or subendocardial ischemia is present. In patients with new onset of acute heart failure, myocarditis may contribute to elevated cardiac enzyme levels. Tests of neuroendocrine activation (e.g., norepinephrine, angiotensin II, plasma renin activity) are technically difficult and are influenced by drugs that modulate these systems; therefore, they are not routinely recommended for diagnostic or prognostic purposes in individual patients. Serial measurements of one or more biomarkers may ultimately help guide therapy in heart failure, but are not currently recommended.

CHEST X-RAY AND ELECTROCARDIOGRAM. The chest x-ray has a long tradition in cardiology for assessing the size and shape of the heart, as well as for studying the structure and perfusion of the lung (see Chap. 15). The technique has lost much of its impact with the introduction of echocardiography, because the size and shape of the heart can be much better quantified by ultrasound than by use of the old radiographic technique. Nevertheless, important information can still be gained by examination of the chest x-ray.

Cardiomegaly can be best estimated from the chest x-ray. A cardiothoracic ratio more than 0.5, when the heart reaches half the size of the chest diameter, has been shown to be a valuable parameter in the follow-up of patients with heart failure. The shape of the heart has been divided into pressure- or volume-overloaded ventricles, dilation of the left atrium, and dilation of the ascending aorta. Although patients with *acute* heart failure have evidence of pulmonary hypertension and interstitial and/or pulmonary edema, most patients with *chronic* heart failure do not. Congestion of the lung with Kerley lines—linear densities of interlobular interstitial edema—over the lower lobes are the typical findings in acute heart failure. These changes are expressions of the interstitial and perivascular edema at the base of the lung, where hydrostatic pressure is higher. The absence of these findings in patients with chronic heart failure reflects the increased capacity of the lymphatics to remove interstitial and/or pulmonary fluid and is consistent with the absence of rales in most patients with chronic heart failure, despite elevated pulmonary artery pressures. The presence and extent of pleural effusion are helpful information in the evaluation of heart failure patients and are still best determined with x-rays or CT scans.

The diagnostic impact of the electrocardiogram (ECG) is rather low but the therapeutic impact is rather high. A normal ECG almost completely excludes the diagnosis of heart failure. Hence, electrocardiographic changes are common in heart failure, such as pathological Q waves, LV hypertrophy with strain, right or left bundle branch block, AV block, or T wave changes. Rhythm disorders such as supraventricular tachyarrhythmias and atrial fibrillation are also common. Ventricular extrasystoles occur frequently and do not portend a poor prognosis, whereas nonsustained and sustained ventricular tachycardia may be considered as potentially harmful. These types of arrhythmias are usually not detected in the resting ECG but may be detected with 24- or 48-hour Holter monitoring (Fig. 23-3). In patients with depressed LV function (LV ejection fraction less than 35 percent), use of an implantable cardioverter-defibrillator (ICD) may be considered (see Chap. 34 and Heart Failure Guidelines). In those patients with a QRS width of more than 120 milliseconds and signs of LV dyssynchrony in the echocardiogram, the implantation of a biventricular pacemaker may also be considered (see Chap. 34 and Heart Failure Guidelines).[11]

EXERCISE TESTING. Exercise testing is of limited value for the diagnosis of heart failure; however, normal maximal exercise test results in an untreated patient almost completely exclude the diagnosis of heart failure. The true value for exercise testing in heart failure is the functional assessment and prognostic stratification. Functional capacity is determined during a progressively increasing load until the patient cannot proceed further. At the time point of maximal exercise, the maximal oxygen uptake ($\dot{V}O_2max$) is measured. This parameter has been shown to reflect the aerobic capacity of the patient and is directly correlated to cardiovascular mortality in patients with heart failure.[12] The exercise test also allows the determination of the anaerobic threshold, where the respiratory quotient rises more than during the lower levels of exercise. This time point indicates that the patient switches from an aerobic to anaerobic metabolism, with production of excess lactate. A practical guideline can be formulated; the exercise test should be stopped when (1) $\dot{V}O_2$ does not increase with further increases in exercise and (2) the patient stops the exercise test because of severe symptoms such as dyspnea or fatigue. Exercise testing has prognostic importance. A peak $\dot{V}O_2$ less than 10 ml/kg per min identifies high-risk patients, whereas a peak $\dot{V}O_2$ more than 18 ml/kg per min identifies low-risk patients. Values between these cutoff limits define a gray zone of medium-risk patients who cannot be stratified further by $\dot{V}O_2$. The available prognostic data for peak $\dot{V}O_2$ in women are limited. Thus, the $\dot{V}O_2max$ level has been used as a limit to determine the time point in the progression of heart failure when cardiac transplantation should be considered (see Chap. 27).[13] Nonetheless, it should be recognized that peak $\dot{V}O_2max$ can be affected by age, gender, muscle mass, and aerobic training status. This may explain why some patients with a low

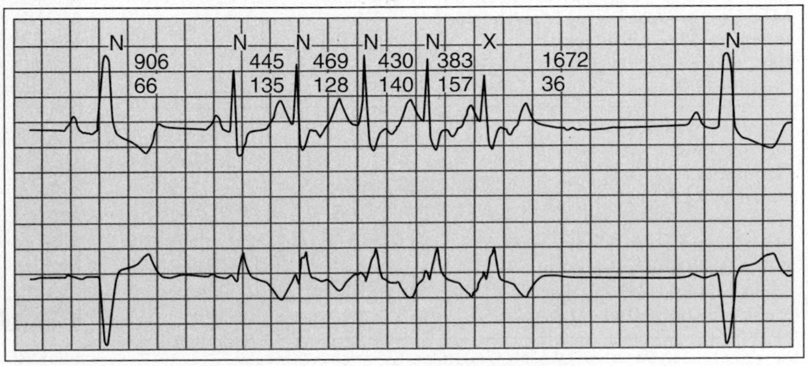

FIGURE 23–3 Nonsustained ventricular tachycardia in a patient with heart failure. Five extrasystoles occur with a heart rate of approximately 150 to 180 bpm.

VO_2max (less than 14 ml/kg/min) still have a fair prognosis.[14] Accordingly, some investigators have proposed using the percentage of predicted VO_2 rather than the absolute VO_2max.[15,16]

Because heart failure patients are often limited and the maximal exercise test is not well tolerated by many patients, a submaximal or symptom-driven exercise test has become popular for routine evaluation, namely the 6-minute walk test. This test measures the distance walked within 6 minutes on a level corridor where the patient can walk at his or her speed, slow down, speed up, or stop as desired. This test is predictive of peak VO_2max and is independently correlated to cardiovascular morbidity and mortality.[14] Because of its simplicity, this test is being used more frequently in large multicenter trials to assess the efficacy of an intervention.

ECHOCARDIOGRAPHY (see Chap. 14). Echocardiography has emerged as the preferred diagnostic method for assessing the anatomy and function of the heart, studying the myocardium and pericardium, and evaluating regional wall motion at rest and during pharmacological stress in heart failure. The technique is noninvasive, applicable at the bedside, excellent for serial studies, and allows an assessment of both global and regional LV function. In the assessment of heart failure, echocardiography is a reliable, reproducible, and safe technique with many important features, such as Doppler echocardiography, Doppler tissue imaging, and strain rate imaging, as well as cardiac motion analysis.[17] The most important features in the evaluation of heart failure patients are the assessment of the LV ejection fraction (LVEF), severity of LV remodeling, and changes in diastolic inflow properties (Table 23-5). The exact features of the method with regard to technology, anatomical and functional properties, Doppler principles, and flow measurements, as well as specific features and findings in different cardiovascular disease entities, are described in Chapter 14. As discussed later, two-dimensional echocardiography is invaluable in the assessment of systolic and diastolic function in patients with heart failure.

RADIONUCLIDE ANGIOGRAPHY (see Chap. 16). Radionuclide angiography has been mainly used to diagnose or exclude coronary artery disease. One major advantage of the technique is its ability to measure myocardial perfusion and function not only at rest, but also under exercise conditions. Radionuclide angiography can determine changes in radioactivity of the left and right ventricle over the cardiac cycle, generating time-activity curves for quantification of regional and global ejection fraction. The technique uses a gamma camera and electrocardiographic gating for temporal synchronization of the measurements. The global measurements are basically three dimensional and highly accurate. A major advantage is the ability to measure cardiac function during exercise, which may help identify individuals with an increase or decrease in LV ejection fraction. An increase has been associated with a maintained recruitable stroke work, whereas those with a decrease in ejection fraction have lost this compensatory mechanism. It has been shown that the lower the LV ejection fraction, and the more LV dysfunction is present, the worse is the clinical outcome with respect to survival.[18] Despite these clear advantages, radionuclide angiography is only rarely used in the diagnostic and prognostic evaluation of patients with heart failure, mainly because there is little added information compared with echocardiography.

COMPUTED TOMOGRAPHY IMAGING (see Chap. 18). CT scanning permits rapid and accurate investigation of the heart and adjacent vessels. Three different techniques are used to assess cardiac anatomy and function.

Spiral CT scanning uses multiple rotations of the CT gantry while the patient moves continuously through the x-ray source. Computer reconstructions allow determination of multiple transaxial scans with 4- to 8-mm thickness during a single breath-hold. For improvement of image quality and better delineation of vascular structures, 20 to 40 ml of radiographic contrast material is injected intravenously and CT acquisitions are performed 10 to 15 seconds after injection, when peak contrast concentration is reached in the left heart (Fig. 23-4). With this technique intra-cardiac volumes and myocardial perfusion can be determined.

Multislice CT scanning has gained a lot of interest. Scanning the heart and its vessels, first 8 to 16, and then 32 to 64, imaging planes (and soon more), have been used. For an accurate assessment of cardiac dimensions and volumes, fast CT scanners are combined with electrocardiographic triggering and breath-holding to avoid motion artifacts.

TABLE 23–5	Echocardiographic Findings in Heart Failure
General Findings	
Size and shape of the ventricle	
LV ejection fraction (LVEF)	
Regional wall motion; synchronicity of ventricular contraction	
LV remodeling (concentric versus eccentric)	
LV or RV hypertrophy (DD—hypertension, COPD, valve disease)	
Morphology and severity of valve lesions	
Mitral inflow and aortic outflow properties; RV pressure gradient	
Output state (low or high)	
Systolic Dysfunction	
Reduced LVEF (<45%)	
Enlarged left ventricle	
Thin LV wall	
Eccentric LV remodeling	
Mild or moderate mitral regurgitation*	
Pulmonary hypertension*	
Reduced mitral filling*	
Signs of increased filling pressure*	
Diastolic Dysfunction	
Normal LVEF (≥45%-50%)	
Normal LV size	
Thick LV wall, dilated atria	
Concentric LV remodeling	
No or minimal mitral regurgitation	
Pulmonary hypertension*	
Abnormal mitral filling pattern*	
Signs of increased filling pressure	

DD = diastolic dysfunction; LV = left ventricular; RV = right ventricular; COPD = chronic obstructive pulmonary disease.
*Indicates Doppler-echocardiographic finding.

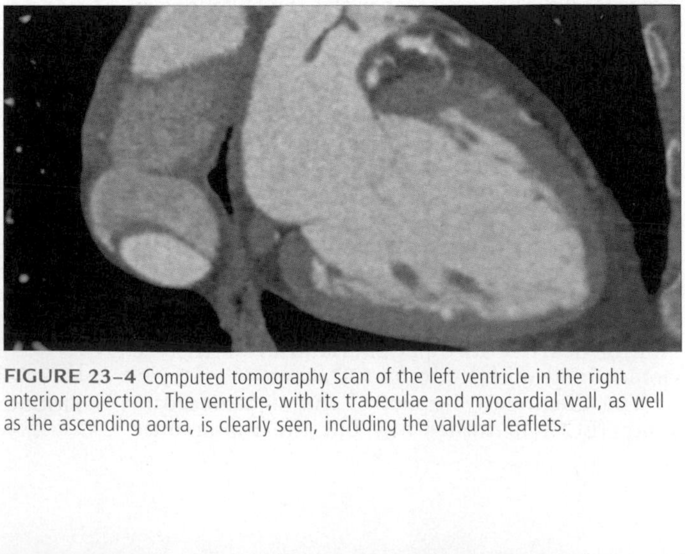

FIGURE 23–4 Computed tomography scan of the left ventricle in the right anterior projection. The ventricle, with its trabeculae and myocardial wall, as well as the ascending aorta, is clearly seen, including the valvular leaflets.

Ultrafast *electron beam tomography* (EBT) uses an electron gun to produce a stream of electrons that are magnetically focused and directed into different target rings, each of which emits two x-ray beams. This technology allows complete cardiac imaging in 50 milliseconds without the need for electrocardiographic gating or breath-holding. Contrast enhancement by intravenous injection of contrast medium permits accurate delineation of intracardiac chambers and vessels at end-diastole and end-systole. However, the infrastructure of this technique is expensive and radiation exposure is relatively high. Therefore, EBT has not gained wide application and has been replaced by multislice CT scanning.

CT scanning has been used in cardiology to diagnose pulmonary embolism, aortic dissections, and pericardial or tumor disease (see Chap. 69). Volumetric and functional evaluations have been done almost exclusively by echocardiography, which is cheaper, feasible at the bedside, and not associated with exposure to radiation. However, the high temporal and spatial resolution of CT technology allows the evaluation of coronary anatomy and morphology (Fig. 23-5), although even the best images are susceptible to artifacts caused by the rapid movement of the coronary arteries, tortuosity of the vessels, calcifications of the arteries, and presence of intracoronary stents or clips after bypass surgery. Nevertheless, CT technology is increasingly being used for noninvasive imaging of the coronary arteries. Multislice CT imaging for the patient with severe heart failure is limited because of the larger dose of contrast needed and the need for beta blockade in patients with a high heart rate (more than 80 bpm) caused by the inverse relationship of heart rate and coronary image quality using current CT methods. These limitations may soon disappear with the advent of the next generation of CT technology.

MAGNETIC RESONANCE IMAGING (see Chap. 17). Magnetic resonance imaging (MRI) has seen many changes over the years of its evolution into a highly sophisticated technology, perhaps the cornerstone of medical imaging in the future. This technique has been shown to be of considerable use in the morphological and functional assessment of the heart but, as with multislice CT scanning, this technology is mainly used to gain additional information (Table 23-6). Cardiac MR imaging requires acquisition of multiple oblique planes relative to the heart. The imaging techniques are designed to render blood dark or bright and to depict various aspects of motion, flow, and perfusion (see Table 23-6). However, cardiac and respiratory motion must be taken into consideration and their effects must be minimized. Electrocardiographic gating has been used prospectively (R wave trigger for data collection) or retrospectively (continuous data collection and retrospective image assignment). The major advantage of retrograde gating is that blood flow can be measured continuously, whereas prospective gating is used for dimensional and functional imaging. Correction for respiration has been done by breath-holding during short sequences (up to 12 to 14 seconds) or by navigator techniques using the position of the diaphragm as a marker for data collection.

Different techniques (Fig. 23-6) have been used for assessing cardiac function with MRI. New MRI sequences allow the assessment of three-dimensional cardiac motion (myocardial tagging; see Chap. 17), blood flow velocity (phase contrast method), or myocardial infarct size (late enhancement technique). Assessment of myocardial viability is of utmost importance to detect ischemic but viable myocardium for potential therapeutic interventions. In heart failure, where 60 to 70 percent of all patients suffer from coronary artery disease, these techniques are helpful for therapeutic and prognostic stratification. Late enhancement MRI has become useful for determination of infarct size in patients with myocardial infarction. Twenty to 40 ml of MR contrast material is injected intravenously and late (after 10 to 12 minutes) MRI scans are obtained. The contrast material is accumulated in the scar tissue and the location and extent of the scar can be determined (Fig. 23-7). Patients with a scar larger than 30 gm have been shown to have poor clinical outcomes.

MR coronary angiography is still not yet a competitive modality for routine use in the heart failure patient. However, the promise of MRI is that it may become part of

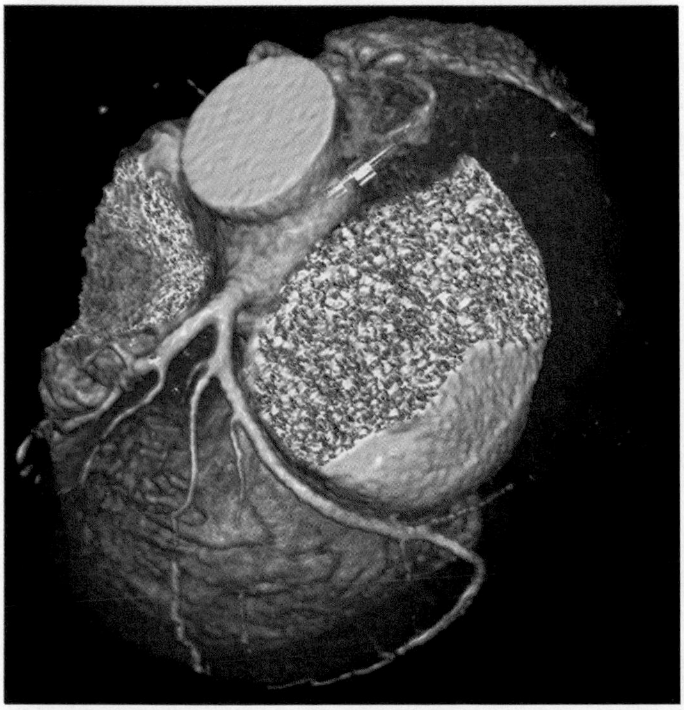

FIGURE 23–5 Three-dimensional reconstructed computed tomography–coronary angiography image in a patient with normal left coronary artery. *(Courtesy of Prof. Juergen Triller, Institute of Radiology, University Hospital, Bern, Switzerland.)*

TABLE 23–6 Cardiac Magnetic Resonance Imaging

Techniques	Indications
Dark blood imaging	Wall thickness, morphology of the myocardium, tumor masses
Bright blood imaging	Wall thickness, geometry of the ventricle
Myocardial tagging	Cardiac rotation, shear motion, torsion, myocardial twist
Phase contrast imaging	Blood flow velocity, cardiac output, pressure gradients
Contrast enhancement	Myocardial fibrosis, ischemic zone, infarct size
MR coronary angiography	Coronary anatomy, coronary plaques
Stress imaging	Wall motion abnormalities, recruitable stroke work, ischemic territory
Perfusion and diffusion imaging	Perfusion abnormalities, territory, ischemic zone
Spectroscopy	Viability, energy-rich phosphosphate

a comprehensive examination of cardiac patients that provides additional information, more than any other technique (e.g., cardiac function, cardiac output, myocardial viability, myocardial energy consumption, coronary flow and anatomy).

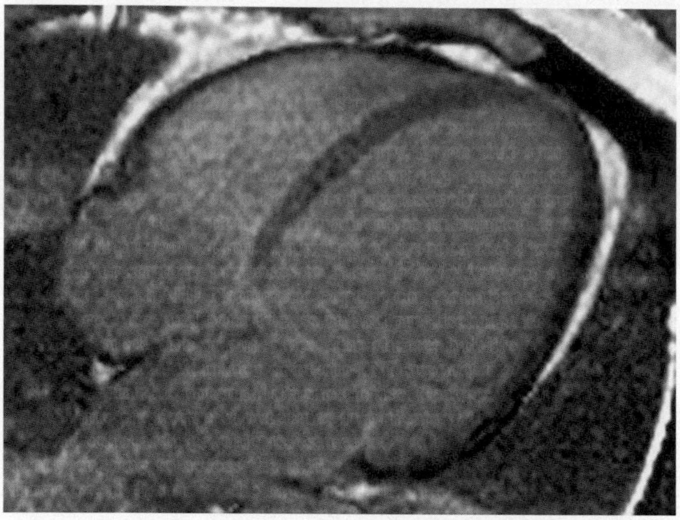

FIGURE 23–6 Magnetic resonance image of the left and right ventricle (apical two-chamber view) in a patient with severe heart failure. The left ventricular ejection fraction is 25 percent and there is eccentric left ventricular remodeling.

CORONARY ANGIOGRAPHY (see Chaps. 19 and 20). Coronary artery disease is the underlying cause in approximately two thirds of patients with heart failure with depressed systolic function (see Chaps. 25 and 54), and may also contribute to the progression of heart failure through endothelial dysfunction, recurrent ischemia, and/or myocardial infarction (MI). Moreover, although coronary artery disease is often evident on angiography or at autopsy in patients with heart failure with a normal EF, there is less often a history of prior MI in these patients. Therefore, it may be useful to define the presence, anatomical characteristics, and functional significance of coronary artery disease in selected heart failure patients who present with signs and symptoms of coronary artery disease. The difficulty lies in identifying appropriate candidates. Heart failure patients with coronary artery disease are often asymptomatic with regard to ischemic symptoms. The best candidates for revascularization are those with the largest amount of viable but jeopardized myocardium and the most severe ischemia (see Chap. 27). However, angina may be missing and dyspnea may be the leading symptom, which is misinterpreted as heart failure symptom rather than an ischemic equivalent. Furthermore, heart failure patients are often elderly and show severe comorbidities and thus may not be optimal candidates for surgical and percutaneous coronary revascularization. Of those patients who are potential candidates and amenable to such an intervention, those with symptomatic angina probably have the most to gain from such a therapy with regard to symptoms and prognosis. For these patients, coronary angiography may be the most cost-

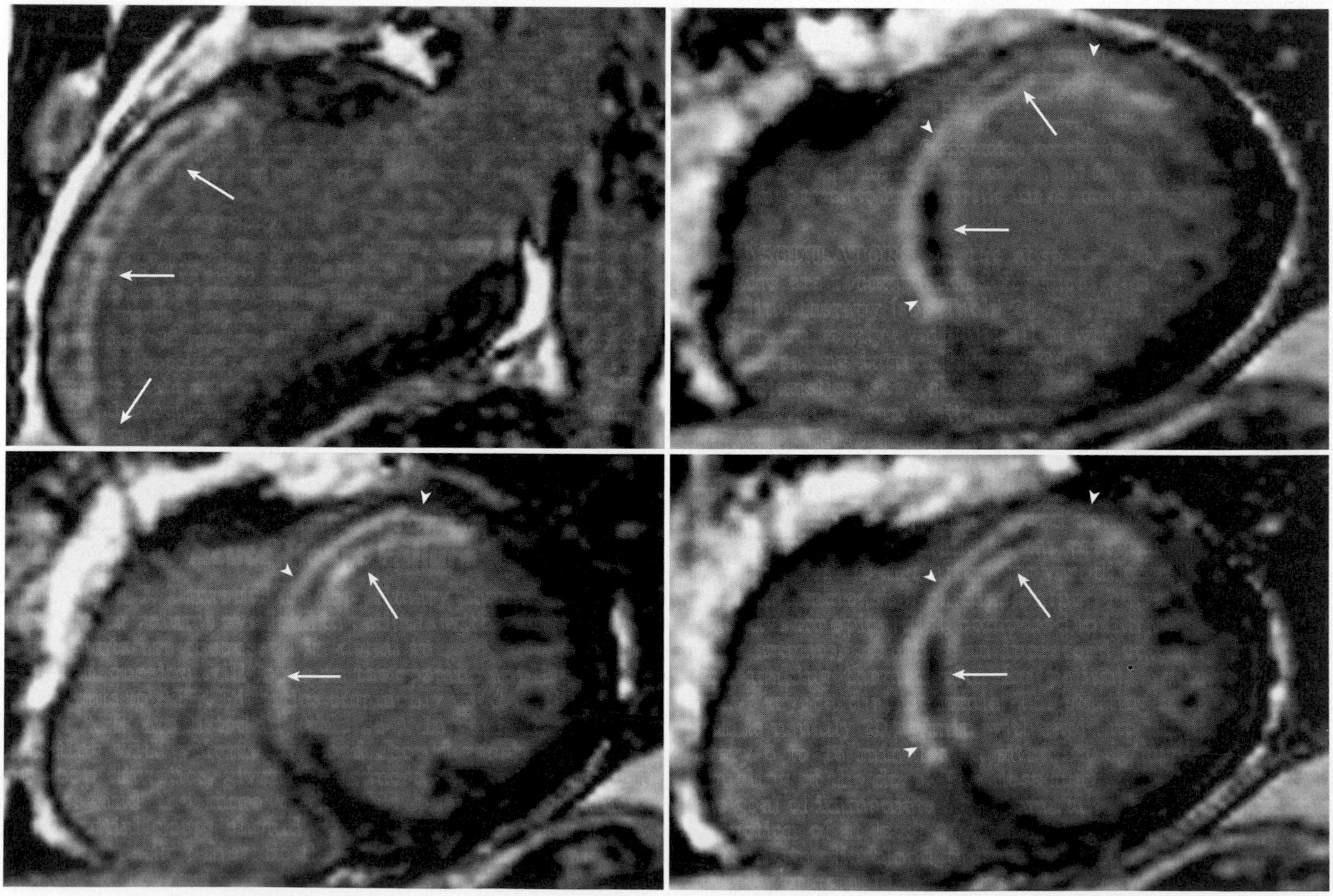

FIGURE 23–7 Late enhancement of the left ventricle in four different projections in a patient with subacute myocardial infarction. Arrows indicate zones with contrast enhancement caused by myocardial ischemia. There are subepicardial and subendocardial layers of enhancement (arrowheads, representing microvascular obstructions), with a central black region (possibly edema).

TABLE 23–7	Current Indications for Coronary Angiography in Patients with Heart Failure
Heart failure patients with angina	
Patients with prior myocardial infarction or known coronary artery disease	
Patients (younger than 65 yr) with unexplained heart failure*	
Positive exercise test in patients with cardiovascular risk factors	
Heart failure patients with positive scintigraphy, stress echocardiography, or positron emission tomography results	
Heart failure patients with severely dyskinetic myocardium	

*Is reasonable to consider.

effective therapy. Coronary angiography should also be considered for patients with acute or acutely decompensated heart failure and patients with severe heart failure (e.g., shock or acute pulmonary edema) who are not responding to initial treatment. Coronary angiography should be performed in patients with angina pectoris or any other evidence of myocardial ischemia, particularly if they are not responding to appropriate antiischemic treatment. For heart failure patients with coronary artery disease, the optimal test for detecting myocardial ischemia remains controversial. The current indications for coronary angiography in patients with heart failure are summarized in Table 23-7.

POSITRON-EMISSION TOMOGRAPHY (PET). PET has been used to determine myocardial perfusion and metabolism noninvasively. The radiotracers used are labeled with positron-emitting isotopes that have chemical and physical properties identical to those of naturally occurring elements such as carbon, oxygen, nitrogen, and fluorine. Image acquisition is done with circular-oriented PET detectors similar to CT scanners. Emission data are displayed as tomograms in a horizontal and vertical axis. Myocardial perfusion can be assessed quantitatively using rubidium or ammonia as tracer. Myocardial metabolism can be studied by using palmitate for assessing fatty acid metabolism or fluoro-2-deoxyglucose for assessing myocardial viability.

Assessment of myocardial blood flow is important for imaging myocardial infarction and infarct size and for detecting stress-induced myocardial ischemia. Myocardial perfusion studies are used for diagnostic purposes to confirm coronary artery disease as the cause of heart failure. Patients with flow alterations may undergo coronary angiography and myocardial revascularization for improving cardiac function. Assessment of myocardial viability is important in patients with heart failure for therapeutic reasons. Glucose uptake–positive regions may qualify for coronary revascularization, whereas glucose uptake–negative regions indicate nonviable tissue with no potential for improving cardiac function. These patients may qualify for heart transplantation rather than myocardial revascularization with percutaneous intervention (PCI) or bypass surgery.

ASSESSMENT OF NORMAL AND ABNORMAL CARDIAC FUNCTION

The fundamental task of the cardiovascular system is to supply the peripheral organs with adequate quantities of oxygenated blood. The performance of the heart requires the complex interplay among the properties of the myocardium, influences of neural and humoral factors, circulating

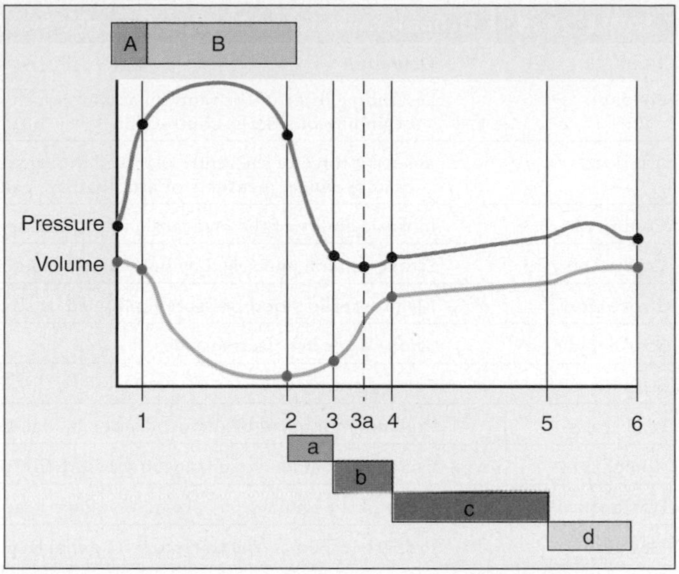

FIGURE 23–8 The cardiac cycle is shown in this schematic with both the left ventricular LV pressure waveform and a plot of LV volume. The time landmarks during the cardiac cycle include the following: 1, aortic valve opening and the beginning of ejection; 2, aortic valve closure; 3, mitral valve opening; 3a, pressure nadir; 4, end of rapid early diastolic filling; 5, onset of atrial contraction; and 6, end-diastole. The phases of the cardiac cycle are denoted by the shaded rectangles displaying the timing of each phase. The two systolic phases are noted above the waveforms—A = isovolumic contraction; B = ejection. The four diastolic phases are noted below the waveforms—a = isovolumic relaxation; b = early diastolic filling; c = diastasis; d = atrial filling.

blood volume, and peripheral vascular compliance and resistance.

Systolic Function in Heart Failure

An important determinant of cardiac performance is LV systolic function, which in turn is determined by preload, afterload, myocardial contractility, and heart rate (Table 23-8). These four determinants allow the heart to adapt its performance to the changing requirements of the peripheral organs, as well as to compensate for a loss of myocardial mass and/or function, such as in heart failure.[19] Cardiac performance is evaluated primarily by assessing LV systolic function. Systole begins with the onset of depolarization and contraction and ends at the cessation of muscle contraction (Fig. 23-8).

PRELOAD. The stretch of the individual sarcomere regulates the performance of the heart. In the words of physiologists of the 19th century, preload is the property of cardiac muscle such that "the larger the quantity of blood which reaches the ventricles, the larger the quantity will be which it throws out."[20] Surrogates of the degree of sarcomere stretch at the onset of contraction include the ventricular end-diastolic volume, diameter, and end-diastolic pressure.

AFTERLOAD. This is the force against which muscle contracts. It is more challenging to quantify afterload in the intact circulation than in isolated cardiac muscle. Two approaches have been followed. The first focuses on the vascular load and uses descriptors such as peripheral vascular resistance or the more complex input impedance (see later), which includes the pulsatile load. The second focuses on the tension in the ventricular wall and considers pressure and cavity size in a more complex formulation, the Laplace law, which considers wall tension to be the product of pressure and radius, whereas the force (or tension) per

TABLE 23–8 Definitions of Terms Used to Describe Systolic and Diastolic Function

Term	Definition
Preload	Distending force of the ventricular wall, which is highest at end-diastole and is responsible for sarcomere length at the beginning of systolic contraction
Afterload	Resisting force of the ventricular wall during systolic ejection, which is necessary to overcome peripheral vascular resistance or impedance; measures of afterload are peak-systolic, mean-systolic, or end-systolic wall stress
Contractility	Intrinsic ability of the myocardium to generate force at a certain rate and time (controlled for loading conditions)
Cardiac output	Stroke volume multiplied by heart rate output
Stroke work	Mean systolic blood pressure multiplied by stroke volume
Stroke force	Stroke work per ejection time
Stress	Force per area
Wall stress	Pressure multiplied by radius, divided by wall thickness × 2
Compliance	Change in volume per change in pressure (dV/dP) or distensibility
Elastance	Slope of the end-systolic pressure-volume relationship
Elasticity	Property of a material to restore its initial length or geometry after distending force has been removed
Strain	Length change in percentage of initial length; two definitions are used: Lagrangian strain, $e = (l - l_0)/l_0$, and natural strain, $e = \ln(l/l_0)$
Stiffness	Pressure per volume change (dP/dV). Ventricular stiffness is a measure for changes of the ventricle as a whole; myocardial stiffness is a measure for changes of the myocardium itself. Ventricular properties are characterized by instantaneous pressure-volume relationships, whereas myocardial properties are best described by stress-strain relations.
Creep	Time-dependent lengthening of a material in the presence of a constant force
Stress relaxation	Time-dependent decrease of stress in the presence of a constant length
Viscoelasticity	Resistance of a material to length changes (strain) or the velocity of length changes (strain rate)

unit of muscle is expressed in three dimensions—circumferential, meridional, and radial (Fig. 23-9).

CONTRACTILITY. This is the intrinsic ability of heart muscle to generate force and to shorten. In the intact circulation, it is manifest as the rate of pressure development and shortening from any given preload. Contractility is normally modulated by various factors, including the neurohumoral milieu. Measures of systolic function and contractility are often considered together and include stroke volume, ejection fraction, maximum rate of pressure increases during isovolumic contraction, and various more sophisticated measurements that attempt to control for loading conditions.[21]

FILLING PRESSURES. The determination of systolic function should be placed in the framework of the ventricular filling pressure that reflects preload; the latter, in turn, is influenced importantly by the status of the circulating blood volume. Filling pressures are also related to both the contractility and diastolic properties of the ventricle (see later). Filling pressures such as ventricular end-diastolic pressure, atrial pressure, and pulmonary capillary wedge pressure (for the left ventricle) and central venous pressure (for the right ventricle) provide valuable clinical information that aids in the differentiation between disparate conditions causing hypotension—for example, hypovolemia versus myocardial failure.

LV end-diastolic pressure (LVEDP) is measured routinely in the cardiac catheterization laboratory during retrograde left heart catheterization (see Chap. 19). It may be difficult to measure LVEDP precisely at rapid heart rates using fluid-filled catheters, especially when there is no distinctive plateau after atrial contraction. The measurement of LVEDP during invasive and interventional procedures provides a simple and often useful indicator of cardiac function. Several common clinical examples demonstrate the usefulness of this measurement. An elevated LVEDP in the presence of a normal LV ejection fraction (LVEF) suggests the presence of diastolic dysfunction (see later). A low LVEDP after a percutaneous coronary intervention suggests volume depletion that should be corrected before the development of hypotension. A markedly elevated LVEDP may be a strong contraindication to the injection of contrast dye and suggests that diuresis is needed.

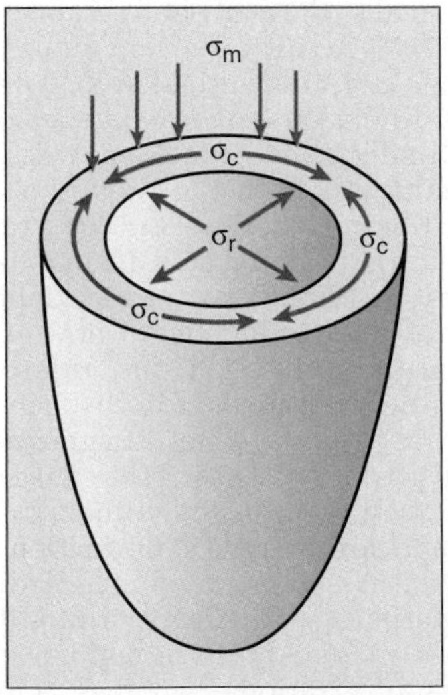

FIGURE 23–9 Circumferential (σ_c), meridional (σ_m), and radial (σ_r) components of left ventricular wall stress from an ellipsoid model. The three components of wall stress are mutually perpendicular. *(With permission from Fifer MA, Grossman W: Measurement of ventricular volumes, ejection fraction, mass, and wall stress.* In *Grossman W [ed]: Cardiac Catheterization and Angiography. 5th ed. Philadelphia, Lea & Febiger, 1996, p 34.)*

Calculations and Measurements of Systolic Function

Clinical parameters for assessing left ventricular systolic function include the following:

- Cardiac index (liter/min/m²): heart rate × stroke volume per body surface area
- Stroke volume index (ml/m²)
- Stroke work index: stroke volume index × mean systolic blood pressure (ml × mm Hg/m²)
- Stroke force index: stroke work index per ejection period in seconds
- Preload recruitable stroke work = relationship between stroke work and end-diastolic volume

CARDIAC OUTPUT AND RELATED MEASURES. Cardiac output is commonly measured by the thermodilution technique (see Chap. 19). Saline injected into the right atrium is detected as a temperature change at a thermistor at the tip of a catheter in the pulmonary artery. The thermodilution catheter transmits the temperature data to a small computer that calculates cardiac output. To improve accuracy, the determination is usually repeated several times and the results are averaged. This technique is less accurate when flow is severely reduced, especially in the presence of tricuspid regurgitation, which leads to dissipation of the "temperature bolus." The presence of intracardiac shunts also introduces potential errors and misinterpretation, because right- and left-sided flows are not equal. The Fick method of measuring cardiac output has greater accuracy than the thermodilution method when oxygen consumption is actually measured, rather than estimated. Measured cardiac output is usually expressed relative to body size (i.e., cardiac index), which is calculated as cardiac output divided by body surface area, expressed in meters squared.

Cardiac output (and index) can be divided by the heart rate to yield stroke volume (and index). An alternative method of deriving stroke volume is by calculating the difference between LV volume at end-diastole and end-systole. This approach is limited by the accuracy of the imaging modality in determining chamber volumes. Accuracy is greatest with a three-dimensionally determined volume with high-resolution imaging, but it may be impaired by the normal beat-to-beat variation in chamber size that occurs during respiration and is accentuated in atrial fibrillation and other arrhythmias. The product of pressure generation and stroke volume equals stroke work; when related to the time interval during which the stroke volume is ejected from the left ventricle (i.e., the ejection time) stroke force may be determined.

VENTRICULAR FUNCTION CURVES. Reduced values of stroke parameters (e.g., volume, work, force, and their indices, corrected for body surface area) are often associated with depressed myocardial contractility, but because these parameters are highly dependent on the loading conditions (preload and afterload), these two variables must also be assessed. The dependency of stroke volume on preload was described more than 100 years ago by Otto Frank and E.H. Starling, and since then has been called the Frank-Starling mechanism.[22] Using this relationship between preload and stroke volume or stroke work, a *ventricular function curve* can be constructed by plotting stroke work at various levels of preload; the latter may be expressed as ventricular end-diastolic volume, end-diastolic pressure, or end-diastolic wall stress (Fig. 23-10). Preload can be altered by volume loading (leg elevation, volume infusion) and unloading (vena caval balloon occlusion).

LV afterload can be estimated from the mean or end-systolic arterial or ventricular pressure or, more accurately, by calculating mean systolic, peak systolic, or end-systolic wall stress. The most reliable method for determination of LV contractility represents the end-systolic pressure-volume relationship (ESPVR; maximum elastance), which is nearly independent of preload and afterload. The slope of this relationship is a measure of LV contractility (Figs. 23-10 and 23-11). The use of ventricular function curves in assessing LV function is limited by technical difficulties in performing measurements in patients, spontaneous variability over the time it takes to make measurements, and interpretation, because these curves are also dependent on gender, age, and afterload. Furthermore, changes in right ventricular (RV) filling pressure can affect the position of the interventricular septum and alter LV diastolic pressure, thereby altering the position of the ventricular function curve as well.

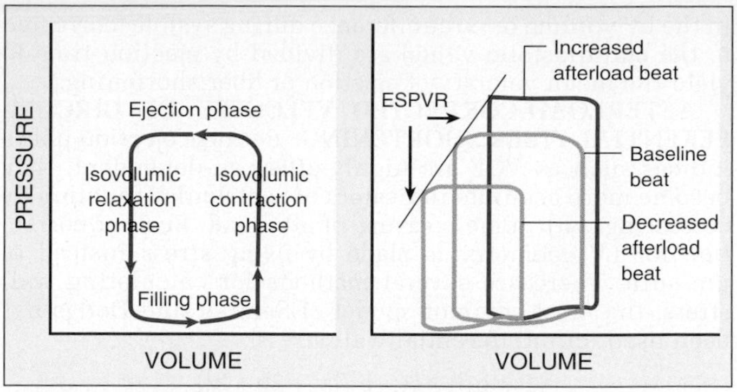

FIGURE 23–10 Left, Left ventricular pressure-volume relationship is shown, with the four phases of the cardiac cycle. **Right,** The graph shows how two additional pressure-volume loops appear with an acute increase and decrease in afterload. Changes in preload can also be used to generate the coordinates. In the clinical setting, it is difficult to generate the end-systolic pressure-volume relationship (ESPVR) free of changes in reflex-mediated variations in contractility. It also requires a means to measure pressure and volume accurately and simultaneously. The end-systolic pressure-volume coordinates form a linear relationship, ESPVR. The slope of the ESPVR line is end-systolic elastance.

Specific Indices of Left Ventricular Systolic Function

There are several indices of global LV systolic function and contractility.[28] Each one is variably dependent on preload and afterload and can be modified by ventricular volume and myocardial mass. The ease of application to the clinical setting is an important feature.

EJECTION FRACTION. The ejection fraction is defined as the ratio of stroke volume to end-diastolic volume. It is most often computed as follows:

$$EF = \frac{(EDV - ESV)}{EDV} \times 100\,(\%)$$

where EF = ejection fraction, EDV = end-diastolic volume, and ESV = end-systolic volume.

Normal values of the left ventricular ejection fraction (LVEF) are 0.55 to 0.75 when determined by cineangiography and echocardiography but may be lower when determined by radionuclide angiography (0.45 to 0.65). There are no gender differences, but the ejection fraction normally declines with age. An acute increase in afterload, such as occurs during acute pressure loading, may decrease the ejection fraction to 0.45 or 0.50 in normal subjects. However, a reduction of the LVEF below 0.45 indicates impaired myocardial function, independent of loading conditions.

The widespread applicability of the ejection fraction in clinical practice is a result of a number of factors, including the conceptual simplicity of its derivation, the ability to determine it easily and reproducibly using different imaging techniques, and an extensive documentation of its clinical usefulness.[21] This parameter has been shown to be of great prognostic value over the short and long term in patients with various heart diseases. However, it is limited in that it depends not only on myocardial contractility but also on preload and afterload, as well as heart rate and synchronicity of contraction. This parameter is also a global parameter and major regional differences in contractility are presented as an average. Therefore, it measures much more than contractility.

END-SYSTOLIC VENTRICULAR VOLUME OR DIMENSION. The clinical usefulness of end-systolic volume or dimension is its relative *independence* of preload. Although strongly afterload-dependent, it is of particular value in assessing left ventricular function in patients with valvular regurgitation.

VELOCITY OF CIRCUMFERENTIAL FIBER SHORTENING. This ejection phase index of systolic function, the velocity of circumferential fiber (VCF) shortening, has been used primarily in research studies. Typically, the changes in the LV volume or circumference during systole (corrected to the end-diastolic value) are divided by ejection time to yield the mean velocity of ejection or fiber shortening.

AFTERLOAD-CORRECTED VELOCITY OF CIRCUMFERENTIAL FIBER SHORTENING. Because ejection phase indices such as VCF are highly afterload-dependent, they become more accurate indicators of ventricular function by correcting with some measure of afterload. Further correction for LV geometry is made by using stress instead of pressure. There are several methods for calculating wall stress; the most common model of Sandler and Dodge has been used (circumferential wall stress):

$$P = b/h \times (1 - b^2/[a^2 + 2b + h])$$

where P = pressure, h = LV wall thickness, b = short half-axis, and a = long half-axis. Patients with reduced left ventricular contractility have a downward shift of the systolic shortening–mean systolic wall stress relationship.

SLOPE OF END-SYSTOLIC PRESSURE-VOLUME RELATIONSHIP (END-SYSTOLIC ELASTANCE). The most reliable index for assessing myocardial contractility in the intact circulation is the end-systolic pressure-volume relationship, ESPVR, which is almost *insensitive* to changes in preload, afterload, and heart rate (see Fig. 23-11). This is widely used in animal studies and occasionally clinically. This relationship can be determined from instantaneous end-systolic pressure-volume coordinates from different cardiac contractions at varying preload and afterload conditions. Using a linear regression analysis for assessing the end-systolic pressure-volume curve, the following equation is used:

$$E(t) = P(t)/V(t) - V_0(t)$$

where E = maximum elastance (mm Hg/ml), P = pressure (mm Hg), V = volume (ml), and V_0 = extrapolated volume at pressure 0 (ml). The slope of this relationship represents the end-systolic elastance, which is a sensitive parameter for assessing myocardial contractility. Assessment of elastance is difficult under clinical conditions, because it requires simultaneous pressure-volume relationships, as well as changes in preload or afterload for construction of the ESPVR. However, this measurement is facilitated by the use of techniques such as radionuclide angiography or conductance catheters, which allow continuous measurements of LV volume while LV volume is changed such as by caval occlusion (see Fig. 23-10).

END-SYSTOLIC STIFFNESS. This index of contractile function is derived from the exponential constant of the end-systolic relationship between wall stress and the natural logarithm of the reciprocal of wall thickness.[28]

PRELOAD RECRUITABLE STROKE WORK. The relation between LV stroke work and LV end-diastolic volume is a representation of systolic function.[29] Like the end-systolic elastance, it is difficult to assess this index in patients because preload needs to be varied to generate this parameter.

MAXIMAL RATE OF PRESSURE RISE. The maximal rate of ventricular pressure rise (max dP/dt) is analogous to the maximal rate of tension development of isolated cardiac muscle, a well-established index of myocardial contractility. However, the concept of a true isovolumic contraction period in the intact heart is no longer correct, because it has been shown with myocardial tagging that during isovolumic contraction, there is systolic rotation (reflecting myocardial shortening) without a change in volume (see later). As a further limitation, max dP/dt is dependent not only on LV contractility but also on heart rate, preload and afterload, synchronicity of contraction, and myocardial hypertrophy. Because this isovolumic index of systolic function is preload-dependent, the relationship between ventricular end-diastolic volume and dP/dt is a more accurate index of contractility than dP/dt alone.

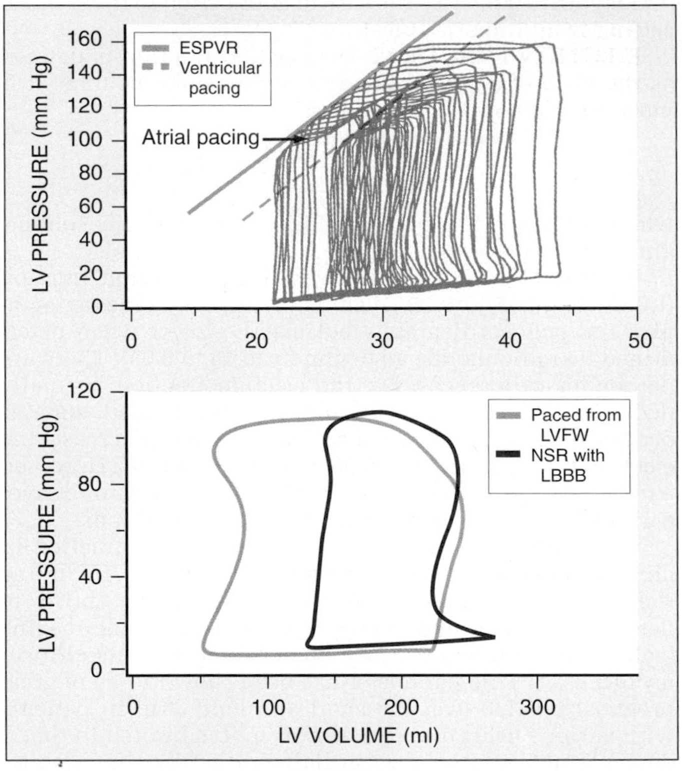

FIGURE 23–11 Top, Left ventricular (LV) pressure-volume loops in an experimental animal during transient caval occlusions. The upper left corners of the loops define the LV end-systolic pressure-volume relation (ESPVR). During atrial pacing producing normal LV activation, the ESPVR is shifted leftward in a parallel fashion, compared with ventricular pacing that produces dyssynchronous LV activation and contraction. **Bottom,** Steady-state LV pressure-volume loop recorded using the conductance catheter in a patient with dilated cardiomyopathy and dyssynchronous LV activation caused by left bundle branch block (LBBB). A decrease in dyssynchronous contraction produced by LV free wall (LVFW) pacing produced loops with greater width (stroke volume) as the end-systolic pressure-volume point shifted toward the left. NSR = normal sinus rhythm. *(**Top,** With permission from Park RC, Little WC, O'Rourke RA: Effect of alteration of left ventricular activation sequence on the left ventricular end-systolic pressure-volume relation in closed-chest dogs. Circ Res 57:711, 1985; and **bottom,** from Kass DA, Chen DH, Curry C, et al: Improved left ventricular mechanics from acute VDD pacing in patients with dilated cardiomyopathy and ventricular conduction delay. Circulation 99:1570, 1999.)*

Regional Indices of Left Ventricular Function

Global measures of LV function, such as those described earlier, lose accuracy when the disease process affects regions of the ventricle differentially; this occurs most notably in coronary artery disease. Chronic myocardial ischemia (i.e., stunning or hibernation; see Chap. 54), and acute or old myocardial infarction may be associated with regional wall motion abnormalities with hypokinesis (reduced shortening) and akinesis (absent shortening) or dyskinesis (systolic elongation or bulging). Often, the nonischemic portion of the ventricle is hyperkinetic or hypercontractile, leading to normal *global* LV function in the presence of impairment of regional function.

The most widely used technique for assessing regional wall motion is the center line method (Fig. 23-12), which demonstrates that shortening at the apex normally is less than at the base. For normalization, systolic shortening may be divided by ejection time. This approach to quantifying regional LV function was initially used in contrast angiograms and then extended to echocardiograms. These measures of endocardial motion and changes in wall thickness are afterload-dependent but do allow comparisons of different regions of the ventricle. As discussed later, MRI with myocardial tagging provides the most comprehensive assessment of regional wall motion. More recently, tissue Doppler strain rates and motion analysis (see Chap. 14) have been used experimentally and clinically.

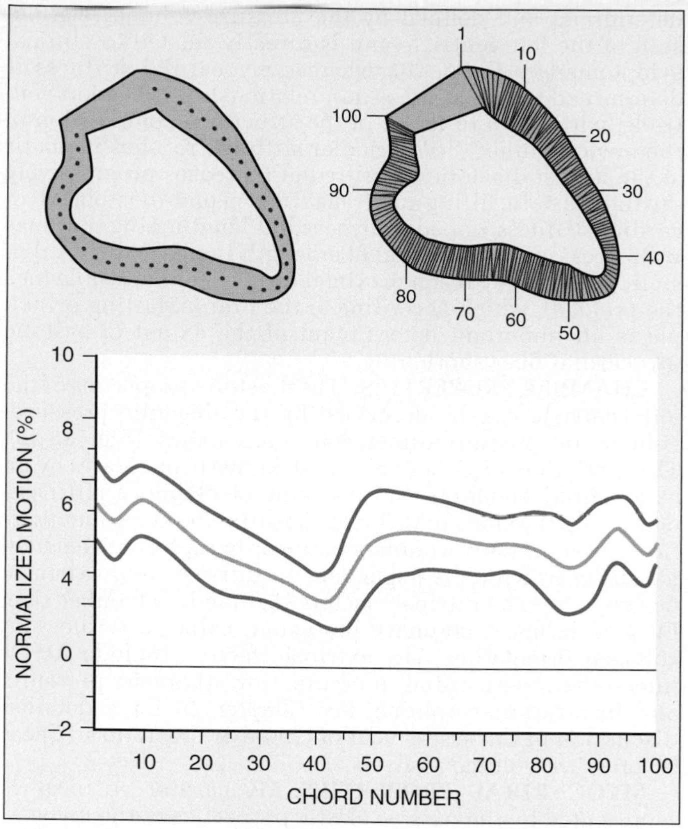

FIGURE 23–12 Assessment of regional left ventricular (LV) function using the center line method. Regional wall motion is determined along 100 chords drawn perpendicular to a center line constructed midway between the end-diastolic and end-systolic contours. Calculated wall motion of the 100 chords **(bottom)** is normalized for heart size by dividing each chord by the length of the end-diastolic perimeter. The normal range is indicated by the dotted lines (mean ± 1 SD). *(With permission from Sheehan FH, Bolson EL, Dodge HT, et al: Advantages and applications of the center line method for characterizing regional ventricular function. Circulation 74:293, 1986.)*

Left Ventricular Dysfunction in Heart Failure

LV dysfunction is characterized by a change in preload and afterload, decrease in myocardial contractility, and increase in diastolic filling pressures.[19] Changes in preload and afterload have been characterized by LV remodeling with an increase in the size of left ventricle and a change in LV geometry. Generally, LV diastolic wall stress is used as parameter for preload and LV end-systolic or mean-systolic wall stress as measure for afterload. Normal values of wall stress depend on the model of calculation (e.g., Laplace, Sandler-Dodge), the orientation of wall stress (e.g., circumferential, meridional, longitudinal; see Fig. 23-9), and the use of a thin wall or a thick wall model. Changes in LV contractility have been determined from pressure-derived indices such as the maximum rate of pressure (max dP/dt) and the slope of the end-systolic pressure-volume relationship (end-systolic elastance). The end-systolic elastance is probably the most reliable index for assessing myocardial contractility, but is difficult to assess using instantaneous end-systolic pressure-volume relationships at varying preload and afterload conditions. Thus, in daily life, this index is only rarely used and mainly for scientific purposes.

More commonly, the volume-derived contractility parameters are used, such as cardiac index, stroke work index, or preload recruitable stroke work. Because these variables are highly dependent on loading conditions, ventricular function curves have been constructed by plotting stroke work at various levels of preload and afterload. The most useful parameter in daily practice is the LVEF fraction, which is the parameter used most frequently for differentiating between systolic and diastolic dysfunction. An ejection fraction of more than 50 percent is considered to be normal, an ejection fraction between 35 to 50 percent is moderately depressed, and an ejection fraction below 35 percent represents a severely depressed systolic pump function. Many of the large clinical heart failure trials are based on these definitions and different therapeutic interventions are dependent on the LVEF, such as the implantation of an ICD. Furthermore, LVEF has become a prognostic parameter although others, such as VO_2max, may be more reliable than a simple parameter of LV pump function. Various regional shortening parameters have been developed in the past but the clinical usefulness of these parameters is limited (velocity of circumferential fiber shortening) and have not reached a wide application for assessing LV dysfunction. Regional indices of LV function are useful in patients with coronary artery disease and regional wall motion abnormalities. Generally, reductions of more than 50 percent of the normal value are considered to represent a reduced regional function.

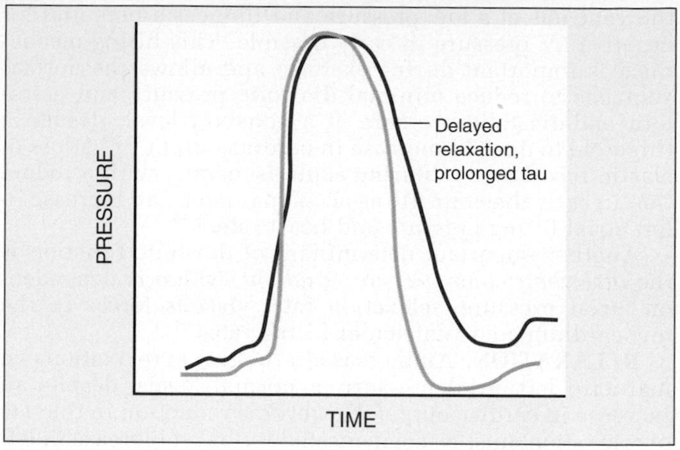

FIGURE 23–13 Two left ventricular (LV) pressure waveforms show a normal contour and then a waveform with delayed relaxation producing a prolonged time constant of relaxation (tau). The pressure coordinates from aortic valve closing to mitral valve opening, i.e., during the isovolumic relaxation period, can be plotted and the negative reciprocal of the log plot is the calculated relation value (tau).

Diastolic Dysfunction in Heart Failure

The assessment of cardiac performance has focused traditionally on systolic function, whereas diastole was considered of secondary importance. However, diastolic function has also been found to play an important role in cardiac morbidity and mortality of heart failure patients and to influence both preload and afterload (see Table 23-8). Diastolic function, its assessment, and factors that influence diastolic function are also discussed in detail in Chapter 26.

Diastolic function is influenced by several factors, such as myocardial relaxation (Fig. 23-13), ventricular filling, and the ventricle's passive elastic properties, but one of the major determinants is heart rate, which determines how much time is available for ventricular filling (see Chap. 26). Thus, impaired diastolic function can be aggravated by tachycardia.

In the normal left ventricle, the end-systolic volume is smaller than its elastic equilibrium and thus it generates *elastic recoil,* which varies inversely with the end-systolic volume. The elastic recoil causes diastolic suction that fills the ventricle at a low pressure and induces a potential for negative LV pressure in early diastole. This filling mechanism is important during exercise and allows the normal ventricle to reduce minimal diastolic pressure and maintain end-diastolic pressure at a constant level, despite a threefold to fivefold increase in cardiac output.[23,24] A loss of elastic recoil occurs during acute ischemia, with a reduction in early diastolic filling accompanied by an increase in left atrial filling pressure and heart rate.[25,26]

Another important determinant of diastolic function is the *atrioventricular pressure gradient,* which is dependent on atrial pressure, relaxation rate, viscous forces in the myocardium, and ventricular filling rates.[23-25]

RELAXATION. An increase in the rate of relaxation can maintain left atrial pressure at normal levels, despite an increase in cardiac output. However, a reduction in the rate of relaxation must be compensated for by an increase in left atrial pressure, if filling, and thus stroke volume is to be maintained. The assessment of relaxation by invasive and noninvasive modalities, the factors that regulate LV relaxation, and the evidence that LV relaxation impairment affects filling pressures are reviewed in Chapter 26.

PASSIVE ELASTIC PROPERTIES. It is necessary to distinguish between ventricular (chamber) and myocardial (muscle) properties (Fig. 23-14).[22-24,27] Ventricular stiffness is determined and defined by the pressure-volume relationship of the left ventricle and is directly related to clinical symptoms (see Chap. 26), whereas myocardial stiffness is determined by the stress-strain relationship of the left ventricle, which is a function of the structural composition of the myocardium.[28-31] Ventricular stiffness reaches its nadir at the lowest diastolic pressure but increases progressively during diastolic filling and is maximal at end-diastole. Myocardial stiffness impedes myocardial lengthening. Because wall stress and myocardial fiber length increase during diastolic filling, they reach maximal levels at end-diastole (i.e., the preload), which according to the Frank-Starling principle is an important determinant of the extent of systolic myocardial fiber shortening.

CHAMBER PROPERTIES. The diastolic properties of the left ventricle can be described by the diastolic pressure-volume or pressure-dimension relationship (Fig. 23-15). Those relationships can be described mathematically by an exponential equation, the constant of chamber stiffness, defined by the slope of this relationship. The slope and position of the pressure-volume relationship represent *ventricular stiffness,* which is dependent on intrinsic and extrinsic factors.[23,24,27] The intrinsic factors include LV chamber size, LV muscle mass, coronary perfusion, collagen tissue, and collagen orientation. The extrinsic factors include RV-LV interaction, pericardial pressure, intrathoracic pressure, and intravascular volume. See Chapter 26 for a detailed discussion of the assessment of chamber diastolic stiffness by pressure volume analysis.

MYOCARDIAL PROPERTIES. Myocardial stiffness is represented by the passive elastic properties of the myocardium that are influenced by the cardiac interstitium and by the structural composition of the myocytes themselves.[28,30,32] Histomorphometric examinations have shown that disorientation of the collagen fibers in experimental heart failure contributes to the increase in myocardial stiffness. The slope of the diastolic stress-strain relationship has been termed the *constant of myocardial stiffness* (see Fig. 23-14). This constant is dependent on the properties, quantity, and

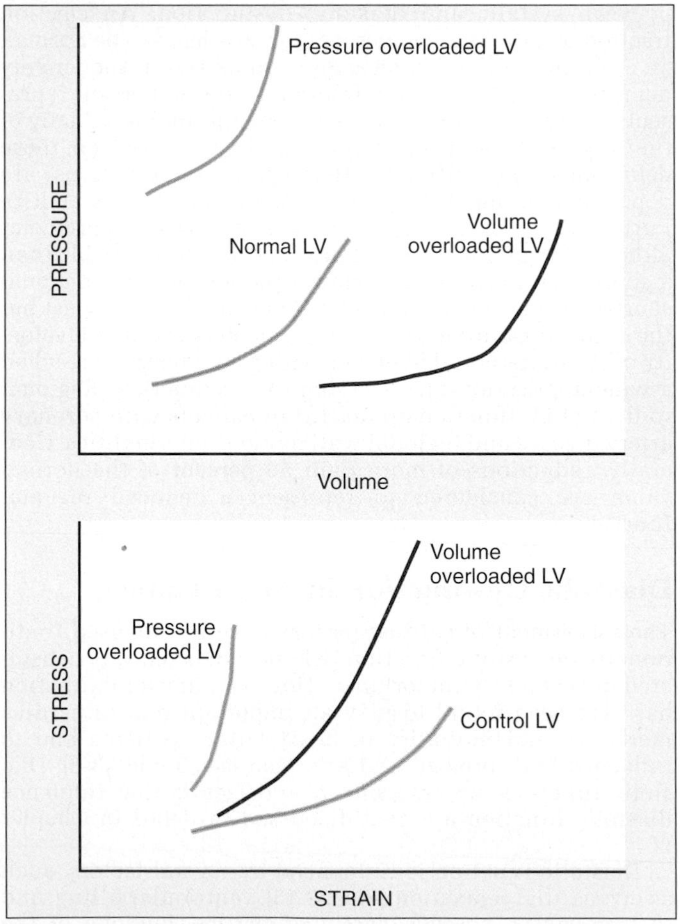

FIGURE 23–14 Schematic representation of the diastolic left ventricular (LV) pressure-volume **(top)** and LV stress-strain relationship **(bottom).** The pressure-volume relationship is dependent on changes of the left ventricle as a whole associated with chronic pressure (upward shift) or volume-overload (rightward shift), whereas the LV stress-strain relationship represents changes of the myocardium. The slope of the stress-strain relationship has been called *stiffness constant of the myocardium*—that is, the steeper the slope, the stiffer the muscle. Muscle stiffness is influenced by the composition of the myocardium—that is, the ratio of the muscular tissue to the extracellular matrix.

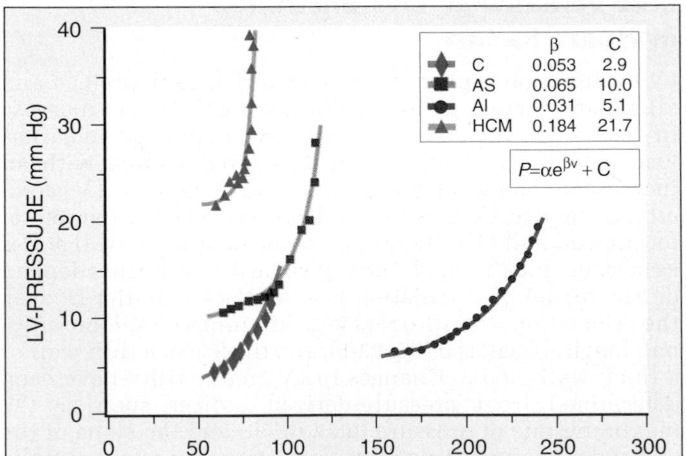

FIGURE 23–15 Left ventricular (LV) pressure-volume relationship during diastole in a control subject (C) and patients with aortic stenosis (AS), aortic regurgitation (AI), and hypertrophic cardiomyopathy (HCM). There is a parallel upward shift in the HCM and a small upward shift in the AS patient caused by the increase in diastolic stiffness. The constant of chamber stiffness (β) is 0.184 in HCM and 0.065 in AS compared with 0.053 in the control patient. However, there is a rightward shift in the AI patient caused by the increase in LV diastolic volume, with a minimal increase in diastolic filling pressure (i.e., caused by a low diastolic chamber stiffness). In this patient, β = 0.031. *(From Mandinov L, Eberli FR, Seiler C, Hess OM: Diastolic heart failure. Cardiovasc Res 45:813, 2000.)*

orientation of the collagen fibers, as well as on myocardial perfusion and temperature.[27,28,31]

LV myocardial stiffness is calculated by plotting instantaneous LV wall stress against LV midwall strain from the lowest diastolic to end-diastolic pressure or from the end of the rapid filling phase to the peak of the a wave. The calculation of stress involves a geometric model of the left ventricle, whereas the calculation of strain requires some assumption of the unstressed LV volume. The most commonly used equation for assessing myocardial stiffness is

$$S = \alpha e^{\beta E} + C$$

where S = wall stress, α = intercept, e = base of the natural logarithm, β = slope of the stress-strain relationship (muscle stiffness constant), E = strain, and C = stress asymptote. Again, a nonlinear curve-fitting procedure is used. *Muscle stiffness* is the slope of the myocardial stress-strain relationship. Average normal values for the muscle stiffness constant are 12, ranging between 5 and 20.[27]

PERICARDIAL PROPERTIES. The pericardium forms a strong, purely elastic sac with extensions that enclose the origins of the ascending aorta, venae cavae, and proximal and distal ends of the pulmonary artery and veins (see Chap. 70). The pericardium consists of two layers, the fibrous outer and the serous inner layers, with up to 30 ml of fluid normally in the sac. The pericardium acts as a barrier to reduce friction between the heart and the surrounding organs. The normal pericardium is relatively stiff[33,34] and the relationship between intrapericardial volume and pressure is a steep monoexponential curve. A small increase in intrapericardial volume leads to a rapid augmentation of intrapericardial pressure and thereby an increase in ventricular pressures. Normal intrapericardial pressure is zero or negative. However, when the volume of the heart increases and exceeds the elastic limit of the pericardial sac, intracavitary pressures in all four chambers of the heart increase. An acute increase in the right- or left-sided volume affects the filling of the contralateral chamber by increasing its diastolic pressure (i.e., through ventricular interaction). The pericardium contributes to diastolic coupling of the atria and ventricles, so that RV and LV filling pressures are closely correlated in the presence of an intact pericardium but are lower in the absence of the pericardium.[33] Cardiac distensibility without the pericardium is influenced primarily by the properties of the myocardium. Elevations of intrapericardial volume and pressure over days to weeks (i.e., chronically) lead to an increase in the volume of the pericardial sac with a fall in pressure as the sac stretches and changes its compliance.[33,34] The volume of intrapericardial fluid may be as high as 1000 to 1200 ml in chronic pericardial effusion, with little constraint on cardiac chambers.

Assessment of Diastolic Function

Several noninvasive techniques are useful for the diagnosis of diastolic dysfunction and quantification of various diastolic parameters. Cardiac catheterization–based techniques, alone or combined with noninvasive techniques such as echocardiography, with simultaneous pressure and volume measurements, still represent the gold standard for quantitative studies and for research requiring calculation of chamber compliance and myocardial stiffness. These techniques are reviewed in detail in Chapter 26.

Imaging Techniques

Although intraventricular pressure and volume measurements are still most widely used for the assessment of diastolic function, a number of noninvasive techniques have been used for the clinical assessment of diastolic function in patients with coronary, valvular, or myocardial heart disease. Doppler echocardiography is frequently used to assess diastolic function in humans; this technique is reviewed in Chapter 26. Cardiac MRI is a newer modality to assess diastolic function and may offer unique insights into myocardial relaxation that are not possible with tissue Doppler studies.

MAGNETIC RESONANCE IMAGING. This technique has been shown to be of considerable use in the morphological and functional assessment of the heart. Additional information may be gained from newer techniques such as magnetic resonance myocardial tagging, which allows for the labeling of specific myocardial regions (Fig. 23-16).[35-38] From these tags, the rotational and translational motion of the left ventricle can be determined; it is characterized by a systolic twisting motion with a clockwise rotation at the base and a counterclockwise rotation at the apex during systole (Fig. 23-17). This motion can best be described as the wringing of a wet towel. The untwisting motion occurs very early in diastole and is directly related to myocardial relaxation. Untwisting may be used as a measure of the rate and completeness of relaxation and may serve as an estimate of early diastolic filling. In the normal left ventricle, systolic rotation begins at end-diastole and continues during isovolumic contraction (see Fig. 23-18), whereas shortening starts during systolic ejection after the aortic valve has opened. Diastolic backrotation starts at end-systole and continues during isovolumic relaxation, whereas diastolic lengthening begins with mitral valve opening and ends with the next end-diastole. Thus, the normal left ventricle performs a rectangular twisting-shortening (i.e., systole) and untwisting-lengthening (i.e., diastole) loop that occurs in opposite directions at the apex and base (Fig. 23-18), resulting in a wringing motion. This motion is determined by the orientation of the muscle fibers within the myocardium. The relationship between myocardial rotation and/or twisting and changes in chamber size provide a unique insight into LV systolic and diastolic function and their interaction.

A loss of myocardial tissue, as in myocardial infarction, or the occurrence of LV asynchrony, as in left bundle branch block, leads to a loss of the normal rotation-relaxation pattern associated with an increase in myocardial energy requirements. The normal systolic wringing motion allows the heart to work economically at a low-energy threshold because the wringing motion requires less energy than the "squeezing" motion. The traditional physiological concept of an isovolumic contraction and relaxation period has to be revised because the concept of an isometrically contracting or isometrically relaxing ventricle is no longer valid. The shortening of the muscle fibers within the LV wall induces systolic rotation during isovolumic contraction and the relaxation of the fibers during isovolumic relaxation causes diastolic backrotation (untwisting). Athletes (with physiological hypertrophy) have a normal rotation-diastolic relaxation pattern, whereas patients with aortic stenosis (with pathological hypertrophy) show a delayed systolic rotation-diastolic relaxation pattern (see Fig. 23-18).

Right Ventricular Function

PATHOPHYSIOLOGY. RV function plays a central role in the clinical outcome in a wide variety of cardiopulmonary disorders. The right ventricle is pivotal in many specific congenital cardiac malformations, and its significance continues into adulthood. Examples are the adaptation to chronic volume overload from residual pulmonary regurgitation in repaired tetralogy of Fallot and to shunting from left to right because of an untreated atrial septal defect. In addition, acquired diseases such as primary and secondary pulmonary hypertension produce a remodeling of the right ventricle that resembles the remodeling of the left ventricle with pressure overload.

The right ventricle differs from the left ventricle regarding the type of work normally performed. Stroke volume is, of course, equal for the two ventricles, but the left ventricle must generate a high pressure to overcome higher gravitation effects and allow appropriate distribution of flow to multiple beds with differences in local resistance. The right ventricle, on the other hand, ejects into a more uniform and compliant pulmonary vascular bed and, therefore, has a

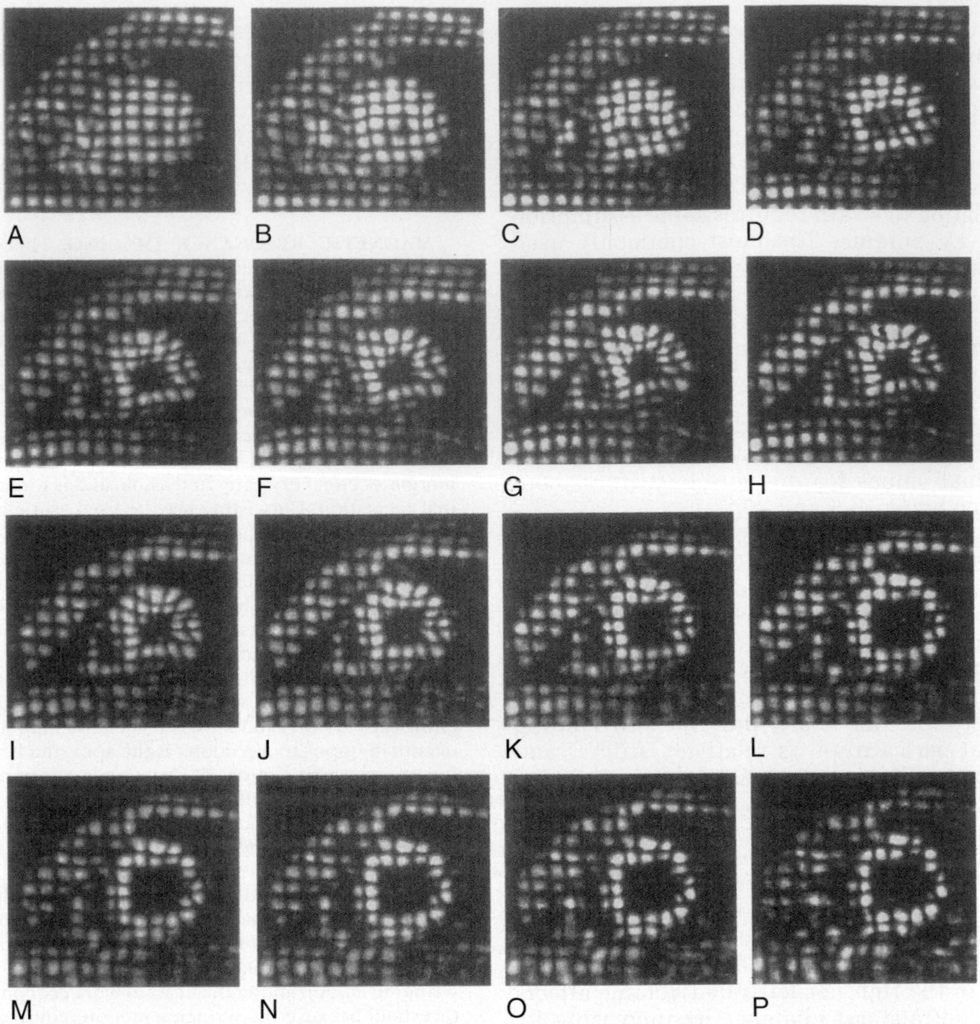

FIGURE 23–16 A-P, Series of magnetic resonance (MR) images in a control patient with normal left ventricular (LV) function (temporal resolution, 35 milliseconds). The MR images show horizontal and vertical lines (myocardial tags) superimposed on the conventional MR image. From the movement of the grid crossing points, the contraction and relaxation behavior of the left ventricle can be determined. During isovolumic contraction, there is a counterclockwise rotation at the apex followed by systolic shortening. During isovolumic relaxation, there is a clockwise rotation ("untwisting") followed by diastolic lengthening. This systolic-diastolic contraction-relaxation behavior is altered in patients with diastolic dysfunction, with prolongation of diastolic backrotation. *(From Mandinov L, Eberli F, Seiler C, Hess OM: Diastolic heart failure. Cardiovasc Res 45:813, 2000.)*

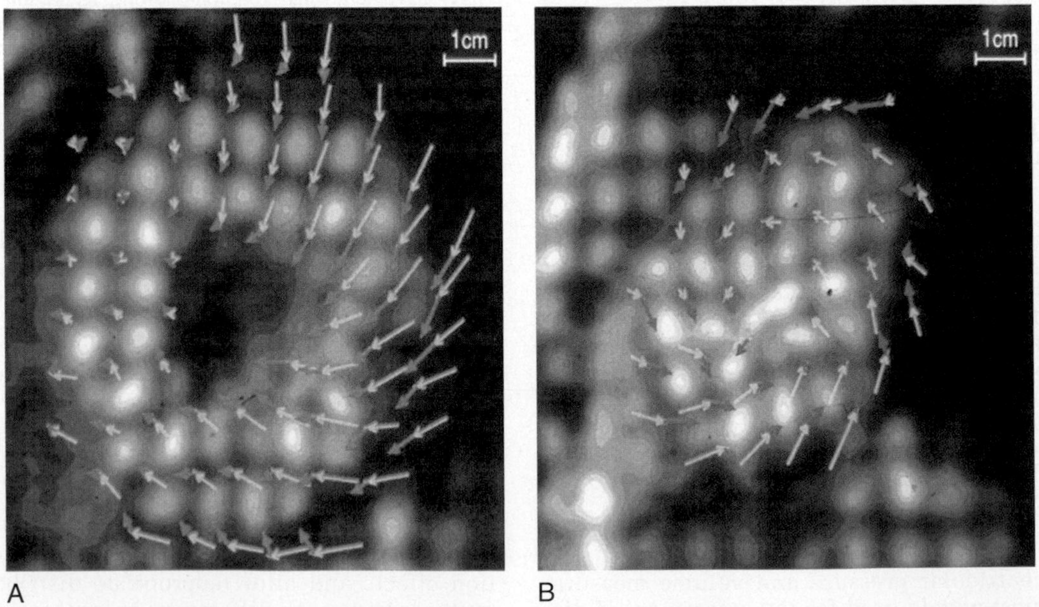

FIGURE 23–17 Ejection phase of the left ventricle at the apex **(A)** and base **(B)** of a healthy subject. End-systolic acquisitions are overlaid with corresponding local trajectories. There is a clockwise rotation at the base and counterclockwise rotation at the apex. This motion pattern has been described as a systolic wringing motion and provides a more sophisticated approach to quantifying regional left ventricular systolic function versus the traditional methods of endocardial shortening and simple wall thickening. *(With permission from Stuber M, Scheidegger MB, Fischer SE, et al: Alterations in the local myocardial motion pattern in patients suffering from pressure overload due to aortic stenosis. Circulation 100:361, 1999.)*

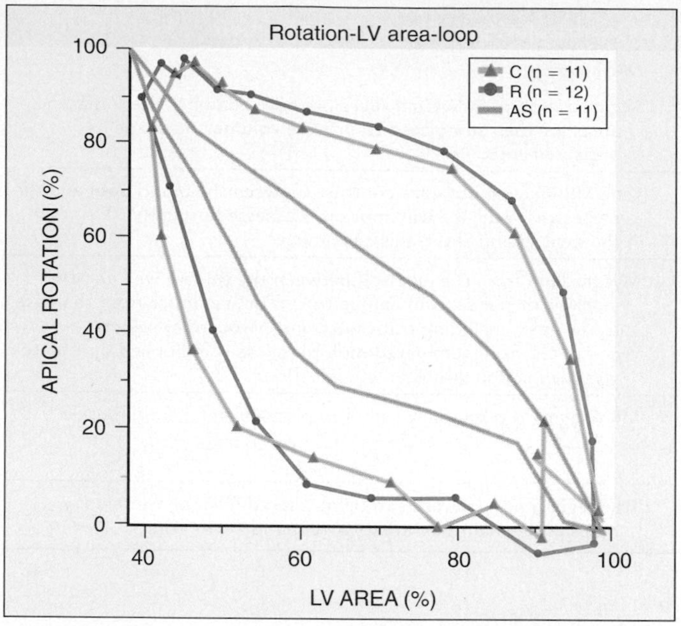

FIGURE 23–18 Tagged magnetic resonance imaging–derived averaged patient data presented as a rotation-area loop in controls (C; $n = 11$), professional rowers (R; $n = 12$), and patients with severe aortic stenosis (AS; $n = 11$). In the rowing athletes, the rotation-area loop has a rectangular shape, as in controls, but in patients with severe hypertrophy (AS), delayed systolic rotation and relaxation are observed. This abnormal rotation-relaxation behavior in pathological hypertrophy reflects changes in LV afterload and myocardial hypertrophy. *(With permission from Stuber M, Scheidegger MB, Fischer SE, et al: Alterations in the local myocardial motion pattern in patients suffering from pressure overload due to aortic stenosis. Circulation 100:361, 1999.)*

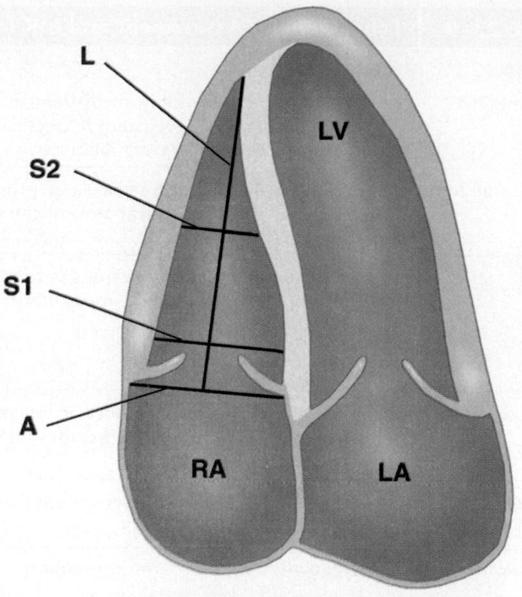

FIGURE 23–19 The right ventricle is schematically illustrated in this echocardiographic apical four-chamber view. From this view, RV size can be quantified along its major axis (L) and two minor axes (S1 and S2) of the right ventricle. Tricuspid annular diameter (A) may also be measured. The important additional measurements of the outflow tract are not shown. The two-dimensional images of the right ventricle from echocardiography are suboptimal in assessing chamber volume and function and provide an impetus for three-dimensional techniques based on ultrasound or other modalities, such as magnetic resonance imaging and computed tomography scanning. LV = left ventricle; RA = right atrium; LA = left atrium. *(With permission from Reynertson S, Kundur R, Mullen G, et al: Asymmetry of right ventricular enlargement in response to tricuspid regurgitation. Circulation 100:465, 1999.)*

thinner wall than the left ventricle to generate this lower pressure. The right ventricle also fills differently. It takes in systemic venous return at very low pressures, including the inspiratory creation of negative intrathoracic pressures, which further sucks venous return into this chamber.

Although the prognostic significance of RV adaptation to pressure or volume overload is widely recognized, the methods for studying this chamber have been slow to develop. A central problem has been in the imaging of this unusually shaped chamber, which normally wraps around the interventricular septum and functions primarily as a component of the left ventricle (Fig. 23-19). The thin-walled RV free wall reduces the feasibility of studying wall thickening during systole and thinning during diastole by echocardiography, as is done in the assessment of LV function. In the future, routine cardiac MRI may allow the assessment of RV free wall motion more appropriately.

ASSESSMENT OF RIGHT VENTRICULAR FUNCTION. Traditional two-dimensional echocardiography allows assessment of RV shape, size, and changes in size during the cardiac cycle. More recently, MRI has advanced the study of RV function by providing images of this eccentric chamber and information on blood flow, regional function, and wall characteristics. A summary of the parameters assessed by MRI imaging and ultrasonography is provided in Table 23-9. Contrast angiography, nuclear angiography, and the conductance catheter have their roles in special focused applications for assessing RV function.

Function and Remodeling of the Right Ventricle: Four Paradigms

An understanding of RV function is best illustrated by considering four examples of the response of this chamber to different pathophysiological conditions, as discussed in the following sections.

CHRONIC VOLUME OVERLOAD. Tricuspid regurgitation from damage to the valve apparatus by frequent endomyocardial biopsy in some heart transplantation patients provides a model of the evolution of RV volume overload.[39] Two- dimensional echocardiography (see Fig. 23-19) allows quantification of the progressive enlargement of the RV end-diastolic cavity area with a change toward a more spherical chamber, as reflected in an increased ratio of midchamber minor dimension to the long axis of 0.5 to 0.7.

Atrial septal defect before and after closure provides another example of the chronic remodeling of the right ventricle and the extent of reversed remodeling following percutaneous closure.[40] Within 1 month of closure, the right ventricle undergoes important electrical and mechanical remodeling with a subsequent plateau at 6 months. The four-chamber two-dimensional echocardiographic views of the RV inflow and outflow tracts demonstrate that all patients have a decrease in chamber size, but 29 percent have some residual chamber enlargement at 1 year. Accompanying this structural remodeling is a significant reduction in QRS duration.[40]

Both RV and LV function, including chamber compliance, are major determinants of the degree and direction of shunting through the atrial septal defect and ultimately may influence RV remodeling after closure.[41] Left-to-right shunting may increase in adulthood as the left ventricle becomes less compliant from acquired diseases. Shunting can, on the other hand, become bidirectional as the right ventricle loses its more compliant nature or develops frank failure.

CHRONIC PRESSURE OVERLOAD. The right ventricle undergoes extensive hypertrophy in primary pulmonary hypertension and leads to progressive RV dilation, reduced systolic performance, secondary tricuspid regurgitation, and overt RV failure with peripheral edema and ascites (see Chap. 73).[42] Although regression of RV hypertrophy has been described as a result of vasodilator therapy, the progressive nature of the primary disease process is unremitting for most patients. Direct (catheter-based) measurement of pressure and cardiac output is an important complement to noninvasive imaging to characterize the stage of the disease in the individual patient.

A more reversible form of pressure overload hypertrophy of the right ventricle is seen in pulmonary hypertension secondary to chronic thromboembolism.[43] After surgical thromboembolectomy, two-dimensional echocardiography has quantified a significant reduction in end-diastolic (30 ± 7 to $21 \pm 5\ cm^2$) and end-systolic (24 ± 6 to

TABLE 23–9 Echo/Doppler Assessment and MR Imaging of Right Ventricular Size, Shape, and Function

Parameter	Echo/Doppler	MR Imaging
RV volume	Standard 2D views allow measurement of multiple dimensions. The parasternal long-axis view shows the outflow tract diameter.	Segmentation of individual slices provides chamber size. Adjacent areas are then summated to provide volume and shape measurements.
Regional wall motion	Free RV wall and interventricular septum are imaged and paradoxical motion can easily be detected	Cine MR imaging provides contrast between the blood pool and the myocardial wall. RV wall motion is assessed using RVOT cines in the sagittal and short-axis cine images
RV mass	Approximated by wall thickness determinations along with chamber size measurements	Myocardium from the junction between the RV free wall and the interventricular septum can be traced on each slice from the base to the apex, including trabeculations. Myocardial volume computed from summated multiple slices is multiplied by 1.05 to give the mass in grams.
RV wall composition	Not well studied in transthoracic images. Intracardiac ultrasound provides higher resolution data.	MR imaging is potentially useful to distinguish fat from muscle.
Regurgitant fraction	Doppler profiles provide semiquantitative approach.	True regurgitant volumes can be measured from phase velocity maps in the main pulmonary artery and aortic root.

RV = right ventricular; RVOT = RV outflow tract; 2D = two-dimensional.

14 ± 4 cm²) cavity area in the four-chamber view.[44] RV fractional shortening increased and tricuspid regurgitation decreased. Furthermore, there was a resultant normalization of interventricular septal motion, improved diastolic filling, and rise in cardiac output.

Valvular pulmonic stenosis produces RV hypertrophy that appears reversible after successful balloon valvuloplasty.[45] The secondary relief of a subvalvular pressure gradient in the RV outflow tract also occurs, presumably from regression of infundibular hypertrophy.[45]

ACUTE ISCHEMIC DYSFUNCTION (see Chap. 50). The acute deterioration in RV function during acute myocardial infarction has been studied by two-dimensional echocardiography and invasively determined pressures and cardiac output.[46,47] Motion of the RV free wall may be dramatically decreased with chamber dilation and an acute elevation of right-sided filling pressures resulting from increased chamber stiffness, mediated in part by an acute pericardial restraining influence.[39] Enlargement of the RV cavity may develop rapidly, with a reversal of septal curvature and paradoxical movement during systole. The derangement of RV function, if severe enough, can result in right-sided heart failure, clear lung fields, and a low cardiac output, despite nearly normal LV function.

CHRONIC VENTRICULAR DYSFUNCTION. Preliminary studies have shown that resynchronization with RV pacing improves function in patients with chronic RV dysfunction, as reflected in RV maximum positive dP/dt and cardiac output.[21,48]

Left Atrial Function

In the last decade, Doppler echocardiography has provided a large experience in functional assessment of the left atrium whereas MR imaging and CT scanning now provide in-depth three-dimensional anatomical assessment of this chamber. Various new interventional techniques require more intensive study of the left atrium. For example, catheter-based ablation of atrial fibrillation, left atrial appendage occlusion devices, atrial septal closure devices, and emerging mitral valve interventions have stimulated an interest in the left atrium, whereas there also has been a new appreciation of the importance of left atrial size and function in a broad spectrum of cardiac disease states.[49-51]

LEFT ATRIAL APPENDAGE. Pulsed-Doppler interrogation of left atrial appendage flow is a major component of the functional assessment of this chamber. The function of the left atrial appendage is determined by factors well studied in the past for LV function.[52-55] Removal of the appendage as well as insertion of devices into the left atrial appendage to block thrombus formation may make the remaining left atrial chamber less compliant.[55]

LEFT ATRIAL CHAMBER SIZE AND SHAPE. The relationships between body size, gender, age, and left atrial volume have been detailed in a reference population using ultrasound techniques.[56] The normal left atrial volume is 42 ± 12 ml. The three-dimensional reconstruction of the left atrium has been developed with ultrasound.[57] CT scanning and MRI have been applied to left atrial size and shape. Images of the left atrium and distal pulmonary veins using multidetector helical CT with multidimensional reconstruction provide accurate, detailed information of these structures.[58]

COMPONENTS OF LEFT ATRIAL FUNCTION. Conceptually, left atrial function can be described as having three components: (1) a distensible reservoir during ventricular systole as blood enters this chamber from the pulmonary veins, while the mitral valve is closed; (2) a passive conduit of blood in early ventricular diastole after mitral valve opening; and (3) a booster pump function occurring during late ventricular diastole and involving atrial contraction.

To understand its function, the volume of the left atrium is determined at three points in time during the cardiac cycle. Immediately before mitral valve opening the left atrium is at its maximal volume, reflecting its reservoir function. With mitral valve opening, the left atrium decompresses rapidly, in part caused by a suction effect from the normal left ventricle during early diastole. The second time point is reached immediately before atrial systole, when the left atrial pre-A wave (ECG) of LV volume is determined. With subsequent atrial contraction, there is further emptying of the left atrium until ventricular end-diastole is reached, and this minimum left atrial volume is measured immediately after atrial contraction. Hoit and Gabel have shown that left atrial conduit function represents 35 percent of all flow through the chamber.[59] The relative roles of active atrial contraction versus atrial conduit function have been clarified in animal studies, demonstrating that the conduit function can compensate for atrial myocardial failure as long as LV function is normal. Left atrial function studied by transmitral flow, as well as pulmonary venous flow patterns and left atrial appendage emptying flow, are Doppler-based techniques that are widely available and can be applied clinically. Multiple factors influence the triphasic and quadriphasic pattern of the pulmonary venous flow pattern (Table 23-10).[49] The systolic or booster pump function of the left atrium can be characterized in many ways that are parallel to LV systolic function assessment.[60-64]

TABLE 23–10 Left Atrial and Ventricular Function Influences on the Pulmonary Venous Flow Velocity Profile

Pulmonary Venous Wave	Function	Left Ventricular (LV) Function
First systolic wave	Atrial relaxation	
Second systolic wave	Reservoir function Atrial compliance	LV contraction Right ventricular contraction
Early diastolic wave	Conduit function	Ventricular relaxation, Ventricular chamber stiffness
Atrial reversal wave	Booster pump	Ventricular chamber stiffness

Modified from Tabata T, Thomas JD, Klein AL: Pulmonary venous flow by Doppler echocardiography: Revisited 12 years later. J Am Coll Cardiol 41:1243, 2003.

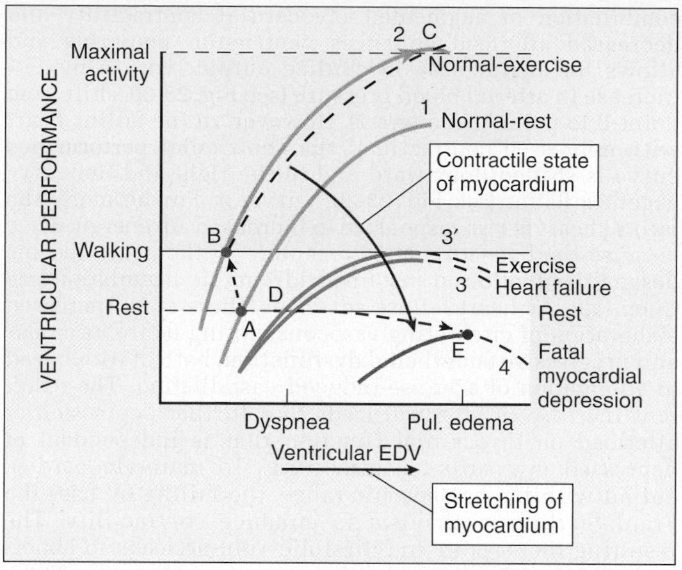

FIGURE 23–20 Ventricular function curves in normal and failing myocardium during exercise. The level of ventricular performance (ordinate) is depicted as a function of the left ventricular (LV) end-diastolic volume (EDV), or preload, which is shown on the abscissa. Curve 1 depicts the interrelationship between LV EDV and ventricular function in a normal heart, and curve 2 depicts the effect of exercise in the normal heart. As shown, the ventricular function curve is shifted upward and to the left as a result of increased heart rate and contractility, as well as peripheral vasodilation in exercising skeletal muscle beds. Curves 3 and 4 show the ventricular function curves in failing hearts, which are shifted progressively downward and to the right and are somewhat flatter. *(Modified from Braunwald E, Ross J Jr, Sonnenblick EH: Mechanisms of Contraction of the Normal and Failing Heart. Boston, Little Brown, 1979.)*

CLINICAL APPLICATION OF ASSESSMENT OF THE LEFT ATRIUM. Doppler-based techniques have been applied to obtain a better understanding of the timing and extent of left atrial myocardial dysfunction, or stunning, after conversion to sinus rhythm from atrial fibrillation[65] and the return of left atrial contractile function following the maze operation.[66] Pharmacological modification of LV diastolic properties that enhance chamber distensibility can augment the atrial contribution to LV filling.[67] A reduction in left atrial size and an increase in left atrium–mediated passive filling of the left ventricle have been observed after modification of LV systolic and diastolic properties following alcohol ablation of the septum in hypertrophic obstructive cardiomyopathy.[68]

EXERCISE AND CARDIAC FUNCTION

Physical exercise is associated with increases in heart rate, venous return, cardiac output, stroke volume, and systolic pressure. Arterial diastolic pressure remains relatively unchanged or decreases slightly and thus pulse pressure increases during exercise, whereas the ejection period shortens. Hemodynamic adaptation depends largely on the type of exercise (i.e., dynamic or isometric exercise), as well as on the severity of exercise and the mass of exercising muscles. Exercise capacity is determined by many factors, such as body position, gender, age, body mass, level of exercise training, and environmental factors, such as temperature, humidity, and ambient oxygen concentration. Adaptation of cardiac function is largely dependent on the level of exercise and the response of the cardiovascular system, as well as the magnitude of adrenergic stimulation. For instance, dynamic exercise (e.g., running, swimming, cycling) is associated with a large increase in cardiac output achieved mainly by increases in heart rate and in stroke volume,[69] whereas isometric exercise (e.g., hand grip, weight lifting, body building) is associated with a moderate increase in cardiac output but a large increase in arterial pressure consequent to enhanced sympathetic stimulation (*pressure loading*). In daily living, both forms of exercise are frequently used and are often combined.

DEFINITION OF ABNORMAL CARDIAC FUNCTION DURING EXERCISE. Most noninvasive exercise studies are carried out in the upright position (treadmill, bicycle ergometer), but invasive (catheter-based) studies are usually performed in the supine position. Because venous return is increased in the supine position, diastolic filling pressure, stroke volume, and cardiac output in the resting state are higher in the supine than in the upright position. Assessment of cardiac function during dynamic or isometric exercise has been carried out by hemodynamic monitoring of the right heart using a Swan-Ganz catheter or a fluid-filled catheter in the left heart and LV angiography. However, most data on exercise have been obtained from right heart catheterization in the supine position. Higher cardiac outputs are reached during maximal exercise in the erect position, but because of technical limitations of most measuring techniques, submaximal exercise has been preferred, to allow a short steady state for measuring hemodynamic data. Increasingly, noninvasive techniques, including two-dimensional echocardiography, radionuclide angiography, and MRI, have been used to study the response to exercise.

Abnormal cardiac function during *maximal* exercise has been based on pulmonary capillary wedge pressure or LVEDP exceeding 20 mm Hg, the cardiac output failing to reach 15 liters/ min, and the ejection fraction failing to rise.

SYSTOLIC FUNCTION DURING EXERCISE. Hemodynamic adaptation of the ventricles to exercise is regulated by an increase in sympathetic activity and the resultant increases in heart rate and cardiac contractility. In the normal heart, when exercise is carried out in the supine position, both LV and RV end-diastolic volumes increase slightly, whereas end-systolic volumes decrease significantly. Both stroke volume and systolic ejection fraction increase and contribute to the augmentation of cardiac output (Fig. 23-20, shift from point A on curve 1 to point B on curve 2). Because end-diastolic volume exhibits little change during exercise, the Frank-Starling mechanism does not play a major role in cardiac adaptation during sustained exercise in the healthy heart. In addition, vasodilation typically occurs in exercising skeletal muscles, which leads to a decrease in peripheral vascular resistance (afterload). This combination of augmented myocardial contractility and decreased afterload enhances ventricular emptying and allows for an increase in cardiac output, with a modest increase in arterial blood pressure (see Fig. 23-20, shift from point B to point C in curve 2). However, in the failing heart with depressed contractility, the ventricular performance curve is shifted downward and to the right and the curve becomes flatter (see Fig. 23-20, curve 3). Furthermore, the failing heart is less responsive to increased adrenergic drive because the beta-adrenergic receptors in the heart become desensitized followed sustained adrenergic stimulation (see Chap. 22). As heart failure advances, there is an increased elaboration of circulating vasoconstricting neurohormones and progressive endothelial dysfunction, both of which lead to attenuation of exercise-induced vasodilation. The resultant increase in afterload leads to a further depression of afterload on myocardial function that is independent of depressed myocardial contractility. To maintain cardiac output within a homeostatic range, the failing LV uses the Frank-Starling mechanism to enhance contractility. The resulting increase in end-diastolic volume leads to abnormally high pulmonary capillary pressures (see Fig. 23-20, point D on curve 3), which can contribute to the dyspnea experienced by patients with heart failure. Over time, the contractile state of the LV deteriorates further as a result of progressive end-organ changes in the heart and the peripheral circulation. The ventricular function curve then becomes further depressed and flatter, so that further increases in end-diastolic volume and adrenergic drive are insufficient to maintain cardiac output (see Fig. 23-20, point E on curve 4) and blood pressure, and the patient dies of "pump failure."

DIASTOLIC FUNCTION DURING EXERCISE. Most studies of the effects of exercise have focused on systolic function; less is known about diastolic function of the normal heart during exercise. There is general agreement that LV end-systolic volume is smaller during exercise because of the enhanced contractile state. At the same time, the rate of relaxation is increased, which allows more rapid filling. These two mechanisms lead to an increase in elastic recoil that enhances ventricular filling at high heart rates when diastolic filling time is abbreviated.[70] These mechanisms maintain stroke volume and prevent undue elevation of ventricular diastolic pressures, even at very high workloads, and thus preload reserve is not needed in the normal heart to achieve maximal cardiac output.

In summary, LV diastolic function during exercise is characterized by the following:

1. Enhanced elastic recoil with a small LV end-systolic volume
2. Rapid LV relaxation caused by enhanced inotropic stimulation
3. Low early diastolic pressures (even negative pressures may occur) because of enhanced diastolic suction
4. Rapid diastolic filling that starts after mitral valve opening; one third of the stroke volume enters the left ventricle when its pressure is still falling

SUMMARY AND FUTURE PERSPECTIVES

The development of new imaging technologies and biomarkers has enabled clinicians to assess heart failure patients accurately and to stratify them with regard to the underlying disorder and the required treatment. An ongoing challenge for clinicians and investigators will be to use newer imaging modalities and biomarkers to help guide optimal therapy and/or necessary cardiac interventions. Recent insights in the field have emphasized that cardiac structure and function can be quantified from different perspectives. Our understanding of the biology of cardiac function will likely advance rapidly during the next decade. Accordingly, the assessment of cardiac structure and function will remain a critical component of the clinical evaluation of patients with heart failure, as well as an invaluable investigative technique to determine the efficacy of newer modalities of therapy.

REFERENCES

Clinical Examination

1. Givertz M, Colucci WS, Braunwald E: Clinical aspects of heart failure: High-output failure, pulmonary edema. *In* Zipes DP, Libby P, Bonow RO, Braunwald E (eds): Braunwald's Heart Disease. 7th ed. Philadelphia, Elsevier, 2005, pp 539-568.
2. Harlan WR, Oberman A, Grimm R, et al: Chronic congestive heart failure in coronary artery disease. Clinical criteria. Ann Intern Med 86:133, 1977.
3. Task Force for the Diagnosis and Treatment of Chronic Heart Failure of the European Society of Cardiology: Guidelines for the diagnosis and treatment of chronic heart failure: Executive summary (update 2005). Eur Heart J 26:1115, 2005.
4. Joshi N: The third heart sound. South Med J 92:756, 1999.
5. Massie BM, Yamani MH: Chronic heart failure: Diagnosis and management. *In* Poole-Wilson PA, Colucci WS, Massie BM, et al (eds): Heart Failure: Scientific Principles and Clinical Practice. New York, Churchill Livingstone, 1997, pp 551-566.

Laboratory Testing

6. Silverberg DS, Wexler D, Sheps D, et al: The effect of correction of mild anemia in severe, resistant congestive heart failure using subcutaneous erythropoietin and intravenous iron: A randomized controlled study. J Am Coll Cardiol 37:1775, 2001.
7. Hillege H, Girbes AR, de Kann PJ, et al: Renal function, neurohormonal activation, and survival in patients with chronic heart failure. Circulation 102:205, 2000.
8. Kuster GM, Tanner H, Printzen G, et al: B-type natriuretic peptide for diagnosis and treatment of congestive heart failure. Swiss Med Wkly 132:623, 2002.
9. Redfield MM, Rodeheffer RJ, Jacobsen SJ, et al: Plasma brain natriuretic peptide concentration: Impact of age and gender. J Am Coll Cardiol 40:976, 2002.
10. Dao Q, Krishnaswamy P, Kazanegra R, et al: Usefulness of B-type natriuretic peptide in the diagnosis of congestive heart failure in an urgent-care setting. J Am Coll Cardiol 37:379, 2001.
11. Cleland JG, Daubert JC, Erdmann E, et al: The effect of cardiac resynchronization on morbidity and mortality in heart failure. N Engl J Med 352:1539, 2005.
12. Likoff MG, Chandler SL, Kay HR: Clinical determinants of mortality and chronic congestive heart failure secondary to idiopathic dilated or to ischemic cardiomyopathy. Am J Cardiol 559:634, 1987.
13. Mancini DM, Eisen H, Kussmaul W, et al: Value of in ambulatory patients with heart failure. Circulation 83:778, 1991.
14. Bittner V, Weiner DH, Yusuf S, et al: Prediction of morbidity and mortality with a 6-minute walk test in patients with left ventricular dysfunction. SOLVD Investigators. JAMA 270:1702, 1993.
15. Stelken AM, Younis LT, Jennison SH, et al: Prognostic value of cardiopulmonary exercise testing using percent achieved of predicted peak oxygen uptake for patients with ischemic and dilated cardiomyopathy. J Am Coll Cardiol 27:345, 1996.
16. Elmariah S, Goldberg LR, Allen M, Kao A: Effects of gender on peak oxygen consumption and the timing of cardiac transplantation. J Am Coll Cardiol 47:2237, 2006.
17. Troughton RW, Prior DL, Frampton CM, et al: Usefulness of tissue Doppler and color M-mode indexes of left ventricular diastolic function in predicting outcomes in systolic left ventricular heart failure (from the ADEPT study). Am J Cardiol 96:257, 2005.
18. Lee KI, Pryor DB, Pieper KS, et al: Prognostic value of radionuclide angiography in medically treated patients with coronary artery disease. A comparison with clinical and catheterization variables. Circulation 82:1706, 1990.

Systolic Function

19. Grossman W: Evaluation of systolic and diastolic function of the myocardium. *In* Baim DS (ed): Cardiac Catheterization, Angiography, and Intervention. 7th ed. Baltimore, Williams & Wilkins, 2006, pp 315-320.
20. Katz A: Ernest Henry Starling: His predecessors, and the "law of the heart." Circulation 106:2986, 2002.
21. Carabello B: Evolution of the study of left ventricular function: Everything old is new again. Circulation 105:2701, 2002.
22. Karunanithi M, Feneley M: Single-beat determination of preload recruitable stroke work relationship: Derivation and evaluation in conscious dogs. J Am Coll Cardiol 35:502, 2000.

Diastolic Function

23. Zile M, Brutsaert D: New concepts in diastolic dysfunction and diastolic heart failure: I. Diagnosis, prognosis, and measurements of diastolic function. Circulation 105:1387, 2002.
24. Zile M, Brutsaert D: New concepts in diastolic dysfunction and diastolic heart failure: II. Causal mechanisms and treatment. Circulation 105:1503, 2002.
25. Bell SP, Nyland L, Tischler MD, et al: Alterations in the determinants of diastolic suction during pacing tachycardia. Circ Res 87:235, 2000.

26. Hess OM, Osakada G, Lavelle J, et al: Diastolic myocardial wall stiffness and ventricular relaxation during partial and complete coronary occlusion in the conscious dog. Circ Res 52:387, 1983.
27. Mandinov L, Eberli FR, Seiler C, Hess OM: Diastolic heart failure. Cardiovasc Res 45:813, 2000.
28. Neumann T, Vollmer A, Schaffner T, et al: Diastolic dysfunction and collagen structure in canine pacing-induced heart failure. J Am Coll Cardiol 31:179, 1999.
29. Spinale FG, Coker ML, Thomas CV, et al: Time-dependent changes in matrix metalloproteinase activity and expression during the progression of congestive heart failure: Relation to ventricular and myocyte function. Circ Res 82:482, 1998.
30. Hein S, Gaasch W, Schaper J: Giant molecule titin and myocardial stiffness. Circulation 106:1303, 2002.
31. Weber KT: Targeting pathological remodeling: Concepts of cardioprotection and reparation. Circulation 102:1342, 2000.
32. Zile MR, Baicu CF: Alterations in ventricular function: diastolic heart failure. *In* Mann DL (ed): Heart Failure: A Companion to Braunwald's Heart Disease. Philadelphia, Saunders, 2003, pp 209-227.
33. Hess OM, Bhargava V, Ross J, Shabetai R: The role of the pericardium in interactions between the cardiac chambers. Am Heart J 106:1377, 1983.
34. Hoit B: Management of effusive and constrictive pericardial heart disease. Circulation 105:2939, 2002.
35. Kudelka AM, Turner DA, Liebson PR, et al: Comparison of cine magnetic resonance imaging and Doppler echocardiography for evaluation of left ventricular diastolic function. Am J Cardiol 80:384, 1997.
36. Stuber M, Schedegger MB, Fischer SE, et al: Alterations in the local myocardial motion pattern in patients suffering from pressure overload caused by aortic stenosis. Circulation 100:361, 1999.
37. Maier SE, Fischer SE, McKinnon GC, et al: Evaluation of left ventricular segmental wall motion in hypertrophic cardiomyopathy with myocardial tagging. Circulation 86:1919, 1992.
38. Fischer SE, McKinnon GC, Maier SE, Boesiger P: Improved myocardial tagging contrast. Magn Reson Med 31:401, 1994.

Right Ventricular Function

39. Reynertson S, Kundur R, Mullen G, et al: Asymmetry of right ventricular enlargement in response to tricuspid regurgitation. Circulation 100:465, 1999.
40. Veldtman G, Razack V, Siu S, et al: Right ventricular form and function after percutaneous atrial septal defect device closure. J Am Coll Cardiol 37:2108, 2001.
41. Brickner M, Hillis L, Lang R: Congenital heart disease in adults: I. N Engl J Med 342:256, 2000.
42. Rubin L: Primary pulmonary hypertension. N Engl J Med 336:111, 1997.
43. Fedullo P, Auger W, Kerr K, Rubin L: Chronic thromboembolic pulmonary hypertension. N Engl J Med 345:1465, 2001.
44. Menzel T, Wagner S, Kramm T, et al: Pathophysiology of impaired right and left ventricular function in chronic embolic pulmonary hypertension: Changes after pulmonary thromboendarterectomy. Chest 118:897, 2000.
45. Chen C, Cheng T, Huang T, et al: Percutaneous balloon valvuloplasty for pulmonic stenosis in adolescents and adults. N Engl J Med 335:21, 1996.
46. Goldstein J: Pathophysiology and management of right heart ischemia. J Am Coll Cardiol 40:841, 2002.
47. Bowers T, O'Neill W, Pica M, Goldstein J: Patterns of coronary compromise resulting in acute right ventricular ischemic dysfunction. Circulation 106:1104, 2002.
48. Dubin A, Feinstein J, Reddy M, et al: Electrical resynchronization: A novel therapy for the failing right ventricle. Circulation 107:2287, 2003.

Left Atrium

49. Grigioni F, Avierinos JF, Ling LH, et al: Atrial fibrillation complicating the course of degenerative mitral regurgitation. J Am Coll Cardiol 40:84, 2002.
50. Rossi A, Cicoira M, Zanolla L, et al: Determinants and prognostic value of left atrial volume in patients with dilated cardiomyopathy. J Am Coll Cardiol 40:142, 2002.
51. Moller J, Hillis GS, Oh JK, et al: Left atrial volume: A powerful predictor of survival after acute myocardial infarction. Circulation 107:2207, 2003.
52. Hoit BD, Shao Y, Gabel M: Influence of acutely altered loading conditions on left atrial appendage flow velocities. J Am Coll Cardiol 24:1117, 1994.
53. Hondo T, Okamoto M, Yamane T, et al: The role of the left atrial appendage: A volume loading study in open-chest dogs. Jpn Heart J 36:225, 1995.
54. Hoit BD, Shao Y, Tsai LM, et al: Altered left atrial compliance after atrial appendectomy: Influence on left atrial and ventricular filling. Circ Res 72:167, 1993.
55. Agmon Y, Khanderia K, Gentile F, Seward JB: Echocardiographic assessment of the left atrial appendage. J Am Coll Cardiol 34:1867, 1999.
56. Pritchett AM, Jacobsen SJ, Mahoney DW, et al: Left atrial volume as an index of left atrial size: A population-based study. J Am Coll Cardiol 41:1036, 2003.
57. Szili-Torok T, Kimman GJ, Scholten HF, et al: Interatrial septum pacing guided by three-dimensional intracardiac echocardiography. J Am Coll Cardiol 40:2139, 2002.
58. Schwartzman D, Lacomis J, Wigginton W: Characterization of left atrium and distal pulmonary vein morphology using multidimensional computed tomography. J Am Coll Cardiol 41:1349, 2003.
59. Hoit BD, Gabel M: Influence of left ventricular dysfunction on the role of atrial contraction: An echocardiographic-hemodynamic study in dogs. J Am Coll Cardiol 36:1713, 2000.
60. Manning WJ, Silverman DI, Katz SE, Douglas PS: Atrial ejection force: A noninvasive assessment of atrial systolic function. J Am Coll Cardiol 22:221, 1993.
61. Alexander J Jr, Sunagawa K, Chang N, Sagawa K: Instantaneous pressure-volume relation of the ejecting canine left atrium. Circ Res 61:209, 1987.
62. Hoit BD, Shao Y, Gabel M, Walsh RA: In vivo assessment of left atrial contractile performance in normal and pathological conditions using a time-varying elastance model. Circulation 89:1829, 1994.
63. Stefanadis C, Dernellis J, Tsiamis E, Toutouza P: Effects of pacing-induced and balloon coronary occlusion ischemia on left atrial function in patients with coronary artery disease. J Am Coll Cardiol 33:687, 1999.
64. Nakatani S, Garcia MJ, Firstenberg MS, et al: Noninvasive assessment of left atrial maximum dP/dt by a combination of transmitral and pulmonary venous flow. J Am Coll Cardiol 34:795, 1999.
65. Sparks P, Jayaprakash S, Mond HG, et al: Left atrial mechanical function after brief duration atrial fibrillation. J Am Coll Cardiol 33:342, 1999.
66. Yuda S, Nakatani S, Kosakai Y, et al: Long-term follow-up of atrial contraction after the maze procedure in patients with mitral valve disease. J Am Coll Cardiol 37:1622, 2001.
67. Sakai H, Kunichika H, Murata K, et al: Improvement of afterload mismatch of left atrial booster pump function with positive inotropic agent. J Am Coll Cardiol 37:270, 2001.
68. Nagueh S, Lakkis NM, Middleton KJ, et al: Changes in left ventricular filling and left atrial function six months after nonsurgical septal reduction therapy for hypertrophic obstructive cardiomyopathy. J Am Coll Cardiol 34:1123, 1999.

Exercise

69. Weber KT, Janicki JS, McElroy PA, Reddy HK: Concepts and applications of cardiopulmonary exercise testing. Chest 93:843, 1988.
70. Nonogi H, Hess OM, Ritter M, Krayenbuehl HP: Diastolic properties of the normal left ventricle during supine exercise. Br Heart J 60:30, 1988.

CHAPTER 24

Diagnosis and Management of Acute Heart Failure

John R. Teerlink

INTRODUCTION

The past two decades have witnessed dramatic advances in the treatment of chronic heart failure (CHF) with the development of novel therapies that have significantly improved the survival of large populations. Despite exceedingly high in-hospital mortality and rehospitalization rates, acute heart failure had initially been ignored. However, during the last decade, there has been growing interest in this field of research with the publication of the first randomized, placebo-controlled AHF trials in 2002.[1,2] New data obtained through these and other randomized, controlled trials of novel therapies, as well as national registries, have provided new insights into AHF and a growing literature has evolved in this area. Accordingly, this chapter will focus on the epidemiology, diagnosis, and management of AHF. The diagnosis and management of chronic heart failure with depressed ejection fraction is discussed in Chaps. 23 and 25, respectively, whereas Chapter 26 discusses these areas for patients with heart failure and normal ejection fraction.

DEFINITION AND CLASSIFICATION OF ACUTE HEART FAILURE

Acute heart failure (AHF) is a multifactorial and heterogeneous syndrome that defies concise classification. For the purpose of this chapter, AHF is defined as the rapid or gradual onset of signs and symptoms of heart failure that result in urgent unplanned hospitalizations or office or emergency department visits.[3] This functional definition of AHF has three crucial elements. The first is temporal: the onset of signs or symptoms must occur relatively rapidly, although the actual deterioration may have been ongoing for a longer period. The second element is the signs and symptoms of heart failure, which are dominated by symptoms of congestion and fluid retention, discussed in detail later. The third element is severity: the symptoms and signs must be significant enough to result in the need for urgent intervention. Although patients may present with the signs and symptoms of AHF in the setting of other diseases, such as myocardial infarction, acute valvular regurgitation or renal failure, the underlying pathology (i.e., myocardial infarction) usually dominates the selection of therapies and, consequently, such etiologies are addressed in other chapters (see Chap. 50).

A number of complementary classification schemes have been developed for AHF. One system classifies patients based on the presence of a history of heart failure or cardiac dysfunction.[4] Patients without such a history are considered *acute de novo heart failure,* whereas those with known disease or history have *acute decompensation of chronic heart failure (ADCHF).* Patients with decompensation of chronic heart failure usually have a less dramatic clinical presentation because the chronic nature of the disorder has allowed for recruitment of compensatory mechanisms and remodeling, such as increased pulmonary lymphatic drainage. In acute *de novo* heart failure, sympathetic activation is more pronounced and the clinical picture is complicated by redistribution of intravascular fluid and marked systemic vasoconstriction. This classification has defined groups of differing risk, but has the limitation that the *de novo* heart failure group is enriched for patients with acute coronary syndromes (ACS), including ST segment elevation myocardial infarctions (STEMI).

Another classification that has been incorporated into guidelines[4,5] categorizes patients based on their clinical presentation. Based on work by Cotter,[6] Gheorghiade and colleagues,[3] the European Society of Cardiology (ESC) guidelines on the diagnosis and treatment of acute heart failure[4] describe six types of patients with typical clinical and hemodynamic characteristics (Table 24-1). The first three categories of patients (acute decompensated heart failure, hypertensive AHF, and AHF with pulmonary edema) compose more than 90 percent of AHF presentations. The *acute decompensated heart failure (ADHF)* patient typically presents with mild to moderate signs and symptoms of congestion and does not meet criteria for other categories. *Hypertensive AHF* cases are characterized by their relatively preserved left ventricular (LV) systolic function, markedly elevated blood pressure, and signs and symptoms of acute pulmonary edema. The third group of patients, *AHF with pulmonary edema,* has a clinical presentation that is dominated by severe respiratory distress orthopnea, signs of pulmonary edema (verified by rales on

TABLE 24–1 Classification and Common Clinical Characteristics of Patients with Acute Heart Failure

Clinical Classification	Symptom Onset	Signs and Symptoms	Hemodynamics	Other Diagnostics
I Acute decompensated congestive heart failure	Usually gradual	Peripheral edema (often significant), dyspnea, usually well-perfused extremities	SBP: Low normal/high CI: Low normal/high PCWP: Mildly increased	CXR: Normal or mild interstitial edema, possible pleural effusion
II Acute heart failure with hypertension/hypertensive crisis	Often very rapid	Dyspnea, altered mental status, possible oliguria/anuria	SBP: High (>180/100 mm Hg) CI: Usually normal PCWP: >18 mm Hg	CXR: Normal or interstitial edema
III Acute heart failure with pulmonary edema	Rapid or gradual	Severe dyspnea, tachypnea, tachycardia	SBP: Low normal	SaO_2: <90% CXR: Alveolar edema
IVa Cardiogenic shock/low output syndrome	Usually gradual	Evidence of hypoperfusion; oliguria	SBP: Low normal CI: Low, <2.2 liters/min/m^2 PCWP: >16 mm Hg	
IVb Severe cardiogenic shock	Often rapid	Marked hypoperfusion; oliguria/anuria	SBP: <90 mm Hg CI: Very low, <1.8 liters/min/m^2 PCWP: >18 mm Hg	Usually in presence of severe LV systolic dysfunction
V High output failure	Rapid or gradual	Well-perfused extremities; often tachycardic	SBP: Variable CI: Increased PCWP: Normal or increased	
VI Right-sided acute heart failure	Rapid or gradual	Edema, markedly elevated neck veins, often poor perfusion, but clear lungs	SBP: Low CI: Low PCWP: Low	CXR: often clear lung fields with evidence of pulmonary hypertension; BNP may be elevated in pulmonary embolus

BNP = B-type natriuretic peptide; CI = cardiac index; CXR = chest x-ray; PCWP = pulmonary capillary wedge pressure; SBP = systolic blood pressure.
Based on Nieminen MS, Bohm M, Cowie MR, et al: Executive summary of the guidelines on the diagnosis and treatment of acute heart failure: The Task Force on Acute Heart Failure of the European Society of Cardiology. Eur Heart J 26:384-416, 2005; and Gheorghiade M, Zannad F, Sopko G, et al: Acute heart failure syndromes: Current state and framework for future research. Circulation 112:3958-3968, 2005.

examination and chest x-ray), and hypoxemia (O_2 saturation usually <90 percent on room air prior to treatment). *Low-output syndrome* in patients with AHF is defined as evidence of tissue hypoperfusion because of heart failure despite adequate preload and represents a continuum of severity ranging from a low-output state to cardiogenic shock to severe cardiogenic shock. The dominant factor in these cases is the degree of global hypoperfusion and the impending risk of end organ damage from decreased cardiac output. *High output failure* remains an uncommon cause of AHF and generally manifests with warm peripheral extremities, pulmonary congestion, and at times, low blood pressure (i.e., sepsis) with high cardiac output and usually an elevated heart rate. Underlying conditions include arrhythmias, anemia, thyrotoxicosis, and Paget disease. *Right-sided AHF* is increasingly recognized as patients with chronic obstructive lung disease develop cor pulmonale and as there is a greater appreciation for the prevalence of pulmonary hypertension. Patients present with increased jugular venous pressure, evidence of right-sided congestion (hepatomegaly, edema), and evidence of a low-output syndrome with hypotension. This classification system provides a useful basis on which specific therapeutic strategies can be developed; it also provides a useful research tool for future trials.

Another clinically relevant and widely used classification system was developed by Stevenson and colleagues.[7] This system evaluates patients based on the clinical presence or absence of hypoperfusion (cold versus warm) and congestion at rest (wet versus dry) (see later; Fig. 24-6). Patients with clinical profile A (dry and warm) had a 6-month mortality of 11 percent compared to 40 percent for profile C (wet and cold) in one study[7] demonstrating that these clinical profiles can have prognostic significance. As will be discussed later, these profiles also have been used to guide therapy.[8,9]

EPIDEMIOLOGY OF ACUTE HEART FAILURE

In the United States, there were 1,093,000 hospital discharges with a primary diagnosis of heart failure in 2003, representing a 174 percent increase since 1979 (Fig. 24-1), and approximately 3 million hospitalizations with heart failure as one of the discharge diagnoses. Estimated costs for primary heart failure hospitalizations in 2006 are $15.4 billion, representing more than one-half of all heart failure-related expenditures. In addition, there were more than 3 million urgent outpatient visits for heart failure.[10] The magnitude of this problem is even greater in Europe, where the ESC estimates that more than 10 million people within their population of 900 million have heart failure.[11] Heart failure consumes 1 to 2 percent of total health expenditures in Europe, and hospital management of AHF represents 67 to 74 percent of this cost.[12] Thus, AHF represents a substantial social and financial burden that will continue to grow as successful treatments for previously fatal cardiovascular diseases are implemented.

International data from the European Union and North and South America demonstrate that the demographics of patients with AHF (Table 24-2) are similar to those with chronic HF. The mean age of patients with AHF is 70 to 75 years old, and they are almost evenly split between the sexes. Approximately one-half of the patients have moderately to severely reduced LV systolic function, and 50 to 76 percent of patients admitted with AHF had a prior history of HF. The EuroHeart Failure Survey II (EHFS II)[13] enrolled 3580 patients hospitalized in 133 centers in 30 European countries for AHF with dyspnea and verification of heart failure based on signs and symptoms, 63 percent of whom were admitted with acute decompensation of chronic heart failure (ADCHF), compared to 37 percent with *de novo* AHF.

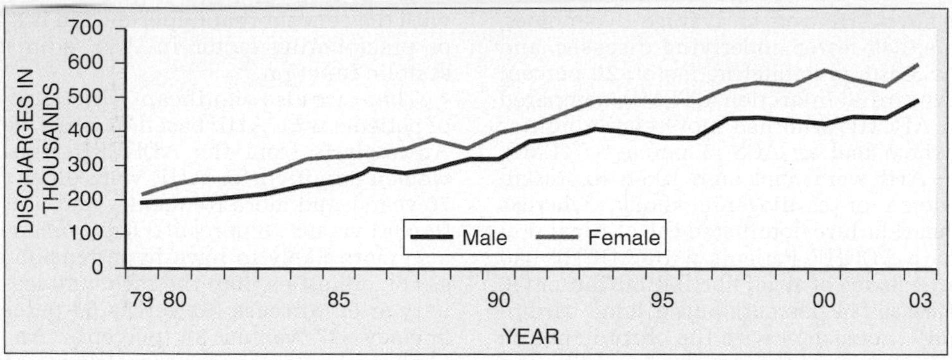

FIGURE 24–1 Hospital discharges for heart failure (HF) by sex (United States: 1970-2003). Total hospital discharges for HF rose from 399,000 in 1979 to 1,093,000 in 2003—an increase of 174 percent. Note: Hospital discharges include people discharged alive and dead. Source: National Hospital Discharge Survey, CDC/NCHS and NHLBI. Data from: Thom T, Haase N, Rosamond W, et al: Heart disease and stroke statistics—2006 update: A report from the American Heart Association Statistics Committee and Stroke Statistics Subcommittee. Circulation 113:e85-151, 2006.

TABLE 24–2 Demographics and Comorbidities of Patients Hospitalized with Acute Heart Failure from Selected Studies

	ADHERE (n = 32,229)	OPTIMIZE-HF (n = 48,612)	Argentina (n = 2974)	EHFS I* (n = 11,327)	EHFS II (n = 3580)	EFICA† (n = 599)	Italian AHF (n= 2807)
Age (y)	75	73	68	71	70	73	73
Pts >75 yo (%)	50	52	N/A	34	N/A	48	46
Male (%)	48	48	59	53	61	59	60
LVEF <40% or mod/sev dysfunction (%)	47	49	74	46	48	55	66
Prior HF (%)	76	88	50	65	63	66	56
Coronary artery disease	57	50		68	54	46	
Myocardial infarction	30		22	39		22	36
Hypertension	74	71	66	53	62	60	66
Dyslipidemia	36	32	26			30	
Stroke/transient ischemic attack	17	16		19	13	10	9 (Stroke)
Atrial fibrillation	31	31‡	27	42	39	25 (on ECG at admission)	21
Pacemaker/ICD	21	15		8	9		17
Peripheral vascular disease	18	14				22	12
Chronic renal insufficiency	30	20	10	17	17	10	25
Chronic dialysis	5	3					
Diabetes	44	42	23	27	33	27	38
COPD/asthma	31	34	15	32	19	21	30

*Included patients with a history of heart failure admitted for other causes.

†Only enrolled patients from the ICU/CCU.

‡ Includes all atrial arrhythmias.

ADHERE and OPTIMIZE-HF are U.S.-based studies, EHFS I & II are from the European Union, and EFICA is from France.

COPD = chronic obstructive pulmonary disease; ECG = electrocardiogram; ICD = implantable cardioverter defibrillator; LVEF = left ventricular ejection fraction; mod/sev = moderate/severe; Pts = patients; yo = years old.

Data from: ADHERE: ADHERE Scientific Advisory Committee. Acute Decompensated Heart Failure National Registry (ADHERE) Core Module Q1 2006 Final Cumulative National Benchmark Report: Scios, Inc.; July, 2006. OPTIMIZE-HF: Gheorghiade M, Abraham WT, Albert NM, et al: Systolic blood pressure at admission, clinical characteristics, and outcomes in patients hospitalized with acute heart failure. JAMA 296:2217-2226, 2006, and personal communication with Dr. Mihai Gheorghiade. Argentina: Perna ER, Barbagelata A, Grinfeld L, et al: Overview of acute decompensated heart failure in Argentina: Lessons learned from five registries during the last decade. Am Heart J 151:84-91, 2006. EHFS I: Cleland JG, Swedberg K, Follath F, et al: The EuroHeart Failure survey programme—a survey on the quality of care among patients with heart failure in Europe. Part 1: Patient characteristics and diagnosis. Eur Heart J 24:442-463, 2003. EHFS II: Nieminen MS, Brutsaert D, Dickstein K, et al: EuroHeart Failure Survey II (EHFS II): A survey on hospitalized acute heart failure patients: Description of population. Eur Heart J 27:2725-2736, 2006. EFICA: Zannad F, Mebazaa A, Juilliere Y, et al: Clinical profile, contemporary management and one-year mortality in patients with severe acute heart failure syndromes: The EFICA study. Eur J Heart Fail 8:697-705, 2006. Italian AHF: Tavazzi L, Maggioni AP, Lucci D, et al: Nationwide survey on acute heart failure in cardiology ward services in Italy. Eur Heart J 27:1207-1215, 2006.

The patients with de novo AHF were on average 1 year older, less likely to be male, had fewer underlying diseases, and 42 percent had an ACS as a precipitating factor, 20 percent with ST-elevation myocardial infarction (STEMI), compared to the patients with ADCHF, who had more comorbidities and 23 percent of whom had an ACS (6 percent STEMI). Patients with de novo AHF were much more likely to present with pulmonary edema or cardiogenic shock, whereas decompensation of heart failure dominated the clinical presentation of those with ADCHF. Patients with ADCHF had a remarkably high prevalence of atrial fibrillation/flutter (46 percent), valvular disease (44 percent), and dilated cardiomyopathy (25 percent)—consistent with the chronic nature of their underlying heart failure.

The ESC AHF guidelines[4] provide a classification for different clinical conditions with which patients in AHF may present (see Table 24-1) and the EHFS II was the first major study to apply this classification scheme to a large population. In this survey, the majority of patients presented with decompensated heart failure (65 percent), whereas pulmonary edema (16 percent) and hypertensive HF (11 percent) were the next most prevalent classes. Despite the fairly liberal definition of cardiogenic shock in the guidelines, which include "low-output state," few patients (4 percent) were classified as being admitted with cardiogenic shock. Right heart failure was also relatively rare (3 percent) and high output failure was not recorded in this survey. Thus, low-output heart failure is relatively rare, although it is surprising that so few patients were classified as having hypertensive HF. Other studies have found similar results with a low proportion of patients classified as hypertensive AHF, yet a high percentage of patients with high blood pressure as a trigger[14,15]—suggesting that the role of hypertension may be underestimated by this classification system. An extraordinarily valuable resource in AHF research is the Acute Decompensated Heart Failure National Registry (ADHERE), an industry-sponsored, large, national (United States), observational, multicenter study of the characteristics, patterns of care, and outcomes of patients hospitalized with ADHF. As of March 31, 2006, 309 representative hospitals from across the United States have enrolled patients who were admitted to an acute care hospital and had a discharge diagnosis of heart failure. In the most recent ADHERE National Benchmark report,[16] 50 percent of 187,565 patients presented with a systolic blood pressure greater than 140 mm Hg and only 2 percent with a systolic blood pressure less than 90 mm Hg, supporting the concept that cardiogenic shock is relatively rare and presentations with hypertension are common.

Most studies have also analyzed patients on the basis of their systolic function as assessed by ejection fraction, and have found that about 50 percent of patients admitted with AHF have systolic dysfunction (left ventricular ejection fraction <40 percent or moderate/severe dysfunction; see Table 24-2), suggesting that one-half of the patients have preserved ejection fraction (see Chap. 26). For many, these data required a significant rethinking of the "typical" presentation of the patient with AHF as usually having decreased systolic function. In the ADHERE registry,[17] the characteristics of the 26,323 patients with preserved systolic function were compared to the 25,865 patients with reduced systolic function. Because of the size of the database, nearly all variables were statistically different, but from a clinical perspective, patients with preserved systolic function were more likely to be older, women, and hypertensive, whereas those patients with reduced systolic function were more likely to have coronary artery disease and a history of myocardial infarction or heart failure. The difference between systolic blood pressure on admission (preserved: 153 mm Hg versus reduced: 139 mm Hg) is consistent with the concept that hypertension is a common underlying or precipitating factor in AHF admissions, regardless of systolic function.[18]

There are also significant differences in the presentation of patients with AHF based on other demographic features. An analysis from the ADHERE registry[19] suggested that women admitted for AHF were older than men (74 versus 70 years), and more frequently had preserved systolic function (51 versus 28 percent). The women in this registry were also more likely to have hypertension and thyroid disease as comorbidities than the men, and less likely to have coronary artery disease (51 versus 64 percent) and renal insufficiency (27 versus 33 percent). An analysis of 34,587 Medicare patients more than the age of 65 years[20] defined a population with a median age of 79 years, 58 percent of whom were women, and 31 percent had an EF >40 percent. Although comorbidities were common (hypertension, 61 percent of patients; coronary artery disease, 56 percent; diabetes, 38 percent; COPD, 33 percent; atrial fibrillation, 30 percent), they seemed roughly similar to that seen in the other registries, reflecting the dominance of the elderly in the overall population. These comorbidities become less frequent in older age cohorts, perhaps because of survival bias, with the exceptions of renal failure, atrial fibrillation, stroke, and dementia. The worsening of renal function with age poses a special problem in the setting of AHF, and is a major impediment in effectively treating the elderly with AHF.

Differences in ethnic groups have been studied most extensively in the United States. In a study based on a nationwide sample of 29,732 U.S. Medicare beneficiaries,[21] the African-American patients with AHF were slightly younger (77 versus 80 years), more likely to be women (64 percent versus 59 percent), had higher blood pressure and heart rate, and more frequently had a history of heart failure, hypertension, and diabetes, compared to white patients. The white patients in this study were much more likely to have coronary artery disease, myocardial infarction, coronary revascularization, and aortic stenosis. In the Organized Program to Initiate Lifesaving Treatment in Hospitalized Patients with Heart Failure (OPTIMIZE-HF) registry,[22] African-American patients (8608/47,189) admitted with AHF were younger (64 versus 75 years), more likely to have left ventricular systolic dysfunction (57 versus 51 percent) with a lower mean EF (35 versus 40 percent), hypertensive etiology for heart failure (39 versus 19 percent), renal dysfunction and diabetes, compared to the non-African-American group. The finding of worse LV dysfunction in the African-Americans is a bit counterintuitive, given the higher incidence of coronary artery disease and myocardial infarction in the non-African-Americans. Lower crude mortality rates have been reported for African-Americans compared to non-African-American patients, but when adjustments are made for these differences in comorbidities, mortality rates are similar.[23] Hispanic-Americans admitted with AHF were more likely to be male, and to have diabetes and hyperlipidemia than both the African-Americans and white Americans.[24] The risks of age, tobacco use, ischemic cardiomyopathy, and renal insufficiency were intermediate for Hispanic-Americans, compared to African-Americans or white Americans. These ethnic differences, as well as possible differences with other ethnic groups, need further investigation to assess the relative contributions of genetics, access to care, and other healthcare factors on AHF.

Concomitant diseases are very common in patients admitted with AHF (see Table 24-2). These comorbidities not only represent diseases that are risk factors for the development of heart failure, but also are reflective of the advanced age of this population. Hypertension is the most prevalent of the concurrent conditions, present in approximately two-thirds of the patients, whereas coronary artery disease is present in about one-half and dyslipidemia more than one-third of patients. Other conditions that are the result of the vascular injury produced by these diseases, such as stroke, peripheral vascular disease, and chronic renal insufficiency are also very common in patients with AHF. Diabetes mellitus is present in more than 40 percent of U.S. patients, most likely related to increasing incidence of obesity, and ranges from 27 to 38 percent in Europe. Chronic obstructive pulmonary disease is also present in approximately 30 percent, confounding the presenting symptoms of dyspnea. Atrial fibrillation appears to be more common in Europe (up to 42 percent, compared to 31 percent in the U.S. patients with AHF), and can precipitate AHF and complicate its management. These other diseases have significant impact on the treatment and clinical course of patients with AHF, and as the patient population ages, they will become only more common.

PATHOPHYSIOLOGY OF ACUTE HEART FAILURE

The pathophysiology of AHF (Fig. 24-2) is as diverse and complicated as its clinical presentations and precipitating factors. However, an understanding of these distinct pathophysiologies provides guidance for management. As noted above, acute cardiovascular emergencies, such as acute coronary syndrome, myocardial infarction, acute valvular insufficiency, ventricular wall rupture (free wall or ventricular septal defect), and pulmonary embolism, can precipitate AHF, but these specific etiologies are discussed elsewhere in detail. AHF also shares many of the basic pathophysiological principles that are prominent in chronic HF (see Chaps. 22 and 25), so this discussion will focus on aspects specifically relevant to AHF.

Cardiac Dysfunction

The traditional paradigm of heart failure caused by a defect in systolic cardiac function has dominated most approaches to AHF, although cardiac function clearly plays a role, it is the dominant feature in a minority of the cases. AHF may be related to either permanent or transient decreases in systolic performance. Preexisting permanent systolic dysfunction creates the milieu in which other triggers can incite AHF. For example, chronic neurohormonal activation increases sodium and water avidity, making the patient much more susceptible to volume overload because of dietary indiscretions. Additional decreases in systolic function can be transiently caused by this neurohormonal and inflammatory stimulation, as well as through myocardial ischemia because of acute coronary syndromes, reduced coronary perfusion from hypotension, or relative ischemia caused by myocardial distention and increased myocardial oxygen demand from increased wall stress. This decreased LV systolic function initiates a series of events that ultimately produce pulmonary edema and end organ dysfunction (see Fig. 24-2). Because of the recursive and highly interdependent nature of these cascades, a perturbation of any element can produce the clinical syndrome of AHF. Although relatively few patients present with the clinical profile of overt cardiogenic shock (approximately 4 percent[4]), systolic dysfunction is present in approximately one-half of the patients who present with AHF (see Table 24-2), suggesting that improving systolic function remains an important potential target for therapies to treat AHF.

As is implied by the above statement, approximately one-half of the patients who present with AHF have preserved systolic function (see Chap. 26), as defined by an LV ejection fraction 40 percent or greater or only mild to no systolic dysfunction by qualitative assessment. Applying a generous cut-off of ≥ 50 percent for a normal EF, recent studies have found that only 24 to 34 percent have a near normal EF[25,26] and even patients with normal ejection fractions can have detectable systolic abnormalities.[27] However, the degree of systolic dysfunction in these patients is unlikely to make a major contribution to the development of AHF. Some have contended that AHF with preserved ejection fraction is actually the result of significant transient decreases in systolic function that subsequently resolve. However, this hypothesis is not supported in studies that performed acute and subsequent assessments of LV function.[28] Thus, the predominant cardiac abnormality in the presentation of patients with AHF and preserved systolic function is diastolic dysfunction,[29,30] resulting in *diastolic heart failure.* The pathophysiology of diastolic heart failure is discussed in detail elsewhere (see Chap. 26), but the fundamental defects are abnormalities in the active relaxation and passive stiffness of the left ventricle.[31] These abnormalities of LV diastolic properties result in a sensitivity to changes in preload and

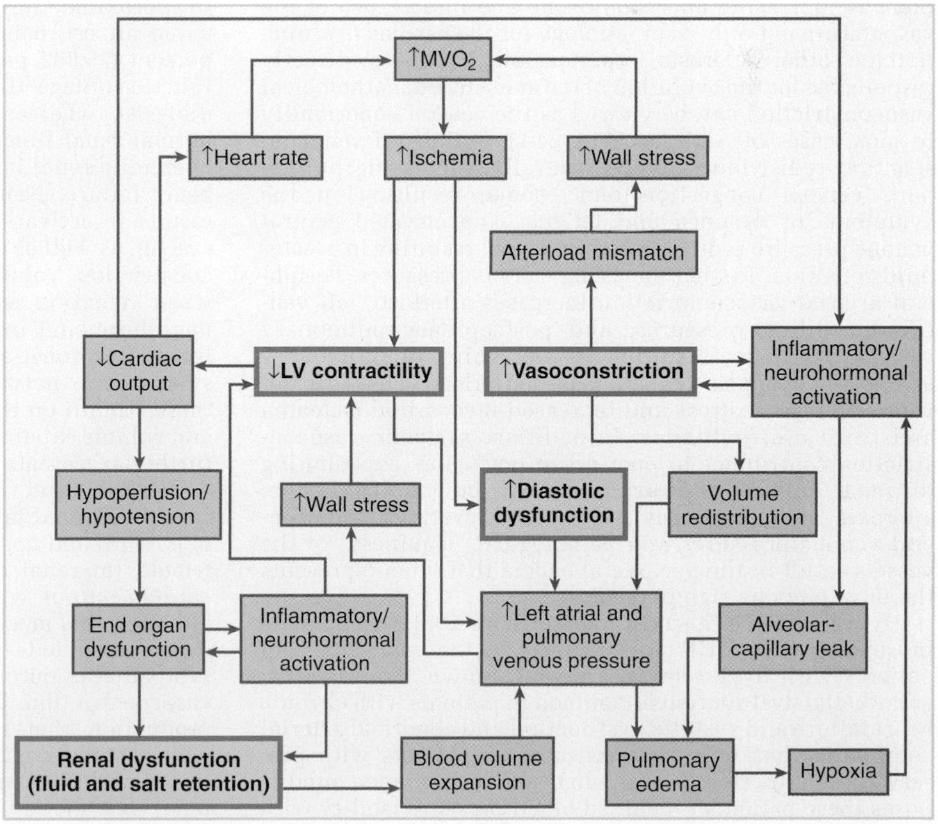

FIGURE 24–2 A schematic representation of the pathophysiology of acute heart failure. Cardiac (decreased contractility or increased diastolic dysfunction), vascular or renal abnormalities are central to the pathophysiology and each can independently cause acute heart failure (ACF). *(MVO_2 = myocardial oxygen consumption.)*

afterload, such that relatively small changes in volumes can result in significant increases in LV filling pressures with consequent increased pulmonary congestion. Myocardial ischemia, tachycardia, arrhythmias, and other factors can exacerbate this diastolic dysfunction and readily precipitate an episode of AHF.

The large majority of patients with AHF present with LV failure, but many of the symptoms and pathophysiology are related to abnormalities of the right ventricle (RV). Only 3 percent of patients in EHFS II were classified as presenting with right heart failure,[13] and these patients had a higher prevalence of chronic obstructive pulmonary disease, atrial fibrillation, and valvular disease (more than 53 percent with moderate or severe tricuspid regurgitation) as comorbidities and fewer had coronary artery disease, compared to the other AHF groups. The pathophysiology of right heart failure is determined by the anatomy of the RV, a thin-walled, crescent-shaped structure readily influenced by changes in intrathoracic pressures. The RV is susceptible to failure with relatively modest increases in afterload, as with pulmonary embolism or acute mitral regurgitation, and in the presence of ischemia or infarction, the RV can fail under normal filling pressures. In the presence of these increased loads, the thin-walled RV rapidly develops markedly increased wall tensions with the commensurate increases in myocardial oxygen demand and ischemia, reducing systolic function and increasing end-diastolic volumes, resulting in even greater wall stresses. In most patients, the intact pericardium restrains the expansion of the RV, often at the expense of the LV, ultimately producing decreased LV output.

Vascular Dysfunction

Although abnormalities in cardiac function have traditionally held the central position in the pathogenesis of AHF, there is increasing appreciation for the importance of the vasculature not only as an etiology for the cardiac dysfunction (i.e., atherosclerosis, hypertension), but also as directly responsible for the evolution of the acute event. Pathological vasoconstriction can be viewed as the central abnormality in most cases of AHF (see Fig. 24-2). Peripheral venoconstriction redistributes blood centrally, increasing pulmonary venous congestion and edema, resulting in the symptoms of dyspnea and fatigue. The elevated central venous pressure reduces renal function, resulting in greater fluid retention, further elevating venous pressures. Peripheral arterial vasoconstriction increases afterload, left ventricular filling pressures, and postcapillary pulmonary venous pressures, resulting in worsening of pulmonary edema and dyspnea. This increased afterload causes greater ventricular wall stress and increased myocardial ischemia and cardiac arrhythmias. In addition, systemic vasoconstriction contributes to poor organ perfusion, contributing to renal failure and symptoms of fatigue, confusion, anorexia, and abdominal discomfort. Elevations in peripheral venous pressures and pathological "leakiness" of the vessels result in the peripheral edema that often represents the most obvious sign of AHF.

Hypertension is the most common comorbidity in patients presenting with AHF, and changes in the vasculature of patients with hypertension are well known. Additionally, endothelial dysfunction is common in patients with chronic heart failure and systolic dysfunction and abnormal arterial compliance has been demonstrated in patients with preserved LV function.[27] This abnormal compliance predisposes these patients to marked blood pressure lability with relatively minor changes in intravascular volume, causing precipitous increases in afterload and ultimately in LV filling pressures resulting in pulmonary congestion. The effects of this vascular abnormality are obviously amplified by LV diastolic dysfunction.

The clinical presentation and treatment of patients with hypertensive AHF reflect this pathophysiology with marked increases in systolic blood pressure (usually greater than 160 mm Hg), relatively minimal volume overload, and rapidly progressive pulmonary edema. The therapies that are effective in the treatment of acute heart failure are predominantly directed at the vasculature. Diuretics such as furosemide reduce central venous pressures through diuresis and possibly direct vasodilating properties, not via any direct effect on the heart. The other commonly used agents, nitroglycerin, nitroprusside and, more recently, nesiritide, are all vasodilators, achieving symptom relief through their actions on the vasculature, without significant direct myocardial effects. Positive inotropes are used in a minority of patients with AHF (about 8 percent[16]), but even the positive inotropes in common use, such as dobutamine, milrinone, and levosimendan, have significant vasodilating effects. Thus, the main therapeutic target of the current therapies has been the vasculature via nonspecific vasodilation, supporting the important role that the vasculature plays in the pathogenesis of AHF.

Renal Dysfunction

As the main organ responsible for volume homeostasis, the kidney is intimately involved in the pathophysiology of AHF (see Fig. 24-2). Intrinsic renal disease can cause volume overload because of the impaired function of existing nephrons or to the loss of nephrons, as in diabetic and hypertensive kidney disease. A remarkably high percentage of patients with AHF have hypertension (74 percent) and diabetes mellitus (44 percent), resulting in at least 30 percent with chronic renal insufficiency.[16] In ADHERE,[32] although investigators reported that renal insufficiency was present in approximately 30 percent of patients admitted with AHF, using an estimated glomerular filtration rate (eGFR), 64 percent (75,382 patients) had at least moderate renal dysfunction (Stage III-V: GFR <60 ml/min/1.73 m^2 or chronic dialysis), whereas only 9 percent (10,660 patients) had normal renal function (Stage I: GFR = 90 ml/min/1.73 m^2). Even mild renal insufficiency can result in a propensity for heart failure. Neurohormonal stimulation of the kidney results in activation of the renin-angiotensin-aldosterone-system, as well as endothelin production, resulting in vasoconstriction. Volume expansion through increased salt and water retention is also mediated by the kidney through neurohormonal inputs, including angiotensin II, endothelin, aldosterone, arginine, vasopressin, epinephrine, and sympathetic nervous system stimulation. The results of these stimuli on the kidney are increased vasoconstriction and volume expansion, causing a positive feedback loop and further exacerbating AHF.

The heart and vasculature are also involved in the pathogenesis of renal failure (see Fig. 24-2). Using the construct of *forward* and *backward* failure, *forward* heart failure contributes to renal dysfunction directly through decreased cardiac output with resultant reduced renal perfusion—although this mechanism may not be as important as commonly assumed—or indirectly by stimulating increased sympathetic output and neurohormones with resultant vasoconstriction. These neurohormones, and the cytokine production that they induce (i.e., transforming growth factor-beta), have also been implicated in direct glomerular injury and sclerosis. *Backward* heart failure contributes to renal dysfunction by increasing central venous pressures, which independently can reduce glomerular filtration rate, as well as free water and sodium excretion.[33] The combined effect of these factors results in a decreased ability of patients with HF to excrete sodium loads, making them more susceptible to dietary indiscretions. In addition, many of the therapies used to treat heart failure can have adverse renal effects. Diuretics can produce hypovolemia, decreasing renal perfusion and glomerular filtration rate, as well as inducing hypertrophy and hyperplasia of the epithelial cells in the distal convoluted tubule, which further increases sodium reabsorption, causing diuretic resistance. These cardiovascular abnormalities can significantly worsen renal dysfunction, exacerbating the volume overload state and increasing heart failure with a positive feedback mechanism. The ultimate result of this potentiating interaction is the *cardiorenal syndrome,* which may be clinically defined as the state wherein the volume overload of heart failure is resistant or refractory to treatment because of progressive renal dysfunction.

PULMONARY EDEMA (see also Chapter 24 Online Supplement: Pathophysiology of Pulmonary Edema)

The normal lung has a limited amount of fluid leakage into the alveolar interstitium. This leakage is limited by the protein osmotic pressure gradient in the capillaries, relatively tight junctions of the capillary endothelium, and by active sodium transport. The remaining interstitial fluid is returned to the systemic circulation via lymphatics. *Cardiogenic pulmonary edema*[34] is the result of an imbalance in fluid resorption and accumulation in the pulmonary interstitium and alveolar space that can be described by a sequence of three stages, progressing from *pulmonary venous engorgement* to *interstitial edema* to *alveolar edema.* Marked dyspnea, tachypnea, anxiety, and sympathetic stimulation accompany severe hypoxemia because of profound reductions in gas exchange.

Progressive volume overload and acute vasoconstriction are the most common causes of pulmonary edema in AHF (see Fig. 24-2). Patients with acute decompensation of chronic heart failure typically develop progressive increases in total body water, resulting in a gradual rise in left ventricular filling pressures and pulmonary edema with symptoms of dyspnea, often accompanied by other signs and symptoms of vascular congestion and volume overload. Acute vasoconstriction or hypertension can also cause cardiogenic pulmonary edema. A number of studies have strongly supported the hypothesis that diastolic dysfunction with afterload mismatch are the central factors in these patients, even in the absence of ischemia. Increases in sympathetic stimulation and in other vasoconstricting signals result in a marked increase in afterload, worsening the afterload mismatch. This vasoconstriction also results in central redistribution of volume to the pulmonary venous circulation, with additional elevations of left ventricular volumes, leading to rapid increases in LV filling pressures, marked pulmonary venous hypertension, and ultimately flash pulmonary edema. Myocardial ischemia potentiates this cycle by further increasing diastolic dysfunction and possibly reducing systolic function, as well as by inducing acute ischemic mitral regurgitation.[35] Hypoalbuminemia, producing a low colloid osmotic pressure, can also facilitate the development of pulmonary edema.[36]

Although cardiogenic edema is predominantly a manifestation of an imbalance of alveolar capillary Starling forces, damage to the alveolar-capillary barrier may also play a role, induced by proinflammatory cytokines, reactive oxygen species, and endothelin. Increases in plasma concentrations of surfactant protein-B (SP-B), a small protein normally confined to the alveolar space with a short half-life, have been demonstrated in patients with AHF and pulmonary edema, and these levels remain elevated for at least 3 days after resolution of the inciting increase in blood pressure and volume overload, suggestive of significant alveolar capillary structural damage.[37] This aspect of the pathophysiology of pulmonary edema in AHF may represent a future therapeutic target.

MYOCARDIAL INJURY

Myocardial injury may also play an important role in the pathogenesis of AHF, both as an instigating factor for cardiac decompensation and as an adverse result of the AHF itself. In Etude Française de l'Insuffisance Cardiaque Aiguë (EFICA),[38] 42 percent of the patients admitted to the intensive care unit with AHF had at least one elevated biomarker of myocardial injury. Heart failure is a known complication of ACS and portends a poor clinical outcome,[39] suggesting that an aggressive evaluation of ischemic etiologies should be performed with the potential goal of earlier revascularization. Myocardial injury has also been found to be associated with AHF in the absence of an acute coronary syndrome. Several studies with serial measurements of troponins have demonstrated significant and sustained increases,[40,41] confirming that ongoing myocardial necrosis in the absence of acute coronary syndrome occurs in AHF. The magnitude of this myocardial injury and its impact on the clinical course of AHF are unknown at this time, but these findings raise the concern that early and rapid intervention in the setting of AHF may be important to prevent further myocardial injury and that some of our interventions may exacerbate myocardial injury, especially if they induce hypotension or increase myocardial oxygen demand.

INFLAMMATORY/NEUROHORMONAL ABNORMALITIES

The role of neurohormonal activation in AHF remains to be fully defined. Increased plasma concentrations of norepinephrine, renin activity, aldosterone, and endothelin-1 have all been reported in patients with AHF,[42,43] resulting in significant vasoconstriction and perhaps mediating the same deleterious pathways as described for CHF (see Chaps. 22 and 25), including increasing atrial and ventricular arrhythmias[44] and exacerbating renal insufficiency. The combination of vasoconstriction and fluid retention mediated by these neurohormones is central to the pathophysiology of AHF.

Inflammatory activation may also play a role. Relative lymphocytopenia, a marker of neurohormonal and inflammatory activation, has been demonstrated in patients with AHF and shown to be a factor for long-term mortality.[45] Concentrations of interleukin-6 (IL-6), tumor necrosis factor, c-reactive protein, and endotoxin have been noted in patients with AHF and have prognostic value.[43,46-48] In addition to direct effects, this activation stimulates the release of other factors, such as the potent procoagulant tissue factor and endothelin-1, which can cause myocardial suppression (worsening LV systolic function), disruption of the pulmonary alveolar capillary barrier (contributing to pulmonary edema), and increased platelet aggregation and coagulation (potentially worsening ischemia). The latter mechanism is supported by a significant correlation between IL-6 levels and increased levels of tissue factor, whereas increases in von Willebrand factor and soluble E-selectin in patients with AHF are indicative of endothelial injury.[49] Further research will be required to define the extent to which these changes are involved in the pathogenesis of AHF or merely a marker.

Precipitants of Acute Heart Failure

AHF is episodic in nature and specific precipitating factors for these episodes can be identified (see also Chapter 24 Online Supplement: Precipitating Factors and Chapter 25). Although at times they remain unknown, it is imperative that these precipitants are actively defined and treated, and that an effective intervention is developed to prevent recurrence. The prevalence of specific triggers varies greatly, depending on the study population (Tables 24-3 and 24-4) and the ascertainment methods within the study. For example, more than 42 percent of patients admitted in EHFS II[13] with de novo AHF had an acute coronary syndrome (ACS) and almost 20 percent of all patients had a STEMI, whereas ACS was considered to be the precipitating factor in 23 percent of patients with acute decompensated CHF and only 6 percent had a STEMI. Not only is there great variability in the known precipitants, but studies have often found that 40 to 50 percent of AHF episodes have no known precipitant.[50-53]

CLINICAL MANIFESTATIONS OF ACUTE HEART FAILURE

Acute heart failure is a clinical syndrome comprising multiple symptoms and signs related to the pathophysiologies described earlier. The rapid and accurate assessment of these patients is critical to providing appropriate therapy, and the history and physical examination, which may elicit the symptoms and signs crucial to diagnosis, are the first steps in this assessment. The foregoing discussion will

TABLE 24–3 Characteristics on Admission by Clinical Classification of EHFS II Patients

Characteristics	Total	Decompensated HF	Pulmonary Edema	Cardiogenic Shock	Hypertensive HF	Right HF
No. of patients (% of total)	3580	2340 (65.4)	581 (16.2)	139 (3.9)	407 (11.4)	113 (3.2)
Age (years), mean (SD)	69.9 (12.5)	69.7 (12.8)	71.2 (11.5)	67.3 (12.7)	69.8 (11.2)	69.6 (13.4)
Age, IQR	62.6-78.7	62.3-78.7	64.6-79.7	59.5-77.2	61.9-78.4	63.0-79.5
Male (%)	61.3	62.1	59.4	67.6	60.4	50.4
Body mass index (kg/m²)	26.8	26.5	26.9	26.4	28.0	26.6
New-onset AHF (%)	37.1	29.7	59.6	64.7	37.3	39.8
Hospitalization for HF within last 12 months (%)	44.5	48	3.7	29.3	45.1	46.4
Underlying diseases (%)						
CHD	53.6	54.0	54.9	52.5	53.8	38.1
Hypertension	62.5	56.0	70.1	54.0	94.6	52.2
Diabetes mellitus	32.8	30.9	39.4	34.3	34.5	29.2
Atrial fibrillation/flutter	38.7	41.3	28.1	24.6	37.7	58.4
Previous stroke or TIA	13.3	12.4	15.7	11.8	16.0	13.3
Valvular disease	34.4	37.5	26.2	18.0	31.7	43.8
Renal failure	16.8	16.6	15.8	18.1	18.7	17.7
Anemia	14.7	15.0	15.7	14.4	11.3	16.8
Chronic obstructive pulmonary disease	19.3	19.2	19.3	18.1	18.0	27.4
Pacemaker implanted	9.1	10.6	5.9	10.8	4.9	8.8
Dilated cardiomyopathy	19.3	21.8	11.4	10.2	20.2	15.9
Precipitating factors (on admission)						
ACS (%)	30.2	24.7	49.4	71.9	24.4	14.2
STEMI	11.1	8.4	17.0	55.4	4.7	6.2
Non-STEMI	10.0	7.7	22.4	12.9	5.4	5.3
Unstable angina	9.1	8.6	10.0	3.6	14.3	2.7
Arrhythmia (%)	32.4	32.9	29.3	29.7	34.5	33.9
Atrial	29.4	30.1	25.7	18.8	34.0	33.0
Ventricular	4.1	3.7	5.2	13.0	2.0	2.7
Valvular cause (%)	26.8	30.2	24.1	17.4	12.6	32.7
Infection (%)	17.6	18.5	17.1	11.8	15.6	17.1
Noncompliance with therapy (%)	22.2	24.6	16.9	7.9	21.9	18.1

Renal failure defined as any of the following: patient's serum creatinine recurrently >0.177 mmol/liter (>2.0 mg/dL) at present or in the past or patient on dialysis or with renal transplant; anemia as reported.

ACS = acute coronary syndrome; AHF = acute heart failure; CHD = coronary heart disease; COPD = chronic obstructive pulmonary disease; HF = heart failure; EHFS II = EuroHeart Failure Survey II; IQR = interquartile range; SD = standard deviation; STEMI, ST-elevation myocardial infarction; TIA = transient ischemic attack.

Data from Nieminen MS, Brutsaert D, Dickstein K, et al: EuroHeart Failure Survey II (EHFS II): A survey on hospitalized acute heart failure patients: Description of population. Eur Heart J 27:2725-2736, 2006.

predominantly focus on aspects specifically pertinent to AHF (see also Chaps. 11 and 22).

Symptoms in Patients Presenting with Acute Heart Failure

The most common reasons for patients to seek medical care for AHF are symptoms related to congestion, and less often hypoperfusion. A list of the more common presenting symptoms is provided in Table 24-5. In ADHERE,[16] of the 187,565 discharges, 89 percent of patients presented with dyspnea, 34 percent with dyspnea at rest, and 31 percent presented with fatigue, clearly establishing the primacy of dyspnea as a presenting symptom in these patients. In the registry associated with the U.S.-based Initiation Management Predischarge Assessment of Carvedilol Heart Failure (IMPACT-HF), many different symptoms were specifically queried, and symptoms related to dyspnea and signs related to volume overload dominate the clinical presentation (Fig. 24-3).[54] A small single-center study[55] used timeline follow-back interviews to also assess the time course of these symptoms and noted that in this small cohort of patients, 63 percent of whom had documented ejection fraction ≤40 percent, symptoms gradually increased over days to weeks prior to admission with more than 62 percent of the patients noting symptoms for more than 1 week prior to hospitalization (Fig. 24-4), suggesting that some of these hospitalizations could be prevented by earlier intervention.

Underlying comorbidities will modify the clinical presentation of patients with AHF. The same proportion of patients with preserved and reduced left ventricular systolic function present with dyspnea at rest (34 percent), although a slightly higher percentage of patients with preserved systolic function had peripheral edema (69 versus 63 percent) and rales (69 versus 67 percent) compared to those with reduced systolic function. Although the symptoms may be similar, there is evidence from a number of trials that the severity of dyspnea, functional limitation, and reductions in quality of life were worse in patients with reduced systolic function. In addition, psychological and social factors, such as depression, fatigue, and overall health perception, also influence the perception of dyspnea.[56]

Patients may also present with symptoms related to systemic venous congestion, including edema, weight gain, increasing abdominal girth, and discomfort, although most practicing clinicians have been surprised by the degree of *peripheral edema* patients can ignore. Significant edema can

TABLE 24–4 Common Precipitants of Acute Heart Failure

Potentially Preventable Precipitants	Preventive Measures/Comments
Poor dietary compliance	Education on salt content; nutritionist consult
Poor medical compliance	Education on indications, side effects, dosing of medications; pharmacist consult
Inappropriate discontinuation/reduction of HF therapy by physician	Careful assessment of volume status
Use of medications known to worsen HF, such as: Nonsteroidal antiinflammatory drugs Calcium antagonists (i.e. verapamil, diltiazem) Thiazolidinediones Antiarrhythmic agents (all class I agents, sotalol) Beta-blockers Anti-TNF antibodies	Physician and patient education In patients with HF, may increase risk of hospitalization 10-fold. Cause increases in peripheral edema Unusual cause now that more physicians have experience
Inadequately treated hypertension	
Anemia	Probably underappreciated as a contributing cause
Excessive alcohol consumption	
Not Readily Preventable Precipitants	
Acute myocardial ischemia/infarction	
Arrhythmias (tachycardia or bradycardia), infection	Especially atrial fibrillation with rapid ventricular response
Acute valvular insufficiency	
Endocrine abnormalities	Improve control of diabetes mellitus, hyperthyroidism/thyrotoxicosis, etc.)

TABLE 24–5 Common Symptoms and Signs of Decompensated Heart Failure

Symptoms	Signs
Predominantly Related to Volume Overload	
Dyspnea (exertional, paroxysmal nocturnal dyspnea, orthopnea, or at rest); cough; wheezing	Rales, pleural effusion
Foot and leg discomfort	Peripheral edema (legs, sacral)
Abdominal discomfort/ bloating; early satiety or anorexia	Ascites/increased abdominal girth; right upper quadrant pain or discomfort; hepatomegaly/splenomegaly; scleral icterus Increased weight Elevated jugular venous pressure, abdominojugular reflux Increasing S_3, accentuated P_2
Predominantly Related to Hypoperfusion	
Fatigue	Cool extremities
Altered mental status, daytime drowsiness, confusion, or difficulty concentrating	Pallor, dusky skin discoloration, hypotension
Dizziness, presyncope, or syncope	Pulse pressure (narrow)/ proportional pulse pressure (low) Pulsus alternans
Other Signs and Symptoms of Acute Heart Failure	
Depression	Orthostatic hypotension (hypovolemia)
Sleep disturbances	S_4
Palpitations	Systolic and diastolic cardiac murmurs

occur centrally, so reports of *abdominal discomfort* and *increasing abdominal girth* may represent decompensation. The abdominal discomfort may be described as early satiety, a sense of bloating or fullness, diffuse nondescript aching, or even right upper quadrant pain (because of liver congestion). Inquiring about changes in belt size or observation of the belt can provide clues to the extent and rapidity of onset of the increased bowel edema and ascites.

Patients with AHF may also present with other symptoms, including fatigue, depression, altered mental status, and sleep disorders. It is unclear how frequent these symptoms may be, given that they are often not recognized as being related to heart failure and are often not specifically elicited. Despite likely underreporting, almost one-third of patients report *fatigue* on presentation with AHF.[16,54] Initially, it was believed that fatigue was the direct result of decreased cardiac output, but the presence of fatigue in patients with preserved LV systolic function and recent research revealing significant metabolic abnormalities, especially of skeletal muscle, have suggested that other mechanisms play an important role in the pathogenesis of fatigue. *Depression* is estimated to be present in about one-third of heart failure patients and major depression is present in 40 percent of hospitalized patients with NYHA class IV heart failure.[57] Depression is a major concern for patients and is one of the most important factors affecting quality of life, contributing to the patient's perception of other symptoms, such as dyspnea, and independently increasing mortality.[58] Although depression may be an unusual primary cause of admission in AHF patients, recognition and treatment of the condition may hasten and improve recovery from the acute episode. *Altered mental status* or *confusion* may also be present in patients with severe AHF. Multiple potential mechanisms may contribute, including hypotension, impaired cerebral circulation, vascular remodeling with abnormal endothelial function, silent cerebral infarction, atrial fibrillation, hypercoagulable state, and advanced age.[59]

Sleep disturbances are a common problem in patients with chronic heart failure and can result in symptoms of marked *drowsiness* and *fatigue*. *Palpitations* are a frequent symptom in patients with heart failure, although it is unclear how often they are the presenting symptoms in patients with AHF. Associated symptoms, including dizziness, presyncope and syncope, should be specifically elicited, and may be indicative of a more malignant arrhythmia, but none of these symptoms is specific enough to establish a diagnosis. Atrial fibrillation is a well-known precipitant of acute decompensation, and given its high preva-

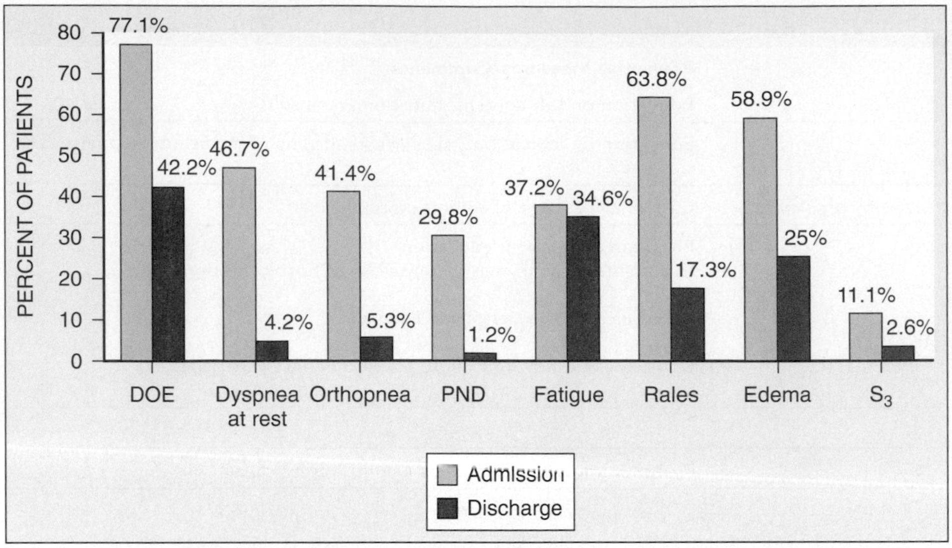

FIGURE 24–3 Heart failure signs and symptoms at admission and discharge in 567 patients enrolled in The Initiation Management Pre-discharge Assessment of Carvedilol Heart Failure (IMPACT-HF) registry. Signs and symptoms of congestion and volume overload dominate the presentation of these patients and many patients remain symptomatic at discharge. DOE = dyspnea on exertion; PND = paroxysmal nocturnal dyspnea; S_3 = third heart sound. *(Data from O'Connor CM, Stough WG, Gallup DS, et al: Demographics, clinical characteristics, and outcomes of patients hospitalized for decompensated heart failure: Observations from the IMPACT-HF registry. J Card Fail 11:200-205, 2005.)*

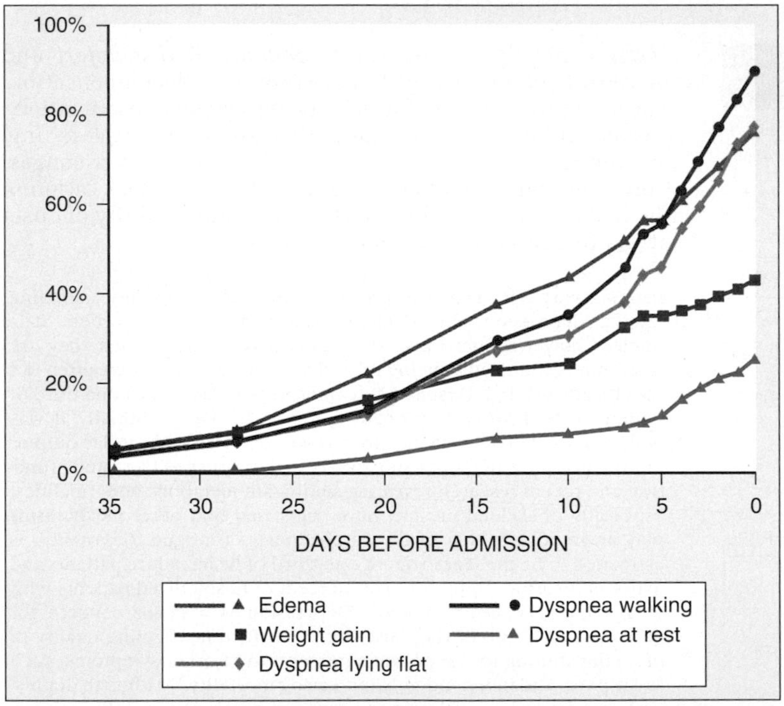

FIGURE 24–4 Number of days from onset of worsening of selected symptoms of heart failure to admission to hospital in 83 patients admitted with heart failure. Most symptoms were present 1 week prior to admission, suggesting that earlier outpatient intervention might reduce hospitalizations. *(Data from Schiff GD, Fung S, Speroff T, McNutt RA: Decompensated heart failure: Symptoms, patterns of onset, and contributing factors. Am J Med 114:625-630, 2003.)*

lence in the heart failure population, should be actively sought as a contributing factor.

Physical Examination of the Acute Heart Failure Patient

The physical examination has previously been discussed (Chaps. 11 and 23) and consequently, this section will address issues specific to the examination of the patient with AHF (see Table 24-5).

General Inspection

General inspection of the patient while obtaining the history is an efficient way to begin the physical examination. The presence of bitemporal wasting may alert the physician to cachexia and concomitant loss of true body weight which accompanies chronic HF. Marked truncal obesity may suggest the possibility of obstructive sleep apnea, associated with pulmonary hypertension and acute right heart failure. Total body anasarca and scleral icterus are other easily visible clues to the presence of increased hepatic venous congestion. Many patients with AHF will have difficulty completing a full history because of dyspnea, either at rest or developing during the interview. Orthopnea may be evident during examination as well, and patients may become visibly anxious as they change position. Pallor or a dusky discoloration of the skin may be suggestive of severely decreased cardiac output and cardiogenic shock. A low-grade increase in body temperature (≥38.0° C) can occur in the setting of marked cutaneous vasoconstriction or myocardial infarction, but persistence of this low-grade increase in temperature after treatment for heart failure or development of a true fever (≥38.5° C) requires further diagnostic evaluation.

Blood Pressure

Measuring the blood pressure is a critical part in the evaluation of patients with AHF; hypotension is one of the strongest predictors of poor outcomes[18,54] and helps to define the clinical profile of the patient and appropriate therapeutic interventions. The examiner is encouraged to obtain the blood pressure personally, given potential inaccuracies in measurement technique and recording.

Systolic blood pressure (SBP) is typically normal or elevated in patients with AHF, with almost 50 percent presenting with SBP >140 mm Hg.[16,18] The combination of underlying hypertension and the marked increase in sympathetic stimulation that accompanies AHF can result in elevations of SBP consistent with hypertensive urgencies or emergencies (12 percent of patients had an SBP over 180 mm Hg on admission[14]). Patients with very low SBP are uncommon, with only 2 percent of patients in ADHERE presenting with an SBP <90 mm Hg.

Diastolic blood pressure (DBP) is an important measure, as well. Increased DBP is suggestive of significant neurohormonal and sympathetic stimulation, whereas low DBP may indicate marked peripheral vasodilation as in sepsis or vasodilator-induced pseudosepsis or severe aortic regurgitation.

Pulse pressure (the difference between systolic and diastolic blood pressure) and the *proportional pulse pressure* (the pulse pressure divided by the systolic blood pressure) are useful derived measures. A low pulse pressure is a marker of a low cardiac output and confers a relative risk of death of 2.5 in patients admitted with AHF.[60] The proportional pulse pressure correlates well with cardiac index and when less than 25 percent had high sensitivity and specificity for a cardiac index of less than 2.2 liter/min/m^2.[61] A high pulse pressure may alert the physician to a high output state including the possibility of unrecognized thyrotoxicosis or anemia.

Changes in blood pressure with specific maneuvers can also provide important information. *Orthostatic hypotension,* a postural decline in blood pressure >10 mm Hg, most often signals volume depletion, but the possibility of an autonomic neuropathy in a patient with diabetes or suspected amyloidosis should be considered. Measuring the blood pressure while the patient performs a *Valsalva maneuver* has been useful to discriminate whether dyspnea is related to a pulmonary process or elevated left-sided filling pressures. In patients with heart failure there is little decrease in pulse pressure in phase 2 of the Valsalva maneuver and no overshoot in phase 4. An accentuated decrease in systolic blood pressure (>10 mm Hg) during normal inspiration *(pulsus paradoxus)* raises the concern of cardiac tamponade which may mimic AHF.

Jugular Venous Pressure

The *jugular venous pressure (JVP)* is literally a barometer of systemic venous hypertension and can be elevated in response to either volume overload or venous vasoconstriction or both. It is perhaps the most useful physical examination finding for evaluating AHF, although it is highly dependent on examiner skill.

The JVP reflects the right atrial pressure, but an elevated JVP is also associated with elevated left-sided filling pressures as measured by the PCWP in patients with chronic heart failure. Additionally, changes in the right atrial pressure correlated with changes in the PCWP during intensive medical therapy. Severe tricuspid regurgitation can be detected by recognizing prominent *v* waves and *y* descents in the jugular venous pulsation. The presence of severe tricuspid regurgitation (TR) may impact the relationship of JVP and PCWP (leading the physician to overestimate the right atrial pressure and, therefore, the left-sided filling pressure), and although severe tricuspid regurgitation is associated with elevated PCWP in advanced heart failure, in patients with right heart failure out of proportion to left, the JVP will not be a reliable indicator of PCWP.

There are several caveats to using the JVP as a noninvasive measure of the PCWP. First, comorbidities such as obesity or lung disease can affect right ventricular (RV) function and, therefore, distort the relationship between right-sided and left-sided filling pressures. Second, 20 percent of patients referred for transplant have discordance between the JVP and PCWP. When the clinical response to therapy guided by the JVP is unanticipated (e.g., development of hypotension and renal failure with diuresis in a patient with persistently elevated JVP), these data remind us that the JVP may not be reflective of the PCWP. Third, although the JVP and PCWP usually track together in chronic heart failure, in the setting of myocardial infarction, they often do not. Whether the JVP reflects the PCWP in heart failure in the setting of intact left ventricular ejection fraction (LVEF) (i.e., diastolic heart failure) is not known. *Abdominojugular* or *hepatojugular reflux,* or the response of the JVP to abdominal pressure, is also informative because it also correlates with elevated left-sided filling pressures.

Cardiac Examination

Visual inspection and palpation of the precordium, followed by careful auscultation, provide important clues to the presence of cardiac dysfunction. *S_3 gallops* or *third heart sounds* are detected in approximately 11 to 34 percent of patients admitted with AHF.[15,54,62] An S_3 is fairly specific as an indicator of LV systolic dysfunction, and correlates with BNP levels.[63] In patients with symptomatic heart failure, it is independently associated with adverse outcomes including heart failure hospitalization and death from pump failure. Other auscultatory findings, such as *S_4 gallops* or *fourth heart sounds, accentuation of P_2* and *systolic and diastolic murmurs* can provide additional clues to the etiology of the AHF.

OTHER PHYSICAL EXAMINATION FINDINGS

Rales or *inspiratory crackles* are the most common physical examination finding[54] and have been noted in 66 to 87 percent of patients admitted for AHF.[15,16] However, rales are often not heard in patients with chronic heart failure and pulmonary venous hypertension because of increased lymphatic drainage, reinforcing the caution that the absence of rales does not necessarily imply normal LV filling pressures.

Other pulmonary signs include *rhonchi* and *wheezes* and evidence of *pleural effusion* or *hydrothorax.* The latter is usually associated with decompensation of chronic heart failure with subacute or chronic elevations of the pulmonary or systemic venous pressures or both. Effusions caused by heart failure are bilateral in more than 85 percent of the cases, with a majority of the unilateral effusions evident on the right-side.

Cool extremities, such as the lower leg with a palpable dorsalis pedis or posterior tibialis pulse (to rule out peripheral vascular disease), suggest decreased peripheral perfusion consistent with a marginal cardiac index, marked vasoconstriction, or both. Of note, the temperature should be assessed at the lower leg as opposed to the foot, and this assessment is relative to the temperature of the examiner hands.

Edema is another classic sign of decompensated CHF. Peripheral edema is present in up to 65 percent of patients admitted with AHF,[16] and is less common in patients presenting with predominantly low output heart failure or cardiogenic shock.[38] The presence of edema has a reasonable positive predictive value for ADHF but a low sensitivity, so its absence does not exclude that diagnosis. Edema caused by AHF is usually dependent, symmetrical, and pitting. It is estimated that a minimum of 4 liters of extracellular fluid is accumulated to produce clinically detectable edema.

Hepatomegaly and *splenomegaly* can occur acutely in patients with AHF because of increased central venous pressure, and in these cases often results in significant tenderness, but it is more often the result of chronic systemic venous hypertension, where it is minimally tender, if at all. Severe tricuspid regurgitation can result in a pulsatile liver on examination and in congestive cirrhosis. *Ascites* occurs in response to elevated central venous pressures by retarding emptying of the peritoneal veins and the hepatic veins. Severe tricuspid disease predisposes to ascites, compared to peripheral edema, as does constrictive pericardial disease. *Visceral congestion* may occur independently of ascites and is impossible to detect on routine physical examination. However, it can contribute to symptoms of bloating and early satiety, potentially interfering with intestinal absorption of oral medications, such as furosemide.

DIAGNOSTIC EVALUATION OF THE PATIENT WITH ACUTE HEART FAILURE

The Task Force on Acute Heart Failure of the European Society of Cardiology (ESC[4]) and the Heart Failure Society of America (HFSA[5]) have both recently issued guidelines for the diagnosis and treatment of AHF, and both guidelines stress that the diagnosis of heart failure is dependent on a careful assessment of the symptoms and signs complemented by diagnostic testing. A more detailed discussion of these diagnostic evaluations is also available in the respective chapters pertaining to chronic heart failure and the diagnostic specific modalities.

Common Laboratory Tests

SERUM ELECTROLYTES. Alterations of serum electrolytes in AHF are similar to those found in chronic heart failure. *Hyponatremia* is a common finding in AHF populations, with approximately 25 to 30 percent of patients with serum sodium <135 mEq/L, although severe hyponatremia (<130 mEq/L) is much less frequent (5 percent[16]). Serum potassium concentrations are typically in the normal range in patients with AHF, with a mean of approximately 4.3 to 4.6 mEq/L and hypokalemia (3 percent; <3.6 mEq/L) and hyperkalemia (8 percent; >5.5 mEq/L) surprisingly uncommon on admission.[15]

MEASURES OF RENAL FUNCTION. *Blood urea nitrogen (BUN)* is more directly related to the severity of AHF than creatinine, and is typically elevated on admission. Serum BUN concentrations increase in AHF because of the decreased glomerular filtration rate (GFR) and the increased sodium reabsorption. Serum BUN is roughly proportional to the increased vasoconstriction in response to hemodynamic perturbations and to the neurohormonal activation in AHF. Mean values range from moderately (30 mg/dl[16,54]) to markedly (81 mg/dl[15]) increased, depending on the patient population. These elevations are usually accompanied by increases in *creatinine,* which is a more direct reflection of the decreased GFR. The mean creatinine on admission in most studies is approximately 1.7 mg/dl and about 20 percent of the patients have creatinine above 2.0 mg/dl. Estimated glomerular filtration rates should be calculated because serum creatinine levels may greatly underestimate the degree of renal dysfunction.

LIVER FUNCTION TESTS. In a study of AHF patients admitted to an intensive care unit, 61 percent had laboratory evidence of liver dysfunction,[38] which may necessitate dose adjustments with some medications.

HEMATOLOGICAL STUDIES. More than one-half of patients who are admitted with AHF have *anemia,* as defined by a hemoglobin concentration of less than 12 g/dl, and 8 to 16 percent have hemoglobin concentrations of less than 10.0 g/dl.[14-16,64] This prevalence appears to be greater than in patients with chronic heart failure, suggesting that hemodilution because of increased plasma volume is most likely a mechanism in the patients with AHF. Bone marrow suppression caused by increases in proinflammatory cytokines and worsening renal function may also result in additional decreases in red blood cell mass.

NATRIURETIC PEPTIDES (BNP, nt-pro-BNP, ANP) (see also Chaps. 22 and 23). The natriuretic peptides are counterregulatory hormones with pleiotropic effects. *B-type natriuretic peptide* (*BNP;* formerly brain natriuretic peptide), along with its cleavage remnant *n-terminal-pro-BNP (nt-pro-BNP),* is synthesized and secreted by the ventricular myocardium in response to increases in volume or pressure, and has a relatively low concentration in storage granules. BNP is cleared from the circulation by receptor-mediated endocytosis via the C-type natriuretic peptide receptor, as well as by enzymatic degradation via zinc-containing endopeptidases located on the vascular endothelial cells and in the renal tubules. nt-pro-BNP has a longer half-life and is renally cleared, making it susceptible to significant changes based on alterations in renal function. In the most recent quarterly data (January to March, 2006) from ADHERE,[16] 81 percent of patients had a BNP assessed, and both BNP (median 843) and nt-pro-BNP (mean 3385) were markedly elevated on admission. Both the ESC and HFSA AHF guidelines suggest that BNP assays are a useful adjunct to clinical assessment.[4,5]

Early studies showed that BNP concentrations were excellent predictors of heart failure in patients presenting with dyspnea, but the question of their utility compared to physician assessments remained. The Breathing Not Properly Multinational Study[65,66] demonstrated that BNP was able to distinguish dyspnea caused by heart failure from that caused by pulmonary disease (Fig. 24-5) with a high degree of predictive power, and was the strongest predictor in multiple logistic regression analysis of the diagnosis of heart failure.[65] In addition, this study was able to demonstrate, using a cut-off of 100 mg/dl for a "normal" BNP, that the BNP test alone had a diagnostic accuracy of 81.2 percent, compared to 74.0 percent for clinical judgment alone.[66] Although it may seem disconcerting that the addition of the physician assessment to the BNP measurement only barely improved diagnostic accuracy to 81.5 percent, the standard for diagnosis in this trial remained the clinical assessment by two cardiologists, reviewing the totality of the clinical information. This trial established the role of BNP testing in the assessment of dyspnea in the emergency setting, and in general, a BNP of less than 100 pg/ml is considered to have a high negative predictive value, whereas concentrations greater than 400 pg/ml have high positive predictive value for heart failure as the etiology of the dyspnea.

Assays for nt-pro-BNP have been developed and have also proved to be effective in diagnosing heart failure in the context of a presentation of dyspnea. Studies with nt-pro-BNP[67] demonstrate that an age-independent cut point of less than 300 pg/ml had a 98 percent negative predictive value, and recommended age-related cut points of 450, 900, and 1800 pg/ml for patients of ages <50, 50 to 75, and >75, respectively, with 90 percent sensitivity and 84 percent specificity for AHF. The B-type Natriuretic Peptide for Acute Shortness of Breath Evaluation (BASEL) study,[68] randomized 452 patients with acute dyspnea to a strategy whereby the physicians were aware of the nt-pro-BNP measures in one group, whereas the others were evaluated in the standard manner. Patients assigned to the nt-pro-BNP group were less likely to be hospitalized or to require intensive unit care, had shorter length of hospital stay with commensurate reductions in hospital costs, and had no difference in readmission or mortality rates. BASEL demonstrated that in patients presenting to the emergency department with dyspnea, the use of the nt-pro-BNP assay had substantial clinical benefits.

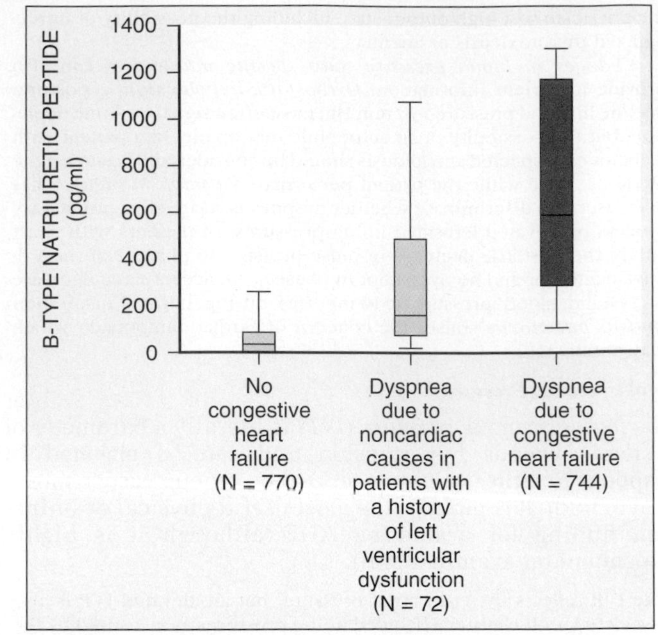

FIGURE 24–5 BNP (B-type natriuretic peptide) concentrations in three groups of patients presenting to the emergency room with dyspnea. Line represents median, boxes show interquartile ranges, and I bars represent highest and lowest values. *(Data from Maisel AS, Krishnaswamy P, Nowak RM, et al: Rapid measurement of B-type natriuretic peptide in the emergency diagnosis of heart failure. N Engl J Med 347:161-167, 2002.)*

The findings of these and other studies have led to widespread adoption of these assays in urgent care settings, but as with all diagnostic tests, BNP assays have important limitations (Table 24-6).[69] The diagnostic accuracy of the assays may be preserved through adjusting the diagnostic cut-off points with respect to specific subgroups. Elevated BNP may also be found in conditions other than primary left ventricular heart failure, including acute coronary syndromes and myocardial infarction, right-sided heart failure with decompensated cor pulmonale or acute pulmonary embolus,[70] and severe sepsis and septic shock.[71] It is important that these diagnoses not be overlooked when interpreting an elevated BNP. Patients with AHF because of systolic heart failure have higher BNP concentrations than those who present with diastolic heart failure,[72] but the extensive overlap of the values limits the usefulness of BNP in distinguishing these forms of heart failure in individual patients.

Atrial natriuretic peptide (ANP) is produced predominantly by the cardiac atrium and is rapidly released from storage granules in response to atrial stretch. Because of this mechanism of release, ANP levels are dynamic, responding to even physiological increases in atrial stretch, as with exercise, although marked pathological increases in atrial pressure or volume produce significantly greater increases. At this time, ANP assessment has not been demonstrated to have significant clinical utility.

BIOMARKERS OF MYOCARDIAL INJURY. Serial measurements of markers of myocardial injury are important in

TABLE 24–6	Conditions that Influence B-Type Natriuretic Peptide (BNP) Concentrations
Increased BNP concentrations may be found in:	
Age (older)	
Sex (female)	
Ethnicity (black)	
Renal dysfunction	
Myocardial infarction/acute coronary syndromes	
Right-sided heart failure (cor pulmonale, acute pulmonary embolus)	
High output failure (cirrhosis, septic shock)	
Decreased BNP concentrations may be found in:	
Obesity	
Early acute heart failure (less than 1 hr)	
Acute mitral regurgitation	
Mitral stenosis (in the absence of right ventricular failure)	
Stable NYHA Class I patients with decreased LV ejection fraction	

Modified from Maisel AS: The diagnosis of acute congestive heart failure: Role of BNP measurements. Heart Fail Rev 8:327-334, 2003.

diagnosing possible acute coronary syndromes or myocardial infarction as a precipitant of AHF. These diagnoses require different treatment strategies and have significant prognostic implications. Therefore, routine serial measurements of troponins (or CK-MB) are recommended.

OTHER POTENTIAL LABORATORY TESTS. *C-reactive protein (CRP)* is a recommended test in the ESC Guidelines as a means to detect underlying infectious processes. Although other markers of inflammation have been shown to be elevated in the setting of AHF, their clinical utility has been limited. *D-dimers* may be useful in diagnosing pulmonary embolism, and *arterial blood gases* are recommended in patients with severe AHF.

Common Diagnostic Tests

CHEST RADIOGRAPHY. Chest radiography was performed in more than 90 percent of patients in ADHERE and there was evidence of congestion in more than 80 percent of these patients.[73]

ELECTROCARDIOGRAM. The *electrocardiogram (ECG)* is an essential diagnostic tool in the evaluation of the patient with AHF. In EFICA,[38] only 13 percent of ECGs were normal, with ischemic changes evident in 29 percent and atrial fibrillation in 25 percent. Of note, noncardiogenic pulmonary edema has been associated with giant, diffuse, symmetrical inverted T waves with QT prolongation, a finding also reported in pulmonary embolism and hypercatecholamine states.

ECHOCARDIOGRAM. An *echocardiogram* may be the single most useful test in evaluating the etiology of the patient with AHF because of its ability to assess global systolic and diastolic function, regional wall motion abnormalities, valvular function, hemodynamics, and pericardial disease. In EHFS II,[13] moderate or severe systolic dysfunction (66 percent), diastolic dysfunction (56 percent), mitral regurgitation (43 percent) and tricuspid regurgitation (30 percent) were noted. The *tissue Doppler* ratio of peak early diastolic transmitral blood flow velocity (E) to the peak early diastolic mitral annular tissue velocity (Ea) (E : Ea ratio) has been shown to be additive to BNP measures in diagnosing AHF inpatients presenting with dyspnea.[74] *Myocardial contrast echocardiography* has also recently been used in patients with AHF to evaluate the presence of coronary artery disease and decreased myocardial flow reserve as an etiology of the decompensation.[75]

PULMONARY ARTERY CATHETER. The *pulmonary artery catheter (PAC)* provides important and clinically relevant hemodynamic data in selected patients, especially those with shock or other severe hemodynamic compromise, with oliguria or anuria, or with unclear hemodynamics and poor response to therapy. Central venous, pulmonary artery and pulmonary capillary wedge pressures are measured directly, and cardiac output can be assessed either through thermodilution or oxygen consumption techniques. From these measures a variety of useful derived values may be calculated, including systemic and pulmonary vascular resistance and stroke work. In skilled hands, this diagnostic tool can enable exquisite tailoring of therapy to specific hemodynamic goals. In EHFS II,[13] only 5 percent of patients had a PAC during hospitalization, with the overwhelming number being used in the patients with cardiogenic shock (25 percent). Therefore, despite the potential benefits, PAC use has decreased substantially in recent years, largely because of safety concerns.

The PAC is an invasive diagnostic tool, associated with the risks of an invasive procedure, including bleeding, infection, arrhythmias and rare catastrophic events, such as pulmonary artery rupture or infarction. A number of studies in patients with a variety of diagnoses have suggested that PAC use is associated with increased complications, length of stay, and mortality. However, it is difficult to isolate the effect of the PAC itself from the increased risk and disease severity of the patients in whom they are used. A recent meta-analysis of trials with PAC use suggested that there is no increased risk of mortality or prolonged hospitalization stay.[76]

The Evaluation Study of Congestive Heart Failure and Pulmonary Artery Catheterization Effectiveness (ESCAPE)[8] was a controlled trial of 433 patients with severe symptomatic heart failure despite recommended therapies randomized to receive therapy guided by clinical assessment and a PAC or by clinical assessment alone. The patients in the study were very ill, but were more representative of an advanced chronic heart failure cohort than AHF. In these patients, use of PAC did not significantly affect the days alive and out of hospital during the first 6 months (133 versus 135 days), mortality (43 versus 38 patients) or the number of days hospitalized (8.7 versus 8.3 days), compared to clinical assessment alone. There were more adverse events, but there were no deaths related to PAC use. This randomized study demonstrated that the PAC is relatively safe in experienced centers, and suggests that this important diagnostic tool may be used in patients in whom the diagnosis of cardiogenic versus noncardiogenic pulmonary edema is in question or when management of the patient's circulatory status is critical.

OTHER POTENTIAL DIAGNOSTIC MODALITIES

A number of additional tests may assist in the diagnosis and management of patients with AHF in the future. Although not new in principle, *phonocardiography* may be a specific indicator of left ventricular dysfunction[63] and has already been demonstrated to improve diagnostic accuracy in patients presenting with dyspnea to the emergency department.[77] *External impedance cardiography (ICG)* is another technology that has promise in providing clinically relevant hemodynamic data in a noninvasive manner. The current generation of ICG measures thoracic impedance via four dual sensors applied to the neck and thorax. ICG has been shown to be as accurate as thermodilution measures of cardiac output and to be additive to clinical assessments and BNP in the diagnosis of AHF in patients with dyspnea, as well as to be predictive of the short-term risk of developing decompensated heart failure.[78] With the proliferation of implantable devices (such as biventricular pacemakers and implantable cardioverter devices), there has been considerable interest in adding monitoring functions to these devices. *Internal thoracic impedance* is a technology already being implemented in a number of these devices.[79] *Implantable hemodynamic monitors* may also provide important information in the diagnosis and management of patients with AHF.

MANAGEMENT OF THE PATIENT WITH ACUTE HEART FAILURE

Stages of Treatment

A central aspect of AHF is the need for urgent care beyond that which may be given in the outpatient setting. Unfortunately, therapies for acute heart failure have rarely been systematically evaluated, and much of the initial approach to these patients has been developed empirically. The management of these patients may be considered in the context of three stages of treatment,[3] and different treatment strategies and the specifics of each therapy will be presented later.

STAGE 1: URGENT/EMERGENT CARE. The initial goals in the management of a patient presenting with AHF are to expeditiously establish the diagnosis, identify the etiology and precipitating factors of the heart failure, treat the life-threatening abnormalities, and initiate therapies to rapidly provide symptom relief. The first point of contact at the admitting hospital for most patients (80 percent) is the emergency department.[16] Although only 1 percent of heart failure patients are initially treated in an emergency department heart failure observation unit, these specialized care centers may be effective in decreasing hospitalizations, ICU and critical care unit admissions, and related health care costs while maintaining the quality of patient care.[80] Most of the diagnostic tests discussed earlier can be rapidly applied to the urgent care setting to guide etiology-specific therapies (i.e., for acute coronary syndromes or atrial fibrillation with rapid ventricular response) and to reveal underlying abnormalities (i.e., hyperkalemia). Immediate noninvasive monitoring of patients is essential, as well as ensuring venous and, if necessary, arterial access.

Initial therapies may follow the algorithm in Figure 24-6. Morphine may relieve anxiety, distress, and dyspnea, although noncontrolled, retrospective observational studies suggest that it may also increase the likelihood of intubation, admission to intensive care unit, and prolong hospital stay. Although not studied rigorously, in the presence of hypoxemia (SaO_2 <95 percent), administration of supplemental oxygen is recommended, although in the absence of hypoxemia, it may cause hyperoxia-induced vasoconstriction, with reduced coronary flow and increased peripheral vascular resistance.

Noninvasive ventilatory support, such as continuous positive airway pressure (CPAP), bilevel positive pressure support (BiPAP) or noninvasive positive pressure ventilation (NIPPV), significantly reduces in-hospital mortality (approximately 40 percent) and markedly decreases intubation rates (more than 50 percent) in patients treated with noninvasive ventilation compared to standard medical therapy.[81-83] There are no apparent differences between CPAP and NIPPV with respect to in-hospital mortality and intubation rate.[82,83] In Europe,[13] more than 30 percent of admissions with pulmonary edema received some type of ventilatory support. Although gaining popularity in the United States, use of these modalities is highly variable[84]; given the dramatic improvement in outcomes, broader adoption of these techniques has the potential to greatly benefit patients. Mechanical ventilation with endotracheal intubation is performed in about 4 to 5 percent of all patients, especially in the setting of respiratory failure from muscle fatigue or in the presence of a high-risk ACS (positive troponin or ST elevation).[13,16]

Atrial fibrillation with rapid ventricular response is the most common tachyarrhythmia requiring treatment. Although it may respond to relief of dyspnea, intravenous digoxin, beta blocker, or diltiazem—or even emergent cardioversion—may be required. In the absence of hypotension, vasodilators play an important role in the initial therapy of patients with pulmonary edema and poor oxygenation, whereas the role of diuretics is more controversial. Systemic volume overload is rarely an emergent issue, although therapy is typically initiated in the emergency department. Most patients (75 percent) in the emergency department receive intravenous diuretics, with a mean door to first intravenous administration time of 2.2 hours in ADHERE.[16] Cardiogenic shock is an unusual presentation of AHF, occurring in less than 4 percent of the patients in EHFS II,[13] most of whom had a myocardial infarction. Intravenous ino-

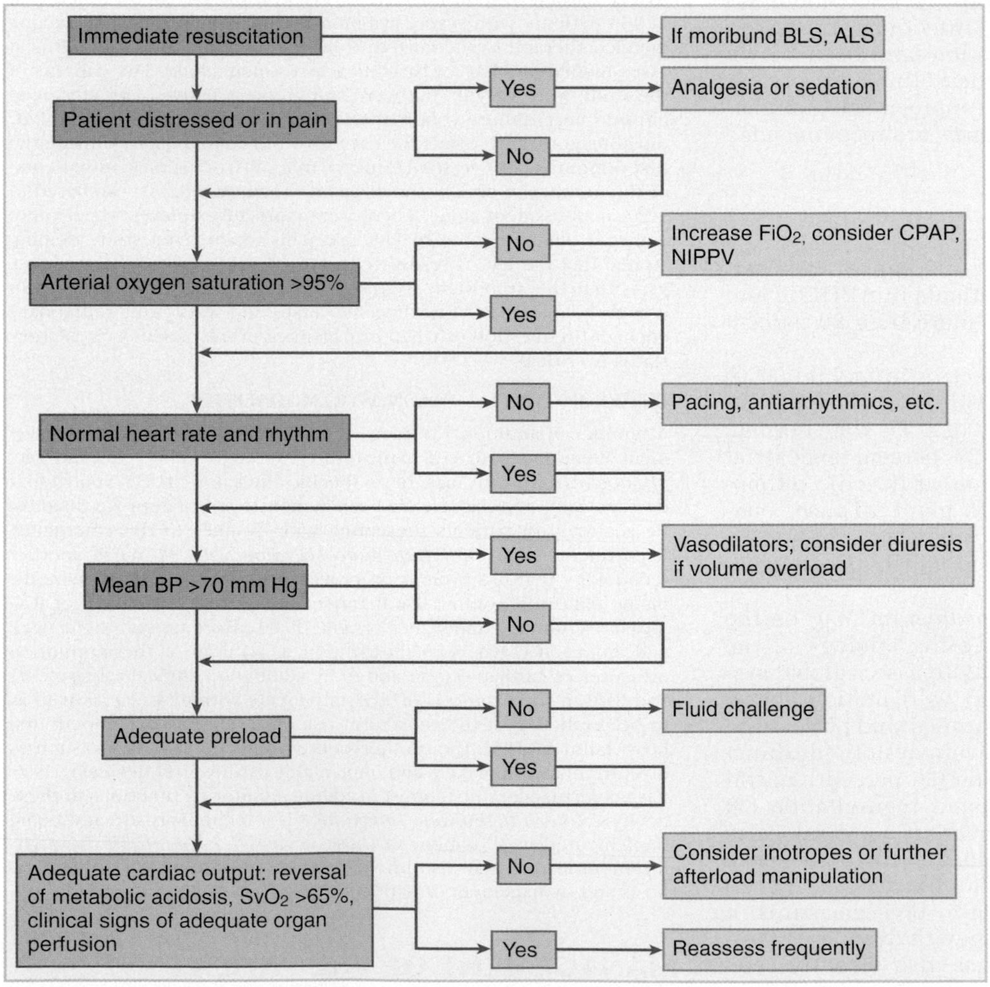

FIGURE 24–6 An algorithm for the immediate management of patients presenting with acute heart failure. ALS = advanced life support; BLS = basic life support; CPAP = continuous positive airway pressure; FiO_2, fractional inspired oxygen concentration; NIPPV = noninvasive positive pressure ventilation; SvO_2 = venous oxygen saturation. *(Modified from Nieminen MS, Bohm M, Cowie MR, et al: Executive summary of the guidelines on the diagnosis and treatment of acute heart failure: The Task Force on Acute Heart Failure of the European Society of Cardiology. Eur Heart J 26:384-416, 2005.)*

tropes or even vasoconstrictors may be required in these patients, with mechanical circulatory support, such as intraaortic balloon pump (IABP) or left ventricular assist device (LVAD), for critical refractory cases.

After the emergent care of the patient, evaluation for triage is performed. In general, hospitalization is recommended for patients with evidence of severe decompensated heart failure, including hypotension (especially if symptomatic), worsening renal function or altered mentation; dyspnea at rest associated with either tachypnea or, less commonly, significant hypoxemia (oxygen saturation <90 percent); hemodynamically significant arrhythmia (most commonly atrial fibrillation either with rapid ventricular response or new onset); and acute coronary syndromes. Hospitalization should be considered in patients with worsened congestion, even in the absence of dyspnea and often reflected by significant weight gain (≥5 kg), other signs or symptoms of pulmonary or systemic congestion, newly diagnosed heart failure, complications of heart failure therapy (such as electrolyte disturbances, frequent ICD firings) or other associated comorbid conditions.[85]

STAGE 2: HOSPITALIZATION. The hospitalization phase goals for the management of a patient with AHF are to complete the diagnostic and acute therapeutic processes that were initiated in the emergency room, to carefully monitor the patient, to optimize the patient's hemodynamic profile, volume status, and clinical symptoms, and to initiate or adjust a maintenance regimen. Ideally, these goals would be met in a manner to minimize intensive care and total hospital length of stay. Most patients (65 percent) are admitted to a telemetry floor, with 13 percent admitted to an ICU/CCU, 9 percent to a step-down unit, and 11 percent to a ward,[16] but regardless of the inpatient unit, careful monitoring is essential. A reliable and reproducible admission weight with daily weights monitoring subsequent changes, daily fluid intake and output, and vital signs, including orthostatic blood pressure, as well as a daily assessment of symptoms and signs, are also crucial. Laboratory monitoring must include daily analysis of electrolytes and renal function, with other tests based on the clinical status. Diagnostic evaluations should include an echocardiogram, if not recently performed, and evaluation of myocardial ischemia, if clinically indicated. Dietary sodium restriction with a low-sodium diet (2 g daily) is useful to restore or maintain euvolemia and fluid restriction (2 liters/day) is recommended for patients with moderate hyponatremia (Na <130 mEq/L) and may be useful in facilitating fluid overload in other patients.[4,85]

Most outpatient medications should be continued during admission, although patients with worsening renal function often have ACE inhibitors withheld. Patients admitted on beta blockers have a lower occurrence of ventricular arrhythmias,[86] a shorter length of stay, and reduced 6-month mortality[87] compared to those not receiving them, and those who were maintained on their therapy had a significantly lower rate of rehospitalization and death within 6 months after discharge, even after adjustments for potential confounders.[87] Therefore, patients should continue their beta blocker therapy during the admission for AHF, unless significant hypotension or cardiogenic shock are present.[4] Other therapeutic interventions are discussed subsequently.

The hospitalization phase of AHF management is also a tremendous opportunity to provide education and behavioral therapies to patients. Patients should receive specific and clear education about the pathophysiology of HF to provide a basis for understanding the indications for drugs, drug counseling from a pharmacist or other provider, outpatient monitoring of fluid status through daily weights, self-adjustment of diuretics, exercise programs, and nutritional counseling, as well as possible consultation with physical and occupational therapy. Comorbidities can be aggressively addressed with education about diabetes, hypertension, coronary artery disease, and other common comorbidities. The hospitalization is also a possible opportunity to enroll the patient in appropriate heart failure disease management programs (see Chap. 25).

STAGE 3: PRE-DISCHARGE. The pre-discharge phase focuses on the goals of optimizing chronic oral therapy, minimizing the side effects of treatments, and ultimately preventing early readmission and improving symptoms and survival. Although there are considerable pressures to rapidly discharge patients in some areas, optimizing their medical regimen[11,88] may prevent subsequent readmissions and improve long-term outcomes. Pre-discharge initiation of a beta blocker, carvedilol, increases the proportion of patients on beta blocker therapy at 60 days (more than 90 percent compared to 73 percent in the post-discharge group), with no increase in adverse events or length of hospitalization.[89] More importantly, pre-discharge initiation of beta blocker therapy may also reduce 60- to 90-day mortality by 54 percent.[90] Despite the overwhelming majority of congestive symptoms on presentation, fewer than 50 percent of the patients were discharged with at least a 5- to 6-lb weight loss.[16,18] Additionally, only one-half of patients were asymptomatic and 27 percent still had edema at discharge, suggesting that there may be room for further improvements in pre-discharge treatment. Some investigators have suggested obtaining pre-discharge BNP in patients, and although these tests have been shown to predict readmission,[91,92] there is no evidence that knowing these values can have an impact on outcomes. A series of studies have also supported the benefits of comprehensive discharge planning with post-discharge support, suggesting that these programs can markedly reduce readmission rates and positively impact quality of life and survival.[93]

The HFSA guidelines[5] suggest the following discharge criteria for all patients: exacerbating factors addressed, at least near optimal volume status achieved, transition from intravenous to oral diuretic completed, patient and family education completed, at least near optimal pharmacological therapy achieved and follow-up clinic visit scheduled, usually within 7 to 10 days. In patients who have advanced HF or have had recurrent admissions, the guidelines also recommend that oral medication regimen be stable for 24 hours, no intravenous vasodilator or inotropic agent for 24 hours, ambulation prior to discharge to assess functional capacity, and plans for post-discharge management (scale present in home, visiting nurse or telephone follow-up within 3 days after discharge).

Treatment Strategies

Treatment strategies for AHF have been largely empirical and limited by an incomplete understanding of the epidemiology and pathophysiology, as well as the relatively blunt nature of the available therapeutic tools.[94]

Stevenson and colleagues developed an approach for the evaluation and treatment of decompensated advanced chronic systolic heart failure on a heart transplant/cardiomyopathy service.[9] This approach, based on the hemodynamic profiles discussed earlier, is predicated on the assumption that hemodynamic abnormalities are the immediate cause of the symptoms and signs of AHF, and that by addressing these derangements, patients will also improve symptomatically. Based on clinical evaluation (described earlier and in Chap. 23), the patient is assigned to one quadrant of a 2 × 2 table, defined by the presence or absence of congestion (wet or dry) and low perfusion (cold or warm) (Fig. 24-7). This strategy emphasizes the importance of ventricular filling pressures as the central component of the heart failure syndrome in these patients, and of tailoring therapy to optimize hemodynamics.[9,95] Another approach, developed by Cotter and colleagues and based on studies of all patients presenting with AHF, emphasizes the importance of the interaction between cardiac function (as assessed by cardiac power) and vascular tone (systemic vascular resistance).[6,96,97] These and other approaches[3] have provided the conceptual framework for the treatment of AHF and informed the development of guidelines.[4,5]

The current general approach incorporates information from three main aspects of the patient's clinical presentation: blood pressure, volume status, and renal function (Table 24-7). *Blood pressure* reflects the interaction between vascular tone and myocardial pump function and is one of the most important prognostic indicators in AHF (see later). Most patients present with elevated blood pressures (see Table 24-2) and consequently will benefit from vasodilator therapy by reducing the vasoconstriction that has resulted in volume redistribution (as in hypertensive AHF) and/or by decreasing preload and afterload with a resultant improvement in cardiac and renal function (as typically occurs in acute decompensated heart failure). Vasodilators are the primary therapy for AHF with pulmonary edema, and for nonhypotensive patients with low cardiac output (poor peripheral or central perfusion with systolic blood pressures above 100 mm Hg). The selection of agent depends on the clinical situation, local practice, and availability. Nitroglycerin and nitroprusside are available in the United States and Europe, whereas nesiritide is approved in the United States.

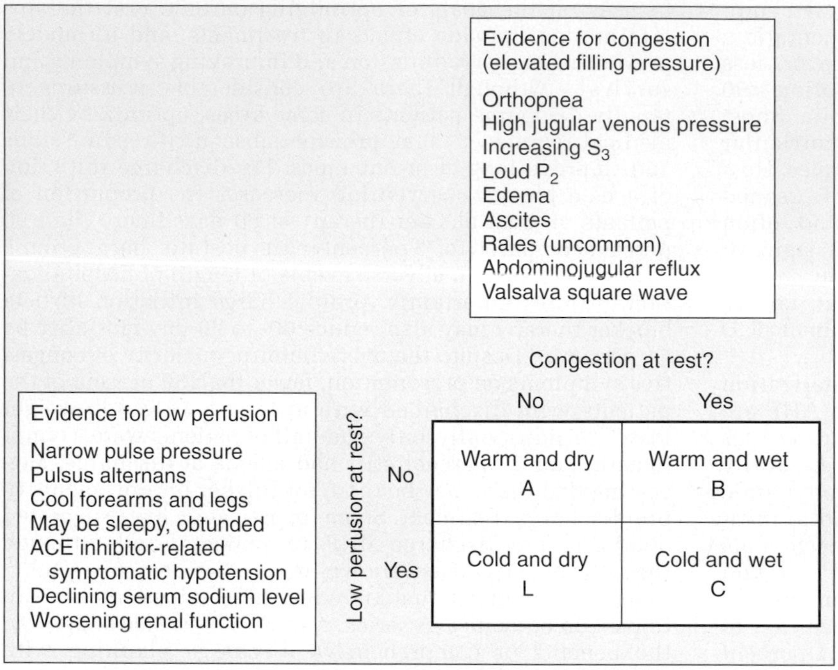

FIGURE 24–7 Hemodynamic profiles of patients presenting with advanced heart failure as described by a 2 × 2 table. Assessment of clinical symptoms and signs allows for classification of patient into a hemodynamic profile and may assist in selecting initial therapy and providing prognostic information. Although this classification scheme was developed for patients with predominantly systolic dysfunction and advanced heart failure, it provides a useful construct for the evaluation of patients with AHF as well. *(Modified from Nohria A, Mielniczuk LM, Stevenson LW: Evaluation and monitoring of patients with acute heart failure syndromes. Am J Cardiol 96:32G-40G, 2005.)*

Hypotension (systolic blood pressure below 90 mm Hg) is a poor prognostic sign in patients with AHF. Treating the potentially reversible, underlying etiologies, such as ACS, pulmonary embolus, and hypovolemia, is essential. Hypovolemic hypotension, usually related to over-diuresis, is unusual in patients presenting with AHF, and unappreciated volume

TABLE 24–7 Treatment Strategies for Acute Heart Failure

Volume Overload*	Worsening Renal Function	Systolic Blood Pressure *>100 mm Hg*	*90-100 mm Hg*	*<90 mm Hg*
Yes	Yes	Vasodilator Diuretics (consider infusion or combination therapy)† Consider ultrafiltration‡	Vasodilator (cautiously)§ and/or inotrope Diuretics (consider infusion or combination therapy)†	Inotrope and/or dopamine Consider norepinephrine or other vasopressor Diuretics (consider infusion or combination therapy)†
Yes	No	Vasodilator Diuretics Consider ultrafiltration‡	Vasodilator (cautiously)§ and/or inotrope	Recheck volume status Inotrope and/or dopamine Consider norepinephrine or other vasopressor Diuretics (consider continuous infusion or combination therapy)†
No	Yes	Vasodilator for hypertensive HF	Vasodilator (cautiously)‡ and/or inotrope	Recheck volume status ? Volume repletion Inotrope and/or dopamine Consider norepinephrine or other vasopressor
No	No	Vasodilator	Consider "normotensive cardiogenic shock" (then treat as if SBP <90 mm Hg)	Recheck volume status ? Volume repletion Inotrope and/or dopamine Consider norepinephrine or other vasopressor

*Volume overload, as characterized by peripheral edema, ascites, or markedly elevated central venous pressures. Pulmonary edema may result from either volume overload or redistribution, and vasodilator therapy should be the primary treatment.

†Increasing intensity of diuretic therapy should be commensurate with clinical response. See text for further description of continuous intravenous infusion or combination diuretic therapy.

‡Ultrafiltration may be considered, especially when large volume of fluid removal is anticipated.

§Many patients with AHF will have improvement in blood pressure and perfusion with the administration of vasodilator therapy, but careful monitoring to prevent hypotension is necessary.

overload may be present, especially in obese patients, in whom neck veins and ascites are difficult to assess. If there is clear evidence of hypovolemia, carefully monitored "fluid challenges" may be attempted. Unless there is symptomatic hypotension or evidence of significant end-organ dysfunction, the fluid replacement should be performed gradually and oral replacement is frequently sufficient; rapid intravenous fluid boluses can precipitate congestive symptoms. Asymptomatic hypotension, as an isolated finding in the absence of congestion and poor peripheral or central perfusion, does not require emergent treatment. Inotropic therapy may be indicated for persistent symptomatic hypotension or hypoperfusion in the setting of advanced systolic dysfunction, especially to improve symptoms, peripheral perfusion and diuresis, although at the expense of increased ischemia and arrhythmias. Dobutamine, dopamine, milrinone, epinephrine, and norepinephrine are the positive inotropic agents available in the United States, whereas levosimendan is additionally available in many other countries. In most patients, invasive pulmonary artery catheter monitoring is not necessary because the functional endpoints of urine output, blood pressure, and end-organ function may be clinically evaluated. The use of vasoconstrictors, such as high-dose dopamine, phenylephrine, epinephrine, norepinephrine, and vasopressin is controversial, although at times necessary, in patients with refractory symptomatic hypotension or hypoperfusion. Rarely, overdosage of afterload-reducing agents can precipitate admissions for AHF with a clinical presentation similar to cardiogenic shock or pseudosepsis. These patients benefit from careful administration of vasoconstrictors.

Most patients with AHF have evidence of volume overload, and for patients in whom this is the dominant presenting feature, such as those with significant peripheral edema or ascites, intravenous diuretics are an important therapy, despite their limitations. These patients typically have 4 to 5 liters of excess volume and amounts greater than 10 liters are not uncommon. The choice of diuretic regimen is influenced by the amount and rapidity of the desired fluid removal and the renal function (see later). Ultrafiltration is another potential option for rapid large-volume removal (see Chap. 25).[98] Diuresis addresses the underlying abnormality and frequently improves symptoms and signs of elevated filling pressures. However, intravenous vasodilator therapy may provide more rapid relief in highly symptomatic patients with evidence of pulmonary congestion. In fact, many patients with hypertensive AHF may require minimal diuretics.

Renal function is the third main aspect of a contemporary approach to treatment of the patient with AHF. Treatment of AHF in the presence of preserved renal function is generally uncomplicated. Diuretics may be given in standard doses, although renal function and volume status must be carefully monitored to prevent hypovolemia. Approximately two-thirds of patients present with at least moderate renal insufficiency.[32] In some patients, this worsening of renal function is a manifestation of the worsening heart failure, and treatment of the heart failure with vasodilators and diuretics may reestablish normal renal function. These patients respond normally to diuretics once the underlying hemodynamic abnormality is addressed and continuing concomitant ACE inhibitors may be helpful. In other patients, the renal insufficiency is an unchanged preexisting condition, which necessitates more intensive diuretic regimens for the diuretic resistance associated with renal insufficiency and has greater likelihood of developing worsening renal function during hospitalization. Comparison of admission renal function to previous values with respect to both the magnitude and rapidity of change will give some indication of which form of renal insufficiency is present. Unfortunately, most patients are admitted with a combination of acute on chronic renal insufficiency, requiring more aggressive treatment regimens to facilitate diuresis, while also placing them at higher risk for complications from such therapies.

Worsening renal function during treatment for AHF occurs in approximately 25 to 45 percent of the patients admitted with AHF, resulting in longer lengths of stay and higher post-discharge mortality.[99] The risk factors associated with this worsening of renal function include older age, lower *baseline creatinine clearance,* presence of atrial fibrillation, concomitant calcium channel blocker use, higher loop diuretic doses, and a history of heart failure, renal dysfunction, diabetes mellitus, or hypertension. Surprisingly, it does not appear to be related to ACE inhibitor use, *baseline serum creatinine,* degree of systolic dysfunction, or because of hemodynamic deterioration, such as lower filling pressures, decreased cardiac output, or estimated renal perfusion pressure.[100,101] These findings have some important implications. First, it is clear that a reliance on absolute serum creatinine concentrations can be misleading, so estimated glomerular filtration rate (eGFR) should be calculated in patients with AHF. Second, over-diuresis or low cardiac output do not appear to be the primary cause of worsening renal function. In fact, in most cases, the filling pressures are elevated at the time of worsening,[101] suggesting that this deterioration is most likely related to the underlying structural renal disease and neurohormonal factors influencing intra- and extrarenal hemodynamics. Although targeted treatments are being investigated, they are currently unavailable, so in the setting of volume overload, intensification of diuretic therapy is indicated, in addition to appropriate vasodilator therapy.

The *cardiorenal syndrome* represents one of the greatest therapeutic challenges in the field of AHF. Although there is no consensus definition to date, one definition of the cardiorenal syndrome is the clinical state wherein the volume overload of heart failure is resistant or refractory to treatment because of progressive renal insufficiency. Although decreases in cardiac output may not be immediately causative, intravenous inotropic therapy can improve renal function and allow effective diuresis. Progressive deterioration of renal function (BUN >80 mg/dl and creatinine >3.0 mg/dl) or hyperkalemia may necessitate discontinuation of ACE inhibitors and spironolactone, although use of other vasodilators should be considered, either intravenous (i.e., nitroglycerin or nitroprusside) or oral (isosorbide dinitrate and hydralazine). Ultimately, more aggressive renal replacement therapy, such as ultrafiltration or even hemodialysis, may be necessary. Discontinuation of these interventions may result in subsequent worsening of function and long-term dialysis or other interventions may need to be considered. The cardiorenal syndrome remains poorly understood and represents a substantial unmet therapeutic need.

INVASIVE HEMODYNAMIC STRATEGY. As described earlier, pulmonary artery catheters (PACs) are a useful tool in the management of some patients with AHF, especially those with unstable or unclear hemodynamics and poor response to therapy, including the development of worsening renal function, oliguria, or anuria. In patients with advanced heart failure in whom PACs are used to tailor therapy, a left ventricular filling pressure as approximated by pulmonary capillary wedge pressure (PCWP) of less than 16 mm Hg, right atrial pressure less than 8 mm Hg, and a systemic vascular resistance between 1000 to 1200 dynes/sec/cm^{-5} are useful targets.[9] Cardiac output is not a direct target, at this time, given that cardiac output often increases in response to vasodilator therapy, agents that directly increase this value are not yet available, and the currently available inotropic agents have considerable adverse effects. Other targets, such as resolution of pulmonary and peripheral edema, as well as ascites, must be addressed in conjunction with these hemodynamic targets. The general principles of the management strategy described earlier apply to (and are based on research from) invasively monitored patients, with the emphasis on reduction of filling pressures and afterload with vasodilators, treatment of volume overload with diuretics, and support of perfusion, when necessary, with inotropes.

OTHER STRATEGIES. Other strategies for guiding therapy in patients with AHF have been proposed. *Symptom improvement* as the sole goal is insufficient to guide therapy, given that symptoms may improve more rapidly than the underlying precipitating factors. However, they do need to be treated aggressively and completely, and assessment of the patient during and after ambulation is essential to confirm improvement in the absence of dyspnea and dizziness.

Another strategy proposes to target *biomarkers* for management of patients with AHF. Natriuretic peptide concentrations correlate with filling pressures and both admission and pre-discharge BNP concentrations are predictive of outcomes. The shorter half-life of BNP and the substantial renal clearance of nt-pro-BNP support the selection of the BNP assay for this potential diagnostic use. Changes in serial measures of BNP are predictive of outcomes in patients with AHF, beyond clinical and echocardiographic assessments,[102] and clinical studies are currently ongoing to assess the utility of serial inpatient BNP measures. However, at this time, the high variability and absence of supportive data argue against routinely using BNP concentrations as a primary therapeutic target, even when baseline "dry weight" BNP values are known.

Another potential target for therapies is *noninvasively measured hemodynamics or volume status.* Changes in the *bioimpedance* to a current applied across the thorax, in conjunction with noninvasive blood pressure and pulse monitoring, provide estimates of hemodynamic variables (such as stroke volume, cardiac output, systemic vascular resistance), cardiac contractility, and thoracic fluid content. Although these measures have been demonstrated to correlate relatively well with thermodilution, cardiac output, and to predict outcomes in the outpatient setting,[78] their utility in the in-hospital setting has not been established. Bioimpedance algorithms have been added to many implantable pacemaker/cardioverter defibrillator devices as well,[79] although they have not been evaluated in the inpatient management of AHF.

Doppler echocardiography (see Chap. 14) can provide estimates of cardiac output, LV filling pressures, pulmonary artery pressures, pulmonary vascular resistance, and right atrial pressures, all of which could guide in-hospital management. The most promising new measure includes the tissue Doppler derived E : Ea ratio (described earlier), where a ratio of >15 predicts a PCWP >15 mm Hg with a sensitivity of 86 percent and specificity of 88 percent and has been demonstrated to be accurate in the emergency room and intensive care settings.[74,103] These and other noninvasive measures will require further validation before they can be adopted broadly for the management of patients with AHF.

Pharmacological Therapies for the Treatment of Acute Heart Failure

DIURETICS. Diuretics are the primary pharmacological treatment for volume overload in patients with heart failure. These agents are discussed in detail in Chap. 25 and the current discussion will focus on the specific application of these agents to AHF. Diuretics commonly used in the treatment of AHF are listed in Table 24-8. In general, patients presenting with volume overload should receive intravenous loop diuretics, given the reduced absorption of oral diuretics and the more predictable pharmacodynamics. Higher initial doses should be administered to those on chronic outpatient diuretic therapy, underlying renal dysfunction, and severe volume overload. Given the steep dose-response curve of these agents, titration should be rapid with doubling of the dose until an effective response is noted. If there is significant volume overload (>5 to 10 liters) or diuretic resistance, a continuous intravenous infusion should be considered. Studies of continuous infusions of loop diuretics suggest a greater diuresis compared to bolus administration with a potentially better safety profile, including less compensatory sodium retention, worsening renal function, ototoxicity, gout symptoms, hypotension, and gastrointestinal complaints. Although there are limited studies, a meta-analysis of two trials suggested a 48 percent reduction in all-cause mortality (relative risk 0.52 [0.38-0.71 95 percent CI]) with continuous intravenous infusions compared to boluses.[104] If additional diuresis is required, administration of a diuretic that blocks the distal tubule can provide significant augmentation of the loop diuretic effect. Intravenous chlorothiazide (500 to 1000 mg) or oral metolazone (2.5 to 10 mg) given prior to the loop diuretic are effective agents, although care must be taken to monitor for hypotension, worsening renal function, and electrolyte abnormalities. Nonsteroidal antiinflammatory drugs can greatly reduce the efficacy of diuretics as well, by reducing renal synthesis of vasodilatory prostaglandins, and these agents should be avoided. If hypokalemia is a persistent problem with marked replacement requirements, administration of a potassium-sparing diuretic, such as spironolactone or eplerenone, should be considered.

The mechanism of action of these agents has been discussed in Chap. 25. Acute administration of furosemide can produce an initial, transient vasoconstriction with resultant deterioration in hemodynamics in patients with AHF. Consequently, concomitant vasodilator therapy is considered important to ameliorate this adverse action. In addition, venodilation with a subsequent decrease in "renal afterload" and pulmonary venous pressure may play an important role in the rapid improvement in renal function and dyspnea, respectively, that is often associated with diuretic administration.

Electrolyte disorders, including hyponatremia, hypokalemia, and hypomagnesemia, are common with intensive diuretic therapy, necessitating daily monitoring with active repletion. In addition to multiple other adverse effects, there is concern that diuretics may contribute to worsening renal function[100] and survival,[105,106] supported by animal studies suggesting that furosemide accelerated the progression of LV dysfunction in a model of chronic heart failure.[107] Thus, there is an increasing trend to limit diuretic use as much as possible.

VASODILATORS. In the absence of hypotension, vasodilators are recommended for most patients with AHF as first line therapy (see Table 24-7). Three types of vasodilators are currently available, all of which cause vasodilation by increasing intracellular cGMP, but each with unique characteristics (see Table 24-8).

Nitrates. Organic nitrates are one of the oldest therapies for AHF. These agents are potent venodilators, producing rapid decreases in pulmonary venous and ventricular filling pressures and improvement in pulmonary congestion, dyspnea, and myocardial oxygen demand at low doses. At slightly higher doses and in the presence of vasoconstriction, nitrates are also arteriolar vasodilators, reducing afterload and increasing cardiac output. Nitrates are relatively selective for epicardial, compared to intramyocardial, coronary arteries, resulting in increased coronary blood flow and making them useful for patients with concomitant active myocardial ischemia. The starting dose of nitroglycerin is usually 20 μg/min with rapid up-titration occurring every 5 to 15 minutes in either 20 μg/min increments or doubling of the dose. The dose may initially be titrated to the goal of immediate symptom relief, but a blood pressure reduction of at least 10 mm Hg in mean arterial pressure with a systolic blood pressure greater than 100 mm Hg is usually preferable. The nitrate dose may need to be reduced if SBP is 90 to 100 mm Hg and will often need to be discontinued with SBP <90 mm Hg.[4] Intravenous nitrates were administered to 38 percent of the patients with AHF in

TABLE 24–8 Intravenous Vasoactive Agents for the Treatment of Acute Heart Failure

Intravenous Medication	Initial Dose	Effective Dose Range*	Comments
Diuretics			
Furosemide	20-80 mg bolus†	20-500 mg bolus	Continuous infusion: 5-40 mg/hr; ototoxicity risk increases with higher (≥240 mg boluses)
Bumetanide	0.5-2 mg bolus†	0.5-4 mg bolus	Continuous infusion: 0.1-0.5 mg/hr
Torsemide	10-40 mg bolus†	20-200 mg bolus	Continuous infusion: 5-20 mg/hr
Vasodilators			
Nitroglycerin, glyceryl trinitrate, 5-mononitrate	20 μg/min	40-400 μg/min	Hypotension, headache; tolerance with continuous use after 24 hr
Isosorbide dinitrate	1 mg/hr	2-10 mg/hr	Hypotension, headache; tolerance with continuous use within 24 hr
Nitroprusside	10 μg/min	30-350 μg/min; 0.3-5 μg/kg/min (usually <4 μg/kg/min)	Caution in patients with active myocardial ischemia Hypotension; cyanide side effects (nausea, dysphoria); thiocyanate toxicity; light sensitive
Nesiritide	2 μg/kg bolus with 0.010-0.030 μg/kg/min infusion‡	0.010-0.030 μg/kg/min§	Uptitration: 1 μg/kg bolus, then increase infusion rate by 0.005 μg/kg/min (no more frequently than every 3 hr, up to a maximum of 0.03 μg/kg/min) Hypotension, headache (less than with organic nitrates); ? worsens renal function, mortality
Inotropes			
Dobutamine	1-2 μg/kg/min	2-20 μg/kg/min	For inotropy and vasodilation; hypotension, tachycardia, arrhythmias; ?mortality
Dopamine	1-2 μg/kg/min	2-4 μg/kg/min	For inotropy and vasodilation; hypotension, tachycardia, arrhythmias; ?mortality
	4-5 μg/kg/min	5-20 μg/kg/min	For inotropy and vasoconstriction; tachycardia, arrhythmias; ?mortality
Milrinone	25-75 μg/kg bolus over 10-20 min‡ followed by infusion	0.10-0.75 μg/kg/min	For vasodilation and inotropy; hypotension, tachycardia, arrhythmias; renal excretion; ?mortality
Enoximone	0.25-0.75 mg/kg	1.25-7.5 μg/kg/min	For vasodilation and inotropy; hypotension, tachycardia, arrhythmias; ?mortality
Levosimendan	12-24 μg/kg bolus over 10 min‡ followed by infusion	0.5-2.0 μg/kg/min	For vasodilation and inotropy; active metabolite present for ~84 hr; hypotension, tachycardia, arrhythmias; ?mortality
Epinephrine		0.05-0.5 μg/kg/min	For vasoconstriction and inotropy; tachycardia, arrhythmias, end-organ hypoperfusion; ?mortality
Norepinephrine		0.2-1.0 μg/kg/min	For vasoconstriction and inotropy; tachycardia, arrhythmias, end-organ hypoperfusion; ?mortality

*In general, titration of medication is accomplished by doubling of dose with careful monitoring for adverse effects.
†Use higher dose range for chronic diuretic use, renal insufficiency, and severe volume overload. Diuretic naïve patients should receive lower doses, initially.
‡Some clinicians do not administer a bolus dose, so as to decrease the risk of hypotension. Bolus not recommended in patients with hypotension.
§Lower doses have also been effective in some small studies.[123]

Europe,[13] but to only 9 percent of patients in the United States.[16] Although part of this difference may be because of the availability of nesiritide in the United States, much of it stems from the predilection of U.S. physicians for high-dose diuretics and positive inotropes. Organic nitrates may also be administered orally, sublingually, or by spray, allowing for convenient emergent treatment prior to establishing intravenous access.

There is limited clinical trial experience with organic nitrates.[108] In a randomized study of 110 patients with fulminant pulmonary edema, patients treated with a high-dose regimen of nitrates compared to low-dose nitrates and high-dose furosemide had fewer myocardial infarctions and less need for mechanical ventilation.[109] Another study,[1] designed to evaluate nesiritide in patients with dyspnea at rest from decompensated heart failure, included a nitroglycerin arm of 143 patients, demonstrated nonsignificant, mild decreases in PCWP (Fig. 24-8) and no significant improvement in patient-assessed dyspnea within 3 hours with nitroglycerin, but the dose was remarkably low (42 μg/min). In a small, single-site substudy[110] where nitroglycerin was aggressively uptitrated to a mean dose of 155 μg/min by 3 hours, there were significant decreases in PCWP (4 to 6 mm Hg decrease from baseline) from 1 to 12 hours, but no difference at 24 hours (Fig. 24-9). There is no information on improvement of dyspnea in this substudy, but clinical experience appears to support the role of these agents in providing rapid symptom relief.

The major limitation of organic nitrates is the tolerance that develops within 24 hours (see Chap. 54). Headache is the most common adverse effect (20 percent within 24 hours[1]) with an increase in abdominal pain also reported. Symptomatic hypotension (5 percent) may also be noted, but resolves rapidly. As with any agent that can reduce preload, administration of nitroglycerin in a patient who is preload dependent (patient with already low or near normal preload or aortic stenosis) can produce significant hypotension.

Sodium Nitroprusside. Sodium nitroprusside (SNP) is one of the most effective, although underutilized therapies for AHF (<1 percent of AHF patients in Europe and the United States[13,16]), particularly in the setting of markedly elevated afterload (e.g., hypertensive AHF) or moderate to severe mitral regurgitation. SNP induces a balanced reduction in afterload and preload that is exquisitely titratable, because of a very short half-life (seconds to a few minutes), resulting in dramatic decreases in filling pressures and forward redistribution of mitral regurgitant flow. Intravenous administration is usually monitored with an indwelling arterial line, although automated blood pressure cuffs are now used in many centers. Titration of the nitroprusside dose to rapidly improve symptoms and to achieve an SBP of 90 to 100 mm Hg are typical goals, and invasive pulmonary artery catheters may assist in meeting other hemodynamic

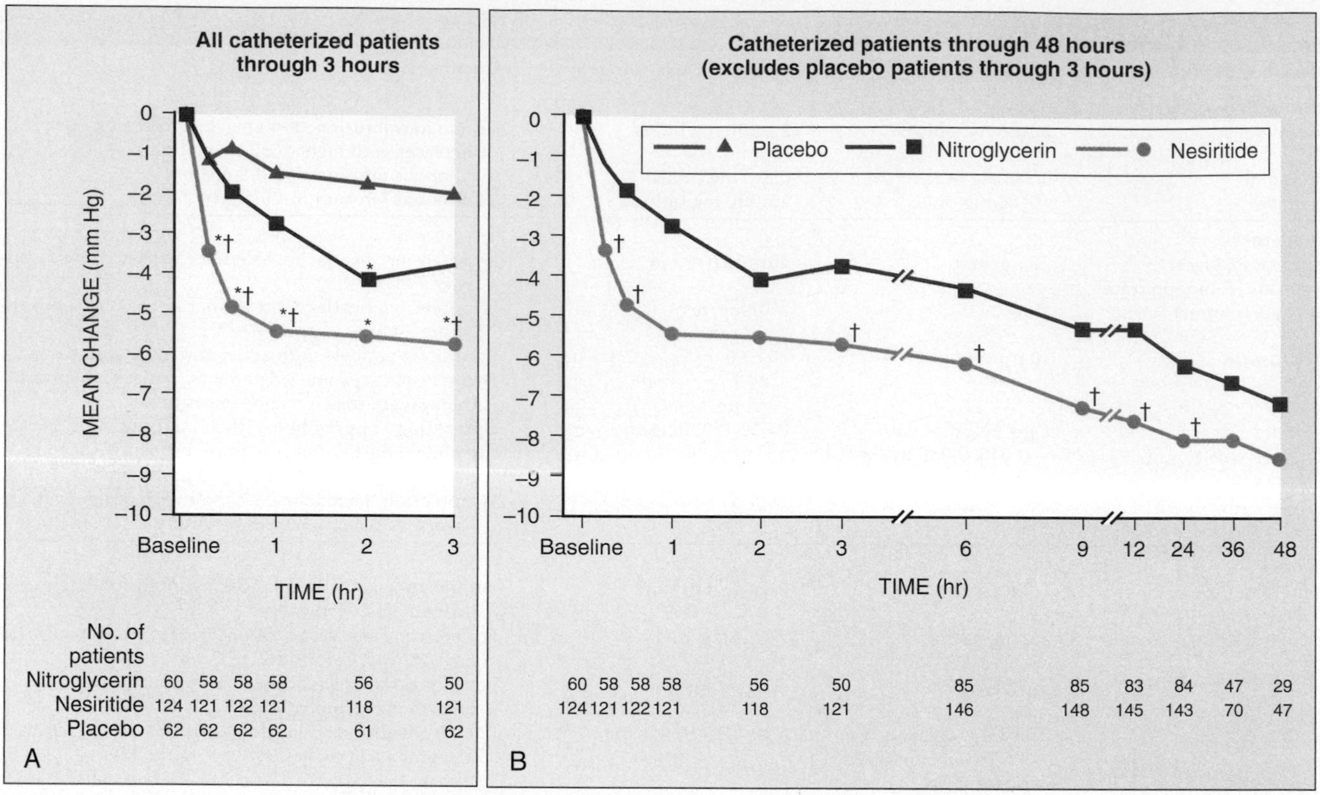

FIGURE 24–8 Changes from baseline in pulmonary capillary wedge pressure in patients with acute heart failure randomized to placebo (triangles), nitroglycerin (squares) and nesiritide (circles). *$p < 0.05$ for nesiritide or nitroglycerin compared with placebo; †$p < 0.05$ for nesiritide compared with nitroglycerin. *(Data from VMAC Investigators: Intravenous nesiritide vs nitroglycerin for treatment of decompensated congestive heart failure: A randomized controlled trial. JAMA 287:1531-1540, 2002.)*

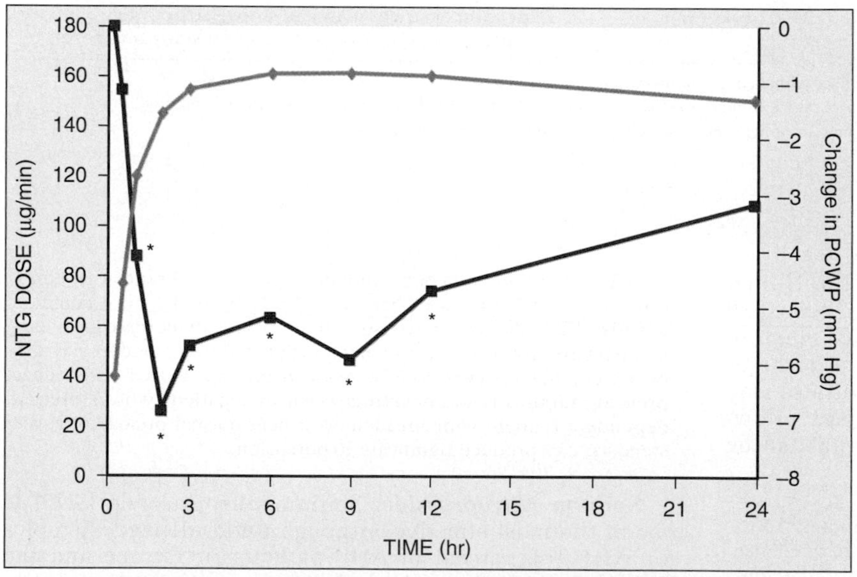

FIGURE 24–9 Change in pulmonary capillary wedge pressure (PCWP; squares) and change in nitroglycerin (NTG; diamonds) dose in a substudy of 12 patients from the VMAC trial. *(Data from Elkayam U, Akhter MW, Singh H, et al: Comparison of effects on left ventricular filling pressure of intravenous nesiritide and high-dose nitroglycerin in patients with decompensated heart failure. Am J Cardiol 93:237-240, 2004.)*

goals. Tapering the dose of nitroprusside prior to discontinuation is advised to avoid the possibility of "rebound hypertension." Physician discomfort with the cyanide metabolites and the historical institutional requirements for invasive arterial monitoring has limited the use of this highly effective therapy.

Nitroprusside, a pro-drug that is rapidly metabolized to nitric oxide and cyanide, has no inherent arrhythmogenic properties, may improve myocardial oxygen demand by reducing afterload and wall stress, creates no significant electrolyte disturbances, and is rarely toxic. Despite its potency, severe hypotension is unusual and rapidly resolves. However, significant vasodilation of the intramyocardial vasculature has been noted, possibly producing a coronary steal phenomenon, and consequently, nitroprusside is not recommended for patients with active myocardial ischemia. The most common complaints with nitroprusside are related to the cyanide metabolite, including nausea, abdominal discomfort, dissociative feelings, and dysphoria. Cyanide rarely accumulates in patients, but impaired hepatic function and doses of >250 µg/min for more than 48 hours increase this risk. Cyanide levels may be measured, but rarely return in a timely fashion to be useful. The thiocyanate metabolite can accumulate in patients with moderate to severe renal insufficiency when exposed to prolonged infusions of high doses (usually >400 µg/min) over days and is usually not relevant in the treatment of AHF.

There are no randomized studies of nitroprusside in patients with AHF,[108] although multiple studies demonstrated dramatic reduction in PCWP (15 mm Hg) and marked increases in cardiac output, associated with increases in diuresis, natriuresis, and decreased neurohormonal activation.[111] One placebo-controlled, postmyocardial infarction trial was stopped early because of a survival benefit of nitroprusside.[112] A larger trial of 812 men with acute myocardial infarction and elevated LV filling pressures (>12 mm Hg) demonstrated beneficial hemodynamic effects of nitroprusside and no difference in 13 week mortality (nitroprusside 17.0 percent versus placebo 19.0 percent).[113] However, in a post-hoc analysis, patients receiving nitroprusside within 9 hours of infarction had a greater mortality compared to placebo (24.2 percent versus 12.7

percent, $p = 0.027$), whereas those receiving study drug after 9 hours had improved survival (14.4 percent versus 22.3 percent, $p = 0.023$). These findings have been interpreted as demonstrating increased mortality with early nitroprusside use and thus, suggesting that nitroprusside is unsafe for patients with ACS or AHF. The post-hoc nature of the analysis makes it highly susceptible to confounding, and it ignores the survival benefit after the acute event, which may be more relevant to the AHF patient. Another study demonstrated the utility of nitroprusside in patients with severe aortic stenosis and LV dysfunction, where nitroprusside rapidly and safely improved hemodynamics, as well as cardiac and renal function.[114]

Nesiritide. B-type natriuretic peptide (BNP), discussed above as a diagnostic tool, may also be used in pharmacological doses for the treatment of AHF. Nesiritide (recombinant human BNP) is identical to the endogenous peptide and causes potent vasodilation in the venous and arterial—including coronary—vasculature; it also produces significant reductions in venous and ventricular filling pressures and mild increases in cardiac output, with subsequent improvement in symptoms of dyspnea. As with other vasodilators, nesiritide may reduce diuretic requirements, but in clinical studies, there is limited evidence for a significant direct "natriuretic" effect. Nesiritide is indicated for treatment of patients with acutely decompensated congestive heart failure who have dyspnea at rest or with minimal activity, but it should not be administered for the indication of replacing diuretics, enhancing diuresis, protecting renal function, or improving survival. A bolus of 2 μg/kg followed by a 0.01 μg/kg/min infusion is the recommended starting dose for nesiritide. There is limited clinical trial experience with uptitration of the drug, but for patients who remain symptomatic with evidence of volume overload and sufficient blood pressure, uptitration may be considered. Nesiritide has clear effects on hemodynamics and is readily administered with limited need for frequent dose adjustments and an absence of tolerance, but its high cost, lack of clear clinical benefit beyond other less expensive and more readily titratable agents, and potential safety concerns, including increased mortality,[115-118] have limited its use.[119]

Nesiritide exerts its activity via guanylyl cyclase-linked natriuretic peptide receptors (NPR A and B) causing cGMP-mediated vasodilation (see Chap. 22, Fig. 22-8). Hypotension, at times prolonged (over 2 hours[1]) despite the relatively short (18 minute) half-life of the peptide, is more common in patients with volume depletion and, consequently, nesiritide is indicated for patients with congestive signs and symptoms. Headache also occurs, although less frequently than with nitroglycerin. Other actions of nesiritide include neurohormonal antagonism with reduction in vasopressin, aldosterone, and sympathetic tone, and alteration of intrarenal hemodynamics and glomerular filtration. Although a reduced diuretic requirement was noted in some clinical trials[1,120] and hemodynamic efficacy has been demonstrated in a subgroup of patients with renal insufficiency and AHF,[121] nesiritide did not improve urine output or renal function in AHF patients with worsening creatinine when studied directly at currently recommended doses.[122] A recent small retrospective review suggests that a low-dose nesiritide regimen (0.0025 to 0.005 μg/kg/min without bolus dosing) produced similar diuresis with fewer diuretics and improved plasma creatinine and BUN compared to standard nesiritide doses and to treatment with other agents.[123] Thus, there remains hope that the theoretical promise of beneficial renal effects may be achieved through different dosing regimens of nesiritide.

The clinical development program for nesiritide was extensive[108] and early studies established its hemodynamic efficacy[120] and the relative absence of arrhythmias compared to dobutamine.[124] The Vasodilation in the Management of Acute CHF (VMAC) trial randomized 489 patients with decompensated CHF and dyspnea at rest to placebo, nitroglycerin, or nesiritide for 3 hours.[1] After 3 hours, patients receiving nesiritide had a significantly greater decrease in PCWP (5.8 mm Hg, change from baseline; see Fig. 24-8) compared to both nitroglycerin (3.8 mm Hg; $p = 0.03$) and placebo (2.0 mm Hg; $p < 0.001$), and improvement in dyspnea compared to placebo ($p = 0.03$; no difference from nitroglycerin). Subsequent publications, based on open-label data with nonrandomized therapies, suggested that nesiritide improved survival compared to dobutamine.[125] However, a pooled-analysis of the randomized, controlled clinical trial data found that nesiritide was associated with over a 45 percent increase in the risk of worsening renal function,[117,118] as well as increased mortality.[116] A recent update to the data suggests there may be a significant doubling of the risk of mortality in the nesiritide-treated patients compared to control treatments (adjusted hazard ratio 1.93 [1.06-3.52 95 percent C.I.]; $p = 0.03$).[115] These analyses are controversial and not conclusive; however, they have provided the context for larger clinical trials to assess the efficacy and safety of nesiritide.

ADRENERGIC AGONISTS. The adrenergic system (see Chap. 22) is central to the regulation of myocardial contractility and vascular tone and adrenergic agonists are potent agents in the treatment of AHF. As noted in Table 24-7, these agents are reserved for use in selected situations of hypoperfusion when other interventions are inappropriate or have failed. If these inotropic agents are initiated (see Table 24-8), a clear target should be established for their discontinuation and allowances made for potential deterioration on withdrawal. Often, readjustment of oral therapies with a reevaluation of the clinical status in the absence of inotropic support is required. At this time, intermittent infusions or "inotrope holidays" cannot be recommended because of the absence of supportive data and the significant risks associated with these agents.[126]

Dobutamine. Dobutamine is the most commonly used positive inotrope in Europe and the United States,[13,16] despite evidence that it increases mortality.[127,128] This prevalence is partially because of practice preferences, as well as clinical necessity. Dobutamine improves cardiac output through direct increases in inotropy and decreases in afterload, as well as increasing chronotropy, and is indicated in patients with low output AHF and SBP less than 85 to 90 mm Hg, often in addition to a vasodilator. Many patients will improve renal perfusion with dobutamine doses of 1 to 2 μg/kg/min, although higher doses (5 to 10 μg/kg/min) may be necessary for more profound hypoperfusion. Tachyphylaxis may occur, partially because of receptor desensitization, with infusions of more than 24 to 48 hours. In general, dobutamine (or dopamine) is the preferred inotrope in patients with significant hypotension and in the setting of significant renal dysfunction, given the renal excretion of milrinone. Beta blocker therapy will result in competitive antagonism of the effects of dobutamine and higher doses of dobutamine (10 to 15 μg/kg/min) will be required to obtain the desired hemodynamic effects. Some investigators report that in the presence of carvedilol, the hemodynamic effects of dobutamine are not only attenuated, but increases in pulmonary pressures and systemic vascular resistance ensue.[129] In cases where the response to dobutamine is insufficient, milrinone may be substituted. The lowest effective dose of dobutamine should be used in the context of continuous blood pressure and rhythm monitoring. The patient should be gradually weaned from dobutamine and clinical status reevaluated with each dose adjustment. Temporary concomitant adjustments to afterload-reducing agents or diuretics may assist in weaning.

As an agonist of both $beta_1$ and $beta_2$ adrenergic receptors with variable effects on the alpha receptors, dobutamine has multiple actions. Beta-receptor stimulation results in increased inotropy and chronotropy through increases in intracellular cAMP and calcium, as well as via direct activation of voltage sensitive calcium channels. At low doses, stimulation of $beta_2$ and alpha receptors causes vasodilation, resulting in decreased aortic impedance and systemic vascular resistance with reduction in afterload and indirect increases in cardiac output. Mitral regurgitant flow is also decreased, providing additional augmentation of forward flow. At higher doses, vasoconstriction can ensue with decreased venous capacitance and increased right atrial pressure. Adverse effects of dobutamine include tachycardia, increasing ventricular response to atrial fibrillation, increased atrial and ventricular arrhythmias,[124] myocardial ischemia and possibly cardiomyocyte necrosis via direct toxic effects and induction of apoptosis.[130] The short half-life of dobutamine can limit some of the sequelae of these effects.

Although the hemodynamic and other effects of dobutamine have been studied, there is only one placebo-controlled, randomized trial in patients with AHF. Although there are some methodological concerns, the CAlcium Sensitzer or Inotrope or NOne in low output heart failure study (CASINO) demonstrated a 42 percent 6-month mortality in patients treated with dobutamine titrated to 10 μg/kg/min compared to 28.3 percent in the placebo group ($p = 0.02$).[127] Such increases in mortality have been demonstrated in other studies of chronic HF and AHF.[128]

Dopamine. In both the United States and Europe,[13,16] dopamine is used as often as dobutamine, presumably as a vasoconstrictor and for its putative effects on renal vasodilation. As a precursor to the synthesis of norepinephrine, an agonist of both adrenergic and dopaminergic receptors, and an inhibitor of norepinephrine uptake, dopamine has complex effects that vary significantly with dose. Initiation of dopamine therapy causes a rapid release of norepinephrine that can precipitate tachycardia, as well as atrial and ventricular arrhythmias. In addition, intermediate to high doses can cause significant vasoconstriction, precipitating heart failure and poor perfusion. Dopamine should be gradually weaned from these doses down to 3 to 5 μg/kg/min and then discontinued to avoid potential hypotensive effects of low-dose dopamine.

Low-dose dopamine (= 2 μg/kg/min) has been proposed to cause selective dilation of renal, splanchnic and cerebral arteries, potentially increasing renal blood flow in a selective manner, as well as promoting natriuresis through direct distal tubular effects. The ESC AHF guidelines[4] suggest that low-dose dopamine may be used to improve renal blood flow and diuresis in patients with AHF, hypotension and oliguria, whereas the word *dopamine* does not appear in the HFSA AHF guidelines.[5] A recent meta-analysis suggests that low-dose dopamine may increase urine output on the first day, associated with no effect on creatinine clearance and a trend toward increased adverse events.[131] If low-dose dopamine therapy is initiated, it should be discontinued in the event of no response.

Intermediate dose dopamine (2 to 10 μg/kg/min) results in enhanced norepinephrine release, stimulating cardiac receptors with an increase in inotropy and mild stimulation of peripheral vasoconstricting receptors. Because the positive inotropic effect is largely dependent on myocardial catecholamine stores, which are often depleted in patients with advanced heart failure, dopamine is a poor inotrope in patients with severe systolic dysfunction.

High-dose dopamine (10 to 20 μg/kg/min) causes peripheral and pulmonary artery vasoconstriction, mediated by direct agonist effects on $alpha_1$ adrenergic receptors. These doses pose a significant risk of precipitating limb and end-organ ischemia and should be used cautiously.

EPINEPHRINE AND NOREPINEPHRINE. Epinephrine is a full beta-receptor agonist and a potent inotropic agent with balanced vasodilator and vasoconstrictor effects. The direct effect of epinephrine on increasing inotropy independent of myocardial catecholamine stores makes epinephrine a useful agent in the treatment of transplant patients with denervated hearts. Norepinephrine is also a potent agonist of the $beta_1$ and the $alpha_1$ receptors, but is a weaker agonist of $beta_2$ receptors, resulting in marked vasoconstriction. Thus, norepinephrine may be more likely to induce end-organ hypoperfusion and tissue necrosis. Both of these agents are usually reserved for profound hypotension or for cardiac resuscitation. Addition of intravenous calcium to the infusion or as a bolus can provide rapid increases in cardiac contractility, although at the expense of significant arrhythmias and myocardial injury.

PHOSPHODIESTERASE INHIBITORS (PDEIs). As described in Chap. 21, cAMP is a ubiquitous signaling molecule that increases inotropy, chronotropy, and lusitropy in cardiomyocytes and causes vasorelaxation in vascular smooth muscle. Phosphodiesterase IIIa is compartmentalized in the cardiac and vascular smooth muscle, where it terminates the signaling activity of cAMP by degrading it to AMP. Many specific inhibitors of PDE IIIa, such as milrinone and enoximone, have been developed to provide organ-specific improvements in hemodynamics through increasing myocardial and vascular smooth muscle cell cAMP. Subcellular localization provides the possibility to stimulate inotropy without increasing heart rate with low doses of highly specific PDEIs. The independence of the mechanism from adrenergic receptors bypasses receptor downregulation, desensitization, and antagonism by beta blockers. Although studies have shown improved hemdoynamic efficacy with PDEIs compared to dobutamine in patients on beta blocker therapy, especially carvedilol,[129] such limitations of dobutamine's effects are not typically clinically relevant. In addition, this mechanism allows for synergistic effects with beta receptor agonists, such as dobutamine. Such combination therapy may be useful in patients with markedly reduced LV systolic function. PDEIs cause significant peripheral and pulmonary vasodilation, reducing afterload and preload, while increasing inotropy. These effects make them well suited for patients with LV dysfunction and pulmonary hypertension or posttransplant patients.

Milrinone is the most commonly used PDEI, but only 3 percent of patients in ADHERE[16] and less than 1 percent in EHFS II[13] received it. Milrinone therapy may be initiated with a 25 to 75 μg/kg bolus over 10 to 20 minutes (in patients with borderline hypotension, this bolus dose is often omitted) and infusions are started at 0.10 μg/kg/min and may be uptitrated to hemodynamic effect. Given the elimination half-life of 2.5 hours and the pharmacodynamic half-life of over 6 hours, effects from uptitration are delayed by at least 15 minutes after dosage adjustment. Because of these pharmacodynamics, patients who have had prolonged administration of milrinone may have delayed deterioration, so they should be observed for at least 48 hours after cessation. Milrinone is renally excreted, necessitating dose adjustment in the presence of renal dysfunction or substitution with dobutamine.

Milrinone has many side effects, including marked hypotension (PAC monitoring is recommended), as well as atrial and ventricular arrhythmias. In OPTIME-CHF (Outcomes of a Prospective Trial of Intravenous Milrinone for Exacerbations of Chronic Heart Failure),[2] 951 patients admitted with exacerbation of systolic heart failure not requiring intravenous inotropic support were randomized to milrinone or placebo infusion. There was no difference in the primary endpoint of days hospitalized for cardiovascular causes with 60 days, but significant increases in sustained hypotension and new atrial arrhythmias were noted in the milrinone-treated patients. In addition, a post-hoc subgroup analysis demonstrated increased mortality in patients with an ischemic etiology of heart failure who received milrinone.[132] This study reinforces the caution that must be exercised in using these agents for the treatment of patients with AHF.

Enoximone. Enoximone is also a PDE IIIa inhibitor that is available in Europe. Dosing is essentially one-tenth that of milrinone, with a bolus dose of 0.25 to 0.75 μg/kg bolus over 10 to 20 minutes, followed by an infusion of 1.25 μg/kg/min. It is extensively metabolized by the liver into renally cleared active metabolites, so doses should be reduced in the setting of either renal or hepatic insufficiency. Otherwise, the above comments apply to this PDEI as well.

CALCIUM SENSITIZERS. Levosimendan is a novel agent that increases myocardial contractility and produces peripheral vasodilation through cardiac myofilament calcium sensitization by calcium-dependent (systolic) troponin C binding and activation of vascular smooth muscle potassium channels, respectively. Levosimendan also has some in vitro PDEI activity, presumably at concentrations much higher than achieved in clinical use.[133] Levosimendan was administered to nearly 4 percent of patients in EHFS II[13] and is available in more than 40 countries, where it is used in patients with reduced LV systolic function and hypoperfusion in the absence of severe hypotension. Although it may be given with a bolus of 12 to 24 μg/kg over 10 minutes, many clinicians directly initiate a continuous infusion at a rate of 0.05 to 0.10 μg/kg/min, which may be uptitrated to 0.2 μg/kg/min. In clinical trials,[108] levosimendan has been shown to significantly increase cardiac output, reduce PCWP and afterload, and improve dyspnea. The potent vasodilating effects of levosimendan can cause significant hypotension, which may be avoided by maintaining filling pressures. Levosimendan has an active, acetylated metabolite with a half-life of more than 80 hours, allowing it to have hemodynamic effects days after discontinuation of the infusion.

Initial clinical studies demonstrated reduced arrhythmias and improved survival with levosimendan compared to placebo[127,134] and dobutamine.[127,128] REVIVE-II (Randomized multicenter evaluation of intravenous levosimendan efficacy versus placebo in the short-term treatment of decompensated heart failure), a recent study of 600 patients, demonstrated significant improvement in the clinical status, serial BNP, and hospital length of stay with levosimendan treatment compared to standard care, but there were also more episodes of hypotension, atrial fibrillation, and ventricular ectopy, as well as a nonsignificant increase in deaths at 14 to 90 days.[135] SURVIVE (Survival of patients with acute heart failure in need of intravenous inotropic support trial) randomized 1327 patients with systolic dysfunction, evidence of low cardiac output, and dyspnea at rest despite diuretics and vasodilators to either levosimendan or dobutamine. An early reduction in mortality was not sustained through 180 days, but levosimendan was associated with a greater incidence of atrial fibrillation and lower incidence of worsening heart failure compared to dobutamine.[135] These studies need to be more completely analyzed before changes in recommendations can be made.[4]

Potential Future Therapies

Milrinone received FDA approval in 1988, but it was not until 2001 that nesiritide was approved. Since then, there has been tremendous activity in the development of new therapeutic agents for the treatment of AHF.[136] Significant advances in engineering and technology have also enabled the development of new approaches to treating AHF with electronic pacing and mechanical circulatory support devices, as well (see Chaps. 25, 28, and 34).

CARDIAC MYOSIN ACTIVATORS. Current inotropic agents increase contractility by mechanisms that require an increase in intracellular cAMP and calcium, which can be arrhythmogenic, increase heart rate, cause hypotension, and may increase myocardial oxygen demand. Cardiac myosin activators may avoid these adverse effects by directly improving the work of the cardiac motor unit. The cardiac myosin ATPase is a structurally distinct component of the molecular motor responsible for myocardial contraction. A number of cardiac myosin activators, including *CK-1827452*, have been developed, which appear to accelerate the strong-binding of the activated myosin to actin, increasing productive mechanical work, as well as inhibiting nonproductive cleavage of ATP by myosin, potentially decreasing ATP consumption. These agents have been shown to increase cardiac contractility without increasing intracellular calcium transients in the in vitro studies or increasing myocardial oxygen demand in the in vivo studies of dogs with heart failure, despite marked increases in cardiac output. In a recent first-in-human study,[137] CK-1827452, administered in an ascending dose protocol with randomized placebo to 34 healthy men, significantly increased LV ejection fraction and fractional shortening, associated with a prolongation of ejection time, consistent with its mechanism of action. CK-1827452 is currently being evaluated in Phase II studies in patients with heart failure.

ISTAROXIME. Calcium cycling is another major component of myocardial contractility and derangements in myocardial calcium cycling are associated with systolic and diastolic dysfunction. Istaroxime is a novel compound, structurally unrelated to digoxin, with a dual mechanism of action: inhibition of the Na^+/K^+-ATPase, which increases intracellular calcium and inotropy, and stimulation of the sarcolemmal calcium pump (SERCA2a), resulting in more rapid calcium uptake into the sarcoplasmic reticulum, which improves myocardial relaxation or lusitropy. As the first agent to specifically target abnormal lusitropy while improving inotropy, istaroxime has shown effects consistent with its mechanism of action in in vitro studies. In studies of animals with heart failure, istaroxime has improved both systolic and diastolic function without increasing myocardial oxygen demand.[138] Similar findings were noted in the first-in-human study,[139] where 19 patients with stable chronic heart failure and LV ejection fraction ≤0.40 received ascending doses of istaroxime with randomized placebo. Istaroxime increased cardiac contractility as measured by impedance cardiography with minimal adverse events. These encouraging results have formed the basis for further studies.

NATRIURETIC PEPTIDES. The extensive scientific background and continuing research in this field has produced a number of potential therapeutic agents. All of these peptides are potent vasodilators and the search continues for an agent that will clearly promote natriuresis and protect or improve renal function in the clinical setting. *Carperitide* is recombinant human atrial natriuretic peptide and has been marketed since 1995 in Japan, where there is extensive clinical experience. *Ularitide* is human recombinant urodilatin, an isoform of atrial natriuretic peptide discovered in human urine. Urodilatin is synthesized by the kidney where it is secreted into the renal tubule and promotes sodium excretion via natriuretic peptide-A receptors. Preclinical and early clinical studies confirmed the ability of ularitide to produce significant vasodilation, as well as natriuresis and diuresis. Two larger studies of ularitide[140,141] demonstrated dose-dependent decreases in PCWP, systemic vascular resistance, and nt-pro-BNP, increases in cardiac output and improvements in patient-assessed dyspnea. There were no significant increases in urine output or decreases in diuretic use and no significant deleterious changes in creatinine. However, dose-dependent decreases in blood pressure were noted, with 16 percent of patients in the high-dose group experiencing hypotension. Ularitide appears to be more potent that nesiritide, but has yet to demonstrate a clinical effect on renal function. These studies have formed the basis for future clinical trials. Other natriuretic peptides are in earlier phases of development, including "designer" natriuretic peptides and fusion products of other proteins with a natriuretic peptide.

ADENOSINE ANTAGONISTS. As noted earlier, agents that can be effective in patients with diuretic resistance or the cardiorenal syndrome are desperately needed. Adenosine, acting via the renal adenosine A_1 receptors, induces afferent arteriolar vasoconstriction, postglomerular vasodilation, and mediates tubuloglomerular feedback, all of which serve to decrease glomerular filtration rate (GFR). In animal and human studies, selective adenosine A_1 inhibition blocked these changes. A small crossover study of *BG9719* in chronic heart failure patients demonstrated that A_1 antagonism could increase both urine output and GFR and could act synergistically with furosemide, producing even greater diuresis with no change in GFR.[142] Another selective adenosine A_1 antagonist, KW-3902, has been investigated in two recently completed Phase II studies.[143] The first study randomized 146 patients with AHF and renal impairment (mean Ccr 45 ml/min) to one of three doses of KW-3902 or placebo and demonstrated a significant increase in 6-hour urine output, as well as a significantly decreased diuretic requirement, more frequent early termination for sufficient diuresis, and a trend toward reduced worsening renal function. The second study demonstrated that three doses of KW-3902 increased urine output with either no change or an increase in creatinine clearance compared to placebo in 33 patients with AHF and renal insufficiency (mean Ccr 35 ml/min) who were refractory to high-dose intravenous diuretics. Phase III trials hopefully will confirm these promising findings.

VASOPRESSIN ANTAGONISTS. Arginine vasopressin, or antidiuretic hormone, is a neurohormone produced by the central nervous system in response to changes in serum osmolality, severe hypovolemia, or hypotension (see Chap. 25). Two types of vasopressin receptors include the V_1 and V_2 receptors, with the V_{1a} receptor mediating vasopressin-induced vasoconstriction and the V_2 receptors mediating water resorption in the kidneys. *Conivaptan* is a combined V_{1a} and V_2 receptor antagonist that has been shown to significantly decrease PCWP and right atrial pressure, as well as increase urine output without changing cardiac index or other hemodynamic variables in patients with stable chronic HF.[108] Conivaptan has been approved by the FDA for treatment of euvolemic hyponatremia.

Another approach to vasopressin antagonism is to selectively block the V_2 receptor, resulting in aquaresis without electrolyte imbalances or neurohormonal stimulation. *Tolvaptan* and lixivaptan are selective V_2 receptor antagonists. The Acute and Chronic Therapeutic Impact of a Vasopressin Antagonist in Congestive Heart Failure (ACTIV-CHF) study demonstrated that tolvaptan treatment of patients with known CHF (EF < 40 percent) hospitalized for AHF and fluid overload significantly reduced body weight and improved serum sodium concentrations.[144] Another recent trial demonstrated that tolvaptan administration to outpatients with euvolemic or hypervolemic hyponatremia improved serum sodium concentrations after 4 and 30 days of treatment, associated with improvement in quality of life indices.[145] The effect of tolvaptan on mortality in patients hospitalized for heart failure was evaluated in the Efficacy of Vasopressin Antagonism in Heart Failure: Outcome Study with Tolvaptan (EVEREST) as discussed in **Chapter 25**.

ENDOTHELIN ANTAGONISTS. Endothelin (ET-1) is one of the most potent vasoconstrictors known. ET-1 concentrations increased with the development of AHF and predicted malignant ventricular arrhythmias and mortality. Early studies demonstrated that the endothelin receptor antagonist, *tezosentan,* would reduce LV filling pressures, decrease afterload, increase cardiac output, and improve symptoms of dyspnea.[108] However, a large Phase III trial was terminated early because of the low probability of demonstrating a difference between tezosentan and placebo with respect to the improvement in patient dyspnea.[135,146] The failure of this development program emphasizes the difficulties of designing trials for new AHF therapies.

CLINICAL OUTCOMES AND PROGNOSIS OF PATIENTS WITH ACUTE HEART FAILURE

Despite advances in therapy for heart failure, improving clinical outcomes of patients with AHF remains a challenge for physicians (Table 24-9).[13-16,18,38,54,147-150] The median length of stay for patients admitted for AHF in Europe ranges from 9 to 11 days and is 15 days for patients initially admitted to an ICU or CCU, where ICU/CCU length of stay ranged from 3 to 7 days. In the United States, median length of stay is 4.3 to 6.4 days, with a median ICU/CCU length of stay of 2.4 days. Rehospitalization within 60 to 90 days occurs in approximately 30 percent of patients. Patients have an in-hospital mortality of approximately 4 to 7 percent, whereas postdischarge mortality at 60 to 90 days varies widely depending on the study, but is approximately 8 to 10 percent, increasing to about 30 percent at 1 year. Some studies suggest even more dramatic figures with 20 percent in-hospital mortality during first heart failure admission and over a 40 percent 1-year mortality.[151] However, this same study suggests that post-discharge cardiovascular survival has improved by 50 percent from 1993/94 to 2000/2001. The in-hospital mortality of AHF is similar to that of an acute myocardial infarction, but the post-discharge mortality of a patient admitted for AHF is approximately fivefold higher.[3]

Many prognostic models have been developed to provide an understanding of these figures, and most predictive models of in-hospital mortality have found that renal dysfunction (usually elevated BUN), lower systolic blood pressure, greater age, and evidence of myocyte necrosis are predictors of increased mortality. The largest analysis[152] found that BUN, systolic blood pressure, heart rate, and age were the main multivariate predictors, and using a different statistical approach with dichotomous variables, suggests that the best single predictor was an elevated admission blood urea nitrogen (BUN ≥ 43 mg/dl), followed by low blood pressure (systolic blood pressure < 115 mm Hg), and then by increased concentrations of serum creatinine (≥2.75 mg/dl). Patients with all three characteristics had an in-hospital mortality of 21.9 percent compared to 2.1 percent in patients with none. Of note, this study had high rates of missing data for admission BNP (82 percent) and cardiac enzymes (45 percent), limiting their contribution to the model. It is clear from this and other analyses that renal dysfunction is one of the most important factors in the outcomes of patients with HF. However, worsening of renal function during hospitalization, even as small as a 0.1 mg/dl increase in creatinine,[153] also predicts longer lengths of stay and increased mortality.[154] In another analysis, a systolic blood pressure below 120 mm Hg was an independent predictor of morbidity and mortality in patients with AHF with either reduced or preserved systolic function.[18] The important implication of these analyses is that relatively minor abnormalities in renal function and blood pressure have tremendous impact on mortality, and physicians may need to readjust their definitions of low blood pressure to include patients with systolic blood pressure less than 115 to

TABLE 24–9 Outcomes in Acute Heart Failure Patients from Selected Studies

			Mortality	
Study	**Patients (n)**	**Rehospitalization**	***Mortality In-Hospital***	***Post-Discharge***
Jong (Ontario; 1994-7)	38,702	N/A	N/A	11.6% 30 d 33.1% 1 yr
Lee (Ontario, 1997-2001)	4,031	N/A	8.7%	10.6% 30 d 31% 1 yr
OPTIME-HF (US)	949	35.2% 60 d*	3.0%	9.6% 60 d
IMPACT-HF Registry (US)	567	25.7% 60 d	2.6%	8.5% 60 d
ADHERE (US)	187,565	N/A	3.8%	N/A
OPTIMIZE-HF (US)	41,267	29.5% 60-90 d	3.8%	8.0% 60-90 d
EHFS I (EU)	11,327	24% 12 wk	6.9%	13.5% 12 wk
Rudiger (Zürich-Helsinki)	312	N/A	8%	11% 30 d 18% 12 wk 29% 1 yr
Tavazzi (Italy)	2,807	38.1% 6 mo	7.3%	12.8% 6 mo
Zannad (France)	581	N/A	N/A	27.4% 4 wk† 46.5% 1 yr†
EHFS II (EU)	3,580	N/A	6.7%	N/A

*Includes death and rehospitalizations.

†Includes only patients who were admitted to ICU/CCU.

120 mm Hg and of worsening renal function to include those with a 0.3 mg/dl increase in creatinine.

As with chronic heart failure, studies of AHF have discovered multiple univariate and independent multivariate predictors of mortality. Increased BNP concentrations have been shown to predict in-hospital outcomes as well as readmission and post-discharge mortality, and even minor increases in markers of myocardial necrosis, such as troponins, can predict in-hospital worsening of heart failure and post-discharge morbidity and mortality. Anemia is another previously underappreciated predictor of poor outcomes in patients with AHF, and it is currently a therapeutic target under investigation in clinical trials (see Chap. 25). Neurohormones, such as endothelin, and markers of inflammation (i.e. C-reactive protein, IL-6), are also strong predictors of mortality.

FUTURE PERSPECTIVES

Acute heart failure will continue to be a growing problem for health care providers. Data from the ongoing registries and studies will provide important information to further define and understand the characteristics of these patients. Although there are many exciting, novel therapeutic approaches under investigation, designing the clinical trials to demonstrate their efficacy will remain a challenge, as long as there is uncertainty in defining meaningful endpoints from both a clinical and regulatory perspective. Currently, effective therapies for the cardiorenal syndrome, cardioprotective strategies, and safe agents for increasing cardiac function appear to be the greatest unmet needs. Targeting specific therapeutic approaches to the underlying pathophysiology and limiting the use of agents known to contribute to poor outcomes will also be possible, as these novel therapies become available. Advances in the care of these patients should be informed by considering AHF a cardiovascular emergency, to be treated as expeditiously as an acute coronary syndrome, with the goal of reducing the persistent high in-hospital mortality. Finally, the admission of a patient for AHF is an opportunity to optimize their outpatient regimen, educate them on the disease process and treatment plan, and involve them in a supportive outpatient management program.[155] Continued research in effective outpatient treatments and management strategies will ultimately be the best way to prevent admissions for acute heart failure.

GENERAL REFERENCES

Mann DL, ed: Heart Failure: A Companion to Braunwald's Heart Disease. Philadelphia, Elsevier, 2004.

O'Connor CM, Stough WG, Gheorghiade M, Adams Jr. (eds): Managing Acute Decompensated Heart Failure. New York, Taylor & Francis, 2005.

REFERENCES

Definition and Classification

1. VMAC Investigators: Intravenous nesiritide vs. nitroglycerin for treatment of decompensated congestive heart failure: A randomized controlled trial. JAMA 287:1531-1540, 2002.
2. Cuffe MS, Califf RM, Adams KF, Jr., et al: Short-term intravenous milrinone for acute exacerbation of chronic heart failure: a randomized controlled trial. JAMA 287:1541-1547, 2002.
3. Gheorghiade M, Zannad F, Sopko G, et al: Acute heart failure syndromes: current state and framework for future research. Circulation 112:3958-3968, 2005.
4. Nieminen MS, Bohm M, Cowie MR, et al: Executive summary of the guidelines on the diagnosis and treatment of acute heart failure: the Task Force on Acute Heart Failure of the European Society of Cardiology. Eur Heart J 26:384-416, 2005.
5. Heart Failure Society of America: Evaluation and management of patients with acute decompensated heart failure. J Card Fail 12:e86-e103, 2006.
6. Cotter G, Moshkovitz Y, Milovanov O, et al: Acute heart failure: a novel approach to its pathogenesis and treatment. Eur J Heart Fail 4:227-234, 2002.
7. Nohria A, Tsang SW, Fang JC, et al: Clinical assessment identifies hemodynamic profiles that predict outcomes in patients admitted with heart failure. J Am Coll Cardiol 41:1797-1804, 2003.
8. Binanay C, Califf RM, Hasselblad V, et al: Evaluation study of congestive heart failure and pulmonary artery catheterization effectiveness: The ESCAPE trial. JAMA 294:1625-1633, 2005.
9. Stevenson LW: Are hemodynamic goals viable in tailoring heart failure therapy? Hemodynamic goals are relevant. Circulation 113:1020-1027; discussion 1033, 2006.

Epidemiology

10. Thom T, Haase N, Rosamond W, et al: Heart disease and stroke statistics—2006 update: A report from the American Heart Association Statistics Committee and Stroke Statistics Subcommittee. Circulation 113:e85-151, 2006.
11. Swedberg K, Cleland J, Dargie H, et al: Guidelines for the diagnosis and treatment of chronic heart failure: Executive summary (update 2005): The Task Force for the Diagnosis and Treatment of Chronic Heart Failure of the European Society of Cardiology. Eur Heart J 26:1115-1140, 2005.
12. Berry C, Murdoch DR, McMurray JJ: Economics of chronic heart failure. Eur J Heart Fail 3:283-291, 2001.
13. Nieminen MS, Brutsaert D, Dickstein K, et al: EuroHeart Failure Survey II (EHFS II): A survey on hospitalized acute heart failure patients: Description of population. Eur Heart J 27:2725-2736, 2006.
14. Rudiger A, Harjola VP, Muller A, et al: Acute heart failure: Clinical presentation, one-year mortality and prognostic factors. Eur J Heart Fail 7:662-670, 2005.
15. Tavazzi L, Maggioni AP, Lucci D, et al: Nationwide survey on acute heart failure in cardiology ward services in Italy. Eur Heart J 27:1207-1215, 2006.
16. ADHERE Scientific Advisory Committee: Acute Decompensated Heart Failure National Registry (ADHERE®) Core Module Q1 2006 Final Cumulative National Benchmark Report: Scios, Inc.; July 2006.
17. Yancy CW, Lopatin M, Stevenson LW, et al: Clinical presentation, management, and in-hospital outcomes of patients admitted with acute decompensated heart failure with preserved systolic function: A report from the Acute Decompensated Heart Failure National Registry (ADHERE) Database. J Am Coll Cardiol 47:76-84, 2006.
18. Gheorghiade M, Abraham WT, Albert NM, et al: Systolic blood pressure at admission, clinical characteristics, and outcomes in patients hospitalized with acute heart failure. JAMA 296:2217-2226, 2006.
19. Galvao M, Kalman J, DeMarco T, et al: Gender differences in in-hospital management and outcomes in patients with decompensated heart failure: Analysis from the Acute Decompensated Heart Failure National Registry (ADHERE). J Card Fail 12:100-107, 2006.
20. Havranek EP, Masoudi FA, Westfall KA, et al: Spectrum of heart failure in older patients: results from the National Heart Failure project. Am Heart J 143:412-417, 2002.
21. Rathore SS, Foody JM, Wang Y, et al: Race, quality of care, and outcomes of elderly patients hospitalized with heart failure. JAMA 289:2517-2524, 2003.
22. Yancy C, Stough WG, Abraham WT, et al: Defining the natural history and improving quality of care for African-Americans hospitalized with heart failure: A report from OPTIMIZE-HF. J Card Fail 11:S190, 2005.
23. Echols MR, Felker GM, Thomas KL, et al: Racial differences in the characteristics of patients admitted for acute decompensated heart failure and their relation to outcomes: Results from the OPTIME-CHF trial. J Card Fail 12:684-688, 2006.
24. Jimenez J, Osorio JM, Andrade S, et al: Decompensated heart failure among Hispanic Americans: A report from the Acute Decompensated Heart Failure National Registry (ADHERE). J Card Fail 10:S93, 2004.

Pathophysiology and Clinical Manifestations

25. Bhatia RS, Tu JV, Lee DS, et al: Outcome of heart failure with preserved ejection fraction in a population-based study. N Engl J Med 355:260-269, 2006.
26. Masoudi FA, Havranek EP, Smith G, et al: Gender, age, and heart failure with preserved left ventricular systolic function. J Am Coll Cardiol 41:217-223, 2003.
27. Kawaguchi M, Hay I, Fetics B, Kass DA: Combined ventricular systolic and arterial stiffening in patients with heart failure and preserved ejection fraction: Implications for systolic and diastolic reserve limitations. Circulation 107:714-720, 2003.
28. Gandhi SK, Powers JC, Nomeir AM, et al: The pathogenesis of acute pulmonary edema associated with hypertension. N Engl J Med 344:17-22, 2001.
29. Baicu CF, Zile MR, Aurigemma GP, Gaasch WH: Left ventricular systolic performance, function, and contractility in patients with diastolic heart failure. Circulation 111:2306-2312, 2005.
30. Redfield MM, Jacobsen SJ, Burnett JC, Jr., et al: Burden of systolic and diastolic ventricular dysfunction in the community: appreciating the scope of the heart failure epidemic. JAMA 289:194-202, 2003.
31. Zile MR, Baicu CF, Gaasch WH: Diastolic heart failure—abnormalities in active relaxation and passive stiffness of the left ventricle. N Engl J Med 350:1953-1959, 2004.
32. Heywood JT, Fonarow GC, Costanzo MR, et al: High prevalence of renal dysfunction and its impact on outcome in 118,465 patients hospitalized with acute decompensated heart failure: A report from the ADHERE® database. J Card Fail 2007 (in press).
33. Firth JD, Raine AE, Ledingham JG: Raised venous pressure: A direct cause of renal sodium retention in oedema? Lancet 1:1033-1035, 1988.
34. Ware LB, Matthay MA: Clinical practice. Acute pulmonary edema. N Engl J Med 353:2788-2796, 2005.
35. Pierard LA, Lancellotti P: The role of ischemic mitral regurgitation in the pathogenesis of acute pulmonary edema. N Engl J Med 351:1627-1634, 2004.

36. Arques S, Ambrosi P, Gelisse R, et al: Hypoalbuminemia in elderly patients with acute diastolic heart failure. J Am Coll Cardiol 42:712-716, 2003.
37. De Pasquale CG, Arnolda LF, Doyle IR, et al: Plasma surfactant protein-B: A novel biomarker in chronic heart failure. Circulation 110:1091-1096, 2004.
38. Zannad F, Mebazaa A, Juilliere Y, et al: Clinical profile, contemporary management and one-year mortality in patients with severe acute heart failure syndromes: The EFICA study. Eur J Heart Fail 8:697-705, 2006.
39. Steg PG, Dabbous OH, Feldman LJ, et al: Determinants and prognostic impact of heart failure complicating acute coronary syndromes: Observations from the Global Registry of Acute Coronary Events (GRACE). Circulation 109:494-499, 2004.
40. Gheorghiade M, Gattis Stough W, Adams KF, Jr., et al: The Pilot Randomized Study of Nesiritide Versus Dobutamine in Heart Failure (PRESERVD-HF). Am J Cardiol 96:18G-25G, 2005.
41. Perna ER, Macin SM, Cimbaro Canella JP, et al: Minor myocardial damage detected by troponin T is a powerful predictor of long-term prognosis in patients with acute decompensated heart failure. Int J Cardiol 99:253-261, 2005.
42. Aronson D, Burger AJ: Neurohormonal prediction of mortality following admission for decompensated heart failure. Am J Cardiol 91:245-248, 2003.
43. Milo O, Cotter G, Kaluski E, et al: Comparison of inflammatory and neurohormonal activation in cardiogenic pulmonary edema secondary to ischemic versus nonischemic causes. Am J Cardiol 92:222-226, 2003.
44. Aronson D, Burger AJ: Neurohumoral activation and ventricular arrhythmias in patients with decompensated congestive heart failure: Role of endothelin. Pacing Clin Electrophysiol 26:703-710, 2003.
45. Rudiger A, Burckhardt OA, Harpes P, et al: The relative lymphocyte count on hospital admission is a risk factor for long-term mortality in patients with acute heart failure. Am J Emerg Med 24:451-454, 2006.
46. Chin BS, Conway DS, Chung NA, et al: Interleukin-6, tissue factor and von Willebrand factor in acute decompensated heart failure: Relationship to treatment and prognosis. Blood Coagul Fibrinolysis 14:515-521, 2003.
47. Mueller C, Laule-Kilian K, Christ A, et al: Inflammation and long-term mortality in acute congestive heart failure. Am Heart J 151:845-850, 2006.
48. Peschel T, Schonauer M, Thiele H, et al: Invasive assessment of bacterial endotoxin and inflammatory cytokines in patients with acute heart failure. Eur J Heart Fail 5:609-614, 2003.
49. Chong AY, Lip GY, Freestone B, Blann AD: Increased circulating endothelial cells in acute heart failure: Comparison with von Willebrand factor and soluble E-selectin. Eur J Heart Fail 8:167-172, 2006.
50. Cohen-Solal A, Desnos M, Delahaye F, et al: A national survey of heart failure in French hospitals. The Myocardiopathy and Heart Failure Working Group of the French Society of Cardiology, the National College of General Hospital Cardiologists and the French Geriatrics Society. Eur Heart J 21:763-769, 2000.
51. Opasich C, Rapezzi C, Lucci D, et al: Precipitating factors and decision-making processes of short-term worsening heart failure despite "optimal" treatment (from the IN-CHF Registry). Am J Cardiol 88:382-387, 2001.
52. Formiga F, Chivite D, Manito N, et al: Hospitalization due to acute heart failure. Role of the precipitating factors. Int J Cardiol 2006.
53. Tsuyuki RT, McKelvie RS, Arnold JM, et al: Acute precipitants of congestive heart failure exacerbations. Arch Intern Med 161:2337-2342, 2001.
54. O'Connor CM, Stough WG, Gallup DS, et al: Demographics, clinical characteristics, and outcomes of patients hospitalized for decompensated heart failure: Observations from the IMPACT-HF registry. J Card Fail 11:200-205, 2005.
55. Schiff GD, Fung S, Speroff T, McNutt RA: Decompensated heart failure: symptoms, patterns of onset, and contributing factors. Am J Med 114:625-630, 2003.
56. Ramasamy R, Hildebrandt T, O'Hea E, et al: Psychological and social factors that correlate with dyspnea in heart failure. Psychosomatics 47:430-434, 2006.
57. Freedland KE, Rich MW, Skala JA, et al: Prevalence of depression in hospitalized patients with congestive heart failure. Psychosomatic Medicine 65:119-128, 2003.
58. de Denus S, Spinler SA, Jessup M, Kao A: History of depression as a predictor of adverse outcomes in patients hospitalized for decompensated heart failure. Pharmacotherapy 24:1306-1310, 2004.
59. Taylor J, Stott DJ: Chronic heart failure and cognitive impairment: Co-existence of conditions or true association? Eur J Heart Fail 4:7-9, 2002.

Physical Examination and Diagnostic Evaluation

60. Aronson D, Burger AJ: Relation between pulse pressure and survival in patients with decompensated heart failure. Am J Cardiol 93:785-788, 2004.
61. Shah MR, Hasselblad V, Stinnett SS, et al: Hemodynamic profiles of advanced heart failure: Association with clinical characteristics and long-term outcomes. J Card Fail 7:105-113, 2001.
62. Perna ER, Barbagelata A, Grinfeld L, et al: Overview of acute decompensated heart failure in Argentina: Lessons learned from 5 registries during the last decade. Am Heart J 151:84-91, 2006.
63. Marcus GM, Gerber IL, McKeown BH, et al: Association between phonocardiographic third and fourth heart sounds and objective measures of left ventricular function. JAMA 293:2238-2244, 2005.
64. Felker GM, Adams KF, Jr., Gattis WA, O'Connor CM: Anemia as a risk factor and therapeutic target in heart failure. J Am Coll Cardiol 44:959-966, 2004.
65. Maisel AS, Krishnaswamy P, Nowak RM, et al: Rapid measurement of B-type natriuretic peptide in the emergency diagnosis of heart failure. N Engl J Med 347:161-167, 2002.
66. McCullough PA, Nowak RM, McCord J, et al: B-type natriuretic peptide and clinical judgment in emergency diagnosis of heart failure: Analysis from Breathing Not Properly (BNP) Multinational Study. Circulation 106:416-422, 2002.
67. Januzzi JL, van Kimmenade R, Lainchbury J, et al: NT-proBNP testing for diagnosis and short-term prognosis in acute destabilized heart failure: An international pooled analysis of 1256 patients: The International Collaborative of NT-proBNP Study. Eur Heart J 27:330-337, 2006.
68. Mueller C, Scholer A, Laule-Kilian K, et al: Use of B-type natriuretic peptide in the evaluation and management of acute dyspnea. N Engl J Med 350:647-654, 2004.
69. Maisel AS: The diagnosis of acute congestive heart failure: Role of BNP measurements. Heart Fail Rev 8:327-334, 2003.
70. Kruger S, Graf J, Merx MW, et al: Brain natriuretic peptide predicts right heart failure in patients with acute pulmonary embolism. Am Heart J 147:60-65, 2004.
71. Rudiger A, Gasser S, Fischler M, et al: Comparable increase of B-type natriuretic peptide and amino-terminal pro-B-type natriuretic peptide levels in patients with severe sepsis, septic shock, and acute heart failure. Crit Care Med 34:2140-2144, 2006.
72. Maisel AS, McCord J, Nowak RM, et al: Bedside B-Type natriuretic peptide in the emergency diagnosis of heart failure with reduced or preserved ejection fraction. Results from the Breathing Not Properly Multinational Study. J Am Coll Cardiol 41:2010-2017, 2003.
73. Collins SP, Lindsell CJ, Storrow AB, Abraham WT: Prevalence of negative chest radiography results in the emergency department patient with decompensated heart failure. Ann Emerg Med 47:13-18, 2006.
74. Huang CH, Tsai MS, Hsieh CC, et al: Diagnostic accuracy of tissue Doppler echocardiography for patients with acute heart failure. Heart 92:1790-1794, 2006.
75. Senior R, Janardhanan R, Jeetley P, Burden L: Myocardial contrast echocardiography for distinguishing ischemic from nonischemic first-onset acute heart failure: Insights into the mechanism of acute heart failure. Circulation 112:1587-1593, 2005.
76. Shah MR, Hasselblad V, Stevenson LW, et al: Impact of the pulmonary artery catheter in critically ill patients: Meta-analysis of randomized clinical trials. JAMA 294:1664-1670, 2005.
77. Collins SP, Lindsell CJ, Peacock WF, et al: The combined utility of an S3 heart sound and B-type natriuretic peptide levels in emergency department patients with dyspnea. J Card Fail 12:286-292, 2006.
78. Packer M, Abraham WT, Mehra MR, et al: Utility of impedance cardiography for the identification of short-term risk of clinical decompensation in stable patients with chronic heart failure. J Am Coll Cardiol 47:2245-2252, 2006.
79. Shochat M, Charach G, Meyler S, et al: Internal thoracic impedance monitoring: A novel method for the preclinical detection of acute heart failure. Cardiovasc Revasc Med 7:41-45, 2006.
80. Peacock WF, Young J, Collins S, et al: Heart failure observation units: Optimizing care. Ann Emerg Med 47:22-33, 2006.
81. Collins SP, Mielniczuk LM, Whittingham HA, et al: The use of noninvasive ventilation in emergency department patients with acute cardiogenic pulmonary edema: A systematic review. Ann Emerg Med 48:260-269, 269 e261-264, 2006.
82. Masip J, Roque M, Sanchez B, et al: Noninvasive ventilation in acute cardiogenic pulmonary edema: Systematic review and meta-analysis. JAMA 294:3124-3130, 2005.
83. Peter JV, Moran JL, Phillips-Hughes J, et al: Effect of non-invasive positive pressure ventilation (NIPPV) on mortality in patients with acute cardiogenic pulmonary oedema: A meta-analysis. Lancet 367:1155-1163, 2006.
84. Maheshwari V, Paioli D, Rothaar R, Hill NS: Utilization of noninvasive ventilation in acute care hospitals: A regional survey. Chest 129:1226-1233, 2006.
85. Heart Failure Society of America: Executive summary: HFSA 2006 Comprehensive Heart Failure Practice Guideline. J Card Fail 12:10-38, 2006.
86. Aronson D, Burger AJ: Concomitant beta-blocker therapy is associated with a lower occurrence of ventricular arrhythmias in patients with decompensated heart failure. J Card Fail 8:79-85, 2002.
87. Butler J, Young JB, Abraham WT, et al: Beta-blocker use and outcomes among hospitalized heart failure patients. J Am Coll Cardiol 47:2462-2469, 2006.
88. Hunt SA: ACC/AHA 2005 guideline update for the diagnosis and management of chronic heart failure in the adult: a report of the American College of Cardiology/American Heart Association Task Force on Practice Guidelines (Writing Committee to Update the 2001 Guidelines for the Evaluation and Management of Heart Failure). J Am Coll Cardiol 46:e1-82, 2005.
89. Gattis WA, O'Connor CM, Gallup DS, et al: Predischarge initiation of carvedilol in patients hospitalized for decompensated heart failure: Results of the Initiation Management Predischarge: Process for Assessment of Carvedilol Therapy in Heart Failure (IMPACT-HF) trial. J Am Coll Cardiol 43:1534-1541, 2004.
90. Fonarow GC, Abraham WT, Albert NM, et al: Carvedilol use at discharge in patients hospitalized for heart failure is associated with improved survival: An analysis from Organized Program to Initiate Lifesaving Treatment in Hospitalized Patients with Heart Failure (OPTIMIZE-HF). Am Heart J 153:82 e81-82 e11, 2007.
91. Hamada Y, Tanaka N, Murata K, et al: Significance of predischarge BNP on one-year outcome in decompensated heart failure—comparative study with echo-Doppler indexes. J Card Fail 11:43-49, 2005.
92. Logeart D, Thabut G, Jourdain P, et al: Predischarge B-type natriuretic peptide assay for identifying patients at high risk of re-admission after decompensated heart failure. J Am Coll Cardiol 43:635-641, 2004.
93. Phillips CO, Wright SM, Kern DE, et al: Comprehensive discharge planning with postdischarge support for older patients with congestive heart failure: A meta-analysis. JAMA 291:1358-1367, 2004.
94. Sharma M, Teerlink JR: A rational approach for the treatment of acute heart failure: Current strategies and future options. Curr Opin Cardiol 19:254-263, 2004.
95. Le Jemtel TH, Alt EU: Are hemodynamic goals viable in tailoring heart failure therapy? Hemodynamic goals are outdated. Circulation 113:1027-1032; discussion 1033, 2006.
96. Cotter G, Moshkovitz Y, Kaluski E, et al: The role of cardiac power and systemic vascular resistance in the pathophysiology and diagnosis of patients with acute congestive heart failure. Eur J Heart Fail 5:443-451, 2003.

97. Tan LB, Williams SG, Wright DJ: Ventriculo-arterial function curves—a new dimension in characterising acute heart failure. Eur J Heart Fail 5:407-410, 2003.
98. Costanzo MR, Guglin ME, Saltzberg MT, et al: Ultrafiltration versus intravenous diuretics for patients hospitalized for acute decompensated heart failure. J Am Coll Cardiol 49:675, 2007.
99. Shlipak MG, Massie BM: The clinical challenge of cardiorenal syndrome. Circulation 110:1514-1517, 2004.
100. Butler J, Forman DE, Abraham WT, et al: Relationship between heart failure treatment and development of worsening renal function among hospitalized patients. Am Heart J 147:331-338, 2004.
101. Weinfeld MS, Chertow GM, Stevenson LW: Aggravated renal dysfunction during intensive therapy for advanced chronic heart failure. Am Heart J 138:285-290, 1999.
102. Gackowski A, Isnard R, Golmard JL, et al: Comparison of echocardiography and plasma B-type natriuretic peptide for monitoring the response to treatment in acute heart failure. Eur Heart J 25:1788-1796, 2004.
103. Dokainish H, Zoghbi WA, Lakkis NM, et al: Optimal noninvasive assessment of left ventricular filling pressures: A comparison of tissue Doppler echocardiography and B-type natriuretic peptide in patients with pulmonary artery catheters. Circulation 109:2432-2439, 2004.
104. Salvador DR, Rey NR, Ramos GC, Punzalan FE: Continuous infusion versus bolus injection of loop diuretics in congestive heart failure. Cochrane Database Syst Rev CD003178, 2005.
105. Ahmed A, Husain A, Love TE, et al: Heart failure, chronic diuretic use, and increase in mortality and hospitalization: An observational study using propensity score methods. Eur Heart J 27:1431-1439, 2006.
106. Eshaghian S, Horwich TB, Fonarow GC: Relation of loop diuretic dose to mortality in advanced heart failure. Am J Cardiol 97:1759-1764, 2006.
107. McCurley JM, Hanlon SU, Wei SK, et al: Furosemide and the progression of left ventricular dysfunction in experimental heart failure. J Am Coll Cardiol 44:1301-1307, 2004.
108. Teerlink JR: Overview of randomized clinical trials in acute heart failure syndromes. Am J Cardiol 96:59G-67G, 2005.
109. Cotter G, Metzkor E, Kaluski E, et al: Randomised trial of high-dose isosorbide dinitrate plus low-dose furosemide versus high-dose furosemide plus low-dose isosorbide dinitrate in severe pulmonary oedema. Lancet 351:389-393, 1998.
110. Elkayam U, Akhter MW, Singh H, et al: Comparison of effects on left ventricular filling pressure of intravenous nesiritide and high-dose nitroglycerin in patients with decompensated heart failure. Am J Cardiol 93:237-240, 2004.
111. Johnson W, Omland T, Hall C, et al: Neurohormonal activation rapidly decreases after intravenous therapy with diuretics and vasodilators for class IV heart failure. J Am Coll Cardiol 39:1623-1629, 2002.
112. Durrer JD, Lie KI, van Capelle FJ, Durrer D: Effect of sodium nitroprusside on mortality in acute myocardial infarction. N Engl J Med 306:1121-1128, 1982.
113. Cohn JN, Franciosa JA, Francis GS, et al: Effect of short-term infusion of sodium nitroprusside on mortality rate in acute myocardial infarction complicated by left ventricular failure: Results of a Veterans Administration cooperative study. N Engl J Med 306:1129-1135, 1982.
114. Khot UN, Novaro GM, Popovic ZB, et al: Nitroprusside in critically ill patients with left ventricular dysfunction and aortic stenosis. N Engl J Med 348:1756-1763, 2003.
115. Aaronson KD, Sackner-Bernstein J: Risk of death associated with nesiritide in patients with acutely decompensated heart failure. JAMA 296:1465-1466, 2006.
116. Sackner-Bernstein JD, Kowalski M, Fox M, Aaronson K: Short-term risk of death after treatment with nesiritide for decompensated heart failure: A pooled analysis of randomized controlled trials. JAMA 293:1900-1905, 2005.
117. Sackner-Bernstein JD, Skopicki HA, Aaronson KD: Risk of worsening renal function with nesiritide in patients with acutely decompensated heart failure. Circulation 111:1487-1491, 2005.
118. Teerlink JR, Massie BM: Nesiritide and worsening of renal function: The emperor's new clothes? Circulation 111:1459-1461, 2005.
119. Hauptman PJ, Schnitzler MA, Swindle J, Burroughs TE: Use of nesiritide before and after publications suggesting drug-related risks in patients with acute decompensated heart failure. JAMA 296:1877-1884, 2006.
120. Colucci WS, Elkayam U, Horton DP, et al: Intravenous nesiritide, a natriuretic peptide, in the treatment of decompensated congestive heart failure. Nesiritide Study Group. N Engl J Med 343:246-253, 2000.
121. Butler J, Emerman C, Peacock WF, et al: The efficacy and safety of B-type natriuretic peptide (nesiritide) in patients with renal insufficiency and acutely decompensated congestive heart failure. Nephrol Dial Transplant 19:391-399, 2004.
122. Wang DJ, Dowling TC, Meadows D, et al: Nesiritide does not improve renal function in patients with chronic heart failure and worsening serum creatinine. Circulation 110:1620-1625, 2004.
123. Riter HG, Redfield MM, Burnett JC, Chen HH: Nonhypotensive low-dose nesiritide has differential renal effects compared with standard-dose nesiritide in patients with acute decompensated heart failure and renal dysfunction. J Am Coll Cardiol 47:2334-2335, 2006.
124. Burger AJ, Horton DP, LeJemtel T, et al: Effect of nesiritide (B-type natriuretic peptide) and dobutamine on ventricular arrhythmias in the treatment of patients with acutely decompensated congestive heart failure: The PRECEDENT study. Am Heart J 144:1102-1108, 2002.
125. Silver MA, Horton DP, Ghali JK, Elkayam U: Effect of nesiritide versus dobutamine on short-term outcomes in the treatment of patients with acutely decompensated heart failure. J Am Coll Cardiol 39:798-803, 2002.
126. Abraham WT, Adams KF, Fonarow GC, et al: In-hospital mortality in patients with acute decompensated heart failure requiring intravenous vasoactive medications: An analysis from the Acute Decompensated Heart Failure National Registry (ADHERE). J Am Coll Cardiol 46:57-64, 2005.
127. Coletta AP, Cleland JG, Freemantle N, Clark AL: Clinical trials update from the European Society of Cardiology Heart Failure meeting: SHAPE, BRING-UP 2 VAS, COLA II, FOSIDIAL, BETACAR, CASINO and meta-analysis of cardiac resynchronisation therapy. Eur J Heart Fail 6:673-676, 2004.
128. Follath F, Cleland JG, Just H, et al: Efficacy and safety of intravenous levosimendan compared with dobutamine in severe low-output heart failure (the LIDO study): A randomised double-blind trial. Lancet 360:196-202, 2002.
129. Metra M, Nodari S, D'Aloia A, et al: Beta-blocker therapy influences the hemodynamic response to inotropic agents in patients with heart failure: A randomized comparison of dobutamine and enoximone before and after chronic treatment with metoprolol or carvedilol. J Am Coll Cardiol 40:1248-1258, 2002.
130. Adamopoulos S, Parissis JT, Iliodromitis EK, et al: Effects of levosimendan versus dobutamine on inflammatory and apoptotic pathways in acutely decompensated chronic heart failure. Am J Cardiol 98:102-106, 2006.
131. Friedrich JO, Adhikari N, Herridge MS, Beyene J: Meta-analysis: low-dose dopamine increases urine output but does not prevent renal dysfunction or death. Ann Intern Med 142:510-524, 2005.
132. Felker GM, Benza RL, Chandler AB, et al: Heart failure etiology and response to milrinone in decompensated heart failure: Results from the OPTIME-CHF study. J Am Coll Cardiol 41:997-1003, 2003.
133. Szilagyi S, Pollesello P, Levijoki J, et al: The effects of levosimendan and OR-1896 on isolated hearts, myocyte-sized preparations and phosphodiesterase enzymes of the guinea pig. Eur J Pharmacol 486:67-74, 2004.
134. Moiseyev VS, Poder P, Andrejevs N, et al: Safety and efficacy of a novel calcium sensitizer, levosimendan, in patients with left ventricular failure due to an acute myocardial infarction. A randomized, placebo-controlled, double-blind study (RUSSLAN). Eur Heart J 23:1422-1432, 2002.
135. Cleland JG, Freemantle N, Coletta AP, Clark AL: Clinical trials update from the American Heart Association: REPAIR-AMI, ASTAMI, JELIS, MEGA, REVIVE-II, SURVIVE, and PROACTIVE. Eur J Heart Fail 8:105-110, 2006.

Future Therapies

136. deGoma EM, Vagelos RH, Fowler MB, Ashley EA: Emerging therapies for the management of decompensated heart failure: From bench to bedside. J Am Coll Cardiol 48:2397-2409, 2006.
137. Teerlink JR, Malik FI, Clarke CP, et al: The selective cardiac myosin activator, CK-1827452, increases left ventricular systolic function by increasing ejection time: Results of a first-in-human study of a unique and novel mechanism. J Card Fail 12:763, 2006.
138. Sabbah HN, Imai M, Cowart D, et al: Hemodynamic properties of a new generation: Positive lusi-inotropic agaent for the acute treatment of advanced heart failure. Am J Cardiol 99:541-546, 2006.
139. Ghali J, Smith W, Torre-Amione G, et al: A Phase 1-2 dose-escalating study evaluating the safety and tolerability of istaroxime on electrocardiographic and hemodynamic parameters in patients with chronic heart failure and reduced systolic function. Am J Cardiol 99:541-546, 2007.
140. Mitrovic V, Luss H, Nitsche K, et al: Effects of the renal natriuretic peptide urodilatin (ularitide) in patients with decompensated chronic heart failure: A double-blind, placebo-controlled, ascending-dose trial. Am Heart J 150:e1231-e1239, 2005.
141. Mitrovic V, Seferovic PM, Simeunovic D, et al: Haemodynamic and clinical effects of ularitide in decompensated heart failure. Eur Heart J 27:2823-2832, 2006.
142. Gottlieb SS, Brater DC, Thomas I, et al: BG9719 (CVT-124), an A1 adenosine receptor antagonist, protects against the decline in renal function observed with diuretic therapy. Circulation 105:1348-1353, 2002.
143. Givertz MM, Fields TK, Pearson L, et al: Effect of the adenosine A_1 receptor antagonist, KW-3902, alone and in combination with furosemide, on diuresis and renal function in hospitalized acutely decompensated heart failure patients with renal impairment or refractory to maximum dose of conventional diuretics: Two randomized, double-blind, placebo-controlled studies. J Card Fail 12:762-763, 2006.
144. Gheorghiade M, Gattis WA, O'Connor CM, et al: Effects of tolvaptan, a vasopressin antagonist, in patients hospitalized with worsening heart failure: A randomized controlled trial. JAMA 291:1963-1971, 2004.
145. Schrier RW, Gross P, Gheorghiade M, et al: Tolvaptan, a selective oral vasopressin V2-receptor antagonist, for hyponatremia. N Engl J Med 355:2099-2112, 2006.
146. Teerlink JR, McMurray JJ, Bourge RC, et al: Tezosentan in patients with acute heart failure: Design of the Value of Endothelin Receptor Inhibition with Tezosentan in Acute heart failure Study (VERITAS). Am Heart J 150:46-53, 2005.

Clinical Outcomes and Prognosis

147. Cleland JG, Swedberg K, Follath F, et al: The EuroHeart Failure survey programme—a survey on the quality of care among patients with heart failure in Europe. Part 1: Patient characteristics and diagnosis. Eur Heart J 24:442-463, 2003.
148. Felker GM, Leimberger JD, Califf RM, et al: Risk stratification after hospitalization for decompensated heart failure. J Card Fail 10:460-466, 2004.
149. Jong P, Vowinckel E, Liu PP, et al: Prognosis and determinants of survival in patients newly hospitalized for heart failure: A population-based study. Arch Intern Med 162:1689-1694, 2002.
150. Lee DS, Austin PC, Rouleau JL, et al: Predicting mortality among patients hospitalized for heart failure: Derivation and validation of a clinical model. JAMA 290:2581-2587, 2003.

151. Blackledge HM, Tomlinson J, Squire IB: Prognosis for patients newly admitted to hospital with heart failure: Survival trends in 12,220 index admissions in Leicestershire 1993-2001. Heart 89:615-620, 2003.
152. Fonarow GC, Adams KF, Jr., Abraham WT, et al: Risk stratification for in-hospital mortality in acutely decompensated heart failure: Classification and regression tree analysis. JAMA 293:572-580, 2005.
153. Gottlieb SS, Abraham W, Butler J, et al: The prognostic importance of different definitions of worsening renal function in congestive heart failure. J Card Fail 8:136-141, 2002.
154. Forman DE, Butler J, Wang Y, et al: Incidence, predictors at admission, and impact of worsening renal function among patients hospitalized with heart failure. J Am Coll Cardiol 43:61-67, 2004.
155. McAlister FA, Stewart S, Ferrua S, McMurray JJ: Multidisciplinary strategies for the management of heart failure patients at high risk for admission: A systematic review of randomized trials. J Am Coll Cardiol 44:810-819, 2004.

CHAPTER 25

Management of Heart Failure Patients with Reduced Ejection Fraction

Douglas L. Mann

EPIDEMIOLOGY

The worldwide prevalence and incidence rates of heart failure (HF) are approaching epidemic proportions, as evidenced by the relentless increase in the number of HF hospitalizations, the growing number of HF-attributable deaths, and the spiraling costs associated with the care of HF patients. Worldwide, HF affects nearly 23 million people. In the United States, HF affects approximately 4.7 million persons (1.5 to 2 percent of the total population), with approximately 550,000 incident cases of HF diagnosed annually.[1] Estimates of the prevalence of symptomatic HF in the general European population are similar to those in the United States and range from 0.4 to 2 percent.[2] The prevalence of HF follows an exponential pattern, rising with age, and affects 6 to 10 percent of people older than 65 years (Fig. 25-1). Data from the Framingham Heart Study have suggested that the overall incidence of HF has declined among women but not among men.[3] However, although the relative incidence of HF is lower in women than in men, women constitute at least half of the cases of HF because of their longer life expectancy. In North America and Europe, the lifetime risk of developing HF is approximately 1 in 5 for a 40-year-old. The overall prevalence of HF is thought to be increasing, in part because our current therapies of cardiac disorders, such as myocardial infarction, valvular heart disease, and arrhythmias, are allowing patients to survive longer. Little is known with respect to the prevalence or risk of developing HF in emerging nations because of the lack of population-based studies in these countries.[4] Although HF was once thought to arise primarily in the setting of a depressed left ventricular (LV) ejection fraction (EF), epidemiological studies have shown that approximately half of patients who develop HF have a normal or preserved EF (EF of 40 to 50 percent or higher). Accordingly, HF patients are now broadly categorized into one of two groups: (1) HF with a reduced or depressed EF (commonly referred to as systolic failure); and (2) HF with a preserved EF (commonly referred to as diastolic failure). The epidemiology of HF with a normal EF is discussed in Chapter 26.

Based on population-attributable risks, hypertension has the greatest impact on the development of HF, accounting for 39 percent of HF events in men and 59 percent in women. Despite its much lower prevalence in the population (3 to 10 percent), myocardial infarction also has a high attributable risk in men (34 percent) and women (13 percent). Valvular heart disease only accounts for 7 to 8 percent of HF cases (Table 25-1).[1] Dyslipidemia characterized by a high total/high-density lipoprotein [HDL] cholesterol ratio, but not the total cholesterol alone was also a risk factor for the development of HF.

Results from the Framingham Study have suggested that obesity is a potential risk factor for the development of HF in men and women (Fig. 25-2).[5] However, although obesity is a risk factor for the development of HF, obese patients with HF seem to have a more favorable clinical prognosis. The association between obesity, a traditional cardiovascular risk factor, and improved clinical outcomes in HF patients (i.e., reverse epidemiology) has been termed the *obesity paradox.*

CAUSATIVE FACTORS

As shown in Table 25-2, any condition that leads to an alteration in LV structure or function can predispose a patient to developing HF. Although the cause of HF in patients with a preserved EF differs from that of patient with depressed EF (see Chap. 26), there is considerable overlap between the causes of these two conditions. In industrialized countries, coronary artery disease (CAD) has become an important cause in men and women, and is responsible for 60 to 75 percent of cases of HF. Hypertension contributes to the development of HF in 75 percent of patients, including most patients with CAD. Both CAD and hypertension interact to augment the risk of HF. Rheumatic heart disease remains a major cause of HF in Africa and Asia, especially in the young. Hypertension is an important cause of HF in the African and African American population. Chagas' disease is still a major cause of HF in South America.[4] Not surprisingly, anemia is a frequent concomitant factor in HF in many developing nations. As developing nations undergo socioeconomic development, the epidemiology of HF is becoming similar to that of Western Europe and North America, with CAD emerging as the single most common cause of HF. Although the contribution of diabetes mellitus to HF is not well understood, diabetes accelerates atherosclerosis and is often associated with hypertension.

In 20 to 30 percent of the cases of HF with a depressed EF, the exact causative basis is not known. These patients are referred to as having nonischemic, dilated, or idiopathic cardiomyopathy if the cause is unknown (see Chap. 64). Prior viral infection (see Chap. 66) or toxin exposure

TABLE 25–1 Risk Factors for Cardiac Failure: Framingham Offspring and Cohort Study*

Risk Factor	Age- and Risk Factor–Adjusted Hazard Ratio		Prevalence (%)		Population-Attributable Risk (%)	
	Men	*Women*	*Men*	*Women*	*Men*	*Women*
High blood pressure (≥140/90 mm Hg)	2.1	3.4	60	62	39	59
Myocardial infarction	6.3	6.0	10	3	34	13
Angina	1.4	1.7	11	9	5	5
Diabetes	1.8	3.7	8	5	6	12
Left ventricular hypertrophy	2.2	2.9	4	3	4	5
Valvular heart disease	2.5	2.1	5	8	7	8

*Subjects aged 40-89 yr; 18-yr follow-up.
From Levy D, Larson MG, Vasan RS, et al: The progression from hypertension to congestive heart failure. JAMA 275:1557, 1996.

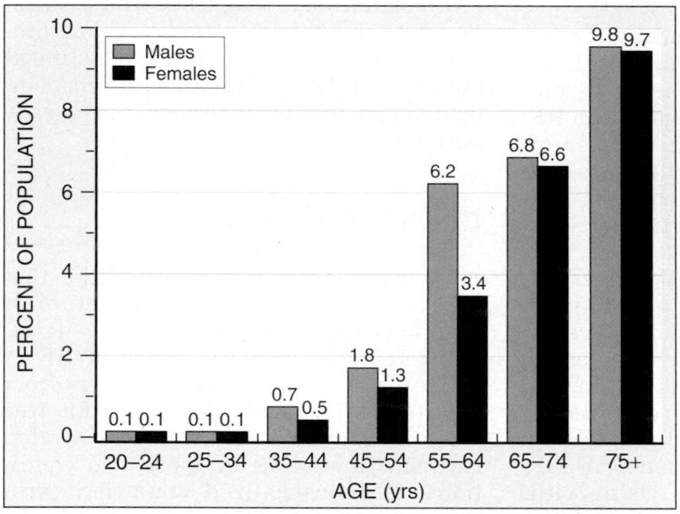

FIGURE 25–1 Prevalence rates of heart failure by gender and age in the United States between 1988 and 1994—the Third National Health and Nutrition Examination Survey (NHANES III). Among men (blue), the prevalence increased from 18 cases per 1000 in those aged 45 to 54 years to 98 cases per 1000 in those aged 75 years and older. Among women (purple), the prevalence increased from 13 cases per 1000 in those aged 45 to 54 years to 97 cases per 1000 in those aged 75 years and older. *(Data from American Heart Association: Heart Disease and Stroke Statistics—2003 Update. Dallas, American Heart Association, 2002.)*

(e.g., alcohol [see Chap. 68] or use of chemotherapeutic agents, see Chap. 85) may also lead to a dilated cardiomyopathy. Although excessive alcohol consumption can promote cardiomyopathy, alcohol consumption per se is not associated with increased risk for HF, and may protect against the development of HF when consumed in moderation.[6] It is also becoming increasingly clear that a large number of cases of dilated cardiomyopathy are secondary to specific genetic defects, most notably those in the cytoskeleton (see Chap. 10). Most forms of familial dilated cardiomyopathy are inherited in an autosomal dominant fashion. Mutations of genes encoding cytoskeletal proteins (desmin, cardiac myosin, vinculin) and nuclear membrane proteins (lamin) have been identified thus far. Dilated cardiomyopathy is also associated with Duchenne, Becker, and limb-girdle muscular dystrophies. Conditions that lead to a high cardiac output (e.g., arteriovenous fistula, anemia) are seldom responsible for the development of HF in a normal heart. However, in the presence of underlying structural heart disease, these conditions often lead to overt congestive failure.

TABLE 25–2 Causes of Chronic Heart Failure (HF)

Myocardial disease
Coronary artery disease Myocardial infarction* Myocardial ischemia*
Chronic pressure overload Hypertension* Obstructive valvular disease*
Chronic volume overload Regurgitant valvular disease Intracardiac (left-to-right) shunting Extracardiac shunting
Nonischemic dilated cardiomyopathy Familial/genetic disorders Infiltrative disorders* Toxic or drug-induced damage Metabolic disorder* Viral or other infectious agents
Disorders of rate and rhythm Chronic bradyarrhythmias Chronic tachyarrhythmias
Pulmonary heart disease
Cor pulmonale
Pulmonary vascular disorders
High-output states
Metabolic disorders Thyrotoxicosis Nutritional disorders (beriberi)
Excessive blood flow requirements Systemic arteriovenous shunting Chronic anemia

*Indicates conditions that can also lead to HF with a preserved ejection fraction.

PROGNOSIS

Although several reports have suggested that the mortality for HF patients is improving, the overall mortality rate remains higher than for many cancers, including those involving the bladder, breast, uterus and prostate. In the Framingham Study, the median survival was 1.7 years for men and 3.2 years for women, with only 25 percent of men and 38 percent of women surviving 5 years.[1] European studies have confirmed a similarly poor long-term prognosis.[2] More recent data from the Framingham Study have examined long-term trends in the survival of patients with HF and shown improved survival for both men and women, with an overall decline in mortality of approximately 12 percent per decade from 1950 to 1999.[3] Moreover, reports from Scotland, Sweden, and the United Kingdom have also suggested that survival rates may be also improving following hospital discharge.[2,7] Of note, the mortality of HF in epidemiological studies is substantially higher than that reported in clinical HF trials involving drug and/or device therapies, in which the mortality figures are often deceptively low because the patients enrolled in trials are younger, are more stable clinically, and tend to be followed more closely clinically.

The role of gender and HF prognosis remains a controversial issue with respect to HF outcomes. Nonetheless, the aggregate data suggest that women with HF have a better overall prognosis than men.[3] However, women appear to have a greater degree of functional incapacity for the same degree of LV dysfunction and also have a higher prevalence of HF with a normal EF (Chap. 26). Controversy has also arisen regarding the impact of race on outcome, with higher mortality rates being reported in blacks in some but not all studies. In the United States, HF affects approximately 3 percent of blacks, whereas in the general population, the prevalence is about 2 percent.[8] Blacks with HF present at an earlier age and have more advanced LV dysfunction and a worse New York Heart Association (NYHA) class at the time of diagnosis. Although the reasons for these differences are not known, differences in HF cause might explain some of these observations. In the registry for the Studies on Left Dysfunction (SOLVD), 73 percent of whites had coronary heart disease as a cause for their HF compared with only 36 percent of black participants. On the other hand, 32 percent of blacks in the SOLVD registry had HF that was attributed to hypertension, with only 4 percent of whites having hypertension as a primary cause. When compared in the SOLVD registry, cardiovascular and total mortality were no different in the black and white cohorts, although the black cohort was younger and had a higher proportion of females than the white group.[9] There may also be additional socioeconomic factors that influence outcomes in black patients, such as geographic location and access to health care. Age is one of the strongest and most consistent predictors of adverse outcome in HF.[3]

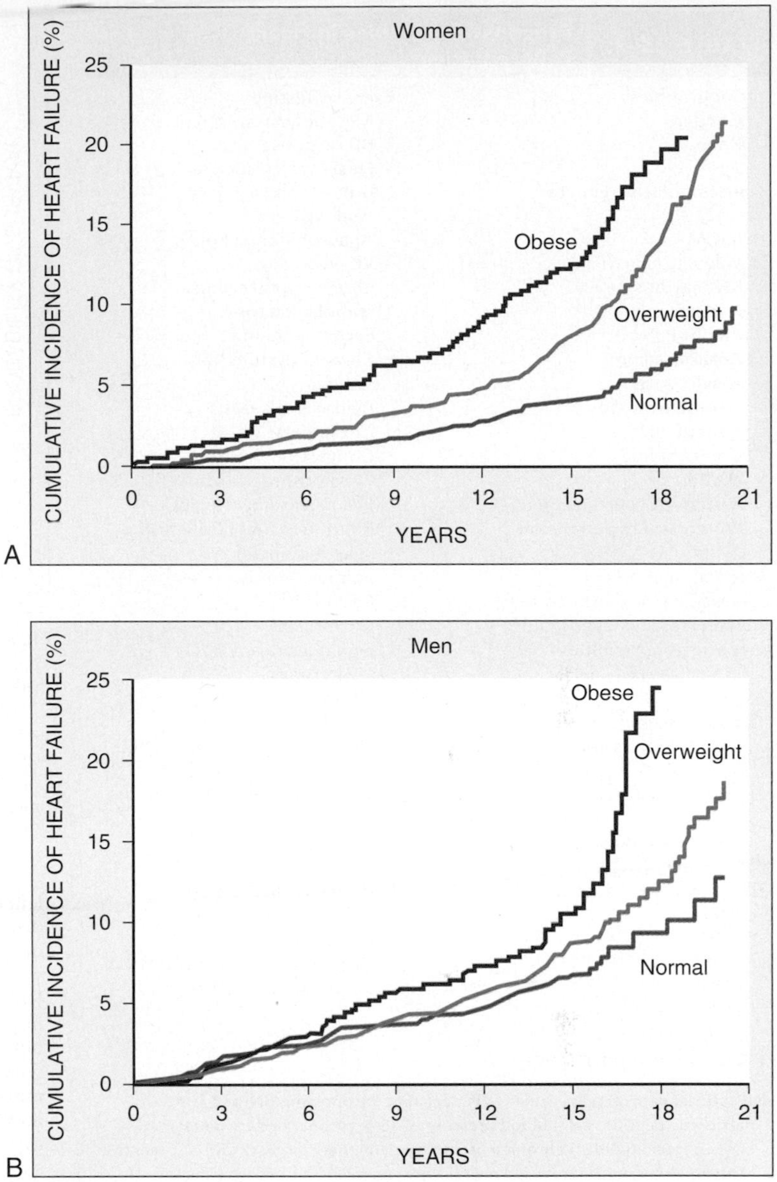

FIGURE 25–2 Cumulative incidence of heart failure in women **(A)** and men **(B)** according to category of body mass index at the baseline examination. The body mass index was 18.5 to 24.9 in normal subjects, 25.0 to 29.9 in overweight subjects, and 30.0 kg/m^2 or more in obese subjects. *(Modified from Kenchaiah S, Evans JC, Levy D, et al: Obesity and the risk of heart failure. N Engl J Med 347:305, 2002.)*

Many other factors have been associated with increased mortality in HF patients (Table 25-3). Most of the factors listed as outcome predictors have survived at least univariate analysis, with many standing out independently when multifactorial analysis techniques are applied. Nonetheless, it is extraordinarily difficult to determine which prognostic variable is most important in predicting an individual patient's outcome in clinical trials or, more importantly, during the daily management of an individual patient. To this end, a multivariate model for predicting the HF prognosis has a been developed and validated. The Seattle Heart Failure Model was derived by retrospectively investigating predictors of survival in HF patients in clinical trials.[10] A stepwise Cox proportional hazard model was used to develop a multivariate risk model, which identified age, gender, ischemic cause, NYHA class, ejection fraction, systolic blood pressure, potassium-sparing diuretic use, statin use, allopurinol use, hemoglobin value, lymphocyte count (percentage), uric acid, sodium, and cholesterol levels, and diuretic dose as significant predictors of survival. The Seattle Heart Failure Model provides an accurate estimate of 1-, 2-, and 3-year survival with the use of easily obtained clinical, pharmacological, device, and laboratory characteristics, and is accessible to all health care providers, with no charge, as an interactive web-based program (http://depts.washington.edu/shfm).

BIOMARKERS AND PROGNOSIS (see Chap. 23). The observation that the renin-angiotensin-aldosterone, adrenergic, and inflammatory systems are activated in HF (see Chap. 22) has prompted the examination of the relationships between various biochemical measurements and clinical outcomes (see Table 25-3). Strong inverse correlations have been reported between survival and plasma levels of norepinephrine (Fig. 25-3), renin, arginine vasopressin, aldosterone, atrial and brain natriuretic peptides (BNPs; see Fig. 23-2), endothelin-1, and inflammatory markers such as tumor necrosis factor (TNF), TNF receptors, C-reactive protein, and erythrocyte sedimentation rate. Markers of

TABLE 25–3 Prognostic Variables in Heart Failure Patients

Demographics	Exercise Testing
Gender	Metabolic assessment
Race	BP response
Age	Heart rate response
Causes of Heart Failure	6-min walk
CAD	Peak VO_2
IDCM	Anaerobic threshold
Valvular heart disease	VE/VCO_2
Myocarditis	Oxygen uptake slope
Hypertrophy	Metabolic Factors
Alcohol	Serum sodium
Anthracyclines	Thyroid dysfunction
Amyloidosis	Anemia
Hemochromatosis	Acidosis, alkalosis
Genetic factors	Chest x-ray
Comorbidities	Congestion
Diabetes	Cardiothoracic ratio
Systemic hypertension	Electrocardiogram (ECG)
Pulmonary hypertension	Rhythm (atrial fibrillation or arrhythmias)
Sleep apnea	Voltage
Obesity, cachexia (body mass)	QRS width
Renal insufficiency	QT interval
Hepatic abnormalities	Signal-averaged ECG (T wave alternans)
COPD	HR variability
Clinical Assessment	Biomarkers
NYHA class (symptoms)	NE, PRA, AVP, aldosterone
Syncope	ANP, BNP, endothelin-1
Angina pectoris	TNF, IL-1, IL-6, IL-10, CRP, ESR
Systolic vs. diastolic dysfunction	Cardiac troponins, hematocrit
Hemodynamic Factors	Endomyocardial Biopsy
LVEF	Inflammatory states
RVEF	Degree of fibrosis
PAP	Degree of cellular disarray
PCWP	Infiltrative processes
CI	
PAP-PCWP	
Exercise hemodynamics	

ANP = atrial natriuretic peptide; AVP = arginine vasopressin; BNP = brain natriuretic peptide; BP = blood pressure; CAD = coronary artery disease; CI = cardiac index; COPD = chronic obstructive pulmonary disease; CRP = C-reactive protein; ESR = erythrocyte sedimentation rate; IDCM = idiopathic dilated cardiomyopathy; IL = interleukin; LVEF = left ventricular ejection fraction; NE = norepinephrine; NYHA = New York Heart Association; PAP = pulmonary artery pressure; PAP-PCWP = gradient across lung; PCWP = pulmonary capillary wedge pressure; PRA = plasma renin activity; RVEF = right ventricular ejection fraction; TNF = tumor necrosis factor; VE = ventilatory exchange.

Modified from Young JB: The prognosis of heart failure. *In* Mann DL (ed): Heart Failure: A Companion to Braunwald's Heart Disease. Philadelphia, Elsevier, 2004, pp 489-506.

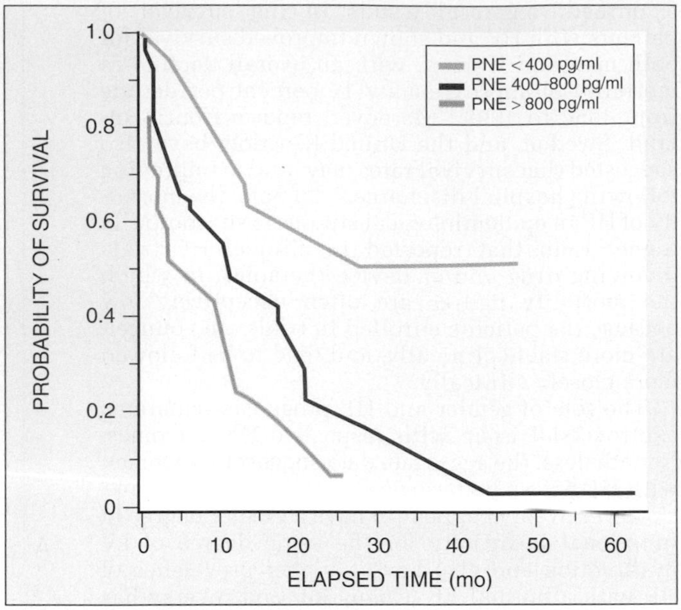

FIGURE 25–3 Life table analysis of survival, according to tercile, based on level of plasma norepinephrine (PNE). Activation of the sympathetic nervous system is a marker of impaired survival in heart failure. Group 1 (blue) (<400 pg/ml) contained 27 patients, group 2 (red) (400 to 800 pg/ml) had 49 patients, and group 3 (yellow) (>800 pg/ml) had 30 patients. The probability of survival in each group was significantly different from the probabilities in the other two groups. *(From Cohn JN, Levine TB, Olivari MT, et al: Plasma norepinephrine as a guide to prognosis in patients with chronic congestive heart failure. N Engl J Med 311:819, 1984.)*

oxidative stress, such as oxidized low-density lipoprotein and serum uric acid, have also been associated with worsening clinical status and impaired survival in patients with chronic HF. Levels of cardiac troponin T and I, sensitive markers of myocyte damage, may be elevated in patients with nonischemic and predict adverse cardiac outcomes. The association between low hemoglobin and hematocrit values and adverse HF outcomes has also long been recognized (Fig. 25-4)[11] but has garnered considerable attention after several recent reports illustrated the independent prognostic value of anemia in patients with HF with reduced or normal EF.[12]

Published estimates of the prevalence of anemia in HF patients vary widely, ranging from 4 to 50 percent, depending on the population studied and definition of anemia that is used [11] In general, the prevalence of anemia is significantly greater in patients with more advanced disease. Furthermore, the severity of anemia may contribute to the increasing severity of HF. In the Framingham study, a lower hematocrit value was a significant risk factor for the development of symptomatic HF.[1] Multiple reports from observational data bases and clinical trial populations have demonstrated a relationship between lower hemoglobin levels and impaired survival in patients.[11] However, it is unclear whether anemia is a cause of decreased survival or simply a marker of more advanced disease. The underlying cause for anemia in HF is likely multifactorial, including reduced sensitivity to erythropoietin receptors, the presence of a hematopoiesis inhibitor, and/or a defective iron supply for erythropoiesis given as possible explanations. Potential treatments for anemia include the use of red blood cell transfusions and treatment with erythropoietin analogues to increase red blood cell production. At present, the role for blood transfusions in patients with cardiovascular disease is controversial. Although a "transfusion threshold" for maintaining the hematocrit higher than 30 percent in patients with cardiovascular disease has generally been accepted, this clinical practice has been based more on expert opinion rather than on direct evidence that documents the efficacy of this form of therapy. Given the risks and costs of red blood cell transfusions and the evanescent benefits of blood transfusions in patients with a chronic anemia, along with the unclear benefit in HF patients, the routine use of blood transfusion cannot be recommended for treating the anemia that occurs in stable HF patients. Of note, several small studies have suggested benefit from the use of erythropoietin analogues and/or iron for treatment of mild anemia in HF.[11] However, there is concern that thromboembolic events may be increased with the former strategy. Treatment of anemic HF patients with the erythropoietin analogue darbepoetin alfa is undergoing further investigation in a large international study, Reduction of Events with Darbepoetin in Heart Failure (RED-HF).[12]

RENAL INSUFFICIENCY. Renal insufficiency is associated with poorer outcomes in patients with HF; however, it is uncertain whether renal impairment is a simply a marker for worsening HF or whether renal impairment might be causally linked to worsening HF. Although more common in patients hospitalized for HF, at least some degree of renal impairment is still present in about half of stable HF outpatients. Patients with renal hypoperfusion or intrinsic renal disease show an impaired response to diuretics and angiotensin-converting enzyme inhibitors (ACEIs) and are at increased risk of adverse effects during treatment with digitalis. In a recent meta-analysis, most HF patients were found to have some degree of renal impairment. These patients represented a high-risk group, with an approximately 50 percent increased relative mortality risk when compared with patients who had normal renal function.[13] Similar findings were observed in the Second Prospective Randomized study of Ibopamine on Mortality and Efficacy, in which impaired renal function was a stronger predictor of mortality than impaired LV function and NYHA class in patients with advanced HF (Fig. 25-5).[14] Thus, renal insufficiency is emerging as a strong independent predictor of adverse outcomes in HF patients.

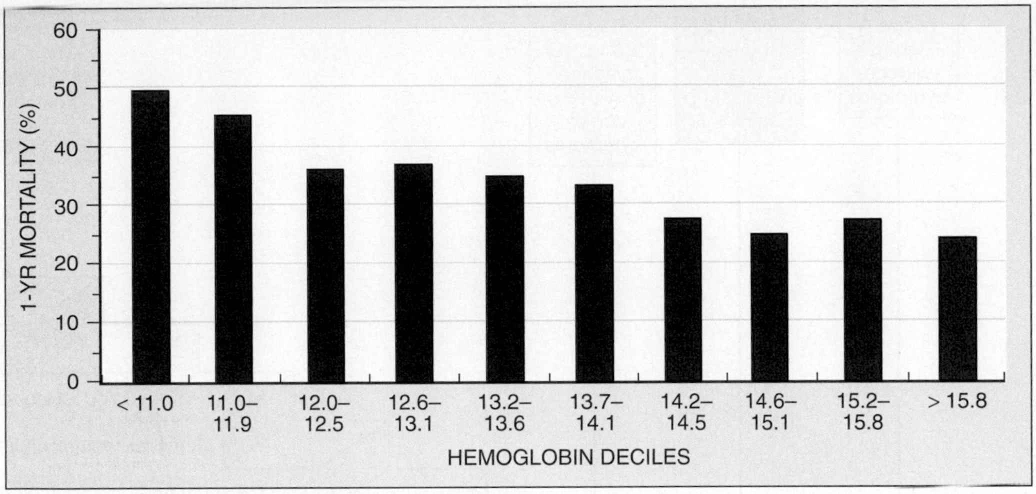

FIGURE 25–4 Anemia is associated with increased mortality in heart failure. In this single-center study, 1061 patients with advanced heart failure were evaluated for cardiac transplantation between 1983 and 1999. At initial presentation, the mean hemoglobin (Hb) level was 13.5 ± 1.9 gm/dl, and the Hb level ranged from 7.1 to 19.0 gm/dl. Lower hemoglobin levels were associated with greater symptoms, reduced exercise capacity, and impaired renal function. One-year mortality rates in the entire cohort divided by decile of Hb level are shown. *(From Horwich TB, Fonarow GC, Hamilton MA, et al: Anemia is associated with worse symptoms, greater impairment in functional capacity and a significant increase in mortality in patients with advanced heart failure. J Am Coll Cardiol 39:1780, 2002.)*

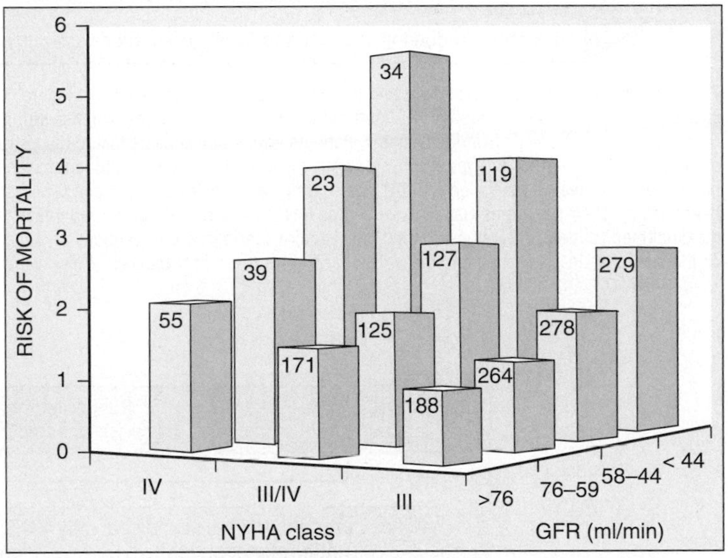

FIGURE 25–5 Effect of renal function on outcomes in heart failure patients. This three-dimensional bar graph shows the risk of mortality (vertical axis) as correlated with decreasing New York heart Association (NYHA) class (horizontal axis) and decreasing quartiles of glomerular filtration rate (GFR; diagonal axis). *(From Hillege HL, Girbes AR, de Kam PJ, et al: Renal function, neurohormonal activation, and survival in patients with chronic heart failure. Circulation 102:203, 2000.)*

APPROACH TO THE PATIENT

Stages of Heart Failure

HF should be viewed as a continuum that is comprised of four interrelated stages (Fig. 25-6).[15] Stage A includes patients who are at high risk for developing HF, but without structural heart disease or symptoms of HF (e.g., patients with diabetes or hypertension). Stage B includes patients who have structural heart disease but without symptoms of HF (e.g., patients with a previous myocardial infarction [MI] and asymptomatic LV dysfunction). Stage C includes patients who have structural heart disease who have developed symptoms of HF (e.g., patients with a previous MI with shortness of breath and fatigue). Stage D includes patients with refractory HF requiring special interventions (e.g., patients with refractory HF who are awaiting cardiac transplantation). A simplified algorithm for approaching patients with HF is illustrated in Figure 25-7. The diagnosis and clinical assessment of patients with HF with a reduced EF are discussed in detail in Chapter 23, and the diagnosis and management of patients with HF with a normal or preserved EF are discussed in detail in Chapter 26.

PATIENTS AT HIGH RISK FOR DEVELOPING HEART FAILURE (STAGE A). For patients at high risk of developing HF, every preventive effort should be made using standard practice guidelines to treat preventable conditions that are known to lead to HF, including hypertension (see Chap. 40), hyperlipidemia (see Chap. 45), and diabetes (see Chap. 43). In this regard, ACEIs are particularly useful in preventing HF in patients who have a history of atherosclerotic vascular disease, diabetes mellitus, or hypertension with associated cardiovascular risk factors.

POPULATION SCREENING. At present, there is limited information available to support the screening of broad populations to detect undiagnosed HF and/or asymptomatic LV dysfunction. One study has suggested that elevated levels of BNP (see Chap. 23) can be used as a cost-effective strategy for screening asymptomatic men and women older than 60 with an EF less than 40 percent.[16] However, screening general populations with BNP is not recommended at this time. Patients who are at very high risk of a developing cardiomyopathy (e.g., those with a strong family history of cardiomyopathy or those receiving cardiotoxic interventions; see Chap. 85) are appropriate targets for more aggressive screening, such as two-dimensional echocardiography to assess LV function. However, the routine periodic assessment of LV function in other patients is not currently recommended. Several sophisticated clinical scoring systems have been developed to screen for HF in population-based studies, including the Framingham Criteria,[17] which screens for HF on the basis of clinical criteria, and the National Health and Nutrition Survey (NHANES),[18] which uses self-reporting of symptoms to identify HF

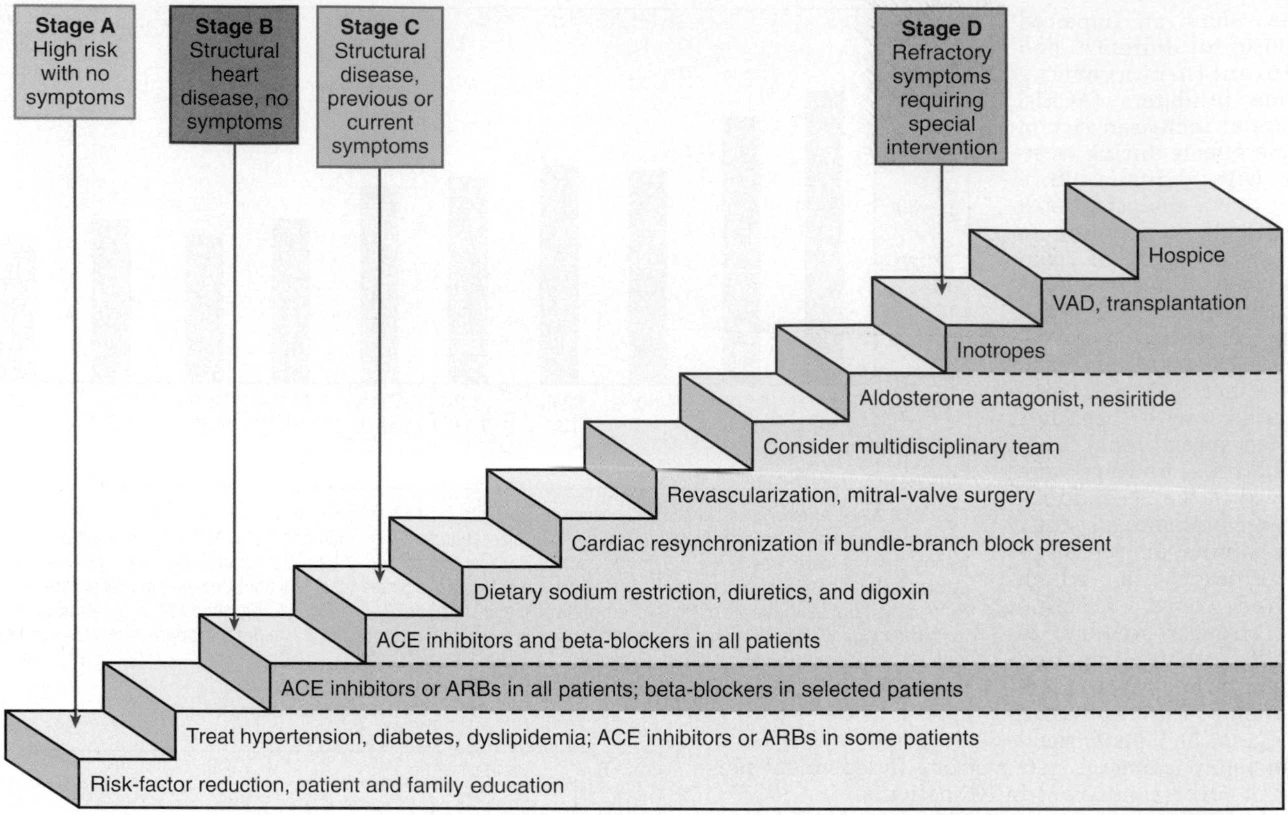

FIGURE 25–6 Stages of heart failure and treatment options for systolic heart failure. Patients with stage A heart failure are at high risk for heart failure but do not have structural heart disease or symptoms of heart failure. This group includes patients with hypertension, diabetes, coronary artery disease, previous exposure to cardiotoxic drugs, or a family hisotry of cardiomyopathy. Patients with stage B heart failure have structural heart disease but have no symptoms of heart failure. This group includes patients with left ventricular hypertrophy, previous myocardial infarction, left ventricular systolic dysfunction, or valvular heart disease, all of whom would be considered to have New York Heart Association (NYHA) class I symptoms. Patients with stage C heart failure have known structural heart disease and current or previous symptoms of heart failure. Their symptoms may be classified as NYHA class I, II, III, or IV. Patients with stage D heart fialure have refractory symptoms of heart failure at rest despite maximal medical therapy, are hospitalized, and require specialized interventions or hospice care. All such patients would be considered to have NYHA class IV symptoms. ACE = angiotensin-converting enzyme; ARB = angiotensin receptor blocker; VAD = ventricular assist device. *(Reprinted from Jessup M, Brozena S: Heart failure. N Eng J Med 348:2007-2018, 2003).*

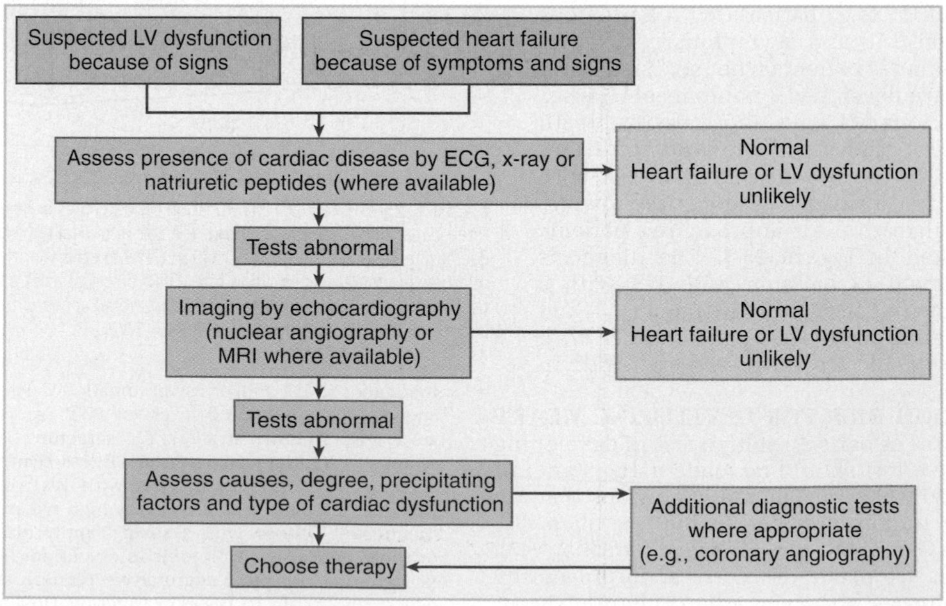

FIGURE 25–7 Relationship between cardiac dysfunction, symptomatic heart failure, and asymptomatic heart failure following appropriate treatment. ECG = electrocardiogram; LV = left ventricular; MRI = magnetic resonance imaging. *(Modified from Swedberg K, Cleland J, Dargie H, et al: Guidelines for the diagnosis and treatment of chronic heart failure: Executive summary [update 2005]: The Task Force for the Diagnosis and Treatment of Chronic Heart Failure of the European Society of Cardiology. Eur Heart J 26:1115, 2005.)*

TABLE 25-4 Diagnostic Criteria for Heart Failure (HF) in Population-Based Studies

Framingham Criteria*		
Major Criteria	*Minor Criteria*	*Major or Minor Criteria*
Paroxysmal nocturnal dyspnea or orthopnea	Ankle edema, night cough	Weight loss >4.5 kg in 5 days in response to treatment
Neck-vein distention	Dyspnea on exertion	
Rales	Hepatomegaly	
Cardiomegaly	Pleural effusion	
Acute pulmonary edema, S_3 gallop	Vital capacity decreased one third from maximal capacity	
Increased venous pressure (>16 cm H_2O)	Tachycardia (rate >120/min)	
Hepatojugular reflux		

NHANES Criteria†		
Category	*Criteria*	
History	Dyspnea	
	On level ground?	1
	On climbing?	1
	Do you stop for breath when walking at an ordinary pace?	2
	Do you stop for breath when after 100 yards on flat ground?	2
Physical examination	Heart rate	
	91-110 beats/min	1
	>110 beats/min	2
	Jugular venous pressure (>6 cm H_2O) alone	1
	plus hepatomegaly or edema	2
	Rales: basilar crackles	1
	Crackles: more than basilar crackles	2
Chest radiography	Upper zone flow redistribution	1
	Interstitial pulmonary edema	2
	Interstitial edema plus pleural fluid	3
	Alveolar pulmonary edema plus pleural fluid	3

*The diagnosis of HF using the Framingham criteria requires the simultaneous presence of at least two major criteria or one major criterion in conjunction with two minor criteria. Minor criteria are acceptable only if they cannot be attributed to another medical condition (e.g., pulmonary hypertension, chronic lung disease, cirrhosis, ascites, nephrotic syndrome).

†NHANES-1 criteria: diagnosis of HF if score ≥3 points.

NHANES = National Health and Nutrition Survey.

Modified from Francis GS, Wilson T: Clinical evaluation of heart failure. *In* Mann DL (ed): Heart Failure: A Companion to Braunwald's Heart Disease. Philadelphia, Elsevier, 2004, pp 507-526.

patients (Table 25-4). However, as discussed in Chapter 23, additional laboratory testing is usually necessary to make the diagnosis of HF definitively when these methodologies are used.

MANAGEMENT OF PATIENTS WITH SYMPTOMATIC AND ASYMPTOMATIC HEART FAILURE

TRANSIENT LV DYSFUNCTION. As noted in Chapter 22, the clinical syndrome of HF with reduced EF begins after an initial index event produces a decline in ejection performance of the heart. However, it is important to recognize that LV dysfunction may develop transiently in different clinical settings that may not invariably lead to the development of the clinical syndrome of HF. Figure 25-8 illustrates the important relationship between LV dysfunction (transient and sustained) and the clinical syndrome of HF (asymptomatic and symptomatic). LV dysfunction with pulmonary edema may develop transiently in patients with previously normal LV structure and function. Most commonly, this occurs postoperatively following cardiac surgery, in the setting of severe brain injury, or after a systemic infection. The general pathophysiological mechanism involved is some form of stunning of functional myocardium (see Chap. 48) or activation of proinflammatory cytokines that are capable of suppressing LV function (see Chap. 22). Emotional stress can also precipitate severe reversible LV dysfunction accompanied by chest pain, pulmonary edema, and cardiogenic shock in patients without coronary disease (tako-tsubo syndrome). In this setting, LV dysfunction is thought to occur secondarily to the deleterious effects of catecholamines following heightened sympathetic stimulation.[19] It is also important to note that exercise-induced LV dysfunction, usually caused by myocardial ischemia, may lead to symptoms by causing a rise in LV filling pressure and a fall in cardiac output in the absence of discernible LV dysfunction at rest. If LV dysfunction persists following the initial cardiac injury, patients may remain asymptomatic for a period of months to years; however, the weight of epidemiological and clinical evidence suggests that at some point. these patients will undergo the transition to overt symptomatic HF.

DEFINING THE APPROPRIATE STRATEGY. The main goals of treatment for HF are to reduce symptoms, prolong survival, improve the quality of life, and prevent disease progression. As will be discussed later, the current pharmacological, device, and surgical therapeutic armamentarium for the management of patients with a reduced EF permits health care providers to achieve each of these goals in the

TABLE 25–5 Pharmacological and Device Therapy in Patients with Chronic Heart Failure (HF)

Indication	ACE inhibitor	Angiotensin Receptor Blocker	Diuretic	Beta Blocker	Aldosterone Antagonist	Cardiac Glycoside	CRT	ICD
Asymptomatic LV dysfunction (NYHA Class I)	Indicated	If ACE intolerant	Not indicated	Post-MI Indicated*	Recent MI	With atrial fibrillation	Not indicated	Not indicated
Symptomatic HF (NYHA Class II)	Indicated	Indicated with or without ACE inhibitor	Indicated if fluid retention	Indicated	Recent MI	1. With atrial fibrillation 2. When improved from more severe HF in sinus rhythm	Not indicated	Indicated
Worsening HF (NYHA Class III or IV)	Indicated	Indicated with or without ACE inhibitor	Indicated, combination of diuretics	Indicated (under specialist's care)	Indicated	Indicated	Indicated if QRS >0.12†	Indicated
End-stage HF (NYHA Class IV)	Indicated	Indicated with or without ACE inhibitor	Indicated, combination of diuretics	Indicated (under specialist's care)	Indicated	Indicated	Indicated if QRS >0.12†	Indicated‡

*Represents expert opinion.[15]

†Patients must be in sinus rhythm.

‡May be indicated in some patients with a prolonged life expectancy.

ACE = angiotensin-converting enzyme; CRT = cardiac resynchronization therapy; ICD = implantable cardioverter-defibrillator; LV = left ventricular; MI = myocardial infarction; NYHA = New York Heart Association.

Modified from Swedberg K, Cleland J, Dargie H, et al: Guidelines for the diagnosis and treatment of chronic heart failure: Executive summary (update 2005): The Task Force for the Diagnosis and Treatment of Chronic Heart Failure of the European Society of Cardiology. Eur Heart J 26:1115, 2005.

great majority of patients. As shown in Table 25-5, once patients have developed structural heart disease (stages B through D), the choice of therapy for patients with HF with a reduced EF depends on their NYHA functional classification (Table 25-6). Although this classification system is notoriously subjective and has large interobserver variability, it has withstood the test of time and continues to be widely applied to patients with HF. For patients who have developed LV systolic dysfunction but who remain asymptomatic (Class I), the goal should be to slow disease progression by blocking neurohormonal systems that lead to cardiac remodeling (see Chap. 22). For patients who have developed symptoms (Classes II to IV), the primary goal should be to alleviate fluid retention, lessen disability, and reduce the risk of further disease progression and death. As will be discussed subsequently, these goals generally require a strategy that combines diuretics (to control salt and water retention) with neurohormonal interventions (to minimize cardiac remodeling).

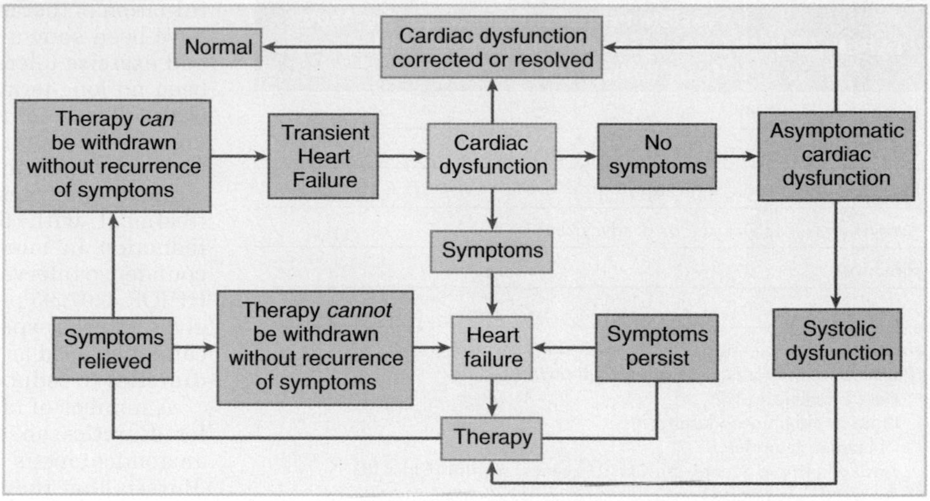

FIGURE 25–8 Algorithm for the diagnosis of heart failure or left ventricular dysfunction. *(Modified from Swedberg K, Cleland J, Dargie H, et al: Guidelines for the diagnosis and treatment of chronic heart failure: Executive summary (update 2005): The Task Force for the Diagnosis and Treatment of Chronic Heart Failure of the European Society of Cardiology. Eur Heart J 26:1115, 2005.)*

TABLE 25–6 New York Heart Association (NYHA) Classification of Cardiac Disease

Functional Capacity	Objective Assessment
Class I	Patients with cardiac disease but without resulting limitation of physical activity. Ordinary physical activity does not cause undue fatigue, palpitations, dyspnea, or anginal pain.
Class II	Patients with cardiac disease resulting in slight limitation of physical activity. They are comfortable at rest. Ordinary physical activity results in fatigue, palpitation, dyspnea, or anginal pain.
Class III	Patients with cardiac disease resulting in marked limitation of physical activity. They are comfortable at rest. Less than ordinary activity causes fatigue, palpitation, dyspnea, or anginal pain.
Class IV	Patients with cardiac disease resulting in inability to carry on any physical activity without discomfort. Symptoms of heart failure or the anginal syndrome may be present, even at rest. If any physical activity is undertaken, discomfort is increased.

Modified from New-York Heart Association: Diseases of the Heart and Blood Vessels, Nomenclature and Criteria for Diagnosis. 6th ed. Boston, Little Brown, 1964, p 114.

General Measures

Identification and correction of the condition(s) responsible for the cardiac structural and/or functional abnormalities are critical (see Table 25-2), insofar as some of the conditions that provoke LV structural and functional abnormalities are potentially treatable and/or reversible. Furthermore, clinicians should aim to carry out aggressive screening for and treatment of comorbidities such as hypertension and diabetes that are believed to underlie the structural heart disease. In addition to searching for reversible causes and comorbidities that contribute to the development of HF, it is equally important to identify factors that lead to worsening HF in stable patients (Table 25-7). Among the most common causes of acute decompensation in a previously stable patient are dietary indiscretion and inappropriate reduction of HF therapy, either from patient self-discontinuation of medication or from physician withdrawal of effective pharmacotherapy (e.g., because of concern over azotemia). HF patients should be advised to stop smoking and to limit alcohol consumption to two drinks per day in men or one drink per day in women. Patients suspected of having an alcohol-induced cardiomyopathy should be advised to abstain from alcohol consumption indefinitely. Excessive temperature extremes and heavy physical exertion should be avoided. Certain drugs are know to make HF worse and should also be avoided. For example, nonsteroidal antiinflammatory drugs (NSAIDs), including cyclooxygenase 2 (COX-2) inhibitors, are not recommended in patients with chronic HF because the risk of renal failure and fluid retention is markedly increased in the setting of reduced renal function and/or ACEI use. Patients should be advised to weigh themselves on a regular basis to monitor weight gain and alert a health care provider or adjust their diuretic dose in the case of a sudden unexpected weight gain of more than 3 or 4 pounds over a 3-day period. Although there is no documented evidence of the effects of immunization in HF patients, they are at high risk of developing pneumococcal pneumonia and influenza. Accordingly, clinicians should consider recommending influenza and pneumococcal vaccines to their HF patient to prevent respiratory infections. It is equally important to educate the patient and family about HF and the importance of a proper diet, as well the importance of compliance with the medical regimen. Supervision of outpatient care by a specially trained nurse or physician assistant and/or specialized HF clinics have all been shown to be helpful, particularly in patients with advanced disease (see later, "Disease Management").

ACTIVITY. Although heavy physical labor is not recommend for HF patients, routine and modest exercise has been shown to be beneficial in patients with NYHA Class I to III HF. For euvolemic patients, regular isotonic exercise such as walking or riding a stationary bicycle ergometer, as tolerated, should be strongly encouraged. Some trials of exercise training have led to encouraging results with reduced symptoms, increased exercise capacity by as much as 15 to 20 percent, and improved quality and quantity of life. The benefits of weight loss by restriction of caloric intake have not been clearly established.

TABLE 25-7	Possible Precipitating Factors for Acute Decompensation in Patients with Chronic Heart Failure (HF)
Dietary indiscretion	
Inappropriate reduction in HF medications	
Myocardial ischemia, infarction	
Arrhythmias (tachycardia or bradycardia)	
Infection	
Anemia	
Initiation of medications that worsen the symptoms of HF Calcium antagonists (verapamil, diltiazem) Beta blockers Nonsteroidal antiinflammatory drugs Thiazolidinediones Antiarrhythmic agents—all Class I agents, sotalol (Class III) Anti-TNF antibodies	
Alcohol consumption	
Pregnancy	
Worsening hypertension	
Acute valvular insufficiency	

TNF = tumor necrosis factor.
From Mann DL: Heart failure and cor pulmonale. *In* Kasper DL, Braunwald E., Fauci AS, et al (eds): Harrison's Principles of Internal Medicine. 17th ed. New York, McGraw-Hill, 2007 (in press).

DIET. Dietary restriction of sodium (2 to 3 gm daily) is recommended in all patients with the clinical syndrome of HF and preserved or depressed EF. Further restriction (less than 2 gm daily) may be considered in moderate to severe HF. Fluid restriction is generally unnecessary unless the patient is hyponatremic (sodium less than 130 mEq/liter), which may develop because of activation of the renin-angiotensin system, excessive secretion of arginine vasopressin (AVP), or loss of salt in excess of water from prior diuretic use. Fluid restriction (less than 2 liters/day) should be considered in hyponatremic patients (sodium less than 130 mEq/liter), or for those patients whose fluid retention is difficult to control despite high doses of diuretics and sodium restriction. Caloric supplementation is recommended for patients with advanced HF and unintentional weight loss or muscle wasting (cardiac cachexia); however, anabolic steroids are not recommended for these patients because of the potential problems with volume retention. The use of dietary supplements (nutraceuticals) should be avoided in the management of symptomatic HF because of the lack of proven benefit and the potential for significant interactions with proven HF therapies.

Management of Fluid Status

Many of the clinical manifestations of HF result from excessive salt and water retention, which leads to an inappropriate volume expansion of the intravascular compartment. Although both digitalis and low doses of ACEIs enhance urinary sodium excretion, few volume-overloaded HF patients can maintain proper sodium balance without the use of diuretic drugs. Indeed, attempts to substitute ACEIs for diuretics have been shown to lead to pulmonary edema and peripheral congestion. In short-term clinical trials, diuretic therapy has led to a reduction in jugular venous pressures, pulmonary congestion, peripheral edema, and body weight, all of which were observed within days of initiation of therapy. In intermediate-term studies, diuretics have been shown to improve cardiac function, symptoms, and exercise tolerance in HF patients.[20] To date, there have been no long-term studies of diuretic therapy in HF; thus, their effects on morbidity and mortality are not clearly known. Although retrospective analyses of clinical trials have suggested that diuretic use is associated with worse clinical outcomes,[21] a meta-analysis has suggested that treatment with diuretic therapy produces a significant reduction in mortality (odds ratio [OR], 0.24; 95 percent confidence interval [CI], 0.07 to 0.83; $P = 0.02$) and worsening HF (OR, 0.07; 95 percent CI, 0.01 to 0.52; $P = 0.01$).[20] However, given the retrospective nature of this review, this analysis cannot be used as formal evidence to recommend the use of diuretics to reduce HF mortality.

A number of classification schemes have been proposed for diuretics on the basis of their mechanism of action, anatomical locus of action within the nephron, and form of diuresis that they elicit (solute versus water diuresis) The most common classification for diuretics uses an admixture of chemical (e.g., thiazide diuretic), site of action (e.g., loop diuretics), and clinical outcomes (e.g., potassium-sparing diuretics). The loop diuretics increase sodium excretion by up to 20 to 25 percent of the filtered load of sodium, enhance free water clearance, and maintain their efficacy unless renal function is severely impaired. In contrast, the thiazide diuretics increase the fractional excretion of sodium to only 5 to 10 percent of the filtered load, tend to decrease free water clearance, and lose their effectiveness in patients with impaired renal function (creatinine clearance less than 40 ml/min). Consequently, the loop diuretics have emerged as the preferred diuretic agents for use in most patients with HF. Diuretics that induce a water diuresis (aquaretics) include demeclocycline, lithium, and vasopressin V_2 receptor antagonists, each of which inhibits the action of AVP on the collecting duct through different mechanisms, thereby increasing free water clearance. Drugs that cause solute diuresis are subdivided into two types—osmotic diuretics, which are nonresorbable solutes that osmotically retain water and other solutes in the tubular lumen, and drugs that selectively inhibit ion transport pathways across tubular epithelia, which constitute most potent, clinically useful diuretics. The classes of diuretics and individual class members are listed in Table 25-8 and their renal sites of action are depicted in Figure 25-9.

Loop Diuretics

The agents classified as loop diuretics, including furosemide, bumetanide, and torsemide, act by reversibly inhibiting the Na^+-K^+-$2Cl^-$ symporter (cotransporter) on the apical membrane of epithelial cells in the thick ascending loop of Henle (see Fig. 25-9). Because furosemide, bumetanide, and torsemide are bound extensively to plasma proteins, delivery of these drugs to the tubule by filtration is limited. However, these drugs are secreted efficiently by the organic acid transport system in the proximal tubule and thereby gain access to their binding sites on the Na^+-K^+-$2Cl^-$ symporter in the luminal membrane of the ascending limb. Thus, the efficacy of loop diuretics is dependent on sufficient renal plasma blood flow and proximal tubular secretion to deliver these agents to their site of action. Probenecid shifts the plasma concentration-response curve for furosemide to the right by competitively inhibiting furosemide excretion by the organic acid transport system. The bioavailability of furosemide ranges from 40 to 70 percent of the oral dose. In contrast, the oral bioavailability of bumetanide and torsemide exceeds 80 percent. Accordingly, these agents may be more effective in advanced HF, albeit at considerably greater cost. Agents in a second functional class of loop diuretics, such as ethacrynic acid, exhibit a

TABLE 25–8 Diuretics for Treating Fluid Retention in Chronic Heart Failure*

Drug	Initial Daily Dose(s)	Maximum Total Daily Dosage	Duration of Action (hr)
Loop diuretic			
Bumetanide	0.5 to 1.0 mg once or twice	10 mg	4 to 6
Furosemide	20 to 40 mg once or twice	600 mg	6 to 8
Torsemide	10 to 20 mg once	200 mg	12 to 16
Thiazide diuretic			
Chlorothiazide	250 to 500 mg once or twice	1000 mg	6 to 12
Chlorthalidone	12.5 to 25 mg once	100 mg	24 to 72
Hydrochlorothiazide	25 mg once or twice	200 mg	6 to 12
Indapamide	2.5 mg once	5 mg	36
Metolazone	5 mg once	20 mg	12 to 24
Potassium-sparing diuretic			
Amiloride	12.5 to 25 mg once	20 mg	24
Triamterene	50 to 75 mg twice	200 mg	7 to 9
AVP antagonist†			
Satavaptan	25 mg once	50 mg once	NS
Tolvaptan	30 mg once	60 mg once	NS
Lixivaptan	125 mg twice	250 mg twice	NS
Conivaptan (IV)	20-mg IV loading dose, followed by 20 mg continuous IV infusion/day	40 IV infusion/day	7 to 9
Sequential nephron blockade			
Metolazone	2.5 to 10 mg once plus loop diuretic		
Hydrochlorothiazide	25 to 100 mg once or twice plus loop diuretic		
Chlorothiazide (IV)	500 to 1000 mg once plus loop diuretic		

*Unless indicated, all dosages are for oral diuretics.

†As of 2007, this class of agents is not FDA-approved for the management of patients with heart failure.

NS = not specified.

Modified from Hunt SA, Abraham WT, Chin MH, JL, et al: ACC/AHA 2005 Guideline Update for the Diagnosis and Management of Chronic Heart Failure in the Adult: A report of the American College of Cardiology/American Heart Association Task Force on Practice Guidelines. Circulation 112:e154, 2005.

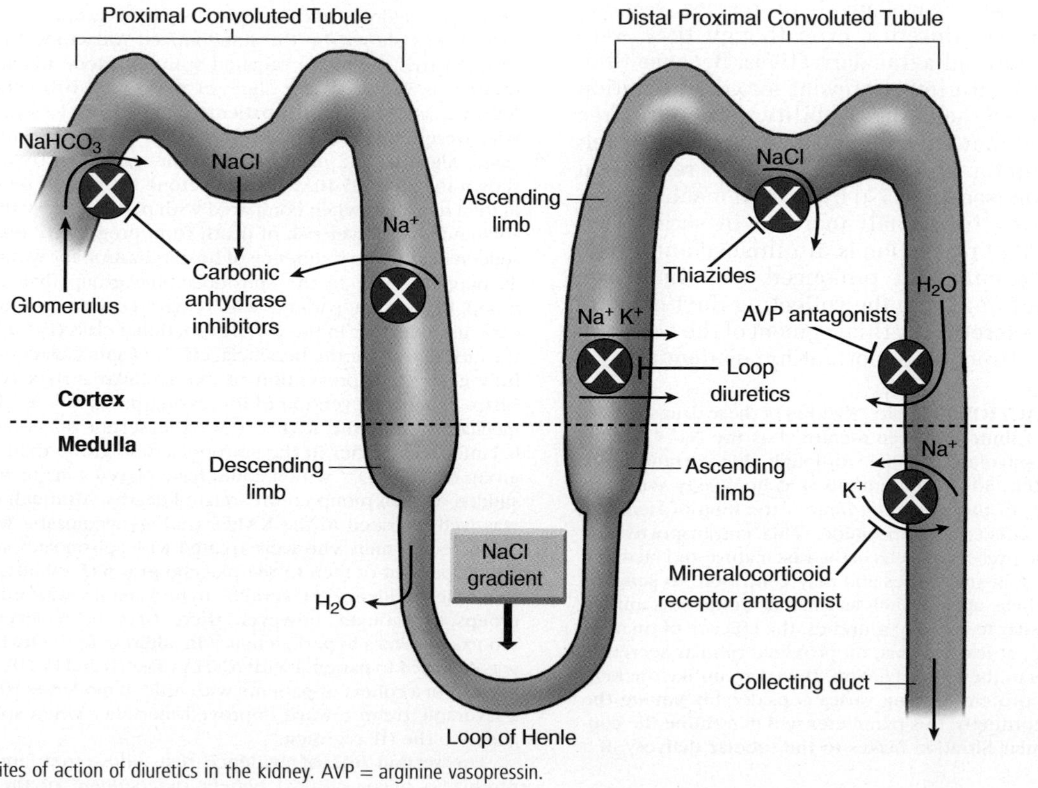

FIGURE 25–9 Sites of action of diuretics in the kidney. AVP = arginine vasopressin.

 slower onset of action and have delayed and only partial reversibility.

MECHANISMS OF ACTION. Loop diuretics are believed to improve symptoms of congestion by several mechanisms. First, loop diuretics reversibly bind to and reversibly inhibit the action of the Na^+-K^+-$2Cl^-$ cotransporter, thereby preventing salt transport in the thick ascending loop of Henle. Inhibition of this symporter also inhibits Ca^{2+} and Mg^{2+} resorption by abolishing the transepithelial potential difference that is the driving force for absorption of these cations. By inhibiting the concentration of solute within the medullary interstitium, these drugs also reduce the driving force for water resorption in the collecting duct, even in the presence of AVP (see Chap. 22). The decreased resorption of water by the collecting duct results in the production of urine that is nearly isotonic with plasma. The increase in delivery of Na^+ and water to the distal nephron segments also markedly enhances K^+ excretion, particularly in the presence of elevated aldosterone levels.

Loop diuretics also exhibit several characteristic effects on intracardiac pressure and systemic hemodynamics. Furosemide acts as a venodilator and reduces right atrial and pulmonary capillary wedge pressures within minutes when given intravenously (0.5 to 1.0 mg/kg). Similar evidence, although not as extensive, has been found for bumetanide and torsemide. This initial improvement in hemodynamics may be secondary to the release of vasodilatory prostaglandins, insofar as studies in animals and humans have demonstrated that the venodilatory actions of furosemide are inhibited by indomethacin. There have also been reports of an acute rise in systemic vascular resistance in response to loop diuretics, which has been attributed to the transient activation of the systemic or intravascular renin-angiotensin system (RAS). The potentially deleterious rise in LV afterload reinforces the importance of initiating vasodilator therapy with diuretics in patients with acute pulmonary edema and adequate blood pressure (see Chap. 24).

Thiazide and Thiazide-like Diuretics

The benzothiadiazides, also known as thiazide diuretics, were the initial class of drugs synthesized to block the Na^+-Cl^- transporter in the distal nephron. Subsequently, drugs that share similar pharmacological properties became known as thiazide-like diuretics, even though they were technically not benzothiadiazine derivatives. Because thiazide and thiazide-like diuretics prevent maximal dilution of urine, they decrease the kidney's ability to increase free water clearance, and may therefore contribute to the development of hyponatremia. Thiazides increase Ca^{2+} resorption in the distal nephron (see Fig. 25-7) by several mechanisms, occasionally resulting in a small increase in serum Ca^{2+} levels. In contrast, Mg^{2+} resorption is diminished and hypomagnesemia may occur with prolonged use. Increased delivery of NaCl and fluid into the collecting duct directly enhances K^+ and H^+ secretion by this segment of the nephron, which may lead to clinically important hypokalemia.

MECHANISMS OF ACTION. The site of action of these drugs within the distal convoluted tubule has been identified as the Na^+-Cl^- symporter of the distal convoluted tubule. Although this cotransporter shares an approximately 50 percent amino acid homology with the Na^+-K+-$2Cl^-$ symporter of the ascending limb of the loop of Henle, it is insensitive to the effects of furosemide. This cotransporter (or related isoforms) is also present on cells in the vasculature and on many cell types in other organs and tissues and may contribute to some of the other actions of these agents, such as their usefulness as antihypertensive agents. Similar to the loop diuretics, the efficacy of thiazide diuretics is dependent, at least in part, on proximal tubular secretion to deliver these agents to their site of action. However, unlike the loop diuretics, the plasma protein binding varies considerably among the thiazide diuretics; accordingly, this parameter will determine the contribution that glomerular filtration makes to the tubular delivery of a specific diuretic.

Mineralocorticoid Receptor Antagonists

Mineralocorticoids, such as aldosterone, cause retention of salt and water and increase the excretion of K^+ and H^+ by binding to specific mineralocorticoid receptors. Early studies indicated that spirolactones block the effects of mineralocorticoids, which subsequently led to the development of specific antagonists for the mineralocorticoid receptor. Spironolactone and eplerenone are synthetic mineralocorticoid receptors that act on the distal nephron to inhibit Na^+ and K^+ excretion at the site of aldosterone action (see Fig. 25-9). Spironolactone has antiandrogenic and progesterone-like effects, which may cause gynecomastia or impotence in men and menstrual irregularities in women. To overcome these side effects, eplerenone was developed by replacing the 17-alpha-thioacetyl group of spironolactone with a carbomethoxy group. As a result of this modification, eplerenone has greater selectivity for the mineralocorticoid receptor than for steroid receptors, and has fewer sex hormone side effects than spironolactone. Eplerenone is further distinguished from spironolactone by its shorter half-life and the fact that it does not have any active metabolites. Although spironolactone and eplerenone are both weak diuretics, clinical trials have shown that both these agents have profound effects on cardiovascular morbidity and mortality (Fig. 25-10) by virtue of their ability to antagonize the deleterious effects of aldosterone in the cardiovascular system (see Chap. 22). Hence, these agents are used in patients with HF more for their ability to antagonize the renin-angiotensin-aldosterone system (see later) than for their diuretic properties.

MECHANISMS OF ACTION. Spironolactone (Table 25-9) and its active metabolite, canrenone, competitively inhibit the binding of aldosterone to mineralocorticoid or type I receptors in many tissues, including epithelial cells of the distal convoluted tubule and collecting duct. These cytosolic receptors are ligand-dependent transcription factors, which on binding of the ligand (e.g., aldosterone) translocate to the nucleus, where they bind to hormone response elements present in the promoter of some genes, including several involved in vascular and myocardial fibrosis, inflammation, and calcification. The first evidence that aldosterone antagonists could produce a major clinical benefit was shown by the Randomized Aldactone Evaluation Study (RALES) trial,[22] which evaluated spironolactone (25 mg/day initially, titrated to 50 mg/day for signs of worsening HF) versus placebo in NYHA Class III or IV HF patients with a LVEF less than 35 percent, who were being treated with an ACEI, a loop diuretic and, in most cases, digoxin. The primary endpoint was death from all causes. As shown in Figure 25-10A, spironolactone led to a 30 percent reduction in total mortality when compared with placebo ($P = 0.001$), which was attributed to a lower risk of death from progressive pump failure and sudden death. The frequency of hospitalization for worsening was also 35 percent lower in the spironolactone group than in the placebo group. In addition, patients who received spironolactone had a significant improvement in the NYHA functional class ($P < 0.001$). Although the mechanism for the beneficial effect of spironolactone has not been fully elucidated, prevention of extracellular matrix remodeling (see Chap. 22) and prevention of increasing potassium levels are plausible mechanisms. In the RALES trial, the serum potassium levels were 0.3 mEq/liter higher in the spironolactone group than in the placebo group ($P = 0.001$),[22] which could have played a major role in reducing sudden or even pump failure–related deaths. Although spironolactone was well tolerated in the RALES trial, gynecomastia was reported in 10 percent of men who were treated with spironolactone as compared with 1 percent of men in the placebo group ($P < 0.001$). In the RALES trial, the incidence of serious hyperkalemia was minimal in both groups of patients, however, there have been several subsequent reports of severe hyperkalemia.[23] In addition to the RALES trial, which was confined to patients with NYHA Class III and IV HF, a retrospective analysis of a cohort of patients with mild to moderate HF has suggested a favorable trend toward improved mortality when spironolactone is added to the HF regimen.[12]

The second line of evidence that aldosterone antagonists could produce a major clinical benefit independent of the their diuretic effects came from the Eplerenone Post-Acute Myocardial Infarction Heart Failure Efficacy and Survival Study (EPHESUS; see Fig. 25-10B), a double-blind, placebo-controlled study that evaluated the effect of eplerenone on morbidity and mortality in patients with acute myocar-

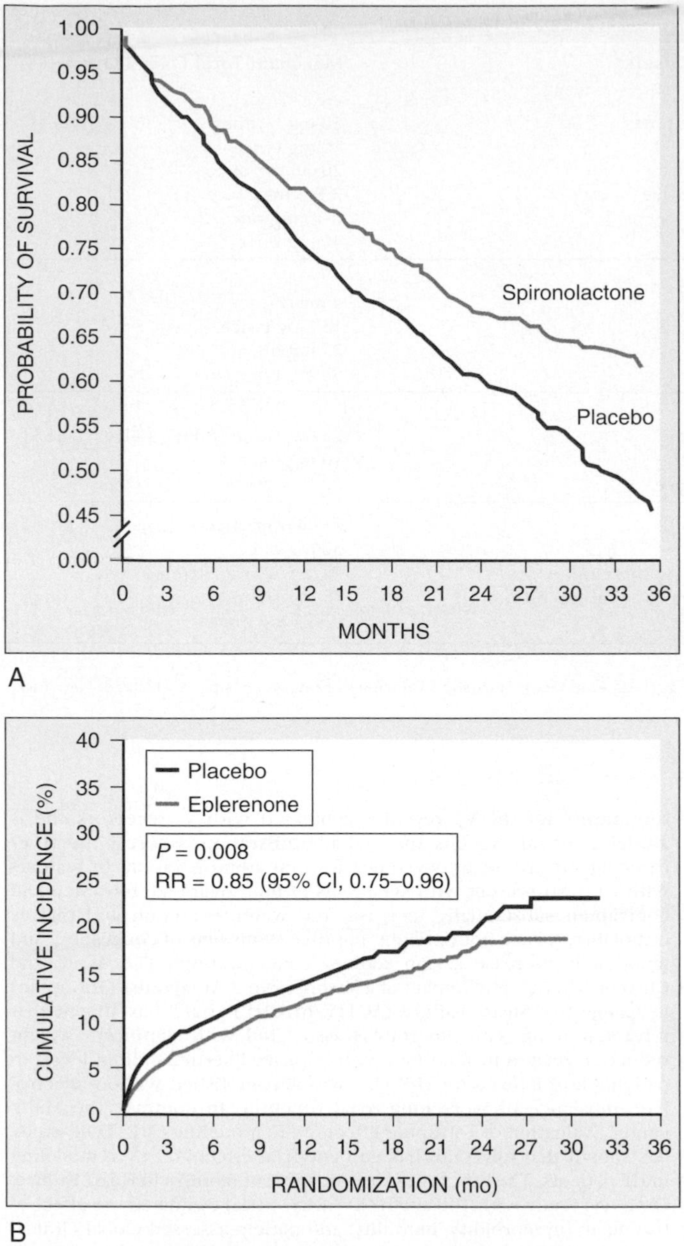

FIGURE 25–10 Kaplan-Meier analysis of the probability of survival among patients in the placebo and treatment groups in the RALES trial **(A)** with spironolactone and the EPHESUS **(B)** trial using eplerenone. EPHESUS = Eplerenone Post-Acute Myocardial Infarction Heart Failure Efficacy and Survival Study; RALES = Randomized Aldactone Evaluation Study; RR = relative risk. *(Modified from Pitt B, Zannad F, Remme WJ, et al: The effect of spironolactone on morbidity and mortality in patients with severe heart failure. Randomized Aldactone Evaluation Study Investigators. N Engl J Med 341:709, 1999; and Pitt B, Remme W, Zannad F, et al: Eplerenone Post-Acute Myocardial Infarction Heart Failure Efficacy and Survival Study Investigators: Eplerenone, a selective aldosterone blocker, in patients with left ventricular dysfunction after myocardial infarction. N Engl J Med 348:1309, 2003.)*

dial infarction complicated by LV dysfunction and HF. Patients were randomly assigned to eplerenone (25 mg/day initially, titrated to a maximum of 50 mg/day) or placebo in addition to optimal medical therapy. The primary endpoints were death from any cause and death from cardiovascular causes or hospitalization for HF, acute myocardial infarction, stroke, or ventricular arrhythmia. As shown in Figure 25-10B, there was a significant decrease in all-cause death in patients who were randomized to receive eplerenone (relative risk [RR], 0.83; 95 percent CI, 0.72 to 0.94; $P = 0.005$). The rate of the other primary endpoint, death from cardiovascular causes or hospitalization for cardiovascular events, was reduced by eplerenone (RR, 0.87; 95 percent CI, 0.79 to 0.95; $P = 0.002$), as was the secondary endpoint of death from any cause or any hospitalization. There was also a reduction in the rate of sudden death from cardiac causes.[24] The role of eplerenone in mild to moderate HF is being examined prospectively in the Eplerenone in Mild Patients Hospitalization and Survival Study in Heart Failure (EMPHASIS) trial.[12]

Potassium-Sparing Diuretics

Triamterene and amiloride are referred to as potassium-sparing diuretics. These agents share the common property of causing a mild increase in NaCl excretion, as well as having antikaluretic properties. Amiloride is a pyrazinoyl guanidine derivative, whereas triamterene is a pteridine derivative. Both drugs are organic bases that are transported into the proximal tubule, where they block Na^+ reabsorption in the late distal tubule and collecting duct. However, because Na^+ retention occurs in more proximal nephron sites in HF, neither amiloride nor triamterene is effective in achieving a net negative Na^+ balance when given alone in HF patients. Both amiloride and triamterene appear to share a similar mechanism of action. Considerable evidence has suggested that amiloride blocks Na^+ channels in the luminal membrane of the principal cells in the late distal tubule and collecting duct, perhaps by competing with Na^+ for negatively charged areas within the pore of the Na^+ channel. Blockade of Na^+ channels leads to hyperpolarization of the luminal membrane of the tubule, which reduces the electrochemical gradient that provides the driving force for K^+ secretion into the lumen. Amiloride and its congeners also inhibit Na^+-H^+ antiporters in renal epithelial cells and in many other cell types, but only at concentrations that are higher than those used clinically.

Carbonic Anhydrase Inhibitors

The zinc metalloenzyme carbonic anhydrase plays an essential role in the $NaHCO_3$ resorption and acid secretion in the proximal tubule. Although weak diuretics, carbonic anhydrase inhibitors (see Table 25-8) such as acetazolamide potently inhibit carbonic anhydrase, resulting in almost complete loss of $NaHCO_3$ resorption in the proximal tubule. The use of these agents in patients with HF is confined to temporary administration to correct the metabolic alkalosis that occurs as a contraction phenomenon in response to the administration of other diuretics. When used repeatedly, these agents can lead to metabolic acidosis as well as severe hypokalemia.

Vasopressin Antagonists

As discussed in Chapter 22, increased circulating levels of the pituitary hormone AVP contribute to the increased systemic vascular resistance and positive water balance in HF patients. The cellular effects of AVP are mediated by interactions with three types of receptors: V_{1a}, V_{1b}, and V_2 (see Chap. 22). Briefly, V_{1a} receptors mediate vasoconstriction, platelet aggregation, and stimulation of myocardial growth factors, V_{1b} modulates adrenocorticotropic hormone (ACTH) secretion from the anterior pituitary, and the V_2 receptor mediates antidiuretic effects by stimulating adenyl cyclase to increase the rate of insertion of water-containing channel vesicles (aquaporins) into the apical membrane (Fig. 25-11). Selective V_{1a} antagonists block the vasoconstricting effects of AVP in peripheral vascular smooth muscle cells, whereas V_2 selective receptor antagonists inhibit recruitment of aquaporin water channels into the apical membranes of collecting duct epithelial cells, thereby reducing the ability of the collecting duct to resorb water (see Fig. 25-11). Combined V_{1a}-V_2 antagonists lead to a decrease in systemic vascular resistance and prevent the dilutional hyponatremia that occurs in HF patients.[25]

TABLE 25–9 Drugs for the Prevention and Treatment for Chronic Heart Failure

Type of Drug	Initial Daily Dose(s)	Maximam Total Daily Dosage
Angiotensin-Converting Enzyme Inhibitor		
Captopril	6.25 mg three times	50 mg 3 times
Enalapril	2.5 mg twice	10 mg twice
Lisinopril	2.5-5.0 mg once	20-35 mg once
Ramipril	1.25-2.5 mg twice	2.5-5 mg twice
Perindopril	2 mg once	8-16 mg once
Fosinopril	5-10 mg once	40 mg once
Angiotensin Receptor Blocker		
Trandolapril	0.5 mg once	4 mg once
Valsartan	40 mg twice	160 mg twice
Candesartan	4 mg once	32 mg once
Losartan	12.5 mg once	50 mg once
Beta Receptor Blocker		
Carvedilol	3.125 mg twice	25 mg twice (50 mg twice if >85 kg)
Bisoprolol	1.25 mg twice	10 mg once
Metoprolol succinate CR/XL	12.5-25 mg once	200 mg once
Spironolactone	12.5-25 mg once	25-50 mg once
Eplerenone	25 mg once	50 mg once
Combination of hydralazine-isosorbide dinitrate	10-25 mg/10 mg three times	75 mg/40 mg 3 times
Fixed dose of hydralazine-isosorbide dinitrate	37.5 mg/20 mg (one tablet) 3 times	75 mg/40 mg (two tablets) 3 times
Digoxin	0.125 mg once	0.375 mg once*

*Trough level should be 0.5-1 ng/ml.

Modified from Mann DL: Heart failure and cor pulmonale. *In* Kasper DL, Braunwald E, Fauci AS, et al (eds): Harrison's Principles of Internal Medicine. 17th ed. New York, McGraw-Hill, 2007 (in press).

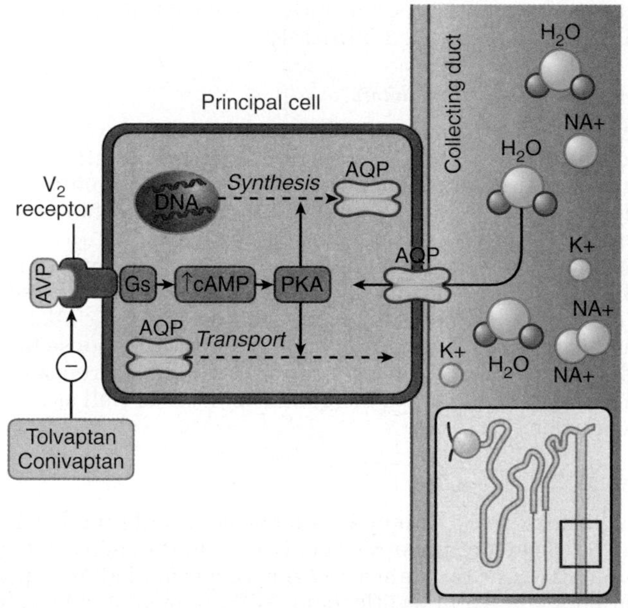

FIGURE 25–11 Mechanism of action of vasopressin antagonists. The binding of arginine vasopressin (AVP) to V_2 receptors stimulates the synthesis of aquaporin (AQP)-2 water channel proteins and promotes their transport to the apical surface. At the cell membrane, aquaporin-2 permits selective free water reabsorption down the medullary osmotic gradient, ultimately decreasing serum osmolarity and increasing fluid balance. V_2 antagonists work by preventing AVP from binding to its cognate receptor. cAMP = cyclic adenosine monophosphate; Gs = G_s protein; PKA = protein kinase A. *(Modified from deGoma EM, Vagelos RH, et al: Emerging therapies for the management of decompensated heart failure: From bench to bedside. J Am Coll Cardiol 48:2397, 2006).*

The AVP antagonists or "vaptans" (see Table 25-8) were developed to block the V_2 receptor (e.g., tolvaptan [OPC-41061], lixivaptan, satavaptan) selectively or block both the V_{1a}-V_2 receptors (e.g., conivaptan) nonselectively. All four AVP antagonists increase urine volume, decrease urine osmolarity, and have no effect on 24-hour sodium excretion. Conivaptan (YM097) is a dual AVP antagonist that has 10 times the affinity for the V_{1a} receptor compared with V_2 receptors and is available for intravenous and oral administration, whereas the other three agents are being developed for oral administration. In patients with HF who present with symptoms of fluid overload, tolvaptan and conivaptan substantially increase free water excretion and plasma osmolality, reduce body weight, improve symptoms of congestion, and moderately increase serum sodium concentrations The Acute and Chronic Therapeutic Impact of a Vasopressin 2 Antagonist (Tolvaptan) in Congestive Heart Failure (ACTIV in CHF) trial[26] has shown that tolvaptan along with diuretics is associated with significant weight reduction related to fluid loss with improved serum sodium levels in patients hospitalized for HF. This was accomplished without electrolyte imbalance or worsening renal function. In contrast, the Multicenter Evaluation of Tolvaptan Effect On Remodeling (METEOR) study has shown that tolvaptan has no beneficial effects on LV remodeling in HF patients. The Efficacy of Vasopressin Antagonism in Heart Failure: Outcome Study with Tolvaptan (EVEREST) trial evaluated the effect of this agent on morbidity, mortality, and patient-assessed global clinical status in NYHA Class III and IV HF patients with an EF less than 40 percent.[27] Results of the EVEREST trial showed that adding oral tolvaptan (30 mg daily) to standard IV therapy in patients hospitalized with acute decompensated heart failure, followed by daily therapy after discharge, had no significant effect on the composite of cardiovascular death or hospitalization for heart failure (hazard ratio, 1.04; 95% CI, 0.95-1.14; $P = .55$), nor a significant effect on the secondary end points of cardiovascular mortality, cardiovascular death or hospitalization, and worsening heart failure. However, treatment with tolvaptan significantly improved secondary end points of day 1 patient-assessed dyspnea, day 1 body weight, and day 7 edema. Tolvaptan caused increased thirst and dry mouth; however, the frequencies of major adverse events were similar in the treatment and control arms.[28] Results of early trials with conivaptan[29] have also demonstrated improvement in fluid status, osmotic balance, and hemodynamic profile in patients with HF presenting with signs and symptoms of decompensation. Intravenous conivaptan is the first AVP antagonist to be approved by the U.S. Food and Drug Administration for the treatment of euvolemic hyponatremia in hospitalized patients. Conivaptan is currently not approved for use in HF patients.

Diuretic Treatment of Heart Failure

Patients with evidence of volume overload or a history of fluid retention should be treated with a diuretic to relieve their symptoms. In symptomatic patients, diuretics should be always used in combination with neurohormonal antagonists that are known to prevent disease progression (see Table 25-9). When patients have moderate to severe HF symptoms or renal insufficiency, a loop diuretic is generally required. Diuretics should be initiated in low doses (see Table 25-8) and then titrated upward to relieve signs and symptoms of fluid overload. A typical starting dose of furosemide for patients with systolic HF and normal renal function is 40 mg, although doses of 80 to 160 mg are often be necessary to achieve adequate diuresis. Because of the steep dose-response curve and effective threshold for loop diuretics (Fig. 25-12), it is critical to find an adequate dose of loop diuretic that leads to a clear-cut diuretic response. One commonly used method for finding the appropriate dose is to double the dose until the desired effect has been achieved or the maximal dose of diuretic has been reached. Once patients have achieved an adequate diuresis, it is important to document their dry weight and make certain that patients weigh themselves daily to maintain this dry weight.

Although furosemide is the most commonly used loop diuretic, the oral bioavailability of furosemide is approximately 40 to 79 percent. Therefore, bumetanide or torsemide may be preferable because of its increased bioavailability. With the exception of torsemide, the commonly used loop diuretics are short-acting (less than 3 hours). For this reason, loop diuretics usually need to be given at least twice daily. Some patients may develop hypotension or azotemia during diuretic therapy. Although the rapidity of diuresis should be slowed in these patients, diuretic therapy should be maintained at a lower level until the patient becomes euvolemic, insofar as persistent volume overload may compromise the effectiveness of some neurohormonal antagonists. Intravenous administration of diuretics may be necessary to relieve congestion acutely (see Fig. 25-12B; see also Chap. 24), and can be done safely in the outpatient setting. After a diuretic effect is achieved with short-acting loop diuretics, increasing administration frequency to twice or even three times daily will provide more diuresis with less physiological perturbation than a larger single dose. Once the congestion has been relieved, treatment with diuretics is continued to prevent the recurrence of salt and water retention to maintain the patient's ideal dry weight.

Complications of Diuretic Use

Patients with HF who are receiving diuretics should be monitored for complications of diuretics on a regular basis. The major complications of diuretic use include electrolyte and metabolic disturbances, volume depletion, and worsening azotemia. The interval for reassessment should be individualized based on severity of illness and underlying renal function, use of concomitant medications such as ACEIs, angiotensin receptor blockers (ARBs), or aldosterone antagonists, past history of electrolyte imbalances, and/or need for more aggressive diuresis.

ELECTROLYTE AND METABOLIC DISTURBANCES. Diuretic use can lead to potassium depletion, which can predispose the patient to significant cardiac arrhythmias. Renal potassium losses from diuretic use can be also exacerbated by increased circulating levels of aldosterone observed in patients with advanced HF, as well by the marked increases in distal nephron Na^+ delivery that follow use of loop or distal nephron diuretics. The level of dietary salt intake may also contribute to the extent of renal K^+ wasting with diuretics.

In the absence of formal guidelines with respect to the level of maintenance of serum K^+ levels in HF patients, many experienced HF clinicians have advocated that the serum K^+ level should be maintained between 4.0 and 5.0 mEq/liter because HF patients are often treated with pharmacological agents likely to provoke proarrhythmic effects in the presence of hypokalemia (e.g., digoxin, type III antiarrhythmics, beta agonists, phosphodiesterase inhibitors). Hypokalemia can be prevented by increasing the oral intake of KCl. The normal daily dietary K^+ intake is approximately 40 to 80 mEq/liter. Therefore, to increase

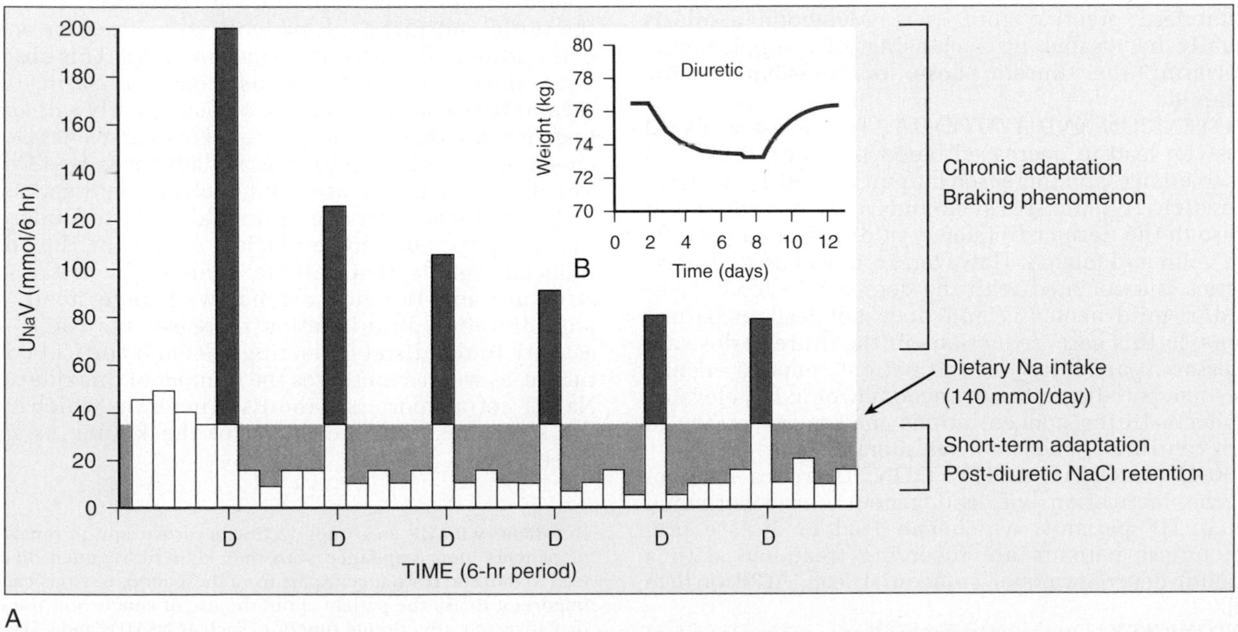

A

FIGURE 25–12 Effects of diuretics on urinary Na excretion and extracellular fluid (ECF) volume. **A,** Effects of a loop diuretic on urinary Na excretion ($U_{Na}V$). Bars represent 6-hour periods before and after doses of loop diuretic (D). Dietary Na intake is noted. The solid portion of the open bars indicates the amount by which Na excretion exceeds intake during natriuresis. The shaded area indicates the amount of positive Na balance after the diuretic effect has worn off. Net Na balance during 24 hours is the difference between the shaded area (postdiuretic NaCl retention) and the solid portion of the open bar (diuretic-induced natriuresis). Chronic adaptation is indicated by progressively smaller peak natriuretic effects (the braking phenomenon) and is mirrored by a return to neutral balance. **Inset (B),** Effect of a diuretic on body weight, taken as an index of ECF volume. Note that steady state is reached within 6 to 8 days despite continued diuretic administration. *(Modified from Ellison DH: Diuretic therapy and resistance in congestive heart failure. Cardiology 96:132, 2001.)*

this by 50 percent requires an additional 20 to 40 mEq/liter K^+ daily. However, in the presence of alkalosis, hyperaldosteronism, or Mg^{2+} depletion, hypokalemia is unresponsive to increased dietary intake of KCl, and more aggressive replacement is necessary. If supplementation is necessary, oral potassium supplements in the form of KCl extended-release tablets or liquid concentrate should be used whenever possible. Intravenous potassium is potentially hazardous and should be avoided except in emergencies. Where appropriate, the use of an aldosterone receptor antagonist may also prevent the development of hypokalemia.

The use of aldosterone receptor antagonists is often associated with the development of life-threatening hyperkalemia, particularly when they are combined with ACEIs and/or ARBs.[23] Potassium supplementation is generally stopped after the initiation of aldosterone antagonists, and patients should be counseled to avoid high potassium–containing foods. However, patients who have required large amounts of potassium supplementation may need to continue receiving supplementation, albeit at a lower dose, particularly when previous episodes of hypokalemia have been associated with ventricular arrhythmias. Diuretics may be associated with a number of other metabolic and electrolyte disturbances, including hyponatremia, hypomagnesemia, metabolic alkalosis, hyperglycemia, hyperlipidemia, and hyperuricemia. Hyponatremia is usually observed in HF patients with excessive activation of the RAS and/or high levels of AVP. Aggressive diuretic use can also lead to hyponatremia. Hyponatremia can usually be treated by more stringent water restriction. Both loop and thiazide diuretics can cause hypomagnesemia, which can aggravate muscle weakness and cardiac arrhythmias. Magnesium replacement should be administered for signs or symptoms of hypomagnesemia (e.g., arrhythmias, muscle cramps), and can be routinely given (with uncertain benefit) to all those receiving large doses of diuretics or requiring large amounts of K^+ replacement. The modest hyperglycemia and/or hyperlipidemia produced by thiazide diuretics is not usually clinically important, and blood glucose and lipid levels are generally easily controlled using standard practice guidelines. Metabolic alkalosis can usually be treated by increasing KCl supplementation, lowering the diuretic dose, or transiently using acetazolamide.

HYPOTENSION AND AZOTEMIA. The excessive use of diuretics can lead to decreased blood pressure, decreased exercise tolerance, and increased fatigue, as well as impaired renal function. Hypotensive symptoms usually resolve after a decrease in the dose or frequency of diuretics in patients who are volume-depleted. However, in most cases, the use of diuretics is associated with the decrease in blood pressure and/or mild azotemia and does not lead to patient symptoms. In this case, reductions in the diuretic dose are not necessary, particularly if the patient remains edematous. In some patients with advanced, chronic HF, elevated BUN and creatinine concentrations may be necessary to maintain control of congestive symptoms.

NEUROHORMONAL ACTIVATION. Diuretics may increase the activation of endogenous neurohormonal systems in HF patients, which can lead to disease progression unless patients are receiving treatment with a concomitant neurohormonal antagonist (e.g., ACEI or beta blocker).

OTOTOXICITY. Ototoxicity, which is more frequent with ethacrynic acid than with the other loop diuretics, can manifest as tinnitus, hearing impairment, and deafness. Hearing impairment and deafness are usually but not invariably reversible. Ototoxicity occurs most frequently with rapid intravenous injections and least frequently with oral administration.

Diuretic Resistance and Management

One inherent limitation of diuretics is that they achieve water loss via excretion of solute at the expense of glomerular filtration, which in turn activates a set of homeostatic mechanisms that ultimately limit their effectiveness. In normal subjects, the magnitude of natriuresis following a given dose of diuretic declines over time as a result of the so-called braking phenomenon (see Fig. 25-12). Studies have shown that the time-dependent decline in natriuresis for a given diuretic dose is critically dependent on reduction of the extracellular fluid volume, which leads to an increase in solute and fluid reabsorption in the proximal tubule. In addition, contraction of the extracellular volume can stimulate efferent sympathetic nerves, which reduces urinary Na^+ excretion by reducing renal blood flow, stimulating renin (and ultimately aldosterone) release, which in turn stimulates Na^+ reabsorption along the nephron (see Chap. 22). The magnitude of the natriuretic effect of potent loop diuretics may also decline in HF patients, particularly as HF progresses. Although the bioavailability of these diuretics is generally not decreased in HF, the potential delay in their rate of absorption may result in peak drug levels in the tubular lumen in the ascending loop of Henle that are insufficient to induce maximal natriuresis (Fig. 25-13). The use of intravenous formulations may obviate this problem (see Chap. 24). However, even with intravenous dosing, a rightward shift of the dose-response curve is observed between the diuretic concentration in the tubular lumen and its natriuretic effect in HF (see Fig. 25-13A). Moreover, the maximal effect (ceiling) is lower in HF. This rightward shift has been referred to as "diuretic resistance" and is likely the result of several factors in addition to the braking phenomenon described earlier. First, most loop diuretics, with the exception of torsemide, are short-acting drugs. Accordingly, after a period of natriuresis, the diuretic concentration in plasma and tubular fluid declines below the diuretic threshold. In this situation, renal Na^+ reabsorption is no longer inhibited and a period of antinatriuresis or postdiuretic NaCl retention ensues. If dietary NaCl intake is moderate to excessive, postdiuretic NaCl retention may overcome the initial natriuresis in patients with excessive activation of the adrenergic nervous system and RAS. This observation forms the rationale for administering short-acting diuretics several times daily to obtain consistent daily salt and water loss. Second, there is a loss of renal responsiveness to endogenous natriuretic peptides as HF advances (see Chap. 22). Third, diuretics increase solute delivery to distal segments of the nephron, causing epithelial cells to undergo both hypertrophy and hyperplasia. Although the diuretic-induced signals that initiate changes in distal nephron structure and function are not well understood, chronic loop diuretic administration increases the Na^+,K^+-ATPase activity in the distal collecting duct and cortical collecting tubule, as well as increases the number of thiazide-sensitive Na^+-Cl^- cotransporters in the distal nephron, which increases the solute resorptive capacity of the kidney as much as threefold.

In patients with HF, an abrupt decline in cardiac and/or renal function or patients' noncompliance with their diuretic regimen or diet may lead to diuretic resistance. Apart from these more obvious causes, it is important to ask the patient about the use of concurrent use of drugs that adversely affect renal function, such as NSAIDs and COX-2 inhibitors (see Table 25-7). The insulin-sensitizing thiazolidinediones have also been linked to increased fluid retention in patients with HF, although the clinical significance of this finding is not known. It has been suggested that thiazolidinediones activate proliferator-activated gamma nuclear receptor expression in the renal collecting duct, which enhances expression of cell surface epithelial Na^+ channels. Moreover, studies in healthy men have shown that pioglitazone stimulates plasma

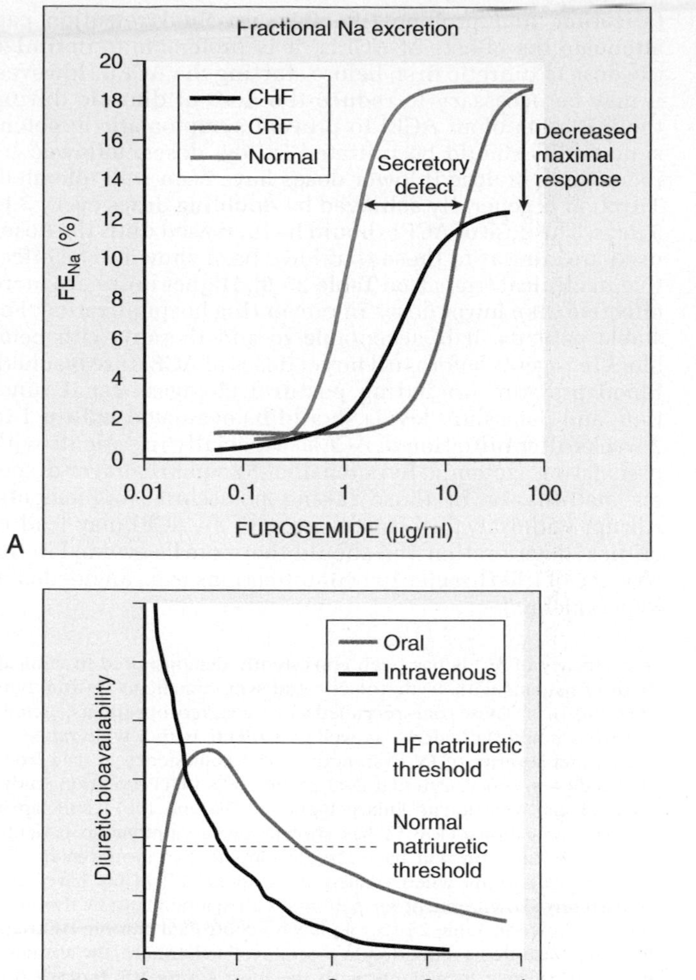

FIGURE 25–13 Dose-response curves for loop diuretics. **A,** Fractional Na excretion (FE_{Na}) as a function of loop diuretic concentration. Compared with normal patients, patients with chronic renal failure (CRF) show a rightward shift in the curve because of impaired diuretic secretion. The maximal response is preserved when expressed as FE_{Na}, but not when expressed as absolute Na excretion. Patients with chronic heart failure (CHF) demonstrate a rightward and downward shift, even when the response is expressed as FE_{Na}, and thus are relatively diuretic resistant. **B,** Comparison of the response to intravenous and oral doses of loop diuretics in normal subjects and HF patients. Diuretic bioavailability is shown for normal and HF patients. The natriuretic threshold necessary to produce a diuresis in shown for normal subjects (dotted line) and for HF patients (solid line). In a normal individual, an oral dose may be as effective as an intravenous dose because the diuretic bioavailability (area under the curve) that is above the natriuretic threshold for intravenous and oral diuretics is approximately equal. However, if the natriuretic threshold increases in a patient with HF, then the oral dose may not provide a high enough serum level to elicit a significant natriuresis. *(Modified from Ellison DH: Diuretic therapy and resistance in congestive heart failure. Cardiology 96:132, 2001.)*

renin activity that may contribute to increased Na^+ retention. Rarely, drugs such as probenecid or high plasma concentrations of some antibiotics may compete with the organic ion transporters in the proximal tubule responsible for the transfer of most diuretics from the recirculation into the tubular lumen. The use of increasing doses of vasodilators, with or without a marked decline in intravascular volume as a result of concomitant diuretic therapy, may lower renal perfusion pressure below that necessary to maintain normal autoregulation and glomerular filtration in patients with renal artery stenosis from atherosclerotic disease. Accordingly, a reduction in renal blood flow may occur despite an increase in cardiac output, thereby leading to a decrease in diuretic effectiveness.

A patient with HF may be considered to be resistant to diuretic drugs when moderate doses of a loop diuretic do not achieve the desired reduction of the extracellular fluid volume. In outpatients, a common and useful method for treating the diuretic-resistant patient is to administer two classes of diuretic concurrently. Adding a proximal tubule diuretic or a distal collecting tubule diuretic to a regimen of loop diuretics is often dramatically effective. As a general rule, when adding a second class of diuretic, the dose of loop diuretic should not be altered because the shape of the dose-response curve for loop diuretics is not affected by the addition of other diuretics, and the loop diuretic must be given at an effective dose for it to be effective. The combination of loop and distal collecting tubule diuretics has been shown to be effective through several mechanisms.[30] One is that distal collecting tubule diuretics have longer half-lives than loop diuretics and may thus prevent or attenuate postdiuretic NaCl retention. A second mechanism by which distal collecting tubule diuretics potentiate the effects of loop diuretics is by inhibiting Na^+ transport along the proximal tubule, insofar as most thiazide diuretics also inhibit carbonic anhydrase and inhibit NaCl transport along the distal renal tubule, which may counteract the increased solute resorptive effects of the hypertrophied and hyperplastic distal epithelial cells.

The selection of a distal collecting tubule diuretic to use as second diuretic is a matter of choice. Many clinicians choose metolazone because its half-life is longer than that of some other distal collecting tubule diuretics, and because it has been reported to remain effective even when the glomerular filtration rate is low. However, direct comparisons between metolazone and several traditional thiazides have shown little difference in natriuretic potency when they are included in a regimen with loop diuretics in HF patients.[30] Distal collecting tubule diuretics may be added in full doses (50 to 100 mg/day hydrochlorothiazide or 2.5 to 10 mg/day metolazone; see Table 25-8) when a rapid and robust response is needed. However, such an approach is likely to lead to excessive fluid and electrolyte depletion if patients are not followed up extremely closely. One reasonable approach to combination therapy is to achieve control of fluid overload by initially adding full doses of distal collecting tubule diuretic on a daily basis and then decreasing the dose of the dose of the distal collecting tubule diuretic to three times weekly to avoid excessive diuresis. An alternate strategy in hospitalized patients is to administer the same daily parenteral dose of a loop diuretic by continuous intravenous infusion, which leads to sustained natriuresis because of the continuous presence of high drug levels in the tubular lumen (see Chap. 24). This approach requires the use of a constant infusion pump but permits more precise control of the natriuretic effect achieved over time, particularly in carefully monitored patients. It also diminishes the potential for a too rapid decline in intravascular volume and hypotension as well as the risk of ototoxicity in patients given large bolus intravenous doses of a loop diuretic. A typical continuous furosemide regimen is initiated with a 20- to 40-mg intravenous loading dose as a bolus injection, followed by a continuous infusion of 5 to 10 mg/hour for a patient who had been receiving 200 mg of oral furosemide/day in divided doses.

Another common reason for diuretic resistance in advanced HF is the development of the cardiorenal syndrome, which is recognized clinically as worsening renal function that limits diuresis in patients with obvious clinical volume overload.[31] In patients with advanced HF, the cardiorenal syndrome is manifested in patients who have repeated HF hospitalizations for worsening volume overload and difficulty in achieving an adequate diuresis because of worsening indices of renal function. This impairment in renal function often is dismissed as pre-renal; however, when measured carefully, neither cardiac output nor renal perfusion pressure have been shown to be reduced in diuretic-treated patients who develop the cardiorenal syndrome. Importantly, worsening indices of renal function contribute to longer hospital stays and predict higher rates of early rehospitalization and death (see Fig. 25-5).[31] The mechanisms for and treatment of the cardiorenal syndrome remain poorly understood.

Device-Based Therapies for Management of Fluid Status

The use of mechanical methods of fluid removal, such as extracorporeal ultrafiltration, may be needed to achieve adequate control of fluid retention, particularly in patients who become resistant and/or refractory to diuretic therapy. Extracorporeal ultrafiltration (UF) removes salt and water isotonically by driving the patient's blood through a highly permeable filter via an extracorporeal circuit in an arteriovenous or venovenous mode. Alternative extracorporeal methods include continuous hemofiltration, continuous hemodialysis, or continuous hemodiafiltration.[32] With slow continuous UF, the patient's intravascular fluid volume remains stable as fluid shifts from the extravascular space into the intravascular space, with the result that there is no deleterious activation of neurohormonal systems. UF has been shown to reduce right atrial and pulmonary artery wedge pressures and increase cardiac output, diuresis, and natriuresis without changes in heart rate, systolic blood pressure, renal function, electrolyte levels, or intravascular volume.[33]

The Relief for Acutely Fluid-Overloaded Patients with Decompensated Congestive Heart Failure (RAPID-CHF) trial, which was the first randomized controlled trial of UF for acute decompensated HF, enrolled 40 patients who were randomized to receive usual care (diuretic) or a single 8-hour UF (using a proprietary device) in addition to usual care. The primary endpoint was weight loss 24 hours after enrollment. Fluid removal after 24 hours was approximately twofold greater in the UF group.[34] The Ultrafiltration versus IV Diuretics for Patients Hospitalized for Acute Decompensated Congestive Heart Failure (UNLOAD) study compared the long-term safety and efficacy of UF therapy (using a proprietary device) with intravenous diuretics in a multicenter trial involving 200 patients who were assessed at entry and at intervals up to 90 days. The primary endpoint of the trial was total weight loss and a change in dyspnea score during the first 48 hours of randomization. Although the two treatments were similar in their ability to relieve dyspnea acutely, UF was associated with significantly greater fluid loss over 48 hours and a lower rate of rehospitalization during the next 90 days.[35]

In addition to extracorporeal methods for relieving volume overload, peritoneal dialysis can be used as a viable alternative therapy for the short-term management of refractory congestive symptoms for patients in whom vascular access cannot be obtained, or for whom appropriate extracorporeal therapies are not available.

Preventing Disease Progression

Drugs that interfere with the excessive activation of the renin angiotensin-aldosterone system and the adrenergic nervous system can relieve the symptoms of HF with a depressed EF by stabilizing and/or reversing cardiac remodeling (see Chap. 22). In this regard ACEIs, ARBs, and beta blockers have emerged as cornerstones of modern HF therapy for patients with a depressed EF (see Table 25-9).

Angiotensin-Converting Enzyme Inhibitors (ACEIs)

There is overwhelming evidence that ACEIs should be used in symptomatic and asymptomatic patients with a reduced EF (less than 40 percent). ACEIs interfere with the RAS by inhibiting the enzyme that is responsible for the conversion of angiotensin I to angiotensin II (see Chap. 22). However, because ACEIs also inhibit kininase II, they may lead to the upregulation of bradykinin, which may further enhance the effects of effects of angiotensin suppression. ACEIs stabilize LV remodeling, improve patient symptoms, prevent hospitalization, and prolong life. Because fluid retention can attenuate the effects of ACEIs, it is preferable to optimize the dose of diuretic first, before starting the ACEI. However, it may be necessary to reduce the dose of diuretic during the initiation of an ACEI to prevent symptomatic hypotension. ACEIs should be initiated in low doses, followed by increments in dose if lower doses have been well tolerated. Titration is generally achieved by doubling doses every 3 to 5 days. The dose of ACEI should be increased until the doses used are similar to those that have been shown to be effective in clinical trials (see Table 25-9). Higher doses are more effective than lower doses in preventing hospitalization. For stable patients, it is acceptable to add therapy with beta-blocking agents before full target doses of ACEIs are reached. Blood pressure (including postural changes), renal function, and potassium levels should be evaluated within 1 to 2 weeks after initiation of ACEIs, especially in patients with preexisting azotemia, hypotension, hyponatremia, or diabetes mellitus, or in those taking potassium supplements. Abrupt withdrawal of treatment with an ACEI may lead to clinical deterioration and should therefore be avoided in the absence of life-threatening complications (e.g., angioedema, hyperkalemia).

The efficacy of ACEIs has been consistently demonstrated in clinical trials of patients with asymptomatic and symptomatic LV dysfunction (Fig. 25-14).[15,36] These trials recruited a broad variety of patients, including women and the elderly, as well as patients with a wide range of causes and severity of LV dysfunction. The consistency of data from the Studies on Left Ventricular Dysfunction (SOLVD) Prevention Study, Survival and Ventricular Enlargement (SAVE) and the Trandolapril Cardiac Evaluation (TRACE) has shown that asymptomatic patients with LV dysfunction will have less development of symptomatic HF and hospitalizations when treated with an ACEI.[15] ACEIs have also consistently shown benefit for patients with symptomatic LV dysfunction. As shown in Table 25-10, all placebo-controlled chronic HF trials have demonstrated a reduction in mortality. Furthermore, the absolute benefit is greatest in patients with the most severe HF. Indeed, the patients with NYHA Class IV HF in the Cooperative North Scandinavian Enalapril Survival Study (CONSENSUS I) had a much larger effect size than the SOLVD Treatment Trial, which in turn had a larger effect size than the SOLVD Prevention Trial. Although only three placebo-controlled mortality trials have been conducted in patients with chronic HF, the aggregate data have suggested that ACEIs reduce mortality in a direct relationship to the degree of severity of chronic HF. The Vasodilator in Heart Failure II (V-HeFT-II) trial has provided evidence that ACEIs improve the natural history of HF through mechanisms other than vasodilation, inasmuch as subjects treated with enalapril have significantly lower mortality than subjects treated with the vasodilatory combination of hydralazine plus isosorbide dinitrate, which does not directly inhibit neurohormonal systems). Although enalapril is the only ACEI that has been used in placebo-controlled mortality trials in chronic HF, as shown in Table 25-10, multiple ACEIs have proved to be more or less equally effective when administered in oral form within the first week of the ischemic event in MI trials. ACEIs markedly enhance survival in patients with signs or symptoms of HF after MI. In addition to these effects on mortality, ACEIs improve the functional status of patients with HF. In contrast, ACEIs only produce small benefits in exercise capacity. Taken together, these observations support the conclusion that the effects of ACEIs on the natural history of chronic HF or post-MI LV dysfunction, or patients at high risk of developing HF, represent class effects of these agents. Nonetheless, it should be emphasized that patients with a low blood pressure (less than 90 mm Hg systolic) or impaired renal function (serum creatinine level higher than 2.5 mg/ml) were not recruited and/or represent a small proportion of patients who participated in these trials.[15] Thus, the efficacy of these agents for these patient populations is less well established.

COMPLICATIONS OF ANGIOTENSIN-CONVERTING ENZYME INHIBITOR USE. Most adverse effects of ACEIs are related to suppression of RAS. The decreases in blood pressure and mild azotemia often seen during the initiation of therapy are, in general, well tolerated and do not require

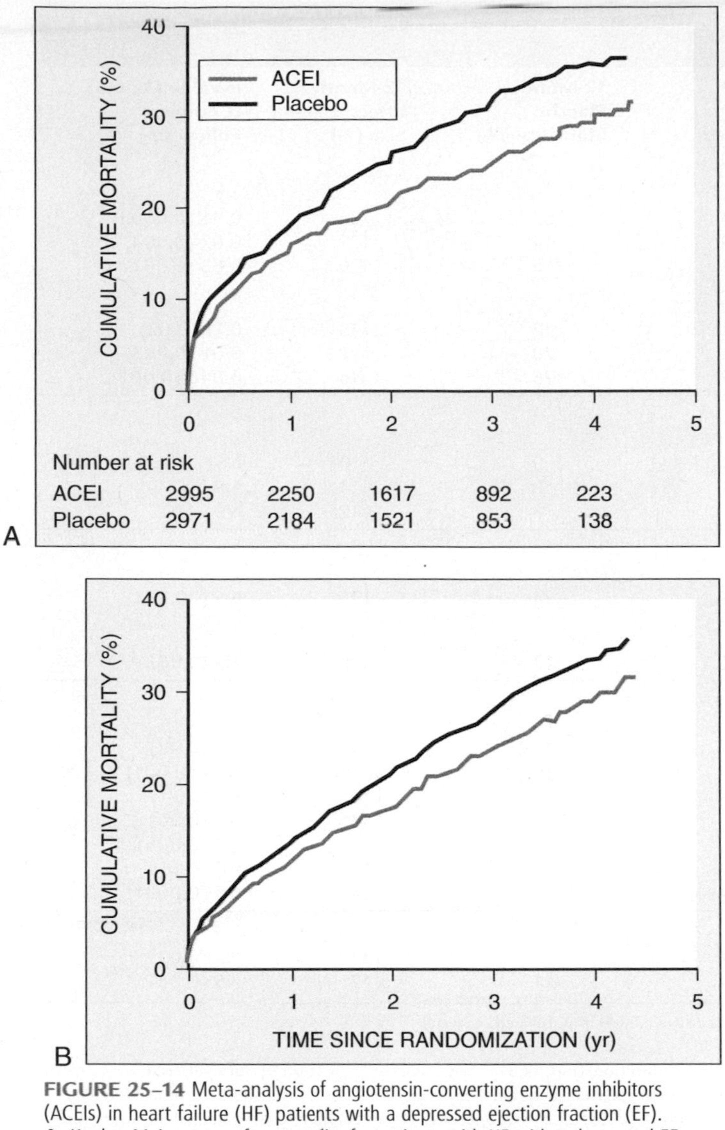

FIGURE 25–14 Meta-analysis of angiotensin-converting enzyme inhibitors (ACEIs) in heart failure (HF) patients with a depressed ejection fraction (EF). **A,** Kaplan-Meier curves for mortality for patients with HF with a depressed EF treated with an ACEI following acute myocardial infarction (three trials). **B,** Kaplan-Meier curves for mortality for patients with HF with a depressed EF treated with an ACEI in five clinical trials, including postinfarction trials. The benefits of ACEIs were observed early and persisted over the long term. *(Modified from Flather MD, Yusuf S, Kober L, et al: Long-term ACE-inhibitor therapy in patients with heart failure or left- ventricular dysfunction: A systematic overview of data from individual patients. ACE-Inhibitor Myocardial Infarction Collaborative Group. Lancet 355:1575, 2000.)*

a decrease in the dose of the ACEI. However, if hypotension is accompanied by dizziness or if the renal dysfunction becomes severe, it may be necessary to decrease the dose of the diuretic if significant fluid retention is not present or decrease the dose of the ACEI if significant fluid retention is present. Potassium retention may also become problematic if the patient is receiving potassium supplements or a potassium-sparing diuretic. Potassium retention that is not responsive to these measures may require a reduction in the dose of ACEI. The side effects of ACEIs that are related to kinin potentiation include a nonproductive cough (10 to 15 percent of patients) and angioedema (1 percent of patients). In patients who cannot tolerate ACEIs because of cough or angioedema, ARBs are the next recommended line of therapy. Patients intolerant to ACEIs because of hyperkalemia or renal insufficiency are likely to experience the same side effects with ARBs. The combination of hydralazine and an oral nitrate should be considered for these latter patients (see Table 25-9).

Angiotensin Receptor Blockers

ARBs are well tolerated in patients who are intolerant of ACEIs because of cough, skin rash, and angioedema and should therefore be used in symptomatic and asymptomatic patients with an EF less than 40 percent who are ACE intolerant for reasons other than hyperkalemia or renal insufficiency (see Table 25-9). Although ACEIs and ARBs inhibit RAS, they do so by a different mechanism. Whereas ACEIs block the enzyme responsible for converting angiotensin I to angiotensin II, ARBs block the effects of angiotensin II on the angiotensin type 1 receptor (see Chap. 22), the receptor subtype responsible for virtually all the adverse biological effects on cardiac remodeling relevant to angiotensin II (see Chap. 22). A number of ARBs are approved for the treatment of hypertension and are now available to clinicians. Three of these—losartan, valsartan, and candesartan—have been extensively evaluated in the setting of HF (see Table 25-9). Some clinical trials have demonstrated that ARBs are as effective as ACEIs in reversing the process of LV remodeling, improving patient symptoms, preventing hospitalization, and prolonging life.[15] Moreover, several studies have shown that there is added therapeutic benefit for the addition of an ARB to an ACEI in patients with chronic HF. ARBs should be initiated with the starting doses shown in Table 25-9, which can be uptitrated every 3 to 5 days by doubling the dose. As with ACEIs, blood pressure, renal function, and potassium levels should be reassessed within 1 to 2 weeks after initiation and followed closely after changes in dose.

In symptomatic HF patients who were intolerant to ACEIs, the aggregate clinical data have suggested that ARBs are as effective as ACEIs in reducing HF morbidity and mortality.[15] Candesartan significantly reduced all-cause mortality, cardiovascular death, or hospital admission for HF in the Candesartan Heart Failure: Assessment of Reduction in Mortality and Morbidity trial (CHARM-Alternative Trial; Fig. 25-15A).[37] Importantly, candesartan reduced all-cause mortality, irrespective of background ACEI or beta blocker therapy. Similar findings were shown with valsartan in the small subgroup of patients not receiving an ACEI in the Valsartan Heart Failure Trial (Val-HeFT).[38] A direct comparison of ACEIs and ARBs was made in the Losartan Heart Failure Survival Study (ELITE-II), which showed that losartan is not associated with improved survival in elderly HF patients when compared with captopril but is significantly better tolerated. Two trials have compared ARBs with ACE inhibition in post-MI patients who developed LV dysfunction or signs of HF. The direct comparison of losartan with captopril indicated that losartan is not as effective as captopril on all-cause mortality, whereas valsartan was shown to be noninferior to captopril on all-cause mortality in the Valsartan in Acute Myocardial Infarction Trial (VALIANT).[39] The combination of captopril and valsartan produced no further reduction in mortality in VALIANT, although the number of adverse events increased. When given in addition to ACEIs in general cohorts of patients with symptomatic HF, the effects of ARBs were shown to have a modest beneficial effect in the CHARM-Added trial (see Fig. 25-15B).[40] However, the addition of valsartan to ACEIs had no beneficial effect on mortality in the Val-HeFT, although the combined endpoint mortality and morbidity was significantly (13.2 percent) lower with valsartan than with placebo because of a reduction in the number of patients hospitalized for HF.[38]

COMPLICATIONS OF ANGIOTENSIN RECEPTOR BLOCKER USE. Both ACEIs and ARBs have similar effects on blood pressure, renal function, and potassium levels. Therefore, the problems of symptomatic hypotension, azotemia, and hyperkalemia will be similar for both of these agents. Although occurring less frequently than with ACEIs, angioedema has also been reported in some patients who receive ARBs. In patients who are intolerant to ACEIs and ARBs, the combined use of hydralazine and isosorbide dini-

TABLE 25–10 Mortality Rates in Placebo-Controlled Trials of Patients with Chronic Heart Failure (EF <40%), with Acute Myocardial Infarction, or at Risk for Heart Failure

Trial Name	Agent	NYHA Class	No. of Subjects Enrolled	12-Month Placebo Mortality (%)	12-Month Effect Size (%)	*P* Value (12 mo) (Complete Follow-up)
Angiotensin-Converting Enzyme Inhibitor						
Heart Failure						
CONSENSUS-1	Enalapril	IV	253	52	↓31	0.01 (0.0003)
SOLVD-Rx	Enalapril	I-III	2569	15	↓21	0.02 (0.004)
SOLVD-Asx	Enalapril	I, II	4228	5	0	0.82 (0.30)
Post–Myocardial Infarction (MI)						
SAVE	Captopril	—	2231	12	↓18	0.11 (0.02)
AIRE	Ramipril	—	1986	20	↓22	0.01 (0.002)
TRACE	Trandolapril	—	1749	26	↓16	0.046 (0.001)
ARBs						
Heart Failure						
Val-HeFT	Valsartan	II-IV	5010	9	0	NS
CHARM-Alternative	Candesartan	II-IV	2028	8	↓14	NS
CHARM-Added	Candesartan	II-IV	2548	8	↓12	NS
Aldosterone Antagonist						
Heart Failure						
RALES	Spironolactone	III, IV	1663	24	↓25	NS (<0.001)
Post-MI						
EPHESUS	Eplerenone	I	6632	12	↓15	NS (0.005)
Beta Blockers						
Heart Failure						
CIBIS-I	Bisoprolol	III, IV	641	11	↓20*	NS (0.22)
U.S. Carvedilol	Carvedilol	II, III	1094	10	↓66*	NS (<0.001)
ANZ-Carvedilol	Carvedilol	I-III	415	6	↓26	NS (>0.1)
CIBIS-II	Bisoprolol	III, IV	2647	13	↓34*	NS (0.001)
MERIT-HF	Metoprolol CR	II-IV	3991	11	↓35*	NS (0.006)
BEST	Bucindolol	III, IV	2708	17	↓10*	NS (0.16)
COPERNICUS	Carvedilol	Severe	2289	18	↓38*	NS (0.0001)
Post-MI						
CAPRICORN	Carvedilol	I	1959	11	↓23*	NS (0.03)
BEAT	Bucindolol	I	343	21	↓12*	NS (0.06)

Twelve-month mortality rates were taken from the survival curves when data were not directly available in published material.

*Effect size at the conclusion of the trial.

AIRE = Acute Infarction Ramipril Efficacy; BEAT = Bucindolol Evaluation in Acute Myocardial Infarction Trial; BEST = Beta-blocker Evaluation of Survival Trial; CAPRICORN = Carvedilol Post-Infarct Survival Control in Left Ventricular Dysfunction; CHARM = Candesartan in Heart Failure-Assessment of Reduction in Mortality and Morbidity; CHF = congestive heart failure; CIBIS = Cardiac Insufficiency Bisoprolol Study; CONSENSUS = Cooperative North Scandinavian Enalapril Survival Study; COPERNICUS = Carvedilol Prospective Randomized Cumulative Survival; EPHESUS = Eplerenone Post-Acute Myocardial Infarction Heart Failure Efficacy and Survival Study; MERIT-HF = Metoprolol CR/XL Randomized Interventional Trial in Congestive Heart Failure; NYHA = New York Heart Association; NS = not specified; RALES = Randomized Aldactone Evaluation Study; SAVE = Survival and Ventricular Enlargement; SOLVD = Studies of Left Ventricular Dysfunction; TRACE = Trandolapril Cardiac Evaluation; Val-HeFT = Valsartan Heart Failure Trial.

Modified from Bristow MR, Linas S, Port DI: Drugs in the treatment of heart failure. *In* Zipes DP, Libby P, Bonow RO, Braunwald E (eds): Braunwald's Heart Disease. 7th ed. Philadelphia, Elsevier, 2004, pp 569-601.

trate may be considered as a therapeutic option (see Table 25-9). However, compliance with this combination has generally been poor because of the large number of tablets required and the high incidence of adverse reactions.

Beta-Adrenergic Receptor Blockers

Beta blocker therapy represents a major advance in the treatment of HF patients with a depressed EF. Beta blockers interfere with the harmful effects of sustained activation of the nervous system by competitively antagonizing one or more adrenergic receptors (beta$_1$-, beta$_2$-, and alpha-adrenergic). Although there are a number of potential benefits to blocking all three receptors, most of the deleterious effects of sympathetic activation are mediated by the beta$_1$-adrenergic receptor.[41] When given in concert with ACEIs, beta blockers reverse the process of LV remodeling, improve patient symptoms, prevent hospitalization, and prolong life. Therefore, beta blockers are indicated for patients with symptomatic or asymptomatic HF and a depressed EF of lower than 40 percent. There are three beta blockers that have been shown to be effective in reducing the risk of death in patients with chronic HF—bisoprolol and sustained-release metoprolol succinate both competitively block the beta$_1$ receptor, and carvedilol competitively blocks the beta$_1$-, beta$_2$-, and alpha-adrenergic receptors. Analogous to the use of ACEIs, beta blockers should be initiated in low doses (see Table 25-9), followed by gradual increments in the dose if lower doses have been well tolerated. The dose of beta blocker should be increased until the doses used are similar to those that have been reported to be effective in clinical trials (see Table 25-9). However, unlike ACEIs, which may be uptitrated relatively rapidly, the dose titration of beta blockers should proceed no sooner than at 2-week intervals because the initiation and/or increased dosing of these agents may lead to worsening fluid retention caused by the abrupt withdrawal of adrenergic support to the heart and circulation. Therefore, it is important to optimize the dose of diuretic before starting therapy with beta blockers.

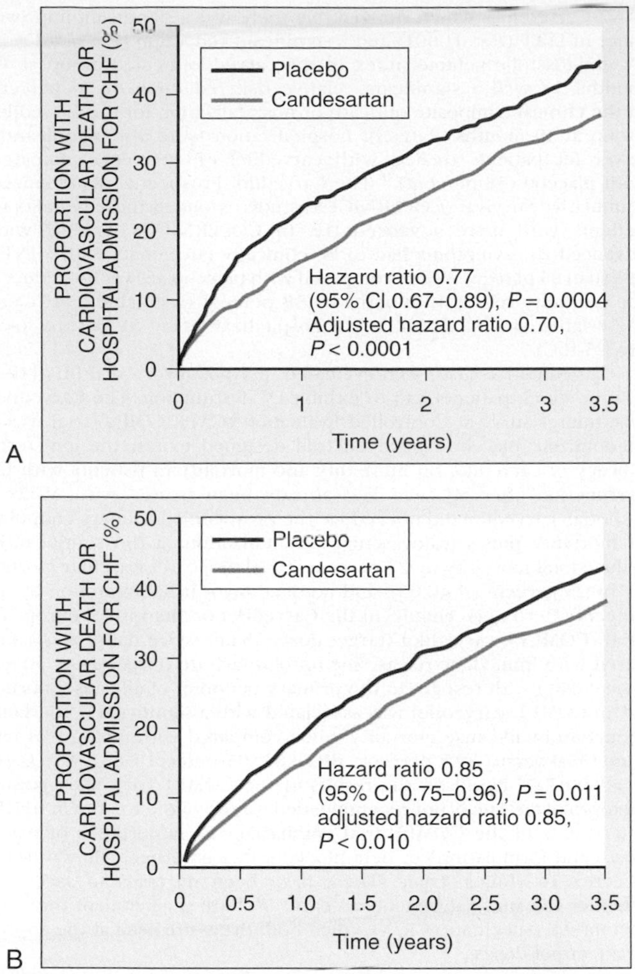

FIGURE 25–15 Effect of candesartan on cardiovascular mortality or hospital admission for heart failure in the CHARM-Alternative **(A)** trial and the CHARM-Added **(B)** trial. Two groups of patients who were randomized to candesartan or placebo are depicted. **A,** Patients who were not receiving an angiotensin-converting enzyme inhibitor (ACEI). **B,** Patients who were receiving an ACEI. The effect size of candesartan was reduced in the group of patients who were receiving an ACEI. CHARM = Candesartan in Heart Failure Assessment of Reduction in Mortality and Morbidity; CHF = congestive heart failure. *(Modified from Granger CB, McMurray JJ, Yusuf S, et al: Effects of candesartan in patients with chronic heart failure and reduced left-ventricular systolic function intolerant to angiotensin-converting-enzyme inhibitors: The CHARM-Alternative trial. Lancet 362:772, 2003; and McMurray JJ, Ostergren J, Swedberg K, et al: Effects of candesartan in patients with chronic heart failure and reduced left-ventricular systolic function taking angiotensin-converting-enzyme inhibitors: The CHARM-Added trial. Lancet 362:767, 2003.)*

If worsening fluid retention does occur, it is likely to occur within 3 to 5 days of initiating therapy and will be manifest as an increase in body weight and/or symptoms of worsening HF. The increased fluid retention can usually be managed by increasing the dose of diuretics. Patients need not be taking high doses of ACEIs before being considered for treatment with a beta blocker, because most patients enrolled in the beta blocker trials were not taking high doses of ACEIs. Furthermore, in patients taking a low dose of an ACEI, the addition of a beta blocker produces a greater improvement in symptoms and reduction in the risk of death than an increase in the dose of the ACEI.

Recent data have shown that beta blockers can be safely started before discharge, even in patients hospitalized for HF, provided that the patients is stable and does not require intravenous HF therapy. Contrary to early reports, the aggregate results of clinical trials have suggested that beta blocker therapy is well tolerated by the great majority of HF patients (more than 85 percent), including patients with comorbid conditions such as diabetes mellitus, chronic obstructive lung disease, and peripheral vascular disease Nonetheless, there is a subset of patients (10 to 15 percent) who remain intolerant to beta blockers because of worsening fluid retention or symptomatic hypotension.

The first placebo-controlled multicenter trial with a beta-blocking agent was the Metoprolol in Dilated Cardiomyopathy (MDC) trial, which used the shorter acting tartrate preparation at a target dose of 50 mg three times a day in symptomatic HF patients with idiopathic dilated cardiomyopathy. Metoprolol tartrate at an average dosage of 108 mg/day reduced the prevalence of the primary endpoint of death or need for cardiac transplantation by 34 percent, which did not quite reach statistical significance ($P = 0.058$).[15] The benefit was entirely the result of a reduction by metoprolol in the morbidity component of the primary endpoint, with no favorable trends in the mortality component of the primary endpoint. A more efficacious formulation of metoprolol was subsequently developed, metoprolol (succinate) CR/XL, which has a better pharmacological profile than metoprolol tartrate because of its controlled-release profile and longer half-life. In the Metoprolol CR/XL Randomized Intervention Trial in Congestive Heart Failure (MERIT-HF), metoprolol CR/XL provided a significant relative risk reduction of 34 percent reduction in mortality in subjects with mild to moderate HF and moderate to severe systolic dysfunction when compared with the placebo group (Fig. 25-16A).[15] Importantly, metoprolol CR/X reduced mortality from both sudden death and progressive pump failure. Furthermore, mortality was reduced across most demographic groups, including older versus younger subjects, nonischemic versus ischemic causes, and lower versus higher ejection fractions.

Bisoprolol is a second-generation $beta_1$ receptor selective blocking agent with approximately 120-fold higher affinity for human $beta_1$ versus $beta_2$ receptors. The first trial performed with bisoprolol was the Cardiac Insufficiency Bisoprolol Study I (CIBIS-I) trial, which examined the effects of bisoprolol on mortality in subjects with symptomatic ischemic or nonischemic cardiomyopathy. CIBIS-I showed a nonsignificant ($P = 0.22$) 20 percentage risk reduction for mortality at 2 years follow-up.[15] Because the sample size for CIBIS-I was based on an unrealistically high expected event rate in the control group, a follow-up trial with more conservative effect size estimates and sample size calculations was conducted. In CIBIS-II, bisoprolol reduced all-cause mortality by 32 percent (11.8 versus 17.3 percent, $P = 0.002$), sudden cardiac death by 45 percent (3.6 versus 6.4 percent, $P = 0.001$), HF hospitalizations by 30 percent (11.9 percent bisoprolol versus 17.6 percent placebo, $P < 0.001$), and all-cause hospitalizations by 15 percent (33.6 versus 39.6 percent, $P = 0.002$) (see Fig. 25-16B).[15] The CIBIS-III trial addressed the important question of whether an initial treatment strategy using the beta blocker bisoprolol was noninferior to a treatment strategy using an ACEI (enalapril) first in patients with newly diagnosed mild to moderate HF. The two strategies were compared in a blinded manner with regard to the combined primary endpoint of all-cause mortality or hospitalization, as well as with regard to each of the components of the primary endpoint individually. In the per-protocol primary endpoint analysis (the most conservative approach with regard to noninferiority), death or rehospitalization occurred in 32.4 percent of the bisoprolol-first strategy and in 33.1 percent of the enalapril-first strategy (hazard ratio [HR], 0.97; 95 percent CI, 0.78 to 1.21; $P = 0.046$ for noninferiority), which missed the prespecified criteria for noninferiority of an HR of 1.17. However, when the data were analyzed using an intent-to-treat analysis, bisoprolol was shown to be noninferior to enalapril (HR, 0.94; 95 percent CI, 0.77 to 1.16; $P = 0.019$ for noninferiority). Although CIBIS-III did not provide clear-cut evidence to justify starting with a beta blocker, the overall safety profile of the two strategies was similar. Current guidelines continue to recommend starting with an ACE inhibitor, followed by the subsequent addition of a beta blocker.

Of the three beta blockers approved for the treatment of HF, carvedilol has been studied most extensively (Table 25-10). The phase III U.S. Trials Program, composed of four individual trials managed by a single Steering and Data and Safety Monitoring Committee, was stopped prematurely because of a highly significant ($P < 0.0001$) 65 percent reduction in mortality by carvedilol that was observed across all four trials. This was followed by a second study, the Australia–New Zealand Heart Failure Research Collaborative Group Carvedilol Trial

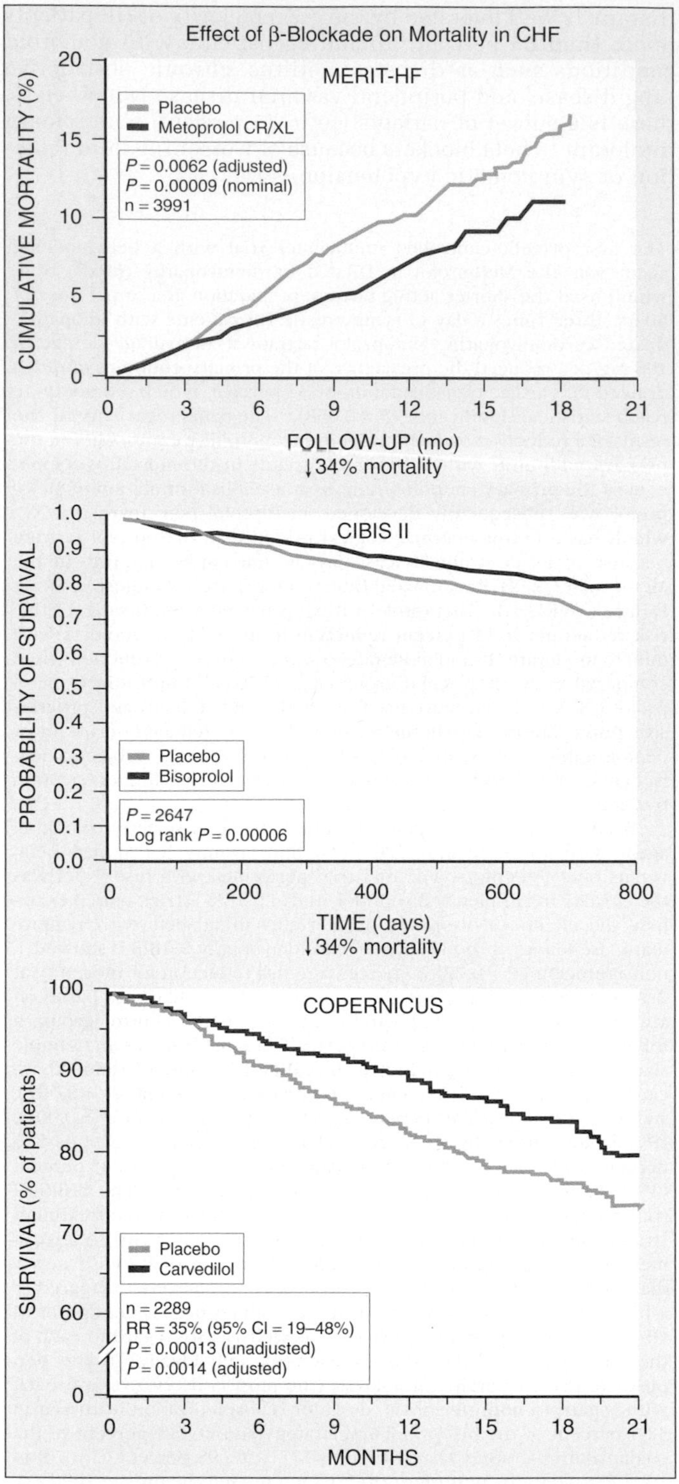

FIGURE 25–16 Kaplan-Meier analysis of the probability of survival in patients in the placebo and beta blocker groups in the MERIT-HF **(top)**, CIBIS II **(middle)**, and COPERNICUS **(bottom)** trials. CHF = chronic heart failure; CI = confidence interval; RR = relative risk. *(Data from The Cardiac Insufficiency Bisoprolol Study II [CIBIS II]: A randomised trial. Lancet 353:9, 1999; Effect of metoprolol in chronic heart failure: Metoprolol CR/XL Randomised Intervention Trial in Congestive Heart Failure [MERIT-HF]. Lancet 353:2001, 1999; and Packer M, Coats AJ, Fowler MB, et al; Carvedilol Prospective Randomized Cumulative Survival Study [COPERNICUS] Group: Effect of carvedilol on survival in severe chronic heart failure. N Engl J Med 344:1651, 2001.)*

(ANZ-Carvedilol), which showed that there was a significant improvement in LVEF ($P < 0.0001$) and a significant reduction ($P = 0.0015$) in LV end-diastolic volume index in the carvedilol-treated group at 12 months, as well a significant relative risk reduction of 26 percent in the clinical composite of death or hospitalization for the carvedilol group at 19 months. Rates of hospitalization were also significantly lower for patients treated with carvedilol (48 percent) compared with placebo (58 percent).[15] The Carvedilol Prospective Randomized Cumulative Survival (COPERNICUS) study extended these benefits to patients with more advanced HF. In COPERNICUS patients with advanced HF, symptoms had to be clinically euvolemic, with a LVEF less than 25 percent. When compared with placebo, carvedilol reduced the mortality risk at 12 months by 38 percent (see Table 25-10) and the relative risk of death or HF hospitalization by 31 percent (see Fig. 25-16C).[15]

Carvedilol has also been evaluated in a postmyocardial infarction trial in which patients had to exhibit LV dysfunction. The Carvedilol Post-Infarct Survival Controlled Evaluation (CAPRICORN) trial was a randomized, placebo-controlled trial designed to test the long-term efficacy of carvedilol on morbidity and mortality in patients with LV dysfunction after MI who had already been treated with ACEIs.[42] Although carvedilol did not reduce the prespecified primary endpoint of mortality plus cardiovascular hospitalization, it did significantly reduce total mortality by 23 percent ($P = 0.03$), cardiovascular mortality by 25 percent ($P < 0.05$), and nonfatal myocardial infarction by 41 percent ($P = 0.014$). Finally, in the Carvedilol or Metoprolol European Trial (COMET), carvedilol (target dose, 25 mg twice daily) was compared with immediate-release metoprolol tartrate (target dose, 50 mg twice daily) with respect to the primary endpoint of all-cause mortality. In COMET, carvedilol was associated with a significant 33 percent reduction in all-cause mortality when compared with metoprolol tartrate (33.9 versus 39.5 percent; HR, 0.83; 95 percent CI, 0.74 to 0.93, $P = 0.0017$).[43] Based on the results of the COMET trial, short-acting metoprolol tartrate is not recommended for use in the treatment of HF. The results of the COMET trial emphasize the importance of using doses and formulations of beta blockers that have been shown to be effective in clinical trials. There have been no trials to ascertain whether the survival benefits of carvedilol are greater than those of metoprolol (succinate) CR/XL when both drugs are used at the appropriate target doses.

Not all studies with beta blockers have been universally successful, suggesting that the effects of beta blockers should not necessarily be viewed broadly as a class effect. Indeed, early studies with the first generation of nonspecific $beta_1$ and $beta_2$ receptors without ancillary vasodilating properties (e.g., propranolol) resulted in significant worsening of HF and death. The Beta-blocker Evaluation of Survival Trial (BEST) evaluated the third-generation beta-blocking agent bucindolol, which is a completely nonselective $beta_1$ and $beta_2$ antagonist with some $alpha_1$ receptor blockade. In the BEST trial, bucindolol produced a statistically nonsignificant ($P = 0.10$) 10 percent reduction in total mortality that was heterogeneous with respect to race. That is, the 76 percent of subjects in BEST who were not black had a statistically significant ($P = 0.01$) 19 percent reduction in mortality, whereas the 24 percent who were black had a nonsignificant trend for an increase (by 17 percent) in mortality (interaction P value <0.05). The differential response of bucindolol in white patients has been suggested to be secondary to a polymorphism (arginine 389) in the $beta_1$-adrenergic receptor (see Chap. 29).[44] Bucindolol is not currently approved for clinical use at this time.

Furthermore, not all antiadrenergic strategies are beneficial in HF patients. For example, moxonidine is a centrally acting imidazoline receptor antagonist that powerfully lowers adrenergic activity. In the Monoxidine in Heart Failure (MOXCON) trial, moxonidine SR or matching placebo was titrated to a target dose of 1.5 mg twice a day.[45] This trial was stopped prematurely because of an early increase in death rate (approximately a 50 percent increase) and adverse events in the moxonidine SR group when compared with placebo. Analysis of norepinephrine (NE) levels showed that NE levels are significantly less in the moxonidine treatment arm, suggesting that generalized sympathetic inhibition (withdrawal) may be deleterious in patients with HF. Nebivolol is a selective $beta_1$ receptor antagonist, not yet approved for the treatment of HF, with ancillary vasodilatory properties that are mediated, at least in part, by nitric oxide. In the Study of Effects of Nebivolol Intervention on Outcomes and Rehospitalization in Seniors with Heart Failure (SENIORS), nebivolol significantly reduced the composite outcome of death or cardiovascular hospitalizations in elderly patients with a known EF less than 35 percent or a previous hospitalization for HF within 1 year (35 percent had an EF more than 35 percent).[46]

SIDE EFFECTS OF BETA BLOCKERS. The adverse affects of beta blockers are generally related to the predictable complications that arise from interfering with the adrenergic nervous system. These reactions generally occur within several days of initiating therapy and are generally responsive to adjusting concomitant medications (see earlier). The problem of fluid retention has been discussed earlier. Treatment with a beta blocker can be accompanied by feelings of general fatigue or weakness. In most cases, the increased fatigue spontaneously resolves within several weeks or months; however, in some patients, it may be severe enough to limit the dose of beta blocker or require the withdrawal or reduction of treatment. Therapy with beta blockers can lead to bradycardia and/or exacerbate heart block. Moreover, beta blockers (particularly those that block the $alpha_1$ receptor) can lead to vasodilatory side effects. Accordingly, the dose of beta blockers should be decreased if the heart rate decreases to less than 50 beats/min and/or second- or third-degree heart block develops, or symptomatic hypotension develops. Beta blockers are not recommended for patients with asthma with active bronchospasm.

Aldosterone Antagonists

Although classified as a potassium-sparing diuretics, drugs that block the effects of aldosterone (e.g., spironolactone) have beneficial effects independent of the effects of these agents on sodium balance (see Fig. 25-10). Although an ACEI may transiently decrease aldosterone secretion, with chronic therapy there is a rapid return of aldosterone to levels similar to those before ACEI administration. The administration of an aldosterone antagonist is recommended for patients with NYHA Class IV or Class III (previously Class IV) HF who have a depressed EF (less than 35 percent), and who are receiving standard therapy, including diuretics, ACEIs, and beta blockers.[15] The dose of aldosterone antagonist should be increased until the doses used are similar to those that have been shown to be effective in clinical trials (see Table 25-9). Spironolactone should be initiated at a dose of 12.5 to 25 mg daily, or occasionally on alternate days. Eplerenone was used after MI in one study at doses of 25 mg per day, increasing to 50 mg daily (see Table 25-10). As noted earlier, potassium supplementation is generally stopped after the initiation of aldosterone antagonists, and patients should be counseled to avoid high potassium–containing foods. Potassium levels and renal function should be rechecked within 3 days and again at 1 week after initiation of an aldosterone antagonist. Subsequent monitoring should be dictated by the general clinical stability of renal function and fluid status but should occur at least monthly for the first 6 months.

SIDE EFFECTS OF ALDOSTERONE ANTAGONISTS. The major problem with the use of aldosterone antagonists is the development of life-threatening hyperkalemia, which is more prone to occur in patients who are receiving potassium supplements or who have underlying renal insufficiency. Aldosterone antagonists are not recommended when the serum creatinine level is higher than 2.5 mg/dl, creatinine clearance is less than 30 ml/min, or the serum potassium level is higher than 5.5 mmol/liter. The development of worsening renal function should lead to consideration of stopping aldosterone antagonists because of the potential risk of hyperkalemia. Painful gynecomastia may develop in 5 to 10 percent of patients who use spironolactone, in which case eplerenone may be substituted.

Management of Patients Who Remain Symptomatic

As noted earlier, an ACEI (or an ARB) plus a beta blocker should be standard background therapy for HF patients with a depressed LVEF. Additional pharmacological therapy (polypharmacy) or device therapy (see later) should be considered in patients who have persistent symptoms or progressive worsening despite optimized therapy with an ACE inhibitor and beta blocker (Fig. 25-17; see also Table 25-9). Agents that may be considered as part of additional therapy include an ARB (NYHA Class II to IV), spironolactone (NYHA Class III or IV), combination of hydralazine and isosorbide dinitrate (NYHA Class II to IV), or digitalis.[15] The optimal choice of additional drug therapy to improve outcome further in patients has not been firmly established. Thus, the choice of specific agent will be influenced by clinical considerations, including renal function, serum potassium concentration, blood pressure, and race (see later). The triple combination of an ACE inhibitor, ARB, and aldosterone antagonist is not recommended because of the risk of hyperkalemia. Digoxin is recommended for patients with symptomatic LV systolic dysfunction who have concomitant atrial fibrillation and should be considered for patients who have signs or symptoms of HF while receiving standard therapy, including ACEIs and beta blockers.

Cardiac Glycosides

Digoxin and digitoxin are the most frequently used cardiac glycosides. Given that digoxin is most commonly used and is the only glycoside that has been evaluated in placebo-controlled trials, there is little reason to prescribe other cardiac glycosides for the management of patients with

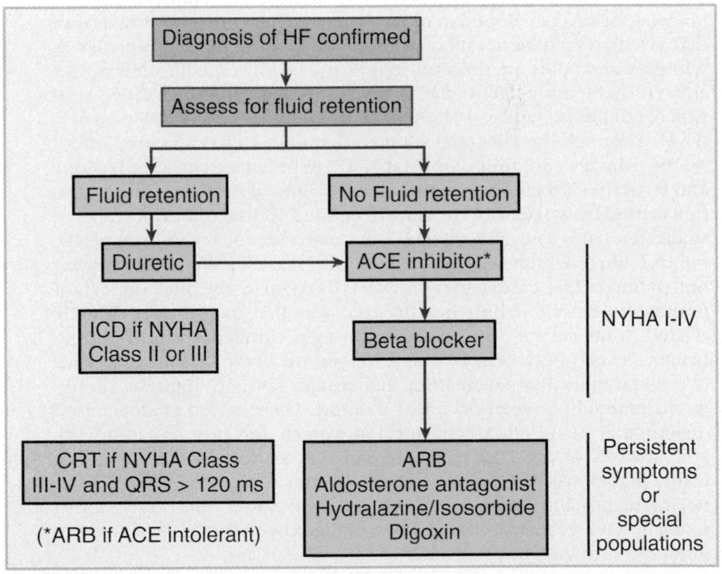

FIGURE 25–17 Treatment algorithm for patients with chronic heart failure (HF) with a reduced ejection fraction (EF). After the clinical diagnosis of HF is made, it is important to treat the fluid retention that the patient experienced before starting an angiotensin-converting enzyme (ACE) inhibitor (or an angiotensin receptor blocker (ARB) if the patient is ACE intolerant). Beta blockers should be started after the fluid retention has been treated and/or the ACE inhibitor has been uptitrated. If the patient remains symptomatic, an ARB, aldosterone antagonist, or digoxin can be added as triple therapy. The fixed-dose combination of hydralazine–isosorbide dinitrate should be added to an ACE inhibitor and beta blocker in African American patients with New York Heart Association (NYHA) Class II, II, or IV HF. Device therapy should be considered in addition to pharmacological therapy for appropriate patients. CRT = cardiac resynchronization therapy; ICD = implantable cardioverter-defibrillator. *(From Mann DL: Heart failure and cor pulmonale.* In *Kasper DL, Braunwald E, Fauci AS, et al (eds): Harrison's Principles of Internal Medicine. 17th ed. New York, McGraw-Hill, 2007 [in press].)*

chronic HF. Digoxin exerts its effects by inhibiting the Na^+,K^+-ATPase pump in cell membranes, including the sarcolemmal Na^+,K^+-ATPase pump of cardiac myocytes (see Chap. 21). Inhibition of the Na^+,K^+-ATPase pump leads to an increase in intracellular calcium concentration and hence increased cardiac contractility, which has led to the suggestion that beneficial effects of digoxin are secondary to its inotropic properties. However, the more likely mechanism of digoxin in HF patients is to sensitize Na^+,K^+-ATPase activity in vagal afferent nerves, leading to an increase in vagal tone that counterbalances the increased activation of the adrenergic system in advanced HF. Digoxin also inhibits Na^+,K^+-ATPase activity in the kidney and may, therefore, blunt renal tubular resorption of sodium. Therapy with digoxin is commonly initiated and maintained at a dosage of 0.125 to 0.25 mg daily. For the great majority of patients, the dosage should be 0.125 mg daily and the serum digoxin level should be less than 1.0 ng/ml, especially in elderly patients, patients with impaired renal function, and patients with a low lean body mass. Higher dosages (e.g., 0.375 to 0.50 mg daily) are rarely used or needed in the management of patients with HF. See Chapter 25 Online Supplement on the website for further details about digitalis, including details about mechanism of action, pharmacokinetics, and interaction with other commonly used drugs.

Although clinicians have used cardiac glycosides to treat patients with chronic HF for well over 200 years, there is still considerable debate regarding the effectiveness of cardiac glycosides in HF patients. Whereas small and medium-sized trials conducted in the 1970s and 1980s yielded equivocal results, two relatively large digoxin withdrawal studies in the early 1990s, the Randomized Assessment of Digoxin and Inhibitors of Angiotensin-Converting Enzyme (RADIANCE) and the Prospective Randomized Study of Ventricular Function and Efficacy of Digoxin (PROVED), have provided strong support for clinical benefit from digoxin.[47] In these studies, worsening HF and HF hospitalizations developed in more patients who were withdrawn from digoxin than in patients who were maintained on digoxin. Insofar as withdrawal studies are difficult to interpret with respect to efficacy of a given therapeutic agent, the Digoxin Investigator Group (DIG) trial was conducted to address the role of digitalis in chronic HF prospectively. Although the DIG trial showed that digoxin has a neutral effect on the primary endpoint of mortality, digoxin reduces hospitalizations and favorably affects the combined endpoints of death or hospitalization caused by worsening HF. Data from the DIG trial indicated a strong trend ($P = 0.06$) toward a decrease in deaths secondary to progressive pump failure, which was offset by an increase in sudden and other non-pump failure cardiac deaths ($P = 0.04$). One of the most important findings to emerge from the DIG trial was that mortality is directly related to the serum digoxin level.[47] In men enrolled in the DIG trial, trough levels between 0.6 and 0.8 ng/ml were associated with decreased mortality, suggesting that trough levels of digitalis should be maintained between 0.5 and 1.0 ng/ml. There is also evidence that digoxin may be potentially harmful in women. In a post hoc multivariable analysis of the DIG trial, digoxin was associated with a significantly higher risk (23 percent) of death from any cause in women but not men, possibly because of the relatively lower body weights in women, who were prescribed doses of digoxin on the basis of a nomogram rather than trough levels.[48]

COMPLICATIONS OF DIGOXIN USE. The principal adverse effects of digoxin are as follows: (1) cardiac arrhythmias, including heart block (especially in the elderly), ectopic and reentrant cardiac rhythms; (2) neurological complaints such as visual disturbances, disorientation, and confusion; and (3) gastrointestinal symptoms such as anorexia, nausea, and vomiting. As noted earlier, these side effects can generally be minimized by maintaining trough levels of 0.5 to 1.0 ng/ml. In patients with HF, overt digitalis toxicity tends to become clinically apparent at serum concentrations greater than 2.0 ng/ml; however, as noted earlier, digitalis toxicity may occur with lower digoxin levels, particularly if hypokalemia or hypomagnesemia coexist. Oral potassium administration is often useful for atrial, atrioventricular (AV), junctional, or ventricular ectopic rhythms, even when the serum potassium level is in the normal range, unless high-grade AV block is also present. However, serum K^+ levels must be monitored carefully to avoid hyperkalemia, especially in patients with renal failure or taking aldosterone receptor antagonists. Potentially life-threatening digoxin toxicity can be reversed by antidigoxin immunotherapy using purified Fab fragments. See Chapter 25 Online Supplement on the website for details. The concomitant use of quinidine, verapamil, spironolactone, flecainide, propafenone, and amiodarone can increase serum digoxin levels and may increase the risk of adverse reactions (see Chap. 25 Online Supplement for details). Patients with advanced heart block should not receive digitalis unless a pacemaker is in place.

Management of Atherosclerotic Disease

The clinical evaluation of atherosclerotic cardiovascular heart disease in HF patients is discussed in Chapter 23. In patients with a prior MI and HF without angina, the use of ACEIs and beta blockers has been shown to decrease the risk of reinfarction and death. Although aspirin has been shown to reduce the risk of major ischemic events in patients without HF, the role of aspirin in patients with HF has not been clearly established.[15] Indeed, prior studies have suggested that the use of aspirin may attenuate the beneficial effects of ACEIs in HF patients. For these reasons, the role of aspirin in preventing ischemic events in patients with chronic HF remains controversial. Alternative antiplatelet agents (e.g., clopidogrel) may not interact adversely with ACEIs and may have superior effects in preventing clinical events; however, their ability to affect outcomes in HF favorably has not been demonstrated Although some clinicians recommend the use of coronary revascularization in patients with HF and coronary artery disease who do not have symptoms of angina, coronary revascularization has not been shown to improve cardiac function or symptoms or prevent reinfarction or death in HF patients without angina. In contrast, coronary artery bypass grafting has been shown to improve symptoms and survival in patients with modestly reduced EF and angina, although patients with clinical HF or markedly depressed ventricular function have generally been excluded from these studies.[15] To this end, an ongoing trial funded by the National Institutes of Health is evaluating the usefulness of surgical revascularization in such patients (see Chapter 27). Until the results of randomized clinical trials are forthcoming, it is reasonable to consider coronary artery revascularization with coronary artery bypass surgery or percutaneous coronary intervention for HF patients who have suitable coronary anatomy and angina, or for patients who have demonstrable evidence of myocardial viability in areas of significant obstructive coronary disease and/or the presence of inducible ischemia.[15] The surgical management of patients with CAD disease and HF is discussed in Chapter 27.

Special Populations

Race

Epidemiological (see earlier) and clinical trial data have raised awareness of potential areas of concern regarding the evaluation and treatment of HF in blacks. A retrospective analysis, the Vasodilator in Heart Failure Trial I (V-HeFT I) trials, has suggested that overall mortality and HF hospitalization is significantly reduced in black patients who receive combination therapy with hydralazine isosorbide, whereas white patients show no treatment effect when compared with placebo. In contrast, in V-HeFT-II, only white patients showed a significant mortality reduction from ACEI therapy (enalapril) when compared with treatment with hydralazine isosorbide, whereas black patients had no apparent treatment benefit from ACEIs.[49] To address the role of hydralazine isosorbide treatment, the African-American Heart Failure Trial (A-HeFT) compared the adjunctive use of a proprietary formulation of isosorbide dinitrate and hydralazine to a standard HF regimen of ACEIs, beta blockers, and diuretics in black patients with NYHA Class III or IV HF.[50] The primary endpoint was a composite score made up of weighted values for death from any cause, a first hospitalization for HF, and change in the quality of life. The study was terminated early because there was a significant 43 percent reduction in the rate of death from any cause (Fig. 25-18) and a significant 33 percent relative reduction in the rate of first hospitalization for HF. The mechanism for the beneficial effect of the hydralazine isosorbide regimen may be related to an improvement in nitric oxide bioavailability; however, the combination therapy group also had a small (but significant) decrease in blood pressure. The effect of this combination of isosorbide dinitrate and hydralazine in other HF patients who are being treated with standard therapy is not known because only blacks were studied in A-HeFT, but there is no reason to believe that this benefit is limited to blacks. The results of the A-HeFT trial have led to the suggestion that the addition of isosorbide dinitrate and hydralazine to a standard medical regimen for HF, including ACEIs and beta blockers, is reasonable and can be effective in blacks with NYHA functional Class III or IV HF (see Fig. 25-17). The emerging field of genomic medicine has begun to suggest that important variances in the expression of certain high-risk, single-nucleotide polymorphisms may be evident along racial lines and may provide a physiological basis for differences in the natural history of HF and differences in drug responsiveness (see Chap. 29).

Elderly Patients

As noted at the beginning of this chapter, the prevalence of HF increases with age (see Fig. 25-1) and HF is the most common reason for hospitalization in elderly patients. Furthermore, unlike other common cardiovascular diseases, the age-adjusted mortality attributed to HF also appears to be increasing. The therapeutic approach to HF with a reduced EF in the elderly should be, in principal, identical to that in younger patients with respect to the choice of pharmacological therapy. However, altered pharmacokinetic and pharmacodynamic properties of cardiovascular drugs in the elderly may require that these therapies be applied more cautiously, with reductions in drug dosages when appropriate (see Chap. 75). Other complicating factors may include blunting of baroreceptor function and orthostatic dysregulation of blood pressure, which may make it difficult to use target doses of some neurohormonal antagonists. Some multidisciplinary HF programs have been successful in decreasing the rate of readmission and associated morbidity in elderly patients (see later).

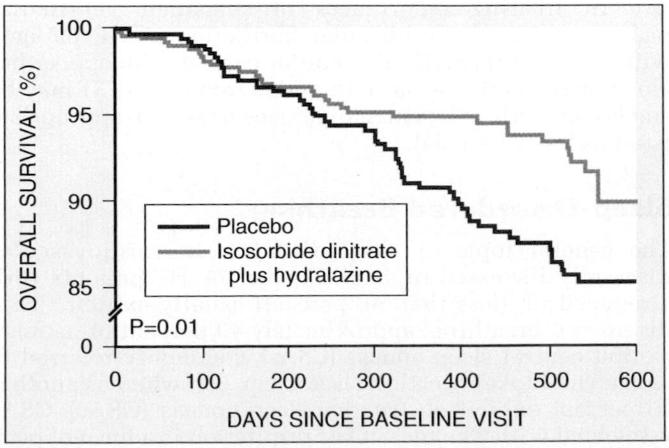

FIGURE 25–18 Kaplan-Meier analysis of the probability of survival in patients in the placebo and isosorbide dinitrate plus hydralazine treatment arms of the A-HeFT (African-American Heart Failure Trial) study. *(Modified from Taylor AL, Ziesche S, Yancy C, et al: Combination of isosorbide dinitrate and hydralazine in blacks with heart failure. N Engl J Med 351:2049, 2004.)*

Cancer Patients

Patients with cancer are particularly predisposed to the development of HF as a result of the cardiotoxic effects of many cancer chemotherapeutic agents. The management of these patients is discussed in Chapter 85.

Anticoagulation and Antiplatelet Therapy

Patients with HF have an increased risk for arterial or venous thromboembolic events. In clinical HF trials, the rate of stroke has ranged from 1.3 to 2.4 percent/year. Depressed LV function is believed to promote relative stasis of blood in dilated cardiac chambers, with increased risk of thrombus formation. Treatment with warfarin (goal international normalized ratio [INR], 2.0 to 3.0) is recommended for all patients with HF and chronic or paroxysmal atrial fibrillation and/or a history of systemic or pulmonary emboli, including stroke or transient ischemic attack. Patients with symptomatic or asymptomatic ischemic cardiomyopathy and documented recent large anterior MI or recent MI with documented LV thrombus should be treated with warfarin (goal INR, 2.0 to 3.0) for the initial 3 months after MI unless there are contraindications. In the absence of these indications, the optimal strategy to prevent stroke in individuals with HF is less certain. There is no compelling evidence that warfarin anticoagulation is beneficial in patients with HF, although it may be considered for selected HF patients after a careful assessment of the potential risks and benefits.[15] To address this important question, the National Institutes of Health is evaluating the usefulness of aspirin and warfarin to determine whether there are differences between warfarin (INR, 2.5 to 3) and aspirin (325 mg) in terms of event-free survival for the composite endpoint of death or stroke (ischemic or hemorrhagic) in patients with an LVEF less than 35 percent who do not have atrial fibrillation or mechanical prosthetic heart valves.[51] Currently, aspirin is recommended for HF patients with ischemic heart disease for the prevention of MI and death. However, lower doses of aspirin (75 or 81 mg) may be preferable because of the concern of worsening of HF at higher doses, as noted earlier.

Management of Cardiac Arrhythmias

The management of atrial arrhythmias is discussed in detail in Chapter 35. Briefly, atrial fibrillation occurs in 15 to 30 percent of patients with HF, and is a frequent cause of cardiac decompensation (see Table 25-7). Most antiarrhythmic agents, with the exception of amiodarone and dofetilide, have negative inotropic effects and are proarrhythmic. Amiodarone is a class III antiarrhythmic that has little or no negative inotropic and/or proarrhythmic effects and is effective against most supraventricular arrhythmias (see Chap. 35). Amiodarone is the preferred drug for restoring and maintaining sinus rhythm, and may improve the success of electrical cardioversion in patients with HF. Amiodarone increases the levels of phenytoin and digoxin and will prolong the INR in patients taking warfarin. Therefore, it is often necessary to reduce the dose of these drugs by as much as 50 percent when initiating therapy with amiodarone. The risk of adverse events, such as hyperthyroidism, hypothyroidism, pulmonary fibrosis, and hepatitis are relatively low, particularly when lower dosages of amiodarone are used (100 to 200 mg/day). Because of the risk of proarrhythmic effects of antiarrhythmic agents in patients with LV dysfunction, it is preferable to treat ventricular arrhythmias with implantable cardioverter-defibrillators (ICDs), either alone or in combination with amiodarone.

Device Therapy

CARDIAC RESYNCHRONIZATION. Cardiac resynchronization therapy (CRT) is discussed in detail in Chapter 34. Briefly, approximately one third of patients with a depressed EF and symptomatic HF (NYHA Class III or IV) manifest a QRS duration longer than 120 milliseconds. This electrocardiographic manifestation of abnormal inter- or intraventricular conduction has been used to identify patients with dyssynchronous ventricular contraction. The mechanical consequences of ventricular dyssynchrony include suboptimal ventricular filling, a reduction in LV contractility, prolonged duration (and therefore greater severity) of mitral regurgitation, and paradoxical septal wall motion. Biventricular pacing, or CRT, stimulates both ventricles nearly simultaneously, thereby improving the coordination of ventricular contraction and reducing the severity of mitral regurgitation. When CRT is added to optimal medical therapy in patients in sinus rhythm, there is a significant decrease in patient mortality and hospitalization, a reversal of LV remodeling, and improved quality of life and exercise capacity (see Table 34-4).[52] In the Cardiac Resynchronization in Heart Failure (CARE-HF) trial, NYHA Class III or IV HF patients with an LVEF less than 35 percent and markers of cardiac dyssynchrony were randomized to medical therapy with or without CRT. CRT resulted in a significant 37 percent reduction (HR, 0.63; 95 percent CI, 0.51 to 0.77; P <0.001) in morbidity and mortality during a mean follow-up of 29.4 months (Fig. 25-19). The benefits of CRT were similar in patients with and without ischemic heart disease and were in addition to those afforded by pharmacological therapy. In addition, CRT reduced the interventricular mechanical delay, the LV end-systolic volume index, and the area of the mitral regurgitant jet and increased the LVEF. Similar overall results with respect to the role of CRT were observed in the Comparison of Medical Therapy, Resynchronization, and Defibrillation Therapies in Heart Failure Trial (COMPANION).[53] Accordingly, based on the aggregate clinical trial experience (see Table 34-4), CRT is recommended for patients in sinus rhythm who have an EF less than 35 percent and a QRS width more than 120 milliseconds and who remain symptomatic (NYHA Class III or IV), despite optimal medical therapy (see Fig. 25-17). The benefits of CRT in patients with atrial fibrillation have not been established.

IMPLANTABLE CARDIOVERTER-DEFIBRILLATOR. ICDs are discussed in detail in Chapters 34 and 36. Briefly, the prophylactic implantation of ICDs in patients with mild to moderate HF (NYHA Class II or III) has been shown to reduce the incidence of sudden cardiac death in patients with ischemic or nonischemic cardiomyopathy.[54] The Sudden Cardiac Death in Heart Failure Trial (SCD-HeFT) evaluated whether amiodarone therapy or single-chamber shock-only ICD therapy would decrease the risk of death from any cause in patients with mild to moderate HF of ischemic or nonischemic cause. SCD-HeFT results have shown that when compared with placebo, amiodarone is associated with a similar risk of death (HR, 1.06; 97.5 percent CI, 0.86 to 1.30; $P = 0.53$), whereas ICD therapy is associated with a 23 percent decreased risk of death (HR, 0.77; 97.5 percent CI, 0.62 to 0.96; $P = 0.007$) (Fig. 25-20). Accordingly, implantation of an ICD should be considered for patients in NYHA Class II or III HF with a depressed EF of less than 30 to 35 percent who are already on optimal background therapy, including an ACEI-ARB, beta blocker, and aldosterone antagonist (see Fig. 25-17). ICDs are also highly effective in treating recurrences of sustained ventricular tachycardia and/or ventricular fibrillation in HF patients with recurrent arrhythmias and/or cardiac syncope, either alone or in combination with amiodarone. An ICD may be combined with a biventricular pacemaker in appropriate patients (see Chap. 34).

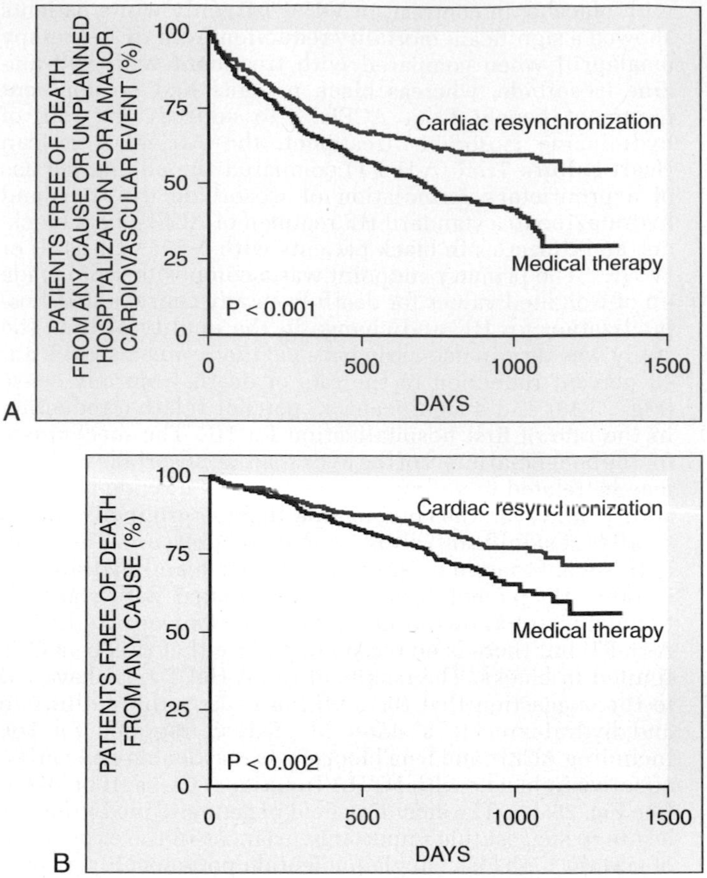

FIGURE 25–19 Kaplan-Meier analysis of the time to death from any cause or an unplanned hospitalization for a major cardiovascular event **(A)** and death from any cause **(B)** in patients receiving standard pharmacological therapy and cardiac resynchronization therapy in the CARE-HF trial (Cardiac Resynchronization in Heart Failure Trial). *(Modified from Cleland JG, Daubert JC, Erdmann E, et al: The effect of cardiac resynchronization on morbidity and mortality in heart failure. N Engl J Med 352:1539, 2005.)*

Sleep-Disordered Breathing

The general topic of sleep disorders in cardiovascular disease is discussed in detail Chapter 74. HF patients with a reduced EF (less than 40 percent) usually exhibit sleep-disordered breathing; approximately 40 percent of patients exhibit central sleep apneas (CSAs), commonly referred to as Cheyne-Stokes breathing (see Chap. 23), whereas another 10 percent exhibit obstructive sleep apneas (OSAs). CSAs associated with Cheyne-Stokes respiration is a form of periodic breathing in which central apneas and hypopneas alternate with periods of hyperventilation that have a waxing-waning pattern of tidal volume. Risk factors for the development of CSA in HF patients include male gender, age older than 60 years, the presence of atrial fibrillation, and hypocapnia.[55] Figure 25-21 illustrates the proposed mechanisms that underlie periodic oscillations in ventilation in HF.

The pattern of Cheyne-Stokes breathing in patients with HF arises because of enhanced chemosensitivity of central and peripheral receptors, as well as increased activity of pulmonary vagal irritant receptors that are stimulated by pulmonary congestion.[56] When HF patients recline, increased venous return from the extremities leads to accumulation of fluid centrally, with a resultant increase in pulmonary congestion that stimulates vagal irritant receptors in the lungs to elicit reflex hyperventilation. Central apnea is usually initiated during sleep by a further acute increase in ventilation and a reduction in $Pa{CO_2}$ that is triggered by a spontaneous arousals. When $Pa{CO_2}$ falls below the threshold level required to stimulate breathing, the central drive to respiratory muscles ceases and central apnea ensues. Apnea will persist until the $Pa{CO_2}$ rises above the threshold required to stimulate ventilation. In contrast to OSA, arousals are not required for the initiation of air flow at the termination of central apneas. Arousals frequently follow the resumption of breathing and thus facilitate periodic breathing by stimulating hyperventilation, thereby further reducing $Pa{CO_2}$ levels below the apneic threshold. Studies have shown that the length of the subsequent ventilatory phase in CSA is inversely proportional to cardiac output, reflecting the delayed transmission of changes in arterial blood gas tensions from the lungs to the peripheral chemoreceptors. Accordingly, HF patients with CSA have a longer ventilatory phase than CSA subjects with normal LV function. However, it bears emphasis that the development of CSA is not dependent on a prolonged circulation time; rather, the influence of the prolonged circulation time in CSA is reflected in the length of the hyperpneic phase and of the total periodic breathing cycle. Once triggered, the pattern of alternating hyperventilation and apnea is sustained by the combination of increased respiratory chemoreceptor drive, pulmonary congestion, arousals, and apnea-induced hypoxia, which cause oscillations in $Pa{CO_2}$ above and below the apneic threshold. Inhalation of a CO_2-enriched gas to raise $Pa{CO_2}$ abolishes CSA.[56]

The main clinical significance of CSA in HF is its association with increased mortality. Whether this is simply because Cheyne-Stokes respiration with CSA is a reflection of advanced disease with poor LV function, or whether its presence constitutes a separate and additive adverse influence on outcomes, is not clear. Nonetheless, multivariate analyses have suggested that CSA remains an independent risk factor for death or cardiac transplantation, even after controlling for potentially confounding risk factors. The potential mechanism(s) for averse out-

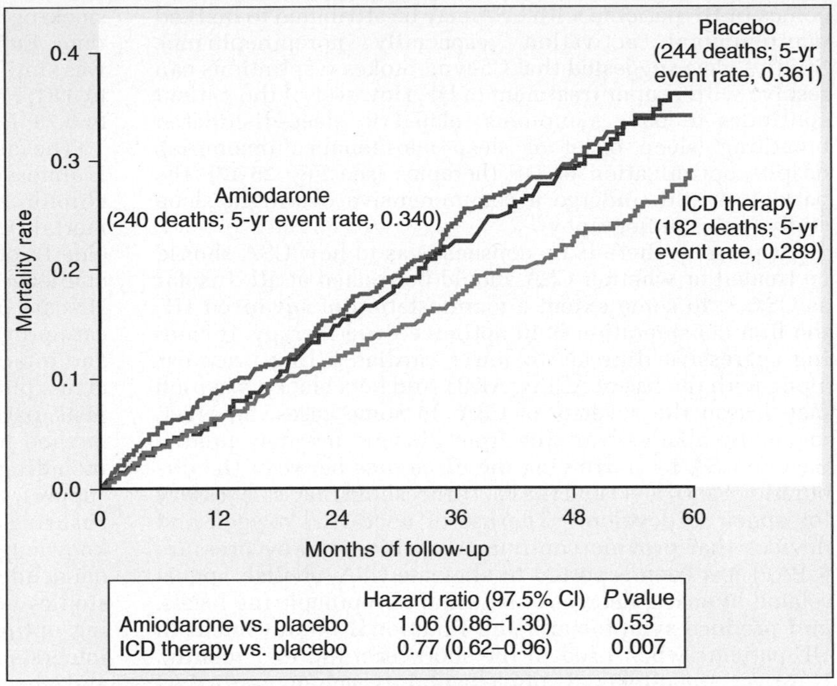

FIGURE 25–20 Kaplan-Meier analysis of the time to death from any cause in patients receiving conventional heart failure therapy, conventional therapy plus amiodarone, or conventional therapy plus a conservatively programmed, shock-only, single-lead implantable cardioverter-defibrillator (ICD) in the SCD-HeFT trial (Sudden Cardiac Death in Heart Failure Trial). *(Modified from Bardy GH, Lee KL, Mark DB, et al: Amiodarone or an implantable cardioverter-defibrillator for congestive heart failure. N Engl J Med 352:225, 2005.)*

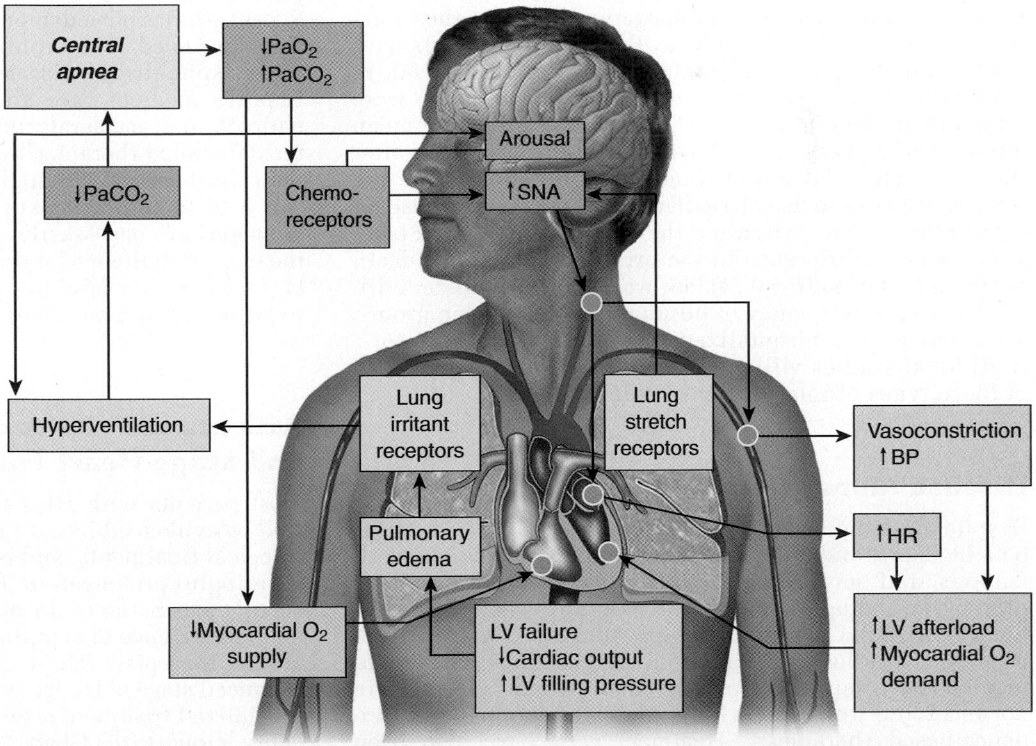

FIGURE 25–21 Pathophysiology of central sleep apnea and Cheyne-Stokes respiration in heart failure (HF). HF leads to increased left ventricular (LV) filling pressure. The resulting pulmonary congestion activates lung vagal irritant receptors, which stimulate hyperventilation and hypocapnia. Superimposed arousals cause further abrupt increases in ventilation and drive the partial pressure of carbon dioxide in arterial blood ($Pa{CO_2}$) below the threshold for ventilation, triggering a central apnea. Central sleep apneas are sustained by recurrent arousal resulting from apnea-induced hypoxia and the increased effort to breathe during the ventilatory phase because of pulmonary congestion and reduced lung compliance. Increased sympathetic activity causes increases in blood pressure (BP) and heart rate (HR) and increases myocardial oxygen (O_2) demand in the presence of reduced supply. SNA = sympathetic nervous system activity; $Pa{O_2}$ = partial pressure of oxygen in arterial blood. *(Redrawn from Bradley TD, Floras JS: Sleep apnea and heart failure. Part II: Central sleep apnea. Circulation 107:1822, 2003.)*

comes in HF patients with CSA may be attributed to marked neurohumoral activation (especially norepinephrine). Studies have suggested that Cheyne-Stokes respirations can resolve with proper treatment of HF. However, if the patient continues to have symptoms related to sleep-disordered breathing (sleep onset or sleep maintenance insomnia), despite optimization of HF therapies (see Fig. 25-17), the patient should undergo a comprehensive overnight sleep study (polysomnography).

At present, there is no consensus as to how CSA should be treated or whether CSA should be treated at all. Insofar as CSA is to some extent a manifestation of advanced HF, the first consideration is to optimize drug therapy, including aggressive diuresis to lower cardiac filling pressure, along with the use of ACEIs, ARBs, and beta blockers, which may lessen the severity of CSA. In some cases, however, metabolic alkalosis arising from diuretic use may predispose to CSA by narrowing the difference between the circulating $Pa{CO_2}$ level and the $Pa{CO_2}$ threshold that is necessary for apnea to develop.[56] The use of nocturnal oxygen and devices that provide continuous positive airway pressure (CPAP) has been reported to alleviate CSA, abolish apnea-related hypoxia, decrease nocturnal norepinephrine levels, and produce symptomatic and functional improvement in HF patients when used in the short term (up to 1 month). However, the effects of supplemental oxygen on cardiovascular endpoints over more prolonged periods have not been assessed.[55,56] Although there is no direct evidence that treatment of sleep-disturbed breathing prevents the development HF, treatment of established LV dysfunction with CPAP breathing has been shown to improve LV structure and function in patients with obstructive or central sleep apnea disturbed breathing syndrome.[55] Despite these objective measurements of improvement with CPAP, this treatment modality did not lead to a prolongation of life in the Canadian Continuous Positive Airway Pressure for Patients with Central Sleep Apnea and Heart Failure (CANPAP) trial. In CANPAP, patients with HF and central sleep apnea were randomly assigned to receive CPAP or no CPAP for a mean duration of 2 years. The trial was discontinued early after the event rate for death or transplantation observed in the trial was too low to detect a difference based on the expected event rate used to determine the sample size for the trial. There was no difference in the primary endpoint of death or transplantation ($P = 0.54$), nor was there a significant difference in the frequency of hospitalization between groups (0.56 versus 0.61 hospitalizations/patient-year; $P = 0.45$).[57] Additional studies will be needed to evaluate the efficacy of these types of interventions in HF patients.

Disease Management

Despite the compelling scientific evidence that ACEIs, ARBs, beta blockers, and aldosterone antagonists reduce hospitalizations and mortality in patients with HF, these life-prolonging therapies continue to be underused outside the highly artificial environment of clinical trials. Indeed, numerous studies in different clinical settings have documented that a significant proportion of patients with HF are not receiving treatment with guideline-recommended, evidence-based therapies.[58] Treatment gaps have also been documented in providing other components of care for patients with HF, especially in the critically important area of patient education. In the CHARM study, "good" adherence, defined as taking more than 80 percent of study medications, was associated with lower all-cause mortality in all patients (HR, 0.65; 95 percent CI, 0.57 to 0.75; $P < 0.0001$), even after adjusting for predictive factors such as demographics, physiological and severity of illness variables, smoking history, and the number of concomitant medications. Furthermore, the clinical outcome for good adherence was similar in the candesartan (HR, 0.66; 95 percent CI, 0.55 to 0.81; $P < 0.0001$) and placebo (HR, 0.64; 95 percent CI, 0.53 to 0.78; $P < 0.0001$) treatment arms.[59]

The failure to deliver optimal medical care to HF patients is almost certainly multifactorial, as it is with other complex chronic conditions that have substantial morbidity and mortality. Furthermore, because many HF patients are elderly, often with have a myriad of comorbidities, a special challenge is also presented to health care providers. Optimal HF care includes the following: a trained network of health care providers involved in the delivery of HF management and interventions, including nurses, case managers, physicians, pharmacists, caseworkers, dietitians, physical therapists, psychologists, and information systems specialists; a method for communicating this knowledge to the patient, including patient education, medication management, peer support, and some form of postacute care and a method of ensuring that the patient has received and understood the knowledge; a system for encouraging adherence to the recommended regimen and patient compliance. Numerous studies have shown that many of the challenges to delivering optimal care to HF patients can be met through an integrated specialized HF clinic approach that uses nurse and physician extenders to deliver and ensure the implementation of care.[59]

Technology-driven strategies that use low-cost telemonitoring also appear promising in terms of improving HF management and outcomes,[60] emphasizing the importance of team management in the care of these complex patients. A disease management approach to HF has been shown to reduce hospitalizations and increase the percentage of patients receiving ideal guideline-recommended therapy.[58] Recent studies have demonstrated that disease management programs need not be confined to the outpatient setting and that hospital-based disease management systems can also improve medical care and education of hospitalized HF patients and accelerate use of evidence-based, guideline-recommended therapies by administering them before hospital discharge.[58] Although disease management strategies can lead to improved survival, it is not clear that these strategies are necessarily more cost-effective. Accordingly, the biggest challenge for disease management programs will be to determine how to support the additional personnel required for this model of care.

Patients with Refractory End-Stage Heart Failure

Most patients with HF caused by reduced LVEF respond well to evidenced-based pharmacological and nonpharmacological treatments, and enjoy a good quality of life with a meaningful prolongation. However, for reasons that are not clear, some patients do not improve or will experience a rapid recurrence of symptoms, despite optimal medical and device therapies. These individuals represent the most advanced stage of HF (stage D) and should be considered for specialized treatment strategies, such as mechanical circulatory support (see Chap. 28), continuous intravenous positive inotropic therapy, referral for cardiac transplantation (see Chap. 27), or hospice care. However, before a patient is considered to have refractory HF, physicians should identify any contributing conditions (see Table 25-7) and ensure that all conventional medical strategies have been optimally used (see Fig. 25-17). When no further therapies are appropriate, careful discussion of the prognosis and options for end-of life care should be initiated (see Chap. 30).

FUTURE PERSPECTIVES

As discussed in this chapter ACEIs, ARBs, aldosterone antagonists, beta blockers, and cardiac devices have substantially improved quality and quantity of life for patients with HF with reduced EF. Unfortunately, we appear to be reaching a ceiling—most recent trials attempting to add additional neurohormone-cytokine inhibition to the background therapy of ACE inhibition and beta blockade have been unsuccessful. This list of failures includes certain endothelin antagonists, tumor necrosis factor antagonists, and neutral endopeptidase inhibitors. This experience indicates the potential limits of neurohormonal inhibitory strategies and strongly signals that different drug development approaches are now needed. Currently, these approaches are under way with trials of new small molecules, cell replacement therapy, and gene therapy, accompanied by growing appreciation of the role pharmacogenetics (see Chap. 6). Some of these emerging therapies are discussed in Chapter 29. Further refinement of device technology and appropriate patient selection may allow device therapies, especially CRT, to be extended to a larger number of eligible patients. It is likely that one or more of these therapies that target maladaptive mechanisms and/or cardiac remodeling will be successful in the near term.

REFERENCES

Epidemiology and Prognosis

1. Kannel WB: Incidence and epidemiology of heart failure. Heart Fail Rev 5:167, 2000.
2. Swedberg K, Cleland J, Dargie H, et al: Guidelines for the diagnosis and treatment of chronic heart failure: Executive summary (update 2005): The Task Force for the Diagnosis and Treatment of Chronic Heart Failure of the European Society of Cardiology. Eur Heart J 26:1115, 2005.
3. Lev D, Kenchaiah S, Larson MG, et al: Long-term trends in the incidence of and survival with heart failure. N Engl J Med 347:1397, 2002.
4. Mendez GF, Cowie MR: The epidemiological features of heart failure in developing countries: A review of the literature. Int J Cardiol 80:213, 2001.
5. Kenchaiah S, Evans JC, Levy D, et al: Obesity and the risk of heart failure. N Engl J Med 347:305, 2002.
6. Walsh CR, Larson MG, Evans JC, et al: Alcohol consumption and risk for congestive heart failure in the Framingham Heart Study. Ann Intern Med 136:181, 2002.
7. Murray-Thomas T, Cowie MR: Epidemiology and clinical aspects of congestive heart failure. J Renin Angiotensin Aldosterone Syst 4:131, 2003.
8. Yancy CW: Heart failure in African Americans: Pathophysiology and treatment. J Card Fail 9:S210, 2003.
9. Young JB:. The prognosis of heart failure. *In* Mann DL (ed): Heart Failure: A Companion to Braunwald's Heart Disease. Philadelphia, WB Saunders, 2003, pp 489-506.
10. Levy WC, Mozaffarian D, Linker DT, et al: The Seattle Heart Failure Model: Prediction of survival in heart failure. Circulation 13:1424, 2006.
11. Tang YD, Katz SD: Anemia in chronic heart failure: Prevalence, cause, clinical correlates, and treatment options. Circulation 113:2454, 2006.
12. Tang WH, Francis GS: The year in heart failure. J Am Coll Cardiol 48:2575, 2006.
13. Smith GL, Lichtman JH, Bracken MB, et al: Renal impairment and outcomes in heart failure: Systematic review and meta-analysis. J Am Coll Cardiol 47:1987, 2006.
14. Hillege HL, Girbes AR, de Kam PJ, et al: Renal function, neurohormonal activation, and survival in patients with chronic heart failure. Circulation 102:203, 2000.
15. Hunt SA, Abraham WT, Chin MH, et al: ACC/AHA 2005 Guideline Update for the Diagnosis and Management of Chronic Heart Failure in the Adult: A report of the American College of Cardiology/American Heart Association Task Force on Practice Guidelines. Circulation 112:e154, 2005.
16. Heidenreich PA, Gubens MA, Fonarow GC, et al: Cost-effectiveness of screening with B-type natriuretic peptide to identify patients with reduced left ventricular ejection fraction. J Am Coll Cardiol 43:1019, 2004.
17. Ho KK, Pinsky JL, Kannel WB, et al: The epidemiology of heart failure: The Framingham Study. J Am Coll Cardiol 22:6A, 1993.
18. Schocken DD, Arrieta MI, Leaverton PE, et al: Prevalence and mortality rate of congestive heart failure in the United States. J Am Coll Cardiol 20:301, 1992.
19. Wittstein IS, Thiemann DR, Lima JA, et al: Neurohumoral features of myocardial stunning due to sudden emotional stress. N Engl J Med 352:539, 2005.

Management of Heart Failure

20. Faris R, Flather MD, Purcell H, et al: Diuretics for heart failure. Cochrane Database Syst Rev (1):CD003838, 2006.
21. Domanski M, Tian X, Haigney M, et al: Diuretic use, progressive heart failure, and death in patients in the DIG study. J Card Fail 12:327, 2006.
22. Pitt B, Zannad F, Remme WJ, et al: The effect of spironolactone on morbidity and mortality in patients with severe heart failure. Randomized Aldactone Evaluation Study Investigators. N Engl J Med 341:709, 1999.
23. Juurlink DN, Mamdani MM, Lee DS, et al: Rates of hyperkalemia after publication of the Randomized Aldactone Evaluation Study. N Engl J Med 351:543, 2004.
24. Pitt B, Remme W, Zannad F: Eplerenone, a selective aldosterone blocker, in patients with left ventricular dysfunction after myocardial infarction. N Engl J Med 348:1309, 2003.
25. Gheorghiade M: The clinical effects of vasopressin receptor antagonists in heart failure. Cleve Clin J Med 73(Suppl 2):S24, 2006.
26. Gheorghiade M, Niazi I, Ouyang J, et al: Vasopressin V2-receptor blockade with tolvaptan in patients with chronic heart failure: Results from a double-blind, randomized trial. Circulation 107:2690, 2003.
27. deGoma EM, Vagelos RH, Fowler MB, et al: Emerging therapies for the management of decompensated heart failure: from bench to bedside. J Am Coll Cardiol 48:2397, 2006.
28. Konstam MA, Gheorghiade M, Burnett JC, Jr, et al: Effects of oral tolvaptan in patients hospitalized for worsening heart failure: The EVEREST Outcome Trial. JAMA 2007 (in press).
29. Udelson JE, Smith WB, Hendrix GH, et al: Acute hemodynamic effects of conivaptan, a dual V(1A) and V(2) vasopressin receptor antagonist, in patients with advanced heart failure. Circulation 104:2417, 2001.
30. Ellison DH: Diuretic therapy and resistance in congestive heart failure. Cardiology 96:132, 2001.
31. Stevenson LW, Nohria A, Mielniczuk L: Torrent or torment from the tubules? Challenge of the cardiorenal connections. J Am Coll Cardiol 45:2004, 2005.
32. Sharma A, Hermann DD, Mehta RL: Clinical benefit and approach of ultrafiltration in acute heart failure. Cardiology 96:144-, 2001.
33. Costanzo MR, Saltzberg M, O'Sullivan J, et al: Early ultrafiltration in patients with decompensated heart failure and diuretic resistance. J Am Coll Cardiol 46:2047, 2005.
34. Bart BA, Boyle A, Bank AJ, et al: Ultrafiltration versus usual care for hospitalized patients with heart failure: The Relief for Acutely Fluid-Overloaded Patients With Decompensated Congestive Heart Failure (RAPID-CHF) trial. J Am Coll Cardiol 46:2043, 2005.
35. Costanzo MR, Guglin ME, Saltzberg MT, et al: Ultrafiltration versus intravenous diuretics for patients hospitalized for acute decompensated heart failure. J Am Coll Cardiol 49:675-683, 2007.
36. Flather MD, Yusuf S, Kober L, et al: Long-term ACE-inhibitor therapy in patients with heart failure or left- ventricular dysfunction: A systematic overview of data from individual patients. ACE-Inhibitor Myocardial Infarction Collaborative Group. Lancet 355:1575, 2000.
37. Granger CB, McMurray JJ, Yusuf S, et al: Effects of candesartan in patients with chronic heart failure and reduced left-ventricular systolic function intolerant to angiotensin-converting-enzyme inhibitors: The CHARM-Alternative trial. Lancet 362:772, 2003.
38. Cohn JN, Tognoni G: A randomized trial of the angiotensin-receptor blocker valsartan in chronic heart failure. N Engl J Med 345:1667, 2001.
39. Pfeffer MA, McMurray JJ, Velazquez EJ, et al: Valsartan, captopril, or both in myocardial infarction complicated by heart failure, left ventricular dysfunction, or both. N Engl J Med 349:1893, 2003.
40. McMurray JJ, Ostergren J, Swedberg K, et al: Effects of candesartan in patients with chronic heart failure and reduced left-ventricular systolic function taking angiotensin-converting enzyme inhibitors: The CHARM-Added trial. Lancet 362:767, 2003.
41. Mann DL, Bristow MR: Mechanisms and models in heart failure: The biomechanical model and beyond. Circulation 111:2837, 2005.
42. Dargie HJ: Effect of carvedilol on outcome after myocardial infarction in patients with left-ventricular dysfunction: The CAPRICORN randomised trial. Lancet 357:1385, 2001.
43. Poole-Wilson PA, Swedberg K, Cleland JG, et al: Comparison of carvedilol and metoprolol on clinical outcomes in patients with chronic heart failure in the Carvedilol Or Metoprolol European Trial (COMET): Randomised controlled trial. Lancet 362:7, 2003.
44. Liggett SB, Mialet-Perez J, Thaneemit-Chen S, et al: A polymorphism within a conserved beta(1) adrenergic receptor motif alters cardiac function and beta-blocker response in human heart failure. Proc Natl Acad Sci U S A 103:11288, 2006.
45. Cohn JN, Pfeffer MA, Rouleau J, et al: Adverse mortality effect of central sympathetic inhibition with sustained-release moxonidine in patients with heart failure (MOXCON). Eur J Heart Fail 5:659, 2003.
46. Flather MD, Shibata MC, Coats AJ, et al: Randomized trial to determine the effect of nebivolol on mortality and cardiovascular hospital admission in elderly patients with heart failure (SENIORS). Eur Heart J 26:215, 2005.
47. Gheorghiade M, Adams KF Jr, Colucci WS: Digoxin in the management of cardiovascular disorders. Circulation 109:2959, 2004.
48. Rathore SS, Wang Y, Krumholz H: M. Sex-based differences in the effect of digoxin for the treatment of heart failure. N Engl J Med 347:1403, 2002.
49. Carson P, Ziesche S, Johnson G, et al: Racial differences in response to therapy for heart failure: Analysis of the vasodilator-heart failure trials. Vasodilator-Heart Failure Trial Study Group. J Card Fail 5:178, 1999.
50. Taylor AL, Ziesche S, Yancy C, et al: Combination of isosorbide dinitrate and hydralazine in blacks with heart failure. N Engl J Med 351:2049, 2004.
51. Pullicino P, Thompson JL, Barton B, et al: Warfarin versus aspirin in patients with reduced cardiac ejection fraction (WARCEF): Rationale, objectives, and design. J Card Fail 12:39, 2006.
52. Cleland JG, Daubert JC, Erdmann E, et al: The effect of cardiac resynchronization on morbidity and mortality in heart failure. N Engl J Med 352:1539, 2005.

53. Bristow MR, Saxon LA, Boehmer J, et al: Cardiac-resynchronization therapy with or without an implantable defibrillator in advanced chronic heart failure. N Engl J Med 350:2140, 2004.
54. Bardy GH, Lee KL, Mark DB, et al: Amiodarone or an implantable cardioverter-defibrillator for congestive heart failure. N Engl J Med 352:225, 2005.
55. Wolk R, Gami AS, Garcia-Touchard A. et al: Sleep and cardiovascular disease. Curr Probl Cardiol 30:625, 2005.
56. Bradley TD, Floras JS: Sleep apnea and heart failure. Part II: Central sleep apnea. Circulation 107:1822, 2003.
57. Bradley TD, Logan AG, Kimoff RJ, et al: Continuous positive airway pressure for central sleep apnea and heart failure. N Engl J Med 353:2025, 20.
58. Fonarow GC: How well are chronic heart failure patients being managed? Rev Cardiovasc Med 7(Suppl 1:S31, 2006.
59. Granger BB, Swedberg K, Ekman I, et al: Adherence to candesartan and placebo and outcomes in chronic heart failure in the CHARM programme: Double-blind, randomised, controlled clinical trial. Lancet 366:2005, 2005.
60. Louis AA, Turner T, Gretton M, et al: A systematic review of telemonitoring for the management of heart failure. Eur J Heart Fail 5:583, 2003.

CHAPTER 26

Heart Failure with Normal Ejection Fraction

Margaret M. Redfield

HISTORICAL PERSPECTIVE

Until the last two decades, the possibility that large numbers of patients with heart failure (HF) might have a normal ejection fraction was not considered. As numerous studies have now demonstrated, heart failure with a normal ejection fraction (HFnlEF) is very common, why it was not previously recognized is unclear. It may be that HFnlEF was always common but that the cardiology community failed to recognize it. It is also possible that the prevalence of HFnlEF has increased over time, leading to more widespread recognition. Support for this concept comes from a recent study, which showed that the prevalence of HFnlEF among patients admitted for HF at a single large institution had increased dramatically over a 15-year period from 1987 to 2001 (Fig. 26-1).[1] The emergence of this "new" form of HF engendered considerable early skepticism, despite growing epidemiological evidence of its importance. Controversy regarding the significance of HFnlEF has largely but not completely abated. This chapter summarizes much of what is currently known regarding HFnlEF, but I have been careful to emphasize that our understanding of this syndrome is incomplete and will continue to evolve as the field advances.

NOMENCLATURE AND CLASSIFICATION

As recognition of the importance of HFnlEF as a public health problem increased, controversy arose over the proper term to use for HFnlEF. Most early studies referred to HFnlEF as diastolic HF, a term implying that diastolic dysfunction is the key pathophysiological mechanism responsible for hemodynamic perturbations and symptoms in these patients. Similarly, systolic HF was commonly used to refer to patients with HF with reduced or depressed EF. Because of the paucity of studies measuring diastolic function in patients with HFnlEF, some have argued that HFnlEF be used. This has been used in current HF management guidelines[2,3] and thus will be used in this chapter. Figure 26-2 serves to define the patient population that is the focus of this chapter and emphasizes consideration of an appropriate differential diagnosis for patients with clinical evidence of HF and normal EF. Additionally, it should be noted that EF is a continuous variable with a fairly normal distribution within the population,[4] and the threshold value to define normal versus reduced EF is arbitrary. Although consensus seems to be building toward use of an EF higher than 50 percent to designate HFnlEF, the approach to patients with borderline reduction in EF (EF, 40 to 50 percent) adds to the complexity of the classification.

EPIDEMIOLOGY

Thirteen epidemiological studies have defined the prevalence of HFnlEF in various HF populations and have documented a prevalence of 50 to 55 percent.[1,5-7] Importantly, the prevalence of HFnlEF among patients with HF varies dramatically with age and gender.[8] The prevalence of HF increases with age (Fig. 26-3A) and is similar in men and women (see Fig. 26-3B). The prevalence of HF with a depressed EF increases with age but is more common in men than in women at any age (see Fig. 26-3D), whereas the prevalence of HFnlEF increases even more dramatically with age (more than HF with a reduced EF) and is much more common in women than in men at any age (see Fig. 26-3C). More data are needed concerning variation in the prevalence of HFnlEF in different regional and ethnic groups.

NATURAL HISTORY

MORTALITY. Most large contemporary studies have now suggested that the mortality for HFnlEF is similar to that of HF with a reduced EF.[1,5-7] Survival curves from two large recent studies comparing survival in HF patients with preserved or reduced EF are shown in Figure 26-4.[7,9] Differences in survival between the two forms of HF are minimal. Although survival has improved over time for patients with HF with a reduced EF, it has not changed for patients with HFnlEF (Fig. 26-5).[9] In the Digitalis Investigation Group (DIG) study, which included patients with HFnlEF,[10] the cause of death was somewhat different in patients with HFnlEF, in whom deaths caused by noncardiovascular and non-HF cardiovascular mechanisms were more frequent (Fig. 26-6).

MORBIDITY. Patients with HFnlEF have comparable morbidity to those with HF with a reduced EF, with similar or

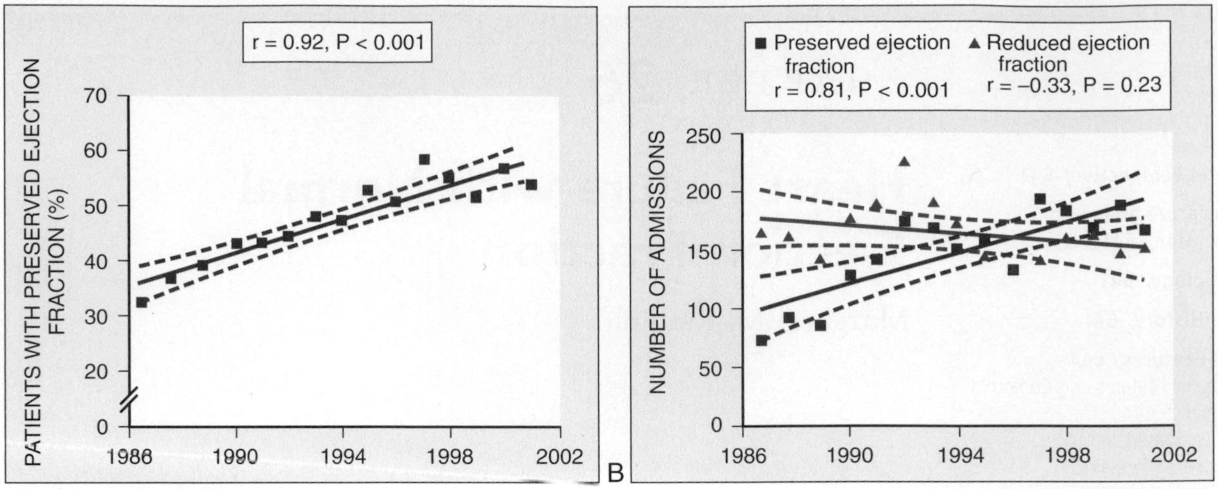

FIGURE 26–1 Increased prevalence of heart failure with normal ejection fraction (HFnlEF). **A,** A large study of patients hospitalized with HF at a single institution over a 15-year period from 1987 to 2001 demonstrated that the percentage of HF patients who have normal EF has increased over time. **B,** This was the result of an increased number of admissions for HFnlEF; the number of admissions for HF with reduced EF remained stable. *(From Owan T, Hodge D, Herges D, et al: Heart failure with preserved ejection fraction: Trends in prevalence and outcomes. N Engl J Med 355:308, 2006.)*

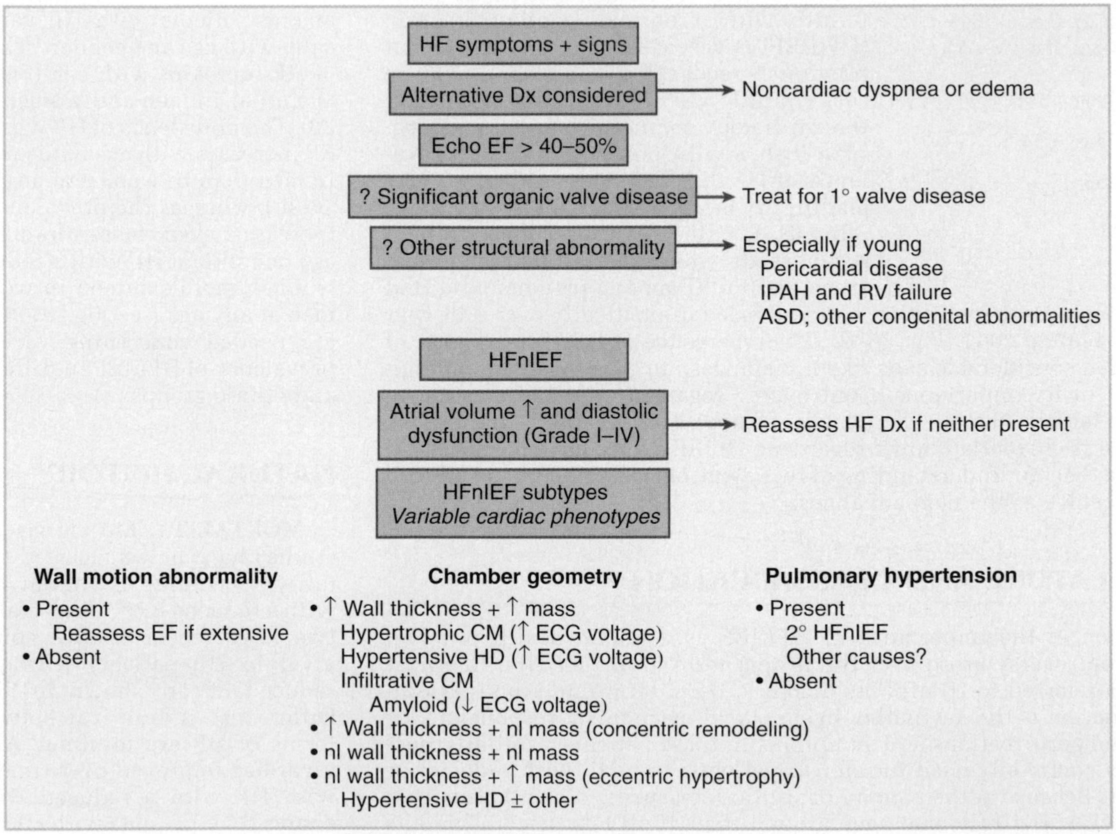

FIGURE 26–2 Heart failure with normal ejection fraction (HFnlEF) classification, differential diagnosis, and variable cardiac phenotype. When using the term *HFnlEF,* care must be taken to exclude conditions attributable to noncardiac processes or to other recognized specific cardiac abnormalities for which effective therapy exists. It must be recognized that the cardiac phenotype in HFnlEF is variable. ASD = atrial septal defect; CM = cardiomyopathy; ECG = electrocardiogram; HD = heart disease; IPAH = idiopathic pulmonary arterial hypertension; nl = normal; RV = right ventricular.

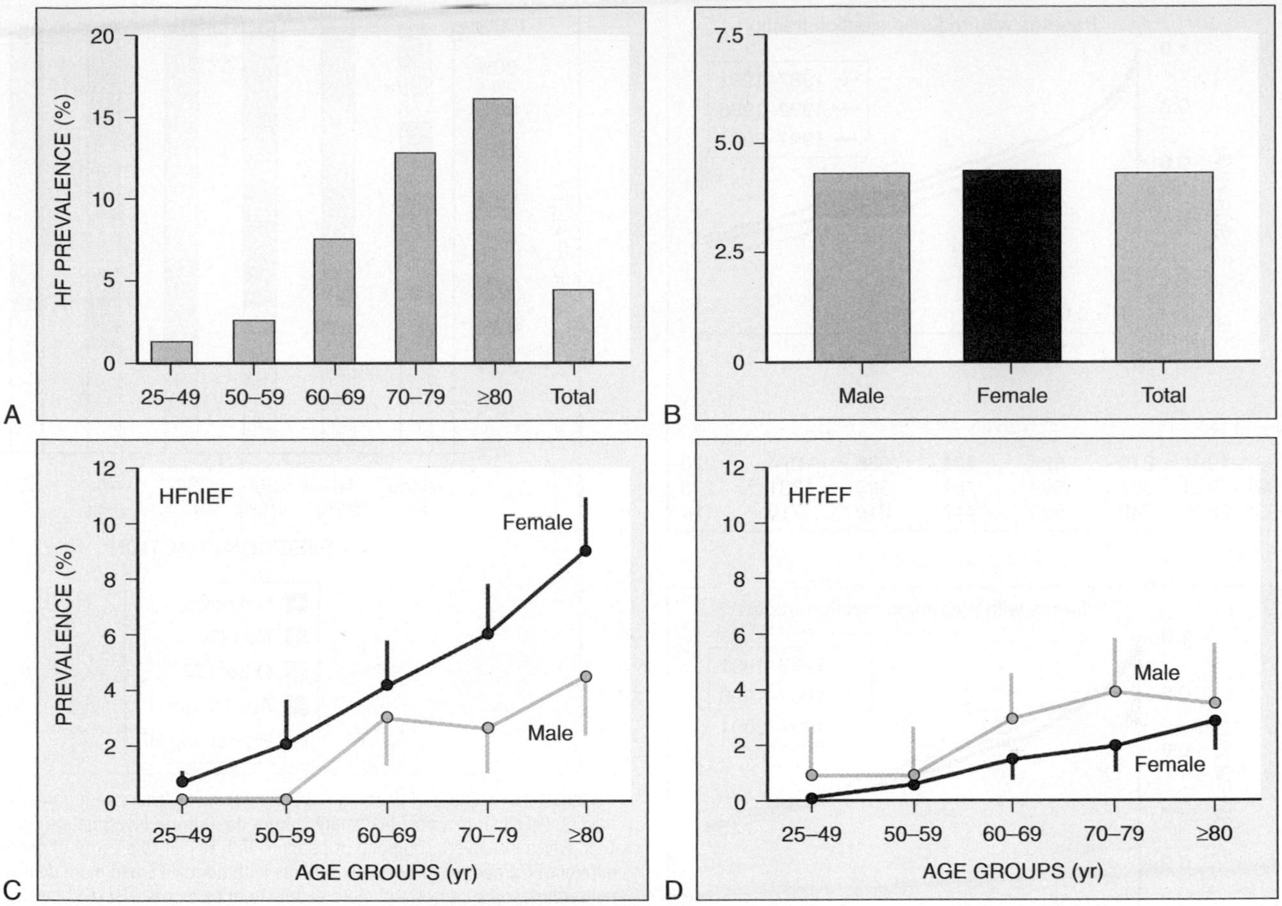

FIGURE 26–3 The age- and gender-specific prevalence of heart failure with normal ejection fraction (HFnlEF) and HF with reduced EF. **A,** HF prevalence by age. **B,** HF prevalence by gender. **C,** HFnlEF prevalence by age. **D,** HF with reduced EF (HFrEF) prevalence by gender. As demonstrated in this study and others,[1,5-7] although the prevalence of both forms of HF increases dramatically with age, the prevalence of HFnlEF increases more steeply with age and, in contrast to HF with reduced EF, is more common in women at any age. *(Modified from Ceia F, Fonseca C, Mota T, et al: Prevalence of chronic heart failure in Southwestern Europe: The EPICA study. Eur J Heart Fail 4:531, 2002.)*

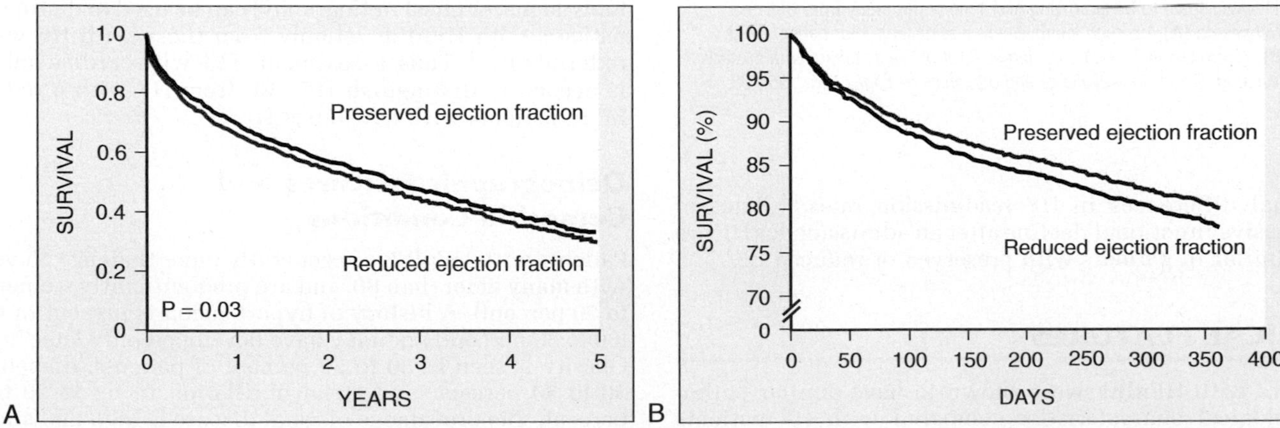

FIGURE 26–4 **A, B,** Kaplan-Meier survival curves comparing survival in patients with heart failure with normal ejection fraction (HFnlEF) with that of patients with HF with reduced EF. As with most previous studies,[5,6] both studies showed only small differences in survival between the two types of HF. Note that the study in **B** compared survival in those patients with an EF less than 40 percent to those with an EF higher than 50 percent, whereas the study in **A** compared survival in those with EF less than or higher than 50 percent. *(**A** from Owan T, Hodge D, Herges D, et al: Heart failure with preserved ejection fraction: Trends in prevalence and outcomes. N Engl J Med 355:308, 2006; **B** from Bhatia RS, Tu JV, Lee DS, et al: Outcome of heart failure with preserved ejection fraction in a population-based study. N Engl J Med 355:260, 2006.)*

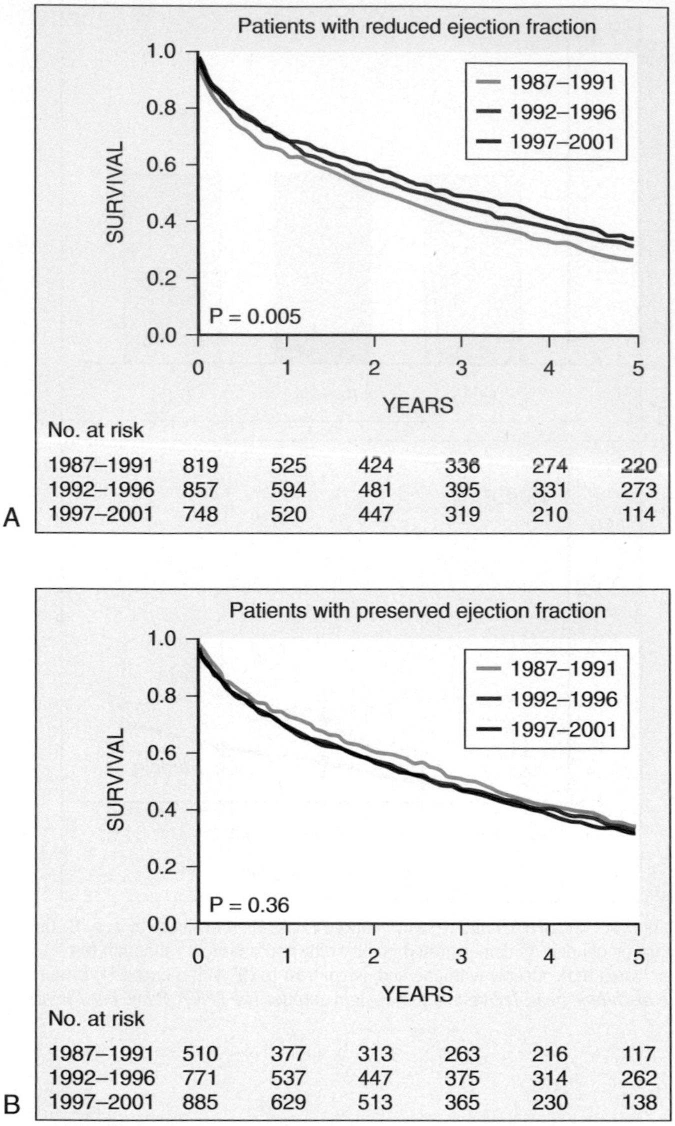

FIGURE 26–5 Survival curves for patients with heart failure with normal ejection fraction (HFnlEF) has not improved. Whereas survival for patients with HF with reduced EF was shown to be improving over time in this study from Olmsted County, Minnesota **(A),** no such improvement was observed for patients with HFnlEF **(B).** *(From Owan T, Hodge D, Herges D, et al: Heart failure with preserved ejection fraction: Trends in prevalence and outcomes. N Engl J Med 355:308, 2006.)*

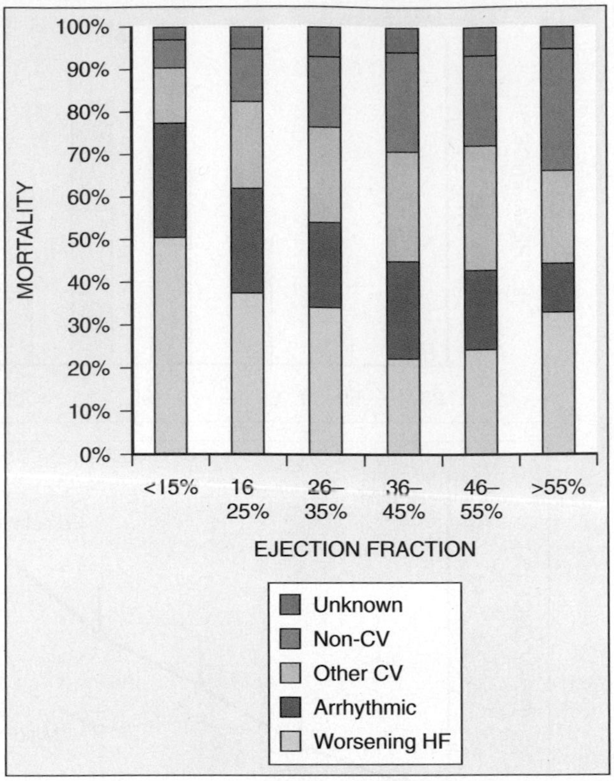

FIGURE 26–6 Cause of death in patients with heart failure with normal ejection fraction (HFnlEF). In a post hoc analysis from the Digoxin Investigation Group (DIG) Trial, which included a subgroup of patients with HFnlEF, the cause of death in different EF groups was assessed. Patients with normal EF had more deaths from noncardiovascular causes and more deaths from cardiovascular (CV) causes other than arrhythmia or HF. *(From Curtis JP, Sokol SI, Wang Y, et al: The association of left ventricular ejection fraction, mortality, and cause of death in stable outpatients with heart failure. J Am Coll Cardiol 42:736, 2003.)*

minimal differences in HF readmission rates.[6,7] Rates of progressive functional decline after an admission for HF are also similar in patients with preserved or reduced EF.[11]

CLINICAL FEATURES

Patients with HFnlEF were shown to have similar pathophysiological characteristics compared with HF patients with a reduced EF including severely reduced exercise capacity, neuroendocrine activation, and impaired quality of life despite normal EF, normal left ventricular (LV) volume, and an increased LV mass-to-volume ratio.[12] Pertinent clinical features in HFnlEF are reviewed in Table 26-1, with particular emphasis on establishing the diagnosis of HF.

Numerous studies have compared clinical features of hospitalized HF patients with normal versus reduced EF. Most have demonstrated minimal differences between clinical symptoms, signs, or radiographic findings and certainly have documented that none of the clinical features (symptoms, signs, or chest radiography) can be used to distinguish patients with HFnlEF reliably from those with HF with a reduced EF.[6,7,13] Thus, assessment of EF with cardiac imaging is needed to distinguish HFnlEF from HF with a reduced EF in patients with new-onset HF.

Demographic Features and Comorbid Conditions

Patients with HFnlEF are generally older than age 65 years, with many older than 80, and are predominantly women (60 to 70 percent). A history of hypertension is present in most (60 to 80 percent) and may have developed only later in life. Obesity is seen in 30 to 50 percent of patients, diabetes in 30 to 50 percent, and atrial fibrillation in up to 20 to 40 percent. The prevalence of renal disease is high and similar to that noted in patients with HF and a reduced EF. The reported medications at diagnosis in patients with HFnlEF have included diuretics, digoxin, angiotensin-converting enzyme (ACE) inhibitors, beta blockers, calcium channel blockers and various other vasodilators, and antihypertensive and antiarrhythmic drugs.[1,5-7,13] The reported prevalence of coronary artery disease varies widely.[14] The demographic features and comorbid conditions, which are highly prevalent in HFnlEF, are discussed in more detail.

TABLE 26–1 Clinical Features of Heart Failure with Normal Ejection Fraction

Parameter	Features
Framingham criteria for diagnosis of heart failure*	
Major criteria	Paroxysmal nocturnal dyspnea or orthopnea Jugular venous distention (or CVP > 16 mm Hg) Rales or acute pulmonary edema Cardiomegaly Hepatojugular reflex Response to diuretic (weight loss >4.5 kg in 5 days)
Minor criteria	Ankle edema Nocturnal cough Exertional dyspnea Pleural effusion Vital capacity < two thirds of normal Hepatomegaly Tachycardia (>120 bpm)
Demographic features	Elderly; female > male
Underlying CV disease	Hypertension, coronary disease, diabetes, atrial fibrillation
Comorbidities	Obesity, renal dysfunction
Doppler echocardiography results	
LV size	Normal to ↓ (small subset with ↑)
LV mass	LVH common but *frequently* absent; ↑ relative wall thickness (>0.45)
Left atrium	Enlarged
Diastolic dysfunction	Grade I-IV (∞ diastolic dysfunction severity, BP, volume status)
Other features	PH, wall motion abnormality, RV enlargement
Pertinent negatives	Rule out valve disease, pericardial disease, ASD
BNP or NT-proBNP	↑ but HFnlEF < HFrEF
Exercise testing	↓ V_{O_2} peak Exaggerated hypertensive response in many Chronotropic incompetence in subset
Chest radiogram	Similar to HFrEF, cardiomegaly, pulmonary venous hypertension, edema, pleural effusion
Electrocardiogram	Variable

*Two major or one major and two minor criteria.

HF = heart failure; HFnlEF = heart failure with normal ejection fraction; CVP = central venous pressure; LV = left ventricular; LVH = left ventricular hypertrophy; BP = blood pressure; PH = pulmonary hypertension; RV = right ventricular; ASD = atrial septal defect; HFrEF = heart failure with reduced ejection fraction; V_{O_2} peak = peak oxygen uptake; bpm = beats per minute; BNP = brain natriuretic peptide; NT-proBNP = N-terminal-pro-BNP.

AGING. Although cardiovascular disease may contribute to diastolic dysfunction in older people, studies have also suggested that diastolic function deteriorates with normal aging.[15] The speed of LV relaxation declines with age in men and women, even in the absence of cardiovascular disease.[15] It also appears that vascular, LV systolic, and LV diastolic stiffness increase with aging.[15,16] Increases in vascular stiffness have been shown to be related to effort intolerance in patients with HFnlEF.[17] Structural cardiac changes with aging (e.g., increased cardiomyocyte size, increased apoptosis with decreased myocyte number, altered growth factor regulation, focal collagen deposition) and functional changes at the cellular level involving blunted beta-adrenergic responsiveness, excitation-contraction coupling, and altered calcium-handling proteins may contribute to diastolic dysfunction with normal aging. Some studies have suggested that prolonged, sustained endurance training may preserve LV compliance with aging and help prevent HF in the elderly.[18]

GENDER. Along with age, female gender is a potent risk factor for HFnlEF, as noted earlier. Indeed, there appears to be important age-gender interactions, such that the prevalence of HFnlEF increases more sharply with age in women than the prevalence of HF with a reduced EF (see Fig. 26-4).[8] The reasons for the female predominance in HFnlEF are not entirely clear, but women have higher vascular and LV systolic and diastolic stiffness than men, and vascular and ventricular stiffness increases more dramatically with age in women.[15] Emerging evidence of unique coronary vascular functional changes in women may play a role in HFnlEF pathophysiology.

HYPERTENSION. Hypertension is the most commonly associated cardiac condition in patients with HFnlEF. Chronically increased blood pressure is an important stimulus for cardiac structural remodeling and functional changes. The resultant hypertensive heart disease is characterized by LV hypertrophy (LVH), increasing vascular and ventricular systolic stiffness, impaired relaxation, and increased diastolic stiffness, all factors linked to the pathogenesis of HFnlEF.[19] In the presence of hypertensive heart disease, ischemia produces exaggerated increases in filling pressures, and hypertensive and ischemic heart disease are often present in combination in patients with HFnlEF. Elucidating which factors mediate transition to HFnlEF in persons with hypertensive heart disease is an area of active investigation.[20,21]

CORONARY ARTERY DISEASE. The reported prevalence of coronary artery disease or myocardial ischemia in patients with HFnlEF varies widely.[5,6,14] Although acute ischemia is known to cause diastolic dysfunction (see later), the role of coronary artery disease and ischemia in contributing to chronic diastolic dysfunction and symptoms in patients with HFnlEF remains speculative. Despite uncertainty regarding the role of ischemia in the pathophysiology of HFnlEF and a lack of data documenting that revascularization improves outcomes in patients with HFnlEF, HF management guidelines recommend revascularization in those HFnlEF patients in whom "ischemia is felt to contribute to diastolic dysfunction."[2,3] Importantly, emerging evidence suggests that unique coronary vascular functional changes are present in women. Whether unique features (e.g., diffuse disease, more endothelial dysfunction) play a role in HFnlEF pathophysiology in women remains to be determined.[14]

ATRIAL FIBRILLATION AND OTHER RHYTHM DISTURBANCES. Atrial fibrillation is recognized as a frequent precipitant of acute decompensation in patients with HFnlEF. Potential mechanisms responsible for this frequent presentation are discussed more fully later. Whereas atrial fibrillation may cause decompensated HF in patients with diastolic dysfunction, diastolic dysfunction (in the absence of HF) is also a risk factor for atrial fibrillation.[22] Thus, diastolic dysfunction, atrial fibrillation, and HFnlEF are common and related conditions that probably share common pathogenic mechanisms in the elderly. The prevalence of ventricular arrhythmias in HFnlEF is poorly defined. Although tachycardia caused by atrial arrhythmias is a recognized precipitant of acute decompensation in HFnlEF, bradycardia and adverse atrioventricular timing caused by first-degree heart block may also adversely affect LV filling in some patients.

OBESITY. Obesity is associated with an increased risk for HF. In general, patients with HFnlEF are more often obese than patients with HF with a reduced EF,[5,6] and the prevalence of diastolic dysfunction is increased in obese persons.[4] Increased adiposity not only imposes an adverse hemodynamic load on the heart but is also a source of a large number of biologically active peptide and nonpeptide mediators, many linked to chronic inflammation by various pathways. Increased body mass index (BMI) is a risk factor for hypertension, diabetes mellitus, coronary artery disease, and atrial fibrillation, all of which are associated with HFnlEF. Studies using tissue Doppler imaging or invasive LV pressure measurement have reported an association between diastolic dysfunction, elevated filling pressures, and obesity.[23]

DIABETES MELLITUS. Diabetes is a potent risk factor for HF, and the prevalence of diabetes is similar in patients with HF and reduced or preserved EF, suggesting that diabetes contributes to the pathophysiology of both forms of HF. Although diabetes predisposes to coronary artery disease, renal dysfunction, and hypertension, numerous direct effects of diabetes and hyperglycemia on myocardial structure and function have been described. The morphological changes in the diabetic heart include myocyte hypertrophy, increased extracellular matrix (fibrosis), and intramyocardial microangiopathy. Functional changes, which may represent a continuum, include endothelial-dependent and endothelial-independent microvascular dysfunction, impaired relaxation, and increased passive diastolic stiffness and contractile dysfunction. Mechanisms contributing to structural and functional coronary vascular and myocardial changes are diverse and include metabolic disturbances, activation of proinflammatory and profibrotic mediators, cardiac autonomic neuropathy, and increases in advanced glycation end-products (AGE), which promote increased collagen accumulation and increased collagen stiffness. AGE accumulation may also play a role in age-related cardiovascular stiffening.

RENAL DYSFUNCTION. The critical impact of renal function on morbidity and mortality in HF is well established. Studies have shown no difference between the severity of renal dysfunction in patients with reduced or preserved EF.[6,7,9] Furthermore, the incidence of worsening renal function during HF therapy is similar in patients with preserved or reduced EF.[24] Although the prevalence of renal vascular disease in HF has been poorly delineated, it is probably high, and bilateral renal artery stenosis with rapid-onset or flash pulmonary edema is a well-recognized cause of HFnlEF. Evaluation of the renal arteries should be considered in patients presenting with the triad of hypertension, renal dysfunction, and HFnlEF.

RARER CAUSES OF HEART FAILURE WITH A NORMAL EJECTION FRACTION. Hypertrophic cardiomyopathy, infiltrative cardiomyopathies such as amyloidosis, valvular disease, and constrictive pericarditis should always be considered in young patients with HFnlEF or patients with other suggestive features (see Fig. 26-2; also see Chaps. 64, 65, and 70). However, these diseases account for a minority of patients with HFnlEF. Idiopathic restrictive cardiomyopathy in young persons without the factors discussed earlier may represent a distinct group, particularly if a family history is present. However, the clinical presentation and echocardiographic appearance in older persons with HFnlEF may be identical to those of patients previously labeled as having restrictive cardiomyopathy. An important consideration in patients with previous malignancy treated with mediastinal radiation is radiation heart disease (see Chap. 85). Radiation can cause pericardial and concomitant myocardial damage, and outcomes after pericardiectomy are frequently poor because of concomitant restrictive myocardial disease. Concomitant valvular disease and premature coronary artery disease are also common in patients with previous mediastinal radiation and may contribute to the pathophysiology of HFnlEF in patients with radiation heart disease.

Factors Associated with Acute Decompensation

It is important to appreciate differences in clinical presentation among patients with acute decompensation or more chronic symptoms.[25,26] Uncontrolled hypertension, dietary or medication noncompliance, atrial arrhythmias, ischemia, and concomitant processes such as infection are common in patients presenting with acutely decompensated HFnlEF. In contrast, patients with chronic, stable HF are likely to have fewer reversible features.

Findings on Doppler Echocardiography

Comprehensive Doppler echocardiography is invaluable in the evaluation of HF patients. Beyond the presence of a normal EF, expected or possible findings in patients with HFnlEF are outlined here and in Table 26-1. Although other cardiovascular imaging techniques may provide as good or even more accurate assessment of cardiac structure or function, the widespread availability and comprehensive functional information provided by echocardiography make it the test of choice for patients with HF.

LV Size. Most patients with HFnlEF have normal chamber dimensions, although a subset will have variable degrees of LV enlargement.[27]

LV Hypertrophy. Although HFnlEF has been thought to occur primarily in patients with LVH, studies that have carefully quantified LV mass report that echocardiographic criteria for LVH are met in less than 50 percent of patients.[12,20,26,28] Patients with HFnlEF have, on average, increased relative wall thickness and an increased mass-to-volume ratio,[12] but these findings often occur in the setting of normal LV mass. Thus, despite traditional teaching, LVH is not invariably present in HFnlEF, in which the cardiac phenotype is variable (see Fig. 26-2). There is some evidence that the prevalence of LVH may be higher in African American HFnlEF patients.[21]

Doppler Echocardiographic Assessment of Diastolic Function and Filling Pressures. The Doppler assessment of diastolic function and filling pressures requires careful acquisition of data and informed interpretation. Early studies focused on the transmitral flow velocity profile. Decreases in the ratio of early to late diastolic filling (E/A), increases in the deceleration time (DT) of the early diastolic filling velocity profile, or increases in the isovolumic relaxation time (IVRT) indicate impaired relaxation. However, in the presence of impaired relaxation, increases in filling pressure progressively modify the transmitral gradient and mitral inflow pattern (Fig. 26-7). A comprehensive Doppler assessment must be used to determine diastolic function and filling pressures.[4] Patients studied at various times during their presentation (e.g., acutely decompensated, after initial treatment of an acute decompensation episode, or as stable outpatients) will display a spectrum of filling patterns, including abnormal relaxation and pseudonormal or restrictive patterns. Such a spectrum has also been reported in patients with HF with a depressed EF and reflects the potent effect of filling pressures, blood pressure, and their interaction with underlying diastolic dysfunction on the Doppler patterns. Thus, depending on their level of compensation and their filling pressures and whether they have exertional or rest symptoms, patients with HFnlEF may display any of the filling patterns outlined in Figure 26-7, although a truly normal profile is uncommon.

Left Atrial Enlargement. Increases in left atrial dimension or volume is commonly, if not almost uniformly, present in patients with HFnlEF.[21,26]

Pulmonary Hypertension. Just as chronic pulmonary venous hypertension leads to pulmonary arterial hypertension in HF with depressed systolic function, the same can occur in HFnlEF, and an elevated tricuspid regurgitant velocity indicative of pulmonary hypertension is common in HFnlEF. Chronic pulmonary venous hypertension in HF has a direct hemodynamic effect on pulmonary pressure and causes reactive pulmonary hypertension, which can be slow to resolve after normalization of LV filling pressures. With time, chronic pulmonary venous hypertension causes pulmonary vascular remodeling (congestive pulmonary vasculopathy) and irreversible pulmonary hypertension. These changes are well described in HF with a reduced EF and mitral valvular disease but can occur in HFnlEF as well. The prevalence of significant pulmonary hypertension in HFnlEF is as high as 50 percent.[25]

Other Doppler Echocardiographic Findings. Regional wall motion abnormalities (with preserved EF) and right ventricular dilation, either because of ischemic disease or pulmonary hypertension, can also be present at echocardiography in patients with HFnlEF.[26] Additional important *negative* findings to be considered at echocardiography include the absence of valvular disease important enough to cause the HF symptoms, pericardial tamponade or constriction, or the presence of congenital heart diseases such as atrial septal defect or other more extensive structural abnormalities (see Fig. 26-2).

Brain Natriuretic Peptide and N-Terminal Pro–Brain Natriuretic Peptide Assays

Numerous studies have now shown that, in general, brain natriuretic peptide (BNP) and N-terminal (NT) pro-BNP assay results are elevated in patients with HFnlEF as compared with results in persons without HF; however, as compared with patients with HF and reduced EF, BNP and NT–pro-BNP values, on average, are lower in HFnlEF.[29] Normal plasma BNP concentrations increase with age and are higher in females. Because patients with HFnlEF are older and more often female than patients with HF and a reduced EF, the standard partition value of 100 pg/ml suggested for the diagnosis of HF may not be appropriate in HFnlEF, because normal elderly women often have BNP values higher than 100 pg/ml.

Exercise Testing

Cardiopulmonary exercise testing (CPET) is useful in the diagnostic evaluation of exercise intolerance of unclear cause and thus, in select patients with suspected HFnlEF in whom concern over pulmonary limitations also exist, CPET may play a role in the diagnostic evaluation. Objective measures of exercise tolerance are similarly impaired in HF (of similar clinical severity) with reduced and preserved

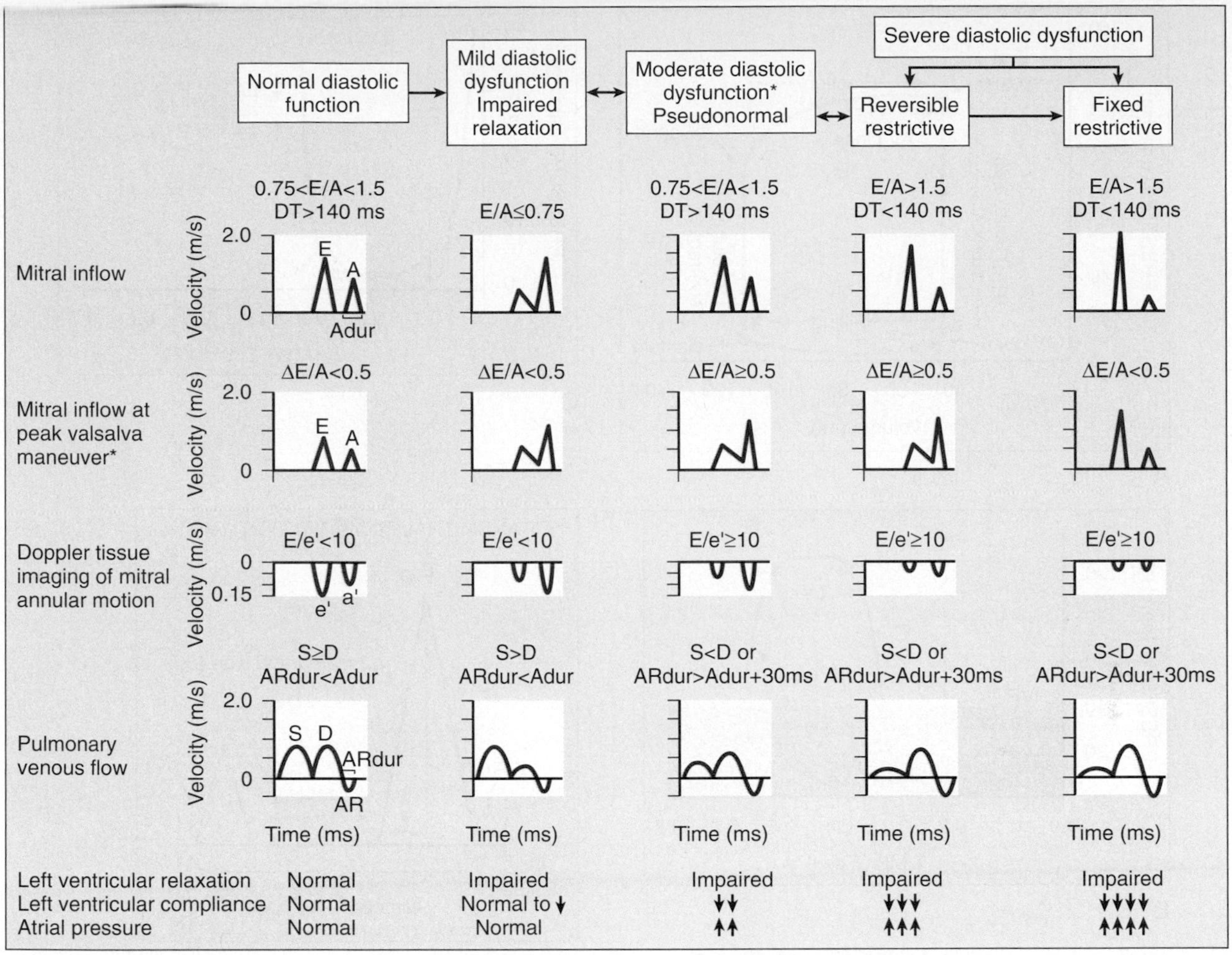

FIGURE 26–7 Proposed progression of diastolic function abnormalities as assessed with comprehensive Doppler echocardiography, with correlation of invasively measured diastolic properties (see text at bottom). A comprehensive Doppler assessment as outlined here can yield useful information regarding relaxation, filling pressures, and (indirectly) diastolic stiffness in most patients but requires careful data acquisition and informed interpretation. A = transmitral flow velocity with atrial contraction; Adur = duration of A above; AR = flow from left atrium to pulmonary veins during atrial contraction; ARdur = duration of AR; D = diastolic; DT = deceleration time; E = early diastolic transmitral flow velocity; e′ = velocity of early diastolic mitral annular motion; S = systolic. *(From Redfield MM, Jacobsen SJ, Burnett JC Jr, et al: Burden of systolic and diastolic ventricular dysfunction in the community: appreciating the scope of the heart failure epidemic. JAMA 289:194, 2003.)*

EF.[12] Although the prognostic features of metabolic stress testing are less well described and less relevant in the HFnlEF population, few of whom are considered for cardiac transplantation, standard exercise stress testing without metabolic measurements may be useful in the evaluation and management of patients with HFnlEF. Exaggerated hypertensive responses to exercise causes load-dependent diastolic dysfunction and recognition, and treatment of exercise-induced hypertension is important in the treatment of HFnlEF. Importantly, stress testing also allows assessment of the heart rate response to exercise. Whereas past recommendations have focused on the potential use of negative chronotropic agents to allow a longer diastolic filling period in patients with impaired relaxation, recent studies have suggested that chronotropic incompetence is also relatively common (higher than 20 percent) in patients with HFnlEF (although not more common than in HF with a reduced EF), even in the absence of beta blocker therapy.[30,31]

PATHOPHYSIOLOGY

Understanding pathophysiological mechanisms in HFnlEF mandates a clear understanding of LV diastolic and systolic function and the manner in which LV function is influenced by volume status, which, together with LV geometry, determines preload, and the arterial system, which, together with LV geometry, affects afterload. Although abnormal diastolic function has long been hypothesized to be the primary factor responsible for hemodynamic perturbations and symptoms in HFnlEF, only recently have studies attempted to prove this hypothesis by studying diastolic function in patients with HFnlEF and relevant control populations (see later). Because LV structure and function are altered by age, gender, and cardiovascular disease in the absence of HF, it is important to understand how LV structure and function differ between persons with HFnlEF and elderly persons with cardiovascular disease but no HF. There is growing evidence confirming that abnormal diastolic function does indeed play a key role in HFnlEF, but the potential for other mechanisms to contribute to the pathophysiology in many patients must also be recognized and will be discussed.

Diastolic Mechanisms (see Chap. 23)

Normal diastolic function allows the ventricle to fill adequately during rest and exercise, without an abnormal increase in diastolic pressures. The phases of diastole are isovolumic relaxation and the filling phase (Fig. 26-8A). The filling phase is divided into early rapid filling, diastasis, and atrial systole (see Fig. 26-8B, C, and D). Early rapid filling

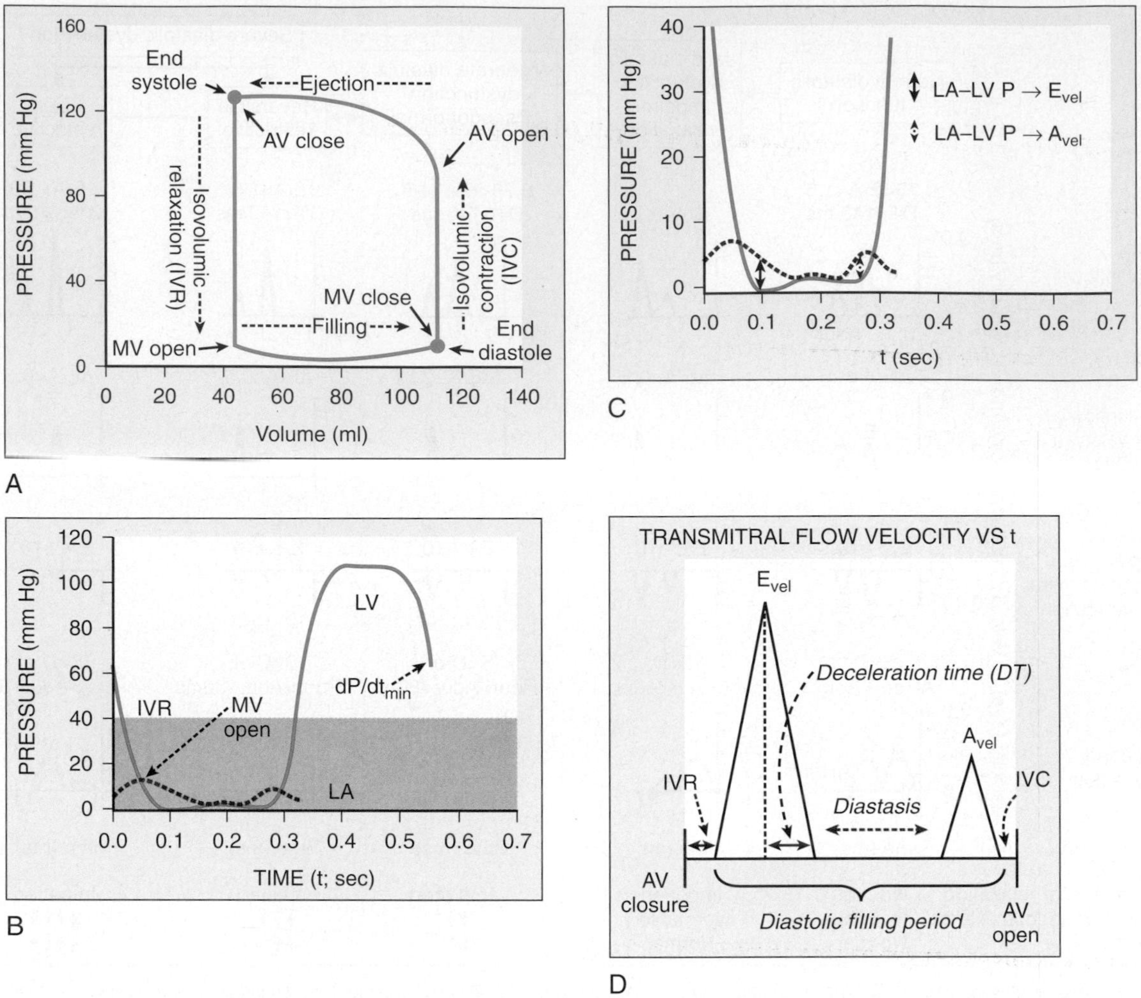

FIGURE 26–8 Assessment of ventricular diastolic function and filling in the pressure (P)-volume, pressure-time, and flow velocity–time domains. **A,** Cardiac cycle in the pressure-volume domain. Diastole includes isovolumic relaxation and the filling phase. **B,** Left ventricular (LV) and left atrial (LA) pressures during diastole, expanded to emphasize diastole **(C)**. **D,** LA to LV pressure gradient determines the velocity of LV filling during early rapid filling, diastasis, and atrial systole. See text for details. A_{vel} = transmitral flow velocity with atrial contraction; AV = aortic valve; E_{vel} = early diastolic transmitral flow velocity; IVC = isovolumic contraction; IVR = isovolumic relaxation; MV = mitral valve; t = time.

contributes 70 to 80 percent of LV filling in normal individuals, and this contribution diminishes with age and various disease states. Early diastolic filling is driven by the left atrial (LA) to LV pressure gradient (see Fig. 26-8C and D), which is dependent on a complex interplay of factors—myocardial relaxation, LV diastolic stiffness, LV elastic recoil, LV contractile state, LA pressures, ventricular interaction, pericardial constraint, LA stiffness, pulmonary vein properties, and mitral orifice area. Diastasis is the period of diastole when the LA and LV pressures are usually almost equal. It contributes less than 5 percent of the LV filling, and its duration shortens with tachycardia. In normal subjects, atrial systole contributes 15 to 25 percent of LV diastolic filling without raising the mean left atrial pressure. This contribution depends on the PR interval, atrial inotropic state, atrial preload, atrial afterload, autonomic tone, and heart rate. Although diastolic function is complex, the most important components are LV relaxation and LV diastolic stiffness.

LV Relaxation

LV relaxation is an active, energy-dependent process that begins during the ejection phase of systole and continues through isovolumic relaxation and the rapid filling phase. In normal hearts, catecholamine-induced enhancement of relaxation during exercise lowers LV pressures in early diastole; thus, enhanced relaxation increases the LA-LV pressure gradient without increasing LA pressures and enhances filling during exercise without the need for elevated LA pressures.

INVASIVE AND NONINVASIVE ASSESSMENT OF LV RELAXATION. The time constant of relaxation (tau, τ) describes the rate of LV pressure decay during isovolumic relaxation. Measurement of tau requires high-fidelity manometer–tipped LV catheters for precise determination. The pressure (P) and time (t) data during the period from end-systole (peak − dP/dt) to the onset of LV filling (determined from LA to LV crossover pressure, or estimated as 5 mm Hg above the end-diastolic pressure) is used to calculate tau (Fig. 26-9). The pressure-time data during isovolumic relaxation are fit to various equations to derive the value of tau. The equations used make different assumptions regarding the LV minimum pressure obtained. The Weiss equation

$$\text{LV P} = P_0 e^{-t/\tau}$$

where P_0 = LV P at end ejection, assumes a zero asymptote (or that the LV minimum pressure must be positive) and thus derives tau as the negative inverse of the slope of the relationship between the natural log (ln) of LV pressure and time during isovolumic relaxation (see Fig. 26-9). The "logistic" equation lets the data drive the asymptote and allows for negative LV minimum pressures, as has been documented in animal studies. With all methods, the larger the value of tau, the longer it takes for the LV to relax and the more impaired is relaxation. A normal value for tau is less than 40 milliseconds in most age groups and relaxation is complete by 3.5 × tau (less than 140 milliseconds).

Doppler echocardiography may also be used to assess relaxation. The transmitral flow velocity versus time profile is affected by impaired relaxation in a variable manner. If relaxation is impaired but LA pressures are not elevated, the slower LV pressure decay and the higher LV minimum pressure associated with impaired relaxation will decrease the early diastolic LA to LV pressure gradient, decrease the velocity of early diastolic filling (E_{vel}), and prolong the duration of early diastolic filling (deceleration time; see Figs. 26-7 and 26-8). Reduced LA emptying during early diastole increases atrial preload and the velocity of filling with atrial contraction (A_{vel}) increases while the E/A ratio decreases. This produces an "impaired relaxation" pattern. However, if LA pressures are elevated, the LA to LV pressure gradient is restored, and the filling velocity profile will resume a normal configuration (pseudonormalization) with a normal E_{vel}, deceleration time, and E/A ratio despite the presence of impaired relaxation. With marked increases in passive LV diastolic stiffness and further elevation of LA pressures, E_{vel} increases further. In this setting, atrial afterload increases (because of the noncompliant LV), A_{vel} decreases, and deceleration time decreases (reflecting rapid equalization of LV diastolic pressures during early diastolic filling), yielding a "restrictive" pattern (see Fig. 26-7). Thus, the transmitral flow pattern alone cannot be used to assess relaxation directly in all patients with HF. Fortunately, measurement of the velocity of mitral annular ascent during early diastole (e'_{vel}) with tissue Doppler imaging (TDI) provides a relatively preload-independent measure of LV relaxation that correlates inversely with tau.[32] Furthermore, the E/e′ ratio is a fairly accurate predictor of the presence of elevated filling pressures. Interpretation of the mitral inflow velocity versus time profile and the mitral annular TDI profile, aided by information gleaned from other parameters (e.g., Valsalva maneuver and pulmonary venous flow velocity profile; see Fig. 26-7) allow assessment of relaxation and filling pressures in most cases.

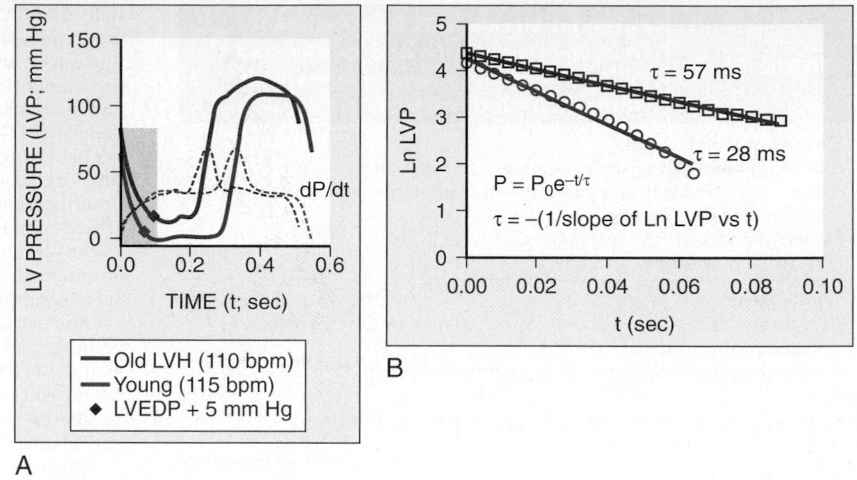

FIGURE 26–9 Invasive assessment of ventricular relaxation—time constant of isovolumic relaxation (tau, τ). **A,** Pressure (P)-time (t) curves starting at the peak negative dP/dt (dotted lines) obtained with a high-fidelity manometer–tipped catheter in a young normal (blue) canine and an elderly canine with chronic hypertension and left ventricular hypertrophy (LVH) (red). Despite similar heart rates and peak positive dP/dt, contraction duration is increased in the elderly dog and filling pressures are increased. **B,** The highlighted area is expanded, and data are graphed as the natural log (ln) of LV pressure versus time during the period from the peak negative dP/dt to 5 mm Hg above the LV end-diastolic pressure (LVEDP). The negative inverse of the slope of this relationship is the time constant of isovolumic relaxation, tau (τ), expressed in milliseconds (ms). Relaxation is impaired (slowed) in the elderly canine. P_0 = LV P at end ejection.

FACTORS REGULATING RELAXATION. LV relaxation is under the triple control of systolic load, myofiber inactivation, and the uniformity of the distribution of load and inactivation in space and time. Thus, the systolic load imposed by increases in blood pressure is a critical factor influencing relaxation and impairment of relaxation, with increases in blood pressure, is referred to as load-dependent impairment in relaxation. Studies have indicated that protein kinase A (PKA)–mediated phosphorylation of troponin I (Tn I) regulates the afterload-relaxation interaction and that reduced PKA-mediated phosphorylation of Tn I contributes to enhanced sensitivity of relaxation to increases in load in heart failure. However, the importance of this mechanism in HFnlEF remains unclear.[33] Uniformity of the distribution of load and inactivation in space and time refers to the fact that increases in systolic load may have different effects, depending on when the load is imposed during systole. Increases in LV pressure late in systole hasten the onset of LV relaxation but relaxation occurs at a slower rate (increased tau).[34] Increases in LV pressure later in systole occur with aging because of age-related vascular stiffening, which alters the timing of reflected pressure wave in the vascular tree so that the reflected wave arrives in late systole rather than diastole. Furthermore, on a myofiber or chamber level, synchrony of relaxation in all segments will enhance LV relaxation, whereas asynchrony (e.g., caused by infarction, ischemia, asymmetry of hypertrophy, or conduction abnormalities) will impair global LV relaxation. Myofiber inactivation refers to the many cellular processes that ultimately influence the rate and extent of detachment of actin myosin cross bridges, allowing myofiber lengthening during diastole, as outlined here (see Table 26-2).[33,35-37]

Actin myosin cross-bridge detachment requires prompt decreases in cytosolic calcium concentrations during diastole. Prolongation of the calcium transient is related to reduced reuptake of calcium into the sarcoplasmic reticulum (SR) by sarcoplasmic reticulum calcium ATPase (SERCA) and its regulatory protein phospholamban, abnormal extrusion of calcium from the myocyte by the sodium calcium exchanger (NCX), or calcium "leak" from the SR in diastole, potentially mediated by abnormalities in the ryanodine-sensitive SR calcium release channel and its modulating protein FKBP-12.6 (see Chap. 21) can result in delayed or incomplete cross-bridge detachment and slowed or incomplete relaxation. Decreases in the amount or activity of SERCA or abnormalities in phospholamban have clearly been shown to regulate relaxation, and gene transfer to enhance myocardial SERCA levels has been shown to improve relaxation in animal models.[33] Beta-adrenergic stimulation results in phosphorylation of phospholamban and enhances relaxation by increasing SERCA activity and the speed of calcium reuptake. Thus, catecholamines are lusitropic (relaxation-enhancing) as well as inotropic agents. As other enzymes or regulatory proteins influencing calcium transients are also regulated by phosphorylation, decreases in the amount or activity of PKA, or increases in protein kinase C, which activates protein phosphatases, and may contribute to impaired relaxation. The importance of rapid decreases in calcium levels in modulating the speed of relaxation is also underscored by studies showing that myocardial gene transfer with parvalbumin, a small intracellular soluble calcium-binding protein found in fast-twitch skeletal muscle fibers, enhances myocyte and LV relaxation.[38]

TABLE 26–2 Potential Mechanisms Responsible for Diastolic Dysfunction and/or Elevated Filling Pressures in Heart Failure with Normal Ejection Fraction

Extramyocardial
Afterload: large artery stiffness, increased resistance
Asynchrony of relaxation caused by conduction abnormalities or right ventricular (RV) pacing
RV–left ventricular (LV) interaction
Pericardial constraint
Whole Heart
Asynchrony of relaxation caused by regional infarction, ischemia, hypertrophy, fibrosis
Concentric remodeling and other geometric changes
Ischemia
Atrial enlargement, atrial systolic and diastolic dysfunction
Rate and rhythm abnormalities
Extracellular Matrix
Increased extracellular matrix (collagen)
Increased collagen stiffness (advanced glycation end products)
Cardiomyocyte
Abnormal calcium homeostasis (↑ diastolic calcium or ↓ rate of calcium reuptake → incomplete or impaired relaxation)
Sarcolemmal calcium channels (sodium-calcium exchanger and calcium pump)
Sarcoplasmic reticulum calcium ATPase (SERCA) abundance and function
Proteins modifying SERCA activity
Phospholamban, calmodulin, calsequestrin abundance and phosphorylation state
Sarcoplasmic reticulum calcium release channels
Myofilaments
Energetics (↓ adenosine triphosphate [ATP] or ↑ adenosine diphosphate [ADP] slows actin myosin cross-bridge release)
ADP/ATP ratio, ADP and inorganic phosphate (P_i) concentration, phosphocreatine shuttle function
Proteins regulating cross-bridge formation and calcium sensitivity
Troponin C calcium binding
Troponin I phosphorylation state
Protein kinase A (PKA) and G protein kinase G (PKG) phosphorylation
Cytoskeletal proteins
Microtubules (increased density) → ↑ diastolic stiffness
Titin isoforms (↑ noncompliant isoform and phosphorylation state) → ↑ diastolic stiffness

Reviewed by Kass DA, Bronzwaer JG, Paulus WJ: What mechanisms underlie diastolic dysfunction in heart failure? Circ Res 94:1533, 2004; Zile MR, Brutsaert DL: New concepts in diastolic dysfunction and diastolic heart failure: Part I: Diagnosis, prognosis, and measurements of diastolic function. Part II: Causal mechanisms and treatment. Circulation 105:1387, 2002; 105:1503, 2002; and Katz AM, Zile MR: New molecular mechanism in diastolic heart failure. Circulation 113:1922, 2006.

As detailed in Chapter 21, contraction and relaxation are regulated by the complex interaction of actin, tropomyosin, myosin, and the regulatory proteins troponin T, I, and C with calcium and phosphorylating protein kinases, as well as adenosine triphosphate (ATP) and adenosine diphosphate (ADP). Whereas binding of calcium to troponin C frees it from inhibition by troponin I, thereby allowing for actin-myosin interactions, phosphorylation of troponin I restores its inhibitory role and hastens relaxation. As noted earlier, troponin I and its phosphorylation state appear to regulate afterload-induced changes in relaxation. Although some evidence of reduced troponin I phosphorylation in HF exists, these observations may also have more important therapeutic implications. This is because methods to enhance the troponin I phosphorylation state may represent a therapeutic strategy, particularly because afterload-induced impairment in relaxation may potently contribute to increased filling pressures and symptoms in HFnlEF (see later).

Energy (ATP) supply can influence relaxation by regulating calcium reuptake via SERCA and by influencing cross-bridge detachment at the myosin heads, where the phosphocreatine shuttle mechanism ensures delivery of ATP from the mitochondria and removal of ADP and inorganic phosphate (P_i) from the site of cross-bridge formation. Inadequate ATP and increased levels of ADP can both impair cross-bridge detachment and slow relaxation. Acute ischemia produces impaired and incomplete relaxation via reduction in ATP and decreases in intracellular pH. Impaired relaxation is the first functional abnormality to occur during acute ischemia; parallel upward shifts of the diastolic pressure-volume relationship (decreased distensibility) have also been described and, along with impairment in relaxation and tachycardia, which enhances the effect of relaxation on filling pressures, contribute to the elevated filling pressures with ischemia. Hypertrophied hearts are more sensitive to ischemia, with greater increases in filling pressures resulting from ischemia.

Abnormalities in the contractile elements themselves, actin and myosin, could also affect cross-bridge detachment. Alterations associated with changes in the myosin isoforms or mutations in genes coding for myosin or actin have been described,[33] although the contribution of altered actin myosin structure and function in HFnlEF remain speculative.

Finally, it must be recognized that diastolic relaxation is coupled to systolic function via the effect of restoring forces. When the LV contracts below its unstressed volume, potential energy is stored, which hastens relaxation during subsequent diastole. This is called elastic recoil, and factors that affect the vigor of systole can therefore affect the speed and extent of relaxation.

EVIDENCE FOR IMPAIRED RELAXATION. Data from studies of humans with HFnlEF,[20,28] elderly hypertensive canines,[39] and mathematical modeling systems[40] have supported the concept that impaired relaxation can contribute to elevated mean LV diastolic pressures in HFnlEF when the heart rate is increased (as during exercise; Fig. 26-10). Furthermore, any other factor that further shortens the diastolic filling period (prolonged contraction or long PR interval) will enhance the effect of impaired relaxation on LV diastolic pressures during filling and thus affect the mean LA pressure needed to fill the LV.[40] Studies in patients with HFnlEF have reported average resting values of tau of approximately 60 milliseconds (heart rate, approximately 70 bpm), with values increasing to approximately 86 milliseconds during exercise.[20,28] Whether therapies to enhance relaxation directly and specifically can be developed, and whether such therapies will relieve symptoms, remains an area of active investigation.

Patients with impaired relaxation and increased dependence on atrial contraction for filling are at risk for developing HF with the onset of atrial fibrillation. The acute reduction in filling associated with loss of atrial systolic activity, coupled with the increased heart rate, mandate acute elevation of LA pressures to maintain filling. In contrast, in normal individuals with normal relaxation and brisk early diastolic filling, dependence on diastasis flow and atrial filling is minimal and rapid atrial fibrillation is much less likely to induce acute pulmonary edema.

Left Ventricular Diastolic Stiffness

Stiffness or elastance is defined as the relationship between the change in stress and the resulting strain. On the chamber level, the elastance of the LV varies over the cardiac cycle (time-varying elastance), and end-systolic and end-diastolic elastance are defined by the changes in systolic or diastolic pressure associated with a change in end-systolic or end-diastolic volume (Fig. 26-11). Increases in LV diastolic stiffness will mandate higher LA pressures to maintain filling and thus promote elevated pulmonary venous pressures and pulmonary congestion when LA pressures are elevated or reduced cardiac output when LA pressures are not elevated.

INVASIVE AND NONINVASIVE ASSESSMENT OF LEFT VENTRICULAR DIASTOLIC STIFFNESS (ELASTANCE). Measurement of LV diastolic stiffness requires the simultaneous assessment of pressure and volume during acute

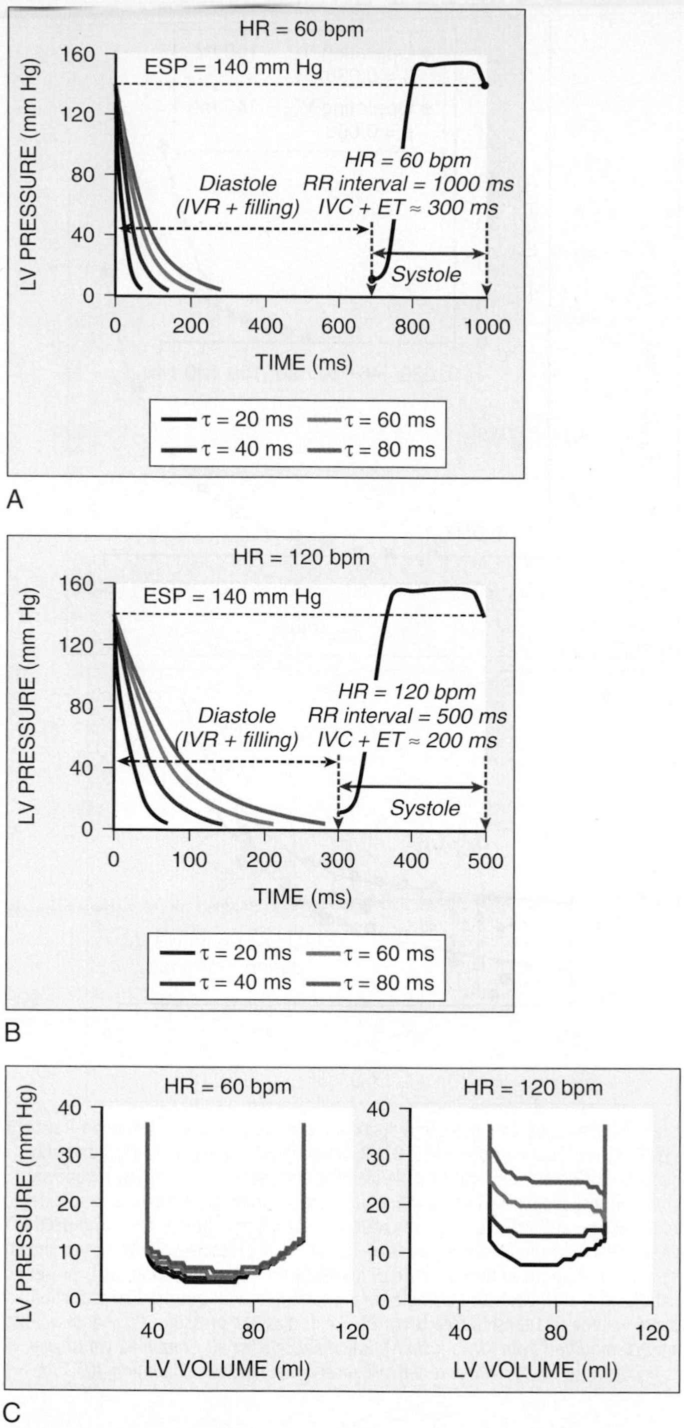

FIGURE 26–10 Impact of impaired relaxation on filling pressures—effect of heart rate (HR). **A, B,** Time course of left ventricular (LV) pressure decay starting at end systole are shown for different degrees of relaxation impairment (τ from 20 to 80 milliseconds). Additionally, the duration of systole and diastole at HRs of 60 bpm **(A)** and 120 bpm **(B)** are shown. At slow heart rates, even marked impairment in relaxation affects only the early diastolic LV pressures. However, at a heart rate of 120 bpm **(B)**, the effect of impaired relaxation on LV diastolic pressures is present throughout most of diastole. **C,** The corresponding diastolic pressure volume profiles for these heart rates and degrees of relaxation impairment were modeled by Hay and colleagues, adjusting for other ventricular and vascular properties. The impact of impaired relaxation on mean LV diastolic filling pressures and the profile of the pressure-volume loop is dramatic at the higher heart rates. ESP = end-systolic pressure; IVR = isovolumic relaxation; IVC = isovolumic contraction; ET = ejection time; bpm = beats per minute. *(***C,** *From Hay I, Rich J, Ferber P, et al: Role of impaired myocardial relaxation in the production of elevated left ventricular filling pressure. Am J Physiol Heart Circ Physiol 288:H1203, 2005.)*

alteration in preload to define the end-diastolic pressure-volume relationship (EDPVR) over a range of preloads, the multiple-beat method (see Fig. 26-11). Alternatively, pressure and volume can be measured over a single-beat, steady-state measurement, and the diastolic portion of the pressure volume curve can be used to estimate stiffness. This single-beat method is subject to three important limitations. First, the EDPVR is curvilinear, and the stiffness measured at a higher operating volume (operant stiffness) will be higher than that obtained when the single beat is taken at a lower operating volume (see Fig. 26-11B). The second limitation is related to the influence of impaired relaxation on the contour of the single-beat diastolic pressure-volume relationship (see Fig. 26-11C). In the normal ventricle, relaxation is brisk and the LV minimum pressure occurs early in diastole, yielding an exponential contour to the mid to late diastolic pressure-volume relationship. Here, only the passive stiffness of the ventricle influences the pressure-volume relationship in mid to late diastole and the pressure and volume data measured over a single cardiac cycle will fit an exponential relationship that allows calculation of a stiffness constant:

$$P = \alpha \times e^{\beta V}$$

where β is the stiffness constant and α is a curve-fitting constant. However, when relaxation is markedly impaired (see Fig. 26-10), relaxation may continue into mid-diastole to an extent determined by the degree of relaxation impairment (tau), heart rate, and duration of contraction (see earlier). Thus, the LV minimum pressure occurs later in diastole, and the diastolic pressure-volume relationship over the single beat is influenced by relaxation and passive stiffness. This limitation is best addressed by using preload reduction to define the EDPVR, avoiding measurements in other portions of diastole that may be influenced by relaxation (see Fig. 26-11C). Alternatively, mathematical methods to correct for the effect of relaxation on diastolic pressures in the single-beat method have been used.[28] Finally, the single-beat method cannot separate the effect of external forces (pericardial constraint and ventricular interdependence) on LV diastolic pressures.

Another important limitation to both the single- and multiple-beat methods for assessment of diastolic stiffness involves the desire to express the position and contour of the exponential EDPVR as a single number and to compare that parameter between groups (i.e., HFnlEF and control populations). In the multiple-beat method, the end-diastolic pressure-volume data points during preload reduction are fitted to one of two frequently used exponential equations:

$$EDP = \alpha \times e^{\beta \times EDV}$$

or

$$EDP = P_0 + \alpha(e^{\beta \times EDV} - 1)$$

In these equations, which relate end-diastolic pressure (EDP) and end-diastolic volume (EDV), a curve fitting constant (α) and a coefficient of stiffness (β) are calculated and the stiffness constant is used to characterize the stiffness of the ventricle. In the second equation, a pressure offset is also calculated (P_0), which allows for quantification of a shift in the position of the EDPVR with or without an accompanying change in the steepness of the relationship. However, because the pressure-volume data acquired in any experiment are not perfectly monoexponential, fitting the data to these equations can often yield very different values for α and β, even when the curves appear similar. Both α and β convey information regarding the stiffness of the ventricle, so if β were not increased but α were increased, one could not conclude that stiffness was normal. Further-

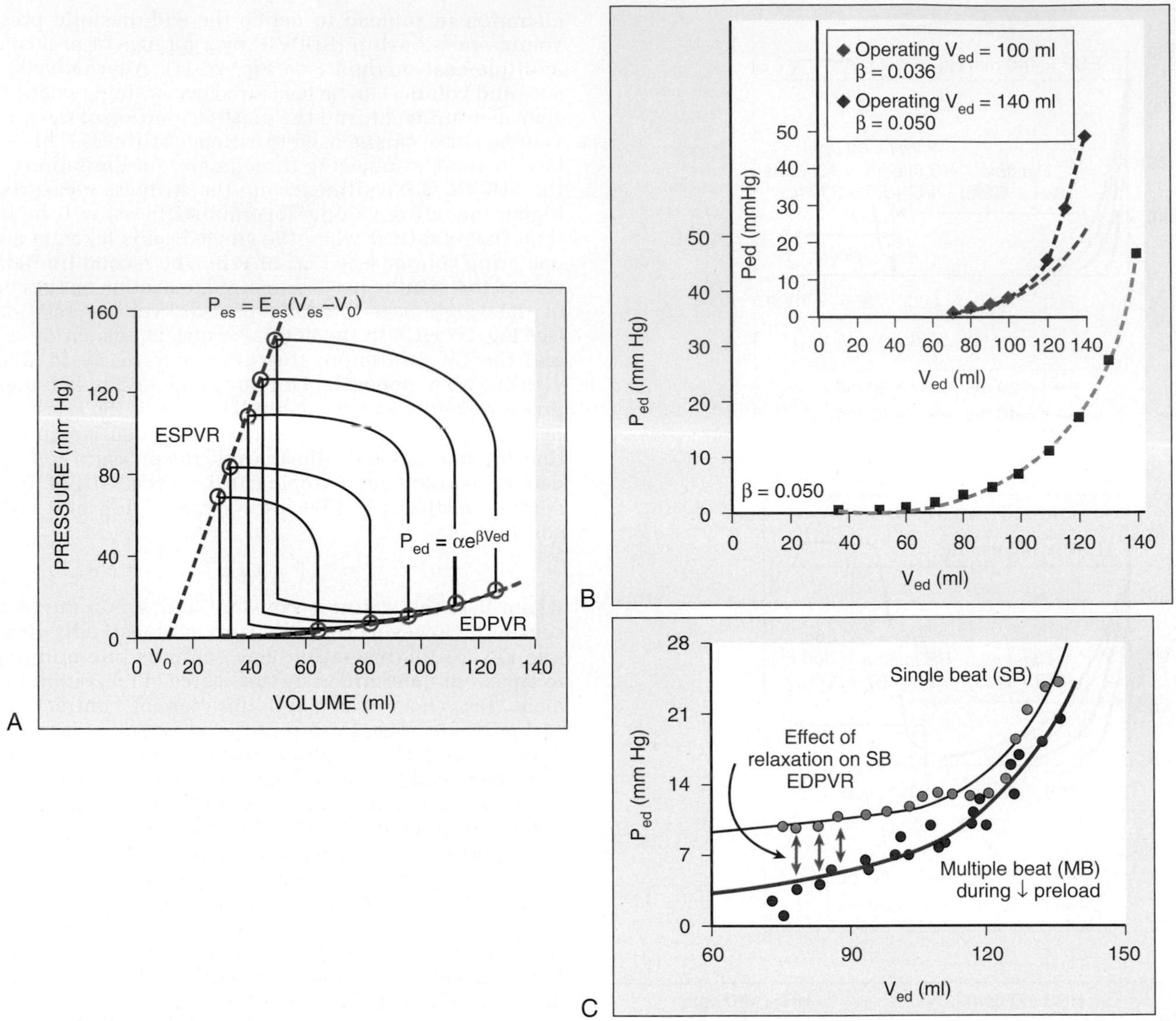

FIGURE 26–11 Invasive assessment of left ventricular (LV) diastolic stiffness. **A,** LV pressure-volume loops during acute reduction in preload produced by sudden transient inferior vena cava occlusion. The relationship between pressure and volume at end systole (ESPVR, red) and end diastole (EDPVR, blue) defines end-systolic (E_{es}) and end-diastolic stiffness. **B,** Curvilinear EDPVR. Thus, at lower operating volumes (insert, blue), diastolic stiffness as reflected by the diastolic stiffness constant (β) will be lower than when stiffness is assessed at higher operating volumes (insert, red). This is true whether stiffness is assessed using a single-beat or multiple-beat method (see text). **C,** Limitations of using the single-beat method of assessing diastolic stiffness. When diastolic pressure and volume data are collected over a single beat (black) and used to calculate stiffness, the pressure data can be affected by relaxation as well as by the passive properties of the ventricle (see text) The diastolic pressure-volume curves shown here were collected with the single-beat (gray) and multiple-beat (red) methods. This effect is most dramatic in the presence of markedly impaired relaxation, as is present in heart failure with normal ejection fraction (HFnlEF) patients. Thus, accurate assessment of diastolic stiffness using a single steady-state beat without preload reduction requires using methods to correct for the effect of impaired relaxation on the diastolic pressure volume relationship (see text). P_{ed} = end-diastolic pressure; P_{es} = end-systolic pressure; V_0 = x intercept of the ESPVR; V_{ed} = end-diastolic volume; V_{es} = end-systolic volume. *(**C** modified from Kawaguchi M, Hay I, Fetics B, et al: Combined ventricular systolic and arterial stiffening in patients with heart failure and preserved ejection fraction: Implications for systolic and diastolic reserve limitations. Circulation 107:714, 2003.)*

more, this can result in considerable variability in group averages for α and β, making it difficult to detect differences between small groups. This limitation can be overcome by converting the exponential pressure-volume relationship to a linear one by plotting the natural log (ln) of EDP versus EDV:

$$\ln EDP = \ln \alpha + \beta(EDV)$$

The slope of this relationship (β) can then be compared, controlling for concomitant changes in the offset (ln α) and for the patient group in multiple linear regression analysis.[41] Alternatively, the measured α and β can be used to calculate the volume at a given EDP (e.g., EDP = 20 mm Hg), and that volume (EDV at 20 mm Hg) can be compared between groups with smaller volumes at a common EDP, reflecting increased diastolic stiffness.[41] More recently, a theoretical method to estimate the EDPVR from a single end-diastolic pressure and volume data point has been described, which may allow estimates of diastolic stiffness from a single beat using invasive or noninvasive data.[42]

A final limitation to either invasive method of characterizing stiffness with pressure-volume data is the considerable difficulty in accurately and instantaneously measuring volume along with pressure, particularly in clinical studies. Use of a conductance catheter allows such instantaneous pressure-volume measurements. Alternatively, invasive LV pressure measurements, coupled with simultaneously acquired echocardiography, contrast ventriculography, and radionuclide angiography, have been used in clinical studies.

Doppler data can provide indirect information regarding LV stiffness. If there is Doppler evidence of elevated filling pressures (increased E/e′ ratio, E/A reversal with Valsalva maneuver, or reduced pulmonary venous systolic flow velocity; see Fig. 26-7) and LV dimension or volume is normal, increased stiffness is inferred. Furthermore, if the deceleration time of the early diastolic transmitral flow velocity profile (see Fig. 26-7) is short, despite evidence of impaired relaxation (reduced early diastolic annular velocity with TDI; see Fig. 26-7), rapid equalization of LV and LA pressures during early diastolic filling and increased LV diastolic stiffness are inferred. Because these Doppler parameters are acquired at a single operating volume, they are subject to the same limitations as single-beat invasive methods; that is, they reflect operating stiffness at a particular diastolic volume and are influenced by external forces.

FACTORS INFLUENCING LEFT VENTRICULAR DIASTOLIC STIFFNESS. As outlined in Table 26-2 and as noted in several studies,[33,35-37] LV diastolic stiffness is affected by a number of factors, which influence the cardiac extracellular matrix, cellular processes at the myocyte level and the myofibers themselves.

The extracellular matrix consists of fibrillar proteins such as collagen type I (predominant form in the myocardium) and type III, elastin, and proteoglycans and basement membrane proteins, such as collagen type IV, laminin, and fibronectin. As outlined in Chapter 21, the myocardial collagen network includes endomysial fibers surrounding individual myocytes and capillaries, perimysial fibers, which interweave muscle bundles, and epimysium fibers, which form a matrix adjacent to the epicardial and endocardial surfaces. The extracellular matrix is dynamic, with the amount regulated by many physical, humoral, and inflammatory mediators that modulate collagen production and breakdown (see Chap. 22). The extracellular matrix is increased in conditions associated with HFnlEF, such as hypertensive heart disease and coronary artery disease. Experimental studies have shown that destruction of perimysial fibers by collagenase perfusion results in decreased LV stiffness. Animal models have demonstrated that interventions associated with increases or decreases in myocardial fibrosis are associated with increased or decreased LV diastolic stiffness. Thus, evidence for the extracellular matrix contributing to diastolic dysfunction by increasing diastolic stiffness or contributing to impairment in relaxation by altering regional loading or uniformity is strong and supports targeting of fibrosis in the therapy of HFnlEF.[33,36,37,50] Also, as mentioned earlier, posttranslational modification of collagen fibers through formation of nonenzymatic collagen cross-linking (advanced glycation end products) has been shown to increase diastolic stiffness.

As discussed in Chapter 21, the giant molecular spring titin also contributes to myocardial diastolic tension. A number of factors, including titin isoform switches (to a less compliant N2B isoform), titin phosphorylation state, titin calcium interactions, and interaction of titin with other signaling molecules and with ion channels, may contribute to the effect of titin on diastolic stiffness. It is believed that alterations in titin may occur in concert with changes in the extracellular matrix, but this interaction is not well defined. Unfortunately, our understanding of the role of alteration in titin and titin interactions in patients with HFnlEF is extremely limited and much remains to be clarified.

Relaxation is clearly recognized to be sensitive in alterations in energetics and is thus characterized as active, whereas diastolic stiffness is characterized as passive. This distinction is probably inaccurate, because reduction in energy supply (as in ischemia) can result in decreased diastolic distensibility, phosphorylation of titin could be acutely regulated, and other factors leading to persistent cross-bridge formation during diastole can occur acutely.

Other structural changes in the myocyte, such as T tubule density, may also occur in disease states associated with hypertrophy and alter diastolic stiffness.

EVIDENCE FOR INCREASED LEFT VENTRICULAR DIASTOLIC STIFFNESS. The difficulties inherent in characterizing LV diastolic stiffness in patients have limited studies characterizing ventricular diastolic stiffness in patients with HFnlEF to only a few. Most[28,43,44] but not all[20] studies have demonstrated increased diastolic stiffness in HFnlEF patients as compared with age-matched (but not always disease-matched) control cohorts without HF.

Other Contributing Factors

Given that HFnlEF develops in elderly patients with a wide spectrum of cardiovascular diseases, the increasingly apparent regional and ethnic variations in the cardiac phenotype in HFnlEF, and the various precipitating factors associated with episodes of acute decompensation in HFnlEF patients, it is likely that factors other than LV diastolic function may also contribute to the pathophysiology and clinical presentation of HFnlEF in some patients.

SYSTOLIC VENTRICULAR VASCULAR STIFFENING. As discussed earlier, previous studies using various indices have established that vascular and ventricular systolic stiffness increases with age and is higher in women.[15,16] The chronic changes in LV systolic stiffness that combine with changes in vascular stiffness may represent cardiovascular adaptations to maintain optimal ventricular-vascular matching and thus optimal cardiac performance. Although ventricular-vascular coupling helps maintain stroke volume and mechanical efficiency, increases in end-systolic elastance (Ees) may have adverse effects. Increases in Ees indicate increased sensitivity of systolic pressure to changes in volume (as demonstrated by the steeper slope of the end-systolic pressure-volume relationship). Thus, volume overload in such individuals could be associated with greater increases in systolic blood pressure. Together, increases in arterial and systolic stiffness promote load-induced impairment in LV relaxation.[20] Thus, age-related systolic ventricular-vascular stiffening could contribute to increases in LV systolic blood pressure, tau, and LV diastolic pressures with exercise and could predispose to HFnlEF, particularly in combination with concomitant alterations in relaxation and diastolic stiffness. Systolic ventricular-vascular stiffening, however, provides a paradigm for understanding exercise-induced or other stress-induced symptoms in HFnlEF patients in whom resting diastolic function does not seem markedly perturbed.

VOLUME OVERLOAD WITHOUT DIASTOLIC DYSFUNCTION. On average, LV cavity dimensions or volumes are normal in patients with HFnlEF. However, the potential for a subgroup of HFnlEF patients to have LV dilation has been previously reported.[26,27] In persons with LV dilation and normal EF, cardiac output is increased, and there may be a high-output subset of patients with HFnlEF who could have increased LV diastolic pressures because of volume overload without underlying diastolic dysfunction. Although the potential for increased volumes in a subset of patients and the importance of volume overload should be acknowledged, most studies have indicated that this represents only a small subset of the HFnlEF population.

ATRIAL DYSFUNCTION. Whereas most discussion has focused on ventricular function in HFnlEF, atrial function may also play an important role in the pathophysiology of HFnlEF. Early- and mid-diastolic LV (and thus LA) pressures, as well as systolic atrial pressures (atrial V wave), are important contributors to mean LA pressure, which is therefore the resistance to filling that the pulmonary venous system faces. LA volumes are increased and LA systolic and diastolic function are impaired in HFnlEF.[21] Indeed, an often forgotten hemodynamic hallmark of restrictive cardiomyopathy is the presence of large V waves in the LA pressure waveform in the absence of mitral regurgitation, reflecting reduced LA compliance. Reduced LA compliance has been shown to have a strong influence on the development of pulmonary arterial hypertension in mitral valve disease and may play a similar role in HFnlEF. Reduced LA systolic function limits LV filling in the setting of impaired relaxation and necessitates higher mean LA pressures to augment early diastolic filling. Thus, enlarged and dysfunctional atria may contribute to the pathophysiology of HFnlEF.

NEUROHUMORAL ACTIVATION. Neurohumoral activation plays a fundamental role in the progression of HF in patients with HF with a reduced EF. Activation of the sympathetic nervous system and the natriuretic peptide system occurs in HF, regardless of EF.[12] Activation of other counter-regulatory hormones, such as renin, angiotensin II, aldosterone, and endothelin, although probable, remains to be established in those with HFnlEF.

LEFT VENTRICULAR SYSTOLIC FUNCTION. By definition, EF is normal in patients with HFnlEF, but some studies have reported that other Doppler indices of contractility are reduced in patients with preclinical diastolic dysfunction or HFnlEF, despite normal EF.[45,46] In contrast, studies measuring these and other indices of contractile function have not found impairment of systolic function in patients with HFnlEF.[20,47,48] Even if subtle changes in systolic performance do exist, their role in contributing to the pathogenesis of HFnlEF remains unclear. More importantly, whether patients with HFnlEF evolve to HF with a reduced EF remains a frequently postulated but unproven and increasingly unlikely theory.

THERAPY

In general, the management of HFnlEF has two objectives. The first is to treat the presenting syndrome of HF—relieve venous congestion and eliminate precipitating factors. The second is to reverse the factors responsible for diastolic dysfunction or other perturbations that lead to HFnlEF. Both nonpharmacological and pharmacological strategies may be used to achieve these objectives. Present treatment strategies for HFnlEF are largely based on assumptions regarding its pathophysiological mechanisms and on extrapolations from proven strategies used in HF with a reduced EF.

Nonpharmacological Therapy

General measures that may be used in the management of patients with chronic HFnlEF are not different from those pursued in patients with HF with a reduced EF. They include daily monitoring of weight, attention to diet and life style, patient education, and close medical follow-up. In patients with HFnlEF, aggressive control of hypertension, tachycardia, and other potential precipitants for HF decompensation should be emphasized. The role of exercise training in patients with HFnlEF has also been explored.[49] Although there are no adequate clinical trials with appropriate outcome endpoints, such as increased longevity, decreased symptoms, or improved quality of life, to prove the benefits of exercise training in patients with HFnlEF definitively, several clinical and experimental studies have suggested that exercise training would be beneficial for such patients.[2,3,18]

Medical and Surgical Therapy

In contrast to the treatment of HF with reduced EF, information to guide the pharmacological therapy of patients with HFnlEF are lacking. Limited available data from clinical studies and randomized controlled clinical trials are reviewed here, followed by largely empirical recommendations regarding therapy.

CLINICAL STUDIES. Small controlled studies have been performed using various standard HF drugs in patients with HFnlEF. The drugs used have included ACE inhibitors, angiotensin receptor antagonists, beta blockers, and calcium channel blockers. These trials have, however, been small or have produced inconclusive results.[50]

RANDOMIZED CONTROLLED CLINICAL TRIALS. The Digitalis Investigators Group (DIG) Trial included a small subgroup of patients with HFnlEF. In the HFnlEF group, digoxin did not alter the primary endpoint of HF hospitalization or cardiovascular mortality (Fig. 26-12A) but did reduce HF hospitalizations.[51] Unfortunately, total cardiovascular hospitalizations were not reduced because of an increased rate of admissions for unstable angina, which completely negated the beneficial effect of reduced HF hospitalizations.

In the CHARM-Preserved Trial,[52] HF patients with an EF higher than 40 percent were randomized to candesartan (an angiotensin receptor antagonist) or placebo in addition to standard therapy. Fewer patients in the candesartan group than in the placebo group reached the primary endpoint of cardiovascular death or HF hospitalization, a finding that reached statistical significance only after adjusting for nonsignificant differences in baseline characteristics (see Fig. 26-12B).

In the PEP-CHF trial, patients older than 70 years with chronic HF and normal or near-normal EF were randomized to perindopril (an ACE inhibitor) or placebo.[53] The primary endpoint was a composite of all-cause mortality or unplanned HF-related hospitalization. Both enrollment and event rates were lower than anticipated and there was a high rate of cessation of blinded therapy, with crossover to open-label ACE inhibitor use in both groups. These factors limited the strength of the study, which did not show significant reduction in the primary endpoint (see Fig. 26-12C). Some trends toward benefit, primarily driven by reduction in HF-related hospitalizations, were observed at 1 year, when crossover therapy rates were lower.

The SENIORS trial tested the effect of the $beta_1$-selective blocker nebivolol in patients with HF.[54] Nebivolol also has vasodilator properties thought to be related to its effects on nitric oxide release. This trial was not restricted to those with normal EF. There was a modest but significant reduction in the primary endpoint of all-cause mortality or cardiovascular hospitalizations which was driven primarily by the effect on hospitalizations. Prespecified subgroup analysis in patients with EF > vs < 35 percent did not detect any trends toward reduced benefit in those with higher EF. Unfortunately, there were very few patients with EF > 50 percent in the trial.

Ongoing clinical trials in HFnlEF are testing the efficacy of the endothelin antagonist, sitaxsentan sodium, irbesartan (I-PRESERVE trial), combinations of diuretics, ramipril, and irbesartan (Hong Kong Diastolic Heart Failure study), aldosterone antagonists (TOPCAT trial), and nesiritide (Use of Nesiritide in the Management of Acute Diastolic Heart Failure trial). (See www.clinicaltrials.gov.)

Current Therapeutic Recommendations

Current recommendations regarding therapy for patients with HFnlEF are outlined in Table 26-3.[2,3] In addition, it is important to treat other contributing comorbidities and risk factors aggressively, such as diabetes, hyperlipidemia, renal dysfunction, and renal vascular disease. One retrospective study has shown that statin use, but not the use of beta blockers, ACE inhibitors, or calcium channel blockers, is associated with improved survival in patients with HFnlEF.[55] Until more clinical trials are performed in patients with HFnlEF, the empirical nature of therapeutic recommendations and their uncertain benefit must be recognized.

FUTURE DIRECTIONS

Great progress has been made in defining the importance of HFnlEF as a public health problem, although better information on regional and ethnic variations in the characteristics and outcomes of patients with HFnlEF is needed. More data regarding outcomes will assist in the definition of endpoints and provide statistical rationales for clinical trials. Design of future clinical studies will need to consider the unique demographics of the HFnlEF population and should include efforts to recruit representative patients from this largely elderly disease cohort. A better understanding of how diastolic dysfunction and other contributing factors (e.g., coronary disease, renal dysfunction, rhythm perturbations, peripheral mechanisms influencing exercise

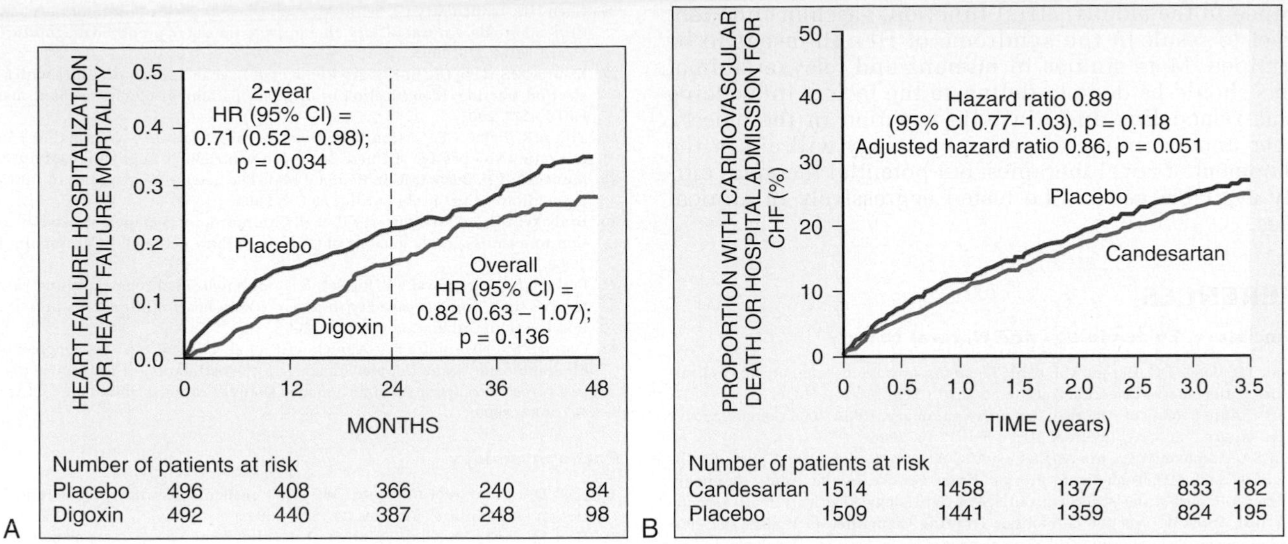

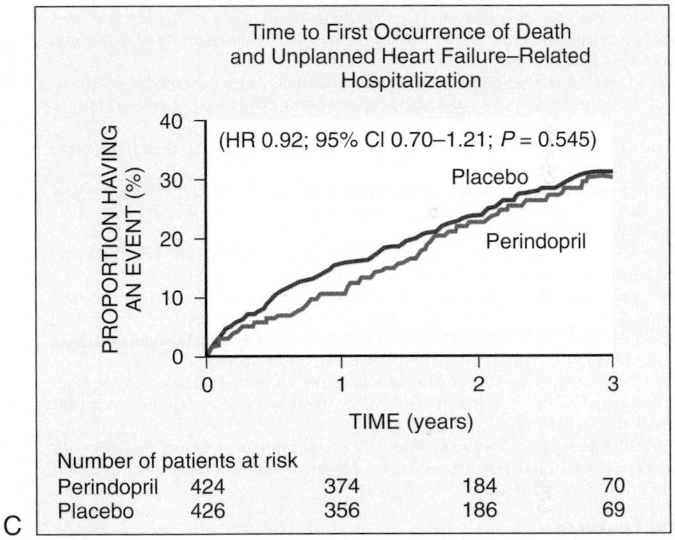

FIGURE 26–12 Kaplan-Meier survival curves for the primary endpoint in the Digitalis Investigators Group (DIG) Trial substudy of patients with heart failure with normal ejection fraction HFnlEF **(A),** the Candesartan in Heart Failure: Assessment of Reduction in Morbidity and Mortality (CHARM)-Preserved Trial **(B),** and the perindopril in elderly people with chronic heart failure (PEP-CHF) trial **(C).** See text for discussion. CI = confidence interval; HR = hazard ratio. *(**A** from Ahmed A, Rich MW, Fleg JL, et al: Effects of digoxin on morbidity and mortality in diastolic heart failure: The ancillary digitalis investigation group trial. Circulation 114:397, 2006; **B** from Yusuf S, Pfeffer MA, Swedberg K, et al: Effects of candesartan in patients with chronic heart failure and preserved left-ventricular ejection fraction: The CHARM-Preserved Trial. Lancet 362:777, 2003; **C** from Cleland JG, Tendera M, Adamus J, et al: The perindopril in elderly people with chronic heart failure (PEP-CHF) study. Eur Heart J 27:2338, 2006.)*

TABLE 26–3 Recommendations for Treatment of Patients with Heart Failure with Normal Ejection Fraction

Class*	Recommendation	Level of Evidence†
I	Physicians should control systolic and diastolic hypertension, in accordance with published guidelines.	A
I	Physicians should control ventricular rate in patients with atrial fibrillation.	C
I	Physicians should use diuretics to control pulmonary congestion and peripheral edema.	C
IIa	Coronary revascularization is reasonable in patients with coronary artery disease in whom symptomatic or demonstrable myocardial ischemia is judged to be having an adverse effect on cardiac function.	C
IIa	Restoration and maintenance of sinus rhythm in patients with atrial fibrillation might be useful to improve symptoms.	C
IIb	The use of beta-adrenergic blocking agents, angiotensin-converting enzyme inhibitors, angiotensin II receptor blockers, or calcium antagonists in patients with controlled hypertension might be effective to minimize symptoms of heart failure.	C
IIb	The use of digitalis to minimize symptoms of heart failure is not well established.	C

*Class I, conditions for which there is evidence and/or general agreement that a given procedure or treatment is beneficial, useful, and effective; class II, conditions for which there is conflicting evidence and/or a divergence of opinion about the usefulness and efficacy of a procedure or treatment, where class IIa is used when the weight of evidence or opinion is in favor of usefulness and efficacy and class IIb is used when the usefulness and efficacy are less well established by evidence or opinion; class III, conditions for which there is evidence and/or general agreement that a procedure or treatment is not useful or effective and in some cases may be harmful.

†Levels of evidence are expressed in the ACC/AHA format as follows: A, data derived from multiple randomized clinical trials or meta-analyses; B, data derived from a single randomized trial, or nonrandomized studies; C, only consensus opinion of experts, case studies, or standard of care.

From Hunt SA, Abraham WT, Chin MH, et al: ACC/AHA 2005 Guideline Update for the Diagnosis and Management of Chronic Heart Failure in the Adult—Summary Article: A Report of the American College of Cardiology/American Heart Association Task Force on Practice Guidelines (Writing Committee to Update the 2001 Guidelines for the Evaluation and Management of Heart Failure): Developed in Collaboration With the American College of Chest Physicians and the International Society for Heart and Lung Transplantation: Endorsed by the Heart Rhythm Society. Circulation 112:1825, 2005.

 tolerance in the elderly, atrial function, vascular function) interact to result in the syndrome of HFnlEF needs to be determined. More studies in humans and relevant animal models should be done to delineate the factors influencing cardiac remodeling and diastolic function in the elderly. Further understanding of pathophysiology will aid in the development of novel therapies, but potential therapies currently available need to be tested aggressively in clinical studies.

REFERENCES

Nomenclature, Epidemiology and Natural History

1. Owan TE, Hodge DO, Herges RM, et al: Trends in prevalence and outcome of heart failure with preserved ejection fraction. N Engl J Med 355:251,, 2006.
2. Heart Failure Society of America: Executive summary: HFSA 2006 Comprehensive Heart Failure Practice Guideline. J Card Fail 12:10, 2006.
3. Hunt SA, Abraham WT, Chin MH, et al: ACC/AHA 2005 Guideline Update for the Diagnosis and Management of Chronic Heart Failure in the Adult—Summary Article: A Report of the American College of Cardiology/American Heart Association Task Force on Practice Guidelines (Writing Committee to Update the 2001 Guidelines for the Evaluation and Management of Heart Failure): Developed in Collaboration With the American College of Chest Physicians and the International Society for Heart and Lung Transplantation: Endorsed by the Heart Rhythm Society. Circulation 112:1825, 2005.
4. Redfield MM, Jacobsen SJ, Burnett JC Jr, et al: Burden of systolic and diastolic ventricular dysfunction in the community: appreciating the scope of the heart failure epidemic. JAMA 289:194, 2003.
5. Owan TE, Redfield MM: Epidemiology of diastolic heart failure. Prog Cardiovasc Dis 47:320, 2005.
6. Hogg K, Swedberg K, McMurray J: Heart failure with preserved left ventricular systolic function; epidemiology, clinical characteristics, and prognosis. J Am Coll Cardiol 43:317, 2004.
7. Bhatia RS, Tu JV, Lee DS, et al: Outcome of heart failure with preserved ejection fraction in a population-based study. N Engl J Med 355:260, 2006.
8. Ceia F, Fonseca C, Mota T, et al: Prevalence of chronic heart failure in Southwestern Europe: The EPICA study. Eur J Heart Fail 4:531, 2002.
9. Owan T, Hodge D, Herges D, et al: Secular trends in renal dysfunction and outcomes in hospitalized heart failure patients. J Card Fail 12:257, 2006.
10. Curtis JP, Sokol SI, Wang Y, et al: The association of left ventricular ejection fraction, mortality, and cause of death in stable outpatients with heart failure. J Am Coll Cardiol 42:736, 2003.
11. Smith GL, Masoudi FA, Vaccarino V, et al: Outcomes in heart failure patients with preserved ejection fraction: Mortality, readmission, and functional decline. J Am Coll Cardiol 41:1510, 2003.

Clinical Features

12. Kitzman DW, Little WC, Brubaker PH, et al: Pathophysiological characterization of isolated diastolic heart failure in comparison to systolic heart failure. JAMA 288:2144, 2002.
13. Thomas JT, Kelly RF, Thomas SJ, et al: Utility of history, physical examination, electrocardiogram, and chest radiograph for differentiating normal from decreased systolic function in patients with heart failure. Am J Med 112:437, 2002.
14. Choudhury L, Gheorghiade M, Bonow RO: Coronary artery disease in patients with heart failure and preserved systolic function. Am J Cardiol 89:719, 2002.
15. Redfield MM, Jacobsen SJ, Borlaug BA, et al: Age- and gender-related ventricular-vascular stiffening: A community-based study. Circulation 112:2254, 2005.
16. Chen CH, Nakayama M, Nevo E, et al: Coupled systolic-ventricular and vascular stiffening with age: Implications for pressure regulation and cardiac reserve in the elderly. J Am Coll Cardiol 32:1221, 1998.
17. Kass DA. Age-related changes in ventricular-arterial coupling: Pathophysiologic implications. Heart Fail Rev 7:51, 2002.
18. Arbab-Zadeh A, Dijk E, Prasad A, et al: Effect of aging and physical activity on left ventricular compliance. Circulation 110:1799, 2004.
19. Diamond JA, Phillips RA. Hypertensive heart disease. Hypertens Res 28:191, 2005.
20. Kawaguchi M, Hay I, Fetics B, et al: Combined ventricular systolic and arterial stiffening in patients with heart failure and preserved ejection fraction: Implications for systolic and diastolic reserve limitations. Circulation 107:714, 2003.
21. Melenovsky V, Borlaug B, Rosen B, et al: Cardiovascular features of heart failure with preserved ejection fraction versus non-failing hypertensive left ventricular hypertrophy in the urban Baltimore community. J Am Coll Cardiol 49:198, 2007.
22. Tsang TS, Gersh BJ, Appleton CP, et al: Left ventricular diastolic dysfunction as a predictor of the first diagnosed nonvalvular atrial fibrillation in 840 elderly men and women. J Am Coll Cardiol 40:1636, 2002.
23. Powell BD, Redfield MM, Bybee KA, et al: Association of obesity with left ventricular remodeling and diastolic dysfunction in patients without coronary artery disease. Am J Cardiol 98:116, 2006.
24. Forman DE, Butler J, Wang Y, et al: Incidence, predictors at admission, and impact of worsening renal function among patients hospitalized with heart failure. J Am Coll Cardiol 43:61, 2004.
25. Klapholz M, Maurer M, Lowe AM, et al: Hospitalization for heart failure in the presence of a normal left ventricular ejection fraction: Results of the New York Heart Failure Registry. J Am Coll Cardiol 43:1432, 2004.
26. Chen HH, Lainchbury JG, Senni M, et al: Diastolic heart failure in the community: Clinical profile, natural history, therapy, and impact of proposed diagnostic criteria. J Card Fail 8:279, 2002.
27. Maurer MS, King DL, El-Khoury Rumbarger L, et al: Left heart failure with a normal ejection fraction: Identification of different pathophysiologic mechanisms. J Card Fail 11:177, 2005.
28. Zile MR, Baicu CF, Gaasch WH: Diastolic heart failure—abnormalities in active relaxation and passive stiffness of the left ventricle. N Engl J Med 350:1953, 2004.
29. Munagala VK, Burnett JC Jr, Redfield MM: The natriuretic peptides in cardiovascular medicine. Curr Probl Cardiol 29:707, 2004.
30. Brubaker PH, Joo KC, Stewart KP, et al: Chronotropic incompetence and its contribution to exercise intolerance in older heart failure patients. J Cardiopulm Rehabil 26:86, 2006.
31. Borlaug BA, Melenovsky V, Russell S, et al: Impaired chronotropic and vasodilator reserve limit exercise capacity in patients with heart failure and a preserved ejection fraction. Circulation 114:2138, 2006.
32. Ommen SR, Nishimura RA, Appleton CP, et al: Clinical utility of Doppler echocardiography and tissue Doppler imaging in the estimation of left ventricular filling pressures: A comparative simultaneous Doppler-catheterization study. Circulation 102:1788, 2000.

Pathophysiology

33. Kass DA, Bronzwaer JG, Paulus WJ: What mechanisms underlie diastolic dysfunction in heart failure? Circ Res 94:1533, 2004.
34. Hori M, Inoue M, Kitakaze M, et al: Loading sequence is a major determinant of afterload-dependent relaxation in intact canine heart. Am J Physiol 249:H747, 1985.
35. Zile MR, Brutsaert DL: New concepts in diastolic dysfunction and diastolic heart failure: Part I: Diagnosis, prognosis, and measurements of diastolic function. Circulation 105:1387, 2002.
36. Zile MR, Brutsaert DL: New concepts in diastolic dysfunction and diastolic heart failure: Part II: Causal mechanisms and treatment. Circulation 105:1503, 2002.
37. Katz AM, Zile MR: New molecular mechanism in diastolic heart failure. Circulation 113:1922, 2006.
38. Huq F, Lebeche D, Iyer V, et al: Gene transfer of parvalbumin improves diastolic dysfunction in senescent myocytes. Circulation 109:2780, 2004.
39. Munagala VK, Hart CY, Burnett JC Jr, et al: Ventricular structure and function in aged dogs with renal hypertension: A model of experimental diastolic heart failure. Circulation 111:1128, 2005.
40. Hay I, Rich J, Ferber P, et al: Role of impaired myocardial relaxation in the production of elevated left ventricular filling pressure. Am J Physiol Heart Circ Physiol 288:H1203, 2005.
41. Burkhoff D, Mirsky I, Suga H: Assessment of systolic and diastolic ventricular properties via pressure-volume analysis: A guide for clinical, translational, and basic researchers. Am J Physiol Heart Circ Physiol 289:H501, 2005.
42. Klotz S, Hay I, Dickstein ML, et al: Single-beat estimation of end-diastolic pressure-volume relationship: A novel method with potential for noninvasive application. Am J Physiol Heart Circ Physiol 291:H403, 2006.
43. Liu C-P, Ting C-T, Lawrence W, et al: Arrhythmias/drugs: Diminished contractile response to increased heart rate in intact human left ventricular hypertrophy: Systolic versus diastolic determinants. Circulation 88:1893, 1993.
44. Borbely A, van der Velden J, Papp Z, et al: Cardiomyocyte stiffness in diastolic heart failure. Circulation 111:774, 2005.
45. Yip G, Wang M, Zhang Y, et al: Left ventricular long axis function in diastolic heart failure is reduced in both diastole and systole: Time for a redefinition? Heart 87:121, 2002.
46. Yu CM, Lin H, Yang H, et al: Progression of systolic abnormalities in patients with "isolated" diastolic heart failure and diastolic dysfunction. Circulation 105:1195, 2002.
47. Aurigemma GP, Zile MR, Gaasch WH: Contractile behavior of the left ventricle in diastolic heart failure: With emphasis on regional systolic function. Circulation 113:296, 2006.
48. Baicu CF, Zile MR, Aurigemma GP, et al: Left ventricular systolic performance, function, and contractility in patients with diastolic heart failure. Circulation 111:2306, 2005.

Therapy

49. Pina IL, Apstein CS, Balady GJ, et al: Exercise and heart failure: A statement from the American Heart Association Committee on exercise, rehabilitation, and prevention. Circulation 107:1210, 2003.
50. Little WC, Brucks S: Therapy for diastolic heart failure. Prog Cardiovasc Dis 47:380, 2005.
51. Ahmed A, Rich MW, Fleg JL, et al: Effects of digoxin on morbidity and mortality in diastolic heart failure: The ancillary digitalis investigation group trial. Circulation 114:397, 2006.
52. Yusuf S, Pfeffer MA, Swedberg K, et al: Effects of candesartan in patients with chronic heart failure and preserved left-ventricular ejection fraction: The CHARM-Preserved Trial. Lancet 362:777, 2003.
53. Cleland JG, Tendera M, Adamus J, et al: The perindopril in elderly people with chronic heart failure (PEP-CHF) study. Eur Heart J 27:2338, 2006.
54. Flather MD, Shibata MC, Coats AJ, et al: Randomized trial to determine the effect of nebivolol on mortality and cardiovascular hospital admission in elderly patients with heart failure (SENIORS). Eur Heart J 26:215, 2005.
55. Fukuta H, Sane DC, Brucks S, et al: Statin therapy may be associated with lower mortality in patients with diastolic heart failure: A preliminary report. Circulation 112:357, 2005.

Management of Heart Failure

A joint task force of the American College of Cardiology and the American Heart Association (ACC/AHA) published guidelines for the evaluation and management of heart failure in 2005.[1] These guidelines updated previous sets of recommendations issued by the ACC/AHA in 2001[2] and 1995,[3] as well as guidelines from the Agency for Health Care Policy and Research in 1994[4] and the Heart Failure Society of America in 1999.[5] New guidelines from the Heart Failure Society were published in 2006.[6] One small but important global change in the ACC/AHA guidelines is the introduction of new nomenclature. Because not all patients have volume overload at the time of initial or subsequent evaluation, the term "heart failure" is now preferred over the older term "congestive heart failure."

Reflecting growing appreciation for the importance of heart failure prevention, the updated ACC/AHA guidelines classify patients according to four stages:

Stage A: patients at high risk for developing heart failure but without structural disorders of the heart

Stage B: patients with a structural disorder of the heart but no symptoms of heart failure

Stage C: patients with past or current symptoms of heart failure associated with underlying structural heart disease

Stage D: patients with end-stage disease who require specialized treatment strategies such as mechanical circulatory support, continuous inotropic infusions, cardiac transplantation, or hospice care.

The advantage of the four-stage system is that it recommends interventions for asymptomatic patients with the goal of preventing signs or symptoms of heart failure. In contrast, the traditional New York Heart Association (NYHA) functional classification system primarily gauges the severity of symptoms in patients who are in stage C or D. Figure 26G-1 summarizes the guideline recommendations for therapy by stage.

As with other ACC/AHA guidelines, these recommendations classify interventions into one of three classes as follows, including two levels of the intermediate group:

Class I: conditions for which there is evidence and/or general agreement that a given procedure/therapy is useful and effective

Class II: conditions for which there is conflicting evidence and/or a divergence of opinion about the usefulness/efficacy of performing the procedure/therapy

Class IIa: weight of evidence and opinion in favor of usefulness/efficacy

Class IIb: usefulness/efficacy is less well established by evidence and opinion

Class III: conditions for which there is evidence and/or general agreement that a procedure or therapy is not useful or effective and in some cases may be harmful

The ACC/AHA guidelines also adopt a convention for rating levels of evidence on which recommendations have been based. Level A recommendations are derived from data from multiple randomized clinical trials; level B recommendations are derived from a single randomized trial or nonrandomized studies; and level C recommendations are based on the consensus opinion of experts. The guidelines emphasize that the strength of evidence does not necessarily reflect the strength of a recommendation. A treatment may be controversial despite having been evaluated in controlled clinical trials; conversely, a strong recommendation may be supported only by historical data or by no data at all.

Initial Patient Evaluation

The ACC/AHA guidelines state that a complete history and physical examination should be the first step in the evaluation of patients with heart failure (Table 26G-1). This evaluation may provide insight into the cause of the patient's heart failure and the presence or absence of structural cardiovascular abnormalities. Other issues to be addressed include presence or absence of history of diabetes, rheumatic fever, chest radiation, exposure to cardiotoxic drugs, and use or abuse of alcohol, illicit drugs, or alternative therapies. The patient's functional and hemodynamic status should also be evaluated to assess prognosis and guide management.

The guidelines recommend that the initial evaluation should include a complete blood count; urinalysis; serum electrolytes, plus calcium and magnesium; renal and hepatic function; fasting blood glucose and HbA_{1c}; lipid profile; thyroid function tests; a chest radiograph; a 12-lead electrocardiogram; two-dimensional echocardiography with Doppler; and coronary arteriography in patients with angina or significant ischemia (unless the patient is ineligible for revascularization).

Measurements of serum ferritin level and transferrin saturation are considered potentially useful for the detection of hemochromatosis, as this condition is a treatable cause of heart failure. Screening for the human immunodeficiency virus, sleep-disturbed breathing, connective tissue diseases, amyloidosis, or pheochromocytoma are also reasonable steps in selected patients.

The updated guidelines reflect recent research on B-type natriuretic peptide. In 2001, the guidelines were noncommittal about routine measurement of this marker. The current ACC/AHA guidelines support its use in the urgent care setting when the diagnosis of heart failure is uncertain, but do not recommend its routine or serial use.

Echocardiography to assess left ventricular function and detect underlying myocardial, valvular, or pericardial disease is considered a more valuable initial test than radionuclide ventriculography or magnetic resonance imaging.

Screening for and assessment of coronary artery disease in patients with heart failure are given considerable attention in these guidelines, reflecting the frequent coexistence of these conditions and the survival benefit of revascularization of patients with severe coronary disease and left ventricular dysfunction. Coronary arteriography is recommended (Class I indication) for patients with angina or significant ischemia and heart failure unless they are not eligible for revascularization. For patients who have chest pain and heart failure, the guidelines provide support for bypassing the step of noninvasive testing and proceeding directly to coronary angiography (Class IIa indication). For patients without chest pain, the guidelines consider coronary angiography "reasonable" for excluding the diagnosis of coronary disease. Maximal exercise testing is also considered "reasonable" to help determine if heart failure is the cause of exercise limitation or for identifying high-risk patients with heart failure who may be candidates for cardiac transplantation or other advanced therapy.

The guidelines offered only weak support for noninvasive testing to define the likelihood of coronary artery disease in patients with heart failure and left ventricular dysfunction and for Holter monitoring in patients with a history of myocardial infarction who might be susceptible to ventricular tachycardia.

Routine use of endomyocardial biopsy, signal-averaged electrocardiography, or routine measurement of circulating levels of neurohormones such as norepinephrine and endothelin is not recommended.

Ongoing Assessment of Patients with Heart Failure

The guidelines support routine assessment of functional and volume status in patients with heart failure, along with assessment of potentially harmful behaviors or habits (see Table 26G-1). They discourage routine serial measurement of ejection fraction at regular intervals, and instead recommend that ejection fraction be reassessed if patients have had a change in clinical status, recovered from a significant

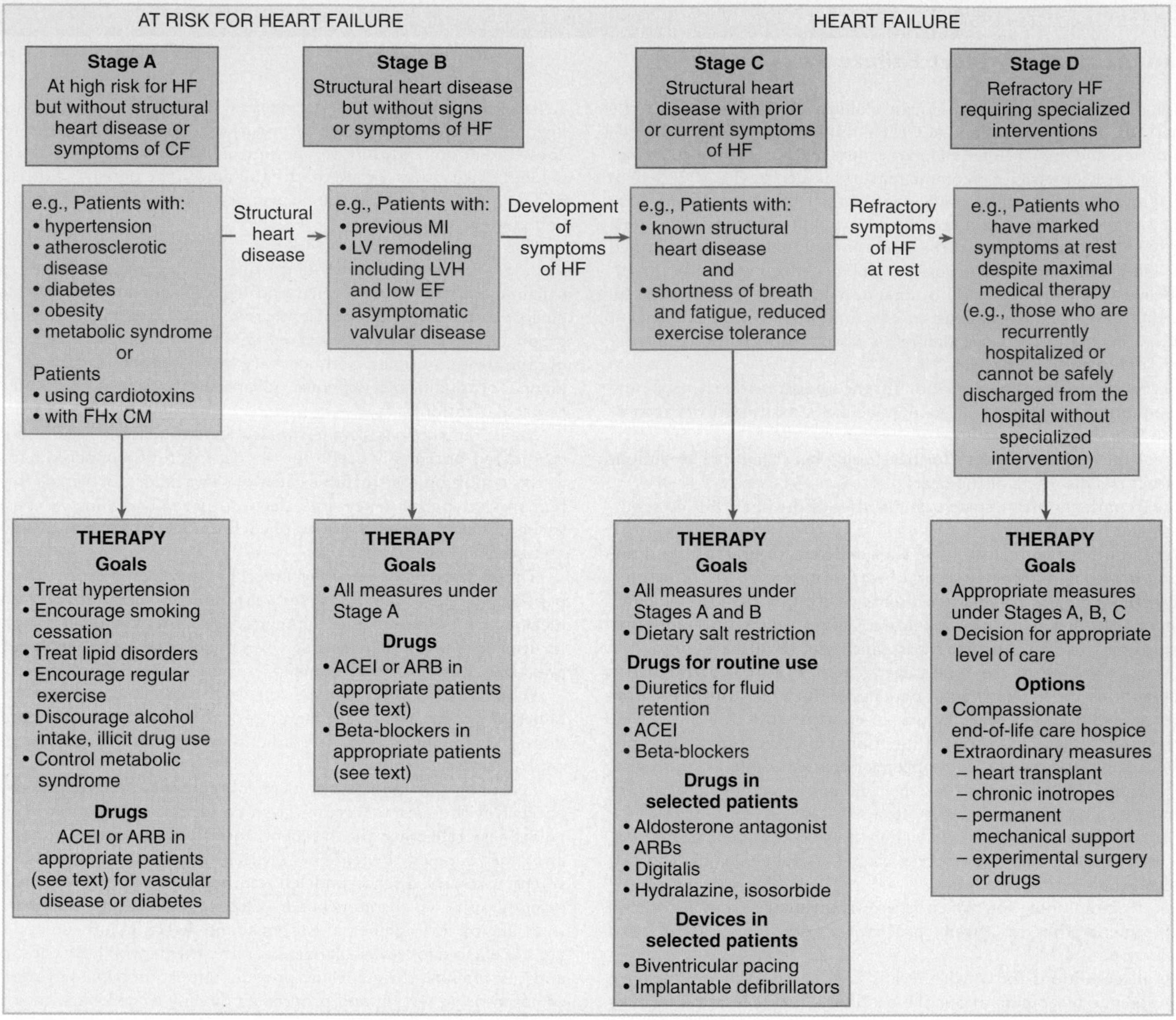

FIGURE 26G-1 Stages in the evolution of heart failure (HF) and recommended therapy by stage. ACEI = angiotensin-converting enzyme inhibitor; ARB = angiotensin receptor blocker; EF = ejection fraction; FHx CM = family history of cardiomyopathy; IV = intravenous; LV = left ventricular; MI = myocardial infarction. *(From Hunt SA, Baker DW, Chin MH, et al: ACC/AHA guidelines for the evaluation and management of chronic heart failure in the adult: A report of the American College of Cardiology/American Heart Association Task Force on Practice Guidelines[Committee to Revise the 1995 Guidelines for the Evaluation and Management of Heart Failure]. J Am Coll Cardiol 104:2996-3007, 2001.)*

clinical event, or received treatment that might affect left ventricular function. The value of serial measurements of B-type natriuretic peptide remains uncertain.

Treatment of Patients at High Risk of Developing Heart Failure (Stage A)

The ACC/AHA guidelines provide strong recommendations (Class I) for control of risk factors for coronary disease and other causes of cardiomyopathy, including hypertension, hyperlipidemia, diabetes, alcohol abuse, cigarette smoking, supraventricular tachycardia, and thyroid disorders (Table 26G-2). Patients at risk for heart failure should also be assessed frequently for evidence that they are developing this condition, particularly those with a strong family history of cardiomyopathy or those receiving cardiotoxic interventions. Attention should be paid to secondary prevention efforts in patients with atherosclerotic vascular disease.

The guidelines suggest a low threshold for use of angiotensin-converting enzyme inhibitors or angiotensin-II receptor blockers (Class IIa). The ACC/AHA task force recommends advising patients not to use nutritional supplements solely to prevent the development of heart failure.

Treatment of Patients with Left Ventricular Dysfunction Who Have Not Developed Symptoms (Stage B)

In this population, the goal of therapy is to reduce the risk of further damage to the left ventricle and to minimize the rate of progression of left ventricular dysfunction. The same risk factor modifications supported for stage A patients are also recommended for stage B patients (Table 26G-3). As is true for virtually all patients with heart failure, no evidence was found to support the use of nutritional supplements.

In the absence of contraindications, beta blockers and ACE inhibitors (or ARBs in those intolerant of ACE inhibitors) are recommended for all patients with histories of myocardial infarction, regardless of

TABLE 26G–1 ACC/AHA Guidelines for Initial Evaluation of Heart Failure

Class	Indication	Level of Evidence*
I (indicated)	1. Thorough history and physical examination to identify cardiac and noncardiac disorders or behaviors that might cause heart failure or accelerate its development or progression	C
	2. Obtain a careful history of current and past use of alcohol, illicit drugs, current or past standard or "alternative therapies," and chemotherapy drugs	C
	3. Initial assessment of the patient's ability to perform routine and desired activities of daily living	C
	4. Initial examination should include assessment of volume status, orthostatic blood pressure changes, measurement of weight and height, and calculation of body mass index	C
	5. Initial laboratory evaluation should include complete blood count, urinalysis, serum electrolytes (including calcium and magnesium), blood urea nitrogen, serum creatinine, fasting blood glucose (glycohemoglobin), lipid profile, liver function tests, and thyroid-stimulating hormone	C
	6. Initial 12-lead electrocardiogram and chest radiograph (PA and lateral)	C
	7. Initial two-dimensional echocardiography with Doppler to assess left ventricular size and ejection fraction, wall thickness, and valve function; radionuclide ventriculography can be performed to assess left ventricular ejection fraction and volumes	C
	8. Coronary arteriography in patients with angina or significant ischemia except those who are not eligible for revascularization	B
IIa (good supportive evidence)	1. Coronary arteriography in patients with chest pain whose coronary anatomy has not been evaluated and who do not have contraindications to coronary revascularization	C
	2. Coronary arteriography in patients with known or suspected coronary artery disease but without angina, except those who are not eligible for revascularization	C
	3. Noninvasive imaging to detect myocardial ischemia and viability in patients with known coronary artery disease and without angina, except those who are not eligible for revascularization	B
	4. Maximal exercise testing with or without measurement of respiratory gas exchange and/or blood oxygen saturation to help determine whether heart failure is the cause of exercise limitation when the contribution of heart failure is uncertain	C
	5. Maximal exercise testing with measurement of respiratory gas exchange to identify high-risk patients who are candidates for cardiac transplantation or other advanced treatments	B
	6. Screening for hemochromatosis, sleep-disturbed breathing, or human immunodeficiency virus in selected patients	C
	7. Tests for rheumatologic diseases, amyloidosis, or pheochromocytoma in patients in whom there is a clinical suspicion of these diseases	C
	8. Endomyocardial biopsy in patients when a specific diagnosis is suspected that would influence therapy	C
	9. Measurement of B-type natriuretic peptide in the urgent care setting when the clinical diagnosis of heart failure is uncertain	A
IIb (weak supportive evidence)	1. Noninvasive imaging to define the likelihood of coronary artery disease in patients with left ventricular dysfunction	C
	2. Holter monitoring in patients with a history of myocardial infarction who are being considered for electrophysiological study to document inducibility of ventricular tachycardia	C
III	1. Routine evaluation with endomyocardial biopsy	C
	2. Routine use of signal-averaged electrocardiography	C
	3. Routine measurement of circulating levels of neurohormones (e.g., norepinephrine or endothelin)	C
ACC/AHA Guidelines for Serial Clinical Assessment of Patients with Heart Failure		
I (indicated)	1. Assess at each visit the patient's ability to perform routine and desired activities of daily living	C
	2. Assess at each visit the patient's volume status and weight	C
	3. Ask at each visit about the patient's current use of alcohol, tobacco, illicit drugs, "alternative therapies," and chemotherapy drugs, as well as about diet and sodium intake	C
IIa (good supportive evidence)	1. Repeat measurements of ejection fraction and structural remodeling in patients who have had a change in clinical status, who have experienced or recovered from a clinical event, or who have received treatment that might have had a significant effect on cardiac function	C
IIb (weak supportive evidence)	1. Serial measurement of B-type natriuretic peptide to guide therapy is not well established	C

ACC = American College of Cardiology; AHA = American Heart Association.
*See guidelines text for definition of level of evidence categories.

ejection fraction; and for all patients with diminished ejection fraction, regardless of history of myocardial infarction. In contrast, the guidelines discourage use of digoxin and calcium-channel blockers with negative inotropic action in this population.

The guidelines support the use of coronary revascularization in appropriate patients, as well as surgery to correct valvular disease in patients with hemodynamically significant valvular stenosis or regurgitation that causes heart failure.

The guidelines indicate that placement of an ICD is reasonable in patients with ischemic cardiomyopathy who have had a recent (>40 days) myocardial infarction, have compromised left ventricular ejection fraction, and have reasonable expectation of survival with good functional status for more than 1 year. There is less evidence supporting ICD placement in similar patients with nonischemic cardiomyopathy.

Treatment of Patients with Left Ventricular Dysfunction and Current or Prior Symptoms (Stage C)

Application of the same measures recommended for preventing or minimizing progression of left ventricular dysfunction for stage A and B patients is supported for stage C patients who have current or prior

TABLE 26G-2 ACC/AHA Guidelines for Treating Patients at High Risk of Developing Heart Failure (Stage A)

Class	Indication	Level of Evidence*
I (indicated)	1. Control of systolic and diastolic hypertension in accordance with contemporary guidelines	A
	2. Treatment of lipid disorders in accordance with contemporary guidelines	A
	3. Control of blood sugar in patients with diabetes mellitus in accordance with contemporary guidelines	C
	4. Avoidance of behaviors that may increase the risk of heart failure, such as smoking, excessive alcohol consumption, and illicit drug use	C
	5. Control of ventricular rate or restoration of sinus rhythm in patients with supraventricular tachyarrhythmias	B
	6. Treatment of thyroid disorders in accordance with contemporary guidelines	C
	7. Perform periodic evaluation for signs and symptoms of heart failure in high-risk patients	C
	8. Follow current guidelines for secondary prevention for patients with known atherosclerotic vascular disease	C
	9. Noninvasive evaluation of left ventricular function in patients with a strong family history of cardiomyopathy or in those receiving cardiotoxic interventions	C
IIa (good supportive evidence)	1. ACE inhibition in patients with a history of atherosclerotic vascular disease, diabetes mellitus, or hypertension with associated cardiovascular risk factors	A
	2. Angiotensin II receptor blockers in patients with a history of atherosclerotic vascular disease, diabetes mellitus, or hypertension with associated cardiovascular risk factors	C
III (not indicated)	1. Use of nutritional supplements to prevent the development of structural heart disease	C

ACC = American College of Cardiology; AHA = American Heart Association.
*See guidelines text for definition of level of evidence categories.

TABLE 26G-3 ACC/AHA Guidelines for Treatment of Asymptomatic Left Ventricular Systolic Dysfunction (Stage B)

Class	Indication	Level of Evidence*
I (indicated)	1. Apply all Class I recommendations for Stage A	A, B, C
	2. Beta-blockade and ACE inhibition in all patients with a recent or remote history of MI regardless of ejection fraction or presence of heart failure	A
	3. Beta-blockade in all patients without a history of MI who have a reduced left ventricular ejection fraction but no heart failure symptoms	C
	4. ACE inhibition in patients with a reduced ejection fraction whether or not they have experienced a myocardial infarction	A
	5. Angiotensin-II receptor blockers (ARBs) for post-myocardial infarction patients without heart failure but with a low left ventricular ejection fraction who are intolerant of ACE inhibitors	B
	6. Treat post-myocardial infarction patients according to contemporary guidelines	C
	7. Recommend coronary revascularization in accordance with contemporary guidelines	A
	8. Valve replacement or repair for patients with hemodynamically significant valvular stenosis or regurgitation	B
IIa (good supportive evidence)	1. ACE inhibition or ARBs for patients with hypertension and left ventricular hypertrophy	B
	2. ARBs for patients with low ejection fraction who are intolerant of ACE inhibitors	C
	3. Placement of an ICD in patients with ischemic cardiomyopathy who are at least 40 days post-myocardial infarction, have a left ventricular ejection fraction ≤30%, are NYHA functional class I on chronic optimal medical therapy, and have reasonable expectation of survival for more than 1 year with a good functional status	B
IIb (weak supportive evidence)	1. Placement of an ICD in patients with nonischemic cardiomyopathy and left ventricular ejection fraction ≤30% who are in NYHA functional class I with chronic optimal medical therapy, and have a reasonable expectation of survival for more than 1 year with good functional status	C
III (not indicated)	1. Use of digoxin in patients with low ejection fraction, sinus rhythm, and no history of heart failure symptoms (risk of harm not balanced by known benefit)	C
	2. Use of nutritional supplements to treat structural heart disease or to prevent the development of symptoms of heart failure	C
	3. Calcium channel blockers with negative inotropic effects may be harmful in asymptomatic patients with low left ventricular ejection fraction after myocardial infarction	C

ACC = American College of Cardiology; AHA = American Heart Association.
*See guidelines text for definition of level of evidence categories.

symptoms attributable to left ventricular dysfunction (Table 26G-4). However, in contrast with the recommendations for stage B patients, the guidelines support use of moderate sodium restriction as well as daily measurement of weight.

Physical activity is recommended for stage C patients. More detailed recommendations are provided in an AHA Scientific Statement on Exercise and Heart Failure, published in 2003.[7] This Scientific Statement noted the absence of large randomized trials of the impact of exercise on outcome for patients with heart failure and observed that most available data on this topic preceded the era of treatment of heart failure with beta blockers. Nevertheless, the authors considered the likely benefit sufficient to support exercise training using an individualized approach. This statement supported use of technologies including gas exchange measurements to provide an objective assessment of functional capacity and direct monitoring (including telemetry monitoring), particularly for initial training sessions. Even fewer data are available on the risks of resistive training in this population, but the Scientific Statement observed that such training seems to offer some physiological benefits and supported the use of small free weights and exercises aimed at strengthening the upper body.

The 2005 ACC/AHA guidelines support the use of beta blockers and ACE inhibitors (ARBs for patients who cannot tolerate ACE inhibitors) for all stage C patients, in the absence of contraindications, and use of diuretics for patients with fluid overload. The risks of initia-

TABLE 26G–4 ACC/AHA Guidelines for Treatment of Symptomatic Left Ventricular Systolic Dysfunction (Stage C)

Class	Indication	Level of Evidence*
I (indicated)	1. Apply all Class I recommendations for Stage A	A, B, C
	2. Diuretics and salt restriction in patients with evidence of fluid retention	C
	3. ACE inhibition in all patients unless agents contraindicated	A
	4. Beta-blockade with one of the three proven to reduce mortality (bisoprolol, carvedilol, or sustained-release metoprolol succinate) in all patients unless contraindicated	A
	5. Angiotensin II receptor blockers approved for the treatment of heart failure (candesartan or valsartan) in patients who cannot tolerate ACE inhibitors	A
	6. Avoid or withdraw drugs known to adversely affect heart failure whenever possible, such as nonsteroidal antiinflammatory drugs, most antiarrhythmic drugs, and most calcium-channel blocking drugs	B
	7. Exercise training as an adjunctive approach to improve clinical status in ambulatory patients	B
	8. Placement of an implantable cardioverter-defibrillator (ICD) for secondary prevention to prolong survival in patients with a history of cardiac arrest, ventricular fibrillation, or hemodynamically destabilizing ventricular tachycardia	A
	9. ICD therapy to prevent sudden cardiac death in patients with ischemic heart disease who are at least 40 days post–myocardial infarction, have a left ventricular ejection fraction ≤30%, with NYHA functional class II or III symptoms while undergoing chronic optimal medical therapy, and who have reasonable expectation of survival for more than 1 year with good functional status	A
	10. ICD therapy to prevent sudden cardiac death in patients with nonischemic cardiomyopathy who have a left ventricular ejection fraction ≤30%, with NYHA functional class II or III symptoms while undergoing chronic optimal medical therapy and who have reasonable expectation of survival for more than 1 year with good functional status	B
	11. Cardiac resynchronization therapy in patients with cardiac dyssynchrony (a QRS duration greater than 0.12 ms), a left ventricular ejection fraction ≤35% who are in sinus rhythm, and are in NYHA functional class III or ambulatory class IV in spite of optimal medical therapy, unless contraindicated	A
	12. Addition of an aldosterone antagonist in selected patients who can be carefully monitored for preserved renal function and normal potassium concentration; creatinine should be ≤2.5 mg/deciliter in men or ≤2.0 mg/deciliter in women and potassium should be ≤5.0 mEq/liter.	B
IIa (good supportive evidence)	1. ARBs are a reasonable alternative to ACE inhibitors as first-line therapy, especially for patients already taking ARBs for other indications	A
	2. Digitalis to decrease hospitalizations for heart failure	B
	3. The addition of a combination of hydralazine and a nitrate for patients who have persistent symptoms in spite of already taking an ACE inhibitor and beta blocker	A
	4. Placement of an ICD in patients with left ventricular ejection fraction between 30% and 35% with NYHA functional class II or III symptoms who are taking chronic optimal medical therapy and who have reasonable expectation of survival for more than 1 year with good functional status	B
IIb (weak supportive evidence)	1. A combination of hydralazine and a nitrate in patients who cannot tolerate an ACE inhibitor or ARB because of drug intolerance, hypotension, or renal insufficiency	C
	2. Adding an ARB in persistently symptomatic patients who are already being treated with conventional therapy	B
III (not indicated)	1. Routinely combining an ACE inhibitor, an ARB, and an aldosterone antagonist	C
	2. Routine use of calcium-channel blocking drugs	A
	3. Long-term use of an infusion of a positive inotropic drug may be harmful and is not recommended except as palliation for patients with end-stage disease who cannot be stabilized with standard medical treatment	C
	4. Use of nutritional supplements as treatment for heart failure	C
	5. Hormonal therapies other than to replete deficiencies may be harmful	C

ACC = American College of Cardiology; AHA = American Heart Association.
*See guidelines text for definition of level of evidence categories.

tion of beta blockers are considered in detail in these guidelines, and three agents proved to reduce mortality in patients with heart failure—bisoprolol, carvedilol, and metoprolol succinate—are recommended for "all stable patients with current or prior symptoms of heart failure and reduced left ventricular dysfunction, unless contraindicated." Addition of an aldosterone antagonist should be considered in patients with moderately severe or severe heart failure symptoms and recent decompensation or with LV dysfunction after MI, who can be carefully monitored for preserved renal function and normal potassium concentration.

Class I recommendations support use of ICDs in stage C patients with a history of cardiac arrest, ventricular fibrillation, or hemodynamically destabilizing ventricular tachycardia; in recent survivors of myocardial infarction with compromised left ventricular ejection fraction, and NYHA functional Class II or III symptoms despite optimal medical therapy; and in similar patients with nonischemic cardiomyopathy. Cardiac resynchronization therapy is recommended in patients with cardiac dyssynchrony and compromised left ventricular ejection fraction who are in sinus rhythm and NYHA functional Class III or ambulatory Class IV despite optimal medical therapy, unless contraindicated. Guidelines covering patient selection for cardiac resynchronization therapy were published in 2005.[8]

The guidelines offer qualified support (Class IIa) for the use of ARBs in place of ACE inhibitors as first-line therapy, especially in patients already taking an ARB for another indication. Digitalis is a reasonable approach to decrease hospitalizations in symptomatic patients. The guidelines also offer support for use of hydralazine/nitrate combinations in patients who continue to have symptoms despite maximal therapy with a beta blocker and ACE inhibitor. There is less support (Class IIb) for using a hydralazine/nitrate combination for patients who cannot take an ACE inhibitor or ARB because of drug intolerance, low blood pressure, or renal insufficiency.

The guidelines explicitly discourage the routine use of a combination of an ACE inhibitor, ARB, and aldosterone antagonist; calcium-channel blockers; long-term infusion of positive inotropic drugs (except as palliation in patients with end-stage disease; Table 26G-5); use of nutritional supplements as treatment; and hormonal therapies other than those needed to replete deficiencies.

TABLE 26G-5 ACC/AHA Guidelines for Treatment of Patients with End-Stage Heart Failure (Stage D)

Class	Indication	Level of Evidence*
I (indicated)	1. Meticulous identification and control of fluid retention	B
	2. Refer potentially eligible patient for cardiac transplantation	B
	3. Refer patient to a heart failure program with expertise in the management of refractory heart failure	A
	4. Discuss options for end-of-life care with the patient and family when severe symptoms persist despite application of all recommended therapies	C
	5. Offer patients with implantable defibrillators and end-stage disease the option to inactivate defibrillation	C
IIa (good supportive evidence)	1. Consider a left ventricular assist device as permanent or "destination" therapy in highly selected patients with refractory end-stage heart failure and an estimated 1-year mortality >50% with medical therapy	B
IIb (weak supportive evidence)	1. Pulmonary artery catheter placement to guide therapy in patients with persistently severe symptoms	C
	2. Mitral valve repair or replacement is not established for severe secondary mitral regurgitation	C
	3. Continuous intravenous infusion of a positive inotropic agent may be considered for palliation	C
III (not indicated)	1. Partial left ventriculectomy is not recommended in patients with nonischemic cardiomyopathy	C
	2. Routine intermittent infusions of positive inotropic agents are not recommended	B

ACC = American College of Cardiology; AHA = American Heart Association.
*See guidelines text for definition of level of evidence categories.

Treatment of Patients with Refractory End-Stage Heart Failure (Stage D)

The ACC/AHA guidelines emphasize the importance of meticulous application of the measures listed as Class I recommendations for patients in stages A, B, and C (see Tables 26G-2 to 26G-4) and consider these patients candidates for specialized treatment strategies, such as referral for cardiac transplantation, mechanical circulatory support, continuous intravenous positive inotropic therapy, or hospice care (see Table 26G-5). The guidelines also endorse the use of team management approaches such as heart failure programs. Detailed specifications of the components of such heart failure programs were provided in an AHA Scientific Statement published in 2000.[9]

The guidelines include explicit cautionary notes about the use of ACE inhibitors and beta blockers in this population. Although consideration of these agents is supported, the guidelines state that "Treatment with either type of drug should not be initiated in patients who have systolic blood pressures less than 80 mm Hg or who have signs of peripheral hypoperfusion. In addition, patients should not be started on a beta-blocker if they have significant fluid retention or if they recently required treatment with an intravenous positive inotropic agent." When these medications are used, very low doses should be prescribed at initiation, and patients should be monitored closely for evidence of intolerance. The guidelines note that spironolactone has been shown to be beneficial in patients with advanced heart failure, but they emphasize that these data are derived from patients with preserved renal function and that spironolactone may induce hyperkalemia in patients with impaired renal function. According to the 2005 guidelines, there is limited evidence to support the placement of a pulmonary artery catheter to guide therapy or mitral valve repair or replacement for severe mitral regurgitation.

The ACC/AHA guidelines recognize the value of continuous intravenous inotropic support for some patients who require a "bridge" strategy while awaiting cardiac transplantation or who cannot otherwise be discharged from the hospital. However, the guidelines directly discourage routine intermittent intravenous infusion of inotropic agents. Similarly, the guidelines did not encourage use of partial left ventriculectomy.

The guidelines also include a summary of indications for cardiac transplantation (Table 26G-6). These indications make explicit that low left ventricular ejection fraction and poor functional status are insufficient indications for transplantation in the absence of demonstrated peak oxygen consumption less than 15 ml/kg/min.

TABLE 26G-6 ACC/AHA Guidelines: Indications for Cardiac Transplantation

Absolute Indications
For hemodynamic compromise due to heart failure
Refractory cardiogenic shock
Documented dependence on IV inotropic support to maintain adequate organ perfusion
Peak VO_2 less than 10 mL/kg/min with achievement of anaerobic metabolism
Severe symptoms of ischemia that consistently limit routine activity and are not amenable to coronary artery bypass surgery or percutaneous coronary intervention
Recurrent symptomatic ventricular arrhythmias refractory to all therapeutic modalities
Relative Indications
Peak VO_2 11 to 14 ml/kg/min (or 55% of predicted) and major limitation of the patient's daily activities
Recurrent unstable ischemia not amenable to other intervention
Recurrent instability of fluid balance/renal function not due to patient noncompliance with medical regimen
Insufficient Indications
Low left ventricular ejection fraction
History of functional Class III or IV symptoms of heart failure
Peak VO_2 greater than 15 ml/kg/min (and greater than 55% of predicted) without other indications

ACC = American College of Cardiology; AHA = American Heart Association; IV, intravenous; VO_2 = oxygen consumption per unit time.

Special Populations and Concomitant Disorders

The ACC/AHA guidelines support consideration of patient-specific needs and coexisting medical conditions. Clinicians are reminded that although heart failure has traditionally been considered to be a disease of men, women—particularly elderly women—make up the majority of the general population with heart failure. Yet women have not been included in sufficient numbers in most large trials to allow for conclusions about the efficacy of the treatments under study. In addition, women, minorities, and the elderly are less likely to receive interventions supported by clinical trials, and differences in the natural history of heart failure and response to treatment exist among various patient subsets.

Patients from high risk ethnic minority groups, such as blacks, as well as from groups underrepresented in clinical trials and those believed to be underserved, should receive the same clinical screening and therapy as received by the broader population, in the absence of specific evidence to the contrary. The guidelines suggest that the addition of isosorbide dinitrate and hydralazine to a standard medical regimen for heart failure that includes ACE inhibition and beta blockade is reasonable and can be effective in blacks with NYHA functional Class III or IV heart failure.

Specific clinical recommendations for the management of patients with concomitant disorders (Table 26G-7) emphasize the importance of meticulous management of hypertension, ischemic heart disease, anticoagulation, and supraventricular and ventricular arrhythmias. The use of digitalis to control the ventricular response rate in patients with atrial fibrillation and amiodarone to decrease the recurrence of atrial arrhythmias and likelihood of an ICD discharge are considered reasonable therapies. There is insufficient evidence to recommend for or against the usefulness of current strategies to restore and maintain sinus rhythm in patients with atrial fibrillation; the usefulness of anticoagulation in patients without atrial fibrillation or a prior myocardial infarction; or improving erythropoiesis in anemia patients. The guidelines do not support routine use of Class I or III antiarrhythmic drugs except amiodarone, or the use of antiarrhythmic drugs as a primary treatment for asymptomatic ventricular arrhythmias.

Heart Failure in Patients with a Normal Ejection Fraction

Recommendations for management of patients with heart failure in the absence of left ventricular systolic dysfunction reflect the lack of conclusive data on effective therapies. The major strategies are control of hypertension, control of ventricular rate in patients with atrial fibrillation, and use of diuretics to control pulmonary congestion and peripheral edema (Table 26G-8). Because myocardial ischemia can cause diastolic dysfunction, the guidelines offer support for consideration of use of coronary revascularization in patients with coronary disease (Class IIa indication). Possibly useful therapies include restoration and maintenance of sinus rhythm in patients with atrial fibrillation, as well as the use of beta blockers, ACE inhibitors, ARBs, or

TABLE 26G-7 ACC/AHA Guidelines for Management of Concomitant Diseases in Patients with Heart Failure

Class	Indication	Level of Evidence*
I (indicated)	1. Apply all other recommendations in the absence of specific exceptions	C
	2. Control systolic and diastolic hypertension and diabetes mellitus in accordance with recommended guidelines	C
	3. Nitrates and beta blockers for the treatment of angina	B
	4. Coronary revascularization according to recommended guidelines in patients with both angina and heart failure	A
	5. Anticoagulants in patients with heart failure who have paroxysmal or persistent atrial fibrillation or a previous thromboembolic event	A
	6. Beta blockade (or amiodarone, if beta blockers are contraindicated or not tolerated) to control the ventricular response rate in patients with atrial fibrillation	A
	7. Treat patients with coronary artery disease and heart failure in accordance with recommended guidelines for chronic stable angina	C
	8. Antiplatelet agents for prevention of myocardial infarction and death in patients with heart failure and underlying coronary artery disease	B
IIa (good supportive evidence)	1. Digitalis to control the ventricular response rate in patients with heart failure and atrial fibrillation	A
	2. Amiodarone to decrease recurrence of atrial arrhythmias and recurrence of ICD discharge for ventricular arrhythmias	C
IIb (weak supportive evidence)	1. Current strategies to restore and maintain sinus rhythm in patients with heart failure and atrial fibrillation is not well established	C
	2. Anticoagulation in patients with heart failure who do not have atrial fibrillation or a previous thromboembolic event is not well established	B
	3. Enhancing erythropoiesis in patients with heart failure and anemia is not established	C
III (not indicated)	1. Class I or III antiarrhythmic drugs are not recommended for the prevention of ventricular arrhythmias	A
	2. Antiarrhythmic medication is not indicated as primary treatment for asymptomatic ventricular arrhythmias or to improve survival	A

ACC = American College of Cardiology; AHA = American Heart Association.
*See guidelines text for definition of level of evidence categories.

TABLE 26G-8 ACC/AHA Guidelines for Treatment of Patients with Heart Failure and Normal Left Ventricular Ejection Fraction

Class	Indication	Level of Evidence*
I (indicated)	1. Control systolic and diastolic hypertension in accordance with published guidelines	A
	2. Control ventricular rate in patients with atrial fibrillation	C
	3. Diuretics to control pulmonary congestion and peripheral edema	C
IIa (good supportive evidence)	1. Coronary revascularization in patients with coronary artery disease in whom symptomatic or demonstrable myocardial ischemia is judged to be having an adverse effect on cardiac function	C
IIb (weak supportive evidence)	1. Restoration and maintenance of sinus rhythm in patients with atrial fibrillation	C
	2. Use of beta-blockade, ACE inhibitors, ARBs, or calcium antagonists may minimize heart failure symptoms	C
	3. Use of digitalis to minimize symptoms is not well established	C

ACC = American College of Cardiology; AHA = American Heart Association.
*See guidelines text for definition of level of evidence categories.

TABLE 26G-9 ACC/AHA Guidelines on End-of-Life Care for Patients with Heart Failure

Class	Indication	Level of Evidence*
I (indicated)	1. Ongoing education of the patient and family regarding prognosis for functional capacity and survival	C
	2. Patient and family education about options for formulating and implementing advance directives and the role of palliative and hospice care services with reevaluation for changing clinical status	C
	3. Discussion regarding the option of inactivating implantable cardioverter-defibrillator	C
	4. Ensure continuity of medical care between inpatient and outpatient settings	C
	5. Palliation at the end of life should include standard components of hospice care, such as opiates for pain control, and should not preclude the use of inotropes and intravenous diuretics	C
	6. Examine current end-of-life processes and work toward improvement in approaches to palliation and end-of-life care	C
III (not indicated)	1. Aggressive procedures performed within the final days of life (including intubation and implantation of a cardioverter-defibrillator) in patients with NYHA functional Class IV symptoms who are not anticipated to experience clinical improvement from available treatments	

ACC = American College of Cardiology; AHA = American Heart Association; IV = intravenous; NYHA = New York Heart Association.
*See guidelines text for definition of level of evidence categories.

calcium-channel blockers to minimize symptoms in patients with controlled hypertension.

END-OF-LIFE CARE

Despite significant advances in the diagnosis and management of heart failure, approximately one-half of individuals die within 5 years of its diagnosis. For many patients, there is an abrupt transition from the period of aggressive intervention to one of palliation and comfort. Addressing end-of-life issues relatively early in the course of heart failure, before the patient becomes unable to participate in decision-making, is important for all involved (Table 26G-9). The guidelines recommend discussing treatment preferences, living wills, and advanced directives. The latter can be more difficult than those for patients with cancer or other conditions. Heart failure can be characterized by periods of good quality of life even after hospitalization for intensive care or the approach of death. In addition to resuscitation, discussions should cover the possible deactivation of an ICD.

Hospice services, once available primarily for cancer patients, are being extended to those dying with heart failure. In such patients, compassionate care may include the use of intravenous diuretics and/or positive inotropic agents, as well as pain medications. The guidelines explicitly discourage the performance of aggressive procedures such as intubation and ICD implantation within the final days of life in patients with severe end-stage symptoms who are not expected to experience clinical improvements.

References

1. Hunt SA: ACC/AHA 2005 guideline update for the diagnosis and management of chronic heart failure in the adult: A report of the American College of Cardiology/American Heart Association Task Force on Practice Guidelines (Writing Committee to Update the 2001 Guidelines for the Evaluation and Management of Heart Failure). J Am Coll Cardiol 46:e1-82, 2005.
2. Hunt SA, Baker DW, Chin MH, et al: ACC/AHA Guidelines for the Evaluation and Management of Chronic Heart Failure in the Adult: Executive Summary: A Report of the American College of Cardiology/American Heart Association Task Force on Practice Guidelines (Committee to Revise the 1995 Guidelines for the Evaluation and Management of Heart Failure): Developed in Collaboration with the International Society for Heart and Lung Transplantation; Endorsed by the Heart Failure Society of America. Circulation 104:2996-3007, 2001.
3. Guidelines for the evaluation and management of heart failure. Report of the American College of Cardiology/American Heart Association Task Force on Practice Guidelines (Committee on Evaluation and Management of Heart Failure). J Am Coll Cardiol 26:1376-1398, 1995.
4. Heart failure: Management of patients with left-ventricular systolic dysfunction. Agency for Health Care Policy and Research. Clin Pract Guidel Quick Ref Guide Clin 1-25, 1994.
5. Heart Failure Society of America (HFSA) practice guidelines. HFSA guidelines for management of patients with heart failure caused by left ventricular systolic dysfunction—pharmacological approaches. J Card Fail 5:357-382, 1999.
6. Heart Failure Society of America: HFSA 2006 Comprehensive Heart Failure Practice Guidelines. J Card Fail 12:e1-e122, 2006.
7. Pina IL, Apstein CS, Balady GJ, et al: Exercise and heart failure: A statement from the American Heart Association Committee on exercise, rehabilitation, and prevention. Circulation 107:1210-1225, 2003.
8. Strickberger SA, Conti J, Daoud EG, et al: Patient selection for cardiac resynchronization therapy: From the Council on Clinical Cardiology Subcommittee on Electrocardiography and Arrhythmias and the Quality of Care and Outcomes Research Interdisciplinary Working Group, in collaboration with the Heart Rhythm Society. Circulation 111:2146-2150, 2005.
9. Grady KL, Dracup K, Kennedy G, et al: Team management of patients with heart failure: A statement for healthcare professionals from The Cardiovascular Nursing Council of the American Heart Association. Circulation 102:2443-2456, 2000.

CHAPTER 27

Surgical Management of Heart Failure

Patrick M. McCarthy

In the current era of modern heart failure management, clinicians frequently encounter optimally treated patients who remain symptomatic from their heart failure. Indeed, despite the variety of available medical therapies and electrophysiological interventions, such as biventricular pacemakers and implantable cardiac defibrillators (see Chap. 25), many heart failure patients are still left with a reduced quality of life and a poor prognosis. In a subpopulation of these patients, surgical intervention may be appropriate for the following: (1) to alleviate ischemia; (2) to attenuate valvular dysfunction: (3) to reverse or reduce mechanical disadvantages caused by ventricular remodeling; and (4) to use cardiac transplantation when all other treatment options have failed.

Although surgical interventions in patients with heart failure and low left ventricular ejection fraction (LVEF) have historically been viewed as high risk, recent studies have suggested that such interventions can be performed with an acceptable early morbidity and mortality and excellent late survival and functional outcomes. In this chapter, we will review each component of potential surgical therapies for heart failure, including coronary artery revascularization, cardiac valve repair, left ventricular (LV) reconstruction, passive cardiac support devices, and cardiac transplantation. In some patients, it may be appropriate to perform just one component (e.g., coronary artery bypass or just a mitral valve repair), whereas in other patients it may be appropriate to perform multiple components together (e.g., coronary artery bypass with mitral and tricuspid valve repair, and LV reconstruction for an LV apical aneurysm) to optimize clinical outcomes.

CORONARY ARTERY REVASCULARIZATION

Ischemic Cardiomyopathy

As discussed in detail in Chapter 54, the term *ischemic cardiomyopathy* is used to describe the myocardial dysfunction that arises secondary to occlusive and/or obstructive coronary artery disease. Although ischemic cardiomyopathy was considered the second most common cause of heart failure (after hypertension) in the Framingham study (see Chap. 25), ischemic cardiomyopathy is now recognized as the most common cause of heart failure in clinical trials. This section focuses on the impact and outcome of surgical coronary artery revascularization in patients with ischemic cardiomyopathy. The medical management for patients with heart failure is reviewed in Chapter 25.

Ischemic cardiomyopathy can be envisioned as three interrelated pathophysiological processes (see Fig. 16-29)—myocardial hibernation, defined as the presence of persistent contractile dysfunction at rest caused by reduced coronary blood flow that can be partially or completely restored to normal by myocardial revascularization; myocardial stunning, wherein the viable myocardium may demonstrate relatively prolonged but transient postischemic contractile dysfunction caused by the generation of oxygen-derived free radicals on reperfusion and by a loss of sensitivity of contractile filaments to calcium; and irreversible myocyte cell death, leading to ventricular remodeling and contractile dysfunction.

Coronary Artery Bypass Grafting

No randomized clinical trials have evaluated the outcomes of revascularization in patients with advanced ischemic cardiomyopathy. As discussed in Chapter 54, the three major randomized clinical trials that have compared coronary artery bypass grafting (CABG) with medical management (the Veterans Administration Cooperative Study, the European Coronary Surgery Study, and the Coronary Artery Surgery Study) have all excluded patients with heart failure or severe LV dysfunction.[1] In the absence of clinical trial data, registries and data bases have been used to guide decision-making for patients with ischemic cardiomyopathy. For example, a report from the Duke database compared CABG with medical therapy over a 25-year period. Medical therapy was used in 1052 patients and CABG in 339.[2] Unadjusted and adjusted survival (Cox proportional hazards model) strongly favored CABG after 30 days and at 10 years. This analysis included all groups by extent of coronary artery disease (Fig. 27-1), as well as by different subgroups (Fig. 27-2). Adjusted overall survival at 1, 5, and 10 years was 83 versus 74 percent, 61 versus 37 percent, and 42 versus 13 percent for CABG versus medical therapy, respectively ($P < 0.0001$).

Because the results of registries and data bases have generally favored coronary artery revascularization over medical therapy, no formal prospective randomize clinical trials of this therapy were initiated until 2002, when the National Institutes for Health (NIH)-funded STICH (Surgical Treatment for Ischemic Heart Failure) trial was initiated. The ongoing STICH trial is a prospective randomized study that will include 2800 patients randomized from 100 centers. Patients with LV dysfunction and coronary artery disease amenable

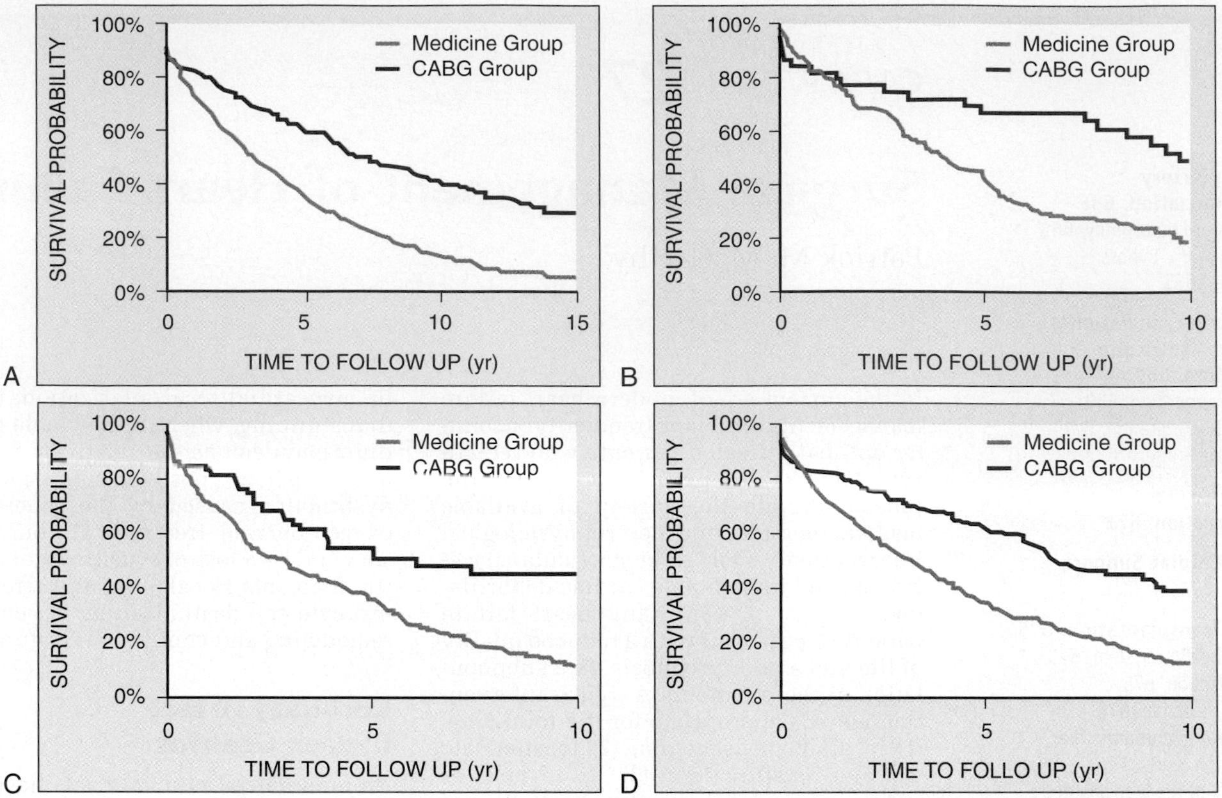

FIGURE 27–1 Coronary artery revascularization versus medical therapy in patients with heart failure. **A,** Overall cohort. **B,** One-vessel disease. **C,** Two-vessel disease. **D,** Three-vessel disease. CABG = coronary artery bypass grafting. *(Modified from O'Connor CM, Velazquez EJ, Gardner LH, et al: Comparison of coronary artery bypass grafting versus medical therapy on long-term outcome in patients with ischemic cardiomyopathy: A 25-year experience from the Duke Cardiovascular Disease Databank. Am J Cardiol 90:101, 2002.)*

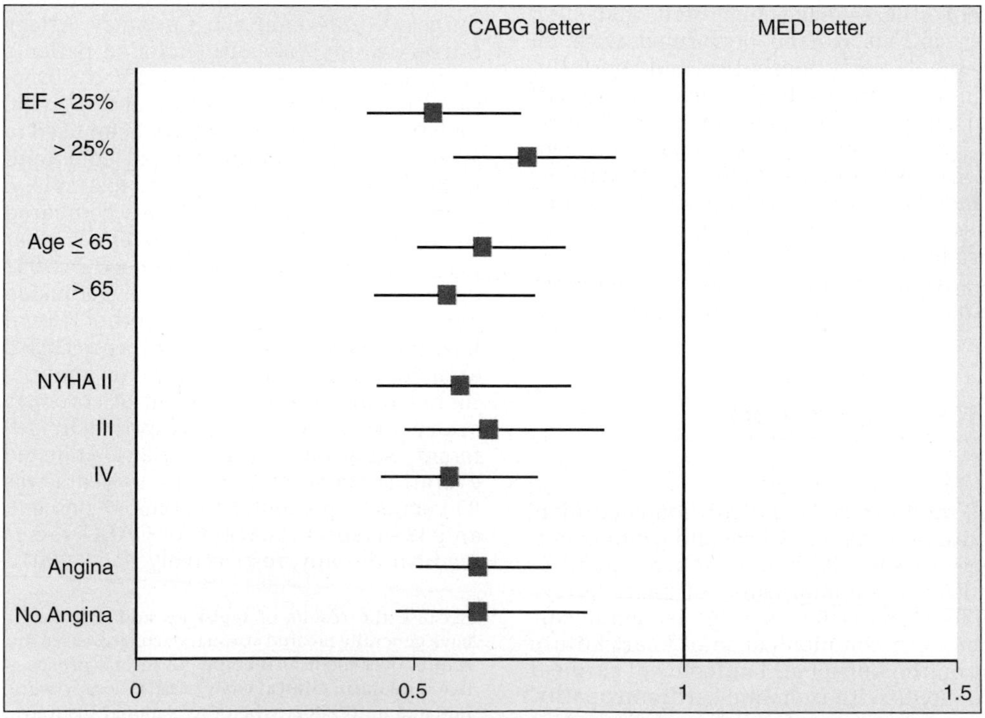

FIGURE 27–2 Subgroup analysis of coronary artery revascularization versus medical therapy in patients with heart failure. Hazard ratios (95 percent confidence interval) for mortality for a number of baseline characteristics all favored CABG. CABG = coronary artery bypass grafting; EF = ejection fraction; MED = medical therapy; NYHA = New York Heart Association. *(Modified from O'Connor CM, Velazquez EJ, Gardner LH, et al: Comparison of coronary artery bypass grafting versus medical therapy on long-term outcome in patients with ischemic cardiomyopathy: A 25-year experience from the Duke Cardiovascular Disease Databank. Am J Cardiol 90:101, 2002.)*

to CABG will be randomized to combinations of three different treatment strategies—CABG, surgical ventricular reconstruction (SVR), and intensive medical therapy. The trial is powered to address two primary hypotheses: (1) CABG combined with medical therapy improves long-term survival when compared with medical therapy alone; and (2) SVR provides an additional long-term survival benefit when combined with CABG and medical therapy alone (Fig. 27-3). Secondary endpoints of the trial include cardiac morbidity and mortality, economic impact of the various treatments, patient quality of life, and usefulness of biochemical and imaging modalities for predicting optimal treatment strategy. Patients will be included in the trial on the basis of an LVEF less than 35 percent and coronary anatomy that is suitable for revascularization.[3]

Patient Selection for Coronary Artery Revascularization

Several clinical factors play a major role in the decision-making process with respect to selecting suitable heart failure patients to undergo coronary artery revascularization, including the presence of angina, the severity of heart failure symptoms, LV dimensions, and the

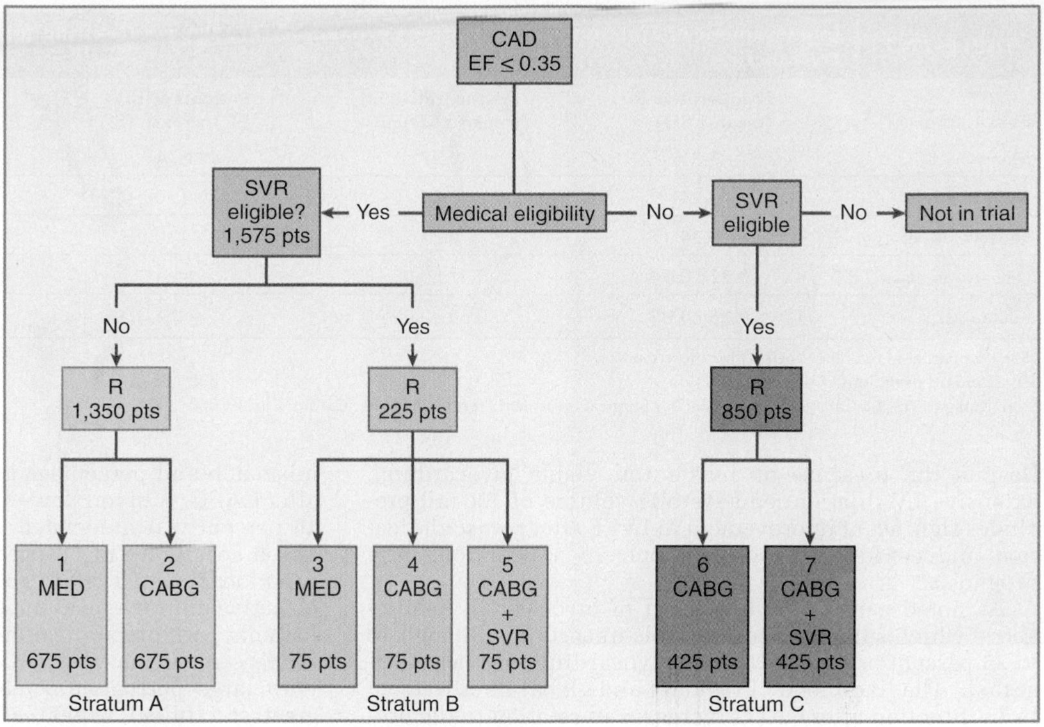

FIGURE 27–3 Treatment strata in the STICH trial. CABG = coronary artery bypass grafting; MED = medical therapy; R = randomized; SVR = surgical ventricular restoration.

degree of hemodynamic compromise. Other major technical issues to be considered are the adequacy of target vessels for revascularization and the extent of jeopardized but still viable myocardium (see Chap. 54). Current studies have suggested that for a significant improvement in heart failure symptoms and LV function to occur after coronary artery revascularization, at least 20 to 25 percent of the myocardium should be viable.[1,4] Most of the earlier studies with coronary artery revascularization included patients whose main symptom was predominantly angina rather than heart failure. However, the absence of angina does not necessarily preclude consideration for surgical revascularization, insofar as individual reports have shown that heart failure patients with large areas of reversible ischemia and no history of angina may demonstrate functional recovery with surgical revascularization. It is therefore critically important to identify patients who have ischemic or hibernating myocardium and adequate target vessels. The noninvasive evaluation of myocardial viability is discussed in Chapter 54.

Risks of Coronary Artery Bypass Grafting

The predicted mortality for an otherwise healthy 70-year-old man with normal LV function undergoing primary CABG in the United States in 2006 was estimated as 0.9 percent according to the Society of Thoracic Surgeons (STS) data base (http://www.sts.org/sections/stsnationaldatabase). The STS-predicted mortality for a 70-year-old patient with no comorbidities but with a 20 percent LVEF was 1.6 percent. However, more recent reports on patients with severe LV dysfunction have indicated that patients undergoing coronary artery bypass grafting with LV systolic dysfunction are at increased risk for perioperative mortality.[5-7] Compared with patients with an LVEF of 40 percent or greater, patients whose LVEFs were between 20 and 39 percent or below 20 percent had 1.5- and 3.4-fold increased perioperative mortality, respectively.[1] Furthermore, mortality rates increase substantially when the LVEF is below 20 percent or when the heart failure is severe (New York Heart Association [NYHA] Class IV). Studies have indicated that for patients with clinical heart failure, perioperative mortality rates will range from approximately 2.6 to 8.7 percent,[5-7] to more than 30 percent in patients older than 70 with severe heart failure and several comorbid conditions.[1] In the CABG Patch trial, patients without angina had a perioperative mortality of 1.3 percent for no angina or no heart failure, 4.8 percent for no angina or NYHA Class I or II heart failure, and 7.4 percent for no angina or NYHA Class III or IV heart failure.[8] Importantly, viability imaging was not used to stratify these outcomes. The impact of heart failure on outcome after CABG was also noted in the SHOCK (Should We Emergently Revascularize Occluded Coronaries for Cardiogenic Shock?) trial.[9] In this randomized trial of revascularization versus medical therapy for cardiogenic shock after myocardial infarction, patients who had undergone CABG had 30-day and 1-year mortality of 42 and 56 percent, respectively. Although this outcome is worse than the results of the CABG Patch trial in patients with compensated heart failure, patients in the medical therapy study arm of the SHOCK trial had worse 30-day and 1-year mortality (56 and 75 percent, respectively) when compared with surgery.[9] Additional determinants of mortality risk include advanced age, female gender, comorbid conditions (e.g., diabetes, clinical cerebrovascular disease, renal dysfunction, significant chronic lung disease), prior coronary bypass surgery, and need for emergent bypass surgery or concomitant valve surgery.[1] Small single center studies have suggested that the surgical risk may be decreased with preoperative balloon pump support or the use of off-pump CABG, but these have not yet been confirmed.

Benefits of Coronary Artery Bypass Grafting

The beneficial effect of revascularization should, theoretically, result from improving blood flow to hypoperfused but viable myocardium, with a subsequent improvement in LV function and clinical outcomes Alleviating ischemia may also lessen the tendency toward proarrhythmias, thereby reducing the incidence of sudden cardiac death. Accordingly, coronary artery revascularization has the potential to improve symptoms of heart failure as well as survival. However, the benefits of coronary artery revascularization need to be balanced against the risks of surgery, which can be substantial in high risk patients, as noted earlier.

IMPROVEMENT IN LV FUNCTION. As shown in Table 27-1, most studies to date have shown that in patients with viable myocardium, an average improvement in LVEF of 8 to 10 percent is likely to occur following coronary artery revascularization.[10] Moreover, these changes are associated with clinical improvement and favorable long-term outcomes.[4] In contrast, when little or no myocardium is viable, LV volumes can continue to increase after coronary artery bypass surgery because of progressive LV remodeling.

TABLE 27–1 Improvement in Ejection Fraction After Coronary Artery Bypass Grafting for Severe Left Ventricular Dysfunction

First Author*	Preoperative EF (mean ± SD)	Postoperative EF (mean ± SD)	Patients with EF Increase (%)	Interval to Postoperative EF	P
Milano et al	0.21	0.27	N/A	N/A	<0.005
Shapira et al	0.24	0.36	73% (>0.07)	5.8 mo	<0.0001
Elefteraides et al	0.24	0.34	70% (≥0.05)	4.6 mo	<0.0001
DeCarlo et al	0.27±0.04	0.38±0.08	N/A	N/A	<0.001
Luciani et al	0.28±0.05	0.38±0.09	N/A	N/A	<0.001

*See Kumpati et al reference (below) for these studies.
SD=standard deviation; EF=ejection fraction.
From Kumpati GS, McCarthy PM, Hoercher KJ: Surgical treatments for heart failure. Cardiol Clin 19:669, 2001.

Despite the presence of substantial viable myocardium, extensive LV dilation (end-systolic volume of 130 ml) precludes significant improvement in LVEF after revascularization and could predispose patients to a poor long-term prognosis.[4]

As noted earlier, the threshold of myocardial viability above which surgery is indicated is uncertain, although 20 to 25 percent or more of the LV myocardium has been suggested.[4] The likelihood of regional and global improvement in LV function after CABG increases in relation to the proportion of dysfunctional but viable myocardium. Thallium-201 single-photon emission computed tomography (SPECT) imaging is a commonly used method for predicting improvement in systolic function following revascularization (see Chap. 16). When patients with ischemic cardiomyopathy were examined by dobutamine stress echocardiography (see Chap. 14) and thallium-201 SPECT before and 3 months after revascularization, the global LVEF at rest rose from 35 to 40 percent after operation.[1] In another study, positron emission tomography (PET) was performed in 12 patients who had irreversible defects by thallium-201 imaging. However, ischemic but viable myocardium was identified by PET in 10 patients, all of whom had successful revascularization, as evidenced by a significant improvement in LVEF from 26 to 36 percent. A study of 20 patients with irreversible thallium defects, 18 of whom had evidence of viability on PET imaging, demonstrated that the LVEF improved from 23 percent before surgery to 39 percent at 1 year of follow-up.[1] Pagano and colleagues found a highly significant correlation ($r = 0.65$; $P = 0.0001$) between the number of viable segments and the changes in LVEF.[11] They noted a significant increase in LVEF from 23 to 32 percent postrevascularization. Most of the gain in function occurred in the group of patients who had at least eight viable segments prior to surgery. These observations suggest that PET can be used to identify patients who may benefit from surgical revascularization, even when myocardial perfusion defects are irreversible by thallium imaging. Thus, recovery of LV function following revascularization is related to the degree of reversible myocardial ischemia, the severity of the LV dysfunction, LV chamber dimensions, and LV geometry. It should be noted that there may be continuing improvements in LVEF as late as 6 to 12 months after surgery.[1]

FUNCTIONAL IMPROVEMENT. Several studies have reported marked improvement in heart failure symptoms following revascularization.[11] However, these results may have been biased by the placebo effect of surgical intervention. In one study, 15 of 21 patients in NYHA Class III or IV heart failure before revascularization had improved to NYHA Class I or II at the end of the 13-month follow-up period.[1] Di Carli and colleagues have studied 36 patients with LVEF of 28 percent using PET imaging.[12] They found a significant correlation between the total extent of a PET mismatch and percentage improvement in functional class after CABG. A blood flow–metabolism mismatch more than 18 percent was associated with a sensitivity of 76 percent and a specificity of 78 percent for predicting a change in functional status after revascularization. A substantial objective improvement in physical activity was noted in patients with presurgical mismatches that occupied at least 20 percent of the ventricular myocardium, Thus, patients with large perfusion-metabolism mismatch exhibited the greatest clinical benefit after revascularization. Another study has shown a similar significant improvement in functional capacity following revascularization, as reflected by a 34 percent increase in exercise capacity from 5.6 to 7.5 METs (metabolic equivalents) in the group of patients with revascularization PET mismatch.[1]

SURVIVAL BENEFIT. A review of the literature for coronary artery disease patients with reduced EF (less than 25 percent) treated with CABG is illustrated in Table 27-2. As shown, late mortality ranged from 10 percent at 1 year to 50 percent at 5 years. Seven studies were identified in which patients were treated medically (Table 27-3), six of which were compared with the surgically treated patients. In all six studies, the surgical group demonstrated improved late survival, with a mortality reduction of 30 to 50 percent. However, it is not clear whether surgery benefits patients whose predominant symptom is heart failure rather than angina. In a meta-analysis of 24 studies involving a total of 3088 patients with ischemic cardiomyopathy, revascularization decreased the risk of death by 79.6 percent in patients with evidence of viable myocardial tissue, yielding an annual mortality of 3.2 percent, compared with 16.0 percent for patients who did not undergo revascularization (Fig. 27-4).[13] In this analysis the type of viability study (thallium perfusion imaging, PET, or dobutamine echocardiography) did not affect the clinical outcomes. Furthermore, the results were more impressive the worse the ventricular function. Patients without evidence of viability showed no benefit with revascularization. However, the reports that comprised this meta-analysis all had individual flaws, and none of the trials analyzed was an ideal randomized clinical trial.

In summary, although coronary artery bypass grafting has been shown to improve symptoms and survival in patients with modestly reduced ejection fraction and angina, patients with clinical heart failure or markedly depressed ventricular function have generally been excluded from these studies (see Chaps. 25 and 54).[14] For patients who present with heart failure secondary to coronary artery disease (i.e., ischemic cardiomyopathy), a coronary angiogram is indicated (see Chap. 23), and viability studies are appropriate for those patients with severe disease. If these tests are positive, the weight of currently available clinical evidence suggests that CABG may improve survival and

TABLE 27–2 Literature Review of Coronary Artery Disease Patients with Severely Reduced Ejection Fraction Treated with Coronary Artery Bypass Grafting

First Author*	Patients (*N*)	Years of Study	Ejection Fraction	Perioperative Mortality (%)	Late Mortality (%)
Vlietstra	10	1966-1972	<0.25	—	60 (2 yr)
Manley	183	1968-1971	Mean, 0.22	16.0	43 (5 yr)
Yatteau	24	1968-1972	<0.25	42	50 (2 yr)
Oldham	11	1969-1972	≤0.25	55	—
Zubiate	140	1969-1975	<0.20	22	41.6 (6 yr)
Faulkner	46	1969-1975	Mean, 0.21	4.0	17 (2 yr)
Mitchel	9	—	<0.20	0.0	11 (1 yr)
Fox	7	1971-1974	<0.20	0.0	14
Jones	41	1973-1977	<0.20	2.5	10 (1 yr)
Alderman	82	1975-1979	≤0.25	8.0	37 (5 yr)
Mochtar	62	1975-1983	Mean, 0.25	4.8	30 (5 yr)
Zubiate	93	1976-1981	<0.20	5.0	50 (5 yr)
Hochberg	51	1976-1982	0.20-0.24	12.0	42 (3 yr)
Hochberg	41	1976-1982	<0.20	37.0	85 (3 yr)
Sanchez	23	1982-1989	Mean, 0.28	9.0	24 (2 yr)
Kron	39	1983-1988	<0.20	2.6	17 (3 yr)
Blakeman	20	1984-1988	Mean, 0.18	15.0	30 (1 yr)
Wong	22	1986-1989	Mean, 0.25	9.0	23 (3 yr)
Christakis	487	1982-1990	<0.20	9.8	—
Hammermeister	251	1987-1990	<0.20	9.2	—
Louie	22	1984-1990	Mean, 0.23	13.6	28 (3 yr)
Milano	118	1981-1991	Mean, 0.21	11.0	42 (5 yr)
Elefteriades	83	1986-1992	Mean, 0.25	8.4	20 (3 yr)
Hausmann	265	1986-1992	Mean, 0.24	7.6	13 (3 yr)
Langenburg	6	1983-1993	≦0.25	8.3	—
Mickleborough	79	1982-1993	<0.20	3.8	32 (5 yr)
Cosgrove	678	1970-1979	<0.20	3.2	—
Cosgrove	610	1980-1982	<0.20	1.6	—

*See Milano et al and Starling et al references (below) for these studies.

From Milano CA, White WD, Smith LR, et al: Coronary artery bypass in patients with severely depressed ventricular function. Ann Thorac Surg 56:487, 1993; and Starling RC, McCarthy PM, Yamini MH: Surgical treatment of chronic congestive heart failure. *In* Mann DL (ed): Heart Failure: A Companion to Braunwald's Heart Disease. WB Saunders, Philadelphia, 2003.

quality of life over medical therapy alone. Current American College of Cardiology/American Heart Association (ACC/AHA) guidelines for CABG in patients with poor LV function attributed a Class I recommendation for those with left main or equivalent disease, Class IIa for those with viable noncontracting muscle, and Class III (not useful, possibly harmful) for those without evidence of ischemia or viability.[15] As noted earlier, the results of the ongoing NIH sponsored STICH trial (see Fig. 27-3) should provide more definitive information with respect to the role of CABG in patients with heart failure.

VALVE SURGERY IN PATIENTS WITH LEFT VENTRICULAR DYSFUNCTION

As discussed in Chapter 62, the surgical treatment of valvular heart disease that leads to LV dysfunction and/or heart failure is now widely accepted. However, patients who have valvular dysfunction *secondary* to a primary cardiomyopathy pose a much more difficult management problem. The following section will focus on the impact and outcome of valve repair or replacement for patients with a dilated cardiomyopathy and secondary mitral and/or regurgitation. The indications for valve replacement in ischemic mitral regurgitation are discussed in Chapter 62.

Mitral Regurgitation

When the failing heart dilates, the papillary muscles are displaced away from the mitral valve annulus, leading to decreased coaptation of the mitral leaflets. This decreased coaptation leads to secondary mitral regurgitation (MR), typically with a central jet of MR recognized on echocardiography (Fig. 27-5). In addition, there is mitral annular dilation, further compounding the problem of mitral valve

TABLE 27–3 Literature Review of Coronary Artery Disease Patients with Severely Reduced Ejection Fraction Treated with Medical Therapy Alone

First Author*	Patients (*N*)	Years of Study	Ejection Fraction	1-Yr Mortality (%)	Late Mortality (%)
Vlietstra	21	1966-1972	<0.25	—	67 (2 yr)
Manley	63	1968-1971	Mean, 0.17	47	90 (6 yr)
Yatteau	42	1968-1972	<0.25	31	38 (2 yr)
Faulkner	70	1968-1975	Mean, 0.20	10	53 (2 yr)
Harris	152	1969-1978	<0.25	30	55 (5 yr)
Zubiate	59	1970-1981	<0.20	50	96 (5 yr)
Alderman	172	1975-1979	<0.25	24	57 (5 yr)

*See Milano et al (below) for actual references.

From Milano CA, White WD, Smith LR, et al: Coronary artery bypass in patients with severely depressed ventricular function. Ann Thorac Surg 56:487, 1993.

leaflet coaptation. Moreover, for patients with ischemic MR, infarction of a papillary muscle with subsequent elongation of the papillary muscle may add another element and a localized eccentric MR jet (see Chap. 62). This secondary (functional) MR leads to a sustained volume overload on the ventricle, which can contribute to worsening LV remodeling and worsening heart failure (see Chap. 22). In a cohort of patients with an LVEF of 35 percent studied at the University of Michigan, 48.6 percent of the patients had 3 to 4+ MR, whereas 36 percent had 3 to 4+ tricuspid regurgitation (TR). In this study, the presence of both MR and TR was associated with decreased survival.[16] Clinically, patients may have a stable course of heart failure for years with only 1 to 2+ MR, and then develop worsening heart failure, with a concomitant worsening of their MR. However, it is not always clear whether the cardiomyopathy caused worsening symptoms and MR, or whether the progression of MR was responsible for the increased symptoms.

The indications for and timing of valve surgery for patients with secondary mitral and/or tricuspid regurgitation are not clear and are currently evolving.[17] The use of a flexible undersized annuloplasty ring was introduced by Bolling and colleagues in 1995 to restore mitral valve competency, to reduce the chronic LV volume overload, and to promote reverse remodeling.[4] For patients with dilated cardiomyopathy and secondary MR, the University of Michigan and other centers have reported low early operative mortality, with good 3- and 5-year survival rates.[18-20] The operation is associated with a remarkable decrease in the severity of symptoms and improvement in quality of life in most cases. Data from the multicenter prospective randomized Acorn trial in heart failure patients with a reduced LVEF (24 ± 9 percent) have demonstrated that the operative mortality was low, 1.6 percent in a group of patients with advanced heart failure.[21] As shown in Figure 27-6, there were favorable changes in LV volumes, LVEF, and quality of life, and NYHA class in the Acorn trial.[21] Freedom from recurrence of MR seems to be related to some extent to the surgical technique used. In particular, the use of completely rigid and small rings appears to have improved the durability of the repair. Moreover, prosthetic rings specifically designed to decrease the septolateral dimension of the mitral annulus have been developed.[22] Preliminary data have suggested that these rings are effective in the elimination of functional MR and favor reverse remodeling, with restoration of an elliptical LV shape and decrease of the sphericity index.[4,22] The current 2006 ACC/AHA guidelines

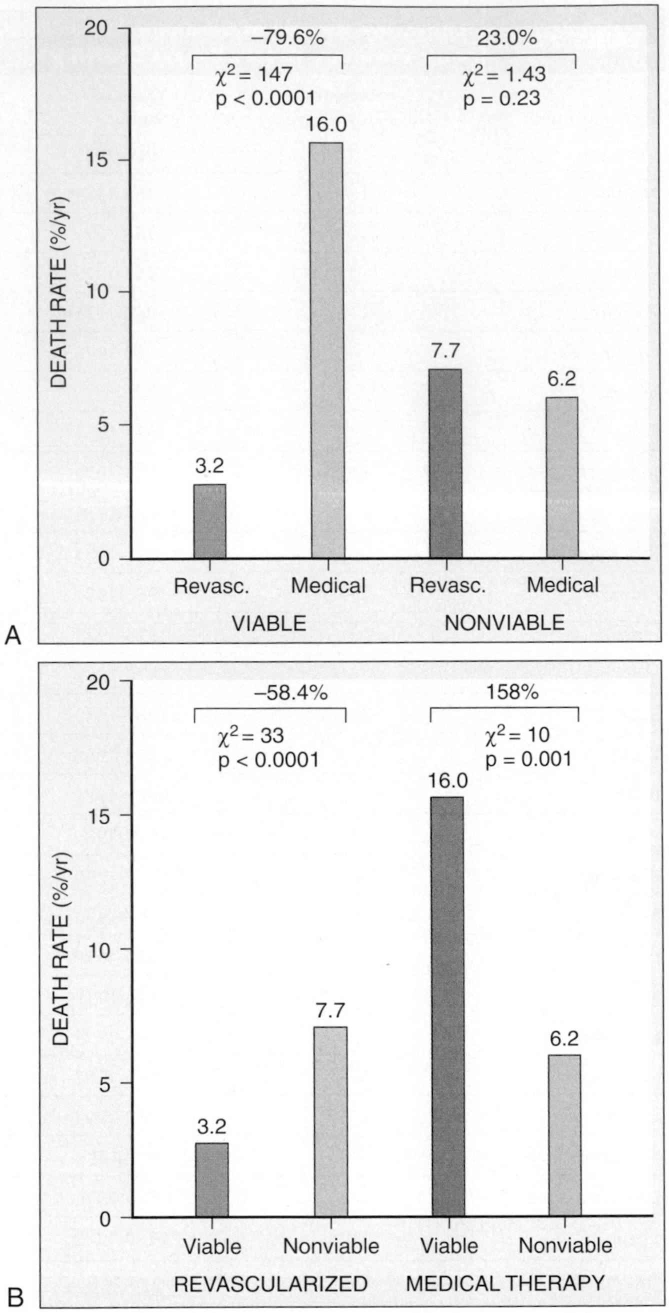

FIGURE 27–4 Meta-analysis of clinical outcomes in patients with and without viable myocardial tissue. **A,** Death rates for patients with and without myocardial viability treated by revascularization or medical therapy. There was a 79.6 percent reduction in mortality for patients with myocardial viability treated by revascularization ($P < 0.0001$). In patients without myocardial viability, there was no significant difference in mortality with revascularization versus medical therapy. **B,** Same data as in **A.** Comparisons are based on treatment strategy in patients with and without myocardial viability. Annual mortality was lower in revascularized patients when viability was present versus absent (3.2 versus 7.7 percent; $P < 0.0001$). Annual mortality was significantly higher in medically treated patients when viability was present versus absent (16 versus 6.2 percent; $P = 0.001$). Revasc. = revascularization. *(From Allman KC, Shaw LJ, Hachamovitch R, et al: Myocardial viability testing and impact of revascularization on prognosis in patients with coronary artery disease and LV dysfunction: A meta-analysis. J Am Coll Cardiol 39:1151, 2002.)*

suggest that mitral valve repair may be considered in this group of patients (Class IIb indication). Patients with structural (myxomatous or rheumatic) valve disease with primary MR and secondary LV dysfunction are generally candidates for valve surgery as well (Class IIa recommendation).[17]

Are there survival benefits for mitral valve surgery in heart failure patients? For patients undergoing coronary artery bypass for ischemic cardiomyopathy, it is difficult to demonstrate improved survival for those patients who have also undergone mitral valve surgery. There have been some studies indicating improved survival versus those undergoing CABG alone.[23,24] However, most series have indicated late survival similar to that of patients undergoing CABG alone.[25-27] A prospective randomized trial has not been done and is clearly needed. Outcomes other than survival have not been well studied in this patient population. For patients with dilated (i.e., nonischemic) cardiomyopathy who undergo mitral valve surgery, the prospective randomized Acorn trial has shown that the patients have a better functional class, ventricular volumes and function, and improved quality of life (see Fig. 27-6)[21]; however, this study was not powered to demonstrate a mortality benefit. The one retrospective study that was designed to assess the effects of mitral valve annuloplasty on mortality in patients with MR and LV systolic dysfunction has shown that mitral valve annuloplasty does not confer a demonstrable mortality benefit.[28] However, this analysis included patients who had undergone a mitral valve annuloplasty using a flexible annuloplasty ring, which subsequent studies have shown is plagued by recurrent MR. Thus, the choice of annuloplasty ring used in this retrospective analysis may have reduced the effectiveness of the mitral valve repair strategy (Steve Bolling, MD, personal communication, December 2006). Again, prospective randomized trials have not been done in this area and are clearly needed. The impact on late outcome of inadequate repair strategies has led to the development and successful launch of rings specifically designed for patients with functional MR, including those with ischemic MR.[22,29]

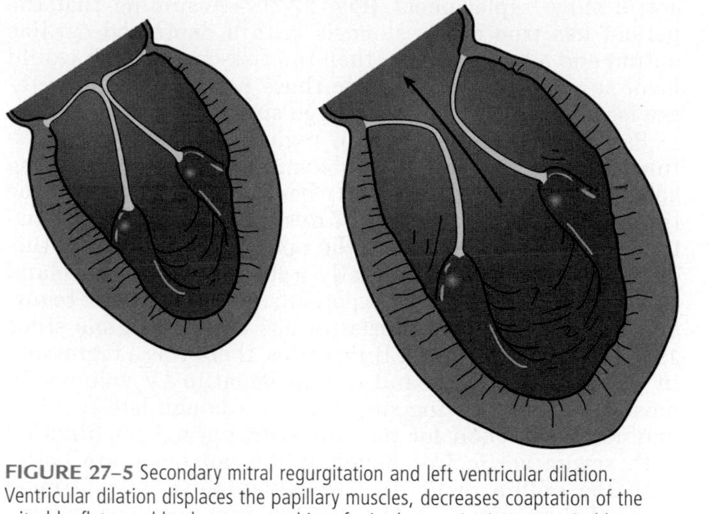

FIGURE 27–5 Secondary mitral regurgitation and left ventricular dilation. Ventricular dilation displaces the papillary muscles, decreases coaptation of the mitral leaflets, and leads to a central jet of mitral regurgitation recognizable on echocardiography. *(From Starling RC, McCarthy PM, Yamini MH: Surgical treatment of chronic congestive heart failure.* In *Mann DL [ed]: Heart Failure: A Companion to Braunwald's Heart Disease. Philadelphia, WB Saunders, p 725.)*

Tricuspid Regurgitation

Surgery for tricuspid valve disease has been relatively ignored. The Carpentier ring, designed specifically for tricuspid valve repair, was released over 30 years ago; however, most tricuspid valve repairs are still either suture-based or done with rings originally released for mitral valve repair. In a series of patients operated on at the Cleveland Clinic from 1990 to 1999, residual tricuspid regurgitation occurred in 14 percent of patients early after operation for all types

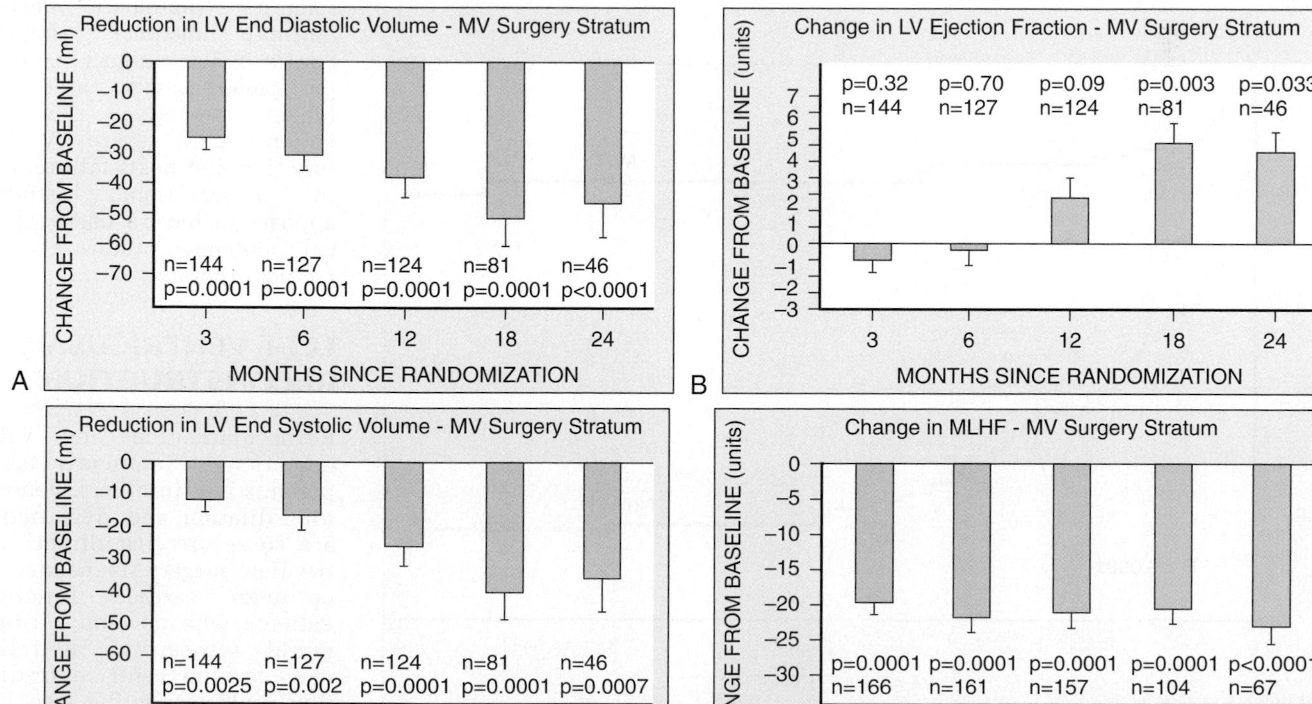

FIGURE 27–6 Clinical outcomes in mitral valve (MV) surgery treatment arm in the Acorn trial. **A,** Change in left ventricular (LV) end-diastolic volume. **B,** Change in LV end-systolic volume. **C,** Change in left ventricular ejection fraction (LVEF). **D,** Change in Minnesota living with heart failure (MLHF) score. *(From Acker MA, Bolling S, Shemin R, et al: Mitral valve surgery in heart failure: Insights from the Acorn clinical trial. J Thorac Cardiovasc Surg 132:568, 2006.)*

of annuloplasty rings, which is a much higher prevalence than after mitral valve repair. Late worsening (beyond 6 months) of tricuspid regurgitation was associated not only with patient comorbidities but also with avoidable causes, such as trans-tricuspid pacing leads and the type of annuloplasty ring used.[30] The indications for and timing of valve surgery for patients with secondary tricuspid regurgitation in heart failure are not clear and are currently evolving.[17] The current 2006 ACC/AHA guidelines suggest that tricuspid repair is beneficial for severe tricuspid regurgitation in patients undergoing mitral valve surgery for MR (Class I indication), and that tricuspid replacement or annuloplasty is reasonable for severe tricuspid regurgitation in patients undergoing mitral valve surgery for MR (Class IIa indication). However, there is no specific mention of tricuspid valve surgery for patients with tricuspid valve regurgitation secondary to dilated cardiomyopathy.[17]

Aortic Valve Surgery

The indications for valve replacement in aortic stenosis and regurgitation are discussed in Chapter 62. This section focuses on aortic valve replacement for patients with aortic valve disease and ventricular dysfunction or heart failure. Patients with aortic stenosis sometimes develop ventricular dysfunction, with a low gradient across the aortic valve (see Chap. 62).[31,32] Aortic valve replacement is warranted in these patients if the LV dysfunction is secondary to the aortic stenosis. Accordingly, it is important to differentiate between pseudo-obstruction, with poor ventricular function leading to reduced opening of the aortic valve, and true aortic stenosis, with a primary valve obstruction that leads to LV dysfunction in patients with aortic stenosis and a low cardiac output. Dobutamine echocardiography is useful to make this determination (see Chaps. 14 and 62). Although some of these patients have been deemed inoperable in the past because of the concern of perioperative mortality, it bears emphasis that the prognosis of these patients, if they do not receive an aortic valve replacement, is extremely poor, with 1-, 5-, and 10-year survival rates of 62, 32, and 18 percent, respectively. Moreover, concomitant pharmacotherapy appears to have had no impact on survival in this series.[33] Nevertheless, studies have indicated that this patient population also can undergo surgery safely, with better outcomes than medical therapy alone. In a study from the Cleveland Clinic, the in-hospital mortality for this group of patients was 8 percent, with 1-year survival of 82 versus 41 percent for those treated with medical therapy alone and 4-year survival of 78 versus 15 percent for those treated with aortic valve replacement (Fig. 27-7).[32] Assuming that the patient has true aortic stenosis with a depressed cardiac output and a low gradient, then the risk-benefit ratio would favor surgical interventions in those patients who are otherwise healthy enough to undergo surgery.[31,32,34]

Patients with severe aortic regurgitation with LV dysfunction pose a different problem. Some patients develop advanced heart failure and have been considered for cardiac transplantation because the LV dysfunction was considered to be irreversible. Although the operative mortality in this group has been high historically, a study from the Cleveland Clinic has indicated that for patients with pure aortic regurgitation, the operative mortality has been negligible since 1985.[35] In the Cleveland Clinic series, there was a regression in LV mass regression and improvement in LV volumes in most patients following surgery.[23,31] Although late survival may not be as good for patients with normal LV function with severe aortic insufficiency, the outcomes are better than the option of cardiac transplantation or continued medical therapy.[35] The ACC/AHA guidelines now endorse surgery in this group (Class I recommendation).[17]

In summary, in experienced centers, mitral valve repair for patients with LV dysfunction and MR may be appropriate in those undergoing CABG, as well as for selected patients with idiopathic dilated cardiomyopathy who remain symptomatic despite optimal medical therapy. Aortic valve surgery can be performed safely, albeit at higher operative risk, in patients with severe LV dysfunction and heart failure, and in observational studies appears to have a better clinical outcome than current medical therapy.

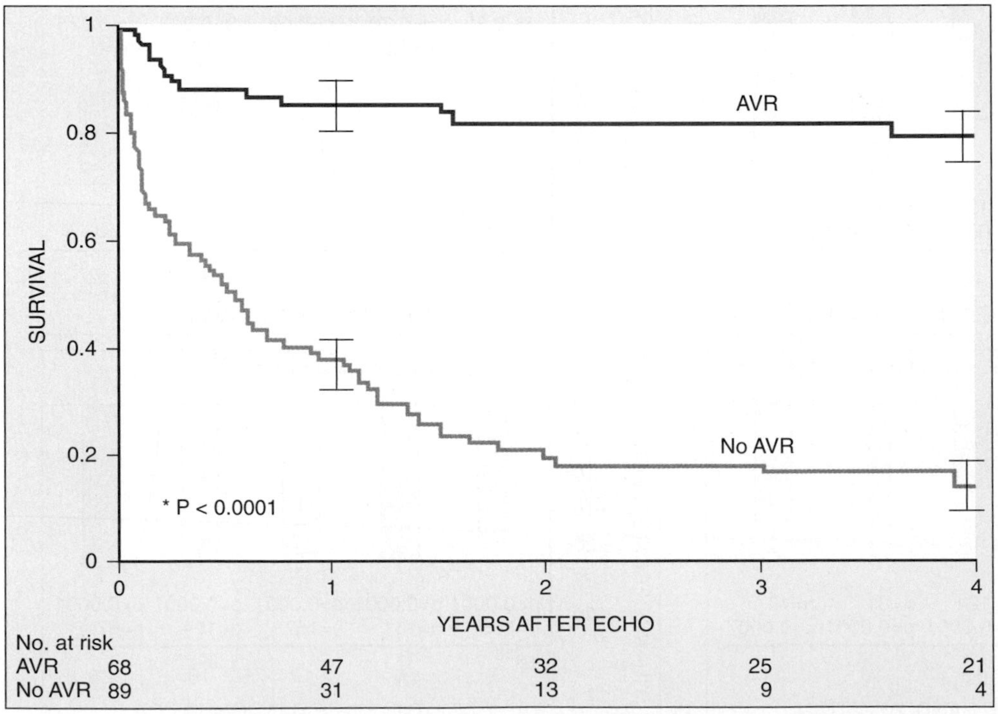

FIGURE 27–7 Kaplan-Meier survival analysis of patients with low gradient aortic stenosis treated with aortic valve replacement (AVR) versus medical therapy (No AVR)($P < 0.0001$). *(From Pereira JJ, Lauer MS, Bashir M, et al: Survival after aortic valve replacement for severe aortic stenosis with low transvalvular gradients and severe LV dysfunction. J Am Coll Cardiol 39:1356, 2002.)*

LEFT VENTRICULAR RECONSTRUCTION

Revascularization and valve operations improve many patients but, in others, ventricular dilation and dysfunction are so severe that direct ventricular surgery is needed to optimize cardiac function. Patients who develop a transmural myocardial infarction may develop ventricular dilation and remodeling (see Fig. 51-6) that leads to changes in increased LV wall stress and LV dysfunction (see Table 22-5).[36] A host of adverse events are initiated, including increased myocardial oxygen consumption secondary to increased wall stress, increased neurohormone and cytokine levels, afterload mismatch, and subendocardial hypoperfusion. In essence, all ventricular reconstruction operations serve to remove or exclude the infarcted segment and work, thereby, to decrease LV volumes, improve LV sphericity, reduce LV wall stress, decrease neurohormonal activation, and improve myocardial oxygen consumption.[37] Concomitant CABG is often necessary and, if more than moderate MR is present, this should also be corrected. This type of operation goes by various names, most commonly termed the *Dor procedure* (after Vincent Dor), in which the aneurysm or akinetic segment is reconstructed, typically with a patch (endoventricular patch plasty), surgical ventricular restoration (SVR), or LV reconstruction. The typical embodiment of this operation is to use a double cerclage creation of a neck between the infarcted and normal myocardium, excision or exclusion of the infarcted segment (depending on the thickness of the residual scar or muscle), and reconstruction without a patch (Fig. 27-8; http://cvbook.nmh.org; see Fig. 11-12 there for a video).[37,38] This operation is currently being studied in stratum B and C of the STICH trial (see Fig. 27-3).

At present, standardized criteria for performing LV reconstruction have not yet been established. At the Northwest Memorial Hospital, the operation is performed for patients with ischemic cardiomyopathy, a dilated heart, and a discrete scar that is transmural, or nearly transmural, and involves a localized segment (usually the anterior wall).[37] Sometimes, this operation is performed as a primary indication for surgery in patients with heart failure. At other times, it is one component of a more complex operation for heart failure. At other times, the patient does not yet have symptomatic heart failure but is undergoing a cardiac operation (e.g., CABG and mitral valve surgery), and the aneurysm is treated secondarily. The risk of the procedure is not high in experienced centers.

The RESTORE (Reconstructive Endoventricular Surgery returning Torsion Original Radius Elliptical shape to the left ventricle) trial was a multicenter study investigating various techniques for LV reconstruction in a registry of 1198 post-anterior infarction heart failure patients operated on between 1998 and 2003. Concomitant procedures included coronary artery bypass grafting in 95 percent, mitral valve repair in 22 percent, and mitral valve replacement in 1 percent. The operative mortality in patients who underwent LV reconstruction was 5.3 percent. At 5 years, the overall survival was 68 ± 2.8 percent and

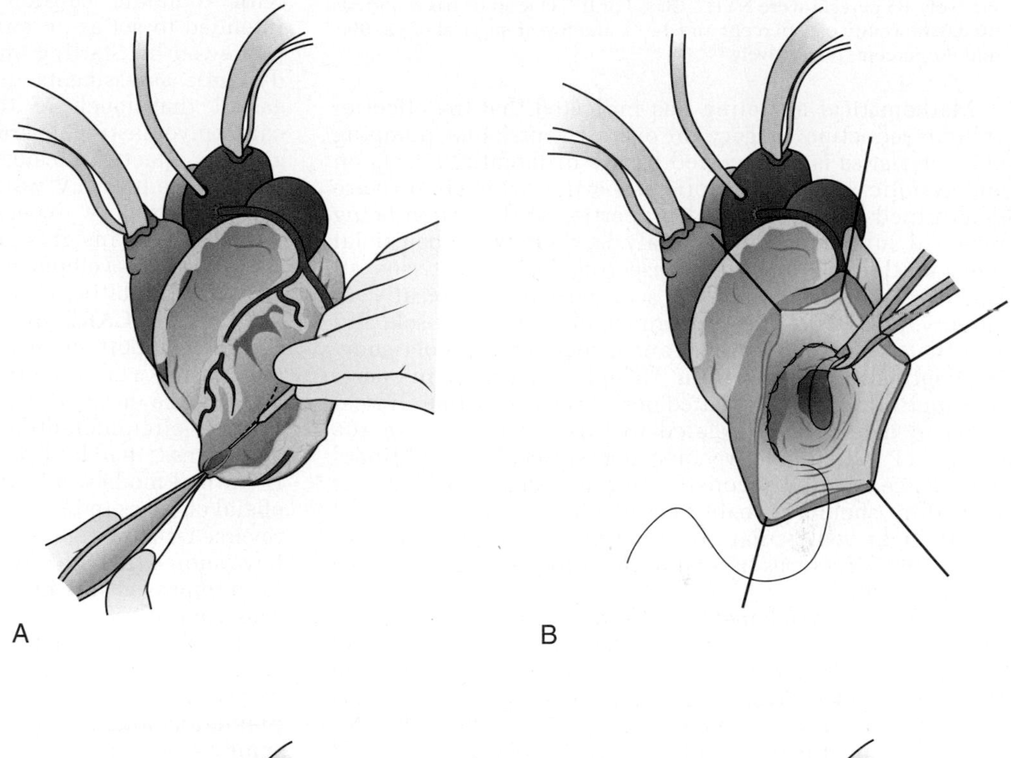

FIGURE 27–8 Left ventricular reconstruction. **A,** The incision for left ventricular reconstruction is typically 2 cm left of the left anterior descending artery (LAD) and extends 3 to 5 cm parallel to the LAD. This is routinely performed with the heart beating and empty **(B)**. Reconstruction begins with a suture placed at the border zone of the infarction, with the suture slightly into the scar. **C,** When the second purse-string suture is tied, the neck of the aneurysm is usually 1 to 3 cm in diameter. Rarely, a patch is used because of heavy calcium on the septum that cannot be removed safely, or concern that the remaining left ventricular cavity will be very small and contribute to diastolic dysfunction. Two strips of felt are positioned on either side of the ventriculotomy. These are sewn in place with horizontal mattress sutures. The mattress sutures should extend all the way down to the prior purse-string sutures. This obliterates the cavity between the aneurysm neck and the left ventricular free wall and minimizes the chances of bleeding. **D,** The ventriculotomy is oversewn superficially in two layers as a final hemostatic layer. *(Modified from McGee EC, Gillinov AM, McCarthy PM: Reverse ventricular remodeling: mechanical options. Curr Opin Cardiol 21:215, 2006.)*

freedom from hospital readmission for heart failure was 78 percent. Logistic regression analysis identified LVEF less than 30 percent, LV end-systolic volume index 80 ml/m^2 or higher, advanced NYHA functional class, and age older than 75 years as risk factors for death. LV reconstruction resulted in a significant decrease in LV end-systolic volume index (from 80.0 ± 51.to 56.0 ± 34.3 ml/m^2) and a significant increase in LVEF (from 29 ± 11.0 to 39 ± 12.3 percent). Preoperatively, 67 percent of patients were in NYHA Class III or IV, whereas postoperatively, 85 percent were NYHA Class I or II.[39] One study has reported 30-day mortality of 1 percent and 1-, 3-, and 5-year survival of 92, 90, and 80 percent, respectively.[40]

Mathematical modeling has indicated that the effect of volume reduction surgery on overall ventricular pumping characteristics is determined by the differential effects on end-systolic and end-diastolic properties, which in turn are determined by the material properties of the region being removed surgically. In this analysis, there was a beneficial effect on this relationship of resecting dyskinetic tissue, an equivocal effect of akinetic scar resection (typically, at surgery, these have the appearance of marbled muscle and scar that are mixed together), and a negative effect of removing contracting myocardium.[41] The heterogeneity in operative mortality and late outcomes observed in the clinical trials to date may be related to this discrepancy in the choice of patients to reconstruct surgically. Additional experience with LV reconstruction has suggested that this procedure should probably be avoided in the presence of severe right ventricular dysfunction and systolic pulmonary artery pressures of 60 mm Hg or higher in the absence of severe MR.[4]

In summary, the benefits of LV reconstruction include a reduction in NYHA functional class, improved LVEF and volumes, and an improvement in neurohormonal activation (Fig. 27-9).[37,40,42,43] Although standardized criteria for performing LV reconstruction have not yet been established for this procedure, the results of the ongoing STICH trial should help determine the role of LV restoration and coronary artery revascularization in patients with heart failure.

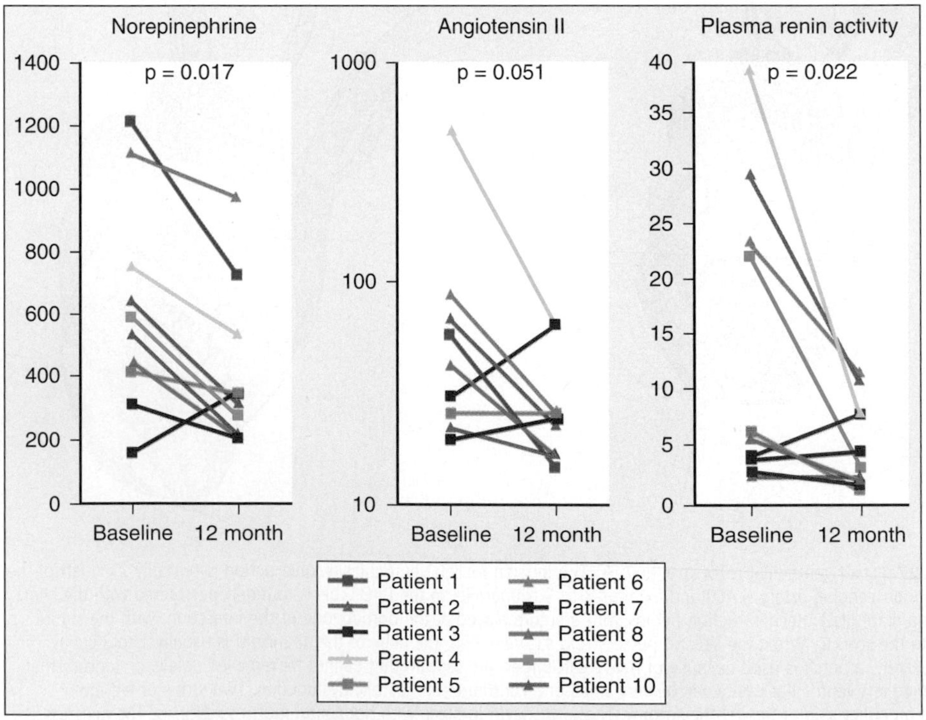

FIGURE 27–9 Improvement in neurohormones after left ventricular reconstruction. Norepinephrine, plasma renin activity, and angiotensin II were measured in 10 patients before and 12 months after left ventricular reconstruction. *(From Schenk S, McCarthy PM, Starling RC, et al: Neurohormonal response to left ventricular reconstruction surgery in ischemic cardiomyopathy. J Thorac Cardiovasc Surg 128:38, 2004.)*

PASSIVE CARDIAC SUPPORT DEVICES

The previous sections have outlined direct surgical reconstruction of coronary arteries, valves, or the LV. This section describes novel surgical approaches to inhibit and/or reverse LV remodeling. The current generation of passive cardiac support devices was developed out of original observations with dynamic cardiomyoplasty, which was originally intended to act as an auxiliary pump for the failing heart (reviewed by Starling and colleagues[1]). Subsequent hemodynamic assessments in animals and humans have suggested that much of the observed benefit of dynamic cardiomyoplasty appeared to be derived from the passive girdling effect of the muscle wrap, which limits ventricular dilation, reduces LV wall stress, and prevents LV remodeling.[1] These early experiences with dynamic cardiomyoplasty and the insights into its biological effects have led to the ongoing development of surgical therapies specifically aimed at inhibiting LV remodeling.

CORCAP CARDIAC SUPPORT DEVICE. The CorCap cardiac support device (CSD; Acorn Cardiovascular, St. Paul, MN) is a fabric mesh device that is surgically implanted around the heart (Fig. 27-10A) The CSD is designed to provide circumferential diastolic support and reduce LV wall stress, thereby leading to reverse cardiac remodeling. In animal models of heart failure, the CSD resulted in beneficial changes in LV structure and function consistent with reverse remodeling (see Fig. 27-10B).[44,45] Early safety studies have shown that the CSD is safe and is associated with long-term improvements in ventricular structure and function.[46] The Acorn trial was a randomized, prospective, multicenter clinical trial involving 300 patients. In this trial, CSD-treated patients had significantly fewer cardiac procedures indicative of worsening heart failure (cardiac transplantation and LV support devices) and experienced an improvement in NYHA class. Treatment with the CSD also led to a decrease in LV end-diastolic and end-systolic volumes, indicative of reverse cardiac remodeling, and an increase in the LV sphericity index (indicative of a more elliptically shaped ventricle). CSD-treated patients also had a significant improvement in quality of life scores. The addition of the CSD device to standard mitral repair or replacement has provided significant additive benefits compared with mitral valve surgery alone and resulted in greater reductions in LV volume and a notable improvement in sphericity index.[21]

PARACOR CARDIAC SUPPORT DEVICE. The Paracor device (Paracor Medical, Sunnyvale, CA) is a nitinol mesh weave that is surgically implanted around the ventricle. The mesh is flexible over a wide range of sizes, which allows it to be collapsed into a delivery system that conforms to the ventricle on deployment. A suction device contained in the delivery system allows for ventricular stabilization and placement of the device through a small minimally invasive thoracotomy. The theoretical and therapeutic concept of the Paracor device is similar to that of the Acorn CSD, but the device has not been as extensively studied as the Acorn CSD. At present, only a small number of patients have been implanted in the

United States and Europe. Planning is underway for a prospective randomized trial.[47]

In summary, the benefits of the passive cardiac restraint include reverse cardiac remodeling (see Fig. 27-10B) and stabilization of disease progression in patients with advanced heart failure, with a significant decrease in the need for major cardiac procedures indicative of worsening heart failure (cardiac transplantation and LV support devices). The device has been most commonly used in patients undergoing mitral valve surgery, but also can be used as stand-alone therapy in medically treated heart failure patients who remain symptomatic despite optimal medical therapy. Future developments will likely entail developing minimally invasive strategies for device implantation, as well as defining the appropriate patient populations for device implantation.

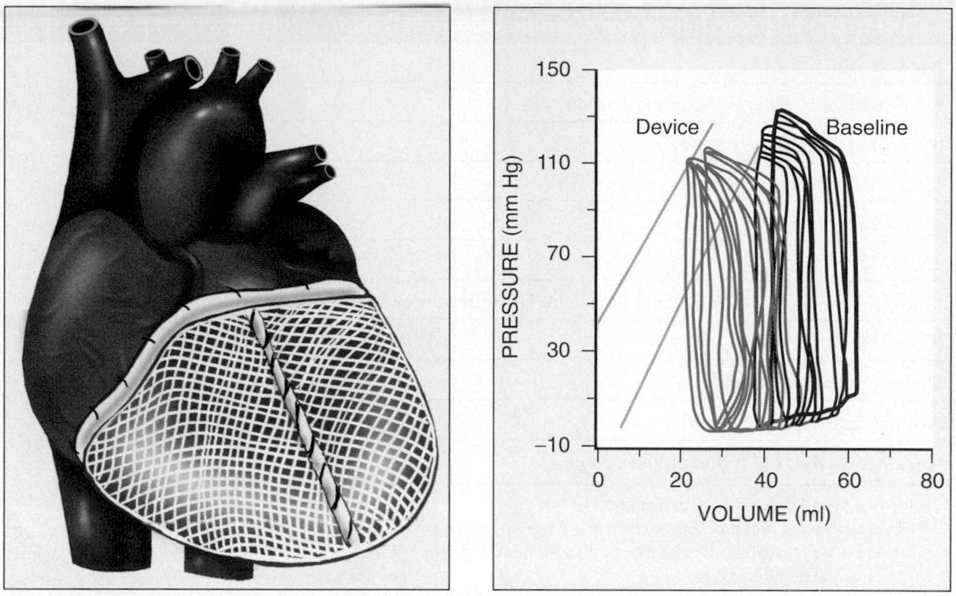

A B

FIGURE 27–10 Passive cardiac support. **A,** CorCap cardiac support device. **B,** Device-induced reduction in chamber size and enhanced systolic performance accompanying this reverse remodeling. The pressure-volume loops generated under different loading states shown in **B** demonstrate end-systolic pressure-volume relationships as well as diastolic chamber properties. These data were obtained in an animal model. *(Modified from Saavedra WF, Tunin RS, Paolocci N, et al: Reverse remodeling and enhanced adrenergic reserve from passive external support in experimental dilated heart failure. J Am Coll Cardiol 39:2069, 2002.)*

CARDIAC TRANSPLANTATION

Cardiac transplantation continues to be the gold standard for the treatment of end-stage cardiac diseases refractory to medical therapy. The clinical success of transplantation has been steadily improving with the refinement of recipient selection, better donor heart management, and the introduction of cyclosporine in the early 1980s, which revolutionized the management of immunosuppression and allograft rejection. This section focuses on the role of cardiac transplantation in the surgical treatment of patients with advanced heart failure.

Donor Allocation System

In the United States, the allocation of donor organs is accomplished under the supervision of the United Network of Organ Sharing (UNOS), a private organization under contract to the federal government. The United States is divided geographically into 11 regions for donor heart allocation. Under UNOS policy, thoracic organs are distributed based on blood type, medical urgency, and time on the waiting list. The physiological limit of approximately 4 hours of ischemic out of body time for hearts precludes a national sharing of donor hearts. Currently, the highest priority is assigned according to the severity of illness.

Each candidate awaiting heart transplantation is assigned a status corresponding to the medical urgency of the candidate who is to receive a heart transplant. For a candidate who is 18 years of age or older at the time of listing, medical urgency is assigned as follows (UNOS policy 3.73). Status 1A refers to patients who are hospitalized and have a left and/or right ventricular assist device(s), a total artificial heart, extracorporeal membrane oxygenation (ECMO), or a balloon pump; this is valid for 30 days unless relisted. Patients have only a one-time window of 30 days after receiving an implantable ventricular assist device unless they develop device-related infection or device failure; a patient with invasive hemodynamic monitoring and two or more inotropic drugs also meets requirement for status 1A. Status 1B refers to hospitalized patients who are being treated with a right or left ventricular circulatory assist device after their initial 30-day window as a status 1A or a continuous intravenous infusion of inotropes. A candidate who does not meet the criteria for status 1A or 1B is listed as status 2; status 2 patients are often those outpatients who are stable on a medical regimen. A candidate who is listed as status 7 is considered temporarily unsuitable to receive a thoracic organ transplant (see also policies of the Organ Procurement and Transplantation network, http://www.optn.org).

Donor Selection

Donor selection is influenced by various factors, including the presence of intrinsic heart disease, ABO blood type compatibility, donor-recipient size disparity, and the presence of transmissible disease. Standard guidelines have been established for cardiac donor selection (Table 27-4). To identify intrinsic cardiac disease. electrocardiography, echocardiography and coronary angiography are used (for male donors older than 45 years and female donors older than 50 years). Donors with a history of active malignancy (excluding basal cell and squamous cell carcinomas of the skin and some isolated brain tumors) are excluded because there is a high probability of transferring malignant cells to the immunosuppressed recipient. To avoid transmitting infectious diseases, serologies for human immunodeficiency virus (HIV), hepatitis B virus (HBV), and hepatitis C virus (HCV) should be negative, although some centers "match" donors who have positive hepatitis serology with seropositive recipients. A recent study using the U.S. Scientific Registry of Transplant Recipients has suggested that patients who receive heart transplants from HCV-positive donors have an increase in posttransplant mortality at 1 year (16.9 versus 8.2 percent in the exposed and unexposed groups, respectively), and at 5 years (41.8 versus 18.5 percent, respectively). Exposed patients are more likely than unexposed patients to die secondary to viral hepatitis or liver failure (13.7 versus 0.4 percent) and coronary artery disease (8.8 versus 3.6 percent), but were less likely to die of graft failure (7.8 versus 16.5 percent). Decreased survival because of HCV

TABLE 27–4 Guidelines for Cardiac Donor Selection
Age<55 yr
No history of chest trauma or cardiac disease
No prolonged hypotension or hypoxemia
Meets hemodynamic criteria
MAP>60 mm Hg
CVP 8-12 mm Hg
Inotropic support <10 μg/kg/min dopamine or dobutamine
Normal ECG
Normal echocardiogram
Normal cardiac angiography*
Negative HBsAg, HCV, and HIV serologies

*Performed as indicated by donor age and history.

CVP=central venous pressure; ECG=electrocardiogram; HBsAg=hepatis B surface antigen; HCV=hepatitis C virus; HIV=human immunodeficiency virus; MAP=mean arterial pressure.

From Hunt SA, Kouretas PC, Balsam LB, Robbins RC: Heart transplantation. *In* Zipes DP, Libby P, Bonow RO, Braunwald E (eds): Braunwald's Heart Disease: A Textbook of Cardiovascular Medicine. Philadelphia, Elsevier Saunders, 2005, p 645.

TABLE 27–5 Indications for Cardiac Transplantation
Presence of
Severe heart failure requiring continuous inotropic therapy
Severe heart failure (NYHA Class III OR IV) with poor short-term prognosis, despite maximal medical therapy
Restrictive or hypertrophic cardiomyopathy with NYHA Class III OR IV symptoms
Refractory angina pectoris with documented cardiac ischemia, despite maximal medical therapy, not amenable to revascularization, with an estimated poor short-term prognosis
Recurrent or refractory ventricular arrhythmias, despite maximal medical and/or device therapy
Complex congenital heart disease with ventricular (systemic or venous) failure that is progressive and not amenable to surgical or percutaneous repair
Hypoplastic left heart syndrome
Low-grade tumors confined to the myocardium, unresectable, and without evidence of metastasis
Absence of
Advanced age
Severe peripheral or vascular disease
Irreversible dysfunction of another organ
History of malignancy with probability of recurrence
Inability to comply with medical regimens
Irreversible pulmonary hypertension (> 4 Wood units)
Active systemic infection.

Modified from Taylor DO: The role of heart transplantation. *In* Young J, McCarthy PM (eds): Heart Failure: A Combined Medical and Surgical Approach. Malden, MA, Blackwell Futura, 2007, pp 228-254.

donor status was significant only in recipients older than 39 years, and occurred irrespective of recipient HCV status.[48]

The actual recovery of hearts from a consented donor is approximately 50 percent, with depressed cardiac function of the donor heart as the main reason that a heart is declined. For cardiac transplantation, height and weight differences up to 20 percent may be tolerated; however, in potential recipients with pulmonary hypertension, a donor whose body size is at least equal to that of the recipient should be chosen to decrease the likelihood of acute right ventricular failure. With the shortage of organ donors, there has been a trend toward liberalizing donor selection criteria, including accepting hearts of older donors, tolerating longer organ ischemic times, and accepting hearts with some structural abnormalities, including mild valvular anomalies, or mild coronary artery disease, or even repairing donor heart defects, such as with coronary artery bypass or valve surgery.[49] The use of older donor hearts (older than 55 years) is now considered in selected high-risk recipients in the absence of other significant risk factors. Recipients of hearts from older donors have a higher perioperative mortality (approximately twofold increase for donors older than 40 years and fourfold for donors older than 50 years), and a higher incidence of cardiac allograft vasculopathy. Nonetheless, the survival of recipients who receive hearts from donors older than 40 years is superior to that of patients who were listed but never transplanted.

Another new direction in heart transplantation is the use of donor hearts with prolonged ischemic time. Although the current guideline that cardiac allograft ischemia time less than 4 hours is safe and has a decreased incidence of posttransplant allograft dysfunction, several transplant centers have reported good clinical outcomes in adults with prolonged donor heart ischemia times longer than 240 minutes. However, none of these studies was able to determine the safe upper limit for allograft ischemic times.[50] ABO compatibility remains an absolute requirement, because hyperacute rejection may occur within minutes when transplantation is performed across ABO barriers.

Recipient Selection

The indications and contraindications for transplantation have been evolving and becoming more refined. The current selection criteria for cardiac recipients are intended to identify the patients with end-stage heart disease who are most likely to have the greatest benefit from the scarce societal resource of a donor heart (Table 27-5). The most important criterion remains the presence of advanced heart disease that cannot be treated by more conservative forms of medical or device therapy (see Chap. 25). In general, optimally treated patients who have NYHA Class IV symptoms, peak oxygen consumption less than 12 to 14 ml/kg/min (or less than 50 percent predicted), and impaired hemodynamics (low cardiac index, elevated filling pressures) are considered possible candidates for transplantation. There are few absolute contraindications to transplantation. Many formerly stringent contraindications, including advanced age, peripheral or cerebral vascular disease, malignancy, irreversible pulmonary hypertension, systemic infection, organ dysfunction and psychosocial issues that affect compliance, are now successfully managed in experienced centers by careful recipient selection.

Age criteria for eligibility were initially rigid; however, over time, it became apparent that chronological and physiological age could be discrepant. There have been a number of single-center reports of excellent post-heart transplant survival in carefully selected older recipients. Although most centers do not have fixed upper age limits, advanced age is a risk factor for reduced long-term survival posttransplant in some, but not all, centers.[50,51] Peripheral and cerebral vascular disease are still contraindications; however, with the wider use of vascular stenting, these are becoming relative contraindications in most centers. Although diabetes itself is no longer a contraindication to transplantation, when a diabetic patient presents with neuropathy, peripheral vascular disease, and renal dysfunction, most programs would not transplant the patient. The institution of chronic immunosuppression, which has been associated with a higher than usual incidence of malignancy, might favor recurrence or more aggressive behavior of a prior or current malignancy. There have been many reports, however, of long-term successful heart transplantation in patients with a remote history of malignancy that is considered to have no probability of recurrence. The practice at Northwestern University is to wait for 5 years until after the malignancy has been successfully treated. In cases in which the malignancy is less remote in history or probability of recurrence less certain, consultation with an oncologist regarding prognosis can be helpful. Systemic infection is still another serious contraindication; however, patients with active LV assist device (LVAD) pocket infections and bacteremia have been successfully transplanted. The source of the infection (the LVAD) is removed, the mediastinum and surgical pocket are extensively débrided, and extensive antibiotics are used perioperatively. Organ dysfunction is also a frequent problem. In some patients, renal dysfunction is simply secondary to low cardiac output and will improve after transplantation. This has been shown repeatedly in patients who had developed acute renal failure, received an LVAD, and then recovered renal function and went on to transplantation.[52] On the other hand, a longstanding elevated serum creatinine level, especially in patients with proteinuria, is of concern. Multiple organ transplants (e.g., heart-kidney, or heart-liver) may be considered for some of these patients.

Psychosocial issues with a history of noncompliance (e.g., continuous alcohol or tobacco abuse for years, despite counseling and repeated attempts to stop) suggest that the patient may not be compliant with the complex medication immunosuppressive regimen (see later). Adolescents are well known for reducing, or discontinuing, their immunosuppression, with disastrous results. These issues require the evaluation of social worker, clinical psychologist, or even psychiatrist, to help assess the patient's suitability for transplantation. Irreversible pulmonary hypertension, with a fixed pulmonary vascular resistance more than 4 Wood units, has long been considered a contraindication to transplantation. However, the reversibility of the pulmonary hypertension in patients with chronic heart failure is now well recognized, and it is believed that if reversibility can be demonstrated acutely with pharmacological maneuvers, the patient will do well with a transplant, because the same reversal could presumably be accomplished in the postoperative setting. Except for the most severely elevated pulmonary pressures, pulmonary hypertension is considered a relative contraindication with gradations of risk to the recipient, depending on the pulmonary artery pressures and the degree of their reversibility. Today, pulmonary hypertension can be managed postoperatively with phosphodiesterase inhibitors, inhaled nitric oxide, and potentially the chronic administration of sildenafil.[53] However, irreversible pulmonary hypertension remains an exclusion from transplant candidacy in most centers unless combined heart and lung transplantation is considered.

Risk factors in recipients now are assessed by the transplantation team on a case by case basis. For example, a 70-year-old patient with no other risk factors may well be a good candidate. A younger patient may tolerate one or two risk factors with a moderate or minimal increase in mortality and still have a good late outcome, especially in experienced centers. Attempts have been made to quantify these various risk factors and their potential impact on morbidity and mortality after transplantation (see Table 27-e1 on website).

Cardiac Transplantation: The Operation

The evolution of the technique for cardiac transplantation evolved from modifications of two different surgical approaches—orthotopic (donor heart implanted in place of the native heart) and heterotopic (donor heart piggy-backed beside the native heart) heart transplantation. Currently, centers attempt to maintain the ischemic time to less than 4 hours to minimize the risk of donor heart failure. However, with complex operations, such as a patient on a ventricular assist device who has extensive adhesions from prior operations, surgical judgment with respect to timing of the operation is critical to keep the ischemic times low. Two orthotopic techniques are used to replace the recipient heart with a donor heart, the classic Shumway-Lower bi-trial transplant technique, in which the donor right atrium is attached directly to the recipient right atrium (Fig. 27-11A) and the increasingly used bicaval technique, in which the superior and inferior vena cava are attached separately and the left atrial anastomosis is done as a cuff (see Fig. 27-11B). The standard biatrial technique results in disruption of normal atrial geometry, and leads to increased atrial size with abnormal or reduced atrial contribution to ventricular filling, right ventricular dysfunction, tricuspid and mitral insufficiency, and sinus node dysfunction.[50]

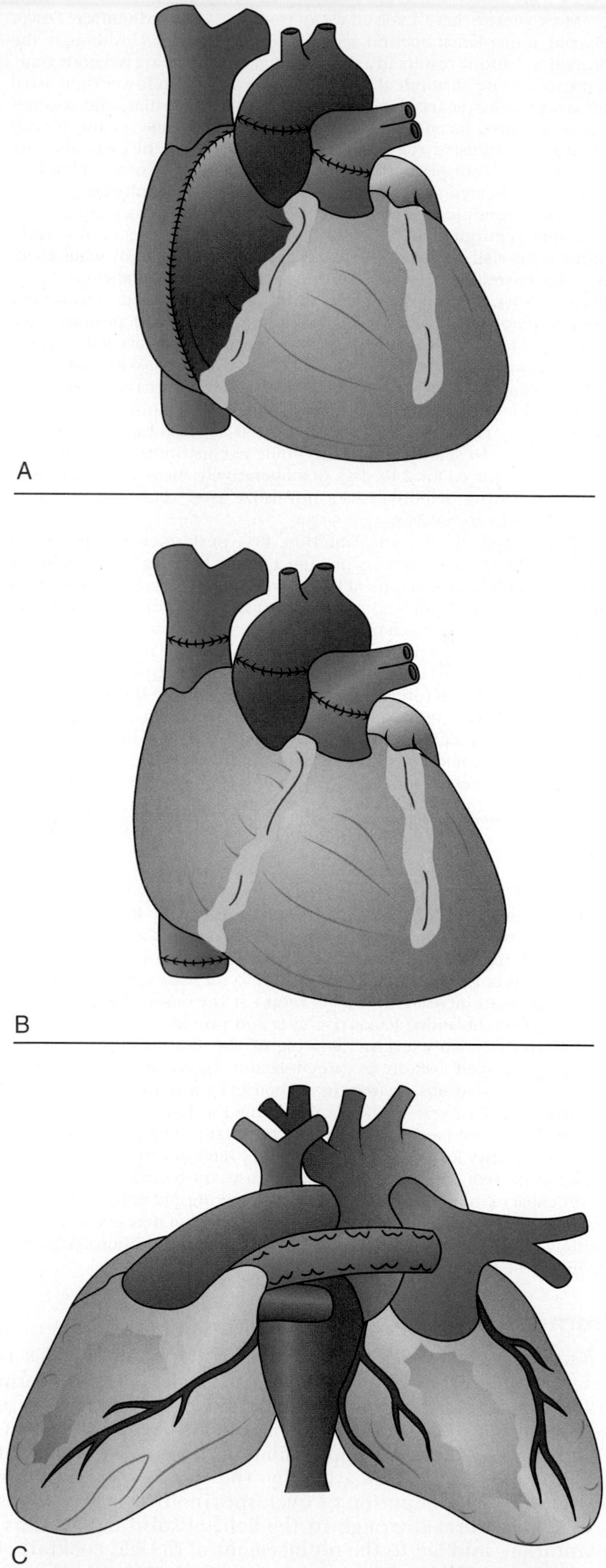

FIGURE 27–11 Surgical techniques for cardiac transplantation. **A,** Standard Lower-Shumway (biatrial) orthotopic heart transplantation. **B,** Bicaval technique of orthotopic heart transplantation. **C,** Heterotopic heart transplantation. *(Modified from Al Khaldi A, Robbins RC: New directions in cardiac transplantation. Annu Rev Med 57:455, 2006.)*

Most centers have evolved away from the classic Shumway-Lower biatrial transplantation and use bicaval anastomosis. Although the bicaval technique results in a slightly longer donor heart ischemia time, it preserves the anatomical integrity of the atria with lower right atrial pressures, a lower incidence of atrial tachyarrhythmias, and less left tricuspid valve incompetence. Despite increasing use of the bicaval technique, tricuspid regurgitation remains a problem early and late after cardiac transplantation. However, experience in a randomized trial has indicated that adding a tricuspid valve annuloplasty to the transplant operation is even more effective in preventing early and late tricuspid regurgitation.[54] Another disadvantage of the bicaval technique is the risk of superior vena cava stenosis, particularly when there is a size mismatch between the donor and recipient. Judicious use of perioperative inotropes, inhaled nitric oxide if needed, intravenous epoprostenol, aerosolized prostaglandins, and careful postoperative intensive care unit (ICU) and ventilator management have led to a generally smooth postoperative course for most patients, with early extubation, short ICU stays, and discharge at 1 week after transplantation. Posttransplantation complications include sinus node dysfunction, which rarely requires a pacemaker, as well as atrial tachycardias that respond well to standard antiarrhythmic agents. Inotropic support is generally required for 2 to days postoperatively. Measures of LV function and resting hemodynamics normalize over time, but may take several weeks to recover.

Heterotopic heart transplantation, first performed by Barnard in 1974 as a LV bypass, involves placing a donor heart in the right lower thorax parallel to the recipient heart, which is left intact. Anastomoses are made in the donor and recipient left atrium, donor and recipient aorta, donor superior vena cava and recipient right atrium or superior vena cava, and donor pulmonary artery and recipient pulmonary artery or right atrium (see Fig. 27-11C). Although rarely performed today, the indications for heterotopic cardiac transplantation include patients with severe fixed pulmonary hypertension, in whom the inability of the naive donor right ventricle to overcome the high pulmonary vascular resistance might result in right heart failure, and a significant size mismatch between a smaller donor and a larger recipient (donor-to-recipient weight ratio less than 75 percent). Heart-lung transplantation may also be considered for patients with severe fixed pulmonary hypertension.

Physiology of the Transplanted Heart

The cardiac allograft is functionally and anatomically denervated, and therefore cannot increase heart rate acutely to increase cardiac output acutely during exercise. Therefore, the transplanted heart relies on the Frank-Starling mechanism (see Chap. 22) to increase cardiac output in response to an increase in venous return at the onset of exercise. Circulating catecholamine levels rise later and provide a delayed chronotropic response to exercise. Slowing of the heart rate occurs in a similarly delayed fashion as catecholamine levels decline. However, cardiac output drops, mainly in response to a reduction in venous return and the reverse of the Frank-Starling mechanism. Despite these atypical adaptive mechanisms, heart transplant recipients have a subnormal capacity for exercise, although they have normal hemodynamic function at rest. Nevertheless, heart transplant recipients have sufficient capacity to perform activities of daily living and at least moderate exercise. Several lines of suggest that reinnervation may occur in some patients late posttransplantation, which may lead to functional improvement of the transplanted heart.[55]

Immunosuppression

Transplantation between members of the same species is referred to as allotransplantation; hence, the use of the term *allograft* to refer to the transplanted heart. Alloantigens are recognized as nonself by the recipient's immune system. Accordingly, immunosuppression is required to prevent destruction of the allograft by the recipient's immune system. The introduction of cyclosporine in the mid-1980s was a major breakthrough in the field of solid organ transplantation, and led to the replacement of the old cocktail of high-dose steroids, azathioprine, and selective use of antithymocyte globulin with a triple-drug therapy regimen that includes a calcineurin inhibitor (cyclosporine or tacrolimus, FK506), steroids (prednisone) and an antiproliferative agent (azathioprine or mycophenolate mofetil, MMF). Based on the results of clinical trials, which showed that MMF is more effective than azathioprine in terms of reducing allograft rejection and mortality, most centers now use MMF as the antiproliferative agent. Although there is no single definitive study that demonstrates the superiority of tacrolimus over cyclosporine, there are certain advantages of tacrolimus: tacrolimus provides rescue therapy in episodes of rejection in cyclosporine-based regimens; tacrolimus may increase mycophenolic acid serum levels, thus potentiating its immunosuppressive effect; and tacrolimus does not cause hirsutism or gingival hyperplasia, which are major side effects with cyclosporine. Signal inhibitor drugs, such as sirolimus or everolimus, are the focus of ongoing clinical research in solid organ transplantation. Sirolimus inhibits cell proliferation in response to cytokines by blocking the proliferation signal mediated by the target of rapamycin (TOR)–dependent pathway. Sirolimus inhibits lymphocyte proliferation induced by cytokines such as interleukin (IL)-2, IL-4, and IL-6, resulting in arrest of the cell cycle in the G1 phase.

Sirolimus or its derivative, everolimus, have three major advantages as immunosuppressive agents: (1) they can be used to treat refractory cardiac rejection; (2) they act downstream of the signal transduction pathway inhibited by calcineurin inhibitors and hence have synergistic effects when combined with these agents; and (3) sirolimus and everolimus inhibit arterial smooth muscle and endothelial cell proliferation, which can prevent the development of transplant arteriopathy.[50] Sirolimus often replaces the calcineurin inhibitor once renal dysfunction develops. Potential adverse effects of sirolimus include impaired wound healing and dyslipidemia. Sirolimus is often changed back to a calcineurin inhibitor or held 1 week prior to any surgical procedure and not restarted until 4 to 6 weeks postoperatively. The basic immunosuppressive regimen can be modified by induction therapy, which consists of the use of powerful antilymphocyte agents such as OKT3 and ATG during the initial period posttransplantation. The concept behind this strategy is that aggressive early immunosuppression could lead to a reduction in the number of episodes of rejection over time. However, this concept has not been uniformly supported by objective data. Although only 45 percent of transplant centers use antilymphocyte therapy, other forms of induction therapy, such as the use of daclizumab (an anti–IL-2 receptor antibody) have been associated with a significant reduction in rejection episodes in cardiac transplantation patients.[56] In addition, today we use "virtual" crossmatch of HLA antibodies in many patients to help predict patients who would be at high risk for rejection and, if possible, avoid using those donors. In summary, there is no longer a specific cocktail for immunosuppression. Different centers use various immunosuppressive agents that are given selectively, based on the crossmatch results, patient comorbidities, and the initial response by the patient to the immunosuppression regimen.

Rejection

Cardiac allograft rejection is an immunological process that left untreated, can lead to destruction of the allograft. The diagnosis of rejection is established by a histological grading system or by a change in clinical parameters, such as hemodynamic deterioration or a decrease in LV systolic function. There are three categories of rejection—hyperacute, antibody-mediated, and acute cellular. Hyperacute rejection takes place within minutes to hours and is caused by preformed antibodies in the recipient. The clinical outcome, without repeat transplantation or use of total artificial heart support, is uniformly fatal. Hyperacute rejection is best avoided by screening the recipient for possible donor-specific antibodies using a panel reactive antibody (PRA) test. Antibody-mediated rejection may manifest as histological evidence of rejection, unexplained cardiac allograft dysfunction, or both. Histologically, antibody-mediated rejection appears as a scant cellular infiltrate with abundant colocalized immunoglobulin and complement components in the allograft microvasculature. The most common form of rejection, acute cellular rejection, occurs in one third to half of heart transplant recipients. Even though the propensity toward allograft rejection decreases over time, and nearly half of the rejection episodes occur in the first 2 to 3 months, late rejection can and does occur. Acute cellular rejection is most frequently diagnosed histologically by endomyocardial biopsy and is graded in accordance with the International Society for Heart and Lung Transplantation (ISHLT) criteria. In 2004, the grading system was revised by an ISHLT multidisciplinary consensus conference, which reclassified acute cellular rejection into four revised (R) categories (Fig. 27-12): grade 0 R—no rejection; grade 1 R—mild rejection (old grade 1A, 1B, and 2); grade 2R—moderate rejection (old grade 3A); and grade 3R—severe rejection (old grade 3B and 4). The new scoring system also recognizes antibody-mediated or humoral rejection as a separate clinical entity.[57] In the absence of clinical deterioration, histological evidence of mild rejection does not typically require changes in therapy, whereas histological evidence of moderate to severe rejection requires treatment, even in the absence of clinical changes. Episodes of rejection occur more frequently during early posttransplantation rather than late.

Although the use of routine surveillance endomyocardial biopsies has changed the long-term survival of heart transplant recipients in the modern era of cyclosporine therapy, the dependence on surveillance endomyocardial biopsy may diminish in the not too distant future. The invasive nature and lack of reproducibility of the endomyocardial biopsy, as well as the inability to diagnose overimmunosuppression, have prompted clinicians to search for other modalities for monitoring cardiac allograft rejection. Given that acute rejection involves the activation of immune cells, it is likely that rejection-induced immune activation will be accompanied by specific changes in the pattern of gene expression in peripheral blood cells before there is any histologically recognizable rejection pattern on endomyocardial biopsy. The Cardiac Allograft Rejection Gene expression Observation (CARGO) study group was formed in 2001 to investigate the usefulness of molecular testing for gene expression in peripheral blood cells for the diagnosis of cardiac rejection.[50] Preliminary results have suggested that there is a good correlation and high predictive value for these molecular fingerprinting techniques with respect to predicting future acute rejection. Molecular testing for gene expression in peripheral blood cells may ultimately replace routine endomyocardial biopsy for rejection surveillance, and might allow for easier tapering of immunosuppression in recipients with better long-term tolerance of the cardiac allograft.

Clinical Outcomes

The ISHLT maintains a registry of information regarding heart transplantations performed worldwide, and generates an annual report that contains data regarding survival, risk factors for mortality, and posttransplantation functional status.[58] The number of reported heart transplants worldwide has continued to decline since the mid-1990s (Fig. 27-13A). This decline has resulted from a decrease in transplantations reported both by non-U.S. and U.S. centers. The age distribution of heart transplant recipients has also changed in recent years. As noted earlier, the proportion of recipients in the 50- to 64-year range and older than 65 years age has increased, whereas the proportion in the 35- to 49-year age range has decreased (see Fig. 27-13B). The age distribution of heart transplant donors, however, has remained relatively stable. The major diagnoses responsible for cardiac transplantation in adults continue to be idiopathic cardiomyopathy and ischemic cardiomyopathy.

Most centers now are able to achieve 85 percent or greater 1-year survival, and survival rates of 90 to 95 percent at 1 year are not uncommon.[58,59] There has been a steady improvement in early survival, which can be seen in the different eras of transplantation as reported by the International Society for Heart and Lung Transplantation (Fig. 27-14). The biggest impact on survival has been in the early perioperative phase and in the first few months after transplantation. Beyond that, there has been a consistent slow steady decline in survival, usually related to the complications of immunosuppression or what is likely a manifestation of chronic rejection, coronary artery vasculopathy (CAV). This steady attrition in survival after the first year is approximately 4 percent/year. Nevertheless, for most recipients today, one can expect a 10-year survival of approximately 50 percent, or perhaps even greater. There is, however, significant variability in centers, and of the 150 heart transplant programs in the United States, only half meet the minimum requirements set by Medicare (12 or more heart transplants/year, with 73 percent 1-year survival). Medicare has recently withdrawn approval of smaller transplantation centers with inadequate patient volume.

According to the ISHLT data base, the following parameters are major risk factors for 1-year mortality posttransplantation: underlying diagnosis of congenital heart disease, patient in hospital and/or on ventilator before transplant, PRA >10 percent, and dialysis. Additional risk factors include older donor age, older recipient age, increased donor heart ischemic time, and elevated recipient bilirubin or creatinine level. Previously, an underlying diagnosis of coronary artery disease, retransplantation, the presence of an intraaortic balloon pump or ventricular assist device at the time of transplantation, or a history of malignancy were risk factors for 1-year mortality; however, they are not risk factors in the most recent cohort of patients. Risk factors that influence 5-year mortality include infection prior to transplantation discharge or during the first posttransplantation year, graft coronary artery disease within the first posttransplantation year, cerebrovascular disease at transplantation, insulin-dependent diabetes, and underlying diagnosis of coronary artery disease.

Although the vast majority of transplant patients report a good functional status after transplantation, less than 40 percent of heart transplant recipients return to work after transplantation. Nonetheless, cardiac transplantation offers independence and a relatively good quality of life for most patients.

Long-Term Complications

The long-term medical complications that occur in heart transplant recipients can be divided into cardiac and noncardiac. The major cardiac long-term complications are the development of coronary artery vasculopathy, also known as transplant coronary artery disease. The major noncardiac complications are malignancy, infection, hypertension, renal failure, and osteoporosis.

ALLOGRAFT CORONARY ARTERY DISEASE (see Chap. 38). Recipients of cardiac allografts are prone to develop a diffuse and often rapidly progressive obliterative pattern of coronary artery disease, referred to as coronary artery vasculopathy (CAV). Indeed, CAV is the main factor limiting the long-term success of heart transplantation. Angiographic evidence of CAV is present by 1 year posttransplantation in 10 percent of patients and is evident in 50 percent by 5 years. The use of intravascular ultrasound has provided earlier and more sensitive diagnosis of the intimal thickening that characterizes the disease (Fig. 27-15).[60] Early reports have suggested that 64-detector computed tomography angiography may also be superior to conventional catheter-based angiography to identify nonobstructive vessel wall disease that may go unrecognized with catheter-based angiography alone.[61] The cause of CAV probably involves immunological

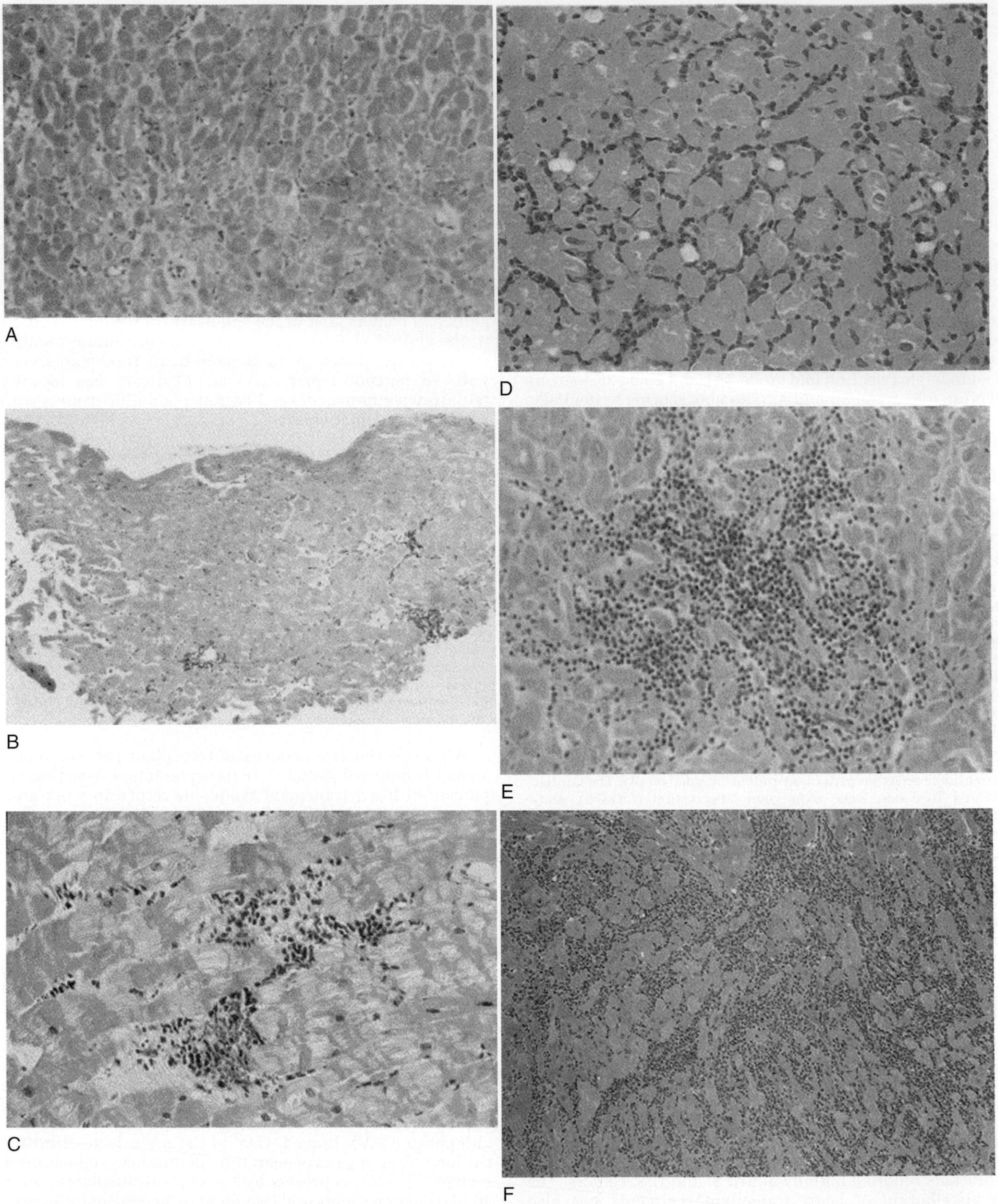

FIGURE 27–12 Histological diagnosis and grading of cardiac allograft rejection. **A,** Grade 0 R—normal endomyocardial biopsy showing no evidence of cellular infiltration. **B,** Grade 1 R—low-power view of endomyocardial biopsy showing three focal perivascular infiltrates without myocyte damage (previously grade 1A). **C,** Grade 1 R—both perivascular and interstitial infiltrates are present but without definite evidence of myocyte damage (previously grade 1A). **D,** Grade 1 R—diffuse mononuclear cell infiltrate with an interstitial pattern of lymphocytes between and around myocytes without associated myocyte damage (previously grade 1B). **E,** Grade 2 R—damaging infiltrate with myocyte damage and architectural distortion (previously grade 3A). **F,** Grade 3 R—diffuse damaging infiltrates with encroachment of myocytes and disruption of normal architecture (previously grade 3B). *(From Stewart S, Winters GL, Fishbein MC, Tazelaar HD, et al: Revision of the 1990 working formulation for the standardization of nomenclature in the diagnosis of heart rejection. J Heart Lung Transplant 24:1710, 2005.)*

and nonimmunological factors. Identifiable risk factors include older donor and recipient age, ischemia-reperfusion injury, human leukocyte antigen (HLA) mismatch, hypertension, hyperlipidemia, insulin resistance, cytomegalovirus infection, and recurrent rejection.[50] These risk factors probably lead directly or indirectly to endothelial injury, with subsequent intimal hyperplasia and vascular smooth muscle proliferation.

A 3-hydroxy-3-methylglutaryl coenzyme A (HMG-CoA) reductase inhibitor is used in most transplant recipients and has been shown to effectively treat posttransplantation hyperlipidemia, as well as to decrease clinically significant posttransplantation rejection. The goal for the low-density lipoprotein cholesterol level is less than 70 to 100 mg/dl. In addition, patients are encouraged to reduce dietary fat intake, to exercise, and to maintain an ideal body weight. It should be recognized that combining an HMG-CoA reductase inhibitor with a calcineurin inhibitor increases the risk of rhabdomyolysis.

As noted earlier, transplant recipients generally have denervation of the afferent and efferent cardiac nerves, and therefore do not experience the subjective sensation of angina pectoris. The sequelae of ischemia in these patients may include arrhythmias, leading to sudden death, and progressive ischemic LV dysfunction, culminating in heart failure. The very diffuseness of the coronary artery disease renders standard revascularization with percutaneous or surgical interventions less useful. Once allograft vasculopathy has led to clinical events, the overall prognosis is very poor in these patients, with a 20 percent survival 1 year after an ischemic clinical event. No drug or agent has clearly been shown to *reverse* this disease, and the only definitive therapy available is retransplantation.

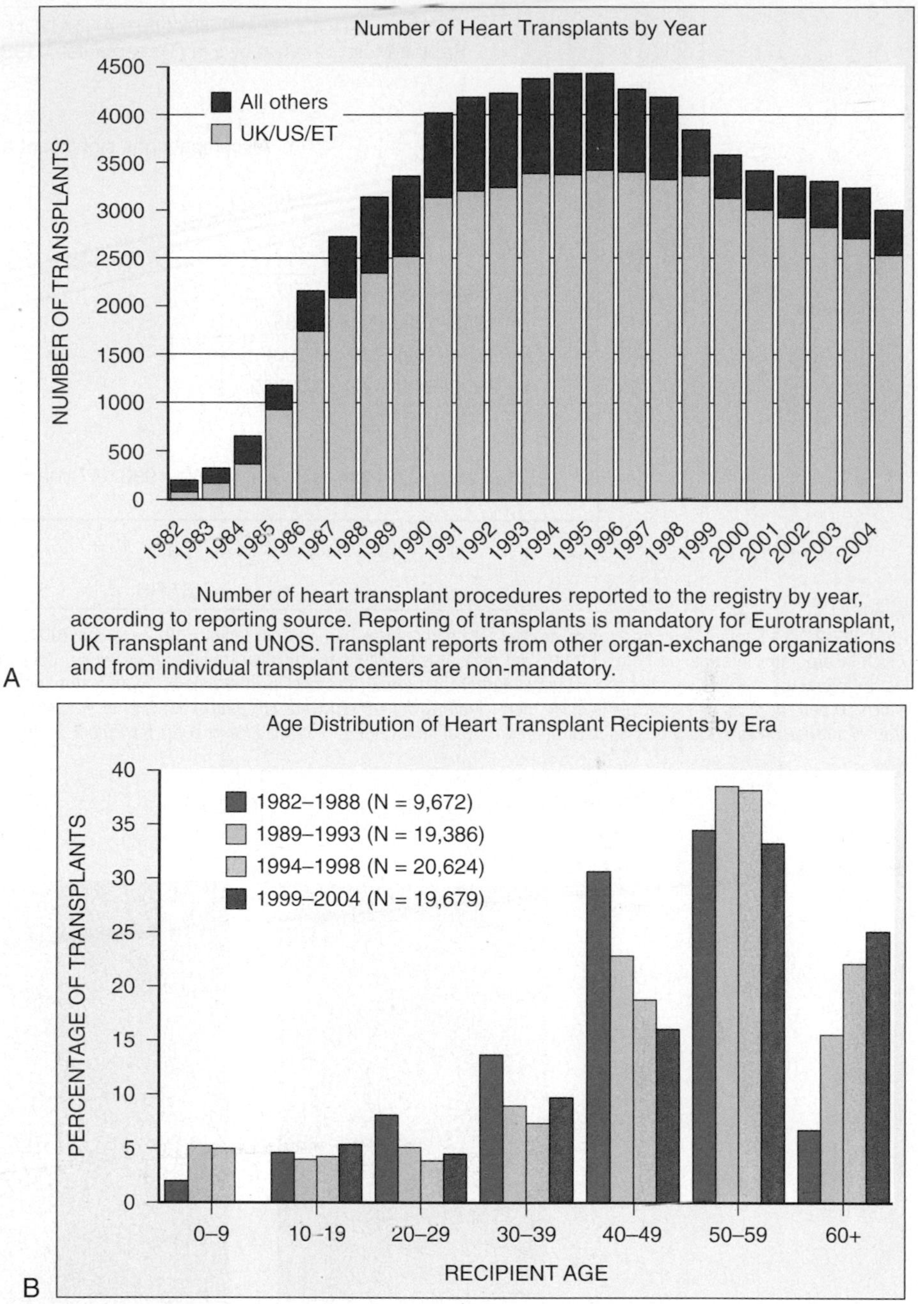

FIGURE 27–13 Number of heart transplants by year **(A)** and age distribution of heart transplant patients by era **(B)**. *(From Taylor DO, Edwards LB, Boucek MM, et al: Registry of the International Society for Heart and Lung Transplantation: Twenty-third official adult heart transplantation report—2006. J Heart Lung Transplant 25:869, 2006.)*

MALIGNANCY. The occurrence of an increased incidence of malignancy is a well-recognized sequela of any program of chronic immunosuppression, and cardiac transplantation is no exception. Lymphoproliferative disorders are among the most frequent posttransplantation complications and, in most cases, seem to be driven by the Epstein-Barr virus. Effective therapy includes reduction of immunosuppression, antiviral agents, and traditional chemoradiation and radiotherapy. Cutaneous malignancies (both basal cell and squamous cell carcinomas) also occur with increased frequency in transplant recipients and can pursue very aggressive courses. The role of decreasing immunosuppression for treatment of these cancers is uncertain. Each annual visit encompasses routine screening for malignancy, including prostate-specific antigen testing, mammography, Pap smear, and dermatological examination. Patients are encouraged to have closer surveillance for colon cancer, with serial colonoscopies every 5 years.

INFECTIONS. The use of immunosuppression to prevent allograft rejection naturally results in an increased susceptibility to infectious complications in transplant recipients. Typically, nosocomial infections occur early posttransplantation, when immunosuppression is the most intense. However, over time, opportunistic infections predominate. Historically, cytomegalovirus and *Pneumocystis carinii* (now known as *P. jiroveci*) infection were seen at a higher frequency, but as a result of aggressive prophylaxis protocols, there has been a significant decline in the appearance of these two agents. Effective management depends on careful surveillance for early signs and symptoms of opportunistic infections.

HYPERTENSION AND RENAL FAILURE. Hypertension occurs in as many as 70 percent of cardiac transplant recipients as a result of the side effects of cyclosporine and

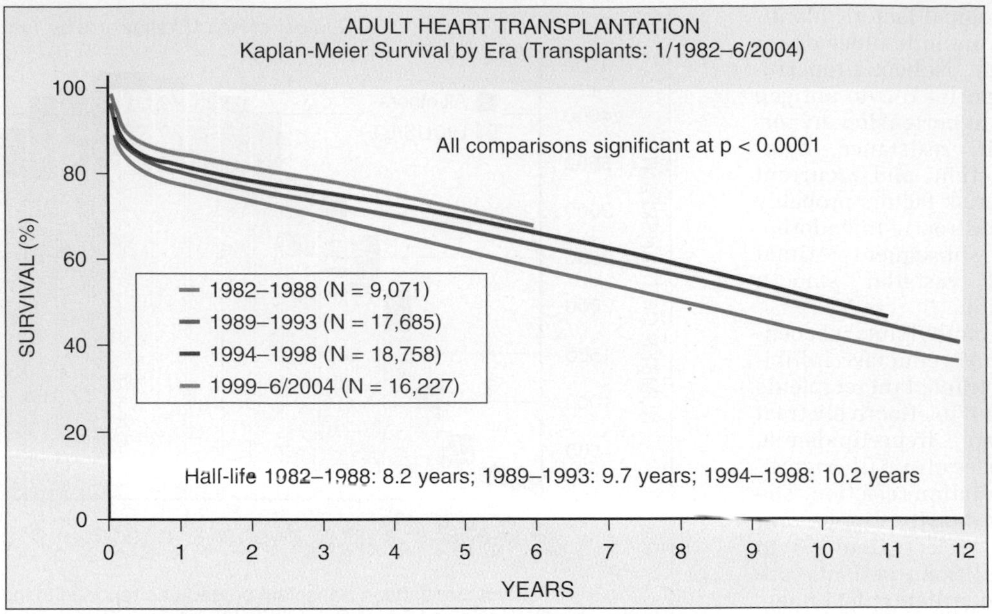

FIGURE 27–14 Kaplan-Meier analysis of survival for heart transplantation from January 1982 to June 2004. Survival was calculated using the Kaplan-Meier method, which incorporates information from all transplant recipients for whom any follow-up has been provided. Because many patients are still alive and some patients have been lost to follow-up, the survival rates are estimates rather than exact rates because the time of death is not known for all patients. The half-life is the estimated time point at which 50 percent of all of the recipients have died. *(From Taylor DO, Edwards LB, Boucek MM, et al: Registry of the International Society for Heart and Lung Transplantation: Twenty-third official adult heart transplantation report—2006. J Heart Lung Transplant 25:869, 2006.)*

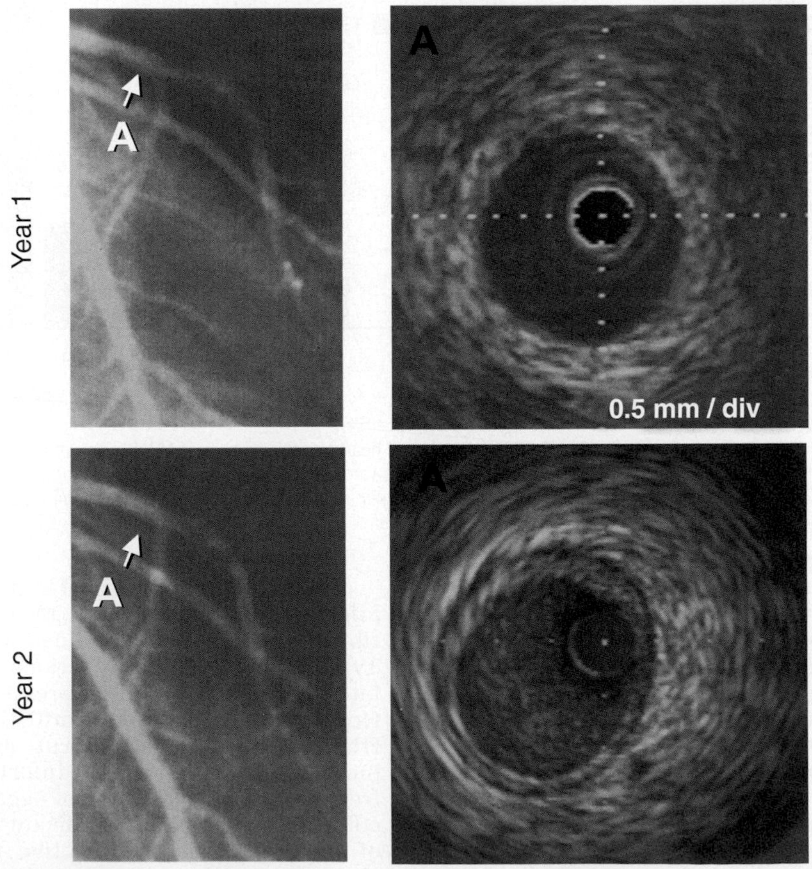

FIGURE 27–15 Graft coronary artery disease—appearance by angiography and intravascular ultrasound. **Left panels,** Angiograms obtained on a transplanted heart at years 1 and 2 following engraftment. **Right panels,** Intravascular ultrasound images obtained at the same time at the points labeled A in the angiograms. Note the progression of concentric intimal thickening that produces narrowing but not the appearance of a focal stenosis on the angiograms. These paired images show that the angiogram can underestimate the degree of intimal thickening in allograft coronary artery disease because of the concentric nature of the intimal expansion. *(From Lee RT, Braunwald E [eds]: Atlas of Cardiac Imaging. Philadelphia, Churchill Livingstone, 1998, p 648.)*

steroids, as well as of preexisting conditions. The treatment of hypertension is no different than in the population at large (see Chap. 40) However, it should be noted that concomitant administration of diltiazem, verapamil, and nicardipine will increase the level of cyclosporine or tacrolimus, and may lead to toxicity unless the dosage of cyclosporine or tacrolimus is reduced. Renal insufficiency occurs in approximately 50 percent of patients and 5 percent of all transplant recipients are either on dialysis or undergo kidney transplantation. Although some renal insufficiency is related to preexisting renal disease, most is acquired. Both tacrolimus and cyclosporine are nephrotoxic and likely account for most renal problems. Sirolimus is less nephrotoxic and can replace a calcineurin inhibitor whenever significant renal dysfunction develops.

OSTEOPOROSIS. The risk of osteoporosis is high in transplant patients because of the underlying inactivity and bed rest. Further bone loss may occur because of prolonged heparin administration and corticosteroid use. Bone loss is most marked in the lumbar spine and may also affect the hip, leading to aseptic necrosis. Treatment with calcium and vitamin D is warranted in all pretransplant and posttransplant patients with evidence of osteoporosis. Bisphosphonates (alendronate sodium) can be safely added to calcium and vitamin D, and effectively increase bone density.

In summary, cardiac transplantation is the most effective treatment for selected patients with end-stage heart failure. Most infections and rejections are preventable or treatable, and the temporary use of mechanical circulatory support pretransplantation no longer augers a poor prognosis following transplantation. Although CAV and malignancy limit long-term survival, the survival at 10 years is approaching 50 percent. Because of the limited availability of donor hearts, care must be taken to ensure that individuals listed as candidates for cardiac transplantation are those who will likely benefit the most. Potentially suitable candidates should be referred early in the course of their end-stage disease to heart failure and transplantation specialists so that transplantation or alternative treatment strategies can be appropriately timed and implemented.

FUTURE PERSPECTIVES

There are many potential surgical targets in heart failure patients, especially in patients with ischemic cardiomyopathy. The most widely used surgery for heart failure is coronary artery bypass grafting and, with the aid of viability studies, this appears to be a very effective therapy for reducing the risks of death as compared with those treated with medical therapy.[13] Overall, heart surgery is not as dangerous as it used to be in this patient population. Furthermore, recent randomized trials in mitral valve surgery and patients with low LVEF would indicate that this is more widely applicable than at just a handful of specialized centers.[21] We think that there is a small discrete segment of patients with localized LV infarction and dilation that may benefit from LV reconstruction.[42] The results of the ongoing STICH trial may provide some insight into this question. As surgical and anesthetic management of heart failure continues to improve, maximizing the surgical options for patients referred for heart transplantation may help diminish the wait times for cardiac transplant candidates who truly have no other surgical or medical options left. Although our early experience suggests that 3-year survival (82 percent) is similar to that of patients who actually received a heart transplant,[62] it will be important to obtain additional outcomes data to be certain that the results in multiple centers are at least equivalent to those currently observed with cardiac transplantation.

REFERENCES

Coronary Artery Revascularization

1. Starling RC, McCarthy PM, Yamini MH: Surgical treatment of chronic congestive heart failure. *In* Mann D (ed): Heart Failure: A Companion to Braunwald's Heart Disease. Philadelphia, WB Saunders, 2003, pp 717-736.
2. O'Connor CM, Velazquez EJ, Gardner LH, et al: Comparison of coronary artery bypass grafting versus medical therapy on long-term outcome in patients with ischemic cardiomyopathy: A 25-year experience from the Duke Cardiovascular Disease Databank. Am J Cardiol 90:101, 2002.
3. Joyce D, Loebe M, Noon GP, et al: Revascularization and ventricular restoration in patients with ischemic heart failure: The STICH trial. Curr Opin Cardiol 18:454, 2003.
4. De Bonis, M.Alfieri, O: Surgery insight: Surgical methods to reverse left ventricular remodeling. Nat Clin Pract Cardiovasc Med 3:507, 2006.
5. Hillis GS, Zehr KJ, Williams AW, et al: Outcome of patients with low ejection fraction undergoing coronary artery bypass grafting: Renal function and mortality after 3.8 years. Circulation 114:I414, 2006.
6. Shapira OM, Hunter CT, Anter E, et al: Coronary artery bypass grafting in patients with severe left ventricular dysfunction—early and mid-term outcomes. J Card Surg 21:225, 2006.
7. Darwazah AK, Abu Sham'a RA, Hussein E, et al: Myocardial revascularization in patients with low ejection fraction < or = 35%: Effect of pump technique on early morbidity and mortality. J Card Surg 21:22, 2006.
8. Argenziano M, Spotnitz HM, Whang W, et al: Risk stratification for coronary bypass surgery in patients with left ventricular dysfunction: Analysis of the coronary artery bypass grafting patch trial database. Circulation 100:II119, 1999.
9. Hochman JS, Sleeper LA, Webb JG, et al: Early revascularization in acute myocardial infarction complicated by cardiogenic shock. SHOCK Investigators. Should We Emergently Revascularize Occluded Coronaries for Cardiogenic Shock. N Engl J Med 341:625, 1999.
10. Kumpati GS, McCarthy PM, Hoercher KJ: Surgical treatments for heart failure. Cardiol Clin 19, 669-681, 2001.
11. Pagano D, Bonser RS,Camici PG: Myocardial revascularization for the treatment of post-ischemic heart failure. Curr Opin Cardiol 14:506, 1999.
12. Di Carli MF, Asgarzadie F, Schelbert HR, et al: Quantitative relation between myocardial viability and improvement in heart failure symptoms after revascularization in patients with ischemic cardiomyopathy. Circulation 92:3436, 1995.
13. Allman KC, Shaw LJ, Hachamovitch R, et al: Myocardial viability testing and impact of revascularization on prognosis in patients with coronary artery disease and left ventricular dysfunction: A meta-analysis. J Am Coll Cardiol 39:1151, 2002.
14. Hunt SA, Abraham WT, Chin MH, et al: ACC/AHA 2005 Guideline Update for the Diagnosis and Management of Chronic Heart Failure in the Adult: A report of the American College of Cardiology/American Heart Association Task Force on Practice Guidelines (Writing Committee to Update the 2001 Guidelines for the Evaluation and Management of Heart Failure): Developed in collaboration with the American College of Chest Physicians and the International Society for Heart and Lung Transplantation: Endorsed by the Heart Rhythm Society. Circulation 112:e154, 2005.
15. Eagle KA, Guyton RA, Davidoff R, et al: ACC/AHA guidelines for coronary artery bypass graft surgery: Executive summary and recommendations : A report of the American College of Cardiology/American Heart Association Task Force on Practice Guidelines (Committee to revise the 1991 guidelines for coronary artery bypass graft surgery). Circulation 100:1464, 1999.

Valve Surgery

16. Koelling TM, Aaronson KD, Cody RJ, et al: Prognostic significance of mitral regurgitation and tricuspid regurgitation in patients with left ventricular systolic dysfunction. Am Heart J 144:524, 2002.
17. Bonow RO, Carabello BA, Chatterjee K, et al: ACC/AHA 2006 guidelines for the management of patients with valvular heart disease: A report of the American College of Cardiology/American Heart Association Task Force on Practice Guidelines (writing Committee to Revise the 1998 guidelines for the management of patients with valvular heart disease) developed in collaboration with the Society of Cardiovascular Anesthesiologists; endorsed by the Society for Cardiovascular Angiography and Interventions and the Society of Thoracic Surgeons. J Am Coll Cardiol 48:e1, 2006.
18. Spoor MT, Geltz A, Bolling SF: Flexible versus nonflexible mitral valve rings for congestive heart failure: differential durability of repair. Circulation 114:I67, 2006.
19. Bishay ES, McCarthy PM, Cosgrove DM, et al: Mitral valve surgery in patients with severe left ventricular dysfunction. Eur J Cardiothorac Surg 17:213, 2000.
20. Shah AS, Hannish SA, Milano CA, et al: Isolated mitral valve repair in patients with depressed left ventricular function. Ann Thorac Surg 80:1309, 2005.
21. Acker MA, Bolling S, Shemin R, et al: Mitral valve surgery in heart failure: Insights from the Acorn Clinical Trial. J Thorac Cardiovasc Surg 132:568, 2006.
22. Maisano F, Redaelli A, Soncini M, et al: An annular prosthesis for the treatment of functional mitral regurgitation: Finite element model analysis of a dog bone-shaped ring prosthesis. Ann Thorac Surg 79:1268, 2005.
23. McCarthy PM: Valve surgery for patients with left ventricular dysfunction. *In* Young J, McCarthy PM (eds): Heart Failure: A Combined Medical and Surgical Approach. Malden, MA, Blackwell Futura, 2006, pp 153-173.

24. Prifti E, Bonacchi M, Frati G, et al: Ischemic mitral valve regurgitation grade II-III: Correction in patients with impaired left ventricular function undergoing simultaneous coronary revascularization. J Heart Valve Dis 10:754, 2001.
25. Thourani VH, Weintraub WS, Guyton RA, et al: Outcomes and long-term survival for patients undergoing mitral valve repair versus replacement: Effect of age and concomitant coronary artery bypass grafting. Circulation 108:298, 2003.
26. Diodato MD, Moon MR, Pasque MK, et al: Repair of ischemic mitral regurgitation does not increase mortality or improve long-term survival in patients undergoing coronary artery revascularization: A propensity analysis. Ann Thorac Surg 78:794, 2004.
27. Wong DR, Agnihotri AK, Hung JW, et al: Long-term survival after surgical revascularization for moderate ischemic mitral regurgitation. Ann Thorac Surg 80:570, 2005.
28. Wu AH, Aaronson KD, Bolling SF, et al: Impact of mitral valve annuloplasty on mortality risk in patients with mitral regurgitation and left ventricular systolic dysfunction. J Am Coll Cardiol 45:381, 2005.
29. Daimon M, Fukuda S, Adams DH, et al: Mitral valve repair with Carpentier-McCarthy-Adams IMR ETlogix annuloplasty ring for ischemic mitral regurgitation: Early echocardiographic results from a multi-center study. Circulation 114:I588, 2006.
30. McCarthy PM, Bhudia SK, Rajeswaran J, et al: Tricuspid valve repair: Durability and risk factors for failure. J Thorac Cardiovasc Surg 127:674, 2004.
31. McCarthy PM: Aortic valve surgery in patients with left ventricular dysfunction. Semin Thorac Cardiovasc Surg 14:137, 2002.
32. Pereira JJ, Lauer MS, Bashir M, et al: Survival after aortic valve replacement for severe aortic stenosis with low transvalvular gradients and severe left ventricular dysfunction. J Am Coll Cardiol 39:1356, 2002.
33. Varadarajan P, Kapoor N, Bansal RC, et al: Clinical profile and natural history of 453 nonsurgically managed patients with severe aortic stenosis. Ann Thorac Surg 82:2111, 2006.
34. Quere JP, Monin JL, Levy F, et al: Influence of preoperative left ventricular contractile reserve on postoperative ejection fraction in low-gradient aortic stenosis. Circulation 113:1738, 2006.
35. Bhudia SK, McCarthy PM, Kumpati GS, et al: Improved outcomes after aortic valve surgery for chronic aortic regurgitation with severe left ventricular dysfunction. J Am Coll Cardiol 49:1465, 2007.

Left Ventricular Reconstruction and Passive Cardiac Support Devices

36. Mann DL: Mechanisms and models in heart failure: A combinatorial approach. Circulation 100:999, 1999.
37. McCarthy PM, McGee EC: Ventricular reconstruction and device therapies for cardiomyopathy patients. *In* Young J, McCarthy PM (eds): Heart Failure: A Combined Medical and Surgical Approach. Malden, MA, Blackwell Futura, 2006, pp 174-191.
38. Caldeira C, McCarthy PM: A simple method of left ventricular reconstruction without patch for ischemic cardiomyopathy. Ann Thorac Surg 72:2148, 2001.
39. George I, Cheng Y, Yi GH, et al: Effect of passive cardiac containment on ventricular synchrony and cardiac function in awake dogs. Eur J Cardiothorac Surg 31:55, 2007.
40. Athanasuleas CL, Buckberg GD, Stanley AW, et al: Surgical ventricular restoration in the treatment of congestive heart failure caused by post-infarction ventricular dilation. J Am Coll Cardiol 44:1439, 2004.
41. Artrip JH, Oz MC, Burkhoff D: Left ventricular volume reduction surgery for heart failure: A physiologic perspective. J Thorac Cardiovasc Surg 122:775, 2001.
42. O'Neill JO, Starling RC, McCarthy PM, et al: The impact of left ventricular reconstruction on survival in patients with ischemic cardiomyopathy. Eur J Cardiothorac Surg 30:753, 2006.
43. Di Donato, M, Sabatier M, Dor V, et al: Effects of the Dor procedure on left ventricular dimension and shape and geometric correlates of mitral regurgitation one year after surgery. J Thorac Cardiovasc Surg 121:91, 2001.
44. Saavedra WF, Tunin RS, Paolocci N, et al: Reverse remodeling and enhanced adrenergic reserve from passive external support in experimental dilated heart failure. J Am Coll Cardiol 39:2069, 2002.
45. Sabbah HN, Sharov VG, Gupta RC, et al: Reversal of chronic molecular and cellular abnormalities caused byheart failure by passive mechanical ventricular containment. Circ Res 93:1095, 2003.
46. Oz MC, Konertz WF, Kleber FX, et al: Global surgical experience with the Acorn cardiac support device. J Thorac Cardiovasc Surg 126:983, 2003.
47. McGee EC, Gillinov AM, McCarthy PM: Reverse ventricular remodeling: Mechanical options. Curr Opin Cardiol 21:215, 2006.

Cardiac Transplantation

48. Gasink LB, Blumberg EA, Localio AR, et al: Hepatitis C virus seropositivity in organ donors and survival in heart transplant recipients. JAMA 296:1843, 2006.
49. Zaroff JG, Rosengard BR, Armstrong WF, et al: Consensus conference report: Maximizing use of organs recovered from the cadaver donor: Cardiac recommendations, March 28-29, 2001, Crystal City, Va. Circulation 106:836, 2002.
50. Al Khaldi A, Robbins RC: New directions in cardiac transplantation. Annu Rev Med 57:455, 2006.
51. Morgan JA, John R, Weinberg AD, et al: Long-term results of cardiac transplantation in patients 65 years of age and older: A comparative analysis. Ann Thorac Surg 76:1982, 2003.
52. Drakos SG, Kfoury AG, Gilbert EM, et al: Multivariate predictors of heart transplantation outcomes in the era of chronic mechanical circulatory support. Ann Thorac Surg 83:62, 2007.
53. George I, Xydas S, Topkara VK, et al: Clinical indication for use and outcomes after inhaled nitric oxide therapy. Ann Thorac Surg 82:2161, 2006.
54. Jeevanandam V, Russell H, Mather P, et al: A one-year comparison of prophylactic donor tricuspid annuloplasty in heart transplantation. Ann Thorac Surg 78:759, 2004.
55. Bengel FM, Ueberfuhr P, Schiepel N, et al: Effect of sympathetic reinnervation on cardiac performance after heart transplantation. N Engl J Med 345:731, 2001.
56. Beniaminovitz A, Itescu S, Lietz K, et al: Prevention of rejection in cardiac transplantation by blockade of the interleukin-2 receptor with a monoclonal antibody. N Engl J Med 342:613, 2000.
57. Stewart S, Winters GL, Fishbein MC, et al: Revision of the 1990 working formulation for the standardization of nomenclature in the diagnosis of heart rejection. J Heart Lung Transplant 24:1710, 2005.
58. Taylor DO, Edwards LB, Boucek MM, et al: Registry of the International Society for Heart and Lung Transplantation: Twenty-third official adult heart transplantation report—2006. J Heart Lung Transplant 25:869, 2006.
59. McCarthy JF, McCarthy PM, Massad MG, et al: Risk factors for death after heart transplantation: Does a single-center experience correlate with multicenter registries? Ann Thorac Surg 65:1574, 1998.
60. Kobashigawa JA. First-year intravascular ultrasound results as a surrogate marker for outcomes after heart transplantation. J Heart Lung Transplant 22:711, 2003.
61. Iyengar S, Feldman DS, Cooke GE, et al: Detection of coronary artery disease in orthotopic heart transplant recipients with 64-detector row computed tomography angiography. J Heart Lung Transplant 25:1363, 2006.
62. Mahon NG, O'Neill JO, Young JB, et al: Contemporary outcomes of outpatients referred for cardiac transplantation evaluation to a tertiary heart failure center: Impact of surgical alternatives. J Card Fail 10:273, 2004.

CHAPTER 28

Assisted Circulation in the Treatment of Heart Failure

Yoshifumi Naka and Eric A. Rose

Although advanced medical therapy benefits increasing numbers of patients with progressive heart failure, the overall survival and quality of life for these patients remain limited. Cardiac transplantation represents the only treatment to provide substantial individual benefit in this setting (see Chap. 27). However, with donor availability limited to only 3000 annually worldwide, the overall impact of transplantation on heart failure has been described as "epidemiologically trivial."[1] Improving the survival and quality of life of patients with end-stage heart disease remains the ultimate goal of mechanical circulatory assistance. Over the past five decades, mechanical circulatory assist devices have evolved substantially. Intraaortic balloon pumps (IABPs) are now used widely in even small community hospitals, and a broad array of sophisticated univentricular, biventricular, short, long-term, and permanent assist devices are used at designated specialized centers. With this evolution, a better understanding of the technological drawbacks limiting current device design has developed, as well as a growing comprehension of appropriate indications for insertion and management. A total artificial heart has obtained. U.S. Food and Drug Administration (FDA) approval for bridging to transplantation[2] and a device whose design specifications allow for its use in neonates, infants, and children is expected to begin clinical trials in the near future.

History

Following the first clinical application of the heart-lung machine by John Gibbon in 1953, cardiopulmonary bypass has become a primary facilitator of modern heart surgery. DeBakey modified a concept first reported by Dennis in 1962, using left heart bypass as a means of extended postoperative support for patients who could not be separated from cardiopulmonary bypass. Development of the theory of counterpulsation as an adjunct allowing for systolic unloading and diastolic augmentation ultimately resulted in Kantrowitz's 1968 report of clinical application of IABP counterpulsation. Initiatives by the National Heart, Lung and Blood Institute (NHLBI), beginning in the 1970s, catalyzed the development of a family of mechanical assist devices, the direct predecessors of current devices. In the 1990s, extensive experience in bridging to transplantation enabled the evolution from bulky extracorporeal devices to smaller, "wearable" designs, which allowed patients to be discharged from the hospital and resume a wide range of activities. The bridging experience set the stage for the REMATCH (Randomized Evaluation for the Treatment of Congestive Heart Failure) trial, which clearly established the survival and quality of life advantage of implanted ventricular assist devices (VADs) in end-stage heart failure patients.[1] Today, VADs exist for a wide variety of conditions (see later). The surgical management of heart failure is discussed elsewhere (see Chap. 27).

INTRAAORTIC BALLOON COUNTERPULSATION

IABP counterpulsation represents one of the most common and widely available methods of mechanical circulatory support, and uses the concepts of systolic unloading and diastolic augmentation (Fig. 28-1). More than 22,000 IABPs were inserted worldwide from 1996 to 2001.[3] IABP counterpulsation has traditionally been used in various surgical and nonsurgical patients in the setting of cardiogenic shock or unstable angina (Table 28-1). It has been estimated that as many as 75 percent of patients who develop cardiogenic shock refractory to medical therapy in the setting of an acute myocardial infarction may improve with IABP use. The goal of IABP application in this setting is to stabilize the patient for revascularization (catheter-based or surgical) or insertion of a more durable VAD. For those undergoing insertion intraoperatively as an adjunct to weaning from cardiopulmonary bypass, IABP counterpulsation is used to offset temporary, reversible myocardial dysfunction.

In a cohort of patients undergoing IABP placement, in-hospital mortality rates varied significantly based on the indication for insertion. Patients receiving IABP support for refractory angina had a 6.4 percent mortality, for intraoperative support a 7.7 percent mortality, for weaning from cardiopulmonary bypass a 25.9 percent mortality, and for cardiogenic shock (without percutaneous or operative intervention) a 38.7 percent mortality.[3] Although the efficacy of IABP use in the setting of unstable or postinfarction angina is controversial, its use for those with ongoing ischemia, unstable angina, deteriorating hemodynamics, or ischemic ventricular tachyarrhythmia refractory to medical management is generally well supported.

The use of IABP is absolutely contraindicated in the setting of aortic insufficiency and aortic dissection. Relative contraindications for use via a femoral arterial approach relate to the vascular consequences of cannulation—significant aortoiliac or iliofemoral disease, and abdominal or descending thoracic aortic aneurysms.

Insertion Technique

The 30- to 50-ml balloon is generally positioned within the thoracic aorta, distal to the left subclavian artery and proximal to the renal arteries (see

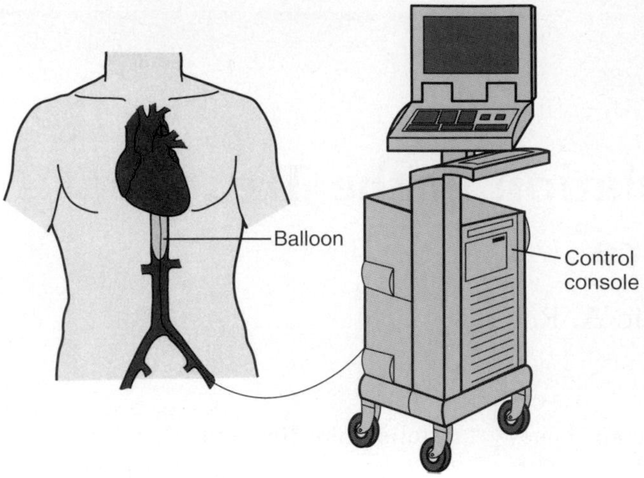

FIGURE 28–1 Intraaortic balloon pump and console, showing the inflated balloon in the descending aorta. *(Modified from Delgado R, Frazier OH, Razeghi P, Taegtmeyer H: Mechanical circulatory support in patients with heart failure.* In *Mann DL [ed]: Heart Failure: A Companion to Braunwald's Heart Disease. Philadelphia, Elsevier, 2004, pp 737-751.)*

TABLE 28–1	Indications for Intraaortic Balloon Pump Counterpulsation
Cardiogenic shock Postcardiotomy Associated with acute myocardial infarction Mechanical complications of myocardial infarction Mitral regurgitation Ventricular septal defect	
In association with coronary artery bypass surgery Preoperative insertion Patients with severe left ventricular dysfunction Patients with intractable ischemic arrhythmias Postoperative insertion Postcardiotomy cardiogenic shock	
In association with nonsurgical revascularization Hemodynamically unstable infarct patients High-risk coronary angioplasty Patients with severe left ventricular dysfunction Complex coronary artery disease	
Stabilization of cardiac transplant recipient before insertion of ventricular assist device	
Postinfarction angina	
Ventricular arrhythmias related to ischemia	

Fig. 28-1). The balloon is typically inserted percutaneously but can be also be placed via direct arterial cannulation from the femoral artery, the axillary artery or, in cases of postcardiotomy shock, through the ascending aorta. With appropriate synchronization, by an arterial blood pressure tracing or electrocardiogram, a set volume of gas is injected into the balloon from a bedside console during cardiac diastole and withdrawn during systole. Balloon inflation thus increases diastolic pressure, thereby augmenting coronary blood flow, whereas deflation reduces the afterload during ventricular contraction, thereby decreasing myocardial energy consumption (see Fig. 19-10). The frequency with which the balloon inflates can be timed to each, every other, or every third cardiac cycle and represents a method by which balloon support may be adjusted. Although IABP assistance affects the myocardial oxygen supply and demand ratio considerably, it has only modest effects on cardiac output, limited by the underlying contractility reserve of the ventricular myocardium.

Removal Technique

The patient may be weaned slowly from balloon support by adjusting the frequency with which the balloon inflates (e.g., 1:1 to 1:3). The patient's coagulation profile and platelet count should be normalized with exogenous blood products, if necessary, prior to balloon removal. Once hemodynamic stability with minimal support is confirmed, balloon inflation is discontinued. Manual pressure is held on the distal femoral artery and the balloon and sheath are removed. The proximal femoral artery is allowed to exsanguinate for 2 to 4 seconds to clear any debris, pressure is transferred to the proximal artery, and the distal artery is allowed to purge its debris. Pressure is then applied to the insertion site for at least 30 minutes.

Complications

The frequency of complications of IABP insertion ranges from 1 to 14 percent.[3] Most of the major morbidities relate to the sequelae of vascular compromise or problems encountered with insertion, which include limb ischemia requiring thrombectomy, revascularization, or amputation, aortic dissection, aortoiliac laceration, femoral artery pseudoaneurysm, retroperitoneal hemorrhage, renal ischemia from malposition, myocardial ischemia from poor timing of balloon augmentation, and deep wound infection requiring operative débridement. The incidence of limb ischemia has diminished slightly with the advent of smaller introducer sheaths and the development of a sheathless balloon technique. Unfortunately, the presence of irreversible limb ischemia from IABP insertion renders most such affected patients poor candidates for later treatment, and thus represents a condition for which ongoing vigilance in its earlier, potentially reversible, stages is mandatory.

VENTRICULAR ASSIST DEVICES

The clinical application of ventricular assist devices (VADs) grew from experience with their application in the operating room. Unlike the IABP, VADs function to reduce myocardial work by reducing ventricular preload while maintaining systemic circulation. They may be used for right ventricular (RVAD), left ventricular (LVAD), or biventricular (BiVAD) support for short-term (less than 1 week) or longer term support, and for permanent (destination therapy) use. The device may be completely extracorporeal, paracorporeal (juxtacorporeal), implantable but with percutaneous power support, or totally implantable, and it may provide continuous or pulsatile flow.

BASIC RATIONALE AND TREATMENT GOALS. Hemodynamic eligibility criteria for mechanical cardiac assistance have traditionally been those representative of cardiogenic shock refractory to medical therapies. In addition, those with intractable cardiac arrhythmias are considered candidates. The patient population has expanded from patients in decompensated chronic heart failure to include a large proportion of acute heart failure patients in cardiogenic shock. Although some reports have demonstrated better outcomes in stable patients awaiting transplantation, acceptable results have been obtained in this emerging acute patient population.[4,5]

There are essentially five therapeutic goals for which patient support with different types of VADs may be targeted, including bridge to recovery, bridge to bridge, bridge to the next decision (triage), bridge to transplant, and destination therapy (Table 28-2).

The first group of patients are those in whom reversibility of ventricular insult is anticipated, the so-called *bridge to recovery* group. Here, patients who may be experiencing postcardiotomy shock despite reasonable preoperative myocardial reserve or who may suffer from a potentially reversible process (e.g., acute myocarditis) benefit from short- to medium-term device support. The management of these patients (even if implanted elsewhere) should be continued at a specialized center experienced in weaning. After a short period of myocardial rest on VAD support, the device is weaned at the bedside or in the operating room, with guidance from transesophageal echocardiography. Resumption of native myocardial function in this setting may

TABLE 28–2 Indications for Ventricular Assist Device Implantation

Intended Use	Therapeutic Goal	Device	Outcomes: Quality of Life	Outcomes: Short-Term Survival (Days to Weeks)	Outcomes: Long-Term Survival (Months)
Bridge to recovery	Temporary support	IABP	+	++	0
		Centrifugal pump	+	+	0
		ECMO	+	+	0
		Abiomed	++	++	+
		HeartMate	+++	+++	+++
		Novacor	+++	+++	+++
Bridge to bridge	Stabilization to LVAD, BiVAD	Abiomed	++	++	+
		Centrifugal Pump	+	+	0
		ECMO	+	+	0
Triage	Bridge to the next decision	TandemHeart	+	+	0
		Impella	+	+	0
Bridge to transplantation	Support to transplantation	HeartMate	+++	+++	+++
		Novacor	+++	+++	+++
		Thoratec BiVAD	++	++	++
		CardioWest TAH	++	+	+
		Axial flow pumps	+++	++	++
Destination therapy	Permanent support	HeartMate	+++	+++	+++
		Novacor	+++	Undocumented—→	
		Axial flow pumps	+++	Undocumented—→	
		Centrifugal flow pumps	+++	Undocumented—→	

BiVAD = biventricular assist device; ECMO = extracorporeal membrane oxygenator; IABP = intraaortic balloon pump; LVAD = left ventricular assist device; TAH = total artificial heart.

allow for device removal (sometimes presaged by viability, as evidenced by positron emission tomography (PET). If hemodynamic decompensation ensues after device removal, a more long-term or permanent device should be considered. Furthermore, as discussed in Chapter 22, a growing number of reports has suggested that VAD support can lead to reverse remodeling at genetic, biochemical, and histological levels; however, only a few centers have achieved a clinically meaningful rate of ventricular recovery leading to the explantation of a device in those with end-stage chronic congestive heart failure.[6] Hon and Yacoub have indicated another possibility, active ventricular remodeling using a supplemental modality to LVAD.[7] At the same time, cell transplantation has gained enthusiasm to treat failing hearts, and several clinical trials have been reported.[8,9]

The second, the *bridge to bridge* cohort, refers to patients who experience acute cardiogenic shock, postcardiotomy or without an operation, at a center that does not offer transplantation or long-term assist devices. In these patients, the efficacious institution of short-term assistance and rapid transfer to a center specialized in ventricular assist support is warranted.[5]

The third group is the *triage* cohort. Patients develop acute critical heart failure caused by massive acute myocardial infarction, fulminant myocarditis, or acute decompensation of stable chronic heart failure. The condition of these patients does not allow thorough assessment of transplant eligibility, reversibility of myocardial function, reversibility of other end-organ function, and mental status. Devices designed for these acute patients are implanted to determine the next step—bridge to long-term device implantation toward heart transplantation, myocardial recovery following interventional or surgical revascularization, or device explantation. The devices are easily and quickly inserted with a minimally invasive technique, such as a percutaneous or peripheral approach.[10,11]

The fourth group of patients is the traditional *bridge to transplant* cohort, who meet the criteria for transplantation and undergo VAD insertion to improve their overall transplantation candidacy.[4] This decision by necessity limits the patient cohort to those younger than 65 years in most cases and often is delineated by blood group; a transplant candidate who is blood type O probably has a protracted waiting time, and thus a lower threshold to device insertion while waiting. Because of concerns regarding infection and the potential need for long-term support, these patients require a more long-term device, preferably implantable, for bridging.

Finally, patients are selected who are *destination therapy* candidates. Several prospective randomized trials including the Randomized Evaluation of Mechanical Assistance for the Treatment of Congestive Heart Failure (REMATCH) and two current studies (Novacor and HeartMate II) are investigating the efficacy of permanent LVAD insertion for patients who are not transplant candidates. REMATCH has demonstrated clear advantages in overall survival and quality of life.[1] Limited survival beyond 2 years of device implantation, as well as a high incidence of adverse device-associated events, have limited the application of destination therapy implants. Extension of destination therapy to more end-stage patients and those with less severe but seriously debilitating heart failure has promoted the ongoing strong interest in the development of simpler, more durable devices, with fewer associated complications.

Indications for Ventricular Assist Device Support

The indications for VAD insertion are in flux. With further experience, the spectrum of disease for which VADs are implanted continues to expand, while our understanding of the timing of implementation and the specific cohorts for which it is appropriate becomes more refined. Broadly speaking, patients in profound shock with end-organ dysfunction and biventricular heart failure need early, efficacious support to avoid permanent end-organ damage and increase their chances of survival. The preferred devices in such a scenario are ones that may provide full ventricular support reestablishing nearly normal hemodynamics, and potentially allowing myocardial recovery. If a prolonged support period is expected, a longer term BiVAD device may be implanted or, if preferred, a longer term LVAD may be used with concomitant use of a short-term RVAD. A total artificial heart (TAH) may in some cases restore end-organ function more quickly, thus providing enhanced survival to transplantation in those who have severe end-organ dysfunction.[2]

POSTCARDIOTOMY SHOCK. Patients undergoing cardiac surgical procedures are at risk for myocardial injury because of myocardial stunning and ischemia, insufficient myocardial protection, reperfusion injury, and cardiac arrhythmias. These patients may be categorized into two groups: (1) those who had persistent or significant dysfunction prior to surgery (and are unlikely to be weaned off device support); and (2) those who had adequate myocardial reserve prior to surgery (and who may only require a few days of temporary support). In general, for those patients who are unable to wean from cardiopulmonary bypass but who maintain otherwise reasonable end-organ function, often the best strategy temporary VAD placement, which may stabilize the patient long enough to be transferred to a center with more experience and more choices of long-term devices should the patient be deemed unweanable.[5] Patients undergoing high-risk cardiac surgery may need mechanical ventricular support if the surgical procedure is not successful. Ideally, such patients should be screened for transplantation candidacy preoperatively and cardiac surgery scheduled with LVAD back-up, in the event that LVAD support and subsequent heart transplantation are needed. Although postcardiotomy shock formerly represented the indication on which early clinical application of VADs was approved, increasing experience with device support in this population has been disappointing. Survival to discharge using short-term extracorporeal devices can be achieved in only 25 percent of patients. Progression to fully implantable devices, if native myocardial recovery does not occur quickly, may enhance outcomes in potentially transplantable patients. Destination therapy experience in this cohort is extremely limited.

CARDIOGENIC SHOCK AFTER ACUTE MYOCARDIAL INFARCTION (see Chap. 50). The survival of patients in cardiogenic shock because of acute myocardial infarction (AMI) often depends on the timely institution of circulatory support.[29] Cardiogenic shock is thought to occur when more than 40 percent of ventricular mass is lost to infarction; without some form of cardiac assistance, this condition is associated with an 80 percent mortality and, even with early revascularization, 1-year survival remains less than 50 percent in these patients.[12] Although controversial, it has been our contention that coronary artery bypass grafting (CABG) may be detrimental to those who suffer acute myocardial infarction with cardiogenic shock if VAD implantation is contemplated. Although LVAD support allows for myocardial rest, in this setting it is highly unlikely that myocardial recovery sufficient to allow for LVAD weaning and explantation would develop. Thus, we advocate early institution of VAD support *without* CABG for this subset of patients. This approach avoids another operation involving cardiopulmonary bypass (for the CABG), as well as additional technical problems of inserting an implantable LVAD with fresh coronary artery bypass grafts in place.[13] The insertion of a minimally invasive VAD, such as TandemHeart or Impella, allows triage of those in cardiogenic shock following acute myocardial infarction (MI) to the next level of care—revascularization and recovery if the myocardium improves spontaneously, bridge to transplant VAD insertion if the myocardium fails but end-organs do recover, or palliative care for comfort in patients whose end-organs continue to deteriorate.

DECOMPENSATED CHRONIC HEART FAILURE

Transplant Eligible. Because of the increase in waiting times, some patients awaiting transplantation deteriorate hemodynamically, with further worsening of end-organ function, and require increasing doses of intravenous inotropes. These patients may not have been listed for transplantation at the time of failure, although often they are followed at transplantation centers. In the absence of an immediately available donor organ, this indication for VAD support allows for the establishment of hemodynamic stability, restoration of end-organ function, and opportunity for nutritional support and rehabilitation pretransplantation. In these patients, long-term support must be considered. Some patients are not deemed candidates for transplantation at the time of LVAD implant because of marginal end-organ function, most commonly renal impairment. For these patients, LVAD support often reverses this injury and allows for full recovery of end-organ function, thereby rendering such patients good transplantation candidates. Other patients in this cohort are those with deteriorating heart failure with a recent history of malignancy in remission. Device therapy restores end-organ function and allows more time to confirm the durability of the remission.

Transplant Ineligible. Other patients are not candidates for transplantation at the time of LVAD implantation on the basis of age or other absolute criteria. When these patients decompensate, LVAD implantation is performed with the anticipation of permanent use for destination therapy. Less than 300 patients have received destination therapy implants since the FDA approval of this indication in 2002. The REMATCH indications for destination therapy remain the standard in this area.

ACUTE MYOCARDITIS AND VENTRICULAR ARRHYTHMIAS (see Chap. 66). LVAD implantation for acute myocarditis, particularly in young patients, sometimes may be used as a bridge to recovery rather than to transplantation. Unfortunately, it is difficult to determine which patients will benefit from short-term support and which will require long-term devices with subsequent transplantation; thus, we believe that one should prepare for long-term support.[14] We advocate initial insertion of a long-term device to allow for expeditious extubation and rehabilitation. After a sufficient degree of rehabilitation has taken place, cardiac function may be evaluated carefully and the device may be explanted if recovery sufficient to sustain reasonable hemodynamics has been documented; if no appreciable recovery has been demonstrated, the patient may be bridged to transplantation. Patients with ventricular arrhythmias represent a unique population in that, aside from the arrhythmia, their contractile function may not be compromised significantly. Nevertheless, if pharmacological therapy and defibrillators have failed, VAD support may be warranted and has successfully been implemented in these cases.[15] Although ventricular decompression often helps control the arrhythmias, persistent ventricular arrhythmias are generally well tolerated in device-supported patients.

Perioperative Risk and Contraindications to Left Ventricular Assist Device Implantation

The selection process for VAD implantation must reach a balance between a too liberal listing of highest risk patients who have unacceptably high mortality rates, and too conservative an approach that overlooks patients who would otherwise have benefited from VAD support. Indeed, judicious use of this resource is essential, because VAD implantation incurs significant social and financial investment. To this end, a scoring system has been devised to determine relative risk and predict which patients would have successful outcomes after LVAD implantation (Table 28-3). With this scoring system, a sum of higher than 5 corresponds to a 47 percent post-LVAD mortality, as opposed to a 9 percent mortality for a score of lower than 5.[16] The acuity of heart failure has also been demonstrated to affect patient survival. In a study by Deng and colleagues, patients receiving emergent LVADs because of acute heart failure had a lower survival to transplantation when compared with those receiving devices for chronic failure or with those who did not need devices while awaiting transplantation.[4] In patients with chronic heart failure advanced age, female gender, diabetes, and a low preoperative albumin level predict poor clinical course.[17]

TABLE 28–3	Revised Risk Factor Summation Score: Left Ventricular Assist Device Screening Score	
Variable	**Relative Risk**	**Weight**
Mechanical ventilation	5.3	4
Postcardiotomy	3.3	2
Prior LVAD	3.3	2
Central venous pressure >16 mm Hg	2.1	1
Prothrombin time > 16 seconds	2.1	1
Excluded by multivariable analysis:		
Prior RVAD	3.2	
Coronary artery disease	2.0	
Acute myocardial infarction	1.7	
Urine output <30 ml/hr	1.2	
Reoperative surgery	1.1	

LVAD = left ventricular assist device; RVAD = right ventricular assist device.
Modified from Rao V, Oz MC, Flannery MA, et al: Revised screening scale to predict survival after insertion of a left ventricular assist device. J Thorac Cardiovasc Surg 125:855, 2003.

Although the contraindications to VAD insertion have diminished substantially, several remain. Most importantly, patients with irreversible end-organ failure are poor device candidates. In particular, those with long-standing renal failure have a prohibitively high morbidity and mortality after VAD insertion because of difficulties in fluid management and the infectious risks of long-term dialysis access. These patients are also unlikely to be transplantation candidates. Irreversible neurological injury also represents a strong contraindication to VAD insertion. Although this may be difficult to assess in the immediate postcardiotomy or acute cardiogenic shock setting, it is important to evaluate prior to VAD insertion. Sedation in obtunded patients should be reduced to confirm the integrity of underlying neurological dysfunction. Overwhelming infection or sepsis represents an absolute contraindication to insertion. Bacteremia may lead to device infection, with the potential for device endocarditis, prolonged sepsis, and multiorgan failure and certainly should be treated prior to LVAD insertion. In a review of device infection, less than 20 percent of patients with infected devices had a successful outcome.[18]

Device Selection

Device selection is invariably influenced by availability and physicians' experiences. Although many studies have been published on individual devices, no study has rigorously compared devices. FDA-approved devices include the following: (1) Abiomed BVS 5000i and AB5000 ventricle for postcardiotomy and post–acute MI (AMI) cardiogenic shock; (2) Thoratec paracorporeal and intracorporeal devices, Novacor LVAS, and pneumatic (model IP) and vented electric (model VE) HeartMate LVAD for bridge to transplantation; and (3) HeartMate XVE LVAD for destination therapy. Various implantable devices, including the Jarvik 2000, HeartMate II, and MicroMed-DeBakey axial flow pumps and the VentrAssist, DuraHeart, and Cor-Aide, implantable centrifugal devices, are being implanted for bridge to transplant or destination therapy under investigational device exemptions (IDEs). In addition to the FDA-approved devices, there are several other VADs in development and clinical use (see later).

Important clinical issues to consider when choosing a device include the expected duration of support, need for biventricular support, cost, device-related risks (e.g., the need for anticoagulation and device failure rates), patient characteristics (especially the size and blood type of the patient), and United Network of Organ Sharing (UNOS) classification rules. Institutional standards of care, ranging from community practice to tertiary heart failure and transplantation centers, also influence device selection. With regard to the size of the patient, the implantable HeartMate XVE and Novacor LVADs require patients' body surface area (BSA) to be more than 1.5 m^2.

Short-Term Devices

EXTRACORPOREAL CENTRIFUGAL PUMPS. Centrifugal pumps were first introduced as alternatives to roller pumps for cardiopulmonary bypass and have been available since the late 1970s for use as short-term cardiac support. These pumps are widely available, relatively inexpensive, and simple to insert and use. They may be used for right, left, or biventricular support and require systemic anticoagulation. One of the most commonly used is the Biomedicus Biopump (Medtronic Biomedicus, Inc., Eden Prairie, MN), which consists of an acrylic pump head with inlet and outlet ports oriented at right angles. The pump is versatile and may be used as an RVAD (from the right atrium or right ventricle to pulmonary artery), as an LVAD (from the left atrium or left ventricular apex to aorta), or as part of an extracorporeal membrane oxygenation (ECMO) circuit.

This device has several disadvantages. First, the need for systemic anticoagulation to an activated clotting time of 200 seconds increases the probability and magnitude of bleeding complications. Second, there is an appreciable amount of interstitial edema potentially created by increased capillary permeability as part of a systemic inflammatory response. Finally, the device requires continuous supervision by specially trained personnel. The centrifugal pump system can incorporate membrane oxygenation in its circuit (ECMO) to provide additional pulmonary support. Although its success has been extensively documented in the neonatal and infant population, the outcomes of its use for adults have been less promising.[19] The main indications for ECMO are the need for mechanical assistance in the face of combined pulmonary failure or pure respiratory failure. When initially used for postcardiotomy cardiogenic shock, survival rates were low (25 percent). Major limitations include a requirement for sedation or paralysis to effect immobilization and full systemic heparinization. Complications are common, including leg ischemia, renal failure, bleeding, and oxygenator failure. Overall, the successful use of ECMO in adults has been limited to selected centers.[19]

ABIOMED BVS 5000i AND AB5000 VENTRICLE. The Abiomed BVS 5000i (Abiomed Cardiovascular, Inc., Danvers, MA) is a short-term univentricular or biventricular support system comprised of external pumps driven by a computer-controlled drive console. Since its initial FDA approval for the setting of postcardiotomy failure, the indications for its use have expanded to include acute myocardial infarction, myocarditis, right ventricular support in conjunction with a long-term LVAD, bridge to recovery, and bridge to transplantation. As a result, the device has become one of the most commonly used means of short-term mechanical cardiac support.[20]

The device is an extracorporeal dual-chamber device composed of two 100-ml polyurethane blood sacs, the inlet and outlet portions of which are guarded by polyurethane valves (see Fig. 28-e1 on website). The device ejects blood by compression of the prosthetic ventricle by a pneumatic drive console. One particular advantage of the BVS 5000i system is its weanability; a hand dial on the console allows the device flow to be weaned manually to off. When used in conjunction with echocardiograms and measures of hemodynamics, this feature allows for easy bedside assessment of return of myocardial function. Other advantages are the ease of insertion and simplicity in operation, obviating the need for a full-time perfusionist at the bedside. The system functions reliably for several days, and has even been used as long as 90 days. Disadvantages of this device include the requirement for continuous anticoagulation, limited mobility, and the requirement of intensive care unit (ICU) monitoring and management.

The Abiomed AB5000 VAD has been recently approved by the FDA (see Fig. 28-e2 on website). The prosthetic ventricle is driven by a fully automatic, vacuum-assisted console, which can be used for both the BVS 5000i and AB5000, and it shares the same cannulas and insertion technique as the BVS 5000i. The important advantage of the AB5000 over the BVS 5000i is its paracorporeal placement, thus allowing ambulation and longer term support.[21]

TANDEMHEART. The TandemHeart (CardiacAssist, Inc., Pittsburgh) is a short-term univentricular assist device intended for use up to 14 days (see Fig. 28-e3 on website). This device can be placed using a percutaneous technique, inserting the inflow cannula in the left atrium through the femoral vein and right atrium and across the interatrial septum. The outflow cannula is placed in the femoral artery, and both cannulas are connected to the extracorporeal miniaturized centrifugal pump. This feature enables rapid and minimally invasive institution of mechanical assistance. It flows up to 4 liters/min and has been shown to reverse severe cardiogenic shock caused by myocardial infarction.[10] The device is commercially available in the United States and has been implanted in more than 500 cases worldwide. Disadvantages of the device include the requirement for continuous anticoagulation and ICU monitoring and management and limited mobility.

IMPELLA. The Impella devices (Abiomed Cardiovascular Inc., Danvers, MA) are minimally invasive catheter-based pumps that can be implanted percutaneously via a cutdown of the femoral or axillary artery or directly to the ascending aorta (see Fig. 28-e4 on website). The system consists of the implantable pump and a mobile console. A microaxial flow pump at the tip of the catheter placed in the left ventricle through the aortic valve propels blood to the outflow portion of the device in the ascending aorta. The placement requires precise adjustment under transesophageal echocardiography (TEE) or fluoroscopic guidance. There are two sizes available; the one that can flow up to 5 liters/min requires surgical insertion via a peripheral artery or a graft on the ascending aorta. This class of device has been shown to help postcardiotomy shock patients[11] and is available in Europe under CE Mark approval. The other can be inserted percutaneously but can flow up to 2.5 liters/min. Advantages and disadvantages of the devices are similar to those of the TandemHeart. The devices are being evaluated in the United States in investigational trials.

ORQIS CANCION SYSTEM. The CANCION system is under clinical investigation in the United States as a novel interventional approach to treat acutely decompensated congestive heart failure (CHF) patients who do not respond adequately to standard medical therapy. The system consists of two catheters, one introduced in the proximal descending thoracic aorta and the other in the femoral artery, and a small blood pump, which draws the blood from the distal part of the aorta and ejects to the proximal part.

Long-Term Support

WITH PULSATILE DEVICES

Several key characteristics apply to the development of long-term device design and are helpful in considering their advantages and disadvantages. First, all pulsatile long-term devices require inflow and outflow valves. In some, these are tissue valves; in others, they are mechanical valves and require long-term anticoagulation. The blood–contact surface of the device also must be addressed with regard to anticoagulation. To overcome the need for anticoagulation, the HeartMate XVE uses an innovative textured surface, which ultimately becomes lined with a pseudoneointima so densely adherent to the surface that embolization is virtually precluded (see Fig. 28-e5 on website).[22] The disadvantage is that its neointima may also act as an immunologically active entity, which can itself promote a form of autoimmunity and immunological reactivity that limits the ultimate transplantability of its recipients.[22-24] Rates of embolization in patients receiving textured surface pulsatile devices have been lower than those with smooth internal surfaces, despite the need for systemic anticoagulation in the latter. However, durability of the single-pusher plate actuation mechanism of the HeartMate LVADs has been substantially less than the double-pusher plate in the Novacor design.[25]

HEARTMATE LEFT VENTRICULAR ASSIST DEVICE (IMPLANTABLE). Devices in the pulsatile HeartMate LVAD family (Thoratec Corporation, Pleasanton, CA) were introduced in 1975 (Fig. 28-2). The system was originally a pneumatic vented (IP) design requiring a large console that limited patients' mobility outside the hospital. In 1991, a clinical trial of the wearable VE model with portable battery units was begun and demonstrated greater mobility, allowing hospital discharge.[26] Since then, both models have demonstrated a 60 to 70 percent rate of survival to transplantation. The worldwide average implant duration is 80 to 100 days, and maximum duration of support has exceeded 2 years. However, in the REMATCH trial, the probability of device failure was demonstrated to be 35 percent at 2 years.[1] Dowling and associates have shown that subsequent modi-

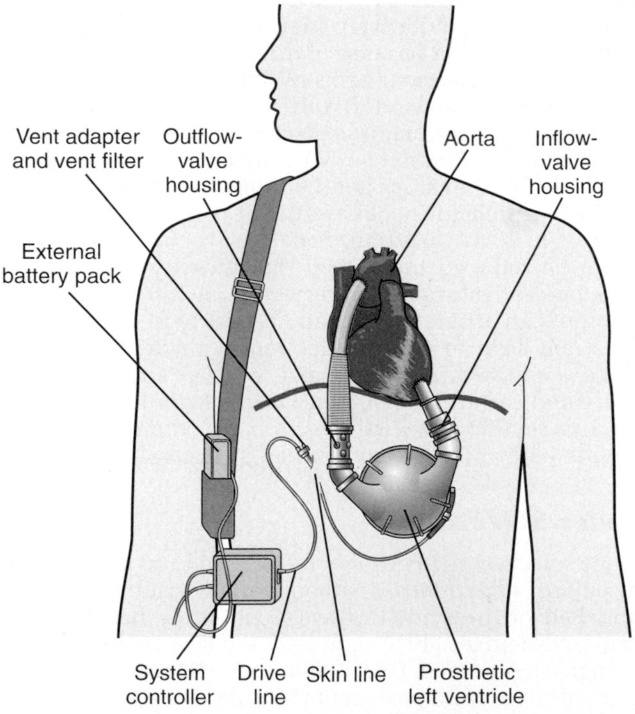

FIGURE 28–2 Components of the left ventricular assist device. The inflow cannula is inserted into the apex of the left ventricle and the outflow cannula is anastomosed to the ascending aorta. Blood returns from the lungs to the left side of the heart and exits through the left ventricular apex and across an inflow valve into the prosthetic pumping chamber. Blood is then actively pumped through an outflow valve into the ascending aorta. The pumping chamber is placed within the abdominal wall or peritoneal cavity. A percutaneous drive line carries the electrical cable and air vent to the battery packs (only the pack on the right side is shown) and electronic controls, which are worn on a shoulder holster or belt, respectively. *(From Rose EA, Gelijns AC, Moskowitz AJ, et al; Randomized Evaluation of Mechanical Assistance for the Treatment of Congestive Heart Failure [REMATCH] Study Group: Long-term mechanical left ventricular assistance for end-stage heart failure. N Engl J Med 345:1435, 2001.)*

fications of the device design may improve durability and reliability.[27]

The HeartMate has a titanium-alloy external housing, with inflow and outflow conduits that use porcine xenograft valves (25 mm). The unique characteristic of the device is its internal blood-contacting surface, which is made of textured titanium on one side and textured polyurethane on the other. This textured surface results in the deposition of a fibrin-cellular matrix that forms a pseudoneointima. The formation of this surface decreases the need for anticoagulation, because embolization is greatly reduced. Patients with these devices take aspirin (for antiinflammation, but not primarily for anticoagulation), with a remarkably low rate of thromboembolic complications and without the need for warfarin (Coumadin). The device has a pumping capacity in excess of 9 liters/min and pulsatile flow is created using a pusher plate system. The device is operated in a fixed-rate or automatic mode; in automatic mode, the pump senses when the chamber is full and activates the pusher plate. The pump is inserted into the left upper quadrant of the abdomen preperitoneally or intraperitoneally. The drive line, consisting of an air vent and power-controller cables, is tunneled subcutaneously and brought out of the skin in the right upper quadrant. Small battery units, worn in a harness, are connected to the cables; battery life is between 4 and 6 hours, depending on the patient's activity level. In case of an emergency, a portable hand pump can be used to activate the device pneumatically.

NOVACOR (IMPLANTABLE). The Novacor (World Heart Corporation, Ottawa, ON, Canada) left ventricular assist system (LVAS) was first successfully used in 1984 as a bridge to transplantation (see Fig. 28-e6 on website). Initially, it was designed as a console-based controller system, but since 1993 has been available with a wearable controller. This system has proven to be reliable, with about 55 to 65 percent of patients surviving to transplantation.[28] The worldwide mean time of support using this system is 85 days, with the device lasting as long as 962 days.

The pump works using dual pusher plates that compress a polyurethane sac. Bioprosthetic valves, 25 mm, are used in the inflow and outflow tracts. The placement of the device is almost identical to that for the HeartMate. However, unlike the HeartMate system, Novacor LVAS patients require anticoagulation with warfarin to avoid embolic events. The prevalence of embolic cerebrovascular events is estimated to be between 27 and 41 percent.[28] An inflow cannula made with Gore-Tex has been introduced, designed to reduce thromboembolic events, with a reported rate of cerebrovascular complications of 10 percent.[29]

PARACORPOREAL PULSATILE DEVICES: THORATEC. The Thoratec paracorporeal VAD is a commonly used system for biventricular support (see Fig. 28-e7 on website). Unlike the Novacor and HeartMate, this paracorporeal system can be applied for univentricular or biventricular support. Because the actual pump chamber is outside the body, this device can be used on patients with a BSA body sizes too small to house the HeartMate or Novacor devices (i.e., smaller than 1.5 m^2). However, a paracorporeal system also limits mobility and thus presents an obstacle for patients in a long-term setting.

The pump consists of a prosthetic ventricle with a maximum stroke volume of 65 ml and cannulas for ventricular or atrial inflow and arterial outflow. Currently, a large pneumatic drive console is available, as well as a smaller, briefcase-sized, power driver unit. Pneumatic drivers provide alternating air pressure to fill and empty the blood pump, and the pump flow rate ranges from 1.3 to 7.2 liters/min. Whereas inflow cannula placement can occur in an atrial or ventricular position, ventricular cannula placement is preferred for left-sided support, because it allows for greater flow rates than atrial cannulation. Anticoagulation with warfarin or heparin is necessary, as in patients with mechanical valves. This device has been used in over 1000 patients for univentricular and biventricular support for both bridge to transplantation and postcardiotomy recovery. Survival to transplantation has been between 60 and 80 percent, depending on which ventricle was supported.[30] Like the BVS 5000i and AB5000 ventricle, the biggest advantage of this system is its versatility; it is easy to place with less surgical dissection and can be used for patients of different sizes, attached to the atrium or ventricle, and used for right and left heart support. However, its paracorporeal location potentially limits the patient's activity and thus limits its use as a permanent device.

THORATEC INTRACORPOREAL VENTRICULAR ASSIST DEVICE. The Thoratec intracorporeal VAD is being designed by the same firm that developed the paracorporeal device . The advantages of this system will be its small size, reliability, implantable right, left, and biventricular systems, and similar technology based on the currently used Thoratec paracorporeal platform. It is targeted toward patients who would benefit from long-term support and the benefits of an implanted device.

TOTAL ARTIFICIAL HEART. The CardioWest TAH (Syncardia, Tucson, AZ) began as the Jarvik-7 TAH that was used in the 1980s. It is a pneumatic, biventricular, orthotopically implanted total artificial heart with an externalized drive line to its console (Fig. 28-3).[31] It consists of two spherical polyurethane chambers with polyurethane diaphragms. Inflow and outflow conduits are constructed of Dacron and contain Medtronic-Hall (Medtronic, Inc., Minneapolis) valves. Despite early obstacles, a new investigational device exemption study began in 1993 and demonstrated support for durations of 12 to 186 days, with a 93 percent survival to transplantation.[31] The device was approved by the FDA as a bridge to transplantation device in 2005 based on 79 percent survival to transplantation of 81 patients.[2] The TAH benefits from the ability to provide complete support and, unlike the other devices, it obviates the presence of the native heart. This is particularly useful in situations in which leaving the native heart in place would be detrimental or impossible (e.g., cardiac tumors). However, adequate intrathoracic space is required to accommodate the TAH. Fitting criteria include a BSA more than 1.7 m^2, anterior-posterior distance more than 10 cm, and combined ventricular volume larger than 1500 ml. Careful intraoperative fitting is critical. In addition to size requirements, strict anticoagulation with warfarin, aspirin, and pentoxifylline is needed. Although rehabilitation and hospital discharge have been an obstacle for the acceptance of this device because of the current design of the large console, the por-

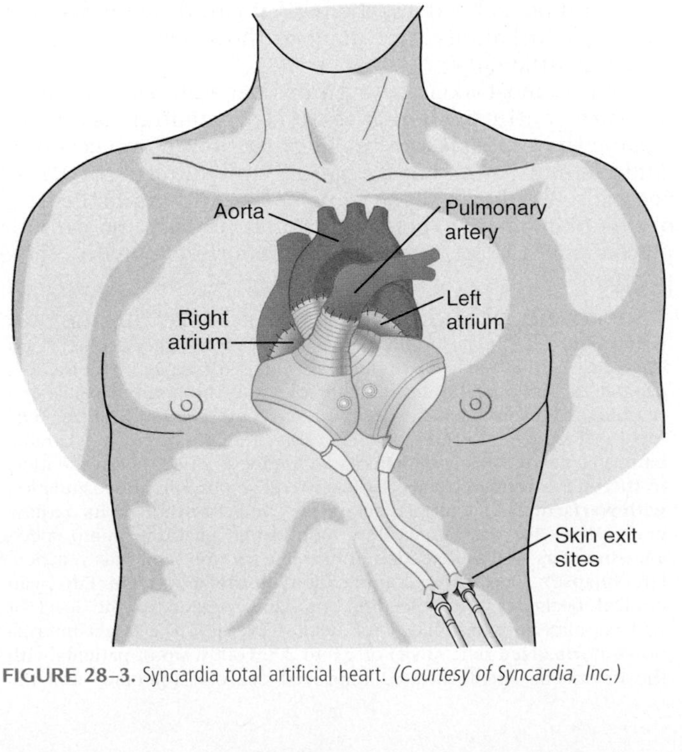

FIGURE 28–3. Syncardia total artificial heart. *(Courtesy of Syncardia, Inc.)*

table console designed for the Berlin Heart Excor device enables this device's recipients to be ambulated.

The AbioCor TAH (Abiomed Cardiovascular Inc., Danvers, MA) consists of an internal thoracic pump, an internal rechargeable battery, internal electronics, and an external battery pack. Clinical trials with the device were halted because of excessive neurological events with the device. An application for Humanitarian Device Exemption approval from the FDA has been recently approved.

TOTALLY IMPLANTABLE PULSATILE DEVICES. There are two devices in this class. One is the Arrow-Lionheart LVD-2000, which is the first system with a transcutaneous energy transmission system and a compliance chamber that allows for complete implantation with no percutaneous lines or connections. The device trial is currently on hold. The other is the Novacor II, which is currently in preclinical testing (see Fig. 28-e8 on website).

NONPULSATILE DEVICES

Axial flow pumps represent one of the newest generations of assist devices. They can provide full cardiac support in a much smaller pump with fewer moving parts and a smaller blood-contacting surface than volume displacement devices. Their small size allows implantation into smaller patients than most pulsatile pumps, with easier device placement and explantation in patients of all sizes compared with larger systems. With fewer moving parts, there are fewer points of friction; therefore, expected durability is increased. However, the bearings of these devices are lubricated with blood, a characteristic that may ultimately limit durability. In addition, shear rates with resultant hemolysis remain a concern.

In addition to their small size, axial flow pumps are notable for nonpulsatile flow. Several studies have demonstrated metabolic and neurohumoral changes in organ perfusion with nonpulsatile flow. However, both clinical and long-term animal studies have failed to demonstrate significant differences in morbidity and mortality with axial flow pumps.[32] Additionally, many patients maintain some native cardiac function during axial pump support and therefore continue to have low-pulsatile patterns of blood flow. Conversely, in the event of a device failure, few options or backup mechanisms exist for axial flow pumps other than replacement and, if device malfunction does occur, because these pumps lack valves, the patient can develop hemodynamic perturbations equivalent to those seen with severe aortic insufficiency.

Finally, most axial flow pumps generate such negative pressure continuously that there is a potential risk of collapsing the ventricle and causing transient pump cessation (and therefore thrombus formation), and fluttering of the left ventricle which can cause ventricular arrhythmia. Because of this phenomenon, both ventricular preload and cannula placement are of paramount importance with these pumps.

MICROMED DEBAKEY VENTRICULAR ASSIST DEVICE. This pump unit is 1.2 inches in diameter, 3 inches long, and weighs 95 gm (Fig. 28-4). It is made of titanium casing with an impeller-inducer capable of pumping 10 liters/min. The rest of the pump consists of a titanium inflow cannula, flowmeter, Dacron outflow graft (Sulzer Inc., Austin, TX), and a percutaneous cable connecting to a wearable battery-control console. The implantation technique is nearly identical to the one described earlier. Patients require chronic anticoagulation with warfarin and an antiplatelet agent. The flow probe on its outflow graft allows for continuous flow monitoring, enabling pump speed adjustment as well as detection of extreme suction (and thus ventricular collapse). The major complication of this device in European clinical trials was late bleeding, probably related to the level of anticoagulation, which has since been decreased to a target international normalized ratio (INR) of 2.0 to 2.5. Follow-up of patients with the device has demonstrated improved exercise tolerance and the

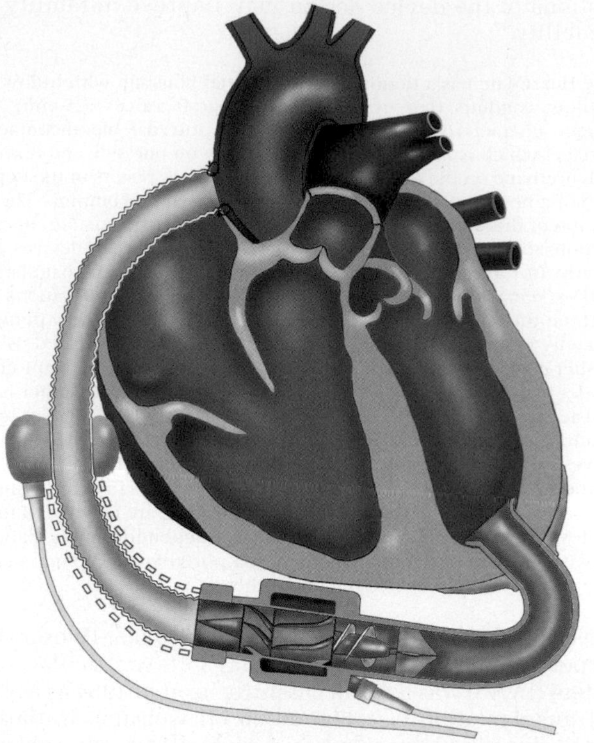

FIGURE 28–4 MicroMed DeBakey axial flow pump. *(Courtesy of MicroMed, Inc.)*

ability to be discharged home with the device while awaiting transplantation.[33] This pump was been implanted in over 300 patients worldwide. An unacceptably high incidence of device thrombosis requiring thrombolysis or device replacement has led to a reevaluation of the pump design.

HEARTMATE II. HeartMate II is an axial flow rotary LVAD made of titanium, capable of producing flow rates more than 10 liters/min at up to 13,000 rpm of the device rotor (see Fig. 28-e9 on website). The implantation technique is almost identical to that of the HeartMate XVE except for its abdominal pocket. Anticoagulation is currently required to keep the INR between 1.5 and 2.5. Power and control are supplied by a percutaneous lead that attaches to a power base unit or portable rechargeable batteries. The pivotal study of the bridge to transplantation arm has now completed enrollment; the destination therapy arm of the trial is actively enrolling patients. The study also has an arm that can provide an option of exchanging a failed HeartMate XVE with a HeartMate II. As of August 2006, this pump has been implanted in over 400 patients.

There are two other axial flow pumps that have been actively tested in the clinical setting, the Jarvik 2000 (Fig. 28-5) and the Incor (see Fig. 28-e10 on website). Unlike the other pumps described in this chapter, the Jarvik 2000 is positioned inside the ventricle, with the outflow graft anastomosed to the descending aorta through a left thoracotomy. Placement of the Incor is identical to the DeBakey and HeartMate II insertion techniques.

Miniaturized Centrifugal Pumps

Years after the invention of centrifugal pumps, researchers are reevaluating these pumps as the third generation of implantable circulatory assist devices. One example is the Levitronix LVAS (Levitronix, Waltham, MA), a pump built on the magnetic levitation concept, which allows the motor to levitate the rotor magnetically so that rotation is achieved without friction, with less thrombogenicity, and with anticipated long-term durability because of lack of metal-to-metal contact (see Fig. 28-e11 on website). The DuraHeart (Terumo, Ann Arbor, MI) (see Fig. 28-e12 on website) and the CorAide device (Arrow International, Cleveland, OH) are based on a similar concept and design. These pumps are currently in clinical trials in Europe and the United States. The VentrAssist (VentraCor, Chatswood, New South Wales,

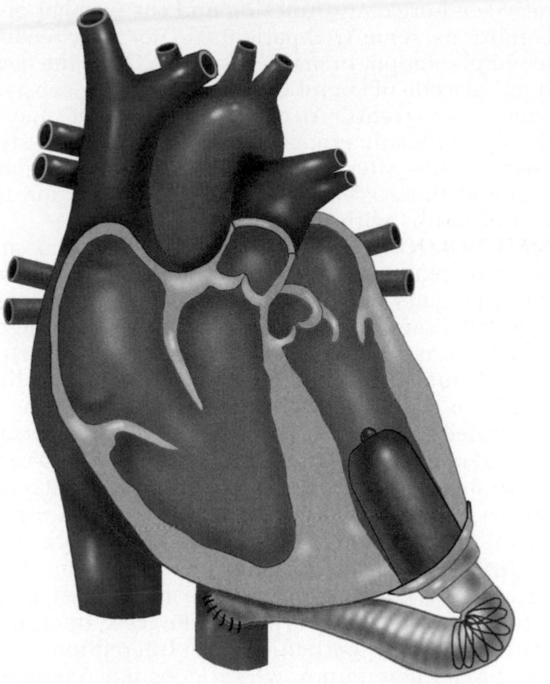

FIGURE 28–5 The Jarvik 2000 axial flow pump. *(Courtesy of Texas Heart Institute, Houston, TX.)*

Australia), unlike the other pumps, has a fluid levitation bearing that enables frictionless impeller rotation without a magnetic system. This device has been implanted in 50 patients in Australia, Europe, and the United States (feasibility trial approved by the FDA).[34] This class of devices may have advantages over axial flow pumps, including durability, better biocompatibility, lower risk of thrombogenesis, and better responsiveness to physiological demands.

Postoperative Management of Left Ventricular Assist Devices

There are several factors important in early postoperative management. Antibiotic prophylaxis is started preoperatively and continues for at least 3 days postimplantation. Right heart failure is immediately or prophylactically treated with milrinone (Primacor) and inhaled nitric oxide. In addition, vasodilatory hypotension is treated with intravenous arginine vasopressin (Pitressin). Aprotinin is continued in the postoperative period until bleeding has stopped. Physical therapy and nutrition are addressed early.

Late postoperative care focuses on rehabilitation and monitoring of the immunological changes induced by the LVAD during the wait for heart transplantation.[35] As discussed earlier in this chapter, the profound ventricular unloading provided by LVAD support can lead to reverse remodeling (see Chap. 22).[36] Although functional recovery allowing LVAD explantation has been reported, our experience has demonstrated that only a small minority of patients can be successfully weaned from their devices.[6,37] The question of which patients are suitable for bridge to recovery and device explantation, and the possibility that myocardial function could be enhanced with drug or cell therapies, are the subjects of intense investigation.

Complications and Adverse Events

BLEEDING. Bleeding is a major complication after implantation of LVADs and can occur in the immediate perioperative period and later postoperatively. Immediate postoperative bleeding requires surgical intervention in 20 to 40 percent of patients. Preoperative heart failure leading to hepatic dysfunction, preoperative anticoagulation, coagulopathy caused by blood-device surface interaction, extensive surgical dissection, and prolonged cardiopulmonary bypass time all contribute to higher rates of bleeding after device implantation. In the immediate postoperative period, coagulation parameters as well as complete blood counts must be monitored closely, and deficiencies in platelet count and coagulation factors must be corrected as necessary. because excessive transfusion of blood products can cause volume overload and subsequently exacerbate right heart failure, care must be taken to avoid unnecessary transfusion. Although meticulous surgical technique is the mainstay of hemostasis, several medications can be used to prevent postoperative bleeding.

It is well established that aprotinin reduces blood loss and blood use in patients receiving assist devices. If excessive bleeding is noted at the time of chest closure, the chest may be left open and packed and the patient taken to the ICU, stabilized, and the chest closed once coagulation has been normalized. Bleeding can also occur late postoperatively. All devices except the pulsatile HeartMate devices require heparin and subsequently warfarin to achieve an ideal INR for each device postoperatively. Aspirin is added to this regimen as an antiplatelet and antiinflammatory agent in all cases. Some rotary pumps require additional antiplatelet medication. Care must be taken to maintain adequate levels of anticoagulation. Because LVADs can activate both coagulation and fibrinolytic pathways, there is the potential to exacerbate bleeding or thrombotic complications, even late postoperatively.[22] Therefore, clinical signs of late bleeding need to be carefully monitored in those patients.

THROMBOEMBOLIC EVENTS. Thromboembolism is a major concern in any patient with mechanical circulatory support, because of the blood-device interface. The prevalence of embolism varies from 2 to 47 percent, with most occurring in the cerebral distribution, although the definition of embolism varies by study.[38,39] The pulsatile HeartMate devices have the lowest thromboembolic rate of all the devices, despite the fact that these patients do not receive warfarin (likely because of the device promoting the formation of a neointimal surface that reduces embolization). All other devices require heparin in the immediate postoperative period and, subsequently, warfarin as well as antiplatelet agents, such as aspirin or clopidogrel.

INFECTION. Infection is one of the most serious complications after LVAD implantation, affecting short- and long-term survival. Although the definition of device-related infection varies by study, LVAD infection, in general, can manifest as drive line, pocket, or bloodstream infections or, ultimately, as device endocarditis.[40] In addition to device-related infections, these patients are susceptible to the common infections seen in critically ill patients such as pneumonia, line sepsis (with multiple catheters and intravenous lines), and urinary tract infections. Therefore, it is sometimes difficult to identify the source of infection when a patient on LVAD support has positive blood cultures. The reported infection rates in these patients are from 12 to 55 percent.[40,41] Pocket infection rates have been reported to be 11 to 24 percent for the pulsatile HeartMate and Novacor systems, whereas the drive line infection rate is even higher, in the range of 18 to 30 percent for the two devices.[18,40,41] Again, there is much variability in these data, because definitions for these infections have not been standardized. Sepsis accounts for 21 to 25 percent of LVAD deaths and occurs at a rate of 11 to 26 percent.[18,40,41]

Various microorganisms are responsible for VAD infections. Gram-positive cocci are most commonly seen, but gram-negative organisms and fungi have been found. If organisms are identified, timely and appropriate systemic and topical management of infection is necessary. Infection itself is not a contraindication to transplantation in this population, and transplantations have successfully been accomplished in infected patients.[41,42] Device endocarditis can be treated with systemic antibiotics as well as emergent heart transplantation, device explantation, or device replacement.[40-42] The interaction between patient and device that occurs after VAD implantation is a topic of much interest. Immunologically, LVAD implantation is accompanied by progressive defects in cellular immunity caused by an aberrant state of T-cell activation and apoptosis. These defects together predispose LVAD patients toward susceptibility to infections.[24]

DEVICE FAILURE. The definition of device failure differs somewhat from device to device; accordingly, it has been difficult to determine the actual rate of device failure among the different devices. Major failures, such as pump diaphragm rupture, require emergent device replacement. Minor failures, such as controller or battery malfunction, usually do not require emergency surgery but do require appropriate treatment, such as replacement of controllers. The probability of device failure was 35 percent at 24 months in the REMATCH trial,[1] which used the HeartMate VE device. However, recent modifications of the system have been aimed at reducing this incidence substantially. The Novacor LVAS has better durability than HeartMate, with a device failure rate between 0 and 2 percent, with devices replaced only after 3 to 4 years of support.

RIGHT HEART FAILURE. In patients with end-stage heart failure, pulmonary vascular resistance (PVR) is usually elevated because of long-standing left heart failure, and is further increased in the early postoperative period by the effects of cardiopulmonary bypass and extensive blood product transfusion. These factors, individually or in combination, can lead to impaired RV contractility, increased RV afterload, and subsequent RV dysfunction.[43] In most cases, unloading and supporting the left ventricle will help decrease PVR and improve RV performance. However, it must be noted that complete LV decompression can also reduce the septal contribution to RV function by causing the interventricular septum to shift toward the left. In this setting, RV contractility may be impaired further by the enhanced preload to the RV from the supplemental LVAD output. Interestingly, two independent analyses have elucidated low preoperative RV stroke work index and low preoperative mean pulmonary artery pressure (PAP) as risk factors for postoperative development of right heart failure or postoperative use of an RVAD.[43,45] Right heart failure has been reported in 10 to 30 percent of patients who received HeartMate or Novacor implantable LVADs, and an RVAD was used in 1 to 11 percent of all patients.[38,43] In patients with Thoratec paracorporeal devices, the incidence of RVAD use was as high as 38 to 42 percent.[44] However, this may be related to differences in patient and device selection criteria and device availability among institutions. Perioperatively, if there is any indication of right heart failure, such as increased central venous pressure (CVP) or decreased LVAD flow with appropriate LV decompression and without tamponade, treatment of right heart failure must be initiated immediately with pulmonary vasodilators (inhaled nitric oxide) and inotropic agents to enhance RV contractility. If RV function does not improve, and the LVAD flow still remains suboptimal (less than 2.4 liters/min/m^2, with CVP higher than 16 mm Hg), RVAD insertion is probably necessary.

MULTISYSTEM ORGAN FAILURE. Multisystem organ failure (MSOF) is another frequent complication in the LVAD population. Because of the significant amount of preoperative end-organ dysfunction and the number of comorbid conditions, some VAD patients do not fully recover after device implantation. In many cases, MSOF is the end result of a long cascade of complications, including sepsis, bleeding, and other events. At other times, MSOF may be the result of significant preoperative multiorgan dysfunction that deteriorates after the insult of surgery. Reflecting the aggregate of these scenarios, MSOF accounts for 11 to 29 percent of deaths with the device.

IMMUNOLOGICAL PERTURBATION. Itescu and colleagues have extensively analyzed the immunological interaction of patients with the pulsatile HeartMate LVAD and demonstrated several important findings.[24] First, significant T-cell activation was noted, both on the LVAD surface and in the circulation, albeit with defective proliferative responses to stimulation. Second, the circulating T-cells demonstrated susceptibility to activation-induced cell death after T-cell receptor engagement. Third, the LVAD recipients demonstrated significant B-cell hyperreactivity. It is believed that these phenomena are responsible for (1) a progressive defect in cellular immunity (thus leading to an increased risk of infection) as well as (2) an increased rate of allosensitization. Few comparable studies have been performed with recipients of other types of devices. Immunological evaluation of the patient-device interaction with the DeBakey axial flow pump, which does not promote a neointimal layer, have demonstrated an initial finding of increased markers of apoptosis. However, these markers declined to normal levels after 7 weeks, and did not appear to confer an increased risk of infection in this cohort.[46]

SENSITIZATION. LVAD implantation is thus associated with an increased risk of developing circulating anti-HLA class I and II antibodies (sensitization), causing as many as 66 percent of patients with an LVAD to be sensitized prior to transplantation.[24] This increased antibody level is associated with a significant risk for early graft failure and poorer patient survival as a result of complement-mediated humoral rejection. Thus, all efforts are made to reduce the number of necessary blood product transfusions (especially platelet) where possible. If the patient has become sensitized, donor-specific cross-matching is mandatory prior to transplantation, resulting in increased waiting time for those patients. Studies have demonstrated that pretransplantation immunomodulatory therapy with intravenously administered cyclophosphamide, together with intravenous immunoglobulin (IV Ig), successfully diminishes serum alloreactivity and reduces waiting list times and the risk of acute rejection in many LVAD recipients.[24]

DESTINATION THERAPY

Because of the constant shortage of available donor organs, the large group of patients who would benefit from circulatory assistance, and the encouraging results from the use of current LVADs as long-term support, a multicenter trial was conducted to evaluate the use of the pulsatile HeartMate LVAD as a permanent device in the treatment of heart failure. REMATCH was undertaken in 1998 and included 129 patients in 20 centers. The patients in the study were randomly assigned to receive either an LVAD or maximal medical therapy, with death as the primary endpoint and several secondary endpoints assessing quality of life, complications, and hospitalizations. The study ended in July 2001 and demonstrated a 48 percent reduction in the risk of death in the group treated with LVADs as compared with those in the medically treated group (Fig. 28-6), with superior quality of life measurements demonstrated in the LVAD treatment group. However, patients with devices were more than twice as likely to develop an adverse event and had a

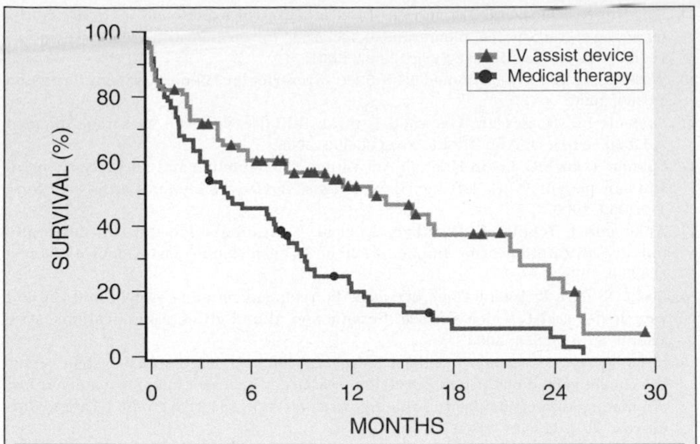

No. at risk						
LV assist device	68	38	22	11	5	1
Medical therapy	61	27	11	4	3	0

FIGURE 28-6 Comparison of actuarial survival curves from REMATCH. LV = left ventricular. *(From Rose EA, Gelijns AC, Moskowitz AJ, et al; Randomized Evaluation of Mechanical Assistance for the Treatment of Congestive Heart Failure (REMATCH) Study Group: Long-term mechanical left ventricular assistance for end-stage heart failure. N Engl J Med 345:1435, 2001.)*

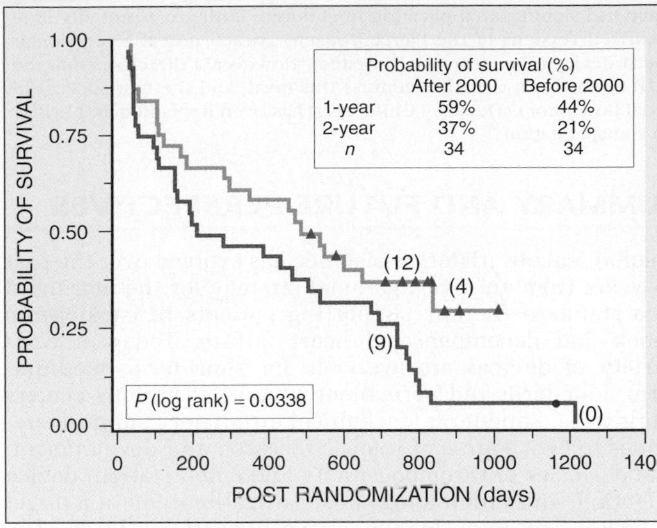

FIGURE 28-7 REMATCH left ventricular assist device learning curve. Actuarial survival curves of those enrolled in REMATCH before and after 2000 are compared in this graphic representation. The upper line (blue) denotes those enrolled after 2000 and the lower line (magenta) denotes those enrolled prior to 2000. *(From Park SJ, Tector A, Piccioni W, et al: Left ventricular assist devices as destination therapy: A new look at survival. J Thorac Cardiovasc Surg 129:9-17, 2005.)*

higher median number of days spent in and out of the hospital.[1]

Further analysis of the REMATCH data after study completion has demonstrated improved outcomes across several phases of the study (Fig. 28-7).[47] Notably, survival in the LVAD cohort was significantly higher for those enrolled after 2000, and 2-year survival demonstrated improvement despite little change in the optimal medical management cohort. Certainly, with the advent of more durable devices, other design improvements, and greater clinical experience, the survival benefit conferred by LVAD destination therapy is likely only to improve further. This trend has been reproduced by a post-REMATCH experience at a group of high-volume centers. This combined experience has shown 60 percent survival at 2 years.[48] Patient selection criteria may also have a major impact on destination therapy outcomes. Lietz and colleagues[49] analyzed the FDA-mandated destination therapy registry data of 208 patients who received the pulsatile HeartMate LVAD after the REMATCH study. A preimplantation risk score using candidates' general conditions, including nutrition, right-ventricular and endorgan function, but not hemodynamic severity of left-ventricular failure, can stratify in-hospital mortality into low-, medium-, high-, and very high-risk classes (Fig. 28-8).[49]

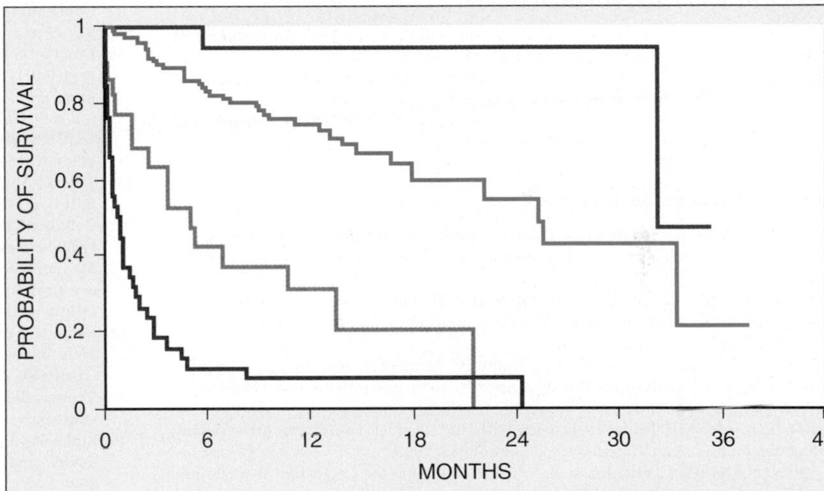

		% Survival			
	N	30 days	6 months	1 year	2 years
Low	21	100	94.4	94.4	94.4
Medium	127	98.4	83.1	74.3	54.5
High	22	77.3	42.2	30.8	0
Very high	38	36.8	10.5	7.9	7.9

FIGURE 28-8 Survival after left ventricular assist device implantation as destination therapy by the cumulative risk score for in-hospital mortality, post-REMATCH experience, $N = 208$.

PEDIATRIC ASSIST DEVICES

Children with end-stage heart failure are at particular risk of dying while awaiting transplantation because of the relative unavailability of donor organs in the pediatric size range. Most clinical experience to date with isolated ventricular assistance has been with children weighing more than 6 kg; the largest experience in smaller children and neonates has been with ECMOs. Several specific requirements for a pediatric assist device make its development difficult. First, the device must be versatile; children with complex heart disease often require biventricular support or might have only a single functional ventricle. In addition, the ability to include an oxygenator in the support circuit may be required. Second, the cannulas must be small enough to allow for ventricular decompression without generating excessive negative pressure (and air entrainment). Third, the device itself must be small enough to be used potentially as an implantable device in larger children and not be cumbersome as a paracorporeal device in smaller infants. Finally, the device must be able to run at flows considered low by adult standards but that will fully support children (e.g., 0.5 to 1.5 liters/min). Worldwide, only the Berlin Heart and Medos pumps have had significant application in children. Both are essentially miniaturized versions of the Pierce-Donachy paracorporeal biventricular assist device (similar to the Thoratec). However, a directive from the NHLBI has been issued to address this need, and the first successful axial flow pump (DeBakey Child VAD) has been implanted as a bridge to transplantation.[50]

SUMMARY AND FUTURE PERSPECTIVES

Mechanical circulatory assistance has evolved over the past 25 years from an investigational strategy for the moribund to a standard therapy supporting patients in cardiogenic shock and decompensated heart failure. Today, a wide variety of devices are available for short-term, medium-term, long-term and permanent support at various centers worldwide. Long-term mechanical circulatory support continues to be a source of intense research and development. The obstacles of thrombogenicity and embolization, device infection, and immunological sensitization remain a target of ongoing research for the currently available VADs. The potential of VADs as destination therapy has further tested the limits of device durability. Finally, the increasing desire to miniaturize pump design to allow for complete implantability and pediatric applications continues to drive development.

REFERENCES

Intraaortic Balloon Counterpulsation

1. Rose EA, Gelijns AC, Moskowitz AJ, et al: Long-term use of a left ventricular assist device for end-stage heart failure. N Engl J Med 345:1435, 2001.
2. Copeland JG, Smith RG, Arabia FA, et al: Cardiac replacement with a total artificial heart as a bridge to transplantation. N Engl J Med 351:859, 2004.
3. Stone GW, Ohman EM, Miller MF, et al: Contemporary utilization and outcomes of intra-aortic balloon counterpulsation in acute myocardial infarction. J Am Coll Cardiol 41:1940, 2003.

Ventricular Assist Devices

4. Deng MC, Weyand M, Hammel D, et al: Selection and outcome of ventricular assist device patients: The Muenster experience. J Heart Lung Transplant 17:817, 1998.
5. Helman DN, Morales DL, Edwards NM, et al: Left ventricular assist device bridge-to-transplant network improves survival after failed cardiotomy. Ann Thorac Surg 68:1187, 1999.
6. Mueller J, Wallukat G, Weng Y, et al: Predictive factors for weaning from a cardiac assist device. An analysis of clinical, gene expression, and protein data. J Heart Lung Transplant 20:202, 2001.
7. Hon JK, Yacoub MH: Bridge to recovery with the use of left ventricular assist device and clenbuterol. Ann Thorac Surg 75(Suppl):S36, 2003.
8. Patel AN, Geffner L, Vina RF, et al: Surgical treatment for congestive heart failure with autologous adult stem cell transplantation: A prospective randomized study. J Thorac Cardiovasc Surg 120:1631, 2005.
9. Menasche P, Hagege AA, Vilquin JT, et al: Autologous skeletal myoblast transplantation for severe postinfarction left ventricular dysfunction. J Am Coll Cardiol 41:1078, 2003.
10. Thiele H, Lauer B, Hambrecht R: Reversal of carcinogenic shock by percutaneous left atrial-to-femoral arterial bypass assistance. Circulation 104:2917, 2001.
11. Jurmann MJ, Siniawski H, Erb M, et al: Initial experience with miniature axial flow ventricular assist devices for postcardiotomy heart failure. Ann Thorac Surg 77:1642, 2004.
12. Hochman JS, Sleeper LA, White HD, et al: One-year survival following early revascularization for cardiogenic shock. JAMA 285:190, 2001.
13. Dang NC, Topkara VK, Leacche M, et al: Left ventricular assist device implantation after acute anterior wall myocardial infarction and cardiogenic shock: Two-center study. J Thorac Cardiovasc Surg 130:693, 2005.
14. Topokara VK, Dang NC, Barili F, et al: Ventricular assist device use for the treatment of acute viral myocarditis. J Thorac Cardiovasc Surg 131:1190, 2006.
15. Swartz MT, Lowdermilk GA, McBride LR: Refractory ventricular tachycardia as an indication for ventricular assist device support. J Thorac Cardiovasc Surg 118:1119, 1999.
16. Rao V, Oz MC, Flannery MA, et al: Revised screening scale to predict survival after insertion of a left ventricular assist device. J Thorac Cardiovasc Surg 125:855, 2003.
17. Dang NC, Topkara VK, Kim BT, et al: Clinical outcomes in patients with chronic congestive heart failure who undergo left ventricular assist device implantation. J Thorac Cardiovasc Surg 130:1302, 2005.
18. Morgan JA, John R, Rao V, Weinberg AD, et al: Bridging to transplant with the HeartMate left ventricular assist device: The Columbia-Presbyterian Twelve-Year Experience. J Thorac Cardiovasc Surg 127:130, 2004.
19. Smedira NG, Moazami N,Golding CM et al: Clinical experience with 202 adults receiving extracorporeal membrane oxygenation for cardiac failure: Survival at five years. J Thorac Cardiovasc Surg 122:92, 2001.
20. Wassenberg PA: The Abiomed BVS 5000 biventricular support system. Perfusion 15:369, 2000.
21. Samuels LE, Homes EC, Garwood P, et al: Initial experience with the Abiomed AB5000 ventricle. Ann Thorac Surg 80:309, 2005.
22. Spanier T, Oz MC, Levin H, et al: Activation of coagulation and fibrinolystic pathways in patients with left ventricular assist devices. J Thorac Cardiovasc Surg 112:1090, 1996.
23. Ankersmit J, Tugulea S, Weinberg A, et al: Activation-induced T-cell death and immune dysfuntion after implantation of left-ventricular assist device. Lancet 354:550, 1999.
24. Itescu S, John R: Interactions between the recipient immune system and the left ventricular assist device surface: Immunological and clinical implications. Ann Thorac Surg 75:S58, 2003.
25. El-Banayosy A, Arusoglu L, Kizner L: Novacor left ventricular assist system versus Heartmate vented electric left ventricular assist system as a long-term mechanical circulatory support device in bridging patients: A prospective study. J Thorac Cardiovasc Surg 119:581, 2000.
26. Frazier OH: First use of an untethered, vented electric left ventricular assist device for long-term support. Circulation 89:2908, 1994.
27. Dowling RD, Park SJ, Pagani FD, et al: HeartMate VE LVAS design enhancements and its impact on device reliability. Eur J Cardiothorac Surg 25:958, 2004.
28. Murali S: Mechanical circulatory support with Novacor LVAS: World-wide clinical results. Thorac Cardiovasc Surg 47:321, 1999.
29. Mussivand T, Hetzer R, Vitali E, et al: Clinical results with an ePTFE inflow conduit for mechanical circulatory support. J Heart Lung Transplant 23:1366, 2004.
30. Farrar DJ: The Thoratec ventricular assist device: A paracorporeal pump for treating acute and chronic heart failure. Semin Thorac Cardiovasc Surg 12:243, 2000.
31. Copeland JG, Arabia FA, Banchy ME, et al: The CardioWest total artificial heart bridge to transplantation: 1993 to 1996 national trial. Ann Thorac Surg 66:1662, 1998.
32. Macha M, Litwak P, Yamazaki K, et al: Survival for up to six months in calves supported with an implantable axial flow ventricular assist device. ASAIO J 43:311, 1997.
33. Goldstein DJ: Worldwide experience with the MicroMed DeBakey ventricular assist device as a bridge to transplantation. Circulation 108(Suppl 1): II272, 2003.
34. Esmore DS, Kaye D, Slamonsen R, et al: First clinical implant of the VentrAssist left ventricular assist system as destination therapy for end-stage heart failure. J Heart Lung Transplant 24:1150, 2005.
35. Morrone TM, Buck LA, Catanese KA, et al: Early progressive mobilization of left ventricular assist device patients is safe and optimizes recovery before heart transplantation. J Heart Lung Transplant 15:423, 1996.
36. Thohan V, Stetson SJ, Nagueh SF, et al: Cellular and hemodynamic responses of falling myocardium to continuous flow mechanical circulatory support using the DeBakey-Noon left ventricular assist device: A comparative analysis with pulsatile-type devices. J Heart Lung Transplant 24:2306, 2005.
37. Mancini DM, Beniaminovitz A, Levin H, et al: Low incidence of myocardial recovery after left ventricular assist device implantation in patients with chronic heart failure. Circulation 98:2383, 1998.
38. McCarthy PM, Smedira NO, Vargo RL, et al: One-hundred patients with the HeartMate left ventricular assist device: Evolving concepts and technology. J Thorac Cardiovasc Surg 115:904, 1998.
39. Thomas CE, Jichici D, Petrucci R, et al: Neurologic complications of the Novacor left ventricular assist device. Ann Thorac Surg 72:1311, 2001.
40. Sinha P, Chen JM, Rajasinghe HR, et al:. Infections during left-ventricular assist device support do not affect posttransplant outcomes. Circulation 102:III194, 2000.
41. Holman WL, Rayburn BK, McGiffin DC: Infection in ventricular assist devices: Prevention and treatment. Ann Thorac Surg 75:S48, 2003.
42. Morgan JA, Park YK, Oz MC, Naka Y: Device-related infections while on left ventricular assist device support do not adversely impact bridging to transplant or posttransplant survival. ASAIO J 49:748, 2003.
43. Kavarana MN, Pessin-Minsley MS, Urtecho J, et al: Right ventricular dysfunction and organ failure in left ventricular assist device recipients: a continuing problem. Ann Thorac Surg 73:745, 2002.
44. McBride LR, Naunheim KS, Fiore AC, et al: Clinical experience with 111 Thoratec ventricular assist devices. Ann Thorac Surg 67:1233, 1999.
45. Schenk S, McCarthy PM, Blackstone EH, et al: Duration of inotropic support after left ventricular assist device implantation: Risk factors and impact on outcome. J Thorac Cardiovasc Surg 131:447, 2006.
46. Ankersmit HJ, Wieselthaler G, Moser B, et al: Transitory immunologic response after implantation of the DeBekey VAD continuous-axial-flow-pump. J Thorac Cardiovasc Surg 123:557, 2002.

Destination Therapy

47. Park SJ, Frazier OH, Piccioni W, et al: Left ventricular assist devices as destination therapy: A new look at survival. J Thorac Cardiovasc Surg 129:9, 2005.
48. Long JW, Kfoury AG, Slaughter MS, et al: Long-term destination therapy with the HeartMate XVE left ventricular assist device: Improved outcomes since the REMATCH study. Congest Heart Fail 11:133, 2005.
49. Lietz K, Long J, Kfoury AG, et al: Risk score for prediction of survival to hospital discharge after left-ventricular assist device implantation as destination therapy. Circulation (submitted).
50. Imamura M, Hale S, Johnson CE, et al: The first successful DeBakey VAD child implantation as a bridge to transplantation. ASAIO J 51:670, 2005.

CHAPTER 29

Emerging Therapies and Strategies in the Treatment of Heart Failure

Stefanie Dimmeler, Douglas L. Mann, and Andreas M. Zeiher

Our current therapeutic approach to the treatment of heart failure (HF) relies on treating patient symptoms using digitalis and diuretics, using neurohormonal antagonists such as angiotensin converting enzyme inhibitors (ACEIs) and/or angiotensin receptor blockers, beta blockers, and aldosterone antagonists to prevent disease (see Chap. 25), as well as the use of biventricular pacemakers and defibrillators in appropriate patient populations (see Chaps. 25 and 34). Despite these pharmacological and device interventions, HF remains a progressive disease with an unacceptably high mortality and morbidity. Thus, there is an ongoing need for new and improved therapeutic approaches for the treatment of HF. In this chapter, we will review some of the new therapeutic approaches that are being evaluated in patients with HF. The organization of this chapter will focus first on new nonpharmacological strategies in HF, including the exciting concept of myocardial repair and regeneration; a review of emerging pharmacological strategies—such as pharmacogenomics; and a discussion of novel targets in HF. New and emerging surgical approaches to HF are reviewed in Chapter 27.

NONPHARMACOLOGICAL STRATEGIES

Myocardial Repair and Regeneration

As noted in Chapter 22, HF may develop as a consequence of myocyte loss or dysfunction, eventually leading to left ventricular remodeling and cardiac decompensation. Replacement of dead or dysfunctional cardiac myocytes through cell-based therapies represents a logical and novel option for the treatment of HF. As will be discussed subsequently, cell-based therapies may achieve true cardiac regeneration by renewing the pool of functionally active cardiac myocytes, or may lead to cardiac repair by supporting neovascularization, supplementing and/or augmenting the cytoprotective mechanisms that occur naturally, or by favorably influencing the remodeling processes. The promise of cellular cardiomyogenesis, neovascularization, and additional cell-mediated beneficial effects, individually or in combination, offers altogether novel opportunities for tailored treatment of the underlying pathobiology.

Stem/Progenitor Cells

In general, two types of stem cells should be discussed separately: embryonic stem cells and adult stem cells (Fig. 29-1). Whereas embryonic stem (ES) cells clearly have the capacity to give rise to all cell types of the body and are able to form tissues and organs, most adult stem cells are more specific (more lineage committed) and the use of adult stem cells for organogenesis has not yet been explored. Embryonic stem cells are derived from the inner cell layer of the early embryonic trophoblast and can be propagated in cell culture in an undifferentiated state infinitely. By changing the cultivation conditions (the so-called *hanging drop technique*), embryonic stem cells aggregate and form embryoid bodies, an early embryonic tissue consisting of all three germ layers. Within an embryoid body, approximately 5 to 10 percent of embryonic stem cells spontaneously differentiate into cardiomyocytes. Functionally active cardiomyocytes (ESC-CM) have been generated from mouse as well as from human ES cells (hESC-CM), although the E-C coupling properties of hESC-CM differ from the adult myocardium.[1] ES cell-derived cardiomyocytes show macromolecular sarcomeric organization, calcium sparks, ionic currents, functional and anatomical integration with surrounding cardiomyocytes, and propagation of electrical activity as well as pacemaker activity.[1] Collectively, these data demonstrate that ES cells spontaneously differentiate into fully functionally active, fetal-like cardiomyocytes in vitro. Although these in vitro data would suggest that ES cells are ideal candidates for in vivo cardiac repair, animal studies have shown a dose-dependent incidence of tumor formation, in particular, teratocarcinoma formation, after transplantation of ES cells into mice. Several strategies aiming to specifically select differentiated cardiomyocytes to exclude highly proliferating ES cells with a tumor-forming capacity are currently being tested. An additional question relates to the immunogenic activity of ES cells in an allogenic setting. It is unclear whether the low immune privilege proposed by experimental studies is maintained when the ES cells are differentiated and functionally integrated into the human heart for a long time. Therefore, the safety of ES cell transplantation remains an unsolved question.[2]

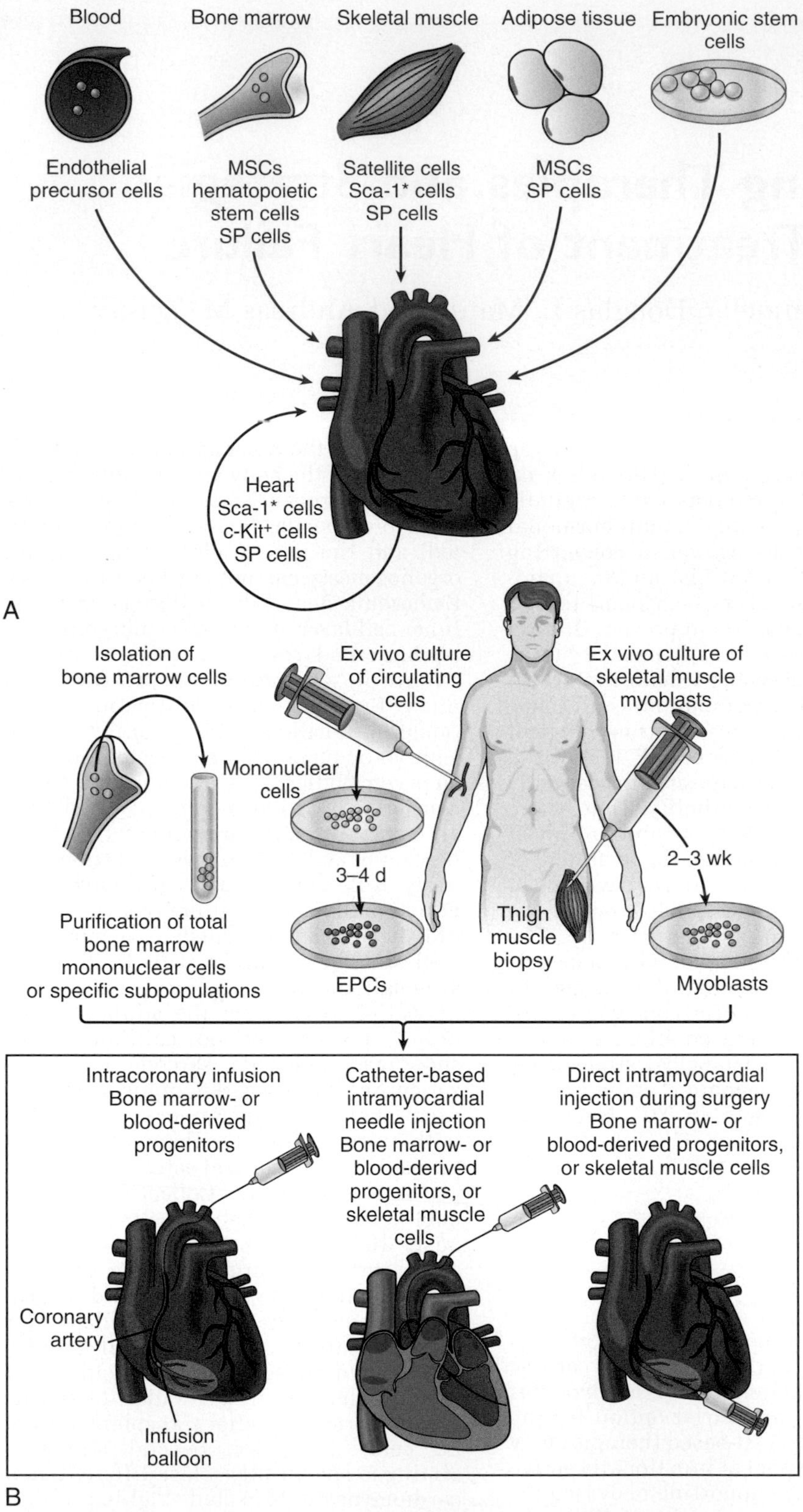

FIGURE 29–1 Cell types and mode of delivery of cells for cardiac repair. **A,** Cell types used for cardiovascular repair. **B,** Delivery strategies used in the clinical setting for cell therapy. MSCs = mesenchymal stem cells. *(From Dimmeler S, Zeiher AM, Schneider MD: Unchain my heart: The scientific foundations of cardiac repair. J Clin Invest 115:572-583, 2005.)*

Adult stem cells comprise at least three different groups: bone marrow-derived stem cells, the circulating pool of stem or progenitor cells (which at least in part are derived from the bone marrow), and tissue-resident stem cells (see Fig. 29-1). Bone marrow-derived stem cells are the best studied and were used in most of the clinical trials performed thus far. Bone marrow contains a complex assortment of progenitor cells, including hematopoietic stem cells (HSCs), the so-called "side population cells" (SP cells, defined by the expression of the Abcg2 transporter allowing export of Hoechst dye),[3] mesenchymal stem cells (MSCs) or stromal cells,[4] and multipotential adult progenitor cells (MAPCs), a subset of MSCs.[5]

Circulating blood-derived progenitor cells were initially discovered when searching for pro-angiogenic cells for therapeutic vasculogenesis. Asahara and Isner isolated "endothelial progenitor cells (EPCs)," which were defined by their ability to form new blood vessels and enhance neovascularization after ischemia (for review see references 6 and 7). Based on the assumption that these cells may represent adult hemangioblasts, those cells were characterized by the expression of hematopoietic markers, such as CD133+ or CD34+, and endothelial markers for VEGF-receptor 2 (KDR or flk-1). However, it is evident that these circulating progenitor cells (particularly when cultured in vitro) comprise several different entities.[6] Individual cells may have clonal potential and stem cell characteristics. Others, including distinct myeloid subpopulations, may preferentially act as pro-angiogenic cells,[8] in addition to their capacity to differentiate to endothelial cells. Myeloid cells also have been shown to contribute to muscle regeneration by fusion, indicating that myeloid subpopulations may act diversely. An interesting source of endothelial progenitor cells is placental cord blood, which is enriched in clonally expandable endothelial progenitor cells.

Mesoangioblasts are vessel-associated multipotent progenitors that express the key marker of angiopoietic progenitors, VEGF-receptor 2, but are distinct from hematopoietic endothelial progenitor cells. In vitro mesoangioblasts differentiate into many mesoderm cell types, such as smooth, cardiac and striated muscle, bone and endothelium, and they improve skeletal muscle dystrophy and heart function.[9,10] Mesoangioblasts may represent not only a source of progenitors for therapeutic applications, but also may establish a lineage relationship between progenitors of vascular and extravascular mesodermal tissues.

The discovery of tissue-resident stem cells in the heart, the "cardiac stem cells," offers the potential to harvest cells, which are primed to acquire a cardiac phenotype and, therefore, might be optimally suited for cardiac repair. Several different populations have been identified and characterized: c-Kit+ cells,[11] Sca-1+ cells,[12] SP cells, and cells expressing the protein Islet-1.[13] Whereas c-Kit+ cells, Sca-1+ cells and cardiac SP cells are isolated from adult hearts, cells expressing Islet-1 so far have only been detected in the postnatal stage. Whether c-Kit+, Sca-1+, and cardiac SP cells comprise three different cell populations is not entirely resolved. At least Sca-1+ cells contain a fraction of SP cells and, among cardiac SP cells, the greatest potential for cardiomyogenic differentiation is restricted to cells positive for Sca-1 expression (but negativo foi CD31)[14]—indicating that the two cell populations may share some common features. Cardiac stem cells also were obtained by growing self-adherent clusters (termed "cardiospheres") from subcultures of murine or human biopsy specimens. Others have generated cardiac SP cell–derived cardiospheres by adapting a method used for creating a neurosphere and claimed that cardiac neural crest cells contribute to cardiac SP cells.[15] Cardiosphere-derived cardiac stem cells as well as c-Kit+ cardiac stem cells are capable of long-term self-renewal and can differentiate into the major specialized cell types of the heart: myocytes and vascular cells (i.e., cells with endothelial or smooth muscle markers). So far, the origin and the mechanisms maintaining the cardiac stem cell pool are unclear. Whereas two recent studies suggested that c-Kit+ and cardiac SP cells may derive from the bone marrow,[16,17] these studies cannot entirely exclude that specific subpopulations of cardiac stem cells originate from distinct sources and may represent remnants from embryonic development in selected niches within the heart.

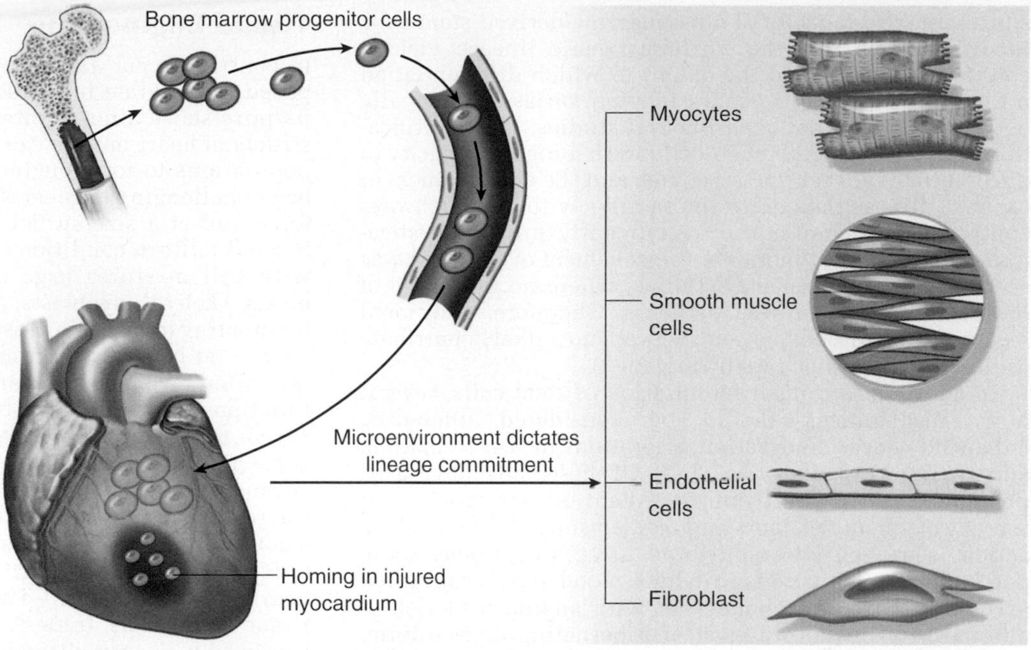

FIGURE 29–2 Homing of bone marrow-derived stem cells to the myocardium. The fate of bone marrow-derived stem cells is determined by the microenvironment that they enter. *(From Anversa P, Leri A: Myocardial rengeneration. In Zipes DP, Libby P, Bonow RO, Braunwald E [eds]: Braunwald's Heart Disease, 7th ed. Philadelphia, Elsevier, 2004, p 1917.)*

Adipose tissue is a rich source of distinct subsets of stem/progenitor cells potentially useful for cardiac repair and neovascularization improvement.[18] Both MSCs and endothelial progenitor cells were isolated after enzymatic digestion of adipose tissue and showed beneficial effects in experimental studies. Very recently, pluripotent spermatogonial stem cells from adult mouse testis have been identified, which possess the capacity to differentiate to fully active cardiac myocytes in vitro.[19]

In summary, the identification and characterization of stem/progenitor cell populations with potential therapeutic properties for the treatment of heart disease is an emerging field. Since direct side-by-side comparisons are missing, it is impossible to estimate what might be the best cell(s) for cardiac repair. Clearly, a ranking will not only be based on the assessment of the functional capacities of the cells to differentiate into cardiac myocytes, but also will include other aspects of progenitor cell functions. Particularly, for the clinical application, the safety of the treatment and the feasibility will be of major importance.

TABLE 29–1 Soluble Factors Influencing Cardiac Stem Cell Differentiation

Factor	Cell Type	Citation
PDGF-AB	Murine BMC	Xaymardan, et al., Circ Res 2004
Wnt3a	Murine PC19 cells	Nakamura, et al., PNAS 2003
Wnt11	Human EPC MSC Murine ES cells	Koyanagi, et al., JBC 2005 Bedada, et al., MCB 2005 Termai, et al., BBRC 2004
5-azacytidine	MSC Murine Sca-1+ cardiac stem cells	Makino, et al., JCI 1999 Oh, et al., PNAS 2003
Oxytocine	Murine PC19 cells Murine Sca-1+ cardiac stem cells	Paquin, et al., PNAS 2002 Matuura, et al., JBC 2004
TGF β	Murine c-Kit+ BMC	Li, et al., Circulation 2005
BMP	Murine P19CL6 cells	Monzen, et al., MCB 1999
Noggin	Murine ES cells	Yauasa, et al., Nat Biotechnology 2005
Ascorbic acid	Murine ES cells	Takahashi, et al., Circulation 2003

BMC = bone marrow mononuclear cells; EPC = endothelial progenitor cells; ES cells = embryonic stem cells; MSC = mesenchymal stem cells.

Mechanisms of Action of Stem Cells

In contrast to ES cells, most adult stem or progenitor cells do not spontaneously differentiate into cardiomyocytes but rather require an adequate stimulus to do so. The local microenvironment plays an important role to induce cell fate changes by physical cell-to-cell interaction and/or by providing paracrine factors (Fig. 29-2). Based on this concept, a co-culture technique was developed whereby stem or progenitor cells are cultured together with rat neonatal ventricular cardiomyocytes to simulate a cardiac-like environment in vitro.[20] Using such a co-culture system to induce differentiation of adult stem or progenitor cells from various species and organs demonstrated that the physical contact with beating neighboring cardiomyocytes is indeed required for the differentiation process to occur. Alternatively, the nonspecific transcriptional activator, the demethylating agent 5'-azacytidine, induced cardiac differentiation in Sca-1+ cardiac stem cells and MSCs suggesting a potential role for epigenetic control of changes in cell fate. The neurohormone oxytocin or cytokines of the Wnt or PDGF family have been employed to induce or enhance differentiation of adult stem cells (Table 29-1). However, experimental studies addressing the capacity of bone marrow-derived stem cells to differentiate into the cardiomyogenic lineage yielded conflicting results, and the extent to which differentiation into cardiac myocytes occurs in vivo varies dramatically between the different experimental studies. The identification of subsets of adult stem cells with a higher capacity to differentiate into cardiac myocytes and the enhancement of cardiac differentiation by interacting with the pathways controlling differentiation are currently under investigation. Interestingly, functional improvement of the heart was seen even in experimental studies, where no formation of new cardiomyocytes was detected. Therefore, additional mechanisms initiated by cell therapy most likely contribute to functional cardiac repair (Fig. 29-3).

In addition to transdifferentiation of stem cells, several other mechanisms should be considered, including enhanced neovascularization, alterations in scar formation, and cytoprotection (see Fig. 29-3). Of these, most obviously, progenitor cells may improve neovascularization and thereby augment nutrients and oxygen supply. This mode of action is expected to contribute to cardiac regeneration, particularly in situations in which blood supply is limited (e.g., as in chronic ischemic HF with angina pectoris), or alternatively in the presence of hibernating myocardium. Neovascularization can be mediated by the physical incorporation of progenitor cells into new capillaries[21] or by perivascular accumulation of cells. Incorporated progenitor cells of most, if not all, types may release growth factors that promote angiogenesis by acting on mature endothelial cells.[22] Paracrine factors may also beneficially influence cardiac repair by protecting cardiac myocytes from apoptotic stimuli or activate cardiac-resident stem cells to enhance the endogenous repair capacity.[22,23] Finally, the release of various cytokines will affect cardiac remodeling processes by altering the development of fibrosis development during scar formation and/or by modulating inflammatory processes. The extent to which progenitor cells contribute to vasculogenesis by becoming physical elements of newly formed vessels versus acting through secreted factors may depend on the environment to which the cells are exposed. Importantly, human bone marrow-derived angioblasts were shown to exert angiogenic as well as paracrine effects.

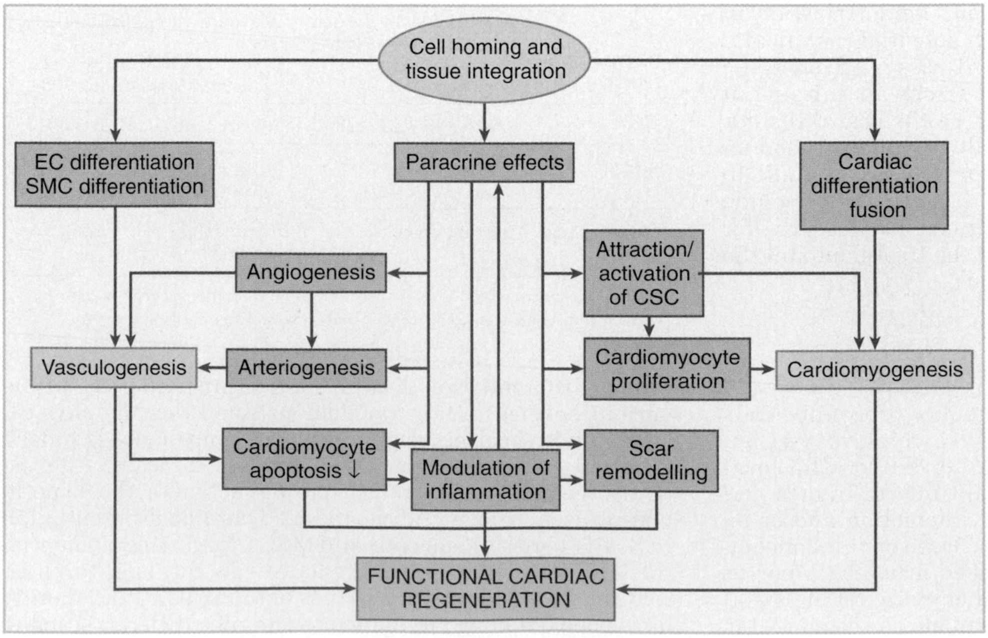

FIGURE 29–3 Proposed mechanisms of action of stem/progenitor cells in cardiovascular repair.

Tissue Engineering

In contrast to cell therapy, where individual cells are supposed to integrate in the scar tissue, tissue engineering in its pure sense aims at providing tissue grafts. Larger constructs of heart muscle can be generated by using heart cell populations to form engineered heart tissue. So far, it has been challenging to generate tissue in vitro with contractile force and at a size sufficient to support the failing heart. Several culture conditions have been used in combination with cell mixtures (e.g., neonatal cardiomyocytes, fibroblasts, skeletal myoblasts, adult and embryonic stem cells) for creating myocardial tissue in vitro. Implantation of engineered rat heart tissue from neonatal rat cardiomyocyte in rats after myocardial infarction improved the contractile function and was shown to be electrically coupled to the native myocardium.[24] Others have used engineered tissue constructs containing skeletal muscle derived cells, and the authors claimed that skeletal muscle cells—in contrast to the results achieved with skeletal muscle cell therapy—are electrically coupled by Gap junctional proteins.[25] Embryonic stem cells are alternative sources for the generation of heart tissue in vitro.[26] The size of the engineered heart tissue constructs (unless vascularized and perfused) is limited by oxygen diffusion. Therefore, researchers have fused several individually cultured single engineered tissue rings.

At the interface between tissue engineering and cell therapy, the development of novel biomaterials has gained increasing interest. Novel biomaterials have been developed to be used as ventricular restraints and to provide scaffolds for in vitro tissue engineering.[27,28] In addition, the injection of new biomaterial such as self-assembling nanofibers can adapt the intramyocardial cellular microenvironments to augment homing and functional integration of cells for in situ tissue engineering and subsequent cardiac regeneration and repair.

Clinical Application of Stem Cells

Clinically Used Cell Types

Currently, a variety of autologous adult progenitor cells are undergoing clinical evaluation. The first clinically relevant cells proposed for cardiac myocytes were skeletal muscle myoblasts—undifferentiated proliferation-competent cells that serve as precursors to skeletal muscle.[29] For clinical use, autologous human myoblasts are isolated from skeletal muscle biopsies, propagated and expanded ex vivo for a few days or weeks, then injected directly into the ventricular wall. Bone marrow is, at present, the most frequent source of stem cells used clinically for cardiac repair. The rapid transition from the bench to the clinic was facilitated by the more than 30 years of clinical experience and the excellent safety profile of infused bone marrow-derived mononuclear cells for bone marrow transplantation. Bone marrow is aspirated under local anesthesia in most of the studies, the entire mononuclear cell fraction is obtained (a heterogeneous mixture of cells with varying percentage of hematopoietic stems cells [HSC], EPC, MSC, and SP cells). So far, isolated bone marrow-derived cells have been injected into the heart without further ex vivo expansion. In a few studies, specific subpopulations such as a fraction of hematopoietic and endothelial progenitor cells expressing the marker protein CD133+ were purified and used. Peripheral blood-derived progenitor cells are used both for clinical cardiac repair and peripheral ischemia. Historically, these circulating "EPCs" are the basis for virtually all clinical studies that have used bone marrow or its circulating derivatives for the treatment of ischemic myocardium. The circulating blood-derived cells that have been used so far are isolated from mononuclear blood cells and selected by culturing the cells in "endothelium-specific" medium for 3 days.[30,31] Alternatively, a specific subfraction, the hematopoietic CD34+ progenitor cell, is enriched from whole blood following G-CSF–mediated mobilization from the bone marrow into the blood (Losordo and colleagues, personal communication).

ROUTES OF APPLICATION. Progenitor cells for cardiac repair can be delivered in different ways (see Fig. 29-1): Intracoronary infusion using standard balloon catheters has been used in all clinical trials treating patients with acute myocardial infarction. This technique offers the advantage that cells can travel directly only into myocardial regions in which nutrient blood flow and oxygen supply are preserved, thereby ensuring a favorable environment for cell survival, a prerequisite for stable engraftment. Conversely, homing of intraarterially applied progenitor cells requires migration out of the vasculature into the surrounding tissue, which may mean that unperfused regions of myocardium will be targeted far less efficiently, if at all. Whereas bone marrow-derived and blood-derived progenitor cells are known to extravasate and migrate to ischemic areas, other cell types may not, and they may even obstruct the microcirculation after intraarterial administration, leading to embolic myocardial damage—thus limiting the use of intracoronary delivery.

Injection of cells into the ventricular wall via a percutaneous endocardial or surgical epicardial approach is an alternative delivery strategy circumventing some of these limitations: Direct delivery of progenitor cells into scar tissue or areas of hibernating myocardium by catheter-based needle injection, direct injection during open-heart surgery, and minimally invasive thoracoscopic procedures are not limited by cell uptake from the circulation or by embolic risk. An offsetting consideration is the risk for ventricular perforation, which may limit direct needle injection into freshly infarcted hearts. In addition, it is hard to envisage that progenitor cells injected into uniformly necrotic tissue—lacking the syncytium of live muscle cells that may furnish instructive signals, and lacking blood flow for the delivery of oxygen and nutrients—would receive the necessary cues and environment to engraft and differentiate. Most cells, if injected directly, simply die. For this reason, electromechanical mapping of viable but "hibernating" myocardium may be useful to pinpoint the preferred regions for injection. Finally, in diffuse disease-like dilated nonischemic cardiomyopathy, focal deposits of directly injected cells might be poorly matched to the underlying anatomy and physiology. Thus, it is likely that nature of the patients' cardiomyopathy will ultimately influence, if not dictate, the source and route chosen among potential progenitor cell therapies. Additional strategies to augment cell homing and promoting homogeneous integration of cells may be required, particularly in patients with chronic healed infarcts or diffuse nonischemic cardiomyopathy lacking active recruitment signals.

Results of Clinical Trials

The results of clinical trials published to date, aiming at progenitor cell-based myocardial repair, are summarized in Tables 29-2 and 29-3. It is essential to distinguish between studies performed in patients with acute myocardial infarction (see Table 29-2) and in patients with chronic HF (see Table 29-3), because fundamentally different pathophysiological processes are targeted. In patients with acute myocardial infarction, progenitor cell transplantation aims to prevent or ameliorate postinfarction left ventricular remodeling, thereby reducing post-infarction HF. Such an effect might be achieved by enhanced neovascularization and reduced cardiomyocyte apoptosis, irrespective of long-term engraftment and transdifferentiation. Conversely, the former two mechanisms acting alone may have limited benefit in patients with long-established scars, absent hibernating myocytes and end-stage HF, where cardiomyogenesis in its pure sense would be desirable.

Cell Therapy in Acute Myocardial Infarction

As summarized in Table 29-2, the published studies overall demonstrate that the infusion of autologous bone marrow mononuclear cells (BMCs) is safe and feasible in patients with acute myocardial infarction. The study by Strauer,[32] the TOPCARE-AMI,[30] the BOOST-trial[33] and the study performed by Fernandez-Aviles[34] reported nearly identical results; that is, an improvement in global LV ejection fraction by 7 to 9 percent, a significant reduction in LV end-systolic volume, and improved perfusion in the infarcted area 4 to 6 months after cell transplantation. Whereas the randomized, controlled trial by Janssens[35] did not reveal a significant effect on global ejection fraction, it did show an increase in regional ejection fraction and a reduction of the infarct size in the BMC group. Only one larger study, the ASTAMI (Autologous Stem-Cell Transplantation in Acute Myocardial Infarction) trial, did not show any benefit.[36] The reason for the failure of the ASTAMI trial to show a benefit of cell therapy is unclear. However, preclinical work has established a fundamental role for cell isolation and processing techniques to determine the functional capacity of progenitor cells used for neovascularization. Because no preclinical functional testing of the cells used for the ASTAMI trial was performed, it is essentially impossible to judge the negative outcome of this trial.

Of note, all of the above cited studies used the total population of bone marrow mononuclear cells, which contain roughly 2 to 3 percent CD34+ cells but also contain SP cells, mesenchymal cells, and potentially other not yet identified cell populations. However, patients after acute myocardial infarction treated with ex vivo expanded circulating blood-derived EPC in one arm of the TOPCARE-AMI trial showed a similar improvement in heart function compared to BMC—indicating that selected subpopulations might have a similar capacity for functional repair at least in the acute myocardial infarction setting.[30] Likewise, the infusion of isolated CD133+ cells, which are enriched for EPC, improved global ejection fraction in patients with acute myocardial infarction.

The beneficial effects seen in most of the pilot phase I/II studies were confirmed in the recent so-far-largest double-blind, randomized, multicenter REPAIR-AMI trial.[37] This study used bone marrow mononuclear cells and demonstrated a significant improvement of global and regional ejection fraction in the BMC group (+5.5 percentage points) compared to placebo (+3 percentage points) 4 months after follow-up (Fig. 29-4). End-systolic volumes significantly increased in the placebo group, but remained unchanged in the BMC group. Interestingly, although the study was not powered to address a potential benefit on clinical endpoints, the incidence of the cumulative endpoints death, myocardial infarction, and rehospitalization for HF was significantly lower in the BMC-treated patients compared to placebo after 1-year follow up.

What variables might influence outcome? The larger number of patients enrolled in the REPAIR-AMI trial allowed for testing several predefined secondary endpoints to generate hypotheses for the next generation trials. There was a significant interaction between the baseline ejection fraction and the improvement seen after BMC therapy. Patients with a lower ejection fraction (<48.9 percent) showed a significant, threefold

TABLE 29–2 Studies with Infusion/Injection of Progenitor Cells in Patients with Acute Myocardial Infarction

Study	Patient No.	Days after AMI	Cell Type	Cell Preparation	Cell Number (×10[6])	Safety	Myocardial Function
Pilot Trials (Phase I/II)							
Strauer, et al.[32]	*N* = 10 (*Nov 03: N* = 40) versus ctrl.	8	BMC	40 ml Ficoll—overnight Teflon	28	+	Regional contractility ⇧ (LVA) End systolic volume ⇩ (LVA) Perfusion ⇧ (Szinti)
TOPCARE= AMI[30]	59	4.9	CPC BMC	250 ml / 3 day culture 50 ml/Ficoll—same day	16 213	+	Global contractility ⇧ (LVA/MRI) End systolic volume ⇩ (LVA/MRI) Viability ⇧ (MRI) Flow reserve ⇧ (Doppler)
Fernandez-Aviles[34]	20	13.5	BMC	50 ml Ficoll—overnight Teflon	78	+	Global contractility ⇧ (MRI) End systolic volume ⇩ (MRI)
Ruan, et al.[56]	10 versus (rand.)	100	BMC versus saline			+	Global contractility ⇧ (LVA)
Bartunek, et al.[57]	12	14	CD133 + BMC	Mouse antibody		Stenosis?	Global contractility ⇧ (LVA)
Chen, et al.[58]	34 versus 35	18	B-MSC versus control	10 day culture		+	Global contractility ⇧ (LVA)
Randomized Trials							
Single/Two Center(s)							
BOOST[33]	60 1 : 1 rand.	4.8	BMC versus rand.	Gelatin control—same day infusion	polysuccinate 2460	+	6 Months: Global contractility ⇧ (MRI) 18 Months: No significant difference (MRI) 18 Months: Diastolic dysfunction ⇩ (Echo)
Janssens, et al.[35]	67 1 : 1 rand.	<24 h	BMC versus i.c. placebo	Ficoll density gradient centrifugation—few hours after acute PCI	304	+	Global contractility no change Infarct size ⇩ (MRI)
ASTAMI[36]	100 1 : 1 rand.	6	BMC versus rand.	Lymphoprep control—next day infusion	87	+	Global contractility no change
Multicenter—Placebo-Controlled, Double-Blind							
REPAIR–204 AMI[37]	1 : 1 rand.	4	BMC versus i.c. placebo	Ficoll density gradient centrifugation—same or next day infusion	234	+	Global contractility ⇧ (QLVA)

AMI = acute myocardial infarction; BMC = bone marrow-derived progenitor cells; CPC = circulating progenitor cells; i.c. = intracoronary; LVA = left ventricular angiography; MRI = magnetic resonance imaging; QLVA = quantitative LVA; rand. = randomized trial.

higher recovery in global ejection fraction indicating that patients with more severe myocardial infarction benefit the most from BMC therapy. Indeed, the beneficial effect on clinical endpoints was also preferentially observed in those patients with a lower baseline ejection fraction after myocardial infarction. This observation confirmed the previous results of the TOPCARE-AMI pilot trial. A second predefined end point addressed the question whether the timing of BMC delivery affects the outcome. Surprisingly, patients who had been treated up to 4 days after the myocardial infarction showed no benefit, whereas later treatment (day 4 to 8) provided an enhanced improvement of ejection fraction during follow-up. Given that several experimental studies demonstrated that the cells provide a cytoprotective activity coinciding with a reduction of cardiomyocyte apoptosis, one would have expected that early timing of cell infusion would have been the most efficient. Based on the data of the REPAIR-AMI trial, one may speculate that the microenvironment after acute myocardial infarction changes during the first week after reperfusion, thereby modulating the homing and/or the subsequent functional activity of the infused cells.[37] It is well known that ischemia/reperfusion induces a transient change in the expression of chemoattractive factors such as VEGF and SDF-1, which are known to be essential for stimulating the recruitment and retention of cells in the tissue. Moreover, the initial edema formation is followed by a transient invasion of different "waves" of cells. Therefore, it is conceivable that cell homing might be best a few days after reperfusion rather than immediately. Further studies are warranted to prospectively address this question.

Overall, the clinical data available indicate that cell therapy with bone marrow-derived cells is feasible and safe at least for the follow-up presently available (up to 5 years in the pioneering studies). None of the studies so far reported an increased incidence of arrhythmias (as has been seen in myoblast trials). Moreover, restenosis, which was considered as a potential side effect by progenitor cell-mediated plaque angiogenesis or plaque inflammation, was increased only in one study using CD133+ cells.[38] Because CD133+ cells were isolated by using a mouse antibody, one may speculate that the remaining antibody might have elicited

TABLE 29–3 Studies with Infusion/Injection of Progenitor Cells in Patients with Old Myocardial Infarction or Chronic Heart Failure

Study	*N*	Status Post MI	Cells	Application	Safety and Functional Assessment
Application with NOGA					
Tse, et al.[59]	*N* = 8	Old MI	BMC	IM with NOGA	Safe Wall motion and thickening ⇧
Fuchs, et al.[50]	*N* = 10 *N* = 21	Old MI	BMC	IM with NOGA	Safe Safe
Perin, et al.[49]	Control *N* = 7 BMC *N* = 14	Old MI	BMC	IM with NOGA	Global contractility ⇧ End systolic volume ⇩
Application During Surgery					
Stamm, et al.[60]	*N* = 12	>10 days after AMI	CD 133⁺ BMC	IM during CABG	Safe Global contractility ⇧ Perfusion ⇧
Hamano, et al.[61]	*N* = 5 *N* = 34	Old MI	BMC	IM during CABG	Safe
Galinanes, et al.[51]	BMC *N* = 11 CABG *N* = 11 CABG + BMC: *N* = 10	Old MI	BMC	IM during CABG	Safe Global contractility ⇧
Intracoronary Administration					
IACT[52]	*N* = 18	Old MI 5 months to 8.5 years	BMC	Intracoronary	Safe Global contractility ⇧ (LVA/MRI) Viability ⇧ (pet)
TOPCARE–CHF[53]	*N* = 92 Control *N* = 23 BMC *N* = 35 CPC *N* = 34	Old MI 3 months-12 years	BMC CPC	Intracoronary	Safe Global contractility ⇧ (BMC better than CPC) (lva)

BMC = bone marrow-derived progenitor cells; CABG = coronary artery bypass graft; CHF = congestive heart failure; CPC = circulating progenitor cells; IM = intramuscularly; MI = myocardial infarction.

a local proinflammatory reaction, despite the failure to detect systemic anti-mouse antibodies in the patients. All other studies did not observe an augmented risk for restenosis; if anything, there was a significantly decreased necessity for revascularization procedures in the REPAIR-AMI trial.

An important issue is whether the improvement seen during the initial 6 months after cell therapy is maintained for a prolonged time. Careful evaluation of the 18 months follow-up data of the BOOST trial indicates that the ejection fraction of the cell therapy group is maintained from 6 to 18 months of follow-up; however, the difference between the cell therapy and the control group was no longer statistically significant because of improvement in ejection fraction in the control group. The small number of patients (30 per group) may preclude detecting a statistical difference between the two groups. The long term 2-year follow-up MRI-derived data of the TOPCARE-AMI trial showed that the ejection fraction is maintained and even further augmented in the treated patients, in parallel with a sustained reduction in NT-proBNP serum levels, suggesting a beneficial effect of long term left ventricular remodeling (S. Dimmeler and A. M. Zeiher, unpublished data). Taken together, these data may provide the rationale to assess the effects of intracoronary BMC infusion on clinical outcome in a large patient cohort with severe acute myocardial infarction.

Mobilization Strategies in Acute Myocardial Infarction

The first evidence that cytokine-induced mobilization might be a viable strategy for augmenting myocardial repair arose from efforts to increase EPC levels for neovascularization. Vascular endothelial growth factor (VEGF) and granulocyte macrophage colony-stimulating factor have been shown to augment EPC levels and to improve peripheral neovascularization.[39] Subsequent experimental reports that bone marrow-derived hematopoietic stem cells could not only augment vascular repair but also promote cardiac regeneration stimulated subsequent studies to use the well-studied cytokine granulocyte colony-stimulating factor (G-CSF) to mobilize bone marrow-derived stem cells for cardiac repair. Additional experimental studies documented beneficial effects by other pro-angiogenic growth factors, including stromal cell-derived factor-1 (SDF-1), angiopoietin-1, placental growth factor, and erythropoietin. Since G-CSF was available for clinical use, this approach was applied most rapidly in clinical studies. Most studies have been performed in patients with acute myocardial infarction who were treated with recombinant G-CSF during the first week after the infarct. The studies have revealed mixed results (Table 29-4), which is likely due to the different timing of G-CSF application. It should be noted that, in experimental studies, G-CSF was given either prior to or simultaneously with the induction of the acute myocardial infarction. In addition, splenectomized animals were used to limit cell clearance.[40,41] Whereas two phase I pilot trials showed a significant improvement of global ejection fraction with G-CSF mobilization,[42,43] two recent larger scale randomized, placebo-controlled studies (STEMMI[44] and REVIVAL[45]) reported no significant influence of G-CSF treatment on heart function in patients after acute myocardial infarction. The recent MAGIC cell-3-DES trial,[46] however, suggests that the combination of G-CSF and additional intracoronary infusion of purified circulating blood-derived progenitor cells may yield better results in patients with acute myocar-

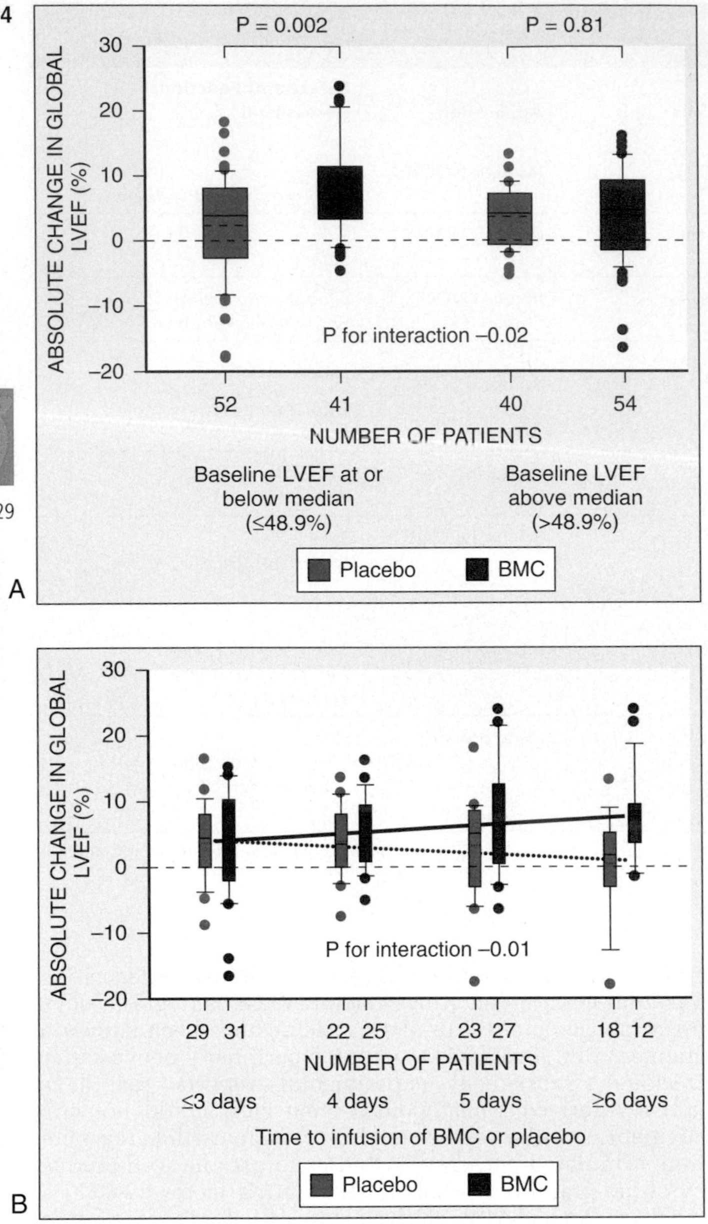

FIGURE 29–4 Principal results of the REPAIR-AMI trial. Interaction between baseline left ventricular ejection fraction and the absolute change in left ventricular ejection fraction (panel **A**) and between the timing of intracoronary infusion of BMC or placebo after reperfusion therapy and the absolute change in left ventricular ejection fraction (panel **B**). In panel **A,** the P value for interaction was determined by analysis of variance. In both panels, the upper and lower edges of each box plot indicate the 25th and 75th percentiles, the "whiskers" the 10th and 90th percentiles, the solid horizontal line the median, and the dashed line the mean. All outliers are shown as individual data points. In panel **B,** the P value for interaction was calculated with the use of a general linear model. The solid line in panel **B** shows the regression curve for the BMC group, and the dotted line shows the regression curve for the placebo group. *(From Schachinger V, Erbs S, Elsasser A, et al: Intracoronary bone marrow-derived progenitor cells in acute myocardial infarction. N Engl J Med 355:1210-1221, 2006.)*

dial infarction. The overall safety of G-CSF treatment in acute myocardial infarction has been reviewed critically. Triggered by the report of Kang and coworkers,[47] who reported a dramatic increase in restenosis after G-CSF treatment for early patients in the MAGIC trial, further studies have provided a detailed analysis of restenosis rates after G-CSF treatment. Importantly, none of the subsequent studies have shown that the short-term treatment with G-CSF had any effect on restenosis. Indeed, a follow-up of the MAGIC study by Kang and coworkers also confirmed that restenosis rates were not augmented in patients when treated with drug-eluting stent.[46] The observed increase in restenosis in the initial MAGIC trial may be partially explained by the study design in which the initial patients were treated with G-CSF before coronary artery stenting. However, the reports of an increased incidence of myocardial infarctions and episodes of angina and arrhythmias during treatment with G-CSF in patients with chronic ischemic cardiomyopathy should continue to raise some concerns as to whether a G-CSF-induced rise in leukocyte number may be responsible for plaque growth or destabilization. Accordingly, in the future, it may be preferable to develop strategies that augment circulating progenitor cells without the simultaneous induction of massive inflammation.

Cell Therapy and Cell Mobilization Strategies in Patients with Chronic Heart Failure

In patients with chronic ischemic heart disease and a prior myocardial infarction, the results of the initial attempts at cell-based myocardial repair have been more heterogeneous, and the number of patients that have been treated has been less when compared to acute myocardial infarction trials. The first cell-based therapy trial used skeletal muscle-derived progenitor cells, which were directly injected into the scarred region of the left ventricle during open heart surgery for coronary artery bypass grafting. Global and regional left ventricular function were significantly and persistently improved. However, the concomitant coronary artery revascularization confounded the assessment of true benefit in these studies. Indeed, in patients not undergoing simultaneous revascularization, the transcatheter injection of myoblasts into the preexisting (5 to 6 year old) postinfarction scar tissue led to a reduction in the symptoms of HF without any objective evidence of an improvement in global left ventricular function. Unfortunately, even though extensive previous animal experiments provided no hint of increased arrhythmias, the enthusiasm for injecting myoblasts into scar tissue for cardiac repair was dampened by development of life-threatening arrhythmias in the patients who were treated.[48] Mechanistically, these arrhythmias may be related to the lack of electrical coupling of skeletal muscle to neighboring cardiac myocytes or, alternatively, it may be contingent on coupling by the few hybrid cells formed by fusion with adjacent cardiac myocytes, which generate spatially heterogeneous calcium transients. Therefore, currently, the implantation of skeletal myoblasts requires the implantation of an implantable cardioverter defibrillator as a mandatory adjunct to therapy.

Bone marrow-derived progenitor cells have been employed in several smaller, nonrandomized trials for chronic ischemic HF using different strategies for cell delivery. Three studies have used electromechanical mapping of the left ventricular endocardial surface to identify sites for injecting cells into areas of myocardial hibernation.[49,50] Each of these studies has shown a significant increase in global left ventricular ejection fraction associated with decreased end-systolic volumes, as well as an improvement in exercise capacity. Although this functional improvement might be secondary to an improved blood supply to hibernating cardiomyocytes, it is also conceivable that hibernating myocardium may provide a more favorable microenvironment for the survival/engraftment of the injected cells when compared to an injection in scar tissue. Others have used a surgical approach to inject bone marrow-derived cells during coronary artery bypass surgery (CABG).

TABLE 29-4 Studies Using Mobilization of Progenitor Cells with Granulocyte Colony-Stimulating Factor

Study	N	Status Post MI	Cells	Safety	Functional Assessment
FIRSTLINE-AMI[42]	N = 50 1 : 1 rand.	Acute MI	G-CSF 10 μg/kg, 6 days	safe	Global contractility ⇧
Kuethe, et al.[43]	N = 14 versus N = 9 control	Acute MI	G-CSF 10 μg/kg, 7 ± 1 days	safe	Global contractility ⇧
STEMMI[44]	N = 78 Rand., double-blind, placebo-controlled	Acute MI	G-CSF 10 μg/kg, 6 days	safe	No change
REVIVAL[45] JAMA 2006	N = 114 Rand., placebo controlled	Acute MI	G-CSF 10 μg/kg, 5 days	safe	No change
Hill, et al.[54] JACC 2005	N = 16	Old MI	G-CSF 10 μg/kg, 5 days	*not* safe (2 × MI)	No change
Huttmann, et al.[55]	N = 16 ICM: N = 9 DCM: N = 7	Old MI DCM	G-CSF 10 μg/kg, 4 times 10 days	Occasional episodes of angina Ventricular fibrillation	Six minute walking distance ⇧
G-CSF with Additional Cell Therapy					
MAGIC[47]	N = 10	Acute and old MI	G-CSF ± CPC (by apheresis)	Restenosis ⇧ (methodological limitations; see text)	Global contractility ⇧
Erbs, et al.[31]	N = 26 Rand., placebo controlled	Old MI	G-CSF plus CPC (cultivation)	safe	Global contractility ⇧
MAGIC cell-3-DES[46]	N = 96 AMI control (N = 25) AMI cell (N = 25) ICM control (N = 16) ICM cell (N = 16)	Acute and old MI	G-CSF plus CPC	safe	AMI: global contractility ⇧ ICM: no change

AMI = acute myocardial infarction; CPC = circulating progenitor cells; DCM = dilated cardiomyopathy; G-CSF = granulocyte colony-stimulating factor; ICM = isolated cardiovascular malformation; MI = myocardial infarction.

Again, an increase in ejection fraction was documented. Although the effect of CABG and BMC cannot be dissociated in these pilot trials, a recent study showed a more profound effect in patients being treated with CABG and cells in comparison to CABG or cells alone.[51] Finally, encouraging preliminary results were recently reported in a controlled safety trial of patients with normal left ventricular ejection fraction, but persistent angina refractory to revascularization procedures (D. Losordo, personal communication). In this trial, blood-derived CD34+ cells were collected following G-CSF mobilization and directly injected into underperfused left ventricular areas by catheter-based electromechanical mapping.

Three published studies addressed the possibility to use intracoronary delivery of BMC by a balloon catheter. The IACT study tested the feasibility of BMC infusion in patients with chronic HF and demonstrated a substantial increase in ejection fraction (+15 percent) in patients with healed (>3 months old) myocardial infarction.[52] Smaller, but significant, improvements were also seen in the randomized controlled trials by Erbs and colleagues and the TOPCARE-CHF study. Erbs and colleagues infused G-CSF mobilized, ex vivo cultivated endothelial progenitor cells in a recanalized coronary artery.[31] Coronary flow reserve in response to adenosine and global ejection fraction were improved in the cell-treated patients compared to recanalization without cell therapy. A smaller, but significant, improvement was also observed in the TOPCARE-CHF study.[53] Interestingly, this study was the first to examine a direct side-by-side comparison of two different cell types in patients with old myocardial infarctions. In this patient cohort, BMCs were shown to be significantly better as compared to circulating progenitor cells. This is in contrast to the TOPCARE-AMI trial, wherein BMC and EPC showed a similar effectiveness in acute myocardial infarction patients.[30] The reason for this discrepancy is unclear. One may speculate that the number and function of circulating cells is further impaired in HF patients and that an additional mobilization step is required to yield a sufficiently high number of functionally active cells (as done by Erbs and colleagues). Another potential explanation may relate to the combination of a lower number of EPC applied (22×10^6 compared to 205×10^6 BMC) and/or a reduced homing capacity in the chronic setting, which might limit the efficiency of EPC.

Finally, as discussed extensively earlier, different cell types may activate different mechanisms which may be more or less beneficial in acute versus chronic ischemic HF. Mobilization of progenitor cells with G-CSF without intracoronary reinfusion did not result in any measurable benefit on left ventricular function, but was associated with adverse coronary events in two studies.[54,55]

Future Perspectives in Myocardial Repair and Regeneration

Cell transplantation has been performed days, months, or years following myocardial infarction. In acute myocardial infarction, the established safety and proof-of-concept studies provide a cogent rationale for larger, randomized trials addressing the question whether cellular therapy aimed at cardiac repair not only improves pump function, but also reduces mortality and morbidity. Several open questions are likely to be answered in the future: (1) what is the optimal time of delivery after acute myocardial infarction? (2) Is there a dose response relationship? and (3) how do different cell types compare? One of the most urgent questions in basic science, to elucidate the mechanism by which stem/progenitor cells achieve a functional improvement, is difficult to test in the clinical scenario. Although clinicians can measure flow reserve and heart function, the underlying detailed mechanism cannot be determined with an ethically applicable technology in the near future. In chronic ischemic HF, a superimposed question is whether identifying hibernating myocardium to direct cell therapy is essential to an effective outcome. For established scar tissue late in the disease, specific strategies might be needed. The treatment of nonischemic heart disease is not yet addressed. An overview of currently ongoing clinical trials of progenitor cell application for cardiac regeneration can be viewed at www.ClinicalTrials.gov.

WHAT IS THE BEST CELL TYPE FOR CARDIAC REPAIR? Direct side by side comparison using different cell types is rare particularly in the clinical setting. Clearly, bone marrow-derived cells have set the stage and have provided beneficial effects in various studies. However, the extent to which ejection fraction is improved, particularly in chronic HF, is limited. Therefore, additional cell types will enter the clinical arena: fat tissue-derived multipotent stem cells, multipotential cells from bone marrow or skeletal muscle (minuscule subpopulations, distinct from the unfractionated bone marrow and the myoblasts in current trials), somatic stem cells from placental cord blood, adipose tissue-derived stem cells and cardiac-resident progenitor cells that have a heightened predisposition to adopt the cardiac muscle fate are on the way for potential clinical application. However, whether the experimentally suggested promise of augmented cardiac myogenesis will translate into enhanced contractile function, when applying cells in patients with chronic HF, is unknown.

More complex and challenging are a series of pathobiological concerns, sending the scientific community from bedside to bench and back again. As long as a patient's own cells are used in the autologous setting, certain of those cells may be unsatisfactory—in their naïve and unmanipulated state—prompting systematic dissection of each step in progenitor cell function. Cell enhancement strategies to improve patient-derived cells by pretreatment with small molecule or genetic modification may contribute to an augmented recruitment as well as in the future may enhance differentiation or other beneficial functions.

Clearly, the use of stem/progenitor cells for cardiac repair is currently not at a stage to be used in routine clinical practice. Despite a wealth of experimental and clinical data suggesting feasibility, safety, and even early clinical efficacy in patients with acute myocardial infarction, progression to widespread clinical application of progenitor cell administration to promote functional cardiac regeneration must be balanced against the inherent risk of testing a novel therapy. As such, attempts of regenerative therapeutic interventions in patients with significant cardiac dysfunction should proceed in controlled trials with the utmost rigorous scientific and ethical standards, paralleled by further extensive in vitro and animal studies. Such a strategy will not only maximize patient safety, which is of paramount interest, but will also generate reciprocal insights into mechanisms and potential shortcomings of cell-based therapies aiming at functional cardiac regeneration. Specific attention should be given to the processing of the cells and to ascertain their functionality for regenerative purposes prior to initiating their clinical application. The promise of functional cardiac regeneration by cell-based therapies offers novel opportunities to address the large, unmet clinical need of treating patients with severe cardiac dysfunction.

GENE THERAPY

Gene therapy represents another emerging therapeutic approach for the treatment of HF. Improvements in gene transfer vectors and gene transfer methodology have enabled recombinant genes to be expressed at robust levels in cardiac myocytes.[56] Further, recent advances in the field of RNA interference (RNAi) suggest that it may also be possible to use gene therapy to "silence" key pathogenetic genes or pathways that are activated in the failing heart.[57,58]

Three elements are necessary for the successful clinical application of any gene therapeutic approach.[59] First a vector or packaging system is necessary to deliver the genetic material. Only a few of the currently available viral vectors are able to achieve efficient, high-level transgene expression in postmitotic cells such as cardiac myocytes. These include recombinant adenoviruses, adeno-associated viruses, and possibly lentivirus. Recombinant adenoviruses have been used most commonly because of their ability to "package" large DNA constructs, as well as their ability to transduce nonreplicating cells. However, the robust immune response these vectors evoke suggests that clinical applications will likely require other vectors or further-refined adenoviral systems. Second, the vector needs to be adequately delivered to the affected tissue(s). The feasibility of in vivo cardiac gene transfer by viral vectors has been consistently demonstrated in experimental studies. As illustrated in Figure 29-5, a number of mechanical approaches have been used to achieve cardiac gene transfer. Intracoronary catheter delivery of an adenovirus encoding the reporter gene beta-galactosidase achieved transduction of approximately 30 percent of the cardiac myocytes in the distribution of the injected coronary artery. Direct injection of adenovirus into the ventricular wall using an epicardial approach has also been shown to induce significant expression of reporter constructs; however, the expression was focal and the needle injections within the heart resulted in myocardial damage. Intramyocardial delivery of adenovirus using an intraventricular approach with retro-infusion of coronary veins has also been used in larger animals, yielding regional areas of transduction. Injection of an adenovirus carrying beta-galactosidase into the pericardial sac transduced only the pericardial cell layers.[59] The third element that is necessary for a successful gene therapeutic approach is to identify the appropriate gene targets to modulate. Table 29-5 summarizes potential targets for gene therapy in HF based on experimental studies. The major promising targets for gene transfer have been those genes that regulate the beta-adrenergic receptor (AR) signaling pathway and genes that regulate calcium handling in the heart.[58]

TABLE 29–5 Potential Therapeutic Targets for Gene Therapy in Heart Failure

Target	Function
Beta-adrenergic receptor kinase inhibitor (βARKct)	Inhibits phosphorylation of β-adrenergic receptor thus preventing its desensitization
Adenylyl cyclase (AC)	Synthesizes cAMP to activate PKA, which then phosphorylates substrates to regulate calcium handling
Sarcoplasmic reticulum Ca^{2+} ATPase (SERCA2)	Responsible for the reuptake of calcium from cytoplasm into the SR lumen. Critical determinant of both relaxation and contractility via calcium sequestration into SR and via controlling SR calcium loading, respectively
Phospholamban (PLN)	Inhibits SERCA2, inactivated by phosphorylation by PKA and CaMKII
Parvalbumin (Parv)	Rapidly removes calcium in myofilaments, naturally abundant in skeletal muscle (not cardiac); results in enhanced relaxation
S100 protein	A calcium binding protein, a positive inotropic regulator of cardiac function that enhances calcium cycling and cardiac contractile performance in vitro and in vivo

CaMKII = Ca^{2+}/calmodulin-dependent protein kinase; PKA = protein kinase A; SR = sarcoplasmic reticulum.

As noted in Chapter 21, the beta-AR signaling pathway is critical for modulating myocardial contractility. Studies have shown that alterations in the myocardial beta-AR both precede and accompany the development of HF in humans, including downregulation of the beta-ARs, functional uncoupling of beta-ARs from second messenger systems, and increased levels of inhibitory G-proteins that blunt beta-AR signaling (see also Chap. 22).[60] Indeed, transgenic mice with cardiac restricted overexpression of the $beta_2$-AR have enhanced myocardial contractility.[61] However, as noted in Chapter 22, excessive and/or sustained stimulation of the beta-AR signaling can also lead to activation of maladaptive signaling pathways in the heart (e.g., activation of the fetal gene program), as well as myocyte death through both necrosis and apoptosis. For example, transgenic mice that overexpress the $beta_1$-AR develop a dilated cardiomyopathy.[62] Viewed together, these types of experimental studies have generated considerable interest in using selective genetic approaches to modulate beta-AR signaling pathways in HF models. Thus far, adenoviral-mediated gene transfer of the human $beta_2$-AR resulted in an improvement in contractility in myocytes isolated from a rabbit model of HF,[59] as well as in myocytes from failing hearts.[58] Similarly, adenoviral-mediated gene transfer of a peptide inhibitor of beta-AR kinase (see Chaps. 21 and 22) resulted in restoration of beta-AR signaling, increased cyclic AMP, and reversal of ventricular dysfunction in rabbit HF models.[59]

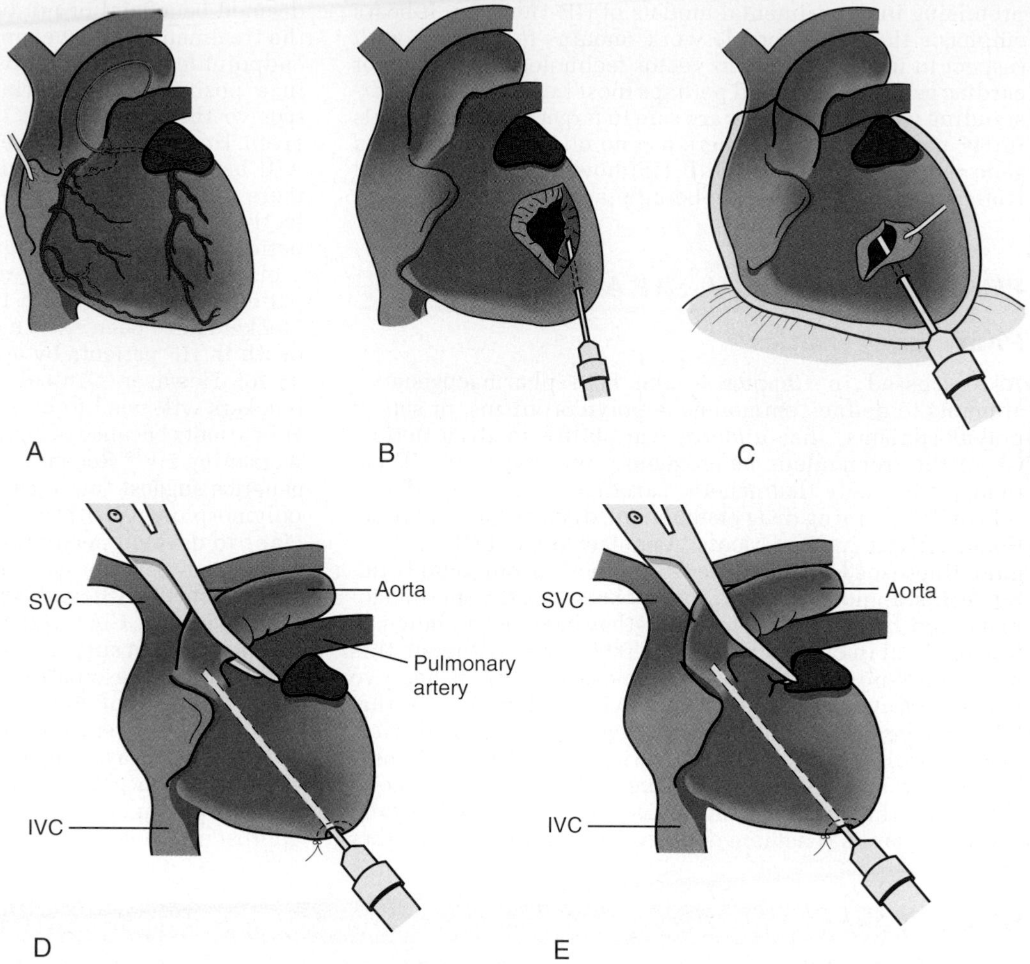

FIGURE 29–5 Different techniques for in vivo cardiac gene transfer. **A,** Coronary perfusion. **B,** Intramyocardial injection. **C,** Pericardial injection. **D,** Aortic clamping. **E,** Cross-clamping of the aorta and pulmonary artery. IVC = inferior vena cava; SVC = superior vena cava. *(Modified from Hajjar RJ, del Monte F, Matsui T, Rosenzweig A: Prospects for gene therapy for heart failure. Circ Res 86:616-621, 2000.)*

Enhancement of myocardial contractility through manipulation of intracellular calcium signaling has garnered considerable enthusiasm as a potential target for gene therapy in HF. Several studies suggest that functional suppression of sarcoplasmic reticulum Ca^{2+}-ATPase (SERCA2a) activity, or an absolute reduction in the amount of SERCA2a protein, may contribute significantly to the abnormalities in Ca^{2+} handling and myocardial contraction observed in failing hearts (see Chap. 22). In an animal model of pressure-overload hypertrophy that transitions to failure, overexpression of SERCA2a by gene transfer in vivo restored both systolic and diastolic function to normal levels.[63] Similarly, overexpression of SERCA2a through gene targeting resulted in normalization of LV volumes, improved energetics, and prolonged survival in an experimental model of pressure-overload hypertrophy.[64] Overexpression of an antisense phospholamban construct or a dominant-negative mutant of phospholamban (see Chap. 21) has recently been shown to enhance SERCA2a activity, consistent with the prior observation that genetic ablation of phospholamban prevents the functional abnormalities otherwise seen in a mouse model of dilated cardiomyopathy.[59] Similar beneficial effects on cardiac contractility, including normalized calcium handling and enhanced SERCA2a activity, have been observed in experimental and human HF models following gene transfer of S100A1 (a calcium binding protein).[65]

In addition to modulating myocardial contractility, gene therapeutic approaches may also be used to target myoycte viability or fibroblast phenotype. Morphological and biological markers of programmed cell death or apoptosis have been identified in human HF, suggesting that these pathways may contribute to cardiomyocyte loss and cardiac dysfunction in HF (see Chap. 22). The potential to block cardiomyocyte apoptosis through somatic gene transfer is, therefore, another area of ongoing investigation.[66] Also, the ability to modulate fibroblast phenotype has been explored in experimental models of myocardial infarction, wherein gene-mediated transfer of myogenic determination gene, MyoD, has been used to transduce cardiac fibroblasts into functional skeletal muscle cells with the intent of reducing infarct size/expansion within the border zones of the infarct.[67]

Future Perspectives in Gene Therapy

Gene transfer strategies that result in improvements in myocardial contractility and/or cardiac remodeling appear promising in experimental models of HF. However, it bears emphasis that considerable work remains to be done with respect to improvements in vector technology, methods for cardiac gene delivery, and perhaps most importantly, understanding what gene targets are safe to target in clinical trials in HF patients. To date, there are no clinical trial data on gene therapy in patients with HF; however, small clinical trials targeting SERCA2 are being planned.

PHARMACOLOGICAL STRATEGIES

Pharmacogenetics

As discussed in Chapter 6, the field pharmacogenetics attempts to define common gene polymorphisms, or sets of polymorphisms, that underlie variability in drug action. Given the tremendous heterogeneity that exists in HF patients, it is likely that genetic variations play a significant role in determining drug metabolism, disposition, and functional activity in HF patients. As noted, current HF practice guidelines (see Heart Failure Guidelines) recommend titrating ACEIs, angiotensin receptor blockers, aldosterone antagonists, and beta blockers to doses that have been shown to be beneficial in clinical trials (see Table 25-9). Although this approach tends to work well for most patients, it has two major shortcomings, the most obvious of which is that basing drug dosing on the doses selected in clinical trials does not allow for dose optimization in patients who may metabolize and/or distribute drug differently. The second problem is that clinical trials are generally designed to yield "binary" results. That is, a drug under investigation is either deemed beneficial or not beneficial because the patients in the treatment arm have, or have not, reached a prespecified endpoint (e.g., death or hospitalization). A beneficial effect in a positive clinical trial implies that all patients will receive the same degree of benefit from the drug that is given. However, a more likely outcome is that a given therapy will have a markedly positive impact for some patients, a more modest effect in others, and may be completely ineffective or perhaps even harmful in a smaller group of treated patients. Thus, even though a drug is deemed beneficial in a clinical trial, there is no guarantee that an individual patient will benefit from the treatment. For example, beta blockers have been shown consistently to reduce the risk of death in HF patients by approximately 35 percent (see Fig. 25-16). However, clinical trials have also shown that beta blockers will need to be discontinued in 8 to 25 percent of HF patients because of significant adverse effects, including worsening HF.[68] Recent advances in the field of pharmacogenetics suggest that a careful analysis of underlying gene polymorphisms within a given patient may enable clinicians to develop personalized therapeutic regimens for HF patients. Given the central role of the renin angiotensin-aldosterone (RAS) and adrenergic systems in the pathophysiology (see Chap. 22) and treatment of HF (see Chap. 25) it is perhaps not surprising that polymorphisms in the genes that regulate these pathways appear to influence the therapeutic efficacy of ACEIs and/or beta blockers. Table 29-6 provides an overview of the major genetic variations in these pathways and the proposed functional impact of these polymorphisms, as well as how these genetic polymorphisms influence traditional pharmacotherapeutic approaches in HF.

TABLE 29–6 Effect of Gene Polymorphisms on the Pharmacological Treatment of Heart Failure

Pathway/Gene	Polymorphism	Functional Impact	Impact on Pharmacological Therapy
Renin-Angiotensin-Aldosterone			
ACE	287 bp insertion (I) or deletion (D) in intron 16	DD genotype has increased ACE activity and worse clinical outcomes in some (but not all studies)	Use of beta blockers and ACEIs attenuates adverse outcomes of DD genotype but has no effect on II/ID genotypes; II/ID genotype predicts reverse LV remodeling in response to spironolactone
Angiotensinogen	Methionine (Met) to threonine (Thr) switch at aa 235	Increased angiotensinogen levels with HTN	Modest risk of hypertension in whites; effect on drug responsiveness in HF not known
Aldosterone synthase	C to T transition at position −344 (T/C)	−344C allele associated with higher aldosterone levels	TT genotype associated with greater impact of fixed combination of isosorbide dinitrate and hydralazine on the event-free survival in the A-HeFT trial
Adrenergic Nervous System			
$Beta_1$-AR	Arginine (Arg), glycine (Gly) switch at aa 389	Arg 389 polymorphism has increased adenylyl cyclase activity in response to agonist 3 × greater than Gly389 variant.	Arg389Arg genotype greatest improvement in EF with beta blockers, and improved mortality with bucindolol treatment in BEST
$Beta_1$-AR	Serine (Ser), glycine (Gly) switch at aa 49	In vitro the Gly49 variant shows decreased receptor expression compared with Ser49 variant after exposure to isoproterenol (24 hours)	Ser49Ser genotype requires higher doses of beta blocker to achieve a mortality benefit
$Beta_2$-AR	Threonine (Thr) to isoleucine Ile switch at aa 164	Ile164 $beta_2$-AR has decreased affinity for catecholamine binding, decreased basal and epinephrine-stimulated adenylyl cyclase activity, and impaired agonist-promoted sequestration; Ile164 transgenic mice display depressed resting and agonist-stimulated contractile function in vivo compared with Thr164 mice	Associated with decreased VO_2 max and worse HF outcomes; effect on drug responsiveness in HF not known
$Alpha_{2C}$-AR	$Alpha_{2C}$ Del322–325	Decreased NE uptake	Increased likelihood of developing HF in patients with the $beta_1$-AR Arg389 polymorphism; effect on drug responsiveness in HF not known

ACE = angiotensin-converting enzyme; AR = adrenergic receptor; HF = heart failure; HTN = hypertension; NE = norepinephrine.

One of the most widely studied genetic variants is the ACE insertion/deletion polymorphism (I/D) that involves a 287-base pair insertion or deletion within intron 16 of the ACE gene. Although the clinical significance of this polymorphism remains controversial, the physiological association with ACE enzymatic activity has consistently been demonstrated. Studies have shown that individuals with the DD genotype have the highest ACE activity and angiotensin II levels, heterozygotes (I/D) have intermediate levels, and individuals who are homozygous for the I allele (I/I) have the lowest levels of ACE activity. The relationship of ACE I/D has been explored in relation to numerous conditions including atherosclerosis, myocardial infarction, left ventricular hypertrophy, hypertrophic cardiomyopathy, and HF. Although the current weight of evidence does not allow for definitive conclusions to be made with respect to the overall contribution of the ACE I/D polymorphism to the clinical outcome in these conditions, there is growing evidence that the ACE I/D polymorphism may predict drug responsiveness to both beta blockers and ACEIs in HF patients. In one study of patients with chronic HF, the ACE DD polymorphism was significantly associated with death or the need for transplantation when compared to patients with II or ID genotypes. Within the ACE DD group, patients treated with beta blockers had significantly improved transplant-free survival when compared to patients not receiving beta blocker therapy, whereas beta blocker treatment had no effect in clinical outcomes in the II or ID groups.[69] In a similar study, patients with the DD genotype had better clinical outcomes when receiving high-dose ACEI therapy when compared to low-dose ACEI therapy, whereas the ACE dose had no effect on clinical outcomes in patients with either the II or ID genotypes. In this study, the regimen of high-dose ACE inhibitors and beta blockers had the greatest impact on transplant-free survival in patients with the DD variant.[69] Taken together these studies suggest a differential clinical response to standard HF therapy based on the ACE I/D polymorphism.

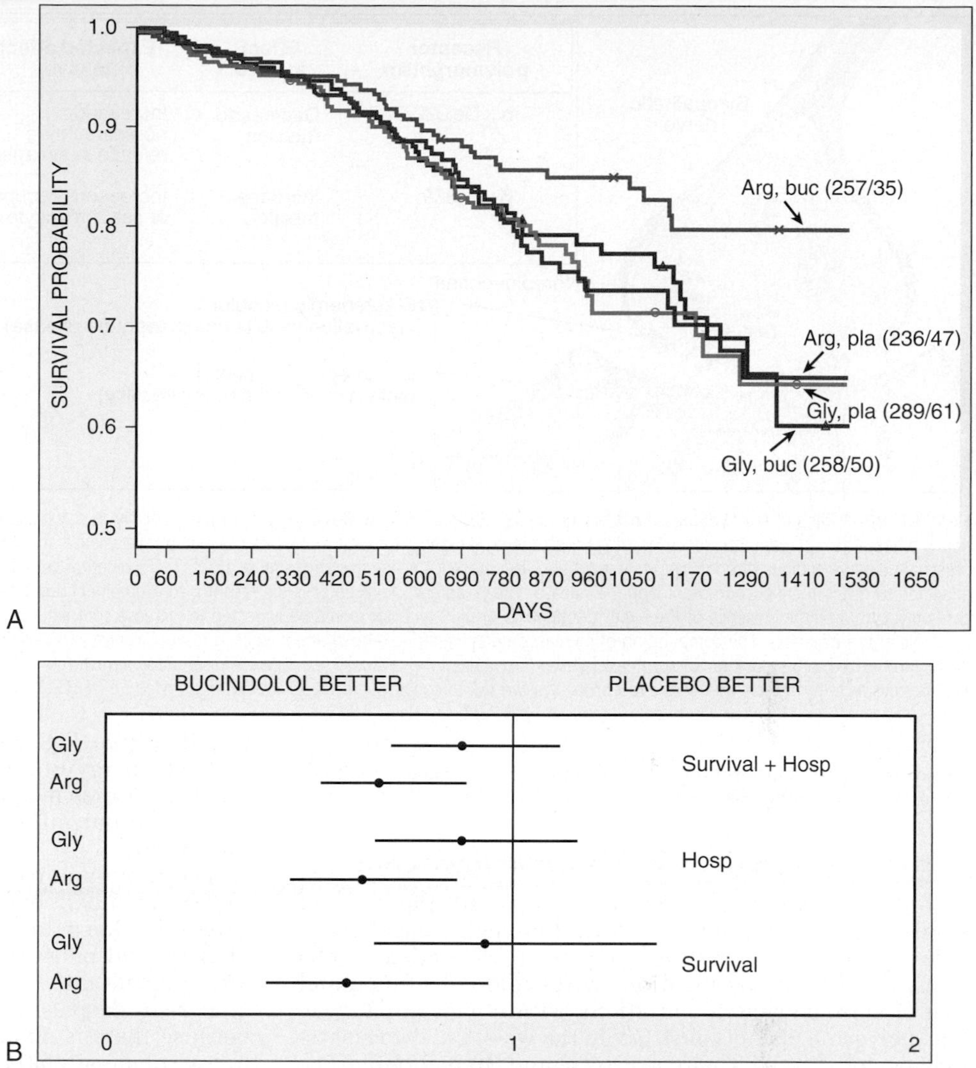

FIGURE 29–6 Kaplan-Meier analysis of endpoints in BEST trial stratified by treatment (placebo or bucindolol) and β_1AR genotype. **A,** For survival, Arg homozygotes had an HR = 0.62, 95 percent CI = 0.40-0.96, $p = 0.03$. In contrast, for $_1$-Gly-389 carriers, the HR = 0.90, 95 percent CI = 0.62-1.30, $p = 0.57$. **B,** Graphical representation of HRs and CIs by bucindolol and placebo is shown. Hosp, hospitalization. *(From Liggett SB, Mialet-Perez J, Thaneemit-Chen S, et al: A polymorphism within a conserved b1-adrenergic receptor motif alters cardiac function and beta blocker response in human heart failure. Proc Natl Acad Sci U S A 103:11288-11293, 2006.)*

Although the impact of genetic heterogeneity on HF outcomes has been extensively studied in predominantly white cohorts, few studies have investigated the impact of genomic variation in blacks. In a genetic substudy of the African-Americans in Heart Failure (A-HeFT) trial (see Chap. 25), a single nucleotide polymorphism within the promoter region of the aldosterone synthase gene (C to T transition at position −344) was shown to predict responsiveness to the fixed combination of hydralazine isosorbide dinitrate (see Chap. 25).[70] In A-HeFT treatment with the fixed combination of hydralazine isosorbide dinitrate was associated with a markedly improved clinical outcome (mortality, HF hospitalization, and change in quality of life at 6 months) in the TT homozygotes, but had no significant impact among subjects with the −344C allele—suggesting that genetic variations in aldosterone production may play an important role in disease progression in blacks with HF.

Polymorphisms that affect the function of beta- or alpha-adrenergic receptors may also influence the pharmacological response in HF patients (see Table 29-6). Patients with a common polymorphism of the beta$_1$-adrenergic receptor (AR) that results in either an arginine (Arg) or glycine (Gly) substitution at amino acid position 389 have different clinical responses to beta blockers. In the Bucindolol Evaluation of Survival Trial (BEST), bucindolol-treated patients who were homozygous for the Arg389 polymorphism (Arg389Arg) had improved clinical outcomes when compared to "glycine carriers" (Arg389Gly and Gly389Gly) who were treated with bucindolol (Fig. 29-6), suggesting that the therapeutic response to beta blockers differs by genotype.[71] The Arg389Arg genotype was also associated with significantly greater reductions in LV end-diastolic and end-systolic diameters following treatment with beta blockers when compared to identically treated Gly389 carriers.[72] The alpha$_{2c}$-adrenergic receptor inhibits norepinephrine release at cardiac presynaptic nerve endings through a negative feedback mechanism. The deletion of four consecutive amino acids in (aa 322-325) in the alpha$_{2c}$-adrenergic receptor results in loss of normal synaptic autoinhibitory feedback mechanism and enhanced presynaptic release of norepinephrine. There appears to be an increased risk of developing HF (Fig. 29-7) when the alpha$_{2c}$Del322-325 and the Arg389 beta$_1$-AR polymorphism are both present (i.e., a diplotype).[73] Although the impact of the alpha$_{2c}$Del322-325 and Arg389 beta$_1$-AR synergism on beta blocker responsiveness is not known, it is likely that patients with this diplotype may have increased responsiveness to beta blockers, based on what has been reported for the Arg389 polymorphism. In addition to contributing to the functional response to beta blockers, genetic polymorphisms that affect drug metabolism may also influence the therapeutic response to beta blockers. For example, genetic variants in the cytochrome P450 (CYP) 2D6 gene have a marked effect on plasma concentrations of metoprolol and carvedilol. In subjects with a nonfunctional CYP2D6 enzyme (poor metabolizers), the peak plasma

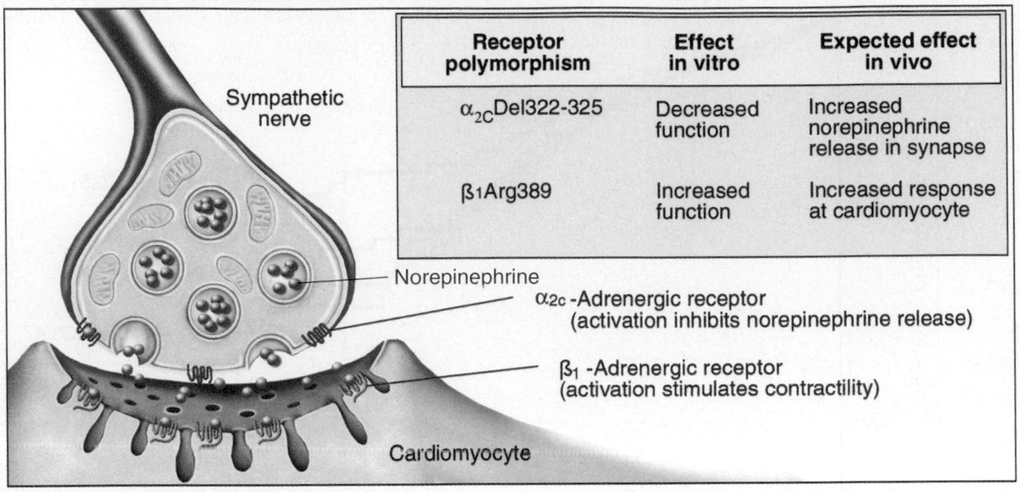

FIGURE 29–7 Basis of the hypothesis that the α_{2c}Del322-325 and β_1Arg389 receptors act synergistically as risk factors for heart failure. The α_{2c}-adrenergic receptor (along with the α_{2a}-adrenergic receptor) inhibits norepinephrine release at cardiac presynaptic nerve endings through negative feedback. The presence of the dysfunctional α_{2c}Del322-325 receptor would be expected to result in enhanced norepinephrine release. The β_1-adrenergic receptor is the receptor for norepinephrine on the cardiomyocyte, and the presence of the hyperfunctional β_1Arg389 receptor would be expected to increase contractile response at the myocytes. The combination of increased norepinephrine release and increased responsiveness of the receptor was hypothesized to be a risk factor for heart failure. *(From Small KM, Wagoner LE, Levin AM, et al: Synergistic polymorphisms of β_1 and α_{2c}-adrenergic receptors and the risk of congestive heart failure. N Engl J Med 347:1135, 2002.)*

concentration of metoprolol is sixfold higher than in subjects with a normally functioning enzyme.[68]

Future Perspectives in Pharmacogenetics

Although previous studies have explored the role of single gene polymorphisms with the renin angiotensin-aldosterone and adrenergic systems in HF patients, it is likely that future investigations will explore the functional role of multiple genetic variations within a given pathway (i.e., polygenic phenotypes). Given the wealth of data emerging from the Human Genome Project and Human Haplotype Mapping Program (HapMap) it will soon be possible to analyze complex phenotypes in relation to drug responsiveness in individual HF patients to better predict outcomes. This statement notwithstanding, it bears emphasis that the concept of personalizing therapeutic approaches in HF based on genetic background is far from fully developed, and will need to be carefully evaluated prospectively in suitable patient populations before this type of information can be used to guide clinical practice.

Metabolic Modulation

Optimization of myocardial energy utilization represents another unique approach for the treatment of HF. As noted in Chapter 22, myocardial high-energy phosphate concentrations are decreased in experimental and clinical HF, leading to the suggestion that the failing heart is "energy starved." In the normal heart, free fatty acids are the preferred fuel for the heart, producing roughly 4 times the ATP per mole of substrate utilized when compared to glucose. However, fatty acid oxidation is less efficient than glucose oxidation, requiring 10 to 12 percent more oxygen consumption to produce equivalent amounts of ATP. In addition, high rates of fatty acid oxidation are also associated with uncoupling of oxidative phosphorylation, an oxygen-wasting phenomenon, leading to an even greater consumption of molecular oxidation. Under conditions wherein oxygen is the limiting substrate, such as occurs in the failing heart (see Chap. 22), glycolysis becomes the more efficient pathway, requiring less oxygen compared with oxidation of free fatty acid. Fatty acid oxidation is physiologically regulated at several levels, including the concentration of circulating free fatty acid substrate, at the level of entry into the mitochondrion, and by the activity of several of the mitochondrial matrix enzymes that comprise the beta-oxidation pathway.[74] On the other hand, the rate of glucose oxidation is regulated primarily, although not exclusively, by the rate of fatty acid oxidation which inhibits the pyruvate dehydrogenase complex (PDH), the activity of which is rate limiting for glucose oxidation (Fig. 29-8A). Inhibition of pyruvate dehydrogenase can lead to increased glucose utilization through conversion of pyruvate to lactate, resulting in progressive tissue acidosis, and impaired myocyte contractility (see Fig. 29-8). From a theoretical perspective, shifting energy utilization from free fatty acids to glucose would optimize metabolic efficiency, reverse abnormalities in the cellular milieu, and improve cardiac function (see Fig. 29-8B).

The prototype partial inhibitors of fatty acid oxidation (pFOX), etomoxir, oxfenicine, and perhexiline, act by inhibiting carnitine palmitoyltransferase I (CPT I), the gatekeeper of fatty acid entry to the mitochondrion (see Fig. 29-8A). These agents shift energy utilization from free fatty acids to glucose by decreasing oxidation of free fatty acids. However, because there is no apparent feedback from CPT I activity to sarcolemmal fatty acid import, CPT I inhibitors can lead to accumulation of unmetabolized lipids in cardiac myocytes, which may lead to lipotoxicity-induced cardiac myocyte cell death. Etomoxir is an oxirane carboxylic acid derivative that indirectly promotes increased glucose oxidation through inhibition of CPT I. In an open-label, uncontrolled trial conducted in 10 patients with NYHA class II-III HF, treatment with etomoxir for 3 months was associated with a significant improvement in LVEF, cardiac output at peak exercise, and clinical status.[75] Subsequent phase II studies with etomoxir were halted because the compound did have the expected efficacy in the treatment of HF (data obtained from MediGene 2002 Annual Report [March 26, 2003]). Although oxfenicine was shown to be beneficial in the canine rapid pacing model of HF, in other animal models treatment with oxfenicine resulted in a dose-related increase in cardiac mass, as well as an increase in liver and kidney weights. Perhexiline is currently in use clinically as an anti-anginal agent. Although there were early reports of hepatotoxicity with this agent, hepatotoxicity occurred in patients with a genetic variant of a cytochrome P450 enzyme (slow hydroxylation), which resulted in drug accumulation, as well as accumulation of phospholipids in the liver and nerves. The risk of toxic effects is virtually eliminated by maintaining plasma concentrations between 150 and 600 ng/ml, at which levels the drug still remains effective.[75] Perhexiline has shown promise as adjunctive therapy for HF in a small short-term randomized double-blind clinical trial in patients with ischemic and nonischemic cardiomyopathy. In this study, 8 weeks of treatment with perhexiline resulted in an increase in the combined primary endpoint of peak oxygen uptake and LVEF, and an improvement in quality of life (Minnesota Living with Heart Failure Questionnaire). Importantly, maximum oxygen uptake increased significantly in both the ischemic and nonischemic groups, suggesting that the benefit of perhexiline was not entirely anti-ischemic.[76] Although there remains some optimism that CPT I inhibitors can be used as adjunctive therapy in HF, other pFOX inhibitors may have fewer side effects.

The pFOX inhibitors trimetazidine and ranolazine were also originally developed as anti-anginal agents. Trimetazidine is a piperazine compound that has been widely used outside of the United States as an anti-anginal agent. Trimetazidine has no discernible vasodilator properties at rest or during dynamic exercise, and has a very favorable side-effect profile. The exact mechanism of trimetazidine is not known, but it appears to work, at least in part, through inhibition of long-chain 3-ketoacyl coenzyme A thiolase, a crucial enzyme in the terminal steps of mitochondrial beta-oxidation. Several small clinical trials have shown improvements in ejection performance, reverse cardiac remodeling, and improvement in NYHA functional class with trimetazidine.[75]

Trimetazidine has been evaluated in a number of small clinical trials in patients with both ischemic and nonischemic cardiomyopathy.[74,75] Two months of treatment with trimetazidine resulted in significant improvement in LVEF at rest and enhanced LV wall motion during a dobutamine stress test compared with placebo in NYHA class II and III HF patients.[74] In two recent small clinical studies trimetazidine was shown to improve systolic LV function in patients with diabetes and ischemic cardiomyopathy when compared with placebo.[74,77] In contrast, another study, which assessed the effects of trimetazidine in patients with HF who were diabetic, demonstrated no significant effect on exercise capacity and only minor effects on LV systolic function.[75] In a study that specifically enrolled elderly patients with CAD and LVEF <50 percent, the group that received 6 months of trimetazidine on top of standard therapy showed a significantly greater improvement in LVEF (~7 percent), as well as smaller LV end-diastolic and systolic dimensions. In addition, the trimetazidine group had improved NYHA functional class and quality-of-life scores (Minnesota Living with Heart Failure Questionnaire). These findings have been confirmed in recent larger trials with longer term follow-up (18 to 24 months), which have also shown improvements in LVEF, reduction in LV volumes, and improvement in NYHA functional class in patients with ischemic cardiomyopathy (LVEF <50 percent).[75] Given the anti-anginal effects of trimetazidine, it is perhaps not surprising that this agent led to improvements in LV function and NYHA functional class in patients with ischemic cardiomyopathy. However, a recent study with trimetazidine also included patients with nonischemic cardiomyopathy, and showed similar increases in LVEF, reductions in LV end-systolic volume, and similar trends for improved quality of life and exercise capacity in both the ischemic and nonischemic groups.[78] Thus, it appears that trimetazidine has both functional and physiological benefits regardless of the HF etiology.

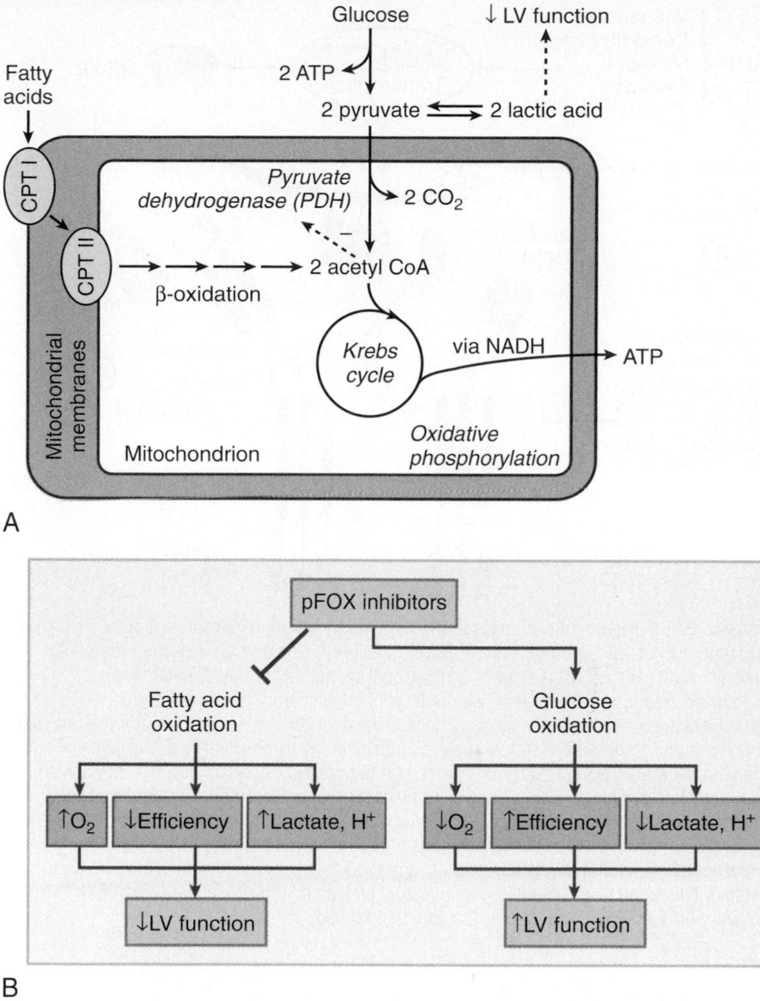

FIGURE 29–8 Metabolism of free fatty acids and glucose. **A,** Metabolic pathway for glucose metabolism and fatty acid oxidation; **B,** Effects switching metabolism from fatty acid beta-oxidation to glucose oxidation (under conditions wherein oxygen supply is rate limiting) using partial inhibitors of fatty acid oxidation (pFOX).

Ranolazine (Ranexa) is a novel anti-ischemic drug that prolongs the QT interval, and is the first FDA-approved pFOX inhibitor for the treatment of angina. The principal mechanism of action for this drug as an antianginal remains controversial, although recent studies suggest that the anti-anginal effects of ranolazine may be related (see Chap. 54) to decreased sodium entry into cells by inhibiting the rapid component of the delayed rectifier K+ current (I_{Kr}[BL3] [see Chap. 31]). Ranolazine also increases the activity of pyruvate decarboxylase, a key regulator of glucose metabolism, most likely due to loss of inhibition of the end-products of the beta-oxidation (NADH, acetyl-CoA). No clinical trials have yet been reported utilizing ranolazine in patients with cardiomyopathy. However, animal studies employing a canine model of chronic HF induced by microembolization have shown that, acutely, ranolazine significantly increased LVEF, peak +dp/dt, stroke volume, and mechanical efficiency.[79]

Future Perspectives in Metabolic Modulation

Switching substrate metabolism using pFOX inhibitors represents an attractive therapeutic target in patients with HF. Conceptually, another means to switch substrate metabolism would be to directly stimulate glucose uptake or pyruvate oxidation; however, pharmacological agents are not currently available for the chronic inhibition of this pathway, nor activation of glucose transport or glycolysis. Although the use of pFOX inhibitors appears promising, it bears emphasis that all of the clinical studies to date are small and have design flaws that are inherent to early phase clinical trials—not the least of which is a lack of long-term outcomes data. Accordingly, additional studies will be required before this therapy can be used in HF patients.

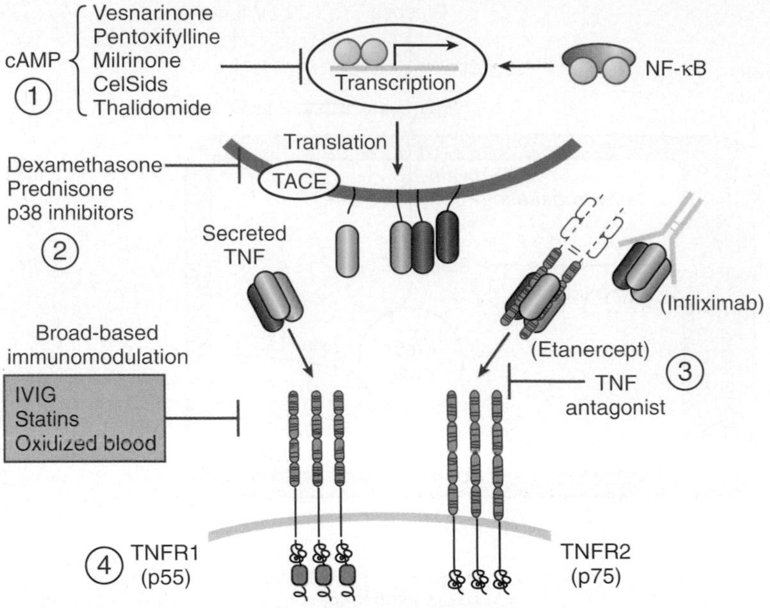

FIGURE 29–9 Therapeutic strategies for antagonizing proinflammatory mediators. TNF gene transcription is mediated, in part, by activation of NF-κB. Agents that increase intracellular levels of cAMP (1) such as vesnarinone, pentoxifylline, milrinone, thalidomide, and thalidomide analogs (CelSids) decrease the level of inflammatory mediators through transcriptional blockade of inflammatory gene expression. Agents such as dexamethasone and prednisone and some p38 inhibitors suppress inflammation by blocking the translation of inflammatory mediators (2). Secreted TNF can be neutralized (3) by soluble TNF antagonists (etanercept) or by neutralizing antibodies (infliximab) that prevent TNF from binding to its cognate type 1 (p55) and type 2 (p75) TNF receptors. In addition to these targeted approaches, broad-based immunomodulatory strategies have been employed (4) using intravenous immunoglobulin (IVIG), statins, and irradiated (oxidized) whole blood (Celacade therapy). *(Modified from Mann DL: Inflammatory mediators and the failing heart: Past, present, and the foreseeable future. Circ Res 91:988-998, 2002.)*

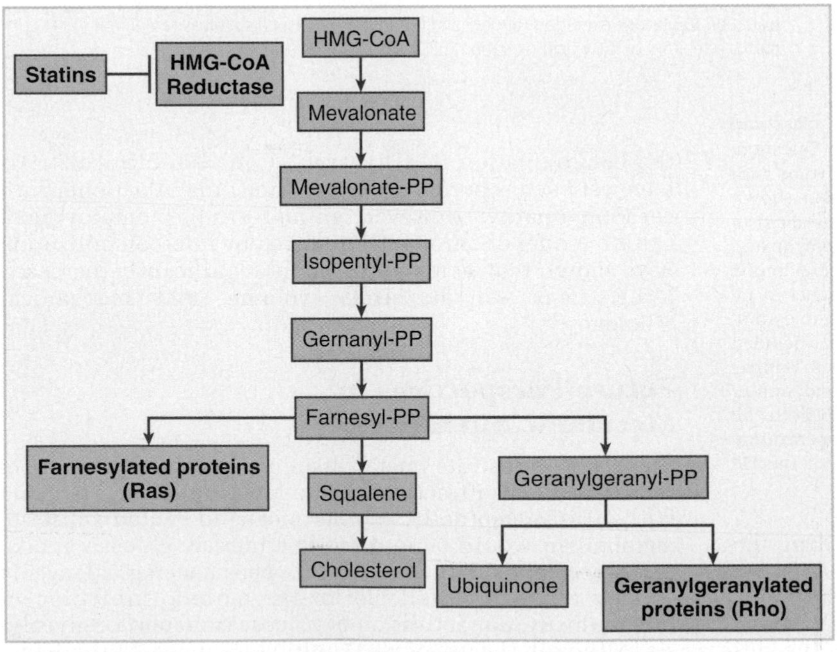

FIGURE 29–10 The mevalonate pathway leads to the synthesis of cholesterol. Important intermediate products in the mevalonate pathway include isoprenoids such as farnesyl pyrophosphate (farnesyl-PP) and geranylgeranyl pyrophosphate (geranylgeranyl-PP), which have been linked to activation Ras- and Rho-mediated signaling. 3-Hydroxy-3-methylglutaryl coenzyme A (HMG-CoA) reductase inhibitors decrease the synthesis of isoprenoids as well as cholesterol, by blocking HMG-CoA reductase. PP = pyrophosphate. *(From Ramasubbu K, Mann DL: The emerging role of statins in the treatment of heart failure. J Am Coll Cardiol 47:342-344, 2006.)*

Immunomodulation

Experimental and clinical studies suggest that inflammation plays a role in the pathogenesis of HF (Chap. 22). Over the past decade a variety of different anti-inflammatory strategies have been tried in small clinical trials in patients with chronic HF (Fig. 29-9; reviewed in references 80, 81). Thus far, two different anti-inflammatory approaches have not favorably impacted morbidity and mortality when examined in phase III clinical trials. The first trial used a targeted anti-cytokine approach with a tumor necrosis factor (TNF) antagonist (RENEWAL [Randomized Etanercept Worldwide Evaluation]),[82] whereas the second trial employed intramuscular injections of autologous blood (ACCLAIM [Advanced Chronic Heart Failure Clinical Assessment of Immune Modulation Therapy]) that had been subjected to oxidative stress ex vivo using a proprietary device (Celacade).[83] Despite these initial disappointing results, there are several emerging antiinflammatory approaches that are currently being evaluated in HF patients. One of the more promising approaches is the use of 3-hydroxy-3-methylglutaryl coenzyme A (HMG-CoA) reductase inhibitors (statins) in patients with chronic HF.

Statins have a variety of pleiotropic effects, including inhibition of inflammatory responses, increased nitric oxide bioavailability, improved endothelial function, and antioxidant properties. In addition to inhibiting cholesterol synthesis, statins also lower intermediate products in the mevalonate pathway including isoprenoids such as farnesyl pyrophosphate (farnesyl-PP) and geranylgeranyl pyrophosphate (geranylgeranyl-PP), which have been linked to activation of downstream signaling pathways mediated by Ras and Rho, respectively (Fig. 29-10). The Ras family of proteins are responsible for cell proliferation and hypertrophy, whereas the Rho family of proteins are important for superoxide generation, inflammation, and cytoskeletal formation. Rho inhibition has also been linked to increased expression of endothelial nitric oxide synthesis, which has a beneficial effect on endothelial function through increased nitric oxide production. Although the mechanism is less clear, statins also activate the phosphatidylinositol 3′-kinase/Akt pathway, which is coupled to cytoprotective signaling pathways.[84] In experimental models statins attenuated LV remodeling and improved LV ejection performance without directly affecting infarct size. The attenuation in LV remodeling was attributed to decreased cardiac myocyte hypertrophy, decreased activation of matrix metalloproteinases, and decreased fibrosis.[84] Importantly, statins have also been shown to promote angiogenesis, mobilize bone-marrow endothelial progenitor cells, and lead to downregulation of angiotensin type 1 receptor—any or all of which may have an additional beneficial effect(s) on cardiac remodeling.[84] Several retrospective analyses of clinical trial data bases have suggested that the use of statins has either reduced the incidence of HF, or reduced mortality in HF patients with known coronary artery disease.[84] Given the known salutary effects of statins on outcomes in coronary artery disease, as well as the high prevalence of ischemic heart disease in HF trials, these findings are perhaps not that surprising. However, several retrospective and prospective trials have shown that HMG-CoA reductase inhibitors may also be beneficial in patients with dilated cardiomyopathy (Fig. 29-11).[84,85]

There have been five prospective trials that have examined the effects of statins in HF patients. Node and coworkers demonstrated that patients with symptomatic nonischemic dilated cardiomyopathy (NYHA class II-III) who were randomized to simvastatin for 14 weeks had an improvement in NYHA functional class, improved LV function, and significant decreases in circulating levels of plasma TNF, interleukin-6 (IL-6), and brain natriuretic peptide.[86] In a smaller study, Laufs and colleagues randomized a small number of patients with nonischemic dilated cardiomyopathy (NYHA II-III) to cerivastatin (0.4 mg) or placebo for an average treatment period of 20 weeks. They observed that statin treatment resulted in an improvement in the quality of life

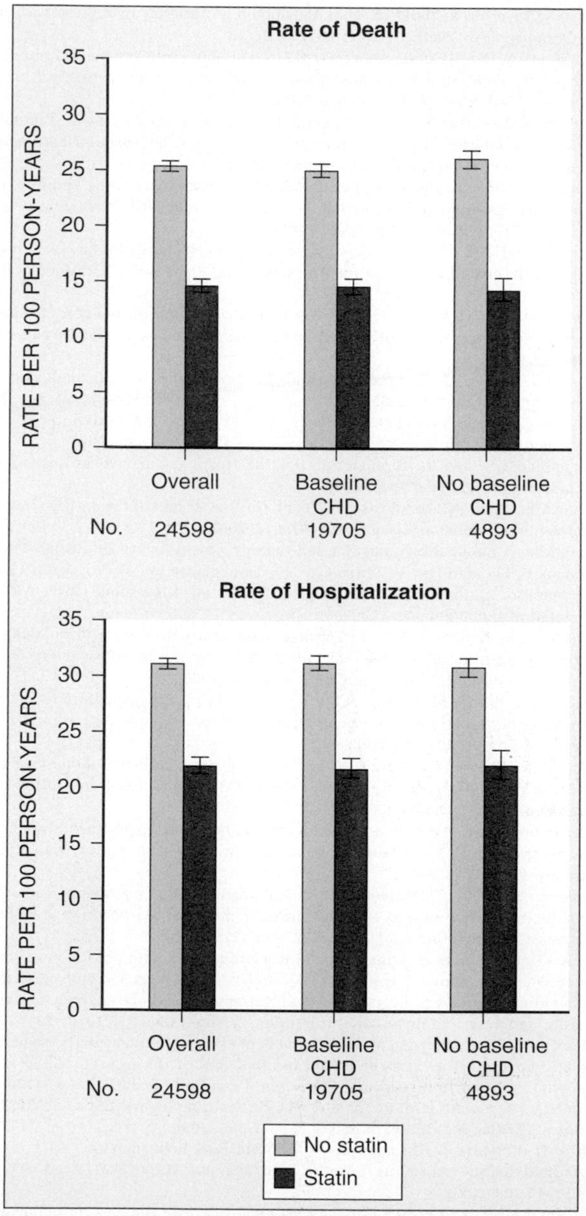

FIGURE 29–11 Age- and sex-adjusted rates of death from any cause and hospitalization for heart failure by incident statin exposure. *(From Go AS, Lee WY, Yang J: Statin therapy and risks for death and hospitalization in chronic heart failure. JAMA 296:2105-2111, 2006.)*

and exercise capacity, as well as decreased plasma concentrations of troponin T, hsCRP, plasminogen activator inhibitor-1, and TNF. In a large (446 patients) prospective nonrandomized trial, statin therapy was associated with a significant decrease in all-cause mortality at 2 years (15 versus 33 percent), as well as a significant decrease in HF hospitalizations (22 versus 38 percent) and nonfatal myocardial infarction (11 versus 15 percent). In this study, statin therapy was associated with a decrease in serum levels of C-reactive protein, IL-6, and the type 2 tumor necrosis factor receptor.[87] Two recent prospective double-blind randomized trials suggested that treatment with atorvastatin (20 to 40 mg/day) is beneficial in patients with nonischemic dilated cardiomyopathy.[87,88] Sola and colleagues studied the effects of 20 mg/day atorvastatin in patients with NYHA class II-IV HF (nonischemic). After 12 months of therapy, there was a significant increase in LVEF (~4 percent) in the atorvastatin group, whereas patients in the placebo group experienced a decline in LVEF during the same period of time (~2 percent). In addition the LV end-diastolic dimensions decreased significantly in the cohort of patients treated with atorvastatin, whereas LV end-diastolic dimension increased in the placebo group. The authors further noted that there was an increase in erythrocyte superoxide dismutase activity and significant reductions in serum levels of high sensitivity C-reactive protein (hsCRP), IL-6, and the type 2 tumor necrosis factor receptor in the atorvastatin group, consistent with a decrease in oxidative stress and inflammation.[90] Similar findings were reported in a small prospective study that examined the effects of 40 mg/day of atorvastatin, wherein statin therapy led to a significant increase in LVEF and a significant decrease in NYHA functional class.[88] However, conflicting results were reported in the UNIVERSE (Rosuvastatin Impact on Ventricular Remodeling Cytokines and Neurohormones) trial.[90] This study examined the effect of rosuvastatin (40 mg/day) on LV remodeling in patients with ischemic and dilated cardiomypathy. Compared to placebo, rosuvastatin was associated with significant reduction of low-density lipoprotein cholesterol, but had no effects on LV dimension, LVEF, or neurohormones. Although the reasons for the discrepant results of the UNIVERSE study are not known, the dose of rosuvastatin used was comparably higher than that used in previous studies with simvastatin and atorvastatin.

There are several theoretical concerns with the use of statins in HF. One is that low circulating levels of cholesterol have been associated with worse outcomes in patients with HF.[91] It has been suggested that circulating lipoproteins bind bacterial endotoxins that have been absorbed from the edematous gut of HF patients (the endotoxin-lipoprotein hypothesis),[92] thereby preventing endotoxin-induced inflammation from occurring. Theoretically, the lipid lowering effect of statins might be deleterious by allowing unbound endotoxin to activate immune cells to produce proinflammatory cytokines. A second theoretical concern is that statins inhibit ubiquinone (CoQ10) synthesis, which might precipitate or aggravate HF by creating problems with mitochondrial respiration **(see Chap. 22)**.

Thalidomide, known for its sedative and antiemetic properties, has been shown to have broad immunomodulatory properties, and is currently used to treat diseases such as multiple myeloma, erythema nodosum leprosum, and rheumatoid arthritis. Three small clinical studies have shown that thalidomide may be beneficial in HF patients.[93,94] The largest of the three studies was a double-blind placebo-controlled study, which showed that treatment with thalidomide (25 mg once daily—increasing to 200 mg once daily) resulted in significant increase in LVEF (~7 percent) along with a significant decrease in LV end-diastolic volumes. Although the results of these small studies appear promising, dose-limiting toxicity has been observed in some HF patients.[93] Accordingly, it will be important to determine the safety and efficacy of thalidomide in larger clinical trials before this therapy can be broadly recommended.

In addition to statin therapy several other immunomodulatory approaches appear to be promising, albeit in selected HF patients. Previous studies have shown that cardiac autoantibodies directed against cardiac cell proteins such as mitochondrial and contractile proteins, cardiac $beta_1$-adrenergic receptors, and muscarinergic receptors may play a pathogenesis of dilated cardiomyopathy. In small nonrandomized noncontrolled studies, immunoadsorption has been shown to improve cardiac function and patient outcomes.[95] However, interpretation of these studies is complicated because patients have also received concomitant therapy with intravenous immunoglobulin (IVIG), which also has immunomodulatory properties. Therapy with IVIG has been evaluated in a wide range of immune-mediated disorders, such as Kawasaki syndrome, idiopathic thrombocytopenic purpura, and multiple sclerosis. Although IVIG had no effect on LVEF in the IMAC trial (Intervention in Myocarditis and Acute Cardiomyopathy), 6 months of treatment with IVIG led to a significant increase in LVEF (~5 percent), independent of HF etiology, in a double-blind placebo-controlled study of NYHA functional Class II to IV HF patients.[81] Although IVIG was safe and well tolerated, the cost of this therapy may limit broader applicability in HF patients.

Future Perspectives in Immunomodulation

Early attempts to target inflammation using specific anticytokine therapies and broad-based immunomodulating approaches have been disappointing when examined in phase III clinical trials. One potential reason for these early failures may be that all currently approved pharamacological therapies for HF have some antiinflammatory effects.[80] Accordingly, in future studies it may be necessary to use biomarkers or a pharmacogenetic approach to select HF patients who have evidence of ongoing inflammation despite optimal medical therapy. Of the current emerging immunomodulatory strategies, statins appear to be the most promising—based on large retrospective and small prospective studies, as well as their well-established safety profile. This statement notwithstanding, it is important to emphasize that our current randomized clinical experience with statins in nonischemic cardiomopathy is limited to several small trials in which fewer than 250 patients have actually been treated. We have no information with respect to the correct dose of statins to use in these HF patients. Accordingly, it is premature to recommend the routine use of statins for all HF patients. There are several ongoing large-scale clinical outcome trials in HF patients, including CORONA (Controlled Rosuvastatin Multinational Trial in Heart Failure) and GISSI-HF (Gruppo Italiano per lo studio della sopravvivenza nell'insufficienza cardiaca [Italian group for the study of the survival in cardiac insufficiency]), which should provide a more definitive answer(s) to the role of statins in HF.

REFERENCES

Myocardial Repair and Regeneration

1. Kehat I., Kenyagin-Karsenti D., Snir M, et al: Human embryonic stem cells can differentiate into myocytes with structural and functional properties of cardiomyocytes. J Clin Invest 108:407-414, 2001.
2. Dai W, Kloner RA: Myocardial regeneration by embryonic stem cell transplantation: present and future trends. Expert Rev Cardiovasc Ther 4:375-383, 2006.
3. Jackson KA, Majka SM, Wang H, et al: Regeneration of ischemic cardiac muscle and vascular endothelium by adult stem cells. J Clin Invest 107:1395-1402, 2001.
4. Toma C, Pittenger MF, Cahill KS, et al: Human mesenchymal stem cells differentiate to a cardiomyocyte phenotype in the adult murine heart. Circulation 105:93-98, 2002.
5. Jiang Y, Jahagirdar BN, Reinhardt RL, et al: Pluripotency of mesenchymal stem cells derived from adult marrow. Nature 418:41-49, 2002.
6. Urbich C, Dimmeler S: Endothelial progenitor cells: Characterization and role in vascular biology. Circ Res 95:343-353, 2004.
7. Rafii S, Lyden D: Therapeutic stem and progenitor cell transplantation for organ vascularization and regeneration. Nat Med 9:702-712, 2003.
8. Grunewald M, Avraham I, Dor Y, et al: VEGF-induced adult neovascularization: Recruitment, retention, and role of accessory cells. Cell 124:175-189, 2006.
9. Galvez BG, Sampaolesi M, Brunelli S, et al: Complete repair of dystrophic skeletal muscle by mesoangioblasts with enhanced migration ability. J Cell Biol 174:231-243, 2006.
10. Galli D, Innocenzi A, Staszewsky L, et al: Mesoangioblasts, vessel-associated multipotent stem cells, repair the infarcted heart by multiple cellular mechanisms: A comparison with bone marrow progenitors, fibroblasts, and endothelial cells. Arterioscler Thromb Vasc Biol 25:692-697, 2005.
11. Beltrami AP, Barlucchi L, Torella D, et al: Adult cardiac stem cells are multipotent and support myocardial regeneration. Cell 114:763-776, 2003.
12. Oh H, Bradfute SB, Gallardo TD, et al: Cardiac progenitor cells from adult myocardium: Homing, differentiation, and fusion after infarction. Proc Natl Acad Sci U S A 100(21):12313-12318, 2003.
13. Laugwitz KL, Moretti A, Lam J, et al: Postnatal isl1+ cardioblasts enter fully differentiated cardiomyocyte lineages. Nature 433:647-653, 2005.
14. Pfister O, Mouquet F, Jain M, et al: Restoration of cardiac progenitor cells after myocardial infarction by self-proliferation and selective homing of bone marrow-derived stem cells. Circ Res 97:52-61, 2005.
15. Tomita Y, Matsumura K, Wakamatsu Y, et al: Cardiac neural crest cells contribute to the dormant multipotent stem cell in the mammalian heart. J Cell Biol 170:1135-1146, 2005.
16. Fazel S, Cimini M, Chen L, et al: Cardioprotective c-kit+ cells are from the bone marrow and regulate the myocardial balance of angiogenic cytokines. J Clin Invest 116:1865-1877, 2006.
17. Mouquet F, Pfister O, Jain M, et al: Restoration of cardiac progenitor cells after myocardial infarction by self-proliferation and selective homing of bone marrow-derived stem cells. Circ Res 97:1090-1092, 2005.
18. Fraser JK, Schreiber R, Strem B, et al: Plasticity of human adipose stem cells toward endothelial cells and cardiomyocytes. Nat Clin Pract Cardiovasc Med 3 Suppl 1: S33-S37, 2006.
19. Guan K, Nayernia K, Maier LS, et al: Pluripotency of spermatogonial stem cells from adult mouse testis. Nature 440:1199-1203, 2006.
20. Condorelli G, Borello U, De Angelis L, et al: Cardiomyocytes induce endothelial cells to trans-differentiate into cardiac muscle: Implications for myocardium regeneration. Proc Natl Acad Sci U S A 98:10733-10738, 2001.
21. Kawamoto A, Tkebuchava T, Yamaguchi J, et al: Intramyocardial transplantation of autologous endothelial progenitor cells for therapeutic neovascularization of myocardial ischemia. Circulation 107:461-468, 2003.
22. Urbich C, Aicher A, Heeschen C, et al: Soluble factors released by endothelial progenitor cells promote migration of endothelial cells and cardiac resident progenitor cells. J Mol Cell Cardiol 39:733-742, 2005.
23. Gnecchi M, He H, Liang OD, et al: Paracrine action accounts for marked protection of ischemic heart by Akt-modified mesenchymal stem cells. Nat Med 11:367-368, 2005.
24. Zimmermann WH, Melnychenko I, Wasmeier G, et al: Engineered heart tissue grafts improve systolic and diastolic function in infarcted rat hearts. Nat Med 12:452-458, 2006.
25. Choi YH, Stamm C, Hammer PE, et al: Cardiac conduction through engineered tissue. Am J Pathol 169:72-85, 2006.
26. Guo XM, Zhao YS, Chang HX, et al: Creation of engineered cardiac tissue in vitro from mouse embryonic stem cells. Circulation 113:2229-2237, 2006.
27. Christman KL, Lee RJ: Biomaterials for the treatment of myocardial infarction. J Am Coll Cardiol 48:907-913, 2006.
28. Davis ME, Hsieh PC, Grodzinsky AJ, et al: Custom design of the cardiac microenvironment with biomaterials. Circ Res 97:8-15, 2005.
29. Menasche P: Skeletal myoblast for cell therapy. Coron Artery Dis 16:105-110, 2005.
30. Assmus B, Schachinger V, Teupe C, et al: Transplantation of Progenitor Cells and Regeneration Enhancement in Acute Myocardial Infarction (TOPCARE-AMI). Circulation 106: 3009-3017, 2002.
31. Erbs S, Linke A, Schuler G, et al: Intracoronary administration of circulating blood-derived progenitor cells after recanalization of chronic coronary artery occlusion improves endothelial function. Circ Res 98:e48, 2006.
32. Strauer BE, Brehm M, Zeus T, et al: Repair of infarcted myocardium by autologous intracoronary mononuclear bone marrow cell transplantation in humans. Circulation 106:1913-1918, 2002.
33. Wollert KC, Meyer GP, Lotz J, et al: Intracoronary autologous bone-marrow cell transfer after myocardial infarction: the BOOST randomised controlled clinical trial. Lancet 364:141-148, 2004.
34. Fernandez-Aviles F, San Roman JA, Garcia-Frade J, et al: Experimental and clinical regenerative capability of human bone marrow cells after myocardial infarction. Circ Res 95:742-748, 2004.
35. Janssens S, Dubois C, Bogaert J, et al: Autologous bone marrow-derived stem-cell transfer in patients with ST-segment elevation myocardial infarction: double-blind, randomised controlled trial. Lancet 367:113-121, 2006.
36. Lunde K, Solheim S, Aakhus S, et al: Intracoronary injection of mononuclear bone marrow cells in acute myocardial infarction. N Engl J Med 355:1199-1209, 2006.
37. Schachinger V, Erbs S, Elsasser A, et al: Intracoronary bone marrow-derived progenitor cells in acute myocardial infarction. N Engl J Med 355:1210-1221, 2006.
38. Mansour S, Vanderheyden M, De Bruyne B, et al: Intracoronary delivery of hematopoietic bone marrow stem cells and luminal loss of the infarct-related artery in patients with recent myocardial infarction. J Am Coll Cardiol 47:1727-1730, 2006.
39. Dimmeler S, Zeiher AM, Schneider MD: Unchain my heart: the scientific foundations of cardiac repair. J Clin Invest 115:572-583, 2005.
40. Orlic D, Kajstura J, Chimenti S, et al: Mobilized bone marrow cells repair the infarcted heart, improving function and survival. Proc Natl Acad Sci U S A 98:10344-10349, 2001.
41. Kuhlmann MT, Kirchhof P, Klocke R, et al: G-CSF/SCF reduces inducible arrhythmias in the infarcted heart potentially via increased connexin43 expression and arteriogenesis. J Exp Med 203:87-97, 2006.
42. Ince H, Petzsch M, Kleine HD, et al: Preservation from left ventricular remodeling by front-integrated revascularization and stem cell liberation in evolving acute

myocardial infarction by use of granulocyte-colony-stimulating factor (FIRSTLINE-AMI). Circulation 112:3097-3106, 2005.
43. Kuethe F, Figulla HR, Herzau M, et al: Treatment with granulocyte colony-stimulating factor for mobilization of bone marrow cells in patients with acute myocardial infarction. Am Heart J 150:115, 2005.
44. Ripa RS, Jorgensen E, Wang Y, et al: Stem cell mobilization induced by subcutaneous granulocyte-colony stimulating factor to improve cardiac regeneration after acute ST-elevation myocardial infarction: Result of the double-blind, randomized, placebo-controlled stem cells in myocardial infarction (STEMMI) trial. Circulation 113:1983-1992, 2006.
45. Zohlnhofer D, Ott I, Mehilli J, et al: Stem cell mobilization by granulocyte colony-stimulating factor in patients with acute myocardial infarction: A randomized controlled trial. JAMA 295:1003-1010, 2006.
46. Kang HJ, Lee HY, Na SH, et al: Differential effect of intracoronary infusion of mobilized peripheral blood stem cells by granulocyte colony-stimulating factor on left ventricular function and remodeling in patients with acute myocardial infarction versus old myocardial infarction: The MAGIC Cell-3-DES randomized, controlled trial. Circulation 114:I145-I151, 2006.
47. Kang HJ, Kim HS, Zhang SY, et al: Effects of intracoronary infusion of peripheral blood stem-cells mobilised with granulocyte-colony stimulating factor on left ventricular systolic function and restenosis after coronary stenting in myocardial infarction: The MAGIC cell randomised clinical trial. Lancet 363:751-756, 2004.
48. Smits PC: Myocardial repair with autologous skeletal myoblasts: A review of the clinical studies and problems. Minerva Cardioangiol 52:525-535, 2004.
49. Perin EC, Dohmann HF, Borojevic R, et al: Transendocardial, autologous bone marrow cell transplantation for severe, chronic ischemic heart failure. Circulation 107:2294-2302, 2003.
50. Fuchs S, Satler LF, Kornowski R, et al: Catheter-based autologous bone marrow myocardial injection in no-option patients with advanced coronary artery disease: A feasibility study. J Am Coll Cardiol 41:1721-1724, 2003.
51. Galinanes M, Loubani M, Davies J, et al: Autotransplantation of unmanipulated bone marrow into scarred myocardium is safe and enhances cardiac function in humans. Cell Transplant 13:7-13, 2004.
52. Strauer BE, Brehm M, Zeus T, et al: Regeneration of human infarcted heart muscle by intracoronary autologous bone marrow cell transplantation in chronic coronary artery disease: The IACT Study. J Am Coll Cardiol 46:1651-1658, 2005.
53. Assmus B, Honold J, Schachinger V, et al: Transcoronary transplantation of progenitor cells after myocardial infarction. N Engl J Med 355:1222-1232, 2006.
54. Hill JM, Syed MA, Arai AE, et al: Outcomes and risks of granulocyte colony-stimulating factor in patients with coronary artery disease. J Am Coll Cardiol 46:1643-1648, 2005.
55. Huttmann A, Duhrsen U, Stypmann J, et al: Granulocyte colony-stimulating factor-induced blood stem cell mobilisation in patients with chronic heart failure—Feasibility, safety and effects on exercise tolerance and cardiac function. Basic ResCardiol 101:78-86, 2006.

Gene Therapy

56. Nayak L, Rosengart TK: Gene therapy for heart failure. Semin Thorac Cardiovasc Surg 17:343-347, 2005.
57. Li CX, Parker A, Menocal E, et al: Delivery of RNA interference. Cell Cycle 5:2103-2109, 2006.
58. Nordlie MA, Wold LE, Simkhovich BZ, et al: Molecular aspects of ischemic heart disease: Ischemia/reperfusion-induced genetic changes and potential applications of gene and RNA interference therapy. J Cardiovasc Pharmacol Ther 11:17-30, 2006.
59. Hajjar RJ, del Monte F, Matsui T, et al: Prospects for gene therapy for heart failure. Circ Res 86:616-621, 2000.
60. Hata JA, Williams ML, Koch WJ: Genetic manipulation of myocardial beta-adrenergic receptor activation and desensitization. J Mol Cell Cardiol 37:11-21, 2004.
61. Milano CA, Allen LF, Rockman HA, et al: Enhanced myocardial function in transgenic mice overexpressing the b2-adrenergic receptor. Science 264:582-586, 1994.
62. Engelhardt S, Hein L, Wiesmann F, et al: Progressive hypertrophy and heart failure in beta1-adrenergic receptor transgenic mice. Proc Natl Acad Sci U S A 96:7059-7064, 1999.
63. Miyamoto MI, del Monte F, Schmidt U, et al: Adenoviral gene transfer of SERCA2a improves left-ventricular function in aortic-banded rats in transition to heart failure. Proc Natl Acad Sci U S A 97:793-798, 2000.
64. Del MF, Harding SE, Dec GW, et al: Targeting phospholamban by gene transfer in human heart failure. Circulation 105:904-907, 2002.
65. Most P, Pleger ST, Volkers M, et al: Cardiac adenoviral S100A1 gene delivery rescues failing myocardium. J Clin Invest 114:1550-1563, 2004.
66. Haunstetter A, Izumo S: Toward antiapoptosis as a new treatment modality. Circ Res 86:371-376, 2000.
67. Murry CE, Wiseman RW, Schwartz SM, et al: Skeletal myoblast transplantation for repair of myocardial necrosis. J Clin Invest 98:2512-2523, 1996.

Pharmacogenetics

68. Muszkat M, Stein CM: Pharmacogenetics and response to beta-adrenergic receptor antagonists in heart failure. Clin Pharmacol Ther 77:123-126, 2005.
69. McNamara DM, Holubkov R, Janosko K, et al: Pharmacogenetic interactions between beta-blocker therapy and the angiotensin-converting enzyme deletion polymorphism in patients with congestive heart failure. Circulation 103:1644-1648, 2001.
70. McNamara DM, Tam SW, Sabolinski ML, et al: Aldosterone synthase promoter polymorphism predicts outcome in African Americans with heart failure: Results from the A-HeFT Trial. J Am Coll Cardiol 48:1277-1282, 2006.
71. Liggett SB, Mialet-Perez J, Thaneemit-Chen S, et al: A polymorphism within a conserved b1-adrenergic receptor motif alters cardiac function and beta-blocker response in human heart failure. Proc Natl Acad Sci U S A 103:11288-11293, 2006.
72. Terra SG, Hamilton KK, Pauly DF, et al: Beta1-adrenergic receptor polymorphisms and left ventricular remodeling changes in response to beta-blocker therapy. Pharmacogenet Genomics 15:227-234, 2005.
73. Small KM, Wagoner LE, Levin AM, et al: Synergistic polymorphisms of beta1- and alpha2C-adrenergic receptors and the risk of congestive heart failure. N Engl J Med 347:1135-1142, 2002.

Metabolic Modulation

74. Stanley WC, Recchia FA, Lopaschuk GD: Myocardial substrate metabolism in the normal and failing heart. Physiol Rev 85:1093-1129, 2005.
75. Abozguia K, Clarke K, Lee L, et al: Modification of myocardial substrate use as a therapy for heart failure. Nat Clin Pract Cardiovasc Med 3:490-498, 2006.
76. Lee L, Campbell R, Scheuermann-Freestone M, et al: Metabolic modulation with perhexiline in chronic heart failure: A randomized, controlled trial of short-term use of a novel treatment. Circulation 112:3280-3288, 2005.
77. Fragasso G, Piatti PM, Monti L, et al: Short- and long-term beneficial effects of trimetazidine in patients with diabetes and ischemic cardiomyopathy. Am.Heart J 146:E18, 2003.
78. Fragasso G, Palloshi A, Puccetti P, et al: A randomized clinical trial of trimetazidine, a partial free fatty acid oxidation inhibitor, in patients with heart failure. J Am Coll Cardiol 48:992-998, 2006.
79. Chandler MP, Stanley WC, Morita H, et al: Short-term treatment with ranolazine improves mechanical efficiency in dogs with chronic heart failure. Circ Res 91:278-280, 2002.

Immunomodulation

80. Mann DL: Inflammatory mediators and the failing heart: Past, present, and the foreseeable future. Circ Res 91:988-998, 2002.
81. Aukrust P, Yndestad A, Ueland T, et al: Anti-inflammatory trials in chronic heart failure. Heart Fail Monit 5:2-9, 2006.
82. Mann DL, McMurray JJV, Packer M, et al: Targeted anti-cytokine therapy in patients with chronic heart failure: Results of the Randomized EtaNcercept Worldwide evALuation (RENEWAL). Circulation 109:1594-1602, 2004.
83. Tang WH, Francis GS: The year in heart failure. J Am Coll Cardiol 48:2575-2583, 2006.
84. Ramasubbu K, Mann DL: The emerging role of statins in the treatment of heart failure. J Am Coll Cardiol 47:342-344, 2006.
85. Go AS, Lee WY, Yang J, et al: Statin therapy and risks for death and hospitalization in chronic heart failure. JAMA 296:2105-2111, 2006.
86. Node K, Fujita M, Kitakaze M, et al: Short-term statin therapy improves cardiac function and symptoms in patients with idiopathic dilated cardiomyopathy. Circulation 108:839-843, 2003.
87. Sola S, Mir MQ, Rajagopalan S, et al: Statin therapy is associated with improved cardiovascular outcomes and levels of inflammatory markers in patients with heart failure. J Card Fail 11:607-612, 2005.
88. Wojnicz R, Wilczek K, Nowalany-Kozielska E, et al: Usefulness of atorvastatin in patients with heart failure due to inflammatory dilated cardiomyopathy and elevated cholesterol levels. Am J Cardiol 97:899-904, 2006.
89. Sola S, Mir MQ, Lerakis S, et al: Atorvastatin improves left ventricular systolic function and serum markers of inflammation in nonischemic heart failure. J Am Coll Cardiol 47:332-337, 2006.
90. Krum H, Ashton E, Reid C, et al: Double-blind, randomized, placebo-controlled study of high-dose HMG CoA reductase inhibitor therapy on ventricular remodeling, pro-inflammatory cytokines and neurohormonal parameters in patients with chronic systolic heart failure. J Card Fail 13:1-7, 2007.
91. Rauchhaus M, Clark AL, Doehner W, et al: The relationship between cholesterol and survival in patients with chronic heart failure. J Am Coll Cardiol 42:1933-1940, 2003.
92. Rauchhaus M, Coats AJ, Anker SD: The endotoxin-lipoprotein hypothesis. Lancet 356:930-933, 2000.
93. Agoston I, Dibbs Z I, Wang F, et al: Preclinical and clinical assessment of the safety and potential efficacy of thalidomide in heart failure. J Card Fail 8:306-314, 2002.
94. Gullestad L, Ueland T, Fjeld JG, et al: Effect of thalidomide on cardiac remodeling in chronic heart failure: Results of a double-blind, placebo-controlled study. Circulation 112:3408-3414, 2005.
95. Mann DL: Autoimmunity, immunoglobulin adsorption and dilated cardiomyopathy: Has the time come for randomized clinical trials? J Am Coll Cardiol 38:184-186, 2001.

CHAPTER 30

Care of Patients with End-Stage Heart Disease

Linda L. Emanuel and Robert O. Bonow

Care for the incurable has been a defining part of medicine from its earliest origins, as reflected in the emphasis on comfort in the writings of fifth century BC Greek physician Hippocrates.[1] In recent history the fields of palliative care and cardiology have developed in parallel and tacit partnership. When English physician William Harvey first described circulation in *Exercitatio anatomica de motu cordis et sanguinis in animalibus* in 1628, hospice meant an almshouse for the poor. However, when French physician Rene Laënnec developed the stethoscope in the early 1800s, two prominent Massachusetts General Hospital physicians were writing on end-of-life care. Jacob Bigelow urged withholding of bloodletting from those for whom it would merely "embitter the approach of death when it is inevitable," and John Warren wrote in "Etherization: with Surgical Remarks" (1848) that ether should be used to relieve the suffering of "mortification." In recent decades, advances in cardiopulmonary resuscitation, cardiovascular surgery, and implantable devices have stimulated medical ethics discussions of who should receive resuscitation, who should undergo life-prolonging procedures, and when life really ends. End-of-life and palliative care more generally remain a defining part of the practice of cardiology. For instance, the primary indication for coronary artery bypass, stents, and other procedures is symptom control and quality of life; in this sense a significant amount of care provided by cardiologists is quality palliative care.

At the same time, consideration of the types of care sought by those who are facing death and dying is beginning to move into the mainstream but clearly needs more attention.[2-4] One study found that of the 15 guidelines on congestive heart failure published up to 2004, none had significant mention of palliative care and only 6 had moderate mention.[5] However, this situation changed with the 2005 ACC/AHA guidelines update on chronic heart failure in the adult,[6] which provides a class I recommendation for educating patients and their families about the role of palliative and hospice care services among the end-of-life recommendations. In addition, a consensus statement[7] prepared by an ad-hoc group of experts in advanced heart failure, palliative medicine, geriatrics, outcome measurement, and health care improvement made similar recommendations and underscored the need for future studies designed to improve end-of-life care in heart failure. By explicitly integrating palliative care considerations into the new patient assessment, treatment decision-making, continuity of care planning, and systems of care delivery, cardiovascular medicine can further advance the quality of care it provides.[8]

EPIDEMIOLOGY

Of the approximately 2.4 million deaths in the United States in 2002, 1.4 million (58 percent) were primarily or secondarily caused by cardiovascular disease.[9] Cardiovascular disease was the primary cause of death in every year of the 20th century except 1918. Although cardiovascular disease is more common with advancing age, particularly in the area of heart failure, it is not restricted to the elderly; more than 152,000 Americans younger than age 65 die from cardiovascular disease each year.[9] The characteristic cardiovascular death is sudden death. However, cardiovascular conditions are also chronic and may afflict children and young adults, as well as the elderly. Roughly 71 million Americans are living with one or more chronic forms of cardiovascular disease: Hypertension afflicts roughly 65 million Americans, coronary artery disease 13.2 million, and congestive heart failure 5 million. Some 5.5 million Americans are living with the aftermath of a stroke.

The site of death has also evolved in an important way. Nearly 60 percent of Americans died as inpatients in hospitals in 1980; by 2000, about 40 percent died in the hospital. Although this trend corresponds with patient and family preferences, patients with cardiovascular disease are least represented among those receiving home care and hospice care. Referrals for hospice care for heart failure are infrequent.[10,11] In 2000, approximately 20 percent of all decedents received hospice care, with cancer patients constituting more than 70 percent of hospice users. Among 9 cancer diagnoses, 15 to 34 percent of decedents used hospice, while among myocardial infarction and congestive heart failure diagnoses, 7 and 8 percent, respectively, of decedents used hospice.[12] In one estimate, only 4 percent of heart failure patients receive palliative care.[10] Patients in need of palliative care may be ambulatory, in long-term care or in the hospital. Consequently, palliative care is necessary in a full range of settings.

PALLIATIVE CARE

Because terminally ill patients have a wide variety of advanced diseases, often with multiple symptoms demanding relief, and require a noninvasive therapeutic regimen to be delivered in a commodious care setting, their care requires some of the most complex and demanding cognitive skills for assessments and interventions. Fundamental to ensuring quality palliative and end-of-life care is a focus on four broad domains of the illness experience: (1) physical symptoms; (2) mental or psychological symptoms; (3) social—relationships, practical issues, and economic—needs; and (4) existential or spiritual needs. Palliative care also provides support for the family, including for their bereavement. Recent empirical studies have confirmed that these domains coincide with the experiences and preferences for care of patients with advanced illness and their families. A whole-person assessment screens for and evaluates needs in each of these four domains. Goals for care are discerned and decided on in discussion with the patient and/or family on the basis of the assessment in each of these domains. Although physicians are responsible for certain, especially technical, interventions and for coordinating the interventions, they depend on an interdisciplinary team and the family to provide all of them. Importantly, failing to address any one of the domains is likely to preclude a good death, and hence a well coordinated, effectively communicating interdisciplinary team takes on special importance in end-of-life care.

ASSESSMENT, GOALS, AND CARE PLANNING

WHOLE-PERSON ASSESSMENT. The assessment of physical and mental symptoms should follow a modified version of the traditional "history and physical" examination that emphasizes symptoms. Questions should discern sources of suffering and how much these symptoms interfere with the patient's life. Standardized assessment questions are available from clinically relevant scales such as the Memorial Symptom Assessment Scale; these have the advantage of ensuring that the assessment is comprehensive. For a patient with late end-stage disease for whom the care goal is quality of being, aspects of the physical examination and tests that are uncomfortable should be carefully evaluated for their benefit-to-burden ratio for the patient. Because a focused physical examination may be all that is reasonable, these skills need to be well developed.

In the area of social needs, health care providers should screen for financial needs, the status of important relationships, care-giving needs, and access to medical care. Relevant questions may include: *How often is there someone to feel close to? How much help do you need with things like getting meals or getting around? How much trouble do you have getting the medical care you need?* In the area of existential needs, providers should assess distress and the patient's sense of being emotionally and existentially settled, and of finding purpose or meaning.[13] Helpful assessment questions can include: *How much are you able to find meaning since your illness began?* Asking about the patient's perception of their care is helpful: *How much do you feel your doctors and nurses respect you? How clear is the information from us about what to expect regarding your illness? How much do you feel that the medical care you are getting fits with your goals?* If concern is detected in any areas, deeper evaluation questions are warranted.[14]

COMMUNICATION. Communication is arguably as powerful an intervention in medicine as any invasive procedure. However, several studies involving patients with advanced heart failure indicate that there is often inadequate communication with patients and their families.[7,10,11,15-17] Compared with patients with cancer, patients with heart failure have less information about their condition and a poorer understanding of its prognosis, in part because of a less certain course of the disease, and they are also less involved in decision making.[17] Continued focus on correcting hemodynamic abnormalities or improving symptoms often takes precedence over communication about prognosis and options for care. Poor communication has significant adverse consequences, and quality communication allows for navigating difficult situations in the best available fashion. Communication requires both effective "signal output" and effective reception, so the clinician must assist the patient and family with their ability to receive difficult information, as well as offer the information in an accessible way.

A seven-step guide for communicating important information has been developed by Buckman[18]: (1) Prepare mentally and physically by (2) setting up a quiet environment with room for face-to-face discussion and accommodating items such as a chair, a box of tissues, a pen and paper to write down information, and a beverage. (3) Begin by asking what the patient and/or family know/understand, and then (4) ask how they prefer to receive new information and how much they want whom to know. (5) Give the new information according to their preferences. (6) Allow for emotional responses. (7) Plan for the next steps in care including identifying the next concrete steps. See Table 30-1 for suggested wording and the rationale behind each step.

PROGNOSIS. Among patients with an equally poor prognosis, 75 percent of cancer patients reported that they knew they would likely die, whereas only 54 percent of noncancer patients, many of whom had cardiac diagnoses, reported the same.[19] The established gap between prognosis in late-stage cardiovascular conditions and the patient's expectation of death, the continuous stream of life-prolonging cardiovascular therapies and devices, the difficulty in establishing accurate prognoses in individual cases, and the need to sustain hope may be only four of multiple factors that conspire to keep poor prognosis from triggering appropriate forms of palliative care.

Clinicians should provide population-based statistics regarding prognosis to patients and families and allow these statistics rather than individual predictions to trigger the kinds of whole-person assessments and continuous goal assessment conversations that follow palliative care guidelines. This in turn will allow patients and families to not only follow plans for care that are appropriate but also achieve the kinds of psychological, social, and existential engagements that people tend to seek when going through the last stages of life.[7,10,16,20-22] Generally, clinicians should share population-based prognosis at the time of diagnosis and then introduce a palliative care framework of whole-person assessment and continuous goal adjustment from the time when clinical indicators suggest a prognosis of 6 months or less. When sharing prognostic information, use language such as: *"Of all the people with your condition in America, about half will go on to live for more than 6 months and about half will die within 6 months"* (or whatever is the appropriate time frame). Go on to say something like: *"We will hope for the best but also plan for the worst so that we are not caught unprepared and you can live your life with a positive attitude."* And further, something such as: *"Many people have special things they want to accom-*

TABLE 30–1 Elements of Communicating Bad News—The P-SPIKES Approach

Acronym	Steps	Aim of the Interaction	Preparations, Questions, or Phrases
P	Preparation	• Mentally prepare for the interaction with the patient and/or family.	• Review what information needs to be communicated. • Plan how you will provide emotional support. • Rehearse key steps and phrases in the interaction.
S	Setting of the interaction	• Ensure the appropriate setting of a serious and emotionally charged discussion.	• Ensure patient, family, and appropriate social supports are present. • Devote sufficient time—do not squeeze in a discussion. • Ensure privacy and prevent interruptions by people or beeper. • Bring a box of tissues.
P	Patient's perception and preparation	• Begin the discussion by establishing the baseline and whether the patient and family can grasp the information. • Ease tension by having the patient and family contribute.	• Start with open-ended questions to encourage participation. • Possible phrases to use: *What do you understand about your illness?* *When you first had symptom X, what did you think it might be?* *What did Dr. X tell you when he sent you here?* *What do you think is going to happen?*
I	Invitation and information needs	• Discover what information needs the patient and/or family have and what limits they want regarding the bad information.	• Possible phrases to use: *If this condition turns out to be something serious, do you want to know?* *Would you like me to tell you the full details of your condition? If not, then whom would you like me to talk to?*
K	Knowledge of the condition	• Provide the bad news or other information to the patient and/or family sensitively.	• Do not just dump the information on the patient and family. • Interrupt and check that the patient and family understand. • Possible phrases to use: *I feel badly to have to tell you this, but ...* *Unfortunately, the tests showed ...* *I'm afraid the news is not good ...*
E	Empathy and exploration	• Identify the cause of the emotions—e.g., poor prognosis. • Empathize with the patient and/or family's feeling. • Explore by asking open-ended questions.	• Strong feelings in reaction to bad news are normal. • Acknowledge what the patient and family are feeling. • Remind them that such feelings are normal even if frightening. • Give them time to respond. • Remind patient and family you will not abandon them. • Possible phrases to use: *I imagine this is very hard for you.* *You must be upset. Tell me how you are feeling.* *I wish the news were different.* *I'll do whatever I can to help you.*
S	Summarize and plan a strategy	• Delineate for the patient and the family the next steps including additional tests or interventions.	• It is the unknown and uncertain that increase anxiety. • Recommend a schedule with goals and landmarks. Provide your rationale for the patient and/or family to accept (or reject). • If the patient and/or family are not ready to discuss the next steps, schedule a follow-up visit.

Modified from Robert Buckman: How to Break Bad News: A Guide for Health Care Professionals. Baltimore, Johns Hopkins University Press, 1992.

plish in this phase of their life—such as a project, a trip, or coming to terms in a personal relationship. I encourage you to think about what that might be for you so that I can do my best to tailor our medical care to your goals." For patients with cardiovascular illnesses, it is often helpful to point out that: *"The good news is that we can expect you to feel well and function pretty normally. Often people with cardiac disease avoid the long phases of disability and suffering that other illnesses can cause. The counterpart is that people sometimes do not engage in the growth that often comes at the end of life or they become overly fearful of dying suddenly. Preparation of the kind we just mentioned can bring the best of both worlds. So let's keep an open discussion about your goals for care."*

CONTINUOUS GOAL ASSESSMENT. Goals for care are numerous. They range from cure of a specific condition, to delaying the course of an incurable disease, to adapting to progressive disability without disrupting the family, to finding peace of mind or personal meaning, to dying in a manner that leaves loved ones with a positive "departure memory." Discernment of goals for care can be approached through a seven-step protocol: (1) Ensure that information is as complete as reasonably possible and understood by all relevant parties (see Whole-Person Assessment and Communication earlier); (2) Explore what the patient and/or family are hoping for; (3) Share all the options with the patient and family. Delineate some relevant goals that are also realistic; (4) Respond empathically to the patient and/or family as they adjust to declining realistic expectations; (5) Make a plan, emphasizing what can be done toward the realistic goals; (6) Follow through with the plan; (7) Review and revise this plan periodically, considering at every encounter whether the goals of care should be reviewed with the patient and/or family. If a patient or family member has difficulty letting go of an unrealistic goal, suggest that while hoping for the best it is still prudent to have a plan for other outcomes as well.

ADVANCE CARE PLANNING. Advance care planning is a process of planning for future medical care in case the patient becomes incapable of making medical decisions. Ideally, it starts before a health care crisis or the terminal phase of an illness. However, although 80 percent of Americans endorse advance care planning, only 20 percent have actually done so. A similarly small proportion of health care providers have completed their own advance care planning. A good first step is for health care providers to start with themselves. Personal planning makes the providers aware of the critical and charged choices in the process and allows them to truthfully tell their patients that they have done this themselves. With experience, advance care planning discussions need not take long.

Steps in effective advance care planning involve: (1) introducing the topic; (2) structuring a discussion; (3) reviewing plans that have been discussed by the patient and family; (4) documenting the plans; (5) updating them periodically; and (6) implementing the advance care directive (Table 30-2). Raising the topic can be done efficiently as a routine matter, analogous to insurance or estate planning, that is recommended for all patients. Structuring a focused discussion (step 2) is the central skill. Identify the health care proxy and recommend his or her involvement in the discussion. Select a worksheet, preferably one that has been evaluated and demonstrated to produce reliable and valid expressions of patient preferences, and orient the patient and proxy to it. Discuss with the patient and proxy one scenario as an example to demonstrate how to think about the issues. Often it is helpful to begin with a scenario in which the patient is likely to have settled preferences, such as being in a persistent vegetative state. Ask the patient and proxy to discuss and complete the worksheet for the other scenarios. If appropriate, suggest they involve family members in the discussion. On a return visit, go over the patient's preferences, checking and resolving any medical or logical inconsistencies. After having the patient and proxy sign the document, place it in the medical chart and be sure that copies are provided to relevant family members and care sites. Because patients' preferences can change, review these documents periodically or after an illness episode or personal experience.

TYPES OF DOCUMENTS. Two broad types of advance care planning documents exist. The first includes living wills or instructional directives; these advisory documents describe the types of decisions that should direct care. Some are specific, delineating scenarios and interventions. Among these, some are for general use and others are for a specific type of disease such as cancer or HIV; some are available in multiple languages.[23] Less specific directives can be general statements or may describe the values that should guide decisions. Health care proxy forms appoint an individual to make decisions. A combined directive that both directs care and designates a proxy is generally recommended, and the directive should clearly indicate whether the patient's preferences or the proxy's choice should take precedence if they conflict.

The U.S. Supreme Court has established that patients have a constitutional right to refuse or terminate life-

TABLE 30–2 Steps in Advance Care Planning

Step	Goals to Be Achieved and Measures to Cover	Useful Phrases or Points to Make
Introducing advance care planning	• Ask the patient what he or she knows about advance care planning and if he or she has already completed an advance care directive. • Indicate that you as a physician have completed advance care planning. • Indicate that you try to perform advance care planning with all patients regardless of prognosis. • Explain the goals of the process as empowering the patient and ensuring you and the proxy understand the patient's preferences. • Provide the patient relevant literature including the advance care directive that you prefer to use. • Recommend the patient identify a proxy decision-maker who should attend the next meeting.	• "I'd like to talk with you about something I try to discuss with all my patients. It's called advance care planning. In fact, I feel that this is such an important topic that I have done this myself. Are you familiar with advance care planning or living wills?" • "Have you thought about the type of care you would want if you ever became too sick to speak for yourself? That is the purpose of advance care planning." • "There is no change in health that we have not discussed. I am bringing this up now because it is sensible for everyone, no matter how well or ill, old or young." • Have many copies of advance care directives available, including in the waiting room, for patients and families.
Structured discussion of scenarios and patient preferences	• Affirm that the goal of the process is to follow the patient's wishes if the patient loses decision-making capacity. • Elicit the patient's overall goals related to health care. • Elicit the patient's preferences for specific interventions in a few salient and common scenarios. • Help the patient define the threshold for withdrawing and withholding interventions. • Define the patient's preference for the role of the proxy.	• Use a structured worksheet with typical scenarios. • Begin the discussion with persistent vegetative state and consider other scenarios, such as recovery from an acute event with serious disability, asking the patient about his or her preferences regarding specific interventions, such as ventilators, nasogastric feedings, and CPR, and then proceeding to less invasive interventions, such as blood transfusions and antibiotics.
Review the patient's preferences	• After the patient has made choices of interventions, review them to ensure they are consistent and medically sensible and that the proxy is aware of them.	
Document the patient's preferences	• Formally complete the advance care directive and have a witness sign it. • Provide a copy for the patient and the proxy. • Insert a copy into the patient's medical record.	
Update the directive	• Periodically, and with major changes in health status, review with the patient the existing choice made and make any modifications.	
Apply the directive	• The directive goes into effect only when the patient becomes unable to make medical decisions for himself or herself. • Reread the directive to be sure about its content. • Discuss your proposed actions on the basis of the directive with the proxy.	

sustaining interventions, and that mentally incompetent patients may do so by having previously provided "clear and convincing evidence" of their advance preferences.[24] As of 2003, all states and the District of Columbia also have living will or health care proxy legislation. State variations exist but are less important than they could be because the Constitution has been interpreted to require states to honor any clear advance care directive. A potentially misleading distinction relates to statutory as opposed to advisory documents. Statutory documents are drafted to fit relevant state statutes. They tend to be written with the goal of protecting clinicians from legal action if they follow the patient's stated wishes. Advisory documents are drafted to reflect the patient's wishes. Both are legal, the first under state law and the second under common or constitutional law. However, it is simpler to honor a statement that complies with all laws, so if a patient is not using a statutory form, it is appropriate to attach a statutory form to the advance care directive being used.

INTERVENTIONS

PHYSICAL AND PSYCHOLOGICAL SYMPTOMS. Many patients with heart failure die with uncontrolled symptoms, often suffering as much as those with advanced forms of cancer.[10,11,22] The most common physical and psychological symptoms among all terminally ill patients include pain, fatigue, insomnia, anorexia, dyspnea, depression, anxiety, and nausea and vomiting. In the last days of life, terminal delirium is also common. Patients with advanced cancer experience an average of 11.5 symptoms including pain, dyspnea, constipation, fatigue, depression, anxiety, and delirium. Such statistics on symptoms for late-stage cardiovascular patients are not available. However, almost one third of cardiovascular deaths have additional causes of death, so the cardiologist managing end-stage disease should be able to manage symptoms from noncardiac conditions as well. Symptom management skills are well described elsewhere.[25]

SOCIAL NEEDS

Financial Burdens. Dying can impose substantial economic strains on patients and families. In the United States, about 20 percent of terminally ill patients and their families have to spend more than 10 percent of family income on health care costs over and above health insurance premiums. Between 10 and 30 percent of families have sold assets, used savings, or taken out a mortgage to pay for the patient's health care costs. Nearly 40 percent of terminally ill patients report that the cost of their illness was a moderate or great economic hardship for their family.

One source of economic burden is related to medical costs. The second, more universal source of economic burden is a decline in the patient's income. In 20 percent of cases, a family member stopped working to provide care. Economic burden is associated with poor physical functioning and needs for housekeeping, nursing, and personal care. That is, more debilitated and less well-off patients experience greater economic burdens. Economic burdens tend to increase the psychological distress of families and patients. Assistance from a social worker, early on if possible, to ensure access to available benefits may be helpful. Many people are unaware of insurance benefits, the Family and Medical Leave Act, and other sources of assistance.

Relationships. Closing the narrative of lived relationships is a nearly universal need. When asked if sudden death or death after an illness is preferable, respondents often initially select the former but soon change to the latter as they reflect on the importance of saying goodbye. Bereaved family members who have not had the chance to say goodbye often have a difficult grief process. Because many of the deaths in cardiology are sudden, this is of particular importance. Patients and their families should be encouraged to settle matters, even though it is more difficult to anticipate the time of death.

Care of seriously ill patients requires efforts to assist the types of encounters and time spent with family and friends that are necessary to meet these needs. Family and close friends may need to be accommodated with unrestricted visiting hours for inpatients including in some cases sleeping near the patient even in institutional settings. Assistance for patients and family members who are unsure about how to create or help preserve memories, whether by providing raw materials such as a scrapbook or memory box or by offering suggestions and informational resources, can be deeply appreciated. Taking photographs and creating videos or audiotapes can be especially helpful to patients with life-shortening illnesses who have younger children.

Family Caregivers. Caring for seriously ill patients places a heavy burden on families.[7,22] Families are required to provide transportation, homemaking, and other services. Typically, paid professionals such as home health nurses and hospice supplement family caregiving; only about a quarter of all caregiving is exclusively paid professional assistance. The trend toward more out-of-hospital deaths will increase reliance on families for end-of-life care. About three quarters of the caregivers of terminally ill patients are female—wives, daughters, and even sisters. Consequently, females tend to be able to rely less on family for caregiving assistance and may need more paid assistance. About 20 percent of terminally ill patients report substantial unmet needs for nursing and personal care.

This makes it imperative to inquire about unmet needs and assist family or paid professional services. Assistance from religious or community groups can often be mobilized by one or two phone calls from the medical team to someone with whom the patient or family identifies.

EXISTENTIAL NEEDS AND THEIR MANAGEMENT. Dying is one of the ultimate existential challenges. Religion and spirituality are important to dying patients.[11] Approximately 70 percent of patients report becoming more religious or spiritual when they become terminally ill, and many find comfort in practices such as prayer. Some studies suggest women and older patients are more likely to experience greater interest in religion and spirituality. On the other hand, about 20 percent of terminally ill patients become less religious, frequently feeling alienated by becoming terminally ill. For other patients, the need is for existential meaning and purpose that is distinct from, and maybe even an antireligious form of, spirituality. Among patients with cardiovascular conditions, clinical experience suggests that fear of sudden death is common. Further, the well-recognized accomplishment of personal growth and relationship resolution characteristic among patients who foresee death in the near future is less apparent among patients with cardiovascular illnesses.[26] This may reflect the rarer recognition of mortality among heart patients than cancer patients.

Health care providers often hesitate to involve themselves in the religious, spiritual, and existential experiences of their patients because the experiences may seem private or related to alternative lifestyles or the providers may seem "soft." But physicians and other members of the interdisciplinary team should be able to at least detect spiritual need. Screening questions have been developed for a physician's spiritual history taking. Spiritual distress can amplify other types of suffering and even masquerade as, for instance, intractable physical pain or anxiety. The screening questions in the whole-person assessment are usually sufficient. Deeper evaluation and intervention is rarely appropriate for the physician unless no other member of the team is available or suitable. Pastors may be helpful, whether from the medical institution or the patient's community.

Precisely how religious practices, spirituality, and existential explorations can be assisted and improve end-of-life care is not well established. In at least one study, only 36 percent of respondents indicated that a clergy member would be comforting. Nevertheless, this increase in religious and spiritual interest among a substantial proportion of dying patients underscores the importance of inquiring how this need can be addressed in individual patients.

MANAGING THE LAST STAGES

WITHDRAWING AND WITHHOLDING LIFESUSTAINING TREATMENT. For centuries, it has been deemed ethical to withhold or withdraw life-sustaining interventions. For patients who are incompetent and terminally ill but have not completed an advance care directive, next-of-kin can exercise this right, although this may be restricted in some states depending on how clear and convincing the evidence is of the patient's preferences. In theory, a patient's right to refuse medical therapy can be limited by four countervailing interests: (1) preservation of life; (2) prevention of suicide; (3) protection of third parties such as children; and (4) preserving the integrity of the medical profession. In practice, these interests almost never override the right of competent patients or incompetent patients who have left explicit advance care directives. Regarding incompetent patients whose wishes are not clear, two criteria can help guide decisions. First, many courts have advocated use of the substituted-judgment criterion, which holds that the proxy decision-makers should try to imagine what the incompetent patient would do if he or she were competent. However, most proxies, even close family members, cannot accurately predict what the patient would have wanted. The second criterion is that of best interests and holds that proxies should decide on the basis of the likely best outcome for the patient. Yet as many family conflicts reveal, different people can have different views of what is in the patient's best interests. As a matter of practice, physicians rely on family members to make decisions that they feel are best and only object if these decisions seem to demand treatments that the physicians consider nonbeneficial.

PHYSICIANS' ORDERS REGARDING RESUSCITATION. In the SUPPORT Project, only 25 percent of patients hospitalized with heart failure recalled having discussions with their physicians about resuscitation preferences.[16] Whenever a patient is a suitable candidate for a Do Not Resuscitate (DNR) order, he or she deserves to have had a comprehensive discussion about goals of care, their plan of care, and possibly also advance care planning. Use of predesigned forms such as the Physicians Orders for Life-Sustaining Treatments in place of limited DNR forms can encourage these more comprehensive and coherent approaches to creating plans of care. In general, an isolated DNR order with no reference to other life-sustaining treatment preferences can be considered a red flag that should prompt a physician to include or return to a whole-person assessment and a comprehensive plan for care with goal-tailored treatment choices.

AUTOMATED IMPLANTABLE CARDIAC DEFIBRILLATORS. With increasing indications for automated implantable cardiac defibrillators (AICDs) in patients with left ventricular dysfunction, the number of patients receiving these devices will undoubtedly increase dramatically in the future.[27] The difficult ethical dilemmas include not only the indications for implanting AICDs and the impact on health care finances but also the issues regarding when these devices should be deactivated.[28] These issues also include the need to discuss these decisions with patients and their families.[6] These discussions should be an essential component of overall advance care planning.

The thorny issues of AICD management are highlighted by a study of family members' views of AICDs in end-of-life care.[29] Among 100 family members of patients who died with AICDs in place, only 27 family members reported discussions of possible deactivation and often only in the last few days of life.

MECHANICAL VENTILATION. Perhaps the most challenging intervention to withdraw is mechanical ventilation. Two approaches are used: "terminal extubation," which is the removal of the endotracheal tube, and "terminal wean," which is the gradual reduction of the FIO_2 or ventilator rate. Some physicians recommend the terminal wean because patients do not develop upper airway obstruction and the distress caused by secretions or stridor, but it is reported that terminal weaning can prolong the dying process. To ensure comfort for conscious or semiconscious patients, a common practice is to inject a bolus of midazolam (2 to 4 mg) before withdrawal followed by 5 to 10 mg of morphine and continuous infusion of morphine (50 percent of the bolus dose per hour). Higher doses will be necessary for patients already receiving anxiolytics and opioids. Caregivers should remove any neuromuscular blocking agents so that patients can show any discomfort that can in turn allow medication titration or additional boluses of morphine or midazolam. Families need to be warned that up to 10 percent of patients unexpectedly survive for 1 day or more after mechanical ventilation is stopped.

FUTILE CARE. Beginning in the late 1980s, some commentators argued that physicians could terminate futile treatments demanded by families of terminally ill patients. No objective definition or standard of futility exists. The term conceals subjective value judgments about when a treatment is not beneficial. A more practical approach acknowledges that many cases in which futility concerns are raised overlie communication gaps or unresolved personal issues that are best dealt with in team or family meetings. Occasionally, true value differences exist; these may be best handled with assistance from an ethics committee.

EUTHANASIA/PHYSICIAN-ASSISTED SUICIDE. Terminating life-sustaining intervention and providing opioids to manage symptoms are not to be confused with euthanasia or physician-assisted suicide. Both the former, unlike the latter, have long been considered ethical by the medical profession and legal by courts.

A growing body of data indicates that depression, hopelessness, and worries about loss of dignity or autonomy are the primary factors motivating a desire for euthanasia or physician-assisted suicide. Although any of these can occur in patients with cardiovascular conditions, there appear to be fewer requests in this population than in cancer and AIDS patients. Perhaps the characteristic sudden death among cardiac patients helps to avoid some of the fears of indignity and dependence associated with a slow, highly symptomatic decline. Nonetheless, multiple symptoms and chronic disability do occur in patients with end-stage heart disease, and requests for physician-assisted suicide or euthanasia also occur. Cardiologists should know how to respond to such requests.

After receiving a request for euthanasia and/or physician-assisted suicide, probe with empathic, open-ended questions to help elucidate the underlying cause for the request such as: "What makes you want to consider this option?" Endorsing either moral opposition or moral support for the act tends to be counterproductive, either lending an impression of being judgmental or of endorsing the worthlessness of the patient's life. Health care providers must reassure the patient of continued care and commitment. Simultaneously, the patient should be educated about: (1) alternative, less controversial options such as symptom management and withdrawing any unwanted treatments; (2) the reality of euthanasia and/or physician-assisted suicide because the patient is likely to have misconceptions about its effectiveness; and (3) the legal implications of the choice. As indicated, depression, hopelessness, and other symptoms of psychological distress, as well as physical suffering and economic burdens, are likely factors motivating the request. Health care providers should identify the factors motivating the request and aggressively treat those factors. Most patients, after these interventions and clarification of options, proceed with a less controversial approach of declining life-sustaining interventions, possibly including refusal of nutrition and hydration.

CARE DURING THE LAST HOURS. Most lay people have limited experiences with the actual dying process and death. They frequently do not know what to expect of the final hours and beyond. Rehearsal and second chances do not occur. Therefore the family and other caregivers must be prepared, especially if the plan is for the patient to die at home.

For patients with heart failure, there may be several last days of life with characteristic pathophysiological changes such as increased orthopnea and nocturnal dyspnea. Patients experience extreme weakness and fatigue and become bed bound. This can lead to bedsores. If the end is near and the sores are causing less distress than dressing changes and frequent turning, it is reasonable to omit these usual types of care. Dry mucosal membranes should be cared for with frequent oral swabbing, lip lubricants, and artificial tears. These activities can provide the family with a form of care to substitute for those that no longer help, such as feeding. With loss of the gag reflex and dysphagia, patients may also accumulate airway and pharyngeal secretions, producing noises during respiration sometimes called "the death rattle." Scopolamine can reduce this. They also have changes in respiration with periods of apnea or Cheyne-Stokes breathing. Decreased intravascular volume and cardiac output cause tachycardia, hypotension, peripheral coolness, and livedo reticularis (skin mottling). Patients can also have urinary and fecal incontinence at death as the sphincters lose their tone. Most importantly, changes occur in consciousness and other neurological functions as brain perfusion falters. Clinical observation indicates that patients have one of two paths to death (Fig. 30-1). In the common clinical course patients become somnolent, then comatose, and die with seeming comfort. In the less common course patients become confused, have hallucinations, delirium, and then seizures before becoming comatose. Management with the help of a palliative care consultant is advisable in the latter case; such difficult deaths can have a profound impact on the family. Reassurance is important that this is a known physiological reaction to decreased brain perfusion and not a personal expression.

Informing families, even by providing an information sheet, about what to expect during the dying process in general can help. For instance, it can be calming to know that patients stop eating because they are dying, not dying because they have stopped eating, or that the "death rattle" is not a sign of suffocation, or that mottling tends to mean that death is near.

People claim that hearing and touch are the last senses to stop functioning. Families should be encouraged to communicate with and touch the patient, even if he or she is unconscious.

When the plan is for the patient to die at home, the family needs to know how to determine when death has occurred including the cardinal signs of cessation of cardiac function and respiration, fixed pupils, coolness, changes in skin color and texture, and incontinence. Remind the family that the eyes may remain open. It helps to have a plan of whom the family and caregivers will contact when the patient is dying or has died. Without a plan, they may panic and call 911, unleashing a cascade of unwanted events from arrival of emergency personnel and resuscitation to hospital admission. Family and caregivers should be instructed to contact hospice, the covering physician, or the on-call member of the palliative care team. Contacting the coroner is unnecessary unless the state requires it for all deaths. Similarly, unless foul play is suspected, the health care team need not contact the coroner either.

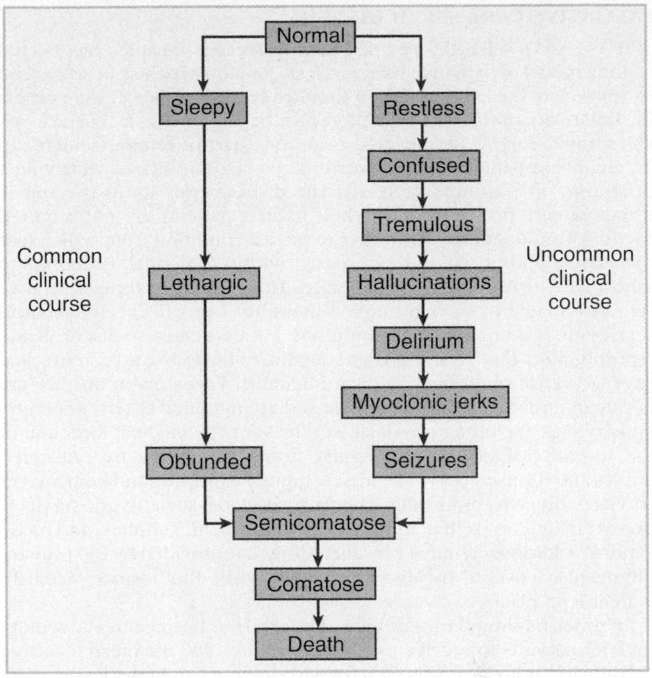

FIGURE 30–1 Common and uncommon clinical courses of the last days of terminally ill patients. *(Modified from Mount Sinai Hospital & Casey House Hospice: Advance planning.* In *Ferris FD, Flannery JS, McNeal HB, et al [eds]: A Comprehensive Guide for the Care of Persons with HIV Disease. Module 4: Palliative Care. Toronto, Mount Sinai Hospital & Casey House Hospice, 1995 [http://www.cpsonline.info/content/resources/hivmodule4.html].)*

Just after the patient dies, even the best-prepared family may experience shock and bereavement and be distraught. They need time to assimilate the event and be comforted. Health care providers should write a bereavement card or letter to the family. It can be appropriate, although it is not obligatory, to attend the funerals of patients in order to lend support to the grieving family and find an opportunity for closure for the physician.

Death is a strong predictor of poor health, and even mortality, for the surviving spouse. It may be important to alert the spouse's physician about the death to be aware of symptoms that might require professional attention.

SUDDEN DEATH. Sudden death may "shortchange" patients from the growth that often happens in the last phase of life and that may make it easier for bereaved family members to go on. Children of patients who have died suddenly may be excessively influenced by the sudden disappearance of their parent, without a chance to say goodbye, and by the fear of suffering the same fate. Preparedness through discussion, planning, and engaging the benefits of the consciously trodden last paths in life can help, as can extended bereavement counseling. The services of a social worker or other professional with expertise in the area should almost always be considered.

HOW AND WHERE. For nearly two decades, hospice has been a leading model of palliative care services. Patients who use hospice tend to appreciate the care, and their families tend to do better than others in similar situations.[30] In 1983 Medicare began paying for hospice services under Part A, the hospital insurance part of reimbursement. To be eligible, a patient must be certified by two physicians as having a prognosis of 6 months or less if the disease runs its usual course. Prognoses are probabilistic by their nature; patients are not required to die within 6 months but rather to have a condition from which half the people with it would be deceased within 6 months. Patients sign a hospice enrollment form that states their intent to forego curative services related to their terminal illness but can still receive medical services for other comorbid conditions. Patients can also disenroll and reenroll later; that is, the hospice Medicare benefit can be reinvoked later to secure traditional Medicare benefits. Payments to hospice are per diem rather than fee-for-service and are intended to cover comprehensive care including physician services for the medical direction of the interdisciplinary team; regular home care visits by registered nurses and licensed practical nurses; home health aide and homemaker services; dietary counseling; chaplain services; social work services; bereavement counseling; and medical equipment, supplies, and medications. Additional clinical care including that provided by the primary physician is covered by Medicare Part B while the hospice Medicare benefit is in place.

Physicians should initiate earlier referrals to hospice to allow more time for patients to receive palliative care. By 1996 the mean length of enrollment in hospice was 65 days with the median being less than 24 days. Since then, the length of enrollment has declined. The hospice length of stay tends to be longer for heart failure patients than for other patients.[31] In two surveys the mean length of stay of patients with heart failure was 43.5 and 60 days.[31,32]

Until relatively recently, hospice had been the main way of securing palliative services for terminally ill patients. Efforts are now directed at ensuring continuity of palliative care across settings and through time. Increasingly, these same types of palliative care services are available as consultative services in hospitals, in day care and other outpatient settings, and nursing homes. For instance, in the United States, although the vast majority of hospice care is provided in residential homes, slightly more than 10 percent now occurs in nursing homes. In addition, palliative care consultations for nonhospice patients can be billed as for other consultations under Medicare Part B, the physician reimbursement part. Many experts believe palliative care should be offered to patients regardless of their prognosis. A patient and his or her family should not have to make an "either curative care or palliative care" choice, in large part because it can be psychologically stressful to embrace mortality. Although provision of palliative care as needed from the onset of illness onward is ideal,[33] discontinuities in care can make this challenging. Documentation of goals, orders for life-sustaining treatment that are comprehensive and standardized,[34] advance care planning, and the date of the most recent update can help coordinate care across care sites, among members of the care team, and along the illness trajectory of changing goals for care.

OUTCOME MEASURES. Care near the end of life cannot be measured by most of the available validated outcome measures because palliative care does not consider death a bad outcome. Similarly, the family and patients receiving end-of-life care may not seek or appreciate the elements of common quality-of-life measurements and may seek different elements of quality that are not included in standard measures when their active engagement is with dying well. Symptom control, enhanced family relationships, and quality of bereavement are difficult to measure and are rarely the primary focus of carefully developed or widely used outcome measures. Nevertheless, outcomes are as important in end-of-life care as in any other field of medical care. Specific end-of-life care instruments are being developed both for assessment, such as The Brief Hospice Inventory and the Needs and the End-of-life Screening Tool (NEST), and for outcome measures, such as the Palliative Care Outcomes Scale (P.O.S.). The field of end-of-life care is ready to enter an era of evidence-based practice and continuous improvement within established institutions.

Acknowledgments

Portions of this chapter are derived from previous writings by Ezekiel and Linda Emanuel.

RESOURCES

The Education in Palliative and End-of-Life Care (EPEC) Project. Northwestern University's Feinberg School of Medicine (http://www.epec.net).

The End of Life/Palliative Education Resource Center (EPERC). Medical College of Wisconsin (http://www.eperc.mcw.edu).

The National Comprehensive Cancer Network (NCCN) Palliative Care Guidelines. NCCN, 2002 (http://www.nccn.org).

REFERENCES

1. Asimov I: Asimov's Biographical Encyclopedia of Science and Technology. 2nd ed. Garden City, NY, Doubleday, 1982.
2. Hanratty B, Hibbert D, Mair F, et al: Doctor's perceptions of palliative care for heart failure: Focus group study. BMJ 325:581, 2002.
3. Easson AM, Crosby JA, Librach SL: Discussion of death and dying in surgical textbooks. Am J Surg 182:34, 2001.
4. Rabow MW, McPhee SJ: Deficiencies in end-of-life care content in medical textbooks. J Am Geriatr Soc 50:397, 2002.
5. Mast KR, Salama MB, Silverman GK, Arnold RM: End-of-life content in treatment guidelines for life-limiting diseases. J Palliat Med 7:754, 2004.
6. Hunt SA, Abraham WT, Chin MH, et al: ACC/AHA 2005 Guideline Update for the Management of Chronic Heart Failure in the Adult: A report of the American College of Cardiology/American Heart Association Task Force on Practice Guidelines (Writing Committee to Update the 2001 Guidelines for the Evaluation and Management of Heart Failure). American College of Cardiology (http://www.acc.org/clinical/guidelines/failure/index.pdf).
7. Goodlin SJ, Hauptman PJ, Arnold R, et al: Consensus statement: Palliative and supportive care in advanced heart failure. J Card Fail 10:200, 2004.
8. Emanuel L, Alexander C, Arnold R, et al: Integrating palliative care into disease management guidelines. J Palliat Med 7:774, 2004.
9. American Heart Association. Heart and Stroke Statistics—2006 Update. Dallas, American Heart Association, 2005 (http://www.americanheart.org).

Palliative Care

10. Gibbs JSR, McCoy ASM, Gibbs LME, et al: Living with and dying from heart failure: The role of palliative care. Heart 88(Suppl):ii36, 2002.
11. Davis PD, Albert NM, Young JB: Palliation of heart failure. Am J Hospice Palliat Med 22:211, 2005.
12. Iwashyna T, Zhang JX, Christakis NA: Disease-specific patterns of hospice and related healthcare use in an incidence cohort of seriously ill elderly patients. J Palliat Med 5:531, 2002.
13. Lo B, Ruston D, Kates LW, et al: Discussing religious and spiritual issues at the end of life: A practical guide for physicians. JAMA 287:749, 2002.

Assessment, Goals, and Care Planning

14. Emanuel LL, Alpert H, Emanuel EJ: Concise screening questions for clinical assessments of terminal care: The needs near the end of life care screening tool (NEST). J Palliat Med 4:465, 2001.
15. Rogers AE, Addington-Hall JM, Abery AJ, et al: Knowledge and communication difficulties for patients with chronic heart failure: Qualitative study. BMJ 321:605, 2000.
16. Krumholtz HM, Phillips RS, Hamel MB, et al: Resuscitation preferences among patients with severe congestive heart failure: Results from the SUPPORT Project. Circulation 98:648, 1998.
17. Murray SA, Boyd K, Kendall M, et al: Dying of lung cancer or cardiac failure: Prospective qualitative interview study of patients and their carers in the community. BMJ 325:929, 2002.
18. Buckman R: How to Break Bad News: A Guide for Health Care Professionals. Baltimore, The Johns Hopkins University Press, 1992, pp 65-97.
19. Lamont EB, Christakis NA: Complexities in prognostication in advanced cancer: "To help them live their lives the way they want to." JAMA 290:98, 2003.
20. Emanuel EJ, Emanuel LL: The promise of a good death. Lancet 351(Suppl): SII21,1998.
21. Singer PA, Martin DK, Kelner M: Quality end-of-life care: Patients' perspectives. JAMA 281:163, 1999.
22. Thorns AR, Gibbs LME, Gibbs JSR: Management of severe heart failure by specialist palliative care. Heart 85:93, 2001.
23. Emanuel LL: The Health Care Directive: Learning how to draft advance care documents. J Am Geriatr Soc 39:1221, 1991 (http://www.medicaldirective.org).
24. President's Commission for the Study of Ethical Issues in Medicine and Biomedical and Behavioral Research, Deciding to Forego Life-Sustaining Treatment. Washington, DC, US Government Printing Office, 1983.
25. An ASCO Curriculum: Optimizing Cancer Care—The Importance of Symptom Management, vols I-II. Dubuque, Iowa, Kendal/Hunt Publishing Company, 2001.
26. Byock I: Dying Well: The Prospect for Growth at the End of Life. New York, Putnam/Riverhead, 1998.
27. McClellan MB, Tunis SR: Medicare coverage of ICDs. N Engl J Med 352:222, 2005.
28. Berger JT: The ethics of deactivating implanted cardioverter defibrillators. Ann Intern Med 142:631, 2005.

29. Goldstein NE, Lampert R, Bradley E, et al: Management of implantable cardioverter defibrillators in end-of-life care. Ann Intern Med 141:835, 2004.
30. Christakis NA, Iwashyna TJ. The health impact of health care on families: A matched cohort study of hospice use by decedents and mortality outcomes in surviving, widowed spouses. Soc Sci Med 57:465, 2003.
31. Christakis N, Escarce J: Survival of Medicare patients after enrollment in hospice programs. N Engl J Med 335:172, 1996.
32. Goodlin SJ, Kutner JS, O'Conner SR, et al: Hospice care for patients with heart failure. J Pain Symptom Manage 29:525, 2005.
33. Goodlin SJ: Palliative care for end-stage heart failure. Curr Heart Fail Rep 2:1550, 2005.
34. Center for Ethics in Health Care: Physician Orders for Life-Sustaining Treatment (POLST) forms. Portland, Ore, Oregon Health Sciences University, 1997.

PART V

Arrhythmias, Sudden Death, and Syncope

CHAPTER 31

Genesis of Cardiac Arrhythmias: Electrophysiological Considerations

Michael Rubart and Douglas P. Zipes

ANATOMY OF THE CARDIAC CONDUCTION SYSTEM

Sinus Node

In humans, the sinus node is a spindle-shaped structure composed of a fibrous tissue matrix with closely packed cells. It is 10 to 20 mm long, 2 to 3 mm wide, and thick, tending to narrow caudally toward the inferior vena cava. It lies less than 1 mm from the epicardial surface, laterally in the right atrial sulcus terminalis at the junction of the superior vena cava and right atrium (Figs. 31-1 and 31-2). The artery supplying the sinus node branches from the right (55 to 60 percent of the time) or the left (40 to 45 percent) circumflex coronary artery and approaches the node from a clockwise or counterclockwise direction around the superior vena cava–right atrium junction.

CELLULAR STRUCTURE. Cells from the sinoatrial node region exhibit a wide variety of morphologies, including spindle- and spider-shaped cells, rod-shaped atrial cells with clear striations, and small round cells corresponding to endothelial cells.[1] Only the spindle- and spider-shaped cells exhibit the typical electrophysiological characteristics of pacemaker cells, including the presence of the hyperpolarization-activated current, I_f,[2] and absence of the inwardly rectifying potassium current, I_{K1}, as well as spontaneous beating under physiological conditions.[3]

GAP JUNCTIONS AND SINOATRIAL COUPLING. The sinoatrial node requires a delicate balance of intercellular electrical coupling to maintain its function as a pacemaker. Excess electrical coupling depresses sinus node automaticity because the sinus node membrane potential is damped by the surrounding atrial myocardium to a more negative potential than the normal maximal diastolic potential, thereby inhibiting spontaneous diastolic depolarization (see Fig. 31-14). Too little coupling may prevent impulse transmission to the adjacent atrial muscle. Restriction of the hyperpolarizing influence of the atrial muscle on the sinus node while maintaining impulse exit into the crista terminalis is achieved by the composition and spatial organization of connexins, proteins that form gap junction channels responsible for intercellular current fluxes (see later "Intercalated Discs"). Connexin40 and connexin45, but not connexin43, are expressed in the central sinus node (Fig. 31-3). The major part of the crista terminalis–sinus node border exhibits a sharp demarcation boundary of connexin43-expressing atrial myocytes and connexin40/connexin45-expressing myocytes. On the endocardial site, a transitional zone exists between the crista terminalis and the peripheral node, in which connexin45 and connexin43 are colocalized This colocalization of different connexin isoforms raises the possibility that individual gap junctional channels in the transitional zone are formed by more than one connexin isoform.[1] These disparate connexin phenotypes may create specific types of hybrid channels with rectifying electrical properties that ensure the maintenance of sinus node pacemaker activity but diminish electrotonic interference from the atrial muscle.[1,4,5]

FUNCTION. Very probably, no single cell in the sinus node serves as *the* pacemaker. Rather, sinus nodal cells function as electrically coupled oscillators that discharge synchronously because of mutual entrainment. Thus, faster discharging cells are slowed by cells firing more slowly, and they themselves speed up so that a "democratically derived" discharge rate occurs. The interaction depends on the degree of coupling and the electrophysiological characteristics of the individual sinoatrial node cell. The resulting rate is not just a simple average of each of the cells. With an individual pacemaker cell coupled to an average of five other cells, each with potentially different electrophysiological properties, the resulting discharge rate is not obvious. In humans, sinus rhythm may result from impulse origin at widely separated sites, with two or three individual wave fronts created that merge to form a single, widely disseminated wave front.

INNERVATION. The sinus node is densely innervated, with postganglionic adrenergic and cholinergic nerve terminals.[6] Discrete vagal efferent pathways innervate both the sinus and

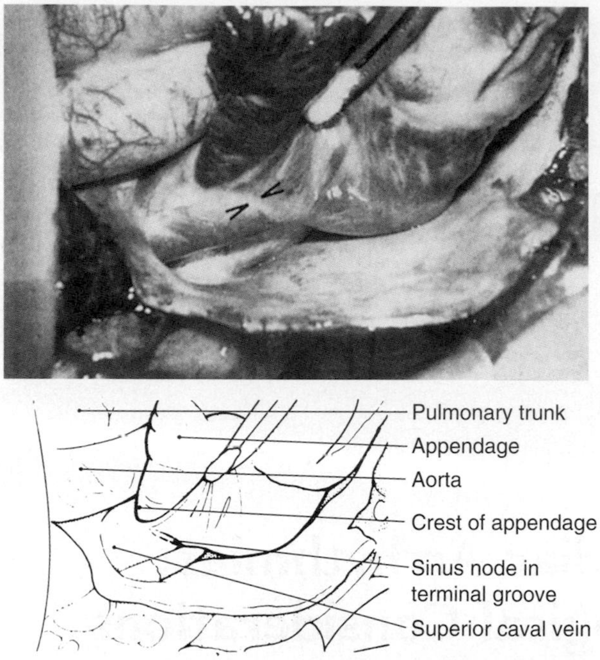

FIGURE 31–1 The human sinus node. This photograph, taken in the operating room, shows the location of the normal cigar-shaped sinus node along the lateral border of the terminal groove at the superior vena cava–atrial junction (arrowheads). *(From Anderson RH, Wilcox BR, Becker AE: Anatomy of the normal heart.* In *Hurst JW, Anderson RH, Becker AE, Wilcox BR [eds]: Atlas of the Heart. New York, Gower, 1988, p 1.2.)*

atrioventricular (AV) regions of the dog and nonhuman primate. Most efferent vagal fibers to the atria appear to converge first at a single fat pad located between the medial portion of the superior vena cava and the aortic root, superior to the right pulmonary artery; the fibers then project onto two other fat pads found at the inferior vena cava-left atrium junction and the right pulmonary vein-atrium junction and subsequently project to both atria. Vagal fibers to the sinus and AV nodes also converge at the superior vena cava-aortic root fat pad before projection to the right pulmonary vein and inferior vena cava fat pads.[6] Although the sinus nodal region contains amounts of norepinephrine equivalent to those in other parts of the right atrium, acetylcholine, acetylcholinesterase, and choline acetyltransferase (the enzyme necessary for the synthesis of acetylcholine) have all been found in greatest concentration in the sinus node, with the next highest concentration in the right and then the left atrium. The concentration of acetylcholine in the ventricles is only 20 to 50 percent of that in the atria.

Neurotransmitters modulate the sinus node discharge rate by stimulation of beta-adrenergic and muscarinic receptors. Both $beta_1$ and $beta_2$ adrenoceptor subtypes are present in the sinoatrial node. Human sinoatrial nodes contain a more than threefold greater density of beta-adrenergic and muscarinic cholinergic receptors than adjacent atrial tissue. The functional significance of beta adrenoceptor subtype diversity in the sinus node is unclear. Binding of receptor agonists released from sympathetic nerve terminals causes a positive chronotropic response through a $beta_1$ receptor-activated pathway involving the stimulatory guanosine triphosphate (GTP) regulatory protein (G_s), activation of adenylyl cyclase, intracellular accumulation of cyclic adenosine monophosphate (cAMP), stimulation of cAMP-dependent protein kinase A, and phosphorylation of target proteins (including the L-type Ca^{2+} channel, the channels underlying I_f, and the ryanodine-sensitive Ca^{2+} release channel [ryanodine receptor] in the sarcoplasmic reticulum membrane[7]). The second messenger pathway underlying $beta_2$ receptor activation–induced heart rate increase and the key target proteins are currently unknown but most likely involve an inhibitory GTP regulatory protein (G_i).[8] The negative chronotropic response of vagal stimulation is mediated by acetylcholine binding to and ensuing activation of M_2 muscarinic receptors. Membrane currents regulated by muscarinic receptor activation include the acetylcholine- and adenosine-sensitive K^+ current ($I_{K(Ach,Ade)}$; see Table 31-3), $I_{Ca.L}$, and I_f. The effect of muscarinic receptor agonist in activating $I_{K(Ach,Ade)}$ is mediated by direct interaction of a G protein subunit with the $K_{(Ach,Ade)}$ channel and does not require second messengers.[9] Activation of $I_{K(Ach,Ade)}$ causes hyperpolarization of the sinoatrial node cell membrane, resulting in a reduced rate of diastolic depolarization. Muscarinic receptor activation–mediated effects on $I_{Ca.L}$ and I_f are primarily caused by a reduction in the intracellular cAMP level, thereby antagonizing the positive chronotropic effects of beta adrenoceptor stimulation.

In addition to its negative chronotropic effect, acetylcholine also prolongs intranodal conduction time, at times to the point of sinus nodal exit block. Acetylcholine increases whereas norepinephrine decreases refractoriness in the center of the sinus node. The phase (timing) in the cardiac cycle at which vagal discharge occurs and the background sympathetic tone importantly influence vagal effects on the sinus rate and conduction (see later). After cessation of vagal stimulation, sinus nodal automaticity may accelerate transiently (postvagal tachycardia). The neurotransmitters neuropeptide Y (NPY) and vasoactive intestinal peptide (VIP) are localized in sympathetic and parasympathetic nerve terminals, respectively. VIP reversibly increases I_f, whereas NPY reversibly decreases I_f.[13] The role of other peripheral neurotransmitters (such as calcitonin gene-related peptide, substance P) in controlling sinus node electrophysiology is unclear.[10]

Internodal and Intraatrial Conduction

Whether impulses travel from the sinus to the AV node over preferentially conducting pathways has been contested. Anatomical evidence has been interpreted to indicate the presence of three intraatrial pathways. The anterior internodal pathway begins at the anterior margin of the sinus node and curves anteriorly around the superior vena cava to enter the anterior interatrial band, called the Bachmann bundle. This band continues to the left atrium, with the anterior internodal pathway entering the superior margin of the AV node. The Bachmann bundle is a large muscle bundle that appears to conduct the cardiac impulse preferentially from the right to the left atrium. The middle internodal tract begins at the superior and posterior margins of the sinus node, travels behind the superior vena cava to the crest of the interatrial septum, and descends in the interatrial septum to the superior margin of the AV node. The posterior internodal tract starts at the posterior margin of the sinus node and travels posteriorly around the superior vena cava and along the crista terminalis to the eustachian ridge and then into the interatrial septum above the coronary sinus, where it joins the posterior portion of the AV node. Some fibers from all three tracts bypass the crest of the AV node and enter its more distal segment. These groups of internodal tissue are best referred to as *internodal atrial myocardium,* not tracts, because they do not appear to be histologically discrete specialized tracts, only plain atrial myocardium.

Preferential internodal conduction—that is, higher conduction velocity between the nodes in some parts of the atrium than in other parts—does exist and may be the result of fiber orientation, size, geometry, or other factors rather than of specialized tracts located between the nodes. Impulse propagation from the atrium to the AV node occurs through multiple preferential input pathways. On the basis of their conduction velocities, these inputs are divided into fast, slow, and intermediate pathways. Notably, the atrial anterosuperior and posteroinferior inputs or approaches to the AV node are the anatomical substrates constituting the fast and slow pathways of AV nodal reentry (see later).[11,12]

Atrioventricular Junctional Area and Intraventricular Conduction System

The normal AV junctional area (Figs. 31-4 and 31-5) can be divided into distinct regions: the transitional cell zone, also called nodal approaches; the compact portion, or the AV node itself; and the penetrating part of the AV bundle (His bundle), which continues as a nonbranching portion. Based on immunohistological analyses, the atrioventricular conduction axis can be segregated into two connecting compartments, one predominantly expressing connexin45 (compact node and transitional cells) and the other predominantly coexpressing connexin43 and connexin45 (His bundle, lower nodal cells, and posterior nodal extension (see Fig. 31-5B through D).[13] The functional role of the new cardiac connexin30.2 in atrioventricular conduction remains to be identified.[14]

TRANSITIONAL CELL ZONE. In the rabbit AV node, the transitional cells or nodal approaches are located in posterior, superficial, and deep groups of cells. They differ histologically from atrial myocardium and connect the latter with the compact portion of the AV node. Some fibers may pass from the posterior internodal tract to the distal portion of the AV node or His bundle and provide the anatomical substrate for conduction to bypass AV nodal slowing. However, the importance of this structure is unclear.

Atrioventricular Node

The compact portion of the AV node is a superficial structure lying just beneath the right atrial endocardium, anterior to the ostium of the coronary sinus, and directly above the insertion of the septal leaflet of the tricuspid valve. It is at the apex of a triangle formed by the tricuspid annulus and the tendon of Todaro, which originates in the central fibrous body and passes posteriorly through the atrial septum to continue with the eustachian valve (see Figs. 31-4 and 31-5A). The term *triangle of Koch,* however, has to be used with caution because histological studies of anatomically normal adult hearts have demonstrated that the tendon of Todaro, which forms one side of the triangle of Koch, is absent in about two thirds of hearts.

The compact portion of the AV node is divided from and becomes the penetrating portion of the His bundle at the point where it enters the central fibrous body. In 85 to 90 percent of human hearts, the arterial supply to the AV node is a branch from the right coronary artery that originates at the posterior intersection of the AV and interventricular grooves (crux). A branch of the circumflex coronary artery provides the AV nodal artery in the remaining hearts. Fibers in the lower part of the AV node may exhibit automatic impulse formation.[15] The main function of the AV node is modulation of atrial impulse transmission to the ventricles, thereby coordinating atrial and ventricular contractions (Fig. 31-6).

Bundle of His (Penetrating Portion of the Atrioventricular Bundle)

This structure connects with the distal part of the compact AV node, perforates the central fibrous body, and continues through the annulus fibrosis, where it is called the nonbranching

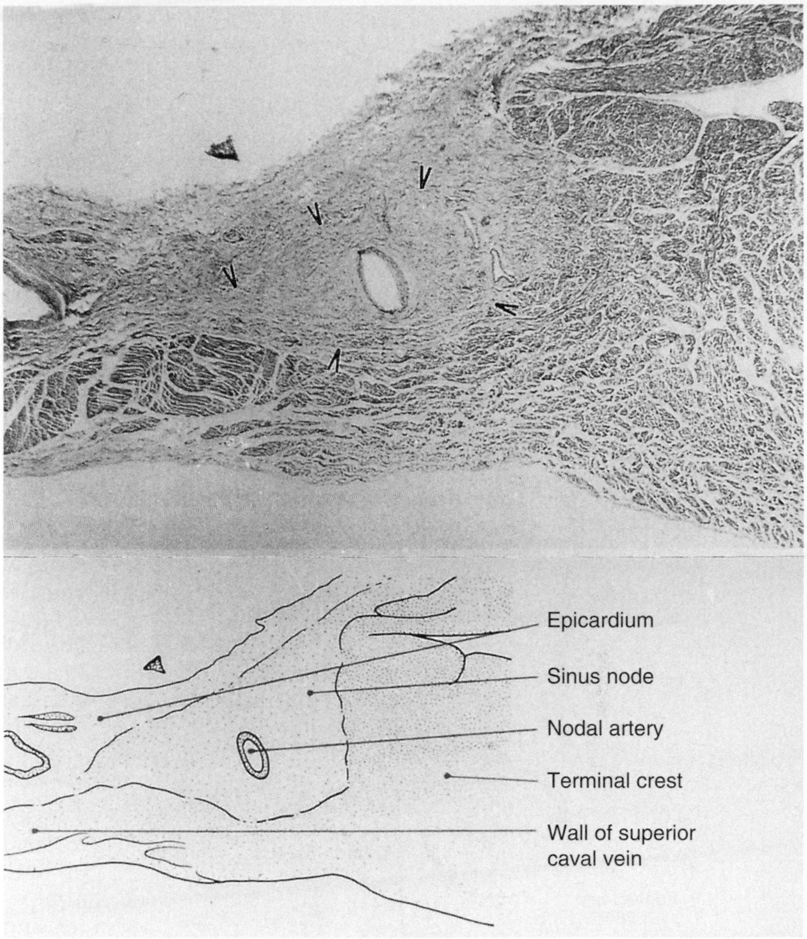

FIGURE 31–2 Histological section taken at right angles to the cigar-shaped sinus node shows that in the short axis, the node is a wedge-shaped structure located between the wall of the superior vena cava and the terminal crest. Discrete boundaries between the sinus node and atrial muscle are noted (arrowheads). The node is penetrated by the sinus nodal artery. *(From Anderson RH, Wilcox BR, Becker AE: Anatomy of the normal heart.* In *Hurst JW, Anderson RH, Becker AE, Wilcox BR [eds]: Atlas of the Heart. New York, Gower, 1988, p 1.2.)*

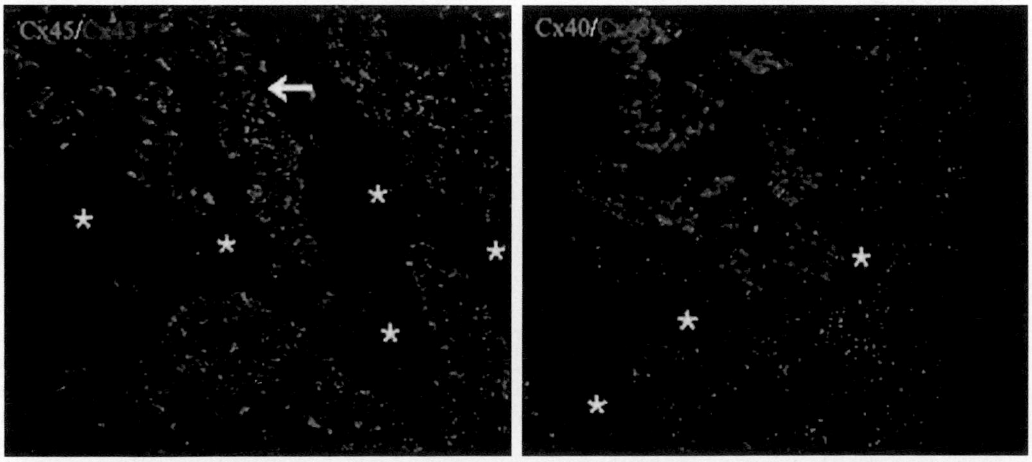

FIGURE 31–3 Sections through the sinoatrial node double-labeled with connexin45 (Cx45) and Cx43 **(left)** and Cx43 with Cx40 **(right)**. Regions positive for Cx40/Cx45 (small punctate green signals) showing no detectable Cx43 signal (red) are sharply demarcated from adjacent Cx43-expressing regions of the crista terminalis. A zone of connective tissue (asterisks) contributes to separation between the zones, although elsewhere (arrow) the zones seem to be more closely approximated. *(From Coppen SR, Kodama I, Boyett MR, et al: Connexin45, a major connexin of the rabbit sino-atrial node, is co-expressed with connexin43 in a restricted zone at the nodal-crista terminalis border. J Histochem Cytochem 47:907, 1999.)*

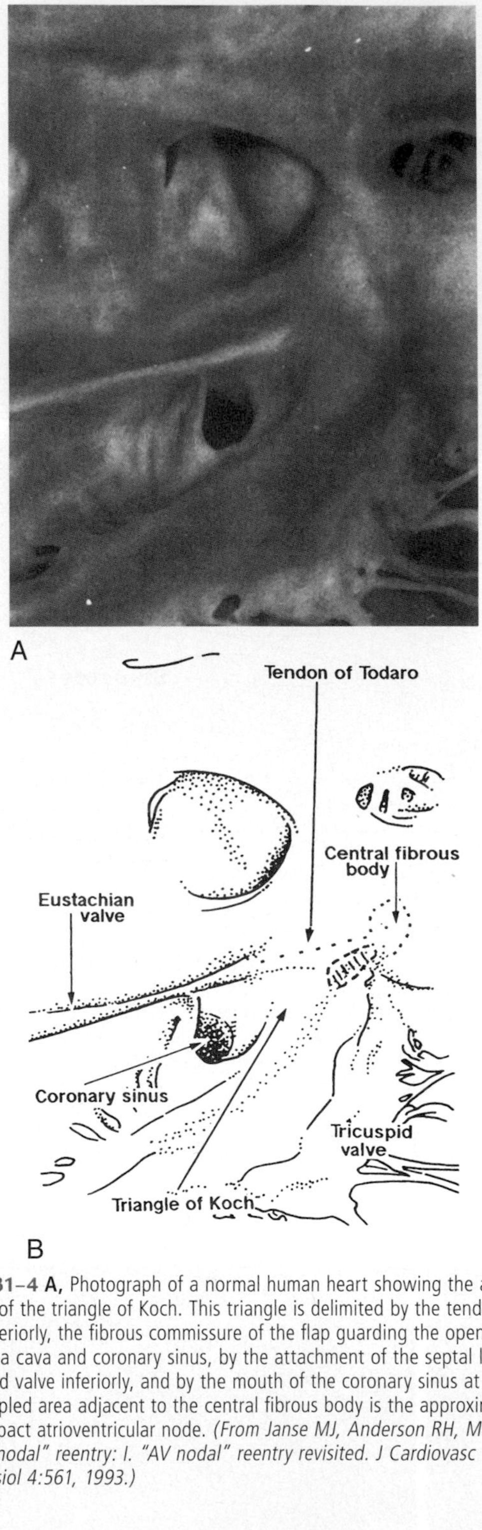

FIGURE 31–4 A, Photograph of a normal human heart showing the anatomical landmarks of the triangle of Koch. This triangle is delimited by the tendon of Todaro superiorly, the fibrous commissure of the flap guarding the openings of the inferior vena cava and coronary sinus, by the attachment of the septal leaflet of the tricuspid valve inferiorly, and by the mouth of the coronary sinus at the base. **B,** The stippled area adjacent to the central fibrous body is the approximate site of the compact atrioventricular node. *(From Janse MJ, Anderson RH, McGuire MA, et al: "AV nodal" reentry: I. "AV nodal" reentry revisited. J Cardiovasc Electrophysiol 4:561, 1993.)*

portion as it penetrates the membranous septum (see Fig. 31-5A). Proximal cells of the penetrating portion are heterogeneous and resemble those of the compact AV node; distal cells are similar to cells in the proximal bundle branches. Connective tissue of the central fibrous body and membranous septum encloses the penetrating portion of the AV bundle, which may send out extensions into the central fibrous body.[16] However, large, well-formed fasciculoventricular connections between the penetrating portion of the AV bundle and the ventricular septal crest are rarely found in adult hearts (see Chap. 35). Branches from the anterior and posterior descending coronary arteries supply the upper muscular interventricular septum with blood, which makes the conduction system at this site more impervious to ischemic damage unless the ischemia is extensive.

Bundle Branches (Branching Portion of the Atrioventricular Bundle)

These structures begin at the superior margin of the muscular interventricular septum, immediately beneath the membranous septum, with the cells of the left bundle branch cascading downward as a continuous sheet onto the septum beneath the noncoronary aortic cusp (Fig. 31-7A). The AV bundle may then give off other left bundle branches, sometimes constituting a true bifascicular system with an anterosuperior branch, in other hearts giving rise to a group of central fibers, and in still others appearing more as a network without a clear division into a fascicular system (see Fig. 31-7B). The right bundle branch continues intramyocardially as an unbranched extension of the AV bundle down the right side of the interventricular septum to the apex of the right ventricle and base of the anterior papillary muscle. In some human hearts, the His bundle traverses the right interventricular crest and gives rise to a right-sided narrow stem origin of the left bundle branch. The anatomy of the left bundle branch system may be variable and may not conform to a constant bifascicular division. However, the concept of a trifascicular system remains useful both to the electrocardiographer and the clinician (see Chap. 12).

Terminal Purkinje Fibers

These fibers connect with the ends of the bundle branches to form interweaving networks on the endocardial surface of both ventricles, which transmit the cardiac impulse almost simultaneously to the entire right and left ventricular endocardium. Purkinje fibers tend to be less concentrated at the base of the ventricle and at the papillary muscle tips. They penetrate the myocardium for varying distances, depending on the animal species. In humans, they apparently penetrate only the inner third of the endocardium, whereas in the pig they almost reach the epicardium. Such variations could influence changes produced by myocardial ischemia—for example, because Purkinje fibers appear to be more resistant to ischemia than ordinary myocardial fibers are.

CELLULAR COMPOSITION OF ATRIOVENTRICULAR JUNCTIONAL AREA AND INTRAVENTRICULAR CONDUCTION SYSTEM. Transitional cells in the rabbit are elongated and smaller than atrial cells, and are separated by numerous strands of connective tissue. They merge at the entrance of the compact portion of the AV node, where the cells are small and spherical, not separated by muscle or connective tissue, and have very few nexuses. They interweave in interconnecting whorls of fasciculi. The AV node is divided on the basis of electrophysiological characteristics into AN, N, and NH regions. In the rabbit, the AN region corresponds to the transitional cell groups of the posterior portion of the node, the NH region to the anterior portion of the bundle of lower nodal cells, and the N region to the small enclosed node where transitional cells merge with midnodal cells. Dead-end pathways, groups of cells that form an apparent electrophysiological cul-de-sac that does not contribute to overall conduction in the node, are also found at several sites. Cells in the penetrating bundle remain similar to compact AV nodal cells.

Purkinje cells are found in the His bundle and bundle branches, cover much of the endocardium of both ventricles (see Fig. 31-7B), and align to form multicellular bundles in longitudinal strands separated by collagen. Although conduction of the cardiac impulse appears to be their major function, free-running Purkinje fibers, sometimes called false tendons, which are composed of many Purkinje cells

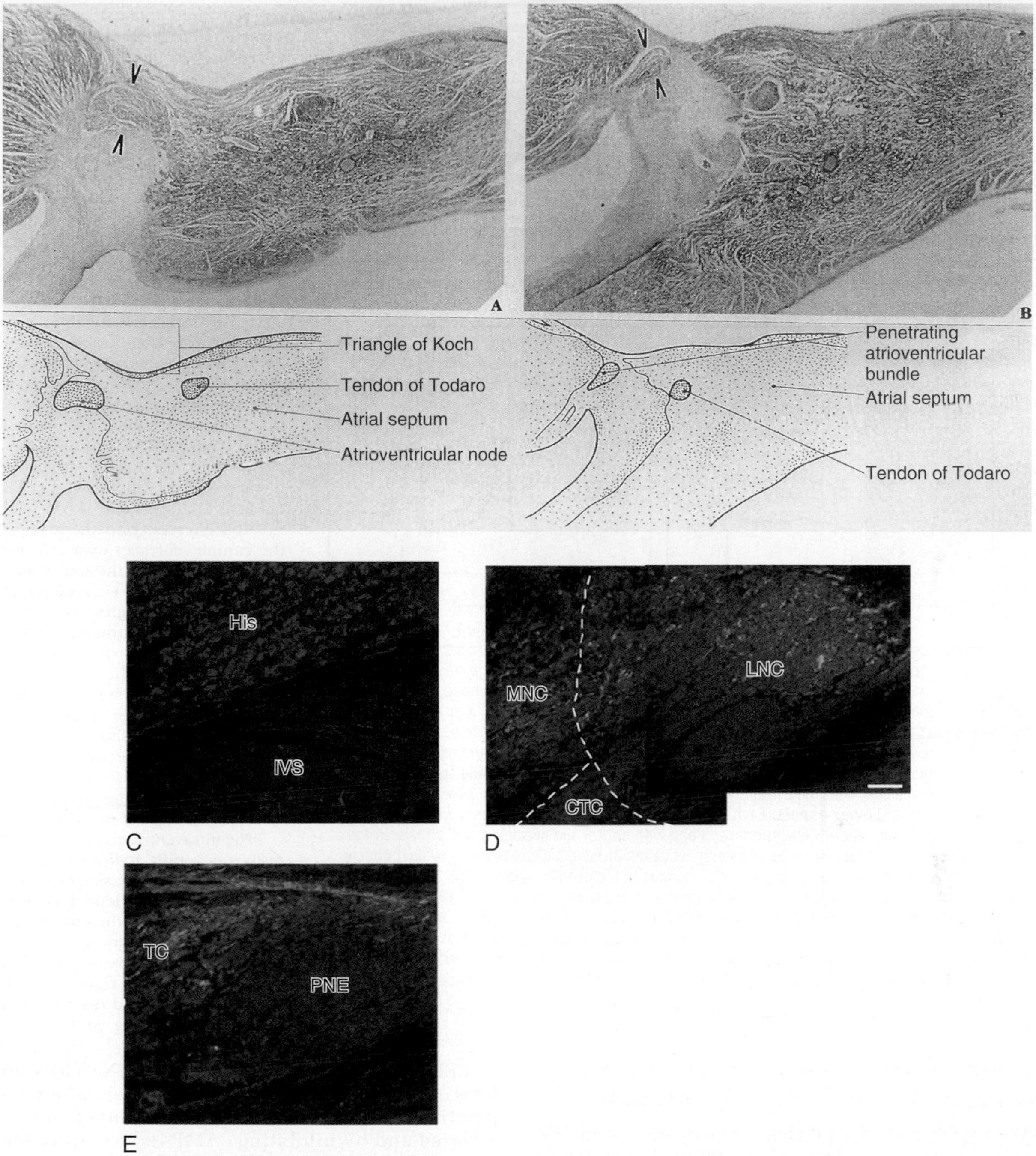

FIGURE 31–5 **A,** Sections through the atrioventricular (AV) junction show the position of the AV node (arrowhead) within the triangle of Koch **(A)** and the penetrating AV bundle of His (arrowheads) within the central fibrous body **(B)**. **C-E,** Sections through the atrioventricular junction labeled with connexin43. **C,** Differential connexin43 labeling patterns within the His bundle and interventricular septum (IVS). **D,** Connexin43-positive lower nodal cells (LNC) contact directly with both connexin43-negative midnodal cells (MNC) and circumferential transitional cells (CTC). **E,** Direct contact between connexin43-negative transitional cells (TC) and connexin43-positive posterior nodal extension (PNE). Green is tissue background fluorescence. *(**A** and **B**, from Anderson RH, Wilcox BR, Becker AE: Anatomy of the normal heart.* In *Hurst JW, Anderson RH, Becker AE, Wilcox BR [eds]: Atlas of the Heart. New York, Gower, 1988, p 1.2; **C-E**, from Ko Y, Yeh H, Ko Y, et al: Three-dimensional reconstruction of the rabbit atrioventricular conduction axis by combining histological, desmin, and connexin mapping data. Circulation 109:1172, 2004. By permission from the American Heart Association.)*

in a series, are capable of contraction. Action potentials propagate within thin Purkinje fiber bundles from base to apex before activation of the surrounding myocytes occurs. Action potential propagation within the His-Purkinje system and the working myocardium is mediated by connexins. Ventricular myocytes express mainly connexin43 and Purkinje fibers express connexin40 and connexin45. The molecular identity of the connexin type that enables impulse transmission at the Purkinje fiber–myocyte junction (PMJ) is unclear. It is also still not clear how the small amount of depolarizing current provided by the thin bundle of Purkinje fibers can activate a much larger mass of ventricular muscle (current to load mismatch).[17] It is possible that individual gap junctional channels at the PMJ are formed by more than one connexin isoform. These disparate connexin phenotypes may create specific types of hybrid channels with unique properties that ensure safe conduction at the PMJ. Because Purkinje cells have markedly longer repolarization times than surrounding myocytes (see Fig. 31-15), these connexin hybrids could also decrease entrainment of repolarization at the PMJ and thereby increase repolarization gradients.

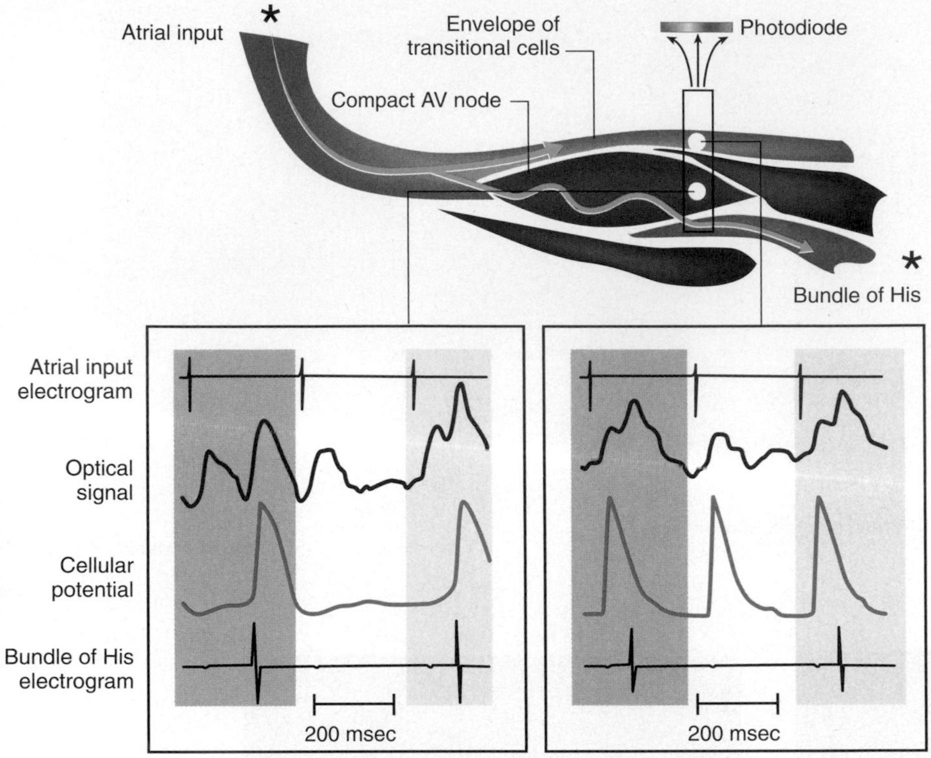

FIGURE 31–6 Multilayer conduction pattern in the atrioventricular (AV) node. Diagram of a cross section through the rabbit AV junction perpendicular to the endocardial atrial surface. The compact node (red) is covered with a superficial layer of transitional cells (blue), providing a connection between the atrial tissue and the compact node. The compact node, in turn, connects to the bundle of His (orange). Connective tissue protrusions are shown in black. Optical recordings of membrane potential changes obtained with a photodiode from the underlying tissue were accompanied by local electrograms from the atrial input to the AV node and from the bundle of His (asterisks). In addition, a microelectrode was used to measure transmembrane potentials at different AV node layers (circles). **Lower panels,** Each illustrates three consecutive heartbeats with simultaneously acquired atrial input and His electrograms, along with optical and microelectrode signals. In the time interval between an atrial input activation and ensuing activation of the bundle of His, two distinct optical action potentials can be identified. The first component corresponds to the depolarization of cells located in the superficial transitional cell layer, whereas the second component reflects the depolarization of cells in the distal portion of the compact AV node. The second beats (white strips) are blocked in the AV node, as indicated by the absence of the signal from the distal portion of the AV node but continued presence of the signal obtained from the transitional cell layer. *(From Efimov IR, Mazgalev TN: High resolution three-dimensional fluorescent imaging reveals multiplayer conduction pattern in the atrioventricular node. Circulation 98:54, 1998. By permission of the American Heart Association.)*

CH 31

Innervation of the Atrioventricular Node, His Bundle, and Ventricular Myocardium

PATHWAYS OF INNERVATION. The AV node and His bundle region are innervated by a rich supply of cholinergic and adrenergic fibers with densities exceeding those found in the ventricular myocardium. Ganglia, nerve fibers, and nerve nets lie close to the AV node. Parasympathetic nerves to the AV node region enter the canine heart at the junction of the inferior vena cava and the inferior aspect of the left atrium, adjacent to the coronary sinus entrance. Nerves in direct contact with AV nodal fibers have been noted, along with agranular and granular vesicular processes, presumably representing cholinergic and adrenergic processes. Acetylcholine release may be concentrated around the N region of the AV node.[6]

In general, autonomic neural input to the heart exhibits some degree of "sidedness," with the right sympathetic and vagal nerves affecting the sinus node more than the AV node and the left sympathetic and vagal nerves affecting the AV node more than the sinus node. The distribution of the neural input to the sinus and AV nodes is complex because of substantial overlapping innervation. Despite the overlap, specific branches of the vagal and sympathetic nerves can be shown to innervate certain regions preferentially. Supersensitivity to acetylcholine follows vagal denervation. Stimulation of the right stellate ganglion produces sinus tachycardia with less effect on AV nodal conduction, whereas stimulation of the left stellate ganglion generally produces a shift in the sinus pacemaker to an ectopic site and consistently shortens AV nodal conduction time and refractoriness, but inconsistently speeds the sinus nodal discharge rate. Stimulation of the right cervical vagus nerve primarily slows the sinus nodal discharge rate, and stimulation of the left vagus primarily prolongs AV nodal conduction time and refractoriness when sidedness is present. Neither sympathetic nor vagal stimulation affects normal conduction in the His bundle. The negative dromotropic response of the heart to vagal stimulation is mediated by activation of $I_{K(Ach,Ade)}$, which results in hyperpolarization of the AV nodal cells, thereby influencing the conductive properties of the node. The positive dromotropic effect of sympathetic stimulation arises as a consequence of activation of the L-type Ca^{2+} current, $I_{Ca.L}$ (see Table 31-3).

Most efferent sympathetic impulses reach the canine ventricles over the ansae subclaviae, branches from the stellate ganglia. Sympathetic nerves then synapse primarily in the caudal cervical ganglia and form individual cardiac nerves that innervate relatively localized parts of the ventricles. On the right side, the major route to the heart is the recurrent cardiac nerve and, on the left, the ventrolateral cardiac nerve. In general, the right sympathetic chain shortens refractoriness primarily of the anterior portion of the ventricles and the left affects primarily the posterior surface of the ventricles, although overlapping areas of distribution occur.

The intraventricular route of sympathetic nerves generally follows coronary arteries. Functional data have suggested that afferent and efferent sympathetic nerves travel in the superficial layers of the epicardium and dive to innervate the endocardium, and anatomical observations have supported this conclusion. Vagal fibers travel intramurally or subendocardially and rise to the epicardium at the AV groove (Fig. 31-8).[6]

EFFECTS OF VAGAL STIMULATION. The vagus modulates cardiac sympathetic activity at prejunctional and postjunctional sites by regulating the amount of norepinephrine released and by inhibiting cAMP-induced phosphorylation of cardiac proteins, such as phospholamban. The latter inhibition occurs at more than one level in the series of reactions constituting the adenylate cyclase–, cyclic AMP–dependent protein kinase system. Neuropeptides released from nerve fibers of both autonomic limbs also modulate autonomic responses. For example, NPY released from sympathetic nerve terminals inhibits cardiac vagal effects.

Tonic vagal stimulation produces a greater absolute reduction in sinus rate in the presence of tonic background sympathetic stimulation, a sympathetic-parasympathetic interaction termed *accentuated antagonism.* In contrast, changes in AV conduction during concomitant sympathetic and vagal stimulation are essentially the algebraic sum of the individual AV conduction responses to tonic vagal and sympathetic stimulation alone. Cardiac responses to brief vagal bursts begin after a short latency and dissipate quickly; in contrast, cardiac responses to sympathetic stimulation commence and dissipate slowly. The rapid onset and offset of responses to vagal stimulation allow dynamic beat-to-beat vagal modulation of heart rate and AV conduction,

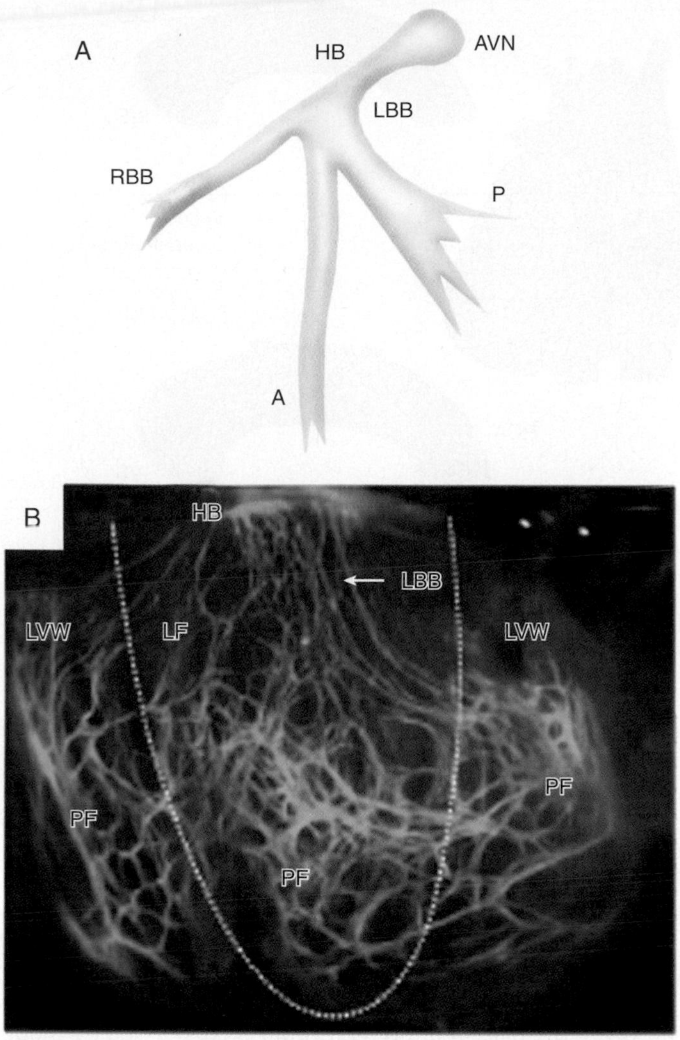

FIGURE 31–7 **A,** Schematic representation of the trifascicular bundle branch system. **B,** Structural organization of the His-Purkinje system in mouse heart. Expression of a green fluorescent protein was specifically targeted to cells of the the His-Purkinje system in mice. Green fluorescent cell networks in the left ventricular chamber are shown. The left ventricular free wall (LVW) was incised from base to apex and then the two parts of the LVW were pulled back to expose the left flank of the interventricular septum (LF). The dotted line demarcates the border between the LF and the LVW. A = anterosuperior fascicle of the left bundle; AVN = atrioventricular node; HB = His bundle; LBB = left bundle branch; P = posteroinferior fascicle of the left bundle branch; RBB = right bundle branch; PF = Purkinje fiber. *(**A** modified from Rosenbaum MB, Elizari MV, Lazzari JO: The Hemiblocks. Oldsmar, Fla, Tampa Tracings, 1970, cover illustration; **B** from Micquerol L, Meysen S, Mangoni M, et al: Architectural and functional asymmetry of the His-Purkinje system of the murine heart. Cardiovasc Res 63:77, 2004.)*

whereas the slow temporal response to sympathetic stimulation precludes any beat-to-beat regulation by sympathetic activity. Periodic vagal bursting, as may occur each time a systolic pressure wave arrives at the baroreceptor regions in the aortic and carotid sinuses, induces phasic changes in sinus cycle length and can entrain the sinus node to discharge faster or slower at periods identical to those of the vagal burst. In a similar phasic manner, vagal bursts prolong AV nodal conduction time and are influenced by background levels of sympathetic tone. Because the peak vagal effects on sinus rate and AV nodal conduction occur at different times in the cardiac cycle, a brief vagal burst can slow the sinus rate without affecting AV nodal conduction or can prolong AV nodal conduction time and not slow the sinus rate.

EFFECTS OF SYMPATHETIC STIMULATION. Stimulation of sympathetic ganglia shortens the refractory period equally in the epicardium and underlying endocardium of the left ventricular free wall, although dispersion of recovery properties occurs—that is, different degrees of shortening of refractoriness occur when measured at different epicardial sites. Nonuniform distribution of norepinephrine may, in part, contribute to some of the nonuniform electrophysiological effects because the ventricular content of norepinephrine is greater at the base than at the apex of the heart, with greater distribution to muscle than to Purkinje fibers. Afferent vagal activity appears to be higher in the posterior ventricular myocardium, which may account for the vagomimetic effects of inferior myocardial infarction.[6]

The vagi exert minimal but measurable effects on ventricular tissue, decreasing the strength of myocardial contraction and prolonging refractoriness. Under some circumstances, acetylcholine can cause a positive inotropic effect. It is now clear that the vagus (acetylcholine) can exert direct effects on some types of ventricular fibers as well as exert indirect effects by modulating sympathetic influences.[6]

Arrhythmias and the Autonomic Nervous System

Alterations in vagal and sympathetic innervation can influence the development of arrhythmias and sudden cardiac death from ventricular tachyarrhythmias.[6,18] Damage to nerves extrinsic to the heart, such as the stellate ganglia, as well as to intrinsic cardiac nerves from diseases that may affect primarily nerves, such as viral infections or, secondarily, from diseases that cause cardiac damage, may produce cardioneuropathy. Such neural changes may create electrical instability through various electrophysiological mechanisms. For example, myocardial infarction can interrupt afferent and efferent neural transmission and create areas of sympathetic supersensitivity that may be conducive to the development of arrhythmias.[6]

Numerous studies have suggested a primary role of altered cardiac sympathetic innervation in arrhythmogenesis. Chronic infusion of nerve growth factor (NGF) to the left stellate ganglion in dogs with chronic myocardial infarction and complete atrioventricular block caused spatially heterogeneous sympathetic cardiac hyperinnervation (nerve sprouting) and dramatically increased the incidence of sudden death from ventricular tachyarrhythmias.[19] A high-cholesterol diet was reported to result in cardiac sympathetic hyperinnervation in rabbits and a marked increase in the incidence of ventricular fibrillation.[18] Explanted human hearts from transplant recipients with a history of arrhythmias exhibited a significantly higher and also more heterogeneous density of sympathetic nerve fibers than those from patients without arrhythmias. Whether neural remodeling also involved parasympathetic nerve fibers in the heart was not examined in these studies. On the other hand, spatially heterogeneous sympathetic denervation was similarly associated with an increased risk of atrial and ventricular arrhythmias. Mutations in genes encoding cardiac ion channel subunits also affect channel function in the central autonomic nervous system,[20] resulting in abnormal firing properties of affected neurons.[21] This observation may partially explain the clinical finding that sudden cardiac death in some variants of the long-QT syndrome (see Chaps. 28 and 32) is typically preceded by a sympathetic arousal.

BASIC ELECTROPHYSIOLOGICAL PRINCIPLES

Physiology of Ion Channels

Electrical signaling in the heart involves the passage of ions through ionic channels. The Na^+, K^+, Ca^{2+}, and Cl^- ions are

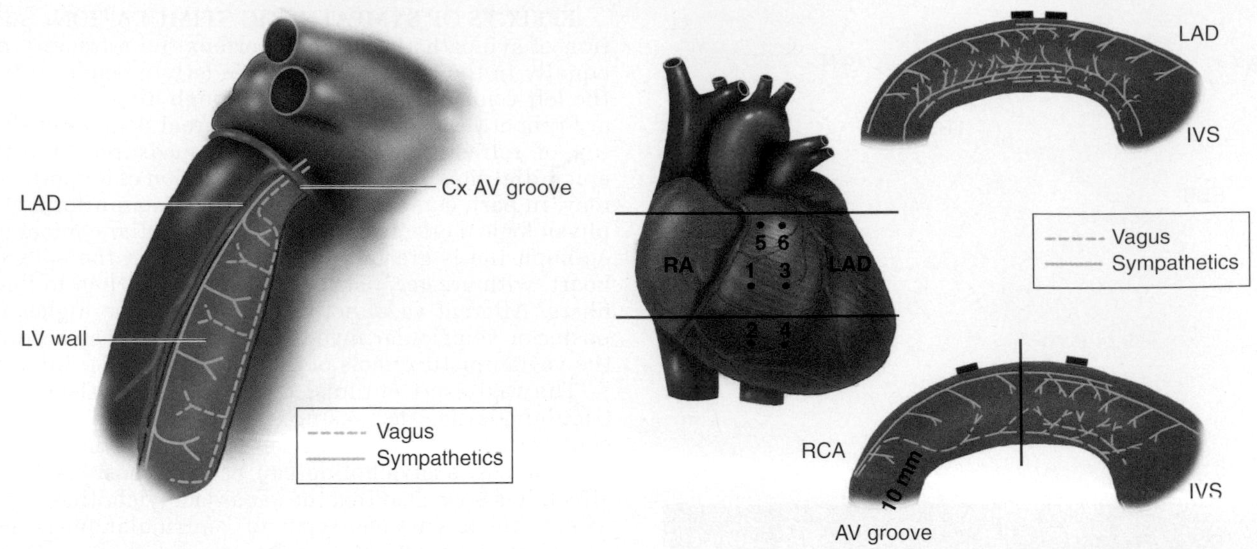

FIGURE 31–8 **Left,** Intraventricular route of sympathetic and vagal nerves to the left ventricle. **Right,** Schematic of the transverse views of the right ventricular (RV) wall showing functional pathways of the efferent sympathetic and vagal nerves. **Top right,** Transverse view of the RV outflow tract at the upper horizontal line on the left. **Bottom right,** Transverse view of the anterolateral wall at the lower horizontal line on the left. The vertical solid line indicates the center of the RV anterolateral wall. Closed circles indicate positions of plunge electrodes (labeled 1 to 6). IVS = interventricular septum; LAD = left anterior descending coronary artery; RA = right atrium; RCA = right coronary artery. *(From Ito M, Zipes DP: Efferent sympathetic and vagal innervation of the canine right ventricle. Circulation 90:1459, 1994. By permission of the American Heart Association.)*

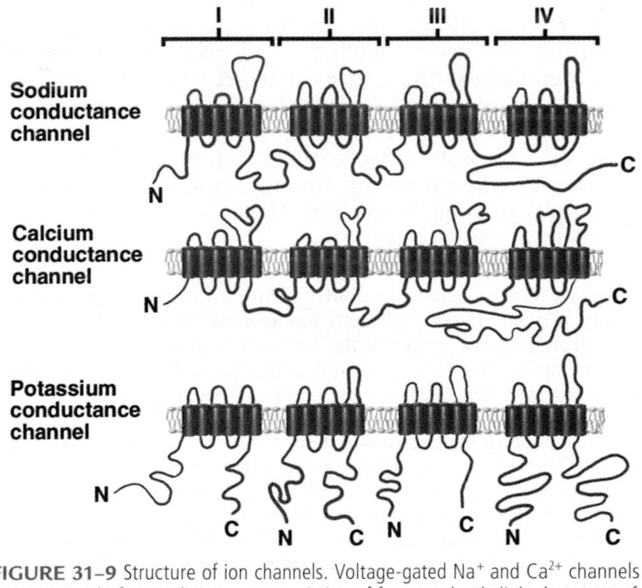

FIGURE 31–9 Structure of ion channels. Voltage-gated Na^+ and Ca^{2+} channels are composed of a *single* tetramer consisting of four covalently linked repeats of the six-transmembrane–spanning motifs, whereas voltage-gated K^+ channels are composed of four *separate* subunits, each containing a single six-transmembrane–spanning motif. Inwardly rectifying K^+ channels are formed by inward rectifier K^+ channel pore-forming (alpha) subunits. In contrast to voltage-gated K^+ channels alpha subunits, the Kir alpha subunits have only two (not six) transmembrane domains. *(Modified from Katz AM: Molecular biology in cardiology, a paradigmatic shift. J Mol Cell Cardiol 20:355, 1988; and from Shivkumar K, Weiss JN: Adenosine triphosphate-sensitive potassium channels.* In *Zipes DP, Jalife J [eds]: Cardiac Electrophysiology: From Cell to Bedside. Philadelphia, WB Saunders, 1999, pp 86-93.)*

the major charge carriers, and their movement across the cell membrane creates a flow of current that generates excitation and signals in cardiac myocytes. Ion channels are macromolecular pores that span the lipid bilayer of the cell membrane (Fig. 31-9). Conformational transitions change (gate) a single ion channel from closed to open, which allows selected ions to flow passively down the electrochemical activity gradient at a very high rate (>10^6 ions/second). The high transfer rates and restriction to "downhill" fluxes not stoichiometrically coupled to the hydrolysis of energy-rich phosphates distinguish ionic channel mechanisms from those of other ion-transporting structures such as the sarcolemmal Na^+,K^+-adenosine triphosphatase (ATPase) or the sarcoplasmic reticular Mg^{2+},Ca^{2+}-ATPase. Ion channels may be gated by extracellular and intracellular ligands, changes in transmembrane voltage, or mechanical stress (see Table 31-3). Gating of single ion channels can best be studied by means of the patch-clamp technique (as discussed by Inoue and Bridge[22]).

Ion channels are usually named after the strongest permeant ion—Na^+, Ca^{2+}, K^+, Cl^-—but some channels are less selective or are not selective, as in gap junctional channels. Channels have also been named after neurotransmitters, as in acetylcholine-sensitive K^+ channels, $I_{K.Ach}$.

The ionic permeability ratio is a commonly used quantitative index of a channel's selectivity. It is defined as the ratio of the permeability of one ion type to that of the main permeant ion type. Permeability ratios of voltage-gated K^+ and Na^+ channels for monovalent and divalent (e.g., Ca^{2+}) cations are usually less than 1 : 10. Voltage-gated Ca^{2+} channels exhibit a more than thousandfold discrimination against Na^+ and K^+ ions (e.g., $P_K/P_{Ca} = 1/3000$) and are impermeable to anions.

Because ions are charged, net ionic flux through an open channel is determined both by the concentration and electrical gradient across the membrane (electrodiffusion). The potential at which the passive flux of ions along the chemical driving force is exactly balanced by the electrical driving force is called the reversal, or Nernst potential, of the channel. In the case of a channel that is perfectly selective for one ion species, the reversal potential equals the thermodynamic equilibrium potential of that ion, E_S, which is given by the Nernst equation in the form

$$E_S = (RT/zF)\ \ln([S_o]/[S_i])$$

where $[S_i]$ and $[S_o]$ are the intracellular and extracellular concentrations of the permeant ion, respectively, z is the valence of the ion, R is the gas constant, F is the Faraday constant, T is the temperature (in kelvin degrees), and ln is the logarithm to the base e. At membrane voltages more positive to the reversal potential of the channel, passive ion movement is outward, whereas it is inward at membrane potentials more negative to the Nernst potential of that channel. If the current through an open channel is carried by more than one permeant ion, the reversal potential becomes a weighted mean of all Nernst potentials.

TABLE 31–1 Intracellular and Extracellular Ion Concentrations in Cardiac Muscle

Ion	Extracellular Concentration (mM)	Intracellular Concentration	Ratio of Extracellular to Intracellular Concentration	E_I (mV)
Na^+	145	15 mM	9.7	+60
K^+	4	150 mM	0.027	−94
Cl^-	120	5-30 mM	4-24	−83 to −36
Ca^{2+}	2	10^{-7} M	2×10^4	+129

Although intracellular Ca^{2+} content is about 2 mM, most of this Ca^{2+} is bound or sequestered in intracellular organelles (mitochondria and sarcoplasmic reticulum).
E_I = equilibrium potential for a particular ion at 37°C.
Modified from Sperelakis N: Origin of the cardiac resting potential. *In* Berne RM, Sperelakis N, Geiger SR (eds): Handbook of Physiology: The Cardiovascular System. Bethesda, Md, American Physiological Society, 1979, p 193.

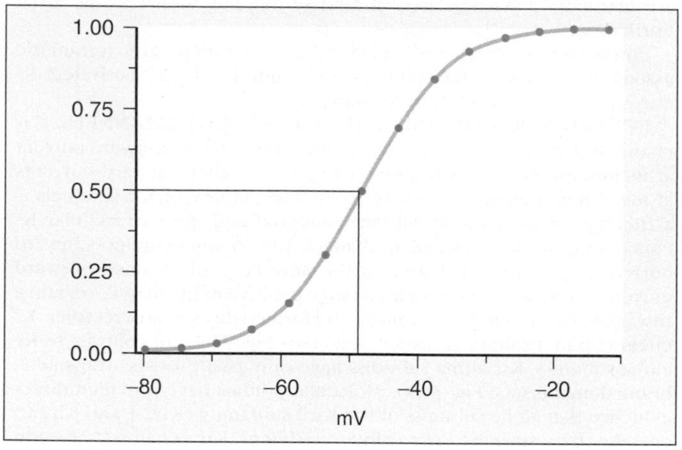

FIGURE 31–10 Voltage dependence of fast Na^+ current activation. Fractional activation (*y* axis) is plotted as a function of membrane potential. Voltage at which activation is half-maximal is demarcated by a vertical line.

Membrane voltages during a cardiac action potential are in the range of −95 to +30 mV. With physiological external K^+ (4 mM; see Table 31-1), E_K is approximately −91 mV, and passive K^+ movement during an action potential is out of the cell. On the other hand, because the calculated reversal potential of a cardiac Ca^{2+} channel is +64 mV (assuming $P_K/P_{Ca} = 1/3000$, $K_i = 150$ mM, $K_o = 4$ mM, $Ca_i = 100$ nM, $Ca_o = 2$ mM), passive Ca^{2+} flux is into the cell. With physiological internal and external chloride concentrations (Table 31-1), E_{Cl} is −80 to −35 mV, and passive movement of Cl^- ions through open chloride channels can be both inward and outward at membrane potentials typically occurring during a cardiac action potential. In more general terms, the direction and magnitude of passive ion flux through a single open channel at any given transmembrane voltage are governed by the reversal potential of that ion and its concentration on the two sides of the membrane, with the net flux being larger when ions move from the more concentrated side.

Ion Flux Through Voltage-Gated Channels

Changes in transmembrane potential determine ion flux through voltage-gated channels, not only through the voltage dependence of the electrochemical driving force on the permeant ion but also through the voltage dependence of channel activation—that is, the fraction of time that a channel permits ions to permeate is determined by the membrane voltage. If the probability of a channel being activated (i.e., the open-state probability of that channel) exhibits voltage dependence, as is the case with the fast Na^+ channel or voltage-dependent K^+ channels in cardiac myocytes, activation increases with membrane depolarization. Note that channels do not have a sharp voltage threshold for opening. The dependence of channel activation on membrane potential is rather a continuous function of voltage and follows a sigmoidal curve (Fig. 31-10). The potential at which activation is half-maximal and the steepness of the activation curve determine the channel's activity during changes in membrane potential. Shifting the activation curve to potentials positive to the midpoint of activation or reducing the steepness of the channel's activation curve, or both, are two possible mechanisms by which ion channel blockers can inhibit ion channel activity.

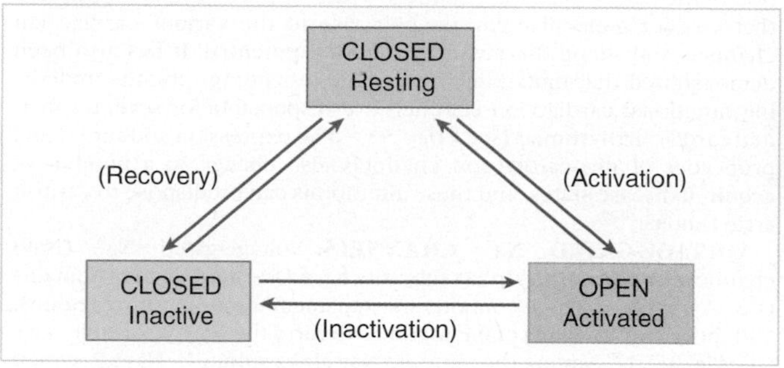

FIGURE 31–11 Simplest scheme for gating of voltage-gated ion channels.

As indicated in Figure 31-11, open channels enter a nonconducting conformation after a depolarizing change in membrane potential, a process termed *inactivation.*[23] If membrane depolarization persists, the channel remains inactivated and cannot reopen. This steady-state inactivation increases with membrane depolarization in a sigmoidal fashion. Inactivation curves of the various voltage-gated ion channel types in the heart differ in their slopes and midpoints of inactivation. For example, sustained cardiomyocyte membrane depolarization to −50 mV (as may occur in acutely ischemic myocardium) causes almost complete inactivation of the fast, voltage-gated Na^+ channel, whereas the L-type Ca^{2+} channel exhibits only little inactivation at this membrane potential.[24] Activation and inactivation curves can overlap, in which case a steady-state or noninactivating current flows. The existence of such a "window" current has been verified for both the voltage-gated Na^+ current[25] and the L-type Ca^{2+} current. The L-type window current has been implicated in the genesis of triggered activity arising from early afterdepolarizations (EADs).

Channels recover from inactivation and then enter the closed state, from which they can be reactivated (see Fig. 31-11). Rates of recovery from inactivation vary among the different types of voltage-dependent channels and usually follow monoexponential or multiexponential time courses, with the longest time constants ranging from a few milliseconds as, for example, for the fast sodium channel, to several seconds, as for some subtypes of K^+ channels (see Table 31-3). Together, the activity of voltage-dependent ion channels in cardiomyocytes over the course of an action potential is tightly regulated by the orchestrated interplay of a number of time- and voltage-dependent gating mechanisms, including activation, inactivation, and recovery from inactivation. All these mechanisms represent potential targets for pharmacological interventions.

Principles of Ionic Current Modulation

The whole-cell current amplitude, I, is the product of the number of functional channels in the membrane available for opening (N), the probability that a channel will open (P_o), and the single-channel current amplitude (i), or $I = N \cdot P_o \cdot i$. Modulation of current amplitudes in single cardiomyocytes therefore results from alterations in N, P_o, i, or any combination of these. Changes in the number of available channels in the cell membrane may result from changes in the expression of ion channel-encoding genes. The magnitude of the single-channel current amplitude is dependent, among other factors, on the ionic concentration gradient across the membrane. For example, an increase in the extracellular Ca^{2+} concentration increases current through a single Ca^{2+} channel. Changes in channel activation can result from phosphorylation or dephosphorylation of the channel protein by second messenger–mediated activation of protein kinases and protein phosphatases, respectively. Channel phosphorylation or dephosphorylation causes a shift in the membrane potential dependence of a channel's activation or availability curve, or both, or modification of the sensitivity of channel activation or inactivation to changes in membrane potential. For example, protein kinase A–mediated potentiation of the cardiac sodium current is partially to the result of a shift of the sodium channel activation curve to more negative potentials.[26]

Molecular Structure of Ion Channels

Electrophysiological studies have detailed the functional properties of Na^+, Ca^{2+}, and K^+ currents in cardiomyocytes, and molecular cloning has revealed a large number of pore-forming (alpha) and auxiliary (beta, delta, and gamma) subunits thought to contribute to the formation of the cell surface ion channels. These studies have demonstrated that distinct molecular entities give rise to the various cardiac ion channels and shape the myocardial action potential. It has also been demonstrated that mutations in the genes encoding subunits underlying functional cardiac ion channels are responsible for several inherited cardiac arrhythmias (see Chap. 9).[27] The expression and functional properties of myocardial ion channels also change in a number of acquired disease states, and these alterations can predispose to cardiac arrhythmias.[28,29]

VOLTAGE-GATED Na^+ CHANNELS. Voltage-gated Na^+ (Nav) channel pore-forming (alpha) subunits have four homologous domains (I to IV), each of which contains six transmembrane-spanning regions, and these four domains come together to form the Na^+ permeable pore (see Fig. 31-9).[30] Among the multiple Nav alpha subunits, Nav1.5 (which is encoded by the *SCN5A* gene) is the prominent Nav alpha subunit expressed in mammalian myocardium. Mutations in the sequence linking domains III and IV in *SCN5A,* associated with the LQT3 syndrome (see Chap. 9), disrupt Nav channel inactivation, which gives rise to a sustained inward Na^+ current during the plateau phase of the action potential and to action potential prolongation. Cases of sudden infant death syndrome (SIDS) in African Americans have been linked to a polymorphism in the *SCN5A* gene, encoding a variant cardiac sodium channel with diminished channel inactivation in the presence of lowered intracellular pH.[31] Mutations in *SCN5A* are also linked to the Brugada syndrome. Brugada syndrome mutations result in reduced Nav current amplitude, which leads to slowing of phase 0 action potential upstroke, reduced action potential amplitude, and altered phase 1 repolarization (see Chap. 9).

Nav1.5 pore-forming alpha subunits coassemble with one to two auxiliary Nav beta subunits to form functional cell surface Nav channels in cardiomyocytes. Nav beta subunits appear to play an important role in anchoring ion channel proteins to the outer cell membrane.

VOLTAGE-GATED Ca^{2+} CHANNELS. Like Nav channels, cardiac voltage-gated Ca^{2+} (Cav) channels are assemblies of four pore-forming alpha subunits and auxiliary Cav beta and/or Cav alpha$_2$-delta subunits (see Fig. 31-9).[30] Among the various alpha subunits, Cav1.2 encoded by the *CACNA1C* gene is the prominent Cav alpha subunit expressed in mammalian myocardium. Cav1.2 channels exhibit many of the time- and voltage-dependent properties and pharmacological sensitivities of cardiac L-type Ca^{2+} currents (see Table 31-3). Accessory subunits modulate the functional properties of Cav channels.

Cav3.1/alpha1G alpha subunits form a Ca^{2+}-selective channel with time- and voltage-dependent characteristics and pharmacological sensitivities that resemble those of the low-voltage activated T-type Ca^{2+} channel. Disruption of the gene encoding Cav3.1/alpha1G alpha subunits (*CACNA1G*) in mice has been demonstrated to slow sinus node rate and atrioventricular conduction consistent with its role in sinus and atrioventricular node function.[32]

VOLTAGE-GATED K^+ CHANNELS. Voltage-gated K^+ channels (Kv) are composed of four *separate* pore-forming (alpha) subunits, each containing six regions (S1 through S6) of hydrophobic amino acids that are thought to form membrane-spanning domains (see Fig. 31-9).[30] Kv alpha subunits expressed in the human heart include members of the Kv1, Kv4, hERG, and KVLQT subfamilies. In addition, Kv channel alpha subunit proteins interact with Kv channel accessory subunits, including minK, KiChIP2, and MiRP1 (see Table 31-3) to form functional cell surface channels with distinct time- and voltage-dependent properties. Coassembly of the Kv4.3 alpha subunits and the accessory subunit KChIP2 give rise to the cardiac transient outward Kv channel, I_{to}. ERG1 alpha subunits, together with MiRP1 accessory subunits, contribute to the generation of functional cardiac I_{Kr} channels. Mutations in the gene encoding ERG1 (*KCNH2*) have been shown to underlie the congenital LQT2 syndrome. These LQT2 syndrome mutations are loss of function mutations and lead to reduced functional I_{Kr} channel expression or to alterations in channel processing or trafficking.[33]

KvLQT1 alpha subunits associate with minK accessory subunits to form functional channels that resemble slowly activating, noninactivating K^+ currents, referred to as I_{Ks}, in human myocardium. Mutations in the minK-encoding gene, *KCNE1,* are associated with the LQT5 syndrome. Mutations in the gene encoding KvLQT1 alpha subunits, *KCNQ1,* have been linked to the LQT1 syndrome. These mutations are all loss of function mutations, resulting in reduced expression of functional I_{Ks} channels in the outer membrane.

Kv1.5 alpha subunits contribute to K^+-selective channels with time- and voltage-dependent characteristics that resemble the rapidly activating and slowly inactivating I_{Kur} in human atrial myocytes. I_{Kur} densities are markedly downregulated in atria of patients with chronic atrial fibrillation.

Small-conductance, Ca^{2+}-sensitive K^+ channels are tetrameric assemblies of SK alpha subunits and underlie a Ca^{2+}-activated K^+ current, $I_{K.Ca}$, in human cardiomyocytes.[34]

INWARDLY RECTIFYING CARDIAC K^+ (Kir) CHANNELS. Kir channels in cardiac myocytes, as in other cells, conduct inward current at membrane potentials negative to E_K and smaller outward currents at membrane potentials positive to E_K. The activity of Kir channels is a function of both the membrane potential and the extracellular K^+ concentration ($[K^+]_o$). As $[K^+]_o$ changes, the channel conducts inward current at potentials negative to the new E_K while a small outward current within a certain potential range positive to the new E_K remains. Inwardly rectifying K^+ channels are formed by inward rectifier K^+ channel pore-forming alpha subunits (see Fig. 31-9). In contrast to Kv alpha subunits, Kir alpha subunits have only two (not six) transmembrane domains (see Fig. 31-9). Molecular studies have provided direct evidence that alpha subunits of the Kir2 subfamily (Kir2.1 and Kir2.2) encode the strongly inwardly rectifying Kir channel, I_{K1}, in cardiomyocytes.

In cardiomyocytes, Kir6.2 alpha subunits assemble with sulfonylurea receptor proteins to form K^+-selective sarcolemmal $I_{K.ATP}$ channels. $I_{K.ATP}$ channels are thought to play a pivotal role in myocardial ischemia and preconditioning. For example, opening of cardiac sarcolemmal $I_{K.ATP}$ channels underlies electrocardiographic ST segment elevation during acute myocardial ischemia. Drugs such as nicorandil and diazoxide open ATP-sensitive K^+ channels, whereas sulfonylurea compounds (such as glibenclamide) inhibit the activity of $I_{K.ATP}$.

The molecular basis of the acetylcholine-activated K^+ channel, $I_{K.Ach}$, is a heteromultimer of two inwardly rectifying potassium channel subunits, Kir3.1 and Kir3.4. Stimulation of $I_{K.Ach}$ by vagally secreted acetylcholine decreases spontaneous depolarization in the sinus node and slows the velocity of conduction in the AV node. Adenosine, through type 1 purinergic receptor–mediated G protein activation, also increases $I_{K.Ach}$ activity in atrial, sinoatrial node, and AV node cells, thus making this compound a treatment of choice for AV reentry tachycardia.

CARDIAC PACEMAKER CHANNEL. The channels underlying the pacemaker ("funny") current, I_f, of sinoatrial myocytes are encoded by the hyperpolarization-activated, cyclic nucleotide–gated (HCN) channel gene family. Of the four known HCN pore-forming alpha subunits, HCN4 is the most highly expressed in the mammalian myocardium.[35] A mutation in the human *HCN4* gene has been linked to familial sinus bradycardia.[36]

Intercalated Discs

Another family of ion channel proteins is that containing the gap junctional channels. These dodecameric channels are found in the intercalated discs between adjacent cells. Three types of specialized junctions make up each intercalated disc. The macula adherens or desmosome and fascia adherens form areas of strong adhesion between cells and may provide a linkage for the transfer of mechanical energy from one cell to the next. The nexus, also called the tight or gap junction, is a region in the intercalated disc where cells are in functional contact with each other. Membranes at these junctions are separated by only about 10 to 20 Å and are connected by a series of hexagonally packed subunit bridges. Gap junctions provide low-resistance electrical coupling between adjacent cells by establishing aqueous pores that directly link the cytoplasm of these adjacent cells. Gap junctions allow movement of ions and small molecules between cells, thereby linking the interiors of adjacent cells.

Gap junctions permit a multicellular structure such as the heart to function electrically like an orderly, synchronized, interconnected unit and are probably responsible in part for the fact that conduction in the myocardium is anisotropic; that is, its anatomical and biophysical properties vary according to the direction in which they are measured. Usually, conduction velocity is two to three times faster longitudinally, in the direction of the long axis of the fiber, than it is transversely, in the direction perpendicular to this long axis.[37] Resistivity is lower longitudinally than transversely. Interestingly, the safety factor for propagation is greater transversely than horizontally. Conduction delay or block occurs more commonly in the longitudinal direction than it does transversely. Cardiac conduction is discontinuous because of resistive discontinuities created by the gap junctions, which have an anisotropic distribution on the cell surface (see Fig. 31-12B).[37] Because of anisotropy, propagation is discontinuous and can be a cause of reentry.

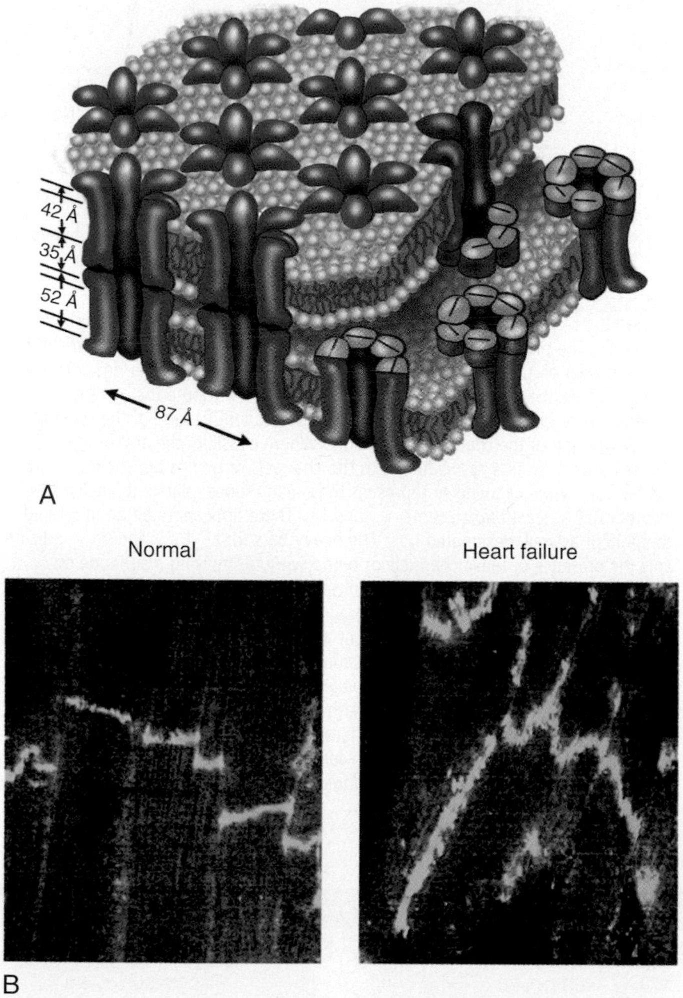

FIGURE 31–12 A, Model of the structure of a gap junction based on results of x-ray diffraction studies. Individual channels are composed of paired hexamers that travel in the membranes of adjacent cells and adjoin in the extracellular gap to form an aqueous pore that provides continuity of the cytoplasm of the two cells. **B,** Sections from a normal dog heart **(left panel)** and a dog heart with experimentally induced dilated cardiomyopathy with anti–connexin43 immune staining **(right panel)**. There is lateralization of connexin43 gap junctions in the myopathic heart. *(**A** from Saffitz JE: Cell-to-cell communication in the heart. Cardiol Rev 3:86, 1995; **B** from Akar FG, Spragg DD, Tunin RS, et al: Mechanisms underlying conduction slowing and arrhythmogenesis in nonischemic dilated cardiomyopathy. Circ Res 95:717, 2004. By permission from the American Heart Association.)*

Gap junctions may also provide "biochemical coupling," which might permit cell to cell movement of ATP or other high-energy phosphates. Gap junctions can also change their electrical resistance. When the intracellular calcium level rises, as in myocardial infarction, the gap junction may close to help seal off the effects of injured from noninjured cells. Acidosis increases and alkalosis decreases gap junctional resistance. Increased gap junctional resistance tends to slow the rate of action potential propagation, a condition that could lead to conduction delay or block. Cardiac-restricted inactivation of gap junctions decreases transverse conduction velocity to a greater degree than longitudinal conduction, resulting in an increased anisotropic ratio that may play a role in premature sudden death from ventricular arrhythmias.[38]

Connexins are the proteins that form the intercellular channels of gap junctions. An individual channel is created by two hemichannels (connexons), each located in the plasma membrane of adjacent cells and composed of six integral membrane protein subunits (connexins). The hemichannels surround an aqueous pore and thereby create a transmembrane channel (Fig. 31-12A). Connexin43, a 43-kDa polypeptide, is the most abundant cardiac connexin, with connexin40 and connexin45 found in smaller amounts. Ventricular muscle expresses connexin43 and connexin45, whereas atrial muscle and components of the specialized conduction system express connexin43, connexin45, and connexin40. Expression of the recently identified connexin30.2 appears to be confined to the cardiac conduction system.[39] Individual cardiac connexins form gap junctional channels with characteristic unitary conductances, voltage sensitivities, and ionic permeabilities. Tissue-specific connexin expression and spatial distribution of gap junctions determine the disparate conduction properties of cardiac tissue. The functional diversity of cardiac gap junctions is further enhanced by the ability of different connexin isoforms to form hybrid gap junctional channels with unique electrophysiological properties. These channel chimeras appear to have a major function in controlling impulse transmission at the sinus node–atrium border, the atrium–AV node transitional zone, and the Purkinje-myocyte border.[5,39]

Alterations in distribution and function of cardiac gap junctions are associated with increased susceptibility to arrhythmias. Conduction slowing and arrhythmogenesis have been associated with redistribution of connexin43 gap junctions from the end of the cardiomyocytes to the lateral borders (see Fig. 31-12B), and with decreased phosphorylation of connexin43 in a dog model of nonischemic dilated cardiomyopathy.[40] Adult mice genetically engineered to express progressively decreasing levels of cardiac connexin43 exhibited increased susceptibility to the induction of fatal tachyarrhythmias.[41,42] Side-to-side electrical coupling between cardiomyocytes from the epicardial border zone of healing infarcts has been shown to be reduced, exaggerating anisotropy and facilitating reentrant activity.[43] Finally, a rare single nucleotide polymorphism in the atrial-specific connexin40 gene has been found to increase the risk of idiopathic atrial fibrillation.[44] Recent studies have suggested that normal electrical coupling of cardiomyocytes via gap junctions depends on normal mechanical coupling via cell-cell adhesion junctions.[45] Defect in cell-cell adhesion or a discontinuity in the linkage between intercellular junctions and the cytoskeleton prevents normal localization of connexins in gap junctions, which in turn could contribute to sudden death from tachyarrhythmias. For example, Carvajal syndrome is caused by recessive mutation in desmoplakin, a protein that links desmosomal adhesion molecules to desmin, a filament protein of the cardiomyocyte cytoskeleton.[46] Naxos disease is caused by a recessive mutation in plakoglobin, a protein that connects N-cadherins to actin and desmosomal cadherins to desmin.[47] In both diseases, remodeling of cardiac gap junctions was observed, and carrier of the mutations have an increased risk of tachyarrhythmias.

Phases of the Cardiac Action Potential

The cardiac transmembrane potential consists of five phases: phase 0, upstroke or rapid depolarization; phase 1, early rapid repolarization; phase 2, plateau; phase 3, final rapid repolarization; and phase 4, resting membrane potential and diastolic depolarization (Figs. 31-13 and 31-14). These phases are the result of passive ion fluxes moving down electrochemical gradients established by active ion pumps and exchange mechanisms. Each ion moves primarily through its own ion-specific channel. Impulses spread from one cell to the next without requiring neural input. The transplanted heart dramatically demonstrates this fact. The following discussion explains the electrogenesis of each of these phases.

GENERAL CONSIDERATIONS. Ionic fluxes regulate membrane potential in cardiac myocytes in the following fashion. When only one type of ion channel opens, assuming that this channel is perfectly selective for that ion, the membrane potential of the entire cell would equal the Nernst potential of that ion. Solving the Nernst equation for the four major ions across the plasma membrane, the following equilibrium potentials are obtained: sodium, +60 mV; potassium, −94 mV; calcium, +129 mV; and chloride, −80 to −35 mV (see Table 31-1). Therefore, if a single K^+-selective channel opens, such as the inwardly rectifying K^+ channel, the membrane potential approaches E_K (−94 mV). If a single Na^+-selective channel opens, the transmembrane potential becomes E_{Na} (+60 mV). A quiescent cardiac myocyte (phase 4) has many more open potassium than sodium channels, and the cell's transmembrane potential is close to E_K (Table 31-2). When two or more types of ion channel open simultaneously, each type tries to make the membrane potential go to the equilibrium potential of that channel. The contribution of each ion type to the overall membrane potential at any given moment is determined by the instantaneous permeability of the plasma membrane to that ion. For example, deviation of the measured resting membrane potential from E_K (see Table 31-1) would predict that other ion types with equilibrium potentials positive to E_K contribute to the resting membrane potential in cardiac myocytes. If it is assumed that Na^+, K^+, and Cl^- are the permeant ions at resting potential, their individual contributions to the resting membrane potential V can be quantified by the GHK *voltage* equation of the form

$$V = (RT/F)\ \ln[(P_K\ [K]_o + P_{Na}\ [Na]_o + P_{Cl}[Cl]_i)/(P_K[K]_I + P_{Na}[Na]P_{Cl}[Cl]_o)]$$

where the symbols have the meanings outlined previously. With only one permeant ion, V becomes the Nernst potential for that ion. With several permeant ion types, V is a weighted mean of all the Nernst potentials.

Intracellular electrical activity can be recorded by inserting a glass microelectrode filled with an electrolyte solution and with a tip diameter smaller than 0.5 μm into a single cell. The electrode produces minimal damage, its entry point apparently being sealed by the cell.

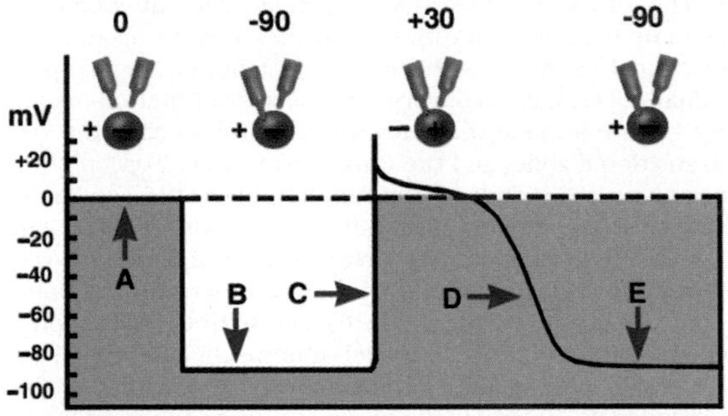

FIGURE 31–13 Demonstration of action potentials recorded during impalement of a cardiac cell. **Upper row,** Shown are a cell (circle), two microelectrodes, and stages during impalement of the cell and its activation and recovery. Both microelectrodes are extracellular (A), and no difference in potential exists between them (0 potential). The environment inside the cell is negative and the outside is positive because the cell is polarized. One microelectrode has pierced the cell membrane (B) to record the intracellular resting membrane potential, which is −90 mV with respect to the outside of the cell. The cell has depolarized (C) and the upstroke of the action potential is recorded. At its peak voltage, the inside of the cell is about +30 mV with respect to the outside of the cell. The repolarization phase (D) is shown, with the membrane returning to its former resting potential (E). *(From Cranefield PF: The Conduction of the Cardiac Impulse. Mount Kisco, NY, Futura, 1975.)*

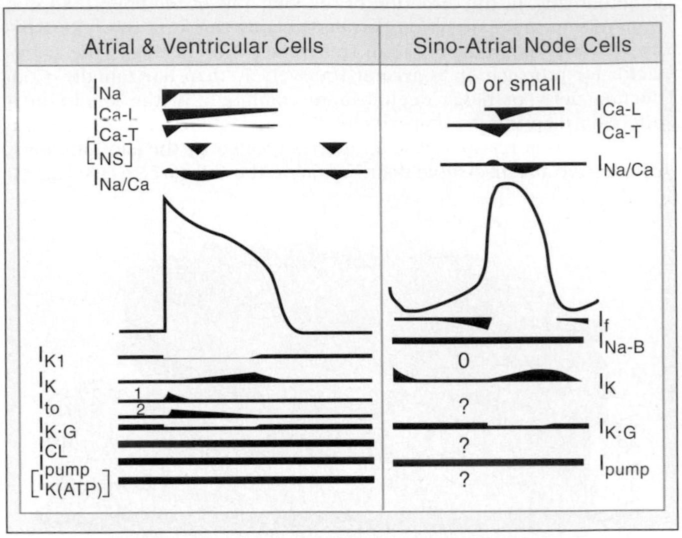

FIGURE 31–14 Currents and channels involved in generating resting and action potentials. The time course of a stylized action potential of atrial and ventricular cells is shown on the left, and that of sinoatrial node cells is on the right. Above and below are the various channels and pumps that contribute the currents underlying the electrical events. See Table 31-3 for identification of the symbols and description of the channels or currents. Where possible, the approximate time courses of the currents associated with the channels or pumps are shown symbolically, without trying to represent their magnitudes relative to each other. I_K incorporates at least two currents, $I_{K\text{-}R}$ and $I_{K\text{-}S}$. There appears to be an ultrarapid component as well, designated $I_{K\text{-}UR}$. The heavy bars for I_{CL}, I_{pump}, and $I_{K(ATP)}$ indicate only the presence of these channels or pump without implying magnitude of currents because that would vary with physiological and pathophysiological conditions. The channels identified by brackets (I_{NS} and $I_{K(ATP)}$) are active only under pathological conditions. I_{NS} may represent a swelling-activated cation current. For the sinoatrial node cells, I_{NS} and I_{K1} are small or absent. Question marks indicate that experimental evidence is not yet available to determine the presence of these channels in sinoatrial cell membranes. Although it is likely that other ionic current mechanisms exist, they are not shown here because their roles in electrogenesis are not sufficiently well defined. *(From Members of the Sicilian Gambit: Antiarrhythmic Therapy: A Pathophysiologic Approach. Mount Kisco, NY, Futura, 1994, p 13.)*

TABLE 31–2 Properties of Transmembrane Potentials in Mammalian Hearts

Property	Sinus Nodal Cell	Atrial Muscle Cell	AV Nodal Cell	Purkinje Fiber	Ventricular Muscle Cell
Resting potential (mV)	−50 to −60	−80 to −90	−60 to −70	−90 to −95	−80 to −90
Action potential					
Amplitude (mV)	60-70	110-120	70-80	120	110-120
Overshoot (mV)	0-10	30	5-15	30	30
Duration (msec)	100-300	100-300	100-300	300-500	200-300
V_{max} (V/sec)	1-10	100-200	5-15	500-700	100-200
Propagation velocity (m/sec)	<0.05	0.3-0.4	0.1	2-3	0.3-0.4
Fiber diameter (μm)	5-10	10-15	1-10	100	10-16

V_{max}=maximal rise of membrane potential.

Modified from Sperelakis N: Origin of the cardiac resting potential. *In* Berne RM, Sperelakis N, Geiger SR (eds): Handbook of Physiology: The Cardiovascular System. Bethesda, Md, American Physiological Society, 1979, p 190.

The transmembrane potential is recorded by using this electrode in reference to an extracellular ground electrode placed in the tissue bath near the cell membrane and represents the potential difference between intracellular and extracellular voltage (see Fig. 31-13). Alternatively, the patch-clamp technique in current clamp mode can be used to measure transmembrane potentials.

Phase 4: The Resting Membrane Potential

The intracellular potential during electrical quiescence in diastole is −50 to −95 mV, depending on the cell type (see Table 31-2). Therefore, the inside of the cell is 50 to 95 mV negative relative to the outside of the cell because of the distribution of ions such as K^+, Na^+, and Cl^-.

Because cardiac myocytes have an abundance of open K^+ channels at rest, the cardiac transmembrane potential (in phase 4) is close to E_K. Potassium outward current through open, inwardly rectifying K^+ channels, I_{K1}, mainly contributes to the resting membrane potential in atrial and ventricular myocytes, as well as in Purkinje cells, under normal conditions. Deviation of the resting membrane potential from E_K is the result of movement of monovalent ions with an equilibrium potential greater than the E_K—for example, Cl^- efflux through activated chloride channels, such as $I_{Cl.cAMP}$, $I_{Cl.Ca}$, and $I_{Cl.swell}$. Calcium does not contribute directly to the resting membrane potential, but changes in intracellular free calcium concentration can affect other membrane conductance values. For example, an increase in sarcoplasmic reticulum Ca^{2+} load can cause spontaneous intracellular Ca^{2+} waves,[48] which in turn activate the Ca^{2+}-dependent chloride conductance $I_{Cl.Ca}$ and thereby lead to spontaneous transient inward currents and concomitant membrane depolarization. Increases in $[Ca^{2+}]_i$ can also stimulate the Na^+/Ca^{2+} exchanger $I_{Na/Ca}$. This protein exchanges three Na^+ ions for one Ca^{2+} ion; the direction is dependent on the sodium and calcium concentrations on the two sides of the membrane and the transmembrane potential difference. At resting membrane potential and during a spontaneous sarcoplasmic reticulum Ca^{2+} release event, this exchanger would generate a net Na^+ influx, possibly causing transient membrane depolarizations (see Fig. 31-25).[48] $[Ca^{2+}]_i$ has also been shown to activate I_{K1} in cardiac myocytes, thereby indirectly contributing to cardiac resting membrane potential.[48] Because of the Na-K pump, which pumps Na^+ out of the cell against its electrochemical gradient and simultaneously pumps K^+ into the cell against its chemical gradient, the intracellular K^+ concentration remains high and the intracellular Na^+ concentration remains low. This pump, fueled by an Na^+,K^+-ATPase enzyme that hydrolyzes ATP for energy, is bound to the membrane. It requires both Na^+ and K^+ to function and can transport three Na^+ ions outward for two K^+ ions inward. Therefore, the pump can be electrogenic and generate a net outward movement of positive charges. The rate of Na^+-K^+ pumping to maintain the same ionic gradients must increase as the heart rate increases because the cell gains a slight amount of Na^+ and loses a slight amount of K^+ with each depolarization. Cardiac glycoside-induced block of the Na^+,K^+-ATPase increases contractility through an increase in intracellular Na^+ concentration, which in turn reduces Ca^{2+} extrusion through the Na^+/Ca^{2+} exchanger (see later), ultimately increasing myocyte contractility.[49]

Phase 0: Upstroke or Rapid Depolarization

A stimulus delivered to excitable tissue evokes an action potential characterized by a sudden voltage change caused by transient depolarization followed by repolarization. The action potential is conducted throughout the heart and is responsible for initiating each heartbeat. Electrical changes in action potential follow a relatively fixed time and voltage relationship that differs according to specific cell types (Fig. 31-15; see Fig. 31-14). In nerve, the entire process takes several milliseconds, whereas action potentials in human cardiac fibers last several hundred milliseconds. Normally, the action potential is independent of the size of the depolarizing stimulus if the latter exceeds a certain threshold potential. Small subthreshold depolarizing stimuli depolarize the membrane in proportion to the strength of the stimulus. However, when the stimulus is sufficiently intense to reduce membrane potential to a threshold value in the range of −70 to −65 mV for normal Purkinje fibers, more intense stimuli do not produce larger action potential responses, and an "all-or-none" response results. In contrast, hyperpolarizing pulses, stimuli that render the membrane potential more negative, elicit a response proportional to the strength of the stimulus.

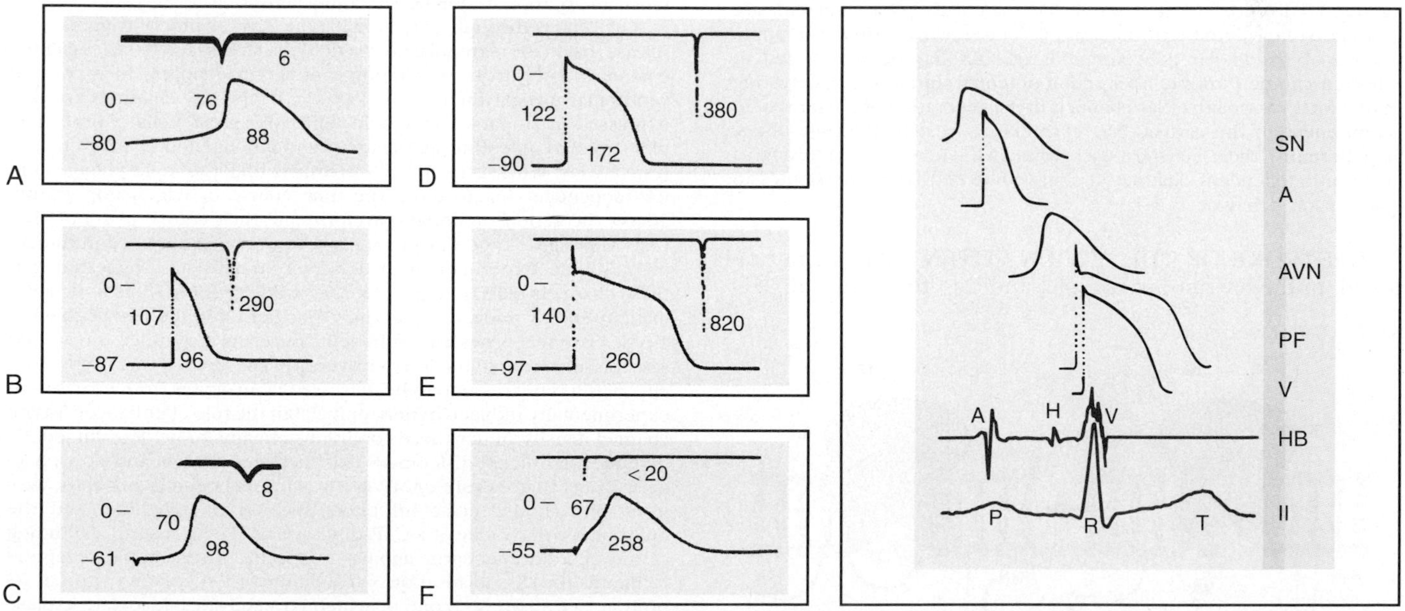

FIGURE 31–15 Action potentials recorded from different tissues in the heart **(left)** remounted along with a His bundle recording and scalar electrocardiogram from a patient **(right)** to illustrate the timing during a single cardiac cycle. In panels **A** to **F**, the top tracing is dV/dt of phase 0 and the second tracing is the action potential. For each panel, the numbers (from left to right) indicate maximum diastolic potential (mV), action potential amplitude (mV), action potential duration at 90 percent of repolarization (milliseconds), and $\dot{V}_{max}$ of phase 0 (V/sec). Zero potential is indicated by the short horizontal line next to the zero on the upper left of each action potential. **A,** Rabbit sinoatrial node. **B,** Canine atrial muscle. **C,** Rabbit atrioventricular node. **D,** Canine ventricular muscle. **E,** Canine Purkinje fiber. **F,** Diseased human ventricle. Note that the action potentials recorded in **A, C,** and **F** have reduced resting membrane potentials, amplitudes, and $\dot{V}_{max}$ when compared with the other action potentials. A = atrial muscle potential; AVN = atrioventricular nodal potential; HB = His bundle recording; II = lead II; PF = Purkinje fiber potential; SN = sinus nodal potential; V = ventricular muscle potential. Horizontal calibration on the left: 50 milliseconds for **A** and **C**, 100 milliseconds for **B, D, E,** and **F;** 200 milliseconds on the right. Vertical calibration on the left, 50 mV. Horizontal calibration on the right, 200 milliseconds. *(Modified from Gilmour RF Jr, Zipes DP: Basic electrophysiology of the slow inward current.* In *Antman E, Stone PH [eds]: Calcium Blocking Agents in the Treatment of Cardiovascular Disorders. Mount Kisco, NY, Futura, 1983, pp 1-37.)*

MECHANISM OF PHASE 0. The upstroke of the cardiac action potential in atrial and ventricular muscle and His-Purkinje fibers is the result of a sudden increase in membrane conductance to Na^+. An externally applied stimulus or a spontaneously generated local membrane circuit current in advance of a propagating action potential depolarizes a sufficiently large area of membrane at a sufficiently rapid rate to open the Na^+ channels and depolarize the membrane further. When the stimulus activates enough Na^+ channels, Na^+ ions enter the cell, down their electrochemical gradient. The excited membrane no longer behaves like a K^+ electrode—that is, exclusively permeable to K^+—but more closely approximates a Na^+ electrode, and the membrane moves toward the Na^+ equilibrium potential.

The rate at which depolarization occurs during phase 0—that is, the maximum rate of change of voltage over time—is indicated by the expression dV/dt_{max} or $\dot{V}_{max}$ (see Table 31-2), which is a reasonable approximation of the rate and magnitude of Na^+ entry into the cell and a determinant of conduction velocity for the propagated action potential. The transient increase in sodium conductance lasts 1 to 2 milliseconds. The action potential, or more properly the Na^+ current (I_{Na}), is said to be regenerative; that is, intracellular movement of a little Na^+ depolarizes the membrane more, which increases conductance to Na^+ more, which allows more Na^+ to enter, and so on. As this process is occurring, however, $[Na^+]_i$ and positive intracellular charges increase and reduce the driving force for Na^+. When the equilibrium potential for Na^+ (E_{Na}) is reached, Na^+ no longer enters the cell; that is, when the driving force acting on the ion to enter the cell balances the driving force acting on the ion to exit the cell, no current flows. In addition, Na^+ conductance is time dependent, so that when the membrane spends some time at voltages less negative than the resting potential, Na^+ conductance decreases (inactivation; see earlier). Therefore, an intervention that reduces membrane potential for a time (acute myocardial ischemia), but not to threshold, partially inactivates Na^+ channels and, if threshold is now achieved, the magnitude and rate of Na^+ influx are reduced, causing the conduction velocity to slow. The process of channel inactivation is thought to be mediated by occlusion of the inner mouth of the pore by the peptide loop that connects domains III and IV (Fig. 31-16).

In cardiac Purkinje fibers and, to a lesser extent, in ventricular muscle, two different populations of Na^+ channels, or two different modes of operation of the same Na^+ channel, exist. One is responsible for the brief Na^+ current of phase 0 and the other, which is longer lasting, participates in the action potential plateau (steady-state or window current).[25] Cardiac voltage-dependent Na^+ (Nav) currents are generally considered tetrodotoxin (TTX)-insensitive. However, application of nanomolar concentrations of TTX has been reported to shorten canine Purkinje fiber action potential durations,[30] suggesting a role for TTX-sensitive Nav channels in the generation of the persistent component of the cardiac Nav currents, at least in Purkinje fibers. Furthermore, there may be a background Na^+ current ($I_{Na\text{-}B}$) through a voltage-independent channel in sinus nodal cells that contributes to pacemaker behavior.

UPSTROKE OF THE ACTION POTENTIAL. In normal atrial and ventricular muscle and in fibers in the His-Purkinje system, action potentials have very rapid upstrokes, with a large $\dot{V}_{max}$, and are called fast responses. Action potentials in the normal sinus and AV nodes and many types of diseased tissue have very slow upstrokes with a reduced $\dot{V}_{max}$ and are called slow responses (Table 31-3; see Fig. 31-15). Upstrokes of slow responses are mediated by a slow inward, predominantly L-type voltage-gated (Cav) Ca^{2+} current ($I_{Ca.L}$) rather than the fast inward I_{Na}. These potentials have been termed *slow response* potentials because the time required for activation and inactivation of the slow inward current ($I_{Ca.L}$) is approximately an order of magnitude slower than that for the fast inward Na^+ current (I_{Na}). Recovery from inactivation also takes longer. Calcium entry and $[Ca^{2+}]_i$ help promote inactivation. The slow channel opens and closes more slowly than the fast channel, remains open for a longer time, and requires more time following a stimulus to be reactivated. In fact, recovery of excitability outlasts full restoration of maximum diastolic potential, which means that even though the membrane potential has returned to normal, the cell has not recovered excitability completely because the latter depends on the elapse of a certain amount of time (i.e., is time-dependent) and not just on recovery of a particular membrane potential (i.e., voltage-dependent), a phenomenon termed *postrepolarization refractoriness*.

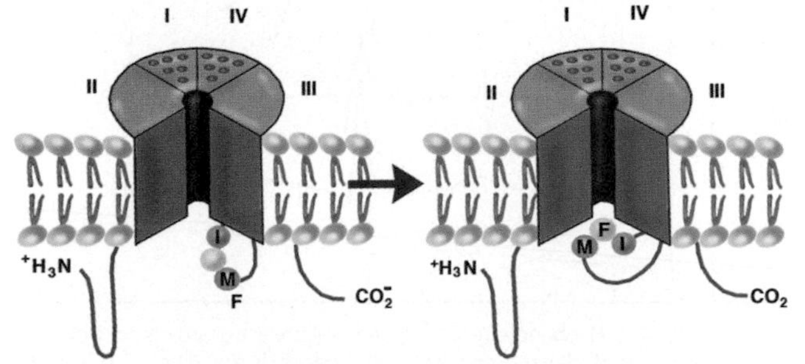

FIGURE 31–16 Mechanism of fast inactivation of sodium channels. The hinged lid mechanism of sodium channel inactivation is illustrated. The intracellular loop connecting domains III and IV of the sodium channel is depicted as forming a hinged lid. The critical residue (Phe1489F) is shown as occluding the intracellular mouth of the pore. *(From Catteral WA: Molecular analysis of voltage-gated sodium channels in the heart and other tissues.* In *Zipes DP, Jalife J [eds]: Cardiac Electrophysiology: From Cell to Bedside. 2nd ed. Philadelphia, WB Saunders, 1994, p 1.)*

The threshold for activation of $I_{Ca.L}$—that is, the voltage that the cell must reach to "turn on" the slow inward current—is about −30 to −40 mV. In fibers of the fast response type, $I_{Ca.L}$ is normally activated during phase 0 by the regenerative depolarization caused by the fast sodium current. Current flows through both fast and slow channels during the latter part of the action potential upstroke. However, $I_{Ca.L}$ is much smaller than the peak Na^+ current and therefore contributes little to the action potential until the fast Na^+ current is inactivated, after completion of phase 0. Thus, $I_{Ca.L}$ affects mainly the plateau of action potentials recorded in atrial and ventricular muscle and His-Purkinje fibers. In addition, $I_{Ca.L}$ may play a prominent role in partially depolarized cells in which the fast Na^+ channels have been inactivated if conditions are appropriate for slow-channel activation.[24]

Ca^{2+} entry through activated L-type Cav channels triggers Ca^{2+} release from the sarcoplasmic reticulum stores and is an essential component of cardiac excitation-contraction coupling in atrial and ventricular myocardium (see Chap. 21). L-type Cav channels are also expressed in sinoatrial and atrioventricular nodal cells, where they play a role in controlling automaticity and action potential propagation, respectively. Cardiac L-type Cav channels undergo rapid voltage- and Ca^{2+}-dependent inactivation, the time course of which importantly affects the action potential waveform and time course of repolarization. Although T-type Cav channels have not been detected in human myocardium, experimental evidence in animals has suggested that these channels play an important role in determining sinus node automaticity and AV nodal conduction.[32] Whether Ca^{2+} influx through open T-type channels provides a sufficient trigger for Ca^{2+} release from the sarcoplasmic reticulum is controversial. The density of T-type Ca^{2+} channels has been found to be increased in myocytes from hearts with experimentally induced hypertrophy,[54] but the role of enhanced T-type channel density under these conditions remains to be determined.

Other significant differences exist between the fast and slow channels. Drugs that elevate cAMP levels, such as beta adrenoceptor agonists, phosphodiesterase inhibitors such as theophylline, and the lipid-soluble derivative of cAMP, dibutyryl cAMP, increase $I_{Ca.L}$. Binding of the beta adrenoceptor agonist to specific sarcolemmal receptors facilitates the dissociation of two subunits of a regulatory protein (G protein; see Chap. 21), one of which (G_s) activates adenylate cyclase and thus increases intracellular levels of cAMP. The latter binds to a regulatory subunit of a cAMP-dependent protein kinase that promotes phosphorylation of specific phosphorylation sites on the channel protein, ultimately resulting in enhanced open-state probability of the channel. Although Nav channels are sensitive to increases in cAMP, the net effect (decrease versus increase) appears to be species-dependent.

Acetylcholine reduces $I_{Ca.L}$ by decreasing adenylate cyclase activity. However, acetylcholine stimulates cyclic guanosine monophosphate (cGMP) accumulation. cGMP has negligible effects on basal $I_{Ca.L}$ but

TABLE 31–3 Synopsis of Ionic Currents in Mammalian Cardiac Myocytes

Current	Subunit	Functional Properties
I_{Na}	Nav1.5 (alpha subunit)	Tetrodotoxin-insensitive voltage-gated Na^+ (Nav) current
$I_{Na.B}$	?	Proposed background Na^+ current through a voltage-independent channel in sinus nodal cells
$I_{Ca.L}$	Cav1.2 (alpha subunit)	L-type (*l*ong lasting, *l*arge conductance) Ca^{2+} currents through voltage-gated Ca^{2+} (Cav) channels blocked by dihydropyridine-type antagonists (e.g., nifedipine), phenylalkylamines (e.g., verapamil), benzothiazepines (e.g., diltiazem), and various divalent ions (e.g., Cd^{2+}); activated by dihydropyridine-type agonists (e.g., Bay K 8644), responsible for phase 0 depolarization and propagation in sinoatrial and AV nodal tissue, and contributing to plateau of atrial, His-Purkinje, and ventricular cells; main trigger of Ca^{2+} release from the sarcoplasmic reticulum (Ca^{2+}-induced Ca^{2+} release); noninactivating or "window" component may underlie early afterdepolarizations
$I_{Ca.T}$	Cav3.1/alpha$_1$ G (alpha subunit)	T-type (*t*ransient current, *t*iny conductance) Ca^{2+} currents through Cav channels blocked by mibefradil but insensitive to dihydropyridines; may contribute inward current to later phase of phase 4 depolarization in pacemaker cells and action potential propagation in AV nodal cells; role in triggering Ca^{2+}-induced Ca^{2+} release uncertain
I_f	HCN4 (alpha subunit)	Hyperpolarization-activated current carried by Na^+ and K^+ in sinoatrial and AV nodal cells and His-Purkinje cells, involved in generating phase 4 depolarization; increases rate of impulse initiation in pacemaker cells
I_{K1}	Kir2.1 (alpha subunit)	K^+ current through inwardly rectifying K^+ (Kir) channels, voltage-dependent block by Ba^{2+} at micromolar concentrations: responsible for maintaining resting membrane potential in atrial, His-Purkinje, and ventricular cells; channel activity is function of both membrane potential and $[K^+]_o$; inward rectification appears to result from depolarization-induced internal block by Mg^{2+}
$I_{K.G}$ ($I_{K.Ach}$, $I_{K.Ade}$)	Kir3.1/Kir3.4 (alpha subunit)	Inwardly rectifying K^+ current activated by muscarinic (M_2) and purinergic (type 1) receptor stimulation via GTP regulatory (G) protein signal transduction; expressed in sinoatrial and AV nodal cells and atrial cells, where it causes hyperpolarization and action potential shortening; activation causes negative chronotropic and dromotropic effects
I_{Ks}	KvLQT1 (alpha subunit)/ minK (beta subunit)	K^+ current carried by a voltage-gated K^+(Kv) channel (delayed rectifier K^+ channel); plays a major role in determining phase 3 of the action potential
I_{Kr}	hERG (alpha subunit)/ MiRP1(beta subunit)	Rapidly activating component of delayed rectifier K^+ current; I_{Kr} specifically blocked by dofetilide and sotalol in a reverse use–dependent manner; inward rectification of I_{Kr} results from depolarization-induced fast inactivation; plays a major role in determining action potential duration
I_{Kur}	Kv1.5 (alpha subunit)	K^+ current through a Kv channel with ultrarapid activation but ultraslow inactivation kinetics; expressed in atrial myocytes; determines action potential duration
$I_{K.Ca}$	SK2 (alpha subunit)	K^+ current through small-conductance Ca^{2+}-activated channels; blocked by apamine and dequalinium chloride; expressed in human atrial myocytes;, determines action potential duration
I_{to} (I_{to1}, I_A)		Kv4.3 (alpha subunit)/KChIP2 (beta subunit); transient outward K^+ current through voltage-gated (Kv) channels; exhibits fast activation and inactivation, and recovery kinetics; blocked by 4-aminopyridine in a reverse use–dependent manner; contributes to time course of phase 1 repolarization
$I_{Cl.Ca}$ (I_{to2})	?	4-Aminopyridine–resistant transient outward current carried by Cl^- ions; activated by increase in intracellular calcium level; blocked by stilbene derivatives (SITS, DIDS); contributes to time course of phase 1 repolarization; may underlie spontaneous transient inward currents under conditions of Ca^{2+} overload; molecular correlate uncertain (Jentsch)
$I_{Cl.cAMP}$	?	Time-independent chloride current regulated by cAMP/adenylate cyclase pathway; slightly depolarizes resting membrane potential and significantly shortens action potential duration; antagonizes action potential prolongation associated with beta-adrenergic stimulation of $I_{Ca.L}$
$I_{Cl.swell}$ or $I_{Cl.vol}$	?	Outwardly rectifying, swelling-activated Cl^- current; inhibited by 9-anthracene carboxylic acid; activation causes resting membrane depolarization and action potential shortening
$I_{K.ATP}$	Kir6.2 (alpha subunit)/SUR	Time-independent K^+ current through Kir channels activated by a fall in intracellular ATP concentration; inhibited by sulfonylurea drugs, such as glibenclamide; activated by pinacidil, nicorandil, cromakalim; causes shortening of action potential duration during myocardial ischemia or hypoxia

Table continues

TABLE 31–3 Synopsis of Ionic Currents in Mammalian Cardiac Myocytes—cont'd

Current	Subunit	Functional Properties
$I_{Cir.swell}$	?	Inwardly rectifying, swelling-activated cation current; permeable to Na^+ and K^+ ($P_{Na}/P_K=8$); inhibited by Gd^{3+}; depolarizes resting membrane potential and prolongs terminal (phase 3) repolarization
$I_{Na/Ca}$	NCX1.1	Current carried by Na^+/Ca^{2+} exchanger; causes net Na^+ outward current and Ca^{2+} inward current (reverse mode) or net Na^+ inward and Ca^{2+} outward current (3 Na^+ for 1 Ca^{2+}); direction of Na^+ flux depends on membrane potential and intracellular and extracellular concentrations of Na^+ and Ca^{2+}; Ca^{2+} influx mediated by $I_{Na/Ca}$ can trigger SR Ca^{2+} release; underlies I_{ti} (transient inward current) under conditions of intracellular Ca^{2+} overload
$I_{Na/K}$	Alpha subunit/beta subunit	Na^+ outward current generated by Na^+,K^+-ATPase (stoichiometry: 3 Na^+ leave and 2 K^+ enter); inhibited by digitalis
Electroneutral Ion-Exchanging Proteins		
Ca^{2+}-ATPase	Extrudes cytosolic calcium	
Na/H	Exchanges intracellular H^+ for extracellular Na^+; cardiac myocytes express isoform NHE 1; specifically inhibited by benzoylguanidine derivatives HOE 694 and HOE 642; inhibition causes intracellular acidification	
Cl^--HCO_3^-	Exchanges intracellular HCO_3^- for external Cl^-; inhibited by SITS	
Na^+-K^+-$2Cl^-$	Cotransporter blocked by amiloride	

ATP = adenosine triphosphate; AV = atrioventricular; cAMP = cyclic adenosine monophosphate; DIDS = 4,4′-diisothiocyanatostilbene-2,2′-disulfonic acid; GTP = guanosine triphosphate; SITS = 4-acetamido-4′-isothiocyanatostilbene-2,2′-disulfonic acid; SR = sarcoplasmic reticulum.

decreases $I_{Ca.L}$ levels that have been elevated by beta adrenoceptor agonists. This effect is mediated by cAMP hydrolysis through a cGMP-stimulated cyclic nucleotide phosphodiesterase.

DIFFERENCES BETWEEN CHANNELS. Fast and slow channels can be differentiated on the basis of their pharmacological sensitivity. Drugs that block the slow channel with a *fair* degree of specificity include verapamil, nifedipine, diltiazem, and D-600 (a methoxy derivative of verapamil). Antiarrhythmic agents such as lidocaine, quinidine, procainamide, and disopyramide (see Chap. 33) affect the fast channel and not the slow channel.

Normal action potentials recorded from the sinus node and the N region of the AV node have a reduced resting membrane potential, action potential amplitude, overshoot, upstroke, and conduction velocity compared with action potentials in muscle or Purkinje fibers (see Fig. 31-15).

Slow-channel blockers suppress sinus and AV nodal action potentials. The prolonged time for reactivation of $I_{Ca.L}$ probably accounts for the fact that sinus and AV nodal cells remain refractory longer than the time that it takes for full voltage repolarization to occur. Thus, premature stimulation immediately after the membrane potential reaches full repolarization leads to action potentials with reduced amplitudes and upstroke velocities. Therefore, slow conduction and prolonged refractoriness are characteristic features of nodal cells. These cells also have a reduced "safety factor for conduction," which means that the stimulating efficacy of the propagating impulse is low and conduction block occurs easily.

INWARD CURRENTS. Thus, I_{Na} and $I_{Ca.L}$ represent two important inward currents. Another important inward current is I_f, also called the pacemaker or "funny" current.[2,50] This current is activated by hyperpolarization and is carried by Na^+ and K^+. It generates phase 4 diastolic depolarization in the sinus node. I_f modulation is one major mechanism whereby beta-adrenergic and cholinergic neurotransmitters regulate cardiac rhythm under physiological conditions. Catecholamines increase the probability of channel opening by shifting the channel's activation curve to more positive potentials, which leads to increased current availability for the generation of diastolic depolarization, hence steepening its rate. Cholinergic action, in general, exerts the opposite effect.[50]

The electrophysiological changes accompanying *acute* myocardial ischemia may represent a depressed form of a fast response in the center of the ischemic zone and a slow response in the border area. Probable slow-response activity has been shown in myocardium resected from patients undergoing surgery for recurrent ventricular tachyarrhythmias (see Fig. 31-15F). Whether and how slow responses play a role in the genesis of ventricular arrhythmias in these patients have not been established.

Phase 1: Early Rapid Repolarization

Following phase 0, the membrane repolarizes rapidly and transiently to almost 0 mV (early notch), partly because of the inactivation of I_{Na} and concomitant activation of several outward currents.

I_{to}. The 4-aminopyridine–sensitive transient outward K^+ current, commonly termed I_{to} (or I_{to1}), is turned on rapidly by depolarization and then rapidly inactivates. Both the density and recovery of I_{to} from inactivation exhibit transmural gradients in the left ventricular free wall, with the density decreasing and reactivation becoming progressively prolonged from epicardium to endocardium.[30] Transmural differences in expression of KChIP2, the auxiliary subunit to Kv4.3 pore-forming alpha-subunits, appears to be the primary determinant of the transmural gradient in I_{to} properties and densities in the human heart.[51] This gradient gives rise to regional differences in action potential shape, with increasingly slower phase 1 restitution kinetics and diminution of the notch along the transmural axis (Fig. 31-17). These regional differences might create transmural voltage gradients, specifically at higher rates, thereby increasing dispersion of repolarization, a putative arrhythmogenic factor (see Brugada syndrome, Chap. 32). However, elimination of the physiological repolarization gradient appears to be similarly arrhythmogenic.[51] Downregulation of I_{to} is at least partially responsible for slowing of phase 1 repolarization in failing human myocytes. Studies have demonstrated that these changes in the phase 1 notch of the cardiac action potential cause a reduction in the kinetics and peak amplitude of the action potential–evoked intracellular Ca^{2+} transient because of failed recruitment and synchronization of the sarcoplasmic reticulum Ca^{2+} release through $I_{Ca.L}$ (Fig. 31-18; see Fig. 31-17C). Thus, modulation of I_{to} appears to play a significant physiological role in controlling cardiac excitation-contraction coupling,[52,53] and it remains to be determined whether transmural dif-

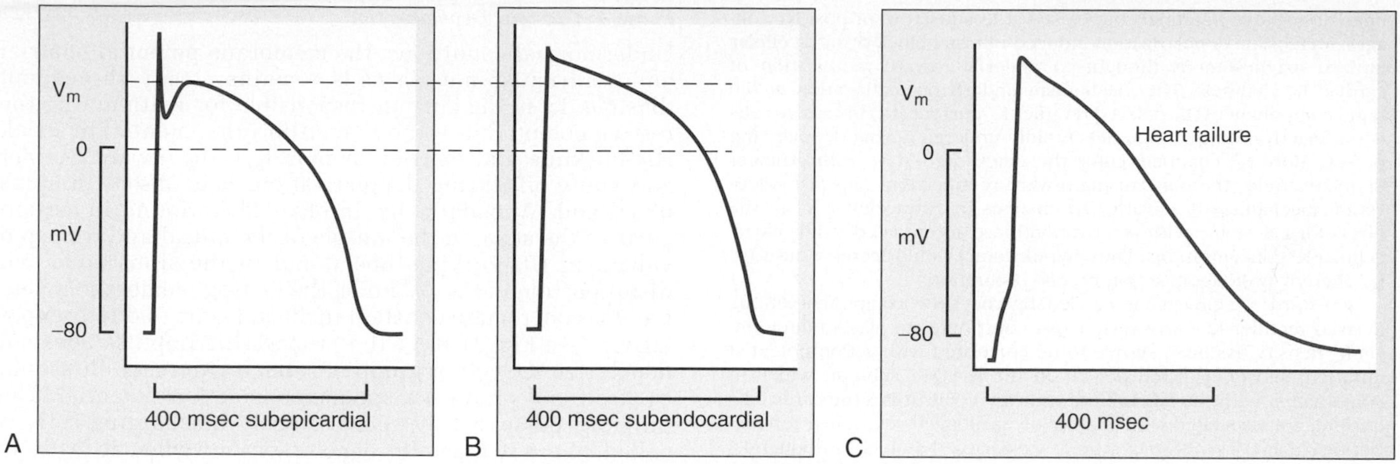

FIGURE 31–17 Action potential plots demonstrating differences in the action potential shape of human ventricular myocytes of subepicardial **(A)** and subendocardial **(B)** origin. Subepicardial myocytes present a prominent notch during phase 1 repolarization of the action potential, most likely caused by a larger I_{to} in these cells. The notch is absent in subendocardial cells. The peak plateau potential is higher in subendocardial than in subepicardial myocytes, and the action potential duration tends to be shorter in subepicardial cells. **C,** Transmembrane action potential in a human ventricular cardiomyocyte of a failing heart. Note loss of the prominent phase 1 notch and delayed repolarization. Recording temperature = 35°C; V_m = membrane potential. *(**A** and **B** from Näbauer M, Beuckelmann DJ, Uberfuhr P, Steinbeck G: Regional differences in current density and rate-dependent properties of the transient outward current in subepicardial and subendocardial myocytes of human left ventricle. Circulation 93:168, 1996. By permission of the American Heart Association; **C** from Priebe L, Beuckelmann DJ: Simulation studies of cellular electrical properties in heart failure. Circ Res 82:1206-1223, 1998.)*

ferences in phase 1 repolarization translate into similar differences in regional contractility.

$I_{Cl.Ca}$. The 4-aminopyridine-resistant, Ca^{2+}-activated chloride current $I_{Cl.Ca}$ (or I_{to2}) also contributes a significant outward current during phase 1 repolarization.[54] This current is activated by the action potential–evoked intracellular Ca^{2+} transient. Therefore, interventions that augment the amplitude of the Ca^{2+} transient associated with the twitch (such as beta-adrenergic receptor stimulation) also enhance outward $I_{Cl.Ca}$. It is not currently known whether human cardiac myocytes express Ca^{2+}-activated chloride channels. Other, time-*independent* chloride currents may also play a role in determining the time course of early repolarization, such as the cAMP- or swelling-activated chloride conductances $I_{Cl.cAMP}$ and $I_{Cl.swell}$.

Na/Ca EXCHANGER. A third current contributing to early repolarization is Na^+ outward movement through the Na^+/Ca^{2+} exchanger operating in reverse mode (see Fig. 31-14).[55] Overexpression of the exchanger in transgenic mice caused accentuation of the early notch in left ventricular myocytes.

Sometimes, a transient depolarization follows phase 1 repolarization. This notch is well defined and separated from phase 2 in Purkinje fibers and left ventricular epicardial and midmyocardial myocytes (see Fig. 31-17).

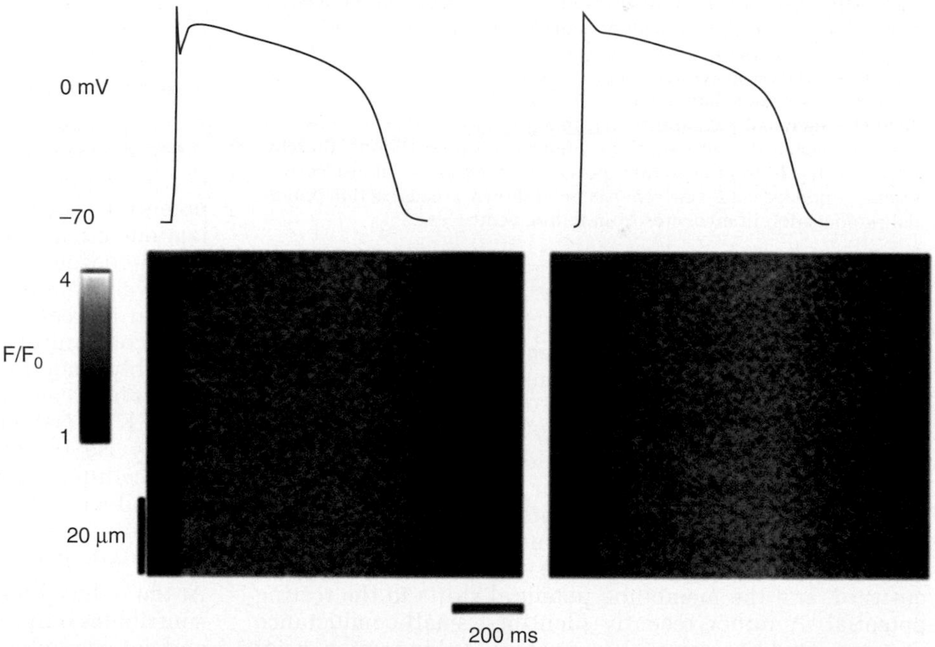

FIGURE 31–18 Diminution of phase 1 amplitude ("notch") causes asynchronous sarcoplasmic reticulum Ca^{2+} release. Normal cardiomyocytes were voltage-clamped with action potential profiles with a normal or congestive heart failure wave shape and local changes in intracellular calcium were recorded simultaneously. When the myocyte was clamped with a normal action potential profile having the early phase 1 repolarization notch **(left),** there was uniform Ca^{2+} release. However, when a congestive heart failure action potential profile without early rapid phase 1 repolarization was used, Ca^{2+} release was dyssynchronous. This dyssynchrony causes a slowing in the rate of rise of the Ca^{2+} transient and a loss of spatial and temporal release uniformity. F/F_0 = fluorescence of Ca^{2+}-indicator normalized to its baseline fluorescence. *(From Harris DM, Mills GD, Chen X, et al: Alterations in early action potential repolarization causes localized failure of sarcoplasmic reticulum Ca^{2+} release. Circ Res 96: 543, 2005. By permission from the American Heart Association.)*

Phase 2: Plateau

During the plateau phase, which may last several hundred milliseconds, membrane conductance to all ions falls to rather low values. Thus, less change in current is required near plateau levels than near resting potential levels to produce the same changes in transmembrane potential. The plateau is maintained by the competition between outward current carried by K^+ and Cl^- ions and inward current carried by Ca^{2+} moving through open L-type Ca^{2+} channels and Na^+ being exchanged for internal Ca^{2+} by the Na^+/Ca^{2+} exchanger operating in forward mode. After depolarization, potassium conductance falls to plateau levels as a result of inward rectification in spite of the large electrochemical driving force on K^+ ions.

Rectification simply means that membrane conductance changes with voltage. Specifically, inward rectification means that K^+ channels are open at negative potentials but closed at less negative or positive voltages. Membrane depolarization-induced internal block by intracellular ionized magnesium is thought to underlie inward rectification of cardiac I_{K1} channels. The mechanism underlying rectification of the rapid component of the delayed rectifier K^+ current (I_{Kr}) in cardiac cells is the inactivation that channels rapidly undergo during depolarizing pulses. More I_{Kr} channels enter the inactivated state with stronger depolarizations, thereby causing inward rectification. This fast inactivation mechanism is sensitive to changes in extracellular K^+ in the physiological range, with inactivation more accentuated at low extracellular K^+ concentrations. Thus, hypokalemia would decrease outward I_{Kr}, thereby prolonging action potential duration.

Outward K^+ movement carried by the slow component of the delayed rectifier K^+ current (I_{Ks}) also contributes to plateau duration: (1) I_{Ks} density has been shown to be correlated with action potential duration; and (2) isolated defects in the KvLQT1 subunit, which in combination with the IsK subunit (minK) reconstitutes the cardiac I_{Ks} current, are associated with abnormally prolonged ventricular repolarization (long-QT syndrome, type 1; see Chaps. 9 and 35). Although I_{Ks} activates slowly compared with action potential duration, it is only slowly inactivated. Therefore, increases in heart rate can cause this activation to accumulate during successive depolarizations, and cumulative activation can determine the contribution to repolarization of K^+ currents that are active during the plateau of the action potential.[23] In conditions of reduced intracellular ATP concentration (e.g., hypoxia, ischemia), K^+ efflux through activated K_{ATP} channels is enhanced, thereby shortening the plateau phase of the action potential. Other ionic mechanisms that control plateau potential and duration include the kinetics of inactivation of the L-type Ca^{2+} current. Reduced efficiency of intracellular free Ca^{2+} to induce Ca^{2+}-dependent inactivation, such as in myocytes from hypertrophic hearts, can result in delayed repolarization. Steady-state components of both I_{Na} and $I_{Ca.L}$ (window currents) can shape the plateau phase.

Na^+,K^+-ATPase generates a net outward current by pumping out three Na^+ ions in exchange for two K^+ ions. Noninactivating chloride currents, such as $I_{Cl.swell}$ and $I_{Cl.cAMP}$, may produce significant outward currents during the plateau phase under certain conditions, thereby significantly shortening action potential duration. A nonselective, swelling-induced cation current has been shown to cause action potential prolongation in myocytes from failing ventricles.

Phase 3: Final Rapid Repolarization

In this portion of the action potential, repolarization proceeds rapidly at least in part because of two currents: time-dependent inactivation of $I_{Ca.L}$, with a decrease in the intracellular movement of positive charges, and activation of repolarizing K^+ currents, including the slow and rapid components of the delayed rectifier K^+ current I_{Ks} and I_{Kr} and the inwardly rectifying K^+ currents I_{K1} and $I_{K.Ach}$, which all cause an increase in the movement of positive charges out of the cell. The net membrane current becomes more outward, and the membrane potential shifts to the resting potential. A rather recently identified small-conductance Ca^{2+}-activated K^+-current, $I_{K.Ca}$, is expressed in human atrial myocytes, where it controls the time course of phase 3 repolarization.[56] Mutations in the human ether-a-go-go–related gene (*HERG*), which is responsible for I_{Kr}, prolong phase 3 repolarization, thereby predisposing to the development of torsades de pointes. Macrolide antibiotics such as erythromycin, antihistamines such as terfenadine, and antifungal drugs such as ketoconazole all inhibit I_{Kr} and have been implicated in the acquired form of long QT syndrome (see Chaps. 9 and 35). A decrease in I_{K1} activity, as is the case in left ventricular myocytes from failing hearts, causes action potential prolongation by slowing of phase 3 repolarization and resting membrane depolarization. Reduction in the outward potassium current through open inward rectifier K^+ channels renders the failing cardiomyocyte more susceptible to the induction of delayed afterdepolarizations triggered by spontaneous intracellular Ca^{2+} release events, and therefore plays a major role in arrhythmogenesis in the failing heart (see Fig. 31-23).

Phase 4: Diastolic Depolarization

Under normal conditions, the membrane potential of atrial and ventricular muscle cells remains steady throughout diastole. I_{K1} is the current responsible for maintaining the resting potential near the K^+ equilibrium potential in atrial, His-Purkinje, and ventricular cells. I_{K1} is the inward rectifier and shuts off during depolarization. It is absent in sinus nodal and AV nodal cells. In other fibers found in certain parts of the atria, in the muscle of the mitral and tricuspid valves, in His-Purkinje fibers, and in the sinus node and distal portion of the AV node, the resting membrane potential does not remain constant in diastole but gradually depolarizes (see Fig. 31-15A). If a propagating impulse does not depolarize the cell or group of cells, it can reach threshold by itself and produce a spontaneous action potential. The property possessed by spontaneously discharging cells is called phase 4 diastolic depolarization; when it leads to initiation of action potentials, automaticity results. The discharge rate of the sinus node normally exceeds the discharge rate of other potentially automatic pacemaker sites and thus maintains dominance of the cardiac rhythm. The discharge rate of the sinus node is normally more sensitive to the effects of norepinephrine and acetylcholine than the discharge rate of ventricular muscle cells. Normal or abnormal automaticity at other sites can cause discharge at rates faster than the sinus nodal discharge rate and can usurp control of the cardiac rhythm for one cycle or many (see Chap. 32).

Normal Automaticity

The ionic basis of automaticity is explained by a net gain in intracellular positive charges during diastole. Contributing to this change is a voltage-dependent channel activated by potentials negative to −50 to −60 mV—that is, a hyperpolarization-activated inward pacemaker current. At this potential, I_f becomes activated and is carried by a channel relatively nonselective for monovalent cations. Hyperpolarization increases its rate of activation and, at −70 mV, the time constant of activation ranges from 2 to 4 seconds. I_f probably underlies the slow diastolic depolarization that occurs between −90 and −60 mV in Purkinje fibers. Although either K^+ or Na^+ ions can serve as ion transporters, I_f carries largely Na^+ at the more negative intracellular voltages. Extracellular K^+ ions activate I_f, but $[Na^+]_o$ does not influence its conductance.

Automaticity in Sinus Nodal Cells

At the reduced membrane potentials of sinus nodal cells, I_f contributes only about 20 percent of the pacemaker current, and automaticity is primarily dependent on I_K and $I_{Ca.L}$ and $I_{Ca.T}$. However, sinus nodal cells exhibit significant I_f current if they are hyperpolarized in the range of −50 to −100 mV. Conversely, I_K in normally polarized Purkinje fibers adds little to the pacemaker current. Deactivation of I_K, the presence of an unidentified background inward current, deactivation of $I_{Ca.T}$, and activation of $I_{Ca.L}$ are the essential processes governing the rate of pacemaker depolarization in sinus and AV nodal cells and in Purkinje fibers whose membrane potential has been depolarized to voltages largely positive to the activation range of I_f.

The sinus nodal discharge rate maintains dominance over latent pacemaker sites because it depolarizes more rapidly and because of overdrive suppression, a mechanism characterized by prolonged suppression of normal pacemakers in proportion to the duration and rate of stimulation by a more rapidly discharging pacemaker. The mechanism may be related to active Na extrusion during the more rapid rate that maintains diastolic depolarization of latent pacemakers at a level more negative than the threshold potential for automatic discharge.

The rate of sinus nodal discharge can be varied by several mechanisms in response to autonomic or other influences. The pacemaker locus can shift within or outside the sinus node to cells discharging faster or more slowly. If the pacemaker site remains the same, alterations in the slope of the diastolic depolarization, maximum diastolic potential, or threshold potential can speed or slow the discharge rate. For example, if the slope of diastolic depolarization steepens and if the resting membrane potential becomes less negative or the threshold potential more negative (within limits), discharge rate increases. Opposite changes slow the discharge rate.

Acetylcholine activates K^+ efflux through acetylcholine-sensitive inward rectifier K^+ channels, which are expressed in both sinus nodal and AV nodal cells, thereby shifting the maximum diastolic potential to more negative values. The same mechanism reduces input resistance at diastolic potentials, which means that a greater depolarizing current would be required to achieve "threshold" for firing an action potential.

Studies using fluorescent calcium-sensitive indicators, combined with imaging and simultaneous measurement of transmembrane action potential, have suggested that cyclic variations in submembrane Ca^{2+} concentration coupled to activation of the Na^+/Ca^{2+} exchange current modulate sinoatrial node cell beating rate and are a factor in establishing dominance of the sinoatrial node cell pacemaker function (Fig. 31-19).[57]

Passive Membrane Electrical Properties

Passive membrane properties, including membrane resistance, capacitance, and cable properties, play an important role in cardiac electrophysiology. Although the cardiac cell membrane is resistant to current flow, it also has capacitative properties, which means that it behaves like a battery and can store charges of opposite signs on its two sides—an excess of negative charges inside the membrane balanced by equivalent positive charges outside the membrane. These resistive and capacitative properties cause the membrane to take a certain amount of time to respond to an applied stimulus, rather than responding instantly, because the charges across the capacitative membrane must be altered first. A subthreshold rectangular current pulse applied to the membrane produces a slowly rising and decaying membrane voltage change rather than a rectangular voltage change. A value called the time constant of the membrane reflects this property. The time constant, tau, is equal to the product of membrane resistance R_m and cell capacitance C_m:

$$\text{tau} = R_m \cdot C_m$$

This is the time taken by the membrane voltage to reach 63 percent of its final value after application of a steady current.

When aligned end to end, cardiac cells, particularly the His-Purkinje system, behave like a long cable in which current flows more easily inside the cell and to the adjacent cell across the gap junction than it does across the cell membrane to the outside. When current is injected at a point, most of it flows along inside the cell, but some leaks out. Because of this loss of current, the voltage change of a cell at a site distant from the point of applied current is less than the change in membrane voltage where the stimulus was given. A measure of this property of a cable is called the space or length constant lambda (λ), which is the distance along the cable from the point of stimulation at which the voltage at steady state is 1/e (37 percent) of its value at the point of introduction.

Restated, λ describes how far current flows before leaking passively across the surface membrane to a value about one third of its initial value. This distance is normally about 2 mm for Purkinje fibers, 0.5 mm for the sinus node, and 0.8 mm for ventricular muscle fibers. λ is about 10 times the length of an individual cell. As an example, if e is approximately 2.7 and a hyperpolarizing current pulse in a Purkinje fiber produces a membrane voltage change of 15 mV at the site of current injection, the membrane potential change one space constant (2 mm) away would be 15/2.7 = 5.5 mV.

Because the current loop in any circuit must be closed, current must flow back to its point of origin. Local circuit currents pass across gap junctions between cells and exit across the sarcolemmal membrane to close the loop and complete the circuit. Inward excitation currents in one area (carried by Na^+ in most regions) flow intracellularly along the length of the tissue (carried mostly by K^+), escape across the membrane, and flow extracellularly in a longitudinal direction. The outside local circuit current is the current recorded on an electrocardiogram (ECG; **see Chap. 9**). Through these local circuit currents, the transmembrane potential of each cell influences the transmembrane potential of its neighbor because of the passive flow of current from one segment of the fiber to another across the low-resistance gap junctions.

As discussed earlier, the speed of conduction depends on active membrane properties such as the magnitude of the Na^+ current, a measure of which is $\dot{V}_{max}$. Passive membrane properties also contribute to conduction velocity and include excitability threshold, which influences the capability of cells adjacent to the one that has been discharged to reach threshold; the intracellular resistance of the cell, determined by the free ions in the cytoplasm; the resistance of the gap junction; and the cross-sectional area of the cell. Direction of propagation is crucial because of the influence of anisotropy, as mentioned earlier.

Loss of Membrane Potential and Arrhythmia Development

Many acquired abnormalities of cardiac muscle or specialized fibers that result in arrhythmias produce a loss of membrane potential; that is, maximum diastolic potential becomes less negative. This change should be viewed as a symptom of an underlying abnormality, analogous to fever or jaundice, rather than as a diagnostic category in and of

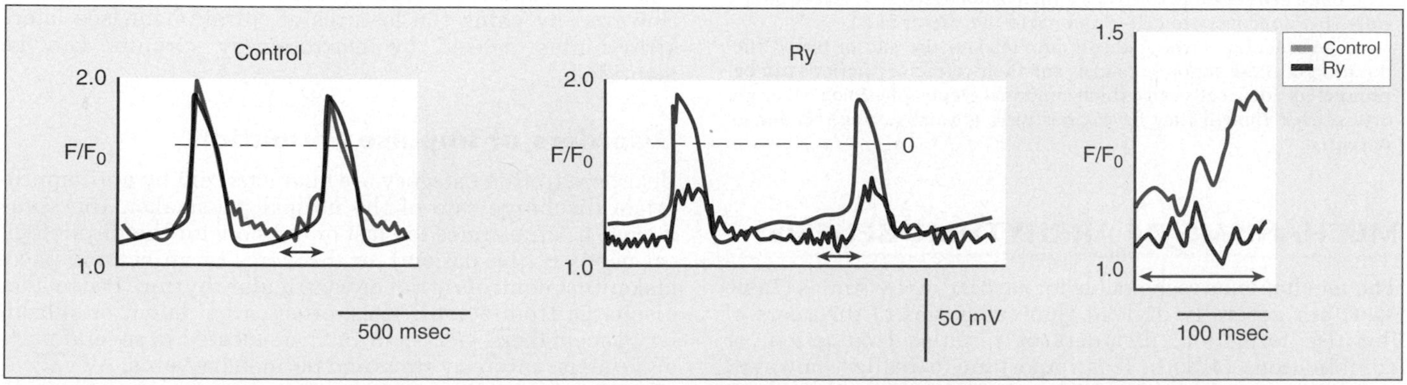

FIGURE 31–19 Ca^{2+} release from the sarcoplasmic reticulum through ryanodine receptors during diastolic depolarization in an isolated rabbit sinoatrial node cell is shown as a plot of variations in intracellular calcium concentration (in blue and magenta, respectively) with simultaneously recorded membrane potential. In the control state, the Ca^{2+} waveform exhibits an increase during the later part of the spontaneous diastolic depolarization that precedes the rapid upstroke of the action potential (bracketed by arrows and shown at greater resolution in the panel on the right). This increase is abolished by the specific blocker of the sarcoplasmic reticulum Ca^{2+} release channel, ryanodine (Ry), concurrent with a slowing of the beating rate by this drug. *(From Lakatta EG, Maltsev VA, Bogdanov KY, et al: Cyclic variation in intracellular calcium. A critical factor for cardiac pacemaker cell dominance. Circ Res 92:e45, 2003.)*

itself, because both the ionic changes resulting in cellular depolarization and the more fundamental biochemical or metabolic abnormalities responsible for the ionic alterations probably have a number of causative factors.

Cellular depolarization can result from elevated $[K^+]_o$ or decreased $[K^+]_i$, an increase in membrane permeability to Na^+ (P_{Na} increases), or a decrease in membrane permeability to K^+ (P_K decreases). Reference to the GHK equation for V (see "Phases of the Cardiac Action Potential: General Considerations") illustrates that these changes alone or in combination make membrane diastolic voltage less negative.

Normal cells perfused by an abnormal milieu (e.g., hyperkalemia), abnormal cells perfused by a normal milieu (e.g., healed myocardial infarction), or abnormal cells perfused by an abnormal milieu (e.g., acute myocardial ischemia and infarction) can exist alone or in combination and reduce resting membrane voltage. Each of these changes can have one or more biochemical or metabolic causes. For example, acute myocardial ischemia results in decreased $[K^+]_i$ and increased $[K^+]_o$, norepinephrine release, and acidosis, which may be related to an increase in intracellular Ca^{2+} and Ca^{2+}-induced transient inward currents and accumulation of amphipathic lipid metabolites and oxygen-free radicals. All these changes can contribute to the development of an abnormal electrophysiological environment and arrhythmias during ischemia and reperfusion. Knowledge of these changes may provide insight into therapy that actually reverses basic defects and restores membrane potential or other abnormalities to normal.

EFFECTS OF REDUCED RESTING POTENTIAL. The reduced resting membrane potential alters the depolarization and repolarization phases of the cardiac action potential. For example, partial membrane depolarization causes a decrease in the steady-state availability of fast sodium channels, thereby reducing the magnitude of peak I_{Na} during phase 0 of the action potential. The subsequent reduction in $\dot{V}_{max}$ and action potential amplitude prolongs the conduction time of the propagated impulse, at times to the point of block.[30]

Action potentials with reduced upstroke velocity resulting from partial inactivation of I_{Na} are called depressed fast responses (see Fig. 31-15F). Their contours often resemble and can be difficult to distinguish from slow responses, in which upstrokes are caused by $I_{Ca.L}$ (see Fig. 31-15F). Membrane depolarization to levels of −60 to −70 mV can inactivate half the Na^+ channels, and depolarization to −50 mV or less can inactivate all the Na^+ channels. At membrane potentials positive to −50 mV, $I_{Ca.L}$ can be activated to generate phase 0 if conditions are appropriate. These action potential changes are likely to be heterogeneous, with unequal degrees of Na^+ inactivation that create areas with minimally reduced velocity, more severely depressed zones, and areas of complete block. These uneven changes are conducive to the development of arrhythmias (Fig. 31-20).

In these cells with reduced membrane potential, refractoriness can outlast voltage recovery of the action potential; that is, the cell can still be refractory or partially refractory after the resting membrane potential returns to its most negative value. Furthermore, if block of the cardiac impulse occurs in a fairly localized area without significant slowing of conduction proximal to the site of block, cells in this proximal zone exhibit short action potentials and refractory periods because unexcited cells distal to the block (still in a polarized state) electrotonically speed recovery in cells proximal to the site of block.

If conduction slows gradually proximal to the site of block, the duration of these action potentials and their refractory periods can be prolonged. Some cells can exhibit abnormal electrophysiological properties, even though they have a relatively normal resting membrane potential.

MECHANISMS OF ARRHYTHMOGENESIS

The mechanisms responsible for cardiac arrhythmias (Table 31-4) are generally divided into categories of disorders of impulse formation, disorders of impulse conduction, or combinations of both. It is important to realize, however, that our currently available diagnostic tools do not permit unequivocal determination of the electrophysiological mechanisms responsible for many clinically occurring arrhythmias or their ionic bases. This is especially true for ventricular arrhythmias. It may be clinically difficult to separate microreentry from automaticity, and often one is left with the consideration that a particular arrhythmia is "most consistent with" or "best explained by" one or the other electrophysiological mechanism. Some tachyarrhythmias can be started by one mechanism and perpetuated by another. An episode of tachycardia caused by one mechanism can precipitate another episode caused by a different mechanism. For example, an initiating tachycardia or premature complex caused by abnormal automaticity can precipitate an episode of tachycardia sustained by reentry. However, by using the features of entrainment (see later), arrhythmias caused by macroreentry circuits can be identified.

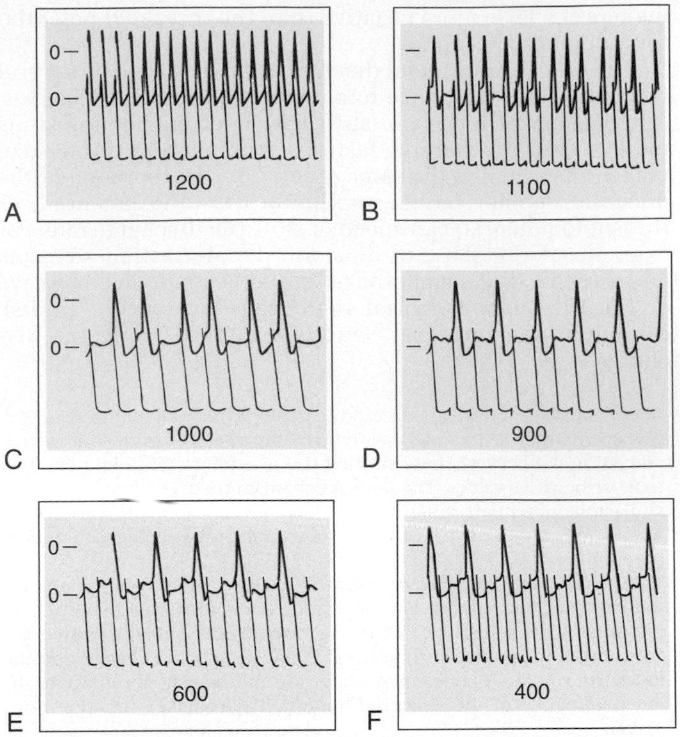

FIGURE 31–20 Rate-dependent conduction from the normal zone into the abnormal zone. **A** to **F,** When the pacing cycle length in the normal zone was shortened from 1200 to 400 milliseconds, increasing degrees of entrance block into the abnormal area occurred and progressed from 1 : 1 conduction at a cycle length of 1200 milliseconds to 4 : 3 conduction at 1100 milliseconds, 3 : 2 conduction at 1000 milliseconds, 2 : 1 conduction at 900 milliseconds, 3 : 1 conduction at 600 milliseconds, and 4 : 1 conduction at 400 milliseconds. Pacing the abnormal zone (not shown) resulted in block to the normal zone (unidirectional propagation). Vertical calibration, 50 mV. Horizontal calibration, 4 seconds in **A** and **B** and 2 seconds in **C** to **F.** *(From Gilmour RF Jr, Heger JJ, Prystowsky EN, et al: Cellular electrophysiologic abnormalities of diseased human ventricular myocardium. Am J Cardiol 51:137, 1983.)*

Disorders of Impulse Formation

Disorders in this category are characterized by an inappropriate discharge rate of the normal pacemaker, the sinus node (e.g., sinus rates too fast or too slow for the physiological needs of the patient), or discharge of an ectopic pacemaker that controls atrial or ventricular rhythm. Pacemaker discharge from ectopic sites, often called latent or subsidiary pacemakers, can occur in fibers located in several parts of the atria, coronary sinus and pulmonary veins, AV valves, portions of the AV junction, and His-Purkinje system. Ordinarily kept from reaching the level of threshold potential because of overdrive suppression by the more rapidly firing sinus node or electrotonic depression from contiguous fibers, ectopic pacemaker activity at one of these latent sites can become manifest when the sinus nodal discharge rate

TABLE 31–4 Mechanisms of Arrhythmogenesis

Disorder	Experimental Examples	Clinical Examples
Disorders of Impulse Formation		
Automaticity		
Normal automaticity	Normal in vivo or in vitro in sinus node; Purkinje fibers, others	Sinus tachycardia or bradycardia inappropriate for clinical situation; possibly ventricular parasystole
Abnormal automaticity	Depolarization-induced automaticity in Purkinje fibers or ventricular muscle	Possibly accelerated ventricular rhythms after myocardial infarction
Triggered activity		
Early afterdepolarizations	EADs produced by barium, hypoxia, high concentrations of catecholamines, drugs such as sotalol, *N*-acetylprocainamide, cesium	Possibly idiopathic and acquired long QT syndromes and associated ventricular arrhythmias
Delayed afterdepolarizations	DADs produced in Purkinje fibers by digitalis	Possibly some digitalis-induced arrhythmias
Disorders of Impulse Conduction		
Block		
Bidirectional or unidirectional without reentry	SA, AV, bundle branch, Purkinje-muscle, others	SA, AV, bundle branch, others
Unidirectional block with reentry	AV node, Purkinje–muscle junction, infarcted myocardium, others	Reciprocating tachycardia in WPW syndrome, AV nodal reentry, VT caused by bundle branch reentry, others
Reflection	Purkinje fiber with area of inexcitability	Unknown
Combined Disorders		
Interactions between automatic foci	Depolarizing or hyperpolarizing subthreshold stimuli speed or slow automatic discharge rate	Modulated parasystole
Interactions between automaticity and conduction	Deceleration-dependent block, overdrive suppression of conduction, entrance and exit block	Similar to experimental

AV = atrioventricular; DAD = delayed afterdepolarization; EAD = early afterdepolarization; SA = sinoatrial; WPW = Wolff-Parkinson-White.

slows or block occurs at some level between the sinus node and the ectopic pacemaker site, which permits *escape* of the latent pacemaker at the latter's normal discharge rate. A clinical example would be sinus bradycardia to a rate of 45 beats/min that permits an AV junctional escape complex to occur at a rate of 50 beats/min.

Alternatively, the discharge rate of the latent pacemaker can speed inappropriately and usurp control of cardiac rhythm from the sinus node, which has been discharging at a normal rate, such as a premature ventricular complex or a burst of ventricular tachycardia. It is important to remember that such disorders of impulse formation can be caused by speeding or slowing of a *normal* pacemaker mechanism (e.g., phase 4 diastolic depolarization that is ionically normal for the sinus node or for an ectopic site such as a Purkinje fiber but occurs inappropriately fast or slow) or by an ionically *abnormal* pacemaker mechanism.

A patient with persistent sinus tachycardia at rest or sinus bradycardia during exertion exhibits inappropriate sinus nodal discharge rates, but the ionic mechanisms responsible for sinus nodal discharge may still be normal, although the kinetics or magnitude of the currents may be altered. Conversely, when a patient experiences ventricular tachycardia during an acute myocardial infarction, ionic mechanisms ordinarily not involved in formation of spontaneous impulses for this fiber type may be operative and generate the tachycardia. For example, although pacemaker activity is not generally found in ordinary working myocardium, the effects of myocardial infarction can perhaps depolarize these cells to membrane potentials at which inactivation of I_K and activation of $I_{Ca.L}$ cause automatic discharge.

Abnormal Automaticity

Mechanisms responsible for normal automaticity were described earlier. Abnormal automaticity can arise from cells that have reduced maximum diastolic potentials, often at membrane potentials positive to −50 mV, when I_K and $I_{Ca.L}$ may be operative.

Automaticity at membrane potentials more negative than −70 mV may be caused by I_f. When the membrane potential is between −50 and −70 mV, the cell may be quiescent. Electrotonic effects from surrounding normally polarized or more depolarized myocardium influence the development of automaticity. Abnormal automaticity has been found in Purkinje fibers removed from dogs subjected to myocardial infarction, in rat myocardium damaged by epinephrine, in human atrial samples, and in ventricular myocardial specimens from patients undergoing aneurysmectomy and endocardial resection for recurrent ventricular tachyarrhythmias.

Abnormal automaticity can be produced in normal muscle or Purkinje fibers by appropriate interventions, such as current passage that reduces diastolic potential. An automatic discharge rate speeds up with progressive depolarization, and hyperpolarizing pulses slow the spontaneous firing. It is possible that partial depolarization and failure to reach normal maximal diastolic potential can induce automatic discharge in most, if not all, cardiac fibers. Although this type of spontaneous automatic activity has been found in human atrial and ventricular fibers, its relationship to the genesis of clinical arrhythmias has not been established.

Rhythms resulting from automaticity may be slow atrial, junctional, and ventricular escape rhythms; certain types of atrial tachycardias (e.g., those produced by digitalis or perhaps those coming from the pulmonary veins), accelerated junctional (nonparoxysmal junctional tachycardia) and idioventricular rhythms, and parasystole (see Chap. 35).

Triggered Activity

Automaticity is the property of a fiber to initiate an impulse spontaneously, without need for prior stimulation, so that electrical quiescence does not occur. Triggered activity is initiated by afterdepolarizations, which are depolarizing oscillations in membrane voltage induced by one or more preceding action potentials. Thus, triggered activity is pacemaker activity that results consequent to a preceding impulse or series of impulses, without which electrical quiescence occurs (Fig. 31-21). This triggering activity is not caused by an automatic self-generating mechanism, and the term *triggered automaticity* is therefore contradictory. These depolarizations can occur before or after full repolarization of the fiber and are best termed *early afterdepolarizations* (EADs), when they arise from a reduced level of membrane potential during phases 2 (type 1) and 3 (type 2) of the cardiac action potential or are termed *late* or *delayed afterdepolarizations* (DADs), when they occur after completion of repolarization (phase 4), generally at a more negative membrane potential than that from which EADs arise (Table 31-5). Not all afterdepolarizations may reach threshold potential but, if they do, they can trigger another afterdepolarization and thus self-perpetuate.

TABLE 31–5 Determinants of Amplitude of Afterdepolarizations

Intervention	Effect on Amplitude of EADs	Effect on Amplitude of DADs
Long cycles (basic and premature)	↑	↓
Long action potential duration	↑	↑
Reduced membrane potential	↑	↓
Na channel blockers	No effect	↓
Ca channel blockers	↓	↓
Catecholamines	↑	↑

↑ = increase amplitude; ↓ = decrease amplitude; DADs = delayed afterdepolarizations; EADs = early afterdepolarizations.

Delayed Afterdepolarizations

DADs and triggered activity have been demonstrated in Purkinje fibers, specialized atrial fibers and ventricular muscle fibers exposed to digitalis preparations, pulmonary veins, normal Purkinje fibers exposed to Na-free superfusates from the endocardium of the intact heart, ventricular myocardial cells from failing hearts (Fig. 31-22) and from mouse hearts with ankyrin-B mutations (see Fig. 31-21) during beta-adrenergic stimulation, and endocardial preparations 1 day after a myocardial infarction.[58,59] When fibers in the rabbit, canine, simian, and human mitral valves and in the canine tricuspid valve and coronary sinus are superfused with norepinephrine, they exhibit the capability for sustained triggered rhythmic activity.

Triggered activity caused by DADs has also been noted in diseased human atrial and ventricular fibers studied in vitro. Left stellate ganglion stimulation can elicit DADs in canine ventricles. In vivo, atrial and ventricular arrhythmias apparently caused by triggered activity have been reported in the dog and possibly in humans. It is tempting to ascribe certain clinical arrhythmias to DADs, such as some arrhythmias precipitated by digitalis or some atrial fibrillations arising from DADs in pulmonary veins. The accelerated idioventricular rhythm 1 day after experimental canine myocardial infarction may be caused by DADs, and some evidence has suggested that certain ventricular tachycardias, such as those arising in the right ventricular outflow tract, may be caused by DADs, whereas other data suggest that EADs are responsible.[60]

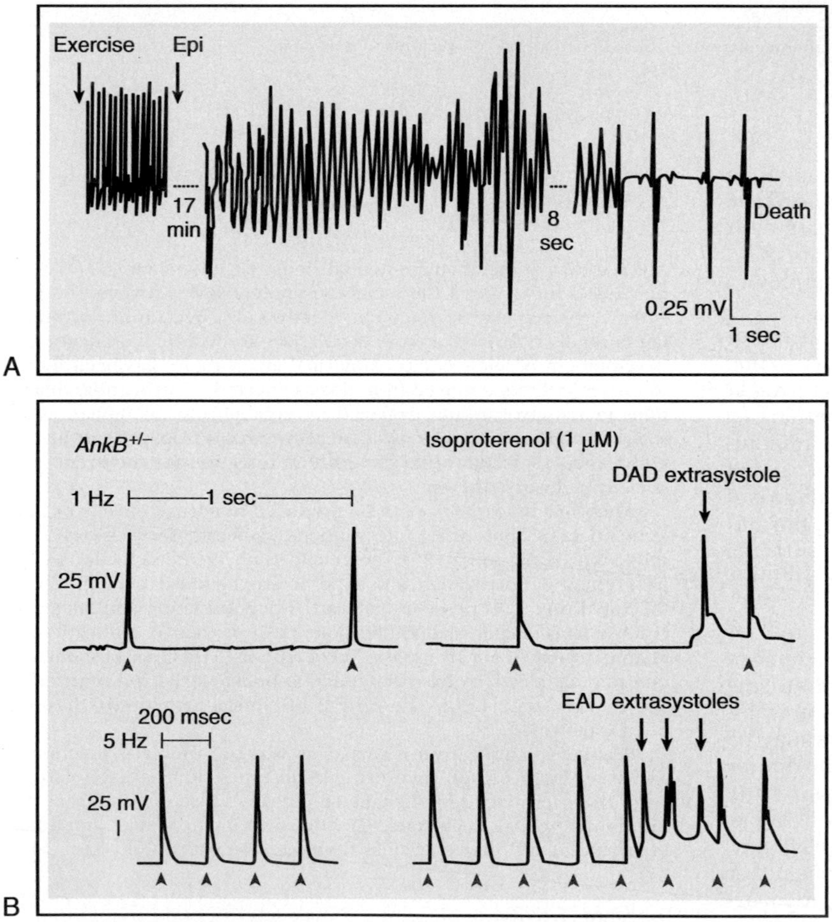

FIGURE 31–21 Polymorphic ventricular tachycardia and sudden death in an animal model of type 4 long QT syndrome. **A,** Electrocardiogram after exercise and administration of epinephrine in a mouse heterozygous for a loss of function mutation in the gene encoding ankyrin-B (*AnkB*⁻). Polymorphic ventricular tachycardia (torsades de pointes) occurred within about 17 minutes of epinephrine administration, followed by marked bradycardia and death 2 minutes after the arrhythmia. **B,** Transmembrane action potentials in single cardiomyocytes from *AnkB*+/− mice at the frequencies indicated. Acute exposure to isoproterenol induced both delayed and early afterdepolarizations that led to extra beats. *(From Mohler PJ, Schott J, Gramolini AO, et al: Ankyrin-B mutation causes type 4 long-QT cardiac arrhythmia and sudden cardiac death. Nature 421:634, 2003.)*

MAJOR ROLE OF INTRACELLULAR Ca^{2+} HANDLING ABNORMALITIES IN DAD GENERATION. It is well recognized that DADs result from activation of a calcium-sensitive inward current elicited by spontaneous increases in intracellular free calcium concentration. Acquired or inherited abnormalities in the properties of the sarcoplasmic reticulum (SR) calcium release channels and/or SR calcium-binding proteins underlie these spontaneous calcium release events.

Rapid mobilization of Ca^{2+} from the SR into the cytosol is mediated by the synchronous opening of ryanodine-sensitive Ca^{2+} release channels (ryanodine receptors, RyRs). The cardiac RyR is composed of four equivalent subunits, each encoded by the *RyR2* gene. During cardiac systole, the small influx of calcium ions through L-type Cav channels triggers a massive release of Ca^{2+} from the SR via synchronous opening of RyR2 channels, a process called Ca^{2+}-induced Ca^{2+} release (see Chap. 21). During diastole, RyR2 channels close and Ca^{2+} is recycled into the SR via calcium pumps, thereby refilling SR Ca^{2+} stores for the next release cycle. The duration and amplitude of Ca^{2+} efflux from the SR are therefore tightly controlled by the gating of RyR2 channels. RyR2 interacts with a number of accessory proteins to form a macromolecular Ca^{2+} release complex (Fig. 31-23). Proteins interact with the RyR2 at multiple sites within the cytosolic domains of RyR2 (e.g., protein phosphatases) or at the SR level (e.g., calsequestrin, the major calcium binding protein in the SR lumen). Among the cytosolic ligands, FKBP-12.6 has been implicated in stabilizing the closed state of the RyR2 channel, preventing diastolic Ca^{2+} leakage.[61]

Mutations in the human *RyR2* gene and in the gene *Casq2* that encodes for calsequestrin (see Fig. 31-23) have been linked to catecholaminergic polymorphic ventricular tachycardia (CPVT). Experimental studies

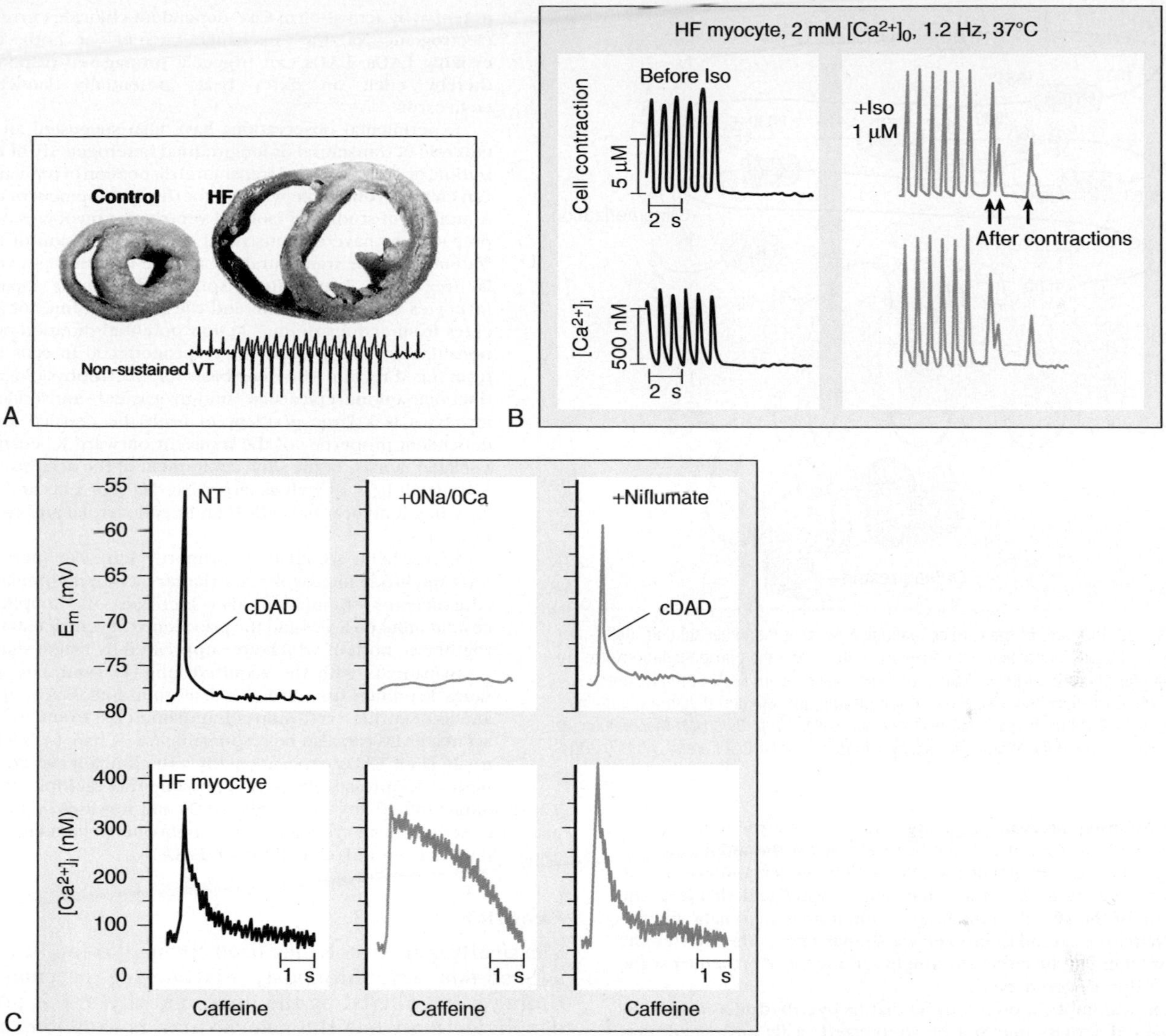

FIGURE 31–22 Ventricular arrhythmia in an animal model of heart failure (aortic constriction-insufficiency in rabbit). **A,** Cross sections of a control and failing heart (HF) and Holter recording of nonsustained ventricular tachycardia (VT) seen in a failing heart. **B,** Spontaneous aftercontractions and increases in $[Ca^{2+}]_i$ in a failing cardiomyocyte after exposure to isoproterenol. **C,** Induction of a delayed afterdepolarization (DAD) by application of caffeine (cDAD) in a cardiomyocyte isolated from a failing rabbit heart. In normal Tyrode's (NT) solution, caffeine causes rapid release of Ca^{2+} from the sarcoplasmic reticulum that leads to increases in intracellular free calcium concentration **(bottom tracing),** which in turn causes membrane depolarization. Blocking the Na^+/Ca^{2+} exchange current in Na^+-free and Ca^{2+}-free solution (0Na/0Ca) abolished DADs despite a similar increase in $[Ca^{2+}]_i$, whereas blocking the Ca^{2+}-activated Cl^- current with niflumate did not prevent DADs. E_m = membrane voltage. *(From Pogwizd SM, Schlotthauer K, Li L, et al: Arrhythmogenesis and contractile dysfunction in heart failure. Circ Res 88:1159, 2001. By permission of the American Heart Association.)*

have revealed that *RyR2* and *Casq2* mutations that underlie CPVT cause an increase in the sensitivity of the RyR2 channel to luminal Ca^{2+} activation on adrenergic stimulation (e.g., from emotional and/or physical stress) and enhance the propensity for spontaneous, diastolic Ca^{2+} release from the SR,[62-66] resulting in DAD-triggered arrhythmias (see later). It is also possible that CPVT mutants exhibit reduced affinity for the binding of the regulatory protein FKBP-12.6, resulting in diastolic Ca^{2+} leakage from the SR.[67] Reduced FKBP-12.6 binding caused by protein kinase A–mediated hyperphosphorylation has been implicated in cardiac arrhythmogenesis associated with heart failure.[68] FKBP-12.6–deficient mice develop polymorphic ventricular tachycardia on adrenergic stimulation.[69] Treatment with the 1,4-benzothiazepine derivative JTV519, which restores FKBP-12.6 affinity for RyR2, has been shown to suppress catecholamine-induced polymorphic ventricular tachycardia in FKBP-12.6–deficient mice.[69]

The inositol 1,4,5-trisphosphate (IP_3) receptor (IP_3R) is a Ca^{2+} release channel that responds to the second messenger IP_3. The type 2 IP_3 receptor (IP_3R2) is the predominant subtype in cardiac myocytes. In atrial myocytes, some IP_3R2 are located near RyR2 channels at the SR Ca^{2+} release sites, and they contribute to altered excitation-contraction coupling and arrhythmogenesis in atria.[70] IP_3-dependent Ca^{2+} signaling has been implied in cardiac arrhythmias attributable to ischemia and reperfusion injury, inflammatory processes, and developing cardiac failure.[71] IP_3 receptors are upregulated in heart failure and atrial fibrillation.[72] In atrial myocytes, IP_3 causes spontaneous $[Ca^{2+}]_i$ transients, Ca^{2+} waves, and Ca^{2+} alternans[73] and facilitates the generation of afterdepolarizations.

The cascade of events linking cellular Ca^{2+} handling abnormalities to cardiac arrhythmias is illustrated in Figure 31-24. Ca^{2+} leaking through SR Ca^{2+} release channels during diastole gives rise to localized increases in the cytosolic calcium level in a single cardiomyocyte. The focally elevated Ca^{2+} then causes a propagating Ca^{2+} wave, which depolarizes the cardiomyocyte membrane, triggering a DAD via transient activation of the inward Na^+/Ca^{2+} exchange current ($I_{Na/Ca}$) (see Fig. 31-24). Inhibitors of calmodulin kinase eliminate transient inward $I_{Na/Ca}$ in isolated rabbit ventricular myocytes, indicating that activation of this enzyme plays an important role in cardiac arrhythmogenesis. In addition, drugs that reduce I_{Na} also reduce the transient inward current, relieve Ca^{2+} overload, and can abolish DADs. DADs most likely play a causative role in arrhythmogenesis in the failing heart, where upregulation of $I_{Na/Ca}$, in combination with downregulation of the inward rectifier K^+ current, I_{K1}, facilitates DAD generation.[48]

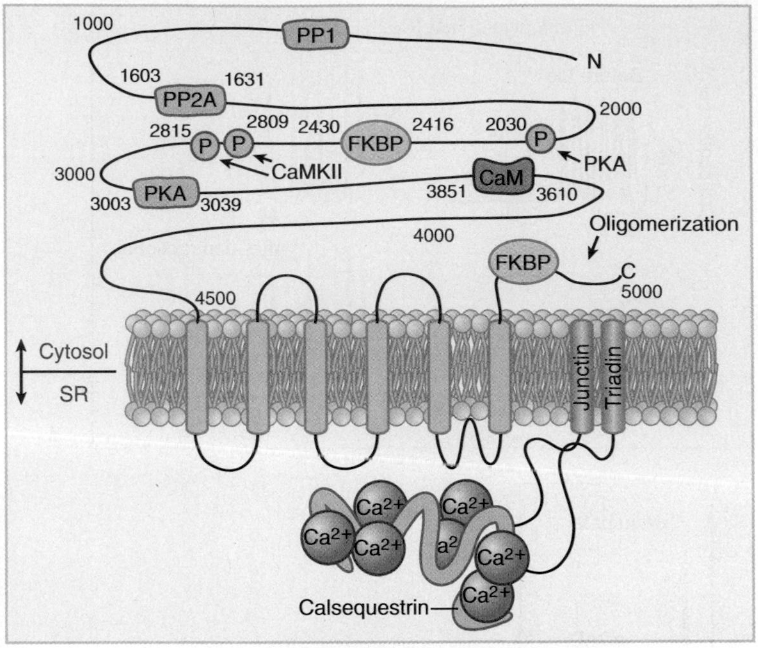

FIGURE 31–23 Structure of the cardiac ryanodine receptor monomer subunit, RyR2, delineating the sites of interaction with auxiliary proteins and the phosphorylation sites (P). PP = protein phosphatase; FKBP = FKBP12.6; CaM = calmodulin; PKA = protein kinase A; CaMKII = calmodulin-dependent kinase II. Calsequestrin, junctin, and triadin are proteins that interact with RyR2 in the sarcoplasmic reticulum (SR). *(From Bers DM: Macromolecular complexes regulating cardiac ryanodine receptor function. J Mol Cell Cardiol 37:417, 2004.)*

Short coupling intervals or pacing at rates more rapid than the triggered activity rate (overdrive pacing) increase(s) the amplitude and shorten(s) the cycle length of the DAD following cessation of pacing (overdrive acceleration), rather than suppressing and delaying the escape rate of the afterdepolarization, as in normal automatic mechanisms. Premature stimulation exerts a similar effect; the shorter the premature interval, the larger the amplitude and the shorter the escape interval of the triggered event.

The clinical implication might be that tachyarrhythmias caused by DAD-triggered activity may not be suppressed easily or, indeed, may be precipitated by rapid rates, either spontaneously (such as a sinus tachycardia) or pacing induced. Finally, because a single premature stimulus can both initiate and terminate triggered activity, differentiation from reentry (see later) becomes difficult. The response to overdrive pacing may help separate triggered arrhythmias from reentrant arrhythmias.

Early Afterdepolarizations

Various interventions, each of which results in an increase in intracellular positivity, can cause EADs. EADs may be responsible for the lengthened repolarization time and ventricular tachyarrhythmias seen in several clinical situations, such as the acquired and congenital forms of the long-QT syndrome (Fig. 31-25; see Chap. 35).[74] Left ansa subclavian stimulation increases the amplitude of cesium-induced EADs in dogs and the prevalence of ventricular tachyarrhythmias more than right ansa subclavian stimulation, possibly because of a greater quantitative effect of the left than that of the right stellate ganglion on the left ventricle.

Patients with the heritable long-QT syndrome have abnormally prolonged cardiac action potential duration and are at increased risk for sudden cardiac death from ventricular tachyarrhythmias (see Chaps. 9 and 35). The genesis of long-QT syndrome–associated ventricular tachycardia or fibrillation is uncertain. There is mounting evidence that increased intracellular Ca^{2+} concentration related to spontaneous Ca^{2+} release from the sarcoplasmic reticulum in cardiomyocytes, coupled with dispersion of repolarization, plays a causative role in long-QT syndrome–associated cardiac arrhythmia and sudden cardiac death (see Figs. 31-21 and 31-25). Action potential prolongation may increase Ca^{2+} influx through L-type Ca^{2+} channels during a cardiac cycle, causing excessive Ca^{2+} accumulation in the sarcoplasmic reticulum and spontaneous sarcoplasmic reticular Ca^{2+} release. The ensuing elevation of intracellular free calcium may depolarize cardiomyocyte membrane potential by activation of Ca^{2+}-dependent chloride currents, the electrogenic Na^+/Ca^{2+} exchange current, or both, thereby evoking EADs. EADs can trigger a propagated response and thereby elicit an extra beat, potentially launching a tachycardia.

Experimental observations have also suggested an important role of transmural or longitudinal heterogeneity of repolarization, or both.[75] Marked transmural dispersion of repolarization can create a vulnerable window for the development of reentry. A number of studies of isolated ventricular myocytes or tissue preparations have demonstrated spatial dispersion of repolarization along the transmural axes of the left and right ventricular free walls. A prominent spike and dome is apparent in myocytes from epicardium and the M region but not in myocytes from endocardium.[76] Action potential duration-rate relationships are considerably more pronounced in cells isolated from the M region. The ionic basis for electrophysiological distinctions among epicardial, midmyocardial, and endocardial myocytes is a large gradient in both the density- and rate-dependent properties of the transient outward K^+ current and a smaller density of the slow component of the delayed rectifier K^+ current I_{Ks},[77] as well as larger late Na^+ currents and inward $I_{Na/Ca}$ in midmyocardial cells than in endocardial and epicardial myocytes.

Sympathetic stimulation, primarily left, can increase the EAD amplitude to provoke ventricular tachyarrhythmias. Alpha adrenoceptor stimulation also increases the amplitude of cesium-induced EADs and the prevalence of ventricular tachyarrhythmias, both of which are suppressed by magnesium.

In patients with the acquired long-QT syndrome and torsades de pointes from drugs such as quinidine, *N*-acetylprocainamide, cisapride, erythromycin, and some class III antiarrhythmic agents, EADs can also be responsible (see Chap. 6). Such drugs easily elicit EADs experimentally and clinically, whereas magnesium suppresses them. It is possible that multiple drugs can cause summating effects to provoke EADs and torsades de pointes in patients. Activators of ATP-dependent potassium channels, such as pinacidil and nicorandil, can eliminate EADs.

Parasystole

Classically, parasystole has been likened to the function of a fixed-rate asynchronously discharging pacemaker—its timing is not altered by the dominant rhythm, it produces depolarization when the myocardium is excitable, and the intervals between discharges are multiples of a basic interval (see Chaps. 34 and 35). Complete entrance block, constant or intermittent, insulates and protects the parasystolic focus from surrounding electrical events and accounts for such behavior. Occasionally, the focus can exhibit exit block, during which it may fail to depolarize excitable myocardium. In fact, the dominant cardiac rhythm may modulate parasystolic discharge to speed up or slow down its rate. Brief subthreshold depolarizations induced during the first half of the cardiac cycle of a spontaneously discharging pacemaker delay the subsequent discharge, whereas similar depolarizations induced in the second half of the cardiac cycle accelerate it (Fig. 31-26).

Disorders of Impulse Conduction

Conduction delay and block can result in bradyarrhythmias or tachyarrhythmias, with the former occurring when the propagating impulse is blocked and is followed by asystole or a slow escape rhythm and the latter when the delay and block produce reentrant excitation (see later). Various factors involving both active and passive membrane properties determine the conduction velocity of an impulse and whether conduction is successful. Among these factors are the stimulating efficacy of the propagating impulse, related to the amplitude and rate of rise of phase 0, the excitability of the tissue into which the impulse is conducted, and the geometry of the tissue.

DECELERATION-DEPENDENT BLOCK. Diastolic depolarization has been suggested as a cause of conduction block at slow rates, so-called bradycardia- or deceleration-dependent block (see Chap. 35). However, excitability *increases* as the membrane depolarizes until about −70 mV, despite a reduction in action potential amplitude and $\dot{V}_{max}$. Evidently, depolarization-induced inactivation of fast Na^+ channels is offset by other factors, such as reduction in the difference between membrane potential and threshold potential and increase in membrane excitability.

PHASE 3 (TACHYCARDIA-DEPENDENT BLOCK). More commonly, impulses are blocked at rapid rates or short cycle lengths as a result of incomplete recovery of refractoriness caused by incomplete time- or voltage-dependent recovery of excitability (see Chap. 32). For example, such incomplete recovery is the usual mechanism responsible for a nonconducted premature P wave or one that conducts with a functional bundle branch block.

DECREMENTAL CONDUCTION. Decremental conduction is a term used commonly in the clinical literature but is often misapplied to describe any Wenckebach-like conduction block—that is, responses similar to block in the AV node during which progressive conduction delay precedes the nonconducted impulse. Correctly used, decremental conduction refers to a situation in which the properties of the fiber change along its length so that the action potential loses its efficacy as a stimulus to excite the fiber ahead of it. Thus, the stimulating efficacy of the propagating action potential diminishes progressively, possibly as a result of its decreasing amplitude and decreasing $\dot{V}_{max}$.

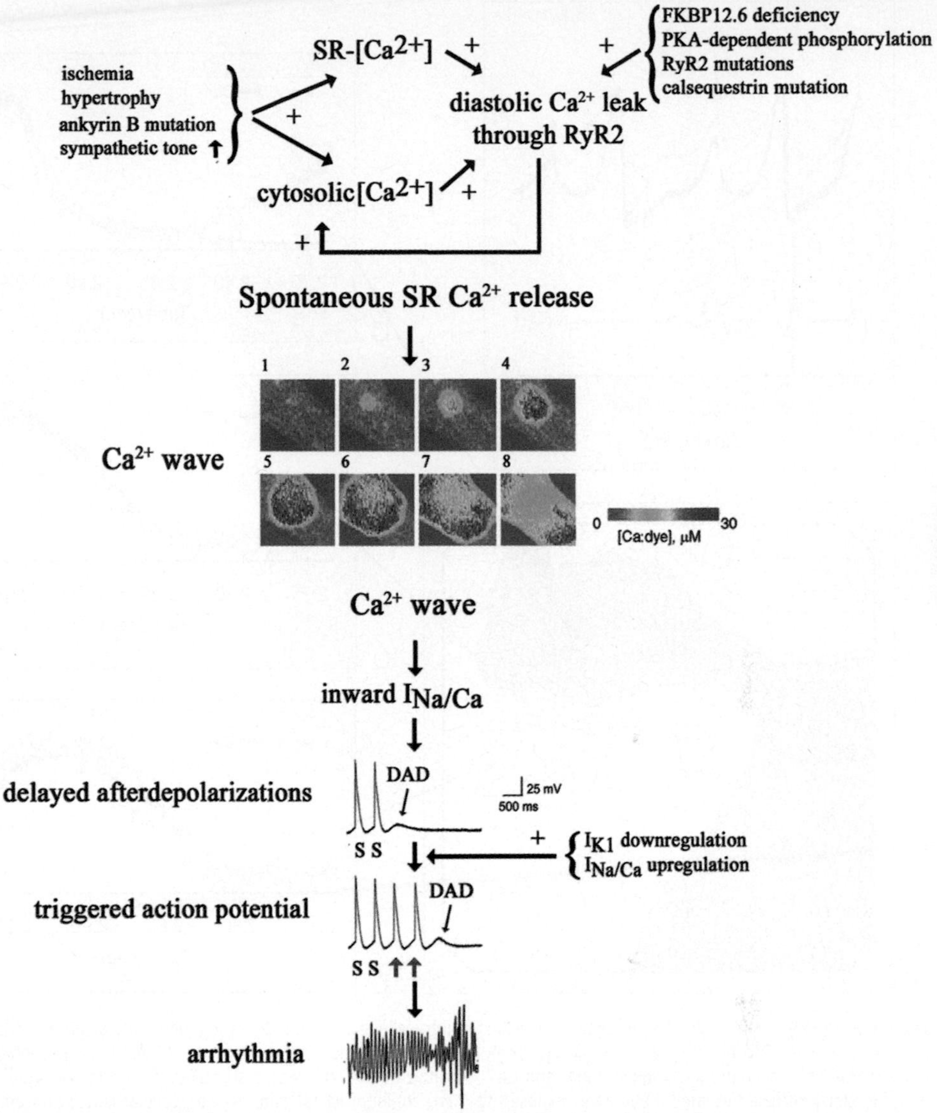

FIGURE 31–24 Proposed scheme of events leading to delayed afterdepolarizations (DADs) and triggered tachyarrhythmia. **Top panel,** Congenital (e.g., gain of function mutations in the *RyR2* or *Casq2* genes) and/or acquired factors (e.g., ischemia, hypertrophy, increased sympathetic tone, heart failure) will cause a diastolic Ca^{2+} leak through RyR2, resulting in localized and transient increases in $[Ca^{2+}]_i$ in cardiomyocytes. **Middle panel,** Representative series of images showing changes in $[Ca^{2+}]_i$ during a Ca^{2+} wave in a single cardiomyocyte loaded with a Ca^{2+}-sensitive fluorescent dye. Images were obtained at 117-ms intervals. Focally elevated Ca^{2+} (2) diffuses to adjacent junctional sarcoplasmic reticulum (SR), where it initiates more Ca^{2+} release events, resulting in a propagating Ca^{2+} wave (3-8). **Bottom panel,** The Ca^{2+} wave, through activation of inward $I_{Na/Ca}$, will depolarize the cardiomyocyte (DAD). If of sufficient magnitude, the DAD will depolarize the cardiomyocyte above threshold, resulting in a single or repetitive premature heartbeat (red arrows), which can trigger an arrhythmia. Downregulation of the inward rectifier potassium current (I_{K1}), or upregulation of $I_{Na/Ca}$ can promote the generation of DAD-triggered action potentials. S = stimulus. *(Modified from Rubart M, Zipes DP: Mechanisms of sudden cardiac death. J Clin Invest 115:2305, 2005. With permission from Journal of Clinical Investigation.)*

Reentry

Electrical activity during each normal cardiac cycle begins in the sinus node and continues until the entire heart has been activated. Each cell becomes activated in turn, and the cardiac impulse dies out when all fibers have been discharged and are completely refractory. During this absolute refractory period, the cardiac impulse has "no place to go." It must be extinguished and restarted by the next sinus impulse. If, however, a group of fibers not activated during the initial wave of depolarization recover excitability in time to be discharged before the impulse dies out, they may serve as a link to reexcite areas that were just discharged and have now recovered from the initial depolarization. Such a process has been given various names, all meaning approximately the same thing—reentry, reentrant excitation, circus movement, reciprocal or echo beat, or reciprocating tachycardia.

ENTRAINMENT. Entraining the tachycardia (i.e., increasing the rate of the tachycardia by pacing), with resumption of the intrinsic rate of the tachycardia when pacing is stopped, establishes the presence of reentry (Fig. 31-27A). Entrainment represents capture or continuous resetting of the reentrant circuit of the tachycardia by the pacing-induced activation. Each pacing stimulus creates a wave front that travels in an anterograde direction (orthodromic) and resets the tachycardia to the pacing rate. A wave front propagating retrogradely in the opposite direction (antidromic) collides with the orthodromic wave front of the previous beat (see Fig. 31-27B). These wave front interactions create electrocardiographic and electrophysiological features that can be explained only by reentry. Therefore, the criteria of entrainment can be used to prove the reentrant mechanism of a clinical tachycardia and form the

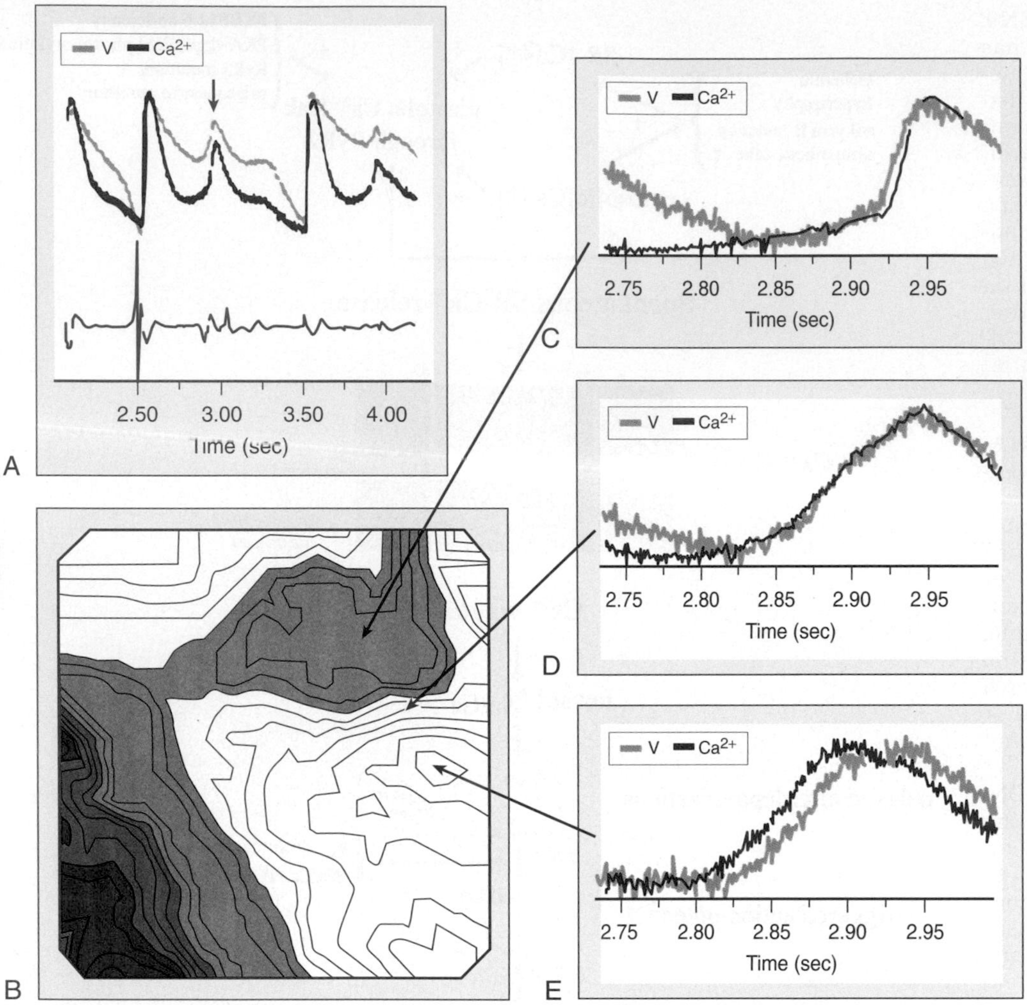

FIGURE 31–25 Primary role of spontaneous increases in intracellular Ca^{2+} $[Ca^{2+}]_i$ in triggering early afterdepolarizations (EADs) in an animal model of type 2 long-QT syndrome. Illustrated is simultaneous mapping of membrane potential (V) and intracellular Ca^{2+} concentration using voltage- and Ca^{2+}-sensitive fluorescent dyes, respectively, from the epicardial surface of a Langendorff-perfused isolated rabbit heart exposed to the I_{Kr} inhibitor E4031 and low extracellular concentrations of K^+ and Mg^{2+}. Under these conditions, action potentials are markedly prolonged and spontaneous EADs develop, causing polymorphic ventricular tachycardia (torsades de pointes). **A,** Recording of V and $[Ca^{2+}]_i$ during an EAD (arrow) and the corresponding depolarizations recorded with bipolar electrogram **(bottom tracing)**. **B,** Activation map of the EAD labeled with an arrow in **A. C** and **D,** Superimposition of V and $[Ca^{2+}]_i$ traces measured at sites remote from the site of origin of the EAD. At those sites, V changes precede or are synchronous with those in $[Ca^{2+}]_i$. **E,** Voltage and $[Ca^{2+}]_i$ traces at the first site to fire an EAD. Here, the rise in $[Ca^{2+}]_i$ precedes the rise of V. *(From Choi B, Burton F, Salama G: Cytosolic Ca²⁺ triggers early afterdepolarizations and torsade de pointes in rabbit hearts with type 2 long QT syndrome. J Physiol [Lond] 543.2:615, 2002.)*

basis for localizing the pathway traveled by the tachycardia wave front. Such localization is essential for ablation therapy.

ANATOMICAL REENTRY. The earliest studies on reentry used models that had anatomically defined separate pathways in which it could be shown that they had (1) an area of unidirectional block, (2) recirculation of the impulse to its point of origin, and (3) elimination of the arrhythmia by cutting the pathway. In models with anatomically defined pathways, because the two (or more) pathways have different electrophysiological properties (e.g., a refractory period longer in one pathway than the other), the impulse is first blocked in one pathway (Fig. 31-28A, site A) and then propagates slowly in the adjacent pathway (see Fig. 31-28A, serpentine arrow, D to C). If conduction in this alternative route is sufficiently depressed, the slowly propagating impulse excites tissue beyond the blocked pathway (see Fig. 31-28A, horizontal lined area) and returns in a reversed direction along the pathway initially blocked (see Fig. 31-28A, B to A) to reexcite tissue proximal to the site of block (see Fig. 31-28A, A to D). A clinical arrhythmia caused by anatomical reentry is most likely to have a monomorphic contour.

For reentry of this type to occur, the time for conduction within the depressed but unblocked area and for excitation of the distal segments must exceed the refractory period of the initially blocked pathway (see Fig. 31-28A, A) and the tissue proximal to the site of block (see Fig. 31-28A, D). Stated another way, continuous reentry requires the anatomical length of the circuit traveled to equal or exceed the reentrant wavelength. The latter is equal to the mean conduction velocity of the impulse multiplied by the longest refractory period of the elements in the circuit. Both values can be different at different points along the reentry pathway, and thus the wavelength value is somewhat contrived.

Conditions for Reentry. The length of the pathway is fixed and determined by the anatomy. Conditions that depress conduction velocity or abbreviate the refractory period promote the development of reentry in this model, whereas prolonging refractoriness and speeding conduction velocity can hinder it. For example, if conduction velocity (0.30 m/sec) and refractoriness (350 milliseconds) for ventricular muscle were normal, a pathway of 105 mm (0.30 m/sec × 0.35 sec) would be necessary for reentry to occur. However, under certain conditions, conduction velocity in ventricular muscle and Purkinje fibers can be very slow (0.03 m/sec) and, if refractoriness is not greatly prolonged (600 milliseconds), a pathway of only 18 mm (0.03 m/sec × 0.60 sec) may be necessary. Such reentry frequently exhibits an excitable gap—that is, a time interval between the end of refractoriness from one cycle and the beginning of depolarization in the next, when tissue in the circuit is excitable. This condition results because the wavelength of the reentrant circuit is less than the pathway length. Electrical stimulation during this time period can invade the reentrant circuit and reset its timing or terminate the tachycardia.

Rapid pacing can entrain the tachycardia—that is, continuously reset it by entering the circuit and propagating around it in the same way as the reentrant impulse—which increases the tachycardia rate to the pacing rate without terminating the tachycardia (see Fig. 31-27). In reentrant circuits with an excitable gap, conduction velocity determines the revolution time of the impulse around the circuit and therefore the rate of the tachycardia. Prolongation of refractoriness, unless it is long enough to eliminate the excitable gap and make the impulse propagate in relatively refractory tissue, does not influence the revolution time around the circuit or the rate of the tachycardia. Anatomical reentry occurs in patients with the Wolff-Parkinson-White syndrome, in AV nodal reentry, in some atrial flutters, in some ventricular tachycardias, and in ventricular fibrillation.[78] For example, mapping studies in isolated swine ventricles have demonstrated key roles of anisotropic anatomic structures (e.g., abrupt changes in fiber orientation) in the maintenance of reentry during ventricular fibrillation.[78]

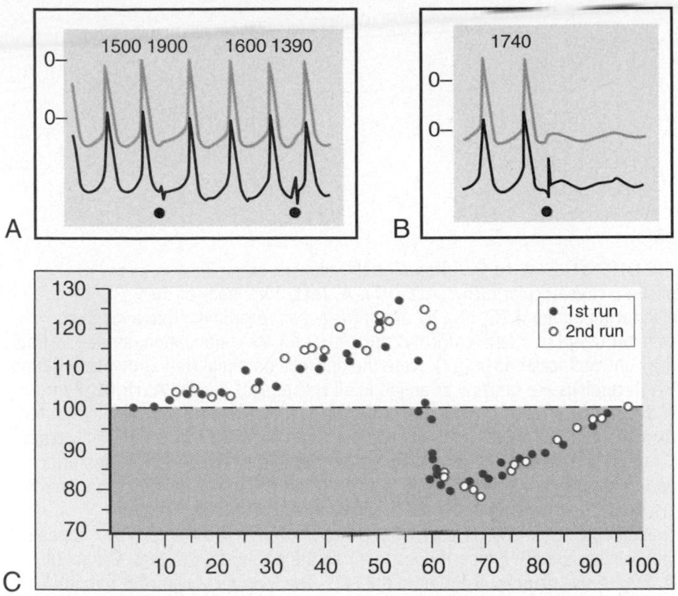

FIGURE 31–26 Modulation of pacemaker activity by subthreshold current pulses in diseased human ventricle. **A,** Two recording sites along the same trabecula in a spontaneously active preparation. Current pulses (indicated by the red dots) of 30 milliseconds in duration were injected through the lower microelectrode at various times. The interval between the spontaneous action potentials is given in milliseconds above each cycle. Injection of a subthreshold current pulse through the lower microelectrode relatively early in the spontaneous cycle (about 680 milliseconds after initiation of the rapid portion of the preceding action potential upstroke) produced a subthreshold depolarization in the upper recording and delayed the next spontaneous discharge by 400 to 1900 milliseconds. This response curve would fall in the first half of the curve indicated in **C.** A current pulse of the same intensity and duration delivered later in the spontaneous cycle (950 milliseconds after the preceding upstroke) accelerated the next discharge by 210 to 1390 milliseconds relative to the previous two action potentials. The response to this current injection falls in the second half of the graph depicted in **C. B,** A stimulus at a precise interval in the cardiac cycle (called the singular point; in this example, 930 milliseconds after the preceding action potential upstroke) abolishes pacemaker activity. **C,** Phase-response curves from experimental data obtained in canine Purkinje fibers in a manner similar to that in the human experiment shown in **A** and **B.** Two different runs are shown. The ordinate in this graph is the percentage increase or decrease in spontaneous cycle length of the "parasystolic focus" (control cycle length equals 100 percent); the abscissa is the percentage of the "parasystolic focus" spontaneous cycle length during which stimulation was performed. The spontaneous cycle length was maximally prolonged (by 26 percent) or shortened (by 20 percent) by subthreshold depolarizations that entered the parasystolic focus after approximately 50 and 60 percent of the cycle had elapsed, respectively. Very similar curves can be plotted for patients with parasystole (e.g., see Figs. 9 and 10 in Zipes DP: Plenary lecture. Cardiac electrophysiology: Promises and contributions. J Am Coll Cardiol 13:1329, 1989). *(**A** and **B** from Gilmour RF Jr, Heger JJ, Prystowsky EN, et al: Cellular electrophysiological abnormalities of diseased human ventricular myocardium. Am J Cardiol 51:137, 1983; **C** from Jalife J, Moe GK: Effect of electronic potentials on pacemaker activity of canine Purkinje fibers and relation to parasystole. Circ Res 39:801, 1976. By permission of the American Heart Association.)*

FUNCTIONAL REENTRY. Functional reentry lacks confining anatomical boundaries and can occur in contiguous fibers that exhibit functionally different electrophysiological properties caused by local differences in transmembrane action potential (e.g., Purkinje-myocyte transition). Dispersion of excitability, refractoriness, or both, as well as anisotropic distributions of intercellular resistance, permit initiation and maintenance of reentry. Functional heterogeneity in the electrophysiological properties of the myocardium has been shown to contribute to the generation and maintenance of tachycardia and fibrillation. These heterogeneities can be fixed, as in the case of spatial redistribution of gap junctions in the failing heart (see Fig. 31-12B)[40] or infarct border zone, or in the case of spatial gradients in the magnitude of the background K^+ current, I_{K1} (Fig. 31-29B; see Table 31-3).[79] They can also change dynamically, as in the acutely ischemic myocardium[80] or in the presence of repolarization-prolonging agents.[81] A very important determinant of the dynamically induced component of heterogeneity has been identified as electrical restitution, the variation of action potential duration and conduction velocity with the diastolic interval.[82] It has been proposed that the breakup of periodic waves is precipitated by oscillations of action potential duration (so-called action potential duration, APD, alternans) of sufficiently large amplitude to cause conduction block along a spiral wave front.

Tachycardias Caused by Reentry

Reentry is probably the cause of many tachyarrhythmias, including various types of supraventricular and ventricular tachycardias, flutter, and fibrillation (see Chap. 35).

Atrial Flutter (see Chap. 35)

Reentry is the most likely cause of the usual form of atrial flutter, with the reentrant circuit confined to the right atrium, where it usually travels counterclockwise in a caudocranial direction in the interatrial septum and in a craniocaudal direction in the right atrial free wall. An area of slow conduction is present in the posterolateral to posteromedial inferior area of the right atrium, with a central area of block that can include an anatomical (inferior vena cava) and functional component. This area of slow conduction is rather constant and represents the site of successful ablation of atrial flutter. Ablation results are consistent with a macroreentry circuit (see Chap. 33).[90-92]

Different reentrant circuits exist in patients with other types of atrial flutter, such as those that occur after surgery or that are associated with an atrial septal defect (see Chap. 61).

Atrial Fibrillation

SPATIOTEMPORAL ORGANIZATION AND FOCAL DISCHARGE (see Chap. 35). According to the multiple-wavelet hypothesis, atrial fibrillation (AF) is characterized by fragmentation of the wave front into multiple daughter wavelets. These wander randomly throughout the atrium and give rise to new wavelets that collide with each other and are mutually annihilated or that give rise to new wavelets in a perpetual activity (for a demonstration of wave front dynamics during fibrillation, see the video from Samie and colleagues[79] on the website).

The randomness of the irregular electrical activity during AF has been disputed on the basis of both statistical methods and experimental studies. A combination of high-resolution video imaging, recordings of the ECG, and spectral analysis was used to demonstrate that reentry in anatomically or functionally determined circuits forms the basis of spatiotemporal periodicity during acute AF. The cycle length of the source in the left atrium determines the dominant peak in the frequency spectra. The underlying periodicity may stem from a repetitive focal source of activity propagated from an individual pulmonary vein to the remainder of the atrium as fibrillating waves. If a single repetitive focal source of activity that undergoes fractionation underlies the maintenance of AF, ablation of this focal source should interrupt AF. Indeed, delivery of radiofrequency energy to discrete sites in the distal pulmonary veins in humans has been shown to eliminate or reduce recurrence of AF.

Several experimental models have been used to study the structural and basic electrophysiological properties of pulmonary veins that are thought to play a role in initiation and maintenance of atrial fibrillation. Morphological studies have demonstrated the presence of complex anatomical structures and phenotypically different cardiomyocytes in pulmonary veins.[85,86] Electrophysiological studies have shown that the combination of reentrant and nonreentrant mechanisms (automaticity and triggered activity) is the underlying arrhythmogenic mechanism for atrial fibrillation initiation from the pulmonary veins.[86,87] Abnormal intracellular calcium handling probably plays a pivotal role in the pulmonary vein electrical activity.[85,86] Dual mapping of cardiomyocyte membrane potential and intracellular free calcium has demonstrated

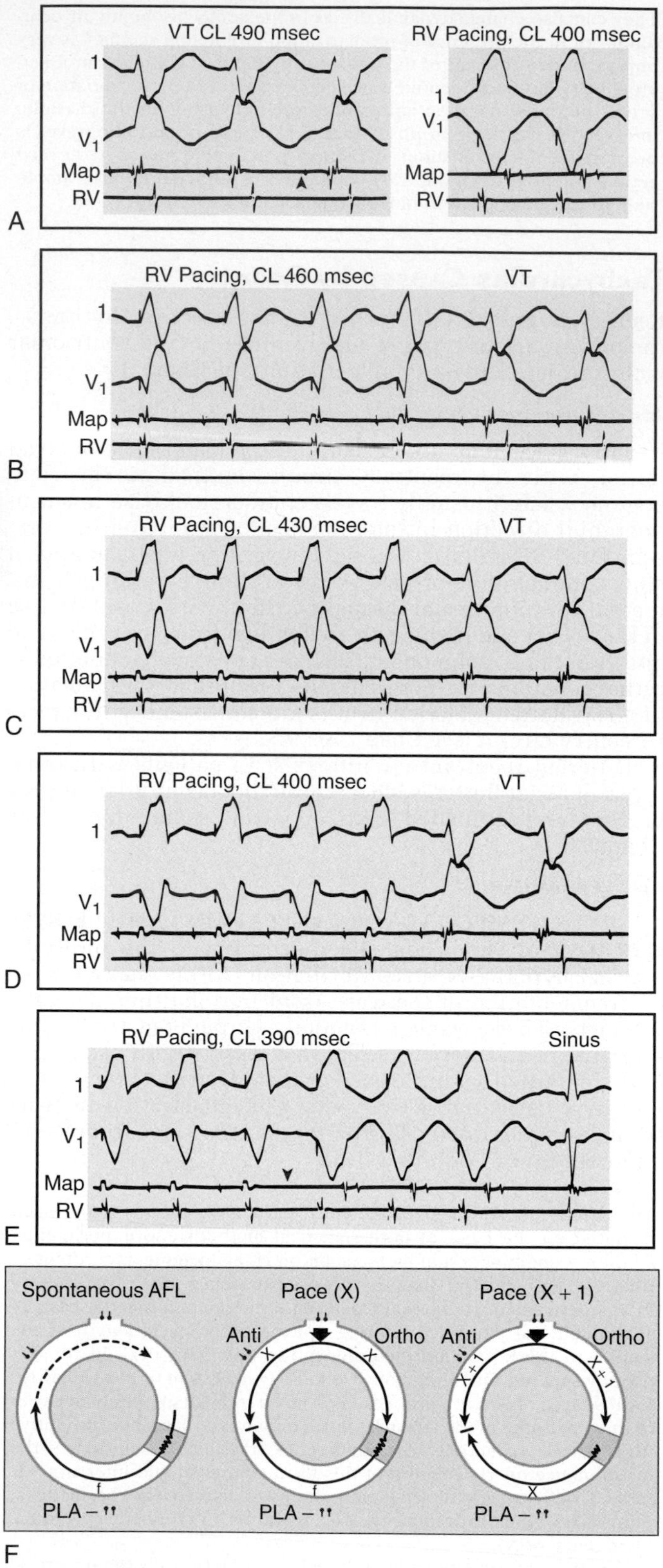

FIGURE 31–27 A to E, Criteria for entrainment exemplified in a case of postinfarct ventricular tachycardia (VT). **A, left,** Two leads of the electrocardiogram (ECG) of a VT and intracardiac recordings from a mapping catheter (Map) at a left ventricular site critical for VT continuation, as well as from the right ventricular apex (RV). Note the diastolic potential (red arrowhead) during VT. Recordings are similarly arranged in all subsequent panels. **A, right,** RV pacing in the setting of sinus rhythm. **B,** RV pacing at a cycle length (CL) slightly shorter than VT produces a QRS complex that is a blend between fully VT and fully paced ("fusion") complexes. All recordings are accelerated to the paced CL and, after pacing ceases, the same VT resumes. Each fused QRS complex is identical and the last beat is entrained, but surface fusion is absent. **C** and **D,** The same phenomena, but at shorter paced CLs. Note that the fused QRS complex appears more similar to pacing than it does to VT as the pacing CL shortens. **B** through **D,** Progressive degrees of fusion in the ECG. The Map recording of **B** through **D** also shows a progression of fusion, with both the morphology and timing of a portion of the electrogram changing with faster pacing. **E,** Finally, a still shorter paced CL results in a sudden change in both the Map electrogram (block in the small diastolic potential, red arrow) and the surface ECG, which is now fully paced. When pacing ceases, VT has been interrupted. **F,** Diagrammatic representation of the reentrant circuit during spontaneous atrial flutter (AFL) and transient entrainment of the AFL. **Left,** The reentrant circuit during spontaneous type I AFL. f = circulating wave front of the AFL. **Center,** Introduction of the first pacing impulse (X) during rapid pacing from a high atrial site during AFL. The large arrow indicates entry of the pacing impulse into the reentrant circuit, whereupon it is conducted orthodromically (Ortho) and antidromically (Anti). The antidromic wave front of the pacing impulse (X) collides with the previous beat, in this case the circulating wave front of the spontaneous AFL (f), which results in an atrial fusion beat and, in effect, terminates the AFL. However, the orthodromic wave front from the pacing impulse (X) continues the tachycardia and resets it to the pacing rate. **Right,** Introduction of the next pacing impulse (X + 1) during rapid pacing from the same high atrial site. The large arrow again indicates the entry of the pacing impulse into the reentrant circuit, whereupon it is conducted orthodromically and antidromically. Once again, the antidromic wave front from the pacing impulse (X + 1) collides with the orthodromic wave front of the previous beat. In this case, it is the orthodromic wave front of the previous paced beat (X), and an atrial fusion beat results. The orthodromic wave front from the pacing impulse (X + 1) continues the tachycardia and resets it to the pacing rate. In all three parts, arrows indicate the direction of spread of the impulses; the serpentine line indicates slow conduction through a presumed area of slow conduction (stippled region) in the reentrant circuit, and the red dots with tails indicate bipolar electrodes at the high atrial pacing site, the posteroinferior portion of the left atrium (PLA), and another atrial site. *(**A-E** from Zipes DP: A century of cardiac arrhythmia: In search of Jason's golden fleece. J Am Coll Cardiol 34:959, 1999; **F** from Waldo AL: Atrial flutter. Entrainment characteristics. J Cardiovasc Electrophysiol 8:337, 1997.)*

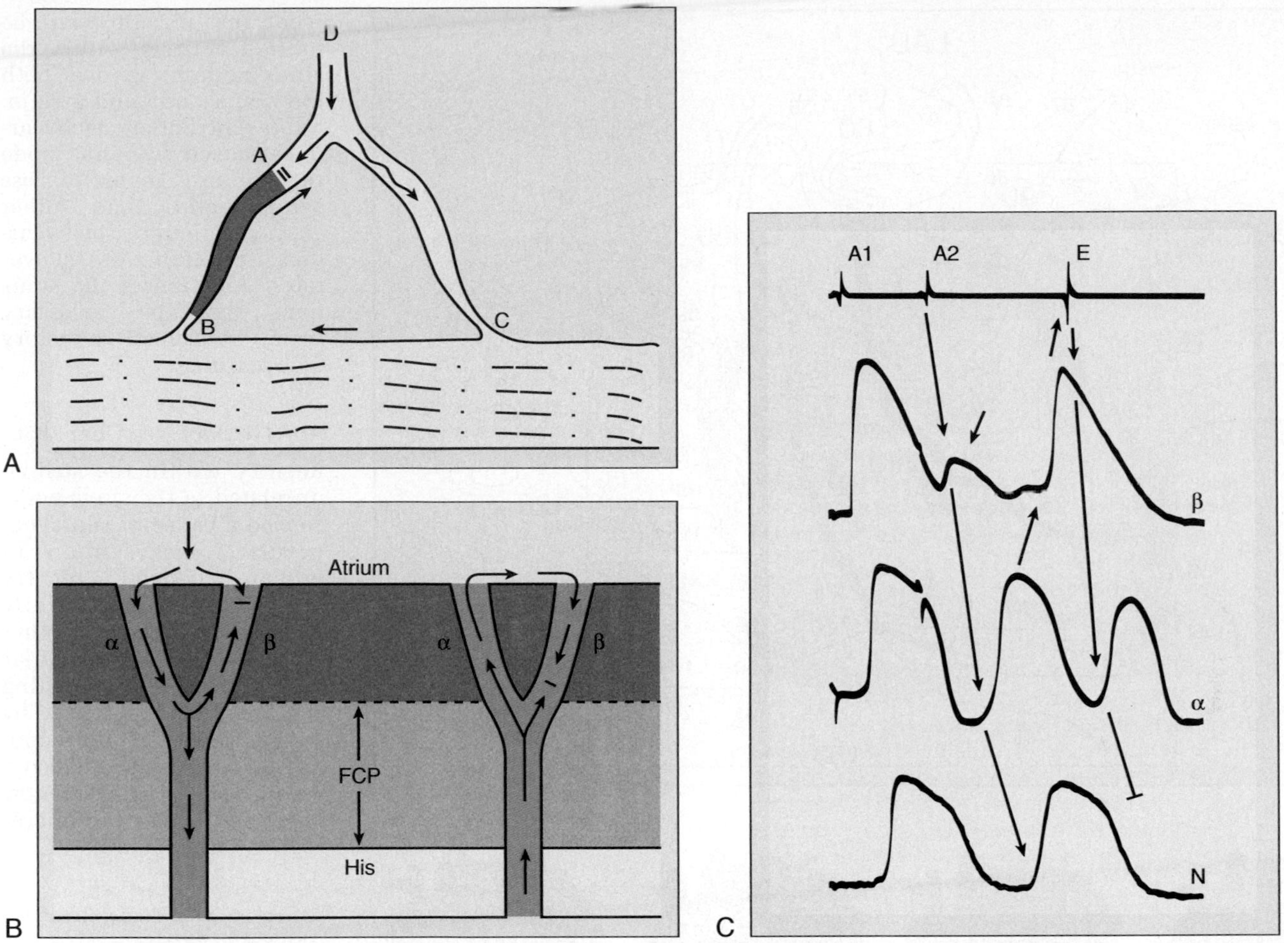

FIGURE 31–28 **A,** Diagram of reentry published by Schmitt and Erlanger in 1928. A Purkinje fiber (D) divides into two pathways (B and C), both of which join ventricular muscle. It is assumed that the original impulse travels down D, is blocked in its anterograde direction at site A (arrow followed by a double bar), but continues slowly down C (serpentine arrow) to excite ventricular muscle. The impulse then reenters the Purkinje twig at B and retrogradely excites A and D. If the impulse continues to propagate through D to the ventricular myocardium and elicits ventricular depolarization, a reentrant ventricular extrasystole results. Continued reentry of this type would produce ventricular tachycardia. **B,** Schematic representation of intranodal dissociation responsible for an atrial echo **(left diagram).** A premature atrial response fails to penetrate the beta (β) pathway, which exhibits a unidirectional block but propagates anterogradely through the alpha (α) pathway. Once the final common pathway (FCP) is engaged, the impulse may return to the atrium through the now-recovered beta pathway to produce an atrial echo. The neighboring **(right)** diagram illustrates the pattern of propagation during generation of a ventricular echo. A premature response in the His bundle traverses the FCP, encounters a refractory beta pathway (unidirectional block), reaches the atrium over the alpha pathway, and returns through a now-recovered beta pathway to produce a ventricular echo. **C,** Actual recordings from the atrium **(top tracing),** with cells impaled in the beta region **(second tracing),** alpha region **(third tracing),** and N portion of the atrioventricular (AV) node **(bottom tracing)** in an isolated rabbit preparation. The basic response to A1 activated both alpha and beta pathways and the N cell (first tier of action potentials). The premature atrial response A2 caused only a local response in the beta cell (short arrow), was delayed in transmission to the alpha cell, and was further delayed in propagation to the N cell. Following the alpha response, a retrograde spontaneous response occurred in the beta cell and propagated to the atrium (E). This atrial response represents an atrial echo. The echo returned to stimulate the alpha cell but was not propagated to the N cell. It is important that although intranodal reentry has been shown to occur within the rabbit AV node, AV nodal reentry in humans probably occurs over extranodal pathways. *(From Mendez C, Moe GK: Demonstrations of a dual AV nodal conduction system in the isolated rabbit heart. Circ Res 19:378, 1966. By permission of the American Heart Association.)*

the appearance of spontaneous Ca release events, resulting in focal discharge.[87] The role of dysfunctions of calcium-handling proteins (e.g., Na^+/Ca^{2+} exchanger, ryanodine receptor calcium release channels) in atrial fibrillation awaits further investigation.

PRIMARY ION CHANNEL ABNORMALITIES IN ATRIAL FIBRILLATION. A number of studies have revealed a primary role of abnormalities in ion channel expression and/or properties in causing atrial fibrillation. Rapid pacing-induced atrial fibrillation in dogs causes a decrease in FKBP-12.6 binding to the ryanodine receptor Ca^{2+} release channel (see Fig. 31-23), resulting in diastolic SR Ca^{2+} leakage, which in turn, through activation of Ca^{2+}-sensitive currents, can initiate electrical instability and contribute to fibrillation.[88] Cav1.3 Ca^{2+} channel–deficient mice exhibit increased susceptibility to inducible atrial flutter and fibrillation.[89] Mice in which the gene encoding KCNE1, an auxiliary subunit of the pore-forming K^+ channel alpha subunit KCNQ1, has been knocked out, display frequent spontaneous episodes of atrial fibrillation.[90] Finally, a human connexin40 gene polymorphism is associated with increased vulnerability to atrial fibrillation induction.[91]

ELECTRICAL REMODELING OF THE ATRIA. Electrical remodeling of the atria appears to be a key determinant for maintenance of AF. Prolonged rapid atrial rates cause electrophysiological alterations of the atria, including shortening and loss of the physiological rate adaptation of refractoriness and decrease in conduction velocity. Because abbreviation of the atrial refractory period is disproportionately larger than reduction of conduction velocity, the wavelength of the reentrant wavelets shortens and thereby promotes reentrant activity (the wavelength is the distance traveled by the depolarization wave front during the duration of its refractory period and equals conduction velocity times refractoriness). The rapid atrial rate also remodels the sinus node.[92]

The ionic basis of shortening of the refractory period and slowing of conduction may be caused by a significant reduction in the density of the L-type Ca^{2+} and the fast Na^+ currents. The electrophysiological changes are paralleled by similar decreases in messenger ribonucleic acid (mRNA) levels of Ca^{2+} and Na^+ channel genes, which suggests alterations in gene expression as the underlying molecular mechanisms

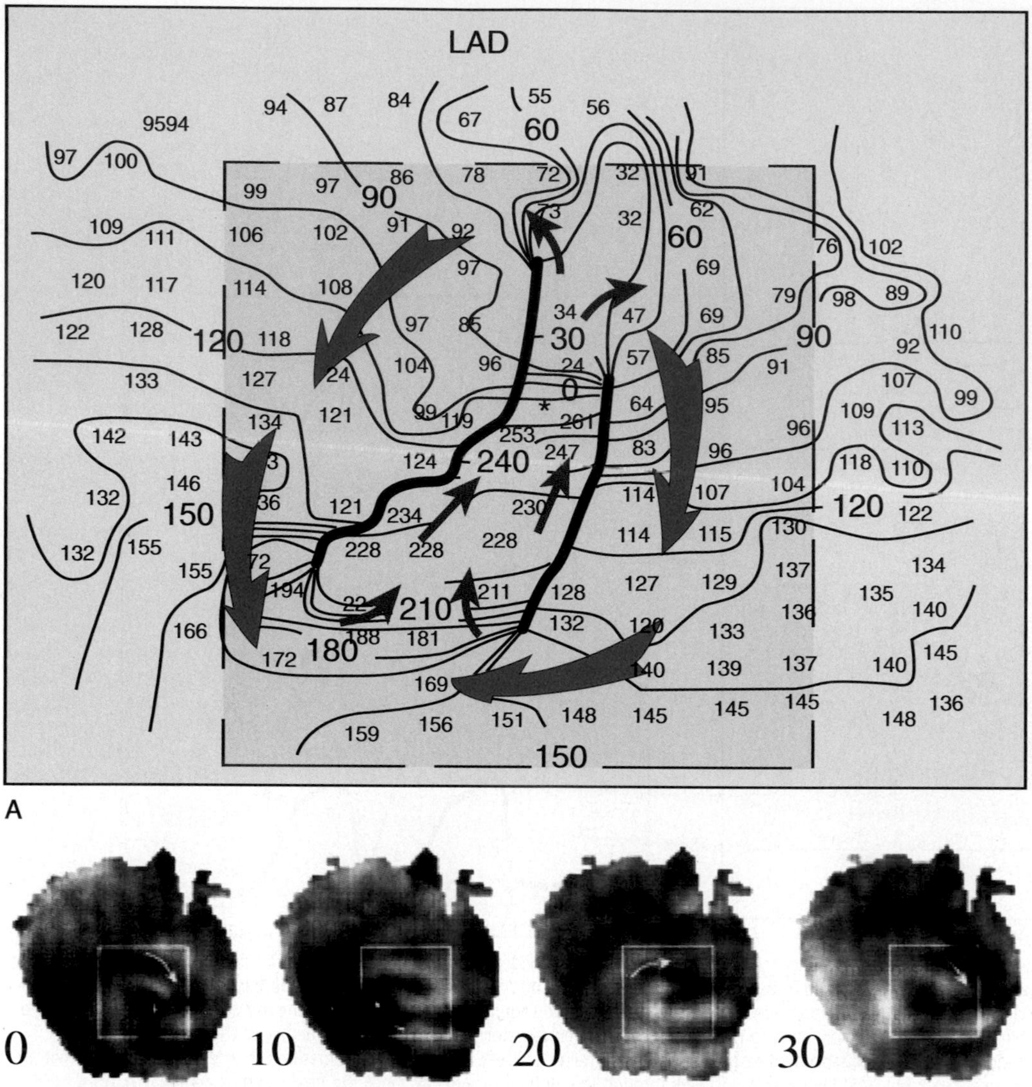

FIGURE 31–29 Functional models of reentry. **A,** Figure-of-8 reentry in anisotropic myocardium. Maps of activation times of a stable reentrant circuit during ventricular tachycardia in the epicardial border zone of a 4-day-old anterior infarct in a dog. The activation times (in milliseconds, small numbers) are shown, as are lines of isochronal activation, at 10-millisecond intervals (larger numbers). The lines of functional block are shown in bold. The circuit consists of clockwise and counterclockwise wave fronts around two functional arcs of block that merge into a central common pathway that usually represents the slow zone of the reentrant circuit. The localization of the functional arcs of block coincides with the spatial disarray of connexin43 gap junctions. **B,** Spiral wave model. Recording of spiral wave reentry during ventricular fibrillation in a Langendorff-perfused guinea pig heart using a potentiometric fluorophore. Shown are the distributions of membrane potentials at four different times during one rotation on the left ventricular epicardial surface, with white and black being the most positive and most negative membrane potentials, respectively. Numbers are time in milliseconds. Arrows denote direction of wave front propagation. *(**A** from Peters NS, Coromilas J, Severs NJ, et al: Disturbed connexin43 gap junction distribution correlates with the location of reentrant circuits in the epicardial border zone of healing canine infarcts that cause ventricular tachycardia. Circulation 95:988, 1997. By permission of the American Heart Association; **B** from Samie FH, Berenfeld O, Anumonwo J, et al: Background potassium current. A determinant of rotor dynamics in ventricular fibrillation. Circ Res 89:1216, 2001. By permission of the American Heart Association.)*

of atrial electrical remodeling. Changes in the density, spatial distribution, or both of various connexin types may also cause alterations in atrial impulse propagation. Autonomic remodeling also appears to play a key role in both triggering and maintaining AF. Long-term selective vagal denervation of the atria and sinus and AV nodes prevents induction of AF. Heterogeneous sympathetic denervation of the atria favors the development of sustained AF.

Sinus Reentry (see Chap. 35)

The sinus node shares with the AV node electrophysiological features such as the potential for dissociation of conduction; that is, an impulse can conduct in some nodal fibers but not in others, thereby permitting reentry to occur. The reentrant circuit can be located entirely within the sinus node or involve both the sinus node and atrium. Supraventricular tachycardias caused by sinus node reentry are generally less symptomatic than other supraventricular tachycardias because of slower rates. Ablation of the sinus node may be necessary in an occasional refractory tachycardia.

Atrial Reentry (see Chap. 35)

Reentry within the atrium, unrelated to the sinus node, can be a cause of supraven tricular tachycardia in humans. Atrial reentry appears to be less frequently encountered than other types of supraventricular tachycardia. Distinguishing atrial tachycardia caused by automaticity or afterdepolarizations from atrial tachycardia sustained by reentry over small areas (i.e., microreentry) is difficult.

Atrioventricular Nodal Reentry (see Chap. 35)

On the basis of conductive properties, multiple AV nodal input pathways, which can be arbitrarily divided into fast, intermediate, and slow pathways (see Fig. 31-31), appear responsible for AV nodal reentrant tachycardia (AVNRT; Figs. 31-30 and 31-31).[11,93] Impulse propagation occurs rapidly over the atrial tissue (red zone in Fig. 31-30D) and slowly toward the AV node through the transitional zone (yellow zone in Fig. 31-30D) surrounding the AV node. All the atrial tissue enveloping Koch's triangle (see Fig. 31-30D) delivered impulses to the AV node, providing direct evidence to support the concept that slow pathway conduction is present in all normal hearts with or without AVNRT. As seen in Figure 31-30C, conduction delay is associated with a progressive decrease in the upstroke velocity of transmembrane action potentials as well as a progressive lengthening of action potential duration as the impulse approaches the AV node area, suggesting that spatial heterogeneity in the passive (density, cellular distribution, and characteristics of gap junctional channels[93]) or active membrane properties (density, characteristics of ion channels, or both) in the transitional zone underlies AV conduction delay. Optical mapping during echo beats reveals the reentrant pathways underlying the various types of AVNRT (see

Fig. 31-31). The reentrant pathway of the slow-fast type starts counterclockwise with block in the fast pathway, delay in conduction across the slow pathway to the compact AV node, exit from the AV node to the fast pathway, and rapid return to the slow pathway through atrial tissue located at the base of Koch's triangle. The reentrant circuit of the fast-slow type is clockwise. In the slow-slow type, anterograde conduction is over the intermediate pathway and retrograde conduction is over the slow pathway. Because slow pathway conduction is involved in each type of AVNRT, this observation explains why ablation of the slow pathway is effective in all types of AVNRT. These results also demonstrate that atrial tissue surrounding Koch's triangle is clearly involved in all three types of AV nodal reentry in these examples (see also Fig. 31-28).

Preexcitation Syndrome (see Chap. 35)

In most patients who have reciprocating tachycardias associated with Wolff-Parkinson-White syndrome, the accessory pathway conducts more rapidly than the normal AV node but takes a longer time to recover excitability; that is, the anterograde refractory period of the accessory pathway exceeds that of the AV node at long cycles. Consequently, a premature atrial complex that occurs sufficiently early is blocked anterogradely in the accessory pathway and continues to the ventricle over the normal AV node and His bundle. After the ventricles have been excited, the impulse is able to enter the accessory pathway retrogradely and return to the atrium. A continuous conduction loop of this type establishes the circuit for the tachycardia. The usual (orthodromic) activation wave during such a reciprocating tachycardia in a patient with an accessory pathway occurs anterogradely over the normal AV node–His-Purkinje system and retrogradely over the accessory pathway, which results in a normal QRS complex (Fig. 31-32).

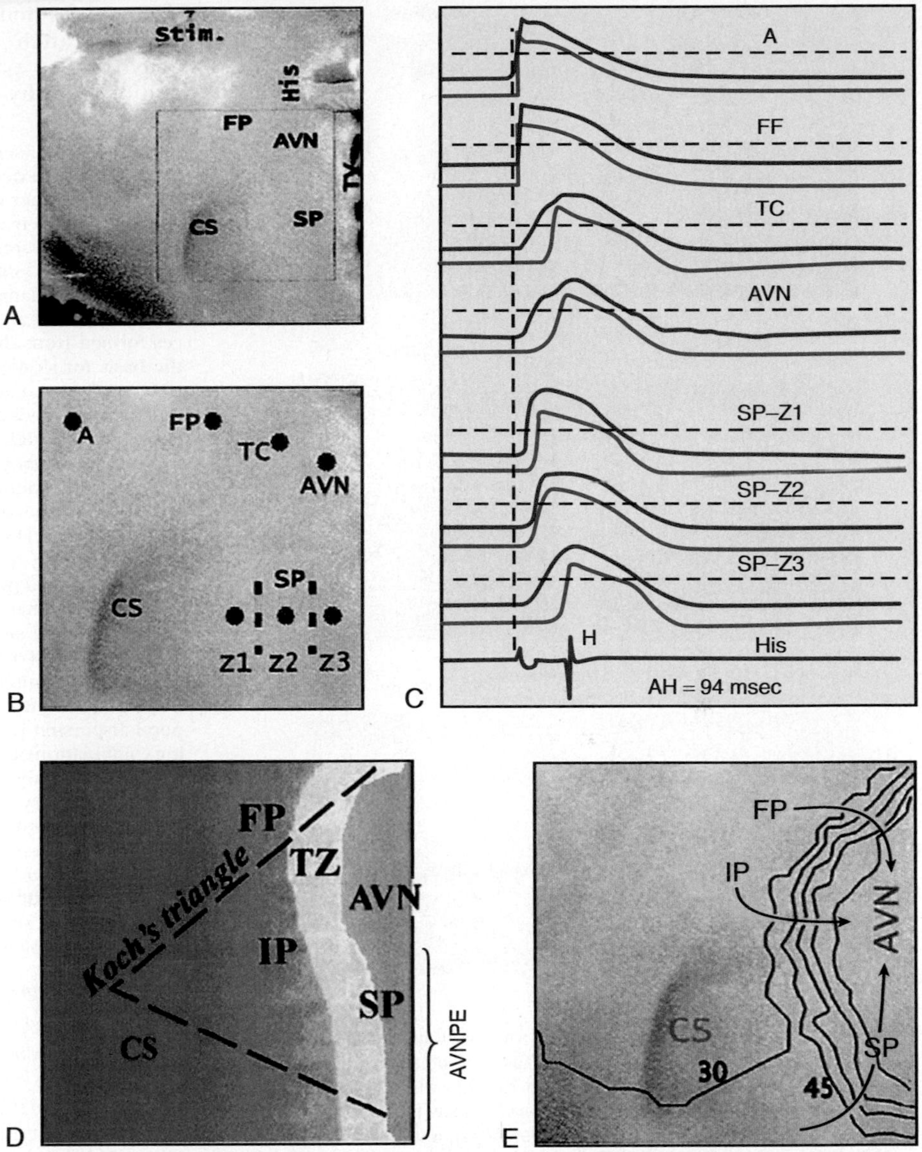

FIGURE 31–30 Atrioventricular (AV) nodal conduction in an isolated, arterially perfused canine preparation. Optical mapping of a potentiometric fluorophore combined with the conventional microelectrode technique was used to delineate the conduction pathways across the AV node. **A,** Endocardial aspect of the preparation. The stimulation electrode (Stim.) and bipolar electrode recording His bundle electrogram (His) are located in the top portion of the picture. The square box next to the tricuspid valve (TV) represents the optical mapping area. AVN = AV node; CS = coronary sinus; FP = fast pathway; SP = slow pathway. **B,** Enlarged picture of optical mapping area to illustrate the sites of microelectrode impalements (dark circles) in atrium (A), fast pathway (FP), transitional cells (TC), AV node (AVN), and three zones (Z1 to Z3) of the slow pathway (SP). **C,** Optical (top, red) and intracellular action potentials (bottom, blue) recorded from different anatomical regions are superimposed and displayed at fast sweep. **D,** Distribution of atrial (red), transitional (yellow), and AV nodal (green) cells in relation to AV nodal inputs (fast [FP], intermediate [IP], and slow [SP] pathways) and posterior extension (AVNPE). **E,** Sketch of the nondiscrete AV nodal input pathways as shown in the optical activation map. *(From Wu J, Zipes DP: Mechanisms underlying atrioventricular nodal conduction and the reentrant circuit of atrioventricular nodal reentrant tachycardia using optical mapping. J Cardiovasc Electrophysiol 13:831, 2002.)*

Because the circuit requires both atria and ventricles, the term *supraventricular tachycardia* is not precisely correct, and the tachycardia is more accurately termed *atrioventricular reciprocating tachycardia* (AVRT). The reentrant loop can be interrupted by ablation of the normal AV node–His bundle pathway *or* the accessory pathway. Occasionally, the activation wave travels in a reverse (antidromic) direction to the ventricles over the accessory pathway and to the atria retrogradely up the AV node. Two accessory pathways can form the circuit in some patients with antidromic AVRT. In some patients, the accessory pathway may be capable of only retrograde conduction ("concealed"), but the circuit and mechanism of AVRT remain the same. Less commonly, the accessory pathway can conduct only anterogradely. The pathway can be localized by analysis of the scalar ECG. Patients can have AF as well as AVRT.

Unusual accessory pathways with AV node–like electrophysiological properties—that is, nodofascicular or nodoventricular fibers—can constitute the circuit for reciprocating tachycardias in patients who have some form of the Wolff-Parkinson-White syndrome. Tachycardia in patients with nodoventricular fibers can be caused by reentry, with these fibers used as the anterograde pathway and the His-Purkinje fibers and a portion of the AV node used retrogradely. In the so-called Lown-Ganong-Levine syndrome (short PR interval and normal QRS complex), conduction over a James fiber

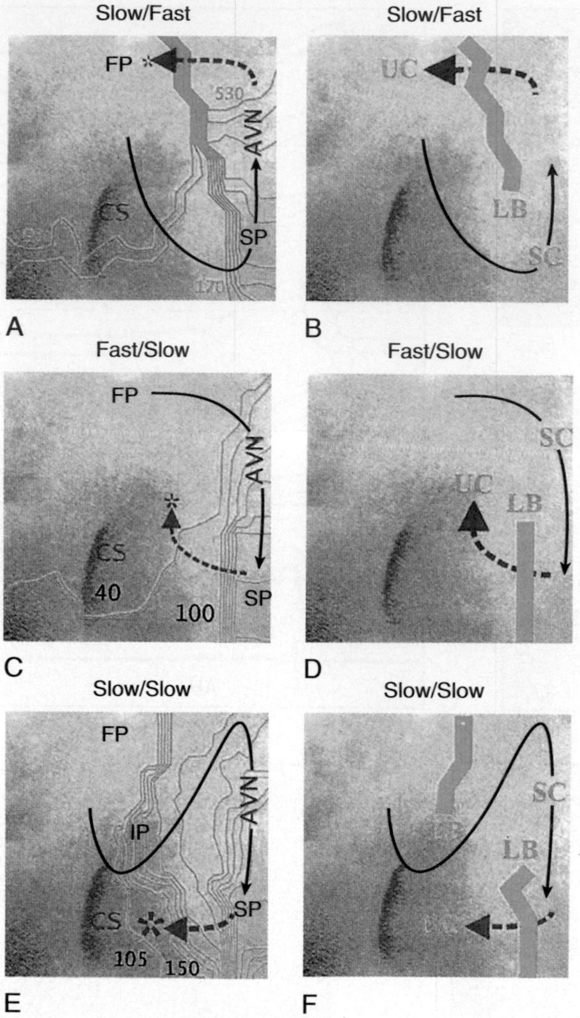

FIGURE 31–31 Reentrant circuits of different types of AV nodal reentrant tachycardia. Pictures of the optical activation maps of A2 obtained from three different experiments at A2 coupling intervals of 190, 220, and 190 milliseconds were merged with the pictures of the mapping area to show the initiation of echo beats in **A** (Slow/Fast), **C** (Fast/Slow), and **E** (Slow/Slow), respectively. The numbers in the maps indicate the activation times in reference to the A2 stimulus. The interrupted black arrow indicates anterograde conduction, and the star and the dashed red arrow represent the site of earliest retrograde atrial activation. The corresponding locations of the lines of block (LB, green), slow anterograde conduction (SC, black arrow), and unidirectional conduction (UC, red) are shown in **B, D,** and **F,** respectively. *(From Wu J, Zipes DP: Mechanisms underlying atrioventricular nodal conduction and the reentrant circuit of atrioventricular nodal reentrant tachycardia using optical mapping. J Cardiovasc Electrophysiol 13:831, 2002.)*

that connects the atrium to the distal portion of the AV node and His bundle has been proposed, although little functional evidence exists to support the presence of this entity.

Ventricular Tachycardia Caused by Reentry (see Chap. 35)

Reentry in the ventricle, both anatomical and functional, as a cause of sustained ventricular tachycardia has been supported by many animal and clinical studies (Fig. 31-33). Reentry in ventricular muscle, with or without contributions from specialized tissue, is responsible for many or most ventricular tachycardias in patients with ischemic heart disease. The area of microreentry appears to be small and, less commonly, a macroreentry is found around the infarct scar. Surviving myocardial tissue separated by connective tissue provides serpentine routes of activation traversing infarcted areas that can establish reentry pathways. Bundle branch reentry can cause sustained ventricular tachycardia, particularly in patients with dilated cardiomyopathy.

Both figure-of-8 (see Fig. 31-29) and single-circle (Fig. 31-34) reentrant loops have been described as circulating around an area of functional block in a manner consistent with the leading circle hypothesis or as conducting slowly across an apparent area of block created by anisotropy. When intramural myocardium survives, it can form part of the reentrant loop. Structural discontinuities that separate muscle bundles—for example, as a result of naturally occurring myocardial fiber orientation and anisotropic conduction, as well as collagen matrices formed from the fibrosis after a myocardial infarction—establish the basis for slowed conduction, fragmented electrograms, and continuous electrical activity, which can lead to reentry. After the infarction, the surviving epicardial border zone undergoes substantial electrical remodeling,[94] including reduced conduction velocity and increased anisotropy associated with the occurrence of reentrant circuits and ventricular tachycardia. Conduction slowing arises from alterations in the spatial distribution and electrophysiological properties of connexin43 gap junctions,[95] as well as from reduced sodium current. During acute ischemia, various factors, including elevated $[K]_o$ and reduced pH, combine to create depressed action potentials in ischemic cells that retard conduction and can lead to reentry. Indeed, optical mapping studies in arterially perfused canine wedge preparations during global no-flow ischemia[80] have demonstrated reentry initiation during initial ischemia and subsequent reperfusion caused by the unidirectional block of conduction resulting from the spatiotemporal dispersion in tissue responses to stimulation. The rapidly changing combination of the transmural dispersion in response to endocardial pacing stimuli and velocity of conduction create a dynamic substrate in which reentry can be initiated and sustained. The results of this study are compatible with previous observations that fibrillation during reperfusion can be caused by intramural reentry. Interestingly, transmural reentry under these experimental conditions could be triggered by epicardial, but not endocardial, stimulation.[77] Clinically, this might facilitate tachycardia induction by a premature ventricular complex arising in the epicardium but not in the endocardium.

Brugada Syndrome

Phase 2 reentry[96] has been implicated in the genesis of ventricular tachycardia-fibrillation associated with the inheritable Brugada syndrome, which is characterized by ST segment elevation (unrelated to ischemia, electrolyte abnormalities, or structural heart disease) in the right precordial (V_1 to V_3) leads of the ECG, often but not always accompanied by an apparent right bundle branch block. The hereditary nature of the syndrome is well established. Approximately 20 percent of Brugada syndrome cases have been linked to mutations in the *SCN5A* gene (see Chap. 9).[97] The gene defect causes acceleration of recovery of the sodium channel from inactivation or a nonfunctional sodium channel. Inhibition of the sodium channel current causes heterogeneous loss of the action potential dome during the plateau phase (phase 2) in the right ventricular epicardium, which leads to a marked dispersion of repolarization and refractoriness and the potential for phase 2 reentry.[98] Whether transmural heterogeneity in Na^+ channel recovery in the right ventricular free wall causes arrhythmia by a similar mechanism remains to be determined.

Ventricular Fibrillation: Initiation and Maintenance (see Chap. 35)

Previous experimental and simulation investigations have suggested that ventricular fibrillation (VF) is maintained solely by reentry. This reentry was thought to be unstable, maintained by wandering wavelets of activation following constantly changing paths of activation and exhibiting frequent conduction block caused by nonuniform dispersion of refractoriness. More recent investigations have suggested other mechanisms of fibrillation maintenance and have introduced the concepts of restitution kinetics, wave front,

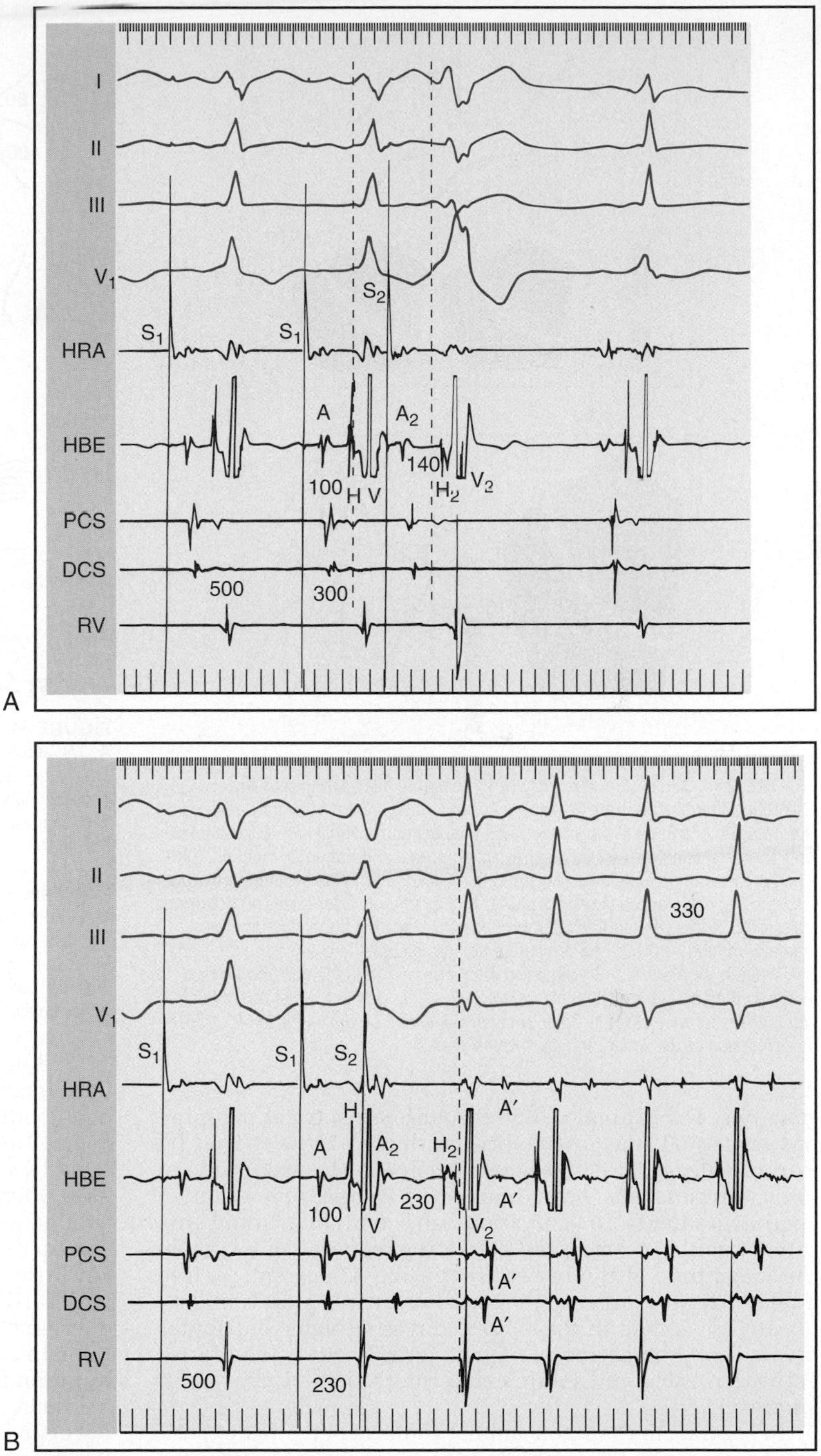

FIGURE 31–32 A, Wolff-Parkinson-White syndrome. Following high right atrial pacing at a cycle length of 500 milliseconds (S_1-S_1), premature stimulation at a coupling interval of 300 milliseconds (S_1-S_2) produces physiological delay in atrioventricular (AV) nodal conduction, resulting in an increase in the A-H interval from 100 to 140 milliseconds but no delay in the AV interval. Consequently, activation of the His bundle occurs following activation of the QRS complex (second interrupted line), and the QRS complex becomes more anomalous in appearance because of increased ventricular activation over the accessory pathway. **B,** Induction of reciprocating atrioventricular tachycardia. Premature stimulation at a coupling interval of 230 milliseconds prolongs the A-H interval to 230 milliseconds and results in anterograde block in the accessory pathway and normalization of the QRS complex (a slight functional aberrancy in the nature of incomplete right bundle branch block occurs). Note that H_2 precedes onset of the QRS complex (interrupted line). Following V_2, the atria are excited retrogradely (A′) beginning in the distal coronary sinus, followed by atrial activation in leads recording from the proximal coronary sinus, His bundle, and high right atrium. A supraventricular tachycardia is initiated at a cycle length of 330 milliseconds. I, II, III, and V_1 indicate scalar ECG leads. DCS = distal coronary sinus electrogram; HBE = His bundle electrogram; HRA = high right atrium; PCS = proximal coronary sinus electrogram; RV = right ventricular electrogram. Time lines are in 50- and 10-millisecond intervals. S_1, stimulus of the drive train; S_2, premature stimulus. A, H-V, atrial His bundle, and ventricular activation during the drive train; A_2, H_2, V_2, atrial His bundle, and ventricular activation during the premature stimulus. *(From Zipes DP, Mahomed Y, King RD, et al: Wolff-Parkinson-White syndrome: Cryosurgical treatment. Indiana Med 89:432, 1986.)*

wave break, and rotor as replacement for the classic reentry theory.[82,99-105]

The hallmark of cardiac fibrillation is ongoing wave break[100] (for a demonstration of wave front dynamics during VF, see the video from Samie and associates[79] on the website; also see Fig. 31-29B). Two hypotheses exist in regard to the genesis of wave breaks during fibrillation. The mother rotor hypothesis states that wave break is related to Wenckebach-like conduction as high-frequency impulses emanating from a relatively stable, intramural mother rotor are unable to sustain 1 : 1 conduction through heterogeneous tissue. In this case, the fastest activating (i.e., dominating) rotor, rather than ongoing wave break, is the engine driving cardiac fibrillation, and wave break only occurs secondarily.[99,103,104,106] Evidence supporting this concept is that frequency analyses have shown the following: (1) single, stable (both in space and time), dominant frequencies in the frequency spectra of membrane voltage signals obtained from various regions of the heart[99,104]; (2) dominant frequencies and the frequency of reentry correlate; (3) relative infrequency of reentry on the surface of the heart during fibrillation, favoring an intramural location of the mother rotor, such as the Purkinje network[99]; and (4) Wenckebach-like conduction at the borders between different dominant frequency domains.[104] These borders can result from preexisting structural and/or functional hetero-

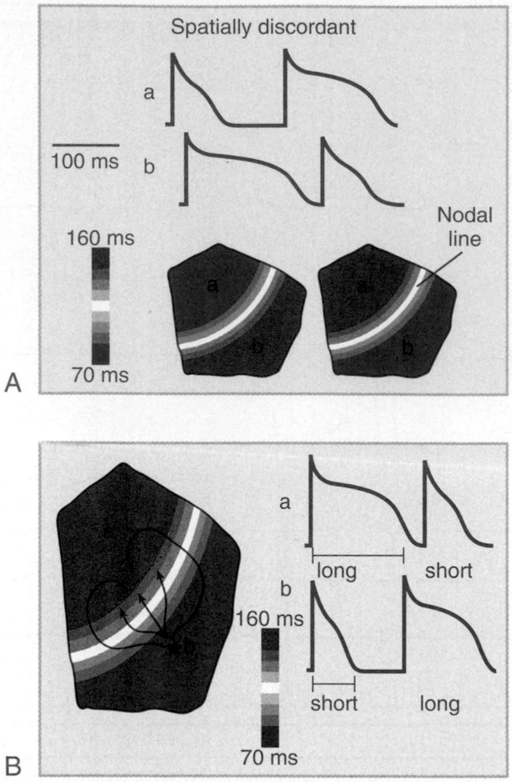

FIGURE 31–33 Initiation of reentry by a premature beat during spatially discordant alternans. **A, upper panel,** At rapid rates, action potentials at site *a* alternate short-long, whereas at the same time action potentials at site *b* alternate long-short, creating a steep gradient of action potential duration distribution, with a nodal line with no action potential duration (APD) alternation separating the out-of-phase regions *a* and *b* **(lower panel). B,** A premature beat (asterisk) occurring in region *b* blocks (dotted line) as it propagates across the nodal line into the region with long APD (*a*). The premature beat propagates laterally along the nodel line, waiting for the long APD region to repolarize and then reenters the blocked region to initiate figure-of-8 reentry. *(From Weiss JN, Karma A, Shiferaw Y, et al: From pulsus to pulseless: The saga of cardiac alternans. Circ Res 98:1244, 2006. By permission of the American Heart Association.)*

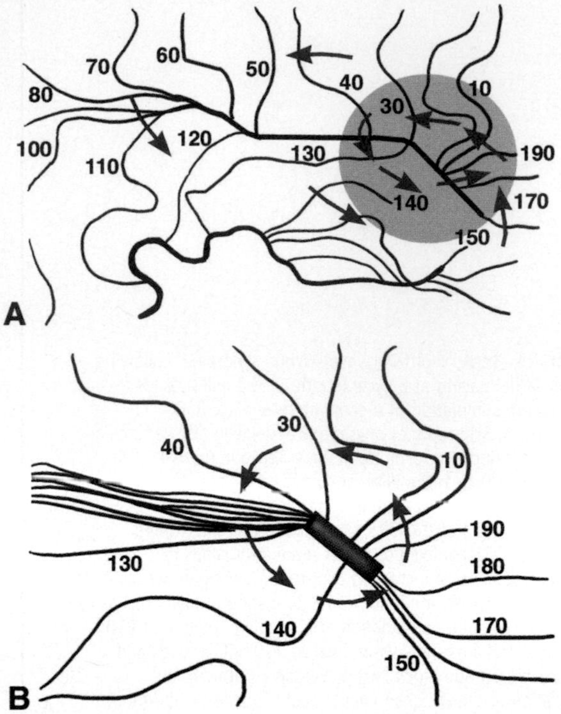

FIGURE 31–34 Model of anisotropic reentry in the epicardial border zone. **A,** The activation map of the single reentrant circuit is shown. The arrows point out the general activation pattern; activation appears to occur around a long line of block. However, parallel isochrones adjacent to the line (isochrones 130 and 140) suggest that activation is also occurring across the line and thereby results in the smaller circuit shown by the arrows in the shaded area. **B,** This circuit is shown enlarged. Rapid activation occurs parallel to the long axis of the fiber orientation (isochrones 10 to 40 and 130 to 150), whereas very slow activation (closely bunched isochrones 50 to 120) occurs transverse to fiber orientation in the circuit. The dark black rectangle is an area of either functional or anatomical block that forms the fulcrum of the circuit. *(From Wit AL, Dillon SM: Anisotropic reentry. In Zipes DP, Jalife J [eds]: Cardiac Electrophysiology: From Cell to Bedside. Philadelphia, WB Saunders, 1990.)*

geneities. For example, high-resolution electrical mapping has suggested that fast activation during VF is driven by Purkinje fibers.[99] Spatial heterogeneity in the magnitude of ionic currents has been implicated in the generation of spatial gradients in activation rates and in maintaining rotor stability in the fastest activating regions. For example, the magnitude of the inward rectifying K^+ current, I_{K1} (see Table 31-2), was larger in the rapidly activating left ventricular myocytes than in the slower activating right ventricular myocytes.[79] Furthermore, regions with larger I_{K1} had faster activation rates and more stable rotors than regions with smaller I_{K1}.[79]

In contrast to the stable mother rotor theory, other experimental evidence has supported the idea that dynamic wave break plays a fundamental role in the initiation and maintenance of VF[100,101,105]: (1) inability to detect a single dominant frequency in frequency analyses from fibrillating hearts; (2) spatiotemporal instability of frequency domain distributions during ventricular fibrillation, with the exception of anatomical borders, such as Purkinje-myocyte transition; (3) failure to demonstrate stable intramural reentry at higher frequencies than at the surface; and (4) boundaries dynamically generated by wavelet behavior rather than by anatomical conduction block. To reproduce the dynamic spatiotemporal instability of dominant frequency domains, a combination of dynamically changing and fixed tissue heterogeneity is required. The most important determinant of the dynamically induced component of heterogeneity has been identified as electrical restitution, the variation of APD and conduction velocity with the diastolic interval.[82] It has been proposed that the breakup of periodic waves is precipitated by oscillations of action potential duration (so-called APD alternans) that are sufficiently large enough to cause conduction block along the spiral wave front. If occurring in a spatially discordant pattern, alternans is considered a key arrhythmogenic factor predisposing the heart to reentry and fibrillation.[107] At the cellular level, the origin of APD alternans appears to be primarily determined by alternations in cardiomyocyte calcium transient amplitude and/or duration (calcium alternans).

During spatially discordant alternans, the APD alternates out of phase in different regions of the heart, thereby increasing dispersion of refractoriness so that ectopic beats have a high probability of inducing reentry. This mechanism is illustrated in Figure 31-33; some regions of the heart alternate in a long-short-long pattern, whereas other regions at the same time alternate in a short-long-short pattern. These out-of-phase regions are separated by a nodal line, in which no alternans is present, but spatial gradients in action potential duration are steepest along this line. Thus, spatially discordant alternans creates gradients in tissue refractoriness, which in turn favor the development of reentry by a premature beat (see Fig. 31-30B). At the cellular level, the steepness of the APD restitution curve (which relates action potential duration to the preceding diastolic interval[82]) and intracellular calcium level ($[Ca^{2+}]_i$) dynamics cause action potential duration and the $[Ca^{2+}]_i$ transient to alternate. Given the bidirectional coupling between changes in $[Ca^{2+}]_i$ and membrane potential—for example, membrane potential determines the activity of L-type Cav channels and, conversely, the $[Ca^{2+}]_i$ transient amplitude strongly modulates action potential duration through its effects on Ca^{2+}-sensitive currents (e.g., $I_{Na/Ca}$) during the action potential plateau—alternation in $[Ca^{2+}]_i$ transient amplitude can cause secondary alternation in action potential duration. Indeed, experimental evidence has strongly suggested that the onset of action potential duration alternans is primarily attributable to instabilities of $[Ca^{2+}]_i$ cycling dynamics, thus defining a causal role of intracellular Ca^{2+} handling abnormalities in initiating electrical instability. At the tissue level, alternans combines with instabilities in conduction velocity to cause alternans to become spatially discordant. T wave alternans is the electrocardiographic manifestation of APD/$[Ca^{2+}]_i$ alternans and thus is a clinical predictor of future arrhythmic events.

Reduction of the slope of the APD restitution curve has prevented the induction of VF in some models. The mass of the tissue appears to be another important factor in the development of fibrillation. In an isolated swine model, it was shown that tissue mass reduction resulted in the termination of VF when a critical mass (19 gm) was reached. In humans, this value appears to be much higher (>111 gm). Similarly, partitioning the atrium into its small segments prevents AF, a concept that has led to a corrective surgical and ablation procedure (see Chap. 33).

Ventricular Tachycardias Caused by Nonreentrant Mechanisms

In some cases of ventricular tachycardia related to coronary artery disease, but especially in patients without coronary artery disease, nonreentrant mechanisms are important causes of ventricular tachycardias. However, in many patients, the mechanism of the ventricular tachycardia remains unknown.

TRIGGERED ACTIVITY. A group of probably nonreentrant ventricular tachycardias occurring in the absence of structural heart disease can be initiated and terminated by programmed stimulation. They are catecholamine-dependent and are terminated by the Valsalva maneuver, adenosine, and verapamil. These ventricular tachycardias are generally, but not exclusively, located in the right ventricular outflow tract and may be caused by triggered activity, possibly DADs that are cAMP-dependent.[108] EADs have been recorded in this tachycardia as well. Left ventricular fascicular tachycardias can be suppressed by verapamil but not generally by adenosine, and some may be caused by triggered activity and others by reentry.[108] EADs and triggered activity may be responsible for torsades de pointes.[75]

AUTOMATICITY. Automatic discharge can be responsible for some ventricular tachycardias and does not appear to be suppressed by adenosine. Unless invasive studies are undertaken, mechanisms of ventricular tachycardia can only be conjectured.

REFERENCES

Anatomy of the Cardiac Conduction System

1. Honjo H, Boyett MR, Coppen SR, et al: Heterogeneous expression of connexins in rabbit sinoatrial node cells: Correlation between connexin isotype and cell size. Cardiovasc Res 53:89, 2002.
2. Altomare C, Terragni B, Brioschi C, et al: Heteromeric HCN1-HCN4 channels: A comparison with native pacemaker channels from the rabbit sinoatrial node. J Physiol (Lond) 549:347, 2003.
3. Dobrzynski H, Billeter R, Greener LD, et al: Expression of Kir2.1 and Kir6.2 transgenes under the control of the alpha-MHC promoter in the sinoatrial and atrioventricular nodes in transgenic mice. J Mol Cell Cardiol 41:855, 2006.
4. Martinez AD, Hayrapetyan V, Moreno AP, et al: Connexin43 and connexin45 form heteromeric gap junction channels in which individual components determine permeability and regulation. Circ Res 90:1100, 2002.
5. Bukauskas FF, Bukaukien A, Verselis VH, et al: Coupling asymmetry of heterotypic connexin 45/connexin 43-EGFP gap junctions: Properties of fast and slow gating mechanisms. Proc Natl Acad Sci U S A 99:7113, 2002.
6. Schwartz PJ, Zipes DP: Autonomic modulation of cardiac arrhythmias. *In* Zipes DP, Jalife J (eds): Cardiac Electrophysiology: From Cell to Bedside. 3rd ed. Philadelphia, WB Saunders, 1999, pp 300-314.
7. Lakatta EG, Maltsev VA, Bogdanov KY, et al: Cyclic variation of intracellular calcium: A critical factor for cardiac pacemaker cell dominance. Circ Res 92:45, 2003.
8. Steinberg SF: The molecular basis for distinct β-adrenergic receptor subtype actions in cardiomyocytes. Circ Res 85:1101, 1999.
9. Ackerman MJ, Clapham DE: G proteins and ion channels. *In* Zipes DP, Jalife J (eds): Cardiac Electrophysiology: From Cell to Bedside. 3rd ed. Philadelphia, WB Saunders, 1999, pp 112-118.
10. Chang F, Yu H, Cohen IS: Actions of vasoactive intestinal peptide and neuropeptide Y on the pacemaker current in canine Purkinje fibers. Circ Res 74:157, 1994.
11. Wu J, Wu J, Olgin J, et al: Mechanisms underlying the reentrant circuit of atrioventricular nodal reentry tachycardia in isolated canine nodal preparations using optical mapping. Circ Res 88:1189, 2001.
12. Nikolski V, Efimov IR: Fluorescent imaging of a dual-pathway atrioventricular nodal conduction system. Circ Res 88:e23, 2001.
13. Ko Y, Yeh H, Ko Y, et al: Three-dimensional reconstruction of the rabbit atrioventricular conduction axis by combining histological, desmin, and connexin mapping data. Circulation 109:1172, 2004.
14. Kreuzberg MM, Schrickel JW, Ghanem A, et al: Connexin30.2-containing gap junction channels decelerate impulse propagation through the atrioventricular node. Proc Natl Acad Sci U S A 103:5959, 2006.
15. Dobrzynski H, Nikolski VP, Sambelashvili AT, et al: Site of origin and molecular substrate of atrioventricular junctional rhythm in the rabbit heart. Circ Res 93:1102, 2003.
16. Wu J, Zipes DP: Mechanisms underlying atrioventricular nodal conduction and the reentrant circuit of atrioventricular nodal reentrant tachycardia using optical mapping. J Cardiovasc Electrophysiol 13:831, 2002.
17. Rohr S, Kucera JP, Fast VG, et al: Paradoxical improvement of impulse conduction in cardiac tissue by partial uncoupling. Science 275:841, 1997.
18. Liu Y, Wu C, Lu L, et al: Sympathetic nerve sprouting, electrical remodeling, and increased vulnerability to ventricular fibrillation in hypercholesterolemic rabbits. Circ Res 92:1145, 2003.
19. Oh YS, Jong AY, Kim DT, et al: Spatial distribution of nerve sprouting after myocardial infarction in mice. Heart Rhythm 3:728, 2006.
20. Hartmann HA, Colom LV, Sutherland ML, Noebels JL: Selective localization of cardiac SCN5A sodium channels in limbic regions of rat brain. Nat Neurosci 2:593, 1999.
21. Shamsuzzaman ASM, Ackerman MJ, Kara T, et al: Sympathetic nerve activity in the congenital long-QT syndrome. Circulation 107:1844, 2003.

Basic Electrophysiological Principles

22. Inoue M, Bridge JHB: Ca^{2+} sparks in rabbit ventricular myocytes evoked by action potentials. Involvement of clusters of L-type Ca^{2+} channels. Circ Res 92:532, 2003.
23. Rasmusson RL, Morales MJ, Wang S, et al: Inactivation of voltage-gated cardiac K^+ channels. Circ Res 82:739, 1998.
24. Rohr S, Kucera JP, Kléber AG: Slow conduction in cardiac tissue, I. Circ Res 83:781, 1998.
25. Sakmann BFAS, Spindler AJ, Bryant SM, et al: Distribution of a persistent sodium current across the ventricular wall in guinea pigs. Circ Res 87:910, 2000.
26. Zhou J, Shin H, Ji Y, et al: Phosphorylation and ER retention signals are required for protein kinase A-mediated potentiation of cardiac sodium current. Circ Res 91:540, 2002.
27. Kass RS, Moss AJ: Long QT syndrome: Novel insights into the mechanisms of cardiac arrhythmias. J Clin Invest 112:810, 2003.
28. Shah M, Akar FG, Tomaselli GF: Molecular basis of arrhythmias. Circulation 112:2517, 2005.
29. Zipes DP, Tomaselli GF: What causes sudden death in heart failure? Circ Res 95:754, 2004.
30. Nerbonne JM, Kass RS: Molecular physiology of cardiac repolarization. Physiol Rev 85:1205, 2005.
31. Plant LD, Bowers PN, Liu Q, et al: A common cardiac sodium channel variant associated with sudden infant death in African Americans, SCN5A S1103Y. J Clin Invest 116:430, 2006.
32. Mangoni ME, Traboulsie A, Leoni AL, et al: Bradycardia and slowing of the atrioventricular conduction in mice lacking CaV3.1/alpha1G T-type calcium channels. Circ Res 98:1422, 2006.
33. Anderson CL, Delisle BP, Anson BD, et al: Most LQT2 mutations reduce Kv11.1 (hERG) current by a class 2 (trafficking-deficient) mechanism. Circulation 113:365, 2006.
34. Xu Y, Tuteja D, Zhang Z, et al: Molecular identification and functional roles of a Ca(2+)-activated K+ channel in human and mouse hearts. J Biol Chem 278:49085, 2003.
35. Baruscotti M, Bucchi A, DiFrancesco D: Physiology and pharmacology of the cardiac pacemaker ("funny") current. Pharmacol Ther 107:59, 2005.
36. Milanesi R, Baruscotti M, Gnecchi-Ruscone T, et al: Familial sinus bradycardia associated with a mutation in the cardiac pacemaker channel. N Engl J Med 354:151, 2006.
37. Kleber A, Rudy Y: Basic mechanisms of cardiac impulse propagation and associated arrhythmias. Physiol Rev 84:431, 2004.
38. Gutstein DE, Morley GE, Tamaddon H, et al: Conduction slowing and sudden arrhythmic death in mice with cardiac-restricted inactivation of connexin43. Circ Res 88:333, 2001.
39. Kreuzberg MM, Söhl G, Kim J: Functional properties of mouse connexin30.2 expressed in the conduction system of the heart. Circ Res 96:1169, 2005.
40. Akar FG, Spragg DD, Tunin RS, et al: Mechanisms underlying conduction slowing and arrhythmogenesis in nonischemic dilated cardiomyopathy. Circ Res 95:717, 2004.
41. Danik SB, Liu F, Zhang F, Suk HJ, et al: Modulation of cardiac gap junction expression and arrhythmic susceptibility. Circ Res 95:1035, 2004.

42. Morley GE, Danik SB, Bernstein S, et al; Reduced intercellular coupling leads to paradoxical propagation across the Purkinje-ventricular junction and aberrant myocardial activation. PNAS 102:4126, 2005.
43. Yao JA, Gutstein DE, Liu F, et al: Cell coupling between ventricular myocyte pairs from connexin43-deficient murine hearts. Circ Res 93:736, 2003.
44. Firouzi M, Ramanna H, Kok B, et al: Association of human connexin40 gene polymorphisms with atrial vulnerability as a risk factor for idiopathic atrial fibrillation. Circ Res 95:e29, 2004.
45. Gard JJ, Yamada K, Green, KG, et al: Remodeling of gap junctions and slow conduction in a mouse model of desmin-related cardiomyopathy. Cardioavasc Res 67:539, 2005.
46. Kaplan SR, Gard JJ, Carvajal-Huerta L, et al: Structural and molecular pathology of the heart in Carvajal syndrome. Cardiovasc Pathol 13:26, 2004.
47. Kaplan SR, Gard JJ, Protonotarios N, et al: Remodeling of gap junctions in arrhythmogenic right ventricular cardiomyopathy due to a deletion in plakoglobin (Naxos disease). Heart Rhythm 1:3, 2004.
48. Rubart M, Zipes DP: Mechanisms of sudden cardiac death. J Clin Invest 115:2305, 2005.
49. Reuter H, Henderson SA, Han T, et al: The Na^+-Ca^{2+} exchanger is essential for the action of cardiac glycosides. Circ Res 90:305, 2002.
50. Baruscotti M, Bucchi A, DiFrancesco D: Physiology and pharmacology of the cardiac pacemaker ("funny") current. Pharmacol Ther 107:59, 2005.
51. Costantini DL, Arruda EP, Agarwal P, et al: The homeodomain transcription factor Irx5 establishes the mouse cardiac ventricular repolarization gradient. Cell 123:347, 2005.
52. Sah R, Ramirez RJ, Backx PH: Modulation of Ca^{2+} release in cardiac myocytes by changes in repolarization rate. Circ Res 90:165, 2002.
53. Sah R, Ramirez RJ, Oudit GY, et al: Regulation of cardiac excitation-contraction coupling by action potential repolarization: Role of the transient outward potassium current (I_{to}). J Physiol (Lond) 546:5, 2003.
54. Zygmunt AC, Goodrow RJ, Weigel CM: I_{NaCa} and $I_{Cl(Ca)}$ contribute to isoproterenol-induced delayed afterdepolarizations in midmyocardial cells. Am J Physiol 275: H1979, 1998.
55. Weber CR, Ginsburg KS, Bers DM: Cardiac submembrane $[Na^+]$ transients sensed by Na^+-Ca^{2+} exchange current. Circ Res 92:950, 2003.
56. Xu Y, Tuteja D, Zhang Z, et al: Molecular identification and functional roles of a Ca(2+)-activated K^+ channel in human and mouse hearts. J Biol Chem 278:49085, 2003.
57. Lakatta EG, Maltsev VA, Bogdanov KY, et al: Cyclic variation in intracellular calcium. A critical factor for cardiac pacemaker cell dominance. Circ Res 92:e45, 2003.

CH 31

Mechanisms of Arrhythmogenesis

58. Patterson E, Po SS, Scherlag BJ, et al: Triggered firing in pulmonary veins initiated by in vitro autonomic nerve stimulation. Heart Rhythm 2:624, 2005.
59. Mohler PJ, Schott J, Gramolini AO, et al: Ankyrin-B mutation causes type 4 long-QT cardiac arrhythmia and sudden cardiac death. Nature 421:634, 2003.
60. Lerman BB, Stein KM, Markowitz SM, et al: Ventricular tachycardia in patients with structurally normal hearts. *In* Zipes DP, Jalife J (eds): Cardiac Electrophysiology: From Cell to Bedside. 3rd ed. Philadelphia, WB Saunders, 1999, pp 640–656.
61. Lehnart SE, Wehrens XH, Marks AR: Calstabin deficiency, ryanodine receptors, and sudden cardiac death. Biochem Biophys Res Commun 322:1267, 2004.
62. Jiang D, Xiao B, Zhang L, et al: Enhanced basal activity of a cardiac Ca^{2+} release channel (ryanodine receptor) mutant associated with ventricular tachycardia and sudden death. Circ Res 91:218, 2002.
63. George CH, Higgs GV, Lai FA: Ryanodine receptor mutations associated with stress-induced ventricular tachycardia mediate increased calcium release in stimulated cardiomyocytes. Circ Res 93:531, 2003.
64. Cerrone MM, Colombi B, Santoro M, et al: Mouse model carrier of a mutation in the cardiac ryanodine receptor bidirectional ventricular tachycardia and fibrillation elicited in a knock-in mouse model carrier of a mutation in the cardiac ryanodine receptor. Circ Res 96:77, 2005.
65. Lahat H, Pras E, Olender T, et al: A missense mutation in a highly conserved region of CASQ2 is associated with autosomal recessive catecholamine-induced polymorphic ventricular tachycardia in Bedouin families from Israel. Am J Hum Genet 69:1378,2001.
66. Terentyev D, Nori A, Santoro M, et al: Abnormal interactions of calsequestrin with the ryanodine receptor calcium release channel complex linked to exercise-induced sudden cardiac death. Circ Res 98:1151, 2006.
67. Wehrens XH, Lehnart SE, Huang F, et al: FKBP12.6 deficiency and defective calcium release channel (ryanodine receptor) function linked to exercise-induced sudden cardiac death. Cell 113:829, 2003.
68. Yano M, Ikeda Y, Matsuzaki M: Altered intracellular Ca^{2+} handling in heart failure. J Clin Invest 115:556, 2005.
69. Wehrens XH, Lehnart SE, Reiken SR, et al: Protection from cardiac arrhythmia through ryanodine receptor-stabilizing protein calstabin2. Science 304:292, 2004.
70. Li X, Zima AV, Sheikh F, et al: Endothelin-1-induced arrhythmogenic Ca2+ signaling is abolished in atrial myocytes of inositol-1,4,5-trisphosphate(IP3)-receptor type 2-deficient mice. Circ Res 96:1274, 2005.
71. Mackenzie L, Bootman MD, Laine M, et al: The role of inositol 1,4,5-trisphosphate receptors in Ca(2+) signalling and the generation of arrhythmias in rat atrial myocytes. J Physiol 541:395, 2002.
72. Yamada J, Ohkusa T, Nao T, et al: Upregulation of inositol 1,4,5-trisphosphate receptor expression in atrial tissue in patients with chronic atrial fibrillation. J Cardiol 39:57, 2002.
73. Zima AV, Blatter LA: Inositol-1,4,5-trisphosphate-dependent Ca(2^+) signalling in cat atrial excitation-contraction coupling and arrhythmias. J Physiol 555:607, 2004.
74. Kass RS, Moss AJ: Long QT syndrome: Novel insights into the mechanisms of cardiac arrhythmias. J Clin Invest 112:810-815, 2003.
75. Choi B, Burton F, Salama G: Cytosolic Ca^{2+} triggers early afterdepolarizations and torsade de pointes in rabbit hearts with type 2 long QT syndrome. J Physiol (Lond) 543.2:615, 2002.
76. Antzelevitch C, Shimizu W, Yan G, et al: The M cell: Its contribution to the ECG and to normal and abnormal electrical function of the heart. J Cardiovasc Electrophysiol 10:1124, 1999.
77. Snyders DJ: Molecular biology of potassium channels. *In* Zipes DP, Jalife J (eds): Cardiac Electrophysiology: From Cell to Bedside. 3rd ed. Philadelphia, WB Saunders, 1999, pp 21–31.
78. Valderrábano M, Lee M, Ohara T, et al: Dynamics of intramural and transmural reentry during ventricular fibrillation in isolated swine ventricles. Circ Res 88:839, 2001.
79. Samie FH, Berenfeld O, Anumonwo J, et al: Background potassium current. A determinant of rotor dynamics in ventricular fibrillation. Circ Res 89:1216, 2001.
80. Wu J, Zipes DP: Transmural reentry triggered by epicardial stimulation during acute ischemia in canine ventricular muscle. Am J Physiol Heart Circ Physiol 283: H2004, 2002.
81. Ueda N, Zipes DP, Wu J Functional and transmural modulation of M cell behavior in canine ventricular wall. Am J Physiol Heart Circ Physiol 287:H2569, 2004.
82. Fox JJ, Riccio ML, Hua F, et al: Spatiotemporal transition to conduction block in canine ventricle. Circ Res 90:289, 2002.
83. Sih HJ, Zipes DP, Berbari EJ, et al: Differences in organization between acute and chronic atrial fibrillation in dogs. J Am Coll Cardiol 36:924, 2000.
84. Haissaguerre M, Jais P, Shah DC, et al: Spontaneous initiation of atrial fibrillation by ectopic beats originating in the pulmonary veins. N Engl J Med 339:659, 1998.
85. Chen Y, Chen S: Electrophysiology of pulmonary veins. J Cardiovasc Electrophysiol 17:220, 2006.
86. Chou CC, Nihei M, Zhou S, et al: Intracellular calcium dynamics and anisotropic reentry in isolated canine pulmonary veins and left atrium. Circulation 111:2889, 2005.
87. Chou CC, Zhou S, Tan AY, et al: High-density mapping of pulmonary veins and left atrium during ibutilide administration in a canine model of sustained atrial fibrillation. Am J Physiol Heart Circ Physiol 289:H2704, 2005.
88. Vest JA, Wehrens XH, Reiken SR, et al: Defective cardiac ryanodine receptor regulation during atrial fibrillation. Circulation 111:2025, 2005.
89. Zhang Z, He Y, Tuteja D, et al: Functional roles of Cav1.3(alpha1D) calcium channels in atria: Insights gained from gene-targeted null mutant mice. Circulation 112:1936, 2005.
90. Temple J, Frias P, Rottman J, et al: Atrial fibrillation in KCNE1-null mice. Circ Res 97:62, 2005.
91. Firouzi M, Ramanna H, Kok B, et al: Association of human connexin40 gene polymorphisms with atrial vulnerability as a risk factor for idiopathic atrial fibrillation. Circ Res 95:e29, 2004.
92. Hadian D, Zipes DP, Olgin JE, et al: Short-term rapid atrial pacing produces electrical remodeling of sinus node function in humans. J Cardiovasc Electrophysiol 13:584, 2002.
93. Nikolski VP, Jones SA, Lancaster MK, et al: Cx43 and dual-pathway electrophysiology of the atrioventricular node and atrioventricular nodal reentry. Circ Res 92:469, 2003.
94. Cabo C, Boyden PA: Electrical remodeling of the epicardial border zone in the canine infarcted heart: A computational analysis. Am J Physiol 284:H372, 2002.
95. Yao J, Hussain W, Patel P, et al: Remodeling of gap junctional channel function in epicardial border zone of healing canine infarcts. Circ Res 92:437, 2003.
96. Morita H, Zipes DP, Lopshire J, et al: T wave alternans in an in vitro canine tissue model of Brugada syndrome Am J Physiol Heart Circ Physiol 291:421, 2006.
97. Chen Q, Glenn E, Zhang D, et al: Genetic basis and molecular mechanism for idiopathic ventricular fibrillation. Nature 392:293, 1998.
98. Antzelevitch C, Brugada P, Brugada J, et al: Brugada syndrome. A decade of progress. Circ Res 91:1114, 2002.
99. Newton JC, Smith WM, Ideker RE: Estimated global transmural distribution of activation rate and conduction block during porcine and canine ventricular fibrillation. Circ Res 94:836, 2004.
100. Valderrábano M, Yang J, Omichi C, et al: Frequency analysis of ventricular fibrillation in swine ventricles. Circ Res 90:213; 2002.
101. Choi B, Nho W, Liu T, et al: Life span of ventricular fibrillation frequencies. Circ Res 91;339, 2002.
102. Nanthakumar K, Huang J, Rogers JM, et al: Regional differences in ventricular fibrillation in the open-chest porcine left ventricle. Circ Res 9:733, 2002.
103. Zaitsev AV, Guha PK, Sarmast F, et al: Wavebreak formation during ventricular fibrillation in the isolated, regionally ischemic pig heart. Circ Res 92:546, 2003.
104. Zaitsev AV, Berenfeld O, Mironov SF, et al: Distribution of excitation frequencies on the epicardial and endocardial surfaces of fibrillating ventricular wall of the sheep heart. Circ Res 86:408, 2000.
105. Roger JM, Huang J, Melnick SB, et al: Sustained reentry in the left ventricle of fibrillating pig hearts. Circ Res 92:539, 2003.
106. Chen J, Mandapati R, Berenfeld O, et al: High-frequency periodic sources underlie ventricular fibrillation in the isolated rabbit heart. Circ Res 86:86, 2000.
107. Weiss JN, Karma A, Shiferaw Y, et al: From pulsus to pulseless: The saga of cardiac alternans. Circ Res 98:1244, 2006.
108. Lerman BB, Stein KM, Markowitz SM, et al: Ventricular tachycardia in patients with structurally normal hearts. *In* Zipes DP, Jalife J (eds): Cardiac Electrophysiology: From Cell to Bedside. Philadelphia, WB Saunders, 1999, pp 640-656.

CHAPTER 32

Diagnosis of Cardiac Arrhythmias

John M. Miller and Douglas P. Zipes

In the management of clinical arrhythmias, the physician must evaluate and treat the whole patient, not just the rhythm disturbance.[1] Some arrhythmias are hazardous to the patient, regardless of the clinical setting (e.g., ventricular fibrillation, VF), whereas others are hazardous because of the clinical setting (e.g., rapidly conducted atrial fibrillation in a patient with severe coronary artery stenoses). Some arrhythmias, such as premature ventricular complexes (PVCs), may be highly symptomatic yet are not associated with any adverse outcome, whereas some patients with atrial fibrillation have no symptoms at all but may still be at significant risk of stroke. Evaluation of the patient begins with a careful history and physical examination and should usually progress from the simplest to the most complex test, from the least invasive and safest to the most invasive and risky, and from the least expensive out-of-hospital evaluations to those that require hospitalization and sophisticated, costly procedures. Occasionally, depending on the clinical circumstances, the physician may wish to proceed directly to a high-risk, expensive procedure, such as an electrophysiological study (EPS), before obtaining a 24-hour electrocardiographic recording.

HISTORY

Patients with cardiac rhythm disturbances can present with various complaints, but commonly symptoms such as palpitations, syncope, presyncope, or congestive heart failure cause them to seek a physician's help. Their awareness of palpitations and of a regular or irregular cardiac rhythm varies greatly.[2] Some patients perceive slight variations in their heart rhythm with uncommon accuracy, whereas others are oblivious even to sustained episodes of ventricular tachycardia (VT); still others complain of palpitations when they actually have regular sinus rhythm.

In assessing a patient with known or suspected arrhythmia, several key pieces of information should be obtained that can help determine a diagnosis or guide further diagnostic testing. The *mode of onset* of an episode may provide clues about the type of arrhythmia or preferred treatment option. For example, palpitations that occur in the setting of exercise, fright, or anger are often caused by catecholamine-sensitive automatic or triggered tachycardias that may respond to adrenergic-blocking agents; palpitations that occur at rest or that awaken the patient may be caused by vagal initiation, such as atrial fibrillation. Lightheadedness or syncope occurring in the setting of a tightly fitting collar, shaving the neck, or turning the head suggests carotid sinus hypersensitivity. The *mode of termination* of episodes may also be helpful: if palpitations can be reliably terminated by breath-holding, Valsalva, or other vagal maneuvers, it is likely that the atrioventricular (AV) node comprises an integral part of a tachycardia circuit; occasionally, focal atrial tachycardias or VTs terminate with vagal maneuvers. Patients should be asked how frequently episodes occur, how long they last, and how severe are their symptoms. These features can help guide how aggressively and quickly the physician needs to pursue a diagnostic or therapeutic plan (a patient with daily episodes associated with near-syncope or severe dyspnea warrants a more expeditious evaluation than one with infrequent episodes of mild palpitations and no other symptoms). Patients can sometimes report the heart rate during an episode (either rapid or slow, regular or irregular) by counting their pulse directly or using an automatic blood pressure or heart rate monitor. Characteristics of mode of onset and frequency of episodes can guide the choice of diagnostic tests (see later).

A careful drug and dietary history should also be sought; some nasal decongestants can provoke tachycardia episodes, whereas beta-adrenergic blocking eye drops for treatment of glaucoma can drain into tear ducts, be absorbed systemically, and precipitate syncope caused by bradycardia. Dietary supplements, particularly those containing ephedrine, can cause arrhythmias. A growing list of drugs can directly or indirectly affect ventricular repolarization and produce long-QT interval-related tachyarrhythmias (see Chap. 6). The patient should be questioned about the presence of systemic illnesses that may be associated with arrhythmias such as chronic obstructive pulmonary disease, thyrotoxicosis (see Chap. 81), pericarditis (see Chap. 70), or congestive heart failure (see Chaps. 24 and 25). A family history of rhythm disturbances is often present in long-QT syndrome (see Chap. 9), hypertrophic cardiomyopathy (see Chap. 65), and muscular or myotonic dystrophies (see Chap. 87).

PHYSICAL EXAMINATION

Examination of the patient during a symptomatic episode can be revealing. Clearly, heart rate and blood pressure are key measurements to make. Assessment of the jugular venous pressure and waveform can disclose the rapid oscillations of atrial flutter or "cannon" A waves indicative of contraction of the right atrium against a closed tricuspid valve in patients with AV dissociation in disorders such as complete heart block or VT. Variations in the intensity of the first heart sound and systolic blood pressure have the same implications.

Physical maneuvers during a tachycardia can have diagnostic and therapeutic value. The Valsalva maneuver or carotid sinus massage causes a transient increase in vagal tone; tachyarrhythmias that depend on the AV node for continuation can terminate or slow with these maneuvers but may also show no change. Focal atrial tachycardias occasionally terminate in response to vagal stimulation, as do rare VTs. Sinus tachycardia slows slightly following vagal stimulation, returning to its original rate soon thereafter; the ventricular response during atrial flutter and fibrillation and other atrial tachycardias can decrease briefly. During wide QRS tachycardias with a 1:1 relationship between P waves and QRS complexes, vagal influence can terminate or slow a supraventricular tachycardia (SVT) that depends on the AV node for perpetuation; on the other hand, vagal effects on the AV node can transiently block retrograde conduction and thus establish the diagnosis of VT by demonstrating AV dissociation. The effect of either of these physical maneuvers typically lasts only seconds; the physician must be ready to observe or record any changes in rhythm on an ECG when the maneuver is performed or the response may not be appreciated.

Carotid massage is performed with the patient supine and comfortable, with the head tipped away from the side being stimulated. Careful auscultation for carotid bruits must always precede any attempt at carotid massage, because there have been reports of embolic events associated with massage. The area of the carotid sinus, at the artery's bifurcation, is palpated with two fingers at the angle of the jaw until a good pulse is felt. Even this minimal amount of pressure may induce a hypersensitive response in affected individuals. If there is no initial effect, a side-to-side or rotating motion of the fingers over the site is performed for up to 5 seconds. A negative response is lack of effect on the electrocardiogram (ECG) after 5 seconds of pressure adequate to cause mild discomfort. Because responses to carotid massage may differ on the two sides, the maneuver can be repeated on the opposite side; however, both sides should never be stimulated simultaneously.

Physical findings can suggest the presence of structural heart disease (and thus generally a clinically more serious situation with a worse overall prognosis), even in the absence of an arrhythmia episode. For example, a laterally displaced or dyskinetic apical impulse, a regurgitant or stenotic murmur, or a third heart sound in an older adult can denote significant myocardial or valvular dysfunction or damage.

ELECTROCARDIOGRAM

The ECG is the primary tool in arrhythmia analysis (see Chap. 12); only an EPS, in which intracardiac catheters are used to record activity from several regions of the heart at one time, is more definitive. Initially, a 12-lead ECG is recorded. In addition, a long continuous recording using the lead that shows distinct P waves is often helpful for closer analysis; most commonly, this is one of the inferior leads (2, 3, aVF) and occasionally V_1 or aVR. The ECG obtained during an episode of arrhythmia may be diagnostic by itself, obviating the need for further diagnostic testing. Figure 32-1 depicts an algorithm for diagnosing specific tachyarrhythmias from the 12-lead ECG (see Chap. 35). A major branch point in the differential diagnosis concerns the QRS duration: wide QRS (more than 0.12 second) tachycardias are often VTs, and narrow QRS (0.12 second or less) tachycardias are almost always SVTs, but there is some overlap (Table 32-1).[3] The next most important questions to answer, regardless of QRS width, concern characteristics of P waves. If P waves are not clearly visible, atrial activity can sometimes be recorded by placing the right and left arm leads in various anterior chest positions to discern P waves (so-called Lewis leads) or by applying esophageal electrodes or obtaining intracavitary right atrial recordings; the latter methods are not readily available in most clinical situations. An echocardiogram showing atrial contraction can be helpful. The long rhythm strip may yield important clues by revealing P waves if perturbations occur during the arrhythmia (e.g., changes in rate, premature complexes, sudden termination, effect of physical maneuvers, as noted earlier).

Each arrhythmia should be approached in a systematic manner to answer the several key questions; as suggested earlier, many of these relate to P wave characteristics and underscore the importance of assessing the ECG carefully for these. If P waves are visible, are the atrial and ventricular rates identical? Are the P-P and R-R intervals regular or irregular? If irregular, is it a consistent, repeating irregularity? Is there a P wave related to each QRS complex? Does the P wave seem to precede ("long RP" interval) or follow ("short RP" interval) the QRS complex (Fig. 32-2)? Are the resultant RP and PR intervals constant? Are all P waves and QRS complexes identical? Is the P wave vector normal or abnormal? Are P, PR, QRS, and QT durations normal? Once these questions have been addressed, one needs to assess the significance of the arrhythmia in view of the clinical setting. Should it be treated and, if so, how? For SVTs with a normal QRS complex, a branching decision tree such as that shown in Figure 32-1 may be useful.

THE LADDER DIAGRAM. The ladder diagram, derived from the ECG, is used to depict depolarization and conduction schematically to aid understanding of the rhythm. Straight or slightly slanting lines drawn on a tiered framework beneath an ECG represent electrical events occurring in the various cardiac structures (Fig. 32-3). Because the ECG and therefore the ladder diagram represent electrical activity against a time base, conduction is indicated by the lines of the ladder diagram sloping in a left-to-right direction. A steep line represents rapid conduction, with more slanting lines depicting slower conduction. A short bar drawn perpendicularly to a sloping line represents blocked conduction. Activity originating in an ectopic site such as the ventricle is indicated by lines emanating from that tier. Sinus nodal discharge and conduction and, under certain circumstances, AV junctional discharge and conduction can only be inferred; their activity is not directly recorded on a scalar ECG.

Most patients have only occasional episodes of arrhythmia and spend most of their time in their baseline rhythm (e.g., sinus, atrial fibrillation). The ECG during the patient's resting rhythm can provide clues about the presence of a substrate for arrhythmia (i.e., structural or physiological abnormalities from which arrhythmias can arise). Several of these are shown in Figure 32-4. In most patients with SVT (aside from those with Wolff-Parkinson-White syndrome), the resting ECG is normal. This is also true for many patients with ventricular tachyarrhythmias. Thus, although capable of showing an abnormality with possible arrhythmic implications, the resting ECG is not a very sensitive tool.

ADDITIONAL TESTS

The following additional tests can be used to evaluate patients who have cardiac arrhythmias. The physician's choice of which test to use depends on the clinical circumstances. For example, a patient with multiple daily episodes of presyncope is likely to have an event recorded on a 24-hour ambulatory ECG (Holter) monitor, whereas in a patient who complains of infrequent anxiety- or exercise-induced palpitations, exercise stress testing may be more likely to provide a diagnosis.

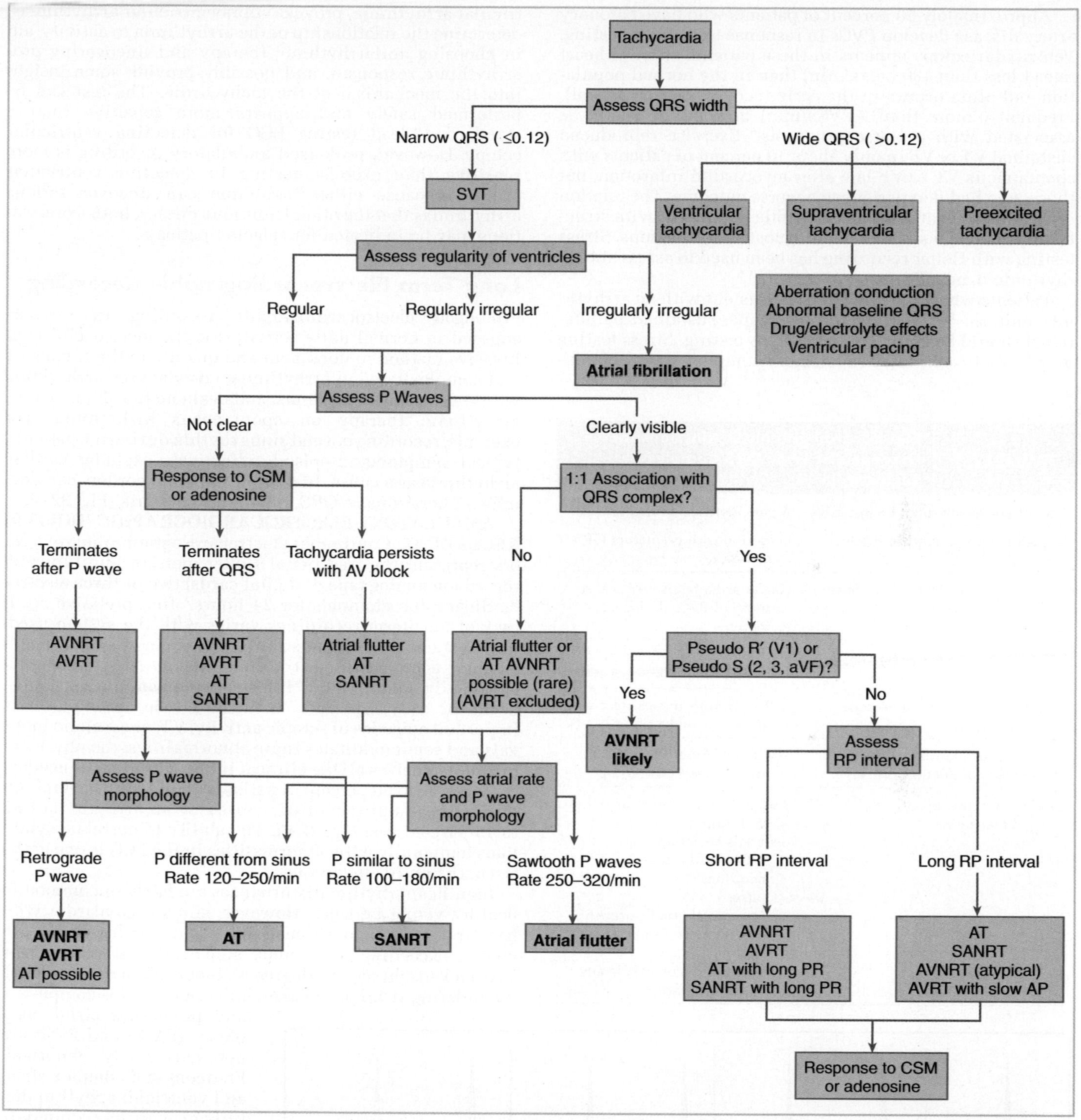

FIGURE 32–1 Stepwise approach to diagnosis of type of tachycardia based on 12-lead electrocardiogram during the episode. The initial step is to determine whether the tachycardia has a wide or narrow QRS complex. For wide-complex tachycardia, see Table 32-1; the remainder of the algorithm is helpful in diagnosing the type of narrow-complex tachycardia. SVT = supraventricular tachycardia; CSM = carotid sinus massage; AV = atrioventricular; AVNRT = AV nodal reentrant tachycardia; AVRT = AV reciprocating tachycardia; AT = atrial tachycardia; SANRT = sinoatrial nodal reentry tachycardia; AP = accessory pathway.

Exercise Testing

Exercise can induce various types of supraventricular and ventricular tachyarrhythmias and, uncommonly, bradyarrhythmias.[4] About one third of normal subjects develop ventricular ectopy in response to exercise testing (see Chap. 13). Ectopy is more likely to occur at faster heart rates, usually in the form of occasional PVCs of constant morphology, or even pairs of PVCs, and is often not reproducible from one stress test to the next. Three to six beats of nonsustained VT can occur in normal patients, especially the elderly, and its occurrence does not establish the existence of ischemic or other forms of heart disease or predict increased cardiovascular morbidity or mortality. Premature supraventricular complexes are often more common during exercise than at rest and increase in frequency with age; their occurrence does not suggest the presence of structural heart disease. A persistent elevation of heart rate after the end of exercise (delay in return to baseline) is associated with a worse cardiovascular prognosis.[5]

Approximately 50 percent of patients who have coronary artery disease develop PVCs in response to exercise testing. Ventricular ectopy appears in these patients at lower heart rates (less than 130 beats/min) than in the normal population and often occurs in the early recovery period as well. Frequent (more than 7 PVCs/min) or complex ectopy is associated with a worse prognosis.[6] Exercise reproduced sustained VT or VF in only about 10 percent of patients with spontaneous VT or VF late after myocardial infarction, but those who had it experienced a worse outcome. The relation of exercise to ventricular arrhythmia in patients with structurally normal hearts has no prognostic implications. Stress testing with Holter recording has been used to assess antiarrhythmic drug efficacy.

Patients who have symptoms consistent with an arrhythmia induced by exercise (e.g., syncope, sustained palpitations) should be considered for stress testing. Stress testing may be indicated to uncover more complex grades of ventricular arrhythmia, provoke supraventricular arrhythmias, determine the relationship of the arrhythmia to activity, aid in choosing antiarrhythmic therapy and uncovering proarrhythmic responses, and possibly provide some insight into the mechanism of the tachycardia. The test can be performed safely and appears more sensitive than a standard 12-lead resting ECG for detecting ventricular ectopy. However, prolonged ambulatory recording is more sensitive than exercise testing in detecting ventricular ectopy. Because either technique can uncover serious arrhythmias that the other technique misses, both examinations may be indicated for selected patients.

TABLE 32–1 Electrocardiographic Distinctions for Diagnosis of Wide QRS Complex Tachycardia

Favor Supraventricular Tachycardia	Favor Ventricular Tachycardia
Initiation with premature P wave	Initiation with premature QRS complex
QRS complexes identical to those in resting rhythm	Tachycardia beats identical to those of PVCs during sinus rhythm
Long-short sequence preceding initiation	Changes in R-R interval precede changes in P-P interval
Changes in P-P interval precede changes in R-R interval	QRS contours inconsistent with aberrant conduction (V_1, V_6)
QRS contours consistent with aberrant conduction (V_1, V_6)	AV dissociation or other non-1:1 AV relationship
Slowing or termination with vagal maneuvers.	Fusion beats, capture beats QRS duration >0.14 sec Left axis deviation (especially −90 to 180 degrees) Concordant R wave progression pattern Contralateral bundle branch block pattern from resting rhythm Absence of rS complex in any precordial lead

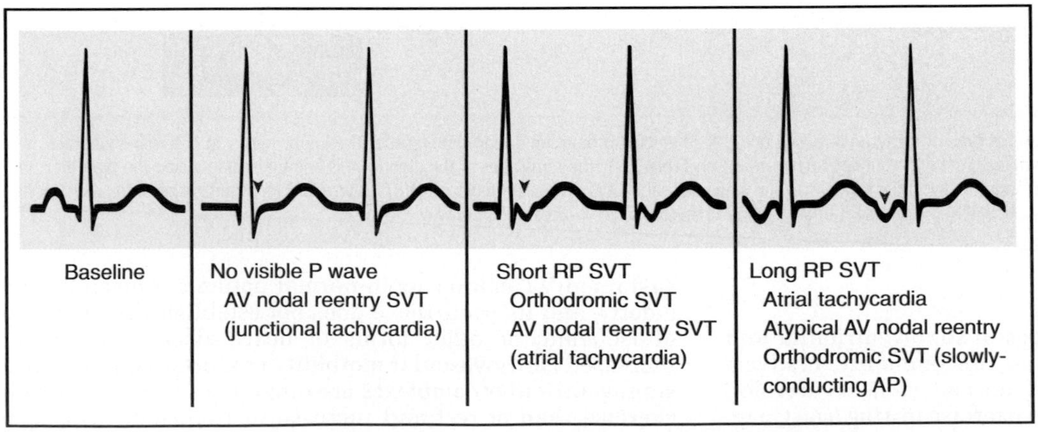

FIGURE 32–2 Differential diagnosis of different types of supraventricular tachycardia (SVT) based on timing of atrial activity (RP and PR intervals). **Left,** Normal beat. Different types of tachycardia are listed below the representative electrocardiographic patterns that they can produce, categorized by P wave position relative to the QRS complex. Red arrow shows the location of the P wave in each example. AV = atrioventricular; AP = accessory pathway.

Long-Term Electrocardiographic Recording

Prolonged electrocardiographic recording in patients engaged in normal daily activities is the most useful noninvasive method to document and quantitate the frequency and complexity of an arrhythmia, correlate the arrhythmia with the patient's symptoms, and evaluate the effect of antiarrhythmic therapy on spontaneous arrhythmia. For example, recording normal sinus rhythm during the patient's typical symptomatic episode effectively excludes cardiac arrhythmia as a cause. In addition, some recorders can document alterations in QRS, ST, and T contours (Fig. 32-5).

AMBULATORY ELECTROCARDIOGRAPHIC (HOLTER) RECORDING. Continuous electrocardiographic tape recorders represent the traditional Holter monitor and typically record (on analog tape or digital cards) two or three electrocardiographic channels for 24 hours.[7] Interpretative accuracy of long-term recordings varies with the system used, but most computers that scan the recording media are sufficiently accurate to meet clinical needs. All systems can potentially record more information than the physician needs or can assimilate. As long as the system detects important episodes of ectopic activity, VT, or asystolic intervals and semiquantitates these abnormalities, the physician probably receives all the clinical information that is needed. Twenty-five to 50 percent of patients experience a complaint during a 24-hour recording, caused by an arrhythmia in 2 to 15 percent (see Fig. 32-6). The ability to correlate symptoms temporally with abnormalities in the ECG is one of the strengths of this technique.

Significant rhythm disturbances are fairly uncommon in healthy young persons. However, sinus bradycardia with heart rates of 35 to 40 beats/min, sinus arrhythmia with pauses exceeding 3 seconds, sinoatrial exit block, type 1 (Wenckebach) second-degree AV block (often during sleep), a wandering atrial pacemaker, junctional escape complexes, and premature atrial complexes (PACs) and PVCs are not necessarily abnormal. Frequent and complex atrial and ventricular rhythm disturbances are less commonly observed, however, and type II second-degree AV conduction disturbances (see Chap. 35) are not recorded in normal patients. Elderly patients (see Chap. 75) may have a higher prevalence of arrhythmias, some of which may be responsible for neurological symptoms (see Fig. 32-6). The long-term prognosis in asymptomatic healthy subjects with frequent and complex PVCs resembles that of the healthy

U.S. population, without an increased risk of death.

Most patients who have ischemic heart disease, particularly those after myocardial infarction (see Chaps. 50 and 51), exhibit PVCs when monitored for 6 to 24 hours. The frequency of PVCs progressively increases over the first several weeks, decreasing at about 6 months after infarction. Frequent and complex PVCs constitute an independent risk factor and are associated with a twofold to fivefold increased risk of cardiac or sudden death in patients after myocardial infarction. Evidence from the Cardiac Arrhythmia Suppression Trial (CAST) raises the possibility that the ventricular ectopy is a marker identifying the patient at risk rather than being causally related to sudden death, because PVC suppression with flecainide, encainide, or moricizine was associated with increased mortality compared with placebo.[8] Thus, the PVC may be an "innocent bystander," unrelated to the tachyarrhythmia producing sudden death. Although the mechanism responsible for the drug-induced exacerbation of mortality is not clear, it may relate to an increase in ischemia-produced conduction delay caused by sodium channel blocking drugs. Holter recordings have been used to determine the efficacy of ablation and antiarrhythmic drug therapy.

Long-term recording of the ECG also has exposed potentially serious arrhythmias and complex ventricular ectopy in patients with left ventricular hypertrophy as well as hypertrophic, dilated, and ischemic cardiomyopathies; in those with mitral valve prolapse (see Chap. 62); in those who have otherwise unexplained syncope (see Chap. 37) or transient vague cerebrovascular symptoms; in those with conduction disturbances, sinus node dysfunction, bradycardia-tachycardia syndrome, Wolff-Parkinson-White syndrome (see Chap. 35), increased QT dispersion, and pacemaker malfunction (see Chap. 34); and after thrombolytic therapy (see Chap. 82). It has been shown that asymptomatic atrial fibrillation occurs far more often than symptomatic episodes in patients with atrial fibrillation.[9] This has important implications for deciding whether a patient needs chronic anticoagulation based only on recurrent symptoms or a single recording of the ECG.

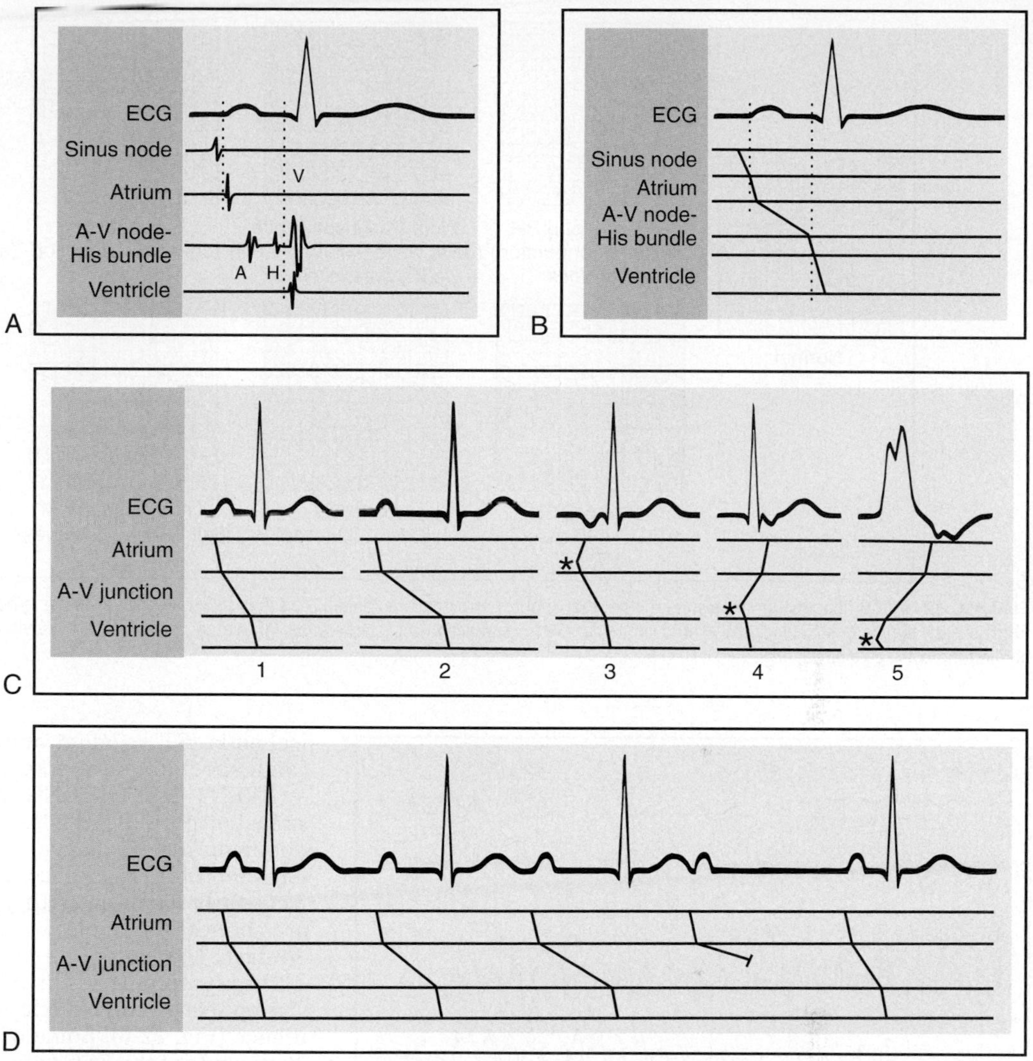

FIGURE 32–3 Intracardiac signals and ladder diagrams. **A,** A single beat is shown with accompanying intracardiac signals from the sinus node, right atrium, atrioventricular (AV) nodal and His bundle regions, and right ventricle. **B,** The same beat is shown with accompanying ladder diagram below. Cardiac regions have been divided into tiers separated by horizontal lines. Vertical dotted lines denote onset of P wave and QRS complexes. Note the relatively steep lines (rapid conduction through atrium, His bundle, and ventricular muscle) and more gently sloping lines as the impulse traverses the sinus and AV nodes (signifying slow conduction). **C,** Several different situations are depicted with accompanying explanatory ladder diagrams. Beat 1 is normal, as in **B**; beat 2 shows first-degree AV delay, with a more gradual slope than normal in the AV nodal tier, signifying very slow conduction in this region. In beat 3, an atrial premature complex is shown (starting in atrial tier as asterisk) producing an inverted P wave on electrocardiogram. In beat 4, an ectopic impulse arises in the His bundle (*) and propagates to the ventricle as well as retrogradely through the AV node to the atrium. In beat 5, a ventricular ectopic complex (*) conducts retrogradely through the His bundle and AV node and eventually to the atrium. **D,** A Wenckebach AV cycle (type 1 second-degree block) is shown. As the PR interval progressively increases from left to right in the figure, the slope of the line in the AV nodal region is progressively less steep until it fails to propagate at all after the fourth P wave (small line perpendicular to sloping AV nodal conduction line), after which the cycle repeats. A = atrial recording; ECG = electrocardiogram; H = His recording; V = ventricular recording.

Variations of Holter recording have been used for particular applications. Repeated 24-hour recording periods may be needed to obtain enough episodes of PAC triggering atrial fibrillation to warrant proceeding to an EPS and catheter ablation. Some monitoring systems are able to reconstruct a full 12-lead ECG from a seven-electrode recording system. This is especially useful when trying to document the electrocardiographic morphology of VT before an ablation procedure or a consistent morphology of PACs that may arise from an ablatable focus of atrial tachycardia or fibrillation. Most Holter recording and analysis systems can place a clearly recognizable deflection on the recording when a pacemaker stimulus is detected. This greatly facilitates diagnosis of potential pacemaker malfunction. Occasion-

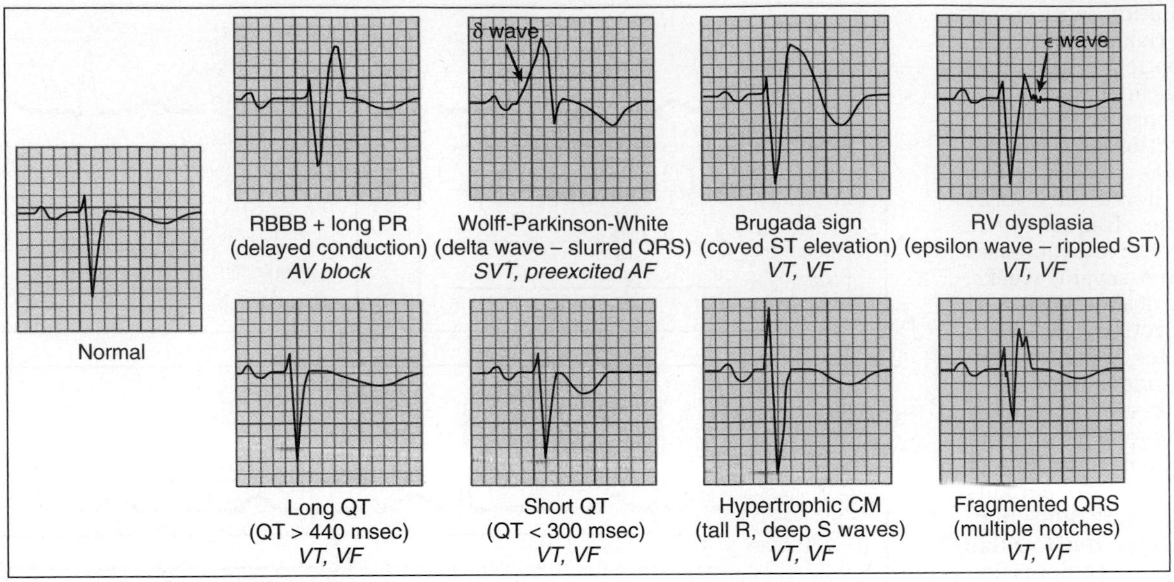

FIGURE 32–4 ECG abnormalities in resting rhythm that suggest arrhythmia potential. Lead V_1 is shown in each example; a normal complex is shown at left for reference. RBBB = right bundle branch block; AV = atrioventricular; SVT = supraventricular tachycardia; AF = atrial fibrillation; VT = ventricular tachycardia; VF = ventricular fibrillation; CM = cardiomyopathy.

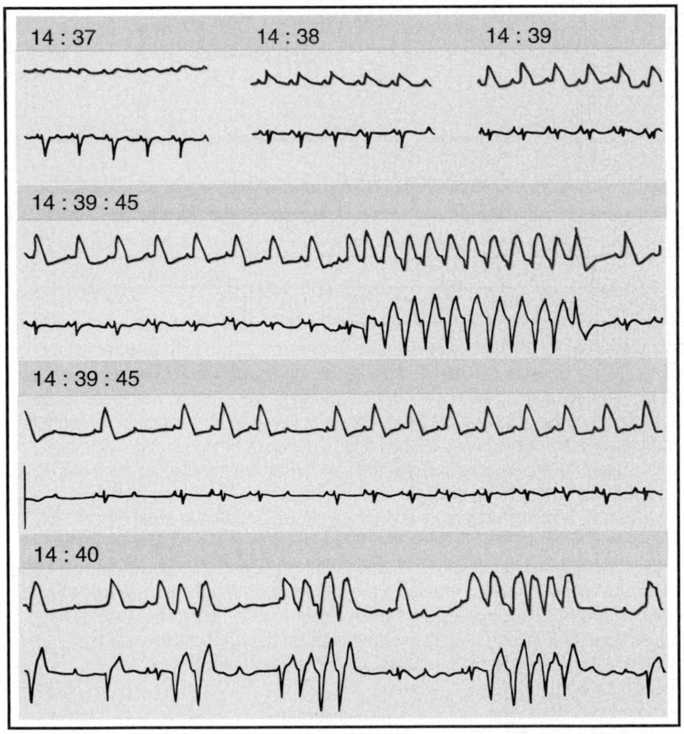

FIGURE 32–5 Long-term electrocardiographic recording in a patient with atypical angina. **Top channel,** Inferior lead. **Bottom channel,** Anterior lead. Note progressive ST segment elevation in the inferior lead, eventually resembling a monophasic action potential. Bursts of nonsustained ventricular tachycardia result. Sinus slowing and Wenckebach atrioventricular (AV) block then occur from a vasodepressor reflex response elicited by ischemia of the inferior myocardial wall or possibly caused by ischemia of the sinus and AV nodes. **Bottom tracing,** Both AV block and ventricular arrhythmias are apparent. Numbers indicate time (e.g., 14:37 = 2:37 P.M.). (Courtesy of D. A. Chilson, MD.)

ally, artifacts in the ECG caused by alterations in tape recording or playback speed can mimic bradycardias or tachycardias and lead to erroneous therapy. Newer digital Holter systems are less subject to this phenomenon. Finally, most systems can also provide heart rate variability data (see later). Use of these systems for detecting myocardial ischemia (ST segment analysis) has yielded mixed results (high specificity but poor sensitivity).

EVENT RECORDING. In many patients, the 24-hour snapshot provided by the Holter recording is incapable of documenting the cause of the patient's symptoms. Longer term monitoring is necessary in these cases, which occur frequently, such as with an event recorder. These devices are about the size of a pager and are kept by the patient for 30 days. During that time, digital recordings can be made during symptomatic episodes and transmitted to a receiving station over standard telephone lines at the patient's convenience (Fig. 32-6). Some of these recorders store more than 30 seconds of the ECG before the patient activates the recording. These loop recorders record continuously, but only a small window of time is present in memory at any time; when the event button is pressed by the patient, the current window is frozen while the device continues recording for another 30 to 60 seconds, depending on how it is configured. Event recorders are highly effective in documenting infrequent events, but the quality of the recordings is more variable than with Holter recorders, and usually only one channel can be recorded. Using some systems, the patient must be able to press the event button to begin recording; if syncope occurs without warning and the patient is not able to actuate the device, it cannot provide diagnostic information. With other systems, the device automatically begins recording the rhythm when the heart rate falls outside predetermined parameters. One system incorporates cell phone technology that automatically notifies a central monitoring facility when certain conditions are met (e.g., extreme bradycardia or tachycardia). In this way, the time between occurrence and effective treatment of serious arrhythmias can be significantly shortened.

Most currently available pacemakers and implantable defibrillators are capable of providing Holter-like data when premature beats or tachycardia episodes occur and can even store electrograms of these events from the implanted leads. The device can then be interrogated later and the electrograms printed for analysis.

IMPLANTABLE LOOP RECORDER. For patients with infrequent and transient symptoms, neither Holter recorders nor 30-day event recorders may yield diagnostic information. In such patients, implantable loop recorders may be used.[10] This device (about the size of a pack of chewing gum) is inserted under the skin at about the second rib on the left front of the chest and is activated by passing a special magnet over the device.[11] It is capable of recording up to 42 minutes of a single channel of the ECG that can be partitioned for one to seven episodes, with up to 20 minutes of the preactivation ECG saved for subsequent downloading to a programming unit for analysis. Both P waves and QRS complexes can usually be identified. The device can be configured to store patient-activated episodes, automatically activated recordings (heart rate outside preset parameters), or a combination of these (Fig. 32-7). In one report, this device was implanted in 24 patients with recurrent syncope who had undergone extensive evaluation without determining a cause of syncope. Over a mean 5-month period after implantation, 21 patients had recurrent syncope; the device was instrumental in establishing the diagnosis in 18 patients.[12,13]

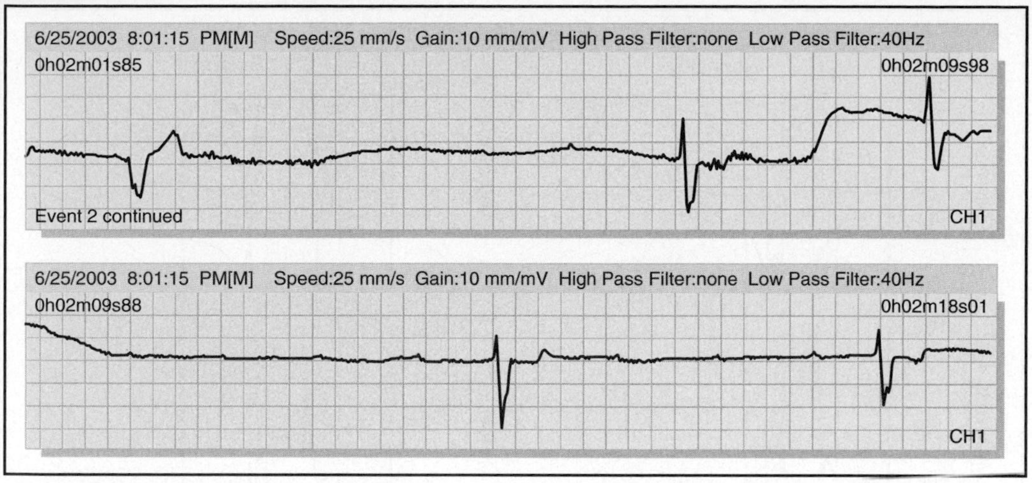

FIGURE 32-6 Continuous electrocardiographic recording from a patient-activated event monitor during an episode of lightheadedness. Sinus rhythm at 75 beats/min with sudden atrioventricular block is present with pauses of longer than 4 seconds and, in the bottom strip, there is an effective heart rate of about 8 beats/min.

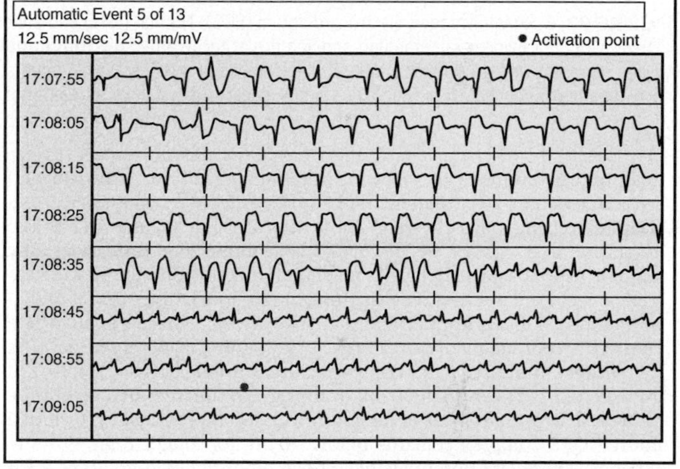

FIGURE 32-7 Recordings from an implantable loop recorder. Each line contains 10 seconds of continuous electrocardiogram from the implanted device. The first four lines show sinus rhythm with premature ventricular complexes; during the fifth line, short runs of atrial tachycardia precede an episode of a faster tachycardia with a different complex (ventricular tachycardia). This episode triggered an automatic activation (red circle) of the device recording (no symptoms associated with the episode).

Heart Rate Variability

Heart rate variability is used to evaluate vagal and sympathetic influences on the sinus node (inferring that the same activity is occurring in the ventricles also) and to identify patients at risk for a cardiovascular event or death.[14,15] Frequency domain analysis resolves parasympathetic and sympathetic influences better than time domain analysis, but both types of analysis are useful. R-R variability predicts all-cause mortality as well as left ventricular ejection fraction or nonsustained VT in patients after myocardial infarction and can be added to other measures of risk to enhance predictive accuracy. Similar results have been obtained in patients with dilated cardiomyopathy (see Chap. 64).[16] High-frequency components of R-R interval variability reflect tonic vagal activity. Reduced RR interval variability, the marker of increased risk, indicates loss or reduction of the physiological periodic sinus node fluctuations, which can be caused by many different influences and may not necessarily represent a particular shift in autonomic modulation. Some investigators have determined that simple heart rate measurement contains as much prognostic information as heart rate variability.[17]

Heart Rate Turbulence

Heart rate turbulence is an index of changes in sinus discharge rate following a PVC that is followed by a compensatory pause.[18] In normal individuals, the sinus rate initially accelerates and then slows; this phenomenon is blunted or absent in patients with various heart diseases.[19] Heart rate turbulence is a measure of reflex vagal control of the heart, whereas heart rate variability is more indicative of overall vagal tone.[20] Abnormal heart rate turbulence is a powerful independent predictor of mortality in patients with coronary artery disease and dilated cardiomyopathy; abnormal indices in some patients can be improved or normalized after treatment with beta blockers and statin drugs.[21]

QT Dispersion

Heterogeneity in refractoriness and conduction velocity is a hallmark of reentrant arrhythmias. One index of heterogeneity of ventricular refractoriness can be found in differences in length of the QT interval in surface leads of the ECG. The most commonly used index to calculate this QT dispersion has been the difference between the longest and shortest QT intervals on the 12-lead ECG, which is often adjusted for heart rate as well as number of leads sampled (when the T wave is flat in some). Other indices have been developed. Abnormally high QT dispersion has been correlated with risk of arrhythmic death in various disorders, although results are not consistent.[22,23] Its mechanism has been characterized in several disease states.[24] QT dispersion has been correlated with efficacy and proarrhythmic potential of drug therapy. Different techniques exist for determining dispersion (including automated algorithms), and the results of one study are often difficult to compare with those of another; in addition, the test is sensitive to age, time of day, season of the year, and even body position.[25] Overall, assessment of QT dispersion (from a standard 12-lead ECG) has not gained popularity as a useful clinical tool.

Signal-Averaged Electrocardiography and Late Potentials

Signal averaging is a method that improves signal-to-noise ratio when signals are recurrent and the noise is random.[26] In conjunction with appropriate filtering and other methods of noise reduction, signal averaging can detect cardiac signals of a few microvolts in amplitude, reducing noise amplitude, such as muscle potentials that are typically 5 to 25 mV, to less than 1 mV. With this method, very low-amplitude electrical potentials generated by the sinus and AV nodes, His bundle, and bundle branches are detectable at the body surface.

One constituent of reentrant ventricular arrhythmias in patients with prior myocardial damage is slow conduction. Direct cardiac

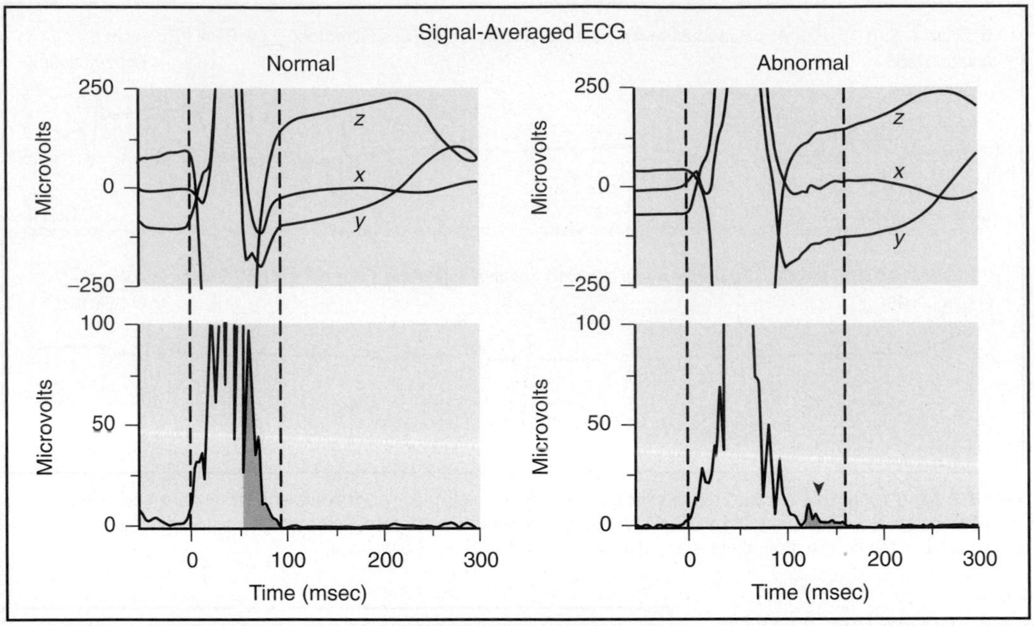

FIGURE 32–8 Signal-averaged electrocardiogram (ECG). Normal **(left)** and abnormal **(right)** results are shown from a patient with prior myocardial infarction and ventricular tachycardia. **Bottom panels,** Shaded blue areas at the end of each tracing represent voltage content of last 40 milliseconds of the filtered QRS integral. The small shaded area in the abnormal study denotes prolonged, slow conduction and suggests the potential for reentrant ventricular arrhythmias.

mapping techniques can record myocardial activation from damaged areas that occurs after the end of the surface electrocardiographic QRS complex during sinus rhythm. These delayed signals have a very low amplitude that cannot be discerned by routine electrocardiography and correspond to the delayed and fragmented conduction in the ventricles recorded with direct mapping techniques (Fig. 32-8). Signal averaging has been applied clinically most often to detect such late ventricular potentials of 1 to 25 mV. Criteria for late potentials are the following: (1) filtered QRS complex duration longer than 114 to 120 milliseconds; (2) less than 20 mV of root mean square signal amplitude in the last 40 milliseconds of the filtered QRS complex; and (3) terminal filtered QRS complex remains below 40 mV for longer than 39 milliseconds. These late potentials have been recorded in 70 to 90 percent of patients with spontaneous sustained and inducible VT after myocardial infarction, in only 0 to 6 percent of normal volunteers, and in 7 to 15 percent of patients after myocardial infarction who do not have VT. Late potentials can be detected as early as 3 hours after the onset of chest pain, increase in prevalence in the first week after myocardial infarction, and disappear in some patients after 1 year. If not present initially, late potentials usually do not appear later. Early use of thrombolytic agents may reduce the prevalence of late potentials after coronary occlusion. Patients with bundle branch block or paced ventricular rhythms already have wide QRS complexes, rendering the technique less useful in these cases.

Late potentials also have been recorded in patients with VT not related to ischemia, such as in dilated cardiomyopathies. Successful surgical resection of the VT can eliminate late potentials but is not necessary to cause tachycardia suppression. The presence of a late potential is a sensitive, but not specific, marker of arrhythmic risk and thus its prognostic use is limited.[27] In specific situations, it can be helpful; for example, a patient with a prior inferior wall myocardial infarction (normally the last portion of the heart to be activated) who has no late potential has a very low likelihood of having VT episodes.

The high-pass filtering used to record late potentials meeting the criteria just noted is called *time domain analysis* because the filter output corresponds in time to the input signal. Because late potentials are high-frequency signals, Fourier transform can be applied to extract high-frequency content from the signal-averaged ECG, called *frequency domain analysis.* Some data suggest that frequency domain analysis provides useful information not available in the time domain analysis.

Signal averaging has been applied to the P wave to determine the risk for developing atrial fibrillation (especially following cardiac surgery) as well as maintenance of sinus rhythm after cardioversion.[28,29] The overall use of the technique remains limited at present.

T Wave Alternans

Beat-to-beat alternation in the amplitude and/or morphology of the electrocardiographic recording of ventricular repolarization, the ST segment and T wave, has been found in conditions favoring the development of ventricular tachyarrhythmias, such as ischemia and long-QT syndrome and in patients with ventricular arrhythmias.[30] The electrophysiological basis appears to be the alternation of repolarization of ventricular myocytes. In the presence of a long QT interval, the cellular basis of alternation has been shown to be caused by beat-to-beat repolarization changes in midmyocardial cells (so called M cells).[31,32] Whether this mechanism applies to different disease states is not known.[33] T wave alternans testing requires exercise or atrial pacing to achieve a heart rate of 100 to 120 beats/min with relatively little atrial or ventricular ectopic activity. The test is less useful in patients with a wide QRS complex (longer than 120 milliseconds). A positive T wave alternans test (Fig. 32-9) is associated with a worse arrhythmic prognosis in various disorders, including ischemic heart disease and nonischemic cardiomyopathy.[34,35] The test's greatest usefulness appears to be in the detection of a group of patients with low risk of developing malignant ventricular arrhythmias (negative T wave alternans test). Although the predictive value of a positive test varies greatly, depending on the population studied, a negative test result strongly predicts freedom from VT and VF in all group studies thus far, at least over a short follow-up period. This has important implications for implantable cardioverter-defibrillator (ICD) use in high-risk patients who have not yet manifested dangerous arrhythmias (primary prevention or prophylactic devices).[36] A significant proportion of these patients will never benefit from these devices (lack of spontaneous VT/VF), and some investigators have suggested that T wave alternans testing may segregate those who are more likely to benefit from ICD use (positive test) from those who are not (negative test), and who should therefore not undergo ICD implantation.[37] Further studies are necessary in this area.[38] T wave alternans may represent a fundamental marker of an electrically unstable myocardium prone to developing VT or VF, and, as such, ST-T wave analysis for alternans may be increasingly useful in the future as a method to risk-stratify patients.

Baroreceptor Reflex Sensitivity Testing

Acute blood pressure elevation triggers a baroreceptor reflex that augments vagal tone to the heart and slows the sinus rate. The increase in sinus cycle length per millimeter of mercury systolic blood pressure increase is a measure of the sensitivity of the baroreceptor reflex and, when reduced, identifies patients susceptible to developing VT and VF.[15] The mechanism of the reduction in baroreceptor reflex sensitivity is not certain. However, this test may be useful to identify patients at risk for developing a serious ventricular arrhythmia after myocardial infarction.

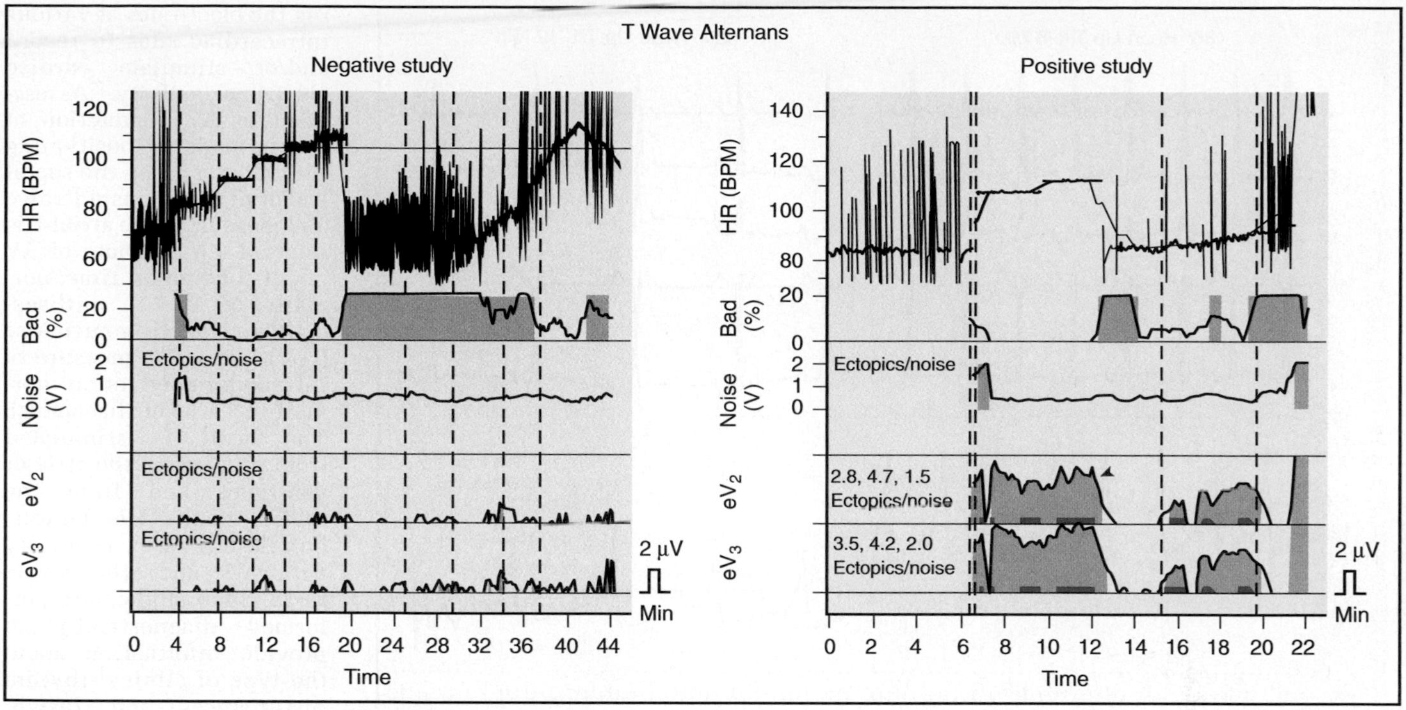

FIGURE 32–9 T wave alternans. Reports of T wave alternans analysis from two patients are shown, displaying heart rate (HR) in beats/min (BPM), proportion of beats rejected from analysis (% Bad), electrocardiogram noise level (in microvolts), and selected precordial leads (V_2 and V_3) as a function of time. **Left panel,** Records from a patient with no structural heart disease; the amplitude of T wave alternans was minimal. **Right panel,** Records from a patient hospitalized for sustained ventricular tachycardia after myocardial infarction shows T wave alternans (blue shaded area, arrow).

Body Surface Mapping

Isopotential body surface maps are used to provide a complete picture of the effects of the currents from the heart on the body surface. The potential distributions are represented by contour lines of equal potential, and each distribution is displayed instant by instant throughout activation, recovery, or both.

Body surface maps have been used clinically to localize and size areas of myocardial ischemia,[39] localize ectopic foci or accessory pathways,[40] differentiate aberrant supraventricular conduction from ventricular origin, recognize the patient prone to developing arrhythmias, and possibly understand the mechanisms involved. Although these procedures are of interest, their clinical usefulness has not yet been established. In addition, the technique is cumbersome and the analysis is complex.

Electrocardiographic Imaging

Another promising technology is electrocardiographic imaging, in which cardiac electrical activity recorded at the skin surface is spatially integrated with imaging data (currently, cardiac CT scanning).[41] Using complex mathematical processing of electrical data collected from 224 electrodes on the skin surface, this technique can plot atrial and ventricular electrical activity on a "shell" of the patient's own heart and thereby follow the course of activation during sinus rhythm or an arrhythmia. Clinical experience is extremely limited thus far.[42]

Upright Tilt-Table Testing

The tilt-table test is used to identify patients who have a vasodepressor and/or cardioinhibitory response as a cause of syncope (see Chap. 37).[43] Patients are positioned on a tilt table in the supine position and are tilted upright to a maximum of 60 to 80 degrees for 20 to 45 minutes, or longer if necessary (Fig. 32-10). Isoproterenol, as a bolus or infusion, may provoke syncope in patients whose initial upright tilt-table test result shows no abnormalities or after just several minutes of tilt to shorten the time of the test necessary to produce a positive response. An initial intravenous isoproterenol dose of 1 mg/min can be increased in 0.5-mg/min steps until symptoms occur or a maximum of 4 mg/min is given. Isoproterenol induces a vasodepressor response in upright susceptible patients, generally consisting of a decrease in heart rate and blood pressure along with near-syncope or syncope. Intravenous edrophonium chloride, nitroglycerin, and esmolol withdrawal have also been used. Atropine can block the early bradycardia but not the hypotension; beta blockers can inhibit the latter. Tilt-table test results are positive in two thirds to three fourths of patients susceptible to neurally mediated syncope and are reproducible in about 80 percent, but have a 10 to 15 percent false-positive response rate. Repeating an initially negative tilt-table test on a subsequent day rarely yields a positive result. A positive test result is more meaningful when it reproduces symptoms that have occurred spontaneously. Positive responses can be divided into cardioinhibitory, vasodepressor, and mixed categories. Therapy with beta blockers, disopyramide, theophylline, selective serotonin reuptake inhibitors, midodrine, and salt loading or fludrocortisone have each been reported to be successful, as has tilt training, in which the patient leans against a wall for prolonged periods to increase tolerance to this body position.

Mechanism. Vasodepressor reactions, which are thought to be caused by activation of unmyelinated left ventricular vagal C fibers, can be triggered by various events, including increased left ventricular pressure (see Chap. 37). Stimulation of C fibers from vigorous left ventricular contraction on a relatively empty cavity reduces efferent sympathetic tone while increasing efferent vagal tone, possibly producing vasodepression caused by vasodilation and paradoxical bradycardia. Isoproterenol increases left ventricular contractility while reducing left ventricular volume. A passive upright tilt exaggerates these responses, because the tilt also reduces venous return and prevents isoproterenol from increasing cardiac output. Some patients may experience profound bradycardia, whereas others may have a prominent vasodepressor component. Dual-chamber pacing has been shown to benefit some patients with refractory neurocardiogenic syncope. Before pacemaker implantation, some investigators have advocated performing a tilt-table test with temporary pacing catheters in place to simulate how a permanent pacing system would perform; however, correlation between this type of acute testing and long-term pacing results has not been proven.

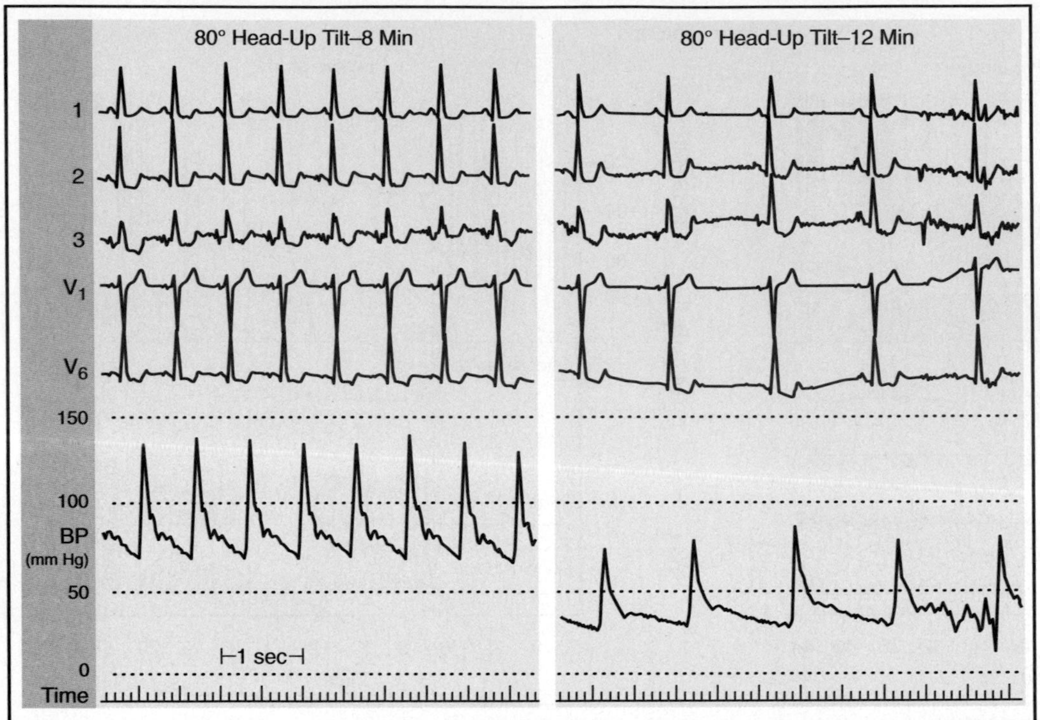

FIGURE 32–10 Head-up tilt-table testing. Surface electrocardiogram leads and an arterial blood pressure (BP) tracing are shown. **Left,** After 8 minutes of head-up tilt at 80 degrees, heart rate and BP were normal and the patient was asymptomatic. **Right,** Four minutes later, systolic BP dropped precipitously to 80 mm Hg, the heart rate fell to 50 beats/min, and the patient lost consciousness. The electrocardiographic artifact at right is seizure activity.

A variant of the neurocardiogenic response, the postural orthostatic tachycardia syndrome (POTS), is characterized by dramatic increases in heart rate during the first 10 minutes of tilt-table testing.[44] POTS appears to be distinct from simple orthostatic hypotension as well as standard neurocardiogenic responses and is thought to be caused by various forms of autonomic imbalance. Relief of symptoms has been effected with fludrocortisone, beta blockers, or combinations.[45]

Esophageal Electrocardiography

Esophageal electrocardiography is a useful noninvasive technique to diagnose arrhythmias. The esophagus is located immediately behind the left atrium, between the left and right pulmonary veins. An electrode in the lumen of the esophagus can record atrial potentials. Bipolar recording is superior to unipolar recording because far-field ventricular events with the former method can lead to possible diagnostic confusion. In addition, atrial and occasionally ventricular pacing can be performed by means of a catheter electrode inserted into the esophagus, and tachycardias can be initiated and terminated. Optimal electrode position for atrial pacing correlates with patient height and is within about 1 cm of the site at which the maximum amplitude of the atrial electrogram is recorded. When recorded simultaneously with the surface ECG, the esophageal atrial electrogram can be used to differentiate SVT with aberrancy from VT and to define the mechanism of SVTs. For example, if atrial and ventricular depolarizations occur simultaneously during a narrow QRS tachycardia, reentry using an accessory AV pathway (Wolff-Parkinson-White syndrome) can be excluded, and AV nodal reentry is the most likely mechanism for the tachycardia. Complications of transesophageal recording and pacing are uncommon, but the technique is not comfortable for most patients and it is therefore not commonly used.

INVASIVE ELECTROPHYSIOLOGICAL STUDIES

An invasive EPS involves introducing multipolar catheter electrodes into the venous and/or arterial system, positioning the electrodes at various intracardiac sites to record and/or stimulate cardiac electrical activity. Assessment of AV conduction at rest is made by positioning the catheter along the septal leaflet of the tricuspid valve and measuring the atrial-His interval (an estimate of AV nodal conduction time; normally, 60 to 125 milliseconds) and the His-ventricular (H-V) interval (a measure of infranodal conduction; normally, 35 to 55 milliseconds). The heart is stimulated from portions of the atria or ventricles and from the region of the His bundle, bundle branches, accessory pathways, and other structures. Such studies are performed diagnostically to provide information about the type of clinical rhythm disturbances and insight into its electrophysiological mechanism. An EPS is used therapeutically to terminate a tachycardia by electrical stimulation or electroshock, to evaluate the effects of therapy by determining whether a particular intervention modifies or prevents electrical induction of a tachycardia or whether an electrical device properly senses and terminates an induced tachyarrhythmia, and to ablate myocardium involved in the tachycardia to prevent further episodes. Finally, these tests have been used prognostically to identify patients at risk for sudden cardiac death. The study may be helpful in patients who have AV block, intraventricular conduction disturbance, sinus node dysfunction, tachycardia, and unexplained syncope or palpitations (see Chap. 35).

The EPS is effective at initiating VT or SVT when these have occurred spontaneously. This enables the use of similar stimulation techniques after an intervention (e.g., drug therapy or surgical or catheter ablation) to assess treatment efficacy. However, false-negative responses—not finding a particular electrical abnormality known to be present—as well as false-positive responses—induction of a nonclinical arrhythmia—may complicate interpretation of the results because many lack reproducibility. Altered autonomic tone in a supine patient undergoing study, hemodynamic or ischemic influences, changing anatomy (e.g., new infarction) after the study, day-to-day variability, and the fact that the test uses an artificial trigger (electrical stimulation) to induce the arrhythmia are several of many factors that may explain the occasional disparity between test results and spontaneous clinical occurrences. Overall, the diagnostic validity and reproducibility of these studies are good, and they are safe when performed by skilled clinical electrophysiologists.

AV BLOCK (see Chap. 35). In patients with AV block, the site of block usually dictates the clinical course of the patient and whether a pacemaker is needed. Generally, the site of AV block can be determined from an analysis of the scalar ECG. When the site of block cannot be determined from such an analysis, and when knowing that the site of block is imperative for patient management, an invasive EPS is indicated. Candidates include symptomatic patients in whom His-Purkinje block is suspected but not established and patients with AV block treated with a pacemaker who continue to be symptomatic, in whom a causal ventricular tachyarrhythmia is sought. Possible candidates are those with second- or third-degree AV block for whom information about the site of block or its mechanism may help direct therapy or assess prognosis and patients suspected of having concealed His bundle extrasystoles. Patients with block in the His-Purkinje system become symptomatic because of periods of bradycardia or asystole and require pacemaker implantation more often than patients who have AV nodal block. Type I (Wenckebach) AV block in older patients may have clinical implications similar to those for type II AV block. The results of EPS for evaluating the conduction system must be interpreted with caution, however. In rare cases, the process of recording conduction intervals alters their values. For example, catheter pressure on the AV node or His bundle can cause a prolongation of the atrial-His or H-V interval and lead to erroneous diagnosis and therapy.

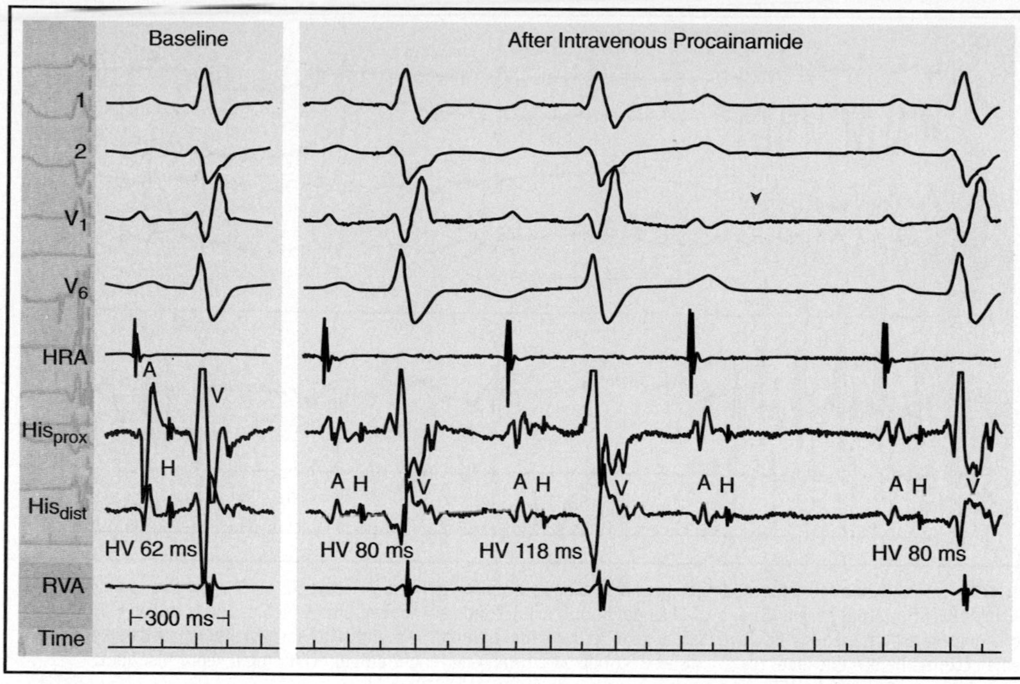

FIGURE 32–11 Testing the His-Purkinje system. A 43-year-old woman with sarcoid underwent electrophysiological study after a syncopal episode. Surface leads 1, 2, V_1, and V_6 are shown, with intracardiac recordings from catheters in the high right atrium (HRA), proximal (His_{prox}), and distal (His_{dist}) electrode pairs of a catheter at the atrioventricular junction to record the His potential, and right ventricular apex (RVA). During baseline recording, the H-V interval is only slightly prolonged (62 milliseconds). After infusion of intravenous procainamide, the H-V interval is longer and infra-His Wenckebach block is present. The arrow denotes the missing QRS complex caused by infra-His block. A = atrial electrogram; H = His potential; V = ventricular electrogram.

INTRAVENTRICULAR CONDUCTION DISTURBANCE. For patients with an intraventricular conduction disturbance, an EPS provides information about the duration of the H-V interval, which can be prolonged with a normal PR interval or normal with a prolonged PR interval. A prolonged H-V interval (longer than 55 milliseconds) is associated with a greater likelihood of developing trifascicular block (but the rate of progression is slow, 2 to 3 percent annually), having structural disease, and higher mortality. Finding very long H-V intervals (longer than 80 to 90 milliseconds) identifies patients at increased risk of developing AV block. The H-V interval has a high specificity (approximately 80 percent) but low sensitivity (approximately 66 percent) for predicting the development of complete AV block. During the study, atrial pacing is used to uncover abnormal His-Purkinje conduction. A positive response is provocation of distal His block during 1 : 1 AV nodal conduction. Again, sensitivity is low but specificity is high. Functional His-Purkinje block caused by normal His-Purkinje refractoriness is not a positive response. Drug infusion, such as that with procainamide or ajmaline, sometimes exposes abnormal His-Purkinje conduction (Fig. 32-11). Ajmaline (not available in the United States) can cause arrhythmias and should be used cautiously.

An EPS is indicated in the patient with symptoms (syncope or presyncope) that appear to be related to a bradyarrhythmia or tachyarrhythmia when no other cause of symptoms is found. For many of these patients, ventricular tachyarrhythmias rather than AV block can be the cause of their symptoms.

SINUS NODE DYSFUNCTION (see Chap. 35). The demonstration of slow sinus rates, sinus exit block, or sinus pauses temporally related to symptoms suggests a causal relationship and usually obviates further diagnostic studies. Carotid sinus pressure that results in several seconds of complete cardiac asystole or AV block and reproduces the patient's usual symptoms exposes the presence of a hypersensitive carotid sinus reflex. Carotid sinus massage must be done cautiously. Rarely, carotid sinus massage can precipitate a stroke. Neurohumoral agents, adenosine, or stress testing can be used to evaluate the effects of autonomic tone on sinus node automaticity and sinoatrial conduction time (SACT). An EPS should be considered in patients who have symptoms attributable to bradycardia or asystole, such as presyncope or syncope, and for whom noninvasive approaches have provided no explanation for the symptoms.

Sinus Node Recovery Time. Sinus node recovery time (SNRT) is a technique that can be useful to evaluate sinus node function. The interval between the last paced high right atrial response and first spontaneous (sinus) high right atrial response after termination of pacing is measured to determine the SNRT. Because the spontaneous sinus rate influences the SNRT, the value is corrected by subtracting the spontaneous sinus node cycle length (before pacing) from the SNRT (Fig. 32-12). This value, the corrected SNRT (CSNRT), is generally shorter than 525 milliseconds. Prolonged CSNRT has been found in patients suspected of having sinus node dysfunction. Direct recordings of the sinus node electrogram have documented that SNRT is influenced by the prolongation of sinoatrial conduction time (the time from the onset of the sinus impulse to the onset of activation of surrounding atrial myocardium), as well as by changes in sinus node automaticity, especially in the first beat after cessation of pacing. After cessation of pacing, the first return sinus cycle can be normal and can be followed by secondary pauses. Secondary pauses appear to be more common in patients whose sinus node dysfunction is caused by sinoatrial exit block (a potential cause of electrocardiographic sinus pauses). Finally, it is important to evaluate AV node and His-Purkinje function in patients with sinus node dysfunction, because many also exhibit impaired AV conduction.

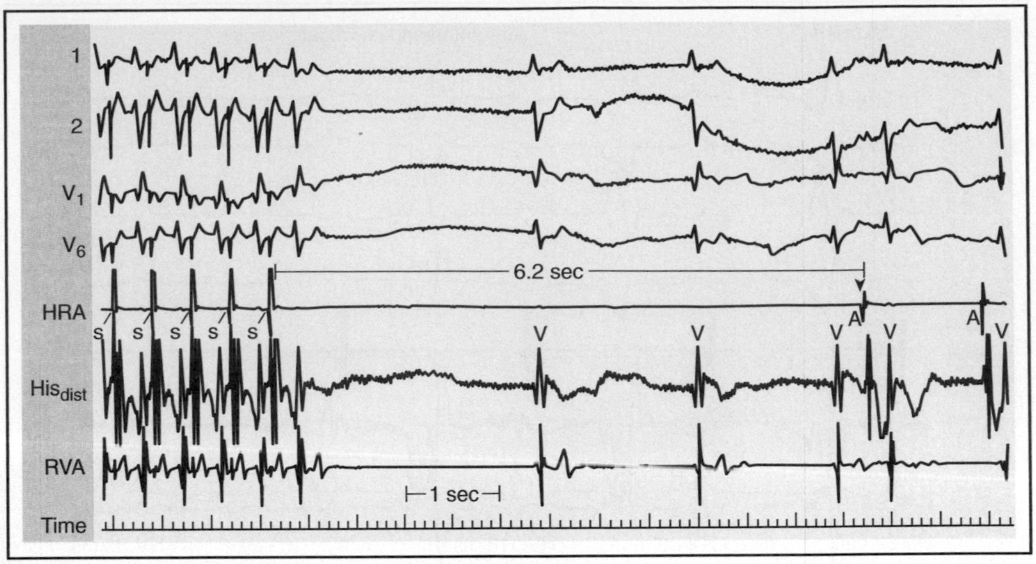

FIGURE 32–12 Abnormal sinus node function. Recordings are similar to those in Figure 32-11. The last five complexes of a 1-minute burst of atrial pacing (S) at a cycle length of 400 milliseconds are shown, after which pacing is stopped. The sinus node does not spontaneously discharge (sinus node recovery time) until 6.2 seconds later (arrow). Three junctional escape beats occurred before this time. His_{dist} = distal electrode pair; HRA = high right atrium; RVA = right ventricular apex.

Sinoatrial Conduction Time. The SACT can be estimated using simple pacing techniques based on the assumptions that (1) conduction times into and out of the sinus node are equal, (2) no depression of sinus node automaticity occurs, and (3) the pacemaker site does not shift after premature stimulation (see Chap. 32). These assumptions can be erroneous, particularly in patients with sinus node dysfunction. SACT can also be measured directly with extracellular electrodes placed in the region of the sinus node. This direct measurement correlates well with the SACT measured indirectly in patients with normal sinus node function. The sensitivity of the SACT and SNRT tests is only about 50 percent for each test alone and about 65 percent when combined. The specificity, when combined, is about 88 percent, with a low predictive value. Thus, if these tests are abnormal, the likelihood of the patient having sinus node dysfunction is great. However, normal results do not exclude the possibility of sinus node disease. Candidates for invasive EPS to evaluate sinus node function are symptomatic patients in whom sinus node dysfunction has not been established as a cause of the symptoms. Potential candidates are those requiring pacemakers to determine the pacing modality, patients with sinus node dysfunction to determine the mechanism and response to therapy, and patients in whom other causes of symptoms (e.g., tachyarrhythmias) are to be excluded.

TACHYCARDIA (see Chap. 35). In patients with tachycardias, an EPS can be used to diagnose the arrhythmia, determine and deliver therapy, determine the anatomical site(s) involved in the tachycardia, identify patients at high risk for developing serious arrhythmias, and gain insights into mechanisms responsible for the arrhythmia. The study can differentiate aberrant supraventricular conduction from ventricular tachyarrhythmias when standard electrocardiographic criteria fail to make the differentiation.

An SVT is recognized electrophysiologically by the presence of an H-V interval equaling or exceeding that recorded during normal sinus rhythm (Fig. 32-13). In contrast, during VT, the H-V interval is shorter than normal or the His deflection cannot be recorded clearly because of superimposition of the larger ventricular electrogram. Only two situations exist in which a consistently short H-V interval occurs, during retrograde activation of the His bundle from activation originating in the ventricle (i.e., PVC or VT) or during conduction over an accessory pathway (preexcitation syndrome). Atrial pacing at rates exceeding the tachycardia rate can demonstrate the ventricular origin of the wide QRS tachycardia by producing fusion and capture beats and normalization of the H-V interval. The only VT that exhibits an H-V interval equal to or slightly exceeding the normal sinus H-V interval is bundle branch reentry, but His activation will be in the retrograde direction.

An EPS should be considered for the following: (1) in patients who have symptomatic, recurrent, or drug-resistant supraventricular or ventricular tachyarrhythmias to help select optimal therapy; (2) in patients with tachyarrhythmias occurring too infrequently to permit adequate diagnostic or therapeutic assessment; (3) in differentiating SVT and aberrant conduction from VT; (4) whenever nonpharmacological therapy, such as the use of electrical devices, catheter ablation, or surgery, is contemplated; (5) in patients surviving an episode of cardiac arrest, occurring 48 hours after an acute myocardial infarction or without evidence of an acute Q wave myocardial infarction; and (6) in assessing the risk of sustained VT in patients with a prior myocardial infarction, ejection fraction of 0.3 to 0.4, and nonsustained VT on an ECG. Generally, EPS is not indicated in patients with long-QT syndrome and torsades de pointes.

The process of initiation and termination of SVT or VT with programmed electrical stimulation to test the potential efficacy of pharmacological, electrical, or surgical therapy represents an important application of EPS in patients with tachycardia. The role of drug therapy in clinically significant arrhythmias continues to diminish; although EPS was once widely used to predict the efficacy of drug therapy in suppressing spontaneous tachycardia recurrences, the technique is now rarely used for this purpose. Noninvasive stimulation from an implanted pacemaker or defibrillator can be used to test the effects of drug therapy given to try to decrease arrhythmia frequency.[46]

UNEXPLAINED SYNCOPE (see Chap. 37). The three common arrhythmic causes of syncope include sinus node dysfunction, AV block, and tachyarrhythmias. Of the three, tachyarrhythmias are most reliably initiated in the electrophysiology laboratory, followed by sinus node abnormalities and His-Purkinje block.[47]

The cause of syncope remains uncertain in up to 50 percent of patients, depending in part on the extent of the evaluation. A careful, accurately performed history and physical examination begin the evaluation,[1] followed by noninvasive tests, including a 12-lead ECG, and can lead to a diagnosis in 50 percent or more of patients. A small percentage (less than 5 percent) of patient develop an arrhythmia coincident with syncope or presyncope during a 24-hour recording of the ECG, whereas a larger percentage (15 percent) have symptoms without an arrhythmia, excluding an arrhythmic cause. Prolonged electrocardiographic monitoring with patient-activated transtelephonic event recorders that have memory loops may increase the yield. Signal averaging has a high sensitivity (approximately 75 percent) and specificity (approximately 90 percent) for predicting patients with syncope in whom VT can be induced at EPS.[27]

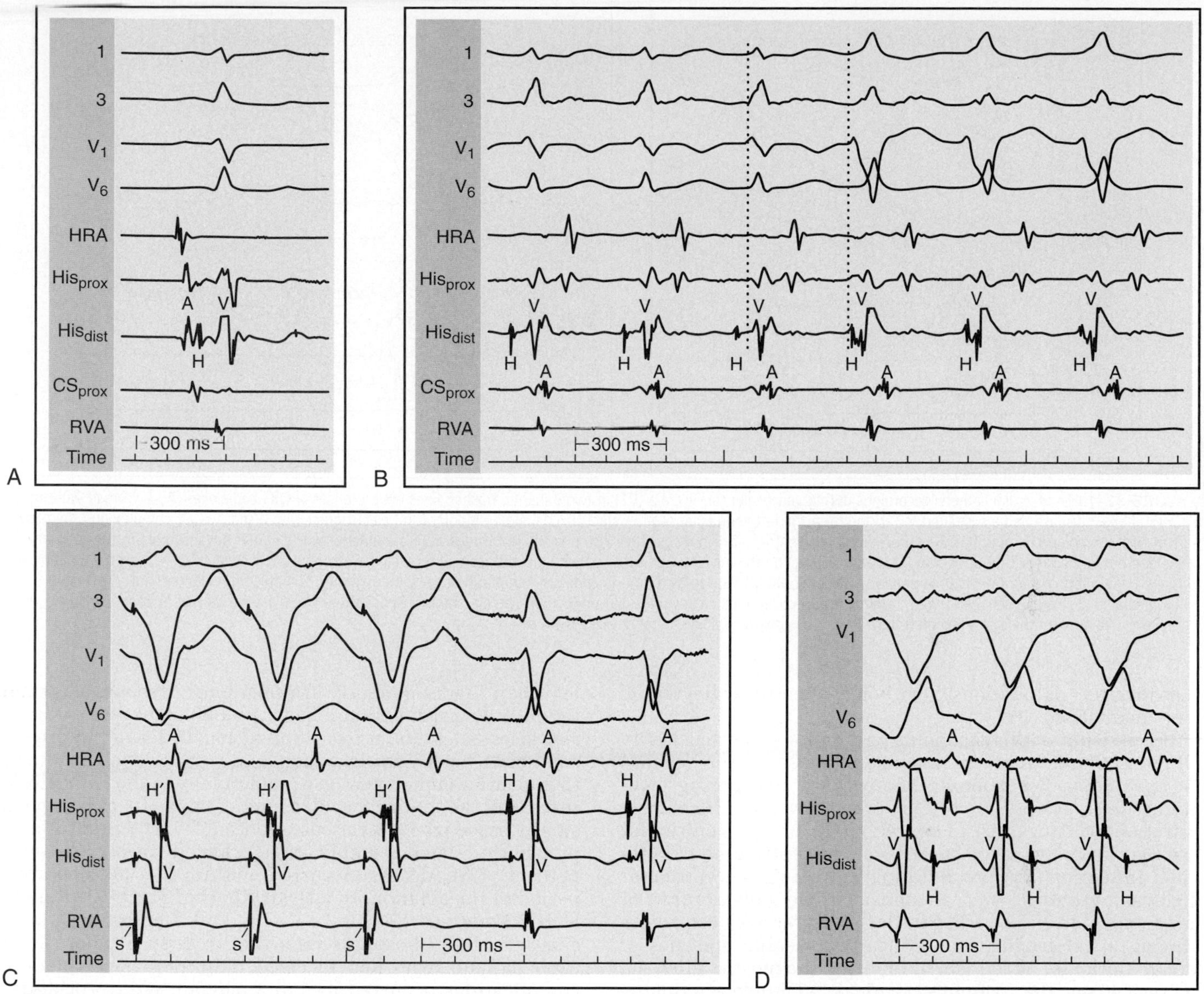

FIGURE 32–13 Bundle of His recordings in different situations similar to those in prior figures (see Figs. 32-11 and 32-12). **A,** Baseline sinus rhythm with normal atrioventricular (AV) conduction. **B,** Orthodromic supraventricular tachycardia with retrograde conduction over a left-sided accessory pathway throughout the tracing. The first three beats have a narrow QRS complex with a normal H-V interval; the last three QRS complexes represent a fusion of conduction over the AV node–His and a slowly conducting right-sided accessory pathway. The His potential occurs after the onset of the wide QRS complex (dashed lines). **C,** Three paced ventricular beats are shown with a retrograde His potential (H′), followed by initiation of AV node reentrant supraventricular tachycardia (atrial depolarization near the end of the QRS complex, as seen in HRA tracing). **D,** Ventricular tachycardia with delayed activation of the His potential and complete retrograde AV node block (dissociated atrial complexes). CS_{prox} = proximal coronary sinus; His_{dist} = distal electrode pair; His_{prox} = proximal electrode pair; HRA = high right atrium; RVA = right ventricular apex.

Tilt-table and stress testing can be useful for some patients, as can long-term electrocardiographic recordings.

The EPS helps explain the cause of syncope or palpitations when it induces an arrhythmia that replicates the patient's symptoms. Syncopal patients with a nondiagnostic EPS have a low incidence of sudden death and an 80 percent remission rate. In those with recurrent syncope, the test is falsely negative in 20 percent because of failure to find AV block or sinus node dysfunction. On the other hand, in many patients with structural heart disease, several abnormalities that could account for syncope can be diagnosed at EPS. Deciding which among these abnormalities is responsible for syncope and therefore requires therapy can be difficult. Mortality and incidence of sudden cardiac death are mainly determined by the presence of underlying heart disease.[48]

Syncopal patients considered for an EPS are those whose spells remain undiagnosed despite general, neurological, and noninvasive cardiac evaluation, particularly if the patient has structural heart disease. The diagnostic yield is about 70 percent in that group but only about 12 percent in patients without structural heart disease.[49] Therapy for a putative cause found during an EPS prevents recurrence of syncope in about 80 percent of patients. Among arrhythmic causes of syncope, intermittent conduction disturbances are the most difficult to diagnose. EPS is poor at establishing this diagnosis, despite an array of provocative tests that can be used. When tachyarrhythmias have been thoroughly sought and excluded and the clinical suspicion of intermittent heart block is high (e.g., bundle branch block or long HV interval), empirical permanent pacing may be justified.

PALPITATIONS. An EPS is indicated in patients with palpitations who have had a pulse documented by medical personnel to be inappropriately rapid without electrocardiographic recording or in those suspected of having clinically

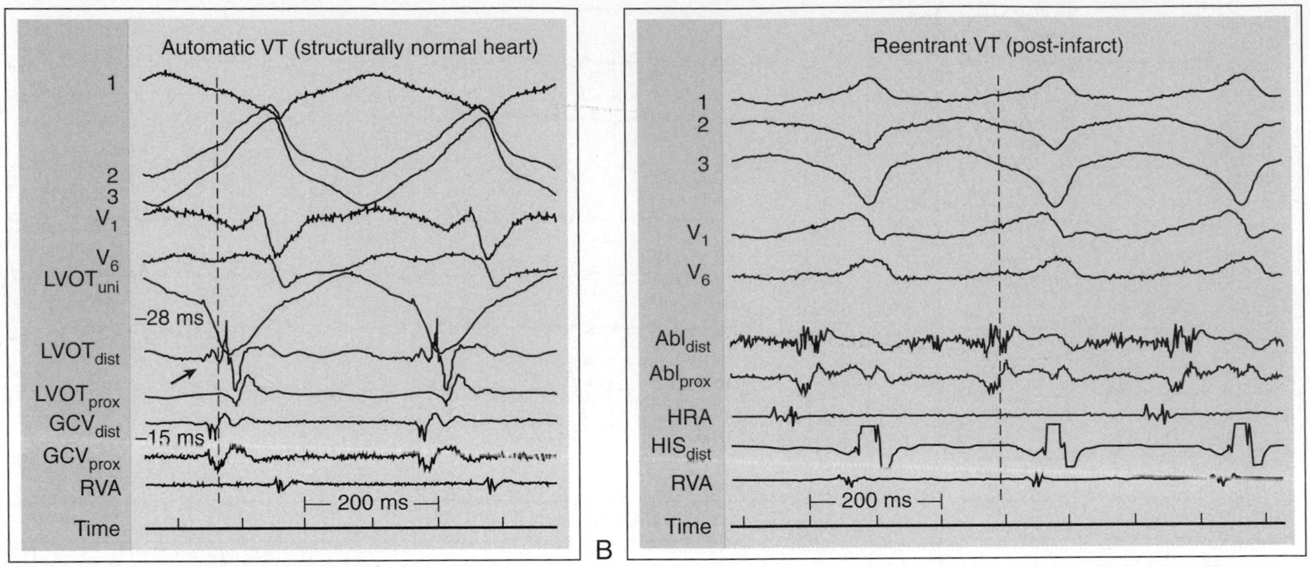

FIGURE 32–14 Endocardial catheter recordings during ventricular tachycardia (VT) in two patients. Dashed lines denote onset of QRS complexes. **A,** A woman without structural heart disease had a sustained VT arising from the left ventricular outflow tract (LVOT). Note unipolar (uni) electrogram with a sharp "QS" complex and the onset (arrow) distal bipolar recording ($LVOT_{dist}$) preceding right ventricular recordings. They also precede recordings from a multielectrode catheter advanced along the coronary sinus and down the great cardiac vein (GCV_{dist} and GCV_{prox}) on the epicardial surface opposite the endocardial recording. Retrograde 1:1 conduction is present. Ablation at this site (LVOT) terminated the VT. **B,** A patient with reentrant VT caused by a prior inferior wall infarction underwent mapping. The ablation catheter (Abl_{dist}) on the inferomedial wall shows a very prolonged, fragmented electrogram indicative of slow conduction. The electrogram spans the entire diastolic interval between QRS complexes. Ablation at this site eliminated the VT. Abl_{prox} = proximal ablation catheter electrodes.

significant palpitations without electrocardiographic documentation.

In patients with syncope or palpitations, the sensitivity of the EPS may be low but may be increased at the expense of specificity. For example, more aggressive pacing techniques (e.g., using three or four premature stimuli), administration of drugs (e.g., isoproterenol), or left ventricular pacing can increase the success rate of ventricular arrhythmia induction by precipitating nonclinical ventricular tachyarrhythmias, such as nonsustained polymorphic or monomorphic VT or VF. Similarly, aggressive techniques during atrial pacing can induce nonspecific episodes of atrial flutter or atrial fibrillation. A diagnostic dilemma arises when the patient's clinical, symptom-producing arrhythmia is one of these nonspecific arrhythmias that can be produced in the normal patient who has no arrhythmia. In most patients, these arrhythmias are regarded as nonclinical (i.e., nonspecific responses to intense stimulation). In other patients, such as those with hypertrophic or dilated nonischemic cardiomyopathy, these may be clinically relevant arrhythmias. However, induction of a sustained SVT (e.g., AV nodal reentry, AV-reciprocating tachycardia) or monomorphic VT is almost never an artifact of intense stimulation. Initiation of these arrhythmias in patients who have not had known spontaneous episodes of these tachycardias is uncommon and provides important information—for example, the induced tachyarrhythmia may be clinically significant and responsible for the patient's symptoms. Generally, other abnormalities, such as prolonged sinus pauses after overdrive atrial pacing or His-Purkinje AV block, are not induced in patients who do not or may not experience these abnormalities spontaneously. Induction of these arrhythmias has a high degree of specificity.

Complications of Electrophysiological Studies

The risks of undergoing only an EPS are small. Because most procedures do not involve left-sided heart access, risk of stroke, systemic embolism, or myocardial infarction is less than that of coronary arteriography. Myocardial perforation with cardiac tamponade, pseudoaneurysms at arterial access sites, and provocation of nonclinical arrhythmias can occur, each with less than 1 in 500 incidence. Adding therapeutic maneuvers (e.g., ablation) to the procedure increases the incidence of complications. In a European survey based on 4398 patients reported from 68 institutions, procedure-related complications ranged from 3.2 to 8 percent. Five deaths occurred within the perioperative period of the ablation. In a Heart Rhythm Society (formerly North American Society of Pacing and Electrophysiology) survey[50] of 164 hospitals reporting in 1998 on more than 3300 patients who had received radiofrequency ablation, complications occurred in 1 to 3 percent, with procedure-related deaths in about 0.2 percent. In a study of 1050 patients undergoing temperature-controlled ablation for supraventricular arrhythmias, 32 (3 percent) had a major complication. Predictors of major complications were ejection fraction less than 0.35 and multiple ablation targets. The improvement in the complication rate probably reflects the learning curve for radiofrequency ablation. In many centers, a diagnostic EPS and even ablation procedures are performed on an outpatient basis. With the increasing use of extensive ablation in the left atrium to treat atrial fibrillation, an increase in systemic thromboembolic complications has been observed, as have pericardial effusion and tamponade, valve damage, and phrenic nerve injury (see Chap. 35).

DIRECT CARDIAC MAPPING: RECORDING POTENTIALS DIRECTLY FROM THE HEART

Cardiac mapping is a method whereby potentials recorded directly from the heart are spatially depicted as a function of time in an integrated manner (Fig. 32-14). The location of recording electrodes (e.g., epicardial, intramural, or endocardial) and the recording mode used (unipolar versus bipolar), as well as the method of display (isopotential versus isochronous maps), depend on the problem under consideration. Special electrodes can record monophasic action potentials.

Direct cardiac mapping by catheter electrodes, or, less commonly, at the time of cardiac surgery, can be used to identify and localize the areas responsible for rhythm disturbances in patients with supraventricular and ventricular tachyarrhythmias for catheter or surgical ablation, isolation, or resection. Disorders amenable to this approach include accessory pathways associated with Wolff-Parkinson-White syndrome, the pathway(s) in AV node reentry, AV node/His bundle ablation, sites of origin of atrial tachycardia and VTs, isolated pathways essential for the maintenance of reentrant atrial tachycardia or VTs, and various substrates responsible for episodes of atrial fibrillation (see Chap. 35). Mapping can also be used to delineate the anatomical course of the His bundle to avoid injury during open-heart surgery, usually for congenital heart surgery or septal accessory pathway ablation.

Early efforts at mapping involved moving an electrode from location to location, acquiring data from a single point at a time, and comparing the timing of local activation with some reference recording as well as other mapped sites. Obtaining enough data points to determine where ablation should be performed relied heavily on the memory of the operator. Specialized mapping systems have now been developed that use computers to log not only the activation times at various points in the heart, but the physical locations from which these were obtained. The mapping information acquired in this way can be displayed on a screen, showing relative activation times in a color-coded sequence. Using such systems, dozens or even hundreds of sites can be sampled relatively quickly, leading to a clear picture of cardiac activation and potential target sites for ablation (Figs. 32-15 and 32-16). Other mapping systems can acquire data from several thousand points simultaneously, using a multipolar electrode array. This is particularly useful for hemodynamically unstable tachycardias or those that terminate spontaneously within seconds, precluding detailed point-to-point mapping.

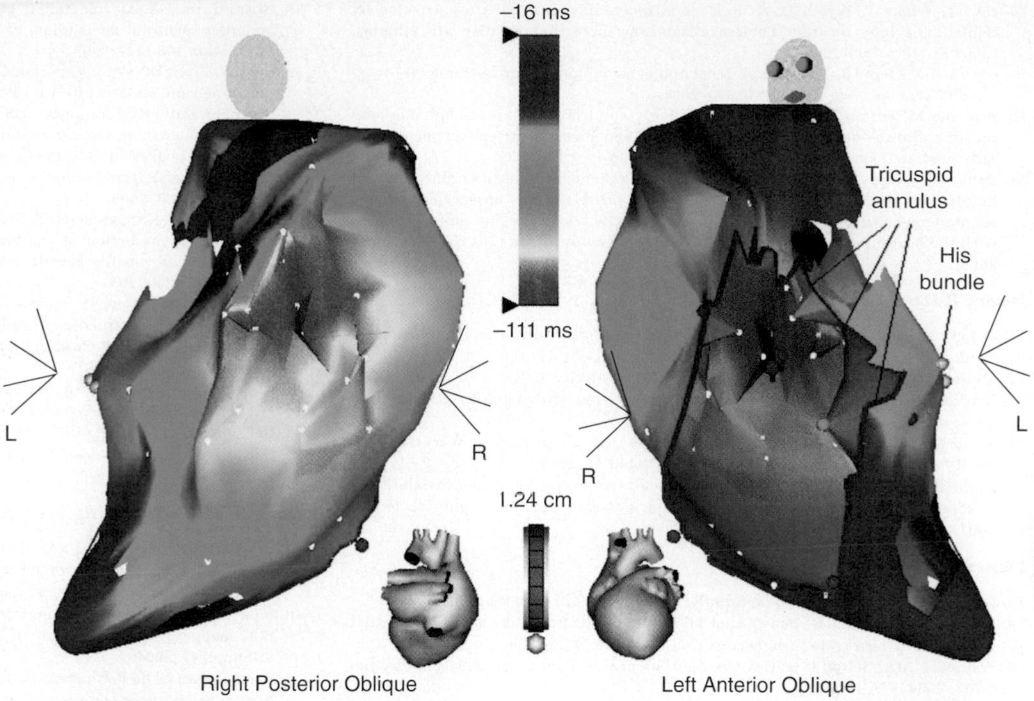

FIGURE 32–15 Electroanatomical map of focal atrial tachycardia. The right atrium is shown in two views (small gray icons at bottom center help with orientation). A color-coded time scale of activation is shown at top center; red indicates earliest activation, purple latest. A distance scale is shown below. This atrial tachycardia arose in the posterolateral right atrium (red spot), with all other areas activated centrifugally. Ablation at this site eliminated the tachycardia.

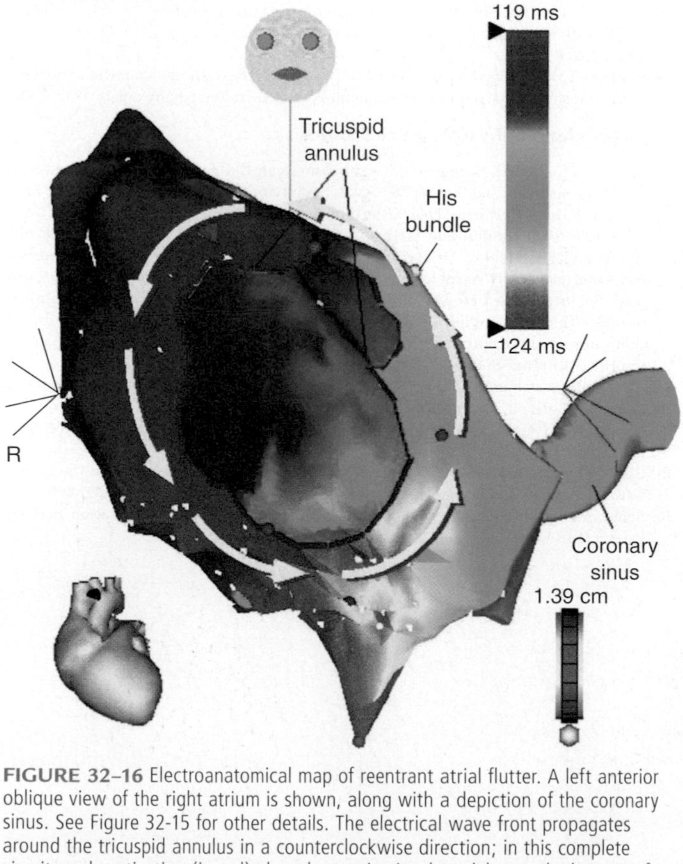

FIGURE 32–16 Electroanatomical map of reentrant atrial flutter. A left anterior oblique view of the right atrium is shown, along with a depiction of the coronary sinus. See Figure 32-15 for other details. The electrical wave front propagates around the tricuspid annulus in a counterclockwise direction; in this complete circuit, early activation (in red) abuts late activation (purple) near the bottom of the tricuspid annulus. The cycle length of the tachycardia was 250 milliseconds, almost completely described by the points shown in the figure (from –124 to +119 milliseconds, a total of 243 milliseconds). A distance scale is shown below.

REFERENCES

1. Zipes DP, Miles WM: Assessment of the patient with a cardiac arrhythmia. *In* Zipes DP, Jalife J (eds): Cardiac Electrophysiology from Cell to Bedside. 4th ed. Philadelphia, WB Saunders, 2004, pp 759-764.
2. Barsky AJ: Palpitations, arrhythmias, and awareness of cardiac activity. Ann Intern Med 134:832, 2001.
3. Miller JM, Das MK, Arora R, et al: Differential diagnosis of wide QRS complex tachycardia. *In* Zipes DP, Jalife J (eds): Cardiac Electrophysiology from Cell to Bedside. 4th ed. Philadelphia, WB Saunders, 2004, pp 747-758.

Exercise Testing

4. Sung RJ, Kuo CT, Lai WT: Exercise-induced cardiac arrhythmias. *In* Zipes DP, Jalife J (eds): Cardiac Electrophysiology from Cell to Bedside. 4th ed. Philadelphia, WB Saunders, 2004, pp 765-771.
5. Cole CR, Blackstone EH, Pashkow FJ, et al: Heart-rate recovery immediately after exercise as a predictor of mortality. N Engl J Med 341:1351, 1999.
6. Frolkis JP, Pothier CE, Blackstone EH, et al: Frequent ventricular ectopy after exercise as a predictor of death. N Engl J Med 348:781, 2003.

Long-Term Electrocardiographic Recording

7. Kennedy HL: Use of long-term (Holter) electrocardiographic recordings. *In* Zipes DP, Jalife J (eds): Cardiac Electrophysiology from Cell to Bedside. 4th ed. Philadelphia, WB Saunders, 2004, pp 772-792.
8. The Cardiac Arrhythmia Suppression Trial (CAST) Investigators: Preliminary report: Effect of encainide and flecainide on mortality in a randomized trial of arrhythmia suppression after myocardial infarction. N Engl J Med 321:406, 1989.
9. Page RL, Tilsch TW, Connolly SJ, et al: Asymptomatic or "silent" atrial fibrillation: Frequency in untreated patients and patients receiving azimilide. Circulation 107:1141, 2003.

10. Ho RT, Wicks T, Wyeth D, et al: Generalized tonic-clonic seizures detected by implantable loop recorder devices: Diagnosing more than cardiac arrhythmias. Heart Rhythm 3:857, 2006.
11. Krahn AD, Klein GJ, Yee R, et al: Detection of asymptomatic arrhythmias in unexplained syncope. Am Heart J 148:326, 2004.
12. Brignole M, Sutton R, Menozzi C, et al: Early application of an implantable loop recorder allows effective specific therapy in patients with recurrent suspected neurally mediated syncope. Eur Heart J 27:1085, 2006.
13. Deharo JC, Jego C, Lanteaume A, et al: An implantable loop recorder study of highly symptomatic vasovagal patients: The heart rhythm observed during a spontaneous syncope is identical to the recurrent syncope but not correlated with the head-up tilt test or adenosine triphosphate test. J Am Coll Cardiol 47:587, 2006.

Heart Rate Variability

14. Tulppo M, Huikuri HV: Origin and significance of heart rate variability. J Am Coll Cardiol 43:2278, 2004.
15. Malik M: Heart rate variability and baroreflex sensitivity. *In* Zipes DP, Jalife J (eds): Cardiac Electrophysiology from Cell to Bedside. 4th ed. Philadelphia, WB Saunders, 2004, pp 823-830.
16. Karcz M, Chojnowska L, Zareba W, et al: Prognostic significance of heart rate variability in dilated cardiomyopathy. Int J Cardiol 87:75, 2003.
17. Abildstrom SZ, Jensen BT, Agner E, et al: Heart rate versus heart rate variability in risk prediction after myocardial infarction. J Cardiovasc Electrophysiol 14:168, 2003.

Heart Rate Turbulence

18. Bauer A, Schmidt G: Heart rate turbulence. J Electrocardiol 36(Suppl):89, 2003.
19. Barthel P, Schneider R, Bauer A, et al: Risk stratification after acute myocardial infarction by heart rate turbulence. Circulation 108:1221, 2003.
20. Watanabe MA, Schmidt G: Heart rate turbulence: A 5-year review. Heart Rhythm 1:732, 2004.
21. Lin LY, Hwang JJ, Lai LP, et al: Restoration of heart rate turbulence by titrated beta-blocker therapy in patients with advanced congestive heart failure: Positive correlation with enhanced vagal modulation of heart rate. J Cardiovasc Electrophysiol 15:752, 2004.

QT Dispersion

22. Padmanabhan S, Silvet H, Amin J, et al: Prognostic value of QT interval and QT dispersion in patients with left ventricular systolic dysfunction: Results from a cohort of 2265 patients with an ejection fraction of < or = 40%. Am Heart J 145:132, 2003.
23. Gang Y, Ono T, Hnatkova K, et al: QT dispersion has no prognostic value in patients with symptomatic heart failure: An ELITE II substudy. Pacing Clin Electrophysiol 26:394, 2003.
24. Antzelevitch C, Oliva A: Amplification of spatial dispersion of repolarization underlies sudden cardiac death associated with catecholaminergic polymorphic VT, long QT, short QT and Brugada syndromes. J Intern Med 259:48, 2006.
25. Kinoshita O, Wakamatsu M, Tomita T, et al: Diurnal variation in QT dispersion in patients with chronic heart failure. Congest Heart Fail 11:262, 2005.

Signal-Averaged Electrocardiography and Late Potentials

26. Berbari E: High-resolution electrocardiography. *In* Zipes DP, Jalife J (eds): Cardiac Electrophysiology from Cell to Bedside. 4th ed. Philadelphia, WB Saunders, 2004, pp 793-802.
27. Kudaiberdieva G, Gorenek B, Goktekin O, et al: Combination of QT variability and signal-averaged electrocardiography in association with ventricular tachycardia in postinfarction patients. J Electrocardiol 36:17, 2003.
28. Budeus M, Hennersdorf M, Perings C, et al: Prediction of the recurrence of atrial fibrillation after successful cardioversion with P wave signal–averaged ECG. Ann Noninvasive Electrocardiol 10:414, 2005.
29. Budeus M, Hennersdorf M, Rohlen S, et al: Prediction of atrial fibrillation after coronary artery bypass grafting: The role of chemoreflex-sensitivity and P wave signal averaged ECG. Int J Cardiol 106:67, 2006.

T Wave Alternans

30. Gold MR, Spencer W: T wave alternans for ventricular arrhythmia risk stratification. Curr Opin Cardiol 18:1, 2003.
31. Akar FG, Yan GX, Antzelevitch C, et al: Unique topographical distribution of M cells underlies reentrant mechanism of torsades de pointes in the long-QT syndrome. Circulation 105:1247, 2002.
32. Ueda N, Zipes DP, Wu J: Functional and transmural modulation of M cell behavior in canine ventricular wall. Am J Physiol Heart Circ Physiol 287:H2569, 2004.
33. Pruvot EJ, Katra RP, Rosenbaum DS, et al: Role of calcium cycling versus restitution in the mechanism of repolarization alternans. Circ Res 94:1083, 2004.
34. Chow T, Kereiakes DJ, Bartone C, et al: Prognostic usefulness of microvolt T-wave alternans in risk stratification of patients with ischemic cardiomyopathy. J Am Coll Cardiol 47:1820, 2006.
35. Hohnloser SH, Klingenheben T, Bloomfield D, et al: Usefulness of microvolt T-wave alternans for prediction of ventricular tachyarrhythmic events in patients with dilated cardiomyopathy: Results from a prospective observational study. J Am Coll Cardiol 41:2220, 2003.
36. Bloomfield DM, Bigger JT, Steinman RC, et al: Microvolt T-wave alternans and the risk of death or sustained ventricular arrhythmias in patients with left ventricular dysfunction. J Am Coll Cardiol 47:456, 2006.
37. Chan PS, Stein K, Chow T, et al: Cost-effectiveness of a microvolt T-wave alternans screening strategy for implantable cardioverter-defibrillator placement in the MADIT-II–eligible population. J Am Coll Cardiol 48:112, 2006.
38. Gehi AK, Stein RH, Metz LD, et al: Microvolt T-wave alternans for the risk stratification of ventricular tachyarrhythmic events: A meta-analysis. J Am Coll Cardiol 46:75, 2005.

Body Surface Mapping and Electrocardiographic Imaging

39. van Dessel PF, van Hemel NM, de Bakker JM, et al: Relation between body surface mapping and endocardial spread of ventricular activation in postinfarction heart. J Cardiovasc Electrophysiol 12:1232, 2001.
40. Sippensgroenewegen A, Natale A, Marrouche NF, et al: Potential role of body surface ECG mapping for localization of atrial fibrillation trigger sites. J Electrocardiol 37(Suppl):47, 2004.
41. Ramanathan C, Jia P, Ghanem R, et al: Activation and repolarization of the normal human heart under complete physiological conditions. Proc Natl Acad Sci U S A 103:6309, 2006.
42. Intini A, Goldstein RN, Jia P, et al Electrocardiographic imaging (ECGI), a novel diagnostic modality used for mapping of focal left ventricular tachycardia in a young athlete. Heart Rhythm 2:1250, 2005.

Upright Tilt-Table Testing

43. Benditt DH, Ermis C, Lui F: Head-up tilt table testing. *In* Zipes DP, Jalife J (eds): Cardiac Electrophysiology from Cell to Bedside. 4th ed. Philadelphia, WB Saunders, 2004, pp 812-822.
44. Brady PA, Low PA, Shen WK: Inappropriate sinus tachycardia, postural orthostatic tachycardia syndrome, and overlapping syndromes. Pacing Clin Electrophysiol 28:1112, 2005.
45. Kanjwal Y, Kosinski D, Grubb BP: The postural orthostatic tachycardia syndrome: Definitions, diagnosis, and management. Pacing Clin Electrophysiol 26:1747, 2003.

Invasive Electrophysiological Studies

46. Zipes DP, Camm AJ, Borggrefe M, et al; American College of Cardiology/American Heart Association Task Force; European Society of Cardiology Committee for Practice Guidelines; European Heart Rhythm Association; Heart Rhythm Society: ACC/AHA/ESC 2006 Guidelines for the Management of Patients With Sudden Cardiac Arrest and Ventricular Arrhythmia: A report of the American College of Cardiology/American Heart Association Task Force on Practice Guidelines and the European Society of Cardiology Committee for Practice Guidelines (writing committee to revise the 2001 Guidelines for the Management of Patients With Atrial Fibrillation): Developed in collaboration with the European Heart Rhythm Association and the Heart Rhythm Society. Circulation 114:e385, 2006.
47. Calkins H: Syncope. *In* Zipes DP, Jalife J (eds): Cardiac Electrophysiology from Cell to Bedside. 4th ed. Philadelphia, WB Saunders, 2004, pp 884-894.
48. Kapoor WN: Current evaluation and management of syncope. Circulation 106:1606, 2002.
49. Goldschlager N, Epstein AE, Grubb BP, et al: Etiologic considerations in the patient with syncope and an apparently normal heart. Arch Intern Med 163:151, 2003.
50. Scheinman MM, Huang S: The 1998 NASPE prospective catheter ablation registry. Pacing Clin Electrophysiol 23:1020, 2000.

CHAPTER 33

Therapy for Cardiac Arrhythmias

John M. Miller and Douglas P. Zipes

The treatment of patients with tachyarrhythmias has evolved dramatically in the last 40 years. In the late 1960s, surgical therapy to cure, not just suppress, tachyarrhythmias became a reality and was replaced by catheter ablation (at first with direct current, and then with radiofrequency current) for cure of tachyarrhythmias in the 1980s. This form of therapy has largely replaced surgical and drug therapy for patients who need treatment for supraventricular tachycardia (SVT) and ventricular tachycardia (VT) in the absence of structural heart disease and has used other forms of energy as well. The implantable cardioverter-defibrillator (ICD) was also developed in the early 1980s and has become standard therapy for patients with serious ventricular arrhythmias in the presence of structural heart disease. Some patients require a combination of these forms of treatment (hybrid therapy, such as an ICD and antiarrhythmic drugs, or surgery and an ICD).[1] Drug therapy of arrhythmias, at one time the only option, now plays a supporting role in many cases.

PHARMACOLOGICAL THERAPY

Principles of clinical pharmacokinetics and pharmacodynamics are discussed in Chapter 6.

General Considerations Regarding Antiarrhythmic Drugs

Most of the available antiarrhythmic drugs (Table 33-1) can be classified according to whether they exert blocking actions predominantly on sodium, potassium, or calcium channels and whether they block receptors. The commonly used Vaughan Williams classification is limited because it is based on the electrophysiological effects exerted by an arbitrary concentration of the drug, generally on normal cardiac tissue. Actually, the actions of these drugs are complex and depend on tissue type, species, degree of acute or chronic damage, heart rate, membrane potential, ionic composition of the extracellular milieu, age (see Chap. 75), and other factors (see Table 33-1). Many drugs exhibit actions that belong in multiple categories or operate indirectly, such as by altering hemodynamics, myocardial metabolism, or autonomic neural transmission. Some drugs have active metabolites that exert effects different from those of the parent compound. Not all drugs in the same class have identical effects (e.g., amiodarone, sotalol and ibutilide). Whereas all class III agents are dramatically different, some drugs in different classes have overlapping actions (e.g., classes IA and IC drugs). In vitro studies on healthy fibers usually establish the properties of antiarrhythmic agents rather than their actual antiarrhythmic properties.

Despite these limitations, the Vaughan Williams classification is widely known and provides a useful communication shorthand, but the reader is cautioned that drug actions are more complex than those depicted by the classification. A more realistic view of antiarrhythmic agents is provided by the Sicilian gambit. This approach to drug classification is an attempt to identify the mechanisms of a particular arrhythmia, determine the vulnerable parameter of the arrhythmia most susceptible to modification, define the target most likely to affect the vulnerable parameter, and then select a drug that will modify the target. This concept provides a framework in which to consider antiarrhythmic drugs (Table 33-2; see Table 33-1).

DRUG CLASSIFICATION (Table 33-3). According to the Vaughan Williams classification, class I drugs predominantly block the fast sodium channel (they can also block potassium channels). They, in turn, are divided into three subgroups, classes IA, IB, and IC.

Class IA. This includes drugs that reduce $\dot{V}_{max}$ (rate of rise of action potential upstroke [phase 0]) and prolong action potential duration (see Chap. 31)—quinidine, procainamide, disopyramide. Their kinetics of onset and offset in blocking the Na^+ channel are of intermediate rapidity (less than 5 seconds).

Class IB. This class of drugs does not reduce $\dot{V}_{max}$ and shortens action potential duration—mexiletine, phenytoin, and lidocaine. Their kinetics of onset and offset in blocking the sodium channel are rapid (less than 500 milliseconds).

Class IC. This class of drugs can reduce $\dot{V}_{max}$, primarily slow conduction, and prolong refractoriness minimally—flecainide, propafenone, and moricizine. These drugs have slow onset and offset kinetics (10 to 20 seconds).

Class II. These drugs block beta-adrenergic receptors, and include propranolol, timolol, and metoprolol.

Class III. This class of drugs predominantly blocks potassium channels (such as I_{Kr}) and prolongs repolarization. Included are sotalol, amiodarone, and bretylium.

Class IV. This class of drugs predominantly blocks the slow calcium channel ($I_{Ca.L}$)—verapamil, diltiazem, nifedipine, and others (felodipine blocks $I_{Ca.T}$).

A newer model has suggested that antiarrhythmic drugs cross the cell membrane and interact with receptors in the membrane channels when the latter are in the rested, activated, or inactivated state (see Table 33-1) (see Chap. 31), and that each of these interactions is characterized by different association and dissociation rate constants. Such interactions are voltage and time dependent. Transitions among rested, activated, and inactivated states are governed by standard Hodgkin-Huxley–

TABLE 33–1 Actions of Drugs Used in Treatment of Arrhythmias

	Channels						Receptors				Pumps	Clinical Effects		
	*Na**			*Ca*	K_r	K_s	*Alpha*	*Beta*	M_2	*P*	*Na-K ATPase*	*LV Function*	*Sinus Rate*	*Extracardiac*
Drug	**Fast**	**Med**	**Slow**											
Quinidine		●A			⊙		○		○			—	↑	⊙
Procainamide		●A			⊙							↓	—	⊙
Disopyramide		●A			⊙				○			↓	—	●
Ajmaline		●A										—	— ↓	○
Lidocaine	○											—	— ↓	○
Mexiletine	○											—	—	○
Phenytoin	○											—	—	⊙
Flecainide			●A		○							↓	—	○
Propafenone		●A			○			⊙				↓	↓	○
Moricizine	●I											↓	—	○
Propranolol	○							●				↓	↓	○
Nadolol								●				↓	↓	○
Amiodarone	○			⊙	●	⊙	⊙	⊙				—	↓	●
Bretylium					●		▣	▣				—	↓	○
Sotalol					●			●				↓	↓	○
Ibutilide					○							—	↓	○
Dofetilide					●							—	—	○
Azimilide					⊙	⊙	○					—	—	○
Verapamil	○			●			⊙					↓	↓	○
Diltiazem				⊙								↓	↓	○
Adenosine										□		—	↓	⊙
Digoxin									○		●	↑	↓	⊙
Atropine									●			—	↑	⊙

*Fast, med (medium), and slow refer to kinetics of recovery from sodium channel blockade.

Relative potency of blockade or extracardiac side effect: ○ = low; ⊙ = moderate; ● = high; □ = agonist; ▣ = agonist/antagonist.

A = activated state blocker; I = inactivated state blocker; — = minimal effect; ↑ = increase; ↓ = decrease; K_r = rapid component of delayed rectifier K^+ current; Ks = slow component of delayed rectifier K^+ current; M_2 = muscarinic receptor subtype 2; P = $alpha_1$-purinergic receptor.

Adapted from Schwartz PJ, Zaza A: Haemodynamic effects of a new multifactorial antihypertensive drug. Eur Heart J 13(Suppl A):26, 1992.

type equations. When the drug is bound (associated) to a receptor site at or very close to the ionic channel (the drug probably does not actually plug the channel), the latter cannot conduct, even in the activated state.

USE-DEPENDENCE. Some drugs exert greater inhibitory effects on the upstroke of the action potential at more rapid rates of stimulation and after longer periods of stimulation, a characteristic called use-dependence. Use-dependence means that depression of $\dot{V}_{max}$ is greater after the channel has been "used" (i.e., after action potential depolarization rather than after a rest period). It is possible that this use-dependence results from preferential interaction of the antiarrhythmic drug with the open or the inactive channel, and there is little interaction with the resting channels of the unstimulated cell. Agents in class IB exhibit fast kinetics of onset and offset or use-dependent block of the fast channel; that is, they bind and dissociate quickly from the receptors. Class IC drugs have slow kinetics, and class IA drugs are intermediate. With increased time spent in diastole (slower rate), a greater proportion of receptors become drug free, and the drug exerts less effect. Cells with reduced membrane potentials recover more slowly from drug actions than cells with more negative membrane potentials.

REVERSE USE-DEPENDENCE. Some drugs exert greater effects at slow rates than at fast rates, a property known as reverse use-dependence. This is particularly true for drugs that lengthen repolarization. The QT interval becomes more prolonged at slow rather than fast rates. This effect is opposite to what the ideal antiarrhythmic agent would do, because prolongation of refractoriness should be increased at fast rates to interrupt or prevent a tachycardia, and should be minimal at slow rates to avoid precipitating torsades de pointes.

MECHANISMS OF ARRHYTHMIA SUPPRESSION (see Table 33-2). Given the fact that enhanced automaticity, triggered activity, or reentry can cause cardiac arrhythmias (see Chap. 31), mechanisms by which antiarrhythmic agents suppress arrhythmias can be postulated. Antiarrhythmic agents can slow the spontaneous discharge frequency of an automatic pacemaker by depressing the slope of diastolic depolarization, shifting the threshold voltage toward zero, or hyperpolarizing the resting membrane potential. Mechanisms whereby different drugs suppress normal or abnormal automaticity may not be the same. In general, however, most antiarrhythmic agents in therapeutic doses depress the automatic firing rate of spontaneously discharging ectopic sites while minimally affecting the discharge rate of the normal sinus node. Slow-channel blockers such as verapamil, beta blockers such as propranolol, and some antiarrhythmic agents such as amiodarone also depress spontaneous discharge of the sinus node, whereas drugs that exert vagolytic effects, such as disopyramide or quinidine, can increase the sinus discharge rate. Drugs can also suppress early or delayed afterdepolarizations and eliminate triggered arrhythmias related to these mechanisms.

TABLE 33–2 Classification of Drug Actions on Arrhythmias Based on Modification of Vulnerable Parameter

Mechanism	Arrhythmia	Vulnerable Parameter (Effect)	Drugs (Effect)
Automaticity			
Enhanced normal	Inappropriate sinus tachycardia Some idiopathic ventricular tachycardias	Phase 4 depolarization (decrease)	Beta-adrenergic blocking agents Na^+ channel blocking agents
Abnormal	Atrial tachycardia	Maximum diastolic potential (hyperpolarization) Phase 4 depolarization (decrease)	Muscarinic receptor subtype 2 (M_2) agonists Ca^{2+} or Na^+ channel blocking agents M_2 agonists
	Accelerated idioventricular rhythms	Phase 4 depolarization (decrease)	Ca^{2+} or Na^+ channel blocking agents
Triggered Activity			
Early afterdepolarization (EAD)	Torsades de pointes	Action potential duration (shorten) EAD (suppress)	Beta-adrenergic agonists; vagolytic agents (increase rate) Ca^{2+} channel blocking agents; Mg^{2+}; beta-adrenergic blocking agents
Delayed afterdepolarization (DAD)	Digitalis-induced arrhythmias	Calcium overload (unload) DAD (suppress)	Ca^{2+} channel blocking agents Na^+ channel blocking agents
	Right ventricular outflow tract ventricular tachycardia	Calcium overload (unload) DAD (suppress)	Beta-adrenergic blocking agents Ca^{2+} channel blocking agents; adenosine
Na^+ Channel–Dependent Reentry			
Long excitable gap	Typical atrial flutter	Conduction and excitability (depress)	Types IA, IC Na^+ channel blocking agents
	Circus movement tachycardia in Wolff-Parkinson-White syndrome (WPW)	Conduction and excitability (depress)	Types IA, IC Na^+ channel blocking agents
	Sustained uniform ventricular tachycardia	Conduction and excitability (depress)	Na^+ channel blocking agents
Short excitable gap	Atypical atrial flutter	Refractory period (prolong)	K^+ channel blocking agents
	Atrial fibrillation	Refractory period (prolong)	K^+ channel blocking agents
	Circus movement tachycardia in WPW	Refractory period (prolong)	Amiodarone, sotalol
	Polymorphic and uniform ventricular tachycardia	Refractory period (prolong)	Type IA Na^+ channel blocking agents
	Bundle branch reentry	Refractory period (prolong)	Type IA Na^+ channel blocking agents; amiodarone
	Ventricular fibrillation	Refractory period (prolong)	
Ca^{2+} Channel-Dependent Reentry			
	Atrioventricular nodal reentrant tachycardia	Conduction and excitability (depress)	Ca^{2+} channel blocking agents
	Circus movement tachycardia in WPW	Conduction and excitability (depress)	Ca^{2+} channel blocking agents
	Verapamil-sensitive ventricular tachycardia	Conduction and excitability (depress)	Ca^{2+} channel blocking agents

From the Task Force of the Working Group on Arrhythmias of the European Society of Cardiology: The Sicilian gambit: A new approach to the classification of antiarrhythmic drugs based on their actions on arrhythmogenic mechanisms. Circulation 84:1831, 1991. Copyright 1991, American Heart Association.

Reentry depends critically on the timing interrelationships between refractoriness and conduction velocity, the presence of unidirectional block in one of the pathways, and other factors that influence refractoriness and conduction, such as excitability (see Chap. 31). An antiarrhythmic agent can stop ongoing reentry that is already present or prevent it from starting if the drug improves or depresses conduction. For example, improving conduction can (1) eliminate the unidirectional block so that reentry cannot begin or (2) facilitate conduction in the reentrant loop so that the returning wave front reenters too quickly, encounter cells that are still refractory, and extinguishes. A drug that depresses conduction can transform the unidirectional block to bidirectional block and thus terminate reentry or prevent it from occurring by creating an area of complete block in the reentrant pathway. Conversely, a drug that slows conduction without producing block or lengthening refractoriness significantly can promote reentry. Finally, most antiarrhythmic agents share the ability to prolong refractoriness relative to their effects on action potential duration (APD); that is, the ratio of effective refractory period (ERP) to APD exceeds 1.0. If a drug prolongs refractoriness of fibers in the reentrant pathway, the pathway may not recover excitability in time to be depolarized by the reentering impulse and the reentrant propagation ceases. The different types of reentry (see Chap. 31) influence the effects and effectiveness of a drug.

When considering the properties of a drug, it is important that the situation, model, or both from which conclusions are drawn be defined with care. Electrophysiological, hemodynamic, autonomic, pharmacokinetic, and adverse effects may all differ in normal subjects compared with patients, in normal tissue compared with abnormal tissue, in cardiac muscle compared with specialized conduction fibers, in atrium as opposed to ventricular muscle, and in different species (Table 33-4).

DRUG METABOLITES. Drug metabolites can add to or alter the effects of the parent compound by exerting similar actions, competing with the parent compound, or mediating drug toxicity. Quinidine has at least four active metabolites but none with a potency exceeding that of the parent drug and none implicated in causing torsades de pointes. About 50 percent of procainamide is metabolized to *N*-acetylprocainamide (NAPA), which prolongs repolarization and is a less effective antiarrhythmic drug but competes with procainamide for renotubular secretory sites and can increase the parent drug's elimination half-life. Lidocaine's metabolite can compete with lidocaine for sodium channels and partially reverse block produced by lidocaine.

PHARMACOGENETICS (see Chap. 6). Genetically determined metabolic pathways account for many of the differences in patients' responses to some drugs. The genetically determined activity of hepatic *N*-acetyltransferase regulates the development of antinuclear antibod-

TABLE 33–3 In Vitro Electrophysiological Characteristics of Antiarrhythmic Drugs

Drug	APD	dV/dt	MDP	ERP	CV	PF Phase 4	SN Auto	Contr	SI Curr	Autonomic Nervous System
Quinidine	↑	↓	0	↑	↓	↓	0	0	0	Antivagal; alpha blocker
Procainamide	↑	↓	0	↑	↓	↓	0	0	0	Slight antivagal
Disopyramide	↑	↓	0	↑	↓	↓	↓ 0 ↑	↓	0	Central: antivagal, antisympathetic
Ajmaline	↑	↓	0	↑	↓	↓	↓ 0	↓	0	Antivagal
Lidocaine	↓	0 ↓	0	↓	0 ↓	↓	0	0	0	0
Mexiletine	↓	0 ↓	0	↓	↓	↓	0	↓	0	0
Phenytoin	↓	↓ 0 ↑	0	↓	0	↓	0		0	0
Flecainide	0 ↑	↓	0	↑	↓ ↓	↓	0	↓	0	0
Propafenone	0 ↑	↓	0	↑	↓ ↓	↓	0	↓	0 ↓	Antisympathetic
Moricizine	↓	↓	0	↓	↓	0	0		0	0
Propranolol	0 ↓	0 ↓	0	↓	0	↓*	↓	↓	0 ↓	Antisympathetic
Amiodarone	↑	0 ↓	0	↑	↓	↓	↓	0 ↑	0	Antisympathetic
Bretylium	↑	0	0	↑	0	0 ↓*	0 ↓	↓	0	Antisympathetic
Sotalol	↑	0 ↓	0	↑	0	0 ↓	↓	↓	0 ↓	Antisympathetic
Ibutilide	↑	0	0	↑	0	0	↓	0	0	0
Dofetilide	↑	0	0	↑	0	0	0	0	0	0
Azimilide	↑	0	0	↑	0	0	0	0	0	0
Verapamil	↓	0	0	0	0	↓*	↓	↓	↓↓	Block alpha receptors (?); enhance vagal
Adenosine	↑	0 ↓	0	↑	0	0 ↓	↓	0	↓	Vagomimetic

*With a background of sympathetic activity.

↑ = increase; ↓ = decrease; 0 = no change; 0 ↑ or 0 ↓ = slight or inconsistent increase or decrease; APD = action potential duration; dV/dt = rate of rise of action potential; MDP = maximum diastolic potential; ERP = effective refractory period (longest S_1-S_2 interval at which S_2 fails to produce a response); CV = conduction velocity; PF = Purkinje fiber; SN Auto = sinus nodal automaticity; Contr = contractility; SI Curr = slow inward current.

ies and development of the lupus syndrome in response to procainamide. Slow acetylator phenotypes appear more prone to develop lupus than rapid acetylators. About 7 percent of subjects lack debrisoquin 4-hydroxylase. The enzyme cytochrome P-450 (CYP450) is needed to metabolize debrisoquin (an antihypertensive drug) and propafenone, hydroxylate several beta blockers, and biotransform flecainide. Lack of this enzyme reduces metabolism of the parent compound, leading to increased plasma concentrations of the parent drug and reduced concentrations of metabolites. Propafenone is metabolized by CYP450 to a compound with slightly less antiarrhythmic and beta-adrenergic blocking effects, as well as fewer central nervous system side effects. Thus, poor metabolizers may experience more heart rate slowing and neurotoxicity than extensive metabolizers.

Understanding stereoselectivity (whereby two compounds with identical atomic composition, but different spatial arrangement, can display different pharmacologic effects) and pharmacogenetics can provide major clues to understanding differences in drug efficacy and toxicity from one patient to the next. Drugs such as rifampin, phenobarbital, and phenytoin induce the synthesis of larger amounts of CYP450, leading to lower concentrations of parent drugs that are extensively metabolized, whereas erythromycin, clarithromycin, fluoxetine, and grapefruit juice inhibit enzyme activity leading to accumulation of the parent compound. This effect is thought to explain why cisapride, an agent that had been used to increase gastric motility, could cause QT interval prolongation and torsades de pointes in isolated cases. Cisapride blocked the delayed rectifier current I_{Kr} but did not prolong the QT interval significantly in most patients, presumably because of extensive metabolism. In patients who take an inhibitor of CYP450 (such as erythromycin) along with cisapride, the latter drug can accumulate, leading to QT prolongation and torsades de pointes.

CLINICAL USE. In treating cardiac rhythm disorders, most drugs are given on a daily basis (in one to three doses) to prevent episodes from occurring or, in the case of atrial fibrillation, control the ventricular rate. Efficacy can be judged in various ways, depending on the clinical circumstances. Symptom reduction (in the case of benign arrhythmias, such as most premature ventricular complexes [PVCs]) and electrocardiographic monitoring (long-term or event; see Chap. 32) are useful; electrophysiologic studies have been used in the past, with suppression of electrical arrhythmia induction as the goal. However, this is rarely used currently. Interrogation of implanted device memory can also provide an indicator of success of drug therapy.

In some patients, tachycardia episodes are infrequent enough (months between occurrences) and symptoms mild enough that reactive drug administration is more reasonable than chronic daily dosing. In this setting, a patient takes a medication only after an episode has started, with the hope that the tachycardia will terminate in response to the drug and a physician's office or emergency room visit can be avoided thereby. This "pill in the pocket" strategy has worked well in patients with atrial fibrillation who have been given one of various medications orally in a monitored setting to ensure safety as well as efficacy before allowing self-medication at home or elsewhere.

SIDE EFFECTS. Antiarrhythmic drugs produce one group of side effects related to excessive dosage and plasma concentrations, resulting in both noncardiac (e.g., neurological defects) and cardiac (e.g., heart failure, some arrhythmias) toxicity, and another group of side effects unrelated to plasma concentrations, which is termed *idiosyncratic.* Examples of the latter include procainamide-induced lupus syndrome and some arrhythmias, such as quinidine-induced torsades de pointes. The latter phenomenon can occur in individuals with a forme fruste of the long QT

TABLE 33–4 Clinical Usage Information for Antiarrhythmic Agents

Drug	Usual Dosage Ranges				Time to Peak Plasma Concentration (Oral) (hr)	Effective Serum or Plasma Concentration (μg/ml)	Half-Life (hr)	Bioavailability (%)	Major Route of Elimination	Pregnancy Class
	Intravenous (mg)		Oral (mg)							
	Loading	*Maintenance*	*Loading*	*Maintenance*						
Quinidine	6 to 10 mg/kg at 0.3 to 0.5 mg/kg/min	—	800 to 1000	300 to 600 q6hr	1.5 to 3.0	3 to 6	5 to 9	60 to 80	Liver	C
Procainamide	6 to 13 mg/kg at 0.2 to 0.5 mg/kg/min	2 to 6 mg/min	500 to 1000	250 to 1000 q4-6hr	1	4 to 10	3 to 5	70 to 85	Kidneys	C
Disopyramide	1 to 2 mg/kg over 15 to 45 min*	1 mg/kg/hr		100 to 300 q6-8hr	1 to 2	2 to 5	8 to 9	80 to 90	Kidneys	C
Lidocaine	1 to 3 mg/kg at 20 to 50 mg/min	1 to 4 mg/min	N/A	N/A	N/A	1 to 5	1 to 2	N/A	Liver	B
Mexiletine	500 mg*	0.5 to 1.0 gm/24 hr	400 to 600	150 to 300 q8-12hr	2 to 4	0.75 to 2	10 to 17	90	Liver	C
Phenytoin	100 mg q5min for ≤1000 mg		1000	100 to 400 q12-24hr	8 to 12	10 to 20	18 to 36	50 to 70	Liver	D
Flecainide	2 mg/kg*	100 to 200 q12hr		50 to 200 q12hr	3 to 4	0.2 to 1.0	20	95	Liver	C
Propafenone	1 to 2 mg/kg		600 to 900	150 to 300 q8-12hr	1 to 3	0.2 to 3.0	5 to 8	25 to 75	Liver	C
Moricizine	N/A	N/A	300	100 to 400 q8hr	1 to 3	0.1	2	40	Liver	B
Propranolol	0.25 to 0.5 mg q5min to ≤0.20 mg/kg			10 to 200 q6-8hr	4	1 to 2.5	3 to 6	35 to 65	Liver	C

Continues

TABLE 33–4 Clinical Usage Information for Antiarrhythmic Agents—cont'd

Drug	Usual Dosage Ranges: Intravenous (mg)		Usual Dosage Ranges: Oral (mg)		Time to Peak Plasma Concentration (Oral) (hr)	Effective Serum or Plasma Concentration (μg/ml)	Half-Life (hr)	Bioavailability (%)	Major Route of Elimination	Pregnancy Class
	Loading	*Maintenance*	*Loading*	*Maintenance*						
Amiodarone	15 mg/min for 10 min, 1 mg/min for 3 hr, 0.5 mg/min thereafter	1 mg/min	800 to 1600 qd for 7-14 days	200 to 600 qd		0.5 to 1.5	56 days	25	Kidneys	D
Bretylium	5 to 10 mg/kg at 1 to 2 mg/kg/min	0.5 to 2 mg/min	N/A	4 mg/kg/day	2 to 4	0.04 to 0.90	8 to 14	20 to 50	Liver	C
Sotalol	10 mg over 1 to 2 min			80 to 320 q12hr	2.5 to 4	2.5	12	90 to 100	Kidneys	B
Ibutilide	1 mg over 10 min	N/A	N/A	N/A	N/A	N/A	6		Kidneys	C
Dofetilide	2- to 5-μg/kg infusion	N/A	N/A	0.125 to 0.5 q12hr			7 to 13	90	Kidneys	C
Azimilide	N/A	N/A	N/A	100 to 200 qd		200 to 1000		90 to 100	Kidneys	—
Verapamil	5 to 10 mg over 1 to 2 min	0.005 mg/kg/min		80 to 120 q6-8hr	1 to 2	0.10 to 0.15	3 to 8	10 to 35	Liver	C
Adenosine	6 to 18 mg (rapidly)	N/A	N/A	N/A	N/A					C
Digoxin	0.5 to 1.0 mg	0.125 to 0.25 qd	0.5 to 1.0	0.125 to 0.25 qd	2 to 6	0.0008 to 0.002	36 to 48	60 to 80	Kidneys	C

*Intravenous use investigational.

N/A = Not applicable.

Results presented may vary according to doses, disease state, and IV or oral administration.

Pregnancy class: A—controlled studies show no fetal risk; B—no controlled studies, but no evidence of fetal risk; fetal harm unlikely; C—fetal risk cannot be excluded; drug should be used only if potential benefits outweigh potential risk; D—definite fetal risk; drug should be avoided unless in a life-threatening situation or safer alternatives do not exist; X—contraindicated in pregnancy.

syndrome (i.e., normal QT interval at rest but markedly prolonged interval in the presence of certain medications). In the future, it is likely that genetic differences will explain many idiosyncratic reactions.[2-4]

Proarrhythmia. Drug-induced or drug-exacerbated cardiac arrhythmias (proarrhythmia) constitute a major clinical problem.[5] Proarrhythmia can be manifested as an increase in frequency of a preexisting arrhythmia, sustaining of a previously nonsustained arrhythmia (even making it incessant), or development of arrhythmias that the patient has not previously experienced. Electrophysiological mechanisms are probably related to prolongation of repolarization, development of early afterdepolarizations to cause torsades de pointes, and alterations in reentry pathways to initiate or sustain tachyarrhythmias (see Chap. 31). Proarrhythmic events can occur in as many as 5 to 10 percent of patients receiving antiarrhythmic agents. Heart failure increases this risk. Patients with atrial fibrillation treated with antiarrhythmic agents had a relative risk of cardiac death of 4.7 if they had a history of heart failure as compared with patients not so treated, who had a relative risk of arrhythmic death of 3.7. Patients without a history of congestive heart failure had no increased risk of cardiac mortality during antiarrhythmic drug treatment. Reduced left ventricular function, treatment with digitalis and diuretics, and longer pretreatment QT interval characterize patients who experience drug-induced ventricular fibrillation (VF). The more commonly known proarrhythmic events occur within several days of beginning drug therapy or changing dosage and are represented by such developments as incessant VT, long QT syndrome, and torsades de pointes. However, in the Cardiac Arrhythmia Suppression Trial (CAST), researchers found that encainide and flecainide reduced spontaneous ventricular arrhythmias but were associated with a total mortality of 7.7 percent, in comparison with 3.0 percent in the group receiving placebo. Deaths were equally distributed throughout the treatment period, raising the important consideration that another type of proarrhythmic response can occur some time after the beginning of drug therapy. Such late proarrhythmic effects may be related to drug-induced exacerbation of regional myocardial conduction delay caused by ischemia and heterogeneous drug concentrations that can promote reentry.

The availability of catheter ablation (see later) and implantable devices (pacemakers and implantable cardioverter-defibrillators [ICDs]; see Chap. 34) to treat a wide variety of arrhythmias has relegated drug therapy to a secondary role. Drugs are still useful to prevent or decrease frequency of recurrences in patients who have relatively infrequent episodes of benign tachycardias, those who have had incomplete success with catheter ablation procedures, and patients with an ICD who have episodes of ventricular arrhythmia, resulting in frequent shocks.

Antiarrhythmic Agents

Class IA Agents

QUINIDINE

Quinidine and quinine are isomeric alkaloids isolated from cinchona bark. Although quinidine shares the antimalarial, antipyretic, and vagolytic actions of quinine, only quinidine has electrophysiological effects.

ELECTROPHYSIOLOGICAL ACTIONS (Table 33-5; see Tables 33-1, 33-2, and 33-3). Quinidine exerts little effect on automaticity of the normal sinus node but suppresses automaticity in normal Purkinje fibers. In patients with the sick sinus syndrome, quinidine can depress sinus node automaticity. Quinidine produces early afterdepolarizations in experimental preparations and in humans, which may be responsible for torsades de pointes. Because of its significant anticholinergic effect and reflex sympathetic stimulation resulting from alpha-adrenergic blockade, which causes peripheral vasodilation, quinidine can increase sinus node discharge rate and can improve atrioventricular (AV) nodal conduction. Quinidine prolongs repolarization, an effect that is more prominent at slow heart rates (reverse use-dependence) because of block of I_{Kr}. Faster rates result in more block of sodium channels and less unblocking because of a smaller percentage of time spent in a polarized state (use-dependence). Isoproterenol can modulate the effects of quinidine on reentrant circuits in humans. Quinidine's effect on I_{to} (but not I_K) varies according to the patient's age and may account for its lower efficacy in children than in adults.

HEMODYNAMIC EFFECTS. Quinidine decreases peripheral vascular resistance and can cause significant hypotension because of its alpha-adrenergic receptor blocking effects. Concomitant administration of vasodilators can exaggerate the potential for hypotension. No significant direct myocardial depressant action occurs with orally administered quinidine.

PHARMACOKINETICS (see Table 33-4). Although orally administered quinidine sulfate and quinidine gluconate exhibit similar systemic availability, plasma quinidine concentrations peak at about 90 minutes after a dose of the sulfate but at 3 to 4 hours after a dose of the gluconate preparation. Quinidine can be given intravenously if it is infused slowly, but intramuscular dosing should be avoided. Approximately 80 percent of plasma quinidine is protein bound, especially to alpha$_1$-acid glycoprotein, which increases in heart failure. Both the liver and the kidneys remove quinidine; dose adjustments may be made according to the creatinine clearance. Metabolism is by means of the CYP450 system. Approximately 20 percent is excreted unchanged in the urine. Because congestive heart failure, hepatic disease, or poor renal function can reduce quinidine elimination and increase plasma concentration, the dosage should be reduced and the drug given cautiously to patients with these disorders while monitoring serum quinidine concentration. Elimination half-life is 5 to 8 hours after oral administration. Quinidine's effect on repolarization and overall efficacy vary directly with left ventricular function; for the same serum concentration, the QT interval is longer in women than in men.[6]

DOSAGE AND ADMINISTRATION (see Table 33-4). The usual oral dose of quinidine sulfate for an adult is 300 to 600 mg four times daily, which results in a steady-state level within about 24 hours. A loading dose of 600 to 1000 mg produces an earlier effective concentration. Oral doses of the gluconate are about 30 percent higher than those of sulfate. Important interactions with other drugs occur.

INDICATIONS. Quinidine is a versatile antiarrhythmic agent, with efficacy in treating premature supraventricular and ventricular complexes and sustained tachyarrhythmias. Its benefits are tempered by adverse effects (see later). It may prevent spontaneous recurrences of AV nodal reentrant tachycardia (AVNRT) and other forms of SVT by prolonging atrial and ventricular refractoriness and depressing conduction in the essential portions of reentrant circuits. Quinidine and other antiarrhythmic agents can also prevent recurrences of tachycardia by suppressing the "trigger" (i.e., PVC or premature atrial complex [PAC]) that initiates a sustained tachycardia (see Chap. 35).

Quinidine successfully terminates atrial flutter or atrial fibrillation in 20 to 60 percent of patients, with higher success rates if the arrhythmia is of more recent onset and if the atria are not enlarged. Before quinidine is administered to these patients, the ventricular response should be slowed sufficiently with a beta or calcium channel blocker because quinidine-induced slowing of the atrial flutter rate (e.g., from 300 to 230 beats/min) and its vagolytic effect on AV nodal conduction can convert a 2:1 AV response (ventricular rate, 150 beats/min) to a 1:1 AV response, with an increase in the ventricular rate (to 230 beats/min). If quinidine is going to be used to try to maintain sinus rhythm after elective cardioversion of patients with atrial fibrillation, it probably should be given for 1 to 2 days before planned cardioversion, because this regimen restores sinus

TABLE 33–5 In Vivo Electrophysiological Characteristics of Antiarrhythmic Drugs

	Electrocardiographic Measurements					Electrophysiologic Intervals					
Drug	*Sinus Rate*	*PR*	*QRS*	*QT*	*JT*	*ERP-AVN*	*ERP-HPS*	*ERP-A*	*ERP-V*	*A-H*	*H-V*
Quinidine	0 ↑	↓ 0 ↑	↑	↑	↑	0 ↑	↑	↑	↑	0 ↓	↑
Procainamide	0	0 ↑	↑	↑	↑	0 ↑	↑	↑	↑	0 ↑	↑
Disopyramide	0 ↑	↓ 0 ↑	↑	↑	↑	↑ 0	↑	↑	↑	↓ 0 ↑	↑
Ajmaline	0	0 ↑	↑	↑	↑	0	↑	↑	↑	↓ 0 ↑	↑
Lidocaine	0	0	0	0 ↓	↓	0 ↓	0 ↑	0	0	0 ↓	0 ↑
Mexiletine	0	0	0	0 ↓	↓	0 ↑	0 ↑	0	0	0 ↑	0 ↑
Phenytoin	0	0	0	0	0	0 ↓	↓	0	0	0 ↑	0
Flecainide	0 ↓	↑	↑	0 ↑	0	↑	↑	↑	↑	↑	↑
Propafenone	0 ↓	↑	↑	0 ↑	0	0 ↑	0 ↑	0 ↑	↑	↑	↑
Moricizine	0 ↓	0 ↑	0 ↑	0	↓	0	0	0 ↑	0 ↑	↑	↑
Propranolol	↓	0 ↑	0	0 ↓	0	↑	0	0	0	0	0
Amiodarone	↓	0 ↑	↑	↑	↑	↑	↑	↑	↑	↑	↑
Bretylium	↓ 0 ↑	0	0	0 ↑	↑	0	↑	↑	↑	↓ 0 ↑	0
Sotalol	↓	0 ↑	0	↑	↑	↑	↑	↑	↑	↑	0
Ibutilide	↓	0 ↓	0	↑	↑	0	0	↑	↑	0	0
Dofetilide	0	0	0	↑	↑	0	0	↑	↑	0	0
Azimilide	0	0	0	↑	↑	0	0	↑	↑	0	0
Verapamil	0 ↓	↑	0	0	0	↑	0	0	0	↑	0
Adenosine	↓ then ↑	↑	0	0	0	↑	0	↓	0	↑	0
Digoxin	↓	↑	0	0	↓	↑	0	↓	0	↑	0

Results presented may vary according to tissue type, drug concentration, and autonomic tone.
↑ = increase; ↓ = decrease; 0 = no change; 0 ↑ or 0 ↓ = slight or inconsistent increase or decrease; A = atrium; AVN = AV node; HPS = His-Purkinje system; V = ventricle; A-H = atrio-His interval (an index of AV nodal conduction); H-V = His-ventricular interval (an index of His-Purkinje conduction); ERP = effective refractory period (longest S_1-S_2 interval at which S_2 fails to produce a response).

rhythm in some patients, thus obviating the need for direct-current cardioversion, and helps maintain sinus rhythm once it has been achieved. In addition, early toxicity or patient's intolerance of the drug may be observed and changes made in drug therapy before attempting cardioversion. However, a meta-analysis of six studies testing the effects of quinidine versus control in maintaining sinus rhythm in patients with atrial fibrillation showed that quinidine-treated patients remain in sinus rhythm longer than the control group but have an increased total mortality over the same period.[7]

Quinidine has limited usefulness in the prevention of ventricular tachycardia and fibrillation; however, patients with primary ventricular fibrillation, as well as those with Brugada syndrome (see Chap. 9), have been treated successfully with this agent.[8] Because it crosses the placenta, quinidine can be used to treat arrhythmias in the fetus.

ADVERSE EFFECTS. The most common adverse effects of chronic oral quinidine therapy are gastrointestinal and include nausea, vomiting, diarrhea, abdominal pain, and anorexia (milder with the gluconate form). Central nervous system toxicity includes tinnitus, hearing loss, visual disturbances, confusion, delirium, and psychosis (cinchonism). Allergic reactions may be manifested as rash, fever, immune-mediated thrombocytopenia, hemolytic anemia and, rarely, anaphylaxis. Side effects may preclude long-term administration of quinidine in 30 to 40 percent of patients.

Quinidine can slow cardiac conduction, sometimes to the point of block, manifested as prolongation of the QRS duration or sinoatrial (SA) or AV nodal conduction disturbances. Quinidine can produce syncope in 0.5 to 2.0 percent of patients, most often the result of a self-terminating episode of torsades de pointes. Quinidine prolongs the QT interval in most patients, whether or not ventricular arrhythmias occur, but significant QT prolongation (QT interval of 500 to 600 milliseconds) is often a characteristic of patients with quinidine syncope. Many of these patients are also receiving digitalis or diuretics or have hypokalemia; women are more susceptible than men. Syncope is unrelated to plasma concentrations of quinidine or duration of therapy, although most episodes occur within the first 2 to 4 days of therapy, often after conversion of atrial fibrillation to sinus rhythm. Therapy requires immediate discontinuation of the drug and avoidance of other drugs that have similar pharmacological effects, because cross-sensitivity exists in some patients. Magnesium given intravenously (2 gm over 1 to 2 minutes, followed by an infusion of 3 to 20 mg/min) is the initial drug treatment of choice. Atrial or ventricular pacing can be used to suppress the ventricular tachyarrhythmia, perhaps acting by suppressing early afterdepolarizations. When pacing is not available, isoproterenol can be given with caution. The arrhythmia gradually dissipates as quinidine is cleared and the QT interval returns to baseline.

Drugs that induce hepatic enzyme production, such as phenobarbital and phenytoin, can shorten the duration of quinidine's action by increasing its rate of elimination. Quinidine can increase plasma concentrations of flecainide by inhibiting the CYP450 enzyme system. Quinidine may elevate serum digoxin and digitoxin concentrations by decreasing total body clearance of digitoxin and by decreasing the clearance, volume of distribution, and affinity of tissue receptors for digoxin.

PROCAINAMIDE

ELECTROPHYSIOLOGICAL ACTIONS (see Tables 33-1, 33-2, 33-3, and 33-5). The cardiac actions of procainamide on automaticity, conduction, excitability, and membrane responsiveness resemble those of quinidine. Procainamide predominantly blocks the inactivated state of I_{Na}. It also blocks I_{Kr} and $I_{K.ATP}$. Like quinidine, procainamide usually prolongs the ERP more than it prolongs the APD and thus may prevent reentry. Procainamide exerts the least anticholinergic effects among type IA drugs. It does not affect normal sinus node automaticity. In vitro, procainamide decreases abnormal automaticity, with less effect on triggered activity or catecholamine-enhanced normal automaticity. The electrophysiological effects of NAPA, procainamide's major metabolite, differ from those of the parent compound. NAPA, a K^+ channel blocker (I_{Kr}), exerts a class III action and prolongs the APD of ventricular muscle and Purkinje fibers in a dose-dependent manner. High levels produce early afterdepolarizations, triggered activity, and torsades de pointes.

HEMODYNAMIC EFFECTS. Procainamide can depress myocardial contractility in high doses. It does not produce alpha blockade but can result in peripheral vasodilation, possibly through antisympathetic effects on brain or spinal cord that can impair cardiovascular reflexes.

PHARMACOKINETICS (see Table 33-4). Oral administration produces a peak plasma concentration in about 1 hour. Approximately 80 percent of oral procainamide is bioavailable; the overall elimination half-life for procainamide is 3 to 5 hours, with 50 to 60 percent of the drug eliminated by the kidney and 10 to 30 percent eliminated by hepatic metabolism. The drug is acetylated to NAPA, which is excreted almost exclusively by the kidneys. As renal function decreases and in patients with heart failure, NAPA levels increase and, because of the risk of serious cardiotoxicity, need to be carefully monitored in these situations. NAPA has an elimination half-life of 7 to 8 hours, but the half-life exceeds 10 hours if high doses of procainamide are used. Small amounts of NAPA are converted back to procainamide by deacetylation. Increased age, congestive heart failure, and reduced creatinine clearance lower the procainamide clearance and necessitate a reduced dosage.

DOSAGE AND ADMINISTRATION (see Table 33-4). Procainamide can be given by the oral, IV, or intramuscular route to achieve plasma concentrations in the range of 4 to 10 mg/ml that produce an antiarrhythmic effect. Several IV regimens have been used to administer procainamide; 25 to 50 mg can be given over a 1-minute period and then repeated every 5 minutes until the arrhythmia has been controlled, hypotension results, or the QRS complex is prolonged more than 50 percent. Doses of 10 to 15 mg/kg at 50 mg/min can also be used. Using this method, the plasma concentration falls rapidly during the first 15 minutes after the loading dose, with parallel effects on refractoriness and conduction. A constant rate IV infusion of procainamide can be given at a dose of 2 to 6 mg/min, depending on the patient's response.

Oral administration of procainamide requires a 3- to 4-hour dosing interval at a total daily dose of 2 to 6 gm, with a steady state reached within 1 day. When a loading dose is used, it should be twice the maintenance dose. Frequent dosing is required because of the short elimination half-life in normal subjects. For the extended-release forms of procainamide, dosing is at 6- to 12-hour intervals. Procainamide is well absorbed after intramuscular injection, with almost 100 percent of the dose bioavailable.

INDICATIONS. Procainamide is used to treat both supraventricular and ventricular arrhythmias in a manner comparable to that of quinidine. Although both drugs have similar electrophysiological actions, either drug can effectively suppress a supraventricular or ventricular arrhythmia that is resistant to the other drug. Procainamide can be used to convert recent-onset atrial fibrillation to sinus rhythm. As with quinidine, prior treatment with beta or calcium channel blockers is recommended to prevent acceleration of the ventricular response during atrial flutter or fibrillation after procainamide therapy. Procainamide can block conduction in the accessory pathway of patients with the Wolff-Parkinson-White syndrome and may be used in patients with atrial fibrillation and a rapid ventricular response related to conduction over the accessory pathway. It can produce His-Purkinje block (see Fig. 32-11) and is sometimes administered during an electrophysiological study (EPS) to stress the His-Purkinje system in evaluating the need for a pacemaker. However, it should be used with caution in patients with evidence of His-Purkinje disease (bundle branch block) in whom a ventricular pacemaker is not readily available. Procainamide is more effective than lidocaine in acutely terminating sustained VT. Most consistently, procainamide slows the VT rate, a change correlated with the increase in QRS duration. The electrophysiological response to procainamide given intravenously appears to predict the response to the drug given orally. It has been used to facilitate VT induction at EPS when the arrhythmia could not be initiated in the baseline state.[9]

ADVERSE EFFECTS. Noncardiac adverse effects from procainamide administration include rashes, myalgias, digital vasculitis, and Raynaud's phenomenon. Fever and agranulocytosis may be the result of hypersensitivity reactions, and white blood cell and differential counts should be assessed at regular intervals. Gastrointestinal side effects are less frequent than with quinidine, and adverse central nervous system side effects are less frequent than with lidocaine. Toxic concentrations of procainamide can diminish myocardial performance and promote hypotension. Various conduction disturbances or ventricular tachyarrhythmias can occur that are similar to those produced by quinidine, including prolonged QT syndrome and polymorphic VT. NAPA can also cause QT prolongation and torsades de pointes. In the absence of sinus node disease, procainamide does not adversely affect sinus node function. In patients with sinus node dysfunction, procainamide can prolong sinus node recovery time and worsen symptoms in some patients who have the bradycardia-tachycardia syndrome.

Arthralgia, fever, pleuropericarditis, hepatomegaly, and hemorrhagic pericardial effusion with tamponade have been described in a systemic lupus erythematosus (SLE)–like syndrome related to procainamide administration. The syndrome occurs more frequently and earlier in patients who are slow acetylators of procainamide and is genetically influenced (see Chap. 6). Acetylating an aromatic amino group on procainamide to form NAPA appears to block the SLE-inducing effect. Sixty to 70 percent of patients who receive procainamide on a chronic basis develop antinuclear antibodies, with clinical symptoms in 20 to 30 percent, but this is reversible when procainamide is stopped. Positive serological test results are not necessarily a reason to discontinue drug therapy; however, the development of symptoms or a positive anti-DNA antibody indicates that drug therapy should be discontinued. Corticosteroid administration in these patients may eliminate the symptoms. In this syndrome, in contrast to naturally occurring SLE, the brain and kidney are spared and there is no predilection for females.

DISOPYRAMIDE

Disopyramide has been approved in the United States for oral administration to treat patients with ventricular and supraventricular arrhythmias.

ELECTROPHYSIOLOGICAL ACTIONS (see Tables 33-1, 33-2, 33-3, and 33-5). Although structurally different from quinidine and procainamide, disopyramide produces similar electrophysiological effects, causing use-dependent block of I_{Na} and non–use-dependent block of I_{Kr}. Disopyramide also inhibits $I_{K,ATP}$; it does not affect calcium-dependent action potentials, except possibly at very high concentrations.

Disopyramide is a muscarinic blocker and can increase the sinus node discharge rate and shorten AV nodal conduction time and refractoriness when the nodes are under cholinergic (vagal) influences. Disopyramide can also slow the sinus node discharge rate by a direct action when given in a high concentration and can significantly depress sinus node activity in patients with sinus node dysfunction. It exerts greater anticholinergic effects than quinidine and does not appear to affect alpha or beta adrenoceptors. The drug prolongs atrial and ventricular refractory periods, but its effect on AV nodal conduction and refractoriness is not consistent. Disopyramide prolongs His-Purkinje conduction time, but infra-His block rarely occurs. It can be administered safely to patients who have first-degree AV delay and narrow QRS complexes.

HEMODYNAMIC EFFECTS. Disopyramide suppresses ventricular systolic performance and is a mild arterial vasodilator. The drug should generally be avoided in patients who have reduced left ventricular systolic function, because they tolerate disopyramide's negative inotropic effects poorly.

PHARMACOKINETICS (see Table 33-4). Disopyramide is 80 to 90 percent absorbed, with a mean elimination half-life of 8 to 9 hours in healthy volunteers but almost 10 hours in patients with heart failure. Renal insufficiency prolongs the elimination time. Thus, in patients who have renal, hepatic, or cardiac insufficiency, loading and maintenance doses need to be reduced. Peak blood levels after oral administration are seen in 1 to 2 hours. It is bound to alpha$_1$-acid glycoprotein and passes through the placenta. About 50 percent of an oral dose is recovered unchanged in the urine, with about 30 percent as the mono-*N*-dealkylated metabolite. The metabolites appear to exert less effect than the parent compound. Erythromycin inhibits its metabolism.

DOSAGE AND ADMINISTRATION (see Table 33-4). Doses are generally 100 to 200 mg orally every 6 hours, with a range of 400 to 1200 mg/day. A controlled-release preparation can be given as 200 to 300 mg every 12 hours.

INDICATIONS. Disopyramide appears comparable to quinidine and procainamide in reducing the frequency of PVCs and effectively preventing recurrence of VT in selected patients. Disopyramide has been combined with other drugs, such as mexiletine, to treat patients who do not respond or only partially respond to one drug.

Disopyramide helps prevent recurrence of atrial fibrillation after successful cardioversion as effectively as quinidine and may terminate atrial flutter. In treating patients with atrial fibrillation, particularly atrial flutter, the ventricular rate must be controlled before administering disopyramide, or the combination of a decrease in atrial rate with vagolytic effects on the AV node can result in 1:1 AV conduction during atrial flutter. Disopyramide may be useful in preventing episodes of neurally mediated syncope. It has been used in patients with hypertrophic cardiomyopathy.

ADVERSE EFFECTS. Three types of adverse effects follow disopyramide administration. The most common effects are related to the drug's potent parasympatholytic properties and include urinary hesitancy or retention, constipation, blurred vision, closed-angle glaucoma, and dry mouth. Symptoms are less with the sustained-release form. Second, disopyramide can produce ventricular tachyarrhythmias that are commonly associated with QT prolongation and torsades de pointes. Some patients can have cross-sensitization to both quinidine and disopyramide and develop torsades de pointes while receiving either drug. When drug-induced torsades de pointes occurs, agents that prolong the QT interval should be used cautiously or not at all. Finally, disopyramide can reduce contractility of the normal ventricle, but the depression of ventricular function is much more pronounced in patients with preexisting ventricular failure. Occasionally, cardiovascular collapse can result.

AJMALINE

Ajmaline, a rauwolfia derivative, has been used extensively to treat patients with ventricular and supraventricular arrhythmias in Europe and Asia but is not available in the United States.

ELECTROPHYSIOLOGICAL ACTIONS (see Tables 33-1, 33-2, 33-3, and 33-5). Like other type IA drugs, ajmaline produces use-dependent block of I_{Na}; it also weakly blocks I_{Kr}. The drug has mild anticholinergic activity.

HEMODYNAMIC EFFECTS. Ajmaline mildly suppresses ventricular systolic performance but does not affect peripheral resistance. It also inhibits platelet activity more potently than aspirin.

PHARMACOKINETICS, DOSAGE AND ADMINISTRATION (see Table 33-4). Ajmaline is well-absorbed, with a mean elimination half-life of 13 min in most patients, making it poorly suited to long-term oral use. The dose for acute arrhythmia termination is generally 50 mg IV over 1 to 2 minutes.

INDICATIONS. Although useful for terminating supraventricular tachycardias by intravenous infusion, other medications have largely supplanted ajmaline for this purpose. The drug's use has evolved to that of a diagnostic tool. When administered IV at doses of 50 mg over 3 min, or 10 mg/minute, to a total dose of 1 mg/kg, ajmaline can have the following effects: (1) delta wave disappearance in patients with Wolff-Parkinson-White syndrome (indicating an accessory pathway anterograde effective refractory period more than 250 milliseconds); (2) ST-T abnormalities and interventricular conduction blocks in patients with occult chagasic cardiomyopathy; (3) heart block in patients with bundle branch block and syncope, but in whom no rhythm disturbance had been discovered; and (4) right precordial ST elevation in patients with suspected Brugada syndrome in whom the resting electrocardiogram (ECG) is normal.[10] It is in this last setting that ajmaline is used most frequently.

ADVERSE EFFECTS. Ajmaline can produce mild anticholinergic side effects as well as mild depression in left ventricular systolic function, and can worsen AV conduction in patients with His-Purkinje disease. Rare occurrences of torsades de pointes have been reported. Ajmaline can cause an increase in the defibrillation threshold.

Class IB Agents

LIDOCAINE

ELECTROPHYSIOLOGICAL ACTIONS (see Tables 33-1, 33-2, 33-3, and 33-5). Lidocaine blocks I_{Na}, predominantly in the open or possibly inactivated state. It has rapid onset and offset kinetics and does not affect normal sinus node automaticity in usual doses but does depress other normal and abnormal forms of automaticity, as well as early and late afterdepolarizations in Purkinje fibers in vitro. Lidocaine has only a modest depressant effect on $\dot{V}_{max}$; however, faster rates of stimulation, reduced pH, increased extracellular K^+ concentration, and reduced membrane potential, all changes that can result from ischemia, increase the ability of lidocaine to block I_{Na}. Lidocaine can convert areas of unidirectional block into bidirectional block during ischemia and prevent development of VF by preventing fragmentation of organized large wave fronts into heterogeneous wavelets.

Except in very high concentrations, lidocaine does not affect slow channel–dependent action potentials, despite its moderate suppression of the slow inward current. Lidocaine has little effect on atrial fibers and does not affect conduction in accessory pathways. Patients with preexisting sinus node dysfunction, abnormal His-Purkinje conduction, or junctional or ventricular escape rhythms can develop depressed automaticity or conduction. Part of its effects may involve inhibition of cardiac sympathetic nerve activity.

HEMODYNAMIC EFFECTS. Clinically significant adverse hemodynamic effects are rarely noted at usual drug concentrations unless left ventricular function is severely impaired.

PHARMACOKINETICS (see Table 33-4). Lidocaine is used only parenterally because oral administration results in extensive first-pass hepatic metabolism and unpredictable low plasma levels, with excessive metabolites that can produce toxicity. Hepatic metabolism of lidocaine depends on hepatic blood flow; severe hepatic disease or reduced hepatic blood flow, as in heart failure or shock, can markedly decrease the rate of lidocaine metabolism. Beta adrenoceptor blockers can decrease hepatic blood flow and increase lidocaine serum concentration. Prolonged infusion can reduce lidocaine clearance. Its elimination half-life averages 1 to 2 hours in normal subjects, longer than 4 hours in patients after uncomplicated myocardial infarction, longer than 10 hours in patients after myocardial infarction complicated by cardiac failure, and even longer in the presence of cardiogenic shock. Maintenance doses should be reduced by one third to one half for patients with low cardiac output. Lidocaine is 50 to 80 percent protein bound and binds to alpha$_1$-acid glycoprotein.

DOSAGE AND ADMINISTRATION (see Table 33-4). Although lidocaine can be given intramuscularly, the IV route is most commonly used. Intramuscular lidocaine is given in doses of 4 to 5 mg/kg (250 to 350 mg), resulting in effective serum levels at about 15 minutes and lasting for about 90 minutes. Intravenously, lidocaine is given as an initial bolus of 1 to 2 mg/kg body weight at a rate of 20 to 50 mg/min, with a second injection of half the initial dose 20 to 40 minutes later. Patients treated with an initial bolus followed by a maintenance infusion may experience transient subtherapeutic plasma concentrations 30 to 120 minutes after initiation of therapy. A second bolus of about 0.5 mg/kg without increasing the maintenance infusion rate reestablishes therapeutic serum concentrations.

If recurrence of arrhythmia appears after a steady state has been achieved (e.g., 6 to 10 hours after starting therapy), a similar bolus should be given and the maintenance infusion rate increased. Increasing the maintenance infusion rate alone without an additional bolus results in a very slow increase in plasma lidocaine concentrations and is therefore not recommended. Another recommended IV dosing regimen is 1.5 mg/kg initially and 0.8 mg/kg at 8-minute intervals for three doses. Doses are reduced by about 50 percent for patients with heart failure.

If the initial bolus of lidocaine is ineffective, up to two more boluses of 1 mg/kg may be administered at 5-minute intervals. Patients who require more than one bolus to achieve a therapeutic effect have arrhythmias that respond only to higher lidocaine plasma concentrations, and a higher maintenance dose may be necessary to sustain these higher concentrations. Maintenance infusion rates in the range of 1 to 4 mg/min produce steady-state plasma levels of 1 to 5 mg/ml in patients with uncomplicated myocardial infarction, but these rates must be reduced during heart failure or shock because of concomitant reduced hepatic blood flow.

INDICATIONS. Lidocaine has moderate efficacy against ventricular arrhythmias of diverse causes; it is generally ineffective against supraventricular arrhythmias. Although once commonly used to try to prevent VF in the first 2 days following acute myocardial infarction, its efficacy was not great and, because it can produce side effects and a possible increase in the risk of developing asystole, this use is not recommended. Lidocaine has been effective in patients after coronary revascularization and in patients resuscitated from out-of-hospital VF, although amiodarone has been shown to yield higher rates of survival, at least to hospital admission.[11]

ADVERSE EFFECTS. The most commonly reported adverse effects of lidocaine are dose-related manifestations of central nervous system toxicity: dizziness, paresthesias, confusion, delirium, stupor, coma, and seizures. Occasional sinus node depression and His-Purkinje block have been reported. Rarely, lidocaine can cause malignant hyperthermia. Both lidocaine and procainamide can elevate defibrillation thresholds.

MEXILETINE

Mexiletine, a local anesthetic congener of lidocaine with anticonvulsant properties, is used for the oral treatment of patients with symptomatic ventricular arrhythmias.

ELECTROPHYSIOLOGICAL ACTIONS (see Tables 33-1, 33-2, 33-3, and 33-5). Mexiletine is similar to lidocaine in many of its electrophysiological actions. In vitro, mexiletine shortens the APD and ERP of Purkinje fibers and, to a lesser extent, of ventricular muscle. It depresses $\dot{V}_{max}$ of phase 0 by blocking I_{Na}, especially at faster rates, and depresses automaticity of Purkinje fibers but not of the normal sinus node. Its onset and offset kinetics are rapid. Hypoxia or ischemia can increase its effects.

Mexiletine can result in severe bradycardia and abnormal sinus node recovery time in patients with sinus node disease, but not in patients with a normal sinus node. It does not affect AV nodal conduction and can depress His-Purkinje conduction, but not greatly, unless conduction was abnormal initially. Mexiletine does not appear to affect human atrial muscle. It does not affect the QT interval.

HEMODYNAMIC EFFECTS. Mexiletine exerts no major hemodynamic effects on ventricular contractile performance or peripheral resistance.

PHARMACOKINETICS (see Table 33-4). Mexiletine is rapidly and almost completely absorbed after oral ingestion by volunteers, with peak plasma concentrations attained in 2 to 4 hours. Elimination half-life in healthy subjects is approximately 10 hours, but 17 hours in patients after myocardial infarction. Therapeutic plasma levels of 0.5 to 2 mg/ml are maintained by oral doses of 200 to 300 mg every 6 to 8 hours. Absorption with less than a 10 percent first-pass hepatic effect occurs in the upper small intestine and is delayed and incomplete in patients who have myocardial infarction and in patients receiving narcotics, antacids, or atropine-like drugs that retard gastric emptying. About 70 percent of the drug is protein bound. The apparent volume of distribution is large, reflecting extensive tissue uptake. Normally, mexiletine is eliminated metabolically by the liver, with less than 10 percent excreted unchanged in the urine. Doses should be reduced in patients with cirrhosis or left ventricular failure. Renal clearance of mexiletine decreases as the urinary pH increases. Known metabolites exert no electrophysiological effects. Metabolism can be increased by phenytoin, phenobarbital, and rifampin and reduced by cimetidine.

DOSAGE AND ADMINISTRATION (see Table 33-4). The recommended starting dose is 200 mg orally every 8 hours when rapid arrhythmia control is not essential. Doses may be increased or decreased by 50 to 100 mg every 2 to 3 days and are better tolerated when given with food. Total daily dose should not exceed 1200 mg. In some patients, administration every 12 hours can be effective.

INDICATIONS. Mexiletine is a moderately effective antiarrhythmic agent for treating patients with acute and chronic ventricular tachyarrhythmias, but not SVTs. Success rates vary from 6 to 60 percent and can be increased in some patients if mexiletine is combined with other drugs such as procainamide, beta blockers, quinidine, disopyramide, propafenone, or amiodarone. Most studies show no clear superiority of mexiletine over other class I agents. Mexiletine may be very useful in children with congenital heart disease and serious ventricular arrhythmias. In treating patients with a long QT interval, mexiletine may be safer than drugs such as quinidine that increase the QT interval further. Limited experience in treating subsets of patients with long-QT syndrome (LQT3, which is related to the *SCN5A* gene for the cardiac sodium channel) suggests a beneficial role (see Chap. 9).

ADVERSE EFFECTS. Up to 40 percent of patients may require a change in dose or discontinuation of mexiletine therapy as a result of adverse effects, including tremor, dysarthria, dizziness, paresthesia, diplopia, nystagmus, mental confusion, anxiety, nausea, vomiting, and dyspepsia. Cardiovascular side effects are rare but include hypotension, bradycardia, and exacerbation of arrhythmia. Adverse effects of mexiletine appear to be dose related, and toxic effects occur at plasma concentrations only slightly higher than therapeutic levels. Therefore, effective use of this antiarrhythmic drug requires careful titration of dose and monitoring of plasma concentration. Lidocaine should be avoided, or the dose reduced, in patients also receiving lidocaine congeners such as mexiletine.

Phenytoin was used originally to treat seizure disorders. Its value as an antiarrhythmic agent remains limited.

ELECTROPHYSIOLOGICAL ACTIONS (see Tables 33-1, 33-2, 33-3, and 33-5). Phenytoin effectively abolishes abnormal automaticity caused by digitalis-induced delayed afterdepolarizations in cardiac Purkinje fibers and suppresses certain digitalis-induced arrhythmias in humans. The rate of rise of action potentials initiated early in the relative refractory period is increased, as is membrane responsiveness, possibly reducing the chance for impaired conduction and block. Phenytoin minimally affects sinus discharge rate and AV conduction in humans. Some of phenytoin's antiarrhythmic effects may be neurally mediated because it can modulate both sympathetic and vagal efferent activity. It has no peripheral cholinergic or beta-adrenergic blocking actions, and minimal hemodynamic effect.

PHARMACOKINETICS (see Table 33-4). The pharmacokinetics of phenytoin are less than ideal. Absorption after oral administration is incomplete and varies with the brand of drug. Plasma concentrations peak 8 to 12 hours after an oral dose; 90 percent of the drug is protein bound. Phenytoin has limited solubility at physiological pH, and intramuscular administration is associated with pain, muscle necrosis, sterile abscesses, and variable absorption. Therapeutic serum concentrations of phenytoin (10 to 20 mg/ml) are similar for treating cardiac arrhythmias and epilepsy. Lower concentrations can suppress certain digitalis-induced arrhythmias.

METABOLISM. Over 90 percent of a dose is hydroxylated in the liver to presumably inactive compounds; significant genetically determined variation can occur. Elimination half-time is about 24 hours and can be slowed in the presence of liver disease or when phenytoin is administered concomitantly with drugs such as warfarin, isoniazid, and phenothiazines, which compete with phenytoin for hepatic enzymes. Because of the large number of medications that can increase or decrease phenytoin levels during chronic therapy, phenytoin plasma concentration should be determined frequently when changes are made in other medications. Phenytoin has concentration-dependent kinetics for elimination that can cause unexpected toxicity, because disproportionately large changes in plasma concentration can follow dose increases.

DOSAGE AND ADMINISTRATION (see Table 33-4). To achieve a therapeutic plasma concentration rapidly, 100 mg of phenytoin should be administered intravenously every 5 minutes until the arrhythmia is controlled, 1 gm has been given, or adverse side effects result. Generally, 700 to 1000 mg controls the arrhythmia. A large central vein should be used to avoid pain and development of phlebitis produced by the drug's alkalotic vehicle. Orally, phenytoin is given as a loading dose of 1000 mg the first day, 500 mg on the second and third days, and 300 to 400 mg daily thereafter. Maintenance doses can generally be given once daily because of the long half-life of elimination.

INDICATIONS. Phenytoin has been used successfully to treat atrial and ventricular arrhythmias caused by digitalis toxicity but is much less effective in treating ventricular arrhythmias in patients with ischemic heart disease or with atrial arrhythmias not caused by digitalis toxicity. It may be useful in some patients with the long-QT syndrome.

ADVERSE EFFECTS. The most common manifestations of phenytoin toxicity are central nervous system effects of nystagmus, ataxia, drowsiness, stupor, and coma and correlate with increases in plasma drug concentration. Nausea, epigastric pain, and anorexia are also relatively common effects of phenytoin. Long-term administration can result in hyperglycemia, hypocalcemia, rashes, megaloblastic anemia, gingival hypertrophy, lymph node hyperplasia (a syndrome resembling malignant lymphoma), peripheral neuropathy, pneumonitis, and drug-induced SLE. Birth defects can also result.

Class IC Agents

FLECAINIDE

Flecainide is approved by the U.S. Food and Drug Administration (FDA) to treat patients with life-threatening ventricular arrhythmias as well as various supraventricular arrhythmias.

ELECTROPHYSIOLOGICAL ACTIONS (see Tables 33-1, 33-2, 33-3, and 33-5). Flecainide exhibits marked use-dependent depressant effects on the rapid sodium channel, decreasing $\dot{V}_{max}$, with slow onset and offset kinetics. Drug dissociation from the sodium channel is slow, with time constants of 10 to 30 seconds (compared with 4 to 8 seconds for quinidine and less than 1 second for lidocaine). Thus, marked drug effects can occur at physiological heart rates. Flecainide shortens the duration of the Purkinje fiber action potential but prolongs it in ventricular muscle, actions that, depending on the circumstances, could enhance or reduce electrical heterogeneity and create or suppress arrhythmias. Flecainide profoundly slows conduction in all cardiac fibers and, in high concentrations, inhibits the slow Ca^{2+} channel (see Chap. 31). Conduction time in the atria, ventricles, AV node, and His-Purkinje system is prolonged. Minimal increases in atrial or ventricular refractoriness or in the QT interval result. Anterograde and retrograde refractoriness in accessory pathways can increase significantly in a use-dependent fashion. Sinus node function remains unchanged in normal subjects but may be depressed in patients with sinus node dysfunction. Flecainide can facilitate or inhibit reentry and may transform atrial fibrillation to flutter. Pacing and defibrillation thresholds are characteristically slightly increased.[12]

HEMODYNAMIC EFFECTS. Flecainide depresses cardiac performance, particularly in patients with compromised ventricular systolic function and should be used cautiously, or not at all, in patients with moderate or severe ventricular systolic dysfunction.

PHARMACOKINETICS (see Table 33-4). Flecainide is at least 90 percent absorbed, with peak plasma concentrations in 3 to 4 hours. Elimination half-life in patients with ventricular arrhythmias is 20 hours, with 85 percent of the drug being excreted unchanged or as an inactive metabolite in urine. Two major metabolites exert fewer effects than the parent drug. Elimination is slower in patients with renal disease and heart failure, and doses should be reduced in these situations. Therapeutic plasma concentrations range from 0.2 to 1.0 mg/ml. About 40 percent of the drug is protein bound. Increases in serum concentrations of digoxin (15 to 25 percent) and propranolol (30 percent) result during coadministration with flecainide. Propranolol, quinidine, and amiodarone may increase flecainide serum concentrations. Five to 7 days of dosing may be required to reach a steady state in some patients.

DOSAGE AND ADMINISTRATION (see Table 33-4). The starting dose is 100 mg every 12 hours, increased in increments of 50 mg twice daily, no sooner than every 3 to 4 days, until efficacy is achieved, an adverse effect is noted, or to a maximum of 400 mg/day. Cardiac rhythm and QRS duration should be monitored after dose changes.

INDICATIONS. Flecainide is indicated for the treatment of life-threatening ventricular tachyarrhythmias, SVTs, and paroxysmal atrial fibrillation. Some experts have suggested that therapy should begin in the hospital while the electrocardiogram is being monitored because of the possibility of proarrhythmic events (see later). Serum concentration should not exceed 1.0 mg/ml. Flecainide is particularly effective in almost totally suppressing PVCs and short runs of nonsustained VT. As with other class I antiarrhythmic drugs, there are no data from controlled studies to indicate that the drug favorably affects survival or sudden cardiac death, and data from the CAST study have indicated increased mortality in patients with coronary artery disease. Flecainide produces a use-dependent prolongation of VT cycle length that can improve hemodynamic tolerance. Flecainide is also useful in various SVTs, such as atrial tachycardia, flutter, and atrial fibrillation (including oral loading to terminate episodes acutely[13]). When administered chronically, isoproterenol can reverse some of these effects. It is important to slow the ventricular rate before treating atrial fibrillation with flecainide to avoid 1:1 AV conduction. Flecainide has been used to treat fetal arrhythmias and arrhythmias in children. Flecainide administration may produce ST elevation in lead V_1 characteristic of Brugada syndrome (see Chap. 9) and has been used as a diagnostic tool in patients suspected of having this disorder.[14]

ADVERSE EFFECTS. Proarrhythmic effects are some of the most important adverse effects of flecainide. Its marked slowing of conduction precludes its use in patients with second-degree AV block without a pacemaker and warrants cautious administration in patients with intraventricular conduction disorders. Worsening of existing ventricular arrhythmias or onset of new ventricular arrhythmias can occur in 5 to 30 percent of patients, especially in patients with preexisting sustained VT, cardiac decompensation, and higher doses of the drug. Failure of the flecainide-related arrhythmia to respond to therapy, including electrical cardioversion-defibrillation, may result in mortality as high as 10 percent in patients who develop proarrhythmic events. Negative inotropic effects can cause or worsen heart failure. Patients with sinus node dysfunction may experience sinus arrest, and those with pacemakers may develop an increase in pacing threshold. In the CAST study, patients treated with flecainide had 5.1 percent mortality or nonfatal cardiac arrest compared with 2.3 percent in the placebo group over 10 months. Mortality was highest in those with non–Q-wave infarction, frequent PVCs, and faster heart rates, raising the possibility of drug interaction with ischemia and electrical instability. Exercise can amplify the conduction slowing in the ventricle produced by flecainide and in some cases can precipitate a proarrhythmic response. Therefore, exercise testing has been recommended to screen for proarrhythmia. Central nervous system complaints, including confusion and irritability, represent the most frequent noncardiac adverse effects. The safety of flecainide during pregnancy has not been determined although, as noted previously, it is occasionally used to treat fetal arrhythmias.[15] It is concentrated in breast milk to a level 2.5- to 4-fold higher than in plasma.

PROPAFENONE

Propafenone has been approved by the FDA for treatment of patients with life-threatening ventricular tachyarrhythmias as well as atrial fibrillation.

ELECTROPHYSIOLOGICAL ACTIONS (see Tables 33-1, 33-2, 33-3, and 33-5). Propafenone blocks the fast sodium current in a use-dependent manner in Purkinje fibers and to a lesser degree in ventricular muscle. Use-dependent effects contribute to its ability to terminate atrial fibrillation. The dissociation constant from the receptor is slow, similar to that of flecainide. Effects are greater in ischemic than normal tissue and at reduced membrane potentials. Propafenone decreases excitability and suppresses spontaneous automaticity and triggered activity. The drug is a weak blocker of I_{Kr} and beta-adrenergic receptors. Although ventricular refractoriness increases, conduction slowing is the major effect. Propafenone has several active metabolites that exert electrophysiologic effects. It depresses sinus node automaticity and A-H, H-V, PR, and QRS intervals increase, as do refractory periods of the atria, ventricles, AV node, and accessory pathways. The QT interval increases only as a function of increased QRS duration.

HEMODYNAMIC EFFECTS. Propafenone and 5-hydroxypropafenone exhibit negative inotropic properties at high concentrations. In patients with left ventricular ejection fractions exceeding 40 percent, the negative inotropic effects are well tolerated, but patients with preexisting left ventricular dysfunction and congestive heart failure may have symptomatic worsening of their hemodynamic status.

PHARMACOKINETICS (see Table 33-4). With more than 95 percent of the drug absorbed, propafenone's maximum plasma concentration occurs in 2 to 3 hours. Systemic bioavailability is dose dependent and ranges from 3 to 40 percent because of variable presystemic clearance. Bioavailability increases as the dose increases, and plasma concentration is therefore nonlinear. A threefold increase in dosage (300 to 900 mg/day) results in a 10-fold increase in plasma concentration, presumably because of saturation of hepatic metabolic mechanisms. Propafenone is 97 percent bound to alpha$_1$-acid glycoprotein, with an elimination half-life of 5 to 8 hours. Maximum therapeutic effects occur at serum concentrations of 0.2 to 1.5 mg/ml. Marked interpatient variability of pharmacokinetics and pharmacodynamics may be the result of genetically determined differences in metabolism (see Chap. 6). About 7 percent of the population are poor metabolizers, who have an elimination half-life of 15 to 20 hours for the parent compound and almost no 5-hydroxypropafenone. The (+)-enantiomer provides nonspecific beta-adrenergic receptor blockade with 2.5 to 5 percent of the potency of propranolol, but because plasma propafenone concentrations may be 50 times or more higher than propranolol levels, these beta-blocking properties may be relevant. Poor metabolizers have a greater beta-adrenergic receptor blocking effect than extensive metabolizers.

DOSAGE AND ADMINISTRATION (see Table 33-4). Most patients respond to oral doses of 150 to 300 mg every 8 hours, not exceeding 1200 mg/day. Doses are similar for patients of both metabolizing phenotypes. A sustained-release form is available for treatment of atrial fibrillation; dosing is 225 to 425 mg twice daily.[16] Concomitant food administration increases bioavailability, as does hepatic dysfunction. No good correlation between plasma propafenone concentration and arrhythmia suppression has been shown. Doses should not be increased more often than every 3 to 4 days. Propafenone increases plasma concentrations of warfarin, digoxin, and metoprolol.

INDICATIONS. Propafenone is indicated for the treatment of paroxysmal SVT, atrial fibrillation, and life-threatening ventricular tachyarrhythmias, and effectively suppresses spontaneous PVCs and nonsustained and sustained VT. Acute termination of atrial fibrillation episodes occurred with a single 600-mg oral dose of propafenone in 76 percent of patients given the drug (twice the rate of those given placebo).[17] It has been used effectively in the pediatric age group. Propafenone increases the pacing threshold but minimally affects the defibrillation threshold. Sinus rate during exercise is reduced. Propafenone use is associated with higher mortality in cardiac arrest survivors than with use of an implantable defibrillator.

ADVERSE EFFECTS. Minor noncardiac effects occur in about 15 percent of patients, with dizziness, disturbances in taste, and blurred vision the most common and gastrointestinal side effects next. Exacerbation of bronchospastic lung disease can occur because of mild beta-blocking effects. Cardiovascular side effects occur in 10 to 15 percent of patients, including AV block, sinus node depression, and worsening of heart failure. Proarrhythmic responses, which occur more often in patients with a history of sustained VT and decreased ejection fractions, appear less commonly than with flecainide (approximately 5 percent). The applicability of data from the CAST study about flecainide to propafenone is not clear, but limiting propafenone's application in a manner similar to that of other class IC drugs seems prudent. Its beta-blocking actions may make it different, however. The safety of propafenone administration during pregnancy has not been established (class C).

MORICIZINE (ETHMOZINE)

Moricizine is a phenothiazine derivative indicated for treatment of patients with ventricular tachyarrhythmias; it has also been used for atrial fibrillation. It was formerly discussed as a class IB antiarrhythmic drug because it shortens Purkinje fiber action potential. However, the intensity of its effect on the Na^+ channel is more like that of a class IA antiarrhythmic drug, whereas the time constants for onset and offset resemble those of class IC agents.

ELECTROPHYSIOLOGICAL ACTIONS. Moricizine decreases I_{Na} predominantly in the inactivated state, with a resultant decrease in $\dot{V}_{max}$ of phase 0 and action potential amplitude (see Tables 33-1, 33-2, 33-3, and 33-5). Moricizine blocks $I_{Ca.L}$ and I_K and prolongs AV node and His-Purkinje conduction times and QRS duration. The JT interval shortens slightly, whereas the QTc is prolonged by 5 percent because of QRS prolongation. Ventricular refractoriness is prolonged slightly, with no consistent atrial change. No alterations in sinus node automaticity result. Moricizine minimally raises the defibrillation threshold.

HEMODYNAMIC EFFECTS. Moricizine exerts minimal effects on cardiac performance in patients with impaired left ventricular function; an occasional patient with significant left ventricular dysfunction may have worsening of heart failure.

PHARMACOKINETICS (see Table 33-4). After oral ingestion, moricizine undergoes extensive first-pass metabolism, resulting in 35 to 40 percent bioavailability. Peak plasma concentrations are reached in 0.5

to 2 hours, later if the drug is taken after meals. Protein binding is 95 percent to alpha$_1$-acid glycoprotein and albumin. Antiarrhythmic and electrophysiological actions do not relate to its plasma concentrations or to any of its more than 20 metabolites. Plasma elimination half-life is 1.5 to 3.5 hours, with roughly 50 percent of the drug excreted in the feces and the rest in the urine.

DOSAGE AND ADMINISTRATION (see Table 33-4). The usual adult dose is 600 to 900 mg/day, given every 8 hours in divided doses, with increments of 150 mg/day at 3-day intervals. Some patients may be treated every 12 hours. Dosage should be reduced in patients with hepatic or renal disease, AV conduction disturbances, or sinus node dysfunction without a pacemaker, and with significant congestive heart failure.

INDICATIONS. Moricizine is indicated for prevention of life-threatening ventricular arrhythmias and has an efficacy about comparable to those of quinidine and disopyramide. Moricizine can have proarrhythmic effects; in the CAST study, it caused an increase in mortality compared with placebo during initial treatment of patients who had symptomatic or minimally symptomatic ventricular arrhythmias after myocardial infarction. Risk was greater in patients taking diuretics.

ADVERSE EFFECTS. Usually, the drug is well tolerated. Noncardiac adverse effects primarily involve the nervous system and include tremor, mood changes, headache, vertigo, nystagmus, and dizziness. Gastrointestinal side effects include nausea, vomiting, and diarrhea. Worsening of congestive heart failure may rarely occur. Proarrhythmic effects have been reported in 3 to 15 percent of patients, more commonly in patients with severe ventricular arrhythmias. Advancing age increases the susceptibility to adverse effects. Moricizine appears to be relatively safe to use during pregnancy (class B) and is present in small amounts in breast milk.

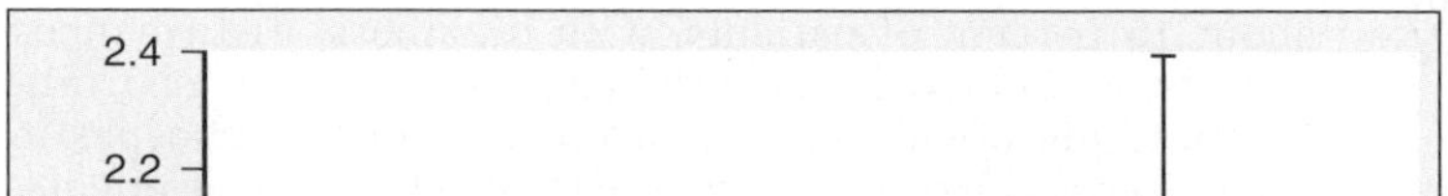

FIGURE 33–1 Meta-analytical data from randomized clinical trials of antiarrhythmic drugs in survivors of acute myocardial infarction. The relative risk is compared with placebo therapy (mean and 95 percent confidence interval) for death during therapy with various electrophysiological classes of compounds. Class I agents, particularly IC, and sotalol increase mortality, whereas beta blockers and amiodarone decrease mortality. Numbers under each drug class refer to number of patients involved in the trials. Amio = amiodarone; Sota = sotalol. (Modified from Teo KK, Yusuf S: *In* Singh BN, Dzau VJ, Vanhoutte PM, Woosley RL [eds]: Cardiovascular Pharmacology and Therapeutics. New York, Churchill Livingstone, 1994, pp 631-643; and Waldo AL, Camm AJ, deRuyter H, et al: Effect of *d*-sotalol on mortality in patients with left ventricular dysfunction after recent and remote myocardial infarction: The SWORD Investigators. Survival With Oral *d*-Sotalol. Lancet 348:7, 1996.)

Class II Agents

BETA ADRENOCEPTOR BLOCKING AGENTS

Although many beta adrenoceptor blocking drugs have been approved for use in the United States, metoprolol, carvedilol, atenolol, propranolol and esmolol have been most widely used to treat supraventricular and ventricular arrhythmias. Acebutolol, nadolol, timolol, betaxolol, pindolol, and bisoprolol have been less extensively used for treatment of arrhythmias. Metoprolol, atenolol, carvedilol, atenolol, timolol, and propranolol decrease overall mortality and sudden death after myocardial infarction (see Chap. 36). It is generally considered that beta blockers possess class effects and that, when titrated to the proper dose, all can be used effectively to treat cardiac arrhythmias, hypertension, or other disorders. However, differences in pharmacokinetic or pharmacodynamic properties that confer safety, reduce adverse effects, or affect dosing intervals or drug interactions influence the choice of agent. Also, some beta blockers, such as sotalol, pindolol, and carvedilol, exert unique actions.

Beta receptors can be separated into those that affect predominantly the heart (beta$_1$) and those that affect predominantly blood vessels and the bronchi (beta$_2$). In low doses, selective beta blockers can block beta$_1$ receptors more than they block beta$_2$ receptors and might be preferable for treating patients with pulmonary or peripheral vascular diseases. In high doses, the "selective" beta$_1$ blockers also block beta$_2$ receptors. Carvedilol also exerts alpha blocking effects and is used primarily in patients with heart failure (see Chaps. 23 through 25).

Some beta blockers exert intrinsic sympathomimetic activity; that is, they slightly activate the beta receptor. These drugs appear to be as efficacious as beta blockers without intrinsic sympathomimetic actions and may cause less slowing of heart rate at rest and less prolongation of AV nodal conduction time. They have been shown to induce less depression of left ventricular function than beta blockers without intrinsic sympathomimetic activity. Only nonselective beta blockers without intrinsic sympathomimetic activity have been demonstrated to reduce mortality in patients after myocardial infarction (Fig. 33-1; see Chaps. 50 and 51).

The following discussion concentrates on the use of propranolol as a prototypical antiarrhythmic agent but is generally applicable to other beta blockers.

ELECTROPHYSIOLOGICAL ACTIONS. Beta blockers exert an electrophysiological action by competitively inhibiting catecholamine binding at beta adrenoceptor sites, an effect almost entirely to the result of the (−)-levorotatory stereoisomer, or by their quinidine-like or direct membrane-stabilizing action (see Tables 33-1, 33-2, 33-3, and 33-5). The latter is a local anesthetic effect that depresses I_{Na} and membrane responsiveness in cardiac Purkinje fibers, occurs at concentrations generally 10 times that necessary to produce beta blockade, and most likely plays an insignificant antiarrhythmic role. Thus, beta blockers exert their major effects in cells most actively stimulated by adrenergic actions. At a beta-blocking concentration, propranolol slows spontaneous automaticity in the sinus node or in Purkinje fibers that are being stimulated by adrenergic tone, producing I_f block (see Chap. 31). Beta blockers also block $I_{Ca.L}$ stimulated by beta agonists. In the absence of adrenergic stimulation, only high concentrations of propranolol slow normal automaticity in Purkinje fibers, probably by a direct membrane action.

Concentrations that cause beta receptor blockade but no local anesthetic effects do not alter the normal resting membrane potential, maximum diastolic potential amplitude, $\dot{V}_{max}$, repolarization, or refractoriness of atrial, Purkinje, or ventricular muscle cells in the absence of catecholamine stimulation. However, in the presence of isoproterenol, a relatively pure beta receptor stimulator, beta blockers reverse isoproterenol's accelerating effects on repolarization. Propranolol reduces the amplitude of digitalis-induced delayed afterdepolarizations and suppresses triggered activity in Purkinje fibers.

Concentrations exceeding 3 mg/ml are required to depress $\dot{V}_{max}$ action potential amplitude, membrane responsiveness, and conduction in normal atrial, ventricular, and Purkinje fibers without altering resting membrane potential. These effects probably result from depression of I_{Na}. Long-term administration of propranolol may lengthen APD. As with the effects of lidocaine, acceleration of repolarization of Purkinje fibers is most marked in areas of the ventricular conduction system in which the APD is greatest. At least one beta blocker, sotalol, markedly increases the time course of repolarization in Purkinje fibers and ventricular muscle.

Propranolol slows the sinus discharge rate in humans by 10 to 20 percent, although severe bradycardia occasionally results if the heart is particularly dependent on sympathetic tone or if sinus node dysfunction is present. The PR interval lengthens, as do AV nodal conduction time and AV nodal effective and functional refractory periods (at a constant heart rate), but refractoriness and conduction in the normal His-Purkinje system remain unchanged, even after high doses of propranolol. Therefore, therapeutic doses of propranolol in humans do not exert a direct depressant or "quinidine-like" action but influence cardiac electrophysiology through a beta-blocking action. Beta blockers do not affect conduction or repolarization in normal ventricular muscle, as evidenced by their lack of effect on the QRS complex and QT interval, respectively.

Because administration of beta blockers that do not have direct membrane action prevents many arrhythmias resulting from activation of the autonomic nervous system, it is thought that the beta-blocking action is responsible for their antiarrhythmic effects. Nevertheless, the possible importance of the direct membrane effect of some of these drugs cannot be discounted totally, because beta blockers with direct membrane actions can affect transmembrane potentials of diseased cardiac fibers at much lower concentrations than are needed to affect normal fibers directly. However, indirect actions on arrhythmogenic effects of ischemia are probably most important. Beta blockers reduce myocardial injury during experimental cardiopulmonary resuscitation.

HEMODYNAMIC EFFECTS. Beta blockers exert negative inotropic effects and can precipitate or worsen heart failure. However, beta blockers clearly improve survival in patients with heart failure (see Chap. 29). By blocking beta receptors, these drugs may allow unopposed alpha-adrenergic effects to produce peripheral vasoconstriction and exacerbate coronary artery spasm or pain from peripheral vascular disease in some patients.

PHARMACOKINETICS (see Table 33-4). Although various types of beta blockers exert similar pharmacological effects, their pharmacokinetics differ substantially. Propranolol is almost 100 percent absorbed, but the effects of first-pass hepatic metabolism reduce bioavailability to about 30 percent and produce significant interpatient variability of plasma concentration for a given dose. Reduction in hepatic blood flow, as in patients with heart failure, decreases the hepatic extraction of propranolol; in these patients, propranolol may further decrease its own elimination rate by reducing cardiac output and hepatic blood flow. Beta blockers eliminated by the kidney tend to have longer half-lives and exhibit less interpatient variability of drug concentration than beta blockers metabolized by the liver.

DOSAGE AND ADMINISTRATION (see Table 33-4). The appropriate dose of propranolol is best determined by a measure of the patient's physiological response, such as changes in resting heart rate or prevention of exercise-induced tachycardia, because wide individual differences exist between the observed physiological effect and plasma concentration. For example, IV dosing is best achieved by titrating the dose to a clinical effect, beginning with doses of 0.25 to 0.50 mg, increasing to 1.0 mg if necessary, and administering doses every 5 minutes until either a desired effect or toxicity is produced or a total of 0.15 to 0.20 mg/kg has been given. In many cases, the short-acting effects of esmolol are preferred. Orally, propranolol is given in four divided doses, usually ranging from 40 to 160 mg/day to more than 1 gm/day. Some beta blockers, such as carvedilol and pindolol, need to be given twice daily; many are available as once-daily long-acting preparations. Generally, if one agent in adequate doses proves to be ineffective, other beta blockers are also ineffective. Conversely, if one agent produces the desired physiologic effect but a side effect develops, another beta blocker can often be substituted successfully.

INDICATIONS. Arrhythmias associated with thyrotoxicosis, pheochromocytoma, and anesthesia with cyclopropane or halothane or arrhythmias largely related to excessive cardiac adrenergic stimulation, such as those initiated by exercise, emotion, or cocaine, often respond to beta blocker therapy. Beta-blocking drugs usually do not convert chronic atrial flutter or atrial fibrillation to normal sinus rhythm but may do so if the arrhythmia is of recent onset and in patients who have recently undergone cardiac surgery.[18] The atrial rate during atrial flutter or fibrillation is not changed, but the ventricular response decreases, because beta blockade prolongs AV nodal conduction time and refractoriness. Esmolol can be used IV for rapid control of heart rate. For reentrant SVTs using the AV node as one of the reentrant pathways, such as AVNRT and orthodromic reciprocating tachycardias in the Wolff-Parkinson-White syndrome or inappropriate sinus tachycardia, or for ATs, beta blockers can slow or terminate the tachycardia and can be used prophylactically to prevent a recurrence. Combining beta blockers with digitalis, quinidine, or various other agents may be effective when the beta blocker as a single agent fails. Metoprolol and esmolol may be useful in patients with multifocal AT. These agents must be used with caution in this arrhythmia, however, because a common setting for it is advanced lung disease, often with a bronchospastic component.

Beta blockers can be effective for digitalis-induced arrhythmias such as AT, nonparoxysmal AV junctional tachycardia, PVCs, or VT. If a significant degree of AV block is present during a digitalis-induced arrhythmia, lidocaine or phenytoin may be preferable to propranolol. Beta blockers can also be useful to treat ventricular arrhythmias associated with the prolonged QT interval syndrome (see Chap. 9) and with mitral valve prolapse (see Chap. 62). For patients with ischemic heart disease, beta blockers generally do not prevent episodes of recurrent monomorphic VT that occur in the absence of acute ischemia. It is well accepted that several beta blockers reduce the incidence of overall death and sudden cardiac death after myocardial infarction (see Chaps. 50 and 51). The mechanism of this reduction in mortality is not entirely clear and may be related to reduction of the extent of ischemic damage, autonomic effects, a direct antiarrhythmic effect, or combinations of these factors. Beta blockers may have been protective against proarrhythmic responses in CAST.

ADVERSE EFFECTS. Adverse cardiovascular effects from beta blockers include unacceptable hypotension, bradycardia, and congestive heart failure. The bradycardia may be caused by sinus slowing or AV block. Sudden withdrawal of propranolol in patients with angina pectoris can precipitate or worsen angina and cardiac arrhythmias and cause an acute myocardial infarction, possibly because of heightened sensitivity to beta agonists caused by previous beta blockade (receptor upregulation). Heightened sensitivity may begin several days after cessation of beta blocker therapy and may last 5 or 6 days. Other adverse effects of beta blockers include worsening of asthma or chronic obstructive pulmonary disease, intermittent claudication, Raynaud's phenomenon, mental depression, increased risk of hypoglycemia in insulin-dependent diabetic patients, easy fatigability, disturbingly vivid dreams or insomnia, and impaired sexual function. Many of these side effects were noted less frequently when using $beta_1$-selective agents, but even so-called cardioselective beta blockers can exacerbate asthma or diabetic control in individual patients.

AMIODARONE

Amiodarone is a benzofuran derivative approved by the FDA for the treatment of patients with life-threatening ventricular tachyarrhythmias when other drugs are ineffective or are not tolerated. Dronedarone, a noniodinated derivative of amiodarone, is being studied as a potentially less toxic alternative to amiodarone; it appears to have equivalent efficacy and probably superior safety compared to amiodarone.[19] As of this writing, it has not been approved for use in the United States.[20]

ELECTROPHYSIOLOGICAL ACTIONS (see Tables 33-1, 33-2, 33-3, and 33-5). When chronically given orally, amiodarone prolongs APD and refractoriness of all cardiac fibers without affecting resting membrane potential (see Chap. 31). When acute effects are evaluated, amiodarone and its metabolite, desethylamiodarone, prolong the APD of ventricular muscle but shorten the APD of Purkinje fibers. Injected into the sinus and AV node arteries, amiodarone reduces sinus and junctional discharge rates and prolongs AV nodal conduction time. It depresses $\dot{V}_{max}$ in ventricular muscle in a rate- or use-dependent manner by blocking of inactivated sodium channels, an effect that is accentuated by depolarized, and reduced by hyperpolarized, membrane potentials. Amiodarone depresses conduction at fast rates more than at slow rates (use-dependence), not only by depressing $\dot{V}_{max}$ but also by increasing resistance to passive current flow. It does not prolong repolarization more at slow than fast rates (i.e., does not demonstrate reverse use-dependence) but does exert time-dependent effects on refractoriness, which may in part explain the high antiarrhythmic efficacy and low incidence of torsades de pointes.

CH 33

Desethylamiodarone has relatively greater effects on fast-channel tissue and probably contributes notably to antiarrhythmic efficacy. The delay in building up adequate concentrations of this metabolite may in part explain the delay in amiodarone's antiarrhythmic action.

Amiodarone noncompetitively antagonizes alpha and beta receptors and blocks conversion of thyroxine (T_4) to triiodothyronine (T_3), which may account for some of its electrophysiological effects. Amiodarone exhibits slow-channel blocking effects, and chronic oral therapy has been found to slow the spontaneous sinus node discharge rate in anesthetized dogs even after pretreatment with propranolol and atropine. With oral administration, it slows the sinus rate by 20 to 30 percent and prolongs the QT interval, at times changing the contour of the T wave and producing U waves.

ERPs of all cardiac tissues are prolonged. His-Purkinje conduction time increases and QRS duration lengthens, especially at fast rates. Amiodarone given intravenously modestly prolongs the refractory period of atrial and ventricular muscle. The PR interval and AV nodal conduction time lengthen. The duration of the QRS complex lengthens at increased rates but less than after oral amiodarone. Thus, far less increase in prolongation of conduction time (except for the AV node), duration of repolarization, and refractoriness occur after IV administration compared with the oral route. Considering these actions, it is clear that amiodarone has class I (blocks I_{Na}), class II (antiadrenergic), and class IV (blocks $I_{Ca.L}$) actions in addition to its class III effects (blocks I_K). Amiodarone's actions approximate those of a theoretically ideal drug that exhibits use-dependent Na^+ channel blockade with fast diastolic recovery from block and use-dependent prolongation of APD. It does not increase and may decrease QT dispersion. Catecholamines can partially reverse some of the effects of amiodarone.

HEMODYNAMIC EFFECTS. Amiodarone is a peripheral and coronary vasodilator. When administered intravenously (150 mg over 10 min, then 1-mg/min infusion) amiodarone decreases heart rate, systemic vascular resistance, left ventricular contractile force, and left ventricular dP/dt. Oral doses of amiodarone sufficient to control cardiac arrhythmias do not depress the left ventricular ejection fraction, even in patients with reduced ejection fractions, and ejection fraction and cardiac output may increase slightly. However, because of antiadrenergic actions of amiodarone and because it does exert some negative inotropic action, it should be given cautiously, particularly when given intravenously, to patients with marginal cardiac compensation.

PHARMACOKINETICS (see Table 33-4). Amiodarone is slowly, variably, and incompletely absorbed, with a systemic bioavailability of 35 to 65 percent. Plasma concentrations peak 3 to 7 hours after a single oral dose. There is a minimal first-pass effect, indicating little hepatic extraction. Elimination is by hepatic excretion into bile with some enterohepatic recirculation. Extensive hepatic metabolism occurs with desethylamiodarone as a major metabolite. Both accumulate extensively in the liver, lung, fat, "blue" skin, and other tissues. Myocardium develops a concentration 10 to 50 times that found in the plasma. Plasma clearance of amiodarone is low, and renal excretion is negligible. Doses need not be reduced in patients with renal disease. Amiodarone and desethylamiodarone are not dialyzable. The volume of distribution is large but variable, averaging 60 liter/kg. Amiodarone is highly protein bound (96 percent), crosses the placenta (10 to 50 percent), and is found in breast milk.

The onset of action after IV administration is generally within 1 to 2 hours. After oral administration, the onset of action may require 2 to 3 days, often 1 to 3 weeks, and, on occasion, even longer. Loading doses reduce this time interval. Plasma concentrations relate well to oral doses during chronic treatment, averaging about 0.5 mg/ml for each 100 mg/day at doses between 100 and 600 mg/day. Elimination half-life is multiphasic, with an initial 50 percent reduction in plasma concentration 3 to 10 days after cessation of drug ingestion (probably representing elimination from well-perfused tissues), followed by a terminal half-life of 26 to 107 days (mean, 53 days), with most patients in the 40- to 55-day range. To achieve steady state without a loading dose takes about 265 days. Interpatient variability of these pharmacokinetic parameters mandates close monitoring of the patient. Therapeutic serum concentrations range from 1 to 2.5 mg/ml. Greater suppression of arrhythmias may occur up to 3.5 mg/ml, but the risk of side effects increases.

DOSAGE AND ADMINISTRATION (see Table 33-4). An optimal dosing schedule for all patients has not been achieved. One recommended approach is to treat with 800 to 1200 mg/day for 1 to 3 weeks, reduced to 400 mg/day for the next several weeks and finally, after 2 to 3 months of treatment, a maintenance dose of 300 mg or less per day. Maintenance drug can be given once or twice daily and should be titrated to the lowest effective dose to minimize the occurrence of side effects. Doses as low as 100 mg/day can be effective in some patients. Regimens must be individualized for a given patient and clinical situation. Amiodarone can be administered intravenously to achieve more rapid loading and effect in emergencies, at initial doses of 15 mg/min for 10 minutes, followed by 1 mg/min for 6 hours, and then 0.5 mg/min for the remaining 18 hours and for the next several days, as necessary. Supplemental infusions of 150 mg over 10 minutes can be used for breakthrough VT or VF. IV infusions can be continued safely for 2 to 3 weeks. IV amiodarone is generally well tolerated, even in patients with left ventricular dysfunction. Patients with depressed ejection fractions should receive IV amiodarone with great caution because of hypotension. High-dose oral loading (800 to 2000 mg/day to maintain trough serum concentrations of 2 to 3 mg/ml) may suppress ventricular arrhythmias in 1 to 2 days.

INDICATIONS. Amiodarone has been used to suppress a wide spectrum of supraventricular and ventricular tachyarrhythmias in utero, in adults, and in children, including AV node and AV entry, junctional tachycardia, atrial flutter and fibrillation, VT and VF associated with coronary artery disease, and hypertrophic cardiomyopathy. Success rates vary widely, depending on the population of patients, arrhythmia, underlying heart disease, length of follow-up, definition and determination of success, and other factors. In general, however, amiodarone's efficacy equals or exceeds that of all other antiarrhythmic agents and may be in the range of 60 to 80 percent for most supraventricular tachyarrhythmias and 40 to 60 percent for ventricular tachyarrhythmias. Amiodarone may be useful in improving survival in patients with hypertrophic cardiomyopathy, nonischemic dilated cardiomyopathy, asymptomatic ventricular arrhythmias after myocardial infarction, and ventricular tachyarrhythmia during and after resuscitation from cardiac arrest. Amiodarone given before open-heart surgery, as well as postoperatively, has been shown to decrease the incidence of postoperative atrial fibrillation.[21] Amiodarone is superior to class I antiarrhythmic agents and sotalol in maintaining sinus rhythm in patients with recurrent atrial fibrillation.

Patients who have an ICD receive fewer shocks if they are treated with amiodarone compared with conventional drugs.[22] Amiodarone has little effect on pacing threshold but typically increases the electrical defibrillation threshold slightly.

Several prospective, randomized, controlled trials, and a meta-analysis[23] have demonstrated improved survival with amiodarone therapy compared with placebo; however, amiodarone has been proved to result in inferior survival compared with ICD therapy and, in the SCD-HeFT population (class II or III heart failure; ejection fraction, 35 percent), survival of amiodarone-treated patients was no different than those treated with placebo.[24] The drug may still be used adjunctively in ICD-treated patients to decrease the frequency of shocks from VT and VF episodes or to control supraventricular tachyarrhythmias that elicit device therapy (see Chap. 35). The drug may slow the rate of spontaneous VT episodes beneath the detection rate of the device; careful patient assessment and, occasionally, device reprogramming and testing are necessary.

Because of the serious nature of the arrhythmias being treated, the unusual pharmacokinetics of the drug, and its adverse effects, amiodarone therapy should generally be started with the patient hospitalized and monitored for at least several days. Combining other antiarrhythmic agents with amiodarone may improve efficacy in some patients.

ADVERSE EFFECTS. Adverse effects are reported by about 75 percent of patients treated with amiodarone for 5 years, but these compel stopping the drug in 18 to 37 percent.[25] The most frequent side effects requiring drug discontinuation involve pulmonary and gastrointestinal complaints. Most adverse effects are reversible with dose reduction or cessation of treatment. Adverse effects are more common when therapy is continued in the long term and at higher doses. Of the noncardiac adverse reactions, pulmonary toxicity is the most serious; in one study, it occurred in 33 of 573 patients between 6 days and 60 months of treatment, with three deaths.[26] The mechanism is unclear but may involve a hypersensitivity reaction, widespread phospholipidosis, or both. Dyspnea, nonproductive cough, and fever are common symptoms, with crackles on examination, hypoxia, a positive gallium scan, reduced diffusion capacity, and radiographic evidence of pulmonary infiltrates. Amiodarone must be discontinued if such pulmonary inflammatory changes occur. Corticosteroids can be tried, but no controlled studies have been done to support their use. A 10 percent mortality results in patients with pulmonary inflammatory changes, often in patients with unrecognized pulmonary involvement that is allowed to progress. Chest radiography and pulmonary function testing, including carbon monoxide diffusion capacity (DLCO), at 3-month intervals for the first year and then twice a year for several years have been recommended. At maintenance doses less than 300 mg/day, pulmonary toxicity is uncommon but can occur.[27] Advanced age, high drug maintenance dose, and reduced predrug diffusion capacity are risk factors for developing pulmonary toxicity. An unchanged DLCO on therapy may be a negative predictor of pulmonary toxicity.

Although asymptomatic elevations of liver enzyme levels are found in most patients, the drug is not stopped unless values exceed two or three times normal in a patient with initially abnormal values. Cirrhosis occurs uncommonly but may be fatal. Neurological dysfunction, photosensitivity (perhaps minimized by sunscreens), bluish skin discoloration, gastroenterological disturbances, and hyperthyroidism (1 to 2 percent) or hypothyroidism (2 to 4 percent) can occur.[28] Amiodarone appears to inhibit the peripheral conversion of T_4 to T_3 so that chemical changes result; these are characterized by a slight increase in T_4, reverse T_3, and thyroid-stimulating hormone (TSH) and a slight decrease in T_3 levels. Reverse T_3 concentration has been used as an index of drug efficacy. During hypothyroidism, the TSH level increases greatly, whereas the level of T_3 increases in hyperthyroidism. Thyroid function tests should be performed approximately every 3 months for the first year, while amiodarone is taken, and once or twice yearly thereafter, sooner if symptoms develop that are consistent with thyroid dysfunction. Corneal microdeposits occur in almost 100 percent of adults receiving the drug longer than 6 months. More serious ocular reactions, including optic neuritis, atrophy with visual loss, or both, have been reported[29] but are rare, and causation by amiodarone has not been established.[30]

Cardiac side effects include symptomatic bradycardias in about 2 percent of patients, worsening of ventricular tachyarrhythmias, with occasional development of torsades de pointes in 1 to 2 percent, possibly higher in women, and worsening of congestive heart failure in 2 percent. Possibly because of interactions with anesthetics, complications after open-heart surgery, including pulmonary dysfunction, hypotension, severe bradycardia, hepatic dysfunction, and low cardiac output, have been noted by some investigators.

In general, the lowest possible maintenance dose of amiodarone that is still effective should be used to avoid significant adverse effects. Many supraventricular arrhythmias can be successfully managed with daily dosages of 200 mg or less, whereas ventricular arrhythmias generally require higher doses. Adverse effects are uncommon at dosages of 200 mg/day or less but still occur. Because of potential toxicity in various organ systems, special multidisciplinary amiodarone clinics have been used by some to attempt to prevent adverse outcomes when using the drug.

Important interactions with other drugs occur and, when given concomitantly with amiodarone, the doses of warfarin, digoxin, and other antiarrhythmic drugs should be reduced by one third to one half and the patient observed closely. Drugs with synergistic actions, such as beta blockers or calcium channel blockers, must be given cautiously. Amiodarone's safety during pregnancy has not been established, and it should be used in the pregnant patient only if no alternatives exist.

BRETYLIUM TOSYLATE

Bretylium is a quaternary ammonium compound that had been used parenterally in patients with life-threatening ventricular tachyarrhythmias (see Chap. 36); it is no longer manufactured in the United States.

ELECTROPHYSIOLOGICAL ACTIONS (see Tables 33-1, 33-2, 33-3, and 33-5). Bretylium is selectively concentrated in sympathetic ganglia and their postganglionic adrenergic nerve terminals. After initially causing norepinephrine release, bretylium prevents norepinephrine release by depressing sympathetic nerve terminal excitability without depressing preganglionic or postganglionic sympathetic nerve conduction, impairing conduction across sympathetic ganglia, depleting the adrenergic neuron of norepinephrine, or decreasing the responsiveness of adrenergic receptors. It produces a state resembling chemical sympathectomy. Initial catecholamine release can exacerbate some arrhythmias, such as those caused by digitalis excess or myocardial infarction. Bretylium has little if any effect on sustained VT but can prevent recurrences of VF. It is not clear whether the chemical sympathectomy-like state alone or together with other actions exerts the antifibrillatory effect.

HEMODYNAMIC EFFECTS. Bretylium does not depress myocardial contractility. After an initial increase in blood pressure, the drug can cause significant hypotension by blocking the efferent limb of the baroreceptor reflex. Hypotension results most commonly when patients are sitting or standing, but can also occur in the supine position in seriously ill patients. Bretylium reduces the extent of the vasoconstriction and tachycardia reflexes during standing, effects that can persist for several days after the drug has been discontinued.

PHARMACOKINETICS (see Table 33-4). Bretylium is usually given intravenously; bioavailability may be less than 50 percent and elimination is almost exclusively by renal excretion, without significant metabolism or active metabolites being recognized. Elimination half-life is 5 to 10 hours but variable (longer in cardiac arrest survivors). Doses should be reduced in patients with renal insufficiency. Onset of action after IV administration occurs within several minutes, but full antiarrhythmic effects may not be seen for 30 minutes to 2 hours.

DOSAGE AND ADMINISTRATION (see Table 33-4). Bretylium can be given intravenously in doses of 5 to 10 mg/kg body weight, diluted in 50 to 100 ml of D_5W, and administered over 10 to 20 minutes or more quickly in a life-threatening state. This dose can be repeated in 1 to 2 hours if the arrhythmia persists. The total daily dosage probably should not exceed 30 mg/kg. A similar initial dose, but undiluted, can be given intramuscularly. The maintenance IV dose is 0.5 to 2.0 mg/min. Intramuscular injection during cardiopulmonary resuscitation from cardiac arrest and in shock states should be avoided because of unreliable absorption during reduced tissue perfusion.

INDICATIONS. Bretylium is used in patients who are in an intensive care setting and who have life-threatening, recurrent ventricular tachyarrhythmias that have not responded to other antiarrhythmic drugs. Bretylium has been effective in treating some patients with drug-resistant tachyarrhythmias and in treating victims of out-of-hospital VF.

ADVERSE EFFECTS. Hypotension, most prominently orthostatic but also supine, is the most significant side effect and can be prevented with tricyclic drugs, such as protriptyline. Transient hypertension, increased sinus rate, and worsening of arrhythmias, often those related to ischemia, may follow initial drug administration and may be caused by initial release of catecholamines. Bretylium should be used cautiously or not at all in patients who have a relatively fixed cardiac output, such as those with severe aortic stenosis. Vasodilators or diuretics can enhance hypotensive effects. Nausea and vomiting can occur after parenteral administration.

SOTALOL

Sotalol is a nonspecific beta adrenoceptor blocker without intrinsic sympathomimetic activity that prolongs repolarization. It is approved by the FDA to treat patients with life-threatening ventricular tachyarrhythmias and those with atrial fibrillation.

ELECTROPHYSIOLOGICAL ACTIONS (see Tables 33-1, 33-2, 33-3, and 33-5). Both *d* and *l* isomers have similar effects on prolonging repolarization, whereas the *l* isomer is responsible for almost all the beta-blocking activity. Sotalol does not block alpha adrenoceptors and does not block the sodium channel (no membrane-stabilizing effects), but does prolong atrial and ventricular repolarization times by reducing I_{Kr}, thus prolonging the plateau of the action potential. Action potential prolongation is greater at slower rates (reverse use-dependence). Resting membrane potential, action potential amplitude, and $\dot{V}_{max}$ are not significantly altered. Sotalol prolongs atrial and ventricular refractoriness, A-H and QT intervals, and sinus cycle length (see Chap. 35).

HEMODYNAMICS. Sotalol exerts a negative inotropic effect only through its beta-blocking action. It can increase the strength of contraction by prolonging repolarization, which occurs maximally at slow heart rates. In patients with reduced cardiac function, sotalol can decrease cardiac index, increase filling pressure, and cause overt heart failure. Therefore, it must be used cautiously in patients with marginal cardiac compensation but appears to be well tolerated in patients with normal cardiac function.

PHARMACOKINETICS (see Table 33-4). Sotalol is completely absorbed and not metabolized, making it 90 to 100 percent bioavailable. It is not bound to plasma proteins, is excreted unchanged primarily by the kidneys, and has an elimination half-life of 10 to 15 hours. Peak plasma concentrations occur 2.5 to 4 hours after oral ingestion, with a steady state attained after five or six doses. Effective antiarrhythmic plasma concentration is in the range of 2.5 mg/ml. There is little intersubject variability in plasma levels. Over the dose range of 160 to 640 mg, sotalol displays dose proportionality with plasma concentration. The dose must be reduced in patients with renal disease. The beta-blocking effect is half-maximal at 80 mg/day and maximal at 320 mg/day. Significant beta-blocking action occurs at 160 mg/day.

DOSAGE (see Table 33-4). The typical oral dose is 80 to 160 mg every 12 hours, allowing 2 to 3 days between dose adjustments to attain a steady state and to monitor the electrocardiogram for arrhythmias and QT prolongation. Doses exceeding 320 mg/day can be used in patients when the potential benefits outweigh the risk of proarrhythmia.

INDICATIONS. Approved by the FDA to treat patients with ventricular tachyarrhythmias and atrial fibrillation, sotalol is also useful to prevent recurrence of a wide variety of SVTs, including atrial flutter, AT, AV node reentry, and AV reentry (see Chap. 35). It also slows the ventricular response to atrial tachyarrhythmias. It appears to be more effective than conventional antiarrhythmic drugs and may be comparable to amiodarone in treating patients with ventricular tachyarrhythmias, as well as prevention of atrial fibrillation recurrences after cardioversion.[31] It has been used successfully to decrease the incidence of atrial fibrillation following cardiac surgery. Sotalol is useful in patients with arrhythmogenic right ventricular dysplasia. Sotalol may be effective in fetal and pediatric patients.[32] Unlike most other antiarrhythmic drugs, it may decrease the frequency of ICD discharges and reduce the defibrillation threshold.

ADVERSE EFFECTS. Proarrhythmia is the most serious adverse effect. Overall, new or worsened ventricular tachyarrhythmias occur in about 4 percent of patients, and this response is the result of torsades de pointes in about 2.5 percent. The incidence of torsades de pointes increases to 4 percent in patients with a history of sustained VT and is dose related, reportedly only 1.6 percent at 320 mg/day but 4.4 percent at 480 mg/day. This proarrhythmic effect was probably the cause of excess mortality in patients given *d*-sotalol (the enantiomer lacking a beta-blocking effect) after an acute myocardial infarction in the Survival With Oral *d*-Sotalol (SWORD) trial. Other adverse effects commonly seen with other beta blockers also apply to sotalol. Sotalol should be used with caution or not at all in combination with other drugs that prolong the QT interval. However, such combinations have been used successfully.

IBUTILIDE

Ibutilide is an agent released for use in acutely terminating episodes of atrial flutter and fibrillation (see Chap. 35).

ELECTROPHYSIOLOGICAL ACTIONS (see Tables 33-1, 33-2, 33-3, and 33-5). Like other class III agents, ibutilide prolongs repolarization. Although it is similar to other class III agents that block outward potassium currents, such as I_{Kr}, ibutilide is unique in that it also activates a slow inward sodium current. Administered intravenously, ibutilide causes mild slowing of the sinus rate and has minimal effects on AV conduction or QRS duration, but the QT interval is characteristically prolonged. Ibutilide has no significant effect on hemodynamics.

PHARMACOKINETICS (see Table 33-4). Ibutilide is administered intravenously and has a large volume of distribution. Clearance is predominantly renal, with a drug half-life averaging 6 hours, but with considerable interpatient variability. Protein binding is approximately 40 percent. One of the drug's metabolites has weak class III effects.

DOSAGE AND ADMINISTRATION (see Table 33-4). Ibutilide is given as an IV infusion of 1 mg over 10 minutes. It should not be given in the presence of a QTc interval longer than 440 milliseconds or other drugs that prolong the QT interval or when uncorrected hypokalemia or bradycardia exists. A second 1-mg dose may be given after the first dose is finished if the arrhythmia persists. Patients must have continuous electrocardiographic monitoring throughout the dosing period and for 6 to 8 hours thereafter because of the risk of ventricular arrhythmias. Pretreatment with IV magnesium may decrease ventricular arrhythmia risk.[33] Up to 60 percent of patients with atrial fibrillation and 70 percent of those with atrial flutter convert to sinus rhythm after 2 mg of ibutilide has been administered.

INDICATIONS. Ibutilide is indicated for termination of an established episode of atrial flutter or fibrillation. It should not be used in patients with frequent short paroxysms of atrial fibrillation because it merely terminates episodes and is not useful for prevention. Patients whose condition is hemodynamically unstable should proceed to direct-current cardioversion. Ibutilide has been used safely and effectively in patients who were already taking amiodarone or propafenone.[34] Ibutilide has been administered at the time of transthoracic electrical cardioversion to increase the likelihood of termination of atrial fibrillation. In one study, all 50 patients given ibutilide before attempted electrical cardioversion achieved sinus rhythm, whereas only 34 of 50 who did not receive the drug converted to sinus rhythm. Of note, all 16 patients who did not respond to electrical cardioversion without ibutilide were successfully electrically cardioverted to sinus rhythm when a second attempt was made after ibutilide pretreatment.[35]

Ibutilide prolongs accessory pathway refractoriness and can temporarily slow the ventricular rate during preexcited atrial fibrillation. The drug can also terminate episodes of organized atrial tachycardia,[36] as well as sustained uniform morphology VT.

ADVERSE EFFECTS. The most significant adverse effects of ibutilide are QT prolongation and torsades de pointes, which occur in approximately 2 percent of patients given the drug (twice as often in women as in men[37]). The adverse effect occurs within the first 4 to 6 hours of dosing, after which the risk is negligible. Thus, patients in whom the drug is used must undergo electrocardiographic monitoring for up to 8 hours after dosing. This requirement can make ibutilide's use in emergency departments or private offices problematic. Ibutilide's safety during pregnancy has not been well studied. Its use should be restricted to patients in whom no safer alternative exists.

DOFETILIDE

Dofetilide is approved for acute conversion of atrial fibrillation to sinus rhythm, as well as chronic suppression of recurrent atrial fibrillation.

ELECTROPHYSIOLOGICAL ACTIONS (see Tables 33-1, 33-2, 33-3, and 33-5). The sole electrophysiological effect of dofetilide appears to be block of the rapid component of the delayed rectifier potassium current (I_{Kr}), which is important in repolarization. This effect is more prominent in the atria than in the ventricles—30 percent increase in atrial refractory period versus 20 percent in the ventricle; see Chap. 31. Dofetilide's effect on I_{Kr} prolongs refractoriness without slowing conduction, which is believed to be largely responsible for its antiarrhythmic effect. It is also responsible for the prolongation of the QT interval on the electrocardiogram, which averages 11 percent but can be much greater. This effect on the QT interval is dose dependent and linear. No other important electrocardiographic changes are observed with the drug. It has no significant hemodynamic effects. Dofetilide is more effective than quinidine at converting atrial fibrillation to sinus rhythm.

PHARMACOKINETICS (see Table 33-4). Orally administered dofetilide is absorbed well, with over 90 percent bioavailability. Fifty to 60 percent of the drug is excreted unchanged in urine, with a mean elimination half-life of 7 to 13 hours. The remainder of the drug undergoes hepatic metabolism to inert compounds. Significant drug-drug interactions have been reported in patients using dofetilide; cimetidine, verapamil, ketoconazole, and trimethoprim, alone or in combination with sulfamethoxazole, cause a significant elevation in the dofetilide serum concentration and should not be used with this drug.

DOSAGE AND ADMINISTRATION (see Table 33-4). Dofetilide is available only as an oral preparation. Dosing is from 0.125 to 0.5 mg twice daily and must be initiated in a hospital setting with continuous electrocardiographic monitoring to ensure that inordinate QT prolongation and torsades de pointes do not develop. Physicians must be specially certified to prescribe the drug. Dosage must be decreased in the presence of impaired renal function or an increase in the QT interval of more than 15 percent, or 500 msec. The drug should not be given to patients with a creatinine clearance less than 20 ml/min or a baseline corrected QT interval longer than 440 milliseconds.

INDICATIONS. IV dofetilide has been used on an investigational basis for termination of an established episode of atrial flutter, fibrillation, or other types of SVT. Oral dofetilide is indicated for prevention of episodes of supraventricular tachyarrhythmias, particularly atrial flutter and fibrillation. Dofetilide's role in therapy for ventricular arrhythmias is less clear. Dofetilide has been shown to have a neutral effect on mortality when given to patients after myocardial infarction.

ADVERSE EFFECTS. The most significant adverse effect of dofetilide is QT interval prolongation with torsades de pointes, occurring in 2 to 4 percent of patients given the drug. Risk is highest in patients with a baseline prolonged QT interval, those who are hypokalemic, those taking some other agent that prolongs repolarization, and after conversion from atrial fibrillation to sinus rhythm. The drug is otherwise well tolerated, with few side effects. Its use in pregnancy has not been studied extensively, and it should probably be avoided in this setting if possible.

AZIMILIDE

Azimilide is a new agent for use in the treatment of atrial flutter and fibrillation; it has not yet approved by the FDA (at the time of this writing).

ELECTROPHYSIOLOGICAL ACTIONS (see Tables 33-1, 33-2, 33-3, and 33-5). Unlike dofetilide, which blocks the rapid component of the delayed rectifier potassium current, azimilide produces a more balanced blockade of both rapid and slow components of I_K.[38] It is presumed that this effect is responsible for the lower rate of proarrhythmia and better preservation of drug efficacy at higher heart rates with this agent compared with pure I_{Kr} blockers. Azimilide produces a mild prolongation of the QT interval but no other meaningful electrocardiographic changes. Unlike dofetilide and sotalol, which have greater effects on atrial than ventricular refractoriness, azimilide exerts a similar effect on each.

PHARMACOKINETICS (see Table 33-4). Azimilide's pharmacokinetic profile is relatively simple and predictable. It can be taken orally once daily, and its absorption is nearly complete and unaffected by food intake. Few drug-drug interactions have been reported to date. Azimilide is cleared by the kidney; some metabolism of the drug to inactive compounds occurs. The drug has no significant adverse hemodynamic effects.

DOSAGE AND ADMINISTRATION (see Table 33-4). Azimilide can be taken by mouth once daily at a dosage of 100 to 200 mg. The drug is well tolerated, and dosing need not be adjusted in the presence of renal or hepatic disease.

INDICATIONS. Azimilide is likely to be indicated for long-term prevention of atrial flutter and fibrillation. The drug has been given safely and was well tolerated in a group of postinfarction patients.[39] Studies are under way to evaluate its efficacy in ventricular arrhythmias; it has decreased the rate of ICD shocks.[40]

ADVERSE EFFECTS. The drug is generally well tolerated. As with other class III agents, the most significant adverse effect of azimilide is torsades de pointes, although this arrhythmia appears to be less common with this agent than with other class III medications, occurring in approximately 1 percent of patients given the drug. Azimilide's safety in pregnancy is not known; its use should probably be avoided, if possible.

CALCIUM CHANNEL ANTAGONISTS: VERAPAMIL AND DILTIAZEM

Verapamil, a synthetic papaverine derivative, is the prototype of a class of drugs that block the slow calcium channel and reduce $I_{Ca.L}$ in cardiac muscle (see Chap. 31). Diltiazem has electrophysiological actions similar to those of verapamil. Nifedipine and other dihydropyridine agents exhibit minimal electrophysiological effects at clinically used doses; these drugs are not discussed here.

ELECTROPHYSIOLOGICAL ACTIONS (see Tables 33-1, 33-2, 33-3, and 33-5). By blocking $I_{Ca.L}$ in all cardiac fibers, verapamil reduces the plateau height of the action potential, slightly shortens muscle action potential, and slightly prolongs total Purkinje fiber action potential. It does not appreciably affect the action potential amplitude, $\dot{V}_{max}$ of phase 0, or resting membrane voltage in cells that have fast-response characteristics related to I_{Na} (e.g., atrial and ventricular muscle, the His-Purkinje system). Verapamil suppresses slow responses elicited by various experimental methods, as well as sustained triggered activity and early and late afterdepolarizations. Verapamil and diltiazem suppress electrical activity in the normal sinus and AV nodes. Verapamil depresses the slope of diastolic depolarization in sinus node cells, $\dot{V}_{max}$ of phase 0, maximum diastolic potential, and prolongs conduction time and refractory periods of the AV node. The AV node blocking effects of verapamil and diltiazem are more apparent at faster rates of stimulation (use-dependence) and in depolarized fibers (voltage-dependence). Verapamil slows the activation and delays recovery from inactivation of the slow channel.

CH 33

Verapamil does exert some local anesthetic activity because the dextrorotatory stereoisomer of the clinically used racemic mixture exerts slight blocking effects on I_{Na}. The levorotatory stereoisomer blocks the slow inward current carried by calcium, as well as other ions, traveling through the slow channel. Verapamil does not modify calcium uptake, binding, or exchange by cardiac microsomes, nor does it affect calcium-activated adenosine triphosphatase. Verapamil does not block beta receptors but may block alpha receptors and potentiate vagal effects on the AV node. Verapamil may also cause other effects that indirectly alter cardiac electrophysiology, such as decreasing platelet adhesiveness or reducing the extent of myocardial ischemia.

In humans, verapamil prolongs conduction time through the AV node (the A-H interval) without affecting the P wave or QRS duration or H-V interval, and lengthens AV nodal anterograde and retrograde refractory periods. The spontaneous sinus rate may decrease slightly, an effect only partially reversed by atropine. More commonly, the sinus rate does not change significantly because verapamil causes peripheral vasodilation, transient hypotension, and reflex sympathetic stimulation that mitigates any direct slowing effect that verapamil exerts on the sinus node. If verapamil is given to a patient who is also receiving a beta blocker, the sinus node discharge rate may slow because reflex sympathetic stimulation is blocked. Verapamil does not exert a significant direct effect on atrial or ventricular refractoriness or on anterograde or retrograde properties of accessory pathways. However, reflex sympathetic stimulation following IV verapamil administration may increase the ventricular response over the accessory pathway during atrial fibrillation in patients with the Wolff-Parkinson-White syndrome.

HEMODYNAMIC EFFECTS. Because verapamil interferes with excitation-contraction coupling, it inhibits vascular smooth muscle contraction and causes marked vasodilation in coronary and other peripheral vascular beds. Propranolol does not block the vasodilation produced by verapamil. Reflex sympathetic effects may reduce the marked negative inotropic action of verapamil on isolated cardiac muscle, but the direct myocardial depressant effects of verapamil may predominate when the drug is given in high doses. In patients with well-preserved left ventricular function, combined therapy with propranolol and verapamil appears to be well tolerated, but beta blockade can accentuate the hemodynamic depressant effects produced by oral verapamil. Patients who have reduced left ventricular function may not tolerate the combined blockade of beta receptors and slow channels; thus, in these patients, verapamil and propranolol should be used in combination either cautiously or not at all. Verapamil decreases myocardial oxygen demand while decreasing coronary vascular resistance. Such changes may be antiarrhythmic.

Peak alterations in hemodynamic variables occur 3 to 5 minutes after completion of a verapamil injection, with the major effects dissipating within 10 minutes. Systemic resistance and mean arterial pressure decrease, as does left ventricular dP/dt_{max}, and left ventricular end-diastolic pressure increases. Heart rate, cardiac index, left ventricular minute work, and mean pulmonary artery pressure do not change significantly. Thus, afterload reduction produced by verapamil significantly counterbalances its negative inotropic action, so that the cardiac index may not be reduced. In addition, when verapamil slows the ventricular rate in a patient with a tachycardia, hemodynamics may also improve. Nevertheless, caution should be exercised when giving verapamil to patients with severe myocardial depression or those receiving beta blockers or disopyramide, because hemodynamic deterioration may progress in some patients.

PHARMACOKINETICS (see Table 33-4). After single oral doses of verapamil, measurable prolongation of AV nodal conduction time occurs in 30 minutes and lasts 4 to 6 hours. After IV administration, AV nodal conduction delay occurs within 1 to 2 minutes and AH interval prolongation is still detectable after 6 hours. After oral administration, absorption is almost complete, but an overall bioavailability of 20 to 35 percent suggests substantial first-pass metabolism in the liver, particularly of the *l*-isomer. The elimination half-life of verapamil is 3 to 7 hours, with up to 70 percent of the drug excreted by the kidneys. Norverapamil is a major metabolite that may contribute to verapamil's electrophysiological actions. Serum protein binding is approximately 90 percent. With diltiazem, the percentage of heart rate reduction in atrial fibrillation is related to plasma concentration.

DOSAGE AND ADMINISTRATION (see Table 33-4). For acute termination of SVT or rapidly achieving ventricular rate control during atrial fibrillation, the most commonly used IV dose of verapamil is 10 mg infused over 1 to 2 minutes while cardiac rhythm and blood pressure are monitored. A second injection of an equal dose may be given 30 minutes later. The initial effect achieved with the first bolus injection, such as slowing of the ventricular response during atrial fibrillation, may be maintained by a continuous infusion of the drug at a rate of 0.005 mg/kg/min. The oral dose is 240 to 480 mg/day in divided doses. Diltiazem is given intravenously at a dose of 0.25 mg/kg as a bolus over 2 minutes, with a second dose in 15 minutes if necessary; because it is generally better tolerated (less hypotension) for long-term administration, such as for control of ventricular rate during atrial fibrillation, diltiazem is preferred over verapamil in this setting. Orally, doses must be adjusted to the patient's needs, with a 120- to 360-mg range. Various long-acting preparations (once daily) are available for verapamil and diltiazem.

INDICATIONS. After simple vagal maneuvers have been tried and adenosine given, IV verapamil or diltiazem is the next treatment of choice for terminating sustained sinus node reentry, AV node reentry, or orthodromic AV reciprocating tachycardia associated with an accessory pathway (see Chap. 35). Verapamil is as effective as adenosine for termination of these arrhythmias. Verapamil should definitely be tried before attempting termination by digitalis administration, pacing, electrical direct-current cardioversion, or acute blood pressure elevation with vasopressors. Verapamil and diltiazem terminate 60 to 90 percent or more episodes of paroxysmal SVTs within several minutes. Verapamil may also be of use in some fetal SVTs. Although IV verapamil has been given along with IV propranolol, this combination should be used only with great caution.

Verapamil and diltiazem decrease the ventricular response over the AV node during atrial fibrillation or atrial flutter, possibly converting a small number of episodes to sinus rhythm, particularly if the atrial flutter or fibrillation is of recent onset. In addition, verapamil may prevent early recurrence of atrial fibrillation after cardioversion.[41] Some patients with atrial flutter may develop atrial fibrillation after verapamil administration. As noted earlier, in patients with preexcited ventricular complexes during atrial fibrillation associated with the Wolff-Parkinson-White syndrome, IV verapamil may accelerate the ventricular response; therefore, the IV route is contraindicated in this situation. Verapamil can terminate some ATs. Even though verapamil can often terminate an idiopathic left septal VT, hemodynamic collapse can occur if IV verapamil is given to patients with the more common forms of VT because they generally occur in the setting of decreased left ventricular systolic function. A general rule for avoiding complications, however, is not to administer IV verapamil to any patient with wide QRS tachycardia unless one is absolutely certain of the nature of the tachycardia and its likely response to verapamil.

Orally, verapamil or diltiazem can prevent the recurrence of AV node reentrant and orthodromic AV reciprocating tachycardias associated with an accessory pathway, as well as help maintain a decreased ventricular response during atrial flutter or atrial fibrillation in patients without an accessory pathway. Verapamil generally has not been effective in treating patients who have recurrent ventricular tachyarrhythmias, although it may suppress some forms of VT, such as a left septal VT (noted earlier). It may also be useful in about two thirds of patients with idiopathic VT that has a left bundle branch block morphology (right ventricular outflow tract origin), patients with hypertrophic cardiomyopathy who have experienced cardiac arrest, patients with a short-coupled variant of polymorphic ventricular tachycardia, and patients with ventricular arrhythmias related to coronary artery spasm. Calcium channel blockers have not been shown to reduce mortality or prevent sudden cardiac death in patients after acute myocardial infarction, except for diltiazem in patients with non–Q-wave infarctions.

ADVERSE EFFECTS. Verapamil must be used cautiously in patients with significant hemodynamic impairment or in those receiving beta blockers, as noted earlier. Hypotension, bradycardia, AV block, and asystole are more likely to occur when the drug is given to patients who are already receiving beta-blocking agents. Hemodynamic collapse has been noted in infants, and verapamil should be used cautiously in patients younger than 1 year. Verapamil should also be used with caution in patients with sinus node abnormalities, because marked depression of sinus node function or asystole can result in some of these patients. Intravenous isoproterenol, calcium, glucagon, dopamine, or atropine, which may be only partially effective, or temporary pacing may be necessary to counteract some of the adverse effects of verapamil. Isoproterenol may be more effective for treating bradyarrhythmias and calcium may be used for treating hemodynamic dysfunction secondary to verapamil. AV node depression is common in overdoses. Contraindications to the use of verapamil and diltiazem include the presence of advanced heart failure, second- or third-degree AV block without a pacemaker in place, atrial fibrillation and anterograde conduction over an accessory pathway, significant sinus node dysfunction, most VTs, cardiogenic shock, and other hypotensive states. Although these drugs probably should not be used in patients with overt heart failure, if it is caused by one of the supraventricular tachyarrhythmias noted earlier, verapamil or diltiazem may restore sinus rhythm or significantly decrease the ventricular rate, leading to hemodynamic improvement. Finally, it is important to note that verapamil can decrease the excretion of digoxin by about 30 percent. Hepatotoxicity may occur on occasion. Verapamil crosses the placental barrier; its use in pregnancy has been associated with impaired uterine contraction, fetal bradycardia and, possibly, fetal digital defects. It should therefore be used only if no effective alternatives exist.

Other Antiarrhythmic Agents

ADENOSINE

Adenosine is an endogenous nucleoside present throughout the body and has been approved by the FDA to treat patients with SVTs.

ELECTROPHYSIOLOGICAL ACTIONS (see Tables 33-1, 33-2, 33-3, and 33-5). Adenosine interacts with A_1 receptors present on the extracellular surface of cardiac cells, activating K^+ channels ($I_{K.Ach}$, $I_{K.Ade}$) in a fashion similar to that produced by acetylcholine. The increase in K^+ conductance shortens atrial APD, hyperpolarizes the membrane potential, and decreases atrial contractility. Similar changes occur in the sinus and AV nodes. In contrast to these direct effects mediated through the guanine nucleotide regulatory proteins G_i and G_o, adenosine antagonizes catecholamine-stimulated adenylate cyclase to decrease cyclic adenosine monophosphate accumulation and to decrease $I_{Ca.L}$ and the pacemaker current I_f in sinus node cells, along with a decrease in $\dot{V}_{max}$. Shifts in pacemaker site within the sinus node and sinus exit block may occur. Adenosine slows the sinus rate in humans, which is followed by a reflex increase in sinus rate. In the N region of the AV node, conduction is depressed, along with decreases in action potential amplitude, duration, and $\dot{V}_{max}$. Transient prolongation of the AH interval results, often with transient first-, second-, or third-degree AV node block. Delay in AV nodal conduction is rate dependent. His-Purkinje conduction is generally not directly affected. Adenosine does not affect conduction in normal accessory pathways. Conduction may be blocked in accessory pathways that have long conduction times or decremental conduction properties. Patients with heart transplants exhibit a supersensitive response to adenosine. Adenosine may mediate the phenomenon of ischemic preconditioning.

PHARMACOKINETICS (see Table 33-4). Adenosine is removed from the extracellular space by washout, enzymatically by degradation to inosine, by phosphorylation to adenosine monophosphate, or by reuptake into cells through a nucleoside transport system. The vascular endothelium and the formed blood elements contain these elimination systems, which result in very rapid clearance of adenosine from the circulation. Elimination half-life is 1 to 6 seconds. Most of adenosine's effects are produced during its first passage through the circulation. Important drug interactions occur; methylxanthines are competitive antagonists, and therapeutic concentrations of theophylline totally block the exogenous adenosine effect. Dipyridamole is a nucleoside transport blocker that blocks reuptake of adenosine, delaying its clearance from the circulation or interstitial space and potentiating its effect. Smaller adenosine doses should be used in patients receiving dipyridamole.

DOSAGE AND ADMINISTRATION (see Table 33-4). To terminate tachycardia, a bolus of adenosine is rapidly injected intravenously at doses of 6 to 12 mg, followed by a flush. Pediatric dosing should be 0.1 to 0.3 mg/kg. When given into a central vein and in patients after heart transplantation or those receiving dipyridamole, the initial dose should be reduced to 3 mg. Transient sinus slowing or AV node block results, lasting less than 5 seconds. Doses of more than 18 mg are unlikely to revert a tachycardia and should not be used.

INDICATIONS. Adenosine has become the drug of first choice to terminate an SVT acutely, such as AV node or AV reentry (see Chap. 35). It is useful in pediatric patients and to judge the effectiveness of ablation of accessory pathways. Adenosine can produce AV block or terminate ATs and sinus node reentry. It results in only transient AV block during atrial flutter or fibrillation and is thus useful only for diagnosis, not therapy. Adenosine terminates a group of VTs whose maintenance depends on adrenergic drive, which is most often located in the right ventricular outflow tract but found at other sites as well; idiopathic left septal VT rarely responds, however. Adenosine has less potential than verapamil for lowering the blood pressure should tachycardia persist after injection.

Doses as low as 2.5 mg terminate some tachycardias; doses of 12 mg or less terminate 92 percent of SVTs, usually within 30 seconds. Successful termination rates with adenosine are comparable to those achieved with verapamil. Because of its effectiveness and extremely short duration of action, adenosine is preferable to verapamil in most cases, particularly in patients who have previously received IV beta adrenoceptor blockers, in those having poorly compensated heart failure or severe hypotension, and in neonates. Verapamil might be chosen first in patients receiving drugs such as theophylline, which is known to interfere with adenosine's actions or metabolism, in patients with active bronchoconstriction, and in those with inadequate venous access.

Adenosine may be useful to help differentiate among causes of wide QRS tachycardias because it terminates many SVTs with aberrancy or reveals the underlying atrial mechanism, and it does not block conduction over an accessory pathway or terminate most VTs. Adenosine in rare cases terminates some VTs, characteristically those of right ventricular outflow tract origin, and therefore tachycardia termination is not completely diagnostic for an SVT. This agent may predispose to the development of atrial fibrillation and might increase the ventricular response in patients with atrial fibrillation conducting over an accessory pathway. Adenosine may also be useful in differentiating conduction over the AV node from that over an accessory pathway during ablative procedures designed to interrupt the accessory pathway. However, this distinction is not absolute because adenosine can block conduction in slowly conducting accessory pathways and does not always produce block in the AV node. Endogenously released adenosine may be important in ischemia and hypoxia-induced AV node block and in postdefibrillation bradyarrhythmias.

ADVERSE EFFECTS. Transient side effects occur in almost 40 percent of patients with SVT given adenosine and are most commonly flushing, dyspnea, and chest pressure. These symptoms are fleeting, lasting less than 1 minute, and are well tolerated. PVCs, transient sinus bradycardia, sinus arrest, and AV block are common when an SVT abruptly terminates. Atrial fibrillation is occasionally observed (12 percent in one study) with adenosine administration, perhaps because of the drug's effect in shortening atrial refractoriness. Induction of atrial fibrillation can be problematic in patients with the Wolff-Parkinson-White syndrome and rapid AV conduction over the accessory pathway.

DIGOXIN

Cardiac actions of digitalis glycosides have been recognized for centuries. Digoxin is used for control of supraventricular arrhythmias, mainly control of ventricular rate during atrial fibrillation. The use of digoxin has decreased because of the availability of agents with greater potency and a wider therapeutic to toxic drug concentration range.

ELECTROPHYSIOLOGICAL ACTIONS (see Tables 33-1, 33-2, 33-3, and 33-5). Digoxin acts mainly through the autonomic nervous system, in particular by enhancing both central and peripheral vagal tone. These actions are largely confined to slowing the sinus node discharge rate, shortening atrial refractoriness, and prolonging AV nodal refractoriness. Electrophysiological effects on the His-Purkinje system and ventricular muscle are minimal, except in toxic concentrations. In studies of denervated hearts, digoxin has relatively little effect on the AV node and causes a mild increase in atrial refractoriness.

The sinus rate and P wave duration are minimally changed in most patients taking digoxin. The sinus rate may decrease in patients with heart failure whose left ventricular performance is improved by the drug; individuals with significant underlying sinus node disease also have slower sinus rates or even sinus arrest. Similarly, the PR interval is generally unchanged, except in patients with underlying AV node disease. QRS and QT intervals are unaffected. The characteristic ST and T wave abnormalities seen with digoxin use do not represent toxicity.

PHARMACOKINETICS (see Table 33-4). Intravenously administered digoxin yields some electrophysiological effect within minutes, with a peak effect occurring after 1.5 to 3 hours. After oral dosing, the peak effect occurs in 4 to 6 hours. The extent of digoxin absorption after oral administration varies depending on the preparation; tablet forms are 60 to 75 percent absorbed, whereas encapsulated gel forms are almost completely absorbed. Ingestion of cholestyramine or an antacid preparation at the same time as digoxin ingestion decreases its absorption. The serum half-life of digoxin is 36 to 48 hours, and the drug is excreted unchanged by the kidneys.

DOSAGE AND ADMINISTRATION (see Table 33-4). In acute loading doses of 0.5 to 1.0 mg, digoxin may be given intravenously or by mouth. Chronic daily oral dosing should be adjusted on the basis of clinical indications and the extent of renal dysfunction. Most patients require from 0.125 to 0.25 mg/day as a single dose. However, as little as 0.125 mg every other day is needed in some patients receiving renal dialysis, whereas young patients may require as much as 0.5 mg/day. Serum digoxin levels may be used to monitor compliance with therapy as well as to determine whether digitalis toxicity is the cause of new symptoms compatible with the diagnosis. However, routine monitoring of digoxin levels is not warranted in patients whose ventricular rate is controlled during atrial fibrillation and who have no symptoms of toxicity.

A large number of pharmacokinetic interactions have been described for digoxin; the most important is with quinidine, which increases serum digoxin concentrations by displacing the drug from tissue binding sites and decreasing renal clearance.

INDICATIONS. Digoxin can be used intravenously to slow the ventricular rate during atrial fibrillation and flutter; it was formerly used to attempt to convert SVTs to sinus rhythm, but its onset of action is much slower and its success rate less than that of adenosine, verapamil, or beta blockers. Thus, it is now rarely used in this way. Digoxin is more commonly used orally to control the ventricular rate in chronic atrial fibrillation. When the patient with atrial fibrillation is at rest and vagal tone predominates, the ventricular rate can be maintained between 60 and 100 beats/min in 40 to 60 percent of cases. However, when the patient begins to exercise, the decrease in vagal tone and increase in adrenergic tone combine to diminish digoxin's beneficial effects on AV nodal conduction. Patients may experience a marked increase in ventricular rate with even mild exertion. Digoxin is therefore rarely used as a single agent to control the ventricular rate in chronic atrial fibrillation. The drug has little ability to prevent episodes of paroxysmal atrial fibrillation or to control ventricular rate during the episodes. Finally, digoxin is no more effective than placebo at terminating episodes of acute- or recent-onset atrial fibrillation.

ADVERSE EFFECTS. One major reason why digoxin use has decreased is its potential for serious adverse effects and the narrow window between therapeutic and toxic concentrations. Digitalis toxicity produces various symptoms and signs, including headache, nausea and vomiting, altered color perception, halo vision, and generalized malaise. More serious than these are digitalis-related arrhythmias, which include bradycardias related to a markedly enhanced vagal effect (e.g., sinus bradycardia or arrest, AV node block) and tachyarrhythmias that may be caused by delayed afterdepolarization-mediated triggered activity (e.g., atrial, junctional, and fascicular or ventricular tachycardia). Worsening renal function, advanced age, hypokalemia, chronic lung disease, hypothyroidism, and amyloidosis increase a patient's sensitivity to digitalis-related arrhythmias. The diagnosis can be confirmed by determining the serum digoxin level. Therapy for most bradycardias consists of withdrawal of digoxin; atropine or temporary pacing may be needed in symptomatic patients. Phenytoin can be used for control of atrial tachyarrhythmias, whereas lidocaine has been successful in treating infranodal tachycardias. Life-threatening arrhythmias can be treated with digoxin-specific antibody fragments. Electrical direct-current cardioversion should be performed only when absolutely necessary in the digitalis-toxic patient because life-threatening VT or VF can result, which can be very difficult to control.

ELECTROTHERAPY OF CARDIAC ARRHYTHMIAS

Direct-Current Electrical Cardioversion

Electrical cardioversion offers obvious advantages over drug therapy in terminating tachycardia. Under conditions optimal for close supervision and monitoring, a precisely regulated "dose" of electricity can restore sinus rhythm immediately and safely. The distinction between supraventricular and ventricular tachyarrhythmias, crucial to the proper medical management of arrhythmias, becomes less significant, and the time-consuming titration of drugs with potential side effects is obviated.

MECHANISMS. Electrical cardioversion appears most effective in terminating tachycardias related to reentry, such as atrial flutter and many cases of atrial fibrillation, AV node reentry, reciprocating tachycardias associated with the Wolff-Parkinson-White syndrome, most forms of VT, ventricular flutter, and VF. The electrical shock, by depolarizing all excitable myocardium and possibly by prolonging refractoriness, interrupts reentrant circuits and establishes electrical homogeneity, which terminates reentry. The mechanism by which a shock successfully terminates VF has not been completely explained. If the precipitating factors are no longer present, interrupting the tachyarrhythmia for only the brief time produced by the shock may prevent its return for long periods, even though the anatomical and electrophysiological substrates required for the tachycardia are still present.

Tachycardias thought to be caused by disorders of impulse formation (automaticity) include parasystole, some forms of AT, ectopic junctional tachycardia (with or without digitalis toxicity), accelerated idioventricular rhythm, and rare forms of VT (see Chaps. 31 and 35). An attempt to cardiovert these tachycardias electrically is not indicated in most cases because they typically recur within seconds after the shock; release of endogenous catecholamines consequent to the shock may further exacerbate the arrhythmia. It has not been established whether cardioversion can terminate tachycardias caused by enhanced automaticity or triggered activity.

TECHNIQUE. Before *elective* cardioversion, a careful physical examination, including palpation of limb pulses, should be performed. A 12-lead ECG is obtained before and after cardioversion, as well as a rhythm strip during the electroshock. The patient, who should be informed completely about what to expect, is in a fasting state and metabolically balanced; that is, blood gases, pH, and electrolytes should be normal, with no evidence of drug toxicity. Withholding digitalis for several days before elective cardioversion in patients without clinical evidence of digitalis toxicity is not necessary, although patients in whom digitalis toxicity is suspected should not be electrically cardioverted until this situation has been corrected. Maintenance antiarrhythmic drug administration 1 to 2 days before electrical cardioversion of patients with atrial fibrillation can revert some patients to sinus rhythm, help prevent recurrence of atrial fibrillation once sinus rhythm is restored, and help determine the patient's tolerance for the drug. There is also evidence that angiotensin-converting enzyme inhibitor and receptor blockers may prevent recurrence of fibrillation, especially in patients with ventricular dysfunction.[42]

Self-adhesive pads applied in the standard apicoanterior or apicoposterior paddle positions have transthoracic impedances similar to those of paddles and are useful in elective cardioversions or other situations in which there is time for their application. Paddles 12 to 13 cm in diameter can be used to deliver maximum current to the heart, but the benefits of these paddles compared with those of paddles 8 to 9 cm in diameter have not been clearly established. Larger paddles may distribute the intracardiac current over a wider area and may reduce shock-induced myocardial injury.

A synchronized shock (i.e., one delivered during the QRS complex) is used for all cardioversions except for very rapid ventricular tachyarrhythmias, such as ventricular flutter or VF (Fig. 33-2). Although generally minimal, shock-related myocardial damage increases directly with increases in applied energy, and so the minimum effective shock should be used. Therefore, shocks are "titrated" when the clinical situation permits. Except for atrial fibrillation, shocks in the range of 25 to 50 J successfully terminate most SVTs and should be tried initially. If unsuccessful, a second shock of higher energy can be delivered. The starting level to terminate atrial fibrillation with older monophasic machines should be no less than 100 J but, with newer biphasic systems, a shock as low as 25 J may succeed. Delivered energy can be increased in a stepwise fashion; up to 360 J can be used safely. Anteroposterior pads may have a higher efficacy rate by placing more of the atrial mass in the shock vector than is the case for apicoanterior pads. If a shock of 360 J fails to convert the rhythm, repeated shocks at the same energy may succeed by decreasing chest wall impedance; reversing pad polarity can occasionally help as well. Administration of ibutilide has been shown to facilitate electrical cardioversion of atrial fibrillation to sinus rhythm.[35] Intracardiac defibrillation can be tried if all attempts at external cardioversion fail. For patients with stable VT, starting levels in the range of 25 to 50 J can be used. If there is some urgency to terminate the tachyarrhythmia, one can begin with higher energies. To terminate VF, 100 to 200 J (biphasic; 200 to 360 J with monophasic machines) is generally used, although much lower energies (less than 50 J) terminate VF when the shock is delivered soon after the onset of the arrhythmia—for example, using adhesive pads in the electrophysiology laboratory.[43]

During elective cardioversion, a short-acting barbiturate such as methohexital, a sedative such as propofol, or an amnesic such as diazepam or midazolam can be used. A physician skilled in airway management should be in attendance, an IV route should be established, and pulse oximetry, the electrocardiogram, and blood pressure should be monitored. All equipment necessary for emergency resuscitation should be immediately accessible. Before cardioversion, 100 percent oxygen may be administered for 5 to 15 minutes by nasal cannula or face mask and is continued throughout the procedure. Manual ventilation of the patient may be necessary to avoid hypoxia during periods of deepest sedation. Adequate sedation of the patient undergoing even urgent cardioversion is essential; some patients who have needlessly

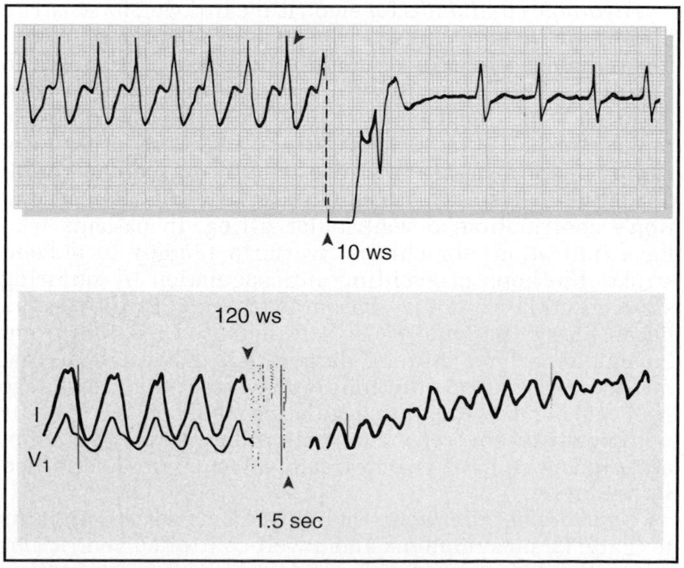

FIGURE 33–2 **Top,** A synchronized shock (note synchronization marks in the apex of the QRS complex (arrow) during ventricular tachycardia is followed by a single repetitive ventricular response and then normal sinus rhythm. **Bottom,** A shock synchronized to the terminal portion of the QRS complex (arrow) in a patient with atrial fibrillation and conduction to the ventricle over an accessory pathway (Wolff-Parkinson-White syndrome) resulted in ventricular fibrillation that was promptly terminated by a 400-J shock. Recording was lost for 1.5 seconds (arrow) because of baseline drift after the shock. ws = watt seconds.

been shocked while awake, perhaps because of uneasiness of the physician with the arrhythmia, have declined further medical care for their arrhythmias because of concern that they would again undergo cardioversion without appropriate sedation.

In up to 5 percent of patients with atrial fibrillation, sinus rhythm cannot be restored by external countershock despite all the preceding measures, including ibutilide pretreatment and biphasic shocks. It is important to distinguish between inability to attain sinus rhythm, indicating inadequate energy delivery to the atria, and inability to maintain sinus rhythm following transient termination of fibrillation; the latter condition (early reinitiation of atrial fibrillation) does not respond to higher energy shocks because fibrillation has already been terminated, but quickly recurs. Pretreatment with an antiarrhythmic drug may help maintain sinus rhythm after subsequent shocks. Patients in whom atrial fibrillation simply cannot be terminated with external shock tend to be very obese or have severe obstructive lung disease. In such cases, internal cardioversion can be performed using specially configured catheters, with multiple large electrodes covering several centimeters of the distal portion of the catheter for distributing shock energy. Using standard percutaneous access, these catheters can be situated in the lateral right atrium and coronary sinus to achieve a shock vector across most of the atrial mass. With such configurations, internal shocks of 2 to 15 J can terminate atrial fibrillation in more than 90 percent of patients whose arrhythmia is refractory to transthoracic shock. Esophageal cardioversion has also been reported.

INDICATIONS. As a rule, any tachycardia that produces hypotension, congestive heart failure, mental status changes, or angina and does not respond promptly to medical management should be terminated electrically. Very rapid ventricular rates in patients with atrial fibrillation and Wolff-Parkinson-White syndrome are often best treated by electrical cardioversion. In almost all cases, the patient's hemodynamic status improves after cardioversion. Rarely, a patient may experience hypotension, reduced cardiac output, or congestive heart failure after the shock. This problem may be related to complications of the cardioversion, such as embolic events, myocardial depression resulting from the anesthetic agent or the shock itself, hypoxia, lack of restoration of left atrial contraction despite return of electrical atrial systole, or postshock arrhythmias. Direct-current countershock of digitalis-induced tachyarrhythmias is contraindicated.

Favorable candidates for electrical cardioversion of atrial fibrillation include patients who (1) have symptomatic atrial fibrillation of less than 12 months' duration; (2) continue to have atrial fibrillation after the precipitating cause has been removed (e.g., after treatment of thyrotoxicosis); (3) have a rapid ventricular rate that is difficult to slow; or (4) have symptoms of decreased cardiac output (e.g., fatigue, lightheadedness, dyspnea) attributable to lack of atrial contraction's contribution to ventricular filling. In patients who have indications for chronic warfarin therapy to prevent stroke, the hope of avoiding anticoagulation by restoring sinus rhythm is not a reason to attempt cardioversion, because these patients are still at increased risk for thromboembolic events. Several large trials have shown that maintenance of sinus rhythm confers no survival advantage over rate control and anticoagulation; thus, not all patients with newly discovered atrial fibrillation warrant an attempt at restoring sinus rhythm. Treatment must be determined individually.

Unfavorable candidates include patients with (1) digitalis toxicity; (2) no symptoms and a well-controlled ventricular rate without therapy; (3) sinus node dysfunction and various unstable supraventricular tachyarrhythmias or bradyarrhythmias—often the bradycardia-tachycardia syndrome—who finally develop and maintain atrial fibrillation, which in essence represents a cure for the sick sinus syndrome; (4) little or no symptomatic improvement with normal sinus rhythm who promptly revert to atrial fibrillation after cardioversion despite drug therapy; (5) a large left atrium and longstanding atrial fibrillation; (6) infrequent episodes of atrial fibrillation that revert spontaneously to sinus rhythm; (7) no mechanical atrial systole after the return of electrical atrial systole; (8) atrial fibrillation and advanced heart block; (9) cardiac surgery planned in the near future; and (10) antiarrhythmic drug intolerance. Atrial fibrillation is more likely to recur after cardioversion in patients who have significant chronic obstructive lung disease, congestive heart failure, mitral valve disease (particularly mitral regurgitation), atrial fibrillation present longer than 1 year, and an enlarged left atrium (echocardiographic diameter more than 4.5 cm).

In patients with atrial flutter, slowing the ventricular rate by administering beta or calcium channel blockers or terminating the flutter with an antiarrhythmic agent may be difficult, and electrical cardioversion is often the initial treatment of choice. For the patient with other types of SVT, electrical cardioversion may be used when (1) vagal maneuvers or simple medical management (e.g., IV adenosine and verapamil) has failed to terminate the tachycardia and (2) the clinical setting indicates that fairly prompt restoration of sinus rhythm is desirable because of hemodynamic decompensation or electrophysiological consequences of the tachycardia. Similarly, in patients with VT, the hemodynamic and electrophysiological consequences of the arrhythmias determine the need for and urgency of direct-current cardioversion. Electrical countershock is the initial treatment of choice for ventricular flutter or VF. Speed is essential (see Chap. 36).

If, after the first shock, reversion of the arrhythmia to sinus rhythm does not occur, a higher energy level should be tried. When transient ventricular arrhythmias result after an unsuccessful shock, a bolus of lidocaine can be given before delivering a shock at the next energy level. If sinus rhythm returns only transiently and is promptly supplanted by the tachycardia, a repeated shock can be tried, depending on the tachyarrhythmia being treated and its consequences. Administration of an antiarrhythmic agent intravenously may be useful before delivering the next cardioversion shock (such as ibutilide in resistant atrial fibrillation). After cardioversion, the patient should be monitored, at least until full consciousness has been restored and preferably for several hours thereafter, depending on the duration of recovery from the particular form of sedation or anesthesia used. If ibutilide has been given, the ECG should be monitored for up to 8 hours because torsades de pointes can develop in the first few hours after administration.

RESULTS. Cardioversion restores sinus rhythm in 70 to 95 percent of patients, depending on the type of tachyarrhythmia. However, sinus rhythm remains after 12 months in less than one third to one half of patients with chronic atrial fibrillation. Thus, maintenance of sinus rhythm, once established, is the difficult problem, not the immediate termination of the tachycardia. The likelihood of maintaining sinus rhythm depends on the particular arrhythmia, the presence of underlying heart disease, and the response to antiarrhythmic drug therapy. Atrial size often decreases after termination of atrial fibrillation and restoration of sinus rhythm, and functional capacity improves.

COMPLICATIONS. Arrhythmias induced by electrical cardioversion are generally caused by inadequate synchronization, with the shock occurring during the ST segment or T wave. Occasionally, a properly synchronized shock can produce VF (see Fig. 33-2). Postshock arrhythmias are usually transient and do not require therapy. Embolic episodes are reported to occur in 1 to 3 percent of patients converted from atrial fibrillation to sinus rhythm. Prior therapeutic anticoagulation (international normalized ratio, 2.0 to 3.0) consistently for at least 3 weeks should be used for patients who have no contraindication to such therapy and have had atrial fibrillation present for longer than 2 to 3 days or of indeterminate duration. This approach is particularly valid for those who are at high risk for emboli, such as those with mitral stenosis and atrial fibrillation of recent onset, a history of recent or recurrent emboli, a prosthetic mitral valve, an enlarged heart (including left atrial enlargement), or congestive heart failure. It is important to note that 3 weeks of therapeutic anticoagulation is not the same as simply administering warfarin for 3 weeks. Anticoagulation with warfarin for at least 4 weeks afterward is recommended, because restoration of atrial mechanical function lags behind that of electrical systolic function and thrombi can still form in largely akinetic atria, although they are electrocardiographically in sinus rhythm. Exclusion of left atrial thrombus by transesophageal echocardiography immediately prior to cardioversion may not always preclude embolism days or weeks after cardioversion of atrial fibrillation. Atrial thrombi may be present in patients with nonfibrillation atrial tachyarrhythmias, such as atrial flutter[44] and AT in patients with congenital heart disease. The same precardioversion and postcardioversion anticoagulation recommendations apply to these patients, as well as to those with atrial fibrillation. Although direct-current shock has been demonstrated in animals to cause myocardial injury, studies in humans have indicated that elevations of myocardial enzymes after cardioversion are not common. ST segment elevation, sometimes dramatic, can occur immediately after elective direct-current cardioversion and last for 1 to 2 minutes, although cardiac enzymes and myocardial scintigraphy may be unremarkable. ST elevation lasting longer than 2 minutes usually indicates myocardial injury unrelated to the shock. A decrease in serum K^+ and Mg^{2+} levels can occur after cardioversion of VT.

Cardioversion of VT can also be achieved by a chest thump.[45] Its mechanism of termination is probably related to a mechanically induced PVC that interrupts a tachycardia and may be related to commotio cordis (see Chap. 78). The thump cannot be timed very well and is probably effective only when delivered during a nonrefractory part of the cardiac cycle. The thump can alter a VT and possibly induce ventricular flutter or VF if it occurs during the vulnerable period of the T wave. Because there may be a slightly greater likelihood of converting a stable VT to VF than of terminating VT to sinus rhythm, chest thump cardioversion should not be attempted unless a defibrillator is simply unavailable.

Implantable Electrical Devices for Treatment of Cardiac Arrhythmias

Implantable devices that monitor the cardiac rhythm and can deliver competing pacing stimuli and low- and high-energy shocks have been used effectively in selected patients (see Chap. 34).

Ablation Therapy for Cardiac Arrhythmias

The purpose of catheter ablation is to destroy myocardial tissue by delivering electrical energy through electrodes on a catheter placed next to an area of the myocardium integrally related to the onset or maintenance of the arrhythmia, or both. For tachycardias with an apparent focal origin (e.g., automatic, triggered activity, microreentry), the focus itself is targeted. In macroreentrant atrial and ventricular tachycardias, inexcitable scar tissue typically separates strands of remaining myocardium and wave fronts propagate around these scars. The target for ablation is a narrow portion of myocardium between inexcitable areas (e.g., scar, valve annulus; Fig. 33-3). The first catheter ablation procedures were performed using direct-current shocks, but this energy source has been supplanted by radiofrequency (RF) energy, which is delivered from an external generator and destroys tissue by controlled heat production.[46] Lasers and

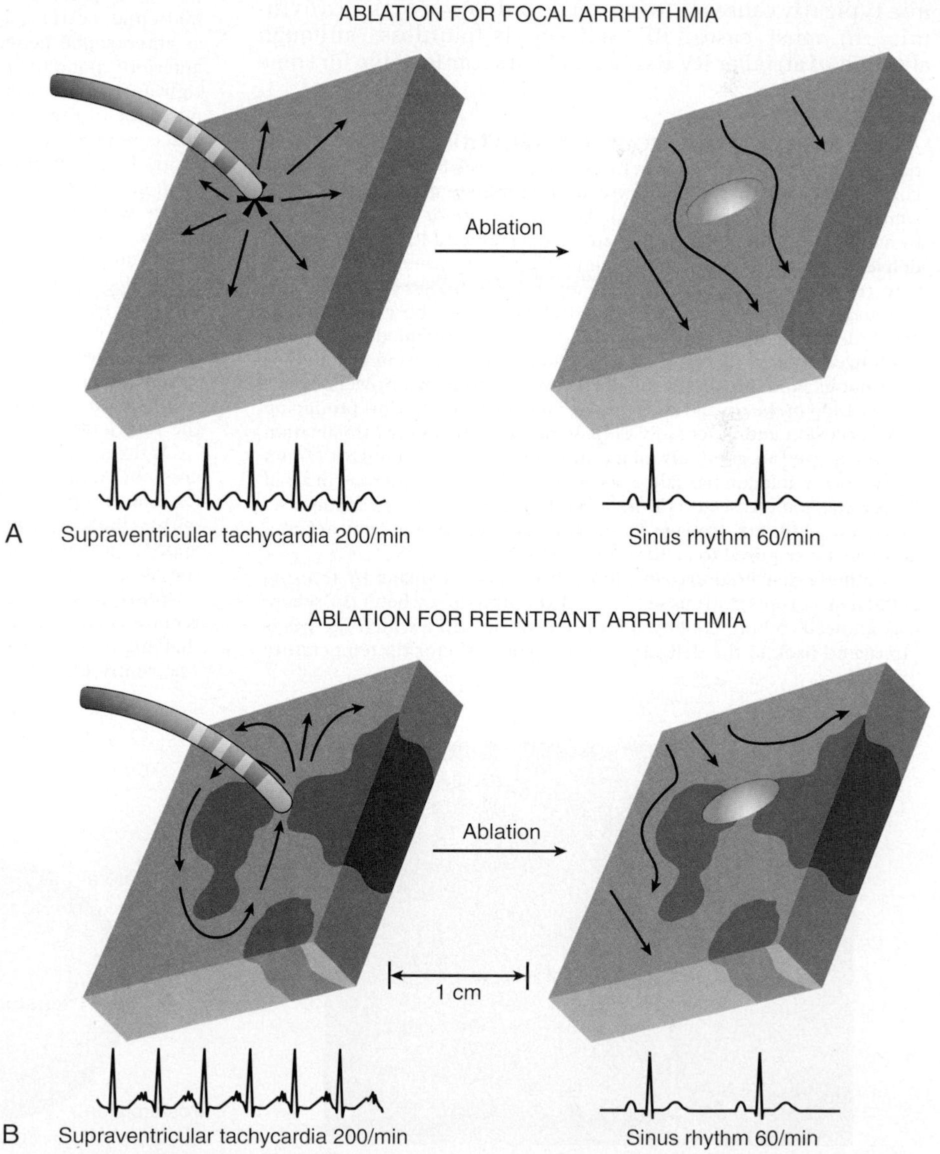

FIGURE 33–3 Strategies for catheter ablation. **A,** Focal tachycardia. At left, supraventricular tachycardia (SVT) is caused by an atrial focus, with activation emanating in all directions. Ablation of the focus (right) eliminates the arrhythmia with minimal disruption of normal activation. **B,** Macroreentrant SVT in setting of prior atrial damage, resulting in scar formation. During SVT (left), a wave front circulates around a scarred area and through a narrow isthmus between this and another area of scar. Ablation at this critical site (right) prevents further reentry.

microwave energy sources have been used, but not commonly; cryothermal catheter ablation has been approved for use in humans. When a target tissue has been identified by an EPS, the tip of the ablation catheter is maneuvered into apposition with this tissue. After stable catheter position and recordings have been ensured, RF energy is delivered between the catheter tip and an indifferent electrode, usually an electrocautery-type grounding pad on the skin of the patient's thigh. Because energies in the RF portion of the electromagnetic spectrum are poorly conducted by cardiac tissue, RF energy instead causes resistive heating in the cells close to the catheter tip (i.e., these cells transduce the electrical energy into thermal energy). When the tissue temperature exceeds 50°C, irreversible cellular damage and tissue death occur. An expanding front of conducted heat emanates from the region of resistive heating while RF delivery continues, resulting in production of a homogeneous, roughly hemispheric lesion of coagulative necrosis 3 to 5 mm in diameter (Fig. 33-4). RF-induced heating of tissue that has inherent automaticity (e.g., His bundle, foci of automatic tachycardias) results in initial acceleration of a rhythm, whereas RF delivery during a reentrant arrhythmia typically causes slowing and termination of the arrhythmia. In most cases, RF delivery is painless, although ablation of atrial or RV tissue can be uncomfortable for some patients.

COOLED-TIP RADIOFREQUENCY ABLATION. There are situations in which the catheter can be delivered to the correct location but conventional RF energy delivery cannot eliminate the tachycardia. In some of these cases, the amount of damage—depth or breadth—caused by standard RF energy is inadequate. Using standard RF energy, power delivery is usually regulated to maintain a preset catheter tip temperature (typically, 55° to 70°C). Tip temperatures higher than 90°C are associated with coagulation of blood elements on the electrode that preclude further energy delivery and could also become detached and embolize. Cooling the catheter tip by internal circulation of liquid or continuous fluid infusion through the tip electrode can prevent excessive heating of the tip and allow greater power delivery, thus producing a larger lesion and potentially enhancing efficacy. Cooled-tip ablation has been used to good advantage in cases in which standard (4-mm tip) catheter ablation has failed, as well as for primary therapy in atrial flutter and some cases of VT associated with structural heart disease, in which additional damage to already diseased areas is not harmful and may be required to achieve the desired result.

Catheter-delivered cryoablation causes tissue damage by freezing cellular structures. Nitrous oxide is delivered to the catheter tip, where it is allowed to boil, cooling the tip electrode, after which the gas is circulated back to the delivery console. The catheter tip temperature can be regulated, cooling to as low as −80°C. Cooling to 0°C causes reversible loss of function and can be used as a diagnostic test (i.e., termination of a tachycardia when the catheter is in contact with a group of cells critical to its perpetuation). The catheter tip can then be cooled more deeply to produce permanent damage and thus cure of the arrhythmia.[47] Cryoablation appears to cause less endocardial damage than RF and may thus engender less risk of thromboemboli following ablation.

RADIOFREQUENCY CATHETER ABLATION OF ACCESSORY PATHWAYS

Location of Pathways. The safety, efficacy, and cost-effectiveness of RF catheter ablation of an accessory AV pathway have made ablation the treatment of choice in most adult and many pediatric patients who have AV reentrant tachycardia (AVRT) or atrial flutter or fibrillation associated with a rapid ventricular response over the accessory pathway (see Chap. 35). When RF energy is delivered to an immature heart, the lesion size can increase as the heart grows; however, this has not been shown to cause problems later in life.

An EPS is performed initially to determine that the accessory pathway is part of the tachycardia circuit or capable of rapid AV conduction during atrial fibrillation and to localize the accessory pathway, the optimal site for ablation. Pathways can exist in the right or left free wall or septum of the heart (Fig. 33-5). Septal accessory pathways are further classified as anteroseptal, midseptal, and posteroseptal. Rare parahisian pathways can be distinguished from anteroseptal pathways. Midseptal locations are true septal pathways, whereas those classified as anteroseptal generally have no septal connection but are located anteriorly along the central fibrous body or right fibrous trigone at the right anterior free wall. Pathways classified as posteroseptal are located posterior to the central fibrous body within the so-called pyramidal space, which is bounded by the posterior superior process of the left ventricle and inferomedial aspects of both atria. Anteroseptal pathways are found near the His bundle, and accessory pathway activation potential as well as His bundle potential can be recorded simultaneously from a catheter placed at the His bundle region. Midseptal pathways are located close to the AV node and can usually be ablated from a right-sided approach; rarely, a left atrial approach is needed. Right posteroseptal pathways insert along the tricuspid ring in the immediate vicinity of the coronary sinus ostium, whereas left posteroseptal pathways are further into the coronary sinus and may be located at a subepicardial site around the proximal coronary sinus, within a middle cardiac vein or coronary sinus diverticulum, or subendocardially along the ventricular aspect of the mitral annulus.

Pathways at all locations and in all age groups can be ablated successfully. Multiple pathways are present in about 5 percent of patients. Occasional epicardial locations may be more easily approached from within the coronary sinus. Rarely, pathways may connect an atrial appendage with adjacent ventricular epicardium, 2 cm or more from the AV groove.

Ablation Site. The optimal ablation site can be found by direct recordings of the accessory pathway (Fig. 33-6), although deflections that mimic accessory pathway potentials can be recorded at other sites. The ventricular insertion site can be determined by finding the site of

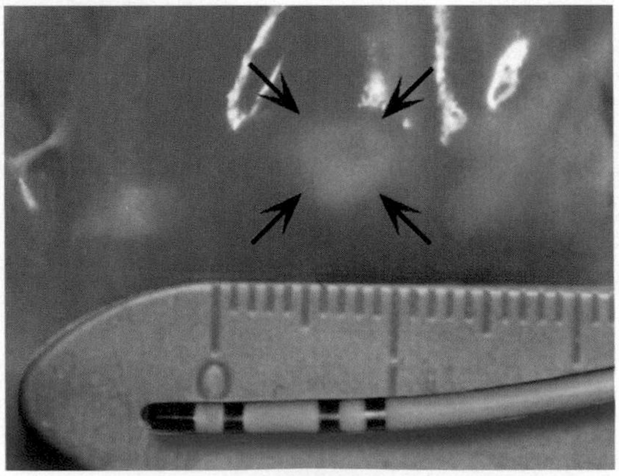

FIGURE 33–4 Radiofrequency lesion in human ventricular myocardium (explanted heart at the time of transplantation). A 30-second application of energy was made at the location denoted by arrows using the tip of the catheter shown. The lesion is 5 mm in diameter and has a well-demarcated border. A central depression in the lesion results from partial desiccation of tissue.

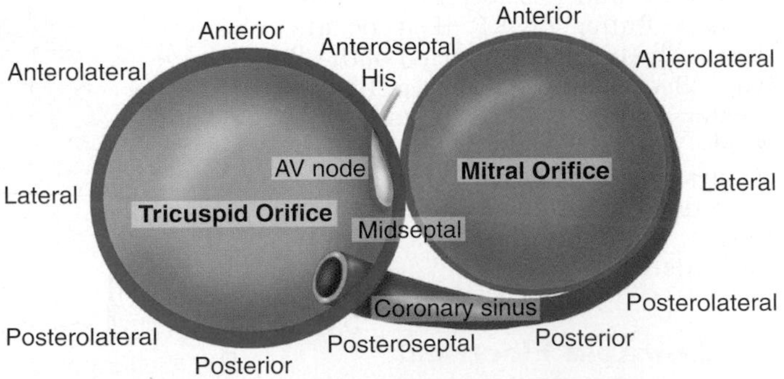

FIGURE 33–5 Locations of accessory pathways by anatomical region. Tricuspid and mitral valve annuli are depicted in a left anterior oblique view. Locations of coronary sinus, atrioventricular node, and bundle of His are shown. Accessory pathways may connect atrial to ventricular myocardium in any of the regions shown. AV = atrioventricular.

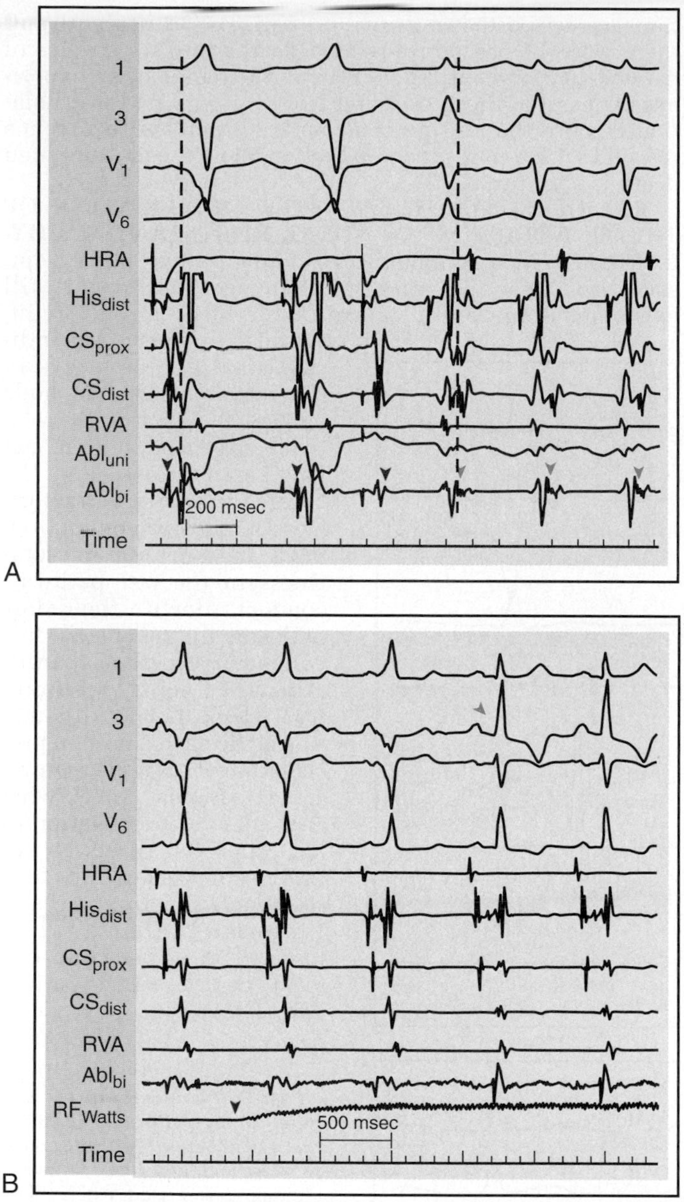

FIGURE 33–6 Wolff-Parkinson-White syndrome. Surface ECG leads 1, 3, V_1, and V_6 are shown, with intracardiac recordings from high right atrium (HRA), distal His (His_{dist}) bundle region, proximal (CS_{prox}) and distal (CS_{dist}) coronary sinus, right ventricular apex (RVA), and unipolar (Abl_{uni}) and bipolar (Abl_{bi}) tip electrodes of ablation catheter. Radiofrequency power in watts (RF_{Watts}) is also shown. **A,** Two beats of atrial pacing are conducted over the accessory pathway (blue arrows in Abl_{bi} recording, from the site of the accessory pathway), resulting in a delta wave on the electrocardiogram; a premature atrial stimulus (center) encounters accessory pathway refractoriness (red arrow), instead conducting over the atrioventricular (AV) node and bundle of His, resulting in a narrow QRS complex and starting an episode of AV reentrant tachycardia. After each narrow QRS complex is an atrial deflection, the earliest portion of which is recorded at the ablation site (green arrows). **B,** Ablation of this pathway is accomplished by delivery of radiofrequency (RF) energy from the ablation catheter tip. The blue arrow denotes onset of radiofrequency energy delivery; two QRS complexes later, the delta wave is abruptly lost (green arrow in lead 3) because of elimination of conduction over the accessory pathway.

the earliest onset of the ventricular electrogram in relation to the onset of the delta wave. Other helpful guidelines include unfiltered unipolar recordings that register a QS wave and the shortest AV conduction time during maximal preexcitation. A major ventricular potential synchronous with the onset of the delta wave can be a target site in left-sided preexcitation, whereas earlier ventricular excitation in relation to the delta wave can be found for right-sided preexcitation. The atrial insertion site of manifest or concealed pathways (i.e., delta wave present or absent, respectively) can be found by locating the site showing the earliest atrial activation during retrograde conduction over the pathway. Reproducible mechanical inhibition of accessory pathway conduction during catheter manipulation and subthreshold stimulation has also been used to determine the optimal site. Accidental catheter trauma should be avoided, however, because it can hide the target for prolonged periods. Intracardiac echocardiography can be helpful at times in delineating unusual anatomy, guiding atrial septal puncture for left-sided access, and determining adequacy of catheter contact at ablation sites.

Left-sided accessory pathways often cross the mitral annulus obliquely. Consequently, the earliest site of retrograde atrial activation and the earliest site of anterograde ventricular activation are not directly across the AV groove from each other. Identification of the earliest site of atrial activation is usually performed during orthodromic AVRT or relatively rapid ventricular pacing, so that retrograde conduction using the AV node does not confuse assessment of the location of the earliest atrial activation.

Successful ablation sites should exhibit stable fluoroscopic and electrical characteristics. During sinus rhythm, the local ventricular activation at the successful ablation site precedes the onset of the delta wave on the ECG by 10 to 35 milliseconds; during orthodromic AVRT, the interval between the onset of ventricular activation in any lead and local atrial activation is usually 70 to 90 milliseconds (see Fig. 33-5). When temperature-measuring ablation catheters are used, a stable rise in catheter tip temperature is a helpful indicator of catheter stability and adequate contact between the electrode and tissue. In such a case, the tip temperature generally exceeds 50°C. The retrograde transaortic and transseptal approaches have been used with equal success to ablate accessory pathways located along the mitral annulus. A routine EPS performed weeks after the ablation procedure is generally not indicated but may be considered in patients who have recurrent delta wave or symptoms of tachycardia. Catheter-delivered cryoablation can be useful in patients with septal accessory pathways, located near the AV conduction system. Using this system, the catheter tip and adjacent tissue can be reversibly cooled to test a potential site. If the accessory pathway conduction fails while normal AV conduction is preserved, deeper cooling can be performed at the site to complete the ablation. If, however, normal AV conduction is worsened, allowing the catheter to rewarm results in no permanent damage.

Atriofascicular accessory pathways have connections consisting of a proximal portion, responsible for conduction delay and decremental conduction properties, and a long distal segment located along the endocardial surface of the right ventricular free wall that has electrophysiological properties similar to those of the right bundle branch. The distal end of the right atriofascicular accessory pathway can insert into the apical region of the right ventricular free wall, close to the distal right bundle branch, or can actually fuse with the latter. Right atriofascicular accessory pathways might represent a duplication of the AV conduction system and can be localized for ablation by recording potentials from the rapidly conducting distal component, which crosses the tricuspid annulus (analogous to the His bundle) and extends to the apical region of the right ventricular free wall. Ablation attempts should be performed more proximally to avoid inadvertently ablating the distal right bundle branch, which could actually be proarrhythmic and create incessant tachycardia by lengthening the reentrant circuit.

Indications. Ablation of accessory pathways is indicated in patients with symptomatic AVRT that is drug resistant or who are drug intolerant or do not desire long-term drug therapy. It is also indicated in patients with atrial fibrillation, or other atrial tachyarrhythmias, and a rapid ventricular response by means of an accessory pathway when the tachycardia is drug resistant or who are drug intolerant or do not desire long-term drug therapy. Other potential candidates include the following: (1) patients with AVRT or atrial fibrillation with rapid ventricular rates identified during an EPS for another arrhythmia; (2) asymptomatic patients with ventricular preexcitation whose livelihood, profession, important activities, insurability, mental well-being, or the public safety would be affected by spontaneous tachyarrhythmias or by the presence of the electrocardiographic abnormality; (3) patients with atrial fibrillation and a controlled ventricular response by means of the accessory pathway; and (4) patients with a family history of sudden cardiac death. Controversy remains as to whether all patients with accessory pathways need treatment; however, ablation has such a high success rate and low complication rate that in most centers, patients who need any form of therapy are referred for catheter ablation.[48]

Results. From the results of an early survey conducted by the North American Society of Pacing and Electrophysiology (now the Heart Rhythm Society),[49] successful ablation of left free wall accessory pathways was achieved in 2312 of 2527 patients (91 percent); of septal accessory pathways, in 1115 of 1279 (87 percent); and of right free wall accessory pathways, in 585 of 715 (82 percent). Significant complications were reported in 94 of 4521 patients (2.1 percent), and there were 13 procedure-related deaths in 4521 studies of patients (0.2 percent). Currently, in the hands of an experienced operator, the success rate for accessory pathway ablation is more than 95 percent, with a 2 percent recurrence rate and a 1 to 2 percent complication rate. Procedure-related death is very rare.

RADIOFREQUENCY CATHETER MODIFICATION OF THE AV NODE FOR AV NODAL REENTRANT TACHYCARDIAS. AV node reentry is a common cause of SVT episodes (see Chaps. 31 and 35). Although controversy still exists about the exact nature of the tachycardia circuit, abundant evidence has indicated that two pathways in the region of the AV node participate, one with relatively fast conduction but long refractoriness and the other with shorter refractoriness but slower conduction. PACs can encounter refractoriness in the fast pathway, conduct down the slow pathway, and reenter the fast pathway retrogradely, initiating AV nodal reentrant SVT (Fig. 33-7). Although this is the most common presentation of AV node reentry, some patients have what appears to be propagation in the opposite direction in this circuit (anterograde fast, retrograde slow), as well as a "slow-slow" variant. Two or more of these variants can exist in the same patient (Fig. 33-8).

Fast-Pathway Ablation. Ablation can be performed to eliminate conduction in the fast pathway or the slow pathway. Although rarely used, when ablating the fast pathway, the electrode tip is positioned along the AV node–His bundle axis in the anterosuperior portion of the tricuspid annulus. The catheter is gradually withdrawn until the atrial electrogram amplitude equals or exceeds that of the ventricular electrogram and the His bundle recording is absent or extremely small (0.05 mV). During energy delivery, the electrocardiogram is monitored for PR prolongation, the occurrence of AV block, or both. If accelerated junctional rhythm is noted during delivery of RF energy, the atrium can be paced at a faster rate to ensure integrity of AV conduction. The initial RF pulse is delivered at 15 to 20 W for 10 to 15 seconds and gradually increased. Endpoints are PR prolongation, elimination of retrograde fast-pathway conduction, and noninducibility of AVNRT. An alternative approach is to apply RF current at the site of earliest retrograde atrial activa-

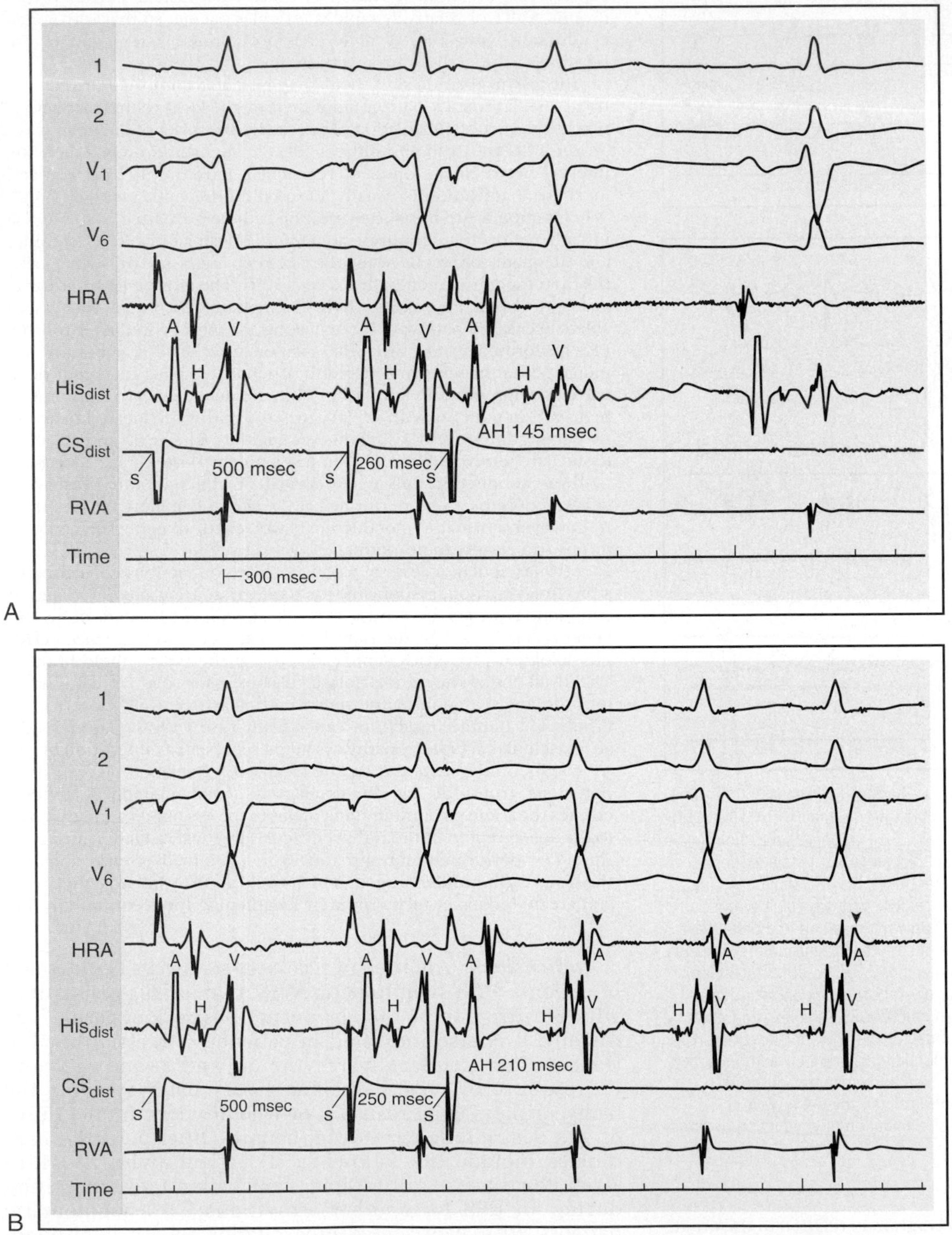

FIGURE 33–7 Atrioventricular (AV) node reentry. **A,** Two atrial paced complexes from the coronary sinus (CS) are followed by an atrial premature stimulus at a coupling interval of 260 milliseconds, resulting in an A-H interval of 145 milliseconds. **B,** The same atrial drive train is followed by an atrial extrastimulus 10 milliseconds earlier than before (250 milliseconds). This results in a marked increase in the A-H interval to 210 milliseconds, after which AV nodal reentrant tachycardia ensues because the extrastimulus encounters block in a "fast" AV node pathway, conducts down a "slow" pathway, and then conducts back up the fast pathway in a repeating fashion. Red arrows denote atrial electrograms coincident with QRS complexes, characteristic of the most common type of AV node reentry. Recording was done as in prior figures.

tion during tachycardia. RF current should be discontinued if the PR interval is prolonged by more than 50 percent or if AV block results. Currently, fast-pathway ablation is rarely performed because it is associated with a prolonged PR interval, a higher recurrence rate (10 to 15 percent), and a slightly higher risk of complete AV block (2 to 5 percent) compared with slow-pathway ablation. One uncommon situation in which fast-pathway ablation may be preferred is for patients who have a markedly prolonged PR interval at rest and no evidence of anterograde fast-pathway conduction. In such cases, ablation of the anterograde slow pathway may produce complete AV block, whereas retrograde fast-pathway ablation can eliminate SVT without altering AV conduction.

Slow-Pathway Ablation. The slow pathway can be located by mapping along the posteromedial tricuspid annulus close to the coronary sinus os. Electrographic recordings are obtained with an atrial-to-ventricular electrogram ratio less than 0.5 and either a multicomponent atrial electrogram or a recording of possible slow-pathway potential. In the anatomical approach, target sites are selected fluoroscopically. A single RF application suffices in many cases but, in others, serial RF lesions may be needed, starting at the most posterior site (near the coronary sinus os) and progressing to the more anterior locus (closer to the His bundle recording site). An accelerated junctional rhythm (Fig. 33-9) usually occurs when RF energy is applied at a site that will result in successful elimination of SVT. The success rate with the anatomical or electrographic mapping approach is equivalent and, most often, combinations of both are used, yielding success rates approaching 100 percent, with less than a 1 percent chance of complete heart block. Catheter-delivered cryoablation has been used for treatment of AVNRT with excellent results. The ability to carry out cryomapping—test potential sites for slow-pathway block with moderate, reversible cooling—should almost entirely eliminate the risk of AV block with ablation.

Slow-pathway ablation results in an increase in the anterograde AV block cycle length and AV node ERP without a change in the AH interval or retrograde conduction properties of the AV node. Patients in whom slow-pathway conduction is completely eliminated almost never have recurrent SVT episodes; approximately 40 percent of patients can have evidence of residual slow-pathway function after successful elimination of sustained AVNRT, usually manifested as persistent dual AV node physiology and single AV node echoes during atrial extrastimulation. The surest endpoint for slow-pathway ablation is the elimination of sustained AVNRT, with and without an infusion of isoproterenol.

AVNRT recurs in about 5 percent of patients after slow-pathway ablation. In some patients, the ERP of the fast pathway decreases after slow-pathway ablation, possibly because of electrotonic interaction between the two pathways. Atypical forms of reentry can result after ablation, as can apparent parasympathetic denervation, resulting in inappropriate sinus tachycardia.

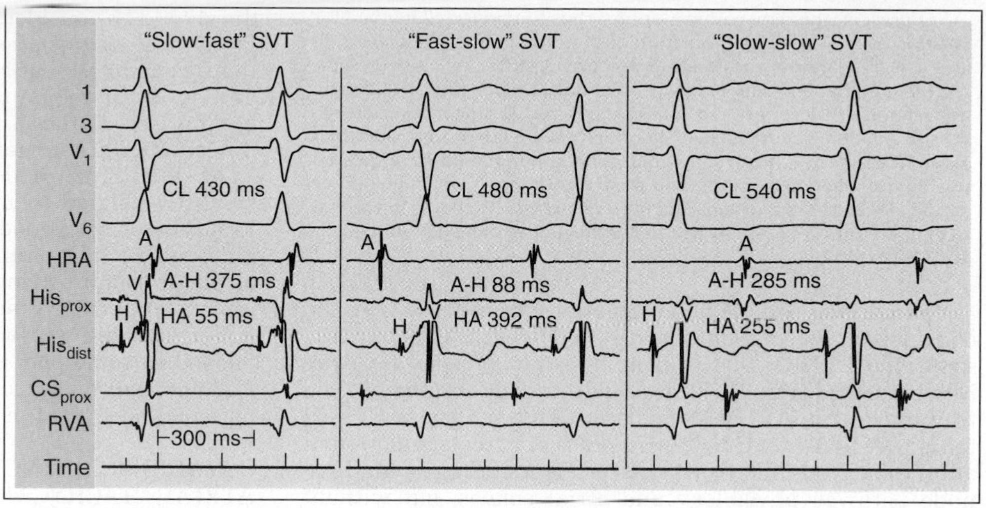

FIGURE 33–8 Three variants of atrioventricular (AV) node reentrant supraventricular tachycardia (SVT) in the same patient. Recordings as in other figures. **Left panel,** Most common type of AV node SVT (anterograde slow pathway, retrograde fast); atrial activation is coincident with ventricular activation. **Center panel,** "Atypical" AV node reentry, with anterograde fast-pathway conduction and retrograde conduction over a slow pathway. **Right panel,** Rare variety is shown, with anterograde conduction over a slow pathway and retrograde conduction over a second slow pathway. Note the similar atrial activation sequences in the latter two (coronary sinus before right atrium), as distinct from that of slow-fast AV node reentry (coronary sinus and right atrial activation nearly simultaneous). Note also the different P-QRS relationships, from simultaneous activation (left, short RP interval) to P in front of the QRS (middle, long RP interval) and P midway in the cardiac cycle (right). Recording was done as in prior figures. CL = cycle length.

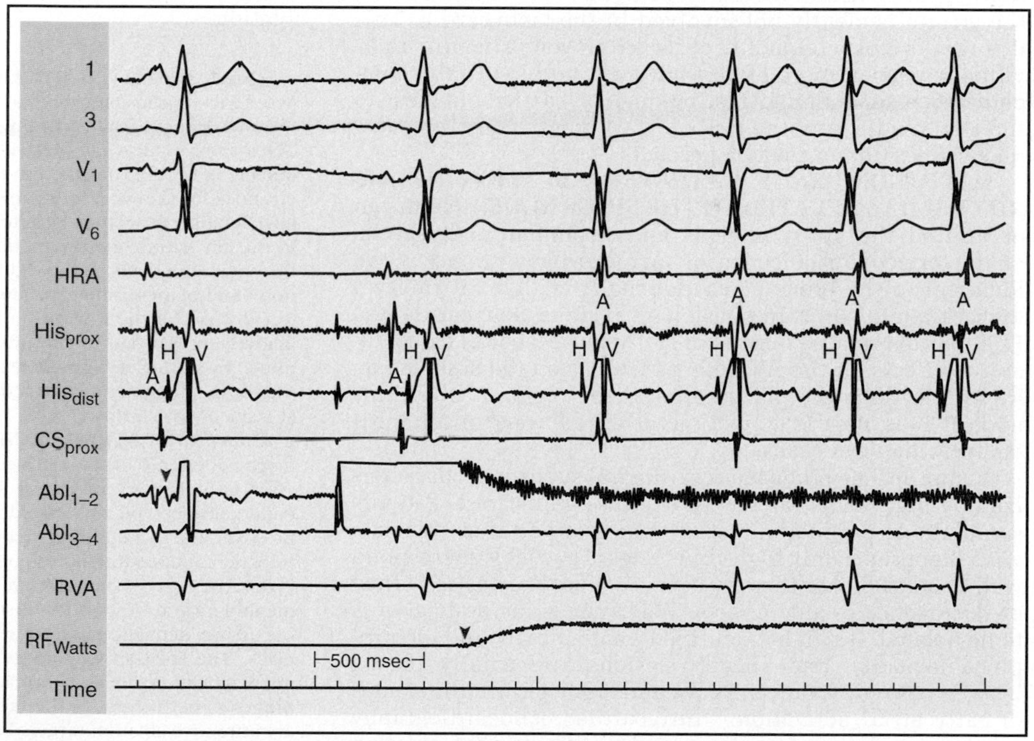

FIGURE 33–9 Atrioventricular (AV) node slow-pathway modification for cure of AV node reentrant supraventricular tachycardia. The ablation recording (arrow in $Abl_{1\text{-}2}$) shows a slurred deflection between atrial and ventricular electrogram components; this may represent the AV node slow-pathway deflection (but it is not the bundle of His deflection, which is instead recorded from a separate catheter 15 mm away). Shortly after the onset of radiofrequency delivery (arrow in RF_{Watts}), an accelerated junctional rhythm begins and gradually speeds up further. Retrograde conduction is present during the junctional rhythm. $Abl_{3\text{-}4}$ = proximal electrode recording from ablation catheter. Recording was done as in prior figures.

At present, the slow-pathway approach is the preferred method for ablation of typical AVNRT. Ablation of the slow pathway is also a safe and effective means for treating atypical AVNRT. In patients with AVNRT undergoing slow-pathway ablation, junctional ectopy during application of RF energy is a sensitive but nonspecific marker of successful ablation, occurring in longer bursts at effective target sites than at ineffective sites. Ventriculoatrial conduction should be expected during the junctional ectopy, and poor ventriculoatrial conduction or actual block may herald subsequent *anterograde* AV block. Junctional ectopic rhythm is caused by heating of the AV node and does not occur with cryoablation.

Indications. RF catheter ablation for AVNRT can be considered for patients with recurrent, symptomatic, sustained AVNRT that is drug resistant or who are drug intolerant or do not desire long-term drug treatment. The procedure can also be considered for a patient with sustained AVNRT identified during EPS or catheter ablation of another arrhythmia, or when there is a finding of dual AV node pathway physiology and atrial echoes, but without AVNRT during EPS in a patient suspected of having AVNRT clinically.

Results. Most centers currently use slow-pathway ablation, resulting in a procedural success rate of 98 percent, recurrence rate less than 2 percent, and incidence of heart block requiring permanent pacing less than 1 percent.

ECTOPIC JUNCTIONAL TACHYCARDIA. Ectopic junctional tachycardia is a rare form of SVT in which the electrocardiogram resembles that in AVNRT but is distinct in that (1) the mechanism is automatic, not reentrant, and (2) the atrium is clearly not involved in the tachycardia. This disorder is most commonly observed in young healthy individuals, women more often than men, and is usually catecholamine dependent. Ablation must be carried out close to the His bundle, and the risk of heart block requiring pacemaker insertion exceeds 5 percent.

RADIOFREQUENCY CATHETER ABLATION OF ARRHYTHMIAS RELATED TO THE SINUS NODE. Reentry in or around the sinus node is an uncommon arrhythmia, characterized by episodes of tachycardia with a P wave identical to the sinus P wave, usually with a PR interval longer than in sinus; in physiological sinus tachycardia, the PR interval remains normal or shortens because of catecholamine effects on the AV node as well as on the sinus node. RF applications are placed around the region of the sinus node at sites of early activation, prior to P wave onset, until tachycardia terminates.

Inappropriate sinus tachycardia is a syndrome characterized by high sinus rates with exercise and at rest. Patients complain of palpitations at all times of day that correlate with inappropriately high sinus rates. They may not respond well to beta blocker therapy because of lack of desired effect or occurrence of side effects. When the sinus node area is to be ablated, it can be identified anatomically and electrophysiologically, and ablation lesions are usually placed between the superior vena cava and crista terminalis at sites of early atrial activation.[50] Intracardiac echocardiography can help in defining anatomy and positioning the ablation catheter. Isoproterenol may be helpful in "forcing" the site of impulse formation to cells with the most rapid discharge rate. Care must be taken to apply RF energy at the most cephalad sites first; initial ablation performed further down the crista terminalis does not alter the atrial rate at the time, but can damage subsidiary pacemaker regions that may be needed after the sinus node has been eventually ablated.

Indications. Catheter ablation for sinus node reentrant tachycardia can be performed in patients with recurrent symptomatic episodes of sustained SVT that is drug resistant or who are drug intolerant or do not desire long-term drug treatment. Patients with inappropriate sinus tachycardia should be considered for ablation only after clear failure of medical therapy, because ablation results are often less than completely satisfactory. Whenever ablation is performed in the region of the sinus node, the patient should be apprised of the risk of needing a pacemaker after the procedure. Phrenic nerve damage is also a possibility.

Results. Sinus node reentrant tachycardia can be successfully ablated in more than 90 percent of candidates. Results are not as good for inappropriate sinus tachycardia; although a good technical result may be obtained at the time of the procedure, symptoms often persist because of recurrence of rapid sinus rates (at or near preablation rates) or for nonarrhythmic reasons. Multiple ablation sessions are needed in some patients, and about 20 percent eventually undergo pacemaker implantation; however, not all these patients have relief of palpitations, despite a normal heart rate.

RADIOFREQUENCY CATHETER ABLATION OF ATRIAL TACHYCARDIA (see Chap. 35). ATs are a heterogeneous group of disorders; causative factors include rapid discharge of a focus (focal tachycardia) and reentry. The former can occur in anyone, irrespective of the presence of structural abnormalities of the atria, whereas reentrant ATs almost always occur in the setting of a structurally damaged atria. Symptoms vary from none, in relatively infrequent or slow ATs in patients without heart disease, to syncope (rapid AT with compromised cardiac function) or heart failure (incessant AT over a period of weeks or months). All forms of AT are amenable to catheter ablation.

FOCAL ATRIAL TACHYCARDIA. In focal ATs (automatic or triggered foci or micro-reentry), activation mapping is used to determine the site of the AT by recording the earliest onset of local activation. These tachycardias can behave capriciously and be practically noninducible in an EPS, despite the patient's complaining of multiple daily episodes for the week prior to EPS. Ten to 15 percent of patients can have multiple atrial foci. Sites tend to cluster near the pulmonary veins in the left atrium and the mouths of the atrial appendages, and along the crista terminalis on the right (Fig. 33-10A; see Fig. 32-15).[51,52] Activation times of these sites typically occur only 15 to 40 milliseconds prior to the onset of the P wave on the ECG. Care must be taken to avoid inadvertent damage to the phrenic nerve; its location can be determined by pacing at high current at a potential site of ablation, observing for diaphragmatic contraction. Ablation should not be performed at a site at which this is seen, if at all possible.

REENTRANT ATRIAL TACHYCARDIA. As noted, these ATs occur more commonly in the setting of structural heart disease, especially after prior surgery involving an atrial incision. The region of slow conduction is typically related to an end of an atriotomy scar; this is, however, not in a constant anatomical location but varies from patient to patient, depending on the operation performed. Therefore, preprocedural review of operative reports and careful electrophysiological mapping are essential. Because reentry within a complete circuit is occurring, activation can be recorded throughout the entire cardiac cycle. The ablation strategy is to identify regions with mid-diastolic atrial activation during tachycardia that can be proved by pacing techniques to be integral to the tachycardia (see Fig. 33-10B).[53] Such sites are attractive ablation targets because they are composed of relatively few cells—hence, electrical silence on the surface ECG in diastole—and are thus more easily ablated by a typical application of RF energy than other areas. Focal ablation of these sites can then be performed, but often tachycardia can still be initiated (usually at a slower rate) or recurs after the procedure. Because these sites are typically located at a relatively narrow zone between the ends of prior scars or surgical incisions and another nonconducting barrier (e.g., another scar, caval orifice, valve annulus), another technique is to make a line of ablation lesions from the end of the scar to the nearest electrical barrier. Reentry can thereby be prevented. This technique is analogous to that used in curing atrial flutter (see later). Because these patients often have extensive atrial disease with islands of scar that could serve as barriers for additional ATs, specialized mapping techniques may be needed to locate these regions and preemptively connect them with ablation lesions to prevent future AT episodes.

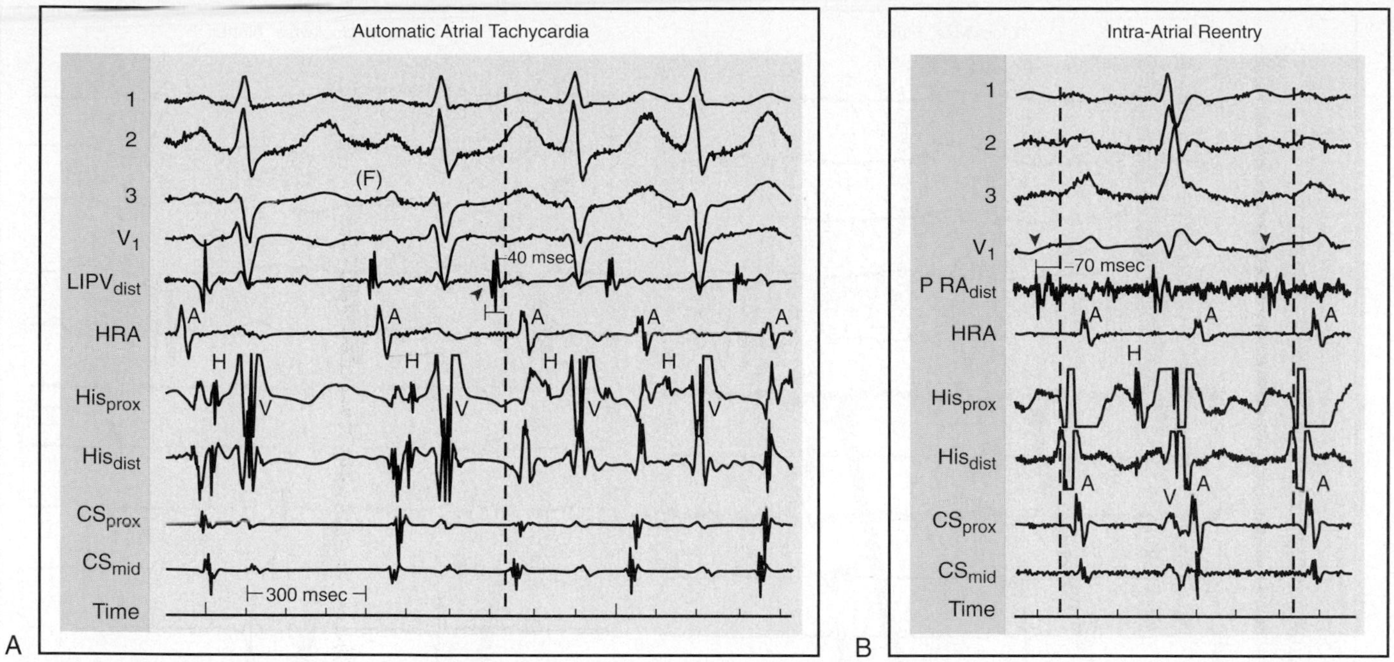

FIGURE 33–10 Atrial tachycardias. **A,** Automatic atrial tachycardia arising in the left inferior pulmonary vein (LIPV). A sinus beat is shown at left, followed by a fusion beat (F) of sinus and tachycardia activation. The last three beats in the panel are atrial tachycardia. The ablation catheter was within the LIPV and recorded a sharp potential (arrow) 40 milliseconds before the P wave onset (dashed line). Ablation at this site terminated the tachycardia. **B,** Intraatrial reentrant tachycardia in a patient who had undergone atrial septal defect repair years earlier. The ablation catheter is in the posterior right atrium (PRA), where a fragmented signal is recorded. A portion of this electrogram (arrows) precedes the P wave onset during tachycardia (dashed line) by 70 milliseconds. Ablation at this site terminated the tachycardia. Recording was done as in prior figures.

Indications. Catheter ablation for ATs should be considered for patients with recurrent episodes of symptomatic sustained ATs that are drug resistant or who are drug intolerant or do not desire long-term drug treatment.

Results. Success rates for ablation of focal AT range from 80 to 95 percent, largely depending on the ability to induce episodes at EPS; when episodes can be initiated with pacing, isoproterenol, or other means, AT can usually be ablated. Reentrant ATs, although more readily induced by an EPS, are often harder to eliminate completely; initial success rates are high (90 percent) but recurrences are seen in up to 20 percent of patients, necessitating drug therapy or another ablation procedure. Complications, occurring in 1 to 2 percent of patients, include phrenic nerve damage, cardiac tamponade, and heart block, with rare perinodal ATs.

RADIOFREQUENCY CATHETER ABLATION OF ATRIAL FLUTTER (see Chap. 35). Atrial flutter may be defined electrocardiographically (most typically, negative sawtooth waves in leads II, III and aVF, at a rate of about 300 beats/min) or electrophysiologically (a rapid, organized macro-reentrant AT, the circuit for which is anatomically determined). Understanding the reentrant pathway for all forms of atrial flutter is essential for developing an ablation approach. Reentry in the right atrium, with the left atrium passively activated, constitutes the mechanism of the typical electrocardiographic variety of atrial flutter, with caudocranial activation along the right atrial septum and craniocaudal activation of the right atrial free wall (Fig. 33-11A). In some cases, a zone of slow conduction exists in the low right atrium, which is typically bounded by the tricuspid annulus, inferior vena cava, and coronary sinus. In other cases, conduction velocity is more uniform throughout the large circuit. Placing an ablative lesion between any two anatomical barriers that transects a portion of the circuit necessary for perpetuation of reentry can be curative. Typically, this is across the isthmus of atrial tissue between the inferior vena caval orifice and tricuspid annulus (the cavotricuspid isthmus), a relatively narrow point in the circuit. Successful ablation can be accomplished where the advancing flutter wave front enters this zone in the low inferolateral right atrium, near the exit of this zone at the inferomedial right atrium, or in between these sites. Locations for RF delivery can be guided anatomically or electrophysiologically. Less commonly, the direction of wave front propagation in this large right atrial circuit is reversed (clockwise flutter proceeding cephalad up the right atrial free wall and caudad down the septum, with upright flutter waves in the inferior leads; see Fig. 33-11A). This arrhythmia, which has been called *atypical atrial flutter,* may also be ablated using the same techniques as with more typical atrial flutter. These two arrhythmias constitute cavotricuspid isthmus–dependent flutter and are distinct from other rapid atrial arrhythmias that may have a similar appearance on the ECG but use different (and often multiple) circuits in other parts of the right or left atrium. Ablation can be more difficult in these cases, which often occur in the setting of advanced lung disease or prior cardiac surgery. A common theme in these complex reentrant arrhythmias is the presence of an anatomically determined zone of inexcitability, around which an electrical wave front can circulate. Specialized mapping tools and skills are necessary to produce successful ablation in these cases.

In patients with atrial fibrillation, an antiarrhythmic drug can slow intraatrial conduction to such an extent that atrial flutter results and fibrillation is no longer observed. In some of these patients, ablation of atrial flutter and having them continue to take the antiarrhythmic drug can prevent recurrences of these atrial arrhythmias.

The endpoint of atrial flutter ablation procedures was initially termination of atrial flutter, with RF application accompanied by noninducibility of the arrhythmia. However, using these criteria, up to 30 percent of patients had recurrent flutter because of lack of complete and permanent conduction block in the cavotricuspid isthmus. In the last several years, the endpoint of ablation has changed to ensuring a line of bidirectional block in this region by pacing from opposite sides of the isthmus (see Fig. 33-11B) or the use of other techniques. Using these criteria, recurrence rates have fallen to less than 5 percent.

Indications. Candidates for RF catheter ablation include patients with recurrent episodes of atrial flutter that are drug resistant, those who are drug intolerant, and those who do not desire long-term drug therapy.

Results. Regardless of circuit location, atrial flutter can be successfully ablated in more than 90 percent of cases, although patients with complex right or left atrial flutters require more extensive and complex procedures.[54] Recur-

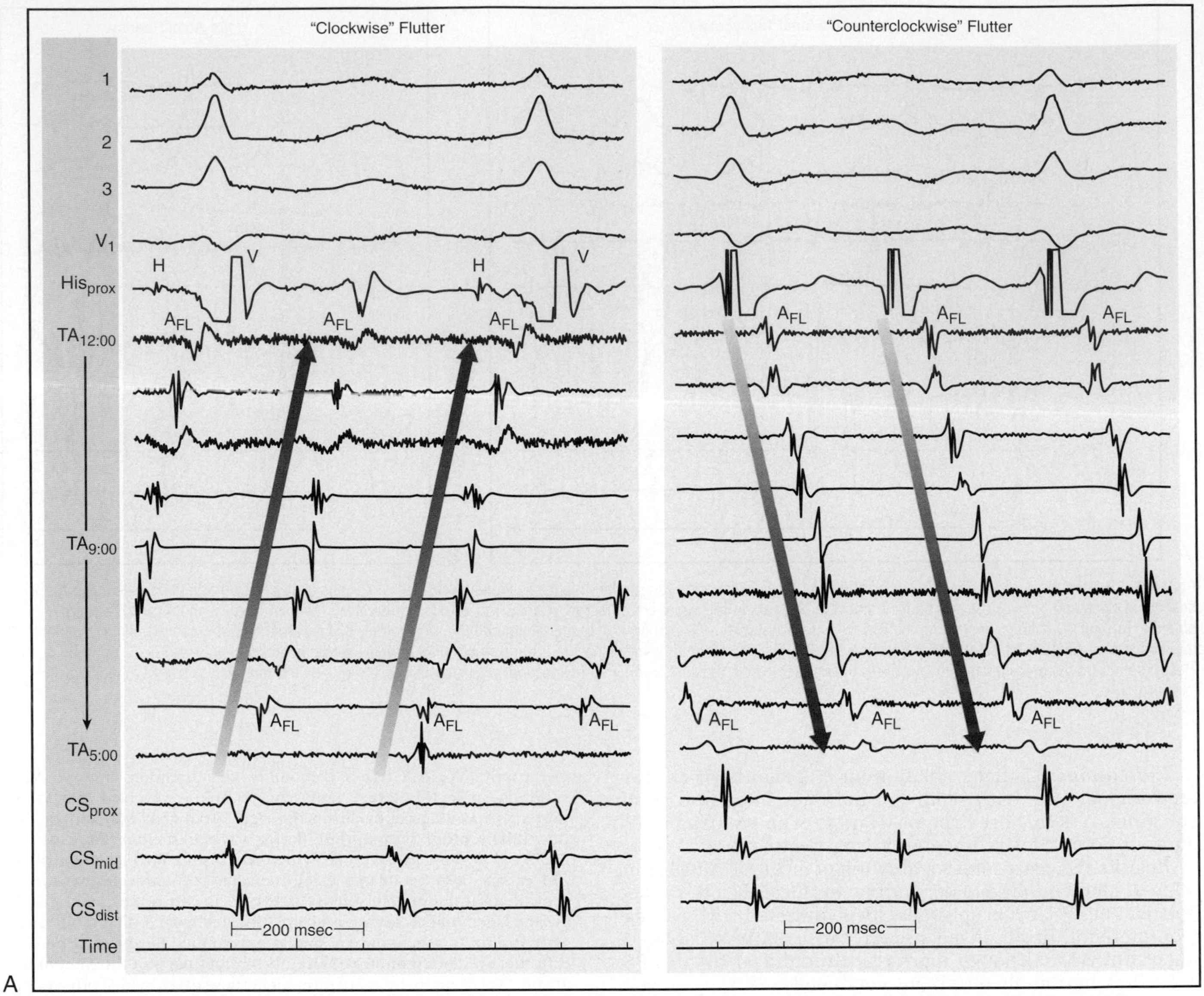

FIGURE 33–11 A, Two forms of atrial flutter in the same patient are shown. A "halo" catheter with 10 electrode pairs is situated on the atrial side of the tricuspid annulus (TA), with recording sites displayed from the top of the annulus (12:00) to the inferomedial aspect (5:00), as shown in fluoroscopic views in **B.** On the left, the wave front of atrial activation proceeds in a clockwise fashion (arrows) along the annulus, whereas at the right the direction of propagation is the reverse.

rence rates are less than 5 percent, except in patients with extensive atrial disease, in whom new circuits can develop over time as new areas of conduction delay and block form. Complications are rare and include inadvertent heart block and phrenic nerve paralysis.

ABLATION AND MODIFICATION OF ATRIOVENTRICULAR CONDUCTION FOR ATRIAL TACHYARRHYTHMIAS. In some patients with atrial tachyarrhythmias who have rapid ventricular rates despite optimal drug therapy, RF ablation can be used to eliminate or modify AV conduction to control the ventricular rates. To achieve RF catheter ablation of AV conduction, a catheter is placed across the tricuspid valve and positioned to record the largest His bundle electrogram associated with the largest atrial electrogram. RF energy is applied until complete AV block has been achieved and is continued for an additional 30 to 60 seconds. If no change in AV conduction is observed after 15 seconds of RF ablation, the catheter is repositioned and the attempt repeated. In occasional patients, attempts at RF ablation using this right-sided heart approach fail to achieve heart block. These patients can undergo an attempt from the left ventricle with a catheter positioned along the posterior interventricular septum, just beneath the aortic valve, to record a large His bundle electrogram. Energy is applied between the catheter electrode and skin patch or between catheters in the left and right ventricles. Success rates currently approach 100 percent, with recurrence of AV conduction in less than 5 percent of cases. Improved left ventricular function can result from control of ventricular rate during atrial fibrillation and withdrawal of rate-controlling medications with negative inotropic action. Permanent ventricular or AV pacing is required after ablation.

In some cases, the AV junction can be modified to slow the ventricular rate without producing complete AV block by ablation in the region of the slow pathway, as described in connection with AV node modification for AV node reentry. Initial success rates for slowing the ventricular response are good; however, long-term results are less consistent. Some patients have a gradual increase in ventricular rate to near-preablation levels, whereas late complete heart block may occur in others. Nonetheless, this procedure can be tried before producing complete AV block.

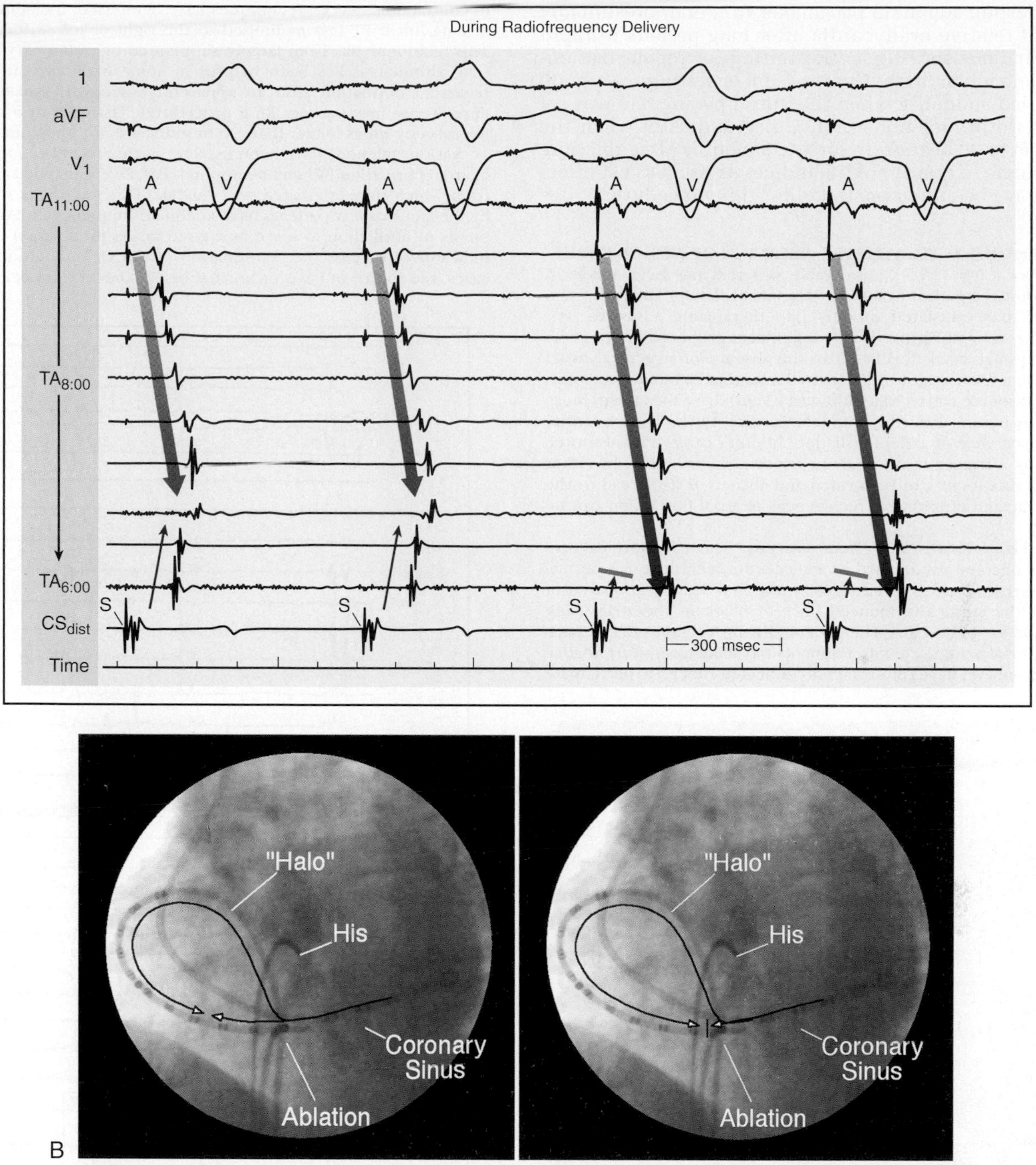

FIGURE 33–11, cont'd B, Ablation of the isthmus of atrial tissue between the tricuspid annulus and inferior vena caval orifice for cure of atrial flutter. Recordings are displayed from the multipolar catheter around much of the circumference of the tricuspid annulus (see left anterior oblique fluoroscopy images). Ablation of this isthmus is performed during coronary sinus pacing. In the two beats on the left, atrial conduction proceeds in two directions around the tricuspid annulus, as indicated by arrows and recorded along the halo catheter. In the two beats on the right, ablation has interrupted conduction in the floor of the right atrium, eliminating one path for transmission along the tricuspid annulus. The halo catheter now records conduction, proceeding all the way around the annulus. This finding demonstrates unidirectional block in the isthmus; block in the other direction may be demonstrated by pacing from one of the halo electrodes and observing a similar lack of isthmus conduction. (The bundle of His recording in the right panel is lost because of catheter movement.)

Indications. Ablation and modification of AV conduction can be considered in the following: (1) patients with symptomatic atrial tachyarrhythmias who have inadequately controlled ventricular rates unless primary ablation of the atrial tachyarrhythmia is possible; (2) similar patients when drugs are not tolerated or patients do not wish to take them, even though the ventricular rate can be controlled; (3) patients with symptomatic, nonparoxysmal, junctional tachycardia that is drug resistant or in whom drugs are not tolerated or are not desired; (4) patients resuscitated from sudden cardiac death related to atrial flutter or atrial fibrillation with a rapid ventricular response in the absence of an accessory pathway; and (5) patients with a dual-chamber pacemaker and a pacemaker-mediated tachycardia that cannot be treated effectively by drugs or by reprogramming the pacemaker. The last three situations are rarely encountered.

Results. Results from a U.S. survey have indicated that the procedure was successful in producing complete AV block in 95 percent of 1600 patients, with significant complications occurring in 21 (1.3 percent) and two procedure-related deaths (0.1 percent).[49] In early studies, up to 4 percent of patients had an episode of sudden death after AV junction ablation despite adequate pacemaker function, presumably because of relative bradycardia after long periods of rapid ventricular rates serving as the setting for repolarization-related ventricular arrhythmias.[55] In one study, 6 of 100 patients died suddenly when the initial pacing rate was set to 60 beats/min, but none of 135 died suddenly when the rate was set to 90 beats/min for 1 to 3 months after ablation. Improvements in quality of life indices as well as cost-effectiveness have been demonstrated for this procedure.

RADIOFREQUENCY CATHETER ABLATION OF ATRIAL FIBRILLATION (see Chap. 35). Considerable progress has been made in understanding the pathophysiology of atrial fibrillation. The use of this information has translated directly into therapeutic advances. For example, it is now recognized that a significant proportion of patients with paroxysmal atrial fibrillation in the absence of structural heart disease have a focal origin of the arrhythmia; that is, rapid discharges from a focal source (often in a pulmonary vein) drive the atrium more rapidly than it can uniformly conduct, leading to the electrocardiographic appearance of atrial fibrillation. In other cases, a focal source can serve as a trigger that initiates episodes of fibrillation. In either scenario, if this focus can be located and ablated or its spread to the rest of the atrium eliminated, recurrences of atrial fibrillation can be prevented.

Location and Ablation of Focal Sources. The maze surgical procedure has become established as a successful technique for permanently restoring sinus rhythm. In 1994, the first reports appeared of replicating the surgically induced lines of block in the atria using catheter ablation in humans. The intent of the procedure is to compartmentalize the atrial muscle into segments too small to support fibrillation wave fronts yet have the segments connected enough to participate in contraction. Several techniques have been used, including creation of long linear RF lesions limited to the right or left atrium, or both. This technique has been largely supplanted by pulmonary vein isolation, although it has been helpful in some patients who have had recurrent fibrillation after an apparently successful isolation procedure. These may be very long procedures, lasting 5 to 8 hours, and fluoroscopy times longer than 90 minutes are not uncommon.

Various methods have been used to locate and ablate focal sources of atrial fibrillation. When first applied, PACs were mapped and the site from which they originated was ablated. This technique was limited by the fact that few patients have adequate frequency of PACs or short bursts of fibrillation to serve as a good target for ablation or a useful indicator of success (i.e., elimination of PACs). In addition, in many cases, the source of PACs or fibrillation was up to 3 cm deep within a

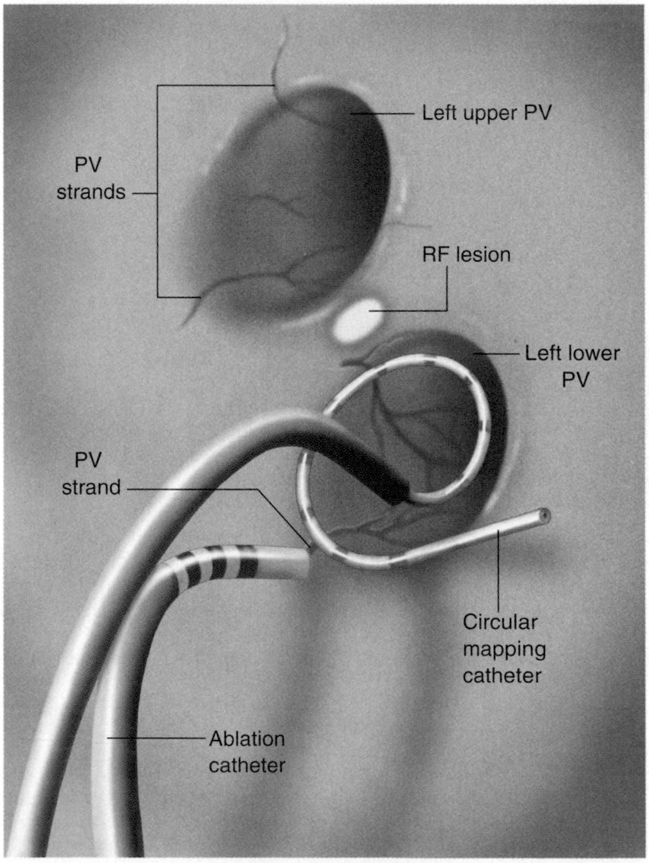

FIGURE 33–12 Depiction of catheters for pulmonary vein (PV) isolation. Both left PVs are illustrated with strands of atrial muscle connecting PV to left atrium at discrete points. A circular mapping catheter is shown resting in the ostium of the left lower PV and an ablation catheter with a large-tip electrode is shown adjacent to electrodes of the circular catheter that are recording a PV potential from the nearby strand. A radiofrequency (RF) lesion, between the two venous ostia, is at the site of a previously ablated strand.

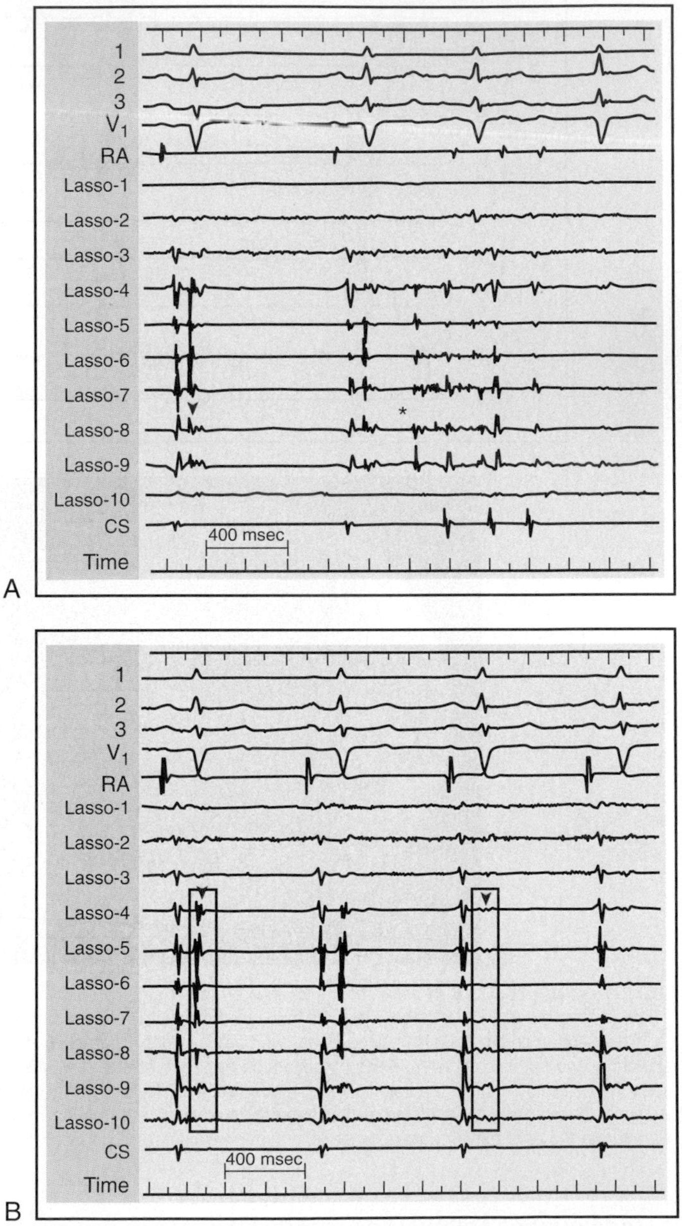

FIGURE 33–13 Sharp pulmonary vein potentials (PVPs). Surface electrocardiographic leads and intracardiac recordings from the right atrium (RA), coronary sinus (CS), and a 10-electrode circular catheter (Lasso) are situated in the ostium of a pulmonary vein. **A,** Lasso recordings show left atrial electrograms followed by sharp PV potentials in recordings Lasso-4 through Lasso-10 during a sinus beat (arrow points to earliest PVP at Lasso-8 as wave front enters vein); an asterisk marks an ectopic beat from this vein that initiates a very short episode of atrial fibrillation. **B,** Recorded during radiofrequency ablation near Lasso-8 recording site; the same sharp PVPs are seen in the first two beats (left arrow) but are absent during the last two beats (right arrow), leaving only the left atrial recordings. This vein has thus been electrically isolated from the left atrium.

pulmonary vein; ablation at these sites could result in pulmonary vein stenosis.[56] As experience grew, it became clear that most cases of paroxysmal atrial fibrillation originated within pulmonary veins; muscular sleeves extend from the left atrium for several centimeters along the pulmonary vein.[57] Efforts then shifted to electrical isolation of the pulmonary veins to prevent spread of impulses from the sites of initiation to the remainder of the atrium. There are several advantages of this strategy over focal ablation: (1) there is a greater likelihood of eliminating fibrillation, because multiple veins may be arrhythmogenic; (2) the patient need not have PACs to perform the ablation; and (3) the risk of pulmonary vein stenosis may be lower. Although strands of atrial muscle enshroud the pulmonary veins, actual electrical connections to atrium may exist at only two or three discrete points. The pulmonary vein isolation strategy can be carried out with mapping of the pulmonary veins to locate and ablate the discrete points of electrical connection between vein and atrium, or with a purely anatomical approach. Mapping uses a circular electrode catheter (Fig. 33-12) or a multipolar "basket" catheter situated within the ostium of the vein. Pulmonary vein potentials, which might be the origin of fibrillation, appear as sharp potentials (Fig. 33-13) or as complex fragmented signals following the nearby left atrial recording (Fig. 33-14).

Ablation is performed on the atrial side of the venoatrial junction until the pulmonary vein potentials are eliminated ("entrance block" into the vein).[58] Ablation can be performed during sinus rhythm or atrial pacing, or even during atrial fibrillation, which often terminates during RF application. Some have advocated pacing from within the vein to demonstrate the more relevant exit block from vein to atrium (see Fig. 33-14). Using the anatomical approach, continuous lines of ablation are made that surround venous orifices. This method requires sophisticated mapping tools to be able to record the sites that have already been ablated and the areas that remain (Fig. 33-15). In some cases, gaps in a line of ablation can be proarrhythmic by providing a path for macroreentry in the left atrium.[59] Some electrophysiologists make an additional line of ablation between the left inferior pulmonary vein and the mitral annulus to forestall this possibility. In many cases, a flutter lesion in the floor of the right atrium is also made, because many patients undergoing a purely left atrial procedure have subsequent episodes of flutter. Each method of isolation requires left atrial access using a patent foramen ovale or the septal puncture technique, with full anticoagulation. This approach increases the risk of bleeding complications[60] and still has not entirely prevented thromboemboli related to the procedure.[61,62] The pulmonary vein isolation approach has been used primarily in younger patients with paroxysmal atrial fibrillation in the absence of structural heart disease; an anatomical method may be more beneficial in patients with permanent atrial fibrillation[63] or in those with structural heart disease,[64] because success rates with ostial isolation are not as high in this group. Other methods, including elimination of parasympathetic ganglionic reflex responses, which can provoke fibrillation episodes,[65] or ablation of complex fractionated atrial electrograms,[66] have also been used with success. A comparison of currently used techniques for ablation of atrial fibrillation is presented in Table 33-6; some are depicted in Figure 33-16. Before the ablation procedure, it is useful to carry out some type of noninvasive study for a better definition of pulmonary venous anatomy, such as a high-resolution computed tomography or magnetic resonance imaging study (Fig. 33-17). This study aids the operator in planning the procedure so that anomalous venous anatomy does not interfere with successful ablation.

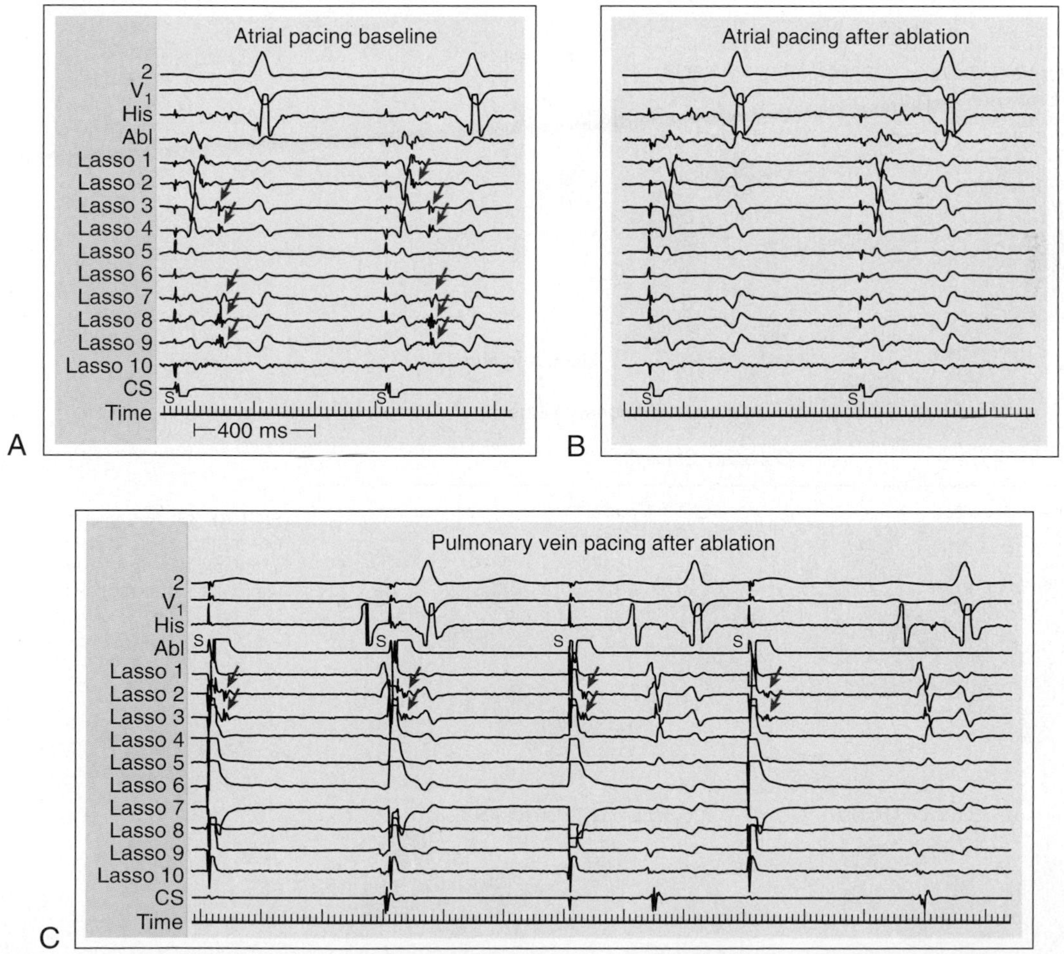

FIGURE 33–14 Pulmonary vein entrance and exit block demonstrated by recording pulmonary vein potentials (PVPs). Recordings during coronary sinus pacing are similar to those in Figure 33-13. **A,** Pre-ablation recordings from PV during atrial pacing; note low-amplitude fragmented PVPs (arrows). **B,** Postablation recordings during atrial pacing. The PVPs are absent, signifying *entrance* block from atrium into the PV. **C,** Pacing from within the PV following ablation, showing capture of PVPs (arrows) but no conduction to the atrium, which remains in sinus rhythm, unaffected by PV pacing and capture. This demonstrates *exit* block from the vein, which is now completely electrically isolated from the atrium. S = stimulus artifact.

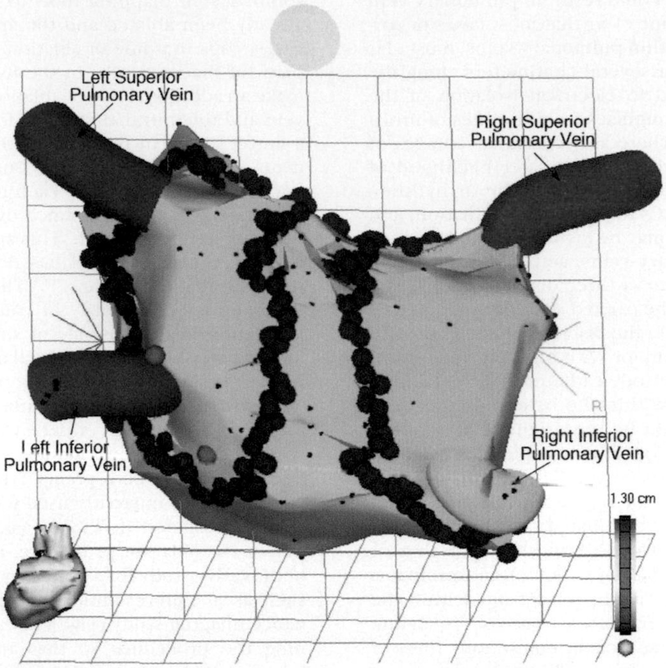

FIGURE 33–15 Circumferential pulmonary vein (PV) ablation. Electroanatomical map of left atrium (aqua shape) viewed from behind. Structures are as noted. Dark red circles denote sites of ablation attempting to surround PV ostia.

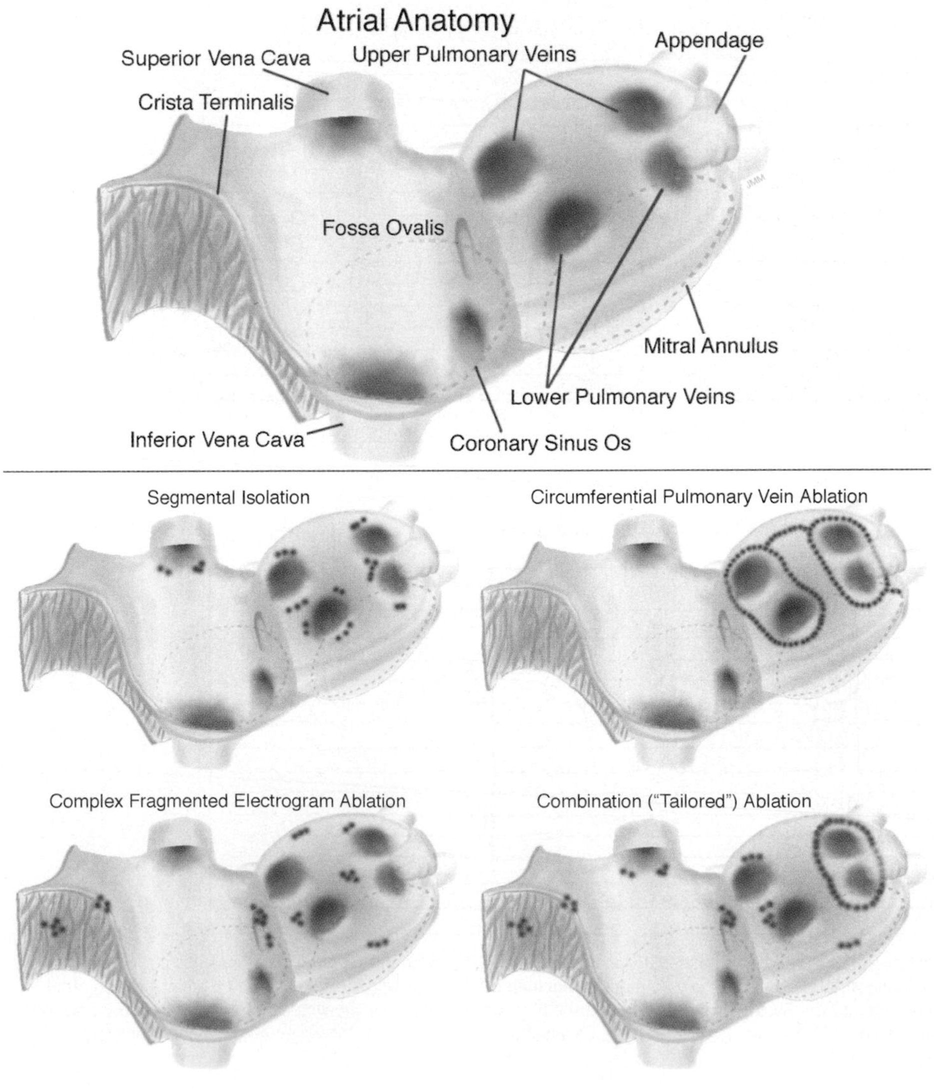

FIGURE 33–16 Catheter ablation procedures for treatment of atrial fibrillation. Atrial anatomy is shown at top; red dots denote sites of ablation according to the ablation strategy. See text for details.

TABLE 33–6 Comparison of Methods of Ablation of Atrial Fibrillation

Method	Strategy	Mechanisms of Success	Advantages	Disadvantages	Extent of Ablation
Catheter Ablation					
Ostial PV isolation	Electrical isolation of PVs from the left atrium	Elimination of spread of AF-inciting impulses from PV foci to atrium Elimination of drivers/triggers at PV/atrial junction	Good success rate; "hard" endpoint; less extensive ablation	Requires mapping; can be tedious; possibility of PV stenosis	+ to ++
Circumferential PV ablation	Wide-area encirclement of PV ostia	PV isolation Ablation of extra-PV drivers/triggers Ablation of autonomic ganglia Disruption of PV-atrial interactions	Good success rate; no mapping needed; low likelihood of PV stenosis	"Soft" endpoint; macroreentrant atrial tachycardias/flutters	++++
Complex fractionated electrogram ablation	Ablation of highly fractionated atrial electrograms during AF	Elimination of drivers, rotors, autonomic ganglia	Good success rate; often less extensive ablation	Requires mapping; patient must be in AF	+ to +++
Trigger ablation	Ablation of triggering arrhythmias (SVT)	Elimination of arrhythmias that trigger AF (without which AF cannot start or sustain)	Good success rate; "hard" endpoint; less extensive ablation	Not applicable in most cases	+
Autonomic ablation	Ablation to eliminate sites of bradycardia/hypotension response	Elimination of autonomic (vagal) triggers for AF	Good success rate; less extensive ablation	Requires mapping; can be tedious; not applicable in all cases	++
Surgical Ablation					
Maze procedure (incisional)	Compartmentalization of atria to prevent ability to sustain AF	Isolation of PVs and extra-PV drivers/triggers Disruption of PV-atrial interactions	High success rate; can excise left atrial appendage; can be performed at time of other cardiac procedures	Requires sternotomy; occasional akinetic atrium	++++
Maze procedure (nonincisional—RF/MW/cryo)	Compartmentalization of atria to prevent ability to sustain AF	Isolation of PVs and extra-PV drivers/triggers Disruption of PV-atrial interactions	High success rate; can excise left atrial appendage; can be performed at time of other cardiac procedures	Technically demanding; cannot be performed at time of other cardiac procedures	++++
Micromaze	Electrical isolation of PVs from the left atrium	Elimination of spread of AF-inciting impulses from PV foci to atrium	Good success rate; minimally invasive		++++

AF = atrial fibrillation; cryo = cryoablation; MW = microwave; PV = pulmonary vein; RF = radiofrequency; SVT = supraventricular tachycardia; + = minimal; ++ = mild; +++ = moderate; ++++ = extensive.

As noted earlier, some patients with atrial fibrillation show a transformation to stable atrial flutter when given antiarrhythmic drugs, particularly sodium channel blocking agents. In these patients, performing a flutter ablation and having the patient continue to take the same drug may prevent arrhythmia recurrence.

Indications. Candidates for focal atrial fibrillation ablation have paroxysmal atrial fibrillation in the absence of structural heart disease and include those whose atrial fibrillation is refractory to medications or who prefer not to take medications. Patients in whom anatomically based linear ablation for atrial fibrillation might be considered include the following: (1) those with some degree of structural heart disease and persistent or chronic atrial fibrillation, for whom maintenance of sinus rhythm is important and in whom atrial fibrillation recurs despite standard antiarrhythmic drugs; and (2) those for whom drug therapy is not tolerated or preferred.

Results. Success rates of ablation for atrial fibrillation range from 70 to 90 percent. Currently, there does not seem to be a preferred technique; mapping-guided segmental isolation of pulmonary venous ostia versus purely anatomically based ablation remains the most widely applied, and many electrophysiologists use several strategies in the same procedure.[67] Reasons for failure of ablation include (1) incomplete isolation of an arrhythmogenic vein, (2) restitution of conduction after apparently successful isolation,[68] (3) nonpulmonary venous sources of fibrillation, and (4) formation of new arrhythmogenic substrate by the ablation (left atrial macroreentry).[69] Pericarditis, pericardial effusion, and cardiac tamponade occur in 1 percent or more of cases.[60] The risk of stroke related to extensive left atrial ablation is approximately 2 percent, even with rigorous anticoagulation regimens.[70] Pulmonary vein stenosis, more likely if ablation is performed within the vein itself rather than at the ostium, can cause dyspnea and pulmonary arterial

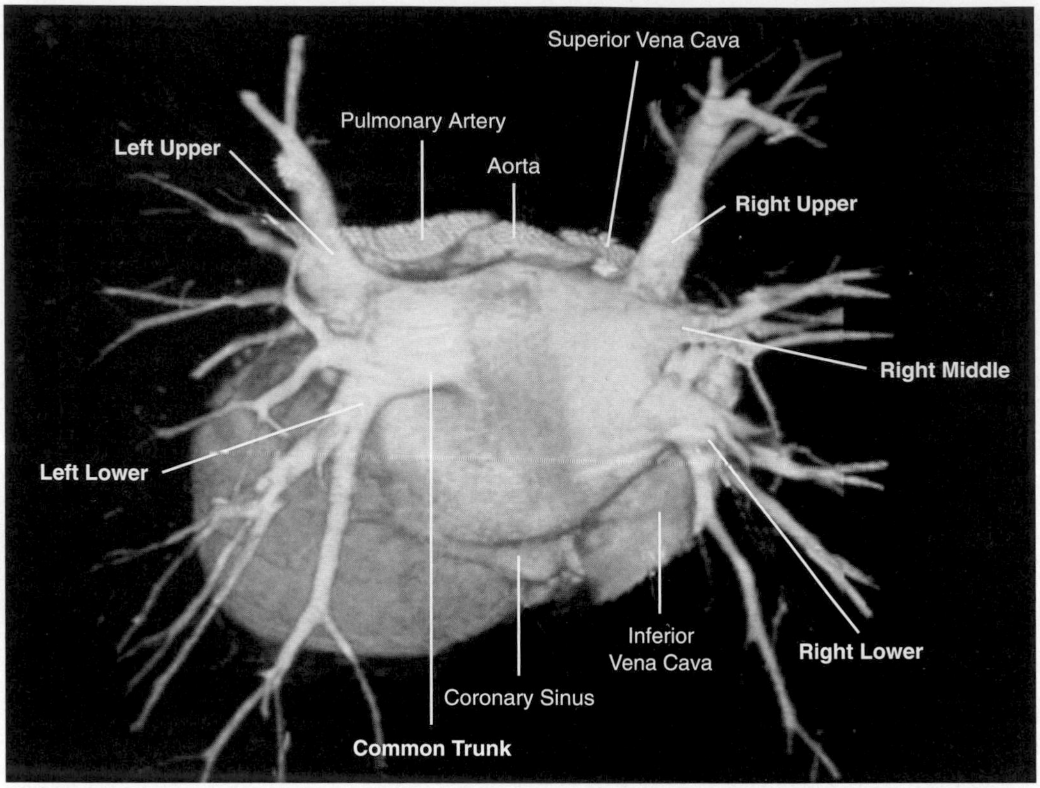

FIGURE 33–17 High-resolution computed tomography view of the left atrium, viewed from behind to illustrate pulmonary vein (PV) anatomy. Instead of two veins entering the left atrium from each lung, this patient had both left veins emptying into a common trunk before entering the atrium and three veins from the right lung. This information helped plan the pulmonary vein isolation procedure.

hypertension. In some cases, angioplasty and stenting have been necessary.[71] Left atrial-esophageal fistulae have been reported[72]; esophageal temperature monitoring may aid in avoiding this potentially life-threatening complication.[73] Cost-effectiveness of ablation[74] and improvement in patient quality of life[75] have been demonstrated following successful ablation.

Other nonpharmacological modalities for the treatment of atrial fibrillation, such as preventive pacing and implantable atrial defibrillators or atrial rhythm management devices, have been used (see Chap. 34).

RADIOFREQUENCY CATHETER ABLATION OF VENTRICULAR TACHYCARDIA. In general, the success rate for ablation of VTs is lower than that for AV node reentry or AV reentry. This lower success rate may be related to the fact that this procedure is often a last resort in patients with drug-resistant VTs who have extensive structural heart disease, but it is also related to more difficult mapping in the ventricles. Furthermore, in the ideal case, the VT induction must completely be reproducible, uniform in QRS morphology from beat to beat, sustained, and hemodynamically stable, so that the patient can tolerate the VT long enough during the procedure to undergo the extensive mapping necessary to localize optimal ablation target sites. Patients with several electrocardiographically distinct, uniform morphologies of VT can still be candidates for ablation because, in many cases, a common reentrant pathway is shared by two or more VT morphologies.[76] Also, the origin of the VT must be fairly circumscribed and endocardially situated, although cases of successful ablation only from the epicardial aspect have become more common.[77] Very rapid VT, polymorphic VT, and infrequent, nonsustained episodes are less well suited to this form of therapy at this time (see later).

Location and Ablation. RF catheter ablation of VT can be divided into idiopathic VT, which occurs in patients with essentially structurally normal hearts, VT that occurs in various disease settings but without coronary artery disease, and VT in patients with coronary artery disease and usually prior myocardial infarction. In the first group, VTs can arise in either ventricle. Right ventricular tachycardias most commonly originate in the outflow tract and have a characteristic left bundle branch block–like, inferior axis morphology (see Chap. 35); less often, VTs arise in the inflow tract or free wall. Initiation of tachycardia can often be facilitated by catecholamines. Most left ventricular VTs are septal in origin and have a characteristic QRS configuration (i.e., right bundle branch block, superior axis); other VTs occur less commonly and arise from different areas of the left ventricle, including the left ventricular outflow tract and aortic sinuses of Valsalva, and are similar in electrocardiographic appearance and clinical behavior to those arising in the right ventricular outflow tract.[78] Abnormal patterns of sympathetic innervation may be present in some. VTs in abnormal hearts without coronary artery disease can be the result of bundle branch reentry (see Chap. 35), most typically observed in patients with dilated cardiomyopathies. In these patients, ablation of the right bundle branch eliminates the tachycardia. VT can occur in right ventricular dysplasia (see Chap. 9), sarcoidosis,[79] Chagas' disease, hypertrophic cardiomyopathy (see Chap. 65), and a host of other noncoronary disease states.

Activation mapping and pace mapping are effective in patients with idiopathic VTs to locate the site of origin of the VT. In activation mapping, the timing of endocardial electrograms sampled by the mapping catheter is compared with the onset of the surface QRS complex. Sites that are activated before the surface QRS onset are near the origin of the VT (Fig. 33-18; see Fig. 32-14). In idiopathic VT, ablation at a site at which the unipolar electrogram shows a QS complex may yield greater success than if an rS potential is observed (Fig. 33-19). Pace mapping involves stimulation of various ventricular sites to produce a QRS contour that duplicates the QRS contour of the spontaneous VT, thus establishing the apparent site of origin of the arrhythmia (see Fig. 33-18). This technique is limited by several methodological problems, but may be useful when the tachycardia cannot be initiated and when a 12-lead ECG has been obtained during the spontaneous VT. Presystolic Purkinje potentials, as well as very low-amplitude mid-diastolic signals, can be recorded during VT from sites at which ablation cures VT in most patients with left ventricular VTs that have a right bundle branch block superior axis.[80] Localization of optimal ablation sites for VT in patients with coronary artery disease and prior infarction is more difficult than in patients with structurally normal hearts because of the altered anatomy and electrophysiology. Pace mapping has lower sensitivity and specificity than for idiopathic VT. Furthermore, reentry circuits can sometimes be large and resistant to the relatively small lesions produced by RF catheter ablation in scarred endocardium.

In scar-based VT (e.g., postinfarction, cardiomyopathies), finding a protected region of diastolic activation used as a critical part of the reentrant circuit is desirable, because ablation at this site has a good chance of eliminating the tachycardia (Fig. 33-20). Because of the extensive derangement in electrophysiology caused by the previous damage (e.g., infarct, myopathy), many areas of the ventricle may have diastolic activation but may not be relevant to the perpetuation of the VT. These "bystander sites" make activation mapping more difficult. Pacing techniques such as entrainment can be used to test whether a site is actually part of a circuit or a bystander. Entrainment involves pacing for several seconds during a tachycardia at a rate slightly faster than the VT rate; after pacing is stopped and the same tachycardia resumes, the timing of the first complex relative to the last paced beat is an indicator of how close the pacing site is to a part of the VT circuit. During entrainment, part of the ventricle is activated by the paced wave front and part by the VT wave front being forced to exit earlier than it ordinarily would, resulting in a fusion complex on the ECG. Pacing from within a critical portion of the circuit itself produces an exact QRS match with the VT; fusion occurs only within the circuit and is "concealed" on the surface electrocardiogram. Sites with a low-amplitude, isolated, mid-diastolic potential that cannot be dissociated from the tachycardia by pacing perturbations, at which entrainment with concealed fusion can be demonstrated, are highly likely to be successful ablation sites.[81-84]

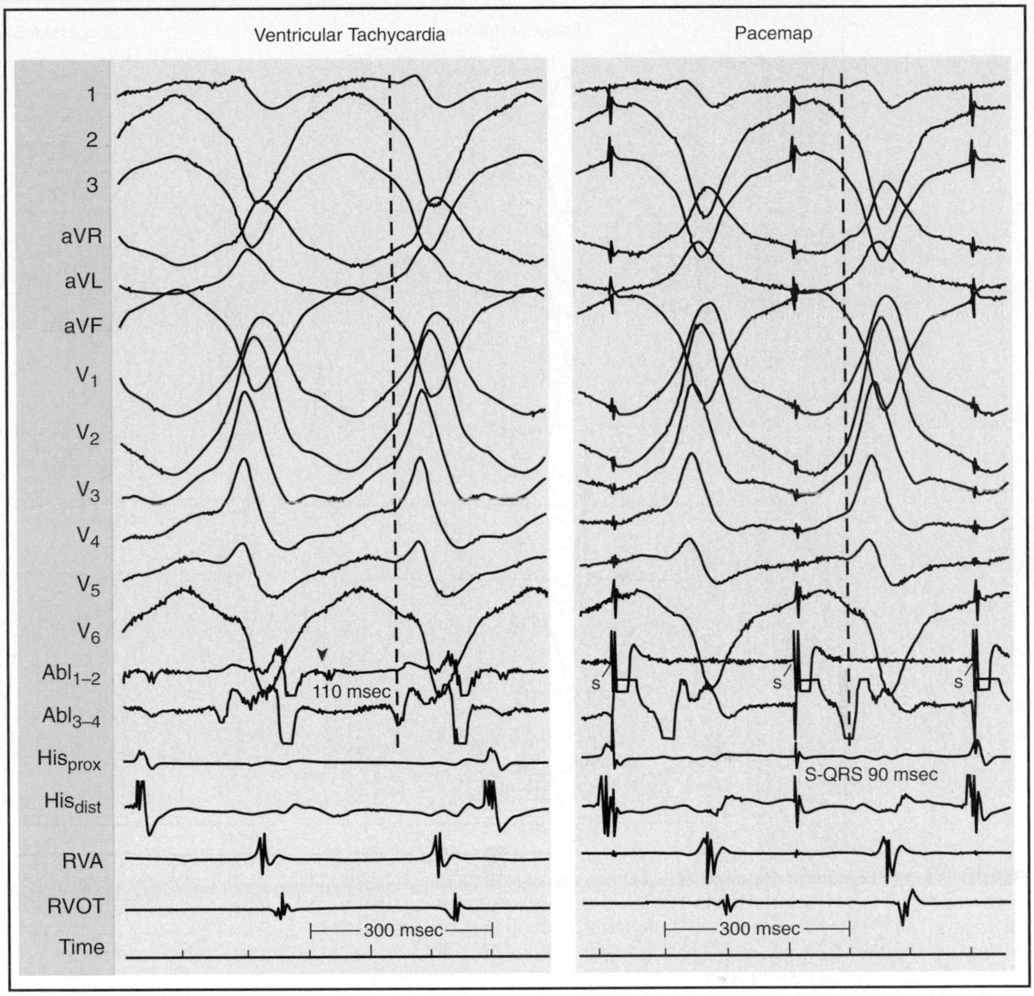

FIGURE 33–18 Ventricular tachycardia and pace mapping. All 12 surface electrocardiographic leads are shown, along with intracardiac recordings during ventricular tachycardia (VT). The Abl_{1-2} recording shows a small deflection occurring early in electrical diastole (arrow) 110 milliseconds before the onset of the QRS (dashed line). In the right panel, pacing is performed from this site. This produces an identical QRS complex in each lead, with a stimulus-QRS onset interval similar to the electrogram-QRS onset interval during VT. Ablation at this site eliminated VT in 2 seconds. RVOT = right ventricular outflow tract.

In a significant proportion of patients with VT in the presence of structural heart disease, activation mapping and entrainment cannot be performed because of poor hemodynamic tolerance of the arrhythmia or inability to initiate sustained tachycardia during an EPS. In these situations, additional methods can be used that are categorized as *substrate mapping,* in which areas of low electrical voltage or from which very delayed potentials are recorded during sinus rhythm,[85] or at which pacing closely replicates a known VT 12-lead ECG morphology (pace mapping),[86] are targeted for ablation without performing any mapping during VT. These methods have yielded very good results in many cases.[87]

In patients without structural heart disease, only a single VT is usually present, and catheter ablation of that VT is most often curative. In patients with extensive structural heart disease, especially those with prior myocardial infarction, multiple VTs are usually present. Catheter ablation of a single VT in such patients may be only palliative and may not eliminate the need for further antiarrhythmic therapy. The genesis of multiple tachycardia morphologies is not clear, although in some cases they are merely different manifestations of one circuit (e.g., different directions of wave front propagation or exit to the ventricle as a whole), and ablation of one may prevent recurrence of others. The presence of multiple VT morphologies contributes to the difficulties in mapping and ablation of VT in these patients, because pacing techniques used to validate recordings at potential sites of ablation may result in a change in morphology to another VT that does not arise in the same region.

After ablation of VT, ventricular stimulation is repeated to assess efficacy. In some cases, rapid polymorphic VT or fibrillation is initiated. The clinical significance of these arrhythmias is unclear, but some evidence has suggested that they have a low likelihood of spontaneous occurrence during follow-up.

As noted earlier, most cases of polymorphic VT and VF are not currently amenable to ablation because of hemodynamic instability and beat-to-beat changes in activation sequence. However, some cases appear to have a focal source (similar to focal sources of atrial fibrillation) and, if the focus can be identified and ablated, further arrhythmia episodes can be prevented. In such cases, repeated episodes of arrhythmia have constant electrocardiographic features of the initiating beat or beats suggesting a consistent source, which may be in either ventricle.[88-90] The electrogram at sites of successful ablation often has very sharp presystolic potentials reminiscent of Purkinje potentials, with a 50- to 100-millisecond delay to the QRS onset.[91]

Indications. Patients considered for RF catheter ablation of VT in the absence of structural heart disease are those with symptomatic, sustained, monomorphic VT when the tachycardia is drug resistant, when the patient is drug intolerant, or when the patient does not desire long-term drug therapy. Patients with structural heart disease who are candidates for ablation include those with bundle branch reentrant VT and those with sustained monomorphic VT and an ICD who are receiving multiple shocks not manageable by reprogramming or concomitant drug therapy. Occasionally, nonsustained VT or even severely symptomatic PVCs require RF catheter ablation. In some of these cases, in which the ventricular ectopy occurs frequently, significant left ventricular systolic dysfunction has occurred (presumably a form of tachycardia-related cardiomyopathy). After successful ablation, ventricular function may significantly improve or even normalize.[92,93]

CH 33

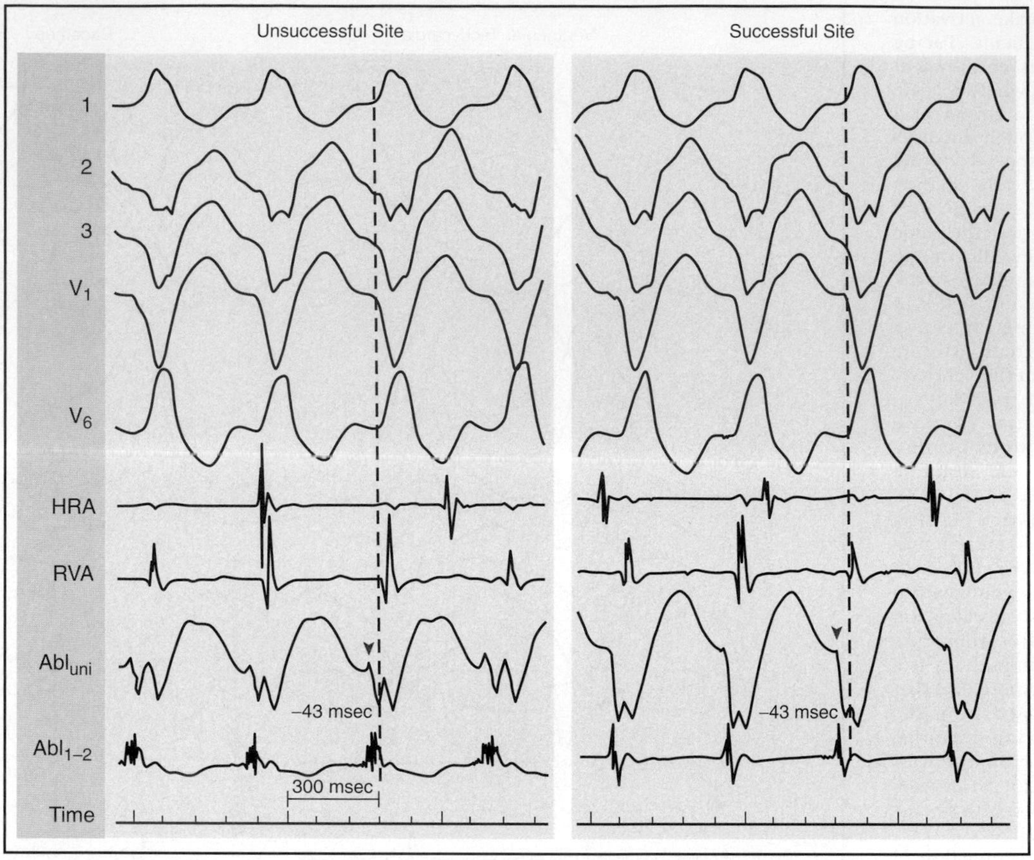

FIGURE 33–19 Recordings from unsuccessful and successful ablation sites in a patient with idiopathic ventricular tachycardia arising in the inferior right ventricular wall. In the recordings from the unsuccessful ablation site, the unipolar signal (arrow) has a small r wave, indicating that a portion of the wave front from the focus of tachycardia was approaching the site from elsewhere. At the successful site, the unipolar recording has a QS configuration, indicating that all depolarization was emanating from this site. In each site, the bipolar recording (Abl_{1-2}) occurs an identical 43 milliseconds before QRS onset (dashed lines).

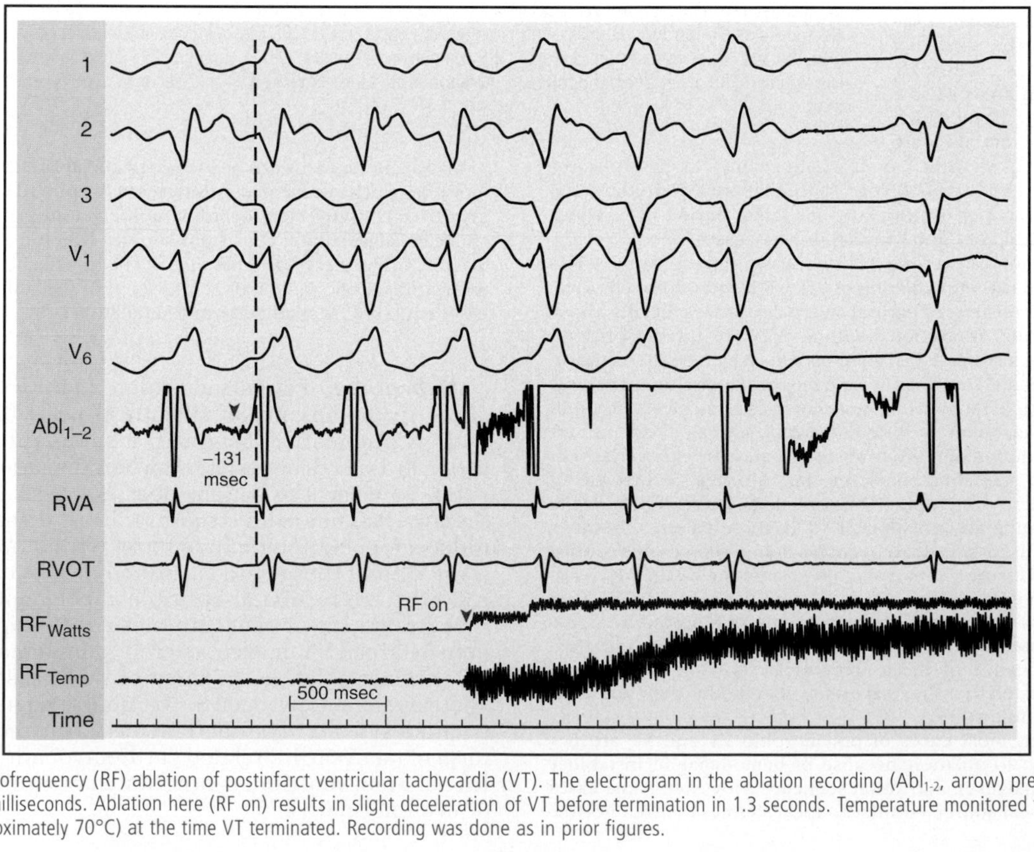

FIGURE 33–20 Radiofrequency (RF) ablation of postinfarct ventricular tachycardia (VT). The electrogram in the ablation recording (Abl_{1-2}, arrow) precedes the QRS onset (dashed line) by 131 milliseconds. Ablation here (RF on) results in slight deceleration of VT before termination in 1.3 seconds. Temperature monitored from the catheter tip had just peaked (approximately 70°C) at the time VT terminated. Recording was done as in prior figures.

Results. In the U.S. survey,[10] the overall success rate of VT ablation was 71 percent. In patients with structurally normal hearts, the success rate was 85 percent. More recent series of patients with postinfarct VT have suggested a 30 percent cure rate for patients (no inducible ventricular arrhythmia of any type, no recurrences), whereas more than 70 percent of patients no longer have recurrences of VT after the procedure, despite inducibility of rapid VT or VF. Almost all these patients have an ICD, regardless of outcome. Significant complications occur in up to 3 percent, including vascular damage, heart block, cardiac tamponade, stroke, and valve damage; death is rare but can occur in patients with severe coronary artery disease and systolic dysfunction.

NEW MAPPING AND ABLATION TECHNOLOGIES FOR PREMATURE VENTRICULAR COMPLEXES

Multielectrode Mapping Systems. As noted earlier, many limitations of ablation are related to inadequate mapping. These problems include only isolated premature complexes during the EPS as opposed to sustained tachycardias (in idiopathic atrial and ventricular tachycardias), nonsustained episodes of VT, poor hemodynamic tolerance of VT, and multiple VT morphologies. Standard mapping techniques sample single sites sequentially and are poorly suited to these situations. New mapping systems are available that enable sampling of many sites simultaneously and incorporate sophisticated computer algorithms for analysis and display of global maps. These mapping systems use various technologies, ranging from multiple electrodes situated on each of several splines of a basket catheter, to the use of low-intensity electrical or magnetic fields to localize the catheter tip in the heart and record and plot activation times on a contour map of the chamber, to the use of complex mathematics to compute "virtual" electrograms recorded from a mesh electrode situated in the middle of a chamber cavity. Some of these systems are capable of generating activation maps of an entire chamber using only one cardiac complex, an obvious advantage in patients with only rare premature complexes, nonsustained arrhythmias, or poor hemodynamic tolerance of sustained arrhythmias.

Epicardial Catheter Mapping. Although most VTs can be ablated from the endocardium, occasional cases are resistant to this therapy. In some of these, epicardial ablation may be successful. Much of the work in this area has been performed in patients with VT related to Chagas' disease, in whom most appear to require epicardial mapping and ablation; it is less frequently necessary in postinfarct or cardiomyopathy patients and those without structural heart disease references.

The technique for gaining access to the epicardium differs slightly from that for pericardiocentesis. A long spinal anesthesia needle is introduced from a subxiphoid approach under fluoroscopic guidance. As the pericardial surface is approached, a small amount of a radiocontrast agent is injected. If the needle tip is still outside the pericardium, the dye stays where injected; when the pericardial space has been entered, the dye disperses, outlining the heart. A guidewire is introduced through the needle and a standard vascular introducer sheath exchanged over the wire. The pericardial space is accessible for a standard mapping ablation catheter. Standard mapping techniques can then be applied. When a site is selected for possible ablation, coronary arteriography may be warranted to avoid delivery of RF energy near a coronary artery. This is less important in cases of postinfarct VT because the VT substrate is typically in a region of prior transmural infarction. The technique can be used for patients who have had prior cardiac surgery, although adhesions may obliterate portions of the pericardial space. The most frequent complication is pericarditis re-lated to the ablation; cardiac tamponade is rare.

Chemical Ablation. Chemical ablation with alcohol or phenol of an area of myocardium involved in a tachycardia has been used to create AV block in patients not responding to catheter ablation and to eliminate atrial and ventricular tachycardias. Recurrences of tachycardia several days after apparently successful ablation are common. Excessive myocardial necrosis is the major complication, and alcohol ablation should be considered only when other ablative approaches fail or cannot be done.

SURGICAL THERAPY FOR TACHYARRHYTHMIAS

The objectives of a surgical approach to treating a tachycardia are to excise, isolate, or interrupt tissue in the heart critical for the initiation, maintenance, or propagation of the tachycardia while preserving or even improving myocardial function. In addition to a direct surgical approach to the arrhythmia, indirect approaches such as aneurysmectomy, coronary artery bypass grafting, and relief of valvular regurgitation or stenosis can be useful for selected patients by improving cardiac hemodynamics and myocardial blood flow. Cardiac sympathectomy alters adrenergic influences on the heart and has been effective in some patients, particularly those who have recurrent VT with the long-QT syndrome.

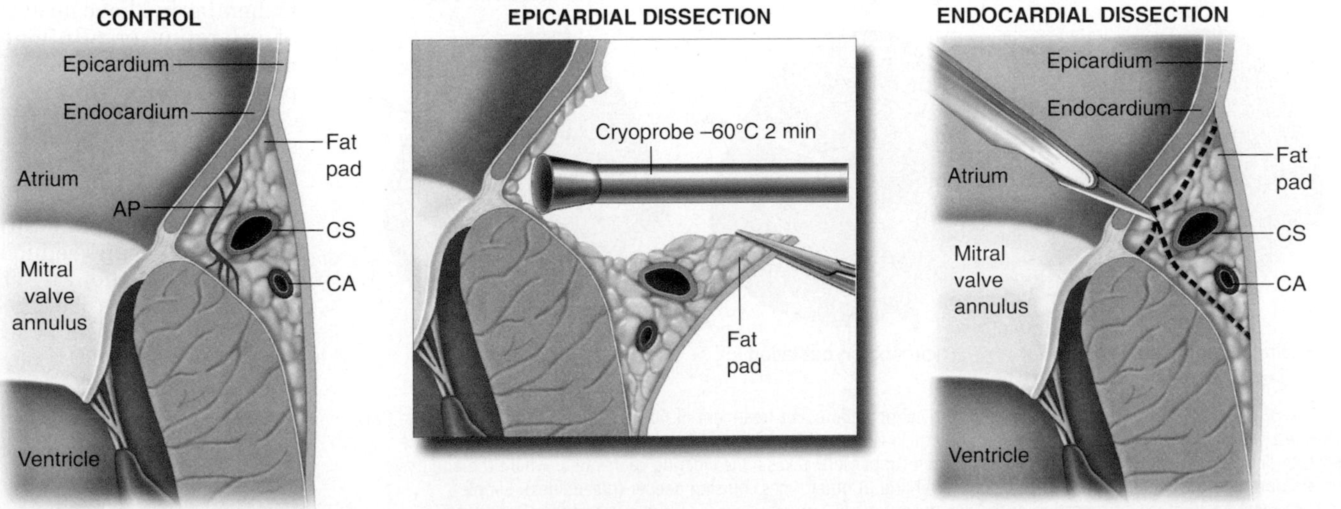

FIGURE 33–21 Schematic diagram showing the two approaches for surgical interruption of an accessory pathway. **Left panel,** Left atrioventricular groove and its vascular contents, the coronary sinus (CS) and circumflex coronary artery (CA). Multiple accessory pathways (APs) course through the fat pad. **Middle panel,** Epicardial dissection approach. **Right panel,** Endocardial dissection. Both approaches clear out the fat pad and interrupt any accessory pathways. (From Zipes DP: Cardiac electrophysiology: Promises and contributions. J Am Coll Cardiol 13:1329, 1989. Reprinted by permission of the American College of Cardiology.)

Surgical procedures exist for patients (adults and children) with ATs, atrial flutter, AV node reentry, and AV reentry (Fig. 33-21). RF catheter ablation adequately treats the vast majority of these patients and has thus replaced direct surgical intervention, except for the occasional patient in whom RF catheter ablation fails or who is having concomitant cardiovascular surgery. In some cases, a prior attempt at RF catheter ablation complicates surgery by obliterating the normal tissue planes that exist in the AV groove of the heart or by rendering tissues very friable. Occasionally, patients with ATs have multiple foci that require surgical intervention.

The maze procedure, developed to treat patients with atrial fibrillation, eliminates the arrhythmia by reducing atrial tissue mass to a size at any instant in time too small to perpetuate the reentrant circuits responsible for atrial fibrillation. It forces atrial activation to proceed along a surgically determined pathway, thus maintaining sinus rhythm with AV nodal conduction. The maze procedure permits organized electrical depolarization of the atria and restores atrial transport function and, in so doing, decreases the risk of thromboembolism. Maintenance of sinus rhythm more than 3 months after the procedure approaches 100 percent, although up to 10 percent of patients require pacemakers because of chronotropic incompetence of the sinus node, related to the surgery or to the preexisting atrial pathology. The advent of minimally invasive endoscopic and endovascular techniques has made it possible to perform an equivalent of the maze procedure without thoracotomy, although success rates are not as good as with the incisional technique. The maze procedure or a variation is now most commonly performed concomitantly with mitral valve surgery rather than as a primary indication. In many centers, intraoperative RF, a microwave procedure, or cryoablation has replaced surgical incisions for performing the maze procedure, although significant complications such as esophageal erosion have been reported.[94] The left atrial appendage, the source for most thromboemboli in patients with atrial fibrillation, can often be removed or ligated during these procedures. Various characteristics of these procedures are compared in Table 33-6.

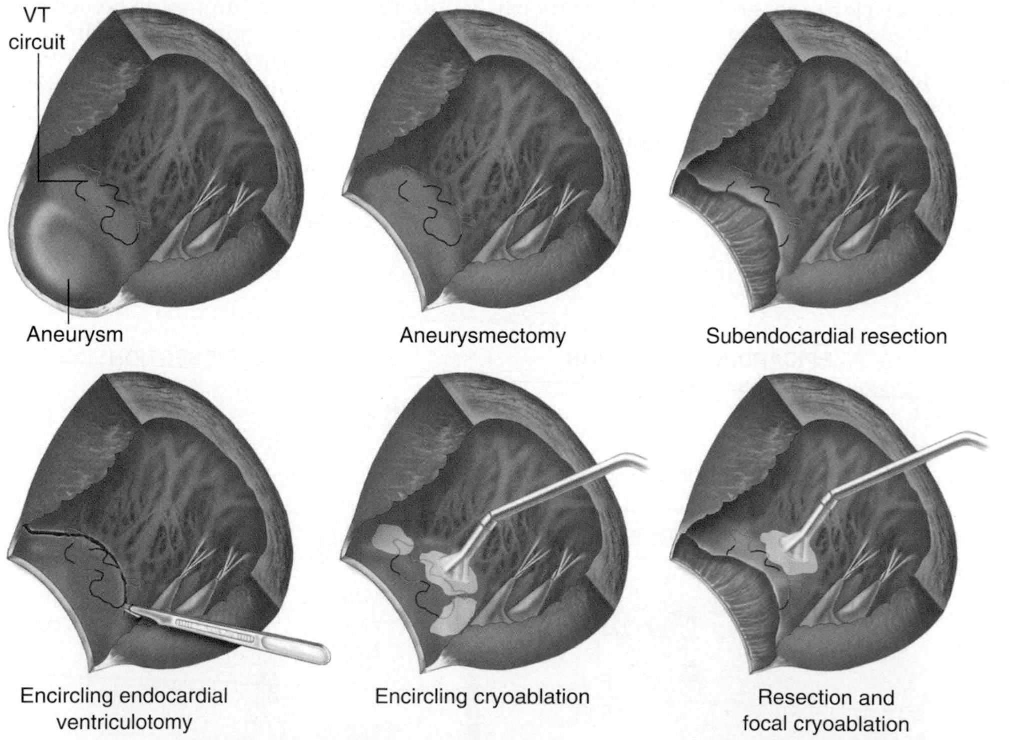

FIGURE 33–22 Schematic diagram showing surgical procedures for treatment of postinfarct ventricular tachycardia (VT) with left ventricular aneurysm. A damaged left ventricle is depicted as opened along the lateral wall and viewing the septum and papillary muscles. The tachycardia circuit (upper left) takes a meandering course near where the aneurysm meets normal myocardium and at times is superficial and at other times coursing deeper (green lines). Simple aneurysmectomy that leaves a portion of the aneurysm for suturing often misses the circuit and thus does not cure the arrhythmia. Using subendocardial resection, a layer of endocardium and subjacent tissue is removed, including at least some of the tachycardia circuit. This resection results in elimination of tachycardia. Encircling endocardial ventriculotomy attempts to isolate the circuit electrically without removing tissue, but it probably actually works by incising portions of the circuit. Cryoablation can be used to encircle the infarct zone or in combination with resection to damaged tissue too deep in the wall to be resected safely.

Ventricular Tachycardia

In contrast to patients with supraventricular arrhythmias, candidates for surgical therapy for ventricular arrhythmias often have severe left ventricular dysfunction, generally the result of coronary artery disease. The cause of the underlying heart disease influences the type of surgery performed. Candidates are patients with drug-resistant, symptomatic, recurrent ventricular tachyarrhythmias who ideally have a segmental wall motion abnormality (scar or aneurysm) with preserved residual left ventricular function, have not benefited from prior attempts at catheter ablation, or are not candidates for catheter ablation because of hemodynamic instability during VT or the presence of left ventricular thrombus. Poorer surgical results are obtained in patients with nonischemic cardiomyopathy.

ISCHEMIC HEART DISEASE. In almost all patients who have VT associated with ischemic heart disease, the arrhythmia, regardless of its configuration on the surface ECG, arises in the left ventricle or on the left ventricular side of the interventricular septum. The ECG contour of the VT can change from a right bundle branch block to a left bundle branch block pattern without a change in the site of earliest diastolic activation, suggesting that the site of the circuit within the left ventricle remains the same, often near the septum, but its exit pathway is altered.

Indirect surgical approaches, including cardiothoracic sympathectomy, coronary artery revascularization, and ventricular aneurysm or infarct resection with or without coronary artery bypass grafting, have been successful in no more than 20 to 30 percent of reported cases. Coronary artery bypass grafting as a primary therapeutic approach has generally been successful only in patients who experience rapid VT during ischemia, as well as patients with ischemia-related VF, but can sometimes be useful in patients with coronary disease resuscitated from sudden death who have no inducible arrhythmias at EPS. These patients generally have a clear relationship between episodes of ventricular arrhythmia and immediately antecedent severe ischemia, and have no evidence of infarction or minimal wall motion abnormalities, with preserved overall left ventricular function. Patients with sustained monomorphic VT or only polymorphic VT rarely have their arrhythmias affected by coronary bypass surgery, although it can reduce the frequency of the arrhythmic episodes in some patients and prevent new ischemic events. In most cases, an ICD is required after the surgical procedure (see Chap. 34).

Surgical Techniques

Generally, two types of direct surgical procedures are used, resection and ablation (Fig. 33-22).[95] The first direct surgical approach to VT was encircling endocardial ventriculotomy, using a transmural ventriculotomy to isolate areas of endocardial fibrosis that were recognized visually; this procedure is rarely used now. The second procedure, subendocardial resection, is based on animal and clinical data indicating that arrhythmias after myocardial infarction arise mostly at the subendocardial borders between normal and infarcted tissues. Subendocardial resection entails peeling off a 1- to 3-mm-thick layer of endocardium, often near the rim of an aneurysm, that has been demonstrated by means of mapping procedures to contain the site of earliest activation recorded during the VT. Some VTs can arise from the epicardium. Tachycardias arising from near the base of the papillary muscles are treated using a cryoprobe cooled to −70°C. Cryoablation can also be used to isolate areas of the ventricle that cannot be resected and is often combined with resection. The neodymium:yttrium-aluminum-garnet laser has also been used with good success, but the equipment is expensive and difficult to work with.

RESULTS. For ventricular tachyarrhythmias, operative mortality ranges from 6 to 23 percent, with success rates, defined as absence of recurrence of spontaneous ventricular arrhythmias, ranging from 59 to 98 percent. In experienced centers, operative mortality can be as low as 5 percent in stable patients undergoing elective procedures, with 85 to 95 percent of survivors free of inducible or spontaneous ventricular tachyarrhythmias. Long-term recurrence rates range from 2 to 15 percent and correlate with results of the patient's postoperative electrophysiological stimulation study. Operative survival is strongly influenced by the degree of left ventricular dysfunction.

Operative mortality for nonthoracotomy ICD implantation is less than 1 percent, with an annual sudden cardiac death mortality rate less than 1 percent. Because of the difference in operative survival and shorter hospital stay with ICD therapy compared with direct surgery for VT and the success rates for catheter ablation in patients who have an ICD but experience frequent episodes of VT, few curative surgical procedures are now performed.

Electrophysiological Studies

PREOPERATIVE ELECTROPHYSIOLOGICAL STUDY. In patients for whom direct surgical therapy for VT is planned, a preoperative EPS is usually warranted. This study involves initiation of the VT and electrophysiological mapping to localize the area to be resected, as is done with catheter ablation. A resolution of 4 to 8 cm^2 of ventricular endocardium is thereby achieved, although more accurate anatomical localization of the mapping electrode tip in the ventricle may be possible. Tachycardias that are too rapid, short in duration, or polymorphic cannot be mapped accurately unless multiple catheters or a multielectrode array is used. Administering a drug such as procainamide may slow the VT and transform a nonsustained polymorphic VT into a sustained VT of uniform contour that can be mapped. Preoperative catheter mapping is contraindicated in patients who have known left ventricular thrombus that might be dislodged by the mapping catheter.

INTRAOPERATIVE VENTRICULAR MAPPING. Electrophysiological mapping is also performed at the time of surgery, with the surgeon using a handheld probe or an electrode array coupled with computer techniques that instantaneously provide an overall activation map, cycle by cycle. The sequence of activation during VT can be plotted and the area of earliest activation determined. Resection or cryoablation of tissue from which these recordings are made usually cures the VT, indicating that they represent a critical portion of the reentrant circuit. However, it is clear that such electrical activity can be late following the preceding cycle or early in advance of the next cycle. When the earliest recordable endocardial electrical activity occurs less than 30 milliseconds before the onset of the QRS complex, the critical portions of the circuit may be in the interventricular septum or near the epicardium of the free wall. In some patients, intramural mapping using a plunge needle electrode can be useful. Most centers now use a strategy of "sequential" subendocardial resection, in which VT is initiated, mapped, and ablated (resected or cryoablated) while the heart is warm and beating and stimulation is immediately repeated. If VT can still be initiated, mapping and resection are also repeated until VT can no longer be initiated. Reentry around an inferior scar, with a critical diastolic pathway confined to an isthmus of ventricular muscle between the scar and mitral valve annulus, can be cured by cryoablation of this isthmus. Cure rates in this situation exceed 93 percent.

REFERENCES

General Considerations Regarding Antiarrhythmic Drugs

1. Murgatroyd FD: "Pills and pulses": Hybrid therapy for atrial fibrillation. J Cardiovasc Electrophysiol 13:S40, 2002.
2. Sarkozy A, Dorian P: Advances in the acute pharmacologic management of cardiac arrhythmias. Curr Cardiol Rep 5:387, 2003.
3. Naccarelli GV, Wolbrette DL, Khan M, et al: Old and new antiarrhythmic drugs for converting and maintaining sinus rhythm in atrial fibrillation: Comparative efficacy and results of trials. Am J Cardiol 91:15D, 2003.
4. Kowey PR, Yan GX, Winkel E, et al: Pharmacologic and nonpharmacologic options to maintain sinus rhythm: Guideline-based and new approaches. Am J Cardiol 91:33D, 2003.
5. Naccarelli GV, Wolbrette DL, Luck J: Proarrhythmia. Med Clin North Am 85:503, 2001.

Quinidine

6. El-Eraky H, Thomas SH: Effects of sex on the pharmacokinetic and pharmacodynamic properties of quinidine. Br J Clin Pharmacol 56:198, 2003.
7. Coplen SE, Antman EM, Berlin JA, et al: Efficacy and safety of quinidine therapy for maintenance of sinus rhythm after cardioversion. A meta-analysis of randomized control trials. Circulation 82:1106, 1990.
8. Belhassen B, Glick A, Viskin S: Efficacy of quinidine in high-risk patients with Brugada syndrome. Circulation 110:1731, 2004.

Procainamide

9. Schreibman DS, McPherson CA, Rosenfeld LE, et al: Usefulness of procainamide challenge for electrophysiologic arrhythmia risk stratification. Am J Cardiol 94:1435, 2004.

Ajmaline

10. Hong K, Brugada J, Oliva A, et al: Value of electrocardiographic parameters and ajmaline test in the diagnosis of Brugada syndrome caused by SCN5A mutations. Circulation 110:3023, 2004.

Lidocaine

11. Dorian P, Cass D, Schwartz B, et al: Amiodarone as compared with lidocaine for shock-resistant ventricular fibrillation. N Engl J Med 346:884, 2002.

Flecainide

12. Kang TS, Yoon YW, Park S, et al: A case of acute ventricular capture threshold rise associated with flecainide acetate. Yonsei Med J 47:152, 2006.
13. Khan IA: Oral loading single dose flecainide for pharmacological cardioversion of recent-onset atrial fibrillation. Int J Cardiol 87:121, 2003.
14. Gasparini M, Priori SG, Mantica M, et al: Flecainide test in Brugada syndrome: A reproducible but risky tool. Pacing Clin Electrophysiol 26:338, 2003.
15. Nakata M, Anno K, Matsumori LT, et al: Successful treatment of supraventricular tachycardia exhibiting hydrops fetalis with flecainide acetate. A case report. Fetal Diagn Ther 18:83, 2003.

Propafenone

16. Pritchett EL, Page RL, Carlson M, et al: Efficacy and safety of sustained-release propafenone (propafenone SR) for patients with atrial fibrillation. Am J Cardiol 92:941, 2003.
17. Capucci A, Villani GQ, Piepoli MF: Reproducible efficacy of loading oral propafenone in restoring sinus rhythm in patients with paroxysmal atrial fibrillation. Am J Cardiol 92:1345, 2003.

Beta Blockers

18. Connolly SJ, Cybulsky I, Lamy A, et al: Double-blind, placebo-controlled, randomized trial of prophylactic metoprolol for reduction of hospital length of stay after heart surgery: The beta-Blocker Length Of Stay (BLOS) study. Am Heart J 145:226, 2003.

Amiodarone

19. Doggrell SA, Hancox JC: Dronedarone: An amiodarone analogue. Expert Opin Invest Drugs 13:415, 2004.
20. Kathofer S, Thomas D, Karle CA: The novel antiarrhythmic drug dronedarone: Comparison with amiodarone. Cardiovasc Drug Rev 23:217, 2005.
21. Mitchell LB, Exner DV, Wyse DG, et al: Prophylactic oral amiodarone for the prevention of arrhythmias that begin early after revascularization, valve replacement, or repair: PAPABEAR: A randomized controlled trial. JAMA 294:3093, 2005.
22. Connolly SJ, Dorian P, Roberts RS, et al: Comparison of beta-blockers, amiodarone plus beta-blockers, or sotalol for prevention of shocks from implantable cardioverter defibrillators: The OPTIC Study: A randomized trial. JAMA 295:165, 2006.
23. Amiodarone Trials Meta-Analysis Investigators: Effect of prophylactic amiodarone on mortality after acute myocardial infarction and in congestive heart failure: Meta-analysis of individual data from 6500 patients in randomised trials. Lancet 350:1417, 1997.
24. Bardy GH, Lee KL, Mark DB, et al: Amiodarone or an implantable cardioverter-defibrillator for congestive heart failure. N Engl J Med 352:225, 2005.
25. Bokhari F, Newman D, Greene M, et al: Long-term comparison of the implantable cardioverter defibrillator versus amiodarone: Eleven-year follow-up of a subset of patients in the Canadian Implantable Defibrillator Study (CIDS). Circulation 110:112, 2004.
26. Dusman RE, Stanton MS, Miles WM, et al: Clinical features of amiodarone-induced pulmonary toxicity. Circulation 82:51, 1990.
27. Ott MC, Khoor A, Leventhal JP, et al: Pulmonary toxicity in patients receiving low-dose amiodarone. Chest 123:646-651, 2003.

28. Erdogan MF, Gulec S, Tutar E, et al: A stepwise approach to the treatment of amiodarone-induced thyrotoxicosis. Thyroid 13:205, 2003.
29. Chen D, Hedges TR: Amiodarone optic neuropathy—review. Semin Ophthalmol 18:169, 2003.
30. Johnson LN, Krohel GB, Thomas ER: The clinical spectrum of amiodarone-associated optic neuropathy. J Natl Med Assoc 96:1477, 2004.

Sotalol

31. Singh BN, Singh SN, Reda DJ, et al: Amiodarone versus sotalol for atrial fibrillation. N Engl J Med 352:1861, 2005.
32. Oudijk MA, Ruskamp JM, Ververs FF, et al: Treatment of fetal tachycardia with sotalol: transplacental pharmacokinetics and pharmacodynamics. J Am Coll Cardiol 42:765, 2003.

Ibutilide

33. Kalus JS, Spencer AP, Tsikouris JP, et al: Impact of prophylactic i.v. magnesium on the efficacy of ibutilide for conversion of atrial fibrillation or flutter. Am J Health Syst Pharm 60:2308, 2003.
34. Fragakis N, Papadopoulos N, Papanastasiou S, et al: Efficacy and safety of ibutilide for cardioversion of atrial flutter and fibrillation in patients receiving amiodarone or propafenone. Pacing Clin Electrophysiol 28:954, 2005.
35. Oral H, Souza JJ, Michaud GF, et al: Facilitating transthoracic cardioversion of atrial fibrillation with ibutilide pretreatment. N Engl J Med 340:1849, 1999.
36. Eidher U, Freihoff F, Kaltenbrunner W, et al: Efficacy and safety of ibutilide for the conversion of monomorphic atrial tachycardia. Pacing Clin Electrophysiol 29:358, 2006.
37. Gowda RM, Khan IA, Punukollu G, et al: Female preponderance in ibutilide-induced torsade de pointes. Int J Cardiol 95:219, 2004.

Azimilide

38. Karam R, Marcello S, Brooks RR, et al: Azimilide dihydrochloride, a novel antiarrhythmic agent. Am J Cardiol 81:40D, 1998.
39. Pratt CM, Singh SN, Al-Khalidi HR, et al: The efficacy of azimilide in the treatment of atrial fibrillation in the presence of left ventricular systolic dysfunction: results from the Azimilide Postinfarct Survival Evaluation (ALIVE) trial. J Am Coll Cardiol 43:1211, 2004.
40. Dorian P, Borggrefe M, Al-Khalidi HR, et al: Placebo-controlled, randomized clinical trial of azimilide for prevention of ventricular tachyarrhythmias in patients with an implantable cardioverter defibrillator. Circulation 110:3646, 2004.

Verapamil

41. De Simone A, Turco P, De Matteis C, et al: Effect of verapamil on secondary cardioversion in patients with early atrial fibrillation recurrence after electrical cardioversion. Am J Cardiol 90:185, 2002.

Other Antiarrhythmic Agents

42. Healey JS, Baranchuk A, Crystal E, et al: Prevention of atrial fibrillation with angiotensin-converting enzyme inhibitors and angiotensin receptor blockers: a meta-analysis. J Am Coll Cardiol 1832, 2005.

Direct-Current Electrical Cardioversion

43. Fuster V, Ryden LE, Cannom DS, et al; American College of Cardiology/American Heart Association Task Force on Practice Guidelines, European Society of Cardiology Committee for Practice Guidelines, European Heart Rhythm Association, Heart Rhythm Society: ACC/AHA/ESC 2006 Guidelines for the Management of Patients with Atrial Fibrillation: A report of the American College of Cardiology/American Heart Association Task Force on Practice Guidelines and the European Society of Cardiology Committee for Practice Guidelines (Writing Committee to Revise the 2001 Guidelines for the Management of Patients With Atrial Fibrillation): Developed in collaboration with the European Heart Rhythm Association and the Heart Rhythm Society. Circulation 114:e257, 2006.
44. Gronefeld GC, Wegener F, Israel CW, et al: Thromboembolic risk of patients referred for radiofrequency catheter ablation of typical atrial flutter without prior appropriate anticoagulation therapy. Pacing Clin Electrophysiol 26:323, 2003.
45. Caldwell G, Millar G, Quinn E, et al: Simple mechanical methods for cardioversion: Defense of the precordial thump and cough version. Br Med J (Clin Res Ed) 291:627, 1985.

Ablation Therapy for Cardiac Arrhythmias

46. Morady F: Radio-frequency ablation as treatment for cardiac arrhythmias. N Engl J Med 340:534, 1999.
47. Gaita F, Haissaguerre M, Giustetto C, et al: Safety and efficacy of cryoablation of accessory pathways adjacent to the normal conduction system. J Cardiovasc Electrophysiol 14:825, 2003.
48. Pappone C, Santinelli V, Manguso F, et al: A randomized study of prophylactic catheter ablation in asymptomatic patients with the Wolff-Parkinson-White syndrome. N Engl J Med 349:1803, 2003.
49. Scheinman MM, Huang S: The 1998 NASPE prospective catheter ablation registry. Pacing Clin Electrophysiol 23:1020, 2000.

Ablation of Supraventricular Tachyarrhythmias

50. Shen WK: Modification and ablation for inappropriate sinus tachycardia: current status. Card Electrophysiol Rev 6:349, 2002.
51. Higa S, Tai CT, Lin YJ, et al: Focal atrial tachycardia: new insight from noncontact mapping and catheter ablation. Circulation 109:84, 2004.
52. Tang K, Ma J, Zhang S, et al: Unipolar electrogram in identification of successful targets for radiofrequency catheter ablation of focal atrial tachycardia. Chin Med J (Engl) 116:1455, 2003.
53. Nakagawa H, Jackman WM: Catheter ablation of macroreentrant atrial tachycardia in patients following atriotomy. Eur Heart J 23:1566, 2002.
54. Calkins H, Canby R, Weiss R, et al: Results of catheter ablation of typical atrial flutter. Am J Cardiol 94:437, 2004.
55. Ozcan C, Jahangir A, Friedman PA, et al: Sudden death after radiofrequency ablation of the atrioventricular node in patients with atrial fibrillation. J Am Coll Cardiol 40:105, 2002.
56. Saad EB, Rossillo A, Saad CP, et al: Pulmonary vein stenosis after radiofrequency ablation of atrial fibrillation: Functional characterization, evolution, and influence of the ablation strategy. Circulation 108:3102, 2003.
57. Tagawa M, Higuchi K, Chinushi M, et al: Myocardium extending from the left atrium onto the pulmonary veins: A comparison between subjects with and without atrial fibrillation. Pacing Clin Electrophysiol 24:1459, 2001.
58. Jaïs P, Hocini M, Sanders P, et al: Long-term evaluation of atrial fibrillation ablation guided by noninducibility. Heart Rhythm 3:140-145, 2006.
59. Deisenhofer I, Estner H, Zrenner B, et al: Left atrial tachycardia after circumferential pulmonary vein ablation for atrial fibrillation: Incidence, electrophysiological characteristics, and results of radiofrequency ablation. Europace 8:573-582, 2006.
60. Hsu LF, Jais P, Hocini M, et al: Incidence and prevention of cardiac tamponade complicating ablation for atrial fibrillation. Pacing Clin Electrophysiol 28(Suppl 1): S106, 2005.
61. Ren JF, Marchlinski FE, Callans DJ, et al: Increased intensity of anticoagulation may reduce risk of thrombus during atrial fibrillation ablation procedures in patients with spontaneous echo contrast. J Cardiovasc Electrophysiol 16:474, 2005.
62. Kok LC, Mangrum JM, Haines DE, et al: Cerebrovascular complication associated with pulmonary vein ablation. J Cardiovasc Electrophysiol 13:764, 2002.
63. Oral H, Pappone C, Chugh A, et al: Circumferential pulmonary-vein ablation for chronic atrial fibrillation. N Engl J Med 354:934, 2006.
64. Hsu LF, Jais P, Sanders P, et al: Catheter ablation for atrial fibrillation in congestive heart failure. N Engl J Med 351:2373, 2004.
65. Pappone C, Santinelli V, Manguso F, et al: Pulmonary vein denervation enhances long-term benefit after circumferential ablation for paroxysmal atrial fibrillation. Circulation 109:327, 2004.
66. Nademanee K, McKenzie J, Kosar E, et al: A new approach for catheter ablation of atrial fibrillation: mapping of the electrophysiologic substrate. J Am Coll Cardiol 43:2044, 2004.
67. Oral H, Chugh A, Good E, et al: A tailored approach to catheter ablation of paroxysmal atrial fibrillation. Circulation 113:1824, 2006.
68. Callans DJ, Gerstenfeld EP, Dixit S, et al: Efficacy of repeat pulmonary vein isolation procedures in patients with recurrent atrial fibrillation. J Cardiovasc Electrophysiol 15:1050, 2004.
69. Mesas CE, Pappone C, Lang CC, et al: Left atrial tachycardia after circumferential pulmonary vein ablation for atrial fibrillation: Electroanatomic characterization and treatment. J Am Coll Cardiol 44:1071, 2004.
70. Oral H, Chugh A, Ozaydin M, et al: Risk of thromboembolic events after percutaneous left atrial radiofrequency ablation of atrial fibrillation. Circulation 114:759, 2006.
71. Qureshi AM, Prieto LR, Latson LA, et al: Transcatheter angioplasty for acquired pulmonary vein stenosis after radiofrequency ablation. Circulation 108:1336, 2003.
72. Pappone C, Oral H, Santinelli V, et al: Atrio-esophageal fistula as a complication of percutaneous transcatheter ablation of atrial fibrillation. Circulation 109:2724, 2004.
73. Redfearn DP, Trim GM, Skanes AC, et al: Esophageal temperature monitoring during radiofrequency ablation of atrial fibrillation. J Cardiovasc Electrophysiol 16:589, 2005.
74. Chan PS, Vijan S, Morady F, et al: Cost-effectiveness of radiofrequency catheter ablation for atrial fibrillation. J Am Coll Cardiol 47:2513, 2006.
75. Weerasooriya R, Jais P, Hocini M, et al: Effect of catheter ablation on quality of life of patients with paroxysmal atrial fibrillation. Heart Rhythm 2:619, 2005.

Ablation of Ventricular Tachyarrhythmias

76. Costeas C, Peters NS, Waldecker B, et al: Mechanisms causing sustained ventricular tachycardia with multiple QRS morphologies: results of mapping studies in the infarcted canine heart. Circulation 96:3721, 1997.
77. Sosa E, Scanavacca M: Epicardial mapping and ablation techniques to control ventricular tachycardia. J Cardiovasc Electrophysiol 16:449, 2005.
78. Ouyang F, Fotuhi P, Ho SY, et al: Repetitive monomorphic ventricular tachycardia originating from the aortic sinus cusp: Electrocardiographic characterization for guiding catheter ablation. J Am Coll Cardiol 39:500, 2002.
79. Koplan BA, Soejima K, Baughman K, et al: Refractory ventricular tachycardia secondary to cardiac sarcoid: electrophysiologic characteristics, mapping, and ablation. Heart Rhythm 3:924, 2006.
80. Ouyang F, Cappato R, Ernst S, et al: Electroanatomic substrate of idiopathic left ventricular tachycardia: unidirectional block and macroreentry within the purkinje network. Circulation 105:462, 2002.
81. Delacretaz E, Stevenson WG: Catheter ablation of ventricular tachycardia in patients with coronary heart disease. Part I: Mapping. Pacing Clin Electrophysiol 24:1261, 2001.
82. Delacretaz E, Stevenson WG: Catheter ablation of ventricular tachycardia in patients with coronary heart disease. Part II: Clinical aspects, limitations, and recent developments. Pacing Clin Electrophysiol 24:1403, 2001.

83. Bogun F, Kim HM, Han J, et al: Comparison of mapping criteria for hemodynamically tolerated, postinfarction ventricular tachycardia. Heart Rhythm 3:20, 2006.
84. El-Shalakany A, Hadjis T, Papageorgiou P, et al: Entrainment/mapping criteria for the prediction of termination of ventricular tachycardia by single radiofrequency lesion in patients with coronary artery disease. Circulation 99:2283, 1999.
85. Bogun F, Bender B, Li YG, et al: Analysis during sinus rhythm of critical sites in reentry circuits of postinfarction ventricular tachycardia. J Interv Card Electrophysiol 7:95, 2002.
86. Brunckhorst CB, Delacretaz E, Soejima K, et al: Identification of the ventricular tachycardia isthmus after infarction by pace mapping. Circulation 110:652, 2004.
87. Soejima K, Stevenson WG, Maisel WH, et al: Electrically unexcitable scar mapping based on pacing threshold for identification of the reentry circuit isthmus: Feasibility for guiding ventricular tachycardia ablation. Circulation 106:1678, 2002.
88. Bänsch D, Ouyang F, Antz M, et al: Successful catheter ablation of electrical storm after myocardial infarction. Circulation 108:3011, 2003.
89. Li YG, Gronefeld G, Israel C, et al: Catheter ablation of frequently recurring ventricular fibrillation in a patient after aortic valve repair. J Cardiovasc Electrophysiol 15:90, 2004.

90. Marrouche NF, Verma A, Wazni O, et al: Mode of initiation and ablation of ventricular fibrillation storms in patients with ischemic cardiomyopathy. J Am Coll Cardiol 43:1715, 2004.
91. Haïssaguerre M, Shoda M, Jaïs P, et al: Mapping and ablation of idiopathic ventricular fibrillation. Circulation 106:962, 2002.
92. Grimm W, Menz V, Hoffmann J, et al: Reversal of tachycardia-induced cardiomyopathy following ablation of repetitive monomorphic right ventricular outflow tract tachycardia. Pacing Clin Electrophysiol 24:166, 2001.
93. Yarlagadda RK, Iwai S, Stein KM, et al: Reversal of cardiomyopathy in patients with repetitive monomorphic ventricular ectopy originating from the right ventricular outflow tract. Circulation 112:1092, 2005.

Surgical Ablation

94. Gillinov AM, Wolf RK: Surgical ablation of atrial fibrillation. Prog Cardiovasc Dis 48:169, 2005.
95. Miller JM, Mahomed Y: Antiarrhythmic surgery. *In* Camm AJ and Saksena S (eds): Electrophysiological Disorders of the Heart. Philadelphia, Elsevier, 2005, pp 981-991.

GUIDELINES *Thomas H. Lee*

Ambulatory Electrocardiographic and Electrophysiological Testing

Guidelines for the appropriate use of ambulatory electrocardiography (ECG) were first published by the American College of Cardiology/American Heart Association (ACC/AHA) in 1989[1] and updated in 1999.[2] In conjunction with other professional societies, the ACC/AHA issued a statement of requirements for clinical competence in ambulatory ECG in 2001.[3] Guidelines for performance of electrophysiology testing were first published in 1989[4] and updated in 1995.[5] A clinical competence statement was issued by the ACC/AHA for electrophysiology studies and catheter ablation in 2000[6]; this was updated by a statement on training in electrophysiology, cardiac pacing, and arrhythmia management in 2006.[7] The AHA and the North American Society of Pacing and Electrophysiology (NASPE, now the Heart Rhythm Society) made recommendations on safety-related issues, such as restrictions on driving, for patients with arrhythmia in 1996[8] (these are covered in the Guidelines to Chap. 34). Since then, efforts to update guidelines have focused on appropriateness of the use of pacemakers and implantable cardioverter-defibrillators (ICDs),[9] reflecting rapid advances in knowledge about the ability of ICDs to improve survival for patients with arrhythmia with or without electrophysiological testing. Guidelines on the latter topic are addressed in Chapter 34.

As with other ACC/AHA guidelines, these use the standard ACC/AHA classification system for indications:

Class I: Conditions for which there is evidence and/or general agreement that the test is useful and effective
Class II: Conditions for which there is conflicting evidence and/or a divergence of opinion about the usefulness or efficacy of performing the test
Class IIa: Weight of evidence or opinion is in favor of usefulness or efficacy
Class IIb: Usefulness or efficacy is less well established by evidence or opinion
Class III: Conditions for which there is evidence and/or general agreement that the test is not useful or effective and in some cases may be harmful

Three levels are used to rate the evidence on which recommendations have been based. Level A recommendations are derived from data from multiple randomized clinical trials, level B recommendations are derived from a single randomized trial or nonrandomized studies, and level C recommendations are based on the consensus opinion of experts.

Ambulatory Electrocardiography

The evolution of guidelines for use of ambulatory ECG from 1989 to 1999 reflected important progress in several areas, including the following:

Understanding of the limited usefulness of suppression of ventricular ectopy with drug therapy
Solid-state digital technology that facilitates transtelephonic transmission of electrocardiographic data
Technical advances in long-term event recorders
Improved signal quality and interpretation
Improved computer arrhythmia interpretation
Increasingly sophisticated monitoring capacity of pacemakers and implantable cardioverter-defibrillators (ICDs)

As a result of progress in these areas, with increased knowledge about arrhythmias, ambulatory ECG is now considered to be of uncertain appropriateness for many indications for which it was once an accepted strategy.

Diagnosis

In the assessment of symptoms that may be caused by arrhythmias, ambulatory ECG is clearly established for the evaluation of syncope (Table 33G-1). A 2006 American Heart Association/American College of Cardiology Foundation scientific statement on the evaluation of syncope stipulates that the type and duration of ambulatory ECG monitoring is dictated by the frequency of symptoms.[10] Holter monitors (24 to 48 hours) are appropriate for episodes that occur at least daily and event recorders (30 to 60 days) for episodes that occur at least monthly. Implantable loop recorders inserted subcutaneously can record bipolar ECG signals for up to 14 months. In patients with unexplained syncope, use of an implantable loop recorder for 1 year is more likely to identify the mechanism of syncope than is a conventional approach that uses Holter or event monitors and electrophysiological testing and is cost-effective.

Ambulatory ECG is also supported for the evaluation of recurrent palpitations, particularly if the frequency of these symptoms makes it reasonably likely that they can be correlated with the tracings obtained during a 24-hour monitoring period. The guidelines comment that data on the use of ambulatory ECG for near-syncope or dizziness are insufficient to describe the diagnostic performance of this technology for patients with such symptoms.

The ACC/AHA guidelines explicitly discourage ambulatory ECG for patients with syncope or palpitations if other causes have been identified during the clinical evaluation and for patients with cerebrovascular accidents and no other evidence of arrhythmia. The guidelines seek to reduce performance of ambulatory ECG "for completeness" in such cases. Little support is provided for use of ambulatory ECG in cases in which the cause of the patient's symptoms is unclear but in which the likelihood of detecting an unsuspected arrhythmia is low (Class IIb indications).

TABLE 33G-1 ACC/AHA Guidelines for Ambulatory Electrocardiography for Assessment of Symptoms and Arrhythmias

Indication	Class I (Indicated)	Class IIa (Good Supportive Evidence)	Class IIb (Weak Supportive Evidence)	Class III (Not Indicated)
Assessment of symptoms possibly related to rhythm disturbances	Patients with unexplained syncope, near-syncope, or episodic dizziness in whom the cause is not obvious Patients with unexplained recurrent palpitation		Patients with episodic shortness of breath, chest pain, or fatigue that is not otherwise explained Patients with neurological events when transient atrial fibrillation or flutter is suspected Patients with symptoms such as syncope, near-syncope, episodic dizziness, or palpitation in whom a probable cause other than an arrhythmia has been identified but in whom symptoms persist despite treatment of this other cause	Patients with symptoms such as syncope, near-syncope, episodic dizziness, or palpitation in whom other causes have been identified by history, physical examination, or laboratory tests Patients with cerebrovascular accidents, without other evidence of arrhythmia
Arrhythmia detection to assess risk for future cardiac events in patients without symptoms from arrhythmia			Post-MI patients with LV dysfunction (ejection fraction <40%) Patients with CHF Patients with idiopathic hypertrophic cardiomyopathy	Patients who have sustained myocardial contusion Systemic hypertensive patients with LV hypertrophy Post-MI patients with normal LV function Preoperative arrhythmia evaluation of patients for noncardiac surgery Patients with sleep apnea Patients with valvular heart disease
Measurement of heart rate variability to assess risk for future cardiac events in patients without symptoms from arrhythmia			Post-MI patients with LV dysfunction Patients with CHF Patients with idiopathic hypertrophic cardiomyopathy	Post-MI patients with normal LV function Diabetic subjects to evaluate for diabetic neuropathy Patients with rhythm disturbances that preclude HRV analysis (e.g., atrial fibrillation)
Assessment of antiarrhythmic therapy	To assess antiarrhythmic drug response in individuals in whom baseline frequency of arrhythmia has been characterized as reproducible and of sufficient frequency to permit analysis	To detect proarrhythmic responses to antiarrhythmic therapy in patients at high risk	To assess rate control during atrial fibrillation To document recurrent or asymptomatic nonsustained arrhythmias during therapy in the outpatient setting	

ACC/AHA = American College of Cardiology/American Heart Association; CHF = congestive heart failure; HRV = heart rhythm variability; LV = left ventricular; MI = myocardial infarction.

Assessment of Risk

The ACC/AHA guidelines discouraged the use of ambulatory ECG for either arrhythmia detection or analysis of heart rhythm variability for the purpose of risk assessment in patients without symptoms of arrhythmia, even if they had cardiovascular conditions such as myocardial contusions, left ventricular hypertrophy, or valvular heart disease (see Table 33G-1). Routine use for patients in whom arrhythmia is a common cause of death (left ventricular dysfunction, hypertrophic cardiomyopathy) was considered a Class IIb indication. These recommendations preceded data demonstrating the beneficial impact of ICDs for patients with left ventricular dysfunction after acute myocardial infarction even without symptoms of arrhythmia.[11] These more recent findings are leading to an expanded role for ambulatory ECG in determining which asymptomatic patients most need these expensive devices.

Efficacy of Antiarrhythmic Therapy

In the absence of data demonstrating that oral antiarrhythmic therapy can improve survival through control of ventricular arrhythmias, ambulatory ECG has a diminished role as a test for evaluation of the efficacy of treatment (see Table 33G-1). Oral antiarrhythmic agents are important for control of supraventricular arrhythmias, but most patients with such arrhythmias do not have episodes every day. Event recorders can be useful for documenting the relationship between symptoms and recurrent arrhythmia and the interval between episodes, which can help guide therapy.

The guidelines provide some support for the use of ambulatory ECG for detection of proarrhythmia during initiation of drug therapy, but patients at high risk for such complications tend to have initiation of these medications as inpatients.

TABLE 33G–2 ACC/AHA Guidelines for Ambulatory Electrocardiography for Assessment of Pacemaker and Implantable Cardioverter-Defibrillator Function

Class	Indication
Class I (indicated)	Evaluation of frequent symptoms of palpitations, syncope, or near-syncope to assess device function to exclude myopotential inhibition and pacemaker-mediated tachycardia and to assist in the programming of enhanced features, such as rate responsivity and automatic mode switching Evaluation of suspected component failure or malfunction when device interrogation is not definitive in establishing a diagnosis To assess the response to adjunctive pharmacological therapy in patients receiving frequent ICD therapy
Class IIa (good supportive evidence)	
Class IIb (weak supportive evidence)	Evaluation of immediate postoperative pacemaker function after pacemaker or ICD implantation as an alternative or adjunct to continuous telemetric monitoring Evaluation of the rate of supraventricular arrhythmias in patients with implanted defibrillators
Class III (not indicated)	Assessment of ICD or pacemaker malfunction when device interrogation, ECG, or other available data (e.g., chest radiograph) are sufficient to establish an underlying cause or diagnosis Routine follow-up in asymptomatic patients

ACC/AHA = American College of Cardiology/American Heart Association; ECG = electrocardiographic; ICD = implantable cardioverter-defibrillator.

Assessment of Pacemaker and Implantable Cardioverter-Defibrillator Function

Ambulatory ECG was considered to be appropriate for evaluation of function of pacemakers and ICDs, but the role of ambulatory ECG is being eroded by increasing diagnostic and monitoring functions being built into these devices. Ambulatory ECG can provide useful information by correlating symptoms with device activity and by detecting abnormalities in sensing and capture during chronic follow-up (Table 33G-2). However, the ACC/AHA guidelines emphasize that ambulatory ECG should not be used when data available from device interrogation are sufficient to guide clinical management.

Monitoring for Myocardial Ischemia

The 1999 ACC/AHA guidelines do not provide strong support for any indications for routine clinical use of ambulatory ECG monitoring for myocardial ischemia (Table 33G-3). The only indication for which the task force felt there was good supportive evidence was for patients with suspected variant angina. This technology was not considered a first-choice alternative to exercise testing for patients who are unable to exercise.

Clinical Competence

The ACC/AHA statement on clinical competence recommended that trainees interpret at least 150 ambulatory electrocardiograms under supervision to acquire minimal competence with this technology.[3] A minimum of 25 test interpretations per year was recommended to maintain competence.

Electrophysiological Procedures for Diagnosis

The ACC/AHA guidelines for use of intracardiac electrophysiological procedures from 1989[4] and 1995[5] reflect the emerging role of catheter ablation as a therapeutic strategy but do not fully reflect the reduced importance of antiarrhythmic medications and the growing role of ICDs that have occurred. Nevertheless, most of the basic themes of these guidelines remain valid today.

These guidelines, which are older than most of the ACC/AHA guidelines, use a simpler, three-category system for assessment of appropriateness, in which Class II indications are not subdivided into indications with more and less support.

TABLE 33G–3 ACC/AHA Guidelines for Ischemia Monitoring

Class	Indication
Class I (indicated)	
Class IIa (good supportive evidence)	Patients with suspected variant angina
Class IIb (weak supportive evidence)	Evaluation of patients with chest pain who cannot exercise Preoperative evaluation for vascular surgery of patients who cannot exercise Patients with known CAD and atypical chest pain syndrome
Class III (not indicated)	Initial evaluation of patients with chest pain who are able to exercise Routine screening of asymptomatic subjects

ACC/AHA = American College of Cardiology/American Heart Association; CAD = coronary artery disease.

Evaluation of Sinus Node Function

Clinical evaluation of sinus node dysfunction is often difficult because of the episodic nature of symptomatic abnormalities and the wide variability in sinus node function in asymptomatic individuals. Invasive tests of sinus function can test the ability of the sinus node to recover from overdrive suppression and assess sinoatrial conduction by introducing atrial extrastimuli or by atrial pacing.

The ACC/AHA guidelines consider electrophysiological studies of sinus node function most appropriate for patients in whom dysfunction is suspected but not proved after a noninvasive evaluation (Table 33G-4). In contrast, the guidelines consider such studies inappropriate when a documented bradyarrhythmia has been found to be correlated with the patient's symptoms and management is unlikely to be influenced by an electrophysiological study. Studies are also considered inappropriate in asymptomatic patients and those who have sinus pauses only during sleep. When bradyarrhythmias were recognized as the cause of the patient's symptoms, electrophysiological studies were considered to have possible but uncertain appropriateness (Class II) if such data might refine treatment choices.

TABLE 33G–4 ACC/AHA Guidelines for Clinical Intracardiac Electrophysiological Studies for Evaluation of Specific Electrocardiographic Abnormalities

Indication	Class I (Appropriate)	Class II (Equivocal)	Class III (Inappropriate)
Evaluation of sinus node function	Symptomatic patients in whom sinus node dysfunction is suspected as the cause of symptoms but a causal relation between an arrhythmia and the symptoms has not been established after appropriate evaluation	Patients with documented sinus node dysfunction in whom evaluation of atrioventricular (AV) or ventriculoatrial (VA) conduction or susceptibility to arrhythmias may aid in selection of the most appropriate pacing modality Patients with electrocardiographically documented sinus bradyarrhythmias to determine whether abnormalities are caused by intrinsic disease, autonomic nervous system dysfunction, or effects of drugs to help select therapeutic options Symptomatic patients with known sinus bradyarrhythmias to evaluate potential for other arrhythmias as the cause of symptoms	Symptomatic patients in whom an association between symptoms and a documented bradyarrhythmia has been established and choice of therapy would not be affected by results of an electrophysiological study Asymptomatic patients with sinus bradyarrhythmias or sinus pauses observed only during sleep, including sleep apnea
Acquired AV block	Symptomatic patients in whom His-Purkinje block, suspected as a cause of symptoms, has not been established Patients with second- or third-degree AV block treated with a pacemaker who remain symptomatic and in whom another arrhythmia is suspected as cause of symptoms	Patients with second- or third-degree AV block in whom knowledge of the site of block or its mechanism or response to pharmacological or other temporary intervention may help direct therapy or assess prognosis Patients with premature, concealed junctional depolarizations suspected as a cause of second- or third-degree AV block pattern (e.g., pseudo-AV block)	Symptomatic patients in whom the symptoms and presence of AV block are correlated by ECG findings Asymptomatic patients with transient AV block associated with sinus slowing (e.g., nocturnal type I second-degree AV block)
Chronic intraventricular conduction delay	Symptomatic patients in whom the cause of symptoms is not known	Asymptomatic patients with bundle branch block in whom pharmacological therapy that could increase conduction delay or produce heart block is contemplated	Asymptomatic patients with intraventricular conduction delay Symptomatic patients whose symptoms can be correlated with or excluded by ECG events
Narrow QRS tachycardia (QRS complex <0.12 sec)	Patients with frequent or poorly tolerated episodes of tachycardia who do not adequately respond to drug therapy and for whom information about site of origin, mechanism, and electrophysiological properties of pathways of the tachycardia is essential for choosing appropriate therapy (e.g., drugs, catheter ablation, pacing, or surgery) Patients who prefer ablative therapy to pharmacological treatment	Patients with frequent episodes of tachycardia requiring drug treatment for whom there is concern about proarrhythmia or effects of the antiarrhythmic drug on the sinus node or AV conduction	Patients with tachycardias easily controlled by vagal maneuvers and/or well-tolerated drug therapy who are not candidates for nonpharmacological therapy
Wide-complex tachycardias	Patients with wide QRS complex tachycardia in whom correct diagnosis is unclear after analysis of available ECG tracings and for whom knowledge of the correct diagnosis is necessary for care	None	Patients with VT or supraventricular tachycardia with aberrant conduction or preexcitation syndromes diagnosed with certainty by ECG criteria and for whom invasive electrophysiological data would not influence therapy; however, data obtained at baseline electrophysiological study in these patients might be appropriate as guide for subsequent therapy
Prolonged QT interval syndrome	None	Identification of proarrhythmic effect of a drug in patients experiencing sustained VT or cardiac arrest while receiving the drug Patients who have equivocal abnormalities of QT interval duration or TU wave configuration, with syncope or symptomatic arrhythmias, in whom catecholamine effects may unmask a distinct QT abnormality	Patients with clinically manifest congenital QT prolongation, with or without symptomatic arrhythmias Patients with acquired prolonged QT syndrome with symptoms closely related to an identifiable cause or mechanism

TABLE 33G–4 ACC/AHA Guidelines for Clinical Intracardiac Electrophysiological Studies for Evaluation of Specific Electrocardiographic Abnormalities—cont'd

Indication	Class I (Appropriate)	Class II (Equivocal)	Class III (Inappropriate)
Wolff-Parkinson-White syndrome	Patients being evaluated for catheter ablation or surgical ablation of an accessory pathway Patients with ventricular preexcitation who have survived cardiac arrest or who have unexplained syncope Symptomatic patients in whom determination of the mechanism of arrhythmia or knowledge of the electrophysiological properties of the accessory pathway and normal conduction system would help in determining appropriate therapy	Asymptomatic patients with a family history of sudden cardiac death or with ventricular preexcitation but no spontaneous arrhythmia who engage in high-risk occupations or activities and in whom knowledge of the electrophysiological properties of the accessory pathway or inducible tachycardia may help determine recommendations for further activities or therapy Patients with ventricular preexcitation who are undergoing cardiac surgery for other reasons	Asymptomatic patients with ventricular preexcitation, except those in Class II
Ventricular premature complexes, couplets, and nonsustained ventricular tachycardia	None	Patients with other risk factors for future arrhythmic events, such as a low ejection fraction, positive signal-averaged electrocardiogram, and nonsustained VT on ambulatory ECG recordings in whom electrophysiological studies will be used for further risk assessment and for guiding therapy in patients with inducible VT Patients with highly symptomatic, uniform morphology premature ventricular complexes, couplets, and nonsustained VT who are considered potential candidates for catheter ablation	Asymptomatic or mildly symptomatic patients with premature ventricular complexes, couplets, and nonsustained VT without other risk factors for sustained arrhythmias

ACC/AHA = American College of Cardiology/American Heart Association; ECG = electrocardiographic.

Acquired Atrioventricular Block

The ACC/AHA guidelines emphasize that electrophysiological studies are inappropriate (Class III) when ECG findings correlate with symptoms and the findings from electrophysiological studies are unlikely to alter management (e.g., documentation of His bundle conduction rarely improves management for a patient whose other clinical data indicate that placement of a permanent pacemaker is warranted because of symptomatic advanced atrioventricular [AV] block). Similarly, electrophysiological studies are not appropriate for asymptomatic patients with mild degrees of AV block who are not likely to warrant pacemaker implantation. According to these guidelines, electrophysiological studies of AV conduction should be performed when a relationship between symptoms and AV block has not been proved; in such patients, another arrhythmia could be the cause of symptoms.

Chronic Intraventricular Delay

According to ACC/AHA guidelines, the main role of electrophysiological testing in patients with prolonged H-V intervals is not to predict future complications but to determine whether the symptoms of arrhythmia are caused by conduction delay or block versus some other arrhythmia. The only Class I (clearly appropriate) indication for electrophysiological testing is in symptomatic patients for whom the cause of symptoms is not known. The guidelines specifically discourage such testing of asymptomatic patients and provide only equivocal support for asymptomatic patients with bundle branch block in whom treatment with drugs that might increase conduction delay is being considered.

Narrow and Wide Complex QRS Tachycardia. The ACC/AHA guidelines define different roles for electrophysiological testing in patients with narrow- and wide-complex tachycardias. In narrow QRS tachycardia, the site of abnormal impulse formation or the reentry circuit can often be determined from information from the 12-lead electrocardiogram. Thus, electrophysiological testing was considered more appropriate as a guide to therapy in this setting than as a tool for diagnosis. Class I indications for electrophysiological testing include patients with recurrent tachycardia for whom data from testing may help clinicians choose among drug therapy, catheter ablation, pacing, and surgery. However, testing is not considered useful for patients whose tachycardias are controlled by vagal maneuvers or medications and who are not candidates for nonpharmacological therapy.

In wide-complex tachycardias, identification of the site of origin is frequently impossible from ECG tracings alone. However, electrophysiological testing permits accurate diagnosis in virtually all patients. Because knowledge of the mechanism of the arrhythmia is essential for selection of optimal therapy, electrophysiological testing was considered appropriate (Class I) for the diagnosis of wide-complex tachycardias in these guidelines. However, when the diagnosis is clear from other data and electrophysiological testing is not likely to influence therapy, the guidelines consider it inappropriate.

Prolonged QT Intervals. The ACC/AHA guidelines do not consider electrophysiological testing for any indications for routine use in patients with prolonged QT intervals. Whether catecholamine infusion during testing is useful for revealing patients who are at high risk for complications or whether electrophysiological testing can be used to evaluate proarrhythmic effects in this population is considered uncertain.

Wolff-Parkinson-White Syndrome. Electrophysiological testing is useful for patients with this syndrome for both diagnosis and planning of therapy. The ACC/AHA guidelines consider electrophysiological testing appropriate for patients who are candidates for catheter or surgical ablation, for those who have had cardiac arrests or unexplained syncope, or for patients whose management might be altered by knowledge of the electrophysiological properties of the accessory pathway and normal conduction system. For asymptomatic patients, however, electrophysiological studies are deemed inappropriate except in special situations, such as patients with high-risk occupations or those with a family history of sudden cardiac death. More recently recognized entities such as Brugada syndrome, catecholaminergic tachycardia, and right ventricular cardiomyopathy were not considered.

Nonsustained Ventricular Tachycardia. For patients with ventricular premature complexes, couplets, and nonsustained ventricular tachycardia, the usefulness of electrophysiological testing is compromised by the lack of therapeutic strategies that have been shown to improve outcomes. There are no clearly appropriate indications for electrophysiological studies in these patients, and the guidelines discourage testing in patients without other risk factors for sustained arrhythmias. Research published since these guidelines suggests that exceptions would include patients who fit the Multicenter Automatic Defibrillator Implantation Trial (MADIT) or Multicenter Unsustained Tachycardia Trial (MUSTT) criteria. For certain patients with other data suggesting an adverse prognosis, electrophysiological testing is believed to have possible but unproven appropriateness (Class II).

Unexplained Syncope

In patients with unexplained syncope and structural heart disease, recent ACC/AHA guidelines on the evaluation of syncope[10] recommend a low threshold for the use of electrophysiological testing (Table 33G-5). In patients without structural heart disease, the yield of electrophysiological testing is low. Thus, the guidelines recommend a higher threshold for use of electrophysiological studies in such patients and suggest that head-up tilt testing may be a more useful test. However, given the low risk of electrophysiological testing, and the high risk of potentially harmful recurrent syncope, electrophysiological testing may be beneficial for patients with a malignant episode of syncope.[10]

Survivors of Cardiac Arrest

The ACC/AHA guidelines consider electrophysiological testing appropriate for patients who are survivors of cardiac arrest other than in the earliest phase of acute myocardial infarction (see Table 33G-5). Since publication of these guidelines, acceptance of the usefulness of ICDs has become more widespread, and many of these patients receive such a device without electrophysiological testing or receive limited electrophysiological testing at device implantation. The guidelines consider electrophysiological studies inappropriate when cardiac arrest has occurred within the first 48 hours of myocardial infarction or when the cardiac arrest results from clearly definable specific causes.

Unexplained Palpitations

The procedure of choice to determine the cause of palpitations is ambulatory ECG, according to the ACC/AHA guidelines. The guidelines suggest that electrophysiological testing should be reserved for patients with palpitations that are associated with syncope or for those in whom electrocardiograms have failed to capture a cause of the palpitations but who have been noted to have a rapid pulse rate by medical personnel (see Table 33G-5). Electrophysiological testing is considered of equivocal value in patients with symptoms so sporadic that they cannot be documented while ambulatory ECGs are performed.

Electrophysiological Studies for Therapeutic Intervention

The 1995 ACC/AHA guidelines for appropriateness of electrophysiological studies for guidance of drug therapy and implantable electrical devices do not fully reflect the decline in the role of oral antiarrhythmic therapy and the rise in the use of ICDs for treatment of patients who have had cardiac arrests (Table 33G-6). However, the guideline recommendations for the role of catheter ablation are still largely valid. The characteristics that are common among appropriate indications include supraventricular arrhythmias that are symptomatic, that cannot be controlled with medications because of limited effectiveness, side effects, or inconvenience, or that have caused sudden cardiac death. Catheter ablation is also useful for some patients with ventricular tachycardia, although patients with extensive structural heart disease tend to have multiple sites of origin of their arrhythmia and may therefore be poor candidates for this procedure. Ablation is sometimes useful as an adjunct to ICD implantation to limit the episodes of ventricular tachycardia requiring ICD treatment.

Clinical Competence

The ACC/AHA statement on clinical competence from 2006[7] describes three levels of training—level 1 for every cardiology trainee, level 2 for those wishing to acquire advanced training in arrhythmia management, and level 3 for those intending to specialize in invasive diagnostic and therapeutic cardiac electrophysiology. The level 3 guidelines recommend a minimum of 1 year of specialized training in electrophysio-

TABLE 33G-5 ACC/AHA Guidelines for Clinical Intracardiac Electrophysiological Studies for Evaluation of Clinical Syndromes

Indication	Class I (Appropriate)	Class II (Equivocal)	Class III (Inappropriate)
Unexplained syncope	Patients with suspected structural heart disease and syncope that remain unexplained after appropriate evaluation	Patients with recurrent unexplained syncope without structural heart disease and a negative head-up tilt test	Patients with known cause of syncope for whom treatment will not be guided by electrophysiological testing
Survivors of cardiac arrest	Patients surviving cardiac arrest without evidence of an acute Q wave MI Patients surviving cardiac arrest occurring more than 48 hr after acute phase of MI in absence of recurrent ischemic event	Patients surviving cardiac arrest caused by bradyarrhythmia Patients surviving cardiac arrest thought to be associated with a congenital repolarization abnormality (long-QT syndrome) in whom results of noninvasive diagnostic testing are equivocal	Patients surviving a cardiac arrest that occurred during the acute phase (<48 hr) of MI Patients with cardiac arrest resulting from clearly definable specific causes such as reversible ischemia, severe valvular aortic stenosis, or noninvasively defined congenital or acquired long-QT syndrome
Unexplained palpitations	Patients with palpitations who have pulse rate documented by medical personnel as inappropriately rapid and in whom ECG recordings fail to document cause of the palpitations Patients with palpitations preceding a syncopal episode	Patients with clinically significant palpitations, suspected to be of cardiac origin, in whom symptoms are sporadic and cannot be documented; studies performed to determine mechanisms of arrhythmias, direct or provide therapy, or assess prognosis	Patients with palpitations documented to be caused by extracardiac causes (e.g., hyperthyroidism)

ACC/AHA = American College of Cardiology/American Heart Association; ECG = electrocardiographic; MI = myocardial infarction.

TABLE 33G–6 ACC/AHA Guidelines for Clinical Intracardiac Electrophysiological Studies for Therapeutic Intervention

Indication	Class I (Appropriate)	Class II (Equivocal)	Class III (Inappropriate)
Guidance of drug therapy	Patients with sustained VT or cardiac arrest, especially those with prior MI Patients with AVNRT, AV reentrant tachycardia using an accessory pathway, or atrial fibrillation associated with an accessory pathway, for whom chronic drug therapy is planned	Patients with sinus node reentrant tachycardia, atrial tachycardia, atrial fibrillation, or atrial flutter without ventricular preexcitation syndrome, for whom chronic drug therapy is planned Patients with arrhythmias not inducible during controlled electrophysiological study for whom drug therapy is planned	Patients with isolated atrial or ventricular premature complexes Patients with ventricular fibrillation with a clearly identified reversible cause
Patients who are candidates for or who have implantable electrical devices	Patients with tachyarrhythmias, before and during implantation, and final (predischarge) programming of an electrical device to confirm its ability to perform as anticipated Patients with an implanted electrical antitachyarrhythmia device in whom changes in status or therapy may have influenced the continued safety and efficacy of the device Patients who have a pacemaker to treat a bradyarrhythmia and receive a cardioverter-defibrillator to test for device interactions	Patients with previously documented indications for pacemaker implantation to test for most appropriate long-term pacing mode and sites to optimize symptomatic improvement and hemodynamics	Patients who are not candidates for device therapy
Indications for catheter ablation procedures	Patients with symptomatic atrial tachyarrhythmias who have inadequately controlled ventricular rates unless primary ablation of the atrial tachyarrhythmia is possible Patients with symptomatic atrial tachyarrhythmias such as those above but in whom drugs are not tolerated or the patient does not wish to take them, even though the ventricular rate can be controlled Patients with symptomatic nonparoxysmal junctional tachycardia that is drug-resistant or the patient is drug-intolerant or does not wish to take it Patients resuscitated from sudden cardiac death caused by atrial flutter or atrial fibrillation with a rapid ventricular response in the absence of an accessory pathway	Patients with a dual-chamber pacemaker and pacemaker-mediated tachycardia that cannot be treated effectively by drugs or by reprogramming the pacemaker	Patients with atrial tachyarrhythmias responsive to drug therapy acceptable to the patient
Radiofrequency catheter ablation for AVNRT	Patients with symptomatic sustained AVNRT that is drug-resistant or the patient is drug-intolerant or does not desire long-term drug therapy	Patients with sustained AVNRT identified during electrophysiological study or catheter ablation of another arrhythmia Finding of dual AV nodal pathway physiology and atrial echoes but without AVNRT during electrophysiological study in patients suspected of having AVNRT clinically	Patients with AVNRT responsive to drug therapy that is well tolerated and preferred by the patient to ablation Finding of dual AV nodal pathway physiology (with or without echo complexes) during electrophysiological study in patients in whom AVNRT is not suspected clinically
Ablation of atrial tachycardia, flutter, and fibrillation: atrium/atrial sites	Patients with atrial tachycardia that is drug-resistant or the patient is drug-intolerant or does not desire long-term drug therapy Patients with atrial flutter that is drug-resistant or the patient is drug-intolerant or does not desire long-term drug therapy	Atrial flutter or atrial tachycardia associated with paroxysmal atrial fibrillation when the tachycardia is drug-resistant or the patient is drug-intolerant or does not desire long-term drug therapy Patients with atrial fibrillation and evidence of a localized site(s) of origin when the tachycardia is drug-resistant or the patient is drug-intolerant or does not desire long-term drug therapy	Patients with atrial arrhythmia responsive to drug therapy, well tolerated, and preferred by the patient to ablation Patients with multiform atrial tachycardia

Continues

TABLE 33G-6 ACC/AHA Guidelines for Clinical Intracardiac Electrophysiological Studies for Therapeutic Intervention—cont'd

Indication	Class I (Appropriate)	Class II (Equivocal)	Class III (Inappropriate)
Ablation of atrial tachycardia, flutter, and fibrillation: accessory pathways	Patients with symptomatic AV reentrant tachycardia that is drug-resistant or the patient is drug-intolerant or does not desire long-term drug therapy Patients with atrial fibrillation (or other atrial tachyarrhythmia) and a rapid ventricular response through the accessory pathway when the tachycardia is drug-resistant or the patient is drug-intolerant or does not desire long-term drug therapy	Patients with AV reentrant tachycardia or atrial fibrillation with rapid ventricular rates identified during electrophysiological study of another arrhythmia Asymptomatic patients with ventricular preexcitation whose livelihood or profession, important activities, insurability, or mental well-being or public safety would be affected by spontaneous tachyarrhythmias or the presence of the ECG abnormality Patients with atrial fibrillation and a controlled ventricular response through the accessory pathway Patients with a family history of sudden cardiac death	Patients who have accessory pathway-related arrhythmias responsive to drug therapy, well tolerated, and preferred by the patient to ablation
Ablation of VT	Patients with symptomatic sustained monomorphic VT when the tachycardia is drug-resistant or the patient is drug-intolerant or does not desire long-term drug therapy Patients with bundle branch reentrant ventricular tachycardia Patients with sustained monomorphic VT and an ICD who are receiving multiple shocks not manageable by reprogramming or concomitant drug therapy	Nonsustained VT that is symptomatic when the tachycardia is drug-resistant or the patient is drug-intolerant or does not desire long-term drug therapy	Patients with VT responsive to drug, ICD, or surgical therapy that is well tolerated and preferred by the patient to ablation Unstable, rapid, multiple, or polymorphic VT that cannot be adequately localized by current mapping techniques Asymptomatic and clinically benign nonsustained VT

ACC/AHA = American College of Cardiology/American Heart Association; AV = atrioventricular; AVNRT = AV nodal reentrant tachycardia; ECG = electrocardiographic; ICD = implantable cardioverter-defibrillator; MI = myocardial infarction; VT = ventricular tachycardia.

logical studies, during which the physician should be the primary operator and analyze 100 to 150 initial diagnostic studies, at least 50 of which should involve patients with supraventricular arrhythmias. Because antiarrhythmic devices constitute a major part of current electrophysiology practice, the guidelines suggest that a trainee should be the primary operator during at least 25 electrophysiological evaluations of implantable antiarrhythmic devices. For maintenance of competence, a minimum of 100 diagnostic electrophysiological studies per year is recommended. The statement also recommends that specialists in electrophysiology attend at least 30 hours of formal continuing medical education every 2 years to remain abreast of changes in knowledge and technology.

For physicians who perform catheter ablation, the NASPE Ad Hoc Committee on Catheter Ablation has recommended that training should include at least 75 catheter ablations, of which at least 10 are accessory pathway ablations and 30 to 50 are mentored ablations.[7] The ACC/AHA statement recommends that physicians who perform ablations carry out at least 20 to 50 ablations per year.

Individuals receiving training in pacemaker implantation must participate as the primary operator (under direct supervision) in at least 50 primary implantations of transvenous pacemakers and 20 pacemaker system revisions or replacements. At least half of the implantations should involve dual-chamber pacemakers. The trainee must also participate in the follow-up of at least 100 pacemaker patient visits and acquire proficiency in advanced pacemaker electrocardiography, interrogation, and programming of complex pacemakers.[7]

References

1. Knoebel SB, Crawford MH, Dunn MI, et al: Guidelines for ambulatory electrocardiography. A report of the American College of Cardiology/American Heart Association Task Force on Assessment of Diagnostic and Therapeutic Cardiovascular Procedures (Subcommittee on Ambulatory Electrocardiography). Circulation 79:206, 1989.
2. Crawford MH, Bernstein SJ, Deedwania PC, et al: ACC/AHA guidelines for ambulatory electrocardiography: executive summary and recommendations. A report of the American College of Cardiology/American Heart Association task force on practice guidelines (committee to revise the guidelines for ambulatory electrocardiography). Circulation 100:886, 1999.
3. Kadish AH, Buxton AE, Kennedy HL, et al: ACC/AHA clinical competence statement on electrocardiography and ambulatory electrocardiography: A report of the ACC/AHA/ACP-ASIM task force on clinical competence (ACC/AHA Committee to develop a clinical competence statement on electrocardiography and ambulatory electrocardiography) endorsed by the International Society for Holter and Noninvasive Electrocardiology. Circulation 104:3169, 2001.
4. Zipes DP, Akhtar M, Denes P, et al: Guidelines for clinical intracardiac electrophysiology studies. A report of the American College of Cardiology/American Heart Association Task Force on Assessment of Diagnostic and Therapeutic Cardiovascular Procedures (Subcommittee to Assess Clinical Intracardiac Electrophysiologic Studies). J Am Coll Cardiol 14:1827, 1989.
5. Zipes DP, DiMarco JP, Gillette PC, et al: Guidelines for clinical intracardiac electrophysiological and catheter ablation procedures. A report of the American College of Cardiology/American Heart Association Task Force on Practice Guidelines (Committee on Clinical Intracardiac Electrophysiologic and Catheter Ablation Procedures), developed in collaboration with the North American Society of Pacing and Electrophysiology. J Am Coll Cardiol 26:555, 1995.
6. Tracy CM, Akhtar M, DiMarco JP, et al: American College of Cardiology/American Heart Association clinical competence statement on invasive electrophysiology studies, catheter ablation, and cardioversion. A report of the American College of Cardiology/American Heart Association/American College of Physicians—American Society of Internal Medicine Task Force on clinical competence. J Am Coll Cardiol 36:1725, 2000.
7. Naccarelli GV, Conti JB, DiMarco JP, et al: Task Force 6: Training in specialized electrophysiology, cardiac pacing, and arrhythmia management: endorsed by the Heart Rhythm Society. J Am Coll Cardiol 47:904, 2006.
8. Epstein AE, Miles WM, Benditt DG, et al: Personal and public safety issues related to arrhythmias that may affect consciousness: implications for regulation and physician recommendations. A medical/scientific statement from the American Heart Association and the North American Society of Pacing and Electrophysiology. Circulation 94:1147, 1996.
9. Gregoratos G, Abrams J, Epstein AE, et al: ACC/AHA/NASPE 2002 guideline update for implantation of cardiac pacemakers and antiarrhythmia devices: summary article: A report of the American College of Cardiology/American Heart Association Task Force on Practice Guidelines (ACC/AHA/NASPE Committee to Update the 1998 Pacemaker Guidelines). Circulation 106:2145, 2002.
10. Strickberger SA, Benson DW, Biaggioni I, et al: AHA/ACCF scientific statement on the evaluation of syncope: From the American Heart Association Councils on Clinical Cardiology, Cardiovascular Nursing, Cardiovascular Disease in the Young, and Stroke, and the Quality of Care and Outcomes Research Interdisciplinary Working Group; and the American College of Cardiology Foundation In Collaboration With the Heart Rhythm Society. J Am Coll Cardiol 47:473, 2006.
11. Moss AJ, Zareba W, Hall WJ, et al: Prophylactic implantation of a defibrillator in patients with myocardial infarction and reduced ejection fraction. N Engl J Med 346:877, 2002.

CHAPTER 34

Cardiac Pacemakers and Cardioverter-Defibrillators

David L. Hayes and Douglas P. Zipes

Implantable devices to manage cardiac arrhythmias have evolved rapidly since the inception of cardiac pacing in the late 1950s. The number of devices implanted continues to increase dramatically with expanded indications for implantable cardioverter-defibrillator (ICD) therapy and the explosion of cardiac resynchronization therapy (CRT). The evolution of ICD and CRT technology has been staggering. The technology for ICDs and CRT has evolved, supported by clinical trials to prove safety and efficacy.

CARDIAC PACEMAKERS

Pacemaker Nomenclature

Pacemaker nomenclature, established in 1974, is necessary to understand the discipline of cardiac pacing (Table 34-1).[1]

- The first position (I) refers to the chamber or chambers in which stimulation occurs: A, atrium; V, ventricle; and D, dual chamber, or both A and V.
- The second position (II) refers to the chamber or chambers in which sensing occurs. The letters are the same as those for the first position. ("S" in both the first and second positions is used to indicate generically that the device is capable of pacing only a single cardiac chamber.)
- The third position (III) refers to the mode of sensing, or how the pacemaker responds to a sensed event. An "I" indicates that a sensed event inhibits the output pulse and causes the pacemaker to recycle for one or more timing cycles. "T" means that an output pulse is triggered in response to a sensed event. "D" means that both "T" and "I" responses can occur. This designation is restricted to dual-chamber systems. An event sensed in the atrium inhibits the atrial output but triggers a ventricular output. Unlike a single-chamber-triggered mode (VVT or AAT), in which an output pulse is triggered immediately on sensing, a dual-chamber mode has a delay between the sensed atrial event and the triggered ventricular output to mimic the normal PR interval. If a native ventricular signal or R wave is sensed, the ventricular output and possibly even the atrial output are inhibited, depending on where sensing occurs.
- The fourth position (IV) of the code indicates both programmability and rate modulation. An "R" in the fourth position indicates that the pacemaker incorporates a sensor to modulate the rate independently of intrinsic cardiac activity, such as with motion or respiration. From a practical standpoint, "R" is the only indicator commonly used in the fourth position.
- The fifth position (V) of the code is used to indicate whether multisite pacing is present in none of the cardiac chambers (0), one or both atria (A), one or both ventricles (V), or any combination of atria and ventricles (D). To describe a patient with a DDDR (dual-chamber rate-adaptive) pacemaker with biventricular stimulation, the code would be DDDRV. (The fifth position of the code is not commonly used.)

Indications for Cardiac Pacing

A joint committee of the American College of Cardiology (ACC), the American Heart Association (AHA), and the Heart Rhythm Society (HRS) has established indications for pacing into categories of class I (generally indicated), class II (may be indicated), and class III (generally not indicated).[2] Although some indications for permanent pacing are relatively certain or unambiguous, others require considerable expertise and judgment. The clinical need for pacing and appropriate objective data, such as electrocardiographic tracings, must be documented clearly in the patient's medical record to ensure reimbursement.

Indications are considered in categories of atrioventricular (AV) block, both acquired and congenital, bifascicular and trifascicular block, sinus node dysfunction, and neurocardiogenic syndromes. Sinus node dysfunction is the most frequent indication for pacing, followed by AV node disease. Pacing for tachyarrhythmias and miscellaneous indications comprises a relatively small percentage of patients receiving pacemakers.

Acquired AV Block

Traditionally, AV block is classified into first-, second-, and third-degree (or complete) heart block (see Chap. 35). Alternatively, it can be defined anatomically as supra-Hisian, intra-Hisian, or infra-Hisian. If the QRS complex is prolonged more than 0.12 second, there is a greater probability that the conduction disturbance is infra-Hisian. Acquired AV block is most commonly idiopathic and related to aging, but it has many potential causes. Indications for permanent pacing in acquired AV block are listed in Table 34-2.

Permanent pacing for AV block that occurs with an acute myocardial infarction (see Chaps. 50 and 51) is required less frequently because of more aggressive and earlier intervention at the time of threat-

TABLE 34–1 Revised NASPE/BPEG Generic Code For Antibradycardia Pacing*

	Position				
	I	*II*	*III*	*IV*	*V*
Category	Chamber(s) paced: O = None A = Atrium V = Ventricle D = Dual (AV)	Chamber(s) sensed: O = None A = Atrium V = Ventricle D = Dual (AV)	Response to sensing: O = None T = Triggered I = Inhibited D = Dual (TI)	Rate modulation: O = None R = Rate modulation	Multisite pacing: O = None A = Atrium V = Ventricle D = Dual (AV)
Manufacturers' designation only	S = Single (A or V)	S = Single (A or V)			

*See text for explanation of use of the code.
BPEG = British Pacing and Electrophysiology Group; NASPE = North American Society of Pacing and Electrophysiology.
From Bernstein AD, Daubert JC, Fletcher RD, et al, North American Society of Pacing and Electrophysiology/British Pacing and Electrophysiology Group: The revised NASPE/BPEG generic code for antibradycardia, adaptive-rate, and multisite pacing. Pacing Clin Electrophysiol 25:260, 2002.

TABLE 34–2 Indications for Permanent Pacing in Atrioventricular (AV) Block

Type of AV Block	Pacemaker Necessary	Pacemaker Probably Necessary	Pacemaker Not Necessary
Third	Symptomatic congenital heart block (CHB) Acquired symptomatic atrioventricular (AV) block Atrial fibrillation with CHB Acquired asymptomatic CHB Neuromuscular diseases with AV block, with or without symptoms		AV block of any degree that is expected to resolve and unlikely to recur (e.g., drug toxicity, Lyme disease, sleep apnea) without treatment
Second	Symptomatic second-degree AV block, regardless of type Asymptomatic advanced second-degree AV block with asystole > 3.0 sec or escape rate < 40 beats/min in awake patients	Asymptomatic, type I, at intra-His or infra-His level* Hemodynamically symptomatic caused by loss of AV synchrony Neuromuscular diseases with AV block, with or without symptoms	Asymptomatic, type I, at supra-His (AV node) level
First		Hemodynamically symptomatic caused by loss of AV synchrony with markedly prolonged PR interval (e.g., >300 msec)	Asymptomatic

*From Shaw DB, Gowers JI, Kekwick CA, et al: Is Mobitz type I atrioventricular block benign in adults? Heart 90:169, 2004.

ened myocardial infarction. A permanent pacemaker is generally considered indicated if complete AV block, Mobitz type II block, or bilateral or alternating bundle branch block persists longer than 72 hours after the acute event.

Congenital Complete Heart Block

Although some controversy remains regarding when to pace patients who have congenital complete heart block, there is a growing tendency to pace most patients who have congenital complete heart block and to do so at earlier ages, even if they are asymptomatic, because of a high incidence of unpredictable syncope with significant mortality from initial attacks, a gradual decrease in heart rate, and a high incidence of acquired mitral regurgitation.[3] In pediatric patients with congenital complete heart block, pacemaker implantation is recommended for congestive heart failure, average heart rate of less than 50 beats/min in the awake infant, history of syncope or presyncope, significant ventricular ectopy, or exercise intolerance.

Chronic Bifascicular and Trifascicular Block

If bifascicular or trifascicular block is associated with transient complete heart block, whether symptomatic or not, pacing is indicated. Pacing in a patient with bifascicular or trifascicular block and syncope that cannot be attributed to any other cause is a class II American College of Cardiology/American Heart Association (ACC/AHA) indication. If the patient is asymptomatic and there is no evidence of AV block, pacing is not indicated.

Sinus Node Dysfunction

There are a number of variants of sinus node dysfunction, and the terms used to describe these variants are often used synonymously, including tachycardia-bradycardia syndrome, sick sinus syndrome, symptomatic sinus bradycardia, sinus arrest, sinus pauses, and chronotropic incompetence (see Chap. 35). The degree of bradycardia at which to consider pacing is controversial but is generally accepted to be a rate of less than 40 beats/min during waking hours, especially if associated with symptoms of fatigue or lightheadedness. There is disagreement about the absolute cycle length at which pacing should be considered. Although every patient needs to be considered individually, sinus pauses exceeding 3 seconds during waking hours are often considered abnormal and may warrant pacing if the patient has symptoms consistent with bradycardia. Pauses that occur during sleep are more difficult to categorize. Because of vagal influences, many normal persons display pauses significantly longer than 3 seconds during sleep. Permanent pacing should be considered for any patient who has a symptomatic bradyarrhythmia if the cause of the bradyarrhythmia is not reversible or the patient requires a medication that produces symptomatic bradycardia. Examples of reversible conditions include transient AV block secondary

TABLE 34–3 Indications for Permanent Pacing in Sinus Node Dysfunction (SND)

Pacemaker Necessary	Pacemaker Probably Necessary	Pacemaker Not Necessary
Symptomatic sinus bradycardia	Symptomatic patients with SND who have documented rates of <40 beats/min without a clear-cut association between significant symptoms and bradycardia	Asymptomatic SND
Symptomatic sinus bradycardia caused by long-term drug therapy of a type and at a dose for which there is no accepted alternative	Syncope of unexplained origin when major abnormalities of SND are discovered or provoked in electrophysiological studies	

to an infectious disease that will respond to appropriate treatment (e.g., Lyme disease), untreated sleep disorder with secondary conduction abnormalities, and hypervagal states.

Permanent pacing for patients with sinus node dysfunction after myocardial infarction is reserved for those who have symptoms during bradycardia. If drug therapy results in symptomatic bradycardia, criteria for permanent pacing should follow the guidelines given for sinus node dysfunction in Table 34-3.

Neurocardiogenic Syncope

Permanent pacing may be indicated for some of the several types of neurally mediated syncope. Neurally mediated syncope includes carotid sinus hypersensitivity and vasovagal syncope (see Chaps. 35 and 89).

The carotid sinus reflex is the physiological response to pressure applied to the carotid sinus. Although this reflex is physiological, some persons have an exaggerated or even pathological response. This reflex has two components, cardioinhibitory and vasodepressor. A cardioinhibitory response results predominantly from increased parasympathetic tone and may be manifested by sinus bradycardia, PR prolongation, or advanced AV block. The vasodepressor response is predominantly caused by sympathetic withdrawal and secondary hypotension. Although a pure cardioinhibitory or pure vasodepressor response can occur, a mixed response is most common. Tilt-table testing can provide the physiological environment for reproducing vasovagal syncope. It is important to document whether the predominant cause of symptoms is cardioinhibitory or vasodepressor, because therapy differs. Tilt-table testing is often helpful in determining the predominant cause (see Chap. 32).

Drugs such as beta blockers are commonly used as first-line therapy for neurally mediated syncope. Although some controversy persists, vasovagal syncope can often be aborted or blunted by dual-chamber pacing and, even if syncope does occur, pacing can prolong consciousness to avoid injury. In the North American Vasovagal Pacemaker Study I (VPS-I),[4] patients with recurrent syncope and a positive tilt test were randomized to dual-chamber pacemaker therapy with "rate drop" or to no pacemaker therapy—that is, no pacemaker implanted. The rate drop algorithm allows the pacemaker to pace at a faster rate if bradycardia suddenly occurs. The study was stopped prematurely because of the benefit observed with pacemaker therapy and showed that only 17 percent of paced patients had recurrent syncope, compared with 59 percent of patients without pacing.

A similar reduction in syncopal episodes was seen in the Vasovagal Syncope International Study (VASIS).[5] As part of the study inclusion criteria, this group of patients had experienced multiple episodes of vasovagal syncope. In the North American Vasovagal Pacemaker Study II (VPS-II),[6] all patients received a pacemaker implant and were then programmed to no pacing (ODO mode) or DDD with rate drop response. In contrast to the initial trial,[4] there was no statistically significant improvement in the group of patients programmed to active pacing with rate drop response.

Guidelines for permanent pacemaker implantation in carotid sinus hypersensitivity and neurocardiogenic syncope are given in Table 34G-7 (see Guidelines at the end of the chapter).

Pacing for the Prevention of Tachyarrhythmias

Permanent pacing is rarely used as the sole method to prevent ventricular tachyarrhythmias, because pacing therapies for ventricular rhythm disorders would most commonly be incorporated in an ICD. However, the guidelines include pacing for pause-dependent ventricular tachycardia (VT), with or without long-QT syndrome, when pacing efficacy is demonstrated as a class I indication for pacing. Pacing for congenital long-QT syndrome is considered a class IIa indication.

Pacing for the termination of AV reentrant or AV nodal reentrant supraventricular tachycardia not responsive to pharmacological or ablative therapy is a class IIb indication. Given the success of ablative and pharmacological approaches, pacing is almost never used for this indication.

Pacing to Prevent Atrial Fibrillation

Multisite and alternate site atrial pacing have been used to prevent recurrent atrial tachyarrhythmias (see Chap. 35). These techniques are thought to decrease the dispersion of refractoriness in the atrium.[7] Various techniques have been used to reduce or prevent atrial tachyarrhythmias. The designation of *dual-site atrial pacing* has generally been used to describe one lead in a standard right atrial position and the other lead in the coronary sinus or near the coronary sinus ostium (Fig. 34-1). With both leads connected to the same port, there is simultaneous pacing at both sites. In one randomized clinical trial, dual-site pacing decreased the number of episodes of paroxysmal atrial fibrillation and flutter and increased the time to recurrent atrial arrhythmias.[8] When no pacing was compared with dual-site or single-site atrial pacing, dual-site pacing was better, but single-site atrial pacing also resulted in significant improvement over no pacing. Single-site atrial septal pacing[9] and Bachmann's bundle pacing[10] have also been assessed. The experience with Bachmann's bundle pacing is very limited, but pacing this site was shown in a multicenter randomized study to shorten P wave duration compared with RAA pacing and, at 1 year, patients had a higher ($p < 0.05$) rate of survival (75 percent) free from chronic atrial fibrillation (AF) with Bachmann's bundle pacing than patients with pacing in the right atrial appendage (47 percent).[10]

Trials of atrial septal pacing have been inconsistent, although at least two prospective randomized studies have shown septal pacing to reduce the recurrence of paroxysmal AF and burden and progression to chronic AF when compared with pacing the right atrial appendage.[9,11,12]

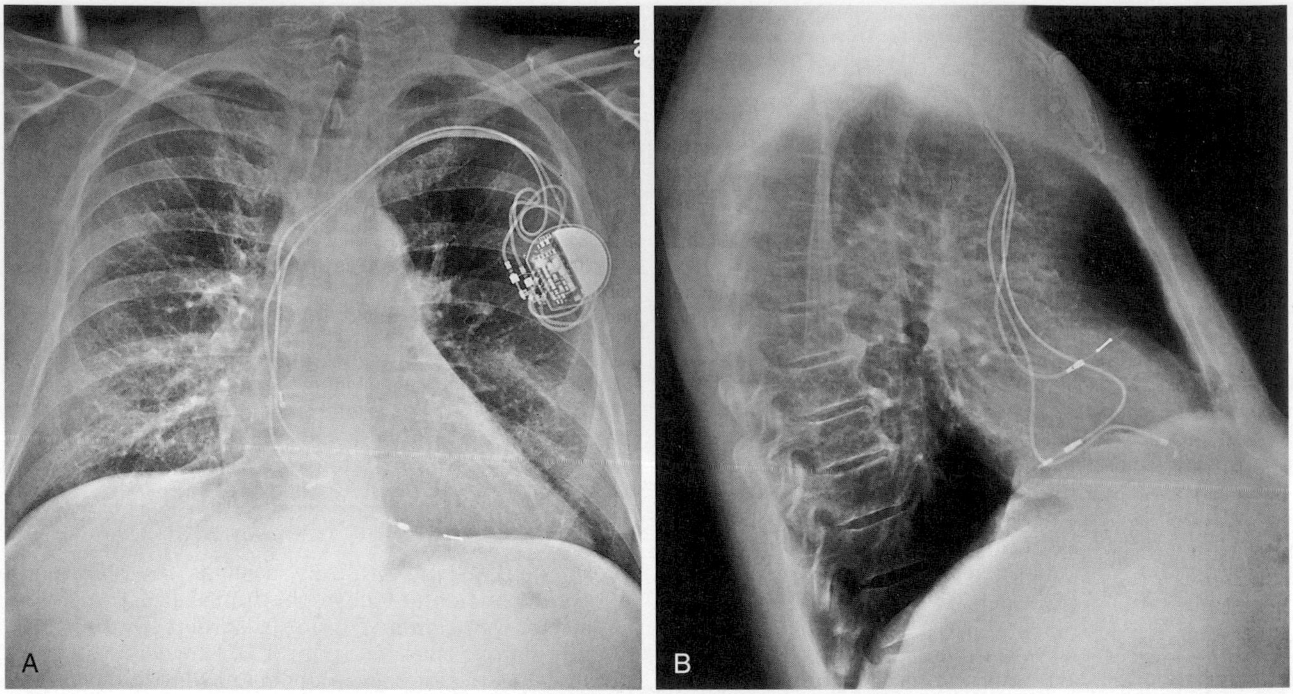

FIGURE 34–1 Posteroanterior **(A)** and lateral **(B)** chest radiographs in a patient with a dual-site atrial pacing system for the prevention of paroxysmal atrial fibrillation. Leads are positioned in the right atrium, near the coronary sinus ostium, and in the right ventricular apex.

Pacing algorithms have been incorporated into pacemakers in an effort to decrease the number of premature atrial complexes and to maintain consistent atrial pacing. Multiple algorithms have been developed, and some pacemakers include as many as four different algorithms. A schematic representation of an algorithm that alters atrial pacing rate as a result of an atrial sensed event is shown in Figure 34-2.

Clinical trials assessing atrial pacing algorithms have demonstrated mixed results. A reduction in AF burden was demonstrated in the Atrial Dynamic Overdrive Pacing Trial (ADOPT).[13]

In the ASPECT trial, the combination of three atrial prevention pacing algorithms did not decrease the frequency or burden of atrial tachyarrhythmias, as classified by the device, during a 3-month crossover period in bradycardic patients regardless of atrial lead position (i.e., septal or nonseptal). However, with the atrial septal pacing site and prevention algorithms "on," there was a decreased frequency of premature atrial contractions and fewer symptomatic atrial tachyarrhythmias.[11]

Even though the advantages of atrial pacing algorithms have yet to be shown definitively, the diagnostic data related to such algorithms have provided important information regarding AF-onset scenarios.[12] Several additional trials are under way, and it is likely that atrial pacing algorithms will be made available in most future dual-chamber pacemakers.

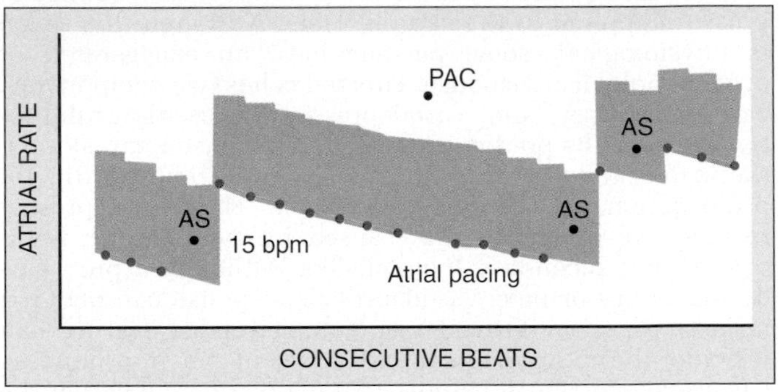

FIGURE 34–2 Schematic representation of an atrial pacing algorithm that increments the atrial pacing rate when a sensed atrial beat (AS) is detected to overdrive the intrinsic atrial rhythm consistently. The pacing rate would decrease after a specified period if no additional AS events were detected. bpm = beats/min; PAC = premature atrial complex.

Cardiac Resynchronization Therapy

Cardiac resynchronization therapy is the term applied to reestablishing synchronous contraction between the left ventricular free wall and ventricular septum in an attempt to improve left ventricular efficiency and, subsequently, to improve functional class. Generally, CRT has been used to describe biventricular ventricular pacing (Fig. 34-3), but cardiac resynchronization can be achieved by left ventricular pacing only in some patients. CRT-P devices are those that provide pacing support only, and CRT-D represents devices also capable of cardioversion and defibrillation (see Fig. 34-3A).[14]

Multiple randomized clinical trials have demonstrated the safety and efficacy of CRT. To date, more than 4000 patients have been included in completed randomized clinical trials of CRT.[15-24]

The inclusion criteria for clinical trials have been relatively narrow. This has resulted in convincing data for the criteria included, such as New York Heart Association (NYHA) functional Class III and IV, wide QRS complex, normal sinus rhythm, and biventricular pacing configuration.

Most trials have relied on primary endpoints reflecting functional status, specifically the 6-minute walk test, NYHA functional class, and quality of life. More recent trials have used composite endpoints, including outcomes such as cardiac mortality, all-cause mortality, and hospitalization for congestive heart failure.

Randomized clinical trials have been consistent in demonstrating improvement in the 6-minute walk, NYHA functional class, and quality of life assessed with the Minnesota Living With Heart Failure questionnaire. Some exceptions exist and will be detailed by individual trial.

Relative consistency in some secondary endpoints has also been found. In the studies assessing peak $\dot{V}O_2$, with the exception of InSync ICD II, in which only patients in NYHA Class II were enrolled, there has been a consistent improvement in this endpoint. Echocardiographic variables, specifically left ventricular end-diastolic dimension, have consistently shown a decrease in left ventricular dimensions, suggesting reverse left ventricular remodeling. When mitral regurgitation has been assessed, it has decreased after CRT. CRT trials are summarized in Table 34-4.

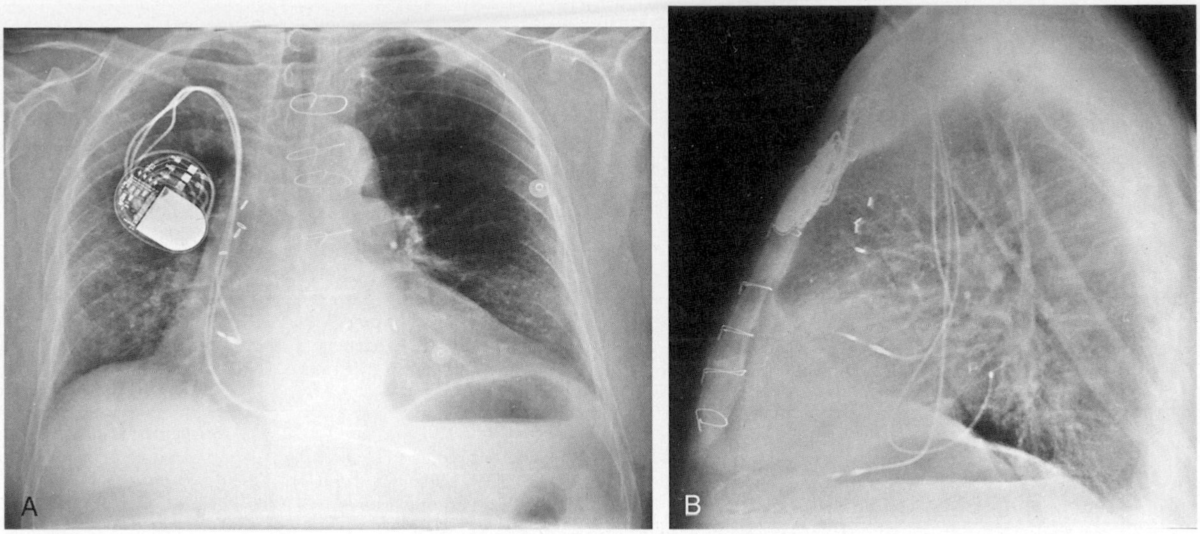

FIGURE 34–3 Posteroanterior **(A)** and **(B)** lateral chest radiographs demonstrating a biventricular pacing system. There are three leads—the first is positioned in the right atrium, the second is positioned in the right ventricular apex, and the third courses posteriorly in the coronary sinus and into the posterolateral cardiac vein.

On the basis of clinical trial results, the U.S. Food and Drug Administration labeling criteria for CRT are the following: NYHA functional Class III or IV, QRS longer than 120 milliseconds, left ventricular ejection fraction of 0.35, optimized medical therapy, and normal sinus rhythm.

Hypertrophic Obstructive Cardiomyopathy (see Chap. 65)

Dual-chamber pacing has been used to treat patients who have severe, symptomatic, medically refractory hypertrophic obstructive cardiomyopathy (HCM),[25-27] based on the concept that the altered septal activation caused by right ventricular apical pacing results in less narrowing of the left ventricular outflow tract and a subsequent decrease in the Venturi effect responsible for systolic anterior motion of the mitral valve.

Pacing in HCM has been the subject of several clinical trials. In general, the trials have demonstrated a decrease in left ventricular outflow gradient but no significant differences in exercise capacity, quality of life score, treadmill exercise time, and peak oxygen consumption.[25-27] Therefore, pacing should not be regarded as a primary treatment for HCM in the absence of an indication for antibradycardia pacing and is currently a class IIb indication according to ACC/AHA guidelines.[2] However, ICD therapy is increasingly used in this subset of patients (see later).

Selection of the Appropriate Pacing Mode

After an indication for pacing has been identified, the next step should be to select the most appropriate pacing mode for the patient. Factors to consider when choosing the pacing mode include the following: underlying rhythm disturbance, including chronotropic response to exercise, overall physical condition, associated medical problems, and exercise capacity.

The effect of pacing mode on morbidity and mortality has been the basis of multiple randomized clinical trials (Table 34-5). In patients with sinus node dysfunction randomized to AAI or VVI pacing, Andersen and colleagues[28] demonstrated a higher incidence of AF in the VVI group and a higher incidence of thromboembolism in the VVI group than in the AAI group ($p = 0.0083$). Although no difference in mortality could be detected with the initial analysis at 3.3 years, subsequent analysis at 5.5 years showed improved survival and less heart failure in the AAI group.[28] In addition, there was a persistent decrease in the incidences of AF and thromboembolic events. This trial stands alone in demonstrating a lower mortality with physiological pacing, perhaps because the physiological pacing mode implemented was AAI mode. With AAI pacing, the patient maintains intrinsic AV conduction and avoids the abnormal depolarization pattern of right ventricular pacing that would occur with VVI or DDD pacing.

The Pacemaker Selection in the Elderly (PASE) trial, a prospective, randomized, single-blind trial, compared DDDR and VVIR pacing modes[29] and found no statistically significant difference in quality of life between DDDR and VVIR pacing modes, but there was a trend toward improved quality of life in patients with sinus node dysfunction randomized to dual-chamber pacing. Perhaps more significant was a crossover of 26 percent of patients intolerant of ventricular pacing to dual-chamber pacing.

The Canadian Trial of Physiologic Pacing (CTOPP)[30] compared VVIR with DDDR or AAIR and had primary endpoints of overall mortality and cerebrovascular accidents and secondary endpoints of AF, hospitalizations for congestive heart failure, and death resulting from a cardiac cause. CTOPP demonstrated that physiological pacing (DDD/AAI) was associated with a reduced incidence of chronic AF but no difference in quality of life or mortality.

The Mode Selection Trial (MOST) also randomized patients with sinus node dysfunction to VVI or DDD pacing, with primary endpoints of all-cause mortality and cerebrovascular accidents.[31] MOST failed to demonstrate any difference in mortality but did demonstrate a lower incidence of AF with physiological pacing and also reduced signs and symptoms of heart failure and slightly improved quality of life. The study concluded that, overall, dual-chamber pacing offers significant improvement compared with ventricular pacing.

The United Kingdom Pacing and Cardiovascular Events (UKPACE) trial compared DDD with VVI pacing modes in patients 70 years and older who required permanent pacing for second- or third-degree AV block.[32] This trial showed no significant difference between pacing modes in the primary endpoint of all-cause mortality or in the composite secondary endpoint of cardiovascular deaths, AF, heart failure hospitalizations, cerebrovascular accidents or thromboembolic events, and reoperation.

The DAVID (Dual Chamber and VVI Implantable Defibrillator) trial was designed to assess the effect of dual-chamber pacing versus backup ventricular pacing in patients with an ICD indication but no indication for antibradycardia pacing, no history of recurrent atrial arrhythmias, and a left ventricular ejection fraction of 0.40.[34] Patients were randomized to DDDR pacing with a lower rate of 70 beats/min versus VVI-backup pacing at 40 beats/min. Dual-chamber pacing offered no advantage and actually increased the combined endpoint of death or hospitalization for heart failure.

Further evidence of the adverse effects of right ventricular apical pacing when no ventricular pacing was required was demonstrated by substudies of the MOST trial.[35] Investigators from this trial demonstrated that in patients with a normal baseline QRS duration, the cumulative percentage of ventricular pacing is a strong predictor of

TABLE 34–4 CRT-P AND CRT-D Randomized Clinical Trials

Study	Design	No. of Patients	End Points: *Primary*	End Points: *Secondary*	Results
PATH-CHF[14]	Crossover	41	Peak $\dot{V}O_2$, 6-min walk	Hospitalizations, NYHA class, QOL	Chronic improvement in 6-min walk, QOL, NYHA class
MUSTIC-SR[15]	Crossover	58	6-min walk	NYHA class, QOL	Sustained improvement in 6-min walk, NYHA class, QOL, peak $\dot{V}O_2$, hospitalizations reduced with CRT at $p < 0.05$
MUSTIC-AF[16]	Crossover	43	6-min walk	NYHA class, QOL, peak $\dot{V}O_2$, worsening CHF, patient preference, total mortality	Sustained improvement in 6-min walk, NYHA class, QOL, peak $\dot{V}O_2$, fewer hospitalizations with CRT
MIRACLE[17]	Parallel arms	453	6-min walk, NYHA class, QOL	Peak $\dot{V}O_2$ Exercise time, LVEF, LVEDD, MR, QRS duration, clinical composite response	Sustained improvement in all three primary endpoints
MIRACLE-ICD[18]	Parallel arms	555	6-min walk, NYHA class, QOL	Peak $\dot{V}O_2$, exercise time, clinical composite response	Improvement in QOL and functional class No improvement in 6-min walk
COMPANION[19]	Parallel arms	1520	Primary composite endpoint was time to death or hospitalization for any cause	All-cause mortality, cardiac morbidity, maximal exercise	CRT and CRT-D reduced risk of primary endpoint
CARE-HF[20]	Open label randomization to control versus CRT device	813	All-cause mortality	All-cause mortality; all-cause mortality and unplanned hospitalizations for or with CHF; days alive and not in hospital for unplanned cardiovascular cause during the minimum period of follow-up; days alive and not in hospital for any reason during minimum period of follow-up; NYHA class at 90 days; QOL at 90 days; patient status at end of study	CRT (without defibrillation) improved symptoms and QOL and reduced complications and risk of death
PATH-CHF II[21]	Crossover (no pacing versus LV pacing)	86	$\dot{V}O_2$ peak, $\dot{V}O_2$ anaerobic, 6-min walk	QOL, NYHA class	Exercise tolerance, 6-min walk, and QOL improved
MIRACLE-ICD II[22]	Parallel arms	186	$\dot{V}O_2$	$\dot{V}E/\dot{V}O_2$, NYHA class, QOL, 6-min walk, LV volume, LVEF, composite clinical response	Improvement in QOL, functional status, exercise capacity
CONTAK-CD[23]	Crossover and parallel controlled	490	6-min walk, NYHA class, QOL	Composite of mortality, CHF, hospitalizations, VT, VF	Trend toward decreased morbidity and mortality end point Improvement in exercise capacity, QOL, and NYHA class
RD-CHF[24]	Crossover in patients already paced with class III or IV CHF (RV versus biventricular pacing)	44	6-min walk, NYHA class, QOL	QRS width, hospitalizations	In previously paced patients, upgrading from RV to biventricular pacing significantly improves symptoms and exercise tolerance

CARE-HF = Cardiac Resynchronization in Heart Failure; CHF = congestive heart failure; COMPANION = Comparison of Medical Therapy, Pacing, and Defibrillation in Heart Failure; CONTAK-CD = Contak Cardioverter-Defibrillator; CRT = cardiac resynchronization therapy; CRT-D = CRT with defibrillator; CRT-P = CRT-pacing only; ICD = implantable cardioverter-defibrillator; LV = left ventricular; LVEDD = left ventricular end-diastolic dimension; LVEF = left ventricular ejection fraction; MIRACLE = Multicenter InSync Randomized Clinical Evaluation; MIRACLE-ICD = Multicenter InSync Randomized Clinical Evaluation-Implantable Cardioverter-Defibrillator; MR = mitral regurgitation; MUSTIC-AF = Multisite Stimulation in Cardiomyopathy-Atrial Fibrillation; MUSTIC-SR = Multisite Stimulation in Cardiomyopathy-Sinus Rhythm; NYHA = New York Heart Association; PATH-CHF = Pacing Therapy in Congestive Heart Failure; QOL = quality of life; RV = right ventricular; VF = ventricular fibrillation; VT = ventricular tachycardia.

TABLE 34–5 Trials Assessing the Effect of Pacing Mode on Morbidity and Mortality

Study	Patient Inclusion Criteria	Endpoints	Treatment Arms	Results
Danish study[28]	Sick sinus syndrome requiring pacing	Mortality, cardiovascular death, AF, TE events, heart failure, AV block	AAI pacing (n = 110) versus VVI pacing (n = 115)	Cumulative incidence of CV death, PAF, chronic AF, and TE events lower with AAI pacing; less severe heart failure with AAI; multivariate analysis—AAI associated with freedom from TE events, survival from CV death
PASE[29]	Age ≥65 yr, need for PPM for prevention or treatment of bradycardia	QOL, all-cause mortality, first nonfatal CVA or death, first hospitalization for CHF, AF, PM syndrome	Single-blind, randomized, controlled comparison; VVIR pacing versus DDDR pacing	QOL improved significantly, but no difference between pacing modes; 26% of patients with VVIR cross over to DDDR because of PM syndrome; trends of borderline statistical significance in endpoints favoring DDDR in patients with SND
CTOPP[30]	Initial PM, life expectancy >1 yr, not in chronic AF	Cardiovascular mortality or stroke, paroxysmal or chronic AF, hospitalization for CHF, QOL, 6-min walk	DDDR or AAIR pacing versus VVIR pacing	No difference in QOL, VI versus DDD/AAI, no statistically significant difference in mortality or stroke, no difference in hospitalizations, 24% decreased incidence of chronic or paroxysmal AF with DDD/AAI
MOST[31]	SND requiring PM, NSR or atrial standstill at time of implantation	Stroke, health status, cost-effectiveness, total mortality, CV mortality, AF, HF score, PM syndrome	DDDR versus VVIR	Lower incidence of AF with DDDR No difference in any other endpoint
UKPACE[32]	AV block requiring PM, age ≥70 yr	All-cause mortality, composite endpoint of CV deaths, HF hospitalization, AF, CVA or events, reoperation	DDDR versus VVI or VVIR	No difference in any endpoint
DANPACE[33]	Tachycardia-bradycardia syndrome with normal AV conduction	All-cause mortality, CV mortality, incidence of AF and TE events, QOL, cost-effectiveness	AAIR versus DDDR	In progress

AF = atrial fibrillation; AV = atrioventricular; CHF = congestive heart failure; CTOPP = Canadian Trial of Physiologic Pacing; CV = cardiovascular; CVA = cardiovascular accident; DANPACE = Danish Pacing Trial; HF = heart failure; MOST = Mode Selection Trial; NSR = normal sinus rhythm; PAF = paroxysmal atrial fibrillation; PASE = Pacemaker Selection in the Elderly; PM = pacemaker; PPM = permanent pacemaker; QOL = quality of life; SND = sinus node dysfunction; TE = thromboembolic; UKPACE = United Kingdom Pacing and Cardiovascular Events.

hospitalization for heart failure, and the risk of AF also increases linearly with the cumulative percentage of ventricular pacing. This occurs even when AV synchrony is preserved.

These findings have led to pacing algorithms that avoid ventricular pacing. Rather than placing a pacemaker capable only of atrial pacing, dual-chamber pacemakers, which dynamically alter the AV interval to allow intrinsic ventricular depolarization, and other pacemakers may allow one or more P waves to occur without a subsequent pacemaker output in an effort to promote intrinsic ventricular depolarization (Fig. 34-4).

Modes and Timing Cycles

The advantages and disadvantages of each pacing mode cannot be comprehended completely unless the timing cycle of each is understood.

Single-Chamber Triggered Pacing

Single-chamber triggered pacing (AAT and VVT) releases an output pulse every time a native event is sensed. This feature increases the current drain on the battery, accelerating its rate of depletion, and deforms the inscription of the intrinsic spontaneous complex on the electrocardiogram (ECG). However, it can serve as an excellent marker for the site of sensing within an intrinsic complex and can prevent inappropriate inhibition from oversensing when the patient does not have a stable escape rhythm. Triggered pacing is used infrequently.

Ventricular-Inhibited Pacing

VVI is a pacing mode that incorporates sensing on the ventricular channel, enabling a sensed ventricular event to inhibit pacemaker output (Fig. 34-5). VVI pacemakers are refractory for an interval after a paced or sensed ventricular event, the ventricular refractory period (VRP). Any ventricular event occurring within the VRP is not sensed and does not reset timing.

VVI pacing protects the patient from lethal bradycardias, but it does not restore or maintain AV synchrony and does not provide rate responsiveness in the patient who is chronotropically incompetent—that is, the patient in whom the spontaneous sinus heart rate does not increase in response to a physiological demand. In addition, some patients with VVI pacing experience symptomatic hemodynamic deterioration during ventricular pacing. Adverse hemodynamics associated with a normally functioning pacing system that cause overt symptoms or limit the patient's ability to achieve optimal functional status is referred to as *pacemaker syndrome.* This syndrome was initially recognized with VVI pacing but can occur with any pacing mode if there is AV dissociation. The most common symptoms of pacemaker

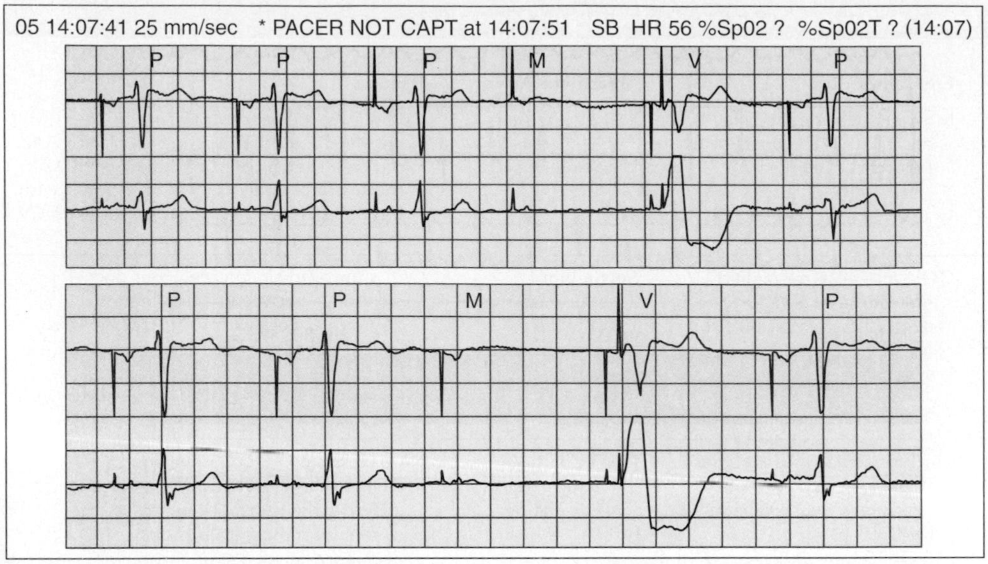

FIGURE 34–4 Example of ventricular avoidance pacing. The MVP Pacing Mode (Medtronic) provides functional AAIR pacing with the ventricular pacing support in the presence of transient or persistent loss of conduction. This promotes atrioventricular conduction by reducing unnecessary right ventricular pacing and decreases the cumulative percentage of right ventricular pacing.

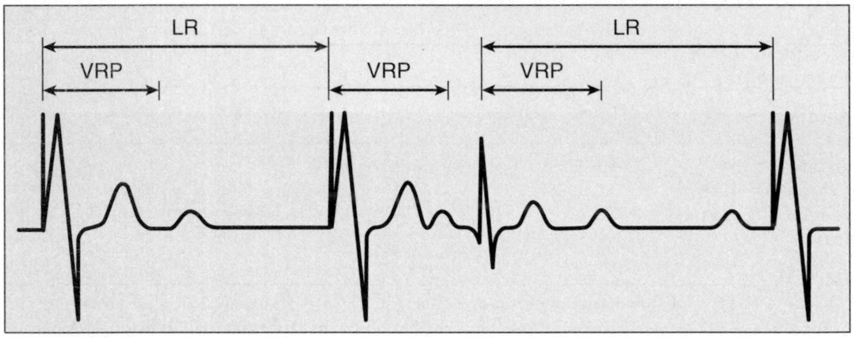

FIGURE 34–5 The VVI timing cycle consists of a defined lower rate limit (LR) and a ventricular refractory period (VRP). When the LR timer is complete, a pacing artifact is delivered in the absence of a sensed intrinsic ventricular event. If an intrinsic QRS occurs, the LR timer is started from that point. A VRP begins with any sensed or paced ventricular activity.

syndrome include general malaise, shortness of breath, dizziness, fatigue, pulsations in the neck or abdomen, cough, and atypical chest pain. The incidence of pacemaker syndrome is difficult to determine and depends on how the syndrome is defined.

Atrial-Inhibited Pacing

AAI pacing mode incorporates the same timing cycles, with the obvious difference that pacing and sensing occur from the atrium and pacemaker output is inhibited by a sensed atrial event (Fig. 34-6). An atrial-paced or sensed event initiates a refractory period during which no spontaneous event is sensed by the pacemaker. When the atrial timing cycle ends, the atrial pacing artifact is delivered regardless of ventricular events because an AAI pacemaker should not sense ventricular events. The single exception to this rule is far-field sensing; that is, the ventricular signal is large enough to be inappropriately sensed by the atrial lead. In this situation, the atrial timing cycle is reset by events sensed in the ventricle. Sometimes this abnormality can be corrected by making the atrial channel less sensitive or by lengthening the refractory period.

AAI pacing is appropriate for patients with sinus node dysfunction and normal AV conduction. The obvious disadvantage of atrial pacing is lack of ventricular support should AV block occur. If the patient with sinus node dysfunction is assessed carefully for AV node disease at the time of pacemaker implantation, the occurrence of clinically significant AV node disease is very low (less than 2 percent per year). Assessment before use of an AAI system should include incremental atrial pacing at the time of pacemaker implantation. Although criteria vary among institutions and implanting physicians, the adult patient should be capable of 1:1 AV node conduction to rates of 120 to 140 beats/min.

Dual-Chamber Pacing

AV SEQUENTIAL, NON-P-SYNCHRONOUS PACING. AV sequential, non-P-synchronous pacing (DDI) is a pacing mode with dual-chamber sensing that incorporates atrial sensing as well as ventricular sensing, which prevents competitive atrial pacing (Fig. 34-7). The DDI mode of response is inhibition only; that is, no tracking of P waves can occur. Therefore, the programmed rate, which by definition is the lower rate because only a single rate exists, is the fastest paced rate that can be seen. DDI is rarely the preimplantation mode of choice but remains a programmable option in most dual-chamber pacemakers. The DDI pacing mode could be considered for patients with intermittent atrial tachyarrhythmias, but a mode that maintains P-wave tracking (e.g., DDD or DDDR) with mode switching is preferable.

ATRIAL SYNCHRONOUS PACING. Atrial synchronous (VDD) pacemakers pace only in the ventricle, sense in both chambers, and respond by inhibition of ventricular output caused by intrinsic ventricular activity and by ventricular tracking of P waves. VDD pacing can be accomplished with a single-lead pacing system in which the lead is capable of pacing in the ventricle in response to sensing atrial activity by way of a remote electrode situated on the intra-atrial portion of the ventricular pacing lead.

In the VDD mode, sensed atrial events initiate the AV interval (AVI). If an intrinsic ventricular event occurs before the termination of the AVI, ventricular output is inhibited and the lower rate timing cycle is reset (Fig. 34-8). If a paced ventricular beat occurs at the end of the AVI, this beat resets the lower rate. If no atrial event occurs, the pacemaker escapes with a paced ventricular event at the lower rate limit—that is, the pacemaker displays VVI activity in the absence of a sensed atrial event. VDD pacing may be appropriate for the patient with normal sinus node function and conduction disease of the AV node.

DUAL-CHAMBER PACING AND SENSING WITH INHIBITION AND TRACKING. In the dual-chamber pacing and sensing with inhibition and tracking (DDD) mode, the basic timing circuit associated with lower rate pacing is divided into two intervals: the ventriculoatrial (VA) interval and the AVI. The AVI may be defined as AV sequential pacing initiated by pacing with subsequent intrinsic ventricular conduction or by a native P wave with subsequent ventricular pacing (Fig. 34-9).

The postventricular atrial refractory period (PVARP) is the period after a sensed or paced ventricular event during which the atrial sensing circuit is refractory. Any atrial event occurring during the PVARP is not sensed by the atrial sensing circuit. If a P wave occurs after the PVARP and is sensed, no atrial pacing artifact is delivered at the end of the VA interval (see Fig. 34-9). Because the maximum tracking rate of the pacemaker is determined by the total atrial refractory period (TARP), the PVARP is a significant determinant of the upper rate limit. *The PVARP is especially important for the prevention of endless loop, or pacemaker-mediated, tachycardia.*

Normal DDD function can appear electrocardiographically as (1) normal sinus rhythm, (2) atrial pacing only, (3) AV sequential pacing, or (4) P-synchronous pacing.

DDD pacing mode is most appropriate for patients with normal sinus node function and AV block. DDD pacing has limitations in the patient with sinus node dysfunction, because P-synchronous pacing is not possible in chronic AF or in patients with a paralyzed or nonexcitable atrium. Also, DDD pacing does not restore rate response in the patient who is chronotropically incompetent. The vast majority of dual-chamber pacing systems implanted are DDDR devices. Even if the patient is chronotropically competent at the time of implantation, the DDDR device allows the greatest long-term flexibility to meet any subsequent needs of the patient.

In any pacemaker capable of P-synchronous pacing, endless loop tachycardia, also called *pacemaker reentrant tachycardia* or *pacemaker-mediated tachycardia,* can result. If AV synchrony is dissociated by any event, most commonly a premature ventricular complex (PVC), retrograde VA conduction can result in a retrograde P wave (Fig. 34-10). If the retrograde P wave is sensed by the atrial sensing circuit of the pacemaker, the AVI is initiated, resulting in a paced ventricular complex at a cycle length approximately equal to the maximum tracking rate. The paced ventricular event can again result in retrograde VA conduction, perpetuating this rapid reentrant circuit. Endless loop tachycardia can be prevented by a PVARP that is long enough to prevent sensing of the retrograde P wave. Most pacemakers also have specific algorithms that attempt to recognize and abort endless loop tachycardia.

Indications for Rate-Adaptive Pacing

Rate-adaptive pacemakers have the ability to increase the pacing rate through sensors that monitor one or more physiological parameters, such as activity and minute ventilation. Single-chamber rate-adaptive pacing (AAIR, VVIR) has timing cycles that are not significantly different from those of its non–rate-adaptive counterparts. The difference lies in the potential variability of the paced rate. Depending on the sensor incorporated and the level of exertion of the patient, the basic interval shortens from the programmed lower rate limit to an upper rate limit programmed to define the absolute shortest cycle length allowable.

VVIR pacing, like VVI, is generally contraindicated if ventricular pacing results in retrograde (VA) conduction or a decrease in blood pressure. Also, if the sinus node is normal, P-synchronous pacing should be considered the optimal method to achieve rate responsiveness.

AAIR pacing can be considered for the patient with sinus node dysfunction and

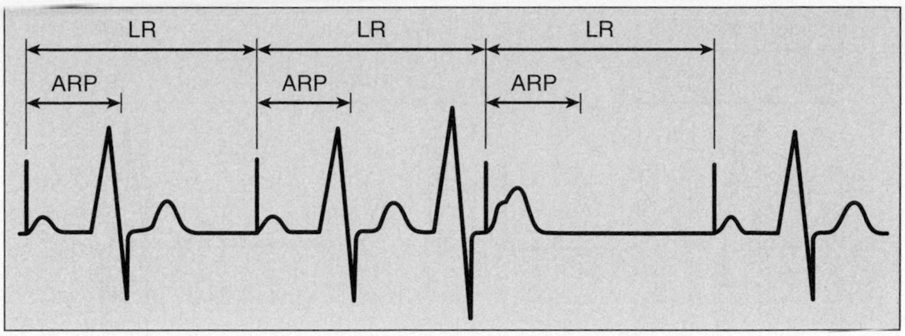

FIGURE 34–6 The AAI timing cycle consists of a defined lower rate (LR) limit and an atrial refractory period (ARP). When the LR cycle is complete, a pacing artifact is delivered in the atrium in the absence of a sensed atrial event. If an intrinsic P wave occurs, the LR timer is started from that point. An ARP begins with any sensed or paced atrial activity. The AAI timing cycle should not be affected by events in the ventricle. In this schematic example, a premature ventricular contraction (PVC) occurs. Appropriately, it is not sensed by the AAI pacemaker, and the atrial pacing artifact occurs in the T wave of the PVC. Even though atrial capture presumably would occur, there is no ventricular event after the paced atrial event because the ventricle is still refractory. However, the timing cycle will be reset by anything that is sensed on the atrial sensing circuit. In this schematic example, a PVC occurs. Appropriately, it is not sensed, and the pacing artifact is delivered after the PVC. Even though there appears to be atrial depolarization, no intrinsic ventricular depolarization occurs because the ventricle is refractory.

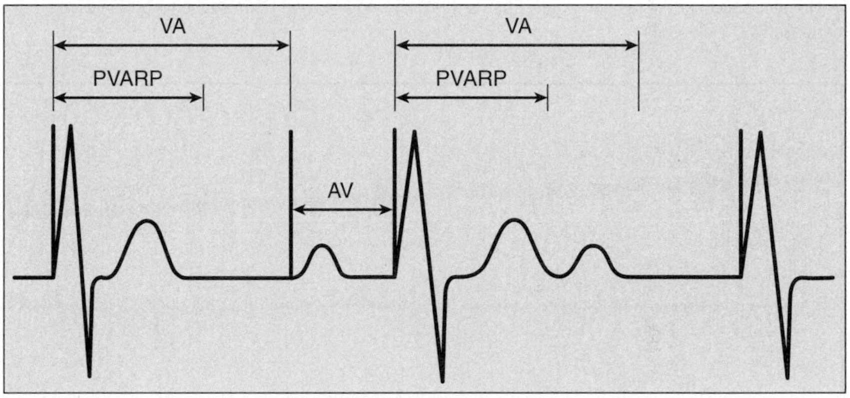

FIGURE 34–7 The timing cycle in DDI pacing consists of a lower rate limit, an atrioventricular (AV) interval, a ventricular refractory period, and an atrial refractory period. The ventricular refractory period is initiated by any sensed or paced ventricular activity, and the atrial refractory period is initiated by any sensed or paced atrial activity. The lower rate limit cannot be violated, even if the sinus rate is occurring at a faster rate. PVARP = postventricular atrial refractory period; VA = ventriculoatrial.

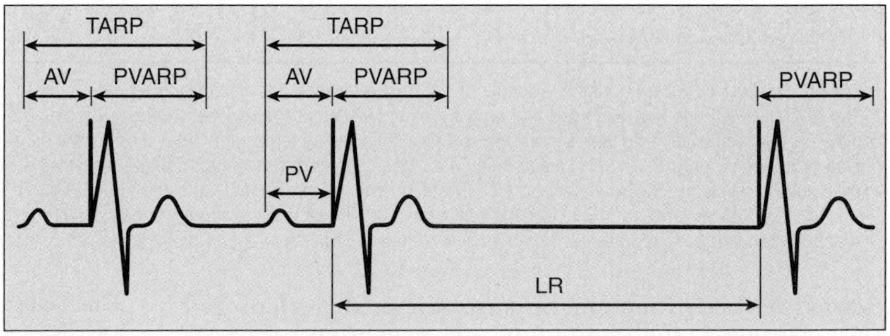

FIGURE 34–8 The timing cycle of VDD consists of a lower rate (LR) limit, an atrioventricular (AV) interval, a ventricular refractory period, a postventricular atrial refractory period (PVARP), and an upper rate limit. A sensed P wave initiates the AV interval (during the AV interval, the atrial sensing channel is refractory). At the end of the AV interval, a ventricular pacing artifact is delivered if no intrinsic ventricular activity has been sensed; this represents P wave tracking pacing. Ventricular activity, paced or sensed, initiates the PVARP and the ventriculoatrial interval (the LR limit interval minus the AV interval). If no P wave activity occurs, the pacemaker escapes with a ventricular pacing artifact at the LR limit. PV = interval from intrinsic atrial event to paced ventricular event; TARP = total atrial refractory period.

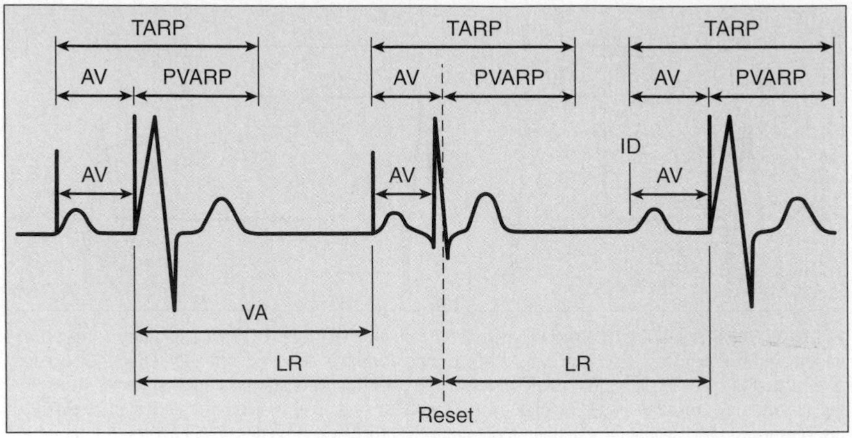

FIGURE 34–9 The timing cycle in DDD consists of a lower rate (LR) limit, an atrioventricular (AV) interval, a postventricular atrial refractory period (PVARP), and an upper rate limit. The AV interval and PVARP together comprise the total atrial refractory period (TARP). If intrinsic atrial and ventricular activity occur before the LR times out, both channels are inhibited and no pacing occurs. If no intrinsic atrial or ventricular activity occurs, there is AV sequential pacing (first sequence). If no atrial activity is sensed before the ventriculoatrial (VA) interval is completed, an atrial pacing artifact is delivered, which initiates the AV interval. If intrinsic ventricular activity occurs before the termination of the AV interval, the ventricular output from the pacemaker is inhibited—that is, atrial pacing (second sequence). If a P wave is sensed before the VA interval is completed, output from the atrial channel is inhibited. The AV interval is initiated and, if no ventricular activity is sensed before the AV interval terminates, a ventricular pacing artifact is delivered—that is, P-synchronous pacing (third sequence). ID = intrinsic deflection.

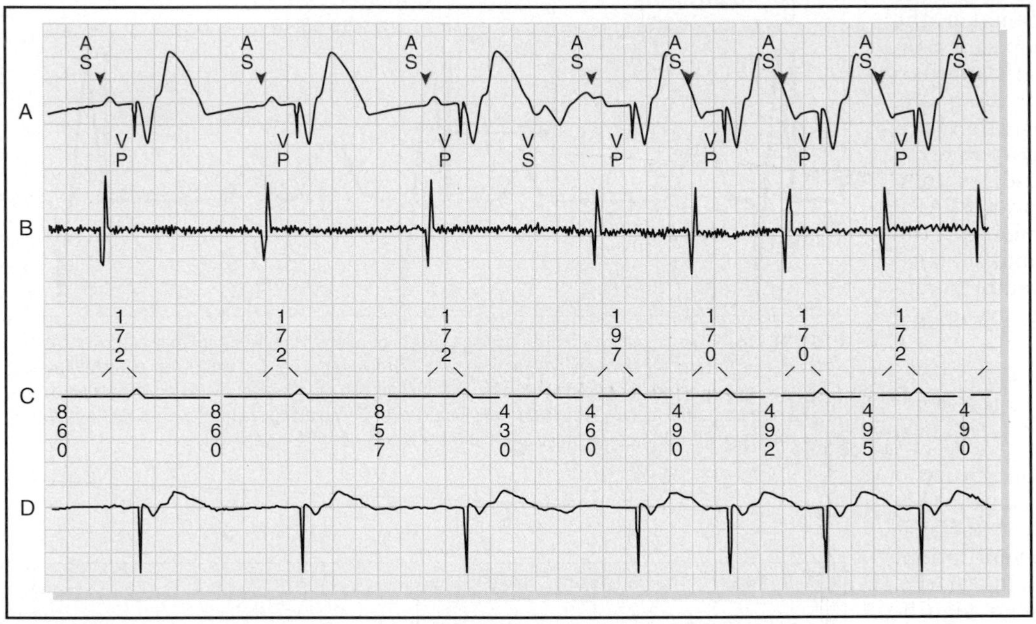

FIGURE 34–10 Electrocardiographic example of pacemaker-mediated tachycardia in a patient whose device is programmed to the DDD pacing mode. The electrocardiographic tracing **(A)** demonstrates P-synchronous pacing. The third paced QRS complex is followed by a ventricular-sensed event that is followed by retrograde atrial sensing and subsequent ventricular pacing at a rate of approximately 115 beats/min. This appearance is consistent with pacemaker-mediated tachycardia, or endless loop tachycardia. **B,** Atrial electrogram. **C,** Marker channel. **D,** Ventricular electrogram. AS = atrial sensed event; VP = ventricular paced event; VS = ventricular sensed event. Arrows indicate sensed or paced events. Numbers above the line indicate milliseconds between events. Numbers below the line indicate milliseconds between ventricular events.

normal AV node function, because this mode restores rate responsiveness and maintains AV synchrony. If AAIR pacing is contemplated, normal AV node conduction must first be determined, as discussed earlier for AAI pacing.

DDDR pacemakers are capable of all the variations described for DDD pacemakers. In addition to using P-synchronous pacing as a method for increasing heart rate, the sensor incorporated in the pacemaker can also drive the increase in heart rate. The resulting rhythm can be sinus driven or sensor driven. The ideal patient for DDDR pacing is one with combined sinus node and AV node dysfunction, because this mode allows restoration of rate responsiveness and AV synchrony.

Algorithms for determining the appropriate pacing mode for patients with sinus node disease and AV node disease are shown in Figure 34-11. The first and more complex algorithm (see Fig. 34-11A) considers most of the available pacing modes. The second algorithm (see Fig. 34-11B) is simpler and assumes that a pacemaker capable of rate adaptation is used. Because the cost has narrowed between DDD and DDDR and VVI and VVIR pacemakers, devices with rate-adaptive capability have dominated the U.S. market.

Selecting the Appropriate Sensor for Rate Adaptive Pacing

Although a number of sensors have been used clinically (some with clinical potential), only activity sensors, minute ventilation sensors, and stimulus-T (QT interval) sensors have achieved clinical acceptance.[36]

ACTIVITY SENSORS. Activity sensing with vibration detection (piezoelectric crystal or accelerometer) has been the most widely used form of rate adaptation because it is simple, easy to apply clinically, and rapid in onset of rate response. Accelerometers have become the activity sensor of choice, having been shown to have a slightly more physiological response than piezoelectric crystal sensors.[37]

MINUTE VENTILATION SENSORS. The minute ventilation (respiratory rate × tidal volume) sensor has an excellent correlation with metabolic demand. In a rate-adaptive pacing system, minute volume is determined by emission of a small charge of known current from the pacemaker and measurement of the resulting voltage at the lead tip. When both current and voltage are known, transthoracic impedance can be measured between the ring electrode and the pacemaker. Because transthoracic impedance varies with respiration and its amplitude varies with tidal volume, the impedance measurement can be used to determine respiratory rate and tidal volume. A pacing algorithm uses the minute volume measurements to alter pacing rate. Long-term reliability of the minute ventilation sensor has been excellent.

STIMULUS-T OR QT-SENSING PACEMAKER. The interval from the onset of a paced QRS complex to the end of the T wave has been used successfully for rate adaptation for many years. Autonomic activity and heart rate affect the stimulus-T interval, and the relationship allows measurement of the stimulus-T interval to be used for rate adaptation.

DUAL-SENSOR COMBINATIONS. The overall performance of market-approved, single-sensor rate-adaptive systems has been excellent. However, sensors have been combined in an effort to mimic more

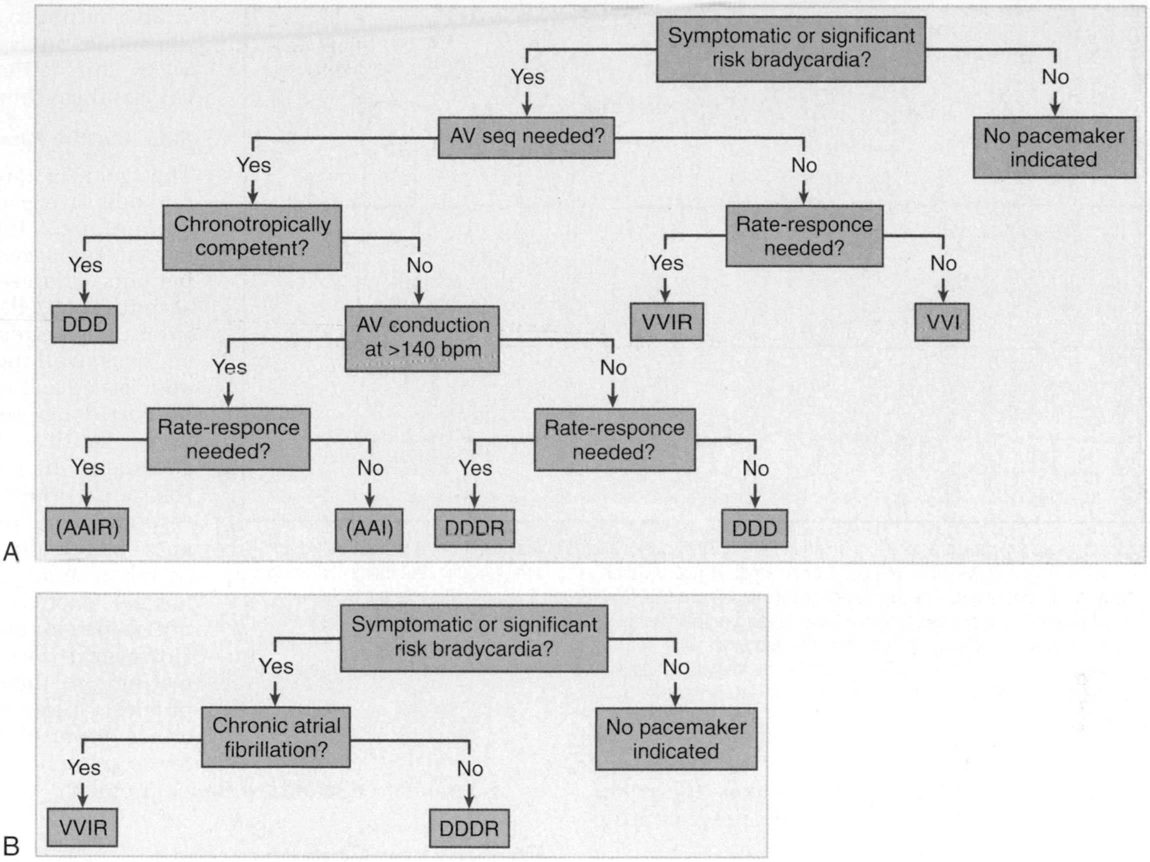

FIGURE 34–11 Algorithms for pacemaker mode selection. **A,** Choice of VVI, VVIR, AAI, AAIR, DDD, or DDDR is allowed. **B,** Only VVIR or DDDR is selected. AV = atrioventricular; bpm = beats/min; seq = sequence.

closely the normal sinus node at all levels of activity and during emotional stress.[37]

The perfect sensor would be resistant to nonphysiological stimuli. A multisensor rate-adaptive pacing system can improve specificity by having one sensor verify or cross-check the other. For example, if one sensor indicates a rate increase and the other does not, a rate increase would not occur. Both sensors would have to be concordant for a sensor-driven rate increase to be allowed.

Pulse Generator Implantation

Only qualified physicians should undertake pacemaker or ICD implantation. The recommended training requirements for pacemaker implantation are as follows[38]: a base of core knowledge for pacemaker follow-up; participation in at least 100 pacemaker follow-up visits; participation in at least 50 initial transvenous pacemaker implantations as the primary operator (it is recommended that at least 50 percent of these be dual-chamber); participation in at least 20 revisions of pacing systems; exposure to lead extraction techniques (suggested); and thorough knowledge of recognition and treatment of pacemaker and surgical complications and emergencies.

Almost all pacemakers and defibrillators are implanted transvenously, with the pulse generator placed in the upper anterior portion of the chest, just anterior to the pectoralis major muscle. Epicardial pacing is usually considered only in persons without venous access—that is, no access to the right ventricle because of an associated congenital anomaly, a prosthetic tricuspid valve, occlusion of central veins used for lead placement, or an intracardiac shunt that could predispose the patient to systemic thromboembolic events if a transvenous lead were present.

Although multiple venous routes have been used for lead placement, the axillary, subclavian, and cephalic veins are most commonly used. The subclavian approach involves a subclavian puncture and the use of one or more peel-away introducers. A lateral approach to the subclavian vein, often lateral enough to be the axillary vein, is preferred to minimize the risk of pneumothorax and to avoid subclavian crush injury to the lead, which is more common when a medial approach is used. The cephalic vein is often large enough to accept one or two pacing leads, and this approach avoids the risks associated with subclavian puncture. Potential complications of subclavian puncture include pneumothorax, hemopneumothorax, subclavian artery puncture, brachial nerve plexus injury, and thoracic duct injury.

Specific electrical measurements must be obtained at the time of pacemaker or ICD implantation, including the following: threshold of stimulation in each chamber paced; determination of intrinsic amplitude of P wave for atrial sensing and QRS for ventricular sensing; impedance values; Wenckebach point if AAI(R) pacing system is implanted; defibrillation threshold for ICD implantation; and assessment for extracardiac pacing at 10-V stimulation.

After placement of the pulse generator, posteroanterior and lateral chest radiographs must be obtained to exclude pneumothorax and also to ensure adequate lead positioning. Before hospital dismissal, the pulse generator should be programmed to determine pacing and sensing thresholds for final programming. If the pulse generator is being programmed to a rate-adaptive pacing mode, this should be assessed to be certain that the rate response is indeed appropriate for a given level of activity.

Pacemaker Programming

All contemporary pacemakers have many programmable parameters that can be altered to optimize and troubleshoot pacemaker function. A detailed description of pacemaker programming is beyond the scope of this text. A few of the most critical parameters merit mention here, but any

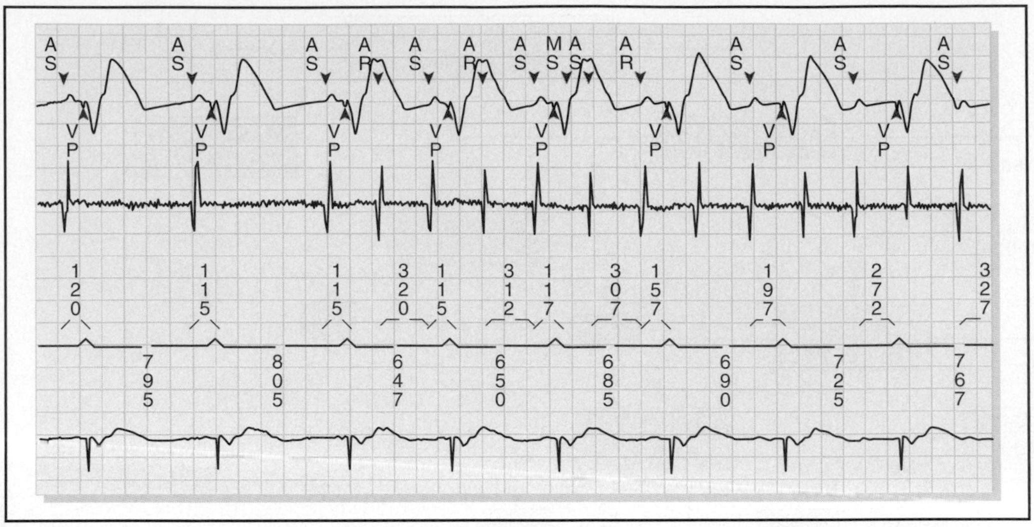

FIGURE 34–12 Electrocardiographic tracing from a patient with a DDD pacemaker. In the initial portion of the tracing, the pacing is in sinus rhythm. This is followed by the onset of an atrial tachyarrhythmia with initial tracking, but mode switching causes reversion to a DDI pacing mode. The top tracing is the marker channel, the second tracing represents the atrial electrogram, the third is the timing channel, and the lower tracing represents the surface electrocardiogram. Arrowheads indicate paced or sensed events or change in operation (mode switch, MS). AR = atrial event in refractory period; AS = atrial sensed event; VP = ventricular paced event. Numbers above the line indicate milliseconds from one event to another (e.g., AS to VP). Numbers below the line indicate milliseconds between ventricular events.

caregiver taking responsibility for pacemaker follow-up should have a thorough knowledge of all programming options.

Pulse Width and Voltage Amplitude

Output programming is probably the most important aspect of programming and should be performed routinely. The output must be high enough to allow an adequate pacing margin of safety but should also be programmed with the intent of maximizing pacemaker longevity. There is no consensus about the best way to program output parameters, but options include doubling the voltage amplitude at threshold, tripling the pulse width at threshold, determining the threshold, or programming output parameters to achieve triple the threshold (determined in microjoules). Some pacemakers automatically determine output parameters and others continually carry out surveillance of the capture threshold and automatically adjust output parameters.

Atrioventricular Interval

In dual-chamber pacemakers, the interval corresponding to the intrinsic PR interval (i.e., the interval between a paced or sensed atrial event and paced ventricular event) must be programmed. As mentioned earlier, there is evidence to support maintenance of intrinsic ventricular activation to avoid the potential adverse effects of right ventricular apical pacing (see Fig. 34-4).

Mode Switching

Mode switching is the ability of the pacemaker to change automatically from a P-synchronous tracking mode to a nontracking mode in response to an inappropriately rapid atrial rhythm (Fig. 34-12). In the DDD(R) or VDD(R) pacing modes, if a supraventricular rhythm disturbance occurs and the pacemaker senses the pathological atrial rhythm, rapid ventricular pacing can occur. Any pacing mode that eliminates tracking of the pathological rhythm (e.g., DDI or DDIR) also eliminates the ability to track normal sinus rhythm, which is usually the predominant rhythm. Mode switching avoids this limitation by switching from DDD or DDDR during sinus rhythm to a nontracking mode, such as DDIR or VVIR, during the pathological atrial rhythm.

Rate-Adaptive Parameters

The goal of programming rate-adaptive pacemakers is to optimize the patient's chronotropic response. For patients who are limited to activities of daily living, informal exercise testing, such as walking at casual and brisk paces in the hospital corridor or in the outpatient facility, is usually adequate. In determining the appropriate heart rate response, the patient's age and "usual activities" must be taken into consideration. Formal exercise testing is not needed for most patients. However, if formal exercise testing is done for this purpose, a low-intensity exercise protocol that allows for a gradual increase may be preferable to a standard Bruce protocol.

Pacemaker Complications

Complications can be divided into those related to implantation and those related to failure of a component of the pacing system. Many complications are related directly to the experience of the implanting physician.

Implant-Related Complications

Most patients undergoing pacemaker implantation have some discomfort at the site of the incision in the early postoperative period. Mild analgesics may be required. Mild ecchymoses around the incision are not uncommon. As noted earlier, if subclavian puncture is used for lead placement, several potential complications can occur, including the possibility of traumatic pneumothorax and hemopneumothorax, inadvertent arterial puncture, air embolism, arteriovenous fistula, thoracic duct injury, subcutaneous emphysema, and brachial plexus injury.

Hematoma formation at the pulse generator site occurs most commonly when anticoagulant therapy is initiated or reinstituted prematurely. A hematoma must be dealt with on the basis of its secondary consequences. Aspiration generally is not advised, and evacuation of the hematoma should be considered only if there is continued bleeding, potential compromise of the suture line or skin integrity, or pain refractory to analgesics.

Usually, introduction of the lead(s) into the subclavian artery, aorta, and left ventricle is readily recognized because of the pulsatile flow of saturated blood. A pacing lead can also be placed in the left ventricle by passing it across an unsuspected atrial or ventricular septal defect (Fig. 34-13). Once the lead is within the subclavian artery, passage into the left ventricle is as easy as passage into the right ventricle via the venous system. Left ventricular lead placement should be recognized if lateral fluoroscopy is used or a lateral chest radiograph is obtained, because the lead is in the posterior aspect of the heart. During right ventricular pacing, the ECG usually has a left bundle branch block (LBBB) pattern, and during left ventricular pacing, a right bundle branch block (RBBB) pattern is most common.

Although thresholds may be adequate, lead placement in the arterial circulation is associated with thrombus formation, embolization and, consequently, stroke. The management of inadvertent left

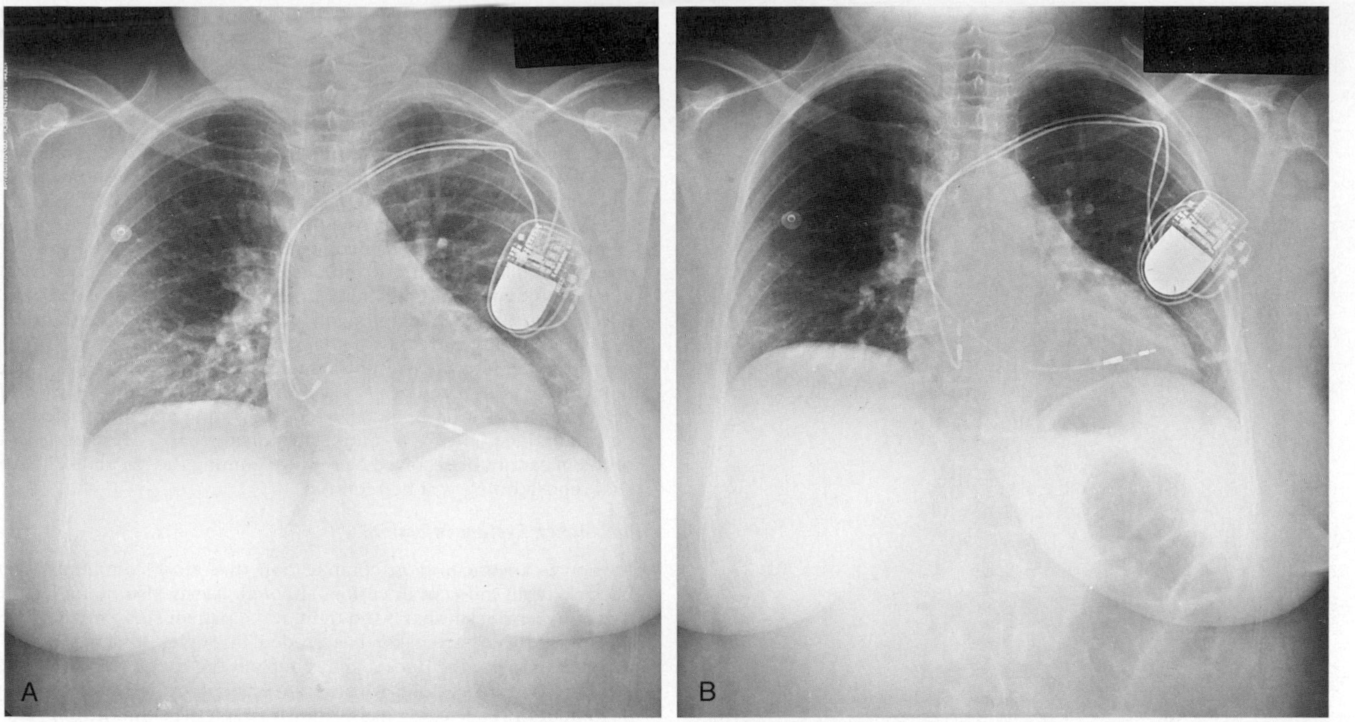

FIGURE 34–13 Posteroanterior chest radiographs of a dual-chamber pacemaker. **A,** Ventricular lead is passing through an atrial septal defect into the left ventricle. **B,** The lead is repositioned in the right ventricular apex.

ventricular lead placement is dependent on the time it is discovered after implantation and individual patient needs and associated comorbidities.

Patients undergoing device implantation should be made aware of the potential for lead perforation. Although cardiac tamponade is the most dramatic outcome from perforation, lack of symptoms after ventricular perforation by a lead is not uncommon. The only sign may be an increasing stimulation threshold. In other patients, the signs can include an RBBB pattern from a lead placed in the right ventricle, intercostal muscle or diaphragmatic contraction, friction rub after implantation, and pericarditis, pericardial effusion, or cardiac tamponade. (Depending on lead position, a RBBB pattern is also possible when the lead is within the right ventricular cavity.)

Ventricular perforation may be suggested by radiography, electrocardiography, and echocardiography. Once perforation has been identified, lead withdrawal and repositioning are usually uncomplicated, although pericardial bleeding or tamponade results rarely.

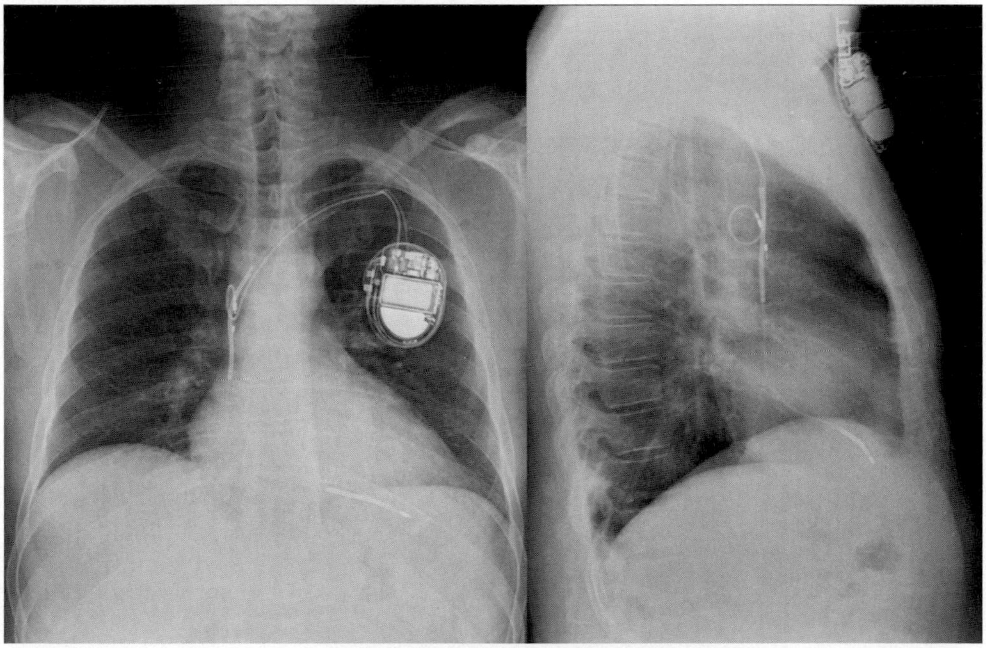

FIGURE 34–14 A, Posteroanterior chest radiograph of a patient with a dual-chamber pacemaker. The atrial lead, originally positioned in a right atrial appendage position, is clearly no longer positioned in the right atrial appendage. **B,** Lateral view also shows definite dislodgment of the atrial lead.

Partial or silent inconsequential venous thrombosis of the subclavian vein is not uncommon after transvenous lead placement and is usually clinically insignificant. Such partial or silent thrombosis may limit venous access at the time of pacing system revision. Symptomatic thrombosis of the subclavian vein, with an edematous, painful, upper extremity, is a relatively rare but recognized complication. Again, management must be individualized. Anticoagulation will be necessary for some patients.

LEAD-RELATED COMPLICATIONS. Several lead-related complications deserve attention, including lead dislodgment (Fig. 34-14), loose connector pin (Fig. 34-15), conductor coil (lead) fracture (Fig. 34-16), and insulation break.

Acceptable dislodgment rates should probably be less than 1 percent for ventricular leads and no more than 2 to 3 percent for atrial leads. Dislodgment may be radiographically evident (macrodislodgment) or not detectable radiographically (microdislodgment). Adequate lead position is assessed with posteroanterior and lateral chest radiographs and comparison with any previous chest radiographs.

Intermittent or complete failure of output can occur because of a loose connection at the interface of the lead and connector block (see Fig. 34-15), usually because the lead was inadequately secured at the time of pacemaker implantation. When a connection is loose, manipu-

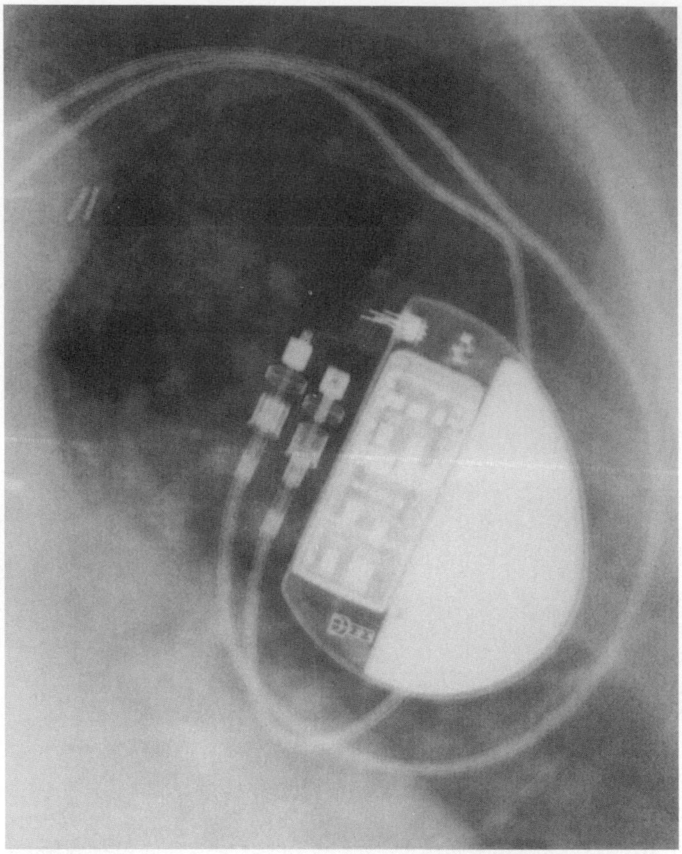

FIGURE 34–15 Close-up of a DDD pacemaker and bipolar leads shows that the lower connector pin (ventricular lead) is not securely in the connector block.

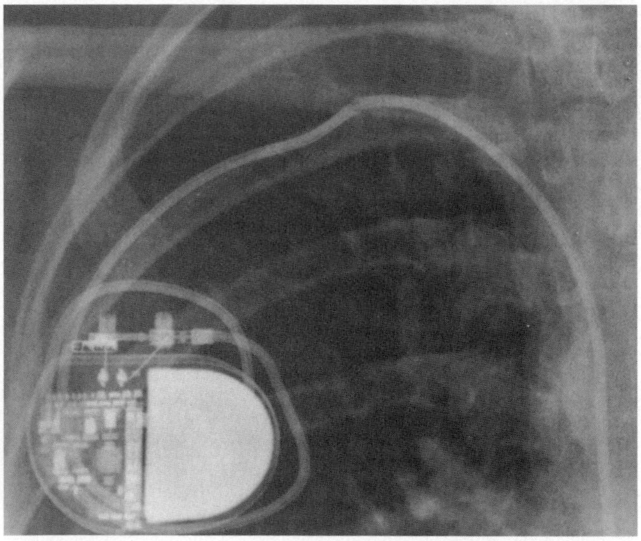

FIGURE 34–16 Close-up view of a portion of the posteroanterior chest radiograph of a patient with a single-chamber pacemaker. The lead has fractured where it passes below the clavicle. The patient presented with intermittent ventricular failure to capture and intermittent failure to output on the ventricular lead. Impedance was intermittently measured at more than 9999 Ω.

lating the pulse generator or pocket may reproduce the problem. The poor connection may be evident radiographically.

Loss of integrity of the insulating material is also uncommon and clinically can present as sensing or pacing abnormalities, or both. Both insulation defects and conductor fractures (see Fig. 34-16) can be caused by crush injury, specifically at the costoclavicular space when placement is by the subclavian puncture technique.

Various arrhythmias can occur after implantation. Supraventricular and ventricular arrhythmias, often encountered during pacemaker implantation, are usually inconsequential.

Extrasystoles can be seen in the early postimplantation period and are usually morphologically similar to the paced beats because they originate at the same site as the paced beats, but are not preceded by a pacemaker stimulus. Such extrasystoles occur most often during the first 24 to 48 hours after implantation, usually resolve spontaneously, and almost never require pharmacological suppression.

Extracardiac stimulation usually involves the diaphragm or pectoral or intercostal muscles. Diaphragmatic stimulation may be caused by direct stimulation of the diaphragm (usually stimulation of the left hemidiaphragm) or stimulation of the phrenic nerve (usually stimulation of the right hemidiaphragm). Diaphragmatic stimulation occurring during the early postimplantation period may be caused by microdislodgment or macrodislodgment of the pacing lead. Stimulation can be minimized or alleviated by decreasing the voltage output or pulse width, or both, but an adequate pacing margin of safety must be maintained after the output parameters are decreased. If the problem cannot be resolved by reprogramming the pacemaker output, lead repositioning will be required.

Pacemaker System Infection

Erosion is an uncommon complication that most commonly occurs because of an indolent infection, although it may also be the result of a pacemaker pocket that is too tight. If the patient seeks medical attention before the pacemaker has eroded through the skin, it may be possible to revise the pocket and reimplant the pacemaker. Impending erosion should be dealt with as an emergency because, once any portion of the pacemaker has eroded through the skin, the only choice is removal of the pacemaker system and placement of a new system in another site.

The incidence of infection after pacemaker implantation should be less than 2 percent and, in most series, has been less than 1 percent. Careful attention to surgical details and sterile procedures is of paramount importance in avoiding pacemaker site infection. Irrigation of the pacemaker pocket with an antibiotic solution at the time of pacemaker implantation is probably more important in the prevention of infection.

Pacemaker infection may appear as local inflammation or abscess formation in the pacemaker pocket, erosion of part of the pacing system with secondary infection, or sepsis with positive blood culture findings with or without a focus of infection elsewhere. The most common clinical presentation is localized pocket infection; septicemia is uncommon. Many infectious agents can be responsible, but early infections are most commonly caused by *Staphylococcus aureus,* are aggressive, and are often associated with fever and systemic symptoms. Late infections commonly are caused by *Staphylococcus epidermidis* and are more indolent, usually without fever or systemic manifestations. Treatment of pacemaker-related septicemia requires removal of the entire infected pacing system, pacemaker, and leads.

Troubleshooting Electrocardiographic Abnormalities

ECG abnormalities in the paced patient can be grouped broadly into failure to capture, failure to output, and sensing abnormalities (undersensing or oversensing).

FAILURE TO CAPTURE. Failure to capture indicates that a pacing artifact is present without subsequent cardiac depolarization (Fig. 34-17). The possible causes of failure to capture are high thresholds with an inadequately programmed output, partial conductor coil fracture, insulation defect, lead dislodgment or perforation, impending total battery depletion, functional noncapture, poor or incompatible connection at the connector block, circuit failure, air in the pulse generator pocket (unipolar pacemaker), and elevated thresholds from drugs or metabolic abnormality.

FAILURE TO OUTPUT. Failure to output (i.e., failure to deliver an appropriate pacing stimulus) is often caused by oversensing and inhibition of output but could also be caused by true failure to output from the pacemaker or circuit interruption that prevents the electrical signal from reaching the heart (Fig. 34-18). The reasons for failure to output are circuit failure, complete or intermittent conductor coil fracture, intermittent or permanently loose set screw, incompatible lead or header, total battery depletion, internal insulation failure (bipolar lead), oversensing of any noncardiac activity, crosstalk (Fig. 34-19), and lack of anodal connector contact (e.g., unipolar lead in bipolar generator, bipolar lead in pacemaker programmed in unipolar mode, air in the pocket of a unipolar device, unipolar pacemaker not in the pocket).

The differential diagnoses of failure to capture and failure to pace obviously overlap somewhat. For example, electrocardiographic manifestations of a conductor coil fracture may include failure to capture because of significant leakage of current at the incomplete fracture site and not enough current remaining to result in stimulation. Nonetheless, the pacemaker stimuli can appear. Alternatively, escaping current can be sensed by the pacemaker and inhibit pacemaker output. If the conductor coil is completely fractured, rendering the circuit incomplete, no pacemaker output will be detected on the ECG. Insulation defects can also be signaled by oversensing and failure to pace or by failure to capture, although the most common consequences of insulation failure are sensing abnormalities.

As the pacemaker battery reaches end stages of depletion, either failure to capture because of decreasing voltage output or failure to pace because of total battery depletion can occur. This degree of battery depletion should be avoided by appropriate pacemaker follow-up.

Apparent failure to capture is noted if a pacemaker stimulus occurs during the refractory period of a spontaneous beat. This is referred to as *functional noncapture.*

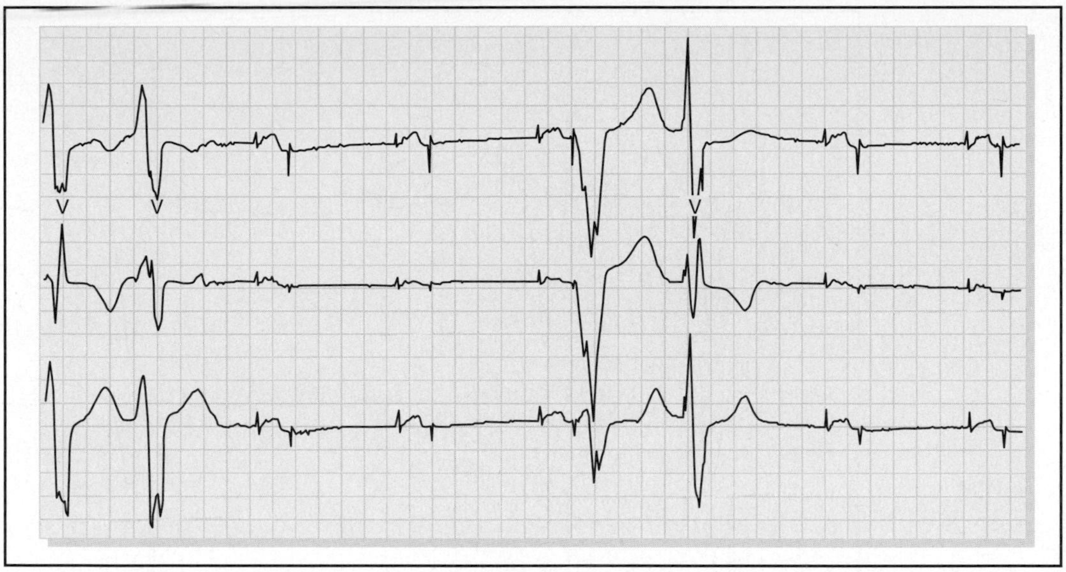

FIGURE 34–17 Electrocardiographic tracing from a patient with a DDDR pacemaker. All ventricular pacing artifacts but one failed to result in ventricular depolarization—that is, failure to capture. In this patient, intermittent ventricular failure to capture was caused by lead dislodgment.

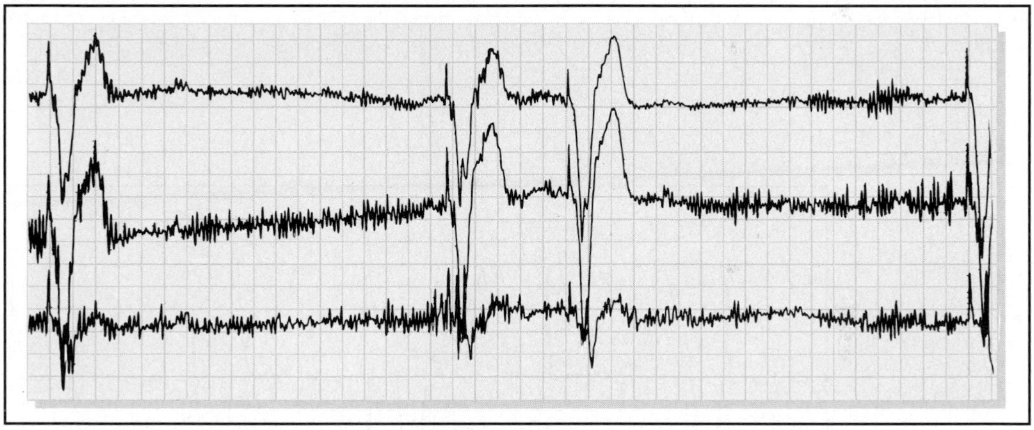

FIGURE 34–18 Electrocardiographic tracings from a patient with a VVIR pacemaker, with a lower rate of 70 beats/min. After an initial paced ventricular beat, there is a pause of approximately 2.8 seconds, with significant baseline artifact. After two additional paced beats, another pause of approximately 2.8 seconds occurs. This patient had a pacemaker programmed to a unipolar sensing configuration. The sensing of myopotentials led to symptomatic pauses, and reprogramming the pacemaker to a bipolar sensing configuration prevented subsequent myopotential oversensing.

SENSING ABNORMALITIES. Sensing abnormalities can be divided into *true abnormalities,* including undersensing (a failure to recognize normal intrinsic cardiac activity; Fig. 34-20) and oversensing (unexpected sensing of an intrinsic or extrinsic electrical signal; see Fig. 34-18), and *functional sensing abnormalities.* The possible causes of sensing abnormalities are lead dislodgment or poor lead positioning, lead insulation failure, circuit failure, magnet application, malfunction of the reed switch, electromagnetic interference (EMI), and battery depletion. The morphology of the intrinsic event is different from that measured at implantation.

True undersensing is most commonly caused by lead dislodgment or inadequate initial lead placement. Sensing abnormalities can commonly be seen secondary to insulation defects and to intermittent "make-or-break" conductor fracture. A normally functioning pacing system at times fails to detect atrial or ventricular extrasystoles. The intrinsic events measured at the time of implantation generate an electrogram at the electrode tip. If an extrasystole is occurring elsewhere in the heart, the sensing vector is different from that of the normal intrinsic beat, and the resulting voltage generated may not be high enough to be sensed by the pacemaker. This anomaly cannot be anticipated unless extrasystoles of the same morphology occur during implantation and can be measured. It is reasonable to attempt reprogramming the sensitivity to allow the extrasystoles to be sensed but, if this is unsuccessful, it is rarely if ever necessary to reposition the lead for this abnormality.

Functional undersensing is present when an intrinsic cardiac event is not sensed because it falls within a programmed refractory period. For example, if an intrinsic atrial event occurs within the PVARP, the event is not, and should not be, sensed. However, without a thorough understanding of the timing cycle, it may appear as though there is true undersensing.

Fusion and pseudofusion beats occur as a result of superimposition of an ineffective pacemaker stimulus on a spontaneously occurring P wave or QRS complex (Fig. 34-21). (*Fusion* is present when the morphology of the cardiac event is a hybrid of the intrinsic morphology and the paced morphology. *Pseudofusion* is present when the pacemaker artifact occurs late enough that the intrinsic morphology is not deformed, but it may appear so because of distortion on the ECG by the superimposed pacing artifact.) Pseudofusion is usually the consequence of pacemaker discharge during the refractory period of intrinsic P or QRS before sufficient intracardiac voltage has been generated to activate the sensing circuit. This is most likely to occur when the pacing rate and the intrinsic rate are similar. Also, pseudofusion beats can be the result of a delayed activation caused by intraventricular conduction abnormalities.

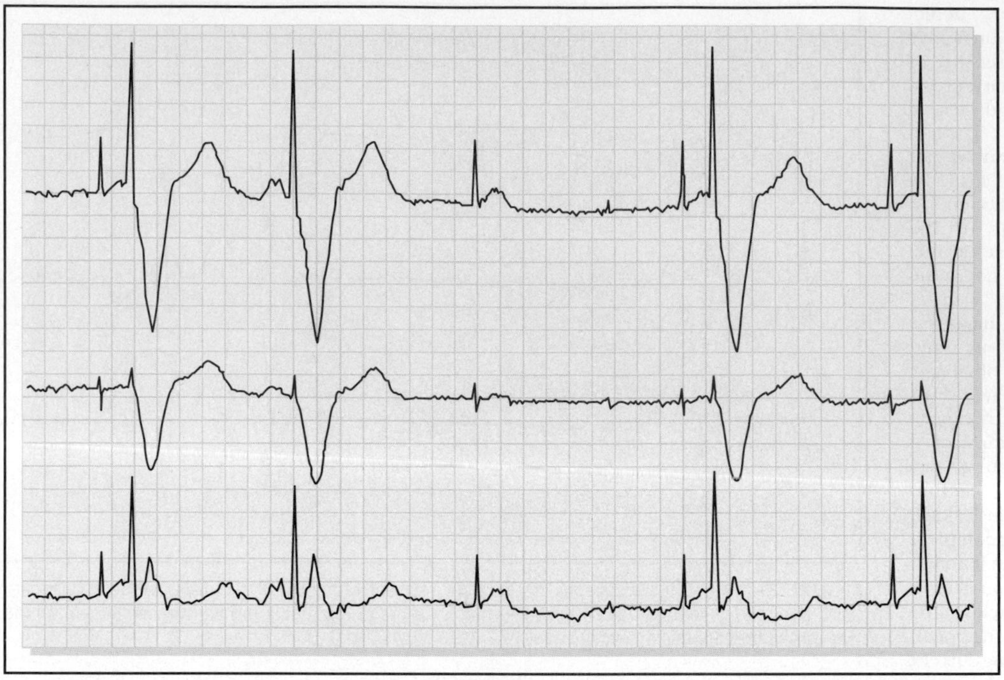

FIGURE 34–19 Patient with a DDD pacemaker. After the third atrial pacing artifact, there is evidence of atrial depolarization, but there is no ventricular pacing output. Failure to deliver the ventricular pacing artifact is caused by crosstalk—that is, the atrial pacing output is sensed by the ventricular sensing circuit, with subsequent inhibition.

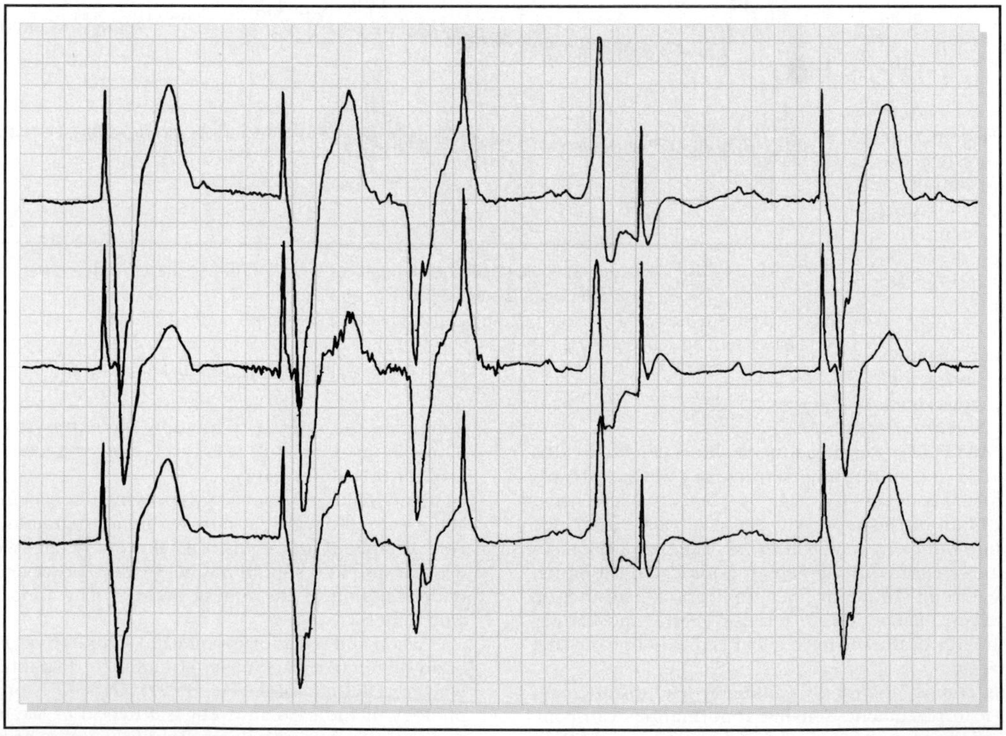

FIGURE 34–20 Electrocardiographic tracing from a patient with a VVI pacemaker with a programmed rate of 70 beats/min. After two paced ventricular complexes, a premature ventricular complex occurs. In approximately 260 milliseconds, a ventricular pacing artifact occurs. This is followed by a P wave with intrinsic atrioventricular nodal conduction and native QRS complex. A pacemaker artifact follows in approximately 220 milliseconds. This represents ventricular undersensing. In this patient, the abnormality occurred because of an insulation failure of the ventricular pacing lead.

IMPLANTABLE CARDIOVERTER-DEFIBRILLATOR THERAPY

Indications for ICD Therapy

The ACC/AHA/HRS guidelines for pacemakers and ICDs are summarized in Table 34-6.

RANDOMIZED CLINICAL TRIALS OF ICD THERAPY

Secondary Prevention Trials. Prevention of sudden cardiac death by ICD therapy was first demonstrated in multiple secondary prevention trials (i.e., patients who had already experienced out-of-hospital cardiac arrest or demonstrated spontaneous sustained ventricular tachycardia or ventricular fibrillation). Secondary prevention trials that have demonstrated reduced mortality with ICD therapy include the Antiarrhythmics Versus Implantable Defibrillators (AVID),[39] Canadian Implantable Defibrillator Study (CIDS),[40] and Cardiac Arrest Study Hamburg (CASH).[41] An exception to this trend was the absence of a significant difference in overall survival seen with ICD therapy in the CIDS trial. (Some have questioned whether this trial was underpowered; see Table 32-5.)

Subset analyses of the secondary prevention trials have demonstrated that individuals with an ejection fraction between 0.20 and 0.34 receive the highest benefit with ICD therapy.[42]

Primary Prevention Trials. Primary prevention ICD trials that identified patients who had not yet experienced a clinically significant ventricular tachyarrhythmia but were at increased risk for such a rhythm disturbance include the following: Multicenter Automatic Defibrillator Implantation Trial (MADIT) I,[43] Coronary Artery Bypass Graft (CABG) PATCH trial,[44] Multicenter Unsustained Tachycardia Trial (MUSTT),[45] MADIT-II,[43] Defibrillators in Non-Ischemic Cardiomyopathy Treatment Evaluation (DEFINITE),[46] Sudden Cardiac Death in Heart Failure Trial (SCD-HeFT),[47] and Defibrillator in Acute Myocardial Infarction Trial (DINAMIT).[48]

MADIT I included patients with a previous myocardial infarction, left ventricular ejection fraction of 0.35, nonsustained VT, and inducible, nonsuppressible VT on electrophysiological study. Patients were randomized to ICD or amiodarone. Over a follow-up of 27 months, there was a 54 percent relative risk reduction in the ICD group.

MADIT II required that patients had a myocardial infarction 1 month before study entry and advanced left ventricular dysfunction (left ventricular ejection fraction, 0.30). Inducibility of ventricular tachyarrhythmia was not part of the inclusion criteria. Approximately 70 percent of patients were in NYHA functional Class I or II heart failure. There was a 31 percent relative risk reduction in the ICD group versus that in the conventional therapy group.

CABG-PATCH should probably be considered separately because it randomized patients who were to undergo coronary artery bypass grafting to either ICD implantation at the time of bypass surgery or postoperative antiarrhythmic treatment. The study was terminated prematurely when the interim analysis failed to show a survival differ-

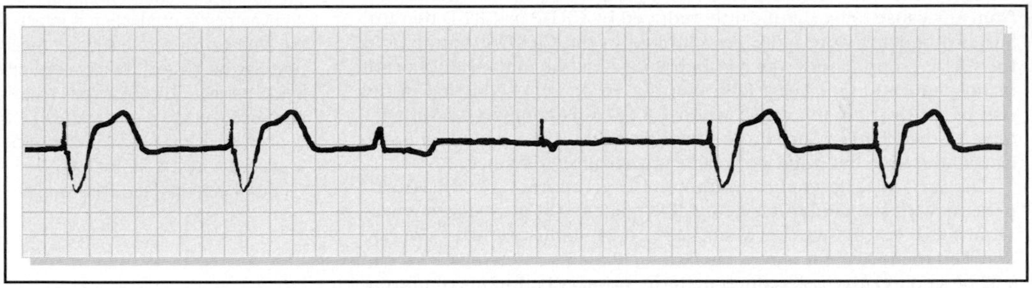

FIGURE 34–21 Electrocardiographic tracing from a patient with a VVI pacemaker. The first two complexes represent fully paced ventricular depolarizations. The third ventricular event is an intrinsic QRS complex, and the fourth event represents a fusion beat. This is followed by two paced ventricular complexes.

TABLE 34–6 Implantable Cardioverter-Defibrillator Indications

Class I	Class II	Class III
Cardiac arrest caused by VF or VT not resulting from a transient or reversible cause Spontaneous sustained VT associated with structural heart disease Syncope of undetermined origin with clinically relevant, hemodynamically significant sustained VT or VF induced at EP study when drug therapy is ineffective, not tolerated, or not preferred Nonsustained VT in patients with coronary disease, prior MI, LV dysfunction, and inducible VF or sustained VT at EP study not suppressible by an NYHA Class I antiarrhythmic drug Spontaneous sustained VT in patients without structural heart disease not amenable to other treatments	Patients with LVEF ≤0.30 at least 1 mo post MI and 3 mo post coronary artery revascularization surgery Cardiac arrest presumed to be caused by VF when EP testing was precluded by other medical conditions Severe symptoms (e.g., syncope) attributable to sustained ventricular tachyarrhythmias while awaiting cardiac transplantation Familial or inherited conditions with a high risk for life-threatening ventricular tachyarrhythmias, such as long-QT syndrome or hypertrophic cardiomyopathy Nonsustained VT with coronary artery disease, prior MI, and LV dysfunction, and inducible sustained VT or VF at EP study Recurrent syncope of undetermined cause in presence of ventricular dysfunction and inducible ventricular arrhythmias at EP study when other causes of syncope have been excluded Syncope of unexplained origin or family history of unexplained sudden cardiac death associated with typical or atypical right bundle branch block and ST-segment elevation (Brugada syndrome) Syncope in patients with advanced structural heart disease in whom thorough invasive and noninvasive investigations have failed to define a cause	Syncope of undetermined cause in patients without inducible ventricular tachyarrhythmias and without structural heart disease Incessant VT or VF VF or VT resulting from arrhythmias amenable to surgical or catheter ablation (e.g., atrial arrhythmias associated with WPW, RVOT VT, idiopathic LV tachycardia, or fascicular VT) Ventricular tachyarrhythmias caused by transient or reversible disorder (e.g., AMI, electrolyte imbalance, drugs or trauma) when correction of the disorder is considered feasible and likely to reduce the risk of recurrent arrhythmia substantially Significant psychiatric illnesses that may be aggravated by device implantation or may preclude systematic follow-up Terminal illnesses with projected life expectancy <6 mo Patients with coronary artery disease with LV dysfunction and prolonged QRS duration in absence of spontaneous or inducible sustained or nonsustained VT who are undergoing coronary bypass surgery NYHA Class IV drug-refractory congestive heart failure in patients who are not candidates for cardiac transplantation

AMI = acute myocardial infarction; EP = electrophysiologic; LV = left ventricular; LVEF = left ventricular ejection fraction; MI = myocardial infarction; NYHA = New York Heart Association; RVOT = right ventricular outflow tract; VF = ventricular fibrillation; VT = ventricular tachycardia; WPW = Wolff-Parkinson-White syndrome.

ence between the two study groups. The deaths in both groups were perioperative and, therefore, could not have been prevented by antiarrhythmic therapy. Analysis of subgroups showed the benefits of the ICD in patients at risk for life-threatening ventricular tachyarrhythmia.[44]

DINAMIT enrolled patients with reduced left ventricular function, left ventricular ejection fraction less than 0.35, and impaired autonomic function who were 6 to 40 days postmyocardial infarction. The primary endpoint was mortality from any cause. Investigators found that ICD therapy in this high-risk group of patients with recent myocardial infarction did not reduce overall mortality. Although ICD therapy was associated with a decrease in the rate of death caused by arrhythmia, the decrease was offset by an increase in the rate of death from nonarrhythmic causes.[48] Primary prevention ICD trials are summarized in Table 35-5.

RELEVANT CRT-D TRIALS. CRT trials have further expanded ICD indications and have provided more information specific to the heart failure population (see Table 34-4). The Comparison of Medical Therapy, Pacing, and Defibrillation Heart Failure (COMPANION trial),[19] designed as a mortality trial, was the first trial to evaluate the effects of CRT on death and hospitalization. This parallel, open-label trial randomized patients to optimized pharmacological therapy (OPT), OPT plus CRT, and OPT plus CRT-D. All patients met the standard criteria for CRT. The trial demonstrated the risk of death or hospitalization from any cause to be significantly reduced by CRT-P or CRT-D therapy. Survival benefits were more pronounced in the CRT-D group than in the CRT-P group. There was a 40 percent reduction in the risk of death or hospitalization for heart failure and a 36 percent reduction in the risk of death from any cause when CRT-D was compared with OPT only. In the CRT-P group, there was a trend toward a reduction in all-cause mortality, but it did not reach statistical significance.

In the Cardiac Resynchronization in Heart Failure (CARE-HF) trial,[20] patients with standard criteria for CRT (evidence of dyssynchrony was required if the QRS was between 120 and 149 milliseconds) were randomized to medical therapy versus CRT-P. Patients receiving CRT-P had a 37 percent relative risk reduction in the primary endpoint (composite of all-cause death and hospitalization for a cardiovascular event) and a 36 percent reduction in all-cause mortality compared with patients receiving medical therapy only.

Inherited arrhythmia conditions include long-QT syndrome,[49] Brugada syndrome,[50] right ventricular arrhythmogenic dysplasia,[51] hypertrophic cardiomyopathy[52] (see Chaps. 9 and 35), and others for which an ICD is often recommended.

ICD Design

The basic components of the ICD are electronic circuitry, power source, and memory, with a microprocessor coordinating the various parts of the system. High-voltage capacitors transform the battery-provided voltage into discharges ranging from less than 1 V for pacing to 750 V for defibrillation. (This is in contrast to the voltage amplifier used in pacemakers, which multiplies the voltage output by storing the electrical output until the appropriate amount of energy is stored and then releasing it.) ICDs incorporate a different sensing circuit than most pacemakers. Because of the need to sense low-amplitude signals reliably during ventricular fibrillation and to avoid sensing extracardiac noise and cardiac signals other than ventricular tachycardia or fibrillation, the sensing circuit is designed to adjust the sensing requirements automatically.

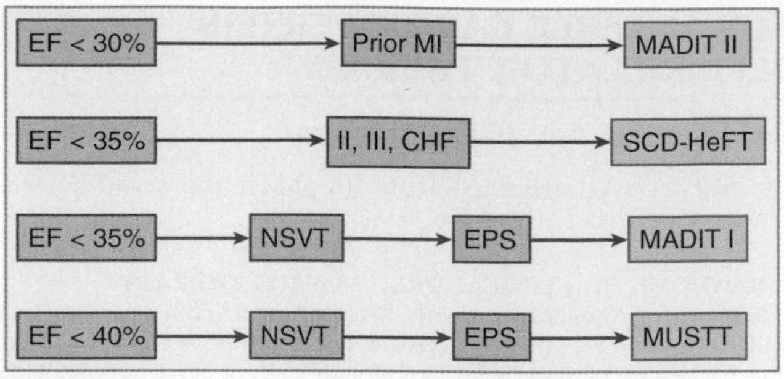

FIGURE 34–22 Diagram showing the need for an implantable cardioverter-defibrillator (ICD) based on randomized clinical trial criteria (MADIT I and II,[43] MUSTT,[45] SCD-HeFT[47]) Once the decision has been made that the patient meets the criteria and should receive an ICD, a decision should be made about single- versus dual-chamber ICD. If the patient meets the criteria for permanent pacing—that is, there is a demonstrable conduction abnormality that would require bradycardia support and the patient's predominant rhythm is normal sinus rhythm—then dual-chamber pacing support is reasonable. If the patient will probably not require bradycardia support with the exception of "postshock" support or if the patient is in chronic atrial fibrillation and requires pacing support, a single-chamber ICD should be selected. Even for patients who meet criteria for pacing, if atrioventricular conduction is intact, the approach currently favored is to program the bradycardia pacing support to minimize or avoid ventricular pacing, when possible, because of the potential adverse effects from chronic right ventricular apical pacing. CHF = congestive heart failure; EF = ejection fraction; EPS = electrophysiological study; MADIT I and II = Multicenter Automatic Defibrillator Implantation Trial I and II; MI = myocardial infarction; MUSTT = Multicenter Sustained Tachycardia Trial; NSVT = nonsuppressible VT; SCD-HeFT = Sudden Cardiac Death in Heart Failure Trial.

Almost all ICD systems are implanted transvenously and include antitachycardia pacing (ATP) and ventricular bradycardia pacing (single- and dual-chamber ICDs with programmable pacing and rate-adaptive options are widely available). CRT-D devices, as noted earlier, incorporate resynchronization therapy with ICD capabilities (Fig. 34-22).

The longevity of ICDs depends on the frequency of shock delivery, the degree of pacemaker dependency, and other programmable options, but most are expected to last from 5 to 9 years. The ICD functions by continuously monitoring the patient's cardiac rate and delivering therapy when the rate exceeds the programmed rate "cutoff." For example, if the ICD is programmed to treat ventricular tachyarrhythmias at a rate cutoff of 175 beats/min, once the ICD detects a rate greater than 175 beats/min, it delivers ATP or charges and delivers a shock, depending on the programmed therapy. A distinction must be made between "sensing," or interpreting the cardiac events correctly, thus allowing the device to respond appropriately, and "detection" of an arrhythmia. Detection refers to the ability of the device to recognize certain types of arrhythmias and to respond appropriately—that is, detection guides and controls delivery of therapies.

ATP has the advantage of terminating a rhythm disturbance without delivery of a shock. ICDs capable of ATP have significant programming flexibility to adjust many aspects of tachycardia detection and therapy, thereby customizing therapy for the individual patient. Different zones, or tiers, of therapy can be programmed to detect ventricular tachyarrhythmias to allow slower arrhythmias to be treated with ATP before a shock is delivered, but still to allow faster tachycardias to be treated more aggressively. The programming for a hypothetical patient is outlined in Table 34-7. In this patient, slower ventricular tachycardia in the range of 126 to 190 beats/min is treated with ATP therapies in zone 1. If initial ATP therapy (ATP-1) is unsuccessful, a second and different ATP therapy (ATP-2) is automatically delivered. If this is unsuccessful, lower energy shocks are attempted before high-energy shocks are delivered. Shocks are synchronized during ventricular tachycardia (cardioversion) or are asynchronous during ventricular fibrillation (defibrillation). A second zone of therapy is determined for a faster VT, and still faster VT or ventricular fibrillation is treated aggressively with a high-energy shock.

It should be noted that although the intent of ATP is to interrupt VT, the tachycardia possibly could be accelerated and degenerate into a faster VT that is not hemodynamically tolerated or into ventricular fibrillation requiring defibrillation.

The zones, detection rates of the different zones, specifics of the different therapies, and bradycardia pacing options all are programmable, and programming flexibility varies significantly from device to device.

TABLE 34-7	Implantable Cardioverter-Defibrillator Therapy	
Zone	Tachycardia Rate (Beats/Min)*	Sequence of Therapy Delivered
1	140-160	ATP-1, ATP-2, 1 J, 5 J, 34 J
2	161-200	ATP, 10 J, 34 J
3	>200	34 J

*All ranges may require adjustment in specific patients.

ATP = antitachycardia pacing therapy; ATP-1 = first ATP; ATP-2 = second (and different) ATP.

Device Selection

Considerations about the type of ICD to select for a given patient include whether the patient has bradycardia requiring pacing support, has associated atrial tachyarrhythmias, or would benefit from CRT (or a combination of these). The need for bradycardia support requires a choice between single- and dual-chamber ICDs based on the mode selection algorithm already described (see Fig. 34-22).

After the DAVID trial, there was a transient reversal of the existing trend to implant more single-chamber ICDs.[34] However, once again, the trend is to implant dual-chamber ICDs that include a pacing algorithm that will minimize ventricular pacing (i.e., maintain intrinsic ventricular depolarization whenever possible, but have back-up ventricular pacing if needed).

If the patient has associated atrial tachyarrhythmias, a dual-chamber ICD capable of detecting and treating atrial tachyarrhythmias should be considered. Some devices also provide the ability to cardiovert atrial tachyarrhythmias. For patients who meet criteria for both CRT and ICD therapy, a CRT-D should be considered.

Issues Unique to ICD Implantation

When the ICD is placed transvenously with the pulse generator in the prepectoral position, the implantation technique and related complications are the same as those for pacemaker implantation, with the exception that complications can arise as a result of determining the defibrillation threshold (DFT). (DFT can be defined as the minimal energy that terminates ventricular fibrillation.) Most ICD procedures are performed with conscious sedation and local anesthesia and deep anesthesia, with mask-supported ventilation during DFT testing. When DFT determination is completed, the patient can be allowed to recover from deeper anesthesia as the pocket is closed.

An acceptable DFT is a value that ensures an adequate safety margin for defibrillation, usually being at least 10 J less than the maximum output of the ICD, which ranges from 30 to 41 J of stored energy. Ideally the DFT would be 14 J. Frequency and type of follow-up may be individualized in some institutions on the basis of the final DFT value.

Generally, the preference is to implant the ICD in the left pectoral region because of a more favorable vector for delivery of the shock. Although successful defibrillation can usually be accomplished with a right-sided implant, the shocking vector may be less than optimal in some patients and could have an effect on achievable DFT. Regardless of whether the ICD is placed on the right or the left side, it is usually possible to achieve excellent DFTs in most patients. Some have advocated eliminating routine ventricular fibrillation induction and DFT testing as part of a routine ICD implantation procedure.[53] However, an adequate defibrillation safety margin of pacing cannot be obtained in a small percentage of patients, estimated as up to 6 percent,[54] and there is an occasional patient in whom an acceptable DFT cannot be achieved with standard lead placement. These outliers make the case for continued routine DFT assessment. In patients in whom no acceptable DFT can be obtained, options include repositioning the ventricular lead to an alternative site or adding another lead in a subcutaneous position or within the superior vena cava. Coronary sinus placement of the ICD lead could also be considered as an approach to a high DFT and/or when there is limited venous access to the right ventricle.

If the ICD lead is being implanted near a redundant or abandoned pacing lead, noise from the other lead may result in interference with the functioning ICD lead. An attempt should be made to implant the new lead at a distance from the existing lead or leads.

Complications

Any of the complications that may occur with pacemaker implantation may also occur with implantation of an ICD. However, two major concerns unique to ICD therapy are the failure to deliver appropriate therapy when indicated and the delivery of inappropriate therapy.

If the patient presents with a symptomatic event and does not believe that any therapy was delivered—that is, he or she experienced no "shock," after the history and physical—the device should be investigated. Although many specific factors should be assessed, the basic considerations would be to determine the following: (1) whether a tachyarrhythmia did occur, through device interrogation, and whether or not therapies of any type were delivered; (2) whether sensing is normal (i.e., could the ventricular tachyarrhythmia have been "undersensed" and thus no arrhythmia met detection criteria); (3) whether settings were appropriate (i.e., therapies were turned "on" and there were no other active parameters that could have prevented appropriate arrhythmia detection); and (4) whether lead integrity is intact.

Frequent ICD discharges may represent a clinical emergency. These discharges may be appropriate or inappropriate (Table 34-8). Appropriate discharges represent frequently occurring VT or fibrillation or an electrical storm (see Chap. 35). If the device is discharging frequently because the defibrillation is unsuccessful, the device may have been programmed to an inappropriately low shock output or the DFT may have increased (e.g., in response to a drug such as amiodarone; see Chap. 33).

Inappropriate discharges are usually the result of detection of a supraventricular tachyarrhythmia, most commonly AF (see Chap. 35). Inappropriate discharge can also be the result of device failure (e.g., lead fracture with generation of make-or-break signals).

Interference

Electromagnetic Interference

Electromagnetic interference (EMI) is defined as any signal, biological or nonbiological, that is within a frequency spectrum detectable by the sensing circuitry of the pacemaker or ICD. EMI can result in rate alteration, sensing abnormalities, asynchronous pacing, noise reversion, or reprogramming.[55] EMI can also cause failure to deliver antibradycardia pacing, inappropriate delivery of antitachycardia therapy, resetting of programmed parameters, and damage to the pulse generator or myocardial interface.

Other cardiac and extracardiac signals that can be falsely interpreted as a P wave or QRS complex and result in oversensing include T waves (Fig. 34-23), myopotential interference, afterpotential delay, and P waves.

Although multiple sources of EMI in the nonhospital environment can potentially result in single-beat inhibition, few, if any, of these are clinically significant and truly represent a threat to the paced patient.

TABLE 34–8 Differential Diagnosis and Management of Multiple Implantable Cardioverter-Defibrillator (ICD) Shocks

Clinical Finding	Management
Frequent ventricular tachycardia or ventricular fibrillation (electrical storm)	Reassess antiarrhythmic therapy and programmed ICD therapy; possible radiofrequency ablation.
Unsuccessful ICD therapy because of inappropriately low-output shock or elevation of defibrillation threshold	Reprogram ICD. Assess potential causes of defibrillation threshold increase (e.g., drugs, recurrent infarction, recurrent ischemia).
Lead fracture	Replace fractured lead.
Lead dislodgment	Reposition lead.
Rapid ventricular rates arising from supraventricular arrhythmias	Reassess antiarrhythmic therapy. Reprogram ICD parameters. Ablate supraventricular arrhythmic focus.
Oversensing separate pacing system	Reprogram pacemaker or ICD (or both). Reposition pacemaker or ICD leads (or both). Remove pacemaker and replace ICD with another ICD with more sophisticated bradycardia support.
Oversensing electromagnetic interference	Avoid source. Reprogram ICD.
Oversensing intracardiac signals	Reprogram ICD. Reposition sensing lead.

Modified from Pinski SL, Fahy GJ: Implantable cardioverter-defibrillators. Am J Med 106:446, 1999.

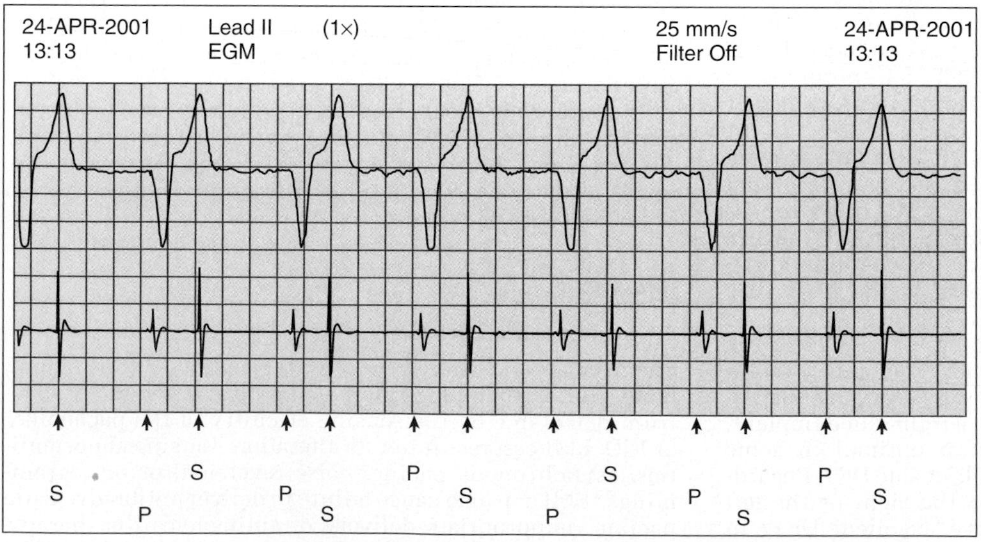

FIGURE 34–23 T-wave oversensing as noted on telemetered tracing with surface ECG **(top)**, ventricular electrogram **(middle)**, and marker annotation **(bottom)**. The paced (P) ventricular rate is approximately 60 beats/min. However, the ventricular electrogram also corresponds to a sensed event (S) that corresponds to the T wave on the surface ECG = electrocardiogram; EMG = electromyogram.

Several potential sources of EMI merit should be mentioned here because of their real potential for causing significant EMI or because of existing confusion or controversy. Industrial strength welding equipment, certain degaussing equipment, and induction ovens are identified sources of EMI that can cause significant pacemaker or ICD interference. Most welding equipment used for hobby welding should not cause any significant problems. For the pacemaker-dependent patient who does hobby welding or any other activity that raises the clinician's concerns about EMI, the environment should be determined safe for the patient before the activity is approved.

Commercially available cell phones are safe for the patient with a device as long as simple measures are followed.[56] The patient should avoid having the activated cell phone directly over the pacemaker or ICD, either from random motion of the phone or by carrying the activated phone in a breast pocket over the device. Although probably not critical, additional safety may be gained by using the phone with the ear contralateral to the implanted device.

Antitheft devices also have potential for pacemaker interference.[57] Practical suggestions are for patients with pacemakers or ICDs to be aware of electronic equipment for article surveillance and to avoid leaning on or lingering near such devices. If the patient passes through the equipment at a normal pace, adverse effects are unlikely. Any patient who feels unusual in any way when near electronic surveillance equipment should move away.

Hospital sources of potentially significant EMI are electrocautery, cardioversion, defibrillation, magnetic resonance imaging (MRI), lithotripsy, radiofrequency ablation, electroshock therapy, and diathermy. The most important aspect of pacemaker or ICD care after exposure to any of these sources of EMI is to reassess the device to be certain that programmed parameters have not been changed.

One of the most frequently asked questions is how to manage the patient with a pacemaker or ICD during an operative procedure, given the potential effects of electrocautery and guidelines for cardioversion and defibrillation.[55] Routine interrogation of the device and deactivation of ICD therapy should be accomplished before the operation. After the procedure, the device should be reinterrogated and ICD therapy reinitiated. (During the time that ICD therapy is "off," the patient must be monitored.) For pacemaker-dependent patients, it is reasonable to program the pacemaker to an asynchronous pacing mode, VOO or DOO, or to achieve the same effect by placing a magnet over the pacemaker throughout the procedure. The potential effects of exposure to electrocautery include reprogramming, permanent damage to the pulse generator, pacemaker inhibition, reversion to a fall-back mode, noise reversion mode, or electrical reset, and myocardial thermal damage. There are guidelines for cardioversion and defibrillation in the patient with a pacemaker or ICD. Ideally, place paddles in the anteroposterior position, try to keep the paddles at least 4 inches from the pulse generator, have the appropriate pacemaker programmer available, and interrogate the pacemaker after the procedure.

With increasing use of MRI, potential interference with implantable devices should be noted. MRI is still considered a relative contraindication for patients with a pacemaker or ICD because of the potential for induction of rapid hemodynamically unstable ventricular rhythms and the theoretical possibility of heating of the conductor coil and thermal damage at the electrode-myocardial interface. Although there have been reports of MRI being performed safely in non–pacemaker-dependent patients,[58,59] there have also been reports of deaths resulting from MRI-induced rhythm disturbances.[60]

Interference from Drugs and Metabolic Abnormalities

Drugs can affect sensing thresholds, pacing thresholds, and DFTs and result in abnormalities in the ECG. Although many drugs have been reported to affect pacing thresholds, class 1C agents are the only drugs that usually cause a problem. Flecainide and propafenone have the potential to increase pacing thresholds and sensing thresholds. If these drugs are administered to the patient with a pacemaker, especially a pacemaker-dependent patient, thresholds should be monitored for change. Amiodarone does not consistently affect pacing thresholds. Changes in drug therapy must also be monitored closely in the patient with an ICD.[61] In addition to altering pacing thresholds and increasing DFTs, certain drugs have the potential for interaction by altering the detection of ventricular tachycardia and producing proarrhythmic effects. Drug-induced slowing of the rate of ventricular tachycardia can result in inadequate detection of the arrhythmia. The DFT can increase from the administration of amiodarone.[62] Other drugs can theoretically increase the DFT or have been reported to do so in single case reports, but a clinically significant change does not often result.[61]

Electrolyte and metabolic abnormalities can affect pacing and sensing thresholds. Hyperkalemia is the most common electrolyte abnormality to cause clinically significant problems, but severe acidosis or alkalosis, hypercapnia, severe hyperglycemia, hypoxemia, and hypothyroidism can also alter thresholds.

Device Follow-up

Patients with pacemakers and ICDs must be followed on a regular schedule. There are different follow-up methods, depending on clinician and institutional preference. For pacemaker follow-up, some caregivers prefer regular office assessment, others prefer transtelephonic follow-up, and still others prefer a combination of the two techniques. Transtelephonic assessment should include collection of a nonmagnet electrocardiographic strip, an electrocardiographic strip with magnet applied to the pacemaker, and measurement of magnet rate and pulse duration (pulse duration on both atrial and ventricular channels should be measured for a dual-chamber pacemaker). The same assessment should be done during an office visit.

Follow-up of the patient with an ICD must include periodic visits during which specific information is collected and assessed. In addition, patients may require interim assessment if there are concerns about the appropriateness of delivered therapy or other changes in the patient's medical status or drug regimen that could affect ICD therapy.

The electrophysiologist or an allied professional with ICD expertise and immediate access to the electrophysiologist should perform follow-up procedures. Aspects of follow-up include the following: history, with specific emphasis on awareness of delivered therapy and any tachyarrhythmic events; device interrogation; assessment of battery status and charge time; retrieval and assessment of stored diagnostic data; periodic radiographic assessment; and periodic arrhythmic induction in the electrophysiology laboratory to assess DFTs and efficacy.

Diagnostic information that can be retrieved varies with different ICDs. ICDs provide information about the cycle length or rate of the detected tachyarrhythmias (Fig. 34-24) and stored electrograms of detected arrhythmias (Fig. 34-25).

Follow-up protocols for patients with ICDs vary. Many caregivers are comfortable with follow-up every 3 to 6 months for the first 3 to 4 years, after which follow-up frequency increases. Internet-based retrieval is available and being used with increasing frequency.

Frequency of DFT testing may depend on the type of ICD system and DFT at implantation or change in medications.

Remote Monitoring

Internet-based device follow-up has been introduced and marks the first major change in device follow-up in many years.[63,64]

Remote monitoring can be loosely defined as the ability to gather incremental device and patient-related data from a remote location. Potential benefits of remote monitoring include the ability to reduce paperwork and directly interact with the electronic medical record, maintain year-round contact with patients, triage patients more effectively and possibly prevent a trip to the emergency department or

EPISODE #3 - JUL 19, 2006 17:51:14

Episode summary

Type:	VT
V. median cycle:	390 ms
V. average cycle:	390 ms
V. interval stability:	0 ms–10 ms
Last therapy:	VT Rx 1–burst, successful
VT/VF duration:	8 sec

SVT criteria triggered prior to VT/VF detection

None

Therapy sequence

VT Rx 1–burst Seq 1
↓
Episode termination

Parameter settings

VF	On	320 ms (188 bpm)
FVT	via VF	260 ms (231 bpm)
VT	On	400 ms (150 bpm)

	NID initial	NID redetect
VF	18/24	12/16
VT	16	12

Sensitivity

V. sensitivity 0.3 mV

	EGM 1	EGM 2
EGM source	HVA to HVB	Vtip to Vring
EGM range	± 8 mV	± 8 mV

Ventricular SVT criteria

VT stability	Off
EGM width	Off

FIGURE 34–24 Example of telemetry information from an implantable cardioverter-defibrillator (ICD). When interrogated, the device provides a large quantity of stored information. In this example, the data include details about an episode that occurred, namely, ventricular tachycardia, at a cycle length of 390 milliseconds, that was terminated successfully with burst pacing. The printout shows the "therapy sequence" as well as the parameter settings, programmed sensitivity, electrograms stored, and the criteria that are programmed "on" or "off" for distinguishing a ventricular tachyarrhythmia from a supraventricular tachyarrhythmia.

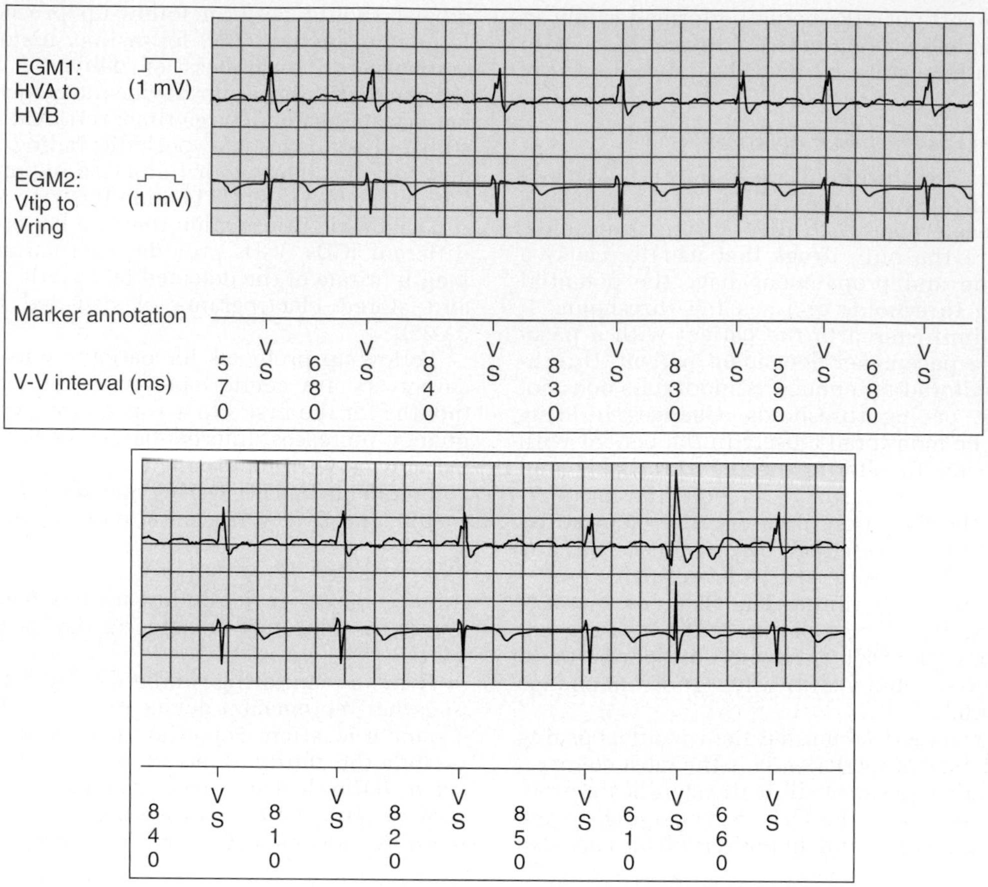

FIGURE 34–25 Example of electrograms stored in an implantable cardioverter-defibrillator (ICD). **Top tracing,** Electrogram 1 (EGM1) recorded from HVA to HVB; EGM2, ventricular EGM recorded from the tip (Vtip) to the ring (Vring) of the ventricular lead. Below this is the marker annotation that explains how each beat on the ventricular EGM was interpreted by the device. **Bottom tracing,** Calculated interval between successive sensed ventricular events (V-V interval).

office, and assimilate the incremental data delivered from increasingly complex devices more efficiently.[65-68]

Currently available systems vary significantly among manufacturers. The general approach is to transfer data from the patient's device to some type of monitoring or programmer-like device. The data are sent from this device to a secure Internet server. The data can then be accessed from this server by the caregiver for analysis and action.

Different systems offer different levels of information remotely and may include full interrogation, real-time electrograms, and different levels of "alerts." In addition, the frequency with which the information is collected varies among systems and, in addition to routine collection, the patient can electively download information if there is some concern about new symptom or symptoms.

Abnormalities may be categorized into different levels of alerts. For example, the service from one manufacturer includes the following as urgent alerts: battery depletion, abnormal lead impedance, abnormal shock impedance, low-amplitude intrinsic R wave, programming change, and notification if ICD therapies are not programmed "on."

It is hoped that remote monitoring will detect device malfunction earlier, asymptomatic brief episodes of device malfunction and/or rhythm disturbances, and potentially the burden of specific dysrhythmias, such as AF. Remote monitoring is gaining acceptance by patients and physicians. Studies of the benefits of remote monitoring are limited, but this approach generally has been well accepted by patients and has detected some rhythm disturbances and device malfunctions that would otherwise have gone undetected until a later date, possibly obviating more significant consequences.[65-68]

REFERENCES

Pacemaker Nomenclature and Indications for Pacing

1. Bernstein AD, Daubert JC, Fletcher RD, et al: North American Society of Pacing and Electrophysiology/British Pacing and Electrophysiology Group: The revised NASPE/BPEG generic code for antibradycardia, adaptive-rate, and multisite pacing. Pacing Clin Electrophysiol 25:260, 2002.
2. Gregoratos G, Abrams J, Epstein AE, et al: American College of Cardiology/American Heart Association Task Force on Practice Guidelines/North American Society for Pacing and Electrophysiology Committee to Update the 1998 Pacemaker Guidelines: ACC/AHA/NASPE 2002 guidelines update for implantation of cardiac pacemakers and antiarrhythmia devices: Summary article. Circulation 106:2145, 2002.
3. Michaelsson M, Jonzon A, Riesenfeld T: Isolated congenital complete atrioventricular block in adult life: A prospective study. Circulation 92:442, 1995.
4. Connolly SJ, Sheldon R, Roberts RS, Gent M: The North American Vasovagal Pacemaker Study (VPS): A randomized trial of permanent cardiac pacing for the prevention of vasovagal syncope. J Am Coll Cardiol 33:16, 1999.
5. Sutton R, Brignole M, Menozzi C, et al: The Vasovagal Syncope International Study (VASIS) Investigators: Is dual-chamber pacing efficacious in treatment of neurally-mediated tilt positive cardioinhibitory syncope? Pacemaker versus no therapy: A multicentre randomised study. Eur J Card Pacing Electrophysiol 3:169, 1993.
6. Connolly SJ, Sheldon R, Thorpe KE, et al; VPS II Investigators: Pacemaker therapy for prevention of syncope in patients with recurrent severe vasovagal syncope: Second Vasovagal Pacemaker Study (VPS II): a randomized trial. JAMA 289:2224, 2003.
7. Gissil AM, Kerr CR, Crystal E: Pacing for the prevention of atrial fibrillation. Can J Cardiol 21:41B, 2005.
8. Saksena S, Prakash A, Ziegler P, et al; DAPPAF Investigators: Improved suppression of recurrent atrial fibrillation with dual-site right atrial pacing and antiarrhythmic drug therapy. J Am Coll Cardiol 40:1140, 2002.
9. Padeletti L, Michelucci A, Pieragnoli P, et al: Atrial septal pacing: A new approach to prevent atrial fibrillation. Pacing Clin Electrophysiol 27:850, 2004.
10. Bailin SJ, Adler S, Giudici M: Prevention of chronic atrial fibrillation by pacing in the region of Bachmann's bundle: Results of a multicenter randomized trial. J Cardiovasc Electrophysiol 12:912, 2001.
11. Padeletti L, Purerfellner H, Adler SW, et al: Worldwide ASPECT Investigators: Combined efficacy of atrial septal lead placement and atrial pacing algorithms for prevention of paroxysmal atrial tachyarrhythmia. J Cardiovasc Electrophysiol 14:1189, 2003.

12. Hoffmann E, Sulke N, Edvardsson N, et al; Atrial Fibrillation Therapy Trial Investigators: New insights into the initiation of atrial fibrillation: A detailed intraindividual and interindividual analysis of the spontaneous onset of atrial fibrillation using new diagnostic pacemaker features. Circulation 113:1933, 2006.
13. Carlson MD, Ip J, Messenger J, et al; Atrial Dynamic Overdrive Pacing Trial (ADOPT) Investigators: A new pacemaker algorithm for the treatment of atrial fibrillation: Results of the Atrial Dynamic Overdrive Pacing Trial (ADOPT). J Am Coll Cardiol 42:627, 2003.

Cardiac Resynchronization Therapy

14. Auricchio A, Stellbrink C, Sack S, et al; Pacing Therapies in Congestive Heart Failure (PATH-CHF) Study Group: Long-term clinical effect of hemodynamically optimized cardiac resynchronization therapy in patients with heart failure and ventricular conduction delay. J Am Coll Cardiol 39:2026, 2002.
15. Cazeau S, Leclercq C, Lavergne T, et al; Multisite Stimulation in Cardiomyopathies (MUSTIC) Study Investigators: Effects of multisite biventricular pacing in patients with heart failure and intraventricular conduction delay. N Engl J Med 344:873, 2001.
16. Linde C, Leclercq C, Rex S, et al: Long-term benefits of biventricular pacing in congestive heart failure: Results from the MUltisite STimulation in cardiomyopathy (MUSTIC) study. J Am Coll Cardiol 40:111, 2002.
17. Abraham WT, Fisher WG, Smith AL, et al; MIRACLE Study Group: Multicenter InSync Randomized Clinical Evaluation. Cardiac resynchronization in chronic heart failure. N Engl J Med 346:1845, 2002.
18. Young JB, Abraham WT, Smith AL, et al; Multicenter InSync ICD Randomized Clinical Evaluation (MIRACLE ICD) Trial Investigators: Combined cardiac resynchronization and implantable cardioversion defibrillation in advanced chronic heart failure: The MIRACLE ICD Trial. JAMA 289:2685, 2003.
19. Bristow MR, Saxon LA, Boehmer J, et al; Comparison of Medical Therapy, Pacing, and Defibrillation in Heart Failure (COMPANION) Investigators: Cardiac-resynchronization therapy with or without an implantable defibrillator in advanced chronic heart failure. N Engl J Med 350:2140, 2004.
20. Cleland JG, Daubert JC, Erdmann E, et al; Cardiac Resynchronization-Heart Failure (CARE-HF) Study Investigators: The effect of cardiac resynchronization on morbidity and mortality in heart failure. N Engl J Med 352:1539, 2005.
21. Auricchio A, Stellbrink C, Butter C, et al; Pacing Therapies in Congestive Heart Failure II Study Group; Guidant Heart Failure Research Group: Clinical efficacy of cardiac resynchronization therapy using left ventricular pacing in heart failure patients stratified by severity of ventricular conduction delay. J Am Coll Cardiol 42:2109, 2003.
22. Abraham WT, Young JB, Leon AR, et al; Multicenter InSync ICD II Study Group: Effects of cardiac resynchronization on disease progression in patients with left ventricular systolic dysfunction, an indication for an implantable cardioverter-defibrillator, and mildly symptomatic chronic heart failure. Circulation 110:2864, 2004.
23. Higgins SL, Hummel JD, Niazi IK, et al: Cardiac resynchronization therapy for the treatment of heart failure in patients with intraventricular conduction delay and malignant ventricular tachyarrhythmias. J Am Coll Cardiol 42:1454, 2003.
24. Leclercq C, Cazeau S, Lellouche D, et al: Upgrading from right-ventricular pacing to biventricular pacing in previously paced patients with advanced heart failure: a randomized controlled study [abstract]. Eur Heart J 24(Suppl):364, 2003.
25. Nishimura RA, Hayes DL, Ilstrup DM, et al: Effect of dual-chamber pacing on systolic and diastolic function in patients with hypertrophic cardiomyopathy: Acute Doppler echocardiographic and catheterization hemodynamic study. J Am Coll Cardiol 27:421, 1996.
26. Kappenberger L, Linde C, Daubert C, et al; PIC Study Group: Pacing in hypertrophic obstructive cardiomyopathy: A randomized crossover study. Eur Heart J 18:1249, 1997.
27. Maron BJ, Nishimura RA, McKenna WJ, et al: Assessment of permanent dual-chamber pacing as a treatment for drug-refractory symptomatic patients with obstructive hypertrophic cardiomyopathy: A randomized, double-blind, crossover study (M-PATHY). Circulation 99:2927, 1999.

Selection of the Appropriate Pacing Mode

28. Andersen HR, Nielsen JC, Thomsen PE, et al: Long-term follow-up of patients from a randomised trial of atrial versus ventricular pacing for sick-sinus syndrome. Lancet 350:1210, 1997.
29. Lamas GA, Orav EJ, Stambler BS, et al; Pacemaker Selection in the Elderly Investigators: Quality of life and clinical outcomes in elderly patients treated with ventricular pacing as compared with dual-chamber pacing. N Engl J Med 338:1097, 1998.
30. Connolly SJ, Kerr CR, Gent M, et al; Canadian Trial of Physiologic Pacing Investigators: Effects of physiologic pacing versus ventricular pacing on the risk of stroke and death caused by cardiovascular causes. N Engl J Med 342:1385, 2000.
31. Lamas GA, Lee KL, Sweeney MO, et al; Mode Selection Trial in Sinus-Node Dysfunction: Ventricular pacing or dual-chamber pacing for sinus-node dysfunction. N Engl J Med 346:1854, 2002.
32. Toff WD, Camm AJ, Skehan JD; United Kingdom Pacing and Cardiovascular Events Trial Investigators: Single-chamber versus dual-chamber pacing for high-grade atrioventricular block. N Engl J Med 353:145, 2005.
33. Andersen HR, Svendsen JH; DANPACE Investigators: The Danish Multicenter Randomized Study on Atrial Inhibited versus Dual-Chamber Pacing in Sick Sinus Syndrome (the DANPACE Study). Heart Drug 1:67, 2001.
34. Wilkoff BL, Cook JR, Epstein AE, et al; Dual Chamber and VVI Implantable Defibrillator Trial Investigators: Dual-chamber pacing or ventricular backup pacing in patients with an implantable defibrillator: The Dual Chamber and VVI Implantable Defibrillator (DAVID) Trial. JAMA 288:3115, 2002.

Modes and Timing Cycles, Rate-Adaptive Pacing, and Pulse Generator Implantation

35. Sweeney MO, Hellkamp AS, Ellenbogen KA; MOde Selection Trial Investigators: Adverse effect of ventricular pacing on heart failure and atrial fibrillation among patients with normal baseline QRS duration in a clinical trial of pacemaker therapy for sinus node dysfunction. Circulation 107:2932, 2003.
36. Leung SK, Lau CP: Developments in sensor-driven pacing. Cardiol Clin 18:113, 2000.
37. Israel CW, Hohnloser SH: Current status of dual-sensor pacemaker systems for correction of chronotropic incompetence. Am J Cardiol 86:86K, 2000.
38. Hayes DL, Naccarelli GV, Furman S, et al; North American Society of Pacing and Electrophysiology: NASPE training requirements for cardiac implantable electronic devices: selection, implantation, and follow-up. Pacing Clin Electrophysiol 26:1556, 2003.

Implantable Cardioverter-Defibrillator Therapy

39. The Antiarrhythmics versus Implantable Defibrillators (AVID) Investigators: A comparison of antiarrhythmic-drug therapy with implantable defibrillators in patients resuscitated from near-fatal ventricular arrhythmias. N Engl J Med 337:1576, 1997.
40. Connolly SJ, Gent M, Roberts RS, et al; Canadian Implantable Defibrillator Study (CIDS): A randomized trial of the implantable cardioverter defibrillator against amiodarone. Circulation 101:1297, 2000.
41. Siebels J, Cappato R, Ruppel R, et al; CASH Investigators: Preliminary results of the Cardiac Arrest Study Hamburg (CASH). Am J Cardiol 72:109F, 1993.
42. Oseroff O, Retyk E, Bochoeyer A; Antiarrhythmics Versus Implantable Defibrillators (AVID); Canadian Implantable Defibrillator Study (CIDS); and Cardiac Arrest Study Hamburg (CASH): Subanalyses of secondary prevention implantable cardioverter-defibrillator trials. Curr Opin Cardiol 19:26, 2004.
43. Moss AJ, Zareba W, Hall WJ, et al: Prophylactic implantation of a defibrillator in patients with myocardial infarction and reduced ejection fraction. N Engl J Med 346:877, 2002.
44. Bigger JT Jr, Coronary Artery Bypass Graft (CABG) Patch Trial Investigators: Prophylactic use of implanted cardiac defibrillators in patients at high risk for ventricular arrhythmias after coronary-artery bypass graft surgery. N Engl J Med 337:1569, 1997.
45. Buxton AE, Fisher JD, Josephson ME, et al; Multicenter Unsustained Tachycardia Trial (MUSTT): Prevention of sudden death in patients with coronary artery disease. Prog Cardiovasc Dis 36:215, 1993.
46. Kadish A, Dyer A, Daubert JP, et al; Defibrillators in Non-Ischemic Cardiomyopathy Treatment Evaluation (DEFINITE) Investigators: Prophylactic defibrillator implantation in patients with nonischemic dilated cardiomyopathy. N Engl J Med 350:2151, 2004.
47. Bardy GH, Lee KL, Mark DB, et al: Amiodarone or an implantable cardioverter-defibrillator for congenital heart failure. N Engl J Med 352:225, 2005.
48. Hohnloser SH, Kuck KH, Dorian P, et al; DINAMIT Investigators: Prophylactic use of an implantable cardioverter-defibrillator after acute myocardial infarction. N Engl J Med 351:2481, 2004.
49. Zareba W, Moss AJ, Daubert JP, et al: Implantable cardioverter defibrillator in high-risk long QT syndrome patients. J Cardiovasc Electrophysiol 14:337, 2003.
50. Cannom DS: Prevention of sudden cardiac death. J Cardiovasc Electrophysiol. 16: S21, 2005.
51. Piccini JP, Dalal D, Roguin A, et al: Predictors of appropriate implantable defibrillator therapies in patients with arrhythmogenic right ventricular dysplasia. Heart Rhythm 2:1188, 2005.
52. Maron BJ, Shen WK, Link MS, et al: Efficacy of implantable cardioverter-defibrillators for the prevention of sudden death in patients with hypertrophic cardiomyopathy. N Engl J Med 342:365, 2000.

ICD Implantation, Complications, and Follow-Up

53. Strickberger SA, Klein GJ: Is defibrillation testing required for defibrillator implantation? J Am Coll Cardiol 44:88, 2004.
54. Russo AM, Sauer W, Gerstenfeld EP, et al: Defibrillation threshold testing: Is it really necessary at the time of implantable cardioverter-defibrillator insertion? Heart Rhythm 2:456, 2005.
55. Atlee JL, Bernstein AD: Cardiac rhythm management devices (part I): Indications, device selection, and function. Anesthesiology 95:1265, 2001.
56. Hayes DL, Wang PJ, Reynolds DW, et al: Interference with cardiac pacemakers by cellular telephones. N Engl J Med 336:1473, 1997.
57. Groh WJ, Boschee SA, Engelstein ED, et al: Interactions between electronic article surveillance systems and implantable cardioverter-defibrillators. Circulation 100:387, 1999.
58. Roguin A, Zviman MM, Meininger GR, et al: Modern pacemaker and implantable cardioverter/defibrillator systems can be magnetic resonance imaging safe: In vitro and in vivo assessment of safety and function at 1.5 T. Circulation 110:475, 2004.
59. Martin ET, Coman JA, Shellock FG, et al: Magnetic resonance imaging and cardiac pacemaker safety at 1.5-tesla. J Am Coll Cardiol 43:1315, 2004.
60. Irnich W, Irnich B, Bartsch C, et al: Do we need pacemakers resistant to magnetic resonance imaging? Europace 7:353, 2005.
61. Carnes CA, Mehdirad AA, Nelson SD: Drug and defibrillator interactions. Pharmacotherapy 18:516, 1998.
62. Huang J, Skinner JL, Rogers JM, et al: The effects of acute and chronic amiodarone on activation patterns and defibrillation threshold during ventricular fibrillation in dogs. J Am Coll Cardiol 40:375, 2002.

63. Theuns DA, Res JC, Jordaens LJ: Home monitoring in ICD therapy: Future perspectives. Europace 5:139, 2003.
64. Chun SH, Friday KJ, Chan A, Liem LB: Clinical benefit and technical accuracy evaluation of wireless home monitoring pacemaker system: Multicenter clinical trial data. J Am Coll Cardiol 41:139A, 2003.
65. Varma N, Stambler B, Chun S: Detection of atrial fibrillation by implanted devices with wireless data transmission capability. Pacing Clin Electrophysiol 28:S133, 2005.
66. Wildau HJ: Wireless remote monitoring for patients with atrial tachyarrhythmias. J Electrocardiol 37:53, 2004.
67. Joseph GK, Wilkoff BL, Dresing T, et al: Remote interrogation and monitoring of implantable cardioverter defibrillators. J Interv Card Electrophysiol 11:161, 2004.
68. Schoenfeld MH, Compton SJ, Mead RH, et al: Remote monitoring of implantable cardioverter defibrillators: a prospective analysis. Pacing Clin Electrophysiol 27:757, 2004.

GUIDELINES *Thomas H. Lee*

Cardiac Pacemakers and Cardioverter-Defibrillators

Guidelines for implantation of cardiac pacemakers and antiarrhythmia devices were published by the American College of Cardiology/American Heart Association (ACC/AHA) and the North American Society for Pacing and Electrophysiology (NASPE) in 1998[1] and updated in 2002.[2] More recent recommendations have been made in guidelines on heart failure in 2005,[3] a scientific statement on atrial pacing in 2005,[4] and updated guidelines in 2006 for management of patients with ventricular arrhythmias and prevention of sudden cardiac death.[5]

As with other ACC/AHA guidelines, these use the standard ACC/AHA classification system for indications:

Class I: Conditions for which there is evidence and/or general agreement that the test is useful and effective

Class II: Conditions for which there is conflicting evidence and/or a divergence of opinion about the usefulness or efficacy of performing the test

Class IIa: Weight of evidence/opinion is in favor of usefulness or efficacy

Class IIb: Usefulness or efficacy is less well established by evidence/opinion

Class III: Conditions for which there is evidence and/or general agreement that the test is not useful or effective and in some cases may be harmful

Three levels are used to rate the evidence upon which recommendations have been based. Level A recommendations are derived from data from multiple randomized clinical trials, level B recommendations are derived from a single randomized trial or nonrandomized studies, and level C recommendations are based on the consensus opinion of experts.

INDICATIONS FOR PERMANENT PACING

(Tables 34G-1 to 34G-10)

Acquired AV Block. For patients with complete or second-degree atrioventricular (AV) block, the ACC/AHA guidelines consider permanent pacing to be appropriate when the abnormality causes complications and is not precipitated by a drug that can be discontinued (see Table 34G-1). Examples of complications include symptomatic bradycardia, congestive heart failure, and confusional states. For asymptomatic patients with complete or advanced second-degree AV block, permanent pacing is considered appropriate for patients at high risk for development of complications, such as those with periods of asystole of 3 seconds or longer or an escape rate less than 40 beats/min, or patients who have had interventions or neuromuscular diseases that have damaged the AV node.

These recommendations differed from those in the prior ACC/AHA guidelines by supporting a lower threshold for use of pacemakers in patients with asymptomatic advanced second-degree heart block and by emphasizing the prognostic importance of the site of origin of the escape rhythm in cases of advanced AV block. For example, when type II second-degree AV block occurs with a wide QRS, pacing now becomes a Class I recommendation, whereas this was a Class IIa recommendation in the prior guidelines.

In addition, heart failure is now considered a complication of AV block that justifies a lower threshold for use of permanent pacing. This theme is also apparent in the Class IIa recommendations, which consider evidence to be generally supportive for the use of pacing in asymptomatic patients with third-degree AV block and ventricular rates or escape rates of 40 beats/min or more, especially if they have cardiomegaly or left ventricular dysfunction.

The guidelines do not support pacing for patients with asymptomatic first-degree or type I second-degree AV block, and they do not support the use of pacing for patients with hypoxia and sleep apnea syndrome in the absence of symptoms. The guideline authors considered support for routine use of atrial pacing for patients with sleep apnea syndrome to be premature, a conclusion supported by recent randomized trials.[6,7]

Chronic Bifascicular and Trifascicular Block. Syncope is common in patients with slowing of conduction below the AV node in the fascicles of the right and left bundles, but the risk of sudden death or progression to complete heart block varies in patient subsets. The ACC/AHA guidelines for pacing in these settings (see Table 34G-2) now include alternating bundle branch block as a Class I indication for pacing, because this finding is recognized as a reflection of abnormal conduction in all three fascicles. The guidelines also provide some support for pacing in patients with findings of markedly abnormal conduction at electrophysiological studies, even if patients are asymptomatic (Class IIa). Pacing is not supported for fascicular block without more than first-degree AV block or symptoms.

Acute Myocardial Infarction. Symptoms do not play a role in appropriateness for pacing in patients with acute myocardial infarction because of the high risk for sudden death in postinfarction patients with conduction system disturbances (see Table 34G-3). The guidelines emphasize that the requirement for temporary pacing after acute myocardial infarction does not automatically indicate a need for permanent pacing. However, permanent pacemakers are supported for use in patients with persistent advanced-degree AV block or transient infranodal AV block and associated bundle branch block. The usefulness of permanent pacemakers for patients with advanced AV block at the AV node level is less clear (Class IIb). Permanent pacing is discouraged if the only indication is transient AV conduction disturbances or left anterior hemiblock.

Sinus Node Dysfunction. As noted in the recommendations for pacing for patients with acquired AV block, the ACC/AHA guidelines support pacing for patients with symptoms caused by bradycardia that is not the result of a drug that can be discontinued. This theme is apparent in the indications for pacing in patients with sinus node dysfunction (see Table 34G-4). Pacing is discouraged in asymptomatic patients, even when resting heart rates are lower than 40 beats/min, and in symptomatic patients when symptoms cannot be proved to be caused by bradycardia. A new Class IIa recommendation is included in the 2002 guidelines that supports pacing in patients with syncope of unexplained origin when major abnormalities of sinus node function are demonstrated at electrophysiological testing.

Prevention and Termination of Tachyarrhythmias. In some patients with long-QT syndrome, continuous pacing can prevent recurrent tachyarrhythmias. In addition, paroxysmal reentrant tachyar-

TABLE 34G-1 ACC/AHA Guidelines for Permanent Pacing in Acquired Atrioventricular Block in Adults

Class	Indication	Level of Evidence
Class I (indicated)	Third-degree and advanced second-degree AV block at any anatomical level, associated with any one of the following conditions:	C
	1. Bradycardia with symptoms (including heart failure) presumed to be caused by AV block	C
	2. Arrhythmias and other medical conditions requiring drugs that result in symptomatic bradycardia	B, C
	3. Documented periods of asystole of 3.0 sec or any escape rate <40 beats/min in awake, symptom-free patients	B, C
	4. After catheter ablation of the AV junction; there are no trials to assess outcome without pacing, and pacing is virtually always planned in this situation unless the operative procedure is AV junction modification	C
	5. Postoperative AV block that is not expected to resolve after cardiac surgery	B
	6. Neuromuscular diseases with AV block, such as myotonic muscular dystrophy, Kearns-Sayre syndrome, Erb dystrophy (limb-girdle), and peroneal muscular atrophy, with or without symptoms, because there may be unpredictable progression of AV conduction disease	B
	Second-degree AV block regardless of type or site of block, with associated symptomatic bradycardia	B
Class IIa (good supportive evidence)	Asymptomatic third-degree AV block at any anatomical site with average awake ventricular rates of ≥40 beats/min, especially if cardiomegaly or LV dysfunction is present	B, C
	Asymptomatic type II second-degree AV block with a narrow QRS; when type II second-degree AV block occurs with a wide QRS, pacing becomes a Class I recommendation	B
	Asymptomatic type I second-degree AV block at intra-His or infra-His levels found at electrophysiological study performed for other indications	B
	First- or second-degree AV block with symptoms similar to those of pacemaker syndrome	B
Class IIb (weak supportive evidence)	Marked first-degree AV block (>0.30 sec) in patients with LV dysfunction and symptoms of congestive heart failure in whom a shorter AV interval results in hemodynamic improvement, presumably by decreasing left atrial filling pressure	C
	Neuromuscular diseases such as myotonic muscular dystrophy, Kearns-Sayre syndrome, Erb dystrophy (limb-girdle), and peroneal muscular atrophy with any degree of AV block (including first-degree AV block), with or without symptoms, because there may be unpredictable progression of AV conduction disease	B
Class III (not indicated)	Asymptomatic first-degree AV block	B
	Asymptomatic type I second-degree AV block at the supra-His (AV node) level or not known to be intrahisian or infrahisian	B, C
	AV block expected to resolve and/or unlikely to recur (e.g., drug toxicity, Lyme disease, or during hypoxia in sleep apnea syndrome in absence of symptoms)	B

ACC = American College of Cardiology; AHA = American Heart Association; AV = atrioventricular; LV = left ventricular.

TABLE 34G-2 ACC/AHA Guidelines for Permanent Pacing in Chronic Bifascicular and Trifascicular Block

Class	Indication	Level of Evidence
Class I (indicated)	Intermittent third-degree AV block	B
	Type II second-degree AV block	B
	Alternating bundle branch block	C
Class IIa (good supportive evidence)	Syncope not demonstrated to be caused by AV block when other likely causes have been excluded, specifically VT	B
	Incidental finding at electrophysiological study of markedly prolonged HV interval (≥100 msec) in asymptomatic patients	B
	Incidental finding at electrophysiological study of pacing-induced infra-His block that is not physiological	B
Class IIb (weak supportive evidence)	Neuromuscular diseases such as myotonic muscular dystrophy, Kearns-Sayre syndrome, Erb dystrophy (limb-girdle), and peroneal muscular atrophy with any degree of fascicular block, without symptoms, because there may be unpredictable progression of AV conduction disease	C
Class III (not indicated)	Fascicular block without AV block or symptoms	B
	Fascicular block with first-degree AV block without symptoms	B

ACC = American College of Cardiology; AHA = American Heart Association; AV = atrioventricular; VT = ventricular tachycardia.

TABLE 34G–3 ACC/AHA Guidelines for Permanent Pacing after the Acute Phase of Myocardial Infarction

Class	Indication	Level of Evidence
Class I (indicated)	Persistent second-degree AV block in the His-Purkinje system with bilateral bundle branch block or third-degree AV block within or below the His-Purkinje system after AMI	B
	Transient advanced (second- or third-degree) infranodal AV block and associated bundle branch block; if site of block is uncertain, electrophysiological study may be necessary	B
	Persistent and symptomatic second- or third-degree AV block	C
Class IIb (weak supportive evidence)	Persistent second- or third-degree AV block at the AV node level	B
Class III (not indicated)	Transient AV block in the absence of intraventricular conduction defects	B
	Transient AV block in the presence of isolated left anterior fascicular block	B
	Acquired left anterior fascicular block in the absence of AV block	B
	Persistent first-degree AV block in the presence of bundle branch block that is old or age-indeterminate	B

ACC = American College of Cardiology; AHA = American Heart Association; AMI = acute myocardial infarction; AV = atrioventricular.

TABLE 34G–4 ACC/AHA Guidelines for Permanent Pacing in Sinus Node Dysfunction

Class	Indication	Level of Evidence
Class I (indicated)	Sinus node dysfunction with documented symptomatic bradycardia, including frequent sinus pauses that produce symptoms; in some patients, bradycardia is iatrogenic and will occur as a consequence of essential long-term drug therapy of type and dose for which there are no acceptable alternatives	C
	Symptomatic chronotropic incompetence	C
Class IIa (good supportive evidence)	Sinus node dysfunction occurring spontaneously or as a result of necessary drug therapy, with heart rate <40 beats/min when a clear association between significant symptoms consistent with bradycardia and the actual presence of bradycardia has not been documented	C
	Syncope of unexplained origin when major abnormalities of sinus node function are discovered or provoked in electrophysiological studies	C
Class IIb (weak supportive evidence)	In minimally symptomatic patients, chronic heart rate <40 beats/min while awake	C
Class III (not indicated)	Sinus node dysfunction in asymptomatic patients, including those in whom substantial sinus bradycardia (heart rate <40 beats/min) is a consequence of long-term drug treatment	
	Sinus node dysfunction in patients with symptoms suggestive of bradycardia that are clearly documented as not associated with a slow heart rate	
	Sinus node dysfunction with symptomatic bradycardia caused by nonessential drug therapy	

ACC = American College of Cardiology; AHA = American Heart Association.

TABLE 34G–5 ACC/AHA Guidelines for Permanent Pacemakers that Automatically Detect and Pace to Terminate Tachycardias

Class	Indication	Level of Evidence
Class I (indicated)	None	
Class IIa (good supportive evidence)	Symptomatic recurrent supraventricular tachycardia reproducibly terminated by pacing in the unlikely event that catheter ablation and/or drugs fail to control the arrhythmia or produce intolerable side effects	C
Class IIb (weak supportive evidence)	Recurrent supraventricular tachycardia or atrial flutter reproducibly terminated by pacing as an alternative to drug therapy or ablation	C
Class III (not indicated)	Tachycardias frequently accelerated or converted to fibrillation by pacing	
	Presence of accessory pathways with capacity for rapid anterograde conduction whether or not the pathways participate in the mechanism of the tachycardia	

ACC = American College of Cardiology; AHA = American Heart Association.

TABLE 34G-6 ACC/AHA Guidelines for Pacing Recommendations to Prevent Tachycardia

Class	Indication	Level of Evidence
Class I (indicated)	Sustained pause-dependent VT, with or without prolonged QT, in which the efficacy of pacing is thoroughly documented	C
Class IIa (good supportive evidence)	High-risk patients with congenital long-QT syndrome	C
Class IIb (weak supportive evidence)	AV reentrant or AV node reentrant supraventricular tachycardia not responsive to medical or ablative therapy	C
	Prevention of symptomatic, drug-refractory, recurrent atrial fibrillation in patients with coexisting sinus node dysfunction	B
Class III (not indicated)	Frequent or complex ventricular ectopic activity without sustained VT in the absence of the long-QT syndrome	
	Torsades de pointes VT from reversible causes	

ACC = American College of Cardiology; AHA = American Heart Association; AV = atrioventricular; VT = ventricular tachycardia.

TABLE 34G-7 ACC/AHA Guidelines for Permanent Pacing in Hypersensitive Carotid Sinus Syndrome and Neurocardiogenic Syncope

Class	Indication	Level of Evidence
Class I (indicated)	Recurrent syncope caused by carotid sinus stimulation; minimal carotid sinus pressure induces ventricular asystole of >3 sec duration in absence of any medication that depresses the sinus node or AV conduction	C
Class IIa (good supportive evidence)	Recurrent syncope without clear provocative events and with a hypersensitive cardioinhibitory response	C
	Significantly symptomatic and recurrent neurocardiogenic syncope associated with bradycardia documented spontaneously or at the time of tilt-table testing	B
Class III (not indicated)	Hyperactive cardioinhibitory response to carotid sinus stimulation in the absence of symptoms or in the presence of vague symptoms such as dizziness, lightheadedness, or both	C
	Recurrent syncope, lightheadedness, or dizziness in the absence of a hyperactive cardioinhibitory response	C
	Situational vasovagal syncope in which avoidance behavior is effective	C

ACC = American College of Cardiology; AHA = American Heart Association; AV = atrioventricular.

TABLE 34G-8 ACC/AHA Guidelines for Pacing in Patients with Cardiomyopathy

Indication	Class I (Indicated)	Class IIa (Good Supportive Evidence)	Class IIb (Weak Supportive Evidence)	Class III (Not Indicated)
Hypertrophic cardiomyopathy	Class I indications for sinus node dysfunction or AV block as described previously		Medically refractory, symptomatic hypertrophic cardiomyopathy with significant resting or provoked LV outflow obstruction	Patients who are symptomatic or medically controlled Symptomatic patients without evidence of LV outflow obstruction
Dilated cardiomyopathy	Class I indications for sinus node dysfunction or AV block as described previously	Biventricular pacing in medic lly refractory, symptomatic NYHA Class III or IV patients with idiopathic dilated or ischemic cardiomyopathy, prolonged QRS interval (≥130 msec), LV end-diastolic diameter ≥55 mm, and ejection fraction ≤35%		Asymptomatic dilated cardiomyopathy Symptomatic dilated cardiomyopathy when patients are rendered asymptomatic by drug therapy Symptomatic ischemic cardiomyopathy when the ischemia is amenable to intervention
After cardiac transplantation	Symptomatic bradyarrhythmias-chronotropic incompetence not expected to resolve and other Class I indications for permanent pacing		Symptomatic bradyarrhythmias-chronotropic incompetence that, although transient, may persist for months and require intervention	Asymptomatic bradyarrhythmias after cardiac transplantation

ACC = American College of Cardiology; AHA = American Heart Association; AV = atrioventricular; LV = left ventricular; NYHA = New York Heart Association.

TABLE 34G-9 ACC/AHA Guidelines for Choice of Pacemaker

Type of Pacemaker	Sinus Node Dysfunction	AV Block	Neurally Mediated Syncope or Carotid Sinus Hypersensitivity
Single-chamber atrial	No suspected abnormality of AV conduction and not at increased risk for future AV block Maintenance of AV synchrony during pacing desired Rate response available if desired	Not appropriate	Not appropriate
Single-chamber ventricular	Maintenance of AV synchrony during pacing not necessary Rate response available if desired	Chronic atrial fibrillation or other atrial tachyarrhythmia or maintenance of AV synchrony during pacing not necessary Rate response available if desired	Chronic atrial fibrillation or other atrial tachyarrhythmia Rate response available if desired
Dual-chamber	AV synchrony during pacing desired Suspected abnormality of AV conduction or increased risk for future AV block Rate response available if desired	Rate response available if desired AV synchrony during pacing desired Atrial pacing desired	Sinus mechanism present Rate response available if desired
Single-lead, atrial-sensing ventricular	Not appropriate	Normal sinus node function and no need for atrial pacing Desire to limit number of pacemaker leads	Not appropriate

ACC = American College of Cardiology; AHA = American Heart Association; AV = atrioventricular.

rhythmias can be terminated in some patients through programmed stimulation and short bursts of rapid pacing. However, the ACC/AHA guidelines do not provide support for the routine use of antitachycardia pacemakers without extensive testing before implantation (see Table 34G-5). The 2002 guidelines actually raise the threshold for use of antitachycardia pacemakers by downgrading its Class I indication for pacing in patients whose recurrent supraventricular tachycardia is unresponsive to antiarrhythmic drugs. This change reflects the committee consensus that drugs and/or ablation therapy should be first-line therapies for most patients. The guidelines continue to consider pacing appropriate (Class I indication) for patients with sustained pause-dependent ventricular tachycardia, with or without prolonged QT, if the efficacy of pacing has been demonstrated (see Table 34G-6).

Prevention of Atrial Fibrillation. Although many pacemakers and ICDs have features designed to prevent atrial fibrillation and to terminate it with rapid atrial pacing, the evidence to support the use of permanent atrial pacing to prevent atrial fibrillation is limited. An American Heart Association Science Advisory, published in 2005, did not support the use of alternative single-site atrial pacing, multisite right atrial pacing, biatrial pacing, overdrive pacing, or antitachycardia atrial pacing to prevent atrial fibrillation in patients who have a bradycardia indication for pacing and also have atrial fibrillation.[4] There is even less evidence to support the role of permanent pacing in the management of atrial fibrillation in patients without symptomatic bradycardia.

Carotid Sinus Syndrome and Neurocardiogenic Syncope. The only Class I indication for permanent pacing in the ACC/AHA guidelines in patients with hypersensitive carotid sinus syndrome is recurrent syncope caused by carotid sinus stimulation in the absence of any drug that depresses the sinus node or AV conduction (see Table 34G-7). However, the guidelines added a new Class IIa indication with support for pacing in patients with recurrent neurocardiogenic syncope associated with bradycardia, reflecting clinical trials showing the benefit of pacing in this setting. Pacing is discouraged in patients without symptoms or who have syncope without bradycardia.

Cardiomyopathy and after Cardiac Transplantation. For patients with hypertrophic or dilated cardiomyopathy or who have had a cardiac transplant, Class I indications for permanent pacing are similar to those in other patient populations (see Table 34G-8). The guidelines do not provide much support for the routine use of pacing in patients with hypertrophic cardiomyopathy for the purpose of reducing left ventricular outflow obstruction (Class IIb indication). However, the 2002 guidelines add a new Class IIa indication of biventricular pacing for patients with dilated cardiomyopathy and prolonged QRS intervals, reflecting multiple trials that have shown clinical and structural benefits from this intervention.

Selection of Pacemakers

The ACC/AHA guidelines provide recommendations (see Table 34G-9) and decision trees to help physicians choose the most appropriate type of pacemaker. These guidelines are aimed at helping physicians match patients' needs to the technology implanted and to anticipate future needs of the patient. Elderly patients should receive devices according to the same indications as younger patients, according to the guidelines.

Follow-up of Patients with Pacemakers

The ACC/AHA guidelines do not directly address follow-up of patients with pacemakers but instead refer physicians to guidelines from other organizations.[8-11] Examples of reasonable follow-up schedules include twice in the first 6 months after implant of single-chamber pacemakers and then once every 12 months and, for dual-chamber pacemakers, twice in the first 6 months and then once every 6 months. Guidelines for transtelephonic monitoring focus on content, not frequency.

Implantable Cardioverter-Defibrillator Therapy

The 2006 guidelines on management of ventricular arrhythmias and prevention of sudden death reflect progress in understanding the role of implantable cardioverter-defibrillators (ICDs),[12,13] which are considered clearly appropriate for several subsets of high-risk patients who are receiving chronic optimal therapy and who have reasonable expectations of survival with a good functional status for more than 1 year (see Table 34G-10). Although the guidelines note that ICD therapy is effective in patients with sustained ventricular tachycardia and impaired left ventricular performance, studies have been inconsistent in enrollment and in findings for patient subsets with different ejection fractions. Acknowledging these inconsistencies, the 2006 ACC/AHA guidelines provide recommendations for ranges of ejection

TABLE 34G-10 ACC/AHA Recommendations for ICD Therapy

Class	Indication	Level of Evidence
Class I (indicated in patents who are receiving chronic optimal therapy and who have reasonable expectation of survival with a good functional status for more than 1 year)	Patients resuscitated from VF who have evidence of prior MI and significant LV dysfunction in whom coronary revascularization cannot be carried out	A
	Patients with LV dysfuncation due to prior MI who are at least 40 days post-MI, with LVEF < 30-40%, and are NYHA functional class II or III	A
	Patients with LV dysfunction due to prior MI who present with hemodynamically unstable sustained VT	A
	Patients with congenital heart disease who are survivors of cardiac arrest after evaluation to define the cause of the event and exclude any reversible causes	B
	Patients with non-ischemic dilated cardiomyopathty and significant LV dysfunction who have sustained VT or VF	A
	Patients with nonischemic dilated cardiomyopathy, how have an LVEF < 30-35% and are NYHA functional class II or III	B
	Patients with hypertrophic cardiomyopathy who have sustained VT and/or VF	B
	Patients with arrhythmogenic right ventricular cardiomyopathy (ARVC) with documented sustained VT or VF	B
	Patients who survived VF or hemodynamically unstable VT, or VT with syncope and who have LVEF < 40%	A
	Long QT syndrome patients with previous cardiac arrest	A
	Brugada syndrome patients with previous cardiac arrest	C
	Patients with catecholaminergic polymorphic ventricular tachycardia who are survivors of cardiac arrest	C
Class IIa (good supportive evidence in patients who are receiving chronic optimal therapy and who have reasonable expectation of survival with a good functional status for more than 1 year)	Patients with LV dysfunction due to prior MI who are least 40 days post-MI, have an LVEF of <30-35%, and are NYHA functional class I	B
	Recurrent VT in patients post-MI with normal or near normal ventricular function	C
	Patients with congenital heart disease and unexplained syncope and impaired ventricular function	B
	Patients with life-threatening ventricular arrhythmias who are not in the acute phase of myocarditis	C
	Patients with unexplained syncope, significant LV dysfunction, and nonischemic dilated cardiomyopathy	C
	Patients with sustained VT and normal or near normal ventricular function and nonischemic dilated cardiomyopathy	C
	Patients with hypertrophic cardiomyopathy who have one or more major risk factors for sudden cardiac death (cardiac arrest; spontaneous sustained VT, family history of premature sudden death, unexplained syncope, LV thickness >30 mm, abnormal exercise blood pressure, or nonsustained spontaneous VT)	C
	Patients with ARVC with extensive disease, including those with LV involvement, one or more affected family members with sudden cardiac death, or undiagnosed syncope when VT or VF has not been excluded as the cause of syncope	C
	In combination with biventricular pacing, or patients in sinus rhythm with a QRS complex of at least 120 ms, with heart failure and NYHA functional class III or IV	B
	Long QT syndrome patients experiencing syncope and/or VT while receiving beta blockers	B
	Brugada syndrome patients with spontaneous ST-segment elevation in V_1, V_2, or V_3, who have had syncope with or without mutations demonstrated in the *SCN5A* gene	C
	Brugada syndrome patients with documented VT that has not resulted in cardiac arrest	C
	Patients with catecholaminergic polymorphic ventricular tachycardia syncope and/or documented sustained VT while receiving beta blockers	C
	Patients with sustained VT and normal or near-normal ventricular function and no structural heart disease	C
Class IIb (weak supportive evidence in patients who are receiving chronic optimal therapy and who have reasonable expectation of survival with a good functional status for more than 1 year)	Patients with nonischemic dilated cardiomyopathy, LVEF < 30-35%, who are NYHA functional class 1	C
	Patients in categories possibly associated with higher risk of cardiac arrest such as long QT2 and long QT3	B
Class III (not indicated)	Acute phase of myocarditis	C

ACC = American College of Cardiology; AHA = American Heart Association; ICD = implantable cardioverter-defibrillator; LV = left ventricular; LVEF = left ventricular ejection fraction; MI = myocardial infarction; NYHA = New York Heart Association; RV = right ventricular; VF = ventricular fibrillation; VT = ventricular tachycardia.

fractions in the context of patient functional status and other clinical data.

The strongest evidence for use of ICDs exists among patients with left ventricular dysfunction who have been resuscitated from VF or hemodynamically unstable VT, or FT with syncope; and for patients who are at least 40 days post-myocardial infarction (MI) and have depressed LV function with ejection fractions less than 30 to 40 percent. On the basis of softer evidence, the 2006 guidelines support use of ICDs in survivors of cardiac arrest or life-threatening arrhythmias with conditions including congenital heart disease, hypertrophic cardiomyopathy, arrhythmogenic right ventricular cardiomyopathy, Brugada syndrome, and catecholaminergic polymorphic ventricular tachycardia. Patients with nonischemic dilated cardiomyopathy who have an ejection fraction less than 30 to 35 percent are also considered appropriate for ICDs.

The 2006 guidelines on heart failure consider it reasonable (Class IIa) to place an ICD in patients with ischemic cardiomyopathy who are at least 40 days post-MI, have a left ventricular ejection fraction of 30 to 35 percent or less, and are NYHA functional class I. ICDs are also considered reasonable for patients with a wide range of cardiac conditions and life-threatening arrhythmias or high-risk histories.

The 2006 guidelines indicate that ventricular arrhythmias that develop in a wide range of noncardiac or systemic diseases that have cardiac implications should be treated according to the same management strategies used in other patients, assuming that the underlying conditions are being treated optimally. These conditions include infiltrative cardiomyopathy; endocrine disorders (e.g., thyroid disorders, pheochromocytoma); end-stage renal failure, especially in patients awaiting renal transplantation; obesity; anorexia; pericardial disease; and neuromuscular conditions.

These guidelines suggest that placement of an ICD might be considered (Class IIb) in patients without heart failure who have nonischemic cardiomyopathy and a left ventricular ejection fraction less than

TABLE 34G-11 AHA/NASPE Guidelines for Safe Resumption of Activities (Classes of Restriction)

Arrhythmia	Private	Commercial
Nonsustained ventricular tachycardia	B_3 if symptoms of impaired consciousness with arrhythmia before treatment A if no impairment of consciousness with arrhythmia	B_6 if symptoms of impaired consciousness with arrhythmia before treatment A if no impairment of consciousness with arrhythmia
Sustained ventricular tachycardia	B_6 B_3 if idiopathic ventricular tachycardia (normal coronary arteries, normal ventricular function) and no impairment of consciousness	C B_6 if idiopathic ventricular tachycardia (normal coronary arteries, normal ventricular function) and no impairment of consciousness
Ventricular fibrillation	B_6	C
Asymptomatic or minimally symptomatic SVT (including WPW syndrome)	A	A
Symptomatic (evidence of hemodynamic compromise) SVT	B until after initiation of therapy that eliminates symptoms	B until after initiation of therapy that eliminates symptoms
Atrial fibrillation treated by catheter ablation of AV node	B	B
SVT with uncontrolled symptoms	C	C
Bradycardia without a pacemaker—no symptoms	A	A
Bradycardia without a pacemaker—syncope or near-syncope	C	C
Bradycardia with a pacemaker—not pacemaker-dependent*	A	A
Bradycardia with a pacemaker—pacemaker-dependent*	B—1 wk	B—4 wk
Vasovagal syncope, mild	A	B_1
Vasovagal syncope, severe		
Treated vasovagal syncope	B_3	B_6
Untreated vasovagal syncope	C	C
Carotid sinus syncope, mild	A	A
Carotid sinus syncope, severe, treated with control	B_1	B_1
Carotid sinus syncope, severe, treated with uncertain control	B_3	B_6
Untreated	C	C

*Patients who are pacemaker-dependent are defined as those who have lost consciousness in the past because of bradyarrhythmias. This group may also include patients immediately after atrioventricular junction ablation or any other patient in whom sudden pacemaker failure would be likely to result in alteration of consciousness.

AHA/NASPE = American Heart Association/North American Society of Pacing and Electrophysiology; AV = atrioventricular; SVT = supraventricular tachycardia; WPW = Wolff-Parkinson-White.

class A = no restriction; class B = restricted for months (in subscript); class C = total restriction.

From Epstein AE, Miles WM, Benditt DG, et al: Personal and public safety issues related to arrhythmias that may affect consciousness: Implications for regulation and physician recommendations. Circulation 94:1147, 1996.

30 to 35 percent who are in NYHA functional class I. ICDs are not considered indicated for long-term prevention of sudden death for patients in the acute phase of myocarditis.

Personal and Public Safety Issues

The AHA and the NASPE published a medical-scientific statement in 1996 that addressed many of the common issues regarding personal and public safety that arise in the care of patients with arrhythmias.[14] This publication summarized guidelines from other organizations, such as the U.S. Federal Aviation Administration, and the limited data available to estimate the risk of injury to the patient and others related to arrhythmias; it provided recommendations about acceptable activities for patients with arrhythmias that may impair consciousness.

The AHA/NASPE guidelines divide patients into three classes (Table 34G-11):

Class A patients should have no restrictions.

Class B patients are restricted for a defined time without arrhythmia recurrence, usually after a therapeutic intervention. This time period is usually expressed as a subscript indicating the number of months of restriction (e.g., B_3).

Class C patients should have total restriction of potentially hazardous activities.

Restrictions were divided into two categories—personal or noncommercial driving and commercial driving or flying. Except where stated otherwise, recommendations for flying were the same as those for commercial drivers. The guidelines noted that recommendations for restriction for commercial drivers might also be relevant to people in other potentially hazardous occupations, such as operators of heavy equipment.

The restrictions imposed by the guidelines vary depending on the severity of the arrhythmia and accompanying symptoms (see Table 34G-11). The duration of the restriction is shorter for patients who do not have impairment of symptoms with their arrhythmias but increases for patients who do have such symptoms and who have ventricular fibrillation or sustained ventricular tachycardia. Patients who have either of these arrhythmias should be totally restricted from commercial driving or flying, according to these guidelines.

These recommendations are for patients who were treated with antiarrhythmic drugs or ICDs. The guidelines recommend that noncommercial drivers should be prohibited from all driving for the first 6 months after ICD implantation; after this period, driving can be resumed if ICD discharge has not occurred. The guidelines recommend that all commercial driving be prohibited permanently after ICD implantation.

Special mention is made of patients with long-QT syndromes. When the QT prolongation is acquired and caused wholly or in part by reversible factors such as electrolyte abnormalities, most patients can be allowed to drive after correction of these factors. Patients who have symptomatic long-QT syndromes should not have driving privileges; those who are asymptomatic with or without treatment can receive driving privileges after a 6-month symptom-free interval.

For patients with supraventricular tachycardias, the guidelines do not impose harsher restrictions on commercial than on private drivers. No restrictions are recommended for patients with minimal or no symptoms with supraventricular tachycardia. For patients who have symptoms suggestive of hemodynamic compromise (e.g., syncope, presyncope, chest pain, or dyspnea), the guidelines recommend restrictions until after initiation of therapy that eliminates symptoms. Patients with supraventricular tachycardia that appears to be successfully ablated can drive after recovery from the procedure. Patients treated with drug therapy should as a minimum have a 1-month symptom-free period before resuming driving, depending on the pretherapy frequency of tachycardia. If symptoms cannot be controlled, permanent full restrictions are recommended.

No restrictions are recommended for patients with bradyarrhythmias who are asymptomatic or who have a pacemaker but are not pacemaker dependent—that is, patients who have lost consciousness in the past because of bradyarrhythmias. "Pacemaker dependent" also includes patients immediately after AV junction ablation or any other patient in whom sudden pacemaker failure would be likely to result in alteration of consciousness. Patients who are pacemaker dependent and have received a pacemaker should be restricted for 1 to 4 weeks, depending on whether they are private or commercial drivers. Patients who have had syncope or presyncope related to bradyarrhythmias who have not received a pacemaker should have full permanent restrictions.

No or only mild restrictions are recommended for patients with mild vasovagal syncope or carotid sinus syncope. The guidelines as written (see Table 34G-11) allow the clinician considerable leeway in determining the duration of restriction.

References

1. Gregoratos G, Cheitlin MD, Conill A, et al: ACC/AHA guidelines for implantation of cardiac pacemakers and antiarrhythmia devices: A report of the American College of Cardiology/American Heart Association Task Force on Practice Guidelines (Committee on Pacemaker Implantation). J Am Coll Cardiol 31:1175, 1998.
2. Gregoratos G, Abrams J, Epstein AE, et al: ACC/AHA/NASPE 2002 guideline update for implantation of cardiac pacemakers and antiarrhythmia devices: Summary article: A report of the American College of Cardiology/American Heart Association Task Force on Practice Guidelines (ACC/AHA/NASPE Committee to Update the 1998 Pacemaker Guidelines). Circulation 106:2145, 2002.
3. Hunt SA, Abraham WT, Chin MH, et al: ACC/AHA 2005 guideline update for the diagnosis and management of chronic heart failure in the adult. Circulation 112: e154, 2005.
4. Knight BP, Gersh BJ, Carlson MD, et al: Role of permanent pacing to prevent atrial fibrillation: Science advisory from the American Heart Association Council on Clinical Cardiology (Subcommittee on Electrocardiography and Arrhythmias) and the Quality of Care and Outcomes Research Interdisciplinary Working Group, in collaboration with the Heart Rhythm Society. Circulation 111:240, 2005.
5. Zipes DP, Camm AJ, Boggrefe M, et al: ACC/AHA/ESC 2006 guidelines for management of patients with ventricular arrhythmias and the prevention of sudden cardiac death: A report of the American College of Cardiology/American Heart Association Task Force and the European Society of Cardiology Committee for Practice Guidelines. Circulation 114:e385, 2006.
6. Krahn AD, Yee R, Erickson MK, et al: Physiologic pacing in patients with obstructive sleep apnea: A prospective, randomized crossover trial. J Am Coll Cardiol 47:379, 2006.
7. Simantirakis EN, Schiza SE, Chrysostomakis SI, et al: Atrial overdrive pacing for the obstructive sleep apnea-hypopnea syndrome. N Engl J Med 353:2568, 2005.
8. Bernstein AD, Irwin ME, Parsonnet V, et al: Report of the NASPE Policy Conference on antibradycardia pacemaker follow-up: Effectiveness, needs, and resources. North American Society of Pacing and Electrophysiology. Pacing Clin Electrophysiol 17:1714, 1994.
9. Levine PA, Belott PH, Bilitch M, et al: Recommendations of the NASPE Policy Conference on pacemaker programmability and follow-up. Pacing Clin Electrophysiol 6:1222, 1983.
10. Fraser JD, Gillis AM, Irwin ME, et al: Guidelines for pacemaker follow-up in Canada: A consensus statement of the Canadian Working Group on Cardiac Pacing. Can J Cardiol 16:355, 2000.
11. Levine PA: Proceedings of the policy conference of the North American Society of Pacing and Electrophysiology on programmability and pacemaker follow-up programs. Clin Prog Pacing Electrophysiol 2:145, 1984.
12. Moss AJ, Zareba W, Hall WJ, et al: Prophylactic implantation of a defibrillator in patients with myocardial infarction and reduced ejection fraction. N Engl J Med 346:877, 2002.
13. Desai AS, Fang JC, Maisel WH, et al: Implantable defibrillators for the prevention of mortality in patients with nonischemic cardiomyopathy: A meta-analysis of randomized controlled trials. JAMA 292:2874, 2004.
14. Epstein AE, Miles WM, Benditt DG, et al: Personal and public safety issues related to arrhythmias that may affect consciousness: Implications for regulation and physician recommendations. A medical/scientific statement from the American Heart Association and the North American Society of Pacing and Electrophysiology. Circulation 94:1147, 1996.

CHAPTER 35

Specific Arrhythmias: Diagnosis and Treatment

Jeffrey E. Olgin and Douglas P. Zipes

NORMAL SINUS RHYTHM

Normal sinus rhythm is arbitrarily limited to impulse formation beginning in the sinus node at rates between 60 and 100 beats/min. Infants and children generally have faster heart rates than adults, both at rest and during exercise. The P wave is upright in electrocardiographic leads I, II, and aVG and negative in lead aVR, with a vector in the frontal plane between 0 and +90 degrees. In the horizontal plane, the P vector is directed anteriorly and slightly leftward and can therefore be negative in leads V_1 and V_2 but positive in V_3 to V_6. The PR interval exceeds 120 milliseconds and can vary slightly with the rate. If the pacemaker site shifts, a change in morphology of the P wave can occur. The rate of sinus rhythm varies significantly and depends on many factors, including age, gender, and physical activity.

The sinus nodal discharge rate responds readily to autonomic stimuli and depends on the effect of the two opposing autonomic influences. Steady vagal stimulation decreases the spontaneous sinus nodal discharge rate and predominates over steady sympathetic stimulation, which increases the spontaneous sinus nodal discharge rate. Single or brief bursts of vagal stimulation can speed, slow, or entrain sinus nodal discharge. A given vagal stimulus produces a greater absolute reduction in heart rate when the basal heart rate has been increased by sympathetic stimulation, a phenomenon known as accentuated antagonism.

Rates below 50 beats/min are considered to be bradycardia and rates greater than 100 beats/min are considered to be tachycardia. As described in Chapter 31, the normal sequence of electrical activation of the heart is from the sinus node through the atria to the atrioventricular (AV) node and His-Purkinje system and to the ventricular myocardium. Arrhythmias resulting in bradycardia or tachycardia can be thought of as specific disorders of each of these components. In this chapter, specific tachyarrhythmias and bradyarrhythmias presented as disorders of this electrophysiologic hierarchy and their characteristics are summarized in Table 35-1.

TACHYARRHYTHMIAS

Tachyarrhythmias are broadly characterized as being a supraventricular tachycardia (SVT), defined as a tachycardia in which the driving circuit or focus originates, at least in part, in tissue above the level of the ventricle (i.e., sinus node, atria, AV node, or His bundle) or a ventricular tachycardia (VT), defined as a tachycardia in which the driving circuit or focus solely originates in ventricular tissue or Purkinje fibers. Because of differences in prognosis and management, the distinction between an SVT and VT is a critical distinction to make early in the acute management of a tachyarrhythmia. In general, VT carries a much graver prognosis, usually implies the presence of significant heart disease, results in more profound hemodynamic compromise, and therefore requires immediate attention and measures to revert to sinus rhythm. On the other hand, SVT is usually not lethal, often does not result in hemodynamic collapse, and therefore more conservative measures can be applied initially to convert to sinus rhythm.

The distinction between an SVT and VT can usually be made on the basis of the electrocardiogram (ECG) obtained during tachycardia. It is important to obtain a 12-lead ECG during tachycardia if possible and to obtain 12-lead (or at least multilead) rhythm strips during any intervention aimed at terminating the tachycardia, because this information is the best way to identify the specific arrhythmia (discussed below) at the bedside. In general, if the QRS is narrow (shorter than 120 milliseconds) during the tachycardia, then the ventricle is being activated via the normal His-Purkinje system and thus the origin of the tachycardia is supraventricular. Therefore, these tachycardias are also often referred to as narrow complex tachycardias. In contrast, whereas a wide QRS (120 milliseconds) during tachycardia suggests a ventricular tachycardia, there are common scenarios in which an SVT can produce a wide QRS complex; thus a more descriptive term, *wide-complex tachycardia,* is often used when the precise arrhythmia mechanism cannot be determined. For example, an SVT with a concurrent bundle branch block (BBB) or intraventricular conduction defect (IVCD) can produce wide-complex tachycardias despite a supraventricular origin. In addition, preexcited tachycardias (tachycardias in which the ventricle is activated in whole or in part over an accessory pathway) produce wide QRS complexes, despite their being supraventricular in origin.

TABLE 35–1 Arrhythmia Characteristics*

Type of Arrhythmia	P Waves			QRS Complexes		
	Rate (beats/min)	*Rhythm*	*Contour*	*Rate (beats/min)*	*Rhythm*	*Contour*
Sinus rhythm	60-100	Regular[†]	Normal	60-100	Regular	Normal
Sinus bradycardia	<60	Regular	Normal	<60	Regular	Normal
Sinus tachycardia	100-180	Regular	May be peaked	100-180	Regular	Normal
AV nodal reentry	150-250	Very regular except at onset and termination	Retrograde; difficult to see; lost in QRS complex	150-250	Very regular except at onset and termination	Normal
Atrial flutter	250-350	Regular	Sawtooth	75-175	Generally regular in absence of drugs or disease	Normal
Atrial fibrillation	400-600	Grossly irregular	Baseline undulation, no P waves	100-160	Grossly irregular	Normal
Atrial tachycardia with block	150-250	Regular; may be irregular	Abnormal	75-200	Generally regular in absence of drugs or disease	Normal
AV junctional rhythm	40-100[§]	Regular	Normal	40-60	Fairly regular	Normal
Reciprocating tachycardias using an accessory (WPW) pathway	150-250	Very regular except at onset and termination	Retrograde; difficult to see; monitor the QRS complex	150-250	Very regular except at onset and termination	Normal
Nonparoxysmal AV junctional tachycardia	60-100[¶]	Regular	Normal	70-130	Fairly regular	Normal
Ventricular tachycardia	60-100[¶]	Regular	Normal	110-250	Fairly regular; may be irregular	Abnormal, >0.12 sec
Accelerated idioventricular rhythm	60-100[¶]	Regular	Normal	50-110	Fairly regular; may be irregular	Abnormal, >0.12 sec
Ventricular flutter	60-100[¶]	Regular	Normal; difficult to see	150-300	Regular	Sine wave
Ventricular fibrillation	60-100[¶]	Regular	Normal; difficult to see	400-600	Grossly irregular	Baseline undulations; no QRS complexes
First-degree AV block	60-100[**]	Regular	Normal	60-100	Regular	Normal
Type I second-degree AV block	60-100[**]	Regular	Normal	30-100	Irregular[††]	Normal
Type II second-degree AV block	60-100[**]	Regular	Normal	30-100	Irregular[††]	Abnormal, >0.12 sec
Complete AV block	60-100[¶]	Regular	Normal	<40	Fairly regular	Abnormal, 0.12 sec
Right bundle branch block	60-100	Regular	Normal	60-100	Regular	Abnormal, 0.12 sec
Left bundle branch block	60-100	Regular	Normal	60-100	Regular	Abnormal, >0.12 sec

AV = atrioventricular; DC = direct current; WPW = Wolff-Parkinson-White.

Modified from Zipes DP: Arrhythmias, *In* Andreoli K, Zipes DP, Wallace AG, et al (eds): Comprehensive Cardiac Care. 6th ed. St Louis, CV Mosby, 1987.

*In an effort to summarize these arrhythmias in tabular form, generalizations have to be made. For example, the response to carotid sinus massage may be slightly different from what is listed. Acute therapy to terminate a tachycardia may be different from chronic therapy to prevent recurrence. Some of the exceptions are indicated in the footnotes; the reader is referred to the text for a complete discussion.

†P waves initiated by sinus node discharge may not be precisely regular because of sinus arrhythmia.

‡Often, carotid sinus massage fails to slow a sinus tachycardia.

§Any independent atrial arrhythmia may exit or the atria may be captured retrogradely.

Ventricular Response to Carotid Sinus Massage	Physical Examination			Treatment
	Intensity of S_1	*Splitting of S_2*	*a Waves*	
Gradual slowing and return to former rate	Constant	Normal	Normal	None
Gradual slowing and return to former rate	Constant	Normal	Normal	None, unless symptomatic; atropine
Gradual slowing[‡] and return to former rate	Constant	Normal	Normal	None, unless symptomatic; treat underlying disease
Abrupt slowing caused by termination of tachycardia, or no effect	Constant	Normal	Constant cannon *a* waves	Vagal stimulation, adenosine, verapamil, digitalis, propranolol, DC shock, pacing
Abrupt slowing and return to former rate; flutter remains	Constant; variable if AV block changing	Normal	Flutter waves	DC shock, digitalis, quinidine, propranolol, verapamil, adenosine
Slowing; gross irregularity remains	Variable	Normal	No *a* waves	Digitalis, quinidine, DC shock, verapamil, adenosine
Abrupt slowing and return to normal rate; tachycardia remains	Constant; variable if AV block changing	Normal	More *a* waves than *c-v* waves	Stop digitalis if toxic; digitalis if not toxic; possibly verapamil
None; may be slight slowing	Variable[¶]	Normal	Intermittent cannon waves	None, unless symptomatic; atropine
Abrupt slowing caused by termination of tachycardia, or no effect	Constant but decreased	Normal	Constant cannon waves	See AV nodal reentry earlier
None; may be slight slowing	Variable[¶]	Normal	Intermittent cannon waves[¶]	None, unless symptomatic; stop digitalis if toxic
None	Variable[¶]	Abnormal	Intermittent cannon waves[¶]	Lidocaine, procainamide, DC shock, quinidine, amiodarone
None	Variable[¶]	Abnormal	Intermittent cannon waves[¶]	None, unless symptomatic; lidocaine, atropine
None	Soft or absent	Soft or absent	Cannon waves	DC shock
None	None	None	Cannon waves	DC shock
Gradual slowing caused by sinus	Constant, diminished	Normal	Normal	None
Slowing caused by sinus slowing and an increase in AV black	Cyclic decrease, then increase after pause	Normal	Normal; increasing *a-c* interval; *a* waves without *c* waves	None, unless symptomatic; atropine
Gradual slowing caused by sinus slowing	Constant	Abnormal	Normal; constant *a-c* interval; *a* waves without *c* waves	Pacemaker
None	Variable**	Abnormal	Intermittent cannon waves**	Pacemaker
Gradual slowing and return to former rate	Constant	Wide	Normal	None
Gradual slowing and return to former rate	Constant	Paradoxical	Normal	None

[¶]Constant if the atria are captured retrogradely.

**Atrial rhythm and rate may vary, depending on whether sinus bradycardia, sinus tachycardia, or another abnormality is the atrial mechanism.

[††]Regular or constant if block is unchanging.

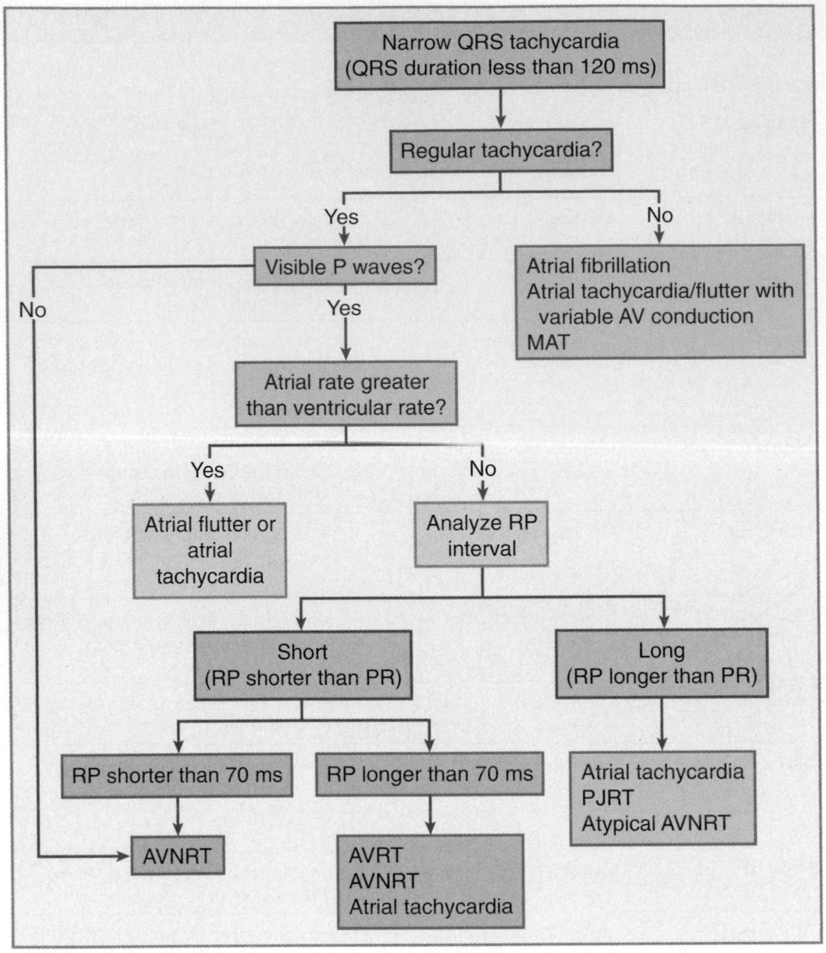

FIGURE 35–1 Algorithm for diagnosing a normal QRS tachycardia. AV = atrioventricular; AVRT = AV reentrant tachycardia; AVNRT = AV nodal reentrant tachycardia; MAT = multifocal atrial tachycardia; PJRT = permanent form of AV junctional reciprocating tachycardia. (From Blomstrom-Lundqvist C, Scheinman MM, Aliot EM, et al: ACC/AHA/ESC guidelines for the management of patients with supraventricular arrhythmias—executive summary: A report of the American College of Cardiology/American Heart Association Task Force on Practice Guidelines and the European Society of Cardiology Committee for Practice Guidelines [Writing Committee to Develop Guidelines for the Management of Patients With Supraventricular Arrhythmias]. Circulation 108:1871, 2003.)

Therefore, although a narrow complex tachycardia almost always makes the diagnosis of an SVT, a wide-complex tachycardia can be supraventricular or ventricular. The presence of fusion or capture beats and of AV dissociation are diagnostic of VT (discussed later, "Ventricular Tachycardia; Electrocardiographic Recognition"), but are often not present or are difficult to detect. Criteria have been developed based on the 12-lead ECG (Fig. 35-1; Table 35-2) that can be helpful in determining whether a wide-complex tachycardia is more likely to be SVT or VT.[1]

Sinus Tachycardia

ELECTROCARDIOGRAPHIC RECOGNITION. Tachycardia (Fig. 35-2) in an adult is defined as a rate of 100 beats/min. During sinus tachycardia, the sinus node exhibits a discharge frequency between 100 and 180 beats/min, but it may be higher with extreme exertion and in young individuals. The maximum heart rate achieved during strenuous physical activity decreases with age from about 200 beats/min at age 20 years to less than 140 beats/min at age 80. Sinus tachycardia generally has a gradual onset and termination. The P-P interval can vary slightly from cycle to cycle, especially at slower rates. P waves have a normal contour, but a larger amplitude can develop and the wave can become peaked. They appear before each QRS complex with a stable PR interval unless concomitant AV block ensues.

Accelerated phase 4 diastolic depolarization of sinus nodal cells (see Chap. 31) is generally responsible for sinus tachycardia and is usually caused by elevated adrenergic tone and/or withdrawal of parasympathetic tone. Carotid sinus massage and Valsalva or other vagal maneuvers gradually slow sinus tachycardia, which then accelerates to its previous rate on cessation of enhanced vagal tone. More rapid sinus rates can fail to slow in response to a vagal maneuver, particularly those driven by high adrenergic tone.

CLINICAL FEATURES. Sinus tachycardia is common in infancy and early childhood and is the normal reaction to various physiological or pathophysiological stresses, such as fever, hypotension, thyrotoxicosis, anemia, anxiety, exertion, hypovolemia, pulmonary emboli, myocardial ischemia, congestive heart failure, or shock. Drugs such as atropine, catecholamines, and thyroid medications, as well as alcohol, nicotine, caffeine, and inflammation, can produce sinus tachycardia. Persistent sinus tachycardia can be a manifestation of heart failure.

In patients with structural heart disease, sinus tachycardia can result in reduced cardiac output or angina or can precipitate another arrhythmia, in part related to the abbreviated ventricular filling time and compromised coronary blood flow. Sinus tachycardia can be a cause of inappropriate defibrillator discharge in patients with an implantable cardioverter-defibrillator (ICD; see Chap. 34). Chronic inappropriate sinus tachycardia (also known as the syndrome of inappropriate sinus tachycardia) has been described in otherwise healthy persons, possibly secondary to increased automaticity of the sinus node or an automatic atrial focus located near the sinus node.[2-4] The abnormality can result from a defect in either sympa-

TABLE 35–2 Major Features in the Differential Diagnosis of Wide QRS Beats Versus Tachycardia

Supports SVT	Supports VT
Slowing or termination by vagal tone	Fusion beats
Onset with premature P wave	Capture beats
RP interval ≤100 msec	AV dissociation
P and QRS rate and rhythm linked to suggest that ventricular activation depends on atrial discharge, e.g., 2 : 1 AV block rSR′ V_1	P and QRS rate and rhythm linked to suggest that atrial activation depends on ventricular discharge, e.g., 2 : 1 VA block
Long-short cycle sequence	"Compensatory" pause Left-axis deviation; QRS duration >140 msec Specific QRS contours (see text)

AV = atrioventricular; SVT = supraventricular tachycardia; VA = ventriculoatrial; VT = ventricular tachycardia.

thetic or vagal nerve control of sinoatrial (SA) automaticity, or an abnormality of the intrinsic heart rate. Postural orthostatic tachycardia syndrome (POTS) is a related syndrome with orthostatic hypotension and sinus tachycardia, in which hypovolemia or drugs are not the cause of the orthostatic decrease in blood pressure. Both syndromes can result from autonomic neuropathy (either peripheral, as seen in diabetics, or central, from spinal cord injury).[2,3] Sinus node reentry (Fig. 35-3) is an atrial tachycardia originating from tissue near the sinus node and thus has a P wave morphology similar to sinus rhythm.[4] The mechanism and management of this tachycardia are discussed later in more detail in the section on focal atrial tachycardias.

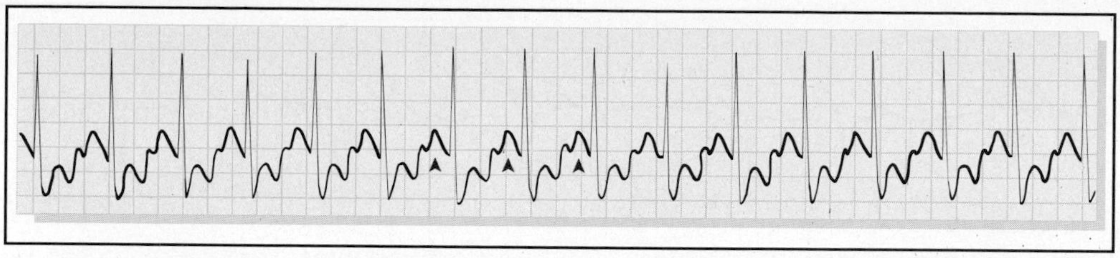

FIGURE 35–2 Sinus tachycardia (150 beats/min) in a patient during acute myocardial ischemia; note the ST segment depression. P waves are indicated by arrowheads.

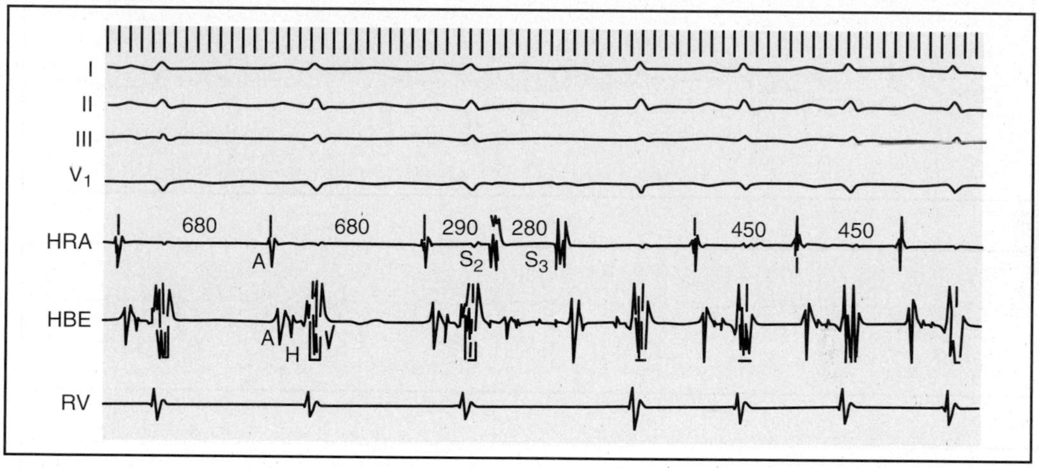

FIGURE 35–3 Sinus node reentry. After three spontaneous sinus-initiated beats, premature stimulation of the high right atrium (S_2, S_3) initiates a sustained tachycardia at a cycle length of 450 milliseconds that has the identical high-low atrial activation sequence characteristic of sinus node discharge. This is sinus node reentry. Leads I, II, III, and V_1 are scalar leads. A = atrial electrogram; H = His electrogram; HBE = His bundle electrogram; HRA = high right atrial electrogram; RV = right ventricular electrogram. Numbers are milliseconds.

MANAGEMENT. Management should focus on the cause of the sinus tachycardia. In the hospital inpatient setting, this is usually obvious (e.g., hemorrhage, sepsis, agitation). In the outpatient setting, the cause may be more elusive. The most common reversible causes include hyperthyroidism, anemia, diabetes (autonomic neuropathy), and hypovolemia. Elimination of tobacco, alcohol, coffee, tea, or other stimulants, such as the sympathomimetic agents in nose drops, may be helpful. Drugs such as propranolol or verapamil, or fluid replacement in a hypovolemic patient or fever reduction in a febrile patient, can be used to help slow the sinus nodal discharge rate. Treatment of inappropriate sinus tachycardia requires beta blockers or calcium channel blockers, alone or in combination. In severe cases, sinus node radiofrequency or surgical ablation may be indicated; however, these approaches are usually only temporarily palliative (see Chap. 33). A specific blocker of the pacemaker current (I_f), ivabradine, has been developed (currently available in some European countries and Australia) and may be useful treatment in some patients with inappropriate or refractory sinus tachycardia.[5]

Premature Atrial Complexes

Premature complexes are among the most common causes of an irregular pulse. They can originate from any area in the heart—most frequently from the ventricles, less often from the atria and the AV junctional area, and rarely from the sinus node. Although premature complexes arise commonly in normal hearts, they are more often associated with structural heart disease and increase in frequency with age.

ELECTROCARDIOGRAPHIC RECOGNITION. The diagnosis of premature atrial complexes (PACs) (Fig. 35-4) is made on the ECG by the presence of a premature P wave with a PR interval of 120 milliseconds (except in Wolff-Parkinson-White [WPW] syndrome, in which case the PR interval is usually shorter than 120 milliseconds). Although the contour of a premature P wave can resemble that of a normal sinus P wave, it generally differs. Whereas variations in the basic sinus rate can at times make the diagnosis of prematurity difficult, differences in the contour of the P waves are usually apparent and indicate a different focus of origin. When a PAC occurs early in diastole, conduction may not be completely normal. The AV junction may still be refractory from the preceding beat and prevent propagation of the impulse (blocked or nonconducted premature atrial complex; see Fig. 35-4A) or cause conduction to be slowed (PAC with a prolonged PR interval). As a general rule, the RP interval is inversely related to the PR interval; thus, a short RP interval produced by an early PAC occurring close to the preceding QRS complex is followed by a long PR interval. When PACs occur early in the cardiac cycle, the premature P waves can be difficult to discern because they are superimposed on T waves. Careful examination of tracings from several leads may be necessary before the PAC is recognized as a slight deformity of the T wave. Often, such PACs are blocked before reaching the ventricle and can be misinterpreted as a sinus pause or sinus exit block (see Fig. 35-4A).

The length of the pause following any premature complex or series of premature complexes is determined by the interaction of several factors. If the PAC occurs when the sinus node and perinodal tissue are not refractory, the impulse can be conducted into the sinus node, discharge it prematurely, and cause the next sinus cycle to begin from that time. The interval between the two normal P waves flanking a PAC that has reset the timing of the basic sinus rhythm is less than twice the normal P-P interval, and the pause after the PAC is said to be "noncompensatory" (see Fig. 35-4E and F). Reset (noncompensatory pause) occurs when the A_1-A_2 interval plus the A_2-A_3 interval is less than two times the A_1-A_1 interval and the A_2-A_3 interval is greater than the A_1-A_1 interval. The interval between the PAC (A_2) and the following sinus-

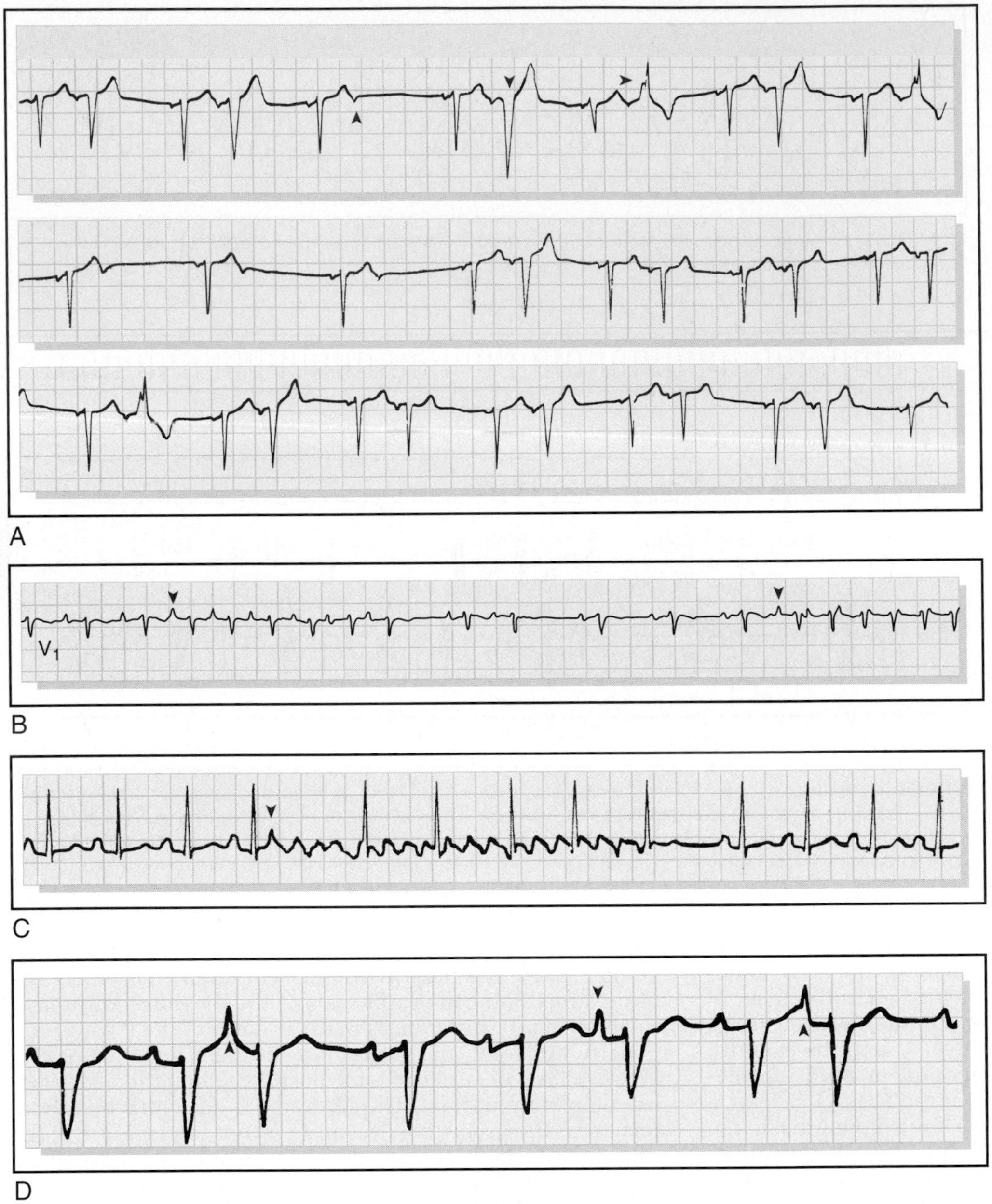

FIGURE 35–4 A, Premature atrial complexes (PACs) that block conduction entirely or conduct with a functional right or functional left bundle branch block. Depending on the preceding cycle length and coupling interval of the PAC, the latter blocks conduction entirely in the atrioventricular (AV) node (arrowhead ↑) or conducts with a functional left bundle branch block (arrowhead ↓) or functional right bundle branch block (arrowhead →). **B,** A PAC on the left (arrowhead) initiates AV nodal reentry that is caused by reentry anterogradely and retrogradely over two slow AV nodal pathways, with a retrograde P wave produced midway in the cardiac cycle. On the right, a PAC (arrowhead) initiates AV nodal reentry as a result of anterograde conduction over the slow pathway and retrograde conduction over the fast pathway (see Fig. 35-13A), which produces a retrograde P wave in the terminal portion of the QRS complex that simulates an r′ wave. **C** and **D,** A PAC (arrowhead ↓) initiating a short run of atrial flutter **(C)** and a PAC (arrowhead ↑) depressing return of the next sinus nodal discharge **(D).** A slightly later PAC (arrowhead ↓) in **D** does not depress sinus nodal automaticity. **B** to **D,** Monitor leads.

initiated P wave (A_3) exceeds one sinus cycle but is less than "fully compensatory" (see later), because the A_2-A_3 interval is lengthened by the time that it takes the ectopic atrial impulse to conduct to the sinus node and depolarize it and then for the sinus impulse to return to the atrium. These factors lengthen the return cycle—that is, the interval between the PAC (A_2) and the following sinus-initiated P wave (A_3) (see Fig. 35-4E and F). Premature discharge of the sinus node by an early PAC can temporarily depress sinus nodal automatic activity and cause the sinus node to beat more slowly initially (see Fig. 35-4D). Often, when this happens, the interval between the A_3 and the next sinus-initiated P wave exceeds the A_1-A_1 interval.

Less commonly, the PAC encounters a refractory sinus node or perinodal tissue (see Fig. 35-4F), in which case the timing of the basic sinus rhythm is not altered, because the sinus node is not reset by the PAC, and the interval between the two normal, sinus-initiated P waves flanking the PAC is twice the normal P-P interval. The interval following this premature atrial discharge is said to be a "full compensatory pause"—that is, of sufficient duration so that the P-P interval bounding the PAC is twice the normal P-P interval. However, sinus arrhythmia can lengthen or shorten this pause. Rarely, an interpolated PAC may occur. In this case, the pause after the PAC is very short, and the interval bounded by the normal sinus-initiated P waves on each side of the PAC is only slightly longer than or is equal to one normal P-P cycle length. The interpolated PAC fails to affect the sinus nodal pacemaker, and the sinus impulse following the PAC is conducted to the ventricles, often with a slightly lengthened PR interval. An interpolated atrial or ventricular premature complex of any type represents the only type of premature systole that does not actually replace the normally conducted beat. Premature atrial complexes can originate in the sinus node and are identified by premature P waves that have a contour identical to that of the normal sinus P wave.

On occasion, when the AV node has had sufficient time to repolarize and conduct without delay, the supraventricular QRS complex initiated by the PAC can be aberrant in configuration, because the His-Purkinje system or ventricular muscle has not completely repolarized and conducts with a functional delay or block (see Fig. 35-4A). The refractory period of cardiac fibers is directly related to cycle length. (In an adult, the AV nodal effective refractory period is prolonged at shorter cycle lengths.) A slow heart rate (long cycle length) produces a longer His-Purkinje refractory period than a faster heart rate. As a consequence, a PAC that follows a long R-R interval (long refractory period) can result in a functional bundle branch block (BBB; aberrant ventricular conduction). Because the right bundle branch at long cycles has a longer refractory period than the left bundle branch, aberration with a right bundle branch block pattern at slow rates occurs more commonly than aberration with a left bundle branch block pattern. At shorter cycles, the refractory period of the left bundle branch exceeds that of the right bundle branch, and a left bundle branch block pattern may be more likely to occur.

CLINICAL FEATURES. Premature atrial complexes can occur in various situations, such as during infection, inflammation, or myocardial ischemia, or they can be provoked by various medications, tension states, or tobacco, alcohol, or caffeine. Premature atrial complexes can precipitate or presage the occurrence of sustained supraventricular (see Fig. 35-4B and C) and, rarely, ventricular tachyarrhythmias.

MANAGEMENT. Premature atrial complexes generally do not require therapy. In symptomatic patients or when the PACs precipitate tachycardias, treatment with a beta blocker or a calcium antagonist can be tried.

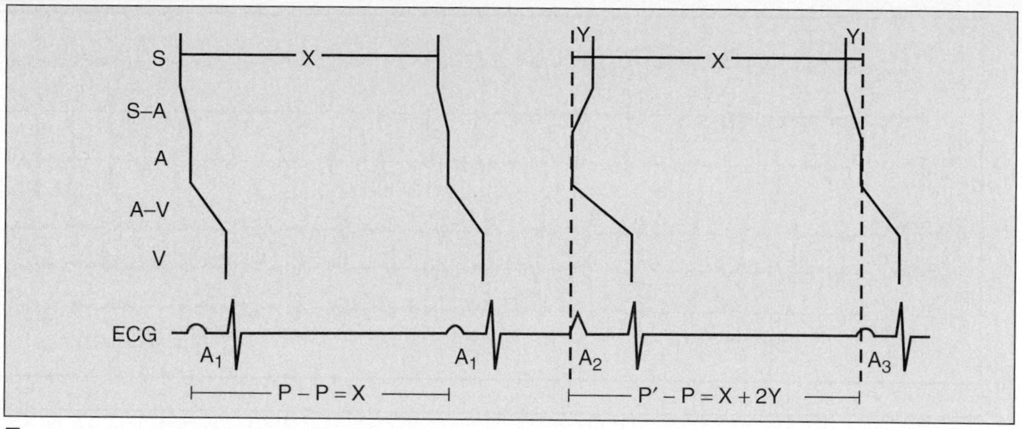

E

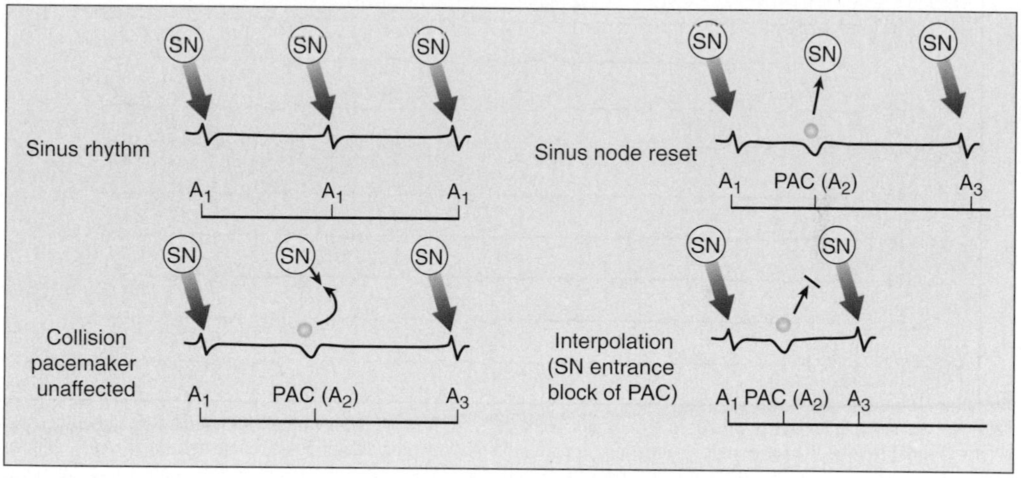

F

FIGURE 35–4, cont'd E, Diagrammatic example of the effects of a PAC. The sinus interval (A_1-A_1) equals X. The third P wave represents a PAC (A_2) that reaches and discharges the sinoatrial (SA) node, which causes the next sinus cycle to begin at that time. Therefore, the P-P (A_2-A_3) interval equals X + 2Y milliseconds, assuming no depression of SA nodal automaticity. **F,** Diagram of interactions of a PAC (yellow circles indicate origin; QRS complexes omitted) with the sinus node (SN) depending on the degree of prematurity. The top represents spontaneous sinus rhythm. The bottom is a late coupled PAC that collides with the exiting sinus impulse and therefore does not affect (or reset) the sinus pacemaker. The next sinus impulse (S_3) occurs at exactly twice the sinus interval. An early coupled PAC in the next diagram is able to penetrate the sinus node and resets the pacemaker, thereby resulting in resetting of the sinus node (as depicted in **E**). An even earlier coupled PAC in the lower figure reaches refractory tissue around the sinus node and is thus unable to penetrate the sinus node (SN entrance block); therefore, it does not affect sinus node discharge. The next spontaneous sinus beat (S_3) arrives exactly at the sinus interval. (**E,** Modified from Zipes DP, Fisch C: Premature atrial contraction. Arch Intern Med 128:453, 1971.)

Atrial Fibrillation

ELECTROCARDIOGRAPHIC RECOGNITION. Atrial fibrillation (Figs. 35-5 and 35-6) is an arrhythmia characterized by seemingly disorganized atrial depolarizations without effective atrial contraction. It was once thought that all atrial fibrillation was caused by a single mechanism of multiple wavelets propagating in random fashion throughout the atria. It is now apparent that there are likely several mechanisms and that there may be some organization to atrial fibrillation. For example, in many patients, atrial fibrillation is caused by a focal discharge at rapid rates and fibrillatory conduction (heterogeneous conduction caused by rapidity of activation) through the atria. Nonetheless, all these potential mechanisms of atrial fibrillation have a common appearance on the ECG. During atrial fibrillation, electrical activity of the atrium can be detected on the ECG as small, irregular baseline undulations of variable amplitude and morphology, called f waves, at a rate of 350 to 600 beats/min. At times, small, fine, rapid f waves can occur and are detectable only by right atrial leads or by intracavitary or esophageal electrodes. The ventricular response is grossly irregular (irregularly irregular) and, in an untreated patient with normal AV conduction, is usually between 100 and 160 beats/min. In patients with WPW syndrome, the ventricular rate during atrial fibrillation can at times exceed 300 beats/min and lead to ventricular fibrillation. Atrial fibrillation should be suspected when the ECG shows supraventricular complexes at an irregular rhythm and no obvious P waves. The recognizable f waves probably do not represent total atrial activity but depict only the larger vectors generated by the multiple wavelets of depolarization that occur at any given moment.

Each recorded f wave is not conducted through the AV junction, so a rapid ventricular response comparable to the atrial rate does not occur. Many atrial impulses are concealed (not recorded in the ECG) because of a collision of wave fronts, or they are blocked in the AV junction without reaching the ventricles (i.e., concealed conduction, which accounts for the irregular ventricular rhythm). The refractory period and conductivity of the AV node are determinants of the ventricular rate. When the ventricular rate is very rapid or very slow, it may appear to be more regular. Even though conversion of atrial fibrillation to atrial flutter is accompanied by slowing of the *atrial* rate, an increase in the ventricular response can result, because more atrial impulses are transmitted to the ventricle as a result of less concealed conduction. Also, it is easier to slow the ventricular rate during atrial fibrillation than during atrial flutter with drugs such as digitalis, calcium antagonists, and beta blockers, because the increased concealed conduction makes it easier to produce an AV block.

CLINICAL FEATURES. Atrial fibrillation is a common arrhythmia that is found in 1 percent of persons older than

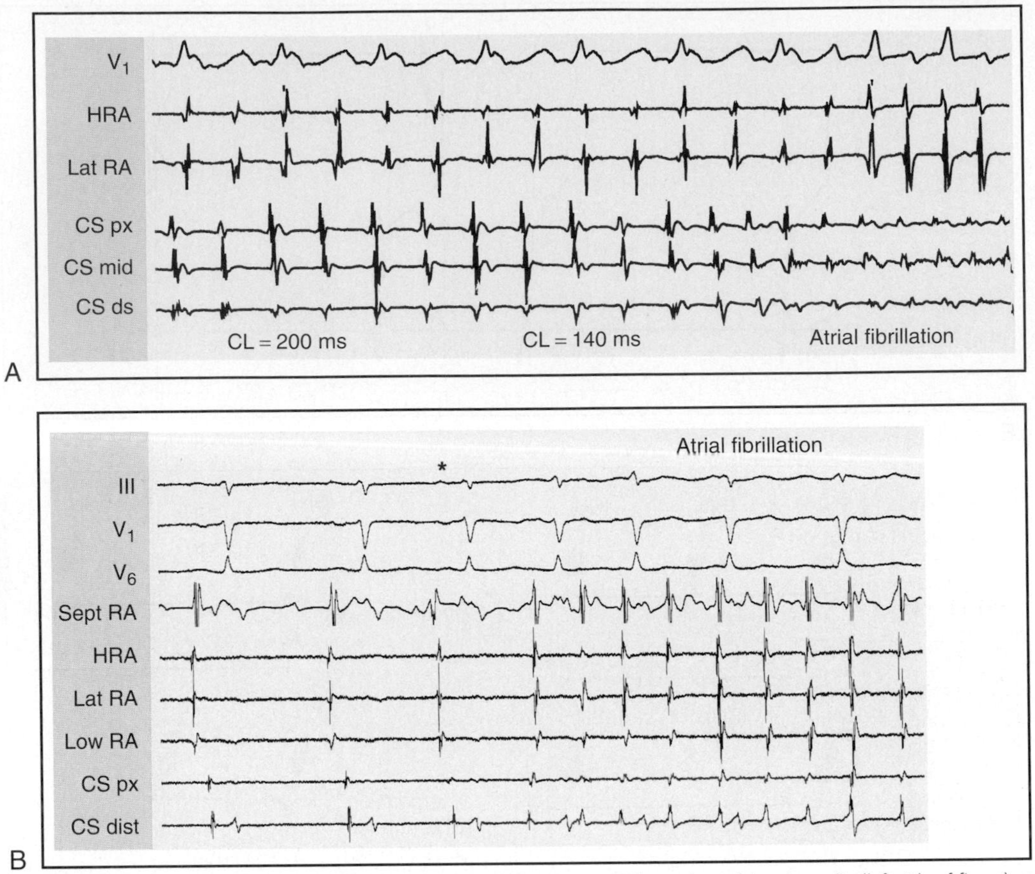

FIGURE 35–5 Atrial fibrillation produced by "focal" mechanisms. **A,** A rapid, regular atrial tachycardia (left side of figure) at a cycle length (CL) of 200 milliseconds degenerates into atrial fibrillation (right side of figure) characterized by rapid, irregular atrial depolarizations. **B,** A premature atrial complex (marked by the asterisk) induces atrial fibrillation (right side of figure). Elimination of these focal triggers for atrial fibrillation can eliminate the atrial fibrillation. CS = coronary sinus; HRA = high right atrial electrogram; RA = right atrium.

60 years to more than 5 percent of patients older than 69 years. From the Framingham data, the lifetime risk of developing atrial fibrillation after age 40 has been found to be 26.0 percent (95 percent confidence interval [CI], 24.0 to 27.0 percent) for men and 23.0 percent (21.0 to 24.0 percent).[6] Estimates are that 2.2 million Americans have atrial fibrillation, which occurs more commonly in men than in women. A history of congestive heart failure, valvular heart disease and stroke, left atrial enlargement, abnormal mitral or aortic valve function, treated systemic hypertension, and advanced age are independently associated with the prevalence of atrial fibrillation. Most recently, obesity has been found as an additional risk factor for developing atrial fibrillation.[7] Four important aspects of atrial fibrillation are treatable contributing factors, control of the ventricular rate, prevention of recurrences, and prevention of thromboembolic episodes. Occult or manifest thyrotoxicosis should be considered in patients with recent-onset atrial fibrillation. Atrial fibrillation can be intermittent or chronic and may be influenced by autonomic activity. Atrial fibrillation, whether it is persistent or intermittent, predisposes to stroke. Symptoms as a result of atrial fibrillation are determined by multiple factors, including the underlying cardiac status, the rapidity and irregularity of ventricular rate, and loss of atrial contraction.

Physical findings include a slight variation in intensity of the first heart sound, absence of *a* waves in the jugular venous pulse, and an irregularly irregular ventricular rhythm. Often, with fast ventricular rates, a significant pulse deficit appears (i.e., the auscultated apical rate is faster than the rate palpated at the wrist, pulse deficit, because each contraction is not sufficiently strong to open the aortic valve or transmit an arterial pressure wave through the peripheral artery). If the ventricular rhythm becomes regular in patients with atrial fibrillation, conversion to sinus rhythm, atrial tachycardia, or atrial flutter with a constant ratio of conducted beats or the development of junctional tachycardia or VT should be suspected.

EMBOLIZATION AND ANTICOAGULATION. In addition to hemodynamic alterations, the risk of systemic emboli, probably arising in the left atrial cavity or appendage as a result of circulatory stasis, is an important consideration (see Chap. 82). Nonvalvular atrial fibrillation is the most common cardiac disease associated with cerebral embolism. In fact, almost half of cardiogenic emboli in the United States occur in patients with nonvalvular atrial fibrillation. The risk of stroke in patients with nonvalvular atrial fibrillation is five to seven times greater than that in controls without atrial fibrillation. Overall, 20 to 25 percent of ischemic strokes are caused by cardiogenic emboli.

Many studies have evaluated the risk of stroke in patients with atrial fibrillation and the benefits of anticoagulation and antiplatelet therapy.[8-12] Patients with mitral stenosis and atrial fibrillation have a 4 to 6 percent incidence of embolism per year. Risk factors that predict stroke in patients with nonvalvular atrial fibrillation include a history of previous stroke or transient ischemic attack (relative risk, 2.5), diabetes (relative risk, 1.7), history of hypertension (relative risk, 1.6), and increasing age (relative risk, 1.4 for each decade). Patients with any of these risk factors have an annual stroke risk of at least 4 percent if untreated. Patients whose only stroke risk factor is congestive heart failure or coronary artery disease have stroke rates approximately three times higher than patients without any risk factors. Left ventricular (LV) dysfunction and a left atrial size larger than 2.5 cm/m^2 on echocardiographic examination are associated with thromboembolism. Patients younger than 60 to 65 years of age who have a normal echocardiogram and no risk factors have an extremely low risk for stroke (1 percent per year). Therefore, the risk of stroke in patients with lone atrial fibrillation—that is, idiopathic atrial fibrillation in the absence of any structural heart disease or any of the risk factors discussed previously—is relatively low. A scoring system to predict risk of stroke accounting for all these clinical risks has been proposed from an analysis of the Framingham Heart Study.[8]

The annual rate of stroke for the unanticoagulated control group in five large anticoagulation trials was 4.5 percent but was reduced to 1.4 percent (68 percent risk reduction) for the warfarin-treated group (60 percent risk reduction in men; 84 percent risk reduction in women). Aspirin, 325 mg/day, produced a risk reduction of 44 percent. The annual rate of major hemorrhage was 1 percent for the control group, 1 percent for the aspirin group, and 1.3 percent for the warfarin group. No difference in stroke risk occurs between paroxysmal (intermittent) atrial fibrillation and sustained (chronic) atrial fibrillation. Anticoagulation therapy is approximately 50 percent more effective than aspirin therapy for the prevention of ischemic stroke in patients with atrial fibrillation. Risk factors for anticoagulant-associated intracranial hemorrhage include excessive anticoagulation and poorly controlled hypertension. Elderly individuals are at increased risk for anticoagulant-associated brain hemorrhage, especially if overanticoagulated.

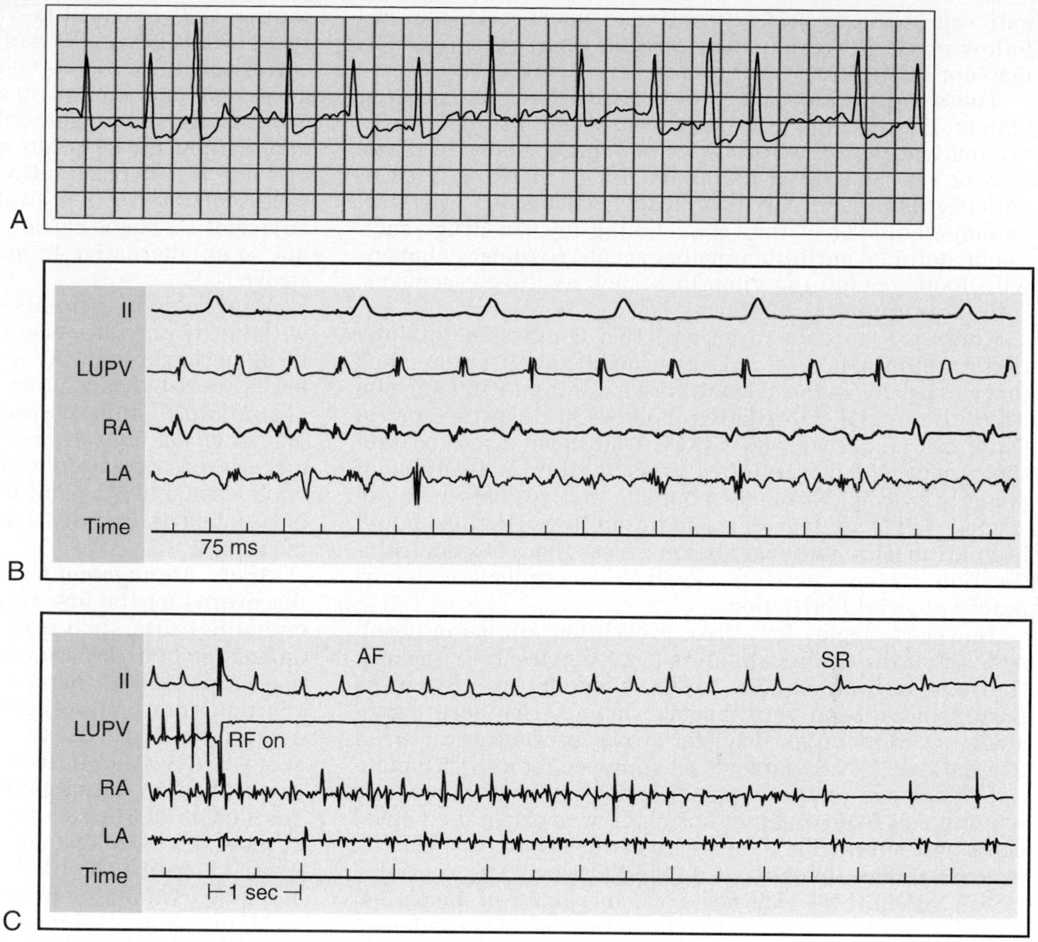

FIGURE 35–6 A, Scalar ECG of atrial fibrillation. Note fibrillatory waves and irregular ventricular response. **B, C,** Focal atrial fibrillation arising from the left upper pulmonary vein (LUPV). **B,** During atrial fibrillation, irregular activity is recorded in the left atrium (LA) and the right atrium (RA). However, with a catheter at the focus in the LUPV, a regular sharp electrogram is recorded. **C,** During radiofrequency (RF) ablation at the site in **A,** the atrial fibrillation terminates within 7 seconds and sinus rhythm ensues.

From these and other data, it appears that individuals younger than 60 years of age without any clinical risk factors or structural heart disease (lone atrial fibrillation) do not require antithrombotic therapy for stroke prevention because of their low risk. The stroke rate is also low (less than 2 percent/year) in patients between the ages of 60 and 75 years with lone atrial fibrillation. These patients may be adequately protected from stroke by aspirin therapy. In very elderly (older than 75 years) patients with atrial fibrillation, anticoagulation should be used with caution and carefully monitored because of the potentially increased risk of intracranial hemorrhage. Nevertheless, elderly patients with atrial fibrillation are still likely to benefit from anticoagulation because they are at particularly high stroke risk. Food and drugs such as antibiotics and antiarrhythmics (e.g., amiodarone) can influence the effects of warfarin (see Chap. 33).

Recommendations for antithrombotic therapy can be made. Any patient with atrial fibrillation who has risk factors for stroke (prior stroke or transient ischemic attack, significant valvular heart disease, hypertension, diabetes, age older than 65 years, left atrial enlargement, coronary artery disease, or congestive heart failure) should be treated with warfarin anticoagulation to achieve an international normalized ratio (INR) of 2.0 to 3.0 for stroke prevention if the individual is a good candidate for oral anticoagulation. Patients with contraindications to anticoagulation and unreliable individuals should be considered for aspirin treatment. Patients with atrial fibrillation who do not have any of the preceding risk factors have a low stroke risk (2 percent/year or less) and can be protected from stroke with aspirin. In patients older than 75 years, anticoagulation should be used with caution and monitored carefully to keep the INR less than 3.0 because of the risk of intracranial hemorrhage.

The risk of embolism following cardioversion to sinus rhythm in patients with atrial fibrillation varies from 0 to 7 percent, depending on the underlying risk factors. This risk is independent of the mode of cardioversion, either by chemical (drug) or direct current (DC) shock. Patients at high risk are those with prior embolism, a mechanical valve prosthesis, or mitral stenosis. Low-risk patients are those younger than 60 years without underlying heart disease. The high-risk group should receive chronic anticoagulation (see later), regardless of whether they will undergo cardioversion. Patients not in the low-risk group who have atrial fibrillation longer than 2 days should receive warfarin to achieve an INR of 2.0 to 3.0 for 3 weeks before elective cardioversion and for 3 to 4 weeks after reversion to sinus rhythm. An alternative strategy is to obtain a transesophageal echocardiogram to exclude the presence of an atrial thrombus. It appears that this technique predicts a group at low risk for the development of thromboembolism following cardioversion, provided that the patients are immediately treated with heparin followed by therapeutic doses of warfarin.[13] Anticoagulation with heparin has been recommended for emergency cardioversion when 3 weeks of anticoagulation or a transesophageal echocardiogram cannot be obtained. No matter which strategy is used, anticoagulation should be continued for at least 4 weeks following cardioversion, because atrial contractile function may not fully return until then.[14,15]

These suggestions must be individualized for a given patient. For example, patients at risk of trauma by virtue of occupation, participation in sports, and episodes of dizziness or syncope are at increased risk of bleeding if given anticoagulants and should probably not receive warfarin. Patients should be warned about taking any new drugs, such as nonsteroidal antiinflammatory agents, or dietary changes with foods containing vitamin K such as leafy vegetables, if they are receiving warfarin.

There are no data to suggest that conversion to sinus rhythm eliminates the risk of thromboembolism and thus this should not be the sole purpose for doing so. In fact, data from the Atrial Fibrillation Follow-Up Investigation of Rhythm Management (AFFIRM) trial have suggested that the strategy of maintaining sinus rhythm is insufficient alone to prevent thromboembolism, and patients who are treated with a strategy of maintaining sinus rhythm should be continued on anticoagulation unless there is a contraindication.[12] Many patients can have asymptomatic recurrences of atrial fibrillation.

Newer strategies for stroke prevention are being developed. Oral thrombin inhibitors (e.g., ximelagatran, melagatran) have been shown to be effective in preventing postoperative deep vein thrombosis and have been evaluated in a randomized trial for stroke prevention in atrial fibrillation.[16-19] Although not yet approved for use, the potential advantage of these agents is their wider therapeutic window not requiring monitoring, like warfarin. Left atrial occlusion, surgically[20,21] or with a catheter-based system,[22,23] is also being evaluated as a method for stroke prevention.

MANAGEMENT. The goals of management of the patient with atrial fibrillation are to reduce the risk of thromboembolism (described earlier) and to control symptoms. The latter is accomplished by controlling the ventricular rate during atrial fibrillation and/or restoring and maintaining sinus rhythm. Currently, no clear benefit has been ascribed to one treatment strategy over the other (rate control versus rhythm control), particularly because antiarrhythmic drugs are only 50 to 70 percent effective and carry risks of proarrhythmia (see later).[24] Data from large clinical studies (e.g., AFFIRM, Pharmacologic Intervention in Atrial Fibrillation [PIAF], and Rate Control versus Electrical Cardioversion [RACE]) all have demonstrated that both treatment strategies are reasonable.[12,25,26] In the largest of these studies, AFFIRM, 4060 patients with atrial fibrillation and risk factors for thromboembolism were randomized to either rhythm control or rate control treatment strategy, using standard pharmacological approaches. The study found no differences in mortality or quality of life between the two groups. In both groups, thromboembolic events occurred in those patients in whom anticoagulation was stopped. These studies compared treatment strategies and did not compare sinus rhythm to atrial fibrillation with rate control. In the AFFIRM trial, only 60 percent of the patients in the rhythm control arm were in sinus rhythm at follow-up, and patients were not rigorously monitored for atrial fibrillation recurrences between visits.

The overall treatment strategy (i.e., ventricular rate control or restoration and maintenance of sinus rhythm) should be individualized for each patient and based on whether patients are symptomatic from uncontrolled ventricular rates or from atrial fibrillation itself (i.e., loss of AV synchrony and atrial contraction) and risk for side effects from drugs. It can sometimes be difficult to determine whether a patient's symptoms are caused by rapid ventricular rates or the loss of atrial contraction. As a general rule, asymptomatic patients found to have atrial fibrillation on a routine ECG are not likely to require rhythm control, and rate control is usually sufficient. Ambulatory monitoring correlating the patient's ventricular response and rhythm to symptoms and exercise testing can be useful to this end. Trials of aggressive rate control or, conversely, cardioversion and maintenance of sinus rhythm are sometimes necessary to make this determination. Intolerance to medications or excessive risk in one strategy may necessitate switching strategies. As stated earlier, a rhythm control strategy should not be an alternative to anticoagulation therapy to reduce stroke risk.

Many elderly patients tolerate atrial fibrillation well without therapy, because the ventricular rate is slow as a result of concomitant AV nodal disease. These patients often have associated sick sinus syndrome, and the development of atrial fibrillation represents a cure of sorts. Such patients may demonstrate serious supraventricular and ventricular arrhythmias or asystole after cardioversion, so the likelihood of establishing and maintaining sinus rhythm should be weighed against the risks of cardioversion or other forms of therapy.

Acute Management. A patient with atrial fibrillation discovered for the first time should be evaluated for a precipitating cause, such as thyrotoxicosis, mitral stenosis, pulmonary emboli, or pericarditis. The patient's clinical status determines initial therapy, the objectives being to slow the ventricular rate and/or restore atrial systole. If sudden onset of atrial fibrillation with a rapid ventricular rate results in acute cardiovascular decompensation, electrical cardioversion is the initial treatment of choice. For other patients, the decision to cardiovert is largely based on the individual clinical situation. The need to restore sinus rhythm must be weighed against the likelihood of successful cardioversion and long-term maintenance of sinus rhythm.

Maintenance of sinus rhythm after cardioversion is influenced by the duration of atrial fibrillation and, in some adults, atrial dilation. Animal studies have indicated that atrial fibrillation begets atrial fibrillation—the longer the patient has atrial fibrillation, the greater the likelihood that it will remain because of a process called electrophysiological remodeling. Similar electrophysiological abnormalities can be demonstrated in patients following short episodes of atrial fibrillation, but the mechanism(s) and clinical significance remain unknown.[27-31] Although parameters such as atrial size and duration of atrial fibrillation predict the success of cardioversion in population studies, enlarged atria and atrial fibrillation of long duration are not absolute contraindications to attempted cardioversion. Internal cardioversion via intracavitary catheters can be effective when transthoracic shocks fail, particularly in obese patients or in those with significant pulmonary disease.[32,33] However, with the advent of biphasic external defibrillators, the success rates and the energy requirement for cardioversion have improved and the need to perform internal cardioversions has decreased.[34-36] Alternatively, antiarrhythmic drugs that lower defibrillation thresholds such as ibutilide can be used to pretreat the patient and increase the success of DC cardioversion.[37] Because atrial contraction may not return immediately after restoration of electrical systole, clinical improvement may be delayed. DC cardioversion establishes normal sinus rhythm in more than 90 percent of patients, but sinus rhythm remains for 12 months in only 30 to 50 percent. Patients with atrial fibrillation of less than 12 months' duration have a greater chance of maintaining sinus rhythm after cardioversion. For patients who do not require emergent cardioversion, chemical cardioversion with IV antiarrhythmic drugs is effective in 35 to 75 percent of patients, depending on the population studied.[38-41] Although procainamide has been used extensively for years, no well-controlled studies have been performed to determine its efficacy. Outside the United States, IV flecainide has been used with good results.[42] IV amiodarone appears to be less effective, with no difference in conversion rates from placebo. IV ibutilide is also effective in about 35 to 75 percent of patients, depending on the population studied.[42,43] In the absence of decompensation, the patient can be treated with drugs such as digitalis, beta blockers, or calcium antagonists to maintain a resting apical rate of 60 to 80 beats/min that does not exceed 100 beats/min after slight exercise. The combined use of digitalis and a beta blocker or calcium antagonist can be helpful in slowing the ventricular rate. Digitalis may be more effective if associated LV dysfunction is present; without such dysfunction, a beta blocker may be preferable to control the ventricular rate.

Long-Term Management. For the rate control strategy, digitalis, calcium channel blockers (diltiazem and verapamil) and beta blockers can be used alone or in combination. For chronic management, digitalis is usually insufficient for adequate rate control during periods of exertion. One should not rely on a resting heart rate during an office visit as the sole evaluation of the adequacy of rate control. Ambulatory monitoring and/or exercise testing can be useful to confirm adequate rate control during activity. In some patients with frequent recurrence and rapid ventricular rates not controlled by drugs or in patients intolerant to drugs, modification or elimination of AV nodal conduction by radiofrequency catheter ablation and implantation of a rate-adaptive VVI pacemaker (VVIR) is acceptable rate control therapy (see Chap. 34). Whenever possible, atrial or dual-chamber pacing is preferable, because the incidence of atrial fibrillation and stroke appears to be reduced compared with VVI pacing.

If a decision to maintain sinus rhythm has been made, class IA, IC, and III (amiodarone, sotalol) agents can be used to terminate acute-onset atrial fibrillation and prevent recurrences of atrial fibrillation (see Chap. 33). No one drug appears clearly superior, and selection is often based on the side effect profile and risk of proarrhythmia.[38,44,45] This appears to be true for newer drugs such as azimilide and dofetilide as well, although comparative trials have not yet been done. Most antiarrhythmic drugs increase the likelihood of maintaining sinus rhythm from about 30 to 50 percent to 50 to 70 percent of patients per year after cardioversion. Some rather recent data suggest that sotalol is less effective than amiodarone or 1C agents.[46,47] Class IA agents are often poorly tolerated and are rarely used in the long-term management of atrial fibrillation. As a general rule, for patients without structural heart disease, IC agents (propafenone and flecainide) are well-tolerated and reasonable first-line agents for maintenance of sinus rhythm. For patients with structural heart disease, amiodarone, dofetilide, or sotalol may be reasonable first-line therapies to maintain sinus rhythm. Occasionally, these agents (especially class IC agents) can "convert" the atrial fibrillation to atrial flutter, which can be slower than usual because of the drug. In these patients, a strategy of an atrial flutter ablation (see later) and continuation of the antiarrhythmic drug can be effective for maintaining sinus rhythm, with up to an 80 percent efficacy. Before electrical cardioversion, an antiarrhythmic agent is often administered for a few days to help prevent relapse of atrial fibrillation, as well as to convert some patients to sinus rhythm. In patients with occasional episodes of persistent atrial fibrillation (requiring cardioversion), a "pill in the pocket" approach can be effective.[48] In these patients, either flecainide or propafenone, usually at high doses, is administered only after the onset of atrial fibrillation to convert the atrial fibrillation. For those patients who fail drug therapy, catheter ablation approaches have been applied successfully. Radiofrequency ablation aimed at electrical isolation of the pulmonary veins or wide area ablation of the posterior left atrium around the pulmonary veins is 70 to 85 percent effective in patients with paroxysmal atrial fibrillation and 50 to 70 percent effective in patients with persistent atrial fibrillation in short-term follow-up studies.[49-52] The surgical maze procedure has been used to eliminate atrial fibrillation, particularly in combination with valve surgery, with a high success rate (see Chap. 33).[53] Newer surgical techniques using specially designed tools (e.g., radiofrequency [RF] clamp, cryoablation, RF pen, high-intensity ultrasound) to replace the traditional cut-and-sew maze procedure enable the procedure to be done faster and through more limited incisions.

Atrial Tachycardias

Three types of atrial tachycardias have been distinguished experimentally—automatic, triggered, and reentrant. Entrainment,[54] resetting curve patterns in response to overdrive pacing, the patient's response to adenosine, and recording of monophasic action potentials may suggest the presence of one of these mechanisms. However, in most cases, no clear identification of the mechanism can be made clinically, because the clinical presentations and electrophysiologic features can overlap, especially when the reentrant circuit is small (i.e., microreentry). For example, adrenergic stimulation can initiate automatic and triggered atrial tachycardias and burst pacing may initiate triggered and microreentrant atrial tachycardias. Therefore, because it determines the approach to mapping and ablation, as well as management, atrial tachycardias are more broadly characterized as being focal (originating from a small area of the atrium with atrial excitation emanating from this focus) or macroreentrant (a relatively large reentrant circuit using conduction barriers to create the circuit). Atrial flutter is the most common type of macroreentrant atrial tachycardia.

Macroreentrant Atrial Tachycardias

Atrial flutter is the prototypic macroreentrant atrial rhythm. Typical atrial flutter (sometimes called type I) is a reentrant rhythm in the right atrium constrained anteriorly by the tricuspid annulus and posteriorly by the crista terminalis and eustachian ridge.[55,56] The flutter can circulate in a counterclockwise direction around the tricuspid annulus in the frontal plane (typical flutter, counterclockwise flutter) or in a clockwise direction (atypical, clockwise, or reverse flutter).[56,57] Because both these forms of atrial flutter use the same circuit and are constrained by the same anatomical structures, their rates and flutter wave morphology on the surface ECG are consistent and predictable (see later). Other forms of atrial flutter are now recognized as distinct types and include atrial macroreentry caused by incisional scars from prior atrial surgery,[58,59] prior atrial ablation, idiopathic fibrosis in areas of the atrium, or other anatomical or functional conduction barriers in the atria. Atrial flutters originating in the left atrium (e.g., circulating around the mitral annulus, involving prior ablation lesions from atrial fibrillation ablations or surgical scars from maze procedures) have also been described.[60-62] Because the barriers that constrain these atrial flutters are variable, the electrocardiographic pattern of these so-called atypical atrial flutters can be varied. Often, flutter wave morphology changes during the same episode of flutter, which indicates multiple circuits and/or nonfixed conduction barriers.

ELECTROCARDIOGRAPHIC RECOGNITION. The atrial rate during typical atrial flutter is usually 250 to 350 beats/min, although it is occasionally slower, particularly when the patient is treated with antiarrhythmic drugs, which can reduce the rate to about 200 beats/min. If such slowing occurs, the ventricles can respond in a 1:1 fashion to the slower atrial rate. Ordinarily, the atrial rate is about 300 beats/min and, in untreated patients, the ventricular rate is half the atrial rate—that is, 150 beats/min (Fig. 35-7A and F). A significantly slower ventricular rate (in the absence of drugs) suggests abnormal AV conduction. In children, in patients with the preexcitation syndrome, occasionally in patients with hyperthyroidism, and in those whose AV nodes conduct rapidly, atrial flutter can conduct to the ventricle in a 1:1 fashion and produce a ventricular rate of 300 beats/min.

In typical atrial flutter, the ECG reveals identically recurring, regular, sawtooth flutter waves (see Figs. 35-4C and 35-7B and F) and evidence of continual electrical activity (lack of an isoelectric interval between flutter waves), often best visualized in leads II, III, aVf, or V_1 (Fig. 35-8). In some cases, transient slowing of the ventricular response, either with carotid sinus massage (see Fig. 35-7B) or adenosine (see Fig. 35-7F), is necessary to visualize the flutter waves. The flutter waves for (type I) typical atrial flutter are inverted (negative) in these leads because of a counterclockwise reentrant pathway, and sometimes they are upright (positive) when the reentrant loop is clockwise (see Fig. 35-8). When the flutter waves are upright from clockwise rotation, they are often notched. If the AV conduction ratio remains constant, the ventricular rhythm will be regular; if the ratio of conducted beats varies (usually the result of a Wenckebach AV block), the ventricular rhythm will be irregular. The irregular ventricular response is frequently caused by Wenckebach periodicity. Recurrent alternation of short and long ventricular intervals can be the result of concealed conduction. Various degrees of penetration into the AV junction by flutter impulses can also influence AV conduction. The ratio of flutter waves to conducted ventricular complexes is most often an even number (e.g., 2:1, 4:1).

As mentioned earlier, because the circuits for atypical flutters (not involving the cavotricuspid isthmus) can be variable, the electrocardiographic features of these

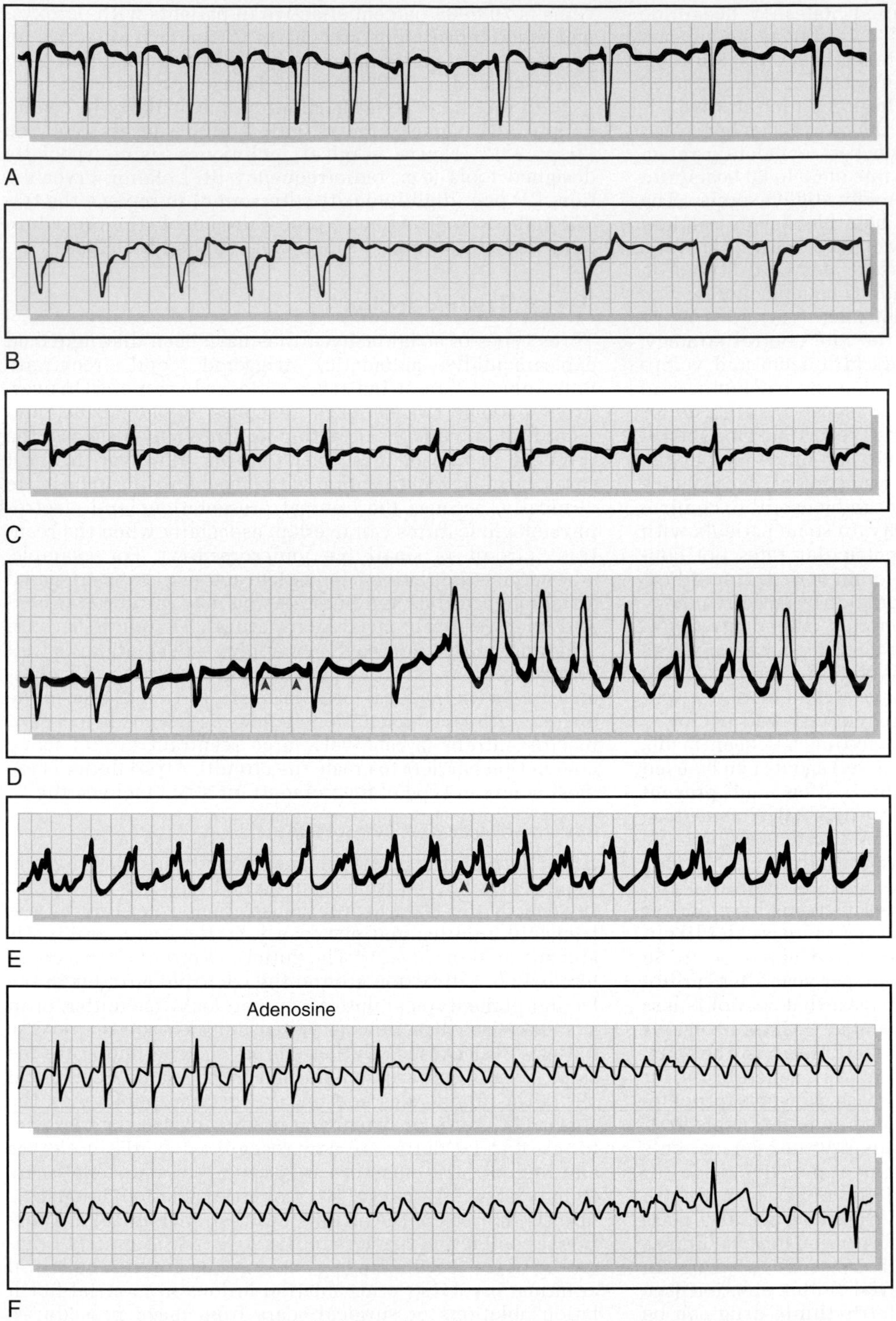

FIGURE 35–7 Various manifestations of atrial flutter. **A,** Atrial flutter at a rate of 300 beats/min conducting impulses to ventricles with a 2:1 block. In the midportion of the tracing, carotid sinus massage converts the block to 4:1, and the ventricular rate slows to 75 beats/min. **B,** Carotid sinus massage produces a transient period of atrioventricular (AV) block, clearly revealing the flutter waves. **C,** Quinidine has slowed the atrial flutter rate to approximately 188 beats/min. The block is variable. **D,** Wide QRS complexes with an rSR′ configuration in V_1 begin after a short cycle that follows a long cycle in the midportion of the electrocardiogram strip. This pattern represents a functional right bundle branch block. Arrowheads indicate flutter waves. **E,** The QRS complexes are 0.12 second in duration and have a regular interval at a rate of 200 beats/min. Atrial activity is also regular at a rate of 300 beats/min and independent of ventricular activity (arrowheads). Thus, atrial flutter is present with a probable ventricular tachycardia, an example of complete AV dissociation. **F,** Adenosine injection given to a patient with a supraventricular tachycardia (SVT) at a rate of 150 beats/min reveals underlying atrial flutter, thus diagnosing the SVT as atrial flutter with 2:1 AV conduction; the flutter waves are obscured within the T waves. Monitor leads are in **A, B, C, E,** and **F.**

macroreentrant atrial tachycardias are highly variable, without consistent rates or flutter wave contours (Fig. 35-9). However, these tachycardias often have a flutter rate similar to that of typical flutter (250 to 350 beats/min).

CLINICAL FEATURES. Atrial flutter is less common than atrial fibrillation. It can occur as a result of atrial dilation from septal defects, pulmonary emboli, mitral or tricuspid valve stenosis or regurgitation, or chronic ventricular failure but can also (rarely) occur without underlying heart disease. Toxic and metabolic conditions that affect the heart, such as thyrotoxicosis, alcoholism, and pericarditis, can cause atrial flutter. Occasionally, it can be congenital, follow surgery for congenital heart disease, or even occur in utero. When it follows reparative surgery of congenital heart disease, most patients will be able to have both typical flutter and an atypical flutter involving the atriotomy that often occurs years after the surgery. In children, continued episodes of atrial flutter are associated with an increased possibility of sudden death.

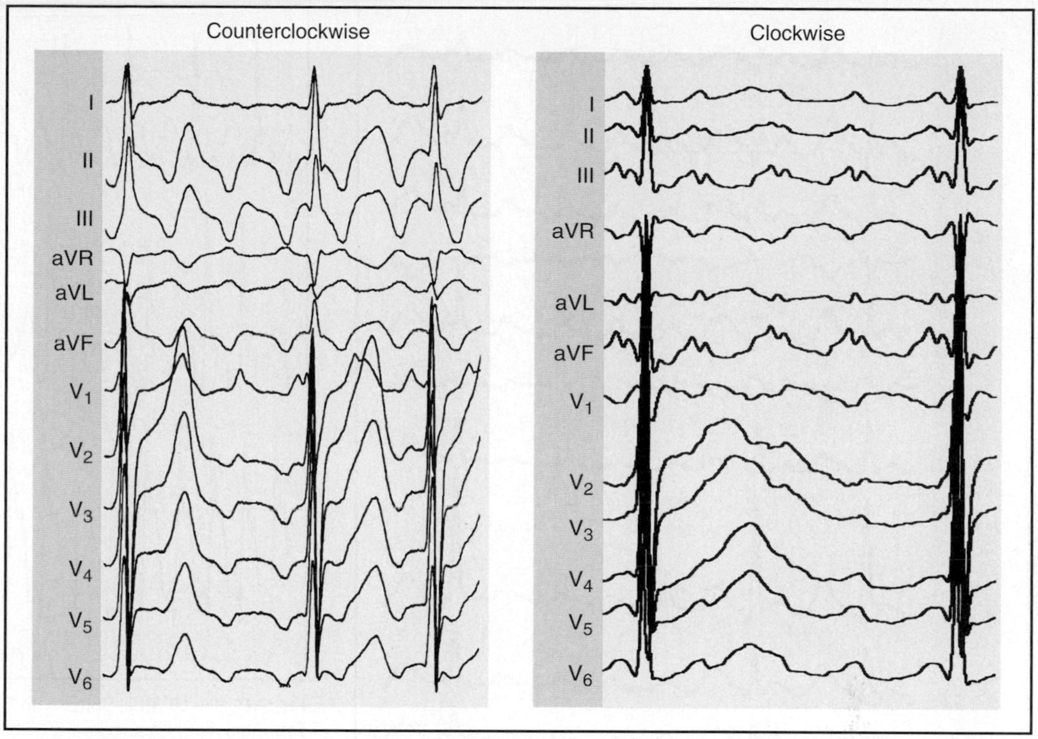

FIGURE 35–8 Twelve-lead ECG of counterclockwise and clockwise atrial flutter. In counterclockwise atrial flutter, the flutter waves are negative in leads II, III, aVL, and V_6 and upright in V_1. In clockwise atrial flutter, the flutter waves are upright in leads II, III, and aVF and often notched.

Atrial flutter usually responds to carotid sinus massage with a decrease in the ventricular rate in stepwise multiples and returns in reverse manner to the former ventricular rate at the termination of carotid massage (see Fig. 35-7A). Physical examination may reveal rapid flutter waves in the jugular venous pulse. If the relationship of flutter waves to conducted QRS complexes remains constant, the first heart sound will have a constant intensity. Occasionally, sounds caused by atrial contraction can be auscultated.

MANAGEMENT. Cardioversion (see Chap. 33) is commonly the initial treatment of choice for atrial flutter because it promptly and effectively restores sinus rhythm. Cardioversion can be accomplished with synchronous DC, which often requires relatively low energies (approximately 50 J). If the electrical shock results in atrial fibrillation, a second shock at a higher energy level is used to restore sinus rhythm or, depending on clinical circumstances, the atrial fibrillation can be left untreated. The latter can revert to atrial flutter or sinus rhythm. The short-acting antiarrhythmic medication ibutilide can also be given IV to convert atrial flutter. Ibutilide appears to successfully cardiovert about 60 to 90 percent of episodes of atrial flutter. However, because this medication prolongs the QT interval, torsades de pointes is a potential complication during and shortly after the infusion. Other medications such as procainamide can be given to convert atrial flutter chemically. Rapid atrial pacing with a catheter in the esophagus or the right atrium can effectively terminate type I (counterclockwise and clockwise) and some forms of atypical atrial flutter in most patients and produce sinus rhythm or atrial fibrillation, with a slowing of the ventricular rate and concomitant clinical improvement. Although the risk of thromboembolism is lower than that for atrial fibrillation, patients with atrial flutter do appear to have a risk of thromboembolism immediately after conversion to sinus rhythm.[63-66] In general, indications for anticoagulation in patients with atrial flutter are similar to those with atrial fibrillation.

Verapamil (see Chap. 33) given as an initial bolus of 5 to 10 mg IV, followed by a constant infusion at a rate of 5 mg/kg/min, or diltiazem 0.25 mg/kg to slow the ventricular response, can be tried. Adenosine produces a transient AV block and can be used to reveal flutter waves if diagnosis of the arrhythmias is in doubt. It will not generally terminate the atrial flutter and can provoke atrial fibrillation. Esmolol, a beta-adrenergic blocker with a 9-minute elimination half-life, can be used to slow the ventricular rate.

If the flutter cannot be electrically cardioverted, terminated by pacing, or slowed by the drugs noted, a short-acting digitalis preparation (digoxin) can be tried alone or with a calcium antagonist or beta blocker. The dose of digitalis necessary to slow the ventricular response varies and at times can result in toxic levels because it is often difficult to slow the ventricular rate during atrial flutter. Frequently, atrial fibrillation develops after digitalis administration and can revert to normal sinus rhythm on withdrawal of digitalis treatment; occasionally, normal sinus rhythm may occur without intervening atrial fibrillation. IV amiodarone has been shown to slow the ventricular rate as effectively as digoxin. As a general rule, atrial flutter is much more difficult to rate-control than atrial fibrillation.

If the atrial flutter persists, class IA or IC drugs (see Chap. 33) can be tried in an attempt to restore sinus rhythm and prevent recurrence of atrial flutter. Amiodarone, especially in low doses of 200 mg/day, can also prevent recurrences. Side effects of these drugs, especially proarrhythmic responses, must be carefully considered and are dealt with at length in Chapter 33. Sometimes, treatment of the underlying disorder, such as thyrotoxicosis, is necessary to effect conversion to sinus rhythm. In many cases, atrial flutter can continue despite antiarrhythmic drugs and, in many cases,

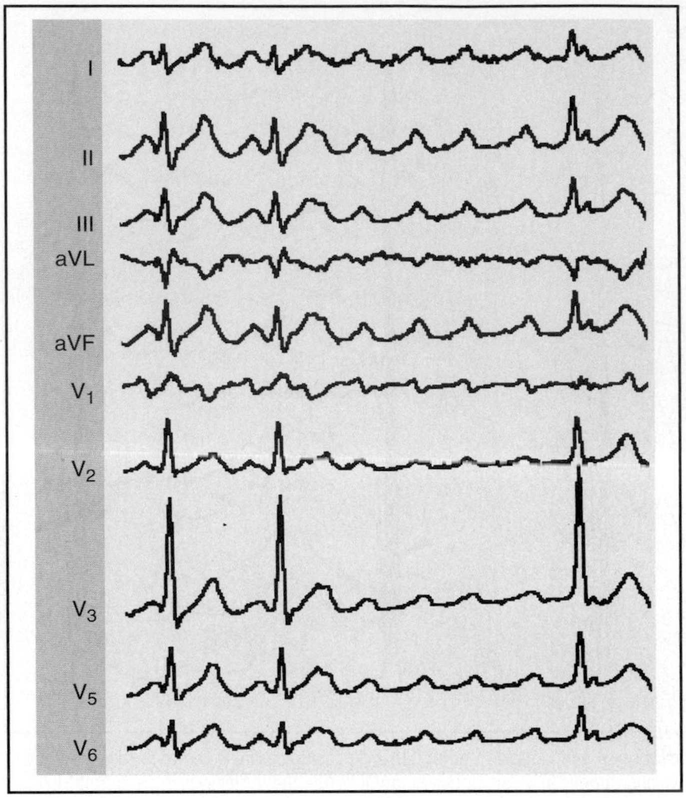

FIGURE 35–9 Macroreentrant atrial tachycardia in a patient who underwent atrial septal defect repair 10 years earlier. This tachycardia uses a reentrant circuit established by the atriotomy on the lateral atrial wall. Ablation to extend the scar to the tricuspid annulus eliminated this tachycardia.

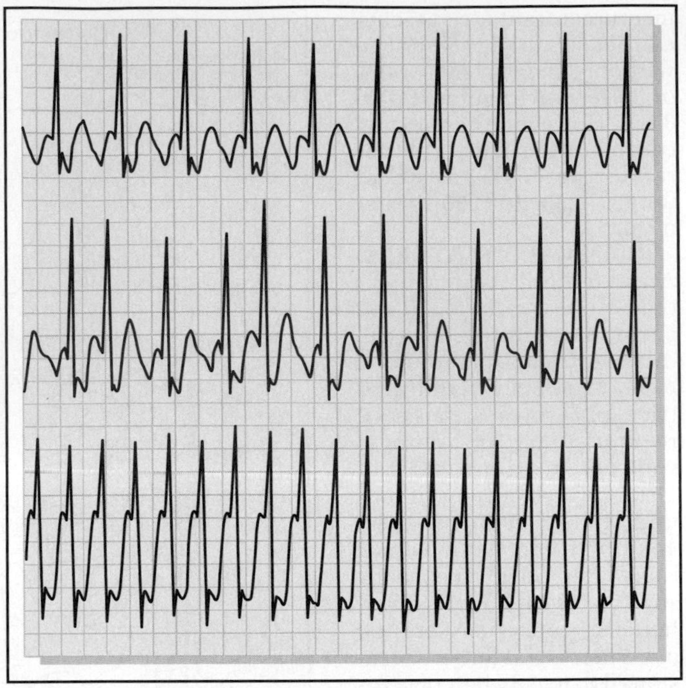

FIGURE 35–10 Atrial flutter with 1:1 conduction caused by flecainide. **Top,** Atrial flutter occurs with 2:1 conduction. **Middle,** 2:1 conduction alternates with 3:2 conduction. **Bottom,** Flecainide administration has been started, and the atrial flutter rate slows, with subsequent 1:1 conduction.

the flutter rate will slow in response to the antiarrhythmic drug. It is important to reemphasize that class I or III drugs should not be used unless the ventricular rate during atrial flutter has been slowed with digitalis, calcium antagonist, or beta-blocking drug. Because of the ability of class I drugs to slow the flutter rate, AV conduction can be facilitated sufficiently to result in a 1:1 ventricular response to the atrial flutter (Fig. 35-10).

Prevention of recurrent atrial flutter is often difficult to achieve medically but should be approached as outlined for atrial fibrillation (see earlier; also see Chap. 33). RF catheter ablation should be considered in patients refractory to medical therapy. RF catheter ablation of typical flutter (counterclockwise and clockwise) is highly effective at curing atrial fibrillation and has a long-term success rate of 90 to 100 percent. Because ablation of atrial flutter is so effective, with little risk, it can be offered as an alternative to drug therapy. Ablation of other forms of macroreentrant atrial tachycardias is also effective, although success rates are somewhat lower and more variable. Increasing evidence has indicated that the risk of emboli in atrial flutter may be more significant than once thought.[63] Because of this, and because many patients with atrial flutter also have atrial fibrillation, anticoagulation is usually warranted. However, carefully controlled studies to determine the degree of embolic risk in patients with only atrial flutter are lacking. Long-term anticoagulation, as in atrial fibrillation, should probably be considered until more definitive data are available.

Focal Atrial Tachycardias

ELECTROCARDIOGRAPHIC RECOGNITION. Focal atrial tachycardias (Fig. 35-11) generally have atrial rates of 150 to 200 beats/min, with a P wave contour different from that of the sinus P wave. However, atrial tachycardias, with foci near the sinus node, can have P wave contours very similar to those in sinus rhythm. At onset, there may be some warming up of the rate, resulting in a slight increase in heart rate over the initial several complexes. Frequently, atrial tachycardias occur in short, recurrent bursts with spontaneous terminations. However, more incessant forms of atrial tachycardias do occur. P waves are usually found in the second half of the tachycardia cycle (long RP–short PR tachycardia). If the atrial rate is not excessive and AV conduction is not depressed, each P wave can conduct to the ventricles. If the atrial rate increases and AV conduction becomes impaired, a Wenckebach (Mobitz type I) second-degree AV block can ensue. This aberration is sometimes called atrial tachycardia with block. When caused by digitalis, other manifestations of digitalis excess are present, such as PVCs. In nearly half the cases of atrial tachycardia with block, the atrial rate is irregular. Characteristic isoelectric intervals between P waves, in contrast to atrial flutter, are usually present in all leads. However, at rapid atrial rates, the distinction between atrial tachycardia with block and atrial flutter can be difficult. Analysis of P wave configuration during tachycardia indicates that a positive or biphasic P wave in V_1 predicts a right atrial focus, whereas a negative P wave in V_1 predicts a left atrial focus.

CLINICAL FEATURES. Although atrial tachycardia occurs commonly in patients with significant structural heart disease such as coronary artery disease, with or without myocardial infarction, cor pulmonale, or digitalis intoxication, it is also seen in patients without structural heart disease. Potassium depletion can precipitate the arrhythmia in patients taking digitalis. The signs, symptoms, and prognosis are usually related to the underlying cardiovascular status and the rate of the tachycardia. Atrial tachycardias often occur in short recurrent bursts but on occasion can be incessant. When incessant, tachycardia-induced cardiomyopathy can result. This can be partially or totally reversible with elimination of the tachycardia. In some patients, exercise or stress can provoke the tachycardia and in others the tachycardia can be positional. Stimulants such as caffeine, chocolate, and ephedrine can also provoke episodes.

Physical findings during a variable rhythm include variable intensity of the first heart sound and systolic blood pressure as a result of the varying AV block and PR interval. An excessive number of *a* waves can be seen in the jugular venous pulse. Carotid sinus massage or administration of adenosine increases the degree of AV block by slowing the ventricular rate in stepwise fashion without terminating the tachycardia, as in atrial flutter. It should be performed cautiously in patients with digitalis toxicity, because serious ventricular arrhythmias can result. Occasionally, carotid sinus massage or adenosine can terminate some forms of atrial tachycardia.

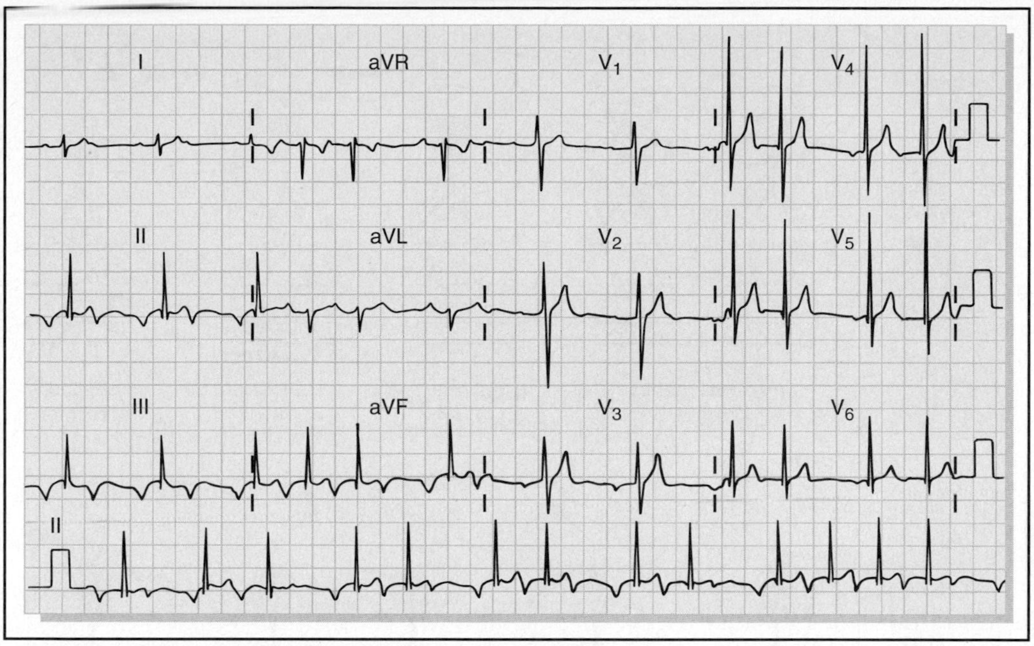

FIGURE 35–11 Atrial tachycardia. This 12-lead electrocardiogram and rhythm strip (bottom) demonstrate an atrial tachycardia at a cycle length of approximately 520 milliseconds. Conduction varies between 3 : 2 and 2 : 1. Note the negative P waves in leads II, III, and aVF and, when consecutive P waves are conducted, that the RP interval exceeds the PR interval. Note also that the tachycardia persists despite the development of atrioventricular (AV) block, an important finding that excludes the participation of an AV accessory pathway and sharply differentiates this tachycardia from the one shown in Figure 35-26.

MANAGEMENT. Atrial tachycardia in a patient not receiving digitalis is treated in a manner similar to the treatment of other atrial tachyarrhythmias. Depending on the clinical situation, digitalis, a beta blocker, or a calcium channel blocker can be administered to slow the ventricular rate; if atrial tachycardia remains, class IA, IC, or III drugs can be added. Catheter ablation procedures are usually effective at eliminating the atrial tachycardia, depending on the mechanism and underlying heart disease.[67] However, atrial tachycardias can occasionally recur at a different site following a successful ablation. If atrial tachycardia appears in a patient receiving digitalis, the drug should initially be assumed to be responsible for the arrhythmia. Therapy includes cessation of digitalis and administration of digitalis antibodies or potassium, if the level is low. Often, the ventricular response is not excessively fast, and simply withholding digitalis is all that is necessary.

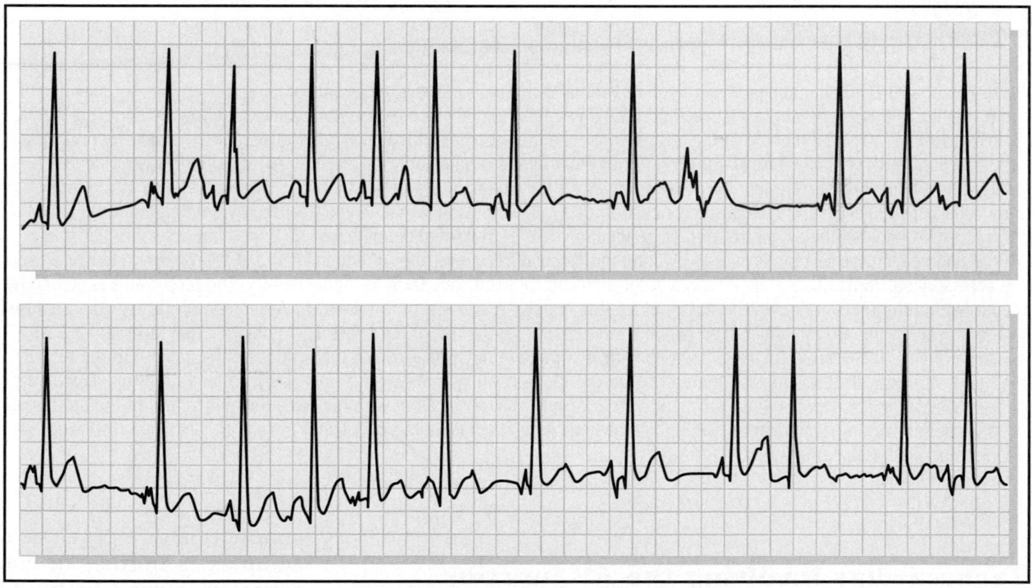

FIGURE 35–12 Chaotic (multifocal) atrial tachycardia. Premature atrial complexes occur at varying cycle lengths and with differing contours.

Chaotic Atrial Tachycardia

Chaotic (sometimes called multifocal) atrial tachycardia is characterized by atrial rates between 100 and 130 beats/min, with marked variation in P wave morphology and totally irregular P-P intervals (Fig. 35-12). Generally, at least three P wave contours are noted, with most P waves conducted to the ventricles, although often with variable PR intervals. This tachycardia occurs commonly in older patients with chronic obstructive pulmonary disease and congestive heart failure, and may eventually develop into atrial fibrillation. Digitalis appears to be an unusual cause, and theophylline administration has been implicated. Chaotic atrial tachycardia can occur in childhood.

MANAGEMENT. Management is primarily directed toward the underlying disease. Antiarrhythmic agents are often ineffective in slowing either the rate of the atrial tachycardia or the ventricular response. Beta-adrenoreceptor blockers should be avoided in patients with bronchospastic pulmonary disease but can be effective if tolerated. Verapamil and amiodarone have been useful. Potassium and magnesium replacement may suppress the tachycardia.

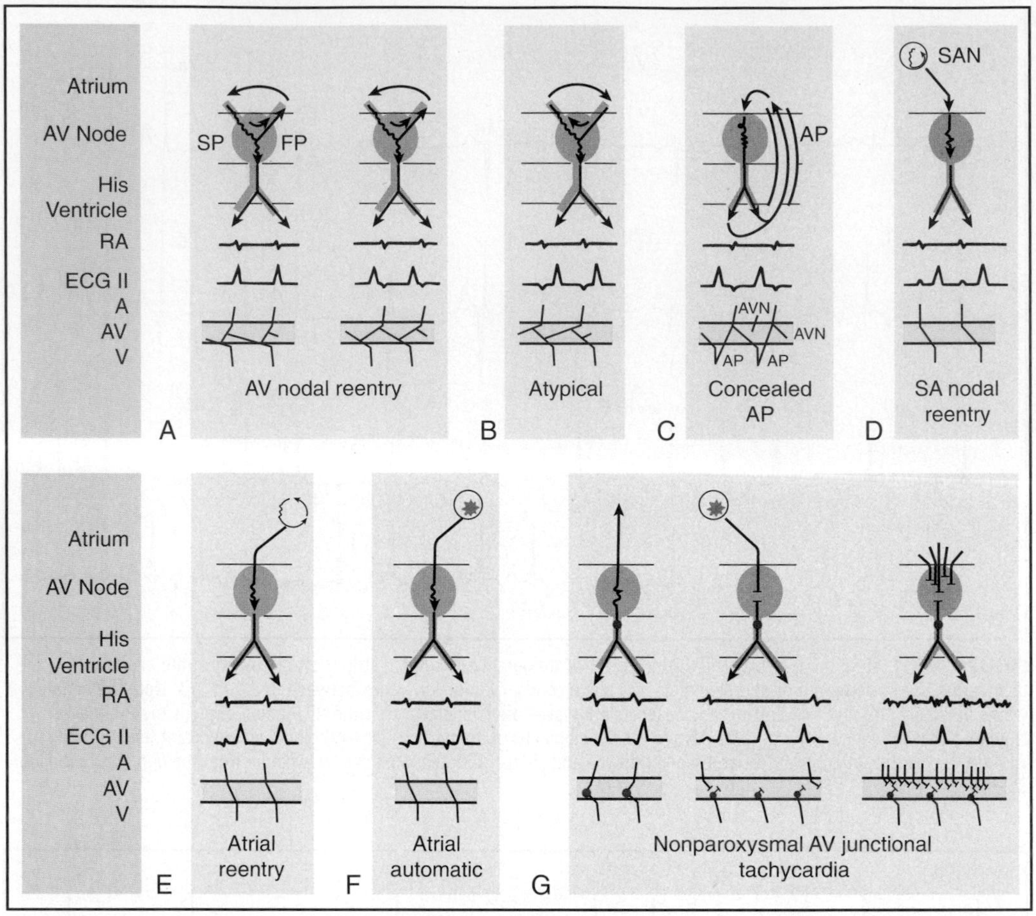

FIGURE 35–13 Diagrammatic representation of various tachycardias. In the upper portion of each example, a schematic of the presumed anatomical pathways is shown; in the lower half, the ECG and explanatory ladder diagram are depicted. **A,** Atrioventricular (AV) nodal reentry. In the left example, reentrant excitation is drawn with retrograde atrial activity occurring simultaneously with ventricular activity as a result of anterograde conduction over the slow AV nodal pathway (SP) and retrograde conduction over the fast AV nodal pathway (FP). In the right example, atrial activity occurs slightly later than ventricular activity because of retrograde conduction delay. **B,** Atypical AV nodal reentry caused by anterograde conduction over a fast AV nodal pathway and retrograde conduction over a slow AV nodal pathway. **C,** Concealed accessory pathway (AP). Reciprocating tachycardia is caused by anterograde conduction over the AV node (AVN) and retrograde conduction over the accessory pathway. Retrograde P waves occur after the QRS complex. **D,** Sinus nodal reentry. The tachycardia is caused by reentry within the sinus node, which then conducts the impulse to the rest of the heart. **E,** Atrial reentry. Tachycardia is caused by reentry within the atrium, which then conducts the impulse to the rest of the heart. **F,** Automatic atrial tachycardia (star indicates origin). Tachycardia is caused by automatic discharge in the atrium, which then conducts the impulse to the rest of the heart; it is difficult to distinguish from atrial reentry. **G,** Nonparoxysmal AV junctional tachycardia. Various manifestations of this tachycardia are depicted with retrograde atrial capture, AV dissociation with the sinus node in control of the atria, and AV dissociation with atrial fibrillation. Star indicates sinus node discharge. Red circles indicate site of junctional discharge. SA = sinoatrial; SAN = sinoatrial node.

Tachycardias Involving the AV Junction

Much confusion exists regarding the nomenclature of tachycardias characterized by a supraventricular QRS complex, a regular R-R interval, and no evidence of ventricular preexcitation. Because it is now apparent that various electrophysiological mechanisms can account for these tachycardias (Fig. 35-13), the nonspecific term *paroxysmal supraventricular tachycardia* has been proposed to encompass the entire group. This term may be inappropriate because some tachycardias in patients with accessory pathways (see later) are no more supraventricular than they are ventricular in origin. That is, they may require participation of both the atria and the ventricles in the reentrant pathway and exhibit a QRS complex of normal contour and duration, only because anterograde conduction occurs over the normal AV node–His bundle pathways (see Fig. 35-13C). If conduction over the reentrant pathway reverses direction and travels in an "antidromic" direction (i.e., to the ventricles over the accessory pathway and to the atria over the AV node–His bundle), the QRS complex exhibits a prolonged duration, although the tachycardia is basically the same. The term *reciprocating tachycardia* has been offered as a substitute for paroxysmal supraventricular tachycardia, but use of such a term presumes the mechanism of the tachycardia to be reentrant, which is probably the case for many supraventricular tachycardias. Reciprocating tachycardia is probably the mechanism of many VTs as well. Thus, no universally acceptable nomenclature exists for these tachycardias, but rather descriptive labels for specific arrhythmias, as used throughout this chapter.

AV Nodal Reentrant Tachycardia

ELECTROCARDIOGRAPHIC RECOGNITION. Reentrant tachycardia involving the AV node is characterized by a tachycardia with a QRS complex of supraventricular origin, with sudden onset and termination generally at rates between 150 and 250 beats/min (usually 180 to 200 beats/min in adults) and with a regular rhythm. Uncommonly, the rate may be as low as 110 beats/min and occasionally, especially in children, may exceed 250 beats/min. Unless functional aberrant ventricular conduction or a previous conduction defect exists, the QRS complex is normal in contour and duration. P waves are generally buried in the QRS complex. Often, the P wave occurs just prior to or just after the end of the QRS and causes a subtle alteration in the QRS complex that results in a pseudo-S or pseudo-r′, which may be recognized only on comparison with the QRS complex in normal sinus rhythm (Fig. 35-14). AV nodal reentry recorded at the onset begins abruptly, usually following a PAC that conducts with a prolonged PR interval (see Figs. 35-13A and 35-4B). The R-R interval can shorten over the course of the first few beats at the onset or lengthen during the last few beats preceding termination of the tachycardia. Variation in cycle length, particularly at the onset of tachycardia or just prior to termination, is usually caused by variation in anterograde AV nodal conduction time. Cycle length and/or QRS alternans can occur, usually when the rate is very fast. Carotid sinus massage can slow the tachycardia slightly prior to its termination or, if termination does not occur, can produce only slight slowing of the tachycardia.

ELECTROPHYSIOLOGICAL FEATURES. An atrial complex that conducts with a critical prolongation of AV nodal conduction time generally precipitates AV nodal reentry (Figs. 35-15 and 35-16). Premature ventricular stimulation can also induce AV nodal reentry in about one third of patients. Data from RF catheter ablation results and mapping support the presence of differential atrial inputs into the AV node, the fast and slow pathways, to explain this tachycardia (see Chaps. 27 and 29). In Figure 35-13A and B, the atria are shown as a necessary link between the fast and slow pathways. Whether these pathways are discrete pathways (perhaps caused by anisotropy) or are functional in nature is not known. In most examples, the retrograde P wave occurs at the onset of the QRS complex, clearly excluding the possibility of an accessory pathway. If an accessory pathway in the ventricle were part of the tachycardia circuit, the ventricles would have to be activated anterogradely before the accessory pathway could be activated retrogradely and depolarize the atria, thus placing the retrograde P wave no earlier than during the ST segment.

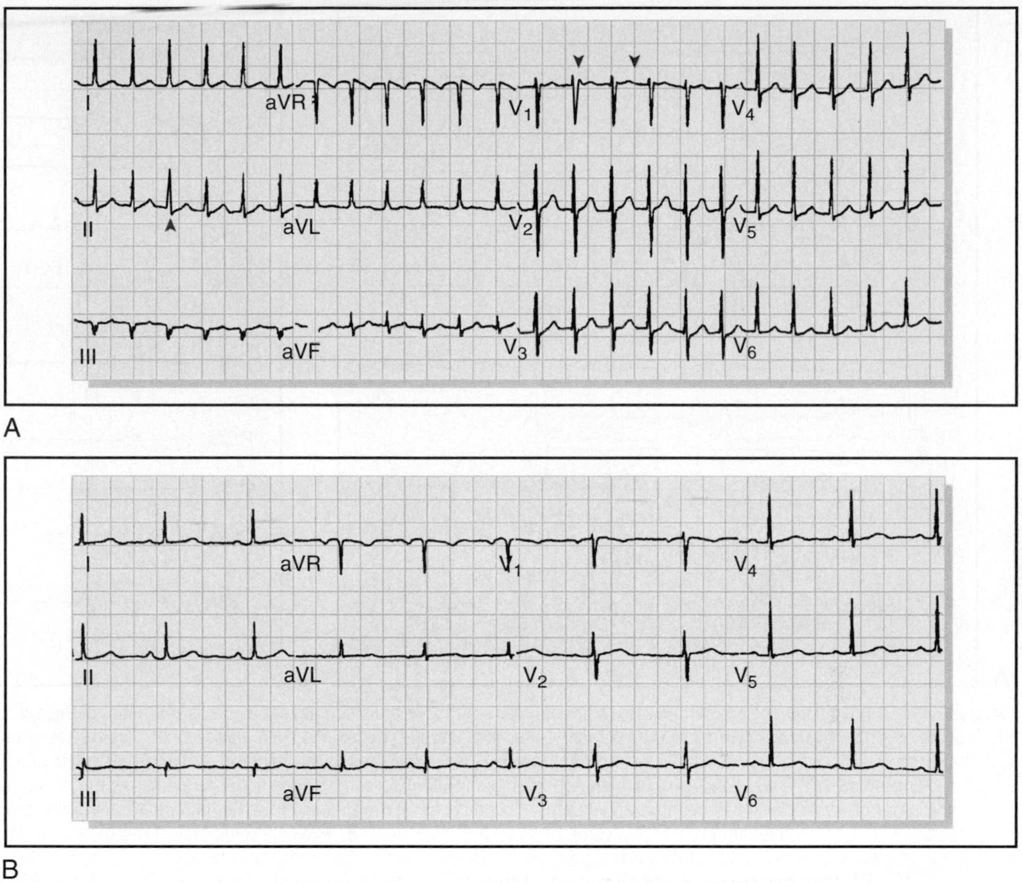

FIGURE 35–14 Twelve-lead electrocardiogram of atrioventricular nodal reentrant tachycardia. **A,** During tachycardia, a pseudo-r′ is seen in lead V_1 (arrowhead) and pseudo-S waves (arrowhead) are seen in leads II, III, and aVF. **B,** These waves become more obvious when compared with the QRS complexes during sinus rhythm.

In approximately 30 percent of cases, atrial activation begins at the end of or just after the QRS complex and gives rise to a discrete P wave on the scalar ECG (often appearing as a nubbin of an R in V_1; see Fig. 35-13A), whereas in most patients, P waves are not seen because they are buried within the inscription of the QRS complex. In the most common variety of AV nodal reentrant tachycardia, the ventriculoatrial (VA) interval (i.e., the interval between the onset of QRS and the onset of atrial activity) is less than 50 percent of the R-R interval, and the ratio of the AV to the VA interval exceeds 1.0. These VA intervals are longer in patients with tachycardia related to accessory pathways, as well as in atypical forms of AV nodal reentry (see Fig. 35-13B).

Slow and Fast Pathways. In most patients, anterograde conduction to the ventricle occurs over the slow pathway and retrograde conduction occurs over the fast pathway (see Chap. 31 and Fig. 35-13A and B). To initiate tachycardia, an atrial complex blocks conduction in the fast pathway anterogradely, travels to the ventricle over the slow pathway, and returns to the atrium over the previously blocked fast pathway ("slow-fast" form). The proximal and distal final pathways for this circus movement appear to be located within the AV node so, as currently conceived, the circus movement occurs over the two atrial approaches and the AV node (see Fig. 35-13A and B). The reentrant loop for typical AV nodal reentry is the anterograde slow AV nodal pathway to the final distal common pathway (probably the distal AV node), to the retrograde fast AV nodal pathway, and then to atrial myocardium. In atypical AV node reentry, the reentry occurs in the opposite direction. In some patients, the His bundle may be incorporated into the reentrant circuit. Less commonly, the reentry pathway can be over two slow pathways or over a slow and intermediate pathway, the so-called slow-slow AV node reentry (see Fig. 35-4B). Some data are consistent with intranodal activity.

The cycle length of the tachycardia generally depends on how well the slow pathway conducts, because the fast pathway usually exhibits excellent capability for retrograde conduction and has the shorter refractory period in the retrograde direction. Therefore, conduction time in the anterograde slow pathway is a major determinant of the cycle length of the tachycardia.

Dual AV Nodal Pathway Concept. Evidence supporting the dual-pathway concept derives from several observations, the most compelling of which is that radiofrequency catheter ablation of either the slow pathway or the fast pathway eliminates AV nodal reentry without eliminating AV nodal conduction. Other observations provide supporting proof. For example, in these patients a plot of the A_1-A_2 versus the A_2-H_2 or the A_1-A_2 versus the H_1-H_2 interval shows a discontinuous curve (Fig. 35-16). The explanation is that at a crucial A_1-A_2 interval, the impulse is suddenly blocked in the fast pathway and is conducted with delay over the slow pathway, with sudden prolongation of the A_2-H_2 (or H_1-H_2) interval. Generally, the A-H interval increases at least 50 milliseconds, with only a 10- to 20-millisecond decrease in the coupling interval of the PAC. Less commonly, dual pathways may be manifest by different PR or A-H intervals during sinus rhythm or at identical paced rates or by a sudden jump in the A-H interval during atrial pacing at a constant cycle length. Two QRS complexes in response to one P wave provide additional evidence (see Fig. 35-15B).

Some patients with AV nodal reentry may not have discontinuous refractory period curves, and some patients who do not have AV nodal reentry can exhibit discontinuous refractory curves. In the latter patients, dual AV nodal pathways can be a benign finding. Many of these patients also exhibit discontinuous curves retrogradely. Similar mechanisms of tachycardia can occur in children. Triple AV nodal pathways can be demonstrated in occasional patients. Virtually irrefutable proof of dual AV nodal pathways is the simultaneous propagation in opposite directions of two AV nodal wave fronts without collision (see Chap. 31) or the production of two QRS complexes from one P wave (see Fig. 35-15B) or two P waves from one QRS complex.

In less than 5 to 10 percent of patients with AV nodal reentry, anterograde conduction proceeds over the fast pathway and retrograde conduction over the slow pathway (termed the unusual form of "fast-

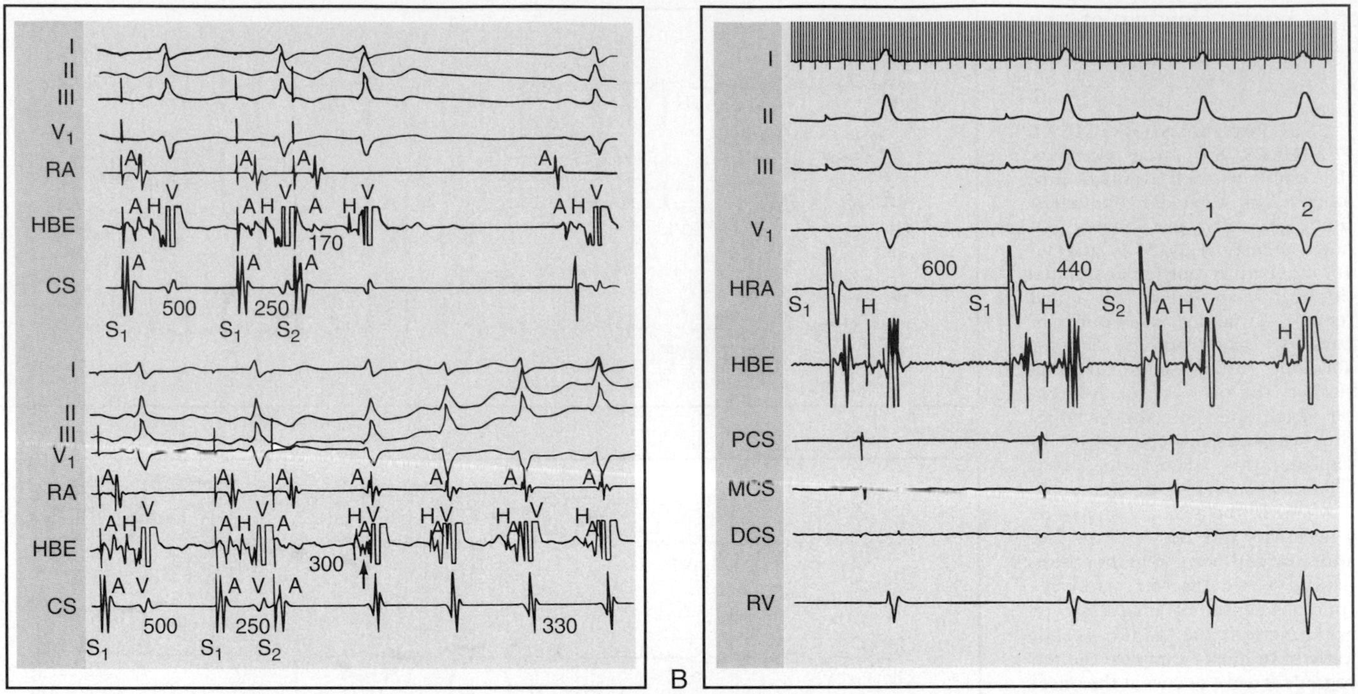

FIGURE 35–15 A, Initiation of atrioventricular (AV) nodal reentrant tachycardia in a patient with dual AV nodal pathways. **Upper** and **lower** panels show the last two paced beats of a train of stimuli delivered to the coronary sinus at a pacing cycle length of 500 milliseconds. The results of premature atrial stimulation at an S_1-S_2 interval of 250 milliseconds on two occasions are shown. **Upper panel,** S_2 was conducted to the ventricle with an A-H interval of 170 milliseconds and was then followed by a sinus beat. **Lower panel,** S_2 was conducted with an A-H interval of 300 milliseconds and initiated AV nodal reentry. Note that the retrograde atrial activity occurs (arrow) prior to the onset of ventricular septal depolarization and is superimposed on the QRS complex. Retrograde atrial activity begins first in the low right atrium (HBE lead) and then progresses to the high right atrium (RA) and coronary sinus (CS) recordings. **B,** Two QRS complexes in response to a single atrial premature complex. After a basic train of S_1 stimuli at 600 milliseconds, an S_2 at 440 milliseconds is introduced. The first QRS complex in response to S_2 occurs after a short A-H interval (95 milliseconds) caused by anterograde conduction over the fast AV nodal pathway. The first QRS complex is labeled 1 (in lead V_1). The second QRS complex in response to the S_2 stimulus (labeled 2) follows a long A-H interval (430 milliseconds) caused by anterograde conduction over the slow AV nodal pathway.

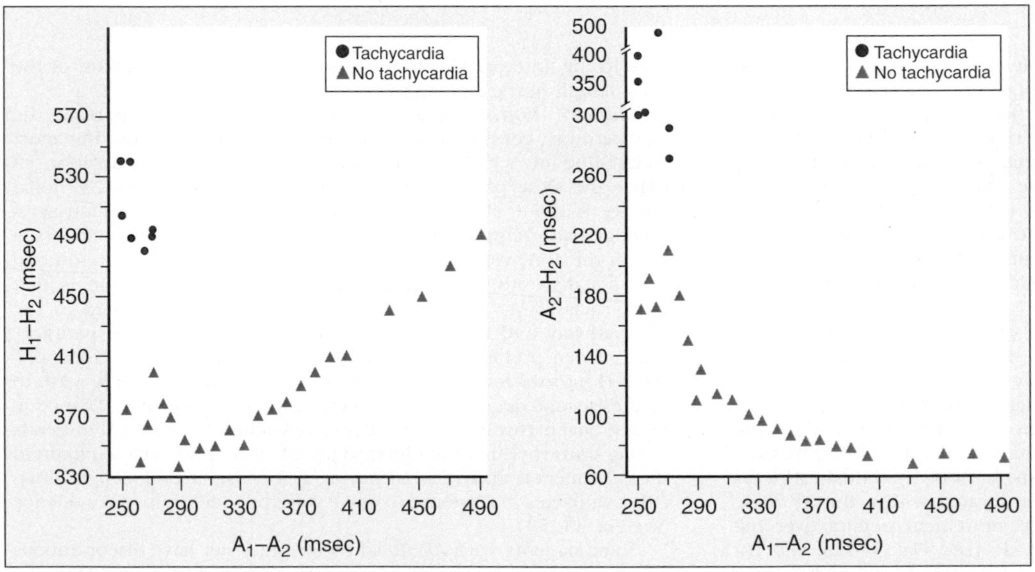

FIGURE 35–16 H_1-H_2 intervals (left) and A_2-H_2 intervals (right) at various A_1-A_2 intervals with a discontinuous atrioventricular (AV) nodal curve. At a critical A_1-A_2 interval, the H_1-H_2 and the A_2-H_2 intervals increase markedly. At the break in the curves, AV nodal reentrant tachycardia is initiated.

slow" AV node reentry), with production of a long VA interval and a relatively short AV interval (generally AV/VA less than 0.75; see Fig. 35-13B). The least common form ("slow-slow") exhibits a retrograde P wave midway in the cardiac cycle. Finally, it is possible to have tachycardias that use the anterograde slow or fast pathways and conduct retrogradely over an accessory pathway (see later).

The ventricles are not needed to maintain AV nodal reentry in humans, and spontaneous AV block has been noted on occasion, particularly at the onset of the arrhythmia. Such block can take place in the AV node distal to the reentry circuit, between the AV node and bundle of His, within the bundle of His, or distal to it (see Chap. 31). Rarely, the block can be located between the reentry circuit in the AV node and the atrium. Most commonly, when block appears, it is below the bundle of His. Termination of the tachycardia generally results from a block in the anterogradely conducting slow pathway (weak link), so a retrograde atrial response is not followed by a His or ventricular response. Functional bundle branch block during AV nodal reentrant tachycardia does not modify the tachycardia significantly.

Retrograde Atrial Activation. The sequence of retrograde atrial activation is normal during AV nodal reentrant supraventricular tachycardia, which means that the earliest site of atrial activation during retrograde conduction over the fast pathway is recorded in the His bundle electrogram, followed by electrograms recorded from the os of the coronary sinus and then spreading to depolarize the rest of the right and left atria. During retrograde conduction over the slow pathway in the atypical type of AV nodal reentry, atrial activation recorded in the proximal coronary sinus precedes atrial activation recorded in the low right atrium, which suggests that the slow and fast pathways can enter the atria at slightly different positions.

TABLE 35-3	Drugs That Slow Conduction in, and Prolong Refractoriness of, Accessory Pathway and AV Node
Affected Tissue	**Drugs**
Accessory pathway AV node	Class IA Class II Class IV Adenosine Digitalis
Both	Class IC Class III (amiodarone)

AV = atrioventricular.

CLINICAL FEATURES. AV nodal reentry commonly occurs in patients who have no structural heart disease and, in the adult population, frequently presents in the third or fourth decade of life. Symptoms frequently accompany the tachycardia and range from feelings of palpitations, nervousness, and anxiety to angina, heart failure, syncope, or shock, depending on the duration and rate of the tachycardia and the presence of structural heart disease. Tachycardia can cause syncope because of the rapid ventricular rate, reduced cardiac output, and cerebral circulation or because of asystole when the tachycardia terminates as a result of tachycardia-induced depression of sinus node automaticity. The prognosis for patients without heart disease is usually good.

MANAGEMENT

Acute Attack. Management of AV nodal reentrant tachycardia depends on the underlying heart disease, how well the tachycardia is tolerated, and the natural history of previous attacks in the individual patient. For some patients, rest, reassurance, and sedation may be all that are required to abort an attack. Vagal maneuvers, including carotid sinus massage, the Valsalva and Müller maneuvers, gagging, and occasionally exposure of the face to ice water, serve as the first line of therapy. These maneuvers may slightly slow the tachycardia rate, which then can speed up to the original rate following cessation of the attempt, or can terminate it. If vagal maneuvers fail, adenosine is the initial drug of choice. Digitalis, calcium antagonists, beta-adrenoceptor blockers, and adenosine normally depress conduction in the anterogradely conducting slow AV nodal pathway, whereas class IA and IC drugs depress conduction in the retrogradely conducting fast pathway (Table 35-3).

ADENOSINE. Adenosine (see Chap. 33), 6 to 12 mg given rapidly IV, is the initial drug of choice and is successful at terminating the tachycardia in about 90 percent of cases.[68] Verapamil (see Chap. 33), 5 to 10 mg IV, or diltiazem, 0.25 to 0.35 mg/kg IV, terminates AV nodal reentry successfully in about 2 minutes in approximately 90 percent of cases and is given when simple vagal maneuvers and adenosine fail.

DIGITALIS. Although it may be effective for longer-term management, digitalis has a slower onset of action than the agents described earlier and thus is not as useful in the acute management. If digitalis is used, digoxin can be given, 0.5 to 1 mg IV, over a period of 10 to 15 minutes, followed by 0.25 mg every 2 to 4 hours, with a total dose less than 1.5 mg within any 24-hour period. Oral digitalis administration to terminate an acute attack is not generally indicated. Vagal maneuvers that were previously ineffective can terminate the tachycardia following digitalis administration and should therefore be repeated.

BETA-ADRENOCEPTOR BLOCKERS. Beta-adrenoreceptor blockers can be effective in treating episodes, but generally are not used as first-line therapy to treat an acute episode because alternatives (adenosine, verapamil, or diltiazem) are more effective and faster acting. Beta-adrenoceptor blockers must be used cautiously, if at all, in patients with heart failure, chronic lung disease, or a history of asthma, because their beta-adrenoceptor blocking action depresses myocardial contractility and can produce bronchospasm.

DC CARDIOVERSION. Rarely, AV nodal reentrant tachycardia (AVNRT) results in hemodynamic compromise and is refractory to adenosine. In such cases of hemodynamic compromise, DC cardioversion may be indicated. DC shock administered to patients who have received excessive amounts of digitalis can be dangerous and result in serious postshock ventricular arrhythmias (see Chap. 33). Particularly if signs or symptoms of cardiac decompensation occur, DC electrical shock should be considered early. DC shock, synchronized to the QRS complex to avoid precipitating ventricular fibrillation, successfully terminates AV nodal reentry, with energies in the range of 10 to 50 J; higher energies may be required in some cases.

PACING. If DC shock is contraindicated or if pacing wires are already in place (postoperatively, or if the patient has a permanent pacemaker), competitive atrial or ventricular pacing can restore sinus rhythm. In some cases, esophageal pacing can be useful (see Chap. 34).

Classes IA, IC, and III drugs are not usually required to terminate AV nodal reentry. Unless contraindicated, DC cardioversion should generally be attempted before using these agents, which are more often administered to prevent recurrence.

Pressor drugs can terminate AV nodal reentry by inducing reflex vagal stimulation mediated by baroreceptors in the carotid sinus and aorta when systolic blood pressure is acutely elevated to levels of about 180 mm Hg, but they are rarely needed unless the patient is also hypotensive.

Prevention of Recurrences. Initially, one must decide whether the frequency and severity of the attacks warrant long-term therapy. If the attacks of paroxysmal tachycardia are infrequent, well-tolerated, and short-lasting, and either terminate spontaneously or are easily terminated by the patient, no prophylactic therapy may be necessary. If the attacks are sufficiently frequent and/or long-lasting to necessitate therapy, the patient can be treated with drugs empirically. If empirical testing is desirable, a long-acting calcium antagonist, a long-acting beta-adrenoceptor blocker, or digitalis are reasonable initial choices. The clinical situation and potential contraindications, such as beta blockers in an asthmatic, usually dictate the selection. If digitalis is used, rapid oral digitalization can be accomplished in 24 to 36 hours with digoxin at an initial dose of 1 to 1.5 mg, followed by 0.25 to 0.5 mg every 6 hours, for a total dose of 2 to 3 mg. A less rapid oral regimen induces digitalization in 2 to 3 days with an initial dose of 0.75 to 1 mg, followed by 0.25 to 0.5 mg every 12 hours, for a total dose of 2 to 3 mg. Alternatively, digoxin administered as a maintenance dose of 0.125 to 0.5 mg achieves digitalization in about 1 week. If any of these drugs are ineffective when taken singly, combinations can be attempted.

RADIOFREQUENCY ABLATION. RF ablation is more than 95 percent effective at curing patients long term, with a low incidence of complications. Because it is preferable to cure the patient of the tachycardia rather than use potentially toxic drugs to suppress it or to implant an antitachycardia device that terminates the tachycardia only after its onset (see Chap. 33), RF catheter ablation should be considered early in the management of patients with symptomatic recurrent episodes of AV node reentry. The procedure can be offered as an alternative to drug therapy in patients with frequent symptomatic episodes. For patients who do not wish to take drugs, patients who are drug intolerant, or those in whom drugs are ineffective, RF catheter ablation is the treatment of choice. It should be considered before long-term therapy with class IA, IC, or III antiarrhythmic drugs. Ablation has replaced surgery in virtually all cases and may be considered the initial treatment of choice in many symptomatic patients.

Accessory AV Pathways

Accessory pathways are fibers that connect the atrium or AV node to the ventricle outside the normal AV nodal–His-Purkinje conduction system. These pathways can conduct impulses in the forward (anterograde from atrium to ventricle) and/or reverse (retrograde from ventricle to atrium) direction and are potential substrates for reentrant tachycardias (AV reciprocating tachycardia). When the pathway is capable of anterograde conduction, the ventricle can be depolarized in part by the accessory pathway (outside of the normal His-Purkinje system) and produces a QRS complex that is preexcited (i.e., with a delta wave; see later). When a ventricular preexcitation is present and the patient has symptoms compatible with tachycardia, he or she is said to have the Wolff-Parkinson-White syndrome. In some cases, the pathways are only able to conduct in the retrograde direction; thus, they do not produce any ventricular preexcitation and are said to be concealed.

REENTRY OVER A CONCEALED (RETROGRADE-ONLY) ACCESSORY PATHWAY

ELECTROCARDIOGRAPHIC RECOGNITION. The presence of an accessory pathway that conducts unidirectionally from the ventricle to the atrium but not in the reverse direction is not apparent by analysis of the scalar ECG during sinus rhythm because the ventricle is not preexcited (Fig. 35-17). Therefore, electrocardiographic manifestations of WPW syndrome are absent, and the accessory pathway is said to be concealed. Because the mechanism responsible for most tachycardias in patients who have WPW syndrome is macroreentry caused by anterograde conduction over the AV node–His bundle pathway and retrograde conduction over an accessory pathway, the latter, even if it only conducts retrogradely, can still participate in the reentrant circuit to cause an AV reciprocating tachycardia. Electrocardiographically, a tachycardia resulting from this mechanism can be suspected when the QRS complex is normal and the retrograde P wave occurs after completion of the QRS complex, in the ST segment, or early in the T wave (see Fig. 35-13C).

The P wave follows the QRS complex during tachycardia because the ventricle must be activated before the propagating impulse can enter the accessory pathway and excite the atria retrogradely. Therefore, the retrograde P wave must occur after ventricular excitation, in contrast to AV nodal reentry, in which the atria are usually excited during ventricular activation (see Fig. 35-13A). Also, the contour of the retrograde P wave can differ from that of the usual retrograde P wave because the atria may be activated eccentrically—that is, in a manner other than the normal retrograde activation sequence, which starts at the low right atrial septum as in AV nodal reentry. This eccentric activation occurs because the concealed accessory pathway in most cases is left-sided, (i.e., inserts into the left atrium), which makes the left atrium the first site of retrograde atrial activation and causes the retrograde P wave to be negative in lead I (see Fig. 35-17).

Finally, because the tachycardia circuit involves the ventricles, if a functional bundle branch block occurs in the same ventricle in which the accessory pathway is located, the VA interval and cycle length of the tachycardia can become longer (Fig. 35-18). This important change ensues because the bundle branch block lengthens the reentrant circuit (see "Preexcitation Syndrome"). For example, the normal activation sequence for a reciprocating tachycardia circuit with a left-sided accessory pathway but without a functional bundle branch block progresses from the atrium to the AV node–His bundle, to the right and left ventricles, to the accessory pathway, and then to the atrium.

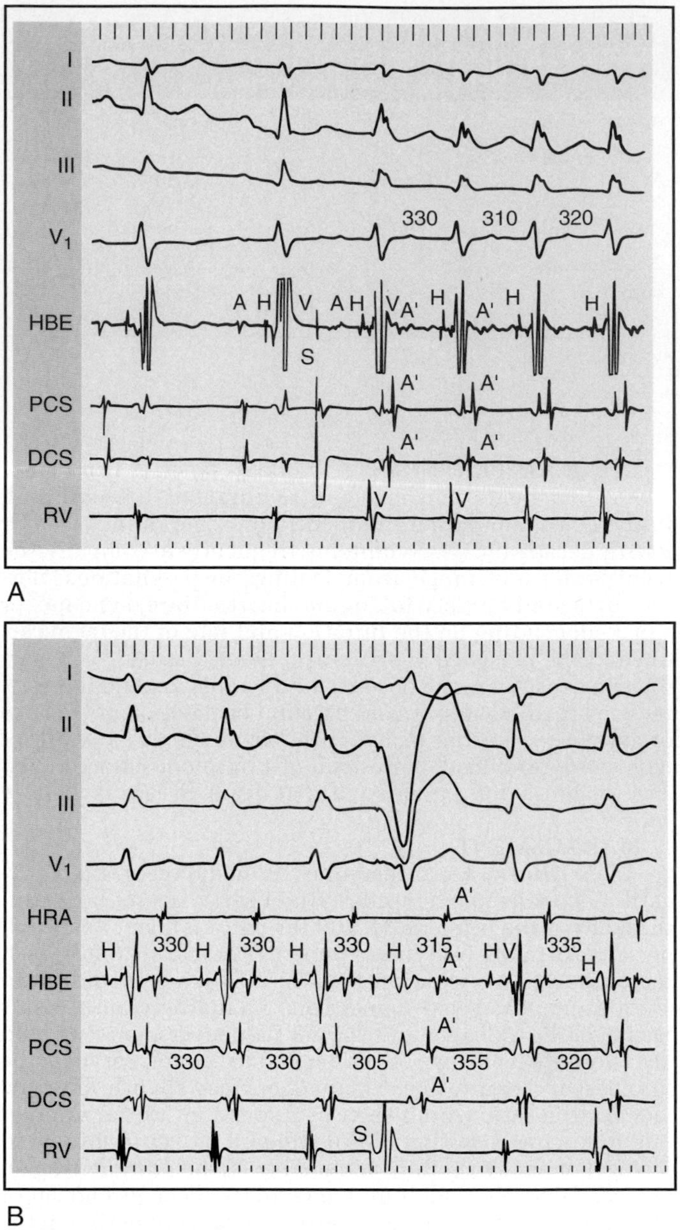

FIGURE 35–17 Atrial preexcitation during atrioventricular (AV) reciprocating tachycardia in a patient with a concealed accessory pathway. No evidence of accessory pathway conduction is present in the two sinus-initiated beats shown in **A.** A premature stimulus in the coronary sinus (S) precipitates a supraventricular tachycardia at a cycle length of approximately 330 milliseconds. The retrograde atrial activation sequence begins first in the distal coronary sinus (A′, DCS), followed by activation recorded in the proximal coronary sinus (PCS), low right atrium (HBE), and then the high right atrium (not shown). The QRS complex is normal and identical to the sinus-initiated QRS complex. (The terminal portion is slightly deformed by superimposition of the retrograde atrial recording.) Note that the RP interval is short and the PR interval is long. The shortest ventriculoatrial (VA) interval exceeds 65 milliseconds, consistent with conduction over a retrogradely conducting AV pathway. **B,** Premature ventricular stimulation at a time when the His bundle is still refractory from anterograde activation during tachycardia shortens the A-A interval from 330 to 305 milliseconds without a change in the retrograde atrial activation sequence. (Note that no change occurs in the H-H interval when the right ventricular stimulus, S, is delivered. H-H intervals are in milliseconds in the HBE lead.) Thus the ventricular stimulus, despite His bundle refractoriness, still reaches the atrium and produces an identical retrograde atrial activation sequence. The only way that this finding can be explained is via conduction over a retrogradely conducting accessory pathway. Therefore, the patient has a concealed accessory pathway with the Wolff-Parkinson-White syndrome. HRA = high right atrium; RV = right ventricle.

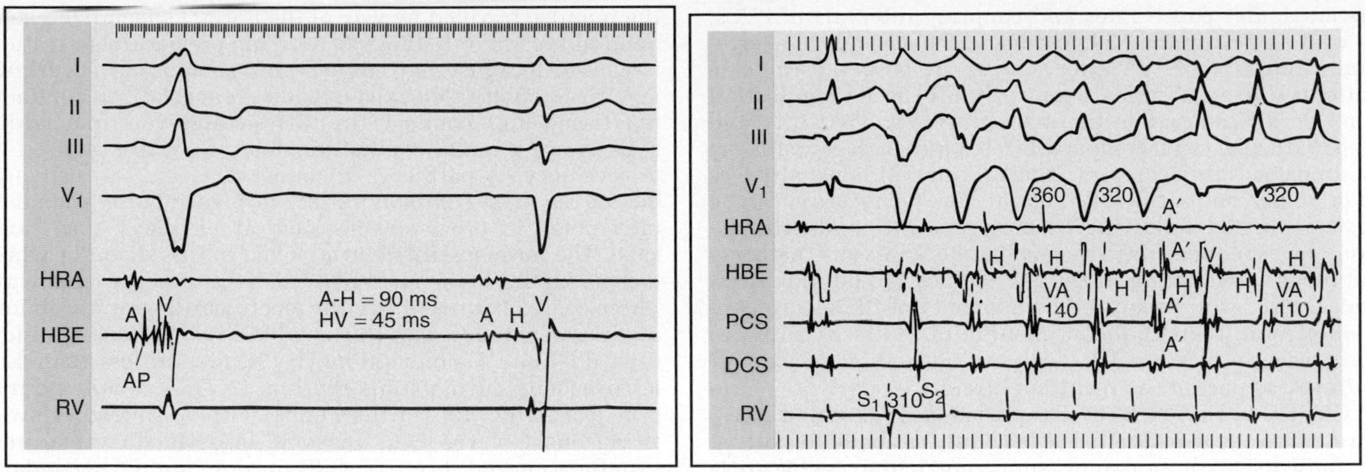

A B

FIGURE 35–18 A, Recording of depolarization of an accessory pathway (AP) with a catheter electrode. The first QRS complex illustrates conduction over the AP. In the scalar ECG, a short P-R interval and delta wave (best seen in leads I and V_1) are apparent. His bundle activation is buried within the ventricular complex. In the following complex, conduction has blocked over the AP and a normal QRS complex results. His bundle activation clearly precedes the onset of ventricular depolarization by 45 milliseconds. The A-H interval for this complex is 90 milliseconds. **B,** Influence of functional ipsilateral bundle branch block on the VA interval during an atrioventricular reciprocating tachycardia. Partial preexcitation can be noted in the sinus-initiated complex (first complex). Two premature ventricular stimuli (S_1, S_2) initiate a sustained supraventricular tachycardia that persists with a left bundle branch block for several complexes before finally reverting to normal. The retrograde atrial activation sequence is recorded first in the proximal coronary sinus lead (arrowhead, PCS), then in the distal coronary sinus lead (DCS) and low right atrium (HBE), and then high in the right atrium (HRA). During the functional bundle branch block, the ventriculoatrial interval in the PCS lead is 140 milliseconds, which shortens to 110 milliseconds when the QRS complex reverts to normal. Such behavior is characteristic of a left-sided accessory pathway with prolongation of the reentrant pathway by the functional left bundle branch block. (**A,** From Prystowsky EN, Browne KF, Zipes DP: Intracardiac recording by catheter electrode of accessory pathway depolarization. J Am Coll Cardiol 1:468, 1983.)

However, during a functional left bundle branch block, for example, the tachycardia circuit travels from the atrium to the AV node–His bundle, to the right ventricle, to the septum, to the left ventricle, to the accessory pathway, and then back to the atrium. This increase in the VA interval provides definitive proof that the ventricle and accessory pathway are part of the reentry circuit. The additional time required for the impulse to travel across the septum from the right to the left ventricle before reaching the accessory pathway and atrium lengthens the VA interval, which lengthens the cycle length of the tachycardia by an equal amount, assuming that no other changes in conduction times occur within the circuit. Thus, lengthening of the tachycardia cycle length by more than 35 milliseconds during an ipsilateral functional bundle branch block is diagnostic of a free wall accessory pathway if the lengthening can be shown to be caused by VA prolongation only and not to prolongation of the H-V interval (which can develop with the appearance of a bundle branch block). In an occasional patient, the increase in cycle length because of prolongation of VA conduction can be nullified by a simultaneous decrease in the PR (A-H) interval.

The presence of an ipsilateral bundle branch block can facilitate reentry and cause an incessant AV reentrant tachycardia. A functional bundle branch block in the ventricle contralateral to the accessory pathway does not lengthen the tachycardia cycle if the H-V interval does not lengthen.

Septal Accessory Pathway. An exception to these observations occurs in a patient with a concealed septal accessory pathway. First, retrograde atrial activation is normal because it occurs retrogradely up the septum. Second, the VA interval and cycle length of the tachycardia increase 25 milliseconds or less with the development of an ipsilateral functional bundle branch block.

Vagal maneuvers, by acting predominantly on the AV node, produce a response on AV reentry similar to AV nodal reentry, and the tachycardia can transiently slow and sometimes terminate. Generally, termination occurs in the anterograde direction, so the last retrograde P wave fails to conduct to the ventricle.

ELECTROPHYSIOLOGICAL FEATURES. Electrophysiological criteria supporting the diagnosis of tachycardia involving reentry over a concealed accessory pathway include the fact that initiation of tachycardia depends on a critical degree of AV delay (necessary to allow time for the accessory pathway to recover excitability so that it can conduct retrogradely), but the delay can be in the AV node or His-Purkinje system; that is, a critical degree of A-H delay is not necessary. Occasionally, a tachycardia can start with little or no measurable lengthening of AV nodal or His-Purkinje conduction time. The AV nodal refractory period curve is smooth, in contrast to the discontinuous curve found in many patients with AV nodal reentry. Dual AV nodal pathways can occasionally be noted as a concomitant but unrelated finding.

DIAGNOSIS OF ACCESSORY PATHWAYS. Diagnosis can be made by demonstrating that during ventricular pacing, premature ventricular stimulation activates the atria before retrograde depolarization of the His bundle, thus indicating that the impulse reached the atria before it depolarized the His bundle and therefore must have traveled a different pathway. Also, if the ventricles can be stimulated prematurely during tachycardia at a time when the His bundle is refractory and the impulse still conducts to the atrium, retrograde propagation traveled to the atrium over a pathway other than the bundle of His (see Fig. 35-17B). If the PVC depolarizes the atria without lengthening the VA interval and with the same retrograde atrial activation sequence, one assumes that the stimulation site (i.e., ventricle) is within the reentrant circuit without intervening His-Purkinje or AV nodal tissue that might increase the VA interval and therefore the A-A interval. In addition, if a PVC delivered at a time when the His bundle is refractory terminates the tachycardia without activating the atria retrogradely, it most likely invaded and blocked conduction in an accessory pathway.

The VA interval (a measurement of conduction over the accessory pathway) is generally constant over a wide range of ventricular paced rates and coupling intervals of PVCs, as well as during the tachycardia in the absence of aberration. Similar short VA intervals can be observed in some patients during AV nodal reentry, but if the VA conduction time or RP interval is the same during tachycardia and ventricular pacing at comparable rates, an accessory pathway is almost certainly present. The VA interval is usually less than 50 percent of the R-R interval. The tachycardia can be easily initiated following premature ventricular stimulation that conducts retrogradely in the accessory pathway but blocks conduction in the AV node or His bundle. Atria and ventricles are required components of the macroreentrant circuit; therefore, continuation of the tachycardia in the presence of AV or VA block excludes an accessory AV pathway as part of the reentrant circuit.

CLINICAL FEATURES. The presence of concealed accessory pathways is estimated to account for about 30 percent of patients with apparent supraventricular tachycardia referred for electrophysiological evaluation. The great majority of these accessory pathways are located between the left ventricle and left atrium or in the posteroseptal area, less commonly between the right ventricle and right atrium. It is important to be aware of a concealed accessory pathway as a possible cause of apparently routine supraventricular tachycardia because the therapeutic response may at times not follow the usual guidelines. Tachycardia rates tend to be somewhat faster than those occurring in AV nodal reentry (200 beats/min), but a great deal of overlap exists between the two groups.

Syncope can occur because the rapid ventricular rate fails to provide adequate cerebral circulation or because the tachyarrhythmia depresses the sinus pacemaker and causes a period of asystole when the tachyarrhythmia terminates. Physical examination reveals an unvarying, regular ventricular rhythm, with constant intensity of the first heart sound. Jugular venous pressure can be elevated (large A wave), but the waveform generally remains constant.

MANAGEMENT. The therapeutic approach to terminate this form of tachycardia acutely is as outlined for AV nodal reentry, because the AV node is a critical part of the circuit here as well. It is necessary to achieve block of a single impulse from atrium to ventricle or ventricle to atrium. Generally, the most successful method is to produce a transient AV nodal block; therefore, vagal maneuvers, IV adenosine, verapamil or diltiazem, digitalis, and beta blockers are acceptable choices. RF catheter ablation and conventional antiarrhythmic agents that prolong the activation time or refractory period in the accessory pathway need to be considered for chronic prophylactic therapy, similar to that discussed for reciprocating tachycardias associated with the preexcitation syndrome. RF catheter ablation is curative, has low risk, and should be considered early for symptomatic patients (see Chap. 33). The presence of atrial fibrillation in patients with a concealed accessory pathway should not be a greater therapeutic challenge than in patients who do not have such a pathway, because anterograde AV conduction occurs only over the AV node and not over an accessory pathway. IV verapamil and digitalis are not contraindicated. However, under some circumstances, such as catecholamine stimulation, anterograde conduction can occur in the apparently concealed accessory pathway.

Preexcitation Syndrome

ELECTROCARDIOGRAPHIC RECOGNITION. Preexcitation, or the WPW abnormality on the ECG, occurs when the atrial impulse activates the entire or some part of the ventricle, or the ventricular impulse activates the entire or some part of the atrium earlier than would be expected if the impulse traveled by way of the normal specialized conduction system only (Fig. 35-19). This premature activation is caused by muscular connections composed of working myocardial fibers that exist outside the specialized conducting tissue and connect the atrium and ventricle while bypassing AV nodal conduction delay. They are referred to as accessory AV pathways or connections and are responsible for the most common variety of preexcitation (incidentally noted in other species such as monkeys, dogs, and cats). The term *syndrome* is attached to this disorder when tachyarrhythmias occur as a result of the accessory pathway. Three basic features typify the electrocardiographic abnormalities of patients with the usual form of WPW conduction caused by an AV connection: (1) PR interval less than 120 milliseconds during sinus rhythm; (2) QRS complex duration exceeding 120 milliseconds with a slurred, slowly rising onset of the QRS in some leads (delta wave) and usually a normal terminal QRS portion; and (3) secondary ST-T wave changes that are generally directed in an opposite direction to the major delta and QRS vectors. Analysis of the scalar ECG can be used to localize the accessory pathway (see Fig. 35-19D).[69]

In the WPW syndrome, the most common tachycardia is characterized by a normal QRS, a regular rhythm, ventricular rates of 150 to 250 beats/min (generally faster than AV nodal reentry), and sudden onset and termination, in most respects behaving like the tachycardia described for conduction over a concealed pathway (see earlier). The major difference between the two is the capacity for anterograde conduction over the accessory pathway during atrial flutter or atrial fibrillation (see later).

Variants

Various other anatomical substrates exist and provide the basis for different electrocardiographic manifestations of several variations of the preexcitation syndrome, as summarized in Table 35-4 (Fig. 35-20). Fibers from the atrium to the His bundle bypassing the physiological delay of the AV node are called atriohisian tracts (see Fig. 35-20B) and are associated with a short PR interval and a normal QRS complex. Although demonstrated anatomically (see later), the electrophysiological significance of these tracts in the genesis of tachycardias with a short PR interval and a normal QRS complex (so-called Lown-Ganong-Levine [LGL] syndrome) remains to be established. Indeed, evidence does not support the presence of a specific LGL syndrome consisting of a short PR interval, normal QRS complex, and tachycardias related to an atriohisian bypass tract.

Another variant of accessory pathway conduction is that caused by atriofascicular or nodofascicular accessory pathways. These fibers result in a unique AV conduction pattern, sometimes referred to as Mahaim conduction, characterized by the development of ventricular preexcitation (widened QRS and short H-V interval) with a progressive increase in the AV interval in response to atrial overdrive pacing, as opposed to the behavior of the usual accessory pathway, in which preexcitation occurs with short AV intervals (Fig. 35-21). Because the accessory pathways responsible for this conduction pattern usually insert into the right bundle branch, preexcitation generally results in a left bundle branch block pattern. This phenomenon can be caused by fibers passing from the AV node to the ventricle, called nodoventricular fibers (or nodofascicular if the insertion is into the right bundle branch rather than ventricular muscle; see Fig. 35-20C). For nodoventricular connections, the PR interval may be normal or short, and the QRS complex is a fusion beat. This pattern of preexcitation can also result from atriofascicular accessory pathways. These fibers almost always represent a duplication of the AV node and the distal conducting system and are located in the right ventricular free wall. The apical end lies close to the lateral tricuspid annulus and conducts slowly, with AV node–like properties. After a long course, the distal portion of these fibers, which conducts rapidly, inserts into the distal right bundle branch or the apical region of the right ventricle. No preexcitation is generally apparent during sinus rhythm but can be exposed by premature right atrial stimulation. The usual absence of retrograde conduction in these pathways produces only an antidromic AV reentry tachycardia ("preexcited" tachycardia), characterized by anterograde

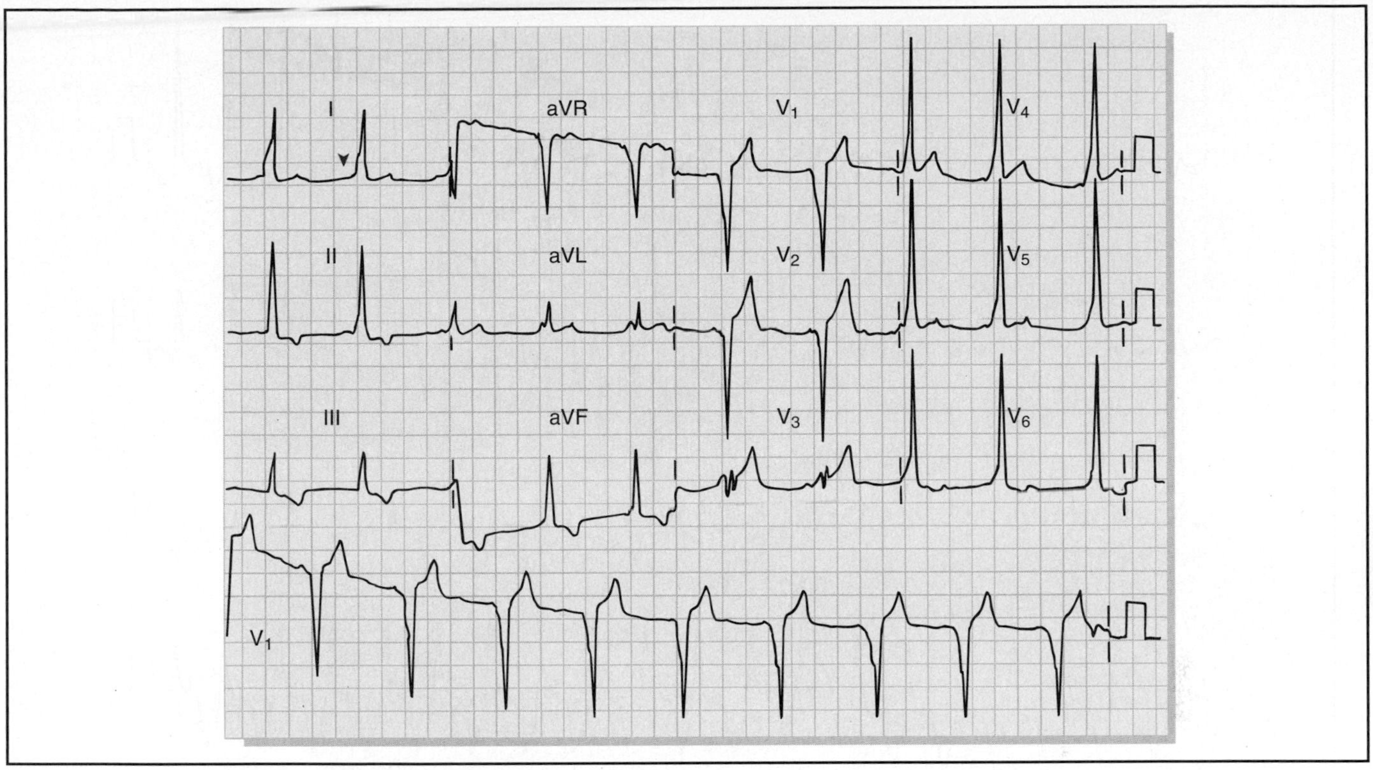

A

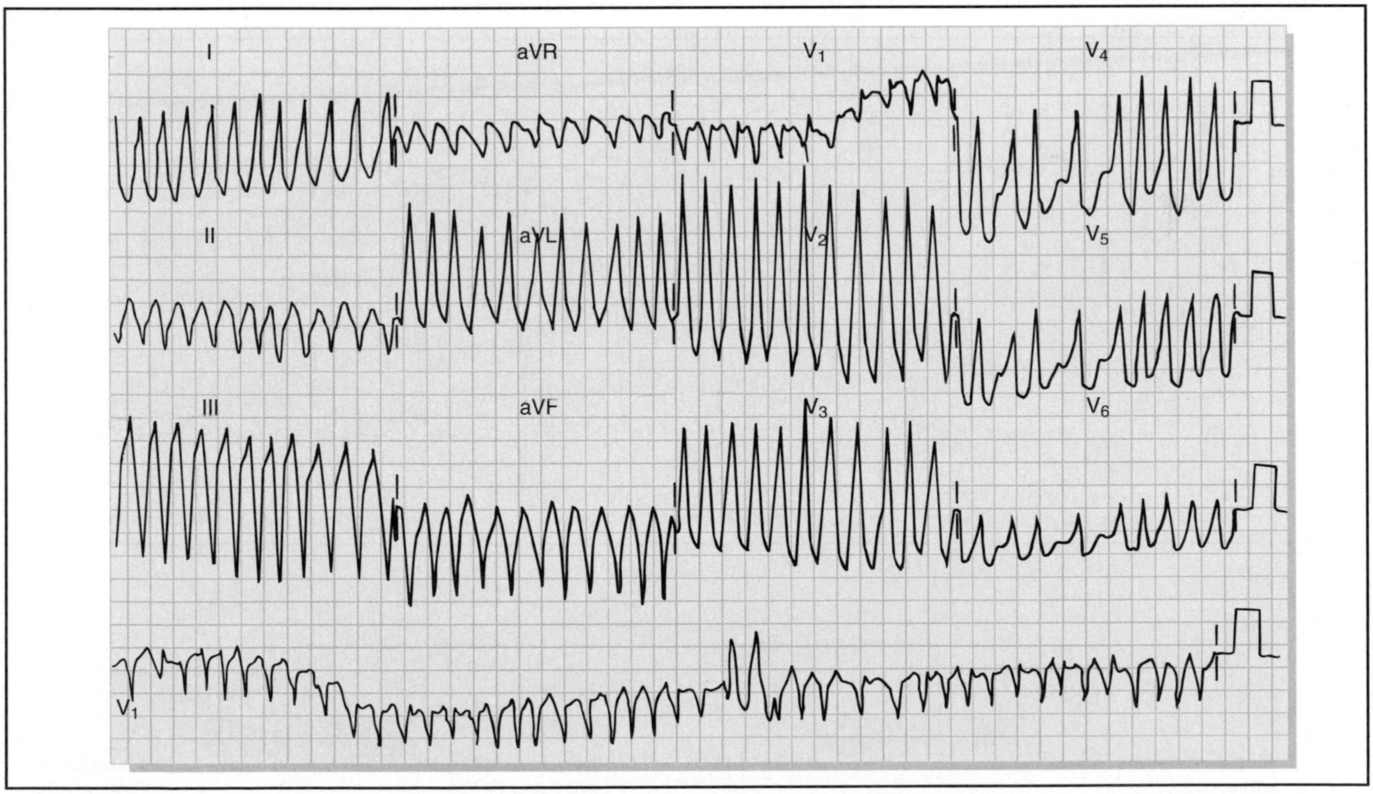

B

FIGURE 35–19 A, Right anteroseptal accessory pathway. The 12-lead electrocardiogram characteristically exhibits a normal to inferior axis. The delta wave is negative in V_1 and V_2, upright in leads I, II, aVL, and aVF, isoelectric in lead III, and negative in aVR. Location was verified at surgery. The arrowhead indicates a delta wave (lead I). **B,** Right posteroseptal accessory pathway. Negative delta waves in leads II, III, and aVF, upright in I and aVL, localize this pathway to the posteroseptal region. The negative delta wave in V_1 with sharp transition to an upright delta wave in V_2 pinpoints it to the right posteroseptal area. Atrial fibrillation is present. The location was verified at surgery. *Figure continues on next page.*

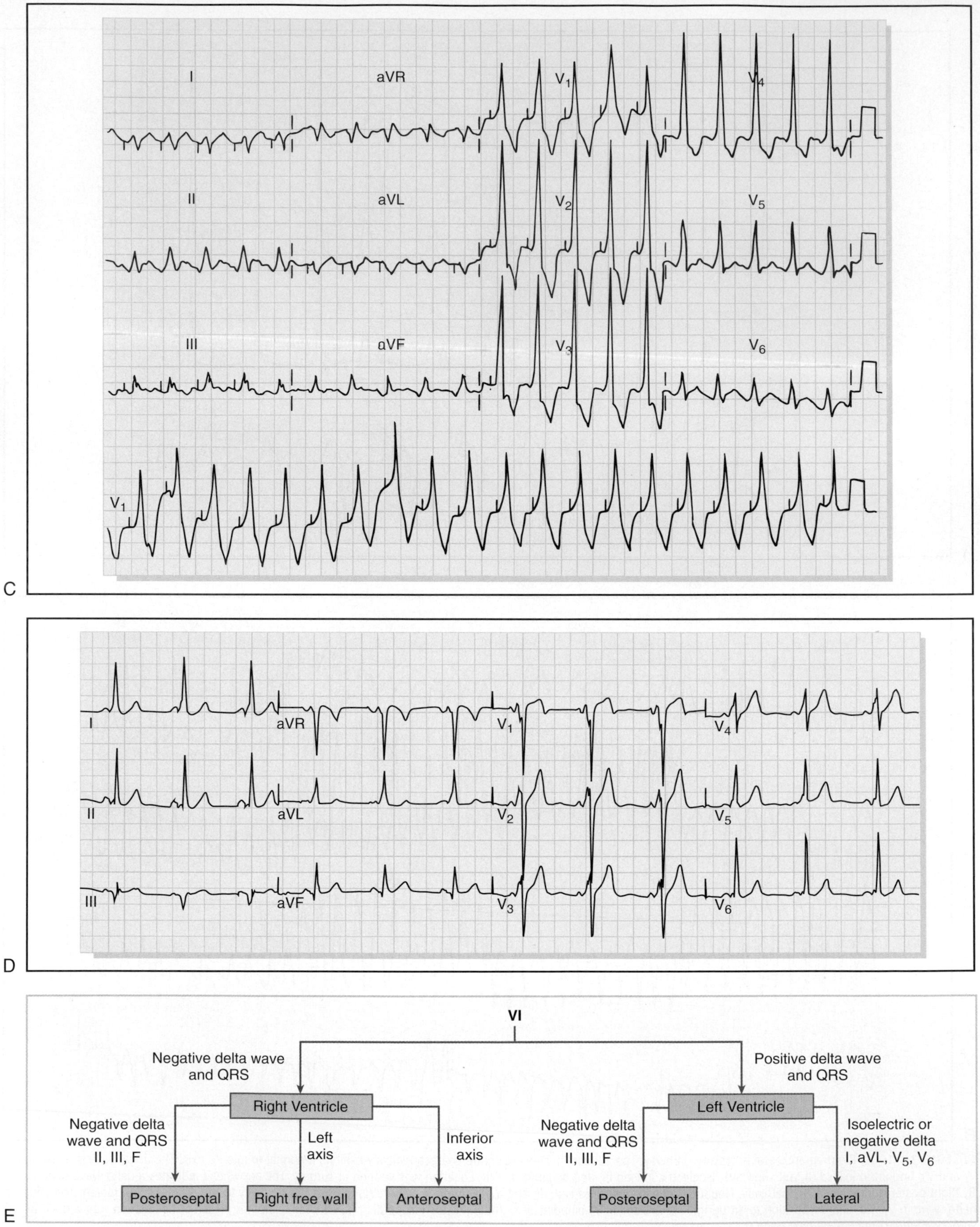

FIGURE 35–19, cont'd C, Left lateral accessory pathway. A positive delta wave in the anterior precordial leads and in leads II, III, and aVF, positive or isoelectric in leads I and aVL, and isoelectric or negative in leads V_5 and V_6 is typical of a left lateral accessory pathway. Rapid coronary sinus pacing (450-millisecond cycle length) was used to enhance preexcitation (negative P wave in leads I, II, III, aVF, and V_3 through V_6). The location was verified at surgery. **D,** Right free wall accessory pathway. The predominantly negative delta wave in V_1 and the axis more leftward than in **A** indicate the presence of a right free wall accessory pathway. **E,** Logic diagram to determine the location of accessory pathways. Begin with analysis of V_1 to determine whether the delta wave and the QRS complex are negative or positive. That establishes the ventricle in which the accessory pathway is located. Next, determine whether the delta wave and QRS complex are negative in leads II, III, and aVF. If so, the accessory pathway is located in a posteroseptal position. If the accessory pathway is located in the right ventricle, an inferior axis indicates an anteroseptal location, whereas a left axis indicates a right free wall location. If the accessory pathway is located in the left ventricle, an isoelectric or negative delta wave and QRS complex in leads I, aVL, V_5, and V_6 indicate a left lateral (free wall) location.

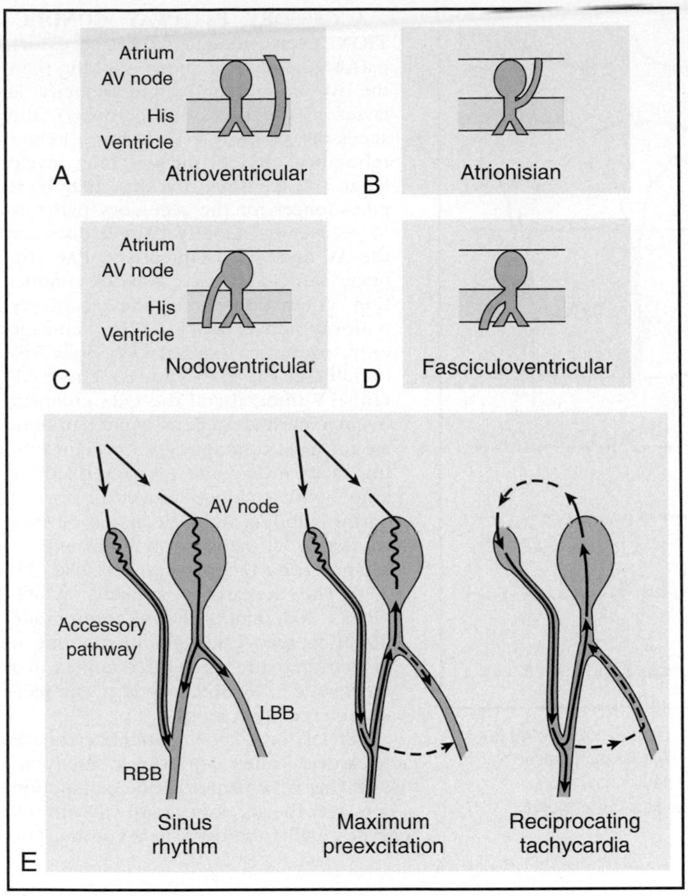

FIGURE 35–20 Schematic representation of accessory pathways. **A,** The "usual" atrioventricular (AV) accessory pathway giving rise to most clinical manifestations of tachycardia associated with Wolff-Parkinson-White (WPW) syndrome. **B,** The very uncommon atriohisian accessory pathway. If Lown-Ganong-Levine syndrome exists, it would have this type of anatomy, which has been demonstrated on occasion histopathologically. **C,** Nodoventricular pathways, original concept, in which anterograde conduction travels down the accessory pathway with retrograde conduction in the bundle branch–His bundle–AV node (see below). **D,** Fasciculoventricular connections, which are not thought to play an important role in the genesis of tachycardias. **E,** The current concept of nodofascicular accessory pathway, in which the accessory pathway is an AV communication with AV node–like properties. Sinus rhythm results in a fusion QRS complex, as in the usual form of WPW syndrome shown in **A.** Maximum preexcitation results in ventricular activation over the accessory pathway, and the His bundle is activated retrogradely. During reciprocating tachycardia, anterograde conduction occurs over the accessory pathway, with retrograde conduction over the normal pathway. LBBB = left bundle branch block; RBBB = right bundle branch block. (**E,** From Benditt DG, Milstein S: Nodoventricular accessory connection: A misnomer or a structural/functional spectrum? J Cardiovasc Electrophysiol 1:231, 1990.)

conduction over the accessory pathway and retrograde conduction over the right bundle branch–His bundle–AV node, thus making the atrium a necessary part of the circuit. The preexcited tachycardia has a left bundle branch block pattern, long AV interval (because of the long conduction time over the accessory pathway), and short VA interval. A right bundle branch block can be proarrhythmic by increasing the length of the tachycardia circuit (the VA interval is prolonged because of a delay in retrograde activation of the His bundle), and the tachycardia can become incessant.

In patients who have an atriohisian tract, theoretically, the QRS complex would remain normal and the short A-H interval fixed or show very little increase during atrial pacing at more rapid rates. This response is uncommon. Rapid atrial pacing in patients who have nodoventricular or nodofascicular connections shortens the H-V interval and widens the QRS complex, with production of a left bundle branch block contour but, in contrast to the situation in patients who have an AV connection (Fig. 35-22), the AV interval also lengthens. In patients who have fasciculoventricular connections, the H-V interval remains short and the QRS complex unchanged and anomalous during rapid atrial pacing.

ELECTROPHYSIOLOGICAL FEATURES OF PREEXCITATION. If the accessory pathway is capable of anterograde conduction, two parallel routes of AV conduction are possible, one subject to physiological delay over the AV node and the other passing directly without delay from the atrium to the ventricle (Figs. 35-20 through 35-28; also see Fig. 35-18). This direct route of conduction produces the typical QRS complex that is a fusion beat as a result of depolarization of the ventricle, in part by the wave front traveling over the accessory pathway and in part by the wave front traveling over the normal AV node–His bundle route. The delta wave represents ventricular activation from input over the accessory pathway. The extent of the contribution to ventricular depolarization by the wave front over each route depends on their relative activation times. If AV nodal conduction delay occurs because of a rapid atrial pacing rate or PAC, for example, more of the ventricle becomes activated over the accessory pathway and the QRS complex becomes more anomalous in contour. Total activation of the ventricle over the accessory pathway can occur if the AV nodal conduction delay is sufficiently long. In contrast, if the accessory pathway is relatively far from the sinus node, for example, a left lateral accessory pathway, or if the AV nodal conduction time is relatively short, more of the ventricle may be activated by conduction over the normal pathway (see Fig. 35-22). The normal fusion beat during sinus rhythm has a short H-V interval or His bundle activation actually begins after the onset of ventricular depolarization, because part of the atrial impulse bypasses the AV node and activates the ventricle early, at a time when the atrial impulse traveling the normal route just reaches the His bundle. This finding of a short or negative H-V interval occurs only during conduction over an accessory pathway or from retrograde His activation during a complex originating in the ventricle, such as a VT.

Pacing the atrium at rapid rates, at premature intervals, or from a site close to the atrial insertion of the accessory pathway accentuates the anomalous activation of the ventricles and shortens the H-V interval even more (His activation may become buried in the ventricular electrogram, as in Fig. 35-22B). The position of the accessory pathway can be determined by careful analysis of the spatial direction of the delta wave in the 12-lead ECG in maximally preexcited beats (see Fig. 35-19). T wave abnormalities can occur after the disappearance of preexcitation, with orientation of the T wave according to the site of preexcitation (T wave memory).

TABLE 35–4 Accessory Pathway Variants

Pathway Type	PR	QRS	Tachycardia	Comments
Atriohisian	Short	Normal	Unlikely	
Atriofascicular	Normal	Preexcitation (LBBB, superior axis)	Antidromic AVRT	Preexcitation with fast atrial rates or atrial extrastimuli
Nodofascicular	Normal	Preexcitation (LBBB, superior axis)	Antidromic AVRT; AVNRT with bystander activation of AP	Preexcitation with fast atrial rates or atrial extrastimuli
Fasciculoventricular	Normal	Anomalous (short H-V)	?	

AP = accessory pathway; AVRT = atrioventricular reentrant tachycardia; AVNRT = atrioventricular nodal reentrant tachycardia; LBBB = left bundle branch block.

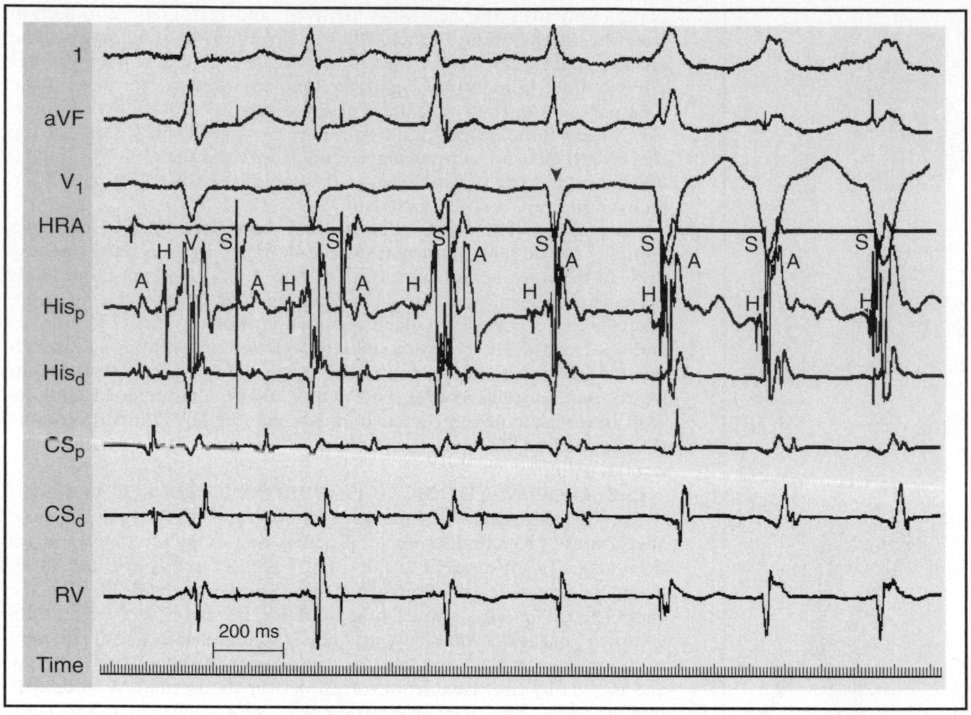

FIGURE 35–21 Development of preexcitation over an atriofascicular accessory pathway. During atrial pacing (S) on the left side of the figure, conduction occurs down the atrioventricular node as evidenced by a normal-appearing QRS complex and a normal H-V interval. The stimulus marked by the arrowhead conducts the impulse down an atriofascicular fiber, which results in a preexcited QRS, as evidenced by a widened QRS and short H-V interval.

ACCESSORY PATHWAY CONDUCTION. Even though the accessory pathway conducts more rapidly than the AV node (conduction velocity is faster in the accessory pathway), the accessory pathway usually has a longer refractory period during long cycle lengths (e.g., sinus rhythm); that is, it takes longer for the accessory pathway to recover excitability than it does for the AV node. Consequently, a PAC can occur sufficiently early to block conduction anterogradely in the accessory pathway and conduct to the ventricle only over the normal AV node–His bundle (see Fig. 35-23A and B). The resultant H-V interval and the QRS complex become normal. Such an event can initiate the most common type of reciprocating tachycardia, one characterized by anterograde conduction over the normal pathway and retrograde conduction over the accessory pathway (orthodromic AV reciprocating tachycardia) (see Fig. 35-23). The accessory pathway, which blocks conduction in an anterograde direction, recovers excitability in time to be activated after the QRS complex in a retrograde direction, thereby completing the reentrant loop.

Much less commonly, patients can have tachycardias called antidromic tachycardias, during which anterograde conduction occurs over the accessory pathway and retrograde conduction over the AV node. The

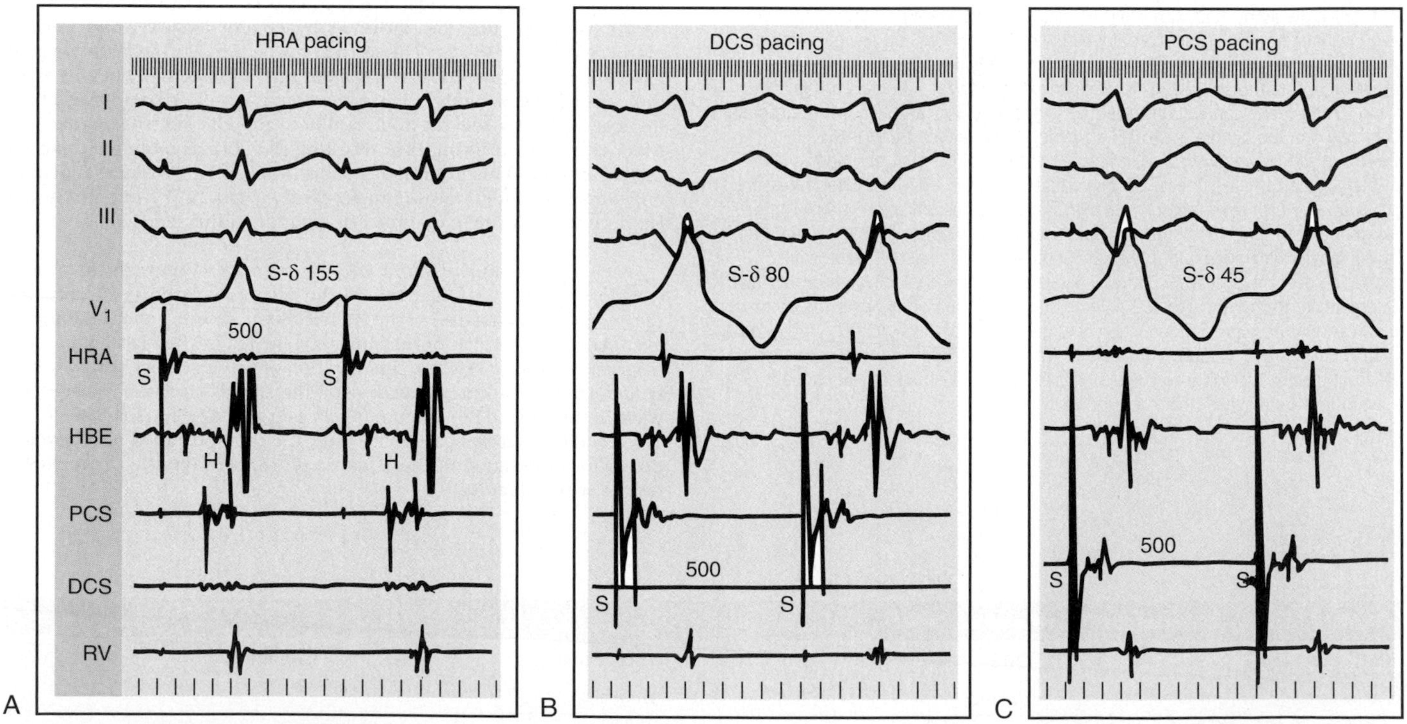

FIGURE 35–22 Atrial pacing at different atrial sites illustrating different conduction over the accessory pathway. **A,** High right atrial pacing at a cycle length of 500 milliseconds produces anomalous activation of the ventricle (note the upright QRS complex in V_1) and a stimulus-delta interval of 155 milliseconds (S-δ 155). This interval indicates that the time from the onset of the stimulus to the beginning of the QRS complex is relatively long, because the stimulus is delivered at a fairly large distance from the accessory pathway. Note that His bundle activation (H) occurs at about the onset of the QRS complex. **B,** Atrial pacing occurs through the distal coronary sinus electrode (DCS). At the same pacing cycle length, DCS pacing results in more anomalous ventricular activation and a shorter stimulus-delta interval (80 milliseconds). His bundle activation is now buried within the inscription of the ventricular electrogram in the HBE lead. **C,** Pacing from the proximal coronary sinus electrode (PCS) results in the shortest stimulus-delta interval (45 milliseconds); such an interval indicates that the pacing stimulus is being delivered very close to the atrial insertion of the accessory pathway, which is located in the left posteroseptal region of the atrioventricular groove.

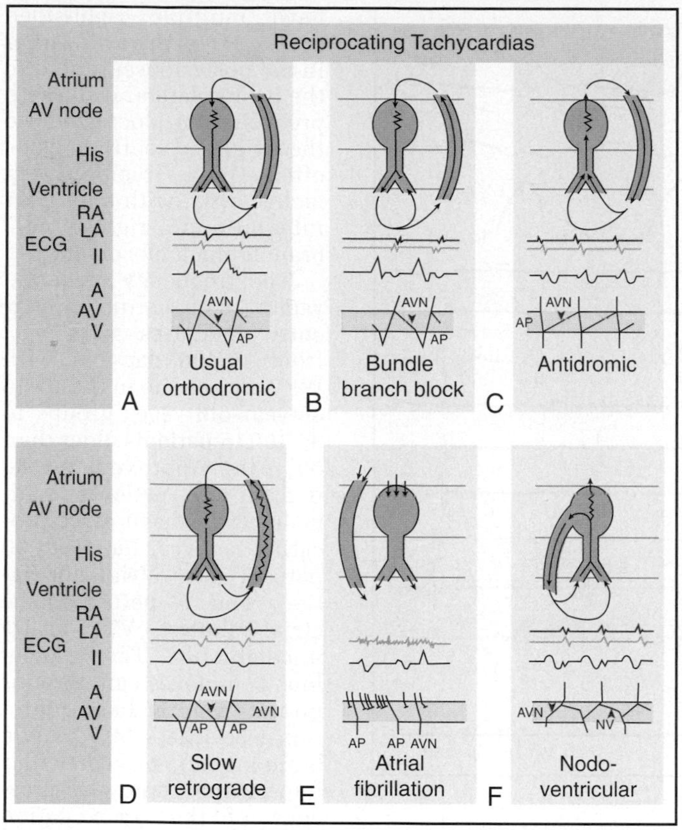

FIGURE 35–23 Schematic diagram of tachycardias associated with accessory pathways. **A,** Orthodromic tachycardia with anterograde conduction (arrowhead) over the atrioventricular (AV) node–His bundle route and retrograde conduction over the accessory pathway (left-sided for this example, as depicted by left atrial activation preceding right atrial activation). **B,** Orthodromic tachycardia and ipsilateral functional bundle branch block. **C,** Antidromic tachycardia with anterograde conduction over the accessory pathway and retrograde conduction (arrowhead) over the AV node–His bundle. **D,** Orthodromic tachycardia with a slowly conducting accessory pathway (arrowhead). **E,** Atrial fibrillation with the accessory pathway as a bystander. **F,** Anterograde conduction over a portion of the AV node and a nodoventricular (NV) pathway and retrograde conduction over the AV node (arrowheads). AP = accessory pathway; AVN = atrioventricular node.

resultant QRS complex is abnormal because of total ventricular activation over the accessory pathway (see Figs. 35-23C and 35-24). In both tachycardias, the accessory pathway is an obligatory part of the reentrant circuit. In patients with bidirectional conduction over the accessory pathway, different fibers can be used anterogradely and retrogradely.

A small percentage of patients have multiple accessory pathways, often suggested by various clues on the ECG and, on occasion, tachycardia can be caused by a reentrant loop conducting anterogradely over one accessory pathway and retrogradely over the other. Fifteen to 20 percent of patients may exhibit AV nodal echoes or AV nodal reentry after interruption of the accessory pathway.

PERMANENT FORM OF AV JUNCTIONAL RECIPROCATING TACHYCARDIA (PJRT). An incessant form of supraventricular tachycardia has been recognized that generally occurs with a long RP interval that exceeds the PR interval (see Figs. 35-25 and 35-26). Usually, a posteroseptal accessory pathway (most often right ventricular, but other locations as well) that conducts very slowly, possibly because of a long and tortuous route, appears responsible. Tachycardia is maintained by anterograde AV nodal conduction and retrograde conduction over the accessory pathway (see Fig. 35-23D). Although anterograde conduction over this pathway has been demonstrated, the long anterograde conduction time over the accessory pathway ordinarily prevents electrocardiographic manifestations of accessory pathway conduction during sinus rhythm. Therefore, during sinus rhythm, the QRS duration is prolonged from conduction over this accessory pathway only when conduction times through the AV node–His bundle exceed those in the accessory pathway.

RECOGNITION OF ACCESSORY PATHWAYS. When retrograde atrial activation during tachycardia occurs over an accessory pathway that connects the left atrium to the left ventricle, the earliest retrograde activity is recorded from a left atrial electrode usually positioned in the coronary sinus (see Fig. 35-17). When retrograde atrial activation during tachycardia occurs over an accessory pathway that connects the right ventricle to the right atrium, the earliest retrograde atrial activity is generally recorded from a lateral right atrial electrode. Participation of a septal accessory pathway creates the earliest retrograde atrial activation in the low right portion of the atrium situated near the septum, anterior or posterior, depending on the insertion site. These mapping techniques provide an accurate assessment of the position of the accessory pathway, which can be anywhere in the AV groove except in the intervalvular trigone between the mitral valve and the aortic valve annuli. Recording electrical activity directly from the accessory pathway obviously provides precise localization.

It may be difficult to distinguish AV nodal reentry from participation of a septal accessory connection using the retrograde sequence of atrial activation, because activation sequences during both tachycardias are similar. Other approaches to demonstrate retrograde atrial activation over the accessory pathway must be tried and can be accomplished by inducing PVCs during tachycardia to determine whether retrograde atrial excitation can occur from the ventricle at a time when the His bundle is refractory (see Fig. 35-17B). VA conduction cannot occur over the normal conduction system because the His bundle is refractory, so an accessory pathway must be present for the atria to become excited. No patient with a reciprocating tachycardia from an accessory AV pathway has a VA interval of less than 70 milliseconds; this is measured from the onset of ventricular depolarization to the onset of the earliest atrial activity recorded on an esophageal lead or a VA interval of less than 95 milliseconds when measured to the high right part of the atrium. In contrast, in most patients with reentry in the AV node, intervals from the onset of ventricular activity to the earliest onset of atrial activity recorded in the esophageal lead are less than 70 milliseconds.

Other Forms of Tachycardia in Patients with Wolff-Parkinson-White Syndrome

Patients can have other types of tachycardia during which the accessory pathway is a bystander—that is, uninvolved in the mechanism responsible for the tachycardia, such as AV nodal reentry or an atrial tachycardia that conducts to the ventricle over the accessory pathway. In patients with atrial flutter or atrial fibrillation, the accessory pathway is not a requisite part of the mechanism responsible for tachycardia, and the flutter or fibrillation occurs in the atrium unrelated to the accessory pathway (see Fig. 35-23E). Propagation to the ventricle during atrial flutter or atrial fibrillation can therefore occur over the normal AV node–His bundle or accessory pathway. Patients with WPW syndrome who have atrial fibrillation almost always have inducible reciprocating tachycardias as well, which can develop into atrial fibrillation (see Fig. 35-27). In fact, interruption of the accessory pathway and elimination of AV reciprocating tachycardia usually prevent recurrence of the atrial fibrillation. Atrial fibrillation presents a potentially serious risk because of the possibility for very rapid conduction over the accessory pathway. At more rapid rates, the refractory period of the accessory pathway can shorten significantly and permit an extremely rapid ventricular response during atrial flutter or atrial fibrillation (see Fig. 35-19B). The rapid ventricular response can exceed the ability of the ventricle to follow in an organized manner; it can result in fragmented, disorganized ventricular activation and hypotension and lead to ventricular fibrillation (see Fig. 35-28). Alternatively, a supraventricular discharge bypassing AV nodal delay can activate the ventricle during the vulnerable period of the antecedent T wave and precipitate ventricular fibrillation. Patients who have had ventricular fibrillation have ventricular cycle lengths during atrial fibrillation in the range of 240 milliseconds or less.

Patients with preexcitation syndrome can have other causes of tachycardia, such as AV nodal reentry, sometimes with dual AV nodal curves, sinus nodal reentry, or even VT unrelated to the accessory pathway. Some accessory pathways can conduct anterogradely only; more commonly, pathways conduct retrogradely only. If the pathway conducts only anterogradely, it cannot participate in the usual form of reciprocating tachycardia (see Fig. 35-23A). It can, however, participate in antidromic tachycardia (see Fig. 35-23C), as well as conduct to the ventricle during atrial flutter or atrial fibrillation (see Fig. 35-23E). Some data suggest that the accessory pathway demonstrates automatic activ-

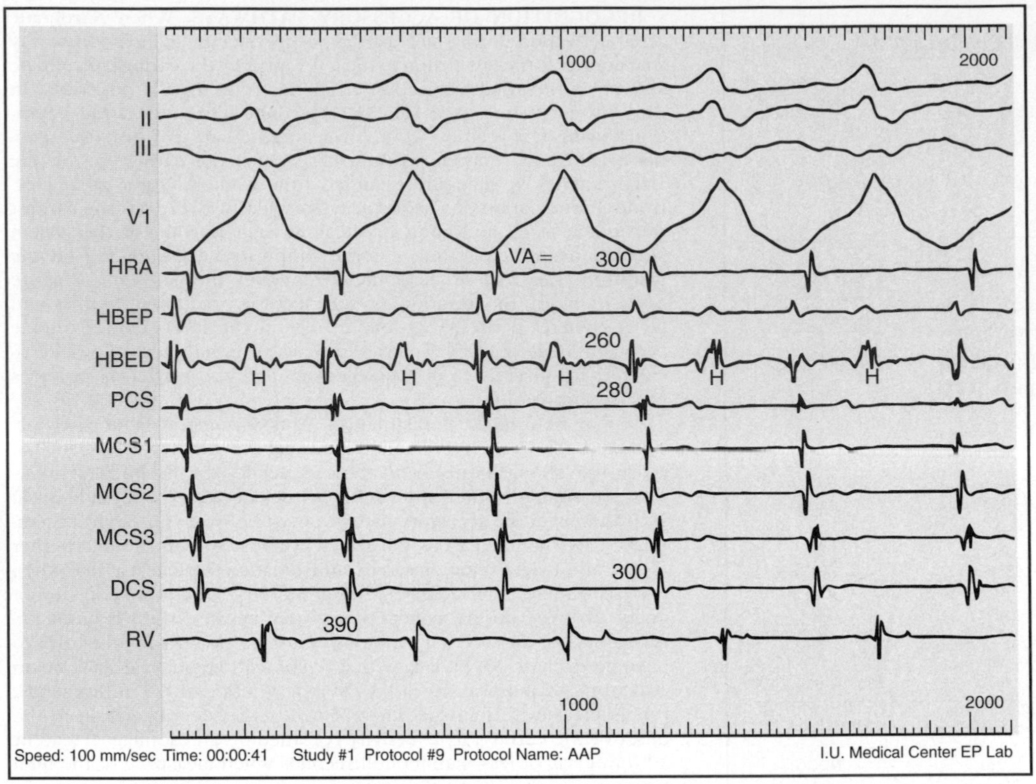

FIGURE 35–24 Antidromic atrioventricular (AV) reciprocating tachycardia. Tachycardia in this example is caused by anterograde conduction over the accessory pathway (note the abnormal QRS complex of a left posterior accessory pathway) and a normal retrograde atrial activation sequence (beginning first in the HBED lead), which is caused by retrograde conduction over the AV node. Tachycardia cycle length is 390 milliseconds, with a ventriculoatrial (VA) interval of 300 milliseconds measured in the high right atrial lead, 260 milliseconds in the distal His lead, and 280 milliseconds in the proximal coronary sinus lead. I, II, III, and V_1 are scalar leads. DCS = distal coronary sinus lead; HBEP and HBED leads = His bundle electrogram, proximal and distal; HRA = high right atrial electrogram; MCS1-3 = midcoronary sinus leads; PCS = proximal coronary sinus; RV = right ventricular electrogram.

CH 35

ity, which could conceivably be responsible for some cases of tachycardia.

"WIDE-QRS" TACHYCARDIAS. In patients with preexcitation syndrome, so-called wide-QRS tachycardias can be caused by multiple mechanisms, including sinus or atrial tachycardias, AV nodal reentry, and atrial flutter or fibrillation with anterograde conduction over the accessory pathway; orthodromic reciprocating tachycardia with functional or preexisting bundle branch block; antidromic reciprocating tachycardia; reciprocating tachycardia with anterograde conduction over one accessory pathway and retrograde conduction over a second one; tachycardias using nodofascicular or atriofascicular fibers; and VT.

CLINICAL FEATURES. The reported incidence of preexcitation syndrome depends in large measure on the population studied and varies from 0.1 to 3/1000 in apparently healthy subjects, with an average of about 1.5/1000. The incidence of the electrocardiographic pattern of WPW conduction in 22,500 healthy aviation personnel was 0.25 percent, with a prevalence of documented tachyarrhythmias of 1.8 percent. Left free wall accessory pathways are most common, followed in frequency by posteroseptal, right free wall, and anteroseptal locations. WPW syndrome is found in all age groups from the fetal and neonatal periods to the elderly, as well as in identical twins. The prevalence is higher in men and decreases with age, apparently because of loss of preexcitation. Most adults with preexcitation syndrome have normal hearts, although various acquired and congenital cardiac defects have been reported, including Ebstein anomaly, mitral valve prolapse, and cardiomyopathies. Patients with Ebstein anomaly (see Chap. 61) often have multiple right-sided accessory pathways, either in the posterior septum or in the posterolateral wall, with preexcitation localized to the atrialized ventricle. They often have reciprocating tachycardia, with a long VA interval and a right bundle branch block morphology.

The frequency of paroxysmal tachycardia apparently increases with age, from 10/100 patients with WPW syndrome in the 20- to 39-year-old age group to 36/100 in patients older than 60 years. Approximately 80 percent of patients with tachycardia have a reciprocating tachycardia, 15 to 30 percent have atrial fibrillation, and 5 percent have atrial flutter. VT occurs uncommonly. The anomalous complexes can mask or mimic myocardial infarction (see Chap. 50), bundle branch block, or ventricular hypertrophy, and the presence of the preexcitation syndrome can suggest an associated cardiac defect. Although the prognosis was once thought to be excellent in patients without tachycardia or an associated cardiac anomaly, data from Italy suggest that there exists some risk, albeit rare, of ventricular fibrillation in asymptomatic children and adults with electrocardiographic evidence of preexcitation.[70,71] For most patients with recurrent tachycardia, the prognosis is good but sudden death occurs rarely, with an estimated frequency of 0.1 percent.

It is highly likely that an accessory pathway is congenital, although its manifestations can be detected in later years and appear to be acquired. Relatives of patients with preexcitation, particularly those with multiple pathways, have an increased prevalence of preexcitation, thus suggesting a hereditary mode of acquisition. Some children and adults can lose their tendency for the development of tachyarrhythmias as they grow older, possibly as a result of fibrotic or other changes at the site of the accessory pathway insertion. Pathways can lose their ability to conduct anterogradely. Tachycardia beginning in infancy can disappear but frequently recurs. Tachycardia still present after 5 years of age persists in 75 percent of patients, regardless of accessory pathway location. Intermittent preexcitation during sinus rhythm and abrupt loss of conduction over the accessory pathway after intravenous procainamide and with exercise suggest that the refractory period of the accessory pathway is long, and that the patient is not at risk for a rapid ventricular rate should atrial flutter or fibrillation develop. These approaches are relatively specific, but not very sensitive, with a low positive predictive accuracy. Exceptions to these safeguards can occur; the only way to be certain of the accessory pathways properties and propensity for rapid conduction is via an electrophysiology study.

TREATMENT. Patients with ventricular preexcitation who have only the electrocardiographic abnormality, without tachyarrhythmias or history of palpitations, do not generally require electrophysiological evaluation or therapy. Data from randomized trials have, however, questioned this paradigm.[70,71] However, for patients with frequent episodes of symptomatic tachyarrhythmia, therapy should be initiated.

Two therapeutic options exist, catheter ablation and pharmacological therapy. Drugs are chosen to prolong conduction time and/or refractoriness in the AV node, the accessory pathway, or both to prevent rapid rates from occurring. If successful, this therapy prevents maintenance of an AV reciprocating tachycardia or a rapid ventricular response to atrial flutter or atrial fibrillation. Some drugs can suppress premature complexes that precipitate the arrhythmias.

Adenosine, verapamil, propranolol, and digitalis all prolong conduction time and refractoriness in the AV node. Verapamil and propranolol do not directly affect conduction in the accessory pathway, and digitalis has had variable effects. Because digitalis has been reported to shorten refractoriness in the accessory

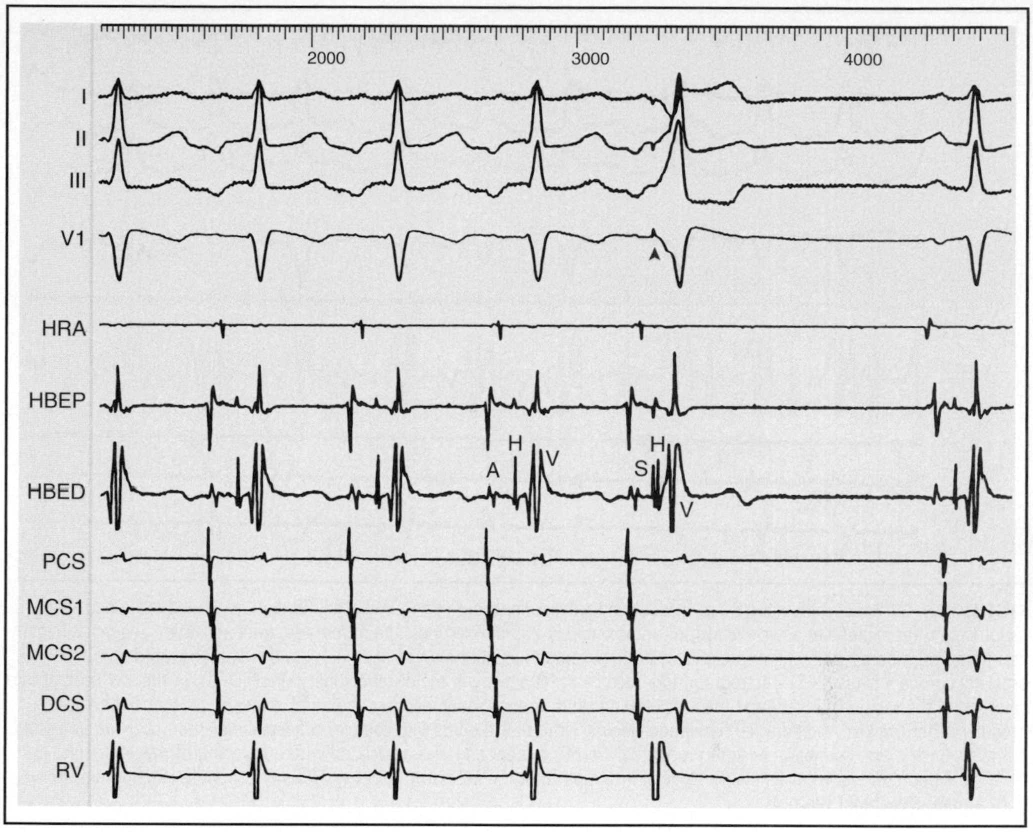

FIGURE 35–25 Termination of the permanent form of atrioventricular (AV) junctional reciprocating tachycardia (PJRT). In the left portion of this example, PJRT is present. The atrial activation sequence is indistinguishable from atypical AV nodal reentry and atrial tachycardia originating in the low right atrium. The response to premature stimulation identifies the tachycardia as PJRT. Premature ventricular stimulation (arrowhead) occurs at a time when the His bundle is refractory from depolarization during the tachycardia (second labeled H). Therefore, premature ventricular stimulation cannot enter the AV node. Furthermore, premature ventricular stimulation does not reach the atrium. Premature ventricular stimulation, however, terminates the tachycardia. This detail can be explained only by the PVC invading and blocking in a retrogradely conducting accessory pathway. I, II, III, and V_1 are scalar electrocardiographic leads. DCS = distal coronary sinus electrograms; HBEP, HBED = His bundle electrogram, proximal and distal; HRA = high right atrial electrogram; MCS1, MCS2 = midcoronary sinus electrograms; PCS = proximal coronary sinus electrogram; RV = right ventricular electrogram.

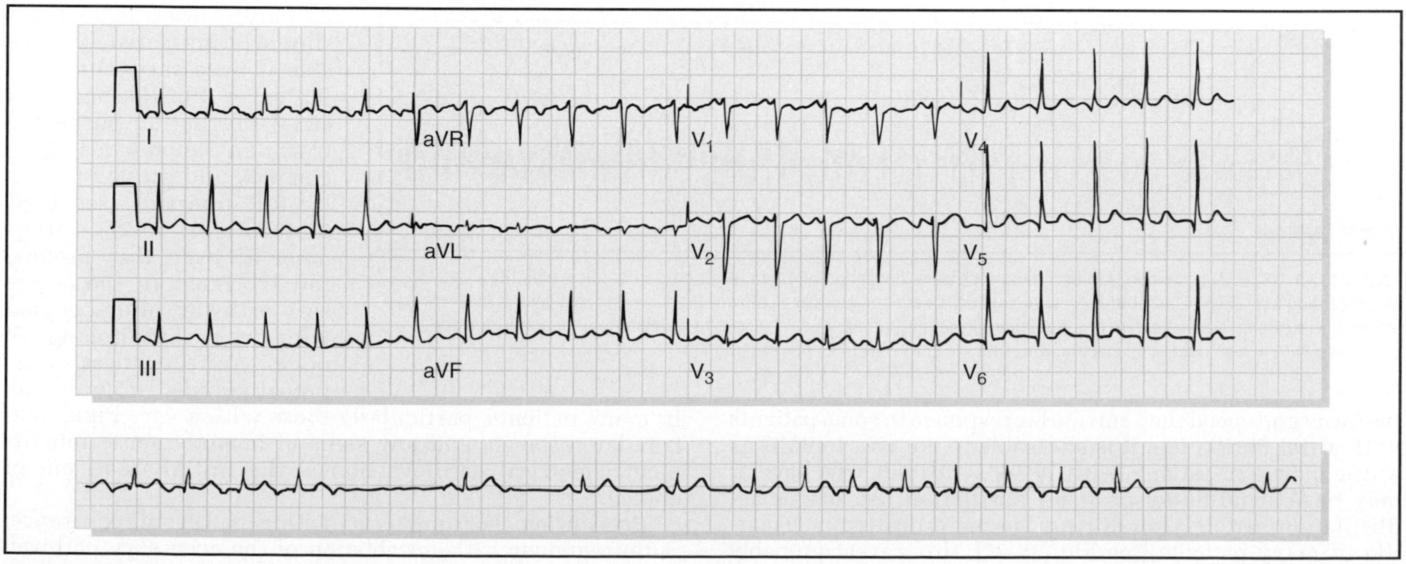

FIGURE 35–26 Permanent form of junctional reciprocating tachycardia (PJRT) in a patient with a left-sided accessory pathway. The 12-lead electrocardiogram demonstrates a long RP interval–short PR interval tachycardia, which in contrast to the usual form of PJRT, exhibits negative P waves in leads I and aVL. The rhythm strips below (lead I) indicate that whenever a nonconducted P wave occurs, the tachycardia always terminates, only to begin again after several sinus beats. This pattern is in marked contrast to that in Figure 35-7, in which the tachycardia continues despite nonconducted P waves.

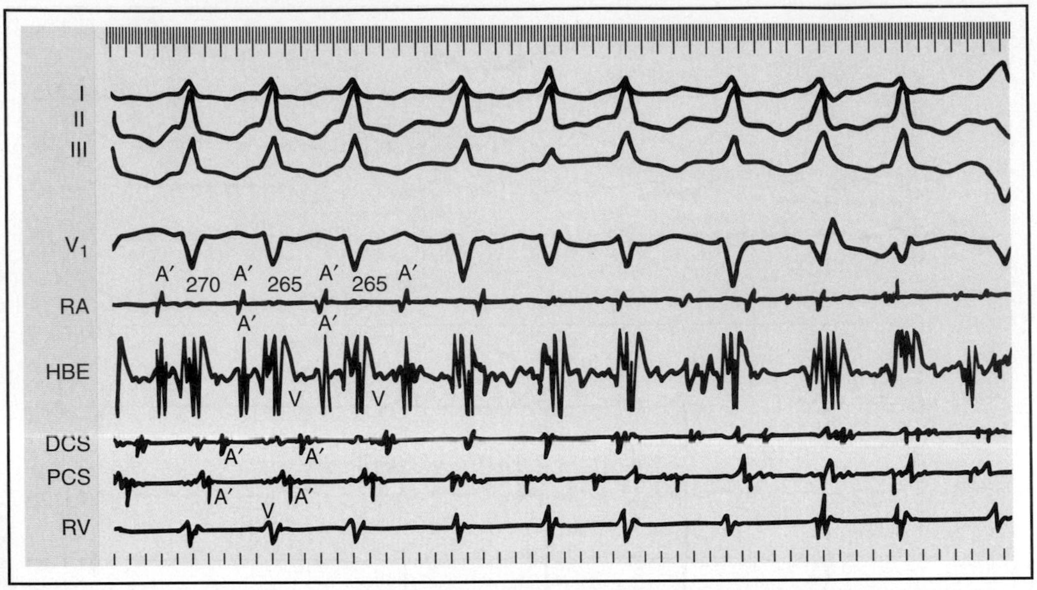

FIGURE 35–27 Atrioventricular (AV) reciprocating tachycardia disorganizing into atrial fibrillation. During sustained AV reciprocating tachycardia at a cycle length of approximately 265 milliseconds, the retrograde atrial activation sequence began first in the right paraseptal region (not shown in this example; location proved at surgery) and was then recorded in the proximal coronary sinus (PCS) electrogram, followed by atrial activity in the distal coronary sinus (DCS), in the low right atrium recorded in the His bundle lead, and then in the high right atrium. Spontaneously, the atrial activation sequence becomes irregular (after the last A′) and atrial fibrillation begins. Note that the last QRS complex reflects conduction over the accessory pathway. Such a transformation occurred repeatedly in this patient and was associated with quickening of the ventricular rate. Atrial fibrillation did not recur following surgical interruption of the accessory pathway. HBE = His bundle electrogram; RA = right atrium; RV = right ventricle.

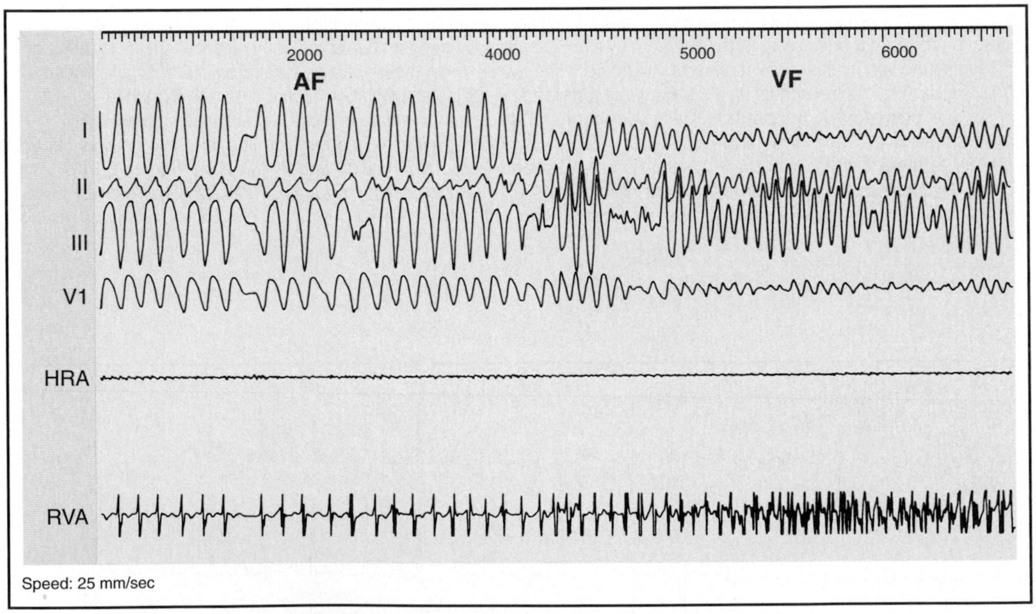

FIGURE 35–28 Atrial fibrillation (AF) becoming ventricular fibrillation (VF). In the left portion of this panel, the electrocardiogram (ECG) demonstrates AF with conduction over an accessory pathway producing a rapid ventricular response, at times in excess of 350 beats/min. In the midportion of the tracing, VF can be seen to develop. I, II, III, and V_1 are scalar ECG leads. HRA = high right atrial electrogram; RVA = right ventricular apex electrogram.

pathway and speed the ventricular response in some patients with atrial fibrillation, it is advisable to not use digitalis as a single drug in patients with WPW syndrome who have or may have atrial flutter or atrial fibrillation. Because atrial fibrillation can develop during the reciprocating tachycardia in many patients (see Fig. 35-27), this caveat probably applies to all patients who have tachycardia and WPW syndrome. Rather, drugs that prolong the refractory period in the accessory pathway should be used, such as classes IA and IC drugs (see Chap. 33).

Class IC drugs, amiodarone, and sotalol can affect both the AV node and the accessory pathway. Lidocaine does not generally prolong refractoriness of the accessory pathway. Verapamil and IV lidocaine can increase the ventricular rate during atrial fibrillation in patients with WPW syndrome. IV verapamil can precipitate ventricular fibrillation when given to a patient with WPW syndrome who has a rapid ventricular rate during atrial fibrillation. This effect does not seem to occur with oral verapamil. Catecholamines can expose WPW syndromes, shorten the refractory period of the accessory pathway, and reverse the effects of some antiarrhythmic drugs.

Termination of an Acute Episode. Termination of an acute episode of reciprocating tachycardia, suspected electrocardiographically from a normal QRS complex, regular R-R intervals, a rate of about 200 beats/min, and a retrograde P wave in the ST segment, should be approached similarly to AV nodal reentry. After vagal maneuvers, adenosine followed by IV verapamil or diltiazem is the initial treatment of choice. Atrial fibrillation can occur after drug administration, particularly adenosine, with a rapid ventricular response. An external cardioverter-defibrillator should be immediately available if necessary. For atrial flutter or fibrillation, with atrial fibrillation suspected from an anomalous QRS complex and grossly irregular R-R intervals (see Figs. 35-19B and 35-27), drugs must be used that prolong refractoriness in the accessory pathway, often coupled with drugs that prolong AV nodal refractoriness (e.g., procainamide, propranolol). In many patients, particularly those with a very rapid ventricular response and any signs of hemodynamic impairment, electrical cardioversion is the initial treatment of choice.

Prevention. For long-term therapy to prevent recurrence, radiofrequency catheter ablation of the accessory pathway has become the first-line therapy for most patients. For those patients with frequent symptomatic arrhythmias that are not fully controlled by drugs or are drug-intolerant, or for those who do not wish to take drugs, ablation is advisable.

This option should be considered early in the course of treatment of a symptomatic patient because of its high success rate, low frequency of complications, and potential cost-effectiveness. Ablation is the treatment of choice in those patients with atrial fibrillation and rapid conduction over an accessory pathway. Whereas transvenous catheter ablation is generally very effective, epicardial ablations via a pericardial approach or surgical interruption of the accessory pathway may be necessary in rare cases.

Drug therapy is an alternative to ablation, but it is not always possible to predict which drugs may be most effective for an individual patient. Some drugs can actually increase the frequency of episodes of reciprocating tachycardia by prolonging the duration of anterograde and not retrograde refractory periods of the accessory pathway, thereby making it easier for a PAC to block conduction anterogradely in the accessory pathway and initiate tachycardia. Oral administration of two drugs, such as flecainide and propranolol, to decrease conduction capability in both limbs of the reentrant circuit can be beneficial. Class IC drugs, amiodarone, or sotalol, which prolong refractoriness in both the accessory pathway and the AV node, can be effective. Depending on the clinical situation, empirical drug trials or serial electrophysiological drug testing can be used to determine optimal drug therapy for patients with reciprocating tachycardia. For patients who have atrial fibrillation with a rapid ventricular response, induction of atrial fibrillation while the patient is receiving therapy is essential to be certain that the ventricular rate is controlled. Exercise or isoproterenol can be superimposed to be certain that the rate is controlled. Patients who have accessory pathways with very short refractory periods may be poor candidates for drug therapy, because the refractory periods may be insignificantly prolonged in response to the standard agents.

SUMMARY OF ELECTROCARDIOGRAPHIC DIAGNOSIS OF SUPRAVENTRICULAR TACHYCARDIAS. Electrocardiographic clues that permit differentiation among the various supraventricular tachycardias are often present. P waves during tachycardia that are identical to sinus P waves and occur with a long RP interval and a short PR interval are most likely caused by sinus nodal reentry, sinus tachycardia, or an atrial tachycardia arising from the right atrium near the sinus node. Retrograde (inverted in leads II, III, and aVF) P waves generally represent reentry involving the AV junction, either AV nodal reentry or reciprocating tachycardia using a paraseptal accessory pathway. Tachycardia without manifest P waves is probably caused by AV nodal reentry (P waves buried in QRS), whereas a tachycardia with an RP interval exceeding 90 milliseconds may be caused by an accessory pathway. AV dissociation or AV block during tachycardia excludes the participation of an AV accessory pathway and makes AV nodal reentry less likely. Multiple tachycardias can occur at different times in the same patient. QRS alternans, thought to be a feature of AV reciprocating tachycardia, is more likely a rapid rate-related phenomenon independent of the tachycardia mechanism. RP-PR relationships (Table 35-5) help differentiate supraventricular tachycardias. QRS voltage can increase during supraventricular tachycardia.

TABLE 35-5 Supraventricular Tachycardias

Short RP/Long PR Internal	Long RP/Short PR Internal
AV node reentry	Atrial tachycardia
AV reentry	Sinus node reentry Atypical AV node reentry AVRT with a slowly conducting accessory pathway (e.g., PJRT)

AV = atrioventricular; AVRT = AV reciprocating tachycardia; PJRT = paroxysmal junctional reciprocating tachycardia.

VENTRICULAR RHYTHM DISTURBANCES

Premature Ventricular Complexes

ELECTROCARDIOGRAPHIC RECOGNITION. A PVC is characterized by the premature occurrence of a QRS complex that is abnormal in shape and has a duration usually exceeding the dominant QRS complex, generally longer than 120 milliseconds. The T wave is usually large and opposite in direction to the major deflection of the QRS. The QRS complex is not preceded by a premature P wave but can be preceded by a nonconducted sinus P wave occurring at its expected time. The diagnosis of a PVC can never be made with unequivocal certainty from the scalar ECG because a supraventricular beat or rhythm can mimic the manifestations of ventricular arrhythmia (Fig. 35-29). Retrograde transmission to the atria from the PVC occurs fairly frequently but is often obscured by the distorted QRS complex and T wave. If the retrograde impulse discharges and resets the sinus node prematurely, it produces a pause that is not fully compensatory. More commonly, the sinus node and atria are not discharged prematurely by the retrograde impulse because interference of impulses frequently occurs at the AV junction in the form of a collision between the anterograde impulse conducted from the sinus node and the retrograde impulse conducted from the PVC. Therefore, a fully compensatory pause usually follows a PVC—the R-R interval produced by the two sinus-initiated QRS complexes on either side of the PVC equals twice the normally conducted R-R interval. The PVC may not produce any pause and may therefore be interpolated (see Fig. 35-29E). Conversely, it may produce a postponed compensatory pause when an interpolated premature complex causes PR prolongation of the first postextrasystolic beat to such a degree that the P wave of the second postextrasystolic beat occurs at a very short RP interval and is therefore blocked.

Interference within the ventricle can result in ventricular fusion beats caused by simultaneous activation of the ventricle by two foci, one from the supraventricular impulse and the other from the PVC. Occasionally, a fusion beat can be narrower than the dominant sinus beat, as when a right bundle branch block pattern of a PVC arising in the left ventricle fuses with the sinus-initiated left bundle branch block complex conducting through the AV junction (see Fig. 35-23), or when a sinus beat with a right bundle branch block pattern fuses with a right ventricular paced beat with a left bundle branch block pattern. Narrow PVCs have also been explained as originating at a point equidistant from each ventricle in the ventricular septum and by arising high in the fascicular system. Whether a compensatory or noncompensatory pause, retrograde atrial excitation, or an interpolated complex, fusion complex, or echo beat occurs (see Fig. 35-29D) is merely a function of how the AV junction conducts and the timing of the events taking place.

The term *bigeminy* refers to pairs of complexes and indicates a normal and premature complex, *trigeminy* indicates a premature complex following two normal beats, a premature complex following three normal beats is called *quadrigeminy*, and so on. Two successive PVCs are known as a pair or a couplet, whereas three successive PVCs are called a triplet. Arbitrarily, three or more successive PVCs are termed *ventricular tachycardia*. PVCs can have different contours and are often called multifocal (Fig. 35-30). More properly, they should be called multiform, polymorphic, or

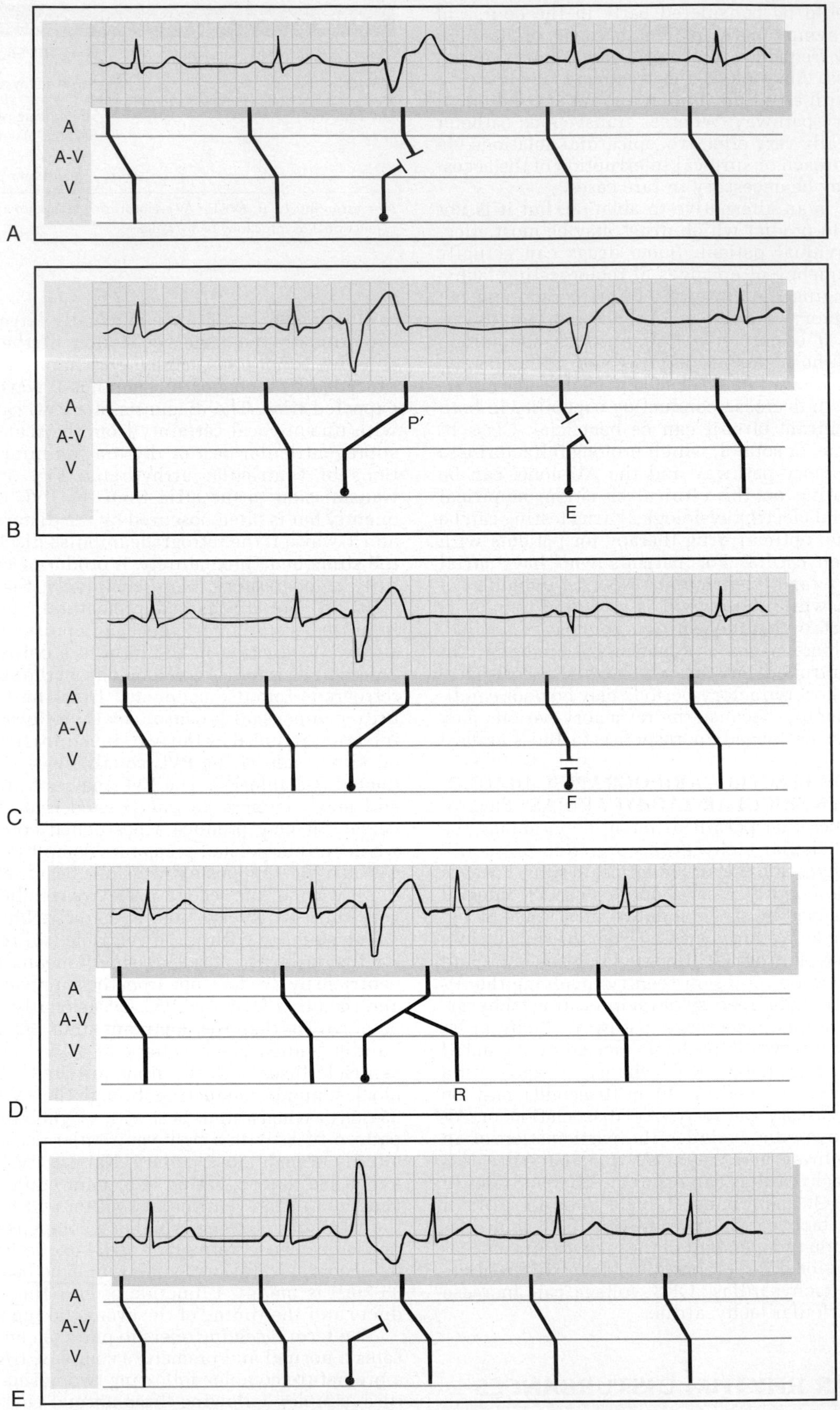

FIGURE 35–29 Premature ventricular complexes (PVCs). **A** to **D** were recorded in the same patient. **A,** A late PVC results in a compensatory pause. **B,** A slower sinus rate and a slightly earlier premature ventricular complex result in retrograde atrial excitation (P′). The sinus node is reset, followed by a noncompensatory pause. Before the sinus-initiated P wave that follows the retrograde P wave can conduct the impulse to the ventricle, ventricular escape (E) occurs. **C,** Events are similar to those in **B** except that a ventricular fusion beat (F) results after the PVC because of a slightly faster sinus rate. **D,** The impulse propagating retrogradely to the atrium reverses its direction after a delay and returns to reexcite the ventricles (R) to produce a ventricular echo. **E,** An interpolated PVC is followed by a slightly prolonged PR interval of the sinus-initiated beat. Lead II. ECG is shown. Red circles indicate origin of PVCs.

pleomorphic because it is not known whether multiple foci are discharging or whether conduction of the impulse originating from one site is merely changing.

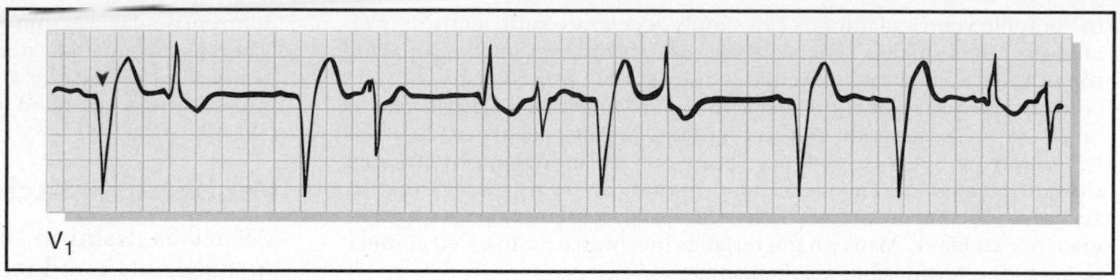

FIGURE 35–30 Multiform premature ventricular complexes (PVCs). The normally conducted QRS complexes exhibit a left bundle branch block contour (arrowhead) and are followed by PVCs with three different morphologies.

PVCs can exhibit fixed or variable coupling; that is, the interval between the normal QRS complex and the PVC can be relatively stable or variable. Fixed coupling can be caused by reentry, triggered activity (see Chap. 31), or other mechanisms. Variable coupling can be caused by parasystole, changing conduction in a reentrant circuit, or changing discharge rates of triggered activity. Usually, it is difficult to determine the precise mechanism responsible for the PVC based on constant or variable coupling intervals.

CLINICAL FEATURES. The prevalence of premature complexes increases with age; they are associated with male gender and a reduced serum potassium concentration. PVCs are more frequent in the morning in patients after myocardial infarction, but this circadian variation is absent in patients with severe LV dysfunction. Symptoms of palpitations or discomfort in the neck or chest can result because of the greater than normal contractile force of the postextrasystolic beat or the feeling that the heart has stopped during the long pause after the premature complex. Long runs of frequent PVCs in patients with heart disease can produce angina, hypotension, or heart failure. Frequent interpolated PVCs actually represent a doubling of the heart rate and can compromise the patient's hemodynamic status. In some patients, frequent PVCs alone can cause heart failure that is reversed when the PVC site is ablated. Activity that increases the heart rate can decrease the patient's awareness of the premature systole or reduce their number. Exercise can increase the number of premature complexes in some patients. Premature systoles can be uncomfortable in patients who have aortic regurgitation because of the large stroke volume. Sleep is usually associated with a decrease in the frequency of ventricular arrhythmias, but some patients can experience an increase.

PVCs occur in association with various stimuli and can be produced by direct mechanical, electrical, and chemical stimulation of the myocardium. Often, they are noted in patients with LV false tendons, during infection, in ischemic or inflamed myocardium, and during hypoxia, anesthesia, or surgery. They can be provoked by various medications, electrolyte imbalance, tension states, myocardial stretch, and excessive use of tobacco, caffeine, or alcohol. Both central and peripheral autonomic stimulation have profound effects on the heart rate and can produce or suppress premature complexes.

Physical examination reveals the presence of a premature beat followed by a pause that is longer than normal. A fully compensatory pause can be distinguished from one that is not fully compensatory, in that the former does not change the timing of the basic rhythm. The premature beat is often accompanied by a decrease in intensity of the heart sounds, often with auscultation of just the first heart sound, which can be sharp and snapping, and a decreased or absent peripheral (e.g., radial) pulse. The relationship of atrial to ventricular systole determines the presence of normal *a* waves or giant *a* waves in the jugular venous pulse, and the length of the PR interval determines the intensity of the first heart sound. The second heart sound can be abnormally split, depending on the origin of the ventricular complex.

The importance of PVCs depends on the clinical setting. In the absence of underlying heart disease, the presence of PVCs usually has no impact on longevity or limitation of activity; antiarrhythmic drugs are not indicated.[71] Patients should be reassured if they are symptomatic (see Chap. 33).

In patients suffering from acute myocardial infarction, PVCs once considered to presage the onset of ventricular fibrillation, such as those occurring close to the preceding T wave, more than five or six per minute, bigeminal or multiform complexes, or those occurring in salvoes of two, three, or more, do not occur in about 50% of patients in whom ventricular fibrillation develops, and ventricular fibrillation does not develop in about 50% of patients who have these PVCs. Thus, these PVCs are not particularly helpful prognostically. The presence of 1 to 10 or more ventricular extrasystoles/hour can identify patients at increased risk for VT or sudden cardiac death after myocardial infarction, but is similarly nonspecific.

MANAGEMENT. In most patients, PVCs (occurring as single PVCs, bigeminy, or trigeminy but excluding nonsustained VT; see later) do not need to be treated, particularly if the patient does not have an acute coronary syndrome, and treatment is usually dictated by the presence of symptoms attributable to the PVCs. Both fast and slow heart rates can provoke the development of PVCs. PVCs accompanying slow ventricular rates can be abolished by increasing the basic rate with atropine or isoproterenol or by pacing, whereas slowing the heart rate in some patients with sinus tachycardia can eradicate PVCs. In hospitalized patients, IV lidocaine (see Chap. 33) is generally the initial treatment of choice to suppress PVCs. If maximum dosages of lidocaine are unsuccessful, IV procainamide can be tried. Propranolol is suggested if other drugs have been unsuccessful. IV magnesium can be useful. For long-term oral maintenance, various class I, II, and III drugs can be useful to prevent VT. Class IC drugs seem particularly successful in suppressing PVCs, but flecainide and moricizine have been shown to increase mortality in patients treated after myocardial infarction. Amiodarone can be effective. Athletes with structural heart disease and ventricular extrasystoles who are in high-risk groups can participate in low-intensity sports only.[72] Thrombolysis therapy does not influence the frequency of ventricular extrasystoles, which are related to residual LV pump performance after myocardial infarction. Low levels of serum potassium and magnesium are associated with higher prevalence rates of ventricular arrhythmias.

Accelerated Idioventricular Rhythm

ELECTROCARDIOGRAPHIC RECOGNITION. The ventricular rate, commonly between 60 and 110 beats/min, usually hovers within 10 beats of the sinus rate, so control of the cardiac rhythm shifts between these two competing pacemaker sites. Consequently, fusion beats often occur at the onset and termination of the arrhythmia as the pacemakers vie for control of ventricular depolarization (Fig. 35-31). Because of the slow rate, capture beats are common. The onset of this arrhythmia is generally gradual (nonparoxysmal) and occurs when the rate of the VT exceeds the sinus rate because of sinus slowing or SA or AV block. The ectopic mechanism can also begin after a PVC, or the ectopic ventricular focus can simply accelerate sufficiently to overtake the sinus rhythm. The slow rate and nonparoxysmal onset avoid the problems initiated by excitation during the vulnerable period, and consequently precipitation of more rapid ventricular arrhythmias is rarely seen. Termination of the rhythm generally occurs gradually as the dominant sinus rhythm accelerates or as the ectopic ventricular rhythm decelerates. The ventricular rhythm can be regular or irregular and can occasionally show sudden doubling, which suggests the presence of exit block. Many characteristics incriminate enhanced automaticity as the responsible mechanism.

The arrhythmia occurs as a rule in patients who have heart disease, such as those with acute myocardial infarction or with digitalis toxicity. It is transient and intermittent, with episodes lasting a few seconds to a minute, and does not appear to seriously affect the patient's clinical course or the prognosis. It commonly occurs at the moment of reperfusion of a previously occluded coronary artery, and can be found during resuscitation.

MANAGEMENT. Suppressive therapy is rarely necessary because the ventricular rate is generally less than 100 beats/min, but such therapy may be considered when AV dissociation results in loss of sequential AV contraction, an accelerated idioventricular rhythm occurs together with a more rapid VT, an accelerated idioventricular rhythm begins with a PVC discharging in the vulnerable period of the preceding T wave, the ventricular rate is too rapid and produces symptoms, or if ventricular fibrillation develops as a result of the accelerated idioventricular rhythm. This last event appears to be fairly rare. Therapy, when indicated, should be as noted earlier for VT. Often, simply increasing the sinus rate with atropine or atrial pacing suppresses the accelerated idioventricular rhythm.

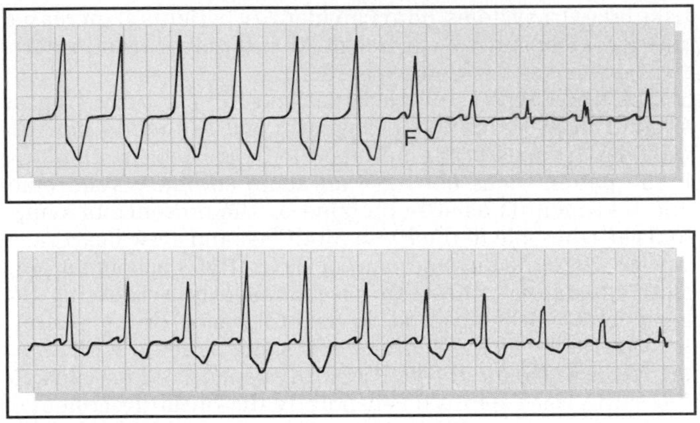

FIGURE 35–31 Accelerated idioventricular rhythm. In this continuous monitor lead recording, an accelerated idioventricular rhythm competes with the sinus rhythm. Wide QRS complexes at a rate of 90 beats/min fuse (F) with the sinus rhythm, which takes control briefly, generates the narrow QRS complexes, and then yields once again to the accelerated idioventricular rhythm as the P waves move "in and out" of the QRS complex. This example of isorhythmic atrioventricular dissociation may be caused by hemodynamic modulation of the sinus rate via the autonomic nervous system.

Ventricular Tachycardia

VT arises distal to the bifurcation of the His bundle in the specialized conduction system, ventricular muscle, or combinations of both tissue types. Mechanisms include disorders of impulse formation (enhanced automaticity or triggered activity) and conduction (reentry) considered earlier (see Chap. 31). In general, the specific type, prognosis, and management of ventricular tachycardia depend on whether underlying structural heart disease is present. With the exception of those patients with inherited VT–sudden cardiac death (SCD) syndromes (see Chap. 9) if structural heart disease is absent, the prognosis in patients with VT and PVCs is generally very good, whereas in the presence of structural heart disease the subsequent risk of SCD is high.

ELECTROCARDIOGRAPHIC RECOGNITION. The electrocardiographic diagnosis of VT is suggested by the occurrence of a series of three or more consecutive, abnormally shaped PVCs whose duration exceeds 120 milliseconds, with the ST-T vector pointing opposite the major QRS deflection. The R-R interval can be exceedingly regular or can vary. Patients can have VTs with multiple morphologies originating at the same or closely adjacent sites, probably with different exit paths. Others have multiple sites of origin. Atrial activity can be independent of ventricular activity, or the atria can be depolarized by the ventricles retrogradely (VA association). Depending on the particular type of VT, rates range from 70 to 250 beats/min, and the onset can be paroxysmal (sudden) or nonparoxysmal. QRS contours during the VT can be unchanging (uniform, monomorphic), and can vary randomly (multiform, polymorphic, or pleomorphic), in a more or less repetitive manner (torsades de pointes), can vary in alternate complexes (bidirectional VT), or in a stable but changing contour (i.e., right bundle branch contour changing to a left bundle branch contour). VT can be sustained, defined arbitrarily as lasting longer than 30 seconds or requiring termination because of hemodynamic collapse, or nonsustained, when it stops spontaneously in less than 30 seconds. Most commonly, very premature stimulation is required to initiate VT electrically, whereas late coupled ventricular complexes usually initiate its spontaneous onset (Fig. 35-32).

Making the electrocardiographic distinction between supraventricular tachycardia with aberration and VT can be difficult at times because features of both arrhythmias overlap and, under certain circumstances, a supraventricular tachycardia can mimic the criteria established for VT.[1] Ventricular complexes with an abnormal and prolonged configuration indicate only that conduction through the ventricle is abnormal, and such complexes can occur in supraventricular rhythms as a result of preexisting bundle branch block, aberrant conduction during

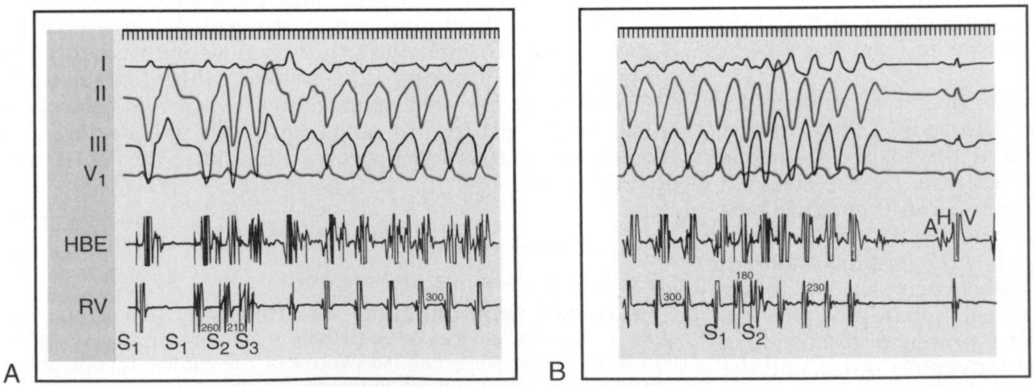

FIGURE 35–32 Initiation and termination of ventricular tachycardia by means of programmed ventricular stimulation. The last two ventricular-paced beats at a cycle length of 600 milliseconds are shown in **A.** A premature stimulus (S_2) at an S_1-S_2 interval of 260 milliseconds and another premature stimulus (S_3) at a cycle length of 210 milliseconds initiate a sustained monomorphic ventricular tachycardia at a cycle length of 300 milliseconds. **B,** Two premature ventricular stimuli (S_1-S_2) create an unstable ventricular tachycardia that persists for several beats at a shorter cycle length (230 milliseconds) and then terminates, followed by sinus rhythm. HBE = His bundle electrogram; RV = right ventricle.

incomplete recovery of repolarization, conduction over accessory pathways, and several other conditions. These complexes do not necessarily indicate the origin of impulse formation or the reason for the abnormal conduction. Conversely, ectopic beats originating in the ventricle can uncommonly have a fairly normal duration and shape. However, VT is the most common cause of tachycardia with a wide QRS complex. A past history of myocardial infarction makes the diagnosis even more likely.

During the course of a tachycardia characterized by wide, abnormal QRS complexes, the presence of fusion beats and capture beats provides maximum support for the diagnosis of VT (Fig. 35-33; see Table 35-2). Fusion beats indicate activation of the ventricle from two different foci, with the implication that one of the foci had a ventricular origin. Capture of the ventricle by the supraventricular rhythm with a normal configuration of the captured QRS complex at an interval shorter than the tachycardia in question indicates that the impulse has a supraventricular origin, and thus excludes a supraventricular origin of the tachycardia. AV dissociation has long been considered a hallmark of VT. However, retrograde VA conduction to the atria from ventricular beats occurs in at least 25 percent of patients, and therefore VT may not exhibit AV dissociation. AV dissociation can occur uncommonly during supraventricular tachycardias. Even if a P wave appears to be related to each QRS complex, it is at times difficult to determine whether the P wave is conducted anterogradely to the next QRS complex (i.e., supraventricular tachycardia with aberrancy and a long PR interval) or retrogradely from the preceding QRS complex (i.e., a VT). As a general rule, however, AV dissociation during tachycardia with a wide QRS is strong presumptive evidence that the tachycardia is of ventricular origin.

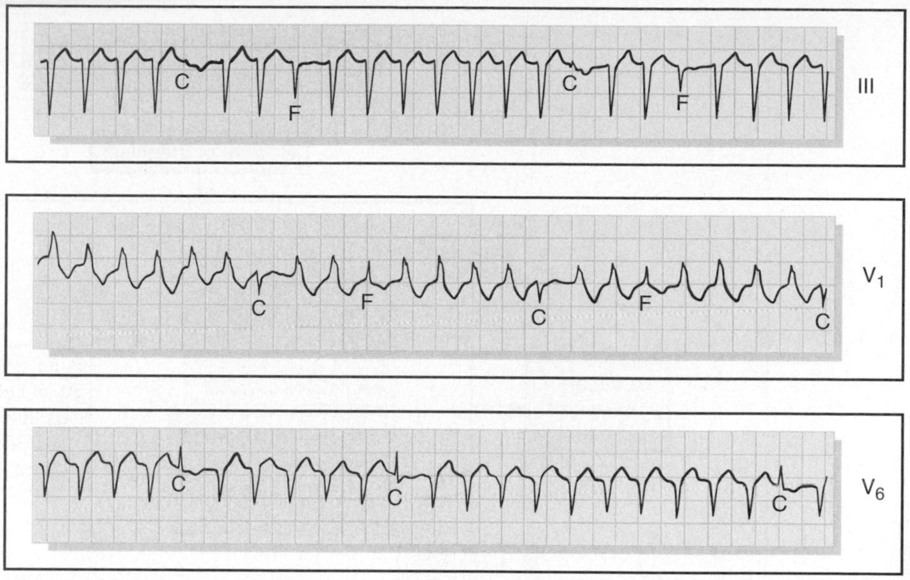

FIGURE 35–33 Fusion and capture beats during ventricular tachycardia. The QRS complex is prolonged, and the R-R interval is regular except for occasional capture beats (C) that have a normal contour and are slightly premature. Complexes intermediate in contour represent fusion beats (F). Thus, even though atrial activity is not clearly apparent, atrioventricular dissociation is present during ventricular tachycardia and produces intermittent capture and fusion beats.

Differentiation Between Ventricular and Supraventricular Tachycardia. Although fusion and capture beats and AV dissociation provide the strongest electrocardiographic evidence for differentiating VT from supraventricular tachycardia with aberrant conduction, these features are not always present. Therefore, other clues from the ECG may be required to help with this differentiation; features characterizing supraventricular arrhythmia with aberrancy include the following: (1) consistent onset of the tachycardia with a premature P wave; (2) a very short RP interval (0.1 second), often requiring an esophageal recording to visualize the P waves; (3) a QRS configuration the same as that occurring from known supraventricular conduction at similar rates; (4) P wave and QRS rate and rhythm linked to suggest that ventricular activation depends on atrial discharge (e.g., an AV Wenckebach block); and (5) slowing or termination of the tachycardia by vagal maneuvers.

Analysis of specific QRS contours can also be helpful in diagnosing VT and localizing its site of origin. For example, QRS contours suggesting VT include left-axis deviation in the frontal plane and a QRS duration exceeding 140 milliseconds, with a QRS of normal duration during sinus rhythm. In precordial leads with an RS pattern, the duration of the onset of the R to the nadir of the S exceeding 100 milliseconds suggests VT as the diagnosis. During VT with a right bundle branch block appearance, (1) the QRS complex is monophasic or biphasic in V_1, with an initial deflection different from that of the sinus-initiated QRS complex, (2) the amplitude of the R wave in V_1 exceeds the R′, and (3) a small R and large S wave or a QS pattern in V_6 may be present. With a VT having a left bundle branch block contour, (1) the axis can be rightward, with negative deflections deeper in V_1 than in V_6, (2) a broad prolonged (more than 40 milliseconds) R wave can be noted in V_1, and (3) a small Q–large R wave or QS pattern in V_6 can exist. A QRS complex that is similar in V_1 through V_6, either all negative or all positive, favors a ventricular origin, as does the presence of a 2 : 1 VA block. (An upright QRS complex in V_1 through V_6 can also occur from conduction over a left-sided accessory pathway.) Supraventricular beats with aberration often have a triphasic pattern in V_1, an initial vector of the abnormal complex similar to that of the normally conducted beats, and a wide QRS complex that terminates a short cycle length following a long cycle (long-short cycle sequence). During atrial fibrillation, fixed coupling, short coupling intervals, a long pause after the abnormal beat, and runs of bigeminy rather than a consecutive series of abnormal complexes all favor a ventricular origin of the premature complex, rather than a supraventricular origin with aberration. A grossly irregular, wide QRS tachycardia with ventricular rates exceeding 200 beats/min should raise the question of atrial fibrillation with conduction over an accessory pathway (see Fig. 35-28). In the presence of a preexisting bundle branch block, a wide QRS tachycardia with a contour different from the contour during sinus rhythm is most likely a VT. Based on these criteria, several algorithms for distinguishing VT from supraventricular tachycardia with aberrancy have been suggested, one of which is shown in Figure 35-34. Exceptions exist to all the aforementioned criteria, especially in patients who have preexisting conduction disturbances or preexcitation syndrome; when in doubt, one must rely on sound clinical judgment and consider the ECG only as one of several helpful ancillary tests.

Termination of a tachycardia by triggering vagal reflexes is considered diagnostic of supraventricular tachycardias. However, VT, especially if originating in the right ventricular outflow tract, can be stopped in a similar manner.

ELECTROPHYSIOLOGICAL FEATURES. Electrophysiologically, VT can be distinguished by a short or negative H-V interval (i.e., H begins after the onset of ventricular depolarization) because of retrograde activation from the ventricles (see Chap. 31). His bundle deflections are not usually apparent during VT because they are obscured by simultaneous ventricular septal depolarization or inadequate catheter position. The latter must be determined during supraventricular rhythm before the onset or after the termination of VT (see Fig. 35-32). His bundle deflections dissociated from ventricular activation are diagnostic, with rare exceptions. VT can produce QRS complexes of narrow duration and short H-V interval, most likely when the site of origin is close to the His bundle in the fascicles.

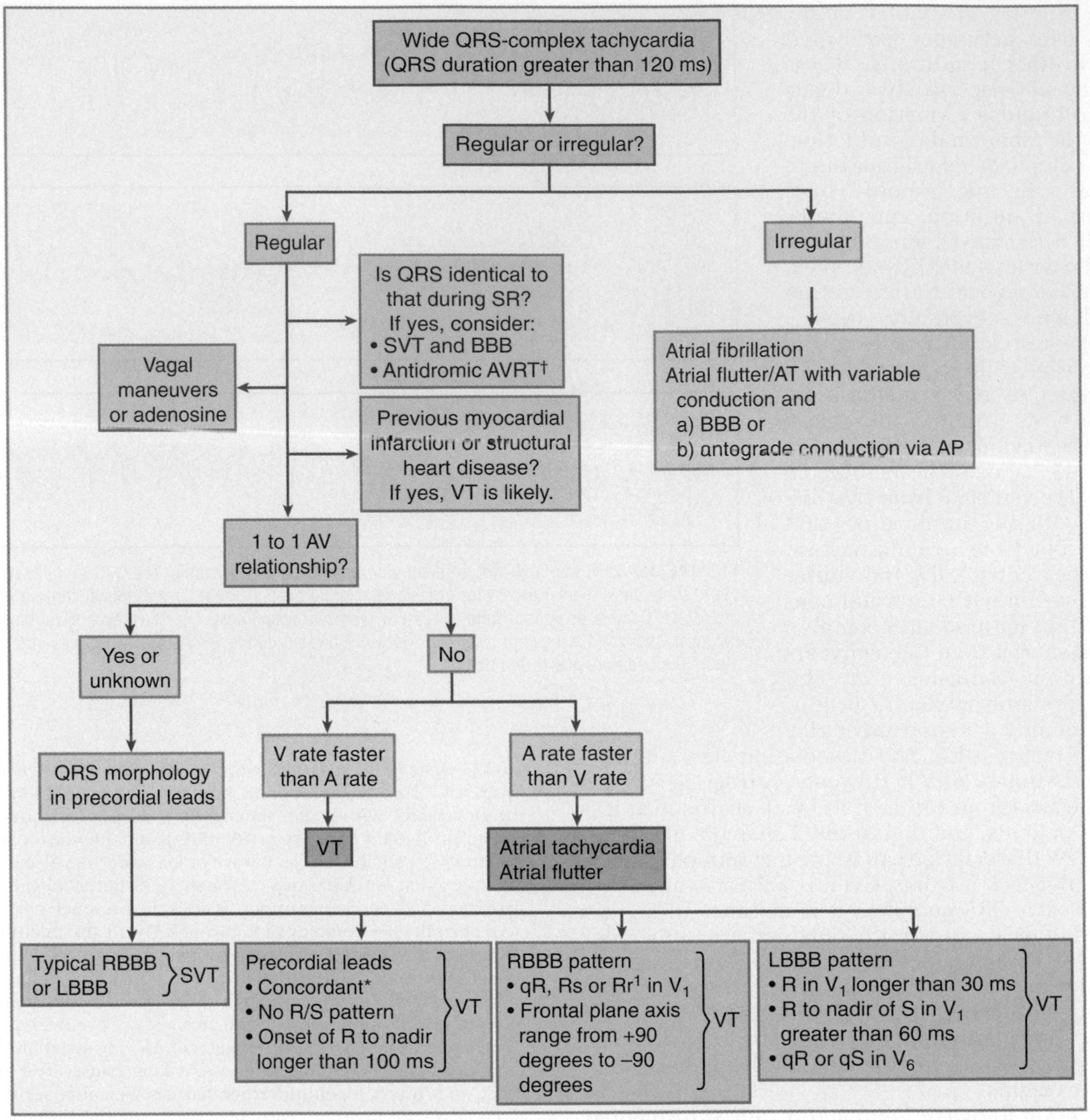

FIGURE 35–34 Algorithm for diagnosing a wide QRS tachycardia. AV = atrioventricular; AVRT = AV reentrant tachycardia; LBBB = left bundle branch block; RBBB = right bundle branch block; SVT = supraventricular tachycardia; VT = ventricular tachycardia. (From Blomstrom-Lundqvist C, Scheinman MM, Aliot EM, et al: ACC/AHA/ESC guidelines for the management of patients with supraventricular arrhythmias—executive summary: A report of the American College of Cardiology/American Heart Association Task Force on Practice Guidelines and the European Society of Cardiology Committee for Practice Guidelines (Writing Committee to Develop Guidelines for the Management of Patients With Supraventricular Arrhythmias). Circulation 108:1871, 2003.)

Successful electrical induction of VT by premature ventricular stimulation (see Fig. 35-32) depends on the characteristics of the VT and the anatomical substrate. Patients with sustained, hemodynamically stable VT and VT secondary to chronic coronary artery disease have monomorphic VT induced more frequently (90 percent) than patients with nonsustained VT, VT from non–coronary-related causes or acute ischemia, and cardiac arrest (40 to 75 percent). In general, it is more difficult to induce VT with late premature ventricular stimuli than with early premature stimuli, during sinus rhythm than during ventricular pacing, and with one premature stimulus than with two or three stimuli. The specificity of VT induction using more than two premature ventricular stimuli begins to decrease, while the sensitivity increases, and nonsustained polymorphic VT or ventricular fibrillation can be induced in patients who have no history of VT. Of patients with stable VT who have inducible sustained monomorphic VT, the latter is induced in about 25 percent with a single extra stimulus, in 50 percent with double extra stimuli, and in 25 percent with triple extra stimuli. Occasionally, VT can be initiated only from the left ventricle or from specific sites in the right ventricle. Multiple premature stimuli reduce the need for LV stimulation. Drugs such as isoproterenol can facilitate the induction of VT. Coughing during VT that causes hypotension can help maintain blood pressure.

Termination by pacing depends significantly on the rate of the VT and the site of pacing. Slower VTs are terminated more easily and with fewer stimuli than are more rapid ones. An increasing number of stimuli are required to terminate more rapid VTs, which increases the risks of pacing-induced acceleration of the VT. Subthreshold stimulation and transthoracic stimulation can terminate VT. Atrial pacing, at times, can also induce and terminate VT (see Chap. 31).

CLINICAL FEATURES. Symptoms occurring during VT depend on the ventricular rate, duration of tachycardia, and presence and extent of the underlying heart disease and peripheral vascular disease. VT can occur in several forms: short, asymptomatic, nonsustained episodes; sustained, hemodynamically stable events, generally occurring at slower rates or in otherwise normal hearts; or unstable runs, often degenerating into ventricular fibrillation. In some patients who have nonsustained VTs initially, sustained episodes or ventricular fibrillation later develop(s). The location of impulse formation and therefore the way in which the depolarization wave spreads across the myocardium can also be important. Physical findings depend in part on the P-to-QRS relationship. If atrial activity is dissociated from the ventricular contractions, the findings of AV dissociation are present. If the atria are captured retrogradely, regularly occurring cannon a waves appear when atrial and ventricular contractions occur simultaneously and signs of AV dissociation are absent.

More than 50% of patients treated for symptomatic recurrent VT have ischemic heart disease. The next largest group has cardiomyopathy (both congestive and hypertrophic), with lesser percentages divided among those with primary electrical disease, such as inherited ion channel abnormalities (see Chap. 9), mitral valve prolapse, valvular heart disease, congenital heart disease, and miscellaneous causes. LV hypertrophy can lead to ventricular arrhythmias. Coronary artery spasm can cause transient myocardial ischemia with severe ventricular arrhythmias in some patients, during ischemia as well as during the apparent reperfusion period. Complex ventricular arrhythmias can occur after coronary artery bypass grafting. In patients resuscitated from sudden cardiac death (see Chap. 36), most (75 percent) have severe coronary artery disease, and ventricular tachyarrhythmias can be induced by premature ventricular stimulation in approximately 75 percent. When VT occurs in an ambulatory patient, it is uncommonly induced by R-on-T PVCs. Patients who have sustained VT are more likely to have a reduced ejection fraction (EF), slowed intraventricular conduction and electrographic abnormalities, LV aneurysm, and previous myocardial infarction than patients who have ventricular fibrillation, thus indicating different electrophysiological and anatomical substrates. Young patients can also suffer cardiac arrest from VT or ventricular fibrillation, and persistent electrical inducibility of arrhythmias in these patients connotes a poor prognosis. In patients with coronary artery disease, sustained VT displays a circadian variation, with peak frequency in the morning.

Many approaches have been used to assess prognosis in patients with ventricular arrhythmias. Reduced baroreceptor sensitivity and heart rate variability apparently caused by reduced vagal activity may indicate an increased risk of VT or sudden cardiac death. The presence of nonsustained VT after myocardial infarction often presages sudden cardiac death. Electrophysiological study findings of reduced LV function, spontaneous ventricular arrhythmias, late potentials on signal-averaged ECG, QT interval dispersion, T wave alternans,[73,74] prolonged QRS duration, heart rate turbulence, and inducible sustained VTs all carry increased risk. Currently, however, no noninvasive technique reliably predicts outcome better than assessment of LV function. LV function and inducibility of VT during electrophysiological study are the two strongest predictors of poor outcome. Some early studies have suggested that T wave alternans may be a good risk-stratifying modality, but randomized trials are pending.[73-75] New risk factors such as an elevated C-reactive protein level, various cytokines, and genotypes may provide useful information in the future. In general, the prognosis for patients with idiopathic VT (see later), in the absence of structural heart disease or a prolonged QT interval, is good and warrants less aggressive treatment than for patients with structural heart disease. Patients with inherited ion channel abnormalities are an exception to that statement (see Chap. 9).

MANAGEMENT. The dramatic changes in the management of VT and aborted sudden death over the past several years have been fueled by several large clinical trials (Table 35-6) and development of the ICD. Management decisions can be stratified into those involved in acute management (or termination) and those involved in long-term therapy (or prevention of recurrence or sudden death; see Chap. 36).

Acute Management of Sustained Ventricular Tachycardia. VT that does not cause hemodynamic decompensation can be treated medically to achieve acute termination by administering IV amiodarone, lidocaine, or procainamide, followed by an infusion of the successful drug. In Europe, ajmaline is often used. Lidocaine is often ineffective; amiodarone, sotalol, and procainamide appear to be superior. In patients in whom procainamide is ineffective or in whom procainamide may be problematic (severe heart failure, renal failure), IV amiodarone is often effective. In general, an initial amiodarone loading dose of 15 mg/min is given over a 10-minute period. This dose is followed by an infusion of 1 mg/min for 6 hours and then a maintenance dose of 0.5 mg/min for the remaining 18 hours and for the next several days, as necessary. If VT does not terminate, or if it recurs, a repeat loading dose can be given. Rarely, sinus bradycardia or AV block can be seen with IV amiodarone. The hypotension associated with IV amiodarone, caused largely by the diluent used in earlier formulations, does not seem to be as frequent a problem and is usually related to the rate of infusion.

If the arrhythmia does not respond to medical therapy, electrical DC cardioversion can be used. VT that precipitates hypotension, shock, angina, congestive heart failure, or symptoms of cerebral hypoperfusion should be treated promptly with DC cardioversion (see Chaps. 33 and 36). Very low energies can terminate VT, beginning with a synchronized shock of 10 to 50 J. Digitalis-induced VT is best treated pharmacologically. After conversion of the arrhythmia to a normal rhythm, it is essential to institute measures to prevent recurrence.

Striking the patient's chest, sometimes called "thumpversion," can terminate VT by mechanically inducing a PVC that presumably interrupts the reentrant pathway necessary to support it. Chest stimulation at the time of the vulnerable period during the arrhythmia can accelerate the VT or possibly provoke ventricular fibrillation.

In some cases, such as VT associated with a remote myocardial infarction (which is caused by reentry), ventricular pacing via a pacing catheter inserted into the right ventricle or transcutaneously at rates faster than the tachycardia can terminate the tachycardia. This procedure incurs the risk of accelerating the VT to ventricular flutter or ventricular fibrillation. In patients with recurrent VT, competitive ventricular pacing can be used to prevent recurrence. Intermittent VT, interrupted by several supraventricular beats, is generally best treated pharmacologically.

A search for reversible conditions contributing to the initiation and maintenance of VT should be made and the conditions corrected, if possible. For example, VT related to ischemia, hypotension, or hypokalemia can at times be terminated by antianginal treatment, vasopressors, or potassium, respectively. Correction of heart failure can reduce the frequency of ventricular arrhythmias. Slow ventricular rates caused by sinus bradycardia or AV block can permit the occurrence of PVCs and ventricular tachyarrhythmias, which can be corrected by administering atropine, temporary isoproterenol administration, or transvenous pacing. Supraventricular tachycardia can initiate ventricular tachyarrhythmias and should be prevented, if possible.

Long-Term Therapy for Prevention of Recurrences. The goal of long-term therapy is to prevent sudden cardiac death and recurrence of symptomatic VT. Asymptomatic nonsustained ventricular arrhythmias in low-risk populations (i.e., preserved LV function) often need not be treated. In patients with symptomatic nonsustained tachycardia, beta blockers are frequently effective in preventing recurrences. In patients refractory to beta blockers, class IC agents, sotalol, or amiodarone can be effective. However, class IC agents should be avoided in patients with structural heart disease,

TABLE 35–6 Clinical Trials in the Treatment of Ventricular Tachycardia and Prevention of Cardiac Arrest

Study	Patient Inclusion	Endpoints	Treatment Arms	Key Results
Primary Prevention Studies				
BHAT[1]	• Post MI	• Total mortality • Sudden cardiac death	• Propranolol • Placebo	Total mortality, sudden cardiac death reduced in treatment arm
CAST[2,3]	• Post MI • ≥6 PVC/hr • LVEF ≤40%	• Arrhythmic death	• Flecainide • Encainide • Moricizine • Placebo	Arrhythmic death increased with all treatment arms
SWORD[4]	• Post MI • LVEF <40% or • Remote MI • NYHA Class II-III	• Total mortality	• D-Sotalol • Placebo	Increased mortality in treatment arm
EMIAT[5]	• Post MI • LVEF <40%	• Total mortality • Arrhythmic death	• Amiodarone • Placebo	Amiodarone reduced arrhythmic death but not total mortality
CAMIAT[6]	• Post MI • ≥10 PVC/hr or NSVT	• Arrhythmic death • Total mortality	• Amiodarone • Placebo	Amiodarone reduced arrhythmic death but not total mortality
GESICA[7]	• CHF • LVEF ≤35%	• Total mortality	• Amiodarone • Best therapy	Amiodarone reduced mortality; patients with NSVT had higher mortality
CHF-STAT[8]	• CHF • LVEF ≤40% • ≥10 PVCs/hr (asymptomatic)	• Total mortality	• Amiodarone • Placebo	No effect in ischemic cardiomyopathy but trend toward reduced mortality in nonischemic cardiomyopathy
CABG-PATCH[9]	• CAD undergoing CABG • LVEF <36% • Positive SAECG	• Total mortality	• CABG • CABG + ICD	No difference in total mortality
MADIT[10]	• Post MI • NSVT • LVEF ≤35% • NYHA Class I-III • Inducible VT not suppressed by procainamide	• Total mortality	• ICD • Antiarrhythmic drug (80% amiodarone)	ICD reduced mortality
MUSTT[11]	• Post MI • LVEF <40% • NSVT	• Arrhythmic death or cardiac arrest	• ICD in nonsuppressible group • Antiarrhythmic drug in suppressible group • No therapy	Improved survival in ICD group; no difference between no therapy and antiarrhythmic group
MADIT II[12]	• Post MI • EF ≤30% • >10 PVC/hr or couplets	• Total mortality	• ICD • No ICD	Improved survival in ICD arm
DINAMIT[13]	• Immediate post MI • EF ≤35%	• Total mortality • Arrhythmic mortality	• ICD • No ICD	No improvement in survival with ICD
COMPANION[14]	• Ischemic or nonischemic CM • NYHA Class III-IV • QRS ≥120 msec	• Total mortality	• Medical therapy • PM-CRT • ICD-CRT	Improved survival in ICD-CRT group > PM-CRT > medical therapy
DEFINITE[15]	• Nonischemic CM • EF ≤36% • PVCs or NSVT	• Total mortality • Arrhythmic mortality	• ICD • No ICD	Improved survival in the ICD arm
SCD-HeFT[16]	• CHF • LVEF ≤35% • NYHA Class II-III	• Total mortality • Arrhythmic mortality • Cost • Quality of life	• ICD • Amiodarone • Placebo	Improved survival with ICD; no effect of amiodarone on survival
Secondary Prevention Studies				
ESVEM[17,18]	• Cardiac arrest, sustained VT, or syncope • ≥10 PVCs/hr • Inducible VT	• Recurrence of arrhythmia	• EP-guided antiarrhythmics (imipramine, mexiletine, procainamide, quinidine, sotalol, pirmenol, propafenone) • Holter-guided antiarrhythmics	No difference between Holter- and EP-guided groups; sotalol group had lowest recurrence rate of VT, arrhythmic death, total death

TABLE 35-6 Clinical Trials in the Treatment of Ventricular Tachycardia and Prevention of Cardiac Arrest—cont'd

Study	Patient Inclusion	Endpoints	Treatment Arms	Key Results
CASCADE[19]	• Cardiac arrest • Not associated with acute MI	• Cardiac mortality • Aborted cardiac arrest	• EP- or Holter-guided conventional drug therapy • Empirical amiodarone	Amiodarone survival better than conventional guided drug therapy
CASH[20]	• Cardiac arrest • Not associated with acute MI	• Total mortality	• Empirical amiodarone • Metoprolol • Propafenone • ICD	Sudden cardiac death mortality lowest in ICD arm; increased mortality in propafenone arm
AVID[21]	• Cardiac arrest or sustained VT	• Total mortality • Cost • Quality of life	• ICD • Drug therapy (empirical amiodarone, or EP- or Holter-guided sotalol)	Survival better in ICD group, with most benefit occurring in first 9 mo; benefit most pronounced in patients with EF <35%.
CIDS[22,23]	• Cardiac arrest or sustained VT	• Total mortality	• ICD • Amiodarone	Survival trended better in ICD group

CABG = coronary artery bypass graft; CAD = coronary artery disease; CHF = congestive heart failure; CM = cardiomyopathy; CRT = cardiac resynchronization therapy; EF = ejection fraction; EP = electrophysiology study; ICD = implantable cardioverter-defibrillator; LVEF = left ventricular ejection fraction; MI = myocardial infarction; NSVT = nonsustained ventricular tachycardia; NYHA = New York Heart Association; PM = pacemaker; PVC = premature ventricular complex; SAECG = signal-averaged electrocardiogram; VT = ventricular tachycardia.

1. A randomized trial of propranolol in patients with acute myocardial infarction. I. Mortality results. JAMA 247:1707, 1982.
2. Echt DS, Liebson PR, Mitchell LB, et al: Mortality and morbidity in patients receiving encainide, flecainide, or placebo. The Cardiac Arrhythmia Suppression Trial [see comments]. N Engl J Med 324:781, 1991.
3. The Cardiac Arrhythmia Suppression Trial II Investigators: Effect of the antiarrhythmic agent moricizine on survival after myocardial infarction. N Engl J Med 327:227, 1992.
4. Waldo AL, Camm AJ, deRuyter H, et al: Effect of d-sotalol on mortality in patients with left ventricular dysfunction after recent and remote myocardial infarction. The SWORD Investigators. Survival With Oral d-Sotalol [see comments]. Lancet 348:7, 1996.
5. Julian DG, Camm AJ, Frangin G, et al: Randomised trial of effect of amiodarone on mortality in patients with left-ventricular dysfunction after recent myocardial infarction: EMIAT. European Myocardial Infarct Amiodarone Trial Investigators [see comments]. Lancet 349:667, 1997.
6. Cairns JA, Connolly SJ, Roberts R, Gent M: Randomised trial of outcome after myocardial infarction in patients with frequent or repetitive ventricular premature depolarisations: CAMIAT. Canadian Amiodarone Myocardial Infarction Arrhythmia Trial Investigators [see comments]. Lancet 349:675, 1997.
7. Doval HC, Nul DR, Grancelli HO, et al: Nonsustained ventricular tachycardia in severe heart failure. Independent marker of increased mortality due to sudden death. GESICA-GEMA Investigators [see comments]. Circulation 94:3198, 1996.
8. Singh SN, Fletcher RD, Fisher SG, et al: Amiodarone in patients with congestive heart failure and asymptomatic ventricular arrhythmia. Survival Trial of Antiarrhythmic Therapy in Congestive Heart Failure [see comments]. N Engl J Med 333:77, 1995.
9. Bigger JT Jr, Whang W, Rottman JN, et al: Mechanisms of death in the CABG Patch trial: A randomized trial of implantable cardiac defibrillator prophylaxis in patients at high risk of death after coronary artery bypass graft surgery. Circulation 99:1416, 1999.
10. Moss AJ, Hall WJ, Cannom DS, et al: Improved survival with an implanted defibrillator in patients with coronary disease at high risk for ventricular arrhythmia. Multicenter Automatic Defibrillator Implantation Trial Investigators. N Engl J Med 335:1933, 1996.
11. Buxton AE, Lee KL, Fisher JD, et al: A randomized study of the prevention of sudden death in patients with coronary artery disease. Multicenter Unsustained Tachycardia Trial Investigators. N Engl J Med 341:1882, 1999.
12. Moss AJ, Zareba W, Hall WJ, et al: Prophylactic implantation of a defibrillator in patients with myocardial infarction and reduced ejection fraction. N Engl J Med 346:877, 2002.
13. Hohnloser SH, Kuck KH, Dorian P, et al: Prophylactic use of an implantable cardioverter-defibrillator after acute myocardial infarction. N Engl J Med 351:2481, 2004.
14. Bristow MR, Saxon LA, Boehmer J, et al: Cardiac-resynchronization therapy with or without an implantable defibrillator in advanced chronic heart failure. N Engl J Med 350:2140, 2004.
15. Kadish A, Dyer A, Daubert JP, et al: Prophylactic defibrillator implantation in patients with nonischemic dilated cardiomyopathy. N Engl J Med 350:2151, 2004.
16. Bardy GH, Lee KL, Mark DB, et al: Sudden Cardiac Death in Heart Failure Trial (SCD-HeFT) Investigators: Amiodarone or an implantable cardioverter-defibrillator for congestive heart failure. N Engl J Med 352:225, 2005.
17. Mason JW: A comparison of electrophysiologic testing with Holter monitoring to predict antiarrhythmic-drug efficacy for ventricular tachyarrhythmias. Electrophysiologic Study versus Electrocardiographic Monitoring Investigators [see comments]. N Engl J Med 329:445, 1993.
18. Mason JW: A comparison of seven antiarrhythmic drugs in patients with ventricular tachyarrhythmias. Electrophysiologic Study versus Electrocardiographic Monitoring Investigators [see comments]. N Engl J Med 329:452, 1993.
19. Greene HL: The CASCADE Study: Randomized antiarrhythmic drug therapy in survivors of cardiac arrest in Seattle. CASCADE Investigators. Am J Cardiol 72:70F, 1993.
20. Siebels J, Cappato R, Ruppel R, et al: Preliminary results of the Cardiac Arrest Study Hamburg (CASH). CASH Investigators. Am J Cardiol 72:109F, 1993.
21. The Antiarrhythmics versus Implantable Defibrillators (AVID) Investigators: A comparison of antiarrhythmic-drug therapy with implantable defibrillators in patients resuscitated from near-fatal ventricular arrhythmias [see comments]. N Engl J Med 337:1576, 1997.
22. Connolly SJ, Gent M, Roberts RS, et al: Canadian Implantable Defibrillator Study (CIDS): Study design and organization. CIDS Co-Investigators. Am J Cardiol 72:103F, 1993.
23. Cappato R: Secondary prevention of sudden death: The Dutch Study, the Antiarrhythmics Versus Implantable Defibrillator Trial, the Cardiac Arrest Study Hamburg, and the Canadian Implantable Defibrillator Study. Am J Cardiol 83:68D, 1999.

especially those with coronary artery disease because of the increased mortality associated with these drugs caused by proarrhythmia. Sotalol should be used cautiously because of its potential for prolonging the QT interval and producing torsades de pointes. Patients with nonsustained VT after myocardial infarction and poor LV function are at significant risk for sudden death. The Multicenter Automatic Defibrillator Trial (MADIT)[76] found that patients with prior myocardial infarction and an EF of 0.35 or less who had inducible VT that was not suppressed with drugs had better survival if treated with an ICD, with a hazard ratio of 0.46. In the Multicenter Unsustained Tachycardia Trial (MUSTT),[77] patients with an EF of 0.40 or less with coronary disease and asymptomatic nonsustained VT who had inducible sustained VT at electrophysiological study had a significant reduction in mortality if treated with an ICD. These studies have suggested that patients with nonsustained VT and an EF of 0.35 to 0.40 or less should undergo electrophysiological study and, if they have inducible VT (i.e., not suppressed with procainamide), should have an ICD.[76] More recently, the MADIT-II study[78] found that patients with ischemic cardiomyopathy (prior myocardial infarction) with an EF of 0.30 or less and no requirement for ventricular arrhythmia had improved survival if treated with an ICD (hazard ratio, 0.69). The Sudden Cardiac Death Heart Failure Trial (SCD-HeFT) found that patients with nonischemic and ischemic cardiomyopathy, NYHA class II or III heart failure, and an EF of 35 percent had no mortality benefit from amiodarone compared with placebo, but those randomized to receive an ICD had a significant mortality benefit.[79] Multiple ICD trials have demonstrated the superiority of the ICD over drugs as primary prevention of sudden cardiac death in patients at risk for a life-threatening ventricular arrhythmia (see Chaps. 33 and 36).[80] Whether additional risk stratifiers (such as T wave alternans) are beneficial is being investigated.

For secondary prevention of sustained VT or cardiac arrest (see Table 35-6 and Chaps. 33 and 36) in patients with structural heart disease, it is now clear from several clinical trials that (1) class I antiarrhythmic drugs produce a worse outcome than class III antiarrhythmic drugs,[81-83] (2) empirical amiodarone results in better survival than electrophysiology-guided antiarrhythmic drugs,[83,84] and (3) ICDs provide better survival than amiodarone, particularly in patients with a left ventricular ejection fraction (LVEF) less than 0.35.[85] Therefore, in patients who have survived a cardiac arrest or who have sustained VT resulting in hemodynamic compromise and poor LV function, an ICD is the treatment of choice. In patients who refuse an ICD, empirical amiodarone is the next best therapy. The optimal therapy for patients with coronary disease who have preserved LV function with sustained VT is not currently known. Empirical amiodarone appears to be the safest therapy, although Holter-guided sotalol has been advocated.[81,82] Some patients who receive ICDs have frequent shocks because of recurrent VT. In these patients, concomitant therapy with amiodarone may be required to reduce the frequency of VT or slow the rate of the VT to allow it to be pace-terminated. Other drugs such as sotalol, procainamide, mexiletine, or flecainide may be required if amiodarone is not effective. Occasionally, a combination of drugs may be effective when a single drug is not. Ablation may also be considered in this situation. Although radiofrequency ablation (see Chap. 33) of certain types of idiopathic VT (see later) is very effective, ablation for postinfarct VT or that associated with dilated cardiomyopathy is somewhat less effective. In addition, because of the significant mortality associated with these arrhythmias in patients with structural heart disease and depressed LV function, ablation is generally used as an adjunct to ICD placement to reduce the frequency of VT and ICD shocks. However, in patients with well-tolerated postinfarct VT and well-preserved LV function or in patients refractory to drugs, it may be used as first-line therapy.[86,87]

Specific Types of Ventricular Tachycardia

A number of fairly specific types of VT have been identified, and distinction is based on either a constellation of distinctive electrocardiographic and electrophysiological features or a specific set of clinical events. Although our understanding of the electrophysiological mechanisms responsible for clinically occurring VTs is still developing (see Chap. 31), being able to identify different types of VTs is the first step toward understanding their mechanisms. These different types of VT often carry different prognoses and responses to different therapy. They are distinct from VTs associated with remote myocardial infarction or dilated cardiomyopathies.

VENTRICULAR ARRHYTHMIAS IN PATIENTS WITH CARDIOMYOPATHIES (see also Chaps. 64 and 65)

ISCHEMIC CARDIOMYOPATHY

Patients with previous myocardial infarction are at risk for developing ventricular tachycardia. In the setting of a remote MI, the mechanism of VT is reentry, involving the infarct scar and in particular the border zone or other areas of the scar with deranged conduction. As a result, the VT in this setting is typically monomorphic. In some cases, more than one morphology can be seen as a result of "reverse" direction reentry or other circuits existing in the infarct scar. Polymorphic VT or VF in the setting of ischemic heart disease usually occurs during active ischemia or infarction. Treatment for VT in the setting of ischemic heart disease follows the recommendations described earlier. In general, ICDs are indicated to prevent SCD from VT in this patient group, especially in those with depressed LV function. Monomorphic VT in this setting is often amenable to pace termination. In patients with preserved LV function and no hemodynamic compromise, optimal long-term treatment is still controversial. Primary suppression with antiarrhythmic drugs (e.g., amiodarone), implantation with an ICD, anti-tachycardia pacing, and ablation are options. Newer approaches to ablation of VT caused by a prior infarct scar have increased the efficacy, but there is a high recurrence rate because of multiple circuits and is in general reserved for refractory VT or very well-tolerated VT (see Chap. 33). Surgical endocardial resection of the scarred area is also an effective treatment for refractory VT caused by prior infarction.

DILATED CARDIOMYOPATHY

Both dilated and hypertrophic cardiomyopathies can be associated with VTs and an increased risk of sudden cardiac death. Induction of VT by programmed stimulation does not reliably identify high-risk patients, whereas T wave alternans may be a useful means of risk stratifying patients with dilated cardiomyopathy.[88,89] Because it is difficult to predict patients at risk of sudden death or those who might respond favorably to an antiarrhythmic drug, ICDs have been advocated for patients with life-threatening ventricular arrhythmias and dilated cardiomyopathy. This recommendation has been supported by a large multicenter randomized trial (see Table 35-6) comparing amiodarone with ICDs in patients with poor ventricular function and symptomatic sustained VT; the study found improved survival in patients who received a defibrillator.[85] Bundle branch reentry may be the basis of some VTs in this population and can be treated by ablating the right bundle branch. Asymptomatic ventricular arrhythmias are common. The role of antiarrhythmic drugs and ICDs in the primary prevention of sudden cardiac death in patients with dilated cardiomyopathy may be warranted in certain high-risk patients, as discussed earlier. However, ongoing clinical trials will further clarify which patient population will benefit the most and which modality is most effective.

HYPERTROPHIC CARDIOMYOPATHY

The risk of sudden death in patients with hypertrophic cardiomyopathy (see Chap. 65) is increased by the presence of syncope, a family history of sudden death in first-degree relatives, septal thickness more than 3 cm, or the presence of nonsustained VT on 24-hour ECG recordings. Asymptomatic or mildly symptomatic patients with brief and infrequent episodes of nonsustained VT have a low mortality. The use of electrophysiological testing to identify patients at increased risk of ventricular arrhythmias and sudden death is controversial. Amiodarone has been useful in some patients with mildly symptomatic, nonsustained VT but not in improving survival. QT dispersion is increased in those with ventricular arrhythmias and sudden death, as is T wave alternans.[90] Dual chamber pacing has been useful in reducing the outflow gradient, but its role in affecting ventricular arrhythmia has not been established. Currently, no totally acceptable way to risk-stratify patients with hypertrophic cardiomyopathy in terms of VT has been identified. In patients believed to be at high risk of sudden death or those with sustained VT or frequent nonsustained VT, an ICD may be indicated.[91] Alcohol ablation of the septum via direct injection into the septal branches of the coronary circulation has been used to improve outflow gradients, but its potential effect on ventricular arrhythmias and sudden cardiac death is of concern.

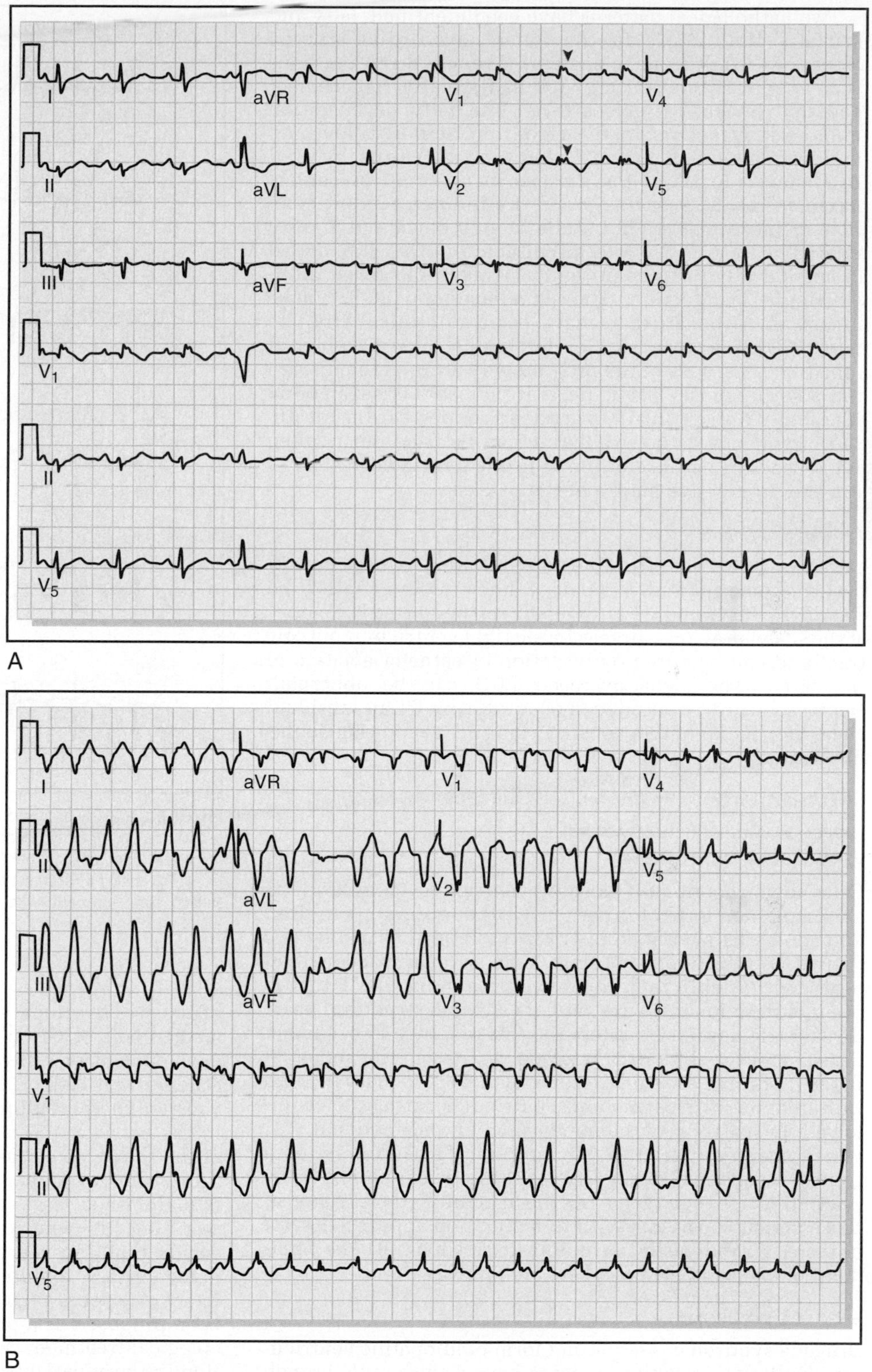

FIGURE 35–35 **A,** Normal sinus rhythm in a patient with arrhythmogenic right ventricular dysplasia. The arrowheads in V_1 and V_2 point to late right ventricular activation called an *epsilon wave.* **B,** Ventricular tachycardia in the same patient with right ventricular dysplasia.

ARRHYTHMOGENIC RIGHT VENTRICULAR CARDIOMYOPATHY

Patients with arrhythmogenic right ventricular cardiomyopathy have VT that generally has a left bundle branch block contour (because the tachycardia arises in the right ventricle), often with right-axis deviation and T waves inverted over the right precordial leads (Fig. 35-35A). The VT may be caused by reentry. Supraventricular arrhythmias can also occur, and exercise can induce the VT in some patients.

Arrhythmogenic right ventricular cardiomyopathy is caused by a type of cardiomyopathy, possibly familial in some patients, with hypokinetic areas involving the wall of the right ventricle. Although genetic abnormalities in desmosomal proteins (plakoglobin, desmoplakin and plakophilin), the ryanodine receptor and transforming growth factor-beta 3 (TGF-β3) have been identified, the precise pathway and pathogenesis remain unknown (see Chaps. 9 and 31).[92] Arrhythmogenic right ventricular cardiomyopathy can be an important cause of ventricular arrhythmia in children and young adults with apparently normal hearts, as well as in older patients. Initial findings can be subtle and often mimic those of outflow tract VT (see later)—that is, manifested only by tachycardia and no symptoms of right-sided heart failure. Right-sided heart failure or asymptomatic right ventricular enlargement can be present with normal pulmonary vasculature. Males predominate, and most patients usually show an abnormal right ventricle by echocardiography, computed tomography, right ventricular angiography, or magnetic resonance imaging, although this abnormality may not be apparent on initial evaluation.

Two pathological patterns have been identified, fatty and fibrofatty infiltration. In the latter, myocardial atrophy appears to result from injury and myocyte death (perhaps from apoptosis) and culminates in fibrofatty replacement mediated by patchy myocarditis. The fatty degeneration preferentially occurs in the right ventricular inflow and outflow tracts and the apex. The left ventricle can be involved in advanced forms of the disease in up to 60 percent of patients. The ECG during sinus rhythm can exhibit complete or incomplete right bundle branch block and T wave inversions in V_1 to V_3. A terminal notch in the QRS, called an epsilon wave, can be present as a result of slowed intraventricular conduction. The signal-averaged ECG can be abnormal. Although there have been no clinical trials to date, ICDs are generally preferable to pharmacological approaches because of the progressive nature of the disease and poor prognosis, particularly if the patients have poorly tolerated VT, resulting in syncope or sudden cardiac death. Radiofrequency catheter ablation can be tried but is often not successful because of the multiple morphologies of VT and the progressive nature of the disease.

Tetralogy of Fallot

Chronic serious ventricular arrhythmias can occur in patients some years after repair of the tetralogy of Fallot (see Chap. 61). Sustained VT after repair can be caused by reentry at the site of previous surgery in the right ventricular outflow tract and can be cured by resection or catheter ablation of this area. The signal-averaged ECG can be abnormal. Decreased cardiac output can occur during VT and residual right ventricular outflow obstruction and lead to ventricular fibrillation.

Inherited Arrhythmia Syndromes (see Chap. 9)

CATECHOLAMINERGIC POLYMORPHIC VENTRICULAR TACHYCARDIA

Catecholaminergic polymorphic ventricular tachycardia is an uncommon form of inherited VT that occurs in children and adolescents without any overt structural heart disease. Patients typically present with syncope or aborted sudden death with highly reproducible, stress-induced VT that is often bidirectional. These patients have no structural heart disease and normal QT intervals. A family history of sudden death or stress-induced syncope is present in about 30 percent of cases. During exercise, typical responses include initial sinus tachycardia and ventricular extrasystoles followed by salvoes of monomorphic or bidirectional VT, which eventually lead to polymorphic VT as exercise continues. A genetic abnormality resulting in a mutation of the ryanodine receptor gene has been identified in many of these patients; patients with this mutation appear to have a higher risk and earlier symptoms (see Chap. 9). The treatment of choice is beta blockers and an ICD.

BRUGADA SYNDROME

Brugada syndrome is a distinct form of idiopathic ventricular fibrillation in which patients have right bundle branch block and ST segment elevation in the anterior precordial leads, without evidence of structural heart disease (Fig. 35-36). Mutations in a gene responsible for the sodium channel *(SCN5A)* have been identified in many families with Brugada syndrome. Although the mutations are on the same gene as that responsible for one form of long-QT syndrome (long-QT-3; see Chap. 9), the site of mutation is different and does not result in a prolonged QT interval. Mutations in the Brugada syndrome result in acceleration of sodium channel recovery or in nonfunctional sodium channels. This syndrome, common in apparently healthy young Southeast Asians, probably accounts for approximately 40 to 60 percent of all cases of idiopathic ventricular fibrillation. The precise mechanism of the electrocardiographic changes and the development of ventricular fibrillation is not known. It is thought that loss of the action potential dome in the right ventricular epicardium, but not in the endocardium, results in the persistent ST segment elevation. Heterogeneous loss of the action potential dome in the right ventricular epicardium leads to propagation of the dome from sites where it is maintained to sites at which it is lost (phase 2 reentry), resulting in ventricular arrhythmias.[93] Among several agents that can reproduce this electrocardiographic phenomenon are sodium channel blockers. They can expose latent electrocardiographic forms of the syndrome and have been proposed as a provocative test. Currently, no pharmacological treatment can reliably prevent ventricular fibrillation in these patients. ICDs are the only effective treatment for preventing sudden death. Electrophysiology studies to determine inducibility of ventricular arrhythmias have been advocated by some as a means to risk stratify; however, this approach remains controversial.

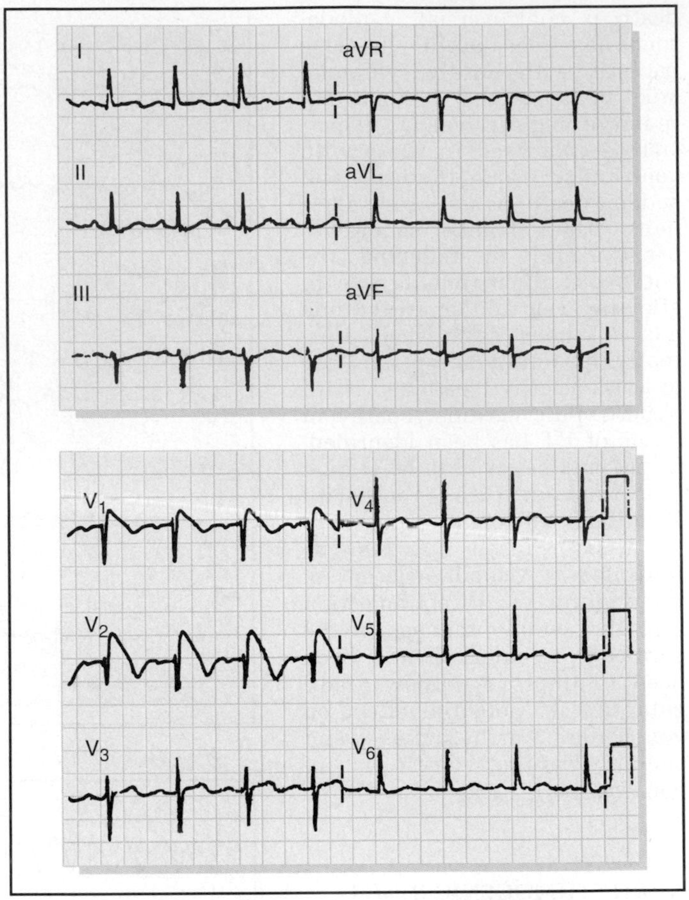

FIGURE 35–36 Twelve-lead ECG of a patient with Brugada syndrome. The ECG is characterized by a right bundle branch block pattern and persistent ST elevation in leads V_1 through V_3. (From Brugada J, Brugada R, Brugada P: Right bundle branch block and ST segment elevation in leads V_1 through V_3: A marker for sudden death in patients without demonstrable structural heart disease. Circulation 97:457, 1998.)

Torsades de Pointes

ELECTROCARDIOGRAPHIC RECOGNITION. The term *torsades de pointes* refers to a VT characterized by QRS complexes of changing amplitude that appear to twist around the isoelectric line and occur at rates of 200 to 250/min (Fig. 35-37A). Originally described in the setting of bradycardia caused by complete heart block, torsades de

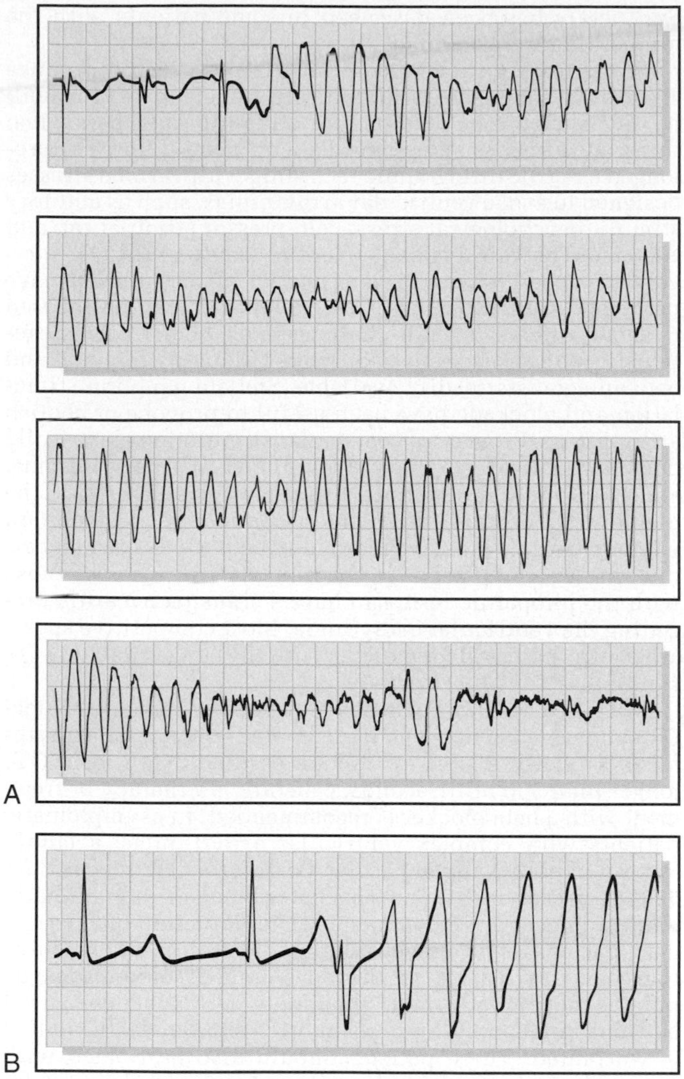

FIGURE 35–37 Torsades de pointes. **A (top four panels),** Continuous monitor lead recording. A demand ventricular pacemaker (VVI) had been implanted because of type II second-degree atrioventricular block. After treatment with amiodarone for recurrent ventricular tachycardia, the QT interval became prolonged (about 640 milliseconds during paced beats), and episodes of torsades de pointes developed. In this recording, the tachycardia spontaneously terminates and a paced ventricular rhythm is restored. Motion artifact is noted at the end of the recording as the patient lost consciousness. **B,** Tracing from a young boy with congenital long-QT syndrome. The QTU interval in the sinus beats is at least 600 milliseconds. Note TU wave alternans in the first and second complexes. A late premature complex occurring in the downslope of the TU wave initiates an episode of ventricular tachycardia.

pointes is usually used to connote a syndrome, not simply an electrocardiographic description of the QRS complex of the tachycardia. It is characterized by prolonged ventricular repolarization, with QT intervals generally exceeding 500 milliseconds. The U wave can also become prominent and merge with the T wave, but its role in this syndrome and in long-QT syndrome is not clear. The abnormal repolarization need not be present or at least prominent in all beats, but may be apparent only on the beat prior to the onset of torsades de pointes (i.e., following a PVC). Long-short R-R cycle sequences commonly precede the onset of torsades de pointes from acquired causes. Relatively late PVCs can discharge during termination of the long T wave and precipitate successive bursts of VT, during which the peaks of the QRS complexes appear successively on one side and then on the other side of the isoelectric baseline; these give the typical twisting appearance, with continuous and progressive changes in QRS contour and amplitude. Torsades de pointes can terminate with progressive prolongation in cycle length and larger and more distinctly formed QRS complexes and culminate in a return to the basal rhythm, a period of ventricular standstill, and a new attack of torsades de pointes or ventricular fibrillation.

A less common form, the short-coupled variant of torsades de pointes, is a malignant disease with a high mortality rate and shares several characteristics with idiopathic ventricular fibrillation. The ventricular arrhythmia in this setting is initiated with a close-coupled PVC and usually does not involve preceding pauses or bradycardia.

VT that is similar morphologically to torsades de pointes and occurs in patients without QT prolongation, whether spontaneous or electrically induced, should generally be classified as polymorphic VT, not as torsades de pointes. The distinction has important therapeutic implications (see later).

ELECTROPHYSIOLOGICAL FEATURES. The electrophysiological mechanisms responsible for torsades de pointes are not completely understood. Most data suggest that early afterdepolarizations (see Chap. 31) are responsible for both long-QT syndrome and the torsades de pointes, or at least its initiation. Perpetuation may be caused by triggered activity, reentry resulting from dispersion of repolarization produced by the early afterdepolarizations, or abnormal automaticity. However, most data currently point to transmural reentry as the most likely mechanism of perpetuation. A distinct group of cells, called M cells, located in the midmyocardium, have prolonged repolarization and may play a role in the genesis of torsades de pointes. The dispersion of repolarization caused by these M cells creates phase 2 reentry, maintaining the torsades de pointes.[94]

CLINICAL FEATURES. Although many predisposing factors have been cited, the most common causes are congenital, severe bradycardia, potassium depletion, and use of antiarrhythmic medications (such as class IA or III antiarrhythmic drugs). More than 50 drugs have been noted to prolong the QT interval (see later, "Long-QT Syndrome"). Clinical features depend on whether the torsades de pointes is caused by the acquired or congenital (idiopathic) long-QT syndrome (see later). Symptoms from the tachycardia depend on its rate and duration, as with other VTs, and range from palpitations to syncope and death. Women, perhaps because of a longer QT interval, are at greater risk for torsades de pointes than men.

MANAGEMENT. The approach to VT with a polymorphic pattern depends on whether it occurs in the setting of a prolonged QT interval. For this practical reason, and because the mechanism of the tachycardia can differ depending on whether a long-QT interval is present, it is important to restrict the definition of torsades de pointes to the typical polymorphic VT in the setting of a long QT and/or U wave in the basal complexes. In all patients with torsades de pointes, administration of class IA, possibly some class IC, and class III antiarrhythmic agents (e.g., amiodarone, dofetilide, sotalol) can increase the abnormal QT interval and worsen the arrhythmia. IV magnesium is the initial treatment of choice for torsades de pointes from an acquired cause, followed by temporary ventricular or atrial pacing. Isoproterenol, given cautiously because it can exacerbate the arrhythmia, can be used to increase the rate until pacing is instituted. Lidocaine, mexiletine, or phenytoin can be tried. The cause of the long QT should be determined and corrected, if possible. When the QT interval is normal, polymorphic VT resembling torsades de pointes is diagnosed, and standard antiarrhythmic drugs can be given. In borderline cases, the clinical context may help determine whether treatment should be initiated with antiarrhythmic drugs. Torsades de pointes resulting from congenital long-QT syndrome is treated with beta blockade, surgical sympathetic interruption, pacing, and ICDs (see later). ECGs obtained from close relatives can help secure the diagnosis of long-QT syndrome in borderline cases.

Long-QT Syndrome

ELECTROCARDIOGRAPHIC RECOGNITION. The upper limit for duration of the normal QT interval corrected for heart rate (QTc) is often given as 0.44 second (see Fig. 35-37B). However, the normal corrected QT interval may actually be longer (0.46 second for men and 0.47 second for women), with a normal range of plus or minus 15 percent of the mean value. The nature of the U wave abnormality and its relationship to long-QT syndrome is not clear. M cells may be responsible for the U wave (see Chap. 31). The probable risk of life-threatening ventricular arrhythmias developing in patients with idiopathic long-QT syndrome is related to the length of the QTc interval. T wave "humps" in the ECG can suggest the presence of long-QT syndrome and may be caused by early afterdepolarizations. A point score system has been suggested to aid in the diagnosis. Unique T wave contours have been ascribed to specific genotypes causing long-QT syndrome.

CLINICAL FEATURES. Long-QT syndrome can be divided into congenital and acquired forms. The congenital form is a familial disorder that can be associated with sensorineural deafness (Jervell and Lange-Nielsen syndrome, autosomal recessive) or normal hearing (Romano-Ward syndrome, autosomal dominant). Most forms of congenital long-QT syndrome are caused by inherited channelopathies created by mutations in one or more genes (see Chap. 9).

The acquired form has a long-QT interval caused by various drugs, such as quinidine, procainamide, *N*-acetylprocainamide, sotalol, amiodarone, disopyramide, phenothiazines, tricyclic antidepressants, erythromycin, pentamidine, some antimalarials, cisapride, and probucol; electrolyte abnormalities, such as hypokalemia and hypomagnesemia; the effects of a liquid protein diet and starvation; central nervous system lesions; significant bradyarrhythmias; cardiac ganglionitis; and mitral valve prolapse. A more comprehensive list that is regularly updated can be found on the Internet (http://www.torsades.org/medical-pros/drug-lists/drug-lists.htm#). In some cases, the acquired long-QT syndrome may be a forme fruste of the inherited form, resulting from polymorphisms in some of the same genes responsible for the acquired syndrome, which becomes manifest when a person takes a drug impairing repolarization.

Patients with congenital long-QT syndrome can initially have syncope, at times misdiagnosed as epilepsy, from torsades de pointes. Sudden death can occur in this group of patients; it occurs in about 10 percent of pediatric patients without preceding symptoms. It is obvious that in some patients, the ventricular arrhythmia becomes sustained and probably results in ventricular fibrillation. Patients with idiopathic long-QT syndrome who are at increased risk for sudden death include those with family members who died suddenly at an early age and those who have experienced syncope. It also appears that the specific mutations carry different risks, with long-QT-1 and long-QT-2 carrying the highest risk for arrhythmias. Although patients with the long-QT-3 mutation tend to have fewer cardiac events, they tend to be more lethal ones. Thus, the cumulative mortality appears to be the same for long-QT-1, long-QT-2, and long-QT-3. Ventricular tachyarrhythmias commonly develop during periods of adrenergic stimulation, such as fright or exertion for long-QT-1 and long-QT-2 mutations, whereas long-QT-3 patients tend to have more events during sleep. Syndactyly has been described in some patients with the idiopathic form (see Chap. 9).

Stress testing can prolong the QT interval and produce T wave alternans, the latter indicative of electrical instability. ECGs should be obtained for all family members when the propositus has symptoms. Patients should undergo prolonged electrocardiographic recording with various stresses designed to evoke ventricular arrhythmias, such as auditory stimuli, psychological stress, cold pressor stimulation, and exercise. The Valsalva maneuver can lengthen the QT interval and cause T wave alternans and VT in patients who have prolonged QT syndromes. Catecholamines can be infused in some patients, but this challenge must be performed cautiously, with resuscitative equipment along with alpha- and beta-antagonists readily available. Stellate ganglion stimulation and blockade have been useful to provoke or abolish arrhythmias. Premature ventricular stimulation electrically does not generally induce arrhythmias in this syndrome, and electrophysiology studies are usually not helpful in the diagnosis. Torsades do pointes commonly develops in patients with the acquired form during periods of bradycardia or after a long pause in the R-R interval, whereas those with the idiopathic form can have a sinus tachycardia preceding the ventricular arrhythmia. Most competitive sports are contraindicated for patients with the congenital long-QT syndrome.[95]

MANAGEMENT. For patients who have idiopathic long-QT syndrome but not syncope, complex ventricular arrhythmias, a family history of sudden cardiac death, or a QTc longer than 500 milliseconds, generally no therapy or treatment with a beta blocker is recommended. In asymptomatic patients with complex ventricular arrhythmias, a family history of early sudden cardiac death or a QTc longer than 500 milliseconds, beta-adrenoceptor blockers at maximally tolerated doses are recommended. Implantation of a permanent pacemaker to prevent the bradycardia and/or pauses that may predispose to the development of torsades de pointes may be indicated. In patients with syncope caused by ventricular arrhythmias or aborted sudden death, an ICD is warranted. These patients should also be treated with concomitant beta blockers and perhaps overdrive atrial pacing (via the ICD) to minimize the frequency of ICD discharges. The ICD is beneficial in these patients, not simply because of the shocking capabilities but because of the ability to pace continually to prevent bradycardia-induced torsades and because of algorithms to prevent post-PVC pauses. The use of an ICD in patients without syncope but with a long-QT interval and a strong family history of sudden death is still controversial but may be warranted in these high-risk patients. For patients who continue to have syncope despite maximum drug therapy, left-sided cervicothoracic sympathetic ganglionectomy that interrupts the stellate ganglion and the first three or four thoracic ganglia may be helpful. For patients with the acquired form and torsades de pointes, IV magnesium and atrial or ventricular pacing are initial choices. Class IB antiarrhythmic drugs or isoproterenol (cautiously) to increase the heart rate can be tried. Avoidance of precipitating drugs is mandatory.

Idiopathic Ventricular Tachycardias

OUTFLOW TRACT TACHYCARDIAS

Idiopathic VTs with monomorphic contours can be divided into at least three types. Two types, paroxysmal VT and repetitive monomorphic VT, appear to originate from the region of the right ventricular outflow tract (Figs. 35-38 and 35-39). Right ventricular outflow tract VTs have a characteristic electrocardiographic appearance of a left bundle branch block contour in V_1 and an inferior axis in the frontal plane. Vagal maneuvers, including adenosine, terminate the VT, whereas exercise, stress, isoproterenol infusion, and rapid or premature stimulation can initiate or perpetuate the tachycardia. Beta blockers and verapamil can suppress this tachycardia as well. The mechanism responsible may be cyclic adenosine monophosphate–triggered activity resulting from early or delayed afterdepolarizations. The paroxysmal form is exercise or stress-induced, whereas the repetitive monomorphic type occurs at rest with sinus beats interposed between runs of nonsustained VT that may be precipitated by transient increases in sympathetic activity unrelated to exertion. In a small number of patients, the tachycardia seems to arise in the inflow tract or apex of the right ventricle. A similar tachycardia has been identified in the left ventricular outflow tract (LVOT) and may mimic that of right ventricular outflow tract tachycardia. A distinguishing feature on ECG is the presence of an S wave in lead I and an early precordial R wave transition (V_1-V_2) during LVOT VT.[96] More recently, it has been recognized that these foci can also occur along the mitral annulus.[97] In some cases, the VT focus can be in the cusp of the aortic valve.[98,99] The prognosis for most patients with outflow tract (right ventricular outflow tract [RVOT] or LVOT) VT is good. Radiofrequency catheter ablation effectively eliminates this focal tachycardia in symptomatic patients. In others, antiarrhythmic drugs can be effective.

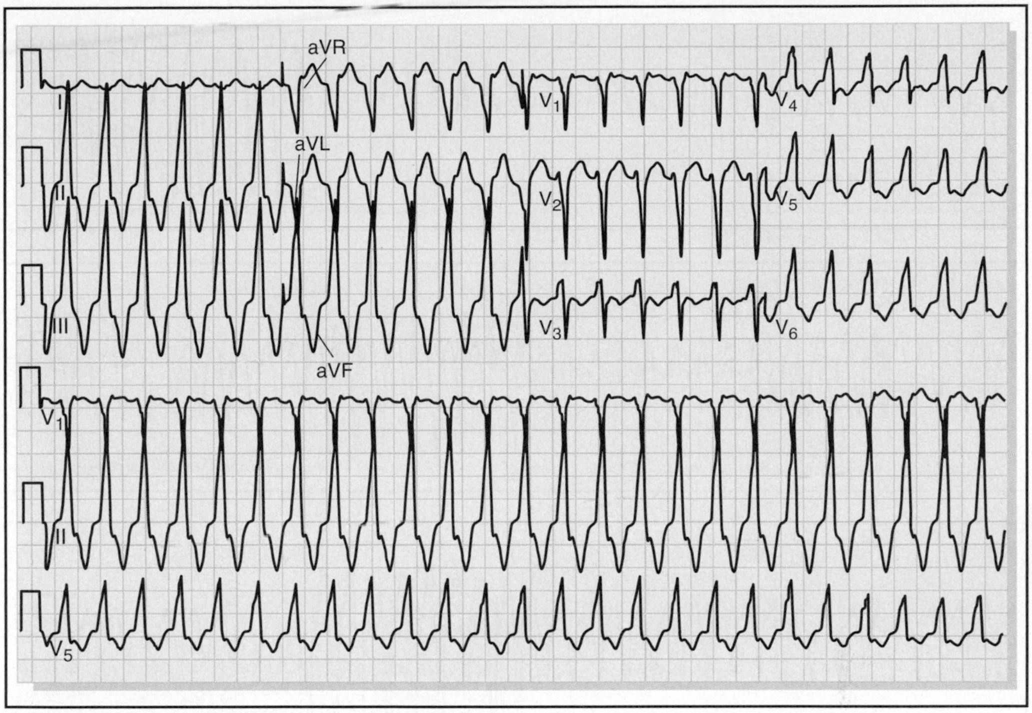

FIGURE 35–38 Ventricular tachycardia originating from the right ventricular outflow tract. This tachycardia is characterized by a left bundle branch block contour in lead V_1 and an inferior axis.

A

B

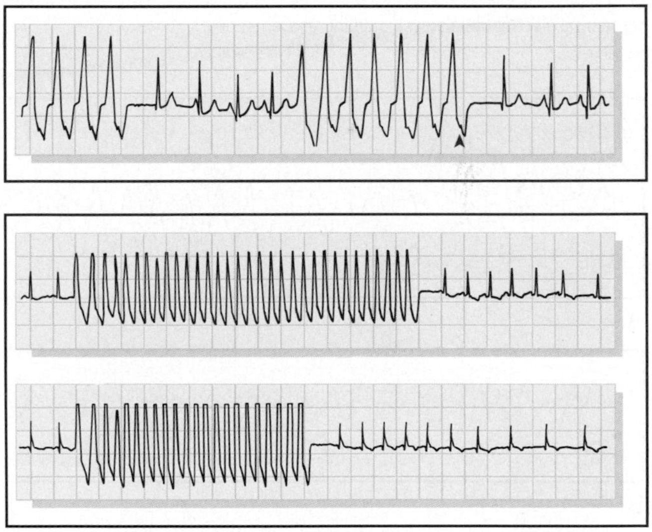

FIGURE 35–39 A, Repetitive monomorphic ventricular tachycardia. Short episodes of a monomorphic ventricular tachycardia at a rate of 160 beats/min repeatedly interrupt the normal sinus rhythm. Retrograde atrial capture probably occurs (the arrowhead points to the deflection in the ST segment), and the retrograde P wave of the last complex of the repetitive monomorphic ventricular tachycardia conducts over the normal pathway to produce a QRS complex with a normal contour. **B,** Short runs of a very rapid (260 beats/min) ventricular tachycardia of uniform contour. They probably provoke a compensatory sympathetic response because each is followed by a brief period of sinus tachycardia. The sinus pacemaker appears unstable, because changes in P wave morphology result.

FASCICULAR VENTRICULAR TACHYCARDIA (LEFT SEPTAL VENTRICULAR TACHYCARDIA)

A left septal VT has been described as arising in the left posterior septum, often preceded by a fascicular potential, and is sometimes called a fascicular tachycardia (Fig. 35-40). Entrainment has been demonstrated, which suggests reentry as a cause of some of the tachycardias. Verapamil or diltiazem suppresses this tachycardia, whereas adenosine does so only rarely. The response to verapamil suggests that the slow inward current may be important, possibly in a reentrant circuit or via delayed afterdepolarizations. Several mechanisms may be operative, and the group may not be homogeneous. Oral verapamil is not as effective as IV verapamil. Once initiated, the tachycardia is paroxysmal and sustained. It can be started by rapid atrial or ventricular pacing and sometimes by exercise or isoproterenol. Generally, the prognosis is good. Radiofrequency catheter ablation is effective in symptomatic patients.

Idiopathic Ventricular Fibrillation

Idiopathic ventricular fibrillation can occur in about 1 to 8 percent of cases of out-of-hospital ventricular fibrillation. Cardiovascular evaluation is normal, except for the arrhythmia. Monomorphic VT is rarely induced at electrophysiological study. The natural history is incompletely known, but recurrences are not uncommon. It is important in this entity, as well as in patients with idiopathic VTs (see later), to remember that the arrhythmia may at times be an early manifestation of a developing cardiomyopathy, at least in some patients. An ICD is a useful therapeutic choice.

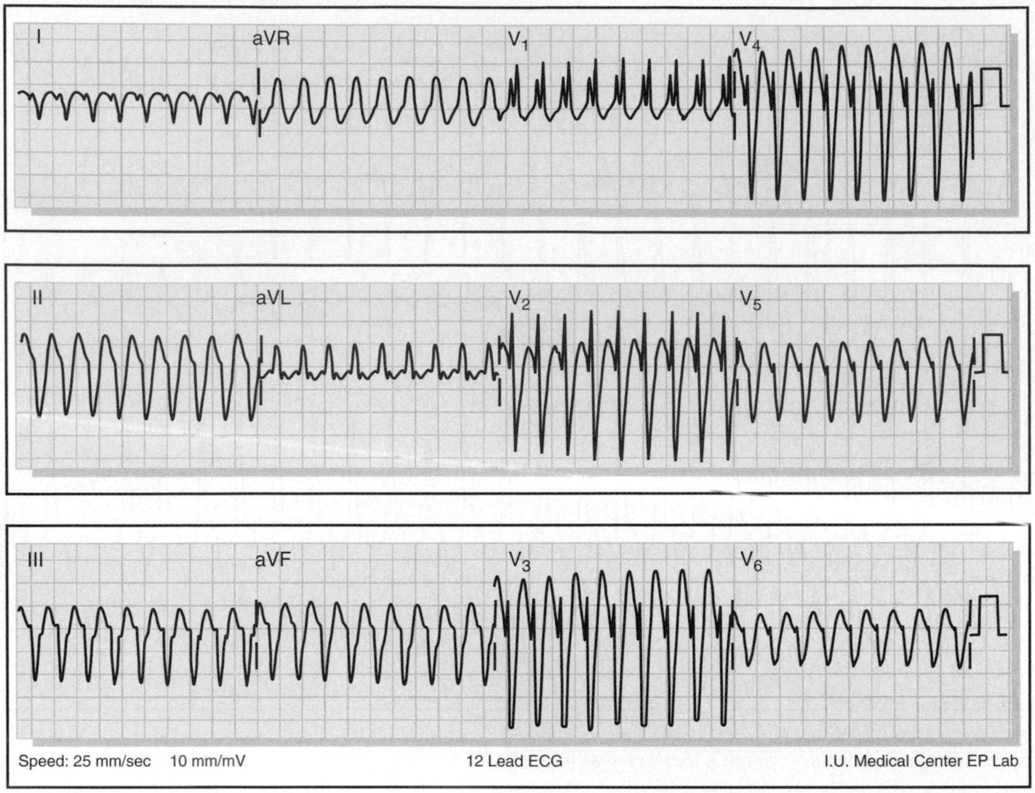

FIGURE 35-40 Left septal ventricular tachycardia. This tachycardia is characterized by a right bundle branch block contour. In this instance, the axis was rightward. The site of the ventricular tachycardia was established to be in the left posterior septum by electrophysiological mapping and ablation.

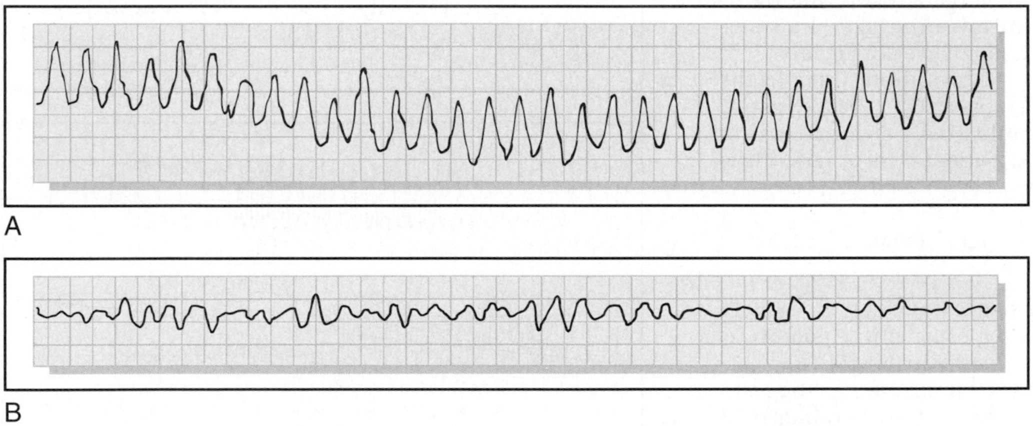

FIGURE 35-41 Ventricular flutter and ventricular fibrillation. **A,** The sine wave appearance of the complexes occurring at a rate of 300 beats/min is characteristic of ventricular flutter. **B,** The irregular undulating baseline typifies ventricular fibrillation.

Bidirectional Ventricular Tachycardia

Bidirectional VT is an uncommon type of VT characterized by QRS complexes with a right bundle branch block pattern, alternating polarity in the frontal plane from −60 to −90 degrees to +120 to +130 degrees, and a regular rhythm. The ventricular rate is between 140 and 200 beats/min. Although the mechanism and site of origin of this tachycardia have remained somewhat controversial, most evidence supports a ventricular origin.

Bidirectional VT can be a manifestation of digitalis excess, typically in older patients and in those with severe myocardial disease. When the tachycardia is caused by digitalis, the extent of toxicity is often advanced, with a poor prognosis. Catecholaminergic polymorphic VT can present as bidirectional VT.

In addition to digoxin-binding antibodies (digoxin immune Fab, Digibind), drugs useful to treat digitalis toxicity such as lidocaine, potassium, phenytoin, and propranolol should be considered if excessive digitalis administration is suspected. Otherwise, the usual therapeutic approach to VT is recommended.

Bundle Branch Reentrant Ventricular Tachycardia

VT secondary to bundle branch reentry is characterized by a QRS morphology determined by the circuit established over the bundle branches or fascicles. Retrograde conduction over the left bundle branch system and anterograde conduction over the right bundle branch create a QRS complex with a left bundle branch block contour and constitute the most common form. The frontal plane axis may be about +30 degrees. Conduction in the opposite direction produces a right bundle branch block contour. Reentry can also occur over the anterior and posterior fascicles. Electrophysiologically, bundle branch reentrant complexes are started after a critical S_2-H_2 or S_3-H_3 delay. The H-V interval of the bundle branch reentrant complex equals or exceeds the H-V interval of the spontaneous normally conducted QRS complex.

Bundle branch reentry is a form of monomorphic sustained VT usually seen in patients with structural heart disease, such as dilated cardiomyopathy. During follow-up, congestive heart failure is the most common cause of death in this population. Myocardial VTs can also be present. Uncommonly, bundle branch reentry can occur in the absence of myocardial disease.

The therapeutic approach is as for other types of VT. In the acute setting, pace termination is frequently effective. Long-term catheter ablation effectively eliminates this form of VT.

Ventricular Flutter and Fibrillation

(see also Chap. 36)

ELECTROCARDIOGRAPHIC RECOGNITION. These arrhythmias represent severe derangements of the heartbeat that usually terminate fatally within 3 to 5 minutes unless corrective measures are undertaken promptly. Ventricular flutter is manifested as a sine wave in appearance—regular large oscillations occurring at a rate of 150 to 300/min (usually about 200) (Fig. 35-41A). The distinction between rapid VT and ventricular flutter can be difficult and is usually of academic interest only. Hemodynamic collapse is present with both. Ventricular fibrillation is recognized by the presence of irregular undulations of varying contour and amplitude (see Fig. 35-41B). Distinct QRS complexes, ST segments, and T waves are absent. Fine-amplitude fibrillatory waves (0.2 mV) are present with prolonged ventricular fibrillation. These fine waves identify patients with worse survival rates and are sometimes confused with asystole.

MECHANISMS. Ventricular fibrillation occurs in various clinical situations but is most commonly associated with coronary artery disease and as a terminal event (see Chap. 31). Thrombolytic agents reduce the incidence of ventricular arrhythmias and inducible VT after myocardial infarction. Cardiovascular events, including sudden cardiac death from ventricular fibrillation, but not asystole, occur most frequently in the morning. Ventricular fibrillation can occur during antiarrhythmic drug administration, hypoxia, ischemia, atrial fibrillation, and very rapid ventricular rates in the preexcitation syndrome, after electrical shock administered during cardioversion (see Chaps. 33 and 34) or accidentally by improperly grounded equipment, and during competitive ventricular pacing to terminate VT.

CLINICAL FEATURES. Ventricular flutter or ventricular fibrillation results in faintness, followed by loss of consciousness, seizures, apnea and eventually, if the rhythm continues untreated, death. The blood pressure is unobtainable, and heart sounds are usually absent. The atria can continue to beat at an independent rhythm for a time or in response to impulses from the fibrillating ventricles. Eventually, electrical activity of the heart ceases.

In patients resuscitated from out-of-hospital cardiac arrest, 75 percent have ventricular fibrillation. Bradycardia or asystole, which can occur in 15 to 25 percent of these patients, is associated with a worse prognosis than ventricular fibrillation and is usually associated with more advanced LV dysfunction. VT commonly precedes the onset of ventricular fibrillation, although frequently no consistent premonitory patterns emerge. Heart rate variability may be decreased.

Although 75 percent of resuscitated patients exhibit significant coronary artery disease, acute transmural myocardial infarction develops in only 20 to 30 percent. Those in whom myocardial infarction does not develop have an increased recurrence rate for sudden cardiac death or ventricular fibrillation. Predictors of death for resuscitated patients include a reduced EF, abnormal wall motion, history of congestive heart failure, history of myocardial infarction but no acute event, and presence of ventricular arrhythmias. Patients discharged after an anterior myocardial infarction complicated by ventricular fibrillation appear to represent a subgroup at high risk of sudden death. Ventricular fibrillation can occur in infants, young people, athletes, and persons without known structural heart disease.

MANAGEMENT. Management should follow basic life support and advanced cardiac life support guidelines (see Chap. 36). Immediate nonsynchronized DC electrical shock using 200 to 400 J is mandatory therapy for ventricular fibrillation and for ventricular flutter that has caused loss of consciousness. Automatic external defibrillators have facilitated the ability to defibrillate early. Cardiopulmonary resuscitation is used only until the defibrillation equipment is readied. Time should not be wasted with cardiopulmonary resuscitation maneuvers if electrical defibrillation can be done promptly. Defibrillation requires fewer joules if done early. If the circulation is markedly inadequate despite return to sinus rhythm, closed-chest massage with artificial ventilation as needed should be instituted. The use of anesthesia during electrical shock is obviously dictated by the patient's condition and is generally not required. After conversion of the arrhythmia to a normal rhythm, it is essential to monitor the rhythm continuously and institute measures to prevent recurrence. Metabolic acidosis quickly follows cardiovascular collapse. If the arrhythmia is terminated within 30 to 60 seconds, significant acidosis does not occur. Judicious use of sodium bicarbonate to reverse the acidosis may be necessary, but its use should not delay administration of defibrillation shocks (see Chap. 36).

If the resuscitation time is short, artificial ventilation by means of a tightly fitting rubber face mask and an Ambu bag is satisfactory and eliminates the delay attending intubation by inexperienced personnel. If such a mask and bag are not available, mouth-to-mouth or mouth-to-nose resuscitation is indicated. It is important to reemphasize that there should be no delay in instituting electrical shock. If the patient is not monitored and it cannot be established whether asystole or ventricular fibrillation caused the cardiovascular collapse, the electrical shock should be administered without wasting precious seconds attempting to obtain an ECG. The DC shock may cause the asystolic heart to begin discharging and also terminate ventricular fibrillation, if the latter is present.

A search for conditions contributing to the initiation of ventricular flutter or fibrillation should be made and the conditions corrected, if possible. Initial medical approaches to prevent recurrence of ventricular fibrillation include IV administration of amiodarone, lidocaine, or procainamide. Amiodarone tends to be the most effective and does not produce the ventricular dysfunction and hypotension often seen with procainamide. Ventricular fibrillation rarely terminates spontaneously, and death results unless countermeasures are instituted immediately. Subsequent therapy is necessary to prevent recurrence. ICDs have become the mainstay of chronic therapy in patients at continued risk for ventricular fibrillation or VT from nonreversible causes (see Chap. 33).

BRADYARRHYTHMIAS

Bradyarrhythmias are arbitrarily defined as a heart rate below 60 beats/min. In some cases, bradyarrhythmias are physiologic, as in well-conditioned athletes with low resting heart rates or type I AV block during sleep, and in other cases are pathological. As with tachyarrhythmias, bradyarrhythmias can be categorized based on the level of disturbance in the hierarchy of the normal impulse generation and conduction system (from sinus node to AV node to His-Purkinje system).

Sinus Bradycardia

ELECTROCARDIOGRAPHIC RECOGNITION. Sinus bradycardia (Fig. 35-42A) exists in an adult when the sinus node discharges at a rate slower than 60 beats/min. P waves have a normal contour and occur before each QRS complex, usually with a constant PR interval longer than 120 milliseconds. Sinus arrhythmia often coexists.

CLINICAL FEATURES. Sinus bradycardia can result from excessive vagal and/or decreased sympathetic tone, as an effect of medications, or from anatomical changes in the sinus node. In most cases, symptomatic sinus bradycardia is caused by the effects of medication. Asymptomatic sinus bradycardia frequently occurs in healthy young adults, particularly well-trained athletes, and decreases in prevalence with advancing age. During sleep, the normal heart rate can fall to 35 to 40 beats/min, especially in adolescents and young adults, with marked sinus arrhythmia sometimes producing pauses of 2 seconds or longer. Eye surgery, coronary arteriography, meningitis, intracranial tumors, increased intracranial pressure, cervical and mediastinal tumors, and certain disease states such as severe hypoxia, myxedema, hypothermia, fibrodegenerative changes, convalescence from some infections, gram-negative sepsis, and mental depression can produce sinus bradycardia. Sinus bradycardia also occurs during vomiting or vasovagal syncope (see Chap. 37) and can be produced by carotid sinus

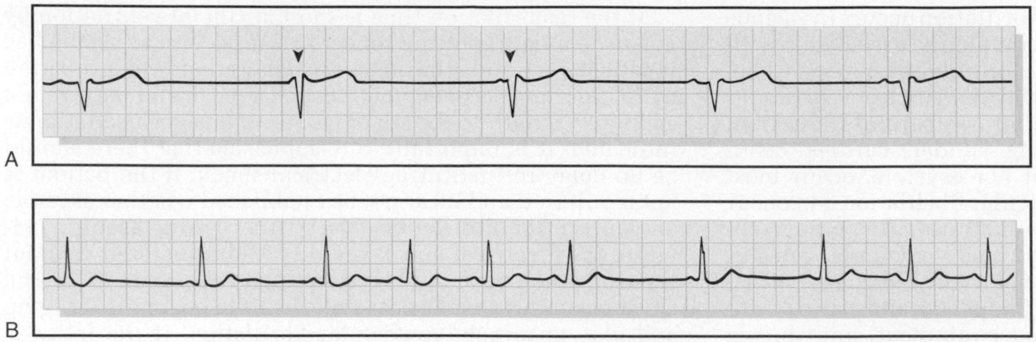

FIGURE 35–42 **A,** Sinus bradycardia at a rate of 40 to 48 beats/min. The second and third QRS complexes (arrowheads) represent junctional escape beats. Note the P waves at the onset of the QRS complex. **B,** Nonrespiratory sinus arrhythmia occurring as a consequence of digitalis toxicity. Monitor leads.

stimulation or by the administration of parasympathomimetic drugs, lithium, amiodarone, beta-adrenoceptor blocking drugs, clonidine, propafenone, or calcium antagonists. Conjunctival instillation of beta blockers for glaucoma can produce sinus or AV nodal abnormalities, especially in the elderly.

In most cases, sinus bradycardia is a benign arrhythmia and can actually be beneficial by producing a longer period of diastole and increasing the ventricular filling time. It can be associated with syncope caused by an abnormal autonomic reflex (cardioinhibitory; see Chap. 37). Sinus bradycardia occurs in 10 to 15 percent of patients with acute myocardial infarction and may be even more prevalent when patients are seen in the early hours of infarction. Unless accompanied by hemodynamic decompensation or arrhythmias, sinus bradycardia is generally associated with a more favorable outcome following myocardial infarction than is the presence of sinus tachycardia. It is usually transient and occurs more commonly during inferior than anterior myocardial infarction; it has also been noted during reperfusion with thrombolytic agents (see Chap. 52). Bradycardia following resuscitation from cardiac arrest is associated with a poor prognosis.

MANAGEMENT. Treatment of sinus bradycardia per se is not usually necessary. For example, if a patient with acute myocardial infarction is asymptomatic, it is probably best to not speed up the sinus rate. If cardiac output is inadequate or if arrhythmias are associated with the slow rate, atropine (0.5 mg IV as an initial dose, repeated if necessary) is usually effective. Lower doses of atropine, particularly when given subcutaneously or intramuscularly, can exert an initial parasympathomimetic effect, possibly via a central action. For symptomatic episodes of sinus bradycardia that are more than momentary or are recurrent (e.g., as during a myocardial infarction), temporary pacing via a transvenous electrode is usually preferable to repeated or prolonged drug therapy. In some patients who experience congestive heart failure or symptoms of low cardiac output as a result of chronic sinus bradycardia, permanent pacing may be needed (see Chap. 34). Atrial pacing is usually preferable to ventricular pacing to preserve sequential AV contraction and is preferable to drug therapy for long-term management of sinus bradycardia. As a general rule, no available drugs increase the heart rate reliably and safely over long periods without important side effects.

Sinus Arrhythmia

Sinus arrhythmia (see Fig. 35-42B) is characterized by a phasic variation in sinus cycle length during which the maximum sinus cycle length minus the minimum sinus cycle length exceeds 120 milliseconds, or the maximum sinus cycle length minus the minimum sinus cycle length divided by the minimum sinus cycle length exceeds 10 percent. It is the most frequent form of arrhythmia and is considered to be a normal event. P wave morphology does not usually vary, and the PR interval exceeds 120 milliseconds and remains unchanged because the focus of discharge remains relatively fixed within the sinus node. Occasionally, the pacemaker focus can wander within the sinus node, or its exit to the atrium may change and produce P waves of a slightly different contour (but not retrograde) and a slightly changing PR interval that exceeds 120 milliseconds.

Sinus arrhythmia commonly occurs in the young, especially those with slower heart rates or following enhanced vagal tone, such as after the administration of digitalis or morphine, and decreases with age or with autonomic dysfunction, such as in diabetic neuropathy. Sinus arrhythmia appears in two basic forms. In the respiratory form, the P-P interval cyclically shortens during inspiration, primarily as a result of reflex inhibition of vagal tone, and slows during expiration; breath-holding eliminates the cycle length variation (see "Heart Rate Variability," Chap. 32). Efferent vagal effects alone have been suggested as being responsible for respiratory sinus arrhythmias. Nonrespiratory sinus arrhythmia is characterized by a phasic variation in the P-P interval unrelated to the respiratory cycle and may be the result of digitalis intoxication. Loss of sinus rhythm variability is a risk factor for sudden cardiac death (see Chap. 36).

Symptoms produced by sinus arrhythmia are uncommon but, on occasion, if the pauses between beats are excessively long, palpitations or dizziness may result. Marked sinus arrhythmia can produce a sinus pause sufficiently long to produce syncope if not accompanied by an escape rhythm.

Treatment is usually unnecessary. Increasing the heart rate by exercise or drugs generally abolishes sinus arrhythmia. Symptomatic individuals may experience relief from palpitations with sedatives, tranquilizers, atropine, ephedrine, or isoproterenol administration, as for the treatment of sinus bradycardia.

VENTRICULOPHASIC SINUS ARRHYTHMIA. The most common example occurs during complete AV block and a slow ventricular rate, when P-P cycles that contain a QRS complex are shorter than P-P cycles without a QRS complex. Similar lengthening can be present in the P-P cycle that follows a PVC with a compensatory pause. Alterations in the P-P interval are probably caused by the influence of the autonomic nervous system responding to changes in ventricular stroke volume.

SINUS PAUSE OR SINUS ARREST. Sinus pause or sinus arrest (Fig. 35-43) is recognized by a pause in the sinus rhythm. The P-P interval delimiting the pause does not equal a multiple of the basic P-P interval. Differentiation of sinus arrest, which is thought to be caused by slowing or cessation of spontaneous sinus nodal automaticity and therefore a disorder of impulse formation, from SA exit block (see later) in patients with sinus arrhythmia can be difficult without direct recordings of sinus node discharge.

Failure of sinus nodal discharge results in the absence of atrial depolarization and in periods of ventricular asystole if escape beats initiated by latent pacemakers do not occur (see Fig. 35-43). Involvement of the sinus node by acute myocardial infarction, degenerative fibrotic changes, effects of digitalis toxicity, stroke, or excessive vagal tone can produce sinus arrest. Transient sinus arrest may have no clinical significance by itself if latent pacemakers promptly escape to prevent ventricular asystole or the genesis of other arrhythmias precipitated by the slow rates. Sinus arrest and AV block have been demonstrated in as many as 30 percent of patients with sleep apnea (see Chap. 74).

Treatment is as outlined earlier for sinus bradycardia. In patients who have a chronic form of sinus node disease characterized by marked sinus bradycardia or sinus arrest, permanent pacing is often necessary. However, as a general rule, chronic pacing for sinus bradycardia is indicated only in symptomatic patients or those with a sinus pause exceeding 3 seconds.

SINOATRIAL EXIT BLOCK. This arrhythmia is recognized electrocardiographically by a pause resulting from absence of the normally expected P wave (Fig. 35-44). The duration of the pause is a multiple of the basic P-P interval. SA exit block is caused by a conduction disturbance during which an impulse formed within the sinus node fails to depolarize the atria or does so with delay (Fig. 35-45). An interval without P waves that equals approximately two, three, or four times the normal P-P cycle characterizes type II second-degree SA exit block. During type I (Wenckebach) second-degree SA exit block, the P-P interval progressively shortens prior to the pause, and the duration of the pause is less than two P-P cycles. (See Chap. 31 for further discussion of Wenckebach intervals.) First-degree SA exit block cannot be recognized on the ECG because SA nodal discharge is not recorded. Third-degree SA exit block can be manifested as a complete absence of P waves and is difficult to diagnose with certainty without sinus node electrograms.

Excessive vagal stimulation, acute myocarditis, infarction, or fibrosis involving the atrium, as well as drugs such as quinidine, procainamide, or digitalis, can produce SA exit block. SA exit block is usually transient. It may be of no clinical importance except to prompt a search for the underlying cause. Occasionally, syncope can result if the SA block is prolonged and unaccompanied by an escape rhythm. SA exit block can occur in well-trained athletes.

Therapy for patients who have symptomatic SA exit block is as outlined earlier for sinus bradycardia.

WANDERING PACEMAKER. This variant of sinus arrhythmia involves passive transfer of the dominant pacemaker focus from the sinus node to latent pacemakers that have the next highest degree of automaticity located in other atrial sites (usually lower in the crista terminalis) or in AV junctional tissue. The change occurs in a gradual fashion over the duration of several beats; thus, only one pacemaker at a time controls the rhythm, in sharp contrast with AV dissociation. The ECG (Fig. 35-46) displays a cyclical increase in the R-R interval—a PR interval that gradually shortens and can become less than 120 milliseconds and a change in the P wave contour, which becomes negative in lead I or II (depending on the site of discharge) or is lost within the QRS complex. Generally, these changes occur in reverse as the pacemaker shifts back to the sinus node. Wandering pacemaker is a normal phenomenon that often occurs in the very young and particularly in athletes, presumably because of augmented vagal tone. Persistence of an AV junctional rhythm (Figs. 35-47 and 35-48) for long periods, however, may indicate underlying heart disease. Treatment is not usually indicated but, if necessary, is the same as that for sinus bradycardia (see earlier).

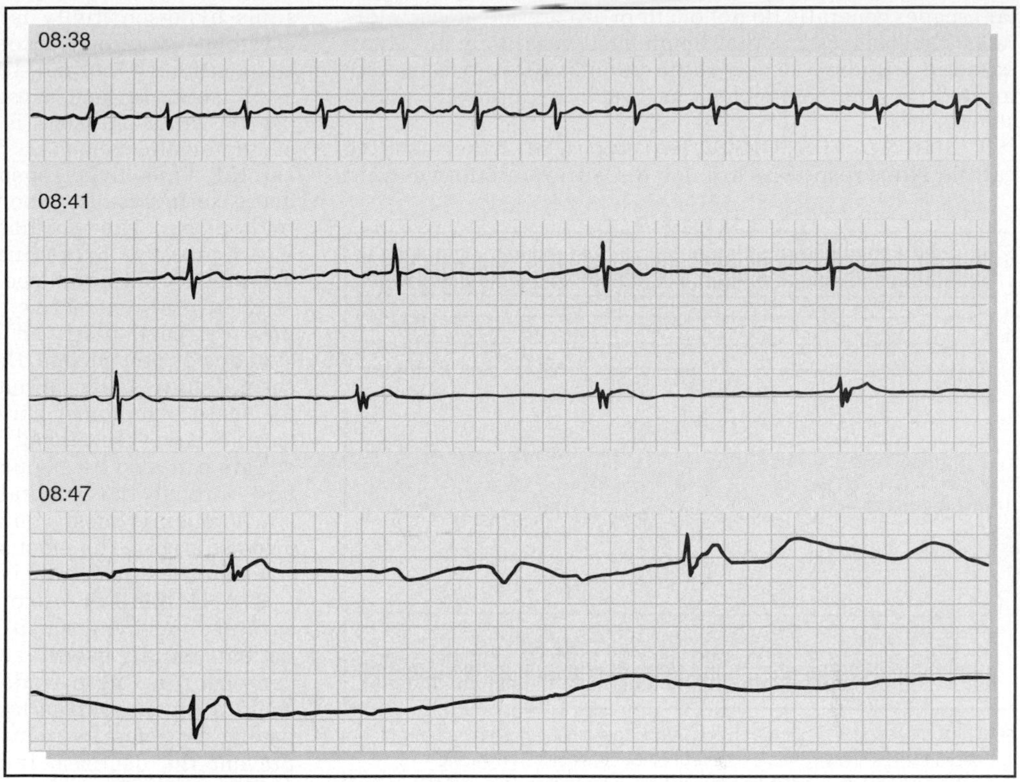

FIGURE 35–43 Sinus arrest. The patient had a long-term electrocardiographic recorder connected when he died suddenly of cardiac standstill. The rhythms demonstrate progressive sinus bradycardia and sinus arrest at 8:41 A.M. The rhythm then becomes a ventricular escape rhythm, which progressively slows and finally ceases at 8:47 A.M. Monitor lead. The double electrocardiographic strips are continuous recordings.

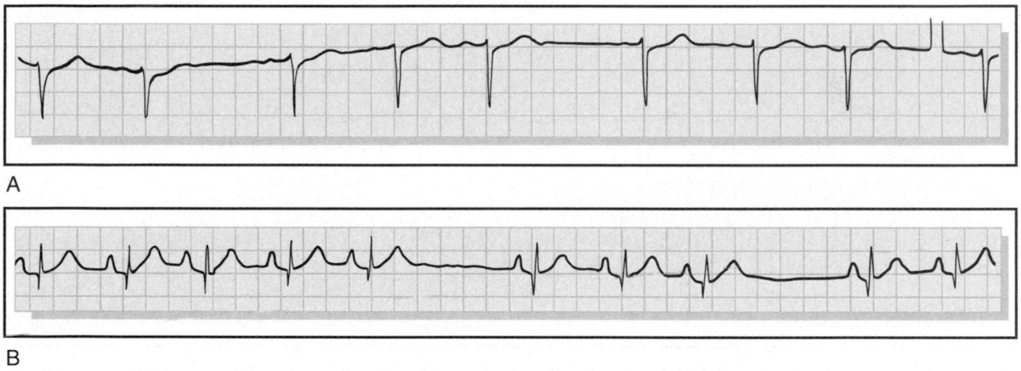

FIGURE 35–44 Sinus nodal exit block. **A,** A type I sinoatrial (SA) nodal exit block has the following features. The P-P interval shortens from the first to the second cycle in each grouping, followed by a pause. The duration of the pause is less than twice the shortest cycle length, and the cycle after the pause exceeds the cycle before the pause. The PR interval is normal and constant. Lead V_1. **B,** The P-P interval varies slightly because of sinus arrhythmia. The two pauses in sinus nodal activity equal twice the basic P-P interval and are consistent with a type II 2 : 1 SA nodal exit block. The PR interval is normal and constant. Lead III.

Hypersensitive Carotid Sinus Syndrome

(see also Chap. 37)

ELECTROCARDIOGRAPHIC RECOGNITION. Hypersensitive carotid sinus syndrome (Fig. 35-49) is characterized most frequently by ventricular asystole caused by cessation of atrial activity from sinus arrest or SA exit block. AV block is observed less frequently, probably in part because the absence of atrial activity from sinus arrest precludes the manifestations of AV block. However, if an atrial pacemaker maintained an atrial rhythm during the episodes, a higher prevalence of AV block would probably be noted. In symptomatic patients, AV junctional or ventricular escapes generally do not occur or are present at very slow rates, thus suggesting that heightened vagal tone and sympathetic withdrawal can suppress subsidiary pacemakers located in the ventricles, as well as supraventricular structures.

CLINICAL FEATURES. Two types of hypersensitive carotid sinus responses are noted. Cardioinhibitory carotid sinus hypersensitivity is generally defined as ventricular asystole exceeding 3 seconds during carotid sinus stimulation, although normal limits have not been definitively established. In fact, asystole exceeding 3 seconds during carotid sinus massage is not common but can occur in asymptomatic subjects (see Fig. 35-49). Vasodepressor carotid sinus hypersensitivity is generally defined as a decrease in systolic blood pressure of 50 mm Hg or more without associated cardiac slowing or a decrease in systolic blood pressure exceeding 30 mm Hg when the patient's symptoms are reproduced.

Even if a hyperactive carotid sinus reflex is elicited in patients, particularly in older patients who complain of syncope or presyncope, the hyperactive reflex elicited with carotid sinus massage may not necessarily be responsible for these symptoms. Direct pressure or extension of the carotid sinus from head turning, neck tension, and tight collars can also be a source of syncope by reducing blood flow through the cerebral arteries. Hypersensitive carotid sinus reflex is most commonly associated with coronary artery disease. The mechanism responsible for hypersensitive carotid sinus reflex is not known.

MANAGEMENT. Atropine abolishes cardioinhibitory carotid sinus hypersensitivity. However, most symptomatic patients require pacemaker implantation. Because AV block can occur during periods of hypersensitive carotid reflex, some form of ventricular pacing, with or without atrial pacing, is generally required. Atropine and pacing do not prevent the decrease in systemic blood pressure in the vasodepressor form of carotid sinus hypersensitivity, which may result from inhibition of sympathetic vasoconstrictor nerves and possibly from activation of cholinergic sympathetic vasodilator fibers. Combinations of vasodepressor and cardioinhibitory types can occur, and vasodepression can account for continued syncope after pacemaker implantation in some patients. Patients who have a hyperactive carotid sinus reflex that does not cause symptoms require no treatment. Drugs such as digitalis, methyldopa, clonidine, and propranolol can enhance the response to carotid sinus massage and be responsible for symptoms in some patients. Elastic support hose and sodium-retaining drugs may be helpful in patients with vasodepressor responses.

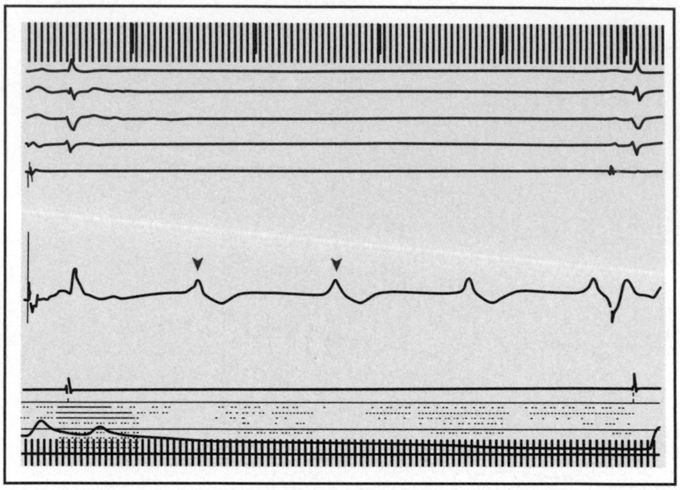

FIGURE 35–45 Sinus node exit block. After a period of atrial pacing (only the last paced cycle is shown), sinus node exit block developed. The tracing demonstrates sinus node potentials (arrowheads), recorded with a catheter electrode, not conducting to the atrium until the last complex. Recordings are leads I, II, III, and V_1, right atrial recording, sinus node recording, and right ventricular apical recording. The bottom tracing is femoral artery blood pressure.

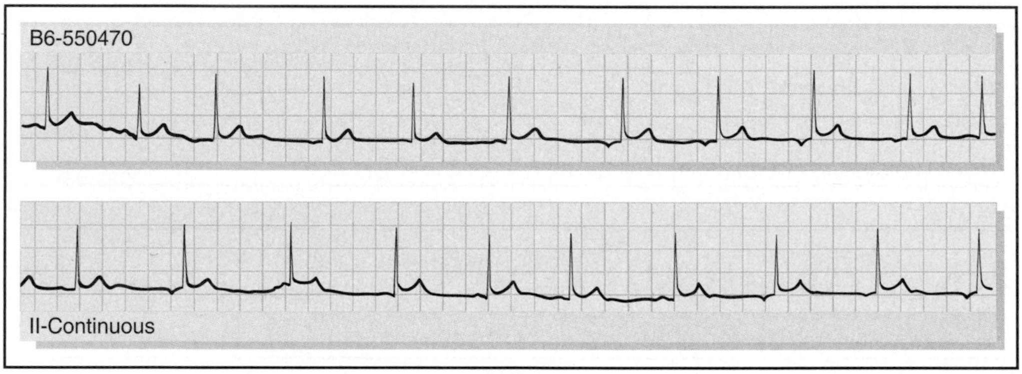

FIGURE 35–46 Wandering atrial pacemaker. As the heart rate slows, the P waves become inverted and then gradually revert toward normal when the heart rate speeds up again. The PR interval shortens to 0.14 second with the inverted P wave and is 0.16 second with the upright P wave. This phasic variation in cycle length with varying P wave contour suggests a shift in pacemaker site and is characteristic of wandering atrial pacemaker.

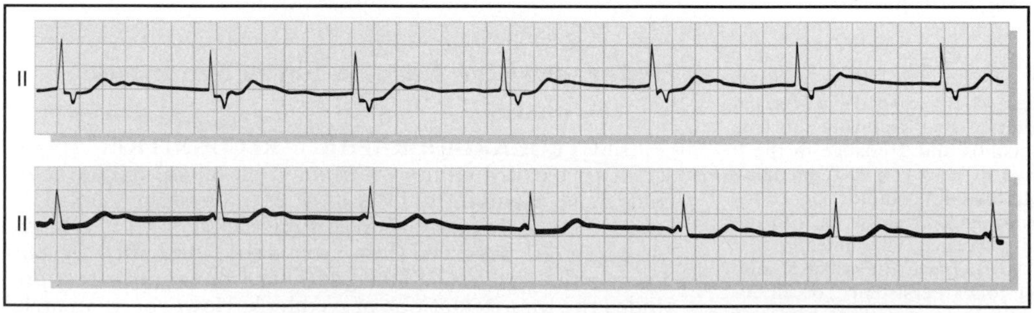

FIGURE 35–47 Atrioventricular (AV) junctional rhythm. **Top,** AV junctional discharge occurs fairly regularly at a rate of approximately 50 beats/min. Retrograde atrial activity follows each junctional discharge. **Bottom,** Recording made on a different day in the same patient. The AV junctional rate is slightly more variable, and retrograde P waves precede onset of the QRS complex. The positive terminal portion of the P wave gives the appearance of AV dissociation, which was not present.

Sick Sinus Syndrome

ELECTROCARDIOGRAPHIC RECOGNITION. *Sick sinus syndrome* is a term applied to a syndrome encompassing a number of sinus nodal abnormalities, including the following: (1) persistent spontaneous sinus bradycardia not caused by drugs and inappropriate for the physiological circumstance; (2) sinus arrest or exit block (Fig. 35-50); (3) combinations of SA and AV conduction disturbances; or

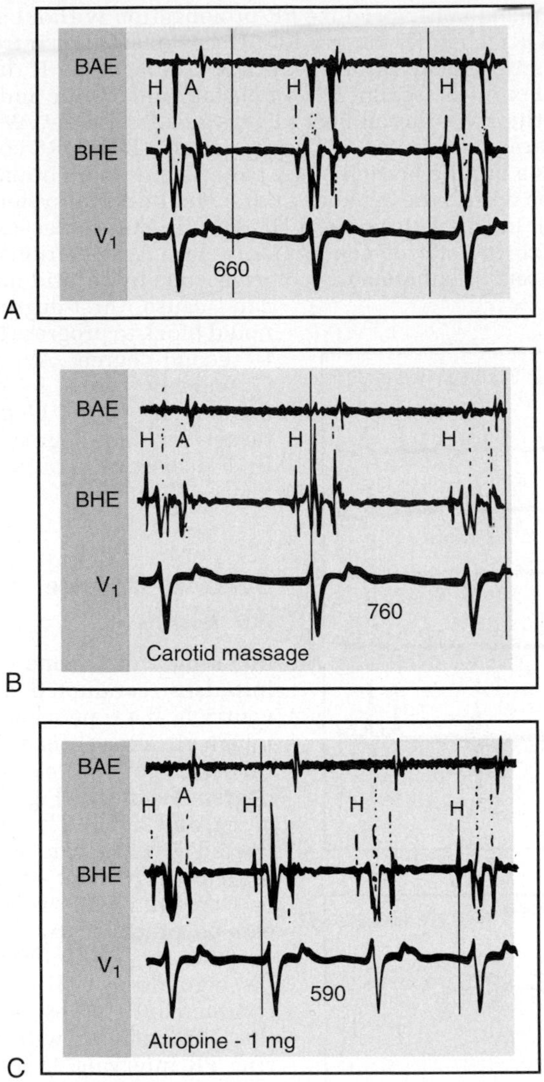

FIGURE 35–48 Nonparoxysmal atrioventricular (AV) junctional tachycardia. **A,** Control. **B,** Response to carotid sinus massage. **C,** Response to atropine 1 mg IV. Note that His bundle depolarization is the earliest recordable electrical activity in each cycle. The atria are depolarized retrogradely (low right atrial activity recorded in the BHE precedes high right atrial activity recorded in the BAE). Note also that carotid sinus massage slows the junctional discharge rate whereas atropine speeds it up. From these tracings alone, one could not distinguish the rhythm from some other types of supraventricular tachycardia. However, the onset and termination of this tachycardia were typical of nonparoxysmal AV junctional tachycardia. BAE = bipolar atrial electrogram; BHE = bipolar His electrogram.

(4) alternation of paroxysms of rapid regular or irregular atrial tachyarrhythmias and periods of slow atrial and ventricular rates (bradycardia-tachycardia syndrome; Fig. 35-51). More than one of these conditions can be recorded in the same patient on different occasions, and often their mechanisms can be shown to be causally interrelated and combined with an abnormal state of AV conduction or automaticity.

Patients who have sinus node disease can be categorized as having intrinsic sinus node disease unrelated to autonomic abnormalities or combinations of intrinsic and autonomic abnormalities. Symptomatic patients with sinus pauses and/or SA exit block frequently show abnormal responses on electrophysiological testing and can have a relatively high incidence of atrial fibrillation. In children, sinus node dysfunction most commonly occurs in those with congenital or acquired heart disease, particularly following corrective cardiac surgery. Sick sinus syndrome can occur in the absence of other cardiac abnormalities. The course of the disease is frequently intermittent and unpredictable because it is influenced by the severity of the underlying heart disease. Excessive physical training can heighten vagal tone and produce syncope related to sinus bradycardia or AV conduction abnormalities in otherwise normal individuals.

The anatomical basis of sick sinus syndrome can involve total or subtotal destruction of the sinus node, areas of nodal-atrial discontinuity, inflammatory or degenerative changes in the nerves and ganglia surrounding the node, and pathological changes in the atrial wall. Fibrosis and fatty infiltration occur, and the sclerodegenerative processes generally involve the sinus node and the AV node or the bundle of His and its branches or distal subdivisions. Occlusion of the sinus node artery may be important.

MANAGEMENT. For patients with sick sinus syndrome, treatment depends on the basic rhythm problem but generally involves permanent pacemaker implantation when symptoms are manifested (see Chap. 34). Pacing for the bradycardia, combined with drug therapy to treat the tachycardia, is required in those with bradycardia-tachycardia syndrome.

ATRIOVENTRICULAR BLOCK (HEART BLOCK)

Heart block is a disturbance of impulse conduction that can be permanent or transient, depending on the anatomical or functional impairment. It must be distinguished from interference, a normal phenomenon that is a disturbance of impulse conduction caused by physiological refractoriness resulting from inexcitability caused by a preceding impulse. Interference or block can occur at any site where impulses are conducted, but they are recognized most commonly between the sinus node and atrium (SA block), between the atria and ventricles (AV block), within the atria (intraatrial block), or within the ventricles (intraventricular block). SA exit block is discussed earlier (see "Sinus Bradycardia"). An AV block exists when the atrial impulse is conducted with delay or is not conducted at all to the ventricle when the AV junction is not physiologically refractory. During AV block, the block can occur in the AV node, His bundle, or bundle branches. In some cases of bundle branch block, the impulse may only be delayed and not completely blocked in the bundle branch, yet the resulting QRS complex may be indistinguishable from a QRS complex generated by a complete bundle branch block.

The conduction disturbance is classified by severity into three categories. During first-degree heart block, conduction time is prolonged but all impulses are conducted. Second-degree heart block occurs in two forms, Mobitz type I (Wenckebach) and type II. Type I heart block is characterized by a progressive lengthening of the conduction time until an impulse is not conducted. Type II heart block denotes occasional or repetitive sudden block of conduction of an impulse, without prior measurable lengthening of conduction time. When no impulses are conducted, complete or third-degree block is present. The degree of block may depend in part on the direction of impulse propagation. For unknown reasons, normal retrograde conduction can occur in the presence of advanced anterograde AV block. The reverse can also occur. Some electrocardiographers use the term *advanced heart block* to indicate blockage of two or more consecutive impulses.

First-Degree AV Block

During first-degree AV block, every atrial impulse conducts to the ventricles and a regular ventricular rate is produced, but the PR interval exceeds 0.20 second in adults. PR intervals as long as 1.0 second have been noted and can at times exceed the P-P interval, a phenomenon known as "skipped" P waves. Clinically important PR interval prolongation can result from a conduction delay in the AV node (A-H interval), in the His-Purkinje system (H-V interval), or at both sites. Equally delayed conduction over both bundle branches can uncommonly produce PR prolongation without significant QRS complex aberration. Occasionally, an intraatrial conduction delay can result in PR prolongation. If the QRS complex in the scalar ECG is normal in contour and duration, the AV delay almost always resides in the AV node, and rarely within the His bundle itself. If the QRS complex shows a bundle branch block pattern, the conduction delay may be within the AV node and/or His-Purkinje system (Fig. 35-52). In this latter case, a His bundle ECG is necessary to localize the site of conduction delay. Acceleration of the atrial rate or enhancement of vagal tone by carotid massage can cause first-degree AV nodal block to progress to type I second-degree AV block. Conversely, type I second-degree AV nodal block can revert to first-degree block with deceleration of the sinus rate.

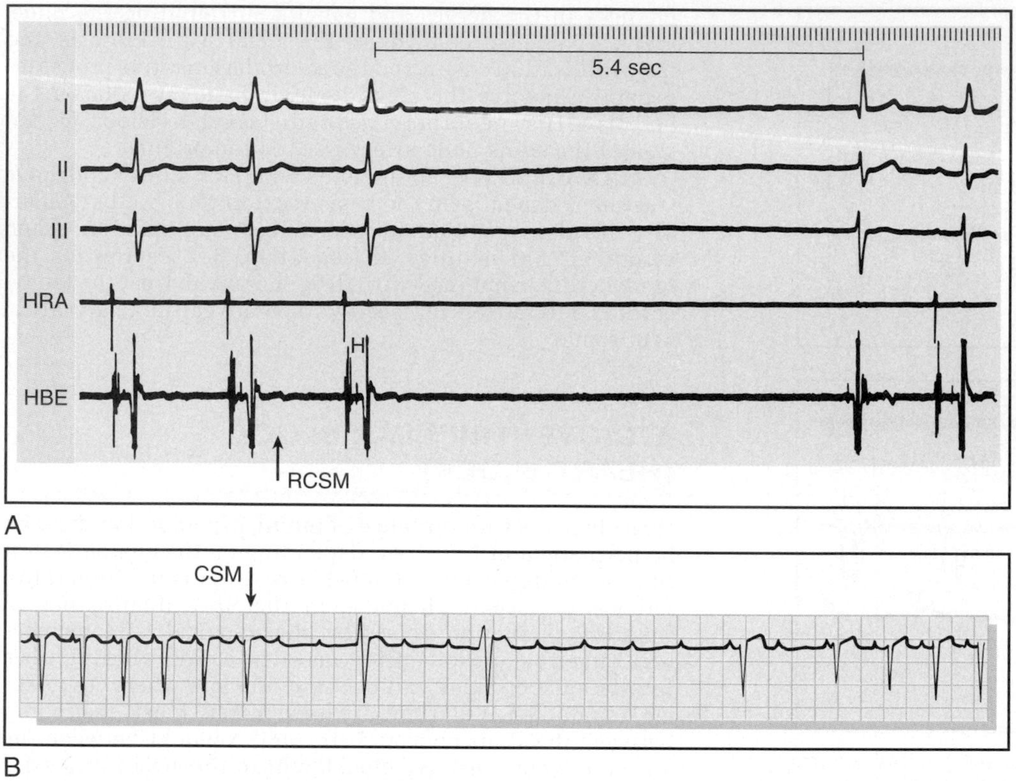

FIGURE 35-49 A, Right carotid sinus massage (RCSM) (arrow) results in sinus arrest and a ventricular escape beat (probably fascicular) 5.4 seconds later. Sinus discharge then resumes. **B,** Carotid sinus massage (CSM) (arrow; monitor lead) results in slight sinus slowing but, more importantly, advanced atrioventricular block. Obviously, an atrial pacemaker without ventricular pacing would be inappropriate for this patient.

Second-Degree AV Block

Blocking of some atrial impulses conducted to the ventricle at a time when physiological interference is not involved constitutes second-degree AV block (Figs. 35-53, 35-54, and 35-55). The nonconducted P wave can be intermittent or frequent, at regular or irregular intervals, and can be preceded by fixed or lengthening PR intervals. A distinguishing feature is that conducted P waves relate to the QRS complex with recurring PR intervals; that is, the association of P with QRS is not random. Electrocardiographically, typical type I second-degree AV block is characterized by progressive PR prolongation culminating

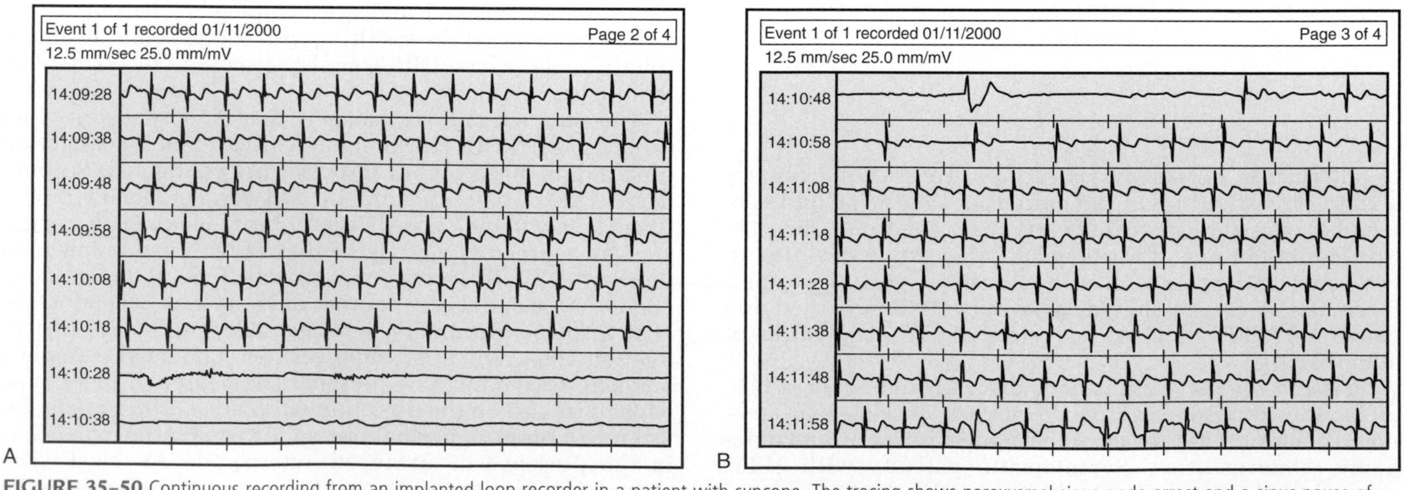

FIGURE 35-50 Continuous recording from an implanted loop recorder in a patient with syncope. The tracing shows paroxysmal sinus node arrest and a sinus pause of nearly 30 seconds. The preceding sinus cycle length appears to lengthen just prior to the pause, suggesting an autonomic component to the pause. There is also a single ventricular escape complex at 14:10:48.

in a nonconducted P wave (see Fig. 35-54), whereas in type II second-degree AV block, the PR interval remains constant prior to the blocked P wave (Fig. 35-56A). In both cases, the AV block is intermittent and generally repetitive and can block several P waves in a row. Often, the eponyms Mobitz type I and Mobitz type II are applied to the two types of block, whereas Wenckebach block refers to type I block only. A Wenckebach block in the His-Purkinje system in a patient with a bundle branch block can resemble an AV nodal Wenckebach block very closely (see Fig. 35-56B).

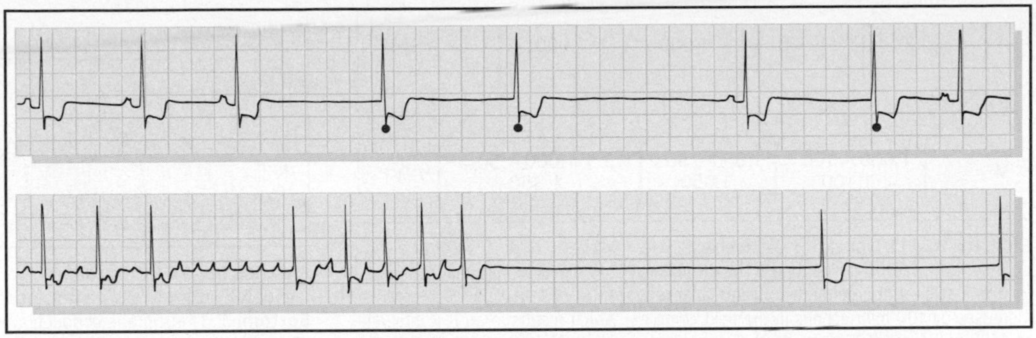

FIGURE 35–51 Sick sinus syndrome with bradycardia-tachycardia. **Top,** Intermittent sinus arrest is apparent with junctional escape beats at irregular intervals (red circles). **Bottom,** In this continuous monitor lead recording, a short episode of atrial flutter is followed by almost 5 seconds of asystole before a junctional escape rhythm resumes. The patient became presyncopal at this point.

Certain features of type I second-degree block deserve special emphasis because when actual conduction times are not apparent on the ECG—for example, during SA, junctional, or ventricular exit block (see Fig. 35-53)—a type I conduction disturbance can be difficult to recognize. During a typical type I block, the increment in conduction time is greatest in the second beat of the Wenckebach group, and the absolute increase in conduction time decreases progressively over subsequent beats. These two features serve to establish the characteristics of classic Wenckebach group beating: (1) the interval between successive beats progressively decreases, although the conduction time increases (but by a decreasing function); (2) the duration of the pause produced by the nonconducted impulse is less than twice the interval preceding the blocked impulse (which is usually the shortest interval); and (3) the cycle following the nonconducted beat (beginning the Wenckebach group) is longer than the cycle preceding the blocked impulse. Although much emphasis has been placed on this characteristic grouping of cycles, primarily to be able to diagnose a Wenckebach exit block, this typical grouping occurs in fewer than 50 percent of patients who have a type I Wenckebach AV nodal block.

Differences in these cycle length patterns can result from changes in pacemaker rate (e.g., sinus arrhythmia), in neurogenic control of conduction, and in the increment of conduction delay. For example, if the PR increment in the last cycle increases, the R-R cycle of the last conducted beat can lengthen rather than shorten. In addition, because the last conducted beat is often at a critical state of conduction, it can become blocked and produce a 5:3 or 3:1 conduction ratio instead of a 5:4 or 3:2 ratio. During a 3:2 Wenckebach structure, the duration of the cycle following the nonconducted beat will be the same as the duration of the cycle preceding the nonconducted beat.

Although it has been suggested that types I and II AV blocks are different manifestations of the same electrophysiological mechanism that differ only quantitatively in the size of the increments, clinically separating second-degree AV block into types I and II serves a useful function and, in most cases, the differentiation can be made easily and reliably from the surface ECG. Type II AV block often antedates the development of Adams-Stokes syncope and complete AV block, whereas type I AV block with a normal QRS complex is generally more benign and does not progress to more advanced forms of AV conduction disturbance. In older people, type I AV block with or without bundle branch block has been associated with a clinical picture similar to that seen in type II AV block.

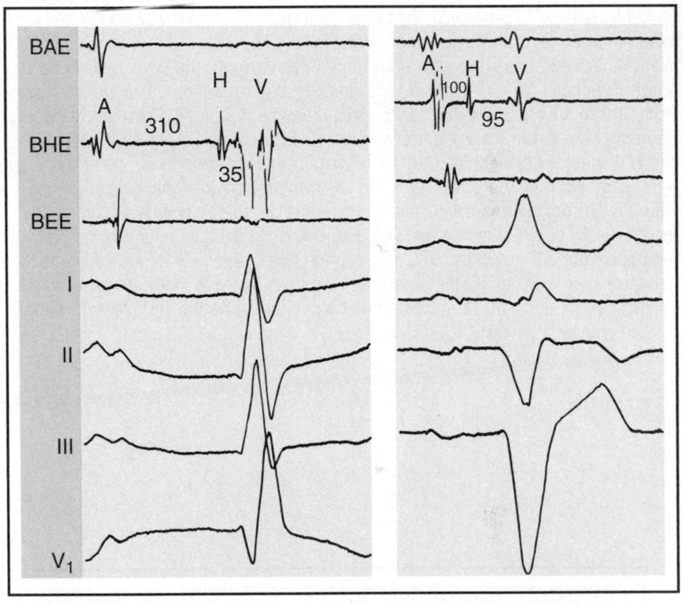

FIGURE 35–52 First-degree atrioventricular (AV) block. One complex during sinus rhythm is shown. **Left panel,** The PR interval measured 370 milliseconds (PA = 25 milliseconds; A-H = 310 milliseconds; H-V = 35 milliseconds) during a right bundle branch block. Conduction delay in the AV node causes the first-degree AV block. **Right panel,** The PR interval is 230 milliseconds (PA = 35 milliseconds; A-H = 100 milliseconds; H-V = 95 milliseconds) during a left bundle branch block. The conduction delay in the His-Purkinje system causes the first-degree AV block. BAE = bipolar atrial electrogram; BE = bipolar electrogram; BHE = bipolar His electrogram.

In a patient with an acute myocardial infarction, type I AV block usually accompanies inferior infarction (perhaps more often if a right ventricular infarction also occurs), is transient, and does not require temporary pacing, whereas type II AV block occurs in the setting of an acute anterior myocardial infarction, can require temporary or permanent pacing, and is associated with a high rate of mortality, generally from pump failure. A high degree of AV block can occur in patients with acute inferior myocardial infarction and is associated with more myocardial damage and a higher mortality rate than in those without AV block.

Although type I conduction disturbance is ubiquitous and can occur in any cardiac tissue in vivo, as well as in vitro, the site of block for the usual forms of second-degree AV block can usually be determined from the surface ECG with sufficient reliability to permit clinical decisions without requiring invasive electrophysiological studies.

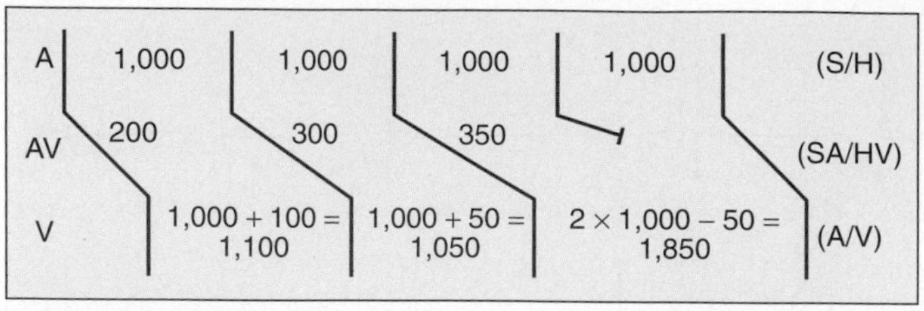

FIGURE 35–53 Typical 4:3 Wenckebach cycle. P waves ("A" tier) occur at a cycle length of 1000 milliseconds. The PR interval ("AV" tier) is 200 milliseconds for the first beat and generates a ventricular response ("V" tier). The PR interval increases by 100 milliseconds in the next complex, which results in an R-R interval of 1100 milliseconds (1000 + 100). The increment in the PR interval is only 50 milliseconds for the third cycle, and the PR interval becomes 350 milliseconds. The R-R interval shortens to 1050 milliseconds (1000 + 50). The next P wave is blocked, and an R-R interval is created that is less than twice the P-P interval by an amount equal to the increments in the PR interval. Thus, the Wenckebach features explained in the text can be found in this diagram. If the increment in the PR interval of the last conducted complex increased rather than decreased (e.g., 150 milliseconds rather than 50 milliseconds), the last R-R interval before the block would increase (1150 milliseconds) rather than decrease and thus become an example of an atypical Wenckebach cycle (see Fig. 35-38). If this were a Wenckebach exit block from the sinus node to the atrium, the sinus node cycle length (S) would be 1000 milliseconds, and the sinoatrial interval would increase from 200 to 300 to 350 milliseconds and culminate in a block. These events would be inapparent in the scalar electrocardiogram (ECG). However, the P-P interval in the ECG would shorten from 1100 to 1050 milliseconds and, finally, there would be a pause of 1850 milliseconds (A). If this rhythm were a junctional rhythm arising from the His bundle and conducting to the ventricle, the junctional rhythm cycle length would be 1000 milliseconds (H) and the H-V interval would progressively lengthen from 200 to 300 to 350 milliseconds, whereas the R-R interval would decrease from 1100 to 1050 milliseconds and then increase to 1850 milliseconds (V). The only clue to the Wenckebach exit block would be the cycle length changes in the ventricular rhythm.

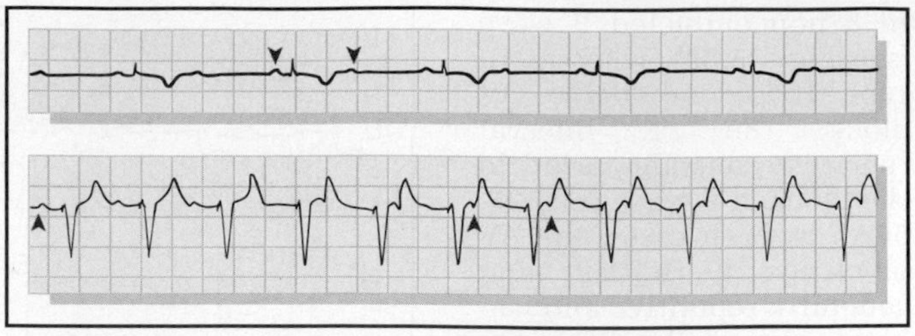

FIGURE 35–54 Unidirectional block. **Top,** During spontaneous sinus rhythm at a rate of 68 beats/min, 2:1 anterograde atrioventricular conduction occurs. **Bottom,** 1:1 retrograde conduction is seen during ventricular pacing at a rate of 70 beats/min. P waves are indicated by arrowheads.

Type I AV block with a normal QRS complex almost always takes place at the level of the AV node, proximal to the His bundle. An exception is the uncommon patient with type I intrahisian block. Type II AV block, particularly in association with a bundle branch block, is localized to the His-Purkinje system. Type I AV block in a patient with a bundle branch block can be caused by a block in the AV node or in the His-Purkinje system. Type II AV block in a patient with a normal QRS complex can be caused by an intrahisian AV block, but the block is likely to be a type I AV nodal block, which exhibits small increments in AV conduction time.

Differentiating Type I from Type II AV Block

The preceding generalizations encompass the vast majority of patients with second-degree AV block. However, certain caveats must be heeded to avoid misdiagnosis because of subtle electrocardiographic changes or exceptions:

1. The 2:1 AV block can be a form of type I or type II AV block (Fig. 35-57). If the QRS complex is normal, the block is more likely to be type I and located in the AV node, and one should search for transition of the 2:1 block to a 3:2 block, during which the PR interval lengthens in the second cardiac cycle. If a bundle branch block is present, the block can be located in the AV node or His-Purkinje system.
2. AV block can occur simultaneously at two or more levels and cause difficulty in distinguishing between types I and II.
3. If the atrial rate varies, it can alter conduction times and cause a type I AV block to stimulate a type II block or change a type II AV block into type I. For example, if the shortest atrial cycle length that has just achieved 1:1 AV nodal conduction at a constant PR interval is decreased by as little as 10 or 20 milliseconds, the P wave of the shortened cycle can block conduction at the level of the AV node without an apparent increase in the antecedent PR interval. An apparent type II AV block in the His-Purkinje system can be converted to type I in the His-Purkinje system in some patients by increasing the atrial rate.
4. Concealed premature His depolarizations can create electrocardiographic patterns that simulate those of type I or II AV block.

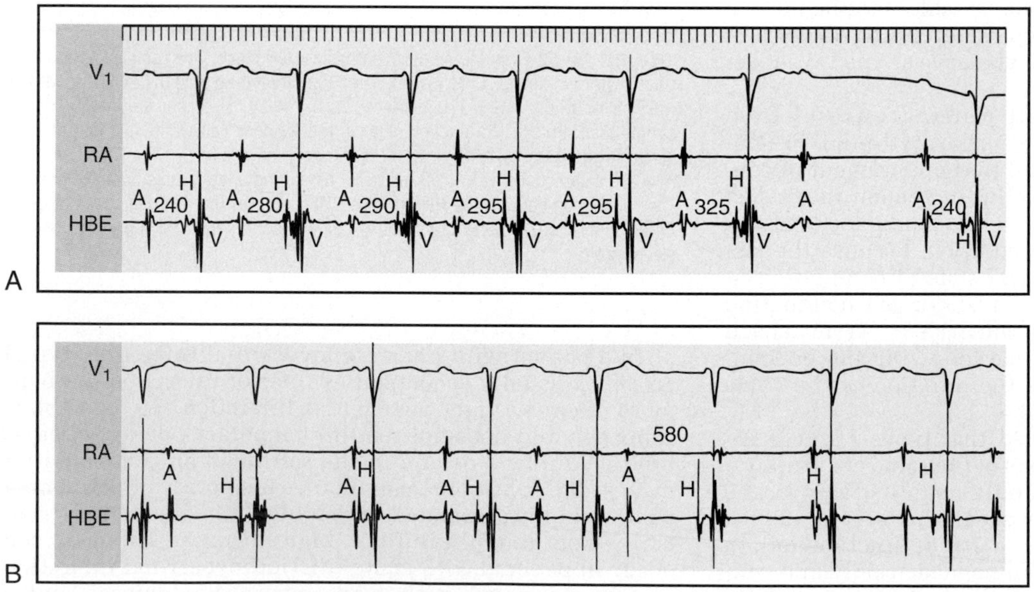

FIGURE 35–55 A, Type I (Wenckebach) atrioventricular (AV) nodal block. During spontaneous sinus rhythm, progressive PR prolongation occurs and culminates in a nonconducted P wave. From the His bundle recording (HBE), it is apparent that the conduction delay and subsequent block occur within the AV node. Because the increment in conduction delay does not consistently decrease, the R-R intervals do not reflect the classic Wenckebach structure. **B,** Recorded 5 minutes after the administration of atropine 0.6 mg IV. Atropine has had its predominant effect on sinus and junctional automaticity by this time, with little improvement in AV conduction. Consequently, more P waves are blocked and AV dissociation, caused by a combination of AV block and an enhanced junctional discharge rate, is present. At 8 minutes (not shown), when atropine finally improved AV conduction, 1:1 AV conduction occurred. RA = right atrium.

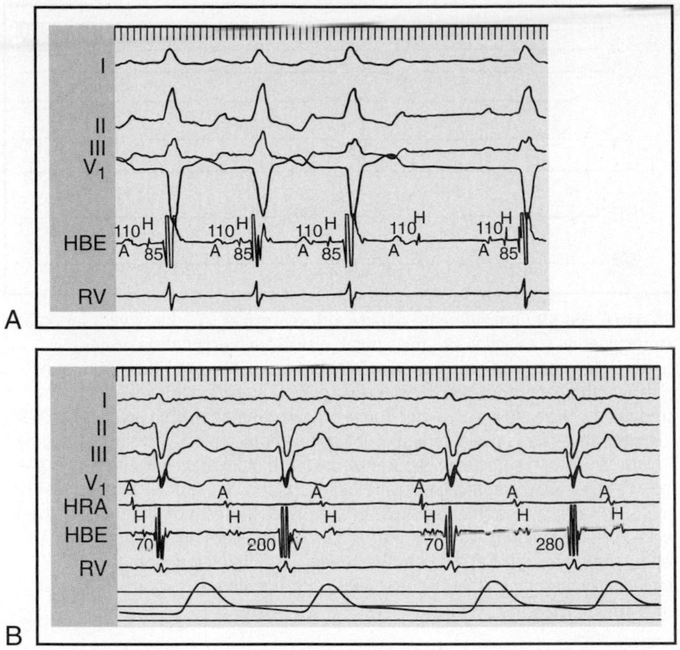

FIGURE 35–56 Type II atrioventricular (AV) block. **A,** The sudden development of a His-Purkinje block is apparent. The A-H and H-V intervals remain constant, as does the PR interval. Left bundle branch block is present. **B,** Wenckebach AV block in the His-Purkinje system. The QRS complex exhibits a right bundle branch block morphology. However, note that the second QRS complex in the 3 : 2 conduction exhibits a slightly different contour from the first QRS complex, particularly in V_1. This finding is the clue that the Wenckebach AV block might be in the His-Purkinje system. The H-V interval increases from 70 to 280 milliseconds, and then block distal to the His bundle results. HBE = His bundle electrogram; HRA = high right atrium; RV = right ventricle.

5. Abrupt transient alterations in autonomic tone can cause sudden block of one or more P waves without altering the PR interval of the conducted P wave before or after the block. Thus, an apparent type II AV block would be produced at the AV node. Clinically, a burst of vagal tone usually lengthens the P-P interval, as well as producing an AV block.
6. The response of the AV block to autonomic changes, either spontaneous or induced, to distinguish type I from type II AV block can be misleading. Although vagal stimulation generally increases and vagolytic agents decrease the extent of type I AV block, such conclusions are based on the assumption that the intervention acts primarily on the AV node and fail to consider rate changes. For example, atropine can minimally improve conduction in the AV node and markedly increase the sinus rate, which results in an increase in AV nodal conduction time and the degree of AV block as a result of the faster atrial rate (see Fig. 35-55B). Conversely, if an increase in vagal tone minimally prolongs AV conduction time but greatly slows the heart rate, the net effect on type I AV block may be to improve conduction. In general, however, carotid sinus massage improves and atropine worsens AV conduction in patients with His-Purkinje block, whereas the opposite results are to be expected in patients who have AV nodal block. Similarly, exercise or isoproterenol is likely to increase the sinus rate and improve AV nodal block, but worsen His-Purkinje block. These interventions can help differentiate the site of block without invasive study, although damaged His-Purkinje tissue may be influenced by changes in autonomic tone.
7. During type I AV block with high ratios of conducted beats, the increment in PR interval can be quite small and suggest a type II AV block if only the last few PR intervals before the blocked P wave are measured. By comparing the PR interval of the first beat in the long Wenckebach cycle with that of the beats immediately preceding the blocked P wave, the increment in AV conduction becomes readily apparent.
8. The classic AV Wenckebach structure depends on a stable atrial rate and a maximal increment in AV conduction time for the second PR interval of the Wenckebach cycle, with a progressive decrease in subsequent beats. Unstable or unusual alterations in the increment of AV conduction time or in the atrial rate, often seen with long Wenckebach cycles, result in atypical forms of type I AV block in which the last R-R interval can lengthen because the PR increment increases; these alterations are common.
9. Finally, it is important to remember that the PR interval in the scalar ECG is made up of conduction through the atrium, AV node, and His-Purkinje system. An increment in H-V conduction, for example, can be masked in the scalar ECG by a reduction in the A-H interval, and the resulting PR interval will not reflect the entire increment in His-Purkinje conduction time. Very long PR intervals (200 milliseconds) are more likely to result from AV nodal conduction delay (and block), with or without concomitant His-Purkinje conduction delay, although an H-V interval of 350 milliseconds is possible.

First-degree and type I second-degree AV block can occur in normal healthy children, and a Wenckebach AV block can be a normal phenomenon in well-trained athletes, as noted earlier, probably related to an increase in resting vagal tone. Occasionally, progressive worsening of the Wenckebach AV conduction disorder can result and the athlete becomes symptomatic and has to decondition. In patients who have chronic second-degree AV nodal block (proximal to the His bundle) without structural heart disease, the course is relatively benign (except in older age groups), whereas in those who have structural heart disease the prognosis is poor and related to the underlying heart disease.

Third-Degree (Complete) AV Block

Third-degree or complete AV block occurs when no atrial activity is conducted to the ventricles and therefore the atria

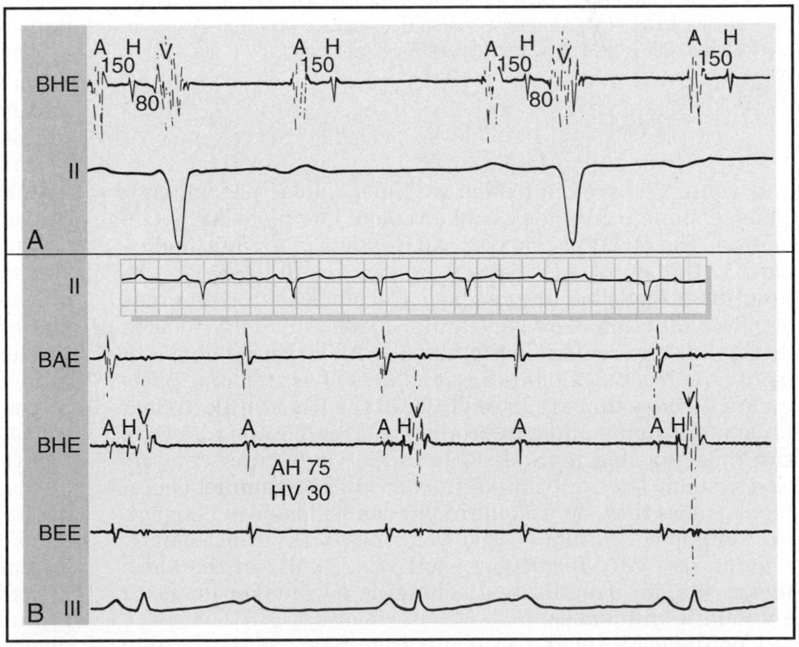

FIGURE 35–57 A 2 : 1 atrioventricular (AV) block proximal and distal to the His bundle deflection in two different patients. **A,** A 2 : 1 AV block seen in the scalar electrocardiogram occurs distal to the His bundle recording site in a patient with right bundle branch block and anterior hemiblock. The A-H interval (150 milliseconds) and H-V interval (80 milliseconds) are both prolonged. **B,** A 2 : 1 AV block proximal to the bundle of His in a patient with a normal QRS complex. The A-H interval (75 milliseconds) and the H-V interval (30 milliseconds) remain constant and normal. BAE = bipolar atrial electrogram; BE = bipolar electrogram; BHE = bipolar His electrogram.

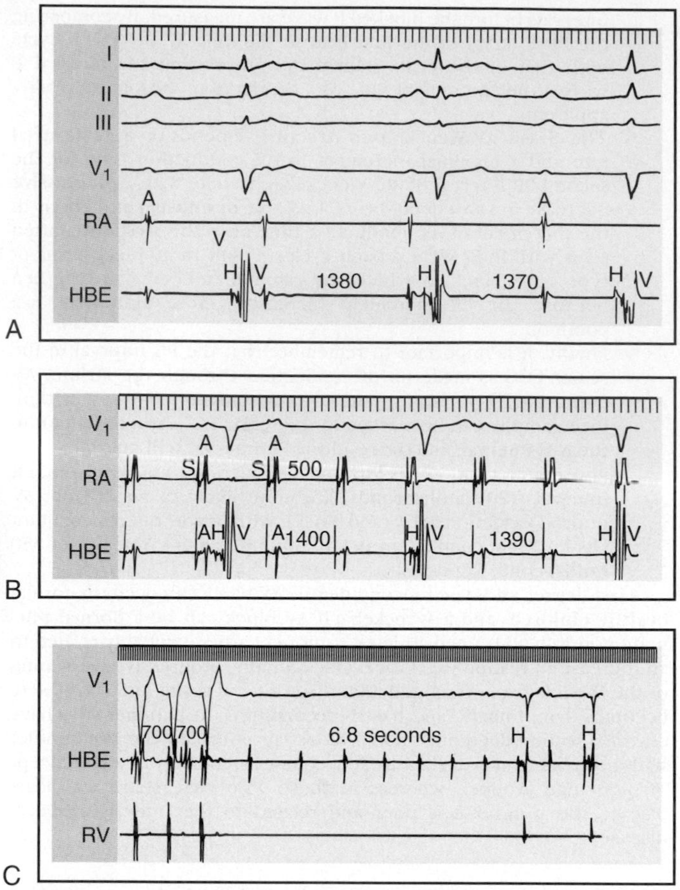

FIGURE 35-58 Congenital third-degree atrioventricular (AV) block. **A,** Complete AV nodal block is apparent. No P wave is followed by a His bundle potential, whereas each ventricular depolarization is preceded by a His bundle potential. **B,** Atrial pacing (cycle length of 500 milliseconds) fails to alter the cycle length of the functional rhythm. Still, no P wave is followed by a His bundle potential. **C,** After 30 seconds of ventricular pacing (cycle length of 700 milliseconds), suppression of the junctional focus results for almost 7 seconds (overdrive suppression of automaticity). HBE = His bundle electrogram; RA = right atrium; RV = right ventricle.

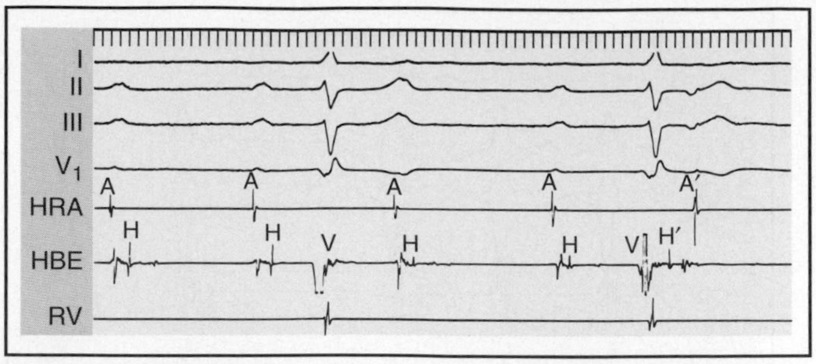

FIGURE 35-59 Complete anterograde atrioventricular (AV) block with retrograde ventriculoatrial conduction. All the sinus P waves are blocked distal to the His bundle, consistent with acquired complete AV block. The ventricles escape at a cycle length of approximately 1800 milliseconds (33 beats/min) and are not preceded by His bundle activation. The ventricular escape rhythm produces a QRS contour with left axis deviation and right bundle branch block, possibly caused by impulse origin in the posterior fascicle of the left bundle branch. Of interest is the fact that the second ventricular escape beat conducts retrogradely through His (H) and to the atrium (note the low-high atrial activation sequence and the negative P wave in leads II and III). The first ventricular complex does not conduct retrogradely, probably because the His bundle is still refractory from the immediately preceding atrial impulse. HBE = His bundle electrogram; HRA = high right atrium; RV = right ventricle.

and ventricles are controlled by independent pacemakers. Thus, complete AV block is one type of complete AV dissociation. The atrial pacemaker can be sinus or ectopic (tachycardia, flutter, or fibrillation) or can result from an AV junctional focus occurring above the block with retrograde atrial conduction. The ventricular focus is usually located just below the region of the block, which can be above or below the His bundle bifurcation. Sites of ventricular pacemaker activity that are in or closer to the His bundle appear to be more stable and can produce a faster escape rate than can those located more distally in the ventricular conduction system. The ventricular rate in acquired complete heart block is less than 40 beats/min but can be faster in congenital complete AV block. The ventricular rhythm, usually regular, can vary in response to PVCs, a shift in the pacemaker site, an irregularly discharging pacemaker focus, or autonomic influences.

Complete AV block can result from block at the level of the AV node (usually congenital) (Fig. 35-58), within the bundle of His, or distal to it in the Purkinje system (usually acquired) (Fig. 35-59). Block proximal to the His bundle generally exhibits normal QRS complexes and rates of 40 to 60 beats/min because the escape focus that controls the ventricle arises in or near the His bundle. In complete AV nodal block, the P wave is not followed by a His deflection, but each ventricular complex is preceded by a His deflection (see Fig. 35-58). His bundle recording can be useful to differentiate AV nodal from intrahisian block because the latter may carry a more serious prognosis than the former. Intrahisian block is recognized infrequently without invasive studies. In patients with AV nodal block, atropine usually speeds both the atrial and ventricular rates. Exercise can reduce the extent of AV nodal block. Acquired complete AV block occurs most commonly distal to the bundle of His because of trifascicular conduction disturbance. Each P wave is followed by a His deflection, and the ventricular escape complexes are not preceded by a His deflection (see Fig. 35-59). The QRS complex is abnormal, and the ventricular rate is usually less than 40 beats/min. A hereditary form caused by degeneration of the His bundle and bundle branches has been linked to the *SCN5A* gene that is also responsible for long-QT-3 (see Chap. 9).

Paroxysmal AV block in some cases can be caused by hyperresponsiveness of the AV node to vagotonic reflexes. Surgery, electrolyte disturbances, myoendocarditis, tumors, Chagas' disease, rheumatoid nodules, calcific aortic stenosis, myxedema, polymyositis, infiltrative processes (e.g., amyloidosis, sarcoidosis, scleroderma), and an almost endless assortment of common and unusual conditions can produce AV block. In adults, rapid rates can sometimes be followed by block, an event known as overdrive suppression of conduction. This form of block may be important as a cause of paroxysmal AV block after cessation of a tachycardia.

In children, the most common cause of AV block is congenital (see Chap. 61). Under such circumstances, the AV block can be an isolated finding or associated with other lesions. Connective tissue disease and the presence of anti-Rh_0 antibodies in the maternal sera of patients with congenital complete AV block raise the possibility that placentally transmitted antibodies play a role in some cases. Anatomical disruption between the atrial musculature and peripheral parts of the conduction system and nodoventricular discontinuity are two common histological findings. Children are most often asymptomatic; however, in some children, symptoms develop that require pacemaker implantation. Mortality from congenital AV block is highest in the neonatal period, is much lower during childhood and adolescence, and increases slowly lator in life. Adams-Stokes attacks can occur in patients with congenital heart block at any age. It is difficult to predict the prognosis in an individual patient. A persistent heart rate at rest of 50 beats/min or less correlates with the incidence of syncope, and extreme bradycardia can contribute to the frequency of Adams-Stokes attacks in children with congenital complete AV block. The site of block may not distinguish symptomatic children who have congenital or surgically induced complete heart block from those without symptoms. Prolonged recovery times of escape foci following rapid pacing (see Fig. 35-58C) and slow heart rates on 24-hour ECG recordings, and the occurrence of paroxysmal tachycardias may be predisposing factors to the development of symptoms.

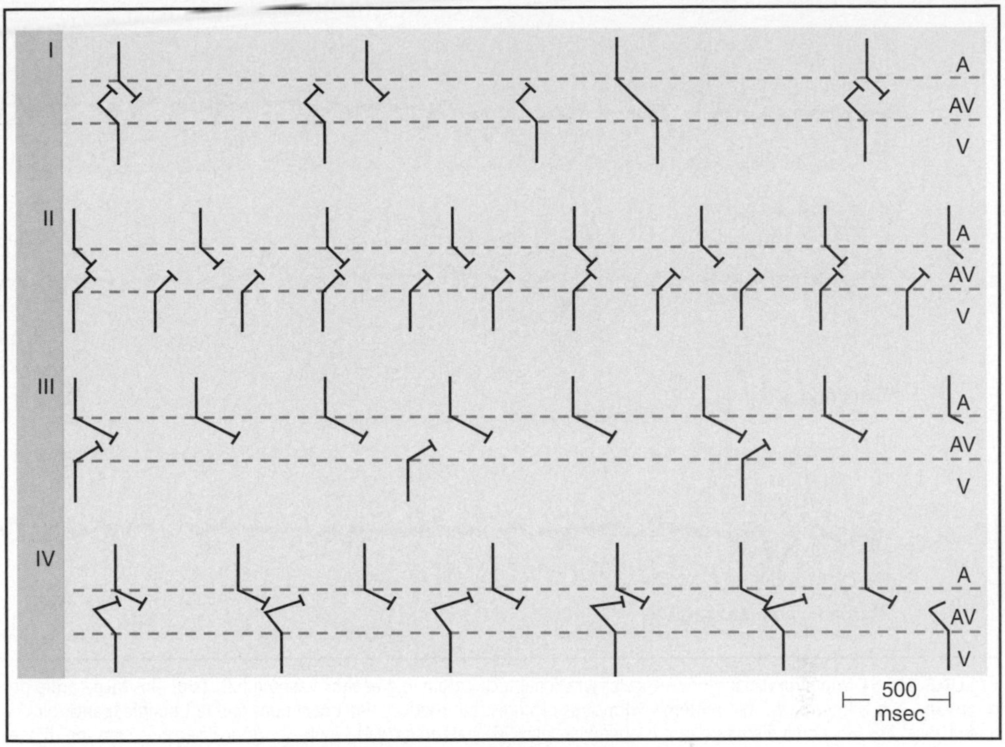

FIGURE 35–60 Diagrammatic illustration of the four causes of atrioventricular (AV) dissociation. **Top panel,** A sinus bradycardia allowing escape of an AV junctional rhythm that does not capture the atria retrogradely illustrates cause I. Intermittent sinus captures occur (third P wave) and produce incomplete AV dissociation. For cause II, ventricular tachycardia without retrograde atrial capture produces complete AV dissociation (see Figs. 35-33 and 35-61). As the third cause, complete AV block with a ventricular escape rhythm is diagrammed (see Figs. 35-58 and 35-59). **Bottom panel,** The combination of causes II and III is shown, which represents a nonparoxysmal AV junctional tachycardia and some degree of AV block.

CLINICAL FEATURES. Many of the signs of AV block are evidenced at the bedside. First-degree AV block can be recognized by a long a-c wave interval in the jugular venous pulse and by diminished intensity of the first heart sound as the PR interval lengthens. In type I second-degree AV block, the heart rate may increase imperceptibly with gradually diminishing intensity of the first heart sound, widening of the a-c interval, terminated by a pause, and an a wave not followed by a v wave. Intermittent ventricular pauses and a waves in the neck not followed by v waves characterize type II AV block. The first heart sound maintains a constant intensity. In complete AV block, the findings are the same as those in AV dissociation (see later).

Significant clinical manifestations of first- and second-degree AV block usually consist of palpitations or subjective feelings of the heart "missing a beat." Persistent 2:1 AV block can produce symptoms of chronic bradycardia. Complete AV block can be accompanied by signs and symptoms of reduced cardiac output, syncope or presyncope, angina, or palpitations from ventricular tachyarrhythmias. It can occur in twins.

MANAGEMENT. For patients with transient or paroxysmal AV block who present with presyncope or syncope, the diagnosis can be elusive. Ambulatory monitoring (Holter or external loop recorders) can be useful, but on occasion monitoring for longer periods may be necessary and thus an implantable loop recorder may be needed to establish the diagnosis. Drugs cannot be relied on to increase the heart rate for more than several hours to several days in patients with symptomatic heart block without producing significant side effects. Therefore, temporary or permanent pacemaker insertion is indicated for patients with symptomatic bradyarrhythmias. For short-term therapy, when the block is likely to be evanescent but still requires treatment or until adequate pacing therapy can be established, vagolytic agents such as atropine are useful for patients who have AV nodal disturbances, whereas catecholamines such as isoproterenol can be used transiently to treat patients who have heart block at any site (see "Sinus Bradycardia"). Isoproterenol should be used with extreme caution or not at all in patients who have acute myocardial infarction. The use of transcutaneous or temporary transvenous pacing is preferable. For symptomatic AV block or high-grade AV block (e.g., infrahisian, type II AV block, third-degree heart block not caused by congenital AV block), permanent pacemaker placement is the treatment of choice.

AV DISSOCIATION

CLASSIFICATION. As the term *AV dissociation* indicates, dissociated or independent beating of the atria and ventricles defines AV dissociation. AV dissociation is never a primary disturbance of rhythm but is a "symptom" of an underlying rhythm disturbance produced by one of three causes or a combination of causes (Fig. 35-60) that prevent the normal transmission of impulses from atrium to ventricle:

1. Slowing of the dominant pacemaker of the heart (usually the sinus node), which allows escape of a subsidiary or latent pacemaker. AV dissociation by default of the primary pacemaker to a subsidiary one in this manner is often a normal phenomenon. It may occur during sinus arrhythmia or sinus bradycardia and permit an independent AV junction rhythm to arise (see Fig. 35-42A).
2. Acceleration of a latent pacemaker, which usurps control of the ventricles. An abnormally enhanced discharge rate of a usually slower subsidiary pacemaker is pathological and commonly occurs during nonparoxysmal AV junctional tachycardia or VT

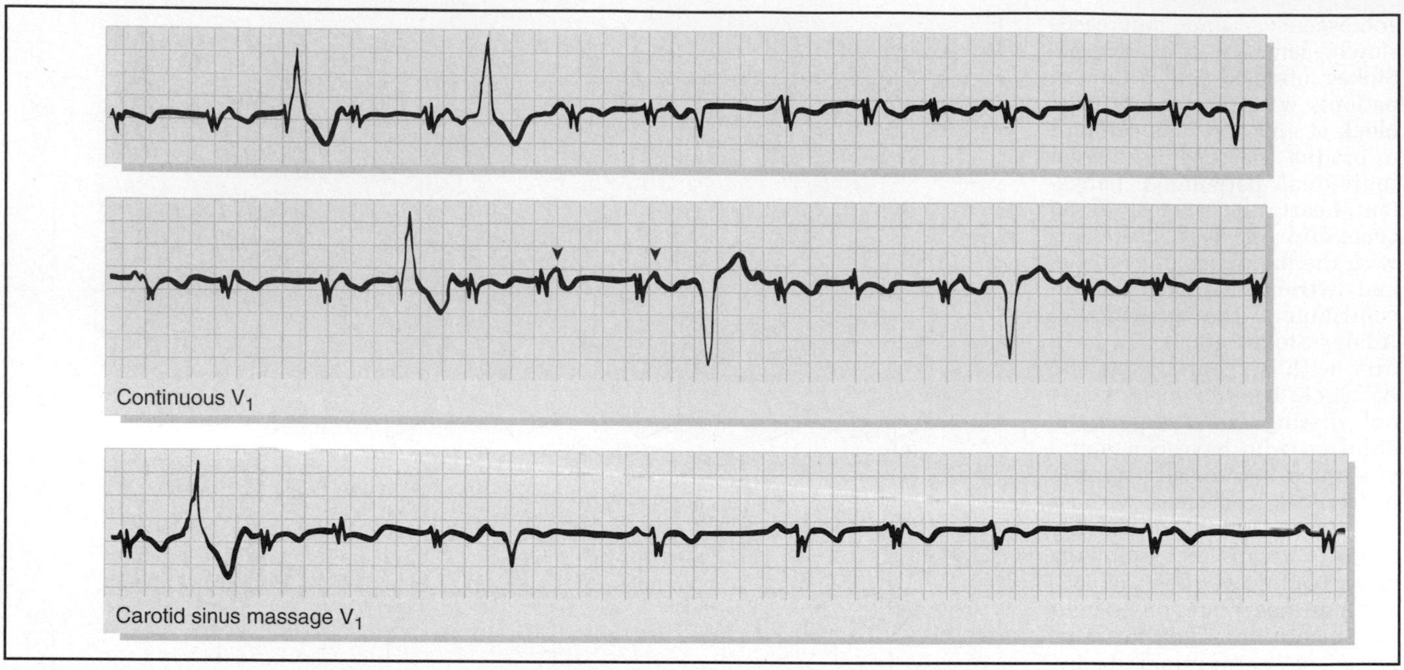

FIGURE 35–61 Nonparoxysmal atrioventricular junctional tachycardia in a healthy young adult. **Top,** This tachycardia occurs at a fairly regular interval (W-shaped complexes) and is interrupted intermittently with sinus captures that produce functional right and left bundle branch blocks. **Middle,** Two P waves are indicated by arrowheads. The junctional discharge rate is approximately 120 beats/min (cycle length = 500 milliseconds) and the rhythm is irregular, sometimes shortened by sinus captures or delayed by concealed conduction that resets and displaces the junctional focus. **Bottom,** Carotid sinus massage slows the junctional as well as the sinus discharge rates.

without retrograde atrial capture (Fig. 35-61; also see Fig. 35-33).

3. Block, generally at the AV junction, which prevents impulses formed at a normal rate in a dominant pacemaker from reaching the ventricles and allows the ventricles to beat under the control of a subsidiary pacemaker. Junctional or ventricular escape rhythm during AV block, without retrograde atrial capture, is a common example in which block gives rise to AV dissociation. Complete AV block is not synonymous with complete AV dissociation. Patients who have complete AV block have complete AV dissociation, but patients who have complete AV dissociation may or may not have complete AV block (see Figs. 35-58 and 35-59).
4. A combination of causes—for example, when digitalis excess results in the production of nonparoxysmal AV junctional tachycardia associated with SA or AV block.

MECHANISMS. With this classification in mind, it is important to emphasize that AV dissociation is not a diagnosis and is used in a similar manner as jaundice or fever. One must state that "AV dissociation is present and is caused by . . ." and then give the cause. An accelerated rate of a slower, normally subsidiary pacemaker or a slower rate of a faster, normally dominant pacemaker that prevents conduction because of physiological collision and mutual extinction of opposing wave fronts (interference) or the manifestations of AV block are the basic disturbances producing AV dissociation. The atria in all these cases beat independently from the ventricles, under control of the sinus node or ectopic atrial or AV junctional pacemakers, and can exhibit any type of supraventricular rhythm. If a single pacemaker establishes control of both atria and ventricles for one beat (capture) or a series of beats (e.g., sinus rhythm, AV junctional rhythm with retrograde atrial capture [see Figs 35-47 and 35-48], VT with retrograde atrial capture), AV dissociation is abolished for that period. Conversely, as stated earlier, whenever the atria and ventricles fail to respond to a single impulse for one beat (PVC without retrograde capture of the atrium) or a series of beats (VT without retrograde atrial capture), AV dissociation exists for that period. The interruption of AV dissociation by one or a series of beats under the control of one pacemaker, anterogradely or retrogradely, indicates that the AV dissociation is incomplete. Complete or incomplete dissociation can also occur in association with all forms of AV block. Commonly, when AV dissociation occurs as a result of AV block, the atrial rate exceeds the ventricular rate. For example, a subsidiary pacemaker with a rate of 40 beats/min can escape in the presence of a 2:1 AV block when the atrial rate is 78 beats/min . If the AV block is bidirectional, AV dissociation results.

ELECTROCARDIOGRAPHIC AND CLINICAL FEATURES. The ECG demonstrates the independence of P waves and QRS complexes. The P wave morphology depends on the rhythm controlling the atria—sinus, atrial tachycardia, junctional, flutter, or fibrillation. During complete AV dissociation, both the QRS complex and the P waves appear regularly spaced without a fixed temporal relationship to each other. When the dissociation is incomplete, a QRS complex of supraventricular contour occurs early and is preceded by a P wave at a PR interval exceeding 0.12 second and within a conductible range. This combination indicates ventricular capture by the supraventricular focus. Similarly, a premature P wave with retrograde morphology and a conductible RP interval may indicate retrograde atrial capture by the subsidiary focus.

Physical findings include a variable intensity of the first heart sound as the PR interval changes, atrial sounds, and a waves in the jugular venous pulse lacking a consistent relationship to ventricular contraction. Intermittent large (cannon) a waves may be seen in the jugular venous pulse when atrial and ventricular contractions occur simultaneously. The second heart sound can split normally or paradoxically, depending on the manner of ventricular activation.

A premature beat representing ventricular capture can interrupt a regular heart rhythm. When the ventricular rate exceeds the atrial rate, a cyclical increase in intensity of the first heart sound is produced as the PR interval shortens, climaxed by a very loud sound (bruit de canon). This intense sound is followed by a sudden reduction in intensity of the first heart sound and the appearance of giant a waves as the PR interval shortens and P waves "march through" the cardiac cycle.

MANAGEMENT. Management is directed toward the underlying heart disease and precipitating cause. The individual components producing the AV dissociation, not the AV dissociation per se, determine the specific type of antiarrhythmic approach.

REFERENCES

Supraventricular Arrhythmias

1. Blomstrom-Lundqvist C, Scheinman MM, Aliot EM, et al: ACC/AHA/ESC guidelines for the management of patients with supraventricular arrhythmias—executive summary: A report of the American College of Cardiology/American Heart Association Task Force on Practice Guidelines and the European Society of Cardiology Committee for Practice Guidelines (Writing Committee to Develop Guidelines for the Management of Patients With Supraventricular Arrhythmias). Circulation 108:1871, 2003.
2. Brady PA, Low PA, Shen WK: Inappropriate sinus tachycardia, postural orthostatic tachycardia syndrome, and overlapping syndromes. Pacing Clin Electrophysiol 28:1112, 2005.
3. Yusuf S, Camm AJ: Deciphering the sinus tachycardias. Clin Cardiol 28:267, 2005.
4. Olgin JE: Inappropriate sinus tachycardia and sinus node reentry. *In* Zipes D, Jalife J (eds): Cardiac Electrophysiology: From Cell to Bedside. 3rd ed. Philadelphia, WB Saunders, 1999, pp 459-468.
5. Yusuf S, Camm AJ: Sinus tachyarrhythmias and the specific bradycardic agents: A marriage made in heaven? J Cardiovasc Pharmacol Ther 8:89, 2003.

Atrial Fibrillation

6. Lloyd-Jones DM, Wang TJ, Leip EP, et al: Lifetime risk for development of atrial fibrillation: the Framingham Heart Study. Circulation 110:1042, 2004.
7. Wang TJ, Parise H, Levy D, et al: Obesity and the risk of new-onset atrial fibrillation. JAMA 292:2471, 2004.
8. Wang TJ, Massaro JM, Levy D, et al: A risk score for predicting stroke or death in individuals with new-onset atrial fibrillation in the community: the Framingham Heart Study. JAMA 290:1049, 2003.
9. Fang MC, Singer DE: Anticoagulation for atrial fibrillation. Cardiol Clin 22:47, 2004.
10. Rockson SG, Albers GW: Comparing the guidelines: anticoagulation therapy to optimize stroke prevention in patients with atrial fibrillation. J Am Coll Cardiol 43:929, 2004.
11. Fuster V, Ryden LE, Asinger RW, et al; American College of Cardiology/American Heart Association Task Force on Practice Guidelines; European Society of Cardiology Committee for Practice Guidelines and Policy Conferences (Committee to Develop Guidelines for the Management of Patients With Atrial Fibrillation); North American Society of Pacing and Electrophysiology: ACC/AHA/ESC Guidelines for the Management of Patients With Atrial Fibrillation: Executive Summary. A Report of the American College of Cardiology/American Heart Association Task Force on Practice Guidelines and the European Society of Cardiology Committee for Practice Guidelines and Policy Conferences (Committee to Develop Guidelines for the Management of Patients With Atrial Fibrillation) Developed in Collaboration With the North American Society of Pacing and Electrophysiology. Circulation 104:2118, 2001.
12. Wyse DG, Waldo AL, DiMarco JP, et al: A comparison of rate control and rhythm control in patients with atrial fibrillation. N Engl J Med 347:1825, 2002.
13. Joglar JA, Kowal RC: Electrical cardioversion of atrial fibrillation. Cardiol Clin 22:101, 2004.
14. Omran H, Jung W, Luderitz B: Left atrial appendage function after internal atrial defibrillation. J Cardiovasc Electrophysiol 9(Suppl):S97, 1998.
15. Escudero EM, San Mauro M, Laugle C: Bilateral atrial function after chemical cardioversion of atrial fibrillation with amiodarone: An echo-Doppler study. J Am Soc Echocardiogr 11:365, 1998.
16. Francis CW, Berkowitz SD, Comp PC, et al: Comparison of ximelagatran with warfarin for the prevention of venous thromboembolism after total knee replacement. N Engl J Med 349:1703, 2003.
17. Schulman S, Wahlander K, Lundstrom T, et al: Secondary prevention of venous thromboembolism with the oral direct thrombin inhibitor ximelagatran. N Engl J Med 349:1713, 2003.
18. Fiessinger JN, Huisman MV, Davidson BL, et al: Ximelagatran vs low-molecular-weight heparin and warfarin for the treatment of deep vein thrombosis: A randomized trial. JAMA 293:681, 2005.
19. Albers GW, Diener HC, Frison L, et al: Ximelagatran vs warfarin for stroke prevention in patients with nonvalvular atrial fibrillation: A randomized trial. JAMA 293:690, 2005.
20. Healey JS, Crystal E, Lamy A, et al: Left Atrial Appendage Occlusion Study (LAAOS): Results of a randomized controlled pilot study of left atrial appendage occlusion during coronary bypass surgery in patients at risk for stroke. Am Heart J 150:288, 2005.
21. Crystal E, Lamy A, Connolly SJ, et al: Left Atrial Appendage Occlusion Study (LAAOS): A randomized clinical trial of left atrial appendage occlusion during routine coronary artery bypass graft surgery for long-term stroke prevention. Am Heart J 145:174, 2003.
22. Ostermayer SH, Reisman M, Kramer PH, et al: Percutaneous left atrial appendage transcatheter occlusion (PLAATO system) to prevent stroke in high-risk patients with non-rheumatic atrial fibrillation: Results from the international multi-center feasibility trials. J Am Coll Cardiol 46:9, 2005.
23. Sievert H, Lesh MD, Trepels T, et al: Percutaneous left atrial appendage transcatheter occlusion to prevent stroke in high-risk patients with atrial fibrillation: Early clinical experience. Circulation 105:1887, 2002.
24. de Denus S, Sanoski CA, Carlsson J, et al: Rate vs rhythm control in patients with atrial fibrillation: A meta-analysis. Arch Intern Med 165:258, 2005.
25. Hohnloser SH, Kuck KH, Lilienthal J: Rhythm or rate control in atrial fibrillation—Pharmacological Intervention in Atrial Fibrillation (PIAF): A randomised trial. Lancet 356:1789, 2000.
26. Saxonhouse SJ, Curtis AB: Risks and benefits of rate control versus maintenance of sinus rhythm. Am J Cardiol 91:27, 2003.
27. Tieleman RG, Van Gelder IC, Crijns HJ, et al. Early recurrences of atrial fibrillation after electrical cardioversion: A result of fibrillation-induced electrical remodeling of the atria? J Am Coll Cardiol 31:167, 1998.
28. Franz MR, Karasik PL, Li C, et al: Electrical remodeling of the human atrium: similar effects in patients with chronic atrial fibrillation and atrial flutter. J Am Coll Cardiol 30:1785, 1997.
29. Daoud EG, Knight BP, Weiss R, et al: Effect of verapamil and procainamide on atrial fibrillation-induced electrical remodeling in humans. Circulation 96:1542, 1997.
30. Olgin JE, Rubart M: Remodeling of the atria and ventricle caused byrate. *In* Zipes D, Jalife J (eds): Cardiac Electrophysiology: From Cell to Bedside. 3rd ed. Philadelphia, WB Saunders, 1999, pp 364-378.
31. Sopher SM, Camm AJ: New trials in atrial fibrillation. J Cardiovasc Electrophysiol 9(Suppl):S211, 1998.
32. Alt E, Ammer R, Schmitt C, et al: A comparison of treatment of atrial fibrillation with low-energy intracardiac cardioversion and conventional external cardioversion [see comments]. Eur Heart J 18:1796, 1997.
33. Levy S, Ricard P, Lau CP, et al: Multicenter low energy transvenous atrial defibrillation (XAD) trial results in different subsets of atrial fibrillation. J Am Coll Cardiol 29:750, 1997.
34. Mittal S, Ayati S, Stein KM, et al: Transthoracic cardioversion of atrial fibrillation: comparison of rectilinear biphasic versus damped sine wave monophasic shocks. Circulation 101:1282, 2000.
35. Page RL, Kerber RE, Russell JK, et al: Biphasic versus monophasic shock waveform for conversion of atrial fibrillation: the results of an international randomized, double-blind multicenter trial. J Am Coll Cardiol 39:1956, 2002.
36. Benditt DG, Samniah N, Iskos D, et al: Biphasic waveform cardioversion as an alternative to internal cardioversion for atrial fibrillation refractory to conventional monophasic waveform transthoracic shock. Am J Cardiol 88:1426, 2001.
37. Oral H, Souza JJ, Michaud GF, et al: Facilitating transthoracic cardioversion of atrial fibrillation with ibutilide pretreatment [see comments]. N Engl J Med 340:1849, 1999.
38. Viskin S, Barron H, Olgin JE, et al: The treatment of atrial fibrillation. Pharmacologic and non-pharmacological strategies. Curr Prob Cardiol 22:44, 1997.
39. Wijffels MC, Crijns HJ: Recent advances in drug therapy for atrial fibrillation. J Cardiovasc Electrophysiol 14(Suppl):S40, 2003.
40. Haghi D, Schumacher B: Current management of symptomatic atrial fibrillation. Am J Cardiovasc Drugs 1:127, 2001.
41. Purerfellner H: Recent developments in cardiovascular drug therapy: Treatment of atrial arrhythmias with new class III drugs and beyond. Curr Med Chem Cardiovasc Hematol Agents 2:79, 2004.
42. McNamara RL, Tamariz LJ, Segal JB, Bass EB: Management of atrial fibrillation: Review of the evidence for the role of pharmacologic therapy, electrical cardioversion, and echocardiography. Ann Intern Med 139:1018, 2003.
43. Das MK, Cheriparambil K, Bedi A, et al: Cardioversion of atrial fibrillation with ibutilide: When is it most effective? Clin Cardiol 25:411, 2002.
44. Naccarelli GV, Wolbrette DL, Khan M, et al: Old and new antiarrhythmic drugs for converting and maintaining sinus rhythm in atrial fibrillation: Comparative efficacy and results of trials. Am J Cardiol 91:15D, 2003.
45. Olgin JE, Viskin S: Management of intermittent atrial fibrillation: Drugs to maintain sinus rhythm. J Cardiovasc Electrophysiol 10:433, 1993.
46. AFFIRM First Antiarrhythmic Drug Substudy Investigators: Maintenance of sinus rhythm in patients with atrial fibrillation: An AFFIRM substudy of the first antiarrhythmic drug. J Am Coll Cardiol 42:20, 2003.
47. Singh BN, Singh SN, Reda DJ, et al: Amiodarone versus sotalol for atrial fibrillation. N Engl J Med 352:1861, 2005.
48. Alboni P, Botto GL, Baldi N, et al: Outpatient treatment of recent-onset atrial fibrillation with the "pill-in-the-pocket" approach. N Engl J Med 351:2384, 2004.
49. Pappone C, Rosanio S, Augello G, et al: Mortality, morbidity, and quality of life after circumferential pulmonary vein ablation for atrial fibrillation: Outcomes from a controlled nonrandomized long-term study. J Am Coll Cardiol 42:185, 2003.
50. Oral H, Chugh A, Good E, et al: A tailored approach to catheter ablation of paroxysmal atrial fibrillation. Circulation 113:1824, 2006.
51. Hsu LF, Jais P, Sanders P, et al: Catheter ablation for atrial fibrillation in congestive heart failure. N Engl J Med 351:2373, 2004.

52. Oral H, Pappone C, Chugh A, et al: Circumferential pulmonary-vein ablation for chronic atrial fibrillation. N Engl J Med 354:934, 2006.
53. Jessurun ER, Van Hemel NM, Defauw JJ, et al: A randomized study of combining maze surgery for atrial fibrillation with mitral valve surgery. J Cardiovasc Surg (Torino) 44:9, 2003.

Atrial Flutter

54. Waldo AL: Atrial flutter: Entrainment characteristics. J Cardiovasc Electrophysiol 8:337, 1997.
55. Kalman JM, Olgin JE, Saxon LA, et al: Activation and entrainment mapping defines the tricuspid annulus as the anterior barrier in typical atrial flutter. Circulation 94:398, 1996.
56. Olgin JE, Kalman JM, Fitzpatrick AP, Lesh MD: Role of right atrial endocardial structures as barriers to conduction during human type I atrial flutter. Activation and entrainment mapping guided by intracardiac echocardiography. Circulation 92:1839, 1995.
57. Kalman JM, Olgin JE, Saxon LA, et al: Electrocardiographic and electrophysiologic characterization of atypical atrial flutter in man: Use of activation and entrainment mapping and implications for catheter ablation. J Cardiovasc Electrophysiol 8:121, 1997.
58. Kalman JM, VanHare GF, Olgin JE, et al: Ablation of 'incisional' reentrant atrial tachycardia complicating surgery for congenital heart disease. Use of entrainment to define a critical isthmus of conduction. Circulation 93:502, 1996.
59. Tai CT, Liu TY, Lee PC, et al: Non-contact mapping to guide radiofrequency ablation of atypical right atrial flutter. J Am Coll Cardiol 44:1080, 2004.
60. Jais P, Shah DC, Haissaguerre M, et al: Mapping and ablation of left atrial flutters. Circulation 101:2928, 2000.
61. Jais P, Sanders P, Hsu LF, et al: Flutter localized to the anterior left atrium after catheter ablation of atrial fibrillation. J Cardiovasc Electrophysiol 17:279, 2006.
62. Ishii Y, Gleva MJ, Gamache MC, et al: Atrial tachyarrhythmias after the maze procedure: Incidence and prognosis. Circulation 110(Suppl 1):II164, 2004.
63. Ghali WA, Wasil BI, Brant R, et al: Atrial flutter and the risk of thromboembolism: a systematic review and meta-analysis. Am J Med 118:101, 2005.
64. Weiss R, Marcovitz P, Knight BP, et al: Acute changes in spontaneous echo contrast and atrial function after cardioversion of persistent atrial flutter. Am J Cardiol 82:1052, 1998.
65. Kontos MC, Paulsen WH: Impairment of left atrial appendage function after spontaneous conversion of atrial flutter. Clin Cardiol 21:769, 1998.
66. Sparks PB, Jayaprakash S, Vohra JK, et al: Left atrial "stunning" following radiofrequency catheter ablation of chronic atrial flutter. J Am Coll Cardiol 32:468, 1998.

Atrial Tachycardia

67. Lee B, Olgin JE: Ablation of focal atrial tachycardias. *In* Wood M, Huang S (eds): Catheter Ablation of Cardiac Arrhythmias: Principles and Practical Approach. 8th ed. Philadelphia, WB Saunders, 2005, pp 181-194.

AV Nodal Reentry

68. Glatter KA, Cheng J, Dorostkar P, et al: Electrophysiologic effects of adenosine in patients with supraventricular tachycardia. Circulation 99:1034, 1999.

Wolff-Parkinson-White Syndrome

69. Arruda MS, McClelland JH, Wang X, et al: Development and validation of an ECG algorithm for identifying accessory pathway ablation site in Wolff-Parkinson-White syndrome. J Cardiovasc Electrophysiol 9:2, 1998.
70. Pappone C, Manguso F, Santinelli R, et al: Radiofrequency ablation in children with asymptomatic Wolff-Parkinson-White syndrome. N Engl J Med 351:1197, 2004.
71. Pappone C, Santinelli V, Manguso F, et al: A randomized study of prophylactic catheter ablation in asymptomatic patients with the Wolff-Parkinson-White syndrome. N Engl J Med 349:1803, 2003.

Ventricular Rhythm Disturbances

72. Maron BJ, Zipes DP: Introduction: Eligibility recommendations for competitive athletes with cardiovascular abnormalities-general considerations. J Am Coll Cardiol 45:1318, 2005.
73. Bloomfield DM, Steinman RC, Namerow PB, et al: Microvolt T-wave alternans distinguishes between patients likely and patients not likely to benefit from implanted cardiac defibrillator therapy: A solution to the Multicenter Automatic Defibrillator Implantation Trial (MADIT) II conundrum. Circulation 110:1885, 2004.
74. Chow T, Kereiakes DJ, Bartone C, et al: Prognostic utility of microvolt T-wave alternans in risk stratification of patients with ischemic cardiomyopathy. J Am Coll Cardiol 47:1820, 2006.
75. Tanno K, Ryu S, Watanabe N, et al: Microvolt T-wave alternans as a predictor of ventricular tachyarrhythmias: a prospective study using atrial pacing. Circulation 109:1854, 2004.
76. Moss AJ, Hall WJ, Cannom DS, et al: Improved survival with an implanted defibrillator in patients with coronary disease at high risk for ventricular arrhythmia. Multicenter Automatic Defibrillator Implantation Trial Investigators. N Engl J Med 335:1933, 1996.
77. Buxton AE, Lee KL, Fisher JD, et al: A randomized study of the prevention of sudden death in patients with coronary artery disease. Multicenter Unsustained Tachycardia Trial Investigators. N Engl J Med 341:1882, 1999.
78. Moss AJ, Zareba W, Hall WJ, et al: Prophylactic implantation of a defibrillator in patients with myocardial infarction and reduced ejection fraction. N Engl J Med 346:877, 2002.
79. Bardy GH, Lee KL, Mark DB, et al; Sudden Cardiac Death in Heart Failure Trial (SCD-HeFT) Investigators: Amiodarone or an implantable cardioverter-defibrillator for congestive heart failure. N Engl J Med 352:225, 2005.
80. European Heart Rhythm Association; Heart Rhythm Society; Zipes DP, Camm AJ, Borggrefe M, et al; American College of Cardiology; American Heart Association Task Force; European Society of Cardiology Committee for Practice Guidelines: ACC/AHA/ESC 2006 guidelines for management of patients with ventricular arrhythmias and the prevention of sudden cardiac death: A report of the American College of Cardiology/American Heart Association Task Force and the European Society of Cardiology Committee for Practice Guidelines (Writing Committee to Develop Guidelines for Management of Patients With Ventricular Arrhythmias and the Prevention of Sudden Cardiac Death). J Am Coll Cardiol 48:e247, 2006.
81. Mason JW: A comparison of electrophysiologic testing with Holter monitoring to predict antiarrhythmic-drug efficacy for ventricular tachyarrhythmias. Electrophysiologic Study versus Electrocardiographic Monitoring Investigators [see comments]. N Engl J Med 329:445, 1993.
82. Mason JW: A comparison of seven antiarrhythmic drugs in patients with ventricular tachyarrhythmias. Electrophysiologic Study versus Electrocardiographic Monitoring Investigators [see comments]. N Engl J Med 329:452, 1993.
83. Siebels J, Cappato R, Ruppel R, et al: Preliminary results of the Cardiac Arrest Study Hamburg (CASH). CASH Investigators. Am J Cardiol 72:109F, 1993.
84. Cappato R: Secondary prevention of sudden death: The Dutch Study, the Antiarrhythmics Versus Implantable Defibrillator Trial, the Cardiac Arrest Study Hamburg, and the Canadian Implantable Defibrillator Study. Am J Cardiol 83:68D, 1999.
85. The Antiarrhythmics versus Implantable Defibrillators (AVID) Investigators: A comparison of antiarrhythmic-drug therapy with implantable defibrillators in patients resuscitated from near-fatal ventricular arrhythmias [see comments]. N Engl J Med 337:1576, 1997.
86. Rothman SA, Hsia HH, Cossu SF, et al: Radiofrequency catheter ablation of postinfarction ventricular tachycardia: long-term success and the significance of inducible nonclinical arrhythmias. Circulation 96:3499, 1997.
87. Miller JM, Engelstein ED, Groh WJ, et al: Radiofrequency catheter ablation for postinfarct ventricular tachycardia. Curr Opin Cardiol 14:30, 1999.
88. Sakabe K, Ikeda T, Sakata T, et al: Comparison of T-wave alternans and QT interval dispersion to predict ventricular tachyarrhythmia in patients with dilated cardiomyopathy and without antiarrhythmic drugs: A prospective study. Jpn Heart J 42:451, 2001.
89. Sakabe K, Ikeda T, Sakata T, et al: Predicting the recurrence of ventricular tachyarrhythmias from T-wave alternans assessed on antiarrhythmic pharmacotherapy: A prospective study in patients with dilated cardiomyopathy. Ann Noninvasive Electrocardiol 6:203, 2001.
90. Kuroda N, Ohnishi Y, Yoshida A, et al: Clinical significance of T-wave alternans in hypertrophic cardiomyopathy. Circ J 66:457, 2002.
91. Almquist AK, Montgomery JV, Haas TS, Maron BJ: Cardioverter-defibrillator implantation in high-risk patients with hypertrophic cardiomyopathy. Heart Rhythm 2:814, 2005.
92. Dokuparti MV, Pamuru PR, Thakkar B, et al: Etiopathogenesis of arrhythmogenic right ventricular cardiomyopathy. J Hum Genet 50:375, 2005.
93. Morita H, Zipes DP, Lopshire J, et al: T wave ALTERNANS in an in vitro canine tissue model of Brugada syndrome. Am J Physiol Heart Circ Physiol 291:H421, 2006.
94. Antzelevitch C, Shimizu W: Cellular mechanisms underlying the long QT syndrome. Curr Opin Cardiol 17:43, 2002.
95. Maron BJ, Zipes DP: Introduction: Eligibility recommendations for competitive athletes with cardiovascular abnormalities—general considerations. J Am Coll Cardiol 45:1318, 2005.
96. Gerstenfeld EP, Dixit S, Callans DJ, et al: Quantitative comparison of spontaneous and paced 12-lead electrocardiogram during right ventricular outflow tract ventricular tachycardia. J Am Coll Cardiol 41:2046, 2003.
97. Kumagai K, Yamauchi Y, Takahashi A, et al: Idiopathic left ventricular tachycardia originating from the mitral annulus. J Cardiovasc Electrophysiol 16:1029, 2005.
98. Ouyang F, Fotuhi P, Ho SY, et al: Repetitive monomorphic ventricular tachycardia originating from the aortic sinus cusp: electrocardiographic characterization for guiding catheter ablation. J Am Coll Cardiol 39:500, 2002.
99. Storey J, Iwasa A, Feld GK: Left ventricular outflow tract tachycardia originating from the right coronary cusp: Identification of location of origin by endocardial noncontact activation mapping from the right ventricular outflow tract. J Cardiovasc Electrophysiol 13:1050, 2002.

Atrial Fibrillation

Guidelines for the management of atrial fibrillation (AF) were first published by the American Heart Association (AHA), American College of Cardiology (ACC), European Society of Cardiology, and North American Society of Pacing and Electrophysiology (now the heart Rhythm Society) in 2001.[1] These were updated in 2006.[2] In between, the American College of Chest Physicians developed guidelines specifically for the prevention and management of postoperative atrial fibrillation after cardiac surgery.[3]

As with other ACC/AHA guidelines, these use the standard ACC/AHA classification system for indications:

Class I: Conditions for which there is evidence and/or general agreement that the test is useful and effective

Class IIa: Weight of evidence or opinion is in favor of usefulness/efficacy

Class IIb: Usefulness or efficacy is less well established by evidence or opinion

Class III: Conditions for which there is evidence and/or general agreement that the test is not useful or effective and in some cases may be harmful

Three levels are used to rate the evidence on which recommendations have been based. Level A recommendations are derived from data from multiple randomized clinical trials, level B recommendations are derived from a single randomized trial or nonrandomized studies, and level C recommendations are based on the consensus opinion of experts.

Classification of Atrial Fibrillation

The guidelines point out that determination of the type of AF is an essential feature of patient evaluation. After two or more episodes, AF is considered recurrent. If recurrent atrial fibrillation resolves spontaneously, it is designated as paroxysmal; if it is sustained beyond 7 days it is termed persistent. Persistent AF also encompasses long-standing AF (generally classified as longer than 1 year), which usually leads to permanent AF.

Management of Atrial Fibrillation

The guidelines identify three primary objectives for the management of atrial fibrillation: rate control, rhythm control, and prevention of thromboembolism. Data from large trials, such as the Atrial Fibrillation Follow-up Investigation of Rhythm Management (AFFIRM)[4] and Rate Control versus Electrical cardioversion for persistent atrial fibrillation (RACE)[5] trials, indicate similar outcomes for rate control and rhythm control. Treatment must be tailored to each individual, depending on the nature, intensity, and frequency of symptoms, patient preferences, comorbid conditions, and ongoing response to treatment. Rate control may be a reasonable initial approach in older patients with persistent AF who have hypertension or heart disease, whereas rhythm control may be a better initial approach for younger individuals, especially those with paroxysmal lone AF.

For rhythm control, drugs are typically the first choice and left atrial ablation is a second-line choice. In some patients, particularly younger individuals with highly symptomatic AF, radiofrequency ablation may be preferred over years of drug therapy. For patients scheduled for coronary bypass or valve surgery, the Cox maze III procedure or left atrial ablation techniques may be effective options for halting AF.

Regardless of the approach to rhythm control, the need for anticoagulation should be based on stroke risk, not whether sinus rhythm is maintained. Clinically silent recurrences of AF in asymptomatic patients treated with antiarrhythmic drugs may be responsible for thromboembolic events after withdrawal of anticoagulation. Hence, the guidelines indicate that patients at high risk for stroke may require long-term anticoagulation.

Rate Control. Symptomatic patients with rapid ventricular rates during AF require prompt medical management. Cardioversion should be considered if symptomatic hypotension, angina, or heart failure is present; intravenous infusion of medications to slow ventricular response is appropriate for less acutely ill patients. In the absence of evidence of preexcitation, intravenous beta blockers or nondihydropyridine calcium blockers can be used; for patients who may have an accessory pathway, intravenous digoxin or amiodarone is preferred.

For patients with persistent or permanent AF, rate control with a beta blocker or nondihydropyridine calcium channel antagonist is recommended (Table 35G-1). Digoxin may also be indicated for patients with heart failure or left ventricular dysfunction, but should not be used as a sole agent for patients with paroxysmal AF. Ablation of the atrioventricular (AV) node or an accessory pathway may be a reasonable approach for controlling heart rate when drug therapy is ineffective or associated with negative side effects. The guidelines caution against using catheter ablation of the AV node without a prior trial of medication.

Rhythm Control. The ACC/AHA guidelines recommend immediate direct-current cardioversion for patients with AF and ongoing myocardial ischemia, symptomatic hypotension, angina, or heart failure when a rapid ventricular response does not respond promptly to pharmacological measures, or for those with AF involving preexcitation when very rapid tachycardia or hemodynamic instability occurs (Table 35G-2). Elective electrical cardioversion is appropriate in patients without hemodynamic instability when AF symptoms are unacceptable.

The guidelines note that restoration of sinus rhythm may be attempted with drugs or direct-current cardioversion. Electrical cardioversion (with biphasic shocks) is more effective than pharmacological cardioversion, but it requires conscious sedation or anesthesia. Pharmacological cardioversion tends to be more convenient and acceptable for patients. Disadvantages include the risk of drug-induced torsades de pointes or other serious arrhythmias.

Repeated cardioversions are considered a reasonable option for the management of symptomatic or recurrent AF in selected patients who prefer this option. The guidelines recommend against frequent repetition of direct-current cardioversion for patients who have relatively short periods of sinus rhythm between relapses of AF after multiple cardioversion procedures, despite prophylactic antiarrhythmic drug therapy. Electrical cardioversion is not indicated for patients with digitalis toxicity or hypokalemia.

Pharmacological cardioversion appears to be most effective when initiated within 7 days after the onset of an episode of AF. The guidelines recommend administration of flecainide, dofetilide, propafenone, or ibutilide; administration of amiodarone is considered a reasonable option (see Table 35G-2). For selected patients without sinus or AV node dysfunction, bundle branch block, QT interval prolongation, the Brugada syndrome, or structural heart disease, a single oral bolus dose of propafenone or flecainide ("pill-in-the-pocket") may be used to terminate persistent AF outside the hospital, once this treatment has been shown to work in a hospital setting. Digoxin and sotalol are not recommended for pharmacological cardioversion.

The guidelines emphasize that anticoagulation prophylaxis should be initiated prior to cardioversion when the arrhythmia has been present for more than 48 hours; immediate cardioversion without anticoagulation is supported when AF has lasted less than 48 hours (see Table 35G-2). The risk of thromboembolism or stroke appears to be similar for pharmacological and electrical methods of cardioversion; thus, the recommendations for anticoagulation are the same for both methods (see Table 35G-2).

TABLE 35G–1 ACC/AHA Recommendations for Pharmacological Rate Control of Atrial Fibrillation (AF)

Class	Indication	Level of Evidence
Class I (indicated)	Control of heart rate using pharmacological agents (either a beta blocker or nondihydropyridine calcium channel antagonist, in most cases) for patients with persistent or permanent AF	B
	In the absence of preexcitation, intravenous administration of beta blockers (esmolol, metoprolol, or propranolol) or nondihydropyridine calcium channel antagonists (verapamil, diltiazem) to slow the ventricular response to AF in the acute setting, exercising caution in patients with hypotension or heart failure (HF)	B
	Intravenous administration of digoxin or amiodarone to control heart rate in patients with AF and HF who do not have an accessory pathway	B
	In patients who experience AF symptoms during activity, for assessing adequacy of heart rate control during exercise, and adjusting drug therapy as needed to keep rate in the physiological range	C
	Digoxin effective following oral administration to control heart rate at rest in patients with AF; indicated for patients with HF, left ventricular (LV) dysfunction, or for sedentary individuals.	C
Class IIa (strong supportive evidence)	Combination of digoxin and beta blocker or nondihydropyridine calcium channel antagonist is reasonable to control the heart rate at rest and during exercise in patients with AF; individualize medication choice and modulate dose to avoid bradycardia	B
	Ablation of the atrioventricular (AV) node or accessory pathway reasonable for rate control when pharmacological therapy is insufficient or associated with side effects	B
	Intravenous amiodarone can be useful to control heart rate in patients with AF when other measures are unsuccessful or contraindicated	C
	In patients with AF and an accessory pathway, intravenous procainamide or ibutilide is reasonable alternative when electrical cardioversion is not necessary	C
Class IIb (weak supportive evidence)	Oral amiodarone may be used when ventricular rate cannot be adequately controlled at rest and during exercise using beta blocker, nondihydropyridine calcium channel antagonist, or digoxin, alone or in combination	C
	Intravenous procainamide, disopyramide, ibutilide, or amiodarone may be considered for hemodynamically stable patients with AF involving conduction over accessory pathway	B
	Catheter-directed ablation of the AV node may be considered when heart rate cannot be controlled with pharmacological agents or tachycardia-mediated cardiomyopathy is suspected.	C
Class III (not indicated)	Digitalis not to be used as sole agent to control rate of ventricular response in patients with paroxysmal AF	B
	Catheter ablation of the AV node should not be attempted without prior trial of medication to control ventricular rate in patients with AF	C
	In patients with decompensated HF and AF, intravenous administration of nondihydropyridine calcium channel antagonist may exacerbate hemodynamic compromise; not recommended	C
	Intravenous administration of digitalis glycosides or nondihydropyridine calcium channel antagonists to patients with AF and a preexcitation syndrome may accelerate the ventricular response; not recommended	C

ACC/AHA = American College of Cardiology/American Heart Association.

TABLE 35G–2 ACC/AHA Recommendations for Cardioversion of Atrial Fibrillation (AF)

Class	Indication	Level of Evidence
Pharmacological Cardioversion		
Class I (indicated)	Administration of flecainide, dofetilide, propafenone, or ibutilide is recommended for pharmacological cardioversion of AF	A
Class IIa (strong supportive evidence)	Administration of amiodarone is a reasonable option for pharmacological cardioversion of AF	A
	A single oral bolus dose of propafenone or flecainide (“pill-in-the-pocket”) can be administered to terminate persistent AF outside the hospital once treatment has proved safe in hospital for selected patients without sinus or AV node dysfunction, bundle-branch block, QT-interval prolongation, the Brugada syndrome, or structural heart disease. Before antiarrhythmic medication is initiated, a beta blocker or nondihydropyridine calcium channel antagonist should be given to prevent rapid atrioventricular (AV) conduction in the event atrial flutter occurs.	C
	Outpatient administration of amiodarone can be beneficial for patients with paroxysmal or persistent AF when rapid restoration of sinus rhythm is not deemed necessary.	C
Class IIb (weak supportive evidence)	Administration of quinidine or procainamide may be considered for pharmacological cardioversion of AF.	C
Class III (not indicated)	Digoxin and sotalol may be harmful when used for pharmacological cardioversion of AF and are not recommended.	A
	Quinidine, procainamide, disopyramide, and dofetilide should not be started out of hospital for conversion of AF to sinus rhythm.	B

TABLE 35G–2 ACC/AHA Recommendations for Cardioversion of Atrial Fibrillation (AF)—cont'd

Class	Indication	Level of Evidence
Direct-Current Cardioversion		
Class I (indicated)	Immediate R wave synchronized direct-current cardioversion is indicated when a rapid ventricular response does not respond promptly to pharmacological measures for patients with AF and ongoing myocardial ischemia, symptomatic hypotension, angina, or heart failure.	C
	Immediate direct-current cardioversion is recommended for patients with AF involving preexcitation when very rapid tachycardia or hemodynamic instability occurs.	B
	Cardioversion is recommended for patients without hemodynamic instability when symptoms of AF are unacceptable. In case of early relapse of AF after cardioversion, repeated direct-current cardioversion attempts may be made following administration of antiarrhythmic medication.	C
Class IIa (strong supportive evidence)	Direct-current cardioversion can be useful to restore sinus rhythm as part of a long-term management strategy for patients with AF.	B
	Patient preference is a reasonable consideration in the selection of infrequently repeated cardioversions for the management of symptomatic or recurrent AF.	C
Class III (not indicated)	Frequent repetition of direct-current cardioversion is not recommended for patients who have relatively short periods of sinus rhythm between relapses of AF after multiple cardioversion procedures, despite prophylactic antiarrhythmic drug therapy.	C
	Electrical cardioversion is contraindicated for patients with digitalis toxicity or hypokalemia.	C
Pharmacological Enhancement of Direct-Current Cardioversion		
Class IIa (strong supportive evidence)	Pretreatment with amiodarone, flecainide, ibutilide, propafenone, or sotalol may enhance the success of direct-current cardioversion and prevent recurrent AF.	B
	In patients who relapse to AF after successful cardioversion, repeating the procedure following prophylactic administration of antiarrhythmic medication may be useful.	C
Class IIb (weak supportive evidence)	For patients with persistent AF, administration of beta blockers,disopyramide, diltiazem, dofetilide, procainamide, or verapamil may be considered.	C
	Out-of-hospital initiation of antiarrhythmic medications may be considered for patients without heart disease to enhance the success of cardioversion of AF.	C
	Out-of-hospital administration of antiarrhythmic medications may be considered to enhance the success of cardioversion of AF in patients with certain forms of heart disease once the safety of the drug has been verified for the patient.	C
Prevention of Thromboembolism in Patients with AF Undergoing Cardioversion		
Class I (indicated)	When the duration of AF is 48 hr or longer, or unknown, anticoagulation (international normalized ratio [INR], 2.0 to 3.0) is recommended for at least 3 wk before and 4 wk after cardioversion, regardless of the method used to restore sinus rhythm.	B
	For patients with AF lasting more than 48 hours who require immediate cardioversion because of hemodynamic instability, heparin should be administered concurrently (unless contraindicated) by an initial intravenous bolus injection followed by a continuous infusion in a dose adjusted to prolong the activated partial thromboplastin time to 1.5 to 2 times the reference control value. Thereafter, oral anticoagulation (INR, 2.0 to 3.0) should be provided for at least 4 wk, as for patients undergoing elective cardioversion. Limited data support subcutaneous administration of low-molecular-weight heparin in this indication.	C
	Cardioversion should be performed immediately, without delay, for prior initiation of anticoagulation, for AF lasting less than 48 hr associated with hemodynamic instability (angina pectoris, myocardial infarction, shock, or pulmonary edema).	C
Class IIa (strong supportive evidence)	During the 48 hr after onset of AF, the need for anticoagulation before and after cardioversion may be based on the patient's risk of thromboembolism.	C
	As an alternative to anticoagulation prior to cardioversion of AF, it is reasonable to perform transesophageal echocardiography (TEE) in search of thrombus in the left atrium or left atrial appendage.	B
	a. For patients with no identifiable thrombus, cardioversion is reasonable immediately after anticoagulation with unfractionated heparin (e.g., initiated by intravenous bolus injection and an infusion continued at a dose adjusted to prolong the activated partial thromboplastin time to 1.5 to 2 times the control value until oral anticoagulation has been established with an oral vitamin K antagonist (e.g., warfarin) as evidenced by an INR ≥ 2.0). Thereafter, continuation of oral anticoagulation (INR, 2.0 to 3.0) is reasonable for a total anticoagulation period of at least 4 wk, as for patients undergoing elective cardioversion. (Limited data are available to support the subcutaneous administration of a low-molecular-weight heparin in this indication.)	B
	b. For patients in whom thrombus is identified by TEE, oral anticoagulation (INR, 2.0 to 3.0) is reasonable for at least 3 wk prior to and 4 wk after restoration of sinus rhythm, and a longer period of anticoagulation may be appropriate, even after apparently successful cardioversion, because the risk of thromboembolism often remains elevated in such cases.	C
	For patients with atrial flutter undergoing cardioversion, anticoagulation can be beneficial according to the recommendations for patients with AF.	C

ACC/AHA = American College of Cardiology/American Heart Association.

TABLE 35G-3 ACC/AHA Recommendations for Maintenance of Sinus Rhythm in Patients with Atrial Fibrillation (AF)

Class	Indication	Level of Evidence
Class I (indicated)	Before initiating antiarrhythmic drug therapy, treat precipitating or reversible causes of AF.	C
Class IIa (strong supportive evidence)	Pharmacological therapy can be useful for patients with AF to maintain sinus rhythm and prevent tachycardia-induced cardiomyopathy.	C
	Infrequent, well-tolerated recurrence of AF is reasonable as a successful outcome of antiarrhythmic drug therapy.	C
	Outpatient initiation of antiarrhythmic drug therapy is reasonable for patients with AF who have no associated heart disease when the agent is well tolerated.	C
	In patients with lone AF without structural heart disease, outpatient initiation of propafenone or flecainide can be beneficial for patients with paroxysmal AF who are in sinus rhythm at the time of drug initiation.	B
	Sotalol can be beneficial for outpatients in sinus rhythm with little or no heart disease, prone to paroxysmal AF, if the baseline uncorrected QT interval is shorter than 460 ms, serum electrolyte levels are normal, and risk factors associated with Class III drug-related proarrhythmia are not present.	C
	Catheter ablation is a reasonable alternative to pharmacological therapy to prevent recurrent AF in symptomatic patients with little or no left atrial enlargement.	C
Class III (not indicated)	Antiarrhythmic therapy with a particular drug is not recommended for maintenance of sinus rhythm in patients with AF who have well-defined risk factors for proarrhythmia with that agent.	A
	Pharmacological therapy is not recommended for maintenance of sinus rhythm in patients with advanced sinus node disease or atrioventricular node dysfunction unless they have a functioning electronic cardiac pacemaker.	C

ACC/AHA = American College of Cardiology/American Heart Association.

TABLE 35G-4 ACC/AHA Recommendations for Preventing Thromboembolism in Atrial Fibrillation (AF)

Class	Indication	Level of Evidence
Class I (indicated)	Antithrombotic therapy is recommended to prevent thromboembolism for all patients with AF except those with lone AF or contraindications.	A
	Select the antithrombotic agent based on the absolute risks of stroke and bleeding and the relative risk and benefit for a given patient.	A
	For patients without mechanical heart valves at high risk of stroke, institute chronic oral anticoagulant therapy with a vitamin K antagonist in a dose adjusted to achieve the target intensity international normalized ratio (INR) of 2.0 to 3.0, unless contraindicated. Factors associated with highest risk for stroke in patients with AF are prior thromboembolism (stroke, transient ischemic attack, or systemic embolism) and rheumatic mitral stenosis.	A
	Anticoagulation with a vitamin K antagonist is recommended for patients with more than one moderate risk factor: age ≧ 75 yr, hypertension, heart failure (HF), impaired left ventricular (LV) systolic function (ejection fraction 35% or less or fractional shortening less than 25%), and diabetes mellitus.	A
	INR should be determined at least weekly during initiation of therapy and monthly when anticoagulation is stable.	A
	Aspirin, 81-325 mg daily, is an alternative to vitamin K antagonists in low-risk patients or in those with contraindications to oral anticoagulation.	A
	For patients with AF and mechanical heart valves, the target INR should be based on the type of prosthesis, maintaining an INR of at least 2.5.	B
	Antithrombotic therapy is recommended for patients with atrial flutter as for those with AF.	C
Class IIa (strong supportive evidence)	Antithrombotic therapy with aspirin or a vitamin K antagonist is reasonable to prevent thromboembolism in patients with nonvalvular AF and only a single validated risk factor (age ≧ 75 yr, especially female patients; hypertension; HF; impaired LV function; or diabetes mellitus) based on an assessment of the risk of bleeding complications, ability to safely sustain adjusted chronic anticoagulation, and patient preferences.	A
	Antithrombotic therapy with aspirin or a vitamin K antagonist is reasonable to prevent thromboembolism in patients with nonvalvular AF who have one or more less well-validated risk factors (age 65 to 74 yr, female gender, or coronary artery disease). The choice of agent should be based on the risk of bleeding complications, ability to sustain adjusted chronic anticoagulation safely, and patient preferences.	B
	Antithrombotic therapy can reasonably be selected using the same criteria irrespective of the pattern (i.e., paroxysmal, persistent, or permanent) of AF.	B
	In patients with AF who do not have mechanical prosthetic heart valves, interrupting anticoagulation for up to 1 wk prior to a surgical or diagnostic procedure that carries a risk of bleeding without substituting heparin is reasonable.	C
	The need for anticoagulation should be reevaluated at regular intervals.	C
Class IIb (weak supportive evidence)	A lower INR target of 2.0 (range, 1.6 to 2.5) may be considered for prevention of ischemic stroke and systemic embolism in patients aged 75 yr and older who are at increased risk of bleeding but without frank contraindications to oral anticoagulant therapy, as well as other patients with moderate risk factors for thromboembolism who are unable to safely tolerate anticoagulation at the standard intensity of INR 2.0 to 3.0.	C

TABLE 35G-4 ACC/AHA Recommendations for Preventing Thromboembolism in Atrial Fibrillation (AF)—cont'd

Class	Indication	Level of Evidence
	In high-risk patients, during interruption of oral anticoagulant therapy for longer than 1 wk for surgical procedures, unfractionated heparin may be administered or low-molecular weight heparin given by subcutaneous injection.	C
	Following percutaneous coronary intervention or revascularization surgery in patients with AF, low-dose aspirin (less than 100 mg/d) and/or clopidogrel (75 mg/d) may be given concurrently with anticoagulation to prevent myocardial ischemic events.	C
	In patients undergoing percutaneous coronary intervention, anticoagulation may be interrupted to prevent bleeding at the site of peripheral arterial puncture, but the vitamin K antagonist should be resumed as soon as possible after the procedure and the dose adjusted to achieve an INR in the therapeutic range. Aspirin may be given temporarily during the hiatus, but the maintenance regimen should then consist of the combination of clopidogrel, 75 mg daily, plus warfarin (INR, 2.0 to 3.0). Clopidogrel should be given for a minimum of 1 mo after implantation of a bare metal stent, at least 3 mo for a sirolimus-eluting stent, at least 6 mo for a paclitaxel-eluting stent, and 12 mo or longer in selected patients, following which warfarin may be continued as monotherapy in the absence of a subsequent coronary event. When warfarin is given in combination with clopidogrel or low-dose aspirin, the dose intensity must be carefully regulated.	C
	In AF patients younger than 60 yr without heart disease or risk factors for thromboembolism (lone AF), the risk of thromboembolism is low without treatment and the effectiveness of aspirin for primary prevention of stroke relative to the risk of bleeding has not been established.	C
	In patients with AF who sustain ischemic stroke or systemic embolism during treatment with low-intensity anticoagulation (INR, 2.0 to 3.0), raising the intensity of anticoagulation to a target INR of 3.0 to 3.5 may be a more reasonable approach than addingan antiplatelet agent.	C
Class III (not indicated)	Long-term anticoagulation with a vitamin K antagonist is not recommended for primary prevention of stroke in younger patients (younger than 60 yr) without heart disease (lone AF) or any risk factors for thromboembolism.	C

ACC/AHA = American College of Cardiology/American Heart Association.

TABLE 35G-5 ACC/AHA Recommendations for Special Considerations in Atrial Fibrillation (AF)

Indication	Class I (Indicated) [Level of Evidence]	Class IIa (Strong Supportive Evidence) [Level of Evidence]	Class IIb (Weak Supportive Evidence) [Level of Evidence]	Class III (Not Indicated) [Level of Evidence]
Postoperative atrial fibrillation	Unless contraindicated, treatment with an oral beta blocker to prevent postoperative AF is recommended for patients undergoing cardiac surgery. [A] Administration of atrioventricular (AV) nodal blocking agents is recommended to achieve rate control in patients who develop postoperative AF. [B]	Preoperative administration of amiodarone reduces the incidence of AF in patients undergoing cardiac surgery and represents appropriate prophylactic therapy for patients at high risk for postoperative AF. [A] It is reasonable to restore sinus rhythm by pharmacological cardioversion with ibutilide or direct-current cardioversion in patients who develop postoperative AF, as advised for nonsurgical patients. [B] It is reasonable to administer antiarrhythmic medications in an attempt to maintain sinus rhythm in patients with recurrent or refractory postoperative AF, as recommended for other patients who develop AF. [B] It is reasonable to administer antithrombotic medication in patients who develop postoperative AF, as recommended for nonsurgical patients. [B]	Prophylactic administration of sotalol may be considered for patients at risk of developing AF following cardiac surgery. [B]	
Acute myocardial infarction	Direct-current cardioversion is recommended for patients with severe hemodynamic compromise or intractable ischemia, or when adequate rate control cannot be achieved with pharmacological	Intravenous administration of digitalis is reasonable to slow a rapid ventricular response and improve left ventricular (LV) function in patients with acute MI and AF associated		The administration of class IC antiarrhythmic drugs is not recommended for patients with

Continues

TABLE 35G–5 ACC/AHA Recommendations for Special Considerations in Atrial Fibrillation (AF)—cont'd

Indication	Class I (Indicated) [Level of Evidence]	Class IIa (Strong Supportive Evidence) [Level of Evidence]	Class IIb (Weak Supportive Evidence) [Level of Evidence]	Class III (Not Indicated) [Level of Evidence]
	agents in patients with acute myocardial infarction (MI) and AF. [C] Intravenous administration of amiodarone is recommended to slow a rapid ventricular response to AF and improve left ventricular (LV) function in patients with acute MI. [C] Intravenous beta blockers and nondihydropyridine calcium antagonists are recommended to slow a rapid ventricular response to AF in patients with acute MI who do not display clinical LV dysfunction, bronchospasm, or AV block. [C] For patients with AF and acute MI, administration of unfractionated heparin by continuous intravenous infusion or intermittent subcutaneous injection is recommended in a dose sufficient to prolong the activated partial thromboplastin time to 1.5 to 2 times the control value, unless contraindications to anticoagulation exist. [C]	with severe LV dysfunction and heart failure (HF). [C]		AF in the setting of acute MI. [C]
Management of AF associated with Wolff-Parkinson-White (WPW) preexcitation syndrome	Catheter ablation of the accessory pathway is recommended for symptomatic patients with AF who have WPW syndrome, particularly those with syncope caused by rapid heart rate or those with a short bypass tract refractory period. [B] Immediate direct-current cardioversion is recommended to prevent ventricular fibrillation in patients with a short anterograde bypass tract refractory period in whom AF occurs with a rapid ventricular response associated with hemodynamic instability. [B] Intravenous procainamide or ibutilide is recommended to restore sinus rhythm in patients with WPW syndrome in whom AF occurs without hemodynamic instability in association with a wide QRS complex on the electrocardiogram (ECG) (≥120 ms duration) or with a rapid preexcited ventricular response. [C]	Intravenous flecainide or direct-current cardioversion is reasonable when very rapid ventricular rates occur in patients with AF involving conduction over an accessory pathway. [B]	It may be reasonable to administer intravenous quinidine, procainamide, disopyramide, ibutilide, or amiodarone to hemodynamically stable patients with AF involving conduction over an accessory pathway. [B]	Intravenous administration of digitalis glycosides or nondihydropyridine calcium channel antagonists is not recommended in patients with WPW syndrome who have preexcited ventricular activation during AF. [B]
Hyperthyroidism	Administration of a beta blocker is recommended to control the rate of ventricular response in patients with AF complicating thyrotoxicosis, unless contraindicated. [B] In circumstances in which a beta blocker cannot be used, administration of a nondihydropyridine calcium channel antagonist (diltiazem or verapamil) is recommended to control the ventricular rate in patients with AF and thyrotoxicosis. [B]			

TABLE 35G–5 ACC/AHA Recommendations for Special Considerations in Atrial Fibrillation (AF)—cont'd

Indication	Class I (Indicated) [Level of Evidence]	Class IIa (Strong Supportive Evidence) [Level of Evidence]	Class IIb (Weak Supportive Evidence) [Level of Evidence]	Class III (Not Indicated) [Level of Evidence]
	In patients with AF associated with thyrotoxicosis, oral anticoagulation (international normalized ratio [INR], 2.0 to 3.0) is recommended to prevent thromboembolism, as recommended for AF patients with other risk factors for stroke. [C] Once a euthyroid state is restored, recommendations for antithrombotic prophylaxis are the same as for patients without hyperthyroidism. [C]			
Management of AF during pregnancy	Digoxin, a beta blocker, or a nondihydropyridine calcium channel antagonist is recommended to control the rate of ventricular response in pregnant patients with AF. [C] Direct-current cardioversion is recommended for pregnant patients who become hemodynamically unstable because of AF. [C] Protection against thromboembolism is recommended throughout pregnancy for all patients with AF (except those with lone AF and/or low thromboembolic risk). Therapy (anticoagulant or aspirin) should be chosen according to the stage of pregnancy. [C]		Administration of heparin may be considered during the first trimester and last month of pregnancy for patients with AF and risk factors for thromboembolism. Unfractionated heparin may be administered either by continuous intravenous infusion in a dose sufficient to prolong the activated partial thromboplastin time to 1.5 to 2 times the control value or by intermittent subcutaneous injection in a dose of 10,000 to 20,000 units every 12 hr, adjusted to prolong the midinterval (6 hr after injection) activated partial thromboplastin time to 1.5 times control. [B] Despite the limited data available, subcutaneous administration of low-molecular weight heparin may be considered during the first trimester and last month of pregnancy for patients with AF and risk factors for thromboembolism. [C] Administration of an oral anticoagulant may be considered during the second trimester for pregnant patients with AF at high thromboembolic risk. [C] Administration of quinidine or procainamide may be considered to achieve pharmacological cardioversion in hemodynamically stable patients who develop AF during pregnancy. [C]	

Continues

TABLE 35G-5 ACC/AHA Recommendations for Special Considerations in Atrial Fibrillation (AF)—cont'd

Indication	Class I (Indicated) [Level of Evidence]	Class IIa (Strong Supportive Evidence) [Level of Evidence]	Class IIb (Weak Supportive Evidence) [Level of Evidence]	Class III (Not Indicated) [Level of Evidence]
Management of AF in patients with hypertrophic cardiomyopathy (HCM)	Oral anticoagulation (INR, 2.0 to 3.0) is recommended for patients with HCM who develop AF, as for other patients at high risk of thromboembolism. [B]	Antiarrhythmic medications can be useful to prevent recurrent AF in patients with HCM. Available data are insufficient to recommend one agent over another in this situation, but (1) disopyramide combined with a beta blocker or nondihydropyridine calcium channel antagonist or (2) amiodarone alone is generally preferred. [C]		
Management of AF in patients with pulmonary disease	Correction of hypoxemia and acidosis is the recommended primary therapeutic measure for patients who develop AF during an acute pulmonary illness or exacerbation of chronic pulmonary disease. [C] A nondihydropyridine calcium channel antagonist (diltiazem or verapamil) is recommended to control the ventricular rate in patients with obstructive pulmonary disease who develop AF. [C] Direct-current cardioversion should be attempted in patients with pulmonary disease who become hemodynamically unstable as a consequence of AF. [C]			Theophylline and beta-adrenergic agonist agents are not recommended for patients with broncho-spastic lung disease who develop AF. [C] Beta blockers, sotalol, propafenone, and adenosine are not recommended for patients with obstructive lung disease who develop AF. [C]

ACC/AHA = American College of Cardiology/American Heart Association.

CH 35

Maintenance of Sinus Rhythm. Following cardioversion, drug therapy may help patients with AF maintain sinus rhythm and prevent tachycardia-induced cardiomyopathy. Precipitating or reversible causes of AF should be treated prior to initiating antiarrhythmic drug therapy (Table 35G-3). Outpatient initiation of antiarrhythmic drug therapy is considered to be a reasonable approach for patients without associated heart disease, as long as the agents are well tolerated. The guidelines indicate that sotalol may be beneficial in outpatients in sinus rhythm with little or no heart disease who are prone to paroxysmal AF if the baseline uncorrected QT interval is shorter than 460 milliseconds, serum electrolyte levels are normal, and risk factors associated with Class III drug-related proarrhythmia are not present. Catheter ablation is recommended as a reasonable alternative to pharmacological therapy to prevent recurrent AF in symptomatic patients with little or no left atrial enlargement.

Prevention of Thromboembolism. The ACC/AHA guidelines recommend antithrombotic therapy for all patients with AF, except those with lone AF or contraindications to antithrombotic therapy (Table 35G-4). Choice of therapy should be determined by the patient's absolute risks of stroke and bleeding. The guidelines recommend anticoagulant therapy with a vitamin K antagonist for patients with more than one moderate risk factor (age older than 75 years, hypertension, heart failure, impaired left ventricular systolic function, or diabetes mellitus). The dose should be adjusted to achieve an international normalized ratio (INR) of 2.0 to 3.0, or at least 2.5 in those with a mechanical heart valve. Aspirin (81 to 325 mg daily) is an alternative to warfarin in low-risk patients or in those with contraindications to oral anticoagulation. Antithrombotic therapy with aspirin or a vitamin K antagonist is reasonable in the intermediate-risk group of patients with nonvalvular AF who have only one validated risk factor or one or more less validated risk factors.

Selection of antithrombotic therapy is not dependent on the pattern of AF. Interruption of anticoagulation for up to 1 week is reasonable in patients with AF who do not have mechanical prosthetic heart valves for surgical or diagnostic procedures that carry a risk of bleeding. For those with mechanical heart valves, use of heparin may be needed during this period. The guidelines recommend against long-term anticoagulation with a vitamin K antagonist for primary prevention of stroke in patients younger than 60 years without heart disease (lone AF) or any risk factors for thromboembolism.

Special Considerations

The guidelines include recommendations regarding the management of atrial fibrillation AF following surgery, during acute myocardial infarction, and in patients with the Wolff-Parkinson-White preexcitation syndrome, hyperthyroidism, hypertrophic cardiomyopathy, or pulmonary disease, or during pregnancy (Table 35G-5). These recommendations include avoiding Class IC antiarrhythmic drugs in the setting of acute myocardial infarction and avoiding digitalis glycosides and nondihydropyridine calcium channel antagonists in patients with evidence of bypass tracts.

References

1. Fuster V, Ryden LE, Asinger RW, et al: ACC/AHA/ESC guidelines for the management of patients with atrial fibrillation: Executive summary. A Report of the American

College of Cardiology/ American Heart Association Task Force on Practice Guidelines and the European Society of Cardiology Committee for Practice Guidelines and Policy Conferences (Committee to Develop Guidelines for the Management of Patients With Atrial Fibrillation): Developed in Collaboration With the North American Society of Pacing and Electrophysiology. J Am Coll Cardiol 38:1231, 2001.

2. Fuster V, Ryden LE, Cannom DS, et al: ACC/AHA/ESC 2006 guidelines for the management of patients with atrial fibrillation: A report of the American College of Cardiology/American Heart Association Task Force on Practice Guidelines and the European Society of Cardiology Committee for Practice Guidelines (Writing Committee to Revise the 2001 Guidelines for the Management of Patients With Atrial Fibrillation): Developed in collaboration with the European Heart Rhythm Association and the Heart Rhythm Society. Circulation 114:e257, 2006.
3. McKeown PP, Gutterman D: Executive summary: American College of Chest Physicians guidelines for the prevention and management of postoperative atrial fibrillation after cardiac surgery. Chest 128:1S, 2005.
4. Wyse DG, Waldo AL, DiMarco JP, et al: A comparison of rate control and rhythm control in patients with atrial fibrillation. N Engl J Med 347:1825, 2002.
5. Van Gelder IC, Hagens VE, Bosker HA, et al: A comparison of rate control and rhythm control in patients with recurrent persistent atrial fibrillation. N Engl J Med 347:1834, 2002.

CHAPTER 36

Cardiac Arrest and Sudden Cardiac Death

Robert J. Myerburg and Agustin Castellanos

DEFINITIONS

Sudden cardiac death (SCD) is defined as natural death from cardiac causes, heralded by abrupt loss of consciousness within 1 hour of the onset of an acute change in cardiovascular status. Preexisting heart disease may or may not have been known to be present, but the time and mode of death are unexpected. This definition incorporates the key elements of natural, rapid, and unexpected. It consolidates previous definitions that have conflicted, mainly because the most useful operational definition of SCD in the past differed for the clinician, the cardiovascular epidemiologist, the pathologist, and the scientist attempting to define pathophysiological mechanisms. As epidemiology, causes, and mechanisms began to be understood, these differences faded.[1]

Four elements must be considered in the construction of a temporal description of SCD to satisfy clinical, scientific, legal, and social considerations: (1) prodromes, (2) onset, (3) cardiac arrest, and (4) biological death (Fig. 36-1). Because the proximate cause of SCD is an abrupt disturbance of cardiovascular function, which is incompatible with maintaining consciousness because of abrupt loss of cerebral blood flow, any definition must recognize the brief time interval between the onset of the mechanism directly responsible for cardiac arrest and the consequent loss of consciousness (see Fig. 36-1C). The 1-hour definition, however, refers to the duration of the "terminal event" (see Fig. 36-1B), which defines the interval between the onset of symptoms signaling the pathophysiological disturbance leading to cardiac arrest and the onset of the cardiac arrest itself (see Fig. 36-1B and C).

Premonitory signs and symptoms are often absent, but nonspecific symptoms can occur during the days or weeks before a cardiac arrest. Prodromes (see Fig. 36-1A) are poor predictors of an impending event because of low sensitivity but may be more specific for an imminent cardiac arrest when they begin abruptly. Sudden onset of chest pain, dyspnea, or palpitations and other symptoms of arrhythmias often precede the onset of cardiac arrest. The fourth element, *biological death* (see Fig. 36-1D), was an immediate consequence of the clinical cardiac arrest in the past, usually occurring within minutes. However, since the development of community-based interventions and life support systems, patients may now remain biologically alive for a long period after the onset of a pathophysiological process that has caused irreversible damage and will ultimately lead to death. In this circumstance, the causative pathophysiological and clinical event is the cardiac arrest itself rather than the factors responsible for the delayed biological death. However, because of legal, forensic, and certain social considerations, biological death must continue to be used as the absolute definition of death.

Finally, the forensic pathologist studying unwitnessed deaths may use the definition of sudden death for a person known to be alive and functioning normally 24 hours before, and this remains appropriate within obvious limits. The generally accepted clinicopathophysiological definition of up to 1 hour between onset of the terminal event and biological death requires qualifications for specific circumstances.

The development of community-based intervention systems has also led to inconsistencies in the use of terms considered absolute. Death is defined biologically, legally, and literally as an absolute and irreversible event. Thus, SCD can be aborted, or a patient can survive cardiac arrest or cardiovascular collapse; however, survival after (sudden) death is a contradiction in terms. Table 36-1 provides definitions for events and terms related to the concept of SCD—death, cardiac arrest, and cardiovascular collapse.

TABLE 36–1 Terms Related to Sudden Cardiac Death

Term	Definition	Qualifiers or Exceptions
Death	Irreversible cessation of all biological functions	None
Cardiac arrest	Abrupt cessation of cardiac pump function, which may be reversible but will lead to death in the absence of prompt intervention	Rare spontaneous reversions, likelihood of successful intervention relates to mechanism of arrest, clinical setting, and time to intervention
Cardiovascular collapse	A (sudden) loss of effective blood flow caused cardiac and/or peripheral vascular factors that may revert spontaneously (e.g., vasodepressor or cardioinhibitory syncope) or only with interventions (e.g., cardiac arrest)	Nonspecific term that includes cardiac arrest and its consequences and also events that characteristically revert spontaneously

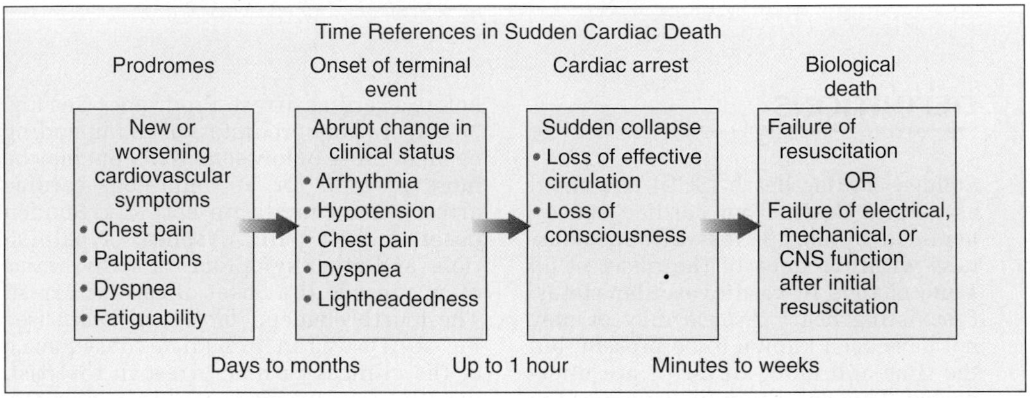

FIGURE 36–1 Sudden cardiac death viewed from four temporal perspectives: (1) prodromes, (2) onset of the terminal event, (3) cardiac arrest, and (4) progression to biological death. Individual variability of the components influences clinical expression. Some victims experience no prodromes, with onset leading almost instantaneously to cardiac arrest; others may have an onset that lasts up to 1 hour before clinical arrest. Some patients may live days to weeks after the cardiac arrest before biological death, often because of irreversible brain damage and dependence upon life support. These factors influence interpretation of the 1-hour definition. The two most relevant clinical factors are onset of the terminal event (2) and the clinical cardiac arrest itself (3); legal and social considerations focus on the time of biological death (4). CNS = central nervous system.

EPIDEMIOLOGY

Epidemiological Overview

Epidemiological studies of SCD are challenging for both theoretical and practical reasons. There are persisting fundamental questions about definition, inconsistencies in access to data, variations in pathophysiological mechanisms and their clinical recognition, and distinctions between population risk and individual risk.[2] In addition, the fact that cardiac arrest leading to SCD has short-term dynamics superimposed on a long-term static or dynamic substrate introduces unusual epidemiological complexities. These include long-term risk prediction based on atherogenesis, myocardial hypertrophy, and ventricular muscle dysfunction, and transient variables such as ischemia, hemodynamic shifts, atherosclerotic plaque disruption and thrombosis, and autonomic variations. The differences between chronic disease evolution and transient events call for different forms of epidemiological modeling. Furthermore, the emerging field of genetic epidemiology adds a new dimension for study, and there is a need for focusing on interventional epidemiology, the latter being a term coined to define the population dynamics of therapeutic outcomes.

Incidence and the Population Burden of Sudden Cardiac Death

The worldwide incidence of SCD is difficult to estimate because it varies largely as a function of coronary heart disease prevalence in different countries (see Chap. 1).[3] Estimates of the annual number of SCDs in the United States, largely based on retrospective death certificate analyses[4,5] and an emergency rescue data base in one study,[6] have ranged from less than 200,000 to more than 450,000 SCDs annually, with the most widely used estimates in the range of 300,000 to 350,000 SCDs annually.[7] These figures suggest an overall incidence between one and two deaths per 1000 persons among the general population. The absence of a uniformly accepted estimate is based in part on the definition of sudden death and inclusion criteria used in individual studies. An accurate number can be found only from a carefully designed prospective epidemiological study.

The temporal definition of sudden death strongly influences epidemiological data. Retrospective death certificate studies have demonstrated that a temporal definition of death less than 2 hours after the onset of symptoms results in 12 to 15 percent of all natural deaths being defined as "sudden" and nearly 90 percent of all natural sudden deaths having cardiac causes. In contrast, the application of a 24-hour definition of sudden death increases the fraction of all natural deaths falling into the sudden category to more than 30 percent but reduces the proportion of all sudden natural deaths resulting from cardiac causes to 75 percent.

Prospective studies have demonstrated that about 50 percent of all coronary heart disease deaths are sudden and unexpected, occurring shortly (instantaneous to 1 hour) after the onset of symptoms. Because coronary heart disease is the dominant cause of both sudden and nonsudden cardiac deaths in the United States, the fraction of total cardiac deaths that are sudden is similar to the fraction of deaths from coronary heart disease that are sudden, although there does appear to be a geographical variation in the fraction of coronary deaths that are sudden.[8] It is also of interest that the age-adjusted decline in coronary heart disease mortality in the United States during the past half-century[9] has not changed the fraction of coronary deaths that are sudden and unexpected,[10] even though there may be a decline in out-of-hospital deaths compared with emergency department deaths. Furthermore, the decreasing age-adjusted mortality does not imply a decrease in absolute numbers of cardiac or sudden deaths because of the growth and aging of the U.S. population and the increasing prevalence of chronic heart disease.[11,12]

Population Pools and Time Dependence of Risk

Three factors are of primary importance for identifying populations at risk and consideration of strategies for prevention of SCD: (1) the absolute numbers and event rates (incidence) among population subgroups (Fig. 36-2A); (2) the

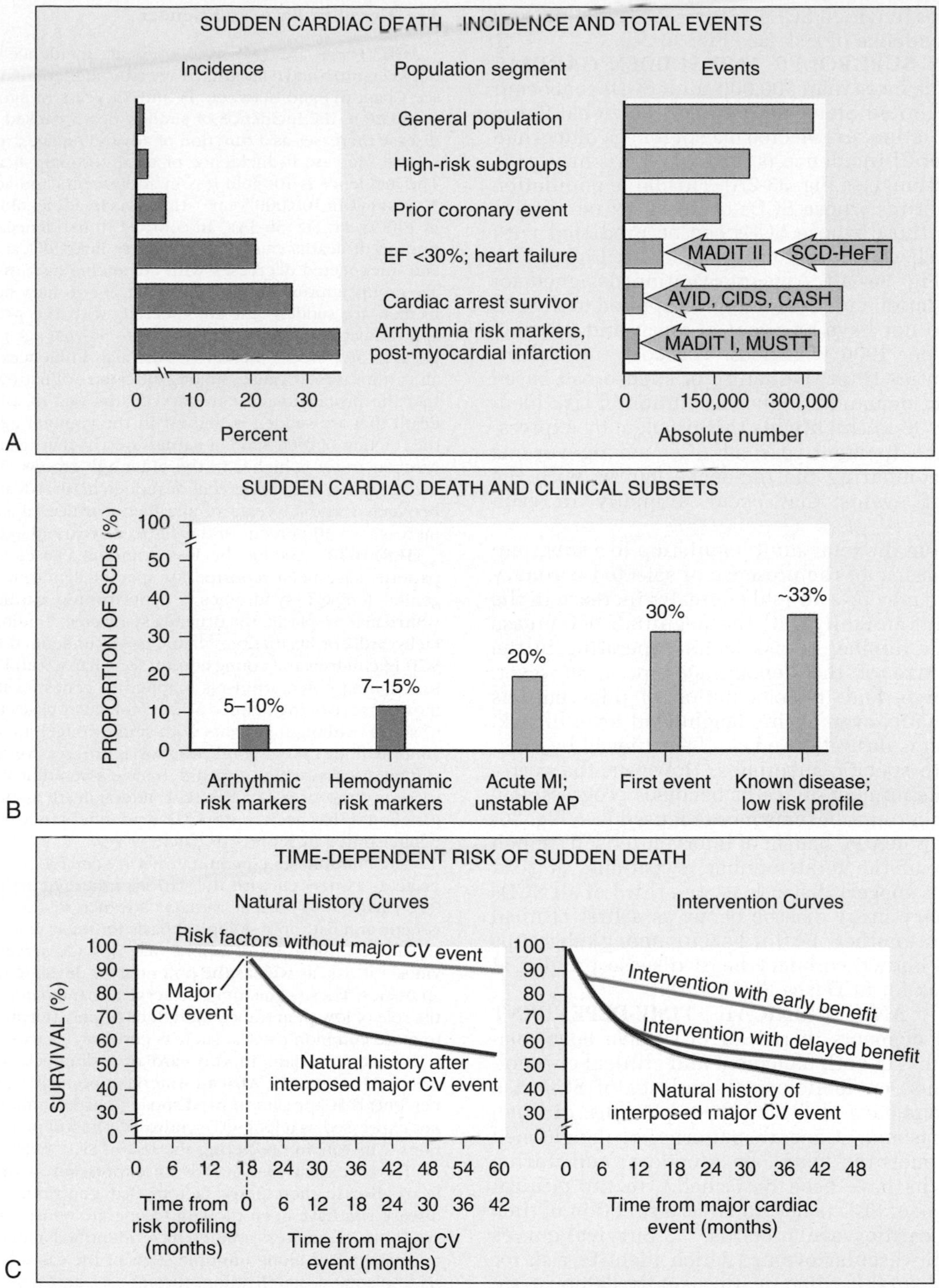

FIGURE 36–2 Impact of population subgroups and time from events on the clinical epidemiology of sudden cardiac death (SCD). **A,** Estimates of incidence (percent/year) and the total number of events per year for the general adult population in the United States and for increasingly high-risk subgroups. The overall adult population has an estimated sudden death incidence of 0.1 to 0.2 percent/year, accounting for a total of more than 300,000 events/year. With the identification of increasingly powerful risk factors, the incidence *increases* progressively, but this is accompanied by a progressive *decrease* in the total number of events represented by each group. The inverse relationship between incidence and total number of events occurs because of the progressively smaller denominator pool in the highest subgroup categories. Successful interventions in larger population subgroups require identification of specific markers to increase the ability to identify specific patients who are at particularly high risk for a future event. (*Note:* The horizontal axis for the incidence figures is not linear and should be interpreted accordingly.) **B,** The distribution of clinical status of victims at the time of SCD. Nearly two thirds of cardiac arrests occur as the first clinically manifest event or in the clinical setting of known disease in the absence of strong risk predictors. Less than 25 percent of the victims have high-risk markers based on arrhythmic or hemodynamic parameters. **C,** SCD risk over time. **Left panel,** The natural history of a population of patients with major risk factors or known cardiovascular disease but at low risk because of freedom from major cardiovascular (CV) events (top curve) is compared with that for patients who have survived a major CV event (bottom curve). Attrition over time is accelerated for the initial 6 to 18 months after the major CV event. After the initial attrition, the slopes of the curves for the high-risk and low-risk populations diverge less, highlighting both the early attrition and attenuation of risk after 18 to 24 months. These relationships have been observed in diverse high-risk subgroups (e.g., cardiac arrest survivors, post–myocardial infarction patients with high-risk markers, recent onset of heart failure). **Right panel,** Shown are two patterns of intervention responses after a major event: a short-term benefit (top), resulting in an early shift of the survival curve without added continuing effect over time, and a delayed but continuing effect over time (bottom). The middle curve illustrates the influence of interventions having delayed benefits on survival curves, without early benefit. AP = angina pectoris; EF = ejection fraction; M.I. = myocardial infarction. *(**A** and **C**, Modified from Myerburg RJ, Kessler KM, Castellanos A: Sudden cardiac death: Structure, function, and time-dependence of risk. Circulation 85(Suppl I):I2, 1992. With permission of the American Heart Association. © 1992 American Heart Association. **B**, Modified from Myerburg RJ: Sudden cardiac death: Exploring the limits of our knowledge. J Cardiovasc Electrophysiol 12:369, 2001.)*

clinical subgroups in which SCDs occur (see Fig. 36-2B); and (3) the time dependence of risk (see Fig. 36-2C).

POPULATION SUBGROUPS AND SUDDEN CARDIAC DEATH. When the more than 300,000 adult SCDs that occur annually in the United States are viewed as a global figure for an adult population, unselected except for age older than 35 years, the overall incidence is 0.1 to 0.2 percent/year (1 to 2/1000 population) (see Fig. 36-2A). This large population base includes victims whose SCDs occur as a first cardiac event as well as those whose SCDs can be predicted with greater accuracy because they are included in higher risk subgroups (see Fig. 36-2B). Any intervention designed for the general population must, therefore, be applied to the 999 per 1000 who do not have an event to reach and possibly influence the 1 per 1000 who does. The cost and risk-to-benefit uncertainties limit the nature of such broad-based interventions and demand a higher resolution of risk identification. Figure 36-2A highlights this problem by expressing the incidence (percent/year) of SCD among various subgroups and comparing the incidence figures with the total number of events that occur annually in each subgroup.

On moving from the total adult population to a subgroup at higher risk because of the presence of selected coronary risk factors, there may be a 10-fold or greater increase in the incidence of events annually, with the magnitude of increase dependent on the number of risk factors operating in the subgroup. The size of the denominator pool, however, remains very large, and implementation of interventions remains problematic, even at this heightened level of risk. Higher resolution is desirable and can be achieved by identification of more specific subgroups. However, the corresponding absolute number of deaths becomes progressively smaller as the subgroups become more focused (see Fig. 36-2A), limiting the potential benefit of interventions to a much smaller fraction of the total number of patients at risk. Various estimates suggest that at least one third of all SCDs related to coronary heart disease occur as a first clinical event. In addition, another one third occur among subgroups of patients with known coronary heart disease profiled at relatively low risk for SCD (see Fig. 36-2B).[9]

BIOLOGICAL AND CLINICAL TIME-DEPENDENT RISK. Temporal elements in risk of SCD have been analyzed in the context of both biological and clinical chronology. In the former, epidemiological analyses of SCD risk among populations have identified three patterns: diurnal, weekly, and seasonal. General patterns of heightened risk during the morning hours, on Mondays, and during the winter months have been described.[13] In the clinical paradigm, the risk of SCD is not linear as a function of time after changes in cardiovascular status.[7,12,14] Survival curves after major cardiovascular events, which identify risk for both sudden and total cardiac death, usually demonstrate that the most rapid rate of attrition occurs during the first 6 to 18 months after the index event (see Fig. 36-2C). Thus, there is a time dependence of risk that focuses the opportunity for maximum efficacy of an intervention during the early period after a conditioning event. Curves that have these characteristics have been generated from among survivors of out-of-hospital cardiac arrest, new onset of heart failure, and unstable angina and from patients having recent myocardial infarction with low ejection fractions and/or heart failure.[15] For the latter, however, early nonarrhythmic deaths also contribute a large proportion of the fatal events. Even though attrition rates decrease over time, an effective intervention can still cause late diversion of treated versus control risk curves, indicating continuing benefit. The addition of time as a dimension for measuring risk may increase the resolution within subgroups.

Age, Heredity, Race, and Gender

AGE. There are two ages of peak incidence of sudden death: between birth and 6 months of age (the sudden infant death syndrome; see Chap. 61) and between 45 and 75 years of age. Among the adult population, the incidence of sudden death caused by coronary heart disease increases as a function of advancing age,[16] paralleling the age-related increase in incidence of total coronary heart disease deaths. The incidence is 100-fold less in adolescents and adults younger than 30 years (1 in 100,000/year)[17] than it is in adults older than 35 years (1 in 1000/year; Fig. 36-3A).[9] In contrast to incidence, however, the proportion of deaths caused by coronary heart diseases that are sudden and unexpected decreases with advancing age. In the 20- to 39-year age group, approximately 75 percent of coronary heart disease deaths in men are sudden and unexpected, with the proportion falling to approximately 60 percent in the 45- to 54-year age group and hovering close to 50 percent thereafter. Age also influences the proportion of all cardiovascular causes among all causes of natural sudden death, in that the proportion of coronary deaths and of all cardiac causes of death that are sudden is highest in the younger age groups, whereas the fraction of total sudden natural deaths that result from any cardiovascular cause is higher in the older age groups. At the other end of the age range, only 19 percent of sudden natural deaths among children between 1 and 13 years of age have cardiac causes; the proportion increases to 30 percent in the 14- to 21-year-old age group.

HEREDITY. Among the less common causes of SCD, hereditary patterns have been reported for specific syndromes such as the congenital long-QT syndromes,[18] hypertrophic cardiomyopathy,[19] right ventricular dysplasia, the Brugada syndrome,[20] "idiopathic" ventricular tachycardia or fibrillation,[21,22] and as yet undefined patterns of familial SCD in children and young adults (see Chaps. 9 and 35). Mutations and functioning polymorphisms mapped to genes located on many chromosomes are being defined as the molecular bases for the entities (see Chap. 9). Although patients with stable congenital conducting system abnormalities have a good prognosis, progressive familial conducting system disease, which appears to have a hereditary pattern, carries an increased risk of SCD.[23] Familial sudden death associated with cardiac ganglionitis has been reported, but an inheritance pattern has not been demonstrated in reports to date.

The multiple specific mutations at gene loci encoding ion channel proteins associated with the various inherited arrhythmia syndromes (see Chap. 9) represent a major advance in the understanding of a genetic and pathophysiological basis for these causes of sudden death. In addition, these observations may provide screening tools for individuals at risk, as well as the potential for devising specific therapeutic strategies. These gene loci also serve as candidates for investigation of the role of low-penetrance mutations or polymorphisms in SCD related to more common causes, such as coronary heart disease. An example is a genetic variant in the cardiac sodium channel gene (*SCN5A*) observed among the African American population (carrier rate = 13.2 percent) that appears to predispose to arrhythmias, even though it is not expressed as a long-QT syndrome phenotype under control conditions.[24] Its role in predicting the risk of SCD awaits clarification.

To the extent that SCD is an expression of underlying coronary heart disease, hereditary factors that contribute to coronary heart disease risk have been thought to operate nonspecifically for the SCD syndrome. However, studies have identified mutations and relevant polymorphisms along multiple steps of the cascade, from atherogenesis to plaque destabilization, thrombosis, and arrhythmogenesis, each of which is associated with increased risk of a coronary event (Fig. 36-4).[25-27] Integration of these individual markers may provide more powerful individual risk prediction in the future. In addition, two population studies have suggested that SCD, as an expression of coronary heart disease, clusters in specific families.[28,29] Whether this familial pattern is genetically or environmentally determined, or both, awaits further clarification.

RACE. A number of studies comparing racial differences in the relative risk of SCD in whites and blacks with coronary heart disease in the United States had yielded conflicting and inconclusive data. However, later studies have demonstrated excess risk of cardiac arrest and SCD among blacks compared with whites (see Fig. 36-3B).[30] SCD rates in Hispanic populations were smaller. The differences were observed across all age groups.

GENDER. The SCD syndrome has a large preponderance in men compared with women during the young adult and early middle-age years because of the protection that women enjoy from coronary atherosclerosis before menopause (see Fig. 36-3B). Various population studies have demonstrated four- to sevenfold excesses of SCD among men compared with women prior to the 65-year-old and older age groups, in which the differences decrease to 2 : 1 or less. As coronary event risk increases in postmenopausal women, SCD risk increases proportionately. Even though the overall risk is much lower in younger women, the classic coronary risk factors are still predictive of events among women,[31] including cigarette smoking, diabetes, use of oral contraceptives, and hyperlipidemia.

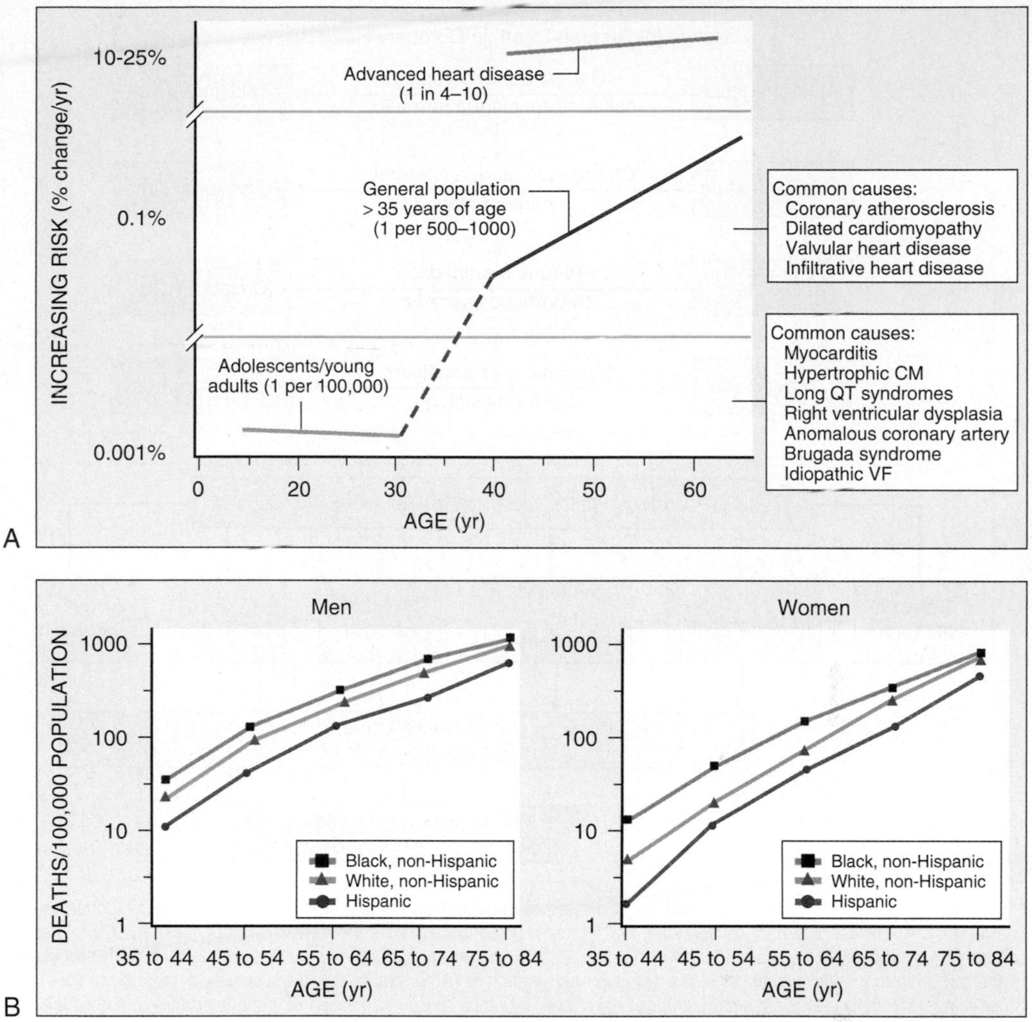

FIGURE 36–3 Age-, gender-, and race-specific risks of sudden cardiac death (SCD). **A,** Age-related and disease-specific risk for SCD. For the general population 35 years of age and older, SCD risk is 0.1 to 0.2 percent/year (1/500 to 1000 population). Among the general population of adolescents and adults younger than 30 years, the overall risk of SCD is 1/100,000 population or 0.001 percent/year. The risk of SCD increases dramatically beyond the age of 35 years and continues to increase past the age of 70 years. The greatest rate of increase is between 40 and 65 years (vertical axis is discontinuous). Among patients older than 30 years, with advanced structural heart disease and markers of high risk for cardiac arrest, the event rate may exceed 25 percent/year, and age-related risk attenuates. Among adolescents and young adults at risk for SCD because of specific identified causes, it is difficult to ascertain risk for individual patients because of variable expression of the disease state. The major risk is electrical, and the competing risk of mechanical heart dysfunction, as in advanced ischemic heart disease or dilated cardiomyopathy, does not contribute significantly to risk in many of these disorders. Therefore, effective electrical interventions are expected to have a better total mortality benefit (see text for details). **B,** SCD risk as a function of age, gender, and race or culture (white, black, and Hispanic). CM = cardiomyopathy; VF = ventricular fibrillation. *(**B,** Modified from Gillum RF: Sudden cardiac death in Hispanic Americans and African Americans. Am J Public Health 87:1461, 1997. Reprinted with permission from the American Public Health Association.)*

Risk Factors for Sudden Cardiac Death

General Profile of Sudden Cardiac Death Risk

Risk profiling for coronary artery disease, by means of the conventional risk factors for coronary atherogenesis, is useful for identifying levels of population risk and individual risk[32] but cannot be used to distinguish individual patients at risk for SCD from those at risk for other manifestations of coronary heart disease. Multivariate analyses of selected risk factors (e.g., age, systolic blood pressure, heart rate, electrocardiographic abnormalities, vital capacity, relative weight, cigarette consumption, and serum cholesterol level) have determined that approximately 50 percent of all SCDs occur among the 10 percent of the population in the highest risk decile, based on multiple risk factors (Fig. 36-5). Thus, the cumulative risk derived from multiple risk factors exceeds the simple arithmetic sum of the individual risks.[32] The comparison of risk factors in the victims of SCD with those in people who develop any manifestations of coronary artery disease does not provide useful patterns, either by univariate or multivariate analysis, to distinguish victims of SCD from the overall pool. In addition, angiographic and hemodynamic patterns discriminate SCD risk from non-SCD risk only under limited conditions. In contrast, familial clustering of SCD as a specific manifestation of the disease may lead to identification of specific genetic abnormalities that predispose to SCD.[28,29]

Hypertension is a clearly established risk factor for coronary heart disease and also emerges as a highly significant risk factor for incidence of SCD.[33,34] However, there is no influence of increasing systolic blood pressure levels on the ratio of sudden deaths to total coronary heart disease deaths. No relationship has been observed between cholesterol concentration and the proportion of coronary deaths that were sudden. Neither the electrocardiographic pattern of left ventricular hypertrophy nor nonspecific ST-T wave abnormalities influence the proportion of total coronary deaths that are sudden and unexpected; only intraventricular conduction abnormalities are suggestive of a disproportionate number of SCDs. The latter is an old observation that is reinforced by data from some device trials that suggest the importance of QRS duration as a risk marker. A low vital capacity also suggests a disproportionate risk for sudden versus total coronary deaths. This is of interest because such a relationship was particularly striking in the Framingham Study in the analysis of data from women who had died suddenly.

The conventional risk factors used in early studies of SCD are the risk factors for the evolution of coronary artery disease. The rationale is based on two facts: (1) coronary disease is the structural basis for 80 percent of SCDs in the

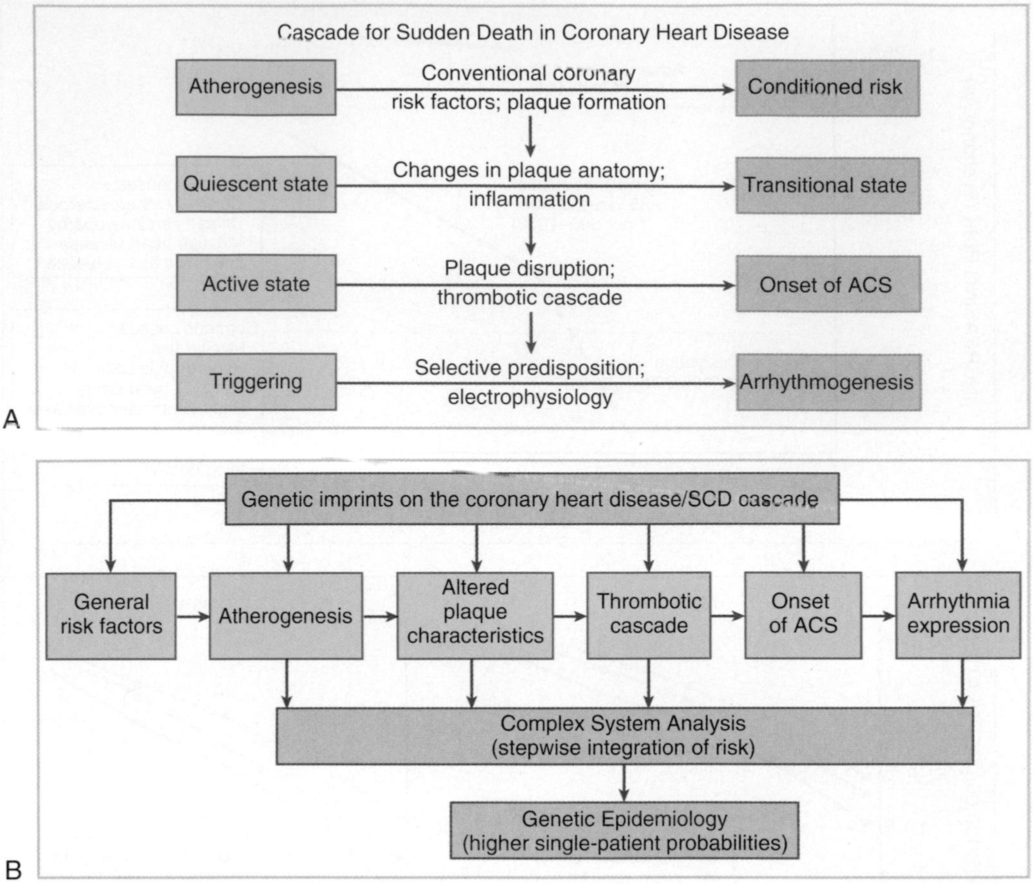

FIGURE 36–4 The coronary atherosclerosis heart disease cascade and genetic imprints on the progression to sudden cardiac death (SCD). **A,** The cascade from conventional risk factors for coronary atherosclerosis to arrhythmogenesis in SCD related to coronary heart disease. The cascade identifies four levels of risk, beginning with lesion initiation and development, progressing to the transition to an active state, then to acute coronary syndromes (ACS), and finally to the specific expression of life-threatening arrhythmias. Multiple factors enter at each level, including specific risk based on genetic profiles of individual patients. **B,** Positions along multiple sites in the cascade from general risk factors for atherosclerosis to arrhythmic expression leading to SCD. Individual risk based on genetic profiles has been identified for atherogenesis, plaque evolution, the thrombotic cascade, and arrhythmia expression. Stepwise integration of these characteristics for individuals through complex analytical methods offers the hope of a field of genetic epidemiology that may lead to higher single-patient probabilities for SCD risk prediction. By integrating the risk associated with each step in the cascade, profiles become more highly specific for individual risk (see text for details). *(Modified from Myerburg RJ: Scientific gaps in the prediction and prevention of sudden cardiac death. J Cardiovasc Electrophysiol 13:709, 2002.)*

United States; and (2) the coronary risk factors are easy to identify because they tend to be present continuously over time (see Fig. 36-4A). However, risk factors specific for fatal arrhythmias are dynamic pathophysiological events and occur transiently.[35] Transient pathophysiological events are being modeled epidemiologically in an attempt to express and use them as clinical risk factors for both profiling and intervention.[2,36] However, data suggest that longitudinal and/or transient risk predictors may have their power blunted by clinical interventions, such as post-myocardial infarction beta blocker therapy.[37]

The identification of specific clinical markers of risk for SCD as a specific expression of both coronary heart disease and other cardiovascular disorders has been a goal for many years.[9,10] Left ventricular ejection fraction has been the most popular of such markers for clinical trials and patient profiling. However, its sensitivity limitations, and inability to identify the large subgroup in which SCD is the first expression of heart disease, have encouraged investigators to seek additional markers. For example, exercise data[23] from a large cohort of males followed for years after a stress test demonstrated that higher resting heart rates, smaller increments in rate during exercise, and a lower decrement in heart rate during the first minute after exercise was a profile that predicted higher risk of SCD during follow-up.[38] In addition, a number of electrocardiographic indicators, such as microvolt T-wave alternans and indices of Q-T duration and dispersion, genetic profiles, and other indices of extent of disease, are also predictive (see Chap. 33).

FUNCTIONAL CAPACITY AND SUDDEN DEATH. The Framingham Study demonstrated a striking relationship between functional classification and death during a 2-year follow-up period. However, the proportion of deaths that were sudden did not vary with functional classification, ranging from 50 to 57 percent in all groups and from those free of clinical heart disease to those in functional class IV. Other studies have also suggested that patients with heart failure with better functional capacity are at lower risk of dying, as expected, but a higher proportion of those deaths are sudden.[10]

LIFE STYLE AND PSYCHOSOCIAL FACTORS

LIFE STYLE. There is a strong association between cigarette smoking and all manifestations of coronary heart disease. The Framingham Study demonstrated that cigarette smokers have a twofold to threefold increase in sudden death risk in each decade of life at entry between 30 and 59 years, and that this is one of the few risk factors in which the proportion of coronary heart disease deaths that are sudden increases in association with the risk factor. In addition, in a study of 310 survivors of out-of-hospital cardiac arrest, the recurrent cardiac arrest rate was 27 percent at 3 years of follow-up among those who continued to smoke after their index event compared with 19 percent in those who stopped ($p < 0.04$).[39] Obesity is a second factor that appears to influence the proportion of coronary deaths that occur suddenly. With increasing relative weight, the percentage of coronary heart disease deaths that were sudden in the Framingham Study increased linearly from a low of 39 percent to a high of 70 percent. Total coronary heart disease deaths increased with increasing relative weight as well.

Associations between levels of physical activity and SCD have been studied with variable results. Epidemiological observations have suggested a relationship between low levels of physical activity and increased coronary heart disease death risk. The Framingham Study, however, showed an insignificant relationship between low levels of physical activity and incidence of sudden death, but a high proportion of sudden to total cardiac deaths at higher levels of physical activity. An association between acute physical exertion and the onset of myocardial infarction has been suggested, particularly among individuals who are habitually physically inactive.[36] A subsequent case-crossover cohort study confirmed this observation for SCD, demonstrating a 17-fold relative increase in SCD associated with vigorous exercise compared with lower level activity or inactive states.[40] However, the absolute risk for events was very low (1 event/1.5 million exercise sessions). Habitual vigorous exercise markedly attenuated risk. In contrast, SCD among young athletes has a higher incidence than among young nonathletic individuals in the same age range (see Chap. 78).[41] Information about physical activity relationships in various clinical settings, such as overt and silent disease states, is still lacking.

PSYCHOSOCIAL FACTORS. The magnitude of recent life changes in the realms of health, work, home and family, and personal and social factors has been related to myocardial infarction and SCD.[42-44] There is an association with significant elevations of life change scores during the 6 months before a coronary event, and the association is particularly striking in victims of SCD. Among women, those who die suddenly are less often married, had fewer children, and had greater educational discrepancies with their spouses than did age-related control subjects living in the same neighborhood as the victims of sudden death. A history of psychiatric treatment, cigarette smoking, and greater quantities of alcohol consumption than the control subjects also characterized the sudden death group. Controlling for other major prognostic factors, risk of sudden and total deaths, and other coronary events is affected by social and economic stresses. Alteration of modifiable life-style factors has been proposed as a strategy for reducing risk of SCD in patients with coronary heart disease,[45] although a study of treatment of depression following myocardial infarction failed to demonstrate an effect on event rates.[46] Acute psychosocial stressors have been associated with a higher risk of cardiovascular events, including SCD.[47-49] The risk appears to cluster around the time of the stress and appears to occur among victims at preexisting risk, with the stressor simply advancing the time of an impending event.[47] The possibility of physical stress-induced coronary plaque disruption also has been suggested.[50]

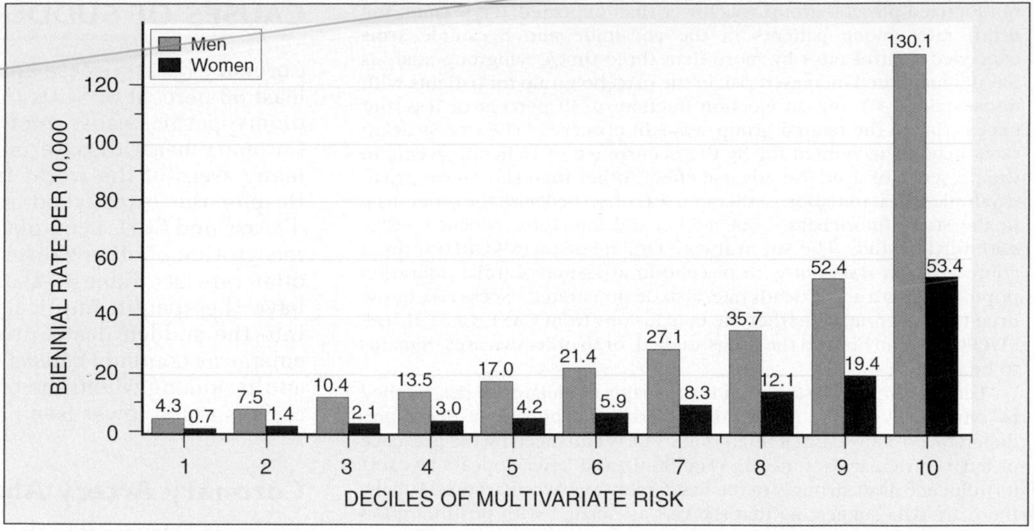

FIGURE 36–5 Risk of sudden death by decile of multivariant risk—26-year follow-up, the Framingham Study. The variables included are age, systolic blood pressure, left ventricular hypertrophy, intraventricular block on the electrocardiogram, nonspecific electrocardiographic abnormalities, serum cholesterol, heart rate, vital capacity, cigarettes consumed daily, and relative weight. *(Modified from Kannel WB, Shatzkin A: Sudden death: Lessons from subsets in population studies. J Am Coll Cardiol 5[Suppl 6]:141B, 1985. Reprinted by permission of the American College of Cardiology.)*

SUDDEN DEATH AND PREVIOUS CORONARY HEART DISEASE. Although SCD is the first clinical manifestation of coronary heart disease in 20 to 25 percent or more of all coronary heart disease patients[1,7,9] and is the first clinical manifestation in more than 30 percent of coronary heart disease-related SCDs (see Fig. 36-2),[9,51] a previous myocardial infarction can be identified in as many as 75 percent of patients who die suddenly. The high incidence of both recognized and unrecognized prior myocardial infarction in victims of SCD has led to a search for predictors of SCD in survivors of myocardial infarction, as well as in patients with other clinical manifestations of coronary heart disease and those with clinically silent disease.

LEFT VENTRICULAR EJECTION FRACTION IN CHRONIC ISCHEMIC HEART DISEASE. A marked reduction of the left ventricular ejection fraction is the most powerful of the known predictors of SCD in patients with chronic ischemic heart disease, as well as those at risk for SCD from other causes (see later). Increased risk, independent of other risk factors, is measurable at ejection fractions higher than 40 percent, but the greatest rate of change of risk is between 30 and 40 percent. An ejection fraction equal to or less than 30 percent is the single most powerful independent predictor for SCD, but has low specificity. Nonetheless, relying on a low ejection fraction as the sole major predictor limits predictive power, because a significant proportion of SCDs may occur among patients with normal or moderately reduced values.[52]

VENTRICULAR ARRHYTHMIAS IN CHRONIC ISCHEMIC HEART DISEASE. Most forms of ambient ventricular ectopic activity (premature ventricular complexes, PVCs, and short runs of nonsustained ventricular tachycardia, VT) have a benign prognosis in the absence of structural heart disease. An exception is polymorphic forms of nonsustained VT that occur in patients without structural heart disease but can have a molecular, functional, drug-related, or electrolyte-related basis for high-risk arrhythmias.[53] When present in subjects in the coronary-prone age groups, however, PVCs select a subgroup with a higher probability of coronary artery disease and of SCD. Exercise-induced PVCs and short runs of nonsustained VT indicate some level of SCD risk,[54] even in the absence of recognizable structural heart disease. However, the data available to support this hypothesis are conflicting, with the possible exception of polymorphic runs of nonsustained VT.[53] Additional data suggest that PVCs and nonsustained VT during both the exercise and recovery phases of a stress test are predictive of increased risk.[55] Arrhythmias in the recovery phase, previously thought to be benign, appear to predict higher risk than arrhythmias in the exercise phase, and there is a gradient of risk with increasing severity of arrhythmias.

The occurrence of PVCs in survivors of myocardial infarction, particularly if frequent and of complex forms such as repetitive PVCs, predicts an increased risk of SCD and total mortality during long-term follow-up. There are conflicting data on the role of measures of frequency and forms of ventricular ectopic activity as discriminators of risk, but most studies have cited a frequency cutoff of 10 PVCs/hour as a threshold level for increased risk. Several investigators have emphasized that the most powerful predictors among the various forms of PVCs are runs of nonsustained VT, although this relationship is now questioned. Many of the reported studies have been based on a single ambulatory monitor sample recorded 1 week to several months after the onset of acute myocardial infarction, and the duration of the samples has ranged from 1 to 48 hours. Other studies have suggested that ambulatory ventricular arrhythmias in patients with heart failure do not specifically predict an increased risk of death.[56]

The results of the Cardiac Arrhythmia Suppression Trial (CAST) (see Chap. 33), designed to test the hypothesis that PVC suppression by antiarrhythmic drugs alters the risk of SCD after myocardial infarction were surprising for two reasons. First, the death rate in the randomized placebo group was lower than expected and second, the death rate among patients in the encainide and flecainide arms exceeded control rates by more than three times. Subgroup analysis has demonstrated increased risk in the placebo group for patients with nonsustained VT and an ejection fraction of 30 percent or less, but excess risk in the treated group was still observed. The excess death rates may be accounted for by the occurrence of ischemic events in the presence of drug. No adverse effect (other than short-term proarrhythmic risk at initiation of therapy) was observed with the other drug in the study (moricizine), but neither did long-term benefit emerge with further study. The Survival with Oral *d*-Sotalol (SWORD) study, a comparison of *d*-sotalol with placebo in a post-myocardial infarction population with a low death rate, also demonstrated excess risk in the drug-treated group. Whether the conclusions from CAST, CAST II, and SWORD extend beyond the drugs studied, or to other diseases, remains to be learned.

Left ventricular dysfunction is the major modulator of risk implied by chronic PVCs after myocardial infarction. The risk of death predicted by post-myocardial infarction PVCs is enhanced by the presence of left ventricular dysfunction (Fig. 36-6); the latter appears to exert its influence most strongly in the first 6 months after infarction. Finally, there are data suggesting that the risk associated with postinfarction ventricular arrhythmias is higher in patients who have non-Q-wave infarctions than in those with transmural infarctions.

CAUSES OF SUDDEN CARDIAC DEATH

Coronary heart disease and its consequences account for at least 80 percent of SCDs in Western countries, and the cardiomyopathies cause another 10 to 15 percent (Table 36-2). Coronary heart disease is also the most common cause in many areas of the world in which its prevalence is lower. Despite the established relation between coronary heart disease and SCD, a complete understanding of SCD requires recognition of other causes that, although less common and often rare (see Table 36-2), may be recognizable before death, have therapeutic implications, and provide broad insight into the sudden death problem.[57,58] Many of these entities emerge as common causes of SCD in adolescents and young adults, among whom the prevalence of coronary atherosclerosis is much lower (see Fig. 36-3A).

Coronary Artery Abnormalities

Although structural abnormalities of coronary arteries other than coronary atherosclerosis are infrequent causes of

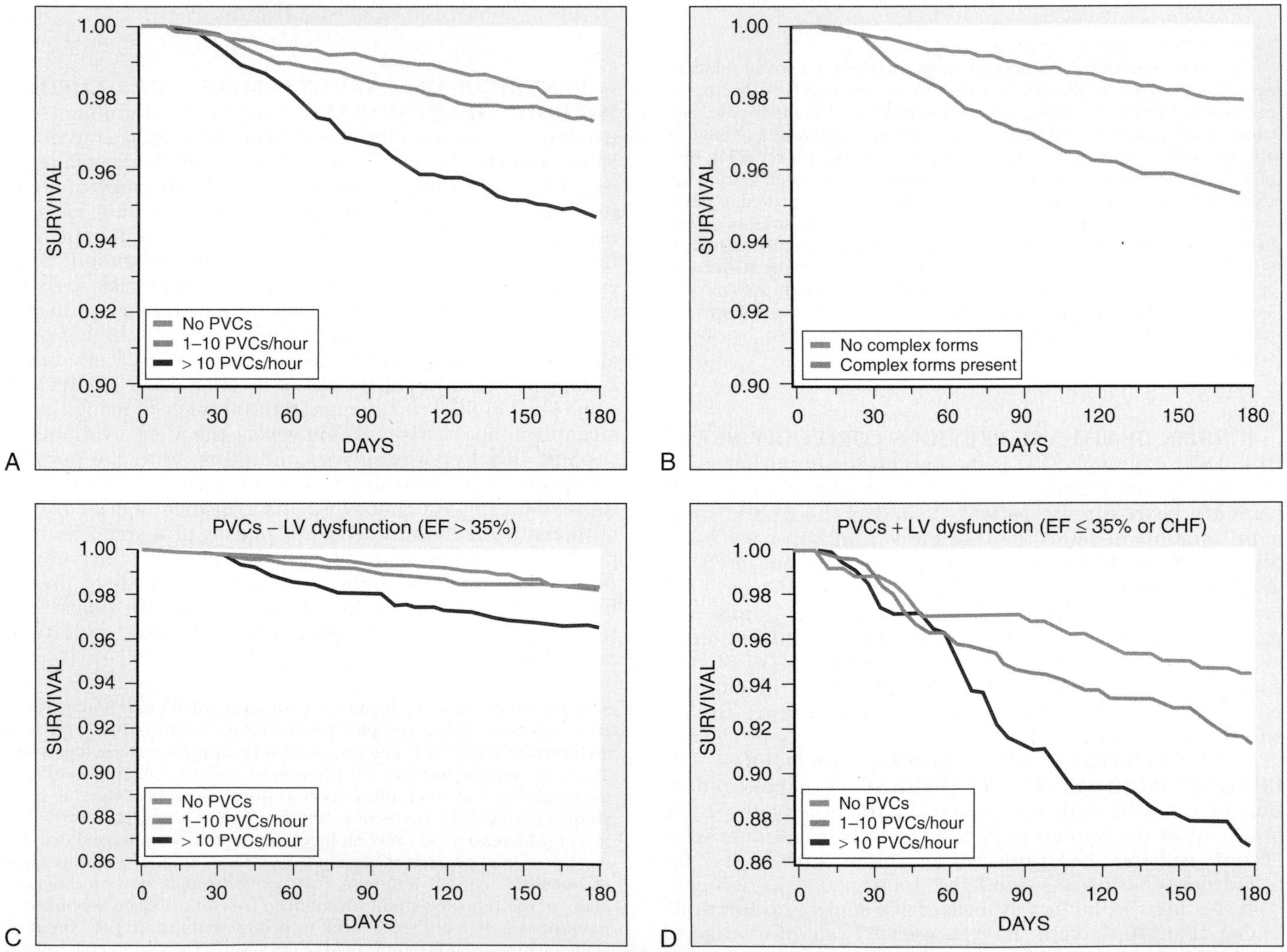

FIGURE 36–6 Prognostic significance of ventricular arrhythmias after myocardial infarction. The Gruppo Italiano per lo Studio della Sopravvivenza nell'Infarto Miocardico (GISSI)-2 data demonstrate that, in the thrombolytic era, frequent premature ventricular complexes (PVCs) carry prognostic information for mortality in the 6 months after an acute myocardial infarction, as previously reported in earlier studies. PVCs occurring at a frequency of more than 10/hour **(A)** and the presence of complex forms **(B)** both have an adverse effect on survival, although the latter did not hold up as an independent predictor on multivariate analysis. **C,** When PVCs occurred in the absence of left ventricular (LV) dysfunction (defined as ejection fraction, EF, less than 35 percent or the occurrence of congestive heart failure, CHF, during the event), the predictive power of frequent PVCs was reduced and, in the presence of LV dysfunction **(D)** it was enhanced. *(From Maggioni AP, Zuanetti G, Franzosi MG, et al: Prevalence and prognostic significance of ventricular arrhythmias after acute myocardial infarction in the fibrinolytic era: GISSI-2 results. Circulation 87:312, 1993.)*

TABLE 36–2 Causes and Contributing Factors in Sudden Cardiac Death

I. Coronary artery abnormalities
  A. Coronary atherosclerosis
    1. Chronic coronary atherosclerosis with acute or transient myocardial ischemia—thrombosis, spasm, physical stress
    2. Acute myocardial infarction, onset and early phase
    3. Chronic atherosclerosis with change in myocardial substrate, including prior myocardial infarction
  B. Congenital abnormalities of coronary arteries
    1. Anomalous origin from pulmonary artery
    2. Other coronary arteriovenous fistula
    3. Origin of a left coronary branch from right or noncoronary sinus of Valsalva
    4. Origin of right coronary artery from left sinus of Valsalva
    5. Hypoplastic or aplastic coronary arteries
    6. Coronary-intracardiac shunt
  C. Coronary artery embolism
    1. Aortic or mitral endocarditis
    2. Prosthetic aortic or mitral valves
    3. Abnormal native valves or left ventricular mural thrombus
    4. Platelet embolism
  D. Coronary arteritis
    1. Polyarteritis nodosa, progressive systemic sclerosis, giant cell arteritis
    2. Mucocutaneous lymph node syndrome (Kawasaki disease)
    3. Syphilitic coronary ostial stenosis
  E. Miscellaneous mechanical obstruction of coronary arteries
    1. Coronary artery dissection in Marfan syndrome
    2. Coronary artery dissection in pregnancy
    3. Prolapse of aortic valve myxomatous polyps into coronary ostia
    4. Dissection or rupture of sinus of Valsalva
  F. Functional obstruction of coronary arteries
    1. Coronary artery spasm with or without atherosclerosis
    2. Myocardial bridges

II. Hypertrophy of ventricular myocardium
  A. Left ventricular hypertrophy associated with coronary heart disease
  B. Hypertensive heart disease without significant coronary atherosclerosis
  C. Hypertrophic myocardium secondary to valvular heart disease
  D. Hypertrophic cardiomyopathy
    1. Obstructive
    2. Nonobstructive
  E. Primary or secondary pulmonary hypertension
    1. Advanced chronic right ventricular overload
    2. Pulmonary hypertension in pregnancy (highest risk peripartum)

III. Myocardial diseases and heart failure
  A. Chronic congestive heart failure
    1. Ischemic cardiomyopathy
    2. Idiopathic dilated cardiomyopathy
      a. Acquired
      b. Hereditary
    3. Alcoholic cardiomyopathy
    4. Hypertensive cardiomyopathy
    5. Postmyocarditis cardiomyopathy
    6. Peripartum cardiomyopathy
  B. Acute and subacute cardiac failure
    1. Massive acute myocardial infarction
    2. Acute myocarditis
    3. Acute alcoholic cardiac dysfunction
    4. Takotsubo syndrome (uncertain sudden death risk)
    5. Ball-valve embolism in aortic stenosis or prosthesis
    6. Mechanical disruptions of cardiac structures
      a. Rupture of ventricular free wall
      b. Disruption of mitral apparatus
        (1) Papillary muscle
        (2) Chordae tendineae
        (3) Leaflet
      c. Rupture of interventricular septum
    7. Acute pulmonary edema in noncompliant ventricles

IV. Inflammatory, infiltrative, neoplastic, and degenerative processes
  A. Viral myocarditis, with or without ventricular dysfunction
    1. Acute phase
    2. Postmyocarditis interstitial fibrosis
  B. Myocarditis associated with the vasculitides
  C. Sarcoidosis
  D. Progressive systemic sclerosis
  E. Amyloidosis
  F. Hemochromatosis
  G. Idiopathic giant cell myocarditis
  H. Chagas' disease
  I. Cardiac ganglionitis
  J. Arrhythmogenic right ventricular dysplasia; right ventricular cardiomyopathy
  K. Neuromuscular diseases (e.g., muscular dystrophy, Friedreich ataxia, myotonic dystrophy)
  L. Intramural tumors
    1. Primary
    2. Metastatic
  M. Obstructive intracavitary tumors
    1. Neoplastic
    2. Thrombotic

V. Diseases of the cardiac valves
  A. Valvular aortic stenosis/insufficiency
  B. Mitral valve disruption
  C. Mitral valve prolapse
  D. Endocarditis
  E. Prosthetic valve dysfunction

VI. Congenital heart disease
  A. Congenital aortic or pulmonic valve stenosis
  B. Right-to-left shunts with Eisenmenger physiology
    1. Advanced disease
    2. During labor and delivery
  C. Late after surgical repair of congenital lesions (e.g., tetralogy of Fallot)

VII. Electrophysiological abnormalities
  A. Abnormalities of the conducting system
    1. Fibrosis of the His-Purkinje system
      a. Primary degeneration (Lenègre's disease)
      b. Secondary to fibrosis and calcification of the "cardiac skeleton" (Lev disease)
      c. Postviral conducting system fibrosis
      d. Hereditary conducting system disease
    2. Anomalous pathways of conduction (Wolff-Parkinson-White syndrome, short refractory period bypass)
  B. Abnormalities of repolarization
    1. Congenital abnormalities of QT interval duration
      a. Congenital long-QT interval syndromes
        (1) Romano-Ward syndrome (without deafness)
        (2) Jervell and Lange-Nielsen syndrome (with deafness)
      b. Congenital short QT interval syndrome
    2. Acquired (or provoked) long QT interval syndromes
      a. Drug effect (with genetic predisposition?)
        (1) Cardiac, antiarrhythmic
        (2) Noncardiac
        (3) Drug interactions
      b. Electrolyte abnormality (response modified by genetic predisposition?)
      c. Toxic substances
      d. Hypothermia
      e. Central nervous system injury; subarachnoid hemorrhage
    3. Brugada syndrome—right bundle branch block and ST segment elevations in the absence of ischemia
  C. Ventricular fibrillation of unknown or uncertain cause
    1. Absence of identifiable structural or functional causes
      a. "Idiopathic" ventricular fibrillation
      b. Short-coupled torsades de pointes, polymorphic ventricular tachycardia
      c. Nonspecific fibrofatty infiltration in previously healthy victim (variation of right ventricular dysplasia?)

Table continues

TABLE 36–2 Causes and Contributing Factors in Sudden Cardiac Death—cont'd

2. Sleep-death in Southeast Asians (see VIIB3, Brugada syndrome) a. Bangungut b. Pokkuri c. Lai-tai	2. After corrective surgery for congenital heart disease 3. Myocarditis 4. Genetic disorders of electrical function (e.g., long-QT interval syndrome) 5. No identified structural or functional cause
VIII. Electrical instability related to neurohumoral and central nervous system influences A. Catecholamine-dependent lethal arrhythmias B. Central nervous system related 1. Psychic stress, emotional extremes 2. Auditory related 3. "Voodoo death" in primitive cultures 4. Diseases of the cardiac nerves 5. Arrhythmia expression in congenital long-QT interval syndrome IX. Sudden infant death syndrome and sudden death in children A. Sudden infant death syndrome 1. Immature respiratory control functions 2. Long-QT interval syndrome 3. Congenital heart disease 4. Myocarditis B. Sudden death in children 1. Eisenmenger syndrome, aortic stenosis, hypertrophic cardiomyopathy, pulmonary atresia	X. Miscellaneous A. Sudden death during extreme physical activity (seek predisposing causes) B. Commotio cordis—blunt chest trauma C. Mechanical interference with venous return 1. Acute cardiac tamponade 2. Massive pulmonary embolism 3. Acute intracardiac thrombosis D. Dissecting aneurysm of the aorta E. Toxic and metabolic disturbances (other than QT-interval effects listed above) 1. Electrolyte disturbances 2. Metabolic disturbances 3. Proarrhythmic effects of antiarrhythmic drugs 4. Proarrhythmic effects of noncardiac drugs F. Mimics sudden cardiac death 1. "Café coronary" 2. Acute alcoholic states ("holiday heart") 3. Acute asthmatic attacks 4. Air or amniotic fluid embolism

SCD, the relative risk of SCD may be high for specific abnormalities. Nonatherosclerotic coronary artery abnormalities include congenital lesions, coronary artery embolism, coronary arteritis, and mechanical abnormalities of the coronary arteries. Among the congenital lesions, anomalous origin of a left coronary artery from the pulmonary artery (see Chaps. 61 and 78) is relatively common and associated with a high death rate in infancy and early childhood without surgical treatment. The early risk for SCD is not excessively high, but patients who survive to adulthood without surgical intervention are at risk for SCD. Other forms of coronary arteriovenous fistulas are much less frequent and associated with a low incidence of SCD.

ANOMALOUS ORIGIN OF CORONARY ARTERIES FROM THE INAPPROPRIATE SINUS OF VALSALVA (see Chap. 78). These anatomical variants are associated with an increased risk of SCD,[59] particularly during exercise. When the anomalous artery passes between the aortic and the pulmonary artery root, the takeoff angle of the anomalous ostium creates a slit-like opening of the vessel, reducing the effective cross-sectional area for blood flow. Congenitally hypoplastic, stenotic, or atretic left coronary arteries are uncommon abnormalities associated with a high risk of myocardial infarction but not of SCD.

EMBOLISM TO THE CORONARY ARTERIES. Coronary artery emboli occur most commonly in aortic valve endocarditis and from thrombotic material on diseased or prosthetic aortic or mitral valves. Emboli can also originate from left ventricular mural thrombi or as a consequence of surgery or cardiac catheterization. Symptoms and signs of myocardial ischemia or infarction are the most common manifestations. In each of these categories, SCD is a risk resulting from the electrophysiological consequences of the embolic ischemic event.

MUCOCUTANEOUS LYMPH NODE SYNDROME (KAWASAKI DISEASE) (see Chap. 84). This syndrome carries a risk of SCD in association with coronary arteritis. Polyarteritis nodosa and related vasculitis syndromes can cause SCD, presumably because of coronary arteritis, as can coronary ostial stenosis in syphilitic aortitis. The latter has become a rare manifestation of syphilis.

MECHANICAL OBSTRUCTION TO CORONARY ARTERIES. Several types of mechanical abnormalities are listed among the causes of SCD. Coronary dissection, with or without dissection of the aorta, occurs in Marfan syndrome (see Chap. 61) and has also been reported after trauma and in the peripartum period of pregnancy. Among the rare mechanical causes of SCD is prolapse of myxomatous polyps from the aortic valve into coronary ostia, as well as dissection or rupture of a sinus of Valsalva aneurysm, with involvement of the coronary ostia and proximal coronary arteries. Finally, deep myocardial bridges over coronary arteries (see Chap. 78) have been reported in association with SCD occurring during strenuous exercise, possibly caused by dynamic mechanical obstruction. However, most myocardial bridges are inconsequential and SCD associated with this anatomy is uncommon.

CORONARY ARTERY SPASM (see Chap. 50). Coronary vasospasm may cause serious arrhythmias and SCD. It is usually associated with some degree of concomitant coronary atherosclerotic disease. Painless myocardial ischemia, associated with either spasm or fixed lesions, is now recognized as a mechanism of previously unexplained sudden death.[60] Different patterns of silent ischemia (e.g., totally asymptomatic, post-myocardial infarction, and mixed silent-anginal pattern) may have different prognostic implications.

Ventricular Hypertrophy and Hypertrophic Cardiomyopathy (see Chaps. 64 and 78)

Left ventricular hypertrophy is an independent risk factor for SCD, accompanies many causes of SCD, and may be a physiological contributor to mechanisms of potentially lethal arrhythmias.[33,34] The underlying states resulting in hypertrophy include hypertensive heart disease with or without atherosclerosis, valvular heart disease, obstructive and nonobstructive hypertrophic cardiomyopathy, primary pulmonary hypertension with right ventricular hypertrophy, and advanced right ventricular overload secondary to congenital heart disease. Each of these conditions is associated with risk of SCD, and it has been suggested that patients with severely hypertrophic ventricles are particularly susceptible to arrhythmic death.

Risk of SCD in obstructive and nonobstructive hypertrophic cardiomyopathy was identified in the early clinical and hemodynamic descriptions of this entity. Among patients who have the obstructive form, up to 70 percent of all deaths are sudden. However, survivors of cardiac arrest in this group may have a better long-term outcome than survivors with other causes, and reports have suggested that the risk of primary cardiac arrest and SCD in hypertrophic cardiomyopathy is lower than previously thought.[61]

A substantial proportion of patients with obstructive and nonobstructive cardiomyopathy have a family history of affected relatives or premature SCDs of unknown cause. Genetic studies have confirmed autosomal dominant inheritance patterns, with a great deal of allele and phenotypic heterogeneity. Most of the mutations are at loci that encode elements in the contractile protein complex, the most common being beta-myosin heavy chain and cardiac troponin T, which together account for more than half of identified abnormalities.[19] In the beta-myosin heavy chain form, there is a relationship between severity of left ventricular hypertrophy and risk of SCD; in the troponin T form, left ventricular hypertrophy is less severe, despite SCD risk. The genetics of hypertrophic cardiomyopathy is characterized by a large number of private mutations in individual families with variable expression. Possible interaction with modifier genes, such as variations in ion channel genes, remains to be clarified.

Specific clinical markers have not been especially predictive of SCD in individual patients, although young age at onset, strong family history of SCD, magnitude of left ventricular mass, ventricular arrhythmias, and worsening symptoms (especially syncope) appear to indicate higher risk.[61-64] Early studies have suggested that a low resting outflow gradient, with a substantial provocable gradient, identifies a high risk of SCD. A more recent study has supported the predictive power of a high resting gradient.[64] The mechanism of SCD in patients with hypertrophic obstructive cardiomyopathy was initially thought to involve outflow tract obstruction, possibly as a consequence of catecholamine stimulation, but later data have focused on lethal arrhythmias as the common mechanism of sudden death in this disease. Risk is also thought to be suggested by PVCs and nonsustained VT on ambulatory recording or the inducibility of potentially lethal arrhythmias during programmed electrical stimulation. However, stable and asymptomatic nonsustained VT has limited predictive power for SCD in these patients. Rapid or polymorphic symptomatic nonsustained tachycardias, or both, have better predictive power.

The question of whether the pathogenesis of the arrhythmias represents an interaction between electrophysiological and hemodynamic abnormalities or is a consequence of electrophysiological derangement of hypertrophied muscle is unanswered. The observation that patients with nonobstructive hypertrophic cardiomyopathy have high-risk arrhythmias and are at increased risk for SCD suggests that an electrophysiological mechanism secondary to the hypertrophied muscle itself plays some role. In athletes younger than 35 years, hypertrophic cardiomyopathy is the most common cause of SCD, in contrast to athletes older than 35, among whom ischemic heart disease is the most common cause.[65]

Dilated Cardiomyopathy and Heart Failure

The advent of therapeutic interventions that provide better long-term control of congestive heart failure has improved long-term survival of these patients (see Chaps. 23 and 25). However, the proportion of patients with heart failure who die suddenly is substantial, especially among those who appear clinically stable (i.e., functional class I or II).[66] The mechanism of SCD (VT or ventricular fibrillation, VF, versus bradyarrhythmia or asystole) appears to be related to cause (i.e., ischemic versus nonischemic). The absolute risk of SCD increases with deteriorating left ventricular function, but the ratio of sudden to nonsudden deaths is related inversely to the extent of functional impairment.[66] Among patients with cardiomyopathy who have good functional capacity (classes I and II), total mortality risk is considerably lower than for those with poor functional capacity (classes III and IV), but the probability that a death will be sudden is higher (Fig. 36-7). Unexplained syncope has been observed to be a powerful predictor of SCD in patients who have functional class III or IV symptoms, regardless of the cause of cardiomyopathy. Ambulatory ventricular arrhythmias do not appear to indicate specific SCD risk in such patients.[56,67,68]

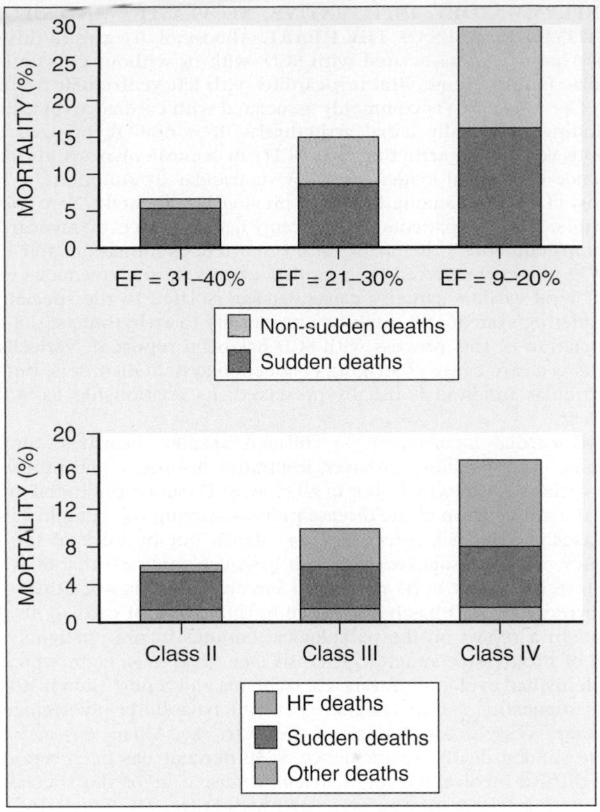

FIGURE 36–7 Risk of sudden cardiac death related to LV ejection fraction (EF) and functional classification in heart failure (HF). The relative probability of death being sudden is higher, and absolute mortality risk lower, among patients with higher ejection fractions and better functional capacity. *(Modified from Cleland JG, Chattopadhyay S, Khand A, et al: Prevalence and incidence of arrhythmias and sudden death in heart failure. Heart Fail Rev 7:229, 2002, with kind permission from Springer Science and Business Media.)*

The interaction between post-myocardial infarction ventricular arrhythmia and depressed ejection fraction in determining risk for SCD has been described. Most studies addressing the relationship between chronic congestive heart failure and SCD have focused on patients with ischemic, idiopathic, alcoholic, and postmyocarditis congestive cardiomyopathy. Peripartum cardiomyopathy (see Chap. 77) may also cause SCD.

Acute Heart Failure

All causes of acute cardiac failure (see Chap. 22), in the absence of prompt interventions, can result in SCD caused by the circulatory failure itself or secondary arrhythmias. The electrophysiological mechanisms involved have been proposed to be caused by acute stretching of myocardial fibers or the His-Purkinje system on the basis of its experimentally demonstrated arrhythmogenic effects. However, the roles of neurohumoral mechanisms and acute electrolyte shifts have not been fully evaluated. Among the causes of acute cardiac failure associated with SCD are massive acute myocardial infarction, acute myocarditis, acute alcoholic cardiac dysfunction, acute pulmonary edema in any form of advanced heart disease, and a number of mechanical causes of heart failure, such as massive pulmonary embolism, mechanical disruption of intracardiac structures secondary to infarction or infection, and ball-valve embolism in aortic or mitral stenosis (see Table 36-2).

INFLAMMATORY, INFILTRATIVE, NEOPLASTIC, AND DEGENERATIVE DISEASES OF THE HEART. Almost all diseases in this category have been associated with SCD, with or without concomitant cardiac failure. Acute viral myocarditis with left ventricular dysfunction (see Chap. 66) is commonly associated with cardiac arrhythmias, including potentially lethal arrhythmias. It is now recognized that serious ventricular arrhythmias or SCD can occur in myocarditis in the absence of clinical evidence of left ventricular dysfunction.[69,70] In a report of 19 SCDs among 1,606,167 previously screened U.S. Air Force recruits, 8 of 19 patients (42 percent) had evidence of myocarditis (5 nonrheumatic, 3 rheumatic) at postmortem examination, and 15 of 19 (79 percent) suffered their cardiac arrests during strenuous exertion. Viral carditis can also cause damage isolated to the specialized conducting system and result in a propensity to arrhythmias; the rare association of this process with SCD has been reported. Varicella in adults is a rare cause of striking conduction system disorders, but left ventricular function is usually preserved; its relationship to SCD is unclear.

Myocardial involvement in collagen-vascular disorders, tumors, chronic granulomatous diseases, infiltrative disorders, and protozoan infestations varies widely, but in all cases SCD can be the initial or terminal manifestation of the disease process. Among the granulomatous diseases, sarcoidosis (see Chap. 64) stands out because of the frequency of SCD associated with it. It has been reported that SCD was the terminal event in 67 percent of sarcoid heart disease deaths; the occurrence of SCD has been related to the extent of cardiac involvement. In a report on the pathological findings in nine patients who died of progressive systemic sclerosis (see Chap. 64), eight who died suddenly had evidence of transient ischemia and reperfusion histologically, suggesting that this might represent Raynaud-like involvement of coronary vessels. Amyloidosis of the heart (see Chap. 64) may also cause sudden death. An incidence of 30 percent has been reported, and diffuse involvement of ventricular muscle or of the specialized conducting system may be associated with SCD.

ARRHYTHMOGENIC RIGHT VENTRICULAR DYSPLASIA OR RIGHT VENTRICULAR CARDIOMYOPATHY (see Chap. 35). This condition is associated with a high incidence of ventricular arrhythmias, including polymorphic nonsustained VT and VF and recurrent sustained monomorphic VT.[71] Although symptomatic monomorphic VT has been well recognized in the syndrome for many years, the risk of SCD was unclear and thought to be relatively low. However, the features of the disease and risks associated with it have now been clarified by a number of studies.[72-74] In a high proportion of victims, perhaps as many as 80 percent, the first manifestation of the disease is "unexplained" syncope or SCD.[72] SCD is often exercise-related and, in some areas of the world where screening for hypertrophic cardiomyopathy has excluded the affected athletes from competition, right ventricular dysplasia has emerged as the most common cause of sports-related SCD.[75]

The genetic basis for right ventricular dysplasia has been explored because a large proportion of the cases (up to an estimated 30 to 50 percent) have a familial distribution.[73,74] The inheritance pattern is autosomal dominant, except in one geographically isolated cluster in which it is autosomal recessive (Naxos disease–plakoglobin locus on chromosome 17). Autosomal dominant mutations have been identified in the ryanodine receptor locus on chromosome 1 [1q42][76] and four loci encoding desmosome structure (plakoglobin, desmoplakin, plakophillin-2, and desmoglein-2).[77-80] The desmosomal loci collectively are the most common known mutations associated with right ventricular dysplasia. Linkage analyses have implicated a heterogeneous distribution of a number of other loci that might contribute to inheritance patterns (see Chap. 9).

VALVULAR HEART DISEASE (see Chap. 62). Before the advent of surgery for valvular heart disease, severe aortic stenosis was associated with a high mortality risk. Approximately 70 percent of deaths were sudden, accounting for an absolute SCD mortality rate of 15 to 20 percent among all affected patients.[81] The advent of safe and effective procedures for aortic valve replacement has reduced the incidence of this cause of sudden death, but patients with prosthetic or heterograft aortic valve replacements remain at some risk for SCD caused by arrhythmias, prosthetic valve dysfunction, or coexistent coronary heart disease.[82] The incidence peaks 3 weeks after operation and then levels off after 8 months. Nonetheless, the risk is still appreciably lower than the historical risk among patients before the advent of valve surgery. A high incidence of ventricular arrhythmia has been observed during follow-up of patients with valve replacement, especially those who had aortic stenosis, multiple valve surgery, or cardiomegaly. Sudden death during follow-up was associated with ventricular arrhythmias and thromboembolism. Hemodynamic variables were less predictive. Stenotic lesions of other valves imply a much lower risk of SCD. Regurgitant lesions, particularly chronic aortic regurgitation and acute mitral regurgitation, may cause SCD, but the risk is also lower than with aortic stenosis.

MITRAL VALVE PROLAPSE (see Chap. 62). This entity is prevalent, but probably less than previously thought,[83] and associated with a high incidence of annoying low-risk cardiac arrhythmias. However, a risk of SCD is apparent, although low.[84] This uncommon complication appears to correlate with nonspecific ST-T wave changes in the inferior leads on the electrocardiogram (ECG). An association with marked redundancy of mitral leaflets on the echocardiogram has also been suggested. Reported associations between QT interval prolongation or preexcitation and SCD in mitral prolapse syndrome are less consistent.

ENDOCARDITIS OF THE AORTIC AND MITRAL VALVES (see Chap. 63). This may be associated with rapid death resulting from acute disruption of the valvular apparatus, coronary embolism, or abscesses of valvular rings or the septum; however, such deaths are rarely true sudden deaths, because conventionally defined tachyarrhythmic mechanisms are uncommon. Coronary embolism from valvular vegetations can trigger fatal ischemic arrhythmia on rare occasions.

CONGENITAL HEART DISEASE. The congenital lesions most commonly associated with SCD are aortic stenosis (see Chap. 61) and communications between the left and right sides of the heart with the Eisenmenger physiology. In the latter, the risk of SCD is a function of the severity of pulmonary vascular disease; also, there is an extraordinarily high risk of maternal mortality during labor and delivery in the pregnant patient with Eisenmenger syndrome (see Chap. 77).[85] Potentially lethal arrhythmias and SCD have been described as late complications after surgical repair of complex congenital lesions, particularly tetralogy of Fallot, transposition of the great arteries, and atrioventricular (AV) canal. These patients should be observed closely and treated aggressively when cardiac arrhythmias are identified, although the late risk of SCD may not be as high as previously thought.

Electrophysiological Abnormalities

Acquired disease of the AV node and His-Purkinje system and the presence of accessory pathways of conduction (see Chap. 35) are two groups of structural abnormalities of specialized conduction that may be associated with SCD. Epidemiological studies have suggested that intraventricular conduction disturbances in coronary heart disease are one of the few factors that can increase the proportion of SCD in coronary heart disease. Several studies from the late 1970s and 1980s had demonstrated increased total mortality and SCD risk during the late in-hospital course and first few months after hospital discharge in patients with anterior myocardial infarctions and right bundle branch or bifascicular block. In one study, 47 percent of patients who had late hospital VF had had the combination of anteroseptal infarction and bundle branch block. This finding corresponded to a VF incidence of 35 percent in a subgroup that represented only 4.1 percent of a total of 966 myocardial infarctions. In a later study, evaluating the impact of thrombolytic therapy on the prethrombolytic era experience, the incidence of pure right bundle branch block was actually higher but that of bifascicular block was lower, as were late complications and mortality.[86] These observations suggest a benefit of thrombolytic therapy, but the principle of increased risk among those who develop advanced conduction abnormalities (probably related to infarct size) is not attenuated by the therapy and the condition still requires aggressive management.

Primary fibrosis (Lenègre's disease) or secondary mechanical injury (Lev's disease) of the His-Purkinje system is commonly associated with intraventricular conduction abnormalities and symptomatic AV block, and less commonly with SCD. The identification of those at risk and the efficacy of pacemakers for preventing SCD, rather than only ameliorating symptoms, have been subjects of debate. However, survival appears to depend more on the nature and extent of the underlying disease than on the conduction disturbance itself.

Patients with congenital AV block (see Chap. 35) or nonprogressive congenital intraventricular block, in the absence of structural cardiac abnormalities and with stable heart rate and rhythm, have been characterized as being at low risk for SCD in the past. In contrast, progressive congenital intraventricular blocks and the coexistence of structural congenital defects predicted a high risk and were considered pacemaker indications. Later data have suggested that patients with the patterns of congenital AV block previously thought to be benign are at risk for a dilated cardiomyopathy,[87] and routine pacemaker implantation in patients older than 15 years, if not indicated sooner, has been suggested by at least one group.[88] Whether there is mortality benefit from pacemakers or a reduction in the incidence of dilated cardiomyopathy is not yet clear. Hereditary forms of AV heart block have also been reported in association with a familial propensity to SCD.[23] Sodium channel gene mutations have been associated with progressive conduction system disturbances, along with aging, and some are variants of Brugada gene expression.[89,90]

The anomalous pathways of conduction, bundles of Kent in the Wolff-Parkinson-White syndrome and Mahaim fibers, are commonly associated with nonlethal arrhythmias. However, when the anomalous pathways of conduction have short refractory periods, the occurrence of atrial fibrillation may allow the initiation of VF during very rapid conduction across the bypass tract (see Chap. 35). The incidence of SCD in patients with short refractory period bypass tracts is unknown because an accurate estimate of its incidence in the general population is not available. Patients who have multiple pathways appear to be at higher risk for SCD, as do patients with a familial pattern of anomalous pathways and premature SCD. Family history is relevant, because a genetic predisposition to Wolff-Parkinson-White syndrome has been suggested.[91]

LONG-QT SYNDROMES (see also Chaps. 9, 31-35). The congenital long-QT syndrome is a functional abnormality caused by hereditary defects of molecular structure in ion channel proteins and is associated with environmental or neurogenic triggers that can initiate symptomatic or lethal arrhythmias. Two hereditary patterns have been described—the much more common autosomal dominant pattern known as the Romano-Ward syndrome and the rare autosomal recessive inheritance pattern, associated with deafness, the Jervell and Lange-Nielsen syndrome. There is a broad range of phenotypical expression, with syncope being the most common expression among symptomatic patients. SCD is less common, although data are limited by the absence of information about the number of undiagnosed carriers in whom fatal cardiac arrest is the first clinical event. Some patients have prolonged QT intervals throughout life without any manifest arrhythmias, whereas others are highly susceptible to symptomatic and potentially fatal ventricular arrhythmias, particularly the torsades de pointes pattern of VT.[92,93] Moreover, genetic studies have demonstrated that penetrance may be low or variable in some families, making electrocardiographic identification of affected members difficult. The relationship between low penetrance and risk of SCD remains undefined, but such patients are likely to be susceptible to QT lengthening effects of drugs or serum electrolyte level variations, expressed clinically as acquired long-QT syndrome (see later).

Higher levels of risk are associated with female gender, greater degrees of QT prolongation or QT alternans, unexplained syncope, family history of premature SCD, and documented torsade de pointes or prior VF. Patients with the syndrome require avoidance of drugs that are associated with QT lengthening and careful medical management, which may include implantable defibrillators.[94] Moreover, efforts to identify and manage relatives medically who carry the mutation is a potentially important preventive strategy, given the familial pattern of expression of the entity (see Chaps. 9, 31-35 for details). A large number of mutations at loci on chromosomes 3, 7, 11, that encode the Na^+ and K^+ channel alpha subunits (*KCNQ1, HERG, SCN5A*), and on chromosome 21 that encode the beta subunits (*KCNE1, KCNE2—minK* and *MiRP*), are implicated in various patterns of the Romano-Ward and Jervell and Lange-Nielsen syndromes. Another form of long-QT syndrome, LQT-4, is associated with a mutation at a locus on chromosome 4 encoding the cytoskeletal element, ankyrin-B[95] (see Chaps. 9 and 31). It has been suggested that ankyrin-B mutations may have arrhythmia implications extending beyond the long-QT syndromes.[96]

From an epidemiological perspective, there is interest in whether QT interval abnormalities, or the propensity thereto, interacting with acquired diseases, predispose to SCD as a specific clinical expression.[2,9,58] In a prospective cohort study of a population having a mean age of 69 years at entry, a prolonged QTc emerged as a powerful risk factor for SCD in the presence of a large burden of cardiovascular disorders, such as myocardial infarction, hypertension, and heart failure.[97]

The acquired form of prolonged QT interval syndrome refers to excessive lengthening of the QT interval and the potential for developing torsade de pointes in response to environmental influences. As with congenital long-QT syndrome, it is more common in women. The syndrome may be caused by drug effects or an individual patient's idiosyncrasies (particularly related to class IA or III antiarrhythmic drugs and psychotropic drugs; see Chap. 75), electrolyte abnormalities, hypothermia, toxic substances, bradyarrhythmia-induced QT adjustments, and central nervous system injury (most commonly, subarachnoid hemorrhage).[98] It has also been reported in intensive weight reduction programs that involve the use of liquid protein diets and in anorexia nervosa. Lithium carbonate can prolong the QT interval and has been reported to be associated with an increased incidence of SCD in cancer patients with preexisting heart disease. Drug interactions have been recognized as a mechanism of prolongation of the QT interval and torsade de pointes.[99,100] A growing body of evidence has suggested that inherited polymorphisms or mutations with low penetrance, involving the same gene loci associated with phenotypically expressed long-QT syndrome, underlie the so-called individual idiosyncrasies to the acquired form in many, if not most, cases.[23,101-103] In acquired prolonged QT syndrome, as in the congenital form, torsade de pointes is commonly the specific arrhythmia that triggers or degenerates into VF.

BRUGADA SYNDROME (see Chaps. 31 and 35). This disorder is characterized by right bundle branch block and an unusual form of nonischemic ST-T wave elevations in the anterior precordial leads (Fig. 36-8), associated with risk of SCD.[104] It is a familial disorder and occurs most commonly in young and middle-aged men. A mutation involving the cardiac Na^+ channel gene (*SCN5A*) has been observed in a minority of cases,[20] and there are compelling data suggesting that other ion channel defects may be a cause.[105] The right bundle branch block and ST-T wave changes may be intermittent and evoked or exaggerated by Na^+ channel blockers (e.g., flecainide). Risk of SCD is difficult to predict. Persistent baseline electrocardiographic changes, syncope, life-threatening arrhythmias, a strong family history of SCD, and inducibility of ventricular tachyarrhythmias during electrophysiological testing, in various combinations, are thought to be the best predictors.[106,107]

Long before the description of the Brugada syndrome, a specific pattern of SCD in young males had been observed in Southeast Asia. Syndromes referred to as *bangungut* in the Philippines, *pokkuri* in Japan, and *lai-tai* in Laos were reported. In each, there was a tendency for death to occur unexpectedly during sleep, and at one time a toxic cause was suspected. Documented cases were reported in Laotians who came to the United States after the Vietnam War. The mechanism was identified as VF in some of these cases. The fact that these cases continue to occur in a new cultural setting has suggested that there might be a hereditary predisposition. Further clinical and genetic observations have led to the conclusion that many, if not all, the subjects had Brugada syndrome.[108,109]

ELECTRICAL INSTABILITY RESULTING FROM NEUROHUMORAL AND CENTRAL NERVOUS SYSTEM INFLUENCES. Catecholamine-dependent lethal arrhythmias in the absence of QT interval prolongation, with control by beta-adrenoceptor blocking agents, have been described. In younger patients, usually men, bidirectional or polymorphic VT associated with SCD risk is related to a genetic disorder involving the ryanodine receptor locus, whereas the syndrome not associated with that genotype appears more likely to occur in older patients, usually women.[110] Several central nervous system–related interactions with cardiac electrical stability have been suggested (see Chap. 87). Epidemiological data have also suggested an association

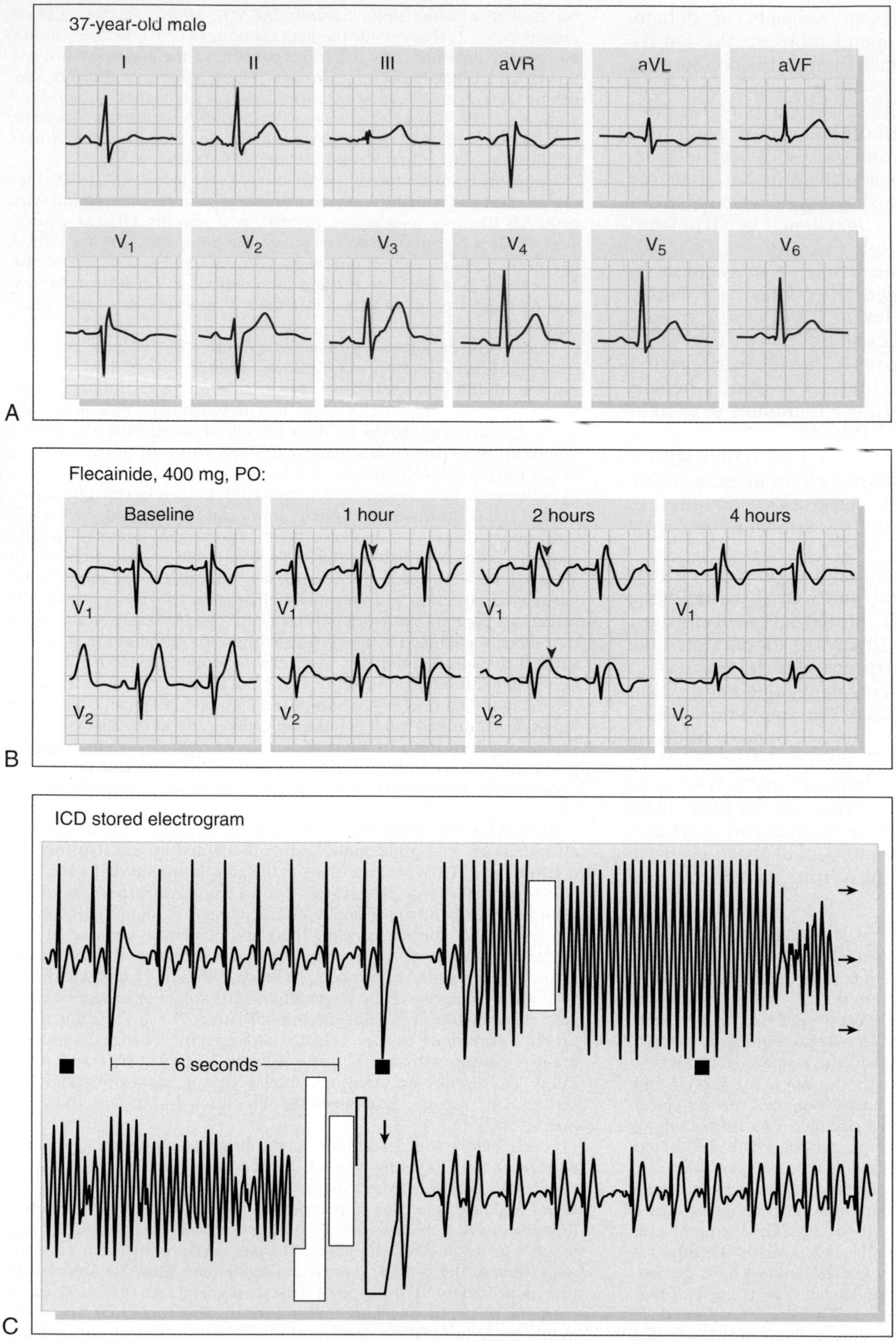

FIGURE 36–8 Electrocardiographic and clinical findings in a 37-year-old man with Brugada syndrome. The patient was resuscitated after out-of-hospital ventricular fibrillation. No structural disease was identified. **A,** The 12-lead electrocardiogram shows an incomplete right bundle branch block pattern, which is not typical for Brugada syndrome. **B,** Typical repolarization changes of Brugada syndrome (arrows) were elicited by a single oral dose of flecainide, 400 mg. The patient received an implantable cardioverter-defibrillator (ICD) and 6 months later had an appropriate shock (arrow) **(C),** as shown on the accompanying electrogram stored in the device.

between behavioral abnormalities and the risk of SCD. Psychological stress and emotional extremes have been suggested as triggering mechanisms for advanced arrhythmias and SCD for many years,[111,112] but there are only limited, largely observational, data supporting such associations. Stress-induced arrhythmias are better supported than stress-induced mortality risk; the latter require further study. Data from the 1994 Los Angeles earthquake have identified an increased rate of fatal cardiac events on that day, but the event rate was reduced over the ensuing 2 weeks, suggesting a triggering of events about to happen rather than independent causation.[113] Associations between auditory stimulation and auditory auras and SCD have been reported. The auditory abnormalities in some forms of congenital QT prolongation have also been observed.

A variant of torsades de pointes, characterized by short coupling intervals between a normal impulse and the initiating impulse, has been described (Fig. 36-9).[114] It appears to have familial trends and to be related to alterations in autonomic nervous system activity. The 12-lead ECG demonstrates normal QT intervals, but VF and sudden death are common (see Chaps. 9 and 35).

Acute emotional stress has been reported as a cause of a specific form of reversible LV dysfunction and heart failure, characterized by ballooning of the apex with a narrow neck at the base of the heart (termed *takotsubo cardiomyopathy,* named for the similarity of this shape to a Japanese octopus fishing pot).[115,116] It is suspected to be catecholamine-mediated and its long-term prognosis is good, but short-term risk of SCD during the acute phase remains uncertain.

The phenomenon of voodoo death has been studied in underdeveloped countries. There appears to be an association between isolation from the tribe, a sense of hopelessness, severe bradyarrhythmias, and sudden death. With cultural changes in many of these areas, the syndrome has become less amenable to observation and study; however, there remain pockets of cultural isolation in which the syndrome may still exist. Limited clinical observations and experimental data modeling voodoo death have suggested a mechanism related to parasympathetic overactivity, as opposed to the evidence for an adrenergic basis for syndromes related to acute emotional stress.

Sudden Infant Death Syndrome and Sudden Cardiac Death in Children

The sudden infant death syndrome (SIDS) occurs between birth and 6 months of age, is more common in male infants, and had an incidence of 0.1 to 0.3 percent of live births prior to widespread publication of appropriate sleep positions in at-risk infants.[117] Because of its abrupt nature, a cardiac mechanism has been suspected for many years, but various causes, with central respiratory dysfunction playing a major role, are considered likely. Many cases of SIDS are believed to represent a form of "sleep apnea" that, if prolonged, can lead to hypoxia, cyanosis, and cardiac arrhythmias. Experiences with near-misses and the results of respiratory monitoring, in conjunction with the propensity of the syndrome to occur in premature infants, have all suggested impaired central nervous system respiratory control reflexes, possibly because of immaturity. There has been interest, however, in the possibility of obstructive apnea as another mechanism. Identification of individual infants at risk is difficult, but the risk does not persist beyond the first 6 months of life. Having infants sleep on their backs was anticipated to reduce the incidence of SIDS and appears to have achieved this goal in some studies, but not all studies have demonstrated this improvement.

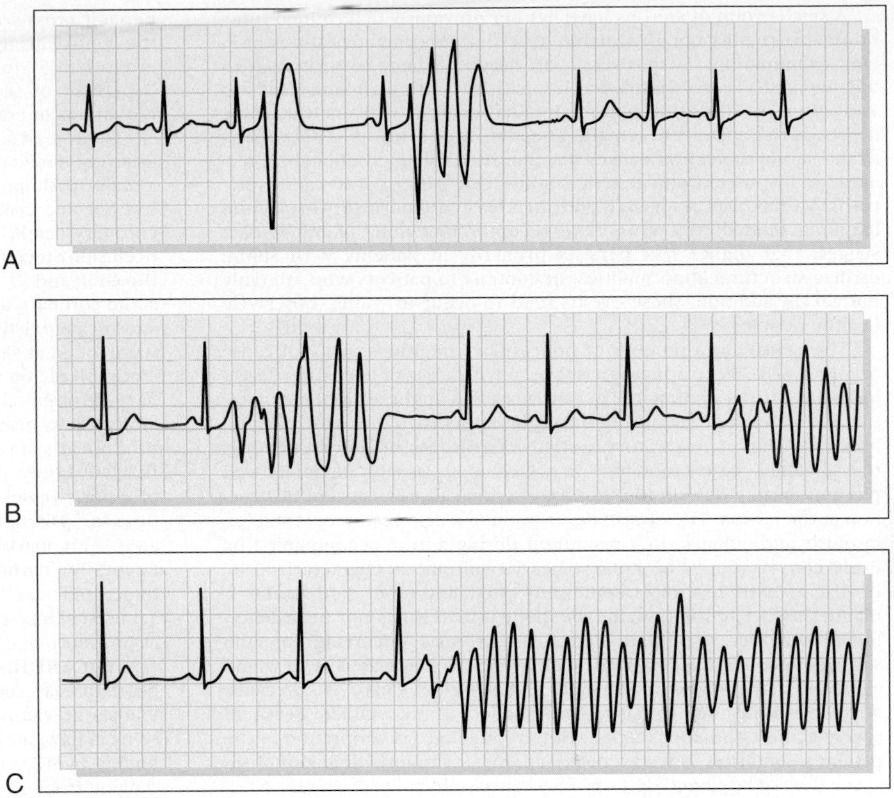

FIGURE 36–9 Short-coupled variant of torsades de pointes. This variant has been observed in people without structural heart disease and normal QT intervals. They are subject to spontaneous episodes of polymorphic ventricular tachycardia (torsades de pointes), which may degenerate into ventricular fibrillation. There is a high risk of sudden death in this uncommon syndrome.

Primary cardiac causes have been considered the basis of this syndrome in some victims, and a large study of ECGs of infants has suggested an association of risk of SIDS with prolonged QT intervals.[118] Subsequently, a near-miss survivor was shown to have a de novo mutation of the Na^+ channel gene (*SCN5A;* chromosome 3), validating the concept that long QT may be one mechanism of SIDS.[119] The combination of the relative incidence of SIDS among victims with the longer QT intervals and documentation of additional long-QT–related arrhythmias in near-misses have supported the notion that a significant fraction of SIDS deaths occur by this mechanism. It does not, however, exclude the respiratory hypothesis as the causative mechanism for most cases. Other cardiac causes have also been reported. Accessory pathways (two cases) and dispersed or immature AV nodal or bundle branch cells in the annulus (four cases) have been described in a group of seven SIDS victims studied by detailed histopathology.

Sudden death in children beyond the age group at risk for SIDS is often associated with identifiable heart disease.[120] Although one earlier study identified cardiac causes in only 25 percent of victims of sudden natural death between the ages of 1 and 21 years, a later report identified cardiac causes in 65 percent, with cardiac causes attributed in 80 percent of older children and adolescents. About 25 percent of SCDs in children occur in those who have undergone previous surgery for congenital cardiac disease. Of the remaining 75 percent, more than half occur in children who have one of four lesions—congenital aortic stenosis, Eisenmenger syndrome, pulmonary stenosis or atresia, or obstructive hypertrophic cardiomyopathy. Neuspiel and Kuller have observed 14 cases of myocarditis among 51 SCDs in children (27 percent).

Other Causes and Circumstances Associated with Sudden Death

SCD can occur during or after extreme physical activity in competing athletes or under special circumstances within the general population. Examples of the latter include intense exercise and basic military training. Among adolescent and young adult competitive athletes, the incidence estimate is in the range of 1/75,000 annually in Italy,[121] compared with less than 1/125,000 for the general nonathlete population in the same age group.[41] However, Maron (see Chap. 78) has reported the frequency of sudden unexpected death related to cardiovascular disease during competitive sports to be 1 in 200,000 individual student athletes per academic year and in 1 in 70,000 over a 3-year high school career. Exercise-related incidence figures are more difficult to ascertain in other populations, but one study reported an incidence of one SCD per 1.5 million exercise sessions in health clubs.[40] The incidence of exercise-related cardiac arrest appears to be lower in women.[122] Most athletes and nonathletes have a previously known or unrecognized cardiac abnormality. In middle-aged and older adults, in whom coronary disease dominates as the cause of SCD, exercise-related deaths appear to be associated with acute plaque disruptions.[50] Whether exercise contributed to the initiation of plaque disruption or preexisting disruption simply set the stage for the fatal response during exercise remains unclear. Among athletes, hypertrophic cardiomyopathy with or without obstruction, occult congenital or acquired coronary artery disease, and valvular aortic stenosis are the most common causes identified after death (see Chap. 78).[65,121,123-127] In a report of a large cohort of U.S. Air Force recruits, a surprisingly large fraction of those who died suddenly during exertion had unsuspected myocarditis. Diseases attributed to molecular structural abnormalities, such as long-QT syndrome and right ventricular dysplasia, are being increasingly recognized as causes of SCD in athletes and exercising nonathletes.[65,124,125] Cardiac trauma (commotio cordis [see Chap. 78]) is the cause in some of these cases.[127]

Sudden death from true cardiac causes in athletes should not be confused with precipitous death related to heat stroke or malignant hyperthermia.[128] In the latter, the victim has usually exercised excessively in hot weather, often with athletic gear that impairs heat dissipation and sometimes in association with the use of substances that cause heat production and vasoconstriction impairing heat exchange. This leads to collapse, with markedly elevated core body temperatures and ultimately irreversible organ system damage. Ingestion of exogenous dietary supplements, particularly ephedrine and caffeine-containing preparations, taken in excess quantities, have been proposed to have a role in precipitating life-threatening arrhythmias, largely based on case report data. As a result, the U.S. Food and Drug Administration (FDA) has banned marketing these substances for athletic performance enhancement or weight loss.

A small group of victims have neither previously determined functional abnormality nor identifiable structural abnormalities at postmortem examination. Such events or deaths, when associated with documented VF, are classified as idiopathic.[129] Although long-term survival after an idiopathic potentially fatal event is still unclear, some degree of risk appears to remain. The idiopathic category is decreasing as the subtle molecular causes become better defined, including recognition by postmortem genetic studies. One pattern of so-called idiopathic VT has been associated with an inherited abnormality in calcium handling related to a ryanodine receptor mutation.[21] Limited data suggest that higher risk persists primarily in patients with subtle cardiac structural abnormalities, in contrast to patients who are truly normal. In addition, these events tend to occur in young, otherwise healthy people.

There also are a number of noncardiac conditions that can cause or mimic SCD. Sleep apnea is associated with a risk of nocturnal death, including deaths attributable to cardiac causes. In these circumstances, the risk of death peaks during the night, rather than the early morning hours.[130] Another respiratory system–based cause of sudden death is the so-called "café coronary," in which food, usually an unchewed piece of meat, lodges in the oropharynx and causes an abrupt obstruction at the glottis. The classic description of a café coronary is sudden cyanosis and collapse in a restaurant during a meal accompanied by lively conversation. The holiday heart syndrome is characterized by cardiac arrhythmias, most commonly atrial, and other cardiac abnormalities associated with acute alcoholic states. It has not been determined whether potentially lethal arrhythmias occurring in such settings account for reported sudden deaths associated with acute alcoholic states. Massive pulmonary embolism (see Chap. 72) can cause acute cardiovascular collapse and sudden death; sudden death in severe acute asthmatic attacks, without prolonged deterioration of the patient's condition, is well recognized. Air or amniotic fluid embolism at the time of labor and delivery may cause sudden death on rare occasions, with the clinical picture mimicking that of SCD. Peripartum air embolism caused by unusual sexual practices has been reported as a cause of such sudden deaths.

Finally, a number of abnormalities that do not directly involve the heart may cause SCD or mimic it. These include aortic dissection (see Chap. 56), acute cardiac tamponade (see Chap. 70), and rapid exsanguination.

PATHOLOGY AND PATHOPHYSIOLOGY

Pathological studies in SCD victims reflect the epidemiological and clinical observations that coronary atherosclerosis is the major predisposing cause. In one report, 81 percent of 220 autopsied victims of SCD had significant coronary heart disease. At least one vessel with more than 75 percent stenosis was found in 94 percent of victims, acute coronary occlusion in 58 percent, healed myocardial infarction in 44 percent, and acute myocardial infarction in 27 percent. These observations are consistent with subsequent studies of the frequency of coronary disease in SCD victims, but the focus has evolved from the simple anatomical presence of coronary lesions to the specific associations with unstable plaques.[50,131] All other causes of SCD (see Table 36-2) collectively account for no more than 15 to 20 percent of cases, but they have provided a large base of enlightening pathological data.

Pathology of Sudden Death Caused by Coronary Heart Disease

CORONARY ARTERIES. Extensive atherosclerosis has long been recognized as the most common pathological finding in the coronary arteries of victims of SCD. The combined results of a number of studies have suggested a general pattern of at least two coronary arteries with 75 percent or greater narrowing in more than 75 percent of the victims. Several studies have demonstrated no specific pattern of distribution of coronary artery lesions that preselect for SCD. In a quantitative analysis comparing coronary artery narrowing at postmortem examination in SCD victims and control subjects, 36 percent of the 5-mm segments of the coronary arteries from the SCD group had 76 to 100 percent cross-sectional area reductions compared with 3 percent in the control group. An additional 34 percent of sections from the SCD group had 51 to 75 percent reductions in cross-sectional area. Only 7 percent of sections from the SCD patients had 0 to 25 percent reductions in cross-sectional area.

The role of active coronary artery lesions, characterized by plaque fissuring, erosion or rupture, platelet aggregation, and thrombosis, as a major pathophysiological mechanism of the onset of cardiac arrest has become clarified.[50,131] Among 100 consecutive victims of sudden coronary death, 44 percent had major (more than 50 percent luminal occlusion) recent coronary thrombi, 30 percent had minor occlusive thrombi, and 21 percent had plaque fissuring. Only 5 percent had no acute coronary artery changes; 65 percent of the thrombi occurred at sites of preexisting high-grade stenoses, and an additional 19 percent were found at sites of more than 50 percent stenosis. In a subsequent study, 50 of 168 victims (30 percent) had occlusive intraluminal coronary thrombi, and 73 (44 percent) had mural intraluminal thrombi. Single-vessel disease, acute infarction at postmortem examination, and prodromal symptoms were associated with the presence of thrombi. In a later study, plaque rupture or erosion was observed in 66 percent of culprit vessel lesions in victims of SCD related to coronary heart disease.[35] Disruption, platelet aggregation, and thrombosis are associated with markers of inflammation and various conventional risk factors for coronary atherosclerosis, such as cigarette smoking and hyperlipidemia.[132] Coronary artery spasm, an established cause of acute ischemia, can also cause SCD[60] and is recognizable in rare cases at postmortem examination.

MYOCARDIUM. Myocardial pathology in SCD caused by coronary heart disease reflects the extensive atherosclerosis usually present. Studies of victims of out-of-hospital SCD and from epidemiological sources have indicated that healed myocardial infarction is a common finding in SCD victims, with most investigators reporting frequencies ranging from 40 to more than 70 percent. In one study, 72 percent of men in the 25- to 44-year age group who died suddenly (24 or fewer hours) with no previous clinical history of coronary heart disease had scars of large (63 percent) or small (less than 1-cm cross-sectional area, 9 percent) areas of healed myocardial necrosis. The incidence of acute myocardial infarction is considerably less, with cytopathological evidence of recent myocardial infarction averaging about 20 percent. This estimate corresponds well with results of studies of out-of-hospital cardiac arrest survivors, who were found to have an incidence of new myocardial infarction in the range of 20 to 30 percent. These pathological observations do not provide insight into the likely possibility that many SCDs occur by acute coronary syndrome mechanisms and progress from ischemia to fatal arrhythmias without time for structural markers to become visible. Even though there is an association between troponin level elevations during chest pain syndromes and risk of subsequent cardiac death,[133] and troponin level increases are seen in a substantial proportion of cardiac arrest survivors, the question of whether the myocardial injury preceded or followed the cardiac arrest is difficult to resolve in individual cases.

VENTRICULAR HYPERTROPHY. Myocardial hypertrophy can coexist and interact with acute or chronic ischemia but appears to confer an independent mortality risk.[33,34] There is no close correlation between increased heart weight and severity of coronary heart disease in SCD victims; heart weights are higher in SCD victims than in those whose death is not sudden, despite similar prevalences of history of hypertension before death. Hypertrophy-associated mortality risk is also independent of left ventricular function and extent of coronary artery disease,[134] and left ventricular hypertrophy itself may predispose to SCD. Experimental data have also suggested increased susceptibility to potentially lethal ventricular arrhythmias in left ventricular hypertrophy with ischemia and reperfusion.[135] A study of massively enlarged hearts (i.e., weighing more than 1000 gm), however, did not indicate an excess incidence of SCD, but the underlying pathology in that study was dominated by lesions that produce volume overload.

SPECIALIZED CONDUCTING SYSTEM IN SUDDEN CARDIAC DEATH

Fibrosis of the specialized conducting system may be observed in SCD victims. Although this process is associated with AV block or intraventricular conduction abnormalities, its role in SCD is uncertain. Lev's and Lenègre's diseases, ischemic injury caused by small-vessel disease, and numerous infiltrative or inflammatory processes can all result in such changes. In addition, active inflammatory processes such as myocarditis and infiltrative processes such as amyloidosis, scleroderma, hemochromatosis, and morbid obesity all may damage or destroy the

AV node, bundle of His, or both, and result in AV block.[136]

Focal diseases such as sarcoidosis, Whipple's disease, and rheumatoid arthritis and fibrotic or fatty infiltration of the AV node or His-Purkinje system with apparent discontinuities[69] can also involve the conducting system (see Chap. 35). These various categories of conducting system disease have been considered as possible pathological substrates for SCD that might be overlooked because of the difficulty in doing careful postmortem examinations of the conducting system routinely. Focal involvement of conducting tissue by tumors (especially mesothelioma of the AV node but also lymphoma, carcinoma, rhabdomyoma, and fibroma) has also been reported, and rare cases of SCD have been associated with these lesions. It has been suggested that abnormal postnatal morphogenesis of the specialized conducting system may be a significant factor in some SCDs in infants and children.

CARDIAC NERVES AND SUDDEN CARDIAC DEATH

Diseases of cardiac nerves have been postulated to have a role in SCD. Neural involvement may be the result of random damage to neural elements within the myocardium (i.e., secondary cardioneuropathy) or may be primary, as in a selective cardiac viral neuropathy. Secondary involvement can be a consequence of ischemic neural injury in coronary heart disease and has been postulated to result in autonomic destabilization, enhancing the propensity to arrhythmias. Nerve sprouting may be important.[137] Some experimental data have supported this hypothesis, and a clinical technique for imaging cardiac neural fibers suggests a changing pattern over time after myocardial infarction. Viral, neurotoxic, and hereditary causes (e.g., progressive muscular dystrophy and Friedreich ataxia) have been emphasized.

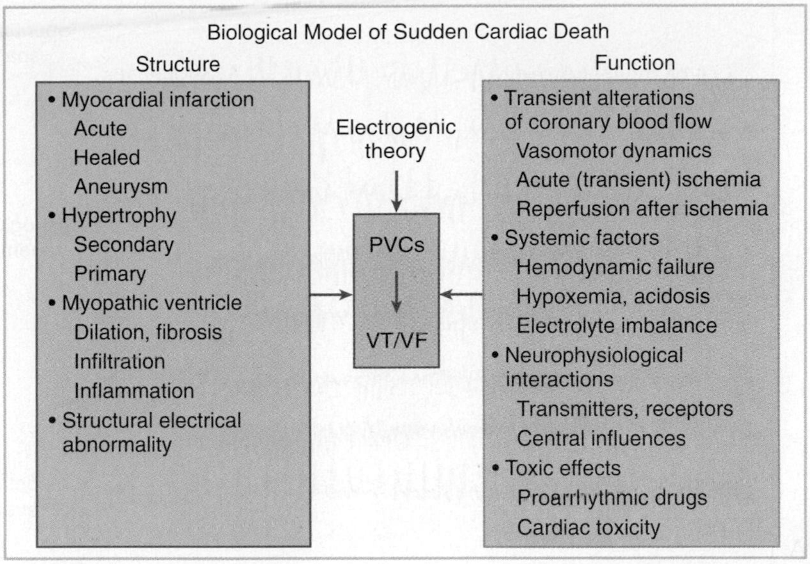

FIGURE 36–10 Biological model of sudden cardiac death (SCD). Structural cardiac abnormalities are commonly defined as the causative basis for SCD. However, functional alterations of the abnormal anatomical substrate are usually required to alter stability of the myocardium, permitting a potentially fatal arrhythmia to be initiated. In this conceptual model, short- or long-term structural abnormalities interact with functional modulations to influence the probability that premature ventricular contractions (PVCs) initiate ventricular tachycardia or fibrillation (VT/VF). *(From Myerburg RJ, Kessler KM, Bassett AL, Castellanos A: A biological approach to sudden cardiac death: Structure, function, and cause. Am J Cardiol 61:1512, 1989.)*

Mechanisms and Pathophysiology

Electrical mechanisms of cardiac arrest are divided into tachyarrhythmic and bradyarrhythmia-asystolic events. The tachyarrhythmias include VF and sustained VT, in which adequate blood flow cannot be maintained and perfusion is inadequate to meet the body's needs. Asystolic events include severe bradyarrhythmias—heart rates slow enough to impede adequate tissue perfusion and inability to generate a mechanical event because of complete absence of electrical activity (asystole) or dissociation between abnormal spontaneous electrical activity and mechanical function (pulseless electrical activity). It is likely that VF, or VT deteriorating to VF, is the initiating event in most cardiac arrests. After a variable period of time, fibrillation may cease and asystole or pulseless electrical activity emerges. In a significant minority of cases, however, the documented initial recording is asystole or pulseless electrical activity, which can continue as such or transform into VF.[138] More commonly, asystolic events or pulseless electrical activity follow(s) an initial tachyarrhythmic event.

The occurrence of potentially lethal tachyarrhythmias, or of severe bradyarrhythmia or asystole, is the end of a cascade of pathophysiological abnormalities that result from complex interactions between coronary vascular events, myocardial injury, variations in autonomic tone, or the metabolic and electrolyte state of the myocardium (see Fig. 36-4).[10,139,140] There is no uniform hypothesis regarding mechanisms by which these elements interact to lead to the final pathway of lethal arrhythmias. However, Figure 36-10 shows a model of the pathophysiology of SCD in which the central event is the initiation of a potentially fatal arrhythmia. The risk of this event is conditioned by the presence of structural abnormalities and modulated by functional variations.[141]

Pathophysiological Mechanisms of Lethal Tachyarrhythmias

CORONARY ARTERY STRUCTURE AND FUNCTION. Among the 80 percent of SCDs associated with coronary atherosclerosis, an extensive distribution of chronic arterial narrowing has been well defined by pathological studies. However, the specific mechanisms by which these lesions lead to potentially lethal disturbances of electrical stability are not simply the consequence of steady-state reductions in regional myocardial blood flow in association with variable demands (see Chap. 38).[9,10,139] A simple increase in myocardial oxygen demand, in the presence of a fixed supply, may be a mechanism of exercise-induced arrhythmias and sudden death during intense physical activity or in others whose heart disease had not previously become clinically manifest. However, the dynamic nature of the pathophysiology of coronary events has led to the recognition that superimposed acute lesions create a setting in which alterations in the metabolic or electrolyte state of the myocardium are the common circumstance leading to disturbed electrical stability. Active vascular events, leading to acute or transient reduction in regional myocardial blood flow in the presence of a normal or previously compromised circulation, constitute a common mechanism of ischemia, angina pectoris, arrhythmias, and SCD.[9,60,139,140] Coronary artery spasm or modulation of coronary collateral flow, predisposed to by local endothelial dysfunction, exposes the myocardium to the double hazard of transient ischemia and reperfusion (Fig. 36-11).[129,139] Neurogenic influences may play a role but do not appear to be a sine qua non for the production of spasm. Vessel susceptibility and humoral factors, particularly those related to platelet activation and aggregation, also appear to be important mechanisms.

Transition of stable atherosclerotic plaques to an "active" state because of endothelial damage, with plaque fissuring leading to platelet activation and aggregation followed by thrombosis, is a mechanism that appears to be present in most SCDs related to coronary heart disease (see Chap. 50). Inflammatory responses in atherosclerotic plaques are now viewed as the condition leading to lesion progression, including erosion, disruption, platelet activation, and thrombosis. In addition to causing subacute or acute critical reduction in regional blood flow, these mechanisms produce a series of biochemical alterations that may enhance or retard susceptibility to VF by means of vasomotor modulation.

The final step in the role of coronary artery pathophysiology leading to ischemia-induced arrhythmias is platelet aggregation and thrombosis (see Fig. 36-4; see Chap. 38). In 1984, Davies and Thomas noted

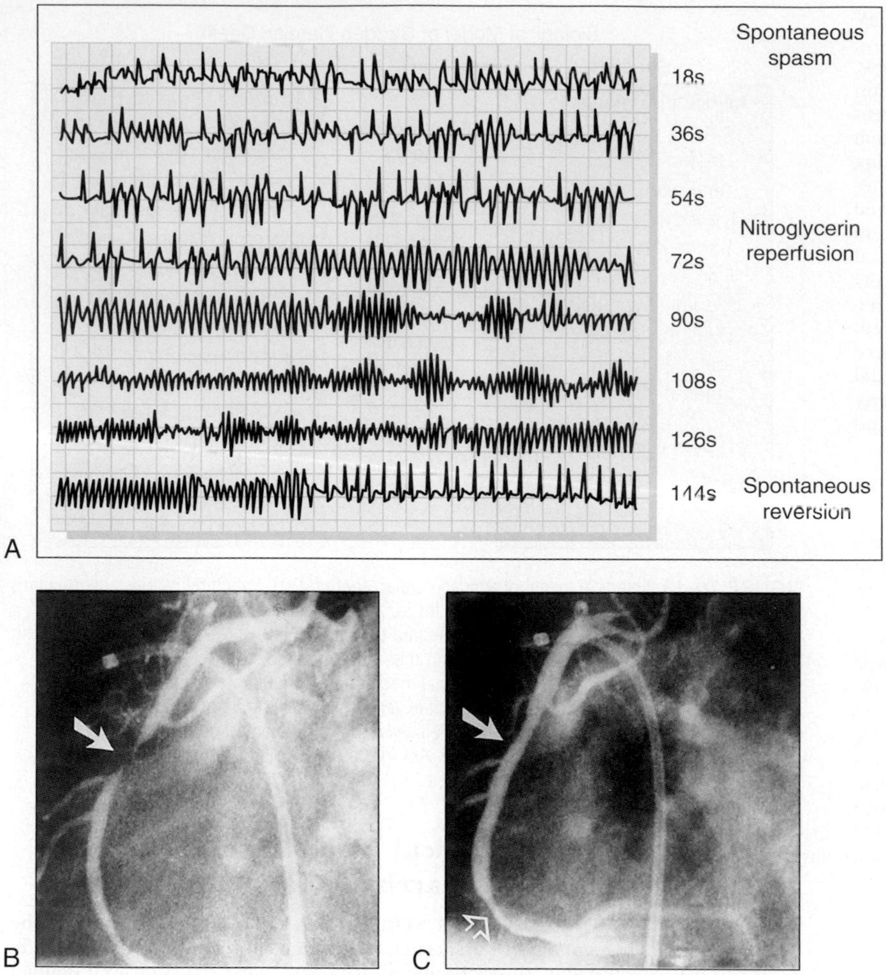

FIGURE 36–11 Life-threatening ventricular arrhythmias associated with acute myocardial ischemia related to coronary artery spasm and with reperfusion. **A,** Continuous lead II electrocardiographic monitor recording during ischemia (time, 0 to 55 seconds) caused by spasm of the right coronary artery **(B)**. There is an abrupt transition (time, 56 to 72 seconds) from repetitive ventricular ectopy to a rapid polymorphic, prefibrillatory tachyarrhythmia (time, 80 to 130 seconds) associated with nitroglycerin-induced reversal of the spasm **(C)**. Closed arrows indicate site of spasm before and after nitroglycerin; open arrow indicates lower grade distal lesion.

that 95 of 100 subjects who died suddenly (less than 6 hours after the onset of symptoms) had acute coronary thrombi, plaque fissuring, or both. This incidence was considerably higher than in many previous reports, but it is noteworthy that only 44 percent of the patients had the largest thrombus occluding 51 percent or more of the cross-sectional area of the involved vessel and only 18 percent of the patients had more than 75 percent occlusion. These findings raised questions about whether mechanical obstruction to flow was dominant or whether the high incidence of nonoccluding thrombi simply reflected the state of activation of the platelets. The discrepancy between the relatively high incidence of acute thrombi in postmortem studies, and the low incidence of evolution of new myocardial infarction among survivors of out-of-hospital VF,[142] highlights this point. Rapid initiation of lethal arrhythmias, spontaneous thrombolysis, a dominant role of spasm induced by platelet products, or a combination of these factors may explain this observation.

ACUTE ISCHEMIA AND INITIATION OF LETHAL ARRHYTHMIAS. The onset of acute ischemia produces immediate electrical, mechanical, and biochemical dysfunction of cardiac muscle (see Figs. 33-10 and 33-11). The specialized conducting tissue is more resistant to acute ischemia than working myocardium, and therefore the electrophysiological consequences are less intense and delayed in onset in specialized conduction tissue. Experimental studies have also provided data on the long-term consequences of left ventricular hypertrophy and healed experimental myocardial infarction. Tissue exposed to chronic stress produced by long-term left ventricular pressure overload and tissue that has healed after ischemic injury both show lasting cellular electrophysiological abnormalities, including regional changes in transmembrane action potentials and refractory periods.[140] Moreover, acute ischemic injury or acute myocardial infarction in the presence of healed myocardial infarction is more arrhythmogenic than the same extent of acute ischemia in previously normal tissue. In addition to the direct effect of ischemia on normal or previously abnormal tissue, reperfusion after transient ischemia can cause lethal arrhythmias (see Fig. 36-11).[60,140] Reperfusion of ischemic areas can occur by three mechanisms: (1) spontaneous thrombolysis, (2) collateral flow from other coronary vascular beds to the ischemic bed, and (3) reversal of vasospasm. Some mechanisms of reperfusion-induced arrhythmogenesis appear to be related to the duration of ischemia before reperfusion. Experimentally, there is a window of vulnerability beginning 5 to 10 minutes after the onset of ischemia and lasting up to 20 to 30 minutes.

ELECTROPHYSIOLOGICAL EFFECTS OF ACUTE ISCHEMIA. Within the first minutes after experimental coronary ligation, there is a propensity to ventricular arrhythmias that abates after 30 minutes and reappears after several hours. The initial 30 minutes of arrhythmias is divided into two periods, the first of which lasts for about 10 minutes and is presumably directly related to the initial ischemic injury. The second period (20 to 30 minutes) may be related either to reperfusion of ischemic areas or to the evolution of different injury patterns in the epicardial and endocardial muscle. Multiple mechanisms of reperfusion arrhythmias have been observed experimentally, including slow conduction and reentry[143] and afterdepolarizations and triggered activity.[135]

At the level of the myocyte, the immediate consequences of ischemia, which include alterations of cell membrane physiology, with efflux of K^+, influx of Ca^{2+}, acidosis, reduction of transmembrane resting potentials, and enhanced automaticity in some tissues, are followed by a separate series of changes during reperfusion. Those of particular interest are the possible continued influx of Ca^{2+}, which may produce electrical instability; responses to alpha or beta adrenoceptor stimulation, or both; and afterdepolarizations as triggering responses for Ca^{2+}-dependent arrhythmias. Other possible mechanisms studied experimentally include formation of superoxide radicals in reperfusion arrhythmias and differential responses of endocardial and epicardial muscle activation times and refractory periods during ischemia or reperfusion. The adenosine triphosphate–dependent K^+ current ($I_{K,ATP}$), which is inactive during normal conditions, is activated during ischemia. Its activation results in a strong efflux of K^+ ions from myocytes, markedly shortening the time course of repolarization and leading to slow conduction and ultimately to inexcitability. The fact that this response is more marked in epicardium than in endocardium leads to a prominent dispersion of repolarization across the myocardium during transmural ischemia. At an intercellular level, ischemia alters the distribution of connexin43, the primary gap junction protein between myocytes.[144] This alteration results in uncoupling of myocytes, a factor that is arrhythmogenic because of altered patterns of excitation and regional changes in conduction velocity.[145]

The importance of the myocardial response to the onset of ischemia has been emphasized on the basis of the demonstration of dramatic cellular electrophysiological changes during the early period after coronary occlusion. However, the state of the myocardium at the time of onset of ischemia is a critical additional factor. Tissue healed after previous injury appears to be more susceptible to the electrical destabilizing effects of acute ischemia, as is chronically hypertrophied muscle. There are data suggesting that remodeling-induced local stretch, regional hypertrophy, or intrinsic cellular alteration may contribute to this vulnerability. Of more direct clinical relevance is the suggestion that K^+ depletion by diuretics and clinical hypokalemia may make ventricular myocardium more susceptible to potentially lethal arrhythmias.

The association of metabolic and electrolyte abnormalities, and neurophysiological and neurohumoral changes, with lethal arrhythmias emphasizes the importance of integrating changes in the myocardial substrate with systemic influences. Most direct among myocardial metabolic changes in response to ischemia are local acute increase in interstitial K^+ levels to values exceeding 15 mM, a decrease in the tissue pH to below 6.0, changes in adrenoceptor activity, and alterations in autonomic nerve traffic, all of which tend to create and maintain electrical instability, especially if regional in distribution. Other metabolic changes such as cyclic adenosine monophosphate elevation, accumulation of free fatty acids and their metabolites, formation of lysophosphoglycerides, and impaired myocardial glycolysis have also been suggested as myocardial destabilizing influences.[146] These local myocardial changes integrate with systemic patterns of autonomic fluctuation that can be observed as patterns of altered heart rate variability and fractal dynamics,[147] potentially identifying subsets of patients predetermined to be at higher risk for SCD during an ischemic event.

TRANSITION FROM MYOCARDIAL INSTABILITY TO LETHAL ARRHYTHMIAS. The combination of a triggering event and a susceptible myocardium is a fundamental electrophysiological concept for the mechanism of initiation of potentially lethal arrhythmias (see Figs. 33-4 and 33-10). The triggering event may be electrophysiological, ischemic, metabolic, or hemodynamic.[141] The endpoint of their interaction is disorganization of patterns of myocardial activation into multiple uncoordinated reentrant pathways (i.e., VF). Clinical, experimental, and pharmacological data have suggested that triggering events in the absence of myocardial instability are unlikely to initiate lethal arrhythmias. Therefore, in the absence of myocardial vulnerability, many triggering events, such as frequent and complex PVCs, may be innocuous.[141]

The onset of ischemia is accompanied by abrupt reductions in transmembrane resting potential and amplitude and in duration of the action potentials in the affected area, with little change in remote areas. When ischemic cells depolarize to resting potentials less than −60 mV, they may become inexcitable and of little electrophysiological importance (see Chap. 31). As they are depolarizing to that range, however, or repolarizing as a consequence of reperfusion, the membranes pass through ranges of reduced excitability, upstroke velocity, and time courses of repolarization. These characteristics result in slow conduction and electrophysiological heterogeneity. When this occurs in ischemic myocardium that is adjacent to nonischemic tissue, it creates a setting for the key elements of reentry, slow conduction and unidirectional block, which makes the myocardium vulnerable to reentrant arrhythmias. When premature impulses are generated in this environment, regardless of their electrical mechanism (e.g., reentrant, triggered activity, automaticity), they may further alter the dispersion of recovery between ischemic tissue, chronically abnormal tissue, and normal cells, ultimately leading to complete disorganization and VF.

The dispersion of refractory periods produced by acute ischemia, which provides the substrate for reentrant tachycardias and VF, may be further enhanced by a healed ischemic injury. The time course of repolarization is lengthened after healing of ischemic injury and shortened by acute ischemia. The coexistence of the two appears to make the ventricle more susceptible to sustained arrhythmias in some experimental models.

Bradyarrhythmias and Asystolic Arrest

The basic electrophysiological mechanism in this form of arrest is failure of normal subordinate automatic activity to assume the pacemaking function of the heart in the absence of normal function of the sinus node, AV junction, or both. Asystolic arrests are more common in severely diseased hearts and with cardiac arrest in patients with a number of end-stage disorders, cardiac and noncardiac. These mechanisms may result, in part, from diffuse involvement of subendocardial Purkinje fibers in advanced heart disease. Systemic influences that increase extracellular K^+ concentration, such as anoxia, acidosis, shock, renal failure, trauma, and hypothermia, can result in partial depolarization of normal or already diseased pacemaker cells in the His-Purkinje system, with a decrease in the slope of spontaneous phase 4 depolarization and ultimate loss of automaticity. These processes can produce global dysfunction of automatic cell activity, in contrast to the regional dysfunction more common in acute ischemia. Functionally depressed automatic cells (e.g., because of increased extracellular K^+ concentration) are more susceptible to overdrive suppression. Under these conditions, brief bursts of tachycardia may be followed by prolonged asystolic periods, with further depression of automaticity by the consequent acidosis and increased local K^+ concentration or by changes in adrenergic tone. The ultimate consequence may be degeneration into VF or persistent asystole.

Pulseless Electrical Activity

Pulseless electrical activity, formerly called electromechanical dissociation, is separated into primary and secondary forms. The common denominator in both is continued electrical rhythmicity of the heart in the absence of effective mechanical function. The secondary form includes the causes that result from an abrupt cessation of cardiac venous return, such as massive pulmonary embolism, acute malfunction of prosthetic valves, exsanguination, and cardiac tamponade from hemopericardium. The primary form is the more familiar; in this form, none of these obvious mechanical factors are present but ventricular muscle fails to produce an effective contraction despite continued electrical activity (i.e., failure of electromechanical coupling). It usually occurs as an end-stage event in advanced heart disease, but can occur in patients with acute ischemic events or, more commonly, after electrical resuscitation from a prolonged cardiac arrest. Although it is not thoroughly understood, it appears that diffuse disease, metabolic abnormalities, or global ischemia provides the pathophysiological substrate. The proximate mechanism for failure of electromechanical coupling may be abnormal intracellular Ca^{2+} metabolism, intracellular acidosis, or perhaps adenosine triphosphate depletion.

CLINICAL FEATURES OF THE PATIENT WITH CARDIAC ARREST

Although the pathological anatomy associated with SCD caused by coronary artery disease reflects the presence of the changes associated with acute coronary syndromes in most cases, only one of five survivors of out-of-hospital VF have clinical evidence of a new transmural myocardial infarction.[142] Nonetheless, many have enzyme level elevations, with nonspecific electrocardiographic changes suggesting myocardial damage, which may be caused by transient ischemia as a triggering event or may be a consequence of the loss of myocardial perfusion during the cardiac arrest. The former supports the concept of transient pathophysiological changes associated with acute coronary syndromes as the trigger for cardiac arrest. The recurrence rate in survivors of out-of-hospital cardiac arrest is low in the subgroup of patients who had documented transmural myocardial infarction. In contrast, early studies have demonstrated a 30 percent recurrence rate at 1 year and 45 percent at 2 years in the survivors who did not have a new transmural myocardial infarction. Recurrence rates decreased subsequently,[142] possibly in part the result of long-term interventions. However, it is not known whether the decrease resulted from a change in the natural history, changes in preventive strategies for underlying disease, or long-term interventions for controlling arrhythmic risk.

Clinical cardiac arrest and SCD can be described in the framework of the same four phases of the event used to establish temporal definitions (see Fig. 36-1)—prodromes, onset of the terminal event, the cardiac arrest, and progression to biological death or survival.

Prodromal Symptoms

Patients at risk for SCD can have prodromes such as chest pain, dyspnea, weakness or fatigue, palpitations, syncope, and a number of nonspecific complaints. Several epidemiological and clinical studies have demonstrated that such symptoms can presage coronary events, particularly myocardial infarction and SCD, and result in contact with the medical system weeks to months before SCD. Among a group of patients successfully resuscitated after out-of-hospital cardiac arrest, 28 percent reported retrospectively that they had had new or changing angina pectoris or dyspnea in the 4 weeks before arrest and 31 percent had seen a physician during this time, but only 12 percent because of these symptoms.

Attempts to identify early prodromal symptoms specific for the patient at risk for SCD have not been successful. Although several studies have reported that 12 to 46 percent of fatalities occur in patients who had seen a physician 1 to 6 months before death, such visits are more likely to presage myocardial infarction or nonsudden deaths, and most complaints responsible for those visits are not heart-related. However, patients who have chest pain as a prodrome to SCD appear to have a higher probability of intraluminal coronary thrombosis at postmortem examination. Fatigue has been a particularly common symptom in the days or weeks before SCD in a number of studies, but this symptom is nonspecific. The symptoms that occur within the last hours or minutes before cardiac arrest are more specific for heart disease and may include symptoms of arrhythmias, ischemia, and heart failure.

Onset of the Terminal Event

The period of 1 hour or less between acute changes in cardiovascular status and the cardiac arrest itself is defined as the "onset of the terminal event." Ambulatory recordings fortuitously obtained during the onset of an unexpected cardiac arrest have indicated dynamic changes in cardiac electrical activity during the minutes or hours before the event.[148] Increasing heart rate and advancing grades of ventricular ectopy are common antecedents of VF. Alterations in autonomic nervous system activity may also contribute to the onset of the event. Studies of short-term variations of heart rate variability, or related measures, have identified changes that correlate with the occurrence of ventricular arrhythmias.[149] Although these physiological properties may be associated with transient electrophysiological destabilization of the myocardium, the extent to which they are paralleled by clinical symptoms or events has been less well documented.[150] SCDs caused by arrhythmias or acute circulatory failure mechanisms correlate with a high incidence of acute myocardial disorders at the onset of the terminal event; such disorders are more likely to be ischemic when the death is caused by arrhythmias and to be associated with low-output states or myocardial anoxia when the deaths are caused by circulatory failure.

Abrupt, unexpected loss of effective circulation can be caused by cardiac arrhythmias or mechanical disturbances, but most such events that terminate in SCD are arrhythmic. Hinkle and Thaler[151] have classified cardiac deaths in 142 subjects who died during a follow-up of 5 to 10 years. Class I was labeled arrhythmic death and class II was death caused by circulatory failure. The distinction between the two classes was based on whether circulatory failure preceded (class II) or followed (class I) the disappearance of the pulse. Among deaths that occurred less than 1 hour after the onset of the terminal illness, 93 percent were caused by arrhythmias; in addition, 90 percent of deaths caused by heart disease were initiated by arrhythmic events rather than circulatory failure. Deaths caused by circulatory failure occurred predominantly among patients who could be identified as having terminal illnesses (95 percent were comatose), were associated more frequently with bradyarrhythmias than with VF as the terminal arrhythmias, and were dominated by noncardiac events as the terminal illness. In contrast, 98 percent of the arrhythmic deaths were associated primarily with cardiac disorders.

Cardiac Arrest

Cardiac arrest is characterized by abrupt loss of consciousness caused by lack of adequate cerebral blood flow. It is an event that uniformly leads to death in the absence of an active intervention, although spontaneous reversions occur rarely. The most common cardiac mechanism is VF, followed by asystole—pulseless electrical activity and sustained VT. Other mechanisms include rupture of the ventricle, cardiac tamponade, acute mechanical obstruction to flow, and acute disruption of a major blood vessel.

The potential for successful resuscitation is a function of the setting in which cardiac arrest occurs, the mechanism of the arrest, and the underlying clinical status of the victim. Closely related to the potential for successful resuscitation is the decision of whether to attempt to resuscitate.[152]

At present, there are fewer low-risk patients with otherwise uncomplicated myocardial infarctions weighting in-hospital cardiac arrest statistics than occurred previously. In one report, only 14 percent of patients receiving in-hospital cardiopulmonary resuscitation (CPR) were discharged from the hospital alive and 20 percent of these patients died within the ensuing 6 months. Although 41 percent of the patients had suffered an acute myocardial infarction, 73 percent had a history of congestive heart failure and 20 percent had had prior cardiac arrests. The mean age of 70 years may have influenced the outcome statistics, but patients with high-risk complicated myocardial infarction and those with other high-risk markers heavily influenced the population of patients at risk for in-hospital cardiac arrest. Noncardiac clinical diagnoses were dominated by renal failure, pneumonia, sepsis, diabetes, and a history of cancer. The strong male preponderance consistently reported in out-of-hospital cardiac arrest studies is not present in in-hospital patients, but the better prognosis of VT or VF mechanisms, compared with pulseless electrical activity (PEA) or asystolic mechanisms, persists (27 percent survival versus 8 percent survival). However, the proportion of arrests caused by in-hospital VT or VF is considerably less (33 percent), with the combination of respiratory arrest, asystole, and PEA dominating the statistics (61 percent). In another report, a 22 percent survival to hospital discharge was observed. Adverse risks were age older than 70 years, prior stroke or renal failure, or heart failure on admission. Better outcomes were predicted by prior angina pectoris or admission because of ventricular arrhythmias.

The important risk factors for death after CPR are listed in Table 36-3. The fraction of out-of-hospital cardiac arrest survivors who are discharged from the hospital alive may now equal or exceed the fraction of in-hospital cardiac arrest victims who are discharged alive, and the postdischarge mortality rate for in-hospital cardiac arrest survivors is higher than that for out-of-hospital cardiac arrest survivors; these are telling clinical statistics. Not only do they emphasize the success of preventive measures for cardiac

TABLE 36–3 Predictors of Mortality After In-Hospital Cardiopulmonary Resuscitation Before Arrest

Before Arrest	
Hypotension (systolic BP<100 mm Hg)	
Pneumonia	
Renal failure (BUN>50 mg/dl)	
Cancer	
Homebound life style	
During Arrest	
Arrest duration >15 min	
Intubation	
Hypotension (systolic BP<100 mm Hg)	
Pneumonia	
Homebound life style	
After Resuscitation	
Coma	
Need for pressors	
Arrest duration>15 min	

BP=blood pressure; BUN=blood urea nitrogen.

Modified from Bedell SE, Delbanco TL, Cook EF, Epstein FH: Survival after cardiopulmonary resuscitation in the hospital. N Engl J Med 309:569, 1983.

arrest in low-risk in-hospital patients, causing those statistics to be dominated by higher risk patients, but also they suggest the need for newer strategies for rapid in-hospital responses,[153] in addition to emphasizing the need for improvement in prehospital and in-hospital care of out-of-hospital cardiac arrest victims.

Among elderly persons, the outcomes after community-based responses to out-of-hospital cardiac arrest are not as good as for younger victims. In one study comparing persons younger than 80 years (mean age, 64 years) with those in their 80s and 90s, survival to hospital discharge among the younger group was 19.4 percent compared with 9.4 percent for octogenarians and 4.4 percent for nonagenarians.[154] However, when the groups were analyzed according to markers favoring survival (e.g., VF, pulseless VT), the incremental benefit was even better for the elderly than for the younger patients (36, 24, and 17 percent, respectively), but the frequency of ventricular tachyarrhythmias compared with nonshockable rhythms was lower among elderly persons.[154] Overall, age is only a weak predictor of an adverse outcome and should not be used in isolation as a reason not to resuscitate. Long-term neurological status and length of hospitalization were similar among older and younger surviving patients.

Progression to Biological Death

The time course for progression from cardiac arrest to biological death is related to the mechanism of the cardiac arrest, the nature of the underlying disease process, and the delay between onset and resuscitative efforts. The onset of irreversible brain damage usually begins within 4 to 6 minutes after loss of cerebral circulation related to unattended cardiac arrest, and biological death follows quickly. In large series, however, it has been demonstrated that a limited number of victims can remain biologically alive for longer periods and may be resuscitated after delays in excess of 8 minutes before beginning basic life support and in excess of 16 minutes before advanced life support. Despite these exceptions, it is clear that the probability of a favorable outcome deteriorates rapidly as a function of time after unattended cardiac arrest. Younger patients with less severe cardiac disease and the absence of coexistent multisystem disease have a higher probability of a favorable outcome after such delays.

Irreversible injury of the central nervous system usually occurs before biological death, and the interval may extend to a period of weeks in patients who are resuscitated during the temporal gap between brain damage and biological death. In-hospital cardiac arrest caused by VF is less likely to have a protracted course between the arrest and biological death, with patients surviving after a prompt intervention or succumbing rapidly because of inability to stabilize cardiac rhythm or hemodynamics.

The patients whose cardiac arrest is caused by sustained VT with cardiac output inadequate to maintain consciousness can remain in VT for considerably longer periods, with blood flow that is marginally sufficient to maintain viability. Thus, there is a longer interval between the onset of cardiac arrest and the end of the period that allows successful resuscitation. The lives of such patients usually end in VF or an asystolic arrest if the VT is not actively or spontaneously reverted. Once the transition from VT to VF or to a bradyarrhythmia has occurred, the subsequent course to biological death is similar to that in patients in whom VF or bradyarrhythmias are the initiating event.

The progression in patients with asystole or PEA as the initiating event is more rapid. Such patients, whether in an in-hospital or out-of-hospital environment, have a poor prognosis because of advanced heart disease or coexistent multisystem disease. They tend to respond poorly to interventions, even if the heart is successfully paced. Although a small subgroup of patients with bradyarrhythmias associated with electrolyte or pharmacological abnormalities may respond well to interventions, most progress rapidly to biological death. The infrequent cardiac arrests caused by mechanical factors such as tamponade, structural disruption, and impedance to flow by major thromboembolic obstructions to right or left ventricular outflow are reversible only in patients in whom the mechanism is recognized and an intervention is feasible. The vast majority of these events lead to rapid biological death, although prompt relief of tamponade will save some lives.

Survivors of Cardiac Arrest

Hospital Course

The conditions of patients who are resuscitated immediately from primary VF associated with acute myocardial infarction usually stabilize promptly, and they require no special management after the early phase of the infarction (see Chap. 51). The management after secondary cardiac arrest in myocardial infarction is dominated by the hemodynamic status of the patient. Survivors of out-of-hospital cardiac arrest may have repetitive ventricular arrhythmias during the initial 24 to 48 hours of hospitalization. These arrhythmias have variable responses to antiarrhythmic therapy, depending on hemodynamic status. The overall rate of recurrent cardiac arrest is low, 10 to 20 percent, but the mortality rate in patients who have recurrent cardiac arrests is about 50 percent. Only 5 to 10 percent of in-hospital deaths after out-of-hospital resuscitation are caused by recurrent cardiac arrhythmias. Patients who have recurrent cardiac arrest have a high incidence of new or preexisting AV or intraventricular conduction abnormalities.[142]

The most common causes of death in hospitalized survivors of out-of-hospital cardiac arrest are noncardiac events related to central nervous system injury.[142,155] These include anoxic encephalopathy and sepsis related to prolonged intubation and hemodynamic monitoring lines. Fifty-nine percent of deaths during index hospitalization after prehospital resuscitation have been reported to be from these causes. Approximately 40 percent of those who arrive in hospital in coma never awaken after admission to the hospital and die after a median survival of 3.5 days. Two thirds of those who regain consciousness have no gross deficits, and an additional 20 percent have persisting cognitive deficits only. Of the patients who do awaken, 25 percent do so by admission, 71 percent by the first hospital day, and 92 percent by the third day. A small number of patients have awakened after prolonged hospitalization. Among those who die in hospital, 80 percent do not awaken before death. Two studies have suggested a potential benefit of therapeutic hypothermia for patients with post-cardiac arrest coma (see later, "Clinical Profile of Survivors of Out-of-Hospital Cardiac Arrest").[156,157]

Cardiac causes of delayed death during hospitalization after out-of-hospital cardiac arrest are most commonly related to hemodynamic deterioration, which accounts for about one third of deaths in hospitals. Among all deaths, those that occurred within the first 48 hours of hospitalization were usually caused by hemodynamic deterioration or arrhythmias regardless of the neurological status; later deaths were related to neurological complications. Admission characteristics most predictive of subsequent awakening included motor response, pupillary light response, spontaneous eye movement, and blood glucose level below 300 mg/dl.

Clinical Profile of Survivors of Out-of-Hospital Cardiac Arrest

The clinical features of survivors of out-of-hospital cardiac arrest are heavily influenced by the type and extent of the underlying disease associated with the event. Causation is dominated by coronary heart disease, which accounts for approximately 80 percent of out-of hospital cardiac arrest in the United States[7] and is commonly extensive. The cardiomyopathies collectively account for another 10 to 15 percent, with all other structural heart diseases plus functional abnormalities and toxic or environmental causes accounting for the remainder (see Table 36-2).[57,158]

Ambient ventricular arrhythmias have been reported in most survivors of prehospital cardiac arrest who had serial ambulatory monitor recordings. These arrhythmias show trends to higher grades of ventricular ectopy in victims of recurrent cardiac arrest compared with long-term survivors. Repetitive PVCs were strongly associated with a history of congestive heart failure or previous myocardial infarction.

LEFT VENTRICULAR FUNCTION. Left ventricular function is abnormal in most survivors of out-of-hospital cardiac arrest, often severely abnormal, but there is a wide variation, ranging from severe dysfunction to normal or near-normal measurements (Fig. 36-12).[159] The severity of myocardial dysfunction estimated shortly after cardiac arrest commonly improves within the first 24 hours of hospitalization.[160] Failure to begin improvement within that time frame is an adverse short-term prognostic sign. In a study of resuscitated out-of-hospital cardiac arrest victims admitted to hospital and subsequently discharged alive and neurologically intact, 47 percent had acute coronary syndromes identified during work-up and had a mean ejection fraction of 42 percent, compared with 32 percent in nonsurvivors.[161] Among survivors to hospital discharge, a reduced ejection fraction is an adverse long-term prognostic sign.

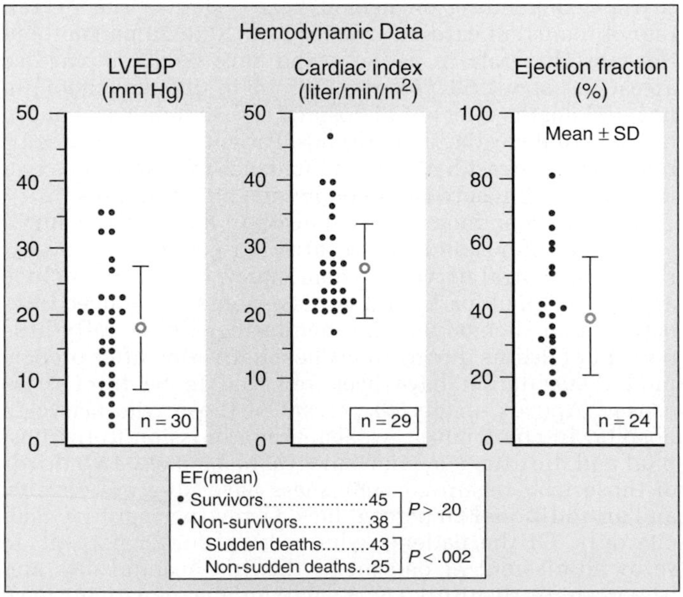

FIGURE 36–12 Hemodynamic data from victims of prehospital cardiac arrest studied during initial postarrest hospitalization. These data indicate a broad range of cardiac function and a statistically insignificant difference between ejection fraction at entry in long-term survivors and in victims of recurrent cardiac arrest. However, patients who died suddenly had a significantly higher ejection fraction than those who died of nonsudden cardiac causes. LVEDP = left ventricular end-diastolic pressure. *(From Myerburg RJ, Conde CA, Sung RJ, et al: Clinical, electrophysiologic and hemodynamic profile of patients resuscitated from prehospital cardiac arrest. Am J Med 68:568, 1980.)*

CORONARY ANGIOGRAPHY. Studies of survivors of out-of-hospital cardiac arrest have shown that as a group, this population tends to have extensive disease but no specific pattern of abnormalities. Acute coronary lesions, usually multifocal, are present in most survivors.[139] Significant lesions in two or more vessels are present in at least 70 percent of patients who have any coronary lesion. Among patients who have recurrent cardiac arrests, the incidence of triple-vessel disease is higher than among those who do not. However, the frequency of moderate to severe stenosis of the left main coronary artery does not differ between cardiac arrest survivors and the overall population of patients with symptomatic coronary heart disease.

EXERCISE TESTING. Exercise testing is no longer commonly used to evaluate the need for, and response to, antiischemic therapy in survivors of out-of-hospital cardiac arrest, except when there is a question of transient ischemia as a mechanism for onset. The probability of a positive test related to ischemia is relatively low, although termination of testing because of fatigue is common.[142] Mortality during follow-up is higher in patients who have angina or failure of a normal rise in systolic blood pressure occurring during exercise.

ELECTROCARDIOGRAPHIC OBSERVATIONS. Among survivors of out-of-hospital cardiac arrest, the 12-lead ECG (see Chap. 12) has proved of value only for discriminating risk of recurrence among those whose cardiac arrest was associated with new transmural myocardial infarction. Patients who develop documented new Q waves in association with a clinical picture suggesting that an acute myocardial infarction began before the cardiac arrest itself are at lower risk for recurrence.[142] In contrast, nonspecific electrocardiographic markers of ischemia, associated with elevations of troponin or creatine kinase MB levels, indicate higher risk of recurrence. A higher incidence of repolarization abnormalities (e.g., ST segment depression, flat T waves, prolonged QT) occurs in out-of-hospital cardiac arrest survivors than in post-myocardial infarction patients, and these might be markers for increased risk. Prolonged QRS duration is associated with increased mortality risk in patients with heart failure,[162] although it is not clear that this observation applies to sudden death specifically or to post-cardiac arrest victims in particular.

BLOOD CHEMISTRY. Lower serum K^+ levels are observed in survivors of cardiac arrest than in patients with acute myocardial infarction or stable coronary heart disease. This finding is probably a consequence of resuscitation interventions rather than a preexisting hypokalemic state because of chronic diuretic use or other causes. Low ionized Ca^{2+} levels, with normal total calcium levels, were also observed during resuscitation from out-of-hospital cardiac arrest. Higher resting lactate levels have been reported in out-of-hospital cardiac arrest survivors than in normal subjects. Lactate levels correlated inversely with ejection fractions and directly with PVC frequency and complexity.

LONG-TERM PROGNOSIS. Studies from the early 1970s have indicated that the risk of recurrent cardiac arrest in the first year after surviving an initial VT-VF event is about 30 percent and at 2 years is 45 percent. Total mortality at 2 years was about 60 percent in both studies. More recent mortality data,[163] including those from the control groups of the secondary prevention implantable cardioverter-defibrillator (ICD) trials,[164-166] have demonstrated 2-year mortality rates between 15 and 25 percent. The apparent improved outcomes, independent of the benefit provided by ICD therapy, are probably attributable to the current interventions used among survivors, such as beta-adrenoceptor blockers, antiischemic procedures, amiodarone, and other therapies that were not available or in general use at the earlier time. Risk of recurrent cardiac arrest and all-cause mortality is higher during the first 12 to 24 months after the index event and relates best to ejection fraction during the first 6 months (Fig. 36-13).

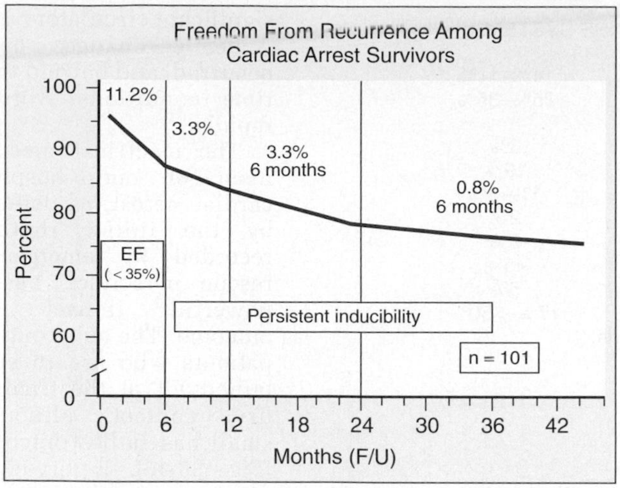

FIGURE 36–13 Time dependence of recurrences among survivors of cardiac arrest. Actuarial analysis of occurrences among a population of 101 cardiac arrest survivors with coronary artery disease is demonstrated. The risk was highest in the first 6 months (11.2 percent) and then fell to 3.3 percent per 6 months for the next three 6-month blocks. After 24 months, the rate fell to 0.8 percent per 6 months. A low ejection fraction (EF) was the most powerful predictor of death during the first 6 months; subsequently, persistent inducibility during programmed stimulation, despite drug therapy or surgery, was the most powerful predictor. F/U = follow-up. *(From Myerburg RJ, Kessler KM, Castellanos A: Sudden cardiac death: Structure, function, and time-dependence of risk. Circulation 85[Suppl I]:I-2, 1992. © 1992 American Heart Association. Modified from Furukawa T, et al: Circulation 80:599, 1989.)*

MANAGEMENT OF CARDIAC ARREST

The response to a cardiac arrest is driven by two urgent principles: (1) restoring a spontaneous circulation as quickly as possible; and (2) maintaining continuous artificial circulatory support until return of a spontaneous circulation has been achieved. To achieve these goals, the management strategy is divided into five elements: (1) initial assessment and summoning an emergency response team; (2) basic life support (BLS); (3) early defibrillation by a first responder (if available); (4) advanced life support; and (5) post-cardiac arrest care. If successful, the algorithm is followed by a sixth element, long-term management. The initial elements can be applied by a broad array of responders, which includes physicians and nurses as well as paramedical personnel, emergency rescue technicians, and laypeople trained in bystander interventions. The requirements for specialized knowledge and skills become progressively more focused as the patient moves through post-cardiac arrest management and into long-term follow-up care.[152,167] These emergency response principles are intended for both in-hospital application and community-based responses.

Community-Based Interventions

The initial systems responding to out-of-hospital cardiac arrests were integrated into fire departments as primary emergency rescue systems. They used paramedical personnel trained in CPR and the use of CPR monitoring equipment, defibrillators, and specific intravenous drug therapy. Although the initial out-of-hospital intervention experience in Miami and Seattle, reported in the mid-1970s, yielded only 14 and 11 percent rates of survival to discharge, respectively, later improvements in the systems saved more lives (Fig. 36-14A).[168] By the early 1980s, both had increased survival rates to about 25 percent,[142,168] and by the late 1980s to 30 percent or more. Improvements correlated with the addition of emergency medical technicians as another tier of responders to provide CPR and earlier defibrillation. Survival rates have decreased since then, presumably because of the extension of rescue systems into less densely populated regions, in addition to increased traffic congestion and "verticalization" of buildings in urban areas (see Fig. 36-14A). Generally, rural areas have lower success rates, and the national success rate for the United States is probably 5 percent or less.

Reports from very densely populated areas (i.e., Chicago and New York City) have also provided disturbing outcome data. The Chicago study has reported that only 9 percent of out-of-hospital cardiac arrest victims survive to be hospitalized and that only 2 percent are discharged alive.[169] Moreover, outcomes in blacks are far worse than in whites (0.8 percent versus 2.6 percent). The fact that a large majority had bradyarrhythmias, asystole, or pulseless electrical activity on initial contact with emergency medical services suggests prolonged times between collapse and emergency medical service arrival, absent or ineffective bystander interventions, or both. The New York City report has indicated a survival-to-hospital discharge rate of only 1.4 percent.[170] Among those who have bystander CPR, the rate increases to 2.9 percent, and bystander CPR plus VF as the initial rhythm yields a further increase to 5.3 percent. Finally, for those whose arrests occurred after the arrival of emergency medical services, the success rate increases further, to 8.5 percent. These trends support the concept that delays and breaks in the "chain of survival"[171] have a major negative impact on results of emergency medical services in densely populated areas.

There are circumstances in which resuscitative efforts in the out-of-hospital setting are deemed futile. The victim found unconscious after an unwitnessed collapse, reasonably assumed to be found after a prolonged interval (e.g., cool skin, rigor mortis) obviously fulfills this classification. However, recent studies have provided markers of futility under less stark circumstances. In a study involving trained responders with automated external defibrillators (AEDs), only 0.5 percent of victims survived if (1) the arrest was not witnessed by Emergency Medical Service (EMS) personnel, (2) there was no return of spontaneous circulation, and (3) no shocks were delivered per protocol. Adding a response time longer than 8 minutes reduced survival to 0.3 percent, and events unwitnessed by a bystander yielded no survivors.[172]

IMPORTANCE OF ELECTRICAL MECHANISMS. Several sources have identified a disturbing trend in initial rhythms recorded by emergency rescue personnel.[5,173,174] Compared with data from the 1970s and 1980s, there has been a decrease in the number of events in which ventricular tachyarrhythmias are the initial rhythm recorded, with a consequent reduction in the proportion of victims who have rhythms amenable to cardioversion-defibrillation (Fig. 36-15). Similar observations have been reported in in-hospital settings.[175] Some studies have now suggested that less than 50 percent of victims have shockable rhythms at initial contact. This fact is associated with a reduction in cumulative survival probabilities from community-based interventions,[5] even though data from studies using nonconventional AED strategies have suggested improvement for outcomes in VT or VF victims.[173,174] Because this finding does not appear to be related to time from the 911 summons to arrival, it is likely that pre-911 delays in recognition and reaction to an event may be playing a role, which suggests a need for more extensive public education programs. Thus, response times may not be as close to true down times as one would hope, impairing the potential for success. The 4- to 6-minute time for a desirable response is not optimal. By 4 minutes,

HISTORY OF COMMUNITY-BASED EMERGENCY RESPONSE SYSTEMS		
1971–1974	Initial Miami/Seattle outcomes	14%, 11%
1978–1985	Peak Miami/Seattle outcomes	25%–35%
1984	Rural outcomes:	
	• Standard basic life support	3%
	• Ambulance-based expanded access	19%
1991	Estimated cumulative U.S. survival	1%–3%
1992–1994	Major metropolitan population centers	2%
1996	Dade county, Florida, current outcomes	9%
1996–1998	Updated U.S. EMS outcomes, cumulative	<5%
1999	"Optimized" EMS systems {OPALS}	5%
2000–2004	Non-conventional responders; Public access sites [Police, security guards, airline personnel, lay persons; airports and airliners, malls, casinos, stadiums]	17%–>50%

A

AED DEPLOYMENT STRATEGIES

Deployment	Examples	Rescuers	Advantages	Limitations
Emergency vehicles	• Police cars • Fire engines • Ambulances	• Trained emergency personnel	• Experienced users • Broad deployment • Objectivity	• Deployment time • Arrival delays • Community variations
Public access sites	• Public buildings • Stadiums, malls • Airports • Airliners	• Security personnel • Designated rescuers • Random lay persons	• Population density • Shorter delays • Lay and emergency personnel access	• Low event rates • Inexperienced users • Panic and confusion
Multi-family dwellings	• Apartments • Condominiums • Hotels	• Security personnel • Designated rescuers • Family members	• Familiar locations • Defined personnel • Shorter delays	• Infrequent use • Low event rates • Geographic factors
Single-family dwellings	• Private homes • Apartments • Neighborhood "Heart watch"	• Family members	• Immediate access • Familiar setting	• Acceptance • Victim may be alone • One-time user; panic

B

FIGURE 36–14 Out-of-hospital cardiac arrest survival and deployment strategies for automated external defibrillators (AEDs). **A,** The history of out-of-hospital cardiac arrest survival statistics demonstrates that standard emergency rescue systems are not sufficient to have a meaningful impact on sudden cardiac death in the community. **B,** Various deployment strategies for nonconventional responders with access to AEDs. For each example, the type of rescuer and the advantages and limitations of each strategy are provided. It is unlikely that any single strategy will dominate; rather, there will be a cumulative benefit from the additive effect of multiple approaches. EMS = emergency medical service; OPALS = Ontario Prehospital Advanced Life Support. *(From Myerburg RJ: Sudden cardiac death: Exploring the limits of our knowledge. J Cardiovasc Electrophysiol 12:369, 2001.)*

CH 36

significant circulatory and ischemic changes have occurred, and beyond that time conditions worsen rapidly.[176]

The electrical mechanism of out-of-hospital cardiac arrest, as defined by the initial rhythm recorded by emergency rescue personnel, has a powerful impact on outcome. The subgroup of patients who are in sustained VT at the time of first contact, although small, has the best outcome (Fig. 36-16). Eighty-eight percent of patients in cardiac arrest related to VT were successfully resuscitated and admitted to the hospital alive, and 67 percent were ultimately discharged alive.[142] However, this relatively low-risk group represents only 7 to 10 percent of all cardiac arrests. Because of the inherent time lag between collapse and initial recordings, it is likely that many more cardiac arrests begin as rapid sustained VT and degenerate into VF before arrival of rescue personnel.

Patients who have a bradyarrhythmia or asystole, or pulseless electrical activity (PEA), at initial contact have the worst prognosis; only 9 percent of such patients in the Miami study were admitted to the hospital alive and none was discharged.[142] In a later experience, there was some improvement in outcome, although the improvement was limited to patients in whom the initial bradyarrhythmia recorded was an idioventricular rhythm that responded promptly to chronotropic agents in the field. In a large prospective observational in-hospital study of cardiac arrests in children and adults, children had a higher probability of asystole or PEA as the initial documented rhythm, but had a better overall survival rate because they had better outcomes of interventions for these rhythms than adults.[175]

Bradyarrhythmias also have adverse prognostic implications after defibrillation from VF in the field. Patients who developed a heart rate lower than 60 beats/min after defibrillation regardless of the specific bradyarrhythmic mechanism had a poor prognosis, with 95 percent of such patients dying before hospitalization or in the hospital. The outcome in the group of patients in whom VF is the initial rhythm recorded is intermediate between the outcomes associated with sustained VT and bradyarrhythmia and asystole. Of such patients, 40 percent were successfully resuscitated and admitted to the hospital alive and 23 percent were ultimately discharged alive (see Fig. 36-16).[142] Later data indicate improvement in outcome. The proportion of each of the electrophysiological mechanisms responsible for cardiac arrest varied among the earlier reports, with VF ranging

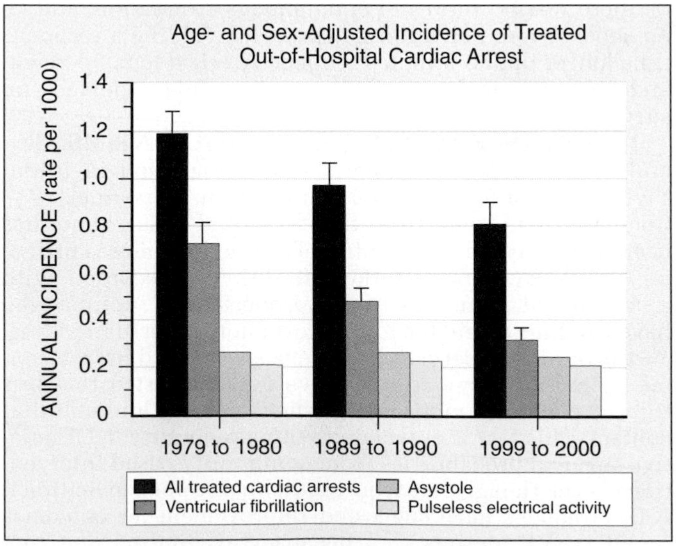

FIGURE 36–15 Changing incidence of ventricular fibrillation in the community. Between 1980 and 2000, there was a progressive decrease in the ventricular fibrillation event rate in the Seattle, Washington, community for unexplained reasons. Of note is the fact that there was no concomitant increase in nonshockable rhythms. The proportion of events with ventricular fibrillation at initial contact is decreasing, as observed in several other studies. *(Modified from Cobb LA, Fahrenbruch CE, Olsufka M, Copass MK: Changing incidence of out-of-hospital ventricular fibrillation, 1980-2000. JAMA 288:3008, 2002.)*

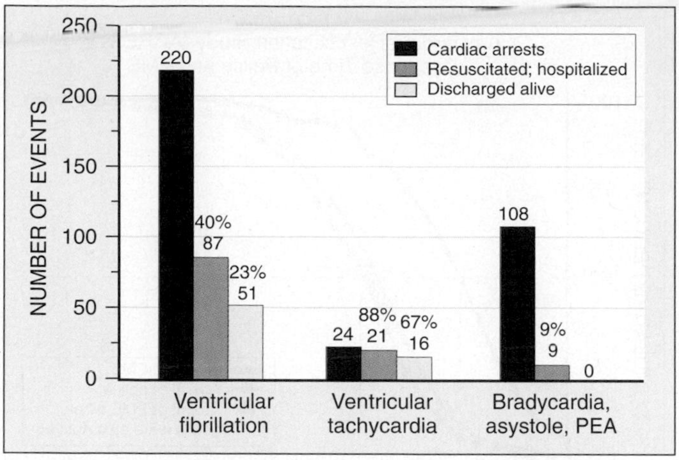

FIGURE 36–16 Survival after out-of-hospital cardiac arrest as a function of the initial electrophysiological mechanism recorded by emergency rescue personnel. The mechanisms among 352 out-of-hospital cardiac arrest victims are separated into three categories: ventricular fibrillation ($n = 220$; 62 percent); ventricular tachycardia ($n = 24$; 7 percent); and bradycardia, asystole, and pulseless electrical activity (PEA) ($n = 108$; 31 percent). The purple bars illustrate the total number of events in each category. The blue bars illustrate the number and percentage of patients who were initially resuscitated in the field and reached the hospital alive in each category, and the yellow bars illustrate the percentage of total events in which patients were discharged from the hospital alive for each category. The data are derived from the Miami, Florida, experience. *(Modified from Myerburg RJ, Kessler KM, Zaman L, et al: Survivors of prehospital cardiac arrest. JAMA 247:1485, 1982.)*

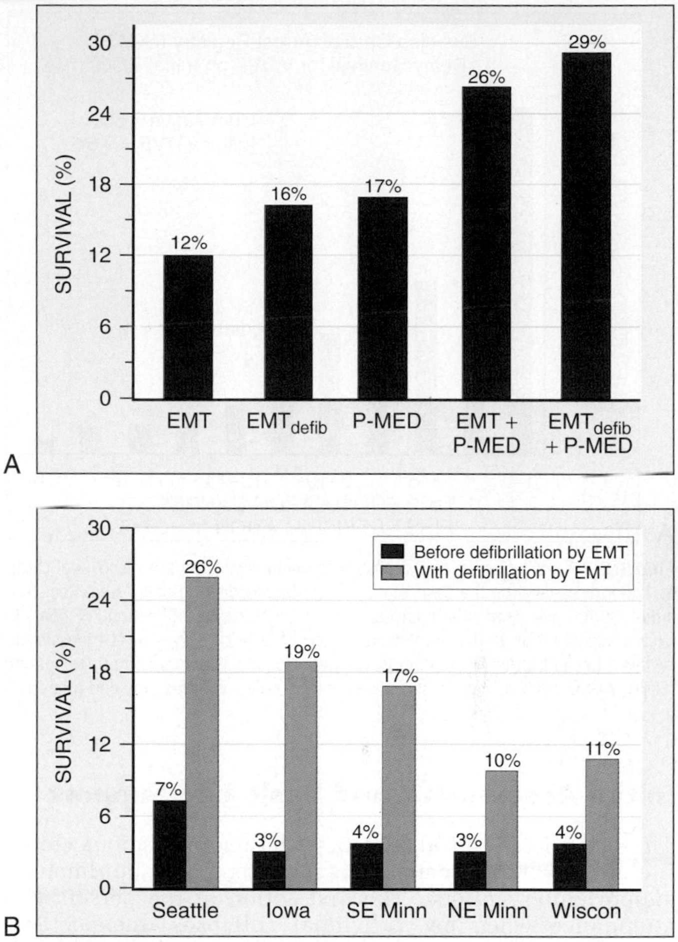

FIGURE 36–17 Impact of emergency rescue system design and immediate defibrillation on out-of-hospital cardiac arrest survival. **A,** Percent survival to hospital discharge with rescue activities by standard emergency medical technician (EMT) trained in cardiopulmonary resuscitation (CPR), EMTs allowed to defibrillate immediately (EMT_{defib}), initial response by paramedics (P-MED), two-tiered system with EMT and P-MED, and two-tiered system with EMTs allowed to defibrillate if they are the first responders plus P-MED. Training of first-responders (EMT_{defib}) and a two-tiered system have the best outcome. **B,** Comparison of outcomes observed in five geographic areas with EMTs providing only CPR (purple) versus EMTs trained to defibrillate as first responders (blue). In each group, there was a marked improvement in outcome when EMT personnel were trained and permitted to defibrillate. *(Modified from Ornato JP, Om A: Community experience in treating out-of-hospital cardiac arrest.* In *Akhtar M, Myerburg RJ, Ruskin JN [eds]: Sudden Cardiac Death: Prevalence, Mechanisms and Approach to Diagnosis and Management. Baltimore, Williams & Wilkins, 1994, p 450.)*

from 65 to more than 90 percent of the study populations and bradyarrhythmia and asystole ranging from 10 to 30 percent. However, in reports from densely populated metropolitan areas, the ratios of tachyarrhythmic to bradyarrhythmic or pulseless activity events were reversed, and outcomes were far worse.[170]

Both improved prehospital care and improvements in in-hospital technology and practices can contribute to better outcomes, as described in the chain of survival concept.[171] Of these two general factors, the influence of prehospital care has been studied in more detail. The importance of early defibrillation for improving outcome has been supported by a number of studies (Fig. 36-17).[176-180] In rural communities, earlier defibrillation by ambulance technicians yielded a 19 percent survival compared with only 3 percent for standard CPR. In another report, an analysis of the relationship between response delay and survival to hospital discharge revealed a 48 percent survival for response times of 2 minutes or less compared with less than 10 percent survival when responses were longer than 10 minutes (Fig. 36-18A).[177] Mean response time was approximately 13 minutes, and overall survival was 5 percent. It was 9.5 percent for those in VT or VF on first contact. These observations have motivated the search for strategies that shorten response times, such as deploying automatic external defibrillators in public places[180] and use by nonconventional responders.[173,178,179] Preliminary data suggest that this strategy may improve outcome by substantial increments based on the rationale of shortening response times (see later and Fig. 36-18B).

A second element in prehospital care that contributes to outcome is the role of bystander CPR by laypeople awaiting the arrival of emergency rescue personnel.[181,182] It has been reported that although there was no significant difference in the percentage of patients successfully resuscitated and admitted to the hospital alive with (67 percent) or without (61 percent) bystander intervention, almost twice as many prehospital cardiac arrest victims were ultimately discharged alive when they had had bystander CPR (43 percent) than when such support was not provided (22 percent). Central nervous system protection, expressed as early regaining of consciousness, is the major protective element of bystander CPR. The rationale for bystander intervention is further highlighted by the relationship between time to defibrillation and survival when analyzed as a function of time to initiation of basic CPR. It has been reported that more than 40 percent of victims whose defibrillation and other advanced life support activities were instituted more than 8 minutes after collapse survived if basic CPR had been initiated less than 2 minutes after onset of the arrest.[168] A period of CPR before defibrillation may also be helpful,[181] particularly if the time to defibrillation exceeds 4 minutes from onset of arrest.[176,183]

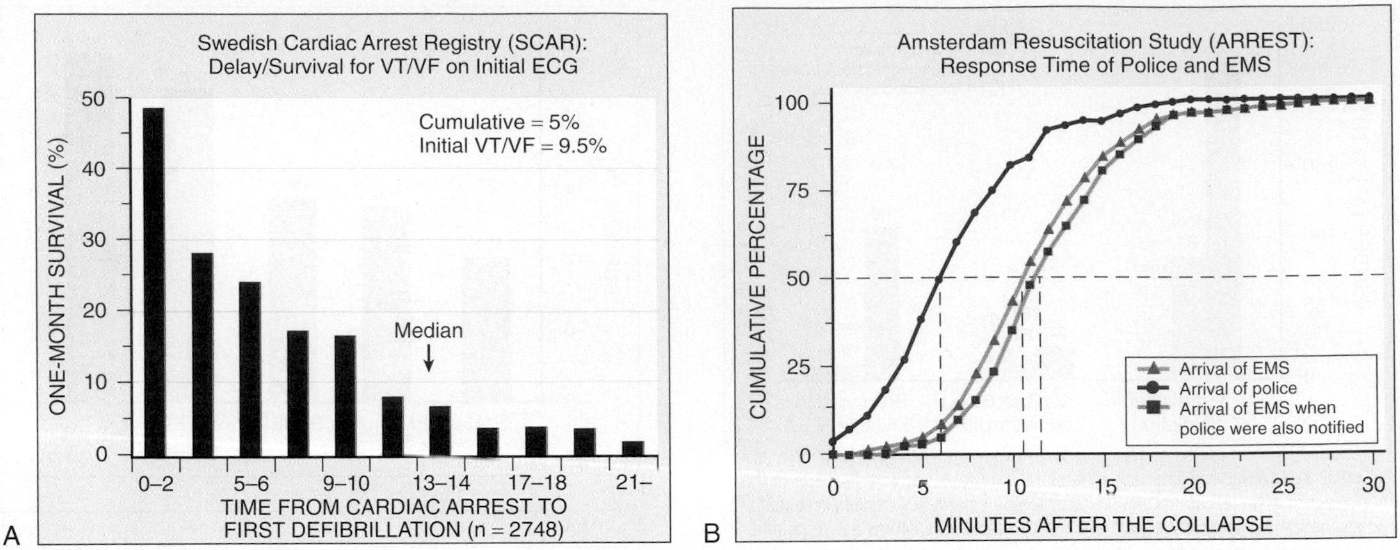

FIGURE 36–18 Influence of response time on survival from out-of-hospital cardiac arrest. **A,** The time from onset of cardiac arrest to initial defibrillation attempt is related to 1-month survival on the basis of data from the Swedish Cardiac Arrest Registry.[177] The cumulative survival rate was 5 percent, and the survival rate for victims whose initial rhythm was ventricular tachycardia (VT) or ventricular fibrillation (VF) was 9.5 percent. The median response time was nearly 13 minutes. Thirty-day survival ranged from a maximum of 48 percent with responses shorter than 2 minutes to less than 5 percent with response time longer than 15 minutes. **B,** The potential for faster response systems, based on the Amsterdam Resuscitation Study, is demonstrated, comparing response times of police vehicles with those of conventional emergency medical systems (EMS). At the 50th percentile of response times, police vehicles provided a nearly 5-minute improvement in arrival time (approximately 6 minutes).[178]

Initial Assessment and Basic Life Support

The activities at initial contact with the unconscious victim include diagnostic maneuvers and basic cardiopulmonary support interventions. The first action of the person(s) in attendance when an individual collapses unexpectedly must be confirmation that collapse is or suspected to be caused by a cardiac arrest. A few seconds of evaluation for response to voice, observation for respiratory movements and skin color, and simultaneous palpation of major arteries for the presence or absence of a pulse yield sufficient information to determine whether a life-threatening incident is in progress. Once a life-threatening incident has been suspected or confirmed, contact with an available emergency medical rescue system (911) for out-of-hospital settings, or a "code" team in-hospital, should be an immediate priority.

The absence of a carotid or femoral pulse, particularly if confirmed by the absence of an audible heartbeat, is a primary diagnostic criterion. For lay responders, the pulse check is no longer recommended.[152,167] Skin color may be pale or intensely cyanotic. Absence of respiratory efforts or the presence of only agonal respiratory efforts, in conjunction with an absent pulse, is diagnostic of cardiac arrest; however, respiratory efforts can persist for 1 minute or longer after the onset of the arrest. In contrast, absence of respiratory efforts or severe stridor with persistence of a pulse suggests a primary respiratory arrest that will lead to a cardiac arrest in a short time. In the latter circumstance, initial efforts should include exploration of the oropharynx in search of a foreign body and the Heimlich maneuver, particularly if the incident occurs in a setting in which aspiration is likely (e.g., restaurant death or café coronary).

CHEST THUMP. When the diagnosis of a pulseless collapse (presumed cardiac arrest) is established, a blow to the chest (precordial thump, "thump-version") may be attempted by a properly trained rescuer. It has been recommended that it be reserved as an advanced life support activity.[152] Caldwell and coworkers[184] have supported its use on the basis of a prospective study in 5000 patients. Precordial thumps successfully reverted VF in 5 events, VT in 11, asystole in 2, and undefined cardiovascular collapse in 2 others in which the electrical mechanism was unknown. In no case was conversion of VT to VF observed. Because the latter is the only major concern about the precordial thump technique and electrical activity can be initiated by mechanical stimulation in the asystolic heart, the technique is considered optional for responding to a pulseless cardiac arrest in the absence of monitoring when a defibrillator is not immediately available. It should not be used unmonitored for the patient with a rapid tachycardia without complete loss of consciousness. For attempted thump-version in cardiac arrest, one or two blows should be delivered firmly to the junction of the middle and lower thirds of the sternum from a height of 8 to 10 inches, but the effort should be abandoned if the patient does not immediately develop a spontaneous pulse and begin breathing. Another mechanical method, which requires that the patient is still conscious, is so-called cough-induced cardiac compression, or cough-version. It is a conscious act of forceful coughing by the patient that may support forward flow by cyclic increases in intrathoracic pressure during VF or may cause conversion of sustained VT. Available data supporting its successful use are limited, and it is not considered an alternative to conventional techniques.

ABCs OF CARDIOPULMONARY RESUSCITATION. The goal of this activity is to maintain viability of the central nervous system, heart, and other vital organs until definitive intervention can be achieved. The activities included in basic life support encompass both the initial responses outlined earlier and their natural flow into establishing ventilation and perfusion. This range of activities can be carried out not only by professional and paraprofessional personnel but also by trained emergency technicians and laypeople. Time is the key issue, and there should be minimal delay between the diagnosis and preparatory efforts in the initial response and the institution of basic life support. This principle has measurable impact for out-of-hospital and in-hospital cardiac arrest. Survival to discharge for in-hospital cardiac arrests, considering all causes and mechanisms, was reported to be 33 percent when CPR was initiated within the first minute compared with 14 percent when the time was longer than 1 minute (odds ratio, 3.06).[153] When VF was the initial rhythm, the corresponding figures were 50 and 32 percent, respectively. In the out-of-hospital setting, if only one witness is present, notification of emergency personnel (calling 911) is the only activity that should precede basic life support.

Airway. Clearing the airway is a critical step in preparing for successful resuscitation. This process includes tilting the head backward and lifting the chin, in addition to exploring the airway for foreign bodies, including dentures, and removing them. The Heimlich maneuver should be performed if there is reason to suspect that a foreign body is lodged in the oropharynx. This maneuver entails wrapping the arms around the victim from the back and delivering a sharp thrust to the upper abdomen with a closed fist. If it is not possible for the person in attendance to carry out the maneuver because of insufficient physical strength, mechanical dislodgment of the foreign body can sometimes be achieved by abdominal thrusts with the unconscious patient in a supine position. The Heimlich maneuver is not entirely benign; ruptured abdominal viscera in the victim have been reported, as has a case in which the rescuer disrupted his own aortic root and died. If there is strong suspicion that respiratory arrest precipitated cardiac arrest, particularly in the presence of a mechanical airway obstruction, a second precordial thump should be delivered after the airway has been cleared.

Breathing. With the head properly placed and the oropharynx clear, mouth-to-mouth resuscitation can be initiated if no specific rescue equipment is available. To a large extent, the procedure used for establishing ventilation depends on the site at which the cardiac arrest occurs. Various devices are available, including plastic oropharyngeal airways, esophageal obturators, the masked Ambu bag, and endotracheal tubes. Intubation is the preferred procedure, but time should not be sacrificed, even in the in-hospital setting, while awaiting an endotracheal tube or a person trained to insert it quickly and properly. Thus, in the in-hospital setting, temporary support with Ambu bag ventilation is the usual method until endotracheal intubation can be carried out and, in the out-of-hospital setting, mouth-to-mouth resuscitation is used while awaiting emergency rescue personnel. The effect of the acquired immunodeficiency syndrome and hepatitis B transmission on attitudes about mouth-to-mouth resuscitation by bystanders and even professional personnel in hospitals is an area of concern, but currently available data assessing risk of infection suggest that it is minimal.[152,167] The impact of this concern on attitudes toward, and outcomes of, resuscitative efforts has not been assessed.

Techniques of CPR based on the hypothesis that increased intrathoracic pressure is the prime mover of blood, rather than cardiac compression itself, have been evaluated, and the guidelines for conventional CPR ventilatory techniques were modified in 2005. For single responders to victims from infancy (excluding newborns) through adulthood, and for adults responded to by two rescuers, a compression-ventilation ratio of 30 : 2 is now recommended.[167] For two-rescuer CPR for infants and children, the former compression-ventilation ratio of 15 : 2 is retained.[152,167]

Circulation. This element of basic life support is intended to maintain blood flow (i.e., circulation) until definitive steps can be taken (Fig. 36-19). The rationale is based on the hypothesis that chest compression allows the heart to maintain an externally driven pump function by sequential emptying and filling of its chambers, with competent valves favoring the forward direction of flow. In fact, the application of this technique has proved successful when used as recommended.[152,167] The palm of one hand is placed over the lower sternum and the heel of the other rests on the dorsum of the lower hand. The sternum is then depressed, with the resuscitator's arms straight at the elbows to provide a less tiring and more forceful fulcrum at the junction of the shoulders and back (see Fig. 36-19). By using this technique, sufficient force is applied to depress the sternum about 4 to 5 cm, with abrupt relaxation, and the cycle is carried out at a rate of about 100 compressions/min. The 2005 changes in CPR recommendations, reducing the number of successive shocks and pulse checks during initial responses, are intended in part to increase the cumulative time of circulatory support during CPR, prior to restoration of a spontaneous pulse.[185]

Despite the fact that this conventional technique produces measurable carotid artery flow and a record of successful resuscitations, the absence of a pressure gradient across the heart in the presence of an extrathoracic arteriovenous pressure gradient has led to the concept that it is not cardiac compression per se, but rather a pumping action produced by pressure changes in the entire thoracic cavity that optimizes systemic blood flow during resuscitation. Experimental work in which the chest is compressed during ventilations rather than between them (simultaneous compression-ventilation) has demonstrated better extrathoracic arterial flow. However, increased carotid artery flow does not necessarily equate with improved cerebral perfusion, and the reduction in coronary blood flow caused by elevated intrathoracic pressures using certain techniques may be too high a price for the improved peripheral flow. In addition, a high thoracoabdominal gradient has been demonstrated during experimental simultaneous compression-ventilation, which could divert flow from the brain in the absence of concomitant abdominal binding. On the basis of these observations, new mechanically assisted techniques, including an active decompression phase (i.e., active compression-

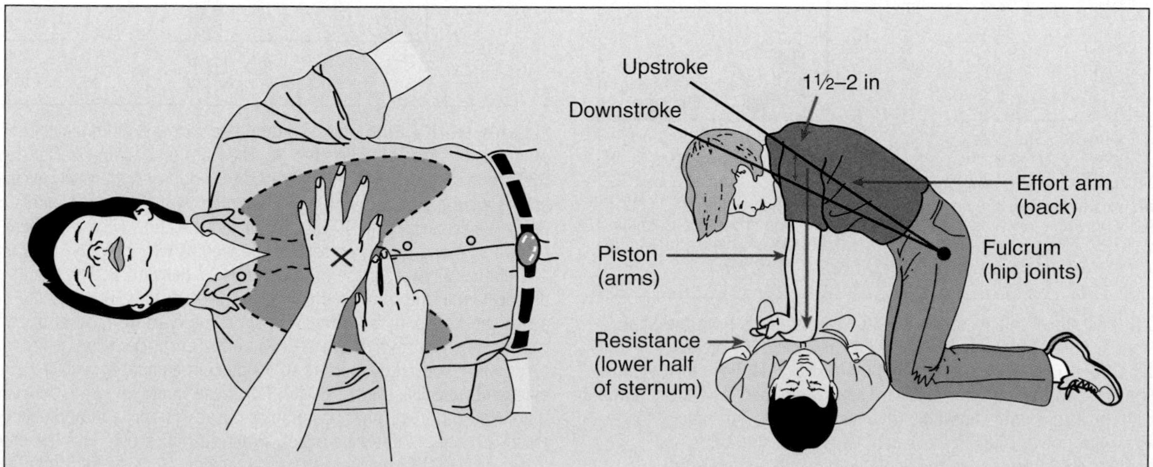

FIGURE 36–19 External chest compression. **Left,** Locating the correct hand position on the lower half of the sternum. **Right,** Proper position of the rescuer, with shoulders directly over the victim's sternum and elbows locked. *(From National Academy of Sciences, National Research Council: Standards and Guidelines for Cardiopulmonary Resuscitation [CPR] and Emergency Cardiac Care [ECC]. JAMA 255:2906, 1986. © 1986, the American Medical Association.)*

decompression), have been evaluated for improved circulation during CPR. More clinical studies are needed before establishing their general clinical applications.

Early Defibrillation by First Responders

The time from onset of cardiac arrest to advanced life support influences outcome statistics. Improvement in both early neurological status and survival occurs in patients defibrillated by first responders, compared with outcomes associated with awaiting the assistance of more highly trained paramedics. The term *first responder* refers to the person on scene providing the initial resuscitative action, and has emerged from minimally trained emergency technicians allowed to carry out defibrillation as part of basic life support to nonconventional responders, such as trained security guards and police, and most recently to laypersons knowledgeable in CRP with access to AEDs. Because the time to defibrillation plays a central role in determining outcome in cardiac arrest caused by VF, the development and deployment of AEDs (see Chap. 34) in the community hold promise for progress in the future.[180] This technology is potentially applicable to a number of different strategic models, each with its own benefits and limitations (see Fig. 36-14B).

Among the strategies that have yielded identifiable survival benefits to date are deployment in police vehicles,[173,174,179] airliners and airports,[186,187] casinos,[188] and more general community-based sites.[174,180,189] Police AED deployment data have been inconsistent in various studies,[173,174,179] possibly because of appropriateness for various types of communities and specific deployment strategies used, but data suggest that there is benefit in large metropolitan areas (Fig. 36-20).[173] Initial airline data were similarly uncertain, but a more recent report on data from a large airline with a well-organized system has suggested benefit (Fig. 36-21A).[186] Similar encouraging results have been reported from deployment of AEDs in the Chicago airport system.[187] Finally, the special circumstance of casinos, in which continuous television monitoring alerts security officers to medical problems immediately, has yielded impressive survival rates (see Fig. 36-21B).[188] For more general community sites, defined as true public access, a large study has suggested a twofold benefit.[189] However, there appears to be a great deal of variability of efficiency on the basis of expected event rates at different types of community sites.[180] No studies have yet provided information on benefit in single family dwellings, despite the fact that this is the most common site of cardiac arrest.[51]

As is the case for any medical device,[190] infrequent malfunctions of AEDs may occur, caused by design or manufacturing defects[191] or by failure to adhere to manufacturers' recommendations for replacement of batteries and leads. It is an obligation of those responsible for maintaining AEDs to remain cognizant of FDA safety alerts and recalls and shelf-lives of batteries and leads.

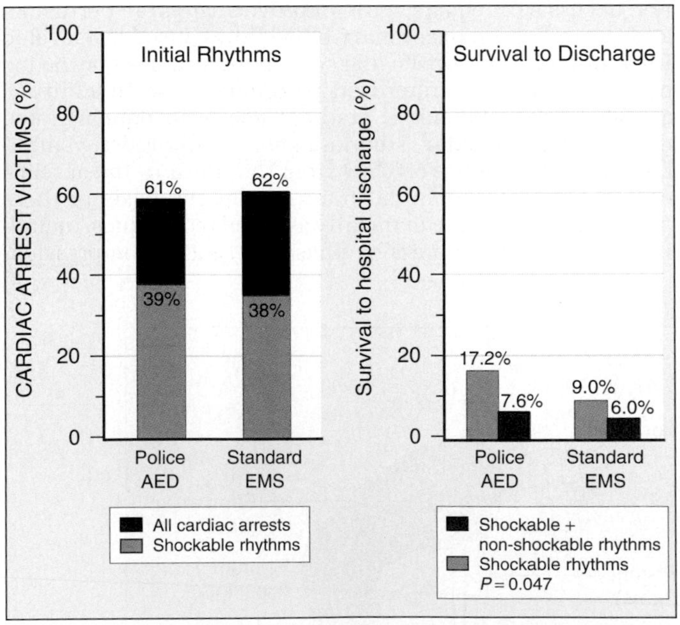

FIGURE 36–20 Rhythms at initial contact and survival statistics from the Miami-Dade County, Florida, police automated external defibrillator (AED) project. Shockable rhythms were observed in just under 40 percent of cardiac arrest victims in both the police AED program and the standard emergency medical system (EMS) historical control data. Those with shockable rhythms had improved survival to hospital discharge, with only a small improvement when both shockable and nonshockable rhythms were included in the analyzed data. *(Modified from Myerburg RJ, Fenster J, Velez M, et al: Impact of community-wide police car deployment of automated external defibrillators on out-of-hospital cardiac arrest. Circulation 106:1058, 2002. Reproduced with permission of the American Heart Association.)*

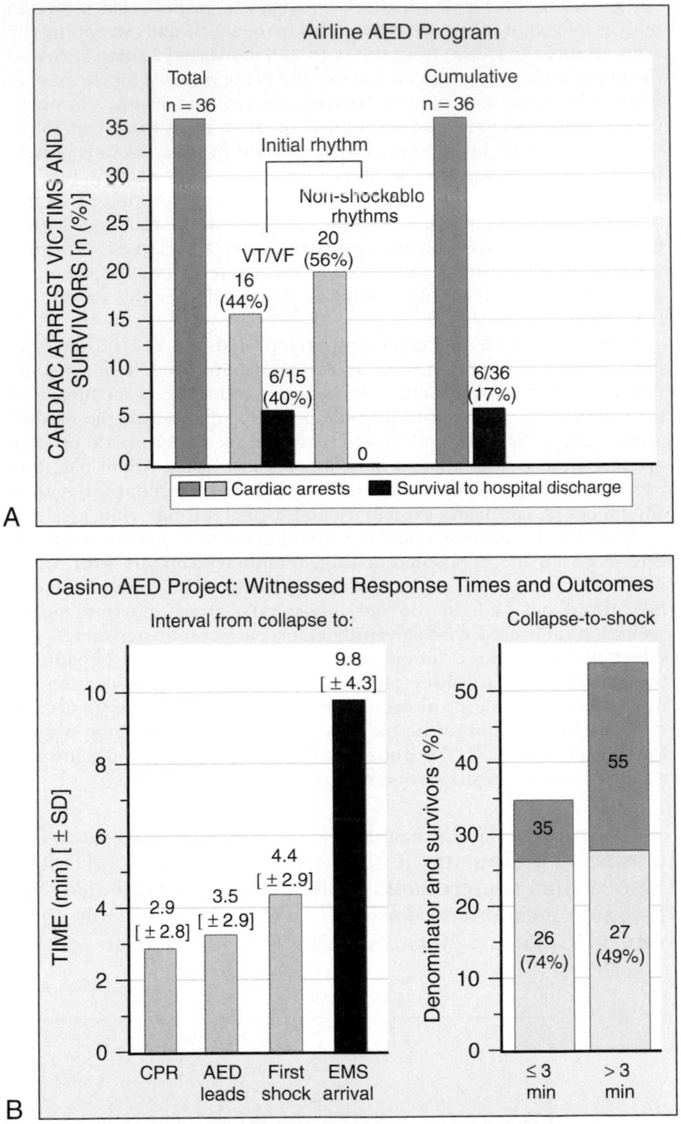

FIGURE 36–21 Outcomes of automated external defibrillator (AED) deployment programs at specific public sites. **A,** The data on outcomes after deployment of AEDs on a major airline demonstrated that approximately 44 percent of the cardiac arrests were associated with a documented ventricular tachycardia or fibrillation (VT/VF) mechanism and 40 percent of those victims survived. There were no survivors among the 56 percent of the victims who had nonshockable rhythms. Cumulative survival for the program was 17 percent. **B,** The results of AED deployment in the controlled environment of casinos. Because the onset of cardiac arrest can frequently be witnessed, short intervals from onset of collapse to cardiopulmonary resuscitation (CPR) and AED shocks were achieved. Response times were reduced by more than 50 percent compared with the standard emergency medical system (EMS). For those found in VT/VF, survival was better than expected from other community-based systems and approached 60 percent for VT/VF with a witnessed onset. When response time was less than 3 minutes, survival for VT/VF was more than 70 percent. *(**A,** Modified from Page RL, Joglar JA, Kowal RC, et al: Use of automated external defibrillators by a U.S. airline. N Engl J Med 343:1210, 2000. **B,** Modified from Valenzuela TD, Roe DJ, Nichol G, et al: Outcomes of rapid defibrillation by security officers after cardiac arrest in casinos. N Engl J Med 343:1206, 2000.)*

Advanced Life Support

This next step in the resuscitative sequence is designed to achieve definitive stabilization of the patient.[152,167] The implementation of advanced life support is not intended to suggest an abrupt cessation of basic life support activities but rather a merging and transition from one level of activity to the next. In the past, advanced life support required judgments and technical skills that removed it from the realm of activity of lay bystanders and even emergency medical technicians, limiting these activities to specifically trained paramedical personnel, nurses, and physicians. With further education of emergency technicians, most community-based CPR programs now permit them to carry out advanced life support activities. In addition, the development and testing of automatic external defibrillators that have the ability to sense and analyze cardiac electrical activity and prompt the user to deliver definitive electrical intervention provides a role for less highly trained rescue personnel (i.e., police, ambulance drivers) and even untrained or minimally trained lay bystanders[180,187,189] for rapid defibrillation.

The general goals of advanced life support are to revert the cardiac rhythm to one that is hemodynamically effective, optimize ventilation, and maintain and support the restored circulation. Thus, during advanced life support, the patient's cardiac rhythm is promptly cardioverted or defibrillated as the first priority if appropriate equipment is immediately available. There is increasing evidence that a short period of closed-chest cardiac compression immediately before defibrillation enhances the probability of survival.[176,181,183] After the initial attempt to restore a hemodynamically effective rhythm, the patient is intubated and oxygenated, if needed, and the heart is paced if a bradyarrhythmia or asystole occurs. An intravenous line is established to deliver medications. After intubation, the goal of ventilation is to reverse hypoxemia and not merely achieve a high alveolar oxygen pressure (P_{O_2}). Thus, oxygen rather than room air should be used to ventilate the patient; if possible, the arterial P_{O_2} should be monitored. Respiratory support in the hospital and an Ambu bag by means of an endotracheal tube, or facemasks in the out-of-hospital setting, are generally used.

DEFIBRILLATION-CARDIOVERSION. Rapid conversion to an effective cardiac electrical mechanism is a key step for successful resuscitation (Fig. 36-22). Delay should be minimal, even when conditions for CPR are optimal. When VF, or VT that is pulseless or accompanied by loss of consciousness, is recognized on a monitor or by telemetry, defibrillation should be carried out immediately. An initial shock of 360 J should be delivered by devices delivering monophasic waveforms and 120 to 200 J using biphasic devices, with the energy depending on the recommendations for individual biphasic devices. Energies delivered through AEDs are generally preprogrammed and vary among available devices. Failure of the initial shock to provide an effective rhythm is a poor prognostic sign. The 2005 updated guidelines[167] have recommended that failure of a single adequate shock to restore a pulse should be followed by continued CPR and a second shock delivered after five cycles of CPR. This supersedes the prior strategy of three successive shocks before resuming CPR.[152] The intent is to maximize circulatory time via chest compressions until a pulse has been restored. If cardiac arrest still persists, the patient is intubated and intravenous access

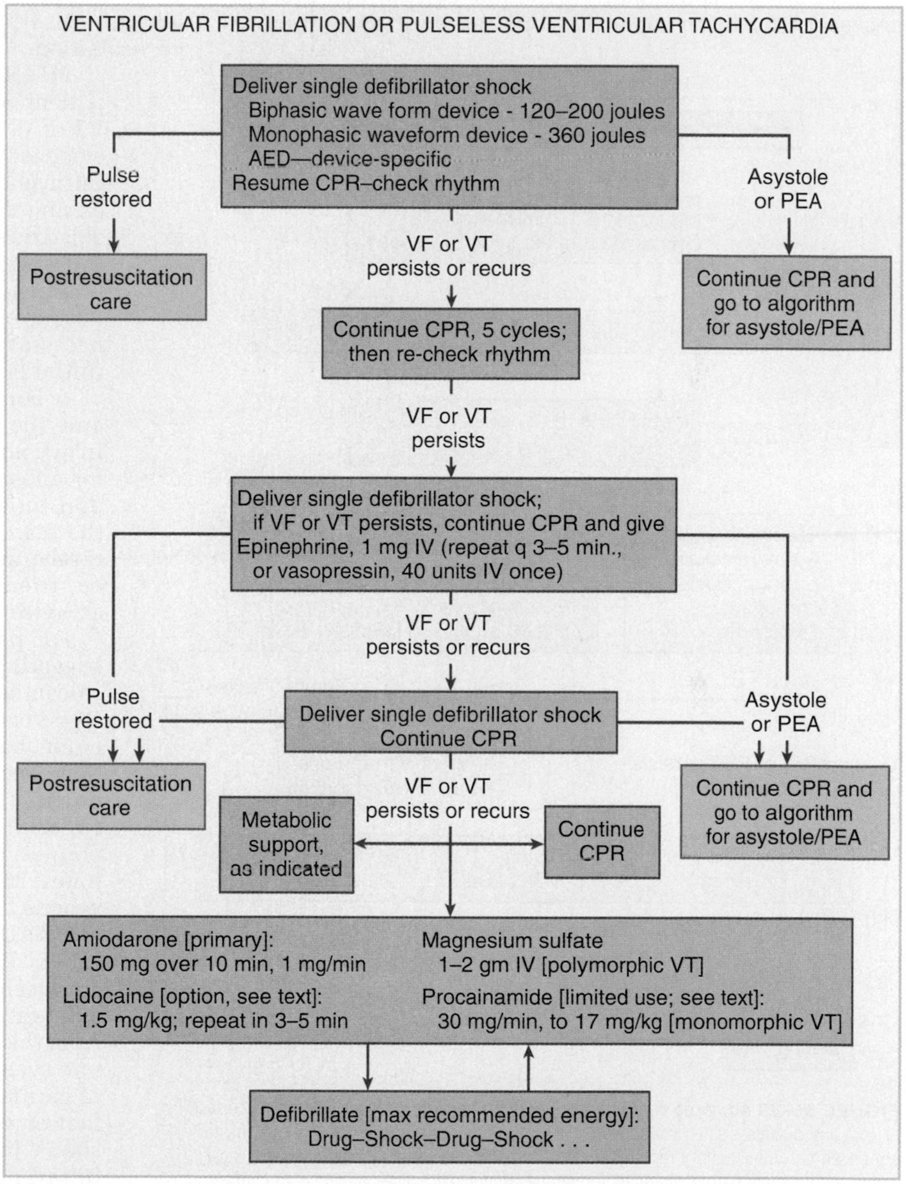

FIGURE 36–22 Advanced life support for ventricular fibrillation (VF) and pulseless ventricular tachycardia (VT). If initial defibrillation fails, the patient should be intubated and intravenous (IV) access immediately established while cardiopulmonary resuscitation (CPR) is continued. Epinephrine, 1 mg intravenously, should be administered and may be repeated several times with additional attempts to defibrillate with 360 J. If the conversion is still unsuccessful, epinephrine may be administered again, although it is unlikely that higher doses would provide any further benefit. Sodium bicarbonate should be administered at this time only if the patient is known to be hyperkalemic, but intravenous antiarrhythmic drugs should be tried (see text). Additional attempts to defibrillate should follow the administration of each drug attempted. Concomitant with all steps, continuation of CPR is paramount. PEA = pulseless electrical activity. *(Modified from ECC Committee, Subcommittees and Task Forces of the American Heart Association: 2005 American Heart Association Guidelines for Cardiopulmonary Resuscitation and Emergency Cardiovascular Care. Circulation 112[Suppl]:IV1, 2005. See original reference for further details.)*

achieved. Epinephrine is administered and followed by repeated defibrillation attempts at 360 J (monophasic) or 200 J or more (biphasic). Epinephrine may be repeated at 3- to 5-minute intervals with a defibrillator shock in between,[152,167] but high-dose epinephrine does not appear to provide added benefit.[192] Vasopressin has been suggested as an alternative to epinephrine.[193]

Simultaneously, the rescuer should focus on ventilation to correct the chemistry of the blood, efforts that render the heart more likely to reestablish a stable rhythm (i.e., improved oxygenation, reversal of acidosis, and improvement of the underlying electrophysiological condition). Although adequate oxygenation of the blood is crucial in the immediate management of the metabolic acidosis of cardiac arrest, additional correction can be achieved, if necessary, by intravenous administration of sodium bicarbonate. Sodium bicarbonate is recommended for circumstances of known or suspected preexisting bicarbonate-responsive causes of acidosis, certain drug overdoses, and prolonged resuscitation runs.[152] The more general role for bicarbonate during cardiac arrest has been questioned but, in any circumstance, much less sodium bicarbonate than was previously recommended is adequate for treatment of acidosis in this setting. Excessive quantities can be deleterious. Although some investigators have questioned the use of sodium bicarbonate because risks of alkalosis, hypernatremia, and hyperosmolality may outweigh its benefits, the circumstances cited may benefit from administration of sodium bicarbonate while CPR is being carried out. Up to 50 percent of the dose may be repeated every 10 to 15 minutes during the course of CPR. When possible, arterial pH, PO_2, and PCO_2 should be monitored during the resuscitation.

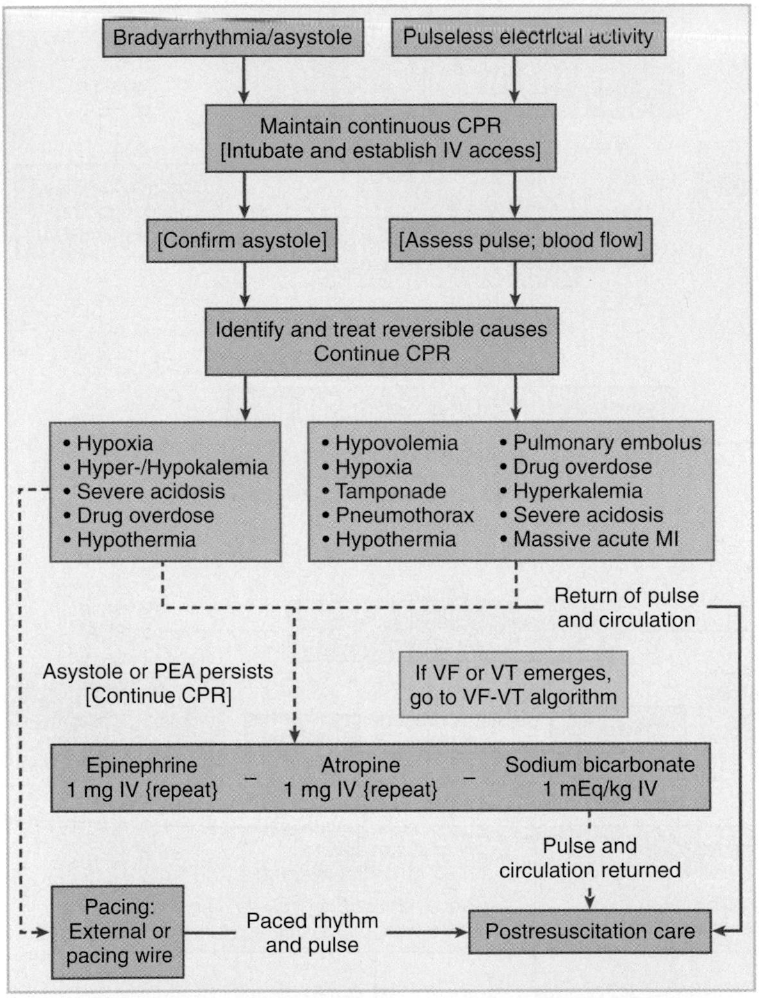

FIGURE 36–23 Advanced cardiac life support for patients with bradyarrhythmic-asystolic arrests and pulseless electrical activity. The patient in any of these states should have continued cardiopulmonary resuscitation (CPR) and be intubated, with intravenous (IV) access established, before pharmacological treatment. The initial activity is to confirm persisting asystole or attempt to assess blood flow in patients thought to have pulseless electrical activity. An immediate attempt should be made to identify and treat reversible or treatable causes of these forms of cardiac arrest. Epinephrine is generally administered first, and atropine or bicarbonate, or both, may be administered subsequently. An attempt to pace the heart with an external device or an intracardiac pacing catheter is advisable, although usually not successful, except for certain reversible bradyarrhythmias. MI = myocardial infarction; PEA = pulseless electrical activity; VF = ventricular fibrillation; VT = ventricular tachycardia. *(Modified from ECC Committee, Subcommittees and Task Forces of the American Heart Association: 2005 American Heart Association Guidelines for Cardiopulmonary Resuscitation and Emergency Cardiovascular Care. Circulation 112[Suppl]: IV1, 2005. See original reference for further details.)*

PHARMACOTHERAPY (see Chap. 33). For the patient who continues to have persistent or recurrent VT or VF despite DC cardioversion after epinephrine, electrical stability of the heart may be achieved by intravenous administration of antiarrhythmic agents during continued resuscitation efforts (see Fig. 36-22). Intravenous amiodarone has emerged as the initial treatment of choice (see Fig. 36-22).[138] Another regimen is amiodarone followed by a maintenance dose over the next 18 hours and for several days, as necessary. Additional bolus dosing can be tried if the initial bolus is unsuccessful.

A bolus of lidocaine may be given intravenously and the dose repeated in 2 minutes for patients in whom amiodarone is unsuccessful and possibly for those who have an acute transmural myocardial infarction as the triggering mechanism for the cardiac arrest. Intravenous procainamide is rarely used in this setting any longer, but may be tried for persisting, hemodynamically stable arrhythmias.

For patients in whom acute hyperkalemia is the triggering event for resistant VF or who have hypocalcemia or are toxic from Ca^{2+} entry blocking drugs, 10 percent calcium gluconate may be helpful.[152] Calcium should not be used routinely during resuscitation, even though ionized Ca^{2+} levels may be low during resuscitation from cardiac arrest. Some resistant forms of polymorphic VT or torsades de pointes, rapid monomorphic VT or ventricular flutter (rate ≥ 260/min), or resistant VF may respond to intravenous beta blocker therapy or IV $MgSO_4$.

BRADYARRHYTHMIC AND ASYSTOLIC ARREST; PULSELESS ELECTRICAL ACTIVITY. The approach to the patient with bradyarrhythmic or asystolic arrest or pulseless electrical activity differs from the approach to the patient with a tachyarrhythmic event (VT or VF; Fig. 36-23).[152,167] When this form of cardiac arrest is recognized, efforts should focus first on establishing control of the cardiorespiratory status (i.e., continue CPR, intubate, and establish intravenous access), reconfirming the rhythm (in two leads if possible), and finally taking actions that favor the emergence of a stable spontaneous rhythm or attempt to pace the heart. Possible reversible causes, particularly for bradyarrhythmia and asystole, should be considered and excluded (or treated) promptly. These include hypovolemia, hypoxia, cardiac tamponade, tension pneumothorax, preexisting acidosis, drug overdose, hypothermia, and hyperkalemia. Epinephrine and atropine are commonly used in an attempt to elicit spontaneous electrical activity or increase the rate of a bradycardia. These have had only limited success, as have intravenous isoproterenol infusions in doses up to 15 to 20 μg/min. In the absence of an intravenous line, epinephrine, 1 mg (10 ml of a 1 : 10,000 solution) may be given by the intracardiac route, but there is danger of coronary or myocardial laceration. Sodium bicarbonate, 1 mEq/kg, may be tried for known or strongly suspected preexisting hyperkalemia or bicarbonate-responsive acidosis.

Pacing of the bradyarrhythmic or asystolic heart has been limited in the past by the unavailability of personnel capable of carrying out such procedures at the scene of cardiac arrests. With the development of more effective external pacing systems, the role of pacing and its influence on outcome must now be reevaluated. Unfortunately, all data to date have suggested that the asystolic patient continues to have a very poor prognosis, despite new techniques.

The published standards for CPR and emergency cardiac care[167] include a series of teaching algorithms to be used as guides to appropriate care. Figures 33-22 and 33-23 provide the algorithms for VF and pulseless VT, asystole (or cardiac standstill), and pulseless electrical activity. These general guides are not to be interpreted as inclusive of all possible approaches or contingencies. The special circumstance of CPR in pregnant women requires additional attention to effects of drugs on the gravid uterus and the fetus, mechanical and physiological influences of pregnancy on the efficacy of CPR, and risk of complications, such as ruptured uterus and lacerated liver.

STABILIZATION. As soon as electrical resuscitation from VT, VF, bradycardia, asystole, or pulseless electrical activity has been achieved, the focus of attention shifts to maintaining a stable electrical, hemodynamic, and central nervous system status. If frequent PVCs and runs of nonsustained VT persist after restoration of a sinus mechanism, a continuous infusion of an effective antiarrhythmic drug is used. Intravenous amiodarone is the preferred agent. Lidocaine, depending on size and clinical factors, is an option for arrhythmias caused by acute ischemic events, and intravenous procainamide may be considered if the others fail. Occasionally, a continuous infusion of propranolol or esmolol is used.

Catecholamines are used in cardiac arrest not only in an attempt to achieve better electrical stability (e.g., conversion from fine to coarse VF, or increasing the rate of spontaneous contraction during bradyarrhythmias) but also for their inotropic and peripheral vascular effects. Epinephrine is the first choice among the catecholamines for use in cardiac arrest because it increases myocardial contractility, elevates perfusion pressure, may convert electromechanical dissociation to electromechanical coupling, and improves chances for defibrillation. Because of its adverse effects on renal and mesenteric flow, norepinephrine is a less desirable agent, despite its inotropic effects. When the chronotropic effect of epinephrine is undesirable, dopamine or dobutamine is preferable to norepinephrine for inotropic effect. Isoproterenol may be used for the treatment of primary or postdefibrillation bradycardia when heart rate control is the primary goal of therapy intended to improve cardiac output. Calcium chloride is sometimes used in patients with pulseless electrical activity that persists after administration of catecholamines. The efficacy of this intervention is uncertain. Stimulation of alpha adrenoceptors may be important during definitive resuscitative efforts. For example, the alpha adrenoceptor–stimulating effects of epinephrine and higher dosages of dopamine, producing elevation of aortic diastolic pressures by peripheral vasoconstriction with increased cerebral and myocardial flow, have been reemphasized.

Post-Cardiac Arrest Care

For successfully resuscitated cardiac arrest victims, whether the event occurred in or out of hospital, post-cardiac arrest care includes admission to an intensive care unit and continuous monitoring for a minimum of 48 to 72 hours. Some elements of postarrest management are common to all resuscitated patients, but prognosis and certain details of management are specific for the clinical setting in which the cardiac arrest occurred. The major management categories include (1) primary cardiac arrest in acute myocardial infarction, (2) secondary cardiac arrest in acute myocardial infarction, (3) cardiac arrest associated with noncardiac disorders, and (4) survival after out-of-hospital cardiac arrest.

Primary Cardiac Arrest in Acute Myocardial Infarction

VF in patients with acute myocardial infarction free of concomitant hemodynamic complications (i.e., primary VF; see Chap. 51) is now less common in hospitalized patients than the 15 to 20 percent incidence before the availability of cardiac care units. The events that do occur are almost always successfully reverted by prompt interventions in properly equipped emergency departments or cardiac care units. If ventricular arrhythmias persist after successful resuscitation, a lidocaine infusion is used. Antiarrhythmic support is usually discontinued after 24 hours if sustained arrhythmias do not recur (see Chap. 33). The occurrence of VF during the early phase of acute myocardial infarction (i.e., first 24 to 48 hours) is not an indication for subsequent electrophysiological testing or long-term antiarrhythmic or device therapy. Pulseless VT, producing the clinical picture of cardiac arrest in acute myocardial infarction, is treated similarly; its intermediate- and long-term implications are the same as those of VF. Cardiac arrest caused by bradyarrhythmias or asystole in acute inferior wall myocardial infarction, in the absence of primary hemodynamic deterioration, is uncommon and may respond to atropine or pacing. The prognosis is good, with no special long-term care required in most cases. Rarely, symptomatic bradyarrhythmias that require permanent pacemakers persist in survivors. In contrast to inferior myocardial infarction, bradyarrhythmic cardiac arrest associated with large anterior wall infarctions (and AV or intraventricular block) has a poor prognosis.

Secondary Cardiac Arrest in Acute Myocardial Infarction

This condition is defined as cardiac arrest occurring in association with, or as a result of, hemodynamic or mechanical dysfunction. The immediate mortality among patients in this setting ranges from 59 to 89 percent, depending on the severity of the hemodynamic abnormalities and size of the myocardial infarction. Resuscitative efforts commonly fail in such patients and, when they are successful, the post-cardiac arrest management is often difficult. When secondary cardiac arrest occurs by the mechanisms of VT or VF, aggressive hemodynamic or antiischemic measures may help achieve rhythm stability. Intravenous amiodarone has emerged as the antiarrhythmic therapy of choice.[138] Lidocaine may also be tried if the mechanism appears to be ischemic but is less likely to be successful in this setting than in primary VF. The success of interventions and prevention of recurrent cardiac arrest are related closely to the success in managing the hemodynamic status. The incidence of cardiac arrest caused by bradyarrhythmias or asystole, or by electromechanical dissociation, is higher in the secondary form of cardiac arrest in acute myocardial infarction. Such patients usually have large myocardial infarctions and major hemodynamic abnormalities, and may be acidotic and hypoxemic. Even with aggressive therapy, the prognosis after asystolic arrest in such patients is poor, and patients are resuscitated only rarely from PEA. All patients in circulatory failure at the onset of arrest are in a high-risk category, with only a 2 percent survival rate among hypotensive patients in one study.

CARDIAC ARREST AMONG IN-HOSPITAL PATIENTS WITH NON-CARDIAC ABNORMALITIES. These patients fall into two major categories: (1) those with life-limiting diseases, such as malignancies, sepsis, organ failure, end-stage pulmonary disease, and advanced central nervous system disease, and (2) those with acute toxic or proarrhythmic states that are potentially reversible. In the former category, the ratio of tachyarrhythmic to bradyarrhythmic cardiac arrest is low and the prognosis for surviving cardiac arrest is poor. Although the data may be somewhat skewed by the practice of assigning "do not resuscitate" orders to patients with end-stage disease, available data for attempted resuscitations show a poor outcome. Only 7 percent of cancer patients, 3 percent of renal failure patients, and no patients with sepsis or acute central nervous system disease were successfully resuscitated and discharged from the hospital. For the few successfully resuscitated patients in these categories, postarrest management is dictated by the underlying precipitating factors.

Most antiarrhythmic drugs (see Chap. 33), a number of drugs used for noncardiac purposes, and electrolyte disturbances can precipitate potentially lethal arrhythmias and cardiac arrest. The class IA and class III antiarrhythmic drugs can cause proarrhythmic responses by lengthening the QT interval and generating torsades de pointes. The class IC drugs rarely cause torsades de pointes but cause excess SCD risk in patients with recent myocardial infarction, possibly by interacting with transient ischemia. Among other categories of drugs, the phenothiazines, tricyclic antidepressants, lithium, terfenadine interacting with ketoconazole (or other blockers of enzymes in the hepatic P450 system), pentamidine, cocaine, erythromycin, and cardiovascular drugs that are not antiarrhythmics, such as lidoflazine, are recognized causes. Beyond these, a broad array of pharmacological and pathophysiological-metabolic causes has been reported. Hypokalemia, hypomagnesemia, and perhaps hypocalcemia are the electrolyte disturbances most closely associated with cardiac arrest. Acidosis and hypoxia can potentiate the vulnerability associated with electrolyte disturbances. Proarrhythmic effects are often prewarned by prolongation of the QT interval, although this electrocardiographic change is not always present.[98]

Impending or manifest cardiac arrest caused by torsades de pointes is managed by intravenous administration of magnesium, pacing, or treatment with isoproterenol and removal of the offending agent. When QT prolongation is the basis, magnesium may effectively control the arrhythmia without shortening the QT interval. Class IC drugs may cause a rapid, sinusoidal VT pattern, especially in patients with poor left ventricular function. This VT has a tendency to recur repetitively after cardioversion until the drug has begun to clear and has been controlled by propranolol in some patients. When the patient's condition can be stabilized until the offending factor is removed (e.g., proarrhythmic drugs) or corrected (e.g., electrolyte imbalances, hypothermia), the prognosis is excellent. The recognition of torsades de pointes (see Chap. 35) and the identification of its risk by prolongation of the QT interval in association with the offending agent are helpful in managing these patients.

POST-CARDIAC ARREST CARE IN SURVIVORS OF OUT-OF-HOSPITAL CARDIAC ARREST. The initial management of survivors of out-of-hospital cardiac arrest centers on stabilizing the cardiac electrical status, supporting hemodynamics, and providing supportive care for reversal of organ damage that has occurred as a consequence of the cardiac arrest. The in-hospital risk of recurrent cardiac arrest is relatively low, and arrhythmias account for only 10 percent of in-hospital deaths after successful prehospital resuscitation. However, the mortality rate during the index hospitalization is 50 percent, indicating that nonarrhythmic mortality dominates the mechanisms of early postresuscitation deaths (30 percent hemodynamic, 60 percent central nervous system–related). Antiarrhythmic therapy, usually intravenous amiodarone, is used in an attempt to prevent recurrent cardiac arrest among patients who demonstrate recurrent arrhythmia during the first 48 hours of postarrest hospitalization. Patients who have preexisting or new AV or intraventricular conduction disturbances are at particularly high risk for recurrent cardiac arrest. The routine use of temporary pacemakers has been evaluated in such patients but has not been found to be helpful for preventing early recurrent cardiac arrest. Invasive techniques for hemodynamic monitoring are used in patients whose condition is unstable but are not used routinely for those whose condition is stable on admission.

Anoxic encephalopathy is a strong predictor of in-hospital death. A suggested addition to the management of this condition is the use of induced mild hypothermia to reduce metabolic demands and cerebral edema.[156,157] When this strategy is applied promptly to the postarrest survivor who remains unconscious on hospital admission, there is a modest but measurable survival benefit. During the later convalescent period, continued attention to central nervous system status, including physical rehabilitation, is of primary importance for an optimal outcome. Respiratory support by conventional methods is used as necessary. Management of other organ system injury (e.g., renal, hepatic), as well as early recognition and treatment of infectious complications, also contributes to ultimate survival.

Long-Term Management of Survivors of Out-of-Hospital Cardiac Arrest

When the survivor of an out-of-hospital cardiac arrest has awakened and achieved electrical and hemodynamic stability, usually within a few days, if it is to occur at all, decisions must be made regarding the nature and extent of the work-up required to establish a long-term management strategy. The goals of the work-up are to identify the specific causative and triggering factors of the cardiac arrest, clarify the functional status of the patient's cardiovascular system, and establish long-term therapeutic strategies. The extent of the work-up is largely dictated by the degree of central nervous system recovery and the factors already known to have contributed to the cardiac arrest. Patients who have limited return of central nervous system function usually do not undergo extensive work-ups, and patients whose cardiac arrests were triggered by an acute transmural myocardial infarction have work-ups similar to those for other patients with acute myocardial infarction (see Chap. 51).

Survivors of out-of-hospital cardiac arrest not associated with acute myocardial infarction who have good return of neurological function appear to have a long-term survival probability commensurate with their age, gender, and extent of disease when treated according to existing guidelines.[161,194] These patients should undergo diagnostic work-ups to define the cause of cardiac arrest and tailor long-term therapy, the latter targeted to the underlying disease and strategies for prevention of recurrent cardiac arrests or SCD. The work-up includes cardiac catheterization with coronary angiography, if coronary atherosclerosis is known or considered to be the possible cause of the event,[195] an evaluation of the functional significance of coronary lesions by stress-imaging techniques, if indicated, determination of functional and hemodynamic status, and an assessment of whether the life-threatening arrhythmic event was caused by a transient risk associated with acute myocardial infarction or there is persisting risk based on clinical characteristics.

GENERAL CARE. The general management of survivors of cardiac arrest is determined by the specific cause and the pathophysiology of the underlying process. For patients with ischemic heart disease (see Chaps. 53 and 54), who constitute approximately 80 percent of cardiac arrest victims, interventions to prevent myocardial ischemia, optimization of therapy for left ventricular dysfunction, and attention to general medical status are all addressed. Although there are limited data suggesting that revascularization procedures may improve the recurrence rate and total mortality rates after survival from out-of-hospital cardiac arrest, no properly controlled prospective studies have validated this impression for bypass surgery or percutaneous interventions. Moreover, a randomized trial of prophylactic implantable defibrillators versus usual therapy in patients with low ejection fractions undergoing coronary bypass surgery in the absence of a history of cardiac arrest or other life-threatening arrhythmia or arrhythmia markers (the Coronary Artery Bypass Graft Patch Trial [CABG-Patch]) revealed no mortality benefit of implantable defibrillators after revascularization.[196] The indications for revascularization after a cardiac arrest are limited to those who have a generally accepted indication for angioplasty or surgery, including (but not limited to) a documented ischemic mechanism for the cardiac arrest.

Although no data from placebo-controlled trials are available to define a benefit of various antiischemic strategies (including beta blockers or other medical antiischemic therapy) for long-term management after out-of-hospital cardiac arrest, medical, catheter interventional, or surgical antiischemic therapy, rather than antiarrhythmic drug therapy, is generally considered the primary approach to long-term management of the subgroup of prehospital cardiac arrest survivors in whom transient myocardial ischemia was the inciting factor. Moreover, in an uncontrolled observation comparing cardiac arrest survivors who had ever received beta blockers after the index event with those who had not received the drug, a significant improvement in long-term outcome was observed among those who had received beta blockers.[197] Further evaluation of the specific role of revascularization procedures and antiischemic medical therapy after out-of-hospital cardiac arrest is needed.

The long-term management of the consequences of left ventricular dysfunction by conventional means, such as digitalis preparations and chronic diuretic use, has been evaluated in several studies. Data from the Multiple Risk Factor Intervention Trial (MRFIT) have suggested a higher mortality rate in the special intervention group, presumably related to diuretic use and K^+ depletion, and other data regarding the relation between K^+ depletion and arrhythmias have focused attention on the routine use of such drugs. Although the facts are currently far from conclusive, it is advisable that diuretic use be accompanied by careful monitoring of electrolyte levels. The use of digoxin in survivors of out-of-hospital cardiac arrest should be tailored to specific indications for left ventricular dysfunction.

The various pharmacological strategies (e.g., angiotensin-converting enzyme inhibitors, carvedilol and other beta-adrenergic blocking agents, and spironolactone) that have been shown to provide a clinical and mortality benefit in patients with left ventricular dysfunction, with or without heart failure, provide an SCD benefit in conjunction with total mortality benefit. The extent to which there is a specific SCD benefit for cardiac arrest survivors is uncertain, although some primary prevention trials have suggested that such benefit occurs.

PREVENTION OF CARDIAC ARREST AND SUDDEN CARDIAC DEATH

Therapeutic strategies to prevent SCD can be classified into five categories: (1) prevention of recurrent events in survivors of cardiac arrest or pulseless VT (secondary prevention), or otherwise symptomatic tachycardias considered life-threatening; (2) prevention of an initial event among patients at high risk because of advanced heart disease with ejection fractions less than or equal to 35 percent (primary prevention); (3) primary prevention in patients with less advanced common or uncommon structural heart diseases and ejection fractions greater than 35 percent; (4) primary prevention in patients with structurally normal hearts, subtle or minor structural abnormalities, or molecular disorders associated with electrophysiological properties that establish risk for ventricular arrhythmias; and (5) primary prevention among the general population (Table 36-4). The last category includes the substantial proportion of SCDs that occur as a first cardiac event among victims previously free of known disease (see earlier).[140]

Four modes of antiarrhythmic therapy, which are not mutually exclusive, may be considered for patients at risk for cardiac arrest—antiarrhythmic drug therapy, surgery, catheter ablation, and implantable defibrillator therapy. The choice of therapy is based on estimation of the potential benefit determined by evaluation of the individual patient and available efficacy and safety data.

Antiarrhythmic Drug Strategies

Historically, the earliest approach to the management of risk of out-of-hospital cardiac arrest and VT with hemodynamic compromise was the use of membrane-active antiarrhythmic agents. This approach was based initially on the assumption that the high frequency of ambient ventricular arrhythmias constituted a triggering mechanism for potentially lethal arrhythmias, and that the electrophysiological abnormalities or instability of the myocardium that predisposed to potentially lethal arrhythmias could be modified by these drugs. The therapeutic strategy for the former was the suppression of ambient ventricular arrhythmias by antiarrhythmic drugs, and the strategy for the latter was the suppression of inducibility of VT or VF during programmed electrical stimulation studies. Observational data have suggested that suppression of ambient arrhythmias, identified on ambulatory recorders, can be achieved by the empirical use of amiodarone, beta-adrenergic blocking agents, or membrane-active antiarrhythmic drugs. On the basis of historical expectations, it was suggested, but not proved, that such suppressive techniques would improve mortality risk. For the membrane-active drugs, the observations that post-cardiac arrest survivors who had been treated with class I antiarrhythmic drugs had a worse outcome than those who were not treated challenged the concept of benefit.[197] That skepticism was definitively reinforced by the results of CAST, which demonstrated that certain class I antiarrhythmic drugs were neutral or harmful. In contrast, beta blocker therapy might have some benefit in such patients.[197] and amiodarone might also be effective for some patients.[198] Ultimately, affirmative data have defined the superiority of ICD therapy for most survivors of tachyarrhythmic cardiac arrest.

Another study, the Electrophysiologic Study Versus Electrocardiographic Monitoring (ESVEM) trial, has suggested

TABLE 36–4 Categories of Therapeutic Strategies for Prevention of Recurrent Cardiac Arrest and Sudden Cardiac Death (SCD)

Prevention Targets	Clinical Examples	Estimate of Risk	Data Sources
Secondary*	Survivors of cardiac arrest; VF/VT	High	Observational; RCT: (+) control
Primary			
Advanced structural cardiac disease	CAD/DCM, EF < 35%	High	Observational; RCT: (+) control RCT: (−) control
Lower grade structural disease	CAD/DCM, EF > 35% RVD, sarcoidosis, HCM	Variable	Observational; RCT: subgroup analyses
Functional cardiac disorders†	Long-QT syndrome, Brugada syndrome	Variable	Observational
SCD as primary event in CAD†	Family history of SCD, risk factors for CAD	Low	Epidemiological, genetic (?)

*Much of the data for secondary prevention, identified as a high-risk population because of the occurrence of a prior cardiac arrest, has derived from observational data and, more recently, from randomized controlled trials (RCTs), all of which have used an active therapy control group—(+) control—comparing outcomes between groups treated with implantable cardioverter defibrillators (ICDs) and antiarrhythmic drugs (see Table 36-5). (−) control indicates the placebo group.

†RCTs are not feasible for primary prevention in patients with these lower risk conditions. However, some information can be acquired from subgroup analysis of larger studies. Decisions for ICD implantation in these patients must be judgment-based rather than evidence-based. Suggestions of familial clustering of sudden death, as a specific expression of coronary artery disease (CAD), raise the question of primary prevention in patients at risk for SCD using epidemiological and perhaps genetic markers in the future.

DCM=dilated cardiomyopathy; EF=ejection fraction; HCM=hypertrophic cardiomyopathy; RVD=right ventricular dysplasia; VF=ventricular fibrillation; VT=ventricular tachycardia.

that the class III antiarrhythmic drug sotalol is superior to class I membrane-active antiarrhythmic agents for patients with ventricular tachyarrhythmias assumed to be life-threatening[199] but provides no comparison with amiodarone or beta blockers. In summary, ambient arrhythmia suppression as a strategy for reduction of risk enjoyed a short period of popularity for VT-VF survivors but, in time, yielded to the apparently greater benefits of amiodarone, and perhaps beta blockers, prescribed empirically. The combination of amiodarone and beta blocker therapy in the post-myocardial infarction patient has been suggested as a strategy that provides greater benefit than either drug alone from subgroup analysis of the European Myocardial Infarct Amiodarone Trial (EMIAT) and Canadian Amiodarone Myocardial Infarction Trial (CAMIAT),[200] and another study reinforced the benefit of beta blockers for the specific prevention of SCD in unselected post-myocardial infarction patients.[37]

Ambulatory Electrocardiographic Recording and Empirical Therapy

The development of reliable methods of analysis of ambulatory recordings has led some investigators to study the usefulness of such recordings for profiling risk of sustained tachyarrhythmic events and to measure suppressibility of ambient arrhythmias as a specific and individualized means of evaluating drug therapy for prevention of SCD. This strategy is now obsolete as a primary approach in the cardiac arrest survivor, but ambulatory monitoring is still used for profiling the risk of developing life-threatening sustained arrhythmias in individuals with certain forms of structural or electrophysiological disease who are considered at high risk. For example, the strategies used in the Multicenter Automatic Defibrillator Implantation Trial (MADIT)[201] and the Multicenter Unsustained Tachycardia Trial (MUSTT)[202] used identification of nonsustained VT in post-myocardial infarction patients with other risk markers for early mortality. Although the ambient arrhythmias were not a target for therapy in the design of the studies, they have established the usefulness of this technique for identifying risk. Similarly, ambulatory recordings, particularly among patients with symptoms, are used as an aid to risk profiling in disorders such as hypertrophic cardiomyopathy, long-QT syndrome, and right ventricular dysplasia and in patients with dilated cardiomyopathy or heart failure.

Finally, empirical antiarrhythmic therapy, predominantly amiodarone, for the prevention of recurrent cardiac arrest or other life-threatening arrhythmias has been observed to have a relative benefit in several studies. Whether it has an absolute mortality benefit can be determined only with data from placebo-controlled trials, which are not available. Moreover, several controlled trials have now suggested that empirical amiodarone is less effective than implantable defibrillators in reducing risk of death among survivors of life-threatening arrhythmic events (Antiarrhythmics Versus Implantable Defibrillators [AVID], Canadian Implantable Defibrillator Study [CIDS], and the Cardiac Arrest Study Hamburg [CASH]), particularly when the ejection fraction is less than 35 percent (see Chap. 34).[164-166] It also failed to perform as well as implantable defibrillators in a controlled trial studying primary SCD prevention in patients with class II and Class III heart failure (Sudden Cardiac Death in Heart Failure Trial [SCD-HeFT]).[203]

PROGRAMMED ELECTRICAL STIMULATION

The second major antiarrhythmic strategy was based on suppression of inducibility of sustained ventricular arrhythmias, considered to be a marker of risk during electrophysiological testing. The use of programmed electrical stimulation to identify benefit on the basis of suppression of inducibility by an antiarrhythmic drug gained popularity for evaluating long-term therapy among survivors of out-of-hospital cardiac arrest. It has evolved as the preferred method of management, despite concerns about the sensitivity and specificity of the various pacing protocols and the extent to which the myocardial status at the time of the programmed electrical stimulation study reflects that present at the time of the clinical cardiac arrest. Nonetheless, most studies have demonstrated limitations based on observations that a relatively small fraction of cardiac arrest survivors (an average of less than 50 percent on the basis of multiple studies) had inducible arrhythmias.

Drug suppression of inducibility during electrophysiological testing as an endpoint for secondary prevention of SCD or primary prevention in high-risk post-myocardial infarction patients has yielded to the benefits of ICD therapy in most subgroups, with a few exceptions among primary prevention categories. It still has use, however, for risk profiling in a number of clinical circumstances.[201,202,204] Despite a large, albeit somewhat conflicting, data base on the role of electrophysiological testing for risk profiling, results of the secondary prevention trials among cardiac arrest survivors have suggested that routine electrophysiological testing among such individuals is no longer necessary, particularly if ICD therapy is available to the patient. All the secondary prevention trials demonstrated a benefit of the ICD over antiarrhythmic therapy, usually using amiodarone, without a determination that risk profiling by electrophysiological testing offered any benefit.[164-166] Under conditions in which a potentially reversible trigger for cardiac arrest can be identified, and perhaps among some cardiac arrest survivors in whom transient ischemia was the initiating mechanism and the ejection fraction is higher than 40 percent, there might be a persistent limited role for such testing as a guide to therapy. In contrast, several primary prevention trials, such as MADIT[201] and MUSTT,[202] used electrophysiological testing to profile risk and demonstrated large benefits. MADIT II,[205] which enrolled patients with lower ejection fractions than MADIT or MUSTT and did not use arrhythmia markers, also demonstrated a survival benefit of ICD therapy. The extent to which MADIT II differs from MADIT and MUSTT and the question of whether the electrophysiological testing criteria in the latter are necessary have yet to be resolved. Until then, electrophysiological testing is used as the indicator leading to ICD use among candidates defined by MADIT and MUSTT criteria.

The implications of induced nonsustained forms of VT are more controversial. Although it has been suggested that induction of nonsustained ventricular rhythms may indicate risk, it is generally considered nonspecific in the absence of structural heart disease or when an aggressive protocol is used. The use of the suppression of nonsustained arrhythmias as an endpoint of therapy is not considered valid.

The reliability of *non*inducibility at baseline electrophysiological stimulation testing for predicting risk and guiding long-term management is also questioned. In the past, opinions ranged from the conclusion that potentially high-risk patients free of inducible ventricular arrhythmias were electrophysiologically stable and required no long-term antiarrhythmic therapy to the other extreme, that such patients remained at risk but did not have an objective endpoint of therapy by this method and therefore must be treated by other techniques. Despite these conflicting opinions, it is generally accepted now that survivors of cardiac arrest without clearly identifiable transient and treatable causes remain at high risk, regardless of inducibility status. Some out-of-hospital cardiac arrests can be clearly demonstrated to result from transient ischemia, and this subgroup appears to achieve benefit from antiischemic therapy.[161]

SURGICAL INTERVENTION STRATEGIES

The previously popular antiarrhythmic surgical techniques now have limited applications. Intraoperative map-guided cryoablation techniques may be used for patients who have inducible, hemodynamically stable sustained monomorphic VT during electrophysiological testing and have suitable ventricular and coronary artery anatomy, amenable to catheter ablation. However, they have little applicability to survivors of out-of-hospital cardiac arrest because the type of arrhythmia favoring this surgical approach is infrequently observed in cardiac arrest survivors. It can be used as adjunctive therapy for ICD recipients whose arrhythmia burden requires frequent shocks. In addition, coronary revascularization procedures have a clearly defined role for cardiac arrest survivors in whom an ischemic mechanism was responsible for the event and suitable surgical anatomy is present.

CATHETER ABLATION THERAPY

The use of catheter ablation techniques to treat ventricular tachyarrhythmias has been most successful for the benign focal tachycardias that originate in the right ventricle or left side of the interventricular septum (see Chap. 33) and for some reentrant VTs. With rare exceptions, catheter ablation techniques are not used for the treatment of higher risk ventricular tachyarrhythmias or for definitive therapy in patients at risk for progression of the arrhythmic substrate. For VT caused by bundle branch reentrant mechanisms, which occur in cardiomyopathies as well as other structural cardiac disorders, ablation of the right bundle branch to interrupt the reentrant cycle has been successful. However, this has limited applicability to the large number of patients with structural heart disease at risk for SCD or those who have survived a cardiac arrest. Nonetheless, catheter ablation is an appropriate adjunctive treatment strategy[206] for patients with ICDs who are having multiple tachyarrhythmic events.

IMPLANTABLE DEFIBRILLATORS

The development of the ICD added a new dimension to the management of patients at high risk for cardiac arrest (see Chap. 34). After the early reports by Mirowski and coworkers[207] and Echt and colleagues,[208] a number of observational studies have confirmed that ICDs can achieve rates of sudden death consistently less than 5 percent at 1 year and total death rates in the 10 to 20 percent range in populations who have high mortality risks, as predicted by mortality surrogates such as historical controls or time to first appropriate shock. However, determination of the mortality benefit of ICDs remained uncertain and were debated for many years.[211] More than 16 years elapsed between the first clinical use of an implanted defibrillator[212] and publication of the first major randomized clinical trial comparing implantable defibrillator therapy with antiarrhythmic drug therapy.[201] During that period, reports had documented the ability of implantable devices to revert potentially fatal arrhythmias, but could not identify a valid relative or absolute mortality benefit because of confounding factors, such as competing risks for sudden and nonsudden death and determination of whether appropriate shocks represented the interruption of an event that would have been fatal. Despite these limitations, ICD therapy continued to increase its relative position among other forms of therapy for survivors of out-of-hospital cardiac arrest and, to a lesser extent, for those considered to be at high risk for a primary cardiac arrest on the basis of specific clinical markers.

With publication of the results of MADIT,[201] information on the relative benefit of defibrillators over antiarrhythmic drug therapy (largely amiodarone) for primary prevention of SCD in a very high-risk population became available (Table 36-5; see also Fig. 36-24). The outcome demonstrated a 59 percent reduction in relative risk of total mortality at 2 years of follow-up (54 percent cumulative) and a 19 percent reduction in absolute risk of dying at 2 years of follow-up. One year later, the first adequately powered secondary prevention trial of ICDs versus antiarrhythmic drugs was published. This study, the AVID trial, demonstrated a 27 percent reduction in relative risk of total

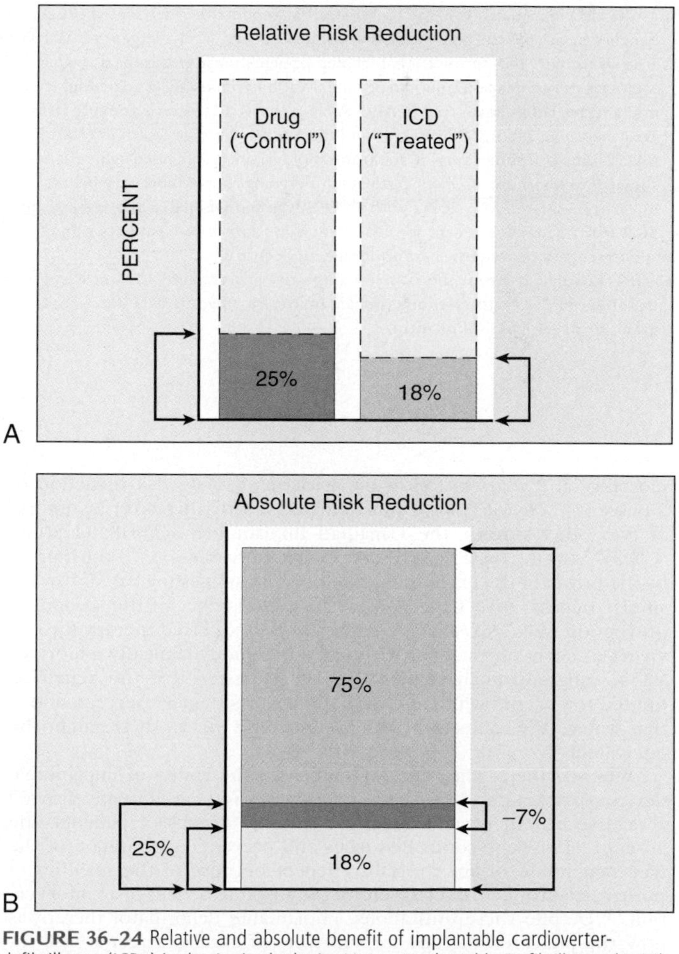

FIGURE 36–24 Relative and absolute benefit of implantable cardioverter-defibrillators (ICDs) in the Antiarrhythmics Versus Implantable Defibrillators (AVID) study. **A,** The ICD-treated subgroup had 18 percent mortality at 2 years versus 25 percent in the drug-treated group, a 27 percent *relative* reduction in the population having events. **B,** When relative reduction is extrapolated to the total target population, the *absolute* reduction of fatal events in the total population is 7 percent. *(From Myerburg RJ, Mitrani R, Interian A Jr, Castellanos A: Interpretation of outcomes of antiarrhythmic clinical trials: Design features and population impact. Circulation 97:1514, 1998. © 1998, American Heart Association.)*

TABLE 36–5 Summary of Major Implantable Cardioverter-Defibrillator Trials for Prevention of Sudden Cardiac Deaths

Trial	Study Group	2-Year Outcomes (%) Control	ICDs	Rel RR	Abs RR
Secondary prevention*					
AVID[164] (n=1061)	VF, VT-syncope VT: EF≤40%	25	18	−27	−7
CIDS[165] (n=659)	VF, VT-syncope VT: EF≤35% and CL<400 ms	21	15	−30	−6
CASH[166] (n=346)	Cardiac arrest survivors (VF, VT)	20 (combined)	12	−37	−8
		2-Yr (MADIT, CABG-Patch, MADIT-2, DEFINITE) and 5-Yr (MUSTT, SCD-HeFT) Outcomes (%) Control	ICDs	Rel RR	Abs RR
Primary prevention†					
MADIT[201] (n=196)	Prior MI, EF≤35%, NS VT, inducible VT, failed IV PA	32	13	−59	−19
MUSTT[202] (n=704)	Prior MI, EF≤40%, NS VT, inducible VT	55	24	−58	−31
CABG-Patch[196] (n=900)	Coronary bypass surgery, EF<36%, SAECG (+)	18	18	0	0
MADIT-II[205] (n=1232)	Prior MI (>1 mo), EF≤30%	22	16	−28	−6
DEFINITE[216] (n=458)	Nonischemic cardiomyopathy, EF≤35%	14	8	−35	−6
SCD-HeFT[203] (n=2521)‡	Class II-III CHF, EF≤35%	36	29	−23	−7

*Three major randomized trials for secondary prevention among survivors of out-of-hospital cardiac arrest, or high-risk ventricular tachycardia (VT), have been completed: the Antiarrhythmics Versus Implantable Defibrillators (AVID) trial, the Canadian Implantable Defibrillator Study (CIDS), and the Cardiac Arrest Study of Hamburg (CASH). Each used an active control, randomized design, comparing ICDs with antiarrhythmic drug (AAD) therapy, primarily amiodarone. The cumulative data, as well as the individual data from the larger studies, support the idea that the ICD is preferable to drug therapy for this high-risk population. However, the large relative benefits translated to more modest absolute benefits, with a large residual risk among the ICD-treated groups in each study.

†These six primary prevention trials included patients presumed to be at high risk but who have not had spontaneous life-threatening ventricular arrhythmias: the Multicenter Automatic Defibrillator Implantation Trial (MADIT), the Multicenter Unsustained Tachycardia Trial (MUSTT), the coronary artery bypass surgery/implantable defibrillator trial (CABG-Patch), the Multicenter Automatic Defibrillator Implantation Trial-2 (MADIT-2), Defibrillators in Non-Ischemic Cardiomyopathy Treatment Evaluation (DEFINITE), and the Sudden Cardiac Death in Heart Failure Trial (SCD-HeFT). MADIT showed an advantage of ICD therapy over AAD therapy, MUSTT showed superiority of electrophysiologically (EP) guided evaluation leading to ICD therapy compared with that leading to drug therapy, and CABG-Patch showed no benefit of ICDs for patients undergoing routine coronary bypass surgery. MADIT-2 showed a benefit of ICD therapy compared with usual therapy for post-myocardial infarction patients with an EF≤30% and DEFINITE showed a strong trend toward statistically significant benefit in nonischemic cardiomyopathy patients. SCD-HeFT showed a benefit for Class II and III heart failure patients with EF<35%.

‡No difference shown between amiodarone and control.

Abs RR=absolute risk reduction; CHF=congestive heart failure; CL=cycle length; EF=ejection fraction; EP=electrophysiological; ICD=implantable cardioverter-defibrillator; IV PA=intravenous procainamide; MI=myocardial infarction; NS=nonsustained; Rel RR=relative risk reduction; SAECG=signal-averaged electrocardiogram; VF=ventricular fibrillation.

mortality at 2 years of follow-up, with an absolute risk reduction of 7 percent.[164] The AVID trial was followed shortly thereafter by reports of two other studies, the Canadian Implantable Defibrillator Study (CIDS)[165] and the Cardiac Arrest Study Hamburg (CASH),[166] both limited by the power of the enrollment numbers but suggesting trends toward similar benefits (see Table 36-5). As a consequence of the secondary prevention trials, ICDs have emerged as the preferred therapy for survivors of out-of-hospital cardiac arrest or hemodynamically important VT. A subgroup analysis of AVID has suggested that the benefit is limited to patients with ejection fractions less than 35 percent; above that value, the outcome with amiodarone or an ICD might be equivalent.[198]

Whereas the studies cited documented the ability of implantable devices to revert potentially fatal arrhythmias and subsequently showed a relative benefit over amiodarone in some groups of patients, the absence of placebo-controlled trials still prevents quantitation of the true magnitude of any mortality benefit because of the inability of positive-controlled trials to identify the absolute benefit of an intervention.[213] Despite these limitations, implantable defibrillator therapy is now the preferred therapy for survivors of cardiac arrest at risk for recurrences and for primary prevention in patients in a number of high-risk categories. Major questions still unanswered include the relative benefit of amiodarone versus defibrillators among lower risk subgroups of survivors of out-of-hospital cardiac arrest, the role of beta blockers, and the role of antiischemic surgical and medical therapy as definitive approaches.

A much larger issue, and one that has not yet been defined, is the use of implantable defibrillators for primary prevention of cardiac arrest in patients thought to be at intermediate levels of risk. Studies of cost-effectiveness, in addition to medical efficacy, are needed.

Application of Therapeutic Strategies to Specific Groups of Patients

SECONDARY PREVENTION AFTER SURVIVING CARDIAC ARREST. As populations of cardiac arrest survivors began to accumulate from community-based emergency rescue activities, long-term therapeutic strategies intended to reduce recurrent cardiac arrest rates and total mortality risks emerged as a mandate for clinical investigators. The problem that affects all long-term strategies for cardiac arrest survivors, however, is the lack of a reliable concurrent natural history denominator against which to compare the results of interventions. This lack is a consequence of ethical concerns about withholding therapy in a placebo-controlled study model for patients at such high risk for dying,[213] in conjunction with the likelihood that general therapies used in such patients may also improve total mortality risk. Earlier approaches to long-term therapy centered on the use of antiarrhythmic drug therapy, largely guided by the results of electrophysiological testing or the empirical use of antiarrhythmic drugs, particularly amiodarone. During the evolution of therapeutic strategies, various observational and positive-controlled studies have suggested first that suppression of inducible ventricular arrhythmias yields a better outcome than failure of suppression, that amiodarone is better than class I antiarrhythmic drugs, and finally that ICDs are better than amiodarone.

Therefore, ICD therapy has emerged as preferred therapy, absent absolute benefit data. Electrophysiological testing for secondary prevention, once routine, is now considered of questionable necessity and is commonly not performed.

Anatomically based antiarrhythmic surgery enjoyed a short period of popularity for secondary prevention, limited by the observation that surgical antiarrhythmic procedures appear to provide benefit to only a small subset of such patients. As the implantable defibrillator came into wider use, it also began to supplant pharmacological antiarrhythmic approaches, with the possible exception of amiodarone, even before the randomized clinical trials demonstrated relative ICD benefit. In the late 1990s, information from randomized clinical trials—AVID, CIDS, and CASH—provided compelling support for the use of ICDs as preferred therapy for secondary prevention of cardiac arrest related to ventricular tachyarrhythmias (Fig. 36-24).

PRIMARY PREVENTION OF OUT-OF-HOSPITAL CARDIAC ARREST WITH ADVANCED HEART DISEASE. Because SCD is frequently the initial clinical expression of underlying structural heart disease or occurs in identified patients profiled to be at low risk (see Fig. 36-2), there has been a longstanding interest in therapeutic strategies targeted to primary prevention. After the disappointing outcome of CAST and the disturbing suggestions of lack of efficacy or adverse effects of the class I antiarrhythmic drugs generally when used for primary or secondary prevention of SCD,[197] interest shifted to the use of amiodarone and implantable defibrillators. Two major trials of amiodarone in post-myocardial infarction patients,[214,215] one of which required ejection fractions less than 40 percent, demonstrated no total mortality benefit, even though both trials demonstrated antiarrhythmic benefit, expressed as a reduction in arrhythmic deaths or resuscitated VF. Subgroup analyses have suggested that the concomitant use of beta blockers does confer a mortality benefit.[200]

In parallel with the amiodarone trials, the first randomized controlled trial comparing antiarrhythmic therapy (primarily amiodarone) with ICD therapy (MADIT) was carried out (see Table 36-5).[201] The randomized patients had ejection fractions less than 35 percent, nonsustained VT during ambulatory recording, and inducible VT that was not suppressible by procainamide. This very high-risk group demonstrated a 54 percent reduction in total mortality with ICD therapy compared with drug therapy, primarily amiodarone. At the same time, a trial comparing ICD implantation with no specific therapies for arrhythmias among patients with ejection fractions less than 36 percent who were undergoing coronary bypass surgery (CABG-Patch) demonstrated no benefit of defibrillators for total mortality.[196] The only marker for arrhythmic risk required for entry into the study was a positive signal-averaged ECG. A third trial, MUSTT,[202] was a complex study designed to determine whether electrophysiologically guided therapy would lead to an improved outcome in patients with nonsustained VT, inducible VT, and a history of prior myocardial infarction. The results demonstrated that although a statistically significant beneficial effect on total mortality was achieved by guiding therapy according to the results of electrophysiological testing, compared with patients with inducible tachycardia who did not receive therapy, the subgroup of patients who received ICDs because they failed to respond to drug therapy accounted for all the benefit. There was 24 percent mortality among ICD-treated patients at 5 years of follow-up compared with 55 percent among those receiving electrophysiologically guided drug therapy and 48 percent among those randomly assigned to no therapy. MADIT II was next among the post-myocardial infarction primary prevention trials reported.[205] In this study, ICD therapy provided a mortality benefit compared with conventional therapy among patients with prior myocardial infarction and ejection fractions less than 30 percent.

A study designed to determine whether patients with nonischemic cardiomyopathy benefit from prophylactic ICD therapy, DEFINITE, was underpowered to achieve statistical significance ($p = .08$). However, the results reported demonstrated a strong trend for benefit, with a 35 percent relative risk reduction and a 6 percent absolute risk reduction over 2 years of follow-up.[216] Finally, the Sudden Cardiac Death-Heart Failure Trial (SCD-HeFT) was designed to test the potential benefit of ICDs versus amiodarone, compared with placebo, in patients with functional class II or III congestive heart failure and ejection fractions less than 35 percent. The results of this study demonstrated a 23 percent reduction in relative risk and an absolute risk reduction of 7 percent over 5 years.[203] Amiodarone provided no added benefit to conventional therapy.

PRIMARY PREVENTION IN PATIENTS WITH LESS ADVANCED COMMON HEART DISEASES OR UNCOMMON DISEASES. Primary prevention trials have been designed to enroll populations of patients with advanced heart disease who were estimated to be at very high risk for SCD and total mortality as a consequence of the severity of the underlying disease. Most clinical trials testing the question of relative efficacy of antiarrhythmic versus ICD therapy have used the ejection fraction as the marker for advanced disease, with the qualifying criteria in the range of 30 to 40 percent or less. Moreover, in the secondary prevention trial, AVID, a subgroup analysis suggested that there is no benefit of ICD therapy over amiodarone for patients with ejection fractions between 36 and 40 percent; all the benefits accrued to those with ejection fractions of 35 percent or less.[198] This observation is important because it raises a question about therapeutic options, for both primary and secondary prevention strategies, when ejection fractions are greater than 35 percent. However, as a retrospective analysis, the observation calls for confirmation in a controlled trial.

Whereas the risk for SCD and total mortality is highest among patients with advanced structural heart disease and low ejection fractions, impaired functional capacity, or both, a substantial portion of the total SCD burden occurs among patients with coronary heart disease or the various nonischemic cardiomyopathies with ejection fractions between 35 and 40 percent and higher. In addition, among patients with heart failure related to various forms of cardiomyopathy, whereas the total mortality risk is considerably lower in patients in functional class I or early class II than in those with late class III or class IV status, the probability of a death being sudden is higher in the former group[66,217] (see Fig. 36-7). Despite this observation, there are no data available to guide therapy for primary prevention of cardiac arrest in such patients.[10,140] This limitation is confounded by the fact that patients in these categories generally have low event rates but cumulatively account for large numbers of SCDs (see Fig. 36-2A). In addition, certain other structural entities associated with some elevation of risk of sudden death in the absence of a severely reduced ejection fraction, such as some patterns of viral myocarditis, hypertrophic cardiomyopathy, right ventricular dysplasia, and sarcoidosis, are managed without the benefit of clinical trials to guide therapeutic decisions (see Table 36-4). Patients with symptomatic ventricular arrhythmias related to structural disorders such as right ventricular dysplasia, in which most of the mortality risk is arrhythmic, are often advised to have an ICD, even in the absence of a prior cardiac arrest or hemodynamically significant VT. Whether antiarrhythmic therapy would be just as effective remains unknown, but the judgment of using defibrillators in patients with a disorder whose fatal expression is primarily arrhythmic carries the strength of logic, often supported by risk profiling based on observational data on clinical markers. Among the entities in which family history is helpful for defining risk, clinical judgment is made easier when there is a strong family history of SCD. Specific support for this approach derives from genetic studies in hypertrophic cardiomyopathy, in which a limited number of the known mutations appear to be associated with a specific risk of SCD.[19] In addition, clinical observational data have supported the use of ICDs in high-risk subsets of patients with hypertrophic cardiomyopathy.[218]

PRIMARY PREVENTION IN PATIENTS WITH STRUCTURALLY NORMAL HEARTS OR MOLECULAR DISORDERS OF CARDIAC ELECTRICAL ACTIVITY. A category of expanding interest in primary preventive therapy has emerged. Clinically subtle or inapparent structural disorders or entities with pure electrophysiological expression, such as the congenital long-QT syndromes, Brugada syndrome, and idiopathic VF, are receiving increasing attention. The decision-making process for secondary prevention strategies for patients with the long-QT syndrome is relatively easy. Individuals who have survived a cardiac arrest or potentially fatal arrhythmic event, especially when there is a family history of SCD, are generally treated with an ICD. Beta blockers are still considered useful for affected family members who have not had an event and perhaps for some subgroups with patients with syncope of undocumented mechanism.[93,94] In contrast, individuals who express the electrocardiographic phenotype of long-QT syndrome without a family history of SCD, absence of symptomatic arrhythmias, or both are generally treated with beta blocker therapy at this time. Between these extremes are the asymptomatic affected family members of patients with symptomatic long-QT syndrome. Given the complexity of the pathophysiology of potentially fatal arrhythmias among such patients, the threshold for considering ICD therapy is decreasing.[93] Genetic screening may ultimately prove useful for identifying specific risk, particularly if individual arrhythmic risk is demonstrated to be determined by one or more modifier genes interacting with the defect responsible for an ion channel pore defect.[58] Currently, many such clinical therapeutic decisions remain judgment-based rather than data-driven. In this context, a family history of premature SCD in affected relatives appears to be useful for the decision-making process for preventive therapy in this general category of patients (see Chaps. 9 and 33).

Among the other molecular arrhythmia syndromes, the Brugada syndrome is one for which management strategies remain problematic and debated.[127,197] The ICD is accepted as the preferred secondary prevention strategy in cardiac arrest survivors and symptomatic affected individuals, even though it is based solely on observational data. However, primary prevention approaches for affected relatives, especially if asymptomatic, are unclear. Studies have suggested that syncope associated with electrocardiographic changes suggestive of the disorder at baseline is a marker of risk sufficient to warrant ICD therapy[127] and that baseline electrocardiographic changes associated with inducibility of ventricular tachyarrhythmias during electrophysiological testing are also a marker of risk.[219] Conversely, the absence of right bundle branch block and ST-T wave changes without provocation suggests lower risk. However, a family history of SCD remains an important factor in judgment-based decisions. Similar arguments, but supported by even less data, apply to affected family members of patients with right ventricular dysplasia.

PRIMARY PREVENTION AMONG THE GENERAL POPULATION. To have a major impact on the problem of SCD in the general population, including adolescents and young adults, we need to move beyond the identification of high-risk patients who have specific clinical entities, advanced or subtle, that predict a high risk of SCD. Rather, it is necessary to find small subgroups of patients at specific risk for SCD in the general population as a manifestation of underlying heart disease, if and when that disease becomes manifest. As an example, the studies that have demonstrated familial clustering of SCD as the first expression of underlying coronary artery disease suggesting genetic or behavioral predisposition may provide some help for the future.[28,29] The report of a common genetic "variant" in the cardiac Na^+ channel gene (*SCN5A* on chromosome 3) among blacks with apparent susceptibility to arrhythmias and proarrhythmic responses to antiarrhythmic drugs[24] supports this concept. With a population frequency of affected individuals in the range of 13 percent, a valuable marker of risk may be offered if further genetic epidemiological studies support the possibility that this is a marker of specific SCD risk during pathophysiological events. If highly specific markers can be found, related to electrophysiological properties or along multiple points in the cascade of coronary events (see Fig. 36-4), preventive therapy before the first expression of an underlying disease may have a major effect on the population problem of SCD. Short of that, successes will be limited to community-based intervention and to the subgroups that are easier to identify and in whom it is more justifiable to use prophylactic interventional therapy on the basis of population size and magnitude of risk.[7,10,141,220]

Adolescents and young adults, including athletes (see Chap. 78), constitute a group for special consideration. The SCD risk in these groups is an order of magnitude of 1 percent of that of the general adult population older than 35 years (see Fig. 36-3A).[65,125,158,221] However, most causes of SCD in these populations are not characterized by advanced life-limiting structural heart disease, and therefore surviving cardiac arrest victims can, with appropriate long-term therapy, be expected to have significant extensions of life. Because most deaths are arrhythmic, the ability to identify individuals at risk in advance of a life-threatening arrhythmic event offers more long-term impact than for older populations. For both the general young population and athletes, identification of individuals at risk may lead to prevention of events triggered by physical activity.[222] In the United States, strategies for screening adolescents, young adults, and athletes to identify the entities that create a risk have largely been limited to questionnaires and a physical examination. The European approach of adding EKG screening for athletes[223] has met with limited acceptance despite some data indicating both feasibility[124] and suggestions of cost-effectiveness.[222] Electrocardiographic screening of the general adolescent population, including athletes, can identify many of those at potential risk because of congenital long-QT syndrome, hypertrophic cardiomyopathy, right ventricular dysplasia, and Brugada syndrome. Although electrocardiographic screening in the adolescent and athletic subgroups is imperfect and usually accompanied by depolarization and repolarization patterns that may be difficult to interpret, this strategy can lead to further testing in appropriate individuals. Echocardiography has also been suggested as a screening method, but it is more expensive and less cost-efficient and does not recognize conditions such as long-QT syndrome and Brugada syndrome. One study has demonstrated a reduction in SCDs in athletes with the use of widespread screening.[121]

SCD risk must be evaluated in competitive athletes with previously known cardiovascular disorders, or those discovered during preparticipation screening, as well as in those with known disorders who wish to participate in recreational sports. Recommendations for the latter, based on intensity of exercise and nature of disease, are available.[224] Issues for competing athletes are more complex, including both medical and legal considerations.[225]

SUDDEN DEATH AND PUBLIC SAFETY

The unexpectedness of SCD has raised questions concerning secondary risk to the public created by people in the throes of a cardiac arrest. There are no data from controlled studies available to guide public policy regarding people at high risk for potentially lethal arrhythmias and for abrupt incapacitation. In a report of observations on 1348 sudden deaths caused by coronary heart disease in people 65 years of age or younger during a 7-year period in Dade County, Florida, 101 (7.5 percent) of the deaths occurred in people who were engaged in activities at the time of death that were potentially hazardous to the public (e.g., driving a motor vehicle, working at altitude, piloting aircraft), and 122 (9.1 percent) of the victims had occupations that could create potential hazards to others if an abrupt loss of consciousness had occurred while they were at work. There were no catastrophic events as a result of these cardiac arrests, only minor property damage in 19 and minor injuries in 5.

Other studies have also led to the conclusion that risk to the public is low. In specific reference to private automobile drivers, most data have shown that sudden death at the wheel usually involves enough of a prodrome to allow the driver to get to the roadside before losing consciousness. An analysis of recurrent VT-VF events among cardiac arrest survivors has suggested limitation of driving privileges for the first 8 months after the index event on the basis of the clustering of recurrent event rates early after the index event.[14,226] Therefore, although there are likely to be isolated cases in which cardiac arrest causes public hazards in the future, the risk appears to be small and, because it is difficult to identify specific individuals at risk, sweeping restrictions to avoid such risks appear unwarranted. The exceptions are people with multisystem disease, particularly senility, and individual circumstances that require specific consideration, such as high-risk patients who have special responsibilities—school bus drivers, aircraft pilots, train operators, and truck drivers.[14,226]

REFERENCES

Definitions

1. Torp-Pedersen C, Kober L, Elming H, Burchart H: Classification of sudden and arrhythmic death. Pacing Clin Electrophysiol 20:245, 1997.

Epidemiology

2. Myerburg RJ, Castellanos A: Emerging paradigms of the epidemiology and demographics of sudden cardiac arrest. Heart Rhythm 3:235, 2006.
3. Priori SG, Aliot E, Blomstrom-Lundqvist C, et al: Task Force on Sudden Cardiac Death of the European Society of Cardiology. Eur Heart J 22:1374, 2001.
4. Escobedo LG, Zack MM: Comparison of sudden and nonsudden coronary deaths in the United States. Circulation 93:2033, 1996.
5. Zheng ZJ, Croft JB, Giles WH, Mensah GA: Sudden cardiac death in the United States, 1989 to 1998. Circulation 104:2158, 2001.
6. Cobb LA, Fahrenbruch CE, Olsufka M, Copass MK: Changing incidence of out-of-hospital ventricular fibrillation, 1980-2000. JAMA 288:3008, 2002.
7. Myerburg RJ, Kessler KM, Castellanos A: Sudden cardiac death: Epidemiology, transient risk, and intervention assessment. Ann Intern Med 119:1187, 1993.
8. Myerburg RJ, Wellens HJJ: Epidemiology of cardiac arrest and sudden cardiac death. *In* Priori S, Zipes D (eds): Sudden Cardiac Death: A Handbook for Clinical Practice. Oxford, UK. Blackwell Publishing, 2006, pp 3-19.
9. Myerburg RJ: Sudden cardiac death: Exploring the limits of our knowledge. J Cardiovasc Electrophysiol 12:369, 2001.
10. Huikuri H, Castellanos A, Myerburg RJ: Sudden death due to cardiac arrhythmias. N Engl J Med 345:1473, 2001.
11. Braunwald E: Cardiovascular medicine at the turn of the millennium: Triumphs, concerns, and opportunities. N Engl J Med 337:1360, 1997.
12. Myerburg RJ, Kessler KM, Castellanos A: Sudden cardiac death: Structure, function, and time-dependence of risk. Circulation 85(Suppl I):I-2, 1992.
13. Arntz HR, Willich SN, Schreiber C, et al: Diurnal, weekly and seasonal variation of sudden death. Population-based analysis of 24,061 consecutive cases. Eur Heart J 21:315, 2000.
14. Larsen GC, Stupey MR, Wallace CG, et al: Recurrent cardiac events in survivors of ventricular fibrillation or tachycardia: Implications for driving restrictions. JAMA 271:1335, 1994.
15. Solomon SD, Zelenkofske S, McMurray JJV, et al; The Valsartan in Acute Myocardial Infarction Trial (VALIANT) Investigators: Sudden death in patients with myocardial infarction and left ventricular dysfunction, heart failure or both. N Engl J Med 352:2581, 2005.
16. Holmberg M, Holmberg S, Herlitz J: Incidence, duration and survival of ventricular fibrillation in out-of-hospital cardiac arrest patients in Sweden. Resuscitation 44:7, 2000.
17. Wren C, O'Sullivan JJ, Wright C: Sudden death in children and adolescents. Heart 83:410, 2000.
18. Schwartz PJ, Priori SG, Spazzolini C, et al: Genotype-phenotype correlation in the long-QT syndrome: Gene-specific triggers for life-threatening arrhythmias. Circulation 103:89, 2001.
19. Marian AJ, Roberts R: Molecular genetic basis of hypertrophic cardiomyopathy: Genetic markers for sudden cardiac death. J Cardiovasc Electrophysiol 9:88, 1998.
20. Chen Q, Kirsch GE, Zhang D, et al: Genetic basis and molecular mechanism for idiopathic ventricular fibrillation. Nature 392:293, 1998.
21. Priori SG, Napolitano C, Memmi M, et al: Clinical and molecular characterization of patients with catecholaminergic polymorphic ventricular tachycardia. Circulation 106:69, 2002.
22. Lahat H, Pras E, Olender T, et al: A missense mutation in a highly conserved region of CASQ2 is associated with autosomal recessive catecholamine-induced polymorphic ventricular tachycardia in Bedouin families from Israel. Am J Hum Genet 69:1378, 2001.
23. Brookfield L, Bharati S, Denes P, et al: Familial sudden death: Report of a case and review of the literature. Chest 94:989, 1988.
24. Splawski I, Timothy KW, Tateyama M, et al: Variant of *SCN5A* sodium channel implicated in risk of cardiac arrhythmia. Science 297:1333, 2002.
25. Boerwinkle E, Ellsworth DL, Hallman DM, Biddinger A: Genetic analysis of atherosclerosis: A research paradigm for the common chronic diseases. Hum Mol Genet 5:1405, 1996.
26. Faber BC, Cleutjens KB, Niessen RL, et al: Identification of genes potentially involved in rupture of human atherosclerotic plaques. Circ Res 89:547, 2001.
27. Spooner PM, Albert C, Benjamin EJ, et al: Sudden cardiac death, genes, and arrhythmogenesis: Consideration of new population and mechanistic approaches from a National Heart, Lung, and Blood Institute Workshop, Parts I and II. Circulation 103:2361 (Pt I), 2447 (Pt II), 2001.
28. Friedlander Y, Siscovick DS, Weinmann S, et al: Family history as a risk factor for primary cardiac arrest. Circulation 97:155, 1998.
29. Jouven X, Desnos M, Guerot C, Ducimetiere P: Predicting sudden death in the population: The Paris Prospective Study I. Circulation 99:1978, 1999.
30. Gillum RF: Sudden cardiac death in Hispanic Americans and African Americans. Am J Public Health 87:1461, 1997.
31. Albert CM, Chae CU, Grodstein F, et al: Prospective study of sudden cardiac death among women in the United States. Circulation 107:2096, 2003.
32. Grundy SM, Balady GJ, Criqui MH, et al: Primary prevention of coronary heart disease: Guidance from Framingham: A statement for healthcare professionals from the AHA Task Force on Risk Reduction. Circulation 97:1876, 1998.
33. Verdecchia P, Schillaci G, Borgioni C, et al: Prognostic significance of serial changes in left ventricular mass in essential hypertension. Circulation 97:48, 1998.
34. Haider AW, Larson MG, Benjamin EJ, Levy D: Increased left ventricular mass and hypertrophy are associated with increased risk for sudden death. J Am Coll Cardiol 32:1454, 1998.
35. Taylor AJ, Burke AP, O'Malley PG, et al: A comparison of the Framingham risk index, coronary artery calcification, and culprit plaque morphology in sudden cardiac death. Circulation 101:1243, 2000.
36. Mittleman MA, Maclure M, Tofler GH, et al: Triggering of acute myocardial infarction by heavy physical exertion: Protection against triggering by regular exertion. N Engl J Med 329:1677, 1993.
37. Huikuri HV, Tapanainen JM, Lindgran K, et al: Prediction of sudden cardiac death after myocardial infarction in the beta-blocking era. J Am Coll Cardiol 42:652, 2003.
38. Jouven X, Empana JP, Schwartz PJ, et al: Heart-rate profile during exercise as a predictor of sudden death. N Engl J Med 352:1951, 2005.
39. Hallstrom AP, Cobb LA, Ray R: Smoking as a risk factor for recurrence of sudden cardiac arrest. N Engl J Med 314:271, 1986.
40. Albert CM, Mittleman MA, Chae CU, et al: Triggering of sudden death from cardiac causes by vigorous exertion. N Engl J Med 343:1355, 2000.
41. Thiene G, Basso C, Corrado D: Is prevention of sudden death in young athletes feasible? Cardiologia 44:497, 1999.
42. Rozanski A, Blumenthal JA, Kaplan J: Impact of psychological factors on the pathogenesis of cardiovascular disease and implications for therapy. Circulation 99:2192, 1999.
43. Krantz DS, Sheps DS, Carney RM, Natelson BH: Effects of mental stress in patients with coronary artery disease: Evidence and clinical implications. JAMA 283:1800, 2000.
44. Irvine J, Basinski A, Baker B, et al: Depression and risk of sudden cardiac death after acute myocardial infarction: Testing for the confounding effects of fatigue. Psychosom Med 61:729, 1999.
45. de Vreede-Swagemakers JJ, Gorgels AP, Weijenberg MP, et al: Risk indicators for out-of-hospital cardiac arrest in patients with coronary artery disease. J Clin Epidemiol 52:601, 1999.
46. The Enhancing Recovery in Coronary Heart Disease Patients (ENRICHD) Randomized Trial Writing Committee: Effects of treating depression and low perceived social support on clinical events after myocardial infarction. JAMA 289:3106, 2003.
47. Leor J, Poole WK, Kloner RA: Sudden cardiac death triggered by an earthquake. N Engl J Med 334:413, 1996.
48. Lampert R, Joska T, Burg MM, et al: Emotional and physical precipitants of ventricular arrhythmia. Circulation 106:1800, 2002.
49. Kloner RA: Natural and unnatural triggers of myocardial infarction. Prog Cardiovasc Dis 48:285, 2006.
50. Burke AP, Farb A, Malcom GT, et al: Plaque rupture and sudden death related to exertion in men with coronary artery disease. JAMA 281:921, 1999.
51. de Vreede-Swagemakers JJ, Gorgels AP, Dubois-Arbouw WI, et al: Out-of-hospital cardiac arrest in the 1990's: A population-based study in the Maastricht area on incidence, characteristics and survival. J Am Coll Cardiol 30:1500, 1997.
52. Stecker EC, Vickers C, Waltz J, et al: Population -based analysis of sudden cardiac death with and without left ventricular systolic dysfunction. J Am Coll Cardiol 47:1161, 2006.
53. Viskin S, Belhassen B: Polymorphic ventricular tachyarrhythmias in the absence of organic heart disease: Classification, differential diagnosis, and implications for therapy. Prog Cardiovasc Dis 41:17, 1998.
54. Jouven X, Zureik M, Desnos M, et al: Long-term outcome in asymptomatic men with exercise-induced premature ventricular depolarizations. N Engl J Med 343:826, 2000.
55. Frolkis JP, Pothier CE, Blackstone EH, Lauer MS: Frequent ventricular ectopy after exercise as a predictor of death. N Engl J Med 348:781, 2003.
56. Teerlink JR, Jalaluddin M, Anderson S, et al: Ambulatory ventricular arrhythmias in patients with heart failure do not specifically predict an increased risk of sudden death. PROMISE (Prospective Randomized Milrinone Survival Evaluation) Investigators. Circulation 101:40, 2000.

Causes of Sudden Cardiac Death

57. Myerburg RJ, Interian A Jr, Mitrani RM, et al: Frequency of sudden cardiac death and profiles of risk. Am J Cardiol 80:10F, 1997.
58. Myerburg RJ: Scientific gaps in the prediction and prevention of sudden cardiac death. J Cardiovasc Electrophysiol 13:709, 2002.
59. Frescura C, Basso C, Thiene G, et al: Anomalous origin of coronary arteries and risk of sudden death: A study based on an autopsy population of congenital heart disease. Hum Pathol 29:689, 1998.
60. Myerburg RJ, Kessler KM, Mallon SM, et al: Life-threatening ventricular arrhythmias in patients with silent myocardial ischemia due to coronary artery spasm. N Engl J Med 326:1451, 1992.
61. Maron BJ, Casey SA, Poliac LC, et al: Clinical course of hypertrophic cardiomyopathy in a regional United States cohort. JAMA 281:650, 1999.

62. McKenna WJ, Behr ER: Hypertrophic cardiomyopathy: Management, risk stratification, and prevention of sudden death. Heart 87:169, 2002.
63. Elliott PM, Gimeno Blanes JR, Mahon NG, et al: Relation between severity of left-ventricular hypertrophy and prognosis in patients with hypertrophic cardiomyopathy. Lancet 357:420, 2001.
64. Maron MS, Olivotto I, Betocchi S, et al: Effect of left ventricular outflow tract obstruction on clinical outcome in hypertrophic cardiomyopathy. N Engl J Med 348:295, 2003.
65. Maron BJ, Shirani J, Poliac LC, et al: Sudden death in young competitive athletes. Clinical, demographic, and pathological profiles. JAMA 276:199, 1996.
66. Cleland JG, Chattopadhyay S, Khand A, et al: Prevalence and incidence of arrhythmias and sudden death in heart failure. Heart Fail Rev 7:229, 2002.
67. Middlekauff HR, Stevenson WG, Stevenson LW, et al: Syncope in advanced heart failure: High sudden death risk regardless of syncope etiology. J Am Coll Cardiol 21:110, 1993.
68. Knight BP, Goyal R, Pelosi F, et al: Outcome of patients with nonischemic dilated cardiomyopathy and unexplained syncope treated with an implantable defibrillator. J Am Coll Cardiol 33:1964, 1999.
69. Corrado D, Basso C, Thiene G: Sudden cardiac death in young people with apparently normal heart. Cardiovasc Res 50:399, 2001.
70. Theleman KP, Kuiper JJ, Roberts WC: Acute myocarditis (predominately lymphocytic) causing sudden death without heart failure. Am J Cardiol 88.1078, 2001
71. Corrado D, Basso C, Nava A, Thiene G: Arrhythmogenic right ventricular cardiomyopathy: Current diagnostic and management strategies. Cardiol Rev 9:259, 2001.
72. Thiene G, Nava A, Corrado D, et al: Right ventricular cardiomyopathy and sudden death in young people. N Engl J Med 318:129, 1988.
73. Fontaine G, Fontaliran F, Hebert JL, et al: Arrhythmogenic right ventricular dysplasia. Annu Rev Med 50:17, 1999.
74. Corrado D, Basso C, Thiene G, et al: Spectrum of clinicopathologic manifestations of arrhythmogenic right ventricular cardiomyopathy/dysplasia: A multicenter study. J Am Coll Cardiol 30:1512, 1997.
75. Furlanello F, Bertoldi A, Dallago M, et al: Cardiac arrest and sudden death in competitive athletes with arrhythmogenic right ventricular dysplasia. Pacing Clin Electrophysiol 21:331, 1998.
76. Tiso N, Stephan DA, Nava A, et al: Identification of mutations in the cardiac ryanodine receptor gene in families affected with arrhythmogenic right ventricular cardiomyopathy type 2 (ARVD2). Hum Mol Genet 10:189, 2001.
77. Rampazzo A, Nava A, Malacrida S, et al: Mutation in human desmoplakin domain binding to plakoglobin causes a dominant form of arrhythmogenic right ventricular cardiomyopathy. Am J Hum Genet 71:1200, 2002.
78. Pilichou K, Nava A, Basso C, et al: Mutations in desmoglein-2 gene are associated with arrhythmogenic right ventricular cardiomyopathy. Circulation 113:1171, 2006.
79. Norman M, Simpson M, Mogensen Jet al: Novel mutation in desmoplakin causes arrhythmogenic left ventricular cardiomyopathy. Circulation 112:636, 2005.
80. Sen-Chowdhry S, Syrris P, McKenna WJ: Genetics of right ventricular cardiomyopathy. J Cardiovasc Electrophysiol 16:927, 2005.
81. Sorgato A, Faggiano P, Aurigemma GP, et al: Ventricular arrhythmias in adult aortic stenosis: Prevalence, mechanisms, and clinical relevance. Chest 113:482, 1998.
82. McGiffin DC, O'Brien MF, Galbraith AJ, et al: An analysis of risk factors for death and mode-specific death after aortic valve replacement with allograft, xenograft, and mechanical valves. J Thorac Cardiovasc Surg 106:895, 1993.
83. Freed LA, Levy D, Levine RA, et al: Prevalence and clinical outcome of mitral valve prolapse. N Engl J Med 341:1, 1999.
84. Chugh SS, Kelly KL, Titus JL: Sudden cardiac death with apparently normal heart. Circulation 102:649, 2000.
85. Weiss BM, Hess OM: Pulmonary vascular disease and pregnancy: Current controversies, management strategies, and perspectives. Eur Heart J 21:104, 2000.
86. Melgarejo-Moreno A, Galcera-Tomas J, Garcia-Alberola A, et al: Incidence, clinical characteristics, and prognostic significance of right bundle-branch block in acute myocardial infarction: A study in the thrombolytic era. Circulation 96:1139, 1997.
87. Udink ten Cate FE, Breur JM, Cohen MI, et al: Dilated cardiomyopathy in isolated congenital complete atrioventricular block: Early and long-term risk in children. J Am Coll Cardiol 37:1129, 2001.
88. Balmer C, Fasnacht M, Rahn M, et al: Long-term follow up of children with congenital complete atrioventricular block and the impact of pacemaker therapy. Europace 4:345, 2002.
89. Tan HL, Bink-Boelkens MT, Bezzina CR, et al: A sodium-channel mutation causes isolated cardiac conduction disease. Nature 409:1043, 2001.
90. Probst V, Allouis M, Sacher F, et al: Progressive cardiac conduction defect is the prevailing phenotype in carriers of a Brugada syndrome *SCN5A* mutation. J Cardiovasc Electrophysiol 17:270, 2006.
91. Gollob MH, Green MS, Tang AS, et al: Identification of a gene responsible for familial Wolff-Parkinson-White syndrome. N Engl J Med 344:1823, 2001.
92. Priori SG, Schwartz PJ, Napolitano C, et al: Risk stratification in the long-QT syndrome. N Engl J Med 348:1866, 2003.
93. Moss AJ, Zareba W, Hall WJ, et al: Effectiveness and limitations of beta-blocker therapy in congenital long-QT syndrome. Circulation 101:616, 2000.
94. Zareba W, Moss AJ, Schwartz PJ, et al: Influence of genotype on the clinical course of the long-QT syndrome. N Engl J Med 339:960, 1998.
95. Mohler PJ, Schott JJ, Gramolini AO, et al: Ankyrin-B mutation causes type 4 long-QT cardiac arrhythmia and sudden cardiac death. Nature 421:634, 2003.
96. Mohler PJ, Splawski I, Napolitano C, et al: A cardiac arrhythmia syndrome caused by loss of ankyrin-B function. Proc Natl Acad Sci U S A 101:9137, 2004.
97. Straus SMJM, Kors JA, De Bruin ML, et al: Prolonged QTc interval and risk of sudden cardiac death in a population of older adults. J Am Coll Cardiol 47:362, 2006.
98. Fu EY, Clemo HF, Ellenbogen KA: Acquired QT prolongation: Mechanisms and implications. Cardiol Rev 6:319, 1998.
99. Woosley RL, Chen Y, Freiman JP, Gillis RA: Mechanism of cardiotoxic actions of terfenadine. JAMA 269:1532, 1993.
100. Ray WA, Murray KT, Meredith S, et al: Oral erythromycin and the risk of sudden death from cardiac causes. N Engl J Med 2004; 351:1089-1096.
101. Sesti F, Abbott GW, Wei J, et al: A common polymorphism associated with antibiotic-induced cardiac arrhythmia. Proc Natl Acad Sci U S A 97:10613, 2000.
102. Napolitano C, Schwartz PJ, Brown AM, et al: Evidence for a cardiac ion channel mutation underlying drug-induced QT prolongation and life-threatening arrhythmias. J Cardiovasc Electrophysiol 11:691, 2000.
103. Makita N, Horie M, Nakamura T, et al: Drug-induced long-QT syndrome associated with a subclinical *SCN5A* mutation. Circulation 106:1269, 2002.
104. Brugada J, Brugada R, Brugada P: Right bundle-branch block and ST-segment elevation in leads V_1 through V_3: A marker for sudden death in patients without demonstrable structural heart disease. Circulation 97:457, 1998.
105. Alings M, Wilde A: "Brugada" syndrome: Clinical data and suggested pathophysiological mechanism. Circulation 99:666, 1999.
106. Priori SG, Napolitano C, Gasparini M, et al: Natural history of Brugada syndrome: Insights for risk stratification and management. Circulation 105:1342, 2002.
107. Brugada J, Brugada R, Antzelevitch C, et al: Long-term follow-up of individuals with the electrocardiographic pattern of right bundle-branch block and ST-segment elevation in precordial leads V1 to V3. Circulation 105:73, 2002.
108. Nademanee K, Veerakul G, Nimmannit S, et al: Arrhythmogenic marker for the sudden unexplained death syndrome in Thai men. Circulation 96:2595, 1997.
109. Vatta M, Dumaine R, Varghese G, Richard TA, et al.: Genetic and biophysical basis of sudden unexplained nocturnal death syndrome (SUNDS), a disease allelic to Brugada syndrome. Hum Mol Genet 11:337, 2002.
110. Priori SG, Napolitano C, Memmi M, et al: Clinical and molecular characterization of patients with catecholaminergic polymorphic ventricular tachycardia. Circulation 106:69, 2002.
111. Krantz DS, Sheps DS, Carney RM, Natelson BH: Effects of mental stress in patients with coronary artery disease: Evidence and clinical implications. JAMA 283:1800, 2000.
112. Lampert R, Joska T, Burg MM, et al: Emotional and physical precipitants of ventricular arrhythmia. Circulation 106:1800, 2002.
113. Leor J, Poole WK, Kloner RA: Sudden cardiac death triggered by an earthquake. N Engl J Med 334:413, 1996.
114. Leenardt A, Glaser E, Burguera M, et al: Short-coupled variant of torsades de pointes: A new electrocardiographic entity in the spectrum of idiopathic ventricular tachyarrhythmias. Circulation 89:206, 1994.
115. Akashi YJ, Nakazawa K, Sakakibara M, Miyake F, et al: The clinical features of takotsubo cardiomyopathy. Quart J Med 96:563, 2003.
116. Sharkey SW, Lesser JR, Zenovich AG, et al: Acute and reversible cardiomyopathy provoked by stress in women from the United States. Circulation 111:472, 2005.
117. Hauck FR, Hunt CE: Sudden infant death syndrome in 2000. Curr Probl Pediatr 30:237, 2000.
118. Schwartz PJ, Stramba-Badiale M, Segantini A, et al: Prolongation of the QT interval and the sudden infant death syndrome. N Engl J Med 338:1709, 1998.
119. Schwartz P, Priori S, Dumaine R, et al: A molecular link between the sudden infant death syndrome and the long-QT syndrome. N Engl J Med 343:262, 2000.
120. Topaz O, Edwards JE: Pathologic features of sudden death in children, adolescents, and young adults. Chest 87:476, 1985.
121. Corrado D, Basso C, Schiavon M, Thiene G: Screening for hypertrophic cardiomyopathy in young athletes. N Engl J Med 339:364, 1998.
122. Whang W, Manson JE, Hu FB, et al: Physical exertion, exercise, and sudden cardiac death in women. JAMA 295:1399, 2006.
123. Virmani R, Burke AP, Farb A, Kark JA: Causes of sudden death in young and middle-aged competitive athletes. Cardiol Clin 15:439, 1997.
124. Maron BJ, Thompson PD, Puffer JC, et al: Cardiovascular preparticipation screening of competitive athletes. A statement for health professionals from the Sudden Death Committee (clinical cardiology) and Congenital Cardiac Defects Committee (cardiovascular disease in the young), American Heart Association. Circulation 94:850, 1996.
125. Myerburg RJ, Mitrani R, Interian A Jr, Castellanos A: Identification of risk of cardiac arrest and sudden cardiac death in athletes. *In* Estes NAM, Salem DN, Wang PJ (eds): Sudden Cardiac Death in the Athlete. Armonk, NY, Futura, 1998, pp 25-55.
126. Basso C, Maron BJ, Corrado D, Thiene G: Clinical profile of congenital coronary artery anomalies with origin from the wrong aortic sinus leading to sudden death in young competitive athletes. J Am Coll Cardiol 35:1493, 2000.
127. Maron BJ, Link MS, Wang PJ, Estes NA 3rd: Clinical profile of commotio cordis: An underappreciated cause of sudden death in the young during sports and other activities. J Cardiovasc Electrophysiol 10:114, 1999.
128. Armstrong LE, Maresh CM: Effects of training, environment, and host factors on the sweating response to exercise. Int J Sports Med 19(Suppl 2):S103, 1998.
129. Joint Steering Committees of the Unexplained Cardiac Arrest Registry of Europe and of the Idiopathic Ventricular Fibrillation Registry of the United States: Survivors of out-of-hospital cardiac arrest with apparently normal heart: Need for definition and standardized clinical evaluation. Circulation 95:265, 1997.
130. Gami AS, Howard DE, Olson EJ, Somers VK. Day-night pattern of sudden death in obstructive sleep apnea. N Engl J Med 351:1206, 2005.

Pathology and Pathophysiology

131. Farb A, Burke AP, Tang AL, et al: Coronary plaque erosion without rupture into a lipid core: A frequent cause of coronary thrombosis in sudden coronary death. Circulation 93:1354, 1996.
132. Burke AP, Farb A, Malcom GT, et al: Coronary risk factors and plaque morphology in men with coronary disease who died suddenly. N Engl J Med 336:1276, 1997.
133. Antman EM, Tanasijevic MJ, Thompson B, et al: Cardiac-specific troponin I levels to predict the risk of mortality in patients with acute coronary syndromes. N Engl J Med 335:1342, 1996.
134. Cooper RS, Simmons BE, Castaner A, et al: Left ventricular hypertrophy is associated with worse survival independent of ventricular function and number of coronary arteries severely narrowed. Am J Cardiol 65:441, 1990.
135. Furukawa T, Bassett AL, Furukawa N, et al: The ionic mechanism of reperfusion-induced early afterdepolarizations in the feline left ventricular hypertrophy. J Clin Invest 91:1521, 1993.
136. Cohle SD, Suarez-Mier MP, Aguilera B: Sudden death resulting from lesions of the cardiac conduction system. Am J Forensic Med Pathol 23:83, 2002.
137. Liu YB, Wu CC, Lu LS, et al: Sympathetic nerve sprouting, electrical remodeling, and increased vulnerability to ventricular fibrillation in hypercholesterolemic rabbits. Circ Res 92:1145, 2003.
138. Dorian P, Cass D, Schwartz B, et al: Amiodarone as compared with lidocaine for shock-resistant ventricular fibrillation. N Engl J Med 347:368, 2002.
139. Mehta D, Curwin J, Gomes JA, Fuster V: Sudden death in coronary artery disease: Acute ischemia versus myocardial substrate. Circulation 96:3215, 1997.
140. Myerburg RJ, Kessler KM, Kimura S, Castellanos A: Sudden cardiac death: Future approaches based on identification and control of transient risk factors. J Cardiovasc Electrophysiol 3:626, 1992.
141. Myerburg RJ, Kessler KM, Bassett AL, Castellanos A: A biological approach to sudden cardiac death: Structure, function, and cause. Am J Cardiol 63:1512, 1989.
142. Myerburg RJ, Kessler KM, Zaman L, et al: Survivors of prehospital cardiac arrest. JAMA 247:1485, 1982.
143. Coronel R, Wilms-Schopman FJG, Opthof T, et al: Reperfusion arrhythmias in isolated perfused pig hearts: Inhomogeneities in extra-cellular potassium, ST and QT potentials, and transmembrane action potentials. Circ Res 71:1131, 1992.
144. Beardslee MA, Lerner DL, Tadros PN, et al: Dephosphorylation and intracellular redistribution of ventricular connexin43 during electrical uncoupling induced by ischemia. Circ Res 87:656, 2000.
145. Yao JA, Hussain W, Patel P, et al: Remodeling of gap junctional channel function in epicardial border zone of healing canine infarcts. Circ Res 92:437, 2003.
146. McLennan PL: Myocardial membrane fatty acids and the antiarrhythmic actions of dietary fish oil in animal models. Lipids 36(Suppl):S111, 2001.
147. Makikallio TH, Koistinen J, Jordaens L, et al: Heart rate dynamics before spontaneous onset of ventricular fibrillation in patients with healed myocardial infarcts. Am J Cardiol 83:880, 1999.

Clinical Characteristics of the Patient with Cardiac Arrest

148. Bayes de Luna A, Coumel P, Leclercq JF: Ambulatory sudden death: Mechanisms of production of fatal arrhythmia on the basis of data from 157 cases. Am Heart J 117:151, 1989.
149. Huikuri HV, Seppanen T, Koistinen MJ, et al: Abnormalities in beat-to-beat dynamics of heart rate before the spontaneous onset of life-threatening ventricular tachyarrhythmias in patients with prior myocardial infarction. Circulation 93:1836, 1996.
150. Huikuri HV, Makikallio TH, Raatikainen MJ, et al: Prediction of sudden cardiac death: Appraisal of the studies and methods assessing the risk of sudden arrhythmic death. Circulation 108:110, 2003.
151. Hinkle LE, Thaler HT: Clinical classification of cardiac deaths. Circulation 65:457, 1982.
152. American Heart Association: International Guidelines 2000 for CPR and ECC. Circulation 102(Suppl I):I1, 2000.
153. Herlitz J, Bang A, Alsen B, Aune S: Characteristics and outcome among patients suffering from in hospital cardiac arrest in relation to the interval between collapse and start of CPR. Resuscitation 53:21, 2002.
154. Kim C, Becker L, Eisenberg MS: Out-of-hospital cardiac arrest in octogenarians and nonagenarians. Arch Intern Med 160:3439, 2000.
155. Kette F, Sbrojavacca R, Rellini G, et al: Epidemiology and survival rate of out-of-hospital cardiac arrest in northeast Italy: The F.A.C.S. study. Friuli Venezia Giulia Cardiac Arrest Cooperative Study. Resuscitation 36:153, 1998.
156. The Hypothermia after Cardiac Arrest Study Group: Mild therapeutic hypothermia to improve the neurologic outcome after cardiac arrest. N Engl J Med 346:549, 2002.
157. Bernard SA, Gray TW, Buist MD, et al: Treatment of comatose survivors of out-of-hospital cardiac arrest with induced hypothermia. N Engl J Med 346:557, 2002.
158. Myerburg RJ: Sudden cardiac death in persons with normal (or near normal) hearts. Am J Cardiol 79(Suppl 6A):3, 1997.
159. Gorgels AP, Gijsbers C, de Vreede-Swagemakers J, et al: Out-of-hospital cardiac arrest—the relevance of heart failure. The Maastricht Circulatory Arrest Registry. Eur Heart J 24:1204, 2003.
160. Laurent I, Monchi M, Chiche JD, et al: Reversible myocardial dysfunction in survivors of out-of-hospital cardiac arrest. J Am Coll Cardiol 40:2110, 2002.
161. Bunch TJ, White RD, Gersh BJ, et al: Long-term outcomes of out-of-hospital cardiac arrest after successful early defibrillation. N Engl J Med 348:2626, 2003.
162. Iuliano S, Fisher SG, Karasik PE, et al: QRS duration and mortality in patients with congestive heart failure. Am Heart J 143:1085, 2002.
163. Pell JP, Corstorphine M, McConnachie A, et al: Post-discharge survival following pre-hospital cardiopulmonary arrest due to cardiac aetology: Temporal trends and impact of changes in clinical management. Eur Heart J 27:406, 2006.
164. The Antiarrhythmics versus Implantable Defibrillators (AVID) Investigators: A comparison of antiarrhythmic-drug therapy with implantable defibrillators in patients resuscitated from near-fatal ventricular arrhythmias. N Engl J Med 337:1576, 1997.
165. Connolly SJ, Gent M, Roberts RS, et al; Canadian Implantable Defibrillator Study (CIDS): A randomized trial of the implantable cardioverter defibrillator against amiodarone. Circulation 101:1297, 2000.
166. Kuck KH, Cappato R, Siebels J, Ruppel R: Randomized comparison of antiarrhythmic drug therapy with implantable defibrillators in patients resuscitated from cardiac arrest: The Cardiac Arrest Study Hamburg (CASH). Circulation 102:748, 2000.

Management of Cardiac Arrest

167. ECC Committee, Subcommittees and Task Forces of the American Heart Association: 2005 American Heart Association Guidelines for Cardiopulmonary Resuscitation and Emergency Cardiovascular Care. Circulation 112(Suppl):IV1, 2005.
168. Cobb LA, Weaver WD, Fahrenbrush CE: Community-based interventions for sudden cardiac death: Impact, limitations, and charges. Circulation 85(Suppl I): I98, 1992.
169. Becker LB, Han BH, Mayer PM, et al: Racial differences in the incidence of cardiac arrest and subsequent survival. N Engl J Med 329:600, 1993.
170. Lombardi G, Gallagher J, Gennis P: Outcome of out-of-hospital cardiac arrest in New York City: The Pre-Hospital Arrest Survival Evaluation (PHASE) Study. JAMA 271:678, 1994.
171. Cummins RO, Ornato JP, Thies WH, Pepe PE: Improving survival from sudden cardiac arrest: The "chain of survival" concept: A statement for heart professionals from the Advanced Cardiac Life Support Subcommittee and the Emergency Cardiac Care Committee, American Heart Association. Circulation 83:1832, 1991.
172. Morrison LJ, Visentin LM, Kiss A, et al; for the TOR Investigators: Validation of a rule for termination of resuscitation in out-of-hospital cardiac arrest. N Engl J Med 355:478, 2006.
173. Myerburg RJ, Fenster J, Velez M, et al: Impact of community-wide police car deployment of automated external defibrillators on out-of-hospital cardiac arrest. Circulation 106:1058, 2002.
174. Capucci A, Aschiere D, Piepoli MF, et al: Tripling survival from sudden cardiac arrest via early defibrillation without tranditional education in cardiopulmonary resuscitation. Circulation 106:1065, 2002.
175. Nadkarni VM, Larkin GL, Peberdy MA, et al; National Registry of Cardiopulmonary Resuscitation Investigators: First documented rhythm and clinical outcome from in-hospital cardiac arrest among children and adults. JAMA 295:50, 2006.
176. Weisfeldt ML, Becker LB: Resuscitation after cardiac arrest: A three-phase time-sensitive model. JAMA 288:3035, 2002.
177. Holmberg M, Holmberg S, Herlitz J: The problem of out-of-hospital cardiac arrest: Prevalence of sudden death in Europe today. Am J Cardiol 83:88D, 1999.
178. Waalewijn RA, de Vos R, Koster RW: Out-of-hospital cardiac arrests in Amsterdam and its surrounding areas: Results from the Amsterdam resuscitation study (ARREST) in "Utstein" style. Resuscitation 28:157, 1998.
179. White RD, Hankins DG, Bugliosi TF: Seven years' experience with early defibrillation by police and paramedics in an emergency medical services system. Resuscitation 39:145, 1998.
180. Becker L, Eisenberg M, Fahrenbruch C, Cobb L: Public locations of cardiac arrest: Implications for public access defibrillation. Circulation 97:2106, 1998.
181. Cobb LA, Fahrenbruch CE, Walsh TR, et al. Influence of cardiopulmonary resuscitation prior to defibrillation in patients with out-of-hospital ventricular fibrillation. JAMA 281:1182, 1999.
182. Dowie R, Campbell H, Donohoe R, Clarke P: "Event tree" analysis of out-of-hospital cardiac arrest data: Confirming the importance of bystander CPR. Resuscitation 56:173, 2003.
183. Wik L, Hansen TB, Fylling F, et al: Delaying defibrillation to give basic cardiopulmonary resuscitation to patients with out-of-hospital ventricular fibrillation: A randomized trial. JAMA 289:1389, 2003.
184. Caldwell G, Miller G, Quinn E, et al: Simple mechanical methods for cardioversion: Defense of the precordial thump and cough version. Br Med J (Clin Res Ed) 291:627, 1985.
185. Valenzuela TD, Kern KB, Clark LL, Berg RA, et al: Interruptions of chest compressions during emergency medical systems resuscitation. Circulation 112:1259, 2005.
186. Page RL, Joglar JA, Kowal RC, et al: Use of automated external defibrillators by a U.S. airline. N Engl J Med 343:1210, 2000.
187. Caffrey SL, Willoughby PJ, Pepe PE, Becker LB: Public use of automated external defibrillators. N Engl J Med 347:1242, 2002.
188. Valenzuela TD, Roe DJ, Nichol G, et al. Outcomes of rapid defibrillation by security officers after cardiac arrest in casinos. N Engl J Med 343:1206, 2000.
189. Hallstrom AP, Ornato JP, Weisfeldt M, et al: Public-access defibrillation and survival after out-of-hospital cardiac arrest. N Engl J Med 351:637, 2004.
190. Myerburg RJ, Feigal DW, Lindsay BD: Life-threatening malfunction of implantable cardiac devices. N Engl J Med 354:2309, 2006.
191. Shah JS, Maisel WH: Recalls and safety alerts affecting automated external defibrillators. JAMA, 296:655, 2006.
192. Gueugniaud PY, Mols P, Goldstein P, et al: A comparison of repeated high doses and repeated standard doses of epinephrine for cardiac arrest outside the hospital: European Epinephrine Study Group. N Engl J Med 339:1595, 1998.

193. Wenzel V, Lindner KH: Arginine vasopressin during cardiopulmonary resuscitation: Laboratory evidence, clinical experience and recommendations, and a view to the future. Crit Care Med 30(4 Suppl):S157, 2002.
194. Zipes DP, Camm AJ, Borggrefe M, et al; ••: ACC/AHA/ESC Guidelines for Management of Patients with Ventricular Arrhythmias and the Prevention of Sudden Cardiac Death. ••: ••, 2006.
195. Spaulding CM, Joly LM, Rosenberg A, et al: Immediate coronary angiography in survivors of out-of-hospital cardiac arrest. N Engl J Med 336:1629, 1997.
196. Bigger JT Jr,: Prophylactic use of implanted cardiac defibrillators in patients at high risk for ventricular arrhythmias after coronary-artery bypass graft surgery. Coronary Artery Bypass Graft (CABG) Patch Trial Investigators. N Engl J Med 337:1569, 1997.
197. Hallstrom AP, Cobb LA, Yu BH, et al: An antiarrhythmic drug experience in 941 patients resuscitated from an initial cardiac arrest between 1970 and 1985. Am J Cardiol 68:1025, 1991.

Prevention of Cardiac Arrest and Sudden Cardiac Death

198. Domanski MJ, Sakseena S, Epstein AE, et al: Relative effectiveness of the implantable cardioverter-defibrillator and antiarrhythmic drugs in patients with varying degrees of left ventricular dysfunction who have survived malignant ventricular arrhythmias. AVID Investigators. Antiarrhythmics Versus Implantable Defibrillators. J Am Coll Cardiol 34:1090, 1999.
199. Mason JW: A comparison of electrophysiologic testing with Holter monitoring to predict antiarrhythmic-drug efficacy for ventricular tachyarrhythmias. Electrophysiologic Study versus Electrocardiographic Monitoring Investigators. N Engl J Med 329:445, 1993.
200. Boutitie F, Boissel JP, Connolly SJ, et al: Amiodarone interaction with beta-blockers: Analysis of the merged EMIAT (European Myocardial Infarct Amiodarone Trial) and CAMIAT (Canadian Amiodarone Myocardial Infarction Trial) databases. The EMIAT and CAMIAT Investigators. Circulation 99:2268, 1999.
201. Moss AJ, Hall WJ, Cannom DS, et al: Improved survival with an implanted defibrillator in patients with coronary disease at high risk for ventricular arrhythmia. Multicenter Automatic Defibrillator Implantation Trial Investigators. N Engl J Med 335:1933, 1996.
202. Buxton AE, Lee KL, Fisher JD, et al: A randomized study of the prevention of sudden death in patients with coronary artery disease. Multicenter Unsustained Tachycardia Trial Investigators. N Engl J Med 341:1882, 1999.
203. Bardy GH, Lee KL, Mark DB, Poole JE, et al: Amiodarone or an implantable cardioverter-defibrillator for congestive heart failure. Sudden Cardiac Death in Heart Failure Trial (SCD-HeFT) Investigators. N Engl J Med 352:225, 2005.
204. Priori SG, Aliot E, Blomstrom-Lundqvist C, et al: Update of the guidelines on sudden cardiac death of the European Society of Cardiology. Eur Heart J 24:13, 2003.
205. Moss AJ, Zareba W, Hall WJ, et al: Prophylactic implantation of a defibrillator in patients with myocardial infarction and reduced ejection fraction. N Engl J Med 346:877, 2002.
206. Strickberger SA, Man KC, Daoud EG: A prospective evaluation of catheter ablation of ventricular tachycardia as adjuvant therapy in patients with coronary artery disease and an implantable cardioverter-defibrillator. Circulation 96:1525, 1997.
207. Mirowski M, Reid PR, Winkle RA, et al: Mortality in patients with implanted automatic defibrillators. Ann Intern Med 98:585, 1983.
208. Echt DS, Armstrong K, Schmidt P, et al: Clinical experience, complications, and survival in 70 patients with the automatic implantable cardioverter/defibrillator. Circulation 71:289, 1985.
209. Tchou PJ, Kadri N, Anderson J, et al: Automatic implantable cardioverter-defibrillators and survival of patients with left ventricular dysfunction and malignant ventricular arrhythmias. Ann Intern Med 109:529, 1988.
210. Myerburg RJ, Luceri RM, Thurer R, et al: Time to first shock and clinical outcome in patients receiving automatic implantable cardioverter-defibrillators. J Am Coll Cardiol 14:508, 1989.
211. Myerburg RJ, Castellanos A: Clinical trials of implantable defibrillators. N Engl J Med 337:1621, 1997.
212. Mirowski M, Reid PR, Mower MM, et al: Termination of malignant ventricular arrhythmias with an implanted automatic defibrillator in human beings. N Engl J Med 303:322, 1980.
213. Myerburg RJ, Mitrani R, Interian A Jr, Castellanos A: Interpretation of outcomes of antiarrhythmic clinical trials: Design features and population impact. Circulation 97:1514, 1998.
214. Julian DG, Camm AJ, Frangin G, et al: Randomised trial of effect of amiodarone on mortality in patients with left-ventricular dysfunction after recent myocardial infarction: EMIAT. European Myocardial Infarct Amiodarone Trial Investigators. Lancet 349:667, 1997.
215. Cairns JA, Connolly SJ, Roberts R, Gent M: Randomised trial of outcome after myocardial infarction in patients with frequent or repetitive ventricular premature depolarisations: CAMIAT. Canadian Amiodarone Myocardial Infarction Arrhythmia Trial Investigators. Lancet 349:675, 1997.
216. Kadish A, Dyer A, Daubert JP, Quigg R, et al: Prophylactic defibrillator implantation in patients with nonischemic dilated cardiomyopathy. Defibrillators in Non-Ischemic Cardiomyopathy Treatment Evaluation (DEFINITE) Investigators. N Engl J Med 350:2151, 2004.
217. MERIT-HF Study Group: Effect of metoprolol CR/XL in chronic heart failure: Metoprolol CR/XL Randomised Intervention Trial in Congestive Heart Failure (MERIT-HF). Lancet 353:2001, 1999.
218. Maron BJ, Shen WK, Link MS, et al: Efficacy of implantable cardioverter-defibrillators for the prevention of sudden death in patients with hypertrophic cardiomyopathy. N Engl J Med 342:365, 2000.
219. Brugada J, Brugada R, Antzelevitch C, et al: Long-term follow-up of individuals with the electrocardiographic pattern of right bundle-branch block and ST-segment elevation in precordial leads V_1 to V_3. Circulation 105:73, 2002.
220. Yusuf S, Sleight P, Pogue J, et al: Effects of an angiotensin-converting enzyme inhibitor, ramipril, on cardiovascular events in high-risk patients. The Heart Outcomes Prevention Evaluation Study Investigators. N Engl J Med 342:748, 2000.
221. Van Camp SP, Bloor CM, Mueller FO, et al: Nontraumatic sports death in high school and college athletes. Med Sci Sports Exerc 27:641, 1995.
222. Fuller CM: Cost effectiveness analysis of screening of high school athletes for risk of sudden cardiac death. Med Sci Sports Exerc 32:887, 2000.
223. Corrado D, Pelliccia A, Bjornstad HH, Vanhees L, et al: Cardiovascular preparticipation screening of young competitive athletes for prevention of sudden death: Proposal for a common European protocol. Eur Heart J 26:516, 2005.
224. Maron BJ, Chaitmen BR, Ackerman MJ, et al: Recommendations for physical activities and recreational sports participation for young patients with genetic cardiovascular diseases. Circulation 109:2807, 2004.
225. Paterick TE, Paterick TJ, Fletcher GF, Maron BJ: Medical and legal issues in the cardiovascular evaluation of competitive athletes. JAMA 294:3011, 2005.

Sudden Death and Public Safety

226. Epstein AE, Miles WM, Benditt DG, et al: Personal and public safety issues related to arrhythmias that may affect consciousness: Implications for regulation and physician recommendations. A medical/scientific statement from the American Heart Association and the North American Society of Pacing and Electrophysiology. Circulation 94:1147, 1996.

CHAPTER 37

Hypotension and Syncope

Hugh Calkins and Douglas P. Zipes

DEFINITION

Syncope is a sudden transient loss of consciousness and postural tone with spontaneous recovery. Loss of consciousness results from a reduction of blood flow to the reticular activating system located in the brain stem and does not require electrical or chemical therapy for reversal. The metabolism of the brain, in contrast to that of many other organs, is exquisitely dependent on perfusion. Consequently, cessation of cerebral blood flow leads to loss of consciousness within approximately 10 seconds. Restoration of appropriate behavior and orientation after a syncopal episode is usually immediate. Retrograde amnesia is uncommon. Syncope is an important clinical problem because it is common, costly, often disabling, may cause injury, and may be the only warning sign before sudden cardiac death (see Chap. 36).[1] Patients with syncope account for 1 percent of hospital admissions and 3 percent of emergency department visits. Elderly persons have a 6 percent annual incidence of syncope (see Chap. 75). Surveys of young adults have revealed that up to 50 percent report a prior episode of loss of consciousness; most of these episodes are isolated events that never come to medical attention. The Framingham Study, in which biennial examinations were performed on 7814 individuals, reported the incidence of a first report of syncope to be 6.2/1000 person-years follow-up.[2] Patients who experience syncope also report a markedly reduced quality of life. The prognosis of patients with syncope varies greatly with the diagnosis. In the Framingham Study, for example, participants with syncope, including those with syncope of unknown origin, had increased mortality compared with participants without syncope. The highest mortality was observed among those with a cardiac cause of syncope. In contrast, the subgroup of participants with neurally mediated syncope (including orthostatic hypotension and medication-related syncope) did not experience increased mortality.[2]

Classification

The causes of apparent syncopal episodes can be separated initially into two groups—true syncope, in which the transient loss of consciousness results from cerebral hypoperfusion, and nonsyncopal conditions, with real or apparent loss of consciousness from other causes.[1] Table 37-1 shows the differential diagnosis of syncope and nonsyncopal conditions, which are indicated by an asterisk. Vascular causes of syncope are most common, followed by cardiac causes. Among cardiac causes of syncope, arrhythmias are most common. The importance of considering nonsyncopal conditions when evaluating a patient with apparent loss of consciousness cannot be underestimated. These nonsyncopal conditions include conditions in which consciousness is lost as a result of metabolic disorders, epilepsy, or alcohol, as well as conditions in which consciousness is only apparently lost (i.e., conversion reaction). These psychogenic causes of syncope are now being recognized with increased frequency.

Although knowledge of the common conditions that can cause syncope is essential and allows the clinician to arrive at a probable cause of syncope in most patients, it is equally important to be aware of several of the less common but potentially lethal causes of syncope, such as the long-QT syndrome, arrhythmogenic right ventricular cardiomyopathy, Brugada syndrome, idiopathic ventricular fibrillation, catecholaminergic polymorphic ventricular tachycardia, short-QT syndrome (see Chap. 9), hypertrophic cardiomyopathy (see Chap. 65), and pulmonary emboli (see Chap. 72).[3-10] It is also important to recognize that distribution of the causes of syncope varies with age.

In young individuals, neurally mediated syncope is the most common, but is an unusual type of syncope in elderly persons.[11] Common causes of syncope in elderly persons include orthostatic hypotension, postprandial hypotension, medication, aortic stenosis (see Chap. 62), carotid sinus hypersensitivity, and bradyarrhythmias (e.g., sick sinus syndrome, heart block; see Chap. 35).

Vascular Causes of Syncope

Vascular causes of syncope, particularly reflex-mediated syncope and orthostatic hypotension, are the most common causes, accounting for at least one third of all syncopal episodes.[1,2,11] In contrast, vascular steal syndromes are exceedingly uncommon causes of syncope.

Orthostatic Hypotension

When a person stands, 500 to 800 ml of blood is displaced to the abdomen and lower extremities, resulting in an abrupt drop in venous return to the heart. This drop leads to a decrease in cardiac output and stimulation of aortic, carotid, and cardiopulmonary baroreceptors, which trigger a reflex increase in sympathetic outflow. As a result, heart rate, cardiac contractility, and vascular resistance increase to maintain a stable systemic blood pressure on standing. Orthostatic hypotension, which is defined as a 20-mm Hg drop in systolic blood pressure or a 10-mm Hg drop in diastolic blood pressure within 3 minutes of standing, results from a defect in any portion of this blood pressure control system. Orthostatic hypotension can be asymptomatic or associated with symptoms such as lightheadedness, dizziness, blurred vision, weakness, palpi-

TABLE 37–1 Causes of Syncope

Vascular
Anatomical
Vascular steal syndromes
Orthostatic
Autonomic insufficiency
Idiopathic
Volume depletion
Drug- and alcohol-induced
Reflex-mediated
Carotid sinus hypersensitivity
Neurally mediated syncope
Glossopharyngeal syncope
Situational (cough, sneeze, swallow, micturition, postprandial)
Cardiac
Anatomical
Obstructive cardiac valvular disease
Aortic dissection
Atrial myxoma
Pericardial disease, tamponade
Hypertrophic obstructive cardiomyopathy
Myocardial ischemia, infarction
Pulmonary embolus
Pulmonary hypertension
Arrhythmias
Bradyarrhythmias
Sinus node dysfunction, bradycardia
Atrioventricular block
Tachyarrhythmias
Supraventricular arrhythmias
Ventricular arrhythmias (including long-QT and Brugada syndromes)
Implanted pacemaker or implantable cardioverter-defibrillator malfunction
Neurological and cerebrovascular*
Arnold-Chiari malformation
Migraine
Seizure (partial complex, temporal lobe)
Vertebrobasilar insufficiency/transient ischemic attack
Metabolic*
Drugs, alcohol
Hyperventilation (hypocapnia)
Hypoglycemia
Hypoxemia
Psychogenic syncope*
Anxiety, panic disorder
Somatization disorders
Syncope of unknown origin

*Disorders resembling syncope.

TABLE 37–2 Causes of Orthostatic Hypotension

Drugs
Diuretics
Alpha-adrenergic blocking drugs—terazosin (Hytrin), labetalol
Adrenergic neuron blocking drugs—guanethidine
Angiotensin-converting enzyme inhibitors
Antidepressants
Monoamine oxidase inhibitors
Alcohol
Diuretics
Ganglion-blocking drugs—hexamethonium, mecamylamine
Tranquilizers—phenothiazines, barbiturates
Vasodilators—prazosin, hydralazine, calcium channel blockers
Centrally acting hypotensive drugs—methyldopa, clonidine
Primary Disorders of Autonomic Failures
Pure autonomic failure (Bradbury-Eggleston syndrome)
Multisystem atrophy (Shy-Drager syndrome)
Parkinson disease with autonomic failure
Secondary Neurogenic Causes
Aging
Autoimmune disease
Guillain-Barré syndrome, mixed connective tissue disease, rheumatoid arthritis
Eaton-Lambert syndrome, systemic lupus erythematosus
Carcinomatosis autonomic neuropathy
Central brain lesions
Multiple sclerosis, Wernicke encephalopathy
Vascular lesions or tumors involving the hypothalamus and midbrain
Dopamine β-hydroxylase deficiency
Familial hyperbradykininism
General medical disorders—diabetes, amyloidosis, alcoholism, renal failure
Hereditary sensory neuropathies, dominant or recessive
Infections of the nervous system—human immunodeficiency virus infection, Chagas' disease, botulism, syphilis
Metabolic disease—vitamin B_{12} deficiency, porphyria, Fabry disease, Tangier disease
Spinal cord lesions

Adapted from Bannister SR (ed): Autonomic Failure, 2nd ed. Oxford, Oxford University Press, 1988, p 8.

tations, tremulousness, and syncope. These symptoms are often worse immediately on arising in the morning or after meals or exercise. Syncope that occurs after meals, particularly in elderly people, can result from a redistribution of blood to the gut. A decline in systolic blood pressure of about 20 mm Hg approximately 1 hour after eating has been reported in up to one third of elderly nursing home residents. Although usually asymptomatic, it can result in lightheadedness or syncope.

Drugs that cause volume depletion or result in vasodilation are the most common cause of orthostatic hypotension (Table 37-2). Elderly patients are particularly susceptible to the hypotensive effects of drugs because of reduced baroreceptor sensitivity, decreased cerebral blood flow, renal sodium wasting, and an impaired thirst mechanism that develops with aging. Orthostatic hypotension can also result from neurogenic causes, which can be subclassified into primary and secondary autonomic failure.[12] Primary causes are generally idiopathic, whereas secondary causes are associated with a known biochemical or structural anomaly or are seen as part of a particular disease or syndrome. There are three types of primary autonomic failure (see Chap. 89). Pure autonomic failure (Bradbury-Eggleston syndrome) is an idiopathic sporadic disorder characterized by orthostatic hypotension, usually in conjunction with evidence of more widespread autonomic failure, such as disturbances in bowel, bladder, thermoregulatory, and sexual function. Patients with pure autonomic failure have reduced supine plasma norepinephrine levels. Multiple system atrophy (Shy-Drager syndrome) is a sporadic, progressive, adult-onset disorder characterized by autonomic dysfunction, parkinsonism, and ataxia in any combination. The third type of primary autonomic failure is Parkinson disease with autonomic failure. A small subset of patients with Parkinson disease may also experience autonomic failure, including orthostatic hypotension. In addition to these forms of chronic autonomic failure is a rare acute panautonomic neuropathy. This neuropathy generally occurs in young people and results in widespread severe sympathetic and parasympathetic failure, with orthostatic hypotension, loss of sweating, disruption of bladder and bowel function, fixed heart rate, and fixed dilated pupils.

Postural orthostatic tachycardia syndrome (POTS) is a milder form of chronic autonomic failure and orthostatic intolerance characterized by the presence of symptoms of orthostatic intolerance, an increase of 28 beats/min or more in heart rate, and absence of a significant change in blood pressure within 5 minutes of standing or upright tilt.[10] POTS appears to result from a failure of the peripheral vasculature to vasoconstrict appropriately under orthostatic stress. POTS can also be associated with syncope related to neurally mediated hypotension (see later).

Reflex-mediated Syncope

There are many reflex-mediated syncopal syndromes (Table 37-3). In each case, the reflex is composed of a trigger (the afferent limb) and a response (the efferent limb). This group of reflex-mediated syncopal syndromes has in common the response limb of the reflex, which consists of increased vagal tone and a withdrawal of peripheral sympathetic tone and leads to bradycardia, vasodilation and, ultimately, hypotension, presyncope, or syncope. What distinguishes these causes of syncope are the specific triggers. For example, micturition syncope results from activation of mechanoreceptors in the bladder, defecation syncope results from neural inputs from gut wall tension receptors, and swallowing syncope results from afferent neural impulses arising from the upper gastrointestinal tract. The two most common types of reflex-mediated syncope, carotid sinus hypersensitivity and neurally mediated hypotension, are discussed later.

NEURALLY MEDIATED HYPOTENSION OR SYNCOPE. The term *neurally mediated hypotension* or *syncope* (also known as neurocardiogenic, vasodepressor, and vasovagal syncope and as "fainting") has been used to describe a common abnormality of blood pressure regulation characterized by the abrupt onset of hypotension with or without bradycardia. Triggers associated with the development of neurally mediated syncope are those that reduce ventricular filling or increase catecholamine secretion.[1,14] They include the sight of blood, pain, prolonged standing, a warm environment or hot shower, and stressful situations. In these types of situations, patients with this condition experience severe lightheadedness, syncope, or both. It has been postulated that these clinical phenomena result from a paradoxical reflex that is initiated when ventricular preload is reduced by venous pooling. This reduction leads to a reduction in cardiac output and blood pressure, which is sensed by arterial baroreceptors. The resultant increased catecholamine levels, combined with reduced venous filling, lead to a vigorously contracting volume-depleted ventricle. The heart itself is involved in this reflex by virtue of the presence of mechanoreceptors, or C-fibers, consisting of nonmyelinated fibers found in the atria, ventricles, and pulmonary artery. It has been proposed that vigorous contraction of a volume-depleted ventricle leads to activation of these receptors in susceptible individuals. These afferent C-fibers project centrally to the dorsal vagal nucleus of the medulla, leading to a "paradoxical" withdrawal of peripheral sympathetic tone and an increase in vagal tone, which, in turn, causes vasodilation and bradycardia. The ultimate clinical consequence is syncope or presyncope.

Not all neurally mediated syncope results from the activation of mechanoreceptors. In humans, it is well known that the sight of blood or extreme emotion can trigger syncope. These observations suggest that higher neural centers can also participate in the pathophysiology of vasovagal syncope. In addition, central mechanisms can contribute to the production of neurally mediated syncope.

CAROTID SINUS HYPERSENSITIVITY. Syncope caused by carotid sinus hypersensitivity results from stimulation of carotid sinus baroreceptors, located in the internal carotid artery above the bifurcation of the common carotid artery. Carotid sinus hypersensitivity is diagnosed by applying gentle pressure over the carotid pulsation just below the angle of the jaw, where the carotid bifurcation is located. Pressure should be applied for 5 to 10 seconds. It is important to perform carotid sinus massage in both the supine and upright positions. The main complications associated

TABLE 37–3 Differentiating Syncope Caused by Neurally Mediated Hypotension, Arrhythmias, and Seizures

Parameter	Neurally Mediated Hypotension	Arrhythmia	Seizure
Demographics, clinical setting	Female>male gender Younger age (<55 yr) More episodes (more than two) Standing, warm room, emotional upset Family history of sudden death	Male>female gender Older age (>54 yr) Fewer episodes (less than three) During exertion, or supine	Younger age (<45 yr) Any setting
Premonitory symptoms	Longer duration (>5 sec) Palpitations Blurred vision Nausea Warmth Diaphoresis Lightheadedness	Shorter duration (<6 sec) Palpitations less common	Sudden onset or brief aura (déjà vu, olfactory, gustatory, visual)
Observations during the event	Pallor Diaphoretic Dilated pupils Slow pulse, low blood pressure Incontinence—may occur Brief clonic movements—may occur	Blue, not pale Incontinence can occur. Brief clonic movements can occur.	Blue face, no pallor Frothing at the mouth Prolonged syncope (duration> 5 min) Tongue biting Horizontal eye deviation Elevated pulse and blood pressure Incontinence more likely* Tonic-clonic movements if grand mal
Residual symptoms	Residual symptoms common Prolonged fatigue common (>90%) Oriented	Residual symptoms uncommon (unless prolonged unconsciousness) Oriented	Residual symptoms common Aching muscles Disoriented Fatigue Headache Slow recovery

*May be observed with any of these causes of syncope but more common with seizures.

with performing carotid sinus massage are neurological. Because of this, carotid sinus massage should be avoided in patients with prior transient ischemic attacks, strokes within the past 3 months, and carotid bruits.

A normal response to carotid sinus massage is a transient decrease in the sinus rate, slowing of atrioventricular (AV) conduction, or both. Carotid sinus hypersensitivity is defined as a sinus pause longer than 3 seconds in duration and a fall in systolic blood pressure of 50 mm Hg or more. The response to carotid sinus massage can be classified as cardioinhibitory (asystole), vasodepressive (fall in systolic blood pressure), or mixed. Carotid sinus hypersensitivity is detected in approximately one third of elderly patients who present with syncope or after falls.[1,15] It is important to recognize, however, that carotid sinus hypersensitivity is also commonly observed in asymptomatic elderly patients.[16] Thus, the diagnosis of carotid sinus hypersensitivity should be approached cautiously after excluding alternative causes of syncope. Once diagnosed, dual-chamber pacemaker implantation is recommended for patients with recurrent syncope or falls resulting from carotid sinus hypersensitivity.[17,18]

Cardiac Causes of Syncope

Cardiac causes of syncope, particularly tachyarrhythmias and bradyarrhythmias, are the second most common causes, accounting for 10 to 20 percent of syncopal episodes (see Chap. 35). Ventricular tachycardia (VT) is the most common tachyarrhythmia that can cause syncope. Supraventricular tachycardia can also cause syncope, although the great majority of patients with supraventricular arrhythmias present with less severe symptoms, such as palpitations, dyspnea, and lightheadedness. Bradyarrhythmias that can result in syncope include sick sinus syndrome as well as AV block. Anatomical causes of syncope include obstruction to blood flow, such as a massive pulmonary embolus, an atrial myxoma, or aortic stenosis.

Neurological Causes of Apparent Syncope

Neurological causes of apparent syncope, including migraines, seizures, Arnold-Chiari malformations, and transient ischemic attacks, are surprisingly uncommon, accounting for less than 10 percent of all cases of syncope. Most patients with an apparent neurological cause of syncope have seizures rather than true syncope.

Metabolic Causes of Apparent Syncope

Metabolic causes of syncope are rare, accounting for less than 5 percent of syncopal episodes. The most common metabolic causes of syncope are hypoglycemia, hypoxia, and hyperventilation. Establishing hypoglycemia as the cause of an apparent loss of consciousness requires demonstration of hypoglycemia during the syncopal episode. Although hyperventilation-induced syncope has been generally considered to be caused by a reduction in cerebral blood flow, this remains an area of debate. Hyperventilation-induced syncope may also have a psychological component. Psychiatric disorders may also cause syncope. Up to 25 percent of patients with syncope of unknown origin may have psychiatric disorders for which apparent syncope is one of the presenting symptoms.[1]

Relationship Between Prognosis and Cause of Syncope

The prognosis for patients with syncope varies greatly with the diagnosis. Syncope of unknown origin or syncope with a noncardiac cause (including reflex-mediated syncope) is generally associated with a benign prognosis. In contrast, syncope with a cardiac cause is associated with up to 30 percent mortality at 1 year.[1,2]

EVALUATION

Identification of the precise cause of syncope is often challenging. Because syncope usually occurs sporadically and infrequently, it is extremely difficult to examine a patient or obtain an electrocardiogram (ECG) during an episode of syncope. For this reason, the primary goal in the evaluation of a patient with syncope is to arrive at a presumptive determination of the cause of syncope.

History and Physical Examination

The history and physical examination are the most important components of the evaluation of a patient with syncope (see Chap. 11). It is well established that the probable cause of syncope can be identified on the basis of the history and physical examination alone in more than 25 percent of patients.[1,11] Maximal information can be obtained from the clinical history when it is approached in a systematic and detailed fashion. Initial evaluation should begin by determining whether the patient did, in fact, experience a syncopal episode. Every effort should be made to differentiate true syncope from apparent syncope with alterations in consciousness resulting from conditions such as metabolic and psychiatric disorders. Although falls can be differentiated from syncope by the absence of loss of consciousness, an overlap between symptoms of falls and syncope has been reported.[1,18] This overlap may reflect the fact that elderly individuals may experience amnesia for the episode of loss of consciousness. When evaluating a patient with syncope, particular attention should then be focused on the following: (1) determining whether the patient has a history of cardiac disease or a family history of cardiac disease, syncope, or sudden death; (2) identifying medications that may have played a role in syncope; (3) quantifying the number and chronicity of prior syncopal and presyncopal episodes; (4) identifying precipitating factors, including body position; and (5) quantifying the type and duration of prodromal and recovery symptoms. It is also useful to obtain careful accounts from witnesses who may have been present. The features of the clinical history most helpful in determining whether syncope resulted from neurally mediated hypotension, an arrhythmia, or a seizure are summarized in Table 37-3.

History

The clinical histories obtained from patients with syncope related to an arrhythmia such as atrioventricular (AV) block or ventricular tachycardia (VT) are similar. In each case, syncope typically occurs with less than 5 seconds of warning and few if any prodromal or recovery symptoms. Demographic features suggesting that syncope results from an arrhythmia such as VT or AV block include male gender, less than three prior episodes of syncope, and increased age. Features of the clinical history that indicate a diagnosis of neurally mediated syncope include palpitations, blurred vision, nausea, warmth, diaphoresis, or lightheadedness before syncope and the presence of nausea, warmth, diaphoresis, or fatigue after syncope.

The clinical history is also valuable in distinguishing seizures from syncope. Features of the clinical history useful in distinguishing seizures from syncope include disorientation following an event, a blue face or not becoming pale during the event, frothing at the mouth, aching muscles, feeling sleepy after the event, and unconsciousness lasting longer than 5 minutes. Tongue biting strongly indicates a seizure rather than syncope as the cause of loss of consciousness. Other findings suggestive of a seizure as a cause of the syncopal episode include (1) an aura before the episode, (2) horizontal eye deviation during the episode, (3) an elevated blood pressure and pulse during the episode, and (4) a headache following the event. Urinary or fecal incontinence can be observed in association with a seizure or a syncopal episode but occurs more commonly in association with a seizure. Grand mal seizures are usually associated with tonic-clonic movements. It is important to note that syncope caused by cerebral ischemia can result in decorticate rigidity, with clonic movements of the arms. Akinetic or petit mal seizures can be recognized by the patient's lack of responsiveness in the absence of a loss of postural tone. Temporal lobe seizures can also be confused with syncope. These seizures last several minutes and are characterized by confusion, changes in the level of consciousness, and autonomic signs, such as flushing. Vertebral basilar insufficiency should be considered as the cause of syncope if syncope occurs in association with other symptoms of brain stem ischemia (e.g., diplopia, tinnitus, focal weakness or sensory loss, vertigo, dysarthria). Migraine-mediated syncope is often associated with a throbbing unilateral headache, scintillating scotomata, and nausea.

In one study, a standardized questionnaire was administered to 102 patients with seizure and 569 patients with syncope.[19] The clinical symptoms reported by patients with syncope were compared with those reported by patients with seizures. Patients with seizures are more likely to have had a cut tongue, bed-wetting, prodromal déjà vu, preoccupation, mood changes, hallucinations or trembling before loss of consciousness, postictal confusion, muscle pain, headaches, observed convulsive movements, head turning, unresponsiveness during loss of consciousness, and blue skin observed by a bystander. Patients with syncope are more likely to experience presyncope, have syncope associated with prolonged sitting or standing, or have presyncope with prolonged sitting or standing, warm environments, and exercise. Patients with syncope are also more likely to experience diaphoresis, dyspnea, chest pain, palpitations, warmth, nausea, and vertigo. The authors of the questionnaire then developed a simple point score of diagnostic criteria that distinguishes seizures from syncope with 85 percent accuracy.[19]

Physical Examination

After obtaining a careful history, evaluation should continue with a physical examination (see Chap. 11). In addition to a complete cardiac examination, particular attention should be focused on determining whether structural heart disease is present, defining the patient's level of hydration, and detecting the presence of significant neurological abnormalities suggestive of a dysautonomia or a cerebrovascular accident. Orthostatic vital signs are a critical component of the evaluation. The patient's blood pressure and heart rate should be obtained while he or she is supine and then obtained each minute for approximately 3 minutes. The two abnormalities that should be sought are (1) early orthostatic hypotension, defined as a 20-mm Hg drop in systolic blood pressure or a 10-mm Hg drop in diastolic blood pressure within 3 minutes of standing, and (2) POTS, defined as an increase of 28 beats/min or more within 5 minutes of standing, with symptoms of orthostatic intolerance. The significance of POTS lies in its close overlap with neurally mediated syncope.[1,13]

Diagnostic Tests

Blood Tests

Blood tests, such as determination of serum electrolyte, cardiac enzyme, glucose, and hematocrit levels, are of low diagnostic value.[1,11] As a result, the routine use of laboratory tests is not recommended for patients with syncope. Under rare circumstances, aspects of the patient's clinical presentation may suggest the diagnostic value of this type of testing.

Tilt-Table Testing

The tilt-table test is a standard and widely accepted diagnostic test for evaluating patients with syncope[1,20] (see Chap. 32). To the extent that upright tilt-table testing provides diagnostic evidence indicating susceptibility to neurally mediated syncope, it is considered the gold standard for establishing this diagnosis. Upright tilt-table testing is generally performed for 30 to 45 minutes at an angle between 60 and 80 degrees (usually 70 degrees). The sensitivity of the test can be increased, with an associated fall in specificity, by the use of longer tilt durations, steeper tilt angles, and provocative agents, such as isoproterenol or nitroglycerin. When isoproterenol is used as a provocative agent, it is recommended that the infusion rate be increased incrementally from 1 to 3 μg/min to increase the heart rate to 25 percent greater than baseline. When nitroglycerin is used, a fixed dose of 400 μg nitroglycerin spray should be administered sublingually, with the patient in the upright position. These two provocative approaches are equivalent in diagnostic accuracy. In the absence of pharmacological provocation, the specificity of the test has been estimated to be 90 percent. It is important to recognize, however, that the specificity of tilt-table testing decreases significantly when provocative agents are used.

There is general agreement that upright tilt-table testing is indicated in patients with recurrent syncope, in high-risk patients with a single syncopal episode for whom there is no evidence of structural heart disease or other causes of syncope have been excluded, and in the evaluation of patients for whom the cause of syncope has been determined (i.e., asystole) but the presence of neurally mediated syncope on upright tilt would influence treatment.[1] There is also general agreement that upright tilt-table testing is not necessary for patients who have experienced only a single syncopal episode that was highly typical for neurally mediated syncope and during which no injury occurred.

Echocardiography

Echocardiograms are commonly used in the evaluation of patients with syncope (see Chap. 14). However, it is not recommended that all patients with syncope undergo echocardiography.[1,11] Current guidelines suggest that an echocardiogram be performed when the patient has clinical features suggestive of a cardiac cause of syncope, such as syncope with exertion or while supine, a family history of sudden death, and/or syncope of abrupt onset. Findings on echocardiography of diagnostic and/or prognostic value include the presence of valvular heart disease (see Chap. 62), atrial myxoma (see Chap. 69), impaired ventricular function (see Chap. 23), evidence of RV overload or pulmonary hypertension (pulmonary emboli; see Chaps. 72 and 73), or the presence of hypertrophic cardiomyopathy (see Chap. 65). An echocardiogram is a valuable screening test for underlying heart disease, including valvular disease (see Chap. 62) and hypertrophic cardiomyopathy.

Stress Tests and Cardiac Catheterizations

Myocardial ischemia is an unlikely cause of syncope and, when present, is usually accompanied by angina (see Chaps.

48 and 49). The use of stress tests in the evaluation of patients with syncope is best reserved for those in whom syncope or presyncope occurred during or immediately after exertion, in association with chest pain, or in a patient at high risk for coronary artery disease.[1,11] It should be noted that even among patients with syncope during exertion, exercise stress testing is highly unlikely to trigger another event (see Chap. 13). Patients suspected of having severe aortic stenosis or obstructive hypertrophic cardiomyopathy should not undergo exercise stress testing because it may precipitate a cardiac arrest. Coronary angiography is recommended in patients with syncope suspected to be caused, directly or indirectly, by myocardial ischemia (see Chap. 19).

Electrocardiography

The 12-lead ECG is another important component in the work-up of a patient with syncope (see Chap. 12). The initial ECG results in establishment of a diagnosis in approximately 5 percent of patients and suggests a diagnosis in another 5 percent of patients. Specific findings that can identify the probable cause of syncope include QT prolongation (long-QT syndrome), the presence of a short PR interval

and a delta wave (Wolff-Parkinson-White syndrome), the presence of a right bundle branch block pattern with ST segment elevation (Brugada syndrome), high-grade AV block, or T wave inversion in the right precordial leads (arrhythmogenic right ventricular cardiomyopathy; see Chap. 35) and evidence of an acute myocardial infarction (see Chap. 50). Any abnormality of the baseline ECG is an independent predictor of cardiac syncope or increased mortality and suggests the need to pursue an evaluation of cardiac causes of syncope.[1] Most patients with syncope have a normal ECG. This finding is useful, because it suggests a low likelihood of a cardiac cause of syncope and is associated with an excellent prognosis, particularly when observed in a young patient with syncope. Despite the low diagnostic yield of electrocardiography, the test is inexpensive and risk free. For these reasons, an ECG is considered a standard part of the evaluation of almost all patients with syncope.[1,11]

SIGNAL-AVERAGED ELECTROCARDIOGRAPHY. Signal-averaged electrocardiography (SAECG) is a noninvasive technique used for the detection of low-amplitude signals in the terminal portion of the QRS complex (late potentials), which are a substrate for ventricular arrhythmias (see Chap. 32). In contrast to a standard ECG, the role of SAECG in the evaluation of patients with syncope is not well established. At present, SAECG testing is not recommended as a standard part of the evaluation of patients with syncope.[1,11] In fact, one of the few situations in which the SAECG is of diagnostic value is when a diagnosis of arrhythmogenic right ventricular dysplasia is being considered.[4]

HOLTER RECORDING. Continuous electrocardiographic monitoring using telemetry or Holter monitoring, or both, is commonly performed in patients with syncope but is unlikely to identify the cause of syncope (see Chap. 32). The information provided by electrocardiographic monitoring at the time of syncope is extremely valuable because it allows an arrhythmic cause of syncope to be established or excluded. However, because of the infrequent and sporadic nature of syncope, the diagnostic yield of Holter monitoring in the evaluation of patients with syncope and presyncope is extremely low. Another clinically useful finding is the detection of symptoms in the absence of an arrhythmia. This finding is observed in up to 15 percent of patients undergoing continuous electrocardiographic monitoring. It is important to emphasize that the absence of an arrhythmia and symptoms during continuous electrocardiographic monitoring may not exclude an arrhythmia as the cause of syncope. In patients suspected of having an arrhythmia as the cause of syncope, additional evaluation such as electrophysiological (EP) testing or event monitoring should be considered (see Chap. 32). Current guidelines recommend that Holter monitoring be used in patients who have clinical or electrocardiographic features suggestive of an arrhythmic syncope or a history of recurrent syncope with injury or suggestive of an arrhythmic syncope to guide subsequent examinations, such as EP testing.[1] Holter monitoring is most likely to be diagnostic when used in the occasional patient with frequent (e.g., daily) episodes of syncope or presyncope.

EVENT RECORDERS. Transtelephonic event monitors are small, portable electrocardiographic recording devices that are carried or worn continuously by the patient and can be activated by the patient to record a rhythm strip. The tracings can be stored and transmitted over telephone lines at a later time. Some event monitors, referred to as continuous loop event monitors, are worn continuously and allow capture of retrospective and prospective electrocardiographic recordings, whereas other types of event monitors record only when activated by the patient. Continuous loop event monitors are preferred when used in the evaluation of a patient with syncope. These devices are often programmed with 4 minutes of retrospective memory and 1 minute of prospective memory on activation. Event monitors are indicated in the evaluation of patients with infrequent but recurrent episodes of presyncope or syncope, particularly when potentially malignant causes of syncope have been excluded.[1,11] When they are used in selected populations of patients, a diagnostic yield as high has 25 percent may be observed. However, a much lower diagnostic yield can be expected in less selected populations.

Implantable Event Recorders. In some patients, episodes of syncope are extremely infrequent, occurring once or twice a year. In this population of patients, a traditional event monitor is unlikely to be diagnostic because of the prolonged length of recording that would be needed to record an event successfully (see Chap. 32). To address this problem, an implantable event monitor has been developed (Medtronic Reveal, Minneapolis). This lightweight and small device (61 × 19 × 8 mm), with a projected longevity of 18 to 24 months, incorporates two electrodes in its can and is implanted in the subcutaneous tissue of the chest. If necessary, the incision can be extended later to allow insertion of a pacemaker or implantable cardioverter-defibrillator. The electrocardiographic signal is stored in a circular buffer capable of recording up to 42 minutes of rhythm. The device can be configured to trigger automatically according to programmed detection criteria as well as with a handheld activator.

The diagnostic value of the implantable event recorder is now well established. Current guidelines recommend that when the mechanism of syncope remains unclear after full evaluation, an implantable event recorder is indicated for patients who have clinical or electrocardiographic features suggesting arrhythmic syncope or a history of recurrent syncope with injury.[1] One recent study has reported that early application of an implantable event monitor in patients with recurrent severe syncopal episodes suspected to be caused by neurally mediated hypotension results in the identification of a subset of patients in whom specific therapy was instituted (e.g., pacemaker to treat asystole, catheter ablation for supraventricular tachycardia) and resulted in a very low 1-year recurrence of syncope.[21] As a result of this and other studies, current guidelines recognize that an implantable event recorder may also be appropriate in the initial phase of a syncope work-up, instead of completion of conventional investigations, for patients with preserved cardiac function who have clinical or electrocardiographic features suggestive of an arrhythmic syncope. An implantable event recorder can also be used to assess the contribution of bradycardia before implanting a permanent pacemaker in patients with suspected or certain neurally mediated syncope who present with frequent or traumatic syncopal episodes.

Electrophysiological Testing

EP testing can provide important diagnostic and prognostic information in patients presenting with syncope (see Chaps. 32 and 33). The results of EP testing can be useful in establishing a diagnosis of sick sinus syndrome, carotid sinus hypersensitivity, heart block, supraventricular tachycardia, or VT. The indications for EP testing in the evaluation of patients with syncope have been outlined in the American College of Cardiology/American Heart Association Statement on the Evaluation of Syncope.[11] These indications have been further refined in the update of the European Guidelines on Management of Syncope.[1] There is general agreement that EP testing should be performed in patients when the initial evaluation suggests an arrhythmic cause of syncope but should not be performed in patients with a known cause of syncope for whom treatment would not be influenced by the findings of the test. EP testing is also indicated to determine the cause of an arrhythmia that has already been determined to be the cause of syncope. It is also indicated in patients in high-risk occupations or other situations in which it is thought that every effort to exclude a cardiac cause of syncope is warranted, despite the low diagnostic yield of an EP study.

Sinus node function is evaluated during EP testing primarily by determining the sinus node recovery time (SNRT) (see Chap. 32). Identification of sinus node dysfunction as the cause of syncope is uncommon during EP testing (less than 5 percent). The absence of evidence of sinus node dysfunction during EP testing does not exclude a bradyarrhythmia as the cause of syncope.

During EP testing, AV conduction is assessed to establish AV block as the probable cause of syncope. Among studies that have reported the results of EP testing in evaluating patients with syncope, AV block was identified as the probable cause of syncope in approximately 10 to 15 percent of patients. Donateo and colleagues reported the results of a systematic evaluation of patients with syncope in the setting of a bundle branch block on their baseline ECG.[22] Of 347 patients referred for evaluation of syncope, 55 had a baseline bundle branch block pattern. Systematic evaluation of these patients, including EP testing, resulted in a diagnosis of cardiac syncope in 25 patients (45 percent)—AV block in 20, sick sinus syndrome in 2, VT in 1, and aortic stenosis in 2. Neurally mediated syncope was diagnosed in 22 patients (40 percent) and syncope remained unexplained in 8 (15 percent).

It is uncommon for a supraventricular tachycardia to cause syncope unless the patient has underlying heart disease, an extremely rapid rate, or a propensity for the development of neurally mediated syncope. The typical pattern observed is the development of syncope or near-syncope at the onset of the supraventricular arrhythmia because of an initial drop in blood pressure (see Chap. 35). The patient often regains consciousness despite the continuation of the arrhythmia because of the activation of a compensatory mechanism. Completion of a standard EP test allows accurate identification of most types of supraventricular arrhythmias that may have caused syncope. The study should be repeated during an isoproterenol infusion to increase the sensitivity of the study, particularly for detecting idiopathic VT or AV nodal reentrant tachycardia. A supraventricular arrhythmia is diagnosed as the probable cause of syncope in less than 5 percent of patients who undergo EP testing for evaluation of syncope of unknown origin.

VT is the most common abnormality uncovered during EP testing in patients with syncope. Among studies that have reported the results of EP testing in evaluating patients with syncope, VT has been identified as the probable cause of syncope in approximately 20 percent of patients. In the past, an EP test has been interpreted as positive for VT when sustained monomorphic VT was induced. The induction of polymorphic VT and ventricular fibrillation were considered to represent nonspecific responses to EP testing. The diagnostic and prognostic importance of the induction of polymorphic VT and/or ventricular fibrillation (VF) remains uncertain.

According to the update of the European Guidelines on Management of Syncope,[1] an EP study is considered diagnostic of the cause of syncope when the following abnormalities are identified: (1) sinus bradycardia and a prolonged corrected sinus node recovery time; (2) bifascicular block and a baseline His-ventricular (H-V) interval longer than 100 milliseconds, or demonstration of second- or third-degree His-Purkinje block during incremental atrial pacing or provoked by an infusion of procainamide; (3) induction of sustained monomorphic VT; and (4) induction of a rapid supraventricular arrhythmia that reproduces hypotensive or spontaneous symptoms. According to these guidelines, findings on EP testing with less certain diagnostic value include an H-V interval longer than 70 but shorter than 100 milliseconds and the induction of polymorphic VT or VF in patients with Brugada syndrome or arrhythmogenic right ventricular cardiomyopathy or in patients resuscitated from a cardiac arrest. These guidelines also note that the induction of polymorphic VT or VF in patients with ischemic or dilated cardiomyopathy has low predictive value. Overall, approximately one third of patients with syncope referred for EP testing to evaluate syncope of unknown origin have a presumptive diagnosis established.

Screening for Neurological Causes of Syncope

Syncope as an isolated symptom rarely has a neurological cause. As a result, widespread use of tests to screen for neurological conditions is rarely diagnostic. In many institutions, computed tomography (CT) scans (see Chap. 18), electroencephalograms (EEGs), and carotid duplex scans are overused, being obtained for more than 50 percent of patients with syncope. A diagnosis is almost never uncovered that was not first suspected on the basis of a careful history and neurological examination. Transient ischemic attacks that result from carotid disease are not accompanied by loss of consciousness. No studies have suggested that carotid Doppler ultrasonography is beneficial in patients with syncope. EEGs should be obtained only when there is a relatively high likelihood of epilepsy. CT and magnetic resonance imaging should be avoided in patients with uncomplicated syncope.

Approach to the Evaluation of Patients with Syncope

Figure 37-1 outlines the approach to the diagnostic evaluation of a patient presenting with syncope, as proposed by the European Society of Cardiology Task Force on Syncope.[1] The initial evaluation begins with a careful history, physical examination, supine and upright blood pressure, and a 12-lead ECG (Table 37-4). Based on this initial evaluation, patients can be classified into those with true syncope and those who have not experienced true syncope. Patients with syncope can be further divided into three main groups: (1) those in whom a certain diagnosis has been established;

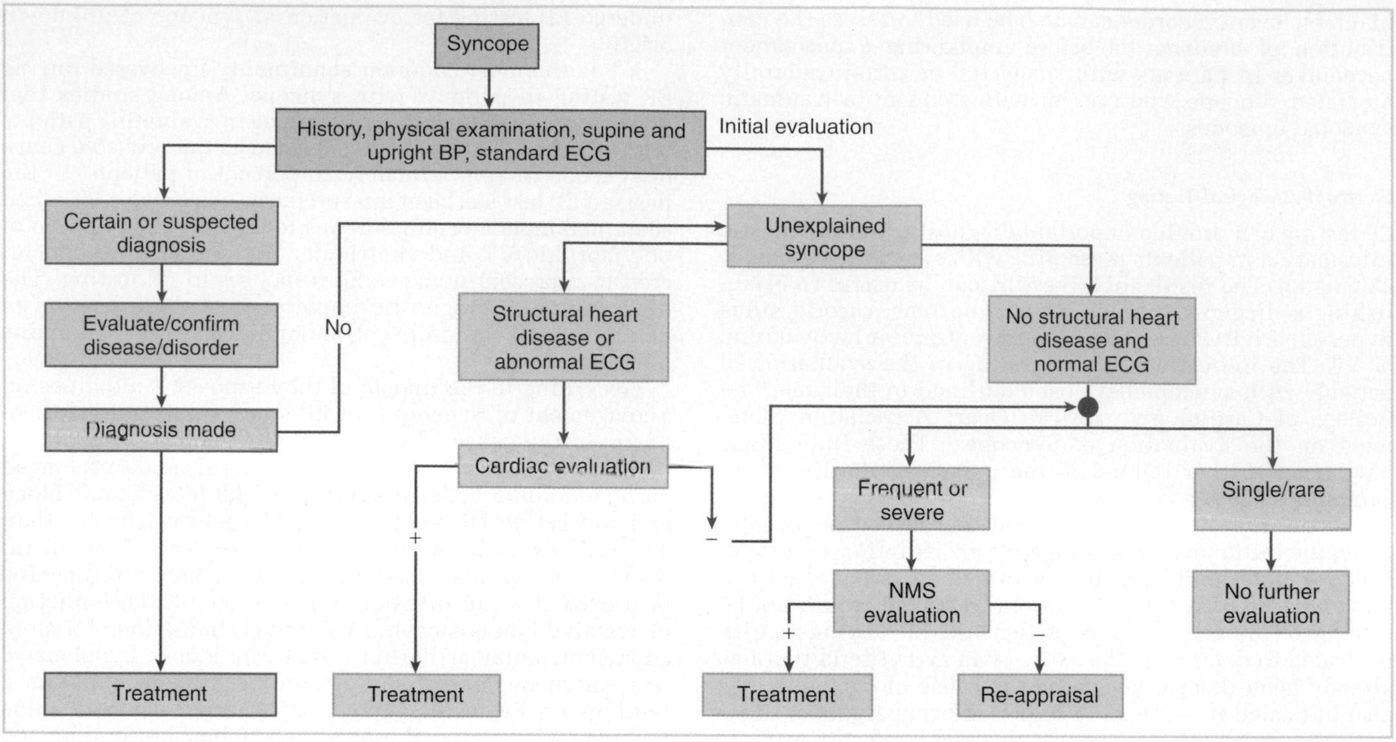

FIGURE 37–1 Diagnostic evaluation of syncope. BP = blood pressure; ECG = electrocardiogram; NMS = neurally mediated syncope.

(2) those with a suspected diagnosis; and (3) those with unexplained syncope. The subsequent use of further diagnostic testing and/or initiation of treatment can then be determined. On the basis of this initial evaluation, performed in an emergency department or outpatient setting, the probable cause of syncope can be identified in up to 50 percent of patients. When this diagnostic approach has been completed, a probable cause of syncope can be determined in more than 75 percent of patients.

The updated European Guidelines on Management of Syncope have called attention to the importance of a structured care pathway in the evaluation of patients with syncope.[1] Other studies have reported favorable outcomes when a syncope evaluation unit or standardized approach to the evaluation of syncope is used.[23-25] Brignole and associates, for example, used decision-based software to standardize the evaluation of syncope in the emergency departments of 11 general hospitals.[24] A diagnostic work-up consistent with the guidelines was carried out in 86 percent of patients, and resulted in a presumptive diagnosis in nearly 100 percent of patients. Hospitalization was deemed appropriate for evaluation of syncope in 25 percent of patients. Another study has randomized patients to a syncope evaluation unit or a standard evaluation. The syncope evaluation unit resulted in a diagnosis in 67 percent of patients versus 10 percent of patients who underwent a standard evaluation.[25]

MANAGEMENT

The approach to treatment of a patient with syncope depends largely on the established diagnosis. For example, the appropriate treatment of a patient with syncope related to AV block or sick sinus syndrome would probably involve placement of a permanent pacemaker (see Chap. 34), with syncope related to Wolff-Parkinson-White syndrome would probably involve catheter ablation (see Chap. 33), and with syncope related to VT or in the setting of an ischemic or nonischemic cardiomyopathy would probably involve placement of an implantable cardioverter-defibrillator (see Chap. 34). For other types of syncope, optimal management may involve discontinuation of an offending pharmacological agent (see Chap. 6), an increase in salt intake, or education of the patient.

Other issues that need to be considered include the indication for hospitalization of a patient with syncope and duration of driving restrictions. Current guidelines recommend that patients with syncope be hospitalized when there is known or suspected heart disease, abnormalities on the ECG suggestive of arrhythmic syncope, syncope with severe injury or during exercise, and syncope when there is a family history of sudden death.[1]

Physicians who care for patients with syncope are often asked to address the issue of driving risk. Patients who experience syncope while driving pose a risk both to themselves and others. Although some would argue that all patients with syncope should never drive again because of the theoretical possibility of a recurrence, this is an impractical solution that would be ignored by many patients. Factors that should be considered when making a recommendation for a particular patient include the following: (1) the potential for recurrent syncope; (2) presence and duration of warning symptoms; (3) whether syncope occurs while seated or only when standing; (4) how often and in what capacity the patient drives; and (5) whether any state laws may be applicable. When considering these issues, physicians should note that acute illnesses, including syncope, are unlikely to cause a motor vehicle accident. The American Heart Association and the Canadian Cardiovascular Society have published guidelines concerning this issue.[26,27] For noncommercial drivers, it is generally recommended that driving be restricted for several months. If the patient remains asymptomatic for several months, driving can then be resumed.

TABLE 37–4	Clinical Features Suggestive of Specific Causes of Syncope
Symptom or Finding	**Diagnostic Consideration**
After sudden unexpected pain, unpleasant sight, sound, or smell	Vasovagal syncope
During or immediately after micturition, cough, swallow, or defecation	Situational syncope
With neuralgia (glossopharyngeal or trigeminal)	Bradycardia or vasodepressor reaction
On standing	Orthostatic hypotension
Prolonged standing at attention	Vasovagal syncope
Well-trained athlete after exertion	Neurally mediated
Changing position (from sitting to lying, bending, turning over in bed)	Atrial myxoma, thrombus
Syncope with exertion	Aortic stenosis, pulmonary hypertension, pulmonary embolus, mitral stenosis, idiopathic hypertrophic subaortic stenosis, coronary artery disease, neurally mediated
With head rotation, pressure on carotid sinus (as in tumors, shaving, tight collars)	Carotid sinus syncope
Associated with vertigo, dysarthria, diplopia, and other motor and sensory symptoms of brain stem ischemia	Transient ischemic attack, subclavian steal, basilar artery migraine
With arm exercise	Subclavian steal
Confusion after episode	Seizure

Neurally Mediated Syncope

Because neurally mediated syncope is so common, treatment options are reviewed here. Treatment of syncope caused by neurally mediated hypotension begins with a careful history, with particular attention focused on identifying precipitating factors, quantifying the degree of salt intake and current medication use, and determining whether the patient has a prior history of peripheral edema, hypertension, asthma, or other conditions that may alter the approach used for treatment. For most patients with neurally mediated syncope, particularly those with infrequent episodes associated with an identifiable precipitant, education and reassurance are sufficient.[1,12,14] Patients should be educated about common precipitating factors, such as dehydration, prolonged standing, alcohol, and medications such as diuretics and vasodilators. Patients should also be taught to sit or lie down at the onset of symptoms or to cross their legs (if sitting) and squeeze them together. Volume expansion by salt supplementation is also commonly recommended. Several studies have reported that ingestion of approximately 500 ml of water acutely improves orthostatic tolerance to tilt in healthy subjects and may be of value as prophylaxis for syncope in blood donors.[28,29] The effectiveness of water ingestion for the management of patients with recurrent neurally mediated syncope has not been well studied.

A rather recent important shift in the approach used for treatment of neurally mediated syncope results from the effectiveness of physical measures and maneuvers in the treatment of patients with this condition.[12,30-32] It is notable that the revised European Guidelines on Management of Syncope have identified the following physical measures as class 2 treatments for neurally mediated syncope: (1) tilt training; (2) head-up tilt sleeping (more than 10 degrees); (3) isometric leg and arm counterpressure maneuvers; and (4) moderate aerobic and isometric exercise.[1] One study, for example, has reported that 2 minutes of an isometric hand grip maneuver initiated at the onset of symptoms during tilt testing rendered two thirds of patients asymptomatic.[31] Other studies have demonstrated that tilt (standing) training, which involves standing against a wall for 40 minutes twice daily, is effective in the treatment of neurally mediated syncope. Despite its effectiveness, this treatment strategy is limited by poor long-term compliance.

In contrast to physical maneuvers, which are now generally accepted as valuable in the management of patients with neurally mediated syncope, the value of pharmacological agents is less certain. The medications that are generally relied on to treat neurally mediated syncope include beta blockers, fludrocortisone, serotonin reuptake inhibitors, and midodrine. Despite the widespread use of these agents, none of these pharmacological agents has been demonstrated to be effective according to the results of a number of large prospective randomized clinical trials. A small study has reported that midodrine is effective.[33] Although beta blockers are considered by many as first-line therapy, several studies have reported that the beta blockers metoprolol, propranolol, and nadolol are no more effective than placebo.[34,35]

Although pacemakers have also been found to be valuable in the treatment of some patients with neurally mediated syncope in several clinical trials, one large controlled trial, in which all subjects received pacemakers but pacing was activated in 50 percent of patients, showed no benefit of pacing.[36] Because of the variable results of these clinical trials and the profound implications of pacemaker implantation, considerable restraint should be exercised when considering the implantation of a pacemaker for treatment of neurally mediated syncope. The development of asystole during tilt-table testing is not considered to be an absolute indication for pacemaker implantation. In fact, one recent study has reported that the heart rhythm observed at the time of a positive tilt-table test does not correlate with the patient's heart rhythm at the time of a subsequent episode of syncope.[37] The European Guidelines on Management of Syncope[1] have stated that cardiac pacing is indicated in the treatment of patients with neurally mediated syncope who have a cardioinhibitory form, more than five episodes/year or severe physical injury or accident, and age older than 40 years (classes 1 and 2).

REFERENCES

Definition and Classification

1. Brignole M, Alboni P, Benditt DG, et al: Guidelines on management (diagnosis and treatment) of syncope—update 2004. Eur Heart J 25:2054, 2004.
2. Soteriades ES, Evans JC, Larson MG, et al: Incidence and prognosis of syncope. N Engl J Med 12:878, 2002.
3. Priori SG, Schwartz PJ, Napolitan C, et al: Risk stratification in the long-QT syndrome. N Engl J Med 348:1866, 2003.
4. Dalal D, Nasir K, Bomma C, et al: Arrhythmogenic right ventricular dysplasia: A United States experience. Circulation 25:3823, 2005.
5. Antzelevitch C, Brugada P, Borggrefe M, et al: Brugada syndrome: Report of the second consensus conference. Heart Rhythm 4:429, 2005.
6. Maron BJ: Hypertrophic cardiomyopathy: A systematic review. JAMA 10:1308, 2002.

7. Calder Kirsten K, Berbert M, Henderson SO: The mortality of untreated pulmonary embolism in emergency department patients. Ann Emerg Med 45:302, 2005.
8. Priori SG, Napolitano C, Memmi M, et al: Clinical and molecular characterization of patients with catecholaminergic polymorphic ventricular tachycardia. Circulation 106:69, 2002.
9. Takashi N, Shimizu W, Taguchi A, et al: Malignant entity of idiopathic ventricular fibrillation and polymorphic ventricular tachycardia initiated by premature extrasystoles origination from the right ventricular outflow tract. J Am Coll Cardiol 4:1288, 2005.
10. Bjerregaard P, Gussak I: Short QT syndrome: Mechanisms, diagnosis and treatment. Nat Clin Pract Cardiovasc Med 2:84, 2005.
11. Strickberger SA, Benson DW, Biaggioni I, et al: AHA/ACCF Scientific Statement on the Evaluation of Syncope. Circulation 113:316, 2006.

Vascular Causes of Syncope

12. Grubb BP: Neurocardiogenic syncope and related disorders of orthostatic intolerance. Circulation 111:2997, 2005.
13. Grubb BP, Kanjwal Y, Kosinski D: The postural tachycardia syndrome: A concise guide to diagnosis and management. J Cardiovasc Electrophysiol 17:108, 2006.
14. Grubb BP: Neurocardiogenic syncope. N Engl J Med 352:1004, 2005.
15. Parry SW, Steen IN, Baptist M, Kenny RA: Amnesia for loss of consciousness in carotid sinus syndrome. J Am Coll Cardiol 45:1840, 2005.
16. Kerr SR, Pearce MS, Brayne C, et al: Carotid sinus hypersensitivity in asymptomatic older persons. Arch Intern Med 166:515, 2006.
17. Gregoratos G, Abrams J, Epstein AE, et al; American College of Cardiology/American Heart Association Task Force on Practice Guidelines/North American Society for Pacing and Electrophysiology Committee to Update the 1998 Pacemaker Guidelines: ACC/AHA/NASPE 2002 guideline update for implantation of cardiac pacemakers and antiarrhythmia devices: Summary article: A report of the American College of Cardiology/American Heart Association Task Force on Practice Guidelines (ACC/AHA/NASPE Committee to Update the 1998 Pacemaker Guidelines). Circulation 106:2145, 2002.
18. Kenny RA, Richardson DA, Bexton RS, et al: Carotid sinus syndrome: A modifiable risk factor for nonaccidental falls in older adults (SAFE PACE). J Am Coll Cardiol 38:1491, 2001.

Causes of Syncope

19. Sheldon R, Rose S, Ritchie D, et al: Historical criteria that distinguish syncope from seizures. J Am Coll Cardiol 40:142, 2002.
20. Benditt DG, Sutton R: Tilt-table testing in the evaluation of syncope. J Cardiovasc Electrophysiol 16:356, 2005.
21. Brignole M, Sutton R, Menozzi C, et al: Early application of an implantable loop recorder allows effective specific therapy in patients with recurrent suspected neurally mediated syncope. Eur Heart J 27:1085, 2005.
22. Donateo P, Brignole M, Alboni P, et al: A standardized conventional evaluation of the mechanism of syncope in patients with bundle branch block. Europace 4:357, 2002.
23. Bartoletti A, Fabiani P, Adriani P, et al: Hospital admission of patients referred to the emergency department for syncope: A single-hospital prospective study based on the application of the European Society of Cardiology Guidelines on syncope. Eur Heart J 27:83, 2006.
24. Brignole M, Menozzi C, Bartoletti A, et al; Evaluation of Guidelines in Syncope Study 2 (EGSYS-2) Group: A new management of syncope: Prospective systematic guideline-based evaluation of patients referred urgently to general hospitals. Eur Heart J 27:76, 2006.
25. Shen WK, Decker WW, Smars PA, et al: Syncope evaluation in the emergency department study (SEEDS). A multidisciplinary approach to syncope management. Circulation 110:3636, 2004.

Management of Patients

26. Epstein AE, Miles WM, Benditt DG: Personal and public safety issues related to arrhythmias that may affect consciousness: Implications for regulation and physician recommendations: An AHA/NASPE Medical Scientific Statement. Circulation 94:1147, 1996.
27. Consensus Conference, Canadian Cardiovascular Society: Assessment of the cardiac patient for fitness to drive. Can J Cardiol 8:406, 1992.
28. Lu C, Diedrich A, Tung C, et al: Water ingestion as prophylaxis against syncope. Circulation 108:2660, 2003.
29. Schroeder C, Bush VE, Norcliffe LJ, et al: Water drinking acutely improves orthostatic tolerance in healthy subjects. Circulation 106:2806, 2002.
30. Abe H, Kondo S, Kohshi K, Nakashima Y: Usefulness of orthostatic self-training for the prevention of neurocardiogenic syncope. Pacing Clin Electrophysiol 25:1454, 2002.
31. Brignole M, Croci F, Menozzi C, et al: Isometric arm counter-pressure maneuvers to abort impending vasovagal syncope. J Am Coll Cardiol 40:2054, 2002.
32. Krediet P, van Dijk N, Linzer M, et al: Management of vasovagal syncope: Controlling or aborting faints by leg crossing and muscle tensing. Circulation 106:1684, 2002.
33. Kaufmann H, Saadia D, Voustianiouk A: Midodrine in neurally mediated syncope: A double-blind randomized, crossover study. Ann Neurol 52:342, 2002.
34. Sheldon R, Connolly S, Rose S, et al; POST Investigators: Prevention of syncope trial (POST): A randomized, placebo-controlled study of metoprolol in the prevention of vasovagal syncope. Circulation 113:1164, 2006.
35. Flevari P, Livanis EG, Theodorakis GN, et al: Vasovagal syncope. A prospective, randomized, crossover evaluation of the effect of propranolol, nadolol and placebo on syncope recurrence and patients' well-being. J Am Coll Cardiol 40:499, 2002.
36. Connolly SJ, Sheldon R, Thorpe K, et al; VPS II Investigators: Pacemaker therapy for prevention of syncope in patients with recurrent severe vasovagal syncope. Second Vasovagal Pacemaker Study (VPSII): A randomized trial. JAMA 289:2224, 2003.
37. Deharo J, Jego C, Lanteaume A, Dijane P: An implantable loop recorder study of highly symptomatic vasovagal patients. J Am Coll Cardiol 47:587, 2006.

PART VI

Preventive Cardiology

CHAPTER 38

The Vascular Biology of Atherosclerosis

Peter Libby

The 20th century witnessed a remarkable evolution in concepts concerning the pathogenesis of atherosclerosis. This disease has a venerable history, having left traces in the arteries of Egyptian mummies. Apparently uncommon in antiquity, atherosclerosis became epidemic as populations increasingly survived early mortality caused by communicable diseases and malnutrition. Economic development and urbanization promoted habits of diet (e.g., a surfeit of saturated fats) and diminished physical activity that can favor atherogenesis (see Chaps. 1, 39, and 42). Such environmental factors have now become globalized, such that we face an epidemic of atherosclerosis that reaches far beyond Western societies (see Chap. 1).

Until very recently most viewed arteries as inanimate tubes rather than living, dynamic tissue. In the mid-nineteenth century, Virchow recognized the participation of cells in atherogenesis. A controversy raged between Virchow, who viewed atherosclerosis as a proliferative disease, and Rokitansky, who believed that atheroma derived from healing and resorption of thrombi. Experiments performed in the early part of the 20th century used dietary modulation to produce fatty lesions in the arteries of rabbits and ultimately identified cholesterol as the culprit. These observations, followed by the characterization of human lipoprotein particles at mid-century, promoted the concept of insudation of lipids as a cause for atherosclerosis. We now recognize that elements of all of these pathogenic theories participate in atherogenesis. This chapter summarizes evidence from human studies, animal experimentation, and in vitro work and presents a synoptic view of atherogenesis, taking into account advances in vascular biology that have deepened our understanding of the process.

Acquaintance with the vascular biology of atherosclerosis should prove useful to the practitioner. Our daily contact with this common disease lulls us into a complacent belief that we understand it better than we actually do. For example, we have just begun to learn why atherosclerosis affects certain regions of the arterial tree preferentially, and why its clinical manifestations occur only at certain times. Atherosclerosis can involve both large and mid-sized arteries diffusely. Post mortem and intravascular ultrasound studies have revealed widespread intimal thickening in patients with atherosclerosis. Many asymptomatic individuals have intimal lesions in their coronary or carotid arteries even in the early decades of life. At the same time, atherosclerosis is a focal disease that produces stenoses in certain areas of affected vessels much more than others. An understanding of the biological basis of the predilection of certain sites to develop atheroma has begun to emerge.

Atherosclerosis also displays heterogeneity in time: this disease has both chronic and acute manifestations. Few human diseases have a longer "incubation" period than atherosclerosis, which begins to affect arteries of many North Americans in the second and third decades of life (Fig. 38-1). Indeed, one in six American teenagers has abnormal thickening of the coronary arteries.[1] Yet typically, symptoms of atherosclerosis do not occur until several decades later, characteristically occurring even later in women. Despite this indolent time course and prolonged period of clinical inactivity, the dreaded complications of

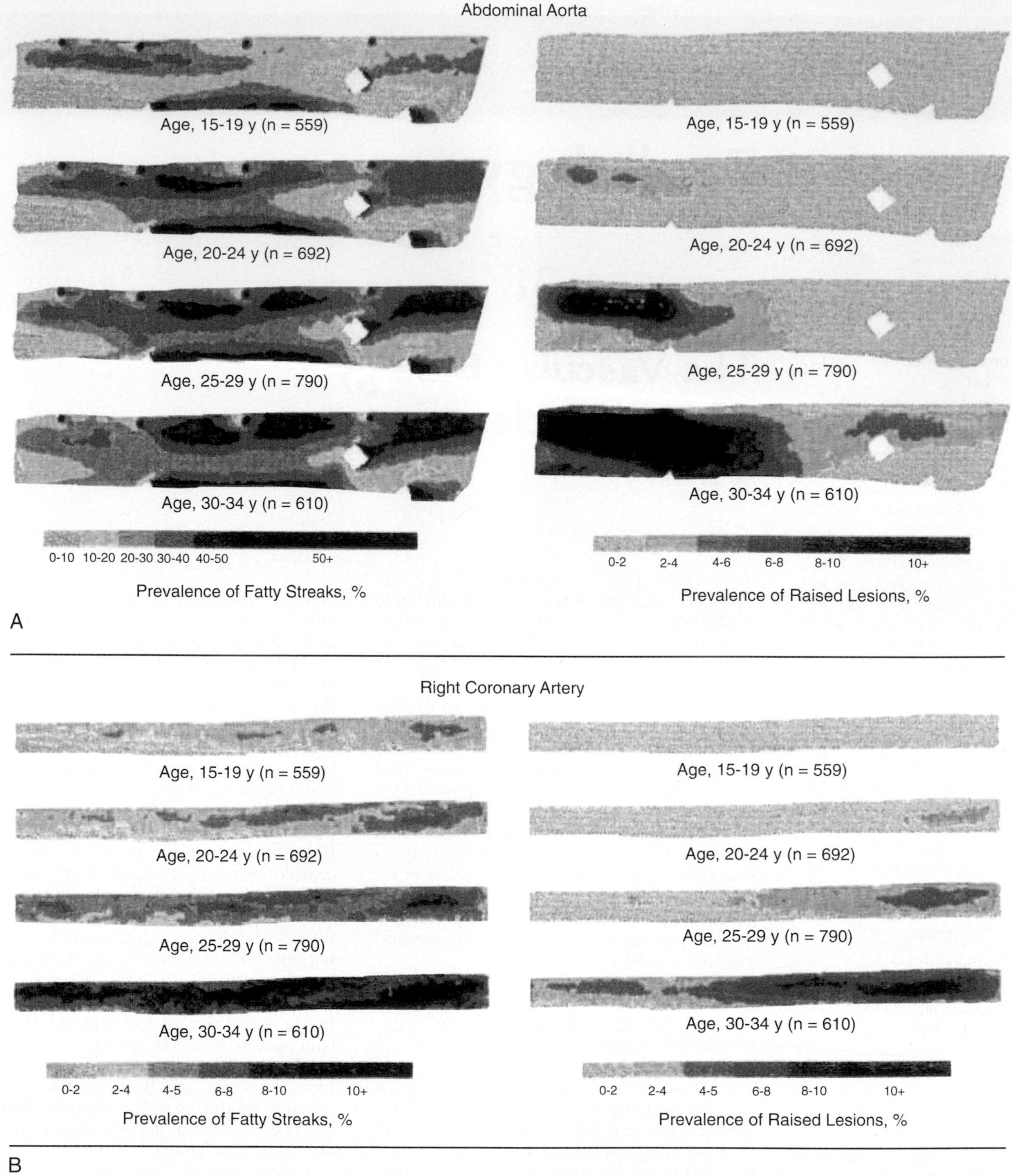

FIGURE 38–1 Prevalence maps of fatty streaks and raised lesions in the abdominal aorta. Composite data from the Pathobiological Determinants of Atherosclerosis In Youth (PDAY) study show pseudocolored representation of morphometric analysis of over 2800 aortas from Americans younger than 35 years of age who succumbed for noncardiac reasons. **A,** Note the early involvement of the dorsal surface of the infrarenal abdominal aorta by fatty streaks followed by raised lesions. **B,** A similar but slightly slower progression of lesions affects the right coronary artery. The scales at the bottoms of the panels show the coding of the pseudocoloring. *(From Strong JP, Malcolm GJ, McMahan CA, et al: Prevalence and extent of atherosclerosis in adolescents and young adults. JAMA 281:727, 1999.)*

atheroma such as myocardial infarction, unstable angina, or stroke typically occur suddenly.

Another poorly understood issue regarding atherogenesis is its role in causing narrowing, or stenosis, of some vessels and ectasia of others. Typically, we fear stenoses in coronary atherosclerosis. However, aneurysm is a common manifestation of this disease in other vessels, including the aorta. Even in the life history of a single atherosclerotic lesion, a phase of ectasia known as positive remodeling, or compensatory enlargement, precedes the formation of stenotic lesions.[2,3] Contemporary vascular biology has begun to shed light on some of these puzzling aspects of atherosclerosis.

STRUCTURE OF THE NORMAL ARTERY

The Cell Types That Comprise the Normal Artery

Endothelial Cells

The endothelial cell of the arterial intima constitutes the crucial contact surface with blood. Arterial endothelial cells possess many highly regulated mechanisms of capital importance in vascular homeostasis that often go awry during the pathogenesis of arterial diseases.[4] For example, the endothelial cell provides one of the only surfaces, either natural or synthetic, that can maintain blood in a liquid state during protracted contact (Fig. 38-2). This remarkable blood compatibility derives in part from the expression of heparan sulfate proteoglycan molecules on the surface of the endothelial cell. These molecules, like heparin, serve as a co-factor for antithrombin III, causing a conformational change that allows this inhibitor to bind to and inactivate thrombin. The surface of the endothelial cell also contains thrombomodulin, which binds thrombin molecules and can exert antithrombotic properties by activating proteins S and C. Should a thrombus begin to form, the normal endothelial cell possesses potent fibrinolytic mechanisms associated with its surface. The endothelial cell can produce both tissue and urokinase-type plasminogen activators. These enzymes catalyze the activation of plasminogen to form plasmin, a fibrinolytic enzyme. (For a complete discussion of the role of endothelium in hemostasis and fibrinolysis, see Chap. 82).

Endothelial cells have a common origin but acquire bed-specific characteristics during development. The endothelial cells that form the inner lining of all blood vessels arise during embryogenesis from regions known as the blood islands, located on the embryo's periphery. Angioblasts, the predecessors of the endothelial cells, share this site with the precursors of blood cells. Despite arising from the same site, cells display considerable heterogeneity even during embryological and early postnatal development. Although endothelial cells presumably derive from a common precursor, the signals they encounter during vessel development differ. As rudimentary blood vessels begin to form, endothelial precursors interact with surrounding cells. The interchange permits spatial and temporal gradients of various stimuli and their receptors on the endothelial cells, leading to this cell type's heterogeneity in the adult. Endothelial cell heterogeneity depends on both environmental stimuli and epigenetic features acquired during development.[5]

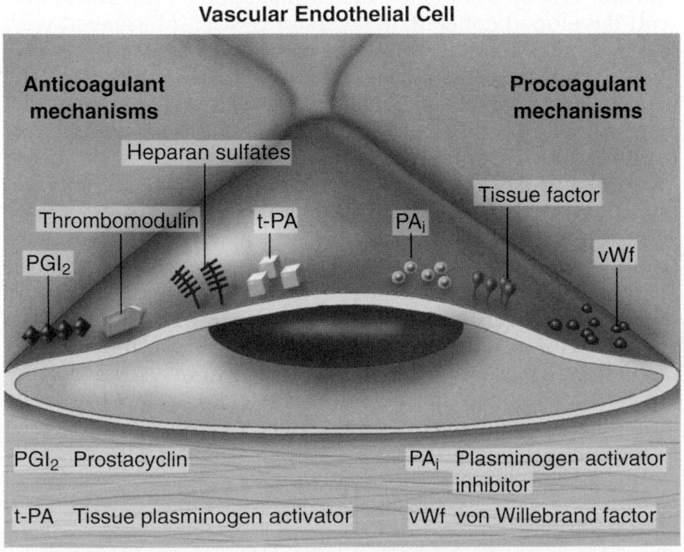

FIGURE 38–2 The endothelial thrombotic balance. This diagram depicts the anticoagulant profibrinolytic functions of the endothelial cell **(left)** and certain procoagulant and antifibrinolytic functions **(right)**. HSPG = heparan sulfate proteoglycan; PAI-1 = plasminogen activator inhibitor-1; PGI_2 = prostacyclin; tPA = tissue type plasminogen activator; uPA = urokinase type plasminogen activator; vWf = von Willebrand factor.

Recent evidence has indicated that the cells that make up various compartments of the arterial wall can originate from bone marrow during postnatal life as well as from their traditional embryological sources. In particular, peripheral blood appears to contain endothelial precursor cells that may help the repair of areas of endothelial desquamation. Moreover, in injured or transplanted arteries, smooth muscle cells of apparent bone marrow origin can take up residence in the intima or media (see later). The endothelial progenitor cells (EPCs) bear characteristic markers such as CD133, CD34, and vascular endothelial growth factor receptor-2. Circulating numbers of EPCs, as assayed in vitro, vary among individuals. Those with a higher burden of risk factors for atherosclerosis have fewer EPCs. EPC number may correlate with prognosis in atherosclerotic patients.[6] More aged individuals may have impaired EPC numbers and hence less ability to repair breaches in intimal integrity.[7]

Differential expression of endothelial genes in various types of blood vessels depends on transcriptional regulation by the local environment. For example, the promoter region of the gene that encodes von Willebrand factor directs expression in the endothelium of brain and heart microvessels but not in larger arteries. Co-culture of endothelial cells with cardiac myocytes, but not other cell types, could selectively activate a von Willebrand factor gene promoter construct. Likewise, endothelial nitric oxide synthase gene activity in the heart shows bed-specific regulation. Members of the EPH family of tyrosine kinase receptors and their ligands, known as ephrins, display heterogeneous expressions in arterial versus venous endothelial cells during development. In the adult, arterial endothelial and SMCs, but not venous vascular cells, express ephrinB2. This finding supports a stable lineage difference between cells that make up arteries and veins. These examples illustrate the molecular diversity of cell location in the circulation.[8] Phage display and proteomic techniques have begun to substantiate the in vivo significance of vascular cell heterogeneity in atherogenesis.[9]

Arterial Smooth Muscle Cells

The second major cell type of the normal artery wall, the smooth muscle cell (SMC) has many important functions in normal vascular homeostasis, as a target of therapies in cardiovascular medicine, and in the pathogenesis of arterial diseases. These cells contract and relax and thus control blood flow through the various arterial beds, generally at the level of the muscular arterioles. In the larger types of arteries involved in atherosclerosis, however, abnormal smooth muscle contraction may cause vasospasm, a complication of atherosclerosis that may aggravate the embarrassment of blood flow. SMCs synthesize the bulk of the complex arterial extracellular matrix that plays a key role in normal vascular homeostasis as well as the formation and complication of atherosclerotic lesions. These cells also can migrate and proliferate, contributing to the formation of intimal hyperplastic lesions including atherosclerosis and restenosis or in stent stenosis following percutaneous intervention, or anastomotic hyperplasia complicating vein grafts. Death of SMC may promote destabilization of atheromatous plaques or favor ectatic remodeling and ultimately aneurysm formation.

In contrast to endothelial cells thought to derive from a common precursor, SMC can arise from many sources. After endothelial cells form tubes, the rudimentary precursor of blood vessels, they recruit the cells that will become smooth muscle, or pericytes (smooth muscle-like cells associated with microvessels). In the descending aorta and arteries of the lower body, the regional mesoderm serves as the source of smooth muscle precursors. The mesodermal cells in somites give rise to the SMCs that invest much of the distal aorta and its branches. In arteries of the upper body, however, SMCs can actually derive from a completely different germ layer, neurectoderm rather than mesoderm. Before the neural tube closes, neurectodermal cells migrate and become the precursors of SMCs in the ascending aorta and some of its branches, including the carotid arteries (Fig. 38-3). SMCs in the coro-

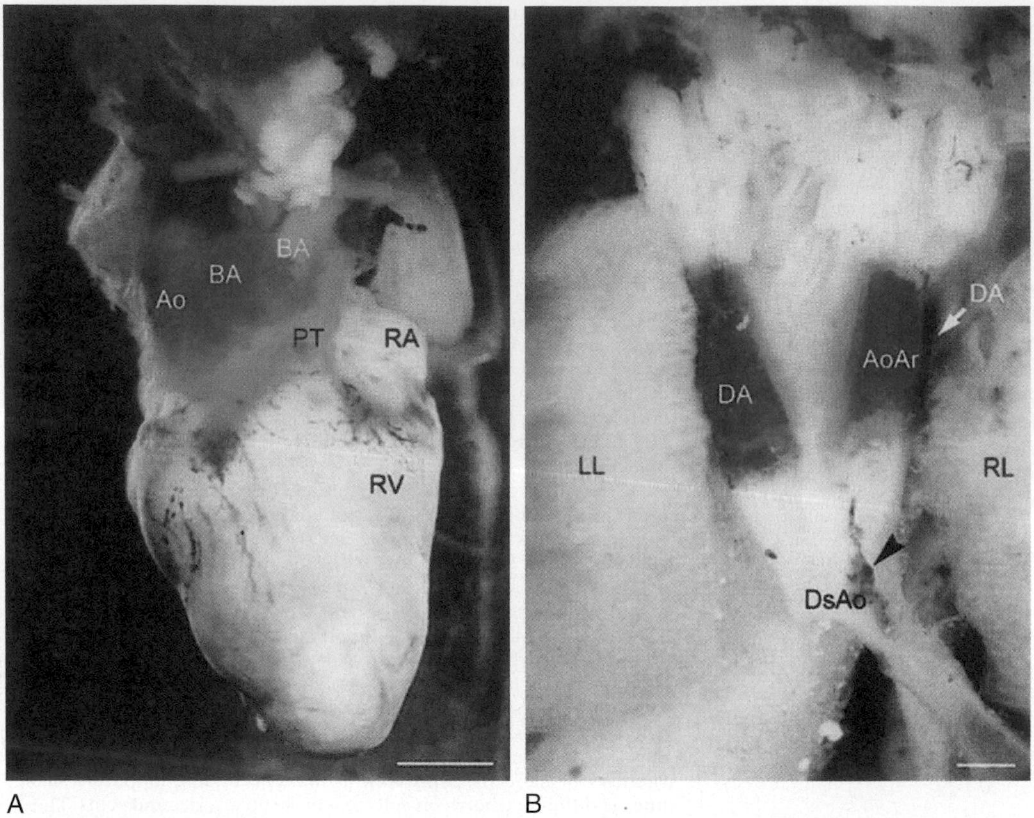

FIGURE 38–3 **Left,** Anterior view of an embryonic chick heart in which cells of neural crest origin stain blue. Note the focal localization of cells derived from neural crest in the great arteries as well as the cardiac innervation plexus spread over the ventricles. Ao = aorta; BA = brachiocephalic artery; PT = pulmonary trunk; RA = right atrium; RV = right ventricle. Bar = 750 μm. **Right,** Posterior view of a chicken embryo heart-lung whole-mount similarly tagged. Note the sharp demarcation in the localization of the blue neural crest-derived cells in the aortic arch (AoAr) and dorsal aorta (DA) before they unite to form the descending aorta (DsAo). The arrowhead indicates neural crest-derived neural tissue. LL and RL indicate left and right lung, respectively. Bar = 250 μm. *(From Bergwerff M, Verberne ME, DeRuiter MC, et al: Neural crest cell contribution to the developing circulatory system. Circ Res 82:221, 1998.)*

nary arteries derive from mesoderm, but in a special way. The precursors of coronary artery SMCs arise from yet another embryological source, a structure known as the proepicardial organ.

As in the case of endothelial cells, SMCs show molecular heterogeneity early during development.[10-12] For example, the promoter of a characteristic smooth muscle gene, known as SM22, drives gene expression in venous, but not arterial, SMCs during embryogenesis. A specific transcription factor known as dHAND signals the recruitment of mesenchyme by endothelial cells in an anatomically heterogeneous manner during development. In particular, dHAND regulation participates selectively in recruitment of mesenchyme in upper body blood vessels versus those of the more caudal portions of the embryo. A CArG box-dependent enhancer within the regulatory regions of the cysteine-rich protein 1 gene directs this protein's expression in arterial, but not venous or visceral, SMCs. Differential dependence on CArG elements in the control of SMC gene transcription furnishes a molecular basis for SMC heterogeneity in different arterial beds.[12] These findings illustrate molecular distinctions between the cells that comprise different types of vessels.

The Intima

Understanding the pathogenesis of atherosclerosis first requires knowledge of the structure and biology of the normal artery as well as its indigenous cell types. Normal arteries have a well-developed tri-laminar structure (Fig. 38-4). The innermost layer, the tunica intima, is thin at birth in humans and many nonhuman species. Although often depicted as a monolayer of endothelial cells abutting directly on a basal lamina, the structure of the adult human intima is actually much more complex and heterogeneous. The endothelial monolayer resides on a basement membrane containing nonfibrillar collagen types, such as type IV collagen, laminin, fibronectin, and other extracellular matrix molecules. With aging, human arteries develop a more complex intima containing arterial SMCs and fibrillar forms of interstitial collagen (types I and III). The SMC produces these extracellular matrix constituents of the arterial intima. The presence of a more complex intima, known by pathologists as diffuse intimal thickening, characterizes most adult human arteries. Some locales in the arterial tree tend to develop thicker intimas than other regions, even in the absence of athorosclerosis (Fig. 38-5). For example, the proximal left anterior descending coronary artery often contains an intimal cushion of SMCs more fully developed than that in typical arteries. The diffuse intimal thickening process does not necessarily go hand in hand with lipid accumulation, and may occur in individuals without substantial burden of atheroma. The internal elastic membrane bounds the tunica intima abluminally, and serves as the border between the intimal layer and the underlying tunica media.

The Tunica Media

The tunica media lies under the media and internal elastic lamina. The media of elastic arteries such as the aorta have well-developed concentric layers of SMCs, interleaved with layers of elastin-rich extracellular matrix (see Fig. 38-4A). This structure appears well adapted to the storage of the kinetic energy of left ventricular systole by the walls of great arteries. The lamellar structure also doubtless contributes to the structural integrity of the arterial trunks. The media of smaller muscular arteries usually have a less stereotyped organization (see Fig. 38-4B). SMCs in these smaller arteries generally embed in the surrounding matrix in a more continuous than lamellar array. The SMCs in normal arteries seldom proliferate. Indeed, rates of both cell division and cell death are quite low under usual circumstances. In the normal artery, a state of homeostasis of extracellular matrix also typically prevails. Because extracellular matrix neither accumulates nor atrophies, rates of arterial matrix synthesis and dissolution usually balance each other. The external elastic lamina bounds the tunica media abluminally, forming the border with the adventitial layer.

The Adventitia

The adventitia of arteries has typically received little attention, although appreciation of its potential roles in arterial homeostasis and pathology has recently increased. The adventitia contains collagen fibrils in a looser array than is usually encountered in the intima. Vasa vasorum and nerve endings localize in this outermost layer of the arterial wall.

The cellular population in the adventitia is more sparse than in other arterial layers. Cells encountered in this layer include fibroblasts and mast cells (see Fig. 38-4). Emerging evidence suggests a role for mast cells in atheroma and aneurysm formation in animal models, but their importance in humans remains speculative.

ATHEROSCLEROSIS INITIATION

Extracellular Lipid Accumulation

The first steps in atherogenesis in humans remain largely conjectural. However, integration of observations of tissues obtained from young humans with the results of experimental studies of atherogenesis in animals provides hints in this regard. On initiation of an atherogenic diet, one typically rich in cholesterol and saturated fat, small lipoprotein particles accumulate in the intima (Fig. 38-6, 1 and 2). These lipoprotein particles appear to decorate the proteoglycan of the arterial intima, and tend to coalesce into aggregates (Fig. 38-7).[13] Detailed kinetic studies of labeled lipoprotein particles indicate that a prolonged residence time characterizes sites of early lesion formation in rabbits. The binding of lipoproteins to proteoglycan in the intima captures and retains these particles, accounting for their prolonged residence time. Lipoprotein particles bound to proteoglycan have increased susceptibility to oxidative or other chemical modifications, considered by many investigators to be an important component of the pathogenesis of early atherosclerosis (see Fig. 38-6, 2).[14] Other studies suggest that permeability of the endothelial monolayer increases at sites of lesion predilection to LDL. Contributors to oxidative stress in the nascent atheroma could include NADH/NADPH oxidases expressed by vascular cells, lipoxygenases expressed by infiltrating leukocytes, or the enzyme myeloperoxidase.[15-18]

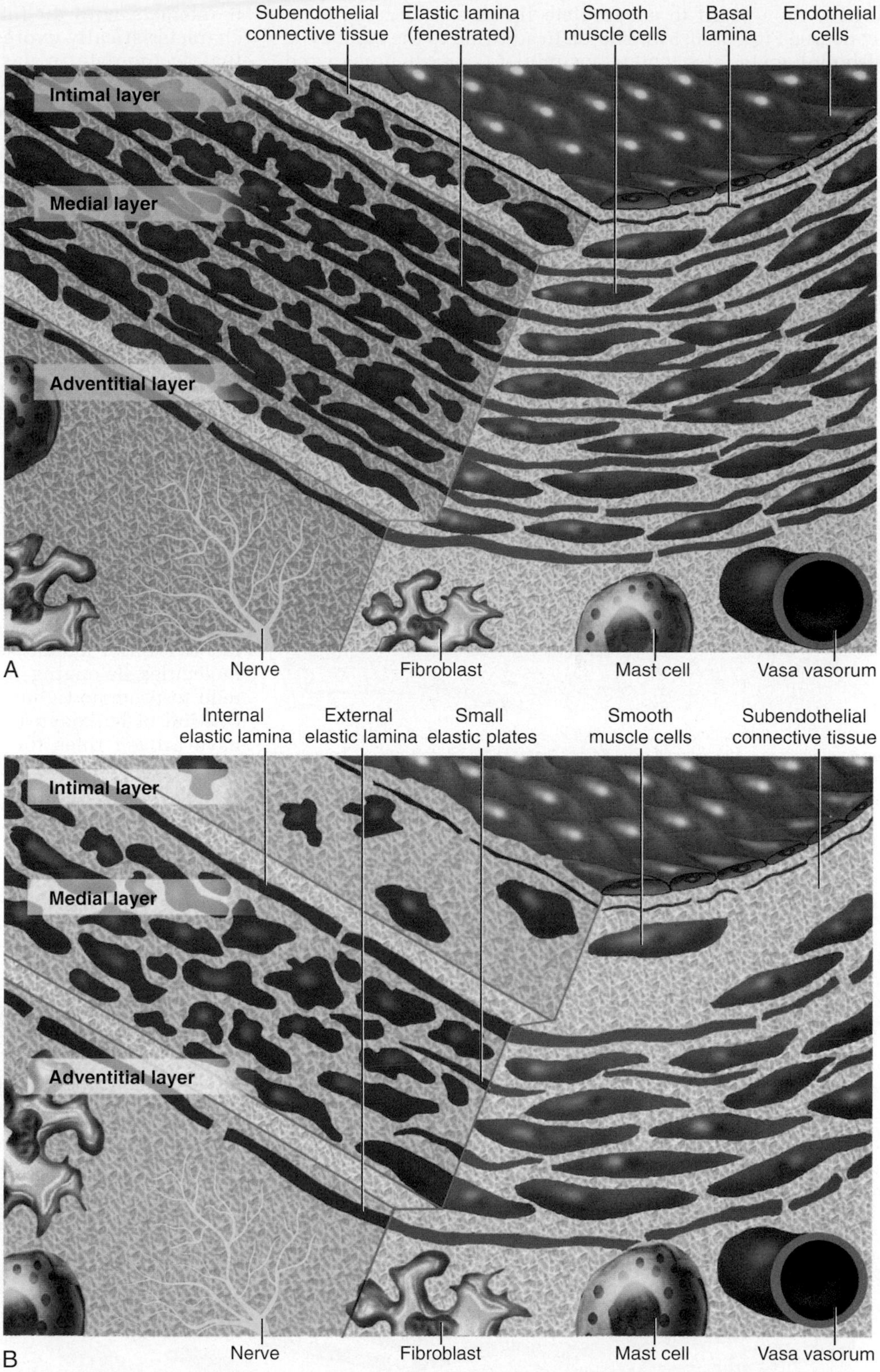

FIGURE 38–4 The structures of normal arteries. **A,** Elastic artery. Note the concentric laminae of elastic tissue that form sandwiches with successive layers of smooth muscle cells (SMCs). Each level of the elastic arterial tree has a characteristic number of elastic laminae. **B,** Muscular artery. The muscular artery, the SMCs, are surrounded by a collagenous matrix but lack the concentric rings of well-organized elastic tissue characteristic of the larger arteries.

Leukocyte Recruitment

Another hallmark of atherogenesis, leukocyte recruitment and accumulation, also occurs early in lesion generation (see Fig. 38-6, 4; Fig. 38-8).[19] The normal endothelial cell generally resists adhesive interactions with leukocytes. Even in inflamed tissues, most recruitment and trafficking of leukocytes occurs in postcapillary venules, not in arteries. However, very early after initiation of hypercholesterolemia, leukocytes adhere to the endothelium and diapedese between endothelial cell junctions to enter the intima, where they begin to accumulate lipids and become foam cells (see Figs. 38-6, 5 and 38-8). In addition to the monocyte, T-lymphocytes also tend to accumulate in early human and animal atherosclerotic lesions. The expression of certain leukocyte adhesion molecules on the surface of the endothelial cell regulates the adherence of monocytes and T-cells to the endothelium. Two broad categories of leukocyte adhesion molecules exist. Members of the immunoglobulin superfamily include structures such as vascular cell adhesion molecule-1 (VCAM-1). This adhesion molecule has particular interest in the context of early atherogenesis because it interacts with an integrin (very late antigen-4, VLA-4) characteristically expressed by those classes of leukocytes that accumulate in nascent atheroma, monocytes, and T-cells. Studies in rabbits and mice have shown expression of VCAM-1 on endothelial cells overlying very early atheromatous lesions. Other members of the immunoglobulin superfamily of leukocyte adhesion molecules include intercellular adhesion molecule-1 (ICAM-1). This molecule is more promiscuous, both in the types of leukocytes it binds and because of its wide and constitutive expression at low levels by endothelial cells in many parts of the circulation.

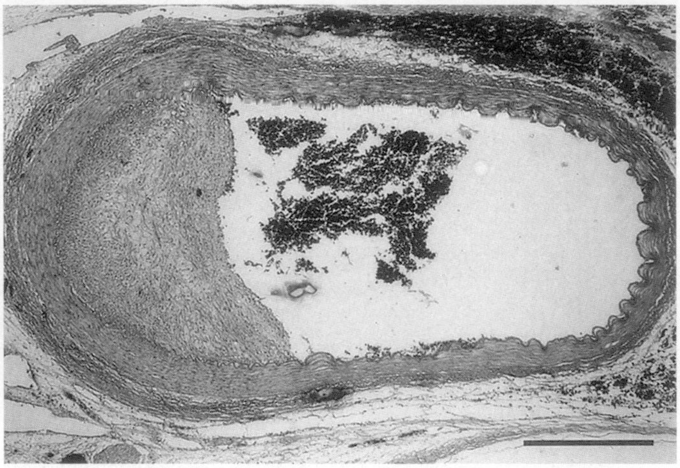

FIGURE 38–5 An intimal cushion shown in a cross-section through the internal carotid artery of a 10-week-old male infant. Areas where intimal cushions form in early life tend to develop atheromas more commonly in later years. The bar shows 0.5 mm. *(From Weniger WJ, Muller GB, Reiter C, et al: Intimal hyperplasia of the infant parasellar carotid artery: A potential developmental factor in atherosclerosis and SIDS. Circ Res 85:970, 1999.)*

Selectins constitute the other broad category of leukocyte adhesion molecules. The prototypical selectin, E-selectin (E for "endothelial," the cell type that selectively expresses this particular family member) probably has little to do with early atherogenesis. E-selectin preferentially recruits polymorphonuclear leukocytes, a cell type seldom, if ever, found in early atheroma (but an essential protagonist in acute inflammation and host defenses against bacterial pathogens).[20] Endothelial cells overlying atheroma do not express high levels of this adhesion molecule. Other members of this family, including P-selectin (P for "platelet," the original source of this adhesion molecule) may play a greater role in leukocyte recruitment in atheroma because endothelial cells overlying human atheroma do express this adhesion molecule. Selectins tend to promote saltatory or rolling locomotion of leukocytes over the endothelium. Adhesion molecules belonging to the immunoglobulin superfamily tend to promote tighter adhesive interactions and immobilization of leukocytes. Studies in genetically altered mice have proven roles for VCAM-1 and P-selectin (including both platelet- and endothelial-derived P-selectin) in experimental atherosclerosis.[19] Increasing evidence supports the accumulation in atheromas of mononuclear phagocytes of distinct subtypes. The functional consequences of this

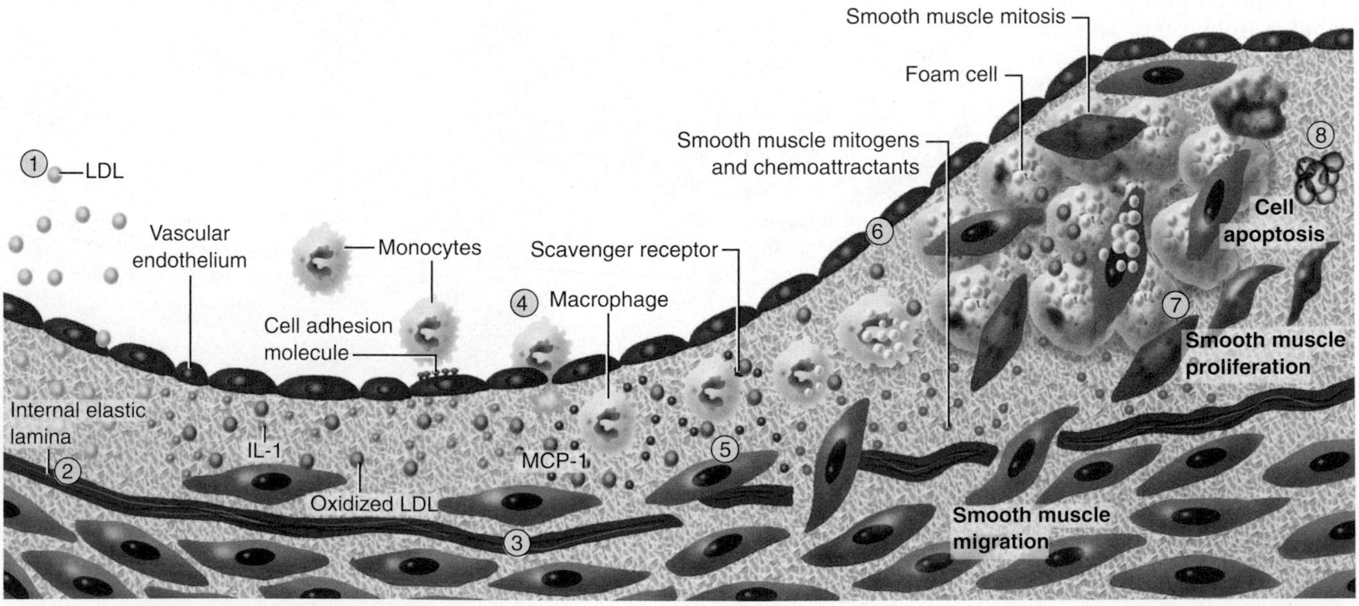

FIGURE 38–6 Schematic of the evolution of the atherosclerotic plaque. **1,** Accumulation of lipoprotein particles in the intima. The modification of these lipoproteins is depicted by the darker color. Modifications include oxidation and glycation. **2,** Oxidative stress including products found in modified lipoproteins can induce local cytokine elaboration. **3,** The cytokines thus induced increase expression of adhesion molecules for leukocytes that cause their attachment and chemoattractant molecules that direct their migration into the intima. **4,** Blood monocytes, on entering the artery wall in response to chemoattractant cytokines such as monocyte chemoattractant protein 1 (MCP-1), encounter stimuli such as macrophage colony-stimulating factor (M-CSF) that can augment their expression of scavenger receptors. **5,** Scavenger receptors mediate the uptake of modified lipoprotein particles and promote the development of foam cells. Macrophage foam cells are a source of mediators such as more cytokines and effector molecules such as hypochlorous acid, superoxide anion (O_2^-), and matrix metalloproteinases. **6,** SMCs in the intima divide, other SMCs migrate into the intima from the media. **7,** SMCs can then divide and elaborate extracellular matrix promoting extracellular matrix accumulation in the growing atherosclerotic plaque. In this manner, the fatty streak can evolve into a fibro-fatty lesion. **8,** In later stages, calcification can occur (not depicted), and fibrosis continues, sometimes accompanied by SMC death (including programmed cell death, or apoptosis) yielding a relatively acellular fibrous capsule surrounding a lipid-rich core that may also contain dying or dead cells and their detritus. IL-1 = interleukin-1; LDL = low-density lipoprotein, SMCs = smooth muscle cells.

selectivity of macrophage populations in plaques requires further study, especially in humans.[21-23]

Once adherent to the endothelium, leukocytes must receive a signal to penetrate the endothelial cells and enter the arterial wall (see Fig. 38-6, 4). The current concept of directed migration of leukocytes involves the action of protein molecules known as chemoattractant cytokines, or chemokines. Two groups of chemokines have particular interest in recruiting the mononuclear cells characteristic of the early atheroma. One such molecule, known as monocyte chemoattractant protein-1 (MCP-1), is produced by the endothelium in response to oxidized lipoprotein and other stimuli. Cells intrinsic to the normal artery, including endothelium and smooth muscle cells, can produce this chemokine when stimulated by inflammatory mediators, as do many other cell types. MCP-1 selectively promotes the directed migration, or chemotaxis, of monocytes. Studies conducted with genetically modified mice lacking MCP-1 or its receptor CCR-2 have delayed and attenuated atheroma formation when placed on an atherosclerosis-prone hyperlipidemic genetic background. Human atherosclerotic lesions express increased levels of MCP-1 compared to uninvolved vessels. Thus, several chemokines appear causally to contribute to monocyte recruitment during atherogenesis in vivo.[21] Interleukin-8, a chemokine that binds to CXCR2 on leukocytes, also participates in experimental atherosclerosis. Another unique cell-surface-bound chemokine, fractalkine, also appears to contribute to atherogenesis.[24] Another group of chemoattractant cytokines may heighten lymphocyte accumulation in plaques as well. Atheromas express a trio of lymphocyte-selective chemokines (IP-10, I-TAC, and MIG). Gamma interferon, a cytokine known to be present in atheromatous plaques, induces the genes encoding this family of T-cell chemoattractants.[25]

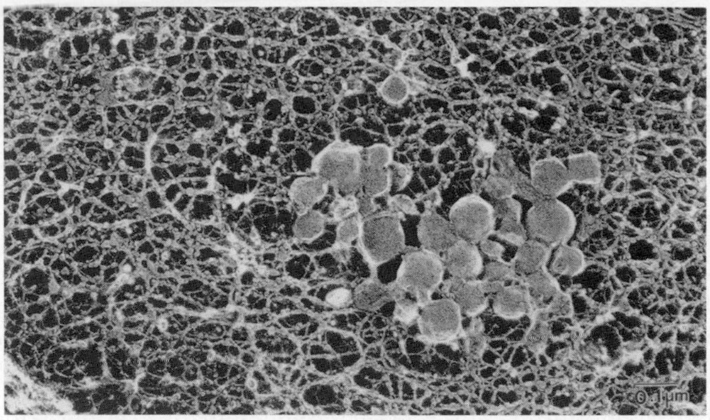

FIGURE 38–7 Scanning electron micrograph of a freeze-etch preparation of rabbit aorta that received an intravenous injection of human low-density lipoprotein. Round LDL particles decorate the strands of proteoglycan found in the subendothelial region of the intima. By binding LDL particles, proteoglycan molecules can retard their traversal of the intima and promote their accumulation. Proteoglycan-associated LDL appears particularly susceptible to oxidative modification. Accumulation of extracellular lipoprotein particles is one of the first morphological changes noted after initiation of an atherogenic diet in experimental animals. *(Reproduced from Nievelstein PF, Fogelman AM, Mottino G, Frank JS: Lipid accumulation in rabbit aortic intima 2 hours after bolus infusion of low-density lipoprotein. A deep-etch and immunolocalization study of ultrarapidly frozen tissue. Arterioscler Thromb 11:1795-1805, 1991.)*

The Focality of Lesion Formation

The spatial heterogeneity of atherosclerosis has proved challenging to explain in mechanistic terms. Equal concentrations of blood-borne risk factors such as lipoproteins bathe the endothelium throughout the vasculature. It is difficult to envisage how injury caused by inhaling cigarette smoke could produce any local rather than global effect on arteries. Yet, atheromas typically form focally, as revealed by studies of morphology, lipid accumulation, and adhesion molecule expression. Some investigators have invoked a multicentric origin hypothesis of atherogenesis, positing that atheromas arise as benign leiomyomata of the artery wall. The monotypia of various molecular markers such as glucose-6-phosphate dehydrogenase isoforms in individual atheroma supports this "monoclonal hypothesis" of atherogenesis. However, the location of sites of lesion predilection at proximal portions of arteries after branch points or bifurcations at flow dividers suggests a hydrodynamic basis for early lesion development. Arteries without many branches (e.g., the internal mammary or radial arteries) tend not to develop atherosclerosis.

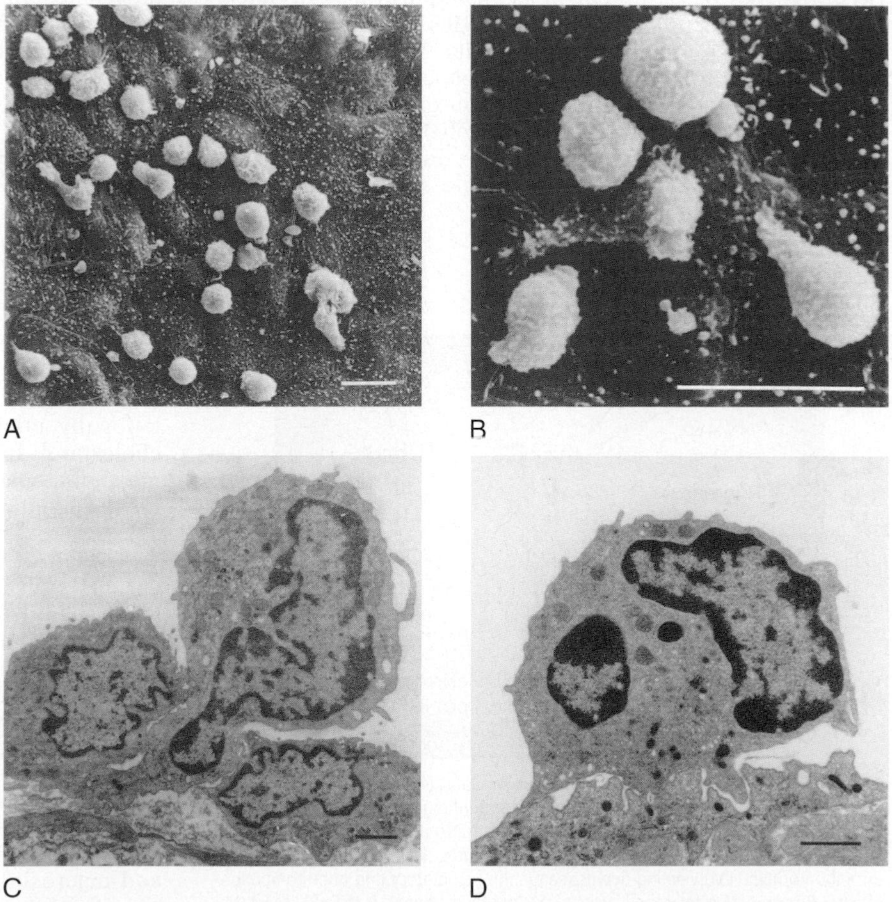

FIGURE 38–8 Electron microscopy of leukocyte interactions with the artery wall in hypercholesterolemic nonhuman primates. Panels **A** and **B,** show scanning electron micrographs that demonstrate the adhesion of mononuclear phagocytes to the intact endothelium 12 days after initiating a hypercholesterolemic diet in rabbits. **C** and **D** are transmission electron micrographs. Note the abundant interdigitations and intimate association of the monocyte with the endothelium in **C.** In **D,** a monocyte appears to diapedese between two endothelial cells to enter the intima. *(Reproduced from Faggiotto A, Ross R, Harker L: Studies of hypercholesterolemia in the nonhuman primate. I. Changes that lead to fatty streak formation. Arteriosclerosis 4:323-340, 1984.)*

Two concepts can help one to understand how local flow disturbances might render certain foci sites of lesion predilection. Locally disturbed flow could induce alterations that promote the steps of early atherogenesis. Alternatively, the laminar flow that usually prevails at sites that do not tend to develop early lesions may elicit antiatherogenic homeostatic mechanisms (atheroprotective functions).[26] The endothelial cell experiences the laminar shear stress of normal flow and the disturbed flow (usually yielding decreased shear stress) at predilected sites. In vitro data suggest that laminar shear stress can augment the expression of genes that may protect against atherosclerosis, including forms of the enzymes superoxide dismutase, or nitric oxide synthase. Superoxide dismutase can reduce oxidative stress by catabolizing the reactive and injurious superoxide anion. Endothelial nitric oxide synthase produces the well-known endogenous vasodilator, nitric oxide (•NO). However, beyond its vasodilating actions, •NO can resist inflammatory activation of endothelial functions such as expression of the adhesion molecule VCAM-1. Nitric oxide appears to exert this antiinflammatory action at the level of gene expression by interfering with the transcriptional regulator nuclear factor kappa B (NFκB). Nitric oxide actually increases the production of IκBα, an intracellular inhibitor of this important transcription factor. NFκB regulates numerous genes involved in inflammatory responses in general, and in atherogenesis in particular.[27]

Recent studies also implicate a transcription factor (Krupple-like factor-2, KLF-2) as an important regulator of endothelial antiinflammatory properties.[28] KLF2 can induce eNOS expression and KLF2 inhibits NFκB function by sequestering co-factors needed to boost NFκB transcriptional activity, resulting in inhibition of the expression of the cassette of KFκB-dependent genes involved in the inflammatory pathways that operate during atherogenesis (Fig. 38-9). Laminar shear stress can also limit expression of another regulator of endothelial function: thioredoxin-interacting protein (Txnip).[29] Txnip inhibits the action of thioredoxin. Increased thioredoxin in regions of laminar shear stress caused by decreased Txnip levels in turn augments activity of apoptosis signal-regulating kinase 1 (ASK1), an activator of JNK and p38. This pathway attenuates JNK and p38 activation by proinflammatory cytokines including tumor necrosis factor (see Fig. 38-9). Thus, several separate athero-protective mechanisms operate such that under usual conditions of laminar shear stress in normal arteries, the endothelium tonically expresses locally acting antiinflammatory functions.[27]

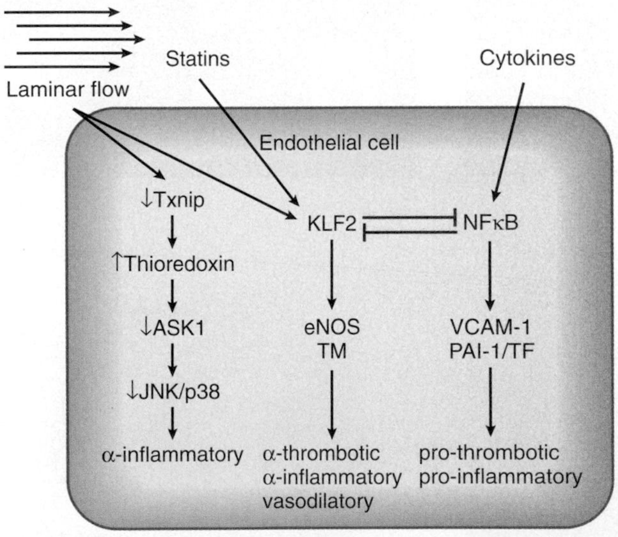

FIGURE 38–9 Novel transcriptional mechanisms that link shear stress to altered expression of genes that influence thrombosis and inflammation. Laminar shear stress can activate Krupple-like factor 2 (KLF2), a transcription factor that activates endothelial nitric oxide synthase (eNOS) that generates nitric oxide as well as thrombomodulin (TM) yielding downstream antiinflammatory and antithrombotic effects. By competing for coactivators of nuclear factor kappa B (NFκB), KLF2 activation attenuates its downstream proinflammatory, prothrombotic, and antifibrinolytic effects mediated by adhesion molecules such as vascular cell adhesion molecule-1 (VCAM-1), plasminogen activator inhibitor-1 (PAI-1) and tissue factor procoagulant (TF). Laminar flow also activates Txnip (thioredoxin interacting protein) that, in turn, augments thioredoxin function, attenuating apoptosis-signal regulating kinase 1 (ASK1), and hence, suppressing Jun kinase (JNK) and the kinase p38, ultimately leading to reduced inflammation. α denotes "anti."

These examples show how basic vascular biology has yielded insights into previously obscure yet important aspects of atherogenesis. Future study of the molecular regulation of vascular cell function by mechanical stimuli should clarify the mechanisms of lesion formation at particular sites in the circulation. Likewise, study of vascular developmental biology may aid understanding of the tendency of certain arteries to develop atherosclerosis at different rates and in different ways. As noted earlier, SMCs vary in embryologic origin in different regions.[12,30] For example, upper body arteries can recruit smooth muscle from neurectoderm, whereas in the lower body SMCs derive principally from mesoderm (see Fig. 38-3). Coronary artery SMCs arise from an anlage known as the proepicardial organ. After injury or transplantation, arteries can repopulate with SMCs derived from bone marrow.[31] How this heterogeneity in the origin of SMCs might affect human atherosclerosis and how it may help to explain some of the poorly understood issues regarding dispersion of atheroma in time and space is intriguing yet speculative.

Intracellular Lipid Accumulation: Foam-Cell Formation

The monocyte, once recruited to the arterial intima, can there imbibe lipid and become a foam cell, or lipid-laden macrophage (see Fig. 38-6, 5 and 6). While most cells can express the classic cell surface receptor for low-density lipoprotein, that receptor does not mediate foam cell accumulation (see Chap. 42). This is evident clinically because patients lacking functional LDL receptors (familial hypercholesterolemia homozygotes) still develop tendinous xanthomata filled with foamy macrophages. The LDL receptor does not mediate foam cell formation because of its exquisite regulation by cholesterol. As soon as a cell collects enough cholesterol from low-density lipoprotein capture for its metabolic needs, an elegant transcriptional control mechanism quenches expression of the receptor (see also Chap. 42).

Instead of the classic low-density lipoprotein receptor, various molecules known as "scavenger" receptors appear to mediate the excessive lipid uptake characteristic of foam cell formation.[32,33] The longest studied of these receptors belongs to the scavenger receptor-A family. These surface molecules bind modified, rather than native, lipoproteins and apparently participate in their internalization. Atherosclerosis-prone mice with mutations that delete functional scavenger receptor-A have less exuberant fatty lesion formation than those with functional scavenger receptor-A molecules. Other receptors that bind modified lipoprotein and that may participate in foam cell formation include CD36 and macrosialin, the latter exhibiting preferential binding specificity for oxidized forms of LDL. (See Chap. 42 for a table of scavenger receptors.)

Once macrophages have taken up residence in the intima and become foam cells, they replicate. The factors that trigger macrophage cell division in the atherosclerotic plaque likely include macrophage-colony stimulating factor (M-CSF). This co-mitogen and survival factor for mononuclear phagocytes exists in human and experimental atheromatous lesions. Again, atherosclerosis-prone mice that lack functional M-CSF have retarded fatty lesion development as well. Other candidates for macrophage mitogens or co-mitogens include interleukin 3 (IL-3) and granulocyte-macrophage colony stimulating factor (GM-CSF).[25] Up to this point in the development of the nascent atheroma, the lesion consists primarily of lipid-engorged macrophages. Complex features such as fibrosis, thrombosis, and calcification do not characterize the fatty streak—the precursor lesion of the complex atheroma. Several lines of evidence suggest that such fatty streaks may be reversible, at least to some extent.

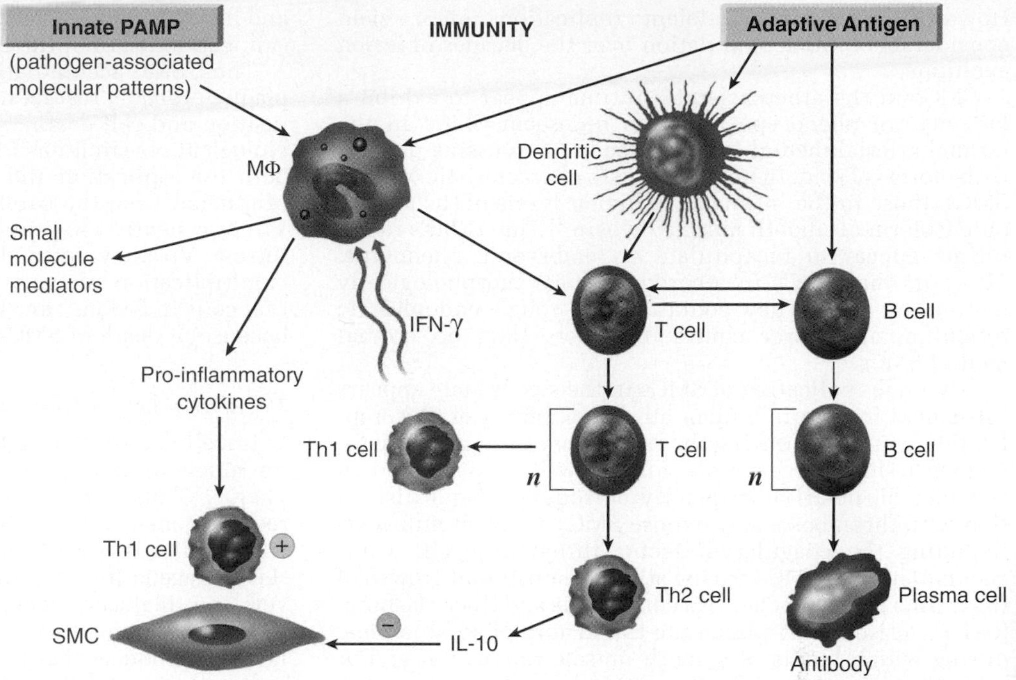

FIGURE 38–10 Innate and adaptive immunity in atherosclerosis. A diagram of the pathways of innate **(left)** and adaptive **(right)** immunity operating during atherogenesis. MΦ = macrophage, IFN-γ = interferon gamma, Th = T helper. *(Adapted from Hansson G, Libby P, Schoenbeck U, Yan Z-Q: Innate and adaptive immunity in the pathogenesis of atherosclerosis. Circ Res 91:281-291, 2002.)*

THE EVOLUTION OF ATHEROMA

Innate and Adaptive Immunity: Mechanisms of Inflammation in Atherogenesis

Over the last decade, basic evidence and clinical evidence have converged, demonstrating a fundamental role for inflammation in atherogenesis (see also Chap. 39).[34-38] The macrophage foam cells recruited to the artery wall early in this process serve as a reservoir for excess lipid. In the established atherosclerotic lesion, these cells also provide a rich source of proinflammatory mediators—proteins such as cytokines and chemokines and various eicosanoids and lipids such as platelet-activating factor. These phagocytic cells also can elaborate large quantities of oxidant species such as superoxide anion in the milieu of the atherosclerotic plaque. This ensemble of mediators can promote inflammation in the plaque and thus contribute to the progression of lesions. The term *innate immunity* describes this type of amplification of the inflammatory response that does not depend on antigenic stimulation (Fig. 38-10).

In addition to innate immunity, mounting evidence supports a prominent role for antigen-specific or adaptive immunity in plaque progression.[34,35] In addition to the mononuclear phagocytes, dendritic cells in atherosclerotic lesion can present antigens to the T cells that constitute an important minority of the leukocytes in the atherosclerotic lesion. Candidate antigens for stimulating this adaptive immune response include modified lipoproteins, heat shock proteins, beta$_2$ glycoprotein Ib, and infectious agents. The antigen-presenting cells (macrophages, dendritic cells, or endothelial cells) allow the antigen to interact with T cells in a manner that triggers their activation. The activated T cells then can secrete copious quantities of cytokines that can modulate atherogenesis.

The T helper cells (bearing CD4) fall into two general categories. Cells of the T helper 1 subtype elaborate proinflammatory cytokines such as interferon gamma, lymphotoxin, CD40 ligand, and tumor necrosis factor-alpha. This panel of Th1 cytokines can, in turn, activate vascular wall cells and orchestrate alterations in plaque biology that can lead to plaque destabilization and heightened thrombogenicity. On the other hand, helper T cells slanted toward the production of Th2 cytokines such as interleukin 10 can inhibit inflammation in the context of atherogenesis.[39] Cytolytic T cells (bearing CD8) can express *fas* ligand and other cytotoxic factors that can promote cytolysis and apoptosis of target cells including smooth muscle and endothelial cells, and macrophages (see Fig. 38-6, 8).[40,41] The death of all three of these cell types can occur in the atherosclerotic lesion and may contribute to plaque progression and complication. Regulatory T cells (Treg) can elaborate transforming growth factor (TGF)-β as well as IL-10. Treg lymphocytes bear the markers CD4 and CD25. Both TGF-β and IL-10 can exert antiinflammatory effects.[42] Several experimental preparations suggest an antiatherosclerotic function of Treg cells in vivo.[37] The role of B cells and antibody in atherosclerosis remains incompletely explored. Humoral immunity may have either atheroprotective or atherogenic properties depending on the circumstances.

Smooth Muscle Cell Migration and Proliferation

The early events in atheroma initiation involve primarily altered endothelial function and recruitment and accumulation of leukocytes, whereas the subsequent evolution of atheroma into more complex plaques involves SMCs as well (see Fig. 38-6, 6 and 7). SMCs in the normal arterial tunica media differ considerably from those in the intima of an evolving atheroma.[10,43] While some SMCs likely arrive in the arterial intima early in life, others that accumulate in advancing atheroma likely arise from cells that have migrated from the underlying media into the intima. The chemoattractants for SMCs likely include molecules such as platelet-derived growth factor (PDGF), a potent SMC chemoattractant secreted by activated macrophages and overexpressed in human atherosclerosis. These SMCs in the atherosclerotic intima can also multiply by cell division. Estimated rates of division of SMCs in the human atherosclerotic lesion are on the order of less than 1 percent.

However, even such indolent replication might yield considerable SMC accumulation over the decades of lesion evolution.

SMCs in the atherosclerotic intima appear to exhibit a less mature phenotype than the quiescent SMCs in the normal arterial medial layer. Instead of expressing primarily isoforms of smooth muscle myosin characteristic of adult SMCs, those in the intima have higher levels of the embryonic isoform of smooth muscle myosin.[43] Thus, SMCs in the intima appear to recapitulate an embryonic phenotype. These intimal SMCs in atheroma appear morphologically distinct as well. They contain more rough endoplasmic reticulum and fewer contractile fibers than do normal medial SMCs.

Although replication of SMCs in the steady state appears infrequent in mature human atheroma, bursts of SMC replication may occur during the life history of a given atheromatous lesion. For example, and as will be discussed in considerable detail subsequently, episodes of plaque disruption with thrombosis may expose SMCs to potent mitogens, including the coagulation factor thrombin itself. Thus, accumulation of SMCs during atherosclerosis and growth of the intima may not occur in a continuous and linear fashion. Rather, "crises" may punctuate the history of an atheroma, during which bursts of smooth muscle replication and/or migration may occur (Fig. 38-11).

Smooth Muscle Cell Death During Atherogenesis

In addition to SMC replication, death of these cells may also participate in complication of the atherosclerotic plaque (see Fig. 38-6, 8). At least some SMCs in advanced human atheroma exhibit fragmentation of their nuclear DNA characteristic of programmed cell death, or apoptosis.[40,41] Apoptosis may occur in response to inflammatory cytokines present in the evolving atheroma. In addition to soluble cytokines that may trigger programmed cell death, the T cells in atheroma may participate in eliminating some SMCs. In particular, certain T cell populations known to accumulate in plaques can express *fas* ligand on their surface. *Fas* ligand can engage *fas* on the surface of SMCs, and in conjunction with soluble proinflammatory cytokines, can lead to death of the SMC.[40,44,45]

Thus, SMC accumulation in the growing atherosclerotic plaque probably results from a tug-of-war between cell replication and cell death.[40] Contemporary cell and molecular biological research has identified candidates for mediating both the replication and attrition of SMCs, a concept that originated from the careful morphological observations of Virchow nearly 150 years ago. Referring to the SMCs in the intima, Virchow noted that early atherogenesis involves a "multiplication of their nuclei." However, he recognized that cells in lesions can "hurry on to their own destruction" because of death of SMCs.

The Arterial Extracellular Matrix

Extracellular matrix rather than cells themselves makes up much of the volume of an advanced atherosclerotic plaque. Thus, extracellular constituents of plaque also require consideration. The major extracellular matrix macromolecules that accumulate in atheroma include interstitial collagens (types I and III) and proteoglycans such as versican, biglycan, aggrecan, and decorin.[46] Elastin fibers may also accumulate in atherosclerotic plaques. The vascular SMC produces these matrix molecules in disease, just as it does during development and maintenance of the normal artery (see Fig. 38-6, 7). Stimuli for excessive collagen production by SMCs include platelet-derived growth factor and TGF-β, a constituent of platelet granules, and a product of many cell types found in lesions including regulatory T cells (Treg).

Much like the accumulation of SMCs, extracellular matrix secretion also depends on a balance, as noted earlier. In this case, the biosynthesis of the extracellular matrix molecules is balanced by breakdown catalyzed in part by catabolic enzymes known as matrix metalloproteinases (MMPs). Dissolution of extracellular matrix macromolecules undoubtedly plays a role in migration of SMCs as they penetrate into the intima from the media through a dense extracellular matrix, traversing the elastin-rich internal elastic lamina. In injured arteries, overexpression of such proteinase inhibitors (known as tissue inhibitors of metalloproteinases, or TIMPs) can delay smooth muscle accumulation in the intima of injured arteries.[47]

Extracellular matrix dissolution also likely plays a role in arterial remodeling that accompanies lesion growth. During the first part of the life history of an atheromatous lesion, growth of the plaque is outward, in an abluminal direction, rather than inward in a way that would lead to luminal stenosis. This outward growth of the intima leads to an increase in caliber of the entire artery. This so-called *positive* remodeling or *compensatory enlargement* must involve turnover of extracellular matrix molecules to accommodate the circumferential growth of the artery. Luminal stenosis tends to occur only after the plaque burden exceeds about 40 percent of the cross-sectional area of the artery.

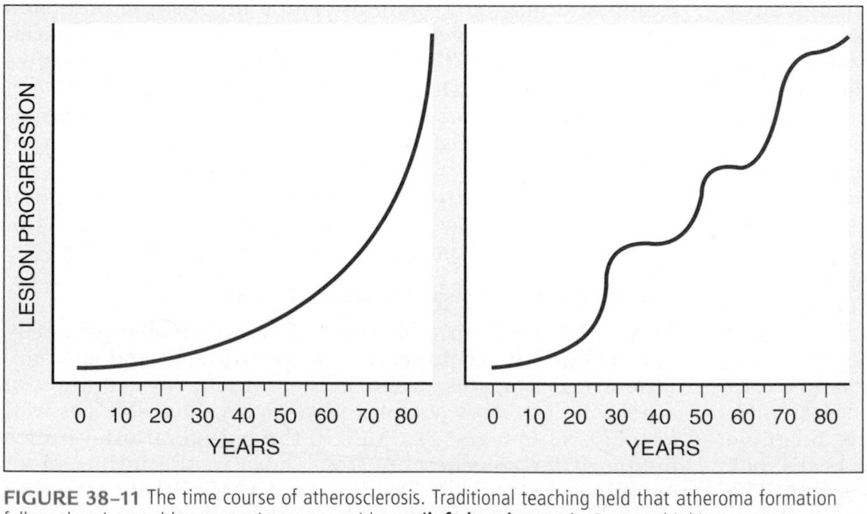

FIGURE 38–11 The time course of atherosclerosis. Traditional teaching held that atheroma formation followed an inexorably progressive course with age **(left-hand curve).** Current thinking suggests an alternative model, a step function rather than a monotonically upward course of lesion evolution in time **(right hand curve).** According to this latter model, "crises" can punctuate periods of relative quiescence during the life history of a lesion. Such crises might follow an episode of plaque disruption, with mural thrombosis, and healing, yielding a spurt in smooth muscle proliferation and matrix deposition. Intraplaque hemorrhage caused by rupture of a friable microvessel might produce a similar scenario. Such episodes might usually be clinically inapparent. Extravascular events such as an intercurrent infection with systemic cytokinemia or endotoxemia could elicit an "echo" at the level of the artery wall, evoking a round of local cytokine gene expression by "professional" inflammatory leukocytes resident in the lesion. The episodic model of plaque progression shown on the **right** fits human angiographic data better than the continuous function, depicted on the **left.**

Angiogenesis in Plaques

The SMC is not alone in its proliferation and migration within the evolving atherosclerotic plaque. Endothelial migration and replication also occur as plaques develop a microcirculation, characterized by plexi of newly formed vessels. Such plaque neovessels usually require special stains for visualization. However, histological examination with appropriate markers for endothelial cells reveals a rich neovascularization in evolving plaques. These microvessels likely form in response to angiogenic peptides overexpressed in atheroma. These angiogenesis factors include acidic and basic fibroblast growth factors, vascular endothelial growth factor (VEGF), placental growth factor (PlGF), and oncostatin M.[48,49]

These microvessels within plaques probably have considerable functional significance. For example, the abundant microvessels in plaques provide a relatively large surface area for the trafficking of leukocytes, which could include both entry and exit of leukocytes. Indeed, in the advanced human atherosclerotic plaque, microvascular endothelium displays the mononuclear-selective adhesion molecules such as VCAM-1 much more prominently than does the macrovascular endothelium overlying the plaque. The microvascularization of plaques may also allow growth of the plaque overcoming diffusion limitations on oxygen and nutrient supply, in analogy with the concept of tumor angiogenic factors and growth of malignant lesions. Consistent with this view, administration of inhibitors of angiogenesis to mice with experimentally induced atherosclerosis limits lesion expansion. Finally, the plaque microvessels may be friable and prone to rupture similar to the neovessels in the diabetic retina.[50] Hemorrhage and thrombosis in situ could promote a local round of SMC proliferation and matrix accumulation in the area immediately adjacent to the microvascular disruption (Fig. 38-12). This scenario illustrates a special case of one of the "crises" described earlier in the evolution of the atheromatous plaque (see Fig. 38-11). Attempts to augment myocardial perfusion by enhancing new vessel growth by transfer of angiogenic proteins, or their genes, might have adverse effects on lesion growth or clinical complications of atheroma by these mechanisms.

Plaque Mineralization

Plaques often develop areas of calcification as they evolve. Indeed, both Virchow and Rokitansky recognized morphological features of bone formation in atherosclerotic plaques in early microscopic descriptions of atherosclerosis. In recent years, understanding of the mechanism of mineralization during evolution of atherosclerotic plaques has advanced. Some subpopulations of SMCs may foster calcification by enhanced secretion of cytokines such as bone morphogenetic proteins, homologues of TGF-β.[51] Atheromatous plaques may also contain proteins with gamma carboxylated glutamic acid residues specialized in sequestering calcium and thus promoting mineralization.

COMPLICATIONS OF ATHEROSCLEROSIS

Arterial Stenoses and Their Clinical Implications

The previous sections have discussed the initiation and evolution of the atherosclerotic plaque. These phases of the atherosclerotic process generally last many years, during which the affected individual often has no symptoms. After the plaque burden exceeds the capacity of the artery to remodel outward, encroachment on the arterial lumen begins. During the chronic asymptomatic or stable phase of lesion evolution, growth probably occurs discontinuously, with periods of relative quiescence punctuated by episodes of rapid progression (see Fig. 38-11). Human angiographic studies support this discontinuous growth of coronary artery stenoses. Eventually the stenoses may progress to a degree that impedes blood flow through the artery. Lesions that produce stenoses of greater than 60 percent can cause flow limitations under conditions of increased demand. This type of athero-occlusive disease commonly produces chronic stable angina pectoris or intermittent claudication on increased demand. Thus, the symptomatic phase of atherosclerosis usually occurs many decades after lesion initiation.

In many cases of myocardial infarction, however, no history of stable angina heralds the acute event. Several kinds of clinical observation suggest that many myocardial infarctions result not from high-grade stenoses, but from lesions that do not limit flow. For example, in individuals who have undergone coronary arteriography in the months preceding myocardial infarction, the culprit lesion most often shows less than 50 percent stenosis. In a compilation of four such serial angiographic studies, only approximately 15 percent of acute myocardial infarctions arise from lesions

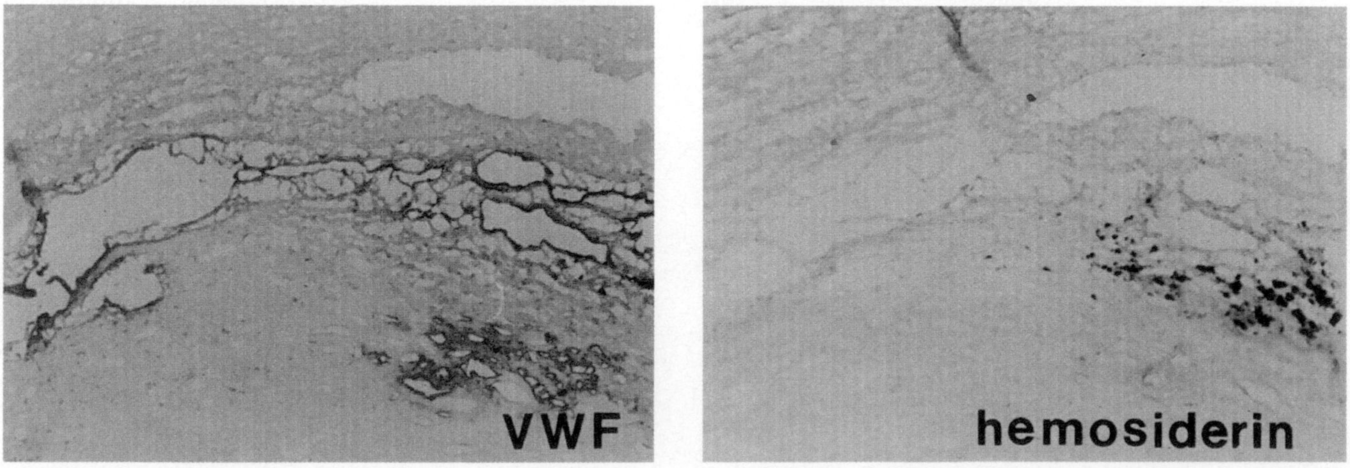

FIGURE 38–12 Intraplaque hemorrhage. A typical human atherosclerotic plaque stained for von Willebrand factor **(left)** and iron by Prussian blue **(right).** The von Willebrand factor stains the endothelial cells that line the microvascular channels and lakes. Note the extravasated von Willebrand factor, that colocalizes with iron deposition, indicating hemosiderin deposition consistent with an intraplaque hemorrhage. *(After Brogi E, Winkles JA, Underwood R, et al: Distinct patterns of expression of fibroblast growth factors and their receptors in human atheroma and non-atherosclerotic arteries: Association of acidic FGF with plaque microvessels and macrophages. J Clin Invest 92:2408-2418, 1993.)*

with degrees of stenosis greater than 60 percent on an antecedent angiogram.[52]

Instead of progressive growth of the intimal lesion to a critical stenosis, we now recognize that thrombosis, complicating a not necessarily occlusive plaque, most often causes episodes of unstable angina or acute myocardial infarction. Angiographic studies performed in individuals undergoing thrombolysis support this view. In one such study, almost one-half of patients undergoing thrombolysis for a first myocardial infarction had an underlying stenosis of less than 50 percent after the acute thrombus was lysed.

These findings do not imply that small atheroma cause most myocardial infarctions. Indeed, culprit lesions of acute myocardial infarction actually may be sizeable. However, they may not produce a critical luminal narrowing because of the phenomenon of compensatory enlargement.[53] Of course, critical stenoses do cause myocardial infarctions. In fact, the high-grade stenoses are more likely to cause acute myocardial infarction than nonocclusive lesions. However, because the noncritical stenoses by far outnumber the tight focal lesions in a given coronary tree, the lesser stenoses cause more infarctions, even though high-grade stenoses have a greater individual probability of causing myocardial infarction.

Thrombosis and Atheroma Complication

This evolution in our view of the pathogenesis of the acute coronary syndromes places new emphasis on thrombosis as the critical mechanism of transition from chronic to acute atherosclerosis. Understanding of the mechanisms of coronary thrombosis has advanced considerably. We now appreciate that a physical disruption of the atherosclerotic plaque commonly causes acute thrombosis. Several major modes of plaque disruption provoke most coronary thrombi.[52,54] The first mechanism, accounting for nearly two-thirds of acute myocardial infarctions, involves a fracture of the fibrous cap of the plaque (Fig. 38-13). Another mode involves a superficial erosion of the intima (Fig. 38-14), accounting for up to one-quarter of acute myocardial infarctions in highly selected referral cases from medical examiners on individuals who have succumbed to sudden cardiac death. Superficial erosion appears more frequently in women than in men as a mechanism of sudden cardiac death.[54]

Plaque Rupture and Thrombosis

The rupture of the plaque's fibrous cap probably reflects an imbalance between the forces that impinge on the plaque's cap and the mechanical strength of the fibrous cap. Interstitial forms of collagen provide most of the biomechanical resistance to disruption to the fibrous cap. Hence, the metabolism of collagen probably participates in regulating the propensity of a plaque to rupture (Fig. 38-15). Factors that decrease collagen synthesis by SMCs can impair their ability to repair and maintain the plaque's fibrous cap. For example, on the one hand the T cell–derived cytokine interferon gamma potently inhibits SMC collagen synthesis. On the other hand, as already noted, certain mediators released from platelet granules during activation can increase SMC collagen synthesis, tending to reinforce the fibrous structure of the plaque. Such mediators include TGF-β and PDGF.

In addition to reduced de novo collagen synthesis by SMCs, increased catabolism of the extracellular matrix macromolecules that comprise the fibrous cap can also contribute to weakening this structure and rendering it susceptible to rupture, and hence thrombosis. The same matrix-degrading enzymes thought to contribute to smooth muscle migration and arterial remodeling may contribute to weakening of the fibrous cap as well (see Fig. 38-15). Macrophages in advanced human atheroma overexpress matrix metalloproteinases and elastolytic cathepsins that can break down the collagen and elastin of the arterial extracellular matrix. Thus, the strength of the plaque's fibrous cap is under dynamic regulation, linking the inflammatory response in the intima with the molecular determinants of plaque stability and hence, thrombotic complications of atheroma. The thinning of the plaque's fibrous cap, a result of reduced collagen synthesis and increased degradation, probably explains why pathological studies have shown that the thin fibrous cap characterizes atherosclerotic plaques that have ruptured and caused fatal myocardial infarction.

Another feature of the so-called *vulnerable* atherosclerotic plaque defined by pathological analysis is a relative lack of SMCs (see Fig. 38-13B). As explained

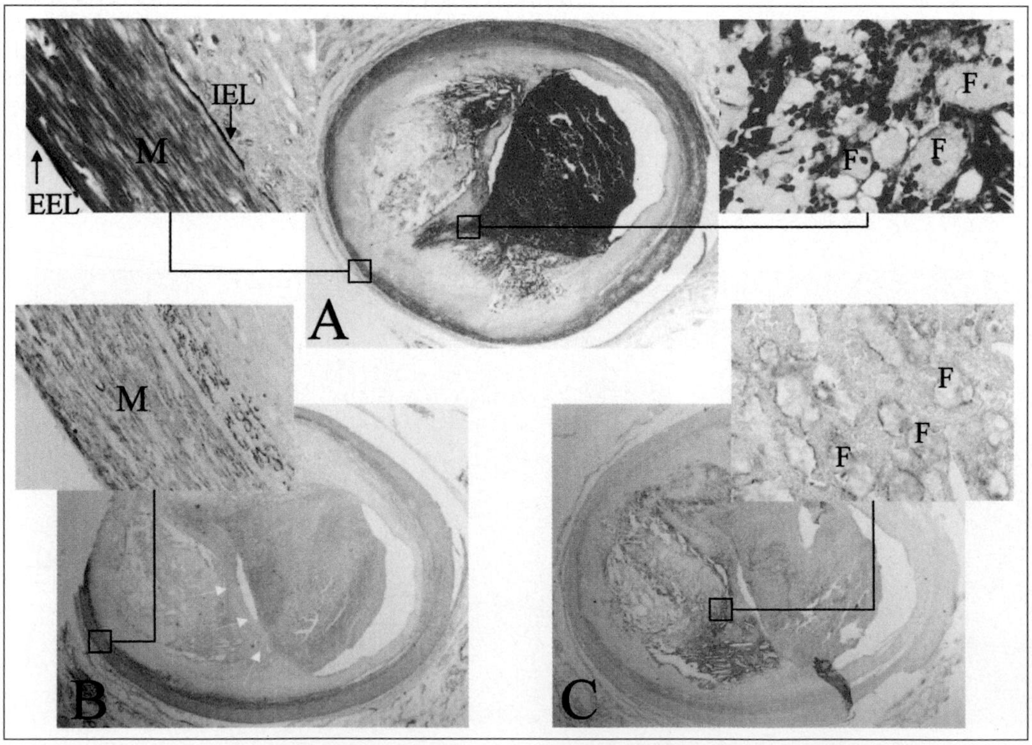

FIGURE 38–13 An example of a ruptured plaque that caused a fatal thrombosis. **A,** Movat stain. **B,** Immunostaining with HHF-35 discloses SMCs. Note the paucity of SMCs in the fibrous cap (white arrowheads), in contrast with the abundant SMCs in the medial layer (inset, M denotes the tunica media). **C,** Macrophage staining (CD-68) shows accumulation of the inflammatory cells near the fibrous cap (inset, F denotes foam cell). EEL = external elastic lamina; IEL = internal elastic lamina. *(Reproduced from Bezerra HG, Higuchi ML, Gutierrez PS, et al: Atheromas that cause fatal thrombosis are usually large and frequently accompanied by vessel enlargement. Cardiovasc Pathol 10:189-196, 2001.)*

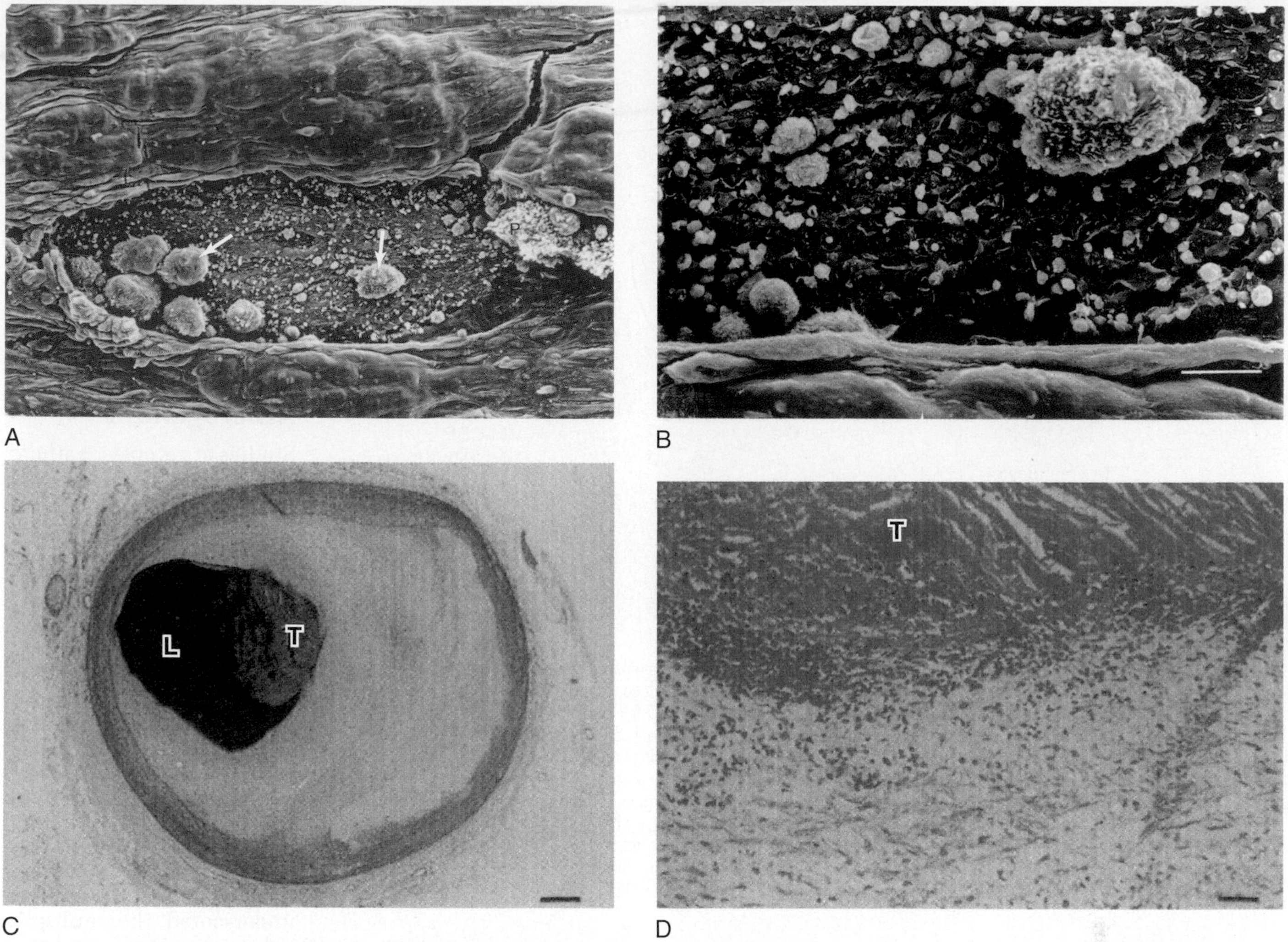

FIGURE 38–14 Superficial erosion of experimental atherosclerotic lesions shown by scanning electron microscopy. Advanced atherosclerotic plaques can promote thrombosis by superficial erosion of the endothelial layer exposing the blood and platelets to the subendothelial basement membrane containing collagen platelet activation and thrombosis. **A,** In the low power view, the rent in endothelium is evident. Leukocytes have adhered to the subendothelium, which is beginning to be covered with a carpet of platelets. **B,** The high power view shows a field selected from the center of **A** that shows the leukocytes and platelets adherent to the subendothelium. **C,** A low-power histological section through a coronary artery thrombosed because of superficial erosion. L = lumen; T = thrombus. **D,** A higher power histological section through a coronary artery thrombosed because of superficial erosion. *(**A** and **B** reproduced from Faggiotto A, Ross R: Studies of hypercholesterolemia in the nonhuman primate. II. Fatty streak conversion to fibrous plaque. Arteriosclerosis 341-356, 1984; **C** and **D** reproduced from Farb A, Burke AP, Tang AL, et al: Coronary plaque erosion without rupture into a lipid core: A frequent cause of coronary thrombosis in sudden coronary death. Circulation 93:1354, 1996.)*

earlier, inflammatory mediators—both soluble and associated with the surface of T-lymphocytes—can provoke programmed cell death of SMCs. "Dropout" of SMCs from regions of local inflammation within plaques probably contributes to the relative lack of SMCs at places where plaques rupture.[40,45] Because these cells are the source of the newly synthesized collagen needed to repair and maintain the matrix of the fibrous cap, the lack of SMCs may contribute to weakening of the fibrous cap and, hence, the propensity of that plaque to rupture.

A prominent accumulation of macrophages and a large lipid pool is a third microanatomical feature of the vulnerable atherosclerotic plaque. From a strictly biomechanical viewpoint, a large lipid pool can concentrate biomechanical forces on the shoulder regions of plaques, common sites of rupture of the fibrous cap. From a metabolic standpoint, the activated macrophage characteristic of the plaque's core region produces the cytokines and the matrix-degrading enzymes thought to regulate aspects of matrix catabolism and SMC apoptosis in turn. Apoptotic macrophages as well as SMCs can generate particulate tissue factor, a potential instigator of microvascular thrombosis after spontaneous or iatrogenic plaque disruption. The success of lipid-lowering therapy in reducing the incidence of acute myocardial infarction or unstable angina in patients at risk may result from a reduced accumulation of lipid and decrease in inflammation and plaque thrombogenicity. Recent animal studies and monitoring of peripheral markers of inflammation in humans support this concept (see also Chaps. 50, 51, and 53).[55,56]

Thrombosis Caused by Superficial Erosion of Plaques

The foregoing section discusses the pathophysiology of rupture of the plaque's fibrous cap. The pathobiology of superficial erosion is much less well understood. In experimental atherosclerosis in the nonhuman primate, areas of endothelial loss and platelet deposition occur in the more advanced plaques (see Fig. 38-14). In humans, superficial erosion appears more likely to cause fatal acute myocardial infarction in women and in individuals with hypertriglyceridemia and diabetes mellitus. However, the underlying

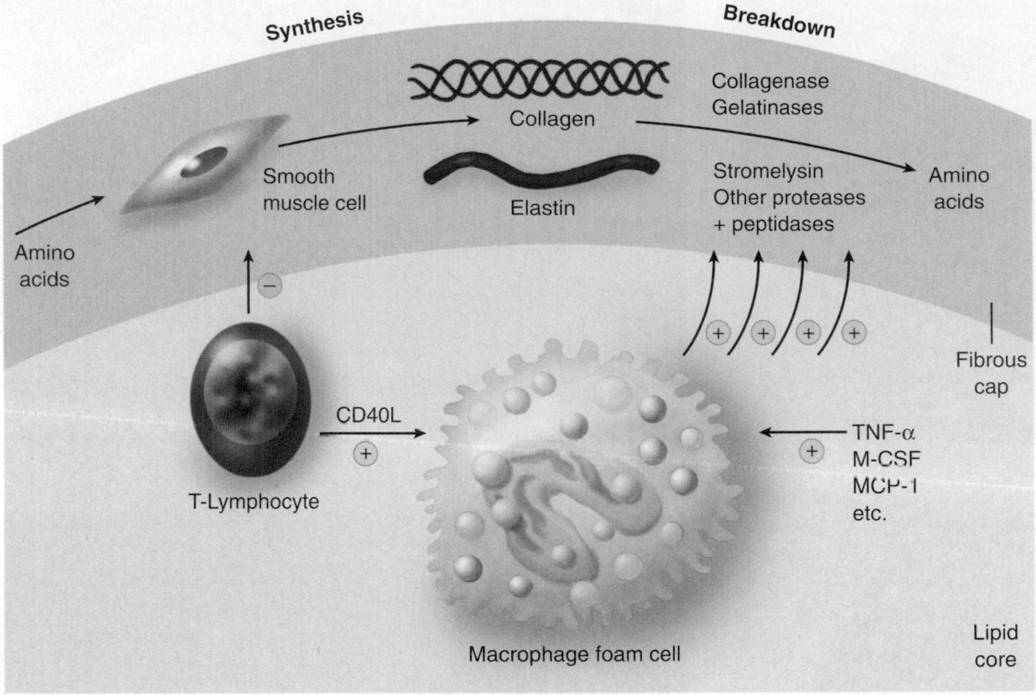

FIGURE 38–15 A schematic relating extracellular matrix metabolism to intimal inflammation during atherogenesis. The lymphocyte can elaborate gamma interferon (IFN-γ) that inhibits SMC collagen production. The lymphocyte can also signal either by elaboration of soluble mediators or by contact activation of macrophages. Other cytokines produced in response to products of oxidized lipoproteins, among other stimuli, can further activate the macrophage. The activated phagocyte can release collagen degrading matrix metalloproteinases, and elastolytic enzymes including certain nonmetalloenzymes, such as cathepsins S and K. These enzymes promote matrix catabolism. Thus, in states characterized by heightened intimal inflammation, the extracellular matrix that confers biomechanical strength to the plaque's fibrous cap is under double attack: decreased synthesis and increased degradation. This results in a weakening and thinning of the fibrous cap, features associated in pathological studies with fatal atheromatous plaque disruptions and thrombosis. TNF-α = tumor necrosis factor-alpha; M-CSF = macrophage colony stimulating factor; MCP-1 = monocyte chemoattractant protein-1. *(Reproduced from Libby P: The molecular bases of the acute coronary syndromes. Circulation 91:2844-2850, 1995.)*

molecular mechanisms remain obscure. Apoptosis of endothelial cells could contribute to desquamation of endothelial cells in areas of superficial erosion. Likewise, matrix metalloproteinases such as certain gelatinases specialized in degrading the nonfibrillar collagen found in the basement membrane (e.g., collagen type IV), might also sever the tetherings of the endothelial cell to the subjacent basal lamina and promote their desquamation.[57]

Most plaque disruptions do not give rise to clinically apparent coronary events. Careful pathoanatomical examination of hearts obtained from individuals who have succumbed to noncardiac death have shown a surprisingly high incidence of focal plaque disruptions with limited mural thrombi. Moreover, hearts fixed in patients immediately after explantation from individuals with severe but chronic stable coronary atherosclerosis and who had undergone transplantation for ischemic cardiomyopathy show similar evidence for ongoing but asymptomatic plaque disruption. Experimentally, in atherosclerotic nonhuman primates, mural platelet thrombi can complicate plaque erosions without causing arterial occlusion. Therefore, repetitive cycles of plaque disruption, thrombosis in situ, and healing probably contribute to lesion evolution and plaque growth. Such episodes of thrombosis and healing constitute one type of "crisis" in the history of a plaque that may cause a burst of SMC proliferation, migration, and matrix synthesis (see Fig. 38-11). The TGF-β and PDGF released from platelet granules stimulate collagen synthesis by SMCs as noted above. Thrombin, generated at sites of mural thrombosis, potently stimulates SMC proliferation. The late stage or "burned out" fibrous and calcific atheroma may repre-sent a late stage of a plaque previously lipid-rich and vulnerable but now rendered fibrous and hypocellular because of a wound-healing response mediated by the products of thrombosis.

The Diffuse and Systemic Nature of Plaque Vulnerability and Inflammation in Atherogenesis

Studies at autopsy of atherosclerotic plaques that caused fatal thrombosis brought the notion of vulnerable high-risk plaque to the fore. This stimulated many investigators to seek ways of identifying and treating such high risk atherosclerotic lesions. Current evidence, however, suggests that more than one such high risk plaque often resides in a given coronary tree.[58] Moreover, the inflammation thought to characterize the so-called *vulnerable* plaque appears widespread. Studies using various imaging modalities have underscored the multiplicity of such high-risk plaques. Careful analysis of angiograms of individuals with acute coronary syndromes has demonstrated evidence for plaque ulceration or thrombosis in more than one lesion in many cases. Individuals with multiple unstable lesions by angiographic criteria tend to have worse outcomes during follow-up. Angioscopic studies have also shown multiple sites of intracoronary thrombosis in patients with acute coronary syndromes. Systematic studies by intravascular ultrasound of the coronary arterial system in individuals with acute coronary syndromes have revealed that more than 80 percent of such individuals have more than one disrupted atherosclerotic plaque.

Several concordant lines of evidence support the systemic and diffuse nature of inflammation in individuals with acute coronary syndromes. Maseri's group demonstrated a transmyocardial gradient in the inflammatory marker myeloperoxidase when sampling from the great cardiac vein (draining the left coronary territory) in individuals with both left and right coronary artery culprit lesions.[59,60] Multiple studies have shown that various systemic markers of inflammation such as C-reactive protein increase in patients at risk for acute coronary syndromes. This is so even in the absence of biochemical evidence of myocardial injury (e.g., elevated troponin levels) that might elicit a secondary acute phase response.[60] Thus, a combination of imaging studies and investigations using inflammatory markers support the diffuse and systemic nature of instability of atheromas in individuals with or at risk for acute coronary syndromes.[36] This recognition has important therapeutic implications. In addition to appropriately deployed local revascularization strategies, such individuals should also have systemic therapy aimed at stabilizing the usually multiple high-risk lesions that may cause recurrent events.

SPECIAL CASES OF ARTERIOSCLEROSIS

Restenosis After Arterial Intervention

The problem of restenosis after percutaneous arterial intervention (see also Chap. 55) represents a special case of arteriosclerosis. After balloon angioplasty, luminal narrowing recurs in approximately one-third of cases within 6 months. Initially, work on the pathophysiology of restenosis after angioplasty focused on smooth muscle proliferation. A good deal of the thinking regarding the pathobiology of restenosis depended on extension to the human situation of the results of withdrawal of an overinflated balloon in a previously normal rat carotid artery. Study of this very well standardized preparation promoted precise understanding of the kinetics of intimal thickening after this type of injury. However, the attempts to transfer this information to human restenosis met with considerable frustration. This disparity between the balloon withdrawal injury of animal arteries and human restenosis is not surprising. The substrate of the animal studies was usually a normal rather than atherosclerotic artery, with all the attendant cellular and molecular differences highlighted earlier. Moreover, a high pressure inflation of an angioplasty balloon resembles only vaguely the overinflated balloon withdrawal injury commonly practiced in rats.

Although SMC proliferation appears prominent in the simple experimental models of intimal thickening, observations on human specimens showed relatively low rates of SMC proliferation and called into question therapeutic targeting of this process. Intravascular ultrasound studies in humans, and considerable evidence from animal experimentation, suggested that a substantial proportion of the loss of luminal caliber after balloon angioplasty resulted from a constriction of the vessel from the adventitial side (so-called *negative remodeling*). These observations renewed interest in adventitial inflammation with scar formation and wound contraction as a mechanism of arterial constriction following balloon angioplasty.[61]

The widespread introduction of stents has changed the face of the restenosis problem. The process of in-stent stenosis, in contrast with restenosis after balloon angioplasty, depends uniquely on intimal thickening, as opposed to negative remodeling. The stent provides a firm scaffold that prevents constriction from the adventitia. Histological analyses reveal that a great deal of the volume of the in-stent restenotic lesion is made up of myxomatous tissue, comprising occasional stellate SMCs embedded in a loose and highly hydrated extracellular matrix. The introduction of stents has reduced the clinical impact of restenosis because of the very effective increase in luminal diameter achieved by this technique. Even if a considerable degree of lumen loss occurs because of intimal thickening, the luminal caliber remains sufficient to alleviate the patient's symptoms because of the excellent dilatation achieved. Currently, stents that elaborate antiproliferative and antiinflammatory substances have shown great benefit in terms of preventing in-stent stenosis, albeit with a potential for augmenting late stent thrombosis (see Chap. 55).[62-64]

Accelerated Arteriosclerosis Following Transplantation

Since the advent of effective immunosuppressive therapy such as cyclosporin, the major limitation to long-term survival of cardiac allografts is the development of an accelerated form of arterial hyperplastic disease (see also Chap. 27). We favor the term arteriosclerosis (hardening of the arteries) rather than atherosclerosis (gruel-hardening) to describe this process because of the inconstant association with lipids (the "gruel" in atherosclerosis).[65] This form of arterial disease often presents a diagnostic challenge. The patient may not experience typical anginal symptoms because of the interruption of cardiac denervation posttransplantation. In addition, graft coronary disease is concentric and diffuse, affecting not only the proximal epicardial coronary vessels, but also penetrating smaller intramyocardial branches (Fig. 38-16). For this reason, the angiogram, well suited to visualize focal and eccentric stenoses, consistently underestimates the degree of transplantation arteriosclerosis.[66]

In most centers, a majority of patients undergoing transplantation have atherosclerotic disease and ischemic cardiomyopathy. However, a sizeable minority undergo heart transplantation for idiopathic dilated cardiomyopathy and may have few, if any, risk factors for atherosclerosis. Even in the absence of traditional risk factors, this latter group of individuals shares the risk of developing accelerated arteriosclerosis. This observation suggests that the pathophysiology of this form of accelerated arteriosclerosis differs from usual atherosclerosis.

The selective involvement of the engrafted vessels with sparing of the host's native arteries suggests that accelerated arteriopathy does not merely result from the immunosuppressive therapy or other systemic factors in the transplantation recipient. Rather, these observations suggest that the immunological differences between the host and the recipient vessels might contribute to the pathogenesis of this disease. Considerable evidence from both human and experimental studies currently supports this viewpoint. Endothelial cells in the transplanted coronary arteries express histocompatibility antigens that can engender an allogeneic immune response from host T cells. The activated T cells can secrete cytokines (e.g., IFN-γ) that can augment histocompatibility gene expression, recruit leukocytes by induction of adhesion molecules, and activate macrophages to produce SMC chemoattractants and growth factors. Interruption of IFN-γ signaling can prevent experimental graft coronary disease in mice. This disease appears to occur despite cyclosporin therapy because this immunosuppressant is relatively ineffective as a suppressor of the endothelial allogeneic response. Indeed, immunosuppressive agents that more effectively suppress the endothelial

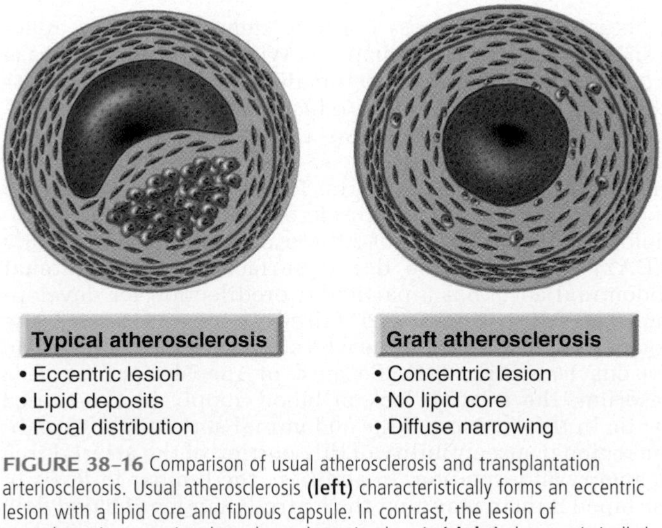

FIGURE 38–16 Comparison of usual atherosclerosis and transplantation arteriosclerosis. Usual atherosclerosis **(left)** characteristically forms an eccentric lesion with a lipid core and fibrous capsule. In contrast, the lesion of transplantation-associated accelerated arteriosclerosis **(right)** characteristically has a concentric intimal expansion without a clear central lipid core.

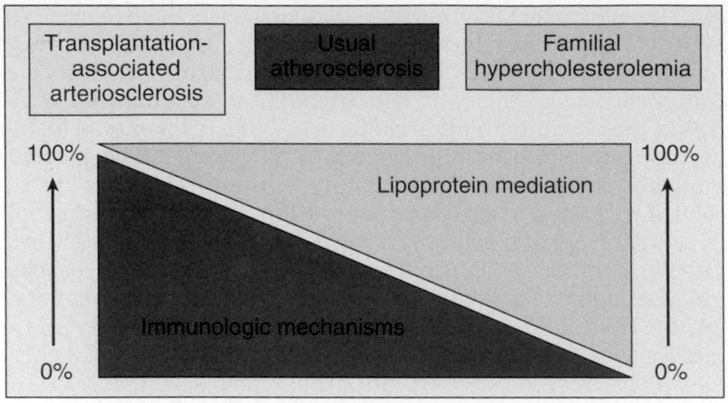

FIGURE 38–17 A multifactorial view of the pathogenesis of atherosclerosis. This diagram depicts two extreme cases of atherosclerosis. One **(far left side)** represents accelerated arteriosclerosis that can occur in the transplanted heart in the absence of traditional coronary risk factors. This disease likely represents primarily immune-mediated arterial intimal disease. The other extreme **(far right side)** depicts the case of a child who may succumb to rampant atherosclerosis in the first decade of life caused solely by an elevated low-density lipoprotein as a result of a mutation in the LDL receptor (homozygous familial hypercholesterolemia). Between these two extremes lie the vast majority of patients with atherosclerosis—probably involving various mixtures of immune and inflammatory and/or lipoprotein-mediated disease. One can further consider that this diagram extends to a third dimension that would involve other candidate risk factors such as homocysteine, Lp(a), infection, tobacco abuse, and so on.

allogeneic response appear effective in retarding graft arteriosclerosis.

The data summarized above suggest that graft arteriosclerosis represents an extreme case of immunologically driven arterial hyperplasia (Fig. 38-17) that can happen in the absence of other risk factors. On the other extreme, patients with homozygous familial hypercholesterolemia can develop fatal atherosclerosis in the first decade of life solely because of an elevation in LDL. The vast majority of patients with atherosclerosis fall somewhere between these two extremes. Analysis of usual atherosclerotic lesions shows evidence for a chronic immune response and lipid accumulation. Therefore, by studying the extreme cases, such as transplantation arteriopathy and familial hypercholesterolemia, one can gain insight into elements of the pathophysiology that contribute to the multifactorial form of atherosclerosis that affects the majority of patients.

Aneurysmal Disease

Atherosclerosis produces not only stenoses but also aneurysmal disease (see also Chap. 56). Why does a single disease process manifest in a directionally opposite manner—for example, most commonly producing stenoses in the coronary arteries, but causing ectasia of the abdominal aorta? In particular, aneurysmal disease characteristically affects the infrarenal abdominal aorta. This region is highly prone to the development of atherosclerosis. Data from the Pathobiological Determinants of Atherosclerosis in Youth Study (PDAY) show that the dorsal surface of the infrarenal abdominal aorta has a particular predilection for development of fatty streaks and raised lesions in Americans younger than 35 years of age who succumbed for noncardiac reasons (see Fig. 38-1). Because of the absence of vasa vasorum, the relative lack of blood supply to the tunica media in this portion of the abdominal aorta might explain the regional susceptibility of this portion of the arterial tree to aneurysm formation. In addition, the lumbar lordosis of the biped human may alter the hydrodynamics of blood flow in the distal aorta, yielding flow disturbances that may promote lesion formation.

Histological examination shows considerable distinction between occlusive atherosclerotic disease and aneurysmal disease. In typical coronary artery atherosclerosis, expansion of the intimal lesion produces stenotic lesions. The tunica media underlying the expanded intima is often thinned, but its general structure remains relatively well preserved. In contrast, transmural destruction of the arterial architecture occurs in aneurysmal disease. In particular, the usually well-defined laminar structure of the normal tunica media disappears with obliteration of the elastic laminae. The medial SMCs, usually well preserved in typical stenotic lesions, are notable for their paucity in the media of advanced aortic aneurysms.

Study of the pathophysiology that underlies these anatomical pathological findings has proved frustrating. Faithful animal models are not available. The human specimens obtainable for analysis generally represent the late stages of this disease. Nonetheless, recent work has identified several mechanisms that may underlie the peculiar pathology of aneurysmal disease. Widespread destruction of the elastic laminae suggests a role for degradation of elastin, collagen, and other constituents of the arterial extracellular matrix.[67] Many studies have documented overexpression of matrix-degrading proteinases, including matrix metalloproteinases in human aortic aneurysm specimens. Current clinical trials are testing the hypothesis that MMP inhibitors can reduce the expansion of aneurysms. Recent experimental work has implicated angiotensin II as a potentiator of aneurysm formation in mice.[68,69] Alterations in TGF-β signaling can predispose to aneurysm formation. Mutations in TGF-β receptors can cause arterial ectasia.[70,71]

Heightened elastolysis may explain the breakdown of the usually ordered structure of the tunica media in this disease. A slant toward T helper cell (Th2) populations in aneurysmal versus occlusive disease may contribute to the overexpression of certain elastolytic enzymes.[72,73] In addition, aortic aneurysms show evidence for considerable inflammation, particularly in the adventitia. The lymphocytes that characteristically abound on the adventitial side of aneurysmal tissue suggest that apoptosis of SMCs triggered by inflammatory mediators including soluble cytokines and *fas* ligand, elaborated by these inflammatory cells, may contribute to SMC destruction, and promote aneurysm formation. Although extracellular matrix degradation and SMC death also occur in sites where atherosclerosis causes stenosis, they appear to predominate in regions of aneurysm formation and to affect the tunica media much more extensively, for reasons that remain obscure.

Infection and Atherosclerosis

Interest persists in the possibility that infections may cause atherosclerosis. A considerable body of sero-epidemiological evidence supports a role for certain bacteria, notably *Chlamydia pneumoniae,* and certain viruses, notably cytomegalovirus (CMV), in the etiology of atherosclerosis. The sero-epidemiological studies have spurred a number of in vivo and in vitro experiments that lend varying degrees of support to this concept. In evaluating the sero-epidemiological evidence, several caveats apply. First, confounding factors should be carefully considered. For example, smokers may have a higher incidence of bronchitis caused by *C. pneumoniae.* Therefore, evidence for infection with *C. pneumoniae* may merely serve as a marker for tobacco use, a known risk factor for atherosclerotic events. Additionally, a strong bias favors publication of positive studies as opposed to negative studies. Meta-analyses of sero-epidemiological studies may be slanted toward the positive merely because of under-reporting of negative studies. Atherosclerosis is a common and virtually ubiquitous disease in developed countries. In most societies, many adults have serological evidence of prior infections with *Herpes viridae,* such as CMV, and respiratory pathogens, such as *C. pneumoniae.* It is difficult to sort out coincidence from causality when the majority of the population studied has evidence of both infection and atherosclerosis.

Although proof that bacteria or viruses can cause atherosclerosis remains elusive, it is plausible that infections may potentiate the action of traditional risk factors, such as hypercholesterolemia. Based on the vascular biology of atherosclerosis discussed in this chapter, a number of scenarios might apply.[74] First, cells within the plaque itself may be a site for infection (e.g., macrophages existing in an established atherosclerotic lesion might become infected with *C. pneumoniae*), which could spur their activation and accelerate the inflammatory pathways that we currently believe operate within the atherosclerotic intima. Specific microbial products, such as lipopolysaccharides, heat shock proteins, or other virulence factors, might act locally at the level of the artery wall to potentiate atherosclerosis in infected lesions.

Extravascular infection might also influence the development of atheromatous lesions and provoke their complication. For example, circulating endotoxin or cytokines produced in response to a remote infection can act locally at the level of the artery wall to promote the activation of vascular cells and of leukocytes in preexisting lesions, producing an "echo" at the level of the artery wall of a remote infection. Also, the acute phase response to an infection in a nonvascular site might affect the incidence of thrombotic complications of atherosclerosis by increasing fibrinogen, plasminogen activator inhibitor, or otherwise altering the balance between coagulation and fibrinolysis. Such disturbance in the prevailing prothrombotic, fibrinolytic balance may critically influence whether a given plaque disruption will produce a clinically inapparent transient or nonocclusive thrombus, or sustained and occlusive thrombi that could cause an acute coronary event.

Acute infections might also produce hemodynamic alterations that could trigger coronary events (e.g., the tachycardia and increased metabolic demands of fever could augment the oxygen requirements of the heart), precipitating ischemia in an otherwise compensated individual. These various scenarios illustrate how infectious processes, either local in the atheroma or extravascular, might aggravate atherogenesis, particularly in preexisting lesions or in concert with traditional risk factors. However, sufficiently powered clinical trials have not shown that treatment with macrolide or fluoroquinolone antibiotics can reduce recurrent coronary events in survivors of myocardial infarction.[75] Even if such studies had been positive, they would not establish a role for a particular infectious agent, nor could they prove that the antibiotic effect of the agents tested, rather than some other action not related to their antimicrobial effect, could produce benefit. However plausible, current clinical evidence does not support a role for bacterial infection in recurrent coronary events.

REFERENCES

1. Tuzcu EM, Kapadia SR, Tutar E, et al: High prevalence of coronary atherosclerosis in asymptomatic teenagers and young adults: Evidence from intravascular ultrasound. Circulation 103:2705, 2001.
2. Pasterkamp G, Galis ZS, de Kleijn DP: Expansive arterial remodeling: Location, location, location. Arterioscler Thromb Vasc Biol 24:650, 2004.
3. Shimizu K, Mitchell RN, Libby P: Inflammation and cellular immune responses in abdominal aortic aneurysms. Arterioscler Thromb Vasc Biol 26:987, 2006.

Structure of the Normal Artery

4. Arnout J, Hoylaerts MF, Lijnen HR: Haemostasis. Handb Exp Pharmacol:1, 2006.
5. Aird WC: Mechanisms of endothelial cell heterogeneity in health and disease. Circ Res 98:159, 2006.
6. Werner N, Kosiol S, Schiegl T, et al: Circulating endothelial progenitor cells and cardiovascular outcomes. N Engl J Med 353:999, 2005.
7. Zhu S, Liu X, Li Y, et al: Aging in the atherosclerosis milieu may accelerate the consumption of bone marrow endothelial progenitor cells. Arterioscler Thromb Vasc Biol 27:113, 2007.
8. Chi JT, Chang HY, Haraldsen G, et al: Endothelial cell diversity revealed by global expression profiling. Proc Natl Acad Sci U S A 100:10623, 2003.
9. Durr E, Yu J, Krasinska KM, et al: Direct proteomic mapping of the lung microvascular endothelial cell surface in vivo and in cell culture. Nat Biotechnol 22:985, 2004.
10. Mulvihill ER, Jaeger J, Sengupta R, et al: Atherosclerotic plaque smooth muscle cells have a distinct phenotype. Arterioscler Thromb Vasc Biol 24:1283, 2004.
11. Bochaton-Piallat ML, Gabbiani G: Modulation of smooth muscle cell proliferation and migration: Role of smooth muscle cell heterogeneity. Handb Exp Pharmacol 170:645, 2005.
12. Yoshida T, Owens GK: Molecular determinants of vascular smooth muscle cell diversity. Circ Res 96:280, 2005.

Atherosclerosis Initiation

13. Kruth HS: Sequestration of aggregated low-density lipoproteins by macrophages. Curr Opin Lipidol 13:483, 2002.
14. Williams KJ, Tabas I: Lipoprotein retention—and clues for atheroma regression. Arterioscler Thromb Vasc Biol 25:1536, 2005.
15. Heinecke JW: Oxidative stress: new approaches to diagnosis and prognosis in atherosclerosis. Am J Cardiol 91:12A, 2003.
16. Griendling KK: Novel NAD(P)H oxidases in the cardiovascular system. Heart 90:491, 2004.
17. Griendling KK: ATVB in focus: Redox mechanisms in blood vessels. Arterioscler Thromb Vasc Biol 25:272, 2005.
18. Lyle AN, Griendling KK: Modulation of vascular smooth muscle signaling by reactive oxygen species. Physiology (Bethesda) 21:269, 2006.
19. Cybulsky MI, Won D, Haidari M: Leukocyte recruitment to atherosclerotic lesions. Can J Cardiol 20 Suppl B:24B, 2004.
20. Ley K: The role of selectins in inflammation and disease. Trends Mol Med 9:263, 2003.
21. Tacke F, Alvarez D, Kaplan TJ, et al: Monocyte subsets differentially employ CCR2, CCR5, and CX3CR1 to accumulate within atherosclerotic plaques. J Clin Invest 117:185, 2007.
22. Swirski FK, Libby P, Aikawa E, et al: Ly-6C monocytes dominate hypercholesterolemia-associated monocytosis and give rise to macrophages in atheromata. J Clin Invest 117:195, 2007.
23. Gordon S: Macrophage heterogeneity and tissue lipids. J Clin Invest 117:89, 2007.
24. Charo IF, Ransohoff RM: The many roles of chemokines and chemokine receptors in inflammation. N Engl J Med 354:610, 2006.
25. Libby P: Inflammation in atherosclerosis. Nature 420:868, 2002.
26. Parmar KM, Larman HB, Dai G, et al: Integration of flow-dependent endothelial phenotypes by Kruppel-like factor 2. J Clin Invest 116:49, 2006.
27. Libby P, Aikawa M, Jain MK: Vascular endothelium and atherosclerosis. Handb Exp Pharmacol:285, 2006.
28. SenBanerjee S, Lin Z, Atkins GB, et al: KLF2 is a novel transcriptional regulator of endothelial proinflammatory activation. J Exp Med 199:1305, 2004.
29. Yamawaki H, Pan S, Lee RT, et al: Fluid shear stress inhibits vascular inflammation by decreasing thioredoxin-interacting protein in endothelial cells. J Clin Invest 115:733, 2005.
30. Majesky MW: Vascular smooth muscle diversity: Insights from developmental biology. Curr Atheroscler Rep 5:208, 2003.
31. Shimizu K, Mitchell RN: Stem cell origins of intimal cells in graft arterial disease. Curr Atheroscler Rep 5:230, 2003.
32. Miller YI, Chang MK, Binder CJ, et al: Oxidized low density lipoprotein and innate immune receptors. Curr Opin Lipidol 14:437, 2003.
33. van Berkel TJ, Out R, Hoekstra M, et al: Scavenger receptors: Friend or foe in atherosclerosis? Curr Opin Lipidol 16:525, 2005.

The Evolution of Atheroma

34. Hansson GK, Libby P, Schonbeck U, et al: Innate and adaptive immunity in the pathogenesis of atherosclerosis. Circ Res 91:281, 2002.
35. Binder CJ, Chang MK, Shaw PX, et al: Innate and acquired immunity in atherogenesis. Nat Med 8:1218, 2002.
36. Libby P, Ridker PM: Inflammation and atherothrombosis: From population biology and bench research to clinical practice. J Am Coll Cardiol 48:A33, 2006.
37. Hansson GK: Inflammation, atherosclerosis, and coronary artery disease. N Engl J Med 352:1685, 2005.
38. Hansson GK, Libby P: The immune response in atherosclerosis: a double-edged sword. Nat Rev Immunol 6:508, 2006.
39. Pinderski LJ, Fischbein MP, Subbanagounder G, et al: Overexpression of interleukin-10 by activated T lymphocytes inhibits atherosclerosis in LDL receptor-deficient Mice by altering lymphocyte and macrophage phenotypes. Circ Res 90:1064, 2002.
40. Geng YJ, Libby P: Progression of atheroma: A struggle between death and procreation. Arterioscler Thromb Vasc Biol 22:1370, 2002.
41. Littlewood TD, Bennett MR: Apoptotic cell death in atherosclerosis. Curr Opin Lipidol 14:469, 2003.
42. Hansson GK, Robertson AK: TGF-beta in atherosclerosis. Arterioscler Thromb Vasc Biol 24:e137, 2004.
43. Manabe I, Nagai R: Regulation of smooth muscle phenotype. Curr Atheroscler Rep 5:214, 2003.

44. Boyle JJ, Weissberg PL, Bennett MR: Tumor Necrosis Factor-α Promotes Macrophage-Induced Vascular Smooth Muscle Cell Apoptosis by Direct and Autocrine Mechanisms. Arterioscler Thromb Vasc Biol 23:1553, 2003.
45. Clarke MC, Figg N, Maguire JJ, et al: Apoptosis of vascular smooth muscle cells induces features of plaque vulnerability in atherosclerosis. Nat Med 12:1075, 2006.
46. Wight TN, Merrilees MJ: Proteoglycans in atherosclerosis and restenosis: key roles for versican. Circ Res 94:1158, 2004.
47. Dollery CM, Libby P: Atherosclerosis and proteinase activation. Cardiovasc Res 69:625, 2006.
48. Pipp F, Heil M, Issbrucker K, et al: VEGFR-1-selective VEGF homologue PlGF is arteriogenic: Evidence for a monocyte-mediated mechanism. Circ Res 92:378, 2003.
49. Moulton KS: Angiogenesis in atherosclerosis: Gathering evidence beyond speculation. Curr Opin Lipidol 17:548, 2006.
50. Kolodgie FD, Gold HK, Burke AP, et al: Intraplaque Hemorrhage and progression of coronary atheroma. N Engl J Med 349:2316, 2003.
51. Doherty TM, Asotra K, Fitzpatrick LA, et al: Calcification in atherosclerosis: Bone biology and chronic inflammation at the arterial crossroads. Proc Natl Acad Sci U S A 100:11201, 2003.

Complications of Atherosclerosis

52. Libby P, Theroux P: Pathophysiology of coronary artery disease. Circulation 111:3481, 2005.
53. Schoenhagen P, Stone GW, Nissen SE, et al: Coronary plaque morphology and frequency of ulceration distant from culprit lesions in patients with unstable and stable presentation. Arterioscler Thromb Vasc Biol 23:1895, 2003.
54. Virmani R, Burke AP, Farb A, et al: Pathology of the vulnerable plaque. J Am Coll Cardiol 47:C13, 2006.
55. Libby P, Aikawa M: Stabilization of atherosclerotic plaques: New mechanisms and clinical targets. Nat Med 8:1257, 2002.
56. Aikawa M: Lipid lowering therapy in atherosclerosis. Semin Vasc Med 4:357, 2004.
57. Sugiyama S, Kugiyama K, Aikawa M, et al: Hypochlorous acid, a macrophage product, induces endothelial apoptosis and tissue factor expression: Involvement of myeloperoxidase-mediated oxidant in plaque erosion and thrombogenesis. Arterioscler Thromb Vasc Biol 24:1309, 2004.
58. Libby P: Act local, act global: Inflammation and the multiplicity of "vulnerable" coronary plaques. J Am Coll Cardiol 45:1600, 2005.
59. Buffon A, Biasucci LM, Liuzzo G, et al: Widespread coronary inflammation in unstable angina. N Engl J Med 347:5, 2002.
60. Libby P, Ridker PM, Maseri A: Inflammation and atherosclerosis. Circulation 105:1135, 2002.

Special Cases of Arteriosclerosis

61. Libby P, Simon DI, Rogers C: Inflammation and arterial injury. *In* Topol EJ (ed): Textbook of Interventional Cardiology, 4th ed. Philadelphia, Elsevier Science, 2003, p. 381.
62. Maisel WH: Unanswered questions—Drug-eluting stents and the risk of late thrombosis. N Engl J Med 356:981, 2007.
63. Marks AR: Sirolimus for the prevention of in-stent restenosis in a coronary artery. N Engl J Med 349:1307, 2003.
64. Bennett MR: In-stent stenosis: Pathology and implications for the development of drug eluting stents. Heart 89:218, 2003.
65. Libby P, Zhao DX: Allograft arteriosclerosis and immune-driven angiogenesis. Circulation 107:1237, 2003.
66. Mitchell RN, Libby P: Vascular remodeling in transplant vasculopathy. Circ Res. In Press, 2007.
67. Thompson RW: Reflections on the pathogenesis of abdominal aortic aneurysms. Cardiovasc Surg 10:389, 2002.
68. Manning MW, Cassi LA, Huang J, et al: Abdominal aortic aneurysms: fresh insights from a novel animal model of the disease. Vasc Med 7:45, 2002.
69. Habashi JP, Judge DP, Holm TM, et al: Losartan, an AT1 antagonist, prevents aortic aneurysm in a mouse model of Marfan syndrome. Science 312:117, 2006.
70. Neptune ER, Frischmeyer PA, Arking DE, et al: Dysregulation of TGF-beta activation contributes to pathogenesis in Marfan syndrome. Nat Genet 33:407, 2003.
71. Loeys BL, Schwarze U, Holm T, et al: Aneurysm syndromes caused by mutations in the TGF-beta receptor. N Engl J Med 355:788, 2006.
72. Schonbeck U, Sukhova GK, Gerdes N, et al: Th2 predominant immune responses prevail in human abdominal aortic aneurysm. Am J Pathol 161:499, 2002.
73. Shimizu K, Shichiri M, Libby P, et al: Th2-predominant inflammation and blockade of IFN-gamma signaling induce aneurysms in allografted aortas. J Clin Invest 114:300, 2004.
74. Kalayoglu MV, Libby P, Byrne GI: *Chlamydia pneumoniae* as an emerging risk factor in cardiovascular disease. JAMA 288:2724, 2002.
75. Andraws R, Berger JS, Brown DL: Effects of antibiotic therapy on outcomes of patients with coronary artery disease: A meta-analysis of randomized controlled trials. JAMA 293:2641, 2005.

CHAPTER 39

Risk Factors for Atherothrombotic Disease

Paul M. Ridker and Peter Libby

Atherothrombosis can no longer be considered a disease of the developed world, because myocardial infarction and stroke are increasingly prevalent worldwide, across all socioeconomic strata. By 2025, cardiovascular mortality on a worldwide scale will likely surpass that of every major disease group, including infection, cancer, and trauma.[1,2] This shift in disease burden has also been reported in China where, accompanying rapid economic development, vascular disease has become a leading cause of death.[3]

Given our current understanding of atherothrombosis, it is historically surprising that the formal conceptual basis for considering specific "cardiovascular risk factors" only emerged when the initial findings of the Framingham Heart Study began to appear in the early 1960s. From an epidemiological perspective, a risk factor is a characteristic or feature of an individual or population that is present early in life and is associated with an increased risk of developing future disease. The risk factor of interest may be an acquired behavior (e.g., smoking), an inherited trait (e.g., familial hyperlipidemia), or a laboratory value (e.g., cholesterol, C-reactive protein). For a risk factor to have clinical usefulness, the marker of interest must predate the onset of disease. Most risk factors used in daily practice have demonstrated a consistent graded-response effect in large prospective epidemiological studies in broad populations. Several risk factors, such as hyperlipidemia and hypertension, are modifiable, and trials have demonstrated that lowering these factors reduces vascular risk. For other risk factors such as smoking, the attributable risk and assumed pathways of effect make trials unethical. It should be recognized, however, that a biomarker need not be proved causal for it to have substantial clinical usefulness. For example, although it remains controversial as to whether markers of inflammation are directly or indirectly associated with atherothrombosis, several inflammatory biomarkers have proved highly effective in clinical practice for evaluating vascular risk.

This chapter reviews the epidemiological evidence underlying risk factors for atherothrombosis in three parts. The first section describes the conventional risk factors of smoking, hypertension, hyperlipidemia, insulin resistance and diabetes, physical activity, and obesity, as well as general strategies for reducing risk related to these disorders. It also briefly reviews evidence relating mental stress and depression, focusing on how they affect traditional measures of vascular risk.

Not all coronary events occur in individuals with multiple traditional risk factors, however, and in some individuals abnormalities of inflammation, hemostasis, and/or thrombosis appear to contribute decisively. In particular, nearly half of all myocardial infarctions and strokes occur among individuals without hyperlipidemia. Thus, the second section of the chapter reviews atherothrombotic risk factors, including high-sensitivity C-reactive protein (hsCRP) and other markers of inflammation, as well as homocysteine and lipoprotein(a). Also reviewed are data regarding hemostatic and thrombotic markers of risk, including fibrinogen, D-dimer, and abnormalities of intrinsic fibrinolysis. In each case, we present the evidence that describes whether these novel risk indicators add to risk prediction over and above conventional factors. Because of its clinical prominence, the use of hsCRP to evaluate global risk more effectively, further delineate the metabolic syndrome, and improve targeting of statin therapy is also reviewed. The third section presents brief overviews of imaging techniques and emerging genetic approaches that may contribute to risk evaluation in the future. The chapter concludes with a discussion of a novel approach to overall risk prediction that can be applied immediately and that allows emerging concepts of inflammatory and heritable risk to play an appropriately greater role in global risk detection.[4,5]

It is important to recognize that for patients with favorable levels of the major risk factors, rates of incident cardiovascular disease, as well as all-cause mortality, are low.[6] Furthermore, with the exception of diabetes and obesity, the prevalence of most cardiovascular risk factors has declined in the United States over the past 40 years.[7] These favorable U.S. trends suggest that interventions to reduce risk can be highly effective when applied in appropriate settings, as evidenced not only by reductions in coronary disease but also by reductions in stroke.[8] Prevention on an international scale is thus a feasible goal. Adherence to a healthy life style may prevent many cases of coronary heart disease. Therefore, targeting risk reduction by life style modification for individuals who have clusters of risk factors seems a sensible primary goal for outpatient preventive cardiovascular practice.[9]

Smoking

Other than advanced age, smoking is the single most important risk factor for coronary artery disease. Cigarette consumption is the leading preventable cause of death in the United States, where it accounts for more than 450,000 deaths annually.[10] Ischemic heart disease causes 35 to 40 percent of all smoking-related deaths, with an additional 8 percent attributable to second-hand smoke exposure. Despite the relative stability in prevalence of current smokers in the United States, rates of tobacco use are increasing among adolescents, young adults, and women. Although increased recognition of the hazards of smoking might be hoped to slow these trends, almost 1 billion individuals now smoke worldwide. Smoking has a particularly large impact in the developing world and annually accounts for 1.17 million deaths worldwide.[11] Even among nonsmokers, inhaled smoke, whether from passive exposure or from cigar or pipe consumption, increases coronary risk. Passive smoking exposure can cause endothelial dysfunction in the coronary circulation as well as increased bronchial responsiveness and concomitant pulmonary dysfunction.

Landmark studies in the early 1950s first reported strong positive associations between cigarette smoke exposure and coronary heart disease. Over the next 50 years, an exceptionally consistent series of prospective studies have documented the effects of smoking on coronary risk. These studies suggest that, compared with nonsmokers, persons who consume 20 or more cigarettes daily have a two- to threefold increase in total coronary heart disease. Moreover, these effects depend on dose; consumption of as few as one to four cigarettes daily increases coronary artery disease risk. Such "light" levels of smoking have a major impact on myocardial infarction and all-cause mortality, even among smokers who do not report inhalation. Smoking acts synergistically with oral contraceptive agents, placing younger women taking these agents at even higher relative risk. In addition to myocardial infarction, cigarette consumption directly relates to increased rates of sudden death, aortic aneurysm formation, symptomatic peripheral vascular disease, and ischemic stroke. As for coronary disease, risk directly increases with the number of cigarettes consumed. Prospective evidence has linked cigarette consumption to an elevated risk of hemorrhagic stroke, including intracranial hemorrhage and subarachnoid hemorrhage, again in a dose-response manner.[12] Continued smoking is also a major risk factor for recurrent myocardial infarction.

Historically, cigarette consumption was prevalent in men before women and, at least in the United States, smoking prevalence remains lower in women than men. However, this gender gap has markedly narrowed, with overall consumption rates in women now in excess of 20 percent. Native Americans and those with less education have higher rates, whereas black and Hispanic women appear to smoke less than white women (Fig. 39-1). Because of adverse synergy with oral contraceptives, young female smokers who take oral contraceptives have particularly elevated risks of premature coronary disease and stroke. Smoking is especially hazardous for women with diabetes.[13]

Beyond acute unfavorable effects on blood pressure and sympathetic tone, and a reduction in myocardial oxygen supply, smoking affects atherothrombosis by several other mechanisms. In addition to accelerating atherosclerotic progression, long-term smoking may enhance oxidation of low-density lipoprotein (LDL) cholesterol and impair endothelium-dependent coronary artery vasodilation. This latter effect has been linked to dysfunctional endothelial nitric oxide biosynthesis following chronic as well as acute cigarette consumption.[14] In addition, smoking has adverse hemostatic and inflammatory effects, including increased levels of CRP, soluble intercellular adhesion molecule-1 (ICAM-1), fibrinogen, and homocysteine.[15] Additionally, smoking is associated with spontaneous platelet aggregation, increased monocyte adhesion to endothelial cells, and adverse alterations in endothelial derived fibrinolytic and antithrombotic factors, including tissue-type plasminogen activator and tissue pathway factor inhibitor. Compared with nonsmokers, smokers have an increased prevalence of coronary spasm and reduced thresholds for ventricular arrhythmia. Accruing evidence has suggested that insulin resistance represents an additional mechanistic link between smoking and premature atherosclerosis.[16]

Cessation of cigarette consumption overwhelmingly remains the single most important intervention in preventive cardiology. In a major overview, smoking cessation was found to reduce coronary heart disease mortality by 36 percent as compared with mortality in subjects who continued smoking, an effect that did not vary by age, gender, or country of origin.[17] In this analysis, the reduction in nonfatal myocardial reinfarction among those who stopped smoking (relative risk, RR, 0.68; 95 percent confidence interval, CI, 0.57 to 0.82) paralleled the overall drop in total cardiovascular mortality (RR, 0.64; 95 percent CI, 0.58 to 0.71). These 35 to 40 percent risk reductions equal or exceed other secondary prevention interventions that have received more attention from physicians and the pharmaceutical industry, including the use of aspirin, statins, beta-blocking agents, and angiotensin-converting enzyme inhibitors.

Reductions in smoking from any mechanism improve health outcomes, particularly when linked to life style changes, including exercise and dietary control. Trials of nicotine replace-

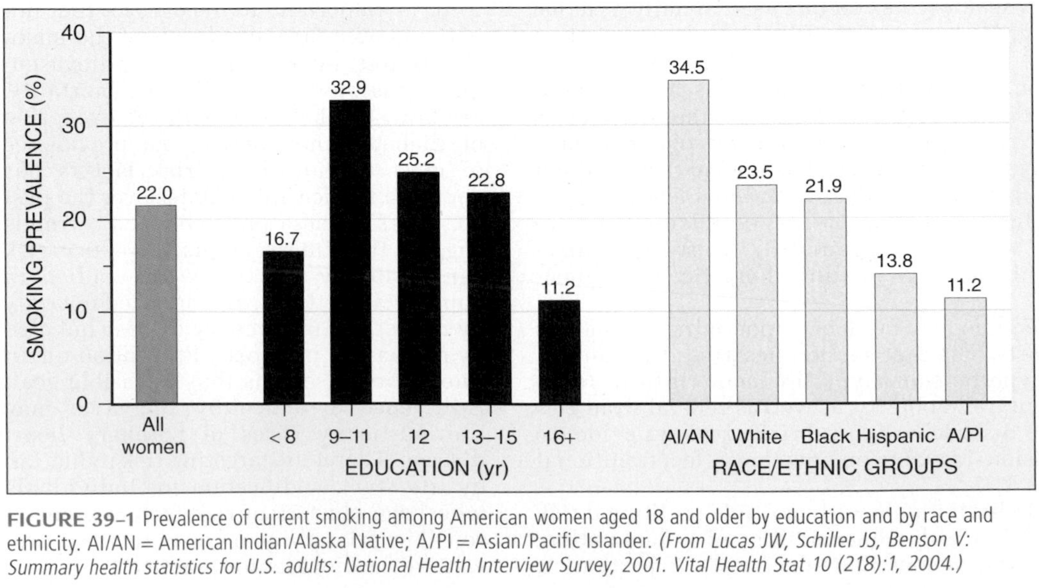

FIGURE 39-1 Prevalence of current smoking among American women aged 18 and older by education and by race and ethnicity. AI/AN = American Indian/Alaska Native; A/PI = Asian/Pacific Islander. *(From Lucas JW, Schiller JS, Benson V: Summary health statistics for U.S. adults: National Health Interview Survey, 2001. Vital Health Stat 10 (218):1, 2004.)*

ment therapy using transdermal nicotine or nicotine chewing gum increase abstention rates after cessation. Such pharmacological programs, as well as physician-guided counseling, are cost-effective and should be provided as standard prevention services. "Low-yield" cigarettes do not appear to reduce the risks of myocardial infarction. Although the elevated cardiovascular risks associated with smoking decrease significantly after cessation, the risks of cancer of the lungs, pancreas, and stomach persist for more than a decade, as do the risks of developing chronic obstructive pulmonary disease. Smoking cessation has clear benefit, but smoking reduction alone appears to have only a marginal effect.[18]

Poor patient understanding of the importance of smoking cessation continues, particularly in the developing world. The observation that smoking predicts better outcome following various reperfusion strategies (the so-called "smoker's paradox") is not because of any benefit of smoking but simply because smokers are likely to undergo such procedures at a much younger age and hence have on average lower comorbidity. Despite public health legislation, the tobacco industry continues its aggressive targeting of young adults, who are most susceptible to new addiction.[19] Thus, community education and physician-based primary prevention remain the most important components of any smoking reduction strategy.

Hypertension (see Chaps. 40 and 41)

High blood pressure often confers silent cardiovascular risk, and its prevalence is steadily increasing. Of the estimated 50 million Americans with high blood pressure, almost one third evade diagnosis and only one fourth receive effective treatment.[20] In the National Health and Nutrition Examination Survey, 28.7 percent of subjects evaluated had a measured blood pressure greater than 140/90 mm Hg or reported use of antihypertensive medications, an increase of almost 4 percent from similar survey data a decade earlier.[21] Hypertension prevalence was highest in non-Hispanic blacks (33.5 percent), increased with age (reaching more than 65 percent after the age of 60 years), and tended to be more prevalent in women than men. Although 68 percent of the study participants were aware of their hypertension, only 58 percent received therapy and only 31 percent had their hypertension controlled (Fig. 39-2). Thus, in contrast to hyperlipidemia, hypertension prevalence is increasing and treatment rates remain poor, highlighting the need for programs targeting prevention. These trends are even more worrisome in Europe, where the prevalence of hypertension exceeds that in the United States and Canada by 60 percent. In sample surveys from nine nations, an average blood pressure observed in the European centers was 136/83 mm Hg, compared with an average blood pressure of 122/77 mm Hg in U.S. and Canadian centers.[22] In 2000, the estimated number of adults worldwide with hypertension was 972 million, 333 million in economically developed countries and 639 million in developing countries; by 2025, the total number of adults with hypertension is anticipated to exceed 1.5 billion (Fig. 39-3).[23]

Part of the complexity of hypertension as a risk factor relates to changing definitions of risk and an understanding that systolic blood pressure and pulse pressure may have greater importance than diastolic blood pressure, contrary to decades of clinical teaching. Most epidemiological studies now recognize the joint contributions of systolic *and* diastolic blood pressure to the development of cardiovascular risk, an issue that has markedly changed strategies for risk detection. Isolated systolic hypertension, in particular, has at least as much importance as diastolic blood pressure for the outcomes of total cardiovascular mortality and stroke. Treatment of systolic hypertension is well supported, even in the elderly.[24] Isolated systolic hypertension thus appears to represent a distinct pathophysiological state in which elevated blood pressure reflects reduced arterial elasticity not necessarily associated with increased peripheral resistance or an elevation in mean arterial pressure. In the Framingham Heart Study, even high-normal blood pressure (systolic blood pressure, 130 to 139 mm Hg, diastolic blood pressure 85 to 89 mm Hg, or both) augments risk of cardiovascular disease twofold compared with lower levels.[25]

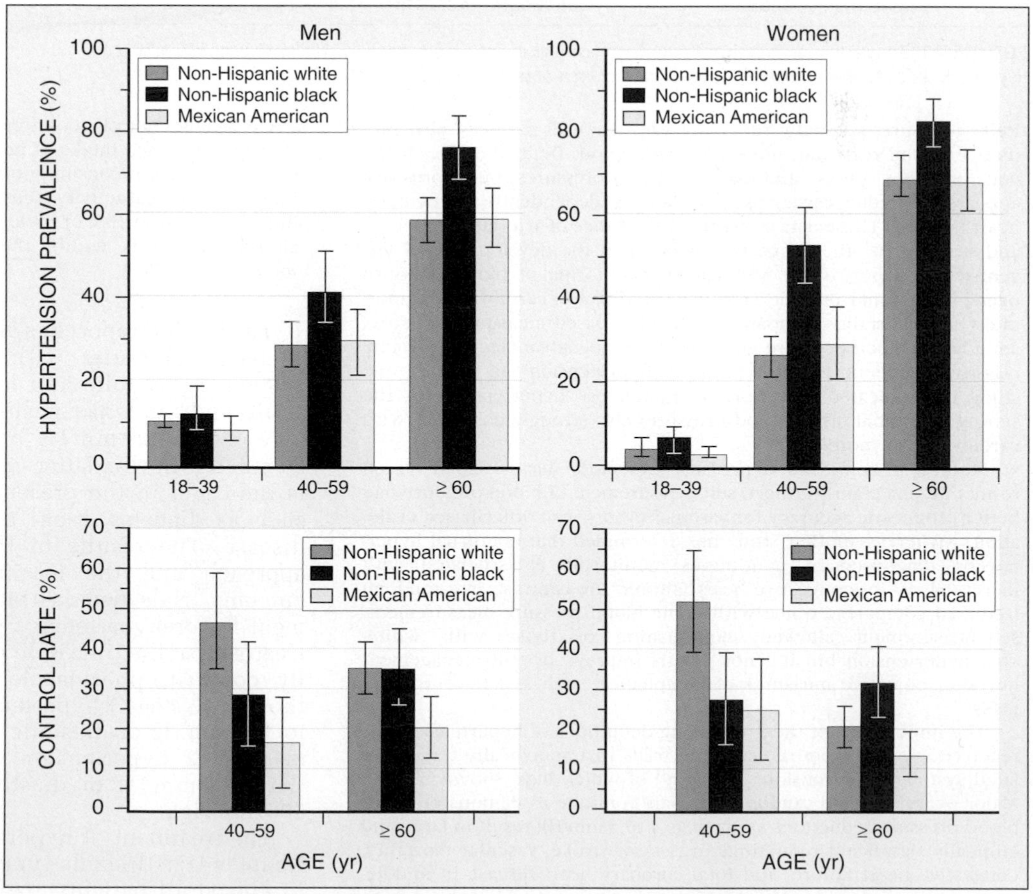

FIGURE 39–2 Hypertension prevalence **(top)** and hypertension control rates **(bottom)** by age and ethnicity among American men and women. *(From Hajjar I, Kotchen TA: Trends in prevalence, awareness, treatment, and control of hypertension in the United States, 1988-2000. JAMA 290:199, 2003.)*

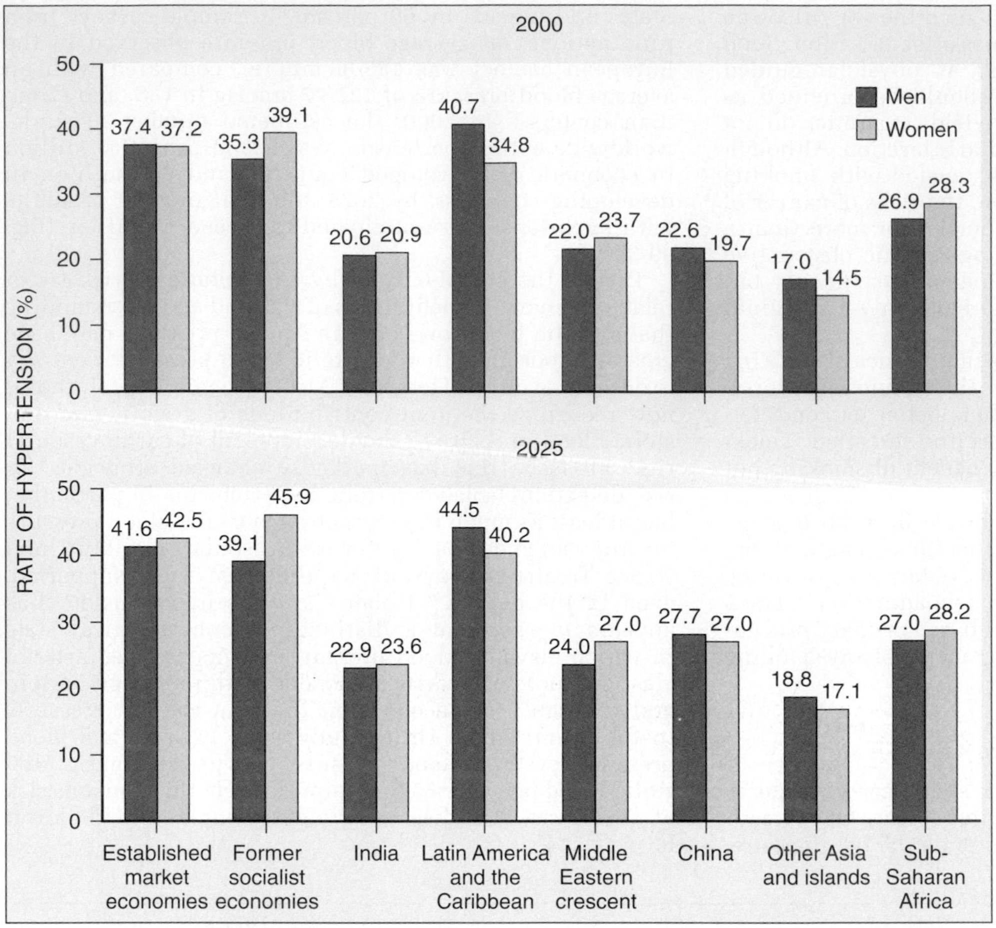

FIGURE 39–3 Hypertension prevalence rates by geographic region, 2000 and 2025. *(From Kearney PM, Whelton M, Reynolds K, et al: Global burden of hypertension: Analysis of worldwide data. Lancet 365:217, 2005.)*

Pulse pressure, generally reflecting vascular wall stiffness, also predicts first and recurrent myocardial infarction. Defined as the difference between systolic and diastolic blood pressures, pulse pressure appears to predict cardiovascular events independently, particularly heart failure.[26] These data stress the importance of arterial compliance and stiffness in atherogenesis as well as in the development of left ventricular hypertrophy. Ambulatory monitoring of blood pressure over 24 hours may provide a stronger predictor of cardiovascular morbidity and mortality compared with office-based measures. Whereas ambulatory blood pressure monitoring has the advantage of correctly classifying patients with "white-coat hypertension" as normal, one study has indicated that isolated ambulatory hypertension (in the setting of normal office blood pressure) also strongly correlates with cardiovascular morbidity.[27]

Studies of home blood pressure evaluation have yielded mixed results. In one elderly cohort, self-measurement of blood pressure had better prognostic accuracy for vascular events than office-based evaluation,[28] whereas another study has determined that nocturnal hypertension diagnosed by continuous monitoring is associated with increased risk of congestive heart failure.[29] By contrast, in a randomized trial comparing office with home blood pressure measurement, self-measurement allowed identification of those with white-coat hypertension but did not greatly improve overall management nor alter objective measures of compliance, such as left ventricular mass.[30]

The importance of these changing definitions of hypertension has received support from intervention trials that specifically target isolated systolic hypertension, almost all of which have shown benefit. Major overviews and randomized trials continue to demonstrate that blood pressure reductions as small as 4 to 5 mm Hg result in large and clinically significant reductions in risk for stroke, vascular mortality, congestive heart failure, and total coronary heart disease in middle-aged subjects, the elderly, and high-risk groups, such as those with diabetes and peripheral arterial disease.[31,32] Among compliant patients, sodium reduction and weight loss can lower blood pressure. However, not all patients respond to such measures, and the long-term success of nonpharmacological approaches to hypertension control has often proven disappointing. By contrast, relatively simple therapies such as low-dose diuretics can have major public health benefit. In an overview of 42 clinical trials that included 192,000 patients, low-dose diuretics compared with placebo yielded reductions of 21 percent in total coronary heart disease, 49 percent in congestive heart failure, 29 percent in stroke, and 19 percent in cardiovascular mortality.[33] In this meta-analysis, although combined therapy was often superior, none of the other first-line therapies for hypertension, including beta blockers, angiotensin-converting enzyme inhibitors, angiotensin receptor blockers, or calcium channel blockers yielded more significant benefits beyond those of low-dose diuretics. Combined low-dose therapies, however, have considerable efficacy in terms of both blood pressure reduction and event prevention. In an analysis of 354 randomized trials, regimens of multiple drugs given at low doses were estimated capable of reducing systolic blood pressure by 20 mm Hg and diastolic blood pressure by 11 mm Hg, effects that could result in stroke reductions of 63 percent and coronary heart disease risk reductions of 46 percent.[34]

The most recent report from the Joint National Committee on Prevention, Detection, Evaluation, and Treatment of High Blood Pressure (JNC VII) has continued appropriately to stress weight control, adoption of the DASH diet with sodium restriction and increased intake of potassium- and calcium-rich foods, moderation of alcohol consumption to fewer than two drinks daily, and increased physical activity (see Chap. 44). Higher folate intake may also link to decreased risk of incident hypertension,[35] whereas increased aldosterone levels within the physiological range predispose to increased risk.[36]

The JNC VII report has also suggested a new classification of blood pressure, with normal defined as less than 120 mm Hg systolic and less than 80 mm Hg diastolic for adults and "prehypertension" defined as systolic blood pressure 120 to 139 mm Hg or diastolic blood pressure 80 to 89 mm Hg. In this latter category, pharmacological therapy is indicated in the presence of other major comorbidities such as diabetes, renal dysfunction, or known vascular disease. The results of the TROPHY trial support this approach and the feasibility of treatment.[37] However, outcome trials demonstrating that the initiation of treatment for prehypertensive patients is superior to initiating treatment at the time of hypertension diagnosis are lacking. By contrast, pharmacological therapy is mandated for those with stage 1 hypertension (systolic blood pressure 140 to 159 mm Hg or diastolic blood pressure 90 to 99 mm Hg) or stage 2 hypertension (systolic blood pressure higher than 160 mm Hg or diastolic blood pressure higher than 100 mm Hg).

The treatment of hypertension is discussed at length in Chapter 41; a thiazide-type diuretic should be the first drug in almost all patients, except those with hyponatremia or gout, and the diuretic should be the cornerstone of any multidrug combination.[38,39] This appears to be true despite the fact that thiazides may have modest adverse effects on insulin resistance, fibrinolysis, and inflammation. Most patients with overt hypertension will require two or more medications to achieve JNC VII target goals for blood pressure reduction. In this regard, angiotensin receptor blocker monotherapy appears to reduce high-sensitivity C-reactive protein (hsCRP) levels and these agents neutralize any adverse effects on hsCRP associated with thiazide diuretics.[40] A number of studies have indicated that adherence to evidence-based prescribing guidelines results not only in improved care but substantial savings.[41] In another trial, attaining blood pressure control was associated with significant benefits, regardless of drug type.[42]

According to JNC VII, patients with chronic renal insufficiency (creatinine level higher than 1.3 mg/dl for women and higher than 1.5 mg/dl in men, or a glomerular filtration rate below 60 ml/m^2) also merit blood pressure reduction, both for the prevention of cardiovascular disease and to slow progression to end-stage renal disease. Patients with obesity, the metabolic syndrome, and frank diabetes represent high-risk groups. For all these patients, target blood pressure should be in the "optimal" range of lower than 120/80 mm Hg[43] (see Chap. 43). Although antihypertensive treatment targeting regression of left ventricular hypertrophy and left ventricular mass has suggested blood pressure–independent effects, the clinical impact of these observations remains uncertain.[44,45]

Hyperlipidemia and Elevated Low-Density Lipoprotein Cholesterol (see Chap. 42)

Although the relationship between cholesterol and atherosclerosis currently enjoys wide acceptance, this has not always been the case, illustrating how difficult changing physician behavior and beliefs can be when dealing with risk detection and disease prevention. In the 1850s, the German pathologist Virchow recognized in human atheromata "numerous plates of cholesterine . . . which display themselves even to the naked eye as glistening lamellae . . . which lie together in large numbers . . . and altogether produce a glittering reflection." In 1913, the Russian experimentalists Anitschkov and Chalatov observed that rabbits fed an egg-rich diet developed lipid-laden arterial lesions reminiscent of human atheromata. Later experiments identified cholesterol as the constituent of eggs that produced arterial lesions.

The biochemistry of cholesterol metabolism advanced throughout the 20th century. The advent of the ultracentrifuge enabled the characterization of lipoprotein fractions in blood and provided the foundation for the detailed study of lipid metabolism. Armed with the ability to assay lipoproteins and cholesterol, translational investigators began to make clinical correlations. Cross-sectional studies of geographically dispersed populations revealed a relationship between serum cholesterol levels and coronary heart disease (CHD) death. A comparative study of ethnic Japanese living in Japan, the Hawaiian Islands, and the continental United States showed that in this relatively genetically homogeneous population, CHD death rates tracked with the environmentally induced augmentation in total serum cholesterol levels.

Confounding factors, however, limit the validity of such cross-sectional studies. Thus, the emergence of data from prospective cohort studies, such as that begun in Framingham in the 1950s, bolstered the relationship between cholesterol and CHD. This study, as well as others performed with different populations around the world, established the concept of cholesterol more firmly as a culprit in coronary heart disease. Substantiation of the relationship between total cholesterol and CHD risk emerged from the Multiple Risk Factor Intervention Trial (MRFIT), studies in the United Kingdom and Europe such as the Northwick Park Study and the Prospective Cardiovascular Munster (PROCAM) Cohort and, more recently, the Atherosclerosis Risk in Communities (ARIC) study. The ARIC cohort has particular relevance to current clinical practice in the United States because it included substantial numbers of women and members of racial minority groups.

Although based on more than a century of experimental and clinical observation, doubt lingered regarding the role of cholesterol in atherosclerosis until surprisingly recently. Through the beginning of the 1990s, controversy enveloped the role of cholesterol-lowering therapy in CHD risk reduction. Despite evidence that high cholesterol levels correlated with coronary death, the proposition that cholesterol-lowering therapy could reduce CHD morbidity remained unproven. Critics pointed to the "J-shaped curve," which apparently described the relationship of serum cholesterol with mortality. Advocates of the cholesterol hypothesis countered that the heightened risk for all-cause death in individuals with low levels of cholesterol might reflect comorbidities such as cancer, inanition, or liver disease. The goal of reducing CHD mortality by drug therapy eluded convincing proof for decades. Indeed, some cholesterol-lowering medications appeared to cause an increase in the incidence of some events, including noncoronary death. In the pioneering coronary drug project, estrogen treatment led to excess mortality in the cohort of men studied. The World Health Organization study of clofibrate showed an increased incidence of noncoronary death. Dietary interventions to lower cholesterol often proved ineffective and, together, such results seemed to challenge the validity of cholesterol as a therapeutic target.

In the 1980s, clinical trial evidence first established a protective effect of pharmacological cholesterol reduction on coronary morbidity. The Lipid Research Clinic study showed that bile acid-binding resins could lower cholesterol levels in individuals with high baseline levels, and a decrease in coronary morbidity accompanied the drop in the serum cholesterol level. However, total mortality did not change significantly. Conclusive evidence regarding the cholesterol hypothesis awaited clinical trials of cholesterol lowering using the hydroxymethylglutaryl coenzyme A (HMG-CoA) reductase inhibitors, agents that lowered LDL cholesterol much more efficiently than previously available drugs. We now possess unassailable clinical trial evidence that lowering of LDL cholesterol levels reduces coronary events in broad segments of the population (see Chap. 42). First shown in survivors of myocardial infarction with relatively high cholesterol levels, clinical trials have extended the benefits of HMG-CoA reductase inhibitors to individuals without known atherosclerotic disease and with average levels of cholesterol. The ensemble of large clinical trials of HMG-CoA reductase inhibitors have substantiated a decrease in total mortality in virtually all major study populations. As a group, placebo-controlled trials of HMG-CoA reductase inhibitors lowered LDL cholesterol levels by 20 to 60 percent and reduced coronary events by up to one third over a 5-year period, with no evidence of an increase in nonvascular mortality.

As demonstrated in the contemporary Heart Protection Study, the HMG-CoA reductase inhibitors can reduce stroke as well as coronary events among individuals with pre-existing vascular disease.[46] More recently, several head-to-head trials comparing different statin regimens have shown that even more aggressive LDL reduction is associated with greater clinical improvements. Such studies include the REVERSAL trial, which monitored intravascular coronary ultrasound,[47] and the PROVE-IT, A-to-Z, and TNT trials, all of which support more aggressive use of statin therapy for reduction in hard clinical endpoints.[48-50]

The case for LDL cholesterol as a coronary heart disease risk factor thus meets most of the criteria established by Koch in the 19th century to establish a causative agent in a disease. High cholesterol levels consistently predict risk of future cardiovascular events in human populations. Animal studies in multiple species have shown a causal relationship between hypercholesterolemia and atherosclerosis. Knowledge of the LDL receptor pathway (see Chap. 42) plus emerging understanding of the vascular biology of atherosclerosis (see Chap. 38) provides biological plausibility for the involvement of LDL in atherogenesis. The human mutations in the LDL receptor produce hypercholesterolemia on a monogenic basis that causes accelerated atherosclerosis as early as the first decade of life in individuals with homozygous familial hypercholesterolemia. Finally, intervention in large clinical trials to lower LDL cholesterol levels by various pathways (e.g., bile acid-binding resins, intestinal bypass surgery, HMG-CoA reductase inhibitors) have shown a reduction in cardiovascular events. Thus, LDL cholesterol fulfills the criteria of modified Koch's postulates as one causative agent in atherosclerosis.

Several independent lines of evidence have suggested that what is regarded as "normal" cholesterol levels in Western society exceed levels that good health requires.[51] In particular, certain rural agrarian societies with very low rates of atherothrombosis have total cholesterol levels well below those accepted as normal in Western societies. Another line of evidence derives from phylogeny. Contemporary humans have much higher total cholesterol levels than those of many other species of higher organisms that thrive nonetheless. As described earlier, clinical trials have shown that LDL cholesterol levels as low as 70 mg/dl provide optimal outcomes, at least for those with established disease. In certain high-risk groups, such as those with diabetes, statin therapy appears effective, even in the absence of overt hyperlipidemia.[52]

Cholesterol levels measured early in life influence long-term cardiovascular risk. In the Bogalusa Heart Study, the burden of risk factors for atherosclerosis, including hypercholesterolemia, were found to correlate with autopsy-proven fatty streak and raised lesion formation in the arterial tree. Studies performed on Johns Hopkins medical students on matriculation, with long-term follow-up, have suggested that cholesterol levels in the third decade correlate with long-term risk of myocardial infarction. Thus, substantial evidence suggests that the burden of risk for cardiovascular disease begins in young adulthood. Autopsy studies from the Korean and Vietnam conflicts, and recent explorations of coronary anatomy by intravascular ultrasonography, have suggested that atherosclerosis affects adolescents in our society. In very high-risk children, clinical trial evidence has demonstrated the efficacy of statin therapy for the treatment of familial hypercholesterolemia.[53]

High-Density Lipoprotein Cholesterol, Apolipoproteins, and Other Lipid Subclasses

As is the case with LDL cholesterol, abundant prospective cohort studies have demonstrated a strong inverse relationship between HDL cholesterol and vascular risk. In general, each increase of HDL cholesterol by 1 mg/dl is associated with a 2 to 3 percent decrease in risk of total cardiovascular disease. Indeed, patients with angiographically proven coronary artery disease more often have low levels of HDL than high levels of LDL, as defined by current criteria. The process of reverse cholesterol transport may explain in part the apparent protective role of HDL against coronary death. According to this concept, HDL could ferry cholesterol from the vessel wall, augmenting peripheral catabolism of cholesterol.[54] HDL can also carry antioxidant enzymes that may reduce the levels of oxidized phospholipids in atheromatous lesions, which might enhance atherogenesis (see Chaps. 38 and 42). Furthermore, overexpressing the apolipoprotein A-I gene in transgenic mice and infusing complexes of apolipoprotein A-I and phospholipids into hyperlipidemic rabbits not only increases HDL cholesterol levels but also decreases atherosclerotic development. However, in contrast to LDL cholesterol, we currently lack a consistent body of clinical trial data on interventions to raise HDL cholesterol levels. Nonetheless, the consistency of the observational data, both cross-sectional and prospective, strongly supports the HDL level as a "negative" risk factor, as incorporated in the Adult Treatment Panel (ATP-III) guidelines, and supports the aggressive search for agents that can directly increase HDL levels.[55] This recognition by the ATP-III—that a biomarker can be useful without fulfilling Koch's postulates—has importance for clinical practice and has implications for several other emerging risk factors (see later).

Several investigators have suggested that measurement of apolipoproteins A-I and B-100 would predict cardiovascular risk better than HDL and LDL cholesterol in clinical practice. Indeed, two recent prospective cohort studies have shown this to be the case for men[56] and women.[57] However, both these studies also found that non-HDL cholesterol (defined as total cholesterol minus HDL cholesterol) provided clinical risk information as least as strong as that of apolipoprotein B-100, an observation that is not surprising, because non-HDL cholesterol correlates very closely with apolipoprotein B-100 levels. Furthermore, both these studies found that the total cholesterol to HDL cholesterol ratio remained a very strong predictor of risk, superior even to the ratio of apolipoprotein B-100 to apolipoprotein A-I (Fig. 39-4). Thus, despite evidence favoring apolipoproteins A-I and B-100 in univariate analyses as replacements for HDL and LDL cholesterol, there remain little clinical data that use of these measures improves overall risk prediction compared with standard lipid testing. Apolipoproteins may, however, have particular use in the monitoring of statin therapy.[58]

Beyond standard chemical measures of total, LDL, and HDL cholesterol, which appropriately form the basis of current lipid screening and reduction guidelines, the amount of cholesterol carried by different classes of lipoprotein particles may influence function and vary widely among individuals. Therefore, measures of core lipid composition and lipoprotein particle size have been hypothesized to provide better measures for risk prediction. Several lines of evidence have indicated that small LDL particles may be more atherogenic than large particles and contribute particularly to the dyslipidemia of diabetes (see Chap. 43). Currently, a number of technologies are available for evaluation of LDL subclasses and particle size. Studies using density gradient ultracentrifugation and gradient gel electrophoresis have generally found that lipoprotein subclass identifies individuals at higher risk for coronary disease and have successfully shown a preferential benefit of lipid-lowering therapy for patients with small, dense LDL particles as compared to large LDL particles. Studies have also found LDL particle concentration, as measured by nuclear magnetic resonance studies, to correlate well with coronary arterial lumen diameter after statin therapy and to have predictive value for future vascular events. For example, in both the Women's Health Study and the Cardiovascular Health Study, LDL particle concentration measured by nuclear magnetic resonance studies predicted incident vascular events better than standard measurement of LDL cholesterol. These relationships remain complex, however, and have not always been consistent.[59] In addition, standardization across technologies available for lipoprotein subclassification has remained problematic. Thus, although intriguing pathophysiological information regarding lipid reduction with statins and gemfibrozil has come from nuclear magnetic resonance spectroscopy studies, as well as density gradient studies,[60,61] it remains unclear whether these novel methods of lipid evaluation add importantly to standard lipid screening in routine practices or should remain specialized tools for research and lipid clinics.

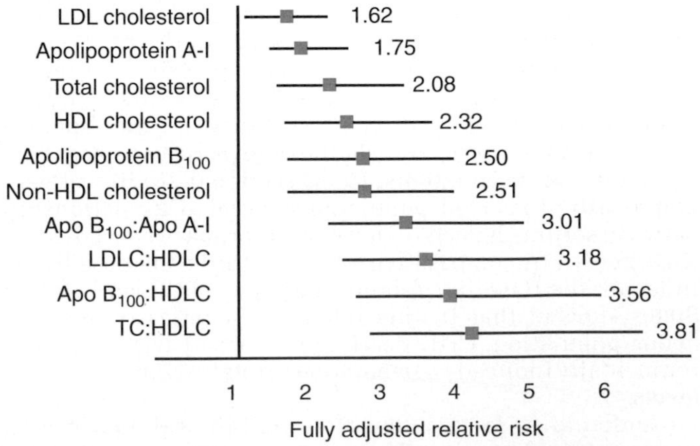

FIGURE 39–4 Adjusted relative risks of future cardiovascular events for selected lipid fractions and lipid ratios. LDLC = low-density lipoprotein cholesterol; HDLC = high-density lipoprotein cholesterol; Apo A-I = apolipoprotein A-I; Apo B_{100} = apolipoprotein B-100; TC = total cholesterol. *(From Ridker PM, Rifai N, Cook NR, et al: Non-HDL cholesterol, apolipoproteins A-1 and B100, standard lipid measures, lipid ratios, and CRP as risk factors for cardiovascular disease in women. JAMA 294:326, 2005.)*

Triglyceride-Rich Lipoproteins and Cardiovascular Risk

In contrast to the compelling evidence favoring a causal role for LDL cholesterol in atherogenesis, the role of triglycerides remains controversial. A number of issues add to this confusion. First, because triglyceride levels tend to vary inversely with HDL cholesterol levels, demonstration of an unequivocal effect of triglycerides on cardiovascular events and mortality independent of HDL levels has proved elusive. Second, the level of triglycerides in the blood depends exquisitely on diet. Sampling serum for triglyceride levels in the fasting state avoids some of the variability in this measurement. However, most humans are in the postprandial state much of the day. The actual exposure of the artery wall to triglyceride-rich lipoprotein particles, such as very-low-density lipoproteins, may constitute a factor that promotes atherosclerosis that would be missed by the fasting lipid profile. For these reasons, among others, current guidelines do not establish a target value of triglycerides. However, some studies have suggested that triglycerides do provide important information about risk in certain populations.[62,63] In view of the tight link of triglyceride levels with known risk factors for atherosclerosis (e.g., low HDL cholesterol level, uncontrolled diabetes, hypothyroidism), the finding of marked and persistently elevated triglyceride levels should enter into the overall risk assessment for an individual and stimulate consideration of the reason for triglyceride level elevation[64] (see Chap. 42). A cautious approach to triglyceride reduction would seem prudent, because randomized trial data using fenofibrate among diabetic patients with elevated triglyceride levels have failed to find significant reductions in risk using this approach.[65]

Metabolic Syndrome, Insulin Resistance, and Diabetes (see Chap. 43)

Insulin resistance and diabetes rank among the major cardiovascular risk factors; in one major survey, the presence of diabetes conferred an equivalent risk to aging 15 years, an impact greater than that of smoking.[66] Almost 35 million Americans have some degree of abnormal glucose tolerance, a condition along with obesity that markedly increases the risk for type 2 diabetes and premature atherothrombosis. Patients with diabetes have two- to eightfold higher rates of future cardiovascular events as compared with age- and ethnically matched nondiabetic individuals, and 75 percent of all deaths in diabetic patients result from coronary heart disease. Compared with unaffected individuals, diabetic patients have a greater atherosclerotic burden, both in the major arteries and in the microvascular circulation. Not surprisingly, diabetic patients have substantially increased rates of atherosclerotic complications in the settings of primary prevention and after coronary interventional procedures (see Chap. 60). Insulin resistance alone confers an elevated risk of congestive heart failure and probably explains the association of obesity with this common vascular complication.[67] Moreover, the risk of cardiovascular disease starts to increase long before the onset of clinical diabetes. In an analysis of data from the Nurses Health Study of women who eventually developed type 2 diabetes, the relative risk of myocardial infarction was elevated threefold *before* the diagnosis of diabetes, a cardiovascular event rate almost as high as the rate in patients with frank diabetes at study entry.[68] These effects are magnified in ethnic minority populations and in patients with other concomitant risk factors.

Although hyperglycemia is associated with microvascular disease, insulin resistance itself promotes atherosclerosis even before it produces frank diabetes, and available data corroborate the role of insulin resistance as an independent risk factor for atherothrombosis. This finding has prompted recommendations for increased surveillance for the metabolic syndrome, a cluster of glucose intolerance and hyperinsulinemia accompanied by hypertriglyceridemia, low HDL levels, hypofibrinolysis, hypertension, microalbuminuria, a predominance of small dense LDL particles, and central obesity. Although several formal definitions of the metabolic syndrome have been proposed, the definition adopted by the National Cholesterol Education Program Adult Treatment Panel[69] requires at least three of the following five criteria: (1) waist circumference larger than 102 cm in men and 88 cm in women; (2) serum triglyceride levels of at least 150 mg/dl; (3) HDL cholesterol less than 40 mg/dl in men and less than 50 mg/dl in women; (4) blood pressure of at least 130/85 mm Hg; and (5) serum glucose concentration of at least 110 mg/dl. Using these criteria, the prevalence of metabolic syndrome in the United States is almost 25 percent, or nearly 50 million persons.

Despite controversy over definitions, several studies have documented that individuals with the metabolic syndrome have elevated vascular event rates. In the Kuopio Ischaemic Heart Disease Risk Factor Study, patients with metabolic syndrome showed markedly increased rates of coronary, cardiovascular, and all-cause mortality (Fig. 39-5).[70] However, not all those with metabolic syndrome have similar risk. Most importantly, endothelial inflammation is now recognized as a major component of metabolic syndrome[71] and the most recent definition of metabolic syndrome from the National Heart, Lung, and Blood Institute includes a pro-inflammatory state.[72] Thus, inflammatory biomarkers such as hsCRP may help further stratify clinical risk and improve the prognostic value of metabolic syndrome. For example, data from the Women's Health Study have indicated that an hsCRP level greater than 3 mg/liter adds important prognostic information about cardiovascular risk at all levels of the metabolic syndrome, whereas those with levels less than 1 mg/liter are at substantially lower risk (Fig. 39-6).[73] This observation is important, because levels of C-reactive protein measured with a high-sensitivity assay also predict incident type 2 diabetes.[74,75] Almost identical data regarding the additive value of hsCRP to the metabolic syndrome in terms of future vascular risk prediction have been obtained from the West of Scotland Coronary Prevention Study.[76] Because hsCRP levels correlate with systemic hypofibrinolysis and with basal insulin levels, hsCRP evaluation may well become a routine part of the definition of metabolic syndrome. As reviewed later in this chapter in sections describing inflammatory markers, this conclusion has emerged in part from observations that atherosclerosis and type 2 diabetes share a common inflammatory basis.[77]

In addition to systemic metabolic abnormalities, hyperglycemia causes accumulation of advanced glycation end products associated with vascular damage. Diabetic patients have markedly impaired endothelial and smooth muscle function and appear to have increased leukocyte adhesion to vascular endothelium, a critical early step in atherogenesis. Diabetic nephropathy, detected by microalbuminuria, accelerates these adverse processes. Among individuals with non–insulin-dependent diabetes, microalbuminuria predicts cardiovascular and all-cause mortality. Abnormalities of endogenous fibrinolysis are also prevalent among diabetic and prediabetic patients. The proinflammatory atherogenic mediator–soluble CD40 ligand is elevated in diabetic patients and declines during thiazolidinedione therapy.[78] These effects, in concert with the impaired endothelium-dependent (nitric oxide–mediated) vasodilation

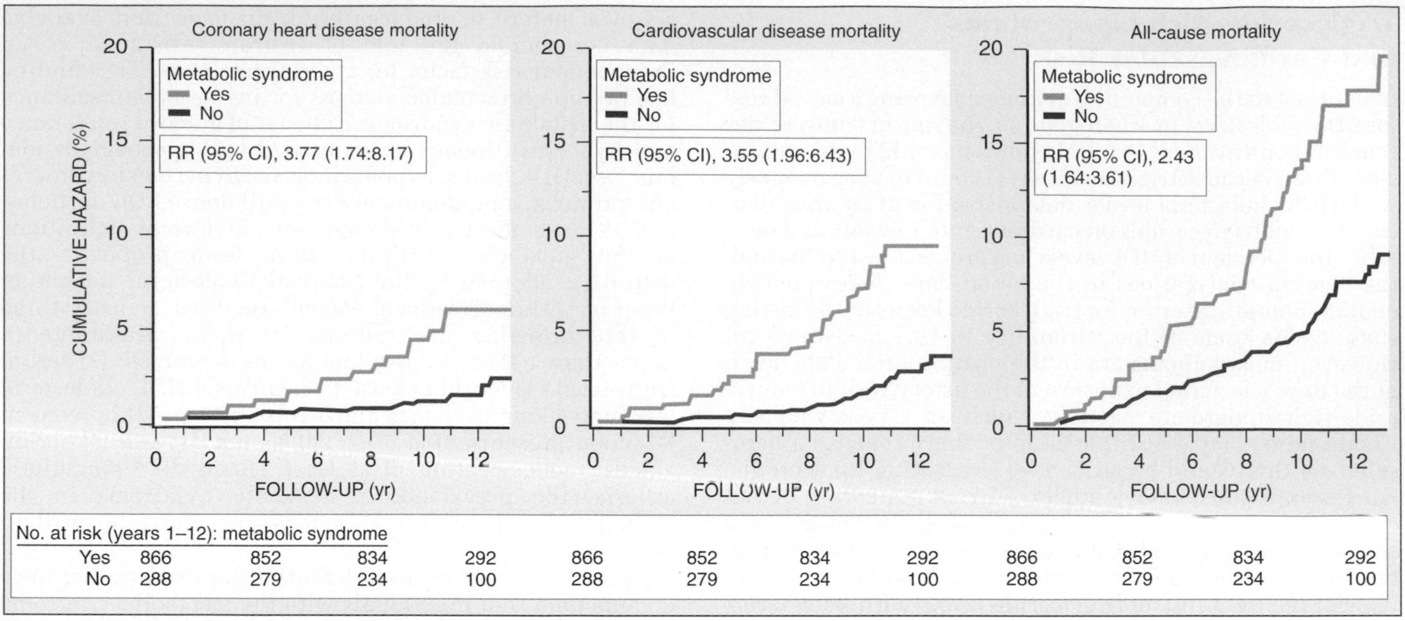

FIGURE 39–5 Cumulative hazard (unadjusted Kaplan-Meier hazard curves) for coronary heart disease, cardiovascular disease, and all-cause mortality among individuals with and without metabolic syndrome. *(From Lakka H, Laaksonen DE, Lakka TA, et al: The metabolic syndrome and total and cardiovascular disease mortality in middle-aged men. JAMA 288:2709, 2002.)*

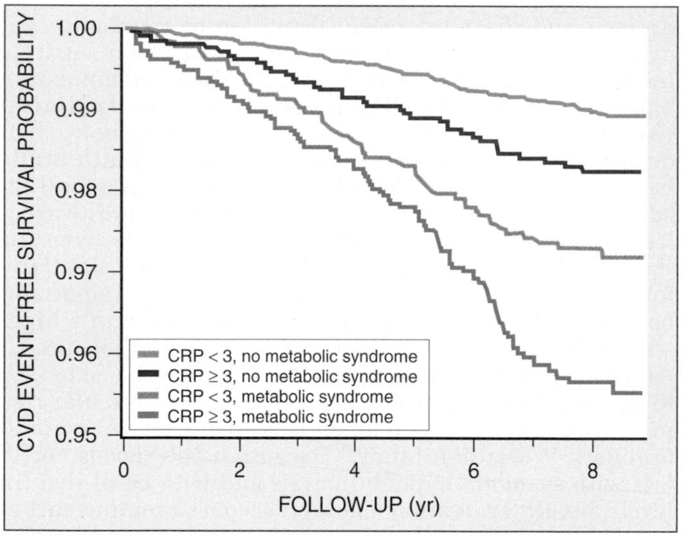

FIGURE 39–6 High-sensitivity C-reactive protein (CRP) adds prognostic information on risk for individuals with and without the metabolic syndrome. CVD = cardiovascular disease. *(From Ridker PM, Buring JE, Cook NR, Rifai N: C-reactive protein, the metabolic syndrome, and risk of incident cardiovascular events: An 8-year follow-up of 14,719 initially healthy American women. Circulation 107:391, 2003.)*

common in diabetic patients, contribute to endothelial cell dysfunction and accelerated atherogenesis.[79]

Chapters 43 and 60 review the data about therapeutic interventions in patients with diabetes or the metabolic syndrome. As recently demonstrated in the Diabetes Control and Complication Trial, intensive treatment of diabetes over a 6.5-year period reduced the risk of cardiovascular disease by 42 percent (95 percent CI, 9 to 63 percent).[80] Unfortunately, poor control of concomitant risk factors in diabetic patients represents a major challenge; in the most recent National Health and Nutrition Examination Survey of the United States, only 31 percent of participants achieved the target goal of HbA_{1C} less than 7.0 percent, only 36 percent achieved the target blood pressure goals of less than 130/80 mm Hg, and more than half had total cholesterol levels in excess of 200 mg/dl; moreover, only 7 percent of all adults with diabetes in the NHANES achieved all three of these crucial target goals.[81] This situation also concerns European general practices, where treatment with diet only remains common and complication rates are very high.[82]

Exercise, Weight Loss, and Obesity

(see Chaps. 44, 46, and 78)

Physical exercise reduces myocardial oxygen demand and increases exercise capacity, both of which correlate with lower levels of coronary risk. The cardioprotective effects of exercise include reduced adiposity and diabetes incidence, lowered blood pressure, and improvement of dyslipidemia, as well as vascular inflammation. Exercise also enhances endothelial dysfunction, insulin sensitivity, and endogenous fibrinolysis.[83] It is thus not surprising that prospective epidemiological studies almost universally demonstrate strong graded associations between levels of physical activity and reduced rates of cardiovascular morbidity and all-cause mortality.

Observational studies have cast doubt on the long-held belief that exercise must be vigorous to be beneficial. Exercise levels achieved with as little as 30 minutes of walking daily provide major coronary benefits. In the Women's Health Initiative, walking briskly for 30 minutes five times/week was associated with a 30 percent reduction in vascular events over a 3.5-year follow-up, an effect that persisted after adjustment for body mass index, age, and ethnicity (Fig. 39-7).[84] In men participating in the Health Professional Follow-Up Study, 30 minutes of daily walking was associated with an 18 percent reduction in coronary risk. In that study, contrary to commonly given medical advice, resistance exercise and weight training also contributed cardiovascular benefit.[85] Accumulated episodes of exercise, even if brief, have further demonstrated benefit, suggesting that risk reduction does not require prolonged vigorous work. Smaller but consistent benefits of modest exercise have been observed for incident stroke, independent of hypertension. A regular exercise program also reduces the transient increase in risk of sudden death that, although extremely rare, can occur during vigorous exercise.[86] Thus, a "no pain, no gain" approach to the prescription of physical activity to reduce vascular risk now appears passé.

On the basis of these data, a joint statement from the Centers for Disease Control and the American College of Sports Medicine has recommended that every American should participate in at least 30 minutes of moderate-intensity physical activity daily. Unfortunately, 7 of 10 American adults fail to meet this very modest level of activity, and one in three has reported no leisure time activity at all. Even though a dose-response relationship between level of exercise and coronary risk exists, many experts worry that even a slightly more aggressive recommendation might discourage motivation to exercise. Nonetheless, the "30 minutes of walking per day" approach to vascular risk reduction may not suffice to reduce weight or maintain a healthy body mass index. In descriptive studies, long-term weight reduction requires more aggressive approaches among formerly obese patients, although one randomized trial has shown short-term benefits of a less aggressive approach.[87]

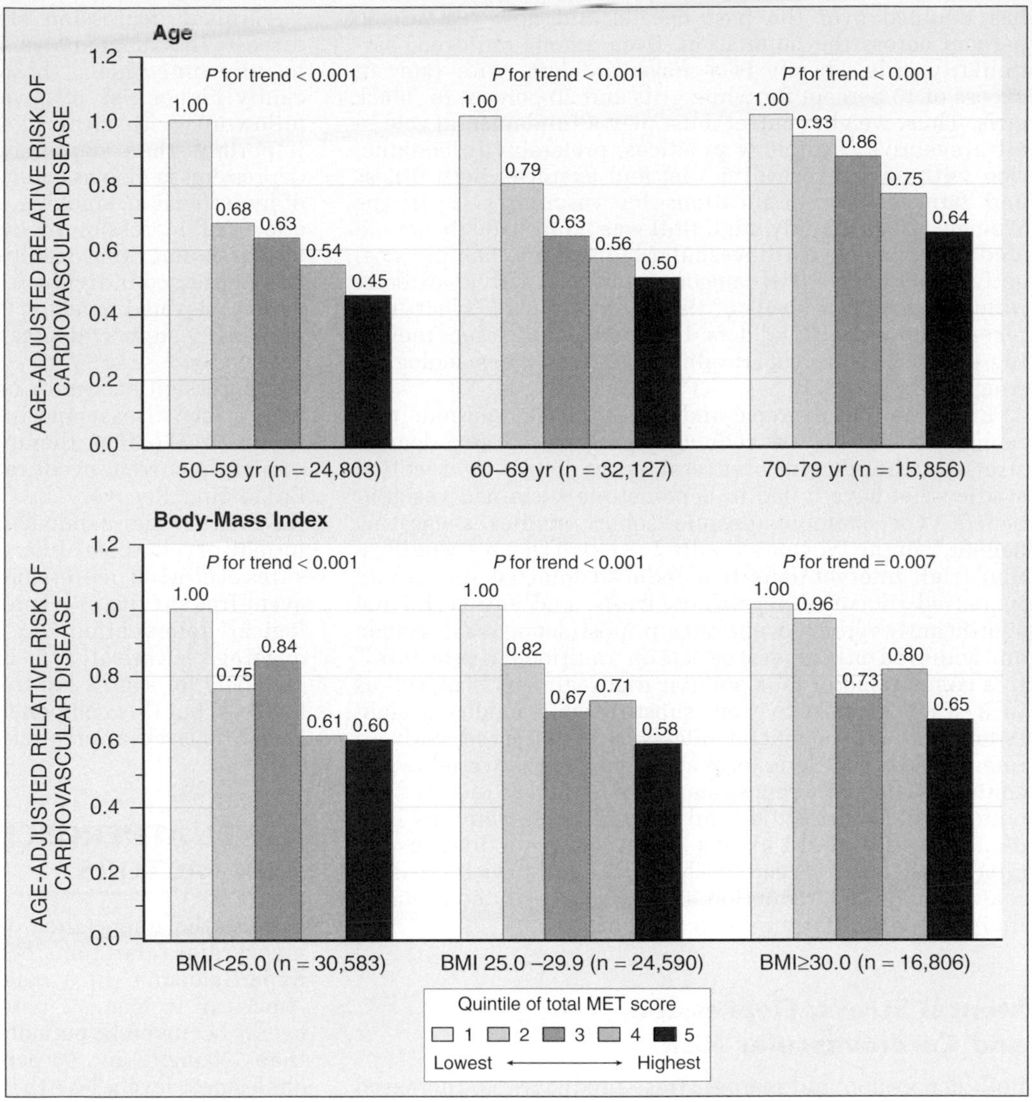

FIGURE 39–7 Relative risks of cardiovascular disease according to quintile of energy expenditure (MET score) from recreational activities stratified by age **(top)** and body mass index **(bottom)**. *(From Manson JE, Greenland P, LaCroix AZ, et al: Walking compared with vigorous exercise for the prevention of cardiovascular events in women. N Engl J Med 347:716, 2002.)*

Regular exercise affects multiple risk factors for atherosclerosis. Aerobic exercise is associated with a mean reduction of systolic blood pressure of 5 mm Hg in hypertensive participants, a level comparable with that of many drug interventions.[88] Although traditionally considered to have only modest effects on total and LDL cholesterol levels, exercise consistently improves HDL cholesterol level and reduces triglycerides. More recent data have indicated that physical activity can increase the average size of LDL particles without a change in plasma LDL concentration.[89] These effects occur even in the absence of clinically significant weight loss and relate more strongly to amount than intensity of exercise. In children, physical activity levels need to substantively exceed 1 hour daily to prevent clustering of cardiovascular risk factors at an early age.[90]

Exercise further improves insulin sensitivity and glycemic control, with major benefits for diabetic patients, including reductions in glycated hemoglobin along with reduced requirements for therapy. These data agree with prospective epidemiological observations that moderate-intensity activity is associated with a reduced incidence of diabetes and with randomized intervention studies, such as the U.S. Diabetes Prevention Program, in which a 58 percent reduction in diabetes risk was observed with modest levels of exercise and a 5 to 7 percent reduction in body weight.[91] Finally, regular exercise lowers C-reactive protein levels, improves coronary endothelial function, and appears to benefit hemostatic variables, including tissue-type plasminogen activator, fibrinogen, von Willebrand factor, fibrin D-dimer, and plasma viscosity.

Controversy remains as to whether obesity itself is a true risk factor for cardiovascular disease or whether its impact on vascular risk is mediated solely through interrelations with glucose intolerance, insulin resistance, hypertension, physical inactivity, and dyslipidemia[92] (see Chap. 44). Midlife obesity, however, strongly presages hospitalization and future complications of coronary heart disease, even among those with few or no other major risk factors.[93] From an epidemiological perspective, obesity alone associates with elevated vascular risk regardless of activity levels, and the waist-to-hip ratio, a surrogate for centripetal or abdominal obesity, independently predicts vascular risk in women and in older men. Among U.S. adults, the prevalence of obesity (defined as a body mass index [BMI] of 30 or higher) has doubled over the past decade and now reaches 30 percent across the population. Even among children, particularly girls, obesity is a major problem, with rates in excess of 10 percent for white girls and 20 percent for black girls. Thus, weight control must play a fundamental role in all preventive cardiology practices, preferably in conjunction with advice regarding diet and exercise. Both fitness and fatness have implications for vascular risk. In the Women's Health Study, high BMI was more strongly associated with adverse cardiovascular biomarkers than physical activity, yet within BMI categories, physical activity directly influenced overall levels of risk.[94] As also made clear from recent randomized trial data, life style modification, including exercise, is a crucial adjunct to any pharmacological weight loss program.[95]

Evidence that exercise and life style interventions will remain crucial for risk reduction programs is also demonstrated by the outcome of several recent dietary intervention studies that have failed to demonstrate sustained vascular benefit. For example, despite cohort studies suggesting benefit,[96] in the Women's Health Initiative Dietary Modification trial, interventions that reduced total fat intake and increased intake of vegetables, fruits, and grains did not significantly reduce event rates in postmenopausal women and achieved only modest effects on traditional risk factors.[97] In a comparison of four popular diet regimens,[98] as well as in a study of carbohydrate substitution,[99] modest weight reductions and beneficial effects were observed with all interventions, but long-term adherence levels were low. By contrast, when adherence rates were higher, as in a study of both Mediterranean diet and life style interventions conducted in the elderly, almost 50 percent reductions in vascular risk were observed.[100] These data will have increasing relevance for risk reduction as rates of obesity continue to increase, particularly in men and children.[101]

Mental Stress, Depression, and Cardiovascular Risk

Both depression and mental stress predispose to increased vascular risk. The adrenergic stimulation of mental stress can augment myocardial oxygen requirements and aggravate myocardial ischemia. Mental stress can cause coronary vasoconstriction, particularly in atherosclerotic coronary arteries, and hence can influence myocardial oxygen supply as well. Studies have further linked mental stress to platelet and endothelial dysfunction, the metabolic syndrome, and the induction of ventricular arrhythmias.

Acute stress, such as that associated with natural disasters, is recognized as a risk factor for acute coronary events. More recently, work-related stress has gained recognition as a source of vascular risk. Work stress has two components—job strain, which combines high work demands and low job control, and effort-reward imbalance, which more closely reflects economic factors in the workplace. Both components are associates with an approximate doubling of risk for myocardial infarction and stroke.[102] Other psychological metrics, including anger and hostility scales, have also been associated with elevated vascular risk. In the INTERHEART study evaluating postinfarction patients from 52 countries, psychosocial stress was found to be associated with vascular risk, with a magnitude of effect similar to that of the major coronary risk factors.[103] The impact of stress reduction has also undergone evaluation in randomized trials. Among patients with stable ischemic heart disease and exercise-induced myocardial ischemia, random allocation to a stress management program reduced emotional distress and improved biomarkers of vascular risk significantly more than usual care.[104]

Clinical depression strongly predicts coronary heart disease. In a meta-analysis of 11 studies involving initially healthy individuals, those with depression had a significantly higher risk of developing coronary disease during follow-up, with clinical depression (RR, 2.7) being more important than depressive mood (RR, 1.5).[105] Although depression is also associated with an increased prevalence of hypertension, smoking, and lack of physical activity, the effects of depression on overall risk remain after adjusting for these and other traditional risk factors. Thus, findings that depressed individuals also have increased platelet activation, elevated levels of hsCRP, and decreased heart rate variability support depression as an independent predictor of events.

Depression occurs in one of five outpatients with coronary artery disease and in one of three patients with heart failure.[106] Whether therapy for postinfarction depression reduces recurrent event rates remains controversial. In the Enhancing Recovery in Coronary Heart Disease Patients (ENRICHD) trial, random allocation between usual care and formal psychosocial intervention modestly improved measures of clinical depression but did not significantly improve event-free survival.[107] Community-based trials of pharmacological intervention for postinfarction depression are ongoing.[108] Clinically, the benefit to both patients and family members for aggressive treatment of depression is likely to be large, but this component of patient care is often ignored in cardiovascular practices.

NOVEL ATHEROSCLEROTIC RISK FACTORS

Despite the importance of blood lipids, 50 percent of all myocardial infarctions occur in individuals without overt hyperlipidemia. In a major prospective study of healthy American women, 77 percent of all future cardiovascular events occurred in patients with LDL cholesterol levels less than 160 mg/dl and 46 percent occurred in those with LDL cholesterol levels less than 130 mg/dl.[109] Although the use of global prediction models like those developed in Framingham greatly improves the detection of heart disease risk, as many as 20 percent of all events occur in the absence of any of the major classic vascular risk factors.

This fact challenges several basic issues related to current screening programs for risk detection and disease prevention. However, clinical data continue to accrue demonstrating the hazard of relying solely on classic risk factors. In one analysis of more than 120,000 patients with coronary heart disease, 15 percent of the women and 19 percent of the men had no evidence of hyperlipidemia, hypertension, diabetes, or smoking and more than 50 percent had only one of these general risk factors.[110] In another large analysis, between 85 and 95 percent of participants with coronary disease had at least one conventional risk factor, but so too did those participants without coronary disease despite follow-up for as long as 30 years.[111] Thus, because of the considerable need to improve vascular risk detection, much research over the past 10 or 15 years has focused on the identification and evaluation of novel atherosclerotic risk factors.[112]

When evaluating any novel risk factor as a potential new screening tool, clinicians need to consider whether (1) there is a standardized and reproducible assay for the marker of interest; (2) there is a consistent series of prospective studies demonstrating that a given parameter predicts future risk; (3) the novel marker adds to the predictive value of lipid screening; and (4) there is evidence that the novel marker adds to global risk prediction scores, such as that in the

Framingham Heart Study. The following section applies these basic epidemiological requirements to a series of novel risk factors, including hsCRP and other markers of inflammation, lipoprotein(a), homocysteine, and markers of fibrinolytic and hemostatic function, such as fibrinogen, D-dimer, tissue plasminogen activator (t-PA), and plasminogen activator inhibitor 1 (PAI-1) antigens (Table 39-1). Physicians should also consider the relative magnitude of novel markers in terms of risk prediction, particularly in comparison with lipid screening. Figure 39-8 shows data describing the relative efficacy of several variables measured at baseline in two large cohorts of initially healthy middle-aged men and women.

High-Sensitivity C-Reactive Protein

Inflammation characterizes all phases of atherothrombosis and provides a critical pathophysiological link between plaque formation and acute rupture, leading to occlusion and infarction[113] (see Chap. 38). Formation of the fatty streak, the earliest phase of atherogenesis, involves recruitment of leukocytes caused by the expression of adhesion molecules on endothelial cells, in turn triggered by inflammatory cytokines such as interleukin-1 and tumor necrosis factor-alpha. Subsequent migration of inflammatory cells into the subendothelial space requires chemotaxis controlled by chemokines induced by the primary cytokines. Mononuclear cells within this initial infiltrate, as well as intrinsic vascular cells, subsequently release growth factors that stimulate proliferation of the smooth muscle cells and lead to plaque progression. The thrombotic complications of plaques often involve physical disruption, usually associated with signs of local and systemic inflammation. Other proinflammatory cytokines such as CD40 ligand can in turn induce tissue factor expression and promote thrombus formation. Moreover, the primary proinflammatory cytokines result in the expression of messenger cytokines such as interleukin-6, which can travel from local sites of inflammation to the liver, where a change in the program of protein synthesis characteristic of the acute phase response is thereby triggered. The acute-phase reactant, CRP, a simple downstream marker of inflammation, has now emerged as a major cardiovascular risk factor.[114]

Composed of five 23-kDa subunits, CRP is a circulating member of the pentraxin family that plays a major role in the human innate immune response. Although derived primarily from the liver, studies have found that cells within human coronary arteries, particularly in the atherosclerotic intima, can also elaborate CRP. More than simply a marker of inflammation, CRP may influence directly vascular vulnerability through several mechanisms, including enhanced expression of local adhesion molecules, increased expression of endothelial PAI-1, reduced endothelial nitric oxide bioactivity, altered LDL uptake by macrophages, and colo-

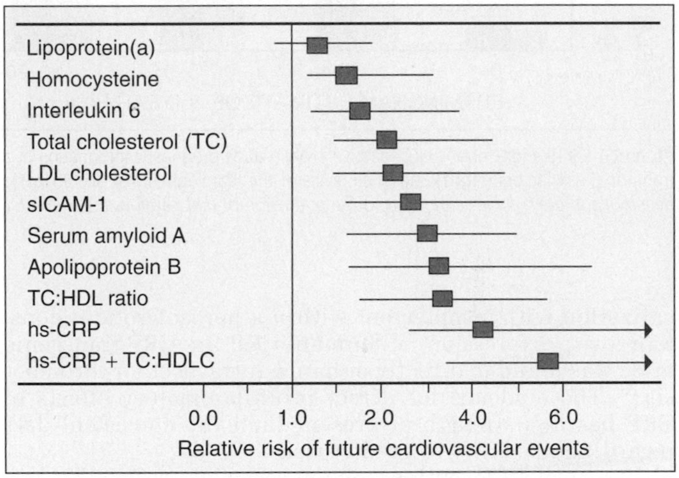

FIGURE 39–8 Relative risks of future myocardial infarction among apparently healthy women according to baseline levels of lipoprotein(a), homocysteine, interleukin-6, total cholesterol, low-density lipoprotein (LDL) cholesterol, soluble intercellular adhesion molecule-1 (sICAM-1), serum amyloid A, apolipoprotein B, ratio of total cholesterol to high-density lipoprotein cholesterol (TC:HDLC), high-sensitivity C-reactive protein (hsCRP), and the combination of hsCRP with the TC:HDLC. *(From Ridker PM: Clinical application of C-reactive protein for cardiovascular disease detection and prevention. Circulation 107:363, 2003.)*

TABLE 39–1 Clinical Epidemiology of Proposed Plasma-Based Biomarkers for Prediction of Future Cardiovascular Events

Biomarker	Prospective Studies Convincing?	Standardized Commercial Assay?	Additive to Lipid Screening?	Additive to Framingham Risk Score?
Inflammation				
hsCRP	++++	+++	+++	+++
sICAM-1	++	±	+	–
SAA	++	–	+	–
IL-6/IL-18	++	–	+	–
Myeloperoxidase	+	–	±	–
sCD40L	+	–	–	–
Altered thrombosis				
t-PA/PAI-1	++	±	–	–
Fibrinogen	+++	±	++	–
Homocysteine	++++	+++	±	–
D-dimer	++	+	–	–
Oxidative stress-oxidized LDL	±	–	–	–
Altered lipids				
Lipoprotein(a)	+++	±	±	–
LDL particle size	++	±	±	–

hsCRP = high-sensitivity C-reactive protein; IL = interleukin; LDL = low-density lipoprotein; PAI-1 = plasminogen activator inhibitor-1; sICAM-1 = intercellular adhesion molecule-1; SAA = serum amyloid A; sCD40L = soluble CD40 ligand; t-PA = tissue plasminogen activator. Plus signs indicate increasing strength of evidence.

Modified from Ridker PM, Brown NJ, Vaughan DE, et al: Established and emerging plasma biomarkers in the prediction of first atherothrombotic events. Circulation 109(25 Suppl 1):IV6, 2004.

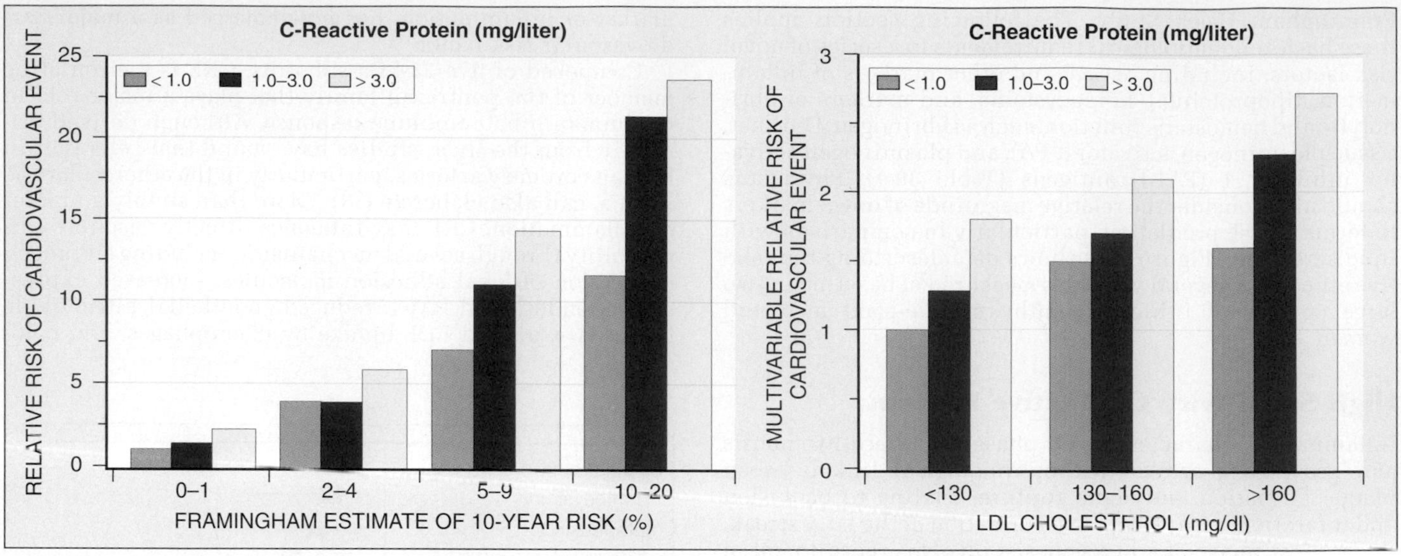

FIGURE 39–9 High-sensitivity C-reactive protein adds prognostic information at all levels of low-density lipoprotein (LDL) cholesterol after multivariate adjustment for traditional risk factors **(right)** and at all levels of the Framingham risk score **(left).** *(From Ridker PM, Rifai N, Rose L, et al: Comparison of C-reactive protein and low-density lipoprotein cholesterol levels in the prediction of first cardiovascular events. N Engl J Med 347:1557, 2002.)*

calization with complement within atherosclerotic lesions. Moreover, expression of human CRP in CRP-transgenic mice was found to directly enhance intravascular thrombosis.[115] The evidence for direct proinflammatory effects of CRP has less strength at present than the consistent data regarding its ability to predict risk.

In primary prevention, a large series of prospective epidemiological studies has demonstrated convincingly that CRP, when measured with high-sensitivity assays, strongly and independently predicts risk of myocardial infarction, stroke, peripheral arterial disease, and sudden cardiac death among apparently healthy individuals. These data apply to women as well as men across all age levels and have been consistent in diverse populations. Most importantly, hsCRP adds prognostic information at all levels of LDL cholesterol and at all levels of risk, as determined by the Framingham Risk Score (Fig. 39-9).[109] In other major studies from the United States and Europe, hsCRP levels predicted subsequent risk better than LDL cholesterol level.[116,117] However, because hsCRP levels reflect a component of vascular risk different from that of cholesterol, the addition of hsCRP to lipid evaluation provides a major opportunity to improve global risk prediction. In clinical terms, absolute vascular risk is higher in individuals with elevated hsCRP levels and low levels of LDL cholesterol than in those with elevated levels of LDL cholesterol but low levels of hsCRP, but current guidelines consider only the latter group to be at high risk (Fig. 39-10). Even in studies that have reported the effect of hsCRP as modest, the magnitude of effect was at least as large as that of hypertension and smoking, data demonstrating the importance of inflammation in atherogenesis.[118]

Largely on the basis of these data, the American Heart Association and the Centers for Disease Control and Prevention issued guidelines in 2003 for the use of hsCRP in clinical practice.[119] Briefly, hsCRP levels less than 1, 1 to 3, and higher than 3 mg/liter should be interpreted as lower, moderate, and higher relative vascular risk, respectively, when considered along with traditional markers of risk. This critical finding has corroborated studies conducted worldwide; all studies of adequate sample size have found the risk of hsCRP to be independent of and additive to traditional risk factors (Fig. 39-11).[57,116,120-124] Screening for hsCRP should be done at the discretion of the physician as part of global risk evaluation, not as a replacement for LDL and HDL testing. Although hsCRP predicts risk across the entire population spectrum, its greatest usefulness is likely to be for those at intermediate risk—that is, individuals with anticipated 10-year event rates between 5 and 20 percent. In a recent analysis of the impact that CRP makes on clinical risk prediction, global risk prediction models that included hsCRP reclassified approximately 20 percent of those otherwise considered to be at intermediate risk; moreover, the impact of hsCRP on risk prediction was at least as large as that of lipid screening.[4] Values of hsCRP in excess of 8 mg/liter may represent an acute-phase response caused by an underlying inflammatory disease or intercurrent infection and should lead to repeat testing in approximately 2 to 3 weeks; consistently high values, however, represent very high risk of future cardiovascular disease, because risk appears to be

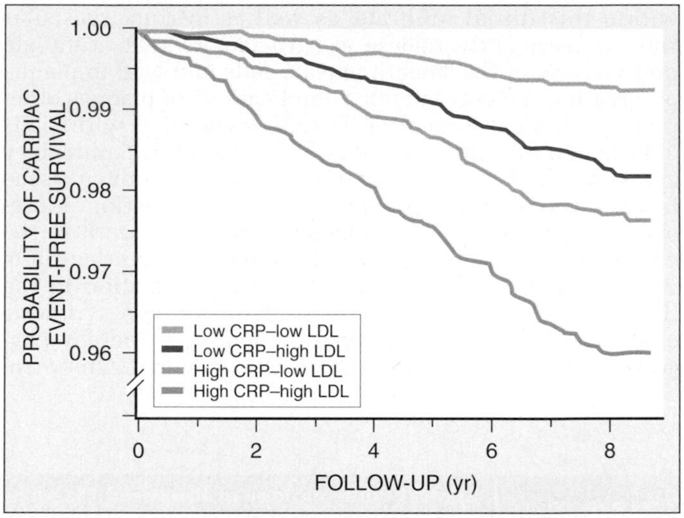

FIGURE 39–10 Cardiovascular event–free survival among apparently healthy individuals according to baseline levels of high-sensitivity C-reactive protein (CRP) and low-density lipoprotein (LDL) cholesterol. *(From Ridker PM, Rifai N, Rose L, et al: Comparison of C-reactive protein and low-density lipoprotein cholesterol levels in the prediction of first cardiovascular events. N Engl J Med 347:1557, 2002.)*

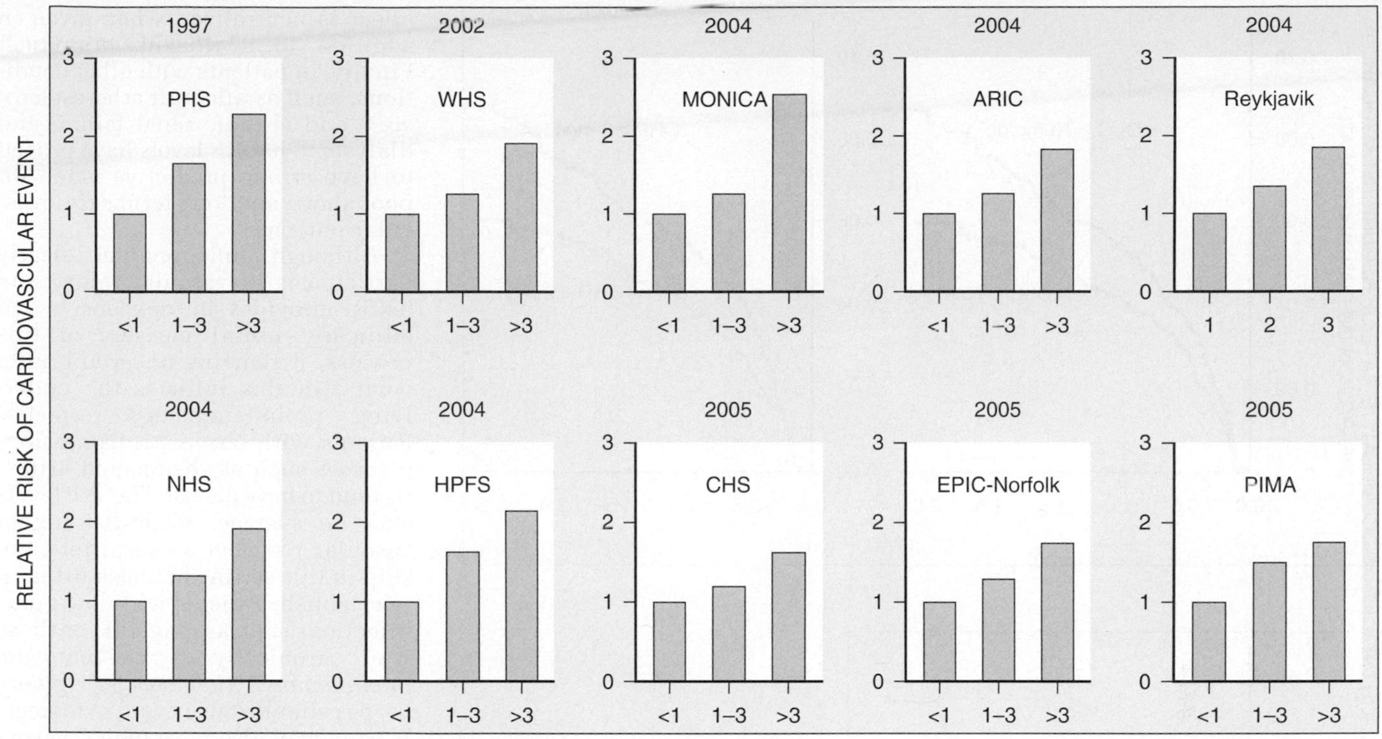

FIGURE 39–11 Framingham-adjusted relative risks of future cardiovascular events according to baseline levels of high-sensitivity C-reactive protein (hsCRP) less than 1, 1 to 3, and more than 3 mg/liter in 10 major prospective cohort studies. PHS = Physicians' Health Study; WHS = Women's Health Study; MONICA = Monitoring Trends and Developments in Cardiovascular Disease; ARIC = Atherosclerosis Risk in Communities Study; NHS = Nurses' Health Study; HPFS = Health Professionals' Follow-up Study; CHS = Cardiovascular Health Study; EPIC-Norfolk = Evaluation for Prevention of Ischemic Complications; PIMA = Pima Indians. *(Modified from Libby P, Ridker PM. Inflammation and atherothrombosis. J Am Coll Cardiol 48:A33, 2006.)*

linear across the full range of hsCRP levels.[125] Because hsCRP levels are stable over long periods, have no circadian variation, and do not depend on prandial state, screening can easily be done on an outpatient basis at the time of cholesterol evaluation.

Levels of hsCRP greater than 3 mg/liter also predict recurrent coronary events, thrombotic complications after angioplasty, poor outcome in the setting of unstable angina, and vascular complications after bypass surgery. All these data support the concept that inflammation plays a critical role throughout the atherothrombotic process. Additionally, hsCRP has prognostic usefulness in cases of acute ischemia, even without troponin level elevation, suggesting that an enhanced inflammatory response at the time of hospital admission can determine subsequent plaque rupture.[126] These findings help explain why individuals with elevated hsCRP levels are also more likely to benefit from aggressive interventions compared with those with low hsCRP levels.

Elevated levels of hsCRP predict not only cardiovascular events but also the onset of type 2 diabetes mellitus,[74,75] perhaps because hsCRP levels correlate with several components of the metabolic syndrome, including those not easily measured in clinical practice such as insulin sensitivity, endothelial dysfunction, and hypofibrinolysis. Thus, hsCRP assessment also adds prognostic information at all levels of the metabolic syndrome.[73,76] Even for individuals with the Adult Treatment Panel (ATP-III) definition of metabolic syndrome, knowledge of hsCRP levels less than 1, 1 to 3, and greater than 3 mg/liter further defines low-, moderate-, and high-risk groups for future vascular events.

Statins lower hsCRP levels in a manner largely unrelated to the magnitude of LDL cholesterol reduction.[127] Data from primary and secondary prevention trials have indicated that the relative benefit of statin therapy in terms of event reduction may be greater in the presence of elevated hsCRP levels. In the AFCAPS/TexCAPS trial, for example, lovastatin appeared to lower cardiovascular event rates, even for those with below-median levels of LDL cholesterol but above-median levels of hsCRP.[128] By contrast, lovastatin did not reduce events in those with neither hyperlipidemia nor inflammation. These observations have led to the hypothesis that statin therapy prevents first vascular events, not only in patients with elevated LDL cholesterol levels, but also in those with elevated levels of hsCRP. This critical hypothesis has been directly investigated.[129] In the PROVE IT-TIMI 22 clinical trial conducted in patients with acute coronary syndromes treated with statin therapy, achieving levels of hsCRP less than 2 mg/liter was as important for long-term event-free survival as was achieving levels of LDL cholesterol less than 70 mg/dl; in fact, the best long-term outcomes were found in those who achieved both these goals (Fig. 39-12).[130] This new concept of "dual goals" for statin therapy, which includes both CRP and LDL level reduction, has been corroborated in the A-to-Z clinical trial,[131] as well as in studies using intravascular ultrasound to monitor disease progression. In this latter setting, only those with CRP reduction had coronary regression with statin therapy, whereas those who achieved both CRP and LDL level reduction had the greatest regression overall.[132] In addition to statins, treatment with fibrates and niacin may also lower hsCRP levels, as does the use of thiazolidinediones. By contrast, oral preparations of hormone replacement therapy tend to increase hsCRP levels. Although aspirin does not lower hsCRP levels directly, the usefulness of aspirin in preventing first vascular events appears to be highest for patients with elevated hsCRP levels.

hsCRP levels correlate only modestly with underlying atherosclerotic disease as measured by carotid intimal medial thickness or by coronary calcification. This observation suggests that hsCRP does not simply reflect the pres-

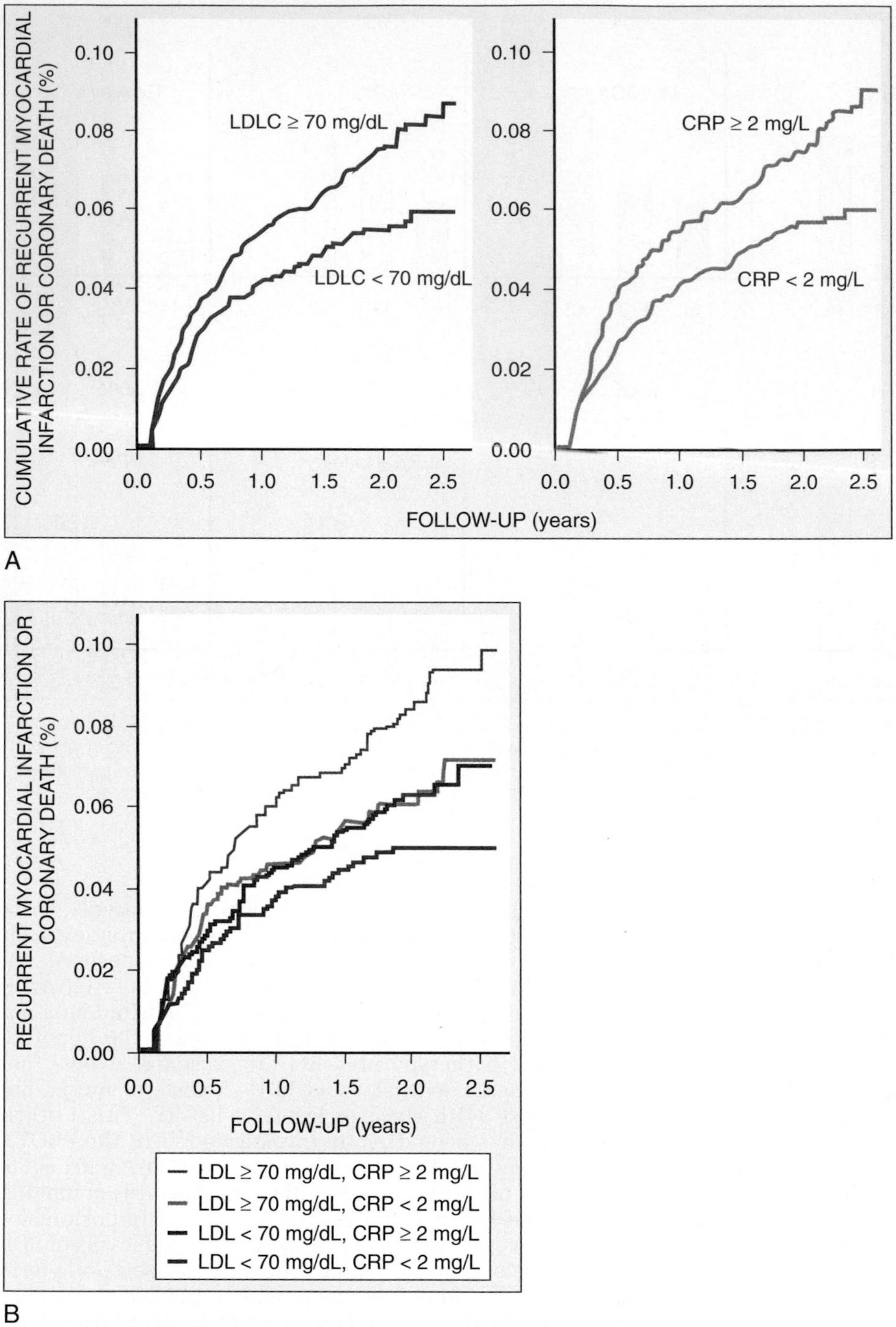

FIGURE 39–12 A, Cumulative rate of recurrent myocardial infarction or death among statin-treated patients according to either levels of LDLC **(left)** or hsCRP **(right)** achieved after 30 days of therapy in the PROVE IT-TIMI 22 trial. **B,** Cumulative rate of recurrent myocardial infarction or death among statin-treated patients according to both levels of LDLC *and* hsCRP achieved after 30 days of therapy in the PROVE IT-TIMI 22 trial. *(From Ridker PM, Cannon CP, Morrow D, et al: C-reactive protein levels and outcomes after statin therapy. N Engl J Med 352:20, 2005.)*

ence of subclinical disease but indicates an increased propensity for plaque disruption and/or thrombosis. Autopsy data support this hypothesis: elevated hsCRP levels occur more often in patients with frankly ruptured plaques than in those with erosive disease or those who died of nonvascular causes. Studies have also indicated that hsCRP levels predict incident hypertension and add prognostic information on vascular risk at all levels of blood pressure.[133,134] These data are of therapeutic interest, because clinical trial data (see earlier) have indicated that angiotensin receptor blockade lowers hsCRP levels, although this effect is neutralized when given in addition to a thiazide diuretic.[40] Finally, in patients with other conditions, such as allograft atherosclerosis[135] and chronic renal failure and dialysis,[136] hsCRP levels have proved to have strong predictive value for poor short- and long-term cardiovascular outcomes.

Although inflammation clearly participates in vascular injury and hsCRP provides an inexpensive and clinically useful measure of this process, it remains uncertain as to what stimulus initiates the underlying proinflammatory response. Patients with chronic inflammatory diseases such as rheumatoid arthritis tend to have elevated hsCRP levels and, on average, somewhat higher vascular risk, but a causal relationship in this setting has been difficult to establish. Patients with low-grade infections such as gingivitis or those who chronically carry *Chlamydia pneumoniae, Helicobacter pylori,* herpes simplex virus, and cytomegalovirus may also have higher vascular risk on the basis of a chronic systemic inflammatory response. However, careful prospective studies of antibody titers directed against these agents have not consistently found evidence of association, and large-scale antibiotic trials have not shown reduced recurrent events in myocardial infarction survivors.[137] Whether novel targeted anti-inflammatory therapies, including specific cytokine inhibitors, can improve coronary outcomes is an active area of research. The potential for direct CRP inhibition has also recently shown promise, at least in mouse models of acute ischemia.[138]

Some have suggested that measurement of hsCRP has only a marginal clinical effect, a conclusion largely based on the observation that the addition of hsCRP to risk prediction models minimally increases the C-statistic, a traditional measure of model fit.[139,140] However, it is important to recognize that once age and smoking are accounted for, neither blood pressure, LDL, nor HDL cholesterol increase the C-statistic, suggesting that this statistical tool lacks sensitivity to major pathophysiological effects.[141] Thus, given the robustness of laboratory and epidemiological data and the low cost of testing, we believe that hsCRP evaluation should become a routine part of coronary risk prediction. In outpatient settings, hsCRP levels should be evaluated at the time of cholesterol screening if the practitioner wishes to use it as an adjunct to global risk prediction. For individuals with an LDL cholesterol level greater than 160 mg/dl, a finding of an elevated hsCRP level should provide an additional impetus for the physician to institute aggressive primary prevention and may help motivate some patients to comply with life style modifications and, when indicated, pharmacotherapy. For individuals with LDL cholesterol levels between 130 and 160 mg/dl, the finding of an elevated hsCRP level indicates substantial risk and, again, should lead to better adherence to preventive efforts and perhaps to earlier use of pharmacological approaches to risk reduction. For individuals with LDL cholesterol levels below 130 mg/dl, an elevated hsCRP value also confers elevated risk. However, although post hoc analyses have suggested that such patients may benefit from statin therapy, clinical trials testing this issue have only recently begun. Such individuals should thus aggressively undergo physical activity, weight loss, and smoking cessation programs. In this setting, an elevated hsCRP level should provide considerable motivation to improve life style, particularly for those previously told that they were not at risk because of an absence of hyperlipidemia. As noted earlier, in patients with acute coronary syndromes, reaching an hsCRP level less than 2 mg/liter appears to be as important for long-term outcomes as reaching an LDL cholesterol level less than 70 mg/dl.

Other Markers of Inflammation

Although hsCRP is by far the best-characterized and most reliable inflammatory biomarker for clinical use, several other markers of inflammation have shown promise in terms of predicting vascular risk. These include cytokines such as interleukin-6, soluble forms of certain cell adhesion molecules such as intercellular adhesion molecule (sICAM-1), P-selectin, or the mediator CD40 ligand, as well as markers of leukocyte activation such as myeloperoxidase. Other inflammatory markers associated with lipid oxidation such as lipoprotein-associated phospholipase A_2 and pregnancy-associated plasma protein A have also shown promise.[142,143] However, each of these biomarkers has analytical issues that need careful evaluation before routine clinical use. For example, some have too short a half-life for clinical diagnostic testing, whereas the ability of others to predict risk in settings of broad populations has proved marginal thus far. Nonetheless, several of these inflammatory biomarkers can shed critical pathophysiological light on the atherothrombotic process, particularly at the time of plaque rupture. For example, soluble CD40 ligand (probably released from activated platelets) may provide insight into the efficacy of specific antithrombotic agents independently of CRP.[144] Similarly, myeloperoxidase may provide prognostic information in cases of acute ischemia over and above that associated with troponin or CRP.[145,146] Thus, continued evaluation of other inflammatory biomarkers may well provide targets for or monitors of therapy, particularly in the setting of acute coronary ischemia.[147]

Homocysteine

Homocysteine is a sulfhydryl-containing amino acid derived from the demethylation of dietary methionine. Patients with rare inherited defects of methionine metabolism can develop severe hyperhomocysteinemia (plasma levels higher than 100 μmol/liter) and have markedly elevated risk of premature atherothrombosis as well as venous thromboembolism. Mechanisms suggested to account for these effects include endothelial dysfunction, accelerated oxidation of LDL cholesterol, impairment of flow-mediated endothelium-derived relaxing factor with subsequent reduction in arterial vasodilation, platelet activation, and oxidative stress. In contrast to severe hyperhomocysteinemia, mild to moderate elevations of homocysteine (plasma levels higher than 15 μmol/liter) are more common in the general population, primarily because of insufficient dietary intake of folic acid. Other patient groups who tend to have elevated levels of homocysteine include those receiving folate antagonists such as methotrexate and carbamazepine and those with impaired homocysteine metabolism caused by hypothyroidism or renal insufficiency.

A common polymorphism in the methylene tetrahydrofolate reductase gene (*MTHFR*) that encodes a thermolabile protein has also been linked to elevated homocysteine levels and to increased vascular risk, at least among individuals homozygous for the variant. Familial association studies have reported higher homocysteine levels in offspring of parents with premature coronary artery disease. However, the clinical importance of the *MTHFR* polymorphism appears modest, and heterozygous individuals display little evidence of elevated homocysteine levels, even in those with low folate intake. In a meta-analysis of 40 observational studies, individuals homozygous for the *MTHFR* 677 TT variant had a 16 percent increase in relative risk (OR, 1.16; 95 percent CI, 1.05-1.28), and this observation was evident only in studies originating in Europe.[148] In populations in whom folate fortification exists, such as in North America, no compelling evidence supports genetic evaluation of *MTHFR* to predict vascular risk. For example, in the large-scale Women's Health Study, *MTHFR* variants were associated with plasma homocysteine levels, which in turn were associated with modest elevation of risk, but there was no independent effect of the gene variants on clinical outcomes.

Reliable immunoassays for total plasma homocysteine (the combination of free homocysteine, bound homocysteine, and mixed disulfides) are now widely available and have largely replaced the use of high-performance liquid chromatography. Despite availability of newer assays, measurement of homocysteine remains controversial and recent guidelines have not advocated their use. This lack of enthusiasm reflects modest overall effects in prospective cohort studies and the publication of several large trials of homocysteine reduction. With regard to epidemiological evidence, the magnitude and strength of association between baseline homocysteine levels and risk of subsequent disease in a meta-analysis was found to be smaller than previously reported.[149] Although there is some heterogeneity between the prospective studies, on average, these meta-analyses have reported a 25 percent lower homocysteine level being associated with an approximate 11 percent lower risk of coronary heart disease, an estimate far smaller than hypothesized. However, at least in the United States, fortification of the food supply has greatly reduced the frequency of low folate and elevated homocysteine levels, particularly for those initially in the moderately elevated range. Thus, the number of individuals potentially identifiable by screening for homocysteine has decreased considerably. On the other hand, investigators in the Framingham Study have found plasma homocysteine levels to be associated with a modest increase in risk for congestive heart failure in adults without prior myocardial infarction.[150]

With regard to clinical trials of homocysteine reduction, several major studies have been completed and none have shown substantive benefit. In the Vitamin Intervention for Stroke Prevention (VISP) trial conducted among 3680 patients with prior stroke allocated to high-dose or low-dose vitamin regimens containing folate and pyridoxine, there was no evidence of differential benefit in the high-dose group, despite greater homocysteine level reduction.[151] In a second trial, of 636 postangioplasty patients treated with folate, vitamin B_6 and vitamin B_{12}, rates of in-stent stenosis were actually higher in most intervention groups compared with those allocated to placebo.[152] This negative trial is clinically important, because it conflicts with prior work that had suggested benefit in this setting. A net harmful effect associated with combined vitamin B supplementation was also observed in the Norwegian Vitamin Trial (NORVIT) involving 3749 participants with recent myocardial infarction. In that trial, mean total homocysteine was lowered by 27 percent in the intervention group, but there was no significant effect on the primary endpoint (hazard ratio [HR], 1.08; 95 percent CI, 0.93 to 1.25), whereas a trend toward increased risk was observed in those allocated to folate, vitamin B_6, and vitamin B_{12} (HR, 1.22; 95 percent CI, 1.00 to 1.50).[153] Finally, in the Heart Outcomes Prevention Evaluation (HOPE-2) trial of 5522 patients with vascular disease or diabetes, 5 years of therapy with folate, vitamin B_6, and vitamin B_{12} resulted in no benefit compared with placebo for total vascular events (HR, 0.95; 95 percent CI, 0.84 to 1.07), cardiovascular mortality (HR, 0.96; 95 percent CI, 0.81 to 1.13), or any of several prespecified secondary endpoints.[154] As a group, these sharply negative trial results conflict with the supposition made from studies of mendelian randomization that had previously argued for a clear causal role between homocysteine concentration and vascular events.[155]

Despite reduced enthusiasm and lack of evidence that homocysteine reduction lowers risk, there remain a few specific patient populations for whom homocysteine evaluation may prove appropriate, including those lacking traditional risk factors, with renal failure, or with markedly premature atherosclerosis or a family history of myocardial infarction and stroke at a young age.[156] It is also crucial to continue folate supplementation in the general population to reduce the risk of neural tube defects, an inexpensive practice that has been in place in the United States for over a decade yet remains a public health challenge for much of Europe and the developing world.[157]

Fibrinogen and Fibrin D-Dimer

Plasma fibrinogen influences platelet aggregation and blood viscosity, interacts with plasminogen binding and, in combination with thrombin, mediates the final step in clot formation and the response to vascular injury.[158] In addition, fibrinogen associates positively with age, obesity, smoking, diabetes, and LDL cholesterol level, and inversely with HDL cholesterol level, alcohol use, physical activity, and exercise level. Fibrinogen, like CRP, is an acute-phase reactant and increases during inflammatory responses.

Given these relationships, it is not surprising that fibrinogen was among the first "novel" risk factors evaluated. Early reports from the Gothenburg, Northwick Park, and Framingham heart studies all found significant positive associations between fibrinogen levels and future risk of cardiovascular events. Since then, a number of other prospective studies have confirmed these findings and, in recent meta-analyses, there was an approximately linear logarithmic association between usual fibrinogen level and the risk of coronary heart disease and stroke. In one analysis, the age- and gender-adjusted hazard ratio per 1-g/liter increase in fibrinogen was 2.4 for coronary heart disease and 2.1 for stroke.[159] Interestingly, these effects were largely unaffected in those studies in which further adjustment for hsCRP was possible. In more recent studies, hsCRP and fibrinogen levels appeared to be additive in their ability to predict risk, although the absolute effect of hsCRP appeared to be larger (Fig. 39-13). Other studies have suggested that the predictive usefulness of fibrinogen is highest in those with other concomitant elevations of lipoprotein(a) or homocysteine.

Despite the consistency of these data, fibrinogen evaluation has found limited use in clinical practice because of suboptimal assay standardization and consistency across reference laboratories remains poor. Fibrates and niacin lower fibrinogen levels but statin therapy does not, an effect different than that observed for hsCRP. Three clinical trials have evaluated the potential benefits of fibrinogen reduction, and all have found disappointing results. The Bezafibrate Infarction Prevention Trial showed no reduction in event rates with active therapy despite a significant reduction in fibrinogen levels and despite evidence that within the study population, baseline fibrinogen levels predicted vascular risk.[160] In a second trial of more than 1500 patients with peripheral vascular disease, bezafibrate reduced fibrinogen levels 13 percent but again had no significant effect on clinical outcomes.[161] Finally, in the HERS trial and in the Women's Health Initiative, hormone replacement therapy lowered fibrinogen levels but did not benefit outcomes.

Fibrin D-dimer reflects the extent of fibrin turnover in the circulation, and epidemiological evidence has found D-dimer levels to have modest predictive value for future vascular events. These studies, when taken together, suggest an approximate relative risk of 1.7 to 1.8 comparing those in the top to bottom thirds of the D-dimer distribution. Following myocardial infarction, D-dimer levels also predict recurrent events and, like CRP, D-dimer predicts poor outcome in troponin-negative ischemia.[162] These studies have pathophysiological interest, and evidence has accumulated that genetic determinants of fibrinogen and D-dimer may lead to altered fibrin clot structure in susceptible individuals. As with fibrinogen, however, the usefulness of D-dimer assessment for arterial thrombosis prediction appears limited in clinical settings. This finding contrasts markedly with the strong clinical usefulness of D-dimer evaluation in the setting of suspected venous thromboembolism.[163]

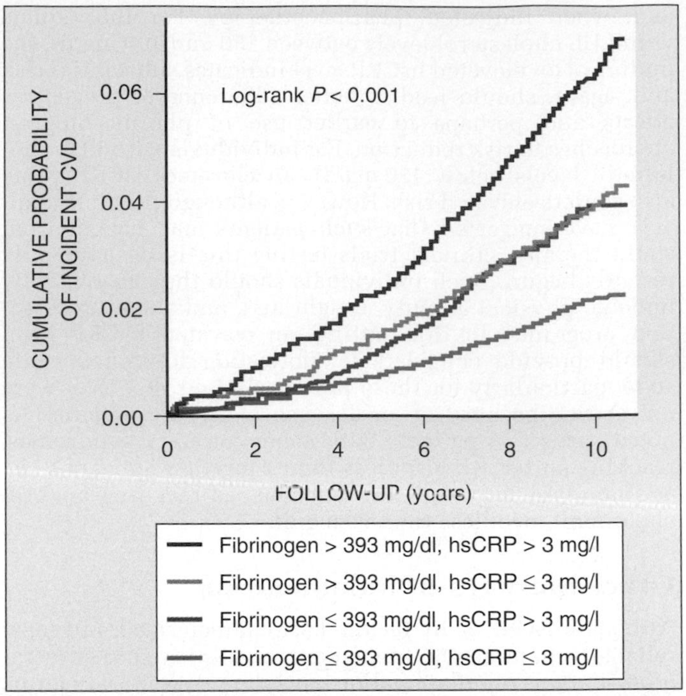

FIGURE 39–13 Cumulative rates of cardiovascular events according to plasma fibrinogen and hsCRP levels. *(Modified from Mora S, Rifai N, Buring JE, Ridker PM: Additive value of immunoassay-measured fibrinogen and high-sensitivity C-reactive protein levels for predicting incident cardiovascular events. Circulation 114:381, 2006.)*

Markers of Fibrinolytic Function

Impaired fibrinolysis can result from an imbalance between the clot-dissolving enzymes t-PA or urokinase-type plasminogen activator and their endogenous inhibitors, primarily PAI-1. Plasma levels of PAI-1 peak in the morning, whereas concentrations of t-PA demonstrate a less prominent circadian variation. On this basis, a relative hypofibrinolytic state may prevail in the morning that, along with increased platelet reactivity, may contribute to the increased risk of myocardial infarction seen during this period. Visceral obesity yields enhanced PAI-1 production from adipocytes, and thus impaired fibrinolysis may help explain how weight gain and obesity influence atherothrombosis. Individuals with the insulin resistance syndrome commonly have impaired fibrinolysis and, in the setting of metabolic syndrome, PAI-1 as well as CRP levels predict adverse vascular outcomes in addition to the onset of type 2 diabetes.[164]

A consistent series of prospective studies has linked abnormalities of fibrinolysis to increased risk of arterial thrombosis. Prospective associations exist between PAI-1 antigen and activity levels and the risk of first and recurrent myocardial infarction. Perhaps paradoxically, individuals at risk for future coronary as well as cerebral thrombosis consistently also have elevated levels of circulating t-PA antigen. These latter effects may represent evidence of underlying endothelial dysfunction in individuals at risk or a direct relationship between t-PA and PAI-1, or they may represent a biological response to impaired fibrinolysis. In this regard, reduced clot lysis time, an overall indicator of net fibrinolytic function, also predicts coronary risk. As reviewed earlier, several studies have indicated that levels of D-dimer, a peptide released by plasmin's action on fibrin, also predicts myocardial infarction, peripheral atherosclerosis, and recurrent coronary events. These observations have been confirmed in studies of women taking and not taking hormone replacement therapy, an important issue because conjugated estrogens decrease PAI-1 antigen concentrations.[165,166] Despite these data, the clinical use of fibrinolytic markers to determine coronary risk offers only marginal value, and no data available suggest that measures of fibrinolysis add to traditional risk scores. Direct measurement of PAI-1 activity is difficult in clinical settings and requires special anticoagulants and precise phlebotomy techniques to avoid degranulation of platelets, a rich source of PAI-1. In addition, markers of fibrinolytic function such as PAI-1 have a wide circadian variation, limiting use in outpatient settings as a risk determinant.

Nonetheless, the recognition that fibrinolytic function contributes to atherothrombosis has yielded several practical applications. For example, PAI-1–resistant thrombolytic agents may provide a means to increase the efficacy of thrombolytic therapy for acute myocardial infarction. Furthermore, the renin-angiotensin system plays an important role in the regulation of fibrinolysis, and angiotensin-converting enzyme inhibitors may favorably affect fibrinolytic balance.[167] Finally, well-described polymorphisms in the PAI-1 promoter and other components of the fibrinolytic system may contribute to interindividual differences in fibrinolytic function.[168]

Lipoprotein(a)

Lipoprotein(a) (Lp[a]) consists of an LDL particle with its apolipoprotein B-100 (apo B-100) component linked by a disulfide bridge to apolipoprotein(a) (apo[a]), a variable-length protein that has sequence homology to plasminogen. The apo(a) component of Lp(a) is a complex molecule composed in part of varying numbers of cysteine-rich kringle IV repeats that result in great heterogeneity. As such, plasma Lp(a) concentrations vary inversely with apo(a) isoform size but also may vary even in isoform size, based on differential levels of production. Underlying its molecular complexity, more than 25 heritable forms of Lp(a) exist, demonstrating the importance of the genome in determining plasma levels, an important issue for risk prediction across different population groups. The close homology between Lp(a) and plasminogen has raised the possibility that this lipoprotein may inhibit endogenous fibrinolysis by competing with plasminogen binding on the endothelium. More recent studies have suggested that Lp(a) binds and inactivates tissue factor pathway inhibitor and may upregulate the expression of plasminogen activator inhibitor, further linking lipoproteins and thrombosis. Lp(a) also colocalizes within atherosclerotic lesions and may have local actions through oxidized phospholipids pathways.[169] Thus, several mechanisms may contribute to a role of Lp(a) in atherothrombosis.

Many but not all prospective cohort studies have supported a role for Lp(a) as a determinant of vascular risk. In a meta-analysis of 27 prospective studies, with a mean follow-up period of 10 years, individuals with Lp(a) levels in the top third of the distribution had a risk 1.6 times higher than those with Lp(a) levels in the bottom third.[170] Adjustment for classic cardiovascular risk factors only modestly attenuated these effects, in part because there is little correlation between Lp(a) and other markers of risk. However, whether the assessment of Lp(a) truly adds prognostic information to overall risk in primary prevention remains uncertain because, in most studies, Lp(a) has been predictive only for those already known to be at high risk because of the presence of other risk factors, in particular elevated levels of LDL cholesterol. Data from the Italian Longitudinal Study on Aging, the Prospective Cardiovascular Munster study, the Bruneck Heart Study, and the PRIME study have suggested that a high serum lipoprotein(a) level is an important risk factor, primarily in individuals with type 2 diabetes or overt hyperlipidemia.[171,172] Other investigators have found that Lp(a) signifies elevated risk in limited situations such as the presence of hyperfibrinogenemia or elevated homocysteine levels, or in the elderly, with multiple other risk factors.[173,174] Several prospective evaluations have shown that lipoprotein(a) predicts risk in a nonlinear manner so that risk increases are very small until Lp(a) levels within the top 5 to 10 percent are reached.[175] Some investigators have advocated lipoprotein(a) assessment in certain patient groups, such as those with established coronary disease or renal failure, although data remain controversial.[176] Evidence that children with recurrent ischemic stroke have elevated Lp(a) levels also supports the potential use of this biomarker in unusual high-risk settings.

Standardization of commercial Lp(a) assays remains problematic and inaccuracy of commercial Lp(a) assays has resulted from the use of techniques sensitive to apo(a) size. However, commercial assays that measure Lp(a) in a manner independent of apo(a) isoform size are now available in some reference laboratories.[177] Using one such assay, investigators in the Women's Health Study have found that extremely high levels of Lp(a) (greater than the 90th percentile, or higher than 65.6 mg/liter) are indeed associated with increased cardiovascular risk, independent of other traditional risk factors.[178] However, this risk increase was nonlinear and limited almost entirely to those with concomitant elevations of LDL cholesterol levels, confirming earlier work (Fig. 39-14). Thus, the presence of threshold effects and interactions with LDL cholesterol do not support the routine measurement of Lp(a) for cardiovascular risk stratification in the general population.

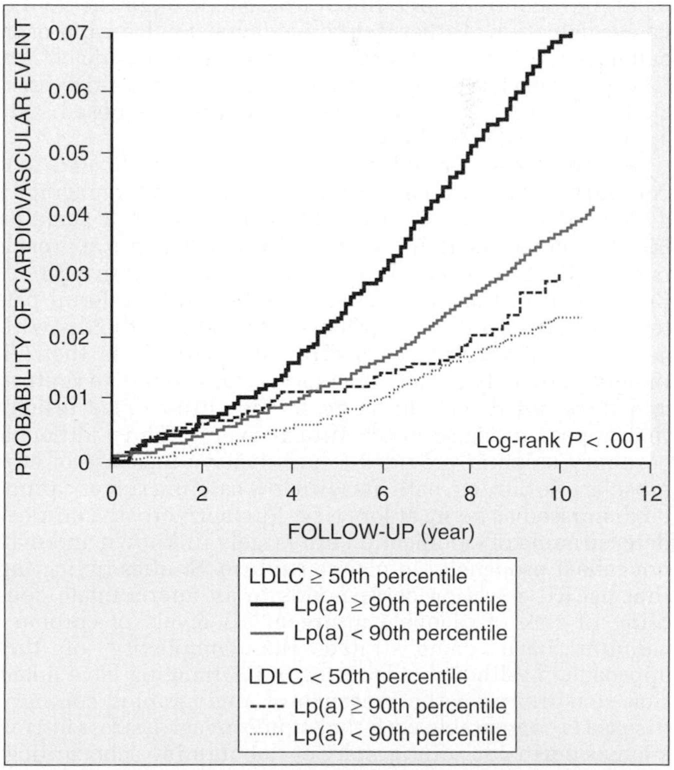

FIGURE 39–14 Cumulative rates of cardiovascular events according to lipoprotein(a) (Lp[a]) levels (higher or lower than the 90th percentile) for those with above or below average levels of low-density lipoprotein cholesterol (LDLC). *(From Suk Danik J, Rifai N, Buring JE, Ridker PM: Lipoprotein(a), measured with an assay independent of apolipoprotein(a) isoform size, and risk of future cardiovascular events among initially healthy women. JAMA 296:1363, 2006.)*

With the exception of high-dose niacin, few interventions lower Lp(a) level and no study has shown that Lp(a) reduction lowers vascular risk. This limitation, as well as the observation that LDL cholesterol reduction markedly reduces any hazard associated with Lp(a), has also dampened enthusiasm for screening. Genetic investigations have suggested important insights into Lp(a) regulation[179] and the development of peptides that inhibit Lp(a) assembly indicate novel pathways for risk reduction that will require direct testing in clinical trials.

FUTURE DIRECTIONS IN CARDIOVASCULAR RISK ASSESSMENT

Some 40 percent of the U.S. adult population is at intermediate risk but do not currently qualify for intensive risk factor intervention, despite the presence of one or more traditional risk factors. In the immediate future, the most important tool to improve risk stratification among these individuals will be the inflammatory biomarker hsCRP as an adjunct to global risk prediction. As reviewed earlier, strong evidence has shown that hsCRP adds prognostic information at all levels of LDL cholesterol, of the Framingham risk score, and of the metabolic syndrome. Thus, hsCRP evaluation, along with standard lipid screening, will likely become common practice in the near future. The pathophysiological implications that follow from the inflammatory hypothesis of atherothrombosis should lead to novel interventions for primary prevention as well as the treatment of acute ischemia.

Direct Plaque Imaging

In addition to the use of inflammatory markers such as hsCRP, strategies to detect vascular disease will likely take several forms. One approach eschews risk factor measurement, but identifies preclinical disease through the noninvasive detection of atherosclerotic plaque. Such an approach can never truly prevent disease, only lead to early detection. However, because many therapies can delay clinical expression of disease once existing lesions are diagnosed, this approach merits consideration.

At this time, a number of studies have indicated that coronary calcification as detected by computed tomography (CT) can detect preclinical atherosclerosis.[180] It remains highly controversial, however, as to whether this approach is cost-effective or has an acceptable false-negative rate.[181] Enrollment in these studies may be biased by referral patterns or self-selection by patients. Part of the difficulty with coronary calcification as a clinical surrogate is that CT imaging probably detects the plaques least likely to rupture and does not detect the noncalcified thin-capped lesions that appear to cause most clinical events. Thus, although coronary calcium provides a noninvasive measure of atherosclerotic burden, patients with low calcium scores cannot be dismissed as being at low risk. Furthermore, the clinical determinants of calcification are largely unknown and may not reflect propensity to plaque rupture. Studies indicating that hsCRP elevation corresponds to an approximate doubling of risk of plaque rupture at all levels of coronary calcium have demonstrated the complexity of this approach.[182] Although advocates of CT imaging have noted that sensitivity for the presence of angiographic coronary disease is comparable with that of noninvasive stress testing such as perfusion scintigraphy or dobutamine echocardiography, the specificity of CT imaging in this setting is low.

Considerable public health concern has also arisen regarding the consequences of overinterpreting the positive and negative predictive values of findings from imaging techniques, such as coronary calcium scores. For example, in one study of currently asymptomatic individuals, 41 percent of all future vascular events occurred in those with a coronary artery calcium score (CACS) less than 100 and 17 percent occurred in those with a CACS of zero.[183] Thus, the absence of a CACS does not preclude risk of coronary events. Moreover, in the same study, those with high Framingham risk scores but low coronary calcium scores remained at high risk.

Relative to simple blood-based biomarkers, imaging tests currently incur considerable expense and thus may be cost-ineffective. One study has shown that provision of calcium scores does not effectively motivate patients' adherence to risk reduction regimens.[184] In other cases, whole-body scans obtained for vascular screening have led to expensive and unnecessary work-ups and biopsies of incidental findings, often requiring repeat imaging at substantial radiation doses. Even when the costs of these false-positive findings are ignored, the quality-adjusted life-year cost estimates for CT screening have been found unfavorable.[185] Several other modalities for the noninvasive assessment of atherosclerosis exist, ranging from those that are well documented and inexpensive (e.g., ankle-brachial index) to those that are exploratory (e.g., thermography and magnetic resonance scanning). Perhaps the best studied noninvasive approach is the ultrasonic measurement of carotid intimal medial thickness. This technique has proved to have strong predictive value in general population studies and minimal additional expense is required, because most centers already have the required sonographic tools in place. Whether any imaging technique will prove cost-effective as a screening tool is currently under study in the Multiethnic Study of Atherosclerosis (MESA) being funded by the National Heart, Lung, and Blood Institute. In the Rotterdam Heart Study, in which simultaneous measures of atherosclerotic burden were obtained, the ankle-brachial index performed as well as carotid intimal medial thickness (IMT) and x-ray evidence of abdominal aortic calcification, but can be performed at no cost at the bedside.[186]

Genetic Determinants of Atherothrombosis

Venous thromboembolism has a major genetic component, and advances in genetic diagnosis (factor V Leiden and the G20210A prothrombin mutation), as well as pharmacogenetic management of warfarin, have already been implemented in many clinical practices (see Chaps. 72 and 82). Similarly, genetic evaluation has found an important role in several well-described heritable disorders that affect cardiac morphology (e.g., those associated with hypertrophic cardiomyopathy) or that cause myocardial conduction defects (e.g., long-QT syndrome; see Chap. 9). By contrast, although clinicians understand that myocardial infarction, stroke, and other forms of arterial disease also have a major heritable component, no genetic screening test for atherothrombosis has yet found a substantive role in routine clinical practice. Nonetheless, with heritability estimates approaching 50 percent in several studies, this situation may well change in the future and has stimulated intensive ongoing investigation.

Deciphering the genetic underpinnings of atherothrombosis presents considerable challenges because of major gene environment interactions. Also, atherothrombosis represents a prototypic complex disease in which multiple small effects accumulate and have a substantial population attributable risk.[187] Some genetic determinants of atherothrombotic cardiovascular disease are well established and have been replicated in multiple cohorts. Perhaps the best known of these is the relationship between polymorphism in the apolipoprotein E (apo E) gene that codes for three common isoforms (E2, E3, and E4), which in turn are associated with differential risks of coronary heart disease. In a meta-analysis of 48 studies incorporating information from over 15,000 affected patients and 33,000 controls, carriers of the apo E e4 allele had a 42 percent higher risk for coronary heart disease (OR, 1.42; 95 percent CI, 1.26 to 1.61) compared with those with the more common e3/3 genotype, whereas carriers of the e4 allele had no significant increase in risk.[188] Other potential genetic determinants of myocardial infarction reported in the cardiovascular literature include polymorphisms in the arachidonate 5-lipooxygenase–activating protein gene and its related pathways,[189,190] in the cyclooxygenase-2 gene,[191] in the proprotein convertase subtilisin-kexin type 9 (*PCSK9*) gene,[192] in the *OX40* ligand gene,[193] and in the *ROS1* gene encoding for tyrosine kinase. Similarly, variation in the beta$_2$-adrenergic receptor gene has been found in two study populations to be associated with an increased risk of sudden death.[194] Other recent observations that ultimately may relate to atherothrombotic risk include the finding of a common genetic variant associated with adult and childhood obesity,[195] polymorphisms associated with an increased risk of diabetes and impaired glucose tolerance,[196] and replicable genetic determinants of CRP.[197] Much of this ongoing work will require careful replication before attaining wide scientific or clinical acceptance. Nonetheless, meta-analysis of available genetic association studies consistently has suggested an important contribution of common variants to the atherothrombotic process.[198]

Although clinically effective genetic screens are not yet available, in daily practice the simple ascertainment of a parental history of early-onset atherosclerosis has proved to be an important predictor of future cardiovascular events. In the Framingham Offspring Study, when compared with those with no parental history of cardiovascular disease, men with at least one parent with premature atherothrombosis (onset younger than age 55 for fathers and younger than age 65 for mothers) had an age-adjusted odds ratio of 2.6 (95 percent CI, 1.7 to 4.1) whereas the similar odds ratio for women was 2.3 (95 percent CI, 1.2 to 3.1).[199] These effects compare in magnitude with those of smoking, hypertension, and hyperlipidemia in the Framingham cohort itself. As noted subsequently, analysis of data from the Women's Health Study has also recently found that a parental history of myocardial infarction before age 60, along with knowledge of CRP levels, can reclassify large numbers of patients as being at higher or lower risk than would have been anticipated on the basis of traditional risk factors alone.

The ultimate promise of an improved genetic understanding of cardiovascular risk is the concept of "personalized medicine," in which targeted interventions can get the right drug to the right patient at the right time. Pharmacogenetic evaluation also has the potential to allow physicians to predict side effects in advance and thus avoid a particular environmental exposure that might adversely interact with a common genetic variant. For example, polymorphism in the HMG-CoA reductase gene is associated with differential effects of statin therapy.[200] A number of investigations are under way to determine whether genetic differences can predict those patients most likely to suffer from statin-associated myopathy. Completion of the Human Genome Project and the International HapMap Project now allows cardiovascular investigators access to vast amounts of DNA-based information that is directly applicable to research subjects with atherothrombotic disease. Optimism regarding the potential for genetic screening is also based in part on rapid technological changes. Currently available genome wide chip products can capture more than 80 percent of all common genetic variation at moderate cost and it is likely that full coverage will be available shortly.[201] Thus, as our understanding of the core genetic basis of atherothrombosis improves, clinicians can anticipate not only new diagnostic tests, but also the possibility for new therapies and new directions in the prevention of atherothrombotic disease and its complications.[202]

Novel Approach to Global Risk Detection

As indicated in the introduction to this chapter, by the mid-1960s, investigators in the Framingham Heart Study had defined the major risk factors of age, hypertension, smoking, and hyperlipidemia, and coined the term *coronary risk factors*. Over time, these four biomarkers, along with gender, have generated global risk prediction scores for the assessment of cardiovascular risk. However, as also described earlier, one vascular event in five occurs in the absence of any of these major risk factors and one in two in the absence of hyperlipidemia. From a research perspective, the past 50 years has seen a remarkable expansion in our understanding of atherothrombosis to include the biology of hemostasis, thrombosis, inflammation, and endothelial dysfunction. Despite this changing view of pathophysiology, the variables in current risk assessment algorithms remain largely unchanged from those evaluated a half-century ago.

An expanded and updated approach to vascular risk detection is needed so that primary care physicians can be guided by the most modern biological constructs. New risk prediction algorithms must involve rigorous evaluation, with particular care given not only to the concepts of discrimination but also calibration and reclassification. This change in focus for prevention must include an understanding that reliance on the C-statistic as a traditional method for selecting variables for inclusion in risk prediction models is outmoded and subject to considerable error.[4] Indeed,

TABLE 39–2 Estimated 10-Year Risk of Atherothrombotic Disease for a 50-Year-Old Nondiabetic Female Smoker*,†

hsCRP (mg/liter)	Parental History?	ATP-III (%)	New Model (%)
0.1	No	11.5	4.9
0.5	No	11.5	6.5
1.0	No	11.5	7.4
3.0	No	11.5	8.9
5.0	No	11.5	9.7
8.0	No	11.5	10.5
10.0	No	11.5	10.9
0.1	Yes	11.5	7.5
0.5	Yes	11.5	9.9
1.0	Yes	11.5	11.2
3.0	Yes	11.5	13.4
5.0	Yes	11.5	14.6
8.0	Yes	11.5	15.8
10.0	Yes	11.5	16.4

*Blood pressure = 155/85 mm Hg; high-density lipoprotein = 35 mg/dl; TC = 240 mg/dl.

†Based on traditional Framingham variables as used in the Adult Treatment Panel (ATP-III) or on new classification that additionally takes into account hsCRP and parental history of myocardial infarction before age 60 years.

hsCRP = high-sensitivity C-reactive protein; TC = total cholesterol.

Modified from Ridker PM, Buring JE, Rifai N, Cook N: Development and validation of improved algorithms for the assessment of global cardiovascular risk in women: The Reynolds Risk Score. JAMA 297:611-619, 2007.

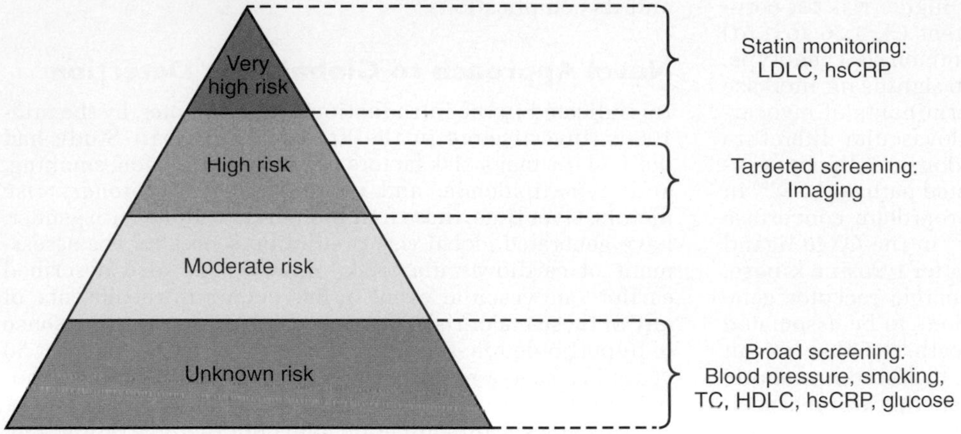

FIGURE 39–15. A cost-effective approach to cardiovascular risk screening. LDLC = low-density lipoprotein cholesterol; HDLC = high-density lipoprotein cholesterol; hsCRP = high-sensitivity C-reactive protein; TC = total cholesterol.

careful investigation has shown that inappropriate reliance on the C-statistic would actually eliminate LDL cholesterol, HDL cholesterol, and blood pressure from most global pre-
CH 39 diction models. Furthermore, continued reliance on 10-year risk estimates rather than estimates of lifetime risk may actually restrain more effective prevention efforts.[203]

In an effort to move beyond traditional risk variables, a few recent investigations have ascertained wide panels of biomarkers in large cohorts of initially healthy individuals who were then followed prospectively for incident vascular events. For example, using such data in the Women's Health Study, nine variables—age, current smoking, systolic blood pressure, hemoglobin A_{1c} among diabetics, hsCRP, apo B-100, apo A-I, Lp(a), and a parental history of premature atherosclerosis—were found to improve risk prediction substantially when compared with traditional Framingham covariates.[204] Importantly, use of this novel algorithm reclassified nearly 50 percent of those otherwise considered to be at intermediate risk on the basis of usual risk factors, an effect that was also seen for a simplified prediction model that substituted non-HDL cholesterol for apo B-100 and HDL cholesterol for apo A-I. Moreover, this reclassification was correct in over 90 percent of cases. For a hypothetical nondiabetic woman with a calculated 10-year Framingham Risk of 10.8 percent, the estimated risks calculated by this updated approach range from a low of 4.7 percent to a high of 16.0 percent (Table 39-2). Application of these newer algorithms could thus have a major impact on personalized medicine and the selection of appropriate patients for pharmacological risk reduction, in particular with statin therapy. This new algorithm, known as the Reynolds Risk Score, can be freely accessed for clinical use at www.reynoldsriskscore.org.[204]

The effective practice of preventive cardiology also requires a careful reevaluation of the core purposes of screening, evaluations of cost-effectiveness, and appropriate use of imaging tests. Figure 39-15 provides a conceptual basis for such an approach. At the bottom of the population pyramid of those at unknown risk, generalized evaluation for smoking status and blood pressure, along with blood measurements of total and HDL cholesterol, hsCRP, and glucose levels, provides a broad basis for ascertaining lifetime risk while simultaneously providing an index of risk for developing incident type 2 diabetes. With this information, most individuals can be categorized as lower, moderate, or higher vascular risk, thus greatly reducing the need in screening for imaging tests that can increase cost and radiation exposure. For those at the top of the risk pyramid who have indications for statin therapy, monitoring of LDL cholesterol levels is needed for application of current guidelines. In this setting, particularly for postinfarction patients, data from several studies have also indicated that achieving a low level of hsCRP, along with a low level of LDL cholesterol, can aid in the assessment of long-term prognosis. Use of such modified methods for global risk prediction holds considerable promise, even if only to heighten interest in prevention. A number of studies continue to find wide underuse of proven preventive interventions, an education gap that will require new and more aggressive approaches to primary and secondary prevention.

REFERENCES

1. Yusuf S, Hawken S, Ounpuu S, et al: Effect of potentially modifiable risk factors associated with myocardial infarction in 52 countries (the INTERHEART study): Case-control study. Lancet 364:937, 2004.
2. Bhatt DL, Steg PG, Ohman EM, et al: Rother J, Wilson PW. International prevalence, recognition, and treatment of cardiovascular risk factors in outpatients with atherothrombosis. JAMA 295:180, 2006.
3. He J, Gu D, Wu X, et al: Major causes of death among men and women in China. N Engl J Med 353:1124, 2005.
4. Cook NR, Buring JE, Ridker PM: The effect of including C-reactive protein in cardiovascular risk prediction models for women. Ann Intern Med 145:21, 2006.
5. Ridker PM, Buring JE, Rifai N, Cook NR: Development and validation of improved algorithms for the assessment of global cardiovascular risk in women: The Reynolds Risk Score. JAMA 297:611-619, 2007.
6. Daviglus ML, Stamler J, Pirzada A, et al: Favorable cardiovascular risk profile in young women and long-term risk of cardiovascular and all-cause mortality. JAMA 292:1588, 2004.
7. Gregg EW, Cheng YJ, Cadwell BL, et al: Secular trends in cardiovascular disease risk factors according to body mass index in U.S. adults. JAMA 293:1868, 2005.
8. Rothwell PM, Coull AJ, Giles MF, et al: Change in stroke incidence, mortality, case-fatality, severity, and risk factors in Oxfordshire, UK from 1981 to 2004 (Oxford Vascular Study). Lancet 363:1925, 2004.
9. Chiuve SE, McCullough ML, Sacks FM, Rimm EB: Healthy life style factors in the primary prevention of coronary heart disease among men: Benefits among users and nonusers of lipid-lowering and antihypertensive medications. Circulation 114:160, 2006.

Smoking

10. Centers for Disease Control and Prevention (CDC): Annual smoking-attributable mortality, years of potential life lost, and economic costs—United States, 1995-1999. MMWR Morb Mortal Wkly Rep 51:300, 2002.
11. Ezzati M, Henley SJ, Thun MJ, Lopez AD: Role of smoking in global and regional cardiovascular mortality. Circulation 112:489, 2005.
12. Kurth T, Kase CS, Berger K, et al: Smoking and the risk of hemorrhagic stroke in men. Stroke 34:1151, 2003.
13. Al-Delaimy WK, Manson JE, Solomon CG, et al: Smoking and risk of coronary heart disease among women with type 2 diabetes mellitus. Arch Intern Med 162:273, 2002.
14. Barua RS, Ambrose JA, Srivastava S, et al: Reactive oxygen species are involved in smoking-induced dysfunction of nitric oxide biosynthesis and upregulation of endothelial nitric oxide synthase: An in vitro demonstration in human coronary artery endothelial cells. Circulation 107:2342, 2003.
15. Bazzano LA, He J, Muntner P, et al: Relationship between cigarette smoking and novel risk factors for cardiovascular disease in the United States. Ann Intern Med 138:891, 2003.
16. Reaven G, Tsao PS: Insulin resistance and compensatory hyperinsulinemia: the key player between cigarette smoking and cardiovascular disease? J Am Coll Cardiol 41:1044, 2003.
17. Critchley JA, Capewell S: Mortality risk reduction associated with smoking cessation in patients with coronary heart disease: a systematic review. JAMA 290:86, 2003.
18. Godtfredsen NS, Holst C, Prescott E, et al: Smoking reduction, smoking cessation, and mortality: A 16-year follow-up of 19,732 men and women from The Copenhagen Centre for Prospective Population Studies. Am J Epidemiol 156:994, 2002.

19. Neuman M, Bitton A, Glantz S: Tobacco industry strategies for influencing European Community tobacco advertising legislation. Lancet 359:1323, 2002.

Hypertension

20. Chobanian AV, Bakris GL, Black HR, et al: The Seventh Report of the Joint National Committee on Prevention, Detection, Evaluation, and Treatment of High Blood Pressure: The JNC 7 report. JAMA 289:2560, 2003.
21. Hajjar I, Kotchen TA: Trends in prevalence, awareness, treatment, and control of hypertension in the United States, 1988-2000. JAMA 290:199, 2003..
22. Wolf-Maier K, Cooper RS, Banegas JR, et al: Hypertension prevalence and blood pressure levels in 6 European countries, Canada, and the United States. JAMA 289:2363, 2003.
23. Kearney PM, Whelton M, Reynolds K, et al: Global burden of hypertension: Analysis of worldwide data. Lancet 365:217, 2005.
24. Chaudhry SI, Krumholz HM, Foody JM: Systolic hypertension in older persons. JAMA 292:1074, 2004.
25. Vasan RS, Larson MG, Leip EP, et al: Impact of high-normal blood pressure on the risk of cardiovascular disease. N Engl J Med 345:1291, 2001.
26. Haider AW, Larson MG, Franklin SS, Levy D: Systolic blood pressure, diastolic blood pressure, and pulse pressure as predictors of risk for congestive heart failure in the Framingham Heart Study. Ann Intern Med 138:10, 2003.
27. Bjorklund K, Lind L, Zethelius B, et al: Isolated ambulatory hypertension predicts cardiovascular morbidity in elderly men. Circulation 107:1297, 2003.
28. Bobrie G, Chatellier G, Genes N, et al: Cardiovascular prognosis of "masked hypertension" detected by blood pressure self-measurement in elderly treated hypertensive patients. JAMA 291:1342, 2004.
29. Ingelsson E, Bjorklund-Bodegard K, Lind L, et al: Diurnal blood pressure pattern and risk of congestive heart failure. JAMA 295:2859, 2006.
30. Staessen JA, Den Hond E, Celis H, et al: Antihypertensive treatment based on blood pressure measurement at home or in the physician's office: A randomized controlled trial. JAMA 291:955, 2004.
31. Mehler PS, Coll JR, Estacio R, et al: Intensive blood pressure control reduces the risk of cardiovascular events in patients with peripheral arterial disease and type 2 diabetes. Circulation 107:753, 2003.
32. Nissen SE, Tuzcu EM, Libby P, et al: Effect of antihypertensive agents on cardiovascular events in patients with coronary disease and normal blood pressure: The CAMELOT study: A randomized controlled trial. JAMA 292:2217, 2004.
33. Psaty BM, Lumley T, Furberg CD, et al: Health outcomes associated with various antihypertensive therapies used as first-line agents: A network meta-analysis. JAMA 289:2534, 2003.
34. Law MR, Wald NJ, Morris JK, Jordan RE: Value of low dose combination treatment with blood pressure lowering drugs: Analysis of 354 randomised trials. BMJ 326:1427, 2003.
35. Forman JP, Rimm EB, Stampfer MJ, Curhan GC: Folate intake and the risk of incident hypertension among US women. JAMA 293:320, 2005.
36. Vasan RS, Evans JC, Larson MG, et al: Serum aldosterone and the incidence of hypertension in nonhypertensive persons. N Engl J Med 351:33, 2004.
37. Julius S, Nesbitt SD, Egan BM, et al: Feasibility of treating prehypertension with an angiotensin-receptor blocker. N Engl J Med 354:1685, 2006.
38. Wassertheil-Smoller S, Psaty B, Greenland P, et al: Association between cardiovascular outcomes and antihypertensive drug treatment in older women. JAMA 292:2849, 2004.
39. Wright JT Jr, Dunn JK, Cutler JA, et al: Outcomes in hypertensive black and nonblack patients treated with chlorthalidone, amlodipine, and lisinopril. JAMA 293:1595, 2005.
40. Ridker PM, Danielson E, Rifai N, Glynn RJ: Valsartan, blood pressure reduction, and C-reactive protein: primary report of the Val-MARC trial. Hypertension 48:73, 2006.
41. Fischer MA, Avorn J: Economic implications of evidence-based prescribing for hypertension: can better care cost less? JAMA 291:1850, 2004.
42. Weber MA, Julius S, Kjeldsen SE, et al: Blood pressure dependent and independent effects of antihypertensive treatment on clinical events in the VALUE Trial. Lancet 363:2049, 2004.
43. Kaplan NM, Opie LH: Controversies in hypertension. Lancet 367:168, 2006.
44. Devereux RB, Wachtell K, Gerdts E, et al: Prognostic significance of left ventricular mass change during treatment of hypertension. JAMA 292:2350, 2004.
45. Okin PM, Devereux RB, Jern S, et al: Regression of electrocardiographic left ventricular hypertrophy during antihypertensive treatment and the prediction of major cardiovascular events. JAMA 292:2343, 2004.

Hyperlipidemia and Elevated LDL Cholesterol

46. Collins R, Armitage J, Parish S, et al: Effects of cholesterol-lowering with simvastatin on stroke and other major vascular events in 20536 people with cerebrovascular disease or other high-risk conditions. Lancet 363:757, 2004.
47. Nissen SE, Tuzcu EM, Schoenhagen P, et al: Effect of intensive compared with moderate lipid-lowering therapy on progression of coronary atherosclerosis: A randomized controlled trial. JAMA 291:1071, 2004.
48. Cannon CP, Braunwald E, McCabe CH, et al: Intensive versus moderate lipid lowering with statins after acute coronary syndromes. N Engl J Med 350:1495, 2004.
49. de Lemos JA, Blazing MA, Wiviott SD, et al: Early intensive vs a delayed conservative simvastatin strategy in patients with acute coronary syndromes: Phase Z of the A to Z trial. JAMA 92:1307, 2004.
50. LaRosa JC, Grundy SM, Waters DD, et al: Intensive lipid lowering with atorvastatin in patients with stable coronary disease. N Engl J Med 352:1425, 2005.
51. Libby P: The forgotten majority: Unfinished business in cardiovascular risk reduction. J Am Coll Cardiol 46:1225, 2005.
52. Colhoun HM, Betteridge DJ, Durrington PN, et al: Primary prevention of cardiovascular disease with atorvastatin in type 2 diabetes in the Collaborative Atorvastatin Diabetes Study (CARDS): Multicentre randomised placebo-controlled trial. Lancet 364:685, 2004.
53. Wiegman A, Hutten BA, de Groot E, et al: Efficacy and safety of statin therapy in children with familial hypercholesterolemia: a randomized controlled trial. JAMA 292:331, 2004.

High-Density Lipoprotein Cholesterol, Apolipoproteins, and Other Lipid Subclasses

54. Brewer HB Jr: Increasing HDL cholesterol levels. N Engl J Med 350:1491, 2004.
55. Forrester JS, Makkar R, Shah PK: Increasing high-density lipoprotein cholesterol in dyslipidemia by cholesteryl ester transfer protein inhibition: An update for clinicians. Circulation 111:1847, 2005.
56. Pischon T, Girman CJ, Sacks FM, et al: Non-high-density lipoprotein cholesterol and apolipoprotein B in the prediction of coronary heart disease in men. Circulation 112:3375, 2005.
57. Ridker PM, Rifai N, Cook NR, et al: Non-HDL cholesterol, apolipoproteins A-I and B100, standard lipid measures, lipid ratios, and CRP as risk factors for cardiovascular disease in women. JAMA 294:326, 2005.
58. Sniderman AD, Furberg CD, Keech A, et al: Apolipoproteins versus lipids as indices of coronary risk and as targets for statin treatment. Lancet 361:777, 2003.
59. Sacks FM, Campos H: Clinical review 163: Cardiovascular endocrinology: Low-density lipoprotein size and cardiovascular disease: a reappraisal. J Clin Endocrinol Metab 88:4525, 2003.
60. Otvos JD, Collins D, Freedman DS, et al: Low-density lipoprotein and high-density lipoprotein particle subclasses predict coronary events and are favorably changed by gemfibrozil therapy in the Veterans Affairs High-Density Lipoprotein Intervention Trial. Circulation 113:1556, 2006.
61. Kathiresan S, Otvos JD, Sullivan LM, et al: Increased small low-density lipoprotein particle number: A prominent feature of the metabolic syndrome in the Framingham Heart Study. Circulation 113:20, 2006.

Triglyceride-Rich Lipoprotein and Cardiovascular Risk

62. Patel A, Barzi F, Jamrozik K, et al: Serum triglycerides as a risk factor for cardiovascular diseases in the Asia-Pacific region. Circulation 110:2678, 2004.
63. Ninomiya JK, L'Italien G, Criqui MH, et al: Association of the metabolic syndrome with history of myocardial infarction and stroke in the Third National Health and Nutrition Examination Survey. Circulation 109:42, 2004.
64. Abdel-Maksoud MF, Hokanson JE: The complex role of triglycerides in cardiovascular disease. Semin Vasc Med 2:325, 2002.
65. Keech A, Simes RJ, Barter P, et al: Effects of long-term fenofibrate therapy on cardiovascular events in 9795 people with type 2 diabetes mellitus (the FIELD study): Randomised controlled trial. Lancet 366:1849, 2005.

Metabolic Syndrome, Insulin Resistance, and Diabetes

66. Booth GL, Kapral MK, Fung K, Tu JV: Relation between age and cardiovascular disease in men and women with diabetes compared with non-diabetic people: A population-based retrospective cohort study. Lancet 368:29, 2006.
67. Ingelsson E, Sundstrom J, Arnlov J, et al: Insulin resistance and risk of congestive heart failure. JAMA 294:334, 2005.
68. Hu FB, Stampfer MJ, Haffner SM, et al: Elevated risk of cardiovascular disease prior to clinical diagnosis of type 2 diabetes. Diabetes Care 25:1129, 2002.
69. Expert Panel on Detection, Evaluation, and Treatment of High Blood Cholesterol in Adults: Executive Summary of The Third Report of The National Cholesterol Education Program (NCEP) Expert Panel on Detection, Evaluation, And Treatment of High Blood Cholesterol In Adults (Adult Treatment Panel III). JAMA 285:2486, 2001.
70. Lakka HM, Laaksonen DE, Lakka TA, et al: The metabolic syndrome and total and cardiovascular disease mortality in middle-aged men. JAMA 288:2709, 2002.
71. Sjoholm A, Nystrom T: Endothelial inflammation in insulin resistance. Lancet 365:610, 2005.
72. Grundy SM, Brewer HB Jr, Cleeman JI, et al: Definition of metabolic syndrome: Report of the National Heart, Lung, and Blood Institute/American Heart Association conference on scientific issues related to definition. Circulation 109:433, 2004.
73. Ridker PM, Buring JE, Cook NR, Rifai N: C-reactive protein, the metabolic syndrome, and risk of incident cardiovascular events: An 8-year follow-up of 14 719 initially healthy American women. Circulation 107:391, 2003.
74. Pradhan AD, Manson JE, Rifai N, et al: C-reactive protein, interleukin 6, and risk of developing type 2 diabetes mellitus. JAMA 286:327, 2001.
75. Hu FB, Meigs JB, Li TY, et al: Inflammatory markers and risk of developing type 2 diabetes in women. Diabetes 53:693, 2004.
76. Sattar N, Gaw A, Scherbakova O, et al: Metabolic syndrome with and without C-reactive protein as a predictor of coronary heart disease and diabetes in the West of Scotland Coronary Prevention Study. Circulation 108:414, 2003.
77. Eckel RH, Grundy SM, Zimmet PZ: The metabolic syndrome. Lancet 365:1415, 2005.
78. Varo N, Vicent D, Libby P, et al: Elevated plasma levels of the atherogenic mediator soluble CD40 ligand in diabetic patients: A novel target of thiazolidinediones. Circulation 107:2664, 2003.
79. Beckman JA, Creager MA, Libby P: Diabetes and atherosclerosis: epidemiology, pathophysiology, and management. JAMA 287:2570, 2002.
80. Nathan DM, Cleary PA, Backlund JY, et al: Intensive diabetes treatment and cardiovascular disease in patients with type 1 diabetes. N Engl J Med 353:2643, 2005.

81. Saydah SH, Fradkin J, Cowie CC: Poor control of risk factors for vascular disease among adults with previously diagnosed diabetes. JAMA 291:335, 2004.
82. Hippisley-Cox J, Pringle M: Prevalence, care, and outcomes for patients with diet-controlled diabetes in general practice: Cross-sectional survey. Lancet 364:423, 2004.

Exercise, Weight Loss, and Obesity

83. Thompson PD, Buchner D, Pina IL, et al: Exercise and physical activity in the prevention and treatment of atherosclerotic cardiovascular disease: A statement from the Council on Clinical Cardiology (Subcommittee on Exercise, Rehabilitation, and Prevention) and the Council on Nutrition, Physical Activity, and Metabolism (Subcommittee on Physical Activity). Circulation 107:3109, 2003.
84. Manson JE, Greenland P, LaCroix AZ, et al: Walking compared with vigorous exercise for the prevention of cardiovascular events in women. N Engl J Med 347:716, 2002.
85. Tanasescu M, Leitzmann MF, Rimm EB, et al: Exercise type and intensity in relation to coronary heart disease in men. JAMA 288:1994, 2002.
86. Whang W, Manson JE, Hu FB, et al: Physical exertion, exercise, and sudden cardiac death in women. JAMA 295:1399, 2006.
87. Irwin ML, Yasui Y, Ulrich CM, et al: Effect of exercise on total and intra-abdominal body fat in postmenopausal women: A randomized controlled trial. JAMA 289:323, 2003.
88. Whelton SP, Chin A, Xin X, He J: Effect of aerobic exercise on blood pressure: a meta-analysis of randomized, controlled trials. Ann Intern Med 136:493, 2002.
89. Kraus WE, Houmard JA, Duscha BD, et al: Effects of the amount and intensity of exercise on plasma lipoproteins. N Engl J Med 347:1483, 2002.
90. Andersen LB, Harro M, Sardinha LB, et al: Physical activity and clustered cardiovascular risk in children: A cross-sectional study (The European Youth Heart Study). Lancet 368:299, 2006.
91. Knowler WC, Barrett-Connor E, Fowler SE, et al: Reduction in the incidence of type 2 diabetes with life style intervention or metformin. N Engl J Med 346:393, 2002.
92. Poirier P, Giles TD, Bray GA, et al: Obesity and cardiovascular disease: Pathophysiology, evaluation, and effect of weight loss: An update of the 1997 American Heart Association Scientific Statement on Obesity and Heart Disease from the Obesity Committee of the Council on Nutrition, Physical Activity, and Metabolism. Circulation 113:898, 2006.
93. Yan LL, Daviglus ML, Liu K, et al: Midlife body mass index and hospitalization and mortality in older age. JAMA 295:190, 2006.
94. Mora S, Lee IM, Buring JE, Ridker PM: Association of physical activity and body mass index with novel and traditional cardiovascular biomarkers in women. JAMA 295:1412, 2006.
95. Wadden TA, Berkowitz RI, Womble LG, et al: Randomized trial of life style modification and pharmacotherapy for obesity. N Engl J Med 353:2111, 2005.
96. He FJ, Nowson CA, MacGregor GA: Fruit and vegetable consumption and stroke: Meta-analysis of cohort studies. Lancet 367:320, 2006.
97. Howard BV, Van Horn L, Hsia J, et al: Low-fat dietary pattern and risk of cardiovascular disease: The Women's Health Initiative Randomized Controlled Dietary Modification Trial. JAMA 295:655, 2006.
98. Dansinger ML, Gleason JA, Griffith JL, et al: Comparison of the Atkins, Ornish, Weight Watchers, and Zone diets for weight loss and heart disease risk reduction: A randomized trial. JAMA 293:43, 2005.
99. Appel LJ, Sacks FM, Carey VJ, et al: Effects of protein, monounsaturated fat, and carbohydrate intake on blood pressure and serum lipids: Results of the OmniHeart randomized trial. JAMA 294:2455, 2005.
100. Knoops KT, de Groot LC, Kromhout D, et al: Mediterranean diet, life style factors, and 10-year mortality in elderly European men and women: The HALE project. JAMA 292:1433, 2004.
101. Ogden CL, Carroll MD, Curtin LR, et al: Prevalence of overweight and obesity in the United States, 1999-2004. JAMA 295:1549, 2006.

Mental Stress, Depression, and Cardiovascular Risk

102. Kivimaki M, Leino-Arjas P, Luukkonen R, et al: Work stress and risk of cardiovascular mortality: prospective cohort study of industrial employees. BMJ 325:857, 2002.
103. Rosengren A, Hawken S, Ounpuu S, et al: Association of psychosocial risk factors with risk of acute myocardial infarction in 11119 cases and 13648 controls from 52 countries (the INTERHEART study): Case-control study. Lancet 364:953, 2004.
104. Blumenthal JA, Sherwood A, Babyak MA, et al: Effects of exercise and stress management training on markers of cardiovascular risk in patients with ischemic heart disease: A randomized controlled trial. JAMA 293:1626, 2005.
105. Rugulies R: Depression as a predictor for coronary heart disease. A review and meta-analysis. Am J Prev Med 23:51, 2002.
106. Whooley MA: Depression and cardiovascular disease: Healing the broken-hearted. JAMA 295:2874, 2006.
107. Berkman LF, Blumenthal J, Burg M, et al: Effects of treating depression and low perceived social support on clinical events after myocardial infarction: The Enhancing Recovery in Coronary Heart Disease Patients (ENRICHD) Randomized Trial. JAMA 289:3106, 2003.
108. Frasure-Smith N, Lesperance F: Depression—a cardiac risk factor in search of a treatment. JAMA 289:3171, 2003.

Novel Atherosclerotic Risk Factors

109. Ridker PM, Rifai N, Rose L, et al: Comparison of C-reactive protein and low-density lipoprotein cholesterol levels in the prediction of first cardiovascular events. N Engl J Med 347:1557, 2002.
110. Khot UN, Khot MB, Bajzer CT, et al: Prevalence of conventional risk factors in patients with coronary heart disease. JAMA 290:898, 2003.
111. Greenland P, Knoll MD, Stamler J, et al: Major risk factors as antecedents of fatal and nonfatal coronary heart disease events. JAMA 290:89, 2003.
112. Hackam DG, Anand SS: Emerging risk factors for atherosclerotic vascular disease: A critical review of the evidence. JAMA 290:932, 2003.

High-Sensitivity C-Reactive Protein (hsCRP)

113. Libby P, Ridker PM: Inflammation and atherothrombosis from population biology and bench research to clinical practice. J Am Coll Cardiol 48:A33, 2006.
114. Ridker PM: Clinical application of C-reactive protein for cardiovascular disease detection and prevention. Circulation 107:363, 2003.
115. Danenberg HD, Szalai AJ, Swaminathan RV, et al: Increased thrombosis after arterial injury in human C-reactive protein-transgenic mice. Circulation 108:512, 2003.
116. Ridker PM, Cushman M, Stampfer MJ, et al: Inflammation, aspirin, and the risk of cardiovascular disease in apparently healthy men. N Engl J Med 336:973, 1997.
117. Boekholdt SM, Hack CE, Sandhu MS, et al: C-reactive protein levels and coronary artery disease incidence and mortality in apparently healthy men and women: The EPIC-Norfolk prospective population study 1993-2003. Atherosclerosis 187:415, 2006.
118. Danesh J, Wheeler JG, Hirschfield GM, et al: C-reactive protein and other circulating markers of inflammation in the prediction of coronary heart disease. N Engl J Med 350:1387, 2004.
119. Pearson TA, Mensah GA, Alexander RW, et al: Markers of inflammation and cardiovascular disease: Application to clinical and public health practice: A statement for healthcare professionals from the Centers for Disease Control and Prevention and the American Heart Association. Circulation 107:499, 2003.
120. Koenig W, Lowel H, Baumert J, Meisinger C: C-reactive protein modulates risk prediction based on the Framingham Score: Implications for future risk assessment: Results from a large cohort study in southern Germany. Circulation 109:1349, 2004.
121. Boekholdt SM, Keller TT, Wareham NJ, et al: Serum levels of type II secretory phospholipase A2 and the risk of future coronary artery disease in apparently healthy men and women: The EPIC-Norfolk Prospective Population Study. Arterioscler Thromb Vasc Biol 25:839, 2005.
122. Pai JK, Pischon T, Ma J, et al: Inflammatory markers and the risk of coronary heart disease in men and women. N Engl J Med 351:2599, 2004.
123. Cushman M, Arnold AM, Psaty BM, et al: C-reactive protein and the 10-year incidence of coronary heart disease in older men and women: the cardiovascular health study. Circulation 112:25, 2005.
124. Laaksonen DE, Niskanen L, Nyyssonen K, et al: C-reactive protein in the prediction of cardiovascular and overall mortality in middle-aged men: a population-based cohort study. Eur Heart J 26:1783, 2005.
125. Ridker PM, Cook N: Clinical usefulness of very high and very low levels of C-reactive protein across the full range of Framingham Risk Scores. Circulation 109:1955, 2004.
126. Lindahl B, Toss H, Siegbahn A, et al: Markers of myocardial damage and inflammation in relation to long-term mortality in unstable coronary artery disease. FRISC Study Group. Fragmin during Instability in Coronary Artery Disease. N Engl J Med 43:1139, 2000.
127. Ridker PM, Rifai N, Pfeffer MA, et al: Long-term effects of pravastatin on plasma concentration of C-reactive protein. The Cholesterol and Recurrent Events (CARE) Investigators. Circulation 100:230, 1999.
128. Ridker PM, Rifai N, Clearfield M, et al: Measurement of C-reactive protein for the targeting of statin therapy in the primary prevention of acute coronary events. N Engl J Med 344:1959, 2001.
129. Ridker PM: Rosuvastatin in the primary prevention of cardiovascular disease among patients with low levels of low-density lipoprotein cholesterol and elevated high-sensitivity C-reactive protein: Rationale and design of the JUPITER trial. Circulation 108:2292, 2003.
130. Ridker PM, Cannon CP, Morrow D, et al: C-reactive protein levels and outcomes after statin therapy. N Engl J Med 352:20, 2005.
131. Morrow DA, de Lemos JA, Sabatine MS, et al: Clinical relevance of C-reactive protein during follow-up of patients with acute coronary syndromes in the Aggrastat-to-Zocor Trial. Circulation 114:281, 2006.
132. Nissen SE, Tuzcu EM, Schoenhagen P, et al: Statin therapy, LDL cholesterol, C-reactive protein, and coronary artery disease. N Engl J Med 352:29, 2005.
133. Blake GJ, Rifai N, Buring JE, Ridker PM: Blood pressure, C-reactive protein, and risk of future cardiovascular events. Circulation 108:2993, 2003.
134. Sesso HD, Buring JE, Rifai N, et al: C-reactive protein and the risk of developing hypertension. JAMA 290:2945, 2003.
135. Labarrere CA, Lee JB, Nelson DR, et al: C-reactive protein, arterial endothelial activation, and development of transplant coronary artery disease: a prospective study. Lancet 360:1462, 2002.
136. Wanner C, Zimmermann J, Schwedler S, Metzger T. Inflammation and cardiovascular risk in dialysis patients. Kidney Int Suppl (80):99, 2002.
137. Andraws R, Berger JS, Brown DL: Effects of antibiotic therapy on outcomes of patients with coronary artery disease: A meta-analysis of randomized controlled trials. JAMA 293:2641, 2005.
138. Pepys MB, Hirschfield GM, Tennent GA, et al: Targeting C-reactive protein for the treatment of cardiovascular disease. Nature 440:1217, 2006.
139. Lloyd-Jones DM, Liu K, Tian L, Greenland P: Narrative review: Assessment of C-reactive protein in risk prediction for cardiovascular disease. Ann Intern Med 145:35, 2006.

140. Folsom AR, Chambless LE, Ballantyne CM, et al: An assessment of incremental coronary risk prediction using C-reactive protein and other novel risk markers: The atherosclerosis risk in communities study. Arch Intern Med 166:1368, 2006.
141. Cook N: Use and misuse of the ROC curve in the medical literature. Circulation 115:928-935, 2007.

Other Markers of Inflammation

142. Zalewski A, Macphee C: Role of lipoprotein-associated phospholipase A2 in atherosclerosis: Biology, epidemiology, and possible therapeutic target. Arterioscler Thromb Vasc Biol 25:923, 2005.
143. Cosin-Sales J, Christiansen M, Kaminski P, et al: Pregnancy-associated plasma protein A and its endogenous inhibitor, the proform of eosinophil major basic protein (proMBP), are related to complex stenosis morphology in patients with stable angina pectoris. Circulation 109:1724, 2004.
144. Heeschen C, Dimmeler S, Hamm CW, et al: Soluble CD40 ligand in acute coronary syndromes. N Engl J Med 348:1104, 2003.
145. Baldus S, Heeschen C, Meinertz T, et al: Myeloperoxidase serum levels predict risk in patients with acute coronary syndromes. Circulation 108:1440, 2003.
146. Brennan ML, Penn MS, Van Lente F, et al: Prognostic value of myeloperoxidase in patients with chest pain. N Engl J Med 349:1595, 2003.
147. Apple FS, Wu AH, Mair J, et al: Future biomarkers for detection of ischemia and risk stratification in acute coronary syndrome. Clin Chem 51:810, 2005.

Homocysteine

148. Klerk M, Verhoef P, Clarke R, et al: MTHFR 677C–>T polymorphism and risk of coronary heart disease: A meta-analysis. JAMA 288:2023, 2002.
149. Ford ES, Smith SJ, Stroup DF, et al: Homocyst(e)ine and cardiovascular disease: A systematic review of the evidence with special emphasis on case-control studies and nested case-control studies. Int J Epidemiol 31:59, 2002.
150. Vasan RS, Beiser A, D'Agostino RB, et al: Plasma homocysteine and risk for congestive heart failure in adults without prior myocardial infarction. JAMA 289:1251, 2003.
151. Toole JF, Malinow MR, Chambless LE, et al: Lowering homocysteine in patients with ischemic stroke to prevent recurrent stroke, myocardial infarction, and death: the Vitamin Intervention for Stroke Prevention (VISP) randomized controlled trial. JAMA 291:565, 2004.
152. Lange H, Suryapranata H, De Luca G, et al: Folate therapy and in-stent restenosis after coronary stenting. N Engl J Med 350:2673, 2004.
153. Bonaa KH, Njolstad I, Ueland PM, et al: Homocysteine lowering and cardiovascular events after acute myocardial infarction. N Engl J Med 354:1578, 2006.
154. Lonn E, Yusuf S, Arnold MJ, et al: Homocysteine lowering with folic acid and B vitamins in vascular disease. N Engl J Med 354:1567, 2006.
155. Casas JP, Bautista LE, Smeeth L, et al: Homocysteine and stroke: Evidence on a causal link from mendelian randomisation. Lancet 365:224, 2005.
156. Loscalzo J: Homocysteine trials—clear outcomes for complex reasons. N Engl J Med 354:1629, 2006.
157. Eichholzer M, Tonz O, Zimmermann R: Folic acid: A public-health challenge. Lancet 367:1352, 2006.

Fibrinogen and Fibrin D-Dimer

158. Kerlin B, Cooley BC, Isermann BH, et al: Cause-effect relation between hyperfibrinogenemia and vascular disease. Blood 103:1728, 2004.
159. Danesh J, Lewington S, Thompson SG, et al; Fibrinogen Studies Collaboration: Plasma fibrinogen level and the risk of major cardiovascular diseases and nonvascular mortality: An individual participant meta-analysis. JAMA 294:1799, 2005.
160. Tanne D, Benderly M, Goldbourt U, et al: A prospective study of plasma fibrinogen levels and the risk of stroke among participants in the bezafibrate infarction prevention study. Am J Med 111:457, 2001.
161. Meade T, Zuhrie R, Cook C, Cooper J: Bezafibrate in men with lower extremity arterial disease: Randomised controlled trial. BMJ 325:1139, 2002.
162. Menown IB, Mathew TP, Gracey HM, et al: Prediction of Recurrent Events by D-Dimer and Inflammatory Markers in Patients with Normal Cardiac Troponin I (PREDICT) Study. Am Heart J 145:986, 2003.
163. Wells PS, Anderson DR, Rodger M, et al: Evaluation of D-dimer in the diagnosis of suspected deep-vein thrombosis. N Engl J Med 349:1227, 2003.

Markers of Fibrinolytic Function

164. Festa A, D'Agostino R Jr, Tracy RP, Haffner SM: Elevated levels of acute-phase proteins and plasminogen activator inhibitor-1 predict the development of type 2 diabetes: The insulin resistance atherosclerosis study. Diabetes 51:1131, 2002.
165. Brown NJ, Abbas A, Byrne D, et al: Comparative effects of estrogen and angiotensin-converting enzyme inhibition on plasminogen activator inhibitor-1 in healthy postmenopausal women. Circulation 105:304, 2002.
166. Pradhan AD, LaCroix AZ, Langer RD, et al: Tissue plasminogen activator antigen and D-dimer as markers for atherothrombotic risk among healthy postmenopausal women. Circulation 110:292, 2004.
167. Pretorius M, Rosenbaum D, Vaughan DE, Brown NJ: Angiotensin-converting enzyme inhibition increases human vascular tissue-type plasminogen activator release through endogenous bradykinin. Circulation 107:579, 2003.
168. Festa A, D'Agostino R Jr, Rich SS, et al: Promoter (4G/5G) plasminogen activator inhibitor-1 genotype and plasminogen activator inhibitor-1 levels in blacks, Hispanics, and non-Hispanic whites: The Insulin Resistance Atherosclerosis Study. Circulation 107:2422, 2003.

Lipoprotein(a)

169. Tsimikas S, Brilakis ES, Miller ER, et al: Oxidized phospholipids, Lp(a) lipoprotein, and coronary artery disease. N Engl J Med 353:46, 2005.
170. Danesh J, Collins R, Peto R: Lipoprotein(a) and coronary heart disease. Meta-analysis of prospective studies. Circulation 102:1082, 2000.
171. Solfrizzi V, Panza F, Colacicco AM, et al: Relation of lipoprotein(a) as coronary risk factor to type 2 diabetes mellitus and low-density lipoprotein cholesterol in patients > or = 65 years of age (the Italian Longitudinal Study on Aging). Am J Cardiol 89:825, 2002.
172. Koschinsky ML, Marcovina SM: The relationship between lipoprotein(a) and the complications of diabetes mellitus. Acta Diabetol 40:65, 2003.
173. Cantin B, Despres JP, Lamarche B, et al: Association of fibrinogen and lipoprotein(a) as a coronary heart disease risk factor in men (the Quebec Cardiovascular Study). Am J Cardiol 89:662, 2002.
174. Ariyo AA, Thach C, Tracy R: Lp(a) lipoprotein, vascular disease, and mortality in the elderly. N Engl J Med 349:2108, 2003.
175. Rifai N, Ma J, Sacks FM, et al: Apolipoprotein(a) size and lipoprotein(a) concentration and future risk of angina pectoris with evidence of severe coronary atherosclerosis in men: The Physicians' Health Study. Clin Chem 50:1364, 2004.
176. Longenecker JC, Klag MJ, Marcovina SM, et al: Small apolipoprotein(a) size predicts mortality in end-stage renal disease: The CHOICE study. Circulation 106:2812, 2002.
177. Marcovina SM, Koschinsky ML, Albers JJ, Skarlatos S: Report of the National Heart, Lung, and Blood Institute Workshop on Lipoprotein(a) and Cardiovascular Disease: Recent advances and future directions. Clin Chem 49:1785, 2003.
178. Suk Danik J, Rifai N, Buring JE, Ridker PM: Lipoprotein(a), measured with an assay independent of apolipoprotein(a) isoform size, and risk of future cardiovascular events among initially healthy women. JAMA 296:1363, 2006.
179. Holmer SR, Hengstenberg C, Kraft HG, et al: Association of polymorphisms of the apolipoprotein(a) gene with lipoprotein(a) levels and myocardial infarction. Circulation 107:696, 2003.

Direct Plaque Imaging

180. Clouse ME: How useful is computed tomography for screening for coronary artery disease? Noninvasive screening for coronary artery disease with computed tomography is useful. Circulation 113:125, discussion, 125, 2006.
181. Chen J, Krumholz HM: How useful is computed tomography for screening for coronary artery disease? Screening for coronary artery disease with electron-beam computed tomography is not useful. Circulation 113:125, discussion, 125, 2006.
182. Park R, Detrano R, Xiang M, et al: Combined use of computed tomography coronary calcium scores and C-reactive protein levels in predicting cardiovascular events in nondiabetic individuals. Circulation 106:2073, 2002.
183. Greenland P, LaBree L, Azen SP, et al: Coronary artery calcium score combined with Framingham score for risk prediction in asymptomatic individuals. JAMA 291:210, 2004.
184. O'Malley PG, Feuerstein IM, Taylor AJ: Impact of electron beam tomography, with or without case management, on motivation, behavioral change, and cardiovascular risk profile: A randomized controlled trial. JAMA 289:2215, 2003.
185. Shaw LJ, Raggi P, Berman DS, Callister TQ: Cost effectiveness of screening for cardiovascular disease with measures of coronary calcium. Prog Cardiovasc Dis 46:171, 2003.
186. van der Meer IM, Bots ML, Hofman A, et al: Predictive value of noninvasive measures of atherosclerosis for incident myocardial infarction: The Rotterdam Study. Circulation 109:1089, 2004.

Genetic Determinants of Atherothrombosis

187. Watkins H, Farrall M: Genetic susceptibility to coronary artery disease: From promise to progress. Nat Rev Genet 7:163, 2006.
188. Song Y, Stampfer MJ, Liu S: Meta-analysis: Apolipoprotein E genotypes and risk for coronary heart disease. Ann Intern Med 141:137, 2004.
189. Helgadottir A, Manolescu A, Thorleifsson G, et al: The gene encoding 5-lipoxygenase activating protein confers risk of myocardial infarction and stroke. Nat Genet 36:233, 2004.
190. Dwyer JH, Allayee H, Dwyer KM, et al: Arachidonate 5-lipoxygenase promoter genotype, dietary arachidonic acid, and atherosclerosis. N Engl J Med 350:29, 2004.
191. Cipollone F, Toniato E, Martinotti S, et al: A polymorphism in the cyclooxygenase 2 gene as an inherited protective factor against myocardial infarction and stroke. JAMA 291:2221, 2004.
192. Cohen JC, Boerwinkle E, Mosley TH Jr, Hobbs HH: Sequence variations in PCSK9, low LDL, and protection against coronary heart disease. N Engl J Med 354:1264, 2006.
193. Wang X, Ria M, Kelmenson PM, et al: Positional identification of TNFSF4, encoding OX40 ligand, as a gene that influences atherosclerosis susceptibility. Nat Genet 37:365, 2005.
194. Sotoodehnia N, Siscovick DS, Vatta M, et al: Beta2-adrenergic receptor genetic variants and risk of sudden cardiac death. Circulation 113:1842, 2006.
195. Herbert A, Gerry NP, McQueen MB, et al: A common genetic variant is associated with adult and childhood obesity. Science 312:279, 2006.
196. Florez JC, Jablonski KA, Bayley N, et al: TCF7L2 polymorphisms and progression to diabetes in the Diabetes Prevention Program. N Engl J Med 355:241, 2006.
197. Miller DT, Zee RY, Suk Danik J, et al: Association of common CRP gene variants with CRP levels and cardiovascular events. Ann Hum Genet 69:623, 2005.
198. Ye Z, Liu EH, Higgins JP, et al: Seven haemostatic gene polymorphisms in coronary disease: Meta-analysis of 66,155 cases and 91,307 controls. Lancet 367:651, 2006.

199. Lloyd-Jones DM, Nam BH, D'Agostino RB Sr, et al: Parental cardiovascular disease as a risk factor for cardiovascular disease in middle-aged adults: A prospective study of parents and offspring. JAMA 291:2204, 2004.
200. Chasman DI, Posada D, Subrahmanyan L, et al: Pharmacogenetic study of statin therapy and cholesterol reduction. JAMA 291:2821, 2004.
201. Pe'er I, de Bakker PI, Maller J, et al: Evaluating and improving power in whole-genome association studies using fixed marker sets. Nat Genet 38:663, 2006.
202. Miller DT, Ridker P, Libby P, Kwiatkowski DJ: Atherosclerosis: The path from genomics to therapeutics. J Am Coll Cardiol 49:1589, 2007.

Novel Approach to Global Risk Detection

203. Ridker PM, Cook N: Should age and time be eliminated from cardiovascular risk prediction models? Rationale for the creation of a new national risk detection program. Circulation 111:657, 2005.
204. Ridker PM, Buring JE, Rifai N, Cook N: Development and validation of improved algorithms for the assessment of global cardiovascular risk in women: The Reynolds Risk Score. JAMA 297:611-619, 2007.

CHAPTER 40

Systemic Hypertension: Mechanisms and Diagnosis

Ronald G. Victor and Norman M. Kaplan

DEFINITION, PREVALENCE, VARIABILITY, AND DETERMINANTS OF HYPERTENSION

Affecting 60 million Americans and 1 billion people worldwide, systemic hypertension remains the most common, readily identifiable, and reversible risk factor for myocardial infarction, stroke, heart failure, atrial fibrillation, aortic dissection, and peripheral arterial disease. Because of escalating obesity and population aging in developed and developing countries, the global burden of hypertension is rising and projected to affect 1.5 billion persons, one third of the world's population, by the year 2025. Thus, hypertension remains the leading cause of death worldwide and one of the world's great public health problems[1] (Fig. 40-1; see Chap. 1).

The asymptomatic nature of the condition delays diagnosis. Effective treatment requires continuity of care by a knowledgeable physician and frequent medical checkups, which are less common in men and low-income minorities. In the vast majority of patients diagnosed with hypertension, a single disease-causing mechanism cannot be identified and treatment remains empirical, often requiring three or more pharmacological agents with complementary mechanisms of action as well as lipid-lowering drugs, antiplatelet drugs, and drugs for concomitant medical conditions, such as diabetes. Pill burden, prescription drug costs, medication side effects, and insufficient time for patient education contribute to nonadherence. Physicians often are slow to initiate and intensify antihypertensive medication. For all these reasons, blood pressure (BP) is controlled to a value below 140/90 mm Hg in less than one third of affected individuals, even in countries with the most advanced systems of health care.[2]

Even among patients whose hypertension is assumed to be well-controlled by current standards, fewer than one in three is protected from subsequent stroke, myocardial infarction, or heart failure.[3] This and the subsequent chapter will review the scientific basis for current recommendations for the diagnosis, evaluation, and treatment of hypertension and will present emerging concepts from clinical and basic research that have begun to affect clinical decision-making.

Definition

Hypertension currently is defined as a usual BP of 140/90 mm Hg or higher, BP levels for which the benefits of pharmacological treatment have been definitively established in randomized placebo-controlled trials.[4] The validity of this conservative definition has been called into question by epidemiological data showing continuous positive relationships between the risk of coronary artery disease (CAD) and stroke deaths with systolic or diastolic BP down to values as low as 115/75 mm Hg (Fig. 40-2).[5] Thus, it has been argued that the artificial dichotomy between hypertension and normotension could delay medical treatment until vascular health has been irreversibly compromised by elevated BP values previously considered to be normal.[6] For certain high-risk patients, such as those with established CAD, emerging data suggest that this may be the case.[7] However, when plotted on standard linear (rather than log-linear) scales (Fig. 40-3), epidemiological data emphasize that the risks of CAD and stroke death increase curvilinearly with increasing systolic BP, most strikingly at values above approximately 140 mm Hg. Moreover, the data emphasize that CAD is the most common cause of death from hypertension; at every level of systolic BP, the absolute risk of CAD death outweighs the risk of stroke death.

Prevalence

In the United States and other developed countries, the prevalence of hypertension increases with age, rising exponentially after age 30 (see Chap. 1). Before age 50, the prevalence of hypertension is somewhat lower in women than in men. After menopause, the prevalence of hypertension increases rapidly in women and exceeds that in men. Eventually, by age 75, below the average lifespan of U.S. men and women, almost 90 percent will have hypertension.[8]

Among U.S. adults, over 40 percent of blacks have hypertension compared with 25 percent of whites and Hispanics. In U.S. blacks, hypertension is not only more prevalent than in other racial and ethnic groups but also starts at a younger age, is more severe, and causes greater target organ damage, leading to greater premature disability and death. In contrast, hypertension prevalence does not vary between blacks and nonblacks in Cuba or in other less developed countries. Furthermore, hypertension is more prevalent in several white European countries than in African Americans and is uncommon among Africans livings in Africa (Fig. 40-4).[9] Although many genetic factors have been postulated to explain the disproportionate burden of hypertension in African Americans, these international data underscore the importance of environment. In 90 to 95 percent of hypertensive patients, a single reversible cause of the elevated BP cannot be identified—hence, the term *primary hypertension.* In the remaining 5 to 10 percent, a more discrete mechanism can be identified, and the condition is termed *secondary* or *identifiable hypertension.*

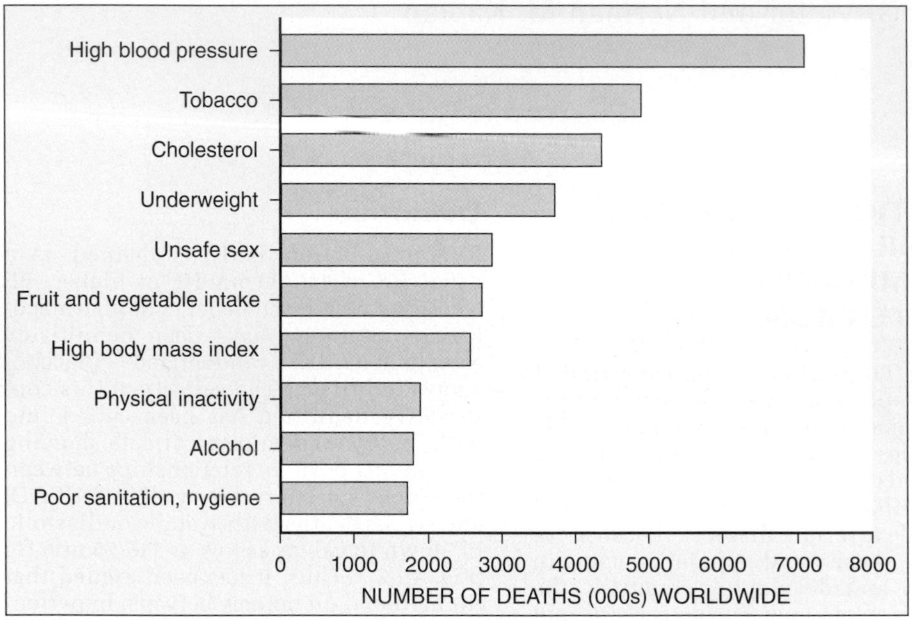

FIGURE 40–1 Potentially preventable causes of death in the world. *(From the World Health Organization: Deaths in 2000 attributable to selected leading risk factors [http://www.who.int/hpr/ NPH/docs/whr_2002_risk_factors.pdf.])*

Blood Pressure Variability and Its Determinants

Behavioral Determinants (see Chap. 39)

In most patients with primary hypertension, readily identifiable behaviors contribute to the elevated BP. The nicotine in cigarette smoke transiently raises BP by 10 to 20 mm Hg with every single cigarette, thereby elevating the average daytime BP in habitual smokers. With alcohol, the risk of hypertension is lower in moderate drinkers (one or two drinks per day) than in teetotalers but increased in heavy drinkers (three or more drinks per day). Caffeine consumption typically causes only a small transient rise in BP which, in some individuals, habituates after the first cup of coffee. Caffeine consumption does not increase the risk of developing hypertension.[10] In normotensive individuals, habitual physical inactivity associates with a markedly increased risk of devel-

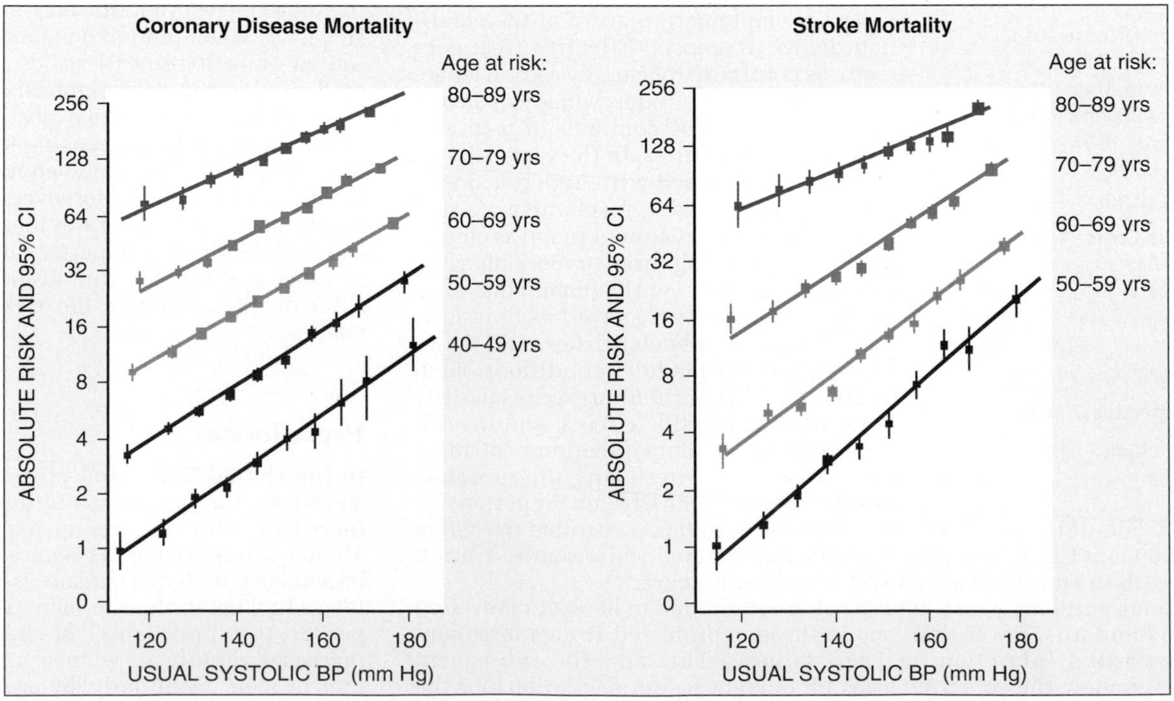

FIGURE 40–2 Absolute risks of coronary artery disease **(left)** and stroke mortality **(right)** for each decade of life (plotted on a logarithmic scale) by usual systolic blood pressure (BP) level (plotted on a linear scale). CI = confidence interval. *(From Prospective Studies Collaboration: Age-specific relevance of usual BP to vascular mortality: A meta-analysis of individual data for one million adults in 61 prospective studies. Lancet 360:1903, 2002.)*

oping hypertension, in part because of weight gain.

Lifetime dietary habits greatly influence the risk of developing hypertension (see Chap. 44). Diets low in fresh fruit may be associated with an increased risk of developing hypertension, perhaps because of lower citrate intake.[11] The two most important behavioral determinants of hypertension, however, are excessive consumption of calories and salt. Across various populations, hypertension prevalence increases linearly with average body mass index. With the unrelenting obesity epidemic, more than 50 percent of all cases of hypertension can be attributed to obesity. The risk of developing hypertension is linearly and tightly related to dietary sodium intake.[12] Interindividual variability in BP responses to dietary sodium loading and sodium restriction indicates an important genetic underpinning.

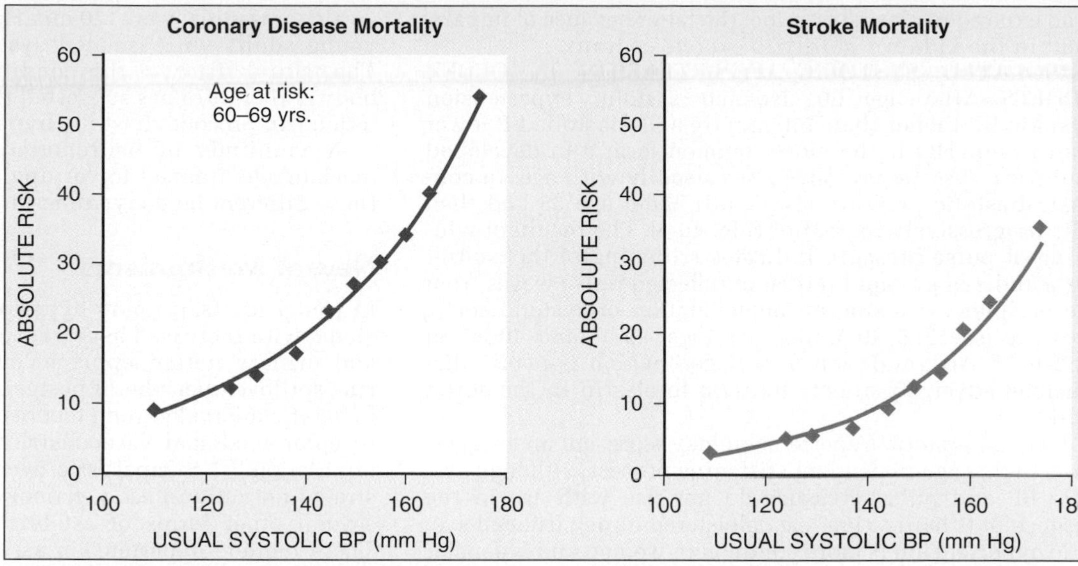

FIGURE 40–3 Curvilinear relation of blood pressure (BP) and cardiovascular risk. Data for 60- to 69-year-olds (the most common age group of study participants in hypertension treatment trials) from Figure 40-2 were replotted on standard linear scales for both abscissa and ordinate. *(From Prospective Studies Collaboration: Age-specific relevance of usual BP to vascular mortality: A meta-analysis of individual data for one million adults in 61 prospective studies. Lancet 360:1903, 2002.)*

Genetic Determinants (see Chap. 8)

Concordance of BPs is higher in families than in unrelated individuals, higher between monozygotic than dizygotic twins, and higher between biological than adoptive siblings living in the same household. As much as 70 percent of the familial aggregation of BP is attributed to shared genes rather than shared environment.

Fourteen genes have been identified that cause mendelian forms of hypertension and nine that cause mendelian forms of hypotension.[13] In every case, the mechanism involves the renal handling of salt and water, thereby emphasizing the pivotal importance of the kidney in human BP regulation. However, these mendelian forms of hypertension together are responsible for only a tiny fraction of the 60 million cases of hypertension in the United States. Mutations in these 23 genes, alone or in combination, do not seem to confer resistance against or sensitivity to the hypertensive effects of the common environmental exposures in the general population. The genetic underpinning of primary hypertension remains conjectural.

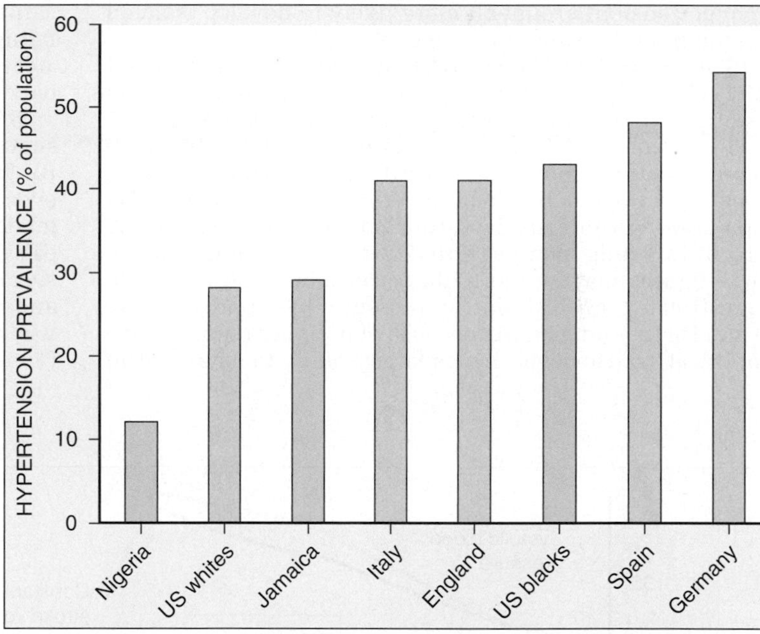

FIGURE 40–4 Geographic variation in hypertension prevalence in populations of African (blue bars) and European (yellow bars) ancestry. *(From Cooper RS, Wolf-Maier K, Luke A, et al: An international comparative study of BP in populations of European vs. African descent. BMC Med 3:1, 2005.)*

MECHANISMS OF PRIMARY (ESSENTIAL) HYPERTENSION

Hemodynamic Subtypes

Mounting evidence indicates that human hypertension can be divided into three distinctly different hemodynamic subtypes that vary sharply by age.

DIASTOLIC HYPERTENSION IN MIDDLE AGE. When hypertension is diagnosed in middle age (typically, 30 to 50 years of age), the most common BP pattern is elevated diastolic pressure with systolic pressure being normal (isolated diastolic hypertension) or elevated (combined systolic-diastolic hypertension). This is classic "essential hypertension." Isolated diastolic hypertension is more common in men and is often associated with middle-age weight gain.[14] Without treatment, isolated diastolic hypertension often progresses to combined systolic-diastolic hypertension. The fundamental hemodynamic fault is an elevated systemic vascular resistance coupled with an inappropriately normal cardiac output. Vasoconstriction at the level of the resistance arterioles results from increased neurohormonal drive and an autoregulatory reaction of vascular smooth muscle to an expanded plasma volume, the latter because of impairment in the kidneys' ability to excrete sodium.

ISOLATED SYSTOLIC HYPERTENSION IN OLDER ADULTS. After age 60, isolated systolic hypertension (systolic BP higher than 140 mm Hg and diastolic BP lower than 90 mm Hg) is the most common form.[15] In developed countries, systolic pressure rises steadily with age; in contrast, diastolic pressure rises until about age 55 and then falls progressively thereafter (Fig. 40-5). The resultant widening of pulse pressure indicates stiffening of the central aorta and a more rapid return of reflected pulse waves from the periphery, causing an augmentation of systolic aortic pressure (see Fig. 40-5; also see Figs. 40-e1 and 40-e2 on website).[16] Accumulation of collagen (which is poorly distensible) adversely affects its ratio to elastin in the aortic wall.

Isolated systolic hypertension may represent an exaggeration of this age-dependent stiffening process, although systolic BP and pulse pressure do not rise with age in the absence of urbanization (e.g., cloistered nuns). Isolated systolic hypertension is more common in women and is a major risk factor for diastolic heart failure, which also is more common in women (see Chaps. 26 and 76).[15] Most cases of isolated systolic hypertension arise de novo after age 60 and are not "burned-out" middle-age diastolic hypertension.[14] Compared with young or middle-aged adults with optimal BP, those with BP in the high-normal range (borderline or prehypertension) are much more likely to develop isolated systolic hypertension after age 60.[14]

ISOLATED SYSTOLIC HYPERTENSION IN YOUNG ADULTS. At the other end of the age spectrum is isolated systolic hypertension in young adults who are typically 17 to 25 years of age. The key hemodynamic abnormalities are increased cardiac output and a stiff aorta, both presumably reflecting an overactive sympathetic nervous system.[17] The population prevalence is estimated to be as high as 25 percent in young men but only 2 percent in young women. These figures may be too high, because brachial artery BP overestimates central aortic pressure by approximately 20 mm Hg in young adults because of peripheral pulse wave amplification. However, in the largest study to date, central aortic pressures were 20 mm Hg higher than normal in young adults with isolated systolic hypertension (ISH).[17] The natural history of this condition is unknown but a large body of literature has suggested that a hyperdynamic circulation can precede diastolic hypertension.

A multitude of neurohormonal, renal, and vascular mechanisms interact to varying degrees in contributing to these different hemodynamic forms of hypertension.

Neural Mechanisms

In young adults, primary hypertension consistently is associated with increased heart rate and cardiac output, plasma and urinary norepinephrine levels, regional norepinephrine spillover, peripheral postganglionic sympathetic nerve firing (by microelectrode recordings), and alpha-adrenergic receptor–mediated vasoconstrictor tone in the peripheral circulation.[18,19] Sympathetic overactivity has been demonstrated not only in early primary hypertension but also in several other forms of established human hypertension. These include hypertension associated with obesity, sleep apnea, early type 2 diabetes mellitus and prediabetes, chronic kidney disease, heart failure, and immunosuppressive therapy with calcineurin inhibitors such as cyclosporine. In these conditions, central sympathetic outflow can be driven by deactivation of inhibitory neural inputs (e.g., baroreceptors), activation of excitatory neural inputs (e.g., carotid body chemoreceptors, renal afferents), or by circulating angiotensin II (A II), which activates pools of excitatory brain stem neurons that are devoid of a blood-brain barrier (Fig. 40-6).

BARORECEPTORS AND HYPERTENSION. In hypertension, the baroreceptors are reset to defend a higher level of BP. Baroreflex control of sinus node function is impaired even in mild hypertension, but baroreflex control of systemic vascular resistance and BP is well preserved. Surgically-implanted carotid baroreceptor pacemakers produce sustained BP reductions in dog models of hypertension[20] and parallel multicenter clinical trials are currently underway in patients with medically refractory hypertension. Complete baroreflex failure (see Chap. 89) is a rare cause of

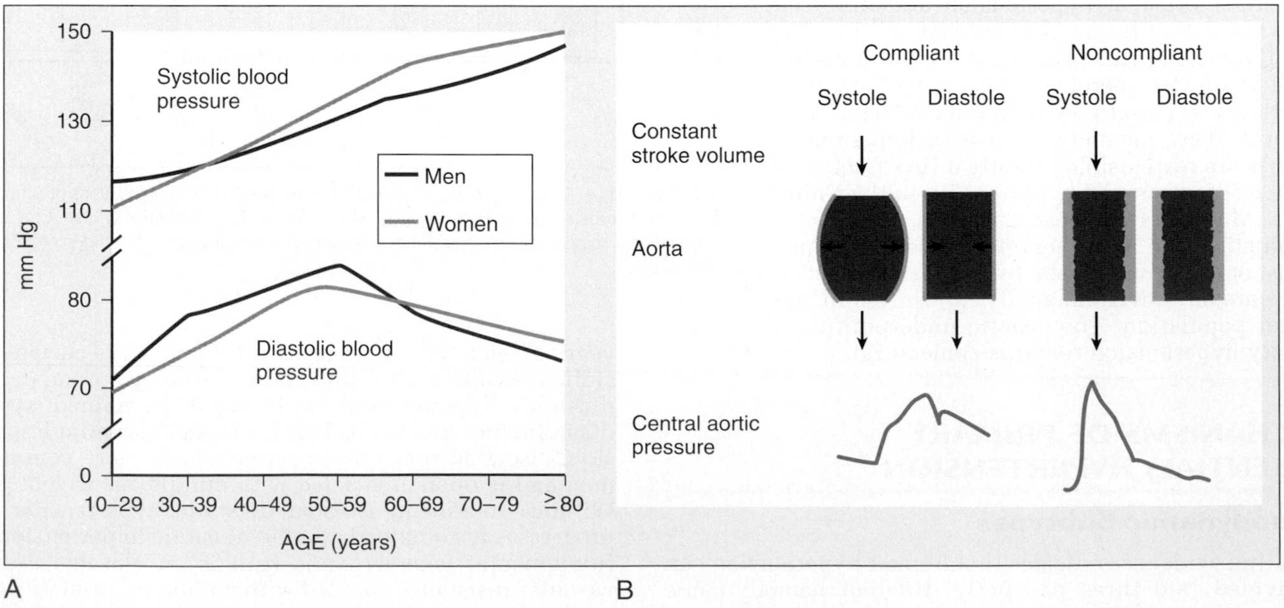

FIGURE 40–5 A, Age-dependent changes in systolic and diastolic blood pressure in the United States. **B,** Schematic representation of the relationship between aortic compliance and pulse pressure. *(**A**, from Burt V, Whelton P, Rocella EJ, et al: Prevalence of hypertension in the U.S. adult population. Results from the Third National Health and Nutrition Examination Survey, 1988-1991. Hypertension 25:305, 1995; and **B**, from Dr. Stanley Franklin, University of California at Irvine, with permission.)*

labile hypertension most often seen in throat cancer survivors as a late complication of radiation therapy, which causes a gradual destruction of the baroreceptor nerves.[21] In contrast, partial baroreceptor dysfunction is common in elderly hypertensives and typically presents with a triad of orthostatic hypotension, supine hypertension, and symptomatic postprandial hypotension, the latter initiated by splanchnic pooling after carbohydrate-rich meals.[22]

OBESITY-RELATED HYPERTENSION. Neural mechanisms of obesity-related hypertension deserve special mention. With weight gain, reflex sympathetic activation is thought to be an important compensation to burn fat but at the expense of sympathetic overactivity in target tissues (i.e., vascular smooth muscle and kidney) that produce hypertension.[23] Near-maximal rates of sympathetic firing are seen in hypertensive patients with the metabolic syndrome with or without new-onset type 2 diabetes. Although the sympathetic activation associates with insulin resistance, the precise stimulus to sympathetic outflow is unknown, with leptin, other adipokines, and A II being potential candidates.

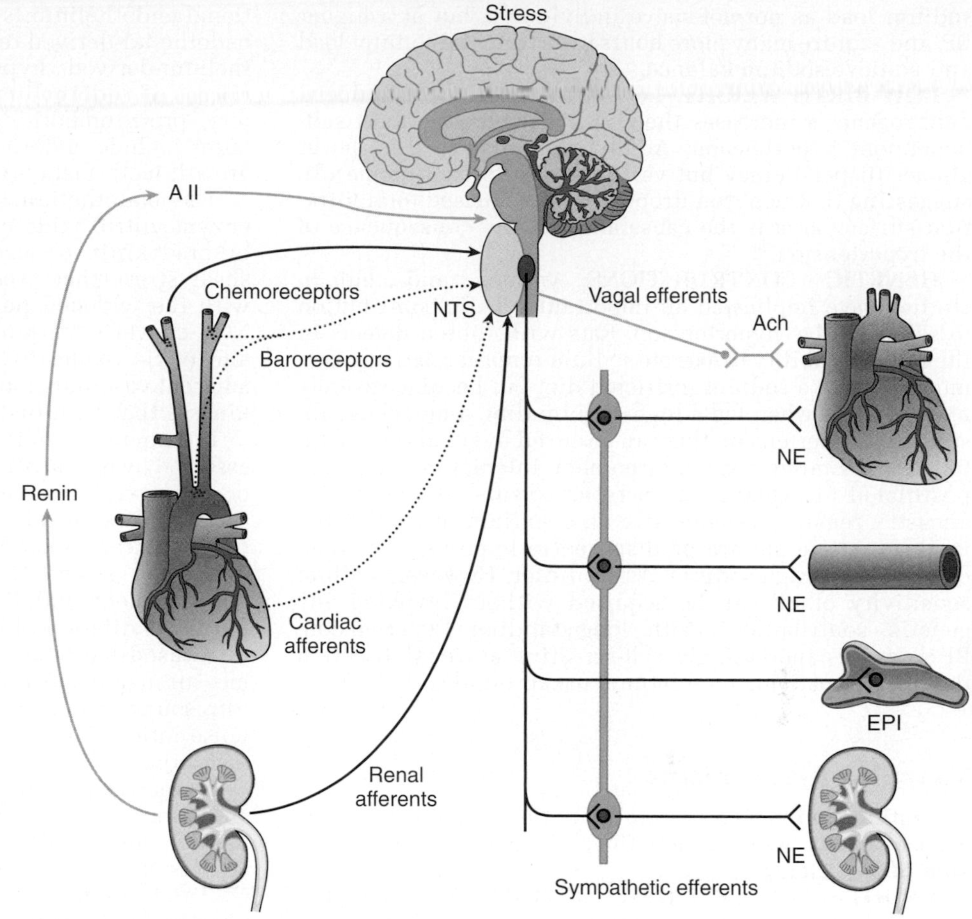

FIGURE 40–6 Sympathetic nervous system. Dotted arrows represent inhibitory neural influences and solid arrows represent excitatory neural influences on sympathetic outflow to the heart, peripheral vasculature, and kidneys. EPI = epinephrine; NTS = nucleus tractus solitarius; NE = norepinephrine; Ach = acetylcholine; A II = angiotensin II.

SLEEP APNEA AS A CAUSE OF NEUROGENIC HYPERTENSION (see Chap. 74). The strongest evidence for sustained neurogenic hypertension in humans is in patients with obstructive sleep apnea. With repeated arterial desaturation during apneas, activation of carotid body chemoreceptors not only causes dramatic pressor episodes throughout the night but also resets the chemoreceptor reflex. Daytime normoxia is misinterpreted as hypoxia, producing sustained reflex sympathetic activation and hypertension, even dur-ing waking hours.[24] Continuous positive airway pressure improves daytime as well as nighttime hypertension, with the fall in BP often paralleling the reduction in sympathetic activity (see Fig. 40-e3 on website).[25] Obstructive sleep apnea not only predisposes to hypertension but also accelerates the risk of several hypertensive complications (e.g., stroke, atrial fibrillation, and cardiovascular death) beyond that explained by BP elevation alone.[26]

LONG-TERM SYMPATHETIC REGULATION OF BLOOD PRESSURE. The sympathetic nervous system is well known to regulate short-term changes in BP, such as transient surges in BP during physical and emotional stress. In addition, sustained sympathetic activation contributes to long-term BP regulation because the renal sympathetic nerves are among the most potent stimuli to renin release by stimulation of $beta_1$ receptors in the juxtaglomerular apparatus and to renal sodium reabsorption by stimulation of $alpha_1$ adrenergic receptors regulating Na-K-ATPase in the collecting duct. In addition, norepinephrine's action on $alpha_1$ adrenoreceptors constitutes a trophic stimulus to cardiac and vascular smooth muscle hypertrophy.[27] In patients with hypertension and left ventricular hypertrophy (LVH), cardiac norepinephrine spillover is increased and may predispose to sudden cardiac death. An increased plasma norepinephrine level is a strong independent predictor of poor survival in chronic hemodialysis patients with hypertension,[28] as has been found in patients with congestive heart failure (see Chap. 22).

Renal Mechanisms

The kidney is the culprit and victim in hypertension, producing a vicious cycle of progressive renal dysfunction and hypertension. In many forms of experimental and human hypertension, the fundamental abnormality is an acquired or inherited defect in the kidneys' ability to excrete the excessive sodium load imposed by a modern high–sodium chloride diet. Renal sodium retention expands the plasma volume, increasing cardiac output and triggering autoregulatory responses that increase systemic vascular resistance. Salt retention also augments the smooth muscle contraction produced by all known endogenous vasoconstrictor substances.

RESETTING OF PRESSURE-NATRIURESIS. In normotensive individuals, BP elevation invokes an immediate increase in renal sodium excretion to shrink plasma volume and return BP to normal. In almost all forms of hypertension, the pressure-natriuresis curve is shifted to the right and, in salt-sensitive hypertension, the slope is reduced. Resetting of the pressure-natriuresis curve leads to nocturia, one of the most common and bothersome symptoms in patients with uncontrolled hypertension. Hypertensive individuals excrete the same amount of a given dietary sodium load as normotensive individuals, but at a higher BP, and require many more hours to excrete the sodium load and achieve sodium balance.

LOW BIRTH WEIGHT. Low birth weight with reduced nephrogenesis increases the risk of developing adult salt-dependent hypertension. Adult hypertensives have fewer glomeruli per kidney but very few obsolescent glomeruli, suggesting that nephron dropout and decreased total filtration surface area is the cause and not the consequence of the hypertension.[29]

GENETIC CONTRIBUTIONS. Animal and human studies have implicated an important genetic contribution to salt-sensitive hypertension. Rats with inbred defects in the kidneys' ability to excrete sodium remain relatively normotensive on a sodium-restricted diet but become severely hypertensive when fed a high-sodium diet, a model of salt-sensitive hypertension that can be cured by renal transplantation. A similar gene-environment interaction has been postulated to explain why persons of sub-Saharan Africa ancestry remain normotensive on a sodium-restricted diet in rural Africa but are predisposed to hypertension when exposed to a high-sodium Western diet. However, sodium sensitivity of BP can be acquired without invoking any genetic contribution. With long-standing hypertension, BP becomes increasingly salt-sensitive as renal function declines in patients of all ethnic backgrounds.

Vascular Mechanisms

Alterations in the structure and function of small and large arteries play a pivotal role in the pathogenesis and progression of hypertension.

ENDOTHELIAL CELL DYSFUNCTION. The endothelial lining of blood vessels is critical to vascular health and constitutes a major defense against hypertension. Dysfunctional endothelium is characterized by impaired release of endothelial-derived relaxing factors (e.g., nitric oxide, endothelium-derived hyperpolarizing factor) and enhanced release of endothelium-derived constricting, proinflammatory, prothrombotic, and growth factors (Fig. 40-7). The latter include endothelin, thromboxane, and transforming growth factor-beta (TGF-β).[30]

The endothelium of all blood vessels expresses the enzyme nitric oxide synthase (NOS), which can be activated by bradykinin or acetylcholine or by the cyclic laminar shear stress that accompanies hypertension, particularly with the widened pulse pressure in ISH. Once activated, NOS converts L-arginine to citrulline, an inert substance, and nitric oxide (NO), a volatile gas that diffuses to the adjacent vascular smooth muscle and activates a series of G kinases that culminate in vasodilation (see Fig. 40-7).

In humans, endothelium-dependent vasodilation can be assessed by measuring increases in the large artery (forearm or coronary) diameter following intraarterial infusion of acetylcholine or release of ischemia (e.g., arrested forearm circulation) or a sudden elevation in BP (cold pressor test; see Chaps. 48 and 57). Competitive inhibitors of NOS specifically block endothelium-dependent dilation but do not block the dilation of these arteries produced by exogenous nitrovasodilators (e.g., nitroglycerin, nitroprusside). These measurements most often are obtained with brachial artery ultrasound, a noninvasive technique with a low-signal-to-noise ratio. More accurate measurements require invasive techniques.

C-reactive protein (CRP) (see Chap. 39) is an easily measured serum biomarker for determining blood vessel inflammation and endothelial dysfunction.[31] Cross-sectional studies have shown strong correlations between elevated CRP and arterial stiffness and elevated pulse pressure. Longitudinal studies have implicated elevated CRP levels as a risk marker (risk factor) for new onset of hypertension and

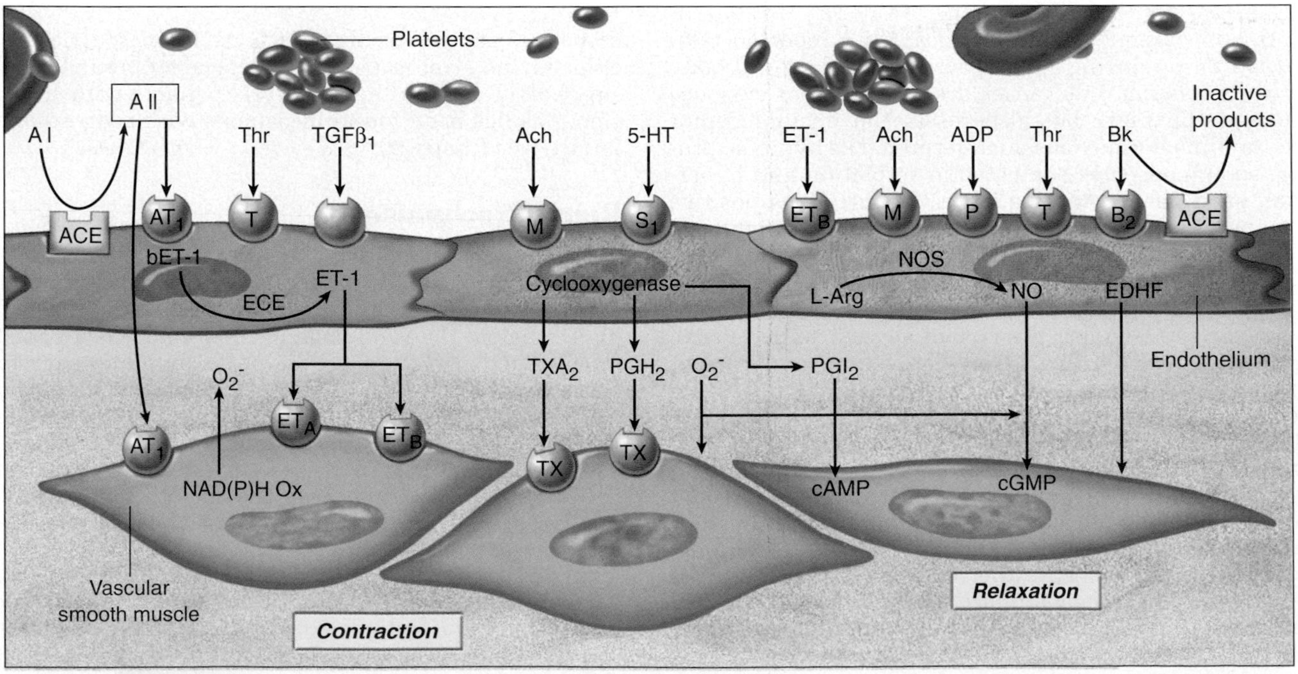

FIGURE 40–7 Endothelium-derived relaxing and constricting factors. Various blood- and platelet-derived substances can activate specific receptors (orange circles) on the endothelial membrane to release relaxing factors such as nitric oxide (NO), prostacyclin (PGI_2), and an endothelium-derived hyperpolarizing factor (EDHF). Contracting factors also are released, such as endothelin (ET-1), angiotensin (A II), and thromboxane A_2 (TXA_2), as well as prostaglandin H_2 (PGH_2). ACE = angiotensin-converting enzyme; 5-HT = serotonin; Bk = bradykinin; ECE = endothelin-converting enzyme; L-Arg = L-arginine; NOS = nitric oxide synthase; O_2^- = superoxide; $TGF\beta_1$ = transforming growth factor beta-1; Thr = thrombin. *(From Ruschitzka F, Corti R, Noll G, et al: A rationale for treatment of endothelial dysfunction in hypertension. J Hypertens 17[Suppl 1]:25, 1999.)*

accelerated progression of hypertensive target organ disease, possibly beyond that explained by BP elevation alone.

One of the principal mechanisms of endothelial cell dysfunction in hypertension is the production of superoxide anion and other reactive oxygen species that quench NO, thereby reducing its bioavailability. There are three main enzymatic sources of vascular superoxide: (1) reduced form of nicotinamide adenine dinucleotide phosphate (NADPH) oxidases, which are universally expressed in all vascular cell types and activated by circulating A II; (2) NOS, which produces superoxide only when an important cofactor (tetrahydrobiopterin) is deficient (a process known as NOS uncoupling); and (3) xanthine oxidase, which produces uric acid.[32] Generation of reactive oxygen species by xanthine oxidase almost certainly accounts for the associations among elevated serum uric acid levels, endothelial dysfunction, and human hypertension.[33] However, uric acid itself is an antioxidant. Thus, the xanthine oxidase inhibitor allopurinol does not consistently lower BP in patients with hypertension because the drug simultaneously reduces both these opposing effects on vascular function.[34]

VASCULAR REMODELING. Over time, endothelial cell dysfunction, neurohormonal activation, and elevated BP cause remodeling of blood vessels, which further perpetuates the hypertension (Fig. 40-8).[35] An increase in the medial thickness relative to lumen diameter (increased media-to-lumen ratio) is the hallmark of hypertensive remodeling in small and large arteries. Small artery remodeling is initiated by vasoconstriction, which normalizes wall stress and averts a trophic response. Normal smooth muscle cells rearrange themselves around a smaller lumen diameter, a process termed *inward eutrophic remodeling*. The media-to-lumen ratio increases but the medial cross-sectional area remains unchanged. By decreasing lumen diameter in the peripheral circulation, inward eutrophic remodeling increases systemic vascular resistance, the hemodynamic hallmark of diastolic hypertension.

In contrast, large artery remodeling is characterized by the expression of hypertrophic genes, triggering increases in medial thickness as well as the media-to-lumen ratio. Such hypertrophic remodeling involves not only an increase in the size of vascular smooth muscle cells but also an accumulation of extracellular matrix proteins such as collagen and fibronectin, because of activation of TGF-β. The resultant large artery stiffness is the hemodynamic hallmark of isolated systolic hypertension.

Antihypertensive therapy may not provide optimal cardiovascular protection unless vascular remodeling is prevented or reversed by normalizing hemodynamic load, restoring normal endothelial cell function, and eliminating the underlying neurohormonal activation.[35]

Hormonal Mechanisms: Renin-Angiotensin-Aldosterone System

(see Fig. 22-3)

Activation of the renin-angiotensin-aldosterone system (RAAS) is one of the most important mechanisms contributing to endothelial cell dysfunction, vascular remodeling, and hypertension (Fig. 40-9). Renin, a protease produced solely by the renal juxtaglomerular cells, cleaves angiotensinogen (renin substrate produced by the liver) to A I, which is converted by angiotensin-converting enzyme (ACE) to A II (see Chap. 88). ACE is most abundant in the lungs but is also present in the heart and systemic vasculature (tissue ACE). Chymase, a serine protease in the heart and systemic arteries, provides an alternative pathway for conversion of A I to A II. The interaction of A II with G protein–coupled AT1 receptors activates numerous cellular processes that contribute to hypertension and accelerate hypertensive end-organ damage (see Fig. 40-9). These include vasoconstriction, generation of reactive oxygen species, vascular inflammation, vascular and cardiac remodeling, and production of aldosterone, the principal mineralocorticoid. There is increasing evidence that aldosterone, A II, and even renin and prorenin activate multiple signaling pathways that can damage vascular health and cause hypertension.

ALDOSTERONE AND EPITHELIAL SODIUM CHANNEL REGULATION. RAAS activation is a major homeostatic mechanism to counter hypovolemic hypotension (as with hemorrhage or salt and water deprivation). Interaction of aldosterone with cytosolic mineralocorticoid receptors in the renal collecting duct cells recruits sodium channels from the cytosol to the surface of the renal epithelium. The epithelial sodium channels (ENaCs) so recruited increase sodium reabsorption, thereby reexpanding plasma volume. Conversely, modern high-salt diets should engender continual feedback inhibition of the RAAS. Suppression of serum aldosterone should trigger sequestration of ENaCs by endocytosis and increased renal sodium excretion, thereby shrinking plasma volume to protect against salt-sensitive hypertension.

Thus, in the setting of high dietary sodium and elevated BP, the RAAS should be completely suppressed, and any degree of RAAS activity is inappropriate. In normotensive

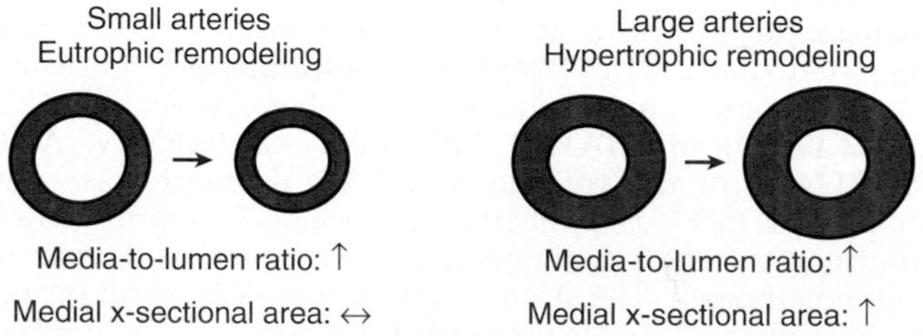

FIGURE 40–8 Vascular remodeling of small and large arteries in hypertension. Diagrams represent arteries in cross section showing the tunica adventitia, tunica media, and tunica intima. *(Modified from Duprez DA: Role of renin-angiotensin-aldosterone system in vascular remodeling and inflammation: a clinical review. J Hypertens 24:983, 2006.)*

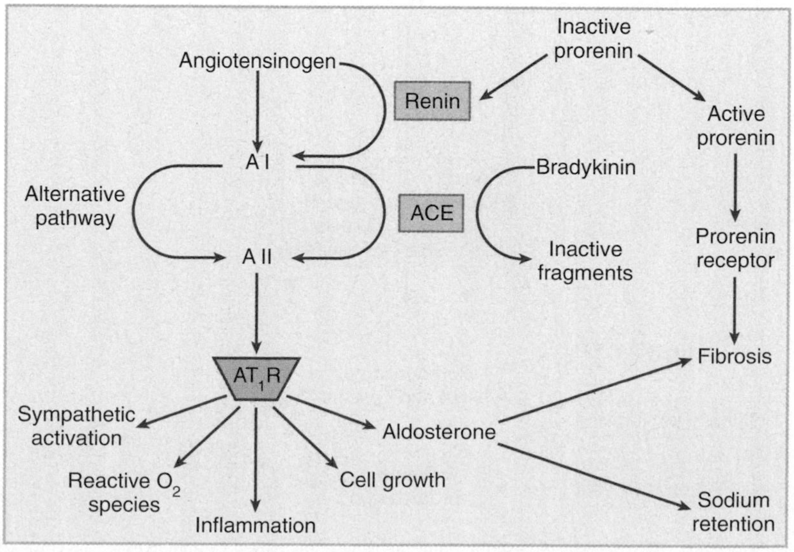

FIGURE 40–9 The renin-angiotensin-aldosterone system. A I = angiotensin I; A II = angiotensin II; ACE = angiotensin-converting enzyme; AT_1R = angiotensin I receptor.

individuals, the risk of developing hypertension increases with increasing levels of serum aldosterone that are well within the normal range.[36] In African Caribbean hypertensives, serum aldosterone levels are higher than in white hypertensives, despite lower plasma renin levels,[37] implicating abnormal aldosterone production by renin-independent mechanisms, a forme fruste of primary aldosteronism. By stimulating mineralocorticoid receptors in the heart and kidney, circulating aldosterone may contribute to the development of cardiac and renal fibrosis in hypertension.[38] By stimulating mineralocorticoid receptors in the brain stem, aldosterone also may contribute to sympathetic overactivity.

RECEPTOR-MEDIATED ACTIONS OF ANGIOTENSIN II. Two main types of angiotensin receptors are known. AT1 receptors are widely expressed in the vasculature, kidney, adrenals, heart, liver, and brain. A I receptor activation explains most of the hypertensive actions of A II. Furthermore, enhanced AT1-mediated signaling provides a central mechanistic explanation for the frequent coexistence of elevated BP with insulin resistance and atherosclerosis and constitutes a major therapeutic target for interrupting every step in cardiovascular disease progression, from vascular remodeling and formation of atherosclerotic plaque to stroke, myocardial infarction (MI), and death (Fig. 40-10).

In contrast, AT2 receptors are widely distributed in the fetus but, in adults, are found only in the adrenal medulla, uterus, ovary, vascular endothelium, and distinct brain regions. In rodents, AT2 receptor activation opposes some of the deleterious effects of AT1 receptors by promoting endothelium-dependent vasodilation by bradykinin and nitric oxide pathways. However, recent animal studies have suggested that AT2 receptors can be profibrotic, but their role in human hypertension remains speculative.

RECEPTOR-MEDIATED ACTIONS OF RENIN AND PRORENIN. In the traditional RAAS, prorenin has been considered to be the inactive precursor of renin, which functions solely to generate A I by enzymatic cleavage of angiotensinogen. These concepts are rapidly evolving as newer studies implicate prorenin and renin as direct cardiac and renal toxins. Prorenin is inactive because a 43–amino acid hinge is closed and prevents it from binding to angiotensinogen. In the kidneys, inactive prorenin is converted to active renin when this inhibitory hinge region is enzymatically cleaved. When circulating prorenin binds to a newly discovered (pro)renin receptor in the heart and kidneys, the hinge is opened (but not cleaved), and this nonenzymatic process fully activates prorenin (see Fig. 40-e4 on website).[39,40] As a result, TGF-β production is accelerated, leading to collagen deposition and fibrosis. This receptor-mediated process is completely independent of A II generation and therefore unaffected by angiotensin-converting enzyme inhibitors (ACEIs) and angiotensin receptor blockers (ARBs). Although ACEIs and ARBs are excellent antihypertensives (see Chap. 41), they trigger large reactive increases in prorenin and renin production that may counter some of the cardiovascular protection afforded by reduced AT1 receptor activation. Of note, prorenin blood levels are 100-fold higher than renin levels.

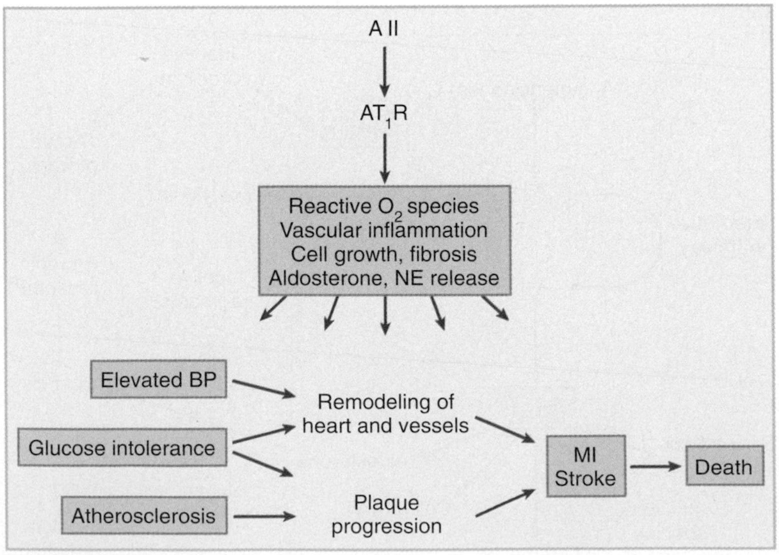

FIGURE 40–10 Schematic representation of the central role played by angiotensin 1 receptor (AT_1R)–mediated signaling in cardiovascular disease progression. A II = angiotensin II; MI = myocardial infarction.

PATHOGENESIS OF HYPERTENSIVE HEART DISEASE

Hypertension is a major risk factor not only for CAD but also for left ventricular hypertrophy and heart failure.

Pressure Overload Hypertrophy

In hypertensive patients, left ventricular hypertrophy is a powerful independent predictor of morbidity and mortality, predisposing to heart failure, ventricular tachyarrhythmia, ischemic stroke, atrial fibrillation, and embolic stroke. There have been tremendous advances in our understanding of the cell and molecular mechanisms underlying pressure overload cardiomyocyte hypertrophy.[41] Moreover, the structural abnormalities in the hypertensive heart are not limited to myocyte hypertrophy. They also include medial hypertrophy of the intramyocardial coronary arteries as well as collagen deposition leading to cardiac fibrosis.[42] These changes result in part from pressure overload and in part from the neurohormonal activation that contributes to hypertension. In animal models, A II, aldosterone, norepinephrine, and prorenin accelerate pressure overload cardiomyocyte hypertrophy and promote cardiac fibrosis, the latter being the hallmark of pathological LVH (in contrast to the physiological hypertrophy of exercise training, which is unaccompanied by fibrosis).

IMPAIRED CORONARY VASODILATOR RESERVE. In the hypertrophied hypertensive heart, coronary blood flow is normal at rest but vasodilator reserve becomes impaired when myocyte mass outstrips the blood supply. Even in the absence of CAD, coronary vasodilator reserve is blunted or absent, leading to subendocardial ischemia under conditions of increased myocardial oxygen demand. The combination of subendocardial ischemia and cardiac fibrosis impairs diastolic relaxation, leading to exertional dyspnea and diastolic heart failure.

Heart Failure

Before the advent of effective drug therapy for hypertension, beginning in the late 1950s, heart failure caused most deaths from hypertension. With better management of hypertension, there has been a dramatic reduction in hypertension-related deaths from heart failure and a significant delay in its onset. Nevertheless, hypertension remains the most common cause of diastolic heart failure. In addition, hypertension indirectly leads to systolic heart failure by virtue of its being a major risk factor for myocardial infarction. It is unclear whether mild or moderate hypertension alone, without myocardial infarction, leads to systolic heart failure.[42]

DIAGNOSIS AND INITIAL EVALUATION OF HYPERTENSION

Hypertension has been termed the *silent killer,* an asymptomatic chronic disorder that, if undetected and untreated, silently damages the blood vessels, heart, brain, and kidneys. Hypertension may not be entirely asymptomatic because, in double-blind placebo-controlled trials, patients' quality of life ratings were often found to improve with successful drug treatment of hypertension. Controlling hypertension can improve exertional dyspnea caused by diastolic dysfunction, nocturia caused by resetting of pressure natriuresis, and possibly even erectile dysfunction caused by endothelial dysfunction.

Initial Evaluation of the Hypertensive Patient

The initial evaluation for hypertension should accomplish three goals: (1) measurement and staging of BP; (2) assessment of the patient's overall cardiovascular risk; and (3) detection of secondary (i.e., identifiable and potentially curable) forms of hypertension.

Measurement of Blood Pressure

STAGING OF OFFICE BP

Currently, BP is staged as normal, prehypertension, or hypertension based on the average of two or more readings taken at two or more office visits. When a person's average systolic and diastolic pressures fall into different stages, the higher stage applies (Table 40-1).[4]

MEASUREMENT TECHNIQUE (see also Chap. 11). In the office, BP should be measured at least twice after 5 minutes of rest, with the patient seated in a chair, the back supported, and the arm bare and at heart level. A large adult-sized cuff should be used to measure BP in overweight adults because the standard-sized cuff can spuriously elevate readings. Tobacco and caffeine should be avoided for at least 30 minutes. BP should be measured in both arms to exclude coarctation of the aorta and after 5 minutes of standing, the latter to exclude a significant postural fall in BP, particularly in older persons and in those with diabetes or other conditions (e.g., Parkinson's disease) that predispose to autonomic insufficiency.

HOME AND AMBULATORY MONITORING

An individual's BP varies widely throughout a 24-hour period and is therefore impossible to characterize accurately except by repeated measurements under various conditions. Out-of-office readings are the only way to obtain a clear picture of a person's usual BP for accurate diagnosis and management. These readings are more predictive of cardiovascular events than office readings and overcome many of the pitfalls of office measurement, including operator errors and alerting (i.e., white coat) reactions.

Many electronic oscillometric monitors are available but few models have been rigorously validated (see dableducational.com). Most oscillometric monitors provide reasonably good estimates of diastolic BP but typically underestimate systolic BP, which is not measured as the first Korotkoff sound but is estimated by applying a multiplier to the pressure corresponding to maximal oscillation (i.e., mean arterial pressure). Each patient's monitor needs to be checked in the office for accuracy and cuff size, because many manufacturers provide only a standard adult cuff. To reduce reporting bias, patients should record their pressures at fixed intervals and keep all readings.

Ambulatory monitoring provides automated measurements of BP over a 24-hour period while patients are engaging in their usual activities, including sleep. Prospective outcome studies in both treated and untreated patients have shown that ambulatory BP measurement predicts fatal and nonfatal myocardial infarction and stroke better than standard office measurement (Fig. 40-11).[43] Recommended normal values include an average daytime BP below 135/85 mm Hg, nighttime BP below 120/70 mm Hg, and 24-hour BP below 130/80 mm Hg.[44] Some experts have recommended a lower cutoff value of 130/80 mm Hg as a more stringent definition of normal daytime BP.

WHITE COAT HYPERTENSION. Up to one third of patients with elevated office BPs have normal home or ambulatory BPs. If the daytime BP is below 135/85 mm Hg (or preferably below 130/80 mm Hg) *and* there is no target organ damage despite consistently elevated office readings, the patient has "office-only" or "white coat" hypertension, presumably caused by a transient adrenergic response to the measurement of BP only in the physician's office. The prog-

TABLE 40–1 Staging of Office Blood Pressure*

Blood Pressure (BP) Stage	Systolic BP (mm Hg)	Diastolic BP (mm Hg)
Normal	<120	<80
Prehypertension	120-139	80-89
Stage 1 hypertension	140-159	90-99
Stage 2 hypertension	≥160	≥100

*Calculation of seated BP is based on the mean of two or more readings on two separate office visits.

From Chobanian AV, Bakris GL, Black HR, et al: The Seventh Report of the Joint National Committee on Prevention, Detection, Evaluation, and Treatment of High Blood Pressure: The JNC 7 report. JAMA 289:2560, 2003.

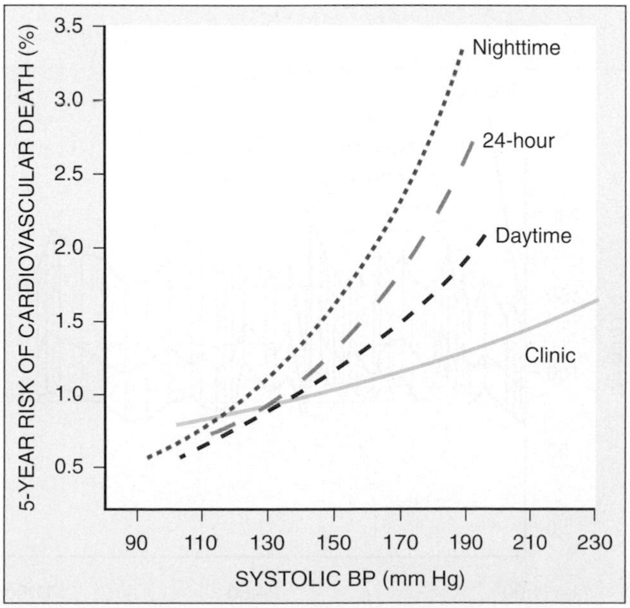

FIGURE 40–11 Superiority of ambulatory over office blood pressure (BP) measurement as a measure of cardiovascular risk. Shown is the adjusted 5-year risk of cardiovascular death (number of deaths per 100 subjects) in the study cohort of 5292 patients for office BP and ambulatory BP. *(From Dolan E, Santon A, Thijs L, et al: Superiority of ambulatory over clinic BP measurement in predicting mortality: The Dublin outcome study. Hypertension 46:156, 2005.)*

nostic importance of white coat hypertension remains unresolved but increasing evidence has suggested that this condition is not as benign as previously assumed. When data from four large prospective studies involving almost 6000 initially untreated patients were combined, the 5-year stroke rate in patients with white coat hypertension was indistinguishable from patients with normal office BPs. However, by the eighth year of follow-up, the stroke rate had increased sharply in the patients with white coat hypertension, equaling or exceeding that in patients with definite hypertension (see Fig. 40-e5 on website).[45]

Many patients do not have pure white coat hypertension but rather white coat aggravation, a white coat reaction superimposed on a milder level of out-of-office hypertension that nevertheless needs treatment (see Fig. 40-e6 on website). In the United States, the only Medicare-approved indication for ambulatory monitoring is elevated office BP with repeatedly normal home readings in the absence of demonstrable target organ damage (ICD 796.2). Recent evidence has suggested that the indications for ambulatory monitoring be expanded. For instance, in up to 30 percent of treated patients with persistently elevated office BP, ambulatory monitoring documents adequate or excessive control of hypertension, eliminating overtreatment.

MASKED HYPERTENSION. Another example of the importance of ambulatory monitoring is in patients in whom office readings underestimate out-of-office BP, presumably because of sympathetic overactivity in daily life caused by job or home stress, tobacco abuse or other adrenergic stimulation that dissipates when coming to the office (Fig. 40-12). Such documentation prevents undertreatment of this masked hypertension, which is present in over 10 percent of patients and clearly increases cardiovascular risk, despite normal office BP readings.[46]

OTHER USES OF AMBULATORY MONITORING. Ambulatory monitoring is the only way to detect hypertension during sleep (see Fig. 40-12). BP normally dips during sleep at night and increases sharply when a person awakens and becomes active in the morning. Nocturnal hypertension (see Fig. 40-12) increases the aggregate hemodynamic load on the cardiovascular system and is a much stronger predictor of cardiovascular outcomes than either daytime ambulatory BP or standard office measurements (see Fig. 40-11).[43] Nocturnal hypertension is particularly common in patients with chronic kidney disease, presumably because of increased cardiac output (centralization of an expanded plasma volume while supine) and increased systemic vascular resistance (failure of sympathetic vasoconstrictor drive to suppress normally during sleep because of persistent activation of an excitatory reflex arising in the diseased kidneys). In addition, ambulatory BP monitoring is particularly useful in diagnosing baroreceptor impairment.

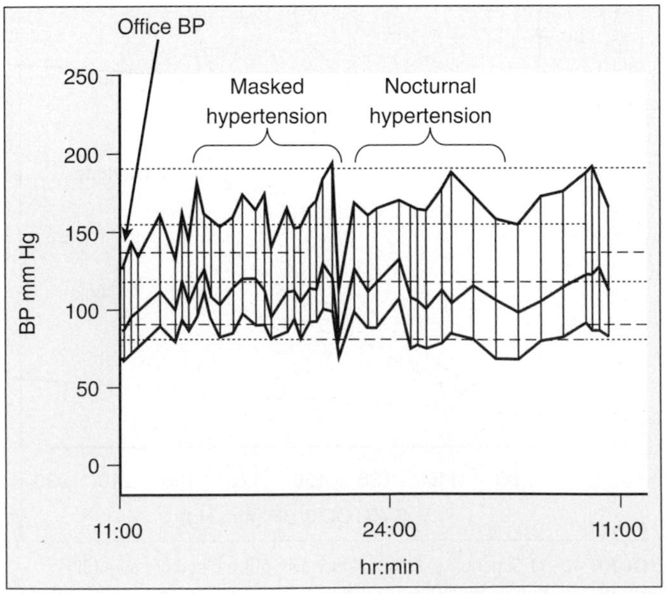

FIGURE 40–12 24-hour ambulatory blood pressure (BP) recording in a patient with apparently normal office BP but with masked hypertension and nocturnal hypertension. *(From Dr. R. G. Victor, University of Texas Southwestern Medical Center, Dallas.)*

Cardiovascular Risk Stratification (see Chap. 39)

In hypertensive individuals, cardiovascular risk increases sharply with BP stage (see Table 40-1), but this is not the only factor to consider. Cardiovascular risk also increases dramatically with hypertensive target organ damage and additional cardiovascular risk factors, the latter being present in almost all patients with hypertension or even prehypertension (Table 40-2).[47,48] In particular, over 75 percent of hypertensive patients meet current criteria for initiation of lipid-lowering medication (low-density lipoprotein [LDL] cholesterol more than 130 mm Hg) and 25 percent have diabetes.[49] Thus, the minimal laboratory testing required for the initial evaluation of hypertension is determination of blood electrolyte, fasting glucose, and serum creatinine levels (with calculated glomerular filtration rate [GFR]), a fasting lipid panel, hematocrit, spot urinalysis

TABLE 40–2	Risks Influencing Prognosis in Patients with Hypertension
Risk Factors for Cardiovascular Disease	
Levels of systolic and diastolic blood pressure	
Age (yr)—men >55; women >65	
Smoking	
Dyslipidemia	
Family history of premature cardiovascular disease	
Abdominal obesity	
Diabetes mellitus	
C-reactive protein ≥1 mg/dl	
Subclinical Target Organ Damage	
Left ventricular hypertrophy	
Ultrasound evidence of arterial wall thickening or atherosclerotic plaque	
Estimated glomerular filtration rate ≤60 ml/min/1.73m^2	
Microalbuminuria	
Clinical Target Organ Damage	
Cerebrovascular disease	
Ischemic stroke	
Cerebral hemorrhage	
Transient ischemic attack	
Heart disease	
Myocardial infarction or acute coronary syndrome	
Angina	
Coronary revascularization	
Congestive heart failure	
Renal disease	
Diabetic nephropathy	
Chronic kidney disease	
Proteinuria (>300 mg/24 hr)	
Peripheral arterial disease	
Advanced retinopathy	
Hemorrhages or exudates	
Papilledema	

Modified from European Society of Hypertension-European Society of Cardiology Guidelines Committee: 2003 European Society of Hypertension-European Society of Cardiology guidelines for the management of arterial hypertension. J Hypertens 21:1011, 2003.

(including urine albumin-to-creatinine ratio), and a resting 12-lead electrocardiogram (ECG).

The gradient between increasing levels of BP and cardiovascular risk becomes progressively steeper as additional risk factors are added (see Fig. 40-e7 on website).[50] For example, in a 50 year-old woman with no other cardiovascular risk factors, her 5-year risk of a cardiovascular complication would be 1 percent if her systolic pressure were 110 mm Hg and only 3 percent if her systolic pressure were as high as 180 mm Hg. If the same woman were a smoker, had a cholesterol level of 240 mg/dl and an HDL cholesterol level of 40 mg/dl, her 5-year cardiovascular risk would increase from 5 percent with a systolic pressure of 110 mm Hg to 18 percent with a systolic pressure of 180 mm Hg. As the overall risks multiply, BP control becomes more important.

DEFINITION OF HIGH RISK

Whereas hypertension is present in 25 percent of adults in the general population, it is present in 75 percent of adults with diabetes and over 90 percent of those with chronic kidney disease. Either of these two comorbidities dramatically increases the cardiovascular risk associated with hypertension, and the presence of hypertension greatly accelerates the progression to end-stage renal disease. Therefore, the 2003 JNC 7 guidelines have recommended a usual BP of 140/90 mm Hg as the threshold for initiating antihypertensive medication in most patients, with a lower threshold of 130/80 mm Hg for high-risk patients with diabetes or chronic kidney disease.[4] Based on more recent data, the operational definition of high-risk patients may be expanded to include those with CAD, stroke, heart failure, or left ventricular hypertrophy (see Chap. 41). In particular, in patients with established CAD, a continuous relationship exists between systolic BP and the rate of progression of coronary atherosclerosis (determined by intravascular ultrasound) over a wide range of systolic pressures, beginning as low as 100 mm Hg (Fig. 40-13).[7]

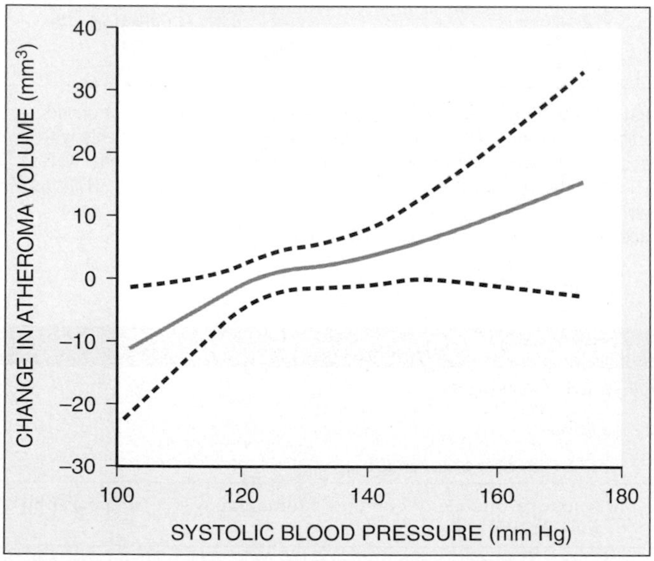

FIGURE 40–13 Relationship between systolic blood pressure (SBP) and the rate of progression of coronary atheroma in 274 patients who completed the intravascular ultrasound substudy of the CAMELOT (Comparison of Amplodipine Versus Enalapril to Limit Occurrences of Thrombosis) trial. A SBP in the 120- to 140-mm Hg range corresponded to no net progression or regression of coronary disease. Values above this range were associated with progression and those below were associated with regression of disease. *(From Sipahi I, Tuzcu EM, Schoenhagen P, et al: Effects of normal, pre-hypertensive, and hypertensive blood pressure levels on progression of coronary atherosclerosis. J Am Coll Cardiol 48:833, 2006.)*

Traditionally, the complications of hypertension are viewed as hypertensive, caused by the increased level of BP per se, or atherosclerotic, caused by concomitant atherosclerosis with BP elevation playing a variable role. However, this view is oversimplified, because both types of complications frequently coexist, as exemplified by hypertensive retinopathy (see Fig. 40-e8 on website)[51] or hypertensive heart disease.

HYPERTENSIVE HEART DISEASE. Hypertension may play an even greater role in causing CAD than is commonly realized because (1) hypertensives have more silent ischemia and unrecognized MIs and (2) patients with acute MI often have preexisting hypertension that has been undetected or untreated. Hypertension status cannot be accurately assessed during an acute coronary syndrome because of pain increasing BP and dysautonomia or pump failure decreasing BP. Preexisting hypertension increases the case-fatality rate associated with an acute MI and substantially increases the risk of hemorrhagic stroke during thrombolytic therapy, especially when systolic BP exceeds 175 mm Hg.

On the ECG, LVH with strain is a serious harbinger of new-onset heart failure and heart failure death.[52] Echocardiography detects LVH more sensitively than electrocardiography. Whereas electrocardiographic LVH is present in 5 to 10 percent of hypertensives, echocardiographic LVH is present in nearly 30 percent of unselected hypertensive adults and in up to 90 percent of patients with severe uncontrolled hypertension. Cardiac magnetic resonance imaging (MRI) is even more sensitive, detecting LVH in 28 percent of white hypertensives but in 62 percent of hypertensive African Americans.[53]

LARGE VESSEL DISEASE. Hypertension also constitutes a major risk factor for and is present in the overwhelming majority of patients with aortic dissection (distal more than proximal dissection), abdominal aortic aneurysm (AAA), and peripheral arterial disease. One-time abdominal ultrasound screening for AAA is recommended after age 65 in smokers and in those with severe systolic hypertension and should be performed if aortic pulsations are detected below the umbilicus, because most AAAs occur below the origin of the renal arteries. Hypertension is present in 50 percent of patients with Takayasu arteritis, a large cell arteritis common in Asia and India.

CEREBROVASCULAR DISEASE. Hypertension is a major risk factor not only for stroke but also for dementia, often the two most dreaded complications of aging. Hypertension accounts for over 50 percent of strokes. In hypertensives, 80 percent of the strokes are ischemic (thrombotic or embolic) and 20 percent hemorrhagic. There is a marked increase in the onset of ischemic stroke on wakening, corresponding to the morning surge in BP. Doppler ultrasonography should be ordered in hypertensive patients with asymptomatic carotid bruits. The risk of stroke is greatest in older patients with isolated systolic hypertension. In middle-aged and elderly hypertensives, asymptomatic cerebral white matter lesions on MRI are remarkably common and are thought to accelerate the brain atrophy and vascular dementia that occurs with aging.

CHRONIC KIDNEY DISEASE. Hypertension is the second most common cause of chronic kidney disease (diabetes is first). With hypertension, the typical pathology of small scarred kidneys (termed *hypertensive nephrosclerosis*) is thought to result from chronic exposure of the renal parenchyma to excessive pressure and flow. Quantitative estimates of urinary albumin excretion and GFR (the latter from www.kdoqi.org) should be obtained from a spot urine collection. Microalbuminuria (defined as a urine albumin to urine creatinine ratio of 30 to 300 μg/mg) is a sensitive early marker of kidney damage and a powerful independent predictor of cardiovascular complications from hypertension, presumably because it reflects systemic vascular disease (see Chaps. 39 and 88).[54] In patients with hypertension, the presence of renal damage dramatically increases the risk of a cardiovascular event. Most patients with hypertensive nephrosclerosis die of heart attack or stroke before renal function deteriorates sufficiently to require chronic hemodialysis.

Identifiable (Secondary) Forms of Hypertension

The third goal of the initial evaluation is to detect identifiable causes of hypertension, thereby offering the possibility of cure in a significant number of patients—particularly those with severe or refractory hypertension (Table 40-3).

RENAL PARENCHYMAL DISEASE (see Chap. 88)

Renal parenchymal disease is the most common cause of secondary hypertension, responsible for 2 to 5 percent of cases. As chronic glomerulonephritis has become less common, hypertensive nephrosclerosis and, to an even greater degree, diabetic nephropathy have become the most common causes of chronic renal disease. The prevalence of chronic renal disease, defined by a reduction in the GFR to less than 60 ml/min/1.73 m^2 or persistent albuminuria of more than 300 mg/day, is estimated to be 11 percent (19.2 million) of the adult U.S. population.[55] The higher prevalence of hypertension among U.S. blacks probably accounts for a significantly higher rate of end-stage renal disease with hypertension as the underlying cause in as many as half of these patients.

As previously noted, microalbuminuria, 30 to 300 mg/day, is closely related to target organ damage and should be determined in every new hypertensive patient by testing a single voided urine specimen. Measurement of the serum creatinine level by itself is an inadequate screening test for significant renal damage, particularly in elderly patients. Therefore, creatinine clearance should be calculated with the Cockcroft-Gault or the modification of diet in renal disease (MDRD) equation, taking age, gender, and body weight into account.[55] Once it begins, renal disease usually progresses, following the concept that a loss of filtration surface leads to both glomerular and systemic hypertension, which engenders more glomerular sclerosis, setting up a cycle of progressive disease. Lowering the level of BP slows the fall in the GFR (Fig. 40-14).[56]

Therefore, it is critical to identify renal damage early, because removal of causal or aggravating factors can prevent the otherwise inexorable progress of renal damage. These factors include obstruction of the urinary tract, depletion of effective circulating volume, nephrotoxic agents, and, most importantly, uncontrolled hypertension.

ACUTE RENAL DISEASES. Hypertension may appear with any sudden, severe insult to the kidneys that markedly impairs excretion of salt and water, which leads to volume expansion, or reduces renal blood flow (e.g., sudden bilateral renal ischemia because of cholesterol emboli), which sets off the RAAS (e.g., bilateral ureteral obstruction). Reversal of hypertension has been particularly striking in men with high-pressure chronic retention of urine, who may manifest renal failure and severe hypertension, both of which may be ameliorated by relief of the obstruction.[57] Some vasculitides also produce rapidly progressive renal damage.

Two commonly used classes of drugs, nonsteroidal anti-inflammatory drugs (NSAIDs) and inhibitors of the renin-angiotensin system, may suddenly worsen renal function in patients with preexisting renal diseases. NSAIDs block the synthesis of prostaglandins, which act as vasodilators within the kidney. Renin-angiotensin inhibitors, both ACEIs and ARBs, may precipitate acute renal failure in patients with bilateral renovascular disease whose renal perfusion depends on high levels of A II.

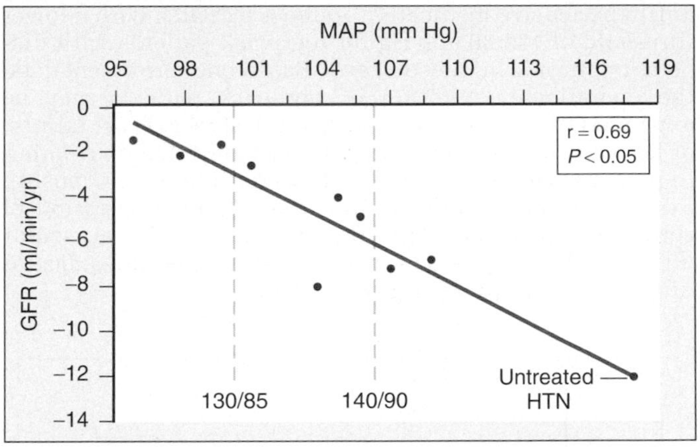

FIGURE 40–14 Relationship between achieved blood pressure control and declines in glomerular filtration rate (GFR) in six clinical trials of patients with diabetic renal disease and three trials of patients with nondiabetic renal disease. HTN = hypertension; MAP = mean arterial pressure. *(From Bakris GL, Williams M, Dworkin L, et al: Preserving renal function in adults with hypertension and diabetes: A consensus approach. Am J Kidney Dis 36:646, 2000.)*

TABLE 40–3 Overall Guide to Work-up for Identifiable Causes of Hypertension

	Diagnostic Procedure	
Diagnosis	***Initial***	***Additional***
Chronic renal disease	Urinalysis, serum creatinine, renal sonography	Isotopic renography, renal biopsy
Renovascular disease	Renal sonography Duplex Doppler sonography	Magnetic resonance or computed tomography (CT) angiography, aortography
Coarctation	Blood pressure in legs	Echocardiography, magnetic resonance imaging or contrast aortography
Primary aldosteronism	Plasma and urinary potassium, plasma renin and aldosterone	Urinary aldosterone after oral salt load, adrenal CT, adrenal venous sampling
Cushing syndrome	Morning plasma cortisol after 1 mg dexamethasone at bedtime	Urinary cortisol after variable doses of dexamethasone, adrenal CT, and scintiscans
Pheochromocytoma	Plasma-free metanephrine Urine metanephrines and catechols	Plasma normetanephrine (basal and after 0.3 mg clonidine) Adrenal CT and scintiscans

CHRONIC RENAL DISEASES. All chronic renal diseases are associated with a higher prevalence of hypertension, and hypertension accelerates the progression of renal damage, regardless of the underlying cause of the renal disease. The control of hypertension can slow or stop the progression of renal diseases and of cardiovascular sequelae (see Fig. 40-14).[58] Uncertainty remains about the goal of antihypertensive therapy in patients with chronic renal disease. In at least three large trials, intensive reduction of BP, down to as low as 125/75 mm Hg, did not slow the rate of decrease of renal function better than achievement of a more standard BP target of 135/85 mm Hg.[59]

With whatever drugs chosen to treat hypertension with chronic kidney disease (CKD), particularly with ACEIs and ARBs, caution is needed in lowering BP in the presence of previously unrecognized bilateral renovascular disease, found in as many as 20 percent of patients with progressive renal damage. However, a modest increase in the serum creatinine level, averaging 30 percent above baseline, predicts a better preservation of renal function, presumably reflecting a successful reduction in intraglomerular pressure.[60]

Patients with diabetic nephropathy (see Chaps. 41 and 88) show particular protection against progressive renal damage by reduction of elevated BP. In patients with diabetes, intensive control of hypertension has proved much more cost-effective than intensive glycemic control or reduction in hypercholesterolemia.[61,62]

Hemodialysis Patients. In patients with end-stage renal disease who are on dialysis, hypertension is a significant risk factor for mortality.[63] Beyond the primary influence of excess fluid volume, hypertension can be accentuated by the accumulation of endogenous inhibitors of nitric oxide synthase and sympathetic overactivity. With neither the vasoconstrictor effects of renal renin nor the vasodepressor actions of various renal hormones, BP may be particularly labile and sensitive to changes in fluid volume. In patients receiving maintenance hemodialysis every 48 hours, elevated BPs tend to fall progressively after dialysis is completed, remain depressed during the remainder of the first 24 hours, and rise again during the second day as a consequence of excessive fluid retention. Only by achieving dry weight, as with 8-hour nocturnal hemodialysis, can BP be controlled.

Renal Transplantation. Although successful renal transplantation may cure primary hypertension, various problems can result, with about 50 percent of recipients becoming hypertensive within 1 year. These problems include stenosis of the renal artery at the site of anastomosis, rejection reactions, high doses of adrenal steroids and cyclosporine or tacrolimus, and excess renin derived from the retained diseased kidneys. ACEI or ARB therapy may obviate the need to remove the native diseased kidneys to relieve hypertension caused by their persistent secretion of renin. The source of the donor kidney may also play a role in the subsequent development of hypertension in the recipient. Hypertension occurs more frequently when donors had a family history of hypertension or when the donors died of subarachnoid hemorrhage and had probably been hypertensive.

RENOVASCULAR HYPERTENSION

Renal artery stenosis is rather easy to find but often difficult to prove to be the cause of reversible hypertension (see Chap. 59). The prevalence of proven renovascular *hypertension* in the overall hypertensive population is unknown, but significant renal artery *stenosis* has been found in 6.8 percent of 824 elderly people in North Carolina (defined as a 60 percent or greater reduction of diameter on duplex sonography) and in 7 percent of hypertensive patients undergoing coronary angiography (defined as a 70 percent or greater stenosis on renal angiography).

Because the presence of renal artery stenosis does not prove that the renovascular lesion is causing the hypertension, screening should focus on those hypertensive patients who have multiple features known to be associated with renovascular hypertension. The greater the number of clues, the more extensive should be the search (Table 40-4).

CLASSIFICATION. In adults, the two major types of renovascular disease tend to appear at different times and affect the genders differently. Atherosclerotic disease affecting mainly the proximal third of the main renal artery is seen mostly in older men. Fibroplastic disease involving mainly the distal two thirds and branches of the renal arteries appears most commonly in younger women. As the population grows older, 90 percent of cases are caused by atherosclerotic disease and only 10 percent by fibroplastic disease. Although the nonatherosclerotic stenoses may involve all layers of the renal artery, the most common is fibromuscular dysplasia.

A number of other intrinsic and extrinsic causes of renovascular hypertension are known, including cholesterol emboli in the renal artery or compression of this vessel by nearby tumors. Most renovascular hypertension develops from partial obstruction of one main renal artery, but only a branch need be involved; segmental disease has been found in about 10 percent of cases. On the other hand, if apparent complete occlusion of the renal artery is slow in developing, enough collateral flow will become available to preserve the viability of the kidney. In this way, the seemingly nonfunctioning kidney may be responsible for continued renin secretion and hypertension. If recognized, such totally occluded vessels can sometimes be repaired, with return of renal function and relief of hypertension.

Renovascular stenosis is often bilateral, although usually one side is clearly predominant. The possibility of bilateral disease should be suspected in those with renal insufficiency, particularly if rapidly progressive oliguric renal failure develops without evidence of obstructive uropathy, and even more so if it develops after the start of ACEI or ARB therapy.

MECHANISMS. The sequence of changes in patients with renovascular hypertension starts with the release of increased amounts of renin when sufficient ischemia is

TABLE 40–4	Clinical Clues for Renovascular Hypertension
History	
Onset of hypertension before 30 or after 50 yr of age	
Abrupt onset of hypertension	
Severe or resistant hypertension	
Symptoms of atherosclerotic disease elsewhere	
Negative family history of hypertension	
Smoker	
Worsening renal function after renin-angiotensin inhibition	
Recurrent flash pulmonary edema	
Examination	
Abdominal bruits	
Other bruits	
Advanced fundal changes	
Laboratory Findings	
Secondary aldosteronism	
Higher plasma renin level	
Low serum potassium level	
Low serum sodium level	
Proteinuria, usually moderate	
Elevated serum creatinine level	
>1.5-cm difference in kidney size on sonography	

induced to diminish pulse pressure against the juxtaglomerular cells in the renal afferent arterioles. A reduction in renal perfusion pressure by 50 percent leads to an immediate and persistent increase in renin secretion from the ischemic kidney, along with suppression of secretion from the contralateral one. With time, an expanded body fluid volume causes renin levels to fall but not to the low level expected from the elevated BP.

DIAGNOSIS. The presence of the clinical features listed in Table 40-4, found in perhaps 5 to 10 percent of all hypertensive persons, indicates the need for a screening test for renovascular hypertension. A positive screening test result or very strong clinical features calls for more definitive confirmatory tests. The initial diagnostic study in most patients should be noninvasive and, if abnormal, followed by a study of renal perfusion to ensure that any renovascular lesion is pathogenic and to decide whether revascularization is indicated (see Fig. 40-15).[64]

All screening studies have limitations. Considerable asymmetry of renal blood flow, 25 percent or more, was found in 148 hypertensive patients whose renal arteries were patent on prior angiography. Such normal asymmetry likely is responsible for the low sensitivity and specificity of captopril-enhanced renal scans. Similarly, the sensitivity of renal duplex sonography for the detection of hemodynamically significant renovascular disease has been reported to be only 50 percent. The accuracy of ultrasonography is

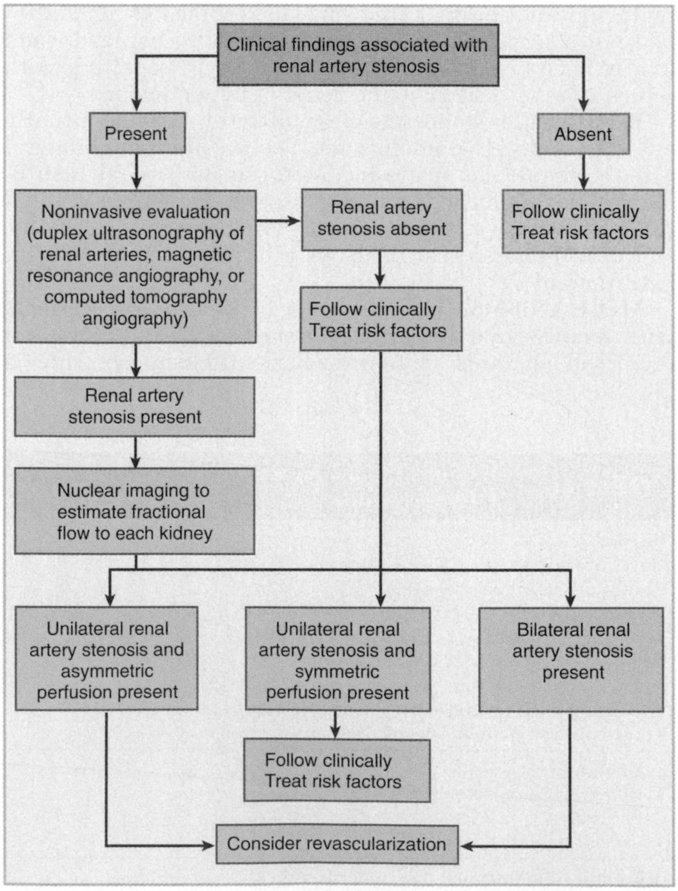

FIGURE 40–15 Algorithm for evaluating patients in whom renal artery stenosis is suspected. Clinical follow-up includes periodic reassessment with duplex ultrasonography, magnetic resonance angiography, and nuclear imaging to estimate fractional blood flow to each kidney. The treatment of risk factors includes smoking cessation and the use of aspirin, lipid-lowering agents, and antihypertensive therapy. (see also Figs. 59-10 and 59-11.) *(Modified from Safian RD, Textor SC: Renal-artery stenosis. N Engl J Med 344:431, 2001.)*

operator-dependent, often requiring scanning times of 1 hour or longer, so its use has been limited. However, a strong association with the outcome of revascularization has been reported with the use of a resistance index to assess flow in renal arteries. Patients with high resistance index values, above 80, reflecting marked intrarenal vascular disease, had generally poor outcomes.[65] Those with lower values had generally good outcomes.

Over the past few years, contrast-enhanced computed tomography and magnetic resonance angiography to screen for renovascular hypertension have become the preferred screening tests because of their excellent sensitivity and specificity (see Fig. 40-e9 on website). With further refinements in image quality, magnetic resonance angiography will likely be more widely used, because it reduces the possibility of contrast-induced nephrotoxicity and avoids exposure to ionizing radiation, as well as its greater potential for an accurate assessment of renal function.[66]

MANAGEMENT. The availability of ACEIs and ARBs can be considered a two-edged sword—one edge provides better control of renovascular hypertension than may be possible with other antihypertensive medications, whereas the other edge exposes the already ischemic kidney to further loss of blood flow by inhibiting the high level of A II that was supporting its circulation. Other antihypertensive drugs may be almost as effective as ACEIs and perhaps safer, but there are no comparative data.

Angioplasty (see Chap. 59). Angioplasty can improve BP (at least transiently) in 60 to 70 percent of patients, more with fibromuscular disease than with atherosclerosis, as is the case for surgery. In three small but controlled trials, balloon angioplasty provided a modest but significantly greater reduction in BP than medical therapy. Stenting has reduced the likelihood of restenosis and is increasingly performed as the initial procedure to preserve renal function.[67]

Surgery. Revascularization by surgery is indicated for patients whose hypertension is not well controlled or whose renal function deteriorates with medical therapy and for those unresponsive to angioplasty or in whom lesions are not amenable to that procedure. Surgery is recommended more to preserve renal function than to relieve hypertension and should be undertaken before the serum creatinine level rises above 3 mg/dl.[64]

RENIN-SECRETING TUMORS

Comprised of juxtaglomerular cells or hemangiopericytomas, renin-secreting tumors occur mostly in young patients with severe hypertension, very high renin levels in both peripheral blood and the kidney harboring the tumor, and secondary aldosteronism manifested by hypokalemia. The tumor can generally be recognized by selective renal angiography, usually performed for suspected renovascular hypertension, although a few are extrarenal. More commonly, children with Wilms tumors (nephroblastoma) may have hypertension and high plasma renin and prorenin levels that revert to normal after nephrectomy.

ADRENAL AND OTHER CAUSES OF HYPERTENSION (see Chap. 81)

Adrenal causes of hypertension include primary excesses of aldosterone, cortisol, and catecholamines; more rarely, excess deoxycorticosterone is present with congenital adrenal hyperplasia. Together, these conditions cause less than 1 percent of all hypertension in general practice, although, as will be noted, primary aldosteronism may be more common than previously thought, especially in patients referred to specialists for the evaluation of refractory hypertension. Each of these adrenal disorders can usually be recognized with relative ease, and patients suspected of having these disorders can be screened by readily available tests.

More of a problem than the diagnosis of these adrenal disorders is the need to exclude their presence because of the increasing identification of incidental adrenal masses when abdominal computed tomography (CT) is done to diagnose intraabdominal pathological conditions. Unsuspected adrenal tumors have been found in about 1 percent of abdominal CT scans obtained for reasons unrelated to the adrenal gland. Screening for hormonal excess should be performed if an adrenal tumor is found (see Table 40-3). Most of these incidentalomas appear to be nonfunctional on the basis of normal basal adrenal hormone levels. When more detailed studies are done, however, a significant number show incomplete suppression of cortisol by dexamethasone—that is, subclinical Cushing disease that does not appear to progress to overt hypercortisolism but may be associated with insulin resistance and osteopenia.[68]

The benign nature of smaller tumors can usually be ensured by appropriate imaging studies. The risk of cancer is low if (1) a noncontrast CT scan shows that the tumor density is less than 10 HU, consistent with low-density lipid, (2) an MRI scan confirms a high lipid content by loss of signal on out-of-phase images, and (3) the tumor is smaller than 4 cm. Tumors 4 cm or larger in size should be resected, because a significant number are malignant.

Primary Aldosteronism and Other Forms of Mineralocorticoid-Induced Hypertension

A number of syndromes with mineralocorticoid excess have been recognized (Table 40-5), with primary aldosteronism being by far the most common. Primary aldosteronism, generally considered relatively rare in unselected populations, has emerged in considerably more patients screened by a plasma aldosterone-to-renin ratio.[69] Moreover, in keeping with the profibrotic effects of aldosterone, many more cardiovascular events are seen in patients with primary aldosteronism than in patients with primary hypertension matched for age, gender, and BP levels.[70]

TABLE 40–5	Syndromes of Mineralocorticoid Excess
Adrenal origin	
Aldosterone excess (primary)	
Aldosterone-producing adenoma	
Bilateral hyperplasia	
Primary unilateral adrenal hyperplasia	
Glucocorticoid-remediable aldosteronism (familial hyperaldosteronism, type 1)	
Adrenal carcinoma	
Extraadrenal tumors	
Deoxycorticosterone excess	
Deoxycorticosterone-secreting tumors	
Congenital adrenal hyperplasia	
11β-hydroxylase deficiency	
17α-hydroxylase deficiency	
Cortisol excess	
Cushing syndrome from ACTH-producing tumor	
Glucocorticoid receptor resistance	
Renal origin	
Activating mutation of mineralocorticoid receptor	
Pseudohypoaldosteronism, type II (Gordon)	
11β-hydroxysteroid dehydrogenase deficiency	
Congenital—apparent mineralocorticoid excess	
Acquired—licorice, carbenoxolone	

PATHOPHYSIOLOGY OF MINERALOCORTICOID EXCESS. Until recently, the most frequently found source of hyperaldosteronism was a solitary aldosterone-producing adenoma. Recently, measurements of plasma renin and aldosterone have identified milder forms of hyperaldosteronism usually associated with bilateral adrenal hyperplasia (BAH).

Aldosterone excess from any source causes hypertension and renal potassium wastage, which should induce hypokalemia (Fig. 40-16). However, most patients with aldosteronism caused by BAH are normokalemic. The lack of overt hypokalemia could be explained in numerous ways: (1) potassium wastage has lowered the serum potassium level, but not yet to hypokalemic levels; (2) with milder degrees of aldosteronism, as are typical with BAH, the excess of aldosterone induces hypertension without causing potassium wastage, a scenario that has never been experimentally or clinically recognized; or (3) the BAH is related to the typical progressive increase in adrenal nodular hyperplasia with age that has no relationship to hypertension. The third explanation would fit with the long-held belief that BAH is simply a form of low-renin hypertension—that is, primary hypertension with plasma renin levels that fall progressively with age while plasma aldosterone levels remain stable.

This third explanation could account for the common findings of an increased aldosterone-to-renin ratio, caused not by increased aldosterone but by decreased renin, and by the presence of BAH in most normokalemic hypertensive patients reported in recent series. In an analysis of the aldosterone-to-renin ratio in 505 patients with primary hypertension, an elevated ratio was found to be a measure of low renin alone, without increased aldosterone, in 36 percent.[69] The positive predictive value of the ratio to identify patients with both increased aldosterone and low renin levels was only 34 percent.

DIAGNOSIS. Despite the recommendation by a few experts that virtually all hypertensive patients be screened by an aldosterone-to-renin ratio measurement, there are good reasons to limit the use of this test. Moreover, if screening is done, rather than using a ratio that could be high only because of a low renin level, a positive result should be based on both an elevated plasma aldosterone level, above 15 ng/dl, as well as a suppressed low renin level. This more conservative view is based on the strong likelihood that only a few normokalemic patients harbor an adenoma that should be resected and that there is no need to identify the presence of BAH in normokalemic patients. This is mainly because distinguishing a unilateral aldosterone-producing adenoma from BAH usually requires an expensive, difficult, and occasionally harmful study: bilateral adrenal venous sampling.

Therefore, screening is recommended only for hypertensive subjects who have a higher likelihood of primary aldosteronism, including those with the following: (1) unprovoked, unexplainable hypokalemia; (2) hypokalemia induced by diuretics but resistant to correction; (3) a family history of aldosteronism; (4) hypertension resistant to appropriate therapy, in which the resistance cannot be explained; or (5) presence of an adrenal mass on CT or MRI. Hyperaldosteronism has been found in as many as 20 percent of patients with resistant hypertension.

If the screening plasma aldosterone and renin levels are suggestive, an oral salt-loading suppression study should be done to document the

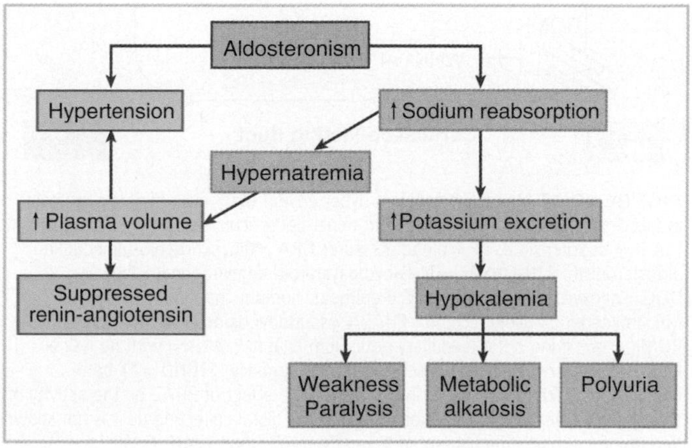

FIGURE 40–16 Pathophysiology of primary aldosteronism.

autonomy of hyperaldosteronism. If the suppression test result is abnormal, a CT or MRI scan is recommended. If a solitary adenoma larger than 1 cm is present and the other gland is clearly normal, the diagnosis of an aldosterone-producing adenoma has been assumed to be reasonably ensured and consideration should be given to laparoscopic adrenalectomy. However, adrenal vein sampling is now strongly recommended before surgery to differentiate unilateral adenoma from bilateral hyperplasia and to confirm exactly which gland, if either, should be removed (see Fig. 40-e10 on website). Because detecting microscopic adenomas may be below the resolution of CT scanning and because minor adrenal nodularity and nonfunctioning adrenal incidentalomas are common, CT findings alone may lead to the wrong conclusion almost 50 percent of the time.[71]

DIFFERENTIAL DIAGNOSIS: MENDELIAN FORMS OF HYPERTENSION. In patients presenting with severe hypertension and hypokalemia, primary aldosteronism needs to be distinguished from rare forms of mineralocorticoid-induced hypertension that are inherited as mendelian traits. Clinical clues of syndromic hypertension are premature onset, often before age 30, severity of the hypertension, which is frequently dramatic, and a compelling family history indicative of mendelian inheritance. All these familial syndromes involve excessive activation of ENaC as a final common mechanism, either caused by gain-of-function mutations of ENaC or of the mineralocorticoid receptor, or to increased production or decreased clearance of the mineralocorticoid receptor ligands—aldosterone as well as deoxycorticosterone, and cortisol (Fig. 40-17).

One type, familial glucocorticoid-remediable aldosteronism, is caused by recombination of genes encoding the aldosterone synthase enzyme (CYP11β2) normally found only in the outer zona glomerulosa and the 11-beta-hydroxylase enzyme (CYP11β1) in the zona fasciculata. The chimeric gene induces an enzyme that catalyzes the synthesis of 18-hydroxylated cortisol in the zona fasciculata. Because this zone is

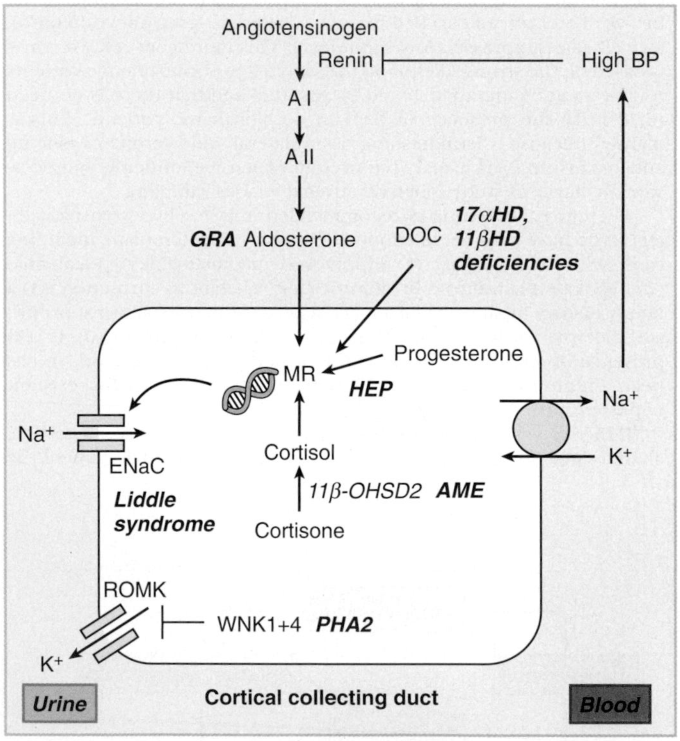

FIGURE 40–17 Mendelian forms of hypertension that cause mineralocorticoid-induced hypertension. AME = apparent mineralocorticoid excess; A I = angiotensin I; A II = angiotensin II; BP = blood pressure; GRA = glucocorticoid-remediable aldosteronism; 11β-OHSD2 = 11-β-hydroxysteroid dehydrogenase type 2; DOC = deoxycorticosterone; ENaC = epithelial sodium channel; MR = mineralocorticoid receptor; PHA2 = pseudohypoaldosteronism type 2; ROMK = rectifying outer medullary potassium channel; WNK = with no lysine kinases; HEP = hypertension exacerbated by pregnancy; 11βHD = 11-beta-hydroxylase; 17αHD = 17-alpha-hydroxylase. The effect of PHA2 on the activity of the thiazide-sensitive Na-Cl cotransporter in the distal collecting duct is not shown. See text for explanation. *(Adapted from Lifton RP, Gharavi AG, Geller DS: Molecular mechanisms of human hypertension. Cell 104:545, 2001.)*

under the control of adrenocorticotropic hormone (ACTH), the glucocorticoid suppressibility of the syndrome is explained. The diagnosis should be made by genetic testing for the chimeric gene and treatment provided with glucocorticoid suppression.

Another rare form is apparent mineralocorticoid excess caused by deficiency of the enzyme 11-beta-hydroxysteroid dehydrogenase type 2 (11β-OHSD2) in the renal tubule, where it normally converts cortisol, which has the ability to act on the mineralocorticoid receptor, to cortisone, which does not. Persistence of high levels of cortisol induces all the features of mineralocorticoid excess. The 11β-OHSD2 enzyme may be congenitally absent (the syndrome of apparent mineralocorticoid excess) or inhibited by the glycyrrhizic acid contained in licorice. Another unusual syndrome with hypertension and hypokalemia but suppressed mineralocorticoid secretion is Liddle syndrome, in which the kidney reabsorbs excess sodium and wastes potassium because of a mutation in the beta or gamma subunits of the epithelial sodium channel.

In most of these cases, volume expansion and severe hypertension cause feedback suppression of plasma renin, and mineralocorticoid receptor activation leads to renal potassium wasting and hypokalemia. One exception is pseudohypoaldosteronism type II, in which the disease-causing mutation produces both low-renin and salt-sensitive hypertension caused by overactivity of the thiazide-sensitive Na-Cl cotransporter in the distal collecting duct and hyperkalemia caused by underactivity of the renal outer medullary potassium channel.

THERAPY. Once the diagnosis of primary aldosteronism is made and the type of adrenal disorder has been established, the choice of therapy is relatively simple. Patients with a solitary adenoma should have the tumor resected by laparoscopic surgery and those with bilateral hyperplasia should be treated with an aldosterone blocker, spironolactone or eplerenone and, if necessary, a thiazide diuretic or other antihypertensive drug. When an adenoma is resected, about half the patients will become normotensive, whereas the others, although improved, remain hypertensive, either from preexisting primary hypertension or from renal damage caused by prolonged secondary hypertension.[72]

Cushing Syndrome (see Chap. 81)

Hypertension occurs in about 80 percent of patients with Cushing syndrome. If left untreated, it can cause marked LVH and CHF. As with hypertension of other endocrine causes, the longer it is present, the less likely it is to disappear when the underlying cause is relieved.

MECHANISM OF HYPERTENSION. BP can increase for a number of reasons. The secretion of mineralocorticoids can also be increased along with cortisol, which itself is a potent activator of the mineralocorticoid receptor. The excess cortisol can overwhelm the ability of renal 11β-OHSD2 to convert it to cortisone, which is not a mineralocorticoid receptor ligand; the excess cortisol overstimulates renal mineralocorticoid receptors to retain sodium and expand plasma volume. Cortisol stimulates the synthesis of renin substrate and the expression of A I receptors, which may be responsible for enhanced pressor effects.

DIAGNOSIS. The syndrome should be suspected in patients with truncal obesity, wide purple striae, thin skin, muscle weakness, and osteoporosis. If clinical features are suggestive, the diagnosis often can be either ruled out or virtually ensured by the measurement of free cortisol in a 24-hour urine sample, the simple overnight dexamethasone suppression test, or determination of late-night salivary cortisol.[73]

THERAPY. In about two thirds of patients with Cushing syndrome, the process begins with overproduction of ACTH by the pituitary, which leads to bilateral adrenal hyperplasia. Although pituitary hyperfunction may reflect a hypothalamic disorder, most patients have discrete pituitary adenomas that can usually be resected by selective transsphenoidal microsurgery.

If an adrenal tumor is present, it should be removed surgically. With earlier diagnosis and more selective surgical therapy, it is hoped that more patients with Cushing syndrome will be cured without a need for lifelong glucocorticoid replacement therapy and with permanent relief of their hypertension. Therapy may require one of a number of drugs[73] temporarily, but rarely permanently.

Congenital Adrenal Hyperplasia

Enzymatic defects may induce hypertension by interfering with cortisol biosynthesis. Low levels of cortisol lead to increased ACTH levels; this increases the accumulation of precursors proximal to the enzymatic block, specifically deoxycorticosterone, which induces mineralocorticoid hypertension. The more common of these is 11-hydroxylase deficiency, which has been attributed to various mutations in the gene and leads to virilization (from excessive androgens) and hypertension with hypokalemia (from excessive deoxycorticosterone). The other is 17-hydroxylase deficiency, which also causes hypertension from excess deoxycorticosterone but, in addition, causes failure of secondary sexual development because sex hormones are also deficient. Affected children are hypertensive, but the defect in sex hormone synthesis may not become obvious until pubertal failure is recognized in adolescence.

Pheochromocytoma (see Chap. 81)

The wild fluctuations in BP and dramatic symptoms of pheochromocytoma usually alert both the patient and physician to the possibility of this diagnosis (Table 40-6). However, such fluctuations may be missed or, as occurs in 50 percent of patients, the hypertension may be persistent. On one hand, the spells typical of a pheochromocytoma, with headache, sweating, and palpitations, may be incorrectly attributed to migraine, menopause, or panic attacks. On the other hand, some patients with severe paroxysmal hypertension do not have a pheochromocytoma but rather marked anxiety. Unfortunately, if the diagnosis of pheochromocytoma is missed, severe complications can arise from exceedingly high BP and damage to the heart by catecholamines.[74] Stroke and hypertensive crises with encephalopathy and retinal hemorrhage may occur, probably because BP levels soar in vessels unprepared by a chronic hypertensive condition. Fortunately, the plasma free metanephrine assay will detect the disease with virtual certainty, so diagnostic indecision should be minimized. See Chapter 81 for details regarding the pathophysiology, diagnosis, and treatment of pheochromocytoma.

Other Causes of Hypertension

A host of other causes of hypertension are known. One that is probably becoming more common is the ingestion of various drugs, prescribed (e.g., cyclosporine, tacrolimus, erythropoietin), purchased over the counter (e.g., ephedra), and illicit (e.g., cocaine, methamphetamine). As previously noted, obstructive sleep apnea has been well characterized as a cause of significant, and often reversible, hypertension.

COARCTATION OF THE AORTA (see Chap. 61). Congenital narrowing of the aorta can occur at any level of the thoracic or abdominal aorta but is typically found just beyond the origin of the left subclavian artery or distal to the insertion of the ligamentum arteriosum. With less severe postductal lesions, symptoms may not appear until the teenage years or later, particularly during pregnancy. Hypertension in the arms, weak or absent femoral pulses, and a loud murmur heard over the back are the classic features of coarctation. The pathogenesis of the hypertension can be more complicated than simple mechanical obstruction, and likely involves a generalized vasoconstrictor mechanism. The lesion can be detected by echocardiography, and MRI or contrast aortography proves the diagnosis. Once repaired, patients may continue to have hypertension that requires careful monitoring and treatment.

HORMONAL DISTURBANCES (see Chap. 81). Hypertension is seen in as many as half of patients with various hormonal disturbances, including acromegaly, hypothyroidism, and hyperparathyroidism. Diagnosis of the latter two conditions has been made easier by readily available blood tests, and affected hypertensive patients can be relieved of their high BP by correction of the hormonal disturbance. Such relief occurs more frequently in patients with hypothyroidism than in those with hyperparathyroidism.

PERIOPERATIVE HYPERTENSION (see Chap. 80). It is uncertain that an elevated preoperative BP is a valid reason to postpone surgery.[75] Preexisting hypertension should be well controlled before elective surgery, with particular attention to correction of diuretic-induced hypokalemia. Antihypertensive agents should not be discontinued perioperatively, in particular to avoid rebound from beta blockers or clonidine. Fortunately, intravenous formulations of most classes are available if oral intake is not possible. Hypertension may appear or worsen in the perioperative period, perhaps more commonly with cardiac than noncardiac surgery (Table 40-7). Patients at high risk for cardiac events have been found to be protected by the use of beta blockers prior to cardiac or noncardiac surgery. Hypertension is of particular concern after heart transplantation, appearing for a number of reasons, including immunosuppression with calcineurin inhibitors (cyclosporine and tacrolimus) and possibly cardiac deafferentation.[76] Reduction of dietary sodium intake and ACEI or ARB therapy should be especially beneficial.

TABLE 40-6 Features Suggestive of Pheochromocytoma
Hypertension—Persistent or Paroxysmal
Markedly variable blood pressures (± orthostatic hypotension)
Sudden paroxysms (± subsequent hypertension) in relation to
Stress: anesthesia, angiography, parturition
Pharmacological provocation—histamine, nicotine, caffeine, beta blockers, glucocorticoids, tricyclic antidepressants
Manipulation of tumors—abdominal palpation, urination
Rare patients persistently normotensive
Unusual settings
Childhood, pregnancy, familial
Multiple endocrine adenomas—medullary carcinoma of the thyroid (MEN-2), mucosal neuromas (MEN-2B)
Von Hippel-Lindau syndrome
Neurocutaneous lesions—neurofibromatosis
Associated Symptoms
Sudden spells with headache, sweating, palpitations, nervousness, nausea, vomiting
Pain in chest or abdomen
Associated Signs
Sweating, tachycardia, arrhythmia, pallor, weight loss

TABLE 40-7 Hypertension Associated with Cardiac Surgery
Preoperative
Anxiety, angina, other manifestations
Discontinuation of antihypertensive therapy
Rebound from beta blockers in patients with coronary artery disease
Intraoperative
Induction of anesthesia—tracheal intubation
Nasopharyngeal, urethral, or rectal manipulation
Before, during, or after cardiopulmonary bypass
Postoperative
Obvious cause—hypoxia, hypercarbia, ventilatory difficulties, hypothermia, shivering, arousal from anesthesia
With no obvious cause—after myocardial revascularization; less frequently after valve replacement; after resection of aortic coarctation

HYPERTENSIVE DISEASES OF WOMEN (see Chap. 76)

Oral Contraceptive Use

The use of estrogen-containing oral contraceptive (OC) pills is probably the most common cause of secondary hypertension in young women. Most women who take them experience a slight rise in BP. Moreover, there is a 1.8-fold increased relative risk of MI and 2.1-fold increased risk of stroke in current users of OCs, but among those who use the low-dose third-generation OCs, only the risk of stroke persists.[77]

These relative risks need to be kept in perspective, because the absolute numbers are low, only 0.4 excess cases of MI and stroke/100,000 women-years of OC use.[78] Most of the risk is seen in women over age 35 who smoke and have other cardiovascular risk factors.

CLINICAL FEATURES. In most women, the hypertension is mild; however, in some, it may accelerate rapidly and cause severe renal damage. When use of the OC is discontinued, BP falls to normal within 3 to 6 months in about 50 percent of patients. Whether the pill caused permanent hypertension in the other half or just uncovered primary hypertension at an earlier time is not clear.

MECHANISMS. Oral contraceptive use probably causes hypertension by volume expansion, because both estrogens and the synthetic progestogens used in oral contraceptive pills cause sodium retention. Although plasma renin levels rise in response to increased levels of angiotensinogen, ACEIs do not alter BP any more in women with OC-induced hypertension than in women with essential hypertension.

MANAGEMENT. The use of estrogen-containing oral contraceptives should be restricted in women older than 35 years, particularly if they also smoke or are hypertensive or obese. Women given the pill should be properly monitored, as follows: (1) the initial supply should be limited; (2) they should be asked to return for a BP check before an additional supply is provided; and (3) if BP has risen, an alternative contraceptive method should be offered. If the pill remains the only acceptable contraceptive method, the elevated BP can be reduced with appropriate therapy. In view of the possible role of aldosterone, use of a diuretic-spironolactone combination seems appropriate. In women who stop taking oral contraceptives, evaluation for secondary hypertensive diseases should be postponed for at least 3 months to allow changes in the RAAS to remit. If the hypertension does not recede, additional work-up and therapy may be needed.

Postmenopausal Hormone Replacement Therapy

Estrogen replacement therapy does not appear to induce hypertension, even though it does induce the various changes in the RAAS seen with oral contraceptive use. In fact, most controlled trials have found a decrease in daytime ambulatory BP and a greater dipping of nocturnal BP in estrogen replacement therapy users.[79] Such lower BPs may reflect a number of effects, including improved endothelium-dependent vasodilation and reduced muscle sympathetic nerve activity.

Hypertension During Pregnancy (see Chap. 77)

In about 12 percent of first pregnancies in previously normotensive women, hypertension appears after 20 weeks (gestational hypertension). In about half of cases, this hypertension will progress to preeclampsia when complicated by proteinuria, edema, or hematological or hepatic abnormalities, which, in turn, increase the risk of progress to eclampsia, defined by the occurrence of convulsions.[80] Women with hypertension predating pregnancy have an even higher incidence of preeclampsia and a greater likelihood of early delivery of small for gestational age babies. Preeclampsia is of unknown cause but occurs more frequently in primigravid women and in pregnancies involving men or women who were the product of a pregnancy complicated by preeclampsia, supporting a genetic role. Additional predisposing factors include young or older age, multiple gestations, concomitant heart or renal disease, and chronic hypertension.[80] The diagnosis is usually based on a rise in pressure of 30/15 mm Hg or more to a level above 140/90 mm Hg. As with other forms of hypertension, the diagnosis is most precisely made by ambulatory BP monitoring.

CLINICAL FEATURES. The features shown in Table 40-8 should help distinguish gestational hypertension and preeclampsia from chronic primary hypertension. The distinction should be made because management and prognosis are different. Gestational hypertension is self-limited and less commonly recurs in subsequent pregnancies, whereas chronic hypertension progresses and usually complicates subsequent pregnancies. Differentiation may be difficult because of a lack of knowledge of the prepregnancy BP and because of the usual tendency for high pressure to fall considerably during the middle trimester, so that hypertension present before pregnancy may not be recognized.

MECHANISMS. The hemodynamic features of gestational hypertension are a further rise in cardiac output than usually seen in normal pregnancy, accompanied by profound vasoconstriction that reduces intravascular capacity even more than blood volume, which may reflect increased central and peripheral sympathetic activity. Increasingly strong evidence has indicated that preeclampsia starts from immune maladaptation leading to inadequate placentation; this results in reduced angiogenic growth factors and increased placental debris entering the maternal circulation, where it provokes a maternal inflammatory response with hypertension.[80] The mother may be particularly vulnerable to encephalopathy because of her previously normal BP. As described in more detail later (see "Hypertensive Crisis"), cerebral blood flow is normally maintained constant over a fairly narrow range of mean arterial pressure,

TABLE 40–8 Differences Between Preeclampsia and Chronic Hypertension

Feature	Preeclampsia	Chronic Hypertension
Age (yr)	Young (<20)	Older (>30)
Parity	Primigravida	Multigravida
Onset	After 20 wk of pregnancy	Before 20 wk of pregnancy
Weight gain and edema	Sudden	Gradual
Systolic blood pressure	<160 mm Hg	>160 mm Hg
Funduscopic findings	Spasm, edema	Arteriovenous nicking, exudates
Left ventricular hypertrophy	Rare	More common
Proteinuria	Present	Absent
Plasma uric acid level	Increased	Normal
Blood pressure after delivery	Normal	Elevated

roughly between 60 and 100 mm Hg in normotensive individuals. In a previously normotensive young woman, an acute rise in BP to 150/100 mm Hg can exceed the upper limit of autoregulation and result in a breakthrough of cerebral blood flow (acute dilation) that leads to cerebral edema and convulsions.

PREVENTION AND TREATMENT. Beyond delay of pregnancy until after the teenage years and better prenatal care, the only other maneuver that has been shown to prevent preeclampsia is the use of low doses of aspirin. The only cure for preeclampsia is delivery, which removes the diseased placenta. To achieve this apparently simple end, the clinician must detect the often symptomless prodromal condition by screening all pregnant women, admitting to hospital those with advanced preeclampsia so as to keep track of an unpredictable situation, and timing preemptive delivery to maximize the safety of mother and baby. Caution is advised in the use of drugs for gestational hypertension, traditionally limited to methyldopa in the United States, but other drugs are used elsewhere. Drug treatment of maternal BP does not improve perinatal outcome and may be associated with fetal growth retardation. Most authorities recommend antihypertensive drugs only if diastolic pressures remain above 100 mm Hg. The only drugs contraindicated are ACEIs and ARBs because of their propensity to induce neonatal renal failure.

CHRONIC HYPERTENSION. If pregnancy begins while a woman is receiving antihypertensive drug therapy, the medications, including diuretics but excluding ACEIs and ARBs, are usually continued in the belief that the mother should be protected and that the fetus will not suffer from any sudden hemodynamic shifts, such as occur when therapy is first begun. However, despite currently available treatment, the incidence of perinatal mortality and fetal growth retardation remains higher in patients with chronic hypertension.

MANAGEMENT OF ECLAMPSIA. With appropriate care of gestational hypertension, eclampsia hardly ever supervenes; when it does, however, maternal and fetal mortality increase markedly. Excellent results have been reported with the use of magnesium sulfate to prevent and treat convulsions.[80] Caution is needed to avoid volume overload, because pulmonary edema is the most common cause of maternal mortality. When compared with women who were normotensive, the overall prognosis for women who had hypertension during pregnancy is not as good, probably because of causes other than preeclampsia, including unrecognized chronic primary hypertension. After delivery, transient or persistent hypertension can develop in the mother. In many cases, early primary hypertension may have been masked by the hemodynamic changes of pregnancy.

HYPERTENSIVE CRISIS

Definitions

A number of clinical circumstances require rapid reduction of BP (Table 40-9). These circumstances can be separated into *emergencies,* which require immediate reduction of BP (within 1 hour), and *urgencies,* which can be treated more slowly. A persistent diastolic pressure exceeding 130 mm Hg is often associated with acute vascular damage; some patients may suffer vascular damage from lower levels of pressure, whereas others are able to withstand even higher levels without apparent harm. The rapidity of the rise may be more important than the absolute level in producing acute vascular damage (see later). Therefore, in practice, all patients with diastolic BP above 130 mm Hg should be treated, some more rapidly with parenteral drugs and others more slowly with oral agents.

TABLE 40–9 Circumstances Requiring Rapid Treatment of Hypertension

Accelerated malignant hypertension with papilledema
Cerebrovascular
Hypertensive encephalopathy
Atherothrombotic brain infarction with severe hypertension
Intracerebral hemorrhage
Subarachnoid hemorrhage
Cardiac
Acute aortic dissection
Acute left ventricular failure
Acute or impending myocardial infarction
After coronary bypass surgery
Renal
Acute glomerulonephritis
Renal crises from collagen-vascular diseases
Severe hypertension after kidney transplantation
Excessive circulating catecholamines
Pheochromocytoma crisis
Food or drug interactions with monoamine oxidase inhibitors
Sympathomimetic drug use (cocaine)
Rebound hypertension after sudden cessation of antihypertensive drugs
Eclampsia
Surgical
Severe hypertension in patients requiring immediate surgery
Postoperative hypertension
Postoperative bleeding from vascular suture lines
Severe body burns
Severe epistaxis
Thrombotic thrombocytopenic purpura

When the rise in pressure causes retinal hemorrhages, exudates, or papilledema, the term *accelerated-malignant hypertension* is used. Hypertensive encephalopathy is characterized by headache, irritability, alterations in consciousness, and other manifestations of central nervous dysfunction with sudden and marked elevations in BP.

Incidence

Fewer than 1 percent of patients with primary hypertension progress to an accelerated-malignant phase. The incidence likely has receded because of more widespread treatment of hypertension. Any hypertensive disease can manifest as a crisis. Some, including pheochromocytoma and renovascular hypertension, do so at a higher rate than that seen with primary hypertension. However, because hypertension is of unknown cause in more than 90 percent of all patients, most hypertensive crises appear in the setting of preexisting primary hypertension.

Pathophysiology

Whenever BP rises and remains above a critical level, various processes set off a series of local and systemic effects that cause further rises in pressure and vascular damage, eventually resulting in accelerated-malignant hypertension. Early studies in animals and humans by Strandgaard and Paulson have elucidated the mechanism of hypertensive encephalopathy.[81] First, they directly measured the caliber of pial arterioles over the cerebral cortex in normotensive cats whose BP was varied over a wide range of infusion by vasodilators or A II. As the pressure fell, the arterioles became dilated; as the pressure rose, they became con-

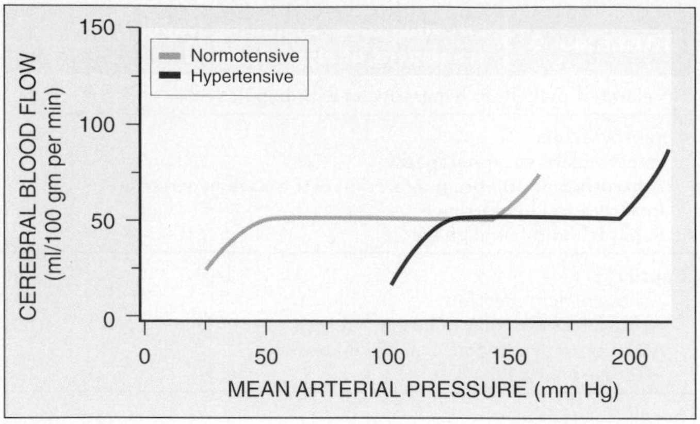

FIGURE 40–18 Idealized curves of cerebral blood flow at varying levels of systemic blood pressure in normotensive and hypertensive subjects. A rightward shift in autoregulation is shown with chronic hypertension. *(Adapted from Strandgaard S, Olesen J, Skinhtoi E, Lassen NA: Autoregulation of brain circulation in severe arterial hypertension. Br Med J 1:507, 1973.)*

stricted. Thus, constant cerebral blood flow was maintained by means of autoregulation, which depends on the cerebral sympathetic nerves. However, when mean arterial pressure rose above 180 mm Hg (i.e., 220/110), the tightly constricted vessels could no longer withstand the pressure and suddenly dilated. This dilation began in an irregular manner, first in areas with less muscle tone and then diffusely, with production of generalized vasodilation. This breakthrough of cerebral blood flow hyperperfuses the brain under high pressure and thereby causes leakage of fluid into the perivascular tissue, resulting in cerebral edema and the syndrome of hypertensive encephalopathy.

In human subjects, cerebral blood flow has been measured repetitively by an isotopic technique while BP was lowered or raised with vasodilators or vasoconstrictors in a manner similar to that used in animal studies. Curves depicting cerebral blood flow as a function of arterial pressure demonstrated autoregulation, with a constancy of flow over mean pressures in normotensive persons from about 60 to 120 mm Hg and in hypertensive patients from about 110 to 180 mm Hg (Fig. 40-18). This shift to the right in hypertensive patients is the result of structural thickening of the arterioles as an adaptation to the chronically elevated pressure. When pressure was raised beyond the upper limit of autoregulation, the same breakthrough with hyperperfusion occurred as was seen in the animal studies. In previously normotensive persons whose vessels have not been altered by prior exposure to high pressure, breakthrough occurred at a mean arterial pressure of about 120 mm Hg (i.e., 140/80 mm Hg); in hypertensive patients, the breakthrough occurred at about 180 mm Hg (i.e., 220/110 mm Hg).

These studies have confirmed clinical observations. In previously normotensive persons, severe encephalopathy occurs with relatively little hypertension. In children with acute glomerulonephritis and in women with eclampsia, convulsions can occur as a result of hypertensive encephalopathy, with BP readings as low as 150/100 mm Hg. Obviously, chronically hypertensive patients withstand such pressures without difficulty; however, when pressure increases significantly, encephalopathy can develop, even in these patients.

Manifestations and Course

The symptoms and signs of hypertensive crises are usually dramatic (Table 40-10), likely reflecting acute damage to endothelium and platelet activation. However, some patients may be relatively asymptomatic, despite markedly elevated pressure and extensive organ damage. Young black men are particularly prone to hypertensive crisis, with severe renal insufficiency. Even in elderly persons, however, hypertension can initially present in an accelerated-malignant phase. If left untreated, patients die quickly of brain damage or more gradually of renal damage. Before effective therapy was available, fewer than 25 percent of patients with malignant hypertension survived 1 year and only 1 percent survived 5 years. With therapy, including renal dialysis, more than 90 percent survive 1 year and about 80 percent survive 5 years.

TABLE 40–10 Clinical Characteristics of Hypertensive Crisis
Blood pressure—usually > 140 mm Hg diastolic
Funduscopic findings—hemorrhages, exudates, papilledema
Cardiac findings—prominent apical impulse, cardiac enlargement, congestive heart failure
Renal findings—oliguria, azotemia
Gastrointestinal findings—nausea, vomiting
Hematological findings—microangiopathic hemolysis

Differential Diagnosis

The presence of hypertensive encephalopathy or accelerated-malignant hypertension demands immediate aggressive therapy to lower BP effectively, often before the specific cause is known. However, certain serious diseases, as well as psychological problems, can mimic a hypertensive crisis, and management of these conditions usually requires different diagnostic and therapeutic approaches. In particular, BP should not be lowered too abruptly, if at all, in a patient with a stroke.[82] See Chapter 41 for specific therapy for hypertensive crises.

FUTURE PERSPECTIVES

The measurement of BP will become more accurate for diagnosis and cardiovascular risk stratification with the greater use of out-of-office measurements and assessments of vascular health using measures of vascular compliance, central aortic pressure, and inflammatory biomarkers. Hopefully, future research on underlying mechanisms of primary hypertension will make treatment less empirical and more effective, as detailed in Chapter 41.

REFERENCES

Epidemiology of Hypertension

1. Campanini B: The World Health Report: Reducing Risks, Promoting Healthy Life. Geneva, World Health Organization, 2002.
2. Wolf-Maier K, Cooper RS, Kramer H, et al: Hypertension treatment and control in five European countries, Canada, and the United States. Hypertension 43:10, 2004.
3. Kaplan NM, Opie LH: Controversies in hypertension. Lancet 367:168, 2006.
4. Chobanian AV, Bakris GL, Black HR, et al: The Seventh Report of the Joint National Committee on Prevention, Detection, Evaluation, and Treatment of High Blood Pressure: The JNC 7 report. JAMA 289:2560, 2003.
5. Lewington S, Clarke R, Qizilbash N, et al: Age-specific relevance of usual blood pressure to vascular mortality: A meta-analysis of individual data for one million adults in 61 prospective studies. Lancet 360:1903, 2002.
6. Giles TD, Berk BC, Black HR, et al: Expanding the definition and classification of hypertension. J Clin Hypertens (Greenwich) 7:505, 2005.
7. Sipahi I, Tuzcu EM, Schoenhagen P, et al: Effects of normal, pre-hypertensive, and hypertensive blood pressure levels on progression of coronary atherosclerosis. J Am Coll Cardiol 48:833, 2006.

8. Vasan RS, Beiser A, Seshadri S, et al: Residual lifetime risk for developing hypertension in middle-aged women and men. The Framingham Heart Study. JAMA 287:1003, 2002.
9. Cooper RS, Wolf-Maier K, Luke A, et al: An international comparative study of blood pressure in populations of European vs. African descent. BMC Med 3:2, 2005.
10. Winkelmayer WC, Stampfer MJ, Willett WC, Curhan GC: Habitual caffeine intake and the risk of hypertension in women. JAMA 294:2330, 2005.
11. Taylor EN, Mount DB, Forman JP, Curhan GC: Association of prevalent hypertension with 24-hour urinary excretion of calcium, citrate, and other factors. Am J Kidney Dis 47:780, 2006.
12. Intersalt Cooperative Research Group: Intersalt: An international study of electrolyte excretion and blood pressure. Results for 24-hour urinary sodium and potassium excretion. BMJ 297:319, 1988.
13. Luft FC: Mendelian forms of human hypertension and mechanisms of disease. Clin Med Res 1:291, 2003.
14. Franklin SS, Pio JR, Wong ND, et al: Predictors of new-onset diastolic and systolic hypertension: The Framingham Heart Study. Circulation 111:1121, 2005.
15. Franklin SS: Hypertension in older people: Part 1. J Clin Hypertens (Greenwich) 8:444, 2006.
16. Mitchell GF: Arterial stiffness and wave reflection in hypertension: Pathophysiological and therapeutic implications. Curr Hypertens Rep 6:436, 2004.
17. McEniery CM, Yasmin, Wallace S, et al: Increased stroke volume and aortic stiffness contribute to isolated systolic hypertension in young adults. Hypertension 46:221-226, 2005.

Pathophysiology of Hypertension

18. Guyenet PG: The sympathetic control of blood pressure. Nat Rev Neurosci 7:335-346, 2006.
19. Smith PA, Graham LN, Mackintosh AF, Stoker JB, et al: Relationship between central sympathetic activity and stages of human hypertension. Am J Hypertens 17:217-222, 2004.
20. Lohmeier TE, Irwin ED, Rossing MA, et al: Prolonged activation of the baroreflex produces sustained hypotension. Hypertension 43:306, 2004.
21. Heusser K, Tank J, Luft FC, Jordan J: Baroreflex failure. Hypertension 45:834, 2005.
22. Vloet LC, Pel-Little RE, Jansen PA, Jansen RW: High prevalence of postprandial and orthostatic hypotension among geriatric patients admitted to Dutch hospitals. J Gerontol A Biol Sci Med Sci 60:1271, 2005.
23. Esler M, Straznicky N, Eikelis N, et al: Mechanisms of sympathetic activation in obesity-related hypertension. Hypertension 48:787, 2006.
24. Baguet JP, Narkiewicz K, Mallion JM: Update on hypertension management: Obstructive sleep apnea and hypertension. J Hypertens 24:205, 2006.
25. Norman D, Loredo JS, Nelesen RA, et al: Effects of continuous positive airway pressure versus supplemental oxygen on 24-hour ambulatory blood pressure. Hypertension 47:840, 2006.
26. Yaggi HK, Concato J, Kernan WN, et al: Obstructive sleep apnea as a risk factor for stroke and death. N Engl J Med 353:2034, 2005.
27. Bleeke T, Zhang H, Madamanchi N, et al: Catecholamine-induced vascular wall growth is dependent on generation of reactive oxygen species. Circ Res 94:37, 2004.
28. Zoccali C, Mallamaci F, Parlongo S, et al: Plasma norepinephrine predicts survival and incident cardiovascular events in patients with end-stage renal disease. Circulation 105:1354, 2002.
29. Keller G, Zimmer G, Mall G, et al: Nephron number in patients with primary hypertension. N Engl J Med 348:101, 2003.
30. August P, Suthanthiran M: Transforming growth factor beta signaling, vascular remodeling, and hypertension. N Engl J Med 354:2721, 2006.
31. Savoia C, Schiffrin EL: Inflammation in hypertension. Curr Opin Nephrol Hypertens 15:152, 2006.
32. Paravicini TM, Touyz RM: Redox signaling in hypertension. Cardiovasc Res 71:247, 2006.
33. Feig DI, Kang DH, Nakagawa T, et al: Uric Acid and hypertension. Curr Hypertens Rep 8:111, 2006.
34. Reyes AJ, Leary WP: Controversies in cardiology. Lancet 367:1314, 2006.
35. Duprez DA: Role of the renin-angiotensin-aldosterone system in vascular remodeling and inflammation: A clinical review. J Hypertens 24:983, 2006.
36. Vasan RS, Evans JC, Larson MG, et al: Serum aldosterone and the incidence of hypertension in nonhypertensive persons. N Engl J Med 351:33, 2004.
37. Stewart AD, Millasseau SC, Dawes M, et al: Aldosterone and left ventricular hypertrophy in Afro-Caribbean subjects with low renin hypertension. Am J Hypertens 19:19, 2006.
38. Schiffrin EL: Effects of aldosterone on the vasculature. Hypertension 47:312, 2006.
39. Huang Y, Wongamorntham S, Kasting J, et al: Renin increases mesangial cell transforming growth factor-beta1 and matrix proteins through receptor-mediated, angiotensin II-independent mechanisms. Kidney Int 69:105, 2006.
40. Danser AH: Prorenin: Back into the arena. Hypertension 47:824, 2006.
41. Frey N, Katus HA, Olson EN, Hill JA: Hypertrophy of the heart: A new therapeutic target? Circulation 109:1580, 2004.
42. Gradman AH, Alfayoumi F: From left ventricular hypertrophy to congestive heart failure: Management of hypertensive heart disease. Prog Cardiovasc Dis 48:326, 2006.
43. Dolan E, Stanton A, Thijs L, et al: Superiority of ambulatory over clinic blood pressure measurement in predicting mortality: The Dublin outcome study. Hypertension 46:156, 2005.
44. O'Brien E, Asmar R, Beilin L, et al: Practice guidelines of the European Society of Hypertension for clinic, ambulatory and self blood pressure measurement. J Hypertens 23:697, 2005.
45. Verdecchia P, Reboldi GP, Angeli F, et al: Short- and long-term incidence of stroke in white-coat hypertension. Hypertension 45:203, 2005.
46. Mancia G, Facchetti R, Bombelli M, et al: Long-term risk of mortality associated with selective and combined elevation in office, home, and ambulatory blood pressure. Hypertension 47:846, 2006.
47. European Society of Hypertension-European Society of Cardiology Guidelines Committee: 2003 European Society of Hypertension-European Society of Cardiology guidelines for the management of arterial hypertension. J Hypertens 21:1011, 2003.
48. Nesbitt SD, Julius S, Leonard D, et al: Is low-risk hypertension fact or fiction? cardiovascular risk profile in the TROPHY study. Am J Hypertens 18:980, 2005.
49. Sever PS, Dahlof B, Poulter NR, et al: Prevention of coronary and stroke events with atorvastatin in hypertensive patients who have average or lower-than-average cholesterol concentrations, in the Anglo-Scandinavian Cardiac Outcomes Trial—Lipid Lowering Arm (ASCOT-LLA): A multicentre randomised controlled trial. Lancet 361:1149, 2003.

Complications of Hypertension

50. Jackson R, Lawes CM, Bennett DA, et al: Treatment with drugs to lower blood pressure and blood cholesterol based on an individual's absolute cardiovascular risk. Lancet 365:434, 2005.
51. Grosso A, Veglio F, Porta M, et al: Hypertensive retinopathy revisited: Some answers, more questions. Br J Ophthalmol 89:1646, 2005.
52. Okin PM, Devereux RB, Nieminen MS, et al: Electrocardiographic strain pattern and prediction of new-onset congestive heart failure in hypertensive patients: The Losartan Intervention for Endpoint Reduction in Hypertension (LIFE) study. Circulation 113:67, 2006.
53. Drazner MH, Dries DL, Peshock RM, et al: Left ventricular hypertrophy is more prevalent in blacks than whites in the general population: The Dallas Heart Study. Hypertension 46:124, 2005.
54. Klausen KP, Scharling H, Jensen G, Jensen JS: New definition of microalbuminuria in hypertensive subjects: Association with incident coronary heart disease and death. Hypertension 46:33, 2005.
55. Stevens LA, Coresh J, Greene T, Levey AS: Assessing kidney function—measured and estimated glomerular filtration rate. N Engl J Med 354:2473, 2006.
56. Bakris GL, Williams M, Dworkin L, et al: Preserving renal function in adults with hypertension and diabetes: a consensus approach. National Kidney Foundation Hypertension and Diabetes Executive Committees Working Group. Am J Kidney Dis 36:646, 2000.
57. Rule AD, Lieber MM, Jacobsen SJ: Is benign prostatic hyperplasia a risk factor for chronic renal failure? J Urol 173:691, 2005.
58. Casas JP, Chua W, Loukogeorgakis S, et al: Effect of inhibitors of the renin-angiotensin system and other antihypertensive drugs on renal outcomes: Systematic review and meta-analysis. Lancet 366:2026, 2005.
59. Pickering TG: Target blood pressure in patients with end-stage renal disease: Evidence-based medicine or the emperor's new clothes? J Clin Hypertens (Greenwich) 8:369, 2006.
60. Palmer BF: Renal dysfunction complicating the treatment of hypertension. N Engl J Med 347:1256, 2002.
61. CDC Diabetes Cost-Effectiveness Group: Cost-effectiveness of intensive glycemic control, intensified hypertension control, and serum cholesterol level reduction for type 2 diabetes. JAMA 287:2542, 2002.
62. Mielniczuk LM, Williams K, Davis DR, et al: Frequency of peripartum cardiomyopathy. Am J Cardiol 97:1765, 2006.
63. Locatelli F, Covic A, Chazot C, et al: Hypertension and cardiovascular risk assessment in dialysis patients. Nephrol Dial Transplant 19:1058, 2004.
64. Textor SC: Stable patients with atherosclerotic renal artery stenosis should be treated first with medical management. Am J Kidney Dis 42:858, 2003.
65. Radermacher J, Chavan A, Bleck J, et al: Use of Doppler ultrasonography to predict the outcome of therapy for renal-artery stenosis. N Engl J Med 344:410, 2001.
66. Dellegrottaglie S, Sanz J, Rajagopalan S: Technology insight: Clinical role of magnetic resonance angiography in the diagnosis and management of renal artery stenosis. Nat Clin Pract Cardiovasc Med 3:329, 2006.
67. White CJ: Catheter-based therapy for atherosclerotic renal artery stenosis. Circulation 113:1464, 2006.
68. Barzon L, Sonino N, Fallo F, et al: Prevalence and natural history of adrenal incidentalomas. Eur J Endocrinol 149:273, 2003.
69. Kaplan NM: The current epidemic of primary aldosteronism: causes and consequences. J Hypertens 22:863, 2004.
70. Milliez P, Girerd X, Plouin PF, et al: Evidence for an increased rate of cardiovascular events in patients with primary aldosteronism. J Am Coll Cardiol 45:1243, 2005.
71. Nwariaku FE, Miller BS, Auchus R, et al: Primary hyperaldosteronism: Effect of adrenal vein sampling on surgical outcome. Arch Surg 141:497, 2006.
72. Sechi LA, Novello M, Lapenna R, et al: Long-term renal outcomes in patients with primary aldosteronism. JAMA 295:2638, 2006.
73. Newell-Price J, Bertagna X, Grossman AB, Nieman LK: Cushing's syndrome. Lancet 367:1605, 2006.
74. Lenders JW, Eisenhofer G, Mannelli M, Pacak K: Phaeochromocytoma. Lancet 366:665, 2005.
75. Casadei B, Abuzeid H: Is there a strong rationale for deferring elective surgery in patients with poorly controlled hypertension? J Hypertens 23:19, 2005.
76. Eisen HJ: Hypertension in heart transplant recipients: more than just cyclosporine. J Am Coll Cardiol 41:433, 2003.

77. Baillargeon JP, McClish DK, Essah PA, Nestler JE: Association between the current use of low-dose oral contraceptives and cardiovascular arterial disease: a meta-analysis. J Clin Endocrinol Metab 90:3863, 2005.
78. Petitti DB: Clinical practice. Combination estrogen-progestin oral contraceptives. N Engl J Med 349:1443, 2003.
79. Morley KJ, Kotchen TA: Impact of female hormones on blood pressure: Review of potential mechanisms and clinical studies. Curr Hypertens Rep 5:505, 2003.
80. Sibai B, Dekker G, Kupferminc M: Pre-eclampsia. Lancet 365:785, 2005.
81. Strandgaard S, Paulson OB: Cerebral blood flow and its pathophysiology in hypertension. Am J Hypertens 2:486, 1989.
82. Adams H, Adams R, Del ZG, Goldstein LB: Guidelines for the early management of patients with ischemic stroke: 2005 guidelines update a scientific statement from the Stroke Council of the American Heart Association/American Stroke Association. Stroke 36:916-923, 2005.

CHAPTER 41

Systemic Hypertension: Therapy

Norman M. Kaplan

Although hypertension is the most common reason for nonpregnant adults to go to a physician in the United States, it remains inadequately treated. There are many reasons, among them physician inertia and the cost of medications being prominent. The main fault, however, resides in the inherent nature of the disease—genetically determined, induced by common but unhealthy life styles, asymptomatic, and persistent, with overt consequences delayed by 10 to 30 years, so that the cost of therapy, both financially and in adverse effects, seems to outweigh benefits to be derived from adherence to the regimen. Furthermore, another disquieting feature of the therapy of most hypertensive patients is that it may not benefit most of those who adhere faithfully to their treatment. Even among elderly patients, such as those enrolled in the Systolic Hypertension in the Elderly Program (SHEP) trial, 111 would need to be treated for 5 years to prevent one cardiovascular death and 19 treated to prevent one cardiovascular event.[1] In view of this relatively small benefit and the cost and side effects of drug therapy, the use of medication for the prevention of hypertension has not been deemed appropriate.

The situation may change for at least three reasons, First, significant increases in cardiovascular morbidity and mortality have now been amply documented,[2] even in those with levels of blood pressure below 140/90 mm Hg; second, blood pressure levels above the assumed "normal" (i.e., 120/80 mm Hg) interact with other cardiovascular risk factors, emphasizing the need to address not only blood pressure but the patients' multiple risk factors[3]; and third, perhaps most important, treatment with drugs having few side effects delay if not prevent the progression of prehypertension into overt hypertension.[4] In addition, the potential for an inexpensive "polypill" with antilipemic, antihypertensive, and antithrombotic components[5] is under investigation.

All these factors are compounded by the realization that the incidence of hypertension, as noted in Chapter 40, continues to increase as the population grows fatter and older.

GENERAL THERAPEUTIC CONSIDERATIONS

Benefits of Therapy

For the largest group of hypertensive patients, those older than 65 years, the benefits of antihypertensive therapy are greater than those for younger subjects, simply because older adults start at so much greater risk[6] (Fig. 41-1). The benefits for those older than 80 years (see Fig. 41-1) are based on few studies, however, and more data will be needed to document how well treatment protects them.

Nonetheless, all those younger than 80 clearly benefit from antihypertensive therapy; the benefit is derived from the extent of blood pressure reduction rather than from how it is reduced.[7] Over the 40 years encompassed by the trials shown in Figure 41-2, benefits of treatment were first documented for patients with severe hypertension, then for those with moderate disease, and only later for those with lesser degrees of hypertension.

The difficulty in showing clear benefits of treatment in the larger part of the hypertensive population, those with stage 1 hypertension or blood pressures from 140/90 to 160/100 mm Hg, should take into account that although their individual risk is relatively low, their large number represents the major contribution to the overall population risk from hypertension. This fact has given rise to two important guidelines for clinical practice: (1) the critical need for prevention of hypertension by population-wide life-style modifications; and (2) the rationale for considering blood pressure in the larger context of overall cardiovascular risk.

Threshold of Therapy

With any blood pressure above 120/80 mm Hg, life-style changes should be strongly emphasized and practical guidance should be provided for achieving the desired changes (see later, "Life-Style Modifications"). Attention must also be given to the other risk factors for cardiovascular disease, described in detail in Chapter 39. Some practitioners use the presence of an overall risk of greater than 10 percent over the next 10 years, based on the Framingham risk score, to begin active drug therapy for elevated blood pressure and blood lipid levels. The use of such risk estimates will likely indicate the need for antihypertensive drug therapy more accurately than blood pressure criteria alone.

The algorithm shown in Figure 41-3 closely follows the one published by the Joint National Committee on Prevention, Detection, Evaluation, and Treatment of High Blood Pressure (JNC-7).[8] Although more liberal than the recommendations of the British Hypertension Society,[9] there may be even lower thresholds for beginning drug therapy if the principle proven by the TROPHY trial in upper range prehypertensives[4] is upheld in larger and longer trials with cardiovascular endpoints. Such trials are now in process but likely will require 6 to 8 years to complete. If drug therapy is not given, close surveillance must still be carried out, because from 10 to 17 percent of the placebo-treated

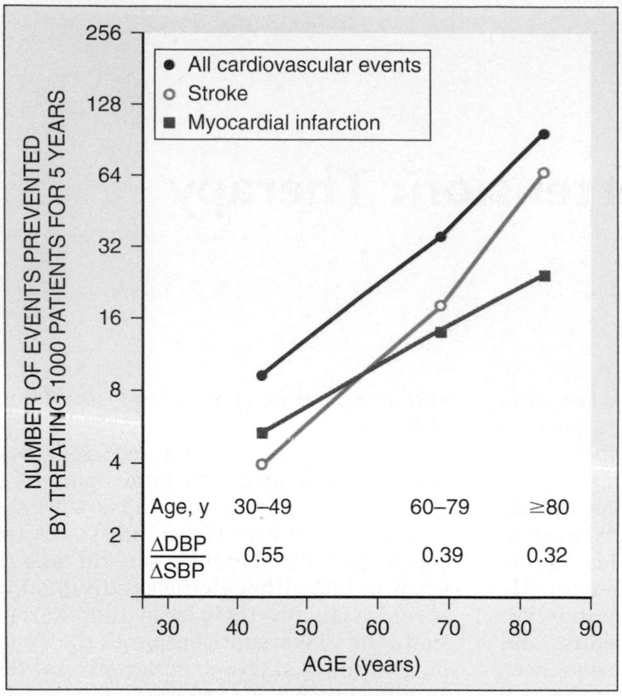

FIGURE 41–1 Absolute benefits for the prevention of fatal and nonfatal cardiovascular events, stroke, and myocardial infarction in three age groups. Symbols represent the number of events that can be prevented by treating 1000 patients for 5 years (y). ΔDBP/ΔSBP = mean ratio of diastolic blood pressure to systolic blood pressure lowering. *(Modified from Wang J-G, Staessen JA, Franklin SS, et al: Systolic and diastolic blood pressure lowering as determinants of cardiovascular outcome. Hypertension 45:907, 2005.)*

patients with an initial blood pressure (BP) from 140/90 to 160/95 mm Hg in various randomized controlled trials (RCTs) had progression of their blood pressure to a level above 170/100. All patients should be strongly advised to use the appropriate life-style modifications (see later).

Systolic Pressure in Elderly Patients

Current guidelines recommend that therapy be given to older adult patients with isolated systolic hypertension (ISH) because they generally have a higher absolute risk of cardiovascular disease and therefore derive greater benefit from treatment. In data from eight RCTs involving elderly patients with ISH, those given drugs achieved impressive reductions in cardiovascular morbidity compared with those given placebo[6] and, in one trial in which cognitive function was specifically monitored, those given drug therapy had a 55 percent reduction in the onset of dementia over an 8-year follow-up.[10] Diagnosis of ISH in these trials was based on a systolic level of 160 mm Hg or higher. A large percentage of elderly persons have systolic blood pressures (SBPs) above 140 but below 160 mm Hg, with diastolic pressures below 90 mm Hg. As of this writing, no studies have documented benefit for this population but, because many of them are inherently at high risk, the JNC-7 report[8] has recommended active drug therapy for those with systolic levels above 140 mm Hg.

THOSE OLDER THAN 80 YEARS. Although the percentage of people in most developed countries older than 80 is increasing faster than any other demographic group, too few of them have been enrolled in therapeutic trials to provide guidance as to the threshold or goal of therapy. From what little is known, caution is needed; in the 1600 patients older than 80 in trials now published, strokes were reduced by antihypertensive drug therapy but mortality tended to

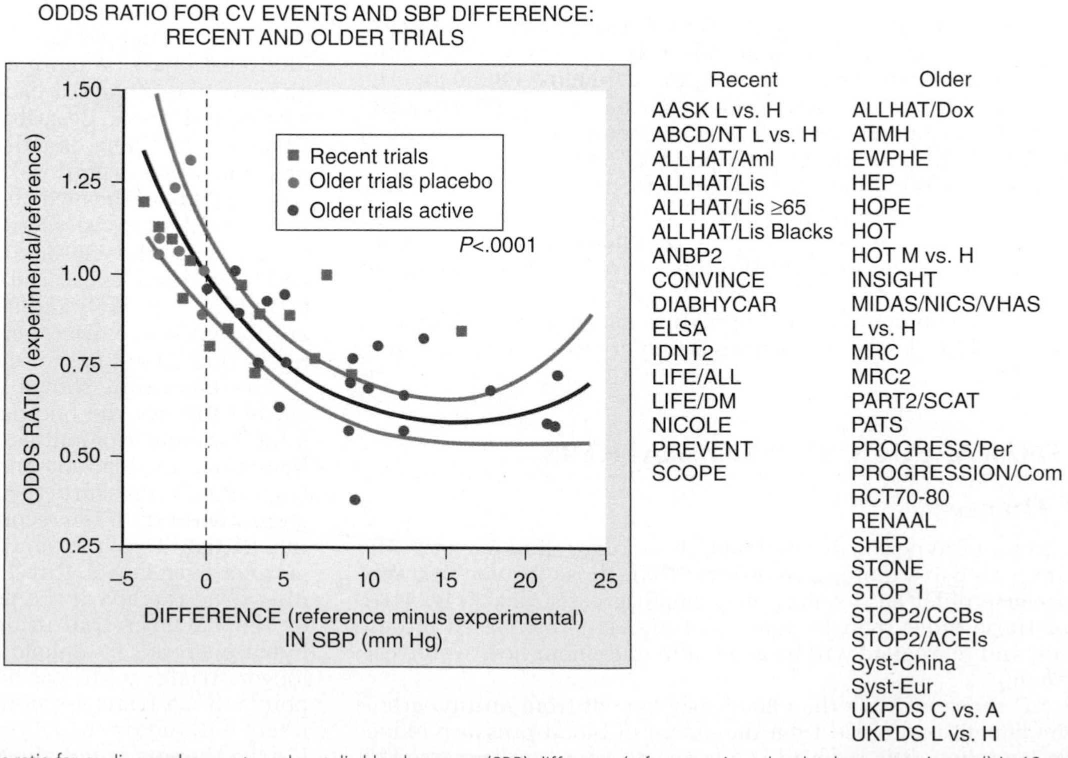

FIGURE 41–2 Odds ratio for cardiovascular events and systolic blood pressure (SBP) difference (reference minus the placebo or experimental) in 16 recent trials and 27 older randomized controlled trials identified by their acronyms. CV = cardiovascular. *(Modified from Staessen JA, Wang J-G, Thijs L: Cardiovascular prevention and blood pressure reduction: A quantitative overview updated until 1 March 2003. J Hypertens 21:1055, 2003.)*

increase.[11] However, in one double-blind parallel group study, a significant slowing of loss of cognitive function was noted among the 600 patients older than 80 whose blood pressure was reduced by an angiotensin II receptor blocker.[12] Until more data become available, a SBP above 160 mm Hg seems an appropriate threshold and the goal should likely be no lower than 150 mm Hg.

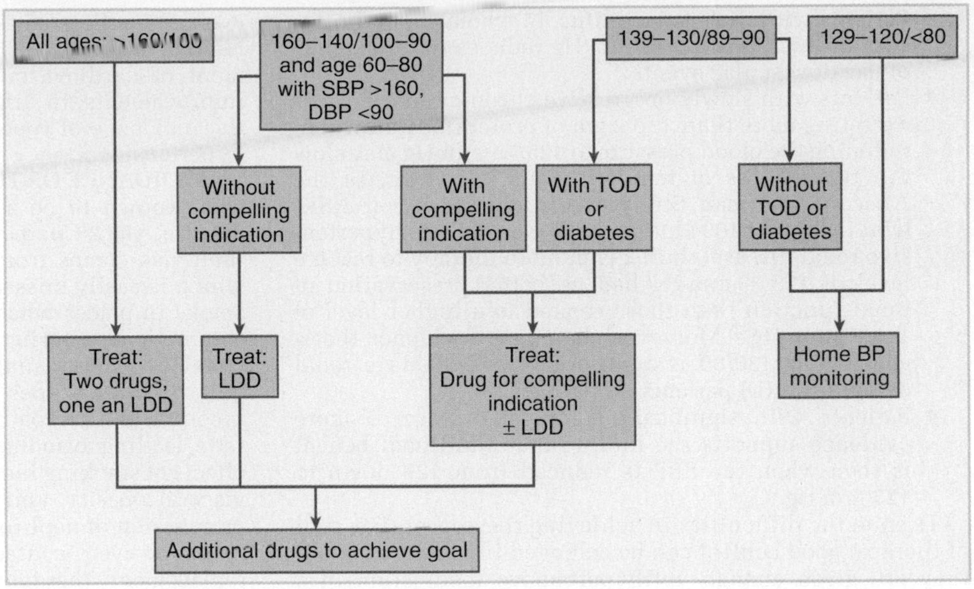

FIGURE 41–3 An algorithm for the decision to manage patients with different average blood pressure (BP) levels, determined by repeated office readings or, preferably, out-of-office readings, with specific attention to those aged 60 to 80 years. The evidence for treatment of those older than 80 is inconclusive. The recommended initial drug choices are indicated. DBP = diastolic blood pressure; LDD = low-dose diuretic; SBP = systolic blood pressure; TOD = target organ damage.

Goal of Therapy

When the decision has been made to treat a patient, the clinician must consider the goal of therapy. In the past, most physicians assumed that the effects of reduction of blood pressure on cardiovascular risk would fit a straight line downward (Fig. 41-4, line A), justifying the saying "the lower, the better." However, data from multiple large trials have indicated a more gradual decline in risk when pressures were reduced to moderate levels (see Fig. 41-4, line B). Subsequently, some evidence has suggested a J curve—that is, a fall in risk until some critical level of pressure is reached, below which the risk goes back up (see Fig. 41-4, line C). The J curve has been found for coronary events with falls in diastolic pressure below 80 mm Hg in patients with diastolic hypertension[13] and, for stroke, with falls of diastolic pressure to below 65 mm Hg in patients with ISH.[14]

Another analysis of evidence for a J curve was based on data for individual patients from seven RCTs involving over 40,000 patients given placebo or drug therapy.[15] A J curve between both systolic and diastolic pressures and cardiovascular mortality was seen, but it occurred in the treated and nontreated groups, with the nadir being 5 mm Hg lower in treated patients. The authors concluded that "The increased risk of events observed with low blood pressure was not related to antihypertensive treatment . . . Poor health conditions leading to low blood pressure and increased risk for death probably explain the J-shaped curve."[15]

Certainly, poor general health may cause low blood pressure and increase the risk for death. Nonetheless, excessive antihypertensive treatment may increase cardiovascular morbidity and mortality. The problem may be even more ominous for elderly patients with ISH, whose diastolic pressures are often low before therapy is started. In the SHEP trial, an increased risk for death and stroke was seen with a fall in diastolic pressure below 65 mm Hg.[14] However, if the diastolic pressure remains above 70 mm Hg, reductions of systolic pressure, even below 120 mm Hg, remain beneficial.[16] Nevertheless, the major clinical problem is not overtreatment but undertreatment. Even in carefully conducted clinical trials in which good control should be at a maximum, systolic blood pressures usually remain above 140 mm Hg, even though diastolic levels can usually be brought down to below 90 mm Hg.

In conclusion, the optimal goal of antihypertensive therapy in most patients with combined systolic and diastolic hypertension who are not at high risk is a blood pressure below 140/90 mm Hg. The greatest benefit is probably derived from lowering the diastolic pressure to 80 to 85 mm Hg. Not only is there no proven benefit with more intensive control, but added cost and probable increased side effects are also associated with more intensive antihypertensive therapy.

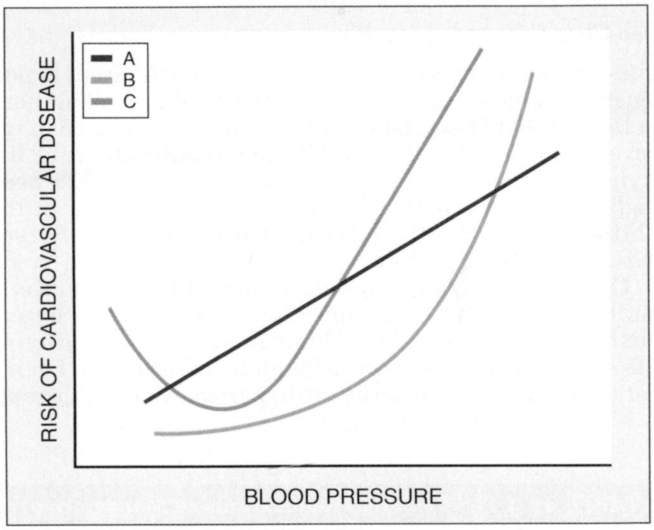

FIGURE 41–4 Graphic representation of three hypothetical relationships between levels of blood pressure and risk of cardiovascular disease. *(See text for details.)*

In elderly patients with ISH, the goal should be a systolic blood pressure of 150 mm Hg; that was the level reached in the RCTs in which benefit was shown. Caution is advised if, inadvertently, diastolic pressures fall below 65 mm Hg. In such an event, less than ideal reductions in systolic levels need to be balanced against the potential for harm if diastolic levels fall below that level.[1]

Although the evidence is scarce, more intensive therapy to attain a diastolic pressure of 80 mm Hg or lower may be desirable in some groups, including the following:

- Black patients, who are at greater risk for hypertensive complications and who may continue to have progressive renal damage, despite a diastolic pressure of 85 to 90 mm Hg.

- Patients with diabetes mellitus, in whom a blood pressure of less than 130/85 mm Hg reduces the incidence of cardiovascular events.
- Patients with slowly progressive chronic renal disease excreting more than 1 to 2 gm of protein/day, in whom reducing the blood pressure to 125/75 mm Hg may slow the rate of loss of renal function. However, in the African American Study of Kidney Disease (AASK) trial involving 1094 blacks with nondiabetic hypertensive renal disease, those given more therapy to reach a level of 128/78 mm Hg had no better preservation of renal function than those treated to a higher level of 141/85 mm Hg.[17] Moreover, there is no evidence that a goal below 130/80 is appropriate for end-stage renal disease (ESRD) patients on dialysis.[18]
- Patients with significant coronary disease, if more evidence supports the finding that additional benefit is seen when the SBP is reduced from 129 down to 125 mm Hg.[19]

Despite the difficulties in achieving the appropriate goal of therapy, good control can be achieved in most patients if they are given enough antihypertensive medication in a progressive manner. Control is enhanced when access to health care is readily available, frequent contact with the same physician is maintained, and physician performance is monitored.

Life-Style Modifications

(see Chaps. 39 and 44 to 46)

Life-style modifications are indicated for virtually all hypertensives (Table 41-1). Adverse life-style habits are ubiquitous in those with hypertension and may play a major role in the development of the disease. Multiple modifications of life style can lower blood pressure, and their use has been highly correlated with the control of hypertension in the Third National Health and Nutrition Examination Survey (NHANES III) population.

Observational and trial data support the importance of multiple simultaneous modifications of life style to accomplish the greatest benefits. Although success in modifying life style may be as or more difficult to achieve than having patients continue long-term antihypertensive drug therapy, even a small persistent reduction in blood pressure can have a major protective effect in regard to the development of cardiovascular disease. Moreover, even modest improvements in life style have been shown to reduce the incidence of type 2 diabetes, a common contributor to hypertension.[20]

AVOIDANCE OF TOBACCO. Smoking cigarettes has long been known to be a major risk factor for cardiovascular disease, yet 25 percent of U.S. adults now smoke. Part of their risk comes from the major pressor effect of tobacco, which is easily missed, because patients are not allowed to smoke in places where blood pressures are recorded. With automatic monitoring, the effect is easy to demonstrate, and blood pressure usually falls immediately when smokers quit. Tolerance does not develop to the pressor effect of nicotine, and sympathetic outflow increases with each cigarette, leading to an increase in arterial stiffness. The noxious effects of smoking include an increase in insulin resistance, visceral obesity, and a particularly detrimental effect on progression of nephropathy. Those who smoke must be told to stop at every contact with a health practitioner. Nicotine replacement therapies are effective and have minimal pressor effects.[21]

WEIGHT REDUCTION. Obesity is growing rapidly in the United States and in all developed and developing societies. Even small amounts of increased weight have impressive consequences. Over 18 years, women with an initial body mass index (BMI) of 24 were five times more likely to have diabetes and twice as likely to have hypertension as women with a BMI of 21 or lower. In many people, most of this increased weight is deposited in the upper body, constituting a major component of the metabolic syndrome (see Chap. 43). Such upper body obesity is a risk factor for hypertension independent of BMI. Upper body obesity is also more commonly associated with obstructive sleep apnea (see Chap. 74). Obstructive sleep apnea can lead to sustained hypertension, and relief of apnea can lower blood pressure. Weight loss is almost always accompanied by a fall in BP, particularly when the degree of weight loss is extensive, as after bariatric surgery.[22]

PHYSICAL ACTIVITY. An increase in physical activity is almost always required for weight reduction. Even without weight loss, however, physical activity can lower the inci-

TABLE 41–1 Life-Style Modifications to Manage Hypertension

Modification	Recommendation	Approximate Systolic Blood Pressure Reduction (range)
Weight reduction	Maintain normal body weight (body mass index 18.5-24.9 kg/m^2)	5-20 mm Hg/10 kg
Adopt DASH eating plan	Consume a diet rich in fruits, vegetables, and low-fat dairy products with a reduced content of saturated and total fat	8-14 mm Hg
Dietary sodium reduction	Reduce dietary sodium intake to no more than 100 mmol/d (2.4 gm sodium or 6 gm sodium chloride)	2-8 mm Hg
Physical activity	Engage in regular aerobic physical activity such as brisk walking (at least 30 min/d, most days of the week)	4-9 mm Hg
Moderation of alcohol consumption	Limit consumption to no more than two drinks (1 oz or 30 ml ethanol; 24 oz beer, 10 oz wine, or 3 oz 80-proof whiskey) per day in most men and to no more than one drink per day in women and lighter weight persons	2.5-4 mm Hg

DASH = Dietary Approaches to Stop Hypertension.

From Chobanian AV, Bakris GL, Black HR, et al; National Heart, Lung, and Blood Institute Joint National Committee on Prevention, Detection, Evaluation, and Treatment of High Blood Pressure; National High Blood Pressure Education Program Coordinating Committee: The Seventh Report of the Joint National Committee on Prevention, Detection, Evaluation, and Treatment of High Blood Pressure: The JNC 7 report. JAMA 289:2560, 2003.

dence of hypertension and diabetes and protect against cardiovascular disease. The blood pressure falls during aerobic exercise and remains lower for the remainder of the day. The overall antihypertensive effect is provided by as little as 30 minutes of aerobic activity three or more times per week.[23]

Dietary Changes

SODIUM REDUCTION. Evidence incriminating the typically high sodium content of the diet of persons living in developed industrialized societies was presented earlier as a cause of hypertension. When hypertension is present, modest salt reduction may help lower the blood pressure. In an analysis by He and MacGregor of 28 well-controlled intervention studies that lasted at least 4 weeks, in which daily intake (based on urinary sodium excretion) was reduced by a median of 78 mmol/24 hours, blood pressures fell an average of 5.0/2.0 mm Hg in 734 hypertensive subjects and 2.0/1.0 mm Hg in 2220 normotensive subjects in a dose-dependent manner (Fig. 41-5).[23a]

Not all hypertensive persons respond to a moderate degree of sodium restriction to the recommended sodium level of 100 mmol or 2.4 gm/day. Nevertheless, even if the blood pressure does not fall with moderate degrees of sodium restriction, patients may still benefit. Multiple cardiovascular and noncardiovascular ill effects have been noted with high sodium intake. In a prospective follow-up of 2400 Finnish men and women, a 100 mmol/24 hour higher sodium excretion was accompanied by a 45 percent increase in the hazard ratio for cardiovascular disease and a 26 percent increase in all-cause mortality.[24] However, rigid degrees of sodium restriction are not only difficult for patients to achieve but also may be counterproductive. The marked stimulation of renin-aldosterone and sympathetic nervous activity that accompanies rigid sodium restriction may prevent the blood pressure from falling and increase the amount of potassium wastage if diuretics are used concomitantly.

Sodium reduction is useful for all persons—as a preventive measure for those who are normotensive and, more certainly, as partial therapy for those who are hypertensive. The easiest way to accomplish moderate sodium reduction is to substitute natural foods for processed foods, because natural foods are low in sodium and high in potassium, whereas most processed foods have had sodium added and potassium removed. It is hoped that those who process food

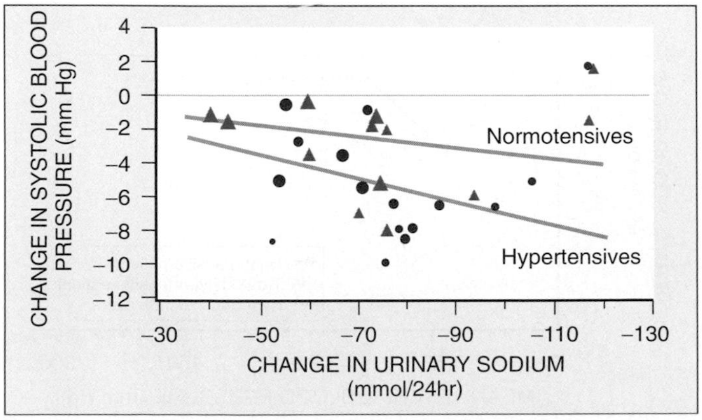

FIGURE 41–5 Relationship between the net change in urinary sodium excretion and systolic blood pressure. The blue triangles represent normotensive subjects and the magenta circles represent hypertensive subjects. The slope is weighted by the inverse of the variance of the net change in systolic blood pressure. The size of the circle is proportional to the weight of the trial. *(Modified from He J, MacGregor GA: Effect of modest salt reduction on blood pressure: A meta-analysis of randomized trials. Implications for public health. J Hum Hypertens 16:766, 2002.)*

will gradually reduce the large amounts of salt often add to these processed foods but, in the meantime, patients should be asked to avoid foods whose label indicates more than 300 mg sodium per portion. Additional guidelines include the following:

- Add no sodium chloride to food during cooking or at the table.
- If a salty taste is desired, use a half–sodium chloride and half–potassium chloride preparation (e.g., Lite-Salt) or a pure potassium chloride substitute.
- Avoid or minimize the use of "fast foods" and processed meats, many of which have high sodium content.
- Recognize the sodium content of some antacids and proprietary medications.

POTASSIUM SUPPLEMENTATION. Some of the advantages of a lower sodium intake may be related to its tendency to increase body potassium content, by a coincidental increase in dietary potassium intake and by a decrease in potassium wastage if diuretics are being used.

Potassium supplements were found to reduce blood pressure an average of 35/2.5 mm Hg in 27 RCTs.[25] Nonetheless, potassium supplements are too costly and potentially hazardous for routine use by normokalemic hypertensive persons. The best source is increased consumption of fruits and vegetables, which reduces the incidence of stroke as well.[26]

CALCIUM SUPPLEMENTS. In 42 mostly short-term studies of either calcium supplements (33) or dietary intervention (9) in 4560 nonpregnant adults, the blood pressure fell 1.44/0.84 mm Hg.[27] Because calcium supplements sometimes raise blood pressure and increase the risk of kidney stones, the best course is to ensure that calcium intake is not inadvertently reduced by reduction of milk and cheese consumption in an attempt to reduce saturated fat and sodium intake.

MAGNESIUM SUPPLEMENTS. A meta-analysis of 20 RCTs of magnesium supplements, averaging 15.4 mmol/24 hours, has found a statistically insignificant fall in blood pressure of 0.6/0.8 mm Hg.[28]

OTHER DIETARY CONSTITUENTS. Significant reductions in blood pressure were observed in a controlled trial of 690 normotensive persons, half of whom ate a diet rich in fruits and vegetables.[29] This fall in blood pressure could reflect increases in fiber, potassium, or other ingredients. Some lowering of the blood pressure has been noted in studies of high fiber intake and high doses of omega-3 fatty acids from fish oil. Higher vegetable protein intake was associated with lower blood pressure.[30] Supplements of vitamin C have had various effects on blood pressure. Caffeine acutely but transiently raises blood pressure, but no association between habitual coffee consumption and the incidence of hypertension has been found.[31] In this same population, sugared or diet cola did increase the risk for hypertension.

MODERATION OF ALCOHOL. Alcohol is a two-edged sword. Too much, particularly in a binge, raises blood pressure and can have lethal effects; too little can deny multiple cardiovascular benefits (see Chap. 39). The "safe" level of regular alcohol consumption with regard to hypertension in men is less than two portions per 24 hours, although even less was found to increase the incidence of hypertension in black men.[32] A portion is defined as about 12 ml of alcohol, the equivalent of 12 oz of beer, 4 oz of wine, or 1.5 oz of liquor. Although regular consumption of moderate amounts of alcohol reduces the risk of coronary disease, heart failure, ischemic stroke, diabetes, and dementia, most experts do not recommend that those with hypertension be encouraged to drink.[33]

RELAXATION TECHNIQUES. Most studies of various cognitive-behavioral therapies have shown transient but not sustained lowering of blood pressure. However, more impressive effects were found in 45 hypertensives who received 10 hours of individualized stress management; after 6 months, ambulatory blood pressure levels were reduced by 6.1/4.3 mm Hg.[34] Perhaps acting in ways beyond relaxation, slow breathing guided by a device has also been found to lower blood pressure.[35] Repeated acupuncture does not lower blood pressure.[36]

COMBINED THERAPIES. When several life-style modifications are combined, additional antihypertensive effects may accrue, but in most trials the extent of changes has been modest. Nonetheless, falls in blood pressure of hypertensives[37] and a decreased incidence of hypertension in prehypertensives[38] have been shown. Despite the need to rely on life-style modifications in the hope of preventing hypertension and in managing the disease once it has developed, the limited success of achieving significant life-style changes in clinical practice must be recognized. Therefore, although life-style changes should be pursued, patients must not be denied the proven benefits of antihypertensive drug therapy.

ANTIHYPERTENSIVE DRUG THERAPY

In the life-style modifications described earlier are not adequate to bring the blood pressure to goal (less than 140/90 mm Hg for most, less than 130/80 mm Hg for those with diabetes or renal insufficiency), or if the level of hypertension at the onset is so high that immediate drug therapy is deemed necessary (more than 160/100 mm Hg), an overall algorithm for treatment should be followed (see Fig. 41-3).

General Guidelines

When drug therapy is decided on, the guidelines presented in Table 41-2 should be followed to provide effective 24-hour control of hypertension in a manner that encourages adherence to the regimen. The approach is based on known pharmacological principles and proven ways to improve adherence.

TABLE 41–2	Guidelines to Improve Maintenance of Antihypertensive Therapy
Be aware of the problem and be alert to signs of inadequate intake of medications: Recognize and manage depression.	
Articulate the goal of therapy: to reduce blood pressure to near-normotension with few or no side effects.	
Educate the patient about the disease and its treatment: Provide individual assessments of current risks and potential benefits of control. Involve the patient in decision-making. Provide written instructions. Encourage family support.	
Maintain contact with the patient: Encourage visits and calls to allied health personnel. Allow the pharmacist to monitor therapy. Give feedback to the patient through home blood pressure readings. Make contact with patients who do not return.	
Keep care inexpensive and simple: Do the least work-up needed to rule out secondary causes. Obtain follow-up laboratory data only yearly unless indicated more often. Use home blood pressure readings. Use nondrug, low-cost therapies. Use once-daily doses of long-acting drugs. Use generic drugs and break larger doses of tablets in half. If appropriate, use combination tablets. Use calendar blister packs (if and when they are marketed). Tailor medication to daily routines. Use detailed clinical protocols monitored by nurses and assistants.	
Prescribe according to pharmacological principles: Add one drug at a time. Start with small doses, aiming for reductions of 5 to 10 mm Hg at each step. Have medication taken immediately on awakening in the morning or after 4 AM if patient awakens to void.	
Be willing to stop unsuccessful therapy and try a different approach.	
Anticipate and address side effects: Adjust therapy to ameliorate side effects that do not disappear spontaneously.	
Continue to add effective and tolerated drugs, stepwise, in sufficient doses to achieve the goal of therapy.	
Provide feedback and validation of success.	

For most patients who do not require more intensive immediate therapy, once the most appropriate agent for initial therapy has been selected (see later), a relatively low dose of a single drug should be started, aiming for a reduction of 5 to 10 mm Hg in blood pressure at each step. Many physicians, by nature and training, wish to control a patient's hypertension rapidly and completely. Regardless of which drugs are used, this approach often leads to undue fatigue, weakness, and postural dizziness, which many patients find intolerable, particularly when they felt well before therapy was begun. Although hypokalemia and other electrolyte abnormalities may be responsible for some of these symptoms, a more likely explanation has been provided by the studies of Strandgaard and Haunso.[39] They have demonstrated the constancy of cerebral blood flow by autoregulation over a range of mean arterial pressures from about 60 to 120 mm Hg in normal subjects and from 110 to 180 mm Hg in patients with hypertension (Fig. 41-6). This shift to the right protects hypertensive patients from a surge of blood flow, which could cause cerebral edema. However, the shift also predisposes hypertensive patients to cerebral ischemia when blood pressure is lowered. The lower limit of autoregulation necessary to preserve a constant cerebral blood flow in hypertensive patients is a mean of about 110 mm Hg. Thus, acutely lowering the pressure from 160/110 mm Hg (mean, 127) to 140/85 mm Hg (mean, 102) may induce cerebral hypoperfusion, without producing hypotension in the accepted sense. This observation provides a probable explanation for what many patients experience at the start of antihypertensive therapy (e.g., fatigue, lethargy, and dizziness), even though blood pressure levels do not seem inordinately low.

Thus, the approach to antihypertensive therapy should be gradual to avoid symptoms related to overly intensive blood pressure reduction. Fortunately, as shown in the middle of Figure 41-6, if therapy is continued for a period, the curve of cerebral autoregulation shifts back toward normal, allowing patients to tolerate greater reductions in blood pressure without experiencing symptoms.

STARTING DOSAGES. The need to start with a fairly small dose also reflects a greater responsiveness of some patients to doses of medication that may be appropriate for most of them. All drugs exert increasing effects with increasing doses, up to a threshold, portrayed by logarithmic and linear dose-response curves (Fig. 41-7).[40] However, different patients require different absolute amounts of drug for their own dose-response.

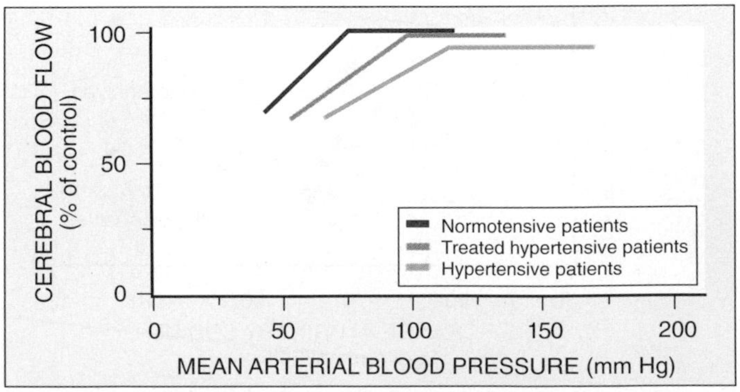

FIGURE 41–6 Mean cerebral blood flow autoregulation curves from normotensive, hypertensive, and effectively treated hypertensive patients. *(Modified from Strandgaard S: Autoregulation of cerebral blood flow in hypertensive patients. The modifying influence of prolonged antihypertensive treatment of the tolerance to acute, drug-induced hypotension. Circulation 53:720, 1976; and Strandgaard S, Haunso S: Why does antihypertensive treatment prevent stroke but not myocardial infarction? Lancet 2:658, 1987.)*

As a hypothetical example, for most patients, 50 mg of the beta blocker atenolol would provide a moderate response, shown as point A on the therapeutic effect curve in Figure 41-7, whereas a dose of 25 mg would provide only a minimal response. At dose A, providing the significant albeit partial response, the side effects would be minimal, as shown by point A′ on the curve of toxic effect. If a starting dose of 100 mg were used, the therapeutic effect would be nearly maximal (point B) but the side effects would be much greater as well (point B′). Therefore, a lower starting dose is preferable for most patients.

However, the response to a given dose is not the same for all patients but rather assumes a bell-shaped curve; some patients are very sensitive to that dose and some very resistant, with most having a moderate response. Therefore, a significant minority of patients (the very sensitive ones) would have a near-maximal response to the 25-mg dose and would better be started on 12.5 mg to achieve a moderate therapeutic effect (point A) with minimal side effects (point A′). Without knowing how individual patients will respond, the safest and easiest approach is to start at a dose that probably is not enough for most patients.

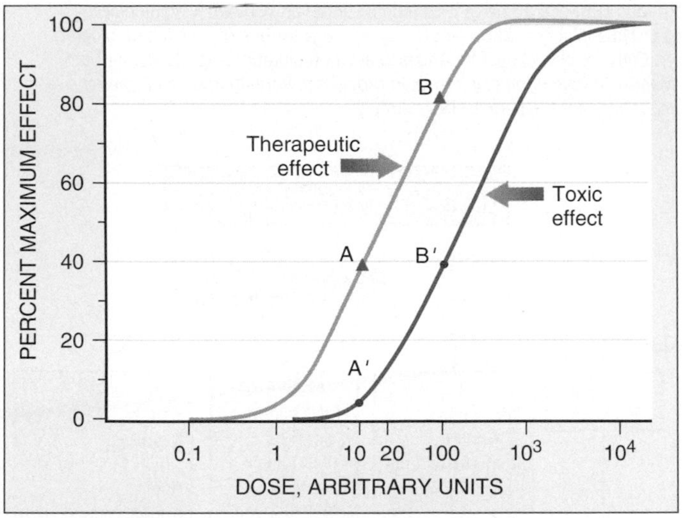

FIGURE 41–7 Theoretical therapeutic and toxic logarithmic and linear dose-response curves. The horizontal axis is the logarithmic scale with arbitrary dose limits. The vertical axis is a linear scale showing percentage of maximum possible response. *(Modified from Fagan TC: Remembering the lessons of basic pharmacology. Arch Intern Med 154:1430, 1994. ©1994 American Medical Association.)*

To allow autoregulation of blood flow to maintain perfusion to vital organs when perfusion pressure is lowered, the decline in pressure should be relatively small and gradual. More precipitous reductions in pressure, as frequently occur with larger starting doses, may induce considerable hypoperfusion, which results in symptoms that are at least bothersome (e.g., fatigue, impotence) and that may be potentially hazardous (e.g., postural hypotension, coronary ischemia). It is far better to start low and go slow.

CHOICE OF INITIAL DRUG. In the past, the choice of initial drug was largely based on perceived differences in the efficacy of lowering blood pressure and the likelihood of side effects. Although comparative trials did show some differences, largely determined by age and race,[41] most found that moderate doses of all classes of drugs provided similar efficacy. This conclusion is hardly surprising because the formulations of almost all antihypertensive drugs are designed to have the same effect—lower the blood pressure by at least 10 percent in most hypertensive patients. More than that would probably be unacceptable to patients; less than that would be unacceptable to practitioners.

Recommendations for the choice of initial therapy have been increasingly based on the compelling indications of other conditions that frequently coexist with hypertension (Table 41-3).[8,9] However, most studies have clearly shown that with equal reductions in achieved blood pressure, all drugs are equally effective in the overall hypertensive population (Fig. 41-8).[42] The one apparent exception showing a significant difference in Figure 41-8, the LIFE trial,[43] compared an angiotensin II receptor blocker (losartan) against a beta blocker (atenolol), but 80 percent of the subjects were also given a diuretic. Moreover, as will be noted later in this chapter, once-daily atenolol has been found to be inferior to all classes of drugs, making it an attractive choice in comparative trials in order to make the other drug look better.[44] This applies to the widely touted Anglo-Scandinavian Cardiac Outcomes Trial–Blood Pressure Lowering Arm (ASCOT-BPLA), which compared a long-acting calcium channel blocker (CCB; amlodipine) to the short-acting atenolol, both given once daily.[45] Moreover, the superior outcomes with the CCB could be ascribed to the lower blood pressures achieved with it.

Another trial, the Antihypertensive and Lipid Lowering Treatment to Prevent Heart Attack Trial (ALLHAT),[46] perhaps the largest ever to be done on the relative value of different antihypertensive drugs, can also be faulted for its inability to achieve equal blood pressure reductions with the comparator drugs. ALLHAT may have shown an equality between a diuretic (chlorthalidone), an angiotensin-converting enzyme (ACE) inhibitor (lisinopril), and a CCB (amlodipine), but the extensive campaign to insist that a thiazide diuretic has thereby been proven to be the best initial choice for therapy may be better justified as a cost-saving maneuver rather than as a rationale based on evidence.

Even some of the compelling indications listed in Table 41-3 do not hold up when large data bases are carefully examined. ACE inhibitors (ACEIs) and angiotensin receptor blockers (ARBs) are widely regarded as being especially renoprotective and they are listed as compelling for diabetic or other nephropathy in Table 41-3. However, in a systemic

TABLE 41–3 Indications and Contraindications for the Use of Antihypertensive Drugs

Class of Drug	Indications	Contraindications
Diuretics	Heart failure Advanced age Systolic hypertension	Gout
Beta blockers	Angina or previous myocardial infarction Heart failure Tachyarrhythmias Migraine	Asthma or chronic obstructive pulmonary disease Heart block
Alpha blockers	Prostatic hypertrophy	Incipient heart failure
Calcium channel blockers	Advanced age Systolic hypertension Cyclosporine-induced hypertension	Heart block (verapamil, diltiazem)
Angiotensin-converting enzyme inhibitors	Heart failure or left ventricular dysfunction Previous myocardial infarction Diabetic or other nephropathy or proteinuria	Pregnancy Bilateral renal artery stenosis Hyperkalemia
Angiotensin receptor blockers	Angiotensin-converting enzyme inhibitor–associated cough Diabetic or other nephropathy Congestive heart failure	Pregnancy Bilateral renal artery stenosis Hyperkalemia

review and meta-analysis of all currently available trials, the conclusion was that "In patients with diabetes, additional renoprotective actions of (ACEIs and ARBs) beyond blood pressure remain unproven, and there is uncertainty about the greater, renoprotection seen in non-diabetic renal disease."[47] Nonetheless, certain classes of drugs may provide special protection for certain classes of patient. Once again, however, the evidence is cloudy; CCBs are widely credited with greater primary protection against stroke,[48] yet in a large RCT of secondary protection, an ARB (eprosartan) was more protective against recurrent strokes than a CCB (nitrendipine), despite equal blood pressure reduction with the two agents.[49]

The achieved blood pressure reduction seems to make the difference. However, in one likely important regard, both ACEIs and ARBs seem definitely to be better than diuretics and beta blockers—protection against the onset of diabetes during the relatively short duration of most trials.[50] Experimental studies have supported the results of multiple clinical trials, so this claim is almost certainly true.

One additional point should be noted. Drugs within a given class may not provide the same long-term cardiovascular-renal protection as others of the same class, even if they provide equal short-term blood pressure reduction.[51] There are and will be very few direct comparisons of drugs in the same class, so caution is advised. As noted later, duration of antihypertensive action may be the major determinant, as appears to be true of the failure of once-daily atenolol compared with other beta blockers.[44]

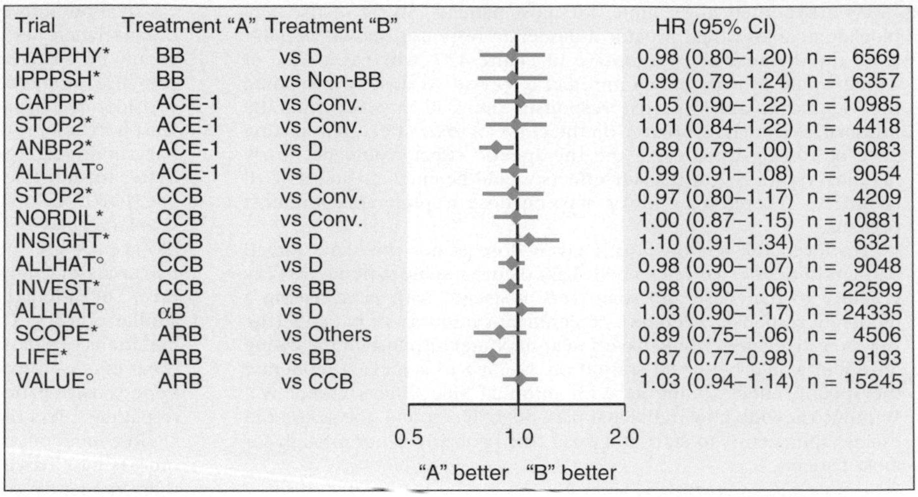

FIGURE 41–8 Trials comparing the effect on primary endpoint of treatments based on different antihypertensive drugs. Primary endpoint was cardiovascular (*) or cardiac (°) morbidity and mortality. Data are shown as differences in hazard ratio (HR) and 95 percent confidence intervals (CI). αB = alpha blocker; ACEI = angiotensin-converting enzyme inhibitor; ARB = angiotensin II receptor blocker; BB = beta blocker; CCB = calcium channel blocker; Conv. = conventional treatment (based on diuretic, beta blocker, or both); D = diuretic. *(Modified from Mancia G: Role of outcome trials in providing information on antihypertensive treatment: Importance and limitations. Am J Hypertens 19:1, 2006.)*

AN OVERALL ALGORITHM. On the basis of these data and in agreement with the JNC-7 report,[8] the algorithm shown in Figure 41-9 seems to represent an appropriate approach to the treatment of stage 1 hypertension. A low-dose thiazide diuretic should be the foundation but is likely to be adequate by itself in only about 30 percent of patients. The remainder should then be given whatever choice seems appropriate for their coexisting conditions (see Table 41-3). On the basis of these short-term efficacy trials, those with only hypertension could logically be given an ACEI if they are younger or nonblack, or a given a CCB if they are older or black.[9] Because the differential responses in blood pressure reduction are largely removed when a diuretic is also given, there seems little reason to favor any drug class in the absence of a specific indication or contraindication.

COMBINATION THERAPY. Because a low dose of a thiazide diuretic potentiates the effect of all other drug classes and because most patients, particularly those with diabetes, renal disease, or levels of blood pressure above 160/100 mm Hg, require two or more drugs for adequate control, a combination of a low-dose diuretic and the appropriate second choice may logically be used at the onset of therapy, as recommended in the JNC-7 report.[8] Other combinations are also available and may improve control of hypertension by lowering the cost and improving adherence to therapy. True polypills may emerge, but the best of such combined formulations remains uncertain.

COMPLETE COVERAGE WITH ONCE-DAILY DOSING. A number of choices within each of the six major classes of antihypertensive drugs now available provide full 24-hour efficacy. Therefore, single daily dosing should be feasible for almost all patients, resulting in improved adherence to therapy. The use of longer acting agents avoids the potential for inducing too great a peak effect to provide an adequate effect at the end of the dosing interval (the trough). Moreover, because many patients occasionally skip a dose of their drugs, there is an additional value in using agents with an inherently long duration of action that covers the skipped dose as well.

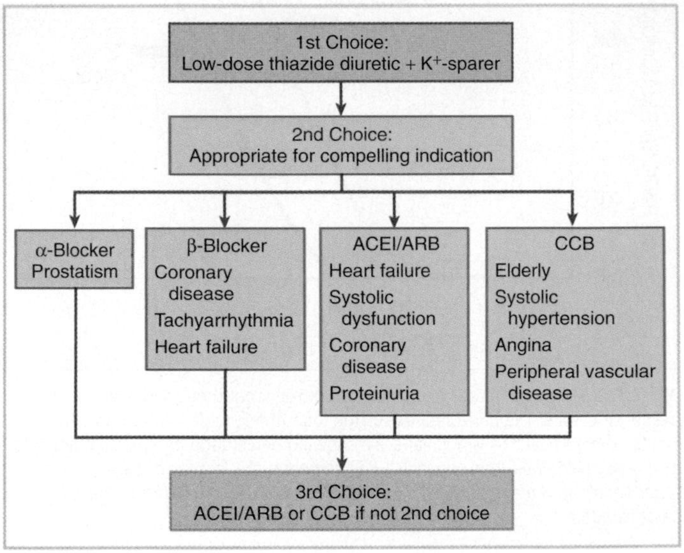

FIGURE 41–9 Algorithm for therapy of hypertension. ACEI = angiotensin-converting enzyme inhibitor; ARB = angiotensin receptor blocker; CCB = calcium channel blocker. Increasing evidence favors an aldosterone blocker as the fourth choice and perhaps as the third choice in many patients.

Long-acting choices are available within each class, such as the beta blocker metoprolol-XL, the alpha blocker doxazosin, the CCB amlodipine, the ACEI trandolapril, and the ARB telmisartan. However, because patients differ not only in terms of degree of response but also in terms of the duration of effect, the prudent course is to document the patient's response at the end of the dosing interval by home or ambulatory monitoring. With this approach, the abrupt surge in blood pressure that occurs on awakening is blunted and, it is hoped, patients can be better protected from the increased incidence of cardiovascular catastrophes at this critical time.

If short-acting medications are taken at bedtime to ensure coverage in the early morning, ischemia to vital organs might be induced by the combination of the maximal effect of the drug within the first 3 to 6 hours after intake and the usual nocturnal decline in pressure. Therefore, the safest course is to take medications with a 24 hour duration of action as early in the morning as possible.

To ensure adequate 24-hour control, home BP monitoring is essential and should be done by all patients. Their management is almost always more effectively based on frequent home readings rather than on occasional office readings.

With the general principles of therapy in mind, particulars about the various classes of drugs available are now covered.

Diuretics

Diuretics may be divided into four major groups by their primary site of action within the tubule, starting in the proximal portion and moving to the collecting duct[1]: agents acting on the proximal tubule, such as carbonic anhydrase inhibitors, which have limited antihypertensive efficacy[2]; loop diuretics[3]; thiazides and related sulfonamide compounds; and potassium-sparing agents[4] (Table 41-4). A thiazide is the usual choice, often in combination with a potassium-sparing agent. An aldosterone blocker is the more logical choice among potassium sparers. Loop diuretics should be reserved for patients with renal insufficiency or resistant hypertension.

MECHANISM OF ACTION. All diuretics initially lower blood pressure by increasing urinary sodium excretion and by reducing plasma volume, extracellular fluid volume, and cardiac output. Within 6 to 8 weeks, the lowered plasma, extracellular fluid volume, and cardiac output return toward but not completely back to normal. At this point and beyond, the lower blood pressure is related to a decline in peripheral resistance, thereby improving the underlying hemodynamic defect of hypertension. However, initial diuresis is needed because diuretics fail to lower the blood pressure when the excreted sodium is returned or when given to patients who have nonfunctioning kidneys. With the shrinkage in blood volume and lower blood pressure, increased secretion of renin and aldosterone retards the continued sodium diuresis. Both renin-induced vasoconstriction and aldosterone-induced sodium retention prevent continued diminution of body fluids and progressive reduction in blood pressure while diuretic therapy is continued.

TABLE 41–4 Representative Diuretics and Potassium-Sparing Agents

Agent	Daily Dose (mg)	Duration of Action (hr)
Thiazides		
Bendroflumethiazide (Naturetin)	1.25-5.0	>18
Hydrochlorothiazide (Esidrix, HydroDIURIL, Oretic)	6.25-50	12-18
Methyclothiazide (Enduron)	2.5-5.0	>24
Trichlormethiazide (Metahydrin, Naqua)	1-4	>34
Related Sulfonamide Compounds		
Chlorthalidone (Hygroton)	12.5-50	24-72
Indapamide (Lozol)	1.25-2.5	24
Metolazone (Mykrox, Zaroxolyn)	0.5-10	24
Loop Diuretics		
Bumetanide (Bumex)	0.5-5	4-6
Ethacrynic acid (Edecrin)	25-100	12
Furosemide (Lasix)	40-480	4-6
Torsemide (Demadex)	5-40	12
Potassium-Sparing Agents		
Amiloride (Midamor)	5-10	24
Eplerenone (Inspra)	50-200	24
Spironolactone (Aldactone)	25-100	8-12
Triamterene (Dyrenium)	50-100	12

CLINICAL EFFECTS. With daily diuretic therapy, systolic pressure usually falls about 10 mm Hg, although the degree depends on various factors, including the initial height of the pressure, quantity of sodium ingested, adequacy of renal function, and intensity of the counterregulatory renin-aldosterone response. Those with initially lower renin or aldosterone levels, including many older adult or black hypertensives, tend to have a greater antihypertensive affect. The antihypertensive effect of the diuretic persists indefinitely, although it may be overwhelmed by excessive dietary sodium intake.

If other antihypertensive drugs are used without diuretics, those that do not block the renin-aldosterone mechanism may have their efficacy blunted by sodium retention. This mechanism probably reflects the success of the drugs in lowering blood initially pressure and involves the abnormal renal pressure-natriuresis relationship that is present in primary hypertension. Just as more pressure is needed to excrete a given load of sodium in a hypertensive individual, so does a lowering of pressure toward normal lead to sodium retention.

Drugs that inhibit the renin-aldosterone mechanism, such as ACEIs, or drugs that induce some natriuresis themselves, such as calcium antagonists, may continue to work without the need for concomitant diuretics. However, a diuretic enhances the effectiveness of all other types of drugs, including calcium antagonists.

DOSAGE AND CHOICE OF AGENT. Most patients with mild to moderate hypertension and a serum creatinine concentration less than 1.5 mg/dl respond to the lower doses of the various diuretics (thiazides and related compounds) listed in Table 41-4. An amount equivalent to 12.5 mg of hydrochlorothiazide is usually adequate for uncomplicated hypertension. A single morning dose of hydrochlorothiazide provides a 24-hour antihypertensive effect but chlorthalidone is stronger and longer acting.[52] With renal damage, manifested by a serum creatinine level exceeding 1.5 mg/dl or creatinine clearance less than 30 ml/min, thiazides are usually ineffective, and two or three daily doses of furosemide, one or two doses of torsemide, or a single dose of metolazone is usually needed. The combination of a thiazide with a loop diuretic may be even more effective by countering the distal nephron hypertrophy seen with loop diuretics alone.

SIDE EFFECTS. A number of biochemical changes often accompany successful diuresis, including a decrease in plasma potassium level and increases in glucose, insulin, and cholesterol levels (Fig. 41-10). Most of these are minimized or absent with low doses of diuretic.

HYPOKALEMIA. The degree of potassium wastage and hypokalemia are directly related to the dose of diuretic; the serum potassium level falls an average of 0.7 mmol/liter with 50 mg of hydrochlorothiazide, 0.4 mmol/liter with 25 mg, and little if any with 12.5 mg. Hypokalemia related to high doses of diuretic may precipitate potentially hazardous ventricular ectopic activity and increase the risk of primary cardiac arrest, particularly in patients known to be susceptible because of concomitant digitalis therapy or myocardial irritability.

The following maneuvers should help prevent diuretic-induced hypokalemia:

- Use the smallest dose of diuretic needed.
- Restrict sodium intake to less than 100 mmol/day.
- Increase dietary potassium intake.
- Use a combination of a thiazide and potassium-sparing agent with caution in patients with renal insufficiency or in association with an ACEI or ARB.
- Use a concomitant beta blocker, ACEI, or ARB, which diminishes potassium loss by blunting the diuretic-induced rise in renin and aldosterone levels.

Hypomagnesemia. In some patients, concomitant diuretic-induced magnesium deficiency prevents restoration of intracellular deficits of potassium, so hypomagnesemia should be corrected.

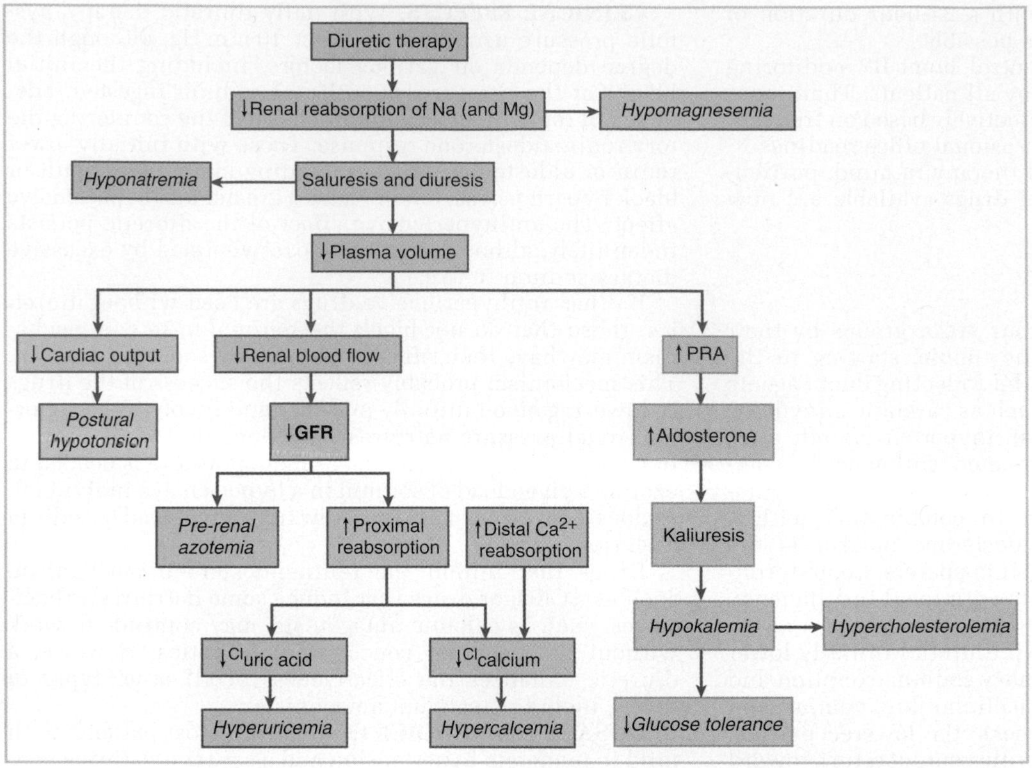

FIGURE 41–10 The mechanisms by which chronic diuretic therapy may lead to various complications. The mechanism for hypercholesterolemia remains in question, although it is shown as arising from hypokalemia. Cl = clearance; GFR = glomerular filtration rate; PRA = plasma renin activity.

Hyperuricemia. The serum uric acid level is elevated in as many as one third of untreated hypertensive patients. With long-term high-dose diuretic therapy, hyperuricemia appears in another third of patients as a consequence of increased proximal tubule reabsorption accompanying volume contraction and may precipitate acute gout. Because asymptomatic hyperuricemia does not cause urate deposition, most investigators agree that it need not be treated.

Hyperglycemia and Insulin Resistance. High doses of diuretics may impair glucose tolerance and precipitate diabetes mellitus, probably because they increase insulin resistance and hyperinsulinemia.

Hypercalcemia. A slight rise in the serum calcium level, less than 0.5 mg/dl, is frequently seen with thiazide diuretic therapy and is accompanied by a 40 to 50 percent decrease in urinary calcium excretion. Thiazide therapy thereby protects against renal stones and osteoporosis.

Hyponatremia. Thiazides may cause insidious hyponatremia, usually in older women.

Erectile Dysfunction. An increase in the incidence of impotence has been noted in men who took 15 mg of chlorthalidone, and this diuretic was the only one of five classes of agents accompanied by this effect.[53]

Renal Cell Carcinoma. A significant but numerically small increase in renal cell carcinoma among diuretic users has been documented.

Sulfa Sensitivity. Ethacrynic acid, the only diuretic that does not have a sulfonamide structure and can be used in those sensitive to sulfas. A slow rechallenge with a sulfonamide diuretic may be successful in overcoming sulfa sensitivity.

LOOP DIURETICS. Loop diuretics are usually needed in the treatment of hypertensive patients with renal insufficiency, defined here as a serum creatinine level exceeding 1.5 mg/dl. Furosemide has been most widely used, although metolazone may be as effective and requires only a single daily dose. When given once or twice daily, furosemide for uncomplicated hypertension provides less antihypertensive action than longer acting diuretics, which better maintain the slight volume contraction needed for the antihypertensive effect of diuretics.

POTASSIUM-SPARING AGENTS. These drugs are normally used in combination with a thiazide diuretic. Of the four currently available, two (eplerenone and spironolactone) are aldosterone antagonists; the other two (triamterene and amiloride) are direct inhibitors of potassium secretion. In combination with a thiazide diuretic, they diminish the amount of potassium wasting. Moreover, low doses of spironolactone have been found to prevent myocardial fibrosis and reduce mortality in patients with heart failure. Eplerenone is a more selective aldosterone antagonist than spironolactone, thereby avoiding the gynecomastia and menstrual irregularities sometimes seen with spironolactone. In view of the increasing evidence that even normal levels of aldosterone induce fibrosis in various tissues, such a selective aldosterone blocker may find much wider use as a potassium sparer.

AN OVERVIEW OF DIURETICS IN HYPERTENSION. A low dose of a thiazide diuretic should almost always be the initial choice of drug therapy for most hypertensives. If not the first choice, a diuretic should certainly be the second drug used. In those with more severe hypertension or renal damage, larger doses of a thiazide or a loop-acting agent are needed. The potential for multiple adverse effects that can be associated with diuretics requires appropriate monitoring but, overall, they remain the least expensive choice and may also provide other benefits, such as protection against osteoporosis.

Adrenergic Inhibitors

A number of drugs that inhibit the adrenergic nervous system are available, including some that act centrally on vasomotor center activity, peripherally on neuronal catecholamine discharge, or by blocking alpha- or beta-adrenergic receptors, or both (Table 41-5); some act at numerous sites. Figure 41-11, a schematic view of the ending of an adrenergic nerve and the effector cell with its receptors, depicts how some of these drugs act. An important aspect of sympathetic activity involves the feedback of norepinephrine to alpha- and beta-adrenergic receptors located on the neuronal surface (i.e., presynaptic receptors). Presynaptic alpha-adrenergic receptor activation inhibits release, whereas presynaptic beta activation stimulates further norepinephrine release.

Drugs That Act on the Neuron

Reserpine, guanethidine, and related compounds act in different ways to inhibit the release of norepinephrine from peripheral adrenergic neurons.

RESERPINE. Reserpine, the most active and widely used of the derivatives of the rauwolfia alkaloids, depletes the postganglionic adrenergic neurons of norepinephrine by inhibiting its uptake into storage vesicles, exposing it to degradation by cytoplasmic monoamine oxidase. The peripheral effect is predominant, although the drug enters the brain and depletes central catecholamine stores as well. This effect probably accounts for the sedation and depression accompanying reserpine use. The drug has certain advantages; only one dose a day is needed and, in combination with a diuretic, the antihypertensive effect is substantial and causes little postural hypotension, and many

TABLE 41-5	Adrenergic Inhibitors Used in Treatment of Hypertension
Peripheral Neuronal Inhibitors	
Reserpine	
Guanethidine (Ismelin)	
Guanadrel (Hylorel)	
Central Adrenergic Inhibitors	
Methyldopa (Aldomet)	
Clonidine (Catapres)	
Guanabenz (Wytensin)	
Guanfacine (Tenex)	
Alpha Receptor Blockers	
Alpha$_1$ and alpha$_2$ receptors	
Phenoxybenzamine (Dibenzyline)	
Alpha$_1$ receptor	
Doxazosin (Cardura)	
Prazosin (Minipress)	
Terazosin (Hytrin)	
Beta Receptor Blockers	
Acebutolol (Sectral)	
Atenolol (Tenormin)	
Betaxolol (Kerlone)	
Bisoprolol (Zebeta)	
Carteolol (Cartrol)	
Metoprolol (Lopressor, Toprol-XL)	
Nadolol (Corgard)	
Penbutolol (Levatol)	
Pindolol (Visken)	
Propranolol (Inderal)	
Timolol (Blocadren)	
Alpha and Beta Receptor Blockers	
Labetalol (Normodyne, Trandate)	
Carvedilol (Coreg)	

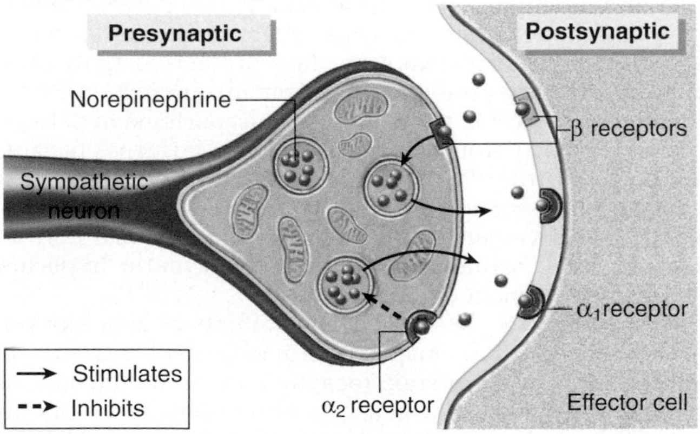

FIGURE 41–11 Simplified schematic view of the adrenergic nerve ending showing that norepinephrine (NE) is released from its storage granules when the nerve is stimulated and enters the synaptic cleft to bind to alpha$_1$ and beta receptors on the effector cell (postsynaptic). In addition, a short feedback loop exists in which NE binds to alpha$_1$ and beta receptors on the neuron (presynaptic) to inhibit or stimulate further release, respectively.

patients experience no side effects. The drug has a relatively flat dose-response curve, so that a dose of only 0.05 mg/day provides almost as much antihypertensive effect as 0.125 or 0.25 mg/day but with fewer side effects. Although it remains popular in some areas and is recommended as an inexpensive choice where resources are limited, use of reserpine has progressively declined because it has no commercial sponsor.

GUANETHIDINE. This agent and a series of related guanidine compounds, including guanadrel, bethanidine, and debrisoquine, act by inhibiting the release of norepinephrine from the adrenergic neurons. Blood pressure is reduced mainly when the patient is upright, as a result of gravitational pooling of blood in the legs, because compensatory sympathetic nervous system–mediated vasoconstriction is blocked. This effect results in the most common side effect, postural hypotension. Unlike reserpine, guanethidine has a steep dose-response curve, so that it can be successfully used in treating hypertension of any degree in daily doses of 10 to 300 mg. As other drugs have become available, guanethidine and related compounds have been relegated mainly to the treatment of severe hypertension unresponsive to all other agents.

Drugs That Act on Receptors

PREDOMINANTLY CENTRAL ALPHA AGONISTS

Of these, only clonidine has much current use, although methyldopa remains one of the few drugs approved for treatment of pregnancy-induced hypertension (see Chap. 77).

METHYLDOPA. The primary site of action of methyldopa is in the central nervous system, where alpha-methylnorepinephrine, derived from methyldopa, is released from adrenergic neurons and stimulates central alpha-adrenergic receptors, reducing the sympathetic outflow from the central nervous system. The blood pressure falls mainly as a result of a decrease in peripheral resistance, with little effect on cardiac output. Renal blood flow is well maintained, and significant postural hypotension is unusual. Methyldopa need be given no more than twice daily, in doses ranging from 250 to 3000 mg/day.

Side effects include some that are common to centrally acting drugs that reduce sympathetic outflow, such as sedation, dry mouth, impotence, and galactorrhea. However, methyldopa causes some unique side effects that are probably of an autoimmune nature because a positive antinuclear antibody test result is obtained in about 10 percent of patients who take the drug, and red cell autoantibodies occur in about 20 percent. Inflammatory disorders in various organs have been reported, most commonly involving the liver (with diffuse parenchymal injury similar to that in viral hepatitis).

CLONIDINE. Although of different structure, clonidine shares many features with methyldopa. It acts at the same central sites, has similar antihypertensive efficacy, and causes many of the same bothersome but less serious side effects (e.g., sedation, dry mouth). It does not, however, induce autoimmune and inflammatory side effects. The drug has a fairly short biological half-life, so that when it is discontinued, the inhibition of norepinephrine release disappears within about 12 to 18 hours and the plasma catecholamine level rises. This effect is responsible for the rapid rebound of the blood pressure to pretreatment levels and the occasional appearance of withdrawal symptoms, including tachycardia, restlessness, and sweating. If the rebound requires treatment, clonidine may be reintroduced or alpha-adrenergic receptor antagonists given. Clonidine is available in a *transdermal* preparation, which may provide smoother blood pressure control for as long as 7 days, with fewer side effects. Bothersome skin rashes preclude its use in perhaps one fourth of patients, however.

GUANABENZ. This drug differs in structure from but shares many characteristics with both methyldopa and clonidine, acting primarily as a central alpha agonist.

GUANFACINE. This drug is also similar to clonidine but is longer acting, which enables once-daily dosing and minimizes rebound hypertension. This agent, although used less than clonidine, is the preferred choice of central alpha agonists.

ALPHA-ADRENERGIC RECEPTOR ANTAGONISTS

These agents may have many attractive features but their use has been limited, initially because of the potential for postural hypotension, and more recently because of a greater likelihood of fluid retention that may provoke congestive heart failure.[46] The first of this class was prazosin but the two that are now used, doxazosin and terazosin, have slower onset and longer duration of action so that they may be given once daily, with less propensity for first-dose hypotension.

Selective alpha blockers are as effective as other antihypertensives.[37] The favorable hemodynamic changes—a fall in peripheral resistance with maintenance of cardiac output—make them an attractive choice for patients who wish to remain physically active. In addition, blood lipids and insulin sensitivity are not adversely altered and may actually improve with alpha blockers, unlike the adverse effects observed with diuretics and beta blockers. The ALLHAT data[46] have clearly indicated the need to use a diuretic with an alpha blocker, particularly in those with left ventricular hypertrophy (LVH) or other risk factors for congestive heart failure. Alpha blockers are now being used primarily for the relief of prostatism. By decreasing the tone of the smooth muscle at the bladder neck and prostate, they relieve the obstructive symptoms of prostatic hypertrophy.

BETA-ADRENERGIC RECEPTOR ANTAGONISTS

In the 1980s, beta-adrenergic receptor blockers became the most popular form of antihypertensive therapy after diuretics, reflecting their relative effectiveness and freedom from many bothersome side effects. Because beta blockers reduce mortality in patients with post-myocardial infarction or heart failure (i.e., secondary prevention), it was assumed they would also provide special protection against initial cardiac events (i.e., primary prevention). However, in multiple large RCTs, the use of beta blockers, particularly atenolol, provided no more protection against the first myocardial infarction (MI) than other drugs and was associated with a statistically significant 16 percent increase in the incidence of stroke.[54] A rationale has long been known but only recently appreciated: beta blockers lower brachial systolic blood pressure equally but lower aortic pressure less well than other drugs. This occurs because they reduce the heart rate so much that the arterial wave reflection from the periphery returns during systole rather than diastole.[55] Therefore, Lindholm and associates have concluded that "beta-blockers should not remain [as] first choice in the treatment of primary hypertension."[54]

DIFFERENCES IN BETA BLOCKERS. Many beta blockers are now available in the United States (Fig. 41-12). Pharmacologically, they differ considerably from one another with respect to degree of absorption, protein binding, and bioavailability. However, the three most important differences affecting their clinical use are cardioselectivity, intrinsic sympathomimetic activity, and lipid solubility. Despite these differences, they all seem to be about equally effective as antihypertensives.

Cardioselectivity. Cardioselectivity refers to the relative blocking effect on the $beta_1$-adrenergic receptors in the heart compared with that on the $beta_2$ receptors in the bronchi, peripheral blood vessels, and elsewhere. Such cardioselectivity has been shown using small doses in acute studies; with the rather high doses used to treat hypertension, much of this selectivity is lost.

Intrinsic Sympathomimetic Activity. Some of these drugs have intrinsic sympathomimetic activity, interacting with beta receptors to cause a measurable agonist response but at the same time blocking the greater agonist effects of endogenous catecholamines.

Lipid Solubility. Atenolol and nadolol are among the least lipid-soluble of the beta blockers, so that they escape hepatic metabolism and are excreted unchanged. Lipid-soluble agents, such as metoprolol and propranolol, are taken up and metabolized in the liver and therefore are more bioavailable after intravenous than oral administration.

MECHANISM OF ACTION. Despite these and other differences, the various beta blockers now available are approximately equipotent as antihypertensive agents. A number of possible mechanisms are likely to be involved in their antihypertensive action. For those without intrinsic sympathomimetic activity, cardiac output falls 15 to 20 percent and renin release is reduced about 60 percent. Central nervous system beta-adrenergic receptor blockade may reduce sympathetic discharge. At the same time that beta blockers lower blood pressure through various mechanisms, their blockade of peripheral beta-adrenergic receptors inhibits vasodilation, leaving alpha receptors open to catecholamine-mediated vasoconstriction. Over time, however, vascular resistance tends to return to normal, which presumably preserves the antihypertensive effect of a reduced cardiac output.

CLINICAL EFFECTS. Even in small doses, beta blockers begin to lower blood pressure within a few hours. Although progressively higher doses have usually been given, careful study has shown a near-maximal effect from smaller doses. Even though beta blockers are less protective than other drugs for primary protection, they remain important for the secondary protection they provide to hypertensive patients with coexisting coronary disease or heart failure.[56] Because beta blockers inhibit sympathetic activity, they have been widely used to reduce the somatic manifestations of stress in people as divergent as violin players and racecar drivers. However, their value in younger, hyperkinetic hypertensives has never been documented.

SIDE EFFECTS. Most of the side effects of beta blockers are related to their major pharmacological action, the blockade of beta-adrenergic receptors. Certain concomitant problems may worsen when beta-adrenergic receptors are blocked, including peripheral vascular disease and bronchospasm. However, in a meta-analysis of 29 studies, cardioselective beta blockers did not have clinically significant adverse respiratory effects in patients with mild to moderate reactive airway disease or chronic obstructive pulmonary disease.[57] The most common side effect is fatigue, probably a consequence of decreased cardiac output. Sexual dysfunction may be increased by beta blockers but depression likely is not.

Beta blockers increase the incidence of diabetes, presumably through a decrease in insulin sensitivity. Diabetic patients may have additional problems with beta blockers, more so with those that are nonselective. The responses to hypoglycemia, both the symptoms (except sweating) and the counterregulatory hormonal changes that raise blood glucose levels, are partially dependent on sympathetic nervous activity. Diabetic patients who are susceptible to hypoglycemia may not be aware of the usual warning signals, except sweating, and may not rebound as quickly.

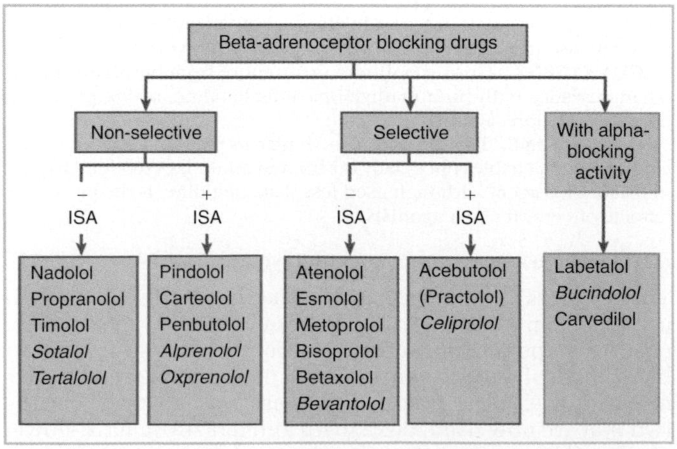

FIGURE 41–12 Classification of beta-adrenoreceptor blockers on the basis of cardioselectivity and intrinsic sympathomimetic activity. Drugs not approved for use in the United States for treatment of hypertension are in italics. ISA = intrinsic sympathomimetic activity. *(Modified from Kaplan NM: Kaplan's Clinical Hypertension, 8th ed. Baltimore, Lippincott Williams & Wilkins, 2002, p 262.)*

Perturbations of lipoprotein metabolism accompany the use of beta blockers. Nonselective agents cause greater rises in triglyceride levels and reductions in cardioprotective high-density lipoprotein cholesterol levels. When a beta blocker is suddenly discontinued, angina pectoris and myocardial infarction may occur. Because patients with hypertension are more susceptible to coronary disease, they should be weaned gradually and given appropriate coronary vasodilator therapy.

Caution is advised in the use of beta blockers for patients suspected of harboring a pheochromocytoma (see Chaps. 40 and 81) because unopposed alpha-adrenergic agonist action might precipitate a serious hypertensive crisis if this disease is present. The use of beta blockers during pregnancy has been clouded by scattered case reports of various fetal problems.

OVERVIEW OF BETA BLOCKERS IN HYPERTENSION. Beta blockers are specifically recommended for hypertensive patients with concomitant coronary disease, particularly after a myocardial infarction, congestive heart failure, or tachyarrhythmia (see Table 41-3). If a beta blocker is chosen, the agents that are more cardioselective offer the likelihood of fewer perturbations of lipid and carbohydrate metabolism and, because of fewer side effects (except for bradycardia), better adherence to therapy. Long-acting formulations are available for once-daily dosing.

ALPHA- AND BETA-ADRENERGIC RECEPTOR ANTAGONISTS

The combination of an alpha and beta blocker in a single molecule is available in the forms of labetalol and carvedilol, with the latter agent approved for treatment of heart failure as well. The fall in pressure results mainly from a decrease in peripheral resistance, with little or no decline in cardiac output. The most bothersome side effects are related to postural hypotension. Both need to be given twice daily. Intravenous labetalol is used to treat hypertensive emergencies.

Vasodilators

In the past, direct-acting arteriolar vasodilators were used mainly as third drugs, when combinations of a diuretic and adrenergic blocker failed to control blood pressure. However, with the availability of vasodilators of different types, such as ACEIs, ARBs, and CCBs, which can be easily tolerated when used as first or second drugs, wider and earlier application of vasodilators in the treatment of hypertension has evolved.

Direct Vasodilators

Hydralazine is the most widely used agent of this type. Minoxidil is more potent but is usually reserved for patients with severe, refractory hypertension associated with renal failure. Nitroprusside and nitroglycerin are given intravenously for hypertensive crises and are discussed later (see "Therapy for Hypertensive Crises").

HYDRALAZINE. Hydralazine, in combination with a diuretic and beta blocker, has been used frequently to treat severe hypertension. The drug acts directly to relax the smooth muscle in precapillary resistance vessels, with little or no effect on postcapillary venous capacitance vessels. As a result, blood pressure falls by a reduction in peripheral resistance but, in the process, a number of compensatory processes, which are activated by the arterial baroreceptor arc, blunt the decrease in pressure and cause side effects. With concomitant use of a diuretic to overcome the tendency for fluid retention and an adrenergic inhibitor to prevent the reflex increase in sympathetic activity and rise in the renin level, the vasodilator is more effective and causes few, if any, side effects.

The drug need be given only twice a day. Its daily dose should be kept below 400 mg to prevent the lupus-like syndrome that appears in 10 to 20 percent of patients who receive more than 400 mg. This reaction, although uncomfortable to the patient, is almost always reversible. The reaction happens seldom with daily doses of 200 mg or less and is more common in slow acetylators of the drug.

MINOXIDIL. This drug vasodilates by opening potassium channels in vascular smooth muscle. Its hemodynamic effects are similar to those of hydralazine, but minoxidil is even more effective and may be used once daily. It is particularly useful for patients with severe hypertension and renal failure. Even more than with hydralazine, diuretics and adrenergic receptor blockers must be used with minoxidil to prevent the reflex increase in cardiac output and fluid retention. Pericardial effusions have appeared in about 3 percent of those given minoxidil, in some without renal or cardiac failure. The drug also causes hair to grow profusely, and the facial hirsutism precludes use of the drug in most women.

Calcium Channel Blockers (see also Chap. 54)

These drugs are among the most popular classes of agents used in the treatment of hypertension. Claims of multiple serious side effects of their use, mostly based on biased observational studies, have been repudiated by data from multiple RCTs, including ALLHAT, in which coronary events were the same for the CCB as for the diuretic or ACEI, and mortality from noncardiovascular causes was significantly lower in the CCB group than in the diuretic or ACEI group.[46]

MECHANISMS OF ACTION. All currently available CCBs interact with the same L-type voltage-gated plasma membrane channel but at different sites and with different consequences. Dihydropyridines (DHPs) have the greatest peripheral vasodilatory action, with little effect on cardiac automaticity, conduction, or contractility. However, comparative trials have shown that verapamil and diltiazem, which do affect these properties, are also effective antihypertensives and may cause fewer side effects related to vasodilation, such as flushing and ankle edema. They induce slight bradycardia and should be used carefully with a beta blocker or in patients with a conduction defect.

CLINICAL USE. CCBs are effective in hypertensive patients of all ages and races. DHP-CCBs reduced cardiovascular events and deaths (Table 41-6) against placebo in RCTs. Compared with other classes of drugs, they may protect better against stroke but less well against heart failure.[58,59] CCBs appear particularly effective in prevention of stroke in older adult hypertensives, perhaps because they tend to have a greater antihypertensive effect than seen in younger patients. They also appear to lower blood pressure in blacks better than in other racial groups[9] but, with equal degrees of blood pressure reduction, they are no better in cardioprotection than a diuretic or ACEI (see Table 41-6).

Calcium antagonists may cause at least an initial natriuresis, probably by producing renal afferent vasodilation, which may lessen the need for concurrent diuretic therapy. In fact, unlike all other antihypertensive agents, they may have their effectiveness reduced rather than enhanced by concomitant dietary sodium restriction, whereas most careful studies show an enhancement of their effect by concomitant diuretic therapy.

The use of CCBs has been questioned in two important groups of hypertensives, those with diabetes and those with nephropathy. Concerning the use of CCBs in patients with type 2 diabetes, a DHP-CCB, nitrendipine, provided excellent protection in those enrolled in the Systolic Hypertension in Europe (Syst-Eur) trial,[60] even better than that provided by a diuretic in the SHEP trial. Therapy based on the DHP-CCB felodipine provided a 51 percent reduction in major cardiovascular events in the 1501 patients with diabetes enrolled in the HOT trial. Among the almost 12,000 diabetics in the ALLHAT trial, the CCB amlodipine was as protective as the ACEI or diuretic.[46]

TABLE 41–6 Comparative Randomized Controlled Trials for Hypertension—Hazard Rate (95% CI)

Therapy	Stroke	Coronary Disease	Heart Failure	CV Events	CV Death	Total Mortality
ACEI versus placebo	0.84 (0.72-0.97)	0.79 (0.71-0.88)	0.82 (0.69-0.96)	0.78 (0.71-0.85)	0.80 (0.68-0.93)	0.88 (0.81-0.96)
CCB versus placebo	0.65 (0.55-0.78)	0.83 (0.67-1.03)	0.99 (0.53-1.86)	0.81 (0.70-0.94)	0.75 (0.59-0.96)	0.88 (0.74-1.04)
ACEI versus D/βB	1.09 (0.96-1.24)	0.97 (0.90-1.05)	0.94 (0.55-1.59)	1.02 (0.97-1.08)	1.03 (0.95-1.11)	0.94 (0.80-1.11)
CCB versus D/βB	0.92 (0.85-0.99)	1.02 (0.96-1.09)	1.27 (1.01-1.61)	1.04 (0.97-1.08)	1.05 (0.97-1.15)	0.95 (0.87-1.03)
ACEI versus CCB	1.08 (0.91-1.28)	0.83 (0.65-1.05)	0.84 (0.75-0.95)	0.95 (0.86-1.04)	1.03 (0.83-1.27)	1.04 (0.94-1.15)

ACEI = angiotensin-converting enzyme inhibitor; CCB = calcium channel blocker; CV = cardiovascular; D/βB = diuretic/beta blocker.

Data from Turnbull F, Neal B, Algert C, et al: Effects of different blood pressure-lowering regimens on major cardiovascular events in individuals with and without diabetes mellitus: Results of prospectively designed overviews of randomized trials. Arch Intern Med 165:1410, 2005; and Verdecchia P, Reboldi G, Angeli F, et al: Angiotensin-converting enzyme inhibitors and calcium channel blockers for coronary heart disease and stroke prevention. Hypertension 46:386, 2005.

The trials included in these two meta-analyses differed somewhat. In the report from Turnbull and colleagues, 27 trials from 1985 to 2003, which included congestive heart failure and mortality endpoints, were included; in the report from Verdecchia and associates, 29 trials comparing ACEIs and CCBs for prevention only of coronary heart disease and stroke from 1996 through 2004 were included.

Concerning the use of CCBs in patients with nephropathy, investigators have agreed that an ACEI or ARB should be the first drug used. However, to provide the degree of blood pressure reduction required to protect such patients maximally, additional drugs are almost always required. A CCB is an appropriate choice as the third drug, with a diuretic as the second. Clearly, a CCB is not as renoprotective as an ACEI[17] or ARB[61] when used as the initial drug but, if needed to achieve the goal of therapy, a CCB is just as clearly an appropriate addition. On the basis of greater reduction in proteinuria seen with non–DHP-CCBs, some researchers think that a non–DHP-CCB should be used. However, the addition of a DHP-CCB does not interfere with the renoprotective effect of ACEIs or ARBs.[61] Moreover, renal function, assessed by estimated glomerular filtration rate, was better preserved by the DHP-CCB than by the diuretic or the ACEI in the ALLHAT study.[46]

SIDE EFFECTS. Side effects preclude the use of these drugs in perhaps 10 percent of patients. Most side effects, such as headaches, flushing, and local ankle edema, are related to the vasodilation for which the drugs are given. With slow-release and longer acting formulations, vasodilative side effects are reduced. It should be no surprise that in a few patients, the antihypertensive effect of the short-acting agents, particularly liquid nifedipine, may be so marked as to reduce blood flow and induce ischemia of vital organs, calling for a moratorium on their use.

A potentially serious adverse effect of the use of calcium antagonists to treat hypertension has been described in a case-control study in which more hypertensive patients who had a myocardial infarction were taking short-acting calcium antagonists than hypertensive patients who had not had an infarct.[62] The most likely explanation for the finding is exclusion bias, which is an inherent problem with case-control studies in which the cases are at greater risk for the complication than the controls; that is, higher risk patients are excluded from the control group but not from the case group. The decrease in coronary events in large RCTs with *long-acting* DHPs is the best proof of the safety of these agents. Similar claims based on case-control studies, that calcium antagonists increase cancer and gastrointestinal bleeding, have also been refuted.[46] Calcium antagonists may be unique in *not* having their antihypertensive efficacy blunted by nonsteroidal antiinflammatory drugs (NSAIDs).[60]

OVERVIEW OF CALCIUM CHANNEL BLOCKERS. CCBs reduce stroke more but heart attacks less than other therapies while having similar effects on overall mortality.[58,59] They work well and are usually well tolerated across the entire spectrum of hypertensives. They have some particular niches—coexisting angina and cyclosporine or NSAID use. If chosen, an inherently long-acting, second-generation DHP such as amlodipine seems the best choice because it maintains better blood pressure control in the critical early morning hours and on throughout the next day if the patient misses a dose. Rate-slowing CCBs, such as verapamil or diltiazem, may be preferable in certain circumstances.

Angiotensin-Converting Enzyme Inhibitors

Activity of the renin-angiotensin system may be inhibited in four ways, all of which can be applied clinically. The first, use of beta-adrenergic receptor blockers to inhibit the release of renin, was discussed earlier. The second, direct inhibition of renin activity by a selective renin inhibitor, aliskiren, has now become available.[63] The third, inhibition of the enzyme that converts the inactive decapeptide angiotensin I (A I) to the active octapeptide angiotensin II (A II), has achieved widespread use with orally effective ACEIs. The fourth, blockade of angiotensin's actions by a competitive receptor blocker, is the basis for the fastest growing class of antihypertensive agents, the ARBs. ARBs may offer additional benefits, but their immediate advantage is the absence of cough that often accompanies ACEIs, as well as less angioedema (see later, "Angiotensin II Receptor Blockers").

MECHANISM OF ACTION. The first of the ACEIs, captopril, was synthesized as a specific inhibitor of the angiotensin-converting enzyme (ACE) that, in the classic pathway, breaks the peptidyl dipeptide bond in angiotensin I. Because A II cannot be formed and A I is inactive, the ACEI paralyzes the classic renin-angiotensin system, thereby removing the effects of most endogenous A II as both a vasoconstrictor and stimulant of aldosterone synthesis.

Interestingly, with long-term use of ACEIs, the plasma A II levels actually return to previous values but the blood pressure remains lowered,[64,65] which suggests that the antihypertensive effect may involve other mechanisms. The same ACE enzyme that converts A I to A II also inactivates the vasodilating hormone bradykinin. By inhibiting the breakdown of bradykinin, ACEIs increase the concentration of a vasodilating hormone while decreasing the concentration of a vasoconstrictor hormone. The increased plasma kinin levels may contribute to the vasodilatory and other beneficial effects of ACEIs, but they are also probably responsible for the most common and bothersome side effects of their use, a dry hacking cough and, less frequently, angioedema.

Regardless of their mechanism of action, ACEIs lower blood pressure mainly by reducing peripheral resistance with little, if any, effect on heart rate, cardiac output, or body fluid volumes, probably reflecting preservation of baroreceptor reflexes. As they restore endothelium-dependent relaxation, resistance arteries become less thickened and more responsive.

CLINICAL USE. In patients with uncomplicated primary hypertension, ACEIs as monotherapy provide antihypertensive effects equal to those of other classes, but they are somewhat less effective in blacks and older adults because of their lower renin levels. Addition of a diuretic, even as little as 6.25 mg of hydrochlorothiazide, enhances the efficacy of an ACEI. More important, ACEI-based therapy has provided significant protection against cardiovascular disease and death when compared against placebo and comparable if not better protection than other classes of drugs (see Table 41-6). In the ALLHAT trial, involving predominantly elderly, high-risk hypertensives, ACEI-based therapy was equal to diuretic-or CCB-based therapies in most respects except against strokes in the black enrollees, probably because of less antihypertensive efficacy.[46] In the Australian National Blood Pressure Study, involving elderly but lower risk hypertensives, ACEI-based therapy provided better protection against cardiovascular events than diuretic-based therapy for the men but not for the women.[65]

ACEIs have proven impressively effective for treatment of hypertensives (and nonhypertensives) with coronary disease or congestive heart failure, as detailed in Chapters 25 and 54. They have become the drug of choice for chronic renal disease, whether diabetic or nondiabetic in origin. The high levels of renin, arising in the juxtaglomerular cells within the renal afferent arterioles, flood the glomeruli and renal efferent arterioles, providing ACEIs (and ARBs) the opportunity to dilate these vessels selectively and lower intraglomerular pressure more effectively than other classes of drugs. These hemodynamic effects may lower renal perfusion and glomerular filtration. However, because acute increases of serum creatinine levels, up to 30 percent, that stabilize within the first 2 months of ACEI therapy are associated with *better* long-term renoprotection, such increased levels should not prompt withdrawal of the drug.[66] On the other hand, renal failure after prolonged use of an ACEI in four patients (and with an ARB in one) that apparently resolved after discontinuation of the ACEI (or ARB) has been reported,[67] so close observation of such patients is needed.

Whether ACEIs and ARBs provide renal and cardiac protection beyond their antihypertensive effects remains in question. The issue has been most intensively studied in patients with proteinuria because it the results are easy to measure. Controlled trials have suggested that the antiproteinuric effect of an ACEI is directly related to its antihypertensive effect, but the data are insufficient. As noted later (see "Angiotensin II Receptor Blockers: Clinical Use"), the potential for an additional antihypertensive effect of an ARB added to an ACEI also remains uncertain.

These drugs have been a mixed blessing for patients with renovascular hypertension. On the one hand, they usually control blood pressure effectively. On the other hand, the removal of the high levels of A II that follow their use may deprive the stenotic kidney of the hormonal drive to its blood flow, thereby causing a marked decline in renal perfusion; consequently, patients with solitary kidneys or bilateral disease may develop acute and sometimes persistent renal failure.

SIDE EFFECTS. Most patients who take an ACEI experience neither the side effects nor biochemical changes often accompanying the use of other drugs that may be of more concern, even though they are not as obvious; neither rises in lipids, glucose, or uric acid levels nor reductions in potassium levels have been noted. To be sure, ACEIs may have specific and nonspecific adverse effects. Specific effects include rare rashes, loss of taste, and leukopenia. In addition, they may cause a hypersensitivity reaction with angioneurotic edema, most frequently in blacks, or a cough, most frequently in Asians.[68] The cough is infrequently associated with pulmonary dysfunction but may not disappear until 3 weeks after the ACEI is discontinued. If a cough appears in a patient who needs an ACEI, an ARB should be substituted.

A more serious problem with ACEIs and ARBs taken by women during pregnancy is their effect on the fetus. The interference with renal development has long been recognized with their use in the second and third trimesters. Even more threatening is the possibility that their use during the first trimester may cause major cardiac and central nervous system malformations.[69] If further documented, this would preclude use of these drugs in virtually all women with child-bearing potential.

The antihypertensive efficacy of ACEIs may be blunted by large (300-mg) doses of aspirin and most NSAIDs. Patients with renal insufficiency or those taking potassium supplements or potassium-sparing agents may not be able to excrete potassium loads and therefore may develop hyperkalemia.

OVERVIEW OF ANGIOTENSIN-CONVERTING ENZYME INHIBITORS. The rationale for the use of ACEIs in the treatment of hypertension has steadily expanded beyond their proven efficacy as antihypertensive agents. In particular, they have proven to provide special advantages in three large groups of patients, those with heart failure, coronary ischemia, or nephropathy. They are the drugs of choice for such patients (see Table 41-3). Moreover, the evidence from the Heart Outcomes Prevention Evaluation (HOPE) trial[70] has led to the recommendation that an ACEI be given to all patients at high risk for coronary disease, whether hypertensive or not. Although an ACEI-based therapy did not outperform a diuretic or a CCB in the ALLHAT trial,[46] their proven special benefits ensure their increased use. Even as ACEIs have become increasingly popular, their position has been threatened by the aggressive marketing of ARBs, agents acting at a more distal site of the renin-angiotensin system.

Angiotensin II Receptor Blockers

MECHANISMS OF ACTION. ARBs displace A II from its specific AT_1 receptor, antagonizing all of its known effects and resulting in a dose-dependent fall in peripheral resistance and little change in heart rate or cardiac output. As a consequence of the competitive displacement, circulating levels of A II increase but, at the same time, the blockade of the renin-angiotensin mechanism is more complete, including any A II that is generated through pathways that do not involve the ACE enzyme. No obvious good or bad effects of the increased A II levels have been proved (along with the higher renin levels, as also seen with ACEIs).

The longest acting ARB, telmisartan, also has been found by in vitro, animal, and limited human studies to have unique (to ARBs) insulin-sensitizing effects, likely because of its structural similarity to PPAR gamma agonists.[71] The major obvious difference between ARBs and ACEIs is the absence of an increase in kinin levels, which may be responsible for some of the beneficial effects of ACEIs and probably more of their side effects. Direct comparisons between the two types of drugs show little difference in antihypertensive efficacy, but cough is not provoked by the ARB, although angioedema has been reported.[72] Losartan has a uricosuric effect that is not seen with other ARBs.[73] As with ACEIs, ARBs have been found to improve endothelial dysfunction and correct the altered structure of resistance arteries in patients with hypertension.[74]

CLINICAL USE. In the recommended doses, all six currently available ARBs have comparable antihypertensive efficacy and all are potentiated by addition of a diuretic. The dose-response curve is fairly flat for all these agents. ARBs have cardiovascular and renal protective effects equal to, if not better than, those of other classes of antihypertensive drugs.[58] The addition of an ARB to a presumed maximal dose of an ACEI has not been shown to increase the antihypertensive effect but did reduce the progression of nondiabetic nephropathy.[75] ARB-based therapy reduces the progress of renal damage in patients with type 2 diabetes with nephropathy; their use in heart failure is described in Chapter 25. Therapy based on the ARB losartan caused LVH to regress and reduced the number of cardiovascular events more than therapy based on the beta blocker atenolol in the LIFE trial of hypertensives with LVH.[43] Potentially important insulin-sensitizing effects of telmisartan await the findings of ongoing outcome trials.

SIDE EFFECTS. Whether or not they are more effective than ACEIs, ARBs are easier to take. In various clinical trials, side effects were generally no greater than with placebo, and the agent was better tolerated than other antihypertensive agents. Fetal toxicity, hyperkalemia, hypotension, and renal impairment are almost certain to be noted occasionally because they are expected consequences of blockade of the renin-angiotensin mechanism but, as yet, no major surprises have surfaced. Their superior side effect profile has prompted the use of one ARB, candesartan, in the TROPHY trial of treating prehypertension.[4]

OVERVIEW OF ANGIOTENSIN II RECEPTOR BLOCKERS. As reflected by the fast growth of the use of ARBs, they are surely being prescribed for many more patients than the 10 percent or so who are intolerant of an ACEI. With the intensely competitive market for the six (or more) of these agents now being heavily promoted, their use will likely continue to grow. However, caution is advised; additional outcome data are needed to determine whether they are as good as the proven ACEIs. All current expert guidelines have recommended ARBs only for those who should receive an ACEI but are intolerant, usually because of cough. Many outcome trials now in progress should provide proof of their special value beyond that found for type II diabetic nephropathy.[61]

Other Agents

Use of the first of the most promising new class of drugs, neutral endopeptidase inhibitors, was curtailed by a high incidence of angioedema. Old vasodilators now used extensively for coronary ischemia, the nitrate isosorbide and transdermal glyceryl trinitrate, are attractive antihypertensive agents but are not likely to be tested properly because of the lack of commercial sponsors. Meanwhile, glitazones, now used for the treatment of diabetes, lower blood pressure in nondiabetic hypertensives, logically as a consequence of improved insulin sensitivity.[76] Statins, sildenafil, progestins with antimineralocorticoid activity, uricosurics, and many more currently used agents may have useful antihypertensive effects. Others now in development will likely be added.

SPECIAL CONSIDERATIONS IN THERAPY

WITHDRAWAL OF DRUGS. As many as 20 percent of treated patients with well-controlled hypertension are able to maintain normotension for as long as 1 year after withdrawal of their drugs. Considering how difficult it may be to achieve adequate control, withdrawal seems inappropriate if the therapy does not cause adverse effects.

RESISTANT HYPERTENSION. There are numerous causes of resistance to therapy, usually defined as the failure of diastolic blood pressure to fall below 90 mm Hg despite the use of three or more drugs (Table 41-7). Patients often do not respond well because they do not take their medications. Often overlooked is physician inertia to modify therapy, a problem that can be overcome particularly in an integrated health care delivery system with appropriate surveillance.[77]

TABLE 41–7 Causes of Inadequate Responsiveness to Therapy

Pseudoresistance	
"White coat" or office elevations	
Pseudohypertension in the elderly	
Nonadherence to Therapy	
Side effects of medication	
Cost of medication	
Lack of consistent and continuous primary care	
Inconvenient and chaotic dosing schedules	
Instructions not understood	
Inadequate education of patients	
Dementia (e.g., memory deficit)	
Drug-Related Causes	
Doses too low	
Inappropriate combinations (e.g., two centrally acting adrenergic inhibitors)	
Rapid inactivation (e.g., hydralazine)	
Drug interactions	
Nonsteroidal anti-inflammatory drugs	Oral contraceptives
Sympathomimetics	Adrenal steroids
Nasal decongestants	Licorice (chewing tobacco)
Appetite suppressants	Cyclosporine
Cocaine	Erythropoietin
Caffeine	Cholestyramine
Antidepressants (monoamine oxidase inhibitors, tricyclics)	
Excessive volume contraction with stimulation of renin and aldosterone	
Hypokalemia (usually diuretic induced)	
Rebound after clonidine withdrawal	
Associated Conditions	
Smoking	
Increasing obesity	
Sleep apnea	
Insulin resistance or hyperinsulinemia	
Ethanol intake more than 1 oz/d (more than three portions)	
Anxiety-induced hyperventilation or panic attacks	
Chronic pain	
Intense vasoconstriction (Raynaud, arteritis)	
Secondary Hypertension	
Renal insufficiency	
Renovascular hypertension	
Pheochromocytoma	
Primary aldosteronism	
Volume Overload	
Excess sodium intake	
Progressive renal damage (nephrosclerosis)	
Fluid retention related to reduction of blood pressure	
Indequate diuretic therapy	

What appears to be a poor response on the basis of office readings of blood pressure may be disclosed to be an adequate response when ambulatory or home readings are done. A number of factors may account for a poor response, even if the medication is taken regularly. Most common is volume overload caused by inadequate diuretic or excessive dietary sodium intake. Larger doses or more potent diuretics often bring resistant hypertension under control.

ANESTHESIA IN HYPERTENSIVE PATIENTS (see Chap. 80). In the absence of significant cardiac dysfunction or other target organ damage, hypertension adds little to the cardiovascular risks of surgery. If possible, however, hypertension should be well controlled by medications before anesthesia and surgery to reduce the risk of myocardial ischemia. Therefore, patients taking antihypertensive medications should continue these drugs, if necessary using dermal or intravenous formulations, as long as the anesthesiologist is aware of their use and takes reasonable precautions to prevent wide swings in pressure. The very short-acting beta blocker esmolol has been successful in preventing surges in blood pressure during intubation, and the use of beta blockers reduced cardiac events in high-risk patients undergoing vascular or nonvascular surgery.

HYPERTENSIVE CHILDREN. Almost nothing is known about the effects of various antihypertensive medications given to children over long periods. In the absence of adequate data, an approach similar to that advocated for adults is advised.[78] Emphasis should be placed on weight reduction in hypertensive children who are obese in the hope of attempting to control hypertension without the need for drug therapy.

HYPERTENSION DURING PREGNANCY. This topic is discussed in Chapters 40 and 77.

HYPERTENSION IN ELDERLY PERSONS (see Chap. 75). A few older adults may have high blood pressure as measured by the sphygmomanometer but may have less or no hypertension when direct intraarterial readings are made—that is, pseudohypertension related to rigid arteries that do not collapse under the cuff.

If the systolic blood pressure alone or both systolic and diastolic levels are elevated, careful lowering of blood pressure with diuretics or DHP calcium antagonists unequivocally reduces cardiovascular morbidity in older hypertensive patients, up to age 80 years.[10] Care is needed because they may have a number of problems with the medications (Table 41-8). In view of the reduced effectiveness of the baroceptor reflex and the failure of peripheral resistance to rise appropriately with standing, postural hypotension should be carefully sought and, if present, addressed before starting antihypertensive therapy. All drugs should be given in slowly increasing doses to prevent excessive lowering of the pressure. Concerns remain about drug treatment of the older old, those over age 80. The small amount of available data shows protection against stroke but possible increases in mortality.[11]

For all older adults, therapy should be started if systolic levels are above 160 mm Hg and slowly increased to bring the level to approximately 150 mm Hg. If the systolic pressure does not go below 160 mm Hg, despite moderate doses of three medications, including a diuretic, attention should be directed to other cardiovascular risk factors but no more antihypertensive drugs given. Caution is advised if the diastolic level goes below 65 mm Hg.[14]

HYPERTENSION IN BLACKS. As noted earlier, blacks have more hypertension and suffer more target organ damage from it, particularly stroke and renal damage. Therapy may need to be started earlier and pursued more vigorously. Blacks, similar to older adults, tend to respond better to diuretics or CCBs as monotherapy, because both groups tend to have lower renin levels and therefore respond less to renin-inhibiting drugs. They also have more angioedema with ACEIs but no more cough than nonblacks.[68]

TABLE 41–8 Possible Causes of Increased Risk from Pharmacological Treatment of Hypertension in Older Adults

Cause	Potential Complications
Diminished baroreceptor activity	Orthostatic hypotension
Decreased intravascular volume	Orthostatic hypotension, dehydration
Sensitivity of hypokalemia	Arrhythmia, muscle weakness
Decreased renal and hepatic function	Drug accumulation
Polypharmacy	Drug interaction
Central nervous system changes	Depression, confusion

PATIENTS WITH HYPERTENSION AND DIABETES (see Chap. 43). Special attention should be given to diabetic patients with hypertension. The two commonly coexist and multiply the cardiovascular risks of each alone. Fortunately, evidence from several trials has now documented the protection provided by *intensive* control of hypertension, in concert with management of the diabetes and dyslipidemia that commonly accompanies the two. Most diabetic hypertensive patients need two or more antihypertensive drugs to bring their pressure to below 130/85 mm Hg, which is probably the highest level that should be tolerated. The benefits of such intensive management were clearly documented in a 7.8-year follow-up of 160 patients with type 2 diabetes and hypertension with microalbuminuria.[79] In the half given more intensive management, the risks of having a cardiovascular event, neuropathy, retinopathy, or autonomic neuropathy were all reduced by 50 percent or more. An ACEI and/or ARB should be included if proteinuria is present. Control will likely require a diuretic and a long-acting DHP.

HYPERTENSIVE PATIENTS WITH IMPOTENCE. Erectile dysfunction is common in hypertensive patients, especially in those who are also diabetic. The problem may be exacerbated by diuretic therapy, even in appropriately low doses. Fortunately, 5-phosphodiesterase inhibitors often return erectile ability, even in the presence of various antihypertensive drugs, with no greater likelihood of adverse events than in those not receiving antihypertensive therapy, with the exception of nitrates.

HYPERTENSION WITH CONGESTIVE HEART FAILURE. Cardiac output may fall so markedly in hypertensive patients who are in heart failure with systolic dysfunction that their blood pressure is reduced, obscuring the degree of hypertension; often, however, the diastolic blood pressure is raised by intense vasoconstriction while the systolic pressure falls as a result of the reduced stroke volume. Lowering the blood pressure may, by itself, relieve the heart failure. Chronic unloading has been most efficiently accomplished with ACEIs, ARBs, aldosterone blockers, and beta blockers, which reduce morbidity and mortality further in ACEI-treated patients in heart failure. As noted in Chapter 40, LVH is frequently found by echocardiography, even in patients with mild hypertension. All antihypertensive drugs except direct vasodilators have been shown to cause LVH to regress, and regression may continue for as long as 5 years of treatment.

HYPERTENSION WITH ISCHEMIC HEART DISEASE. The coexistence of ischemic heart disease makes antihypertensive therapy even more essential because relief of the hypertension may ameliorate the coronary disease. Beta blockers and calcium antagonists are particularly useful if angina or arrhythmia is present. Caution is needed to avoid decreased coronary perfusion, which may be responsible for the J curve seen in several trials (see earlier, "Goal of Therapy").[13,14] The often markedly high levels of blood pressure during the early phase of an acute myocardial infarction may reflect sympathetic nervous hyperreactivity to pain. Antihypertensive drugs that do not decrease cardiac output may be used cautiously in the immediate postinfarction period, whereas beta blockers and ACEIs provide long-term benefit.

HYPERTENSION AND STROKES. As the most direct cause of strokes, hypertension causes even more strokes than heart attacks as people grow older. Reduction of elevated blood pressure protects against stroke much more

TABLE 41–9 Parenteral Drugs for Treatment of Hypertensive Emergency

Drug*	Dose	Onset of Action	Adverse Effects†
Diuretics			
Furosemide	20-40 mg in 1-2 min, repeated and higher doses with renal insufficiency	5-15 min	Volume depletion, hypokalemia
Vasodilators			
Nitroprusside (Nitropress)	0.25-10 µg/kg/min as IV infusion	Immediate	Nausea, vomiting, muscle twitching, sweating, thiocyanate and cyanide intoxication
Nitroglycerin (Nitro-Bid IV)	5-100 µ/min as IV infusion	2-5 min	Headache, vomiting, methemoglobinemia, tolerance with prolonged use
Fenoldopam (Corlopam)	0.1-0.6 µg/kg/min as IV infusion	4-5 min	Reflex tachycardia, increased intraocular pressure, headache
Nicardipine‡ (Cardene I.V.)	5-15 mg/h IV	5-10 min	Headache, nausea, flushing, tachycardia, local phlebitis
Hydralazine (Apresoline)	10-20 mg IV 10-50 mg IM	10-20 min 20-30 min	Tachycardia, flushing, headache, vomiting, worsening of angina
Adrenergic Inhibitors			
Phentolamine	5-15 mg IV	1-2 min	Tachycardia, flushing, headache
Esmolol (Brevibloc)	200-500 mg/kg/min for 4 min, then 50-300 µg/kg/min IV	1-2 min	Hypotension, nausea
Labetalol (Normodyne, Trandate)	20-80 mg IV bolus every 10 min 2 mg/min IV infusion	5-10 min	Vomiting, scalp tingling, burning in throat, dizziness, nausea, heart block, orthostatic hypotension

*In order of rapidity of action.
†Hypotension may occur with any.
‡Intravenous formulations of other calcium channel blockers are also available.

than heart attack.[7] However, if a stroke occurs and blood pressure is high, as it usually is, uncertainty remains about whether to lower it, because lowering pressure could extend cerebral ischemia by lowering cerebral blood flow and perfusion. If the blood pressure is lowered, short-acting parenteral drugs that can be quickly reduced if the stroke progresses have generally been used. Transdermal glyceryl trinitrate may safely lower blood pressure and maintain cerebral blood flow while providing rapid reversibility if there is too much of a decrease in blood pressure.[80] After stroke, reduction of hypertension unquestionably reduces recurrence.

THERAPY FOR HYPERTENSIVE CRISES

When diastolic blood pressure exceeds 140 mm Hg, rapidly progressive damage to the arterial vasculature is demonstrable experimentally, and a surge of cerebral blood flow may rapidly lead to encephalopathy (see Chap. 40). If such high pressures persist or if there are any signs of encephalopathy, the pressures should be lowered using parenteral agents in patients considered to be in immediate danger or with oral agents in those who are alert and in no other acute distress.

A number of drugs for this purpose are currently available (Table 41-9). If diastolic pressure exceeds 140 mm Hg and the patient has any complications, such as an aortic dissection, a constant infusion of nitroprusside is most effective and almost always lowers the pressure to the desired level. Constant monitoring with an intraarterial line is mandatory because a slightly excessive dose may lower the pressure abruptly to levels that induce shock. The potency and rapidity of action of nitroprusside have made it the treatment of choice for life-threatening hypertension. However, because nitroprusside acts as a venous and arteriolar dilator, venous return and cardiac output are lowered and intracranial pressures may increase. Therefore, other parenteral agents are being more widely used, including labetalol and the calcium antagonist nicardipine.

With any of these agents, intravenous furosemide is often needed to lower blood pressure further and prevent retention of salt and water. Diuretics should not be given if volume depletion is initially present. For patients in less immediate danger, oral therapy may be used. Almost every drug has been used and most, with repeated doses, reduce high blood pressure. The prior preference for liquid nifedipine by mouth or sublingually has been diminished because of occasional ischemic complications resulting from too rapid reduction in blood pressure. Oral doses of other short-acting formulations may be used, including furosemide, propranolol, captopril, or felodipine. A safer course for any patients, particularly if their current high blood pressures simply reflect stopping previously effective oral medication and they are asymptomatic, is simply to restart the previous medication and monitor their response closely. If their nonadherence to therapy was caused by side effects, appropriate changes should be made.

Most centers are seeing fewer patients in hypertensive crisis, presumably because more patients are diagnosed and treated before the disease proceeds on this malignant course. The continued successful treatment of many more hypertensive persons will prevent the more frequent long-range cardiovascular complications of hypertension.

FUTURE PERSPECTIVES

The treatment of hypertension will continue to improve, both in quantity and quality. However, because the genetic foundations will elude correction in the near term and the environmental precipitants will probably never be controllable, the management of hypertension will continue to command considerable resources and work. Treatment may become less difficult with more long-acting, easier to take medications, but there will never be a silver bullet to cure the disease. The greatest need is to prevent young people from developing bad habits that predispose them to hypertension. Prevention may only be possible with pills. Perhaps, as in rats, the pills may need to be taken early in life but, without reliable markers to identify those who will become hypertensive before age 60, this seems unlikely. Lastly, the number of older adults will continue to increase and without the ability to prevent atherosclerotic stiffening of their arteries, they will be the most needy and least manageable of those with hypertension.

REFERENCES

General Guidelines

1. Kaplan NM: Treatment of hypertension: Why, when, how far. *In* Kaplan NM: Kaplan's Clinical Hypertension. 9th ed. Philadelphia, Lippincott, Williams & Wilkins, 2006, pp 161-191.
2. Kshirsagar AV, Carpenter M, Bang H, et al: Blood pressure usually considered normal is associated with an elevated risk of cardiovascular disease. Am J Med 119:133, 2006.
3. Jackson R, Lawes CM, Bennett DA, et al: Treatment with drugs to lower blood pressure and blood cholesterol based on an individual's absolute cardiovascular risk. Lancet 365:434, 2006.
4. Julius S, Nesbitt SD, Egan BM, et al: Feasibility of treating prehypertension with an angiotensin-receptor blocker. N Engl J Med 354:1685, 2006.
5. Wald NJ, Law MR: A strategy to reduce cardiovascular disease by more than 80 percent. BMJ 326:1419, 2006.
6. Wang JG, Staessen JA, Franklin SS, et al: Systolic and diastolic blood pressure lowering as determinants of cardiovascular outcome. Hypertension 45:907, 2005.
7. Staessen JA, Wang JG, Thijs L: Cardiovascular prevention and blood pressure reduction: A quantitative overview updated until 1 March 2003. J Hypertens 21:1055, 2003.
8. National High Blood Pressure Education Program Coordinating Committee: Seventh report of the Joint National Committee on Prevention, Detection, Evaluation, and Treatment of High Blood Pressure. Hypertension 42:1206, 2003.
9. Williams B, Poulter NR, Brown MJ, et al: Guidelines for management of hypertension: Report of the fourth working party of the British Hypertension Society, 2004-BHS IV. J Hum Hypertens 18:139, 2004.

Benefits and Targets of Therapy

10. Forette F, Seux ML, Staessen JA, et al: The prevention of dementia with antihypertensive treatment: New evidence from the Systolic Hypertension in Europe (Syst-Eur) study. Arch Intern Med 162:2046, 2002.
11. Bulpitt CJ, Beckett NS, Cooke J, et al: Results of the pilot study for the Hypertension in the Very Elderly Trial. J Hypertens 21:2409, 2003.
12. Skoog I, Lithell H, Hansson L, et al: Effect of baseline cognitive function and antihypertensive treatment on cognitive and cardiovascular outcomes: Study on COgnition and Prognosis in the Elderly (SCOPE). Am J Hypertens 18:1052, 2005.
13. Messerli FH, Mancia G, Conti CR, et al: Dogma disputed: Can aggressively lowering blood pressure in hypertensive patients with coronary artery disease be dangerous? Ann Intern Med 144:884, 2006.
14. Somes GW, Pahor M, Shorr RI, et al: The role of diastolic blood pressure when treating isolated systolic hypertension. Arch Intern Med 159:2004, 1999.
15. Boutitie F, Gueyffier F, Pocock S, et al: J-shaped relationship between blood pressure and mortality in hypertensive patients: New insights from a meta-analysis of individual-patient data. Ann Intern Med 136:438, 2002.
16. Arima H: Lower target blood pressures are safe and effective for the prevention of recurrent stroke: The PROGRESS trial. J Hypertens 24:1201, 2006.
17. Wright JT Jr, Bakris G, Greene T, et al: Effect of blood pressure lowering and antihypertensive drug class on progression of hypertensive kidney disease: Results from the AASK trial. JAMA 288:2421, 2002.
18. Pickering TG: Target blood pressure in patients with end-stage renal disease: Evidence-based medicine or the emperor's new clothes? J Clin Hypertens (Greenwich) 8:369, 2006.
19. Nissen SE, Tuzcu EM, Libby P, et al: Effect of antihypertensive agents on cardiovascular events in patients with coronary disease and normal blood pressure: The CAMELOT study: A randomized controlled trial. JAMA 292:2217, 2004.

Life-Style Modification

20. Diabetes Prevention Program Research Group: Reduction in the incidence of type 2 diabetes with lifestyle intervention of metformin. N Engl J Med 346:393, 2002.
21. Najem B, Houssiere A, Pathak A, et al: Acute cardiovascular and sympathetic effects of nicotine replacement therapy. Hypertension 47:1162, 2006.
22. Sjostrom L, Lindroos AK, Peltonen M, et al: Lifestyle, diabetes, and cardiovascular risk factors 10 years after bariatric surgery. N Engl J Med 351:2683, 2004.
23. Elley CR, Arroll B: Refining the exercise prescription for hypertension. Lancet 366:1248, 2005.

23a. He J, MacGregor GA: Effect of modest salt reduction on blood pressure: A meta-analysis of randomized trials. Implications for public health. J Hum Hypertens 16:766, 2002.

24. Tuomilehto J, Jousilahti P, Rastenyte D, et al: Urinary sodium excretion and cardiovascular mortality in Finland: a prospective study. Lancet 357:848, 2001.
25. Geleijnse J: Blood pressure response to changes in sodium and potassium intake: A metaregression analysis of randomised trials. J Hum Hypertens 17:471, 2003.
26. He FJ, Nowson CA, MacGregor GA: Fruit and vegetable consumption and stroke: Meta-analysis of cohort studies. Lancet 367:320, 2006.
27. Griffith LE, Guyatt GH, Cook RJ, et al: The influence of dietary and nondietary calcium supplementation on blood pressure: An updated meta-analysis of randomized controlled trials. Am J Hypertens 12:84, 1999.
28. Jee SH, Miller ER III, Guallar E, et al: The effect of magnesium supplementation on blood pressure: A meta-analysis of randomized clinical trials. Am J Hypertens 15:691, 2002.
29. John JH, Ziebland S, Yudkin P, et al: Effects of fruit and vegetable consumption on plasma antioxidant concentrations and blood pressure: A randomised controlled trial. Lancet 359:1969, 2002.
30. Elliott P, Stamler J, Dyer AR, et al: Association between protein intake and blood pressure: The INTERMAP Study. Arch Intern Med 166:79, 2006.
31. Winkelmayer WC, Stampfer MJ, Willett WC, et al: Habitual caffeine intake and the risk of hypertension in women. JAMA 294:2330, 2005.
32. Fuchs FD, Chambless LE, Whelton PK, et al: Alcohol consumption and the incidence of hypertension: The Atherosclerosis Risk in Communities Study. Hypertension 37:1242, 2001.
33. Beilin LJ, Puddey IB: Alcohol and hypertension: An update. Hypertension 47:1035, 2006.
34. Linden W, Lenz JW, Con AH: Individualized stress management for primary hypertension: A randomized trial. Arch Intern Med 161:1071, 2001.
35. Rosenthal T, Alter A, Peleg E, et al: Device-guided breathing exercises reduce blood pressure: Ambulatory and home measurements. Am J Hypertens 14:74, 2001.
36. Macklin E, Wayne PM, Kalish LA, et al: Stop Hypertension with the Acupuncture Research Program (SHARP): Results of a randomized, controlled clinical trial. Hypertension 48:838, 2006.
37. Neaton JD, Grimm RH Jr, Prineas RJ, et al: Treatment of Mild Hypertension Study. Final results. Treatment of Mild Hypertension Study Research Group. JAMA 270:713, 1993.
38. Elmer PJ, Obarzanek E, Vollmer WM, et al: Effects of comprehensive lifestyle modification on diet, weight, physical fitness, and blood pressure control: 18-month results of a randomized trial. Ann Intern Med 144:485, 2006.

Pharmacological Therapy

39. Strandgaard S, Haunsø S: Why does antihypertensive treatment prevent stroke but not myocardial infarction? Lancet 2:658, 1987.
40. Fagan TC: Remembering the lessons of basic pharmacology. Arch Intern Med 154:1430, 1994.
41. Brown MJ: Hypertension and ethnic group. BMJ 332:833, 2006.
42. Mancia G: Role of outcome trials in providing information on antihypertensive treatment: importance and limitations. Am J Hypertens 19:1, 2006.
43. Dahlof B, Devereux RB, Kjeldsen SE, et al: Cardiovascular morbidity and mortality in the Losartan Intervention For Endpoint reduction in hypertension study (LIFE): A randomised trial against atenolol. Lancet 359:995, 2002.
44. Psaty BM, Weiss NS, Furberg CD: Recent trials in hypertension: Compelling science or commercial speech? JAMA 295:1704, 2006.
45. Dahlof B, Sever PS, Poulter NR, et al: Prevention of cardiovascular events with an antihypertensive regimen of amlodipine adding perindopril as required versus atenolol adding bendroflumethiazide as required, in the Anglo-Scandinavian Cardiac Outcomes Trial–Blood Pressure Lowering Arm (ASCOT-BPLA): A multicentre randomised controlled trial. Lancet 366:895, 2005.
46. ALLHAT Investigators and Coordinators for the ALLHAT Collaborative Research Group: Major outcomes in high-risk hypertensive patients randomized to angiotensin-converting enzyme inhibitor or calcium channel blocker vs diuretic: The Antihypertensive and Lipid-Lowering Treatment to Prevent Heart Attack Trial (ALLHAT). JAMA 288:2981, 2002.
47. Casas JP, Chua W, Loukogeorgakis S, et al: Effect of inhibitors of the renin-angiotensin system and other antihypertensive drugs on renal outcomes: Systematic review and meta-analysis. Lancet 366:2026, 2005.
48. Turnbull F: Effects of different blood-pressure-lowering regimens on major cardiovascular events: Results of prospectively-designed overviews of randomised trials. Lancet 362:1527, 2003.
49. Schrader J, Luders S, Kulschewski A, et al: Morbidity and Mortality After Stroke, Eprosartan Compared with Nitrendipine for Secondary Prevention: Principal results of a prospective randomized controlled study (MOSES). Stroke 36:1218, 2005.
50. Mancia G, Grassi G, Zanchetti A: New-onset diabetes and antihypertensive drugs. J Hypertens 24:3, 2006.
51. Pickering TG: Class effects and labeling of antihypertensive drugs. J Clin Hypertens (Greenwich) 8:215, 2006.
52. Ernst ME, Carter BL, Goerdt CJ, et al: Comparative antihypertensive effects of hydrochlorothiazide and chlorthalidone on ambulatory and office blood pressure. Hypertension 47:352, 2006.
53. Grimm RH Jr, Grandits GA, Prineas RJ, et al: Long-term effects on sexual function of five antihypertensive drugs and nutritional hygienic treatment in hypertensive men and women. Treatment of Mild Hypertension Study (TOMHS). Hypertension 29:8, 1997.
54. Lindholm LH, Carlberg B, Samuelsson O: Should beta blockers remain first choice in the treatment of primary hypertension? A meta-analysis. Lancet 366:1545, 2005.
55. Williams B, Lacy PS, Thom SM, et al: Differential impact of blood pressure-lowering drugs on central aortic pressure and clinical outcomes: Principal results of the Conduit Artery Function Evaluation (CAFE) study. Circulation 113:1213, 2006.
56. Devereaux PJ, Beattie WS, Choi PT, et al: How strong is the evidence for the use of perioperative beta blockers in non-cardiac surgery? Systematic review and meta-analysis of randomised controlled trials. BMJ 331:313, 2005.
57. Salpeter SR, Ormiston TM, Salpeter EE: Cardioselective beta-blockers in patients with reactive airway disease: A meta-analysis. Ann Intern Med 137:715, 2002.
58. Turnbull F, Neal B, Algert C, et al: Effects of different blood pressure-lowering regimens on major cardiovascular events in individuals with and without diabetes mellitus: Results of prospectively designed overviews of randomized trials. Arch Intern Med 165:1410, 2005.
59. Verdecchia P, Reboldi G, Angeli F, et al: Angiotensin-converting enzyme inhibitors and calcium channel blockers for coronary heart disease and stroke prevention. Hypertension 46:386, 2005.
60. Celis H, Thijs L, Staessen JA, et al: Interaction between nonsteroidal anti-inflammatory drug intake and calcium-channel blocker-based antihypertensive treatment in the Syst-Eur trial. J Hum Hypertens 15:613, 2001.

61. Brenner BM, Cooper ME, de ZD, et al: Effects of losartan on renal and cardiovascular outcomes in patients with type 2 diabetes and nephropathy. N Engl J Med 345:861, 2001.
62. Psaty BM, Heckbert SR, Koepsell TD, et al: The risk of myocardial infarction associated with antihypertensive drug therapies. JAMA 274:620, 1995.
63. Azizi M, Webb R, Nussberger J, et al: Renin inhibition with aliskiren: Where are we now, and where are we going? J Hypertens 24:243, 2006.
64. Forclaz A, Maillard M, Nussberger J, et al: Angiotensin II receptor blockade: Is there truly a benefit of adding an ACE inhibitor? Hypertension 41:31, 2003.
65. Wing LM, Reid CM, Ryan P, et al: A comparison of outcomes with angiotensin-converting enzyme inhibitors and diuretics for hypertension in the elderly. N Engl J Med 348:583, 2003.
66. Bakris GL, Weir MR: Angiotensin-converting enzyme inhibitor-associated elevations in serum creatinine: Is this a cause for concern? Arch Intern Med 160:685, 2003.
67. Onuigbo MA, Onuigbo NT: Late onset renal failure from angiotensin blockade (LORFFAB): A prospective thirty-month Mayo Health System clinic experience. Med Sci Monit 11:CR462, 2005.
68. McDowell SE, Coleman JJ, Ferner RE: Systematic review and meta-analysis of ethnic differences in risks of adverse reactions to drugs used in cardiovascular medicine. BMJ 332:1177, 2006.
69. Cooper WO, Hernandez-Diaz S, Arbogast PG, et al: Major congenital malformations after first-trimester exposure to ACE inhibitors. N Engl J Med 354:2443, 2006.
70. Danchin N, Cucherat M, Thuillez C, et al: Angiotensin-converting enzyme inhibitors in patients with coronary artery disease and absence of heart failure or left ventricular systolic dysfunction: An overview of long-term randomized controlled trials. Arch Intern Med 166:787, 2006.
71. Sugimoto K, Qi NR, Kazdova L, et al: Telmisartan but not valsartan increases caloric expenditure and protects against weight gain and hepatic steatosis. Hypertension 47:1003, 2006.
72. Warner KK, Visconti JA, Tschampel MM: Angiotensin II receptor blockers in patients with ACE inhibitor-induced angioedema. Ann Pharmacother 34:526, 2000.
73. Dang A, Zhang Y, Liu G, et al: Effects of losartan and irbesartan on serum uric acid in hypertensive patients with hyperuricaemia in Chinese population. J Hum Hypertens 20:45, 2006.
74. Brassard P, Amiri F, Schiffrin EL: Combined angiotensin II type 1 and type 2 receptor blockade on vascular remodeling and matrix metalloproteinases in resistance arteries. Hypertension 46:598, 2005.
75. Nakao N, Yoshimura A, Morita H, et al: Combination treatment of angiotensin-II receptor blocker and angiotensin-converting-enzyme inhibitor in non-diabetic renal disease (COOPERATE): A randomised controlled trial. Lancet 361:117, 2003.
76. Sarafidis PA, Lasaridis AN: Actions of peroxisome proliferator-activated receptors-gamma agonists explaining a possible blood pressure-lowering effect. Am J Hypertens 19:646, 2006.
77. Rodondi N, Peng T, Karter AJ, et al: Therapy modifications in response to poorly controlled hypertension, dyslipidemia, and diabetes mellitus. Ann Intern Med 144:475, 2006.
78. National High Blood Pressure Education Program Working Group on Hypertension Control in Children and Adolescents: Update on the 1987 task force report on high blood pressure in choldren and adolescents: A working group report from the National High Blood Pressure Education Program. Pediatrics 98:649, 1996.
79. Gaede P, Vedel P, Larsen N, et al: Multifactorial intervention and cardiovascular disease in patients with type 2 diabetes. N Engl J Med 348:383, 2003.
80. Willmot M, Ghadami A, Whysall B, et al: Transdermal glyceryl trinitrate lowers blood pressure and maintains cerebral blood flow in recent stroke. Hypertension 47:1209, 2006.

GUIDELINES *Thomas H. Lee*

Treatment of Hypertension

The major U.S. guidelines for management of hypertension are issued by the Joint National Committee on Prevention, Detection, Evaluation, and Treatment of High Blood Pressure, a group coordinated by the National Heart Lung and Blood Institute (NHLBI). Its seventh and most recent guidelines were published in 2003, and are known as JNC-7.[1] Other recent recommendations have been published in other countries, such as guidelines from the British Hypertension Society in 2004[2] and the Canadian Hypertension Education Program in 2006.[3,4] In 2003, recommendations regarding blood pressure control in patients with diabetes were issued by the American College of Physicians,[5] and for African Americans by the International Society on Hypertension in Blacks.[6]

Initial Evaluation

JNC-7 updated NHLBI recommendations from prior guidelines issued in 1997[7] in several important ways. First, JNC-7 introduced the concept of "prehypertension," which is systolic blood pressures of 120 to 139 mm Hg or a diastolic blood pressure of 80 to 89 mm Hg. JNC-7 recommended a more aggressive approach to patients with blood pressures in this range, with an emphasis on lifestyle modifications to prevent cardiovascular disease. JNC-7 describes "normal" blood pressure as systolic pressures below 120 mm Hg and diastolic blood pressures below 80 mm Hg. Stage 1 hypertension is systolic blood pressure 140 to 159 mm Hg or diastolic blood pressure 90 to 99 mm Hg. Patients with higher blood pressures have stage 2 hypertension.

Health care providers rarely follow established procedures for measuring blood pressure. In addition, there is increasing evidence that clinical blood pressure measurements made by a trained professional using a mercury sphygmomanometer and the Korotkoff sound technique may lead to the misclassification of large numbers of individuals. Guidelines from the American Heart Association[8] define proper procedures for measuring blood pressure. These include the following:

Allow the patient to sit quietly for 5 minutes before measuring blood pressure.

The patient should be seated comfortably with the back supported and the upper arm bared without constrictive clothing. The legs should not be crossed.

The arm should be supported at heart level, and the bladder of the cuff should encircle at least 80% of the arm circumference. Larger or smaller cuffs must be used as needed.

The mercury column should be deflated at 2 to 3 mm/sec, and the first and last audible sounds should be taken as systolic and diastolic pressure. The column should be read to the nearest 2 mm Hg.

Neither the patient nor the observer should talk during the measurement.

These measurement guidelines recommend a mercury sphygmomanometer as the standard for measurement, but recognize that these devices are being replaced by newer technologies. The "guidelines" recommend ambulatory monitoring for the evaluation of white coat hypertension, and home monitoring in select patients may be useful for predicting cardiovascular events and monitoring the effects of treatment.

JNC-6 gives recommendations for follow-up of patients after initial measurement of blood pressure (Table 41G-1). These recommendations should be guided by the blood pressure and other clinical data, including past blood pressure measurements, other cardiovascular risk factors, or target organ disease. JNC-7 recommends routine laboratory tests before the initiation of therapy that include 12-lead electrocardiography; urinalysis; determination of blood glucose, hematocrit, and serum potassium, creatinine, and calcium levels, and lipid profile. More extensive testing for identifiable causes of hypertension is not indicated routinely.

Initial Management Strategy

The goal of treatment according to JNC-7 is to reduce blood pressure to below 140 mm Hg systolic and 90 mm Hg diastolic; in patients with concomitant diabetes or renal disease, the goal is blood pressure below 130/80 mm Hg.

These guidelines recommend that initial management be based on the patient's blood pressure stage and other medical issues (Table 41G-2). Life style modifications should be encouraged for all patients, including those with normal blood pressures, and should be used as the sole therapy for patients with prehypertension unless they have clinical evidence of "compelling indications." These indications include

TABLE 41G–1 Joint National Committee (JNC)-6 Guidelines for Follow-up Based on Initial Blood Pressure Measurements for Adults

Initial Blood Pressure (mm Hg)*		
Systolic	*Diastolic*	**Follow-up Recommended**
<130	<85	Recheck in 2 yr.
130-139	85-89	Recheck in 1 yr (provide information about life style modifications).
140-159	90-99	Confirm within 2 mo (provide information about life style modifications).
160-179	100-109	Evaluate or refer to source of care within 1 mo.
≥180	≥110	Evaluate or refer to source of care immediately or within 1 wk, depending on clinical situation.

*If systolic and diastolic categories are different, follow recommendations for shorter time follow-up.

TABLE 41G–2 Joint National Committee (JNC)-7 Guidelines for Classification and Management of Hypertension in Adults

				Initial Drug Therapy	
Blood Pressure Classification	**Systolic Blood Pressure (mm Hg)**	**Diastolic Blood Pressure (mm Hg)**	**Life Style Modification**	*Without Compelling Indications*	*With Compelling Indications**
Normal	<120	And <80	Encourage	No antihypertensive drug indicated	Drug(s) for compelling indications†
Prehypertension	120-139	Or 80-89	Yes	No antihypertensive drug indicated	Drug(s) for compelling indications†
Stage 1 hypertension	140-159	Or 90-99	Yes	Thiazide-type diuretics for most	Drug(s) for compelling indications†
Stage 2 hypertension	≥160	Or ≥100	Yes	Two-drug combination for most (usually thiazide-type diuretic plus ACEI, ARB, BB, or CCB)	Other antihypertensive drugs (diuretics, ACEI, ARB, BB, CCB) as needed

*Heart failure, postmyocardial infarction, high coronary artery disease risk, diabetes, chronic kidney disease, recurrent stroke prevention.
†Treat patients with chronic kidney disease or diabetes to blood pressure goal of <130/80 mm Hg.
ACEI = angiotensin-converting enzyme inhibitor; ARB = angiotensin receptor blocker; BB = beta blocker; CCB = calcium channel blocker.

TABLE 41G–3 Joint National Committee (JNC)-7 Guidelines for Recommended Drugs for Patients with Compelling Indications

	Recommended Drugs					
Compelling Indication	*Diuretic*	*Beta Blocker*	*ACE Inhibitor*	*Angiotensin Receptor Blocker*	*Calcium Channel Blocker*	*Aldosterone Antagonist*
Heart failure	+	+	+	+		+
Postmyocardial infarction		+	+			+
High coronary disease risk	+	+	+		+	
Diabetes	+	+	+	+	+	
Chronic kidney disease			+	+		
Recurrent stroke prevention	+		+			

ACE = angiotensin-converting enzyme.

heart failure, postmyocardial infarction, high coronary artery disease risk, diabetes, chronic kidney disease, and need for recurrent stroke prevention.

Recommended life style modifications include:

Weight reduction to maintain normal body weight (body mass index, 18.5 to 24.9 kg/m2)

Adoption of the Dietary Approaches to Stop Hypertension (DASH) eating plan[9]

Dietary sodium reduction to no more than 100 mmol/day (2.4 g sodium or 6 g sodium chloride)

Physical activity—at least 30 minutes per day, most days of the week

Limit alcohol intake to no more than two drinks (1 oz or 30 ml ethanol; e.g., 24 oz beer, 10 oz wine, or 3 oz 80-proof whiskey) per day in most men and to no more than one drink per day in women and lighter weight persons.

Drug Therapy

JNC-7 guidelines recommend thiazide-type diuretics as the initial therapy for most patients with hypertension, either alone or in combination with one of the other classes. Table 41G-3 describes JNC-7's list of "compelling indications" and recommended therapies. The guidelines note that most patients who are hypertensive will require two or more antihypertensive agents to achieve their blood pressure goals. When blood pressure is more than 20/10 mm Hg above goal, the guidelines recommend that clinicians consider initiating therapy with two drugs.

Guidelines from other organizations vary slightly in thresholds for initiating therapy. For example, the British Hypertension Society's guidelines support initiation of drug therapy for all patients with systolic blood pressure of 160 mm Hg or sustained diastolic blood pressure of 100 mm Hg, despite nonpharmacological measures. Drug treatment is also indicated for patients with sustained systolic blood pressures of 140 to 159 mm Hg or diastolic blood pressures of 90 to 99 mm Hg if target organ damage is present, or there is evidence of established cardiovascular disease or diabetes, or the 10-year coronary heart disease risk is greater than 15%. For most patients, these guidelines recommend a target of reducing systolic pressure below 140 mm Hg and diastolic pressure below 85 mm Hg. For patients with diabetes, a lower target is recommended. These guidelines recommend initiation of therapy with a diuretic unless there is a contraindication or a compelling indication for another drug class.

For patients with hypertension and diabetes, the 2003 recommendations from the American College of Physicians include a target blood pressure of no more than 135/80 mm Hg.[5] These guidelines recommend thiazide diuretics or angiotensin-converting enzyme (ACE) inhibitors as first-line agents for blood pressure control in most patients.

Guidelines developed for the treatment of African Americans recommend lower thresholds for drug therapy and more aggressive treatment strategies.[6] These guidelines recommend a lower blood pressure target (130/80 mm Hg) for African Americans with hypertension who also have conditions such as heart disease, kidney disease, or diabetes. This statement notes that physicians should have a low threshold for using more than one drug for treatment of hypertension in African Americans.

FOLLOW-UP AND REFERRAL TO SPECIALISTS

In follow-up, the JNC-7 guidelines recommend that most patients should be seen at approximately monthly intervals until the blood pressure goal is reached. More frequent visits are recommended for patients with stage 2 hypertension or with complicating comorbid conditions. Serum potassium and creatinine levels should be monitored at least once or twice annually. After blood pressure is at goal and stable, follow-up visits can be scheduled at 3- to 6-month intervals. Low-dose aspirin therapy should be considered only after blood pressure is controlled because of risk of hemorrhagic stroke in patients with uncontrolled hypertension.

References

1. Chobanian AV, Bakris GL, Black HR, et al: The seventh report of the Joint National Committee on Prevention, Detection, Evaluation, and Treatment of High Blood Pressure. National Heart, Lung, and Blood Institute, 2003 (http://www.nhlbi.nih.gov/guidelines/hypertension/jnc7full.pdf).
2. Williams B, Poulter NR, Brown MJ, et al: Guidelines for management of hypertension: report of the fourth working party of the British Hypertension Society, 2004-BHS IV. J Hum Hypertens 18:139, 2004.
3. Khan NA, McAlister FA, Rabkin SW, et al: The 2006 Canadian Hypertension Education Program recommendations for the management of hypertension: Part II—therapy. Can J Cardiol 22:583, 2006.
4. Hemmelgarn BR, McAlister FA, Grover S, et al. The 2006 Canadian Hypertension Education Program recommendations for the management of hypertension: Part I—blood pressure measurement, diagnosis and assessment of risk. Can J Cardiol 22:573, 2006.
5. Snow V, Weiss KB, Mottur-Pilson C: The evidence base for tight blood pressure control in the management of type 2 diabetes mellitus. Ann Intern Med 138:587, 2003.
6. Douglas JG, Bakris GL, Epstein M, et al: Management of high blood pressure in African Americans: Consensus statement of the Hypertension in African Americans Working Group of the International Society on Hypertension in Blacks. Arch Intern Med 163:525, 2003.
7. The sixth report of the Joint National Committee on prevention, detection, evaluation, and treatment of high blood pressure. Arch Intern Med 157:2413, 1997.
8. Pickering TG, Hall JE, Appel LJ, et al: Recommendations for blood pressure measurement in humans and experimental animals: Part 1: Blood pressure measurement in humans: A statement for professionals from the Subcommittee of Professional and Public Education of the American Heart Association Council on High Blood Pressure Research. Hypertension 45:142, 2005.
9. Sacks FM, Svetkey LP, Vollmer WM, et al: Effects on blood pressure of reduced dietary sodium and the Dietary Approaches to Stop Hypertension (DASH) diet. DASH-Sodium Collaborative Research Group. N Engl J Med 344:3, 2001.

CHAPTER 42

Lipoprotein Disorders and Cardiovascular Disease

Jacques Genest and Peter Libby

INTRODUCTION

Serum levels of lipids and lipoprotein lipids have proven to be among the most potent and best substantiated risk factors for atherosclerosis in general and coronary heart disease (CHD) in particular. Chapter 38 discusses the biological basis of atherosclerosis. Chapter 39 presents the observational data on lipids as a key component of the palette of cardiovascular risk factors. The present chapter deals with the fundamentals of lipid metabolism, the therapeutic approaches to treatment of lipid disorders, and the evidence base regarding their clinical use.

Although the term *hyperlipidemia* has long been used in clinical practice, the term dyslipoproteinemia more appropriately reflects the disorders of the lipid and lipoprotein transport pathways associated with arterial diseases. Dyslipidemia encompasses disorders often encountered in clinical practice such as low high-density lipoprotein (HDL) cholesterol level and elevated triglyceride level but an average total plasma cholesterol level. Certain rare lipoprotein disorders can cause overt clinical manifestations, but most common dyslipoproteinemias themselves only rarely cause symptoms or produce clinical signs that are evident on physical examination. Rather, they require laboratory tests for detection. Dyslipoproteinemias constitute a major risk factor for atherosclerosis and coronary artery disease, and their proper recognition and management can reduce cardiovascular and total mortality rates. Thus the fundamentals of lipidology presented here have importance for the daily practice of cardiovascular medicine.

LIPOPROTEIN TRANSPORT SYSTEM

Biochemistry of Lipids

The lipid transport system has evolved to carry hydrophobic molecules (fat) from sites of origin to sites of utilization through the aqueous environment of plasma. The proteins (apolipoproteins) that mediate this process are conserved throughout evolution in organisms with a circulatory system. Most apolipoproteins derive from an ancestral gene and contain both hydrophilic and hydrophobic domains. This amphipathic structure enables these proteins to bridge the interface between the aqueous environment of plasma and the phospholipid constituents of the lipoprotein.[1] The major types of lipids that circulate in plasma include cholesterol and cholesteryl esters, phospholipids, and triglycerides (Fig. 42-1).

Cholesterol contributes an essential component of mammalian cell membranes and furnishes substrate for steroid hormones and bile acids. Many cell functions depend critically on membrane cholesterol, and cells tightly regulate cholesterol content. Most of the cholesterol in plasma circulates in the form of cholesteryl esters, in the core of lipoprotein particles. The enzyme lecithin cholesterol acyltransferase (LCAT) forms cholesteryl esters in the blood compartment by transferring a fatty acyl chain from phosphatidylcholine to cholesterol.

Triglycerides consist of a three-carbon glycerol backbone covalently linked to three fatty acids. The fatty acid composition varies in terms of chain length and presence of double bonds (degree of saturation). Triglyceride molecules are nonpolar and hydrophobic; they are transported in the core of the lipoprotein. Hydrolysis of triglycerides by lipases generates free fatty acids (FFAs) used for energy.

Phospholipids, constituents of all cellular membranes, consist of a glycerol molecule linked to two fatty acids. The fatty acids differ in length and in the presence of a single (monounsaturated) or multiple (polyunsaturated) double bonds. The third carbon of the glycerol moiety carries a phosphate group to which one of four molecules is linked: choline (phosphatidylcholine or lecithin), ethanolamine (phosphatidylethanolamine), serine (phosphatidylserine), or inositol (phosphatidylinositol). A related phospholipid, sphingomyelin, has special functions in the plasma membrane in the formation of membrane microdomains, such as rafts and caveolae. The structure of sphingomy-

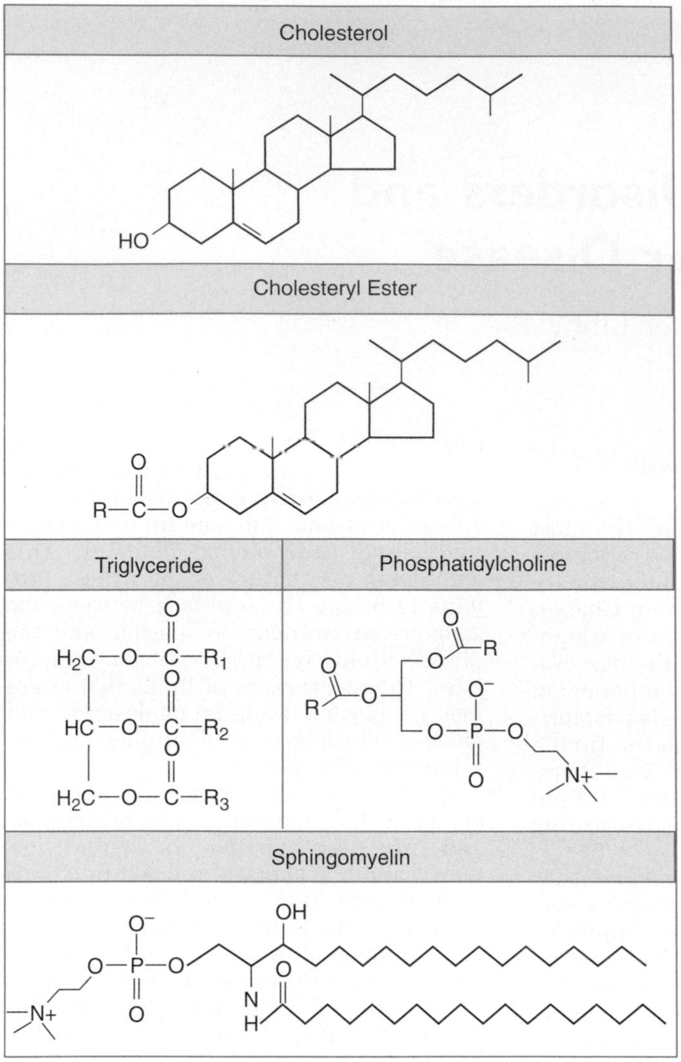

FIGURE 42–1 Biochemical structure of the major lipid molecules: cholesterol, cholesteryl esters, triglycerides, and phospholipids (phosphatidylcholine and sphingomyelin).

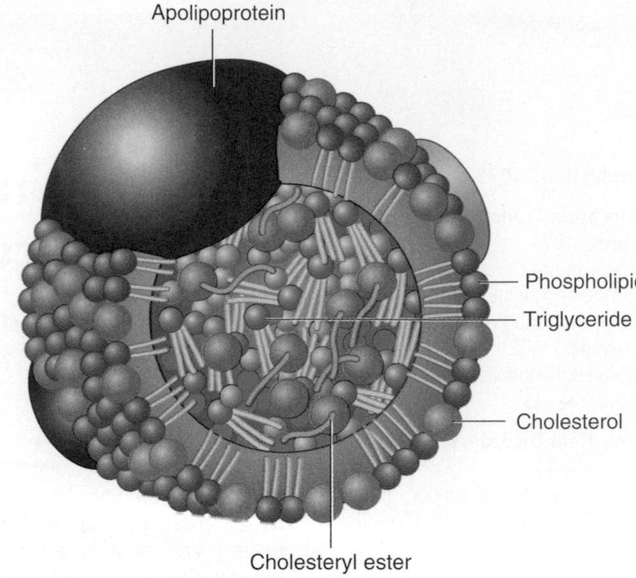

FIGURE 42–2 Structure of lipoproteins. Phospholipids are oriented with their polar group toward the aqueous environment of plasma. Free cholesterol is inserted within the phospholipid layer. The core of the lipoprotein is made up of cholesteryl esters and triglycerides. Apolipoproteins are involved in the secretion of the lipoprotein, provide structural integrity, and act as cofactors for enzymes or as ligands for various receptors.

elin resembles that of phosphatidylcholine. The backbone of sphingolipids uses the amino acid serine rather than glycerol. Phospholipids are polar molecules, more soluble than triglycerides or cholesterol or its esters. Phospholipids participate in signal transduction pathways: Hydrolysis by membrane-associated phospholipases generates second messengers such as diacyl glycerols, lysophospholipids, phosphatidic acids, and FFAs such as arachidonate that can regulate many cell functions.

Lipoproteins, Apolipoproteins, Receptors, and Processing Enzymes

Lipoproteins are complex macromolecular structures, composed of an envelope of phospholipids and free cholesterol, a core of cholesteryl esters, and triglycerides. The apolipoproteins comprise the protein moiety of lipoproteins (Fig. 42-2). Lipoproteins vary in size, density in the aqueous environment of plasma, and lipid and apolipoprotein content (Fig. 42-3, Table 42-1). The classification of lipoproteins reflects their density in plasma (1.006 gm/ml) as gauged by flotation in the ultracentrifuge. The triglyceride-rich lipoproteins consisting of chylomicrons and very-low-density lipoprotein (VLDL) have a density less than 1.006 gm/ml. The rest of the ultracentrifuged plasma consists of low-density lipoprotein (LDL), HDL, and lipoprotein (a) (Lp[a]).

Apolipoproteins have four major roles: (1) assembly and secretion of the lipoprotein (apo B_{100} and B_{48}); (2) structural integrity of the lipoprotein (apo B, apo E, apo AI, apo AII); (3) coactivators or inhibitors of enzymes (apo AI, CI, CII, CIII); and (4) binding or docking to specific receptors and proteins for cellular uptake of the entire particle or selective uptake of a lipid component (apo AI, B_{100}, E) (Table 42-2). The role of several apolipoproteins (AIV, AV, D, and J) remain incompletely understood.

Many proteins regulate the synthesis, secretion, and metabolic fate of lipoproteins; their characterization has provided insight in molecular cellular physiology and provided targets for drug development (Table 42-3). The discovery of the LDL receptor furnished a landmark in understanding cholesterol metabolism and receptor-mediated endocytosis. The LDL receptor regulates the entry of cholesterol into cells, as tight control mechanisms alter its expression on the cell surface, depending on need. Other receptors for lipoproteins include several that bind VLDL but not LDL. The LDL receptor–related peptide, which mediates the uptake of chylomicron remnants and VLDL, preferentially recognizes apolipoprotein E (apo E).[2] The LDL receptor–related peptide interacts with hepatic lipase. A specific VLDL receptor also exists.[3] The interaction between hepatocytes and the various lipoproteins containing apo E is complex and involves cell surface proteoglycans that provide a scaffolding for lipolytic enzymes (lipoprotein lipase and hepatic lipase) involved in remnant lipoprotein recognition.[4-6] Macrophages express receptors that bind modified (especially oxidized) lipoproteins. These scavenger lipoprotein receptors mediate the uptake of oxidized LDL into macrophages. In contrast to the exquisitely regulated LDL receptor, high cellular cholesterol content does not suppress scavenger receptors, enabling the intimal macrophages to accumulate abundant cholesterol, become foam cells, and form fatty streaks. Endothelial cells can also take

TABLE 42–1 Plasma Lipoprotein Composition

	Origin	Density (gm/ml)	Size (nm)	Protein (%)	[Cholesterol] in plasma (mmol/liter)*	[Triglyceride] in fasting plasma (mmol/liter)†	Major apo	Other apo
Chylomicrons	Intestine	<0.95	100-1000	1-2	0.0	0	B48	AI, C's
VLDL	Liver	<1.006	40-50	10	0.1-0.4	0.2-1.2	B100	AI, C's
IDL	VLDL	1.006-1.019	25-30	18	0.1-0.3	0.1-0.3	B100, E	
LDL	IDL	1.019-1.063	20-25	25	1.5-3.5	0.2-0.4	B100	
HDL	Liver, intestine	1.063-1.210	6-10	40-55	0.9-1.6	0.1-0.2	AI, AII	AIV
Lipoprotein(a)	Liver	1.051-1.082	25	30-50			B100, (a)	

*In mmol/liter; for mg/dl, multiply by 38.67.
†In mmol/liter; for mg/dl, multiply by 88.5.
Apo= apolipoprotein; HDL=high-density lipoprotein; IDL=intermediate-density lipoprotein; LDL=low-density lipoprotein; VLDL=very-low-density lipoprotein.

up modified lipoproteins through a specific receptor such as Lox-1.[7]

At least two physiologically relevant receptors bind HDL particles: the scavenger receptor class B (SR-B1; also named CLA-1 in humans)[8] and the adenosine triphosphate–binding cassette transporter A1 (ABCA1).[9] SR-B1 is a receptor for HDL (also for LDL and VLDL, but with less affinity). SR-B1 mediates the selective uptake of HDL cholesteryl esters in steroidogenic tissues, hepatocytes, and endothelium. The ABCA1 mediates cellular phospholipid (and possibly cholesterol) efflux and is necessary and essential for HDL biogenesis.[9]

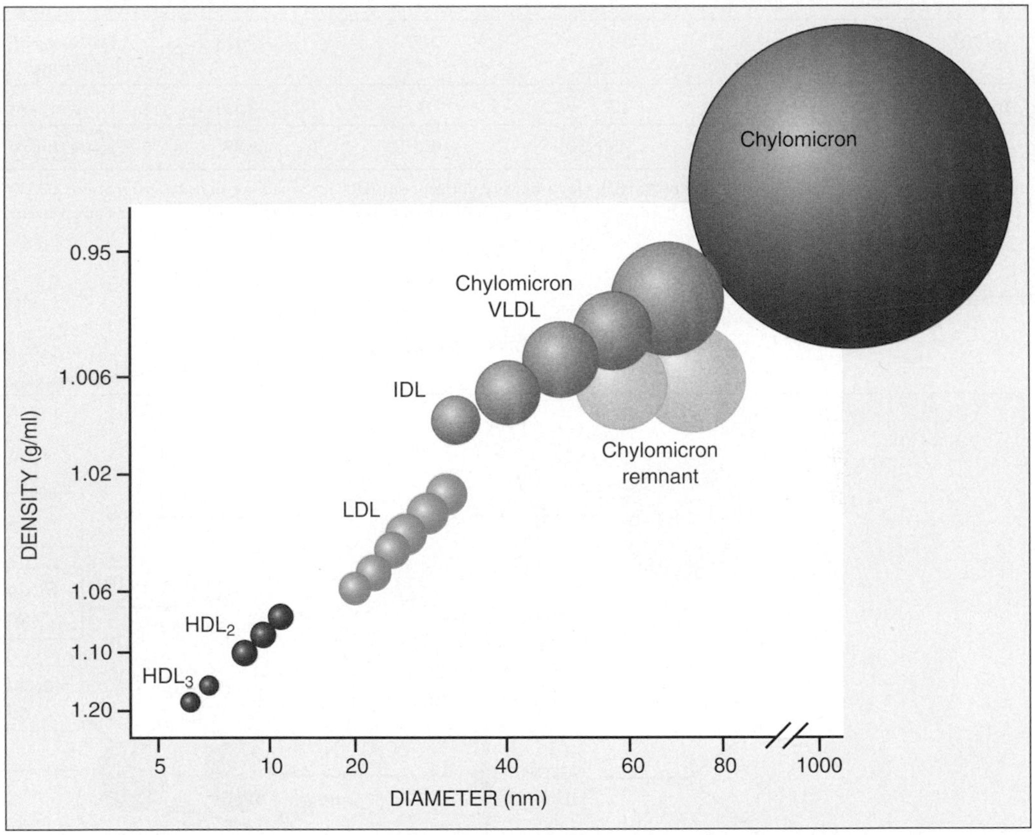

FIGURE 42–3 Relative size of plasma lipoproteins according to their hydrated density. HDL = high-density lipoprotein; IDL = intermediate-density lipoprotein; LDL = low-density lipoprotein.

Lipoprotein Metabolism and Transport

The lipoprotein transport system has two major roles: the efficient transport of triglycerides from the intestine and the liver to sites of utilization (fat tissue or muscle) and the transport of cholesterol to peripheral tissues, for membrane synthesis and steroid hormone production, or to the liver for bile acid synthesis.

INTESTINAL PATHWAY (CHYLOMICRONS TO CHYLOMICRON REMNANTS). Life requires fats. The human body derives essential fatty acids that it cannot make from the diet. Fat typically furnishes 20 to 40 percent of daily calories. Triglycerides comprise the major portion of ingested fats. For an individual consuming 2000 kcal/day, with 30 percent in the form of fat, this represents approximately 66 gm of triglycerides per day and approximately 250 mg (0.250 gm) of cholesterol.

On ingestion, pancreatic lipases hydrolyze triglycerides into FFAs and monoglycerides or diglycerides. Emulsification by bile salts leads to the formation of intestinal micelles. Micelles resemble lipoproteins in that they consist of phospholipids, free cholesterol, bile acids, diglycerides and monoglycerides, FFAs, and glycerol. The mechanism of micelle uptake by the intestinal brush border cells still engenders debate. The Niemann-Pick C1-like 1 (NPC1-L1) protein is part of an intestinal cholesterol transporter complex, as well as the target for the selective cholesterol absorption inhibitor ezetimibe[10] (see later). The advent of inhibitors of cholesterol uptake has rekindled interest in the mechanisms of intestinal fat absorption. After uptake into intestinal cells, fatty acids undergo reesterification to form triglycerides and packaging into chylomicrons inside the intestinal cell and enter the portal circulation (Fig. 42-4). Chylomicrons contain apo B_{48}, the amino-terminal component of apo B_{100}. In the intestine the apo B gene is modified during transcription into mRNA with a substitution of a uracil for a cytosine by an apo B_{48} editing enzyme complex (ApoBec). This

TABLE 42–2	Apolipoproteins					
Name	Predominant Lipoprotein	Molecular Weight (kDa)	Plasma Concentration (mg/dl)	Chromosome	Role	Human Disease
Apo AI	HDL	28.3	90-160	11q23	ACAT activation, structural	HDL deficiency
Apo AII	HDL	17	25-45	1q21-23	Structural	
Apo AIV	HDL	45	10-20	11q23	Structural, absorption	
Apo AV	VLDL, HDL			11q23	TRL metabolism[72]	
Apo B100	LDL, VLDL	512	50-150	2q23-24	Structural, LDL-R binding	Hypobetalipoproteinemia
Apo B48	Chylomicrons	241	0-100	2q23-24	Structural	
Apo CI	Chylomicrons	6.63	5-6	19q13.2	TRL metabolism	
Apo CII	Chylomicrons, VLDL	8.84	3-5	19q13.2	LPL activation	Hyperchylomicronemia
Apo CIII	Chylomicrons, VLDL	8.76	10-14	11q23	LPL inhibition	Hypertriglyceridemia
Apo D	HDL	33	4-7	3q26.2	LCAT	
Apo E	Chylomicron remnant, IDL	34	2-8	19q13.2	LDL-R, ApoE-R binding	Type III
Apo J	HDL	70	10	18p21	Complement system	
Apo(a)	Lipoprotein(a)	250-800	0-200	6q27	Tissue injury?	

Apo=apolipoprotein; ApoE-R=Apo E receptor; HDL=high-density lipoprotein; IDL=intermediate-density lipoprotein; LCAT=lecithin: cholesterol acyltransferase; LDL=low-density lipoprotein; LDL-R=LDL receptor; TRL=triglyceride-rich lipoprotein; VLDL=very-low-density lipoprotein.

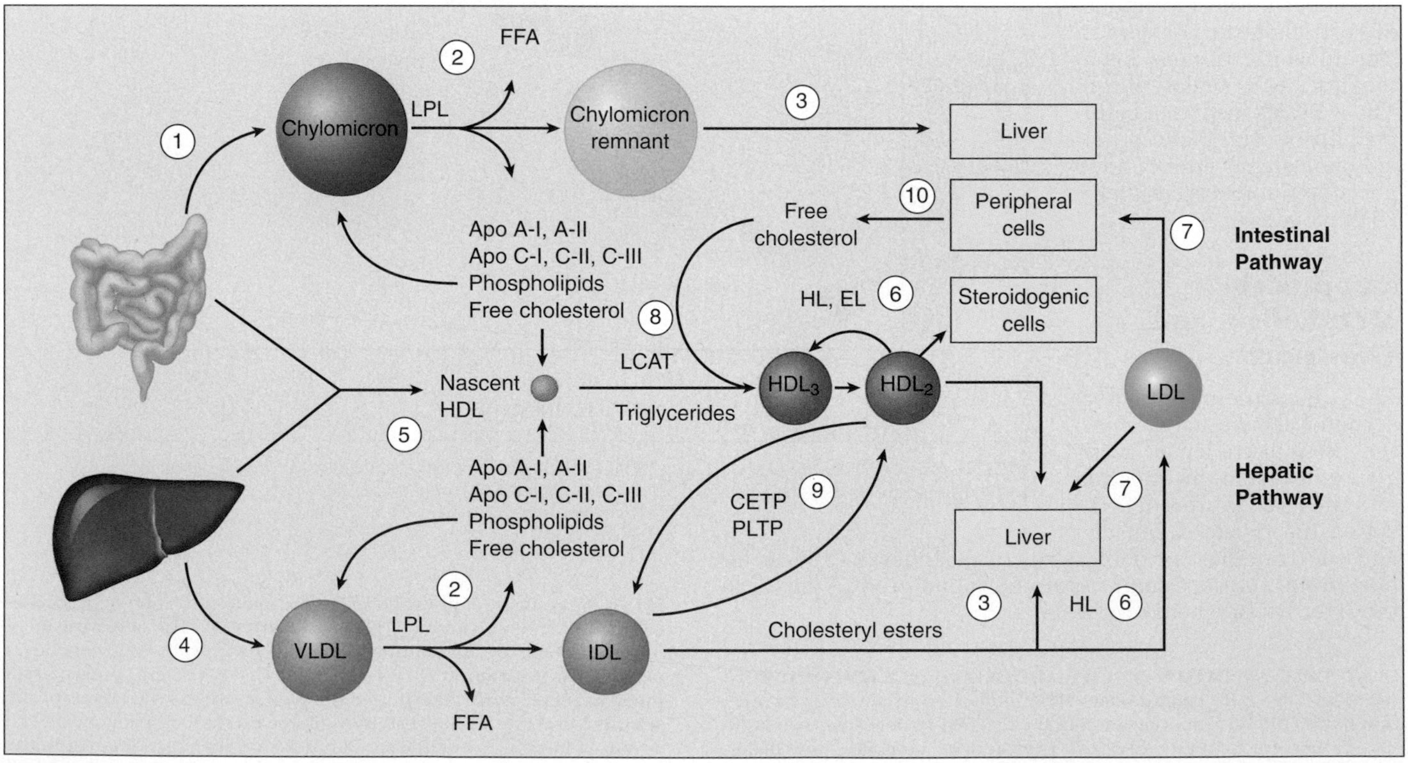

FIGURE 42–4 Schematic diagram of the lipid transport system. Numbers in circles refer to explanation in text. Apo = apolipoprotein; CETP = cholesteryl ester transfer protein; EL = endothelial lipase; FFA = free fatty acids; HL = hepatic lipase; HDL = high-density lipoprotein; IDL = intermediate-density lipoprotein; LCAT = lecithin cholesterol acyltransferase; LDL = low-density lipoprotein; LPL = lipoprotein lipase; PLTP = phospholipid transfer protein; VLDL = very-low-density lipoprotein.

TABLE 42–3 Lipoprotein Processing Enzymes, Receptors, Modulating Proteins

Abbreviation	Name	Role	Chromosome	Human Disease
ABCA1	ATP binding cassette AI	Cellular cholesterol and phospholipid efflux	9q31	Tangier disease
ABCG1	ATP binding cassette GI	Cellular cholesterol efflux	21q22.3	
ABCG5/G8	ATP binding cassette G5 and G8	Intestinal sitosterol transporter	21	Sitosterolemia
ACAT1	acetyl-CoA acetyltransferase 1	Cellular cholesterol esterification	1q22.3	
ACAT2	acetyl-CoA acetyltransferase 2	Cellular cholesterol esterification	6q25.3	
ApoE-R	ApoE containing lipoprotein receptor	TRL uptake	1p34	
CD36	Fatty acid translocase	Fatty acid transport	7q11.2	
CETP	Cholesteryl ester transfer protein	Lipid exchange in plasma	16q21	Elevated HDL cholesterol
EL	Endothelial lipase	PL hydrolysis	18q21.1	
HL	Hepatic lipase	Tg hydrolysis	15q21	Remnant accumulation
HSL (LIPE)	Hormone-sensitive lipase	Fatty acid release from adipocytes	19q13.2	
LCAT	Lecithin : cholesterol acyltransferase	Cholesterol esterification (plasma)	16q22.1	LCAT deficiency, low HDL
LDL-R	Low-density lipoprotein receptor	LDL uptake	19p13	Familial hypercholesterolemia
Lox1	Scavenger receptor	OxLDL uptake, endothelium	12p12-13	Oxidized lipoprotein uptake
LPL	Lipoprotein lipase	Tg hydrolysis	8p22	Hyperchylomicronemia
LRP1	LDL-R–related protein	Protease uptake, many ligands	19q12	
LRP2	LDL-R–related protein 2 (megalin)	Protease uptake, apo J	2q24-31	
MTP	Microsomal triglyceride transfer protein	Apo B assembly	4q22-24	Abetalipoproteinemia
NPC1	Niemann-Pick C gene product	Cellular cholesterol transport	18q11-12	Niemann-Pick type C
NPC1L1	Niemann-Pick C1-like 1 protein	Intestinal cholesterol absorption	7p13	
PLTP	Phospholipid transfer protein	Lipid exchange in plasma	20q12	
PCSK9	Proprotein convertase, subtilisin/kexin-9	Protein cleavage	1p34.1	Hypercholesterolemia
SMPD1	Sphingomyelinase phosphodiesterase	Sphingomyelin hydrolysis	11p15.4	Niemann-Pick types A and B
SRA	Scavenger receptor A	OxLDL uptake, macrophages	8p21	
SR-B1	Scavenger receptor B1	HDL CE uptake	12	
VLDL-R	Very-low-density lipoprotein receptor	VLDL uptake	9q24	

mechanism involves a cytosine deaminase and leads to a termination codon at residue 2153 and a truncated form of apo B. Only intestinal cells express ApoBec.

Chylomicrons rapidly enter the plasma compartment after meals. In capillaries of adipose tissue or muscle cells in the peripheral circulation, chylomicrons encounter lipoprotein lipase (LPL), an enzyme attached to heparan sulfate and present on the luminal side of endothelial cells (see Fig. 42-4, part 2). LPL activity is modulated by apo CII (an activator) and by apo CIII (an inhibitor). Lipoprotein lipase has broad specificity for triglycerides; it cleaves all fatty acyl residues attached to glycerol, generating three molecules of FFA for each molecule of glycerol. Muscle cells rapidly take up fatty acids. Adipose cells can store triglycerides made from fatty acids for energy utilization, a process that requires insulin. Fatty acids can also bind to fatty acid-binding proteins and travel to the liver, where they are repackaged in VLDL. Peripheral resistance to insulin can thus increase the delivery of FFAs to the liver with a consequent increase in VLDL secretion and increased apo B particles in plasma. As discussed later, this is one of the consequences of the metabolic syndrome (see Chap. 43). The remnant particles, derived from chylomicra following LPL action, contain apo E and enter the liver for degradation and reutilization of their core constituents (see Fig. 42-4, part 3).

HEPATIC PATHWAY (VERY-LOW-DENSITY LIPOPROTEIN TO INTERMEDIATE-DENSITY LIPOPROTEIN). Food is not always available, and dietary fat content varies. The body must ensure readily available triglycerides to meet energy demands. Hepatic secretion of

VLDL particles serves this function (see Fig. 42-4, part 4). VLDLs are triglyceride-rich lipoproteins smaller than chylomicrons (see Table 42-1 and Fig. 42-3). They contain apo B_{100} as their main apolipoprotein. As opposed to apo B_{48}, apo B_{100} contains a domain recognized by the LDL receptor (the apo B/E receptor). VLDL particles follow the same catabolic pathway through lipoprotein lipase as chylomicrons (see Fig. 42-4, part 2). During hydrolysis of triglyceride-rich lipoproteins by LPL, an exchange of proteins and lipids takes place: VLDL particles (and chylomicrons) acquire apo Cs and apo E, in part from HDL particles. VLDLs also exchange triglycerides for cholesteryl esters from HDL (mediated by cholesteryl ester transfer protein [CETP]) (see Fig. 42-4, part 9). Such bidirectional transfer of constituents among lipoproteins serves several purposes: acquisition of specific apolipoproteins by lipoproteins that will dictate their metabolic fate; transfer of phospholipids onto nascent HDL particles mediated by phospholipid transfer protein (PLTP) (during the loss of core triglycerides, the phospholipid envelope becomes redundant and is shed off to apo AI to form new HDL particles); and transfer of cholesterol from HDL to VLDL remnants so that it can be metabolized in the liver. This exchange constitutes a major part of the reverse cholesterol transport pathway.

After hydrolysis of triglycerides partly depletes VLDL of triglycerides, VLDL particles have relatively more cholesterol. They shed several apolipoproteins (especially the C apolipoproteins) and acquire apo E. The VLDL remnant lipoprotein, called intermediate-density lipoprotein (IDL), is taken up by the liver via its apo E moiety (see Fig. 42-4, part 3) or further delipidated by hepatic lipase to form an LDL particle (see Fig. 42-4, part 6). At least four receptors exist for triglyceride-rich lipoprotein (TRL), TRL remnants, and apo B-containing lipoproteins: the VLDL receptor, the remnant receptor, the LDL receptor (also called the apo B/E receptor), and the LDL receptor–related peptide. Most hepatic receptors share the ability to recognize apo E, an engagement that mediates uptake of several classes of lipoproteins including VLDL and intermediate-density lipoprotein. The interaction between apo E and its ligand is complex and involves the docking of TRL on heparan sulfate proteoglycans before presentation of the ligand to its receptor.

LOW-DENSITY LIPOPROTEINS. LDL particles contain predominantly cholesteryl esters packaged with the protein moiety apo B_{100}. Normally, triglycerides constitute only 4 to 8 percent of the LDL mass (see Table 42-1). In the presence of elevated plasma triglyceride levels, LDL particles can become enriched in triglycerides and depleted in core cholesteryl esters. LDL particle size variation results from changes in core constituents, with an increase in triglycerides and a relative decrease in cholesteryl esters leading to smaller, denser LDL particles.

The LDL particles in most higher mammals including humans and nonhuman primates serve as the main carriers of cholesterol. In other mammals such as rodents or rabbits, VLDL and HDL particles transport most of the cholesterol. Cells can either make cholesterol from acetate through enzymatic reactions requiring at least 33 steps or obtain it as cholesteryl esters from LDL particles. Cells internalize LDL via the LDL receptor (LDL-R) (Fig. 42-5A). LDL particles contain one molecule of apo B. Although several domains of apo B are highly lipophilic and associate with phospholipids, a region surrounding residue 3500 binds with high affinity and saturability LDL-R. The LDL-R localizes in a region of the plasma membrane rich in the protein clathrin (see Figs. 42-4, part 7 and 42-5A). Once bound to the receptor, clathrin polymerizes and forms an endosome that contains LDL bound to its receptor, a portion of the plasma membrane, and clathrin. These internalized particles then fuse with lysosomes whose catabolic enzymes (cholesteryl ester hydrolase, cathepsins) will in turn release free cholesterol and degrade apo B. The LDL-R will detach itself from its ligand and recycle to the plasma membrane.

Cells tightly regulate cholesterol content by (1) cholesterol synthesis in the smooth endoplasmic reticulum (via the rate-limiting step hydroxymethylglutaryl coenzyme A [HMG-CoA] reductase); (2) receptor-mediated endocytosis of LDL (two mechanisms under the control of the steroid-responsive element binding protein [SREBP]); (3) cholesterol efflux from plasma membrane to cholesterol acceptor particles (predominantly apo AI and HDL) via the ABCA1 transporter; and (4) intracellular cholesterol esterification via the enzyme acyl-CoA: cholesteryl acyltransferase (ACAT) (see Fig. 42-5A and B). The SREBP coordinately regulates the first two pathways at the level of gene transcription. Cellular cholesterol binds to a protein called SCAP (SREPB cholesterol-activated protein), which is located on the endoplasmic reticulum. Cholesterol inhibits the interaction of SCAP with SREPB. In the absence of cholesterol, SCAP will mediate the cleavage of SREBP at two sites by specific proteases and release an amino (NH_2) fragment of SREBP. The SREBP NH_2 fragment will migrate to the nucleus and increase the transcriptional activity of genes involved in cellular cholesterol and fatty acid homeostasis. Cleavage of SREBP depends on a proprotein convertase related to the subtilisin/kexin family of convertases. Another member of the convertase superfamily, proprotein convertase subtilisin/kexin 9 (PCSK9), may participate in the cellular degradation of the LDL-R; gain of function mutations in this gene cause dominant familial hypercholesterolemia, while loss of function increases LDL-R and lowers LDL-C significantly.[11] Cholesterol content in membranes regulates the ACAT pathway at the level of protein regulation.[12] Humans express two separate forms of ACAT. ACAT1 and ACAT2 derive from different genes and mediate cholesterol esterification in cytoplasm and in the endoplasmic reticulum lumen for lipoprotein assembly and secretion.

Regulation of cholesterol efflux depends in part on the ABCA1 pathway, controlled in turn by hydroxysterols (especially 24- and 27-OH cholesterol, which act as ligands for the liver-specific receptor [LXR] family of transcriptional regulatory factors). In conditions of cell cholesterol sufficiency, the cell can decrease its input of cholesterol by decreasing the de novo synthesis of cholesterol. The cell can also decrease the amount of cholesterol that enters the cell via the LDL-R, increase the amount stored as cholesteryl esters, and promote the removal of cholesterol by increasing its movement to the plasma membrane for efflux.

HIGH-DENSITY LIPOPROTEIN AND REVERSE CHOLESTEROL TRANSPORT. Epidemiological studies have consistently shown an inverse relationship between plasma levels of HDL cholesterol and the presence of coronary artery disease. HDL promotes reverse cholesterol transport and can prevent lipoprotein oxidation and exert antiinflammatory actions in vitro.

The metabolism of HDL is complex and incompletely understood. The complexity arises because HDL particles acquire their components from several sources while these components also are metabolized at different sites. Apolipoprotein AI, the main protein of HDL, is synthesized in the intestine and liver. Approximately 80 percent of HDL originates from the liver[13] and 20 percent from the intestine (see Fig. 42-4, part 5).[14] Lipid-free apo AI acquires phospholipids from cell membranes and from redundant phospholipids shed during hydrolysis of triglyceride-rich lipoproteins. Lipid-free apo AI binds to ABCA1 and promotes its phosphorylation via cyclic adenosine monophosphate, which increases the net efflux of phospholipids and cholesterol onto apo AI to form a nascent HDL particle (see Fig. 42-4, part 10).[15,16] This particle, containing apo AI and phospholipids (and little cholesterol), resembles a flattened disk in which the phospholipids form a bilayer surrounded by two molecules of apo AI arranged in a circular fashion at the periphery of the disk (see Fig. 42-5B). These nascent HDL particles will mediate further cellular cholesterol efflux. Currently, standard laboratory tests do not measure these HDL precursors because they contain little or no cholesterol. On reaching a cell membrane, the nascent HDL particles will capture membrane-associated cholesterol and promote the efflux of free cholesterol onto other HDL particles (see Fig. 42-4, part 10). Conceptually, the formation of HDL particles appears to involve two steps: the first ABCA1-dependent, and the second, probably not requiring ABCA1.[17] The efflux of cellular cholesterol from peripheral cells such as macrophages does not contribute importantly to overall HDL-C mass but may have an important effect on export of cholesterol from atheromata. Macrophage can efflux cholesterol onto apo AI and apoE, onto nascent HDL particles via the ABCA1 transporter, or onto spherical HDL particles, via the ABCG1 transporter (see Fig. 42-5E). The plasma enzyme LCAT, an enzyme activated by apo AI, then esterifies the free cholesterol (see Figs. 42-4, part 8, and 42-5B). LCAT transfers an acyl chain (a fatty acid) from the R2 position of a phospholipid to the 3′-OH residue of cholesterol, resulting in the formation of a cholesteryl ester (see Fig. 42-1). In a process called *selective uptake of cholesterol,* HDL also provides cholesterol to steroid hormone-producing tissues and the liver through the scavenger SR-B1 receptor (see Fig. 42-5C).[18]

Because of their hydrophobility, cholesteryl esters move to the core of the lipoprotein and the HDL particle now assumes a spherical configuration (a particle denoted HDL3). With further cholesterol esterification, the HDL particle increases in size to become the more buoyant HDL22. Cholesterol within HDL particles can exchange with triglyceride-rich lipoproteins via cholesteryl ester transfer protein (CETP), which mediates an equimolar exchange of cholesterol from HDL to triglyceride-rich lipoprotein and triglyceride movement from triglyceride-rich lipoprotein onto HDL (see Fig. 42-4, part 9). Inhibition of CETP increases HDL-C in the blood and represents a therapeutic target for cardiovascular disease prevention. Phospholipid transfer protein (PLTP) mediates the transfer of phospholipids between triglyceride-rich lipoprotein and HDL particles. Triglyceride-enriched HDL is denoted as HDL2b. Hepatic lipase can hydrolyze triglycerides and endothelial lipase can hydrolyze phospholipids within these particles, converting them back to HDL_3 particles (see Fig. 42-4, part 6).

One mechanism of reverse cholesterol transport includes the uptake of cellular cholesterol from extra-hepatic tissues such as lipid-laden macrophages and its esterification by LCAT, transport by large HDL particles, and exchange for one triglyceride molecule by CETP. Originally on an HDL particle, the cholesterol molecule can now be taken up by hepatic receptors on a triglyceride-rich lipoprotein or LDL particle. HDL particles therefore act as shuttles among tissue cholesterol, triglyceride-rich lipoprotein, and the liver.

Most HDL originates in the liver[13] and intestines.[14] Reverse cholesterol transport by HDL contributes a small but potentially important portion of the plasma HDL mass. Indeed, selective inactivation of macrophage ABCA1 does not change HDL-C levels in mice, but there is an increase in atherosclerosis.[19] The catabolism of HDL particles has engendered debate among lipoprotein researchers. The protein component of HDL particles exchanges with lipoproteins of other classes. The kidneys appear to be a route of elimination of apolipoprotein AI and other HDL apolipoproteins. The lipid component of HDL particles also follows a different metabolic route (see Fig. 42-5B-C).

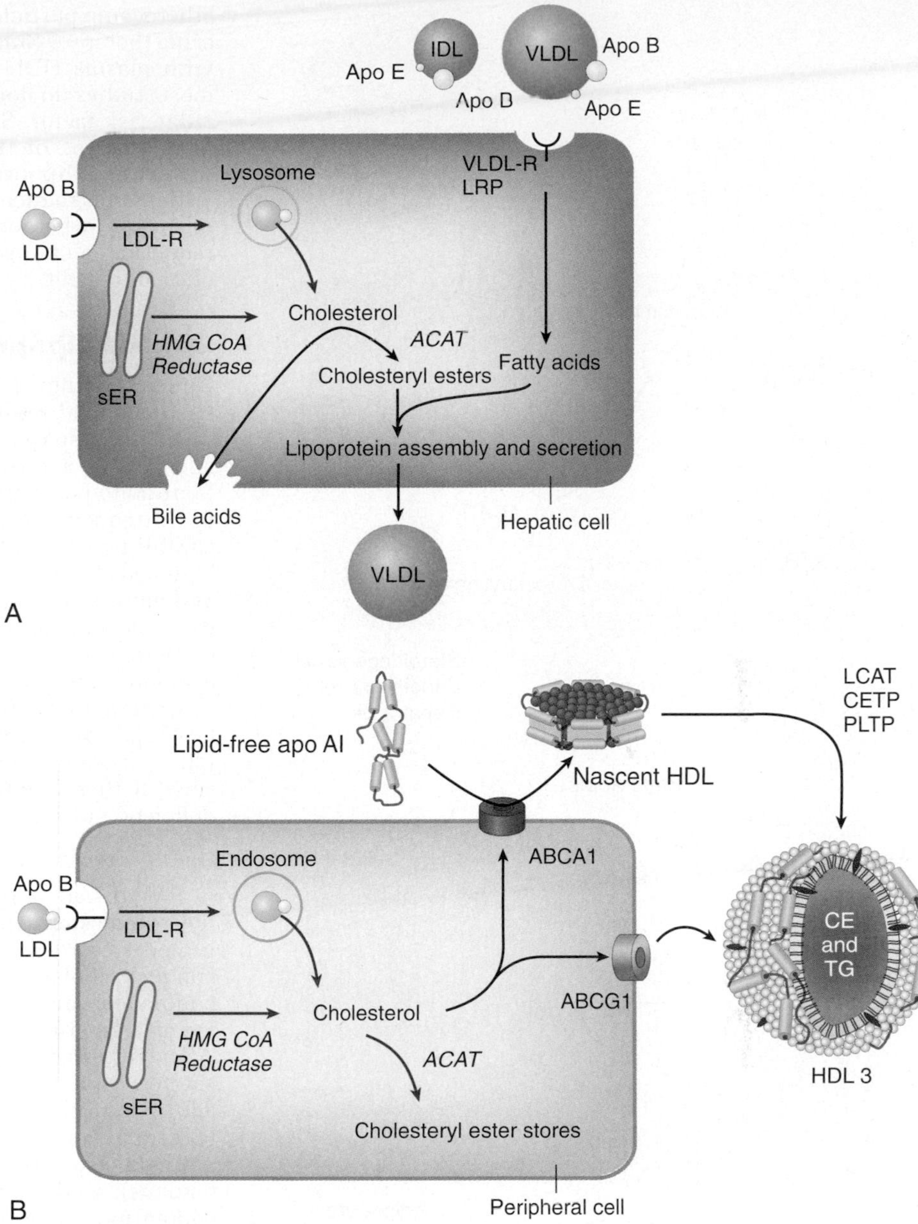

FIGURE 42–5 Cellular cholesterol homeostasis in various tissues. **A,** Cholesterol homeostasis (hepatocytes). **B,** Cellular cholesterol efflux (peripheral cells).

LIPOPROTEIN DISORDERS

Definitions

Time and new knowledge have stimulated necessary changes to the classification of lipoprotein disorders. The original classification of lipoprotein disorders by Fredrickson, Lees, and Levy was based on the measurement of total plasma cholesterol and triglycerides and analyzed lipoprotein patterns after separation by electrophoresis. This classification recognized elevations of chylomicrons (type I), VLDL or pre–beta lipoproteins (type IV), "broad beta" disease (or type III hyperlipoproteinemia), beta lipoproteins (LDL) (type II), and elevations of both chylomicrons and VLDL (type V). In addition, the combined elevations of pre–beta lipoproteins (VLDL) and beta (LDL) lipoproteins was recognized as type IIb hyperlipoproteinemia. Though providing a useful conceptual framework, this classification has some drawbacks: It does not include HDL cholesterol, and it does not differentiate severe monogenic lipoprotein disorders from the more common polygenic disorders. Subsequently, the World Health Organization, the European Atherosclerosis Society and, more recently, the National Cholesterol Education Program have classified lipoprotein disorders on the basis of arbitrary cut points.

A practical approach describes the lipoprotein disorder by the absolute plasma levels of lipids (cholesterol and triglycerides) and lipoprotein cholesterol levels (LDL and HDL cholesterol) and considers clinical manifestations of hyperlipoproteinemia in the context of biochemical characterization. For example, a young patient presenting with eruptive xanthomas and a plasma triglyceride level of 11.3 mmol/liter (1000 mg/dl) likely has familial hyperchylomicronemia. An obese, hypertensive middle-aged man with a cholesterol level of 6.4 mmol/liter (247 mg/dl), a triglyceride level of 3.1 mmol/liter (274 mg/dl), a HDL cholesterol level of 0.8 mmol/liter (31 mg/dl), and a calculated LDL cholesterol level of 4.2 mmol/liter (162 mg/dl) likely has the metabolic syndrome, a finding that should spur evaluation of its other components including hypertension and hyperglycemia.

The clinical usefulness of apolipoprotein levels has stirred debate. Although a useful research tool in general, the measurement of apolipoproteins AI and B may add little substantial information to that provided by the conventional lipid profile. Taken as a single measurement, the apo B level provides information on the number of potentially atherogenic particles and can be used as a goal of lipid-lowering therapy.[20] Similarly, LDL particle size correlates highly with plasma HDL cholesterol and triglyceride levels, and most studies do not show it to be an independent cardiovascular risk factor. Small, dense LDL particles tend to track with features of the metabolic syndrome, which usually involves dyslipoproteinemia with elevated plasma triglycerides and reduced HDL cholesterol levels.[21] It remains uncertain whether, in addition to LDL particle number reduction, a change in LDL particle size will bring further clinical benefit.

Genetic Lipoprotein Disorders

Understanding of the genetics of lipoprotein metabolism has expanded rapidly. Classification of genetic lipoprotein disorders usually requires a biochemical phenotype in addition to a clinical phenotype. With the exception of familial hypercholesterolemia, monogenic disorders tend to be infrequent or rare. Disorders considered heritable on careful family study may be difficult to characterize unambiguously because of age, gender, penetrance, and gene–gene and environmental interactions. Most common lipoprotein disorders encountered clinically result from the interaction of increasing age, lack of physical exercise, weight gain, and a suboptimal diet with individual genetic make-up.

Genetic lipoprotein disorders can affect LDL, lipoprotein (a) (Lp[a]), remnant lipoproteins, triglyceride-rich lipoproteins (chylomicrons and VLDL), or HDL (Table 42-4). Within each of these, genetic disorders can cause an excess or a deficiency of a specific class of lipoprotein.

Low-Density Lipoproteins (Type II Hyperlipidemia)

FAMILIAL HYPERCHOLESTEROLEMIA. Familial hypercholesterolemia is the most thoroughly studied lipoprotein disorder. The elucidation of the pathway by which complex molecules enter the cell by receptor-mediated endocytosis and the discovery of the LDL receptor represent landmarks in cell biology and clinical investigation. Affected subjects have an elevated LDL cholesterol level greater than the 95th percentile for age and gender. In adulthood, clinical manifestations include corneal arcus; tendinous xanthomas over the extensor tendons (metacarpophalangeal joints and patellar, triceps, and Achilles tendons); and xanthelasmas. Transmission is autosomal codominant. Familial hypercholesterolemia affects approximately 1 in 500, although this prevalence is higher in popu-

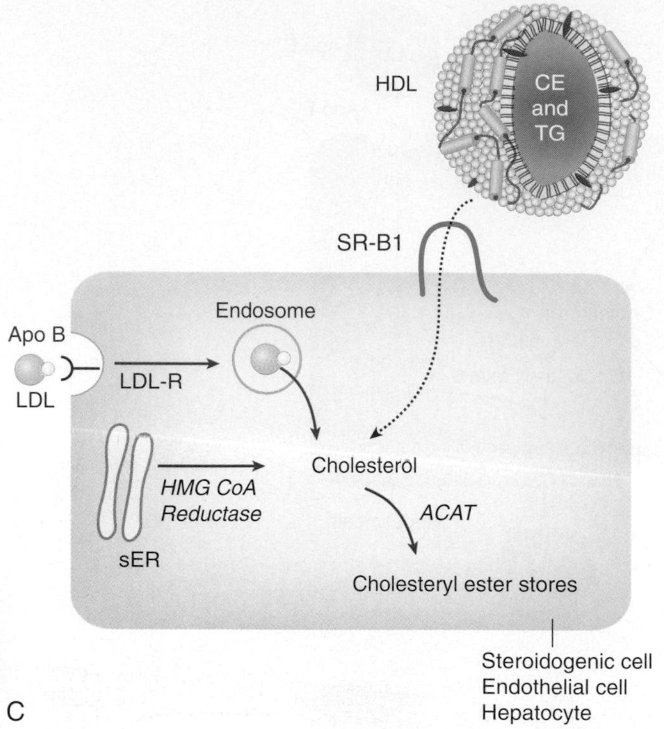

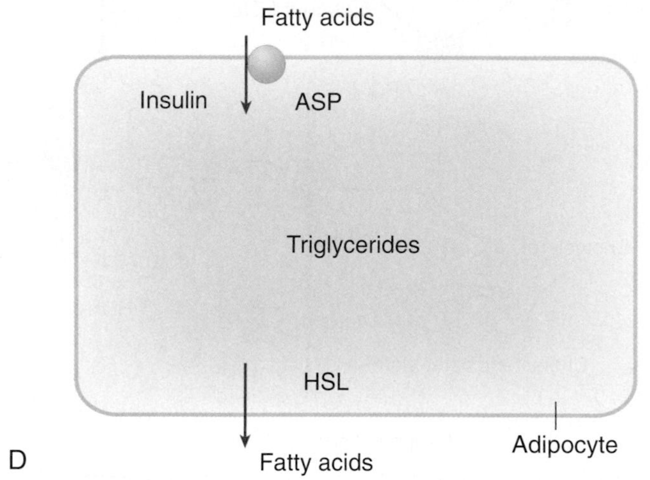

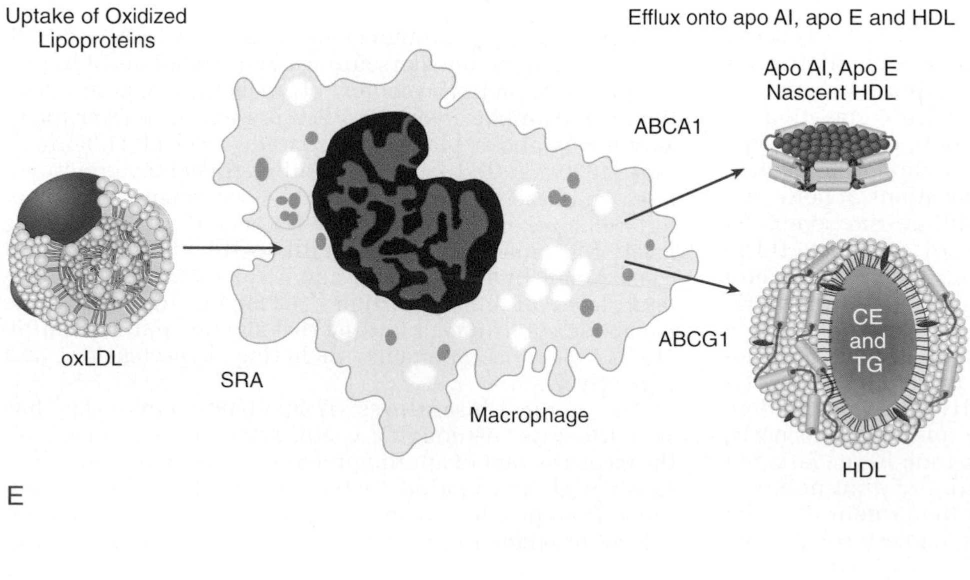

FIGURE 42–5, cont'd C, Selective uptake of cholesterol (adrenal cells, hepatocytes, endothelial cells). **D,** Adipocytes and **E,** macrophages foam cells. ABCA1 = ATP-binding cassette transporter A1; ABCG1 = ATP-binding cassette transporter G1; ACAT = acyl-coenzyme A : cholesterol acyltransferase; Apo = apolipoprotein; ASP = acylation-stimulating protein; CE = cholesterol esters; CETP = cholesteryl ester transfer protein; HDL = high-density lipoprotein; HMG CoA Red = hydroxymethylglutaryl coenzyme A reductase; HSL = hormone-sensitive lipase; IDL = intermediate-density lipoprotein; LCAT = lecithin cholesterol acyltransferase; LDL = low-density lipoprotein; LDL-R = low-density lipoprotein receptor; LRP = low-density lipoprotein receptor–related peptide; PLTP = phospholipid transfer protein; sER = smooth endoplasmic reticulum; SR-B1 = scavenger receptor B1; TG = triglycerides; VLDL = very-low-density lipoprotein; VLDL-R = very-low-density lipoprotein receptor.

TABLE 42–4 Genetic Lipoprotein Disorders

Disorder	Gene	Fig. Part 42-4
LDL Particles		
Familial hypercholesterolemia	LDL-R	7
Familial defective apo B-100	Apo B	7
Autosomal dominant hypercholesterolemia	PCSK9	7
Autosomal recessive hypercholesterolemia	ARH	7
Abetalipoproteinemia	MTP	
Hypobetalipoproteinemia	Apo B	
Familial sitosterolemia	ABCG5/ ABCG8	
Familial lipoprotein(a) hyperlipoproteinemia	Apo (a)	
Remnant Lipoproteins		
Dysbetalipoproteinemia type III	Apo E	3
Hepatic lipase deficiency	HL	6
Triglyceride-Rich Lipoproteins		
Lipoprotein lipase deficiency	LPL	2
Apo CII deficiency	Apo CII	2
Apo AV	Apo AV	
Familial hypertriglyceridemia	Polygenic	
Familial combined hyperlipidemia	Polygenic	
HDL Particles		
Apo AI deficiency	Apo AI	
Tangier disease / Familial HDL deficiency	ABCA1	10
Familial LCAT deficiency syndromes	LCAT	8
CETP deficiency	CETP	9
Niemann-Pick disease types A and B	SMPD1	
Niemann-Pick disease type C	NPC1	

lations with founder effects. Patients with familial hypercholesterolemia have a high risk of developing coronary artery disease (CAD) by the third to fourth decade in men and approximately 8 to 10 years later in women. Diagnosis is based on elevated plasma LDL cholesterol level, family history of premature CAD, and the presence of xanthomas. A molecular diagnosis is sometimes required. Defects of the LDL-R gene cause an accumulation of LDL particles in plasma and thus alter the function of the LDL-R protein and cause familial hypercholesterolemia (see Fig. 42-4, part 7). To date, there are more than 1000 identified mutations of the LDL-R gene (see http://www.ucl.ac.uk/fh/).[22]

FAMILIAL DEFECTIVE APO B. Mutations within the apo B gene that lead to an abnormal ligand-receptor interaction can cause a form of familial hypercholesterolemia clinically indistinguishable from the primary form. Several mutations at the postulated binding site to the LDL-R cause this disorder, familial defective apo B_{100} (see Fig. 42-4, part 7). These consist of apo $B_{Arg3500Gln}$, apo $B_{Arg3500Trp}$, and apo $B_{Arg3531Cys}$.[23] The apo $B_{Arg3500Gln}$ results from a G → A substitution at nucleotide 3500 within exon 26 of the apo B gene. The defective apo B has a reduced affinity (20 to 30 percent of control) for the LDL-R. LDL particles with defective apo B have a plasma half-life threefold to fourfold greater than the half-life of normal LDL. Because of their increased persistence, these LDL particles can more readily undergo oxidative modifications that can enhance their atherogenicity. Affected subjects usually have elevated LDL cholesterol levels up to 400 mg/dl (10.4 mmol/liter) but may also have normal levels. Familial defective apo B 100 has a prevalence similar to that of familial hypercholesterolemia (1/500). In subjects with the classic presentation of familial hypercholesterolemia, the prevalence of familial defective apo B 100 is reported to be 1 in 50 to 1 in 20. The reasons for the variability of plasma LDL cholesterol levels remain unexplained.

An autosomal dominant form of hypercholesterolemia that maps to chromosome 1p34.1 involves a mutation within the proprotein convertase, subtilisin/kexin type 9 gene *(PCSK9)*. *PCSK9* codes for a protein identified as neural apoptosis-regulated convertase 1 (NARC1), a novel proprotein convertase belonging to the subtilase family of convertases. It is related to subtilisin/kexin isoenzyme-1 (site-1 protease), required for cleavage of SREBP.[11] Subjects with loss of function mutation of *PCSK9* have a markedly lower LDL-C than subjects without the mutation. Black Americans have a higher prevalence of this protective mutation than whites. In the Atherosclerosis Risk in Communities study, subjects with life-long low LDL-C because of a mutation at the *PCSK9* gene locus had a marked reduction in coronary events,[24] confirming that genetic low LDL-C states confer cardioprotective advantage. An autosomal recessive form of familial hypercholesterolemia has been identified in kindred from Sardinia and is caused by mutations in the ARH gene that encodes a protein involved in the recycling of the LDL-receptor.[25]

HYPOBETALIPOPROTEINEMIA AND ABETALIPOPROTEINEMIA. Mutations within the apo B gene can lead to truncations of the mature apo B_{100} peptide. Many such mutations cause a syndrome characterized by reduced LDL and VLDL cholesterol but little or no clinical manifestations and no known risk of cardiovascular disease, a condition referred to as *hypobetalipoproteinemia.* Apo B truncated close to its amino terminus loses the ability to bind lipids, producing a syndrome similar to abetalipoproteinemia, a rare recessive lipoprotein disorder of infancy that causes mental retardation and growth abnormalities. Abetalipoproteinemia is caused by a mutation in gene coding for the microsomal triglyceride transfer protein (MTP) required for assembly of apo B-containing lipoproteins in the liver and the intestine. The resulting lack of apo B–containing lipoproteins in plasma causes a marked deficiency of fat-soluble vitamins (A, D, E, and K) that circulate in lipoproteins. In turn, this results in mental and developmental retardation in affected children.

SITOSTEROLEMIA. A rare condition of increased intestinal absorption and decreased excretion of plant sterols (sitosterol and campesterol) can mimic severe familial hypercholesterolemia, with extensive xanthoma formation. Premature atherosclerosis, often apparent clinically well before adulthood, occurs frequently in patients with sitosterolemia. Diagnosis requires specialized analysis of plasma sterols demonstrating an elevation in sitosterol, campesterol, cholestanol, sitostanol, and campestanol. Interestingly, plasma cholesterol is normal or reduced, and triglycerides are normal. Positional cloning techniques have localized the defect to chromosome 2p21. Mutations in the adenosine triphosphate binding cassette G5 and G8 genes (*ABCG5* and *ABCG8*) have been found in patients with sitosterolemia. The gene products of *ABCG5* and *ABCG8* are half ABC transporters and are thought to form a heterodimer characteristic of the full ABC transporters. The complex is located in the villous border of intestinal cells and actively pumps plant sterols back into the intestinal lumen. A defect in either of the genes renders the complex inactive, and absorption of plant sterols (rather than their elimination) ensues. *ABCG5* and *ABCG8* mutations leading to sitosterolemia are rare.[26]

LIPOPROTEIN(a) (see Chap. 39). Lipoprotein(a) (pronounced "lipoprotein little a") consists of an LDL particle linked covalently with one molecule of apo(a). The apo(a) moiety consists of a protein with a high degree of homology with plasminogen. The apo(a) gene appears to have arisen from the plasminogen gene by nonhomologous recombination. The apo(a) gene has multiple repeats of one of the kringle motifs (kringle IV), varying in number from 12 to more than 40 in each individual. Plasma lipoprotein(a) levels depend almost entirely on genetics and correlate inversely with the number of kringle repeats and, therefore, with the molecular weight of apo(a).[27] Few environmental factors or medications modulate plasma lipoprotein(a) levels. The pathogenesis of lipoprotein(a) may result from an antifibrinolytic potential and/or ability to bind oxidized lipoproteins. Some prospective epidemiological studies have shown a positive (albeit weak) association between lipoprotein(a) and coronary artery disease (see Chap. 39).[28]

Triglyceride-Rich Lipoproteins

In subjects with the metabolic syndrome and in diabetic patients, elevation of plasma triglyceride level occurs most often in the presence of visceral (abdominal) obesity and a diet rich in calories, carbohydrates, and saturated fats. Severe elevation of plasma triglycerides can result from genetic disorders of the processing enzymes or apolipoproteins and poorly controlled diabetes.

FAMILIAL HYPERTRIGLYCERIDEMIA (TYPE IV HYPERLIPOPROTEINEMIA). Familial hypertriglyceridemia is not associated with clinical signs such as corneal arcus, xanthoma, and xanthelasmas. Plasma triglycerides, VLDL cholesterol, and VLDL triglycerides are moderately to markedly elevated; LDL cholesterol level is usually low, as is HDL cholesterol. Total cholesterol is normal or elevated, depending on VLDL cholesterol levels. Fasting plasma concentrations of triglycerides are in the range of 2.3 to 5.7 mmol/liter (200 to 500 mg/dl). After a meal, plasma triglycerides may exceed 11.3 mmol/liter (1000 mg/dl). The disorder is found in first-degree relatives, but phenotypic variability is related to gender, age, hormone use (especially estrogens), and diet. Alcohol intake potently stimulates hypertriglyceridemia in these subjects, as does caloric or carbohydrate intake. The relationship with coronary artery disease is not as strong as with familial combined hyperlipidemia and not seen in all studies. Depending on criteria used, the prevalence of familial hypertriglyceridemia ranges from 1 in 100 to 1 in 50. The disorder is highly heterogeneous and likely results from several genes, with a strong environmental influence. An unrelated disorder, familial glycerolemia, a chromosome X-linked genetic disorder, may mimic familial hypertriglyceridemia because most measurement techniques for triglycerides use the measurement of glycerol after enzymatic hydrolysis of triglycerides.[29] The diagnosis of familial hyperglycerolemia requires ultracentrifugation of plasma and analysis of glycerol.

Hepatic overproduction of VLDL causes familial hypertriglyceridemia (see Fig. 42-4, part 4); the catabolism (uptake) of VLDL particles can be normal or reduced. Lipolysis by LPL appears not to be a limiting factor, although the triglyceride load, especially in the postprandial state, may limit processing of VLDL particles. The genetic basis of familial hypertriglyceridemia is unknown, and the candidate approach to find the gene or genes involved (apo B, LDL, apo CIII) has not yielded fruit thus far. Treatment is based first on lifestyle modifications including withdrawal of hormones (estrogens and progesterone), limiting alcohol intake, reducing caloric intake, and increasing exercise. The decision to treat this disorder with medications (see later) depends on global cardiovascular risk.

An infrequent disorder characterized by severe elevation in plasma triglyceride levels (both VLDL and chylomicrons) is associated with a fat-rich diet, obesity, and poorly controlled diabetes. Recognized as type V hyperlipidemia, the pathogenesis is multifactorial and results from overproduction of both VLDL and chylomicrons and from decreased catabolism of these particles.

FAMILIAL HYPERCHYLOMICRONEMIA (TYPE I HYPERLIPIDEMIA). This rare disorder of severe hypertriglyceridemia associates with elevations in fasting plasma triglycerides greater than 11.3 mmol/liter (>1000 mg/dl). These patients have recurrent bouts of pancreatitis and eruptive xanthomas. Interestingly, severe hypertriglyceridemia can also be associated with xerostomia, xerophthalmia, and behavioral abnormalities. The hypertriglyceridemia results from a markedly reduced or absent LPL activity or, more rarely, the absence of its activator, apo CII (see Fig. 42-4, part 2).[30] These defects lead to a lack of hydrolysis of chylomicrons and VLDL and their accumulation in plasma, especially after meals. Extreme elevations of plasma triglycerides (>113 mmol/liter; >10,000 mg/dl) can result.

Plasma from a patient with high triglycerides is milky white, and a clear band of chylomicrons can be seen on top of the plasma after it stands overnight in a refrigerator. Populations with a founder effect can have a high prevalence of LPL mutations. At least 60 LPL mutations can cause LPL deficiency. LPL188, LPLasn291ser, and LPL207 are frequently associated with hyperchylomicronemia. Heterozygotes for the disorder tend to have an increase in fasting plasma triglycerides and smaller, denser LDL particles. Many patients with complete LPL deficiency present in childhood fail to thrive and have recurrent bouts of pancreatitis. To underscore the importance of LPL's role, the LPL-deficient mouse leads to a perinatal lethal phenotype.[31] The treatment of acute pancreatitis includes intravenous hydration and avoidance of fat in the diet (including in parenteral nutrition). Plasma filtration is required only rarely. Chronic treatment includes avoidance of alcohol and dietary fats. To make the diet more palatable, short-chain fatty acids (which are not incorporated in chylomicrons) can be used to supplement the diet.

TYPE III HYPERLIPOPROTEINEMIA. Type III hyperlipoproteinemia, also referred to as *dysbetalipoproteinemia* or *broad beta disease,* is a rare genetic lipoprotein disorder characterized by an accumulation in plasma of remnant lipoprotein particles. On lipoprotein agarose gel electrophoresis, a typical pattern of a broad band between the prebeta (VLDL) and beta (LDL) lipoproteins is observed, hence the name *broad beta disease.* Patients with this disease clearly have increased cardiovascular risk. The clinical presentation consists of pathognomonic tuberous xanthomas and palmar striated xanthomas. The lipoprotein profile shows increased cholesterol and triglyceride levels and reduced HDL cholesterol. Remnant lipoproteins (partly catabolized chylomicrons and VLDL) accumulate in plasma and accumulate cholesterol esters. The defect results from abnormal apo E, which does not bind to hepatic receptors that recognize apo E as a ligand (see Fig. 42-4, part 3).[32] The ratio of VLDL cholesterol to triglycerides, normally less than 0.7 mmol/liter (<0.30 mg/dl), is elevated in patients with type III hyperlipoproteinemia because of cholesteryl ester enrichment of remnant particles. The diagnosis includes plasma ultracentrifugation for lipoprotein separation, lipoprotein electrophoresis, and apo E phenotyping or genotyping. Patients with type III hyperlipoproteinemia have the apo E2/2 phenotype or genotype. Three common alleles for apo E exist: apo E2, E3, and E4. The apo E2 allele has markedly decreased binding to the apo B/E receptor.

In a normal population the prevalence of the apo E2/2 phenotype is approximately 0.7 to 1 percent. Type III hyperlipoproteinemia occurs in approximately 1 percent of subjects bearing the apo E2/2 phenotype. The reasons for the relative rarity of type III dyslipoproteinemia are not fully understood. As discussed previously, a second hit is thought to impart the full expression of the disorder. Other rare mutations of the apo E gene can cause type III hyperlipoproteinemia.[32] In general, type III dyslipoproteinemia responds well to dietary therapy; correction of other metabolic abnormalities (diabetes, obesity); and, in cases requiring drug therapy, fibric acid derivatives or statins. The importance of the apo E gene and protein is underscored by the widespread use of the apo E–deficient mouse, which develops experimental atherosclerosis.[33]

FAMILIAL COMBINED HYPERLIPIDEMIA. One of the most common familial lipoprotein disorders is familial combined hyperlipoproteinemia (FCH). Described initially in survivors of myocardial infarction (MI), the definition of familial combined hyperlipoproteinemia has undergone several refinements. It is characterized by the presence of elevated total cholesterol and/or triglyceride levels based on arbitrary cut points in several members of the same family. Advances in analytical techniques have added the measurement of LDL cholesterol and, in some cases, apo B levels. Because of the lack of a clear-cut clinical or biochemical marker, considerable overlap exists among familial combined hyperlipoproteinemia, familial dyslipidemic hypertension, the metabolic syndrome, and hyperapobetalipoproteinemia. Genetic heterogeneity probably underlies familial combined hyperlipoproteinemia, which has a prevalence of approximately 1 in 50 and accounts for 10 to 20 percent of patients with premature CAD. The condition has few clinical signs; corneal arcus, xanthomas, and xanthelasmas occur infrequently. The biochemical abnormalities include elevation of plasma total and LDL cholesterol levels (>90th to 95th percentile) and/or an elevation of plasma triglycerides (>90th to 95th percentile)—a type IIb lipoprotein phenotype, often in correlation with low HDL cholesterol and elevated apo B levels; small, dense LDL particles are seen frequently. For a diagnosis of familial combined hyperlipoproteinemia, the disorder must be identified in at least one first-degree relative. The underlying metabolic disorder appears to be hepatic overproduction of apo B–containing lipoproteins, delayed postprandial triglyceride-rich lipoprotein clearance, and increased flux of FFAs to the liver.

Experimental data have shown that substrate levels drive hepatic apo B secretion, the most important substrates being FFA and cholesteryl esters. Increased delivery of FFA to the liver, as occurs in states of insulin resistance, leads to increased hepatic apo B secretion (see Chap. 43). Familial combined hyperlipoproteinemia has complex genetics. It was initially considered an autosomal codominant trait; modifying factors include gender, age of onset, and comorbid states such as obesity, lack of exercise, and diet. Initial reports of linkage with the apo AI-CIII-AIV and LPL genes remain unsubstantiated. A novel locus on chromosomes 1 and 16 in Finnish families currently appears to be a promising candidate gene related to familial combined hyperlipoproteinemia.[34]

Reports of the acylation-stimulating protein (ASP), also known as complement *C3desARG,* suggest that abnormal peripheral uptake of FFA may underlie some cases of familial combined hyperlipoproteinemia and the insulin-resistance metabolic syndrome.[35] A putative receptor for ASP has been identified as the orphan receptor C5L2, the complement C5 receptor that also binds complement C3desARG. Abnormal binding of ASP to peripheral cells has been reported in subjects with familial combined hyperlipoproteinemia. Abnormal ASP binding causes decreased uptake of FFAs into adipocytes and subsequent increased flux of FFAs to the liver (see Fig. 42-5D). FFAs are a major substrate for hepatic apo B–containing lipoprotein assembly and secretion.

Reduced plasma levels of HDL cholesterol consistently correlate with the development or presence of CAD (see Chap. 39). Most cases of reduced HDL cholesterol result from elevated plasma triglycerides or apo B levels and often keep company with other features of the metabolic syndrome. Primary forms of reduced HDL cholesterol have been identified in cases of premature CAD and helped shed light on the complex metabolism of HDL particles. Genetic disorders of HDL can result from decreased production or abnormal maturation and increased catabolism.[36] Genetic lipoprotein disorders leading to moderate to severe elevations in plasma triglycerides cause a reduction in HDL cholesterol levels. Familial hyperchylomicronemia, familial hypertriglyceridemia, and familial combined hyperlipoproteinemia are all associated with reduced HDL cholesterol levels. In complex disorders of lipoprotein metabolism such as familial combined hyperlipidemia, the metabolic syndrome, and common forms of hypertriglyceridemia, several factors most likely correlate to low HDL cholesterol level. Plasma triglycerides and HDL cholesterol levels vary inversely. For several reasons, patients with elevated apo B levels also have reduced HDL cholesterol levels. First, decreased lipolysis of triglyceride-rich lipoproteins (each VLDL contains one molecule of apo B) decrease the substrate (phospholipids) available for HDL maturation. Second, triglyceride enrichment of HDL increases their catabolic rate and hence reduces their plasma concentration. Third, exchange of lipids between HDL and triglyceride-rich lipoprotein is reduced, leading to a more rapid disappearance of HDL from plasma.[37] The inverse relationship between HDL cholesterol levels and plasma triglycerides reflects the interdependency of the metabolism of triglyceride-rich lipoproteins and HDL particles.

APO AI GENE DEFECTS. Primary defects affecting production of HDL particles consist predominantly of apo AI-CIII-AIV gene defects. More than 46 mutations affect the structure of apo AI,[38] leading to a marked reduction in HDL cholesterol levels. Not all of these defects are associated with premature cardiovascular disease. Clinical presentations can vary from extensive atypical xanthomatosis and corneal infiltration of lipids to no manifestations at all. Treatment of these apo AI gene defects generally fails to raise HDL cholesterol levels. Other mutations of apo AI lead to an increased catabolic rate of apo AI and may not be associated with cardiovascular disease. One such mutation, apo AI_{Milano} (apo $AI_{Arg173Cys}$), appears to confer longevity despite low HDL levels.[38]

LCAT, CETP DEFICIENCY. Genetic defects in the HDL-processing enzymes give rise to interesting phenotypes. Deficiencies of LCAT, the enzyme that catalyzes the formation of cholesteryl esters in plasma, cause corneal infiltration of neutral lipids and hematological abnormalities due to abnormal constitution of red blood cell membranes. LCAT deficiency can lead to an entity called "fish eye disease" because of the characteristic pattern of corneal infiltration observed in affected individuals.[39]

Patients without CETP have very elevated HDL cholesterol levels, enriched in cholesteryl esters. Because CETP assists the transfer of HDL cholesteryl esters into triglyceride-rich lipoproteins, a deficiency of this enzyme causes accumulation of cholesteryl esters within HDL particles. CETP deficiency is not associated with premature CAD but may not afford protection against CAD.[40]

TANGIER DISEASE AND FAMILIAL HDL DEFICIENCY. A rare disorder of HDL deficiency was identified in a proband from the Chesapeake Bay island of Tangier in the United States. The proband, whose sister was also affected, had markedly enlarged yellow tonsils and nearly absent HDL cholesterol levels, an entity now called *Tangier disease.* The cellular defect in Tangier disease consists of a reduced cellular cholesterol efflux in skin fibroblasts and macrophages from affected subjects.[41] A more common entity, familial HDL deficiency, was also found to result from decreased cellular cholesterol. The genetic defect in Tangier disease and in familial HDL deficiency results from mutations at the ATP binding cassette A1 gene *(ABCA1)* that encodes the ABCA1 transporter (see Fig. 42-5B).[42] At least 100 mutations have been reported within ABCA1, causing Tangier disease (homozygous or compound heterozygous mutations) or familial HDL deficiency (heterozygous mutations). Although subjects with Tangier disease and familial HDL deficiency are at increased risk for CAD, their low levels of LDL cholesterol appear to have a protective effect. ABCA1 appears to shuttle from the late endosomal compartment to the plasma membrane and act as a membrane-bound transporter of phospholipids (and cholesterol) onto acceptor proteins such as apo AI and apo E. Hydroxysterols regulate ABCA1 via the LXR/RXR nuclear receptor pathway. ABCA1 undergoes phosphorylation via protein kinase A and acts as a receptor for apo AI.

OTHER CHOLESTEROL TRANSPORT DEFECTS. Niemann-Pick type C disease is a disorder of lysosomal cholesterol transport. In patients with Niemann-Pick type C disease, mental retardation and neurological manifestations occur frequently. The cellular phenotype involves markedly decreased cholesterol esterification and cellular cholesterol transport defect to the Golgi apparatus. Unlike Tangier disease/familial HDL deficiency, the cellular defect in Niemann-Pick type C disease appears proximal to the transport of cholesterol to the plasma membrane. The gene for Niemann-Pick type C disease *(NPC1)* has been mapped to 18q21 and the gene codes for a 1278-amino acid protein, the role of which appears to be involved in cholesterol shuttling between the late endosomal pathway and the plasma membrane. The *NPC1* gene product shares homology with the morphogen receptor *patched* and the SREBP cleavage activating protein (SCAP).[43] Niemann-Pick type C cells lack NPC1 protein, and cholesterol sequestration within the late endosome compartment prevents up-regulation of *ABCA1.* These patients have impaired cellular cholesterol efflux and HDL assembly.[44] Niemann-Pick type I disease (subtypes A and B), caused by mutations at the sphingomyelin phosphodiesterase-1 *(SMPD-1)* gene, is associated with a low HDL cholesterol level. The *SMPD-1* gene codes for a lysosomal (acidic) and secretory sphingomyelinase. The low HDL cholesterol level in Niemann-Pick A and B patients appears to result from a decrease in LCAT reaction because of abnormal HDL constituents.[45]

Secondary Causes of Hyperlipidemia and the Metabolic Syndrome

Several clinical disorders lead to alterations in lipoprotein status (Table 42-5).

HORMONAL CAUSES. Hypothyroidism, a not infrequent cause of secondary lipoprotein disorders, often manifests with elevated LDL cholesterol, triglycerides, or both. An elevated level of thyroid-stimulating hormone is key to the diagnosis, and the lipoprotein abnormalities often revert to normal after correction of thyroid status. Rarely, hypothyroidism may uncover a genetic lipoprotein disorder such as type III hyperlipidemia. Estrogens can elevate plasma triglycerides and HDL cholesterol levels, probably because of increases in both hepatic VLDL and apo AI production. In postmenopausal women, estrogens may reduce LDL cholesterol by up to 15 percent. The use of estrogens for the

TABLE 42-5	Secondary Causes of Dyslipoproteinemias
Metabolic	Diabetes Lipodystrophy Glycogen storage disorders
Renal	Chronic renal failure Glomerulonephritis
Hepatic	Cirrhosis
Hormonal	Estrogens Progesterones Growth hormone Thyroid disorders (hypothyroidism) Corticosteroids
Lifestyle	Physical inactivity Obesity Diet rich in fats, saturated fats Alcohol intake
Medications	Retinoic acid derivatives Glucocorticoids Exogenous estrogens Thiazide diuretics Beta-adrenergic blockers (selective) Testosterone Immunosuppressive medications (cyclosporine) Antiviral medications (human immunodeficiency virus protease inhibitors)

 treatment of lipoprotein disorders is no longer recommended because of the slight increase in cardiovascular risk with prolonged use of estrogens in the postmenopausal period (see Chaps. 45 and 76).[46] Rarely, pregnancy causes severe increases in plasma triglycerides, on a background of lipoprotein lipase deficiency. Such cases present a serious threat to mother and child and require referral to specialized centers. Male sex hormones and anabolic steroids can increase hepatic lipase activity and have been used in the treatment of hypertriglyceridemia in men. Growth hormone can reduce LDL cholesterol and augment HDL cholesterol but is not recommended in the treatment of lipoprotein disorders.

METABOLIC CAUSES. The most frequent secondary cause of dyslipoproteinemia is probably the constellation of metabolic abnormalities seen in patients with the metabolic syndrome (see Chaps. 39 and 43). The finding of increased visceral fat (abdominal obesity), elevated blood pressure, and impaired glucose tolerance often clusters with increased plasma triglycerides and a reduced HDL cholesterol level. These are the major components of the metabolic syndrome.[21,47] The lack of internationally recognized uniform criteria for the metabolic syndrome among other issues casts doubt on the usefulness of this syndrome as a diagnostic entity.[48] Overt diabetes, especially type II diabetes, frequently elevates plasma triglycerides and reduces HDL cholesterol. These abnormalities have prognostic implications in patients with type II diabetes. Poor control of diabetes, obesity, and moderate to severe hyperglycemia can yield severe hypertriglyceridemia with chylomicronemia and increased VLDL cholesterol levels. Subjects with type 1 diabetes can also have severe hypertriglyceridemia when poorly controlled. Familial lipodystrophy (complete or partial) may be associated with increased VLDL secretion. Dunnigan lipodystrophy, a genetic disorder with features of the metabolic syndrome, is caused by mutations within the Lamin A/C gene and is associated with limb-girdle fat atrophy. Excess plasma triglycerides often accompany glycogen storage disorders.

RENAL DISORDERS. In subjects with glomerulonephritis and protein-losing nephropathies, a marked increase in secretion of hepatic lipoproteins can raise LDL cholesterol levels, which may approach the levels seen in subjects with familial hypercholesterolemia. By contrast, patients with chronic renal failure have a pattern of hypertriglyceridemia with reduced HDL cholesterol. Patients with end-stage renal disease, including those on hemodialysis or chronic ambulatory peritoneal dialysis, have a poor prognosis and accelerated atherosclerosis and should undergo aggressive treatment of lipoprotein disorders. This approach, however, has been recently challenged when a recent trial of statins in diabetic patients on dialysis showed no reduction in cardiovascular endpoints. After organ transplantation, the immunosuppressive regimen (glucocorticoids and cyclosporine) typically elevates triglycerides and reduces HDL cholesterol levels. Because transplant patients generally have an increase in cardiovascular risk, a secondary hyperlipidemia may warrant treatment. Patients receiving the combination of statin plus cyclosporine merit careful dose titrations and monitoring for myopathy.

LIVER DISEASE. Obstructive liver disease, especially primary biliary cirrhosis, may lead to the formation of an abnormal lipoprotein termed *lipoprotein-x*. This type of lipoprotein is found in cases of LCAT deficiency and consists of an LDL-like particle but with a marked reduction in cholesteryl esters. Extensive xanthoma formation on the face and palmar areas can result from accumulation of lipoprotein-x.

LIFESTYLE. Factors contributing to obesity such as an imbalance between caloric intake and energy expenditure, lack of physical activity, and a diet rich in saturated fats and refined sugars contribute in large part to the lipid and lipoprotein lipid levels within a population (see Chaps. 39 and 44).

MEDICATION. Several medications can alter lipoproteins. Thiazide diuretics can increase plasma triglyceride levels. Beta blockers, especially non-beta-1 selective, increase triglycerides and lower HDL cholesterol levels. Retinoic acid and estrogens can increase triglyceride levels, sometimes dramatically. Corticosteroids and immunosuppressive agents can increase plasma triglyceride levels and lower HDL cholesterol levels. Estrogens can increase plasma HDL cholesterol significantly and often increase triglyceride concentrations.

In clinical practice, many dyslipoproteinemias, other than the genetic forms mentioned earlier, share an important environmental cause. Lifestyle changes (diet, exercise, reduction of abdominal obesity) should form the foundation for the treatment of most dyslipidemias. The effects of marked alterations in lifestyle; reduction in dietary fats, especially saturated fats; and exercise can improve cardiovascular prognosis. Translating these findings into practice, however, has been more difficult. For example, dietary manipulations as performed in a physician's office lead to relatively small reductions in plasma lipid and lipoprotein cholesterol levels (see Chaps. 39, 44, and 45).

DRUGS THAT AFFECT LIPID METABOLISM (Table 42-6)

Bile Acid–Binding Resins

The bile acid–binding resins interrupt the enterohepatic circulation of bile acids by inhibiting their reabsorption in the intestine (more than 90 percent of bile acids reabsorbed). Currently, their main use is adjunctive therapy in patients with severe hypercholesterolemia due to increased LDL cholesterol. Because bile acid–binding resins are not absorbed systemically (they remain in the intestine and are eliminated in the stool), they are considered safe in chil-

TABLE 42–6 Current Lipid-Lowering Medications

Generic Name	Trade Name	Recommended Dose Range
Statins		
Atorvastatin	Lipitor	10-80 mg
Fluvastatin	Lescol	20-80 mg
Lovastatin	Mevacor	20-80 mg
Pravastatin	Pravachol	10-40 mg
Rosuvastatin	Crestor	5-40 mg
Simvastatin	Zocor	10-80 mg
Bile Acid Absorption Inhibitors		
Cholestyramine	Questran	4-24 gm
Colestipol	Colestid	5-30 gm
Colesevelam	WelChol	3.8-4.5 gm
Cholesterol Absorption Inhibitors		
Ezetimibe	Zetia (Ezetrol)	10 mg
Fibrates*		
Bezafibrate	Bezalip	400 mg
Fenofibrate	Tricor	67-200 mg (Lipidil Micro, EZ)
Gemfibrozil†	Lopid	600-1200 mg
Niacin‡	Niacin	1-3 gm
Nicotinic acid	Niaspan	1-2 gm

*Avoid in patients with renal insufficiency.
†Not recommended in combination with statins.
‡Use with caution in patients with diabetes or glucose intolerance.

dren. Cholestyramine (Questran) is used in 4-gm unit doses as powder, and colestipol (Colestid) is used in 5-gm unit doses. Effective doses range from 2 to 6 unit doses/day, always taken with meals. The most important side effects are predominantly gastrointestinal, with constipation, a sensation of fullness, and gastrointestinal discomfort. Hypertriglyceridemia can result from the use of these drugs. Decreased drug absorption dictates careful scheduling of medications 1 hour before or 3 hours after the patient takes bile acid–binding resins. Bile acid–binding resins can be used in combination with statins and/or cholesterol absorption inhibitors in cases of severe hypercholesterolemia.

Hydroxymethylglutaryl–Coenzyme A Reductase Inhibitors (Statins)

Statins inhibit HMG-CoA reductase and prevent the formation of mevalonate, the rate-limiting step of sterol synthesis. To maintain cellular cholesterol homeostasis, expression of the LDL-R increases and the rate of cholesteryl ester formation declines. These homeostatic adjustments to HMG-CoA reductase inhibition increase LDL cholesterol clearance from plasma and decrease hepatic production of VLDL and LDL. In addition to blocking the synthesis of cholesterol, statins also interfere with the synthesis of lipid intermediates with important biological effects. In the cholesterol synthetic pathway, intermediate molecules of dimethylallyl pyrophosphate are metabolized by prenyl transferase into geranyl pyrophosphate and subsequently into farnesyl pyrophosphate. This step occurs before the formation of squalenes.[49] These intermediates, geranylgeranyl and farnesyl, are used for protein prenylation, a mechanism by which a lipid moiety attaches covalently to a protein, allowing anchoring into cell membranes and enhancing its biological activity. This is the case for the GTP-binding proteins Rho A, Rac, and Ras. Indeed, statins may increase HDL cholesterol in part by preventing the geranylgeranylation of Rho A and phosphorylation of peroxysome proliferator-activated receptor alpha (PPARα), a factor that regulates apo AI transcription.[49] Altered protein prenylation may also mediate some of the putative effects of statins not related to a reduction in LDL cholesterol levels.

Atherosclerosis is an inflammatory disease. Statins decrease C-reactive protein,[50] induce apoptosis in smooth muscle cells, alter collagen content of atherosclerotic plaques, alter endothelial function, and decrease the inflammatory component of plaques[51,52] (see also Chaps. 38 and 39). Some investigators argue that statins possess effects independent of their inhibition of HMG CoA reductase. Experts remain speculative whether clinically important differences exist in efficacy between statins for a given percentage reduction in LDL cholesterol.

Statins are generally well tolerated; side effects include reversible elevation in transaminases and myositis, which causes discontinuation of the drug in less than 1 percent of patients. The currently available drugs are fluvastatin (Lescol), 20 to 80 mg/day; lovastatin (Mevacor), 20 to 80 mg/day; pravastatin (Pravachol), 20 to 40 mg/day; simvastatin (Zocor), 10 to 80 mg/day; atorvastatin (Lipitor), 10 to 80 mg/day; and rosuvastatin (Crestor), 5 to 40 mg/day. Concomitant drugs that interfere with the metabolism of statins by inhibiting the cytochrome P450 3A4 and 2C9 systems can increase plasma concentrations of statins. These include antibiotics, antifungal medications, certain antiviral drugs, grapefruit juice, cyclosporine, amiodarone, and several others.

Cholesterol Absorption Inhibitors

The development of selective inhibitors of intestinal sterol absorption has significantly advanced the treatment of lipoprotein disorders. Ezetimibe is the first such compound. It appears to limit selective uptake of cholesterol and other sterols by intestinal epithelial cells, by interfering with the Niemann-Pick C1-like 1 protein 1 (NPC1L1).[10] Ezetimibe is particularly indicated for patients with LDL cholesterol levels above target on a maximally tolerated statin dose. Ezetimibe lowers LDL cholesterol by about 18 percent and adds to the effect of statins.[53] Because ezetimibe also prevents the intestinal absorption of sitosterol, it might be the drug of choice in cases of sitosterolemia. The current dose of ezetimibe is 10 mg/day.

Fibric Acid Derivatives (Fibrates)

Two derivatives of fibric acid are currently available in the United States, and two more are available in Canada and Europe. Gemfibrozil (Lopid) is used at a dose of 600 mg twice a day and is indicated in cases of hypertriglyceridemia and in the secondary prevention of cardiovascular diseases in patients with low HDL cholesterol levels. These latter recommendations are based on the Veterans Affairs HDL Intervention Trial (VA-HIT). Fenofibrate (Tricor; Lipidil Micro, EZ) is used to treat hypertriglyceridemia and combined hyperlipoproteinemia. The dose is 200 mg/day, and a new formulation is available to vary the dose from 67 mg (especially in cases of renal failure) to 267 mg/day. Clofibrate (Atromid) is still available in some centers, although its use has declined since the introduction of newer molecules. Ciprofibrate (Lypanthyl, Lipanor) and bezafibrate (Bezalip) are more widely used in Europe. The main indications for the use of fibrates is in the treatment of hypertriglyceridemia when diet and lifestyle changes are not sufficient. Another potential indication is in the prevention of cardiovascular diseases in patients with elevated plasma triglycerides and low HDL cholesterol, although the data supporting their use are weaker than those for statins.

The mechanism of action of fibrates involves interaction with the nuclear transcription factor PPARα that regulates the transcription of the LPL, apo CII, and apo AI genes. The side effects of fibrates include cutaneous manifestations; gastrointestinal effects (abdominal discomfort, increased bile lithogenicity); erectile dysfunction; elevated transaminases; interaction with oral anticoagulants; and elevated plasma homocysteine, especially with fenofibrate and, to a lesser extent, with bezafibrate.[54] Because fibrates increase LPL activity, LDL cholesterol levels may rise in patients with hypertriglyceridemia treated with this class of medications. Fibrates, especially gemfibrozil, can inhibit the glucuronidation of statins and thus retard their elimination. For this reason, combination of gemfibrozil with statins may increase the risk of myotoxicity.

Nicotinic Acid (Niacin)

Niacin has been used for decades for the treatment of dyslipidemias and is particularly effective in increasing HDL cholesterol and lowering triglyceride levels. The effect of niacin on LDL cholesterol is more modest. Effective doses of niacin are in the range of 3000 mg/day, in three separate doses. Using an escalating dose schedule to reach the full dose in 2 to 3 weeks rather than starting with the full dose is preferable. Slow-release forms of niacin including Niaspan (1 to 2 gm/day) decrease the side effect profile of the drug. Skin flushing can be attenuated by taking a daily aspirin. Niacin decreases the hepatic secretion of VLDL from the liver and decreased FFA mobilization for the periphery. Although niacin has been shown in the long-term follow-up of the Coronary Drug Project to decrease mortality at 15 years, significant and common minor side effects and much less frequent serious adverse actions, as well as the development of statins, hamper its use. Side effects of niacin include flushing, hyperuricemia, hyperglycemia, hepatotoxicity, acanthosis nigricans, and gastritis. Close laboratory monitoring of side effects is warranted. Long-acting niacin has the advantage of a once- or twice-daily dosing schedule, but older preparations of slow-release niacin were potentially more hepatotoxic. Niacin effectively raises HDL cholesterol levels and, in combination with low-dose statin, can retard the angiographic progression of CAD and decrease adverse cardiac events.[55] Recent work has identified cell surface receptors for nicotinic acid that belong to the G protein–coupled heptahelical superfamily. This discovery may speed the elucidation of the molecular mechanism of nicotinic acid's effects on lipid metabolism.[56]

Cholesteryl Ester Transfer Protein Inhibitors

The inhibition of cholesteryl ester transfer protein (CETP) by pharmacological agents mimics the genetic heterozygous CETP deficiency state (see Fig. 42-4, part 9). The CETP inhibitor Torcetrapib[57] was removed from clinical trials because of an increase in serious adverse events. A marked increase in larger, more buoyant HDL particles is observed in patients on Torcetrapib; these particles appear to promote cellular cholesterol efflux efficiently. Reported side effects include elevation in hepatic transaminases, an increase in blood pressure, and abdominal symptoms.

Fish Oils

Fish oils are rich in polyunsaturated fatty acids such as eicosapentaenoic acid or docosahexaenoic acid, with the first double bond in the omega-3 position. These fatty acids lower plasma triglyceride levels and have antithrombotic properties. Although employed in the treatment of hypertriglyceridemia, their use is reserved in cases of severe hypertriglyceridemia refractory to conventional therapy. Fish oils decrease VLDL synthesis and decrease VLDL apo B. The response to fish oils depends on dose, requiring a daily intake of up to 10 gm of eicosapentaenoic acid or docosahexaenoic acid for a significant benefit on plasma triglyceride levels. A prescription form of omega-3 fatty acids has become available in the United States, labeled for use in extreme hypertriglyceridemia (>500 mg/dl).

Phytosterols

Phytosterols are derivatives of cholesterol from plants and trees. They interfere with the formation of micelles in the intestine and prevent intestinal cholesterol absorption. They can be obtained as "neutraceuticals" or can be incorporated in soft margarines. The sterols may prove useful for the adjunctive management of lipoprotein disorders and are part of the therapeutic lifestyle change regimen in the current guidelines (see later).

Other Medications

Probucol was used as an antioxidant and had modest effects on plasma lipoprotein levels. The lack of conclusive evidence that probucol has beneficial effects and profound reduction in HDL levels and prolongation of QT interval led to its withdrawal. A study indicates that it may have a role in the prevention of restenosis after coronary angioplasty if used before the procedure.[58] Thyroxine is no longer used as a lipid modulator unless hypothyroidism has been documented.

Monitoring of Lipid Therapy

After initiation of medical therapy, the response should be checked within the first 3 months, along with transaminases and creatinine kinase. Thereafter, clinical judgment should dictate the interval between follow-up visits. Although frequent visits are probably not useful in the detection of serious side effects, they serve to encourage compliance and adherence to diet and lifestyle changes.

CLINICAL TRIALS OF DRUGS AFFECTING LIPID METABOLISM

Numerous pathological, epidemiological, genetic, and interventional trials have validated the central tenet of the lipid hypothesis, which proposes a causal relationship between dyslipidemia and atherogenesis and identifies lipid modification as a risk-reducing strategy for CHD (see Chap. 38). A number of small trials using dietary or drug therapies have demonstrated the angiographic benefit of managing elevated total cholesterol and LDL cholesterol. Early clinical trials using bile-acid sequestrants, fibrates, or nicotinic acid reported modest reductions in coronary risk with modest reductions in LDL cholesterol.

The advent of the HMG-CoA reductase inhibitors, or statins, in the mid-1980s made possible more aggressive reduction of LDL cholesterol. By the late 1990s, several large-scale, prospective randomized trials with these drugs had reported robust reductions in relative cardiovascular risks, compared with placebo.[59-68] This section discusses the more recent trials in this area, specifically in high-risk primary prevention, intensive LDL-C lowering in secondary prevention, the benefits of intensive therapy in acute coronary syndromes, regression studies, and specific subgroup analysis (the elderly and the diabetic patient). The focus on statin trials reflects the widespread clinical success of this category of drugs. Ample reviews have considered the results of the older trials. We refer readers interested in these earlier trials to previous editions of this textbook.

Treating High-Risk (Primary Prevention) Patients (Tables 42-7A and B)

As the interaction of multiple coronary risk factors has received greater clinical importance, recommendations for clinical practice have increasingly embraced the concept of global risk management. This global risk is calculated using an algorithm that considers not only total cholesterol but also HDL cholesterol, smoking, age, hypertension, and gender (see Chap. 39). Adult diabetic subjects are considered to be at high cardiovascular risk, with few exceptions. Cardiovascular risk is determined as cardiovascular death or nonfatal MI in the next 10 years on the basis of the Framingham Heart Study risk score and determines the intensity of lipid intervention. On the basis of evidence from clinical trials, the 2004 U.S. Adult Treatment Panel (ATP III) modified its guidelines, recommending a more aggressive LDL-C target in high-risk subjects.[69] Similar risk stratification and targets are proposed in Europe.[70]

Because global risk assessment shifts emphasis away from abnormal lipids alone to the patient's overall risk profile, it raises an important issue for the future of lipid management. That is, should the decision to initiate lipid modification for cardiovascular risk reduction be based on high risk or high cholesterol? Recent trials have evaluated this question.

TABLE 42–7A	Primary Prevention Trials of Statin Therapy	
	WOSCOPS	**AFCAPS/TexCAPS**
N (% women)	6596 (0)	6605 (15)
Duration (yrs)	4.9	5.2
Intervention	Pravastatin, 40 mg/day	Lovastatin, 20-40 mg/day
Baseline lipids (mg/dl)		
Total cholesterol	272	221
LDL cholesterol	192	150
HDL cholesterol	44	36 men; 40 women
Triglycerides	164	158
% Lipid changes, treatment vs. placebo		
Total cholesterol	−20	−19
LDL cholesterol	−26	−26
HDL cholesterol	+5	+5
Triglycerides	−12	−13
Endpoints (% changes in risk), treatment vs. placebo		
Nonfatal MI/CHD death	**−31**	−25
Fatal/nonfatal MI	—	−40
Acute major coronary events	—	**−37**
Total mortality	−22	+3 (NS)
CHD mortality	−28	too few
Revascularizations	−37	−33
Stroke	−11 (NS)	—

AFCAPS/TexCAPS=Air Force/Texas Coronary Atherosclerosis Prevention Study; CHD=coronary heart disease; HDL=high-density lipoprotein; LDL=low-density lipoprotein; MI=myocardial infarction; NS=nonsignificant; WOSCOPS=West of Scotland Coronary Prevention Study; **bold**=study's primary endpoint; —=not reported.

The Medical Research Council/British Heart Foundation Heart Protection Study (HPS) evaluated the role of statin therapy in at-risk patients for whom guidelines at the time would not have recommended drug intervention.[64] In HPS, however, more than 65 percent of patients had evidence of atherosclerosis (coronary or peripheral) and the remainder had diabetes or multiple risk factors. The broad inclusion criteria of cardiovascular risk and age (40 to 80 years), simple entry criteria (total cholesterol > 135 mg/dl (3.5 mmol/liter), and number randomized (20,536) make this trial a seminal contribution in the field. The two-by-two factorial design of the HPS intended to analyze the effect of simvastatin, 40 mg/day, versus placebo with or without a combination of antioxidant vitamins (600 mg alpha tocopherol, 250 mg ascorbic acid, 20 mg beta carotene) on the risk of major vascular events.

The combination of antioxidant vitamins did not affect morbidity or mortality. Simvastatin treatment, on the other hand, reduced the risk for any major vascular event by 24 percent ($p = 0.0001$), with an absolute risk reduction of 5.4 percent (28.3 percent in the placebo group minus 19.4 percent in the simvastatin group). The all-cause mortality rate fell by 13 percent ($p = 0.0003$), with a significant 17 percent reduction ($p = 0.0001$) in deaths attributed to any vascular cause. No increase occurred in noncardiac causes of mortality such as neoplasia, respiratory disease, or other nonvascular deaths.

Subgroup analysis in HPS had sufficient power to examine women ($n = 5072$), diabetics ($n = 4282$), CHD patients ($n = 7150$), and subjects older than 75 years of age ($n = 1263$). All of these subgroups benefited from the statin therapy.

The Prospective Evaluation of Pravastatin in the Elderly (PROSPER) assessed the impact of treatment with pravastatin 40 mg/day versus placebo in 5804 men and women aged 70 to 82 years of age with a history of vascular disease (coronary, cerebrovascular, or peripheral vascular) or a risk factor profile consistent with high risk (smoking, hypertension, or diabetes).[65] Participants in this study had plasma total cholesterol levels between 155 and 350 mg/dl (4 to 9 mmol/liter) and triglyceride concentrations less than 530 mg/dl (6 mmol/liter). Women accounted for more than half of the individuals in PROSPER. The mean follow-up was 3.2 years, and the composite primary endpoint included

TABLE 42–7B	Trials of Statin Therapy in High-Risk Patients			
	HPS	**ALL-HAT LLT**	**ASCOT LLA**	**PROSPER**
N (% women)	20536 (24.7)	10355 (48.8)	10305 (18.8)	5804 (51.7)
Duration (yrs)	5	4.8	3.3	3.2
Percent with Hx of CVD or CHD	65%	14%	14%	44%
Statin crossover rate	17%	26.1%	9%	10%
Intervention	Simvastatin, 40 mg/day vs. placebo	Pravastatin, 20-40 mg/day vs. usual care	Atorvastatin, 10 mg/day vs. placebo	Pravastatin, 40 mg/day vs. placebo
Baseline lipids, mg/dl (mmol/liter)				
Total cholesterol	228 (5.9)	224 (5.8)	213 (5.5)	221 (5.7)
LDL cholesterol	132 (3.4)	146 (3.8)	132 (3.4)	147 (3.8)
HDL cholesterol	41 (1.06)	48 (1.2)	50 (1.3)	50 (1.3)
Triglycerides	124 (1.4)	152 (1.7)	152 (1.7)	58 (1.5)
% Lipid changes, treatment vs. placebo				
Total cholesterol	−20	−10	−24	NR
LDL cholesterol	−29	−17	−35	−34
HDL cholesterol	+3	+1	0	+5
Triglycerides	−21	—	−17	−13
Endpoints (% changes in risk), treatment versus placebo				
Major cardiovascular events	**−24**	—	—	**+15**
Nonfatal MI/CHD death	−27	NS	**+36**	−19
Fatal/nonfatal MI	—	—	—	—
Total mortality	−13	**NS**	NS	NS
CHD mortality	−17	NS	NS	−24
Revascularizations	−24	—	—	NS
Stroke	−25	NS	−27	NS

ALL-HAT LLT=Antihypertensive and Lipid-Lowering Treatment to Prevent Heart Attack Trial; ASCOT LLA=Anglo-Scandinavian Cardiac Outcomes Trial Lipid Lowering Arm; **bold**=study's primary endpoint; CHD=coronary heart disease; HDL=high-density lipoprotein; HPS=Heart Protection Study; Hx=history; LDL=low-density lipoprotein; MI=myocardial infarction; NS=nonsignificant; PROSPER=Prospective Study of Pravastatin in the Elderly at Risk; —=not reported.

coronary death, nonfatal MI, and fatal or nonfatal stroke. Pravastatin treatment reduced the relative risk for this endpoint significantly by 15 percent ($p = 0.014$) and for CHD death by 24 percent ($p = 0.043$). The treatment showed similar benefit across many subgroups: those with versus those without prior vascular disease; men versus women; tertiles of baseline LDL cholesterol; current smokers versus nonsmokers; and those with and those without a history of hypertension. Participants in the lowest tertile of baseline HDL cholesterol (<1.11 mmol/L or 43 mg/dl) experienced greater benefit than those in the higher tertiles.

Lipid-modifying treatment had no effect on the risk for stroke (see also Chap. 58) or on cognitive function, both of which are important endpoints in an older population.

Hypertensive Patients

The large Antihypertensive and Lipid-Lowering Treatment to Prevent Heart Attack Trial (ALL-HAT) sought to determine whether cholesterol lowering with open-label pravastatin 40 mg/day (plus resin, if needed) would reduce total mortality in 10,355 moderately hypercholesterolemic, hypertensive men and women, aged 55 years or older, with at least one other CHD risk factor, as compared with usual care.[66] The ALL-HAT patients met lipid criteria of an LDL cholesterol level of 120 to 189 mg/dl (3.1 to 5 mmol/liter) (or 100 to 129 mg/dl [2.6 to 3.3 mmol/liter] in those with CHD) and triglycerides less than 350 mg/dl (<3.9 mmol/liter).

In contrast with other large statin studies, ALL-HAT reported no benefit and no harm of statin treatment compared with usual care on any study endpoint. The study may have been underpowered because of difficulties related to patient recruitment. The trial was open labeled, and there was declining adherence in the pravastatin group and a high crossover rate to statin therapy in the usual-care group (by 6 years, more than 25 percent of these patients were receiving a statin). Indeed, the absolute difference in total cholesterol between the pravastatin and the usual-care group by the end of the trial was only 9.6 percent, which was approximately half of the reduction achieved in older statin trials.

The lipid-lowering arm of the Anglo-Scandinavian Cardiac Outcomes Trial (ASCOT) assessed the clinical effect of atorvastatin, 10 mg/day, versus placebo in 10,305 hypertensive patients with a total cholesterol level of less than 250 mg/dl (6.5 mmol/liter) and a high-risk profile.[67] Although the trial excluded individuals with previous MI, current angina, or cerebrovascular disease within 3 months before randomization, the randomized patients had evidence of other vascular disease or CHD risk equivalents (left ventricular hypertrophy, other electrocardiographic abnormalities, peripheral arterial disease, previous cerebrovascular disease, diabetes) or several other CHD risk factors.

Originally planned to have a follow-up period of 5 years, the ASCOT ended early after a median follow-up of 3.3 years, after 100 primary endpoint events had occurred in the atorvastatin group compared with 154 in the placebo group. The relative risk reduction was 36 percent ($p = 0.0005$), and the benefit became apparent within a year of the study's initiation. Benefit was similar across prespecified subgroups. Atorvastatin reduced the relative risk for stroke by 27 percent ($p = 0.024$) and for total cardiovascular events by 21 percent ($p = 0.0005$). Total mortality and adverse events did not differ between the treatment groups.

Diabetic Patients

Because of their high risk for developing CHD, diabetic patients warrant aggressive lipid modification, according to U.S. guidelines (see Chaps. 43 and 45). However, few trials have evaluated the effects of lipid modification on clinical endpoints in this population, and the evidence of benefit derives largely from subgroup analyses. The Collaborative Atorvastatin Diabetes Study (CARDS) examined patients with type II diabetes without manifest CHD.[68] Entry criteria included not only diabetes but also at least one other CHD risk factor: current smoking, hypertension, retinopathy, or microalbuminuria or macroalbuminuria. The trial enrolled individuals with LDL cholesterol levels less than 160 mg/dl (4.14 mmol/liter) and triglycerides less than 600 mg/dl (6.78 mmol/liter). The study included 2838 men and women, 40 to 75 years of age. The trial used a fixed dosage of atorvastatin of 10 mg/day compared with placebo. The primary efficacy parameter is the time from randomization to the occurrence of a first primary endpoint event, which may include major coronary events, revascularizations, stroke, unstable angina, or resuscitated cardiac arrest. The study was stopped prematurely for benefit. A 36 percent reduction occurred ($p = 0.001$) in primary endpoints (CHD death, nonfatal MI, unstable angina, revascularization, and fatal and nonfatal stroke).

The FIELD trial[71] was carried out in Australia, New Zealand, and Finland and examined the effect of fenofibrate, 200 mg/day, on the development of CHD in patients with diabetes for 5 years. The investigators examined 9795 patients, age 50 to 75 years with type II diabetes diagnosed after age 35 years and no clear indication for cholesterol-lowering therapy at baseline at the time of study design. Lipid entry criteria were total cholesterol 116 to 251 mg/dl (3 to 6.5 mmol/liter), plus either total cholesterol to HDL ratio > 4 or triglyceride > 88.6 mg/dl (1 mmol/liter). The primary composite endpoint of CHD death or nonfatal MI was not significantly lower in the fenofibrate group compared with the placebo group (5.2 versus 5.8 percent, $p = 0.16$). Subgroup analysis showed a nonsignificant increase in CHD death (2.2 percent on fenofibrate versus 1.9 percent on placebo, $p = 0.22$), but a significant reduction in nonfatal MI on fenofibrate (3.2 versus 4.2 percent, $p = 0.01$). The secondary composite endpoint of total CV events was significantly lower in the fenofibrate group compared with the placebo group (12.5 versus 13.9 percent, $p = 0.035$). Cardiovascular mortality (2.9 percent fenofibrate versus 2.6 percent placebo, $p = 0.41$), total mortality (7.3 percent fenofibrate versus 6.9 percent placebo, $p = 0.18$), and stroke (3.2 percent fenofibrate versus 3.6 percent placebo, $p = 0.36$) were not significantly different between the fenofibrate and placebo groups. The rate of statin drop-in in the fenofibrate group averaged 8 percent, whereas it averaged 17 percent in the placebo group during the course of the trial.

The CARDS and FIELD trials were similar in several respects including inclusion criteria and baseline lipid levels. On the basis of these trials, prevention of cardiovascular disease in diabetic subjects should include a statin.

Other Fibrate Trials

The Veterans Affairs Cooperative Studies Program High-Density Lipoprotein Cholesterol Intervention Trial (VA-HIT)[72] was a multicenter, randomized study that assessed the effects of gemfibrozil at a dose of 1200 mg/day versus dietary therapy on the incidence of cardiovascular events in 2531 men with known CHD and low baseline HDL cholesterol levels.[73] Enrollment criteria for VA-HIT required an HDL cholesterol level of 40 mg/dl (1.03 mmol/liter) or less or LDL cholesterol level of less than 140 mg/dl (3.6 mmol/liter) and triglycerides at 300 mg/dl (3.4 mmol/liter) or less.

The mean age of subjects in the VA-HIT was 64 years, with more than 75 percent of the patients older than 60 years of age. Baseline lipids in the VA-HIT revealed a total cholesterol level of 175 mg/dl, HDL cholesterol of 32 mg/dl, LDL cholesterol of 111 mg/dl, and triglycerides of 161 mg/dl. Gemfibrozil therapy resulted in essentially minimal alterations in total cholesterol and LDL levels. Total cholesterol was decreased by 4 percent as compared with placebo, and no significant change was demonstrable with LDL cholesterol concentrations. Triglycerides, on the other hand, fell by 31 percent and HDL cholesterol increased by 6 percent. The primary endpoint of the VA-HIT was the combination of CHD death and nonfatal MI. Patients randomized to receive placebo accounted for 275 events, compared with 219 events in the gemfibrozil group. The decline in coronary events represented a 22 percent risk reduction that was statistically significant ($p = 0.006$). The event curves began to diverge at approximately 2 years after the beginning of the trial.

The Bezafibrate Infarction Prevention (BIP)[73] study reported no reduction in fatal and nonfatal MI and CHD death in a cohort of 3090 men and women with CHD, total cholesterol of 180 to 250 mg/dl, HDL cholesterol less than 45 mg/dl (1.2 mmol/liter), triglycerides less than 300 mg/dl (3.4 mmol/liter), and LDL cholesterol less than 180 mg/dl (4.7 mmol/liter) who were treated with either bezafibrate, 400 mg/day, or placebo. Despite producing an increase in HDL cholesterol of 14 percent and reduction in triglycerides of 25 percent compared with placebo, fibrate treatment did not reduce CHD risk. After 6.2 years, the reduction in the cumulative probability of the primary endpoint was 7.3 percent ($p = 0.24$). However, a substantial risk reduction with bezafibrate (5 percent; $p = 0.02$) was observed post hoc in the small subgroup of patients with elevated triglycerides at baseline (>200 mg/dl [2.3 mmol/liter]).

The Action to Control Cardiovascular Risk in Diabetes (ACCORD) study, sponsored by the U.S. National Heart, Lung, and Blood Institute, anticipates enrolling 10,000 patients with type II diabetes mellitus (from www.accordtrial.org). The trial will compare effects on cardiovascular disease events of three strategies: intensive glycemic control; increasing HDL cholesterol and lowering triglycerides (with strict LDL cholesterol and glycemic control); and intensive blood pressure control (in the context of tight glycemic control). The lipid-modification arm of ACCORD will evaluate a fibrate intended to lower triglycerides and increase HDL cholesterol, combined with a statin to lower the LDL cholesterol level. The ACCORD study, therefore, will assess the effect of multiple risk factor intervention in diabetic patients and will also provide valuable information about the use of the statin-fibrate combination in preventing clinical events. In January 2003 the ACCORD main trial began a 30-month recruiting period. Follow-up will continue until 2009.

SECONDARY PREVENTION TRIALS (Table 42-8, see Fig. 42-6)

In the past decade and a half, secondary prevention trials have shown the power of large, well-designed trials examining the effect of statins on cardiovascular events, cardiovascular mortality, and total mortality.

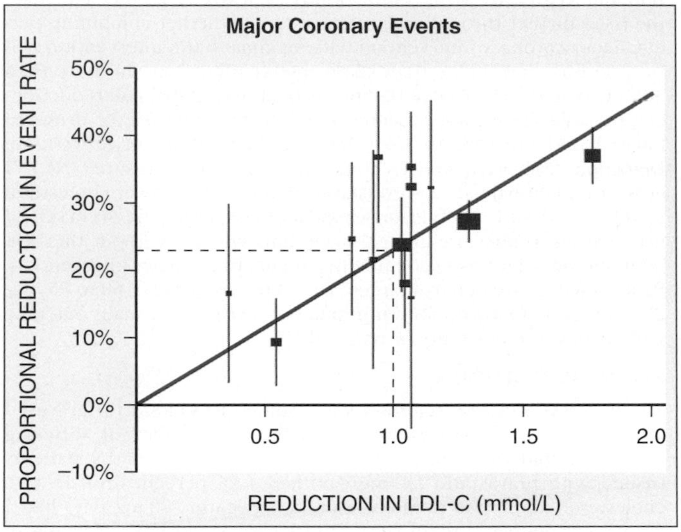

FIGURE 42–6 Clinical trials of statin therapy have demonstrated benefits in patients across the spectrum of coronary disease. *(From Baigent C, Keech A, Kearney PM, et al: Efficacy and safety of cholesterol-lowering treatment: Prospective meta-analysis of data from 90,056 participants in 14 randomised trials of statins. Lancet 366:1267, 2005.)*

The results of the 4S,[63] CARE,[61] LIPID,[62] and HPS[64] have been discussed previously. A recent meta-analysis involving 90,056 subjects in 14 trials of cardiovascular disease prevention with statins, carried by the Cholesterol Treatment Trialists,[74] showed a linear relationship between the absolute decrease in LDL-C and reduction in cardiovascular events (CHD death or nonfatal MI). A 1 mmol/liter (38.67 mg/dl) reduction in LDL-C was associated with a 22 percent reduction in cardiovascular events. Importantly, this magnitude of effect was preserved when the LDL-C was reduced even further (see Fig. 42-6). National guidelines recommended a therapeutic target of 2.6 mmol/liter for LDL-C (100 mg/dl); the results of recent clinical trials have stimulated a revision of this recommendation to less than 1.75 mmol/liter (70 mg/dl). Two recent trials have examined the effect of lowering LDL-C below recommended targets: the Treating to New Targets (TNT) trial[75] and the Incremental Decrease in Endpoints through Aggressive Lipid Lowering (IDEAL) trial.[76]

The TNT trial examined patients with stable CHD and an LDL-C 130 to 250 mg/dl (3.4 to 6.5 mmol/liter) and triglycerides <600 mg/dl (6.8 mmol/liter). From a screening population of more than 18,468 subjects, 15,464 were randomized to atorvastatin 10 mg/day. Patients who did not reach the LDL-C target of less than 130 mg/dl (3.4 mmol/liter) were excluded; 10,001 patients were then randomized to atorvastatin 10 mg/day to reach an average LDL-C of 100 mg/dl (2.6 mmol/liter) or to atorvastatin 80 mg/day to reach a mean LDL-C of 80 mg/dl (2 mmol/liter). The primary outcome measure was CHD death, nonfatal MI, resuscitated cardiac arrest, and fatal or nonfatal stroke. After a mean follow-up of 4.9 years, the primary outcome measure was decreased by 22 percent (HR 0.78, 95 percent CI 0.69, 0.89, $p = 0.0002$). The absolute risk decreased from 8.3 to 6.7 percent events/4.9 years. Cardiovascular mortality was decreased by 20 percent (nonsignificant), from 127 deaths (2.5 percent) on atorvastatin 10 mg versus 101 (2 percent) on atorvastatin 80 mg (HR 0.80, $p = 0.09$). Total mortality was not changed (282 deaths [5.6 percent] on atorvastatin 10 mg versus 284 deaths [5.7 percent]) (HR 1.01, $p = 0.92$). Overall, TNT confirmed that in patients with stable CHD, intensive LDL-C lowering decreased cardiovascular events.

The IDEAL trial evaluated 8888 patients with stable CHD aged 80 years or younger to simvastatin 20 mg/day or atorvastatin 80 mg/day. Patients were followed for an average of 4.8 years. The primary outcome measure was CHD death, nonfatal MI, or resuscitated cardiac arrest. On treatment LDL-C levels were 104 mg/dl (2.6 mmol/liter) in the simvastatin 20 mg group versus 81 mg/dl (2.6 mmol/liter) in the atorvastatin 80 mg group. A major cardiac event occurred in 463 patients on simvastatin (10.4 percent) compared with 411 patients (9.3 percent) in the atorvastatin group (HR 0.89, 95 percent CI 0.78 to 1.01, $p = 0.07$).

TABLE 42–8 Secondary Prevention Trials of Statin Therapy

Study	4S (*n*=4444)	CARE (*n*=4159)	LIPID (*n*=9014)	HPS (*n*=20,536)	TNT (*n*=10,001)†	IDEAL (*n*=8888)
% Men	81	86	83	75	81	81
Age	35-69	21-75	31-75	40-80	29-76 61 yr	30-80 62 yr
% Smokers	26	21	10	14	13	20
% HTN	26	43	41	41	54	33
% DM Medications	4.5	14	9	29	15	12
Aspirin	37	83	82	63	88	79
Beta blocker	57	40	47	26	55	75
Calcium	31	39	35	—	26	19
Baseline LDL-C mg/dl (mmol/liter)	4.9	3.6	3.9	3.4	2.5* (3.9)	3.1
Achieved LDL-C on treatment CHD event rate	122 (3.2)	98 (2.5)	112 (2.9)	89 (2.3)	77 (2.0)	81 (2.1)
Placebo	28.0	13.2	15.9	11.8	8.3	10.4
Treatment	19.4	10.2	12.3	8.7	6.7	9.3*

*Nonsignificant.

†In the TNT study, all patients were initially on atorvastatin 10 mg/day.

Nonfatal MI occurred in 321 patients (7.2 percent) on simvastatin and in 267 patients (6 percent) on atorvastatin (HR 0.87, 95 percent CI 0.77 to 0.98, $p = 0.02$). No changes occurred in total mortality (374 [8.4 percent] in the simvastatin group versus 366 [8.2 percent] in the atorvastatin group [HR 0.98, $p = 0.81$]).

Both the TNT and IDEAL studies show that intensive LDL-C lowering decreases cardiovascular events; neither study was sufficiently powered to evaluate total mortality. The Study of the Effectiveness of Additional Reductions in Cholesterol and Homocysteine (SEARCH)[77] will determine, in 12,000 patients, whether intensive treatment with simvastatin 80 mg, compared with 20 mg, will result in further CHD events. In SEARCH, an additional arm of the trial will investigate the effects of B vitamins to reduce homocysteine on cardiovascular events.

ACUTE CORONARY SYNDROMES (see also Chaps. 51 and 53)

Earlier secondary prevention statin studies generally selected patients who were at least 3 to 6 months post coronary event and stabilized. Substantial interest has turned to the question of statin treatment in the period immediately following an acute coronary syndrome.

The Myocardial Ischemia Reduction and Aggressive Cholesterol Lowering (MIRACL) trial[78] examined the premise that early and intensive treatment with high-dose atorvastatin therapy begun immediately after the onset of an acute coronary event might produce beneficial clinical effects in a much larger cohort ($n = 3086$). The composite primary endpoint of MIRACL included nonfatal acute MI, cardiac arrest, or symptomatic myocardial ischemia. Atorvastatin resulted in a modest albeit statistically significant 16 percent improvement in relative risk for the primary endpoint ($p = 0.048$). The major effect of early atorvastatin was a reduction in recurrent myocardial ischemia, which was decreased by 26 percent ($p = 0.02$). Although statistically significant, the clinical benefits observed in MIRACL were not as robust as those seen in the larger and longer secondary prevention trials (see Table 42-8).

The Aggrastat-to-Zocor (A-to-Z) study[79] randomized patients with acute coronary syndromes (randomized to tirofiban or heparin) to receive either simvastatin, 40 to 80 mg/day, or diet plus simvastatin, 20 mg/day. Overall, the results of this trial were neutral.

The Pravastatin or Atorvastatin Evaluation and Infection Therapy (PROVE-IT) trial[80] compared pravastatin, 40 mg/day, with atorvastatin, 80 mg/day, in 4162 post acute coronary event patients. This study also had an antibiotic treatment arm. The lipid-lowering arm of PROVE-IT showed that in patients who have recently survived an acute coronary syndrome, an intensive statin regimen that yielded a median LDL cholesterol of 62 mg/dl (1.60 mmol/liter) provided greater protection against death or major cardiovascular events than less aggressive therapy that lowered LDL cholesterol to a median of 95 mg/dl (2.5 mmol/liter), a level below the upper limit recommended by ATP-III as a target for this category of patients.

MEDICAL THERAPY VERSUS REVASCULARIZATION

The Atorvastatin versus Revascularization Treatment (AVERT) trial evaluated the potential benefits of aggressive lipid lowering with open-label atorvastatin, 80 mg/day, versus usual care on ischemic events in a cohort of 341 patients with stable atherosclerosis who were scheduled to undergo an elective percutaneous revascularization procedure.[81] Follow-up was 18 months. Qualification requirements included at least one native coronary vessel with 50 percent or greater stenosis and an LDL cholesterol level in excess of 115 mg/dl. Exclusion criteria included triglycerides in excess of 500 mg/dl, ejection fraction less than 40 percent, inability to complete 4 minutes of exercise on a standard Bruce protocol, left main or triple vessel coronary atherosclerosis, or recent unstable angina or MI.

The composite primary endpoint in the AVERT trial encompassed the incidence of ischemic events, defined as cardiac death, resuscitation after cardiac arrest, nonfatal MI, stroke, worsening angina, or revascularization (coronary artery bypass graft or repeat angioplasty). The patients randomized to usual care received percutaneous coronary interventions, and approximately one third of the patients with treated lesions underwent placement of a coronary stent. The patients treated with angioplasty could receive hypolipidemic therapy as part of usual care. Lipid-lowering drugs were administered in 73 percent of patients in this group at some time during the follow-up (71 percent of the total group received statins). Despite this "drop-in" of lipid-lowering therapy, the atorvastatin group had lower total cholesterol, LDL cholesterol, and triglycerides relative to usual care.

A total of 22 ischemic events occurred in the group randomized to receive aggressive lipid-lowering therapy, compared with 37 events in the usual-care group (36 percent reduction; $p = 0.048$). The difference in the treatment arms tended toward statistical significance because the significance level was adjusted to 0.045 because of the performance of two interim analyses. Atorvastatin treatment significantly delayed the time to the first event ($p = 0.027$) compared with usual care, but 54 percent of angioplasty patients compared with 41 percent of atorvastatin patients had improvement of Canadian Cardiovascular Society (CCS) classification of angina symptoms ($p = 0.009$). Seventeen serious adverse events were reported in the atorvastatin group, although none was attributed to atorvastatin. Twenty-eight of the patients in the angioplasty group had serious adverse events; six of these patients had events attributable to the angioplasty.

These results support a strategy of aggressive lipid-lowering therapy to complement revascularization in patients with stable angina. The multicenter, randomized Clinical Outcomes Utilizing Revascularization and Aggressive Drug Evaluation (COURAGE) trial may elucidate the issue further through its investigation of whether combining percutaneous coronary intervention with maximal statin intervention will provide greater benefits than statin intervention alone in more than 3000 patients.[82] The COURAGE protocol targets global risk reduction, emphasizing (1) lifestyle modification; (2) maximal use of drugs to lower blood pressure to Joint National Committee on Prevention, Detection, Evaluation, and Treatment of High Blood Pressure (JNC) VI goals; (3) maximal use of simvastatin, 80 mg/day, to lower cholesterol to below current U.S. goals for secondary prevention; and (4) maximal use of drug to alleviate anginal symptoms with or without the best interventional devices to conduct percutaneous coronary intervention. Patients will be treated to a target LDL cholesterol level of 60 to 85 mg/dl and will be followed for a minimum of 3 years. The main outcome will be all-cause mortality or nonfatal MI.

REGRESSION STUDIES

The Reversal of Atherosclerosis with Lipitor (REVERSAL) trial[83] used intravascular ultrasonography to examine the effect of differing degrees of lipid-lowering on plaque volume. Over 18 months, patients treated with pravastatin (40 mg/day) had a 25 percent drop in LDL cholesterol, and those randomized to atorvastatin (80 mg/day) had a 46 percent decrease, to an average LDL cholesterol level of 79 mg/dl (2.6 mmol/liter). The more aggressive lipid-lowering regimen reduced lesion volume. The primary endpoint was a reduction in the total atheroma volume, which increased by 0.4 percent on pravastatin but decreased by 2.7 percent ($p = 0.02$) on atorvastatin.

The ASTEROID study[84] was designed to evaluate whether 24 months' treatment with rosuvastatin 40 mg would result in regression of coronary atherosclerosis as measured by IVUS in 507 patients. During treatment with rosuvastatin 40 mg, LDL-C decreased from 130 mg/dl (3.4 mmol/liter) to 61 mg/dl (1.6 mmol/liter); HDL-C increased by 14.7 percent. Three hundred and forty-nine patients underwent a follow-up IVUS after 2 years. Several efficacy parameters were used: The median change in percent atheroma volume decreased by 0.79 percent, and the median change in most diseased subsegment decreased by 5.6 percent; both $p < 0.001$. No control or comparator group was used. The ASTEROID showed that rosuvastatin at a dose of 40 mg promotes coronary atherosclerosis regression.

APPROACH TO THE TREATMENT OF LIPOPROTEIN DISORDERS

Patients with lipoprotein disorders should undergo comprehensive evaluation and management in the context of a global risk reduction program (see Chap. 45). Most patients with dyslipoproteinemias lack symptoms, except for those with severe hypertriglyceridemia who can present with acute pancreatitis and those with familial lipoprotein disorders who have cutaneous manifestations (xanthomas, xanthelasmas). In the evaluation of patients with dyslipidemia, secondary causes should be sought and treated. The clinical evaluation should include a thorough history including a complete family history that may reveal clues as to the genetic cause but also to the genetic susceptibility to cardiovascular disease. The physician should seek and address other risk factors (cigarette smoking, obesity, diabetes) and institute a management plan to improve lifestyle such as diet, physical activity, and alcohol intake. Such interventions should make use of nonphysician health professionals (e.g., those with training in diet and nutrition, physical therapy, and smoking cessation). The ATP III Therapeutic Lifestyle Change program offers one such approach. Concomitant medication use in addition to lifestyle change will often be necessary to achieve current guideline goals.

The physical examination should include a search for xanthomas (in extensor tendons including hands, elbows, knees, Achilles tendons, and palmar xanthomas) and the presence of xanthelasmas, corneal arcus, and corneal opacifications. The blood pressure, waist circumference, weight, and height should be recorded, and signs of arterial compromise sought, and a complete cardiovascular examination performed. The evaluation of peripheral pulses and the determination of the ankle-brachial index may reveal important clues for the presence of peripheral vascular disease (see Chap. 57).

The diagnosis of lipoprotein disorders depends on laboratory measurements (Table 42-9). The fasting lipid profile generally suffices for most lipoprotein disorders, and specialized laboratories can refine the diagnosis and provide expertise for extreme cases. Additional tests often involve considerable expense and may not increase the predictive value beyond that of the lipid profile, although they can help in refining the diagnosis. To assess baseline risk in individuals on lipid-lowering therapy, the medication should be stopped for 1 month before a lipid profile is measured. Many advanced lipid tests available in specialized centers (see Table 42-9) seldom add to the clinical assessment specified earlier.

After diagnosis of a lipid disorder (based on at least two lipid profiles), secondary causes should be evaluated by measurement of thyroid-stimulating hormone and glucose. Patients who will receive medications should have measurement of baseline liver function (alanine aminotransferase [ALT]) and creatinine kinase. A decision to treat high-risk subjects (e.g., patients with an acute coronary syndrome or post-MI or coronary revascularization) should start immediately and should commence concomitantly with lifestyle changes.[69]

Target Levels (see Chap. 45)

The National Cholesterol Education Program Adult Treatment Panel III (NCEP ATP III)[69] has recommended treatment of hypercholesterolemia. Target levels depend on overall risk of cardiovascular death or nonfatal MI. Patients with CAD or atherosclerosis of other vascular beds (carotids or peripheral vascular disease), adults with diabetes, and those patients with an estimated 10-year risk of developing CAD of greater than 20 percent fall into a high-risk category and merit aggressive treatment including medications along with lifestyle modifications, exercise, and diet to achieve a primary target of an LDL cholesterol level less than 2.6 mmol/liter (100 mg/dl). In subjects with triglycerides greater than 200 mg/dl, ATP III presents a secondary target of a non-HDL cholesterol level less than 3.4 mmol/liter (130 mg/dl). Many of these individuals have the metabolic syndrome.

Lifestyle Changes

TREATMENT. The therapeutic options consist of lifestyle modifications; treatment of secondary causes; and, if possible, diet and medications.

DIET (see Chap. 44). Individuals with dyslipoproteinemias should always adopt dietary therapy. High-risk subjects should have medications started concomitantly with a diet because, in many cases, diet may not suffice to reach target levels. The diet should have three objectives. First, it should allow the patient to reach and maintain ideal body weight. Second, it should provide a well-balanced diet with fruits, vegetables, and whole grains. Third, it should be restricted in saturated fats and refined carbohydrates. Dietary counseling should involve a professional dietitian. Often, the help of dietitians, weight loss programs, or diabetic outpatient centers can aid sustained weight loss. Currently, the ATP III and the American Heart Association recommend a diet in which protein intake represents 15 to 20 percent of calories, fats represent less than 35 percent, with only 7 percent from saturated fats, and the remaining calories derive from carbohydrates. Cholesterol intake should be less than 300 mg/day.

Treatment of Combined Lipoprotein Disorders

Combined lipoprotein disorders, characterized by an increase in plasma total cholesterol and triglycerides, frequently occur in clinical practice and present difficult challenges. Patients with combined lipoprotein disorders have an increase in LDL cholesterol and LDL particle number (as reflected by an increase in total or LDL apo B); small, dense LDL particles; increased VLDL cholesterol and VLDL triglycerides; and a reduced HDL cholesterol level. Patients with this pattern of combined dyslipidemia often have obesity and the metabolic syndrome. Treatment should begin with lifestyle modifications, with a diet reduced in total calories and saturated fats, weight reduction, and increased physical activity. Drug treatment, when warranted, aims to correct the predominant lipoprotein abnor-

TABLE 42–9 Laboratory Tests for the Diagnosis of Lipoprotein Disorders

Lipid Profile	May Help in Diagnosis	Specialized Centers	Research Tools
Cholesterol	LDL particle size	Lipoprotein separation by UTC*	Molecular diagnosis
Triglycerides	Apo B	LPL assay LCAT assay	
HDL cholesterol	Apo AI	Apo E levels	
LDL cholesterol†	Apo E genotype/phenotype Lipoprotein(a)	Apolipoprotein separation by PAGE Apo CII, CIII LDL-R assay	

*Ultracentrifugation.

†Calculated as LDL cholesterol+Total cholesterol− (triglycerides/2.2+HDL cholesterol) in mmol/liter (or triglycerides divided by 5 mg/dl); valid for triglycerides <4.5 mmol/liter (<400 mg/dl). LDL cholesterol can also be directly measured in plasma.

Apo=apolipoprotein; HDL=high-density lipoprotein; LCAT=lecithin cholesterol acyltransferase; LDL=low-density lipoprotein; LDL-R=LDL receptor; LPL=lipoprotein lipase; PAGE=polyacrylamide gel electrophoresis.

mality. Statins can reduce plasma triglyceride levels, particularly in individuals with high baseline triglyceride levels. Fibrates reduce triglycerides and may change the composition of LDL to larger and less dense particles. The role of fibric acid derivatives in the secondary prevention of cardiovascular diseases in diabetic subjects with low HDL cholesterol levels has been cast into doubt after publication of the FIELD trial.[71] Fibrates can paradoxically increase LDL cholesterol levels (because of increased lipoprotein lipase activity). Plasma total homocysteine levels may increase with fenofibrate and to a lesser extent with bezafibrate. In view of the effects of gemfibrozil on glucuronidation of statins, we advise against gemfibrozil use in combination therapy with statins. The combination of a statin with a fibrate, however, has proved highly effective in correcting the combined dyslipoproteinemias; whether this approach prevents recurrent cardiovascular events remains to be shown by appropriate clinical trials. Patients taking a fibrate plus a statin merit close medical follow-up for evidence of hepatotoxicity or myositis within the first 6 weeks of therapy and every 6 months thereafter. The combined use of a statin and ezetimibe for the treatment of severe hypercholesterolemia or to reach recommended target levels when monotherapy with a statin is either insufficient or causes unwanted side effects has a good rationale, although unsubstantiated by clinical trials.

Other combinations including fibric acid derivatives with bile acid–binding resins and niacin with bile acid–binding resins, have also proved useful in specific cases. The combination of fibrates or statins with niacin requires experience and care because of the risk of hepatotoxicity and myositis. The search for correctable causes (e.g., uncontrolled diabetes, obesity, hypothyroidism, alcohol use) of combined dyslipidemia and the benefit of lifestyle modifications require reemphasis. Often, the help of dietitians, weight loss programs, or diabetic outpatient centers adds considerably to management success.

EXTRACORPOREAL LOW-DENSITY LIPOPROTEIN FILTRATION. Patients with severe hypercholesterolemia, especially those with homozygous familial hypercholesterolemia or severe heterozygous familial hypercholesterolemia, may warrant treatment by extracorporeal LDL elimination. These techniques use selective filtration, adsorption, or precipitation of LDL (or apo B–containing particles) after plasma separation. Specialized centers have LDL-pheresis available. This approach can dramatically reduce the risk of developing cardiovascular disease and improve survival.[85]

Novel Approaches

The development of novel pharmaceutical agents for the treatment of lipoprotein disorders will likely continue because cardiovascular disease due to atherosclerosis represents the largest burden of disease for the near future. Better targeting of high-risk individuals will allow optimization of expensive therapies. The finding that subjects who were previously identified as being at relatively low risk of CAD on the basis of their LDL cholesterol levels but who have an elevated C-reactive protein level derive benefit from a statin in the primary prevention of CAD may radically alter the concept of cardiovascular risk stratification (see also Chaps. 39 and 45).[50] If markers of inflammation in addition to conventional risk factors can better identify cardiovascular risk, physicians' attitudes should embrace these findings. This hypothesis is undergoing rigorous testing in a clinical trial.

Novel therapies to raise HDL-C have received considerable support in a proof-of-concept clinical trial in which patients with an acute coronary syndrome were given weekly injections of apo AI_{Milano}–reconstituted proteoliposomes, in effect nascent HDL particles.[86] Remarkably, a reduction of 4.7 percent of atheroma volume was documented by IVUS after 5 weeks of treatment. Although difficult to apply clinically, this small trial affirmed the benefits of raising HDL-C in patients with CHD.

The burgeoning field of pharmacogenetics might, in the near future, allow treatment of patients on the basis of their genetic make-up. Genetic screening may become a useful clinical tool as technology improves and rapid genotyping for diagnostic and prognostic purposes becomes available for clinicians. Other than cost issues, the ethics of screening for genetic predisposition to disease and access to information represent daunting challenges. The discovery that the apo E4 allele carries the risk of early-onset Alzheimer disease, one of the familial forms of the disorder, illustrates the ethical complexities of genetic testing in the realm of lipoprotein disorders.

Drug Development and Future Directions

Novel proteins that regulate the synthesis of lipids have become therapeutic targets for drug development. The development of competitive inhibitors of HMG-CoA reductase leading to statin drugs provides a good example. These drugs have an important impact on cardiovascular morbidity and mortality reduction in high-risk individuals. Inhibitors of pancreatic lipases are being used to treat obesity. Future potential drug targets might include inhibition of apo B secretion by inhibiting the microsomal triglyceride transfer protein, which is crucial in the assembly of apo B–containing lipoproteins. Hepatic steatosis has limited this therapeutic option in humans. Recent work has shown that selective inhibitors of ACAT do not retard atherosclerosis, and their antiatherogenic role remains unproven. The PCSK9 enzyme associated with genetically low LDL levels represents another potential therapeutic target. Drugs that increase cellular cholesterol efflux to increase HDL cholesterol levels including apo AI mimetics may also prove useful in the treatment of atherosclerosis.

Other therapeutic modalities in the treatment of atherosclerosis by modulating lipoprotein metabolism include the development of new inhibitors of CETP to increase HDL cholesterol levels or modulation of LCAT, as well as inhibitors of bile acid transport to decrease intestinal cholesterol uptake. Pharmacological modulation of HDL cholesterol levels, other than by niacin, has not led to results proportional to those achieved for LDL cholesterol. Potential modulators of HDL cholesterol levels include SR-B1, ABCA1 and ABCG1 pathways, apo AI, and its homologues and mimetics.

Specific Subgroups (Diabetics and the Elderly)

Patients with diabetes should receive a statin. Multiple observational studies have documented a markedly increased risk of CHD in adult diabetics over the long term. Preventive strategies with aspirin, angiotensin convertase inhibitors, tight glycemic control, and statins have all shown benefit. Data from CARDS and TNT support benefits of intensive LDL-C lowering in diabetics.[87]

The elderly represent a unique challenge; most of the attributable risk in patients older than 75 or 80 years old is due to age, and the predictive value of an elevated cholesterol decreases with increasing age.[69] The value of statins and other lipid-lowering drugs in the elderly in primary prevention lacks an evidence base at present, yet the data from PROSPER, HPS, 4S, and several other studies strongly suggest that secondary preventive measures should not be withheld from older patients solely because of age.

Gene Therapy

Severe, homozygous, monogenic disorders may eventually be treated by gene therapy. The initial trials of gene therapy in cases of homozygous familial hypercholesterolemia have not led to a major improvement and have largely been abandoned. However, the lifelong burden of these rare disorders and the potential for cure makes this approach appealing. Other diseases such as abetalipoproteinemia, LPL deficiency, Niemann-Pick type C disease, sitosterolemia, and Tangier disease may become targets for gene therapy. If the approach to correct these disorders is successful, the more widespread applications of gene-based therapies for the purpose of reducing potential cardiovascular risk will become a daunting medical, social, and ethical problem.

REFERENCES

Lipoproteins and Their Trafficking

1. Sorci-Thomas MG, Curtiss L, Parks JS, et al: The hydrophobic face orientation of apolipoprotein A-I amphipathic helix domain 143-164 regulates lecithin : cholesterol acyltransferase activation. J Biol Chem 273:11776, 1998.
2. Hiltunen TP, Luoma JS, Nikkari T, Yla-Herttuala S: Expression of LDL receptor, VLDL receptor, LDL receptor-related protein, and scavenger receptor in rabbit atherosclerotic lesions: Marked induction of scavenger receptor and VLDL receptor expression during lesion development. Circulation 97:1079, 1998.
3. Nimpf J, Schneider WJ: The VLDL receptor: An LDL receptor relative with eight ligand binding repeats, LR8. Atherosclerosis 141:191, 1998.
4. Mahley RW, Ji ZS: Remnant lipoprotein metabolism: Key pathways involving cell-surface heparan sulfate proteoglycans and apolipoprotein E. J Lipid Res 40:1, 1999.
5. Brown ML, Ramprasad MP, Umeda PK, et al: A macrophage receptor for apolipoprotein B_{48}: Cloning, expression, and atherosclerosis. Proc Natl Acad Sci U S A 97:7488, 2000.
6. de Man FH, de Beer F, van der Laarse A, et al: Lipolysis of very low density lipoproteins by heparan sulfate proteoglycan-bound lipoprotein lipase. J Lipid Res 38:2465, 1997.
7. Sawamura T, Kume N, Aoyama T, et al: An endothelial receptor for oxidized low-density lipoprotein. Nature 386:73, 1997.
8. Acton S, Rigotti A, Landschulz KT, et al: Identification of scavenger receptor SR-BI as a high density lipoprotein receptor. Science 271:518, 1996.
9. Krimbou L, Hassan HH, Blain S, et al: Biogenesis and speciation of nascent apo AI–containing particles in various cell lines. J Lipid Res 46:1668, 2005.
10. Altmann SW, Davis HR Jr, Zhu LJ, et al: Niemann-Pick C1 like 1 protein is critical for intestinal cholesterol absorption. Science 303:1201, 2004.
11. Abifadel M, Varret M, Rabes JP, et al: Mutations in *PCSK9* cause autosomal dominant hypercholesterolemia. Nat Genet 34:154, 2003.
12. Willner EL, Tow B, Buhman KK, et al: Deficiency of acyl CoA : cholesterol acyltransferase 2 prevents atherosclerosis in apolipoprotein E-deficient mice. Proc Natl Acad Sci U S A 100:1262, 2003.
13. Timmins JM, Lee JY, Boudyguina E, et al: Targeted inactivation of hepatic ABCA1 causes profound hypoalphalipoproteinemia and kidney hypercatabolism of apoA-I. J Clin Invest 115:1333, 2005.
14. Brunham LR, Kruit JK, Iqbal J, et al: Intestinal ABCA1 directly contributes to HDL biogenesis in vivo. J Clin Invest 116:1052, 2006.
15. Denis M, Haidar B, Marcil M, et al: Molecular and cellular physiology of apolipoprotein A-I lipidation by the ATP binding cassette A1 (ABCA1). J Biol Chem 279:7384, 2004.
16. Haidar B, Denis M, Marcil M, et al: Apolipoprotein A-I activates cellular camp signaling through the ABCA1 receptor. Evidence for molecular interactions between ABCA1 receptor and G protein. J Biol Chem 279:9963, 2004.
17. Chau P, Nakamura Y, Fielding CJ, Fielding PE: Mechanism of prebeta-HDL formation and activation. Biochemistry 45:3981, 2006.
18. Li XA, Titlow WB, Jackson BA, et al: High density lipoprotein binding to scavenger receptor, class B, type I activates endothelial nitric-oxide synthase in a ceramide-dependent manner. J Biol Chem 277:11058, 2002.
19. Van Eck M, Singaraja RR, Ye D, et al: Macrophage ATP-binding cassette transporter A1 overexpression inhibits atherosclerotic lesion progression in low-density lipoprotein receptor knockout mice. Arterioscler Thromb Vasc Biol 26:929, 2006.

Lipoproteins and Cardiovascular Risk

20. Barter PJ, Ballantyne CM, Carmena R, et al: Apo B versus cholesterol in estimating cardiovascular risk and in guiding therapy: Report of the thirty-person/ten-country panel. J Intern Med 259:247, 2006.
21. Grundy SM, Cleeman JI, Daniels SR, et al: American Heart Association; National Heart, Lung, and Blood Institute. Diagnosis and management of the metabolic syndrome: An American Heart Association/National Heart, Lung, and Blood Institute Scientific Statement. Circulation 112:2735, 2005.
22. Wilson DJ, Gahan M, Haddad L, et al: A World Wide Web site for low-density lipoprotein receptor gene mutations in familial hypercholesterolemia: Sequence-based, tabular, and direct submission data handling. Am J Cardiol 81:1509, 1998.
23. Hansen PS, Defesche JC, Kastelein JJ, et al: Phenotypic variation in patients heterozygous for familial defective apolipoprotein B (FDB) in three European countries. Arterioscler Thromb Vasc Biol 17:741, 1997.
24. Cohen JC, Boerwinkle E, Mosley TH Jr, Hobbs HH: Sequence variations in *PCSK9*, low LDL, and protection against coronary heart disease. N Engl J Med 354:1264, 2006.
25. Garuti R, Jones C, Li WP, et al: The modular adaptor protein autosomal recessive hypercholesterolemia (ARH) promotes low density lipoprotein receptor clustering into clathrin-coated pits. J Biol Chem 9:40996, 2005.
26. Berge KE, Tian H, Graf GA, et al: Accumulation of dietary cholesterol in sitosterolemia caused by mutations in adjacent ABC transporters. Science 290:1771, 2000.
27. Mooser V, Mancini FP, Bopp S, et al: Sequence polymorphisms in the apo(a) gene associated with specific levels of Lp(a) in plasma. Hum Mol Genet 4:173, 1995.
28. Danesh J, Collins R, Peto R: Lipoprotein(a) and coronary heart disease: Meta-analysis of prospective studies. Circulation 102:1082, 2000.
29. Sjarif DR, Sinke RJ, Duran M, et al: Clinical heterogeneity and novel mutations in the glycerol kinase gene in three families with isolated glycerol kinase deficiency. J Med Genet 35:650, 1998.
30. Santamarina-Fojo S: The familial chylomicronemia syndrome. Endocrinol Metab Clin North Am 27:551, viii, 1998.
31. Weinstock PH, Bisgaier CL, Aalto-Setala K, et al: Severe hypertriglyceridemia, reduced high density lipoprotein, and neonatal death in lipoprotein lipase knockout mice: Mild hypertriglyceridemia with impaired very low density lipoprotein clearance in heterozygotes. J Clin Invest 96:2555, 1995.
32. Mahley RW, Huang Y, Rall SC Jr: Pathogenesis of type III hyperlipoproteinemia (dysbetalipoproteinemia): Questions, quandaries, and paradoxes. J Lipid Res 40:1933, 1999.
33. Zhang SH, Reddick RL, Piedrahita JA, Maeda N: Spontaneous hypercholesterolemia and arterial lesions in mice lacking apolipoprotein E. Science 258:468, 1992.
34. Pajukanta P, Lilja HE, Sinsheimer JS, et al: Familial combined hyperlipidemia is associated with upstream transcription factor 1 (USF1). Nat Genet 36:371, 2004.
35. Kalant D, MacLaren R, Cui W, et al: C5L2 is a functional receptor for acylation-stimulating protein. J Biol Chem 280:23936, 2005.
36. Dastani Z, Engert JC, Genest J, Marcil M: Genetics of high-density lipoproteins. Curr Opin Cardiol 2006.
37. Lewis GF, Rader DJ: New insights into the regulation of HDL metabolism and reverse cholesterol transport. Circ Res 96:1221, 2005.
38. Sorci-Thomas MG, Thomas MJ: The effects of altered apolipoprotein A-I structure on plasma HDL concentration. Trends Cardiovasc Med 12:121, 2002.
39. Boekholdt SM, Kuivenhoven JA, Hovingh GK, et al: CETP gene variation: Relation to lipid parameters and cardiovascular risk. Curr Opin Lipidol 15:393, 2004.
40. Calabresi L, Pisciotta L, Costantin A, et al: The molecular basis of lecithin : cholesterol acyltransferase deficiency syndromes: A comprehensive study of molecular and biochemical findings in 13 unrelated Italian families. Arterioscler Thromb Vasc Biol 25:1972, 2005.
41. Brooks-Wilson A, Marcil M, Clee SM, et al: Mutations in ABC1 in Tangier disease and familial high-density lipoprotein deficiency. Nat Genet 22:336, 1999.
42. Marcil M, Brooks-Wilson A, Clee SM, et al: Mutations in the *ABC1* gene in familial HDL deficiency with defective cholesterol efflux. Lancet 354:1341, 1999.
43. Carstea ED, Morris JA, Coleman KG, et al: Niemann-Pick C1 disease gene: Homology to mediators of cholesterol homeostasis. Science 277:228, 1997.
44. Choi HY, Karten B, Chan T, et al: Impaired ABCA1-dependent lipid efflux and hypoalphalipoproteinemia in human Niemann-Pick type C disease. J Biol Chem 278:32569, 2003.
45. Lee CY, Lesimple A, Denis M, et al: Increased sphingomyelin content impairs HDL biogenesis and maturation in human Niemann-Pick disease type B. J Lipid Res 47:622, 2006.
46. Anderson GL, Limacher M, Assaf AR: Effects of conjugated equine estrogen in postmenopausal women with hysterectomy: The Women's Health Initiative randomized controlled trial. JAMA 291:1701, 2004.
47. Meigs JB, Wilson PW, Fox CS, et al: Body mass index, metabolic syndrome and risk of type 2 diabetes or cardiovascular disease. J Clin Endocrinol Metab 91:2906, 2006.
48. Kahn R, Buse J, Ferrannini E, et al: The metabolic syndrome: Time for a critical appraisal: Joint statement from the American Diabetes Association and the European Association for the Study of Diabetes. Diabetes Care 28:2289, 2005.
49. Martin G, Duez H, Blanquart C, et al: Statin-induced inhibition of the Rho-singaling pathway activates PPAR alpha and induces apo AI. J Clin Invest 107:1423, 2001.

Treatment of Lipid Disorders

50. Ridker PM, JUPITER Study Group: Rosuvastatin in the primary prevention of cardiovascular disease among patients with low levels of low-density lipoprotein cholesterol and elevated high-sensitivity C-reactive protein: Rationale and design of the JUPITER trial. Circulation 108:2292, 2003.
51. Davignon J: Beneficial cardiovascular pleiotropic effects of statins. Circulation 109(Suppl):III39, 2004.
52. Libby P, Aikawa M: Stabilization of atherosclerotic plaques: New mechanisms and clinical targets. Nat Med 8:1257, 2002.
53. Genest J: Combination of statin and ezetimibe for the treatment of dyslipidemias and the prevention of coronary artery disease. Can J Cardiol 22:863, 2006.

54. Sebestjen M, Keber I, Zegura B, et al: Statin and fibrate treatment of combined hyperlipidemia: The effects on some novel risk factors. Thromb Haemost 92:1129, 2004.
55. Brown BG, Zhao XQ, Chait A, et al: Simvastatin and niacin, antioxidant vitamins, or the combination for the prevention of coronary disease. N Engl J Med 345:1583, 2001.
56. Wise A, Foord SM, Fraser NJ, et al: Molecular identification of high and low affinity receptors for nicotinic acid. J Biol Chem 278:9869, 2003.
57. Brousseau ME, Schaefer EJ, Wolfe ML, et al: Effects of an inhibitor of cholesteryl ester transfer protein on HDL cholesterol. N Engl J Med 350:1505, 2004.
58. Cote G, Tardif JC, Lesperance J, et al: Effects of probucol on vascular remodeling after coronary angioplasty. Multivitamins and Protocol Study Group. Circulation 99:30, 1999.
59. Downs JR, Clearfield M, Weis S, et al: Primary prevention of acute coronary events with lovastatin in men and women with average cholesterol levels: Results of AFCAPS/TexCAPS. Air Force/Texas Coronary Atherosclerosis Prevention Study. JAMA 279:1615, 1998.
60. Shepherd J, Cobbe SM, Ford I, et al: Prevention of coronary heart disease with pravastatin in men with hypercholesterolemia. West of Scotland Coronary Prevention Study Group. N Engl J Med 333:1301, 1995.
61. Sacks FM, Pfeffer MA, Moye LA, et al: The effect of pravastatin on coronary events after myocardial infarction in patients with average cholesterol levels. Cholesterol and Recurrent Events Trial investigators. N Engl J Med 335:1001, 1996.
62. Prevention of cardiovascular events and death with pravastatin in patients with coronary heart disease and a broad range of initial cholesterol levels. The Long-Term Intervention with Pravastatin in Ischaemic Disease (LIPID) Study Group. N Engl J Med 339:1349, 1998.
63. Randomised trial of cholesterol lowering in 4444 patients with coronary heart disease: The Scandinavian Simvastatin Survival Study (4S). Lancet 344:1383, 1994.
64. MRC/BHF Heart Protection Study of cholesterol lowering with simvastatin in 20,536 high-risk individuals: A randomised placebo-controlled trial. Lancet 360:7, 2002.
65. Shepherd J, Blauw GJ, Murphy MB, et al: Pravastatin in elderly individuals at risk of vascular disease (PROSPER): A randomised controlled trial. Lancet 360:1623, 2002.

66. Major outcomes in moderately hypercholesterolemic, hypertensive patients randomized to pravastatin vs usual care: The Antihypertensive and Lipid-Lowering Treatment to Prevent Heart Attack Trial (ALLHAT-LLT). JAMA 288:2998, 2002.
67. Sever PS, Dahlof B, Poulter NR, et al: Prevention of coronary and stroke events with atorvastatin in hypertensive patients who have average or lower-than-average cholesterol concentrations, in the Anglo-Scandinavian Cardiac Outcomes Trial-Lipid Lowering Arm (ASCOT-LLA): A multicentre randomised controlled trial. Lancet 361:1149, 2003.
68. Colhoun HM, Betteridge DJ, Durrington PN, et al: Primary prevention of cardiovascular disease with atorvastatin in type 2 diabetes in the Collaborative Atorvastatin Diabetes Study (CARDS): multicentre randomised placebo-controlled trial. Lancet 364;685, 2004.
69. Grundy SM, Cleeman JI, Merz CNB, et al: Implications of recent clinical trials for the National Cholesterol Education Program Adult Treatment Panel III Guidelines. Circulation 110:227, 2004.
70. de Backer G, Ambrosioni E, Borch-Johnsen K, et al: European guidelines on cardiovascular disease prevention in clinical practice—Third Joint Task Force of European and Other Societies on Cardiovascular Disease Prevention in Clinical Practice (constituted by representatives of eight societies and by invited experts). Atherosclerosis 171:145, 2003.
71. Keech A, Simes RJ, Barter P, et al: Effects of long-term fenofibrate therapy on cardiovascular events in 9795 people with type 2 diabetes mellitus (the FIELD Study): Randomised controlled trial. Lancet 366:1849, 2005.
72. Rubins HB, Robins SJ, Collins D, et al: Gemfibrozil for the secondary prevention of coronary heart disease in men with low levels of high-density lipoprotein cholesterol. Veterans Affairs High-Density Lipoprotein Cholesterol Intervention Trial Study Group. N Engl J Med 341:410, 1999.
73. Secondary prevention by raising HDL cholesterol and reducing triglycerides in patients with coronary artery disease: The Bezafibrate Infarction Prevention (BIP) study. Circulation 102:21, 2000.
74. Baigent C, Keech A, Kearney PM, et al: Efficacy and safety of cholesterol-lowering treatment: Prospective meta-analysis of data from 90,056 participants in 14 randomised trials of statins. Lancet 366:1267, 2005.
75. Larosa JC, Grundy SM, Waters D, et al: Intensive lipid lowering with atorvastatin in patients with stable coronary disease. N Engl J Med 352:1425, 2005.
76. Pedersen TR, Faergeman O, Kastelein JJ, et al: High-dose atorvastatin vs usual dose simvastatin for secondary prevention after myocardial infarction—the IDEAL study: A randomized controlled trial. JAMA 294:2437, 2005.
77. McMahon M, Kirkpatrick C, Cummings CE, et al: A pilot study with simvastatin and folic acid/vitamin B12 in preparation for the Study of the Effectiveness of Additional Reductions in Cholesterol and Homocysteine (SEARCH). Nutr Metab Cardiovasc Dis 10:195, 2000.
78. Schwartz GG, Olsson AG, Ezekowitz MD, et al: Effects of atorvastatin on early recurrent ischemic events in acute coronary syndromes: The MIRACL study: A randomized controlled trial. JAMA 285:1711, 2001.
79. de Lemos JA, Blazing MA, Wiviott SD, et al: Early intensive vs a delayed conservative simvastatin strategy in patients with acute coronary syndromes: Phase Z of the A to Z trial. JAMA 292:1307, 2004.
80. Cannon CP, Braunwald E, McCabe CH, et al: Intensive versus moderate lipid lowering with statins after acute coronary syndromes. N Engl J Med 350:1495, 2004.
81. Pitt B, Waters D, Brown WV, et al: Aggressive lipid-lowering therapy compared with angioplasty in stable coronary artery disease. Atorvastatin versus Revascularization Treatment Investigators. N Engl J Med 341:70, 1999.
82. Chiquette E, Chilton R: Aggressive medical management of coronary artery disease versus mechanical revascularization. Curr Atheroscler Rep 5:118, 2003.
83. Nissen SE, Tuzcu EM, Schoenhagen P, et al: Effect of intensive compared with moderate lipid-lowering therapy on progression of coronary atherosclerosis: A randomized controlled trial. JAMA 291:1071, 2004.
84. Nissen SE, Nicholls SJ, Sipahi I, et al: Effect of very high intensity statin therapy on regression of coronary atherosclerosis: The ASTEROID trial. JAMA 295:1556, 2006.
85. Nishimura S, Sekiguchi M, Kano T, et al: Effects of intensive lipid lowering by low-density lipoprotein apheresis on regression of coronary atherosclerosis in patients with familial hypercholesterolemia: Japan Low-density Lipoprotein Apheresis Coronary Atherosclerosis Prospective Study (L-CAPS). Atherosclerosis 144:409, 1999.
86. Nissen SE, Tsunoda T, Tuzcu EM, et al: Effect of recombinant ApoA-I_{Milano} on coronary atherosclerosis in patients with acute coronary syndromes: A randomized controlled trial. JAMA 290:2292, 2003.
87. Shepherd J, Barter P, Carmena R, et al: Effect of LDL cholesterol lowering substantially below currently recommended levels in diabetic patients with coronary artery heart disease and diabetes. The treating to New Targets (TNT) study. Diabetes Care 29:1220, 2006.

CHAPTER 43

Diabetes Mellitus, the Metabolic Syndrome, and Atherosclerotic Vascular Disease

Joshua A. Beckman, Peter Libby, and Mark A. Creager

Vascular diseases account for most morbidity and mortality in patients with diabetes mellitus.[1] Diabetes causes microvascular diseases, such as nephropathy, neuropathy, and retinopathy, and macrovascular disease (e.g., atherosclerosis). Atherosclerosis of the coronary, cerebral, and peripheral arteries accounts for approximately 80 percent of mortality and for 75 percent of hospitalizations in persons with diabetes (see also Chap. 60).

Approximately 8 percent of the United States population has diabetes, undiagnosed in half the cases.[2] The prevalence of diabetes follows that of obesity, which affected approximately 18 percent of the U.S. population in 1998. Hispanics, blacks, Native Americans, and Asian Indians bear a disproportionate burden of diabetic cardiovascular disease.[3] The predilection for these ethnic groups to develop obesity and glucose intolerance on a Western diet may have a genetic basis, because the ability to store fat may have conferred a survival advantage in populations subject to famine. This selective pressure could enrich these populations with genes that facilitate fat storage, the so-called "thrifty gene" hypothesis.[4]

The prevalence of diabetes is increasing in the United States population (Fig. 43-1) and has grown from approximately 2 million cases in the early 1960s to 15 million in the year 2000. Americans born in 2000 will have an estimated 36 percent chance of developing diabetes in their lifetime.[5] In New York City, from 1990 to 2000, the incidence of diabetes increased 61 and 52 percent in men and women, respectively. Moreover, the prevalence of diabetes in patients with myocardial infarction increased from 21 to 36 percent.[6] Current estimates project 22 million cases by the year 2025. These figures raise the specter of a reversal in the improvement in cardiovascular outcomes over the last two decades when viewed in the light of the rapidly expanding diabetic population. The general population in the United States has enjoyed an impressive decline in the mortality associated with heart disease in the last several decades. However, the decrease in cardiovascular mortality in diabetic men and women has lagged well behind that of the general population.[7]

Cardiovascular disease in diabetes also affects the economic resources of the health care system. Data from a managed care organization on the 1-year costs of treating more than 85,000 patients with diabetes compared with age- and gender-matched nondiabetic counterparts has attributed the largest proportion (17 percent) of the excess costs associated with diabetes to coronary artery disease.[8] For comparison, end-stage renal disease accounted for only 11 percent of the excess costs of treatment.

Better implementation of therapies that reduce cardiovascular risk in diabetic patients will require moving beyond the traditional primary focus on glycemic control. A working knowledge of the effects of diabetes mellitus on the heart and blood vessels will aid physicians caring for these patients.

DIAGNOSTIC CRITERIA FOR DIABETES MELLITUS

In 1997, the American Diabetes Association proposed new criteria for the diagnosis of diabetes mellitus.[9] These criteria use a single blood glucose determination after an 8-hour fast (fasting plasma glucose, FPG) as the major diagnostic criterion (Table 43-1). An FPG level less than 110 mg/dl is considered normal. A new diagnostic category known as impaired fasting glucose (IFG) encompasses FPGs greater than 110 but less than 126 mg/dl. A FPG higher than 126 mg/dl establishes the diagnosis of diabetes mellitus. Type 2 diabetes mellitus, previously known as non–insulin-dependent or adult onset diabetes, represents 90 percent of the diabetic population. Type 1 diabetes, known previously as insulin-dependent or juvenile onset diabetes, accounts for the remaining 10 percent. Both forms of diabetes confer independent risk for cardiovascular events, although patients with type 1 diabetes generally develop cardiovascular disease at a much younger age than those with type 2 diabetes.

EPIDEMIOLOGY OF CARDIOVASCULAR DISEASE IN DIABETES MELLITUS

The clinical manifestations of diabetes-related atherosclerosis occur in every major vascular territory, notably the coronary, cerebral, and peripheral (limb) arteries.

Coronary Artery Disease

Patients with diabetes have a two- to fourfold increase in the risk of coronary artery disease (CAD).[10] In the Multiple Risk Factor Intervention (MRFIT) study, more than

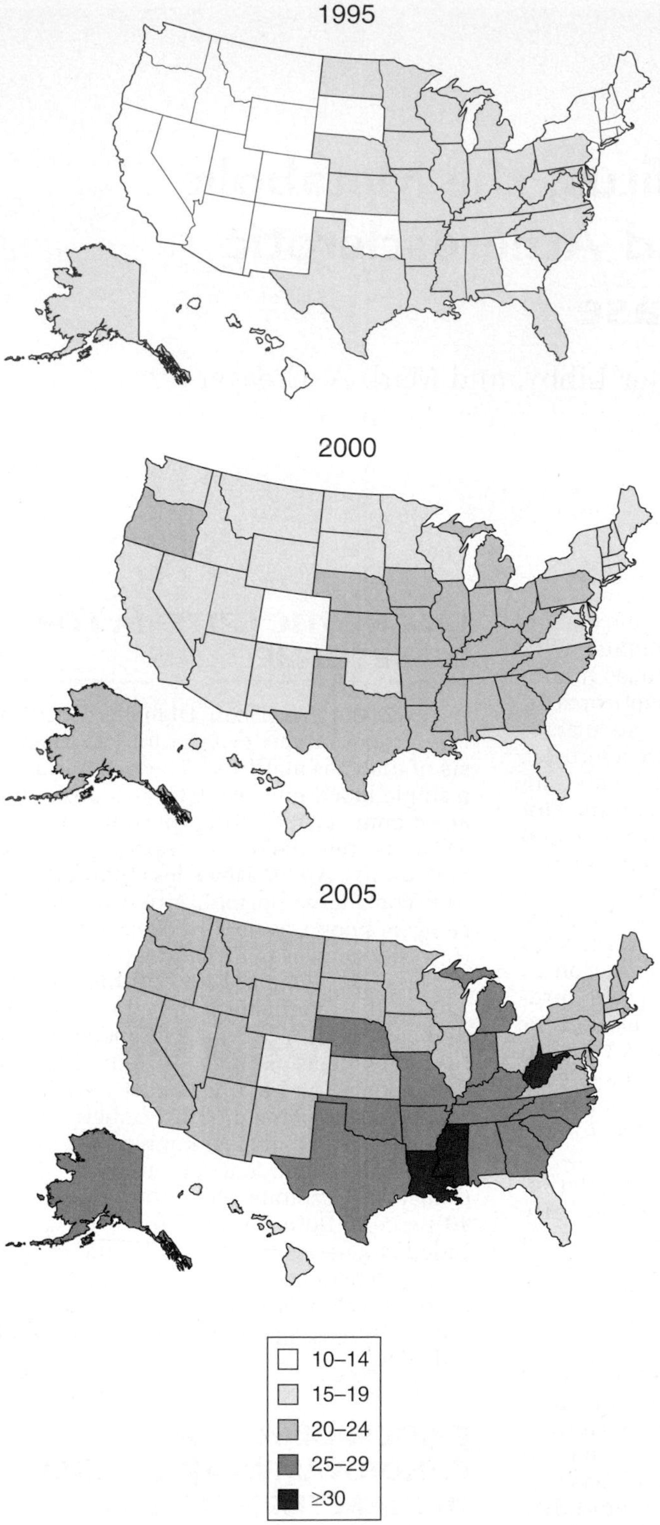

FIGURE 43–1 Obesity in U.S. adults. Over the 10-year period of 1995 to 2005, the prevalence of obesity among U.S. adults increased in every region of the nation. Obesity is associated with the development of type 2 diabetes mellitus and may serve as the root underlying the increase in type 2 diabetes. *(From Centers for Disease Control and Prevention (CDC): State-specific prevalence of obesity among adults—United States, 2005. MMWR Morb Mortal Wkly Rep 55;985, 2006.)*

5000 men (out of approximately 350,000 screened) who reported taking medications for diabetes were followed for an average of 12 years. For every age stratum, ethnic background, and risk factor level, men with diabetes had an absolute risk of CAD death more than three times higher than that in the nondiabetic cohort, even after adjustment

TABLE 43–1 Criteria for the Diagnosis of Diabetes Mellitus

Normal Value	Impaired Fasting Glucose Level	Diabetes Mellitus
FPG <110 mg/dl	FPG ≥110 mg/dl and < 126 mg/dl (IFG)	FPG ≥126 mg/dl
2-hr PG* <140 mg/dl	2-hr PG* ≥140 mg/dl and < 200 mg/dl (IGT)	2-hr PG* ≥200 mg/dl
*2-hr PG 2-hr postload glucose		Symptoms of DM and random plasma glucose concentration ≥ 200 mg/dl

*Rather than using the classic glucose tolerance curve with multiple time points sampled, these criteria use, in parallel to the FPG measurements, a 2-hour postglucose load set of criteria. The plasma sample is obtained 2 hours following an oral administration of 75 gm of anhydrous glucose in aqueous solution.

DM = diabetes mellitus; FPG = fasting plasma glucose; IFG = impaired fasting glucose; IGT = impaired glucose tolerance.

Report of the Expert Committee on the Diagnosis and Classification of Diabetes Mellitus. Diabetes Care 20:1183, 1997.

for established risk factors. Another large cohort of 11,554 white men and 666 black men between the ages of 35 and 64, screened from 1967 to 1973 and followed prospectively for 22 years, showed similar findings.

In the general population, women experience relative protection from myocardial infarction and usually develop CAD approximately 10 years later than men. However, diabetes blunts the cardiovascular benefit of female gender.[1] Diabetic American women of European or African ancestry have this heightened risk. Diabetes increases the risk of death after myocardial infarction in women more than men (see Chap. 60). In the First National Health and Nutrition Examination Survey (NHANES) and the NHANES Epidemiologic Follow-up Survey conducted 10 years apart, age-adjusted mortality decreased in nondiabetic men and women, less so in diabetic men, but increased by 23 percent in diabetic women.[11]

Multiple studies have supported the notion that in patients with diabetes, acute and long-term adverse cardiovascular events substantially increase.[10] A Finnish epidemiological survey compared the rates of myocardial infarction (MI) in nondiabetic and diabetic populations (Fig. 43-2). In this study, patients with diabetes but without prior myocardial infarction had the same level of risk for subsequent acute coronary events as nondiabetics with a history of previous myocardial infarction. In the six-nation Oasis study, diabetic patients presenting with unstable angina or non–Q wave MI had increased rates of stroke, congestive heart failure, and death during the index hospitalization compared with nondiabetic patients. In the Gruppo Italiano per lo Studio della Sopravvivenza nell'Infarto Miocardico-2 (GISSI-2) study of thrombolytic therapy in patients with myocardial infarction, diabetes increased the rate of death in men by 40 percent and women by 90 percent. In the Should We Emergently Revascularize Occluded Coronaries for Cardiogenic Shock (SHOCK) trial,[12] which evaluated a strategy of early revascularization in patients with myocardial infarction complicated by cardiogenic shock, 31.1 percent of the patients had diabetes, a much higher percentage than in the population in general. Moreover, the patients with diabetes experienced a 36 percent excess in mortality compared with patients without diabetes. In the Finnish contribution to the WHO MONICA Project (World Health Organization Multinational Monitor-

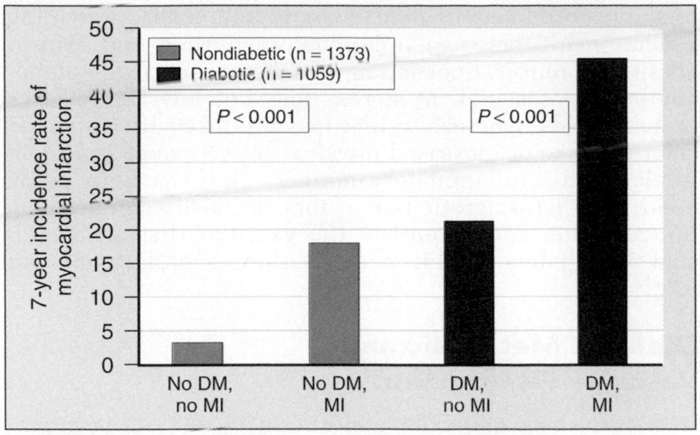

FIGURE 43–2 Marked increase in risk of coronary artery disease in type 2 diabetics. These data show a striking increase in risk of first or recurrent myocardial infarction (MI) in diabetics, compared with nondiabetic subjects, in a population-based study in Finland over a 7-year follow-up period. These data also show that the diabetic without a history of previous myocardial infarction has an approximately equal risk for first myocardial infarction as a nondiabetic subject who has already sustained myocardial infarction. These data support recommendations from the American Diabetes Association to treat diabetic subjects as if they already have established coronary artery disease. DM = diabetes mellitus. *(From Haffner SM, Lehto S, Ronnemaa T, et al: Mortality from coronary heart disease in subjects with type 2 diabetes and in nondiabetic subjects with and without prior myocardial infarction. N Engl J Med 339:229, 1998.)*

ing of Trends and Determinants of Cardiovascular Disease), 1-year mortality was 38 percent higher for diabetic men and 86 percent higher for diabetic women. In a follow-up study of more than 5000 patients who presented to an emergency department with symptoms suggestive of myocardial infarction, diabetic patients had a 53.5 percent 5-year mortality rate compared with 23.3 percent among nondiabetic patients. Younger diabetic patients have an even greater trend toward an increasing risk of death. In a statewide analysis of myocardial infarction, the risk of death in diabetic subjects was 87 percent greater than nondiabetics aged 30 to 49 years but only 17 percent greater in the 70- to 89-year-old age group.

Cerebrovascular Disease

Diabetes mellitus increases the frequency of cerebral atherosclerosis and the risk of stroke.[13] In patients presenting with a stroke, the prevalence of diabetes is three times that of matched controls and diabetes increases the risk of stroke up to fourfold. In the MRFIT study, diabetic subjects who required medication for glucose control were threefold as likely to develop a stroke as nondiabetic subjects. Similarly, in more than 12,000 male and female subjects followed for 6 to 8 years in the Atherosclerosis Risk in Communities Study, the relative risk of an ischemic stroke was increased nearly fourfold by the presence of diabetes. Moreover, insulin resistance varies inversely with the risk of stroke.[14] Diabetic subjects have more severe carotid atherosclerosis as assessed by ultrasonography and a fivefold excess prevalence of calcified carotid atheroma as observed on dental panoramic radiographs.[15]

Diabetes puts younger patients at particular risk for stroke.[13] Diabetes decreases the age at presentation for stroke compared with persons who do not have diabetes. One in 10 stroke victims are younger than 55 years and diabetes increases the stroke risk more than 10-fold in this age group. In the Baltimore-Washington Cooperative Young Stroke Study of 296 cases of incident ischemic stroke subjects aged 18 to 44 years, diabetes markedly increased the risk of stroke. The age-adjusted odds ratio for stroke was 3.3 for black women, 4.2 for black men, 6.2 for white women, and up to as high as 23.1 for white men.

Most studies have found that diabetes increases the risk of stroke more in women than men.[1] In the Renfrew/Paisley Study,[16] a 20-year follow-up study in Scotland of 7052 men and 8354 women aged 45 to 64 years, diabetic women had a nearly threefold excess in stroke, whereas the 52 percent increase in diabetic men did not achieve statistical significance. Furthermore, diabetic women also had a higher risk of death from stroke. In another study of 16,600 patients, diabetes accounted for 16 percent of stroke-related mortality in men and 33 percent in women. Diabetes augments the risk of stroke more in blacks and Caribbean Hispanics than in whites. In the Northern Manhattan Stroke Study, the odds ratio for stroke risk was 1.8 for blacks and 2.1 for Caribbean Hispanics compared with whites.[17] Diabetes also increased the risk of stroke-related dementia more in blacks and Hispanics than in whites.[18]

Diabetes worsens stroke outcome as well. Diabetes doubles the risk of recurrent stroke, more than triples the risk of stroke-related dementia, and markedly increases mortality, both total and stroke-related.[19] In the Renfrew/Paisley study,[16] diabetes raised the relative risk of death after stroke by 290 percent in men and 400 percent in women over 20 years of follow-up.

Peripheral Arterial Disease

Diabetes increases the incidence of peripheral arterial disease (PAD) two- to fourfold.[1] Diabetic patients more often have femoral bruits and absent pedal pulses. The prevalence of peripheral arterial disease (PAD) in unselected persons with diabetes, based on decreased ankle-brachial indices (see Chap. 57), ranges from 12 to 16 percent. In Europeans, the prevalence of peripheral arterial disease is twice as high (26.3 versus 15.3 percent) in asymptomatic outpatients in primary care practices.[20]

The duration of diabetes and the degree of hyperglycemia correlate with the prevalence and severity of PAD (see Chap. 57).[21] In addition to increasing the frequency of PAD, diabetes affects the distribution of atherosclerosis in the lower extremity. PAD in diabetic patients typically affects tibial and peroneal arteries, as well as femoral and popliteal arteries. Moreover, diabetic patients more likely have vascular calcification than nondiabetic cohorts.

In addition to an increased frequency of lower extremity atherosclerosis, diabetes mellitus augments the likelihood of developing the symptomatic forms of PAD. In the Framingham study, diabetes mellitus increased the risk of claudication by 350 percent in men and 860 percent in women. The duration of diabetes was also found to increase the risk of developing claudication in most, but not all, studies. Diabetes also promotes development of critical limb ischemia and tissue loss. Diabetes more than doubles the risk of critical limb ischemia in men and is the most common cause of amputation in the United States.[10] Diabetic patients have a 12.7-fold greater relative risk for amputation than nondiabetic persons in the Medicare population in Minnesota. In the highest risk age group, diabetic persons aged 65 to 74 years, the relative risk of amputation increases 23.5-fold. These trends extend beyond the United States. The Global Lower Extremity Amputation Study Group has reported that the percentage of patients with diabetes may reach as high as 90 percent in patients undergoing their first amputations in populations studied in North America, Europe, and East Asia.[22]

PATHOPHYSIOLOGY OF DIABETIC VASCULAR DISEASE

Adipocyte Biology and Inflammation

We increasingly recognize the role of inflammation in the pathogenesis of diabetes and the metabolic syndrome (Fig. 43-3).[23] In type 1 diabetes, immune injury to the pancreatic islets probably plays a causal role in the development of the disease. In type 2 diabetes, inflammatory mediators released by adipose tissue probably play a key role in the pathogenesis of the cardiovascular complications of this condition. The adipocyte, long regarded as a storage depot for triglycerides, actually can generate substantial quantities of proinflammatory mediators, such as tumor necrosis factor-alpha (TNF-α).[23] TNF-α can cause insulin resistance and can thus causally link adiposity to type 1 diabetes. TNF-α and allied proinflammatory cytokines derived from the adipocyte can activate vascular endothelial and smooth muscle cells to provoke aspects of vascular dysfunction, discussed earlier. In this manner, adipocyte products can directly promote vascular dysfunction and hasten atherogenesis.

Adipocytes can also elaborate chemoattractant molecules, such as monocyte chemoattractant protein, which can recruit inflammatory leukocytes to enter adipose tissue.[24] Once present, these "professional" phagocytes can amplify the production of proinflammatory mediators and perpetuate the inflammatory cycle related to insulin resistance and the vascular complications of diabetes mellitus. Some evidence has suggested that visceral adipose tissue plays a particularly pernicious role in perpetuating proinflammatory pathways by producing proportionately more of these mediators than subcutaneous adipose tissue.[25] Waist circumference and visceral adiposity, as determined by imaging, correlate with C-reactive protein levels, indicating a relationship between inflammatory burden and central obesity. Moreover, liposuction, which evacuates subcutaneous but not visceral fat stores, does not lower C-reactive protein levels, whereas weight loss produced by restricted caloric intake or increased physical activity does diminish levels of this inflammatory marker. Thus, as with many other proatherosclerotic risk factors, adiposity can promote inflammation and potentiate the vascular disease associated with diabetes and its complications (see Chaps. 38 and 39).[25]

Diabetic Metabolic and Vascular Dysfunction

Diabetes causes metabolic abnormalities, including hyperglycemia, dyslipidemia, and insulin resistance, that disrupt normal arterial function and render arteries susceptible to atherosclerosis. It specifically alters the function of vascular endothelium and smooth muscle cells, as well as platelets, in ways that promote atherogenesis. Diabetes impairs the vasodilator function of endothelial cells and decreases the bioavailability of nitric oxide (NO).[26] Moreover, characteristic metabolic disturbances in diabetes, including hyperglycemia, increased free fatty acid concentrations, and insulin resistance, can individually decrease nitric oxide bioavailability and attenuate endothelial function.[27] Endothelial dysfunction also occurs in healthy adult offspring of type 2 diabetic parents, suggesting an inheritable abnormality as well.[28]

Hyperglycemia decreases NO production from endothelial nitric oxide synthase (eNOS) and increases its degradation via generation of reactive oxygen species (ROS). Hyperglycemia triggers the production of ROS in vascular cells through enzymatic (protein kinase C and the reduced form of nicotinamide adenine dinucleotide phosphate [NADPH] oxidases) and nonenzymatic sources of oxidant stress (e.g., the formation of advanced glycation end products, AGEs).[29] As oxidative stress increases, the eNOS cofactor tetrahydrobiopterin becomes oxidized and uncouples eNOS, which cause the enzyme to produce superoxide anion instead of NO.[30] Superoxide anion quenches NO in a diffusion-limited reaction to produce peroxynitrite. Peroxynitrite inhibits prostacyclin synthase and endothelium-dependent hyperpolarizing factor activity. Similar to the effects of hyperglycemia, free fatty acids activate intracellular enzymatic oxidant sources, including protein kinase C, NADPH oxidases, and eNOS, yielding analogous increases in superoxide anion.[30,31]

The excess adipose tissue that usually accompanies type 2 diabetes mellitus releases excess fatty acids. Reduced skeletal muscle uptake of free fatty acids further augments their plasma levels.[32] Increased concentrations of free fatty acids exert deleterious actions in several areas (see earlier). In healthy humans, free

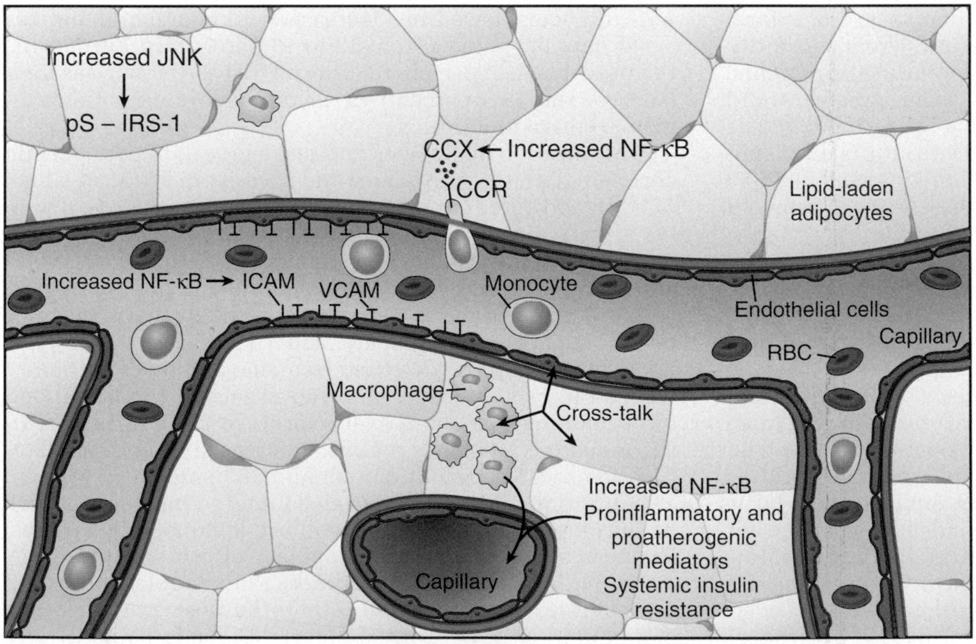

FIGURE 43–3 Obesity, adipose tissue, and inflammation. Obesity-mediated increases in adipose causes a state of cellular stress and activation of mitogenic cell signaling, including JNK and nuclear factor kappa B (NF-κB). These inflammatory signaling pathways increase adipocyte production of proinflammatory cytokines, including tumor necrosis factor-alpha, interleukin-6, leptin, and resistin, chemokines such as monocyte chemoattractant protein-1, and other proatherogenic mediators, for example plasminogen activator inhibitor 1. Overlying endothelial cells express adhesion molecules (e.g., intercellular adhesion molecule 1, ICAM-1, and vascular cell adhesion molecule 1, VCAM-1) and chemoattractant molecules (CCX) that bind monocytes to receptors (CCR) to recruit them to the adipose tissues. There monocytes become macrophages and produce inflammatory cytokines and chemokines to enhance local inflammation and propagate the inflammatory diathesis systemically. pS-IRS-1 = phosphosezine insulin receptor substrate–1; RBC = red blood cell. *(From Shoelson SE, Lee J, Goldfine AB: Inflammation and insulin resistance. J Clin Invest 116:1793, 2006.)*

fatty acid infusion impairs endothelial function and the co-infusion of an antioxidant restores it.[33] Free fatty acids also attenuate prostacyclin bioavailability by inhibiting prostacyclin synthase.[34] Moreover, free fatty acids interfere with intracellular signaling pathways to cause not only muscle and visceral insulin resistance but also vascular insulin resistance.[35]

In diabetes, hyperglycemia and increased free fatty acids increase the concentration in the cell of the metabolite diacylglycerol.[36] Diacylglycerol, in turn, activates a family of enzymes known as protein kinase C (PKC), that perform key regulatory functions by phosphorylating proteins important in metabolic control. Recent work[30] has implicated activation of the PKC family in cardiovascular complications of diabetes. Activation of PKC can inhibit the expression of eNOS, augment cytokine-induced tissue factor gene expression and procoagulant activity in human endothelial cells, and increase the production of proinflammatory cytokines, proliferation of vascular wall cells, and production of extracellular matrix macromolecules that accumulate during atherosclerotic lesion formation.[30] In vivo evidence has supported a role of PKC activation in the pathogenesis of various aspects of vascular dysfunction in vivo. Administration of a selective inhibitor of protein kinase C-beta (PKC-β) prevents impaired endothelial function in healthy humans exposed to hyperglycemia, reduces visual loss in diabetic patients with retinopathy, and may attenuate diabetic neuropathy (Fig. 43-4).[37-39]

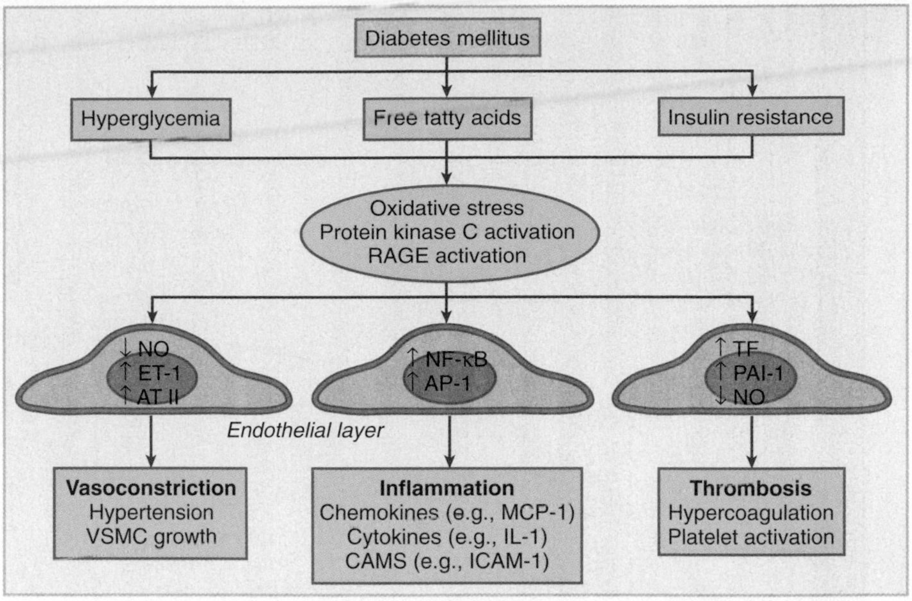

FIGURE 43–4 Endothelial dysfunction in diabetes. Normally, the endothelium maintains vascular homeostasis by promoting vasodilation, minimizing inflammation, and preventing thrombosis. In diabetes, hyperglycemia, excess free fatty acid release, dyslipidemia, and insulin resistance increase reactive oxygen species production, formation of advanced glycation end products (AGE), and activation of protein kinase C, diminishing the bioavailability of nitric oxide and decreasing its potent vasodilatory, antiinflammatory, and antithrombotic effects. Diabetes impairs endothelial function and promotes vasoconstriction, inflammation, and thrombosis. Decreasing nitric oxide and increasing endothelin-1 and angiotensin II concentrations increases vascular tone and VSMC growth and migration. Activation of inflammatory transcription factors nuclear factor kappa B (NF-κB) and activator protein-1 (AP-1) induce liberation of leukocyte-attracting chemokines, production of inflammatory cytokines, and expression of cell adhesion molecules. Attenuated nitric oxide and prostacyclin activate platelets while increases in plasmin activator inhibitor-1 and tissue factor create a prothrombotic milieu. RAGE = receptor for advanced glycation end products; NO = nitric oxide; ET-1 = endothelin-1; AT II = angiotensin II; VSMC = vascular smooth muscle cell; NF-κB = nuclear factor kappa B; AP-1 = activator protein-1; MCP-1 = monocyte chemoattractant protein-1; IL-1 = interleukin-1; CAMS = cell adhesion molecules; TF = tissue factor; PAI-1 = plasminogen activator inhibitor 1. *(From Creager MA, Luscher TF, Cosentino F, Beckman JA: Diabetes and vascular disease: Pathophysiology, clinical consequences, and medical therapy: Part I. Circulation 108:1527, 2003.)*

Although typically associated with impairments in skeletal glucose muscle uptake, many tissues in the diabetic patient demonstrate insulin resistance, including adipose, liver, and endothelial cells.[27] Normal vascular function requires intact endothelial insulin signaling. For example, in genetically engineered mice that lack the endothelial cell insulin receptor, vascular endothelial nitric oxide synthase concentration decreases 60 percent.[40] Endothelial insulin resistance alters the pattern of activation of intracellular signaling pathways, favoring stimulation of mitogen-activated protein (MAP) kinases over phosphatidylinositol 3 (PI-3) kinase. Preferential activation of the MAP kinase pathway decreases nitric oxide production, increases endothelin production, stimulates the transcription of inflammatory genes, and increases the tendency to coagulation.[41] Drug-induced improvement in insulin sensitivity reduces cytokine production and inflammatory transcription factor activation and increases nitric oxide bioavailability.[42,43]

Studies have identified a novel potential mechanism for mediating impaired endothelial-dependent vasodilator function. An endogenous competitive inhibitor of nitric oxide synthase, known as asymmetric dimethylarginine (ADMA), increases directly with insulin resistance in nondiabetic subjects and glycemic control in diabetes[44] and improves with glycemic control.[45] The accumulation of ADMA may result from inhibition of its catabolism because of reduction in activity of the enzyme dimethylarginine dimethylaminohydrolase. Another study has suggested that dysregulation of this enzyme raises levels of ADMA in diabetics.[46] These findings indicate another potential molecular pathway of impaired vascular function in diabetes.

Diabetes also disturbs vascular function through nonenzymatic glycation of macromolecules. In states of hyperglycemia and increased oxidative stress, many proteins and even lipids undergo nonenzymatic glycation. For example, hemoglobin A_{1c}, the glycated form of hemoglobin, provides the clinician with an integrated gauge of hyperglycemia. Glycated proteins can form structures known as AGEs that cause the macromolecule to take on a brown hue, similar to burnt sugar. Numerous chemical studies have characterized the structure of AGEs. AGEs accumulate in the vessel wall and appear to contribute to the pathobiology of complications of diabetes, notably the accelerated vascular disease characteristic of this condition (Fig. 43-5).[47] Phospholipids and apolipoproteins can form AGEs[47] and AGE-modified proteins can accumulate in diabetic subjects. The presence of glycated forms of low-density lipoproteins (LDLs) can engender an immune response and contribute to macrovascular disease. AGE-modified LDL apoprotein and LDL lipid levels increase in diabetic subjects compared with nondiabetics.[48]

Cells have several surface receptors for AGE that mediate their biological effects. Exposure to AGE-modified proteins can elicit the production of inflammatory cytokines from vascular cells, cause impaired endothelium-dependent vasodilator function, and augment endothelial expression of various leukocyte adhesion molecules implicated in atherogenesis in vivo.[49] Experimentally, AGEs in the

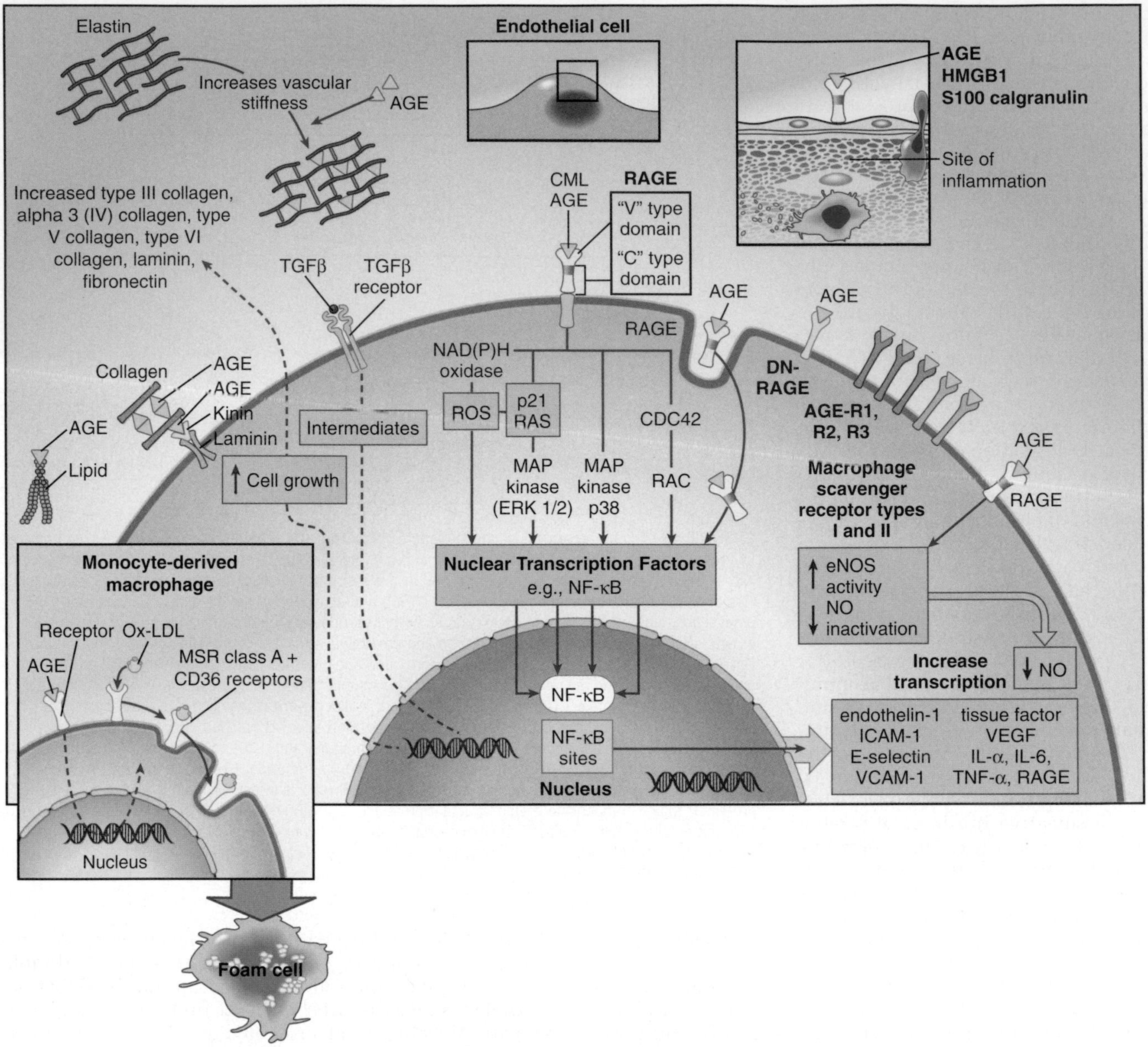

FIGURE 43–5 The vascular effects of advanced glycation end products (AGEs). In the extracellular matrix, AGEs form on lipids, collagen, elastin, and vitronectin, altering the matrix composition and augmenting stiffness. AGE-mediated activation of RAGE stimulates oxygen-derived free radical production, mitogenic pathway stimulation, and activation of the inflammatory transcription factor NF-κB. Activation of NF-κB heightens transcription of vasoconstrictor agents such as endothelin, inflammatory mediators such as cellular adhesion molecules, and prothrombotic substances such as tissue factor. AGEs decrease nitric oxide bioavailability through increases in oxidant stress and modification of eNOS. CML = N-(carboxymethyl) lysine; DN = dominant negative; eNOS = endothelial nitric oxide synthase; HMGB1 = high-mobility group box-1; ICAM-1 = intercellular adhesion molecule-1; IL-α = interleukin-alpha; MAO = monoamine oxidase; MSR = macrophage scavenger receptor; NO = nitric oxide; NF-κB = nuclear factor kappa B; Ox-LDL = oxidated low-density lipoprotein; RAGE = receptor for AGE; ROS = reactive oxygen species; TGF-α = transforming growth factor-alpha; TNF-α = tumor necrosis factor-alpha; VCAM-1 = vascular cell adhesion molecule-1. *(From Goldin A, Beckman JA, Schmidt AM, Creager MA: Advanced glycation end products: Sparking the development of diabetic vascular injury. Circulation 114:597, 2006.)*

subendothelium induce monocyte diapedesis into the vascular wall, mediate their effects through the inflammatory transcription factor nuclear factor kappa B (NF-κB), and augment vascular wall coagulation through attenuation of thrombomodulin activity and upregulation of tissue factor expression.[49] In humans, increased AGE production is associated with reduced nitric oxide bioavailability through impairment of eNOS transcription and activity, production of oxygen-derived free radicals, and activation of NF-κB.

One extensively characterized receptor for AGE is known as the receptor for advanced glycation end products, RAGE.[50] Studies have supported a functional role for RAGE in the development of experimental atherosclerosis. Mice lacking the apolipoprotein E gene are susceptible to atherosclerosis, and administration of an antibody fragment that neutralizes RAGE attenuates atherosclerosis in these mutant mice. This beneficial effect on atherosclerotic lesion development does not depend on a change in blood sugar levels or lipoprotein profile,[51] supporting a role for AGE in atherogenesis.

Through decreases in NO, increases in oxidative stress, AGE production, and activation of its receptor, and insulin resistance, diabetes increases vascular inflammation via the activation and nuclear translocation of intracellular transcription factors, NF-κB and activator protein-1 (AP-1).[27] These factors cause the expression of genes responsible for producing chemokines, cytokines, leukocyte adhesion molecules, and proinflammatory mediators, such as TNF-α.[50] Diabetes further aggravates plaque progression by causing endothelial cells to produce cytokines, which decrease collagen production by vascular smooth muscle cells, and to enhance endothelial cell production of matrix metalloproteinases and tissue factor.[52] These changes may decrease the stability of the atherosclerotic plaque's fibrous cap, increasing the likelihood and severity of plaque rupture (see Chap. 38).

Numerous basic science and clinical studies have indicated an increased level of oxidative stress in diabetes.[53] The reactive oxygen species in turn can augment the formation of reactive carbonyl species. Nonoxidative reactions can also increase the concentrations of reactive carbonyl compounds under hyperglycemic conditions. The reactive carbonyl species can derivatize proteins and lipids. Among the products of reactions of proteins with reactive oxygen and carbonyl species are the AGEs (see later). There is little doubt that products of glycoxidation accumulate in diabetic patients. However, they accumulate in nondiabetic elderly individuals as well. Other studies have suggested that overwhelming the capacity of detoxifying mechanisms for reactive carbonyl groups may account for the increase in oxidant and carbonyl stress in diabetics.

Diabetes impairs vascular smooth muscle function and augments the production of vasoconstrictor mediators, including endothelin-1,[1] which causes vascular smooth muscle growth and inflammation. Levels of other atherogenic mediators, including angiotensin II and vasoconstrictor prostanoids, increase in diabetes as well.[1] Patients with type 2 diabetes have impaired vasodilation, possibly reflecting an abnormality in NO signal transduction.[26] Moreover, diabetic patients have attenuated vasoconstriction to endothelin-1 and angiotensin.[54] Diabetes may alter subcellular calcium distribution in smooth muscle cells,[55] resulting in augmented vasoconstriction in response to norepinephrine and phenylephrine. However, most diabetics have peripheral autonomic impairment at the time of diagnosis, and vascular beds regulated by these nerves have decreased arterial resistance.[1] Similar to endothelial cells, diabetes activates atherogenic mechanisms within vascular smooth muscle cells, including protein kinase C, RAGE, NF-κB and the production of oxidative stress.[30] Diabetes heightens vascular smooth muscle cell migration in atherosclerotic lesions. Advanced atherosclerotic lesions have fewer vascular smooth muscle cells in diabetic patients than nondiabetic patients, possibly resulting in decreased resiliency of the fibrous cap and thereby increasing the risk of rupture and luminal thrombosis.[56]

Platelet abnormalities occur in diabetes that parallel those found in endothelial cells, including activation of protein kinase C, decreased production of platelet-derived nitric oxide, and increased oxidative stress.[57] Diabetes impairs platelet calcium homeostasis, which may contribute importantly to abnormal platelet activity, because calcium regulates platelet shape change, secretion, aggregation, and thromboxane formation. Moreover, platelets from patients with diabetes have increased expression of the adhesive glycoproteins (GP) Ib and GP IIb/IIIa.[1] Patients with type 2 diabetes have attenuated insulin-mediated antagonism of platelet activation and higher levels of prothrombotic platelet microparticles.[58,59] Type 2 diabetes and its associated metabolic abnormalities favor an imbalance in the coagulation and fibrinolytic systems that support clot formation and stability. Type 2 diabetes increases plasminogen activator inhibitor type 1 (PAI-1) levels, impairing fibrinolytic capacity in atherosclerotic lesions.[60] Moreover, diabetes increases the expression of tissue factor and levels of plasma coagulation factors, and decreases levels of endogenous anticoagulants.[60] These various abnormalities may contribute to heightened susceptibility to the thrombotic complications of atherosclerosis.

THERAPEUTIC OPTIONS FOR DIABETIC VASCULAR DISEASE

Since the 1990s, treatment of diabetes has evolved from a focus on hyperglycemia to a broader view encompassing all the metabolic disturbances associated with diabetes, including insulin resistance, dyslipidemia, hypertension, and platelet activation. Each of these abnormalities plays an important role in cardiovascular disease development and progression.

Life Style Modification

Improvements in each dysmetabolic component of diabetes may be acquired through healthy modifications in life style. In the Diabetes Prevention Program, 3324 subjects with impaired glucose tolerance were randomized to intensive life style adjustments or standard life style and placebo or metformin.[61] Both intensive life style changes and metformin significantly reduced the rate of diabetes development by 31 and 58 percent, respectively, in comparison with placebo.[62] Intensive life style changes also reduced the development of other risk factors for cardiovascular disease. At 3 years of follow-up, the need for pharmacological therapy was reduced by 27 to 28 percent for hypertension and by 25 percent for hyperlipidemia.[61]

Pharmacological Therapy

Prevention of Diabetes

Recent clinical trials have demonstrated the potential of pharmacological therapy to decrease the frequency of progression to type 2 diabetes in patients with insulin resistance. The Diabetes Reduction Assessment with Ramipril and Rosiglitazone Medication (DREAM) study investigators randomized 5269 persons 30 years of age or older who had impaired fasting plasma glucose or impaired glucose tolerance to the angiotensin-converting enzyme inhibitor ramipril, up to 15 mg daily,[63] or the thiazolidinedione rosiglitazone, 8 mg daily,[64] in a 2 × 2 factorial randomized trial. At a median follow-up of 3 years, rosiglitazone significantly reduced the rate of diabetes or death by 60 percent from 26 to 11.6 percent, whereas ramipril had no significant effect. Pharmacological improvement in obesity with antagonism of the cannabinoid type 1 receptor increased high-density lipoprotein (HDL) and reduced triglycerides, suggesting that weight loss, either through life style or pharmacological intervention, may also reduce the rate of progression to diabetes in an at-risk population.[65] Ongoing trials are examining the link between intensive life style changes and pharmacological interventions and hard endpoints, such as myocardial infarction and death.

Hyperglycemia and Insulin Resistance

Hyperglycemia, a fundamental component of diabetes, adversely affects vascular function and directly correlates with cardiovascular events (see Chap. 60).[1] In the United Kingdom Prospective Diabetes Study (UKPDS), hemoglobin A_{1c} levels above 6.2 percent indicated an increased risk of macrovascular disease. For each 1 percent elevation in hemoglobin A_{1c}, coronary heart disease risk increased by 11 percent. A meta-analysis of almost 100,000 diabetic patients found that increases in plasma glucose concentration correlated with augmented cardiovascular risk, beginning with glucose concentrations below the diabetic threshold.[66] Data concerning the role of glucose intolerance are inconsistent. In UKPDS, the relative risk of coronary heart disease did not increase until hemoglobin A_{1c} levels exceeded 7 percent, suggesting a threshold.[67]

Several clinical trials have sought to determine whether intensive treatment of blood glucose levels can reduce the risk of CHD associated with diabetes. Large, adequately powered studies, such as UKPDS, have shown a nonsignificant trend in favor of intensive blood glucose control in terms of reduction of MI.[68] This trial randomized 3867 patients with newly diagnosed type 2 diabetes to intensive therapy (diet plus oral therapy or insulin) or to conventional therapy. Patients entered into the study had a low background prevalence of coronary heart disease (CHD) and a low rate of CHD risk factors. Patients were followed for approximately 10 years. As in the Diabetes Control and Complications Trial (DCCT), microvascular endpoints were improved in the intensive therapy arm. There was also a trend for a reduced rate of myocardial infarction in the group receiving intensive blood glucose control ($p = 0.052$).[68]

More recent data have supported the notion that tight glycemic control may decrease the rate of cardiovascular morbidity and mortality. In the Epidemiology of Diabetes Interventions and Complications study, the long-term follow-up study of patients in the DCCT trial, type 1 subjects underwent carotid ultrasound 1 to 2 years after the end of DCCT and again 4 years later.[69] The subjects in the intensive glycemic control arm had significantly less progression of their carotid intima-media thickness (IMT) than the patients in the usual control arm. Over the 17 years of follow-up, intensive therapy reduced the risk of any cardiovascular event by 42 percent, from 7.1 percent (52 of 780 patients) to 4.4 percent (31 of 711 patients), revealing a modest absolute extended benefit of tight control.[70] In the STOP-Noninsulin-Dependent Diabetes Mellitus (NIDDM) trial, patients with impaired glucose tolerance were randomized to acarbose, an alpha-glucosidase inhibitor, or matching placebo and followed for an average of 3.3 years.[71] Patients taking acarbose had significantly fewer cardiovascular events (including MI, new angina, revascularization, cardiovascular death, congestive heart failure, cerebrovascular events, and peripheral arterial disease) than subjects taking placebo. Ongoing clinical trials with more aggressive glycemic control may enable a true evaluation of the hypothesis that glycemic control serves an important role in the prevention of cardiovascular disease.

Insulin resistance may provide the crucial link between hyperglycemia and cardiovascular disease (Table 43-2). This collective occurrence of multiple metabolic abnormalities in an individual patient has been given various names—syndrome X, the insulin resistance syndrome, and cardiovascular dysmetabolic syndrome. The risk cluster of the metabolic syndrome (see Table 43-2) clearly confers excess cardiovascular risk and varies based on ethnic origin. Some have doubted whether the risk of the constellation of components reflects mere additivity or actual synergy in this regard.[72] We believe that the construct of the metabolic syndrome provides a useful framework for patient assessment and management, because it emphasizes the multifaceted pattern of risk factors actually encountered in daily practice and the need to institute life style modification and a global risk modification strategy for optimum prevention.[73] Data from a number of studies have indicated that insulin resistance independently predicts cardiovascular disease risk. In a large triethnic population comprised of equal numbers of subjects with diabetes, hyperglycemia, and normal glucose tolerance, insulin resistance correlated positively with atherosclerosis, as assessed by carotid IMT. Because insulin resistance typically precedes the development of hyperglycemia, these findings may explain, in part, the elevated risk of coronary heart disease in individuals with newly diagnosed type 2 diabetes. Indeed, the severity of insulin resistance directly correlates with rates of myocardial infarction,[74] stroke,[14] and peripheral arterial disease.[21] In UKPDS, improving insulin resistance with metformin decreased macrovascular events; this result has engendered some controversy because the addition of metformin to sulfonylurea therapy seems to increase cardiovascular risk.[75,76]

TABLE 43–2 Components of the Cardiovascular Dysmetabolic Syndrome

	Feature	
Risk Factor	***Men***	***Women***
Hyperglycemia	Glucose >110 mg/dl	Glucose >110 mg/dl
Dyslipidemia		
HDL cholesterol	<40 mg/dl	<50 mg/dl
Triglycerides	>150 mg/dl	>150 mg/dl
Obesity—Ethnic Group, Waist Circumference (inches)		
Subsaharan African	≥37	≥32
South/Central American	≥35	≥32
Chinese	≥35	≥32
Japanese	≥34	≥35
Hypertension	Blood pressure >130/85 mm Hg	Blood pressure >130/85 mm Hg
Age (yr)	>45	>55

The availability of the thiazolidinediones (TZDs) provides a second approach to improve insulin sensitivity and glycemic control. TZDs bind and activate peroxisome proliferator-activated receptor gamma (PPAR gamma), a nuclear receptor that participates in differentiation of adipocytes and modulates functions of vascular cells related to atherogenesis.[77] In addition to improving insulin sensitivity, PPAR gamma agonists may have antiinflammatory activity and directly retard atherogenesis.[77] TZDs also may decrease the concentration of small, dense LDLs and augment LDL resistance to oxidation. However, total, LDL, and high-density lipoprotein (HDL) cholesterol concentrations increase, making the net effect on the lipid profile unclear.[78] TZDs have complex effects, because activation of PPAR gamma may promote macrophage lipid accumulation.[79] In a study of patients with type 2 diabetes, rosiglitazone improved endothelial function and exercise capacity after 4 months of therapy compared with placebo.[80] In another study of patients with type 2 diabetes, pioglitazone reduced insulin resistance and carotid IMT compared with glimepiride, a sulfonylurea.[81] The Prospective Pioglitazone Clinical Trial in Macrovascular Events (PROACTIVE) trial randomized 5238 type 2 diabetic subjects with macrovascular disease to titrated pioglitazone (15 to 45 mg daily) or placebo.[82] Follow-up for a mean of 34.5 months showed a nonsignificant trend toward a 10 percent relative risk reduction and 2 percent absolute risk reduction in the primary endpoint (mortality, nonfatal myocardial infarction, acute coronary syndrome, coronary or peripheral revascularization, above-ankle amputation). The secondary endpoint of the composite of all-cause mortality, nonfatal myocardial infarction and stroke, fell significantly by 16 percent, from 14.0 to 11.9 percent.[82] Ongoing clinical trials will determine whether improvements in insulin resistance with TZDs or other drugs can decrease cardiovascular morbidity and mortality in patients with or at risk for diabetes.

Dyslipidemia

Even though patients with diabetes typically have LDL cholesterol levels in the average range, they often have elevated triglyceride and decreased HDL cholesterol levels and small, dense LDL particles (see Chap. 42). Increased delivery of free fatty acids to the liver caused by adipose efflux and impaired skeletal muscle uptake increases hepatic production of very low-density lipoprotein (VLDL) and cholesteryl ester synthesis (Fig. 43-6).[83] Overproduction of triglyceride-rich lipoproteins and impaired clearance by lipoprotein lipase lead to hypertriglyceridemia in diabetics.[83]

Triglyceride levels tend to vary inversely with HDL levels because cholesteryl ester transfer protein mediates exchanges of cholesterol from the HDL to VLDL form.[83] The combination of elevated triglycerides and low HDL is more common than elevated total and LDL cholesterol in diabetic patients with CAD. In addition to abnormalities of concentration,

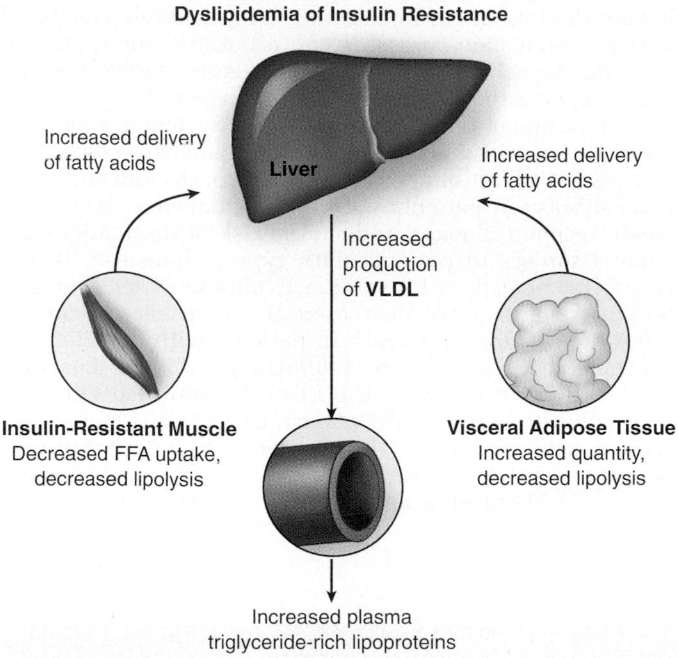

FIGURE 43–6 The pathogenesis of diabetic dyslipidemia. Increased production of very-low-density lipoproteins (VLDLs) from the liver results from increased delivery of fatty acids because of decreased uptake by muscle and increased delivery of fatty acids from visceral abdominal fat to the liver via the portal circulation. Decreased catabolism of postprandial triglyceride-rich lipoprotein particles caused by reduced lipoprotein lipase activity accentuates diabetic dyslipidemia (not shown). FFA = free fatty acid.

functional defects in the HDL of diabetic subjects, and a diminished capacity to prevent LDL oxidation, also may promote atherogenesis. Increased concentrations of small, dense LDL in a diabetic person results from abnormal cholesterol and triglyceride transfer between VLDL and LDL and depends on increased levels of VLDL, particularly when triglyceride concentrations exceed 130 mg/dl.[83] Small, dense LDL particles are proatherogenic. They bind readily to intimal proteoglycans, which enhances their retention in the intima, promoting their oxidative modification and hence uptake by macrophages and smooth muscle cells.[84]

Life style modification should be the first step in management of dyslipidemia in those with diabetes and the metabolic syndrome, as in other populations. Each component of diabetic dysmetabolism improves with weight loss, exercise, and dietary modification. Large clinical trials have demonstrated the benefits of pharmacological intervention. Lipid-lowering therapy, particularly with 3-hydroxy-3-methylglutaryl coenzyme A (HMG-CoA) reductase inhibitors or statins, reduces cardiovascular risk more in diabetic than nondiabetic subjects (Table 43-3).[1] In the Heart Protection Study (HPS), the reduction risk even extended to patients with pretreatment LDL cholesterol levels below 100 mg/dl.[85] In the Anglo-Scandinavian Cardiac Outcomes Trial—Lipid Lowering Arm (ASCOT-LLA), atorvastatin reduced the rate of major cardiovascular events by 23 percent, from 11.9 to 9.3 percent, compared with placebo in the 2532 hypertensive subjects with type 2 diabetes mellitus.[86] In another study, atorvastatin did not reduce death, nonfatal myocardial infarction, and stroke in dialysis patients with type 2 diabetes, indicative of the pernicious effect of end-stage renal disease despite statin treatment.[87]

Fibric acid derivatives address particularly the increased triglyceride and decreased HDL concentrations characteristic of diabetic dyslipidemia (see Chap. 42 for a full discussion). In the Veterans Affairs High Density Lipoprotein Cholesterol Intervention Trial (VA-HIT), treatment with gemfibrozil resulted in a 24 percent risk reduction for myocardial infarction in the diabetic subjects, who represented 25 percent of enrolled subjects, an outcome similar to that observed in nondiabetic subjects.[88] In the Diabetes Atherosclerosis Intervention Study (DAIS), fenofibrate limited angiographic progression of coronary artery lesions in a diabetic cohort, but the event reduction did not achieve statistical significance because of the small sample size in this angiographic trial.[89] These results were amplified in the Fenofibrate Intervention and Event Lowering in Diabetes (FIELD) study, in which 9795 type 2 diabetic subjects aged

TABLE 43–3 Statin Therapy in Diabetes

Study	No. of Patients	Indication	Drug	Duration (yr)	CV Outcome	Risk Reduction (%)
AFCAPS[99]	155	PP, average TC, low HDL	Lovastatin	5.2	FMI, NFMI, SD	43
4S[100]	202	Stable CAD, elevated TC	Simvastatin	5.3	Fatal CHD + NFMI	51
CARE[101]	602	Stable CAD, average TC	Pravastatin	5	Fatal CHD + NFMI + CR	22
LIPID[102]	782	Stable CAD, average TC	Pravastatin	6.1	Fatal CHD + NFMI	17
HPS[85]	5983	Diabetes	Simvastatin	4.8	MI + CVA + CR + NCR	33
ASCOT-LA[86]	2532	Diabetes, hypertension	Atorvastatin	3.3	Death, NFMI, CVA	23
DM and RF[103]	1255	Diabetes, RF	Atorvastatin	4.0	FMI + CVAD + NFMI + NFCVA	8 (NS)

CAD = coronary artery disease; CHD = coronary heart disease; CR = coronary revascularization; CV = cardiovascular; CVA = cerebrovascular accident (stroke); CVAD = stroke death; DM = diabetes mellitus; FMI = fatal myocardial infarction; HDL = high-density lipoprotein; MI = myocardial infarction; NCR = noncoronary revascularization; NFCVA = nonfatal stroke; NFMI = nonfatal myocardial infarction; NS = not significant; PP = primary prevention; RF = renal failure; SD = sudden death; TC = total cholesterol.

50 to 75 years received fenofibrate or placebo.[90] At 5 years of follow-up, the fenofibrate-treated group had a nonsignificant reduction in coronary events and a trend toward higher mortality. Fibrates may have antiatherogenic effects that do not depend on lipid lowering. Fibrates bind to PPAR alpha, which exerts antiinflammatory effects that include the reduction of endothelial cell activation by proinflammatory cytokines and decreased tissue factor production by human macrophages.[91] Evidence supporting the use of fibric acid derivatives as first-line agents is limited in patients with diabetes, as shown in the VA-HIT and FIELD trials. These agents may have value as second-lipid agents in diabetic patients with persistently elevated triglyceride levels and low HDL, a hypothesis undergoing testing in the Action to Control Cardiovascular Risk in Diabetes (ACCORD) trial (see Chap. 42). Combinations of statins and fibrates, particularly gemfibrozil, warrant careful monitoring for muscle injury. Despite concern over worsening glycemic control, nicotinic acid therapy in diabetic persons can increase HDL levels.

Hypertension (see Chap. 41)

Hypertension and insulin resistance frequently occur together as part of the dysmetabolic syndrome (see Table 43-2). The addition of hypertension to the clinical picture of diabetes amplifies the already high cardiovascular disease risk in these patients. Aggressive blood pressure control prevents more cardiovascular events in diabetics than nondiabetics.[1] The Appropriate Blood-Pressure Control in Diabetes (ABCD) trial investigated the effect of aggressive blood pressure control in type 2 diabetic patients with peripheral arterial disease. The intensively treated group (128/75 mm Hg) had no increased risk of cardiovascular events over 4 years of follow-up.[92]

The role of specific classes of antihypertensive drugs in reducing cardiovascular morbidity and mortality in patients with diabetes has engendered controversy.[93] The UKPDS[76] and Systolic Hypertension in Europe Trial (Syst-Eur) have shown beneficial effects for both ACE inhibitors and calcium channel blockers in patients with diabetes (Table 43-4). Also, in the UKPDS, 1148 hypertensive patients with type 2 diabetes responded equally well to captopril or atenolol in terms of achieving blood pressure control, and had similar reductions in the risk of macrovascular disease. Aggressive blood pressure reduction with either agent significantly reduced stroke and deaths caused by diabetes. Myocardial infarction declined 21 percent in the group randomized to tight blood pressure (BP) control, but this change was not statistically significant. Although the blood pressure in the UKPDS subgroup assigned to tight BP control was good (averaging 144/82 mm Hg), data from the Syst-Eur trial and the HOT trial have indicated that achieving even lower blood pressure with calcium channel blockers further lowers the rate of cardiovascular complications compared with moderate blood pressure control. Achieving American Diabetes Association target blood pressure (130/80 mm Hg) almost always requires more than one agent.[94]

Modulation of the renin-angiotensin system has particular importance in diabetic patients. Angiotensin-converting enzyme (ACE) inhibitors reduce nephropathy and end-stage renal disease in patients with type 1 diabetes, and angiotensin receptor blockers reduce the risk of these microvascular disorders in patients with type 2 diabetes.[95] In the Heart Outcomes and Prevention Evaluation (HOPE) study, ramipril significantly decreased the rates of myocardial infarction, stroke, and death in patients with diabetes and a mean blood pressure of 140/80 mm Hg.[96] The Losartan Intervention For Endpoint (LIFE) study[97] enrolled 1195 diabetic subjects as part of the cohort. Participants had hypertension and evidence of left ventricular hypertrophy. Subjects were randomized to losartan or atenolol. Despite equivalent blood pressure lowering, the subjects random-

TABLE 43–4 Treatment of Hypertension in Diabetes

Study	No. of Patients	Population	Drug	Duration (yr)	Blood Pressure Control (mm Hg) *Tight*	*Less Tight*	CV Outcome	Risk Reduction (%)
Placebo-Controlled Trials								
SHEP[104]	583	Elderly, T2	Chlorthalidone	5	143/68	155/72	CHD	56
							CV mortality	34
HOT[105]	1501	T2, 50-80 yr	Felodipine	3	140/81	144/85	CV events	51
							MI	50
Syst-Eur[106]	492	T2	Nitrendipine	2	153/76	182/81	Stroke	69
							CV mortality	70
UKPDS[76]	1148	T2	Captopril or atenolol	8.4	144/82	154/87	Stroke	44
							Death	37
HOPE[96]	3547	T2 + 1 RF	Ramipril	4.5	140/77	143/77	MI	22
							Stroke	33
							Mortality	24
			Initial Therapy		**Drug 1**	**Drug 2**		
Drug Comparison Trials								
CAPP[107]	572	DM	Captopril versus diuretic or beta blocker	7	155/89	153/88	FMI/NFMI + CVA/CVD	41
LIFE[97]	1195	DM + LVH	Losartan versus atenolol	4.8	146/79	148/79	CV events	22
							Mortality	39

T2 = type 2 diabetes; RF = cardiovascular risk factor; DM = diabetes; LVH = left ventricular hypertrophy; CHD = coronary heart disease; CV = cardiovascular; MI = myocardial infarction; FMI = fatal myocardial infarction; NFMI = nonfatal myocardial infarction; CVA = stroke; CVD = fatal stroke.

ized to losartan experienced a 39 percent reduction in all-cause mortality, a 37 percent reduction in cardiovascular mortality, and a 21 percent reduction in stroke.[97]

Comprehensive Risk Factor Modification

Aggressive modification of every risk factor may produce results with greater additive benefit than expected from treatment of each individual risk factor. The Steno-2 trial randomized 160 subjects to intensive multifactorial risk factor modification, including dietary modification (fat intake less than 30 percent of total consumption), light to moderate exercise three to five times per week, smoking cessation courses, ACE inhibitors, multivitamins, aspirin, intensive glucose control, and lipid modification, or to conventional therapy.[98] This combination of interventions significantly and markedly reduced the rate of cardiovascular events, from 85 events among 35 patients in the conventional arm to 33 events among 19 patients in the intensive risk factor modification group. Aggressive therapies to modify the risks of cardiovascular disease will diminish the clinical manifestations of vascular disease and should be implemented (Fig. 43-7).

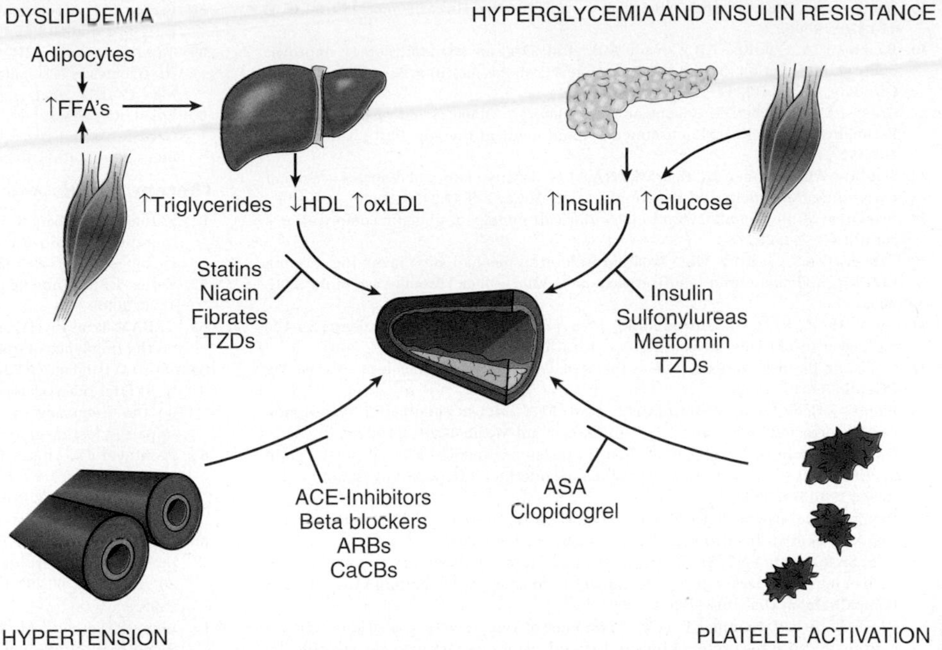

FIGURE 43–7 Antiatherosclerosis therapy in diabetes. To stem the onset and progression of atherosclerosis, patients with diabetes require therapy for each metabolic abnormality. Statins improve the lipid profile and decrease the risk of myocardial infarction and death, whereas the evidence for cardiovascular benefits with fibric acid derivatives is mixed. The first clinical trial of thiazolidinediones (TZDs) for cardiovascular outcomes therapy has been completed and showed a trend toward benefit. Treatment of hypertension decreases the rate of myocardial infarction and stroke in diabetes. Therapy should include angiotensin-converting enzyme (ACE) inhibitors or angiotensin receptor blockers (ARBs) for their microvascular and possible atherosclerosis benefits. The heightened thrombotic potential of the diabetic state supports the use of platelet antagonists, such as aspirin or clopidogrel. Although strict treatment of hyperglycemia does not significantly reduce the incidence of myocardial infarction or death, the improvement in microvascular outcomes itself warrants vigorous pursuit of rigorous glycemic control in diabetes. FFA's = free fatty acids; HDL = high-density lipoprotein; oxLDL = oxidated low-density lipoprotein; CaCBs = calcium channel blockers; ASA = aspirin. *(Modified from Libby P, Plutzky J: Diabetic macrovascular disease: The glucose paradox? Circulation 106:2760, 2002.)*

CONCLUSION

Atherosclerosis and its complications cause most of the death and much of the disability in patients with diabetes mellitus. Intensive treatment of the entire scope of metabolic abnormalities, beyond hyperglycemia alone, significantly reduces the rates of adverse cardiovascular events. As the prevalence of patients with diabetes increases, strategies to ensure the appropriate and aggressive use of life style modification and medical therapy will help stem the tide of death and disability in this high-risk population.

REFERENCES

Epidemiology

1. Beckman JA, Creager MA, Libby P: Diabetes and atherosclerosis: Epidemiology, pathophysiology, and management. JAMA 287:2570, 2002.
2. Mokdad AH, Ford ES, Bowman BA, et al: Prevalence of obesity, diabetes, and obesity-related health risk factors, 2001. JAMA 289:76, 2003.
3. Egede LE, Dagogo-Jack S: Epidemiology of type 2 diabetes: Focus on ethnic minorities. Med Clin North Am 89:viii, 949, 2005.
4. Lazar MA: How obesity causes diabetes: Not a tall tale. Science 307:373, 2005.
5. Narayan KMV, Boyle JP, Thompson TJ, et al: Lifetime risk for diabetes mellitus in the United States. JAMA 290:1884, 2003.
6. Fang J, Alderman MH: Impact of the increasing burden of diabetes on acute myocardial infarction in New York City: 1990-2000. Diabetes 55:768, 2006.
7. Schreinemachers DM: Mortality from ischemic heart disease and diabetes mellitus (type 2) in four U.S. wheat-producing states: A hypothesis-generating study. Environ Health Perspect 114:186, 2006.
8. Peele PB, Lave JR, Songer TJ: Diabetes in employer-sponsored health insurance. Diabetes Care 25:1964, 2002.
9. Report of the Expert Committee on the Diagnosis and Classification of Diabetes Mellitus. Diabetes Care 20:1183, 1997.
10. Luscher TF, Creager MA, Beckman JA, Cosentino F: Diabetes and vascular disease: Pathophysiology, clinical consequences, and medical therapy: Part II. Circulation 108:1655, 2003.
11. Gu K, Cowie CC, Harris MI: Diabetes and decline in heart disease mortality in US adults. JAMA 281:1291, 1999.
12. Shindler DM, Palmeri ST, Antonelli TA, et al: Diabetes mellitus in cardiogenic shock complicating acute myocardial infarction: a report from the SHOCK Trial Registry. Should we emergently revascularize occluded coronaries for cardiogenic shocK? J Am Coll Cardiol 36(Suppl A):109, 2000.
13. Kissela B, Air E: Diabetes: Impact on stroke risk and poststroke recovery. Semin Neurol 26:100, 2006.
14. Kernan WN, Inzucchi SE, Viscoli CM, et al: Insulin resistance and risk for stroke. Neurology 59:809, 2002.
15. Friedlander AH, Garrett NR, Norman DC: The prevalence of calcified carotid artery atheromas on the panoramic radiographs of patients with type 2 diabetes mellitus. J Am Dent Assoc 133:1516, 2002.
16. Sacco RL, Boden-Albala B, Abel G, et al: Race-ethnic disparities in the impact of stroke risk factors: The northern Manhattan stroke study. Stroke 32:1725, 2001.
17. Luchsinger JA, Tang MX, Stern Y, et al: Diabetes mellitus and risk of Alzheimer's disease and dementia with stroke in a multiethnic cohort. Am J Epidemiol 154:635, 2001.
18. Hu G, Sarti C, Jousilahti P, et al: The impact of history of hypertension and type 2 diabetes at baseline on the incidence of stroke and stroke mortality. Stroke 36:2538, 2005.
19. Hart CL, Hole DJ, Smith GD: Comparison of risk factors for stroke incidence and stroke mortality in 20 years of follow-up in men and women in the Renfrew/Paisley Study in Scotland. Stroke 31:1893, 2000.
20. Lange S, Diehm C, Darius H, et al: High prevalence of peripheral arterial disease and low treatment rates in elderly primary care patients with diabetes. Exp Clin Endocrinol Diabetes 112:566, 2004.
21. Marso SP, Hiatt WR: Peripheral arterial disease in patients with diabetes. J Am Coll Cardiol 47:921, 2006.
22. Boulton AJ, Vileikyte L, Ragnarson-Tennvall G, Apelqvist J: The global burden of diabetic foot disease. Lancet 366:1719, 2005.

Pathophysiology of Diabetic Vascular Disease

23. Berg AH, Scherer PE: Adipose tissue, inflammation, and cardiovascular disease. Circ Res 96:939, 2005.
24. Tilg H, Moschen AR: Adipocytokines: Mediators linking adipose tissue, inflammation and immunity. Nat Rev Immunol 6:772, 2006.

25. Shoelson SE, Lee J, Goldfine AB: Inflammation and insulin resistance. J Clin Invest 116:1793, 2006.
26. Beckman JA, Goldfine AB, Gordon MB, et al: Oral antioxidant therapy improves endothelial function in type 1 but not type 2 diabetes mellitus. Am J Physiol Heart Circ Physiol 285:H2392, 2003.
27. Creager MA, Luscher TF, Cosentino F, Beckman JA: Diabetes and vascular disease: Pathophysiology, clinical consequences, and medical therapy: Part I. Circulation 108:1527, 2003.
28. Goldfine AB, Beckman JA, Betensky RA, et al: Family history of diabetes is a major determinant of endothelial function. J Am Coll Cardiol 47:2456, 2006.
29. Brownlee M: Biochemistry and molecular cell biology of diabetic complications. Nature 414:813, 2001.
30. Rask-Madsen C, King GL: Proatherosclerotic mechanisms involving protein kinase C in diabetes and insulin resistance. Arterioscler Thromb Vasc Biol 25:487, 2005.
31. Xu Y, He Z, King GL: Introduction of hyperglycemia and dyslipidemia in the pathogenesis of diabetic vascular complications. Curr Diab Rep 5:91, 2005.
32. Goldstein BJ: Insulin resistance as the core defect in type 2 diabetes mellitus. Am J Cardiol 90:3G, 2002.
33. Pleiner J, Schaller G, Mittermayer F, et al: FFA-induced endothelial dysfunction can be corrected by vitamin C. J Clin Endocrinol Metab 87:2913, 2002.
34. Du X, Edelstein D, Obici S, et al: Insulin resistance reduces arterial prostacyclin synthase and eNOS activities by increasing endothelial fatty acid oxidation. J Clin Invest 116:1071, 2006.
35. Belfort R, Mandarino L, Kashyap S, et al: Dose-response effect of elevated plasma free fatty acid on insulin signaling. Diabetes 54:1640, 2005.
36. Itani SI, Ruderman NB, Schmieder F, Boden G: Lipid-induced insulin resistance in human muscle is associated with changes in diacylglycerol, protein kinase C, and IkappaB-alpha. Diabetes 51:2005, 2002.
37. Vinik AI, Bril V, Kempler P, et al: Treatment of symptomatic diabetic peripheral neuropathy with the protein kinase C beta-inhibitor ruboxistaurin mesylate during a 1-year, randomized, placebo-controlled, double-blind clinical trial. Clin Ther 27:1164, 2005.
38. PKC-DRS2 Group: Effect of ruboxistaurin on visual loss in patients with diabetic retinopathy. Ophthalmology 113:2221, 2006.
39. Beckman JA, Goldfine AB, Gordon MB, et al: Inhibition of protein kinase C beta prevents impaired endothelium- dependent vasodilation caused by hyperglycemia in humans. Circ Res 90:10, 2002.
40. Vicent D, Ilany J, Kondo T, et al: The role of endothelial insulin signaling in the regulation of vascular tone and insulin resistance. J Clin Invest 111:1373, 2003.
41. Montagnani M, Golovchenko I, Kim I, et al: Inhibition of phosphatidylinositol 3-kinase enhances mitogenic actions of insulin in endothelial cells. J Biol Chem 277:1794, 2002.
42. Isoda K, Young JL, Zirlik A, et al: Metformin inhibits proinflammatory responses and nuclear factor-kappaB in human vascular wall cells. Arterioscler Thromb Vasc Biol 26:611, 2006.
43. Davis BJ, Xie Z, Viollet B, Zou MH: Activation of the AMP-activated kinase by antidiabetes drug metformin stimulates nitric oxide synthesis in vivo by promoting the association of heat shock protein 90 and endothelial nitric oxide synthase. Diabetes 55:496, 2006.
44. Paiva H, Lehtimaki T, Laakso J, et al: Plasma concentrations of asymmetric-dimethyl-arginine in type 2 diabetes associate with glycemic control and glomerular filtration rate but not with risk factors of vasculopathy. Metabolism 52:303, 2003.
45. Asagami T, Abbasi F, Stuelinger M, et al: Metformin treatment lowers asymmetric dimethylarginine concentrations in patients with type 2 diabetes. Metabolism 51:843, 2002.
46. Lin KY, Ito A, Asagami T, et al: Impaired nitric oxide synthase pathway in diabetes mellitus: Role of asymmetric dimethylarginine and dimethylarginine dimethylaminohydrolase. Circulation 106:987, 2002.
47. Wendt T, Bucciarelli L, Qu W, et al: Receptor for advanced glycation endproducts (RAGE) and vascular inflammation: Insights into the pathogenesis of macrovascular complications in diabetes. Curr Atheroscler Rep 4:228, 2002.
48. Brownlee M: Negative consequences of glycation. Metabolism 49(Suppl 1):9, 2000.
49. Goldin A, Beckman JA, Schmidt AM, Creager MA: Advanced glycation end products: Sparking the development of diabetic vascular injury. Circulation 114:597, 2006.
50. Wautier JL, Schmidt AM: Protein glycation: A firm link to endothelial cell dysfunction. Circ Res 95:233, 2004.
51. Hudson BI, Wendt T, Bucciarelli LG, et al: Diabetic vascular disease: It's all the RAGE. Antioxid Redox Signal 7:1588, 2005.
52. Uemura S, Matsushita H, Li W, et al: Diabetes mellitus enhances vascular matrix metalloproteinase activity: Role of oxidative stress. Circ Res 88:1291, 2001.
53. Ceriello A: Oxidative stress and diabetes-associated complications. Endocr Pract 12(Suppl 1):60, 2006.
54. Endemann DH, Schiffrin EL: Endothelial dysfunction. J Am Soc Nephrol 15:1983, 2004.
55. Fleischhacker E, Esenabhalu VE, Spitaler M, et al: Human diabetes is associated with hyperreactivity of vascular smooth muscle cells due to altered subcellular Ca^{2+} distribution. Diabetes 48:1323, 1999.
56. Burke AP, Kolodgie FD, Zieske A, et al: Morphologic findings of coronary atherosclerotic plaques in diabetics: a postmortem study. Arterioscler Thromb Vasc Biol 24:1266, 2004.
57. Sudic D, Razmara M, Forslund M, et al: High glucose levels enhance platelet activation: Involvement of multiple mechanisms. Br J Haematol 133:315, 2006.

58. Ferreira IA, Mocking AI, Feijge MA, et al: Platelet inhibition by insulin is absent in type 2 diabetes mellitus. Arterioscler Thromb Vasc Biol 26:417, 2006.
59. Tan KT, Tayebjee MH, Lim HS, Lip GY: Clinically apparent atherosclerotic disease in diabetes is associated with an increase in platelet microparticle levels. Diabet Med 22:1657, 2005.
60. Eckel RH, Wassef M, Chait A, et al: Prevention Conference VI: Diabetes and Cardiovascular Disease: Writing Group II: Pathogenesis of atherosclerosis in diabetes. Circulation 105:e138, 2002.

Therapy for Diabetic Vascular Disease

61. Ratner R, Goldberg R, Haffner S, et al: Impact of intensive life style and metformin therapy on cardiovascular disease risk factors in the diabetes prevention program. Diabetes Care 28:888, 2005.
62. Ratner RE: An update on the Diabetes Prevention Program. Endocr Pract 12(Suppl 1):20, 2006.
63. DREAM Trial Investigators; Bosch J, Yusuf S, Gerstein HC, et al: Effect of ramipril on the incidence of diabetes. N Engl J Med 355:1608, 2006.
64. DREAM (Diabetes REduction Assessment with ramipril and rosiglitazone Medication) Trial Investigators; Gerstein HC, Yusuf S, Bosch J, et al: Effect of rosiglitazone on the frequency of diabetes in patients with impaired glucose tolerance or impaired fasting glucose: A randomised controlled trial. Lancet 368:1096. 2006.
65. Pi-Sunyer FX, Aronne LJ, Heshmati HM, et al: Effect of rimonabant, a cannabinoid-1 receptor blocker, on weight and cardiometabolic risk factors in overweight or obese patients: RIO-North America: A randomized controlled trial. JAMA 295:761, 2006.
66. Coutinho M, Gerstein HC, Wang Y, Yusuf S: The relationship between glucose and incident cardiovascular events. A metaregression analysis of published data from 20 studies of 95,783 individuals followed for 12.4 years. Diabetes Care 22:233, 1999.
67. Libby P, Nathan DM, Abraham K, et al: Report of the National Heart, Lung, and Blood Institute-National Institute of Diabetes and Digestive and Kidney Diseases Working Group on Cardiovascular Complications of Type 1 Diabetes Mellitus. Circulation 111:3489, 2005.
68. UK Prospective Diabetes Study (UKPDS) Group: Intensive blood-glucose control with sulphonylureas or insulin compared with conventional treatment and risk of complications in patients with type 2 diabetes (UKPDS 33). Lancet 352:837, 1998.
69. Nathan DM, Lachin J, Cleary P, et al: Intensive diabetes therapy and carotid intima-media thickness in type 1 diabetes mellitus. N Engl J Med 348:2294, 2003.
70. Nathan DM, Cleary PA, Backlund JY, et al: Intensive diabetes treatment and cardiovascular disease in patients with type 1 diabetes. N Engl J Med 353:2643, 2005.
71. Chiasson JL, Josse RG, Gomis R, et al: Acarbose treatment and the risk of cardiovascular disease and hypertension in patients with impaired glucose tolerance: The STOP-NIDDM trial. JAMA 290:486, 2003.
72. Kahn R, Buse J, Ferrannini E, Stern M: The metabolic syndrome: Time for a critical appraisal: Joint statement from the American Diabetes Association and the European Association for the Study of Diabetes. Diabetes Care 28:2289, 2005.
73. Grundy SM: Does the metabolic syndrome exist? Diabetes Care 29:1689, 2006; discussion, 1693.
74. Hedblad B, Nilsson P, Engstrom G, et al: Insulin resistance in nondiabetic subjects is associated with increased incidence of myocardial infarction and death. Diabet Med 19:470, 2002.
75. Centers for Disease Control and Prevention: Diabetes-related amputations of lower extremities in the Medicare population—Minnesota, 1993-1995. MMWR Morb Mortal Wkly Rep 47:649, 1998.
76. UK Prospective Diabetes Study (UKPDS) Group: Efficacy of atenolol and captopril in reducing risk of macrovascular and microvascular complications in type 2 diabetes (UKPDS 39). BMJ 317:713, 1998.
77. Plutzky J: Inflammation in atherosclerosis and diabetes mellitus. Rev Endocr Metab Disord 5:255, 2004.
78. Campbell IW: The clinical significance of PPAR gamma agonism. Curr Mol Med 5:349, 2005.
79. Nicholson AC: Expression of CD36 in macrophages and atherosclerosis: The role of lipid regulation of PPARgamma signaling. Trends Cardiovasc Med 14:8, 2004.
80. Regensteiner JG, Bauer TA, Reusch JE: Rosiglitazone improves exercise capacity in individuals with type 2 diabetes. Diabetes Care 28:2877, 2005.
81. Langenfeld MR, Forst T, Hohberg C, et al: Pioglitazone decreases carotid intima-media thickness independently of glycemic control in patients with type 2 diabetes mellitus: Results from a controlled randomized study. Circulation 111:2525, 2005.
82. Dormandy JA, Charbonnel B, Eckland DJ, et al: Secondary prevention of macrovascular events in patients with type 2 diabetes in the PROactive Study (PROspective pioglitAzone Clinical Trial In macroVascular Events): A randomised controlled trial. Lancet 366:1279, 2005.
83. Nesto RW: Beyond low-density lipoprotein: Addressing the atherogenic lipid triad in type 2 diabetes mellitus and the metabolic syndrome. Am J Cardiovasc Drugs 5:379, 2005.
84. Carmena R, Duriez P, Fruchart JC: Atherogenic lipoprotein particles in atherosclerosis. Circulation 109(Suppl 1):III2, 2004.
85. Collins R, Armitage J, Parish S, et al: MRC/BHF Heart Protection Study of cholesterol-lowering with simvastatin in 5963 people with diabetes: A randomised placebo-controlled trial. Lancet 361:2005, 2003.
86. Sever PS, Poulter NR, Dahlof B, et al: Reduction in cardiovascular events with atorvastatin in 2,532 patients with type 2 diabetes: Anglo-Scandinavian Cardiac Outcomes Trial—lipid-lowering arm (ASCOT-LLA). Diabetes Care 28:1151, 2005.
87. Wanner C, Krane V, Marz W, et al: Atorvastatin in patients with type 2 diabetes mellitus undergoing hemodialysis. N Engl J Med 353:238, 2005.

88. Rubins HB, Robins SJ, Collins D, et al: Gemfibrozil for the secondary prevention of coronary heart disease in men with low levels of high-density lipoprotein cholesterol. Veterans Affairs High-Density Lipoprotein Cholesterol Intervention Trial Study Group. N Engl J Med 341:410, 1999.
89. Effect of fenofibrate on progression of coronary-artery disease in type 2 diabetes: The Diabetes Atherosclerosis Intervention Study, a randomised study. Lancet 357:905, 2001.
90. Keech A, Simes RJ, Barter P, et al: Effects of long-term fenofibrate therapy on cardiovascular events in 9795 people with type 2 diabetes mellitus (the FIELD study): Randomised controlled trial. Lancet 366:1849, 2005.
91. Lefebvre P, Chinetti G, Fruchart JC, Staels B: Sorting out the roles of PPAR alpha in energy metabolism and vascular homeostasis. J Clin Invest 116:571, 2006.
92. Mehler PS, Coll JR, Estacio R, et al: Intensive blood pressure control reduces the risk of cardiovascular events in patients with peripheral arterial disease and type 2 diabetes. Circulation 107:753, 2003.
93. Vijan S, Hayward RA: Treatment of hypertension in type 2 diabetes mellitus: Blood pressure goals, choice of agents, and setting priorities in diabetes care. Ann Intern Med 138:593, 2003.
94. Nilsson M, Cifkova R, Kjeldsen SE: Treatment of hypertension in patients with type-2 diabetes mellitus. Blood Press 15:62, 2006.
95. Deinum J, Chaturvedi N: The renin-angiotensin system and vascular disease in diabetes. Semin Vasc Med 2:149, 2002.
96. Heart Outcomes Prevention Evaluation Study Investigators: Effects of ramipril on cardiovascular and microvascular outcomes in people with diabetes mellitus: Results of the HOPE study and MICRO-HOPE substudy. Lancet 355:253, 2000.
97. Lindholm LH, Ibsen H, Dahlof B, et al: Cardiovascular morbidity and mortality in patients with diabetes in the Losartan Intervention For Endpoint reduction in hypertension study (LIFE): A randomised trial against atenolol. Lancet 359:1004, 2002.
98. Gaede P, Vedel P, Larsen N, et al: Multifactorial intervention and cardiovascular disease in patients with type 2 diabetes. N Engl J Med 348:383, 2003.
99. Downs JR, Clearfield M, Weis S, et al: Primary prevention of acute coronary events with lovastatin in men and women with average cholesterol levels: Results of AFCAPS/TexCAPS. Air Force/Texas Coronary Atherosclerosis Prevention Study. JAMA 279:1615, 1998.
100. Randomised trial of cholesterol lowering in 4444 patients with coronary heart disease: The Scandinavian Simvastatin Survival Study (4S). Lancet 344:1383, 1994.
101. Sacks FM, Pfeffer MA, Moye LA, et al: Cholesterol and recurrent events trial investigators. The effect of pravastatin on coronary events after myocardial infarction in patients with average cholesterol levels. N Engl J Med 335:1001, 1996.
102. Prevention of cardiovascular events and death with pravastatin in patients with coronary heart disease and a broad range of initial cholesterol levels. The Long-Term Intervention with Pravastatin in Ischaemic Disease (LIPID) Study Group. N Engl J Med 339:1349, 1998.
103. Wanner C, Krane V, Marz W, et al: Atorvastatin in patients with type 2 diabetes mellitus undergoing hemodialysis. N Engl J Med 353:238, 2005.
104. Curb JD, Pressel SL, Cutler JA, et al: Effect of diuretic-based antihypertensive treatment on cardiovascular disease risk in older diabetic patients with isolated systolic hypertension. Systolic Hypertension in the Elderly Program Cooperative Research Group. JAMA 276:1886, 1996.
105. Hansson L, Zanchetti A, Carruthers SG, et al: Effects of intensive blood-pressure lowering and low-dose aspirin in patients with hypertension: Principal results of the Hypertension Optimal Treatment (HOT) randomized trial. HOT Study Group. Lancet 351:1755, 1998.
106. Staessen JA, Fagard R, Thijs L, et al: Randomised double-blind comparison of placebo and active treatment for older patients with isolated systolic hypertension. The Systolic Hypertension in Europe (Syst-Eur) Trial Investigators. Lancet 350:757, 1997.
107. Niskanen L, Hedner T, Hansson L, et al: Reduced cardiovascular morbidity and mortality in hypertensive diabetic patients on first-line therapy with an ACE inhibitor compared with a diuretic/beta-blocker-based treatment regimen: A subanalysis of the Captopril Prevention Project. Diabetes Care 24:2091, 2001.

CHAPTER 44

Nutrition and Cardiovascular Disease

Ronald M. Krauss

Appropriate nutritional practices have central importance in managing risk for atherosclerotic cardiovascular disease. Indeed, many of the current dietary guidelines for the health of the general population aim to prevent cardiovascular disease. These recommendations emerge from considerable evidence for nutritional influences on cardiovascular disease risk and a smaller but compelling number of studies indicating that certain dietary modifications can reduce that risk. Additional dietary interventions can benefit patients at higher risk because of specific conditions such as dyslipidemia, hypertension, and obesity. Because of the complexities of testing specific nutrient effects and the inherent difficulties of conducting randomized, controlled clinical endpoint trials for nutritional interventions, they generally cannot be subjected to the same evidence-based criteria that are used to assess drug treatments. Nevertheless, a body of information supports a number of dietary interventions for reducing cardiovascular disease risk and calls into question others that are promoted without an adequate scientific basis.

Effectiveness of dietary recommendations requires provision to patients in a manner that promotes implementation and long-term adherence. The involvement of dietitians and other trained members of a health care team can greatly aid this goal. Of critical importance is the commitment of the health care provider to nutritional guidance and the ability to convey this in terms that patients can accept and readily integrate into their daily lives. Ensuring the patient's understanding of the principles and the goals of the dietary recommendations is an essential element of this process.

The information in this chapter is consistent with dietary guidelines prepared in recent years by the American Heart Association (AHA)[1]; the Adult Treatment Panel III of the National Cholesterol Education Program[2]; the National Heart, Lung, and Blood Institute (NHLBI) Joint National Committee on Prevention, Detection, Evaluation and Treatment of High Blood Pressure[3]; the NHLBI Clinical Guidelines on the Identification, Evaluation, and Treatment of Overweight and Obesity in Adults[4]; and the 2005 U.S. Dietary Guidelines.

EFFECTS OF OVERALL DIETARY PATTERN AND SPECIFIC FOOD CATEGORIES ON CARDIOVASCULAR DISEASE

Observational Evidence

Numerous epidemiological studies have identified dietary patterns and food categories associated with reduced risk of cardiovascular disease.[5] Although the interpretation of these studies is limited by their observational nature, the imprecision of the dietary information collected, and the difficulty of correcting for confounding effects of other health behaviors, nevertheless they represent the only feasible approach for drawing conclusions regarding the overall impact of dietary pattern and intake of specific food categories on health outcomes. These analyses permit the general conclusion that lower risk for cardiovascular disease is promoted by emphasis on intake of fruits and vegetables, whole grains, nuts and legumes, fish (preferably fatty), poultry and lean meats, low-fat and fat-free dairy products, and liquid vegetable oils. Major nutrient characteristics of these diets include high density of micronutrients and fiber; moderate amounts of unsaturated fats including omega-3 fatty acids; and lower content of saturated and *trans* fatty acids, sugars, and starches with a high glycemic effect. The relation of these nutrients to cardiovascular disease risk is described further later in the chapter. Epidemiological studies have reported that adherence to such patterns is associated with reductions in cardiovascular disease risk of 30 percent or more.[1,6-9] However, it is important to recognize that the nutrient composition of these dietary patterns agrees with current recommended dietary intakes for overall health.

A large number of epidemiological studies have reported relationships of specific food categories within these dietary patterns to cardiovascular disease risk, and these studies have formed the basis for recommended intakes of these foods in current dietary guidelines.[1]

FRUITS AND VEGETABLES. Consumption of fruits and vegetables of three or more servings per day versus less than once per day was associated with a 27 percent reduction in cardiovascular disease risk,[10] consistent with results from other studies in which there was a graded risk reduction associated with higher intakes.[11-13] Data suggest that intake of green leafy vegetables and foods rich in carotenoids and vitamin C contribute particularly strongly to this relationship. Based on these data, together with evidence from the Dietary Approaches to Stop Hypertension (DASH) trial, described further later,[14,15] consumption of at least five portions per day of a variety of fruits and vegetables is generally recommended for maintaining cardiovascular health.[1]

WHOLE GRAINS AND FIBER. Consumption of whole grains has been associated with reduced cardiovascular disease risk in a number of studies.[16,17] Although this effect may be related to fiber intake,[18,19] not all studies have indicated that the relationship with fiber intake is independent of other variables.[20] Indeed, there is reason to implicate effects of other nutrients in whole grains that are shared by other plant foods, particularly vitamins, phytoestrogens, phenols, omega-3 fatty acids, resistant starch, and minerals.

Another issue surrounding intake of whole grains is the potential inverse relationship with consumption of sugars and starches with a high glycemic effect, which may have adverse effects on cardiovascular risk.[21] The magnitude of glycemia, namely the blood glucose elevation following consumption of a dietary carbohydrate, primarily reflects the rate of starch digestion and absorption from the intestine, and this in turn can lead to undesirable metabolic consequences, such as a greater rate of increase in postprandial insulin and an increase in plasma triglycerides.[22] A value ("glycemic index") can be assigned to a food on the basis of the magnitude of blood glucose elevation following consumption of this food in relation to that following a standard food (white bread).[22] However, the reliability of this index as a measure of metabolic effects of meals and the relation of glycemic load (the quantity of foods with high glycemic index) to disease risk has been challenged.[23]

This food category therefore illustrates the general difficulty of statistically dissociating the effects of a single food category from others that are part of an overall dietary pattern. Nevertheless, a meta-analysis indicated an average 27 percent reduction in coronary heart disease (CHD) independently associated with whole grain consumption and suggested an intake of at least three servings per day for cardiovascular health.[24]

LEGUMES. Increased intake of legumes (e.g., peas, beans, soybeans, lentils) has been associated with reduced cardiovascular disease risk in some,[25] but not all,[11] analyses. In the case of soy, earlier reports for beneficial effects of cholesterol-lowering effects of soy protein, as well as vascular effects of soy isoflavones, have recently been challenged[26] and overall there is no direct evidence for reduced cardiovascular risk.

NUTS. Several large studies have indicated an association of nut consumption with reduced cardiovascular disease risk.[27-29] Women who consumed 5 oz. of nuts per week had a 35 percent lower risk of nonfatal myocardial infarction compared with those eating less than 1 oz. per month,[27] whereas men who consumed nuts twice per week or more had a 47 percent reduction in risk for sudden cardiac death and a 30 percent reduction in total CHD mortality compared with those who rarely or never consumed nuts.[28] As with other complex plant foods, it is difficult to determine which components of nuts may be responsible for these beneficial associations. Nuts are good sources of monounsaturated fatty acids, fiber, minerals, and flavonoids. Walnuts are particularly rich in polyunsaturated fatty acids such as linoleic and alpha-linolenic acid.[28] Almond intake has been found to have beneficial effects on plasma lipoproteins,[29] but comparisons with the effects of other nuts have not been reported.

FISH AND OMEGA-3 FATTY ACIDS. A number of studies have reported that consumption of fish, especially species with a high content of omega-3 fatty acids, confers protection from ischemic heart disease[30] and that this relationship is particularly strong for CHD mortality and sudden cardiac death. A recent analysis of the epidemiological data concluded that intake of small quantities of fish is associated with a 17 percent reduction in CHD mortality risk and a 27 percent reduction in risk for nonfatal myocardial infarction, whereas each additional serving per week is associated with a further reduction of 3.9 percent in CHD mortality but no further reduction in risk for myocardial infarction (Fig. 44-1).[31]

Although fish have a number of important nutritive qualities, their major cardiovascular benefit likely derives from their content of the omega-3 fatty acids, eicosapentaenoic acid (EPA) and docosahexanoic acid (DHA). Increased plasma levels of these fatty acids predicted a considerable reduction in sudden cardiac death,[32] a result consistent with that of a report indicating that intake of 5.5 gm/month of EPA plus DHA (equivalent to one portion of fatty fish per week) was associated with a 50 percent lower incidence of primary cardiac arrest compared with individuals consuming no fish.[33] This effect appears to be related to enrichment of membrane phospholipids with omega-3 fatty acids and a resulting reduction in risk for abnormal cardiac electrical conductivity.[33] Other properties of these fatty acids that may benefit risk for CHD include antiplatelet and antiinflammatory effects, as well as reduction in plasma triglycerides at higher doses.[30] On the basis of these studies, as well as results of intervention trials with omega-3 fatty acids described later, the AHA has recommended consumption of two portions of fish per week,[1] particularly those fish rich in omega-3 fatty acids (e.g., salmon, mackerel, albacore tuna, swordfish, herring, sardines, lake trout). Because these fish (particularly predatory fish such as swordfish and some types of tuna) can contain significant quantities of contaminants including methylmercury, polychlorinated biphenyls, and dioxin, the U.S. Environmental Protection Agency and the U.S. Food and Drug Administration (FDA) have provided guidelines for maximal intakes, an issue of particular concern for children and women of childbearing age. In most cases, however, the recommendation of two portions per week falls within these guidelines.

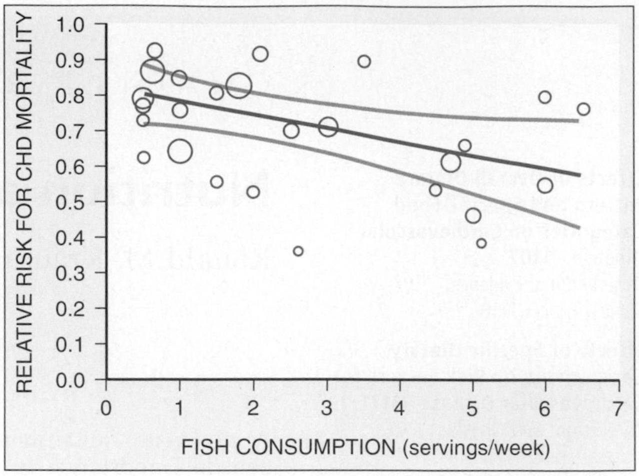

FIGURE 44–1 Regression of coronary heart disease mortality versus fish consumption in the general population. Note that the area of each data point is proportional to its statistical weight. The upper and lower bands denote the confidence interval (95 percent) on mean of the predicted value. CHD = coronary heart disease. *(From Konig A, Bousan C, Cohen JT, et al: A quantitative analysis of fish consumption and coronary heart disease mortality. Am J Prev Med 29:335, 2005.)*

Several clinical trials have supported evidence from epidemiological studies that higher intakes of fish may particularly benefit patients with CHD (Table 44-1).[30] In the Gruppo Italiano per lo Studio della Sopravvivenza nell'Infarto Miocardio (GISSI) secondary prevention trial,[34] a supplement containing a total of 0.85 gm/day of EPA and DHA resulted in reductions of 45 and 30 percent in sudden cardiovascular death. Total mortality and sudden death were reduced after 3 and 4 months of treatment, respectively, consistent with reduction of arrhythmia by the treatment. However, a recent review of 48 randomized clinical trials and 41 cohort studies of omega-3 fatty acid intake did not find evidence for significant cardiovascular benefit.[35]

On the basis of the overall evidence to date, the AHA has recommended that supplemental EPA plus DHA at doses of

TABLE 44–1 Trials of Dietary Interventions and Coronary Events*

Trial	Patients in Intervention Group	Dietary Intervention	Dietary Fat (Energy) in Treatment Group, %	Energy From P and S Fat in Treatment Group, %	Overall Trial Duration, y	Change in Serum Cholesterol Level, %†	Change in CHD, %‡
Low-Fat Approach							
MRC (low fat)	123 male MI patients	Reduce total fat	22	NR	3	−5	+5
DART	1015 male MI patients	Reduce total fat	32	NR	2	−4	−9
WHI	19,541 women	Reduced total fat	29	P = 6; S = 10	8	−1	0
High-Polyunsaturated-Fat Approach							
Finnish Mental Hospital Study	676 men without CHD	Reduce saturated fat, increase polyunsaturated fat	35	P = 13; S = 9	6	−15	−44§
Los Angeles Veteran Study	424 men; most had no evidence of existing CHD	Reduce saturated fat, increase polyunsaturated fat	40	P = 16; S = 9	8	−13§	−20 in CHD, −31§ in cardiovascular events
Oslo Diet-Heart Study	206 male MI patients	Reduce saturated fat, increase polyunsaturated fat	39	P = 21; S = 9	5	−14§	−25§
MRC (soy oil)	199 male MI patients	Reduce saturated fat, increase polyunsaturated fat	46	P:S ratio = 2	4	−15§	−12
Minnesota Coronary Survey	4393 men and 4664 women	Reduce saturated fat, increase polyunsaturated fat	38	P = 15; S = 9	1‖	−14§	0
Increase Omega-3 Fatty Acid							
DART	1015 male MI patients	Fish twice per week or fish oil (1.5 gm/d)	NR	NR	2	NR	−16 on CHD events, −29§ in total mortality
GISSI-Prevenzione	5666 MI patients, primarily men	Fish oil (EPA + DHA, 1 gm/d)	NR	NR	3.5	0	−30§ in cardiovascular death, −45§ in sudden death
Indian Experiment of Infarct Survival 4	242 MI patients, primarily men	Fish oil (EPA,1.08 gm/d) or mustard oil (ALA, 2.9 gm/d)	NR	NR	1	0	−30‡ in fish oil group, −19 in mustard oil group
Whole-Diet Approach							
Lyon Diet Heart Study	302 MI patients, primarily men	High ALA intake and Mediterranean diet	31	P:S ratio = 0.7	3.8	0	−72§
Indian Experiment of Infarct Survival	204 MI patients, primarily men	High intake of fruits, vegetables, nuts, and whole grains	24	P:S ratio = 1.2	1	−9§	−40§

*From Hu FB, Willett WC: Optimal diets for prevention of coronary artery disease: JAMA 288:2569, 2002, and Howard BV, Van Horn L, Hsia J, et al: Low-fat dietary pattern and risk of cardiovascular disease: The Women's Health Initiative Randomized Controlled Dietary Modification Trial. JAMA 295:655, 2006.

†Change in cholesterol level refers to the percentage change in serum cholesterol level in the treatment group compared with the change in the control group.

‡Change in CHD refers to the percentage difference in coronary event rates in the treatment group compared with the control group.

§$p < .05$.

‖The total duration of the study was 4.5 years, but the mean duration of the intervention was only 1 year.

ALA = α-linolenic acid; CHD = coronary heart disease; DART = Diet and Reinfarction Trial; DHA = docosahexaenoic acid; EPA = eicosapentaenoic acid; GISSI = Gruppo Italiano per lo Studio della Sopravvivenza nell'Infarto Miocardico; MI = myocardial infarction; NR = not reported; MRC = Medical Research Council; P = polyunsaturated fat; S, saturated fat; WHI = Women's Health Initiative.

up to 1 gm/day may be considered for risk reduction in patients with CHD in consultation with their physician.[30] Supplements also could be a component of the medical management of hypertriglyceridemia, a setting that requires even larger doses (2 to 4 gm/day). The availability of high-quality omega-3 fatty acid supplements, free of contaminants, is an important prerequisite to their use.

Accumulating epidemiological evidence indicates that alpha-linolenic acid, an omega-3 fatty acid precursor of longer chain EPA and DHA that is found in flaxseed, chia, and a variety of vegetable and nut oils, reduces risk for cardiovascular disease,[36-38] although as with fish oils, the strongest evidence is for reduced cardiovascular mortality,[39] specifically sudden cardiac death,[40] suggesting the primary importance of antiarrhythmic effects. Although there are no clinical trials of alpha-linolenic acid under way, the results of the Lyon Diet Heart Study described later agree with a cardiovascular benefit of supplementing the diet with this fatty acid.

ALCOHOL. Moderate alcohol consumption (one to three alcoholic beverages per day) is strongly and consistently associated with lower risk for CHD than either abstention or higher intakes.[41] Some data have suggested that wine, particularly red varieties, confers particular benefit, possibly due to its content of polyphenols such as resveratrol, which may have direct benefits on vascular reactivity, thrombosis, and oxidative stress.[42] However, most studies have not documented such a differential benefit of red versus white wine, and it appears likely that the major benefit of alcohol consumption is related to an increase in high-density lipoprotein (HDL) cholesterol and perhaps to other effects such as reduced fibrinogen, platelet aggregation, and inflammation.[41-45] Men who consumed alcohol three or four times per week reportedly had a 37 percent reduction in risk for myocardial infarction compared with men who drank less than once per week, and the risk reduction was no greater with more frequent consumption.[46] Current recommendations from the AHA[1] and the U.S. Dietary Guidelines Advisory Committee are that men who drink alcohol may consume up to two alcoholic beverages per day, and women no more than one per day, in part because of alcohol-related breast cancer risk. Because of the potential hazards associated with habituation to alcohol, the potential for adverse effects such as hepatotoxicity and aggravation of hypertriglyceridemia, and the favorable benefit/risk ratio of other dietary practices and therapeutic interventions, individuals should not begin to consume alcohol as a means of reducing coronary disease risk.

Clinical Trials (see Table 44-1)

Relatively few clinical trials have examined the effects of overall dietary patterns or specific food categories on cardiovascular disease endpoints. Early randomized trials (Wadsworth Veterans Affairs Hospital, Oslo Diet-Heart, Finnish Mental Hospital Study) tested the effectiveness of cholesterol-lowering diets enriched in polyunsaturated fatty acids.[47] These trials showed a 25 to 50 percent reduction in cardiovascular disease endpoints over 5 to 12 years in conjunction with a 13 to 15 percent reduction in blood cholesterol levels. Notably, these diets were not low in total fat (30 to 40 percent of calories).

More recently, the Lyon Diet Heart Study tested the effects of a Mediterranean-style diet in 423 patients with documented coronary artery disease who were followed for a mean of 3.8 years.[48] Compared with the control diet, the experimental diet had increased amounts of fruits, vegetables, legumes, and fiber and reductions of meats, butter, and cream (but not cheese). In addition, the diet contained a margarine enriched in alpha-linolenic acid, an omega-3 fatty acid precursor of the longer chain EPA plus DHA found in fatty fish. Total fat was approximately 31 percent in both diets. Despite lower content of dietary saturated fat, there were no differences in plasma lipids, lipoproteins, or other major risk factors between the two diets. However, significant reductions occurred in all outcome measures including all-cause mortality (56 percent), cardiac mortality (65 percent), and nonfatal myocardial infarction (70 percent) (Fig. 44-2).[48] Although many components of the dietary program may have contributed to these results, as discussed earlier, the authors suggested a particularly important role for increased omega-3 fatty acid intake.

The largest long-term randomized dietary intervention trial to date, the Women's Health Initiative (WHI) Randomized Controlled Dietary Modification Trial,[49] was designed to test the hypothesis that a diet low in fat and high in fruit, vegetable, and grain consumption would lead to a reduction of cardiovascular disease events. Nearly 50,000 postmenopausal women were randomized to an intervention group receiving regularly scheduled individualized dietary consultations or to a comparison group receiving diet-related education materials only. Despite achieving a reduction in total fat intake between the intervention and control groups (28.8 percent versus 37 percent of calories ($p < 0.001$), respectively), no significant effects of the intervention on CHD, stroke, or CVD were observed during the 8-year follow-up. The authors suggested that the lack of benefit on CVD endpoints might have been related to the minimal changes in LDL cholesterol observed due to the counterbalancing effects of saturated fat and polyunsaturated fats. Nevertheless, the results of WHI support the increasingly accepted concept that modulation of total dietary fat intake within the range consumed in the general population does not alter CVD risk.

The effects of a much more extreme low-fat diet in the context of an intensive life-style intervention were evaluated in the Life-Style Heart Trial[50] and a more recent multicenter extension of this program.[51] The regimen includes a vegetarian diet with 10 percent total fat, as well as aerobic exercise training, stress management, smoking cessation, and psychosocial support. In the Life-Style Heart Trial, 48 men with coronary artery disease were allocated to intervention and control groups, and 35 completed a 5-year follow-up. In the experimental group, the average percent diameter stenosis at baseline decreased 1.75 absolute percentage points after 1 year (a 4.5 percent relative improvement) and by 3.1 absolute percentage points after 5 years (a 7.9 percent relative improvement). In contrast, the average percent diameter stenosis in the control group increased by 2.3 percentage points after 1 year (a 5.4 percent relative worsening) and by 11.8 percentage points after 5 years (a 27.7 percent relative worsening) ($p = 0.001$ between groups).

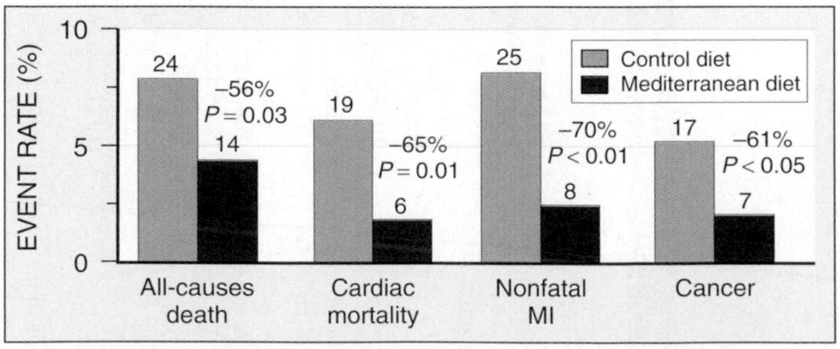

FIGURE 44–2 The effect of a Mediterranean diet on total mortality, coronary disease events, and cancer in men after acute myocardial infarction based on the Lyon Heart Study. *(From Sacks FM, Katan M: Randomized clinical trials on the effects of dietary fat and carbohydrate on plasma lipoproteins and cardiovascular disease. Am J Med 113:13S, 2002.)*

Twenty-five cardiac events occurred in 28 experimental group patients versus 45 events in 20 control group patients during the 5-year follow-up (risk ratio for any event for the control group, 2.47 [95 percent confidence interval, 1.48 to 4.20]). Among major cardiovascular risk factors, the intervention program versus control resulted in a significant 40 percent versus 1 percent reduction of low-density lipoprotein (LDL) cholesterol and a 17 percent versus 4 percent reduction in body weight, with no significant changes in HDL, cholesterol, triglyceride, or blood pressure. Thus this approach offers an effective means of coronary disease risk reduction, although the magnitude of the contribution of the low-fat diet per se, in the context of the overall program and in comparison with more moderate dietary regimens, has not been established.

EFFECTS OF SPECIFIC DIETARY COMPONENTS ON RISK FACTORS FOR CARDIOVASCULAR DISEASE

The effects of dietary patterns and specific food categories on cardiovascular disease risk may operate in part through their effects on risk factors. The major diet-related risk factors are obesity, plasma lipids and lipoproteins, and blood pressure. Other factors for which dietary benefits are less well established include homocysteine, inflammation, and oxidative stress. Other than antiplatelet effects of omega-3 fatty acids, there is little indication of dietary effects on thrombosis.

Overweight and Obesity

Overweight and obesity, defined respectively as body mass index higher than 25 and more than 30 kg/m^2, respectively,[4] are progressively increasing in prevalence in the United States and globally. These conditions are associated with numerous comorbidities affecting cardiovascular disease risk, notably dyslipidemia, hypertension, diabetes, and metabolic syndrome. The underlying guidelines for prevention and treatment of excess body target both diet and physical activity:[52]

1. Match intake of energy (calories) to overall energy needs; limit consumption of foods with a high-caloric density and/or low nutritional quality including those with a high content of sugars.
2. Maintain a level of physical activity that achieves fitness and balances energy expenditure with energy intake; for weight reduction, expenditure should exceed intake (see also Chaps. 46 and 78).

These principles, which agree with those of the NHLBI,[4] recognize that weight reduction requires achieving a negative energy balance. In this regard, carefully controlled metabolic studies have established that at a given level of physical activity, reduced energy intake will result in weight loss irrespective of the macronutrient (carbohydrate, fat, protein) composition of the diet over a rather wide range. Nonetheless, considerable controversy persists as to whether diets with differing macronutrient composition differ in their effectiveness in achieving short-term or long-term weight loss. A detailed discussion of this controversy exceeds the scope of this chapter, but arguments based on observational data or on intervention programs that incorporate dietary change with increases in physical activity and other behavioral changes do not adequately address the question of diet composition per se as a factor that affects the efficacy of weight loss. In fact, studies of individuals who have achieved long-term weight loss indicate that these individuals employ a number of behavioral changes to control dietary fat intake, have higher levels of physical activity (especially strenuous activity), and maintain a greater frequency of self-weighing.[53]

However, even this information does not help to establish whether alternate dietary strategies, such as very-low-carbohydrate and/or high-protein diets may prove even more effective on the basis of either their metabolic effects or their influence on eating behavior. Only recently have studies specifically tested the efficacy of such dietary approaches.[54-57] Results to date suggest that at least over periods up to 6 months, average weight loss is higher for diets with very-low-carbohydrate content (e.g., <35 gm/day) than with diets containing more conventional amounts of carbohydrate that are restricted in total fat (Table 44-2).[58] Possible explanations for this finding include the restricted

TABLE 44–2 Comparison of Low-Carbohydrate and Reduced-Fat Diets

Variable	Low-Carbohydrate Diet*	Reduced-Fat Diet†
Caloric restriction	Not necessary; ketosis may help reduce intake	Necessary
Food choices	Highly restricted	Moderately restricted
Initial rate of weight loss	Rapid, with increased diuresis	Gradual, with some diuresis
Weight loss	Dependent on duration	Dependent on duration
Weight maintenance	Unproven over the long term	Unproven over the long term
Cholesterol		
LDL	No change	Decrease
HDL	Greater increase	Increase
Triglycerides	Greater decrease	Decrease
Potential long-term concerns	Calciuria (renal stones and decreased bone mass) Relatively high-protein content (patients with renal or hepatic disease) Atherogenicity (high saturated fat, trans fat, and cholesterol levels and relative absence of fruits, vegetables, and whole grains	None

*A low-carbohydrate diet is defined as one that provides <35 gm of carbohydrate per day. The Atkins diet begins with a stricter limitation (20 gm/day) for at least the first 2 weeks, with a gradual increase of 5 gm/week to achieve a rate of weight loss of approximately 2 lb (0.9 kg) per week until a weight within 5 to 10 lb (2.3 to 4.5 kg) of the goal is achieved. Carbohydrate intake is then further increased by 10 gm/week until weight loss ceases.

†A reduced-fat diet is defined as one in which fat constitutes <30% of the total caloric intake; under certain circumstances (e.g., in some patients with the metabolic syndrome), fat intake of ≤35% of the total caloric intake is recommended.

LDL = low-density lipoprotein; HDL = high-density lipoprotein.

From Bonow RO, Eckel RH: Diet, obesity, and cardiovascular risk. N Engl J Med 348:2057, 2003.

food choices and the possibility that higher dietary content of protein and/or lower content of carbohydrates, especially simple sugars and rapidly digested starches with lower glycemic effects, increase satiety. Nevertheless, evidence for longer-term efficacy of such diets is lacking, a concern heightened by evidence of declining compliance by the end of one year,[55,56,59] an issue that applies to all dietary programs. Differing effects of these diets on body fat or body composition have not been demonstrated. However, questions remain regarding the long-term safety and overall health effects of such diets, particularly because they lack many of the foods associated with maintaining cardiovascular and overall health including fruits, vegetables, and whole grains. Additionally, they are high in saturated and trans fats and cholesterol, although, as described later, the expected effects of these fats on LDL cholesterol levels appear to be attenuated. Another major concern is whether diets with extreme deviations from conventional food choices (i.e., very low in either carbohydrate or fat) can be effectively sustained over the long term (e.g., years). In the case of low-fat diets, this appears possible at least for highly motivated individuals[53] and for population groups such as East Asians, but it remains undetermined for very-low-carbohydrate/high-protein/high-fat diets, regimens for which little long-term population experience exists. Also of specific concern are the long-term consequences of high-protein intake, particularly in the setting of renal disease or diabetes.[60]

Plasma Lipids (see also Chap. 42)

TOTAL AND LDL CHOLESTEROL. Dietary management of LDL cholesterol remains a major goal of coronary artery disease risk management.[2] Although diet-induced lowering of LDL cholesterol has not been firmly proved to reduce coronary disease risk, this conclusion is reasonable on the basis of both the results of dietary trials designed to lower LDL, described earlier, and the relation of drug-induced reductions in LDL cholesterol to decreases in coronary disease morbidity and mortality. Nutritional factors known to increase LDL cholesterol levels include saturated and *trans* fatty acids, dietary cholesterol, and excess body weight. Although total fat intake tends to correlate with that of saturated fat, there is no evidence that LDL levels rise due to increased dietary total fat intake per se. In fact, as mentioned earlier, trials employing high total and unsaturated fat consumption resulted in lower LDL cholesterol and reduced heart disease risk. Moreover, recent studies have indicated that at least over the short term, very-low-carbohydrate diets with high levels of total fat and protein blunt the expected increases in LDL cholesterol expected from high saturated fat intake.[54-57,61]

Substitution of carbohydrates and/or unsaturated fatty acids for saturated and *trans* fatty acids reduces LDL cholesterol. Many studies have assessed the quantitative effects of these dietary changes on LDL and other lipids and lipoproteins, as recently summarized and reviewed (Fig. 44-3).[62,63] When substituted for carbohydrates, the greatest increases in LDL cholesterol result from C12:0 (lauric), C14:0 (myristic), and C16:0 (palmitic) fatty acids found in dairy fat, meat, and tropical oils, with equivalent changes induced by *trans* monounsaturated fatty acids found in baked goods, stick margarine, and fried "fast foods" such as French fries. In contrast, 18 : 0 fatty acid (stearic), which is found in many of the same foods, generally does not raise LDL cholesterol levels. No increases in LDL cholesterol follow intake of monounsaturated fatty acids, principally 18 : 1 (oleic), a major component of olive and canola oils. Polyunsaturated fatty acids of the omega-6 series, principally 18 : 2 (linoleic), found in vegetable and seed oils such as corn, safflower, and sunflower oils lower plasma total and LDL cholesterol via enhanced receptor-dependent clearance of LDL and decreased LDL production. Availability of linoleic acid modulates the cholesterolemic potential of other fatty acids, such that saturated and *trans* fats exert a more exaggerated effect on LDL cholesterol when linoleic acid concentrations fall below a threshold value (<3 percent of energy).[37]

Recent guidelines from the American Heart Association recommend consumption of less than 7 percent of calories as saturated fat and further limitation for those with a level of LDL cholesterol higher than that recommended for their overall risk status.[1] For *trans* fatty acids, it is recommended that intake be reduced to a minimum, a goal that will be aided by inclusion of *trans* fatty acid content on food labels.

With the exception of egg yolk and shellfish, dietary cholesterol is found in foods of animal origin that are also high in saturated fat. On average, an increase of 100 mg/day of dietary cholesterol increases total serum cholesterol about 2 to 3 mg/dl, of which approximately 70 percent is in the LDL fraction.[63] This effect of added cholesterol varies considerably among individuals and is attenuated at higher cholesterol intakes. The LDL cholesterol increase would predict approximately a 1 to 2 percent increase in CHD risk, possibly offsetting the effects of concomitantly increased HDL cholesterol. An effect of this magnitude is difficult to detect in epidemiological data and may contribute to the reported lack of association of egg yolk intake with coronary disease risk for amounts up to one or more eggs (≈215 mg cholesterol) per day, except in patients with diabetes. On the basis of available data, as well as the infeasibility of consuming diets with markedly restricted cholesterol content, current guidelines[1,2] recommend limiting intake to less than 300 mg/day for the general population and less than 200 mg/day for individuals at increased

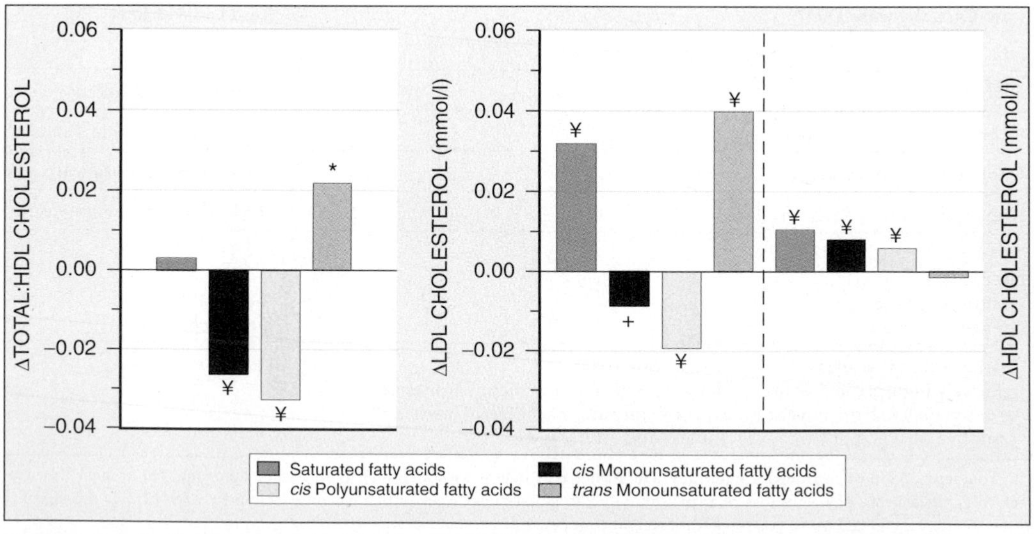

FIGURE 44–3 Predicted changes (Δ) in the ratio of serum total to HDL cholesterol and in LDL- and HDL-cholesterol concentrations when carbohydrates constituting 1 percent of energy are replaced isoenergetically with saturated, *cis* monosaturated, *cis* polyunsaturated, or *trans* monounsaturated fatty acids. *$p < 0.05$; +$p < 0.01$; ¥$p < 0.001$. *(From Mensink RP, Zock PL, Kester AD, Katan MB: Effects of dietary fatty acids and carbohydrates on the ratio of serum total to HDL cholesterol and on serum lipids and apolipoproteins: A meta-analysis of 60 controlled trials. Am J Clin Nutr 77:1146, 2003.)*

risk for heart disease by National Cholesterol Education Program criteria.

Although there is wide interindividual variation in response to these changes,[64] the reductions in LDL cholesterol that may be expected with adoption of diets low in saturated fat and cholesterol are generally in the range of 5 to 10 percent. Near-maximal response of LDL cholesterol to dietary change occurs as early as 3 to 4 weeks, and thereafter it can be determined whether additional therapeutic measures will be required to achieve the desired LDL cholesterol target.

Some epidemiological analyses have shown positive independent associations of saturated fat intake with CHD risk, but the relationships have been relatively weak and inconsistent.[65] This likely reflects several factors including the relatively small average effects of saturated fat on LDL cholesterol and the possible offsetting increases in HDL cholesterol as described later. On the other hand, *trans* fatty acid intake appears to have a stronger relationship with CHD risk,[65] perhaps reflecting the finding that HDL cholesterol levels are not increased by *trans* fat or perhaps the existence of other adverse effects of these fatty acids on disease mechanisms.

The recent OmniHeart trial showed that substitution of either protein or monounsaturated fat for carbohydrate without change in body weight reduced LDL cholesterol, as well as triglyceride.[66] This result agrees with other recent evidence for the benefits on LDL and other components of the lipoprotein profile of substituting protein and/or fat for carbohydrate in the diet.[61,67]

Other nutritional measures that can reduce LDL cholesterol include weight loss, which may be particularly effective on a higher carbohydrate diet,[61] and addition of plant sterol and stanol esters[68,69]; viscous fiber (in particular, beta-glucan, a component of oat fiber)[70]; and nuts.[29] LDL cholesterol has been found to fall by a mean of 28 percent on a diet that combines diet components in amounts (per 1000 kcal) that have been reported to be beneficial individually: plant sterols 1 gm, soy protein 21.4 gm, viscous fibers 9.8 gm, and almonds 14 gm.[71] This reduction was comparable to that achieved by lovastatin 20 mg/day (30.9 percent) and significantly greater than with a diet low in saturated fat (4.5 percent of energy) and cholesterol (8 percent LDL cholesterol reduction).

HDL CHOLESTEROL. Although HDL cholesterol correlates inversely and independently with risk for coronary artery disease, it remains uncertain whether changes in HDL cholesterol, and in particular those induced by diet, predict changes in risk. There are two general categories of nutritional effect on HDL: those due to changes in dietary fatty acid composition and those due to factors that also affect plasma triglyceride levels, as described in the next section. Because dietary fatty acids have major effects on LDL and HDL cholesterol, it is necessary to examine these effects jointly to assess the potential impact of HDL change on coronary disease risk. The ratio of LDL or total cholesterol to HDL cholesterol permits assessment of these joint effects. A review of 60 dietary trials has indicated that the plasma cholesterol–to–HDL cholesterol ratio did not change if saturated fatty acids replaced an isocaloric amount of dietary carbohydrates. However, this ratio decreased if *cis* unsaturated fatty acids replaced saturated fatty acids (see Fig. 44-3).[62] The effect on total HDL-to-cholesterol ratio of replacing *trans* fatty acids with a mix of carbohydrates and *cis* unsaturated fatty acids was almost twice as large as that of replacing saturated fatty acids. Lauric acid greatly increased total cholesterol, but much of its effect was on HDL cholesterol, resulting in a lower ratio of total : HDL cholesterol for oils rich in lauric acid, such as coconut oil. As discussed earlier, the tandem effects of dietary saturated fatty acids, as well as dietary cholesterol on total and HDL cholesterol, may contribute to the relatively weak relationship of these nutrients to CHD risk.

TRIGLYCERIDE AND THE ATHEROGENIC DYSLIPIDEMIA OF OBESITY, DIABETES, AND THE METABOLIC SYNDROME. Elevated plasma triglyceride independently but rather weakly predicts CHD risk. Its principal cardiovascular significance is as a component of, and a marker for, the atherogenic dyslipidemia commonly found in patients with excess adiposity, the metabolic syndrome, and type II diabetes mellitus (see Chaps. 43 and 60). The triad of lipid abnormalities in these conditions consists of elevated plasma triglyceride (>150 mg/dl); reduced HDL cholesterol; and a relative excess of small, dense LDL particles with total LDL cholesterol levels that are generally average.[72] Adiposity itself is the principal nutritionally related influence on atherogenic dyslipidemia. Among nutrients, the major determinant of this dyslipidemic triad is carbohydrate.[73] In general, simple sugars and rapidly hydrolyzed starches have a greater glyceridemic effect than more complex carbohydrates and those consumed in conjunction with higher intake of fiber. The glyceridemic effects of carbohydrates tend to correlate with their glycemic effects.[22] Dietary carbohydrate-induced increases in plasma triglyceride are often accompanied by decreases in HDL cholesterol and increases in levels of small, dense LDL particles.[74] Correspondingly, carbohydrate limitation improves components of the dyslipidemic triad.[54-57,61] Although no direct evidence links these diet-induced changes directly to CHD risk, dietary glycemic load, a measure of the quantity of high glycemic foods related to high plasma triglyceride and low HDL cholesterol, strongly and independently predicts CHD risk.[21] Hence patients with this form of dyslipidemia should restrict consumption of sugars and high glycemic/glyceridemic carbohydrates.

Blood Pressure

Current recommendations for nonpharmacological management of elevated blood pressure include weight reduction, moderation in alcohol consumption, limitation of sodium intake, and increased intake of certain other minerals (see Chap. 41).[1,3,75] Another important therapeutic modality for reducing blood pressure is the DASH combination diet.[14,15] Taken together, the evidence supporting these recommendations described later reinforces the roles of multiple components of an overall dietary pattern in promoting cardiovascular and general health.

BODY WEIGHT. Numerous clinical trials reviewed elsewhere[1,3] have documented a substantial and significant relation between change in weight and change in blood pressure. It has been estimated that a reduction of more than 1 mm Hg in systolic and diastolic blood pressure may occur for each kilogram of weight loss.

DIETARY SODIUM. Numerous observational studies and clinical trials have demonstrated that a high intake of sodium can result in an increase in blood pressure.[76] Meta-analyses of randomized trials have shown that on average, reducing sodium intake by about 80 mmol (1.8 gm)/day yields systolic and diastolic blood pressure reductions of about 4 and 2 mm Hg in hypertensive patients and smaller reductions in normotensive subjects.[77] Although the blood pressure response to change in salt intake varies among individuals, in part because of genetic factors and other variables such as age, classification of individuals as "responders" or "nonresponders" can be difficult.[78]

The Trials of Hypertension Prevention documented that sodium reduction, alone or combined with weight loss, can lower the incidence of hypertension by about 20 percent.[79] In the Trials of Nonpharmacologic Interventions in the Elderly, a reduced salt intake with or without weight loss significantly reduced blood pressure and the need for antihypertensive medication in older persons.[80] In both trials the dietary interventions reduced total sodium intake to about 100 mmol/day. Although the DASH-sodium trial has shown that lowering sodium intake to 50 mmol/day can achieve further blood pressure reduction (see later), such a limitation is extremely difficult to implement because of the high sodium content of many prepared foods. Overall, the available data support the current AHA population guideline of limiting salt intake to 6 gm/day, the equivalent of

100 mmol of sodium (2400 mg) per day.[1,75] Careful selection of foods and limitation of added salt can substantially lower sodium intake, and these measures can have particular benefit in hypertensive patients.

ALCOHOL. Observational data have consistently demonstrated a relationship between heavy drinking (three or more standard drinks per day) and higher blood pressure.[81] Clinical trials of reducing alcohol consumption have yielded less conclusive findings. As stated previously, the totality of the evidence supports a recommendation to limit alcohol intake to no more than two drinks per day for men and one drink per day for women.

POTASSIUM, MAGNESIUM, AND CALCIUM INTAKE. As reviewed elsewhere,[76,82] observational data have provided evidence that increased intakes of these minerals are associated with lower blood pressure. Clinical trials have also documented a beneficial impact of potassium supplements on blood pressure, but the evidence for calcium and magnesium is less consistent.[76,82] A meta-analysis of randomized trials of the effects of potassium supplementation[83] found that, on average, supplementation of diets with 60 to 120 mmol/day reduced systolic and diastolic blood pressure by 4.4 and 2.5 mm Hg in hypertensive patients and by 1.8 and 1 mm Hg in normotensive subjects. Because a high dietary intake of potassium, magnesium, and calcium can be achieved from food sources and because diets rich in these minerals provide a variety of other nutrients, the preferred strategy for increasing mineral intake is through foods rather than supplements.

DIETARY PATTERN. The DASH study[14,84] found that a diet rich in fruits and vegetables (five to nine servings per day) and low-fat dairy products (two to four servings a day), along with reduced saturated and total fat content, reduced systolic and diastolic blood pressure by 5.5 and 3 mm Hg more than did a control diet of equal sodium content that produced no differences in sodium or body weight. As with other interventions, reductions were substantially greater in hypertensive than normotensive subjects, and reductions were larger in black than nonblack subjects. In a second trial in the DASH-sodium study, progressive sodium restriction in the DASH diet (from a daily intake of 150 to 100 mmol and 50 mmol) further reduced blood pressure, such that the DASH diet with the lowest sodium intake led to a mean systolic blood pressure that was 7.1 mm Hg lower in participants without hypertension and 11.5 mm Hg lower in participants with hypertension.[15,85] However, particularly among normotensive and nonblack subjects, most of the blood pressure reduction could be accounted for by the DASH diet rather than additional sodium restriction.

Due to the multifactorial dietary intervention of DASH, its mechanisms of effectiveness cannot be determined. However, the diet was rich in potassium, calcium, and magnesium, and hence the findings are consistent with the possibility that these elements contributed to the observed reductions in blood pressure. A similar conclusion may be drawn from the Vanguard study, a trial that used a dietary regimen based on prepackaged foods.[86]

Prospective observational studies also have supported the influence of overall dietary pattern on blood pressure. In the CARDIA study, 4304 young adults were followed for more than 15 years in a multicenter, population-based, prospective study of CVD risk evolution.[87] Diets rich in whole grains, refined grains, fruits, vegetables, and nuts or legumes were found to be inversely related to blood pressure while positive effects of red and processed meat intake on blood pressure were observed. In a cohort of approximately 1700 persons followed over 7 years, individuals consuming 14 to 42 servings of fruit or vegetables per month had a smaller average increase in blood pressure than those with lower intakes.[88]

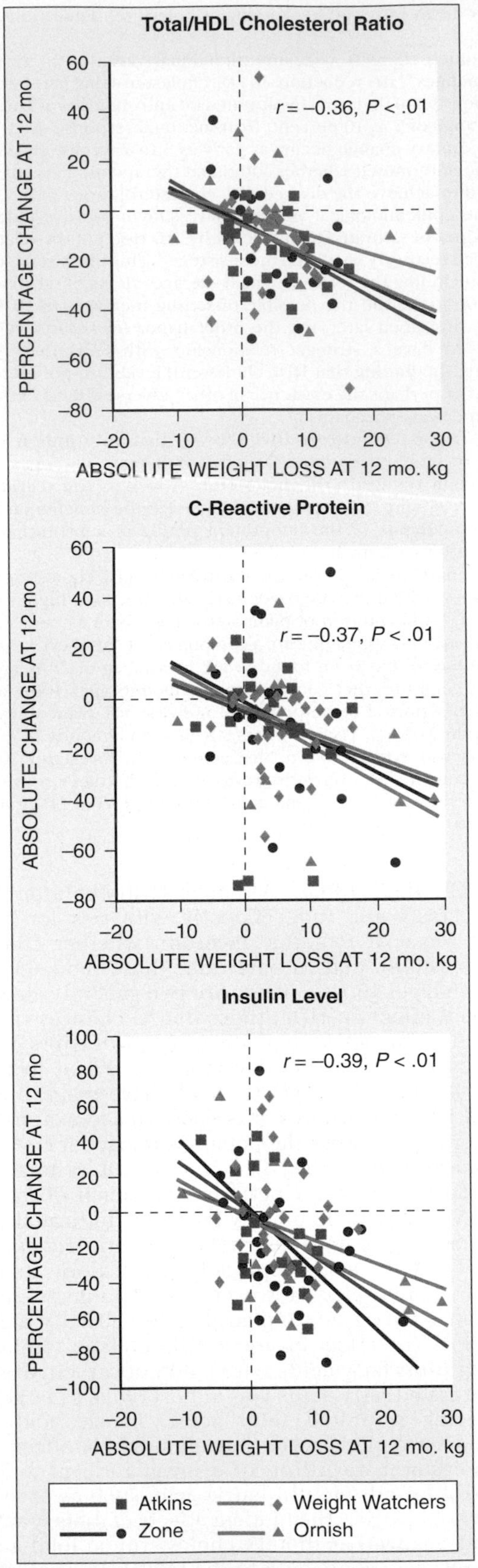

FIGURE 44–4 One-year changes in total/HDL cholesterol ratio, C-reactive protein, and insulin as a function of weight loss. In cases of missing data, baseline values were carried forward. HDL = high-density lipoprotein. The curves in each plot indicate linear regression functions for each diet group. Difference among diet groups: $p = 0.48$ for total/HDL cholesterol ratio; $p = 0.57$ for C-reactive protein; and $p = 0.31$ for insulin level. *(From Dansinger ML, Gleason JA, Griffith JL, et al: Comparison of the Atkins, Ornish, Weight Watchers, and Zone diets for weight loss and heart disease risk reduction: A randomized trial. JAMA 293:43, 2005.)*

OTHER DIETARY EFFECTS ON BLOOD PRESSURE. Limited observational data suggest beneficial effects of additional dietary components on blood pressure. These include fish; alpha-linolenic acid[89]; whole grains (in particular, oats)[90]; and protein (in particular, soy and total vegetable protein).[90-93] The suggestion that soy isoflavone content may contribute to this benefit agrees with a recent report that polyphenols in dark chocolate can also promote blood pressure reduction.[94] Substitution of either protein or monounsaturated fat for carbohydrate substantially decreases blood pressure in prehypertensive and stage 1 hypertensive subjects.[71] Although the role of individual nutrients in lowering blood pressure in this study cannot be ascertained, the results raise the possibility that reduced carbohydrate intake may be a factor.

Other Cardiovascular Risk Factors Related to Diet (see also Chap. 39)

HOMOCYSTEINE. Recent meta-analyses have concluded that elevated plasma homocysteine levels modestly increase the risk for ischemic heart disease and stroke.[95,96] Folic acid, as well as pyridoxine and cyanocobalamin (vitamins B_6 and B_{12}), are the major dietary components influencing plasma homocysteine levels.[97]

Three recent large intervention trials using combinations of folic acid, vitamin B_6, and vitamin B_{12} to lower homocysteine levels found no differences in cardiovascular disease endpoints after 2 to 5 years of follow-up.[98-100] Though marginal trends toward fewer strokes in the vitamin supplementation group were observed in two of the studies,[99,100] there was a nearly significant trend toward more myocardial infarction in the vitamin group in one, the HOPE 2 study.[99]

The lack of efficacy of vitamin supplementation in reducing cardiovascular disease risk through reduction of homocysteine levels speaks to the complexity of the relationship between plasma homocysteine levels and disease risk. For example, elevated plasma homocysteine might mark other pathological factors. In light of these recent clinical trials, recommendations regarding use of folic acid and multivitamin supplements in the prevention of cardiovascular disease are unwarranted.[101]

DIETARY INFLUENCES ON C-REACTIVE PROTEIN. As reviewed recently,[45] a number of nutritional factors influence C-reactive protein (CRP), a well-established coronary artery disease risk factor (see Chap. 39).[102] Chief among these is adiposity.[103] Weight loss is the most effective nutritional intervention for reducing CRP levels.[59,104,105] Indeed, weight loss, when achieved by a variety of specific diets, reduces CRP in parallel with total/HDL cholesterol and insulin levels (Fig. 44-4). CRP associates positively with glycemic load[106] and inversely with intake of alcohol[44] and arginine,[107] but prospective clinical studies of these effects have not been reported. Higher glycemic loads associate with elevated levels of CRP in both normal and overweight women. The "portfolio" diet containing multiple supplements that lowered plasma LDL cholesterol also lowered CRP to a level similar to that obtained with low-dose statin therapy.[71]

ANTIOXIDANT VITAMINS (see also Chap. 45). Despite evidence supporting the role of oxidative stress in atherogenesis and observational data relating antioxidant intake to reduced risk of cardiovascular disease, clinical trials have for the most part shown no benefit.[101,108] A meta-analysis of 15 randomized clinical trials of vitamin E or beta-carotene supplementation ($n = 81{,}788$ and 138,113 persons, respectively) showed no effects of vitamin E supplementation on CVD endpoints and a small but significant increase in total mortality, as well as mortality from CVD in patients receiving beta-carotene supplements (Fig. 44-5).[108] Recently, in the Women's Health Study, supplementation with 600 IU of vitamin E on alternate days also showed no effect on

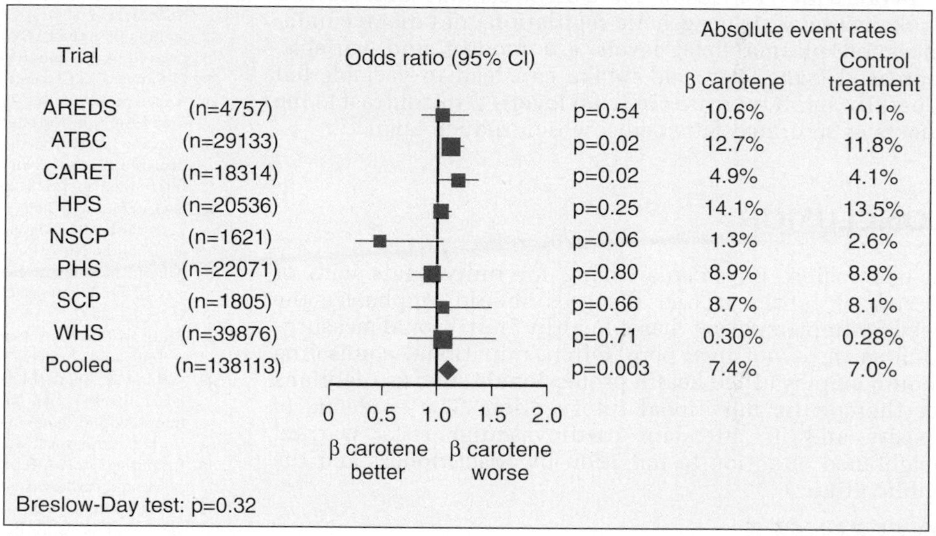

A

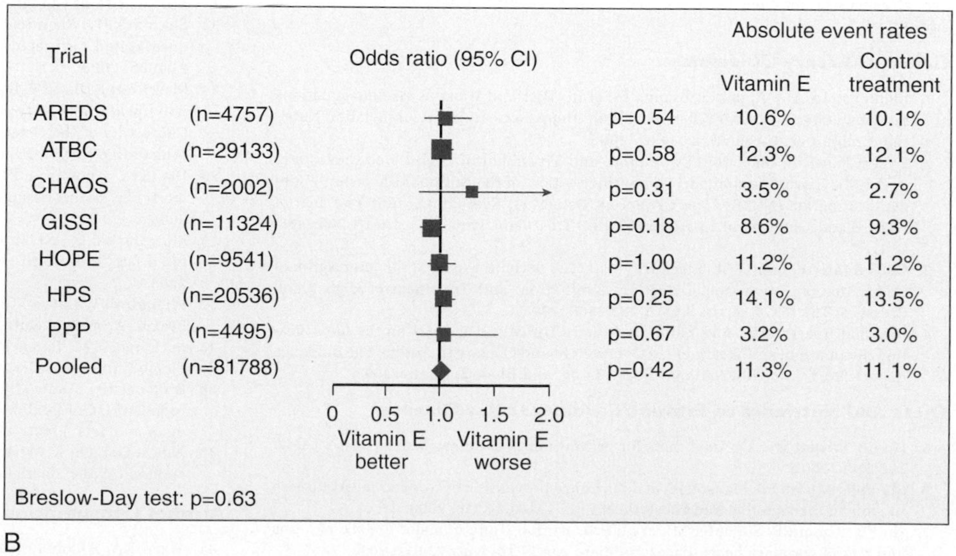

B

FIGURE 44–5 A, Odds ratios (95 percent confidence interval [CI]) of all-cause mortality for individuals treated with beta carotene or control therapy. **B,** Odds ratios (95 percent CI) of all-cause mortality for individuals treated with vitamin E or control therapy. *(From Vivekananthan DP, Penn MS, Sapp SK, et al: Use of antioxidant vitamins for the prevention of cardiovascular disease: Meta-analysis of randomized trials. Lancet 361:2017, 2003.)*

 major CVD events or total mortality, though CVD mortality was significantly lower.[109] The randomized, placebo-controlled Heart Protection Study trial of 20,536 high-risk individuals showed no benefit with a supplement of 600 mg of vitamin E, 250 mg of vitamin C, and 20 mg of beta carotene daily.[110] In a smaller study, the cardiovascular protective effects of statin plus niacin therapy in patients with coronary artery disease were attenuated by coadministration of a mixture of antioxidants that also resulted in reductions of large HDL particles.[111] More recently, treatment with vitamins C and E in conjunction with intense atorvastatin treatment showed no additional benefit on CVD health.[112] Finally, in a study of the effects of hormone and antioxidant therapy in post-menopausal women, antioxidant therapy did not improve coronary angiographic change[113] or vasodilator function.[114] It is possible that the observational studies reflect confounding effects of other dietary or lifestyle practices that correlate with antioxidant consumption either in foods or supplements or that longer-term consumption is necessary to achieve benefits. However, given the available data, no recommendation can be made at this time for the use of antioxidant supplements to reduce cardiovascular disease risk.

LP(a). This risk factor for cardiovascular disease and stroke is under strong genetic regulation, and dietary influences on plasma Lp(a) levels are modest and variable. Increased *trans* fatty acid intake can lead to variable but generally small increases in Lp(a) levels,[115] in contrast to the effects of saturated fatty acids, which reduce Lp(a).[116]

CONCLUSION

In conclusion, physicians caring for individuals with or at risk of cardiovascular diseases should emphasize the need for implementing "heart-healthy" nutritional measures such as those outlined here. Often, nutritional counseling should employ allied health professionals such as dietitians for therapeutic nutritional intervention. The epidemic of obesity and its attendant cardiovascular risks warrant heightened attention to nutrition by practitioners and the public alike.

REFERENCES

For references to the older literature, see Chap. 41 in *Braunwald's Heart Disease*, 7th edition.

General Dietary Guidelines

1. Lichtenstein AH, Appel LJ, Brands M, et al: Diet and lifestyle recommendations revision 2006. A scientific statement from the American Heart Association Nutrition Committee. Circulation 114:82, 2006.
2. Expert Panel on Detection, Evaluation, and Treatment of High Blood Cholesterol in Adults: Executive summary of the third report of the National Cholesterol Education Program (NCEP) Expert Panel on Detection, Evaluation, and Treatment of High Blood Cholesterol in Adults (Adult Treatment Panel III). JAMA 285:2486, 2001.
3. Chobanian AV, Bakris GL, Black HR, et al: The seventh report of the Joint National Committee on Prevention, Detection, Evaluation, and Treatment of High Blood Pressure: The JNC 7 report. JAMA 289:2560, 2003.
4. National Heart, Lung, and Blood Institute: Clinical Guidelines on the Identification, Evaluation, and Treatment of Overweight and Obesity in Adults: The Evidence Report. Rockville, Md, National Heart, Lung, and Blood Institute, 1998.

Diets and Nutrients to Prevent Cardiovascular Disease

5. Hu FB, Willett WC: Optimal diets for prevention of coronary heart disease. JAMA 288:2569, 2002.
6. Stampfer MJ, Hu FB, Manson JE, et al: Primary prevention of coronary heart disease in women through diet and lifestyle. N Engl J Med 343:16, 2000.
7. Hu FB, Rimm EB, Stampfer MJ, et al: Prospective study of major dietary patterns and risk of coronary heart disease in men. Am J Clin Nutr 72:912, 2000.
8. Trichopoulou A, Costacou T, Bamia C, Trichopoulos D: Adherence to a Mediterranean diet and survival in a Greek population. N Engl J Med 348:2599, 2003.
9. Barzi F, Woodward M, Marfisi RM, et al: Mediterranean diet and all-causes mortality after myocardial infarction: Results from the GISSI-Prevenzione trial. Eur J Clin Nutr 57:604, 2003.
10. Bazzano LA, He J, Ogden LG, et al: Fruit and vegetable intake and risk of cardiovascular disease in U.S. adults: The First National Health and Nutrition Examination Survey Epidemiologic Follow-up Study. Am J Clin Nutr 76:93, 2002.
11. Joshipura KJ, Hu FB, Manson JE, et al: The effect of fruit and vegetable intake on risk for coronary heart disease. Ann Intern Med 134:1106, 2001.
12. Liu S, Lee IM, Ajani U, et al: Intake of vegetables rich in carotenoids and risk of coronary heart disease in men: The Physicians' Health Study. Int J Epidemiol 30:130, 2001.
13. Liu S, Manson JE, Lee IM, et al: Fruit and vegetable intake and risk of cardiovascular disease: The Women's Health Study. Am J Clin Nutr 72:922, 2000.
14. Appel LJ, Moore TJ, Obarzanek E, et al: A clinical trial of the effects of dietary patterns on blood pressure. DASH Collaborative Research Group. N Engl J Med 336:1117, 1997.
15. Sacks FM, Svetkey LP, Vollmer WM, et al: Effects on blood pressure of reduced dietary sodium and the Dietary Approaches to Stop Hypertension (DASH) diet. DASH-Sodium Collaborative Research Group. N Engl J Med 344:3, 2001.
16. Liu S, Stampfer MJ, Hu FB, et al: Whole-grain consumption and risk of coronary heart disease: Results from the Nurses' Health Study. Am J Clin Nutr 70:412, 1999.
17. Flight I, Clifton P: Cereal grains and legumes in the prevention of coronary heart disease and stroke: A review of the literature. Eur J Clin Nutr 60:1145, 2006.
18. Bazzano LA, He J, Ogden LG, et al: Dietary fiber intake and reduced risk of coronary heart disease in U.S. men and women: The National Health and Nutrition Examination Survey I Epidemiologic Follow-up Study. Arch Intern Med 163:1897, 2003.
19. Pereira MA, O'Reilly E, Augustsson K, et al: Dietary fiber and risk of coronary heart disease: A pooled analysis of cohort studies. Arch Intern Med 164:370, 2004.
20. Liu S, Buring JE, Sesso HD, et al: A prospective study of dietary fiber intake and risk of cardiovascular disease among women. J Am Coll Cardiol 39:49, 2002.
21. Liu S, Willett WC, Stampfer MJ, et al: A prospective study of dietary glycemic load, carbohydrate intake, and risk of coronary heart disease in U.S. women. Am J Clin Nutr 71:1455, 2000.
22. Jenkins DJ, Kendall CW, Augustin LS, et al: Glycemic index: Overview of implications in health and disease. Am J Clin Nutr 76:266S, 2002.
23. Pi-Sunyer FX: Glycemic index and disease. Am J Clin Nutr 76:290S, 2002.
24. Anderson JW, Hanna TJ, Peng X, Kryscio RJ: Whole-grain foods and heart disease risk. J Am Coll Nutr 19:291S, 2000.
25. Bazzano LA, He J, Ogden LG, et al: Legume consumption and risk of coronary heart disease in U.S. men and women: NHANES I Epidemiologic Follow-up Study. Arch Intern Med 161:2573, 2001.
26. Sacks FM, Lichtenstein A, Van Horn L, et al: Soy protein, isoflavones, and cardiovascular health: An American Heart Association Science Advisory for professionals from the Nutrition Committee. Circulation 113:1034, 2006.
27. Albert CM, Gaziano JM, Willett WC, Manson JE: Nut consumption and decreased risk of sudden cardiac death in the Physicians' Health Study. Arch Intern Med 162:1382, 2002.
28. Feldman EB: The scientific evidence for a beneficial health relationship between walnuts and coronary heart disease. J Nutr 132:1062S, 2002.
29. Jenkins DJ, Kendall CW, Marchie A, et al: Dose response of almonds on coronary heart disease risk factors: Blood lipids, oxidized low-density lipoproteins, lipoprotein(a), homocysteine, and pulmonary nitric oxide: A randomized, controlled, crossover trial. Circulation 106:1327, 2002.
30. Kris-Etherton PM, Harris WS, Appel LJ: Fish consumption, fish oil, omega-3 fatty acids, and cardiovascular disease. Circulation 106:2747, 2002.
31. Konig A, Bouzan C, Cohen JT, et al: A quantitative analysis of fish consumption and coronary heart disease mortality. Am J Prev Med 29:335, 2005.
32. Albert CM, Campos H, Stampfer MJ, et al: Blood levels of long-chain n-3 fatty acids and the risk of sudden death. N Engl J Med 346:1113, 2002.
33. Siscovick DS, Raghunathan T, King I, et al: Dietary intake of long-chain n-3 polyunsaturated fatty acids and the risk of primary cardiac arrest. Am J Clin Nutr 71:208S, 2000.
34. Marchioli R, Barzi F, Bomba E, et al: Early protection against sudden death by n-3 polyunsaturated fatty acids after myocardial infarction: Time-course analysis of the results of the Gruppo Italiano per lo Studio della Sopravvivenza nell'Infarto Miocardico (GISSI)-Prevenzione. Circulation 105:1897, 2002.
35. Hooper L, Thompson RL, Harrison RA, et al: Risks and benefits of omega 3 fats for mortality, cardiovascular disease, and cancer: Systematic review. BMJ 332:752, 2006.
36. Mozaffarian D, Ascherio A, Hu FB, et al: Interplay between different polyunsaturated fatty acids and risk of coronary heart disease in men. Circulation 111:157, 2005.
37. Wijendran V, Hayes KC: Dietary n-6 and n-3 fatty acid balance and cardiovascular health. Annu Rev Nutr 24:597, 2004.
38. de Lorgeril M, Salen P: Alpha-linolenic acid and coronary heart disease. Nutr Metab Cardiovasc Dis 14:162, 2004.
39. Brouwer IA, Katan MB, Zock PL: Dietary alpha-linolenic acid is associated with reduced risk of fatal coronary heart disease, but increased prostate cancer risk: A meta-analysis. J Nutr 134:919, 2004.
40. Albert CM, Oh K, Whang W, et al: Dietary alpha-linolenic acid intake and risk of sudden cardiac death and coronary heart disease. Circulation 112:3232, 2005.

Alcohol Consumption and Cardiovascular Disease

41. Vogel RA: Alcohol, heart disease, and mortality: A review. Rev Cardiovasc Med 3:7, 2002.
42. Goldberg IJ, Mosca L, Piano MR, Fisher EA: AHA science advisory: Wine and your heart: A science advisory for healthcare professionals from the Nutrition Committee, Council on Epidemiology and Prevention, and Council on Cardiovascular Nursing of the American Heart Association. Stroke 32:591, 2001.

43. Sierksma A, van der Gaag MS, Kluft C, Hendriks HF: Moderate alcohol consumption reduces plasma C-reactive protein and fibrinogen levels: A randomized, diet-controlled intervention study. Eur J Clin Nutr 56:1130, 2002.
44. Albert MA, Glynn RJ, Ridker PM: Alcohol consumption and plasma concentration of C-reactive protein. Circulation 107:443, 2003.
45. Basu A, Devaraj S, Jialal I: Dietary factors that promote or retard inflammation. Arterioscler Thromb Vasc Biol 26:995, 2006.
46. Mukamal KJ, Conigrave KM, Mittleman MA, et al: Roles of drinking pattern and type of alcohol consumed in coronary heart disease in men. N Engl J Med 348:109, 2003.

Diet, Lifestyle Modification, Cardiovascular Disease, Obesity, Lipids

47. Sacks FM, Katan M: Randomized clinical trials on the effects of dietary fat and carbohydrate on plasma lipoproteins and cardiovascular disease. Am J Med 113(Suppl 9B):13S, 2002.
48. de Lorgeril M, Salen P, Martin JL, et al: Mediterranean diet, traditional risk factors, and the rate of cardiovascular complications after myocardial infarction: Final report of the Lyon Diet Heart Study. Circulation 99:779, 1999.
49. Howard BV, Van Horn L, Hsia J, et al: Low-fat dietary pattern and risk of cardiovascular disease: The Women's Health Initiative Randomized Controlled Dietary Modification Trial. JAMA 295:655, 2006.
50. Ornish D, Scherwitz LW, Billings JH, et al: Intensive lifestyle changes for reversal of coronary heart disease. JAMA 280:2001, 1998.
51. Koertge J, Weidner G, Elliott-Eller M, et al: Improvement in medical risk factors and quality of life in women and men with coronary artery disease in the Multicenter Lifestyle Demonstration Project. Am J Cardiol 91:1316, 2003.
52. Krauss RM, Eckel RH, Howard B, et al: AHA Dietary Guidelines-revision 2000: A statement for healthcare professionals from the Nutrition Committee of the American Heart Association. Circulation 102:2284, 2000.
53. McGuire MT, Wing RR, Klem ML, Hill JO: Behavioral strategies of individuals who have maintained long-term weight losses. Obes Res 7:334, 1999.
54. Westman EC, Yancy WS, Edman JS, et al: Effect of 6-month adherence to a very low carbohydrate diet program. Am J Med 113:30, 2002.
55. Foster GD, Wyatt HR, Hill JO, et al: A randomized trial of a low-carbohydrate diet for obesity. N Engl J Med 348:2082, 2003.
56. Stern L, Iqbal N, Seshadri P, et al: The effects of low-carbohydrate versus conventional weight loss diets in severely obese adults: One-year follow-up of a randomized trial. Ann Intern Med 140:778, 2004.
57. Nordmann AJ, Nordmann A, Briel M, et al: Effects of low-carbohydrate vs low-fat diets on weight loss and cardiovascular risk factors: A meta-analysis of randomized controlled trials. Arch Intern Med 166:285, 2006.
58. Bonow RO, Eckel RH: Diet, obesity, and cardiovascular risk. N Engl J Med 348:2057, 2003.
59. Dansinger ML, Gleason JA, Griffith JL, et al: Comparison of the Atkins, Ornish, Weight Watchers, and Zone diets for weight loss and heart disease risk reduction: A randomized trial. JAMA 293:43, 2005.
60. St Jeor ST, Howard BV, Prewitt TE, et al: Dietary protein and weight reduction: A statement for healthcare professionals from the Nutrition Committee of the Council on Nutrition, Physical Activity, and Metabolism of the American Heart Association. Circulation 104:1869, 2001.
61. Krauss RM, Blanche PJ, Rawlings RS, et al: Separate effects of reduced carbohydrate intake and weight loss on atherogenic dyslipidemia. Am J Clin Nutr 83:1025, 2006.
62. Mensink RP, Zock PL, Kester AD, Katan MB: Effects of dietary fatty acids and carbohydrates on the ratio of serum total to HDL cholesterol and on serum lipids and apolipoproteins: A meta-analysis of 60 controlled trials. Am J Clin Nutr 77:1146, 2003.
63. National Academy of Sciences and Institute of Medicine: Dietary Reference Intakes: Energy, carbohydrate, fiber, fat, fatty acids, cholesterol, protein, and amino acids. Washington, DC, National Academies Press, 2002.
64. Dreon DM, Krauss RM: Diet-gene interactions in human lipoprotein metabolism. J Am Coll Nutr 16:313, 1997.
65. Hu FB, Manson JE, Willett WC: Types of dietary fat and risk of coronary heart disease: A critical review. J Am Coll Nutr 20:5, 2001.
66. Appel LJ, Sacks FM, Carey VJ, et al: Effects of protein, monounsaturated fat, and carbohydrate intake on blood pressure and serum lipids: Results of the OmniHeart randomized trial. JAMA 294:2455, 2005.
67. Luscombe-Marsh ND, Noakes M, Wittert GA, et al: Carbohydrate-restricted diets high in either monounsaturated fat or protein are equally effective at promoting fat loss and improving blood lipids. Am J Clin Nutr 81:762, 2005.
68. Lichtenstein AH, Deckelbaum RJ: AHA Science Advisory. Stanol/sterol ester-containing foods and blood cholesterol levels: A statement for healthcare professionals from the Nutrition Committee of the Council on Nutrition, Physical Activity, and Metabolism of the American Heart Association. Circulation 103:1177, 2001.
69. Cater NB, Garcia-Garcia AB, Vega GL, et al: Responsiveness of plasma lipids and lipoproteins to plant stanol esters. Am J Cardiol 96:23D, 2005.
70. Van Horn L: Fiber, lipids, and coronary heart disease: A statement for healthcare professionals from the Nutrition Committee, American Heart Association. Circulation 95:2701, 1997.
71. Jenkins DJ, Kendall CW, Marchie A, et al: Effects of a dietary portfolio of cholesterol-lowering foods versus lovastatin on serum lipids and C-reactive protein. JAMA 290:502, 2003.
72. Berneis KK, Krauss RM: Metabolic origins and clinical significance of LDL heterogeneity. J Lipid Res 43:1363, 2002.
73. Parks EJ, Hellerstein MK: Carbohydrate-induced hypertriacylglycerolemia: Historical perspective and review of biological mechanisms. Am J Clin Nutr 71:412, 2000.
74. Krauss RM: Dietary and genetic effects on low-density lipoprotein heterogeneity. Annu Rev Nutr 21:283, 2001.

Dietary Factors and Blood Pressure Control

75. Appel LJ, Brands MW, Daniels SR, et al: Dietary approaches to prevent and treat hypertension: A scientific statement from the American Heart Association. Hypertension 47:296, 2006.
76. Kotchen TA, McCarron DA: Dietary electrolytes and blood pressure: A statement for healthcare professionals from the American Heart Association Nutrition Committee. Circulation 98:613, 1998.
77. Graudal NA, Galloe AM, Garred P: Effects of sodium restriction on blood pressure, renin, aldosterone, catecholamines, cholesterols, and triglyceride: A meta-analysis. JAMA 279:1383, 1998.
78. Obarzanek E, Proschan MA, Vollmer WM, et al: Individual blood pressure responses to changes in salt intake: Results from the DASH-Sodium Trial. Hypertension 42:459, 2003.
79. Trials of Hypertension Prevention Collaborative Research Group. Effects of weight loss and sodium reduction intervention on blood pressure and hypertension incidence in overweight people with high-normal blood pressure: The Trials of Hypertension Prevention, Phase II. Arch Intern Med 157:657, 1997.
80. Whelton PK, Appel LJ, Espeland MA, et al: Sodium reduction and weight loss in the treatment of hypertension in older persons: A randomized controlled trial of nonpharmacologic interventions in the elderly (TONE). TONE Collaborative Research Group. JAMA 279:839, 1998.
81. Klatsky AL: Alcohol and cardiovascular disease-more than one paradox to consider. Alcohol and hypertension: Does it matter? Yes. J Cardiovasc Risk 10:21, 2003.
82. Vaskonen T: Dietary minerals and modification of cardiovascular risk factors. J Nutr Biochem 14:492, 2003.
83. Whelton PK, He J, Cutler JA, et al: Effects of oral potassium on blood pressure: Meta-analysis of randomized controlled clinical trials. JAMA 277:1624, 1997.
84. Svetkey LP Simons-Morton D, Vollmer WM, et al: Effects of dietary patterns on blood pressure: Subgroup analysis of the Dietary Approaches to Stop Hypertension (DASH) randomized clinical trial. Arch Intern Med 159:285, 1999.
85. Vollmer WM, Sacks FM, Ard J, et al: Effects of diet and sodium intake on blood pressure: Subgroup analysis of the DASH-Sodium trial. Ann Intern Med 135:1019, 2001.
86. Resnick LM, Oparil S, Chait A, et al: Factors affecting blood pressure responses to diet: The Vanguard study. Am J Hypertens 13:956, 2000.
87. Steffen LM, Kroenke CH, Yu X, et al: Associations of plant food, dairy product, and meat intakes with 15-y incidence of elevated blood pressure in young black and white adults: The Coronary Artery Risk Development in Young Adults (CARDIA) Study. Am J Clin Nutr 82:1169, 2005.
88. Miura K, Greenland P, Stamler J, et al: Relation of vegetable, fruit, and meat intake to 7-year blood pressure change in middle-aged men: The Chicago Western Electric Study. Am J Epidemiol 159:572, 2004.
89. Djousse L, Arnett DK, Pankow JS, et al: Dietary linolenic acid is associated with a lower prevalence of hypertension in the NHLBI Family Heart Study. Hypertension 45:368, 2005.
90. Saltzman E, Das SK, Lichtenstein AH, et al: An oat-containing hypocaloric diet reduces systolic blood pressure and improves lipid profile beyond effects of weight loss in men and women. J Nutr 131:1465, 2001.
91. Burke V, Hodgson JM, Beilin LJ, et al: Dietary protein and soluble fiber reduce ambulatory blood pressure in treated hypertensives. Hypertension 38:821, 2001.
92. Teede HJ, Dalais FS, Kotsopoulos D, et al: Dietary soy has both beneficial and potentially adverse cardiovascular effects: A placebo-controlled study in men and postmenopausal women. J Clin Endocrinol Metab 86:3053, 2001.
93. Rivas M, Garay RP, Escanero JF, et al: Soy milk lowers blood pressure in men and women with mild to moderate essential hypertension. J Nutr 132:1900, 2002.
94. Taubert D, Berkels R, Roesen R, Klaus W: Chocolate and blood pressure in elderly individuals with isolated systolic hypertension. JAMA 290:1029, 2003.

Homocysteine, Diet, and Cardiovascular Disease

95. Bautista LE, Arenas IA, Penuela A, Martinez LX: Total plasma homocysteine level and risk of cardiovascular disease: A meta-analysis of prospective cohort studies. J Clin Epidemiol 55:882, 2002.
96. Homocysteine Cooperative Research Group. Homocysteine and risk of ischemic heart disease and stroke: A meta-analysis. JAMA 288:2015, 2002.
97. Malinow MR, Bostom AG, Krauss RM: Homocyst(e)ine, diet, and cardiovascular diseases: A statement for healthcare professionals from the Nutrition Committee, American Heart Association. Circulation 99:178, 1999.
98. Toole JF, Malinow MR, Chambless LE, et al: Lowering homocysteine in patients with ischemic stroke to prevent recurrent stroke, myocardial infarction, and death: The Vitamin Intervention for Stroke Prevention (VISP) randomized controlled trial. JAMA 291:565, 2004.
99. Lonn E, Yusuf S, Arnold MJ, et al: Homocysteine lowering with folic acid and B vitamins in vascular disease. N Engl J Med 354:1567, 2006.
100. Bonaa KH, Njolstad I, Ueland PM, et al: Homocysteine lowering and cardiovascular events after acute myocardial infarction. N Engl J Med 354:1578, 2006.
101. Morris CD, Carson S: Routine vitamin supplementation to prevent cardiovascular disease: A summary of the evidence for the U.S. Preventive Services Task Force. Ann Intern Med 139:56, 2003.

102. Pearson TA, Mensah GA, Alexander RW, et al: Markers of inflammation and cardiovascular disease-application to clinical and public health practice: A statement for healthcare professionals from the Centers for Disease Control and Prevention and the American Heart Association. Circulation 107:499, 2003.
103. McLaughlin T, Abbasi F, Lamendola C, et al: Differentiation between obesity and insulin resistance in the association with C-reactive protein. Circulation 106:2908, 2002.
104. Esposito K, Pontillo A, Di Palo C, et al: Effect of weight loss and lifestyle changes on vascular inflammatory markers in obese women: A randomized trial. JAMA 289:1799, 2003.
105. Dietrich M, Jialal I: The effect of weight loss on a stable biomarker of inflammation, C-reactive protein. Nutr Rev 63:22, 2005.
106. Liu S, Manson JE, Buring JE, et al: Relation between a diet with a high glycemic load and plasma concentrations of high-sensitivity C-reactive protein in middle-aged women. Am J Clin Nutr 75:492, 2002.
107. Wells BJ, Mainous AG III, Everett CJ: Association between dietary arginine and C-reactive protein. Nutrition 21:125, 2005.
108. Vivekananthan DP, Penn MS, Sapp SK, et al: Use of antioxidant vitamins for the prevention of cardiovascular disease: Meta-analysis of randomised trials. Lancet 361:2017, 2003.
109. Lee IM, Cook NR, Gaziano JM, et al: Vitamin E in the primary prevention of cardiovascular disease and cancer: The Women's Health Study: A randomized controlled trial. JAMA 294:56, 2005.
110. MRC/BHF Heart Protection Study of antioxidant vitamin supplementation in 20,536 high-risk individuals: A randomised placebo-controlled trial. Lancet 360:23, 2002.
111. Brown BG, Zhao XQ, Chait A, et al: Simvastatin and niacin, antioxidant vitamins, or the combination for the prevention of coronary disease. N Engl J Med 345:1583, 2001.
112. Stone PH, Lloyd-Jones DM, Kinlay S, et al: Effect of intensive lipid lowering, with or without antioxidant vitamins, compared with moderate lipid lowering on myocardial ischemia in patients with stable coronary artery disease: The Vascular Basis for the Treatment of Myocardial Ischemia Study. Circulation 111:1747, 2005.
113. Waters DD, Alderman EL, Hsia J, et al: Effects of hormone replacement therapy and antioxidant vitamin supplements on coronary atherosclerosis in postmenopausal women: A randomized controlled trial. JAMA 288:2432, 2002.
114. Kelemen M, Vaidya D, Waters DD, et al: Hormone therapy and antioxidant vitamins do not improve endothelial vasodilator function in postmenopausal women with established coronary artery disease: A substudy of the Women's Angiographic Vitamin and Estrogen (WAVE) trial. Atherosclerosis 179:193, 2005.
115. Lichtenstein AH: Dietary *trans* fatty acid. J Cardiopulm Rehabil 20:143, 2000.
116. Ginsberg HN, Kris-Etherton P, Dennis B, et al: Effects of reducing dietary saturated fatty acids on plasma lipids and lipoproteins in healthy subjects: The DELTA Study, protocol 1. Arterioscler Thromb Vasc Biol 18:441, 1998.

CHAPTER 45

Primary and Secondary Prevention of Coronary Heart Disease

J. Michael Gaziano, JoAnn E. Manson, and Paul M. Ridker

Both primary and secondary prevention of coronary heart disease (CHD) have indisputable public health importance. Given the prevalence of CHD, preventing even a small proportion of events would save thousands of lives, avoid inestimable suffering, and save billions of health care dollars. In addition, measures that prevent CHD may also mitigate other manifestations of atherosclerosis, such as stroke and peripheral artery disease, and may have an impact on hypertension, diabetes, cognitive function, cancer, depression, and other chronic conditions. Because cardiovascular disease (CVD) has become the number one killer worldwide, widespread deployment of affordable preventive strategies should have high priority in developed and developing countries.

Our ever-increasing knowledge about the pathogenesis of atherosclerosis and our understanding of the interrelationship between life style, biochemical, and even genetic risk factors and heart disease have contributed to significant declines in age-adjusted cardiovascular mortality (Fig. 45-1). The first step toward prevention entails using these factors to predict who is likely to experience atherosclerotic events. Several scores have been developed that use risk factors to estimate an individual's risk of future cardiovascular events (see Chap. 39). However, the process of disease prevention must move beyond using factors to predict future events and identify interventions that definitively reduce risk. Once trials have weighed the benefits of given interventions against their risks and costs, guidelines for health care providers and the general public can be established.

A number of single risk factor guidelines have been developed and have resulted in early success in screening and treatment of several major risk factors, such as smoking, dyslipidemia, and hypertension. Implementing and integrating these guidelines, however, remains a difficult task. The number and complexity of guidelines clearly impedes their implementation. Lack of time for physicians to act on guidelines is also an additional hurdle; delivering only those cardiovascular-related preventive services recommended by the U.S. Preventive Services Task Force (USPSTF) would take the clinician a minimum of 1.5 hours per day.[1] Lack of reimbursement also limits the delivery of certain preventive interventions.

In an attempt to simplify the approach to CVD prevention, this chapter defines risk factors in a novel way. First, we discuss the various types of risk factors and how risk factor information can be used in clinical practice. Then, we provide a simple approach to using risk factors to predict risk. This is followed by a scheme for prioritizing preventive interventions that divides interventions into three categories. The chapter then examines potentially modifiable risk factor domains and interventions, with information on prevalence, associated risk, benefit of treatment, cost efficacy, and recommendations and guidelines for each, followed by a discussion of multiple risk factor intervention strategies. It concludes with a summary of the approach to the patient.

USING RISK FACTOR INFORMATION

When CVD first emerged as the dominant chronic disease in high-income countries, it was thought of as a natural consequence of aging. But cardiovascular disease appears in most cases to be predominantly a "human-made" disease, heavily influenced by the choices we make. The past 50 years have witnessed great progress in identifying a large number of life-style, as well as biochemical and genetic, factors associated with CVD and in disseminating this information to the public.

In the 1950s and 1960s, several types of epidemiological studies helped establish a definitive cause and effect relationship between certain behaviors and CVD. For example, the Seven Countries Study, a large cross-cultural study, clearly demonstrated that CVD rates varied around the world, implicating environmental factors. Migration studies comparing CVD prevalence in those of the same ethnic background living in geographically diverse locations lent further credence to the theory that environmental factors play a key role in the development of CVD. In fact, migration studies described differences in the prevalence of various environmental factors, such as cigarette smoking, that may have contributed to the differences in the rates of disease. By 1961, data from the landmark Framingham Heart Study showed that hypertension, high cholesterol, and smoking all increased the risk of heart disease and, in a report published that year by the Framingham researchers, "factors of risk" associated with the devel-

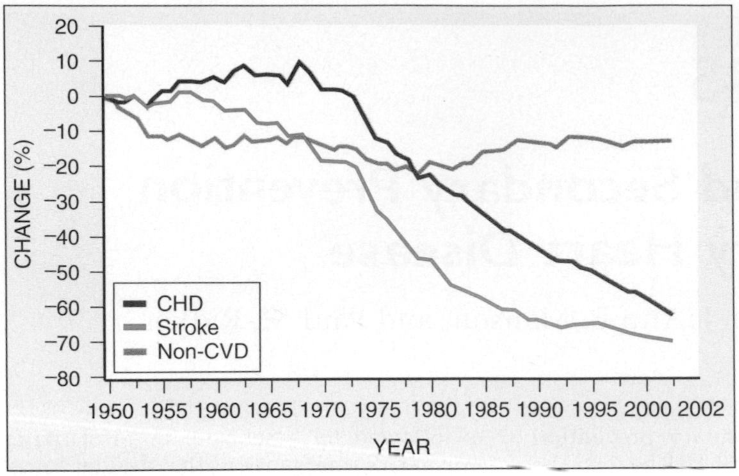

FIGURE 45–1 Change in age-adjusted mortality from coronary heart disease (CHD), stroke, and non-CVD in the United States, 1950 to 2002. CVD = cardiovascular disease. *(From National Heart, Lung, and Blood Institute: Morbidity and Mortality: 2004 Chart Book on Cardiovascular, Lung, and Blood Diseases. Bethesda, MD, National Heart, Lung, and Blood Institute, 2004, p 23.)*

TABLE 45–1	Types of Studies Used in Establishing Preventive Strategies

Basic research
  In vitro studies
  Animal studies	

Human physiological studies	

Epidemiological studies
  Descriptive studies
    Case reports
    Cross-sectional surveys
    Cross-cultural comparison studies
    Temporal trend studies
  Analytical studies
    Observational
      Case-control studies
      Cohort studies
    Intervention (randomized trials)	

Cost-efficacy studies	
Meta-analyses	

opment of CHD were first described. Since then, risk factor has become an integral part of the language of epidemiology, cardiology, and a host of other disciplines. This early work clearly told us that the development of CVD involves a number of factors.

Risk factor generally applies to a variable that can predict a future cardiovascular event, but some of these predictors are also potential targets for intervention. For the purposes of risk estimation, what matters is the predictive value of the risk factor, the feasibility of assessing it, and the cost of assessment. Age, for example, is a useful predictor, because it associates strongly with cardiovascular risk and can be assessed easily and at no cost. However, when trying to identify potential targets for intervention, it is worth considering which factors can be modified to lower risk using safe and effective interventions, such as smoking.

Types of Evidence About Risk Factors

Evidence about risk factors has come from various sources. Autopsy studies have shown that atherosclerosis can begin at an early age if risk factors—the same risk factors that lead to CVD in adults—are present (see Chap. 38).[2,3] The establishment of cause and effect, a crucial step in identifying predictors and developing preventive intervention, requires data from several types of research (Table 45-1). Basic research and human physiological studies have provided insight into the mechanisms underlying atherogenesis and have helped elucidate the biological plausibility of potential interventions to modify these effects. Human observational studies, such as case-control studies and prospective cohorts, are extremely useful in establishing risk attributable to a single factor. Randomized trials can help confirm causation and are essential in establishing interventions to modify the risk.

Each of these strategies has strengths and weaknesses. Descriptive studies (e.g., case reports, case series, cross-sectional surveys, cross-cultural studies, and studies of population-based temporal trends) have considerable value for their ability to generate hypotheses. However, their design prevents adequate control for potential factors that may confound apparent associations. Observational studies (e.g., case-control and prospective cohort studies) give researchers greater control over potential confounders. They are extremely useful in establishing risk attributable to a single factor, particularly when the effect of a given factor is large, as is the case for smoking and lung cancer. When searching for small to moderate effects, however, the amount of uncontrolled confounding in observational studies may be as large as the probable risk itself. In such cases, randomized trials are essential for confirming causation.

Once a factor has been established as causally related to disease, potential interventions to modify the factor must be developed and tested. Even when causality is not in question, trials help quantify the magnitude of an intervention's effect. In addition, when the intervention involves competing risks and benefits, randomized trials are needed to determine the net clinical effect of the intervention. This consideration has critical importance because the magnitude of associated risk does not relate necessarily to the magnitude of benefit derived from the intervention. Such lack of correlation may be a result of the inability of the intervention to achieve the necessary change, or a change in the parameter may not result in the necessary change in risk in a proportional manner. An example is the difference between the observed risk associated with a 1-mm Hg rise in blood pressure and the lower than anticipated benefit on CHD derived from reducing blood pressure by this amount.[4,5] Similarly, even though elevated levels of homocysteine have been implicated as a risk factor for CHD and folic acid reduces homocysteine levels, evidence from randomized trials has indicated that reducing homocysteine levels with folic acid does not reduce vascular risk.

Meta-analyses can provide better estimates of risk associated from a given factor or the benefits of a given intervention. For example, the best estimate of the benefit of aspirin in secondary prevention has come from a large meta-analysis of nearly 300 trials, demonstrating that aspirin reduces the risk of a major CVD event by 25 percent in those with vascular disease.

Once reasonable estimates of benefit and risk have been established for a given factor, cost-effectiveness analyses can help establish guidelines for intervention (see Chap. 3). The common currency used to compare interventions is the quality-adjusted life-year (QALY) or disability-adjusted life-year (DALY). Estimates derived from cost- and risk-benefit analyses depend on the underlying assumptions made in a given analysis. Because prevention measures have a long time horizon (decades or longer), the consequences of initial assumptions may have more impact than those of interventions with a short time horizon. Nonetheless, the cost-effectiveness of interventions to prevent heart disease is important because of the prevalence of CHD and the high cost of treatment.

Cost-effectiveness estimates are calculated as the ratio of net cost to gain in life expectancy. Interventions with an incremental cost-effectiveness ratio less than $40,000 per QALY are comparable to other chronic interventions, such as hypertension management and hemodialysis. Those with a cost-effectiveness ratio under $20,000 per QALY are very favorable, whereas those exceeding $40,000 per QALY tend to be higher than what is generally accepted by most insurers. The economic impact of ineffective primary prevention in persons with two or more modifiable risk factors has been estimated at $13.2 billion annually.[6]

Coronary Heart Disease as a Multifactorial Disease (see Chaps. 39 to 43)

Our knowledge of the biological process of atherosclerosis has led to a working model for the progression of this disease

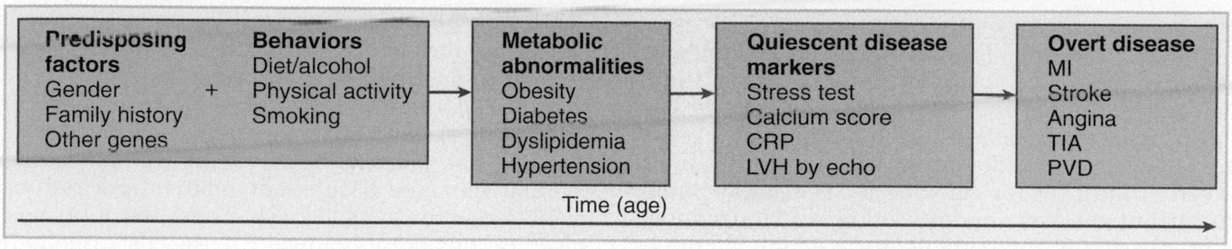

FIGURE 45–2 Progression of atherosclerosis. CRP = C-reactive protein; LVH = left ventricular hypertrophy; MI = myocardial infarction; TIA = transient ischemic attack; PVD = peripheral vascular disease.

and to the many factors that cause it. Coronary heart disease generally results from the convergence of a number of factors. Most people with cardiovascular disease have small, concurrent adverse changes in multiple risk factors rather than extreme deviations in any single risk factor. Left unchecked, atherosclerosis will proceed along a continuum (Fig. 45-2). Predisposing factors such as genes interact with behavioral factors, such as the type of diet an individual follows, whether he or she drinks alcohol, and the amount of exercise he or she gets on a regular basis. This combination of predisposing factors and behaviors can lead to metabolic abnormalities, such as dyslipidemia, hypertension, obesity, and diabetes, which may eventually result in quiescent disease. Clues to this underlying quiescent disease can be obtained by using various diagnostic tests. Some tests that assess physical changes in the artery, such as the intima-media thickness of the carotid artery or a coronary calcium score, can be used to estimate underlying atherosclerotic burden, whereas exercise stress testing can detect coronary stenoses that provoke ischemia. Other tests such as high-sensitivity C-reactive protein (CRP) measurement predict the likelihood of a cardiovascular event, but may not correlate well with plaque burden. Eventually, this quiescent disease may become overt in the form of a transient ischemic attack (TIA), myocardial infarction (MI), or other cardiovascular event. Factors useful in predicting who is at risk can come from any stage in this process, whether they are modifiable or not. For example, a family history of heart disease and a behavior such as smoking are risk factors. A metabolic factor such as high low-density lipoprotein (LDL) is also a risk factor. The existence of disease, such as having a prior MI or stroke, also strongly predicts future events. These distinctions outline the joint usefulness of predisposing risk factors and disease markers, both of which can be important for identifying individuals with an elevated chance of developing clinical complications.

While they may be useful, these distinctions are somewhat arbitrary. At times, it may be difficult to classify a factor in a distinct category. For example, family history could represent an individual's genes *or* behaviors that are passed from one generation to the next. Is hypertension a metabolic risk factor that results in part from the influence of risk-modifying behaviors, such as an atherosclerotic diet or physical inactivity, or is it a manifestation of endothelial dysfunction and thereby a marker of atherosclerosis?

Use of Risk Factors

Regardless of where these factors fit in the progression of the disease, they can be divided into two broad categories based on how we use them in clinical practice—those that are useful for predicting risk (risk predictors) and those that are targets for risk reduction (potential risk-reducing interventions; Fig. 45-3). Some factors such as cigarette smoking and blood pressure fall into both categories. If a given factor has predictive value, we cannot infer that modification of a risk factor will lead to reduced risk. The benefit of intervention must clearly exceed any risks and be worth the cost. Then, it must be implemented in appropriate populations. So, how do we decide on which to use for risk prediction and which to use as targets to lower risk? Approaches for using risk factors for prediction and risk reduction are defined later. This chapter considers only those factors that modify intermediate- or long-term risk. Interventions used acutely to modify short-term risk, such as aspirin or thrombolysis in the setting of an acute myocardial infarction, are considered elsewhere in this text (see Chaps. 51 to 53).

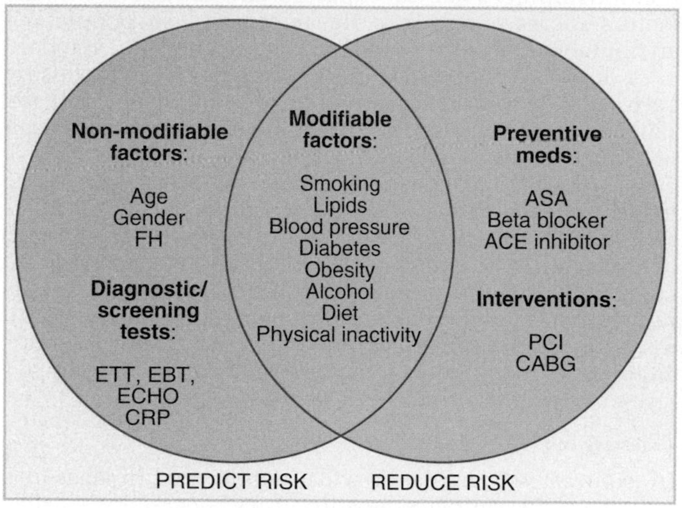

FIGURE 45–3 Risk factors can be divided into those that are useful in predicting risk and those that are useful targets for lowering risk. ACE = angiotensin-converting enzyme; ASA = acetylsalicylic acid; CABG = coronary artery bypass graft; CRP = C-reactive protein; EBT = electron beam tomography; ECHO = echocardiography; ETT = exercise tolerance test; FH = family history; PCI = percutaneous coronary intervention.

Predicting and Assessing Risk

Risk prediction can apply to a population or to an individual. Population information can be gathered on a representative sample of the population to estimate the rates of various risk factors in the population for the purposes of planning public health messages and allocating resources for screening programs. Assessment of individual risk is for the purpose of targeting subsegments of the population with more intensive programs for risk reduction. In this section, we briefly describe the assessment of risk factors and event rates in the overall population, followed by a detailed discussion of assessment of risk in the individual.

Assessing Risk at a Population Level: Incidence, Prevalence, and Population-Attributable Risk

Sound public policy requires evaluation of the impact of different factors on the *population*. Population risk depends not only on the strength of the risk factor–disease association and the benefit of intervention but also on how common the factor is in the general population. These concepts are captured in incidence, prevalence, and population-attributable risk. Although incidence rates reflect the frequency of new cases of disease or a risk factor over a given period, prevalence reflects the proportion of individuals with a given condition or factor at a single point. Population-attributable risk, or how much of the population's risk of disease is attributable to a given factor, is driven by the proportion of the public with a given risk factor and the magnitude of the associated risk.

Population-attributable risk also reflects the shape of the relationship between the exposure and the disease. Many factors increase risk in a linear fashion, so population-attributable risk can be computed against an ideal standard or a low-risk individual. For example, the relationship between hypertension and heart disease and stroke is linear. Thus, lowering blood pressure at any level in the pathological range reduces risk. In contrast, the shape of the risk curve for obesity appears nonlinear, with risk increasing logarithmically. Thus, each incremental pound gained is associated with much more risk in those who are already overweight. Population-attributable risk is an important concept for determining resource allocation among various preventive interventions and in prioritizing public health messages, such as antismoking campaigns. However, in this chapter, we focus more on the assessment of an individual's risk of future cardiovascular events.

Assessing Individual Risk

In contrast to population-wide public health measures, which are disseminated broadly, clinicians are responsible for making recommendations for prevention to an individual. A fundamental step in targeting individual preventive strategies involves assessing the risk of developing a clinically relevant outcome, because the cost efficacy of any intervention varies according to global risk in a given individual or population. Because absolute risk in those with known disease is higher than in those at lower risk, fewer high-risk individuals require treatment to save one life or prevent one event in comparison to those at lower risk, even if relative risk reductions are identical in both groups.

To illustrate this concept, assume that an intervention reduces mortality by 25 percent in both primary and secondary prevention (Fig. 45-4). Furthermore, assume that a high-risk individual with CHD has a 20 percent chance of death from cardiovascular disease over the next 10 years, whereas a low-risk individual has a 1 percent chance of

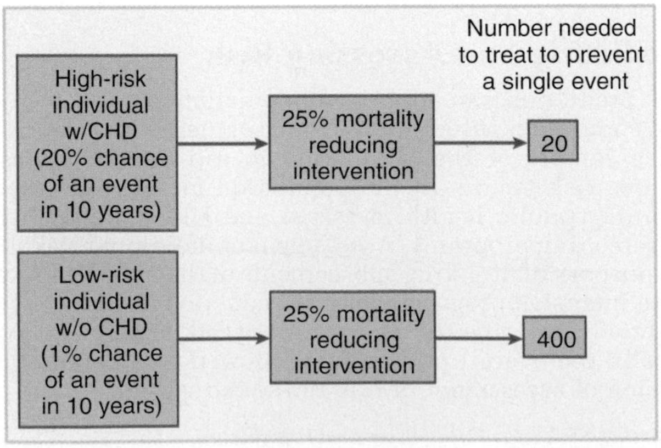

FIGURE 45–4 The cost efficacy of an intervention that reduces risk by 25 percent among those that are high risk and those that are low risk varies by baseline level of risk. In a population with a 20 percent risk of an event over 10 years, only 20 patients need to be treated to prevent a single event compared with 400 low-risk individuals. CHD = coronary heart disease.

death over the same period. To save a life among those at high risk, one would have to treat only 20 patients (4 of whom are destined to die) for 10 years so that a 25 percent relative risk reduction would result in 1 life saved (3 deaths instead of 4). On the other hand, one would have to treat 400 low-risk patients (4 of whom are also destined to die) so that the same 25 percent relative risk reduction would yield 3 deaths instead of 4. Thus, the total cost per lives saved is considerably lower ($^1/_{20}$ the cost) among individuals at higher absolute risk. High-cost interventions are generally cost-effective only in high-risk individuals; however, if the cost of intervention is low, there can be cost-effectiveness even in low-risk subgroups.

When predicting risk, a "perfect" risk factor is one that is prevalent in the population, can be easily and safely measured, and has good predictive value. It must also be inexpensive to measure, a major potential limitation for expensive imaging techniques such as screening with electron beam computed tomography (CT) or magnetic resonance imaging (MRI). Furthermore, the false-positive rate associated with screening must be low to avoid unnecessary and potentially hazardous consequences. Age and gender are examples of nonmodifiable risk factors that meet these criteria; similarly, blood pressure and smoking status are examples of modifiable factors that are easy to assess. The results of diagnostic tests can also serve as predictors of future events.

Global and Individual Risk Scores

Because many risk predictors are correlated, it is often possible to predict risk with information on just a few risk factors. So, although it is possible to assess many factors, in most cases, when conducting an initial screen, a handful of easily measured risk factors suffices to determine an individual's overall risk of CHD. For those who clearly have very low or very high risk after initial screening, measuring and evaluating numerous additional risk factors will provide very little, if any, incremental information helpful in managing the patient; it is largely for those at intermediate risk (see later) that additional screening will provide valuable information. Assessing an individual's absolute risk enables cost-effective targeting of interventions. As evidence of the importance of individual risk assessment, the National Cholesterol Education Program (NCEP) Adult Treatment Panel (ATP) III,[7] the Seventh Joint National Committee on Prevention, Detection, Evaluation, and Treatment of High Blood Pressure (JNC-7),[8] and the U.S. Preventive Services Task Force (USPSTF) have all suggested some assessment of the individual's risk to gauge the intensity of various interventions. The American Diabetes Association also recommends a tiered approach to management based on absolute risk.[9]

A crude way to categorize individuals as being at higher or lower risk is by the presence or absence of established cardiovascular disease. Those with known cardiovascular disease, including coronary, cerebrovascular, or peripheral artery disease, are on average at much higher risk than those without known disease. Approximately 80 percent of those with known cardiovascular disease will die of some form of cardiovascular disease, whereas those without known cardiovascular disease have approximately half that cardiovascular disease mortality rate. As discussed later in this chapter, those with cardiovascular disease generally warrant aggressive preventive interventions. Risk reduction in these individuals is referred to as *secondary prevention,* as opposed to *primary prevention* in those without overt cardiovascular disease.

Individuals with diabetes constitute a second high-risk group. Rates of cardiovascular disease events and mortality in diabetic patients considerably exceed those in the general population; thus, patients with diabetes warrant aggressive preventive interventions. Another group of patients at exceedingly high risk for cardiovascular disease events and death are those with chronic renal failure, many of whom have diabetes.

For those who do not have known CVD or diabetes, several risk prediction strategies have been developed using some of the risk factors outlined in Figure 45-3. Early versions of some guidelines advocated merely counting risk factors. The Framingham Heart Study investigators have developed a useful tool to assess risk of a first cardiovascular event based on age, gender, total or LDL cholesterol, high-density lipoprotein (HDL) cholesterol, systolic and diastolic blood pressure, and history of diabetes and cigarette smoking.[4] Point-based weights are assigned to the presence and/or level of each risk factor. Once the points have been assigned and summed, the total score can be translated to an estimated absolute risk of a CHD event occurring within the next 10 years. The National Heart, Lung, and Blood Institute has made available an online version of this 10-year risk calculator (http://hp2010.nhlbihin.net/atpiii/calculator.asp), as well as versions that can be downloaded to a clinician's desktop computer (http://hp2010.nhlbi.net/atpiii/riskcalc.htm) or handheld device (http://hp2010.nhlbihin.net/atp3palm.htm). Risk assessment scales are also available from the Framingham investigators for the secondary prevention of myocardial infarction and stroke. However, because all patients with prior evidence of cardiovascular disease have high risk for recurrent events and require aggressive preventive efforts, the usefulness of these tools is unclear.

There are a number of alternatives to the Framingham Risk Score. The Heart Systematic Coronary Risk Evaluation project, or HeartScore, was assembled by a European joint task force using data from cohort studies in 12 European countries involving more than 200,000 individuals. HeartScore has replaced earlier risk stratification models promulgated by the European Society of Cardiology and shifted the emphasis from the prevention of CHD to the prevention of CVD.[10] Using age, gender, systolic blood pressure, and total cholesterol, or the HDL-total cholesterol ratio, HeartScore calculates the 10-year risk of CVD death rather than the risk of any cardiovascular event. Diabetes was not included because it was not reliably measured in the cohorts used to develop the scores. Those for whom the risk of a fatal event is 5 percent or greater over the next 10 years are recommended for aggressive management (HeartScore can be accessed at http://www.escardio.org/initiatives/prevention/?hit=redirect).

Another instrument for assessing absolute risk has emerged from the Prospective Cardiovascular Munster (PROCAM) Study, a long-term follow-up study of more than 5000 men aged 35 to 65 years recruited between 1979 and 1985. Risk factors included in the PROCAM algorithm include cigarette smoking, systolic blood pressure, LDL cholesterol, HDL cholesterol, fasting triglyceride levels, diabetes, family history of myocardial infarction, and age. Answers to questions regarding these factors is tallied into a point score, just as with the Framingham algorithm, and this point score is converted into a 10-year absolute risk of fatal or nonfatal myocardial infarction or sudden cardiac death.[11]

Updated in 2003, the New Zealand Guidelines Group has assembled tables that assess risk over 5 rather than 10 years (Fig. 45-5). This model predicts the 5-year total cardiovascular disease risk based on age, gender, ethnicity (Maori or non-Maori), smoking history, lipid and glucose levels, and blood pressure. Patients are categorized as being at very high, high, moderate, or mild risk. Those with known CVD, genetic lipid disorders, or diabetes and renal disease constitute the very high-risk category because most have a greater than 20 percent chance of a subsequent CVD event over the next 5 years. Aggressive management is recommended for those whose total CVD risk is greater than 15 percent.

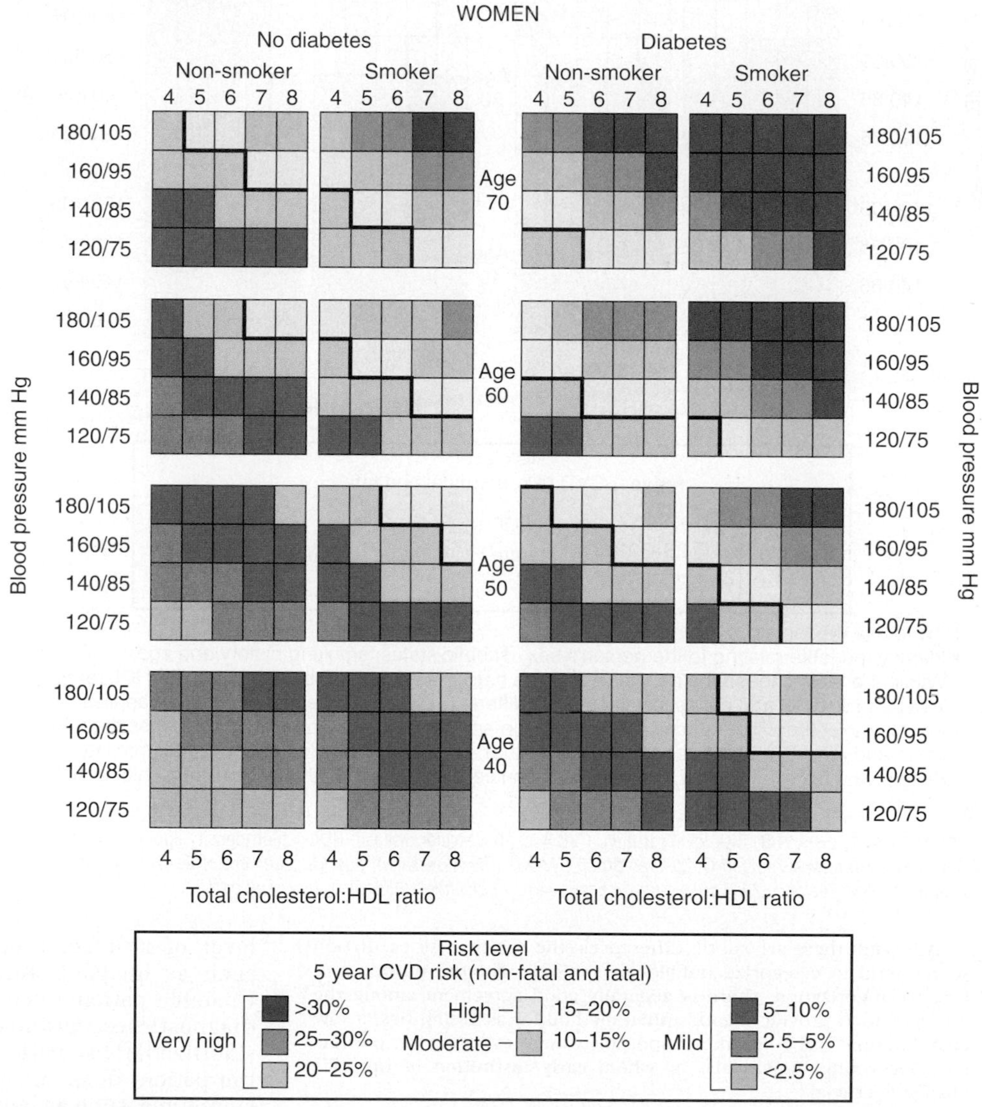

How to use the tables:

- Identify the table relating to the person's sex, diabetic status, smoking history and age.
- Within the table choose the cell nearest to the person's age, blood pressure and TC:HDL ratio. When the systolic and diastolic values fall in different risk levels, the higher category applies.
- For example, the lower left cell contains all non-smokers without diabetes who are less than 45 years and have a TC:HDL ratio less than 4.5 and a blood pressure less than 130/80 mm Hg. People who fall exactly on a threshold between cells are placed in the cell indicating higher risk.

A

FIGURE 45–5 Risk assessment tool devised by a New Zealand task force to determine 5-year total cardiovascular disease risk based on age, gender, ethnicity, smoking history, lipid and glucose levels, and blood pressure. **A,** Risk level for women.

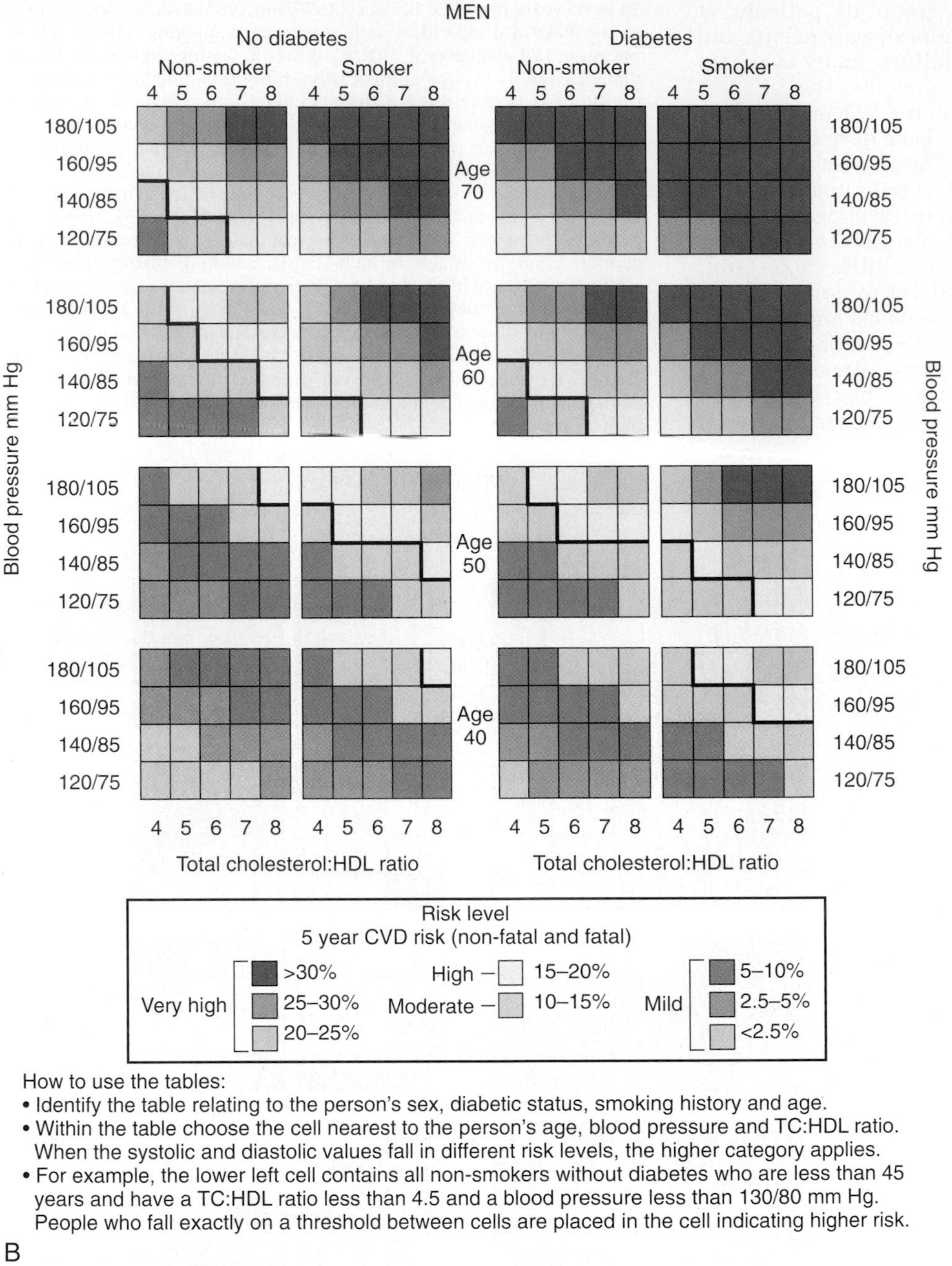

FIGURE 45–5, cont'd B, Risk level for men. CVD = cardiovascular disease; HDL = high-density lipoprotein; TC = total cholesterol. *(From New Zealand Guidelines Group (NZGG): The Assessment and Management of Cardiovascular Risk, Wellington, New Zealand, 2003 [http://www.nzgg.org.nz/guidelines/ 0035/CVD_Risk_Full.pdf].)*

Although there are subtle differences, the various risk prediction scores tend to categorize individuals similarly. For the purposes of broad categorization, there is generally good agreement among the scores, which provide a good initial method for assessing risk at low cost. Lifetime risk is another important way to express risk, particularly for young individuals, in whom early institution of life-style change is crucial.[12]

A number of diagnostic tests that were developed for patients with specific complaints and novel biochemical markers have emerged as potential ways to augment these simple scores. Calcium scores determined by electron beam CT and exercise tolerance tests represent such diagnostic tests for which substantial data are available.[13] Other tests with prognostic information include echocardiography and even cardiac catheterization. Each test adds prognostic information; however, these tests entail substantial costs and potential adverse consequences, and their usefulness in prevention remains controversial.[14]

CRP, a marker of inflammation, holds promise in providing incremental predictive value beyond the initial screen (see Chap. 39). Investigators in the Women's Health Study have recently shown that the addition of simple covariates such as family history, hemoglobin A_{1c} (HbA_{1c}) if diabetic, and CRP can lead to nearly 50 percent of all women at intermediate risk being reclassified to higher or lower risk categories, and that this reclassification is correct in nearly all cases, at least as compared with traditional risk scoring by ATP III criteria.[15] Thus, improved risk prediction algorithms are available for general use that should help ensure that preventive therapies, both life-style and pharmacological based, are applied to the correct group of at-risk individuals

Risk Assessment in the Office

Clinicians can easily classify their patients' long-term risk of a coronary heart disease events, as well as other cardiovascular disease events, as very high, high, intermediate, or low using a few simple questions and office measures, such as blood pressure. We have developed an algorithm that provides a detailed method for categorizing patients according to their overall risk (Fig. 45-6). An individual's cardiovascular disease status is the first question in the algorithm. If the individual has known cardiovascular disease, then we must determine if it is stable. If the patient is stable, no further classification is needed, because this patient is by definition at very high long-term risk and requires the most aggressive level of risk-factor modification. Evidence of instability such as unstable angina indicates high short-term risk. Unstable patients need immediate referral for appropriate diagnostic testing and appropriate interventions. Even when stabilized, these patients have a very high long-term risk. If the patient does not have known CVD but has worrisome symptoms, such as new-onset chest pain that suggests coronary artery or cardiovascular disease, the patient will also require evaluation for potentially high short-term risk with appropriate diagnostic testing. If diagnosed with CVD, this patient will have further testing, such as a catheterization, and interventions as needed, and ultimately will be placed in the very high-risk group. If these test results are negative, they will return to the primary prevention group for risk assessment.

For those without CVD, a key factor is whether the patient is diabetic. If so, long-term risk is clearly high and he or she

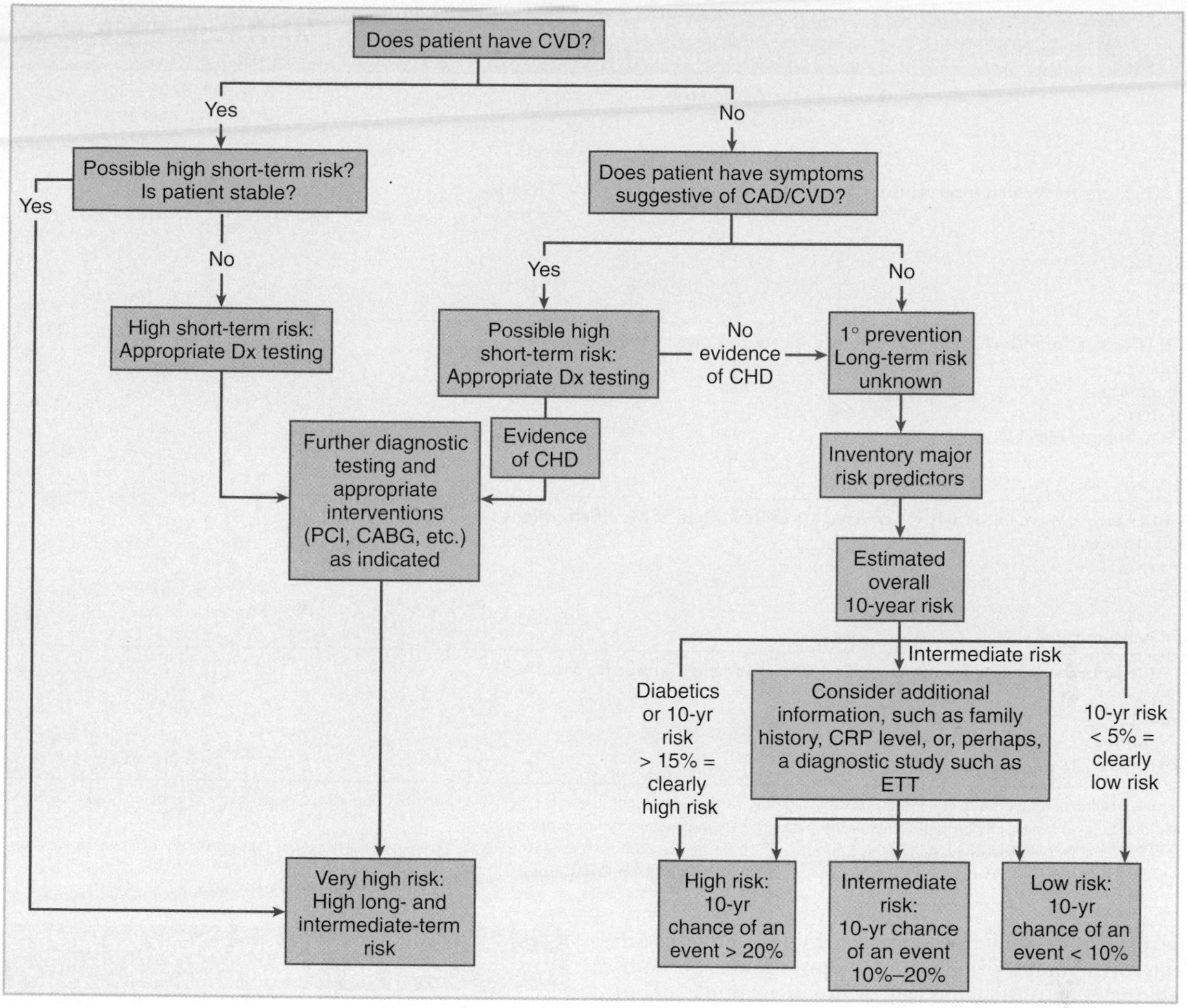

FIGURE 45–6 Cardiovascular disease risk assessment algorithm. By asking a few simple questions, clinicians can determine a patient's long-term risk of a coronary event. CABG = coronary artery bypass graft; CAD = coronary artery disease; CRP = C-reactive protein; CVD = cardiovascular disease; ETT = exercise tolerance test; PCI = percutaneous coronary intervention.

will be classified as high-risk primary prevention. Following the algorithm, patients without overt CVD or diabetes should be evaluated for overall 10-year risk of experiencing a cardiac event using a simple risk prediction tool such as the well-known Framingham Risk Score or another similar tool. Individuals with a very high Framingham Risk Score (20 percent or greater chance of a major CHD event in 10 years) also fall into the high-risk category. At the other end of the spectrum are those who have fewer than two risk factors or a Framingham 10-year risk score of less than 5 percent; they are solidly in the low-risk category. Again, following the algorithm, for those patients who fall into the intermediate-risk category or who are on the cusp between high and intermediate risk once the score is calculated (5 to 15 percent 10-year risk), the clinician may use additional information to stratify the patient better. Other clinical information can be used or the clinician may consider a secondary screen if there is some uncertainty about how aggressive to be with certain risk factor interventions. An inexpensive first step for such patients is measurement of CRP, whereas more expensive and complex options might include an exercise tolerance test (ETT) or electron beam CT to determine calcium score. (The American Heart Association [AHA] and USPSTF have approved the use of an ETT for preventive decision-making.) Each of these tests appears to add prognostic information to the Framingham Risk Score. CRP can be useful in this setting and will less likely result in intervention, the value of which in asymptomatic patients is unknown. The outcome of this process will refine the risk assessment and permit classification into the high-, intermediate-, or low-risk category. This classification of overall risk is helpful when making a decision about whether to intervene and in determining the intensity of the intervention (see later).

Lowering Risk: Interventions at an Individual and Population Level

Three complementary approaches may be used to reduce the population burden of cardiovascular disease: (1) therapeutic interventions for secondary prevention in patients with known cardiovascular disease; (2) identification and targeting of high-risk individuals for primary prevention through mass screening or case finding; and (3) general recommendations disseminated throughout the population. Each of these approaches has merit in different situations, depending on the cost-effectiveness of the intervention and on the overall risk-benefit ratio. For example, targeted interventions such as specialized cardiac rehabilitation and lifestyle programs have shown the greatest efficacy in motivated individuals who hope to avoid a recurrent myocardial infarction (secondary prevention), whereas mass screening

TABLE 45–2 Evidence Supporting Association of Risk Factors with Cardiovascular Disease, Usefulness of Measuring Them, and Responsiveness to Intervention

Risk Factor	Evidence for Association with CVD: *Epidemiological*	*Clinical Trials*	Clinical Measurement Useful?	Response to: *Nonpharmacological Therapy*	*Pharmacological Therapy*
Category I (Factors for Which Interventions Have Been Proved to Lower CVD Risk)					
Cigarette smoking	+++	++	+++	+++	++
LDL cholesterol	+++	+++	+++	+++	+++
High-fat/high-cholesterol diet	+++	++	++	++	–
Hypertension	+++	+++ (stroke)	+++	+	+++
Left ventricular hypertrophy	+++	+	++	–	++
Category II (Factors for Which Interventions Are Likely to Lower CVD Risk)					
Diabetes mellitus	+++	+	+++	++	+++
Physical inactivity	+++	++	++	++	–
HDL cholesterol	+++	+	+++	++	+
Triglycerides; small, dense LDL	++	++	+++	++	+++
Obesity	+++	–	+++	++	+
Postmenopausal status (women)	+++	–	+++	–	+++
Category III (Factors Associated with Increased CVD Risk That, if Modified, Might Lower CVD Risk)					
Psychosocial factors	++	+	+++	+	–
Lipoprotein(a)	+	–	+	–	+
Homocysteine	++	–	+	++	++
Oxidative stress	+	–	–	+	++
No alcohol consumption	+++	–	++	++	–
Category IV (Factors Associated with Increased CVD Risk but Cannot Be Modified)					
Age	+++	–	+++	–	–
Male gender	+++	–	+++	–	–
Low socioeconomic status	+++	–	++	–	–
Family history of early-onset CVD	+++	–	+++	–	–

+ = weak, somewhat consistent evidence; ++ = moderately strong, rather consistent evidence; +++ = very strong, consistent evidence; – = poor or nonexistent evidence; CVD = cardiovascular disease; HDL = high-density lipoprotein; LDL = low-density lipoprotein.

Modified from Pearson TA. McBride PE, Miller NH, Smith SC: 27th Bethesda Conference: Matching the intensity of risk factor management with the hazard for coronary disease events. Task Force 8. Organization of preventive cardiology service. J Am Coll Cardiol 27:1039, 1996.

programs for high blood pressure and hyperlipidemia are cost-effective (primary prevention). Population-wide campaigns against cigarette smoking offer an example of an effective public health approach. Implementation of the first two strategies requires risk assessment at the individual level, whereas the latter requires knowledge of risk at the population level.

If individuals can reduce their risk factor burden before age 50, they may substantially lower their lifetime risk of developing CVD. Framingham Heart Study participants who were free of CVD at 50 and free of any major risk factors had substantially lower lifetime risks (5.2 versus 68.9 percent for men and 8.2 versus 50.2 percent for women) and markedly longer median survival (more than 39 versus 28 years for men and more than 39 versus 31 years for women) than participants who had two or more major risk factors at 50.[16]

TABLE 45–3 Classification Scheme for Modifiable Risk Factors

Class	Definition
1	Basic research and human observational studies indicate a clear causal relationship. Intervention data (typically from randomized trials) demonstrate the magnitude of the benefit and risk. Interventions are cost-effective.
2	Basic research and human observational studies indicate a causal relationship. Intervention data from large-scale trials are limited. Lack of adequate intervention data precludes determination of cost-effectiveness.
3	Basic research and human observational studies demonstrate associations, but the independent nature of a causal relationship is not yet clear. Interventions are not yet available or have not been adequately tested.

Classification of Interventions for Modifiable Risk Factors

Because there are many potential targets for modification, implementation of a preventive strategy for a given patient requires a practical systematic approach to prioritizing interventions and allocating resources. A report from the American College of Cardiology's 27th Bethesda Conference has placed risk factors into four categories according to the likelihood that modification of the factor will result in lower risk.[17] These categories include the following: (1) factors for which interventions have been proved to reduce risk; (2) factors for which interventions are likely to lower the incidence of events; (3) factors clearly associated with CHD risk that, if modified, might lower the incidence of coronary events; and (4) factors associated with CHD risk that cannot be modified or, if modified, are not likely to decrease risk (Table 45-2). Adapting this useful classification scheme to clinical practice requires consideration of cost efficacy. We present a modified classification scheme of interventions for major modifiable risk factors based not only on the strength of the association and evidence of benefit of intervention but also on cost efficacy (Table 45-3).

CLASS 1. Class 1 risk factors have a clear causal relationship with heart disease (Table 45-4). Solid evidence, generally from randomized clinical trials, has demonstrated the magnitude of the benefit associated with intervention, as well as its risks and cost. Cigarette smoking, hypertension, and dyslipidemias are causally related to CHD, and the cor-

TABLE 45–4	Risk Factors and Interventions for Coronary Heart Disease	
Class	Risk Factor	Intervention
1	Smoking Dyslipidemia High blood pressure Preventive medications	Smoking cessation Lipid management Blood pressure management Aspirin, angiotensin-converting enzyme inhibitor, beta blocker
2	Diabetes, prediabetes Physical inactivity Overweight, obesity Unhealthy diet, alcohol	Diabetes management Activity management Weight management Improved diet
3	Menopause, hormone replacement therapy Micronutrients Psychological factors Novel biochemical and genetic markers	

responding interventions—smoking cessation, blood pressure management, and lipid profile management—all are cost-effective in both primary and secondary prevention. For management of hypertension and dyslipidemia, extensive trial and cost efficacy data enable a tiered approach based on absolute risk at baseline. Pharmacological approaches proven to be beneficial and cost-effective in specific situations for secondary prevention include aspirin, beta blockers, and angiotensin-converting enzyme (ACE) inhibitors, and aspirin for higher risk primary prevention.

CLASS 2. Class 2 includes risk factors for which the available evidence (largely basic research and human observational studies) has strongly indicated a causal relationship and suggested that intervention will probably reduce the incidence of events but for which evidence on the benefits, risks, and costs of intervention is limited. Class 2 risk factors that clearly increase the risk of CHD include diabetes and prediabetes, obesity, physical inactivity, and various dietary factors. Trial data on interventions in diabetes are forthcoming. However, data from large-scale, long-term randomized trials on weight management and physical activity with CHD outcomes will likely remain limited. Despite their limitations, class 2 interventions are useful in addressing global risk and have the potential to lower the risk of initial or recurrent CHD. Although it makes sense to invest more resources to modify these factors in individuals at highest risk, guidelines for class 2 interventions do not generally distinguish between high- and low-risk individuals.

CLASS 3. Class 3 risk factors and interventions are currently under active investigation. For many factors in this class, evidence is incomplete and an independent causal relationship with CHD cannot be inferred. For others in which evidence is promising, such as C-reactive protein, specific interventions are not yet available or widely tested, despite clear-cut relationships to risk. Thus, although these factors may be useful for risk assessment, their role in preventing CHD remains uncertain. For these reasons, hormone replacement therapy, dietary practices such as the consumption of nutritional supplements, psychological factors, and several novel biochemical and genetic markers are currently considered as class 3 factors. The identification of high risk may in and of itself provide motivation for better compliance with life-style modifications. For example, individuals with elevated levels of CRP may be more likely to comply with dietary advice and smoking cessation if they understand that they have an elevated cardiovascular risk.

The three following sections provide a summary of interventions followed by a summary of how to implement the specific strategies. The subsequent sections summarize the approach to intervention for each category of factors.

CLASS 1 INTERVENTIONS

In this category are the four primary interventions: smoking cessation, management of dyslipidemia, management of blood pressure, and prophylactic pharmacological interventions in selected patients. Each of these should be seriously considered in those with CVD and diabetes and, when appropriate, in primary prevention patients, and this consideration should be documented.

Cigarette Smoking and Cessation (see Chap. 39)

PREVALENCE. In the United States, per capita cigarette consumption rose dramatically in the first half of the 20th century. More than 65 percent of men born between 1911 and 1920 were smoking by 1945. Annual per capita consumption of cigarettes hit an astonishing 4286 (more than 200 packs/year) in 1963, but has since declined to 1875.[18] The prevalence of smoking among men peaked in 1955 when well over half were smokers; among women, that point came 10 years later, with more than one third smoking. Since then, smoking rates have declined substantially, with 21 percent of Americans smoking. Slightly more men than women are current smokers; approximately 23 percent of men aged 18 and older are smokers, as compared with 18 percent of women.[19] Smoking rates among high school seniors rose from 30 percent in the mid-1980s, with higher rates among females, to approximately 36.5 percent by 1997,[20] but now appear to be on a gradual downward trend. Smoking rates tend to be higher among those with lower socioeconomic status and those with a high school education or less.[21]

ASSOCIATED RISK. Smoking increases the risk of CHD (see Chap. 39). By the middle of the 20th century, seminal studies linking smoking and heart disease had been published. The Surgeon General's report in 1964 reaffirmed the epidemiological relationship between the two and, by 1983, the Surgeon General firmly established cigarette smoking as the leading avoidable cause of cardiovascular disease. The Surgeon General's 1989 report presented definitive data from observational case-control and cohort studies, largely among men, that demonstrated that smoking doubles the incidence of CHD and increases CHD mortality by 50 percent, and that these risks increase with age and the number of cigarettes smoked. Similar increases in the relative risk for CHD have been observed among women.

In the United States, cigarette smoking is the leading preventable cause of death and accounts for an estimated 438,000 deaths each year—35 percent of which result from cardiovascular disease—and more than 5 million years of potential life lost.[22] Worldwide, smoking rates continue to rise, with the greatest increases in the developing world; 1 million more deaths were attributable to tobacco in 2000 than in 1990.[23]

BENEFIT OF INTERVENTION. Although data from large-scale randomized trials concerning the risk reduction associated with smoking cessation are limited, observational studies have demonstrated clear benefits of smoking cessation. Smokers who quit reduce their excess risk of a coronary event by 50 percent in the first year or two after cessation, with much of this gain in the first few months. This period is followed by a more gradual decline, with the risk of former smokers approaching that of never-smokers after 3 to 5 years.

COST EFFICACY. Smoking cessation is highly cost-effective in both primary and secondary prevention. The intervention is usually short term and thus of low cost. In fact, smoking cessation programs generally cost less than continued smoking. The gains in life expectancy are large, and the earlier in life an individual stops smoking, the larger the potential gain; a 35-year-old male smoker may add 3 years to his life expectancy on cessation. Costs vary, depending on the intensity of intervention and the use of pharmacological agents. A Swedish study has found that over a 20-year period, the incremental costs per QALY saved were relatively low for bupropion in comparison to nicotine patches: approximately $660 per QALY gained for men and about $490 per QALY gained for women.[24] Several nonpharmacological approaches have also been found effective.

GUIDELINES AND RECOMMENDATIONS. Clinical practice guidelines from the U.S. Public Health Service recognize that tobacco dependence is a chronic condition that generally requires repeated intervention. They recommend asking patients about tobacco use at every visit, a strategy supported by the U.S. Preventive Services Task Force.[25] The Public Health Service guidelines support a combination of counseling and pharmacological therapy, when necessary. Three types of counseling and behavioral therapies appear to be particularly effective: (1) provision of problem-solving and skills training; (2) provision of social support in treatment; and (3) help securing social support outside of treatment. Six first-line pharmacotherapies that reliably increase long-term smoking abstinence were also identified. These are sustained-release bupropion hydrochloride, nicotine gum, nicotine patch, nicotine inhaler, nicotine nasal spray, and nicotine lozenge.

In view of the addictive nature of smoking and the tendency to increase smoking over time, smoking reduction, as opposed to smoking cessation, is not an acceptable strategy. The efficacy of smoking intervention programs ranges from a 6 percent 1-year success rate for physician counseling to 18 percent for self-help programs and 20 to 40 percent for cessation programs with pharmacological intervention with nicotine gum or patches.[26] Although it is important to counsel patients at all stages about the hazards of smoking and the benefits of quitting, the period soon after a cardiac event is an opportune time to encourage a patient to make an effort to stop smoking.

FUTURE CHALLENGES. In the United States, efforts aimed at cessation need to be maintained but, worldwide, intense public health efforts are needed to reverse the alarming rise in smoking rates occurring in many developing countries—nearly 60 percent of men in China now smoke. Approximately 82 percent of the 1.1 billion people who smoke worldwide reside in low- and middle-income countries.[27] The low rates of success in cessation efforts offer a challenge to clinicians, and greater emphasis must be placed on preventing smoking in the first place.

Hypercholesterolemia and Lipid Control (see also Chap. 42)

PREVALENCE. Mean cholesterol levels have declined modestly in the United States since the early 1960s.[21] Even with this decline, half of all American adults have cholesterol levels greater than 200 mg/dl, and 17 percent have cholesterol levels higher than 240 mg/dl.[21] Low HDL and high triglyceride levels tend to coincide and often result from metabolic phenomena distinct from those leading to high levels of LDL cholesterol. Thus, low HDL and high triglyceride levels can occur alone or in combination with high LDL levels.

ASSOCIATED RISK. Several cholesterol parameters are causally associated with an increased risk of CHD. A 1-mg/dl increase in the serum LDL cholesterol level is associated with a 2 to 3 percent increase in risk for CHD, and elevations earlier in life may be associated with higher increases in risk.[10] HDL cholesterol has emerged as an important independent predictor of CHD; every 1-mg/dl decrease in HDL cholesterol causes a 3 to 4 percent increase in coronary artery disease.[7] Furthermore, the ratio of total or LDL cholesterol to HDL cholesterol may predict CHD risk better than LDL alone. A 1-unit decrease in this ratio (which is easily achievable with statin drugs) reduces the risk of myocardial infarction by more than 50 percent. The TC/HDL ratio may be superior to the ratio of apolipoprotein (apo) A to apo B.[28] Non-HDL also predicts risk well; because non-HDL correlates highly with apo B, evaluation of this apolipoprotein seems unnecessary and cost-ineffective.

Imprecision in triglyceride measurements, intraindividual variability, diet dependence, and complex interactions between triglycerides and other lipid parameters may obscure the impact of triglycerides in the development of CHD. However, fasting triglyceride levels do correlate with CHD risk, particularly when HDL levels are considered.[29] This interdependence suggests that some triglyceride-rich lipoproteins are atherogenic. A number of studies have suggested that elevated triglycerides independently predict CHD risk.[10] The clinical usefulness of nonfasting triglyceride levels remains unclear.

BENEFIT OF INTERVENTION. Clear benefits have been demonstrated for dietary and pharmacological treatments that lower serum cholesterol (see Chap. 42). A number of completed large-scale primary and secondary prevention trials using 3-hydroxy-3-methylglutaryl coenzyme A reductase inhibitors (statins) have demonstrated significant reductions in CHD and stroke in various populations. These include patients with established CHD; those with coronary disease, other occlusive arterial disease, or diabetes but normal cholesterol levels; those without clinically evident atherosclerotic cardiovascular disease and average total and LDL cholesterol levels; elderly individuals at risk of vascular disease; and hypertensive patients with average or lower than average cholesterol levels. A 2005 meta-analysis of 14 randomized trials with 90,056 participants has shown that statin therapy can safely reduce the 5-year incidence of major coronary events, coronary revascularization, and stroke by about 20 percent per mmol/liter reduction in LDL level, irrespective of the pretreatment cholesterol level, age, gender, or preexisting disease and without any increases in cancer.[30] This reduction in risk is linear, resulting in comparable risk reductions across the spectrum of lipid levels (Fig. 45-7).

Long-term daily compliance appears to be far more important in determining outcome efficacy than any demonstrated differences between statins in terms of potency. A recent meta-analysis of four large randomized trials among those with existing disease has found that intensive therapy with high-dose statins has clear benefits over standard-dose therapy in reducing the risk of myocardial infarction, stroke, or any cardiovascular event.[31] Some,[32] but not all,[33] trial data support the early initiation of statin therapy following myocardial infarction or coronary artery bypass grafting.

Gemfibrozil, an agent that increases HDL and lowers triglyceride levels, reduces risk among those with high total and LDL cholesterol. In the Veterans Affairs High-Density Lipoprotein Cholesterol Intervention Trial (VA-HIT), a 22 percent reduction in cardiovascular events was observed with gemfibrozil treatment in a population with low HDL levels (less than 40 mg/dl [1 mmol/liter]).[34] This risk reduction occurred in the absence of any substantial change in

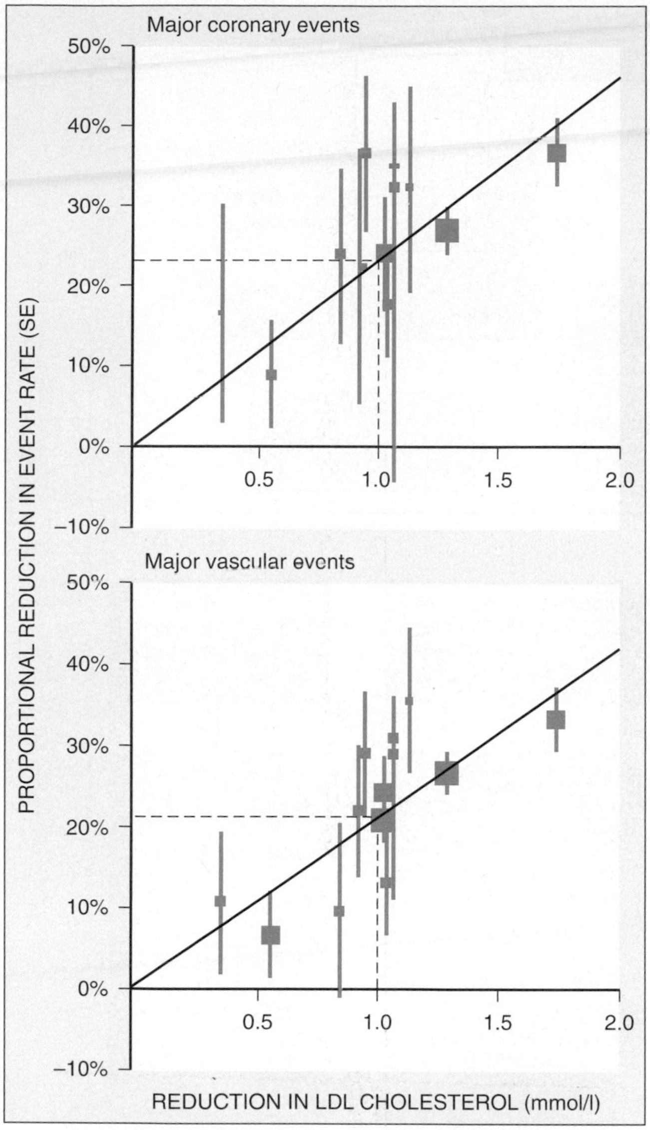

FIGURE 45–7 Graphic representation of meta-analysis demonstrating a linear relationship between the degree of lipid lowering and the degree of reduction in risk of coronary heart disease and cardiovascular disease. LDL = low-density lipoprotein; SE = standard error. *(From Baigent C, Keech A, Kearney PM, et al: Efficacy and safety of cholesterol-lowering treatment: Prospective meta-analysis of data from 90,056 participants in 14 randomised trials of statins. Lancet 366:1267, 2005.)*

LDL cholesterol, data that support the potential for agents targeted at HDL and triglyceride levels. Nicotinic acid can raise HDL levels and reduce CHD events (see Chap. 42). Another class of drugs with the potential to raise HDL levels is now in clinical development. Cholesteryl ester transfer protein (CETP) inhibitors have the potential to increase HDL levels substantially and modestly decrease LDL levels.[35] However, despite hopes that CETP inhibitors would benefit outcomes in conjunction with statins, the recent halt in development of one CETP inhibitor because of apparent hazards underscores the need for long-term clinical trial data in the realm of HDL intervention.[36]

COST EFFICACY. The cost efficacy of nonpharmacological interventions to lower LDL cholesterol is unclear (see Chap. 3). Pharmacological intervention, however, is clearly cost-effective under certain conditions, and available data permit tailoring recommendations to the level of baseline CHD risk. Early analyses of cholesterol reduction for secondary prevention, which used data from cholestyramine trials, have resulted in very costly interventions, largely because the available drugs were relatively ineffective. In contrast, data for statin therapy are remarkably consistent and, with the addition of two more generic statins in 2006, recent analyses have indicated that they may prove cost-effective for a larger number of individuals.

Before the introduction of any generic statins, Prosser and colleagues[37] applied data from several large-scale, long-term, randomized controlled trials of statins to the Coronary Heart Disease Policy. In primary prevention, statins failed to reach a cost-effectiveness ratio of $50,000 per QALY in any of the risk subgroups and ranged as high as $1.4 million per QALY. In secondary prevention, statin therapy was clearly cost-effective, ranging from $1800 per QALY for a man aged 45 to 54 years to $40,000 for a woman aged 35 to 44 years. Statin therapy is also effective and cost-effective for secondary prevention in patients 75 to 84 years of age.[37,38] All these QALY evaluations are highly sensitive to drug cost and can be expected to decline substantially as more statin agents transition into generic drugs. Simvastatin and pravastatin both became available as generics in 2006, joining lovastatin, which has been prescribed in generic form since 1999. A recent analysis has found that a daily dose of 40 mg of generic simvastatin would cost less than $1350/life-year gained for those with an annual risk of major vascular events of 1 percent or more, regardless of their age at the start of treatment.[39]

GUIDELINES AND TREATMENT. All patients with cardiovascular disease should be screened for serum cholesterol levels. In primary prevention, some controversy remains regarding screening. The NCEP recommends routine screening of all adults older than 20 years,[7] the American College of Physicians (ACP) recommends screening only men ages 35 to 65 and women ages 45 to 65,[40] and the USPSTF recommends screening all men aged 35 and older and all women aged 45 and older.[25] Screening of patients with cardiovascular disease should include a full fasting lipid profile, including total cholesterol, HDL, and triglyceride levels. For patients without cardiovascular disease, screening for HDL remains controversial, with the NCEP recommending for screening and the ACP recommending against it. Because HDL levels and the ratio of total cholesterol to HDL cholesterol powerfully predict risk and aid in the detection of individuals who have elevated LDL levels despite moderate levels of total cholesterol, it seems prudent to check HDL along with total cholesterol, although nonfasting levels are sufficient.

To reduce the prevalence of hyperlipidemia in the United States, the NCEP issued its first ATP report in 1988. The latest one was published in 2002,[7] although some elements were updated in 2004. Under the latest NCEP guidelines, the number of U.S. adults eligible for lipid modification has increased from 52 to 65 million for therapeutic life-style changes, and from approximately 13 to 36 million for drug therapy. The goals of intervention are based on the level of CHD risk for an individual (Fig. 45-8).

The updated ATP III guidelines recommend different therapeutic targets depending on a patient's overall risk, which includes calculation of his or her Framingham risk score and consideration of other markers of risk such as elevated triglyceride and CRP levels and family history. Patients with existing CHD (or a CHD risk equivalent, such as diabetes or peripheral vascular disease) are at the highest risk for a cardiovascular event and thus have the lowest LDL target (less than 100 mg/dl), with the option of setting the goal at less than 70 mg/dl for those who have had a recent acute coronary event or who have CVD combined with either diabetes or severe or poorly controlled risk factors (Table 45-5).

In 2006, the AHA/ACC (American Heart Association/American College of Cardiology) updated their secondary

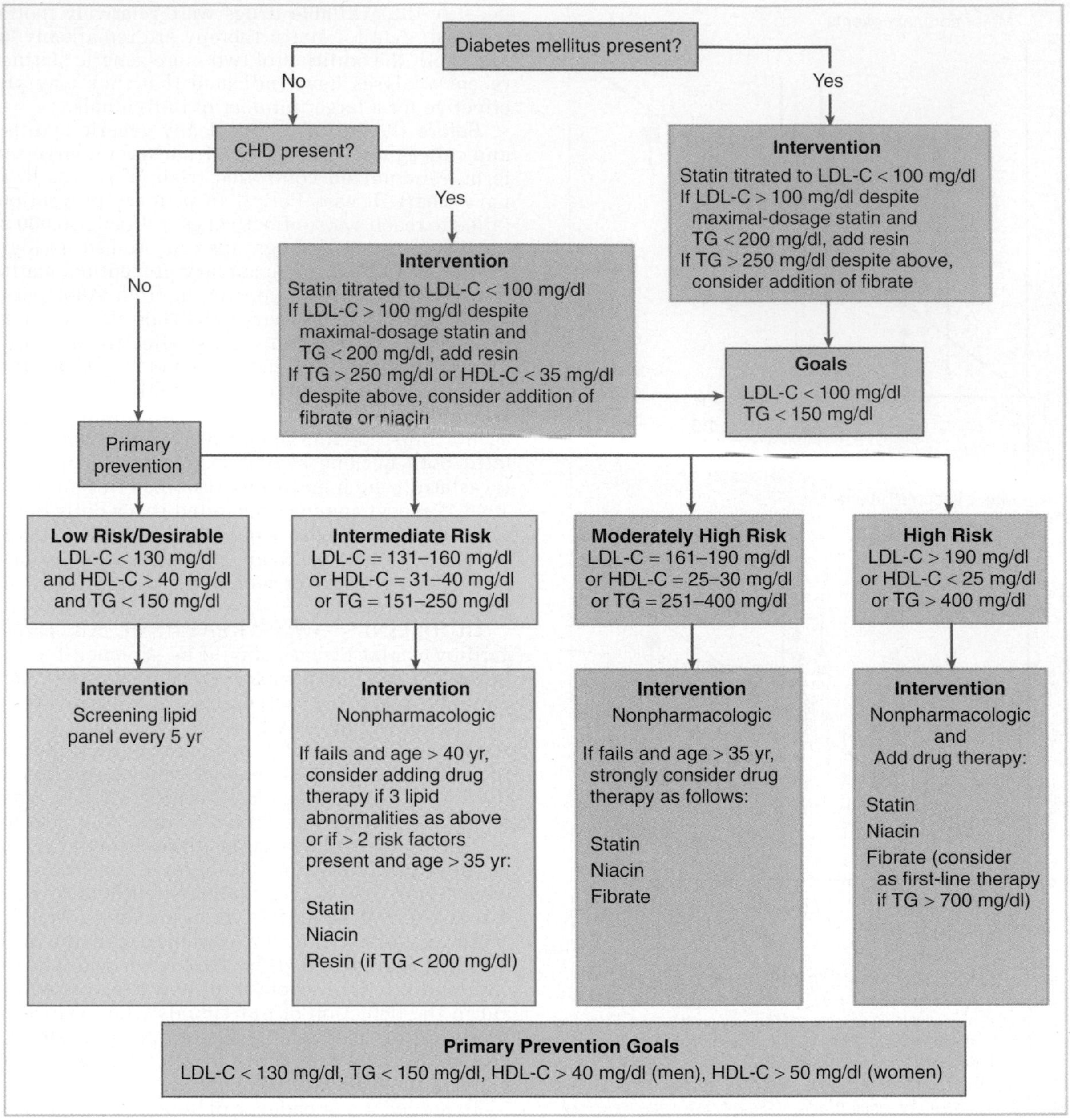

FIGURE 45–8 Algorithm for lipid-lowering therapy based on findings from intervention trials. CHD = coronary heart disease; HDL-C = high-density lipoprotein cholesterol; LDL-C = low-density lipoprotein cholesterol; TG = triglycerides. *(From Third Report of the National Cholesterol Education Program [NCEP] Expert Panel on Detection, Evaluation, and Treatment of High Blood Cholesterol in Adults [Adult Treatment Panel III]: Final report. Circulation 106:3143, 2002;* see also Chap. 42.*)*

TABLE 45–5 Low-Density Lipoprotein (LDL) Goals for Three Risk Levels

Risk Level	LDL Goal (mg/dl)
CHD and CHD risk equivalent*	<100
Multiple (2+) risk factors	<130†
0–1 risk factor	<160

*Diabetes, chronic kidney disease.

†LDL goal for individuals with multiple risk factors and a 10-yr overall risk >20% is <100 mg/dl.

CHD = coronary heart disease.

From Third Report of the National Cholesterol Education Program (NCEP) Expert Panel on Detection, Evaluation, and Treatment of High Blood Cholesterol in Adults (Adult Treatment Panel III) final report. Circulation 106:3143, 2002.

prevention guidelines for lipid management, echoing the recommendations made by the NCEP 2 years earlier and strengthening some of them. As with the NCEP guidelines, the LDL goal remains at less than 100 mg/dl, and less than 70 mg/dl has been added as an optional goal. However, the AHA/ACC extends the less than 70 mg/dl option to all patients with CAD, not just those at very high risk, a view that remains controversial.[41] Also, patients with a triglyceride level of 200 to 499 mg/dl should have a non-HDL cholesterol level less than 130 mg/dl, with a further reduction to less than 100 mg/dl considered reasonable.

According to the NCEP guidelines for primary prevention, patients at moderately high risk of developing CHD—two or more risk factors and a 10-year overall risk of 10 to 20 percent—should be treated to an LDL target less than 130 mg/dl or, optionally, to 100 mg/dl. This is also the target for patients with moderate risk, two or more risk factors, and a less than 10 percent risk for heart attack over the next 10 years. Those at even lower risk should be treated to a target LDL level less than 160 mg/dl. In addition, as part of its first-line therapeutic life-style changes, the NCEP recommends a diet that includes 25 to 35 percent of calories from fat, with saturated fat accounting for less than 7 percent of fat intake and cholesterol intake limited to less than 200 mg/day (see Chap. 44).

Because patients may find it difficult to understand percentage of calories, translating these guidelines into grams of fat, protein, and other dietary constituents may be helpful. Professional counseling with a dietitian may also be helpful. If dietary therapy does not achieve the target LDL level, drug therapy should be started (see Chap. 42). In all cases, drug therapy should be an adjunct to dietary therapy and increased physical activity.

Guidelines from the European Society of Cardiology (ESC) also have tiers.[42] Although the target is identical for all patients (total cholesterol of less than 190 mg/dl [5 mmol/liter] and LDL cholesterol of less than 115 mg/dl [3 mmol/liter]), the timing and intensity of drug therapy are different. In primary prevention, if the absolute 10-year risk of a CHD event or the projected risk at age 60 is 5 percent or greater, life-style modifications are recommended and lipid levels should be checked in 3 months. If the total or LDL cholesterol level is above target at this checkup, drug therapy may be instituted. For high-risk asymptomatic individuals whose total and LDL cholesterol levels are already close to the target levels (5 and 3 mmol/liter, respectively), the treatment goals are total cholesterol less than 4.5 mmol/liter (175 mg/dl) and LDL less than 2.5 mmol/liter (100 mg/dl). These goals are the same for those with established CVD and/or diabetes.

In secondary prevention, individuals with high LDL who also have low HDL or high triglyceride levels should be treated aggressively and consideration given to combination therapy (see Chap. 42). Furthermore, for those with known disease who have low HDL and normal LDL levels, consideration can be given to pharmacological intervention based on the results of VA-HIT. In primary prevention, nonpharmacological interventions are warranted for individuals who have a normal LDL but a low HDL and/or high triglyceride level, because trial data regarding drug therapy in such cases are insufficient. Intervention data regarding patients with isolated elevated triglyceride levels are needed.

FUTURE CHALLENGES. Given the linear relationship between level of cholesterol and risk and the similar linear relationship between lowering risk and change in total or LDL cholesterol level, more attention should be focused on change in LDL cholesterol level rather than on fixed targets. Additional randomized trial data are needed to clarify the role of cholesterol screening and the association between reducing serum cholesterol and stroke prevention. Although cholesterol levels are falling or stable in industrialized countries, they are rising in developing countries as Western diets are increasingly adopted. Low-cost plans for intervention in low- and middle-income countries need to be developed.

Hypertension and Blood Pressure Control (see Chap. 41)

PREVALENCE. As defined by JNC-7,[8] an estimated 65 million Americans are hypertensive and another 59 million fall into a new category termed *prehypertension* (Table 45-6).[21] High blood pressure is more common in blacks than whites and in men than women. The prevalence of hypertension increases with age, from 7 percent of those aged 18 to 39 years to 66 percent of those older than 60 years.[43] Data from the Framingham Heart Study have suggested that normotensive individuals at age 55 have a 90 percent lifetime risk for developing hypertension.[44] In the United States, hypertension prevalence appears to be increasing. Although control of hypertension improved throughout the 1990s, particularly among older patients, control rates remain low (30 percent).[45,46]

ASSOCIATED RISK. Studies have consistently demonstrated that elevated systolic or diastolic blood pressure is associated with an increased risk of CVD (see Chaps. 39 and 40).[5,47] A collaborative meta-analysis of individual participant data from 61 prospective observational studies with 1 million participants has shown a linear risk relationship between blood pressure and the risk of vascular mortality down to a pressure of at least 115/75 mm Hg throughout middle and old age.[47] Hypertension is also associated with increased risk of heart failure, stroke, and kidney disease. The shape of the cardiovascular disease risk curve is linear. For individuals aged 40 to 70 years, each increment of 20 mm Hg in systolic blood pressure or 10 mm Hg in diastolic blood pressure doubles the risk of cardiovascular disease across a blood pressure range from 115/75 to

TABLE 45–6 Classification and Management of Blood Pressure (BP) for Adults

			Management		
				Initial Drug Therapy	
BP Classification	Systolic BP (mm Hg)	Diastolic BP (mm Hg)	Lifestyle Modification	*Without Compelling Indication*	*With Compelling Indication*
Normal	<120	*and* <80	Encourage		
Prehypertension	120–139	*or* 80–89	Yes	None indicated	Drugs for compelling indications* (treat to BP target <130/80)
Stage 1 hypertension	140–159	*or* 90–99	Yes	Thiazide-type diuretics for most. May consider ACEI, ARB, BB, CCB, or combination	Drug(s) for compelling indications* Other antihypertensive drugs (diuretics, ACEI, ARB, BB, CCB) as needed
Stage 2 hypertension	≥160	*or* ≥100	Yes	Two-drug combination for most (usually thiazide-type diuretic and ACEI or ARB or BB or CCB)	

*Patients with chronic kidney disease or diabetes.

ACEI = angiotensin-converting enzyme inhibitor; ARB = angiotensin-receptor blocker; BB = beta blocker; BP = blood pressure; CCB = calcium channel blocker.

From Chobanian AV, Bakris GL, Black HR, et al: The Seventh Report of the Joint National Committee on Prevention, Detection, Evaluation, and Treatment of High Blood Pressure: The JNC 7 Report. JAMA 289:2560, 2003.

185/115 mm Hg. Systolic blood pressure remains the most useful clinical predictor of risk.

BENEFIT OF INTERVENTION. Since the late 1960s, a number of randomized trials have confirmed the protective effect of treating mild to moderate hypertension. Precise estimates of risk reduction have come from meta-analyses reporting that lowering diastolic blood pressure by 5 to 6 mm Hg results in a 42 percent reduction in the risk of stroke and a 15 percent reduction in the risk of CHD events.[48] The Antihypertensive and Lipid-Lowering Treatment to Prevent Heart Attack Trial (ALLHAT) has demonstrated the efficacy of thiazide diuretics compared with other antihypertensive agents.[49] Some of the benefit of the diuretics may have been a result of slightly better reduction in blood pressure.[50] ALLHAT was one of 29 randomized trials included in a 2003 meta-analysis that examined the effects of various blood pressure–lowering regimens on major CVD events. No significant differences were observed between treatment approaches based on ACE inhibitors, calcium antagonists, diuretics, or beta blockers, although ACE inhibitor–based regimens reduced blood pressure less. In addition, this study has demonstrated a linear relationship in that larger reductions in blood pressure produced larger reductions in risk.[51] Two antihypertensive agents will be needed for initial therapy for many patients, particularly those with more severe hypertension.

COST EFFICACY. Detection and management of hypertension are highly cost-effective in both primary and secondary prevention. However, more aggressive management in those at high risk due to the existence of cardiovascular disease or diabetes is warranted based on greater cost-effectiveness. In secondary prevention, for agents such as diuretics and beta blockers, the cost is below $10,000 per QALY for patients with established CHD, even when blood pressure is only mildly elevated.[52] In primary prevention, the cost ranges between $10,000 and $20,000 per QALY in individuals with moderate to severe elevations in blood pressure. However, the cost approaches an unacceptable range of $100,000 per QALY for higher priced medications. Cost-effectiveness decreases with increasing age. Given these issues, careful cost-effective evaluation is needed for recommendations from JNC-7, because this guideline suggests the use of multiple agents and favors intervention for a wider group of individuals, including those with minor elevations of blood pressure.

GUIDELINES AND TREATMENT. The U.S. Preventive Services Task Force (USPSTF) has recommended routine blood pressure testing of all adults.[53] The JNC-7[8] has defined four levels of blood pressure according to the risk imparted (see Table 45-6). Recommendations for intervention from the JNC-7 are based on the level of blood pressure and the level of absolute risk. The absolute risk strata are defined according to the presence or absence of target-organ disease, clinical cardiovascular disease, diabetes, and cardiovascular risk factors, such as smoking, hyperlipidemia, age older than 60 years, gender, and family history of early-onset cardiovascular disease. The JNC-7 has set a blood pressure goal of <140/90 mm Hg for lower risk patients and of <130/80 mm Hg for those with cardiovascular disease, diabetes, or chronic kidney disease. Because the relationship of blood pressure to risk of cardiovascular disease is linear, a significant portion of the population-attributable risk occurs in those with blood pressure in the JNC-7 category of prehypertension—a systolic blood pressure of 120 to 139 mm Hg or a diastolic pressure of 80 to 89 mm Hg.

For all individuals with blood pressure of 120/80 mm Hg or greater, JNC-7 recommends life-style modifications, including smoking cessation, weight reduction if needed, increased physical activity, limited alcohol intake, limited sodium intake, maintenance of adequate potassium and calcium intake, and adoption of the dietary approaches to stop hypertension (DASH) eating plan, a diet with a reduced content of saturated and total fats that is also rich in fruits, vegetables, and low-fat dairy products (see Chap. 44).[54]

Initiation of drug therapy depends on blood pressure and the absolute level of risk. For example, among individuals with stage 1 hypertension but no evidence of end-organ damage, vascular disease, or diabetes and one cardiovascular disease risk factor, life-style modification and drug therapy are recommended. For individuals with stage 2 hypertension, combination therapy that usually includes a thiazide-type diuretic is the starting point for therapy. The guidelines also recommend initiating therapy with two drugs, one of which is a diuretic, when blood pressure is more than 20/10 mm Hg above the target level. The specific therapeutic agents recommended by JNC-7 are discussed at length in Chapter 41. Most patients require more than one agent to achieve their blood pressure goal.

Guidelines from the European Society of Cardiology have stratified initial therapy somewhat differently. High-normal blood pressure is defined as systolic pressure between 130 and 139 mm Hg or diastolic pressure of 85 to 89 mm Hg, and drug therapy is only recommended for individuals in this category who are at very high risk because of a prior MI, TIA, or similar clinical condition.[55] Among patients with grade 1 (systolic pressure of 140 to 159 mm Hg or diastolic pressure of 90 to 99 mm Hg) or grade 2 hypertension (systolic pressure of 160 to 179 mm Hg or diastolic pressure of 100 to 109 mm Hg), drug treatment should be started promptly in those at high risk (three or more risk factors, target organ damage, or diabetes) or very high risk (obvious clinical disease). For patients in these two categories who are at moderate or low risk, life-style modification with monitoring for extended periods (at least 3 months) is recommended. If systolic values are still 140 mm Hg or above or diastolic values remain at 90 mm Hg or above, drug therapy should be initiated in patients at moderate risk and considered for those at lower risk. As with the JNC-7 recommendations, life-style modifications should always be used as an adjunct to drug therapy.

Data from ALLHAT have also indicated that a thiazide-type diuretic may be a good choice for first-line antihypertensive therapy.[49] For primary prevention, the use of beta blockers as a first-line therapy has come under scrutiny. The Anglo-Scandinavian Cardiac Outcomes Trial-Blood Pressure Lowering Arm (ASCOT-BPLA) trial assigned 19,257 hypertensive patients at moderate risk of developing CVD events to one of two regimens; (1) a beta blocker plus, if needed, a thiazide diuretic; or (2) a long-acting calcium channel blocker plus, when needed, an ACE inhibitor.[56] The trial was halted early as it became clear that those on beta blockers were becoming increasingly disadvantaged as time went on. A meta-analysis of 20 trials has concluded that beta blockers should not remain the first choice in treating primary hypertension.[57]

In 2006, the British Hypertension Society updated pharmacological treatment guidelines ahead of schedule to revise its previous recommendation concerning beta blockers as the preferred first-line therapy for hypertension.[58] The working group cited evidence that beta blockers do not work as well as other drugs, particularly in the elderly, and noted increasing evidence that the most frequently used beta blockers at usual doses carry an unacceptable risk of provoking type 2 diabetes. According to the new guidelines, for all patients 55 and over and black patients of any age, a calcium channel blocker or a thiazide-type diuretic is the first choice. If a second drug is required, an ACE inhibitor is preferred (or an angiotensin receptor blocker [ARB] if an ACE inhibitor is not tolerated). In patients younger than 55, the first-choice therapy should be an ACE inhibitor or ARB if needed. A calcium channel blocker or a thiazide-type diuretic should be added if another drug is required. Regardless of age, if three drugs are needed, the guidelines recommend a combination of an ACE inhibitor, a calcium channel blocker, and a thiazide-type diuretic.

FUTURE CHALLENGES. Just like cholesterol, the relationship between risk and increasing levels of blood pressure and risk reduction and degree of blood pressure lowering is linear. Thus, more attention should be focused on changing blood pressure rather than treating to a specific target. In the developed world, the prevalence of hypertension is increasing as populations age. Approximately 40 percent of those with hypertension do not know that they have this condition and are not being treated for it, and only one third of patients treated for hypertension have their blood pressure under control.[8] In developing countries, hypertension rates are rising rapidly with urbanization and changes in life-style habits. A new estimate of the attributable global burden of nonoptimal blood pressure (more than 115 mm Hg) has shown that overall approximately two thirds of the disease burden occurs in the developing world, and that worldwide roughly two thirds of this burden occurs in those 45 to 69 years old.[59]

Cardiac Protection with Aspirin and Other Pharmacological Agents

Several pharmacological interventions have proved highly effective in the prevention of cardiovascular disease. Pharmacological reduction of risk during or immediately after the development of CHD has been demonstrated for aspirin, beta blockers, and ACE inhibitors. Each of these agents has proven efficacy in intermediate and longer term secondary prevention among various subgroups of patients. Aspirin is also an effective primary prevention agent for some groups.

ANTIPLATELET THERAPY: SECONDARY PREVENTION. Aspirin therapy in patients with existing cardiovascular disease (see Chaps. 51, 53, and 54) reduces the risk of subsequent events by 25 percent. Meta-analyses have demonstrated clear reductions in mortality and nonfatal cardiovascular disease events among those with prior myocardial infarction, stroke, bypass surgery, angioplasty, peripheral vascular surgery, or angina.[60] In these meta-analyses, doses above 75 mg/day were shown to be clearly beneficial, with no trend toward increasing benefit at higher doses. In contrast, below 75 mg/day, there was a nonsignificant attenuated risk reduction of only 15 percent. However, the AHA/ACC has recently lowered the recommended prophylactic dose range from 75 to 325 mg/day to 75 to 162 mg/day, based on antiplatelet trials that have shown no difference in benefit with the lower dose but have shown a reduced risk of bleeding.[41] Other antiplatelet agents do not offer much over aspirin. In the Antiplatelet Trialists Collaboration (ATC) analysis, other agents did not offer superiority. Whether or not there is a modest benefit of clopidogrel over aspirin is not clear; despite randomized trials that included thousands of patients and data on comparative cost, efficacy is unclear. A recent trial comparing clopidogrel and aspirin versus aspirin alone in high-risk patients found that overall clopidogrel plus aspirin was not significantly more effective than aspirin alone in reducing the rate of MI, stroke, or death from CVD, but that dual antiplatelet therapy did increase the risk of moderate to severe bleeding.[61] Although evidence supports the addition of clopidogrel to aspirin in certain high-risk patients, such as those with acute ischemia or after stent placement, the increased bleeding risk makes this strategy unacceptable for primary prevention.

Unless contraindicated, aspirin should be used by most patients with known cardiovascular disease. Other antiplatelet agents with demonstrated efficacy, such as clopidogrel, should be limited to patients with aspirin allergy or intolerance. Clopidogrel has a much less favorable cost-effectiveness than aspirin, and the drug is associated with increased hemorrhage, so clopidogrel should not be used instead of aspirin in primary prevention. Data from the Coronary Heart Disease Policy Model have suggested that extending the use of aspirin therapy for secondary prevention from current levels to all eligible patients for 25 years would have an estimated cost-effectiveness ratio of about $11,000 per QALY gained. Clopidogrel alone in all patients or in routine combination with aspirin had an incremental cost of more than $130,000 per QALY gained.[62]

ASPIRIN IN PRIMARY PREVENTION. Six large-scale trials have assessed the benefits of low-dose aspirin in the prevention of cardiovascular disease. Three of the trials were limited to men and one was limited to women. Taken together, these studies have suggested a benefit of prophylactic aspirin in primary prevention of MI and ischemic stroke.[63] The Women's Health Study (WHS) addressed the benefit-to-risk ratio of aspirin therapy for primary prevention of CVD specifically in women. In that study, a 100-mg dose of aspirin every other day lowered the risk of stroke but did not affect the risk of myocardial infarction or death from other cardiovascular causes in this group of initially healthy women who were 45 or older.[64] However, among study participants 65 or older, the 100-mg alternate-day aspirin dose reduced the risk of major cardiovascular events by 26 percent. The WHS also looked at primary prevention using an aspirin dose below 75 mg, which produced a suboptimal effect. The nonsignificant 9 percent reduction in CVD events was consistent with the nonsignificant reduction of 13 percent in the secondary prevention meta-analysis for doses below 75 mg.[60]

In 2002, both the USPSTF[65] and AHA[66] concluded that aspirin decreases the incidence of CHD in adults at increased risk for heart disease. Among individuals with a 10-year risk of CHD of 6 percent or greater, the USPSTF determined that the benefits of taking aspirin outweigh the increased risk of gastrointestinal bleeding or hemorrhagic stroke. In 2004, the AHA offered more specific guidelines for women, recommending aspirin for women whose 10-year risk of a first coronary event exceeds 20 percent and a consideration for using it in women whose 10-year risk is between 10 and 20 percent. The ESC has recommended low-dose aspirin (75 mg) in primary prevention only for men at particularly high risk of CHD.[67]

BETA-ADRENERGIC RECEPTOR BLOCKERS. A number of trials have demonstrated the long-term efficacy of administration of beta-adrenergic receptor blocking agents (beta blockers) after myocardial infarction in reducing mortality, and meta-analyses have suggested a 23 percent mortality reduction with long-term use (see Chaps. 51, 52, and 54).[68] Long-term use of beta blockers also lowers the risk of recurrent cardiovascular events. Cross-trial comparisons have suggested that the higher the level of beta blockade, as measured by heart rate reduction relative to the control group, the greater the benefit. Beta blockade after myocardial infarction and in the setting of congestive heart failure is also extremely cost-effective. Data from the Coronary Heart Disease Policy Model have suggested that implementing beta blocker therapy in all first MI survivors annually over 20 years would prevent 62,000 myocardial infarctions and result in 72,000 fewer CHD deaths; the cost-effectiveness of beta blocker therapy would be less than $11,000 per QALY gained, even under unfavorable assumptions.[69] Beta blockers such as carvedilol and metoprolol have been shown to reduce mortality in those with CHF.

ANGIOTENSIN-CONVERTING ENZYME INHIBITORS. The benefit of ACE inhibitors in individuals at high risk for CHD events is substantial. Following myocardial infarction, the use of an ACE inhibitor is associated with a 7 percent reduction in mortality at 30 days.[70,71] Among individuals with a low ejection fraction after myocardial infarction, total mortality is reduced by 26 percent (see Chap. 51). A meta-analysis of six randomized, controlled trials has suggested that long-term ACE inhibitor therapy reduces the risk of major clinical outcomes by 22 percent.[72] Findings from the Heart Outcomes Prevention Evaluation (HOPE) study have suggested that the benefits of ACE inhibitors extend to those with clinical CHD and diabetes, even in the absence of left ventricular dysfunction.[73] Results from the Candesartan in Heart Failure Assessment of Reduction in Mortality and Morbidity (CHARM) trials have indicated that the use of an angiotensin receptor blocker such as candesartan among patients with heart failure can prevent 1 death for every 63 patients treated, prevent 1 first hospitalization with heart failure for every 23 patients treated, and prevent 1 new case of diabetes for every 71 patients treated.[74]

ORAL ANTICOAGULANTS. Oral anticoagulants (see Chaps. 35, 62, 72, and 82) prevent embolic events in patients with prosthetic heart valves and atrial fibrillation. Less certain is their role, either alone or in combination with aspirin, in the secondary prevention of events in those with CHD. The results of randomized controlled trials are inconsistent, a troubling issue because oral anticoagulants have significant bleeding as a side effect.

A 1999 meta-analysis has provided a comprehensive summary of data on high-, moderate-, and low-intensity oral anticoagulants alone or in combination with aspirin versus placebo or aspirin alone in those with cardiovascular disease.[75] In this analysis, high- and moderate-intensity oral anticoagulation reduced myocardial infarction and stroke rates when compared with placebo but increased the risk of hemorrhage. The combination of low-intensity oral anticoagulation plus aspirin did not appear to confer any benefit over aspirin alone, whereas the combination of moderate- or high-intensity oral anticoagulation plus aspirin did appear to offer promising benefits. However, a more recent analysis, including the results from newer trials (CHAMP, LoWASA, WARIS-II, and ASPECT-2), has concluded that moderate- to high-intensity anticoagulants should not be used routinely as an alternative or supplement to aspirin in high-risk acute coronary syndrome (ACS) patients because of the increased risk of bleeding.[76] Clinical trials comparing anticoagulants with clopidogrel alone or in combination with clopidogrel in ACS patients are needed.

RECOMMENDATIONS. Aspirin should be used for all patients with any form of known ischemic disease. Aspirin in combination with a second antiplatelet agent such as clopidogrel is used in acute settings and should be reserved for the highest risk patients. Beta blockers should be considered after myocardial infarction and in those with heart failure. ACE inhibitors are cost-effective and should be considered standard therapy in patients with a low ejection fraction and in other high-risk patients. All three agents are recommended for secondary prevention by the AHA, ACC, and ESC. The USPSTF has recommended aspirin as primary prevention for those with a 5-year cardiovascular disease risk of 3 percent or higher (equivalent to a 6 percent 10-year risk). Oral anticoagulants, although offering clear benefit in appropriate patients with atrial fibrillation (AF) and certain prosthetic valves, are not recommended for the general prevention of CHD events.

CLASS 2 INTERVENTIONS

Class 2 interventions relate to risk factors that appear to have strong causal associations with CHD risk and the form of CVD, and for which intervention has the potential to reduce risk but for which intervention data are limited (see Table 45-4). Factors in this category include diabetes, obesity, physical inactivity, and alcohol intake. In general, cost-effectiveness data are not available because of a lack of adequate intervention data.

Diabetes and Diabetes Control (see Chaps. 43 and 60)

PREVALENCE. In the United States, nearly 21 million people, 7 percent of the U.S. population, have diabetes mellitus; approximately 90 percent of cases are type 2 diabetes.[77] One third of people with diabetes are not aware that they have the disease. The prevalence of diabetes appears to have increased over the last decade, which may be a reflection of increasing body mass index (BMI). Another alarming trend is the recent increase in type 2 diabetes (formerly called *adult-onset diabetes*) among children, who account for more than 30 percent of new cases in some parts of the United States.[78,79] If current trends continue, more than one in three individuals born in 2000 will develop type 2 diabetes during their lifetime.[80]

ASSOCIATED RISK. Diabetes is a powerful risk factor for atherosclerotic disease, its complications, and cardiovascular disease–related mortality. By age 40, CHD is the leading cause of death in both diabetic men and women, with surveys showing heart disease listed on 69 percent of death certificates in a representative national cohort of adults with diabetes.[81] During 10 years of follow-up in the Health Professionals Follow-Up Study, the multivariate relative risks for fatal CHD were 3.84 (95 percent confidence interval [CI], 3.12 to 4.71) for those with diabetes only, 7.88 (95 percent CI, 6.86 to 9.05) for those with myocardial infarction only, and 13.41 (95 percent CI, 10.49 to 17.16) for those with both diabetes and myocardial infarction compared with those without diabetes or prior myocardial infarction at baseline.[82] Similar although not quite as pronounced associations were observed in women in the Nurses' Health Study over a 20-year period.[83] Diabetes has a stronger effect on the risk of CHD in women compared with men, with diabetic women facing a greater risk of CHD mortality.[84]

Evidence has indicated that individuals with diabetes but without established CHD have as high a risk for fatal CHD as those with established CHD but without diabetes.[85] However, this is subject to debate, with at least one study concluding that in men, established CHD signifies a higher risk for CHD mortality than diabetes, whereas in women, diabetes is associated with greater risk for CHD mortality.[84] The bottom line is that individuals with diabetes must be considered at high risk for CHD, regardless of the presence or absence of other risk factors and, furthermore, diabetic patients with well-controlled levels of hemoglobin A_{1c} (HbA_{1c}) appear to be at lower vascular risk than those with poor control.

BENEFITS OF TREATMENT. Maintaining normoglycemia may reduce the risk of microvascular (renal and eye) disease. However, data demonstrating reduced risk of CHD with tight glycemic control are scant. In the Diabetes Complications and Control Trial (DCCT), an apparent reduction in CHD events among patients with type 1 diabetes assigned to intensive therapy did not achieve statistical significance in an updated analysis, perhaps because of a relatively small number of events in this relatively young cohort.[86] In type 2 diabetes, although oral hypoglycemic agents and insulin can improve glycemic control, their role in the reduction of risk from macrovascular complications remains unclear. Although the ASCOT-BPLA and HOPE trials have suggested that ACE inhibitor therapy may reduce the onset of diabetes,[56,73,87] this was not confirmed in the prospective DREAM trial, which was designed to address this question directly.[88] On the other hand, the same trial found that rosiglitazone, a drug commonly used to treat type 2 diabetes, may delay the onset of frank diabetes, although the long-term benefits of this approach are unknown.[89]

Aggressive multifactorial interventions in diabetics appear to be effective in reducing CHD events. In a trial of 160 patients with type 2 diabetes and microalbuminuria who were allocated to conventional care or intensive therapy (life-style and pharmacological interventions intended to maintain glycated hemoglobin below 6.5 percent, total cholesterol below 175 mg/dl, triglycerides below 150 mg/dl, and blood pressure below 130/80 mm Hg), rates of incident cardiovascular events were reduced by more than 50 percent over an 8-year follow-up period (hazard ratio, 0.47; 95 percent CI, 0.24 to 0.73).[90] Given beneficial results in diabetic patients enrolled in cardiovascular event reduction trials of statins, aspirin, and ACE inhibitors, these data regarding the continued importance of life-style management are important. Improved screening must also be undertaken if the diabetic population is to benefit from these advances; in a study of Medicare beneficiaries with diabetes, half had not undergone lipid evaluation.[91] Most important with regard to cardiovascular disease, subgroup analyses of large placebo-controlled trials of cholesterol- and triglyceride-lowering therapy have indicated that those with diabetes benefit as much from these therapies as nondiabetics.[8]

GUIDELINES AND RECOMMENDATIONS. Diet and exercise are integral components of the treatment strategy for patients with diabetes. In many patients with type 2 diabetes, glycemic control can be achieved by modest weight loss through diet and exercise.

In contrast to patients with type 1 diabetes, those with type 2 diabetes are much more likely to have multiple coronary risk factors than is the case for the general population. Thus, aggressive modification of associated risk factors, including treatment of hypertension, aggressive reduction of serum cholesterol, reduction of weight, and increased physical activity, is of paramount importance in reducing the risk of CHD in people with diabetes.

Guidelines from the American Diabetes Association have recommended treating patients with diabetes and hypertension to a target blood pressure lower than 130/80 mm Hg. Individuals with borderline readings, up to 139 or 89 mm Hg, should receive life-style and behavioral therapy for 3 months. If the follow-up pressures are over 140 mm Hg systolic or 90 mm Hg diastolic, pharmacotherapy is recommended, with one of the medications being an ACE inhibitor or an ARB.[92] Current guidelines from the NCEP consider diabetes to be a CHD equivalent.[7] Thus, even for diabetic patients without previous CHD, the LDL cholesterol level goal is lower than 100 mg/dl.[9] Life-style changes should be attempted first and supplemented with a statin when necessary or if starting LDL levels are higher than 130 mg/dl. If the HDL level is less than 40 mg/dl, a fibrate may also be used. Initial therapy for hypertriglyceridemia is weight loss and improved glycemic control. Additional triglyceride lowering can be achieved with high-dose statins (for subjects with both high LDL and triglyceride levels), a fibrate, or niacin. Administration of a drug that inhibits intestinal absorption of cholesterol, such as ezetimibe, also appears to raise HDL,[93] although there are no event reduction data available for this agent, either in combination or as monotherapy. The American Diabetes Association has also recommended daily low-dose aspirin therapy for diabetics with evidence of large-vessel disease (e.g., those with a history of myocardial infarction, vascular bypass procedure, stroke or transient ischemic attack, peripheral vascular disease, claudication, and/or angina), as well as for those without evidence of CVD but who are over age 40 or at high risk for it based on cardiovascular risk factors, such as smoking, hypercholesterolemia, hypertension, or obesity.[94]

Prediabetes and Metabolic Syndrome

ASSOCIATED RISK. The *metabolic syndrome* is a cluster of metabolic abnormalities that includes insulin resistance, dyslipidemia, hypertension, a proinflammatory state, and excess weight, particularly abdominal adiposity (see Chaps. 39 and 43). The syndrome is common: approximately 27 percent of U.S. adults[95] and 10 percent of adolescents between 12 and 19[96] meet the criteria for metabolic syndrome. Individuals with metabolic syndrome are at increased risk for diabetes and cardiovascular disease and at increased risk of mortality from CVD. Not all patients with metabolic syndrome are at equal risk of developing type 2 diabetes or vascular events, and several studies have suggested that other factors such as inflammation can identify a subgroup of high-risk individuals.

BENEFITS OF TREATMENT. Two randomized clinical trials have demonstrated that patients with metabolic syndrome or impaired glucose tolerance benefit markedly from life-style interventions. In the Finnish Diabetes Prevention Study, 522 overweight individuals with impaired glucose tolerance either received no intervention or received individualized counseling with regard to reducing weight, total fat intake, and increasing physical activity. Over a 3.2-year follow-up period, weight loss was significantly greater in the active intervention group, and the incidence of type 2 diabetes was reduced from 23 to 11 percent, a risk reduction of almost 60 percent ($P < 0.001$).[97] Using this simple intervention, five subjects with impaired glucose tolerance treated for 5 years would prevent one case of type 2 diabetes. Further support for this hypothesis has been derived from the Diabetes Prevention Program, which randomly assigned 3234 nondiabetic American patients with abnormal glucose metabolism to placebo, metformin, or a life-style reduction program targeting weight loss and exercise.[98] In this trial, the life-style intervention reduced the incidence of type 2 diabetes by 58 percent as compared with placebo, whereas metformin reduced risk by 31 percent. Importantly, the life style–induced reduction was significantly greater than that achieved with pharmacological therapy.

Taken together, these two pivotal trials demonstrate that type 2 diabetes can be prevented or delayed, an effect that in turn will likely reduce atherosclerotic complications in this high-risk group. However, precise estimates for reduction in risk of cardiovascular disease events are unknown, and therefore cost-effectiveness data are not available.

Life-style intervention can have a large population impact. In a prospective study of women, more than 90 percent of all incident cases of diabetes occurred in those who failed to exercise, had a BMI greater than 25, smoked, or had poor dietary habits.[82] The impact of exercise cannot be underestimated, because nearly one third of all diabetic patients report a life-long pattern of minimal physical exertion.[99] Moreover, although a 2-hour postchallenge glucose measure provides improved sensitivity for risk detection in nondiabetic patients compared with fasting glucose levels, the clinical usefulness of this approach appears modest.[100]

RECOMMENDATIONS. Both the ATP III[7] and JNC-7[8] guidelines have addressed the metabolic syndrome. Patients are classified as having the metabolic syndrome if they have three or more of the following features:

- Waist size more than 40 inches for men, or more than 35 inches for women
- Blood pressure more than 135/85 mm Hg
- HDL level less than 40 mg/dl for men or 50 mg/dl for women
- Triglyceride levels more than 150 mg/dl
- Fasting blood sugar level more than 100 mg/dl

The main target of therapy is the underlying insulin-resistant state. The safest and most effective strategies for reducing insulin resistance include weight reduction in overweight and obese patients and increased physical activity. Although drugs that can improve insulin resistance are available, there is no clear evidence that they reduce CHD risk in patients with metabolic syndrome. Drug therapy to improve the lipid profile, lower blood pressure, and treat the prothrombotic state reduces cardiac risk in this population.[7]

Overweight, Obesity, and Weight Management (see Chaps. 39 and 44)

PREVALENCE. Over the past four decades, the proportion of the U.S. population considered to be overweight (BMI more than 25.0) and obese (BMI more than 30.0) has risen steadily (Fig. 45-9). In the National Health and Nutrition Examination Survey, NHANES (1960 to 1962), an estimated 31.6 percent of men and women met the definition for overweight (BMI of 25.0 to 29.9 kg/m^2), of whom 13.4 percent were obese (BMI more than 30 kg/m^2).[101] Today, nearly two out of three Americans are overweight or obese,[102] with the 1999 to 2000 NHANES showing 64.5 percent of men and women classified as overweight, of whom 30.5 percent were obese.[103]

The prevalence of overweight and obesity in children and adolescents is rising, paralleling that in adults. An estimated 15 percent of those aged 6 to 19 years and 10.4 percent of those aged 2 to 5 years are considered overweight or obese,[103] an alarming trend, because early obesity strongly predicts later cardiovascular disease. Of considerable concern, excess weight may explain the surprising and dramatic increases in type 2 diabetes in children. In some parts of the United States, more than 30 percent of new cases of type 2 diabetes are in children, and most of these are attributable to obesity.[78,79]

ASSOCIATED RISK. Obesity and overweight are strongly associated with the risk of CHD as well as stroke. Because various measures have been used to define overweight and obesity, reports on the magnitude of their association with CHD are not entirely consistent. Whether excess weight is an independent risk factor for CHD is disputed because its impact on CHD risk may be mediated, at least in part, by other coronary risk factors, such as hypertension, dyslipidemia, glucose intolerance, and inflammatory and hemostatic factors. However, given its strong association with CVD, obesity is an important and easily assessed marker of risk.

Data from numerous cohort and metabolic studies provide consistent evidence linking excess weight and inactivity with impaired health. A recent long-term study of women has looked at the relative importance of obesity and physical activity as predictors of CHD risk. Although BMI, waist-to-hip ratio, and physical inactivity all independently contributed to development of CHD, the study found that obesity confers a greater level of risk than physical inactivity over a 20-year period.[104] Excess weight increases the risk of metabolic disorders such as hypertension, dyslipidemia, insulin resistance, and glucose intolerance. For example, in the Marks and Spencer Cardiovascular Risk Factor Study of 14,077 middle-aged women, highly significant age-adjusted differences were observed across seven categories of BMI (less than 20 to more than 30 kg/m^2) for systolic and diastolic blood pressure, serum total cholesterol, LDL cholesterol, HDL cholesterol, triglycerides, apo A-1, apo B, and fasting blood glucose levels.[105] Excess weight is associated with increases in inflammatory markers such as C-reactive protein and fibrinogen in adults and children, increases that have been associated with elevated risks of cardiovascular disease. Excess weight is also strongly linked to increased risk of CHD, ischemic stroke, type 2 diabetes, and a host of other chronic conditions. The distribution of body fat may also play a role in the development of CHD, with abdominal adiposity posing a substantially greater risk in women and men. A waist circumference more than 35 inches in women and more than 40 inches in men is an easily measured marker of increased CHD risk. Whereas distribution of weight assessed by waist circumference, waist-to-hip ratio, or even CT or MRI scanning adds marginal predictive value, BMI remains the most useful and readily obtained measurement for assessing this metabolic parameter.

Excess weight has enormous personal and economic burdens. Estimates from six large prospective cohorts have suggested that excess weight accounts for an estimated 280,000 to 320,000 deaths a year in the United States, more than 80 percent of which occur among individuals with BMI greater than 30 kg/m^2.[106] Data from a national survey of almost 10,000 U.S. adults have suggested that obesity is associated with more chronic disorders and poorer health-related quality of life than smoking or problem drinking.[107] Medical spending for weight-related conditions accounted for an estimated 9 percent of the total annual U.S. medical expenses in 1998, or $78 billion,[108] an amount that rivals expenditures on smoking-related conditions. A study that examined the impact of weight gain per se in initially overweight men and women between 35 and 65 years old found that the 3-year increase in health care costs was $561 greater for individuals who gained 20 pounds or more during this period than for their weight-stable counterparts.[109]

BENEFITS OF INTERVENTION. No large-scale randomized trials of weight reduction as an isolated intervention are available on which to estimate the benefits of weight loss in lowering risk of CHD. However, sufficient information is available from numerous observational studies and small or short-term randomized clinical trials[110,111] to conclude that weight loss offers substantial health benefits (Table 45-7). Modest weight loss, about 5 to 10 percent, is associated with a significant improvement in blood pressure in individuals with and without hypertension.[110] Modest weight loss improves the lipoprotein profile, yielding lower levels of serum triglycerides, higher levels of HDL cholesterol, and small reductions in total and LDL cholesterol, as well as improvements in glucose tolerance and/or insulin resistance.[110] Weight loss also helps relieve sleep apnea[112] (see Chap. 74).

There is little consensus, however, on the ideal approach to weight reduction. Promoting life-style changes to encourage weight reduction has been disappointing. Although 25 percent of American men and 43 percent of American women may attempt to lose weight in any given year, failure rates are exceedingly high. One reason may be that most individuals who are

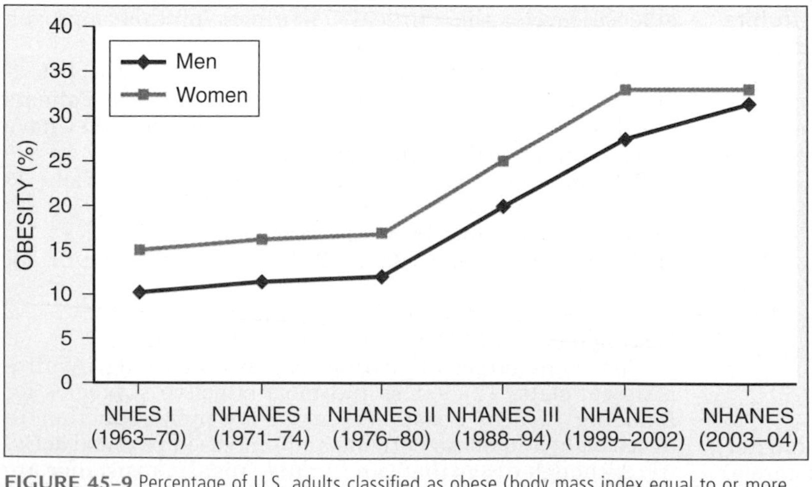

FIGURE 45–9 Percentage of U.S. adults classified as obese (body mass index equal to or more than 30 kg/m^2) in health surveys from 1963 to 2004. NHES = National Health Examination Survey; NHANES = National Health and Nutrition Examination Survey. *(Data from Flegal KM, Carroll MD, Ogden CL, Johnson CL: Prevalence and trends in obesity among U.S. adults, 1999-2000. JAMA 288:1723, 2002; and Ogden CL, Carroll MD, Curtin LR, et al: Prevalence of overweight and obesity in the United States, 1999-2004. JAMA 295:1549, 2006.)*

TABLE 45-7	Weight Loss and Physical Activity Benefits for Those Overweight or Obese (or with Insufficient Daily Activity)	
Disease/Risk Factor	**Weight Loss**	**Physical Activity**
Hypertension	↓↓↓	↓↓↓
Type 2 diabetes mellitus	↓↓↓	↓↓
Lipid profile	Definite improvement	Definite improvement
Coronary heart disease	↓↓	↓↓↓
Stroke	↓	↓↓
Colorectal cancer	↓	↓↓
Breast cancer	↓	↓
Osteoarthritis	↓↓	↓
Osteoporosis	→	↓↓↓
Gallbladder disease	↓	↓
Sleep apnea	↓↓	Unknown
Mental health	Probable improvement	Probable improvement

↓↓↓ = strong decrease in risk; ↓↓ = moderate decrease in risk; ↓ = slight decrease in risk; → = no benefit.

From Manson JE, Skerrett PJ, Greenland P, VanItallie TB: The escalating pandemics of obesity and sedentary lifestyle: A call to action for clinicians. Arch Intern Med 164:249, 2004.

trying to lose weight are not following recommendations to reduce calorie intake and engage in at least 150 minutes of leisure time activity per week. Effective treatment strategies generally involve a multifaceted approach, including dietary counseling, behavioral modification, increased physical activity, and psychosocial support. Recent observational studies and clinical trials have suggested that pharmacotherapy and bariatric surgery may hold some promise in promoting weight loss, but long-term success and long-term risks, as well as cost-effectiveness, have not been fully evaluated.[113]

COST-EFFECTIVENESS. Without precise estimates of the benefit and with substantial variability in intervention strategies, it is currently impossible to estimate the cost-benefit ratio of weight loss programs or interventions.

RECOMMENDATIONS AND GUIDELINES. Numerous options are available for helping patients lose weight. Guidelines produced by the National Heart, Lung, and Blood Institute and the North American Association for the Study of Obesity[110,114] emphasize a three-part strategy for weight loss that includes calorie restriction, structured physical activity, and behavioral therapy for all patients with a BMI greater than 30 kg/m^2 and those with a BMI of 25.0 to 29.9 kg/m^2 and a history of CHD or two or more disease risk factors (see later for discussions of interventions for specific physical activity and diet recommendations). Pharmacotherapy may be appropriate for some individuals, and bariatric surgery can be considered for morbidly obese patients.

Physical Inactivity and Exercise (see Chaps. 39, 46, and 78)

PREVALENCE. Physical inactivity is one of the most common modifiable risk factors for CHD. Data from the National Health Interview Survey have suggested that 70 percent of U.S. adults do not meet the current recommendation of 30 minutes of light to moderate physical activity at least 5 days a week or vigorous activity for at least 20 minutes on 5 or more days of the week.[21] Nearly 25 percent do not engage in any leisure time physical activity at all,[21] with women being more sedentary than men. Lack of sufficient physical activity is also endemic among children. Only a minority of schoolchildren have daily physical education classes,[115,116] and walking and bicycling by children has declined. In contrast, the time spent in sedentary activities such as watching television, playing video games, or using a computer has dramatically increased. Older individuals, who are most at risk for cardiovascular disease, are less likely to be physically active than younger individuals, and women tend to be less active than men. Each of these demographic changes has led to an increase in childhood diabetes, so that type 2 diabetes can no longer be called adult-onset diabetes.

ASSOCIATED RISK. Data from more than 40 observational studies have demonstrated clear evidence of an inverse linear dose-response relationship between physical activity and all-cause mortality rates in younger and older men and women. Data available in the mid-1950s showed that CHD rates were lower in bus conductors and mail carriers than sedentary bus drivers and postal supervisors. By incorporating estimates of leisure time activity in their analyses, these investigators found that civil servants with sedentary jobs who engaged in vigorous sports were half as likely to suffer myocardial infarction as those who did not engage in such activities. Since then, a number of observational studies have reported similar inverse associations between activity level from work or play and CHD. Minimal adherence to current physical activity guidelines, which yield an energy expenditure of about 1000 kcal/week, is associated with a significant 20 to 30 percent reduction in risk of all-cause mortality.[117] A 1990 meta-analysis of 27 observational cohort studies has demonstrated that the risk of CHD in sedentary individuals is almost twice that of active individuals after controlling for other coronary risk factors. Long-term prospective studies of men and women have consistently shown that regular physical activity protects against death from CHD. These benefits apply to activities as simple as brisk walking, which has been shown to reduce the risk of CHD in women[118] and men,[72] as well as the risk of type 2 diabetes.[119] Shifting even late in life from a sedentary life style to a more active one confers a reduction in mortality from CHD.[120,121] Physical activity is also associated with a decreased risk of stroke in men[122] and women,[123] primarily because of its beneficial effects on body weight, blood pressure, serum cholesterol level, and glucose tolerance.

Although no large-scale randomized trials of physical activity are available, numerous trials of moderate size and duration have been conducted in healthy individuals, those at high risk for cardiovascular disease, and those with existing cardiovascular disease. Despite differences in design, these trials have generally demonstrated a cardiovascular benefit. The ideal intensity, frequency, and duration of physical activity, however, have still not been determined.

BENEFIT OF INTERVENTION. Whereas cessation of activity appears to result in increased risk of CHD, the lack of large-scale, randomized, primary prevention trials on the benefits of physical activity makes it difficult to determine the precise magnitude of benefit of exercise in terms of CHD reduction. Physical activity does, however, have clearly demonstrated benefits on cardiovascular risk factors. Exercise increases HDL levels, reduces LDL and triglyceride levels, increases insulin sensitivity, and reduces blood pressure in hypertensive and normotensive individuals. Exercise also improves endothelial function and reduces CRP levels.

In secondary prevention, cardiac rehabilitation programs with an exercise component tend to report benefit in reducing subsequent events. Pooled data from many of these trials have suggested reductions in total and cardiovascular mortality of about 25 percent.[124]

GUIDELINES AND TREATMENT. The American Heart Association has recently issued revised diet and life-style recommendations that offer guidance for anyone over the age of 2, with or without CVD.[125] The recommendations call for 30 minutes or more of physical activity most days of the week, even if it is broken up into smaller increments. In addition, the AHA suggests that Americans need to focus on reducing sedentary activities, such as watching TV and surfing the Web, and instead make "daily choices to move rather than be moved." Previously issued guidelines from the AHA/ACC for secondary prevention have also encouraged patients to be physically active. An exercise prescription might include walking, jogging, cycling, swimming, or other aerobic activity for 30 to 60 minutes on most days of the week, supplemented with an increase in daily life-style activities such as walking up stairs when possible, instead of taking the elevator or using an escalator. Strength training may offer additional cardiovascular and other benefits. Structured exercise programs may enhance long-term compliance. For primary prevention, the U.S. Surgeon General's recommendation is an excellent starting point—every adult should engage in 30 minutes of moderately intense physical activity on most, if not all, days of the week, and more activity if weight loss is desired.[126]

From a practical standpoint, advice on physical activity should begin with an assessment of a patient's current activities, including physical activity at work and during leisure time. If the assessment indicates that activity is less than optimal, an evaluation of the barriers in the way of a good activity life style should be carried out. Common potential barriers include lack of time, energy, and desire and a safe, convenient place to exercise. Other barriers include medical conditions such as osteoarthritis or other physical conditions, such as prior stroke. Patients should be empowered to overcome these barriers. This should be followed by advice to add calorie expenditure to everyday activities, such as walking instead of driving. Advice from a physician should include gradual increase in leisure activity up to 30 or more minutes per day. Also, intensity of exercise should be discussed with those who have made a commitment to the recommended 30 minutes of exercise or more per day.

Diet and Moderate Alcohol Consumption

Diet (see Chap. 44)

Diet has an important impact on CHD risk. Cross-cultural studies have suggested that diet plays a role in CHD as well as other chronic diseases. For example, the Ni-Hon-San study has indicated that Japanese immigrants who moved to Hawaii and California develop CHD and ischemic stroke at rates comparable to lifetime residents of the United States. However, understanding the specific components of the Western diet that impart this risk has been challenging. Dietary research is hampered by the difficulty of measuring dietary components. Nonetheless, several dietary factors have been well studied. In this section, we discuss macronutrients (fats, carbohydrates, and protein sources), as well as alcohol. Supplements, nutraceuticals, and specific foods are discussed later (see "Class 3 Interventions").

OBSERVATIONAL STUDIES. Observational studies have suggested a number of dietary factors that may influence the risk of CHD. One of the key features of the Western life style is an excess of caloric intake relative to caloric expenditure. One of the most consistent findings in observational dietary research is that individuals who consume higher amounts of fruits and vegetables have lower rates of heart disease[127] and stroke.[128] Other components of the Western diet that may increase the risk of CHD include saturated and trans fats, simple carbohydrates that represent a higher glycemic load, and lack of fiber.

Metabolic Trials. Metabolic trials have suggested that diet is an important component of any prevention program. Diet can have a profound effect on weight reduction, which can improve dyslipidemia, hypertension, and diabetes. Even without weight loss, a healthy diet can improve the lipid profile and deliver nutrients that have salutary effects on the cardiovascular system. In the DASH trial, 459 adults with systolic blood pressure lower than 160 mm Hg and diastolic pressure lower than 80 to 95 mm Hg were randomized to one of the following: (1) a control diet low in fruits, vegetables, and dairy products and with a fat content of 37 percent; (2) a diet rich in fruits and vegetables; or (3) a combination diet rich in fruits, vegetables, and low-fat dairy products. Both of the intervention diets substantially reduced systolic and diastolic blood pressure in individuals with and without hypertension.[54]

A review of data from 147 metabolic studies, prospective cohort studies, and clinical trials has suggested that at least three dietary strategies are effective in preventing CHD.[129] These include substituting nonhydrogenated unsaturated fats for saturated and trans fats; increasing consumption of omega-3 fatty acids from fish, fish oil supplements, or plant sources; and adhering to a diet high in fruits, vegetables, nuts, and whole grains and low in refined grain products.

Diet Trials with Coronary Heart Disease Endpoints. Trial data exploring the impact of dietary changes alone on CHD events are very limited. The Lyon Diet Heart Study randomized 605 survivors of a first myocardial infarction to a Mediterranean-type diet or a "prudent Western-type diet." After a mean follow-up of 46 months, the risk of cardiac death or acute myocardial infarction was 65 percent lower for those consuming the Mediterranean diet.[130]

DIETARY RECOMMENDATIONS. Given limited trial data, it is difficult to answer the patient's question, "What should I eat to prevent heart disease?" However, based on observational studies, patients should be advised of some general principles that consistently emerge from the data. To help patients understand these general recommendations, a simple set of rules can be the basis for an improved diet:

- Total caloric intake must be balanced with energy expenditure. If weight reduction is desired, the balance must be fewer calories in than out.
- Simple carbohydrates (sugars and starches) that have a high glycemic load should be avoided in favor of carbohydrate sources that are high in fiber (e.g., whole wheat products, beans) to delay the absorption of sugars and reduce the insulin response.
- Maximize fruit and vegetable intake. The U.S. Department of Agriculture recommends 1 to 2.5 cups of fruit and 1 to 4 cups of vegetables per day.
- Minimize intake of saturated and trans fats. Instead, select monounsaturated and polyunsaturated fats and whole grains. Adequate intake of omega-3 fatty acids also appears to reduce the incidence of cardiovascular disease and especially sudden cardiac death.[131] Inclusion of two or three servings of fish per week (particularly fatty fish) may help prevent cardiovascular events.
- Protein sources that are low in saturated or trans fats should replace those high in these harmful fats.

Added salt should be limited, particularly for those whose blood pressure seems to be more responsive to salt restriction.

Alcohol

Alcohol consumption has complex effects on cardiovascular disease. Observational studies have demonstrated that heavy alcohol intake increases total mortality and cardiovascular disease mortality. In contrast, more than 100 prospective studies have shown an inverse association between light to moderate drinking and risk of heart attack, ischemic stroke, peripheral vascular disease, sudden cardiac death, and death from all cardiovascular causes.[132] The effect is relatively consistent, corresponding to a 20 to 45 percent reduction in risk. Moderate alcohol consumption is associated with decreased cardiovascular risk with regard to primary and secondary prevention and among men and women. Mechanisms underlying the effect of moderate alcohol consumption, defined as one or two drinks daily, include raising HDL levels, improving fibrinolytic capacity, and reducing platelet aggregation and CRP levels.[133] Trials have clearly demonstrated the protective effect of alcohol on HDL. Although some have suggested unique cardioprotective properties associated with red wine consumption, most studies have found equal benefits for all forms of alcohol when consumed in moderation.

RECOMMENDATIONS (see also Chap. 68). Although the association of alcohol and reduced risk for CHD is likely to be causal, any individual or public health recommendation must consider the complexity of alcohol's metabolic, physiological, and psychological effects. With alcohol, the difference between daily intake of small to moderate and large quantities may be the difference between preventing and causing disease. All patients should be counseled to avoid excessive alcohol consumption. For appropriate patients, a discussion of alcohol intake can be part of routine preventive counseling. In general, one or two drinks per day may be safe for men. For women, because of their generally smaller lean body mass and potential differences in liver metabolism, lower levels may be more prudent. However, counseling must be individualized; other medical problems, including other coronary risk factors (particularly hypertension and diabetes), liver disease, tendency toward excess use, family history of alcoholism, and possibly a family history of breast and colon cancer, should be taken into account when discussing alcohol consumption.

CLASS 3 INTERVENTIONS

Class 3 interventions relate to risk factors that are currently under investigation (see Table 45-4) but are not ready for clinical practice. For some of them, a causal relationship with CHD cannot be determined because of limited data. For others, in which causal relationships are apparent, interventions are not yet available or tested. Clinicians need to be prepared to discuss these factors with their patients—they often come up in conversation, because they are areas of active research and often receive considerable media attention.

Menopause and Postmenopausal Estrogen Therapy (see Chap. 76)

RISK ASSOCIATED WITH MENOPAUSE. Before age 45, cardiovascular disease afflicts relatively few women in the United States and other developed countries. By age 60, however, it is the leading cause of death in women.[134] Although men exhibit a higher incidence of CHD at every age, as well as higher mortality rates from it, the gap narrows substantially after natural menopause and bilateral oophorectomy.

A wide range of factors may explain the increased risk of CHD after menopause. These include adverse changes in lipid and glucose metabolism that result in an increase in LDL cholesterol and a decrease in HDL cholesterol levels, an increase in glucose intolerance, and changes in hemostatic factors and vascular function. These changes have long been attributed to the decline in endogenous estrogen that accompanies menopause.

Considerable evidence from observational studies had suggested that the use of postmenopausal hormone therapy reduces the risk of CHD. A meta-analysis of 40 cohort and case-control studies has suggested a 50 percent reduction in the risk of CHD associated with current estrogen use.[135] In an early analysis from the Nurses' Health Study, one of the largest prospective cohort studies to address this question, current users of estrogen had about half the risk of CHD (relative risk, 0.51; 95 percent CI, 0.37 to 0.70) as nonusers. Such data, together with the known favorable effects of oral estrogen on the lipid profile, have provided the foundation for widespread use of postmenopausal hormone therapy to prevent cardiovascular disease.

EFFECTS OF HORMONE REPLACEMENT. Physiological effects of exogenous estrogen are consistent with a cardioprotective effect. Estrogen reduces LDL and increases HDL levels; reduces Lp(a) lipoprotein, plasminogen-activator inhibitor type 1, and insulin levels; inhibits oxidation of LDL; and improves endothelial vascular function. The effects of estrogen on inflammation are complex, because levels of fibrinogen decrease but levels of CRP increase. Many of these effects are pronounced with oral estrogen and minimal when estrogen is given transdermally, suggesting a first-pass effect. Estrogen may also improve glucose tolerance.

Despite observational data and physiological data suggesting benefits of HRT, data from at least seven recent randomized trials (five on secondary prevention and two on primary prevention) have not only failed to support a possible benefit of hormone therapy for CHD but indicate that combined estrogen and progestin may actually *increase* CHD risk.[136] This abrupt about-face with regard to the possible benefits of hormone therapy illustrates the problem of uncontrolled confounding in observational cohort studies and the importance of randomized, controlled trials. Emerging evidence has indicated that age and time since menopause may also modulate the effect of estrogen on cardiovascular risk.

The first secondary prevention trial, the Heart and Estrogen/Progestin Replacement Study (HERS), found no cardiovascular benefit of estrogen-progestin supplementation, even with extended follow-up.[137] Subsequent trials found no beneficial effect of hormone therapy or an increased risk of CHD events.[138-141]

One arm of the large-scale Women's Health Initiative (WHI) was designed to evaluate the relative benefits and risks of estrogen plus progestin in 16,608 postmenopausal women aged 50 to 79 years, with an intact uterus at baseline, over a planned 8.5-year period. However, after a mean of 5.2 years of follow-up, the trial's data and safety monitoring board recommended stopping the trial because the test statistics for invasive breast cancer exceeded the stopping boundary for this adverse effect, and the global index statistics indicated that risks exceeded benefits. At that time, the estimated hazard ratios were 1.29 (95 percent CI, 1.02 to 1.63) for CHD, 1.41 (95 percent CI, 1.07 to 1.85) for stroke, and 2.13 (95 percent CI, 1.39 to 3.25) for pulmonary embolism. The hazard ratio for total cardiovascular disease was 1.22 (95 percent CI, 1.09 to 1.36).[136] The absolute excess cardiovascular risks per 10,000 person-years attributable to estrogen plus progestin were seven more CHD events, eight more strokes, and eight more pulmonary emboli. Benefits included a reduced risk of fracture and colorectal cancer.

More recently, the unopposed estrogen arm of the WHI, which included 10,739 generally healthy postmenopausal women ages 50 to 79 without a uterus, was also halted early because of a slightly increased risk of stroke, particularly in women 60 or older.[142] After 6.8 years of follow-up, the use of estrogen was associated with a 39 percent increase in incidence of stroke, a nonsignificant 9 percent reduction in CHD, and a 30 to 39 percent reduction in fracture rate. A closer examination has suggested that younger and more recently menopausal women had a reduced risk of CHD (MI and coronary revascularization) and a more favorable global index with estrogen than with placebo.[143]

Although menopause clearly increases the risk of CVD, recent trial evidence has indicated that estrogen and progestin replacement do not confer cardiovascular protection, especially for older women. Whether or not other replacement regimens or agents provide CVD protection is being addressed in other trials.

RECOMMENDATIONS. Hormone therapy is no longer recommended as an approach to the prevention of cardiovascular disease by the U.S. Preventive Services Task Force, the North American Menopause Society, the American Heart Association, or other scientific organizations.[144] Furthermore, in 2003, the U.S. Food and Drug Administration revised the labeling for all postmenopausal hormone therapies containing estrogen alone or estrogen plus a progestogen to include a boxed warning that highlights the increased risk for heart disease, myocardial infarction, stroke, and breast cancer.[145] Nonetheless, hormone therapy continues to have a role in clinical practice for the treatment of moderate to severe menopausal symptoms.

Dietary Supplements and Specific Foods and Nutrients

A host of micronutrients and specific foods are under investigation as agents for reducing the risk of cardiovascular disease (see Chap. 44). Common supplements used by many to reduce the risk of heart disease as well as other chronic illnesses include multivitamins, B vitamins and folate, antioxidants such as vitamins E and C, various carotenoids, and ubiquinone (coenzyme Q_{10}), among others. Foods that may limit cardiovascular risk include whole grains, fiber, fish and fish oils, and soy protein. Observational studies tend to report lower rates of CHD events in those who take antioxidant vitamins and folate supplements; however, studies are inconsistent and the effects are modest.

The importance of randomized clinical trials with regard to heart-healthy foods and nutrients is best illustrated by briefly describing the advantages and disadvantages of vitamin E. Basic research has strongly suggested that oxidative stress plays an important role in the development of atherosclerotic disease and that vitamin E may delay or prevent various steps in atherosclerosis. By the mid-1990s, observational data had strongly suggested that high doses of vitamin E reduce the risk of CHD, particularly with regard to secondary prevention. Completed secondary prevention trials, however, have demonstrated that vitamin E supplementation has little impact on CHD risk.[146] The results of two long-running primary prevention trials have echoed this finding. Both the Women's Health Study[147] and the SU.VI.MAX trial,[148] which evaluated a combination of antioxidants including 30 mg of vitamin E, found that vitamin E supplementation conferred no significant reduction in the risk of CVD. In the Women's Antioxidant Cardiovascular Study, a secondary prevention trial, there was no cardiovascular benefit for women who took any of three antioxidants, vitamin E, vitamin C, or beta carotene, over a 9-year period.

In the Gruppo Italiano per lo Studio della Sopravvivenza nell'Infarto Miocardico (GISSI), 11,324 survivors of a recent myocardial infarction were randomized to daily supplements containing 1 gm of omega-3 polyunsaturated fatty acids, 300 mg of vitamin E, both, or neither for 3.5 years. Treatment with the omega-3 polyunsaturated fatty acids, but not vitamin E, lowered the relative risk of the primary endpoint, which included death, nonfatal myocardial infarction, and stroke, by 10 percent (95 percent CI, 1 to 18).[149] This benefit was primarily attributable to a decrease in the risk of death rather than nonfatal myocardial infarction or stroke.

Finally, plasma homocysteine levels have consistently been associated with increased vascular risk in multiple prospective cohort studies and, on that basis, it was hypothesized that homocysteine reduction with folate would reduce vascular event rates. However, multiple trials of folate supplementation in patients with established vascular disease have shown no evidence of clinical benefit.[150-152]

RECOMMENDATIONS. There are generally no trial data supporting supplements in the prevention of CHD or other CVD events. Antioxidants have not demonstrated clear benefits in the prevention of CHD, but observational data have raised the possibility that various micronutrients and specific foods could lower the risk of CHD. However, soy protein and isoflavone supplements lost some popularity in 2006 when the American Heart Association, which had previously recommended soy, reversed itself after reviewing the results of 22 studies, saying that it could not recommend the use of isoflavone supplements in pills or food for the prevention of heart disease.[153] More trials of fish oil supplements are needed before general recommendations can be made. Several recent trials have failed to find benefit with folate supplementation, suggesting that homocysteine reduction is not associated with reduced vascular risk.

Psychosocial Factors and Counseling (see Chap. 86)

RELATIONSHIP OF PSYCHOSOCIAL FACTORS TO CORONARY HEART DISEASE. Like diet, the study of psychosocial factors as potential risk factors for CHD is hampered by imprecision in definitions and widely accepted metrics. Psychosocial factors such as depression, chronic hostility, social isolation, and perceived lack of social support have been consistently linked with risk of CHD. Further data are needed, however, to confirm these relationships and establish the efficacy of interventional strategies. Data are inconsistent regarding associations between vascular risk and other psychological factors, such as work-related stress, type A behavior, and anxiety.

TRIALS. Studies of therapeutic interventions, although not blinded, have suggested a role for improving psychosocial factors as part of prevention programs, particularly in secondary prevention. The strongest evidence comes from post-MI patients.[154] Although abundant data have suggested that stress and depression are prevalent and predict events after myocardial infarction, data on interventions are limited. A meta-analysis of 37 small studies of health education and stress management programs for CHD patients has suggested that such efforts might reduce cardiac mortality by 34 percent and recurrent myocardial infarction by 29 percent, possibly through favorable effects on blood pressure, cholesterol, body weight, smoking behavior, physical activity, and dietary habits.[154]

The Enhancing Recovery in Coronary Heart Disease Patients (ENRICHD) randomized trial recruited 2481 patients (26 percent with perceived low social support, 39 percent with clinical depression, and 34 percent with both low social support and depression) within 4 weeks of myocardial infarction.[155] Half were randomized to cognitive behavioral therapy and drug therapy, if needed, and half to usual medical care. The intervention did not increase event-free survival. It did improve depression and social isolation, although the relative improvement in the intervention group compared with the usual care group was less than expected because of substantial improvement in usual care patients.

Preliminary evidence has suggested that pharmacotherapy for depression following myocardial infarction, revascularization, or the diagnosis of coronary disease may improve morbidity and mortality. The Sertraline Antidepressant Heart Attack Randomized Trial (SADHART) has demonstrated the safety of this selective serotonin reuptake inhibitor as a treatment for recurrent depression in cardiovascular patients. Sertraline had no more impact on left ventricular ejection fraction, treatment-emergent ventricular premature complex runs, or other cardiac measures than placebo.[156] Scores on depression and mood scales were better in the sertraline group, particularly in those who had been depressed before their heart attacks, a group in which postattack depression is especially likely. Of note, rates of second heart attacks, heart failure, episodes of chest pain, or heart-related deaths were lower in the sertraline group than the placebo group. In the ENRICHD trial, antidepressant use was also associated with significantly lower risks of nonfatal myocardial infarction or death.[155]

Novel Biochemical and Genetic Markers

A full discussion of novel biochemical and genetic risk markers for cardiovascular disease is provided in Chapter 39. Broadly, several hemostatic and inflammatory markers, novel lipid parameters, cellular adhesion molecules, indicators of prior infection, and markers of oxidative stress have all been linked to steps in atherogenesis, thrombosis, or cardiovascular disease events. Of these novel risk factors, only the CRP level has been shown to add prognostic information over and above that provided by global risk prediction models, such as the Framingham Risk Score. CRP levels also consistently predict stroke, recurrent coronary events, and cardiovascular mortality. Guidelines from the Centers for Disease Control and Prevention and the American Heart Association have encouraged the use of the CRP level as an adjunct to risk prediction, particularly for those at intermediate risk.[157] In U.S. women, recent data have indicated that 20 to 30 percent of all individuals with ATP III–predicted risk between 5 and 20 percent can be reclassified correctly to higher or lower risk categories when the CRP level is measured. This endorsement of CRP partly reflects the low cost of evaluation, particularly in comparison to other screening approaches based on imaging techniques such as CT scans for coronary calcium. In general, when used as part of global risk prediction algorithms, levels of CRP less than 1, 1 to 3, and more than 3 mg/L correspond to lower, average, and higher relative risks of future vascular disease, respectively. The addition of high CRP level to formal definitions of metabolic syndrome also improves the predictive accuracy for vascular events and incident diabetes. To date, other inflammatory biomarkers such as lipoprotein-associated phospholipase A_2 ($LpPLA_2$), fibrinogen, and sCD40 ligand have shown limited use once levels of CRP are known.

Other novel risk factors such as Lp(a) lipoprotein and homocysteine have more limited use in general screening but may be helpful in settings of premature disease and in families affected by atherosclerosis who lack clusters of traditional risk factors. With regard to Lp(a), the availability of assays independent of apolipoprotein kringle repeats represents a significant advance that helps resolve inconsistencies in prior reports.[158] A common limitation to all these novel markers is that no data yet exist that lowering levels leads to reduced vascular risk, and thus their use is largely limited to risk identification and motivation for life-style change. For example, although statin therapy lowers CRP levels and post hoc analyses of completed statin trials have suggested survival benefits for those with elevated CRP levels, prospective trials directly testing the use of CRP to target statin therapy are only now being initiated. Similarly, although folate lowers homocysteine levels, evidence that this approach lowers vascular risk is lacking. The potential clinical usefulness of these markers[159] and current evidence regarding their modification are covered in Chapter 39.

A number of common genetic polymorphisms have been associated with coronary risk factors. For example, carriers of a common mutation in the *MTHFR* gene have elevated levels of homocysteine, and there are multiple inherited abnormalities of lipid metabolism linked both to hyperlipidemia and elevated vascular risk. Similarly, almost half of the variance in CRP is heritable. However, as discussed in Chapter 39, there is no evidence that screening for any of these polymorphisms substantially adds to information more easily obtained from direct plasma measures of homocysteine, lipid, or CRP levels. This finding for arterial thrombosis is in marked contrast to findings for venous thromboembolism, where evaluation for factor V Leiden and the prothrombin mutation has proven clinically useful (see Chap. 82). Thus, although genetic screening holds great promise for identifying individuals at risk for subsequent events, its role in primary or secondary prevention remains unproven for atherothrombotic disease at this time. However, one can envision a time when genetic assays will play a role in identifying at-risk individuals and targeting therapies to reduce their risk of subsequent events.[160]

Multiple Risk Factor Intervention Programs

Although most prevention studies focus on changing a single factor, several have attempted to measure the impact of simultaneously changing multiple risk factors. In theory, the potential for synergistic effects among risk factors could lead to substantial reductions in risk that are multiplicative and offer the possibility of meaningful reductions in the risk of cardiovascular disease.[161]

Although these multiple risk factor intervention trials (Table 45-8) have made major contributions to our understanding of cardiovascular risk, as well as our knowledge of what makes for effective (and ineffective) intervention strategies, their results have been mixed. It is clear that intervention on multiple levels can reduce risk factors and that this reduction can be sustained over time. In a Belgian study that was part of the World Health Organization (WHO) European Collaborative Trial in the Multifactorial Prevention of Coronary Heart Disease, an intervention program composed of face-to-face counseling about eating habits, smoking, and physical activity substantially reduced predictors of coronary risk when compared with a control program that offered no such advice. The effect was sustained for 5 years.

A common result from multiple risk factor intervention trials is a change in risk factor levels or composite scores for those receiving intervention. However, this change has not always translated into lower event rates. Explanations for this inconsistency include the possibility that the magnitude of intervention was too small or that control patients may also have improved their health habits over time. What is clear from these trials, however, is that multiple simultaneous interventions can reduce cardiovascular risk when the planned interventions are large enough and are adequately implemented.

In an analysis of seven multiple intervention trials, changes in the multiple logistic function of risk were plotted against the reduction in risk of CHD. The strong linear relationship (Fig. 45-10) suggests that as long as risk factors are truly modified, event rates will also be reduced.

SUMMARY OF RECOMMENDATIONS

In this section, we outline a general approach to a patient. This process can be summarized in several easy steps.

STEP 1. The appropriate strategy for any given patient begins with an assessment of the overall risk of a first or subsequent cardiovascular event. Using the algorithm (see Fig. 45-6), patients can be broadly classified into four groups: (1) those with overt cardiovascular disease, including previous myocardial infarction, stroke, peripheral vascular disease, angina, or prior vascular procedure; (2) those without overt cardiovascular disease but with diabetes or high risk based on one of several composite scores; (3) those at moderate risk; and (4) those at low risk. Those with car-

TABLE 45–8 Multiple Intervention Trials

Trial	Population	Intervention	Change in Risk Factor(s)	Impact on Endpoint(s)
Multiple Risk Factor Intervention Trial	12,866 men aged 35-57 yr at high risk for CHD; average 7-yr follow-up	Stepped-care therapy for high BP, counseling for smoking cessation, and dietary advice for high cholesterol; *or* usual care	Coronary risk factors declined in both groups, although to a greater degree in intervention group	Nonsignificant change in CHD death: 17.9/1000 in intervention group, 19.3/1000 in usual care group
Oslo Trial	1232 men aged 40-49 yr with coronary risk in upper quartile; 5-yr follow-up	Diet similar to AHA step 1, counseling to stop smoking; *or* usual care	LDL-C (13%), triglycerides (20%), tobacco consumption (45%), and weight were lower in intervention group than usual care group; in both groups, physical activity and BP unchanged versus baseline	Significant reduction in fatal MI, nonfatal MI, sudden death, and cerebrovascular accidents in intervention versus control; 55% decrease in CHD death and 32% decrease in total mortality
WHO Multifactorial Trial	60,881 men aged 40-59 yr from 80 factories in Belgium, Italy, Poland, and United Kingdom; average 6 yr of intervention and follow-up	Educational materials or individual counseling regarding diet, smoking cessation, physical activity, and BP; drug therapy as needed for BP control; *or* no intervention	Coronary risk predictors significantly lower in intervention group during first 5 yr of trial; by trial's end, differences were statistically significant only for high-risk subjects who received face-to-face counseling	Nonsignificant differences in all-cause mortality (−5.3%), total CHD (−10.2%; $P = 0.07$), fatal CHD (6.9%), and nonfatal MI (−14.8%; $P = 0.06$) for intervention group versus nonintervention group
North Karelia Project	11,992 men and women aged 25-59 yr; 10-yr follow-up	Population-based prevention program with outreach for smoking cessation and for reducing BP, serum cholesterol, and other CVD risk factors	In intervention group, 28% decrease in smoking, 3% decrease in serum cholesterol, and 3% decrease in BP versus reference group	Age-adjusted CHD mortality decreased 22% in intervention group, 12% in reference group, and 11% in all of Finland ($P < 0.05$)
Göteborg Primary Prevention Trial	Random sample of 20,000 men aged 47-55 yr; average 10 yr of intervention and follow-up	Antihypertensive treatment in subjects with SBP > 175 mm Hg or DBP > 115 mm Hg, dietary advice for subjects with serum cholesterol levels >260 mg/dl, and smoking cessation advice; *or* usual care	BP, serum cholesterol, and smoking all decreased markedly in both intervention and control groups	No significant differences in total mortality, stroke, and CHD incidence
Minnesota Heart Health Program	400,000 residents aged 30-74 yr from 6 (3 paired) midwestern communities; 5- to 6-yr intervention program	Individual counseling and community outreach on decreasing BP and serum cholesterol, smoking cessation, and increasing physical activity; *or* no intervention	Generally favorable, although not statistically significant changes in intervention group versus reference group	No significant difference in CAD death rate
Pawtucket Heart Health Program	140,000 residents aged 18-64 yr of Pawtucket, RI, and a reference community; 7-yr intervention program	Community-wide educational programs designed to help individuals lower cholesterol and BP, stop smoking, maintain healthy weight, and increase physical activity	Small, not statistically significant decreases in serum cholesterol and BP in Pawtucket; slightly less smoking in the reference community	Projected CVD rates significantly (16%) less in Pawtucket during education program, but dropped to 8% after education program
Stanford Five-City Project	320,300 residents of five California cities (two intervention, three comparison); 5-yr intervention program	Individual counseling and community outreach regarding decreasing BP and serum cholesterol, smoking cessation, and increasing physical activity	Statistically significant reductions in community averages of plasma cholesterol level (2%), BP (4%), resting pulse rate (3%), and smoking rate (13%) in intervention communities versus reference communities	Decreased composite total mortality risk scores (15%) and CHD risk scores (16%) in intervention communities versus reference communities

Lifestyle Heart Trial	48 men and women aged 35-75 yr with ischemic heart disease; 4-yr intervention and follow-up	Low-fat vegetarian diet, moderate aerobic exercise, stress management training, smoking cessation, and group support; *or* usual care	After 4 yr, participants in intervention group were exercising more, practicing more stress management, and consuming less cholesterol and fewer fat calories than those in usual care group	In intervention group after 4 yr, significant reductions in frequency, duration, and severity of angina; fewer revascularizations (21% vs. 60%); and regression of atherosclerotic lesions (versus continued worsening in usual care group)
Heidelberg Trial	113 men and women recruited after coronary angiography for stable angina pectoris; 6-yr intervention and follow-up	Intervention group: AHA step 3 diet, 30 min of exercise daily, and two 60-min group counseling sessions per week; *or* advice about the AHA step 1 diet and encouragement of moderate aerobic exercise	Nonsignificant reductions in total cholesterol and triglycerides, maintenance of BMI, and significant increase in physical work capacity among those in intervention group	As assessed by coronary arteriography, significantly slower progression of coronary artery stenosis in intervention group, combined with significant improvements in myocardial perfusion
Stanford Coronary Risk Intervention Project	300 men and women < age 75 yr without severe congestive heart failure, pulmonary disease, intermittent claudication, or noncardiac life-threatening illness	Low-fat diet (<20% of calories from fat and <75 mg of cholesterol/d), physical activity, and counseling for smoking cessation, with cholesterol-lowering medication as needed; *or* usual care with personal physician	Significant improvements in percent body fat, weight, BP, LDL-C, triglycerides, HDL-C, and exercise capacity in treatment group versus controls	Although progression of coronary artery disease occurred in both groups, intervention group had a 47% lower rate of progression per individual and a 58% lower rate of progression in diseased vessel segments than reference group

AHA = American Heart Association; BMI = body mass index; BP = blood pressure; CAD = coronary artery disease; CHD = coronary heart disease; CVD = cardiovascular disease; DBP = diastolic BP; HDL-C = high-density lipoprotein cholesterol; LDL-C = low-density lipoprotein cholesterol; MI = myocardial infarction; SBP = systolic BP; WHO = World Health Organization.

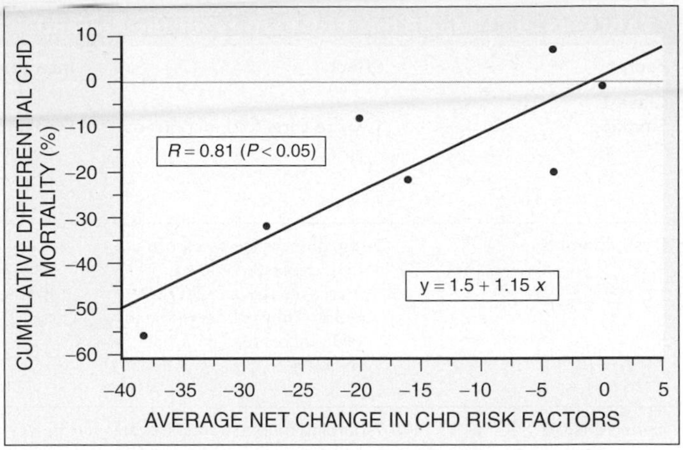

FIGURE 45–10 Difference in a composite risk factor score plotted between treated and untreated groups, which showed a statistically significant correlation between the magnitude of risk factor improvement and coronary heart disease (CHD) mortality. Data were taken from seven trials, four of which made up the World Health Organization European Collaborative Trial in Multifactorial Prevention of Coronary Heart Disease. *(From Kornitzer M: Changing individual behavior.* In *Marmot M, Elliott P [eds]: Coronary Heart Disease Epidemiology: From Aetiology to Public Health. Oxford, Oxford University Press, 1992, p 492.)*

diovascular disease and diabetes are generally straightforward to identify. Stratifying the remaining group requires the use of other predictive risk factor information with a score such as that developed by the Framingham Heart Study, the ESC, or the New Zealand Guidelines Group.

STEP 2. Once patients have been categorized into the respective risk strata, an inventory of the eight class 1 and 2 targets for intervention mentioned earlier should be undertaken.

STEP 3. Table 45-9 summarizes the interventional approaches for all three risk strata. For several risk factors—cigarette smoking, dyslipidemias, and hypertension—the strength and consistency of association with atherosclerotic disease indicate a causal relationship, and the benefits of intervention are well documented for both primary and secondary prevention. Cigarette smoking cessation should be used for all. Drug therapy for dyslipidemia should be instituted for those with a 10-year CHD risk of 10 percent or greater, and the goal should be a substantial lowering in LDL levels. Similarly, pharmacological blood pressure lowering should be instituted in those at moderate risk. There is little doubt that diabetes, physical inactivity, obesity, and certain dietary factors increase the risk of CHD and that light to moderate alcohol consumption reduces the risk, but the precise magnitude of the effect attributable to intervention for these factors has been difficult to document. Low-cost interventions appear warranted for all. Structured programs are cost-effective for those with known disease.

STEP 4. Periodic reassessment of risk factors and their trajectories, as well as overall risk, can be useful in assessing the adequacy of intervention and motivating patients to be compliant with the overall prevention prescription. This prescription should be adjusted depending on which factors are or are not being well modified.

Many of these activities can be undertaken by allied health professionals in a prevention program. Case management models of prevention have been demonstrated as useful in higher risk groups following myocardial infarction or bypass surgery.[162]

SPECIAL POPULATIONS (see Chap. 2). CVD is the leading cause of death in American women as well as in women in most of the developed world. In the United States,

TABLE 45–9 Modifiable Risk Factors for the Prevention of Cardiovascular Disease

Factor	Effect	Intervention	Comment
Class 1			
Smoking	Two- to threefold increased risk	Smoking cessation with behavioral and pharmacological interventions	Smoking cessation results in 60% reduction of CHD risk by 3 yr; about half of that benefit occurs in first 3-6 mo after quitting; interventions cost-effective in both primary, secondary prevention
Dyslipidemias	1-mg/dl increase in serum LDL cholesterol level increases risk of CVD by 2-3%; 1-mg/dl decrease in HDL increases CHD risk by 3-4%	Dietary changes combined with lipid-lowering medications	HDL and triglyceride measures useful markers of CHD risk; limited trial data suggest that intervention reduces risk; lipid-lowering drugs cost-effective in any patient with 10-yr CHD risk >10%: reduction in risk is proportional to amount of LDL lowering, so goal should be substantial reduction in LDL
Hypertension	7-mm Hg increase in BP over baseline increases risk of CVD by 27%	Life-style modifications, weight loss, limited alcohol intake, aerobic exercise, medications	Reduction in BP results in reduction in risk of stroke and CHD proportional to reduction in BP; for moderate-risk patient, pharmacological blood pressure lowering with goal of substantial change in BP should be initiated
Pharmacological Therapies			
Aspirin in secondary prevention	Reduces CVD events by 23%	Daily low-dose aspirin	Reduces risk in those with any form of CVD
Beta blockers following MI	Reduce CVD events by 18% and clearly reduce risk in those with CHF	Daily beta blocker use	Trial data suggest that benefit may increase with increasing dose
ACE inhibitors for patients with low EF and following MI	Reduce CVD events by 22% in those with low EF and by 7% following MI	Daily ACE inhibitor use	Trial data suggest that benefit may increase with increasing dose
Aspirin in primary prevention	Pooled trial data indicate a reduction in risk of first MI and total CVD	Daily or alternate-day low-dose aspirin	Prophylactic aspirin use in higher risk subjects reduces risk of CVD events
Class 2			
Diabetes	Increases risk two- to fourfold in men and three- to sevenfold in women	Maintaining normoglycemia with diet, exercise, weight management, oral agents, insulin, as needed	Type 1—trial data strongly suggest that tight control with insulin reduces risk of microvascular disease, may reduce risk of CVD events; type 2—tight control appears to reduce microvascular disease, but data on risk of CHD not available; NIDDM patients likely to have multiple coronary risk factors that should be aggressively modified
Obesity and physical inactivity	Increase risk	Diet, exercise, weight management programs	In addition to improving other CVD risk factors, maintaining ideal body weight and physically active life style may reduce risk of MI as much as 50%, but trial data limited
Dietary factors	Fruit and vegetable intake, type and amount of fat, type and amount of carbohydrate, fiber, trans fatty acids affect CHD rates		USDA and AHA recommend a diet rich in fruits and vegetables; reduction in saturated and trans fatty acid intake, increase in whole grains also appear to be helpful
Moderate alcohol intake (one drink per day)	Decreases risk of MI by 30-50%	Discussion of alcohol intake with all patients	Risk-benefit ratio for moderate alcohol consumption may vary widely by gender, also based on underlying risk of CHD; recommendations must be made individually, with careful regard for conditions such as hypertension, diabetes, liver disease, history of alcohol abuse, risk of breast cancer
Class 3			
Menopause	Increases CVD risk; large randomized controlled trial results suggest that hormone replacement therapy does not confer cardioprotection, may increase risk of stroke; long-term use associated with increased risk of breast cancer, unopposed estrogen increases risk of endometrial cancer		Neither estrogen alone nor combination of estrogen and progestin recommended as strategy for decreasing CVD risk in postmenopausal women
Dietary supplements	Examples include multivitamins, antioxidant supplements, folate, vitamins B_{12} and B_6, fish oils		Randomized trial results of antioxidant supplements, folic acid, B vitamins have been disappointing

TABLE 45–9 Modifiable Risk Factors for the Prevention of Cardiovascular Disease—cont'd

Specific Factors	Comment	
Psychological factors	Examples include depression, lack of social support, stress, type A personality	Trials of antidepressants for secondary prevention have not demonstrated clear reduction in risk of CHD
Novel biochemical and genetic markers	Examples include fibrinogen, homocysteine, Lp(a), $LpPLA_2$, t-PA, von Willebrand factor, factor VII, C-reactive protein, soluble adhesion molecules (sICAM, sVCAM), antibodies to various infectious agents, measures of oxidative stress	Additional observational data needed to clarify role of these factors in clinical practice; potential genetic markers, therapies emerging at rapid rate

ACE = angiotensin-converting enzyme; BP = blood pressure; CHD = coronary heart disease; CVD = cardiovascular disease; EF = ejection fraction; HDL = high-density lipoprotein; LDL = low-density lipoprotein; Lp(a) = lipoprotein (a); $LpPLA_2$ = lipoprotein-associated phospholipase A_2; MI = myocardial infarction; NIDDM = non-insulin-dependent diabetes mellitus; RCTs = randomized controlled trials; sICAM = soluble intercellular adhesion molecule; sVCAM = soluble vascular cell adhesion molecule; t-PA = tissue plasminogen activator; USDA = U.S. Department of Agriculture.

more than 240,000 women die from CHD, the most common form, each year. However, a study of primary care physicians, obstetrician-gynecologists, and cardiologists found that fewer than one in five physicians were aware that more women than men die of CVD each year.[163] The AHA has published new guidelines for CVD prevention in women,[164] consisting of a set of clinical recommendations tailored to a woman's individual level of risk. The elderly also represent a special population. Interventions described in earlier generally apply to healthy elderly individuals. As is the case with any pharmacological intervention, the starting dose may be lower than for younger individuals. Comorbid conditions and medication interactions must be taken into account. However, beneficial interventions should not be withheld based on age alone. Special attention must be given to improving education to enhance adherence to preventive advice for those of low socioeconomic status.

FUTURE CHALLENGES

Primary and secondary prevention have contributed substantially to the reduction in CHD mortality rates, but challenges remain. First, as the population ages, the number of individuals with factors that put them at risk for cardiovascular disease will increase, because the prevalence of many of these factors increases with age. Similarly, the number of people living with cardiovascular disease will increase, thus necessitating greater secondary preventive efforts.

Second, trends of several modifiable risk factors are troubling. Obesity and physical inactivity are epidemic in all sectors of the population, including children. These factors tend to increase rates of diabetes and hypertension and slow the favorable trends in achieving lower lipid levels. These shifts may lead to slowing of the decline in age-adjusted CHD and stroke rates or even a reversal of these positive trends (see Chap. 1).

Third, in addition to developing a better understanding of the mechanistic and epidemiological determinants of atherosclerotic disease, we must find more effective strategies for establishing priorities for interventions in prevention programs, implementing existing guidelines for risk factor modification, and developing low-cost interventions for factors for which guidelines are not yet available. Many life-style changes are difficult to achieve and even harder to maintain over the long term. Effective interventions need to involve not only those affected but also the family, workplace, school, and even the entire community.

Fourth, for clinicians, identifying a successful strategy for each patient is of critical importance. Further research on cost-benefit and risk-benefit ratios will enable better targeting of interventions for maximal individual and societal benefits. More widespread use of multifaceted self-help and health professional–directed prevention programs should help sustain the decline in cardiovascular disease mortality rates in the United States.

Finally, a unified single set of guidelines for primary and secondary CVD prevention would likely improve the ease of implementation. Both primary and secondary prevention merit increased attention worldwide, especially in low- and middle-income countries (see Chap. 1). The development of country-specific prevention guidelines that take into account the prevalence of various risk factors, cultural beliefs, and health care resources, such as those developed by New Zealand, should be encouraged.

REFERENCES

Basics of Cardiovascular Prevention

1. Yarnall KS, Pollak KI, Ostbye T, et al: Primary care: Is there enough time for prevention? Am J Publ Health 93:635, 2003.
2. Berenson GS, Srinivasan SR, Bao W, et al: Association between multiple cardiovascular risk factors and atherosclerosis in children and young adults. The Bogalusa Heart Study. N Engl J Med 338:1650, 1998.
3. Relationship of atherosclerosis in young men to serum lipoprotein cholesterol concentrations and smoking. A preliminary report from the Pathobiological Determinants of Atherosclerosis in Youth (PDAY) Research Group. JAMA 264:3018, 1990.
4. Wilson PW, D'Agostino RB, Levy D, et al: Prediction of coronary heart disease using risk factor categories. Circulation 97:1837, 1998.
5. MacMahon S, Peto R, Cutler J, et al: Blood pressure, stroke, and coronary heart disease. Part 1, Prolonged differences in blood pressure: Prospective observational studies corrected for the regression dilution bias. Lancet 335:765, 1990.
6. Qureshi AI, Suri MF, Kirmani JF, Divani AA: The relative impact of inadequate primary and secondary prevention on cardiovascular mortality in the United States. Stroke 35:2346, 2004.

Cardiovascular Risk Assessment and Management Targets

7. Third Report of the National Cholesterol Education Program (NCEP) Expert Panel on Detection, Evaluation, and Treatment of High Blood Cholesterol in Adults (Adult Treatment Panel III) final report. Circulation 106:3143, 2002.
8. Chobanian AV, Bakris GL, Black HR, et al: The Seventh Report of the Joint National Committee on Prevention, Detection, Evaluation, and Treatment of High Blood Pressure: The JNC 7 report. JAMA 289:2560, 2003.
9. Haffner SM: Management of dyslipidemia in adults with diabetes. Diabetes Care 26(Suppl 1):S83, 2003.
10. Conroy RM, Pyorala K, Fitzgerald AP, et al: Estimation of ten-year risk of fatal cardiovascular disease in Europe: The SCORE project. Eur Heart J 24:987, 2003 (http://www.escardio.org/initiatives/prevention/?hit=redirect).
11. Assmann G, Cullen P, Schulte H: Simple scoring scheme for calculating the risk of acute coronary events based on the 10-year follow-up of the prospective cardiovascular Munster (PROCAM) study. Circulation 105:310, 2002.
12. Ridker PM, Cook N: Should age and time be eliminated from cardiovascular risk prediction models? Rationale for the creation of a new national risk detection program. Circulation 111:657, 2005.
13. Greenland P, Gaziano JM: Clinical practice. Selecting asymptomatic patients for coronary computed tomography or electrocardiographic exercise testing. N Engl J Med 349:465, 2003.
14. Folsom AR, Chambless LE, Ballantyne CM, et al: An assessment of incremental coronary risk prediction using C-reactive protein and other novel risk markers:

The atherosclerosis risk in communities study. Arch Intern Med 166:1368, 2006.
15. Cook NR, Buring JE, Ridker PM: The effect of including C-reactive protein in cardiovascular risk prediction models for women. Ann Intern Med 145:21, 2006.
16. Lloyd-Jones DM, Leip EP, Larson MG, et al: Prediction of lifetime risk for cardiovascular disease by risk factor burden at 50 years of age. Circulation 113:791, 2006.
17. Pearson TA, McBride PE, Miller NH, Smith SC: 27th Bethesda Conference: Matching the intensity of risk factor management with the hazard for coronary disease events. Task Force 8. Organization of preventive cardiology service. J Am Coll Cardiol 27:1039, 1996.

Tobacco Abuse

18. Federal Trade Commission Cigarette Report for 2001 (http://www.ftc.gov/os/2003/06/2001cigreport.pdf).
19. State-specific prevalence of current cigarette smoking among adults and secondhand smoke rules and policies in homes and workplaces—United States, 2005. MMWR Morb Mortal Wkly Rep 55:1148, 2006.
20. Johnston LD, O'Malley PM, Bachman JG: Monitoring the Future: National Survey Results on Drug Use, 1975-2005, Vol I. Secondary School Students. Rockville, MD, National Institutes of Health, National Institute on Drug Abuse, 2005.
21. Thom T, Haase N, Rosamond W, et al: Heart disease and stroke statistics—2006 update: A report from the American Heart Association Statistics Committee and Stroke Statistics Subcommittee. Circulation 113:e85, 2006.
22. Annual smoking—attributable mortality, years of potential life lost, and productivity losses—United States, 1997-2001. MMWR Morb Mortal Wkly Rep 54:625, 2005.
23. World Health Organization: Reducing Risks, Promoting Healthy Life: World Health Report 2002. Geneva, World Health Organization, 2002.
24. Bolin K, Lindgren B, Willers S: The cost usefulness of bupropion in smoking cessation health programs: Simulation model results for Sweden. Chest 129:651, 2006.
25. U.S. Preventive Services Task Force: Guide to Clinical Preventive Services, 2000-2003: Recommendations of the U.S. Preventive Services Task Force. 3rd ed. Rockville, MD, Agency for Healthcare Research and Quality, 2003.
26. Thomson CC, Rigotti NA: Hospital- and clinic-based smoking cessation interventions for smokers with cardiovascular disease. Prog Cardiovasc Dis 45:459, 2003.
27. Jha P, Chaloupka JM, Moore J, et al: Tobacco addiction. *In* Jamison D, Breman JG, Measham AR, et al (eds): Disease Control Priorities in Developing Countries. 2nd ed. New York, Oxford University Press, 2006, pp 869-885.

Dyslipidemias

28. Ridker PM, Rifai N, Cook NR, et al: Non-HDL cholesterol, apolipoproteins A-I and B100, standard lipid measures, lipid ratios, and CRP as risk factors for cardiovascular disease in women. JAMA 294:326, 2005.
29. Gaziano JM, Hennekens CH, O'Donnell CJ, et al: Fasting triglycerides, high-density lipoprotein, and risk of myocardial infarction. Circulation 96:2520, 1997.
30. Baigent C, Keech A, Kearney PM, et al: Efficacy and safety of cholesterol-lowering treatment: Prospective meta-analysis of data from 90,056 participants in 14 randomised trials of statins. Lancet 366:1267, 2005.
31. Cannon CP, Steinberg BA, Murphy SA, et al: Meta-analysis of cardiovascular outcomes trials comparing intensive versus moderate statin therapy. J Am Coll Cardiol 48:438, 2006.
32. Schwartz GG, Olsson AG, Ezekowitz MD, et al: Effects of atorvastatin on early recurrent ischemic events in acute coronary syndromes: The MIRACL study: A randomized controlled trial. JAMA 285:1711, 2001.
33. Newby LK, Kristinsson A, Bhapkar MV, et al: Early statin initiation and outcomes in patients with acute coronary syndromes. JAMA 287:3087, 2002.
34. Rubins HB, Robins SJ, Collins D, et al: Gemfibrozil for the secondary prevention of coronary heart disease in men with low levels of high-density lipoprotein cholesterol. Veterans Affairs High-Density Lipoprotein Cholesterol Intervention Trial Study Group. N Engl J Med 341:410, 1999.
35. Barter PJ, Kastelein JJ: Targeting cholesteryl ester transfer protein for the prevention and management of cardiovascular disease. J Am Coll Cardiol 47:492, 2006.
36. Schaefer EJ, Asztalos BF: Cholesteryl ester transfer protein inhibition, high-density lipoprotein metabolism and heart disease risk reduction. Curr Opin Lipidol 17:394, 2006.
37. Prosser LA, Stinnett AA, Goldman PA, et al: Cost-effectiveness of cholesterol-lowering therapies according to selected patient characteristics. Ann Intern Med 132:769, 2000.
38. Ganz DA, Kuntz KM, Jacobson GA, Avorn J: Cost-effectiveness of 3-hydroxy-3-methylglutaryl coenzyme A reductase inhibitor therapy in older patients with myocardial infarction. Ann Intern Med 132:780, 2000.
39. Heart Protection Study Collaborative; Mihaylova B, Briggs A, Armitage J, et al: Lifetime cost effectiveness of simvastatin in a range of risk groups and age groups derived from a randomised trial of 20,536 people. BMJ 333:1145, 2006.
40. American College of Physicians: Guidelines for using serum cholesterol, high-density lipoprotein cholesterol, and triglyceride levels as screening tests for preventing coronary heart disease in adults. Part 1. Ann Intern Med 124:515, 1996.
41. Smith SC Jr, Allen J, Blair SN, et al: AHA/ACC guidelines for secondary prevention for patients with coronary and other atherosclerotic vascular disease: 2006 update endorsed by the National Heart, Lung, and Blood Institute. J Am Coll Cardiol 47:2130, 2006.
42. De Backer G, Ambrosioni E, Borch-Johnsen K, et al: European guidelines on cardiovascular disease prevention in clinical practice. Third Joint Task Force of European and Other Societies on Cardiovascular Disease Prevention in Clinical Practice. Eur Heart J 24:1601, 2003.

Hypertension

43. Cheung BM, Ong KL, Man YB, et al: Prevalence, awareness, treatment, and control of hypertension: United States National Health and Nutrition Examination Survey 2001-2002. J Clin Hypertens (Greenwich) 8:93, 2006.
44. Vasan RS, Beiser A, Seshadri S, et al: Residual lifetime risk for developing hypertension in middle-aged women and men: The Framingham Heart Study. JAMA 287:1003, 2002.
45. Hajjar I, Kotchen TA: Trends in prevalence, awareness, treatment, and control of hypertension in the United States, 1988-2000. JAMA 290:199, 2003.
46. Sawicki PT, McGauran N: Have ALLHAT, ANBP2, ASCOT-BPLA, and so forth improved our knowledge about better hypertension care? Hypertension 48:1, 2006.
47. Lewington S, Clarke R, Qizilbash N, et al: Age-specific relevance of usual blood pressure to vascular mortality: A meta-analysis of individual data for one million adults in 61 prospective studies. Lancet 360:1903, 2002.
48. Collins R, Peto R, MacMahon S, et al: Blood pressure, stroke, and coronary heart disease. Part 2, Short-term reductions in blood pressure: Overview of randomised drug trials in their epidemiologic context. Lancet 335:827, 1990.
49. ALLHAT Officers and Coordinators for the ALLHAT Collaborative Research Group: Major outcomes in high-risk hypertensive patients randomized to angiotensin-converting enzyme inhibitor or calcium channel blocker vs diuretic: The Antihypertensive and Lipid-Lowering Treatment to Prevent Heart Attack Trial (ALLHAT). JAMA 288:2981, 2002.
50. Weber MA: New results and analysis expand and modify key interpretations of the ALLHAT trial. Rev Cardiovasc Med 5:164, 2004.
51. Turnbull F: Effects of different blood-pressure-lowering regimens on major cardiovascular events: results of prospectively-designed overviews of randomised trials. Lancet 362:1527, 2003.
52. Pearce KA, Furberg CD, Psaty BM, Kirk J: Cost-minimization and the number needed to treat in uncomplicated hypertension. Am J Hypertens 11:618, 1998.
53. U.S. Preventive Services Task Force: Guide to Clinical Preventive Services, 2006: Recommendations of the U.S. Preventive Services Task Force. AHRQ Publication No. 06-0588. Rockville, MD. Agency for Healthcare Research and Quality, 2006 (http://www.ahrq.gov/clinic/pocketgd/index.html).
54. Appel LJ, Moore TJ, Obarzanek E, et al: A clinical trial of the effects of dietary patterns on blood pressure. DASH Collaborative Research Group. N Engl J Med 336:1117, 1997.
55. European Society of Hypertension-European Society of Cardiology Guidelines Committee: 2003 European Society of Hypertension-European Society of Cardiology guidelines for the management of arterial hypertension. J Hypertens 21:1011, 2003.
56. Dahlof B, Sever PS, Poulter NR, et al: Prevention of cardiovascular events with an antihypertensive regimen of amlodipine adding perindopril as required versus atenolol adding bendroflumethiazide as required, in the Anglo-Scandinavian Cardiac Outcomes Trial-Blood Pressure Lowering Arm (ASCOT-BPLA): A multicentre randomised controlled trial. Lancet 366:895, 2005.
57. Lindholm LH, Carlberg B, Samuelsson O: Should beta blockers remain first choice in the treatment of primary hypertension? A meta-analysis. Lancet 366:1545, 2005.
58. Clinical guideline 34: Hypertension: Management of hypertension in adults in primary care: Partial update. 2006 (http://www.nice.org.uk/cg034guidance).
59. Lawes CM, Vander Hoorn S, Law MR, et al: Blood pressure and the global burden of disease 2000. Part II: Estimates of attributable burden. J Hypertens 24:423, 2006.

Antithrombotics

60. Antithrombotic Trialists' Collaboration: Collaborative meta-analysis of randomised trials of antiplatelet therapy for prevention of death, myocardial infarction, and stroke in high risk patients. BMJ 324:71, 2002.
61. Bhatt DL, Fox KA, Hacke W, et al: Clopidogrel and aspirin versus aspirin alone for the prevention of atherothrombotic events. N Engl J Med 354:1706, 2006.
62. Gaspoz JM, Coxson PG, Goldman PA, et al: Cost effectiveness of aspirin, clopidogrel, or both for secondary prevention of coronary heart disease. N Engl J Med 346:1800, 2002.
63. Berger JS, Roncaglioni MC, Avanzini F, et al: Aspirin for the primary prevention of cardiovascular events in women and men: A sex-specific meta-analysis of randomized controlled trials. JAMA 295:306, 2006.
64. Ridker PM, Cook NR, Lee IM, et al: A randomized trial of low-dose aspirin in the primary prevention of cardiovascular disease in women. N Engl J Med 352:1293, 2005.
65. U.S. Preventive Services Task Force: Aspirin for the primary prevention of cardiovascular events: Recommendation and rationale. Ann Intern Med 136:157, 2002.
66. Pearson TA, Blair SN, Daniels SR, et al: AHA Guidelines for Primary Prevention of Cardiovascular Disease and Stroke: 2002 Update: Consensus Panel Guide to Comprehensive Risk Reduction for Adult Patients Without Coronary or Other Atherosclerotic Vascular Diseases. American Heart Association Science Advisory and Coordinating Committee. Circulation 106:388, 2002.
67. Wood D, De Backer G, Faergeman O, et al: Prevention of coronary heart disease in clinical practice: Recommendations of the Second Joint Task Force of European and other Societies on Coronary Prevention. Eur Heart J 19:1434, 1998.

Secondary Prevention

68. Freemantle N, Cleland J, Young P, et al: Beta blockade after myocardial infarction: Systematic review and meta regression analysis. BMJ 318:1730, 1999.

69. Phillips KA, Shlipak MG, Coxson P, et al: Health and economic benefits of increased beta-blocker use following myocardial infarction. JAMA 284:2748, 2000.
70. ACE Inhibitor Myocardial Infarction Collaborative Group: Indications for ACE inhibitors in the early treatment of acute myocardial infarction: Systematic overview of individual data from 100,000 patients in randomized trials. Circulation 97:2202, 1998.
71. Domanski MJ, Exner DV, Borkowf CB, et al: Effect of angiotensin converting enzyme inhibition on sudden cardiac death in patients following acute myocardial infarction. A meta- analysis of randomized clinical trials. J Am Coll Cardiol 33:598, 1999.
72. Tanasescu M, Leitzmann MF, Rimm EB, et al: Exercise type and intensity in relation to coronary heart disease in men. JAMA 288:1994, 2002.
73. Yusuf S, Sleight P, Pogue J, et al: Effects of an angiotensin-converting-enzyme inhibitor, ramipril, on cardiovascular events in high-risk patients. The Heart Outcomes Prevention Evaluation Study Investigators. N Engl J Med 342:145, 2000.
74. Pfeffer MA, Swedberg K, Granger CB, et al: Effects of candesartan on mortality and morbidity in patients with chronic heart failure: The CHARM-Overall programme. Lancet 362:759, 2003.
75. Anand SS, Yusuf S: Oral anticoagulant therapy in patients with coronary artery disease: a meta-analysis. JAMA 282:2058, 1999.
76. Husted SE, Ziegler BK, Kher A: Long-term anticoagulant therapy in patients with coronary artery disease. Eur Heart J 27:913, 2006.

Diabetes

77. Centers for Disease Control and Prevention: National Diabetes Fact Sheet: General information and national estimates on diabetes in the United States, 2005. Atlanta, U.S. Department of Health and Human Services, Centers for Disease Control and Prevention, 2005 (http://www.cdc.gov/diabetes/pubs/factsheet05.htm).
78. American Diabetes Association: Type 2 diabetes in children and adolescents. Diabetes Care 23:381, 2000.
79. Fagot-Campagna A, Pettitt DJ, Engelgau MM, et al: Type 2 diabetes among North American children and adolescents: an epidemiological review and a public health perspective. J Pediatr 136:664, 2000.
80. Narayan KM, Boyle JP, Thompson TJ, et al: Lifetime risk for diabetes mellitus in the United States. JAMA 290:1884, 2003.
81. Gu K, Cowie CC, Harris MI: Mortality in adults with and without diabetes in a national cohort of the U.S. population, 1971-1993. Diabetes Care 21:1138, 1998.
82. Hu FB, Stampfer MJ, Solomon CG, et al: The impact of diabetes mellitus on mortality from all causes and coronary heart disease in women: 20 years of follow-up. Arch Intern Med 161:1717, 2001.
83. Cho E, Rimm EB, Stampfer MJ, et al: The impact of diabetes mellitus and prior myocardial infarction on mortality from all causes and from coronary heart disease in men. J Am Coll Cardiol 40:954, 2002.
84. Natarajan S, Liao Y, Cao G, et al: Sex differences in risk for coronary heart disease mortality associated with diabetes and established coronary heart disease. Arch Intern Med 163:1735, 2003.
85. Haffner SM, Lehto S, Ronnemaa T, et al: Mortality from coronary heart disease in subjects with type 2 diabetes and in nondiabetic subjects with and without prior myocardial infarction. N Engl J Med 339:229, 1998.
86. Nathan DM, Cleary PA, Backlund JY, et al: Intensive diabetes treatment and cardiovascular disease in patients with type 1 diabetes. N Engl J Med 353:2643, 2005.
87. Gerstein HC, Mann JF, Pogue J, et al: Prevalence and determinants of microalbuminuria in high-risk diabetic and nondiabetic patients in the Heart Outcomes Prevention Evaluation Study. The HOPE Study Investigators. Diabetes Care 23(Suppl 2):B35, 2000.
88. Bosch J, Yusuf S, Gerstein HC, et al: Effect of ramipril on the incidence of diabetes. N Engl J Med 355:1551, 2006.
89. Gerstein HC, Yusuf S, Bosch J, et al: Effect of rosiglitazone on the frequency of diabetes in patients with impaired glucose tolerance or impaired fasting glucose: A randomised controlled trial. Lancet 368:1096, 2006.
90. Gaede P, Vedel P, Larsen N, et al: Multifactorial intervention and cardiovascular disease in patients with type 2 diabetes. N Engl J Med 348:383, 2003.
91. Arday DR, Fleming BB, Keller DK, et al: Variation in diabetes care among states: Do patient characteristics matter? Diabetes Care 25:2230, 2002.
92. Arauz-Pacheco C, Parrott MA, Raskin P: Hypertension management in adults with diabetes. Diabetes Care 27(Suppl 1):S65, 2004.
93. Ballantyne CM, Houri J, Notarbartolo A, et al: Effect of ezetimibe coadministered with atorvastatin in 628 patients with primary hypercholesterolemia: A prospective, randomized, double-blind trial. Circulation 107:2409, 2003.
94. Colwell J: Aspirin therapy in diabetes. Diabetes Care 27(Suppl):72S, 2004.
95. Ford ES, Giles WH, Mokdad AH: Increasing prevalence of the metabolic syndrome among U.S. Adults. Diabetes Care 27:2444, 2004.
96. de Ferranti SD, Gauvreau K, Ludwig DS, et al: Prevalence of the metabolic syndrome in American adolescents: Findings from the Third National Health and Nutrition Examination Survey. Circulation 110:2494, 2004.
97. Tuomilehto J, Lindstrom J, Eriksson JG, et al: Prevention of type 2 diabetes mellitus by changes in lifestyle among subjects with impaired glucose tolerance. N Engl J Med 344:1343, 2001.
98. Knowler WC, Barrett-Connor E, Fowler SE, et al: Reduction in the incidence of type 2 diabetes with lifestyle intervention or metformin. N Engl J Med 346:393, 2002.
99. Nelson KM, Reiber G, Boyko EJ: Diet and exercise among adults with type 2 diabetes: Findings from the Third National Health and Nutrition Examination Survey (NHANES III). Diabetes Care 25:1722, 2002.
100. Smith NL, Barzilay JI, Shaffer D, et al: Fasting and 2-hour postchallenge serum glucose measures and risk of incident cardiovascular events in the elderly: The Cardiovascular Health Study. Arch Intern Med 162:209, 2002.

Obesity

101. Flegal KM, Carroll MD, Kuczmarski RJ, Johnson CL: Overweight and obesity in the United States: Prevalence and trends, 1960-1994. Int J Obes Relat Metab Disord 22:39, 1998.
102. Hedley AA, Ogden CL, Johnson CL, et al: Prevalence of overweight and obesity among U.S. children, adolescents, and adults, 1999-2002. JAMA 291:2847, 2004.
103. Flegal KM, Carroll MD, Ogden CL, Johnson CL: Prevalence and trends in obesity among U.S. adults, 1999-2000. JAMA 288:1723, 2002.
104. Li TY, Rana JS, Manson JE, et al: Obesity as compared with physical activity in predicting risk of coronary heart disease in women. Circulation 113:499, 2006.
105. Ashton WD, Nanchahal K, Wood DA: Body mass index and metabolic risk factors for coronary heart disease in women. Eur Heart J 22:46, 2001.
106. Allison DB, Fontaine KR, Manson JE, et al: Annual deaths attributable to obesity in the United States. JAMA 282:1530, 1998.
107. Sturm R, Wells KB: Does obesity contribute as much to morbidity as poverty or smoking? Public Health 115:229, 2001.
108. Finkelstein EA, Fiebelkorn IC, Wang G: National medical spending attributable to overweight and obesity: How much, and who's paying? Health Aff (Millwood) Suppl Web Exclusives:W3, 219, 2003.
109. Elmer PJ, Brown JB, Nichols GA, Oster G: Effects of weight gain on medical care costs. Int J Obes Relat Metab Disord 28:1365, 2004.
110. National Heart, Lung, and Blood Institute: Clinical Guidelines On The Identification, Evaluation, and Treatment of Overweight and Obesity in Adults. Bethesda, MD, National Institutes of Health, National Heart, Lung, and Blood Institute, Obesity Education Initiative, 1998.
111. Stefanick ML: Exercise and weight loss. *In* Hennekens CH (ed): Clinical Trials in Cardiovascular Disease: A Companion Guide to Braunwald's Heart Disease. Philadelphia, WB Saunders, 1999, pp 375-391.
112. Peppard PE, Young T, Palta M, et al: Longitudinal study of moderate weight change and sleep-disordered breathing. JAMA 284:3015, 2000.
113. Manson JE, Skerrett PJ, Greenland P, VanItallie TB: The escalating pandemics of obesity and sedentary lifestyle. A call to action for clinicians. Arch Intern Med 164:249, 2004.
114. National Heart, Lung, and Blood Institute, North American Association for the Study of Obesity: The Practical Guide: Identification, Evaluation, and Treatment of Overweight and Obesity in Adults. Washington, DC, National Heart, Lung, and Blood Institute, 2000.
115. LaRosa JC, He J, Vupputuri S: Effect of statins on risk of coronary disease: a meta-analysis of randomized controlled trials. JAMA 282:2340, 1999.

Physical Activity

116. Nader PR: Frequency and intensity of activity of third-grade children in physical education. Arch Pediatr Adolesc Med 157:185, 2003.
117. Lee IM, Skerrett PJ: Physical activity and all-cause mortality: What is the dose-response relation? Med Sci Sports Exerc 33:S459; discussion, S493, 2001.
118. Manson JE, Greenland P, LaCroix AZ, et al: Walking compared with vigorous exercise for the prevention of cardiovascular events in women. N Engl J Med 347:716, 2002.
119. Hu FB, Sigal RJ, Rich-Edwards JW, et al: Walking compared with vigorous physical activity and risk of type 2 diabetes in women: a prospective study. JAMA 282:1433, 1999.
120. Gregg EW, Cauley JA, Stone K, et al: Relationship of changes in physical activity and mortality among older women. JAMA 289:2379, 2003.
121. Wannamethee SG, Shaper AG, Walker M: Changes in physical activity, mortality, and incidence of coronary heart disease in older men. Lancet 351:1603, 1998.
122. Lee IM, Hennekens CH, Berger K, et al: Exercise and risk of stroke in male physicians. Stroke 30:1, 1999.
123. Hu FB, Stampfer MJ, Colditz GA, et al: Physical activity and risk of stroke in women. JAMA 283:2961, 2000.
124. Jolliffe JA, Rees K, Taylor RS, et al: Exercise-based rehabilitation for coronary heart disease. Cochrane Database Syst Rev (1):CD001800, 2003.
125. Lichtenstein AH, Appel LJ, Brands M, et al: Diet and lifestyle recommendations revision 2006: A scientific statement from the American Heart Association Nutrition Committee. Circulation 114:82, 2006.
126. Saaddine J: Physical Activity and Health: A Report of the Surgeon General. Washington, DC, U.S. Department of Health and Human Services, Centers for Disease Control and Prevention, 1996.

Diet and Cardiovascular Prevention

127. Ness AR, Powles JW: Fruit and vegetables, and cardiovascular disease: A review. Int J Epidemiol 1997;26:1, 1997.
128. Joshipura KJ, Ascherio A, Manson JE, et al: Fruit and vegetable intake in relation to risk of ischemic stroke. JAMA 282:1233, 1999.
129. Hu FB, Willett WC: Optimal diets for prevention of coronary heart disease. JAMA 288:2569, 2002.
130. de Lorgeril M, Salen P, Martin JL, et al: Mediterranean diet, traditional risk factors, and the rate of cardiovascular complications after myocardial infarction: Final report of the Lyon Diet Heart Study. Circulation 99:779, 1999.
131. Kris-Etherton PM, Harris WS, Appel LJ: Fish consumption, fish oil, omega-3 fatty acids, and cardiovascular disease. Circulation 106:2747, 2002.
132. Goldberg IJ, Mosca L, Piano MR, Fisher EA: AHA Science Advisory: Wine and your heart: A science advisory for healthcare professionals from the Nutrition Committee, Council on Epidemiology and Prevention, and Council on Cardiovascular Nursing of the American Heart Association. Circulation 103:472, 2001.

133. Rimm EB, Williams P, Fosher K, et al: Moderate alcohol intake and lower risk of coronary heart disease: meta-analysis of effects on lipids and haemostatic factors. BMJ 319:1523, 1999.
134. Anderson RN: Deaths: Leading causes for 2000. Natl Vital Stat Rep 50:1, 2002.

Hormone Therapy

135. Grodstein F, Stampfer MJ: The epidemiology of postmenopausal hormone therapy and cardiovascular disease. *In* Goldhaber SZ, Ridker PM (eds): Thrombosis and Thromboembolism. New York, Marcel Dekker, 2002, pp 67-78.
136. Rossouw JE, Anderson GL, Prentice RL, et al: Risks and benefits of estrogen plus progestin in healthy postmenopausal women: Principal results from the Women's Health Initiative randomized controlled trial. JAMA 288:321, 2002.
137. Grady D, Herrington D, Bittner V, et al: Cardiovascular disease outcomes during 6.8 years of hormone therapy: Heart and Estrogen/Progestin Replacement Study follow-up (HERS II). JAMA 288:49, 2002.
138. Herrington DM, Reboussin DM, Brosnihan KB, et al: Effects of estrogen replacement on the progression of coronary-artery atherosclerosis. N Engl J Med 343:522, 2000.
139. Clarke SC, Kelleher J, Lloyd-Jones H, et al: A study of hormone replacement therapy in postmenopausal women with ischaemic heart disease: The Papworth HRT atherosclerosis study. BJOG 109:1056, 2002.
140. Waters DD, Alderman EL, Hsia J, et al: Effects of hormone replacement therapy and antioxidant vitamin supplements on coronary atherosclerosis in postmenopausal women: A randomized controlled trial. JAMA 288:2432, 2002.
141. Cherry N, Gilmour K, Hannaford P, et al: Oestrogen therapy for prevention of reinfarction in postmenopausal women: A randomised placebo controlled trial. Lancet 360:2001, 2002.
142. Anderson GL, Limacher M, Assaf AR, et al: Effects of conjugated equine estrogen in postmenopausal women with hysterectomy: The Women's Health Initiative randomized controlled trial. JAMA 291:1701, 2004.
143. Hsia J, Langer RD, Manson JE, et al: Conjugated equine estrogens and coronary heart disease: The Women's Health Initiative. Arch Intern Med 166:357, 2006.
144. North American Menopause Society: Amended report from the NAMS Advisory Panel on Postmenopausal Hormone Therapy. Menopause 10:6, 2003.
145. U.S. Food and Drug Administration: FDA approves new labels for estrogen and estrogen with progestin therapies for postmenopausal women following review of Women's Health Initiative data. Washington, DC, U.S. Food and Drug Administration, 2003 (http://www.fda.gov/bbs/topics/news/2003/new00843.html).

Antioxidants, Vitamins, and Nutrients

146. Gaziano JM: Vitamin E and cardiovascular disease: Observational studies. Ann N Y Acad Sci 1031:280, 2004.
147. Lee IM, Cook NR, Gaziano JM, et al: Vitamin E in the primary prevention of cardiovascular disease and cancer: the Women's Health Study: A randomized controlled trial. JAMA 294:56, 2005.
148. Hercberg S, Galan P, Preziosi P, et al: The SU.VI.MAX Study: A randomized, placebo-controlled trial of the health effects of antioxidant vitamins and minerals. Arch Intern Med 164:2335, 2004.
149. Gruppo Italiano per lo Studio della Sopravvivenza nell'Infarto miocardico: Dietary supplementation with n-3 polyunsaturated fatty acids and vitamin E after myocardial infarction: results of the GISSI-Prevenzione trial. Lancet 354:447, 1999.
150. Toole JF, Malinow MR, Chambless LE, et al: Lowering homocysteine in patients with ischemic stroke to prevent recurrent stroke, myocardial infarction, and death: the Vitamin Intervention for Stroke Prevention (VISP) randomized controlled trial. JAMA 291:565, 2004.
151. Bonaa KH, Njolstad I, Ueland PM, et al: Homocysteine lowering and cardiovascular events after acute myocardial infarction. N Engl J Med 354:1578, 2006.
152. Lonn E, Yusuf S, Arnold MJ, et al: Homocysteine lowering with folic acid and B vitamins in vascular disease. N Engl J Med 354:1567, 2006.
153. Sacks FM, Lichtenstein A, Van Horn L, et al: Soy protein, isoflavones, and cardiovascular health: An American Heart Association Science Advisory for professionals from the Nutrition Committee. Circulation 113:1034, 2006.

Psychosocial Risk Factors

154. Dusseldorp E, van Elderen T, Maes S, et al: A meta-analysis of psychoeducational programs for coronary heart disease patients. Health Psychol 18:506, 1999.
155. Berkman LF, Blumenthal J, Burg M, et al: Effects of treating depression and low perceived social support on clinical events after myocardial infarction: The Enhancing Recovery in Coronary Heart Disease Patients (ENRICHD) Randomized Trial. JAMA 289:3106, 2003.
156. Glassman AH, O'Connor CM, Califf RM, et al: Sertraline treatment of major depression in patients with acute MI or unstable angina. JAMA 288:701, 2002.

Emerging Risk Factors and Management Strategies

157. Pearson TA, Mensah GA, Alexander RW, et al: Markers of inflammation and cardiovascular disease: Application to clinical and public health practice: A statement for healthcare professionals from the Centers for Disease Control and Prevention and the American Heart Association. Circulation 107:499, 2003.
158. Suk Danik J, Rifai N, Buring JE, Ridker PM: Lipoprotein(a), measured with an assay independent of apolipoprotein(a) isoform size, and risk of future cardiovascular events among initially healthy women. JAMA 296:1363, 2006.
159. Ridker PM: Evaluating novel cardiovascular risk factors: Can we better predict heart attacks? Ann Intern Med 130:933, 1999.
160. Libby P, Ridker PM: Novel inflammatory markers of coronary risk: Theory versus practice. Circulation 100:1148, 1999.
161. Ornish D, Hart JA: Multiple risk factor intervention trials. *In* Hennekens CH (ed): Clinical Trials in Cardiovascular Disease: A Companion Guide to Braunwald's Heart Disease. Philadelphia, WB Saunders, 1999, pp 432-446.
162. DeBusk RF, West JA, Miller NH, Taylor CB: Chronic disease management: Treating the patient with disease(s) vs treating disease(s) in the patient. Arch Intern Med 159:2739, 1999.
163. Mosca L, Linfante AH, Benjamin EJ, et al: National study of physician awareness and adherence to cardiovascular disease prevention guidelines. Circulation 111:499, 2005.
164. Mosca L, Banka CL, Benjamin EJ, et al: Evidence-based guidelines for cardiovascular disease prevention in women: 2007 update. Circulation 115:1481, 2007.

CHAPTER 46

Exercise-Based, Comprehensive Cardiac Rehabilitation

Paul D. Thompson

HISTORICAL PERSPECTIVE

Prolonged hospitalizations lasting several weeks followed by months of restricted physical activity were the standard treatment of myocardial infarction (MI) until the early 1950s. Indeed, as recently as the early 1970s, patients were routinely hospitalized for 3 weeks after an MI. Exercise-based cardiac rehabilitation programs were initiated in the 1950s to reverse the physical deconditioning and reduced exercise capacity produced by such hospitalizations and attendant, restricted physical activity. Exercise training was central to reversing this deconditioning process. Exercise training was also central to cardiac rehabilitation efforts because exercise was one of the few interventions documented to delay the onset of classic angina pectoris before the availability of beta-adrenergic blockers, calcium channel blockers, coronary artery bypass grafting (CABG), and percutaneous transluminal coronary angioplasty (PTCA).[1,2]

Abbreviated hospital stays, as well as effective medicines and procedures to treat myocardial ischemia, have influenced the structure and design of cardiac rehabilitation programs. Exercise training remains the cornerstone of cardiac rehabilitation efforts, but other components including education and counseling to improve psychological well-being, reduce cigarette smoking, and increase adherence to medicines and diet are now key components of the comprehensive rehabilitation effort.[3] These educational components are deemed important enough to be required for accreditation by the American Association of Cardiovascular and Pulmonary Rehabilitation.[4]

Nevertheless, exercise training remains a critical key component of cardiac rehabilitation programs because of its ability to increase exercise capacity; reduce exercise-induced cardiac ischemia and angina; and reduce such cardiac risk factors as serum lipids, blood pressure, and endothelial dysfunction.[5] Consequently, the present chapter addresses the totality of the cardiac rehabilitation effort but emphasizes the use of exercise training in this process.

BASIC PRINCIPLES OF EXERCISE PHYSIOLOGY AND OF EXERCISE TRAINING[5]

MAXIMAL OXYGEN UPTAKE ($\dot{V}O_2$) (see also Chap. 78). Only small amounts of energy are immediately available in skeletal muscle. Consequently, both aerobic and resistance exercise (Table 46-1) increase the body's oxygen requirements to supply energy to the exercising muscle. The amount of energy used during exercise is measured indirectly as the amount of O_2 consumed. This is referred to as the *ventilatory oxygen consumption* or $\dot{V}O_2$. Rearranging the Fick equation: cardiac output ($\dot{Q}$) = $\dot{V}O_2$/the arterial − venous O_2 difference (A-V $O_2\Delta$) demonstrates that $\dot{V}O_2$ is the product of $\dot{Q}$ and A-V $O_2\Delta$. Thus the metabolic demands of exercise are met by increasing O_2 delivery via increases in $\dot{Q}$, which in turn is the product of heart rate (HR) and cardiac stroke volume (SV), as well as by increases in the A-V $O_2\Delta$. The A-V $O_2\Delta$ increases during exercise by blood flow redistribution from nonexercising tissue (e.g., the kidney and splanchnic bed) to exercising muscle, by increased O_2 extraction in the exercising muscle, and by hemoconcentration due to plasma fluid losses into the exercising muscle interstitial space. The increase in $\dot{Q}$ during exercise is tightly coupled to the increase in $\dot{V}O_2$ so that a 1 liter increase in $\dot{V}O_2$ elicits an approximately 6 liter increase in $\dot{Q}$. Maximal exercise capacity is measured as $\dot{V}O_{2max}$ or the maximal amount of oxygen that the individual can transport during exercise before being limited by fatigue or dyspnea. $\dot{V}O_{2max}$ in an individual is a highly stable and reproducible measure of exercise capacity. It is expressed as either an absolute value in liters per minute or relative to body weight (BW) as ml/kg-BW/minute. The maximal increase in the A-V $O_2\Delta$ is fixed at approximately 15 to 17 volume percent. Because the exercise workrate determines $\dot{V}O_2$, which is the product of $\dot{Q}$ and the A-V $O_2\Delta$, and because the maximal A-V $O_2\Delta$ is relatively fixed, maximal exercise capacity or $\dot{V}O_{2max}$ indirectly measures maximal cardiac pump capacity or maximal $\dot{Q}$ and SV.

MYOCARDIAL OXYGEN UPTAKE ($\dot{M}O_2$). Myocardial O_2 demand ($\dot{M}O_2$) can be estimated as the product of HR and systolic blood pressure (SBP) or the so-called double product. Although the absolute exercise workrate determines $\dot{V}O_2$ and $\dot{Q}$, the increases in HR and SBP are determined by the exercise $\dot{V}O_2$ requirement as a percentage of $\dot{V}O_{2max}$. Consequently, for any absolute exercise level, an individual with a larger $\dot{V}O_{2max}$ uses less of his or her maximal capacity and demonstrates a lower HR and SBP exercise response. The key point is that $\dot{M}O_2$ is not determined solely by the external exercise workrate, but by the exercise workrate relative to maximal exercise capacity.

VENTILATORY THRESHOLD (VT). Expired CO_2 ($\dot{V}CO_2$) also increases as the exercise workrate increases. Increases in $\dot{V}O_2$ and $\dot{V}CO_2$ are parallel early during exercise, but the rate of CO_2 expiration increases more rapidly and the coupling of $\dot{V}O_2$ and $\dot{V}CO_2$ diverge at what is termed the *ventilatory threshold* (VT). This divergence is due to

TABLE 46–1 Terms to Describe Exercise

Physical activity—any bodily movement
Exercise—physical activity to stress and train
Aerobic exercise—exercise that primarily stresses the oxygen transport system and includes activities such as walking, jogging, swimming, cycling
Resistance exercise—exercise that primarily stresses the musculoskeletal system and includes weight lifting
Exercise training—exercise performed repetitively in order to increase the performance capacity of the cardiovascular (aerobic exercise training) or muscular skeletal (resistance exercise training) systems

From Thompson PD: Exercise prescription and proscription for patients with coronary artery disease. Circulation 112:2354, 2005.

the production of lactic acid, buffering of the lactic acid H^+ ions by bicarbonate, and the subsequent exhalation of additional CO_2. The VT has also been known as the "anaerobic threshold" and as "OBLA" (onset of blood lactate accumulation). Because CO_2 stimulates respiratory drive, the VT is also associated with a nonlinear increase in the respiratory rate and mild dyspnea. The VT generally occurs at approximately 50 percent of $\dot{V}O_{2max}$ in exercise-untrained individuals but at higher levels of percent $\dot{V}O_{2max}$ in exercise-trained subjects. VT is an important measurement of exercise tolerance because it represents the maximal steady workrate that can be maintained during submaximal exercise.

Effect of Cardiac Disease on Exercise Performance

Exercise performance may be normal for age and gender in individuals with cardiac disease. Alternatively, exercise capacity in cardiac patients may be limited by diseases that limit maximal SV, impair the HR response, or produce myocardial ischemia that produces limiting symptoms or a diminished increase in SV. Medications such as beta-adrenergic blocking agents that limit the HR response to exercise or physical activity restrictions that produce a detraining effect may also contribute to reduced exercise tolerance in cardiac patients.

Effect of Exercise Training on Exercise Performance

The primary effect of exercise training, either aerobic or strength training, is to increase exercise capacity. With strength training the primary adaptation is to increase muscular strength and muscular endurance in the exercise-trained muscle. The principal effect of primarily aerobic exercise training is to increase $\dot{V}O_{2max}$. This increase in maximal exercise capacity means that any submaximal workrate requires a lower percentage of $\dot{V}O_{2max}$, thereby reducing the HR and SBP response and the $\dot{M}O_2$ requirements. Endurance exercise training also increases both the absolute VT and the VT as a percent of $\dot{V}O_{2max}$. Multiple adaptations contribute to the improvement in exercise tolerance after exercise training, including increases in SV and a widening of the A-V $O_2\Delta$, although the magnitude of the later has obvious physiological limits.

The magnitude of the increase in exercise $\dot{V}O_{2max}$ with endurance exercise training depends on multiple factors including the age of the subject, the intensity and duration of the training regimen, genetic factors, underlying disease states, and whether or not testing and training use similar exercises. In general, the magnitude of the improvement in exercise tolerance is greater in young subjects trained intensely. For cardiac rehabilitation patients, reported increases in $\dot{V}O_{2max}$ average 11 to 36 percent,[6] although the response varies with the severity of the underlying disease. For example, individuals with markedly reduced ventricular function may achieve much of their increase in exercise capacity by widening the A-V $O_2\Delta$, whereas increases in cardiac output have been documented with 12 months of exercise training in some cardiac patients.[5] In addition to increasing maximal exercise capacity, endurance exercise training increases endurance capacity by virtue of its effects on VT. This effect is extremely important because increased submaximal exercise endurance capacity reduces dyspnea at submaximal workrates and assists performance of most daily tasks, virtually none of which require maximal effort.

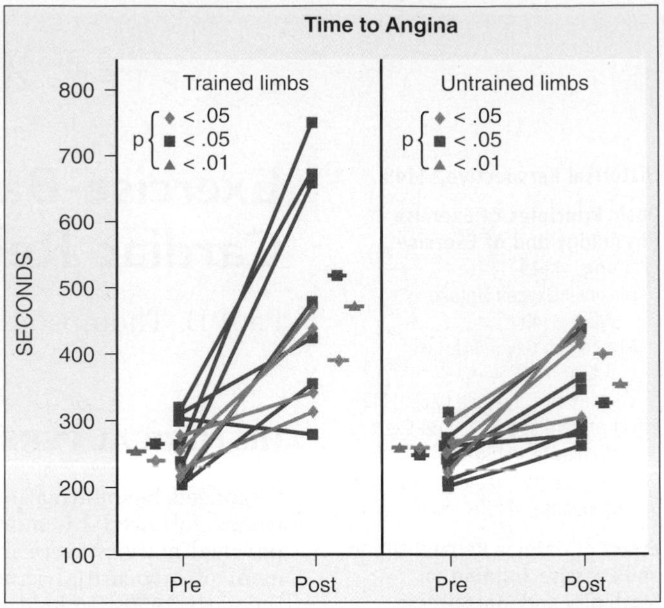

FIGURE 46–1 Time to angina during exercise with trained and untrained limbs before (PRE) and after (POST) 8 weeks of arm ($n = 4$) or leg ($n = 7$) exercise training shows that much of the exercise training effect is specific to the trained muscle groups (training specificity). However, some benefits accrue to untrained limb exercise. Subjects trained under supervision (40 minutes, 3 times weekly at or near their anginal threshold). Nitroglycerin permitted more intense exercise without pain. Barred symbols = mean values; green triangles = mean for all subjects. *(From Thompson PD: Exercise prescription and proscription for patients with coronary artery disease. Circulation 112:2354, 2005.)*

EFFECT OF CARDIAC REHABILITATION AND EXERCISE TRAINING ON MORBIDITY AND MORTALITY IN CARDIAC PATIENTS

Angina Pectoris

Currently, most patients with angina pectoris have their symptoms controlled with medication or by revascularization by PTCA or CABG. Consequently, and with rare exceptions,[7] much of the evidence that exercise training improves effort tolerance in patients with angina pectoris was obtained before 1990 (Fig. 46-1). Exercise training increases the exercise time to the onset of angina or even eliminates angina entirely by at least two mechanisms.

First, exercise training reduces the $\dot{M}O_2$ requirements during submaximal exercise.[5] Endurance exercise training increases $\dot{V}O_{2max}$. Because the HR and SBP response to exercise relate more closely to the percent $\dot{V}O_{2max}$ elicited by an exercise task and not to the absolute exercise work rate, the increase in $\dot{V}O_{2max}$ with exercise training reduces the HR and SBP response to submaximal exercise. This reduction in double product reduces the $\dot{M}O_2$ requirements and delays the onset of angina.

Second, exercise training reduces endothelial dysfunction.[8-10] Normal coronary arteries dilate with exercise, whereas atherosclerotic coronary arteries often demonstrate endothelial dysfunction evidenced by exercise-induced vasoconstriction. Exercise training reduces endothelial dysfunction, as measured by quantitative coronary angiography during infusions of the endothelial agonist acetylcholine.[8] Some patients also demonstrate increases in the rate pressure product at the onset of exercise after only brief periods of exercise training,[5] also supporting the concept of improved endothelial function (Fig. 46-2).

Exercise training in patients with angina, at least in the United States, is primarily relegated to use in patients who are anatomically unsuitable or not amenable to coronary interventions, but recent clinical trial evidence should prompt reevaluation of this approach. Hambrecht and colleagues[7] evaluated changes in exercise performance, coronary artery anatomy, and clinical outcomes in 101 men aged ≤70 years with stable angina pectoris. Subjects were randomized to either a year of exercise training or to PTCA. Subjects were excluded if the coronary lesion was not suitable for PTCA or if they had high-grade stenosis of the left anterior descending artery, greater than 25 percent left main stenosis, valvular disease, an ejection fraction less than 40 percent, an MI within 2 months, or PTCA or CABG within 12 months. The exercise training consisted of 2 weeks of 6 daily 10-minute sessions at 70 percent of their maximal tolerated HR, followed by daily 20-minute home exercise sessions plus a weekly 60-minute supervised session.

Forty-seven subjects in each group completed the trial. The exercise level at the onset of ischemia increased 30 percent in the exercise-trained and 20 percent in the PTCA subjects. These differences were not significant, but increases in maximal exercise capacity (20 versus 0 percent) and $\dot{V}O_{2max}$ (16 versus 2 percent) were significantly greater in the exercise-trained subjects. The potential target lesion did not change in the exercise subjects, and only 15 percent of the PTCA subjects demonstrated restenosis defined as greater than 50 percent luminal narrowing at the PTCA site. Total coronary artery disease (CAD) progression measured by angiographic scoring was less in the exercise-trained group, however, and 88 percent of the PTCA versus only 70 percent of the exercise-trained subjects experienced a major cardiovascular event including an MI, stroke, a revascularization procedure, or hospitalization for angina. This difference was statistically significant (Fig. 46-3). These results require confirmation and, because of the selection criteria, cannot be generalized to all subjects with stable angina pectoris. Nevertheless, these results do document that exercise training can aid the management of selected patients with angina.

Effect of Cardiac Rehabilitation on Morbidity and Mortality in Patients with Coronary Artery Disease

At least four meta-analyses have examined the effect of exercise-based cardiac rehabilitation on clinical outcomes.[5] All provide essentially identical results because they are based on many of the same studies. The most recent analysis examined 48 trials and included 8940 patients randomized to either cardiac rehabilitation or usual care.[11] Total and cardiac mortality were 20 and 26 percent lower, respectively, in the cardiac rehabilitation participants ($p < 0.05$ for

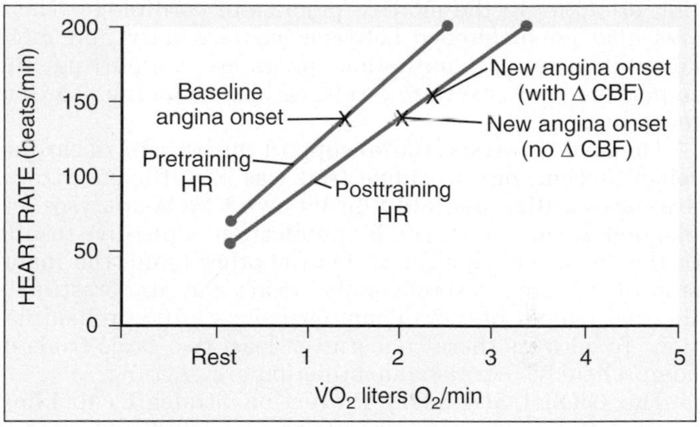

FIGURE 46–2 Changes in exercise tolerance and the onset of angina with exercise training. The heart rate (HR) versus $\dot{V}O_2$ slope is shifted so that any workrate ($\dot{V}O_2$) elicits a slower HR response. Angina is delayed to the same HR if there is no change in coronary blood flow (new angina onset [no Δ CBF]) or delayed to a higher HR if coronary blood flow is increased by improved endothelial function. *(From Thompson PD: Exercise prescription and proscription for patients with coronary artery disease. Circulation 112:2354, 2005.)*

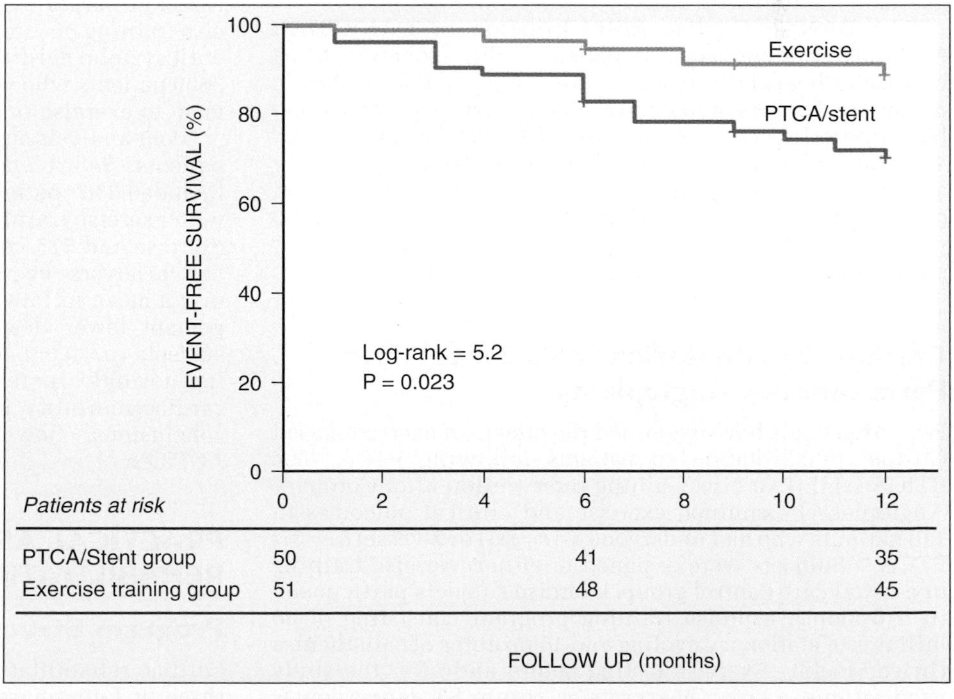

FIGURE 46–3 Event-free survival in 101 carefully selected patients with stable angina randomly assigned to percutaneous transluminal coronary angioplasty intervention (PTCA/stent) or to a year of exercise training. Numbers at figure bottom indicate patients free of events. Event-free survival was significantly better in the exercise training group (88 versus 70 percent, $p = 0.02$ by log-rank test). *(From Hambrecht R, Walther C, Mobius-Winkler S, et al: Percutaneous coronary angioplasty compared with exercise training in patients with stable coronary artery disease: A randomized trial. Circulation 109:1371, 2004.)*

both). Recurrent myocardial infarctions were also 20 percent lower, but this change was not statistically significant.

The majority of the trials in this meta-analysis were performed before modern revascularization strategies, so it is possible that many of the subjects in these early studies had residual coronary stenoses and inducible ischemia. Such patients are now routinely revascularized by PTCA or CABG. Given the beneficial effects of exercise training on cardiac ischemia and the present widespread use of revascularization strategies, it is not certain that similar reductions in cardiac mortality would accrue with present-day cardiac rehabilitation patients. The most recent meta-analysis found no differences in results from studies before and after 1995, suggesting that the benefits of cardiac rehabilitation do apply to the modern practice of cardiology. There was also no difference between exercise only and more comprehensive rehabilitation programs supporting the importance of exercise training in reducing cardiac mortality.

The meta-analysis studies support the benefits of cardiac rehabilitation, but no single trial was of sufficient size to evaluate cardiac mortality on its own.[5] Meta-analyses are plagued by the propensity for publication of positive results or the "positive paper bias." On the other hand, the inclusion of so many "exercise-only" trials may underestimate the real benefit of more comprehensive cardiac rehabilitation. To address these concerns, at least two large trials of comprehensive cardiac rehabilitation are ongoing.

The **Gl**O**bal** **S**econdary **P**revention Strategi**E**s to **L**imit events after myocardial infarction or GOSPEL study has enrolled 3241 patients in 78 Italian centers.[12] All subjects will undergo 3 months of standard cardiac rehabilitation and are then randomized to 3 years of an intensive rehabilitation effort or are returned to the care of their primary physicians. Participants in the intensive rehabilitation arm participate in exercise, lifestyle and risk factor counseling, and clinical assessments monthly for 6 months and then biannually for the rest of the study. The results should be available in 2007.

The **DAN**ish Cardiac **REHAB**ilitation or DANREHAB trial has randomized 770 patients with ischemic heart disease or heart failure or who are at high risk for ischemic disease to 6 weeks of intensive, hospital-based cardiac rehabilitation followed by 12 months of outpatient follow-up.[13] The intervention consists of exercise training, dietary advice, risk factor management, smoking cessation, and clinical support. The recruitment goal for the study is 1800 patients. When these results will be available and whether sufficient subjects can be recruited are unknown.[13]

Cardiac Rehabilitation in Patients After Percutaneous Angioplasty

Few large trials have examined the effects of exercise-based cardiac rehabilitation in patients following PTCA. The ETICA trial (Exercise Training Intervention after Coronary Angioplasty) examined exercise and clinical outcomes in 118 patients who had undergone 1- ($n = 81$) or 2-vessel ($n = 37$) PTCA.[14] Subjects were assigned to either exercise training or a usual care control group. Exercise subjects participated in a 6-month exercise training program consisting of 30 minutes of stationary cycling and 15 minutes of calisthenics thrice weekly. Exercise testing before and after the study used fatigue, a target heart rate or ≥1 mm ST depression as the endpoint.

$\dot{V}O_{2max}$ and quality-of-life measures each improved approximately 26 percent ($p < 0.001$) and only in the exercise-trained subjects. Angiographic restenosis defined as greater than 50 percent luminal narrowing at the angioplasty site did not differ at 6 months between the two groups (29 versus 33 percent), but luminal diameter at the angioplasty site was approximately 30 percent greater in the exercise-trained patients ($p < 0.05$). Disease progression and new lesions in major coronary arteries, both defined as a greater than 20 percent decrease in coronary diameter, were significantly less frequent in the exercise subjects. Cardiac ischemia measured as thallium perfusion defects also improved only in the trained subjects. Subjects were followed for 33 ± 7 months after the end of the protocol. Over this time there were no deaths in either group, but there were 20 percent ($p < 0.008$) fewer PTCAs (4 versus 11), MIs (1 versus 3), and CABGs (2 versus 5) in the exercise-trained subjects.

This study preceded the frequent use of stents during PTCA and the use of drug-eluting stents. Specifically, only 19 of the exercise-trained and 18 of the control subjects received a stent. Also, lipid-lowering therapy was prohibited because a secondary study examined the effect of exercise on lipid levels. Consequently, it is not clear if exercise training would produce similar reductions in atherosclerotic progression and cardiac events in patients treated with more contemporary therapies. Nevertheless, more current therapies should not alter the differences in exercise performance or quality of life measures observed in this trial. Also, it is not clear how much of the improvement in the angiographic appearance of the coronary tree was due to structural change in the atherosclerotic plaque versus functional changes in coronary artery tone due to improved endothelial function.

Cardiac Rehabilitation in Heart Failure

As with CAD, there is no trial of sufficient size to determine conclusively the effect of exercise rehabilitation on survival in patients with heart failure (HF). The HF-ACTION trial or **H**eart **F**ailure and **A** **C**ontrolled **T**rial **I**nvestigating **O**utcomes of Exercise Trai**N**ing) trial has been funded by the National Institutes of Health to examine the effect of exercise training on cardiac morbidity and mortality in patients with systolic cardiac dysfunction. The trial seeks to enroll 3000 patients who will be randomized to receive encouragement to exercise or a formal exercise program.[15]

Meta-analysis support exists for an exercise benefit in HF patients. Smart and Marwick[16] collected 81 studies that included 2387 patients with HF. $\dot{V}O_{2max}$ increased 16 percent with exercise training. Outcome data were available for 622 exercise and 575 control patients. There was no difference in total adverse events between the exercising control groups over a mean follow-up of 5.9 months. On the other hand, 29 percent fewer deaths occurred in the exercise training subjects ($p = 0.06$). Such results suggest that exercise training not only increases exercise capacity but may reduce cardiac mortality in patients with systolic HF. Definitive conclusions, however, must await the results of HF ACTION.

PRACTICAL ASPECTS OF CARDIAC REHABILITATION PROGRAMS

Program Structure

Cardiac rehabilitation programs are generally divided into three or four phases on the basis of the patient's clinical status (Table 46-2). Phase 1 refers to inpatient programs started soon after the acute cardiac event or intervention. Phase 1 programs are less common presently because of the brevity of most hospital stays, although some European countries still have inpatient rehabilitation programs that

TABLE 46-2	Traditional Terminology for the Phases of Cardiac Rehabilitation
Phase 1	Inpatient rehabilitation, usually lasting for the duration of hospitalization. It emphasizes a gradual, progressive approach to exercise and an education program that helps the patient understand the disease process, the rehabilitation process, and initial preventive efforts to slow the progression of disease.
Phase 2	Multifaceted outpatient rehabilitation, lasting 2-3 mo. Emphasizes safe physical activity to improve conditioning with continued behavior modification aimed at smoking cessation, weight loss, healthy eating, and other factors to reduce disease risk. Initiate an exercise prescription.
Phase 3	Supervised rehabilitation, lasting 6-12 mo. Establishes a prescription for safe exercise that can be performed at home or in a community service facility, such as a senior center or YMCA, and continues to emphasize risk factor reduction.
Phase 4	Maintenance, indefinite.

may last several weeks. Even with the short duration of many cardiac hospital admissions, phase 1 programs remain useful in mobilizing elderly patients after complicated cardiac events and in many patients after cardiac surgery. Phase 1 programs in the United States are often directed by physical therapy departments or a dedicated cardiac rehabilitation staff. Phase 1 is also an excellent way to introduce patients to the concept of cardiac rehabilitation and to solicit appropriate referrals.

Phase 2 refers to physician-supervised outpatient programs. Physician supervision is required for reimbursement by most U.S. insurance carriers, as is electrocardiographic monitoring. Historically, patients in phase 2 programs exercise 3 times weekly for 3 months. Other approaches to cardiac rehabilitation include simple home-based, self-supervised programs; home-based, visiting nurse–supervised programs; and home-based programs with telephone electrocardiographic monitoring. Such approaches have been examined in research settings and compare favorably with standard facility-based programs. Indeed, exercise capacity appears to improve more with home-based training,[17] although such improvements may result from the tendency for studied programs to show improvement or "attention bias" alone. Other approaches to program duration have also been examined including one session weekly for a year.[18] Such approaches can increase exercise capacity and may assist adoption of an ongoing exercise program, but the standard facility-based, 12-week programs are most readily recognized and are the only programs to our knowledge covered by insurance carriers.

Phase 3 refers to non-ECG monitored, medically supervised, maintenance programs, which are often provided by the same facilities providing phase 2 programs. Some insurance carriers offer limited reimbursement for phase 3 programs. Phase 4 refers to programs that do not usually provide medical supervision and are usually provided by health clubs and fitness facilities. Phase 4 programs are not covered by medical insurance in the United States.

Staff Coverage

The standard cardiac rehabilitation program has a physician medical director, a staff nurse, plus other nurses or individuals with training in exercise physiology to design the exercise and educational programs and supervise the exercise sessions. To qualify for Medicare reimbursement in the United States, phase 2 cardiac rehabilitation programs must have the supervising physician present during the rehabilitation sessions. Also, for reimbursement, patients must have an ECG strip recorded, interpreted, and mounted in the chart for each session. Definition of the term "present" for the physician is open to interpretation but has generally referred to being in the facility and available within moments for any emergency. All cardiac rehabilitation staff should be trained in advanced cardiac life support. A nurse should be available during the exercise rehabilitation sessions to handle emergencies and administer medications. Staffing levels are recommended at 1 staff member per 5 participants during phase 2 and 1 staff member per 10 to 15 participants during phase 3 to 4 sessions.

Design and Administration of the Exercise Training Program

Patients referred to cardiac rehabilitation should undergo a symptom-limited exercise test before entering the program. The exercise test is required to exclude important symptoms, ischemia, or arrhythmias that might require other interventions before exercise training. The exercise test also serves to establish baseline exercise capacity and to determine maximum heart rate for use in preparing an exercise prescription. These tests are usually done with the patient on his or her usual medications to mimic the heart rate response likely to occur during exercise training.

Typical exercise training sessions for cardiac rehabilitation patients consists of 5 minutes of warm-up followed by at least 20 minutes of aerobic exercise training and 5 to 15 minutes of cool-down. The warm-up session consists of stretching and light calisthenics. Some resistance exercise training using light weights or exercise machines should also be performed, often after the aerobic session and as part of an extended cool-down. Such exercises as biceps curls, triceps extensions, military presses (for patients without shoulder problems), shoulder shrugs, bent-knee pushups, bent-knee "crunches," and quarter squats address most of the major muscle groups and increase the patients' ability to perform the tasks of work and daily living, which often require lifting and carrying activities.

The aerobic exercise training component is generally performed at 60 to 70 percent of $\dot{V}O_{2max}$, which corresponds to approximately 70 to 80 percent of maximum heart rate (Table 46-3). Some patients require lower training intensities. Although 20 minutes of exercise training is standard, shorter periods of exercise training are beneficial and longer sessions almost certainly provide additional benefit. Most cardiac rehabilitation programs recommend other activities such as yard work and walking on days when patients do not attend supervised sessions.

Exercise testing before starting cardiac rehabilitation is useful, but not all patients, especially those after recent MI, undergo such testing. Patients who did not undergo exercise testing before the program can exercise at a heart rate 20 beats faster than their resting value. Another approach is exercising patients at their resting HR plus a specified additional percent of rest. For example, during month 1, the patient might exercise at rest HR + 20 to 30 percent rest HR; month 2, rest HR + 20 to 40 percent rest HR; and month 3, rest HR + 20 to 50 percent rest HR. Alternatively, such patients can exercise to the point of mild dyspnea and maintain that level during the training session. As discussed earlier, the onset of dyspnea approximates the VT and is an adequate intensity for a training stimulus. Finally, patients can exercise to a "somewhat hard" level using number scales designed to estimate the intensity of exertion, such as the modified Borg scale.

TABLE 46–3 Exercise Prescriptions for Coronary Artery Disease (CAD) Patients

Patients	Intensity	Frequency	Duration
Aerobic Exercise			
General CAD	70-85% peak HR	≥3 times weekly	≥20 min per session
With asymptomatic ischemia	70-85% ischemic HR	≥3 times weekly	≥20 min per session
With angina	70-85% ischemic HR or angina onset	≥3 times weekly	≥20 min per session
With angioplasty±stent	As for general CAD patient		
With claudication	Walking to pain tolerance	≥3 times weekly	≥30 min per session
With New York Heart Association Class I-III HF	As for general CAD patient		
Resistance Exercise			
For most CAD patients	30-50% RM	2-3 times weekly	12-15 repetitions

HF=heart failure; HR=heart rate; RM=1-repetition maximal weight.
From Thompson PD: Exercise prescription and proscription for patients with coronary artery disease. Circulation 112:2354, 2005.

Unsupervised Exercise Training

Many patients cannot attend supervised exercise training sessions because a cardiac rehabilitation program is not available or because it is not convenient to attend supervised sessions. Nevertheless, all CAD patients should be advised to exercise for its cardiovascular benefits.

Patients without lower limb orthopedic problems should be encouraged to use brisk walking as their exercise training modality. Patients in unsupervised programs should generally be encouraged to exercise to the onset of mild dyspnea for the reasons mentioned earlier. Such an approach obviates the need for pulse monitoring. Many patients either cannot accurately monitor their heart rate or become unduly concerned about pulse irregularities caused by premature atrial or ventricular contractions. Patients exercising on their own can also be encouraged to judge their exercise intensity using the "talk test" (i.e., exercising at the fastest walking rate that still permits comfortable conversation). This workrate corresponds to the exercising training range recommended for cardiac patients.[5]

OTHER COMPONENTS OF COMPREHENSIVE CARDIAC REHABILITATION

In 1994 the American Heart Association recommended that cardiac rehabilitation programs expand to include other strategies designed to reduce cardiovascular risk.[6] These included nutritional, psychological, and vocational counseling, as well as serum lipid, blood pressure, and smoking risk factor management. These components of secondary CAD prevention are undoubtedly critically important. Lipid reduction with statins, for example, has repeatedly been shown to reduce recurrent cardiac events in CAD patients[19] (see Chaps. 42 and 45). A review of 20 prospective cohort studies suggests that CAD patients who stop smoking experience a 36 percent reduction in total mortality.[20] Addressing such issues often requires a balancing of the roles of the cardiac rehabilitation staff and those of the primary care physician. The cardiac rehabilitation personnel generally focus on counseling aspects of risk factor management. They can also serve as a knowledgeable source to interpret laboratory results and physician instructions and as patient advocates with their primary physicians. With lipid management, for example, the rehabilitation staff may evaluate the results from the patient's physician and suggest that the patient request a more aggressive treatment approach to achieve cholesterol goals.

Programs differ as to how they deliver the counseling and education components of the program. Evaluating the participant's learning style may help to maximize the program's education potential. Many programs use the aerobic exercise time to visit with and educate the patient while he or she is on the exercise apparatus. Some programs simply make printed material available to the participants. Other programs use television monitors and either commercially available or locally prepared video programs to deliver the counseling and risk reduction messages. Some programs have replaced exercise sessions with educational programs, an approach we oppose given the physiological benefits of exercise training. Classroom activities can be scheduled creatively in addition to the exercise sessions, allowing participants to choose what education programs best meet their needs. Ideally, educational programs on nutrition, lipid management, smoking cessation, and psychological issues should be delivered by experts in the field, but such experts are often not available, requiring the rehabilitation staff to provide these sessions or to purchase commercially available programs.

INSURANCE COVERAGE

Insurance coverage of cardiac rehabilitation activities is critically important for patients to be able to receive these services. Starting March 22, 2006,[21] Medicare in the United States began reimbursing patients who are characterized by the following:

1. Have had an acute myocardial infarction (AMI) within the preceding 12 months
2. Have undergone CAGB
3. Have stable angina pectoris
4. Have undergone a cardiac valve repair or replacement
5. Have undergone PTCA
6. Have received a heart or heart-lung transplant

This most recent iteration of the reimbursement policies extended coverage to items 3 through 6, which were not previously covered.[22] This is critically important in the United States because many private insurers follow the Medicare reimbursement procedures. Routine coverage is for a total of 36 exercise sessions. Cardiac rehabilitation is not covered by Medicare for HF but is covered by some insurance carriers. Insurance coverage in other parts of the world varies greatly.

PRESENT PROBLEMS WITH CARDIAC REHABILITATION

The major present problem with exercise-based cardiac rehabilitation is its underutilization. Only some 25 to 30 percent of men and 11 to 20 percent of women eligible for cardiac rehabilitation participate in such programs.[23] Physician endorsement of cardiac rehabilitation is one of the most important predictors of participation.[23] It is unclear why physicians do not routinely refer patients, although physicians' underestimation of the benefits of exercise, health professionals' lack of knowledge about exercise training, and the absence of exercise advocates similar to pharmaceutical representatives may contribute. All physicians should refer eligible patients to cardiac rehabilitation. Even when the physician is not convinced of the benefit, the patient often finds the experience rewarding and reassuring. One of the most effective ways to combat the lack of referral is to include cardiac rehabilitation in standardized order sets for appropriate cardiac patients.

THE FUTURE OF CARDIAC REHABILITATION

Ideally, in the future exercise-based cardiac rehabilitation should be used more widely to improve endothelial dysfunction and to manage angina pectoris and stable coronary artery disease, thereby reducing such costly interventions as PTCA and CABG. Little conclusive information establishes that PTCA saves lives, whereas there is evidence, albeit from a small controlled clinical trial, that exercise training decreases cardiovascular events compared with PTCA in selected patients with angina pectoris.[7] This trial requires confirmation in larger sample sets. Also, ongoing trials are comparing cardiac rehabilitation versus usual care in cardiac patients.[12,13] Even if these trials do not support the routine use of exercise training in cardiac patients, additional trials should be initiated comparing intensive rehabilitation and best available medical therapy to PTCA or CABG in CAD patients. The evidence that CABG is superior to medical therapy in selected CAD patients is decades old and may no longer be valid given the availability of statins and other highly effective pharmacological interventions. Appropriately designed trials may document that comprehensive cardiac rehabilitation including exercise training and aggressive lifestyle and medication management of risk factors obviate the need for such surgical therapy.

Acknowledgments

The author thanks the staff of the Hartford Hospital Cardiac Rehabilitation Program for the years of education they have provided to the author and Lucie Bohannon, MS, PT, for advice on the practical aspects of rehabilitation.

REFERENCES

Exercise Physiology

1. Redwood DR, Rosing DR, Epstein SE: Circulatory and symptomatic effects of physical training in patients with coronary-artery disease and angina pectoris. N Engl J Med 286:959, 1972.
2. Detry JM, Rousseau M, Vandenbroucke G, et al: Increased arteriovenous oxygen difference after physical training in coronary heart disease. Circulation 44:109, 1971.

3. Ades PA: Cardiac rehabilitation and secondary prevention of coronary heart disease. N Engl J Med 345:892, 2001.
4. American Association of Cardiovascular and Pulmonary Rehabilitation (http://www.aacvpr.org/certification/). Accessed May 28, 2006.

Rehabilitation in Coronary Artery Disease

5. Thompson PD: Exercise prescription and proscription for patients with coronary artery disease. Circulation 112:2354, 2005.
6. Leon AS, Franklin BA, Costa F, et al: Cardiac rehabilitation and secondary prevention of coronary heart disease: An American Heart Association scientific statement from the Council on Clinical Cardiology (Subcommittee on Exercise, Cardiac Rehabilitation, and Prevention) and the Council on Nutrition, Physical Activity, and Metabolism (Subcommittee on Physical Activity), in collaboration with the American Association of Cardiovascular and Pulmonary Rehabilitation. Circulation 111:369, 2005.
7. Hambrecht R, Walther C, Mobius-Winkler S, et al: Percutaneous coronary angioplasty compared with exercise training in patients with stable coronary artery disease: A randomized trial. Circulation 109:1371, 2004.
8. Hambrecht R, Wolf A, Gielen S, et al: Effect of exercise on coronary endothelial function in patients with coronary artery disease. N Engl J Med 342:454, 2000.
9. Moyna NM, Thompson PD: The effect of physical activity on endothelial function in man. Acta Physiol Scand 180:113, 2004.
10. Hambrecht R, Adams V, Erbs S, et al: Regular physical activity improves endothelial function in patients with coronary artery disease by increasing phosphorylation of endothelial nitric oxide synthase. Circulation 107:3152, 2003.
11. Taylor RS, Brown A, Ebrahim S, et al: Exercise-based rehabilitation for patients with coronary heart disease: Systematic review and meta-analysis of randomized controlled trials. Am J Med 116:682, 2004.
12. Giannuzzi P, Temporelli PL, Maggioni AP, et al: GlObal Secondary Prevention strategiEs to Limit event recurrence after myocardial infarction: The GOSPEL study. A trial from the Italian Cardiac Rehabilitation Network: Rationale and design. Eur J Cardiovasc Prev Rehabil 12:555, 2005.
13. Zwisler AD, Schou L, Soja AM, et al: A randomized clinical trial of hospital-based, comprehensive cardiac rehabilitation versus usual care for patients with congestive heart failure, ischemic heart disease, or high risk of ischemic heart disease (the DANREHAB trial)—design, intervention, and population. Am Heart J 150:899, 2005.

Exercise Intervention in Heart Failure

14. Belardinelli R, Paolini I, Cianci G, et al: Exercise training intervention after coronary angioplasty: The ETICA trial. J Am Coll Cardiol 37:1891, 2001.
15. Cleland JG, Huan LP, Freemantle N, et al: Clinical trials update from the European Society of Cardiology: SENIORS, ACES, PROVE-IT, ACTION, and the HF-ACTION trial. Eur J Heart Fail 6:787, 2004.
16. Smart N, Marwick TH: Exercise training for patients with heart failure: A systematic review of factors that improve mortality and morbidity. Am J Med 116:693, 2004.

Practical Aspects of Cardiac Rehabilitation Programs

17. Jolly K, Taylor RS, Lip GY, Stevens A: Home-based cardiac rehabilitation compared with centre-based rehabilitation and usual care: A systematic review and meta-analysis. Int J Cardiol 111:343, 2005.
18. Hamm LF, Kavanagh T, Campbell RB, et al: Timeline for peak improvements during 52 weeks of outpatient cardiac rehabilitation. J Cardiopulm Rehabil 24:374, 2004.
19. Gotto AM Jr: Review of primary and secondary prevention trials with lovastatin, pravastatin, and simvastatin. Am J Cardiol 96:34F, 2005.
20. Critchley JA, Capewell S: Mortality risk reduction associated with smoking cessation in patients with coronary heart disease: A systematic review. JAMA 290:86, 2003.
21. Centers for Medicare and Medicaid Services: Medicare coverage database (https://www.cms.hhs.gov/mcd/viewdecisionmemo.asp?id=164). Accessed March 22, 2006 and June 8, 2006.
22. Centers for Medicare and Medicaid Services: New York State Medicare Local Medical Review Policy (http://www.empiremedicare.com/nyorkpolicya/policy/cardiac.htm). Accessed Dec. 28, 2004.
23. Jackson L, Leclerc J, Erskine Y, Linden W: Getting the most out of cardiac rehabilitation: A review of referral and adherence predictors. Heart 91:10, 2005.

CHAPTER 47

Complementary and Alternative Approaches to Management of Patients with Heart Disease

John H. K. Vogel, Rebecca B. Costello, and Mitchell W. Krucoff

GENERAL CONSIDERATIONS

Complementary and alternative medicine (CAM) is the term currently used by the National Institute of Health (NIH) to describe this field of inquiry. Herbs, vitamins, and nonherbal dietary products, as well as therapies involving spirituality, bioenergetics (e.g., acupuncture and energy fields), and mind-body, are all considered to be forms of complementary, alternative, or integrative medicine.

According to the National Center for Complementary and Alternative Medicine (NCCAM) and the National Center for Health Statistics (NCHS),[1] 36 percent of American adults use some form of CAM.[2] When prayer specifically for health reasons is included in the definition of CAM, that figure rises to 62 percent. Of note, CAM is being taught in some 25 medical centers in the country.[3]

Listening, trust, and compassion embody the principles used by great physicians caring for patients on physical, mental, and spiritual levels. Integrating CAM into medicine must be guided by compassion but enhanced by science and must remain meaningful through solid physician-patient relationships, because human caring and relationships are central to the health care process. Physicians must establish trust and a feeling of safe harbor for patients so that we may, by understanding their concerns and discovering their goals and desires, convey accurate and appropriate information when proposing a reasonable, mutually agreeable plan of care. A great majority of our patients have become involved in CAM. It is therefore important, even if the physician has problems accepting CAM, to respect the patient's belief system and continue to have their trust so as not to drive the patient away.

In addition, because patients perceive that many physicians do not care about their involvement in CAM or the herbs or supplements they are taking, they fail to communicate this information to their physicians. This can result in detrimental adverse herbal or supplement allopathic drug interventions. Thus, it is extremely important for the physician to be aware exactly what their patients are taking to avoid these problems.

Successful treatment and prevention of complex chronic disease almost always require multi-component therapy, coupled with life-style modifications. With only modest evidence-based data available to clinicians and their patients regarding the benefits and potential risks of dietary supplements and herbal products, clinicians will need to become more attentive to recognizing and recording use of supplements and responding to patients' inquiries and preferences.

APPLICATIONS OF COMPLEMENTARY AND ALTERNATIVE MEDICINE

Stress Relief

Stress relief is clearly one of the major risk factors in cardiovascular disease, and methods for dealing with stress are very important (see Chap. 86).

IMPACT OF STRESS ON CARDIOVASCULAR DISEASE RISK FACTORS. Stress may lead to hypertension through repeated blood pressure elevations and by increasing the amount of vasoconstricting hormones (see Chap. 40). Stress factors leading to hypertension include job strain, social environment, emotional stress, race, and white coat hypertension. In the Framingham study,[4] hypertension was involved in over 80 percent of all cardiovascular deaths. In addition, hypertension was at least twice as strong a predictor of death as smoking or elevated blood cholesterol level. Over 50 million Americans are currently hypertensive.

Stress Management

PET OWNERSHIP. Pet ownership reduces stress and can convey a sense of companionship and purpose. Pet ownership has been shown to increase heart rate variability (see Chap. 32) in patients with cardiovascular disease.[5]

MINDFULNESS-BASED STRESS REDUCTION. Mindfulness-based stress reduction (MBSR) uses the techniques of mindfulness meditation, gentle yoga, and coordinated deep breathing to decrease pain and anxiety. In a meta-analysis, MBSR has been shown to help individuals alleviate stress and suffering associated with various diseases.[6]

GUIDED IMAGERY. Guided imagery is a therapeutic technique that allows a person to use his or her own imagination to connect body and mind to achieve desirable outcomes, such as decreased pain perception and reduced anxiety. Guided imagery has been studied for patients both pre- and postsurgical intervention. A recent study of cardiothoracic surgery patients demonstrated that both pain and anxiety decreased significantly with guided imagery.[7] An ongoing trial at Scripps Clinic using guided imagery and healing touch pre- and postcardiothoracic surgery has demonstrated a 50 percent reduction in pain and anxiety in the treatment group.

TRANSCENDENTAL MEDITATION. Transcendental meditation (TM) offers a unique technique for meditation and relaxation and is one of the most studied CAM therapies, with research dating back to the 1970s. TM has been shown not only to improve blood pressure but also the insulin resistance components of the metabolic syndrome and cardiac autonomic nervous system tone.[8]

BIOFEEDBACK. Biofeedback is a technique to train people to change habitual reactions to stress. In patients with coronary artery disease, biofeedback increases heart rate variability (HRV).

DIETARY SUPPLEMENTS AND NATURAL PRODUCTS. A number of food components have been recommended and endorsed for lowering the risk of cardiovascular disease, including plant sterols and stanol esters, soluble fibers, omega-3 fatty acids, garlic, soy, tea, and moderate alcohol intake.[9,10] The Dietary Supplement Health and Education Act (DSHEA) of 1994 amended the federal Food, Drug, and Cosmetic Act by defining as a dietary supplement any product (other than tobacco) that contains a vitamin, mineral, herb or other botanical, or amino acid and is intended as a supplement to the diet. In the United States today, products intended to supplement the diet may be marketed as dietary supplements providing that their intended use is not to diagnose, treat, cure, or prevent disease (a claim reserved for conventional drugs) and that they not be represented as conventional foods. The U.S. Food and Drug Administration (FDA) has estimated that there were more than 29,000 different dietary supplement products on the market in 2000, with an average of 1,000 new products being added annually. Several countries (e.g., Germany, France, Sweden, Canada, and Australia) have implemented strategies for licensing herbal remedies, including premarket approval. However, premarket approval and licensing are not required in the United States.

There are a number of approved drug substances that originate from plants, such as digoxin, atropine, reserpine, and amiodarone. However, only a few commercial herbal products available in the United States have been tested for cardiovascular indications: hawthorn (heart failure and coronary insufficiency), garlic (atherosclerosis), ginkgo (arterial occlusive disease), and horse chestnut (chronic venous insufficiency). Few U.S. products benefit from rigorous characterization and standardization necessary for clinical study. Herbal products, unlike most conventional drugs, provide a complex mixture of bioactive entities, which may or may not have therapeutic activity. The active ingredient is frequently not known and complete characterization of all the chemical constituents is lacking (Table 47-1). As with conventional drugs, many herbal products are therapeutic at one dose and toxic at another. Concurrent use of herbs may mimic, magnify, or oppose the effect of drugs. The importance of unrecognized interactions between herbs and conventional drugs is particularly relevant in cardiology because many cardiovascular drugs have a narrow therapeutic window (Table 47-2). Table 47-3 lists sources for more information on dietary supplements and herbal medicines.

Herbal-drug interactions can be characterized as pharmacodynamic or pharmacokinetic. Pharmacodynamic interactions can occur when constituents of herbal products have synergistic or antagonist activity in relation to a conventional drug, thus altering the site of action at the receptor level. Pharmacokinetic interactions result from alterations of absorption, distribution, metabolism, and elimination of a conventional drug by a herbal product or dietary supplement. Herbal products contain several chemicals that are metabolized by phase 1 and phase 2 drug-metabolizing pathways, especially CYP3A4, and also serve as substrates for certain transporters and P-glycoprotein (PGP; see Chap. 6). In vivo and in vitro studies have indicated that PGP-mediated efflux and/or CYP-mediated metabolism is likely to be a potential candidate for drug-herbal interactions, adversely affecting drug efficacy and/or toxicity. Clinical implications of such drug-herbal interactions depend on various factors such as dose, frequency and timing of herbal intake, dosing regimen, route of drug administration, and therapeutic range. Additionally, use of herbal products may significantly alter laboratory results. Abnormal laboratory test results may indicate that clinicians should ascertain a detailed history of the use of herbal products and dietary supplements from their patients. A herbal product can affect clinical laboratory test results by direct assay interference, most commonly with an immunoassay, exert physiologic effects through toxicity or enzyme induction, and interfere by the presence of contaminants.

TABLE 47–1 Herbal versus Synthetic Drugs

Drug	Herbal
Active ingredient known	Active ingredient often not known, marker compounds act as surrogates for consistency
Pure compound available	Pure compound not available, often as mixtures
Composition constant	Composition variable, because of season, temperature, and harvest conditions
Mechanism often known	Mechanism often unknown
Toxicology often known, but at least evaluated	Toxicology often not studied
Typically, a short tradition of use	Typically, a long tradition of use
Frequently, a narrow therapeutic window	Generally, a wide therapeutic window
Adverse effects frequent	Adverse effects rare

Hypertension (see Chap. 41)

Randomized clinical trials for hypertension have been conducted with garlic (*Allium sativum*), ginkgo (*Ginkgo biloba*), hawthorn (*Crataegus*), pycnogenol or French maritime pine bark extract (*Pinus maritima*), olive leaf extract (*Olea europaea*), Asian ginseng (*Panax ginseng*), coenzyme Q1O, calcium, and magnesium. The results have been variable and modest. A meta-analysis has shown that compared with placebo, garlic produced average blood pressure (BP) reductions of 8 mm Hg (systolic) and 5 mm Hg (diastolic).[11] However, an evidence-based review of 27 small, randomized, placebo-controlled trials, all but one in adults and of short duration, reported mixed but never large effects of various garlic preparations on blood pressure outcomes. Most studies have not found significant differences between subjects randomized to garlic compared with those randomized to placebo.[12] Adverse effects of oral ingestion of garlic are objectionable breath and body odor. Other possible but not proven adverse effects have included flatulence, esophageal and abdominal pain, small intestinal obstruction, contact dermatitis, rhinitis, asthma, bleeding, and myocardial infarction.

A systematic review of coenzyme Q10 in hypertension that evaluated eight studies documented a mean decrease in systolic blood pressure of 16 mm Hg and a decrease of 10 mm Hg in diastolic blood pressure, but only half of these studies were placebo-controlled.[13] A recent Cochrane review has confirmed a lack of effect of combined calcium, magnesium, and potassium supplementation for the management of primary hypertension in adults.[14]

Lipid Lowering (see Chap. 42)

Conventional and dietary supplements for hyperlipidemia include products reported to decrease liver production of lipids, such as artichoke extract (*Cynara scolymus*), garlic, policosanol, and red yeast rice (*Monascus purpureus*). Products reported to decrease the absorption of lipids include stanol and sterol esters, chitosan, barley, psyllium, and oat bran fibers. Additionally, fish oils, docosahexaenoic acid (DHA), and eicosapentaenoic acid (EPA) and soy have been extensively studied in clinical trials. Guggulipid (*Commiphora guggul*) and policosanol will be described here.

GUGGULIPID (*Commiphora guggul*). Guggulipid has a long history of use in Ayurvedic medicine. In the first randomized controlled trial of guggulipid in the United States, 103 healthy adults with hypercholesterolemia given 1000 or 2000 mg guggulipid containing 2.5 percent guggulsterones experienced no improvement in their lipid levels. A hypersensitivity rash was reported in a small number of subjects.[15] Effects of guggulipids on high-density lipoproteins (HDLs) were mixed. A standard dose of guggulsterones containing 75 to 150 mg has been given as 1000 to 2000 mg guggulipid two or three times daily. Guggulipids can cause gastrointestinal upset, headache, mild nausea, belching, hiccups, and rash. Concomitant oral administration can

Text continues on p. 1162.

TABLE 47–2 Potential Interactions between Dietary Supplements and Conventional Medications

Supplement	Reported Uses	Active Ingredients	Potential Interactions	Comments and Suggested Guidelines for Use
Aloe, dried juice from leaf, latex	Relief from constipation; used as a laxative or cathartic	Anthracine derivatives from dried leaf juice and latex constituents	May ↓ absorption of other drugs; may ↑ potassium losses with digoxin or cardiac glycosides containing herbs, antiarrhythmics, diuretics, and corticosteroids	Approved in Germany for treatment of constipation—limit use to 2 weeks; side effects—abdominal pain, nausea, vomiting, diarrhea, electrolyte (potassium losses) imbalance at higher doses
Arginine	Improves coronary blood flow; adjuvant therapy for CHF, angina, hypertension, CHD	L-Arginine	May cause additive hypotensive effects if combined with hypertensive drugs or nitrates	L-Arginine is precursor of nitric oxide, has been shown to improve coronary and brachial artery endothelial function; potential side effects include GI symptoms, gout, may exacerbate airway inflammation in asthma; efficacy of oral L-arginine for CHD awaits confirmation
Artichoke leaf extract *(Cynara scolymus)*	Lowers blood cholesterol level	Phenolic acids (chlorogenic acid, cynarin, and caffeic acid), sesquiterpene lactones and flavonoids	No known interactions with herbs and other dietary supplements, drugs, foods or laboratory test results	In the United States, artichoke has GRAS use in foods; few data from rigorous clinical trials exist; beneficial effects reported, but not compelling; potential adverse effects include flatulence, allergic dermatitis
Carnitine	Relief from angina; adjunct therapy for heart failure	L-Carnitine, acetyl-L-carnitine and propionyl-L-carnitine	Concomitant use with acenocoumarol may potentiate (decrease) anticoagulant effects; unknown whether interactions occur with warfarin	L-Carnitine is naturally found in the body. D-or DL-carnitine should not be substituted for L-carnitine; potential side effects include GI upset, diarrhea, body odor, seizures; FDA approved L-carnitine for use in primary carnitine deficiency; CHF clinical trials underway in Italy; monitor INRs in patients on anticoagulant therapies
Coenzyme Q10 (Co-Q10; ubiquinone)	Improves cardiac performance and recovery from ischemic events; adjuvant therapy for lowering blood pressure, reducing symptoms of CHF, and cardiotoxicity associated with chemotherapy	Q10—refers to the 5-carbon isoprenoid units attached to the quinone ring	Use with HMG-CoA reductase inhibitors (statins) and some oral hypoglycemic agents can reduce serum Co-Q10 levels; Co-Q10 may have pro-coagulant properties, may reduce the effects of warfarin and ↑ INR; may have additive blood pressure—lowering effects when used with hypertensive agents	The Japanese government has approved Co-Q10 for treatment of CHF; no reports of significant toxicity in studies lasting up to 30 months; potential side effects include gastritis, loss of appetite, nausea, and diarrhea; data conflicting in patients on anticoagulation; monitor INR in patients taking warfarin
Danshen *(Salvia miltiorhiza)*	Promotes blood flow; treats CVD disorders	Dried root and rhizome contain tanshinones and phenolic compounds	Potential interaction with anticoagulant and antiplatelet drugs and/or supplements; may increase risk of bleeding and ↑ INR; may interfere with serum digoxin measurements	TCM sold over the counter; prescribed by TCM doctors for acute MI, angina, thrombotic disorders; may cause pruritus, upset stomach, reduced appetite; avoid use in patients taking warfarin
Dong quai *(Angelica sinensis)*	Reduces symptoms of menopause; lowers blood pressure	Contains coumarin derivatives	Potential interaction with anticoagulant or antiplatelet drugs and/or supplements; may increase risk of bleeding and ↑ INR	Popular TCM preparation that is generally well tolerated; avoid use in patients taking warfarin
Fenugreek *(Trigonella foenum-graecum)*	Control of blood glucose levels; prevention of CVD; lowers blood cholesterol level	Seed components and constituents; contains anticoagulant coumarins	Theoretically, high mucilage content of fenugreek can ↓ blood sugar levels as well as ↓ or delay absorption of oral drugs; could enhance anticoagulant drug activity and ↑ risk of bleeding	Fenugreek has GRAS status in the United States, therefore likely safe when seed preparations are used in amounts commonly found in foods; potential side effects include diarrhea, flatulence, hypoglycemia with large doses; monitor warfarin levels; monitor insulin levels
Garlic *(Allium sativum)*	Lowers blood cholesterol level; lowers blood pressure	Allyl sulfur compounds, such as alliin, which is rapidly converted to allicin	Interacts with P-450 enzyme system; concomitant use with herbs or drugs that have coumarin constituents or affect platelet aggregation could ↑ INR and risk of bleeding; concomitant use with EPA or fish oils may ↑ anti-thrombotic effects	Has been used in clinical studies up to 4 years without reports of toxicity; additive effects on cholesterol lowering seen when taken with lipid-lowering agents; mixed data for blood pressure; monitor individuals on warfarin; discontinue use prior to surgery

TABLE 47–2 Potential Interactions between Dietary Supplements and Conventional Medications—cont'd

Supplement	Reported Uses	Active Ingredients	Potential Interactions	Comments and Suggested Guidelines for Use
Ginkgo leaf extract (*Ginkgo biloba*)	Aids in circulation to improve cognitive function; relief of pain caused by intermittent claudication	Flavonoids and flavone glycosides (ginkgolides and bilobalides)	Ginkgolides have antiplatelet activity, are PAF receptor antagonists; may have an additive effect with other blood-thinning agents such as herbs and/or drugs with anticoagulant or antiplatelet potential; may ↑ INR and risk of bleeding; may also affect bioavailability of other drugs. Avoid use with insulin and thiazide diuretics	Likely safe when used orally and appropriately; discontinue use prior to surgery; avoid in individuals with diabetes; five cases of cerebral hemorrhage have been reported in those taking prescription anticoagulants; avoid use with warfarin
Ginseng root, Asian (*Panax ginseng*)	Acts as an "adaptogen" to enhance energy levels, relieve stress and ease symptoms of anxiety; antihypertensive; improves control of blood sugar	Ginsenosides—main active components derived from the root	Interacts with P-450 enzyme system; potential to interact with anticoagulants, antiplatelet drugs, corticosteroids, calcium channel blockers, digoxin, methyldopa; interacts with MAO inhibitors, stimulants, phenelzine sulfate (an antidepressant); may enhance effect of hypoglycemics	Ginseng used for medicinal purposes for over 2000 years; safety of long term (>3 mo) use unknown but has been well-tolerated in clinical studies; most common side effect is insomnia; use with caution in individuals with history of CVD or diabetes; monitor individuals on warfarin; monitor insulin levels in insulin-dependent diabetics; discontinue use prior to surgery
Green tea (*Camellia sinensis*)	Lowers blood cholesterol; lowers blood pressure; improves cognitive performance; weight loss	Parts used include leaf bud, leaf, and stem; polyphenols contain flavanols, such as catechins, flavandiols, flavonoids, phenolic acids, caffeine	Green tea contains catechins, caffeine, vitamin K; thus may interfere with anticoagulant and antiplatelet drugs and antagonize effect of warfarin to ↓ INR; verapamil reported to ↑ plasma caffeine concentrations by 25%	Green tea health claim for CVD rejected by FDA; patients on warfarin need to be routinely questioned about intake of vitamin K–containing foods, beverages, dietary supplements; monitor INR in patients who habitually consume green tea and are on warfarin
Hawthorn (*Crataegus*)	Reduces symptoms of mild CHF, ischemic heart disease, reduces risk of arrhythmias and atherosclerosis	Hawthorn leaf extract (leaves and flowers) contain procyanidins, flavonoids, triterpenoids, catechins, aromatic carboxylic acids	May potentiate effects of digitalis, have additive effects when combined with beta blockers, calcium channel blockers, nitrates to ↑ vasodilation	In Germany, hawthorn prescribed for "mild cardiac insufficiency"; generally well tolerated and safe for short-term use; most common side effects are GI upset, fatigue, dizziness
Horse chestnut seed extracts (*Aesculus hippocastanum*)	Reduce swelling and discomfort caused by chronic venous insufficiency, varicose veins, phlebitis	Aescin, triterpene saponin, and aesculin, a glycoside, which is also a hydroxycoumarin	May ↑ effects of anticoagulants and antiplatelet drugs; possibly induces hypoglycemic effects; do not administer with drugs known to cause nephrotoxicity	Most widely prescribed oral antiedema venous remedy in Germany; treatment for 1 to 3 mo may be required before full therapeutic effects are apparent; side effects uncommon but GI irritation and toxic nephropathy may occur; monitor individuals on warfarin; monitor blood glucose levels in diabetics
Magnesium (Mg)	Reduces the risk of CVD, hypertension	Magnesium salts (chloride, citrate, gluconate, hydroxide, oxide, lactate, and sulfate)	Mg may interfere with absorption of digoxin; may ↓ efficacy of oral anticoagulants; long-term use of lasix and thiazide diuretics may deplete body stores of Mg	Safe when used orally and appropriately; not to exceed the UL of 350 mg/day unless prescribed for repletion; diarrhea common side effect at higher doses; individuals with impaired kidney function at higher risk for adverse effects
Omega-3 fatty acids or fish oils	Lowers blood cholesterol and triglyceride levels	DHA (docosahexaenoic acid); EPA (eicosapentaenoic acid)	Long-term use may ↑ risk of vitamin E deficiency; avoid drugs and herbs with anticoagulant-antiplatelet potential, antihypertensive drugs, cyclosporin, etretinate	Fish oils have GRAS status in the United States; safe when used orally and appropriately; clinical trials have shown that fish oils significantly ↓ triglyceride levels by 20%–50%, effective in reducing acute cardiac events; up to 6 gm/day does not appear to interfere significantly with warfarin therapy but monitoring patients on warfarin is recommended; may cause belching, halitosis, heartburn, nosebleeds

Policosanol	Lowers blood cholesterol level; used for peripheral vascular insufficiency, intermittent claudication	Derived from various plant sources; contains mixture of waxy alcohols	Policosanol may inhibit platelet aggregration; use caution with anticoagulant, antiplatelet drugs or supplements such as garlic and ginkgo, high doses of vitamin E	Appears to be well tolerated in some patients; may cause erythema, migraines, insomnia, irritability, dizziness, upset stomach, skin rash; monitor INR in patients on warfarin
Red clover *(Trifolium pratense)*	Reduces menopausal symptoms; helps maintain bone density in lower spine	Leaves and flowers contain isoflavones (formononetin, daidzein, genistein) and coumarins	Interacts with P-450 system; may ↑ effects of digoxin	Labeling of products may be confusing—same amount of isoflavones can differ significantly depending on how isoflavones are calculated (with or without related sugar constituents)
St. John's wort *(Hypericum perforatum)*	Symptoms associated with depression, anxiety; mood disturbances associated with menopause	Hypericin or hyperforin	Interacts with P-450 system (induces CYP34A and P-glycoprotein) and drugs metabolized in liver; may antagonize effect of warfarin and ↓ INR; ↓ plasma levels of simvastatin; ↑ effects of digoxin, MAO inhibitors, or serotonin uptake inhibitors; ↓ effects of anticonvulsants and antidiabetic drugs; ↑ photosensitivity with other such drugs	Likely safe when used orally and appropriately; therapeutic effects may take 2 to 4 wk to achieve; long-term safety unknown; most common side effect is insomnia; photosensitivity at high doses; avoid use with warfarin; discontinue use prior to surgery
Vitamin E	Prevents CVD (CHD, stroke)	Family of eight fat-soluble antioxidants, alpha-tocopherol most active form	Anticoagulant-antiplatelet drugs, herbal medicines with anticoagulant and antiplatelet potential, may ↑ INR; vitamin E may impair hematological reponse to iron therapy in patients with iron deficiency anemia; avoid large doses of vitamin E during treatment of iron deficiency; high doses of vitamin E (>800 units/day) can antagonize effects of vitamin K and ↑ risk of bleeding	Relatively nontoxic; safe when used orally in amounts not exceeding UL of 1000 mg/day; conversion factor: 1 mg = 1.26 IU; RDA of 15 mg = 22 IU (natural form) or 33 IU (synthetic form); possible ↑ risk of bleeding for those on anticoagulants or with vitamin K deficiency; possible ↑ risk of hemorrhage in high-risk groups; monitor INR in patients taking warfarin and vitamin E > 800 IU daily
Vitamin K	Supports normal clotting function	Forms of vitamin K include phytonadione (vitamin K_1), menaquinone (vitamin K_2), dihydrophylloquinone	Antagonizes effects of oral anticoagulants; concomitant use of Co-Q10 or herbs with clotting potential may have additive effects and ↑ risk of clotting; high doses of vitamin E (>800 units/day) can antagonize effects of vitamin K and ↑ risk of bleeding	Primary sources of vitamin K–containing foods are dark green vegetables and oils; other sources include adequate foods; fast foods, some dietary supplements; adequate intake for adult men is 120 µg/day, 90 µg/day for women; oral vitamin K causes few adverse effects
Yohimbine *(Pausinystalia yohimbe)*	All forms of erectile dysfunction	Yohimbine hydrochloride (yohimbe bark)	Taken by itself can cause HTN; lower doses may have favorable effect on orthostatic hypotension induced by tricyclic antidepressants; large doses can cause severe hypotension, cardiac arrhythmias, death	Yohimbine hydrochloride available as FDA-approved drug for treatment of impotence; older forms (e.g., yohimbe bark extracts, yohimbine sold in health food stores) may contain varying amounts of yohimbine and other ingredients; yohimbe bark is on German Commission E's list of unapproved herbs; side effects include HTN, anxiety, headache, GI symptoms; should not be used by older adults or those with HTN, heart, kidney, or liver disease

CHD = coronary heart disease; CHF = congestive heart failure; CVD = cardiovascular disease; EPA = eicosapentaenoic acid; FDA = U.S. Food and Drug Administration; GI = gastrointestinal; GRAS = generally recognized as safe; HMG-CoA = hydroxymethylglutaryl-coenzyme A reductase; HTN = hypertension; INR = international normalized ratio; MAO = monoamine oxidase; NSAIDs = nonsteroidal antiinflammatory drugs; PAD = peripheral arterial disease; PAF = platelet aggregating factor; RDA = recommended daily allowance; TCM = traditional Chinese medicine; UL = upper tolerable limit.

Data from Ang-Lee MK, Moss J, Yuan CS: Herbal medicines and perioperative care. JAMA 286:208, 2001; Chavez ML, Jordon MA, Chevez PI: Evidence-based drug-herbal interactions. Life Sci 78:2146, 2006; Dasgupta A, Bernard DW: Herbal remedies. Effects on clinical laboratory studies. Arch Pathol Lab Med 130:521, 2006; Ernst E: Cardiovascular adverse effects of herbal medicines: A systematic review of the recent literature. J Cardiol 19:818, 2003; Greenblatt DJ, von Moltke LL: Interaction of warfarin with drugs, natural substances, and foods. J Clin Pharmacol 45:127, 2005; Holbrook AM, Pereira JA, Labiris R, et al; Systematic overview of warfarin and its drug and food interactions. Arch Intern Med 165:1095, 2005; Jellin JM (ed): Natural Medicines Comprehensive Database. 8th ed. Stockton CA, Therapeutic Research Faculty. 2006; Izzo AA, Di Carlo G, Borrelli F, Dernst E: Cardiovascular pharmacotherapy and herbal medicines: The risk of drug interaction. Int J Cardiol 98:1, 2005; Nutescu EA, Shapiro NL, Ibrahim S, West P: Warfarin and its interactions with foods, herbs and other dietary supplements. Expert Opin Drug Saf 5:433, 2006; Vall G, Giardina EGV: Benefits, adverse effects and drug interactions of herbal therapies with cardiovascular effects. J Am Coll Cardiol 39 1083, 2002.

reduce propranolol and diltiazem bioavailability and might reduce the therapeutic effects of these drugs. Guggulipid may also exert antiplatelet and anticoagulant effects. Definitive safety and efficacy data are lacking in subjects on Western diets.

POLICOSANOL. Policosanol is derived from a sugar cane extract or wheat germ oil extract that contains a mixture of aliphatic alcohols. Lipid-lowering effects may involve inhibition of cholesterol synthesis in the liver and increasing degradation of low-density lipoprotein (LDL) cholesterol. Over 1000 subjects have been studied for periods of 6 weeks to 1 year in 15 randomized, placebo-controlled trials using policosanol (5 to 20 mg/day) for lipid lowering. At dosages of 10 to 20 mg/day, significant reductions were observed for total cholesterol (17 to 21 percent) and LDL cholesterol (21 to 29 percent), with increases in HDL cholesterol (8 to 15 percent).[16] There are no data on efficacy determined by clinical endpoints. Although policosanol appears to be well tolerated, caution should be exercised when combining policosanol with antiplatelet or anticoagulant agents, including garlic, ginkgo, and high doses of vitamin E,[17] because policosanol has been shown to inhibit platelet aggregation in healthy and diseased patients. Independent verification is needed before its use can be recommended.

Peripheral Vascular Disease and Venous Insufficiency (see Chap. 57)

Compounds studied for a role in moderating peripheral vascular disease include garlic, ginkgo, omega-3 fatty acids, Padma 28 (a herbal mixture containing 22 different ingredients) and vitamin E. Available data from randomized controlled trials, systematic reviews, and meta-analyses have suggested that ginkgo is effective compared with placebo for patients with intermittent claudication. Padma 28 was also found to be effective, although the data are limited.[18] Horse chestnut seed extract has been studied and found to be effective for the relief of venous insufficiency.

GINKGO LEAF EXTRACT *(Ginkgo biloba)*. Ginkgo has been used for relief of intermittent claudication in patients with peripheral arterial occlusive disease (PAD). The reviewed data have suggested that *Ginkgo biloba* extract is effective compared with placebo for patients with intermittent claudication (PAD Fontaine stage II). Dosages used in clinical trials ranged from 120 to 160 mg/day. Pain-free walking distance and maximal walking distance were often the monitored outcomes of interest. Ginkgo leaf and its extracts contain several bioactive constituents including flavonoids, terpenoids, and organic acids. The main active principles are bilobalide and ginkgolides. As with other phytomedicines, several constituents of ginkgo extracts may contribute to its therapeutic effect. Ginkgo does not appear to interact or adversely affect concomitant therapy with cardiac glycosides. Ginkgo appears to provide a small benefit in the treatment of PAD,[19] possibly by free radical scavenging, antiplatelet actions, antiinflammatory actions, vasodilation, and decreased blood viscosity. The most common dosage is 40 mg of standardized extract of ginkgo leaf three times daily. Ginkgo is considered relatively safe, with a few documented adverse effects being mild gastrointestinal upset, nausea, dyspepsia, and headache. Ginkgo has been reported to increase the risk of bleeding. Its concomitant use with aspirin, nonsteroidal antiinflammatory drugs (NSAIDs), and anticoagulants, such as warfarin and heparin, is not advised.[20]

HORSE CHESTNUT *(Aesculus hippocastanum)*. Horse chestnut seed extract (HCSE) contains saponins, coumarins, flavonoids, and tannins. Its biological activity has been shown to be related to the saponins, notably aescin. A systematic review of 17 randomized placebo-controlled trials was recently completed.[21] Leg pain assessed in six trials ($N = 543$) showed significant reduction compared to placebo. Four of five trials ($N = 420$) reported significant reduction in edema in patients treated with HCSE compared with placebo. Calf and ankle circumference was also reduced by HCSE. One trial found HCSE to be as efficacious as treatment with compression stockings. An effective dose of HCSE is standardized to 100 to 150 mg aescin daily. Symptoms such as pruritus and feelings of fatigue and tenseness were also reduced with HCSE. Side effects are uncommon but include gastrointestinal irritation, dizziness, nausea, headache, and pruritus. Two cases of toxic nephropathy have been reported. Contraindications to its use include hypersensitivity to aescin or horse chestnut and renal or hepatic dysfunction. Aescin, the main saponin component in HCSE, binds to plasma protein and may affect the binding of other drugs. HCSE has also been suspected of causing hypoglycemic effects. The German Commission E has approved the use of HCSE in chronic venous insufficiency and commercial preparations are available in the United States.

Heart Failure (see Chap. 29)

Several dietary supplements have been used in patients with mild heart failure. Some of these products may affect or modulate the renin-angiotensin-aldosterone system (e.g., L-arginine), act as diuretics (e.g., dandelion, corn silk, stinging nettle), or as positive inotropes similar to digoxin (e.g., oleander, pheasant's eye, squill) and hawthorn. Lastly, coenzyme Q10 has been used for support of cellular metabolism. Magnesium and thiamine have been used to replenish body stores of these nutrients caused by wasting and polypharmacy common in patients with heart failure. Of those supplements identified here, hawthorn, coenzyme Q10 and L-carnitine have been evaluated in randomized controlled clinical trials.

HAWTHORN *(Crataegus)*. Orally, hawthorn leaf extract has been used for congestive heart failure, cor pulmonale, ischemic heart disease, arrhythmias, blood pressure reduction, atherosclerosis, and cerebral insufficiency. Preparations made from flowers with leaves are sold as prescription medications in parts of Europe and Asia. Hawthorn may have clinical value in congestive heart failure as an adjunct to standard treatment.

Hawthorn has positive inotropic effects and is a peripheral vasodilator. It increases myocardial perfusion and stroke volume and reduces afterload. Hawthorn may offer some advantages over digoxin in mild heart failure. Compared with digitalis, hawthorn has a wider therapeutic range, lower risk in case of toxicity, has less arrhythmogenic potential, is safer to use in renal impairment, and can be safely used with diuretics and laxatives. However, hawthorn could enhance the activity of digitalis and care should be taken when combining it with beta blockers and Class III antiarrhythmics. A recent systematic review has identified 29 clinical studies using single-ingredient hawthorn-containing preparations. Data on adverse effects from 5577 patients noted 166 adverse events, 8 of which were severe, and were associated with one particular branded extract preparation. The daily dosage and duration of treatment ranged from 160 to 1800 mg of extract and from 3 to 24 weeks, respectively. There were, however, no reports of drug interactions noted.[22] Most frequent adverse events associated with hawthorn include dizziness, vertigo, headaches, migraines, and palpitations. A treatment period of at least 6 weeks is recommended to establish efficacy. Hawthorn use should be supervised by a clinician.

COENZYME Q10 (UBIQUINONE). Coenzyme Q10 (Co-Q10) is involved in oxidative phosphorylation and the generation of ATP. In addition, Co-Q10 acts as a free radical scavenger and membrane stabilizer. There have been over 40 controlled trials of the clinical effects of Co-Q10 on cardiovascular disease. Early studies have shown benefit in subjective (e.g., quality of life, decrease in hospitalizations) and objective (e.g., increased left ventricular ejection fraction, LVEF, stroke index) parameters, but more recent studies have been less supportive. A recent review of nine randomized trials of Co-Q10 in heart failure concluded there were nonsignificant trends toward increased ejection fraction and reduced mortality, but there were insufficient numbers of patients for meaningful results. Mortality benefit has not been established. Case reports have associated Co-Q10 therapy with decreased international normalized ratio (INR) in patients on warfarin therapy; however, 100 mg of Co-Q10 daily had no effect on the INR in patients on warfarin in a randomized, double-blind, placebo-controlled crossover trial.[23] Typical doses range from 100 to 200 mg, divided, two to three times daily. Caution is advised if patients take Co-Q10 and warfarin, because Co-Q10 may decrease the effectiveness of warfarin. 3-Hydroxy-3-methylglutaryl–coenzyme A (HMG-CoA) reductase inhibitors may inhibit the natural synthesis of Co-Q10, and reduced levels of Co-Q10 have been documented in small controlled clinical trials in patients on statin therapies.[24,25] Reduced levels of Co-Q10 may place the patient at increased risk for myopathy, but studies of supplemental Co-Q10 for decreasing myalgias and myositis have not been definitive. One unique formulation of Co-Q10 has received FDA orphan drug status for treating mitochondrial disorders.

Interactions with Anticoagulant Therapies (see Chap. 82)

An estimated 4 million patients are receiving long-term antithrombotic therapies (anticoagulants and/or antiplatelet agents) to manage or treat their disease condition and are at highest risk for drug-supplement interactions. Dietary supplements are used by approximately 36 to 52 percent of the general population and are taken concurrently with prescription drugs by approximately 16 percent of the population.[26] Many supplements have been reputed to interact with antithrombotic therapies, although relatively little data are available concerning the scope of the problem.

Supplements that can affect normal coagulation and platelet activity include danshen *(Salvia miltiorhiza)*, garlic, *Ginkgo biloba, Panax ginseng,* and St. John's wort *(Hypericum perforatum)*. Many of these supplements have also been reported to interact with coumarin anticoagulants. In addition to supplement heterogeneity, individual patient responses also reflect specific genetic polymorphisms in the cytochrome P-450 system and other metabolic pathways that can alter the metabolism of warfarin and/or dietary supplements. Given the variety of dietary supplements available, an important aspect of the management of patients on oral anticoagulant therapy remains a regular assessment of supplement use, and physicians should ensure that patients are aware of the potential risks and benefits of taking supplements in conjunction with their prescribed medications.

Herbals can affect the pharmacokinetics of warfarin by decreasing its absorption from the gastrointestinal (GI) tract or by altering its metabolic clearance. Other possible mechanisms include decreased platelet aggregation, decreased serum levels of thromboxane, prostaglandin, or phospholipase A_2, decreased synthesis of cyclooxygenase, inhibition of platelet-activating factor, conversion of fibrin to fibrinogen, and inhibition of CYP2C9 and vitamin K and coumarin content. The main enzyme responsible for S-warfarin metabolism is CYP2C9, and any factor that modifies the expression and activity of this enzyme can influence the anticoagulant response.[27]

Cardiac Catheterization (see Chap. 19)

Patients undergoing invasive diagnostic and interventional percutaneous procedures are generally awake in both the periprocedural and intraprocedural periods. Anticipation leading up to the procedure includes personal concerns about death, stroke, and myocardial infarction, and have been characterized repeatedly for their potential to induce ischemic episodes.[28] The interplay of emotional states with physical discomforts may promote exaggerated reactions that interfere with the conduct of the procedure or, worse, actually result in complications.

Techniques that foster relaxation, support, and spiritual faith could be fertile areas of adjunctive care. Mechanistically, noetic care paradigms that systematically integrate compassion, love, companionship, touch, faith, music, light, and even architectural space have the potential to affect processes mediated at a cellular level through intangible means and could affect perception and comfort, clinical outcomes, or both.

NOETIC THERAPIES. Noetic (e.g., mental or intellectual) therapies include a broad range of healing disciplines metaphorically considered to make use of the human spirit or other intangible human capabilities such as vital energy ("chi"), including qi gong, reiki, healing touch, healing prayer, music, imagery, stress relaxation, and pranayama (relaxed abdominal) breathing techniques, among others. Observational studies of guided imagery, relaxation techniques, and music in conjunction with invasive radiological procedures have reported[29] an analgesic effect measured by a subjective pain scale and reduced use of narcotics, predominantly in conjunction with the arteriotomy itself.

The largest overall published experience with patients in the catheterization laboratory has come from the Monitoring and Actualization of Noetic Trainings (MANTRA) project.[30] In the MANTRA pilot study, 150 patients presenting with acute coronary syndromes who required coronary care unit management and scheduled for urgent but not emergent catheterization and PCI were randomized to five parallel therapies, including standard care, or one of four noetic therapies: guided imagery, healing touch, stress relaxation, or distant intercessory prayer. Patients randomized to standard care and distant prayer remained blinded to their treatment assignment, whereas patients assigned imagery, touch, or stress relaxation interacted with a trained practitioner as open label interventions prior to catheterization and percutaneous intervention (PCI). Based on the limitations of the pilot study (e.g., small denominator, single center, parallel treatment assignments unable to assess synergy), the MANTRA II study[28] was designed with the power to show significance if a 30 percent treatment effect was reproducible. MANTRA II was a multicenter study of 748 patients undergoing elective PCI, followed for 6-month MACE, all-cause hospitalization, and death. Prespecified secondary endpoints examining different temporal periods or mechanistic differences following stenting included in-hospital MACE, 6-month rehospitalization and death, and 6-month mortality. Following the cultural paradigm, in which preprocedural support often consisted of both bedside and distant noetic interventions, a 2 × 2 factorial design was used to provide 1:1 randomization of all patients to double-blinded distant prayer and, in addition, 1:1 randomization of all patients to open label bedside noetic therapy. Thus, 25 percent of patients received both, 25 percent received neither (standard care group), 25 percent received only the bedside intervention, and 25 percent received only the distant blinded noetic intervention. For the bedside intervention, all practitioners were required to have at least healing touch level I certification. Because MANTRA II patients were in elective care settings, a longer period of 45 minutes was allowed. The bedside intervention in MANTRA II incorporated the use of rapport development and relaxed abdominal breathing, with a combination of music, imagery, and touch therapy (MIT). The music imagery script was delivered by Sony Walkman using dual headphones so that patient and practitioner could listen together, followed by the healing touch session with music in the background. If the patient desired, he or she was allowed to wear the headphones and listen to the music in the catheterization laboratory as well.

The prayer intervention for the first two thirds of MANTRA II enrollment was similar to the multiethnic, multi-time zone approach used in the pilot study; however, the number of prayer groups was expanded from 8 to 12. A higher "dose" was established at the two-thirds point by adding a second 12-prayer group, who prayed for the prayers of the first 12 congregations who were praying for the patients by name—a so-called two tiered or amplifier approach. Neither distant double-blinded intercessory prayer, bedside MIT, nor the combination of both showed any effect on the primary composite endpoint, which occurred in 37 percent of patients overall. The authors noted that off-protocol prayer by friends, family, or chaplains increased from 39 percent in the urgent setting of the MANTRA pilot to 89 percent in the elective PCI population of MANTRA II. Although a much smaller sample size was exposed to the high-dose two-tiered prayer, a trend toward out-of-hospital benefit in the secondary 6-month rehospitalization and death endpoint was observed in the high-dose prayer group, possibly suggesting a threshold effect relative to the single-tiered or lower dose prayer therapy.

Opportunities for further understanding and clinical investigations into the optimal catheterization laboratory environment, to enhance qualitative personal comfort or to improve clinical outcomes associated with invasive procedures in patients with heart disease, can be identified by shifting the periprocedural vision from the purely allopathic technical perspective to a more holistic view of the interplay between somatic pathophysiological processes, emotional and spiritual states, often referred to as the mind-body-spirit equilibrium. Influences on pain, vascular tone, platelet activation, and immune-mediated inflammatory responses can be attributed to this entire range of human psychoneurophysiology. Thus, the potential for advancing novel care strategies that systematically use intangible human capacities that are currently more culturally than scientifically integrated into medical practice can be identified.

From a holistic perspective, the question is not how to replace invasive interventional technology with intangible therapeutics, but how to augment our best technology with unique endogenous resources—a vision of optimal catheterization laboratory care as a sanctuary of "high tech-high touch" cardiovascular care. In the absence of any defined mechanisms through which such interventions might measurably exert their effects, however, systematic study of safety and effectiveness will remain critical to the real integration of CAM into the catheterization laboratory.

Intensive Care Units

The idea that an environment of care could affect patients' recovery and staff morale is intuitive but has not been given a proper consideration in our culture. Cardiovascular centers can change to a healing environment by renovating physical space using principles of feng shui, an ancient Chinese art and science of living in harmony with the environment, to direct the flow of chi, or energy. Patients stay in the same area or, at least, are not to be transferred more than once during their hospitalization. In addition, including integrative medicine consultations, massage and reflexology, guided imagery and music therapy, and breathing meditation can aid in recovery, as can a program run by a dedicated staff of holistic nurse practitioners, registered nurses trained in various modalities of CAM, and experienced massage therapists. The use of pain and antianxiety medications can decrease and patient satisfaction scores can increase. The program enables patients to take an active role in their recovery as well as make changes toward life-long wellness and disease prevention, empowering them to enhance their quality of life at present and in the future. In addition to the best medical care, key concepts include nutrition, exercise, stress management, relaxation, and spirituality.

Cardiac Surgery (see Chaps. 27 and 29)

The use of CAM is not only for primary care diseases. As shown by a study of 376 consecutive patients undergoing cardiac surgery, many cardiac surgery patients use some form of CAM but do not discuss its use with their physicians.[31] Among patients surveyed, 75 percent admitted the use of alternative medical therapy (44 percent without prayers and vitamins), but only 17 percent had discussed CAM use with their cardiac physicians, and 48 percent did not want to discuss it with any physicians. The most common CAM practices that cardiac surgeons need to understand are generally grouped into mind-body therapies and vitamin and herbal supplements.

MIND-BODY THERAPIES. The use of these therapies before, during, and after cardiac surgery may occur in roughly 50 percent of patients undergoing surgery. Depression is common in patients with heart disease and cardiac surgery, and is associated with adverse outcomes and increased long-term mortality. In addition, the cost of treating cardiac patients with mild to moderate depression is 41 percent higher in the first year following a major cardiac event, including surgery.[32] Type A behavior is thought to predispose to heart disease. Hostility and anger are associated with increased risk of acute coronary events, as are anxiety, panic symptoms and, perhaps, vital exhaustion. Social isolation and lack of social support are more powerful risk factors than some traditional risk factors, such as smoking. The autonomic nervous system (ANS) is sensitive to thoughts and emotions, with negative reactions creating disorder and imbalance in the ANS and positive feelings such as appreciation creating order and balance.[33] In addition, chronic stress elevates basal cortisol, impairs the body's ability to respond to acute stressors, and can lead to poor healing and recovery following surgery. Thus, many mind-body therapies have potential usefulness following or in conjunction with cardiac surgery. Religious practice, belief patterns, guided imagery during cardiac surgery, and the related social support appear to play a positive role, such as promoting recovery after cardiac surgery and limiting postoperative length of stay.[34]

SPECIFIC HERBALS TO AVOID PERIOPERATIVELY. Significant problems have been associated with the use of ephedra products for weight loss. Ephedra acts as a sympathomimetic, leading to increased arterial blood pressure, increased heart rate, increased oxygen consumption in heart muscle, and vasoconstriction. Dandelion herbal is prototypical of potassium-wasting herbals, of which there have been numerous anecdotal and other reports. Most importantly for cardiac surgeons, over 40 different herbs have anticoagulant effects of their own and thus could increase the risk of adverse bleeding events. Other popular herbs have been associated with decreased activity of warfarin.[2] It is imperative to ask all persons taking aspirin or warfarin about the use of plant-based medicines.

AGING

Much has been written about the aging process (see Chap. 75). Weil[35] has presented a number of suggestions: eating an antiinflammatory diet, using dietary supplements wisely to support the body's defenses and natural healing power, using preventive medicine intelligently, knowing the risks of age-related disease, getting appropriate diagnostic and screening tests and immunizations, treating problems such as hypertension and abnormal lipid levels in the early stages, getting regular physical activity throughout life, getting adequate rest and sleep, learning and practicing methods of stress reduction, exercising the mind as well as the body, maintaining social and intellectual connections throughout life, being flexible in mind and body, learning to adapt to losses and to let go of behaviors no longer appropriate for your age, thinking about and trying to discover the benefits of aging, not denying the reality of aging nor putting energy into trying to stop it, using the experience of aging as a stimulus for spiritual awakening and growth, and keeping records of the lessons learned, the wisdom gained, and the value held. At critical points in life, this list can be revised and shared with loved ones. Vogel[36] has added admonitions about eating less, exercising more, not smoking, slowing one's heart rate, procreating later, taking a statin, and having one drink per day.

In extending the lives of so many patients, we now have millions who have entered a terminal stage of their disease with high mortality rates and considerable torment (see Chap. 30). Thus, it is our responsibility to develop methods, tools, and approaches that can provide a more positive end-of-life experience for our patients. To deal with this, it is important to listen to the patients, develop a discussion, and review their personal desires. The *Five Wishes* document[37] helps people express how they should be treated if seriously ill and unable to speak for themselves. It is unique among living wills and similar forms because it includes all of our needs—medical, personal, emotional, and spiritual. The *Five Wishes* encourages a discussion of the patient's wishes with family and physician. End-of-life directives are imperative. The *Five Wishes* also lets the patient's family and physicians become aware of the following:

1. Who the patient wants to make health care decisions when the patient can't make them.
2. The type of medical treatment that the patient wants or doesn't want.
3. How comfortable the patient wants to be.
4. How the patient wants people to treat him or her.
5. What the patient wants loved ones to know.

Thus, the physician should listen carefully, trying to understand the patient's viewpoint. Listening does not require the physician to agree with the patient or misrepresent his or her own views. Patients and families who believe that the physician understands them and cares about them will result in trust between the physician and patient and thus there will be a more successful conclusion to treatment. By responding to patients' spiritual and religious concerns and needs, physicians may help them find comfort and closure near the end of life.

TABLE 47-3 Reference Sources for Information on Dietary Supplements and Herbal Medicines

BOOKS AND PUBLICATIONS

Barrett M: The Handbook of Clinically Tested Herbal Remedies. Vols. 1 and 2. Binghamton, NY, Haworth Herbal Press, 2004.
ISBN: 0789027232
Description: A thorough, informative, in-depth text for clinicians searching for accurate information on herbal clinical trials.

Fugh-Berman A: The 5-Minute Herb and Dietary Supplement Clinical Consult. Philadelphia, Lippincott Williams & Wilkins, 2003.
ISBN: 0683302736
Description: Includes herbs, minerals, vitamins, amino acids, and enzymes and their uses to treat common problems and improve health.

Blumenthal M, Brinckmann J, Wollschlaeger B: The ABC Clinical Guide to Herbs. Austin, TX, American Botanical Council, 2003.
ISBN: 1588901572
Description: Provides health professionals with information on 29 of the most popular herbs, and other herbal products. Information includes usage, dosage, contraindications, adverse effects, drug interactions, and pharmacological effects.

Coates PM, Blackman MR, Cragg GM, et al (eds): Encyclopedia of Dietary Supplements. New York, Marcel Dekker, 2005.
ISBN: 0824755049
Description: Provides detailed scientific information on over 75 dietary supplements, including description and chemical composition, mechanisms of action, pharmacology, usage and dosage, safety, adverse effects, and regulatory issues.

Katz DL: Nutrition in Clinical Practice. A Comprehensive, Evidence-Based Manual for the Practitioner. 2nd ed. Philadelphia, Lippincott Williams & Wilkins, 2007.
ISBN: 1582558213
Description: Nutrition information provided along with information on supplements (nutraceuticals). Nutrient and supplement reference tables included.

Simon M, Bone K: The Essential Guide to Herbal Safety. New York, Churchill Livingstone, 2004.
ISBN: 0443071713
Description: This guide contains comprehensive reviews, in monograph format, of the published safety data for 125 herbs. Covers issues of quality, interactions, adverse reactions, toxicity, allergic contact sensitivity, and idiosyncratic reactions.

Schulz V, Hansel R, Blumenthal M, Tyler VE: Rational Phytotherapy: A Physician's Guide to Herbal Medicine. 5th ed. New York, Springer Verlag, 2004.
ISBN: 3540408320
Description: Reviews the pharmaceutical aspects of phytotherapy.

Thrombosis Research: Special Issue. Papers from the NIH Conference on Dietary Supplements, Coagulation, and Antithrombotic Therapies. 117(1–2): 2005.

EVIDENCE-BASED REVIEWS

Agency for Healthcare Research and Quality (AHRQ): http://ahrq.gov and http://preventiveservices.ahrq.gov
Description: AHRQ supports research designed to improve the outcomes and quality of health care, reduce its costs, address patient safety and medical errors, and broaden access to effective services.

Available Reviews:

- Effect of Supplemental Antioxidants Vitamin C, Vitamin E, and Coenzyme Q10 for the Prevention and Treatment of Cardiovascular Disease: http://www.ahrq.gov/clinic/epcsums/antioxsum.htm
- Garlic: Effects on Cardiovascular Risks and Disease, Protective Effects Against Cancer, and Clinical Adverse Effects: http://www.ahrq.gov/clinic/epcsums/garlicsum.htm
- Omega-3 Fatty Acids
  - Health Effects: http://www.ahrq.gov/clinic/tp/o3cardtp.htm
  - Risk Factors: http://www.ahrq.gov/clinic/tp/o3cardrisktp.htm
  - Arrhythmias: http://www.ahrq.gov/clinic/tp/o3arrtp.htm
- Effects of Soy on Health Outcomes: http://www.ahrq.gov/clinic/epcsums/soysum.htm
- Multivitamin and Mineral Supplements and Prevention of Chronic Disease: http://www.ahrq.gov/clinic/tp/multivittp.htm

Cochrane Systematic Reviews: http://www.cochrane.org/index.htm
Description: The Cochrane Collaboration is an international nonprofit, independent organization. It produces and disseminates systematic reviews of health care interventions and promotes the search for evidence in the form of clinical trials and other studies of interventions.

Lichtenstein AH, Appel LJ, Brands M, et al: AHA Scientific Statement. Diet and Lifestyle Recommendations Revision 2006. A scientific statement from the American Heart Association Nutrition Committee. Circulation 114:82, 2006.

National Center for Complementary and Alternative Medicine (NCCAM): http://nccam.nih.gov/research/policies/guideonct.htm. NIH Guidance on Designing Clinical Trials of CAM Therapies: Determining Dose Ranges.

Vogel JHK, Bolling SF, Costello RB, et al: Integrating complementary medicine into cardiovascular medicine: A report of the American College of Cardiology Foundation Task Force on Clinical Expert Consensus Documents (Writing Committee to Develop an Expert Consensus Document on Complementary and Integrative Medicine). J Am Coll Cardiol 46:184, 2005.

DATA BASES

AltMedDex System: http://www.micromedex.com/procucts/altmeddex/ (by subscription)
Description: Referenced information on herbals, vitamins, minerals, other dietary supplements, Chinese medicine, acupuncture and more. Includes data on dosing, pharmacokinetics, and clinical applications.

International Bibliographic Information on Dietary Supplements (IBIDS) Database: http://ods.od.nih.gov/Health_Information/IBIDS.aspx.

National Institutes of Health, Office of Dietary Supplements, and the National Agricultural Library, Food and Nutrition Information Center.
Description: IBIDS is a comprehensive bibliographic data base that helps health care providers, researchers, and consumers find credible, scientific literature on dietary supplements. Currently, the data base contains dietary supplement citations and abstracts from MEDLINE, AGRICOLA, and AGRIS, and selected nutrition journals from CAB Abstracts and CAB's Global Health data bases, dating from 1986 to the present.

Natural Medicines Comprehensive Database: www.NaturalDatabase.com (by subscription).

The Pharmacist's Letter/The Prescriber's Letter, updated yearly.
Description: Referenced, peer-reviewed, continuously updated online data base. Search by keyword or by brand name products. Includes drug-herb interactions and conditions.

MEDLINEPlus for Herbal Information: http://www.nlm.nih.gov/medlineplus/herbalmedicine.html
Description: Contains up-to-date, quality health care information on herbs and herbal medicine from the National Library of Medicine at the National Institutes of Health.

MEDLINEPlus for Dietary supplements: http://www.nlm.nih.gov/medlineplus/dietarysupplements.html
Description: Links, including the latest research, on dietary supplements from the National Library of Medicine at the National Institutes of Health.

MONOGRAPHS

American Herbal Pharmacopeia and Therapeutic Compendium (AHP): http://www.herbal-ahp.org.
Description: The American Herbal Pharmacopoeia began developing qualitative and therapeutic monographs in 1994, and will produce 300 monographs on botanicals, including many of the Ayurvedic, Chinese, and Western herbs most frequently used in the United States.

Table continues

TABLE 47–3 Reference Sources for Information on Dietary Supplements and Herbal Medicines—cont'd

The Complete German Commission E Monographs: Therapeutic Guide to Herbal Medicines

Mark Blumenthal, German Federal Institute for Drugs and Medical Devices Commission E, American Botanical Council, Integrative Medicine Communications, Werner R. Busse, J. Klein, Robert Rister (editors) Siegrid Klein, Chance Riggins

Austin, TX, American Botanical Council

Boston, MA: Integrative Medicine Communications, 1998. 685 pp.
ISBN: 096555550X
Web site: www.herbalgram.org.
Description: The German government's Commission E findings regarding the approved uses, contraindications, side effects, dosage, drug interactions, and other therapeutic effects of 300 herbs and phytomedicines.

Health Canada. Natural Health Products Compendium of Monographs: http://www.hc-sc.gc.ca/dhp-mps/prodnatur/applications/licen-rod/monograph./index_e.html

Description: The Health Canada Natural Health Products Directorate, Health Canada, 2003, developed the Compendium of Monographs as a tool for the timely and efficient evaluation of the safety and efficacy of many commonly used medicinal ingredients found in natural health products.

CME PROGRAMS

Sponsor: Archives of Internal Medicine: http://cmejama-archives.ama-assn.org/cgi/hierarchy/amacme_course;archinte165/10/1095
May 25, 2005: Systematic Overview of Warfarin and its Food and Drug Interactions.

Sponsor: College of Pharmacy, University of Illinois at Chicago: http://www.uic.edu/pharmacy/conted
Preceptorship: Antithrombosis Management
Botanicals for Women's and Men's Health

Sponsor: Northwest AHEC, Wake Forest University School of Medicine: https://northwestahec.wfubmc.edu/learn/herbs_ce/index.cfm
Curriculum on Herbs and Dietary Supplements

Acknowledgment

The authors thank Erminia Guarneri, MD, FACC, and Cathy Young, RN, MBA, for their help with this chapter.

REFERENCES

General Considerations

1. Barnes P, Powell-Griner E. McFann K, Nahin R: CDC Advanced Data Report #343, Complementary and alternative medicine use among adults, May 27, 2004.
2. Vogel JH, Bolling SF, Costello RB, et al; American College of Cardiology Foundation Task Force on Clinical Expert Consensus Documents (Writing Committee to Develop an Expert Consensus Document on Complementary and Integrative Medicine): Integrating complementary medicine into cardiovascular medicine. A report of the American College of Cardiology Foundation Task Force on Clinical Expert Consensus Documents (Writing Committee to Develop an Expert Consensus Document on Complementary and Integrative Medicine). J Am Coll Cardiol 46:184, 2005.
3. Vogel JHK, Krucoff MW (eds): Integrative Cardiology. New York, McGraw-Hill, 2007 (in press).

Applications of CAM

4. Kannel WB, Dawber TR, Kagan A, Revotskie J: Factors of risk in the development of coronary heart disease—six-year follow-up experience. The Framingham Study. Ann Intern Med 55:33, 1961.
5. Friedmann E, Thomas SA, Stein PK, Kleiger RE: Relation between pet ownership and heart rate variability in patients with healed myocardial infarcts. Am J Cardiol 91:718, 2003.
6. Grossman P, Niemann L, Schmidt S, Walach H: Mindfulness-based stress reduction and health benefits. A meta-analysis. J Psychosom Res 57:35, 2004.
7. Kshettry VR, Carole LF, Henly SJ, et al: Complementary alternative medical therapies for heart surgery patients: Feasibility, safety, and impact. Ann Thorac Surg 81:201, 2006.
8. Paul-Labrador M, Polk D, Dwyer JH, et al: Effects of a randomized controlled trial of transcendental meditation on components of the metabolic syndrome in subjects with coronary heart disease. Arch Intern Med 166:1218, 2006.
9. American Heart Association Nutrition Committee; Lichtenstein AH, Appel U, Brands M, et al: Diet and lifestyle recommendations revision 2006: A scientific statement from the American Heart Association Nutrition Committee. Circulation 114:82, 2006.
10. Vogel JHK, Bolling SF, Costello RB, et al; American College of Cardiology Foundation Task Force on Clinical Expert Consensus Documents (Writing Committee to Develop an Expert Consensus Document on Complementary and Integrative Medicine): Integrating complementary medicine into cardiovascular medicine: A report of the American College of Cardiology Foundation Task Force on Clinical Expert Consensus Documents (Writing Committee to Develop an Expert Consensus Document on Complementary and Integrative Medicine). J Am Coll Cardiol 46:184, 2005.
11. Ernst E: Complementary/alternative medicine for hypertension: A mini-review. Wien Med Wochenschr 155:386, 2005.
12. Mulrow C, Lawrence V, Ackermann R, et al: Garlic: Effects on cardiovascular risks and disease, protective effects against cancer, and clinical adverse effects. Evid Rep Technol Assess (Summ) (20):1, 2000.
13. Rosenfeldt F, Hilton D, Pepe S, Krum H: Systematic review of effect of coenzyme Q10 in physical exercise, hypertension, and heart failure. Biofactors 18:91, 2003.
14. Beyer FR, Dickinson HO, Nicolson DI, et al: Combined calcium, magnesium, and potassium supplementation for the management of primary hypertension in adults. Cochrane Database System Rev (3):CD004805, 2006.
15. Szapary PO, Wolfe ML, Bloedon LT, et al: Guggulipid for the treatment of hypercholesterolemia: A randomized controlled trial. JAMA 290:765, 2003.
16. Berthold HK, Unverdorben S, Degenhardt R., et al: Effect of the policosanol in lipid levels among patients with hypercholesterolemia or combined hyperlipidemia. A randomized controlled trial. JAMA 295:2262, 2006.
17. Arruzazabala ML, Molina V, Mas R, et al: Antiplatelet effects of policosanol (20 and 40 mg/day) in healthy volunteers and dyslipidemic patients. Clin Exp Pharmacol Physiol 20:891, 2002.
18. Pittler MH, Ernst E: Complementary therapies for peripheral arterial disease: Systematic review. Atherosclerosis 181:1, 2005.
19. Ernst E: The risk-benefit profile of commonly used herbal therapies: Ginkgo, St. John's Wort, Ginseng, Echinacea, Saw Palmetto, and Kava. Ann Intern Med 136:42, 2002.
20. Jellin JM (ed): Natural Medicines Comprehensive Database. 8th ed. Stockton, CA, Therapeutic Research Faculty, 2006.
21. Pittler MH, Ernst E: Horse chestnut seed extract for chronic venous insufficiency. Cochrane Database System Rev (1):CD003230, 2006.
22. Daniele C, Mazzanti G, Pittler MH, Ernst E: Adverse-event profile of *Crataegus* spp. A systematic review. Drug Safety 29:523, 2006.
23. Engelsen J, Nielsen JD, Winther K: Effect of Coenzyme Q10 and Ginkgo biloba on warfarin dosage in stable, long-term warfarin treated outpatients: A randomised, double-blind, placebo-cross-over trial. Thromb Haemost 87:1075, 2002.
24. Rundek T, Naini A, Sacco R, et al: Atorvastatin decrease the coenzyme Q10 level in the blood of patients at risk for cardiovascular disease and stroke. Arch Neurol 61:889, 2004.
25. Silver MA, Langsjoe PH, Szabo S, et al: Effect of atorvastatin on left ventricular diastolic function and ability of coenzyme Q10 to reverse that dysfunction. Am J Cardiol 94:1306, 2004.
26. Kaufman OW, Kelly JP, Rosenberg L, et al: Recent patterns of medication use in the ambulatory adult population of the United States: The Slone Survey. JAMA 287:337, 2002.
27. Greenblatt DJ, von Moltke LL: Interaction of warfarin with drugs, natural substances, and foods. J Clin Pharmacol 45:127, 2005.
28. Bengston A, Herlitz J, Karisson T, et al: Distress correlates with the degree of chest pain: A description of patients awaiting revascularization. Heart 75:257, 1996.
29. Bally K, Campbell D, Chesnick K, Tranmer JE: Effects of the patient-controlled music therapy during coronary angiography on procedural pain and anxiety distress syndrome. Crit Care Nurse 23:50, 2003.
30. Krucoff MW, Crater SW, Gallup D, et al: Imagery, touch, and prayer as adjuncts to interventional cardiac care: The Monitoring and Actualization of Noetic Trainings (MANTRA) II randomized study. Lancet 366:211, 2005.
31. Liu, EH, Turner LM, Lin SX, et al: Use of alternative medicine by patients undergoing cardiac surgery. J Thorac Cardiovasc Surg 120:335, 2000.
32. Hemingway H, Marmot M: Evidence-based cardiology: Psychosocial factors in the aetiology and prognosis of coronary heart disease. Systematic review of prospective cohort studies. BMJ 318:1460, 1999.
33. Luskin FM, Newell KA, Griffith M, et al: A review of mind-body therapies in the treatment of cardiovascular disease. Part 1: Implications for the elderly. Altern Ther Health Med 4:46, 1998.
34. Ai AL, Bolling SF: The use of complementary and alternative therapies among middle-aged and older cardiac patients. Am J Med Qual 17:21, 2002.

Aging

35. Weil A: Healthy Aging. New York, Alfred A Knopf, 2005.
36. Vogel RA: 15-minute lifestyle modification: The TLC for your heart program. Presented at the 20th Annual Cardiovascular Conference. Kohala Coast, Hawaii, February 18, 2005.
37. The Five Wishes document: Aging with Dignity (http://fivewishes.org).

Disclosure Index

The following contributors have indicated that they have a relationship that, in the context of their participation in the writing of a chapter for the Eighth Edition of *Braunwald's Heart Disease,* could be perceived by some people as a real or apparent conflict of interest, but do not consider that it has influenced the writing of their chapter. Codes for the disclosure information (institution[s] and nature of relationship[s]) are provided below.

Relationship Codes

A—Stock options or bond holdings in a for-profit corporation or self-directed pension plan
B—Research grants
C—Employment (full or part-time)
D—Ownership or partnership
E—Consulting fees or other remuneration received by the contributor or immediate family
F—Nonremunerative positions, such as board member, trustee, or public spokesperson
G—Receipt of royalties
H—"Speaker's bureau"

Institution and Company Codes

001—Abbott Labs
002—Accumetrics
003—Acorn Cardiovascular
004—Actelion Pharmaceuticals
005—Active Biotic
006—Adolor
007—AGA Medical
008—Alexion Pharmaceuticals
009—Alnylam
010—Alteon
011—American College of Nutrition
012—American Heart Association
013—Amgen
014—Amorcyte Inc.
015—Anexon
016—Angiodynamics
017—Apotex
018—Arena
019—Armgo Pharma
020—Astellas
021—Astra Zeneca, Inc.
022—Atlas Venture Advisors, Inc.
023—AtheroGenics, Inc.
024—Avanir
025—Aventis
026—Baker Brothers Advisors LLC
027—Barr-Teva Litigation
028—BASS Medical
029—Bayer Italy
030—Bayer Healthcare
031—Beckman-Coulter
032—BGB-New York
033—Biomarin Pharmaceuticals
034—Bioscience Webster
035—Biosite, Inc.
036—BG Medicine
037—Blackwell Publishing
038—Bluhm Cardiovascular Institute
039—BMS
040—BMS-Sanofi
041—Boeringer Ingelheim
042—Boston Scientific Corporation
043—Boston Scientific Inc.
044—Bracco
045—Bristol-Meyers Squibb Company
046—Cardiac Concepts Inc.
047—Cardiac Dimensions
048—CardioDynamics
049—Cardiokine Inc.
050—Cardio DX
051—CardioMems Inc.
052—CDC
053—Centocor
054—CHF Solutions
055—Circulation
056—Cordis Corporation
057—Critical Diagnostics
058—Cryocor
059—Current Protocols in Human Genetics
060—Cytokinetics, Inc.
061—CV Therapeutics, Inc.
062—Dade Behring
063—Daiichi Sankyo
064—Dime
065—Edwards Lifesciences
066—Eisai
067—Eli Lilly and Company
068—Elsevier
069—Emisphere
070—Encysive
071—E Z EM
072—GE Healthcare
073—Genentech
074—Genzyme
075—Geron
076—Gilead Sciences
077—Glaxo Smith Kline
078—GSK
079—Guidant Corporation
080—I3DNL
081—IBM
082—Interleukin Genetics
083—Int'l Life Sciences Health & Environmental Sciences Institute
084—Inverness Medical Inc.
085—ISIS
086—Johnson & Johnson
087—Kowa Research Institute
088—LabCorp
089—Laboratory of Molecular Medicine/HPCGG
090—Lippincott
091—LPath
092—Lung RX
093—Mallinckrodt
094—Medicines Company
095—Medicure
096—Medscape
097—Medtronic, Inc.
098—Merck & Co., Inc.
099—Merck Cardiovascular Scientific
100—Merck/Schering-Plough Corp.
101—MG Medicine
102—Millennium Pharmaceuticals
103—Molecular Insight Pharmaceuticals
104—Myogen
105—National Heart, Lung and Blood Institute
106—NCME
107—Neurological Technologies
108—NIH
109—NIH/Agency for Healthcare Research and Quality
110—Nitromed
111—Northpoint Domain
112—NovaCardia
113—Novartis, Inc.
114—Ortho-Clinical Diagnostics

115—Pfizer, Inc.
116—Philips Medical
117—Physical Logic AG
118—Preventicum
119—Prime
120—Procter and Gamble
121—Protein Design Labs
122—Reliant Pharmaceuticals
123—Regeneron
124—Resmed Foundation
125—Respironics
126—Roche Diagnostics
127—SAB
128—Sanofi-Aventis
129—Sapphire Therapeutics, Inc.
130—Scios, Inc.
131—Servier France
132—Schering
133—Schering Plough Corp.
134—Sciele, Inc.
135—Siemens
136—Siemens Medical Solutions
137—Sigma Tau
138—Stereotaxis
139—St. Jude Medical
140—T2cure
141—Takeda
142—Terumo Heart, Inc.
143—Tethys
144—Thoratec
145—United Therapeutics, Inc.
146—VA
147—Vanderbilt/Genaissance
148—Vascular Biogenics
149—Vasculitis Foundation
150—Ventracor Inc.
151—Vertex
152—Visen Scientific
153—Wyeth
154—Xceed Molecular Scientific Advisory Board
155—Xoma

Contributors

Achenbach, Stephan B-132, B-136, E-44, E-45
Antman, Elliot E-67, E-128
Baim, Donald S. C-42
Beckman, Joshua A.
Bettmann, Michael H-16, H-71
Bonow, Robert O. E-65
Braunwald, Eugene B-21, B-30, B-61, B-67, B-98, B-113, B-115, B-128, B-133, E-63, E-115, E-128, E-133
Calkins, Hugh E-97
Carroll, John D. B-166, H-166
Costello, Rebecca C-108, F-11
Creager, Mark A. B-67, B-98, E-5, E-33, E-45, E-74, E-98, E-128, E-137, H-45, H-128
Dilsizian, Vasken A-72, A-103, B-20, B-72, B-103, E-45, E-103, H-20, H-45, H-72, H-93
Dimmeler, Stefanie D-140, E-74, E-79, E-97, E-115, E-140, H-140
Douglas, Pamela S. A-50, A-102, A-111, B-97, E-72, E-77, E-88, E-98, E-99, E-101, E-111, E-152, E-154
Eagle, Kim B-35, B-45, B-115, B-128, E-108, E-115, E-128
Force, Thomas E-113, H-98
Gersh, Bernard J. F-14, F-21, F-43, F-45, F-61, F-113
Goldhaber, Sam B-41, B-66, B-78, B-128, E-39, E-41, E-69, E-128
Goldstein, Larry B. B-7, B-39, B-41, B-52, B-106, B-108, E-86, E-107, E-115
Hoffman, Gary B-108, B-149, E-53, E-73, E-123
Isselbacher, Eric M. H-115
Kaplan, Norman E-113, H-41, H-115, G-90
LeWinter, Martin B-97, B-113, E-97, H-113, H-141
Libby, Peter E-21, E-23, E-41, E-45, E-77, H-21, H-41, H-45, H-77
Lipshultz, Steve B-77, B-113, B-115, B-126, B-155
Mann, Douglas A-97, E-3, E-97, F-19, F-91
Mark, Daniel B-8, B-95, B-97, B-105, B-109, B-115, B-120, E-21, E-25, E-97, E-113, G-68
McLaughlin, Vallerie B-4, B-70, B-92, B-115, B-145, E-4, E-76, H-4, H-76, H-115
McManus, Bruce B-13, B-81, B-113, E-13, E-116
Miller, John B-42, B-97, B-139, E-34, E-42, E-97, E-138, E-139
Morrow, David E-30, E-31, E-57, E-61, E-62, E-73, E-77, E-114, E-126, E-128
Myerburg, Robert E-43, E-79, E-120, E-122, H-43, H-79
Nesto, Richard W. E-78, E-128, H-78, H-128, H-141
Newby, L. Kristin B-12, B-35, B-36, B-40, B-84, B-126, B-133, E-6, E-61, E-86, E-120, E-130, H-40
Olgin, Jeffrey B-58, B-139
Opie, Lionel E-29, G-68
Pennell, Dudley J. B-17, B-97, B-113, B-135, E-97, E-113, E-118, E-135, H-17, H-113
Priori, Silvia B-79, B-97, H-79, H-97
Pyeritz, Reed E. B-74, E-74, H-74
Redfield, Margaret B-10, B-35, B-47, B-79, B-97, B-130, B-139, G-15
Resnic, Frederic S. B-94, B-139, H-139
Ridker, Paul B-1, B-21, B-128, E-1, E-21, E-62, E-85, E-113, E-148
Roden, Dan E-22, E-24, E-26, E-27, E-49, E-61, E-67, E-78, E-79, E-113, E-115, E-128, E-129, E-147, F-97, H-83
Schwartz, Janice E-134
Seidman, Christine F-89, G-59
Seidman, Jonathan C-89, F-89, G-59
Simon, Daniel I. B-2, B-56, B-86, B-133, E-56, E-86, E-128, E-133, H-56, H-67, H-86, H-94, H-128, H-133
Somers, Virend K. B-124, E-46, E-125
Teerlink, John A-60, B-1, B-4, B-45, B-48, B-54, B-60, B-112, B-130, E-1, E-4, E-20, E-28, E-45, E-60, E-75, E-104, E-121, E-153
Warnes, Carole G-37
Yancy, Clyde W. Jr. B-130, E-77, E-97, E-110, E-113, E-130, H-77, H-113
Yoshifumi, Naka E-51, E-142, E-150, H-144
Zeiher, Andreas M. A-140, B-79, B-128, E-79, H-115
Zipes, Douglas P. A-116, B-97, E-97, E-116, E-153

Index

Note: Page numbers followed by f and t indicate figures and tables, respectively.

B

D

N

O

V

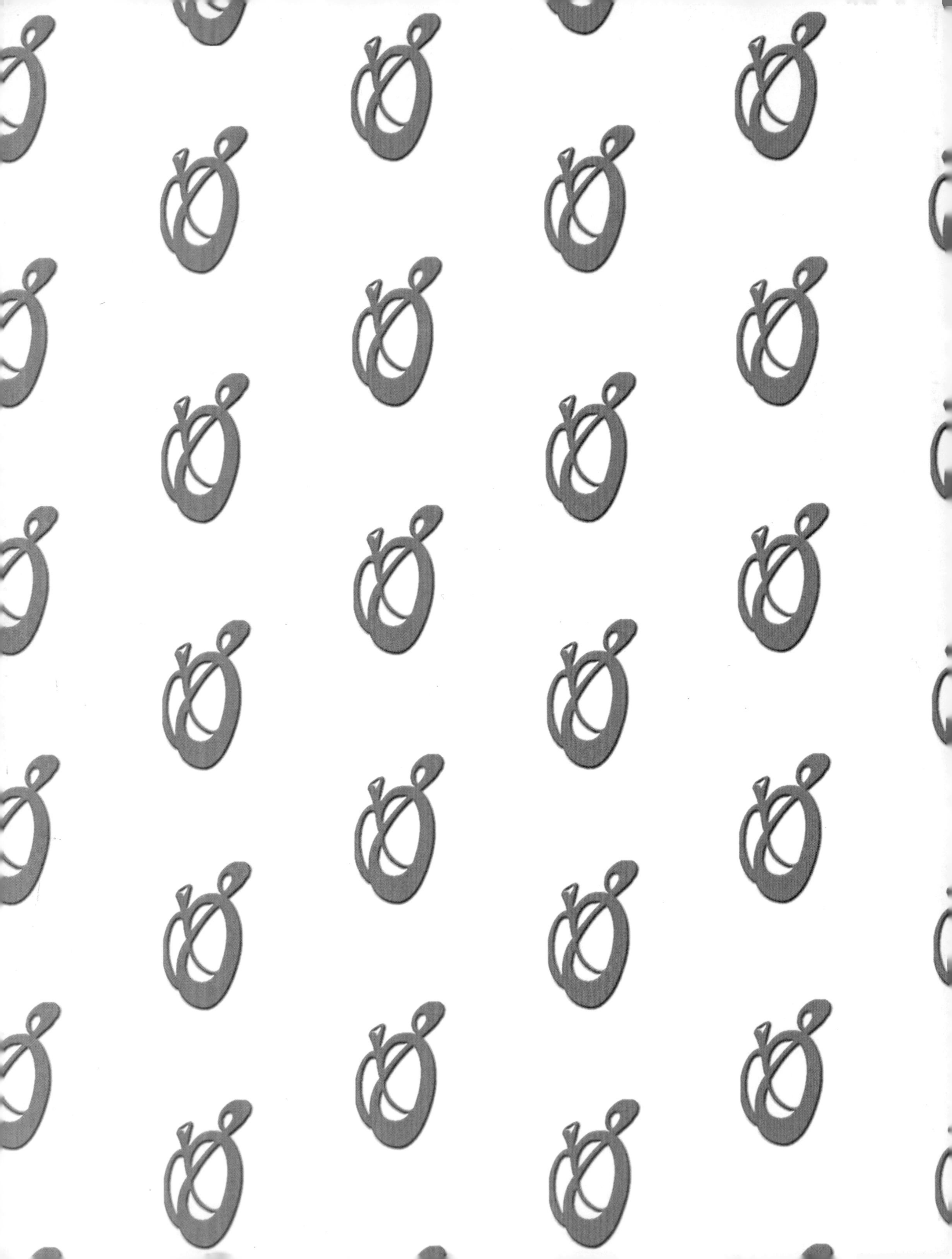